Clinical Environmental Health and Toxic Exposures

Clinical Environmental Health and Toxic Exposures

Second Edition

John B. Sullivan, Jr., M.D.

Associate Dean for Clinical Affairs,
Associate Professor of Emergency Medicine,
University of Arizona Health Sciences Center,
Tucson, Arizona

Gary R. Krieger, M.D., M.P.H., D.A.B.T.

Associate Adjunct Professor of Toxicology,
University of Colorado School of Pharmacy;
Department of Molecular and Environmental Toxicology,
University of Colorado Health Sciences Center,
Denver, Colorado

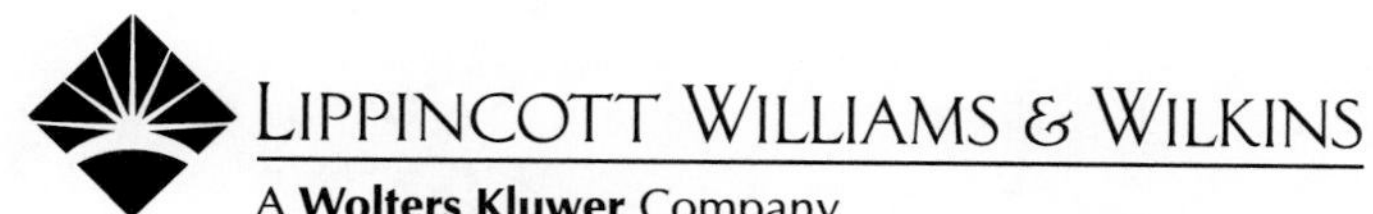

A **Wolters Kluwer** Company

Philadelphia • Baltimore • New York • London
Buenos Aires • Hong Kong • Sydney • Tokyo

Acquisitions Editor: Anne M. Sydor
Developmental Editor: Leah Ann Kiehne Hayes/Sarah Fitz-Hugh
Supervising Editor: Mary Ann McLaughlin
Production Editors: Erica Broennle and Allison Spearman, Silverchair Science + Communications
Manufacturing Manager: Ben Rivera
Cover Designer: Mark Lerner
Compositor: Silverchair Science + Communications
Printer: Courier Westford

530 Walnut Street
Philadelphia, PA 19106 USA
LWW.com

1st edition entitled Hazardous Materials Toxicology: Clinical Principles of Environmental Health, 1992

Library of Congress Cataloging-in-Publication Data
Clinical environmental health and toxic exposures / editors, John B. Sullivan, Jr., Gary R. Krieger. -- 2nd ed.
p. cm.
Rev. ed. of: Hazardous materials toxicology / editors, John B. Sullivan, Jr., Gary R. Krieger. Baltimore : Williams & Wilkins, c1992.
Includes bibliographical references and index.
ISBN 0-683-08027-X
1. Environmental toxicology. 2. Environmental health. I. Sullivan, John B. (John Burke) II. Krieger, Gary R. III. Hazardous materials toxicology.
[DNLM: 1. Hazardous Substances--toxicity. 2. Environmental Exposure. 3. Environmental Health. 4. Risk Factors. WA 465 C641 1999]
RA1226.C56 1999
615.9'02--dc21
DNLM/DLC
for Library of Congress 99-33986
CIP

Care has been taken to confirm the accuracy of the information presented and to describe generally accepted practices. However, the authors, editors, and publisher are not responsible for errors or omissions or for any consequences from application of the information in this book and make no warranty, expressed or implied, with respect to the currency, completeness, or accuracy of the contents of the publication. Application of this information in a particular situation remains the professional responsibility of the practitioner.

The authors, editors, and publisher have exerted every effort to ensure that drug selection and dosage set forth in this text are in accordance with current recommendations and practice at the time of publication. However, in view of ongoing research, changes in government regulations, and the constant flow of information relating to drug therapy and drug reactions, the reader is urged to check the package insert for each drug for any change in indications and dosage and for added warnings and precautions. This is particularly important when the recommended agent is a new or infrequently employed drug.

Some drugs and medical devices presented in this publication have Food and Drug Administration (FDA) clearance for limited use in restricted research settings. It is the responsibility of health care providers to ascertain the FDA status of each drug or device planned for use in their clinical practice.

10 9 8 7 6 5 4 3 2 1

Contents

Contributing Authors

Rodney D. Adam, M.D.
Associate Professor of Medicine and Microbiology/Immunology, University of Arizona College of Medicine, Tucson, Arizona

Robert Anderson, M.D., M.P.H.
Mountain Technical Center, Littleton, Colorado

John S. Andrews, Jr., M.D., M.P.H.
Agency for Toxic Substances and Disease Registry, Atlanta, Georgia

Lidia Artiola i Fortuny, Ph.D.
Tucson, Arizona

Drew Badger, Ph.D.
Professor, Department of Pharmacology and Toxicology, University of Arizona College of Medicine, Tucson, Arizona

Benoit Bailey, M.D., M.Sc., F.R.C.P.C.
Department of Pharmacology and Toxicology, The Hospital for Sick Children, Toronto, Ontario, Canada

Carol M. Baldwin, R.N., Ph.D.
Research Assistant Professor of Medicine, Respiratory Sciences Center, University of Arizona College of Medicine, Tucson, Arizona

Marci Balge, R.N., M.S.
Partner, Newfields, LLC, Denver, Colorado

John R. Balmes, M.D.
Professor, Department of Medicine, University of California, San Francisco; Acting Director, Center for Occupational and Environmental Health, San Francisco, California

Jerry L. Bangert, M.D.
Assistant Professor of Clinical Pathology and Dermatology, University of Arizona College of Medicine, Tucson, Arizona

Cheryl S. Barbanel, M.D., M.B.A., M.P.H.
Associate Professor of Occupational and Environmental Medicine, Boston University School of Medicine, Boston, Massachusetts

Donald G. Barceloux, M.D., F.A.C.E.P., F.A.A.C.T.
Associate Clinical Professor of Medicine, University of California, Los Angeles, UCLA School of Medicine, Los Angeles, California; Pomona Valley Community Medical Center, Pomona, California

Iris R. Bell, M.D., Ph.D.
Associate Professor of Psychiatry, Psychology, and Family and Community Medicine, University of Arizona College of Medicine, Tucson, Arizona

John G. Benitez, M.D., M.P.H.
Associate Professor of Emergency Medicine and Environmental Medicine, Finger Lakes Regional Poison and Drug Information Center, University of Rochester School of Medicine and Dentistry, Rochester, New York

Neal L. Benowitz, M.D.
Professor of Medicine, University of California, San Francisco, School of Medicine; Chief, Division of Clinical Pharmacology, San Francisco General Hospital, San Francisco, California

Alfred M. Bernard, Ph.D.
Professor, Université Catholique de Louvain School of Public Health, Toxicology Department, Brussels, Belgium

Tareg A. Bey, M.D., F.A.C.E.P.
Assistant Clinical Professor of Emergency Medicine, University of California, Irvine, College of Medicine, Orange, California

Steven Black, M.S.
Health Effects Group, Tucson, Arizona

Leslie V. Boyer, M.D.
Department of Pediatrics, University of Arizona Health Sciences Center, Tucson, Arizona

Caryl S. Brailsford, M.D., M.S.
Medical Director, Arizona Poison Center

Alvin C. Bronstein, M.D., F.A.C.E.P.
Assistant Professor of Surgery, University of Colorado School of Medicine; Medical Director, Rocky Mountain Poison and Drug Center, Denver Health and Hospital Authority, Denver, Colorado

Bradford O. Brooks, Ph.D.
IBM Center for Process and Product Toxicology, IBM Corporation, Boulder, Colorado

William B. Bunn III, M.D., J.D., M.P.H.
Associate Professor, Northwestern University Medical School, Vice President, Health Safety and Productivity, Navistar Corporation, Chicago, Illinois

Jefferey L. Burgess, M.D., M.P.H.
University of Arizona Prevention Center, Tuscon, Arizona

Dean E. Carter, Ph.D.
Professor of Pharmacology and Toxicology, University of Arizona College of Pharmacy, Tucson, Arizona

Gerald R. Chase, Ph.D.
Mountain Technical Center, Littleton, Colorado

Kenneth H. Chase, M.D.
Washington Occupational Health Associates, Inc., Washington, D.C.

Charles R. Clark, Ph.D.
Manager, Toxicology and Product Safety, Tosco Corporation, Santa Ana, California

John J. Clary, Ph.D.
BioRisk, Midland, Michigan

Marianne Cloeren, M.D., M.P.H.
Associate, Occupational and Environmental Health, Department of Environmental Health Sciences, The Johns Hopkins School of Hygiene and Public Health, Baltimore, Maryland

Ernesto Cortes-Belen, M.D.
Fellow, Medical Toxicology and Instructor in Emergency Medicine, University of Pittsburgh School of Medicine, Pittsburgh, Pennsylvania

Clifton D. Crutchfield, Ph.D., C.I.H.
Community and Environmental Health, University of Arizona, Tucson, Arizona

Steven C. Curry, M.D.
Department of Medical Toxicology, Good Samaritan Regional Poison Center, Phoenix, Arizona

Rosalind R. Dalefield, B.V.Sc., Ph.D.
Dames & Moore, Inc., Denver, Colorado

Joanne Mary Dalgleish, M.B.
Prahran, Victoria, Australia

John G. Danby, M.S.
Senior Industrial Hygienist, Ergonomics, Health, and Safety, Coherent Auburn Division, Auburn, California

Feroza M. Daroowalla, M.D., M.P.H.
Department of Occupational and Environmental Medicine, Harborview Medical Center, Seattle, Washington

Richard C. Dart, M.D., Ph.D.
Director, Rocky Mountain Poison and Drug Center, Denver, Colorado

Donna L. Dehn, M.S., M.Ph.
Research Assistant, Department of Molecular Toxicology, University of Colorado School of Pharmacy, University of Colorado Health Sciences Center, Denver, Colorado

Jou-Fang Deng, M.D.
Associate Professor of Medicine, Veterans General Hospital, Taipei, Taiwan

Bradley Y. Dennis, M.D.
Medical Director, Brookwood Medical Center, Birmingham, Alabama

Samir M. Douidar, M.D., Ph.D.
Tampa, Florida

Alan M. Ducatman, M.D., M.Sc.
Institute of Occupational and Environmental Health, West Virginia University School of Medicine, Morgantown, West Virginia

Jacek Dutkiewicz, Ph.D.
Professor of Microbiology, Head of Department of Occupational Biohazards, National Institute of Agricultural Medicine, Lublin, Poland

Francis J. Farrell, M.D.
Watertown, New York

Miguel C. Fernández, M.D.
Assistant Professor of Surgery and Emergency Medicine, University of Texas Medical School at San Antonio; Medical Director, South Texas Poison Center, San Antonio, Texas

Christopher M. Filley, M.D.
Professor of Neurology and Psychiatry, University of Colorado School of Medicine; Behavioral Neurology Section, Denver Veterans Affairs Medical Center, Denver, Colorado

Michael L. Fischman, M.D., M.P.H.
Associate Clinical Professor, Division of Occupational and Environmental Medicine, University of California, San Francisco, School of Medicine, Walnut Creek, California

Donald C. Fisher, M.D., M.S.
Occupational Health Network, Albuquerque, New Mexico

Gary Fujimoto, M.D.
Medical Director, Palo Alto Medical Clinic, Palo Alto, California

Lorne K. Garrettson, M.D.
Professor Emeritus, Departments of Pediatrics and Environmental and Occupational Medicine, Emory University School of Medicine, Atlanta, Georgia

Robert J. Geller, M.D.
Associate Professor of Pediatrics, Emory University School of Medicine; Medical Director, Georgia Poison Center, Grady Health System, Atlanta, Georgia

Raquel L. Gibly, M.D.
Instructor of Clinical Surgery, Medical Toxicology Fellow, Department of Surgery, University of Arizona Health Sciences Center, Tucson, Arizona

Peter L. Goering, Ph.D., D.A.B.T.
Research Toxicologist, Center for Devices and Radiological Health, U.S. Food and Drug Administration, Rockville, Maryland

Harriet S. Goldman, D.D.S., M.P.H.
Associate Professor of Clinical Dentistry, Columbia University School of Dental and Oral Surgery; Chairman, Department of Dentistry, Morristown Memorial Hospital, Morristown, New Jersey

Melissa Gonzales, Ph.D.
Epidemiology and Biomarkers Branch, Human Studies Division, National Health and Environmental Effects Research Laboratory, Office of Research and Development, U.S. Environmental Protection Agency, Research Triangle Park, North Carolina

Kimberlie A. Graeme, M.D.
Fellowship Director, Department of Medical Toxicology, Good Samaritan Regional Medical Center, Phoenix, Arizona; Associate Professor of Clinical Emergency Medicine, University of Arizona College of Medicine; Department of Surgery, University Medical Center, Tucson, Arizona

William V. Gustin
Captain, Miami-Dade County Fire and Rescue Department, Wellington, Florida

Christina E. Hantsch, M.D.
Fellow, Center for Clinical Toxicology, Vanderbilt University Medical Center, Nashville, Tennessee

Myron C. Harrison, M.D., M.P.H.
Senior Health Advisor, Safety, Health, and Environment, Exxon Mobil Corporation, Irving, Texas

Robert J. Harrison, M.D., M.P.H.
Associate Clinical Professor, Division of Occupational and Environmental Medicine, University of California, San Francisco, School of Medicine, San Francisco, California

Georgia A. Hart, M.A.
Toxicologist, Department of Health, Safety, and Environment, Johns Manville Corporation, Littleton, Colorado

Thomas W. Hesterberg, Ph.D.
Director, Department of Health, Safety, and Environment, Johns Manville Corporation, Littleton, Colorado

Philip Hewitt, Ph.D.
E. Merk, Institut Für Toxikologic, Darmstadt, Germany

J. Michael Hitt, M.D.
Woodland Park, Colorado

John P. Holland, M.D., M.P.H.
Holland Associates, Olympia, Washington

Monica Lambert Hultquist, R.N., M.P.H.
Health Effects Group, Tucson, Arizona

Katherine L. Hunting, Ph.D., M.P.H.
Center for Risk Science and Public Health, George Washington University Medical Center, Washington, D.C.

Richard D. Irons, Ph.D.
Professor, University of Colorado School of Medicine; Director, Molecular Toxicology and Environmental Health Sciences, University of Colorado Health Sciences Center, Denver, Colorado

Donald W. Kautz, M.P.H., M.B.A.
Health Effects Group, Tucson, Arizona

James P. Kelly, M.D.
Associate Professor of Clinical Neurology, Northwestern University Medical School and Chicago Neurological Institute, Chicago, Illinois

James P. Keogh, M.D.
Occupational Health Project, University of Maryland School of Medicine, Baltimore, Maryland

J. Fergus Kerr, M.D.
Prahran, Victoria, Australia

Janet E. Kester, Ph.D.
Senior Science Advisor, ENVIRON International Corporation, St. Peters, Missouri

Allen G. Kraut, M.D., F.R.C.P.C.
Associate Professor, Department of Community Heath Sciences and Internal Medicine, University of Manitoba Faculty of Medicine, Winnipeg, Manitoba Canada

Edward P. Krenzelok, Pharm.D.
Professor of Pharmacy and Pediatrics, University of Pittsburgh School of Medicine; Director, Pittsburgh Poison Center, Children's Hospital of Pittsburgh, Pittsburgh, Pennsylvania

Gary R. Krieger, M.D., M.P.H., D.A.B.T.
Associate Adjunct Professor of Toxicology, University of Colorado School of Pharmacy; Department of Molecular and Environmental Toxicology, University of Colorado Health Sciences Center, Denver, Colorado

Ken Kulig, M.D.
Toxicology Associates, Denver, Colorado

Donald B. Kunkel, M.D.
Good Samaritan Regional Medical Center, Department of Medical Toxicology, Phoenix, Arizona

Charles E. Lambert, Ph.D., DABT
Senior Staff Toxicologist, Unocal Corporation, Brea, California

Hon-Wing Leung, Ph.D., D.A.B.T., C.I.H.
Associate Director of Applied Toxicology, Department of Health, Safety, and Environment, Union Carbide Corporation, Danbury, Connecticut

Paul J. A. Lever, M.S., Ph.D
Department Head and Associate Professor, Department of Mining and Geological Engineering, University of Arizona, Tucson, Arizona

Robert J. Levine, M.D.
Emergency Department, Mercy Hospital, Miami, Florida

Richard Lewis, M.D., M.P.H.
Moreland Hills, Ohio

Daniel F. Liberman, Ph.D.
Visiting Scientist, Massachusetts Institute of Technology, Cambridge, Massachusetts

Christopher H. Linden, M.D.
Associate Professor of Emergency Medicine, University of Massachusetts Medical School, Worcester, Massachusetts

Michael J. Lipsett, M.D.
Assistant Clinical Professor of Epidemiology and Biostatistics, University of California, San Francisco, School of Medicine, San Francisco, California

Frank A. LoVecchio, D.O.
Medical Director, Poison Control Center, Department of Medical Toxicology, Good Samaritan Regional Medical Center, Phoenix, Arizona

John A. Lowe, C.I.H.
Leader, Human Health Risk Assessment Delivery Center, Dayton, Ohio

Howard Maibach, M.D.
Professor of Dermatology, University of California, San Francisco, School of Medicine, San Francisco, California

Lisa A. Maier, M.D.
Departments of Immunology and Respiratory Diseases, National Jewish Center, Denver, Colorado

Melanie A. Marty, Ph.D.
Chief, Air Risk Assessment Unit, Office of Environmental Health Hazard Assessment, Berkeley, California

Thomas J. Mason, Ph.D.
Professor of Epidemiology, Department of Epidemiology and Biostatistics, University of South Florida College of Public Health, Tampa, Florida

Michael A. McGuigan, M.D., M.B.A.
Associate Professor of Pediatrics, Pharmacology, and Health Administration, University of Toronto Faculty of Medicine; Division of Clinical Pharmacology and Toxicology, The Hospital for Sick Children, Toronto, Ontario, Canada

Jude T. McNally
Assistant Director, Arizona Poison and Drug Information Center, Tucson, Arizona

William J. Meggs, M.D., Ph.D.
Professor of Emergency Medicine, Division of Toxicology, East Carolina University School of Medicine, Greenville, North Carolina

Jacqueline Messite, M.D.
Clinical Professor of Environmental Medicine, New York University School of Medicine, New York, New York

Linda M. Micale, M.S.
Tucson, Arizona

Donald M. Molenaar, M.D., M.P.H.
Brea, California

Chodaesessie Wellesley-Cole Morgan, M.P.H., Ph.D.
Graduate Research Associate, Department of Community and Family Health, University of South Florida College of Public Health, Tampa, Florida

Linda H. Morse, M.D.
Daly City, California

Larry L. Needham, Ph.D.
Chief, Toxicology Branch, Division of Environmental Health Laboratory Sciences, National Center for Environmental Health, Centers for Disease Control and Prevention, Atlanta, Georgia

Lee S. Newman, M.D., M.A.
Head of Division of Environmental and Occupational Health Sciences, National Jewish Medical and Research Center, Denver, Colorado

Robert J. Noecker, M.D.
Assistant Professor of Ophthalmology, University of Arizona College of Medicine, Tucson, Arizona

Mary Kay O'Rourke, Ph.D.
Professor of Medicine and Research Analyst, Health-Related Professions, University of Arizona School of Medicine, Tucson, Arizona

Frederick W. Oehme, Ph.D., D.V.M.
Professor of Toxicology, Pathobiology, Medicine, and Physiology, Comparative Toxicology Laboratories, Kansas State University, Manhattan, Kansas

Herbert H. Ortega, M.D., Ph.D.
El Paso, Texas

Deborah J. Owen, M.D., M.P.H.
Medical Director, San Francisco Fire Department, San Francisco, California

Donald G. Patterson, Jr., Ph.D.
Deputy Chief, Toxicology Branch, Centers for Disease Control and Prevention, Northeast, Atlanta, Georgia

Dennis J. Paustenbach, M.D.
Chemical Risk Division, McLaren Environmental Engineer, Alameda, California

John M. Peters, M.D., Sc.D.
Hastings Professor of Preventive Medicine, University of Southern California School of Medicine, Los Angeles, California

Karen K. Phillips, M.D., M.P.H., F.A.C.O.E.M.
Medical Director, St. Elizabeth Company Care, Lincoln, Nebraska

Paul D. Phillips, J.D.
Partner and Director, Environmental Law Section, Holland & Hart, Denver, Colorado

Scott D. Phillips, M.D., F.A.C.P., F.A.C.M.T.
Associate Clinical Professor of Medicine, University of Colorado School of Medicine; Division of Clinical Pharmacology and Toxicology, University of Colorado Health Sciences Center; Toxicology Associates, Denver, Colorado

Steven Pike, M.D.
President, EnvironMD, Tucson, Arizona

Richard E. Rodriguez, Ph.D.
Department of Chemistry, Texas Wesleyan University, Fort Worth, Texas

Carlisle F. Runge, M.A., Ph.D.
Distinguished McKnight University Professor, Department of Applied Economics and Law, University of Minnesota, St. Paul, Minnesota

Jill Ryer-Powder, Ph.D., D.A.B.T.
Manager of Health Sciences Environ, Irvine, California

Richard S. Schottenfeld, M.D.
Veterans Affairs Medical Center, Psychiatry Service, Tucson, Arizona

Raymond J. Schumacher, M.D., M.P.H.
Tucson, Arizona

Barbara Scolnick, M.D.
Department of Occupational and Environmental Medicine, Cambridge Hospital, Cambridge, Massachusetts

Donna L. Seger, M.D., F.A.C.E.P., F.A.A.C.T.
Assistant Professor of Medicine and Emergency Medicine, Vanderbilt University School of Medicine; Medical Director of Middle Tennessee Poison Center, Nashville, Tennessee

James Seltzer, M.D.
Medical Director, Indoor Hygienic Technologies, San Diego, California

Peter G. Shields, M.D.
Professor of Medicine and Oncology, Georgetown University Medical Center; Associate Director for Population Science, Lombardi Cancer Center; Washington, D.C.

Dennis J. Shusterman, M.D., M.P.H.
Associate Clinical Professor of Medicine, University of California, San Francisco, School of Medicine, San Francisco, California

Claus-Peter Siegers, M.D.
Professor of Pharmacology and Toxicology, Department of Experimental and Clinical Pharmacology and Toxicology, Medical University of Lübeck, Lübeck, Germany

I. Glenn Sipes, Ph.D.
Professor of Medicine, Department of Pharmacology, University of Arizona College of Medicine; Head of Pharmacology and Toxicology, University of Arizona College of Pharmacy, Tucson, Arizona

Dorsett D. Smith, M.D.
Clinical Professor of Medicine, Departments of Respiratory Disease and Critical Care, University of Washington School of Medicine, Seattle, Washington

Wayne R. Snodgrass, M.D., Ph.D.
Assistant Professor of Family and Community Medicine, University of Arizona College of Medicine; Area Medical Director, Concentra Medical Centers, Tucson, Arizona

Daniel A. Spyker, M.D., Ph.D.
Senior Medical Director, Purdue Pharma, LP, Stamford, Connecticut

Charles E. Stewart, M.D.
Colorado Springs, Colorado

Miroslav Styblo, Ph.D.
Research Assistant Professor of Pediatrics and Nutrition, University of North Carolina at Chapel Hill School of Medicine, Chapel Hill, North Carolina

John B. Sullivan, Jr., M.D.
Associate Dean for Clinical Affairs, Associate Professor of Emergency Medicine, University of Arizona Health Sciences Center, Tucson, Arizona

F. William Sunderman, Jr., M.D.
Visitng Scholar, Department of Chemistry and Biochemistry, Middlebury College, Middlebury, Vermont

Sue Sundstrom, Ph.D., D.A.B.T.
Toxicologist, Toxicology and Risk Assessment Consulting Services, Groton, Massachusetts

Ana A. Taras, M.P.H.
Director of Planning, William F. Ryan Community Health Center, New York, New York

David J. Thomas, Ph.D.
Pharmacokinetics Branch, Ecpt. Toxicology Division, NHEERL, ORD, U.S. Environmental Protection Agency, Research Triangle Park, North Carolina

Theodore G. Tong, Pharm.D
Associate Dean for Academic and Student Affairs and Professor of Pharmacy Practice, Pharmacology, and Toxicology, University of Arizona College of Pharmacy, Tucson, Arizona

Richard L. Urie, C.I.H.
Golden, Colorado

Mark D. Van Ert, M.S., Ph.D.
Associate Professor of Public Health, Department of Community and Environmental Health Practice and Policy, University of Arizona College of Public Health, Tucson, Arizona

George L. Voelz, M.D.
Guest Scientist (Retired), Environment, Safety, and Health Division, Los Alamos National Laboratory, Los Alamos, New Mexico

Michael P. Waalkes, Ph.D.
Chief, Inorganic Carcinogenesis Section, Laboratory of Comparative Carcinogenesis, National Cancer Institute at the National Institute of Environmental Health Sciences, Research Triangle Park, North Carolina

Zakaria Z. Wahba, Ph.D.
Senior Pharmacologist, Office of Generic Drugs, U.S. Food and Drug Administration, Rockville, Maryland

Kevin L. Wallace, M.D.
Clinical Associate Professor, Department of Medical Toxicology, University of Arizona; Good Samaritan Regional Medical Center, Phoenix, Arizona

Bridget T. Walsh, D.O.
Associate Professor of Clinical Medicine, University of Arizona College of Medicine, Southern Arizona Veterans Affairs Health Care System, Tucson, Arizona

Frank G. Walter, M.D., F.A.C.E.P., F.A.C.M.T.
Associate Professor of Surgery, Departments of Emergency Medicine and Medical Toxicology, University of Arizona College of Medicine, Tucson, Arizona

Neill K. Weaver, M.D.
Former Clinical Professor of Internal Medicine and Professor of Occupational Medicine and Environmental Hygiene, Tulane University School of Medicine, New Orleans, Louisiana; Former Director, Medicine and Biological Science, American Petroleum Institute, Washington, D.C.; Consultant in Occupational and Environmental Medicine, Arlington, Virginia

Janet S. Weiss, M.D.
Clinical Faculty, Department of Occupational and Environmental Medicine, University of California, San Francisco, School of Medicine, San Francisco, California

Larry W. Welch, E.D.D.
Department of Neurology, Vanderbilt University Medical Center, Nashville, Tennessee

Laura S. Welch, M.D.
Adjunct Professor of Environmental and Occupational Health, Section Director, Department of Occupational Medicine, Washington Hospital Center, Washington, D.C.

John Whysner, M.D., Ph.D.
Chief, Division of Pathology and Toxicology, American Health Foundation, Valhalla, New York

James M. Woolfenden, M.D.
Professor of Radiology, Department of Radiology, University of Arizona College of Medicine, University of Arizona Health Sciences Center, Tucson, Arizona

Luke Yip, M.D.
Clinical Assistant Professor of Pharmaceutical Sciences, University of Colorado School of Pharmacy; Attending Faculty, Rocky Mountain Poison and Drug Center; Department of Medicine, Section of Clinical Toxicology, Denver Health Medical Center, Denver, Colorado

David E. Yocum, M.D.
Professor of Medicine, University of Arizona College of Medicine, Tucson, Arizona

Foreword

Toxicology is the study of the probability, not the possibility, of physical or chemical agents causing effects (i.e., toxicity) at a specific dose and under the conditions of use (i.e., hazards). The methodology for determining this probability is to identify the duration and level of exposure, to quantitate the dose of an agent in the environment (i.e., the external dose), and to estimate the dose that gains entrance into the body by injection, inhalation, ingestion, or dermal exposure (i.e., the internal dose). Once these factors are known, a health professional must review the scientific medical literature to determine whether a causal relationship exists between a particular dose and a specific medical outcome or symptom. A differential diagnosis to rule out other causes for a given condition must also be added, because symptoms may be caused by several different processes.

A toxicology analysis is necessary because a sufficient dose of any agent may cause toxicity. This includes substances such as sugar, water, oxygen, and salt. Too much sugar causes diabetes, but sugar is essential for life. Too much water causes electrolyte imbalances, and too much oxygen damages the lungs. Large doses of salt cause brain damage. Aspirin is a good example of the link between pharmacology and toxicology; at recommended doses it is clinically useful, but at high doses it is life-threatening.

In occupational and environmental toxicology, the distinction between the terms *toxicity* and *hazard* is critical. Toxicity is a fundamental property of all substances that describes a dose-response relationship between a given amount of a substance and its effect on cells, organs, or body systems. *Hazard* refers to the effect on cells, organs, or body systems under the condition of use. For example, for a sealed container of cyanide, there is a known dose-response relationship between a given amount of the contents of the container and its effect on cells, organs, or body systems. While in a closed container, the cyanide poses no risk. The hazard exists only if the cyanide container is opened and used in a manner that causes exposure to doses beyond known safe levels.

A problem exists for the health professional trying to provide clinical environmental health probabilities concerning toxic exposures. With increasing information provided through professional journals, texts, World Wide Web sites, and mass-communication media, it may be difficult to assess the accuracy of environmental toxicology information. For example, scientifically unsound notions concerning the dangers of carcinogens in apples and benzene in bottled water, the potential of coffee to cause pancreatic cancer, and the hazards of electric blankets, dental amalgams, cellular phones, and video display terminals, pose special problems that need resolution.

To fill this scientific gap and meet the need for reliable environmental toxicology information, Drs. Sullivan and Krieger and their colleagues in 1992 published a useful text entitled *Hazardous Materials Toxicology: Clinical Principles of Environmental Health*. I referred to this text many times to help formulate for myself and my patients important questions about risk, toxicity, and hazard. Uniform editing, updated bibliographies, and thorough indexing make this second edition, *Clinical Environmental Health and Toxic Exposures*, extremely useful for health professionals, government employees, poison control center workers, and teachers. Most importantly, this text will help health professionals plan for emergencies and prevent environmental health problems. Although some uncertainty will always exist about environmental toxicology, careful use of this text will help make the field of environmental toxicology educational and exciting.

Charles E. Becker, M.D.
Professor Emeritus
Department of Medicine
University of California, San Francisco, School of Medicine
San Francisco, California

Foreword

As a species, humans are a fragile and vulnerable life form. Unable to tolerate the ordinary changes in weather, climate, and atmospheric perturbations without significant alterations in their immediate environment, they have survived, frequently at the cost of increasing the hostility of their environment.

From the first capture of fire to the latest creation of nuclear energy, humans have attempted to alleviate the ravages of their immediate environment, and, in that process, the technology for the maintenance and improvement of life has become a health menace.

The need for good science in the field of environmental health is even greater than in 1992, when this useful book was first published. As we create new environmental disasters with our technology, and as we encounter risks from deliberate disasters, such as terrorist attacks with nerve agents, the demand for a safe environment increases. How clean is clean? What can we tolerate in our atmosphere without harm, or at least with minimal harm? When we prepare to clean up a contaminated environment, how much do we have to do?

Given the state of evidence on which many of the environmental decisions in our society have been made, it is clear that we have often acted out of panic, theory, untested hypothesis, and political pressure.

Every community has hidden environmental health hazards that do not become apparent until a tragic accident occurs, but, at least since the first edition of this book, there have been increases in the awareness of industrial hazards and in the energy and motivation to prevent the unmanageable, to minimize the necessary costs of industrial wastes, and to attempt to preserve our environment for long-term use.

Much still needs to be done. Without improved monitoring systems and identification methodologies, we are forced to await the recognition of multiple casualties before dealing with sources of disease.

Our public health networks need intensified clearing and recording capabilities, and part of that monitoring must include environmental toxins.

The only way that we can avoid the phobias induced by superstitions, fear of the unknown, and politically driven decisions devoid of common sense is by increasing our level of true scientific knowledge.

Clinical Environmental Health and Toxic Exposures contains precisely the kind of scientific evidence that will help guide our decision making, as well as our management of environmental disasters.

The authors have considerably expanded on the first edition and have incorporated current knowledge in a highly useful and readable way.

It is with great pleasure that I watch the development of the science of this vitally important field. I can only hope and trust that the people most responsible for the decisions that affect our environment will use this text and profit from its wisdom.

Peter Rosen, M.D.
Clinical Professor of Medicine and Surgery
Director, Emergency Medicine Residency Program
University of California, San Diego, School of Medicine
La Jolla, California

Preface

Health is often referred to as a harmony of body and mind. However, a third crucial variable in the health equation is often ignored: the environment. What is the extent to which environmental contamination plays a role in causing disease? Differentiating passion from proof and emotion from evidence is critical, because regulatory policies are often driven by determining the theoretical health risks associated with specific environmental pollutants. However, the connection between environmental hazards and disease causation is sometimes complex and often controversial. For example, there are often acrimonious debates over the relationships between air pollution and respiratory disease rates and hazardous waste sites and cancer.

As life expectancy increases in some western nations, cancer may surpass heart disease as the predominant cause of death. In the United States, one in three people will be diagnosed with some type of cancer during his or her lifetime, and almost one in four will die from it. The role of exposure to hazardous materials as a major factor in these statistics remains highly contentious. Overall, in the United States, when cancers caused by smoking are excluded, there is an upward trend in some specific forms of malignancy. This increased incidence has been attributed to a growing and aging population, improved screening techniques, earlier diagnosis, and the impact of environmental and occupational chemical exposure. Although the technical ability to assay chemicals in air, water, soil, and food has improved, the debate swirling around whether low-level exposure to chemicals causes cancer in humans is a significant twenty-first century issue.

Another area of intense scrutiny is the cost-versus-benefit analysis of environmental regulations. The environmental regulatory process is inextricably intertwined with politics, economics, and the legal system of a given country. Although politicians and economists argue the cost–benefit analyses of environmental decisions, they frequently have difficulty assessing and accounting for the true economic value of the environment as it contributes to human welfare. Unfortunately, policy making is not a controlled laboratory experiment; thus, there are trade-offs and compromises that are not driven by above-the-fray scientific rationalism. Nevertheless, it is critical that health care providers have an accurate and educational basis of what is known and what is simply conjecture or belief without objective foundation.

With these concepts in mind, we present the second edition of *Clinical Environmental Health and Toxic Exposures*. We trust our revisions will provide readers with informative and objective chapters on diverse environmental health topics, while expanding on hazardous materials toxicology in the twenty-first century.

John B. Sullivan, Jr., M.D.
Gary R. Krieger, M.D., M.P.H., D.A.B.T.

SECTION

I

General Principles of Environmental Health

CHAPTER 1

Environment and Health: Going into the Twenty-First Century

John B. Sullivan, Jr., and Gary R. Krieger

PAST IS PROLOGUE

Since the mid-1970s, environmentalism has become an accepted part of the political and economic landscape of every country and major international institution, including banks (1). Although *environmentalism* is a concept universally embraced, the actual meaning of the term and its relationship to health outcomes is not always clear. For example, estimates that environmental factors cause cancer range from 4% to 75% (2). This wide variation of attribution is directly related to the difficulty of defining *environmental factors*.

The collapse of communism in Eastern Europe and the former Soviet Union has provided access to a unique "experiment in nature" on the relationship between pollution, lifestyle, economics, and health. For decades, the Soviet government exploited the natural resources of more than 8 million square miles, leaving hazardous-waste sites and destruction of a once pristine environment. Now, Russia and the other 14 Soviet republics face an ecological shambles while they struggle to develop in a market-oriented global economy (3). While their great rivers served as channels for human and chemical wastes, tons of nuclear waste also were abandoned under Arctic waters, and highly toxic pesticides were indiscriminately spread over agricultural lands. Despite signing an international antidumping treaty in 1976, Soviet authorities continued their extensive dumping of nuclear waste into Arctic waters off the city of Murmansk, 200 miles above the Arctic Circle (3).

Unsound Soviet agricultural practices diverted two rivers, the Syr Darya and Amu Darya, that fed into the Aral Sea in Kazakhstan, to irrigate rice and cotton fields. By 1975, both rivers were not only highly contaminated with chemicals, sewage, and metals; they also were dying. The Aral Sea, once larger than West Virginia, now consists of two shallow bodies of polluted water (3).

As the Soviet Union teetered toward collapse, Kazakhstan's government ordered health studies, which showed high concentrations of toxic metals in soil, immune system abnormalities in 58% of children, and widespread chromosomal damage. Then, on April 26, 1986, in the city of Chernobyl, reactor no. 4 exploded, spewing an estimated 100 million curies of radionuclides, such as cesium 137 and iodine 131, and exposing 4.9 million people in Ukraine, Belarus, and Russia to radioactive fallout. One hundred eighty tons of uranium fuel remain in the rubble of the unsecured sarcophagus (4).

The rest of the world was not without problems. In 1984, 2,000 people died from a hazardous chemical release accident in Bhopal, India. On March 24, 1989, 11 million gallons of North Slope crude oil poured into the unsullied waters of Prince William Sound when the *Exxon Valdez* struck a reef. Contingency plans created for dealing with such a spill failed after 12 years of trouble-free operations. The Prince William Sound has become a laboratory for scientific research in oil pollution of a pristine environment (5).

Across continents and below the equator, deep within the rain forests of Africa, a virus silently made its transition from monkey to human, beginning the catastrophic epidemic of the acquired immunodeficiency syndrome (AIDS). Breaking out from the same rain forests, a hemorrhagic fever virus named *Ebola* frightened the world with its lethal virulence.

War and social disruption, themes throughout human history, continued to exact their toll on populations and the environment throughout the 1990s. The Persian Gulf War resulted in massive environmental pollution. Oily clouds from burning wells rose as high as 22,000 feet. Satellite images from 440 miles above the ground photographed pollutants covering 10,000 square miles. From the blackened burning landscape to the fine mist of oil particles suspended in the air, the Gulf suffered an environmental insult the human health effects of which have yet to be determined. The U.S. military now struggles to understand the cause of an illness termed the *Gulf War syndrome*.

In 1997, feverish political debate in the United States escalated over global warming, regulation of atmospheric particles less than 2.5 μm in diameter, and reauthorization of the Endangered Species Act. A chemical weapons treaty was signed, and xenoestrogens were linked with breast cancer, initiating a "feminization" of the environment debate. Underpinning most of these environmental contamination scenarios are economic and political themes permanently entwined with environmentalism (6,7).

Environmental Health and Political Economics

The media have highlighted the degraded environmental conditions in Central and Eastern Europe and the former Soviet Union. Photographs of soot-covered children and denuded landscapes became symbols of ignoring proper environmental stewardship. The implication of such journalism is that environmentally induced disease is at epidemic levels. Although substantial evidence exists that heavy levels of pollution have affected health in Central and Eastern Europe, a convincing case has not been made that air, water, soil, and food contamination is the sole cause of the observed life expectancy change. In contrast, some studies of acute and subacute geographically localized populations demonstrate changes in morbidity due to environmental exposures.

On examination, there appears to be a widening life expectancy gap between the countries of Central and Eastern Europe and the Western democracies. In general, life expectancy for both men and women is much lower in Central and Eastern Europe than in the West (7,8). This gap emerged in the 1960s and has persisted and widened since the 1970s. Life expectancy differences are most pronounced for the age groups older than 30 years. Similarly, female life expectancy statistics for the East have improved but at a much slower rate than their Western counterparts. According to a 1993 World Bank study, the most significant predictor of a nation's health status is its per capita gross domestic product (GDP) rather than the nature and type of its health services (6). The relationship between GDP per capita and life expectancy at birth is strong and persistent, particularly at lower levels of income. However, income differentials, rather than income levels, seem to be a better predictor of healthiness, implying that "equitable" income distribution is more closely allied with longevity (7). Given the compressed income distribution that was characteristic of the Socialist countries, the rapid and uneven introduction of Capitalism is potentially significant, because market economies tend to accentuate income distribution within populations.

A particularly problematic political economic struggle is the cost of environmental regulations. In 1980, the cost of U.S. environmental regulatory compliance was estimated to be approximately $53 billion. Now these costs exceed $150 billion. Since 1993, the number of regulatory proposals has increased 20%. Business and individuals now conflict with federal regulators over wetlands, mining, hazardous-waste sites, and the effects of greenhouse gases on the environment. However, although the overall cost-effectiveness of environmental regulation is sharply debated, undeniable progress has occurred in the control of toxic exposures and disease prevention.

In 1991, the EPA estimated that cleanup of nonfederal hazardous-waste sites would cost $30 billion. Updated estimates project cleanup costs for all sites through the year 2020 to be closer to $750 billion, with a range of $500 billion to $1 trillion. This estimate covered federal and nonfederal sites and the Environmental Protection Agency's (EPA's) National Priority List (NPL) sites. Regarding the NPL sites, it was estimated that costs through the year 2020 would range from $106 billion to $320 billion dollars (9). At the end of 1995, 1,296 hazardous-waste sites were listed on the EPA's NPL.

The U.S. Congressional Budget Office in 1994 offered different estimates for nonfederal NPL sites, with projected costs ranging from $42 billion to $120 billion. These Congressional Budget Office estimates involved discounted present dollars. In addition to site remediation, the General Accounting Office estimates that $31 billion will be needed for maintenance and monitoring costs at NPL sites over the next 10 years (9).

Environmental justice also became a theme. EPA demographic data from the 1980s indicated that 41 million people live within a 4-mile radius of an NPL site, and 11 million people live within 1 mile of an NPL site. The socioeconomically disadvantaged are reported to be disproportionately located near such sites (10).

In 1992, heads of state attended the United Nations Conference on Environment and Development in Rio de Janeiro, Brazil. This earth summit developed a comprehensive document termed *Agenda 21* to provide a blueprint for actions through the year 2000. *Agenda 21* provided for planning in areas affecting relationships between the environment and the economy (11). *Agenda 21*'s proposal to adopt precautionary approaches in managing the life cycle of toxic chemicals to prevent and reduce risk to human health and the environment involved four programs:

1. Promote the prevention and minimization of hazardous-waste.
2. Promote and strengthen institutional capacities in hazardous-waste management.
3. Promote and strengthen international cooperation in the management of transboundary movements of hazardous-waste.
4. Prevent illegal traffic in hazardous-waste.

More than 350 million tons of hazardous-waste are generated worldwide each year (11). Shipment and disposal of this waste is an economic activity for many industrialized countries, creating concerns about the transboundary importation of hazardous-waste. In 1987, the United Nations Environment Program initiated a study on illegal trafficking of hazardous-waste. Evidence showed that illegal traffic was a threat to both the environment and human health. To date, 90 countries have prohibited the import of hazardous-waste.

Data from the Chemical Manufacturers Association and the U.S. EPA indicate that the amount of industrial hazardous- and toxic waste generation in the United States continues to increase. Source reduction activities may provide economic as well as environmental benefits to industry (Table 1-1). Although the data from Central and Eastern Europe and the former Soviet Union are consistent with the Western experience since the 1970s, several trends expected to dominate twenty-first century environmentalism are emerging (6):

TABLE 1-1. Source-reduction accomplishments by 29 U.S. chemical manufacturing plants, 1985–1992

Concept	Average accomplishment
Amount of waste reduced	1.6 million lb/plant
Percentage of waste stream reduced	71% in the individual targeted waste stream
Medium of waste reduced by plants	49%, wastewater; 44%, solid wastes; and 24%, air emissions
Implementation time	8.2 months (range, 3 mo to >3 y)
Increase in product yields	7% (range, 1%–40%)
Annual savings per source	$351,000 (range, <$6,000 to ≥$1 million)
Capital costs per plant of implementing source-reduction activities	25%, no capital investment; approximately 50%, <$100,000 (paid back in 18 mo); and 13%, between $1 million and $10 million (paid back in ≈2.5 y)
Annual savings per dollar of capital investment	$3.49 (range, $1.0–$10.0)

From ref. 11, with permission from Princeton Scientific Publishing Co., Inc., Princeton, NJ.

- An evolution from workplace exposure studies to community studies, with emphasis on subtle morbidity outcomes rather than mortality
- An expansion of "environmental pollution" to encompass more than industrial sources, such as infectious diseases, global warming, and loss of biodiversity
- International cooperation in preventing illegal international trafficking in hazardous-waste
- A continued debate between advocates of command-and-control regulation and environmental free marketeers
- Promotion of hazardous-waste minimization
- The use of environmental standards by developed countries as ill-disguised trade barriers
- Emphasis on resource conservation and sustainable resource efforts

NEW HAZARDS FROM OLD SOURCES

Air Pollution

Air pollution continues to be a major focus of regulatory controversy. The U.S. EPA's proposed new standards for particles measuring less than 2.5 µm ($PM_{2.5}$) is producing heated debate. These new standards are meant to protect susceptible populations, such as those persons with respiratory disease, children, and the elderly. The Clean Air Act mandates that the EPA set National Ambient Air Quality Standards for six criteria pollutants: ozone, particulate matter under 10 µm and 2.5 µm, nitrogen dioxide, sulfur dioxide, carbon monoxide, and lead. The EPA also is mandated to review standards every 5 years but has failed to do so. Therefore, the American Lung Association, among others, sued the EPA for reconsideration of ozone and particulate standards. As a result, two panels of the Clean Air Scientific Advisory Committee were established, one for ozone and one for particulate matter, and health studies of both pollutants were reviewed, after which the EPA decided that current standards do not adequately protect susceptible populations (12).

After the EPA's proposed particulate standard was released in draft in November 1996, a swell of controversy emerged. These fine particles are currently a fraction of the PM_{10} particles. The EPA's new proposed standards maintain current standards for PM_{10} and add new requirements for $PM_{2.5}$ and ozone. Although both changes are controversial, the particulate change engendered the most intense arguments. Questions arose as to whether the science behind the new air standard was practical and sound and whether the policy was cost-effective or would impose undue hardship on some industries. The EPA suggested that the new standards would have benefits that would total more than $112 billion annually in the form of fewer premature deaths, hospital admissions, and medical care. However, half of all U.S. counties would fail to meet one or both of the newly proposed standards, and bringing every county into compliance would cost at least $6 to $8 billion a year for at least a decade (12). This type of mandate illustrates the disagreement about just what constitutes margins of safety, as the Clean Air Act does not limit expense in setting public health standards.

The EPA has estimated that reducing $PM_{2.5}$ pollution could save 20,000 lives per year among the elderly and those with preexisting pulmonary and cardiac conditions. The organization also estimates that respiratory hospital admissions might drop by 9,000 per year (12). Arguments counter that these epidemiologic correlations do not constitute causation and that the paucity of scientific information concerning $PM_{2.5}$ particles mandates more scientific study before new standards are issued (13). Experts have expressed concern over potential errors in the $PM_{2.5}$ epidemiologic data (13). They argue that the mortality and morbidity studies have been a time series with no personal measures of exposure (13). Analyses of many studies on which the EPA relied have produced contradictory results. Biases and confounding factors from other pollutants, such as sulfur dioxide, ozone, and nitrogen dioxide, exist.

In 1996, in response to the EPA's continued lack of cost-consciousness, Congress passed the Small Business Regulatory Enforcement Fairness Act, which requires federal agencies issuing major rules to submit to Congress a cost-benefit analysis of that rule. Within 60 days, the House and Senate can vote on the rule. If the vote is not taken, then the rule takes effect. The final resolution of these rule changes is, at best, uncertain and likely to dominate regulatory debate well into the twenty-first century.

Disease Emergence

Infectious diseases remain the leading cause of death worldwide. Since international travel has increased, diseases can now be easily spread through traffic routes. Land use changes and zoonotic disease spread caused by urban sprawl and ecological changes are increasing challenges to public health. As an example, destruction of the rain forest in Brazil has been associated with advancing and escalating cases of malaria. Emergence of new diseases and old diseases can be traced to factors of social disruption, war, human behavior, lack of public health infrastructure, and environmental disruption (Table 1-2).

As an example of environmental disruption, the toxic dinoflagellate *Pfiesteria piscicida*, known as the *fish killer*, has been linked with the killing of tens of thousands of fish in Maryland's Pocomoke River. These dinoflagellates release a toxin that causes dermal lesions and short-term memory problems in exposed humans. The dinoflagellate is thought to flourish in waters replete with nitrogen and phosphorus caused by runoff from farms and industrial waste (14).

Climate change is another potential public health challenge that can result in disease emergence. The National Oceanic and

TABLE 1-2. Factors in emergence of diseases

Categories	Examples
Societal events	Economic impoverishment; war or civil conflict; population growth and migration; urban decay
Health care	New medical devices; organ or tissue transplantation; drugs causing immunosuppression; widespread use of antibiotics
Food production	Globalization of food supplies; changes in food processing and packaging
Human behavior	Sexual behavior; drug use; travel; diet; outdoor recreation; use of child-care facilities
Environmental changes	Deforestation and reforestation; changes in water ecosystems; flood and drought; famine; global warming
Public health infrastructure	Curtailment or reduction in prevention programs; inadequate communicable disease surveillance; lack of trained personnel (epidemiologists, laboratory scientists, vector and rodent control specialists)
Microbial adaptation and change	Changes in virulence and toxin production; development of drug resistance; microbes as cofactors in chronic diseases

From Department of Health and Human Services, Centers for Disease Control and Prevention. Emerging infectious disease threats: a prevention strategy for the United States, 1994. *Environ Health Perspect* 1996;(7):104.

Atmospheric Administration estimates that the global temperature has increased between 0.3°C and 0.6°C during the last century and has been strongest at night in the Northern Hemisphere. CO_2, a major "greenhouse" gas, arises from natural sources as well as human-related fuel combustion. Computer modeling predicts that, should the atmospheric CO_2 double over the next 100 years, the global temperature would increase 1.5°C to 4.5°C (3°F to 9°F). Such a temperature change would cause the seas to rise 15 to 90 cm and alter the ecological pattern of infectious diseases such as malaria, yellow fever, encephalitis, cholera, and dengue fever (14). The warming of waters would support the growth of toxic algae, which in turn would result in flooding of coastal areas and rivers and the consequent loss of farmland and furtherance of soil erosion.

Further substantiating the potential of vectorborne disease spread with the advent of global warming, a computer model simulation has predicted a significant increase in the seasonal and geographic distribution of the sandfly, *Phlebotomus papatasii*, and of drought in Southwest Asia (14). The sandfly is a vector for sandfly fever (a viral infection with low mortality) and leishmaniasis (caused by a protozoan that infects skin and viscera).

For centuries, El Niño has appeared as a periodic episode of warm water, changing winds, and shifting ocean currents over much of the equatorial Pacific. Occurring every 7 or 8 years, El Niño is now known to be more than just a warming trend off the Peruvian coast. The El Niño of 1982 through 1983 left 2,000 people dead and $13 billion in economic losses. El Niño causes major climatic changes, floods, droughts, and crop losses. This climate phenomenon cycles between warm and cold and is a powerful influence on global weather patterns. As warm water spreads into other areas of the Pacific Ocean, storms and climate changes follow, with a shift in high-altitude winds (the jet stream) that serve as weather tracks in the Northern and Southern hemispheres. The 1993 Hantavirus outbreak in the southwestern United States may have been an El Niño consequence. One hundred thirty people experienced acute and highly fatal respiratory disease after breathing air contaminated by feces of infected rodents. Hantavirus infection carried a mortality of 50%, and the shifting of the climate from El Niño is speculated to have increased the rodent population through excessive spring rains, which increased food for these animals.

The incidence of dengue fever, a mosquito-borne illness characterized by sudden onset of fever, headaches, arthralgias, myalgia, nausea, and hemorrhages, has dramatically increased worldwide. An average of 29,000 hemorrhagic cases now are reported annually. Hemorrhagic disease is the leading cause of death in children in Southwest Asia and has made a dramatic resurgence in Cuba and other areas of Latin America (14).

A Chinese freighter may have triggered a massive cholera epidemic in 1991 by releasing contaminated ballast water in Lima, Peru. Cholera vibrio can remain dormant inside algae for long periods and can be activated by warm water. In the early 1990s, several El Niños appeared in a row. Also, because Lima's drinking water is not chlorinated, more than 3,500 people were killed and 300,000 became ill (14).

An outbreak of coccidiomycosis after an earthquake in California is an example of how natural disasters can increase the risk of disease. Spores were spread in dust clouds generated by the earthquake and the landslide that followed, exposing residents of Simi Valley to coccidia (15). The disease outbreak corresponded to a point source exposure and was consistent with the incubation period of acute coccidiomycosis.

In spring 1993 in Milwaukee, Wisconsin, contamination of water supply by *Cryptosporidium*, a gastrointestinal parasite, resulted in severe, acute, watery diarrhea, nausea, vomiting, and fever in those who ingested the water. Four hundred thousand people were affected, and 100 deaths were related to ingestion of the oocyst-contaminated water. *Cryptosporidium* is resistant to chlorine, and standard water treatment filters do not capture the micrometer-size parasite.

In the United States, the Centers for Disease Control and Prevention in Atlanta have been preparing for improved disease surveillance and the development of electronic networks for monitoring emerging diseases and pathogen resistance problems. Sentinel networks within hospital emergency departments have been organized to identify such diseases quickly (16).

ECOPOLITICS AND ECONOMICS GOING INTO THE TWENTY-FIRST CENTURY

Politics and economics are inseparable, and because economics tends to control political decisions, cost-benefit analysis will continue to affect environmental regulatory processes. An economic fact is that nothing is free: Everything has an opportunity cost, and unlimited human wants in the face of limited output of goods and services make economic decisions necessary. But while politicians use economics to question environmental policy, who questions whether the contributions of ecosystems are fairly valued in such economic analyses? Because ecosystems are not fully captured in commercial market analyses, their true worth is likely discounted. Such neglect may compromise human welfare (17).

Earth Capital

What is the economic contribution of intact ecosystems to human health and welfare? Estimating the incremental or marginal value of ecosystems should stimulate economic, political, and ethical debates. Nonetheless, without our ecological infrastructure, global economies would grind to a halt. Consequently, an understanding of the concept of *earth capital* is important to economic discussions involving the environment.

Capital is either human or nonhuman. *Nonhuman capital* consists of machines, buildings, land, and infrastructure for production of goods and services. *Human capital* is labor, knowledge, and skills that allow an increased output of goods and services. Economic growth does not occur without increased input of resources. Therefore, output requires investment. Economists define *investment* as the production of new capital. Depending on the definition of nonhuman capital, economists point out that the nonhuman capital per person in developed nations is several factors of ten higher than the same per capita figures in developing countries (17).

Because ecosystems are interdependent, much of the output of ecological goods and services can be viewed as joint ventures of earth capital markets (Table 1-3). These goods and services include atmosphere containing the appropriate amount of oxygen to support human life; carbon dioxide to support plant life; clean water to support aquatic life and human life; wetlands, rivers, oceans, and fertile soil to support human, animal, and plant life; energy flow and cycling of carbon, oxygen, and nitrogen among life systems and nonliving systems; and other natural resources.

The economic value of ecosystems can be defined as being equal to the output of goods and services plus the ecosystems' infrastructure. The use of earth capital, just like any other capital, without regeneration or reinvestment would eventually drain the capital supply (17) and, unlike other forms of capital, earth capital cannot be easily substituted.

TABLE 1-3. Ecosystem services and functions

Number	Ecosystem service	Ecosystem functions	Examples
1	Gas regulation	Regulation of atmospheric chemical composition	CO_2/O_2 balance, O_3 for UVB protection, and SO_x levels
2	Climate regulation	Regulation of global temperature, precipitation, and other biologically mediated climatic processes at global or local levels	Greenhouse gas regulation, DMS production affecting cloud formation
3	Disturbance regulation	Capacitance, damping, and integrity of ecosystem response to environmental fluctuations	Storm protection, flood control, drought recovery, and other aspects of habitat response to environmental variability mainly controlled by vegetation structure
4	Water regulation	Regulation of hydrologic flows	Provisioning of water for agricultural (e.g., irrigation) or industrial (e.g., milling) processes or transportation
5	Water supply	Storage and retention of water	Provisioning of water by watersheds, reservoirs, and aquifers
6	Erosion control and sediment retention	Retention of soil within an ecosystem	Prevention of loss of soil by wind, runoff, or other removal processes, storage of silt in lakes and wetlands
7	Soil formation	Soil formation processes	Weathering of rock and the accumulation of organic material
8	Nutrient cycling	Storage, internal cycling, processing, and acquisition of nutrients	Nitrogen fixation; nitrogen, phosphorus, and other elemental or nutrient cycles
9	Waste treatment	Recovery of mobile nutrients and removal or breakdown of excess or xenobiotics	Waste treatment, pollution control, detoxification
10	Pollination	Movement of floral gametes	Provisioning of pollinators for the reproduction of plant populations
11	Biological control	Trophic-dynamic regulations of populations	Keystone predator control of prey species, reduction of herbivory by top predators
12	Refugia	Habitat for resident and transient populations	Nurseries, habitat for migratory species, regional habitats for locally harvested species, or overwintering grounds
13	Food production	That portion of gross primary production extractable as food	Production of fish, game, crops, nuts, fruits by hunting, gathering, subsistence farming, or fishing
14	Raw materials	That portion of gross primary production extractable as raw materials	Production of lumber, fuel, or fodder
15	Genetic resources	Sources of unique biological materials and products	Medicine, products for materials science, genes for resistance to plant pathogens and crop pests, ornamental species (pets and horticultural varieties of plants)
16	Recreation	Providing opportunities for recreational activities	Ecotourism, sport fishing, and other outdoor recreational activities
17	Cultural	Providing opportunities for noncommercial uses	Aesthetic, artistic, educational, spiritual, and scientific values of ecosystems

From ref. 20, with permission from *Nature*.

A central problem underscoring environmental economics is that the value of earth capital in ecosystem services is not easily traced through classically defined financial markets. Instead, many of the benefits of ecosystems—clean air, clean water, soil, climate, recreational lands—flow directly to humans without passing through market economies. Different individuals place different values on these "aesthetics."

Costanza has estimated that the global ecosystems provide an average value of $33 trillion per year to human welfare in U.S. dollars (17). This is 1.8 times the GDP of all global economies, and most of it is outside of established markets. He estimated that marine ecosystems provided 63% of this value, mostly from coastal areas. Terrestrial ecosystems, forests, and wetlands provided 38% of the value. The value range estimated was between $16 trillion and $54 trillion per year.

Another economic example here in the United States is embodied in the debate over the Endangered Species Act. Passed by Congress and signed by President Nixon in 1973, the Endangered Species Act was drafted on the assumption that each life form may prove valuable in ways that cannot yet be measured and that each life form is entitled to exist for its own sake. It is a bill of rights for nonhumans, protecting not only U.S. species listed as endangered but also more than 500 foreign oceanic species (18). Since 1973, the list of names of endangered or threatened species in the United States has grown from 109 to more than 900. The act is considered to be a potent piece of environmental legislation, reshaping the way American society lives and uses the land. At the same time, it is fueling acrimonious debate about economic balance, property rights, and growth limitations.

The global warming debate is also replete with economic arguments. Critics cite the cost of a 20% reduction in atmospheric CO_2 in the United States to be in the tens of billions of dollars, with costs expected to be in the trillions by 2015. Such costs pose a tough ethical question: Is the benefit of a 30% reduction in global warming by reducing CO_2 emissions 20% worth 1% or less of the nation's gross national product (GNP)? The economic model used to criticize CO_2 reduction was based solely on negative economic consequences to agricultural and water loss up to 1% of the GNP. No economic value was placed on the other ecosystems or other health consequences.

In summary, because ecopolitics and economics will be major influences in the twenty-first century, the environment must be given its true value weight in decision-making processes. If not, human welfare may suffer. Global GDP would have to increase by an estimated $33 trillion in U.S. dollars to cover services (some captured and some uncaptured) in existing economies to replace current ecosystem goods, services, and infrastructure. If ecosystems required payment for their contribution value to both global economy and human welfare, the price of goods, services, and commodities using ecoservices either directly or indirectly would have to be accounted for in current price, labor, and human capital markets. Global GNPs would change drastically. As earth capital is stressed, their value will increase, along with associated costs.

Agendas for the Twenty-First Century

Environmental issues will continue to affect the welfare and health of individuals and populations into the twenty-first century. Politics and economics will either continue to cloud science in the debate on environmental pollution and the interrelated health of humans and ecosystems or will help to clarify the facts and provide answers to pollution problems. However, global economic integration may generate friction among nations that have different environmental standards, thus allowing the potential use of these standards as trade barriers.

A better understanding of how susceptible populations are affected by environmental contamination is necessary to help prevent disease. Reproductive, genotoxic, and xenoestrogenic activities of environmental contaminants also require further research as population pressures on ecosystems increase. Increased focus is needed also on sustainability of resources, resource conservation, innovative procedures for minimizing waste production, and recycling. Partnerships between regulators and industry will be crucial to achieve goals of resource conservation and sustainability. Multidisciplinary research will better define the interdependent relationship between environment and health. Finally, better economic modeling inclusive of natural capital and "silent" ecosystem markets will be critical to reinvesting in the environment. Overall, there is no shortage of agendas.

REFERENCES

1. Costain WD. History and development. In: Krieger GR, ed. *Environmental management: accident prevention manual for business and industry.* Itasca, IL: National Safety Council, 1995.
2. Gochfeld M. Overview of environmental medicine. In: Brooks S, Gochfeld M, Herzstein J, Jackson R, Schenker M, eds. *Environmental medicine.* New York: Mosby, 1995:3–8.
3. Edwards M. Pollution in the former Soviet Union: lethal legacy. *National Geographic* 1994;186(2):70–98.
4. Edwards M. Living with the monster Chernobyl. *National Geographic* 1994;186(2):100–115.
5. Lee D, Fobes N. Tragedy in Alaska waters. *National Geographic* 1989;176(2): 260–263.
6. Jamison DT, Mosley WH, Measham AR, Bobadilla JL, eds. World Bank disease control priorities in developing countries. New York: Oxford University Press, 1993.
7. Wilkinson RG. Income distribution and life expectancy. *BMJ* 1992;304:165–168.
8. Krieger GR. Environmental hazards in the international setting. In: Fleming L, Herzstein J, Bunn W, eds. *Issues in international occupational and environmental medicine.* Beverly, MA: OEM Press, 1997:129–146.
9. Johnson B. Hazardous waste: human health effects. *Toxicol Ind Health* 1997; 13(2/3):121–143.
10. Heitgard J, Burg J, Strickland H. Geographic information systems approach to estimating and assessing national priorities list site demographics: racial and Hispanic origin. *Int J Occup Med Toxicol* 1995;4:343.
11. Cortinas de Nava C. Worldwide overview of hazardous waste. *Toxicol Ind Health* 1996;12(2):127–137.
12. Brown K. A decent proposal? EPA's new clean air standards. *Environ Health Perspect* 1997;105(4):378–383.
13. Gamble J, Lewis J. Health and respirable particulate (PM 10) air pollution: a causal or statistical association? *Environ Health Perspect* 1996;104(8):838–850.
14. Pinholster G. The specter of infection. *Environ Health Perspect* 1996;104(7): 694–699.
15. Schneider E, Hajjeh R, Spiegel R. A coccidiomycosis outbreak following the Northridge, California, earthquake. *JAMA* 1997;277(11):904–908.
16. Lederberg J. Infectious disease—a threat to global health and security [Editorial]. *JAMA* 1996;276(5):417–419.
17. Costanza R, d'Arge R, deGroot R, et al. The value of the world's ecosystem services and natural capital. *Nature* 1997;387:253–260.
18. Chadwick D. The endangered species act. *National Geographic* 1995;187(3):3–41.

CHAPTER 2

Environmental Sciences: Pollutant Fate and Transport in the Environment

John B. Sullivan, Jr., and Gary R. Krieger

Xenobiotic wastes and contaminants travel throughout ecosystems via the complex hydrogeopollution cycle. Along the way, pollutants are transformed into more or less toxic forms through reactions in soil, water, or air or through biodegradation, or they present health hazards to other life-forms through bioaccumulation or contamination of water, soil, and air (1).

The discipline of *chemodynamics*—the study of pollution movement—uses concepts of chemistry, physics, hydrology, geology, toxicology, and engineering to make predictions about the extent of contamination and its risk (1). As such, chemodynamics involves (a) physical and chemical properties that influence pollutant transport; (b) factors that influence persistence of chemicals in the environment; (c) partitioning of chemicals in the media of air, water, and soil; (d) bioaccumulation; and (e) public health and ecological risks from environmental contaminants (1–8).

LINKING POLLUTION, POPULATION, AND DEVELOPMENT

The population of the earth exceeds 5 billion and is expected to double by 2020. Intact, healthy ecosystems contribute to human health by recycling energy, oxygen, carbon, nitrogen, and nutrients to support life-based systems. Ecosystems regulate climate; generate atmosphere; form and maintain soils; provide for growth of crops; control carriers of human, plant, and animal diseases; and are efficient at waste disposal.

The Environmental Continuum

Ecology is the study of the relationships between organisms and their environment. An ecosystem is a diverse biological community together with its natural environment functioning as an intact unit. The components of ecosystems—soil, water, air, and life-forms—are linked in a continuum that allows for the transport and cycling of pollutants. This continuum is linked by physiochemical and biological interfaces, which act as barriers or pathways for contaminant movement:

- Liquid
- Gas-liquid interface (atmosphere and water)
- Liquid-soil interface (water and soil)
- Liquid-liquid interface (streams, rivers, lakes, and oceans)
- Soil-air interface (soil and air)
- Biological interface (bioaccumulation and biodegradation)

The speed and ultimate concentrations across the interface boundary are affected by a variety of processes:

- Physical and chemical properties of the contaminant material
- Bioaccumulative properties of the material
- Physical geography of the setting where the contaminant is introduced (soil types; depth to the water table; proximity of rivers, streams, lakes, or other surface-water bodies)

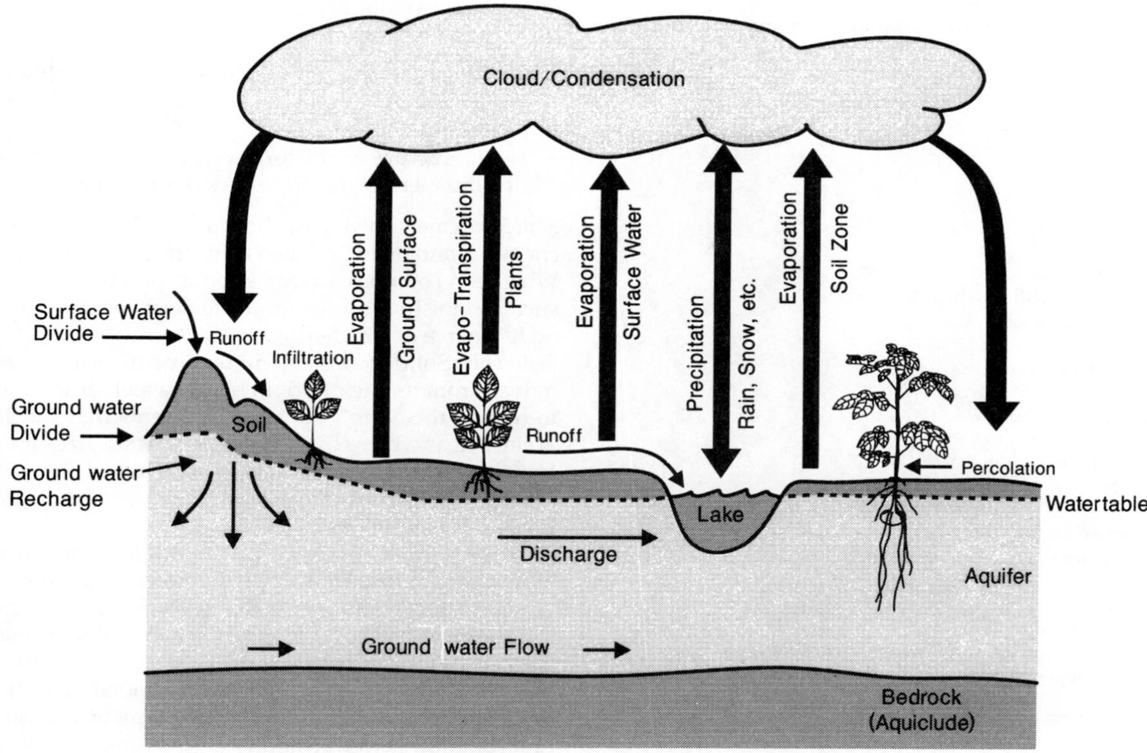

Figure 2-1. The hydrologic cycle. From ref. 5, with permission.

- General climate conditions, such as temperature, wind direction and speed, and general atmospheric stability during and immediately after a release
- Magnitude, volume, and type of contamination (acute or long-term slow release)

THE HYDROGEOPOLLUTION CYCLE

Water evaporates from sources around the globe, including oceans and seas, to form a resource that replenishes these original sources. This cyclic movement of water is termed the *hydrologic cycle* (Fig. 2-1). The geologic cycle involves pollutant movement through soil, sediment, and rock. Contaminants from pollution sources can reach water and soil through a combination of the actions involving the hydrologic cycle and the geologic cycle. Combined, these form the *hydrogeopollution cycle* (Fig. 2-2).

Sources of pollution are either point source or distributed source (Tables 2-1 and 2-2). Point sources of contamination are geographically defined; can be mapped; and are discernible in size, shape, and location. Distributed sources are usually widespread throughout a large area with difficult boundaries to define.

Through a complex interplay of both hydrologic and geologic cycles, pollutants move about the environment through the hydrogeopollution cycle, advancing their spread from either point sources or distributive sources.

Environmental Interfaces

The hydrogeopollution cycle is the framework for understanding contaminant movement throughout the environment. This cycle describes solid, liquid, and vapor phases through which pollutants move. Most pollutants contaminating soil move through groundwater supplies. Thus, characteristics of soil and water movement are important factors in determining pollutant fate and transport. Certain geologic, hydrologic, and physiochemical terms are useful to understand movement of contaminants through the various environmental interfaces.

GEOLOGIC TERMS

Mineral: A naturally occurring solid with a defined crystal structure and a limited range of composition.

Rock: A natural aggregate of one or more minerals. Three major classes of rocks are:

- *Sedimentary rock*: Rock formed by accumulating sediments. Sedimentary rocks are characteristically stratified. They include chemical sedimentary rocks—such as limestone,

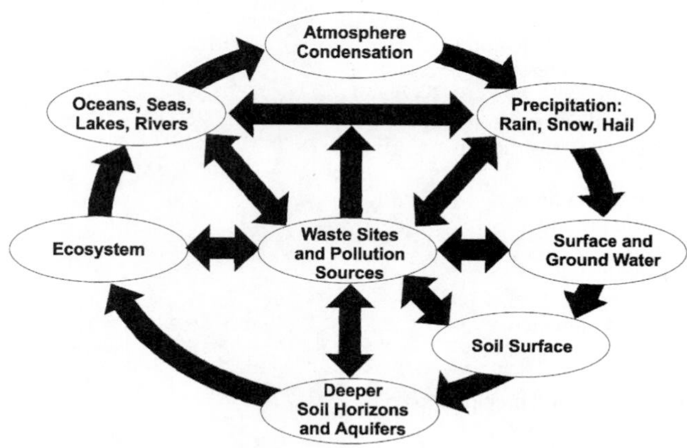

Figure 2-2. Hydrogeopollution cycle.

TABLE 2-1. Point sources of contamination and pollution

Sewage disposal
- Animal and human waste
- Sewage lagoons
- Septic systems
- Barnyards/feed lots

Surface waste disposal sites
- Landfills/garbage dumps
- Surface waste dumps

Underground disposal sites
- Storage tanks (low-, medium-, high-level wastes)
- Pit latrines, tunnels, trenches, caves

Spills, washings
- Waste subsurface injections
- Oil/gas/waste spills
- Auto workshop washings
- Research/laboratory washings
- Seawater/saltwater intrusions
- Mine drainages

Mining
- Gas explosions/seepages
- Mine dumps, tailings
- Tunnels/excavations outflows
- Saline ponds/lakes

Natural mineral/ore deposits
- Hot springs/mineralized waters
- Anhydrite/pyrite deposits/evaporites

gypsum, and salt deposits—as well as physical sedimentary rocks, such as sandstone and shale.

- *Igneous rock*: Rock formed by cooling of a magna or melt. Common igneous rocks include granite, basalt, and tuff.
- *Metamorphic rock*: Rock formed from a preexisting rock or sediment by subjection to heat and/or pressure without complete melting. Metamorphic rocks include gneiss, schist, and marble.

Geologic structures: Features produced by the deformation of rocks. Geologic structures may occur at scales ranging from microscopic to continental (or oceanic). Significant types of geologic structures include:

- *Fold*: Bending or crumpling produced in stratified rocks (and sediments) by compressive stress.
- *Fracture*: Break in rocks.
- *Fault*: Fracture or fracture zone along which there has been displacement of the opposite sides relative to one another.

Soil: Earth material that has been so acted on by natural physical, chemical, and biological agents that it can support rooted plants. Whether a soil does, in fact, support plants depends on factors such as moisture content and chemical composition, as well as on its degree of weathering.

Sediment: Solid material—mineral or organic—that has been moved from its site of origin by air, water, or ice and has come to rest on the earth's surface. Sediments may be classified by grain size as well as by composition. Grain sizes for sediments, from coarse to fine, are gravel, sand, silt, and clay.

TABLE 2-2. Distributed sources of contamination and pollution

Agriculture
- Cropland
- Pasture and rangeland
- Irrigated land
- Woodland
- Feedlots
- Growing stock

Forestry
- Logging, soil erosion
- Road building

Construction
- Urban development
- Highway construction

Mining
- Surface, tailings
- Underground

Terrestrial
- Landfills
- Dumps

Utility maintenance
- Highways and streets
- Deicing

Urban runoff and precipitation
- Floods and snowmelt
- Rainfall and snowfall

HYDROLOGY TERMS

Advection: Process of dissolved chemicals within an aquifer unit moving at the average velocity of the groundwater.

Aquifer: A saturated, permeable geologic unit that can transmit significant or usable quantities of water under ordinary hydraulic gradients.

Aquitard: Geologic unit that inhibits groundwater flow because of its low permeability. Aquitards frequently separate aquifer units but flow across an aquitard is possible. If little flow occurs, the unit is termed an *aquiclude*.

Capillary fringe: Transition zone from the partially saturated vadose zone to the water-table surface.

Confined aquifer: An aquifer that has an overlying layer that does not allow direct contact of the aquifer with the atmosphere. Water in a confined aquifer is under pressure, and wells penetrating into the aquifer will have a water level that reflects the pressure in the aquifer at the point of penetration. Also called an *artesian aquifer*.

Degradation: The transformation of a contaminant to other forms through decay, biodegradation, or other process.

Discharge: The quantity or process of water being lost from the saturated zone.

Dispersion: Spreading of a contaminant source as it flows through an aquifer.

Evapotranspiration: Water that is returned to the atmosphere by evaporation from the surface and by transpiration from plants.

Hydraulic conductivity: A coefficient of proportionality between specific discharge and hydraulic gradient. The hydraulic conductivity is related to the permeability of an earth material for a given fluid at a given degree of saturation. Unless otherwise stated, it is assumed that the hydraulic conductivity is stated for a geologic material that is fully saturated with water. Determined from well-pumping tests.

Hydraulic gradient: The change in hydraulic head between two points divided by the distance between the points. Determined from a water level map.

Hydraulic head: The product of fluid potential and the acceleration that is due to gravity of groundwater in an aquifer. Head is the sum of two components: the elevation head (elevation of the measuring point) and the pressure head (the incremental elevation due to the pressure exerted by the water at the point of measurement).

Infiltration: Percolation of water through earth materials to the saturated zone of the groundwater system.

Perched aquifer: Beds of clay, silt, or other materials of limited extent that present a restriction to flow of downward-moving water in the vadose zone may cause local areas of saturation above the regional water table. An unsaturated zone is present between the bottom of the perching bed and the water table.

Permeability: The ability of an earth material to transmit a fluid (usually taken to be water).

Porosity: The percentage of an earth material that is open space.

Potentiometric surface: The surface to which water in an aquifer would rise under hydrostatic pressure. For an unconfined aquifer, the potentiometric surface is the water-table surface. For a confined aquifer, the potentiometric surface lies above the elevation of the aquifer in which the water is found.

Recharge: The quantity or process of water being added to the saturated zone.

Saturated zone: The zone in earth materials in which the pore space is completely filled with liquid water. In the saturated zone, the pressure head is greater than atmospheric. Sometimes called the *phreatic zone*.

Soil zone: Area in which evaporation and transpiration of water occurs.

Sorption: Transfer process in which dissolved chemicals in the groundwater become attached to sedimentary materials, organic matter, or both.

Specific discharge: Flow rate divided by the cross-sectional area across which the flow occurs.

Storage: The quantity of water that is held in the pore space of an aquifer but that may be released (and begin to flow) when a hydraulic stress is applied to the aquifer.

Unconfined aquifer: An aquifer in which the top of the saturated zone (water table) is in direct contact with the atmosphere through the open pores of the earth material above. Also called a *water-table aquifer*.

Vadose zone: The zone in soils in which the pore space is not completely filled with water, although there is moisture present. Sometimes called the *unsaturated zone*. The pressure head is less in the vadose zone than in the atmosphere.

Water table: The surface at which the water pressure in the pores of the porous geologic materials is exactly atmospheric. The elevation of the water table is identified by determining the elevation of water in a well that penetrates the vadose zone and is open to the top of the saturated zone.

PHYSIOCHEMICAL CHARACTERISTICS

Chemical and physical characteristics dictate how pollutants partition across environmental interfaces:

- Melting point
- Boiling point
- Vapor pressure
- Solubility
- Ionization potential
- Acid–base strengths
- Polarity
- Organic structure
- Degree of halogen substitution
- Oxygen content of xenobiotic

The melting and boiling points determine the physical state of the material at the ambient temperature during a chemical release. A sudden chemical release occurring in winter has different fate and transport characteristics than a chemical spill during a summer rainstorm. The physical state of a chemical can also be predicted based on a knowledge of the ambient temperature conditions and the boiling and melting points. For example, a chemical that is a solid at room temperature but a liquid at 100°F (37.8°C) will behave quite differently if the release occurs during below-freezing conditions or on a hot summer day.

Physical partitioning is the separation of a chemical between two phases in which it is soluble, distributing itself between the two phases in fixed proportions, independent of the quantity of the chemical. The partition coefficient is the ratio of the concentrations in the two phases (1). This relationship can be expressed in general terms as:

$$C_1/C_2 = K^{1-2}$$

C_1 = equilibrium concentration in phase 1
C_2 = equilibrium concentration in phase 2
K^{1-2} = partition coefficient between phases 1 and 2

Depending on the medium, there are physical partitioning properties that are critical for the most common interfaces. The acid–base nature of a chemical determines its tendency to release or accept electrons and affects its solubility and dissociation in a liquid. The organic structure of a xenobiotic influences its fate and transport. Organic compounds may be aliphatic, saturated or unsaturated, aromatic, halogenated, or oxygenated; they may contain metals; or they may be cyclic aliphatics. Lipid solubility and partitioning between interfaces is influenced by structure and physical characteristics.

According to the Environmental Protection Agency (EPA), the following are chemical and physical properties that affect partitioning of chemicals in water, soil, and air (9):

- *Acids and bases*. An acid is a hydrogen-containing substance that dissociates on solution in water to produce one or more hydrogen ions. Acids and bases, though, are defined by different concepts. A base dissociates on solution in water to form hydroxyl ions. According to the Coury-Bronsted definition, an acid is a substance that gives up a proton, and a base is substance that accepts a proton. The strength of an acid depends on its tendency to give up a proton. The Lewis definition states that an acid is a substance that takes up an electron pair to form a covalent bond, whereas a base furnishes an electron pair to form a covalent bond.
- *Adsorption coefficients*. Adsorption coefficients are the distribution between water and a solid [e.g., soils, sediments $K_{(oc)}$ is the most commonly used abbreviation and is the micrograms adsorbed per microgram of organic carbon (soil solid phase) divided by the microgram per milliliter of solution. Kd is unadjusted for dependence on organic carbon. To adjust for the fraction of organic carbon [$F_{(oc)}$], $Kd = K_{(oc)} \times F_{(oc)}$.
- *Advection*. The transport of water flowing in a particular direction (more or less horizontally), such as water flowing because of the current in a stream or river.
- *Bioconcentration factor*. The measure of the extent of chemical partitioning at equilibrium between a biological medium (e.g., fish tissue, plant tissue) and water. The higher the bioconcentration factor, the greater the accumulation.
- *Biodegradation*. Biodegradation transformations are reactions that are due to the metabolic activity of aquatic microbes, primarily bacteria. Depending on the specific chemical, the transformations may be very fast because of the presence of enzymes; for other compounds, the process may be very slow. For chemicals in which the transformation is fast, biodegradation is often the most important transformation process in the aquatic environment.
- *Convection*. The transport of water because of density gradients. In this form of transport, the driving forces of the currents are density gradients resulting from temperature differences in deep lakes, and temperature and salinity differences in estuaries.
- *Dispersion*. The scattering of particles because of the combined effect of shear and diffusion (molecular and turbulent). Usually, the combined effect of shear and transverse diffusion, represented as an effective dispersion, is orders of magnitude greater than other diffusive mechanisms acting in the direction of flow in rivers and estuaries.

- *Henry's Law Constant.* Henry's Law Constant (H) is the air-water partition coefficient and the rate a substance will evaporate from water. The higher H is, the more likely a chemical will move from water to air. H equals the vapor pressure of a substance divided by the aqueous solubility.
- *Hydrolysis.* A decomposition reaction involving the splitting of water into its ions and the formation of a weak acid or weak base. Compounds are altered in a hydrolytic reaction by the replacement of some chemical group with a hydroxyl group. These reactions are commonly catalyzed by the presence of hydrogen or hydroxide ions, hence the reaction rate is strongly dependent on the pH of the system.
- *Ionization.* The process by which neutral atoms or groups of atoms become electrically charged, either positive or negative, by loss or gain of electrons. Organic compounds that are either acids or bases are strongly affected by the concentration of hydrogen ions in water. An organic acid or base that is extensively ionized is different from the neutral molecule in solubility, adsorption, bioconcentration, and toxic characteristics. The ionized species of an organic acid is absorbed by sediments to a much lesser degree than is the neutral form. The solubility of an ionic form of an organic chemical will likely be greater than for the neutral species. Therefore, as a chemical is ionized under environmental conditions, the change in physical properties as well as the chemical reactivity will change with pH.
- *Melting point and boiling point.* Melting point and boiling point describe the physical state at ambient temperature and pressure and provide data relevant for changes in the physical state of a chemical.
- *Molecular diffusion.* The scattering of particles by random molecular motion, commonly characterized by Fick's law of diffusion.
- *Oxidation-reduction.* The transfer of electrons from the reduced species to the oxidized species. The oxidation-reduction potential is an important process in that it can control the oxidation number of the metals present in solution and may also change the oxidation state and structure of organic compounds.
- *Particle deposition.* The settling of particles from the water body to the underlying bed.
- *Particle entrainment.* The picking up or lifting of particles from the underlying bed of a water body by turbulent motion over the bed.
- *Particle settling.* The sinking of particles having densities greater than the fluid of the water body, such as sediments or suspended solids.
- *Partitioning.* Partitioning describes whether substances are water seeking (hydrophilic) or water avoiding (hydrophobic). Partitioning also characterizes the ability of a substance to bioaccumulate, transport through skin, and sorb to soils. Octanol is used as a surrogate for lipids (fats) and can predict bioconcentration in aquatic organisms. $K_{(ow)}$ is the measure of the octanol-water partition coefficient.
- *pH.* The negative log of the hydrogen ion concentration

$$pH = -\log [H^+]$$

- The pH values found in most aquatic systems range from approximately pH 4 to 9, with extreme values as low as pH 2 and as high as pH 11.
- *Photolysis.* The degradation process whereby radiant energy in the form of photons breaks the chemical bonds of a molecule. Direct photolysis involves direct absorption of photons by the molecule. Indirect photolysis involves the absorption of energy by a molecule from another molecule that has absorbed the photons.
- *Shear.* Mixing that is due to variations in the guild velocity at different positions in the water body. One example of this could occur in a lake where a significant decrease in temperature occurs with depth, thereby causing a thermal resistance (resistance of colder and, therefore, denser and lower-lying water to be displaced by warmer, lighter, and higher-lying water). A shear plane divides the surface current that follows the wind from the return currents that run counter to the wind.
- *Sorption.* Sorption is a transfer process whereby dissolved chemicals in the soil become attached to sedimentary materials. Some chemicals may exhibit nonreversible sorption characteristics. Different particle sizes (sand, clay, and silts) exhibit different properties. Salinity affects the sorption process. Some of the compounds that may be strongly affected by sorption include heavy metals and hydrophobic nonpolar compounds.
- *Turbulent diffusion.* Scattering of particles by random turbulent motion (advective transport via turbulent motion in the form of eddies).
- *Vapor pressure.* Vapor pressure determines partitioning to air; the higher the vapor pressure, the more likely a chemical is to exist in a gaseous state. Vapor pressure changes as temperature and pressure change.
- *Volatilization.* A physical transfer process in which a chemical is transferred between the water and the atmosphere at the water-air interface.
- *Water solubility.* Water solubility determines partitioning to water and is temperature dependent.

Soil Structure and Characteristics

Understanding soil is key to understanding pollution movement. Soil is a complex mixture of particulates, organic matter, water, and living organisms. It is the end product of the action of weather, climate, and living organisms on a parent material over a period of time (7). Soil consists of solids, liquids, and gases that maintain an equilibrium with the other two environmental media of water and air. It is responsible for plant nutrition and cycling of nutrients, which maintains the balance of oxygen and carbon dioxide in the atmosphere.

Soil has a biotic phase, containing living microorganisms, and an abiotic—or nonliving—phase. The structure of the soil also determines whether it contains large or small amounts of oxygen and water, as well as organic material. Soil is approximately 95% inorganic and 5% organic by weight (1,7).

The three primary inorganic materials of soil are sand, silt, and clay. The percentages of these three mixtures determine the texture and physiochemical properties. Soil particle size varies: Clay is less than 0.002 mm, silt is 0.002 to 0.02 mm, and gravel is greater than 2 mm in diameter. The various combinations of clays, silts, and gravels create soil textures.

The three primary particulate materials of soil can aggregate into secondary structures known as PEDS. The arrangement of basic soil particles into aggregates, or PEDS, creates voids or pores to be formed in the soil mixture that can be filled with water or organic and plant material. The larger the pore spaces, the easier it is for water and pollutants to move through soil and rock.

The major structural properties of soil include (a) the size of primary and secondary soil particles (PEDS) and (b) the size, distribution, and quantity of pores. These properties—along with texture—affect pollutant absorption and transfer. The conductivity of water, heat, and gases is also altered by pore size and soil pore variability.

Soils that have little or no structure are characterized as "massive" (7) and have little void spaces. Soil pores can be open or closed. Many of these spaces contain microorganisms, fungus, and bacteria—some that use oxygen, others that exist in anaerobic conditions.

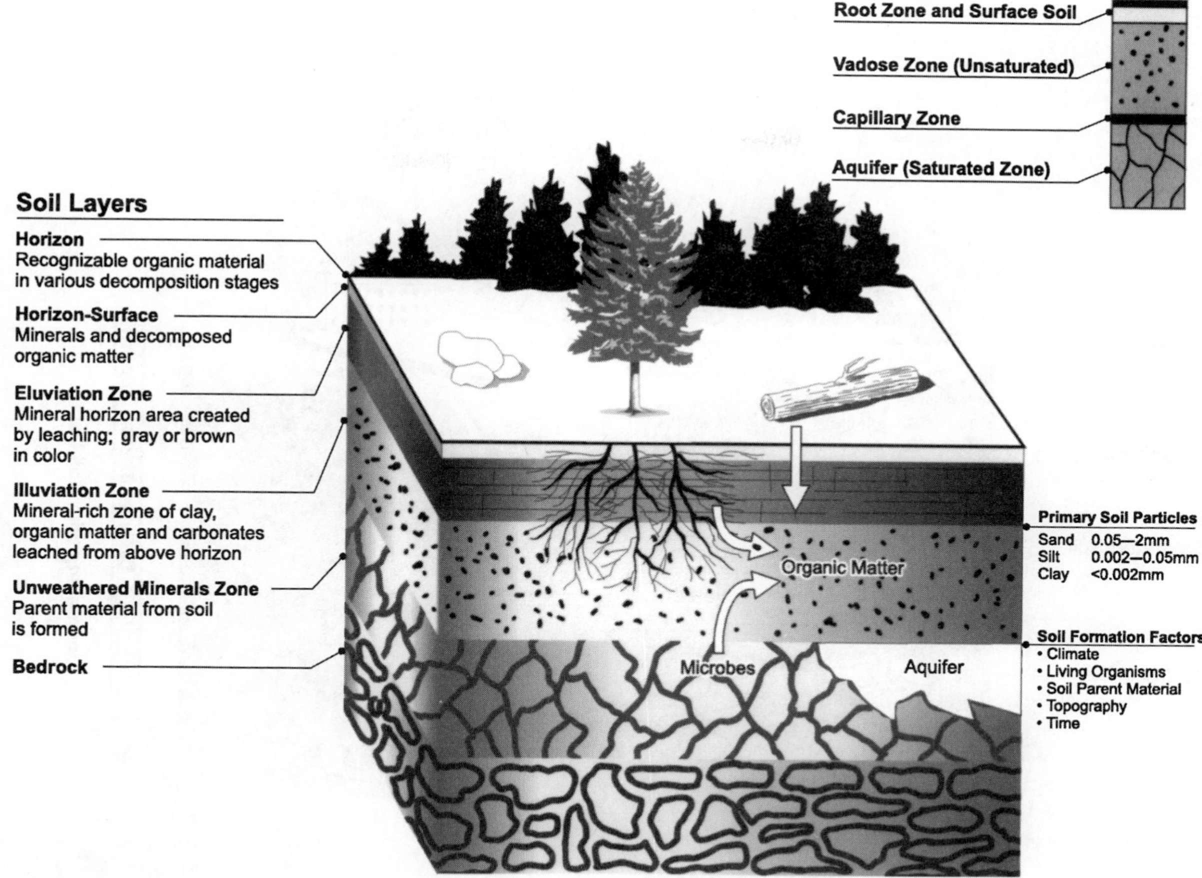

Figure 2-3. The characteristics of soil can be described in its various layers, known as *horizons*.

The soil surface or root zone supports plant growth. The region below this surface layer is the *vadose zone*, a water unsaturated area between groundwater and soil surface layer. The characteristics of soil can be described in its various layers, known as *horizons* (Fig. 2-3). The number and nature of these horizons provide unique characteristics to soil and influence the spread, fate, and transport of pollutants. The three most important horizons are:

1. A horizon: layer of maximum biological activity and of removal of dissolved or suspended materials in water
2. B horizon: layers of suspended materials, including residual oxides, silicate clays, or other transformed materials
3. C horizon: weathered mineral material that is unaffected by soil-forming processes except for the accumulation of salts or oxides of varying solubilities

The concepts of soil horizons and profiles are important terms of reference during environmental investigations of potentially hazardous materials. When soil samples are required, it is common practice to sample the B horizon. This is particularly important when naturally occurring chemicals, such as lead, arsenic, and cadmium, are under investigation at the study site. There is natural variation in the concentration of metals in soils and groundwater; therefore, it is often important to differentiate between naturally occurring levels of metals and man-made or anthropogenic contributions to these media to correctly interpret contaminant spread.

Within the different soil horizons, there is important variability that is due to the presence of clays, silts, and sands. The clay fraction is considered active because it has an extremely large surface area per unit mass of particles and is capable of forming colloids (suspensions of finely divided particles in a continuous medium). In addition, clays have an ability to swell and retain surface ions as a result of adsorption or sorption of pollutants. This ability affects the movement of both water and chemicals in soil.

In contrast to clays, silts generally have smaller surface areas, no swelling properties, and poor capacity to adsorb ions. Finally, the presence of decomposed organic matter (humus) and inorganic compounds—such as iron and aluminum oxides—is critical, because these materials can bind soil particles together and form aggregates that affect the pore size and physical behavior of a particular soil layer.

Physiochemical Properties of Soil

In addition to physical characteristics, soil has physiochemical and biological properties that relate to pollutant retention, fate, and movement:

- Soil and water pH
- Soil electric charges
- Adsorption or sorption properties
- Ion-exchange capacity
- Complex formation of metal pollutants
- Organic content of soil
- Precipitation and retardation properties
- Biodegradation and bioaccumulation of xenobiotics

Organic matter in soil originates from plant material and the action of microbes. The organic makeup of the soil can vary between 1% and 5%. In more humid areas, the organic content of soil is approximately 5%, whereas in more arid areas, it is

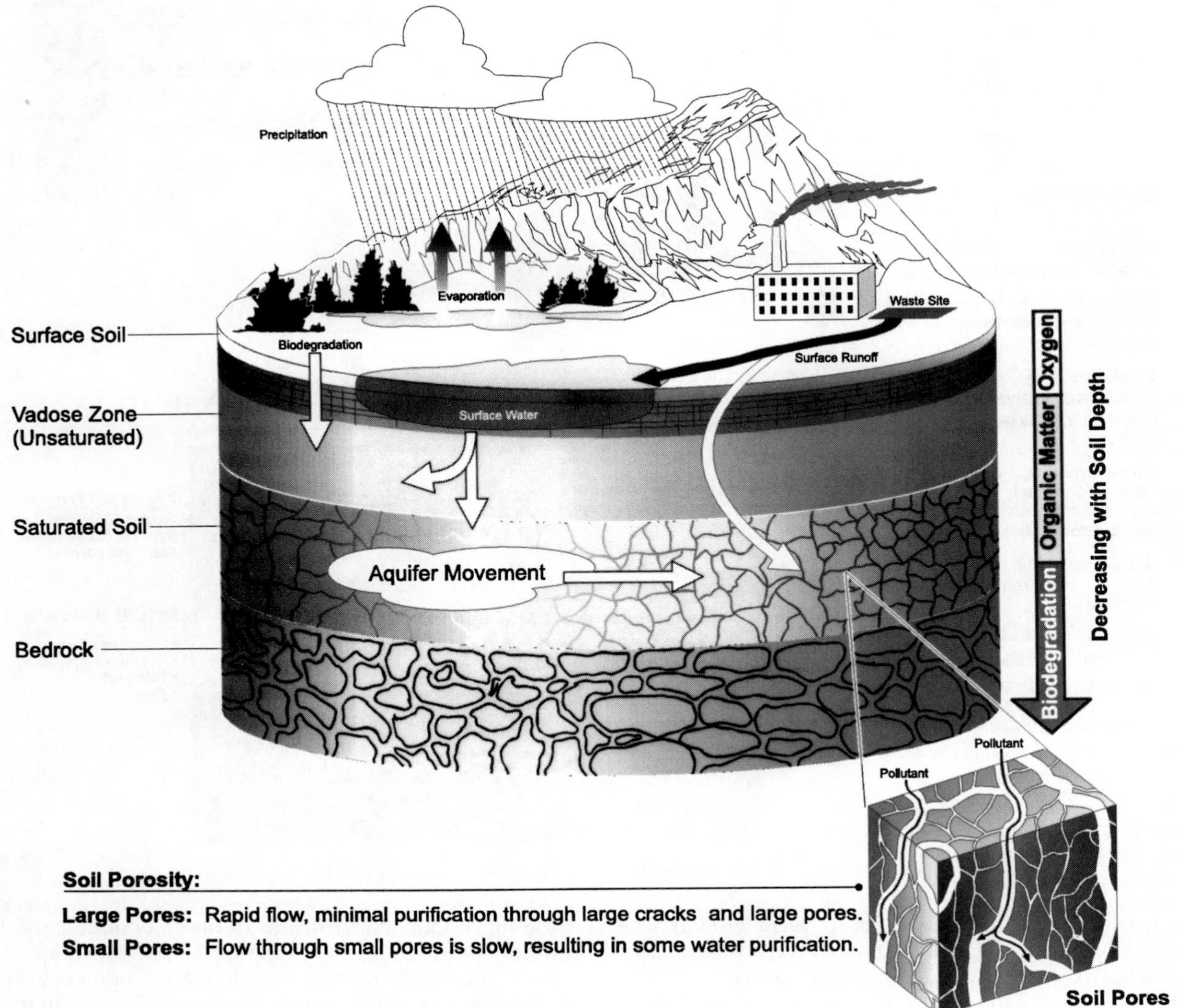

Figure 2-4. Pollutant flow with groundwater through soil.

approximately 1%. The organic matrix of the soil also affects electrical charge, pH, and physical properties of the soil. Organic content of soil decreases with increasing depth below the ground's surface (Fig. 2-4).

The electrical charges associated with clay and soil pH influence pollutant transport. Clay normally carries a negative charge, because its high organic content maintains an overall negative charge. Clay also consists of silicone and aluminum oxides, which can precipitate metals. Soil with high organic content contains carboxyl groups subject to ionization and thus contributes an overall negative charge to the soil.

The presence of negative charges in clay and soil with high organic material allows the process of cation or ion exchange to occur. *Ion exchange* is the process that occurs when a dissolved chemical in soil substitutes itself for another chemical that is already adsorbed onto a mineral or soil surface. The primary ions affected by this process are cations, and the measure of this factor in soil is termed the *cation exchange capacity* (*CEC*). The CEC of a soil varies directly as a function of the amount and distribution of clay and organic matter present. The CEC has a significant impact on the uptake of chemicals into plants. Gain or loss of cations along the surface of clay can lead to the equivalent loss or gain of negative charges.

The adsorption of pollutants to soil materials—either inorganic or organic matter—is an important principle in the movement of pollutants through soil and water. If the pollutant is adsorbed by the soil, then it moves more slowly into groundwater.

Sorption is the retention of pollutant chemicals to soil particles. Inorganic pollutants are attracted to the negative charges of the soil particles. Clay particles with negative charges attract cations such as calcium, magnesium, and sodium potassium, which can precipitate out as salts. Cation exchange at the site of negatively charged soil particles is a mechanism for the retention of heavy metals, such as lead, cadmium, and zinc (1,7).

Anionic contaminants are more mobile because they are not attracted to the highly negatively charged soil mass. The least mobile are cationic pollutants. Xenobiotics can be adsorbed to soil particles with more organic material and soil-sharing chemical hydrocarbon similarities. The more negatively charged organic pollutants, such as phenols, can move more quickly through the soil because of their lack of adsorption to negatively charged soil particles.

Soil pH is another function affecting pollutants. A pH lower than 7 indicates acidic soil; a pH higher than 7 indicates alkaline soil. Soils in areas with high rainfall usually have a higher concentration of organic matter and an acidic pH, because the basic ion charges are leached from the organic material in the clay.

In arid regions, soil tends to be more alkaline because of low organic material and low water content. The pH of soil affects chemical solubility because of the overall influence of charge and ionization; thus, soil pH and electrical charge directly affect the transport and fate of pollutants and contaminants.

Precipitation and complex formation affects trace metals, such as iron (Fe), copper (Cu), zinc (Zn), arsenic (As), lead (Pb), selenium (Se), nickel (Ni), cobalt (Co), and cadmium (Cd). The trace metal cations in a soil solution form complexes and precipitate as a function of the content and type of organic matter, the presence of other oxide minerals (aluminum and iron), soil pH, soil Eh (oxidation-reduction potential), and the CEC. The bioavailability of trace metal and organic chemical uptake is affected by the factors that influence complex formation. These effects have serious impacts when soil treatment options are considered because of chemical contamination.

Retardation is a measure of the lack of movement of a chemical in the soil because of chemical reactions, such as ion exchange and adsorptive processes to soil particles. The *retardation factor* (*Rf*) is a commonly used term and is related to its distribution coefficient, *Kd*.

$$Rf = 1 + Kd \times \frac{Ps}{N}$$

Kd = distribution coefficient
Ps = bulk density of the solid
N = total porosity of soil

Soil has a gaseous phase in equilibrium with the atmosphere. The gases of oxygen, carbon dioxide, nitrogen, and other volatile compounds in the atmosphere are found in soil, but usually at different concentrations. The oxygen content of soil is important, because aerobic microorganisms use oxygen in soil to biodegrade hydrocarbon chemicals. Soil oxygen content is normally approximately 19% to 20%. Carbon dioxide content is approximately 1%. Oxygen in the soil is found either physically dissolved in the soil water or in porous spaces; soil with more pore space generally has more oxygen content. Aerobic soil microbes require both the water and oxygen that is found in these pore spaces. The moisture of the soil controls the amount of oxygen in it. In more saturated soils, oxygen content may be very low. Closed soil spaces and soil pores allow anaerobic microorganisms—which provide key metabolic processes—to flourish. The level of O_2 in soil generally decreases with soil depth.

BIOLOGICAL PHASE OF SOIL

Soil contains populations of microbial organisms important to the fate, transport, and biodegradation of contaminants. Organisms in the soil include bacteria, viruses, fungi, algae, protozoa, and arthropods (Table 2-3).

There are approximately 1×10^8 bacteria per gram of soil. Bacteria are involved in biotransformation of both organic and inorganic compounds. Soil contains both aerobic and anaerobic organisms. Two other important microbes are actinomycetes (1×10^7 per g) and fungi (1×10^6 per g) (1,7).

The biomass of bacteria extends as deep as the root zone, with aerobic bacteria more prevalent than anaerobes. As soil depth increases, the predominant bacteria are anaerobes. The biodegradation properties of soil biomass decrease with soil depth from the ground surface.

The most numerous soil bacteria are *Arthrobacter,* and they are variable in gram-staining characteristics. The second most common are actinomycetes, which share characteristics common to both bacteria and fungi. Actinomycetes are single-cell organisms, but they branch into filaments that resemble mycelia of fungi.

TABLE 2-3. Soil microorganisms

Microorganism	Traits
Arthrobacter	Most numerous bacteria in soil Pleomorphic Gram variable Comprise 40% of soil microbes
Actinomycetes	Have characteristics of bacteria and fungi Aerobic, chemoheterotrophic, single elongated cells with a tendency to form branching hyphaelike filaments Dominated by gram-positive *Streptomyces* 5% to 20% of soil microbes
Pseudomonas	Gram-negative rods comprising 10% to 20% of soil bacteria Vary from aerobic to anaerobic As heterotrophs, involved in organic compound metabolism
Bacillus	Gram-positive rods Aerobic Produce endospores Comprise 10% of bacterial soil population Heterotrophic nutrition
Fungi	Most common genera are *Penicillium, Aspergillus, Fusarium, Alternaria, Rhizopus, Rhizoctonia*

The genus *Streptomyces* is the most common of these gram-positive organisms. Actinomycetes produce conidiospores and hyphae. Actinomycetes metabolize organic compounds, such as phenols, and heterocyclic compounds. The end product is usually an aromatic compound that adds to the humus of the soil. *Geosmin* is the earthy odor associated with soil; it is produced by actinomycetes (7). Actinomycetes are more tolerant in alkaline soils with low moisture.

Fungi are the third major group of soil microorganisms (1×10^6 per g of soil). They are also involved in the degradation of organic compounds. Fungi consist of mold, mildew, yeasts, mushrooms, and rusts. Most are aerobic, except for yeasts. Fungi are eukaryotic and do not contain chlorophyll; thus, they do not photosynthesize. Filamentous fungi are important components of soil that actively biodegrade organic compounds. Fungi contain enzyme systems involved in biodegradation of organic materials. Fungi tolerate more acidic soils and are involved in degradation of organic materials in acidic soils (7). They also tolerate low soil moisture.

The large biodiverse microbial population in soil is stressed by competition for nutrients, water, and growth factors. Soil microbes are also divided according to nutrition (7):

- Autotrophs: obtain energy from inorganic sources and CO_2
- Photoautotrophs: obtain energy from photosynthesis
- Chemoautotrophs: obtain energy from oxidation of inorganic substances
- Heterotrophs: obtain energy from organic substances
- Chemoheterotrophs: obtain energy from oxidation

Chemoautotrophs and chemoheterotrophs tend to be more dominant in soil. Many of the microbes in soil are parasitic or predatory to others. Nonindigenous microbes added to soil usually do not survive long because of this intense competition. Carbon and nitrogen are nutrients found in soils, and the soil bacteria in microorganisms compete for these as nutrients. Humus is an organic nutrient material slowly mineralized (converted to CO_2 and water) by microorganisms. Microorganisms also use organic pollutants as substrates, thus biotransforming these xenobiotics to more or less toxic forms.

Abiotic stressors on soil microorganisms are light, moisture, temperature, pH, nutrient content, soil texture (e.g., clay, sand, and gravel), and the oxidation-reduction potential (7).

Organisms dependent on light are restricted to the uppermost inches of soil. Moisture content of soil also decides oxygen content. Saturated soils are more anaerobic; dry soils are more aerobic.

Soil microbes are also described as psychrophilic (low temperature), mesophilic (mild temperature), or thermophilic (high temperature) dwelling. Most soil microbes are mesophilic dwelling. A soil pH of 6 to 8 is optimal for most microbes.

Surface Water Pollutant Movement

Water movement in soil is influenced by the degree of saturation. Water is attracted by hydrogen bonds to soil particles, thus creating an energy of movement described as a *potential*. Water tends to move from an area of high potential to low potential. Relatively unsaturated soils hold on to water more tightly compared with saturated soil.

The geology of a site provides the physical framework, but it is the hydrology that is the engine that drives the system and moves contaminants from one area to another. This movement is the critical factor that determines whether a spill or leak ultimately affects the underground water supply.

Soil is divided into *saturated* and *unsaturated* in terms of water content. Surface soil is relatively unsaturated, because only the smallest of soil pores contain water. A hole drilled into soil will eventually reach water that accumulates at a certain level in the borehole. This is the *groundwater level*. Soil below the groundwater level is saturated. The area between groundwater table and the surface of the ground is the *unsaturated zone*, or *vadose zone*, the area between the groundwater table and the lowest of the plant root zone (see Figs. 2-3 and 2-4).

In general, as water infiltrates the earth's surface, it moves vertically downward through soil toward the saturated zone. Saturated water moves laterally from areas of greater hydrostatic pressure to areas of lesser hydrostatic pressure. The prime driving force is gravity. Chemicals entering soil move downward through the root zone and the unsaturated area into groundwater. Groundwater moves in a horizontal direction, which causes a dimensional spread that creates diffusion and dispersion of the chemicals.

Underlying most land areas are bodies of water called *aquifers*. An aquifer is a permeable geologic unit that can store and transmit large quantities of water. There are three types of aquifers:

- Confined (artesian): contained in a closed space under pressure
- Perched: have clay or silt beds that restrict water flow in unsaturated vadose zone
- Unconfined: in contact with surface water

Aquifers vary from small to very large. (The Ogalalla aquifer, for example, underlies areas of Kansas, North Texas, and Nebraska.) Water flow in aquifers is basically horizontal because of a difference in pressures and elevation. Terms relating to aquifers describe flow in a groundwater system: *hydraulic conductivity, porosity, transmissivity,* and *storage coefficient*.

The storage coefficient for an unconfined aquifer in contact with surface water is the amount of water that drains from soil as a result of the force of gravity. The storage coefficient for a confined aquifer expresses changes in storage that are due to the elasticity of the soil and compressibility of water. As water percolates from ground surfaces through the unsaturated zone of soil, aquifers can be replenished.

The movement and storage of groundwater are affected by soil porosity, hydraulic conductivity, climate, and gradient. Movement of water in saturated or unsaturated soil and groundwater is described by Darcy's Law:

$$Q = \frac{K\Delta HAt}{Z}$$

K = the hydraulic conductivity in meters per day

ΔH = the energy difference between two points, usually an inlet and an outlet (such as a column of saturated soil) expressed in meters

A = the cross-sectional area of the column in meters^2

t = time (usually days)

Z = length of column (usually meters)

Q = meters^3

In 1856, Henry Darcy reported that the volume of water (Q) moving through a column of soil is proportional to the hydraulic head difference (ΔH) between the inlet and outlet, the cross-sectional area (A) of the column, and time; and is inversely proportional to the length of the column (Z). Darcy's Law is a measure of the average or bulk velocity through a given cross section of a porous medium and is valid for steady flow with constant flux. Turbulence invalidates Darcy's Law.

Darcy's Law is also applied to describe water flow in unsaturated soil, but the hydraulic conductivity is not constant because of loss of water via soil pores. Fortunately, for most groundwater systems—laminar or streamlike—smooth flow rather than turbulent flow is present. Thus, Darcy's Law is the basic groundwater flow equation. Along with contaminant transport processes of advection, dispersion, sorption, or adsorption (retardation) and degradation, Darcy's Law can be used to quantify the nature and extent of potential contaminant movement in water.

For contaminant transport in near-surface aquifers, the primary transport process is advection, which transports most solutes at the velocity of the groundwater flow. This process is augmented by dispersion, which is spreading of contaminants as a result of tortuous flow paths through soil. Dispersion dictates the shape of contaminant plumes but is usually not the primary transport process. Contaminant transport is impeded by adsorption to soil, or transfer of contaminants from groundwater to soil, which is usually a reversible process.

The analysis of pollutant fate and transport in surface-water bodies depends on hydrologic transport processes. The predictive accuracy of fate-transport models is complex because of multiple scales of motion, turbulence flow, boundary-layer effects, and multiple transport mechanisms.

The environmental fate of a pollutant entering a surface-water body is highly dependent on the type of water body: (a) rivers and streams, (b) impoundments, or (c) estuaries and oceans. Rivers and streams exhibit turbulent flow; impoundments offer a near-stagnant environment; and estuaries and oceans involve consideration of tidal and salt- and freshwater effects.

Like groundwater, surface water has its own vocabulary and controlling mathematical equations. Whereas Darcy's equation applies to a steady flow of water through soil, in most real pollution situations, soil and water conditions change constantly. Complex mathematical calculations are needed to describe water moving through soil pores at varying velocities. The concept of pore-water velocity is important, because it is the actual rate at which contaminants move through soil and water. Computer models are used to predict contaminant flow through soil and groundwater. The effects of sinks and other sources—such as discharge from pipes and river runoff—must be considered in such computer modeling.

Groundwater depth is an important factor in the movement of pollutants. The shallower the groundwater depth, the more easily polluted the groundwater can become. Aquifers—

recharged when water moves from the surface through the unsaturated zone into the groundwater—can become contaminated with pollutants not retarded by soil.

The properties of soil, the chemicals, the climate, and the vegetation all affect movement of chemicals throughout soil and into water. The porosity of soil and soil materials affects movement and mass transport of chemicals. Velocity of movement varies through the different pores, fissures, and aggregates of soil, causing chemicals and xenobiotics to move at different rates. The movement of chemicals obeys the physical laws of mass transport and diffusion. Chemical plumes can be mapped in soil showing toxin movements in groundwater.

Movement of Pollutants in the Air-Water Interfaces

The interaction across air-water (gas-liquid) interfaces is a function of four conditions: (a) the solubility of the chemical in liquid versus gas; (b) the nature of the receiving liquid, such as freshwater versus seawater; (c) space confinement, such as a closed space versus an open space; and (d) evaporation, volatilization, and sorption of the chemical.

Evaporation is the transfer of liquid to gas. Solubilization is the transfer between pollutant into a water phase. Volatilization is the transfer between water and gas phases. Sorption is the transfer between water and solid phases (Fig. 2-5).

The solubility of either organic or inorganic pollutants helps determine their transportability into aqueous phases of soil. Solubility is a property of the miscibility of organic compounds and the electrical charges of inorganic compounds. Thus, the solubility of organic compounds in water helps determine their movement and transport. As temperatures increase, the solubility of organic compounds increases. Many environmental pollutants consist of multiple chemical contaminants, which have varying miscibilities and solubilities in groundwater.

Organic solvents also evaporate into the atmosphere from soil or into the soil atmosphere. Organic pollutants volatilize from their water phase into a gaseous phase, which is a mechanism of transport in the vadose zone.

The solubility of pollutants differs when measured in freshwater versus seawater. For example, two common solvents, benzene and toluene, are more soluble in freshwater than in seawater. This has important planning implications for spill-response teams. Assuming constant pressure and temperature, the expected air concentration over an ocean spill tends to be higher compared with a lake or river spill, because more of the solvents are dissolved in the freshwater.

Similarly, when a pure liquid-air interfaces in a closed space, the vapor pressure of the chemical is the dominant predictor of chemical air concentration. As the ambient temperature increases, the rate of vaporization also increases. Thus, the temperature of the liquid surface at the interface has a substantial impact on the vaporization and the measured vapor pressure. It would be expected that a crude oil spill in cold waters would produce different environmental impacts than a warm-water release.

Another common way that air-water (liquid) interfaces are expressed is by Henry's Law. Henry's Law describes the volatilization of a pollutant between water and gas phases and is important in describing pollutant movement in the vadose zone of soil (1,7).

$$\text{Henry's Law: } C_g = HC_w$$

C_g = concentration of pollutant (mg/L) in gas phase (air)
H = Henry's constant
C_w = concentration of pollutant in water phase (mg/L)

Henry's Law describes the partitioning of a contaminant between liquid and gas (water versus air). Henry's constant (H) describes the rate at which a substance evaporates from water and can be calculated by dividing the vapor pressure of a chemical by its aqueous solubility.

As H increases, it becomes more likely that a chemical will move from water to air. For example, the H for benzene is approximately 5 times greater than the value for anthracite and 4,000 times greater than benzo[*a*]pyrene. The knowledge of vapor pressure, solubility, or Henry's Law constant provides a predictor of air-water interface behavior.

Pollutant Movement in Air-Soil and Liquid-Soil Interfaces

Knowledge of the dynamics of air-soil and liquid-soil interfaces is important, because direct spills and leaks to soil are common. The subsequent behavior of the released material is partially a function of a soil-specific property known as *adsorption* or *sorption*. Chemicals may enter soil and water through runoff, sorption to soil, or leaching, then be taken up by plants or volatilize into air (Fig. 2-6).

Sorption is the process of chemicals attaching to the surfaces of minerals and organic matter in soil and rock. Sorption is generally considered a reversible process, although in some circumstances, a material will tightly adhere to the soil, releasing little to either air or water. Mathematically, sorption can be defined by the following equation:

$$K = \frac{C_s}{C_w}$$

where K is the water-soil partition coefficient of the compound for a particular soil, C_s is the mass of the chemical adsorbed on the soil per unit of bulk dry mass, and C_w is the mass of the chemical dissolved in a unit of water that is in contact with the soil.

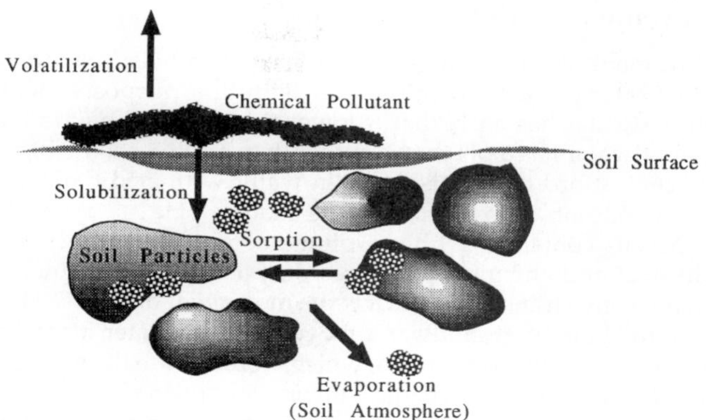

Figure 2-5. Water-air phase pollutant transfer.

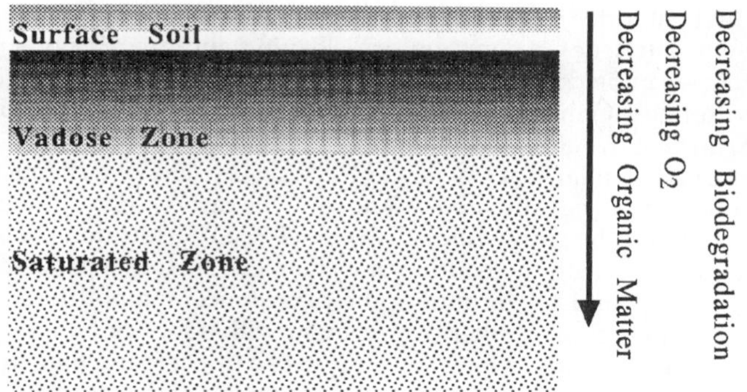

Figure 2-6. Decreasing O_2, biodegradation, and organic content of soil with increasing soil depth.

The degree of adsorption is highly dependent on the organic content of soil, and this is reflected by another commonly used term, the *organic carbon sorption coefficient*—$K_{(oc)}$—used to define the soil retention of an organic compound. Soil organic content less than 1% is considered low, whereas levels of 3% to 5% are more representative of most soils. $K_{(oc)}$ and K can be connected by the formula:

$$K = K_{(oc)} \times C_{(oc)}$$

where $C_{(oc)}$ is the fraction of organic carbon content of soil (grams of organic carbon per grams of soil). This formula is useful for most organic pesticides contaminating soil (1,7). Converting $K_{(oc)}$ to K and knowing $C_{(oc)}$ for the soil, the binding of organic compounds to soil can be obtained using sorption isotherms.

Soil-Water Sorption Isotherms

A quantitative description of the relationship between the concentration of a pollutant adsorbed by soil and the concentration in water can be determined using sorption isotherms (7). Based on Henry's Law, a simple linear isotherm can describe the relationship:

$$S = KC_w$$

S = pollutant concentration sorbed by soil (mg/kg)
K = sorption coefficient (liter/kg or mL/g)
C_w = name of chemical dissolved in water that is in contact with soil

The larger the K value, the greater degree the absorption of pollutant.

Knowledge of either K or $K_{(oc)}$ is useful, because a variety of fate-transport predictions can be made based on the value of these terms. For example, chemicals with a K of less than 1.0 move more easily in a water system. Similarly, a K greater than 10 implies that a chemical is adsorbed to the soil. Chemicals with $K_{(oc)}$ values greater than 10,000 are highly adsorbed to soils, whereas a $K_{(oc)}$ of less than 1,000 is indicative of a more mobile substance. Solvents like benzene are highly mobile in soil, frequently migrate through the soil column, and can contaminate groundwater. This is in contrast to poorly mobile chemicals typified by polyaromatic hydrocarbons, which tend to adhere tightly to the soil and are less likely to move to groundwater at depth.

K is directly related to another descriptive term: the *retardation factor*. In general, as chemical movement is retarded in a soil column, it is potentially subjected to a variety of degradation or transformation processes (e.g., microbial, digestive, hydrolytic) that can convert the starting molecule into a more or less toxic by-product. For example, 1,1,2-trichloroethylene (TCE) is converted under anaerobic soil conditions to dichloroethylene and vinyl chloride (8). Similarly, under certain soil conditions, perchloroethylene—a common dry-cleaning and degreasing solvent—can be converted to TCE. Hence, it is possible to begin with one chemical at the soil surface and find different compounds at the groundwater level.

The potential movement and leaching capacity of a chemical pollutant can be estimated by knowing the carbon sorption coefficient and the compound's half-life ($T\frac{1}{2}$). The sorption coefficient, along with the half-life of a chemical, such as a pesticide, can be useful in determining the persistence of a pollutant in soil. A pesticide or other contaminant with a low carbon-sorption coefficient and a long half-life poses a threat to leaching into groundwater supplies. A contaminant with a high soil-sorption coefficient and a long half-life will remain somewhat immobile in ground soil.

Pesticides with short half-lives and intermediate sorption coefficients are considered the "safest" for the environment (6). Most pesticides tend to stay in biologically active areas of soil and are thus subject to more intense biodegradation.

Pollution Movement in Liquid-Liquid Interfaces

Liquid-liquid interfaces are typified by sudden releases of hydrocarbons (crude oil) into saltwater or freshwater bodies. These pollution problems create an environmental interface between the underside of an oil slick and the water phase. In this situation, the density of the hydrocarbon phase is usually less than the water phase, so the oil floats on the water surface, creating a slick. If the density of the released material is greater than water, the material sinks and creates a different type of liquid-liquid interface problem. When a water-surface oil slick is created, a variety of processes affect the nature of the interface:

- Evaporation
- Photochemical and oxidative reactions
- Dissolution and emulsification
- Biodegradation

These processes are influenced by the ambient air and water temperatures. In addition, rough sea surfaces can significantly alter the interface boundary conditions.

The lower boiling-point organic hydrocarbons in oil evaporate over a period of several hours. The more polar hydrocarbons dissolve quickly in water. In general, the liquid-to-air movement accounts for the majority of the interface transfer, assuming stable sea conditions. There is a mass transfer from the hydrocarbon layer to the water phase, but evaporation is the dominant mechanism of release. Evaporation to air is rapid, and the transfer rate decreases by as many as two orders of magnitude within 8 days (1).

As lighter hydrocarbon fractions evaporate, the residual oil becomes more viscous, which affects the kinetics of further air transfer. At this stage of an oil slick, a film forms on the surface of the unmixed oil and prevents further evaporation of the lighter fractions unless chemical dispersants are used.

At this point, the other physical, mechanical (wave action), chemical, and biological processes become dominant. Heavier oil fractions coalesce and form tar balls, which eventually sink because of the accumulation of sand and shell material. This process results in the creation of a liquid-liquid interface below the water surface. Thus, a crude oil or other type of hydrocarbon spill illustrates the intricate interaction of the different types of interface problems. Ultimately, the role of biodegradation becomes critical to alter an oil spill.

Movement of Metals in Groundwater

Movement of metals in groundwater and soil is a function of soil/water pH and sorption. For definition purposes, acidic groundwater has a pH that is lower than 5.5, and neutralized groundwater has a pH that is higher than 5.5. In general, higher concentrations of metals occur in water with acidic pH, and lower concentrations occur at more alkaline pH.

Metals contained within a plume of water are affected by physical and chemical processes. Physical processes include (a) advective transport, which is the movement of solutes along with the bulk of groundwater movement in a water mass, and (b) hydrodynamic dispersion, which would cause the spread of solute as a result of mechanical mixing and fusion.

Chemical reactions include precipitation and adsorption, which can change the concentration of metals in groundwater.

Calcium carbonate, sodium hydroxide, and aluminum oxide in water cause most metals to precipitate out of solution. Aluminum and ion oxides adsorb cadmium and arsenic. Chemical processes also occur as a result of oxidation reactions and changes in water pH. Changes in water pH are due to the presence of or degassing of carbon dioxide. A higher CO_2 content increases carbonic acid concentrations, which then raise the pH of water. Many metals become insoluble precipitates in acidic water.

Metals in groundwater can adsorb to soil particles or be dissolved in soil water. pH of the water and physical characteristics of the soil are primary factors that control the state of metals and surface soils.

Metals can be removed from surface soils through leaching into deeper soils or groundwater. They can also be lost by surface runoff or wind erosion.

The distribution-of-movement rate of metals in a water plume is controlled by chemical interactions between acidic groundwater and the aquifer matrix. The main chemical parameters controlling mobility include (a) the acidity of the water plume and (b) the neutralization capacity of the aquifer. The neutralization capacity of an aquifer depends on its calcium carbonate content. Chemical reactions between calcium carbonate and the acidic groundwater consume acidity, decreasing hydrogen ion concentration and elevating pH. The neutralization capacity of more alkaline water in an aquifer slows the movement of the metal plume. As acidic groundwater moves through the aquifer, the front of the plume is neutralized by chemical reactions with calcium carbonate. As neutralization raises the pH at the front of the plume, solubility of the metals is exceeded, and metal hydroxides precipitate, which removes metals from the solution. The degree to which the metals precipitate depends on the pH as well as the characteristic of each of the metals. Relatively soluble metal, such as manganese, can migrate past the front of an acidic plume. Both increased metal solubility and adsorption can attenuate the presence of metals in groundwater. As the pH continues to rise along the flow path of an aquifer, the less soluble metals precipitate from solution.

Human exposure to metals in groundwater occurs through wells, ingestion of irrigated vegetables, ingestion of water-fed animal meats, and dermal exposure. The pH of water determines what metals may be at concentrations high enough to produce health risks. Depending on the pollution source, the metals may be more or less toxic. Mining operations, metals leaching from mine waste, and smelting operations result in the most toxic metals, such as lead, mercury, arsenic, cadmium, manganese, chromium, copper, zinc, beryllium, and nickel.

Pollutant Movement Across Biological Interfaces

Assessing chemodynamics across biological interfaces is determined by the extent to which chemicals bioaccumulate and are biodegraded. Living organisms can concentrate chemicals in their tissues at levels significantly greater than the concentration in water or soil.

Although it is difficult to directly measure bioaccumulation, there is an adequate surrogate measure for organic chemicals called the *octanol-water partition coefficient* [$K_{(ow)}$]. Octanol is a reasonably good surrogate for lipid, so the ability of a chemical to preferentially partition into octanol (versus water) is considered a relatively accurate predictor of bioaccumulation. $K_{(ow)}$ is formally defined as the ratio of the concentration of a chemical in the octanol phase to its concentration in the aqueous phase. $K_{(ow)}$ is directly related to the tendency to bioconcentrate and is inversely correlated with water solubility. Highly water-soluble chemicals are very mobile and less likely to volatilize and persist; hence, they are less able to bioconcentrate. Chemicals with large $K_{(ow)}$ values (e.g., polychlorinated biphenyls, DDT, and dioxins) tend to accumulate in soil, sediment, and biota, but not in water. Conversely, chemicals such as solvents (e.g., benzene, toluene) with small $K_{(ow)}$ values tend to preferentially partition to air and water.

The $K_{(ow)}$ numbers are frequently presented as logarithms or log $K_{(ow)}$. For example, the log $K_{(ow)}$ of benzene is 2.12, whereas the log $K_{(ow)}$ for DDT is 6.19. This difference does not appear significant until the log values are transformed into their "natural" values: Benzene is 131.8 and DDT is 1,548,817. The difference is readily apparent, and it is easy to see why DDT is so persistent in living organisms.

Metal bioaccumulation up the food chain to humans occurs from contamination of soil and water, irrigation of crops by contaminated water, and contaminated water fed to consumable animals.

Chemical and metal concentrations in plants are estimated from their concentrations in soil using the following equation (9):

$$C_p = C_s \times B_f \times (1 - f_w)$$

C_p = concentration in plants (μg/kg)
C_s = soil concentration (μg/kg)
B_f = soil/plant biotransfer factor (soil μg/kg)/(water μg/kg)
f_w = water fraction of plant (no units)

The concentration in plants (C_p) is influenced by the type of chemical (organic versus inorganic) and the soil-plant biotransfer factor. This factor is the ratio of dry-weight chemical concentration in plants to the chemical concentration in soil. Inorganic chemicals bioaccumulate in reproductive areas of plants (fruits, seeds, tubers) and in vegetative portions (leaves, stems). Metals also bind to sulfhydryl groups of proteins.

The soil/plant partitioning coefficient of metals varies and is influenced by soil/water pH. As an example, the biotransfer soil/plant partition coefficient for arsenic = 0.04, manganese = 0.25, and cadmium = 0.55 for vegetative portions of plants. For reproductive portions of plants, these values are arsenic = 0.006, manganese = 0.05, and cadmium = 0.25 (10).

Metal bioaccumulation in animals is mainly through water and feed ingestion and can be determined by the EPA using the equation:

$$C_a = C_w \times B_f \times IR_w$$

C_a = concentration in animal (μg/kg)
C_w = concentration in water (μg/L)
B_f = biotransfer factor
IR_w = ingestion rate of water or feed by animal

Some biotransfer factors for inorganic compounds and metals are available. For those not available, assumptions are made (9). The biotransfer factor for beef has been estimated for the following example metals: arsenic = 2×10^{-3}, cadmium = 5.5×10^{-4}, lead = 4×10^{-3}, mercury 2.5×10^{-1}, nickel = 6.0×10^{-3}, thallium 4.0×10^{-2}, manganese = 4.0×10^{-4} (9).

The use of any biotransfer factors is based on conservative assumptions that chemical concentrations in animal tissue accumulate in direct proportion to daily intake of the pollutant. This assumption does not account for normal physiologic regulation of certain metals found normally in animals.

POLLUTANT BIODEGRADATION

The microbiological mass of soil is a potent resource for removal of environmental contaminants through biodegradation. Many organic environmental pollutants serve as substrates for soil microbes. The common chemical classes of these xenobiotics are:

- Aliphatic hydrocarbons (saturated and unsaturated)
- Aromatic hydrocarbons (single and multiple aromatic rings)
- Cyclic aliphatics
- Halogenated hydrocarbons
- Oxygenated organic substances (ketones, esters, ethers, alcohols)

Bioavailability of an organic compound is dependent on the water content of the soil, its oxygen content, the soil nutrients for microorganisms, the biomass of microbes, the proper mixture of microbes, and the physiochemical properties of the xenobiotic.

The important factors of oxygen and organic content of soil among the different areas of surface soil, vadose zone, and groundwater region allow certain predictions to be made relative to biodegradation:

- Biodegradation in aerobic surface soils is rapid.
- Biodegradation in vadose zones is aerobic but slower because of the decreasing oxygen tension and decreasing or more dormant populations of microbes.
- Biodegradation in groundwater is slow and mainly anaerobic.
- Limited nitrogen supplies impede biodegradation, whereas additional nitrogen can enhance the process.

Each step of biodegradation pathways involves catalytic enzymes. The lack of certain biodegrading enzymes is a reason for persistence of some xenobiotics in the environment. The lack of certain biodegrading microorganisms in a contaminated soil also results in persistent contaminant presence. Complete biodegradation of a compound through oxidation would result in carbon dioxide and water. This is termed *mineralization*.

Environmental contaminants that are similar to natural substances in the environment are more easily biodegraded than those that are dissimilar. Biodegradation can also create more toxic compounds that are more stable in the environment than the parent compound. TCE, for instance, is anaerobically biodegraded to vinyl chloride. Elemental mercury can be biotransformed to organic methylmercury.

The following factors influence the biodegradation process in soil:

- Mass of microorganisms
- Soil pH
- Soil temperature
- Presence or absence of water
- Oxygen availability
- Soil organic content
- Nitrogen availability

Environmental contamination usually occurs in surface soils, the vadose zone, and the saturated zone, and the presence of oxygen and organic matter varies among these zones. There is a decreasing rate of biodegradation with decreasing oxygen and decreasing organic matter of soils as soil depth increases.

Biodegradation also proceeds more rapidly in aerobic conditions compared with anaerobic conditions in general. Aliphatic hydrocarbons are generally degraded aerobically more efficiently than anaerobically (7).

Soil contains various areas of both anaerobic and aerobic activity, depending on the presence of water and oxygen. Most aerobic activity occurs in the surface soil layers and in the vadose zone (see Fig. 2-6).

Surface soil is usually rich in organic material, but if there are insufficient numbers of microorganisms in soil, biodegradation will be slow or will not happen at all.

Nitrogen content of organic compounds critically affects biodegradation. Hydrocarbons in oil spills are nitrogen poor. Biodegradation is enhanced when nitrogen is added, because microorganisms use nitrogen in their metabolism (7).

The chemical structure of xenobiotics is a major determining factor in their biodegradation. Compounds that have a propensity for soil sorption are less readily bioavailable and less water soluble, and are thus less biodegradable. Extensive branching of hydrocarbon chains generally impedes biodegradation. The presence of chlorinated groups on hydrocarbons slows or impedes biodegradation.

Anaerobic biodegradation is also a pathway for transformation of environmental pollutants. Highly substituted organochlorine compounds tend to be biodegraded by anaerobic conditions. Aliphatic hydrocarbons are biodegraded slowly under anaerobic conditions. However, oxygen-containing or unsaturated aliphatics are readily biodegraded anaerobically. Oxygenated aromatic compounds can also be biodegraded anaerobically.

Aliphatic Hydrocarbons

Aliphatic hydrocarbons are either straight chained or branched, saturated (alkanes) or unsaturated (alkenes), and may be oxygenated or may contain substituted halogens. Aliphatic hydrocarbons containing oxygen are biodegraded under anaerobic and aerobic conditions. Saturated aliphatics have a higher hydrogen content, whereas the C = C bonds of unsaturated aliphatics decrease hydrogen content.

Ketones, ethers, esters, alcohols, and unsaturated aliphatics are mainly biodegraded under anaerobic conditions in soil (Fig. 2-7). Oxygen is incorporated into the unsaturated C = C bond to form an aldehyde, ketone, or alcohol. Eventually, alkanes and alkenes are metabolized to a fatty acid, which is used in the tricarboxylic acid cycle of cell metabolism (Fig. 2-8).

Halogenated Aliphatics

Aerobic biodegradation of chlorinated aliphatic compounds generally proceeds by either dehalogenation through substitution processes or oxidation. The substitution reaction is nucleophilic—that is, the chlorine is substituted by a hydroxyl group (7). Halogenated aliphatics are biodegraded both aerobically and anaerobically (Fig. 2-9). Anaerobic conditions favor biodegradation of highly halogenated organic compounds. Aerobic conditions favor biodegradation of mono- or dihalogenated organic compounds (7). The process of anaerobic reductive dehalogenation involves formation of an alkyl radical, which scavenges a hydrogen ion and forms an alkene.

Heavily chlorinated organic hydrocarbons are more stable under aerobic conditions. Anaerobic removal of chlorine groups is favored by the increasing chlorine content of organic compounds.

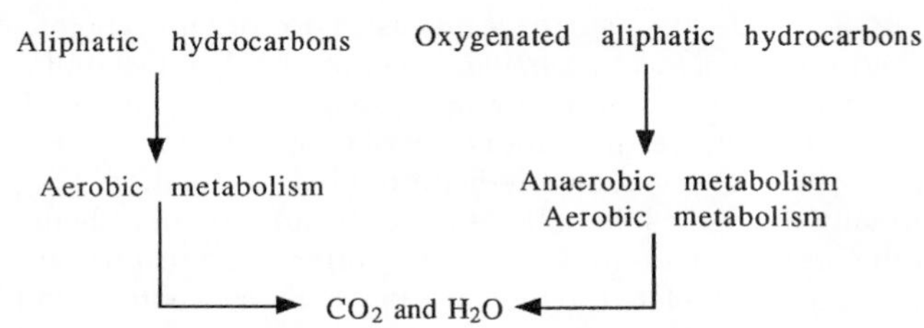

Figure 2-7. Aliphatic biodegradation.

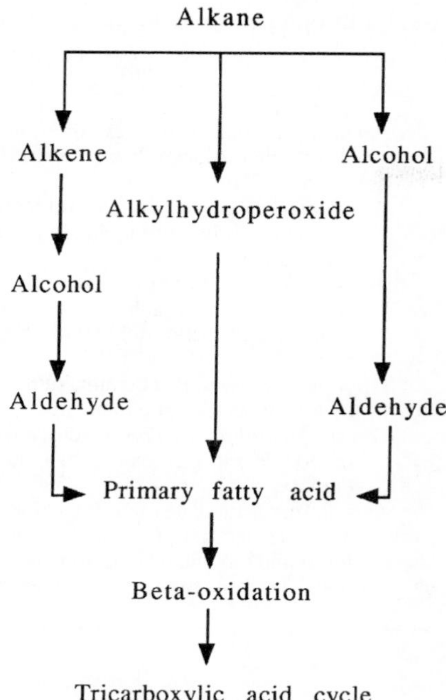

Figure 2-8. Alkane and alkene aerobic biodegradation.

Aromatic Biodegradation

Aromatic hydrocarbons—such as benzene, toluene, ethylbenzene, and polyaromatic hydrocarbons—tend to highly sorb to soil particles and soil with high organic content. This high sorption rate, along with lower water solubility, decreases their availability for biodegradation. Also, as the number of aromatic rings increases, their solubility, bioavailability, and biodegradation decreases.

Transformation of aromatic hydrocarbons by hydroxylation of the aromatic ring is one of the more common biotransformation processes (Fig. 2-10). Dioxygenases and monooxygenases are enzyme systems in bacteria and fungi that biotransform aromatic compounds.

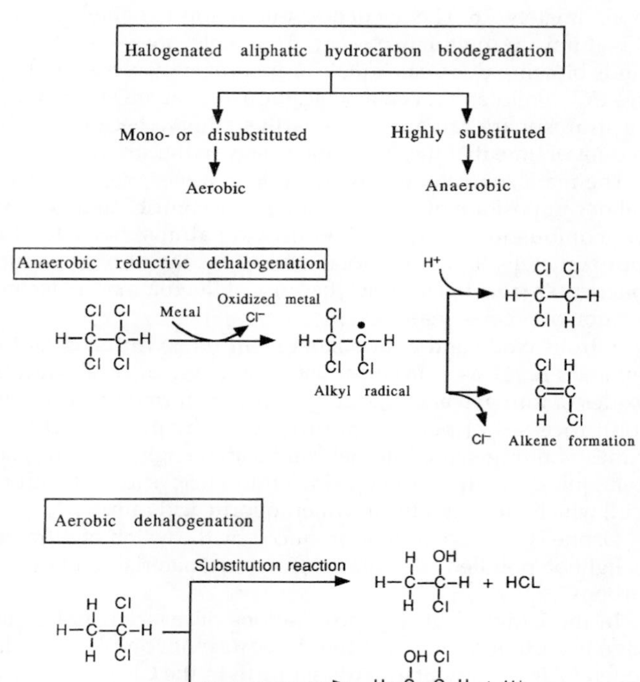

Figure 2-9. Halogenated aliphatic hydrocarbon biodegradation.

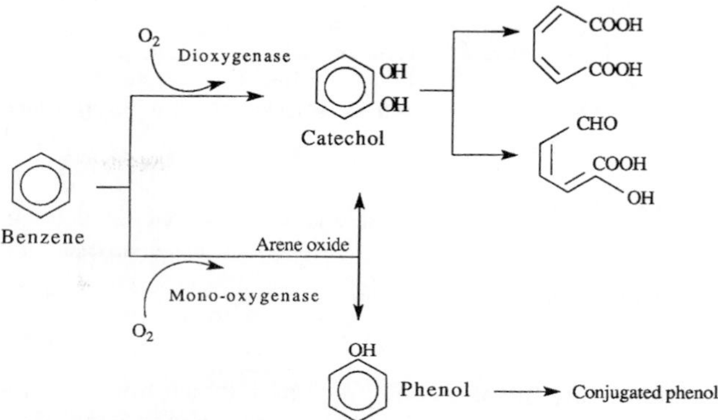

Figure 2-10. Biodegradation of benzene.

As an example, creosols undergo aerobic and anaerobic biodegradation by soil bacteria. Pseudomonads and other bacteria contain a flavocytochrome enzyme that biodegrades creosols (Fig. 2-11). In order of magnitude and efficiency, biodegradation of creosols is in the order of para > meta > ortho, both for aerobic and anaerobic biodegradation.

Cyclic Aliphatic Biodegradation

Cyclic aliphatics, such as cyclohexane, undergo aerobic biodegradation by microorganisms. The biodegradation of these alicyclic hydrocarbon rings requires mixed populations of microorganisms to form first an alcohol, then a hexanone, then a lactone, and finally, breaking of the cyclic ring to form a hexanoic acid (Fig. 2-12).

Metal Biotransformation

Metals undergo environmental transformation. Many examples exist in which metals become more toxic when acted on biologically, such as mercury transformation to methylmercury. Metals of toxic importance include mercury, lead, arsenic, cadmium, manganese, magnesium, chromium, copper, nickel, zinc, tin, beryllium, and selenium. Metals can bioconcentrate up the food chain because of their binding capacity to sulfhydryl groups of protein.

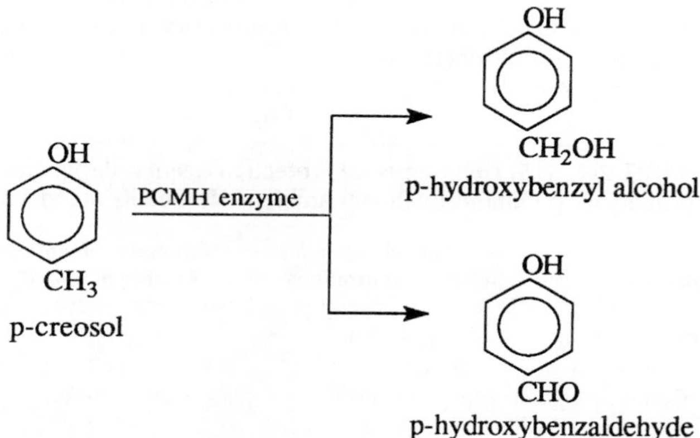

Figure 2-11. PCMH enzyme catalyzes dehydrogenation and hydration of p-creosol to alcohol, then to aldehyde or ketone. O-creosol and m-creosol are biotransformed to hydroxybenzaldehyde, then to hydroxybenzoic acid, and onto phenol or to benzaldehyde.

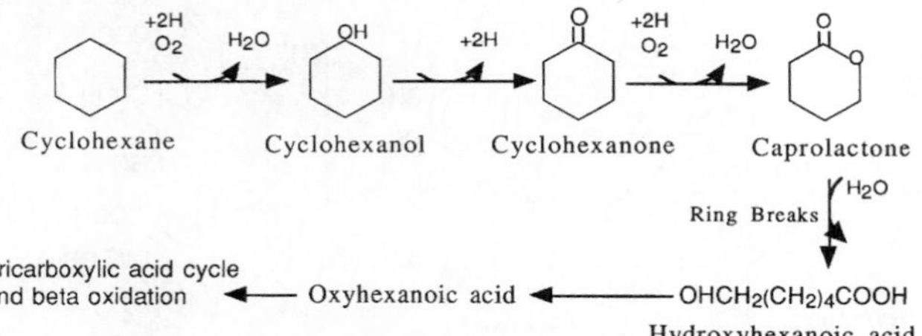

Figure 2-12. Biodegradation of cyclic aliphatic.

Oxidation of metals is one process by which transformation occurs in the environment by microorganisms. Alkylation is another mechanism of microbial transformation of metals, exemplified by the transformation of mercury into methylmercury. The process results in mercury that can bioconcentrate and be more toxic than the parent compound. The formation of organometals is an important biotransformation process.

Transport and Fate of Atmospheric Pollutants

Air pollution is a major public health problem and exacerbates asthma, bronchitis, and chronic obstructive pulmonary disease (11–15). Air pollutants are categorized as primary (Table 2-4) or secondary. Besides affecting human health, atmospheric pollution also affects plants and animals and causes property damage.

In 1963, the Clean Air Act was passed, and the EPA was charged with regulation of outdoor air pollutants from both stationary and mobile sources. In 1970, an amendment to the Clean Air Act established National Ambient Air Quality Standards to protect public health and regulated five primary air pollutants: carbon monoxide, NO_2, SO_2, ozone, PM_{10}, and lead. Individual states were given responsibility for attaining and maintaining the standards set forth in these amendments (see Table 2-4).

Air pollution occurs as a result of human activities and natural phenomena. The air pollutants of most concern are carbon monoxide, nitrogen oxides, sulfur oxides, ozone, volatile hydrocarbons, hydrogen sulfide, and carbon dioxide. These gaseous pollutants are expressed in terms of microgram per meter cubed ($\mu g/m^3$). Other air pollutants are particulate pollutants and suspended dust. These particulates can consist of dust, fumes, mist, smokes, and aerosols.

Controversy rages around stricter EPA rules governing particles of 2.5 micrometers in diameter and less ($PM_{2.5}$). Currently, the EPA regulates particles of 10 micrometers in size (PM_{10}) with a current standard of 150 $\mu g/m^3$ for a 24-hour period. Studies show $PM_{2.5}$ particles increase risk of respiratory disease and the incidence of mortality (11–16).

TABLE 2-4. U.S. Environmental Protection Agency–designated primary air pollutants (National Ambient Air Quality Standard)

Pollutant	Period of averaging for mean concentrations	National Ambient Air Quality Standard
CO	8 h	9 μL/L
	1 h	35 μL/L
NO_2	Annual	0.05 μL/L
O_3	1 h	0.120 μL/L
SO_2	Annual	0.03 μL/L
	24 h	0.14 μL/L
PM_{10}	Annual	50 $\mu g/m^3$
	24 h	150 $\mu g/m^3$

TABLE 2-5. Anthropogenic and natural air pollutants

Pollutant	Source
Anthropogenic pollutants	*Stationary combustion sources*: Ashes, smokes, particulates, sulfur oxides, nitrogen oxides, CO, and CO_2 Acid rain *Transportation sources*: Smoke and particulates, dust, lead, carbon monoxide, nitrogen oxides, volatile hydrocarbons *Industrial sources*: Various acids, acidic, nitric phosphoric, sulfuric, volatile organic solvents and hydrocarbons, chlorine, ammonia gas, a variety of metals
Natural air pollutants	*Erupting volcanoes*: Particulates, sulfur oxides, hydrogen sulfides, methane, dust *Forest fires and prairie fires*: Hydrocarbons, carbon monoxide, nitrogen oxides, ash, dust, and particulates *Dust storms*: Particulate matter of various sizes, plants and trees in forests, CO_2, and a blue haze over forest and mountain areas from atmospheric reactions of volatile organics produced by trees

ANTHROPOGENIC VERSUS NATURAL AIR POLLUTANTS

Anthropogenic pollutants are man-made and originate from three sources: (a) stationary combustion, (b) exhaust emissions from vehicles using fuels, and (c) industrial processes. These sources produce a combination of particulates, sulfur oxides, nitrogen oxides, carbon monoxide, carbon dioxide, and release volatile hydrocarbons into the air (Table 2-5), such as benzene, toluene, trimethylbenzene, heptane, xylene, 2-methylpentane, *n*-hexane, octane, nonane, methane, tetrachloroethylene.

Sulfur oxides released from man-made sources are the main component producing acid rain. Rain normally has a pH of approximately 5.6. The pH of acid rain is approximately 3.

Natural air pollutants occur from volcanoes, forest fires, winds blowing dust, earthquakes, and vegetation that contributes CO_2. Pollutants, such as volcanic ash, that are emitted into the stratosphere can affect the earth's climate because of the amount of time that these pollutants stay in the stratosphere.

The main source of carbon dioxide in atmosphere is microbial decomposition of organic matter. The contribution of fossil fuel combustion to the carbon dioxide atmospheric load is approximately 10% of the total. The CO_2 content of the atmosphere rises from fall to spring because of fluctuations in decomposition of organic matter.

Nitrous oxide and ammonia are natural constituents of the soil and are released from industrial and agricultural sources. Oxides of nitrogen and oxides of sulfur are formed by combustion processes of petroleum products. The main sources of oxides of nitrogen are internal combustion engines. Both gases react quickly with air to be oxidized to nitric acid and sulfuric acid, which then dissolve in water to form acid rain.

Ozone is an air pollutant produced by the action of ultraviolet light on polluted air containing organic materials and hydrocarbons.

In the United States, concentrations of most air pollutants have been in a downward trend because of compliance with Federal Air Quality Standards set forth in the Clean Air Act of 1970. However, many urban areas still cannot meet specific compliance standards for some pollutants such as CO, ozone, or particulates.

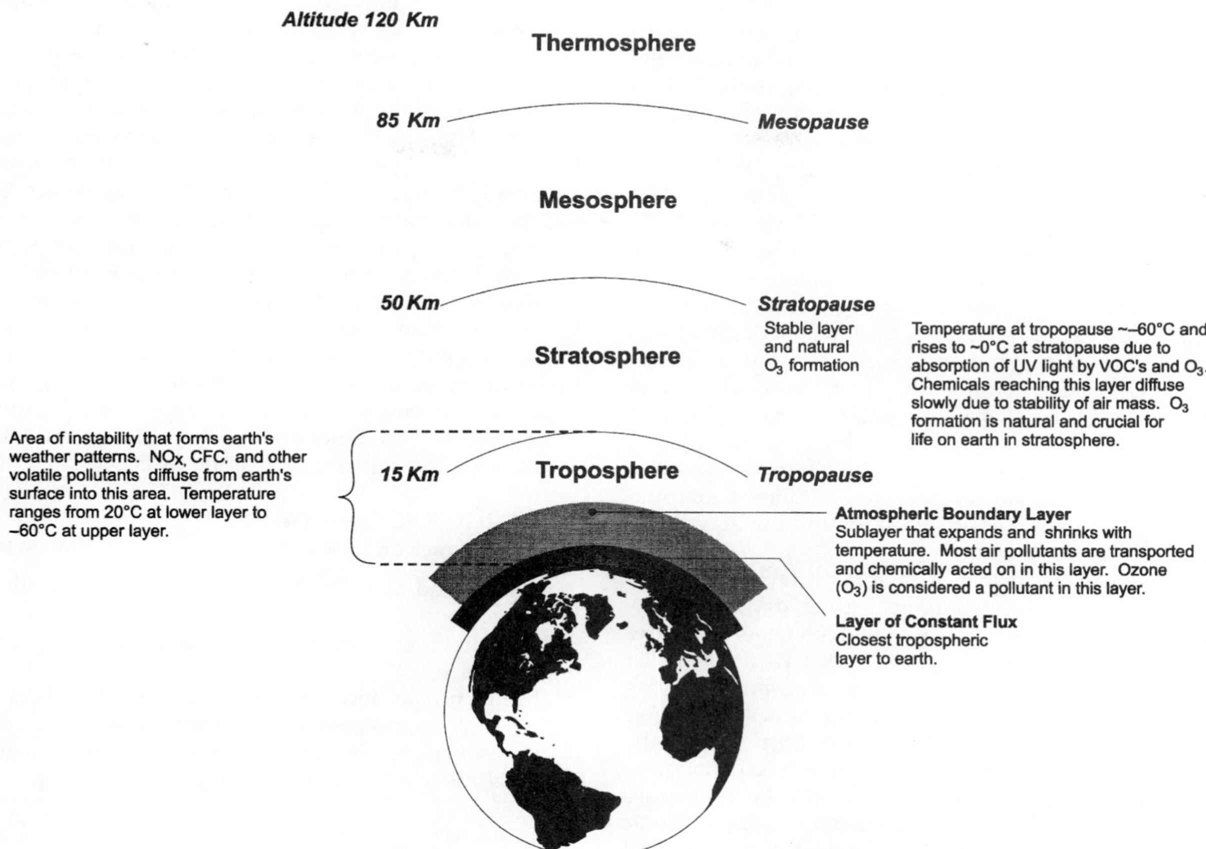

Figure 2-13. Earth atmospheric levels. CFC, chlorofluorocarbon; NO_x, nitrogen oxides; VOC, volatile organic chemical.

Earth's Atmosphere and Pollution

Earth's atmosphere is divided into zones defined by temperature and altitude (Fig. 2-13). The lower atmosphere—the troposphere—extends from the surface of the earth to a height of approximately 15 kilometers. Most weather we experience on earth's surface occurs in the troposphere.

The atmospheric layer at the bottom of the troposphere is called the *atmospheric boundary layer.* In this region, air gradient, temperature, winds, and humidity are most active. The air is turbulent, readily mixes, and is influenced by the time of day and temperature. The atmospheric boundary layer fluctuates in height depending on the time of day. When the temperature is highest, this layer may be as much as 1 kilometer in height; it shrinks to approximately 10% of this by nighttime (1,7). Most transport and transformation of air pollutants occurs within the atmospheric boundary layer. The chemical composition of the atmosphere consists mainly of nitrogen, oxygen, and argon gases. Other atmospheric gases are neon, helium, and krypton. Some atmospheric gases are constant, whereas trace gases are variable in concentration. Midwestern state governors argue that the new particulate standards will throw their states out of compliance, forcing new and more costly controls.

The layer closest to earth is the *surface layer,* approximately one-tenth of the boundary layer in depth. The surface layer is in constant flux.

The upper atmosphere consists of the *stratosphere*, the *mesosphere*, and the *thermosphere*. The stratosphere is a stable layer of atmosphere extending to a height of approximately 50 kilometers. This is a highly stable area. Little mixing of pollutants occurs here, and pollutants that enter it tend to diffuse very slowly toward the higher atmospheric layers.

The stratosphere is where ozone is formed, both naturally and by photochemical processes. Stratospheric ozone is essential to life on earth because it absorbs ultraviolet radiation that would be harmful to biological organisms. In the troposphere, ozone is considered a pollutant, whereas in the stratosphere, it is a critical feature for life to exist on earth. The higher layers of the atmosphere, the mesosphere and thermosphere, have little influence on weather patterns and pollutant transport.

Atmospheric pressure is another factor that influences pollutant movement. The *atmospheric pressure* is the mass pressure and kinetic energy of the molecules in the atmosphere. Horizontal variations of this pressure result in air flow or winds across the earth. The differences in air pressure across the earth's surface depend on the altitude of the surface, such as sea level versus mountain. Even sea level pressures can vary because of heating effects of the sun, water vapor, and cloud cover.

The atmosphere is a dynamic medium with physical properties that determine the fate and transport of environmental contaminants:

- Wind
- Air pressure
- Air density
- Temperature
- Water vapor
- Air mass movement
- Radiant energy

Air movement and climate changes help divert and disperse pollutants, whereas air stability allows pollutants to accumulate. Pollutants, source inversions that inhibit mixing of air, the presence of high ultraviolet intensity and sunlight, the lack of winds for dispersion, and the geographic terrain all influence the movement of pollutants in the atmosphere.

Temperature inversions that concentrate air pollutants are generated by surface cooling of the earth through loss of infrared radiation or evaporation from the surface to the sky, allowing the ground surface to cool. This generally occurs on clear, calm nights (1,7). Such inversions are common in the western United States during fall, winter, and spring, when the air is dry and the skies are clear. Loss of water through evaporation also plays a part in inversion generation. Such evaporative loss can occur over large irrigated crop fields. Inversions can last from days to weeks, resulting in negative health effects to humans and animals.

Environmental contaminates can be transformed via atmospheric chemical reactions in air and in precipitation. Chlorofluorocarbons (CFCs) are not easily acted on and can stay in the atmosphere for many years.

The main mechanisms by which environmental contaminants leave the atmosphere are gravitational setting, dry deposition, and wet deposition (7). Gravitational setting can remove particles with diameters that are larger than 1 micrometer. Particles smaller than 1 micrometer remain suspended in the atmosphere for long periods of time. *Dry deposition* is the adsorption or "sinking" of volatile pollutants by the soil and plants. *Wet deposition* is the removal of pollution by rain and other forms of precipitation.

Rain is naturally acidic—with a pH between 5 and 6—because it absorbs carbon dioxide in the atmosphere, forming carbonic acid. When rain comes into contact with oxides of nitrogen and sulfur, it becomes more acidic, and its pH can drop to less than 4.

The effects of atmospheric releases of air pollutants can be evaluated by analyzing the following information:

- Source characteristics
- Site-specific factors
- Meteorologic conditions
- Geography of area
- Topography of area
- Contaminant properties

SOURCE AND SITE CHARACTERISTICS OF AIR POLLUTANTS

Source characteristics refer to (a) type of source; (b) rate of pollutant release; (c) the plume height, or height of the release source; and (d) a variety of other site-specific parameters. Sources are defined as point, nonpoint, or multiple-release points.

Point sources refer to a specific emission point, such as an industrial stack associated with a refinery or other industrial process. This source can be defined in terms of height above ground, stack diameter, gas velocity, and temperature at the stack opening. *Nonpoint* or *area sources* are several sources distributed over a homogeneous surface area.

Usually, the individual sources within an area are small and are dominated by a point source. If there are multiple overlapping sources along a specified surface area, they are known as *line sources*. An example of a line source is urban traffic within a defined geographic area.

Multiple source refers to the combination of point and nonpoint sources, such as ones typically found in urban or industrial settings. For example, a major highway (line source) may be adjacent to a large refinery composed of both point and nonpoint sources.

For each source type, the rate of release or emission rate must be defined. Multiple-source emission rates must incorporate time and spatial distribution of emissions from all sources.

Plume height is the physical height of the stack adjusted by factors that can either raise (buoyancy or momentum) or lower (downwash or deflection) the plume. Plume height affects the time required for released contaminants to reach ground level. This is important, because peak ground-level exposure concentrations are typically not located close to a point source with a high plume height. Elevated ground-level concentrations from smelter stacks are usually found a significant distance from the source. Other factors that affect plume height include (a) contaminant release temperature (e.g., greater buoyancy and greater rise), (b) stack-tip downwash (i.e., velocity of the stack contaminant emitted is low relative to ambient wind speed, thus effective plume height is lower), and (c) downwash that is due to adjacent structure.

Site-specific factors that affect the source include (a) operational variations in emissions and meteorologic conditions over time; (b) use of emission controls, such as scrubbers; and (c) fugitive emissions from other ground-level sources, such as storage facilities, piping, flanges, valves, and fittings.

METEOROLOGIC CONDITIONS

A variety of meteorologic conditions affect air pollutant transport:

- Wind speed and direction (causing increased dilution and dispersion)
- Precipitation that increases ground pollutant deposition near the source
- Turbulence produced by kinetic and thermal energy transfers between air and the terrain (dispersion is enhanced at lower atmospheric levels, but the reverse may occur at higher atmospheric levels if conditions are stable and wind speed is high).

GEOGRAPHY

Dispersion of contaminants is categorized as a function of distance from the source, either (a) near-field, less than 30 miles (50 km) from the source, or (b) far-field, greater than 30 miles (50 km) from the source. In general, near-field scale exposures are not affected by atmospheric chemical reactions, and the plume is assumed to spread both laterally and vertically in a Gaussian (bell-shaped) distribution under steady-state atmospheric conditions (Fig. 2-14). The EPA has a variety of Gaussian plume models, such as the Industrial Source Complex short- and long-term models, which are used for exposure-point concentration determinations. These models typically assume constant wind

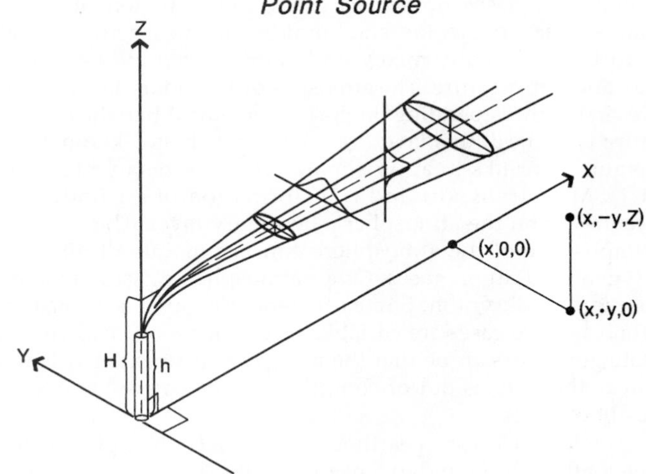

Figure 2-14. Gaussian dispersion model. With permission from U.S. Environmental Protection Agency. Guidelines on air quality models. Research Triangle Park, NC: Office of Air Quality Planning and Standards, 1986. [Rev. ed. publ. no. EPA–450-2–78–027R.]

speed and flat terrain and are accurate within a factor of two versus actual measured value. Far-field calculations and models are more complex and are typically used for radiologic assessment.

TOPOGRAPHY

By definition, the area surrounding a point source ranges from flat to topographically complex. *Flat terrain* is characterized by land and building elevations below the stack height of the source. Topographically complex terrains—either land or building elevations—are greater than stack height or occur where terrain deflects or alters air movement, such as by mountains, valleys, or large bodies of water. For regulatory purposes, most atmospheric fate-transport calculations assume flat terrain.

CONTAMINANT PROPERTIES

As discussed earlier for ground and surface water, the ultimate exposure point concentration can be significantly affected by both chemical and physical processes that affect a given pollutant. Transformational processes, such as photolysis and oxidation, may alter the initial pollutant concentration and produce reactive secondary air pollutants, such as photochemical smog.

Processes such as dissolution, adsorption, settling, and precipitation also significantly affect the ultimate exposure concentration.

Photochemical Smog

Photochemical smog pollution occurs in industrialized urban areas, such as Los Angeles and Mexico City, that are subjected to intense solar radiation effects. This type of smog is a chemical reaction between primary air pollutants and other contaminants in the air catalyzed by sunlight (Fig. 2-15).

Photochemical smog, consisting mainly of oxides of nitrogen and peroxyacetyl nitrate, appears as brown clouds, the result of a reaction of ozone with peroxyacetyl nitrate and nitrous oxides. Brown clouds occur in cities with more intense sunlight, such as the western cities. Smog in eastern cities is mainly gray because of smoke and sulfur dioxides.

Conditions favorable to ozone formation include temperatures greater than 32°C, intense radiation, low precipitation, and low winds (6). Many cities exceed current federal air quality standards for ozone. Volatile hydrocarbons are necessary for ozone buildup. Solar ultraviolet radiation breaks down nitrogen dioxide into nitrous oxide and oxygen, which then combines with O_2 to form O_3. The accumulation of ozone in the environment would not occur if it were not for volatile hydrocarbons disrupting the cycle by reacting with nitrogen oxide and oxygen to form more NO_2. Thus hydrocarbons, from whatever their sources, are important in the role of ozone accumulation in the air. Ozone can also occur from lightning and from its diffusion down from the stratosphere (1,7), where it is naturally occurring.

Ozone and particulates are a component of city smog, can be a human health hazard, and can affect plants and animals. Ozone can cause loss of trees, plants, and forests. Conditions that exacerbate stagnation of air favor photochemical smog: high pressures; calm air; numerous sources of pollutants; inversions that prevent mixing of air; clear skies, which allow ultraviolet ray intensity; low winds that do not disperse pollutants; and mountain terrains, which accumulate pollutants in the cities.

Rural soils have a high nitrogen oxide content, which can emit nitrogen oxides into the atmosphere (1,7) that contribute to air pollution and ozone formation. The concentration of ozone in rural and in more urban atmospheric environments is controlled by reactions involving nitrogen oxides, hydrocarbons, and hydroxyl groups. Trends have shown that those types of air pollutants begin decreasing in the United States once federal air quality standards are met. Improvement in vehicles and mass transportation has helped. Fuel efficiencies with pollution controls have been beneficial. There has also been a marked decrease in atmospheric lead—as well as particulates, sulfur dioxide, volatile hydrocarbons, and carbon monoxide—since 1970 (1,7).

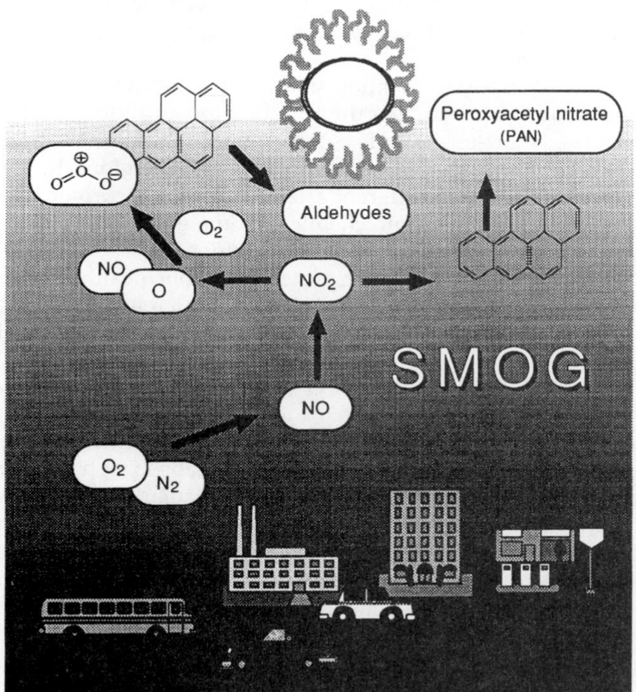

Figure 2-15. Photochemical smog. Nitric oxide (NO) pollutant in the air is catalyzed to generate nitrogen dioxide (NO_2), ozone (O_3), and peroxyacetyl nitrate (PAN) in complex reactions involving ultraviolet light and hydrocarbon pollutants.

ACID RAIN

Normal rain has a pH of 5.6; acid rain has a pH of less than 4. This is mainly a problem in the eastern United States, where sulfuric acids have resulted from industrial pollutants in the atmosphere. In the western United States, acidity of rain is mainly due to nitric acid generated from nitrogen oxides from internal combustion.

There has been concern that North American lakes have become so acidic that some aquatic life is unable to survive. Melting of winter snows that have accumulated acidic substances can produce a form of "acid shock" to water sources as runoff enters rivers, streams, and lakes during the spring, killing aquatic life. The sulfuric acidity of the rain can be neutralized by soil containing magnesium, aluminum, calcium, sodium, and potassium. The alkalinity of the soil is a key factor in preventing runoff acid rain. The soils of the northeastern United States have a lower acid-neutralizing capacity. Acid rain may decrease growth of forests because of leaching of nutrients from the soil, changing the soil's nutrient content.

Climate Changes and the Greenhouse Effect

Atmospheric CO_2 absorbs heat and retards earth's cooling. This is termed the *greenhouse effect* and is a major topic of controversy. Carbon dioxide's main environmental source is natural, from vegetation and forests around the earth. The addition to this natural carbon dioxide by fossil fuel use and petroleum hydrocarbon burning adds extra atmospheric carbon dioxide. But how much and to what effect produces much debate.

The additive effect of this extra human-related generation of carbon dioxide is predicted to add approximately 1°C to global mean temperature by 2025 and 3°C by the end of the twenty-first century. The consequences of global warming for life on earth can only be theorized, and this is a highly politicized issue. This greenhouse effect has been modeled on computer as a looming disaster and criticized by others as unrealistic.

The main greenhouse gas, carbon dioxide, has a natural cycle. Once it is produced, it can be absorbed by water and participate in plant photosynthesis, which removes a significant amount of it from the atmosphere. However, carbon dioxide on the earth's surface is being increased by deforestation and fossil fuel burning. Other gases that contribute to the greenhouse effect are methane, N_2O, CFCs, and ozone (O_3). There is agreement that the average surface air temperature of the earth has increased approximately 0.6°C over this past century. Anthropogenic pollutants and sulfates in the troposphere may be the basis of climatic changes. Analyses also indicate a statistical relationship, whereby temperature in the Northern Hemisphere is influenced by temperature in the Southern Hemisphere.

The greenhouse effect is so designated because all these gases absorb long waves of radiation, which tends to maintain a warmer climate on earth. The concern is that if greenhouse gases continue to increase, then the earth's climate may change. CFCs used as refrigerants are considered to be another significant contributor to the greenhouse effect.

Nitrous oxide (N_2O) absorbs long-wave radiation very efficiently but only accounts for about 5% of the greenhouse effect. However, nitrogen oxide has a very long half-life in the atmosphere—approximately 150 years. Thus, it can build up more significantly and contribute to more of a greenhouse effect in the twenty-first century.

The National Academy of Sciences study on global warming provides the most reliable information and predictions:

- Greenhouse gases include CO_2, water vapor, methane (CH_4), nitrous oxide (N_2O), and CFCs, which absorb ultraviolet radiation and trap radiant energy in the lower atmosphere of the earth.
- 1.5°C warming is likely to be the long-range global temperature response if atmospheric CO_2 doubles. This prediction is the best estimate based on climate models and review of past, ancient climates. The earth has not been more than 1°C to 2°C warmer now than over the past 10,000 years of human civilization. A change in global warming of the magnitude of 1.5°C to 4.5°C could alter global climate with potentially catastrophic results.
- There is a natural greenhouse effect from cloud cover, water vapor, and CO_2 from vegetation that accounts for 33°C of natural earth warming.
- Human activity has added 25% more CO_2; 100% more methane; and other gases, such as CFCs, volatile hydrocarbons, and N_2O to the concentration of natural greenhouse gases.
- The earth has warmed between 0.5°C and 0.6°C over the twentieth century. The 1980s were the warmest decade on record. This warming is unlikely to be from natural causes.
- The average global rate of atmospheric warming has been 1°C for every 1,000 years.
- Predicted human-induced global climate changes range from 1° to 5°C per 100 years.

Uncertainties about global warming remain, fueled by fiery political and economic debates. However, most scientists agree that a 1.5°C to 4.5°C increase in warming is likely if CO_2 doubles over the next 50 years. If this happens, consequences cannot reliably be predicted: Disease outbreak and social disruption from ecological, agricultural, geologic, and hydrologic catastrophes are possible.

ATMOSPHERIC OZONE DEPLETION

Depletion of ozone in the stratosphere is another environmental concern and controversy. Damage to the ozone layer is an economic, environmental, and political concern because of CFCs used as refrigerants and propellants. In 1979, CFC propellants were banned in the United States because of their effect on ozone. Evidence of CFC effects in the decline of ozone over the Antarctic led to the Montreal Protocol, which calls for a phase-out of CFC production by 2000 (7).

Ozone absorbs ultraviolet light, thus decreasing the amount of ultraviolet light penetrating to the earth's surface. A decrease in ozone concentration in the stratosphere would allow more health-damaging ultraviolet radiation to reach the earth's surface. This can result in increased cancer, such as skin cancers and melanomas. Chemicals that cause the destruction of ozone in the stratosphere are nitrogen oxides, moisture, and CFCs.

CFCs are stable in the troposphere, but once in the stratosphere, they can be chemically dissociated by the solar ultraviolet radiation to produce Cl and ClO, which deplete ozone. Fluorine monoxide is a chief cause of ozone depletion in the polar regions (7).

ENVIRONMENTAL TOXICOLOGY

Environmental toxicology as a complement to chemodynamics is the science of the adverse effects of environmental contaminants and pollutants on the biosphere and ecosystems, including humans. Environmental exposure pathways are complex and reflect the environmental continuum throughout air, water, soil, and living organisms (Fig. 2-16).

Exposure-Response Relationship

Characterization of the relationship between an exposure to a substance and the amount absorbed into the body to cause an adverse response is a fundamental objective of toxicology. Subtle toxic effects are prime concerns, in addition to more obvious health effects.

Equally important to understanding a substance's toxicity is the relationship between the rate of exposure/dose and the response: short-term–acute, subchronic, chronic, or long-term exposure. The target organ for toxicity, and therefore the toxic effect, may be quite different after acute versus chronic exposure, even with the same chemical. Some effects are delayed, such as a reproductive toxicity and carcinogenesis.

To set reference limits for protecting public health, the toxicologist focuses on the lowest dose at which adverse effects appear for a specific xenobiotic. The measured endpoint may be lethality using LD_{50} (the lethal dose of a chemical for 50% of the population), or the endpoint may be subtle, such as a small cellular change in a target organ.

Exposure is the amount of a substance with which an organism comes into contact through routes of absorption. *Absorbed dose* is the amount of toxin reaching a particular target receptor. Dose is generally expressed as mg/kg/day. In the case of inhalation exposure, the EPA uses units of milligrams per cubic meter of air (mg/m^3).

The route by which a chemical enters the body greatly influences its toxicity. Metabolic transformation of a chemical by enzymatic processes, such as occur in the liver, can detoxify a xenobiotic or produce a more toxic metabolite. Differing exposure routes may result in different expressions of toxicity.

Dose-response relationships display a variety of characteristics that depend on the toxin being studied, health, age, nutritional state, and physiology of the target organism.

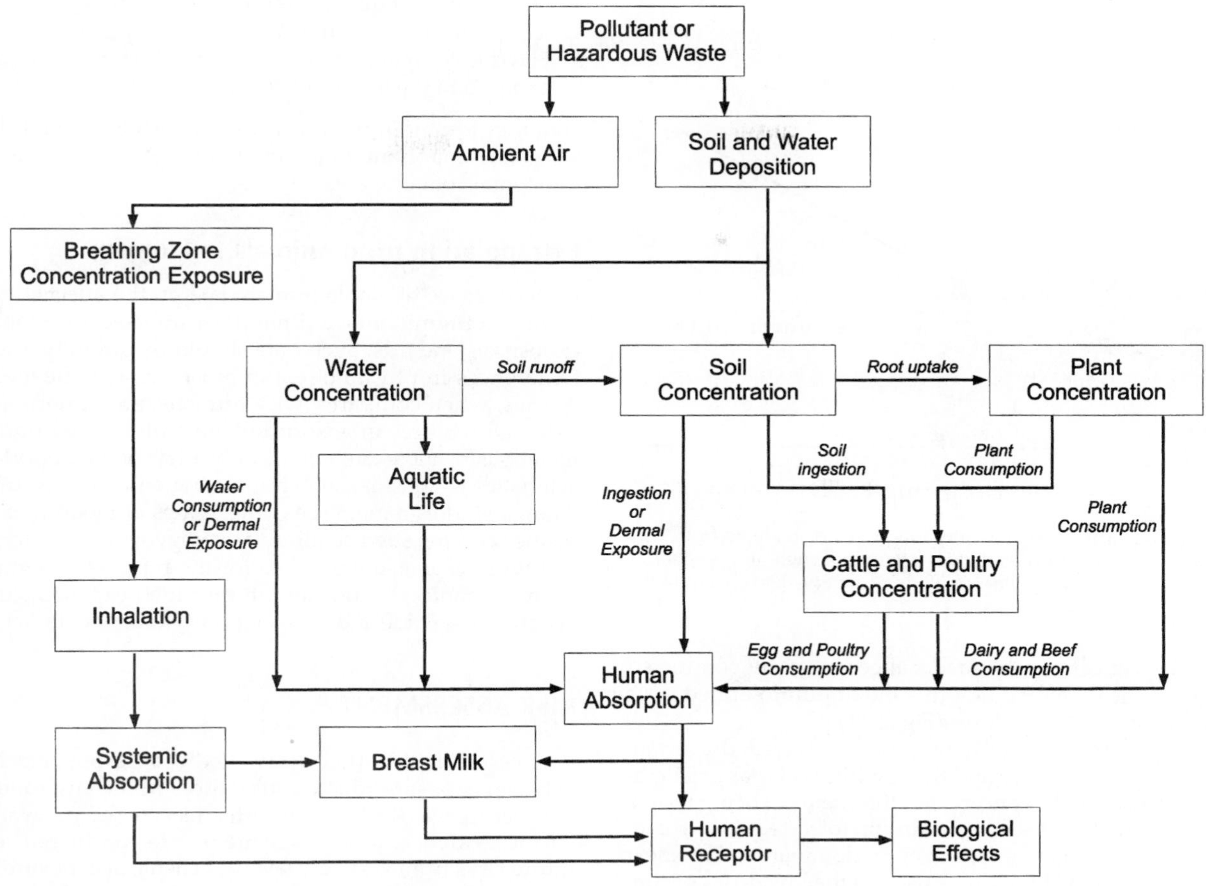

Figure 2-16. Environmental exposure pathways.

The relationship between dose and response for a study using a large population and many doses is a classical sigmoid curve (see Chapter 5). The sigmoidal dose-response relationship shows the normal distribution of biological variance commonly found in living systems. The variance in response shows that members of the population have different susceptibilities to the effects of the toxin.

The slope of the relationship is an important indicator of toxin behavior. A steep slope suggests that toxicity of the chemical may become severe with only a slight increase in dose. By contrast, a shallow dose-response slope indicates that larger increases in dose are necessary to cause a toxic effect and that signs or symptoms that warn of impending toxicity may gradually increase over the range of doses administered.

Threshold Dose

An important assumption in the interpretation of the dose-response relationship is that there is some dose below which no adverse effect is observable. This is the *threshold dose*. A fundamental concept for most systemic (noncancer-causing) toxins is that there is some dose below which the organism repair mechanisms can prevent the onset of adverse effects. Establishing this threshold dose is an objective of toxicologic studies that use experimental animals. The threshold concept has important implications for the regulatory toxicologist and public health officials.

This threshold dose for the most sensitive toxicologic endpoint is used as a point of departure for setting regulatory limits on exposure to environmental toxins. Threshold doses, called the *NOAEL* (no observable adverse effect level), or the next highest dose, *LOAEL* (lowest observable adverse effect level), are used as benchmarks for establishing acceptable contaminant levels in drinking water, soil, foods, and air. The *NOAEL* or *LOAEL* is commonly divided by one or more uncertainty factors to account for possible interspecies and interindividual variability in the toxicity of a chemical.

By setting the acceptable exposure limit through the use of uncertainty factors and modifying factors based on the characteristics of the available information, health professionals and the public can be reasonably assured that no toxicity will occur at the exposure limit set. Such exposure limits for noncancer endpoints through the oral route of exposure are called *reference doses* (*RfDs*) and are presented in units of milligrams per cubic meter (mg/m^3). In contrast to the dose-response relationship for most noncancer-causing toxins, which are curvilinear and display a threshold or NOAEL, cancer-causing chemicals are thought to display linear nonthreshold dose-response relationships. The assumption of linearity in the dose-response for carcinogenic chemicals is controversial.

Assessing Cancer Risk

Assessing potential risk of cancer after exposure to environmental toxins is dominated by the notion that a nominal dose of a carcinogen is assumed by regulators to be directly and linearly proportional to the dose. The EPA employs linear or near-linear extrapolation of data available from animal studies to human exposures. Criticism of this approach focuses on questions regarding the relevance of high-dose experimental studies conducted in rats or mice to human exposures that are likely to be thousands of times lower. Researchers typically determine the highest dose that experimental animals can tolerate over a life-

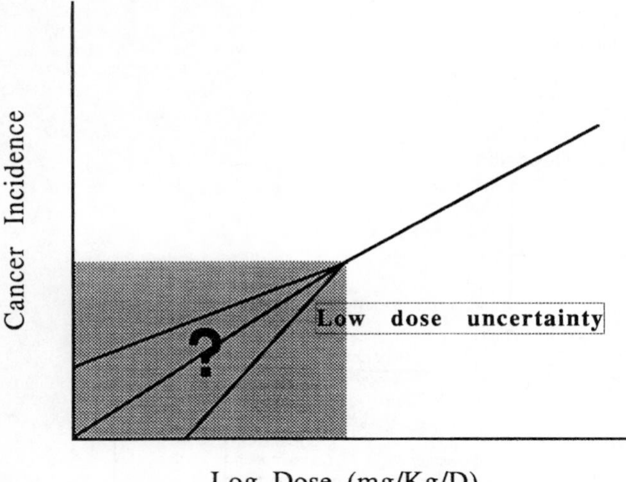

Figure 2-17. Cancer incidence at very low doses is modeled from data collected at much higher doses. Critics argue that such an approach is inaccurate and may result in widely differing cancer risk estimates at the low doses encountered in humans.

time to study cancer causation. A cancer bioassay conducted using rats or mice may include this maximum tolerated dose and only one or two lower doses (Fig. 2-17).

Critics argue that at the high doses delivered during an experiment, cellular toxicity and the resulting cellular proliferation are the causes of the cancer—not the chemical being tested. Beyond criticism of the use of a maximum tolerated dose in cancer bioassays, concern has arisen over predominant use of linear extrapolation from the high doses used to the low doses of concern to the human population.

A commonly employed algorithm for extrapolation of experimental animal data to low dose is the linear multistage model. This mathematical model assumes that cancer develops by multiple steps and that these steps may be additive.

This protective approach assures that the actual probability of encountering cancer under the experimental conditions is likely to be below the estimate obtained and may be as low as zero. The result obtained from this approach is functionally equivalent to the one-hit model, and dose-response linearity is assured.

Implicit in the linear models for cancer risk assessment is the idea that there is a cancer threshold dose for the induction of carcinogenesis and that any dose—no matter how small—has some probability of producing carcinogenesis. Several alternative algorithms that predict cancer risk at low doses are available in the literature.

Epidemiologic Studies

Human data that are of sufficient quality for determining the health risks from chemical exposure can be obtained from appropriate epidemiologic studies. The sensitivity of exposure and risk assessment to predict health consequences declines from rigorously controlled animal studies to clinical observation. Animal studies can identify excess risk in the vicinity of 1 in 100,000, which is the regulatory area of concern. Clinical studies range from 1 in 10 to 1 in 100, and properly conducted epidemiology studies lie between 1 in 1,000 and 1 in 10,000. To identify excess risk, epidemiologic studies must do the following:

- Be conducted on a large enough population to allow meaningful statistics
- Have adequate measures of exposure or dose
- Have sufficient quality control that the study can be scientifically interpreted or repeated by independent investigators
- Have a comparable control population that has not been exposed to the hazard of concern

When epidemiologic studies are conducted well, they are extremely important for learning the effects of exposure to environmental contaminants.

Extrapolation from Animals to Humans

In the absence of viable human data on the effects of environmental contaminants, animal data are used to establish safe exposure standards. Such data should be carefully interpreted. Differences in physiology and biochemistry of experimental species, when compared with humans, are important to consider. Differences in absorption, gastrointestinal transit time, metabolism, and excretion are only a few of the important characteristics to consider in extrapolating animal data to humans. Animal studies remain the cornerstones of modern biomedical science and the subdiscipline toxicology.

EPA interprets animal data for the purpose of setting limits for most nonfood exposures and for food exposures under the Federal Insecticide and Fungicide and Rodenticide Act (FIFRA).

RISK ASSESSMENT

Risk assessment is the study of the possible relationships between exposure to toxic substances in the environment and the occurrence of adverse health effects based on available scientific evidence. Risk assessments are conducted to project future risks from very low levels of chemical exposure that cannot be measured directly. Gaps in health risk assessments (HRA) are bridged by applying health-conservative assumptions. Use of health-conservative methods results in estimated levels of risk that are greater than would actually be experienced as a result of exposure to chemical hazards and are unlikely to underestimate the exposures or risks. The following steps are involved in risk assessment (Fig. 2-18):

1. Hazard identification (collect and evaluate data)—involves data collection and selection of chemicals of greatest health concern
2. Toxicity assessment—involves estimating no-adverse-effects levels and health criteria
3. Exposure assessment—involves the identification of exposed populations, sources, exposure pathways, and estimation of exposure concentrations through those pathways

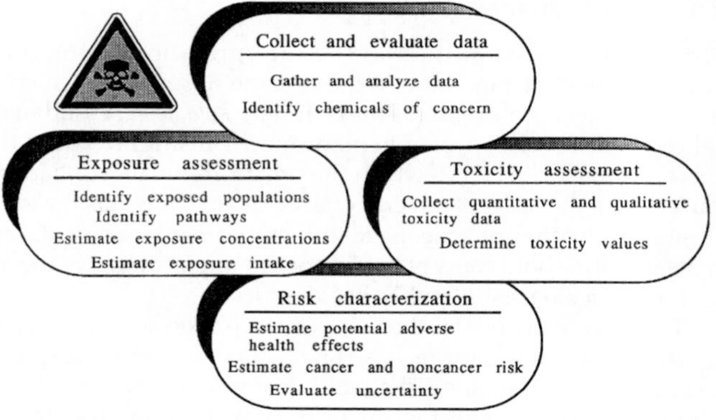

Figure 2-18. Risk assessment summary.

4. Risk characterization—combines the results of the exposure and toxicity assessments to provide numeric estimates of health risks

Toxicity Assessment

The *toxicity assessment* derives the numeric criteria used for evaluating the potential for systemic—or noncarcinogenic—effects and cancer risks associated with exposure to contaminants. An RfD is a health-based criterion often used in evaluating noncarcinogenic effects. RfD levels are developed by the EPA's Environmental Criteria Assessment Office. The RfD is based on the assumption that thresholds exist for certain toxic effects, such as cellular necrosis, but may not exist for other toxic effects, such as carcinogenicity. In general, the RfD is an estimate of a daily exposure to the human population (including sensitive subgroups) that is unlikely to be associated with an appreciable risk of deleterious effects during a lifetime.

Numeric estimates of cancer potency are presented as slope factors (SFs). Under the assumption of dose-response linearity at low doses, the SF defines the cancer risk that is due to continuous constant lifetime exposure of 1 unit of carcinogen concentration, expressed in units of risk per mg/kg/day. Individual cancer risk (a unitless number) is calculated as the product of pollutant intake (in mg/kg/day) and the SF for that pollutant in $(mg/kg/day)^{-1}$. For both carcinogens and noncarcinogens, effects from exposures to multiple chemicals are assumed to be additive; however, noncarcinogens are additive only for similar end-target organs. This appears to be a reasonable approach to addressing effects from exposures to mixture.

Exposure Assessment

Exposure assessment provides the most direct comparison between the historical and epidemiologic information evaluating the significance of certain exposure pathways. *Exposure assessment* is the estimation of the magnitude, frequency, duration, and routes of exposure to humans. The exposure is typically evaluated by estimating the amount of a chemical that could come into contact with the lungs, gastrointestinal tract, or skin during a specific time. The exposure assessment for this site is based on scenarios that define the potentially exposed populations, frequencies and duration of potential exposures, the possible exposure pathways, and the concentrations in air, food, or soil that potentially contact these populations through the pathways delineated in the exposure scenarios.

Exposure assumptions for risk assessments performed for Comprehensive Environmental Responsibility Compensation Liability Act (CERCLA) sites are based on a reasonable maximum exposure (RME) scenario. The RME scenario is defined as the highest exposure that is reasonably expected to occur at a site. The intent of the RME scenario is to develop an estimate of exposure well above an average exposure level that is still within the range of possible exposures. The assumptions used in estimating the RME and the rationale for those assumptions are those that provide a 95% upper confidence limit of the average level of exposure associated with chemicals at a site. Such methods have been developed by the EPA because they are not likely to underestimate the exposures or risks from site contaminants in actuality. Typical assumptions include the following:

- Exposure for a lifetime or near-lifetime duration (ranging from 30 to 70 years, in the absence of other data indicating a different exposure duration)
- Daily exposure, typically for 250 to 365 days per year (in the absence of other data indicating a different frequency of exposure)
- Specified contact rates with contaminated media (50 to 200 mg/day soil ingestion rate, 2 L of drinking water per day ingestion rate)
- Concentrations in environmental media that do not degrade or transform over time

These assumptions invariably overestimate health risks. For example, experience with these methods indicates that they predict the soil-ingestion exposure pathway as providing as significant a contribution to total exposure (hence total estimated risk) as ingestion of contaminated groundwater; however, available epidemiologic evidence has not indicated increased rates of adverse effects associated with soil ingestion, with the exception of childhood lead exposures. Use of these exposure assumptions addresses the EPA's mandate to have remedial actions that primarily protect public health (with cost and feasibility considerations being secondary). However, use of such methods could drastically overestimate health risks (Figs. 2-19 and 2-20).

$$I = C \times \frac{CR \times EFD}{BW} \times \frac{1}{AT}$$

Figure 2-19. Formula for calculating chemical intakes.
- I = intake; the amount of chemical at the exchange boundary (mg/kg body weight day)
- Chemical-related variable
  C = chemical concentration; the average concentration contacted over the exposure period (e.g., mg/L water)
- Variables that describe the exposed population
  CR = contact rate; the amount of contaminated medium contacted per unit time or event (e.g., L/day)
  EFD = exposure frequency and duration; describes how long and how often exposure occurs. Often calculated using two terms (EF and ED):
  BW = body weight; the average body weight over the exposure period (kg)
- Assessment-determined variable
  AT = averaging time; period over which exposure is averaged (days)

(Adapted from ref. 9.)

$$\text{INTAKE (mg / kg / day)} = \frac{CS \times IRSOIL \times CF \times FISOIL \times EF \times ED}{BW \times AT}$$

Figure 2-20. Childhood exposures to a metal in soil are estimated using the calculation table shown. CS, chemical concentration in soil (mg/kg); IRSOIL, ingestion rate (mg soil per day); CF, conversion factor (10^{-6}kg/mg); FISOIL, fraction ingested from contaminated source (unitless); EF, exposure frequency (days/year); ED, exposure duration (years); BW, body weight (kg); AT, averaging time (period over which exposure is averaged in days).
Variable values
CS = Site-specific measured values
IRSOIL = 200 mg/day (children, 1 through 6 years old)
CF = 10^{-6} kg/mg
FISOIL = Pathway-specific value (should consider contaminant location and population activity patterns)
EF = 365 days/year
ED = 6 years, assumed exposure duration for a child
BW = 16 kg (children 1 through 6 years old, fiftieth percentile)
AT = Pathway-specific period of exposure for carcinogenic effects (i.e., 70 years × 365 days/year).

Risk Characterization

Risk characterization provides a quantitative description concerning the existence and magnitude of potential public health concerns related to environmental contamination. Risk characterization involves combining the results of the exposure and toxicity assessments, providing numeric estimates of health risk, and characterizing the magnitude of uncertainty associated with the risk estimates.

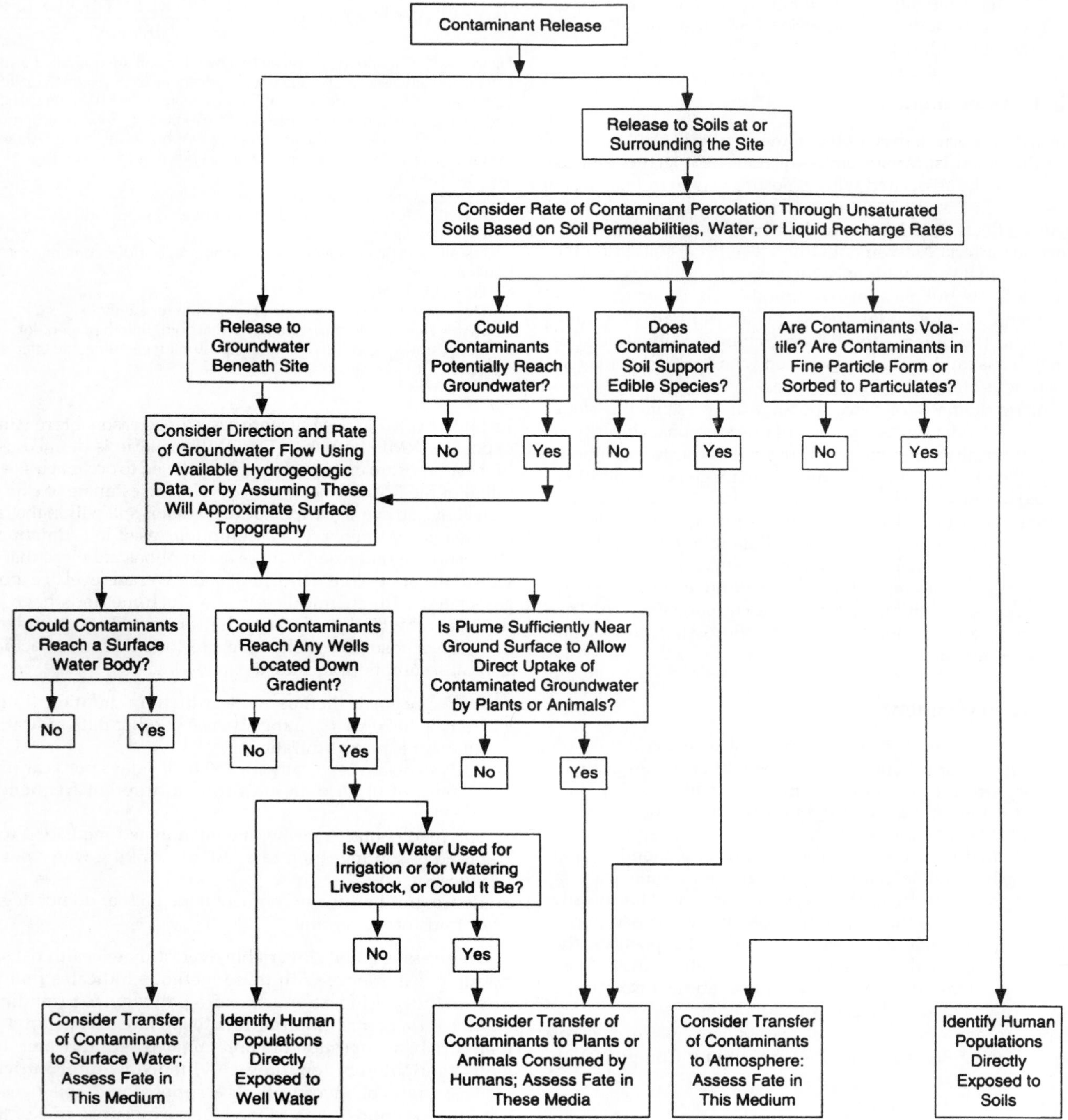

Figure 2-21. Flowchart for fate and transport assessment of soils and groundwater. (Adapted from ref. 9.)

It is reasonable to conclude that the assumptions used in the EPA risk assessment guidance overestimate potential exposures; however, in the absence of data further characterizing the parameters used to express the magnitude, frequency, and duration of exposure, these methods will continue to be employed for estimating health risks.

Ecological Risk Assessment

This is the process of evaluating the probability of adverse effects of contaminants, usually xenobiotics and other stressors on the environment. FIFRA, the Comprehensive Environmental Responsibility Compensation Liability Act, and the Resource Conservation and Recovery Act require such risk amounts as part of remedial investigation and assessment of feasibility of cleanup. In early formulations, ecological risk assessments were designed to model the four steps developed for human risk assessment. However, more recent EPA guidance for ecological risk assessment has stressed the unique considerations specific to ecosystems (e.g., individual species versus population or community level risks).

The uniqueness of this type of study is the identification of ecological stressors and endpoint results of stressors. Two

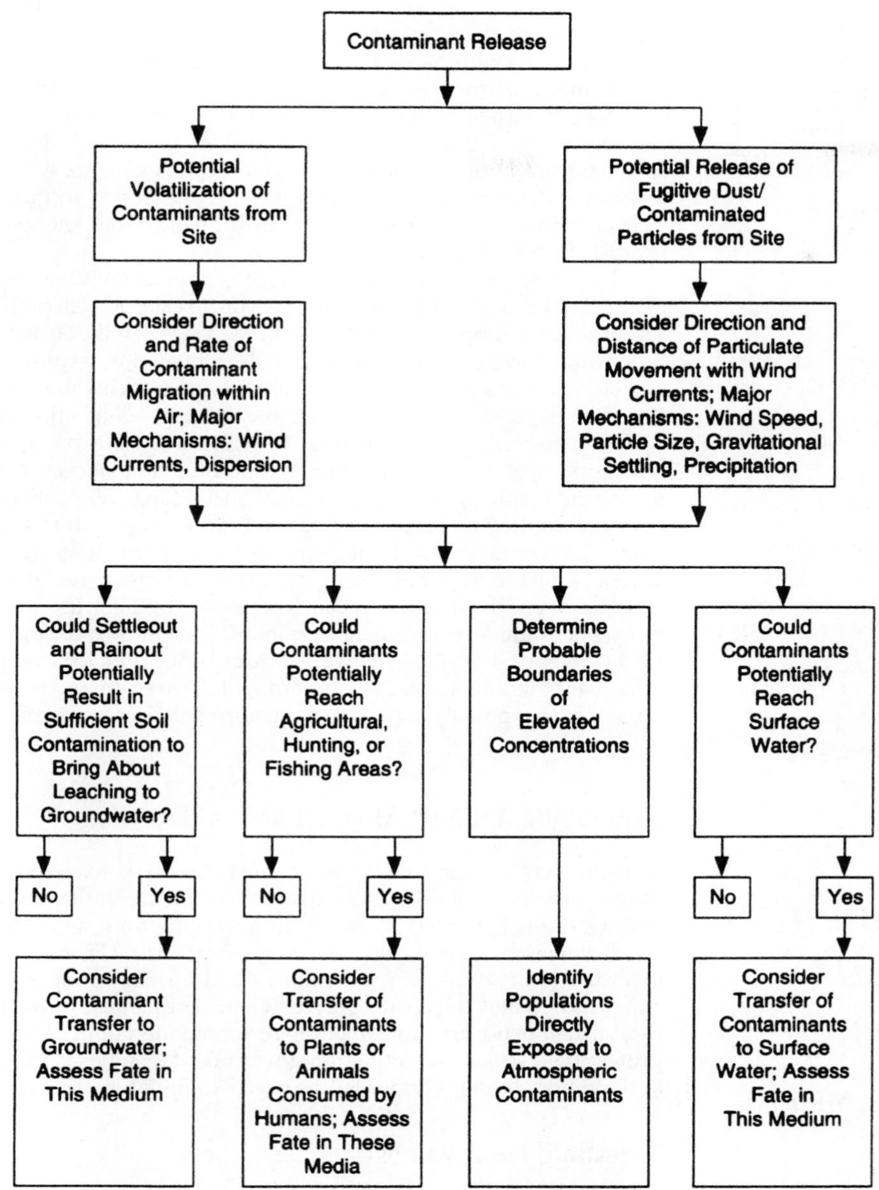

Figure 2-22. Flowchart for fate and transport assessments of the atmosphere. (Adapted with permission from ref. 9.)

types of endpoints are used: *assessment endpoints* and *measurement endpoints* (6). Assessment endpoints reflect recognized environmental values to the public (e.g., clean water, clean air, forests, presence of a certain animal species or plant species). Measurement endpoints are quantifiable factors relating to the environmental assessment that is valued by a public.

Typically, ecological risk assessments evaluate the adverse effect of stressors on biological components of an environment. Matching ecological impact to stressors provides a profile of the adverse effect on air environment. Such stressors as xenobiotics involve careful laboratory analysis and chemodynamic assessment. Models, assumptions, and extrapolations are made, and scientific judgment is applied to the problem.

Basically, the ecological risk assessment may extrapolate to the whole ecosystem from single-species toxicity testing or single-species stressor effects.

SUMMARY

The basic principles of chemodynamics in air, water, and soil are employed to evaluate the potential to be a health or ecological hazard. Summary flowcharts from the EPA's *Risk Assessment Guidance for Superfund* (9) for the environmental media are presented in Figures 2-21 and 2-22 to organize the approach to fate-transport evaluation.

REFERENCES

1. Krieger GR, Logselen MJ, Weis CP, Moreno J. Basic principles of environmental science. In: Krieger GR, ed. *Environmental management, accident prevention manual for business and industry,* 2nd ed. Itasca, IL: National Safety Council, 2000:97–128.
2. VanHouten GL, Cropper ML. *When is a life too costly to save? Policy research working paper 1260.* Washington: World Bank, 1994.

3. Cupta S, VanHouten GL, Cropper ML. The value of superfund cleanups. In: Binley R, ed. *The true state of the planet*. New York: The Free Press, 1995.
4. Shy CM. Chemical contamination of water supplies. *Environ Health Perspect* 1985;62:399–406.
5. Egboka B, Nwankwor G, Orajaka I, Ejiofor A. Principles and problems of environmental pollution of groundwater resources with case examples from developing countries. *Environ Health Perspect* 1989;83:39–68.
6. Levine R, Chitwood DD. Public health investigations of hazardous organic chemical disposal in the United States. *Environ Health Perspect* 1985;62:415–422.
7. Pepper I, Gerba C, Brusseau M, eds. *Pollution science*. New York: Academic Press, 1996.
8. Smith L, Dragun J. Degradation of volatile chlorinated aliphatic priority pollutants in ground water. *Environ Int* 1984;10:291–298.
9. Environmental Protection Agency. Risk assessment guidance for superfund. Volume 1: Human Health Evaluation Manual (Part A) Interior Final. Washington: EPA; December 1989. EPA/540/1–89/002.
10. Baes C, Sharp A, Sjoreen A, Shor R. *A review and analysis of parameters for assessing transport of environmentally released radionuclides through agriculture*. Oak Ridge, TN: Oak Ridge National Laboratory, 1984.
11. Roemer W, Hoek G, Brunekreef B. Effect of ambient winter air pollution on respiratory health of children with chronic respiratory symptoms. *Am Rev Respir Dis* 1993;147:118–124.
12. Neas LM, Dockery DW, Koutrakis P, Tollerud DJ, Speizer FE. The association of ambient air pollution with twice daily peak expiratory flow rate measurements in children. *Am J Epidemiol* 1995;141(2):111–122.
13. Pope CA, Dockery DW, Spengler JD, Raizenne ME. Respiratory health and PM_{10} pollution: a daily time series analysis. *Am Rev Respir Dis* 1991;144:668–784.
14. Braun-Fahrlander C, Ackermann-Liebrich U, Schwartz J, Gnehm HP, Rutishauser M, Wanner HU. Air pollution and respiratory symptoms in preschool children. *Am Rev Respir Dis* 1992;145:42–47.
15. Peters A, Goldstein IF, Beyer U, et al. Acute health effects of exposure to high levels of air pollutants in eastern Europe. *Am J Epidemiol* 1996; 144(6):570–581.
16. Pope CA, Dockery DW. Acute health effects PM_{10} pollution on symptomatic and asymptomatic children. *Am Rev Respir Dis* 1992;145:1123–1128.

CHAPTER 3
Principles of Environmental and Occupational Hazard Assessment

Mark D. Van Ert, Clifton D. Crutchfield, and John B. Sullivan, Jr.

EXPOSURE AND DOSE

A fundamental precept of human toxicology is that the intensity of toxic action is a function of the concentration of the toxic agent that reaches a target organ or tissue. The relationship between concentration and intensity of effect is commonly referred to as the *dose-response relationship* for a given substance. *Dose* is defined as the amount or mass of contaminant that is absorbed or deposited in the body over an increment of time. The *total dose* experienced by an individual refers to the sum of doses resulting from all environmental contact with a contaminant received by a person over a given time interval (1).

Biological measures of a chemical or its metabolites in various matrices, such as blood or urine, are seeing increased application as more direct indicators of dose (i.e., biological exposure indices). But in many instances, it is not practical to assess exposure by using exhaled air, blood, urine, or other biological specimens. It is often necessary to rely on exposure measurement as a surrogate for estimating dose. In the workplace and related environments, exposure measurement serves as a bridge between conditions of work and potential toxic effect (2).

The concept of *exposure* is formally defined as an event that occurs when there is contact between a human and the environment with a contaminant of specific concentration for an interval of time. The unit of expression for exposure is: concentration × time (1,3). Exposure (or dose) profiles describe the exposure concentration (or dose) as a function of time. Expressed differently, concentration and time are used to depict exposure while amount and time characterize dose (3). It is necessary to measure or estimate the exposure (dose) to appreciate the potential health effects from a substance.

To use exposure as a surrogate for dose, certain assumptions are required to relate the duration of an exposure to expected effect (2). The implied assumption, called *Haber's rule*, states that the effect is proportional to cumulative dose. Dose is estimated by exposure concentration times the duration of the exposure (3). This straightforward relationship is used to express exposure as a function of contaminant concentration and time. What is lost in this expression is an appreciation for any variation in concentration that occurred during the averaging time. In an occupational setting, this relationship has resulted in the use of 8- or 40-hour averaging times to express acceptable levels of employee exposure. In certain instances, this concept has been expanded to express cumulative exposure over extended periods, such as parts-per-million (ppm)—years. For example, Haber's rule implies that exposure to 100 ppm for 5 years is dose-equivalent to an exposure of 500 ppm for 1 year. Time-weighted averages (TWAs) are widely used in exposure assessments, especially as part of risk assessments for carcinogens.

EXPOSURE AND HEALTH STANDARDS

Measurement of exposure as a surrogate measure of dose serves as the basis for establishing occupational exposure limits. Most of these limits are based on an 8-hour averaging time, although shorter averaging times also are used. Short-term (15-minute) exposure limits (STELs), are recommended for fast-acting substances or when dose rate may be critical to health impact. Established exposure limits include recommended limits set by professional societies or other nongovernmental bodies, as well as regulatory limits (standards) enforced by regulatory agencies.

Threshold Limit Values

Industrial hygienists employed by governmental agencies formed a group dedicated to the establishment of principles and policies for governing employee exposures to airborne chemicals. This group, named the American Conference of Governmental Industrial Hygienists (ACGIH), composed a list of chemical exposure limits that eventually became accepted as threshold limit values (TLVs) intended to serve as exposure guidelines for worker protection. The ACGIH has defined three categories of TLVs: (a) the TWA (TLV-TWA), (b) the short-term exposure limit (TLV-STEL), and (c) the ceiling limit (TLV-C) (Table 3-1).

TLVs are TWA concentrations of airborne chemicals to which nearly all workers may be exposed, day after day, without adverse effect (4). ACGIH has established these concentrations as guidelines for the control of exposures. The basis on which the TLVs are established varies from substance to substance. It may include protection against impairment of health, reasonable freedom from irritation, narcosis, nuisance, or other forms of stress (4). The TLVs cannot be viewed as a relative index of toxicity but rather as guidelines for "acceptable" exposure to a particular substance over a typical workday or workweek.

The TLV-TWA refers to the airborne concentration of a substance to which workers can be continuously exposed in an

TABLE 3-1. Occupational exposure limits

Value	Abbreviation	Definition
Threshold limit value (three types) (ACGIH)	TLV	Refers to airborne concentrations of substances and represents conditions under which it is believed that nearly all workers may be repeatedly exposed day after day without adverse effect.
Threshold limit value/time-weighted average (ACGIH)	TLV-TWA	The TWA concentration for a normal 8-hour workday and a 40-hour workweek, to which nearly all workers may be repeatedly exposed, day after day, without adverse effect.
Threshold limit value/short-term exposure limit	TLV-STEL	The concentration to which workers can be exposed continuously for a short period without suffering from: (a) irritation; (b) chronic or irreversible tissue damage; or (c) narcosis of sufficient degree to increase the likelihood of accidental injury, impair self-rescue, or materially reduce work efficiency, and provided that the daily TLV-TWA is not exceeded. A STEL is defined as a 15-minute TWA exposure that should not be exceeded at any time during a workday even if the 8-hour TWA is within the TLV-TWA. Exposures above the TLV-TWA up to the STEL should not be longer than 15 minutes and should not occur more than four times per day. There should be at least 60 minutes between successive exposures in this range. An averaging period other than 15 minutes may be recommended when this is warranted by observed biological effects. In the absence of a STEL, which takes precedence, excursions in worker exposure levels may exceed three times the TLV-TWA for no more than a total of 30 minutes during a workday, and under no circumstances should they exceed five times the TLV-TWA for no more than a total of 30 minutes during a workday, provided the TLV-TWA is not exceeded.
Threshold limit value/ceiling (ACGIH)	TLV-C	The concentration that should not be exceeded during any part of the working exposure.
Permissible exposure limit (OSHA)	PEL	Same as TLV-TWA.
Immediately dangerous to life and health (OSHA)	IDLH	A maximum concentration (in air) from which one could escape within 30 minutes without any escape-impairing symptoms or any irreversible health effects.
Recommended exposure limit (NIOSH)	REL	Highest allowable airborne concentration that is not expected to injure a worker; expressed as a ceiling limit or TWA for an 8- to 10-hour workday.

ACGIH, American Conference of Governmental Industrial Hygienists; OSHA, Occupational Safety and Health Administration; NIOSH, National Institute for Occupational Safety and Health.

occupational setting over an 8-hour period or 40-hour workweek (4). The TLV-TWA is calculated as follows:

$$\mathrm{TLV} \approx \mathrm{TWA} = \frac{C_1T_1 + C_2T_2 + \bullet\bullet\bullet + C_nT_n}{8}$$

The TLVs should be viewed as guidelines or recommendations in the control of potential health hazards. They should not be used by anyone untrained in the discipline of industrial hygiene and unaware of their limitations (4). The ACGIH insists that the TLVs are not to be used as fine lines between unsafe and safe levels of exposure. It is acknowledged that a small percentage of workers may experience discomfort from some substances at concentrations at or below the TLV; a smaller percentage may be affected by aggravation of a preexisting condition or by development of an occupational disease (4). Individuals who are hypersusceptible or otherwise unusually responsive to some industrial chemicals because of genetic factors, age, personal habits (e.g., smoking, alcohol or other drugs), or medication may not be adequately protected from adverse health effects from certain chemicals at concentrations at or below the TLVs (4). Known or suspected carcinogens may not be assigned TLVs.

The basis on which certain TLV recommendations have been made has been criticized for being too limited. An analysis of the basis for the TLVs found that many have been developed by ad hoc procedures (5). It was suggested that a more aggressive policy be adopted by the ACGIH regarding TLVs for carcinogens, but not necessarily for substances that produce effects other than cancer. New information regarding the toxicology of chemicals and other agents, especially information pertaining to the human health experience, has provided a better foundation on which to support TLVs and other standards. The annual updating of the TLVs and the publication of recommended exposure limits (RELs) and hazard alert bulletins by the National Institute for Occupational Safety and Health (NIOSH) represent avenues for incorporating and disseminating the most recent information affecting the basis for standards. Health professionals assigned responsibility for the health and welfare of workers should consider all sources of scientific information involved in the standards-setting process when considering acceptable exposure limits for workers.

Conversion of Threshold Limit Values in Parts Per Million to mg/m^3

TLVs for gases and vapors are usually established in terms of ppm of substances in air by volume. TLVs may also be listed in terms of milligrams of substance per cubic meter of air (mg/m^3), where 24.45 = molar volume of air in liters at normal temperature and pressure conditions (25°C and 760 mm Hg), giving a conversion equation of:

$$\text{TLV in mg/m}^3 = \frac{(\text{TLV in ppm})\left(\begin{array}{c}\text{gram molecular}\\ \text{weight of substance}\end{array}\right)}{24.45}$$

Conversely, the equation for converting TLVs in mg/m^3 to ppm is:

$$\text{TLV in ppm} = \frac{(\text{TLV in mg/m}^3)(24.45)}{\text{gram molecular weight of substance}}$$

Values are rounded to two significant figures below 100 and to three significant figures above 100. This is done to avoid increasing or decreasing the TLV significantly by the conversion of units.

When converting TLVs to mg/m^3 for other temperatures and pressures, the reference TLVs should be used as a starting point. When converting values expressed as an element (e.g., as Fe or Ni), the molecular value of the element should be used, not that of the entire compound.

Permissible Exposure Limits

Permissible exposure limits (PELs) are conceptually the same as many TLVs but differ in some specific allowable concentrations. PELs are enforceable standards under the Occupational Safety and Health Administration (OSHA), whereas the TLVs are intended as guidelines. The first occupational safety and health standards were derived from the 1968 TLV list adapted from nearly 400 substances, as well as certain standards of the American National Standards Institute and the Walsh-Healey Public Contracts Act.

Under the authority of the Occupational Safety and Health Act of 1970, the 1968 TLVs and certain American National Standards Institute standards were adopted and promulgated by OSHA as the PELs for all workers covered by the act. The current list of PELs, similar to the ones adopted from the ACGIH, has been expanded by OSHA to include updated regulations for benzene, lead, arsenic, vinyl chloride, acrylonitrile, and asbestos. This expanded group of standards now is used to regulate human exposure in the work environment.

For OSHA to change or add a new PEL, either a lengthy rulemaking procedure or emergency temporary standard process is required. The ACGIH, however, can modify or add new substances listed during its annual updating of the TLV listing. Currently, there are approximately 600 substances listed in the ACGIH's TLV handbook.

Recommended Exposure Limits

NIOSH is the principal federal agency engaged in research at the national level to eliminate on-the-job hazards. Under the authority of the Occupational Safety and Health Act of 1970 (Public Law 91-596), NIOSH continues to develop and periodically revise recommendations for limits of exposure to potentially hazardous substances or conditions in the workplace. The RELs are published annually and transmitted to OSHA or the Mine Safety and Health Administration of the U.S. Department of Labor for use in promulgating legal standards. These published documents specify NIOSH RELs for a variety of chemical agents.

Preventive measures designed to reduce or eliminate health effects of these hazards are also recommended by NIOSH for consideration by OSHA. All known and available scientific information relevant to the potential hazard is evaluated by NIOSH in formulating these recommendations. Exposure limits are based on the best available information from human and animal studies, epidemiologic assessment, and industrial experience. It should be noted that the PELs established by OSHA are not always in agreement with the TLVs proposed by the ACGIH or the RELs recommended by NIOSH.

NIOSH also is involved in preparing documents related to special hazard reviews and occupational hazard assessments. These criteria documents provide safety and health assessments of specific chemical hazards along with recommended control and monitoring methods. NIOSH also evaluates new and emerging occupational health hazard data and publishes bulletins on them. These hazard alert bulletins provide information on previously unrecognized toxic hazards, report updates on current hazards, or disseminate information on hazard control methods and monitoring.

Conditions Immediately Dangerous to Life or Health

Conditions immediately dangerous to life or health (IDLH) are established by NIOSH for the purpose of respirator selection to protect health and life of those entering potentially dangerous situations. IDLH indicates an atmospheric concentration of any toxic corrosive or asphyxiant substance that poses an immediate threat to life or would cause irreversible or delayed effects or would interfere with an individual's ability to escape from a dangerous atmosphere.

Conditions IDLH can be caused by the presence of explosive or flammable materials, a deficiency of oxygen as can occur in a confined space, the presence of a highly toxic compound in high concentration, or the presence of ionizing radiation. Dangerous conditions can also be associated with a variety of processes and reactions involving chemicals as well as physical processes (Table 3-2).

TABLE 3-2. Hazardous processes, reactions, and conditions

Fires and explosions
Flammable liquids
Compressed gases
Confined spaces
Oxygen-deficient areas
Release of chemicals in vapor form
Dust and particulate formation
Fume formation
Release or spill of corrosives
Unknown spilled material
Oxidation reactions
Chemical reactions
Heating chemicals near flashpoints
Release of cryogenic fluids
Sudden release of pressurized gases
Radioactive materials
Thermal reactions
Electrical shock
Loading and unloading processes
Low-pressure operations
Handling large quantities of flammable liquids

Worker Protection

Evaluation of worker exposures is accomplished by determining the concentration of contaminants within the breathing zone of the individual. These concentrations can be compared with established exposure limits (PELs, RELs, TLVs). If detected concentrations are in excess of established limits, engineering or administrative controls can be instituted to control exposures to within acceptable limits. If such controls are not feasible or are unsuccessful in reducing concentrations, personal protective equipment may be required.

EXPOSURE ASSESSMENT

The mere presence of a particular hazard in an environment does not indicate that human exposure has occurred, nor does it provide an adequate basis for determining potential risk. The exposure potential must be assessed for an individual or group to determine the actual risk. The storage of large amounts of chemical solvents in nonleaking containers may constitute a potential hazard to persons or the immediate environment, but is not a potential hazard until human or environmental exposure occurs.

Hazard evaluation involves both the toxicity of the chemical or material and the opportunity for exposure to cause disease. Therefore, the evaluation should include

1. Nature of the chemical or chemicals
2. Quantity of material and its physical form
3. Routes of exposure and potential of multiple exposures
4. Duration of exposure (acute, chronic, long term)
5. Magnitude and frequency of the exposure
6. Representative monitoring data
7. Control measures that limit exposure
8. Toxicity of the material in biological systems
9. Medications used by exposed person that might influence toxicity
10. Exposure-dose-response relationships
11. Prior health status and genetic predisposition

Exposures can be defined using qualitative and quantitative bases. The most useful information is obtained from quantitative data on a specific agent, because these types of data can best be related to established exposure limits (TLVs, PELs, or other reference limits) designed to minimize the occurrence of health effects. Although the intention of most standard-setting bodies is to set exposure limits below which no significant effect is expected to occur over a working lifetime, the difficulty has been the identification of the minimal-risk level for the agent of concern. Standard setting frequently is impeded by the paucity or quality of dose-response information on which decisions regarding appropriate standards are made. Often, the more conservative recommendations or standards are used by practitioners as indices of acceptable exposure.

Exposure Terms

Exposures are generally classified as acute, chronic, or long term. An acute exposure involves a single dose during a short time. Acute exposures can involve either single or multiple chemicals. Health effects may become apparent very quickly. Chronic exposure involves receiving a dose at frequencies over a period that may be days, months, or years. Health effects after chronic exposure are a function of the frequency of the exposure, contaminant concentration, route of exposure, accumulation and metabolism of the chemical, possible synergism among multiple chemicals, and the inherent toxicity of the chemical or material. Chronic exposures usually occur over longer periods and involve lower concentrations. Long-term exposures generally last more than 1 year on a continuous basis.

The biological variability in toxic responses among humans and other animals can be considerable. Toxins may have small or large margins of safety. Exposures may be multiple and erratic in the occupational setting. The overall biological response can be influenced by other environmental exposures that may act synergistically.

DEFINITION OF HAZARD CLASSES

The toxic action of a material is a function of its physical and chemical properties. The form or physical state of a material determines the route of entry as well as the potential hazard associated with a substance. The form of the substance also dictates the method used to monitor or detect the contaminant.

Gas

A gas is defined as a compound that is in the gaseous state at a temperature of 25°C and 760 mm Hg pressure. Normally, a gas is a formless fluid that occupies a space and can be changed to the liquid or solid state only by the combined effort of increased pressure and reduced temperature.

Vapors

Vapors are the gaseous form of substances that are normally in the solid or liquid state at room temperature and pressure (25°C and 760 mm Hg). Vapors can be changed back to the solid or liquid state either by increasing the pressure or decreasing the temperature. Evaporation is the process by which a liquid is changed into the vapor state and mixed with the surrounding atmosphere. Organic solvents with low boiling points volatilize quickly, yielding solvent vapors. Vapors, like gases, diffuse throughout the space they occupy. Concentrations of gases and vapors are typically expressed on a ppm (vol/vol) or mg/m^3 basis. Exposure or area assessments for gases and vapors are generally conducted by using direct reading instrumentation (either grab or continuous monitor types) or indirect (integrative) techniques such as sorbent tubes or passive dosimeters.

Aerosols

Aerosols are liquid or solid particles suspended in air that are of fine enough particle size to remain dispersed for a period. Aerosol concentrations are expressed on a mass per unit volume basis (e.g., mg/m^3) or on a numerical, fiber per cubic centimeter or millions of particles per cubic foot basis. Aerosols include the following contaminant categories:

- Dusts: Solid particles formed from the handling, crushing, grinding, rapid impact, or detonation of organic or inorganic materials such as ores, rocks, metal, coal, wood, or grain. Dusts do not tend to flocculate except under electrostatic forces, but settle under the influence of gravity. Examples include mineral dusts (e.g., asbestos, quartz, or talc) and organic dusts.
- Fumes: Solid particles formed when a volatilized solid, such as a metal, condenses in cool air. This physical change is often accompanied by a chemical reaction, such as oxidation. The solid particles that make up a fume are extremely fine, usually less than 1.0 μm. Fumes flocculate and sometimes coalesce. Examples include lead oxide fumes from smelting and iron oxide fumes from iron welding.
- Smoke: Solid particles generated by incomplete combustion of carbonaceous materials such as coal or oil. Generally, carbon or soot particles are less than 0.1–0.5 μm. Smoke generally contains droplets as well as dry particles. Tobacco, for instance, produces a wet smoke composed of minute, tarry droplets. The size of the particles contained in tobacco smoke is approximately 0.25 μm.
- Mists: Suspended liquid particles generated by condensation from the gaseous to the liquid state or by the breakup of a liquid into a dispersed state by splashing, foaming, or atomizing. Examples of mists include: (a) oil mist produced during cutting and grinding operations, (b) acid mists from electroplating, (c) acid or alkali mist from pickling operations, and (d) paint mists from spraying operations.
- Fog: Liquid particles formed by condensation of water vapor.
- Smog: Mixture of liquid and solid matter in the air generated from the dispersion of incomplete combustion products into a moist atmosphere (the term *smog* is derived from smoke and fog).

Solids

Solids are materials that retain a given shape under standard conditions.

Liquids

A liquid is a state of matter that assumes the shape of its container.

Bioaerosols

Bioaerosols are airborne biological source particles, both viable and nonviable, that include living organisms capable of reproduction or replication, such as bacteria, protozoa, fungi, and viruses. The term includes nonviable components, pieces, and by-products of microorganisms such as endotoxins, toxins, mycotoxins, pollens, spores, and immunogenic macromolecules.

Exposure or area assessments for aerosols are generally accomplished using integrative techniques such as collection on filters either alone or in concert with size-selective precollectors. A less common but convenient approach is the use of direct-reading aerosol monitors.

Solvent Vapor Pressure and Health Hazards

The concept of the vapor pressure of a solvent as it relates to hazards and toxic health effects is important. The vapor pressure of a solvent is directly related to its airborne concentration and its toxic hazard and human exposure. Vapor pressure is the force per unit area exerted by molecules of a vapor that is in equilibrium with a liquid or solid. Vapor pressure is expressed in terms of mm Hg in relation to atmospheric pressure (1 atm = 760 mm Hg). The vapor pressure of a solvent also is directly related to its economical use because of volatilization loss. The toxic hazard of an organic solvent is dependent on its vapor pressure and its intrinsic chemical properties. The vapor pressure directly relates to the concentration of solvent in the breathing zone of exposed individuals.

The vapor pressure of a solvent obeys the same physical laws as other gases:

$$Pv = nRt/V$$

Pv = vapor pressure (mm Hg)
n = moles
V = gas volume (M^3)
R = gas constant (6.236×10^5)
t = absolute gas temperature in K°

Rearrangement of this formula yields an equation that allows the calculation of the vapor concentration from the vapor pressure of a gas (vapor) that is in an equilibrium state:

$$Pv = nRt/V = CRt/MW = (X)(\text{atm})(2 \times 10^6)$$

C = concentration (mg/m^3)
MW = molecular weight
X = concentration in ppm
atm = 760 mm Hg

The vapor hazard ratio of solvents can be compared by this method to help determine the potential of human exposure. The formula expresses the vapor pressure in terms of an equilibrium state or worst-case scenario, as would be achieved in a closed environment. Solvents or chemicals with the same TLV may present two distinctively different health hazards caused by their different vapor pressures. An example of this hazard assessment with two related chemicals is as follows:

Chemical A	TLV = 0.02
	Vapor pressure = 0.00014 at 25°C
Chemical B	TLV = 0.02
	Vapor pressure = 0.00001 at 25°C

Rearranging this equation allows for a calculation of the vapor concentration in ppm of a vapor in an equilibrium state (V_{peq}):

$$V_{peq} = \frac{(Pv) \cdot (1 \cdot 10^6)}{\text{atm}}$$

The equilibrium vapor pressure, as calculated using the above formula, can be used to calculate a vapor hazard ratio (VHR):

$$\text{VHR} = \frac{\text{equilibrium vapor pressure (ppm)}}{\text{threshold limit value (ppm)}}$$

The greater the vapor hazard ratio, the greater the potential hazard for inhalation and dermal contact.

$$V_{peq}\text{ (Chemical B)} = \frac{(1.4 \cdot 10^{-4})(1 \cdot 10^6)}{760\text{ mm Hg}} = 0.184\text{ ppm}$$

$$V_{peq}\text{ (Chemical A)} = \frac{(1.4 \cdot 10^{-5})(1 \cdot 10^6)}{760\text{ mm Hg}} = 0.0132\text{ ppm}$$

$$\text{Chemical A VHR} = \frac{0.184\text{ ppm}}{0.002\text{ ppm}} = 92$$

$$\text{Chemical B VHR} = \frac{0.0132\text{ ppm}}{0.002\text{ ppm}} = 6.6$$

Chemical B would present much less of a hazard than chemical A in terms of vapor exposure. Chemical B also would have a lower air concentration than its TLV.

MONITORING STRATEGIES

The purpose of a monitoring program is to: (a) characterize the nature of the exposure; (b) determine whether the risk of exposure exists; (c) quantify the amount of the exposure; (d) relate the exposure to possible toxic effects; (e) ensure that concentrations of hazardous substances do not exceed established TLVs, RELs, or regulatory standards; and (f) prevent disease. Monitoring helps determine the protection required for a specific activity or site. It also dictates the types of personal protective equipment required when other control measures are not feasible.

Although some monitoring techniques do not yield an immediate determination of airborne contaminant levels because of the need for laboratory analysis, this approach provides a definitive statement about the identity and magnitude of multiple contaminants over a specified sampling period. Mass spectrometric analysis can be used to confirm the identity of contaminants in a mixed exposure environment.

The nature of the environment being monitored dictates the sampling strategies and kinds of instrumentation to be used. Questions to be addressed in any monitoring program are

- What is the purpose of the monitoring?
- What is the suspected chemical or contaminant?
- What kind of instrumentation is required for specificity and sensitivity?
- Where is the monitoring going to be performed? Ambient air? Personal breathing zone?
- When is it to be performed?
- Over what length of time is the monitoring to occur?
- How many samples are to be collected?

Sampling strategies must include a quality assurance program to account for proper calibration of instruments before and after sampling procedures, adequate flow control during sampling, and use of accepted standards and procedures for determining sampled volumes and analyzing collected contaminants.

Area versus Point-Source Monitoring

Personal air monitoring is preferred for evaluating work exposure to airborne chemicals. Typically, air sampling permits one to estimate an employee's 8-hour or 15-minute TWA exposure to a substance by collecting one or more personal samples over a work shift. The collection of multiple samples over the duration of a work shift allows one to measure exposures for individual tasks and still estimate workers' 8-hour TWA exposure.

Area samples are useful in determining background contaminant levels, evaluating the effectiveness of control measures, and identifying possible sources of exposure. But neither area monitoring nor point-source monitoring provides an estimate of worker exposure because environmental conditions at a fixed site frequently do not represent those experienced by the worker. Under certain conditions, workroom samples may reflect a worker's average exposure. But samples must be collected in the immediate vicinity of the worker's breathing zone during his or her various activities to represent his or her actual exposure. Without vigilant observation of the employee's pattern of work, one cannot obtain a representative estimate of the worker's exposure from area monitoring data. Area sampling, even when carefully designed to estimate a worker's exposure, fails to comply with OSHA regulations that require personal monitoring. For obvious reasons, area monitoring in outdoor environments provides little information with which to estimate personal exposures.

RATIONALE FOR AIR MONITORING

Assessment of occupational exposures serves as the primary reason for conducting air monitoring studies. The magnitude of personal exposures to specific chemical, biological, and physical agents is compared to occupational exposure limits for determining the acceptability of the work environment relative to these exposure guidelines. Other reasons exist for conducting air monitoring. Many of these reasons contribute either directly or indirectly to insights regarding the work environment, control of exposure, and protection of human health. Reasons for initiating air monitoring studies are

- Monitoring of personnel to characterize their exposures and determine compliance with consensus, regulatory, or other occupational exposure limits.
- Response to workers' inquiries or complaints regarding the nature of their work environment.
- Evaluation of point-source emissions to determine their potential contribution to employee exposures, area levels, and compliance with emission standards.
- Evaluation of confined spaces for safety and health hazards before entry.
- Evaluation of the effectiveness of engineering or administrative exposure control measures.
- Support of data for epidemiologic investigation, whether prospective or retrospective in nature.
- Research aimed at characterizing the composition, concentration, and form of exposure agents from new processes, products, and so forth.
- Support of evidence for legal actions directed at characterizing an employee's occupational work history.

Regardless of the reason for initiating an air monitoring study, it is incumbent on the environmental and occupational health specialist to define clearly the purposes of a monitoring exercise or program, and establish protocols to achieve these objectives. Information derived from air monitoring may be of little value unless descriptive criteria pertinent to exposure and other assessments are stated clearly by the professional on field sampling sheets or in survey reports. Assuming air samples are collected and analyzed according to standard or other acceptable protocols, it is critical to describe properly the conditions under which air samples were collected. This information imparts meaning and context to monitoring data. Professionals who are properly trained and experienced in the field of environmental and occupational health often are able to deduce the significance of samples with minimal descriptions of the conditions or situations under which air samples were collected. But to the untrained recipient of data, its meaning may be misconstrued. For example, area or point-source data may be interpreted incorrectly as being representative of personal exposure data when the information actually was intended to evaluate a potential source of emission or conditions at a specific location at one point in time. Professionals should be aware that their data may be interpreted incorrectly if its intended purpose is not stated clearly on sampling data sheets or survey reports.

Descriptive information useful in defining the intended purpose and context of monitoring data include the following elements:

- Statement regarding purpose of monitoring
- Type of monitoring (personal, area, point source)
- Individual's job title and description (if data are personal sample)
- Monitoring location (precise information to fix location)
- Task description (multiple activities and duration of each should be described individually)
- Time and duration of monitoring (if multiple samples are collected, time, duration, and description of each activity should be noted)
- Use of personal protective equipment (respirators, clothing, and eye protection, including specifics on type and model)
- Engineering or administrative controls in use during the monitoring period
- Factors that may affect reliability of data

Although exposure assessments are conducted under a variety of schemes, they all have as their goal a statement about potential human exposure. A set of eight good exposure assessment practices has been proposed that are particularly useful in large- and small-scale exposure assessments (5). Good exposure assessment practice components include the writing of a study protocol for conducting a study, consideration of available resources, specification of an exposure assessment model, and a study design. The design should include sampling and analytical methods and data analysis strategies, quality assurance, archiving of all program elements, communication of personal exposure information, and a statement of overall uncertainty in exposure assessment (5,6).

Monitoring Techniques

Two basic techniques are used to evaluate personnel exposures and contaminant levels in an environment. Direct and indirect monitoring devices are used. Direct or real-time devices give a direct readout of pollutant concentration, often on an instantaneous and continuous basis.

Indirect or integrative monitoring devices are used to collect contaminants over extended periods, ranging from 15 minutes to 8 hours or more. They provide a TWA estimate of contaminant levels over a given sampling period. Laboratory analysis is required to determine the mass of contaminant collected, which is then time-weighted to estimate average exposure concentration of the contaminant. The methods used to analyze such samples may provide additional information regarding the identity and concentration of contaminants.

DIRECT MONITORING

Direct or real-time monitoring instruments can be used at various locations to provide instantaneous information concerning

TABLE 3-3. Direct air sampling instruments

Instrument	Detection method	Chemical	Detection limits
Compound-specific instruments	Electrochemical cell	Hydrogen cyanide	0–100 ppm
		Hydrogen sulfide	0–100 ppm
		Oxygen	0–100%
		Nitrogen dioxide	0.01–50.00 ppm
		Carbon monoxide	0–500 ppm
Portable gas chromatograph	Flame ionization	Organic vapors	0.2 ppm
			0–1,000 ppm
	Photoionization	Compounds with ionization potential less than or equal to the output energy of the ultraviolet lamp	0.1 ppb
Aerosol monitor	Light scattering	Aerosols	0.001 mg/m^3
Mercury vapor analyzer	Ultraviolet light	Mercury vapor	0–1 mg/m^3
Combustible gas detector	Catalytic combustion	Vapors of combustible gases	0–100% LEL
Portable photoionization detector	Photoionization	Compounds with ionization potential less than or equal to the output energy of the ultraviolet lamp	0.05–2,000.00 ppm
Portable infrared analyzer	Infrared absorption	Infrared absorbing compounds	0–9,999 ppm
Portable FID	Flame ionization	Organic vapors	0–1,000 ppm
Gamma radiation detector	Scintillation detector	Gamma radiation	Does not detect beta or alpha

FID, flame ionization detector; LEL, lower explosive limit; ppb, parts per billion; ppm, parts per million.

personal and ambient air concentrations of certain chemicals, radioactive materials, or conditions IDLH.

Direct-reading instruments provide an immediate and continuous readout of contaminant levels in a specific work environment. They can be used to detect emission point sources, the effectiveness of control measures, and changes in an environment over time. These capabilities permit checks for compliance with ceiling and short-term exposure limits and estimates of TWA concentrations, when coupled with data processors (e.g., data loggers). One group of direct-reading devices—portable gas chromatographs—can provide not only a direct readout of contaminant concentration, but also more specific information on the identity of airborne contaminants that other methods cannot furnish.

Direct-reading instruments can provide real-time measurement of potentially hazardous environments. But proper data interpretation is dependent on the user's skill and knowledge of the calibration, principle of operation, application, and limitations of the instrument. Users also should be aware of factors such as instrument specificity, especially as it applies to detection of a substance in the presence of potential chemical interferences.

The sensitivity or limits of detection of direct-reading instruments also impact the validity and usefulness of instrument data. Choice of a particular direct-reading instrument is dependent on the physical and chemical state of the contaminant to be detected. For example, many combustible gas detectors do not indicate a combustible atmosphere in the presence of high vapor or gas concentrations devoid of the oxygen needed for instrument response. The types of direct-reading instruments that are available include

Explosimeters and combustible gas indicators
Photoionization detector (UV)
Portable gas chromatograph
Oxygen meters
Radiation detectors
Portable infrared spectrophotometer

Direct-reading instruments are used to provide immediate insights into contaminant levels and, in certain settings, warnings where dangerous airborne contaminants may exist or appear during work (Table 3-3). They are the primary instruments used to initially characterize an unknown hazardous site. They detect organic vapors, various gases, and other contaminants being released into the atmosphere. They also can detect the presence of explosive conditions and flammable gases, a lack of oxygen, and the presence of ionizing radiation. Contemporary real-time monitors are very sensitive, with detection limits in ppm and, in some cases, parts per billion range (e.g., photoionization detector). Because of problems of specificity when multiple chemicals are present, identification and quantitation can become difficult. False readings can occur because of interference from other chemicals.

Direct-reading instruments have certain limitations in their capacity to detect different families of hazardous substances. They can detect or measure certain specific substances or classes of chemicals, so it is possible to miss other hazards when limited information is available on the types of contaminants potentially present in the work environment. In other instances, these instruments are not designed to detect extremely low air concentrations (e.g., <1 ppm).

It is critical that direct-reading instruments be used by highly qualified persons such as certified industrial hygienists or technicians who are skilled at proper instrument selection, calibration, use, and interpretation of information.

GRAB SAMPLING

Direct-reading devices, such as indicator tubes, often are used for collecting grab samples. Grab samples are taken to measure the concentration of a contaminant over a brief sampling time (several minutes or less) to obtain a general appreciation of environmental conditions at a specific operation or location. Before using such devices, it is important to know the identity of the airborne contaminants. Grab or instantaneous air samples also may be collected in evacuated containers (e.g., canisters, bags, and syringes) followed by laboratory analysis.

ELECTROCHEMICAL DEVICES

Electrochemical cells, which operate on the principle of membrane electrolysis, commonly are used to detect gases such as carbon monoxide (Table 3-4). The gas passes through a membrane and reacts with an electrolyte. This reaction produces a flow of electrons proportional to the partial pressure of the gas in the air. With the addition of chemical filtration mechanisms preceding the cells, instruments may be made more sensitive and specific for a variety of gases.

TABLE 3-4. Electrochemical cells for compound detection

Simple paraffins
Halogenated paraffins
Aliphatic ring compounds
Nitrogen-containing compounds
Unsaturated acids and esters
Chlorinated aromatics
Chlorinated olefins
Aromatics
Organometallics
Carbon-oxygen compounds
Sulfur-containing compounds
Phosphorus compounds

Adapted from Transducer Research, Inc., 1228 Olympus Drive, Naperville, IL.

EXPLOSIMETERS

Combustibility or explosivity is generally detected with an instrument that uses a catalytic combustion process. The gaseous contaminant burns on a heated wire, thus altering resistance to flow of an electric current (Fig. 3-1).

A gas (or vapor) sample is drawn into the instrument across a heated filament and ignited. The resulting change in electrical resistance of the filament is detected by conventional bridge measurement techniques. The degree of induced electrical resistance is directly proportional to the gas (or vapor) concentration of the gas (or vapor) being drawn into the instrument. The heat of combustion—a particular physical characteristic of combustible gases—is used for quantitative detection. This procedure is nonspecific when mixtures of gases are being analyzed. Typically, these instruments read in percentage of the LEL so they are not useful in measuring concentrations in the ppm range. They are not to be used in determining concentrations relative to the PELs.

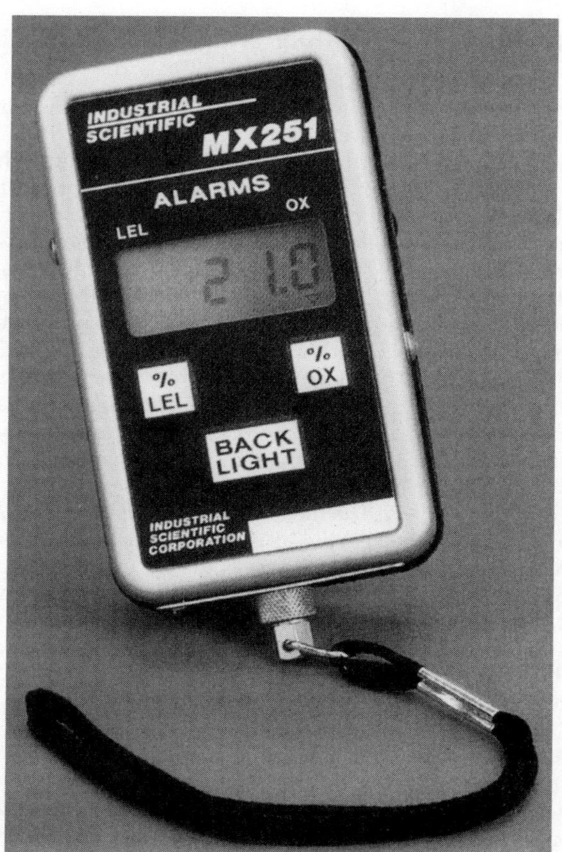

Figure 3-1. Lower explosives limit and O_2 deficiency monitor for conditions immediately dangerous to life or health. (Photograph courtesy of Hazco.)

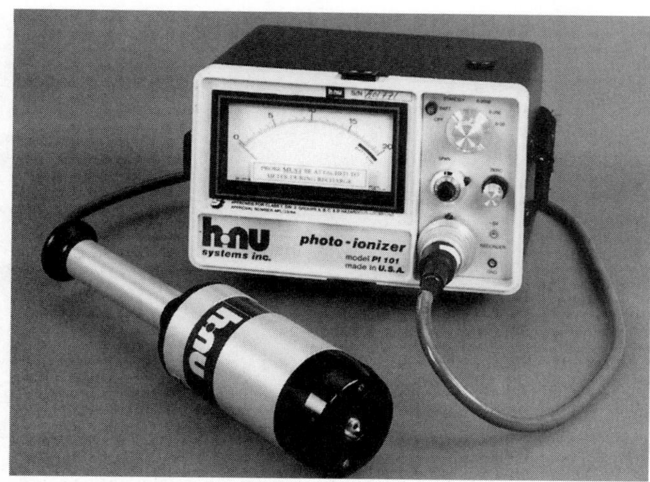

Figure 3-2. Photoionization detector for detection of organic vapors and inorganic gases such as hydrogen sulfide and ammonia. (Photograph courtesy of Hazco.)

ORGANIC VAPOR MONITORS

Monitors with a photoionization detector (PID) represent a nonspecific instrument that uses an ultraviolet lamp (Fig. 3-2). The gas is carried into a ionization chamber and ionized by an ultraviolet beam. The resulting degree of ionization produces an electric signal that can be read on a meter.

Other gas-detecting instruments use a flame ionization detector (FID). These instruments are used to detect a volatile hydrocarbon. The hydrocarbon is drawn into the ionization chamber, and a hydrogen flame ignites the compound. The resulting degree of ionization produces an electrical signal that can be read on a meter. The FID is not as sensitive as other detectors and is less sensitive to compounds containing electronegative atoms such as oxygen, sulfur, and chlorine.

Portable gas chromatographs equipped with FIDs or PIDs can be used to separate and detect multiple gases and vapors (Fig. 3-3). Such instruments greatly increase the specificity of gas and vapor detection.

PID and FID devices are the common direct-reading detection instruments used at industrial and hazardous-materials sites. These instruments do not detect hydrogen sulfide or hydrogen cyanide. Multiple methods of detection are needed at hazardous-materials sites to ensure safety of personnel.

Other instruments use absorption of various wavelengths of infrared energy as a detection method. These may be for personal monitoring also (Fig. 3-4). The gas is drawn into a chamber through which infrared radiation is projected. The gases are selected by adjusting for specific wavelengths of infrared light. The measured absorbance is then converted to a ppm value through appropriate instrument calibration. These instruments allow for the detection of multiple gases such as organic vapors, carbon dioxide, chlorine, hydrogen cyanide, hydrofluoric acid, hydrogen sulfide, formaldehyde, sulfur dioxide, ammonia, and nitrogen dioxide.

MERCURY MONITOR

Elemental mercury, which vaporizes at room temperatures, can be a significant hazard in confined areas. It has no odor. Real-

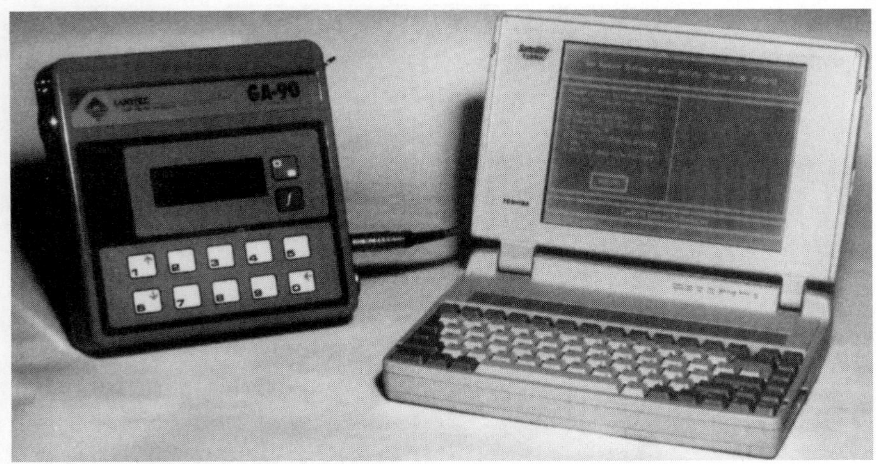

Figure 3-3. GA-90 infrared gas analyzer for portable use at hazardous sites. (Photograph courtesy of Hazco.)

time airborne concentrations can be measured using a gold-film technology mercury-vapor detector with a sensitivity of 0.003 mg/m^3 (Jerome Instruments, Jerome, AZ).

DETECTOR TUBES

Gas detector (indicator) tubes also can be used on site as direct-reading and grab-sampling instruments. These direct-reading colorimetric tubes contain a reagent that reacts with a standard volume of air and the gaseous contaminant drawn through it (Fig. 3-5). The reagent changes color in the presence of specific hazardous gases. The concentration of the contaminant in the air is read directly on the calibrated tube in ppm. The length or intensity of the color band indicates the quantity of hazardous gas present (Table 3-5).

Long-term detector tubes that require the assistance of a low-slow sampling pump provide an integrative approach to evaluating concentration over extended periods such as an entire work shift. At the end of the monitoring period, the length of the color band provides a direct readout of the TWA concentration.

PARTICLE MONITORS

Real-time monitoring for airborne particulate concentrations can be accomplished using portable direct-reading devices. The principle of operation of these monitors involves light scattering, piezoelectric effects, or beta attenuation. Such instruments should be calibrated against standard particulate monitoring methods to validate their performance.

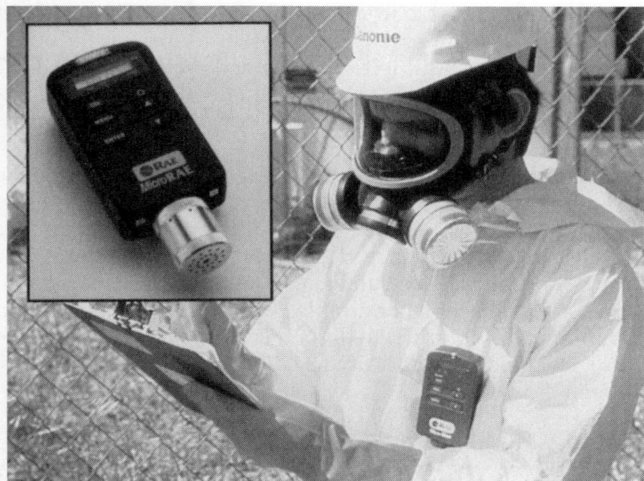

Figure 3-4. Personal monitor for volatile organic chemicals.

METALS

Information derived from real-time particulate monitors may be used other than for estimating particulate concentrations on a direct numerical or mass basis. For example, if one knows the average concentration of metals in a soil matrix or bulk sample, this value, as a percentage, can be applied to a reading obtained by a direct-reading aerosol monitor in mg/m^3 to obtain an approximate airborne concentration of a metal. This method provides only an approximation of the true airborne metal concentration because the metal content of the source material may vary. The analysis of filter samples for specific metal contaminants provides an accurate estimate of exposure to individual metals.

Indirect (Integrative) Monitoring Methods

INDIRECT MONITORING

Indirect or integrative monitoring is useful for measuring air concentrations of chemicals over a period, typically 15 minutes or longer, to better describe a hazardous environment. Although direct-reading instruments are available for a more limited number of specific toxic agents, indirect analytical techniques simultaneously can collect multiple chemicals at very low concentrations for subsequent analysis. Indirect-reading instruments provide a historical assessment of a site that may have changed since the samples were collected because collection occurs over a specified period and analysis occurs off site.

Indirect-reading instruments or integrative samplers, such as charcoal tubes and passive dosimeters or badges, are used to detect low concentrations of chemicals that may be present in occupational environments. Such monitors collect air samples over extended periods and provide estimates of average exposure or concentration. The measured levels represent TWA concentrations over the specified sampling period. An important concept in the use of these devices is the selection of the proper sampling method and medium to be used, both of which depend on the nature of the substance sampled. The analysis of air samples collected using such methods occurs at a later time in a licensed or certified analytical laboratory. Specific monitoring techniques are described in the following sections.

SOLID SORBENT TUBES

Sampling for gases and vapors with solid sorbent tubes typically is accomplished by drawing contaminant-laden air through a bed of granular sorbent (e.g., charcoal, silica gel, tenax) with a vacuum pump. The contaminant is adsorbed on a granular material. Then it is removed by a chemical or thermal desorptive process. The desorbed material is identified and

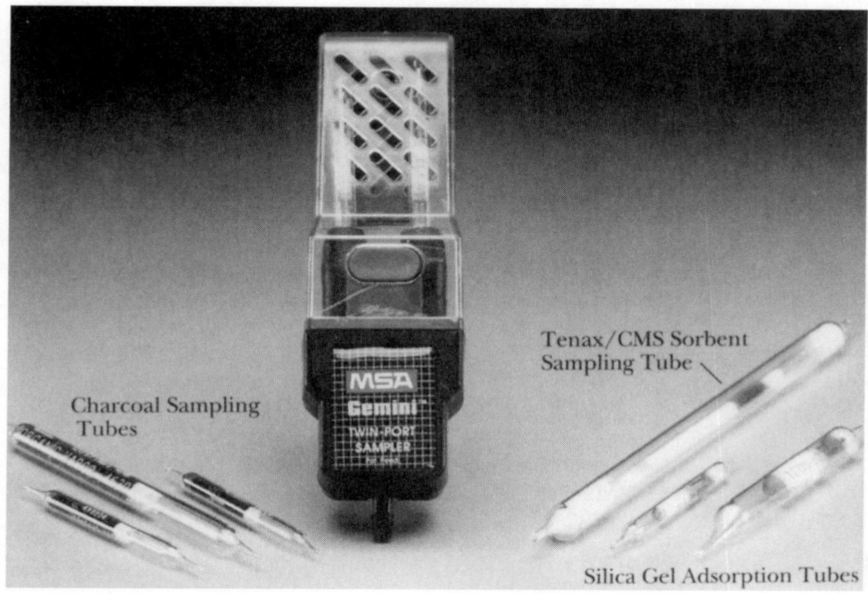

Figure 3-5. Sorbent tube sampling system for airborne chemicals. (Photograph courtesy of Hazco.)

quantified by laboratory procedures. Calibration of pumps before and after monitoring is required to accurately determine the collected air volumes.

PASSIVE DIFFUSIONAL MONITORS

Passive diffusional monitors operate much the same as solid sorbent tubes except that the contaminant is deposited on a sorbent bed by diffusion rather than by actively drawing contaminant-laden air through the collection device. Analysis of the samples is similar to that for solid sorbent tubes.

BUBBLERS (IMPINGERS)

Contaminant-laden air is drawn through a bubbler or impinger containing a liquid media in which the contaminant is soluble. The liquid-media–contaminant matrix then is chemically prepared for laboratory analysis (e.g., spectrophotometry).

ENVIRONMENTAL MONITORING OF BIOLOGICAL AGENTS

Biologicals consist of viable and nonviable agents. Viable agents, which can be grown on culture media or isolated from the environment, include microorganisms such as fungus, bacteria, virus, protozoa, and spores. Nonviable agents are pollen, pieces of microorganisms, and chemical products such as toxins, volatile organic chemicals, mycotoxins, and endotoxins. Biological sampling can be complex and should be performed by professionals for the following reasons:

- The sampling method should be matched to the environmental conditions to characterize the contamination and adverse health effects.
- Sampling should be performed with controls.
- Cultures should be processed by a qualified laboratory.

Bioaerosols are airborne dusts consisting of organic matter, biological material, and inorganic material. Exposure can cause nonallergic and allergic-mediated diseases, including hypersensitivity, pneumonitis, rhinitis, asthma, and airway inflammation.

Indoor biological contamination is defined as the presence of (a) bioaerosols of a kind and concentration likely to cause disease or predispose to disease, (b) inappropriate concentration of outdoor bioaerosols, or (c) microbiological growth that might become aerosolized. Environmental monitoring of bioaerosols usually reveals a diverse mixture of viable and nonviable agents with dynamics of movement determined by

- Particle size related to their diameter
- Shape
- Density
- Hydrophobic or hydrophilic properties
- Electrical charges
- Chemical nature

The primary factors that determine particle aerodynamics are diameter and density. For particles that are more spherical, the aerodynamic properties are related more to the diameter of the sphere. For elongated or spherical particles, the smallest diameter may influence its aerodynamic properties.

Large particles fall faster than smaller ones. Therefore, gravity collection assays may overestimate large particles compared to small. Also, small particles flow around a surface whereas larger particles impact a surface. Hydrophilic particles are collected more easily in a liquid impinger collection method than hydrophobic particles, which pass through the liquid. The electrostatic charge affects particle behavior with respect to surface interaction. Charged particles are more attracted to surfaces with opposite charges. Particle aerodynamics and aerodynamic properties of particles all influence assay systems.

Exposure Guidelines for Biological Agents

No TLVs or PELs exist for interpreting biological contaminants, culturable bioaerosols, countable bioaerosols, or pathogenic agents. Cultural bioaerosols are usually not of a single microbial entity, but rather are complex mixtures. Different sampling methods for bioaerosols can provide different results. Defining human exposure to a single agent or toxin in a bioaerosol is difficult. For these reasons, establishing TLV or PEL standards is not possible currently.

Assays for biochemical markers of biologicals, volatile chemical by-products, mycotoxins, and endotoxins are improving, but field validation is still lacking. The current state-of-the-art biological monitoring and hazard assessment remains professional judgment based on research reports, clinical case studies, and exposure-response relationships.

TABLE 3-5. Detector and indicator tubes

Chemical	Sensitivity/ range (ppm)	OSHA PEL (ppm 1989)
Acetaldehyde	100–1,000	100
Acetic acid	5–80	10
Acetone	100–12,000	750
Acid compounds (air)	Qualitative	—
Acrylonitrile	0.5–20.0	—
	5–700	35 (STEL)
	25–700	35 (STEL)
Aliphatic hydrocarbons	2–23 mg/L	—
Ammonia	2–30	35 (STEL)
Aniline	0.5–10.0	2
Arsenic trioxide	0.2 mg AS/m^3	—
Arsine	0.05–60.00	0.05
Organic arsines	Qualitative	—
Basic compounds (air)	Qualitative	—
Benzene	2–60	1
	0.5–10.0	1
Bromine	0.2–30.0	0.1
n-Butane	0.1–0.8%	800
l-Butylene	1–55 mg/L	—
Carbon dioxide	1–20 vol %	10,000
	0.5–10.0 vol %	10,000
Carbon disulfide	3–95	4
Carbon monoxide	10–3,000	35
Carbon tetrachloride	1–15	2
Carbonyl chloride	0.05–1.50	—
Chlorine	0.2–30.0	0.5
Chlorobenzene	5–200	75
2-Chloro-1,3-butadiene	5–90	10
1-Chloro-2,3-epoxypropane	5–60	2
Chloroformates	0.2–10.0	—
Chloroprene	5–90	10
Chromic acid	0.1–0.5 mg/m^3	0.1 (ceiling)
Cyanogen chloride	0.25–5.00	0.3 (ceiling)
Cyclohexane	100–1,500	300
Cyclohexylamine	2–30	10
Demeton	0.05	0.1
Dimethyldichlorovinylphosphate	Qualitative	0.1 mg/m^3
p-Dichlorobenzene	2–100	75
Dichlorovos	0.05	—
Diethyl ether	100–4,000	400
Dioborane	0.05–3.00	0.1
Dimethyl acetamide	10–40	10
Dimethyl formamide	10–40	10
Dimethyl sulfate	0.005–0.050	0.1
Epichlorhydrin	5–50	2
Ethanol	100–3,000	1,000
Ether	100–4,000	—
Ethyl acetate	200–3,000	400
Ethyl benzene	30–600	100
Ethyl ether	100–4,000	400
Ethyl mercaptan	0.5–5.0	0.5
Ethylene	50–2,500	—
	0.1–5.0	—
Ethylene glycol	10–180 mg/m^3	50 (ceiling)
Ethylene glycol dinitrate	0.25	0.1 mg/m^3 (STEL)
Ethylene oxide	1–30	1
Formaldehyde	0.2–5.0	1
	0.5–10.0	1
Formic acid	1–15	5
n-Hexane	100–3,000	50
Hydrazine	0.2–10.0	0.1
Hydrocarbons	0.1–0.8	—
Hydrochloric acid	0.5–25.0	—
Hydrocyanic acid	2–150	—
Hydrogen fluoride	1.5–15.0	3
Hydrogen peroxide	0.1–3.0	1
Hydrogen sulfide	1–200	10
Isopropyl alcohol	100–3,000	400
Mercaptan	0.5–5.0	—
Mercury vapor	0.1–2.0 mg/m^3	1 mg/m^3 (ceiling)
Methacrylonitrile	1–10	1
Methane	Qualitative	—
Methanol	50–3,000	200
Methyl acrylate	5–200	10
Methyl bromide	3–100	5
Methyl chloroform	50–600	350
Methyl mercaptan	2–100	0.5
Methyl methacrylate	50–50,000	100
Methylene chloride	50–2,000	500
Monostyrene	50–400	—
Nickel (aerosol)	0.25–1.00 mg/m^3	1 mg/m^3
Nickel tetracarbonyl	0.1–1.0	—
Nitric acid	1–50	1 (STEL)
Nitrogen dioxide	0.5–25.0	1 (STEL)
Nitrous fumes	0.5–10.0	1 (STEL)
n-Octane	100–2,500	300
Oil mist	1–10 mg/m^3	5 mg/m^3
Olefins (butylene, propylene)	1–55 mg/L	—
Organic basic nitrogens	Qualitative	—
Oxygen	5–23 vol %	—
Ozone	0.05–1.40	0.1
	10–300	0.1
n-Pentane	100–1,500	600
Perchlorethylene	5–50	25
Phenol	5	5
Phosgene	0.04–1.5	0.1
Phosphine	0.1–40.0	0.3
Propane	0.5–1.3 vol %	1,000
n-Propanol	100–3,000	200
Sulfur dioxide	0.5–25.0	2
Sulfuric acid	1–5 mg/m^3	1 mg/m^3
Toluene	5–400	100
Toluene diisocyanate	0.02–0.20	0.005
o-Toluidine	1–30	5
1,1,1-Trichloroethane	50–600	350
Trichloroethylene	2–200	50
Triethylamine	5–60	10
Vinyl chloride	1–50	1
o-Xylene	10–400	100

OSHA, Occupational Safety and Health Administration; ppm, parts per million; STEL, short-term exposure limit.

Environmental Sampling for Bioaerosols

Before sampling, the environment should be surveyed for contamination sources, dispersion sources, and exposure of individuals to biologicals. Overgrowth of bacteria or fungi cause musty or foul odors. Observations can result in immediate decisions about the health and safety of an environment and the relationship of signs and symptoms to environmental conditions. Inspection involves detection of odors, and noting of water-damaged areas, moisture in ventilation systems, stagnant water sources, or easily observed areas of mold growth.

Assaying for fungi, fungal elements (spores, hyphae), and bacteria involve three basic methods:

1. Air sampling
2. Swab or surface sampling
3. Bulk sampling

SURFACE OR SWAB SAMPLING

Wiping or swabbing an area of suspected biological contamination helps characterize the genus and species of microorganisms predominantly present. Surfaces are swabbed with a sterile, cotton-tip stick moistened with nutrient media such as 0.1% peptone with 0.01% Tween 80. The swabs are placed in a sterile tube and plated on agar.

Another technique is to place the swab into a 250-mL flask with nutrient broth, place the flasks on a rotary shaker for 20 minutes, then inoculate agar plates with a 0.1–0.2-mL aliquot of the suspension (7–9).

BULK SAMPLING

With bulk sampling, a physical sample is collected from a surface or specifically identified biological source such as the dust in a ventilation system. Such sampling helps determine the amount of an agent per gram of dust or contaminated material. But this does not consider the total amount of contaminant in the environment or the amount that might be aerosolized. To have meaning, bulk samples must be collected from the primary source of the causative agent in the environment. Generally, one gram of dust is extracted in sterile water with nutrient broth and agitated. The suspension is serially diluted and an aliquot is inoculated on appropriate agar (7–9).

AIR SAMPLING

Air sampling uses a device to collect a certain amount of air to determine the colony-forming units per cubic meter (CFU/m^3) of viable biologicals. Three basic sampling methods exist for collecting bacteria or fungi (7–9):

1. Drawing a volume of air through sterile microporous filter
2. Impinging air into a liquid
3. Collecting a fixed volume of air with impaction of viable organisms, spores, or hyphae on agar

Air sampling is more representative of human exposure to bioaerosols than wipe sampling or bulk sampling. But there are many variables in air sampling that affect results. First, collecting a representative sample of bioaerosols in a certain space over time to make health hazard determinations is the goal, but is not always representative. Particle aerodynamics and chemical and electrical nature all affect bioaerosol sampling. The sampling device and culture media also are critical to both collection and growth of microorganisms for identification.

Particle size can vary from smaller than 1 μm to more than 100 μm. Characterizing the sample from such a large range and size of particles can be difficult when using a single collecting device. But bioaerosols of concern generally range from 0.1 μm to 10.0 μm. Focusing on the particle size provides a better human exposure representation.

Choice of culture media is critical for growing bacteria and fungi (Table 3-6). Culture media can be general or nutrient-specific (i.e., designed to grow a particular organism). *Aspergillus* and *Penicillium* are hardy and persist in dry conditions. *Botrytis* and *Stachybotrys chartarum* are not as viable. If found in air sampling, their presence should be evaluated carefully as a potential environmental health problem. The selection of culture media is critical because different microbes may grow poorly or not at all in standard culture media and under certain conditions. Living organisms also can be damaged by the collection technique and fail to grow. Air sampling for culture usually underestimates the true bioaerosol concentration (8). For comparison, air sampling should be conducted outdoors in close proximity to the fresh air intakes to serve as controls. Indoor air samples should be collected simultaneously near suspected sources of contamination before and after agitation of sources. Source agitation can produce a 1,000-fold increase in the indoor air bioaerosol concentrations. Gravity or settling Petri dishes with culture media are of no use in sampling because they underestimate or may fail to detect biological contaminants that can remain in the air for lengthy periods. Summarizing, important issues involving air sampling for viable biologicals include

- Detection of viable organisms by culture
- Choice of appropriate culture media
- Timing of sampling to best characterize the biological exposure
- Choice of sampler device
- Identification of the genera and species of microorganism
- Interpreting the results in terms of exposure and health hazards

TABLE 3-6. Culture media for biologicals

Biological	Culture media
Saprotrophic fungi	Malt extract agar
Xerophilic	Malt-salt agar
saprotrophic fungi	Dichloren glycerol agar
Stachybotrys atra	Cellulose agar
Bacteria	Blood agar
	Tryptic soy agar (TSA)
	Aerobic agar
	Nutrient agar
	Sterile peptone water for use with liquid impinger
Actinomycetes	TSA
	Specific culture medium
Legionella bacteria	Buffered charcoal yeast extract (BCYE) agar with antibiotics or BCYE containing L-cysteine

Air Sampling Devices

Devices for sampling air (7) include (a) suction samplers that impact particles on surfaces or into liquid, or trap particles on filters; (b) rotating impact samplers that impact particles on rapidly moving surfaces; (c) electrostatic samplers that attract particles to electrically charged surfaces; and (d) gravity devices that trap particles falling from the air (Table 3-7).

Impactor sampling is more practical for nonindustrial sampling of bioaerosols. In heavily contaminated environments, impinger sampling is more appropriate.

Sampling time is an important variable when sampling for microorganisms. Continuous sampling over an exposure period of interest might be ideal but may not be achievable. Sampling duration often is constrained by desiccation of media by airflow and the potential of overloading media surface with microorganisms, which can lead to overgrowth during incubation.

CENTRIFUGAL SAMPLER

A centrifugal sampler draws in particles from air and impacts them on an agar surface using centrifugal force. The commonly used Reuter Centrifugal Sampler (Biotest, Danville, NJ) samples air at 280 liters per minute. Another model is designed to sample air rates from 1 to 1,000 liters per minute. Bioaerosols are impacted against agar strips that then are incubated for colony growth (7).

ALL GLASS IMPINGER

The all glass impinger (AGI-30, Ace Glass, Vineland, NJ) concentrates air samples of bioaerosols by drawing air through a curved inlet that simulates nasal passages, then through a jet where particles are impinged on a liquid. The AGI-30 is a frequently used device with an air sampling rate of 12.5 liters per minute. The AGI-30 is used to sample air for bacteria, fungi (spores and hyphae), and viruses (7).

TABLE 3-7. Commonly used samplers for collecting indoor bioaerosols

Sampler	Principle of operation	Sampling rate, 1 pm	Recommended sample time	Minimum CFUs detected	Applications/remarks
Slit to agar impactor	Impaction onto agar on rotating plate or stationary plate	30–700 continuous	Variable; 1–60 min or 7 d	—	Provides information on aerosol concentrations over time
Sieve-type impactors					
Single-stage portable	Impaction onto agar on "rodac" plate	90 or 185	0.5 or 0.3 min	22 or 16	Approximately 40% as efficient as slit sampler; portable, useful as probe
Single-stage impactor	Impaction onto agar, 100-mm plates	28	1 min	35	Nearly as efficient as slit, bulky to handle, AC operation
Two-stage impactor	Impaction onto agar, two 100-mm plates	28	1–5 min	35	Same as single-stage impactor but divides samples into respirable and nonrespirable fractions
Filter cassettes	Filtration	1–2	15–60 min or 8 h	8–33	Some desiccation loss; portable, inexpensive, useful as probe
High-volume filtration	Electrostatic collection into liquid	Up to 1,000	Variable	—	—
All glass impingers	Impingement into liquid	12.5	30 min	3	Fungi require wetting agent; useful over wide range of particle concentrations
Centrifugal sampler	Impaction onto agar, plastic strips	40	0.5 min	50	Cannot be calibrated; small, portable, useful as a probe

AC, alternating current; CFUs, colony-forming units; PM, phase modulation.
With permission from U.S. Environmental Protection Agency. Introduction to indoor air quality: a self-paced learning module. Washington: EPA, Office of Air and Radiation; 1991; EPA publication 400/3-91/002.

CYCLONE SCRUBBER

The cyclone scrubber collects aerosols by tangential impingement into thin layer created by a liquid mist that impacts the sampler wall. Collection fluid is delivered by a controlled flow rate through a jet inlet that creates a mist that traps bioaerosols. This device is used to sample for viruses, bacteria, and *Legionella* bacteria (7).

ANDERSEN MULTIHOLE IMPACTOR

Several types of Andersen multihole impactors are available, including single- and multistage. The device works by pulling air through jet holes below which are Petri dishes of agar. Air sampling rate is fixed at 28.3 liters per minute. Some Andersen samplers are multistage with different jet diameters for each stage. This design allows sampling for coarse particles and fine particles. The six-stage impactor is efficient for collecting bacteria and fungi in indoor air (7).

SURFACE AIR SYSTEM SAMPLER

The surface air system sampler is a portable, multiorifice device that collects microorganisms by inertial impaction. Air drawn through a jet is deflected 90% and agar serves as the obstacle to air flow. Larger particles impact on agar while smaller particles follow the jet stream (7).

SPORE TRAPS

A spore trap can provide a continuous recording of spores that collect on a greased tape. It can run for days. This allows for the recording of spore size and type. It can help detect fluctuation in concentrations in nature of spores during a time course.

Other Assays for Characterization of Biological Contamination

Identification of microbe genus and species along with determination of the relative percentages of fungal, bacterial, and spore species is critical to assessing health risks. Analysis of bioaerosols may also include (9,10)

- Microscopy: Visually characterizing spores, pollen, or particles by microscope
- Assaying for antigen content of dust
- Assaying for endotoxin content of dust (gram-negative bacteria)
- Chemical assays for volatile organic compounds of fungi and bacteria
- Assaying for mycotoxins (fungi)
- Assaying for (1→3)-β-glucan in dust samples (fungi)

BACTERIA

Bacteria are single-celled microbes without a nucleus (procaryotic) usually less than 4 μm in diameter. Bacteria possess a thick cell wall and are divided into two main types based on Gram's stain: gram-positive or gram-negative. Some bacteria are pathogenic. All bacteria can cause health problems if they have a nutrient source and amplify indoors. Culture plate impactors are used for bacterial sampling using general media such as nutrient agar, blood agar, or casein soy peptone agar. Specialized media can be used to grow certain types of bacteria. Pathogenic bacteria grow best at approximately 95°F (35°C). Thermophilic organisms grow best at 122°F (50°C) or higher and most other common organisms grow between 25° and 30°C (77° to 86°F).

The presence of more than 1,000 CFU/m^3 of gram-positive or more than 500 CFU/m^3 of gram-negative bacteria in air samples is a health concern. The presence of any species of pathogenic bacteria, such as *Legionella* and *Pseudomonas*, should raise concerns. Gram-negative bacteria are associated with environmental endotoxins. Positive bacteria have a peptidoglycan present in cell walls. Peptidoglycan is an immunomodulator similar to endotoxin but with less potency. Bacteria can produce spores that are temperature and drought resistant.

Stagnant water is a reservoir for gram-negative bacteria. *Legionella* also grows in stagnant water. *Legionella pneumophila* may not be detected in air samples, which makes sampling from potentially contaminated water sources important to detect this organism.

Many gram-negative bacteria are found in agricultural settings. Composting activities are associated with bioaerosols in excess of 10,000 CFU/m^3.

Pseudomonas can grow in metal-cutting machine fluids. Gram-negative bacteria grow on chronically wet building materials. Levels of biological contaminants indoors must be compared to levels found outdoors. For pathogenic contaminants such as *L. pneumophila*, any finding would be abnormal and indicate contamination and potentially serious health consequences.

Indoor bacteria generally originate from activities of the human occupants. Excessive quantities of human-source bacteria, such as *Bacillus subtilis*, indicate overcrowding or poor, ineffective ventilation. The presence of pathogens, such as actinomycetes, *L. pneumophila*, or *Pseudomonas*, or of an endotoxin indicates potentially serious contamination.

Bacterial air-sampled concentrations of less than 1,000 CFU/m^3 generally are not a concern, provided there is not a preponderance of one organism type. Concern is generated by air-sampled concentrations of gram-negative bacteria or pathogenic bacteria that are greater than 500 CFU/m^3.

Muramic Acid (Peptidoglycan)

The cell walls of gram-positive bacteria contain a chemical called *peptidoglycan* that has toxicity similar to endotoxin (11). Gram-positive bacteria containing peptidoglycan may pose a health problem when they accumulate indoors, because peptidoglycans have inflammatory and respiratory health effects.

Muramic acid is a component of peptidoglycan in bacterial cell walls. It is not found anywhere else (7,11). Therefore, muramic acid is a marker for peptidoglycan presence and indicates contaminating presence of gram-positive bacteria.

Tandem gas chromatography and mass spectrometry (GC-MS) have allowed improved specificity of detection of muramic acid but remains a research tool (12). The presence of muramic acid in air concentrations of dust should be correlated with health effects.

Endotoxins

Endotoxins are lipopolysaccharides (LPSs) derived from the outer membrane of gram-negative bacteria and blue-green algae. Endotoxins are composed of proteins, lipids, and LPSs. *LPS* refers to endotoxin material that is free of protein and other cell wall components. LPSs consist of a lipid component and a polysaccharide component. The lipid component—lipid A—is responsible for most of the toxic and adverse properties of endotoxins (13). The polysaccharide component is hydrophilic. It varies considerably between bacterial species while the lipid component is fairly constant on bacterial species. Most endotoxin exposure is caused by gram-negative bacteria in the environment. Endotoxins also are present in organic dust.

Environmental monitoring for endotoxins is performed by the sampling of water or airborne dust with analysis of aqueous extracts by the limulus amebocyte lysate test (LAL) (7,14,15). Although the LAL assay is standard for endotoxin detection by the U.S. Food and Drug Administration (FDA), there is no generally accepted standard for sampling and extraction (16). Standardization of the LAL assay has been attempted. For environmental dust, the use of the quantitative chromogenic modification of the LAL test is recommended (7,13–16). Reagents and endotoxin standards are available in kit form (Kinetic-QCL, Bio Whittaker, Walkersville, MD). Another method using the kinetic turbidimetric approach (KLARE, *k*inetic-turbidimetric *l*imulus *a*ssay with *r*esistant-parallels-line *e*stimate) yields results that are consistent with gas chromatography and mass spectrometry (17).

The FDA has a standard reference for endotoxin that is 50 endotoxin U/mL (EU/mL), which is approximately 5 ng/mL (7,14–18) (Standard Reference Endotoxin EC-5, No. 23550-3 USP, Customer Service Department 1643, 12601 Twinbrook Parkway, Rockville, MD 20852).

The LAL assay has interferences caused by dust. A wide coefficient of variation also exists in some studies using the assay (17).

Recommendations are emerging for the sampling of endotoxin as it relates to interpreting health effects. More recent versions of the LAL assay are proving to be more sensitive, with ranges of 0.01 to 100 EU/mL, or approximately 1 pg/mL to 10 ng/mL. The detection limit of airborne endotoxin for the LAL method is approximately 5 pg/m^3 (0.05 EU/m^3). The absolute measurement of endotoxin is probably inaccurate because it only assays measurements of endotoxins collected within that period of sampling.

Levels of endotoxin as they relate to illness are difficult to ascertain. Some guidelines are emerging (19). The International Commission on Environmental Health has guidelines for endotoxin of 1 μg/m^3 for pneumonitis and 0.001 μg/m^3 for general airway inflammation (7).

It is important to have an internal standard for endotoxin because different LAL test batches can give different results (7). Using standard endotoxins as part of the procedure is recommended. The FDA uses *Escherichia coli*-5 in its standardization procedures. The *E. coli*-5 reference is based on purified lipopolysaccharides from *E. coli* organisms as expressed in endotoxin units measured by LAL test activity. Commercial LAL tests also include a control standard endotoxin based on *E. coli* and sometimes on *Serratia abortus equi*. Caution should be used to ensure that the LAL test is endotoxin-specific, and does not react with (1→3)-β-glucan, which has a reactive affinity for factor G in the LAL test kit reagent.

No occupational exposure standard for endotoxins exists, although recommendations are being made to establish exposure limits (20).

Air sampling for endotoxin uses standard procedures for collection of airborne dust. Water samples should be collected in sterile containers. Filters should be selected that allow for efficient dust extraction. Polyvinyl chloride filters bind endotoxin. Polyvinyl chloride and cellulose acetate filters provide higher extraction efficiencies compared to glass fiber filters (7). Polycarbonate filters also are efficient in capturing endotoxin. A 100-liter air sample is sufficient to determine endotoxin indoors.

The medical literature reflects no adverse effect levels for inhaled endotoxin ranging from 9 ng/m^3 to 170 ng/m^3 (90 to 1,700 EU/m^3). These calculated "no effect" levels are based on epidemiologic studies of exposed populations with a safety factor of two applied (18).

The Dutch Expert Committee on Occupational Standards has proposed a health-based recommended limit of 50 EU/m^3 (4.5 ng/m^3 over an 8-hour exposure period) (13).

3-HYDROXYLATED FATTY ACIDS

An alternative assay method to determine endotoxin is based on detection of 3-hydroxylated (OH) fatty acids of LPS by GC-MS. These 3-OH fatty acids are linked to the glucosamine disaccharide portion of lipid A (7). GC-MS thus allows for determining chemical markers of gram-negative bacterial populations present indoors.

The LAL assay is more sensitive, but the GC-MS analysis of 3-OH fatty acids allows for identification of bacteria. The chiral configuration of the 3-OH fatty acids can be obtained to separate optically active configurations (R and S) (7).

Viruses

Assaying for the presence of viruses requires specialized culture media. Viral-culture media are generally tissue cultures. If collection is delayed more than 1 hour, the samples should be refrigerated.

FUNGUS

Fungi are eukaryotic—they possess a nucleus—and exist as single cells or multiple cells. Fungi are not photosynthetic. Fungi release enzymes that dissolve organic material on which they grow. These chemicals cause the typical musty odor of damp areas indoors. Fungi have hyphae and produce spores. Sampling of fungi can be performed by plating air, bulk, or liquid samples on appropriate culture media such as potato dextrose, Sabouraud-S dextrose, or malt-extract agar. Malt-extract agar has advantages because it does not support bacterial growth and it also is a medium in which *Aspergillus* species grow. *Aspergillus fumigatus* generally grows at 45°C in incubation. All other cultures for fungi are incubated at room temperature.

High-volume-filtration sampling devices can be used to evaluate airborne antigens and mycotoxins. Volumetric sampling with sieve or slit impactors also can be performed over an interval of time in areas of suspected high fungal spore concentrations.

Fungal concentrations in indoor air samples should be equal to or less than outdoor concentrations while distributions of genus and species should be similar. Air concentrations less than 100 CFU/m^3 are generally not a concern. Those higher than 500 CFU/m^3 should be compared to controls because they could be a concern, while those higher than 1,000 CFU/m^3 definitely are a concern. Disturbing a source of fungus or mold elevates spore counts up to 1,000-fold the baseline level in the air. *Penicillium*, *Cladosporium*, and *Alternaria* are the most prevalent fungal spores found in indoor environments.

Fungal Chemical Markers

Fungi produce toxic and immunoreactive chemical by-products that cause inflammation, respiratory irritancy, fatigue, lassitude, and other constitution symptoms:

- Mycotoxins
- Low-molecular-weight volatile compounds: geosmin, 1-octen-3-ol, 3-methylfuran
- (1→3)-β-glucan
- Enzymes
- Ergosterol

VOLATILES GENERATED BY FUNGI

Volatile chemicals generated by fungi can be used to determine fungal presence and the nature of fungal contamination indoors. Detection of 3-methylfuran indicates fungal growth and amplification (7). Detection of 1-octen-3-ol indicates dormant fungal mass. Geosmin presence indicates fungal mass presence and active growth (7).

Air concentrations of ergosterol measurements can be used to assay fungal mass in indoor dust. Ergosterol is a membrane sterol of fungal filaments. Ergosterol is very stable and is found in living and nonviable spores. Air is collected on a microspore titer and spores are extracted with methanol. Analysis is by GC-MS or high-pressure liquid chromatography. One study showed 3.2 μg of ergosterol per milligram of spores. *Aspergillus* and *Penicillium* produce 1.4 μg/mg to 6.0 μg/mg (21–23).

Fungi release volatile organic chemicals while growing. These chemical by-products can be sampled with a portable air sampler (Anasorb 747 carbon tube). Samples should be obtained in areas of concern and near ventilation intakes outdoors with control samples. GC-MS with selected ion detector is used to analyze for volatile chemicals (24).

INTERPRETING RESULTS OF FUNGAL ASSAYS

Components of the fungal cell wall may be responsible for organic toxic dust syndrome and hypersensitivity pneumonitis, and can be responsible for symptoms of chronic fatigue, fever, nausea, arthralgia, and anorexia (25).

Assaying environments for biological contamination should combine air sampling, bulk sampling, and inspection to characterize the extent of contamination and make decisions regarding health hazards. Comparison with outdoor control samples is important. Results of sampling are as follows:

- A predominance of fungal species in indoor air samples that are not dominant outdoors indicates poor indoor air quality and a potential health hazard.
- Many mycoflora are found commonly indoors. *Cladosporium*, *Alternaria*, and *Penicillium* are common indoors. However, air concentrations of total fungal presence should not exceed 1,000 CFU/m^3.
- *Cladosporium*, *Alternaria*, *Epicoccum*, and *Basidiomycetes* are present outdoors seasonally. In naturally ventilated buildings, the outdoor concentration may equal the indoor concentration. Wetness and moisture cause proliferation of fungi.
- Remediation should follow guidelines for removing and decontamination of fungal overgrowth (26,27).
- Presence of pathogenic fungi requires action. Pathogens include *Aspergillus* fungi (*A. fumigatus*, *A. flavus*), histoplasma capsulatum, and *Cryptococcus neoformans*. *A. fumigatus* grows in warm conditions in composting material. *Fusarium* species, particularly *F. moniliform*, may be found in damp or wet ventilation systems, and can infect immunocompromised individuals.

Fungal spore counts are obtained by drawing air in a sampler and impacting them on a moving, sticky surface. The spores can be examined microscopically. Microporous filters also are used to sample spores. Spores are eluted from the filters and counted microscopically.

MYCOTOXINS

Mycotoxins are chemical components of fungal cell walls and can persist for a long time in the environment after the fungus is dead or no longer viable. Mycotoxins can adhere to dust particles, be present in spores, and disperse in air currents. The presence of mycotoxins is not ruled out by the inability to grow mycotoxin-producing fungal species in culture. Identified mycotoxins include the following:

Diacetoxyscirpenol
Sterigmatocystin
Tannins
T2-toxin
Deoxynivalenol
Fumonisin
Zearalenone
Stachybotrys toxins
Mycophenolic acid
Aflatoxin B1, B2, G1, G2, M1
Ochratoxin A
Satratoxin F, G, H
Verrucarin J
Roridin E
Citrinin
Roquefortine
Patulin
Rubratoxin B

Fungi produce mycotoxins under narrow and strict nutrient and climate conditions. The ability to isolate mycotoxins from cultured fungi does not mean that these fungi are producing mycotoxins in the indoor environment. *Stachybotrys atra*, known to produce mycotoxins, cannot compete with other fungi like *Penicillium* in culture. Therefore, *Stachybotrys* may be missed in the environment when cultured.

GLUCANS

(1→3)-β-glucan possesses potent immunostimulatory and inflammatory properties through macrophage activation. Measurement of (1→3)-β-glucan is performed using a glucan-specific limulus lysate assay (7,20,25). This biological assay currently is the only one available for measurement of glucans in environmental samples. Demonstration of airborne glucan requires generating air movements to suspend dust in the environment to obtain relevant assay data.

The LAL assay contains an enzyme that reacts with (1→3)-β-glucan. The enzyme was isolated by Sepharose column chromatography to develop an assay for the glucan with pg/mL sensitivity (28). Release of cytokines, such as tumor necrosis factor-2, from macrophages is induced by (1→3)-β-glucan.

The presence of (1→3)-β-glucan in air correlates with illness. Air concentrations of 0.01 to 100 ng/m^3 of (1→3)-β-glucan are associated with chronic respiratory inflammation. Air samples are collected on a cellulose acetate/nitrate membrane filter. Filters are extracted by cold aqueous 0.3N NaOH (29).

ORGANIC AND COTTON DUSTS

Organic dusts consist of particles of vegetable, animal, and microbial origin. Organic dusts contain bacteria and fungi in the range of 10^4 to 10^{12} CFU/m^3 (30). Allergic alveolitis is caused by organic dusts. Causative species include *A. fumigatus, A. flavus, Aspergillus clavatus, Aspergillus niger, Aspergillus terreus, A. versicolor, Cryptostroma corticale, Eurotium rubrum, Penicillium* spp, *Alternaria* spp., *Cladosporium* spp., and *Didynella* spp. (20). Sampling for cotton dusts has provided the experience with organic dust exposure and health effects.

Continuous exposure to microbial concentrations greater than 1×10^5 CFU/m^3 is associated with respiratory illness (20). The cotton dust standard PEL for lint-free dust is 0.2 mg/m^3 for an 8-hour TWA in yarn manufacturing, 0.75 mg/m^3 in weaving and slashing, and 0.5 mg/m^3 in nontextile industries using cotton (31).

Sampling for organic dusts may also involve detection of toxic and pro-inflammatory components such as endotoxin, mycotoxins, and (1→3)-β-glucan (32).

Allergens and Antigen Load in Dust

Analytical assays are available to determine allergen concentrations in dust and bioaerosol samples indoors. Major allergens tested for are cat, dog, dust mite, and cockroaches. Immunoassays are available for detection of select antigens such as latex and fungal and bacterial by-products.

Sampling devices include vacuum cleaners with high-volume pumps and filters. Immunoassays with monoclonal or polyclonal antibodies are used to detect allergens in dust samples. Collection devices are standard vacuum cleaners with high retention bags with 97% efficiency for particles of a diameter greater than 1 μm. Filter cassettes are used with a 0.45-μm pore size attached to standard vacuum as a nozzle. For many allergens, standards or references exist and are available from the World Health Organization and the FDA (Office of Biologics Research and Review, Center for Drugs and Biologics).

Selecting the site for allergen sampling varies depending on the health complaints and presence of animals, dust mites, or roaches. Most samples are obtained from carpet, upholstery, surface dust, kitchens, cabinets, interior wall spaces, bedding, and ventilation ducts. The sampling objective is to characterize human exposure as close as possible.

Because allergens cause adverse health reactions at very low concentrations in sensitized individuals, there is no TLV or PEL (Table 3-8). Individuals vary in terms of their adverse response to allergens. Thresholds can be used only to provide advice to patients to reduce exposure, warn of potential risk, and point out the need to clean or change an environment.

Samples of 500 mg of dust are recommended as the minimum for testing. The antigen is extracted from the dust sample. This can affect the sensitivity and variability of the immunoassay. Coefficients of variation for these assays are approximately 20% (7).

Tannic acid interferes with analysis of dog and cat allergens by immunoassay. Tannic acid is sometimes recommended as an antiallergen treatment for carpet.

TABLE 3-8. Commercially available tests for environmental allergens in dust samples

Antigen	Type of assay	Thresholds reported by testing laboratories
Cat allergen (*Felis domesticus*)	PAb[a]	Low threshold (<20 μg/g)[c]
Fel d I (*Felis domesticus*)	MAb[b]	Threshold for sensitization (8 μg/g)[d]
Dust mites (*Dermatophagoides farinae* and *Dermatophagoides pteronyssinus*)	PAb	Low threshold (<15 μg/g)[c]
Der p I (from *D. pteronyssinus*)	MAb	Threshold for sensitization (2 μg/g) Dose for symptoms (10 μg/g)[d]
Der f I (from *D. farinae*)	MAb	Threshold for sensitization (2 μg/g) Dose for symptoms (10 μg/g)[d]
Dog allergen (*Canis familiaris*)	PAb	Low threshold (<20 μg/g)[c]
Can f I (*C. familiaris*)	MAb	Threshold for sensitization (10 μg/g)[c]
Cockroach (*Blattella germanica* and *Periplaneta americana*)	PAb	Low threshold (5 μg/g)[c]
Bla g I (from *B. germanica*)	MAb	Threshold for sensitization (2 U/g)[c]

[a]Polyclonal antibody enzyme immunoassay (EIA) with specificity for multiple antigens from the indicated species.
[b]Monoclonal antibody EIA with specificity for individual antigenic determinants from these various organisms.
[c]These low thresholds are based on an arbitrary classification scheme in which allergen concentrations are defined as low, medium, or high.
[d]Thresholds based on epidemiologic studies designed to estimate what level of allergen was likely to result in sensitization in patients with atopic tendencies. For the two mite epitopes (Der f I and Der p I) the dose of allergen that elicited symptoms in clinically sensitive individuals was also determined.
From American Industrial Hygiene Association Biosafety Committee. Allergens. In: Dillon H, Heinsohn P, Miller J, eds. Field guide for the determination of biological contaminants in environmental samples. Fairfax, VA: American Industrial Hygiene Association, 1996:151, with permission.

TABLE 3-9. Guidelines for assessing health hazards of biologicals

Biological agent	No health concern	Health concern	Reference source
Bacteria	<1,000 CFU/m³ (gram-positive)	>1,000 CFU/m³ >500 CFU/m³ (gram-negative)	7, 8, 31
	<500 CFU/m³ (gram-negative)	Presence of pathogenic bacteria	
Fungus	<100 CFU/m³ or less than outdoor control	>1,000 CFU/m³ Concentration of species-specific fungus Presence of pathogenic fungi or mycotoxin-producing fungi	7, 8, 31
Muramic acid	No data	Presence indicates gram-positive bacteria; correlate with symptoms	7, 11, 12
Ergosterol	No data	3.2 µg/mg of spores 1.4-6.0 µg/mg spores, *Aspergillus* and *Penicillium*	7, 23–25
Endotoxin	9–170 ng/m³ (900–1,700 EU/m³)	4.5 ng/m³ 8-h exposure period (50 EU/m³)	Dutch Expert Commission on Occupational Standards
		Endotoxin: 1 µg/m³ for toxic pneumonitis, 0.001 µg/m³ for airway inflammation	International Commission of Occupational Health 11, 13–20
Antigen	Below sensitization threshold	Dust mite (Der p I/g of dust) Low: <2 µg/g Moderate: 2–10 µg/g of dust High: >10 µg/g dust Threshold for sensitization = 2 µg/g Cat allergen Fel D I/g of dust Low: <1 µg/g Moderate: 1–8 µg/g High: >8 µg/g Threshold for sensitization = 2 µg/g Cockroach (*Blattella germanica*) Threshold for sensitization = 2 U/g	7, 8
(1→3)-β-glucan	None detected	0.01–100.00 ng/m³	7, 20, 21, 25, 28, 29
Mycotoxin	Correlate with signs and symptoms	0–10² ng/m³, correlate with signs and symptoms	7, 21, 25, 27, 28
Protozoa	Absent	Any present	8, 9
Organic dust spores	Low levels decrease risk	10^6–10^{10} spores/m³ Allergic alveolitis, hypersensitivity, organic dust toxic syndrome	20, 21
Microorganisms in organic dust	Low levels decrease risk	1 × 10^5 CFU/m³ Allergic alveolitis, hypersensitivity, organic dust toxic syndrome	20, 21

CFU, colony-forming unit.

Integrated Monitoring Strategy for Toxic Chemical Markers of Biologicals

An integrated approach that characterizes chemical biomarkers of biologicals involves assaying for 3-OH fatty acids, muramic acid (peptidoglycan and fungal mass), and ergosterol by tandem GC-MS (7,12).

Assessing the health hazards of biologicals and products of biologicals is difficult because of the lack of standards. However, guidelines exist to assist decision making (Table 3-9).

INORGANIC DUST AND PARTICULATES

Inorganic dusts are broadly classified as

- Mineral dusts (silica and silicates)
- Metallic dusts
- Asbestiform dusts
- Carbon dusts

Health problems secondary to inorganic particulates relate to their size, chemical makeup, airborne concentration, and length of exposure. Inorganic dust and related particulates are derived mainly from silica, silicates, metals, asbestiform minerals, and synthetic crystalline fibers (Fig. 3-6).

Mineral dust health hazards include:

- Silica
- Asbestos
- Silicates
- Talc (magnesium silicate)
- Clay (aluminum silicate)
- Kaolin (aluminum silicate)
- Mica (aluminum silicate)
- Feldspar (potassium silicate, NaCa silicate)

Particulate size determines whether aerosols are respirable. In general, particles approximately 10 µm in diameter lodge in the upper airway. Particles smaller than 5 µm in diameter penetrate to lower areas of the respiratory tract where they can deposit and remain for long periods. Those particles that are smaller than 1 µm in diameter generally are able to penetrate into the lower terminal bronchioles, and those that are smaller than 0.5 µm in diameter may be able to reach the terminal alveolar sacs (Fig. 3-7).

Inorganic particulates are divided broadly into metallic and nonmetallic categories. Nonmetallic particles containing silica are divided further into crystalline or amorphous types.

Metallic particulates exist in the form of dusts or fumes. They range in toxicity. Metal fume fever is the acute febrile respiratory illness caused by inhalation of metal fumes. Metal particulates can also cause dermal lesions such as contact dermatitis, allergic dermatitis, and granulomas. Some metal dusts are systemically

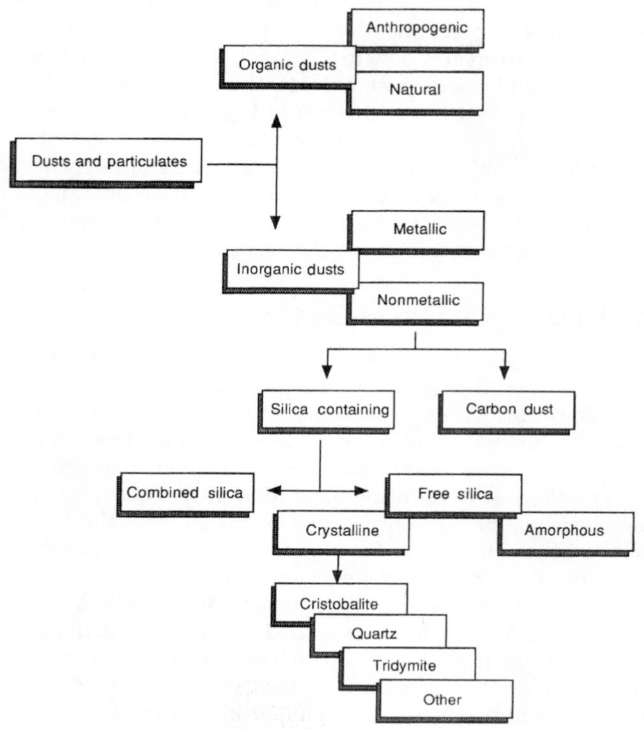

Figure 3-6. Dust and particulates classification.

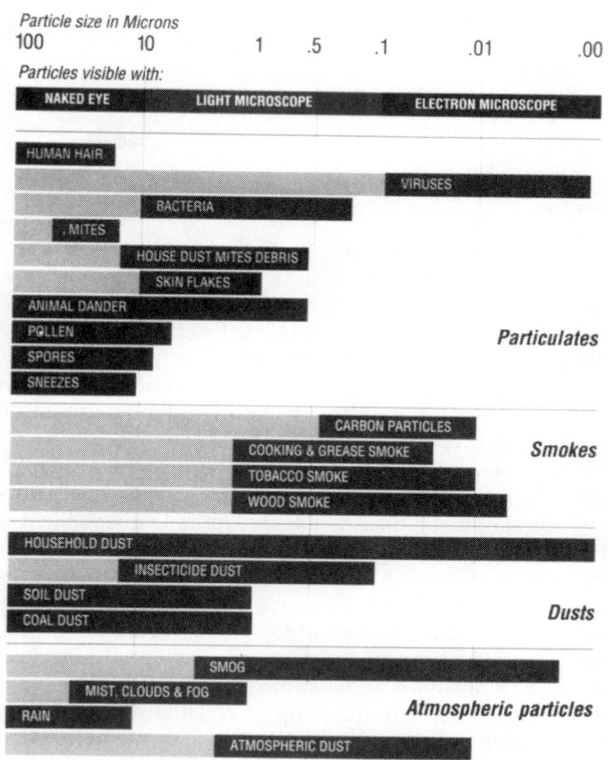

Figure 3-7. Particulate size determines whether aerosols are respirable. (Courtesy: Honeywell, Inc., Home and Building Control, Golden Valley, MN.)

absorbed, resulting in clinical toxicity (e.g., cadmium, manganese, beryllium, lead, arsenic, chromium, and copper).

Particles suspended in air are usually not visible unless they are highly concentrated or approximately 50 μm in diameter. Dust particles settle according to their diameter size. Particles larger than 10 μm settle more quickly than particles that have a diameter smaller than 10 μm. Respirable particles are generally 5 μm or smaller and remain suspended in air for hours. In comparison, pollens have diameters from 18 to 25 μm. Particles of 0.5 μm or smaller in diameter remain airborne for 3 to 6 hours.

The U.S. Environmental Protection Agency (EPA) currently regulates particles of 10-μm diameter (PM_{10}) under National Ambient Air Quality Standards for outdoor air. Health risks from ambient air pollution is associated with particulate pollution 10 μm or smaller in diameter in ambient outdoor air. The PM_{10} standard in the National Ambient Air Quality Standards is 150 mg/m^3, with a yearly average of 50 mg/m^3 (33).

Silica

Silicon refers to the element Si. *Silicon dioxide* (SiO_2) refers to natural amorphous silica (noncrystallized), crystalline silica (quartz), and silicates (clay or aluminum silicate). Silica occurs naturally in either the crystalline or amorphous form. Silica is found in rocks of all varieties. Silicone is synthetic amorphous polymers of SiO_2. Silica is divided into crystalline and noncrystalline forms. Crystalline silica can be further subdivided (see Fig. 3-6). Amorphous SiO_2 is less of a health hazard than crystalline silica (31).

Silicates are composed of silicon and oxygen combined with cations of aluminum, magnesium, sodium, calcium, and potassium. The chemical makeup of silicates also dictates their health risks (fibrous, platy, or granular):

Fiber: Material with length to breadth ratio of at least 3

Platy: Composed of continuous layers of tetrahedral silicate sheets sandwiching octahedral cations such as Al^{+3} or Mg^{+2}

Granule: Large, visible particles such as sand or clay

The crystalline or free silica found in quartz, tridymite, and cristobalite causes silicosis. Crystallized SiO_2 is sand. The percentage of SiO_2 in materials varies (32):

Clay: 0% to 40%
Mica: 0% to 10%
Talc: 0% to 5%
Limestone: 0% to 3%
Feldspar: 12% to 25%
Brick/tile: 10% to 35%
Pottery: 15% to 25%
Sand: 50% to 90%

Clay is a diverse group of hydrated aluminum silicate minerals with a particulate size smaller than 2 μm in diameter. Magnesium silicates are talc. Aluminum silicates are mica and kaolin. Certain silicates, such as talc, may contain crystalline silica and asbestos. Clay minerals include kaolin, bentonite, Fuller's earth, and feldspar. Diatomaceous earth is a gritty amorphous silica made up of skeletons of small aquatic plants (diatoms). Under temperature and pressure, it may contain significant amounts of crystalline tridymite and cristobalite. Therefore, appreciable environmental dust levels should be controlled for crystalline silica.

The OSHA PEL for dusts containing crystalline silica takes into account the percentage of silica present in a sample (31,34):

$$\text{PEL (mg/m}^3\text{) of dust} = \frac{10 \text{ mg/m}^3}{(\% \text{ SiO}_2 + 2)}$$

This formula is based on dust collection by a size-selective sampling device. It represents the fraction of dust that is respirable, which then can penetrate and remain in the alveoli (32). The PEL for the concentration of free dust with less than 1% crystalline silica is 5 mg/m^3 (this is the reason for the constant "2") (31).

The TLV-TWA for crystalline silica is 0.1 mg/m^3 of respirable quartz in air, regardless of the total dust concentration. For other silicas, the TLVs are as follows (34):

Cristobalite = 0.05 mg/m^3
Tridymite = 0.05 mg/m^3

Asbestos

Asbestos refers to a family of fibrous, hydrated mineral silicates that are fire and heat resistant and insoluble in strong acids and alkalis. Asbestos minerals are classified in two groups: amphiboles and serpentines. Asbestos is used in insulation materials of all varieties. The term *asbestiform* refers to fibrous material of 5 µm or longer with a length to width ratio of 3. The adverse health properties of long, thin fibers longer than 5 µm and less than 0.5 µm in breadth have been established.

In an effort to avoid the use of asbestos fibers because of their health effects, newer generations of fibers have been developed: rock wool, slag wool, glass wool, and ceramic fibers. Such synthetic mineral fibers have been found to have their own health effects. These fibers can withstand very high temperatures of approximately 1,000°C. They are amalgamated from silicon dioxide or aluminum silicates with additives such as aluminum oxide, titanium dioxide, zinc oxide, magnesium oxide, lithium oxide, barium oxide, calcium oxide, sodium oxide, and potassium oxide.

Amphibole fibers are made up of crystalline subfibrils consisting of hydrated magnesium silicates. They are held together by electrostatic bonds to form rigid, nearly indestructible log-like fibers. Serpentine chrysotile fibers are made up of subfibrils rolled into scrolls of platy magnesium silicate or chrysotile fibers. Serpentine subfibrils are bound loosely by electrostatic fones, making them pliable and flexible.

Amphiboles are subdivided into:

- Commercial amphiboles
  - Amosite: $(FeMg)SiO_3$
  - Crocidolite: $NaFe[SiO_3][2H_2O]$
- Noncommercial amphiboles
  - Tremolite: $Ca_2Mg_5Si_8O_{22}[OH]_2$
  - Anthophyllite: $[MgFe]_7Si_8O_{22}$
  - Actinolite: $CaO \cdot 3(MgFe)O \cdot SiO_2$

OSHA has regulated asbestos since 1971 (40 *CFR* 763, EPA, 1987) in response to the Asbestos Hazard Emergency Response Act. Asbestos PELs are

0.1 fiber/cc of air (8-hour TWA)
1.0 fiber/cc of air (STEL)

The long, thin fibers (longer than 5-µm length and smaller than 0.5-µm diameter) cause clinical disease. Amphiboles with these physical characteristics cause inflammatory pulmonary reactions.

Scanning and transmission electron microscopy are used to identify and quantify asbestos fiber exposures. EPA requires these methods to be used through protocols developed under the Asbestos Hazard Emergency Response Act.

Other Mineral Dusts

Limestone and marble are other building materials that produce dust when ground. Limestone is mainly calcium carbonate and magnesium carbonate. Limestone arises from natural metamorphosis of the cytoskeletons of crustaceans, corals, and mollusks.

Carbon dusts include coal dust, graphite, lignite, peat, and carbon black. Coal dust contains a variety of organic compounds, such as benzenes, naphthalenes, polynuclear aromatic hydrocarbons, and phenols, in addition to carbon. Coal dust also contains inorganic material components. Anthracite coal has the highest carbon content, approximately 95%. Lignite has the lowest carbon content, approximately 65% to 75%, with a higher percentage of quartz, ash, and volatile material (31). The carbon content of bituminous coal is between anthracite and lignite. Pneumoconiosis occurs with chronic lifetime exposure to respirable coal dust.

Natural graphite is different from synthetic graphite. Natural graphite is composed of crystalline carbon with variable amounts of quartz and impurities such as silicates. Synthetic graphite is produced from coal. Carbon black is hard crystalline carbon.

Particulates Not Otherwise Classified

A number of specific exposure limits have been established for certain classes of organic and inorganic dusts with recognized toxicologic properties. Even in the absence of such properties, it has been shown that substantial burdens of dust deposits in the lungs can have adverse health effects. At lower concentrations, dust particles without recognized toxic properties can impede the clearance of more toxic dust particles from the lung by decreasing the mobility of alveolar macrophages. A potentially fatal condition known as *alveolar proteinosis* can be caused by exposure to high concentrations of such dusts (34). As a consequence, the ACGIH has established TLVs for particulates not otherwise classified (PNOC), which were formerly classified as "nuisance dusts." The shift to the PNOC designation was aimed at emphasizing that all materials are potentially toxic and that, even in the absence of specifically recognized toxic effects, it is dangerous to consider materials harmless at all exposure concentrations. The ACGIH TLV-TWA for total inhalable PNOC currently is set at 10 mg/m^3. The TLV-TWA for respirable PNOC [smaller than 10-µm aerodynamic diameter (a 3.5-µm particle has a 50% chance of deposition)] is set at 3 mg/m^3. The OSHA PEL for total dust is 15 mg/m^3, and a PEL for respirable dust is 5 mg/m^3.

Assessing Particle Exposure

Sometimes it is necessary to sample airborne dust and analyze it for size and chemical composition to evaluate the health hazard it presents. Particles larger than 10 µm in diameter are usually not considered a health hazard because they do not remain suspended in air very long nor do they penetrate airways. Particles smaller than 10 µm are a health hazard.

It is critical to differentiate respirable dust from nonrespirable dust with sampling methods. The cyclone sampler is used to sample for respirable dust. Dust and particulate monitoring is performed using cyclone separators that collect dusts and separate particles by their sizes. The cyclone separator uses a filter and filter cassettes. Air is drawn past the filter with a pump. Particles are collected on the filter membrane. Filter selection depends on the size of particles to be collected. Pore sizes vary:

- Silica and metal fumes (0.8 to 37.0 µm)
- Nuisance dust (5.0 to 37.0 µm)

Horizontal elucidators placed in front of a cyclone sampler remove coarse particles by gravity.

Because particles of 5 µm or smaller deposit and stay in deeper areas of the lung, health concerns are directed at measuring these smaller particles. Gravimetric and chemical analyses usually are performed on the particles to better characterize their health hazards. Atomic absorption is used to identify metals. X-ray diffraction is used to determine inorganic compounds and their crystalline structure.

The total dust concentration by weight in an environment does not provide enough information on its health hazard. To better characterize health risks, it is important to determine both the respirable dust and its chemical and physical nature. Personal-breathing-zone dust analysis provides the best characterization of health risk. It can be performed by personal sampling devices taken over a period, usually 8 hours. The free silica content is important to determine separate from the total dust collected (31).

REFERENCES

1. National Academy of Sciences. *Human assessment for airborne pollutants—advances and opportunities.* Washington: National Academy Press, 1991.
2. Environmental Protection Agency. Guidelines for exposure assessment. *Federal Register* 1992 May 29:57:22888.
3. Lipton S, Lunch J. *Health hazard control in chemical process industry.* New York: John Wiley and Sons, 1987.
4. American Conference of Governmental Industrial Hygienists. *Threshold limit values for chemical substances and physical agents and biological exposure indices for 1996.* Cincinnati: American Conference of Governmental Industrial Hygienists, 1996.
5. Rappaport S. Threshold limit values, permissible exposure limits and feasibility: the basis for exposure limits in the U.S. *Am J Ind Med* 1993;23:683–694.
6. Hawkins NC, Jayjock MA, Lynch J. A rationale and framework for establishing the quality of human exposure assessments. *Am Ind Hyg Assoc J* 1992 Jan;53(1):34–41.
7. Dillion H, Heinsohn P, Miller D. *Field guide for the determination of biological contaminants in environmental samples.* Fairfax, VA: AIHA Publications, 1996.
8. Seltzer J. Biologic contaminants. *Occup Med: State of the Art Reviews* 1995;10(1):1–25.
9. Burge H. Aerobiology of the indoor environment. *Occup Med: State of the Art Reviews* 1995;10(1):27–40.
10. Cox C, Wathes C. *Bioaerosols—handbook of samplers and sampling.* Chelsea, MI: CRC Press/Louis Publications, 1995.
11. Chetty C, Schwab J. Endotoxin-like products of gram positive bacteria. In: Rietschel E, ed. *Handbook of endotoxin.* Amsterdam: Elsevier Science, 1984;1.
12. Fox A, Wright L, Fox K. Gas chromatography–tandem mass spectrometry for trace detection of muramic acid, a peptidoglycan chemical marker, in organic dust. *J Microbiol Methods* 1995;22:11–26.
13. Heederik D, Douwes J. Towards an occupational exposure limit for endotoxins. *Ann Agric Environ Med* 1997;4(1):12–19.
14. Burrell R. Human responses to bacterial endotoxin. *Circ Shock* 1994;43:137–153.
15. Rylander R. Endotoxins in the environment. In: Levin J, Alving C, Munford R, Redl H, eds. *Bacterial endotoxins: lipopolysaccharides from genes to therapy.* New York: John Wiley and Sons, 1995.
16. Douwes J, Bersloot P, Hollander A, et al. Influence of various dust sampling and extraction methods on the measurement of airborne endotoxin. *Appl Environ Microbiol* 1995;61:1763–1769.
17. Hollander A, Heederik D, Versloot P, Douwes J. Inhibition and enhancement in the analysis of airborne endotoxin levels in various occupational environments. *Am Ind Hyg Assoc J* 1993;54(11):647–653.
18. Milton D, Gere R, Feldman H, Greaves I. Endotoxin measurement: aerosol sampling and applications of a new limulus method. *Am Ind Hyg Assoc J* 1990;51(6):331–337.
19. Rylander R. Endotoxins. In: Rylander R, Jacobs RR, eds. *Organic dust: exposure, effects and prevention.* Boca Raton, FL: Lewis Publishers, 1994.
20. Dutkiewicz J. Bacteria and fungi in organic dust as potential health hazards. *Ann Agric Environ Med* 1997;4:11–16.
21. Gessner M, Chauvet E. Ergosterol-to-biomass conversion factors for aquatic *Hyphomycetes. Appl Environ Microbiol* 1993;59:502–507.
22. Setiz L, Sauer R, Burroughs H, et al. Ergosterol as a measure of fungal growth. *Phytopathology* 1979;69:1202–1203.
23. Miller J, Young J. The use of ergosterol to measure exposure to fungal propagules in indoor air. *Am Ind Hyg Assoc J* 1997;58:39–43.
24. Wessen B, Strom G, Scheops K. MVOC profiles—a tool for indoor air quality assessment in indoor air quality—an integrated approach. In: Morawska L, ed. Amsterdam: Elsevier, 1995.
25. Auger P, Gourdeau P, Miller D. Clinical experience with patients suffering chronic fatigue–like syndrome and repeated upper respiratory infections in relation to airborne molds. *Am J Ind Med* 1994;25:41–42.
26. Shaughnessy R, Morey P. Remediation of microbial contamination. In: Macher J, ed. *Bioaerosols: assessment and control.* Cincinnati: ACGIH, 1999.
27. Guidelines on assessment and remediation of fungi in indoor environments. New York: N Y City Department of Health, 2000.
28. Goto H, Yuasa F, Rylander R. (1→3)-β-D-glucan in indoor air—its measurement and *in vitro* activity. *Am J Ind Med* 1994;25:81–83.
29. Rylander R, Persson K, Goto K, et al. Airborne (1→3)-β-D glucan may be related to symptoms in sick buildings. *Indoor Environ* 1992;1:263–267.
30. Jacobs R. Sampling environments containing organic dust. *Am J Ind Med* 1994;25:3–11.
31. Ploy B, Niland J, Quinlan P. *Fundamentals of industrial hygiene*, 4th ed. Itasca, IL: National Safety Council, 1996.
32. Norn S. A possible mechanism in organic dust related diseases. *Am J Ind Med* 1994;25:91–95.
33. Choudhury A, Gordian M, Morris S. Associations between respiratory illness and PM_{10} air pollution. *Arch Environ Health* 1997;52(2):113–117.
34. American Conference of Governmental Industrial Hygienists. *Threshold limit values for chemical substances and physical agents and biological exposure indices for 1997.* Cincinnati, OH: ACGIH, 1997.

CHAPTER 4

Principles of Toxicology

I. Glenn Sipes and Drew Badger

DEFINITION AND SCOPE OF TOXICOLOGY

Toxicology is a broad field of study encompassing multiple scientific disciplines, including biology, chemistry, and environmental sciences. Its primary focus is to determine the adverse effects of chemicals on biological systems. Historically, toxicologic studies were performed to identify those agents that can elicit abnormal physical or behavioral signs of injury. Investigators have extended their efforts to also determine the mechanisms underlying the development of toxicity. Because of the increased awareness of the number and quantities of toxicants generated, and of their potential for causing adverse effects, several subdisciplines of toxicology have emerged (Table 4-1).

Toxicologic Model Systems

To assess the potential toxicity of a chemical, several different model systems have been used. These include whole animal models, isolated perfused organ systems, precision-cut tissue slices, isolated cell cultures, organella subfractions, and so forth. With animal models, toxicity can be assessed by monitoring effects ranging from appetite depression, body weight loss, or behavioral changes to more fatal conditions such as tumor formation or death. Likewise, *in vitro* systems can reveal the potential for toxicity, but are also important in elucidating molecular and cellular mechanisms of toxicity.

In Vitro Model Systems

Several different *in vitro* systems are used to assess toxicity. In such systems, toxicologic endpoints may often be determined readily. For example, chemical-induced toxicity to cells can often be determined easily, either by microscopic evaluation of cells or by measuring biochemical events associated with the cells (e.g., dye exclusion or protein synthesis). *In vitro* systems have also provided important mechanistic information to certain models of injury (1,2).

Animal Models

Although *in vitro* studies are useful for understanding toxicologic mechanisms, animal studies are still required to understand the full range of chemical-mediated effects that can occur in the whole organism. This is because effects seen *in vivo* may not agree with findings established using *in vitro* studies. For example, certain chemicals may cause injury to a particular cell type *in vivo* by eliciting a deleterious inflammatory response. However, this same cell type may be much less susceptible to injury when it is exposed to a chemical as a primary isolated cell culture in which recruitment and activation of inflammatory cells do not occur. On the contrary, *in vitro* studies can show effects that do not occur *in vivo*. For example, several compounds that have been shown to damage DNA in one or more *in vitro* mutagenicity tests (which are indicators of carcinogenicity) do not actually produce tumors in the whole animal. An explanation as to why false-positives occur is not always known, but may be caused by *in vivo* metabolic or detoxification pathways that are not present *in vitro*, or due to an inability of the carcinogen to reach its target site in the body. Collectively, these examples illustrate the requirement of multiple host factors, some of which are independent of the target cell or tissue, for certain compounds to elicit toxicity.

With animal studies, most heterogeneous populations exposed to a toxic agent exhibit a normal or gaussian distribution in which most individuals exhibit a similar degree of susceptibility. Figure 4-1 illustrates a gaussian distribution for the diameter of red blood cells. It shows that, although there are both small and large cells, most of them fall within a given size range. Much like cell size, toxic exposures often cause a similar degree of toxicity to most individuals within the population. In certain instances, however, bimodal or even trimodal distributions are seen, in which two or three distinct populations can be identified (e.g., fast or slow acetylators).

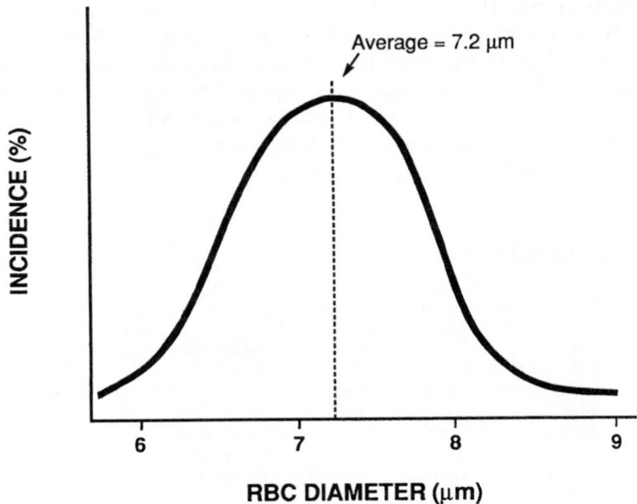

Figure 4-1. Frequency distribution curve for erythrocyte (RBC) diameter shows a normal biological distribution.

DOSE-RESPONSE RELATIONSHIPS

One of the most important concepts in toxicology is the dose-response relationship. The underlying premise is that any compound can be toxic if it is encountered in large enough doses. No matter what the compound's potency (or how little compound is necessary to produce an effect), its respective toxic dose threshold must be surpassed to produce toxicity. This rule, of course, may not hold true when there are extenuating circumstances such as nutritional deficiency or stress. Likewise, the established toxic dose threshold value is questionable when exposures contain multiple chemicals that alter the host's ability to handle potential toxicants. Even so, dose-response relationships are a useful foundation for establishing appropriate threshold limits for toxic exposures.

Figure 4-2 shows a typical sigmoidal dose-response curve in which toxicity is not seen at the lower doses of a chemical exposure. With an increasing dose, toxicity manifests and continues to rise until, ultimately, there is either a 100% response or one or more factors contributing to toxicity are saturated. The critical point that defines the barrier between subtoxic and toxic exposure levels is referred to as the *threshold dose*. It should be noted,

TABLE 4-1. Major subdisciplines of toxicology

Subdiscipline	Description
Clinical	Causation, diagnosis, and management of established poisoning in humans.
Veterinary	Causation, diagnosis, and management of established poisoning in domestic and wild animals.
Forensic	Establishing the cause of death or intoxication in humans by analytical procedures and with particular reference to legal processes.
Occupational	Assessing the potential of adverse effects from chemicals in the occupational environment and the recommendation of appropriate protective and precautionary measures.
Pharmacologic	Assessing the toxicity of therapeutic agents.
Environmental	Assessing the effects of toxic pollutants, usually at low concentrations, released from commercial and domestic sites into their immediate environment and subsequently widely distributed by air and water current and by diffusion through soil. Environmental toxicology can also be broken down into aquatic- and ecotoxicology.
Ecotoxicology	Assessing the effects of toxic pollutants on ecological populations and communities (e.g., plants, microorganisms).
Aquatic toxicology	Assessing the toxicity on aquatic organisms of chemicals discharged into marine and freshwater.
Regulatory	Administrative function concerned with the development of interpretations of mandatory toxicology test programs and with particular reference to controlling the use, distribution, and availability of chemicals used commercially, domestically, and therapeutically.
Laboratory	Design and conduct of *in vivo* and *in vitro* toxicology testing programs; elucidate mechanisms of toxicity.
Analytical	Isolation, identification, and quantification of toxicants and their metabolites.

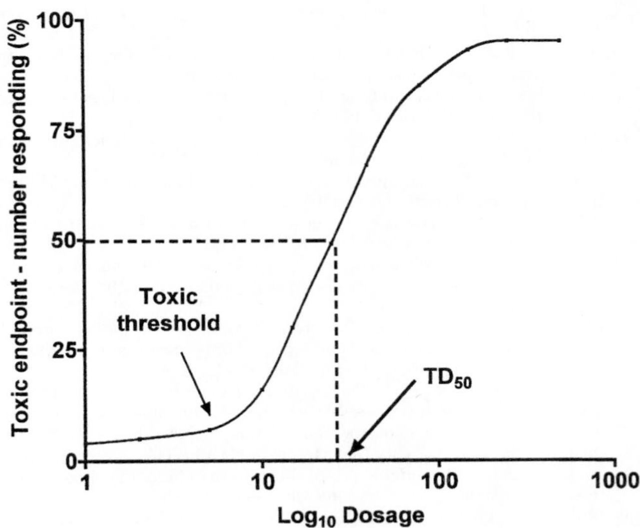

Figure 4-2. Typical sigmoidal cumulative dose-response curve for toxic effect. The slope of a curve is determined by the increase in response as a function of incremental increases in dosage (presented in a logarithmic scale). The TD_{50} is seen as the dose that produces a toxic effect in 50% of the population.

however, that this threshold may vary depending on the sensitivity of the toxicologic endpoint. The dose at which this toxic threshold is reached is also dependent on a number of intrinsic host factors, including the rate of conversion to toxic metabolites, receptor affinity, and availability of detoxification mechanisms, among others. In addition, chemicals cause injury by different mechanisms and therefore do not exhibit the same dose-response characteristics (3).

Even compounds of similar structure can show dramatic differences in toxicity. This is illustrated by the three isomers of dichlorobenzene (DCB), of which 4,5-epoxides are the most toxic metabolites. Both 1,2- and 1,3-DCB can form the 4,5-epoxide, but because 1,4-DCB has a chlorine at the 4-position, it cannot form this metabolite (3). Thus, it appears that the reported DCB isomer-specific toxicity is mediated by two related factors: (a) each isomer generates different metabolites, and (b) different epoxide metabolites of DCB have a differential reactivity for cellular targets. Thus, even structural isomers can produce highly variable toxic responses.

Toxicologic Measurements

Toxicologic endpoints can be classified as either quantal or continuous. Although death is an all-or-none response (a quantal response), other observations, such as altered body weight or blood pressure, may be considered a continuous (or graded) response. With each classification, dose-response curves can be generated and used to determine a median effective dose (ED_{50}), or the dose at which 50% of the population elicits a biochemical or physiologic response to a chemical exposure. The ED_{50} can also be denoted by a name that reflects more precisely the type of endpoint being monitored. For example, the dose of compound that kills 50% of the experimental group is referred to as the *median lethal dose* (LD_{50}) or *median lethal concentration* (LC_{50}) for exposures in which the actual dose is unknown (i.e., air or drinking water exposures). These values reflect the variability in the studied population's susceptibility to the lethal toxicity of the test substance. However, such measurements are relatively crude by today's standards and provide little information in terms of toxicologic mechanism or relevant environmental exposure levels (4). Perhaps a more relevant estimate of toxicity is the median toxic dose (TD_{50}), or the dose at which 50% of the exposed animals elicit signs of nonlethal (generalized or defined) toxicity. By measuring toxic endpoints other than death, investigators are better able to determine the dose range that could lead to symptoms of injury and that would be considered unacceptable from a quality-of-life perspective.

Receptor-Mediated Toxicity

For toxic effects that are mediated by receptor binding, affinities and efficacies may differ between chemicals. Although few environmental chemicals have been shown to elicit toxicity via receptor interaction, pollutants or chemicals such as dioxin (tetrachlorodibenzo-*p*-dioxin), polycyclic aromatic hydrocarbons, and certain polychlorinated and polybrominated biphenyls are known to interact with the endogenous aromatic hydrocarbon (Ah) receptor. With each of these chemicals, interaction with the Ah receptor is thought to initiate a cascade of events underlying their associated toxic effects.

NATURE OF TOXIC EFFECTS

Several protective biological mechanisms prevent or protect the host organism from the (potentially) toxic substance. For example, biotransforming enzymes can convert toxic chemicals to nontoxic products, metallothionein and other biomolecules can chelate and promote the excretion of toxic metals, and transport systems can eliminate chemicals or their metabolites, or both, in the bile or urine. Other protective mechanisms include DNA and tissue repair, phagocytosis of damaged cells, apoptosis, and adaptive responses such as induction or inhibition of biotransforming enzymes. With excessive exposure to chemicals, however, one or more protective mechanisms may become saturated, leading to the accumulation of toxic products. Ultimately, these products can cause extreme physiologic responses, including altered biochemical pathways, altered tissue morphology, oxidative stress (lipid peroxidation), inflammation, and aberrant growth processes.

Altered biochemical pathways can occur when foreign substances of close structural similarity to normal substances become incorporated into biochemical pathways and are then metabolized to a toxic product. A classic example is fluoroacetate, which becomes incorporated in the Krebs cycle as fluoroacetyl coenzyme A (CoA), which combines with oxaloacetate to form fluorocitrate. The latter inhibits aconitase, blocking the tricarboxylic acid cycle, and results, particularly, in cardiac and nervous system toxicity (5).

Altered tissue morphology can be seen when a chemical exposure causes some alteration in the normal tissue architecture. This can be seen as either gross changes and alterations, which are visible at the microscopic level. These include hyperplasia and hypoplasia or hypertrophy and atrophy of parenchymal cells, trans- or dedifferentiation of cells, increased prevalence of necrotic or apoptotic cells, a change in the relative proportions of cells in the tissue or infiltration of leukocytes.

Lipid peroxidation in biological membranes by free radicals starts a chain of events resulting in cellular dysfunction and death. These radicals may be oxygen, nitrogen, or carbon centered. The complex series of events includes oxidation of fatty acids to lipid hydroperoxides, which undergo degradation to various products, including toxic aldehydes. The generation of organic radicals during peroxidation results in a self-propagating reaction (6). For example, carbon tetrachloride is metabolized by a hepatic cytochrome P-450–dependent monooxygenase system to trichloromethyl and trichloromethyl peroxy radicals. These radicals initiate the process of lipid peroxidation. As membrane lipids peroxidize, membranes degrade and cells die. The end result is hepatic necrosis in the centrilobular region caused by the high concentration of cytochrome P-450 in the centrilobular hepatocytes (7).

Inflammation is a local response to irritant chemicals or a component of systemic tissue injury. The inflammatory response may be acute, with irritant or tissue-damaging materials, or chronic, with repetitive exposure to low doses of irritants or the presence of insoluble particulate material. Fibrosis may occur as a consequence of a chronic inflammatory process.

Neoplasia is defined as any new and abnormal cell growth associated with a tissue and in which the growth is uncontrolled and progressive. Tumors are classified as benign when the cells are well differentiated, have a low mitotic index, and when the tissue architecture is at least semimaintained. Malignant tumors, on the other hand, are less differentiated, have a higher mitotic index, cause a disruption in the normal tissue architecture, and can invade surrounding or distant tissues. Tumorigenesis and oncogenesis describe the development of neoplasms; the word *carcinogenesis* should be restricted to malignant neoplasms.

CLASSIFICATIONS OF TOXICITY

If harmful effects occur at the sites where a substance comes into initial contact with the body, they are referred to as *local effects*. If substances are absorbed from the sites of contact, they or their metabolites may produce toxic effects systemically. Also, because toxicity can depend on the number of exposures, an additional classification of toxic effects is the development after a single (acute) exposure or after multiple (repeated) exposures. Repeated exposure can cover a wide time span; however, it is convenient to refer to short-term exposure (not more than 5% life span), subchronic exposure (5% to 20% of life span), and chronic exposure (entire life span or a greater portion of it).

Toxicity also may be described as temporary (reversible or transient) or permanent (persistent). Latent (delayed-onset) toxicity exists when there is a period free from signs after an acute exposure. Cumulative toxicity involves progressive injury produced by successive exposures. Such toxicities can occur because of accumulation of chemical or because of an accumulation of lesions, or both. Substances may also be classified and described by the primary tissue or organ that is the target for toxicity (hepatotoxic, nephrotoxic, neurotoxic, genotoxic, ototoxic, immunotoxic). A pathologic description of the toxicity of a material requires inclusion of whether effects are local, systemic, or mixed; nature and (if known) mechanism of toxicity; organs and tissues affected; and condition of exposure (including chemical species, route, and number or magnitude of exposure).

FACTORS INFLUENCING TOXICITY OF A CHEMICAL

Multiple factors exist that can affect the response of individuals to toxicants and that provide a mechanistic basis for individual variation. Typically, factors that influence toxicity do so by altering either the concentration of toxic forms of the compound at the site of injury (a toxicokinetic effect), or the target tissue's response to toxicant exposure (a toxicodynamic effect). Toxicodynamic effects may be caused by factors that alter tissue repair after a chemical insult, by factors that alter the immune response to xenobiotics, or any other factor that affects the degree of chemical-induced toxicity without affecting the concentration of toxic forms at the site of injury. Toxicokinetic effects are caused by factors that alter the uptake of a compound into the body, its movement within the body, its conversion to toxic or nontoxic species, or its removal from the body. Therefore absorption, distribution, metabolism, and excretion (collectively referred to as *chemical disposition*) are the toxicokinetic factors that govern the amount of ultimate toxicant that reach the site of injury.

Exposure (Dosing) Characteristics

With each route of exposure, the probability of adverse effects developing in response to environmental chemical exposure can be complex and depends particularly on the magnitude, duration, and frequency of exposure. These factors determine the amount of material to which an organism is exposed (the environmental exposure dose) and hence the amount of material that can be absorbed (the absorbed dose). The latter determines the amount of toxic material (parent molecule or metabolite) available for distribution to the target site (i.e., the internal dose). For a given environmental exposure, the probability of inducing toxicity depends on the relationship between rate of absorption, metabolism (activation and detoxification), and elimination of parent compound and metabolites.

The route of chemical exposure can play a significant role in determining the site and degree of toxicity. Chemicals that undergo hepatic activation are likely to exhibit greater toxicity when given orally than if absorbed across the lung or skin. This is owing to the high proportion of material presented directly to the liver via the portal vein, resulting in greater amounts of toxic metabolites formed for presentation to the liver or other tissues. In contrast, chemicals that undergo hepatic detoxification may be less toxic orally than when absorbed percutaneously or across the respiratory tract. For example, after absorption from the lungs, chemicals can be distributed directly to tissues via arterial perfusion. This would reduce the potential for detoxification, resulting in delivery of toxicants to extrahepatic tissues.

In determining the influence of route of absorption on biotransformation and toxicity, both the magnitude and time scale for dosing should be considered. Thus, when a single large dose of a metabolically activated compound is given orally, extensive formation of toxic metabolites overwhelms detoxification mechanisms and may result in the development of acute toxicity. If the same dose of material is given orally over extended time, the amount of material presented to the liver is less at any given time. This results in a favorable balance between activation and detoxification, thereby reducing the release of toxic metabolites present in the liver and released into the systemic circulation.

With repeated exposure, the relative amounts of metabolites and the distribution and elimination of metabolites and parent compound may be different from that after an acute exposure. Repeated exposures may induce and enhance mechanisms of biotransformation of the absorbed material and thus alter the relative proportions of parent compound and metabolites (toxic or nontoxic). For compounds that are poorly biotransformed and excreted, repeated exposure leads to the accumulation of the chemical and hence to a potential for cumulative toxicity. Thus, the mechanisms underlying toxicity may differ appreciably between bolus and repeated exposures, and can explain how different exposure regimens can determine whether toxicity occurs and the nature of the toxicity.

The nature, severity, and likelihood of toxicity is also influenced by the order, magnitude, number, and frequency of dosing. This is best illustrated by the classic model of chemical carcinogenesis. If the promoting agent is given after the initiating agent, an increased incidence of tumors is observed. However, administration of the initiating agent after the promoting agent does not lead to an increased tumor incidence. In some cases, tumor formation may be surpassed. In this model, tumors do not arise in the absence of the initiating agent, or in the absence of a particular order (initiator then promoter), frequency (repeated exposure of promoting agent), and duration (extended exposure to promoting agent) of toxicant exposures.

Environmental Factors

Environmental factors are known to influence the development of toxicity, including temperature, relative humidity, exposure to sunlight, and other environmental stressors (e.g., predators, loud noise). For example, by enhancing blood flow to the skin, elevated external temperatures can increase the percutaneous absorption of chemicals. In addition, stressful stimuli, such as loud noise and cold, can increase aromatic hydroxylation, an effect that alters the disposition and potentially the outcome and degree of toxicity associated with a variety of chemical exposures.

Miscellaneous Factors

A variety of other factors may affect the nature and exhibition of toxicity, depending on the conditions of the study. For example, in animal studies, housing conditions, repeated handling, dosing volume, humidity, and diet can all influence the toxic response. Significant interlaboratory variability may also accompany otherwise standard procedures owing to variability in test conditions and procedures. How diet, stress, living conditions, and other socioeconomic factors influence the toxicologic response in humans needs extensive investigation.

ABSORPTION

Absorption of a substance from the site of exposure results from passive diffusion, facilitated diffusion, active transport, or the formation of transport vesicles (pinocytosis and phagocytosis). With each of these processes, the amount of a chemical in contact with the absorbing surface is one of the principal determinants of absorbed dose. In general, the higher the concentration, the greater the absorbed dose. However, if mechanisms other than simple diffusion across a concentration gradient are operating, a simple proportionate relationship between concentration and absorbed dose may not exist. In such instances, a rate-limiting factor could result in proportionately smaller increases in absorbed dose for incremental increases in concentration at the absorption site. In particular, when there is absorption by active transport, there may be saturation of the absorption process and a ceiling value.

The process of absorption may be facilitated or retarded by a variety of factors. Elevated temperature increases percutaneous absorption by cutaneous vasodilation while surface-active materials facilitate penetration. The integrity of the absorbing surface is an important factor relevant to evaluation of hazards from chemicals contaminating the skin. Absorbing conditions along the gastrointestinal tract are likewise dependent on pH, the amount of food, the nature of microflora, and so forth. In addition, the concentration of the chemical in contact with the surface and the surface area of contact are important features relating to absorption.

ROUTES OF ADMINISTRATION AND EXPOSURE DURATION

The primary route by which a material comes into contact with the body, and from where it may be absorbed to exert systemic toxicity, is the route of exposure. With environmental and occupational exposures the primary routes of exposure occur via contact and subsequent absorption through a body surface such as skin, eye, or mucosa of the alimentary or respiratory tract. These are, respectively, the percutaneous, transocular, oral, and inhalation routes of exposure (Fig. 4-3). Because they provide the barrier between the internal host and the environment, each of these tissues are certainly targets for toxicants. However, each of these tissues may also be targeted via systemic exposure.

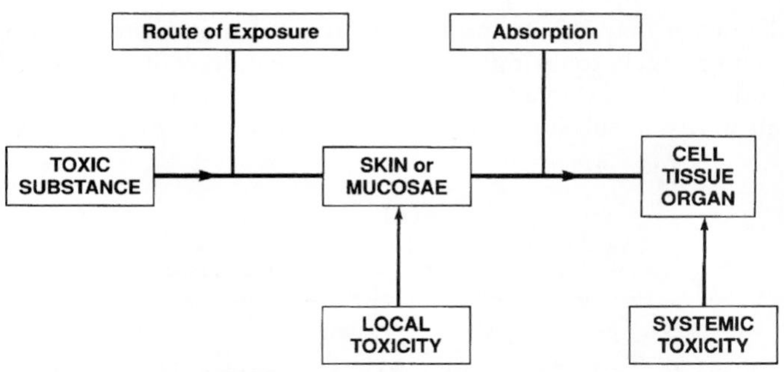

Figure 4-3. Basis for general classification of toxic effects.

Oral

The gastrointestinal tract is an important route by which systemically toxic materials may be absorbed, particularly those that are present in drinking water or food. Even inhaled compounds can undergo some oral absorption. They can be delivered to the gut by the mucociliary escalator. Oral absorption is governed by the physical-chemical properties of the chemical as well as by physiologic or biochemical properties of the host. Although lipophilic chemicals can be absorbed from the stomach, it is the small intestine, with its excessive surface area and microvilli, from which most chemicals are absorbed. Factors such as pH, food, microflora, and intestinal motility can greatly influence the extent of absorption. In addition, both the intestinal mucosa and gut microflora have the capacity to biotransform chemicals. This process can limit absorption or modify the chemical such that new chemical species are presented systemically.

Percutaneous Absorption

The percutaneous absorption of materials can be a significant route for the absorption of toxic materials. Factors influencing the percutaneous absorption of substances include skin site, integrity of skin (i.e., hydration state or abrasions), temperature, formulation, concentration, and physiochemical characteristics such as molecular weight and hydrophilic and lipophilic characteristics of the material. Although small molecular weight lipophilic compounds can be extensively absorbed, volatilization from unoccluded skin tends to reduce their absorption.

Inhalation

The penetration and distribution of fibers and particulates in the respiratory tract are determined principally by their size. Thus, in general, particles having a mass medium aerodynamic diameter larger than 50 mm do not enter the respiratory tract; those larger than 10 mm are deposited in the upper respiratory tract; those having a range of 2 to 10 mm are deposited in the trachea, bronchi, and bronchioles; and only particles with diameters smaller than 1.2 mm reach the alveoli. Thus, larger, insoluble particles are more likely to cause local reactions in the upper respiratory tract. The potential for alveolar injury and absorption is greater with smaller diameter particles (8).

The likelihood for toxicity from atmospherically dispersed materials depends on a number of factors, the most important of which include physical state, size, water solubility, concentration, and time and frequency of exposure. The water solubility of a gas or vapor influences the depth of penetration of a material into the respiratory tract. As water solubility decreases and lipid solubility increases, there is a more effective penetration toward the alveoli. Water-soluble molecules, such as formaldehyde, are deposited in the upper respiratory tract and are capable of causing primary irritation in the nose, upper respiratory tract, and eyes.

The likelihood that inhaled substances may produce local effects in the respiratory tract depends on their physical and chemical characteristics, solubility, reactivity with tissue components, and site of deposition. Dependent on the nature of the material, conditions of exposure, and biological reactivity, the types of response produced include bronchoconstriction, cell necrosis, acute or chronic inflammation, immune-mediated hypersensitivity reactions, and neoplasia, among others. The degree to which inhaled gases, vapors, and particulates are absorbed, and their potential to produce systemic toxicity, depends on molecular weight, solubility in tissue fluids, metabolism by lung tissue, diffusion rate, and ventilation rate.

Transocular

Local and systemic adverse effects in the eye may be produced by exposure to liquids, solids, and atmospherically dispersed materials. Local effects include transient inflammation, permanent injury, and hypersensitivity reactions. Penetration may lead to iritis, glaucoma, and cataract. Systemically active materials targeting the eye may also be absorbed from periocular blood vessels and nasal mucosa after passage down the nasolacrimal duct.

BIODISTRIBUTION

After absorption, chemicals circulate in blood either free or bound to plasma proteins and blood cells. Because it is the unbound form that is available for tissue distribution, the degree of binding and factors that influence the equilibrium between the free and bound forms can have a profound influence on the toxicity (as well as metabolism, storage, or excretion) of a chemical. Within the tissues, there may be binding, storage, metabolic activation, or detoxification. Binding may produce a high tissue to plasma partition ratio and be a source for slow redistribution into the circulation after the cessation of environmental exposure. Examples of storage sites include adipose tissue for lipophilic materials (including chlorinated pesticides), and bone for fluoride, lead, and strontium. The relationship between exposure dose and release rate may be complex. For example, volatile lipophilic materials are generally more rapidly released from tissue sites compared to nonvolatile lipophilic substances because they can be exhaled to reduce blood levels. Tissue permeability may be modified by tissue-specific barriers such as the blood–brain barrier, blood–testis barrier, and placenta.

BIOTRANSFORMATION AND BIOACTIVATION: THE ROLE OF METABOLISM IN CHEMICAL TOXICITY

Once they are delivered to tissues, chemicals often undergo biotransformation, which is defined as metabolism by tissue enzymes. Biotransformation is a critical event in the determination of toxicity: (a) it promotes the elimination of chemicals from the body (prevents accumulation), (b) it can lead to the formation of toxic metabolites or reactive intermediates, and (c) it is a site of chemical-chemical interactions. A large and diverse group of enzymes catalyze biotransformation and are typically classified as either phase I or phase II enzymes, depending on the reactions they catalyze. Phase I reactions modify lipophilic chemicals either by oxidation or hydrolysis to produce or expose polar functional groups. Phase II reactions add polar biomolecules to the substrate to produce very polar metabolites that often are excreted by specific mechanisms. In general, this process of biotransformation is designed to convert lipophilic substances to more hydrophilic derivatives that can be more readily eliminated in aqueous media (bile, urine). The multiplicity and catalytic diversity of phase I and II biotransformation enzymes allow an organism to biotransform an extraordinarily diverse range of chemicals. Typically, the process yields innocuous products with little or no pharmacologic activity. On the other hand, this same metabolic versatility also results in bioactivation of a broad range of chemical toxicants.

Products of biotransformation whose formation can lead to toxicity are termed *toxic metabolites.* In many cases, the toxic metabolites are transient, unstable products called *reactive intermediates* or *reactive metabolites.* Reactive metabolites are therefore the species that ultimately produce molecular damage. The common characteristic of virtually all reactive metabolites is that they have been rendered electron-deficient by metabolism. Such electron-deficient molecules, termed *electrophiles,* tend to react preferentially with electron-rich molecules, termed *nucleophiles.* In a cellular environment, the most prominent nucleophiles are sulfur, nitrogen, and oxygen atoms found on important macromolecules such as proteins and DNA. Electrophiles either add to nucleophiles to produce covalent adducts or remove electrons from nucleophiles to produce oxidation products. In either case, the structure and function of target nucleophiles is changed. These changes amount to molecular damage and can lead to cell and tissue dysfunction.

Nevertheless, bioactivation does not necessarily result in injury for two reasons. First, toxic metabolites may undergo detoxication, a diminishing of chemical reactivity. Detoxication may involve enzyme-catalyzed biotransformation or nonenzymatic chemical reactions. Second, molecular damage to cell macromolecules often can be repaired, or the affected component can be replaced. Consequently, detoxication and repair are often as important as bioactivation in determining the susceptibility of tissues to chemical injury. Tissues in which bioactivation is efficiently balanced by detoxication and repair are resistant to injury. On the other hand, high doses, repeated exposures, or increased bioactivation caused by enzyme induction may drive the relationship between bioactivation and detoxication to a threshold of imbalance and precipitate injury.

CONCEPTS OF PHASE I AND PHASE II METABOLISM

Phase I metabolism can be broadly defined as biotransformation that either adds polar functional groups or exposes latent functional groups in a substrate. Addition of polar groups is almost always achieved by introduction of oxygen into the substrate by oxidases. Exposure of latent polar groups can be accomplished either by oxidases or by hydrolases, which include esterases, decarboxylases, and amidases. Phase II metabolism is the biosynthetic conjugation of substrates with endogenous biomolecules such as amino acids, glucuronic acid, sulfate, and glutathione. Specific transport systems for the conjugates direct their excretion from tissues. Together, phase I and II metabolism convert lipophilic chemicals to more hydrophilic products and direct them to specific excretion pathways. Biotransformation of the leukemogenic solvent benzene is an excellent example of the complementary roles of phase I and II metabolism (Fig. 4-4). Phase I metabolism first introduces polarity by adding a hydroxyl group to convert benzene to phenol. Phase II conjugation with the bulky, polar sulfate group (or glucuronic acid) amplifies the polar characteristics of phenol and produces a very water-soluble product that is readily excreted.

Organs of Biotransformation and Significance of Extrahepatic Bioactivation

The liver is the most important organ of biotransformation, owing largely to its high content and great diversity of phase I and II enzymes. In addition, the splanchnic circulation carries all orally absorbed chemicals through the liver before they

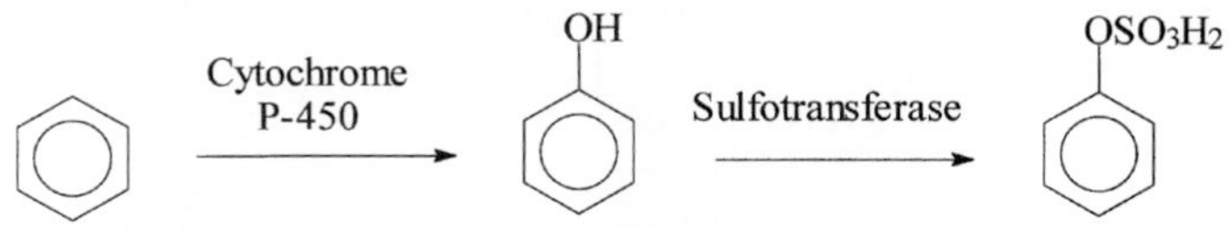

Figure 4-4. Metabolism of benzene to phenol and phenyl sulfate by phase I and phase II enzymes.

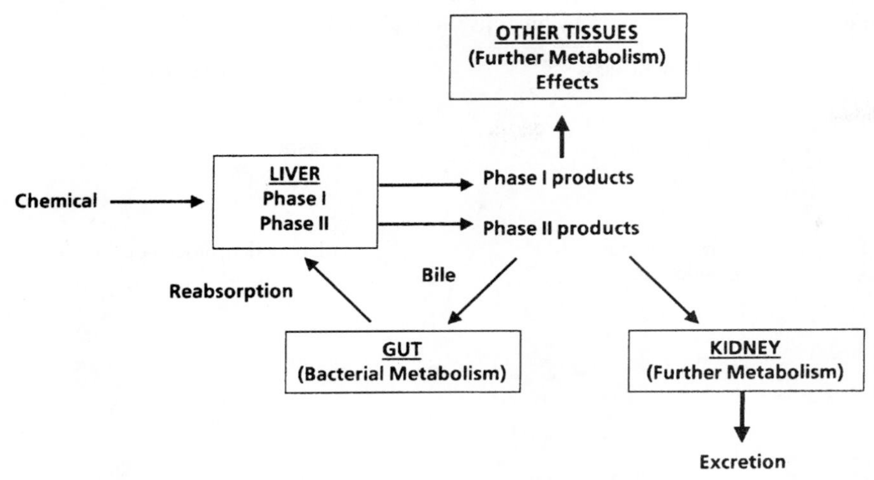

Figure 4-5. Interrelationships between organs involved in biotransformation.

reach the systemic circulation, allowing hepatic "first pass" metabolism to occur. The leaky hepatic capillary network and the extensive surface area provided by hepatocyte microvilli promote efficient hepatic extraction of chemicals at the cellular level. The liver also is the major metabolite-releasing organ (Fig. 4-5). Phase I products released into the systemic circulation may then produce effects in other tissues (9). The liver also releases conjugate products of phase II metabolism into the blood, from which they may be extracted for renal metabolism, and into the bile, from which they may enter cycles of enterohepatic recirculation. Despite this dominant role of hepatic metabolism, other tissues may make critical contributions to bioactivation. The kidney and lung both contain relatively high levels of phase I and II enzymes. The kidney is particularly important because this organ has specific systems for the absorption and catabolism of phase II metabolite conjugates. These and other tissues, including the stomach, intestine, gonads, and skin, may play key roles in local generation of toxic metabolites despite their modest contributions to systemic clearance of xenobiotics (10).

Although hepatic metabolism plays a central role in biotransformation, extrahepatic bioactivation may nonetheless be of great importance in determining many toxic responses. When extrahepatic bioactivation plays a crucial role in toxicity, it does so by generating high levels of reactive metabolites in the susceptible tissue, usually within a specific cell type (11). Some very reactive metabolites may not survive in the circulation at levels sufficient to induce critical injury in extrahepatic tissues, even when hepatic production of the reactive metabolite exceeds that in other tissues. Extrahepatic tissues also may either produce certain toxic metabolites more efficiently, or they may produce different metabolites of greater toxicity than does the liver. Finally, extrahepatic metabolism may be uniquely capable of converting nonreactive toxic metabolites from the liver to reactive metabolites.

Enzymes of Bioactivation: Phase I Enzymes

The remarkable variety of chemicals that undergo bioactivation is a consequence both of the diversity and catalytic versatility of phase I enzymes. Most biotransformation enzymes exist in multiple forms, called *isozymes*, each of which may accept many structurally diverse substrates. Phase I enzymes involved in bioactivation are grouped here by the types of reactions they catalyze: (a) the mixed-function oxygenases: cytochromes P-450 and flavin-containing monooxygenase (FMO), (b) prostaglandin synthetase-hydroperoxidase (PGS) and other peroxidases, (c) alcohol dehydrogenase and aldehyde dehydrogenase, (d) flavoprotein reductases, and (e) epoxide hydrase. Table 4-2 lists representative examples of bioactivation reactions that are catalyzed by phase I enzymes.

Mixed-Function Oxygenases

Cytochromes P-450 and FMO both reside in the endoplasmic reticulum of cells and accept reducing equivalents from reduced nicotinamide adenine dinucleotide phosphate (NADPH) (Fig. 4-6). The P-450s are a large superfamily of enzymes that may be subdivided into several complex multigene families (12). Individual tissues frequently contain several different P-450 isozymes, and tissue-specific forms also occur. The expression of individual enzymes may be subject to genetic polymorphisms, and various isozymes may be induced by drugs, hormones, and environmental chemicals. P-450s are also subject to inactivation by suicide substrates and reactive metabolites (13). P-450 isozymes often display overlapping substrate specificities, so that more than one isozyme may contribute to biotransformation of a chemical, although one isozyme often predominates. P-450s accept electrons from NADPH via the intermediary flavoprotein NADPH-cytochrome P-450 reductase. P-450s are hemoproteins, the levels of which are controlled in part by heme biosynthesis and thus related to iron metabolism. Metabolic alterations, such as starvation, that lower the NADPH to the oxidized form of nicotinamide adenine dinucleotide phosphate ($NADP^+$) ratio can lower enzyme activity. Oxidations by P-450 dominate phase I biotransformation. P-450s catalyze the oxidation of virtually all classes of organic molecules. P-450 substrates range from simple one-carbon molecules, such as chloroform, to steroids and the complex heterocycle cyclosporin. P-450s also catalyze the reductive bioactivation of a limited number of halogenated hydrocarbons, such as carbon tetrachloride and the anesthetic halothane, to produce reactive free radicals (13). This unusual reaction is favored under hypoxic conditions.

In contrast to the vast biochemical diversity of the P-450s, FMOs catalyze the NADPH-dependent oxidation of a more limited range of substrates. These include nitrogen, sulfur, phosphorous, and other heteroatom-containing compounds. In addition, those forms that have been sequenced fall into a family of only five classes (i.e., FMO1, FMO2, FMO3, FMO4, and FMO5), which is much less diverse than the P-450 gene family. FMO expression is both tissue- and species-dependent (14), and, in animal models, FMOs have been shown to be regulated

TABLE 4-2. Examples of reactive intermediates formed by bioactivation: phase I processes

Parent chemical	Reactive intermediate	Generic class	Enzymes involved
$CHCl_3$ chloroform	$Cl\text{-}C(=O)\text{-}Cl$ phosgene[a]	Acyl halide	P-450
$CH_2{=}CH\text{-}CH_2OH$ allyl alcohol	$CH_2{=}CH\text{-}C(=O)\text{-}H$ acrolein	α, β-Unsaturated aldehyde	Alcohol dehydrogenase
$ClCH_2CH_2Cl$ 1,2-dichloroethane	$ClCH_2C(=O)\text{-}H$ 2-chloroacetaldehyde	Aldehyde	P-450
$(CH_3)_2N\text{-}N{=}O$ 1,1-dimethylnitrosamine	$CH_3\text{-}N_2^+$ methyldiazonium ion[a]	Alkyl diazonium ion	P-450
$CH_3(CH_2)_4CH_3$ *n*-hexane	$CH_3\text{-}C(=O)\text{-}(CH_2)_2\text{-}C(=O)\text{-}CH_3$ 2,5-hexanedione	Diketone	1. P-450[b] 2. Alcohol dehydrogenase
$ClCH{=}CH_2$ vinyl chloride	$ClCH\text{-}CH_2$ (epoxide, O bridging) chloroethylene oxide	Epoxide	P-450
benzo[*a*]pyrene	HO, OH benzo[*a*]pyrene diol epoxide	Diol epoxide	1. P-450[b] 2. Epoxide hydrase 3. P-450 or peroxidase
benzene	p-benzoquinone	Quinone	1. P-450[b] 2. Peroxidase
CCl_4 carbon tetrachloride	$\bullet CCl_3$ trichloromethyl radical[a]	Alkyl radical	P-450 (reduction)
H_3C–N⁺–N⁺–CH_3 paraquat	H_3C–N⁺–N–CH_3 paraquat	Cation radical	Flavoprotein reductases
H_2N–C₆H₄–OH p-aminophenol	HN=C₆H₄=O *p*-benzoquinone imine	Quinone imine	Peroxidase
$CH_3C(=S)NH_2$ thioacetamide	$CH_3C(=S(O)_2)NH_2$ thioacetamide-S,S-dioxide	S,S–Dioxide	FMO, P-450

FMO, flavin-containing monooxygenase.
[a]Rearrangement of primary metabolite yields reactive intermediate.
[b]Multiple enzymatic steps are represented in sequence.

by endogenous hormones, dietary influences, and other tissue-specific factors (15). For example, FMO levels in rat liver are positively regulated by testosterone and repressed by estradiol. However, the means by which FMOs are regulated in humans is uncertain.

Prostaglandin Synthetase-Hydroperoxidase and Other Peroxidases

A diverse group of peroxidases catabolize hydrogen peroxide or other hydroperoxides to water and alcohols (see Fig. 4-6).

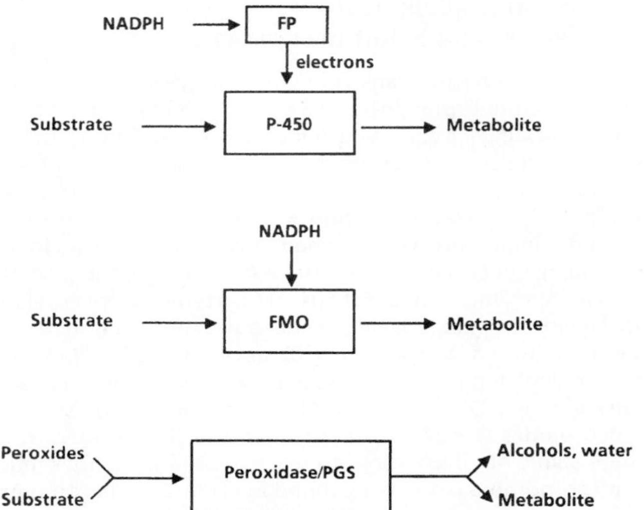

Figure 4-6. Comparison of enzymes and cofactor requirements for phase I bioactivation by P-450 (top), flavin-containing monooxygenase (FMO) (middle), and peroxidases (bottom). FP, flavoprotein reductase; NADPH, nicotinamide adenine dinucleotide phosphate; PGS, prostaglandin synthetase-hydroperoxidase.

Oxidants generated as side products in these reactions may then produce reactive metabolites from many chemicals, including aromatic amines, phenols, hydroquinones, alkenes, and polycyclic aromatic hydrocarbons (16). Peroxidases, such as leukocyte myeloperoxidase, eosinophil peroxidase, and chloroperoxidase, use hydrogen peroxide produced by the leukocyte respiratory burst. PGS, on the other hand, forms prostaglandin hydroperoxides from arachidonic acid as primary products. During the subsequent reduction of these hydroperoxides, other cosubstrates, such as drugs and chemicals, are oxidized. This mechanism, known as *cooxidation*, consumes arachidonic acid and a cosubstrate to produce prostaglandins and oxidized cosubstrates. The wide distribution of PGS in mammalian tissues suggests that it may be involved in a number of extrahepatic bioactivation reactions, particularly in tissues with low P-450 content, such as the renal inner medulla and the urinary bladder endothelium.

Dehydrogenases

Owing to its high content of alcohol and aldehyde dehydrogenases, the liver is the major organ of alcohol metabolism. Alcohol dehydrogenases oxidize primary, secondary, and aromatic alcohols to aldehydes and ketones. Aldehyde dehydrogenases oxidize a variety of aldehydes to the corresponding carboxylic acids. Both enzymes use the oxidized form of nicotinamide adenine dinucleotide (NAD^+) as a cofactor. A specific formaldehyde dehydrogenase uses NAD^+ and reduced glutathione together as cofactors to oxidize formaldehyde to formic acid. Both enzymes exist in multiple forms with overlapping substrate specificities and are ethanol-inducible. Rates of alcohol metabolism reflect not only enzyme levels, but also the disposition of inhibitory aldehyde products and cofactor levels. Substrates of major toxicologic significance are ethanol, methanol, ethylene glycol, and allelic alcohols, whose conversion to reactive aldehydes and ketones often results in tissue injury. Although it generally serves a detoxication role, aldehyde dehydrogenase may participate in bioactivation of ethylene glycol by oxidizing glycolaldehyde to oxalate and of allyl alcohol to acrolein.

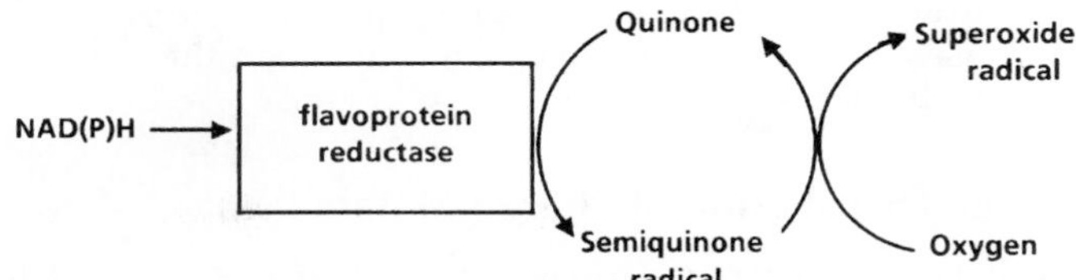

Figure 4-7. Oxygen radical production by flavoprotein-catalyzed redox cycling of a quinone.

Flavoprotein Reductases

The flavoprotein reductases NADPH-cytochrome P-450 reductase and reduced nicotinamide adenine dinucleotide (NADH) dehydrogenase bioactivate certain quinone-containing chemicals, nitroaromatics, and bipyridylium compounds through a single electron transfer to generate radicals (17). These radical intermediates may transfer an electron to molecular oxygen, which regenerates the parent compound and initiates an oxygen radical cascade that may ultimately damage cellular biomolecules (Fig. 4-7). The NAD(P)H-driven oxidation reduction of chemicals, which gives rise to oxygen radicals, is termed *redox cycling* and is largely dependent on the redox potentials of the enzyme and substrate, so not all quinones, nitroaromatics, and bipyridylium compounds are reduced. Chemicals whose bioactivation by this mechanism leads to oxygen radical formation include the bipyridylium herbicide paraquat, the antitumor agent doxorubicin hydrochloride (Adriamycin), a variety of nitroaromatic compounds, including the antibiotic nitrofurantoin, and some iron and copper chelates (17).

Epoxide Hydrases

Like the aldehyde dehydrogenases, epoxide hydrases serve both bioactivation and detoxication functions. Epoxide hydrases catalyze the hydrolytic opening of epoxides to trans-dihydrodiols (18). Microsomal and cytosolic forms of epoxide hydrase have been characterized and require no cofactors or prosthetic groups. The leading example of bioactivation by the microsomal enzyme, hydrolysis of polycyclic aromatic hydrocarbon monoepoxides, would appear at first to be detoxication. However, the dihydrodiol products are then oxidized again by P-450 to reac-

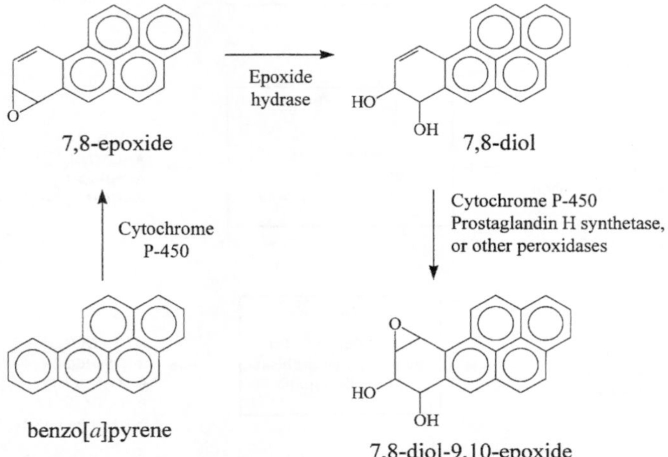

Figure 4-8. Sequential bioactivation of benzo[*a*]pyrene. Multiple enzymes catalyze the bioactivation of benzo[*a*]pyrene to the 7, 8-diol-9, 10-epoxide, the ultimate carcinogenic form. Additional metabolites, not shown, are also formed.

tive diol epoxides, which are poor substrates for epoxide hydrase and are much more carcinogenic than the monoepoxides (19) (Fig. 4-8).

Tissue Distribution of Phase I Metabolism

With the exception of peroxidases, the highest levels of all of the phase I enzymes are in the liver. P-450s are found in many other tissues, including kidney, lung, intestinal mucosa, skin, adrenal cortex, and testis (10). Likewise, FMO messenger RNA (mRNA) levels have been detected in the lung, liver, intestine, kidney, esophagus, and nasal mucosa. Their relative distributions are clearly species- and gender-dependent (15). Peroxidases are widely distributed but probably are important bioactivation enzymes only in tissues where P-450 activities are relatively low, such as bone marrow, renal inner medulla, uterine endometrium, bladder epithelium, and skin (16). Bioactivation by dehydrogenases is limited largely to the liver.

ENZYMES OF BIOTRANSFORMATION OR BIOACTIVATION: PHASE II ENZYMES

Most phase II biotransformation reactions produce inactive metabolites or result in detoxication. Nevertheless, phase II enzymes participate in the bioactivation of certain classes of chemicals. Like phase I biotransformation, phase II processes operate on a structurally diverse range of substrates. This characteristic reflects the relatively broad substrate specificity of individual enzymes and the contributions of multiple enzyme forms to metabolism. Phase II enzymes are grouped here by category: (a) ester or amide-forming enzymes, such as uridinediphosphoglucuronyl transferases (UDPGTs), sulfotransferases, and acetyl-CoA:amine *N*-acetyltransferases (NATs); (b) the glutathione-*S*-transferases (GSTs); and (c) cysteine conjugate β-lyase, which cleaves certain cysteine conjugates to produce reactive metabolites during the renal catabolism of glutathione conjugates.

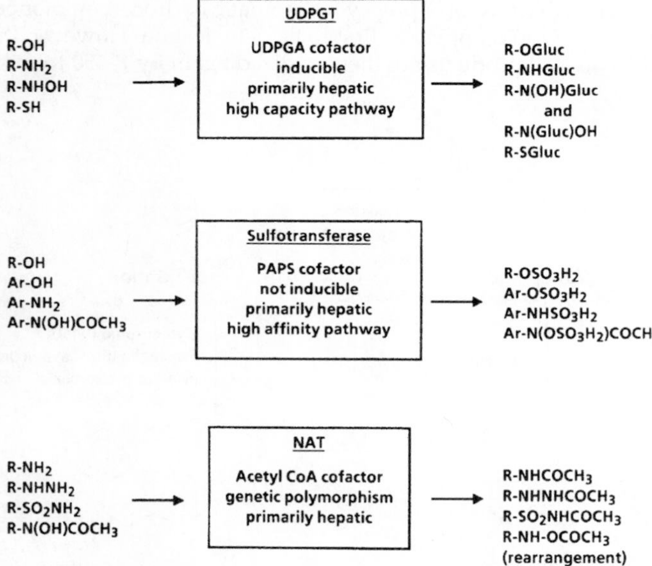

Figure 4-9. Reactions and characteristic features of phase II biotransformation reactions by uridinediphosphoglucuronyl transferase (UDPGT; top), sulfotransferase (middle), and *N*-acetyltransferase (NAT; bottom). CoA, coenzyme A; PAPs, cofactor 3'-phosphoadenosine-5'-phosphosulfate; UDPGA, uridinediphosphoglucuronic acid.

Uridinediphosphoglucuronyl Transferases and Sulfotransferases

UDPGT catalyzes the transfer of glucuronic acid from the cofactor uridinediphosphoglucuronic acid (UDPGA) to nucleophilic carboxylic acids, hydroxyl groups, amines, and thiols on substrates to form esters or ethers (*O*-glucuronides), amides (*N*-glucuronides), and thiolesters (*S*-glucuronides) (20) (Fig. 4-9). Although UDPGTs are less inducible than P-450s, agents such as phenobarbital, polycyclic aromatic hydrocarbons, dioxin, and polyhalogenated biphenyls induce up to fivefold increases in selected enzyme activities. Different isozymes display relative specificity for planar aromatic substrates, bulky aliphatic substrates, bilirubin, and steroids (20). Levels of the UDPGA cofactor are depleted by fasting, which may lower glucuronidation rates *in vivo*. UDPGTs catalyze the formation of both *N*- and *O*-glucuronides from *N*-hydroxyarylamines. The former are the more stable but decompose to reactive products under mildly acidic conditions, such as are found in urine (21). This decomposition to reactive products is thought to explain, in part, the generation of bladder tumors by aromatic amines.

Several different sulfotransferase enzymes transfer sulfate from the cofactor 3'-phosphoadenosine-5'-phosphosulfate (PAPS) to alcohols, phenols, and hydroxysteroids to produce the corresponding sulfate esters (22) (see Fig. 4-9). One of these enzymes, aryl sulfate sulfur transferase, mediates bioactivation of aryl hydroxylamines and arylhydroxamic acids. This enzyme transfers the sulfuryl group from a phenolic sulfuryl donor to an acceptor phenol without the use of PAPS or PAP (23). Although not inducible, the enzyme is inhibited by pentachlorophenol and 2,6-dichloro-4-nitrophenol (22). Sulfotransferases often display a higher substrate affinity than do UDPGTs. The small hepatic PAPS cofactor pool may become depleted and produce a dose-dependent shift from sulfation to glucuronidation. Sulfation is therefore regarded as a high affinity–low capacity system and glucuronidation as a low affinity–high capacity system. Nevertheless, the PAPS cofactor pool and, consequently, sulfotransferase activity is less susceptible to dietary manipulation than is the UDPGA pool.

Acetylcoenzyme A: Amine *N*-Acetyltransferase

NAT catalyzes the acetylation by acetyl-CoA of aromatic primary amines, *N*-hydroxyarylamines, sulfonamides, hydrazines, and hydrazides (see Fig. 4-9). NAT also catalyzes the rearrangement of arylhydroxamic acids to *N*-acetoxyarylamines (Ar-$NHOCOCH_3$), which are reactive alkylating agents (24). A genetic polymorphism in acetylation activity has been characterized in humans and rabbits. In the rabbit model, this polymorphism governs susceptibility to certain arylamine toxicants and carcinogens whose bioactivation involves *N*-acetylation (25). In addition to its role in arylamine and arylhydroxamic acid carcinogenesis, NAT initiates the bioactivation of hydrazine-containing drugs such as isoniazid. Human genetic polymorphisms in acetylation activities are caused by mutations in the gene for NAT2 (26). Work suggests that rapid acetylator phenotype may be a predisposing factor in some human cancers associated with exposure to carcinogenic arylamines (27).

Aryl sulfotransferase and UDPGT, along with NAT, complete the biotransformation of toxic and carcinogenic arylamines (Ar-NH_2) and *N*-acetylarylamides (Ar-$NHCOCH_3$) by converting their phase I metabolites [*N*-hydroxyarylamines (Ar-NHOH) and arylhydroxamic acids (Ar-N(OH)$COCH_3$)] to reactive esters (24) (Fig. 4-10). The *N*,*O*-esters produced by these enzymes differ in stability and in chemical reactivity toward proteins and DNA.

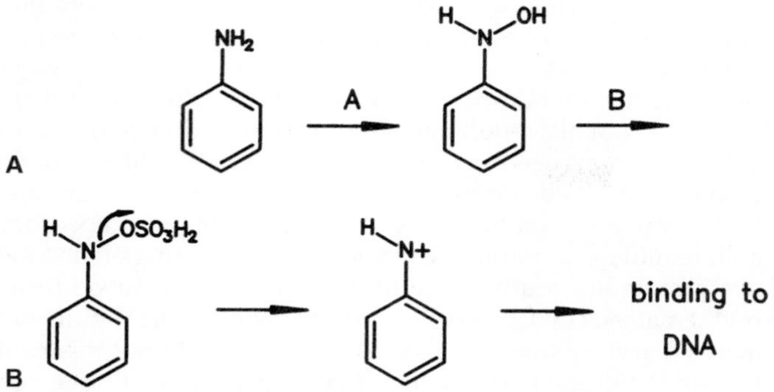

Figure 4-10. Formation of a reactive *N,O*-sulfate ester from an arylamine carcinogen by phase I *N*-hydroxylation **A:** followed by phase II conjugation. **B:** The labile sulfate ester decomposes to produce a reactive *arylnitrenium ion,* which binds to DNA. Decomposition of analogous *N*-acetoxy and *N,O*-glucuronide derivatives also yields arylnitrenium ions.

The *N,O*-sulfates and *N*-acetoxy derivatives of arylhydroxamic acids are much more reactive than the *N,O*-glucuronides and *N*-hydroxy-*N*-glucuronides, which may serve as transport forms of the carcinogens. Consequently, sulfotransferase and NAT are critical mediators of hepatocarcinogenic bioactivation, whereas UDPGT-dependent bioactivation may contribute to extrahepatic carcinogenesis (24).

Glutathione-*S*-Transferases

GSTs catalyze conjugate formation between reduced glutathione (GSH) and electrophilic cosubstrates. Although GSTs are found in virtually all tissues, the liver contains the highest levels, in which GSTs comprise up to 10% of the total hepatic cytosolic protein. GSTs comprise a large enzyme family in which expression of isozymes is often tissue-specific. Many xenobiotics induce GST, and the human enzymes display extensive polymorphism (28). GSH serves many critical functions within cells, including detoxification of reactive chemicals, transport of amino acids, synthesis of leukotrienes, regulation of thiol stores, and protection from oxidative stress, among others. Its depletion by conjugation with reactive metabolites can thus disrupt vital homeostatic mechanisms and increase the vulnerability of cells to toxic insult. For example, GSH can detoxify reactive oxygen species. In the absence of GSH, these species can promote lipid peroxidation and other deleterious events. Although GSTs primarily function as a versatile and effective enzymatic detoxication system, four mechanisms of GST-dependent bioactivation have been identified (29). Depending on the substrate, GSH conjugates can release a toxic metabolite, cyclize to yield a reactive episulfonium ion, or be degraded to toxic sulfhydryl or cysteinyl conjugates (Fig. 4-11).

Cysteine Conjugate β-Lyase

Renal β-lyase is found both in cytosol and in mitochondria. This pyridoxal phosphate-containing enzyme, which is identical to glutamine transaminase K, cleaves cysteine-*S*-conjugates to pyruvate, ammonia, and a thiol fragment (30). Depending on the structure of the conjugated xenobiotic moiety, the thiol fragment may rearrange to a reactive electrophile. The activity of the enzyme is stimulated by α-keto acids, which regenerate the pyridoxal form of the enzyme from the pyridoxamine form. β-Lyase catalyzes the bioactivation of a limited number of halocarbon-cysteine conjugates, which are ultimately derived from glutathione conjugation. This enzyme thus completes a bioactivation process begun by GST in the liver. The roles of GST and β-lyase in the bioactivation of the nephrotoxicant hexachlorobutadiene are summarized in Figure 4-11.

Tissue Distribution of Phase II Metabolism

Phase II enzymes occur in the principal organs of metabolism, including liver, kidney, lung, gut, and skin. However, the liver contains the highest levels of UDPGT, sulfotransferase, and *N*-acetyltransferase activity and probably is the principal site of bioactivation by these enzymes (31). GST-catalyzed bioactivation is potentially important in any tissue where it occurs, because some of the products formed are reactive enough to cause damage at the site where they are formed. Indeed, chemicals such as halogenated aliphatic fumigants, whose bioactivation requires only GST, often produce damage at the site of exposure (32). β-Lyase activity is found in both liver and kidney, but cysteine conjugates that are substrates for this enzyme are generated exclusively in the kidney by renal catabolism of glutathione conjugates.

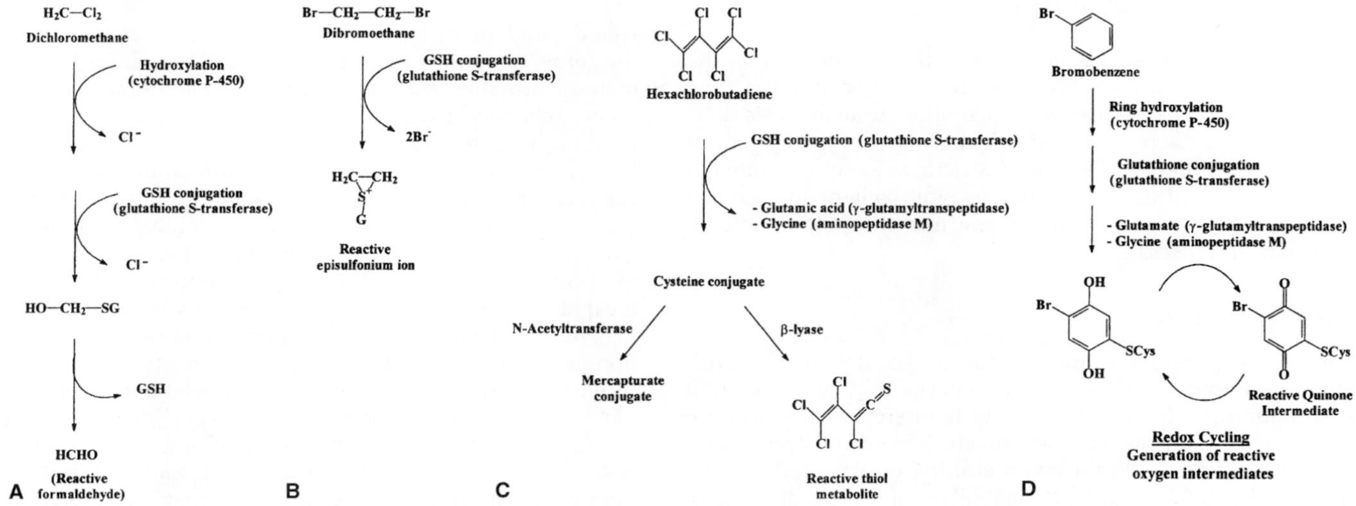

Figure 4-11. Bioactivation of chemicals by glutathione conjugation.

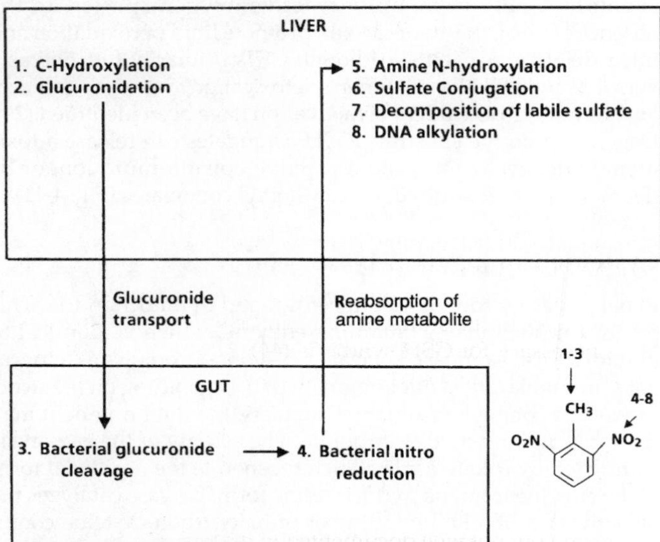

Figure 4-12. Interplay between hepatic and gut bacterial enzymes in the bioactivation of the hepatocarcinogen 2,6-dinitrotoluene. Hepatic metabolism to the glucuronide (steps 1 and 2) presents the molecule to gut bacteria, which reduce the nitro group to an amine (step 4). Reabsorption, hepatic *N*-hydroxylation, and conjugation (steps 5 and 6) produce a labile *N,O*-sulfate ester, which decomposes to a reactive intermediate that alkylates DNA.

Gastrointestinal Bacterial Enzymes

Metabolism of chemicals by bacteria in the gut may cleave phase II metabolites to release their precursors. This is accomplished by bacterial hydrolases that catabolize glucuronides and sulfates. Reabsorption of these completes the cycle of enterohepatic recirculation. In addition, the anaerobic environment of the gut promotes reductive biotransformation of chemicals by bacteria. Bacterial reduction of nitroaromatic compounds yields amines that may be reabsorbed and undergo further hepatic bioactivation (33). Bacterial β-glucuronidase and nitro-reductases play an indispensable role in the multistep bioactivation of 2,6-dinitrotoluene (Fig. 4-12).

FACTORS AFFECTING BIOTRANSFORMATION: THE METABOLIC BASIS OF INDIVIDUAL VARIATION

The ability of tissues to bioactivate chemicals depends on the variety, activities, and levels of biotransformation enzymes they contain. To a great extent, enzyme activities are an intrinsic characteristic for a given tissue and reflect genetic controls, age, and gender. Superimposed on these restrictions are environmental factors that may dramatically alter enzyme content and activity. These extrinsic factors include enzyme induction and inhibition, nutrition, and disease.

Genetic Factors

Subtle differences in enzyme structure and content between different individuals may account for interindividual variation in susceptibility to chemical toxicity. Such differences may produce variations in enzyme activities toward certain substrates. Certain individuals within a given ethnic population display a decreased P-450–dependent metabolism of certain drugs (34). Studies have shown that certain hepatic P-450s in slow metabolizers are structurally altered compared with the corresponding enzymes in normal individuals (35). Slow metabolizers may also lack the isozyme required to catalyze a particular reaction, as has been found in some rat strains that display genetic variation in drug metabolism. This structural alteration of the enzyme probably reflects genetic alterations and could either enhance or suppress bioactivation, depending on the role of the enzyme involved. Polymorphisms in drug metabolism also have been observed for *N*-acetylation of aromatic amine–, aryl sulfonamide–, and aryl hydrazine–containing drugs (36). Slow acetylators are more prone to develop drug-induced lupus erythematosus (36), whereas rapid acetylators more rapidly bioactivate aryl hydrazines. Extensive genetic polymorphisms in human P-450 and GST enzymes (35), which are the most extensively studied human biotransformation enzymes, suggest that genetic diversity in human populations could influence susceptibility to toxicants and carcinogens.

Gender

Large gender differences in monooxygenase activities have been reported in rats and mice and are a result of hormonal regulation of some biotransformation enzymes (37). In humans, such differences are less apparent, because gender-linked variation may be obscured by the superimposition of extensive genetic variation.

Species and Strain

Species and strain differences in susceptibility to chemically induced toxicity may be due to differences in rates of absorption, metabolism, formation of toxic metabolites, and excretion. In some cases, species differences may cause animal studies to give underestimates, and in other instances overestimates, for acute oral toxicity to humans. For example, Sprague-Dawley rats are much less susceptible to the hepatotoxicity caused by 1,2-dichlorobenzene than Fischer-344 rats. It appears that these differences may be attributed to the differential production of reactive oxygenated metabolites as well as the different rates of glutathione depletion between rat strains (38). In addition, because humans generate significantly fewer of the metabolites postulated as being responsible for hepatic injury, their risk after exposure to 1,2-DCB may likely be overestimated when risk assessment is based solely on toxicity studies conducted in the rat.

Age

Age-dependent variation in metabolism is most prominent in the fetus/neonate and in the elderly. That underdeveloped biotransformation enzyme systems in neonates may predispose them to chemical toxicities is well known. These toxicities result from the accumulation of a parent chemical or its toxic metabolites. This could also lead to fetal accumulation of some toxic chemicals from the maternal circulation, despite maternal contributions to clearance. However, to suggest that biotransformation is largely absent in the fetus and the neonate is an oversimplification. Unlike nonprimate species, the human fetus is capable of bioactivating foreign chemicals by the P-450 system (39). In addition, placental enzymes may contribute to bioactivation (40). Biotransformation in the fetus/neonate should therefore be regarded as a dynamic characteristic that reflects the variable states of development of several enzyme systems involved. It should be emphasized that other factors involved with the disposition of chemicals are also altered in the very young and the elderly. These include hepatic and renal blood flow, excretory mechanisms, and possibly other changes which certainly can influence chemical-induced toxicity.

Enzyme Induction

Many drugs, environmental pollutants, and natural products share the ability to induce the synthesis of biotransformation enzymes. This phenomenon, called *induction*, has been extensively studied in animals and has important implications for bioactivation in humans. Induction requires increased *de novo* synthesis of new enzymes as a result of gene activation by the inducing agent. This is reflected by increased levels of mRNA that code for the induced proteins. Some inducers, such as the polycyclic aromatic hydrocarbons and 2,3,7,8-tetrachlorodibenzodioxin, interact with an endogenous cytosolic receptor in target cells referred to as the *aryl hydrocarbon* (*Ah*) receptor. This complex migrates to the nucleus and activates genes for inducible proteins. The mechanism of action of other inducers, such as barbiturates, is not as well understood. Even so, accompanying phenobarbital induction of CYP2B1 is an increased production and stabilization of CYP2B1 mRNA. Inducers may enhance the synthesis of some isozymes within an enzyme class yet suppress the synthesis of others. For example, both phenobarbital and the polychlorinated biphenyl mixture Arochlor 1254 induce several rat P-450s while concomitantly lowering the levels of some P-450s found in uninduced animals. Moreover, inducing agents often affect levels of more than one enzyme system, as illustrated by the ability of phenobarbital, polyhalogenated biphenyls, and polycyclic aromatic hydrocarbons to induce not only P-450 but also UDPGT and GST. Concomitant induction of multiple phase I and II enzymes makes the overall effect of an inducer on bioactivation difficult to predict.

One consequence of enzyme induction is increased enzyme activity in the principal tissues of bioactivation. This is observed, for example, with carbon tetrachloride or bromobenzene bioactivation in the liver. After enzyme induction with phenobarbital, the bioactivation of these two chemicals is dramatically increased, as is the severity of the liver injury they produce. Alternatively, induction can produce such a disproportionate increase in bioactivation in another tissue that the locus of bioactivation shifts to that tissue.

In humans, induction may occur as the result of exposure to chemicals through chronic lifestyle habits (e.g., polycyclic aromatic hydrocarbon ingestion through smoking, alcohol consumption) or through acute treatment with therapeutic agents (e.g., barbiturates, rifampin). Certain environmental pollutants (polyhalogenated biphenyls, dioxins, halogenated insecticides) may induce biotransformation enzymes in humans, as they are potent inducers in animal models (31).

Enzyme Inhibition

Like inducers, inhibitors can potentially enhance or inhibit bioactivation. Bioactivation that involves a particular enzyme can be blocked by inhibiting the enzyme. On the other hand, inhibition may block nontoxic pathways of biotransformation and direct increased amounts of substrate through a toxic pathway, a phenomenon referred to as *metabolic switching*.

There are different types of inhibitors (41): (a) competitive inhibitors, such as alternate substrates; (b) noncompetitive inhibitors, such as alkylating agents that react with enzymes but do not compete with substrates; and (c) noncompetitive inhibitors, which form enzyme-bound, reactive metabolites that inhibit or destroy (suicide inactivators) the enzyme during its catalytic cycle. Other inhibitors may deplete cells of a prosthetic group or cofactor. For example, cobalt depletes cells of the P-450 precursor, heme, by inducing heme oxygenase, its major degradation enzyme, and by inhibiting the rate-limiting enzyme in heme biosynthesis, δ-aminolevulinate synthetase (42). Other agents deplete GSH (43), which is required for GST-dependent conjugation and which provides a protective barrier. Inhibition of bioactivation also can occur with repeated low doses of a chemical that gives rise to reactive metabolites that destroy enzymes. Such low-dose pretreatment has been effective in protecting laboratory animals against several toxic chemicals.

Nutrition and Disease

Biotransformation can be curtailed or altered under conditions of nutritional insufficiency and disease. In laboratory animals, 24- to 36-hour starvation lowers the NADPH/$NADP^+$ ratio, depletes uridine diphosphate-glucuronic acid for glucuronide synthesis, and depletes tissue stores of GSH and sulfur-containing amino acids necessary for GSH synthesis (44). For example, acute oral toxicity of drugs may range significantly, with a higher toxicity in starved animals. This greater acute toxicity in the starved animals may be due to accelerated gastric emptying and increased intestinal absorption. Less severe dietary deficiencies, such as low protein diets, carbohydrate, vitamin, and mineral deficiencies all tend to reduce biotransformation in animals. Similar effects are postulated but not well documented in humans (44). Hepatic diseases, including cirrhosis, hepatitis, and obstructive jaundice retard the hepatic clearance of many drugs and are expected to block the hepatic bioactivation of toxicants. Alternatively, hypothyroidism, hepatic, renal, pulmonary, or gastrointestinal disease may promote bioactivation and toxicity in other tissues by slowing or removing nontoxic clearance pathways. Diet can also markedly influence the natural tumor incidence in animals and modulate carcinogen-induced tumor incidence. The importance of dietary factors in toxicity has been reviewed (45).

TIME OF DOSING

Diurnal and seasonal variations in toxicity may relate to circadian variations in biochemical, physiologic, and hormonal profiles. For example, with nocturnal animals, such as mice, GSH levels are highest in the morning hours, after they have been feeding throughout the night. Because of this, mice are less susceptible to acetaminophen toxicity in the morning (at the end of the dark phase), as opposed to the late afternoon (at the end of the light phase).

REACTIVE METABOLITES AS ULTIMATE CHEMICAL TOXICANTS AND CARCINOGENS

A common misconception regarding reactive metabolites is that they react indiscriminately with cellular components. Due to their electrophilic nature, reactive metabolites either oxidize or form covalent adducts with cellular nucleophiles. Selectivity in electrophile-nucleophile interactions results from mutually reinforcing chemical reactivities of both species (41). Electrophiles preferentially modify nucleophiles with whose chemical properties they are especially compatible. Consequently, reactive metabolites display a considerable degree of target selectivity in their reactions with biomolecules. For example, α, β-unsaturated carbonyl compounds and quinones bind almost exclusively to proteins, whereas carbocations (carbonium ions, R_3C^+) and epoxides extensively modify DNA. Acylating agents, such as isocyanates and acyl halides, form stable adducts with lysine amines in proteins but are not known to react with DNA (41).

Free radicals and related oxidants are ubiquitous products of normal metabolism, and formation of oxidants by certain cell types is essential to health. For example, formation of oxidants by activated phagocytes plays a key role in cell-mediated immunity. However, chemical toxicants may lead to free radical-mediated oxidative damage, either due to direct stimulation of

TABLE 4-3. Cytochrome P-450 isozyme-specific bioactivation of chemicals

CYP 1A2
2-Aminofluorene
2-Aminoanthracene
2-Naphthylamine
4-Aminobiphenyl
CYP 2E1
Benzene
Carbon tetrachloride
Chloroform
Methylene chloride
Trichloroethylene
Ethylene dibromide
Styrene
Vinyl chloride
CYP 1A1
Polycyclic aromatic hydrocarbons (benzo[*a*]pyrene)
CYP 2A6
N-Nitrosodimethylamine
CYP 3A4
Aflatoxin B_1
Aflatoxin G_1
1-Nitropyrene

Adapted from ref. 46.

radical formation or through toxicant inhibition of antioxidant defenses. Free radicals and related oxidants are formed in biological systems ultimately from superoxide and nitric oxide, which react either together or separately to form a variety of radical and nonradical oxidants, including hydrogen peroxide, peroxynitrite, hydroxyl radical, hypochlorous acid, peroxyl radicals, and nitrogen oxides (46). These oxidants display a wide variety of reactivities and may produce frank oxidative damage (e.g., oxidation of membrane lipids, proteins, or DNA) as well as more subtle effects, including perturbations in cellular signaling and gene expression.

The formation of reactive metabolites is typically catalyzed by the phase I and phase II enzymes. Probably the most widely studied reactions are those involving P-450–mediated bioactivation. Table 4-3 illustrates a number of substrates for P-450 and the specific isoforms that catalyze their bioactivation to reactive metabolites. These reactive metabolites may be classified on the basis of their stability, which dictates the distance they may migrate from their site of origin to react with a target (41). The most reactive are the intermediates formed by suicide inactivators, which, by definition, react with the enzyme during its catalytic cycle (13). Suicide inactivators of P-450 include vinyl halides, terminal olefins, acetylenes, dihydropyridines, and cyclopropyl compounds (13). Next are very reactive products that are released from the enzyme, but that react primarily with that protein. A reactive acyl halide metabolite of chloramphenicol and electrophilic sulfur released from parathion are examples of reactive products that inactivate P-450. *N*-Acetoxy arylamine metabolites likewise inactivate the *N*-acetyl transferase isozyme that produces them (24). Less reactive are metabolites that may migrate to other compartments within a cell or tissue. This group may comprise the majority of electrophiles generated by metabolism. These metabolites share the ability to cross biological membranes, a characteristic that has been demonstrated for metabolites of several toxic or carcinogenic chemicals, including benzo[*a*]pyrene, bromobenzene, dimethylnitrosamine, vinyl chloride, 1,1-dichloroethylene, and trichloroethylene (41). Less reactive still are those metabolites that may leave their tissue of origin to produce damage in other tissues. Examples of this class are 2,5-hexanedione, a hepatic hexane metabolite that causes peripheral neuropathy; pyrrolic metabolites of pyrrollizidine alkaloids, which migrate from liver to the lung, where they produce endothelia damage; and epoxides of 4-vinylcyclohexene, which produce ovarian toxicity (11,47).

DETOXICATION

Detoxication refers to all reactions, enzyme-catalyzed or not, that consume toxic metabolites without producing injury. The simplest of the nonenzymatic reactions is hydrolysis, which may be a major detoxication mechanism for very reactive electrophiles, such as acyl halides, some epoxides, carbocations, isocyanates, and episulfonium ions (41). The most important nonenzymic detoxication of radicals is by reaction with biological antioxidants, such as vitamin E and vitamin C, which react with free radicals to produce relatively unreactive antioxidant radicals that do not further propagate radical injury (48).

Enzyme-catalyzed detoxication of nonradical reactive metabolites is accomplished principally by GST and, to a lesser extent, by epoxide hydrase (49). Although GSH reacts nonenzymatically with many electrophiles, GST catalysis greatly increases the rate and efficiency of the reactions. The multiplicity of GST enzymes with broad substrate specificities and their high content in many tissues make GST the most versatile detoxication system known (28). *In vivo*, experimental inhibition of this system is accomplished by GSH depletion rather than by enzyme inhibition *per se*. Depletion of tissue GSH by starvation, by inhibition of GSH synthesis, or by chemical GSH depletion dramatically increases both covalent binding of reactive metabolites to tissue components and tissue injury (49).

The glutathione redox cycle provides GSH-dependent protection against injury (50). Hydrogen peroxide and other hydroperoxides are reduced to innocuous alcohols and water by GSH and the selenoenzyme glutathione peroxidase. The glutathione disulfide produced by this reaction is reduced back to GSH by the NADPH-dependent glutathione reductase. The glutathione redox cycle thus consumes one molecule each of hydroperoxide and NADPH. The cycle can be inhibited by antitumor nitrosoureas, whose isocyanate breakdown products inactivate glutathione reductase, or by severe GSH depletion (50). Dietary selenium deprivation lowers glutathione peroxidase levels and may increase tissue sensitivity to oxidant stress (51). Some GSTs express peroxidase activity and may participate in hydroperoxide metabolism.

Two other enzymes of great significance for free radical detoxication are superoxide dismutase and catalase. Superoxide dismutase catalyzes the dismutation of two superoxide anion radicals to produce one molecule each of oxygen and hydrogen peroxide (52). Found in all tissues, SOD isozymes rely on Cu-Zn or Mn centers for catalytic activity, but require no additional cofactor. Hydrogen peroxide is then further catabolized by the GSH redox cycle, as discussed in the previous paragraph, or by catalase, a peroxisomal enzyme found in many tissues. Catalase requires no cofactor and catabolizes hydrogen peroxide almost exclusively.

Excretion

Substances may be excreted as parent compound, metabolites, and phase II conjugates. A major route of excretion is renal, and in some cases the urinary elimination of parent compound, metabolite, or conjugate may be used as a means for assessing absorbed dose. Some materials may be excreted in bile and feces; in such cases, there may also be enterohepatic recycling of

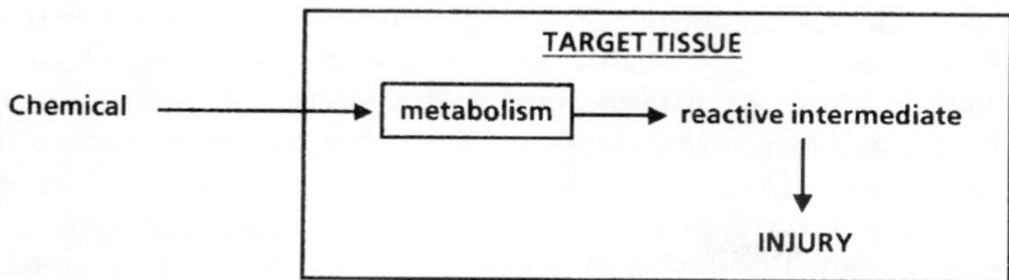

Figure 4-13. Model 1.

the parent compound or metabolite. Certain volatile materials and metabolites may be eliminated in expired air. The excretion of materials in sweat, hair, nails, and saliva is usually quantitatively insignificant, but these routes may be of importance for a forensic or occupational exposure diagnosis of intoxication. A variety of poorly metabolized, lipophilic compounds (polychlorinated biphenyls, polybromated biphenyls, DDE) that are sequestered in adipose tissue can be mobilized during lactation. They are then excreted in milk and thus transferred to the neonate.

MODELS OF TISSUE SUSCEPTIBILITY: CLASSIFYING TOXIC AND CARCINOGENIC CHEMICALS BY PATTERNS OF BIOACTIVATION

Many tissues are targets for injury by toxic metabolites of chemicals. Some of these tissues are capable of extensive biotransformation; others are not. Several enzyme-catalyzed metabolic steps, sometimes by enzymes in more than one tissue, are required to produce reactive metabolites from some chemicals. Others undergo simple, one-step bioactivation. Some toxic metabolites produce injury at the sites where they are formed, whereas others may migrate to produce effects at distant sites. Obviously, the sometimes complicated interplay between these factors dictates how and where bioactivation causes tissue injury.

Models

The following three models provide a framework for classifying chemical toxicants and carcinogens on the basis of how their bioactivation leads to tissue injury.

TABLE 4-4. Classification of toxic chemicals according to the rule of bioactivation: model 1

Chemical class: examples	Target tissue	Bioactivation enzyme(s)	Ultimate toxic metabolites	Effect(s)
Aromatic amines				
Benzidine, 2-naphthylamine	Bladder	Peroxidase	Diamines, radicals?	Carcinogenicity
	Liver	NAT, P-450, NAT or sulfotransferase	*N,O*-Acetoxy or *N,O*-sulfate derivative	Carcinogenicity
Arylhydroxamic acids				
Acetylaminofluorene	Liver	P-450, sulfotransferase	*N,O*-Sulfate ester	Carcinogenicity
Bipyridylium herbicides				
Paraquat, diquat	Lung, liver	Flavoprotein reductases	Cation radicals, oxygen radicals	Toxicity
Furans				
4-Ipomennol, 3-methylfuran	Lung, liver, kidney	P-450	α, β-Unsaturated dicarbonyls, epoxides?	Toxicity
Haloalkanes (a)				
CCl_4, CCl_3Br, halothane	Liver, lung, kidney	P-450	Radicals	Toxicity
Haloalkanes (b)				
$CHCl_3$, 1,1,2-trichloroethane	Liver, kidney	P-450	Acyl halides	Toxicity
Haloalkanes (c)				
1,2-Dibromoethane, 1,2-dichloromethane, 1,2-dibromo-3-chloropropane	Respiratory tract, stomach, esophagus, testis	GST	Episulfonium ion	Carcinogenesis
Haloalkenes				
1,1-Dichloroethylene, trichloroethylene	Liver, lung, kidney	P-450	Acyl halides, aldehydes, epoxides	Toxicity, carcinogenicity
Haloaromatics				
Bromobenzene, chlorobenzene, polyhalogenated biphenyls	Liver, lung, kidney	P-450	Arene oxides, quinones	Toxicity
Hydrazines				
1,2-Dimethyl hydrazine	Colon, liver	P-450, FMO	Diazomethane	Carcinogenesis
1,1-Dimethyl hydrazine	Liver (vasculature)	FMO	Methylradical, dimethyl diazonium ion	Carcinogenesis
Nitroaromatics				
Ronidazole, nitrofurantoin	Lung, liver	Flavoprotein reductases	Anion radicals, oxygen radicals	Toxicity
N-Nitrosamines				
Dimethylnitrosamine	Liver, stomach, lung	P-450	Methyldiazonium ion	Carcinogenesis
Polycyclic aromatic hydrocarbons				
Naphthalene, benzo[*a*]pyrene	Lung, skin, mammary glands	P-450, epoxide hydrase, peroxidase	Arene oxides, quinones	Toxicity, carcinogenesis
Pyrrolines				
Monocrotaline	Liver	P-450	Pyrroles	Carcinogenesis
Thiono-sulfur compounds				
Thioacetamide, α–naphthyl thiourea, carbon disulfide	Liver, lung	FMO, P-450	S-Oxide:S,S-dioxide, atomic sulfur	Carcinogenesis, toxicity

FMO, flavin-containing monooxygenase; GST, glutathione-*S*-transferase; NAT, *N*-acetyltransferase.

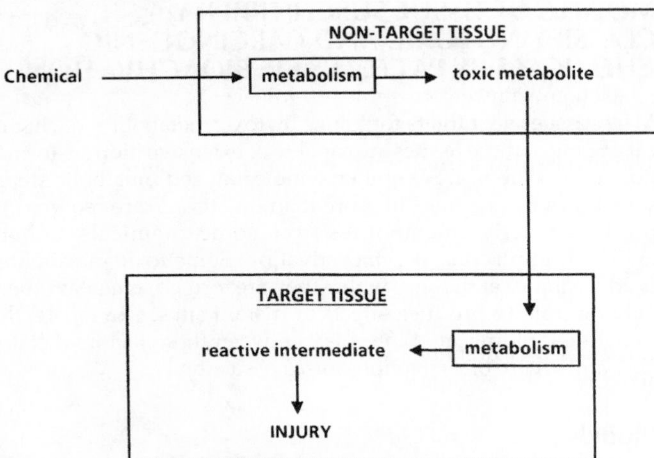

Figure 4-14. Model 2.

MODEL 1

The target tissue contains the necessary enzymes to bioactivate the parent chemical to a reactive metabolite, which produces injury (Fig. 4-13). This is the simplest model and can be applied to many toxicants and carcinogens that produce their effects in tissues with significant bioactivation capacity, such as the liver, lung, and kidney (Table 4-4). This model applies best to chemicals whose toxic metabolites are very reactive and may not migrate far from the cells that produce them.

MODEL 2

The target tissue cannot biotransform the parent chemical to a reactive metabolite *in situ* but can further bioactivate a toxic metabolite produced by another tissue (Fig. 4-14). This model applies mainly to chemicals whose initial metabolism is in the liver (Table 4-5). However, other obligate biotransformation steps may take place in other tissues, such as the gut, in which bacterial biotransformation may produce a toxic metabolite that is reabsorbed and causes toxicity elsewhere. The target tissues contain biotransformation enzymes that are not present in the liver, such as enzymes of glutathione conjugate catabolism in the renal proximal tubules, peroxidases in the renal inner medulla, lymphocyte myeloperoxidase in bone marrow, and extrahepatic tissue-specific forms of P-450. The primary metabolites are chemically unreactive, but the secondary metabolites are reactive enough to produce injury principally in the tissue in which they are formed.

MODEL 3

The target tissue can neither completely nor partially bioactivate the parent chemical but is uniquely susceptible to a reactive metabolite produced by another tissue (Fig. 4-15). This model generally applies to chemicals that produce damage in tissues in which bioactivation either does not occur or may occur to a minimal extent (Table 4-6). Target tissues in this model could range from peripheral nerves, which display little (if any) biotransformation capacity, to lung, which is active in biotransformation. Their common characteristic is that both lack the ability to bioactivate a given chemical yet are damaged by its metabolites from another tissue. The biochemical bases of susceptibility could involve exposure to high levels of a toxic metabolite, inadequate detoxication, a preponderance of targets compatible with a certain reactive metabolite, or inadequate repair. The assignment of a chemical to this model can be made with confidence only when the bioactivation of a chemical and the fate of its reactive metabolites are known. Uncertainty regarding either of these may lead one to incorrect classification under model 3 when a more proper classification would be models 1 or 2.

Toxic Interactions

In real life, exposures do not occur in isolation. Rather, exposures are commonly comprised of multiple chemicals, encountered either by successive exposure or as a chemical mixture.

TABLE 4-5. Classification of toxic chemicals according to the role of bioactivation: model 2

Chemical class: example	Initial bioactivation site: enzyme	Primary toxic metabolite(s)	Target tissue: bioactivation enzyme(s)	Ultimate toxic metabolite	Effect(s)
Aromatic hydrocarbons					
Benzene	Liver: P-450	Phenol, hydroquinones, catechol	Bone marrow stem cells: myeloperoxidase	Quinones	Toxicity, leukemogenesis
Haloalkenes					
Hexachlorobutadiene	Liver: GST	Glutathione conjugate	Renal proximal tubule: γ-Glutamyl transpeptidase Dipeptidase β–Lyase	Thionoacylhalide, thioketone	Toxicity
Nitroaromatics					
2,6-Dinitrotoluene	Liver: P-450 UDPGT	 Dinitrobenzyl alcohol *O*-Glucuronide	Liver: P-450 Sulfotransferase	 Hydroxylaminonitrobenzyl alcohol *N,O*-Sulfate ester	 Carcinogenesis
	Gut: Bacterial β–glucuronidase Bacterial nitroreductase	 Dinitrobenzyl alcohol Aminonitrobenzyl alcohol			

GST, glutathione-*S*-transferase; UDPGT, uridinediphosphoglucuronyl transferase.

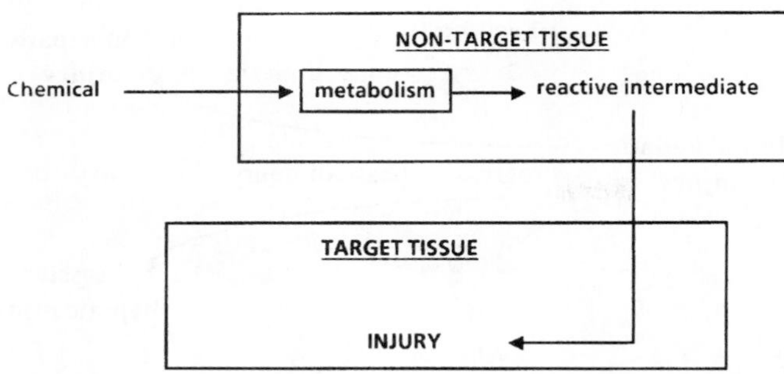

Figure 4-15. Model 3.

When this occurs, toxicity caused by individual chemicals may be modified by prior or simultaneous exposure to others. A convenient descriptive classification of the types of interactions that may occur follows:

- Independent effect: Substances qualitatively and quantitatively exert toxicity independent of each other.
- Additive effects: Materials with similar qualitative toxicity produce a response that is quantitatively equal to the sum of the effects produced by the individual constituents.
- Antagonistic effect: Materials oppose each others' toxicity, or one interferes with the toxicity of another; a particular example is that of antidotal action.
- Potentiating effects: One material, usually of low toxicity, enhances the expression of toxicity by another; the result is more severe injury than that produced by the toxic species alone.
- Synergistic effects: Two materials, given simultaneously, produce toxicity significantly greater than anticipated from that of either material; the effect differs from potentiation in that each substance contributes to toxicity, and the net effect is always greater than additive.

The mechanisms underlying each of these chemical interactions can be described as either *toxicokinetic* or *toxicodynamic*. Toxicokinetic interactions occur when one compound alters the concentration of toxic forms (parent molecule, toxic metabolites, or reactive intermediates) at target sites (Fig. 4-16A). Chemical-induced alterations in the absorption, distribution, biotransformation, and excretion of chemicals are the major causes of toxicokinetic interactions. It is important to emphasize that, independent of the type of chemical interaction, it is the mechanism of toxicity that determines the degree to which chemical interactions result in toxicity. For example, if the toxic form of a chemical is a reactive metabolite, then inhibition of biotransformation by another chemical may result in protection. Conversely, if the parent compound is the toxic form, then inhibition of biotransformation will potentiate, or exacerbate the degree of toxicity.

It is also important to mention that certain chemicals may produce multiple effects that can result in chemical interactions. For example, ethanol elicits a dose-dependent alteration of hepatic P-450 enzymes causing inhibition or induction with acute or chronic exposures, respectively. Thus in certain instances, the nature of chemical-chemical interactions depends not only on the mechanism of toxicity, but also on the chemical exposure characteristics. In addition, whereas phenobarbital induces the concentration and activity of certain P-450 isoforms, it also

TABLE 4-6. Classification of toxic chemicals according to the role of bioactivation: model 3

Chemical class: example	Bioactivation site: enzyme	Toxic metabolite(s)	Target tissue	Determinant of susceptibility	Effect
Alkanes					
Hexane	Liver: a. P-450 b. Alcohol dehydrogenase	2,5-Diketone	Peripheral nerve	Binding to lysine residues in axonal neurofilaments	Toxicity
Aromatic amines					
2-Naphthylamine	Liver: a. P-450 or FMO b. UDPGT	*N*-Glucuronide	Bladder epithelium	Hydrolysis of *N*-glucuronide in acidic urine yields reactive product	Carcinogenesis
Glycols					
Ethylene glycol	Liver: a. Alcohol dehydrogenase b. Aldehyde dehydrogenase	Oxalate	Renal tubules	Calcium oxalate, precipitate blocks, renal tubules	Toxicity
Haloalkenes					
Vinyl chloride	Hepatic parenchymal cell: P-450	Epoxide	Hepatic endothelial cell	Deficient DNA repair in endothelial cell vs. parenchymal cell	Carcinogenesis
Hydrazines					
1,2-Dimethylhydrazine	Hepatic parenchymal cell: P-450	Diazomethane	Hepatic endothelial cell	Deficient DNA repair in endothelial cell vs. parenchymal cell	Carcinogenesis
N-Nitrosamines					
Dimethyl nitrosamine	Hepatic parenchymal cell: P-450	α-Hydroxy–*N*-nitrosamine	Hepatic endothelial cell	Deficient DNA repair in endothelial cell vs. parenchymal cell	Carcinogenesis
Pyrrolines					
Pyrrolizidine alkaloids	Liver: P-450	Pyrroles	Pulmonary endothelium	"First pass" clearance of reactive hepatic metabolites	Toxicity

FMO, flavin-containing monooxygenase; UDPGT, uridinediphosphoglucuronyl transferase.

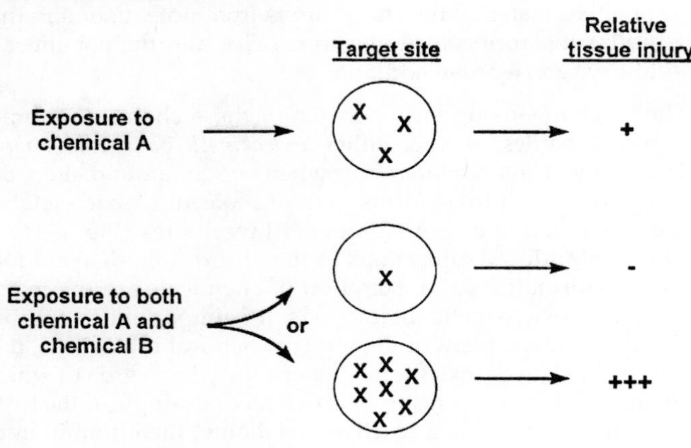

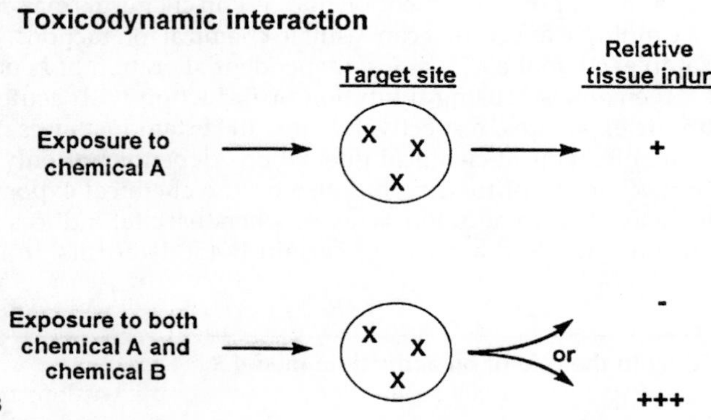

Figure 4-16. Toxicokinetic/toxicodynamic interactions. Panels show the effect one chemical can have on the toxicity of another. Panel **A** demonstrates how chemical B alters the concentration of toxic forms (X) of chemical A at the site of injury and how these alterations modulate the relative tissue injury (toxicokinetic effect). Panel **B** demonstrates how chemical B modulates the relative tissue injury without affecting the concentration of X at the target sight (toxicodynamic effect).

induces the activity of the phase II enzyme, glucuronosyl transferase. Conceivably, therefore, phenobarbital pretreatment could enhance or prevent toxicity caused by subsequent chemical exposures. The nature of this effect depends on the relative importance of P-450–mediated bioactivation and phase II enzyme-catalyzed detoxification.

Toxicodynamic interactions occur when one compound influences the host response to a given toxicant without affecting the concentration of toxic forms at the site of injury (Fig. 4-16B). For example, in rats, large doses of retinol can increase the activation state of Kupffer cells. By enhancing the inflammatory response to xenobiotics (i.e., Kupffer cell activation), retinol promotes the progression of hepatic injury initiated by hepatotoxicant exposure (53,54) (Fig. 4-17). Similarly, injury can progress if chemicals modify cellular repair processes (55). Thus with inhibition of repair, even minimal or moderate exposure to toxicants may result in widespread tissue damage. Based on these and other findings, understanding mechanisms of toxicodynamic interactions is an important area of research.

Most investigations of chemical interactions are designed to study how one chemical influences the toxicity of another. Although such studies can provide important mechanistic information, they do not address the interactive toxicity of complex mixtures or how exposure to complex mixtures can influence the pharmacologic and toxicologic effects of drugs and other chemicals. Complex mixtures are usually poorly defined and, in addition to parent materials, contain degradation products, contaminants, and trace additives. However, the chemical components of a mixture may change over time. Because of this, it is extremely difficult to study the toxicity as a result of exposure to complex mixtures.

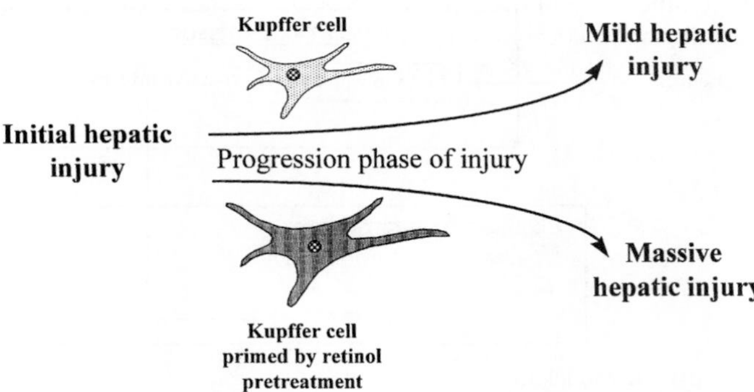

Figure 4-17. Retinol pretreatment increases the activation state of Kupffer cells. On exposure to a hepatotoxic chemical, these "primed" Kupffer cells greatly exacerbate the progressive (inflammatory) component of hepatic injury.

It is likely that mixtures will produce a variety of toxicokinetic and toxicodynamic interactions that will alter the toxicologic response. Of concern is the duration of exposure to chemical mixtures and how these interactions shift the threshold doses with respect to toxic responses. With respect to the inhalation route of exposure, there are potential interactions among chemical mixtures: (a) sensory irritants that can alter the rate and depth of breathing, allowing certain chemicals to penetrate distant respiratory airways, may be present; (b) some substances can cause anosmia, and hence remove an olfactory warning for other inhaled materials; (c) particulates may adsorb other materials, thereby acting as a carrier mechanism to the deep lung; (d) certain compounds can increase the viscosity of others, thereby limiting their removal from the respiratory tract; and (e) some chemicals may induce or inhibit biotransformation enzymes. Taken together, these potential effects caused by chemicals present in a mixture can modify both the local (i.e., pulmonary) and systemic toxicity caused by chemical exposure. Thus, in assessing toxicity from mixtures, it is important to consider the following: (a) chemical and physical interactions of the individual materials, (b) the effect that one chemical may have on the toxicokinetic or toxicodynamic characteristics of another, and (c) the possibility for interaction between parent compound and metabolites.

NATURE, DESIGN, AND CONDUCT OF TOXICOLOGY STUDIES

Toxicology studies attempt to describe and quantify the potential for a chemical, or mixture of chemicals, to produce local and systemic adverse effects and to determine factors that may influence the nature, severity, and reversibility of effects. Specific features that any toxicology testing study should include are the following:

- The nature of the adverse effects or the fundamental pathologic process (pathotoxicology)

- Relationship of the adverse effects to use of the substance in normal and occupational situations
- Dose-response relationships (average, range, hyperreactive groups, no-effects, and minimum-effects doses)
- Modifying factors
- Effects of acute overexposure
- Effects of repeated exposure (short- and long-term)
- Recognition of adverse effects
- Definition of allowable and nonallowable exposures
- Definition of monitoring procedures
- Guidance on protective and restrictive procedures
- Guidance on first aid and medical management
- Definition of at-risk populations (e.g., gender, preexisting disease, genetically susceptible)

Toxicology testing generally begins with single exposure *in vivo* or *in vitro* studies and progresses to evaluating the effects of long-term repeated exposures. Studies having specific endpoints, such as teratology and reproductive effects, are conducted as the emerging toxicology profile and end-use exposure patterns dictate. Toxicology testing procedures can be conveniently subdivided into general and specific. The *general* toxicology studies are those in which animals are exposed to a test material and are examined for a variety of toxic effects that the monitoring procedures permit. *Specific* toxicology studies are those in which exposed animals, or *in vitro* test systems, are monitored for a defined endpoint. Frequently used toxicology studies determine local and systemic inflammatory effects, immune-mediated hypersensitivity reactions, neurologic and behavioral toxicity, teratology, reproductive toxicity, organ-specific toxicity, genotoxicity, and sensory irritation.

HAZARD EVALUATION AND RISK ASSESSMENT

Toxicology is concerned with defining the potential for a material to produce adverse effects, whereas hazard evaluation is a process to determine whether any of the known potential adverse effects will develop under specific conditions of use. Thus, toxicology is but one of the many considerations to be considered in the hazard evaluation process. These considerations include the following:

- Physical and chemical properties of the material
- Patterns of use
- Characteristics of handling materials
- Source of exposure and route of exposure, both normal and possible misuse
- Control measures
- Magnitude, duration, and frequency of exposure
- Physical nature of exposure conditions (solid, liquid, vapor, gas, aerosol)
- Variability in exposure conditions
- Population exposed (number, gender, age, health status)
- Experience and information derived from exposed human populations

An approach to define the probability of adverse health effects developing from long-term, low-dose exposure is that of quantitative risk assessment. This approach attempts to quantify the risk of adverse health effects developing in response to environmental exposure to chemicals and may result in the development and implementation of risk management programs. The quantitative information on which the mathematic analyses are based is commonly derived from laboratory animal studies and occasionally from epidemiologic studies. In deriving risk values for particular exposure situations, many assumptions are made in calculating risks for human exposures. These include similarity between species in metabolism and pharmacokinetic characteristics and validity and relevancy of experimental conditions. In addition, the endpoint must be homogeneous in the population, and thresholds may not exist. Because many of these and other assumptions may be invalid, the calculated risk assessment values may only have partial scientific validity; as such, they are principally used for administrative purposes and guidelines by regulatory agencies. Clearly, the most reliable risk assessments are those based on information derived from both animals and humans with graded dose-response relationships and a knowledge of the comparative metabolism and pharmacokinetics of the material under consideration. Physiologically based pharmacokinetic modeling is a method that enhances the scientific basis and facilitates the intelligent interpretation of data used for risk assessment purposes, thus allowing greater confidence in risk evaluation. Mechanism-based decisions are considered in the classification of chemical carcinogens.

Special Considerations in Human Hazard Evaluation

Laboratory toxicologic studies are conducted under highly controlled conditions using healthy animals of a particular weight range. The extrapolation of such information to a heterogeneous human population, with differing lifestyles and variable states of health, needs to be undertaken with considerable caution, taking into account all possible known and predictable variables.

Quantitative risk assessments are frequently conducted for worktime or lifetime exposure to low concentrations of chemicals. They are based on extrapolating dose-response relationships from animal studies or human data, to determine risk at known or anticipated range of occupational or environmental exposure dosages. The approaches are frequently used to assess risk from carcinogens, teratogens, reproductively active substances, and genotoxic materials. There is insufficient information on mechanisms of toxicity for particular materials to allow scientifically valid, appropriate mathematic models to be developed for a specific toxic effect. The current method of extrapolation makes many assumptions: (a) the existence of thresholds for specific toxic endpoints, (b) linearity of dose-response relationships, (c) comparability of metabolism and pharmacokinetic parameters between species, (d) the interaction between xenobiotics and biological systems at low concentrations, and (e) the statistical reliability and biological variability resulting from the relatively small numbers of animals that may technically and ethically be incorporated into animal studies. Thus, with current mathematical approaches of data extrapolation, quantitative risk assessments should be regarded as best guesses for environmentally safe exposure dosages. The findings from quantitative risk assessment may result in risk management measures being undertaken. This involves the development and implementation of regulatory action, taking into account additional factors, such as available control measures, cost-benefit analyses, and acceptable levels of risk.

REFERENCES

1. Charbonneau M, Perreault F, Greselin E, Brodeur J, Plaa GL. Assessment of the minimal effective dose of acetone for potentiation of the hepatotoxicity induced by trichloroethylene-carbon tetrachloride mixtures. *Fundam Appl Toxicol* 1988;10:431–438.
2. Lieber C. Mechanisms of ethanol-drug-nutrition interactions. *Clin Toxicol* 1994;32(6):631–681.
3. Hissink AM, Oudshoorn MJ, Van Ommen B, Haenen GRMM, Van Bladeren PJ. Differences in cytochrome P-450–mediated biotransformation of 1,2-dichlorobenzene by rat and man: implications for human risk assessment. *Chem Res Toxicol* 1996;9:1249–1256.

4. Zbinden G, Flury-Roversi M. Significance of the LD_{50} test for the toxicologic evaluation of chemical substances. *Arch Toxicol* 1981;47:77–99.
5. Ballantyne B. The comparative short-term mammalian toxicology of phenarsazine oxide and phenoxarsine oxide. *Toxicology* 1978;10:341–361.
6. Horton AA, Fairhurst S. Lipid peroxidation and mechanism of toxicity. *Crit Rev Toxicol* 1987;18:27–79.
7. Albano E, Lott KAK, Slater TF, et al. Spin-trapping studies on the free-radical products formed by metabolic activation of carbon tetrachloride in rat liver microsomal fractions. *Biochem J* 1982;204:593–603.
8. Stanton MF, Layard M, Tegeris A, et al. Relation of particle dimension to carcinogenicity in amphobile asbestosis and other fibrous minerals. *J Natl Cancer Inst* 1981;67:965–975.
9. Boyd MR, Statham CN. The effect of hepatic metabolism on the production and toxicity of reactive metabolites in extrahepatic tissues. *Drug Metab Rev* 1983;14:35–47.
10. Rydstrom J, Montelius J, Bengtsson M, eds. *Extrahepatic drug metabolism and chemical carcinogenesis*. Amsterdam: Elsevier, 1983.
11. Boyd MR. Biochemical mechanisms of chemical-induced lung injury: roles of metabolic activation. *Crit Rev Toxicol* 1980;7:103–176.
12. Nebert DW, Nelson DR, Adesnik M, et al. The P-450 superfamily: update on listing of all genes and recommended nomenclature of the chromosomal loci. *DNA* 1989;8:1–14.
13. Ortiz de Montellano PR, Reich NO. Inhibition of P-450 enzymes. In: Ortiz de Montellano PR, ed. *Cytochrome P-450: structure, mechanism, and biochemistry.* New York: Plenum, 1986:277–314.
14. Shehin-Johnson SE, Williams DE, Larsen-Su S, et al. Tissue-specific expression of flavin-containing monooxygenase (FMO) forms 1 and 2 in the rabbit. *J Pharmacol Exp Ther* 1995;272:1293–1299.
15. Cashman JR. Monoamine oxidase and flavin-containing monooxygenases. In: Sipes IG, McQueen CA, Gandolfi AJ, eds. *Comprehensive toxicology.* Vol 3. In Press.
16. O'Brien PJ. Radical formation during the peroxidase catalyzed metabolism of carcinogens and xenobiotics: the reactivity of these radicals with GSH, DNA, and unsaturated lipid. *Free Radic Biol Med* 1988;4:169–183.
17. Smith MT, Evans CG, Thor H, Orrenius S. Quinone-induced oxidative injury to cells and tissues. In: Sies H, ed. *Oxidative stress*. Orlando, FL: Academic Press, 1985:91–113.
18. Siedegard J, DePierre J. Microsomal eposide hydrase: properties, regulation, and function. *Biochim Biophys Acta* 1983;695:251–270.
19. Levin W, Buening MK, Wood AW, et al. An enantiomeric interaction in the metabolism and mutagenicity of (+)- and (–)-benzo[*a*]pyrene-7,8-oxide. *J Biol Chem* 1980;255:9067–9074.
20. Siest G, Antoine B, Fournel S, Magdalou J, Thommasin J. The glucuronosyltransferases: what progress can pharmacologists expect from molecular biology and cellular enzymology? *Biochem Pharmacol* 1987;36:983–989.
21. Kadlubar FF, Miller JA, Miller EC. Hepatic microsomal *N*-glucuronidation and nucleic acid binding of *N*-hydroxyarylamines in relation to urinary bladder carcinogenesis. *Cancer Res* 1977;37:805–814.
22. Jakoby WB, Duffel MW, Lyon ES, Ramaswamy S. Sulfotransferases active with xenobiotics: comments on mechanism. In: Bridges JW, Chasseaud LF, eds. *Progress in drug metabolism*. Vol 8. Philadelphia: Taylor and Francis, 1984:11–34.
23. Waterman M, Guengerich F. Chapter 3.02. In: Sipes IG, McQueen CA, Gandolfi AJ. *Comprehensive Toxicology.* Vol 3. NY: Pergamon, 1997:7–14.
24. Hanna PE, Banks RB. Arylhydroxylamines and arylhydroxamic acids: conjugation reactions. In: Anders MW, ed. *Bioactivation of foreign compounds*. Orlando, FL: Academic Press, 1985:376–402.
25. Weber WW. Acetylation pharmacogenetics: experimental models for human toxicity. *Fed Proc* 1984;43:2332–2337.
26. Blum M, Demierre A, Grant DM, Heim M, Meyer UA. Molecular mechanism of slow acetylation of drugs and carcinogens in humans. *Proc Natl Acad Sci U S A* 1991;88(12):5237–5241.
27. Kaderlik KR, Kadlubar FF. Metabolic polymorphisms and carcinogen-DNA adduct formation in human populations. *Pharmacogenetics* 1995;5:S108–S117.
28. Ketterer B, Christodoulides LG. Enzymology of cytosolic glutathione S-transferases. *Adv Pharmacol* 1994;27:37–69.
29. Parkinson A. Biotransformation of xenobiotics. In: Klaassen CD, Amdur MO, Doull J, eds. *Casarett and Doull's toxicology: the basic science of poisons*, 5th ed. New York: McGraw-Hill, 1996:113–186.
30. Stevens JL, Ayoubi N, Robbins JD. The role of mitochondrial matrix enzymes in the metabolism and toxicity of cysteine conjugates. *J Biol Chem* 1988;263:3395–3401.
31. Sipes IG, Gandolfi AJ. Biotransformation of toxicants. In: Klaassen CD, Amdur MO, Doull J, eds. *Casarett and Doull's toxicology: the basic science of poisons*, 3rd ed. New York: Macmillan, 1986:64–98.
32. Olson WA, Habermann RT, Weisburger EK, Ward JM, Weisburger JH. Induction of stomach cancer in rats and mice by halogenated aliphatic fumigants. *J Natl Cancer Inst* 1973;51:1993–1995.
33. Goldman P. Role of the intestinal microflora. In: Jakoby WB, Bend JR, Caldwell J, eds. *Metabolic basis of detoxication*. New York: Academic Press, 1982:323–338.
34. Idle JR, Smith RL. Polymorphism of oxidation at carbon centers of drugs and their clinical significance. *Drug Metab Rev* 1979;9:301–317.
35. Guengerich FP, Distlerath LM, Reilly PEB, et al. Human liver cytochromes P-450 involved in polymorphisms of drug oxidation. *Xenobiotica* 1986;16:367–378.
36. Uetrecht JP, Woosley RL. Acetylator phenotype and lupus erythematosus. *Clin Pharmacokinet* 1981;6:118–134.
37. Skett P. Hormonal regulation and sex differences of xenobiotic metabolism. In: Bridges JW, Chasseaud LF, Gibson GG, eds. *Progress in drug metabolism.* Vol. 10. Philadelphia: Taylor and Francis, 1987:86–140.
38. Younis HS, Hoglen NC, Kuester RK, Sipes IG. Hepatocellular glutathione disulfide alterations in male fischer-344 and Sprague-Dawley rats following 1,2-dichlorobenzene administration. *Fundam Appl Toxicol* 1997;36(1):A No. 416.
39. Rane A, Pacifici GM. Formation and metabolism of toxic metabolites in the human fetus. In: Soyka LF, Redmond GP, eds. *Drug metabolism in the immature human*. New York: Raven Press, 1981:29–35.
40. Pelkonen O. Xenobiotic metabolism in human placenta. In: Soyka LF, Redmond GP, eds. *Drug metabolism in the immature human*. New York: Raven Press, 1981:19–27.
41. Guengerich FP, Liebler DC. Enzymatic activation of chemicals to toxic metabolites. *Crit Rev Toxicol* 1985;14:259–307.
42. Maines MD, Kappas A. Regulation of cytochrome P-450–dependent microsomal drug-metabolizing enzymes by nickel, cobalt, and iron. *Clin Pharmacol Ther* 1977;22:780–790.
43. Chasseaud LF. Role of glutathione and glutathione-S-transferases in the metabolism of carcinogens and other electrophilic agents. *Adv Cancer Res* 1979;29:175–274.
44. Guengerich FP. Effects of nutritive factors on metabolic processes involving bioactivation and detoxication of chemicals. *Annu Rev Nutr* 1984;4:207–231.
45. Angeli-Greaves M, McLean AEM. Effect of diet on the toxicity of drugs. In: Gorrod AW, ed. *Drug toxicity.* London: Taylor and Francis, 1981:91–100.
46. Guengerich FP, Shimada T. Oxidation of toxic and carcinogenic chemicals by human cytochrome P-450 enzymes. *Chem Res Toxicol* 1991;4(4):391–407.
47. Doerr JK, Hooser SB, Smith BJ, Sipes IG. Ovarian toxicity of 4-vinylcyclohexene and related olefins in B6C3F1 mice: role of diepoxides. *Chem Res Toxicol* 1995;8:963–969.
48. Machlin LJ, Bendich A. Free radical tissue damage: protective role of antioxidant nutrients. *FASEB J* 1987;1:441–445.
49. Reed DJ. Cellular defense mechanisms. In: Anders MW, ed. *Bioactivation of foreign compounds*. Orlando, FL: Academic Press, 1985:71–108.
50. Reed DJ. Regulation of reductive processes by glutathione. *Biochem Pharmacol* 1986;35:7–13.
51. Sies H. Hydroperoxides and thiol oxidants in the study of oxidative stress in intact cells and organs. In: Sies H, ed. *Oxidative stress*. Orlando, FL: Academic Press, 1985:73–90.
52. Fridovich I. Superoxide dismutases. *Adv Enzymol Relat Area Mol Biol* 1986;58:61–97.
53. ElSisi AE, Earnest DL, Sipes IG. Vitamin A potentiation of carbon tetrachloride hepatotoxicity: role of liver macrophages and active oxygen species. *Toxicol Appl Pharmacol* 1993;119:295–301.
54. Badger DA, Sauer JM, Hoglen NC, Jolley CS, Sipes IG. The role of inflammatory cells and cytochrome P-450 in the potentiation of CCl_4-induced liver injury by a single dose of retinol. *Toxicol Appl Pharmacol* 1996;141:507–519.
55. Calabrese EJ, Mehendele HM. A review of the role of tissue repair as an adaptive strategy: why low doses are often non-toxic and why high doses can be fatal. *Food Chem Toxicol* 1996;34(3):301–311.

CHAPTER 5
Principles of Epidemiology

Mary Kay O'Rourke

Traditional epidemiology is exemplified by Dr. John Snow's investigation of cholera outbreaks in London (1). He plotted the spatial distribution of all cholera deaths during 1848–1849 and 1853–1854 and evaluated characteristics of the dead, including common water companies. He found that a disproportionate number of people living near Broad Street who used water distributed by the Southwark company had died. Three water companies served different populations in London, and the number of deaths were not directly comparable.

Snow calculated frequencies by looking at the number of deaths over the total number of people served by each company. He actively encouraged the cleanup of the water supply by removing the pump handle from the distribution source. When the water system cleanup began, the specific causal agent for cholera was unknown. Yet, the work was done so carefully, and the resulting association was so strong, that remediation began before the specific causal agent was identified. Snow's work defined the essential elements of traditional or classic epidemiology: collection of unbiased data gathered by design (although this was a fortuitous circumstance), consideration of factors outside the disease, calculation using appropriate measures, and eventual changes in public policy.

Before World War II, traditional epidemiology focused on acute outbreaks of epidemic disease, and investigations proceeded similarly to those of Dr. Snow. With the development of vaccines and the science of immunology, epidemics were reduced and epidemiology entered an "epidemic transition" (2,3). Since 1970, modern epidemiology has emerged as an academic field in which chronic, noninfectious disorders are studied as the source of mortality in the developed world. Currently, the widely held working definition of epidemiology is the study of the distribution and determinants of disease in human populations (4). Modern epidemiologists perform this task by focusing on a single disease, exposure, or condition and carefully selecting subjects who are affected and unaffected by the condition. Researchers then observe events. These studies focus on changes in the individuals, and results are projected over the population.

Many believe that this approach to epidemiology has become too narrow (5). They believe that (a) epidemiologists have lost their broad base of medical and general knowledge (6), (b) epidemiology should focus on the conditions of the population as well as the individual, and (c) modern epidemiology has lost its relationship to public health (7,8). Epidemiology serves as the basic science of public health and as such has a contributory role to the public health mission. The subtle difference is evident in the definitions proposed by Last (6). *Epidemiology* is "the study of the distribution and determinants of health-related states or events in specified populations, and the application of this study to the control of health problems," whereas *public health* is ". . . the combination of sciences, skills, and beliefs . . . directed to the maintenance and improvement of the health of all the people through collective or social actions" (9). As scientists, modern epidemiologists report the data, results, and their significance to the communities involved in the study regardless of the outcome. The epidemiologist must remain objective or lose scientific credibility. As a science, epidemiology provides the data that promote either status quo or change. Advocacy of change through collective or social action falls to communities, activists, and policy makers with scientific input from epidemiologists.

There are three basic purposes to epidemiologic studies. These are (a) to elucidate the etiology of specific diseases by considering epidemiologic data in light of data from other disciplines, such as genetics, biochemistry, and microbiology; (b) to examine how consistent epidemiologic data are with hypotheses derived in the laboratory or clinical setting; and (c) to develop and evaluate preventive strategies and public health control practices. Recently, the World Health Organization has focused on purposes of environmental epidemiology (10). The stated purposes parallel those of epidemiology: (a) to evaluate the effects of environmental conditions on health, (b) to evaluate the efficacy of preventive and control measures, and (c) to provide policy makers and public health workers with information for the development of policy and prevention strategies.

Traditional epidemiology attains these purposes primarily through observation. In this regard, epidemiology is analogous to natural history. The epidemiologist cannot introduce a variable into a system while holding other variables constant. Instead, the epidemiologist must measure relative differences among well-characterized groups without introducing change to the system. Experimental epidemiology is more like engineering or toxicology, in which laboratory experiments can be designed to hold all variables constant and change only one condition. Laboratory studies can define direct causal relationships. In traditional epidemiology, statistical associations among variables are identified and inferences are drawn.

Epidemiology is undergoing change. Infectious disease epidemiology and chronic disease epidemiology were separated during the transition years. Today, epidemiologists specialize in areas like molecular epidemiology, clinical epidemiology, psychosocial epidemiology, environmental epidemiology, occupational epidemiology, and injury epidemiology. Each area has its focus and specific study designs, but all areas employ the same fundamentals.

Several excellent reference sources are available for more in-depth study of epidemiology (11,12).

BASIC VOCABULARY USED IN EPIDEMIOLOGY

The brief description of Snow's work can serve as an example to help explain a few commonly used terms in epidemiology. Epidemiology uses statistics to evaluate changes in sickness (*morbidity*) and death (*mortality*). Mortality statistics are much easier to measure than morbidity. A person is born and dies once; these are events that can be counted once in a lifetime. The statistics are compiled for a specific geographic area (city, county, state, nation) over a fixed period of time (usually monthly or yearly). Mortality statistics are compiled from death certificates and published through the National Center for Health Statistics.

Disease, sickness, illness, injury, disorders, and disabilities are alluded to under the term *morbidity*. Epidemiologists evaluate morbidity among different groups. For instance, Snow compared the cholera in one part of London with that in another part. The area served by the Southwark water company had eight times as many people living in it, or potentially affected, as the area served by the Lambeth water company. To standardize the measures for comparison, Snow calculated what amounted to a frequency for each area. The actual percentage (0.5%) would appear very low, even though the disease was an epidemic. Epidemiologists convert the percentage value into human terms to express them. By the end of the epidemic, 5 people per 1,000 people died in the Southwark area (9). This represents the *prevalence* of the disease in Southwark. Prevalence is reported for a single point in time—in this case, the end of the epidemic. The prevalence varies depending on when it is calculated relative to the course of the disease in the community. A closely related measure is *incidence*. The incidence rate indicates how many new cases of a disease are found in a community in a fixed amount of time. Incidence rates indicate whether a disease is growing, declining, or stable in a community. Different public health policies need to be implemented depending on changes in the incidence rate. Growing incidence rates require immediate public action to mitigate the spread of the condition. Snow removed the Broad Street pump handle to prevent the community from consuming the tainted water. Declining and stable conditions require persistent effort among researchers, public health advocates, and policy makers to eradicate the disease or condition. Prevalence and incidence are key measures of morbidity.

Key measures for mortality are related to those of morbidity. One of the most important measures of death is *survival*. Survival is the likelihood of remaining alive for a specified period of time after diagnosis of the disease. Survival is most frequently cited for cancer. Specified time periods are usually presented as 1 or 5 years. The shorter the specified time frame, the more severe the disease. Survival is calculated for a specified time frame as the number of newly diagnosed cases of a disease (A)

minus the number of deaths (D) over the newly diagnosed number of cases during the specified time frame:

$$\text{Survival} = \frac{(A - D)}{A}$$

These statistics are only accurate if the patient can be followed over the entire time period. The opposite of survival is known as case fatality. *Case fatality* is the number of deaths from a disease (D) over the number of diagnosed patients (A):

$$\text{Case fatality} = \frac{D}{A}$$

These measures can be calculated for different age and racial classes to determine differences within the population. Neither survival nor case fatality is rates. The *crude death rate* is the total number of people who died over the total population for a given group or disease. Sometimes these rates need to be refined by examining death for a single age or racial group. Then the standardized mortality rate (SMR) is calculated. The SMR evaluates the actual observed deaths for a group over the expected deaths. Expected deaths are calculated by multiplying the death rates for the general population (p) by the number of deaths for the observed population (g) summed for all population groups [SMR = observed deaths (D) divided by the sum of deaths for each group; where the group expected values is death in the general population (p) × deaths found in the group of concern (g)]:

$$\text{SMR} = \frac{\text{observed deaths } (D)}{\text{expected deaths}[\Sigma(p_x \times g_x)]} \times 100$$

When a person seeks medical aid for a given condition or disease, he or she is a *patient* while receiving care. If a study involves invasive procedures while the person is in a clinical setting, he or she remains a patient. A person being treated by drug therapy (or placebo) and subjected to frequent medical checkups is still a patient.

Epidemiologic studies on patients are sometimes referred to as *clinical epidemiology* or *clinical decision analysis* (6,11). The people evaluated continue to be called patients. These are usually small studies involving experimental procedures. When Snow was treating people for cholera, they were patients; some of his work was etiologic and related to clinical epidemiology. His *post facto* analysis was traditional epidemiology.

Epidemiology studies that recruit from the general population enroll *subjects*. The subject may or may not have the disease, exposure, or trait under consideration. All study participants are subjects. If the subject has the disease (or trait or exposure), then he or she becomes a *case*. If the subject lacks the trait, is unexposed, or fails to contract the disease, then he or she becomes a *control*. Both cases and controls are *subjects*. In Snow's research, people who lived in the area served by the Southwark water district and contracted cholera were cases. People living in the Southwark water district who failed to contract the disease were *positive controls*. They lived in the defined area, they were exposed, and they failed to contract the disease. People served by the Lambeth water company were *negative controls*.

In a few cases, some of the people living in the area of town served by the London water company also became ill and died. What could have killed them? Perhaps they moved from one area to another. Perhaps contaminated foodstuffs were brought from relatives from the other part of town. If questions could be asked of the dead from outside Southwark, other *variables* (or factors) resulting in contraction of cholera might be identified. These factors are *confounding variables* or *confounders*; they mask, confuse, or distort the relationship between the exposure and the disease of interest. Confounders appear to influence the disease, but they are not *causal* determinants of the disease.

Sometimes there is no single causal agent resulting in a disease. This is particularly true in environmental epidemiology, in which exposure can come from multiple sources and through multiple pathways. Some epidemiologists promote the concept of a *web of causation*. The web of causation accurately illustrates the complexity with which epidemiologists are faced.

One way of limiting the influence of confounders is to *match* subjects. Matching can occur at the level of the specific individual (*individual matching*), of controls and cases (*frequency matching*), or by characteristics for a group (*category matching*). Characteristics of the study cases are identified; some of these might be characteristics such as age, race, exposure, and smoking status. Specific confounders will vary among studies. Subjects in the control group will be matched to subjects among the cases based on the confounders identified. Then differences among the groups can be evaluated. *Stratification* is another statistical manipulation of the study groups to control for confounding variables in the data analysis.

Epidemiology is a data-intensive study. Some computer/database jargon creeps into the field. This creates some confusion among the new initiates related to definitions for *case* and *variable*. Databases frequently have measurements listed for subjects, whether they are cases or controls. Once in the database, each subject is referred to as a case, and each measurement (e.g., age, gender, ethnicity) is recorded as a variable. In this instance, two disciplines use the same terms to mean different things.

Frequently, epidemiologic studies are described in temporal terms relative to the formulation of the hypothesis and the initiation of the study. A *retrospective study* examines a disease event or exposure that occurred in the past. One example is a survey of cause of death (mortality) within a community in which information is available through death certificates (a descriptive retrospective study). Retrospective case-control studies are conducted to evaluate exposure and disease in matched patients. Persons unaffected by an exposure are compared with those affected to determine differences (e.g., exposure, behavioral, genetic) related to the disease. Advantages to retrospective studies include comparatively low cost, greater ease in matching and characterizing subjects in comparable groups, well-characterized smaller groups, possibly less conduction time, and simultaneous evaluation of multiple risk factors because all the data is available. Disadvantages to retrospective studies focus on data availability; unknowns related to data quality in terms of collection, transcription interviewer bias, and subject recall; local publicity surrounding the topic under study; differential recollection of events by subjects; and bias in the population selected based on under- or overrepresentation of any group in the initial records.

A *prospective study* enrolls a population to test a hypothesis and then evaluates that population at intervals for specific disease (or wellness) traits. Because of the longitudinal nature of prospective studies, it is important to use standardized measures in the evaluation and examine differences that may be a function of changes in the age of the participants. Today, common usage suggests that the terms *prospective*, *cohort*, *longitudinal*, *follow-up*, *concurrent*, and *incidence* are all synonyms. The advantages of a prospective study include the opportunity to gather complete and accurate information; the potential for change through time in the subject's status relative to the hypothesis being tested or evaluated; the opportunity to develop a relationship with the subjects based on trust, and the increased likelihood of more accurate data as a result; and the potential to evaluate the influence of temporal variations on the data. Disadvantages associated with prospective studies are the following:

- The duration of the study as reflected in the high cost
- The administrative nightmare of subject tracking through time

- The loss of subjects through time because of subject dropout
- Migration from the area and death
- Maintaining consistently high-quality data measurements in spite of staff changes and other factors for the duration of the study

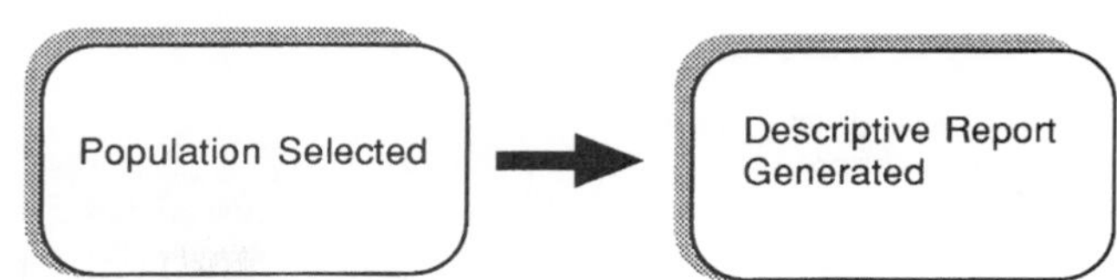

Figure 5-1. The descriptive study.

TYPES OF EPIDEMIOLOGIC STUDIES

Classic epidemiology describes two basic types of studies: observational and experimental. Typically, conditions are not altered in observational studies; investigators merely record and report what they find (observe). Observations are made of (a) the agent (disease/exposure/medication), (b) the host (the person and host characteristics), and (c) the environment (including time, place, and conditions). Experimental epidemiologic studies record baseline conditions; researchers then alter the system (e.g., provide a specific drug, change an environmental condition, remove a contaminant) and reevaluate the conditions after the passage of some predefined time period(s). Differences in the measured values may be attributed to the "intervention" or change.

Observational studies, whether descriptive or analytic, have some advantages over experimental study designs. Foremost among these is their occurrence in natural settings. They are also the most practical to perform because there is no manipulation of the study factor, only persistent observation. Therefore, results have greater impact on local public health and policy. There are also disadvantages. The investigator has only limited control over the study, so the study results tend to be unique to each local area in which a study is conducted. Further replication of results is difficult.

In general, observational studies can be either retrospective or prospective, whereas experimental studies can only be prospective by nature of the intervention. Collection of data at multiple time horizons creates special problems for environmental epidemiologists. They must be careful to never relate symptoms collected at one time with environmental data collected at a different time.

Results for either observational or experimental studies must be compared with a reference population or control group to have any meaning. It describes the most common types of studies undertaken and cites examples of each. Some suggest replacing observational studies with classic epidemiology and experimental studies with clinical epidemiology (11). Such a change would be inappropriate. Today, many epidemiologists work in disciplines in which true experiments are performed. These may address topics such as treatments of carpets against house dust mites (environmental epidemiology), testing different safety equipment used in the workplace (occupational epidemiology), and testing clinical treatments (clinical epidemiology).

Observational Studies—Descriptive

Descriptive studies are implemented when little is known about a disease, exposure, or trait. Study objectives focus on disease prevalence and determining how the disease varies through time (etiology). Descriptive studies generate hypotheses to be tested. The simplest descriptive study is a case report, which communicates the effects of a single toxic agent or disease on an individual patient. The case report alerts the medical community to an unrecognized or special manifestation of disease. It is the first step to determining the disease or exposure prevalence.

Retrospective descriptive studies are conducted on routinely collected data including common demographic variables (e.g., age, gender, ethnicity, education and income levels, occupation, marital status). When agencies such as the Centers for Disease Control and Prevention suspect a public health problem, they analyze incoming data for trends; they employ *passive surveillance* methods. If the problem persists, they actively solicit more complete data and address the issue. This is *active surveillance* and may use a customized survey or questionnaire. Descriptive studies report current conditions but make no attempt to link any of the variables. The report provides rates of behaviors or disease occurrences. The value lies in comparing reports of a variable, such as smoking, from one area with another: Location A has more or less smoking than Location B (Fig. 5-1).

Another important analytic tool is simply graphing the distribution of a measurement and comparing simple statistics, such as mean, median, and range, with published values. Investigators determine the prevalence of samples exceeding levels of concern or threshold values for a toxin.

Observational Studies—Analytic

There are four major types of analytic studies. Analytic studies are conducted when sufficient information is available about the disease, exposure, or trait to form an *a priori* hypothesis. Objectives for analytic studies generally include identification of risk factors, assessment of the influence of each risk factor on the disease or condition, and identification of possible mediation strategies. When the design is appropriate and the study is carefully executed, analytic studies further the identification of cause-effect relationships in evaluating the disease.

ECOLOGICAL STUDIES

These studies examine the relationship between two or more variables at the population level. They are most attractive when using large data sets. For instance, the amount of cholesterol-reducing medication sold might be compared with the number of heart attacks across a number of countries. No effort is used to pair medication with individual health status; medication use is compared with the disease rate. Such analyses are instrumental in refining hypotheses. Because analysis is done on such a broad scale, confounders attain less importance. Unfortunately, many explanations may be possible for the results of these correlational analyses. Further, the association of variables at the group level may not hold when considered in greater detail for the individuals. Projecting the group result on individuals is known as *ecological fallacy* and must be avoided (Fig. 5-2).

CROSS-SECTIONAL STUDIES

Cross-sectional studies measure how commonly diseases occur at a single point in time. They are frequently called *prevalence studies* for this reason. Cross-sectional studies recruit and characterize the population in terms of disease. Instead of waiting for the disease to develop in people lacking the disease (cohort study), the cross-sectional study assesses the prevalence of disease among groups with various characteristics.

One of the strengths of the cross-sectional study is that the population is randomly selected and should be statistically rep-

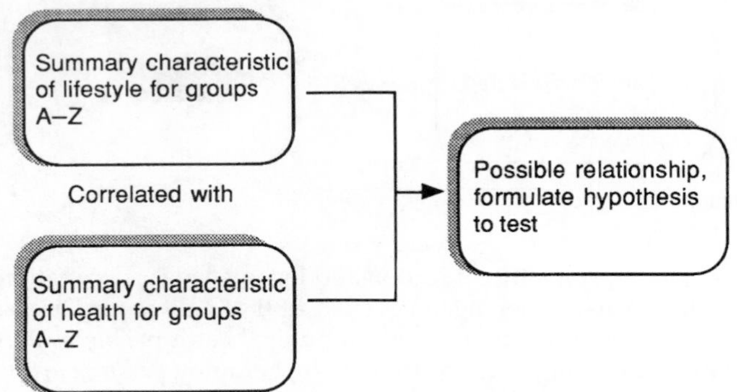

Figure 5-2. An example of an ecological or correlational approach.

resentative of the entire population. Therefore, information obtained in the sample subset can be modeled upward to represent a larger region. The more representative the population, the more accurate the study results. Some countries conduct regular cross-sectional evaluations to determine changes in disease; the survey results are used to assess health care needs for policy makers. Investigation of chronic disease may be well served by the cross-sectional study design; evaluation of acute disease or intermittent exposures may be less well served.

COHORT STUDIES

Cohort studies follow a population recruited for its lack of the disease (or trait or exposure) being evaluated. The population is followed through time, and changes in disease status are measured at intervals. The measurements evaluate change in health status, presumably in response to the factor of interest. Frequently, the age and gender of the subjects are held constant to limit confounders, but such limiting is not essential. Cohort studies can be conducted either prospectively or retrospectively when suitable records are available (Fig. 5-3). Prospective cohort studies are also known as *follow-up*, *incidence*, *panel*, and *longitudinal studies*, and among observational studies they offer the greatest opportunity to implement an experimental design. The goals and hypotheses can be well defined at the onset of the study, and the necessary data can be collected at the appropriate intervals. Statistical data analysis produces the basis of interpretation through inference, and conclusions are drawn. Prospective cohort studies are valuable if the disease or measurable health effect is common.

Because of the follow-up intervals provided by evaluations of a cohort, investigators are able to calculate the incidence of a disease (new cases/total cases per unit time). Incidence can be calculated for specific groups by breaking the cohort into classes (stratifying).

One of the best known cohort studies is the Framingham Heart Study. It continues to evaluate the role of multiple factors (e.g., elevated blood pressure, lipid levels, excess body weight, lack of exercise, pulmonary function, smoking habits) on the etiology of heart disease. In 1948, 5,127 randomly selected adults, initially free from heart disease, were enrolled for the cohort study. Study rationale, methods, and initial findings were reported (13,14). Follow-up and evaluation are still under way, examining extensions of the initial hypotheses for this study (15). With more than 40 years of follow-up and the development of special studies, many opportunities exist to evaluate these data retrospectively.

Through the years, a number of retroprospective studies have used the Framingham study population. A disease or trait of interest was identified while the original cohort was being followed. Data were retrospectively evaluated to identify potential causal agents. After a testable hypothesis was formulated, supplemental measurements were made from that point forward on the population. Such add-on studies were enlightening and cost-effective.

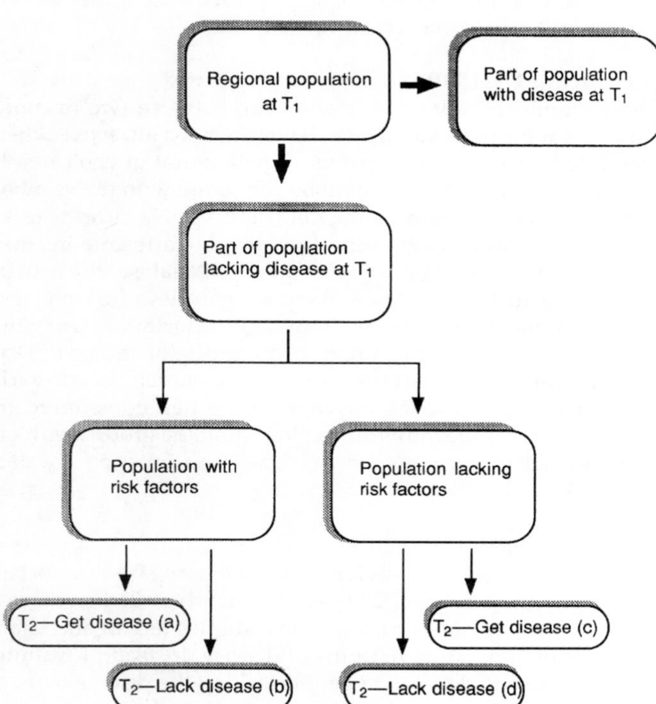

Figure 5-3. Diagram of a prospective cohort study. T_1 indicates the time the study population is recruited. T_2 represents the predetermined follow-up time when the population is reevaluated.

RELATIVE RISK AND ATTRIBUTABLE RISK

Besides incidence, two other common measures are derived from cohort studies. *Relative risk* indicates how much risk an exposed person (or person with some risk factor) has over the unexposed (risk-factor–free) person in terms of contracting a disease or condition. The risk ratio or relative risk is the frequency of disease among those exposed to a risk factor over the frequency of disease for those not exposed to the risk factor:

$$\frac{\frac{a}{(a+b)}}{\frac{c}{(c+d)}}$$

If the relative risk is greater than 1.0, then the risk is greater in the exposed group. How much greater than 1.0 does the value need to be to have any meaning? A report in *Science* suggests that a relative risk lower than 1.55 is probably not meaningful, and that most epidemiologists do not become enthusiastic until a relative risk exceeds 3.0 or even 4.0 (16).

Reputable epidemiologists also desire to see a biological mechanism that supports the statistical association. The article ends with a wonderful quotation by Sander Greenland, who sees no "sin" in gathering the data and evaluating the associations. He states, "The sin comes in believing a causal hypothesis is true because your study came up with a positive result, or believing the opposite because your study was negative" (16).

Another measure to determine how much risk of disease is the result of any one factor is *attributable risk*. Other terms for attributable risk include the *etiologic fraction* when referring to disease, *population attributable risk, population attributable risk percent*, and *attributable fraction*. The attributable risk is the proportion of new disease cases in a fixed time that can be attributed to a single factor (of all the many factors) that is being investigated. Attributable risk can only be measured in a dynamic population with the ability to evaluate incidence. This limits attributable risk to selected cohort and other longitudinal studies. Using the example of Fig. 5-3, the attributable risk is commonly calculated as:

$$[a/(a+c)-b/(b+d)]$$

If considered for a specific time interval, attributable risk is:

$$[a/(a+c)-b/(b+d)]/[1-(b(b+d))]$$

for a given time period (5).

Cohort studies are most successful when the recruited population is large and the disease investigated is common. Cohort studies have less inherent bias, because recruited subjects lack the disease at the time of enrollment. Disease is detected during the follow-up evaluations. Thus, the investigator observes the relationship without biasing the results. Problems in cohort studies include the loss of subjects over time, incomplete follow-up of the entire cohort at each interval, and even intervals of follow-up. Cohort studies are usually conducted in discrete geographic areas. Results among cohort studies can vary considerably.

RETROSPECTIVE COHORT STUDY

Cohort studies are least successful when the disease is rare; the final number of cases will be too low to perform suitable statistical analyses. One solution is a retrospective cohort analysis. Retrospective analysis is difficult because subjects' characteristics or the "causal" factors may have been inadequately characterized. In recent years, investigators have been more creative and moved toward *multicenter studies*. Multicenter studies are commonly used in the evaluation of new drugs and are prospective, but the approach holds promise for the analysis of rare diseases. Several investigators have retrospectively examined multicenter drug trial data to investigate the etiology of selected diseases (17).

HYBRID STUDY DESIGNS

There are many hybrid study designs. As an example, the Tucson Epidemiology Study of Airway Obstructive Diseases began in 1972, and the population continues to be monitored (18,19). This study combines design elements of both the cross-sectional and cohort approaches. A great deal of work goes into recruiting a cross-sectional population that is randomly selected and statistically representative of the general population (i.e., population based). The initial screening questionnaire used in recruitment and baseline evaluation is a point-in-time, cross-sectional evaluation. Tucson researchers chose to follow the cross-sectional population longitudinally. Such designs provide researchers with maximum flexibility.

CASE-CONTROL STUDIES

Case-control studies examine a population made of two groups. One group has the disease, trait, or condition of interest, whereas the comparison group does not. Individuals in the groups may be matched to eliminate confounders.

Case-control studies suffer an identity crisis. The definitions of retrospective and prospective are fairly clear, and they are consistent with the current literature, which defines them in general terms based on data collection relative to study initiation. In the same literature, the terms are disease referent, not data-collection referent. A study is retrospective if the subject has the disease at the time of study initiation—even though the data will be collected longitudinally through future follow-up. According to others, this makes a case-control study a retrospective study, because the group of interest already has the disease (12). Beaglehold et al. suggest that case-control studies can be either (9). Case-control studies are retrospective if the data were gathered in the past or prospective if the data will be obtained in the future.

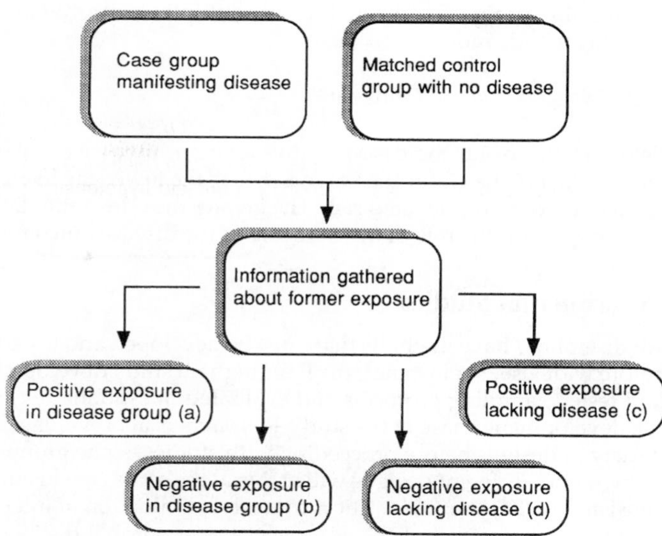

Figure 5-4. A retrospective case-control study. The disease or exposure occurred in the past. Note that the letters (a through d) associated with the outcome groups are used to explain odds ratios.

One common use of the case-control study is the investigation of the role of environmental agents in disease. For instance, several recent studies have recruited a population with a disease outcome thought to be associated with pesticide exposure and compared the exposed group with populations matched by age and gender but lacking the exposure. They indicate elevated risk of disease or symptoms among the exposed subject group (20–23). The case-control approach may not be suitable to evaluate environmental exposures for the following reasons: (a) exposure information is gathered retrospective to the manifestation of the disease; (b) recall may not be particularly good, and subjects may have a bias regarding the causality of their condition; (c) to eliminate the potential of unknown exposure, subjects and controls are usually not drawn from the same population; and (d) pairing or matching is important to ensure comparable groups, but matching introduces its own errors.

Case-control studies do not involve dynamic populations like a cohort study; instead, they are fixed groups defined by the investigator. As a result, neither incidence, prevalence, nor relative or attributable risk can be calculated as a measure. *Relative odds* or *odds ratios* are the best measure to obtain from case-control studies. An odds ratio in a case-controlled study is a simple calculation. The investigator has set up two groups of equal numbers: the cases and the controls (Fig. 5-4). If there is no difference between the two groups, the fraction of each group (exposed and not exposed) expressing the disease or condition should be the same:

$$\left(\frac{a}{b}=\frac{c}{d}\right)$$

Solving this proportion through cross multiplication provides us with an odds ratio:

$$\text{Odds ratio} = \frac{ad}{bc}$$

Below a value of 1.0, there is a negative relationship between the factors. Again, the closer the value is to 1.0, the lower the likelihood of there being elevated risk. The greater the odds ratio, the more important the role of the exposure in the disease outcome.

Experimental Studies

All disciplines have methods that must be developed and tested before wide use. For instance, the Framingham study developed and tested sampling protocols and evaluated questionnaires in the development phase of the study. Researchers also evaluate a variety of designs before proceeding with studies; some groups test whether different designs will arrive at the same conclusion consistently (24). Another critical concern is evaluation of interviewing techniques and the accuracy of one variable (i.e., job title) over another (i.e., job duties) as it relates to exposure or disease endpoint (i.e., exposure to asbestos) (25). Researchers also compare different laboratory analytic tests over large numbers of people to determine efficacy (26). Methods development takes an immense amount of time in epidemiologic studies. Such studies are always incidental to the main goal of the project, and publication of these results facilitates epidemiology as a discipline.

Randomized Controlled Clinical Trials

Randomized controlled clinical trials are routinely used by clinicians to assess the efficacy of drugs not yet on the market or other experimental treatment procedures. Before testing in humans, drugs and procedures are extensively tested in the laboratory and in animal models, and there is a reasonable expectation that the treatment will cause no harm and prove valuable.

The subject pool is usually drawn from patient populations. The patients are selected based on their willingness to participate and their ability to meet predetermined criteria for the study. Patients meeting the criteria are generally homogeneous in terms of disease status and confounding factors. Patients/participants are then randomized and assigned to treatment and control groups. Before initiating the study, the individuals in each group should be evaluated to obtain all baseline measurements of health that will be related to outcome measurements in the study. This study is usually a *double-blind* approach. Neither the clinician nor the patient/participant knows the group assignment.

A mix of biostatistical procedures can be used to evaluate clinical trials. First, graph the data for each group. This is the most obvious method of comparing different rates of outcome measurements. Then move on to simple statistical tests. Chi square contingency tests are a commonly used approach. These do not require a normal distribution of the data; the investigator can define the comparative groups. Variables being evaluated must be normally distributed or transformed to a normal distribution if regression or correlation matrices are calculated. The smartest thing to do is consult a biostatistician before gathering data. This will help the clinician gather appropriate data for evaluation.

One of the most critical issues in clinical trials and case-control studies is finding a population large enough to test. This has led to the multicenter trials used particularly for rare diseases. Clinical trials require a number of special ethical considerations. Like all studies, they require informed consent. Further, the physician is obligated to provide the best possible care. If the experimental procedure is the best possible care, then the clinician cannot withhold the treatment, even though it is experimental. Once the study is initiated, patients must be carefully monitored. Patients suffering severe outcomes either through lack of essential medication or through inappropriate response to the treatment must be withdrawn from the study, and all withdrawals must be carefully documented.

FIELD TRIALS

Field trials are implemented among individuals who are disease free and presumed to be at risk. Field trials are designed to keep people healthy through preventive actions administered to the individual. The most common types of field trials are related to vaccination programs. These studies are hard to evaluate, because they are negative data. Successful field trials result when people continue to be well; it is not always possible to determine whether people in an area would have remained disease free without the intervention. Testing the Salk polio vaccine may have been the largest field trial ever undertaken. The trial involved more than 1 million children. Today, many of the vaccination field trials occur in the third world to seek to abate diseases like malaria and cholera. New field trials address environmental issues. These include programs to screen children's blood for lead and to evaluate other media, such as soil, air, and house dust.

COMMUNITY TRIALS

These address problems with a social or behavioral basis. The best way to address these problems is through changes in group behavior within the community. Community trials have been implemented to alter behaviors that lead to heart disease. Lifestyle changes promoting wellness can be implemented on a community-wide scale (27). Areas needing improvement include exercise, diet, and smoking behavior (28).

Community trials face a variety of limits. When communities are the study unit, only a small number can be evaluated, so any type of statistical evaluation is limited. It would be nearly impossible to develop a single protocol to implement in multiple communities. Social conditions in each community demand a customized approach. Because the protocol cannot be held constant, program effectiveness cannot be compared across communities. Measuring the effectiveness of a program is confounded by potential differences among communities. Finally, in this age of communication, communities are not isolated. Information comes in from other areas that may dilute or negate the message being conveyed. Community trials appear to be a rather imperfect experiment.

TYPES OF ERROR, POWER, AND SOURCES OF BIAS IN EPIDEMIOLOGIC STUDIES

Fatal research errors result when the main study hypothesis is falsely rejected or falsely accepted. The study hypothesis is always phrased as a *null hypothesis* for statistical tests. The null hypothesis states that there is no difference between the groups being analyzed. These errors are divided into two groups. Type I error rejects the null hypothesis when it is actually correct, whereas Type II error accepts the null hypothesis when it is actually incorrect. A number of factors contribute to the probability of committing a Type II error, including the true values of the measured parameter, the level of significance desired by the investigator, whether the hypothesis will be evaluated using a one- or two-tailed test, the standard deviation of the measured value, and the overall number of data points collected. Type II errors will decline the closer that the sample population reflects the value of the true population.

One method of limiting Type II error is by increasing the number of the subjects in a study. This provides added confidence in accepting the null hypothesis. Beyond a certain number of subjects, very little additional power is gained. *Power* is defined as the ability of a study to detect a true effect of a specified magnitude. To keep study costs limited, it is important to appropriately calculate the amount of power required to avoid a Type II error. This provides precision for the study. Standard power calculations are provided in a variety of program packages and texts (29). Complex study designs require more than just the typical type of power calculation; this is particularly evident with randomized clinical trials (29,30).

Associations and Cause

Statistical analyses can be applied to data gathered using appropriate study designs. A common misperception is that because two factors are associated to a significant level, one factor causes the other. This is particularly problematic among students and lay readers. Statistical association is not enough to determine causation.

Ten causality criteria have been described (31). Investigated factors are more likely to be causally related to a disease when these ten factors are maximized:

1. *Consistency*: The risk factors are consistently associated with the disease.
2. *Strength*: Association between the disease and the factors is very strong.
3. *Specificity*: The risk factor appears specific to only a few diseases.
4. *Time relationships*: The factor believed to be causal always precedes the disease.
5. *Congruence*: Other "known" information is consistent with the newly identified factor.
6. *Sensitivity*: The presumed factor is present as each new outbreak of the disease is evaluated.
7. *Biological/medical*: The pathogen or factor is mechanistically capable of causing the disease.
8. *Plausibility*: Causal inferences are not contradicted by other information.
9. *Experiments and research*: In fact, causal inferences are supported by other research.
10. *Analogy*: Similar cause-and-effect associations are parallel and prove useful by analogy.

The cause of disease transmission can be direct or indirect. Swollen prostate glands result in urine retention and are associated with urinary tract infections. The swollen gland might harbor bacteria and serve as a reservoir of urinary tract infection (direct causation), or the failure to completely empty the bladder may result in the infection. One is a direct causal agent; the other is indirect. Cause is not easily defined and should not be readily attributed.

Errors

The more complex the project, the more opportunity for errors. I am currently working to minimize errors at every level in a complex environmental assessment survey called *National Human Exposure Assessment Survey (NHEXAS) Arizona*. This multimedia, multipathway survey is being conducted in the state of Arizona. Unlike most studies, this project has a complete quality assurance plan in place to minimize errors and document occurrences of same. NHEXAS is a field-based project conducted in homes (32). It is cross-sectional and uses a population-based probability design to identify subjects. NHEXAS is broken into several areas: population selection, field recruitment, handling of materials (shipping and receiving), field monitoring, equipment repair and calibration, local laboratory, collaborating laboratories, tracking of samples and results, questionnaire checks, coding, data entry, data verification, data validation, data management, preparation of specific data files for analysis, and statistical analysis and interpretation. We have more than 2,500 pages of procedures and documentation and an independent quality-assurance officer. All of these elaborate plans cannot eliminate errors. Instead, we attempt to minimize the errors and faithfully document errors that occur. This quality-assurance approach is extremely useful, and funded projects will be confronted with this need in the future.

Studies encounter two major types of errors: *random errors* and *systematic errors*. Random errors can be minimized or documented. For instance, certain environmental samples must be kept cold. All refrigerators are checked by a laboratory technician every day. The lab tech documents the maximum and minimum temperature experienced by each unit every day. Recently, a cleaning crew unplugged a refrigerator to use the electric outlet. They forgot to plug in the refrigerator when done. Laboratory spikes were destroyed in the process. They were never used in samples, because the laboratory staff caught the error. Time and money were lost, but study samples were not affected. The problem was recorded in the refrigerator log, and remedial actions were taken. This is an example of the type of random error that can affect a study. These are regrettable, but they rarely affect the study outcome. This same event could have produced a systematic error if the laboratory technician had ignored the problem and used the spikes. Use of compromised spikes would have introduced the same error to each sample, a systematic error. Completing a study with low systematic error results in a study with high precision.

The best way to minimize systematic error is to have well-trained interviewers and field technicians who are unbiased. Interviewers must accept sampling wherever sent in fulfillment of the study design. They must go to all areas and leave only if they feel their personal safety is in immediate danger. The area will then be sampled another day with additional support staff available. The interviewers are trained to place no value judgment on the subject's response. They must be open and accepting of all responses. This also means understanding subjects who speak other languages and having all written materials translated into the appropriate language or dialect.

POPULATION SELECTION BIAS

In some studies, selection of the population is fairly direct. If there is an environmental exposure to a toxic chemical, then those exposed are investigated. The population is characterized, but the cohort definition relates to the event; demographic and physiologic factors do not play a role. This "enrollment by fate" can be contrasted with the study of chronic disease. Some chronic diseases are gender specific, and therefore the study group is limited to that gender. By definition, men do not get ovarian cancer and women do not get testicular cancer. Sometimes there appears to be an association between the disease and one gender. Heart disease in midlife is found far more frequently in men. When designing a new study, the epidemiologist is faced with the following issues when recruiting a cohort: (a) gender is a confounder, (b) it takes longer for the disease to express in women, and (c) lower frequency and longer follow-up require greater cost.

In the 1960s and 1970s, relatively few studies examined heart disease in both sexes. What about women and heart disease? What about men with breast cancer? Our sex sensitivities have seemingly been elevated, and studies can be found for both conditions. The change may only be at an academic and not a clinical level. Breast cancer is generally not recognized in men until the advanced stages of the disease. As for women and heart disease, a study indicates that men suffering myocardial infarction continue to receive more aggressive treatment, both invasive and noninvasive, than women (33). The authors conclude that women receive adequate treatment, and men may be overtreated. This treatment bias illustrates the influence epidemiology can have in medicine; to prevent such bias, the epidemiologist is obligated to study disease across all demographic groups whenever possible.

"HEALTHY WORKER" EFFECT

Another type of bias plagues epidemiologic studies implemented in the workplace. Workers who can tolerate poor environmental quality are generally healthier or less sensitive. This "healthy worker" bias may act as a confounder in some studies. The converse also occurs; sometimes subjects with chronic diseases are more likely to participate in a study. Both are types of self-selection. It is best to recruit populations in a manner that enables the researcher to independently determine the representativeness of the population selected by comparison with other databases (e.g., the U.S. census).

TEST VALIDITY

All tests in a study must be capable of measuring what they are intended to measure, and that measurement must reflect the "truth" of the population being studied. This applies to questionnaire instruments used in the field and laboratory tests. Questionnaires should be reliable and validated before use. Recall bias is a special problem associated with questionnaire administration. Researchers should make certain the time horizons for which they are obtaining information are appropriate relative to a subject's ability to recall the event. Recall is dependent on the detail required. As a rule of thumb, general patterns of activity and behavior may be recalled for as long as 5 months. Specific activities or consumption may be recalled with greatest accuracy for the day. Certain activities may remain in memory for approximately one week, depending on the individual. There are two types of validity: internal and external.

Internal validity applies to the measure being obtained from a population. We readminister questionnaires by phone within a few months of initial administration. This enables us to determine the extent to which general questions are answered consistently and to measure the associated error. We also use internal standards in laboratory analyses to make certain each batch of samples has internal consistency in terms of results.

External validity can be measured by supplying split samples to two different laboratories for independent analysis or, in the case of questionnaires, by having interviewers observed and evaluated by people external to the project.

ETHICAL ISSUES IN EPIDEMIOLOGY

Epidemiology is governed by ethical considerations, as are other medical sciences. Guidelines on professional conduct and ethical responsibilities are outlined in the Declaration of Helsinki and in *Ethics and Epidemiology: International Guidelines* (34). Subjects must be aware that the proposed study may not be helpful to them personally but will add to the scientific knowledge about a disease or circumstance. Free and informed voluntary consent must be obtained for all study participants. Subjects have the right to withdraw from the study at any time without hard feelings. Epidemiologists have an obligation to report specific results to individual participants and summary results to the communities affected. All epidemiologic studies should be reviewed by the appropriate institutional committees before implementation.

Issues of environmental justice, race, and ethnicity must also be carefully considered when selecting a sample. The sample should be representative of the broader population, and the study design should be constructed to evaluate minority groups regardless of cultural and language barriers. The American College of Epidemiologists states, "The health of all racial and ethnic groups, especially of their disadvantaged members, is of critical importance for public health" (35).

SUMMARY

For many years, epidemiology was the almost exclusive domain of the medical profession. In recent years, medicine has lost its dominance, a fact bemoaned by some. The computer age and on-line databases enable people lacking basic knowledge of a specific disease to manipulate data and report results that may be misleading. Therefore, the most critical component of epidemiology is a sound knowledge base. That may mean formulation of a team of scientists with diverse backgrounds.

Because epidemiology deals directly with human health and death, the public is highly interested in the results. This poses a problem when interacting with the lay press. A small elevation of relative risk results in a huge concern within affected communities. The epidemiologist may carefully explain the technical results to a community but must also communicate in a way that can be understood and dealt with appropriately.

REFERENCES

1. Cameron D, Jones IG. John Snow, the Broad Street pump and modern epidemiology. *Int J Epidemiol* 1983;12:393–395.
2. Susser M. Epidemiology in the United States after World War II: the evolution of a technique. *Epidemiol Rev* 1985;7:147–177.
3. Oppenheimer GM. Comment: epidemiology and the liberal arts—toward a new paradigm? *Am J Public Health* 1995;85:918–920.
4. Greenberg RS, Daniels SR, Flanders WD, et al. *Medical epidemiology.* Norwalk, CT: Appleton & Lange, 1993.
5. Holland WW. The hazards of epidemiology. *Am J Public Health* 1995;85:515–517.
6. Last JM. *A dictionary of epidemiology,* 2nd ed. New York: Oxford University Press, 1988.
7. LaPorte RE, Barinas E, Chang YF, Libman I. Global epidemiology and public health in the 21st century. Applications of new technology. *Ann Epidemiol* 1995;5:152–157.
8. Shy CM. The failure of academic epidemiology: witness for the prosecution. *Am J Epidemiol* 1997;145:479–484.
9. Beaglehold R, Bonita R, Kjellstrom T. *Basic epidemiology.* Geneva, Switzerland: World Health Organization, 1994.
10. Phillipp R, Kjellstrom T. Courses in environmental and occupational epidemiology. *World Health Forum* 1994;15:43–47.
11. Jeckel JF, Elmore JG, Katz DL. *Epidemiology, biostatistics and preventive medicine.* Philadelphia: WB Saunders, 1995.
12. Farmer R, Miller D, Lawrenson R. *Lecture notes on epidemiology and public health medicine,* 4th ed. Cambridge, MA: Blackwell Science, 1995.
13. Dawber TR, Meadors GF, Moore FF. Epidemiological approaches to heart disease: the Framingham study. *Am J Public Health* 1951;41:279.
14. Dawber TR, Moore FF, Mann GV. Coronary heart disease in the Framingham study. *Am J Public Health* 1957; 47[Suppl]:4.
15. Goldberg RJ, Larson M, Levy D. Factors associated with survival to 75 years of age in middle-aged men and women: the Framingham study. *Arch Intern Med* 1995;155:505–509.
16. Taubes G. Epidemiology faces its limits. *Science* 1995;259:154–159.
17. Ross DJ, Jordan SC, Nathan SD, et al. Delayed development of obliterative bronchiolitis syndrome with OKT3 after unilateral lung transplantation: a plea for multicenter immunosuppressive trials. *Chest* 1995;109:857–859.

18. Lebowitz MD, Burrows B. Tucson epidemiologic study of obstructive lung diseases. II: Effects of in-migration factors on the prevalence of obstructive lung disease. *Am J Epidemiol* 1975;102:153–163.
19. Lebowitz MD, Sherrill DL, Kaltenborn W, Burrows B. Peak expiratory flow from maximum expiratory flow volume curves in a community population: cross-sectional and longitudinal analyses. *Eur Respir J* 1997;24:29s–38s.
20. Meinert R, Kaatsch P, Kaletsch U, et al. Childhood leukemia and exposure to pesticides: results of a case control study in northern Germany. *Eur J Cancer* 1995;32A:1943–1948.
21. Kiefer M, Rivas F, Moon JD, Checkaway H. Symptoms of cholinesterase activity among rural residents living near cotton fields in Nicaragua. *Occup Environ Med* 1995;53:725–729.
22. Liou HH, Tsai MC, Chen CJ, et al. Environmental risk factors and Parkinson's disease: a case control study in Taiwan. *Neurology* 1997;48:1583–1588.
23. Freyzek JP, Garabrant DH, Harlow SD, et al. A case-control study and self-reported exposures to pesticide and pancreatic cancer in southeast Michigan. *Int J Cancer* 1997:72:52–57.
24. Sears MR, Lewis S, Herbison GP, et al. Comparison of reported prevalences of recent asthma in longitudinal and cross-sectional studies. *Eur Respir J* 1997:10:52–54.
25. Orlowski E, Pohlabeln H, Berrino F, et al. Retrospective assessment of asbestos exposure—II. At the job level: complementary of job-specific questionnaire and job exposure matrices. *Int J Epidemiol* 1993;22[Suppl 2]:S95–S105.
26. Hamar GB, McGeehin MA, Phifer BL, et al. Volatile organic compound testing of a population living near a hazardous waste site. *J Expo Anal Environ Epidemiol* 1995;5:247–255.
27. Leupker RV. Community trials. *Prev Med* 1994:23:502–505.
28. Freedman LS, Gail MH, Green SB, Corle DK. The efficiency of the matched-pairs design of the community intervention trial for smoking cessation (COMMIT). *Control Clin Trials* 1997;18:131–139.
29. Law MG. Sample size calculations for within patient comparisons with a binary or survival endpoint. *Control Clin Trials* 1995;17:221–225.
30. Willan AR. Power function arguments in support of an alternative approach for analyzing management trials. *Control Clin Trials* 1994;15:211–219.
31. Hill AB. The environment and disease: association or causation. *Proc R Soc Med* 1955;58:295–300.
32. Lebowitz MD, O'Rourke MK, Gordon SM, et al. Population-based exposure measurements in Arizona: a phase I field study in support of the National Human Exposure Assessment Survey. *J Expo Anal Environ Epidemiol* 1995;5:297–324.
33. Green LA, Ruffin MT. Differences in management of suspected myocardial infarction in men and women. *J Fam Pract* 1993;35:389–393.
34. Bánkowski Z, Bryant JA, Last JM. *Ethics and epidemiology: international guidelines: proceedings of the XXVth Council for the International Organizations of Medical Sciences conference.* Geneva, Switzerland: CIOMS, 1991.
35. Matanowski GM, Nasca PC, Swanson GM, et al. Statement of principles: epidemiology and minority populations. *Ann Epidemiol* 1995;5:505–508.

CHAPTER 6
Principles of Risk Assessment

Rosalind R. Dalefield, Frederick W. Oehme, and Gary R. Krieger

WHAT IS RISK ASSESSMENT?

Risk assessment, as applied to toxic hazards, is the process of evaluating the nature and likelihood of adverse effects that may occur following exposure to a chemical (1). The risk-assessment process seeks to assign an objective measure of risk to a certain exposure so decisions on chemical exposure are based on reason rather than on fear, prejudice, or the skills of interested parties in manipulating the media or applying political pressure.

Approximately 100,000 chemicals are in commercial use, of which 15,000 are classified as *high production volume,* meaning that more than 10,000 tons of each are produced each year. Some 10,000 chemicals—including 500 high production volume chemicals—in modern industrial use have not yet been adequately tested for risk-assessment purposes (2,3). New chemicals are being produced all the time, and some form of risk assessment is vital to identify and control exposure to those chemicals that pose a threat to human health.

Adequate testing typically costs between $1 million and $2 million and takes 3 to 5 years (4). The cost of compliance with U.S. Environmental Protection Agency (EPA) regulations exceeded $100 billion annually in 1991 and is forecast by the EPA to rise to $200 billion annually by the end of the decade. The cost-effectiveness of these regulations has been the subject of several reviews by the World Bank (5–7).

Despite the enormous cost of risk assessment, current risk-assessment procedures are not held in high regard within the scientific community, interest groups, or the public at large (8). Public perceptions of chemical risks are profoundly negative, even when the risks are extremely small (1). Poor science and sensational reporting can lead to profound anxiety and falls in property values in communities that are not in fact at increased risk of adverse health effects. The conservative nature of current risk-assessment methods is not well publicized. EPA guidelines stress that the agency's numeric estimates of risk are unlikely to be too low and the true risk may be as low as zero, but this caveat is not always communicated prominently to the public (8). Antiregulation critics oppose current risk-assessment methods on the grounds that they exaggerate risk and are excessively expensive, whereas many scientists regard risk assessment as lacking in validation and fraught with assumptions.

Legal challenges to regulatory action are the rule rather than the exception. Therefore, the EPA must be able to defend its decisions in a court of law by providing scientifically valid protocols to the chemical manufacturers and allowing a reasonable time for data collection, analysis, submission, and preparing a risk assessment. Test guidelines, risk-assessment guidelines, risk assessments, and the resulting risk-management decisions are all subject to internal and external scientific review. The EPA is also required to prepare and file a regulator impact statement, which weighs the cost and benefits of the regulation (9).

President Clinton's Executive Order 12866 (Executive Order 1993a) includes the following principles:

- The EPA will consider the degree and nature of the risk.
- Regulations will be designed in a cost-effective manner.
- Both risks and benefits will be assessed.
- The agency will use the best reasonably obtainable scientific, technical, and economic information.
- Regulations will be tailored to pose the least burden, and the agency will consider the costs of cumulative regulations (10).

Risk assessment is expensive, in both time and money, to both chemical manufacturers and regulatory agencies. It is highly desirable that the results of the process are scientifically valid.

CURRENT SYSTEMS FOR RISK ASSESSMENT

Currently, risk-assessment procedures can be divided into (a) risk assessment for noncancer toxic effects, (b) cancer risk assessment, (c) risk assessment for reproductive and developmental toxicity, and (d) neurotoxicity risk assessment. However, in July 1997, the EPA began to develop guidance for cumulative risk assessment. Cumulative risk assessment would represent a shift to a more broadly based approach characterized by consideration of multiple endpoints, sources, pathways, and routes of exposure. The most current information on the agency's evolving position can be found at the EPA Web site (www.epa.gov).

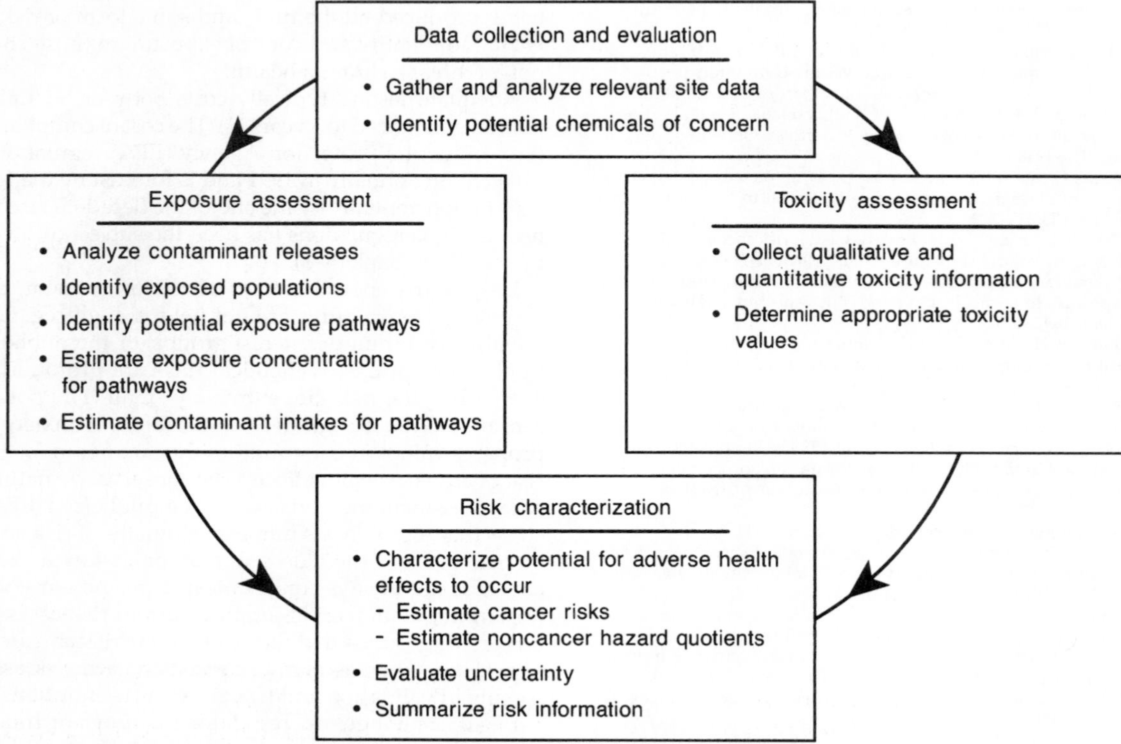

Figure 6-1. Risk-assessment summary. With permission from U.S. Environmental Protection Agency 1989.

RISK ASSESSMENT FOR TOXIC EFFECTS EXCLUDING CANCER

Present Default Process of Risk Assessment

A *default option* is the option chosen on the basis of risk-assessment policy that appears to be the best choice in the absence of data to the contrary (11). The primary default process used by the EPA for quantitative risk assessment of noncancer effects is the reference-dose (RfD) approach. The process aims to identify a safe exposure level that does not cause any adverse effect on human health. RfD, formerly known as an *acceptable daily intake* (8), is measured in mg/kg/day.

The risk-assessment process (Fig. 6-1) for noncancer effects includes the following (12–14):

- Hazard identification is the evaluation of the existing human and animal data to determine whether the chemical is likely to be a hazard. Chemical and physical properties are less often used (15).
- Dose-response assessment and toxicity assessment include the evaluation of dose-response relationships and the determination of the RfD.
- Exposure estimation of likely human exposure range(s) is done via direct monitoring or modeling of exposure scenarios.
- Risk characterization is the integration of the information from all the foregoing steps to determine the potential human risk under particular exposure scenarios (12).

Hazard Identification and Evaluation

Hazard identification qualitatively and quantitatively evaluates whether a hazard is present. This process attempts to determine what substances or chemicals are present, their sources, their pathways of exposure, and whether they have the ability to potentially produce adverse health effects in humans, animals, or the environment (Fig. 6-2).

All data available on the substances present are collected, organized, and evaluated for toxic potential. Data are examined to determine whether there is evidence of carcinogenesis or toxic endpoints, such as functional, physiologic, biochemical, or pathologic alterations.

Toxicity Assessment

Toxicity assessment, also referred to as *dose-response assessment*, defines the relationship between the exposure/dose-response relationship of the chemical and the potential development of adverse health effects. The goal is to determine where on the continuum of the dose-response curve an adverse human health effect is likely to occur. Standard slope factors and RfDs are used. If a compound does not have an EPA-approved RfD value, then procedures are used to calculate these values. RfDs are calculated for acute, subchronic, and chronic exposures, and for different exposure routes. Risk is generally calculated for the most sensitive toxic effect for a given exposure duration. This assumes that protecting against the most sensitive effect protects against all other toxic effects (13). If human data are not available, data from the animal species most sensitive to the toxic effect are used. Animal studies generally include at least three dose rates besides the control group. The highest dose is usually at a level that produces generalized toxic effects. The lowest dose is at a level at which no detectable effect is produced, and this dose is used as the *no observed adverse effects level* (*NOAEL*) (14).

Calculation of the RfD starts from the NOAEL. The NOAEL is divided by a series of uncertainty factors (UFs) to derive the RfD:

$$\text{RfD} = \frac{\text{NOAEL}}{\text{UF}_1 \times \text{UF}_2 \times \text{UF}_n}$$

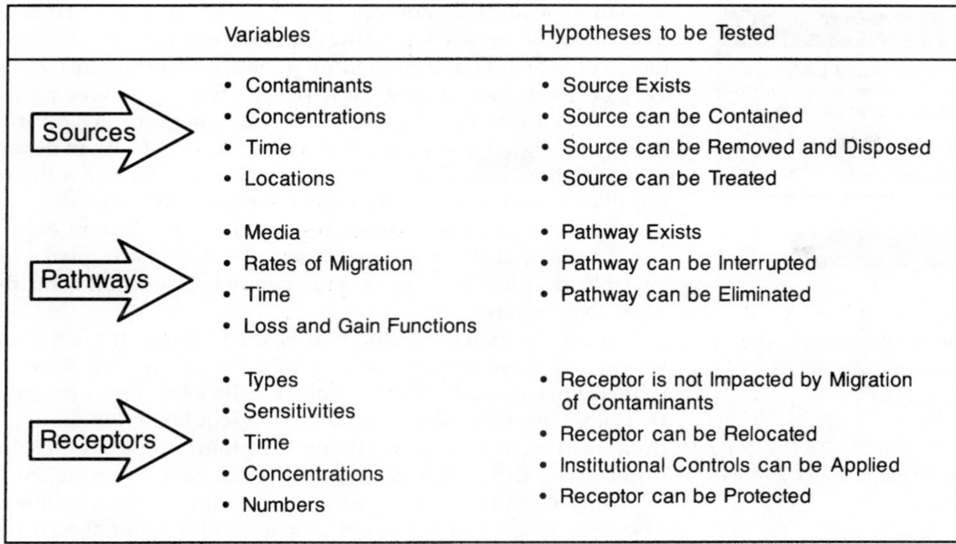

Variables
Hypotheses to be Tested
Sources
• Contaminants
• Concentrations
• Time
• Locations
• Source Exists
• Source can be Contained
• Source can be Removed and Disposed
• Source can be Treated
Pathways
• Media
• Rates of Migration
• Time
• Loss and Gain Functions
• Pathway Exists
• Pathway can be Interrupted
• Pathway can be Eliminated
Receptors
• Types
• Sensitivities
• Time
• Concentrations
• Numbers
• Receptor is not Impacted by Migration of Contaminants
• Receptor can be Relocated
• Institutional Controls can be Applied
• Receptor can be Protected

Figure 6-2. Elements of conceptual evaluation model. With permission from U.S. Environmental Protection Agency 1989.

The NOAEL is available from experimental data on the chemical that most closely approximates a level or concentration at or below which no toxic effects were detected. A safety factor makes allowances for uncertainties or knowledge gaps in the data available on the chemical under consideration. Safety factors are customarily established by the type of data available for the evaluation.

Uncertainty factors may include

- A UF of 10 for extrapolation from animals to humans (10A). This is based on the observation that humans are generally more sensitive to acute chemical toxicity than lab animals on a quantity/body-weight basis (15).
- A UF of 10 for extrapolation from less than chronic effects to chronic exposure (10S) if, for example, only subchronic (90-day) animal data are available rather than the preferred 2 years (5).
- A UF of 10 to allow for variability in susceptibility between humans (10H).

If an NOAEL is not identified, the EPA recommends that the lowest observed adverse effects level (LOAEL) is used as the starting point and that the LOAEL is divided by an uncertainty factor between 1 and 10 to obtain a theoretical NOAEL (Table 6-1) (8).

The assessor may also divide by a modifying factor, not exceeding a value of 10, if in the judgment of the assessor the peculiarities of the database for a particular chemical justify this (16). In theory, a total UF of 100,000 is possible, but in practice, if the total UF is 10,000, the database is considered too uncertain to estimate the RfD (13).

TABLE 6-1. Safety factors used in risk assessment to establish reference doses or acceptable levels of exposure to chemicals

Safety factor	Criteria for application
10	Extrapolating data from long-term human exposure to allow for hypersensitive individuals in the population
10	Additional tenfold factor when extrapolating from chronic animal studies
10	Additional tenfold factor when less than chronic animal studies are available
1–10	Scientific judgment is used to establish any additional safety factor to account for uncertainties not addressed previously

The RfD is used in determining risk by the following equation:

$$\text{Risk} = \text{PF}(\text{CDI} - \text{RfD})$$

CDI = chronic daily intake (mg/kg/day)
PF = potency factor slope of dose-response curve

If the CDI is less than the RfD, then the risk is assessed to be negligible.

The RfD approach assumes that there is a threshold of effect. That is, between zero and the threshold, there is a range over which no toxic effects occur. It is assumed that below the threshold, homeostatic mechanisms can maintain normal health. Because of the inherent uncertainties, the dose-response model that gives the most conservative estimate of the threshold is used (13).

Additional studies may be done to elucidate the nature of chronic toxic effects that may be due to accumulation of the chemical (or a metabolite) or accumulation of damage. To distinguish these, it is necessary to determine whether the chemical accumulates in the body, whether acute dosing causes damage (and, if so, how quickly and effectively it is repaired), and whether the chronic effects are more closely related to total dose or dose rate per day (14).

Exposure Assessment

Exposure assessment is the quantification and evaluation of the dose of chemical incurred from the exposure situation under consideration (Fig. 6-3). This step attempts to determine the type and magnitude of potential human exposures to chemicals.

Data from air, soil, water, and biota are examined. Exposure assessment includes consideration of the population exposed and the magnitude, frequency, duration, and routes of exposure. The susceptible population incurring exposure must be determined. The routes of exposure must be established, whether oral, via ingestion from water or diet; inhalation; dermal contact; or any combination of these. Magnitude, frequency, and duration of exposures must be determined. Exposure doses (EDs) are then calculated to give estimates of chronic daily and lifetime exposures.

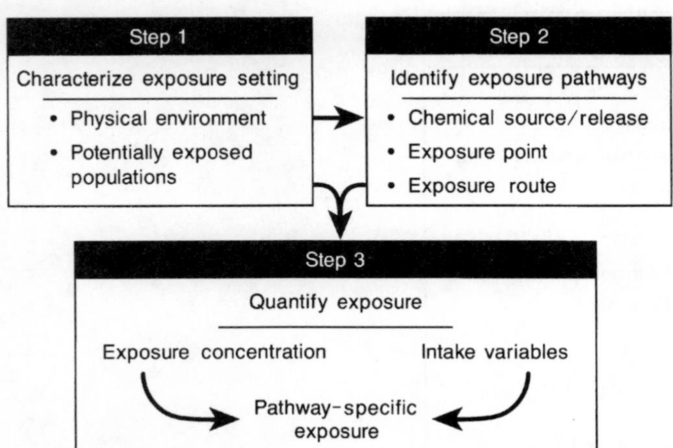

Figure 6-3. Exposure assessment process. With permission from U.S. Environmental Protection Agency 1989.

Risk Characterization

Risk characterization is the final step in the risk-assessment process. This step uses all information and assumptions acquired by the previous three steps. It provides qualitative conclusions regarding the likelihood that a chemical may pose a human health hazard. It also provides a quantitative risk value for exposure to the chemical(s) under consideration. Uncertainties in the data are pointed out and explained or rationalized if not addressed earlier in the process.

The target value of the risk characterization step is determined by the goal of the risk assessment. If the chemical under consideration is a carcinogen, the target is a cancer risk value—that is, how many cases of cancer are expected beyond the background incidence in the unexposed population. If the chemical causes noncarcinogenic effects, the target value is a hazard index (HI). The HI is the ED to RfD ratio. The EPA's equation is

$$\text{Noncancer hazard quotient} = \text{ED/RfD}$$

ED = exposure dose
RfD = reference dose

Where ED and RfD are expressed in the same units and represent the same exposure period (i.e., chronic, subchronic, or shorter terms).

The CDI can be substituted for the ED to establish the HI. If the RfD is less than the CDI or ED, the HI is greater than 1, and the risk is presumed significant.

In the case of a carcinogen, this allows a determination of whether the number of excess cancer deaths likely to occur will be higher than acceptable. In the case of a substance with a toxic endpoint other than cancer, it allows a determination as to whether exposure will result in a significant likelihood of adverse toxic health effects. Both carcinogenic and noncarcinogenic effects can occur with the same substance (e.g., arsenic, benzene); therefore, these effects are separately calculated.

Limitations of Current System

It is widely accepted that the current RfD system has many drawbacks. Animal studies are usually carried out in homogeneous, inbred laboratory strains (3) that bear little resemblance to the highly outbred human population. Exposure is limited to a single agent, which is the exception rather than the rule for human exposures. Xenobiotic chemicals are metabolized and detoxified by enzymatic pathways, the existence or predominance of which is determined by genetics and therefore may vary between species or even between strains. Enzyme pathways that are readily saturated in one species may not be readily saturated in another. The chemical is typically in doses much higher than those actually experienced by the human population and at which human enzymatic pathways may be saturated (3). Most animal studies are done at constant exposure levels; real-life human exposure tends to be in peaks of variable duration. Such peaks are extremely important contributors to exposure (17).

In recognition of these differences, the EPA uses human data whenever these are available. Obviously, however, human data are not available for new chemicals. Even for chemicals that have been in use for some time, adequate epidemiologic data are frequently unavailable. Epidemiologic studies in humans are difficult to conduct. It is not easy to reconstruct exposure conditions or to correct for confounding variables. The effect of coexposures to other chemicals cannot always be excluded. If exposure is rare, the study will be small. Epidemiologic studies are typically very time consuming (3) and expensive, and they usually lack sufficient power to establish cause and effect. Human exposure models that can produce realistic predictions of exposure to chemicals using human activity patterns and source information have yet to be developed and validated (17).

The use of the NOAEL to derive the RfD focuses on the dose that is the NOAEL and essentially ignores the other data. The choice of NOAEL is greatly dependent on the number and spacing of doses in a study. If dose spacing is too large or too few doses are tested, a NOAEL may be underestimated. By the time the NOAEL is divided by UFs, the RfD may be greatly underestimated (14).

The default assumption is that absorption is 100% by all routes, which is unlikely to be true for most chemicals (18).

The default process assumes a linear dose-response relationship, which may not be correct. If chemicals are metabolized to a toxic metabolite or are detoxified by a saturable enzyme pathway, the dose-response curve is modified. Some chemicals have a U-shaped dose-response curve. This may represent overcorrection by homeostatic mechanisms in the face of disturbance (19). Alternatively, a U-shaped curve may occur because the chemical has both negative and positive effects. If this is the case, the balance between the negative and positive effects may vary between individuals and between populations. These are hardly novel concepts to pharmaceutical manufacturers. Many therapeutic drugs are toxic in excess, and the toxicity of therapeutic drugs differs between individuals. For example, many over-the-counter painkillers are not safe for use in young children. However, the balance between negative effects and possible positive effects of environmental chemicals is not generally considered in risk assessment (19).

U-shaped curves need to be carefully assessed (19). If a U-shaped dose-response curve is detected, the curve may be divided into sections (14).

Current methods cannot be used to estimate the frequency or severity of the adverse health effects that may occur in the population if the RfD is exceeded, because they contain no information on the slope of the dose-response curve (5,20).

The current system undoubtedly has limitations. However, retrospective analysis shows that many human tragedies—including those as a result of thalidomide, asbestos, and many others that are less well publicized—could have been prevented, had the testing that is currently in place been done. The use of animals as models for humans has been validated for a wide range of adverse effects affecting the liver, kidneys, lungs, heart, eyes, skin, and gastric mucosa, as well as those that provoke hemolysis. The extent to which the current system has served to prevent human suffering remains unknown. It is very difficult to measure the disease and suffering that have been prevented because regulatory toxicology and risk assessment have been effective (20).

How Can Risk Assessment Be Improved?

Although it is generally acknowledged that the current system can and should be improved, this will take time. Toxicologists are not free to choose their methods of investigation. The experimental approaches currently used are anchored in national and international guidelines and laws (20). Current trends and recommendations for the improvement are discussed in the following sections.

PHYSIOLOGICALLY BASED PHARMACOKINETIC AND PHARMACODYNAMIC MODELS

The accuracy of risk assessment can be improved by the use of physiologically based pharmacokinetic (PBPK) models. PBPK models were first developed for anesthetics (21). Their use was subsequently expanded to other therapeutic drugs, and since the 1980s they have been applied to toxicology.

A PBPK model incorporates physiologic processes to describe the relationship between the dose to which an organism is exposed and the biologically effective dose acting at the level of the target tissue(s). This is in contrast to the traditional RfD, which is based on administered dose, not target organ concentrations or even blood levels (15). The PBPK model takes into account physiologic factors, such as body weight, age, sex, metabolic rate, respiratory rate, cardiac output, and inherited or induced activities of metabolizing enzymes. Characteristics of the chemical in question that determine how readily it is absorbed and distributed are also built into the model (22). An example of this type of model used by the EPA is the integrated uptake biokinetic model for lead exposure.

Physiologically based pharmacokinetic/pharmacodynamic (PBPK/PD) models also address the pharmacodynamics of the chemical—that is, the mechanism(s) by which the dose at the target tissue(s) produces its adverse effect(s) (23). PBPK/PD models may also incorporate data on progression of toxic and repair processes (21). The development and application of pharmacokinetic models are more advanced than of pharmacodynamic or PBPK/PD models (21).

PBPK models have the potential to greatly improve the accuracy of cross-species extrapolation, because they calculate a target tissue dose based on pharmacokinetic and physiologic parameters. Normal human values for physiologic parameters are substituted for the animal parameters in the PBPK equation. PBPK models can also provide accurate estimates of the impact of human variability—for example, the effect of inherited or acquired variations in activity of metabolizing enzymes (22).

PBPK modeling can improve the validity of interspecies extrapolation (24). For example, if the half-life in minutes of styrene is compared between species, rats clear styrene much more rapidly than humans. This gives the impression that the rat may not be a good experimental model for styrene toxicity in humans. However, application of a PBPK model for styrene kinetics that includes physiologic parameters, such as organ volumes, ventilation, and perfusion rates, shows that the disposition of the chemical in the two species is the same (23). Modeling the metabolism of ethylene oxide has served to validate the default equation relating body weight, metabolic rate, and half-life of chemicals in the body (24).

Interspecies extrapolation is simplified by the fact that many common physiologic parameters are already well established for humans and experimental rodents (22). Whereas physiologic parameters change fairly coherently with changes in body size and surface area, metabolic parameters are less predictable, being dependent on the specific enzymes active in different species. However, these can be measured for inclusion in a comprehensive model (21).

PBPK models can be used to estimate the adverse effects over a wide range of dose rates and exposure conditions (18). For example, in the case of an inhaled poison, the effect of increased respiration that is due to physical exertion can be calculated (22).

Route-to-route extrapolation can be undertaken more accurately using PBPK models than by using the default assumption that absorption is 100% by all routes (18). The default process assumes a linear dose-response relationship, which does not allow for the effect of saturation of metabolic or excretory pathways. The capacities of these pathways can be built into a PBPK model (18,23). PBPK modeling does not always produce a higher RfD than the default method, but the result is based on more information (24) and is, therefore, more defensible in scientific terms.

The major limitation in construction of a PBPK model is the availability of sufficient experimental data to construct and validate the model. The complexity of the model is limited by practical considerations (22). It should be borne in mind that the accuracy of the results from a PBPK model can only be as good as the model. If the assumptions used in constructing the model are flawed, the results will be inaccurate. For example, the distribution of toxicants in PBPK models may be described using body *compartments*, which are not an accurate representation of the real body. The movement of a chemical between compartments is often based on linear kinetics rather than the transport mechanisms that really operate. Metabolic kinetics may be oversimplified and not representative of real enzymes. Metabolism is usually treated as a single step, when in reality it is a complex sequence of biochemical reactions that may be altered at numerous points (25). Despite their limitations, it is generally accepted that PBPK and PBPK/PD models are likely to yield more meaningful results than the current system. The more physiologic and biochemical information that can be incorporated, the more realistic the model will be (25).

Although PBPK/PD models may never be able to duplicate the enormous complexity of an intact organism, they constitute the best and most promising tools for improving two essential components of risk assessment: interspecies extrapolations and low-dose extrapolations (21).

BIOMARKERS

There are three different classes of biomarkers: biomarkers of exposure, of effect, and of susceptibility.

A biomarker of exposure is an exogenous substance, its metabolite the product of an interaction between a xenobiotic agent and some target cell (26). Biomarkers of exposure are not routinely used in exposure assessment, but the advantage of using them is that they provide objective evidence of the actual level of the chemical that has been absorbed into the body (27). Biomarkers that directly reflect the cumulative dose of a poison are rare. An example of such a biomarker is polychlorinated biphenyl (PCB) in blood. Most biomarkers have short half-lives and therefore reflect the short-term situation only. This means that they must be measured repeatedly if the cumulative exposure is to be estimated from them (28).

A biomarker of effect is a measurable alteration within the organism that can be recognized as an existing or potential health impairment or disease (26). Individuals show elevated biomarkers of effect before overt disease occurs. In some cases, if the individual is removed from the exposure, overt disease can be avoided, but in other cases, by the time the biomarker is elevated, overt disease is inevitable (27).

A biomarker of susceptibility is an indicator of an inherited or acquired limitation of an organism's ability to cope with exposure to a specific xenobiotic substance (26).

For a biomarker of exposure or effect to be validated, it must be shown to be related to the pharmacokinetics or pharmacodynamics of the chemical in question. Biomarkers can be used to improve the accuracy of extrapolation beyond the tested dose rates and/or species. Biomarkers have other advantages. They can elucidate dose-time–response relationships and mechanisms of toxic action and can also, in some cases, improve the sensitivity of detection of adverse effects (24). Biomarkers of susceptibility have the potential to identify and characterize human subpopulations that are at particular risk (29). Study of mechanisms of toxicity is an increasing trend in the science of toxicology; accordingly, the incorporation of biomarkers into toxic risk assessment is likely to increase. However, at present there are few biomarkers that are sufficiently well validated for use in quantitative risk assessment (29).

INDIVIDUAL SUSCEPTIBILITY

Commonly used strains of laboratory rodents are extensively inbred, in contrast to the human population. Because the focus of toxicity testing has been on establishing causal connections, in-group variability—both genetic and environmental—has been avoided by the use of genetically homogeneous groups of healthy young adult animals maintained with a minimum of variability in environmental factors, such as diet and physiologic stressors. Epidemiologic data from human populations include variables, but their effect may not be reported by the subjects or identified by the epidemiologist (30).

Variability in physiologic and metabolic parameters can be considerable. For example, breathing rates vary 1.8- to 2.5-fold between adults and 65-fold between adults and infants. Enzyme activity levels can show even more variability. For example, 1,000-fold interindividual differences have been found for cytochrome P-450 2D6, which metabolizes tobacco smoke to carcinogenic nitrosamines (30). Similar variations have been found for other metabolizing enzymes. Assigning relative risk factors based on a single genetic polymorphism, even if the carriers are readily identifiable, is not necessarily a solution, because there are often multiple metabolic pathways and detoxification processes for any given chemical. Furthermore, genes do not act in isolation but as part of a series of events in a pathway or cascade. The downstream consequences of alterations upstream may not be well understood or readily predictable (31).

Preexisting disease can be a cause of interindividual variability. For example, in some of the commonly used strains of laboratory rats, males develop nephropathy with age, resulting in a twofold increase in their water intake. This will obviously affect the intake of waterborne chemicals in a long-term study (32). As another example, nutrition has been found to be an important determinant of outcome after toxic liver injury (33).

One area that is attracting increasing attention is developmental variability. Unique features of the fetus, infant, and child make them peculiarly susceptible to some chemicals. For example, the rapidly dividing cells of the fetus are particularly vulnerable to genotoxic damage. Migrating cells can be misdirected or stopped by toxic insults. Some cases of psychomotor retardation are attributed to abnormal neuronal migration in the brain. The particular susceptibility of the fetus to methylmercury is an example of this mechanism. The infant may have a particularly high intake of poisons that are excreted in breast milk, such as PCBs. Newborns and infants are more susceptible to dermal absorption of chemicals than adults. Infants have a higher respiratory rate and a relatively greater pulmonary absorptive area than adults; consequently, many are likely to absorb a greater dose of airborne chemicals. Metabolic and excretion rates are higher in children than adults, reaching a peak approximately between 8 to 10 years of age. Physiologic differences in brain capillary cell function may account for the greater susceptibility of children to acute lead encephalopathy. Behavioral differences, such as the tendency of infants toward oral exploration, may also increase their risk of ingesting toxic chemicals. In general, data on the effects of toxic hazards on the fetus and developing child are lacking. Consideration needs to be given to the distinctive characteristics and vulnerabilities of children, rather than assuming that they are simply small adults (34).

The regulatory community has not yet developed procedures to incorporate quantitative data on variability into decision making. Thus, there is no incentive for the manufacturers of new chemicals to collect data on variability of response or for regulatory agencies to demand them. Data from the most sensitive population has generally been used in those instances in which it was available, but the database remains deficient (30).

There is a growing trend toward the use of Monte Carlo analysis in exposure assessment. In Monte Carlo analysis, a number of potential exposure parameters are randomly sampled from the range of possible exposure parameters. These parameters are then applied to the exposure model to generate an estimate of the distribution of exposures that is likely to occur in a real-life population. The EPA has published guidance in the use of Monte Carlo analysis in risk assessments (35,36). The same approach can be applied to a PBPK model to estimate the results of individual variation in physiologic and metabolic parameters. For example, if the detoxification of a chemical is catalyzed by an enzyme, the activity of which is known to vary between individuals, a hypothetical population with a range of enzyme activities may be generated and then sampled by computer. The sampled enzyme activities may then be applied to the PBPK model to generate a range of possible consequences that may be seen in a real-life population.

The increasing application of biomarkers to determine the internal fate of toxicants will also help to draw attention to biological variability and quantify it.

BENCHMARK APPROACH

An alternative to the use of an NOAEL in risk assessment is the use of a benchmark dose. The *benchmark dose* is the lower confidence limit on a dose, which results in a small but measurable increase in the incidence or severity of an effect—for example, a 10% increase in response (14).

The benchmark dose is determined by using all the available dose-response data. This is in contrast to the NOAEL approach, in which all the dose-response data above the NOAEL are ignored (37). Thus, the benchmark approach incorporates information on the shape of the dose-response curve that the conventional NOAEL does not (14).

One of the disadvantages of the NOAEL approach is that the NOAEL must be one of the doses chosen in the experimental design. If all the doses given have an effect, then the NOAEL must be estimated from the LOAEL, with consequent introduction of yet another uncertainty factor. The benchmark-dose approach does not require an NOAEL to be identified or estimated (14,37).

The accuracy of the NOAEL is affected by the size of the study group and the choice of dose levels. The NOAEL selected can fall anywhere between zero and an incidence just below that detectable as an increase above control level (usually 7% to 10%) (14). In general, the more sensitive the bioassay and the more animals used, the lower the resulting NOAEL. Thus, there is a disincentive for companies that develop chemicals to use experimental designs with a greater sensitivity than absolutely required by regulatory agencies. The benchmark approach, on the other hand, encourages good science, because the benchmark dose is generally higher when it arises from a bioassay with an adequate group size (37).

One important advantage of this approach is that the benchmark dose allows the estimation of the magnitude of adverse effects that may result if the RfD is exceeded (14).

CONSIDERATION OF REPAIR

Understanding of the mechanisms by which toxic chemicals inflict injury has increased greatly since the mid-1980s, but understanding of repair mechanisms has not kept pace. However, some toxicity models have been studied in which the importance of repair mechanisms is illustrated (38).

One well-studied situation is that in which prior exposure to a nontoxic level of chlordecone increases 67-fold the lethality of carbon tetrachloride in rats. It has been found that, ordinarily, a low dose of carbon tetrachloride is not lethal, because tissue repair is stimulated at the same time that tissue injury is inflicted. Cell division occurs in two waves: an early wave, approximately 6 hours after administration of carbon tetrachloride, and another larger wave, 36 to 48 hours after administration. The early wave, which arises from a small number of hepatocytes that are in the G2 phase, is abolished by prior exposure to chlordecone, because the cells lack the energy to divide because of decreased availability of adenosine triphosphate. Abolition of the early wave of cell division means that the biochemical signals required to prime the neighboring cells do not occur. When the second wave of cell division occurs, it is too little and too late to counter the injury, and the animal dies. This model illustrates dramatically the importance of the repair process to the outcome in toxicoses (38).

In some cases, prior exposure to a low dose of a chemical confers a degree of protection against a normally lethal dose of a compound. This phenomenon of autoprotection can be induced in animals in the case of carbon tetrachloride. The underlying mechanism is stimulated tissue repair (38).

Tissue repair is the mechanism behind the existence of a threshold, the level below which no adverse effects occur. Stimulation of tissue repair varies with animal species and between strains within a species, and this is thought to be a significant cause of variations in susceptibility. The accuracy of risk assessment could be increased by the measurement of both tissue injury and stimulated tissue repair (38).

QUANTITATIVE STRUCTURE-ACTIVITY RELATIONSHIPS

The sheer number of new and existing chemicals means that there is a need to improve the process of selecting chemicals for toxicity testing (39).

Many chemicals already in production have not been exhaustively tested for toxicologic effects. New chemicals are being introduced at a rate of as many as 700,000 per year. The potential to create new chemical compounds is colossal. There would be considerable savings of both expense and time if it were possible to accurately predict the toxicity of a new chemical from its structure. Many groups are researching the area of quantitative structure-activity relationships (QSARs). Between 15,000 and 20,000 QSAR studies have been published (40). A number of QSAR models have been developed that relate the toxicity of classes of chemicals to their structures. These models work well when a chemical can be assigned to a single chemical class for which a good QSAR model exists. The models fail in cases in which the chemical is complex, belongs to more than one structural class, or is entirely novel (41).

It is not possible to predict the toxicology of a chemical from its structure (42), so QSARs cannot at present replace standard bioassays. However, the existing database can be used to identify chemicals that are likely to be toxic and can therefore be used to determine priorities in toxicologic testing (32). As the database grows, the potential of QSAR models to provide a useful interim estimate of toxicity should increase. Powerful computer technology will play an important role in the compilation of the database required before accurate predictions will be possible (40).

RISK ASSESSMENT OF CHEMICAL MIXTURES

In the past, most toxicology resources have been devoted to single chemicals. Yet human exposure to chemicals is rarely, if ever, limited to a single chemical. The interest of toxicologists in the toxicology of mixtures is increasing.

The combined effects of chemicals may be less than or more than additive (43–46). Interactions may be chemical interactions—such as the formation of nitrosamines from nitrites and amines—or biological interactions at many levels, including absorption, distribution, excretion, metabolism, and actions at receptor sites or susceptible molecules (44). The nature of the interaction may vary depending on the toxic effect measured. For example, both chlorinated insecticides and halogenated solvents are hepatotoxic, but the insecticide is likely to act as a nervous system stimulant, whereas the solvent is likely to be a nervous system depressant (44).

Systematic investigation of chemical interactions by traditional methods is impractical, if not impossible, because of the enormous number of possible combinations and interactions. Therefore, to target research efforts, there is a desperate need for predictive systems to identify which combinations are likely to interact (45).

Similarly, epidemiologic investigations of chemical mixtures have been limited by the need for large sample sizes. Epidemiologists start with a statistical prediction based on the assumption that effects will be additive and refer to any departure from this statistical prediction as *effect modification*. Effect modification may be due to synergism or antagonism. Standardized criteria for recognition of effect modification have not yet been developed (46).

In risk assessment, the most commonly used method for dealing with chemical mixtures is the HI approach. This approach assumes a purely additive effect with no interaction. It is further assumed that the chemicals in the mixture act by the same mechanism, have identical dose-response curves, and differ only in potency. In short, they are treated as dilutions or concentrations of each other. This approach can lead to substantial errors if synergistic or antagonistic effects occur (43).

The EPA has published guidelines on how to deal with some aspects of mixture toxicology and has compiled a database on known pollutant interactions (44). Present EPA guidelines allow for the use of models other than additivity models if justified by the data (47).

Far more information, particularly in the area of mechanisms of toxicity, is required before it will be possible to predict chemical interactions. PBPK/PD modeling, coupled to Monte Carlo simulation, is likely to be an important method in future efforts to predict toxicity of chemical mixtures (48). Computer technology has reached the point at which PBPK/PD models for individual chemicals could be linked at the pharmacokinetic and/or pharmacodynamic levels to predict toxicologic interactions (45).

The EPA has an ongoing research program investigating PBPK/PD modeling for chemical mixtures. Other areas of EPA research include toxicity thresholds and interaction thresholds for chemical mixtures, identification of optimal experimental designs to estimate joint thresholds, assessment from epidemiologic data as to whether additivity is occurring, mechanisms of interaction, and n-dimensional models of dose-response relationships for recognizing effect modification (49).

RISK ASSESSMENT FOR REPRODUCTIVE AND DEVELOPMENTAL EFFECTS

Human reproduction is a highly emotive area. Most people feel strongly about their own fertility and about the health of the children they produce. In addition, human reproduction is a remarkably inefficient process with high levels of abnormal outcome.

Between 10% and 20% of couples have impaired fertility (50). It is believed that as many as 50% of human conceptions are lost before implantation. Somewhere between 15% and 30% of implanted pregnancies fail before the first missed menstruation and go undetected, unless urinary human chorionic gonadotropin levels are monitored (51). An additional 15% to 20% of pregnancies end in miscarriage before 28 weeks' gestation (50). The causes of 65% to 70% of all miscarriages are unknown (2). Some 10% of pregnancies that continue beyond 28 weeks end in stillbirth, and another 10% end in delivery of a premature infant who may not survive (50).

Approximately 3% of children born in the United States have a major malformation at birth. Many more are later found to have problems of developmental origin—6% to 7% by 1 year of age and 12% to 14% by school age (52).

Between 2% and 25% of all congenital defects are due to a chromosomal, spontaneous, or inherited genetic anomaly. An additional 7% to 10% are due to infection or maternal disease. Approximately 2% can be traced to drugs or environmental chemicals. This leaves 66% to 70% for which no cause can be identified (50). The high proportion of developmental defects for which the cause is unknown makes it difficult to evaluate the developmental risks associated with a chemical exposure (52).

Every component of the reproductive process is susceptible to some exogenous agent (53). Reproductive toxicity and developmental toxicity must be treated as special situations for a number of reasons:

- There are three potential targets: the man, the woman, and the conceptus.
- There are several organ systems—reproductive and neuroendocrine—and numerous individual organs to be considered (54).
- Reproduction occurs intermittently. The adverse effects of reproductive or developmental toxicants may go unnoticed until reproduction is attempted (50).
- Reproductive toxicity not only involves more than one person, it also involves many years of susceptibility.

The relevant time period during which a reproductive toxicant may act begins with the conception of both the child's parents and continues until the child becomes an adult and is ready to become a parent. The window of susceptibility begins at the conceptions of the child's parents because their precursor germ cells, reproductive tracts, and endocrine systems all develop before they are born. The maternal and paternal germ cells are then susceptible throughout the development, childhood, adolescence, and adulthood of the parents. The susceptibility window continues through gametogenesis, mating, sperm transport and fertilization, implantation, and prenatal development. The child continues to be susceptible to toxicants that may affect his or her reproductive success throughout his or her childhood, adolescence, and adulthood (26).

The critical stage of pregnancy during which teratogens may induce structural malformations is the period of organogenesis, which in humans is from 20 to 70 days after the last menstrual period. However, exposure of the mother before this time could still result in malformations if the teratogen or its teratogenic metabolite persists in the mother's body.

During the fetal period, toxic effects include growth retardation, fetal death, functional impairment, and transplacental carcinogenesis. Some forms of structural malformation may also occur during this period.

Toxic exposures during the prenatal and early postnatal periods have been shown to affect functions that include behavior, reproduction, endocrine function, immune competence, xenobiotic metabolism, and certain other physiologic functions (55).

Exposure of the man may also lead to reproductive toxicity, either directly, through damage to sperm, or indirectly, through semen. Many substances are excreted in semen, and some of these may persist in the female long after conception (55). There is growing evidence that exposure of men to exogenous agents may result in abnormal fetal loss, birth defects, and childhood cancer. Epidemiologic studies have shown that for men, some occupations—such as those in the petroleum and chemical industries—are associated with abnormal reproductive outcomes. Furthermore, studies in rodents have conclusively demonstrated that exposure of the male rodent before mating can lead to abnormalities in the offspring. However, the mechanisms are unknown in both mice and humans (26).

There are three major categories of possible mechanism of male reproductive toxicity:

- Nongenetic impairment of the male's fertility (e.g., decreased spermatogenesis). This may result from toxic insults to any of a variety of cells, including Leydig cells, Sertoli cells, epididymal cells, or the cells of the various stages in spermatogenesis.
- *Genetic mechanisms*—damage to the germline DNA leading to chromosomal abnormalities or gene mutations in the offspring. Sperm carrying cytogenetic abnormalities are still capable of fertilization (26). No agent has been demonstrated to induce reproductive cell mutations in humans (13,56), but genetic abnormalities resulting from such induced mutations in human germ cells remain theoretically possible. The fertilized egg has the capacity to repair DNA lesions in sperm, but this capacity varies even between strains of mice (26).
- *Epigenetic mechanisms*—damage to the germline DNA that leads to abnormal outcomes by mechanisms other than mutation (26). An example of an epigenetic mechanism that could, in theory, be affected by toxicants is *imprinting*. This is the term for the phenomenon in which, for certain genes, only the maternal or paternal alleles are expressed during development. Thus, although the zygote has two copies of a given gene, in practical terms it only has one and may not be able to survive if that one does not operate correctly (26).

Although genetic abnormalities resulting from induced mutations in human germ cells have not yet been detected, this may be, at least in part, because they are difficult to detect. Mutations in genes that code for enzymes are mostly recessive. Heterozygous carriers generally possess enzyme activity that is sufficient for normal functioning and, therefore, are not detected unless or until the activity of that enzyme is assayed. Many generations may pass before two carriers produce a homozygous baby with symptoms because of profound deficiency of that enzyme activity. On the other hand, mutations in genes for structural proteins tend to be dominant. They also tend to be incompatible with survival and, therefore, may not come to light because the conceptus is lost early in pregnancy (56).

Present Systems for Assessing Reproductive and Developmental Effects

A variety of animal tests for the study of reproductive toxicity are available (2). Multigenerational studies are the most inclusive and are presently required by most regulatory agencies (54).

THE MULTIGENERATION REPRODUCTION STUDY, OR TWO-GENERATION REPRODUCTION STUDY

The Multigeneration Reproduction Study begins with exposure of animals of both sexes before mating. Exposure continues through pregnancy, the postnatal development of the offspring, and their mating and pregnancies, parturitions, and lactations. Animals of all generations are closely monitored, and histopathologic examinations are performed on parent animals of all generations. This study is designed to test for effects that only become apparent after accumulation over at least one generation (2).

Other tests for measurement of reproductive toxicity include the Study of Fertility and General Reproductive Performance, or One-Generation Reproductive Study. Animals of both sexes are exposed to the test substance well before mating and throughout mating and early pregnancy. Females rear their young to weaning. Observations are made concerning fertility and reproductive toxicity in the parents and concerning morphologic and functional development in the progeny (2).

EMBRYO/FETOTOXICITY STUDY OR TERATOLOGY STUDY

Pregnant animals are exposed to relatively high concentrations of the test chemical during the organogenesis stage of gestation. Pregnant animals are killed 1 day before natural delivery to avoid loss of deformed fetuses as a result of cannibalism. Detailed examinations are made of the fetuses (2).

PERI- AND POSTNATAL TOXICITY STUDY

This study concentrates on possible effects of exposure late in pregnancy or via breast milk on postnatal development. Exposure begins in the last trimester of pregnancy and continues through parturition and lactation. The physical and functional development of the progeny are closely monitored. This includes neurologic, behavioral, and cognitive functions.

SPERM EVALUATION TESTS

Sperm evaluation tests include observations of morphology, motility, vitality, and capacity to penetrate an ovum (2). The EPA's *Guidelines for Developmental Toxicity Risk Assessment* states the following assumptions:

- An agent that produces an adverse effect in experimental animal studies will potentially pose a hazard to humans after sufficient exposure during development. This assumption is based on the observation that in almost all cases, experimental animal data are predictive of a developmental effect in humans.
- All of the four manifestations of developmental toxicity (death, structural abnormalities, growth alterations, and functional deficits) are of concern.
- The types of developmental effects seen in animal studies are not necessarily the same as those that may be produced in humans. The manifestations of developmental toxicity may vary between species (52). Not all species are equally susceptible or sensitive to the teratogenic effects of a given chemical (55). It is impossible to predict which species of animal will show developmental alterations most like those seen in humans (52).
- The most sensitive species is appropriate for use. This is the default assumption in the absence of pharmacokinetic, pharmacodynamic, or other data that could indicate the most appropriate species. This default is justified by the observation that for the majority of known developmental toxicants, humans are as sensitive as, or more sensitive than, the most sensitive animal species tested (52).
- In general, a threshold is assumed for the dose-response curve for agents that produce developmental toxicity. The developing organism is known to have some capacity for repair.

The EPA applies a safety factor of 100 from the maternal or fetal NOAEL to all developmental toxicants. However, California's Safe Drinking Water and Toxic Enforcement Act of 1986 assumes that a 1,000-fold safety factor should be used to protect the fetus (13).

Directions in Reproductive and Developmental Effects

Traditionally, the NOAEL/UF approach has been used in developmental toxicity risk assessment, but the EPA is investigating more quantitative approaches, such as the benchmark-dose approach, and is supporting more research into mechanisms of developmental toxicity (52).

Research into mechanisms of teratogenesis is also required. The mechanism of the primary molecular damage is unknown for all known teratogens (52). Historically, it has been thought that the early conceptus, before organogenesis, is not susceptible to congenital malformations, because all the cells are multipotential; therefore, if some are killed, others can compensate for them. However, there is now strong evidence that teratogens can act during the preorganogenesis period at any time, from sperm entry into the ovum until the late blastocyst stage (52).

In contrast to the situation for developmental toxins—of which in almost all cases experimental animal data are predictive of a developmental effect in humans—there is a need for reliable predictive models of human teratogens. The great majority of human teratogens were discovered in humans before they were discovered in animals, and then largely through case studies rather than epidemiologic studies (55). Animals also tend to be poor models of human reproductive toxicants (57). Reproductive processes vary considerably between species (53).

Multigenerational trials are expensive and time consuming. They are controversial because of the number of animals sacrificed and the need to sacrifice females immediately before parturition. *In vitro* screens are not yet available to replace the *in vivo* tests used to assess developmental toxicity (58). One promising alternative is the use of the chick embryo *in vitro*, which can be used to detect lethality, growth retardation, and interference with differentiation. Embryonic and fetal testing using the chicken embryo *in vitro* eliminates the need to use pregnant animals. The chicken embryo *in vitro* produces better results than the chick *in ovo* test, which has been found to be too sensitive (59).

An international collaboration exists to maintain a worldwide surveillance of approximately 4 million newborn babies each year. One of the goals of this collaboration is to detect changes in the incidence of specific malformations that may be the result of environmental hazards and, if possible, to eliminate these tragedies (55).

RISK ASSESSMENT FOR NEUROTOXIC EFFECTS

Neurotoxicity constitutes a special situation in risk assessment, because serious changes in behavior or cognitive function can occur that cannot be recognized by histopathology. In addition, the central nervous system is complex, highly specialized, and limited in its capacity for repair. For example, after infancy, lost neurons cannot be replaced.

Lifetime rodent bioassays are used to detect neurotoxic effects. Multigenerational studies are used for the detection of developmental neurotoxicity. The recommended neurotoxicity screening procedure published by the EPA includes a functional observational battery, an assessment of motor activity, and neuropathology. Parameters measured include activity, autonomic nervous system function, convulsions, excitability, neuromuscular function, and sensorimotor function. The inclusion of systematic observational methods is a recent development (60).

Behavioral toxicology is a relatively new discipline, and the methods applied are still under development. Studies of lead toxicity have shown that rats and primates develop signs of behavioral toxicity at almost identical exposure levels to those causing behavioral toxicity in humans. These findings validate the use of animal behavior studies in behavioral toxicity risk assessment (61).

Changes in cognitive abilities such as memory and learning have been reported in many human cases of neurotoxic exposure. Many tests have been developed to measure cognitive function in laboratory animals, but there is as yet no consensus of opinion on which of these tests are the best for screening purposes (60).

Developmental Neurotoxicity

The fetus and developing child need special consideration in terms of neurotoxicity (34). Mitotic activity of cerebral neurons occurs prenatally and in the first 2 years of postnatal life. Migration of neurons in the brain occurs prenatally, and disruption of this process can have disastrous consequences. Brain growth includes branching of neuronal dendrites, which determines the number of synapses between neurons and, consequently, the efficiency of brain function. Cognitive development continues well into adolescence. Disruption of any of these processes by a toxicant is generally irreversible, and developmental neurotoxicity may result from a single exposure. Dose and timing of exposure are critical variables in determining which endpoints of neurologic development may be affected.

Comparison between neurotoxic effects occurring during development in humans and those occurring during development in rodents has shown remarkable similarities in the effects of a number of diverse toxicants, including lead, methylmercury, ethanol, PCBs, and phenytoin. In the qualitative sense, rodents are good models for human developmental neurotoxicity in the areas of motor development and function, cognitive function, sensory function, and motivational/arousal behavior. There is insufficient information to determine the suitability of rodents for neurotoxic effects on the development of social function (62).

Because several major events that occur prenatally in the human infant occur postnatally in the rat pup, the investigation of developmental neurotoxicity in rats is extended into postnatal life. This practice also allows study of the effects of exposure through milk (62).

The EPA has developed comprehensive protocols for both a basic developmental neurotoxicity screening battery to be incorporated into any developmental or reproductive toxicity study and a stand-alone developmental neurotoxicity battery (63). These batteries of tests evaluate multiple categories of function. Testing of neurologic functions should extend at least to weaning—if not to adulthood—of animals that are exposed prenatally (62). EPA policy is that in developmental neurotoxicology, transient effects and developmental delays constitute adverse effects (62), because their effects may be far reaching.

RISK ASSESSMENT FOR CANCER

Cancer, a large group of diseases characterized by uncontrolled growth and spread of abnormal cells (64), is very common. One out of every four Americans dies of cancer (5). Carcinogens, as identified by animal tests, are not rare. Approximately 50% of synthetic chemicals and 50% or more of naturally occurring substances are carcinogenic in animal tests (65). Damage to or errors in DNA may occur spontaneously during DNA replication as a result of endogenous DNA-reactive material or after exposure to exogenous carcinogens that are not necessarily human-made (66).

Age is the most important risk factor for developing cancer. Approximately 60% of all cancers occur in people older than 65 years. This century has seen a great extension in life expectancy in the Western world and a consequential increase in the proportion of people older than 65. The overall prevalence of cancer has accordingly increased. Additionally, it is possible that the often lethal infections of childhood that were common in earlier centuries exerted a selection pressure in favor of individuals resistant to infection and also to degenerative diseases such as cancer (67). However, if the proportion of cancer that is associated with tobacco is not included, the overall mortality rate for the remaining cancers has actually declined in many countries from 1970 to 1990 (68). Over the last 50 years, from 1950 to 1999, the incidences (adjusted for age) of prostate cancer, liver cancer, stomach cancer, and uterine cancer have declined. The rates of breast cancer, colon cancer, leukemia, pancreatic cancer, bladder cancer, and rectal cancer have remained unchanged. The rates of lung cancer and melanoma have increased.

Smoking is considered the cause of approximately 50% of cancer deaths (65). Diet is the cause of 35% of cancers, and infection—at 10%—is another significant cause. In short, the vast majority of cancers are caused by exposure to tobacco, diet, and viruses, all of which are naturally occurring substances (68). By comparison, occupational factors are thought to cause 4% of cancers; pollution, 2%; and industrial products, less than 1% (65).

Cancer is believed to result from a series of genetic alterations. It is believed that at least two critical cellular changes are required in its development. For some tumors, there are at least six mutations between the initial mutation and the eventual metastatic tumor (69). *Initiation*, which may involve more than one step, predisposes a cell to malignant transformation. Either an oncogene is activated, or a tumor-suppressor gene is inactivated (66). Cell proliferation is a key factor in initiation and is involved in every step of the cancer process (66).

Genetic alterations are more likely to occur during cell division than in the nondividing cell (70). The potential for mutation in genes that govern growth control is increased during replication, because many of those genes are transcribed and may experience greater exposure to mutagens (66). Increased cell replication may increase the frequency of spontaneous mutations by errors in replication. Also, those genetic alterations that do occur—including errors of replication, endogenous DNA adducts, and exogenous DNA adducts—may be converted to mutations before DNA repair can occur (66,70).

Inactivation of DNA repair pathways is known to increase the likelihood of malignant transformation, and differences in gene-specific and strand-specific repair are associated with increased likelihood of malignant transformation (71). However, little is known about whether repair activity is inducible in mammalian cells.

The term *progression* refers to later stages of cancer development: changes in the number and arrangement of chromosomes associated with increased growth rate, invasiveness, and metastasis (66).

The process of carcinogenesis is quite inefficient. Many preneoplastic lesions, such as mutated cells and altered cell foci, do not ultimately lead to cancer. The estimated probability of an initiated liver cell developing into a malignant tumor is in the order of 1 in 100,000 (72).

How Do Carcinogens Work?

Chemical carcinogens may act by inducing mutations or altering cellular growth control (66). Genotoxic chemicals may react with DNA or alter the structure or number of chromosomes (66). Many chemicals that lead to cancer enter the body as precarcinogens and are metabolized to genotoxic species that bind covalently to specific sites in DNA (73). Because many chemical carcinogens require metabolic activation to genotoxic species, numerous variables in the areas of metabolism and pharmacokinetics may affect the ultimate outcome (74). Most of the reactions that convert precarcinogens to their genotoxic metabolites are carried out by cytochrome P-450 enzymes. Many forms of these enzymes exist, and there are significant differences in their activities between and within species.

Most cytochrome P-450 enzymes are concentrated in the liver, but they are also found in other tissues. Cancer in organs other than the liver may be due to extrahepatic activation or transport of metabolites from the liver to the target tissue (73).

Genotoxic chemicals can generally be identified by assays for reactivity with DNA, inductions or mutations, or induction of DNA repair. Genotoxic chemicals are much more effective carcinogens at doses that also induce cell proliferation (66).

There are two classes of nongenotoxic carcinogens that do not react with DNA. These are *mitogens*, which induce cell proliferation in the target tissue, and *cytotoxins*, which produce cell death followed by regenerative cell proliferation (66).

Cytotoxicants act as carcinogens only at doses that produce cell death and regenerative cell proliferation. Any chemical that kills normal cells is likely to increase the accumulation of mutated cells, because there is always a risk of mutation occurring during regenerative cell division. During replicative DNA synthesis, DNA is unwound and suffers greater exposure to endogenous mutagens. Such mutagens may be produced by the inflammation that accompanies cellular necrosis (75). Cytotoxicants may cause preferential growth of initiated cells, because these cells may be more refractory to lethality or more responsive to growth stimulatory signals (66).

Saccharin is an example of a chemical that induces cytotoxicity and cell proliferation only at massive doses. It is common practice to extrapolate the results of rodent studies at these high doses to humans exposed to doses several orders of magnitude lower (66).

Cocarcinogenesis is the enhancement of tumor induction by an agent that by itself is not genotoxic and that is administered before or together with a carcinogen. Possible mechanisms by which cocarcinogens may operate include increased uptake of the carcinogen, increased activation of the carcinogen, depletion of competing nucleophilic molecules, inhibition of the rate or fidelity of DNA repair, or enhancement of the conversion of DNA lesions to permanent alterations (44).

In contrast to cocarcinogenesis, *promotion* refers to the enhancement of neoplasm induction by a nongenotoxic agent administered after the carcinogen—that is, when initiation is complete (44). Promotion is the biological activity most often attributed to mitogens and cytotoxicants. Promoters accelerate tumor formation by enhancing clonal expansion of preneoplastic cells. Regenerative cell replication may include preferential proliferation of precancerous or cancerous cells (66).

Initiation can take place rapidly, after a single exposure to an initiator, and is a permanent event (44). In contrast, prolonged exposure to a promoter is required before the effect becomes irreversible (44).

It is increasingly difficult to define a chemical rigidly as an initiator or a promoter. Initiation, promotion, and progression are highly dependent on dose rate, total dose at the target tissue, and the experimental species under study (66).

Present System of Cancer Risk Assessment

Chemicals are tested for carcinogenic effect in lifetime rodent bioassays of 2 years' duration, during which time rats and mice of both genders are given the chemical in question at the maximum tolerated dose (MTD) and one-half of the MTD. The MTD is the largest dose that can be applied to animals without causing chronic toxicity (8). This is used to ensure maximum sensitivity to any carcinogenic effect and to limit to a manageable number the number of animals required to detect the effect. If the levels to which humans are exposed were used, millions of test animals would be required to detect an effect and to be sure that it was a significant effect and not a result of chance (65).

The EPA then applies the *linear multistage model* to the results of the lifetime rodent bioassay. The linear multistage model assumes that all carcinogens act by genotoxicity and that if any dose of a toxic substance can cause cancer, then every dose can cause cancer in equal proportion. That is, if 1,000 ppm cause 1,000 cancers, then 1 ppm will cause one cancer (65). Another default assumption is that humans are as sensitive as the most sensitive animal species, strain, and sex (72). Table 6-2 summarizes calculation models that have been used for carcinogen risk assessment. The EPA has used the following carcinogen classification groups:

- Group A: Known human carcinogen.
- Group B: Probable human carcinogen—this is subdivided into B1, for which the evidence includes limited human evidence and some animal evidence, and B2, for which there is animal evidence only.
- Group C: Possible human carcinogen based on limited evidence in animals only.
- Group D: Inadequately tested.
- Group E: Has been tested and apparently is not a carcinogen.

The EPA is proposing to replace this rating system with a narrative statement describing the evidence of carcinogenicity for each chemical (13).

TABLE 6-2. Carcinogenic risk calculations

Model	Lifetime risk (1.0 mg/kg/day of toxin)	Comment
One-hit	6×10^{-5} (1 in 17,000)	Assumes a carcinogenic change induced by one molecule or one radiation interaction.
Linear multistage	6×10^{-6} (1 in 167,000)	EPA's model of choice. Assumes multiple stages for carcinogenesis that involves multiple carcinogens, cocarcinogens, and cancer promoters.
Multihit	4.4×10^{-7} (1 in 2.3 million)	Least conservative model. Assumes several interactions are required to cause carcinogenesis. Produces a linear relationship between hit and dose. The slope of dose-response curve at low dose is called the *potency factor* (PF). Lifetime risk = AD × PF.
Probit	1.9×10^{-9} (1 in 5.3 billion)	Questionable for use in carcinogenesis risk. Appropriate for assessing acute toxicity.

AD, average dose.
Adapted from U.S. Environmental Protection Agency (EPA). Proposed guidelines for carcinogen risk assessment. *Fed Reg* 1996;61:17960–18011.

The EPA is mandated to set a maximum contaminant level at which the risk of cancer is increased by only one in a million over a human lifetime of 70 years. This is over and above the background risk of 250,000 in a million.

EPA guidelines stress that the agency's numeric estimates of risk are unlikely to be too low, and the true risk may be as low as zero. This caveat is always communicated prominently to the public (8).

Limitations of the Current System

Under the current system, human risk is extrapolated from rodent results despite the fact that, even between rats and mice, congruence in results is only 70% (4). In studies conducted by the National Cancer Institute and National Toxicology Program, 50% of chemicals caused cancer in at least one species and gender of rodent. However, only 13.8% of chemicals studied adequately in male and female rats and male and female mice caused cancer in both species and both genders (12).

Many carcinogens show quantitative differences in activity between species (73). These are likely to be due to differences between species in the existence of metabolic pathways, which pathway predominates, and how readily metabolic pathways are saturated (74). It is reasonable to assume that a genotoxic chemical that reacts with rodent DNA will react with human DNA, but only if the absorption and metabolism are such that they are similarly brought into contact with the DNA (13).

Oncogenes and tumor-suppressor genes are often species specific, in some cases even strain specific (17). Some mechanisms by which chemicals cause cancer in rodents do not operate in human beings. For example, trichloracetic acid does not induce peroxisome proliferation in human liver cells as it does in mice (74). Human hepatocytes are minimally sensitive, if at all, to peroxisome proliferators and the phenobarbital-like enzyme inducers that constitute the major classes of nongenotoxic carcinogens in mouse liver (68). Trichloroethylene induces liver tumors in mice by a species-specific pathway that does not operate in rats and is unlikely to operate in humans (68).

Spontaneous tumor incidences differ between rodents and humans. Two of the most prevalent tumors in humans—colorectal and prostate—virtually never occur spontaneously in rodents. In contrast, the liver is by far the dominant target of both spontaneous and induced tumors in rats and mice. Spontaneous human liver cancer is very rare. Liver cancer in humans is almost always associated with cirrhosis, hepatitis B virus infection, or human immunodeficiency virus infection (68).

The use of high doses of chemicals is also controversial. The MTD and one-half the MTD are far in excess of environmental exposure and are given continuously over the animals' lifetimes (66). There is increasing concern that much of the cancer response measure in rodent bioassays is not due to genotoxic mechanisms but is a consequence of the cell proliferation produced only at the high doses of chemicals used in bioassays (66). At such high doses, metabolic pathways are likely to be saturated, whereas at the levels at which humans are exposed, metabolism is often linear and first order (74). In addition, high doses of a test chemical may overwhelm natural detoxification mechanisms (66).

Evaluation of the results of MTD bioassays calls into question the validity of the practice of using the MTD. Some analyses have shown that 43% to 66% of positive bioassays were positive only at the MTD. In those cases in which a carcinogenic effect was observed at a dose lower than the MTD, the lower dose was typically one-half of the MTD. A typical positive result for carcinogenicity in a bioassay is an incidence of cancer in 10% to 100% of the test population. Extrapolation is then made down to an incidence of 1 in 1 million in order to define an MCL, despite the fact that extrapolation beyond a standard curve is not good science. These extrapolations are frequently made from only one data point. A linear dose-response curve passing through zero is assumed (39).

The 2-year exposure of rodents covers most of their life span and thus is likely to greatly overexaggerate the insult to humans who are exposed to a chemical for perhaps only a few years of a 70-year life span. The lifetime rodent bioassay may, therefore, be too sensitive for human risk assessment because of both too high a rate of exposure and too long an exposure period (68).

The linear multistage model treats all carcinogens as genotoxic mutagens and assumes there is no threshold above zero. It does not allow for mechanisms that may act as barriers between the applied dose and the dose at the target tissue, such as absorption barriers, active transport processes, and enzymes of bioactivation or detoxification (66).

The assumption that carcinogens do not have a threshold is debated. The carcinogenicity of cytotoxic, nongenotoxic carcinogens is likely to be conditional on doses high enough to produce cell death and subsequent cell proliferation (66). It is less clear whether mitogens have a dose-response threshold. Many mitogens act through cellular receptors. A certain amount of receptor occupancy is required before a response is triggered. Some receptor-mediated pharmaceuticals trigger a response at very low doses, whereas others acting at the same receptor require a much higher dose to trigger the same response (66).

In 1992, the National Toxicology Program Board of Scientific Counselors identified the following assumptions, which are used to extrapolate from the MTD but do not appear to be valid: Pharmacokinetics are not dose dependent; the dose-response relationship is linear; DNA repair is not dependent on dose; response is not dependent on age; and the test dose need not bear a relationship to human exposure.

Assessment of carcinogenicity also needs to include consideration of pharmacokinetics and metabolism, dose-response relationships, genotoxic versus nongenotoxic mechanisms, and unique susceptibility (39).

The EPA cancer risk-assessment process has other weaknesses. Cancer risk is always based on the most sensitive species tested, a conservative assumption that may not be valid. Estimates are sometimes based on tumors in organs that humans do not have, such as Zymbal's gland, a holocrine sebaceous gland located at the base of the rat ear, for which no equivalent exists in humans. Human equivalent exposures are calculated on the basis of surface area rather than on volume or weight. The final result is not based on the maximum likelihood estimate (MLE) but on the upper bound of the MLE, putting the final risk factor at 2 standard deviations higher than the MLE (65). The linear multistage model does not make allowance for the fact that the body can repair damage to DNA (65).

EPA scientists acknowledge that the current methodology greatly overestimates risk. The standard EPA disclaimer states that the real risk factor lies somewhere between the unit risk factor and zero. An EPA scientist has said that six of the assumptions that the EPA uses may overestimate human risk by up to 10,800 times (65).

In a 1986 revision of the guidelines, EPA authorized departure from the policy default options if justified by scientific data (10). Since then, the EPA has departed from the default options in some cases, including the following: In 1988, the EPA concluded that tumors arising from hormonal imbalance would exhibit a threshold (10), and in 1990 the EPA concluded that tumors related to the alpha-2-gamma-globulin nephropathy in male rats, such as those that arise secondary to exposure to vaporized unleaded gasoline—d-limonene and 1,4-dichlorobenzene—are a species-specific phenomenon that is not predictive of relevance to human risk (10,72).

How Can Cancer Risk= Assessment Be Improved?

Worldwide capacity for conducting long-term animal carcinogenesis assays is limited. The necessary experiments are very expensive, taking 5 or more years to complete from design to publication. Knowledgeable staff and adequate facilities are in short supply. The investigations are time consuming, meticulous, and laborious. Although the search continues for cheaper and more rapid testing procedures, the replacement of long-term *in vivo* carcinogenesis studies is not yet in sight.

A two-staged model termed MVK (Moolgavkar, Venzon, and Knudson) has been proposed, and it shows promise as a model for cancer development. Unlike the linear multistage model, the MVK takes into account the important factors of tissue growth and cellular kinetics. In the interests of simplicity, it describes only two transformational stages (76). Cells are either normal, intermediate (one critical mutation), or malignant (two critical mutations). Division, death, differentiation, and mutation rates for normal and intermediate cell populations are specified. From these, the model calculates the number of cells in each population at a given time. A tumor is assumed to arise from the clonal expansion of a single malignant cell.

The MVK model can easily be linked to models of modes of action. It is consistent with the mechanism of action of tumor-suppressor genes and allows the definition of the three major classes of carcinogen: genotoxic, mitogenic, and cytotoxic. In the two-stage model, genotoxic carcinogens may be initiators or completers. Initiators increase the mutation rate in the first stage, and completers increase the rate of the second stage. In the two-stage model, nongenotoxic carcinogens are promoters, agents that increase the net birth rate of mutated cells. Incorporation of quantitative data on such effects as mutation rates and cell proliferation is essential, and much work is needed to generate these data. Once validated, this and similar models should be able to improve extrapolation between species and between dose rates (66).

Another approach to reducing the time and expense of lifetime rodent bioassays is to identify biomarkers of carcinogenicity and thus circumvent the long lead-in time required for tumors to develop. Considerably more progress has been made in using biomarkers to monitor genotoxicity than in using biomarkers for carcinogenesis induced by nongenotoxic mechanisms. Protein adducts and activated oncogenes are examples of biomarkers for cancer (77).

Many techniques have been developed for identifying genotoxins *in vitro*. However, the sensitivity and specificity of these tests is generally well less than 90%. Furthermore, genotoxicity *in vitro* does not inevitably mean carcinogenicity *in vivo*. The predictive value of *in vitro* genotoxicity tests is still well below that of long-term animal studies (3).

There is also a need for a short-term screening test for nongenotoxic carcinogens. Measurement of the induction of cell proliferation is one possible approach. However, some agents may affect only the growth of preneoplastic cells. Additionally, standardized methodology would be required, because changes in dose, route, or vehicle can have dramatic effects on the induction of cell proliferation (66).

Research attention has also focused on methods to identify carcinogens by their chemical structure. Quantitative structure-activity relationships of carcinogens may be hypothesis driven or knowledge based. Using the hypothesis-driven approach, the chemical is analyzed for structural characteristics known likely to react with DNA. This approach assumes that a given carcinogen is genotoxic. It leads to a rather circular argument if used alone. The knowledge-based approach does not require a mechanistic hypothesis. The expert system is given a set of chemical structures and their known carcinogenicity and asked to identify structural determinants associated with carcinogenicity or lack of carcinogenicity. The significance of those structural determinants must then be interpreted by a human expert. This system can identify genotoxic and nongenotoxic determinants. A number of structural moieties have now been identified that are good predictors of both genotoxic and nongenotoxic carcinogenicity. The challenge now is to identify the mechanisms by which these structures exert their effects (78).

EMERGING ISSUES IN RISK ASSESSMENT

Immunotoxicology

Risk assessment of substances that are toxic to the immune system is a relatively new area. Little information on immunotoxicity is currently available for environmental chemicals. The EPA has an assigned RfD based on immunotoxicity data for only one chemical. The EPA and the Food and Drug Administration are in the process of developing test guidelines for immunotoxic response (13).

Although the immune system is extremely complex and made of many organs and cells, a large number of its parameters can be measured. However, there is no accepted definition of what constitutes an immunotoxic agent in experimental rodents (79). No single test is adequate to measure the immunotoxic effects of chemicals in the entire immune system (13). There is insufficient knowledge to determine whether chemical-induced changes to the immune system are necessarily deleterious to the health of the animal. Some readily measured characteristics of the immune system, such as leukocyte counts, thymus weight, and spleen cellularity, are poor predictors of immunotoxicity. Some parts of the immune system act as negative feedback mechanisms on others to maintain homeostasis. In some cases, therefore, the net effect of an immunotoxic chemical may be immune stimulation. For example, a chemical that inhibits T cells will lead to B-cell proliferation (80).

A number of chemicals—including halogenated polycyclic hydrocarbons, metals, solvents, polycyclic aromatics, and pesticides—have immunomodulative effects. However, it has been difficult to relate these changes to any clearly identifiable health risk or disease process (13).

One area of concern is that immunosuppression may lead to an increase in cancer. The theory of immunosurveillance postulates that selective destruction of aberrant cells by the immune system is important in the prevention of cancer. The demonstration of immunosuppression in animals and people with cancer does not prove this theory, because cancer can lead to immunosuppression. Therefore, epidemiologists have undertaken cohort studies of immunosuppressed patients. These groups include transplant recipients, people with inherited immunodeficiencies, people on immunosuppressive medication for disorders such as rheumatoid arthritis, and people with acquired immunodeficiency syndrome. The studies have shown that people in these groups do have an increased incidence of cancer, but this is largely due to a marked increase in the incidence of a few malignancies, most of which are known or strongly suspected to be viral in origin. Lymphomas, for which strong evidence exists that the Epstein-Barr virus is the initiator, are greatly increased in incidence. Other cancers that are increased in incidence in the immunosuppressed are squamous cell carcinoma and cervical cancer, associated with human papillomavirus; primary liver cancer, for which hepatitis B is known to be a significant risk factor; and Kaposi's sarcoma, which is believed to be initiated by an as yet unidentified virus. In summary, it appears that immune surveillance in healthy people primarily limits the development of those cancers that are of viral origin (80). This means that if an environmental toxicant does cause immunosuppression, it should be apparent by increases in these particular cancers.

Immunosuppression is not the only form of immunotoxicity. The development of hypersensitivity responses, such as allergies, is another form of immunotoxicity.

Both inherited traits and environmental factors determine an individual's risk of developing a hypersensitivity reaction. These reactions tend to affect only a small proportion of the population. For chemicals in the environment, two major targets of immunotoxicity are the respiratory system and the skin. The major concerns are related to allergic immunotoxicity, such as asthma, allergic rhinitis, and allergic dermatitis (13). Immunotoxic responses can have very different dose-response relationships from those seen for other target organs or systems. In the case of allergens, a high dose of an immunotoxin may produce tolerance, whereas a low dose may sensitize (13). Once sensitized, an individual may show a severe reaction to a very small amount of the chemical or any substance that the immune system recognizes as being antigenically similar to the sensitizing chemical.

Alternatives to Animal Testing

Animal testing is part of the mandatory requirements of many regulatory agencies. Nowhere in the world are *in vitro* data used as the sole basis for regulatory decisions (58). However, animal testing is enormously expensive and time consuming and is becoming increasingly unpopular with the general public.

Opponents of animal testing can point to examples of animal testing for which the scientific basis is weak; therefore, scientists should have to justify it either ethically or legally (81). Furthermore, some responses—such as allergies and certain other idiosyncratic responses—are unique to humans and will not be recognized in animal studies, no matter how many species are used (82).

Many cosmetic companies have publicized the fact that they have stopped animal testing, which tends to give the impression that animal testing is easily replaced. In fact, the testing conducted by these companies was in most cases never required by law, but was conducted voluntarily by the companies for common law or product liability considerations. The cessation of such testing has not affected the legally required testing of medicines, pesticides, and industry chemicals, some of which are subsequently used in cosmetics (81).

In vitro assays are unlikely to be accepted by regulatory agencies unless they are at least as informative and predictive as the current *in vivo* tests, regardless of the fact that *in vitro* tests are simpler, cheaper, faster, and more politically acceptable (83). There is a lack of knowledge of *in vivo* mechanisms of toxicity that precludes the selection of appropriate *in vitro* systems on mechanistic grounds (81). Increasing knowledge of mechanisms of toxicity and carcinogenicity should make it increasingly possible to identify valid *in vitro* tests.

In vitro methods are not themselves entirely free from ethical problems. One problem is that normal cell lines cannot be maintained indefinitely *in vitro*. After a maximum of 50 mitoses (the Hayflick limit), normal cell lines die. Only neoplastic cell lines are immortal, and these are not representative of normal cells. Intracellular organization of neoplastic cells is different than that of normal cells (54). Neoplastic cells are also different than normal cells in their response to toxic insults. The greater sensitivity of neoplastic cells to several known chemicals forms the basis of chemotherapy. Therefore, the use of *in vitro* systems still necessitates the killing of animals to allow the harvesting of cells or tissues.

Some people may accept that killing *per se* is not an ethical problem, provided the animals do not suffer (83), but this viewpoint may not be universally acceptable. In addition, cell lines *in vitro* generally need to be maintained in culture medium that contains serum, and this may come from abused animals (83).

One of the strongest arguments for using *in vitro* systems in toxicity testing is that human tissue can be used, thus removing the uncertainty that results from interspecies extrapolation (83). Deriving human cell lines without exploiting human suffering and death is itself a complex ethical area.

Although animal welfare activists have claimed that *in vitro* systems can totally replace animal studies, elimination of whole animal studies appears unlikely. *In vitro* test systems can isolate cellular responses, but they can also alter or eliminate biological functions that may be important for toxicity or repair. The use of isolated cells and tissues circumvents repair processes beyond those of the cell itself (72). *In vitro* systems have the potential to miss a critical toxifying or detoxifying step or even a critical organ or cell. Metabolic activity often changes *in vitro*. Complex physical and biochemical relationships between different cell types may be disrupted or lost, and these relationships may be critical to toxicity (54).

In vitro studies of specific cellular functions may, however, lead to better design and use of *in vivo* studies (54), thus reducing use of animals. *In vitro* systems are likely to be rapid and sensitive tools for identifying the cell type most sensitive to a toxicant (83). Many major chemical companies have already developed *in vitro* tests for use as screening procedures before embarking on animal testing (81).

Short-term *in vitro* assays, including the *Salmonella* mutation and chromosomal aberration tests, are already in use for the detection of genotoxins that may initiate cancer. However, there is increasing evidence that mutagenicity and genotoxicity do not always correlate with carcinogenicity. These short-term tests have other limitations. They do not determine the target organ–specific carcinogenicity and cannot measure promotion potential or carcinogenicity by nongenotoxic mechanisms. A number of medium-term bioassays are under study, involving a range of organs (84), with the aim of reducing the need for expensive, time-consuming lifetime rodent bioassays.

Multispecies testing is required by some regulatory agencies but is often hard to justify (85). In the majority of cases, species' differences are of a quantitative rather than a qualitative nature. Advocates of multispecies testing frequently use the argument that dogs *and* rats should be tested because rats do not vomit and, therefore, cannot be used to detect an emetic effect. However, the use of dogs is going to the other extreme, because dogs vomit very readily, and this response in dogs does not accurately predict the same response in humans. If one test species shows a particular toxicologic response that does not occur in the other, it cannot be determined which species more accurately predicts the human response. In such a case, testing would then be carried out in a nonhuman primate, but this approach has been largely abandoned.

The current approach is to research the mechanistic basis for the difference in response. *In vitro* models are increasingly used in this research. When a plausible hypothesis for the interspecies difference has been established, it is often possible to determine which species is most representative of the human response. *In vitro* studies using human tissue or directed investigations in humans may be used in this determination. As understanding of the physiologic basis for interspecies variations in response has grown, it has become increasingly possible to identify the species most likely to be predictive of the human response (82), thus reducing the need for multispecies testing.

SUMMARY AND CONCLUSIONS

The existing risk-assessment procedures are designed to be conservative—to err on the safe side. They have the disadvantages that they tend to be time consuming, extremely expensive, and hard to defend on scientific grounds. They do not take mechanisms of toxicity or carcinogenicity into account. The backlog of chemicals that have yet to be adequately tested for toxicity and/or carcinogenicity is growing. The flaws in the current approaches are well recognized. Prevailing trends in risk-assessment research are toward predictive tests and models and the incorporation of growing knowledge of the mechanisms of toxicity and carcinogenicity. However, much more work is required to design and validate these tests and models before the current system can be replaced.

REFERENCES

1. Brecher RW. Risk assessment. *Toxicol Pathol* 1997;25(1):23–26.
2. Koeter HBWM. Test guideline development and animal welfare: regulatory acceptance of *in vitro* studies. *Reprod Toxicol* 1993;7:117–123.
3. Meijers JMM, Swaen GMH, Schreiber GH, Sturmans F. Occupational epidemiological studies in risk assessment and their relation to animal experimental data. *Regul Toxicol Pharmacol* 1992;15:215–222.
4. Omenn GS. Assessing the risk assessment paradigm. *Toxicology* 1995;102: 23–28.
5. Gupta S, VanHoutven G, Cropper M. *The value of superfund cleanups: evidence from US Environmental Agency decisions.* Washington: World Bank, Policy Research Department; Environment, Infrastructure, and Agriculture Division, March 1994.
6. Hartman R, Wheeler D, Singh M. *The cost of air pollution abatement.* Washington: World Bank, Policy Research Department; Environment, Infrastructure, and Agriculture Division, December 1994.
7. VanHoutven G, Cropper M. *When is a life too costly to save? Evidence from U.S. Environmental regulations.* Washington: World Bank, Policy Research Department; Environment, Infrastructure, and Agriculture Division, March 1994.
8. Graham JD. Historical perspective on risk assessment in the federal government. *Toxicology* 1995;102:29–52.
9. McMaster SB. Developmental toxicity, reproductive toxicity, and neurotoxicity as regulatory endpoints. *Toxicol Lett* 1993;68:225–230.
10. Barnard RC. Scientific method and risk assessment. *Regul Toxicol Pharmacol* 1994;19:211–218.
11. Lotti M. Mechanisms of toxicity and risk assessment. *Toxicol Lett* 1995;77: 9–14.
12. Fan A, Howd R, Davis B. Risk assessment of environmental chemicals. *Annu Rev Pharmacol Toxicol* 1995;35:341–368.
13. Kimmel CA. Quantitative approaches to human risk assessment for noncancer health effects. *Neurotoxicology* 1990;11:189–198.
14. Schwetz BA. Use of mechanistic and pharmacokinetic data for risk assessment at the National Institute of Environmental Health Sciences (NIEHS). *Toxicol Lett* 1995;79:29–32.
15. Huff J, Hoel D. Perspective and overview of the concepts and value of hazard identification as the initial phase of risk assessment for cancer and human health. *Scand Work Environ Health* 1992;18[Suppl 1]:83–89.
16. Kadry AM, Skowronski GA, Abdel-Rahman MS. Evaluation of the use of uncertainty factors in deriving RfDs for some chlorinated compounds. *J Toxicol Environ Health* 1995;45:83–95.
17. Gregory AR. Uncertainty in health risk assessments. *Regul Toxicol Pharmacol* 1990;11:191–200.
18. Leung H-W, Paustenbach DF. Physiologically based pharmacokinetic and pharmacodynamic modeling in health risk assessment and characterization of hazardous substances. *Toxicol Lett* 1995;79:55–65.
19. Davis JM, Svendsgaard DJ. U-shaped dose-response curves: their occurrence and implications for risk assessment. *J Toxicol Environ Health* 1990;30:71–78.
20. Zbinden G. Predictive value of animal studies in toxicology. *Regul Toxicol Pharmacol* 1991;14:167–177.
21. Andersen ME. Development of physiologically based pharmacokinetic and physiologically based pharmacodynamic models for applications in toxicology and risk assessment. *Toxicol Lett* 1995;79:35–44.
22. Clewell HJ III. The application of physiologically based pharmacokinetic modeling in human health risk assessment of hazardous substances. *Toxicol Lett* 1995;79:207–217.
23. Medinsky MA. The application of physiologically based pharmacokinetic/pharmacodynamic (PBPK/PD) modeling to understanding the mechanism of action of hazardous substances. *Toxicol Lett* 1995;79:185–191.
24. Hattis D. Use of biological markers and pharmacokinetics in human health risk assessment. *Environ Health Perspect* 1991;90:229–238.
25. Kohn MC. Achieving credibility in risk assessment models. *Toxicol Lett* 1995;79:107–114.
26. Wyrobek AJ. Methods and concepts in detecting abnormal reproductive outcomes of paternal origin. *Reprod Toxicol* 1993;7:3–16.
27. Lowry LK. Role of biomarkers in the assessment of health risks. *Toxicol Lett* 1995;77:31–38.
28. Lauwerys RR, Bernard A, Roels H, Buchet JP. Health risk assessment of long-term exposure to non-genotoxic chemicals: application of biological indices. *Toxicol Lett* 1995;77:39–44.
29. Schulte P, Mazzuckelli LF. Validation of biological markers for quantitative risk assessment. *Environ Health Perspect* 1991;90:239–246.
30. Hattis D. Human interindividual variability in susceptibility to toxic effects: from annoying detail to a central determinant of risk. *Toxicology* 1996;111:5–14.
31. Grassman JA. Obtaining information about susceptibility from the epidemiological literature. *Toxicology* 1996;111:253–270.
32. Preston RJ. Interindividual variations in susceptibility and sensitivity: linking risk assessment and risk management. *Toxicology* 1996;111:331–341.
33. Luijckx NBJ, Rao GN, McConnell, Surtzen G, Kroes R. The intake of chemicals related to age in long-term toxicity studies—considerations for risk assessment. *Regul Toxicol Pharmacol* 1994;20:96–104.
34. Chanda S, Mehendale HM. Role of nutrition in the survival after hepatotoxic injury. *Toxicology* 1996;111:163–178.
35. Graeter LJ, Mortensen ME. Lids are different: developmental variability in toxicology. *Toxicology* 1996;111:15–20.
36. Clewell HJ III, Anderson ME. Use of physiologically based pharmacokinetic modeling to investigate individual versus population risk. *Toxicology* 1996;111:315–329.
37. Environmental Protection Agency. *Summary report for the workshop on Monte Carlo analysis.* EPA/630/T–96/010.
38. Environmental Protection Agency. *Guiding principles for Monte Carlo Analysis.* EPA/630/R–97/001.
39. Auton TR. Calculation of benchmark doses form teratology data. *Regul Toxicol Pharmacol* 1994;10:152–167.
40. Mehendale HM. Injury and repair as opposing forces in risk assessment. *Toxicol Lett* 1995;82/83:891–899.
41. Goodman JI. A rational approach to risk assessment requires the use of biological information: an analysis of the National Toxicology Program (NTP), final report of the advisory review by the NTP Board of Scientific Counselors. *Regul Toxicol Pharmacol* 1994;19:51–59.
42. Hansch C, Hoekman D, Lea A, Zhang L, Li P. The expanding role of quantitative structure-activity relationships (QSAR) in toxicology. *Toxicol Lett* 1995;79:45–53.
43. Basak SC, Bertelsen S, Grunwald GD. Use of graph theoretic parameters in risk assessment of chemicals. *Toxicol Lett* 1995;79:239–250.
44. Klopman G, Rosenkranz HS. Toxicity estimation by chemical substructure analysis: the TOX II program. *Toxicol Lett* 1995;79:145–155.
45. Mumtaz MM. Risk assessment of chemical mixtures from a public health perspective. *Toxicol Lett* 1995;82/83:527–532.
46. Calabrese EF. Toxicological consequences of multiple chemical interactions: a primer. *Toxicology* 1995;105:121–135.
47. Yang RSH, El-Masri HA, Thomas RS, Constan AA. The use of physiologically pharmacokinetic/pharmacodynamic dosimetry models for chemical mixtures. *Toxicol Lett* 1995;82/83:497–504.
48. Samet JM. What can we expect from epidemiologic studies of chemical mixtures? *Toxicology* 1995;105:307–314.
49. Feron VJ, Groten JP, Jonker D, Cassee FR, vanBladeren PJ. Toxicology of chemical mixtures: challenges for today and the future. *Toxicology* 1995;105: 415–427.
50. El-Masri HA, Thomas RS, Benjamin SA, Yang RSH. Physiologically based pharmacokinetic/pharmacodynamic modeling of chemical mixtures and possible applications in risk assessment. *Toxicology* 1995;105:275–282.
51. Teuschler LK, Hertzberg RC. Current and future risk assessment guidelines, policy and methods development for chemical mixtures. *Toxicology* 1995; 105:137–144.
52. Mattison DR. An overview of biological markers in reproductive and developmental toxicology: concepts, definitions and use in risk assessment. *Biomed Environ Sci* 1991;4:8–34.
53. Sweeny AM, LaPorte RE. Advances in early fetal loss research: importance for risk assessment. *Environ Health Perspect* 1991;90:165–169.
54. Kimmel CA, Generoso WM, Thomas RD, Bakshi KS. A new frontier in understanding the mechanisms of developmental abnormalities. *Toxicol Appl Pharmacol* 1993;119:159–165.
55. Svitz DA, Harlow SD. Selection of reproductive health endpoints for environmental risk assessment. *Environ Health Perspect* 1991;90:159–164.
56. Lamb JC IV, Chapin RE. Testicular and germ cell toxicity: *in vitro* approaches. *Reprod Toxicol* 1993;7:7–22.
57. Peters PWJ. Risk assessment of drug use in pregnancy: prevention of birth defects. *Ann Ist Super Sanita* 1993;29(1):131–137.
58. Sobels FH. Approaches to assessing genetic risks form exposure to chemicals. *Environ Health Perspect* 1993;101[Suppl 3]:327–332.
59. Briggs GB. Risk assessment policy for evaluating reproductive system toxicants and the impact of responses on sensitive populations. *Toxicology* 1996;111:305–313.
60. Schwetz BA. Utility of *in vitro* assays: summary of international workshop on *in vitro* methods in reproductive toxicology. *Reprod Toxicol* 1993;7:171–173.

61. Schmid BP, Honegger P, Kucera P. Embryonic and fetal development: fundamental research. *Reprod Toxicol* 1993;7:155–164.
62. Moser VC, Becker GC, MacPhail RD, Kulig BM. The IPCS collaborative study on neurobehavioral screening methods. *Fundam Appl Toxicol* 1997;35:143–151.
63. Annau Z. Behavioral toxicology and risk assessment. *Neurotoxicol Teratol* 1990;12:547–551.
64. Francis EZ, Kimmel CA , Rees DC. Workshop on the qualitative and quantitative comparability of human and animal developmental neurotoxicity: summary and implications. *Neurotoxicol Teratol* 1990;12:285–292.
65. Buelke–Sam J, Mactutus CF. Workshop on the qualitative and quantitative comparability of human and animal developmental neurotoxicity, work group II report: testing methods in developmental neurotoxicity for use in human risk assessment. *Neurotoxicol Teratol* 1990;12:269–274.
66. Huff JE. Chemical toxicity and chemical carcinogenesis: is there a causal connection? A comparative morphological evaluation of 1500 experiments. In: Vainio H, Magee PN, McGregor B, MacMichael AJ, eds. *Mechanisms of carcinogenesis in risk identification*. IARC, 1992.
67. Withers BF III, Ferguson PW, Swift DA. Chemicals, cancer and risk assessment. *J La State Med Soc* 1991;143(1):33–40.
68. Butterwork BE, Popp JA, Connolly RB, Goldsworthy TL. Chemically induced cell proliferation in carcinogenesis. In: Vainio H, Magee PN, McGregor DB, MacMichael AJ, eds. *Mechanisms of carcinogenesis in risk identification*. IARC, 1992.
69. Tomatis L. How much of the human disease burden is attributable to environmental chemicals? *Toxicol Lett* 1995;77:1–8.
70. Monro A. How useful are chronic (lifespan) toxicology studies in rodents in identifying pharmaceuticals that pose a carcinogenic risk to humans? *Adverse Drug React Toxicol Rev* 1993;12(1):5–34.
71. Goldstein BD. Risk assessment methodology: maximum tolerated dose and two-stage carcinogenesis models. *Toxicol Pathol* 1994;22(2):194–197.
72. Key TJA, Beral V. Sex hormones and cancer. In: Vainio H, Magee PN, MacGregor DB, MacMichael AJ, eds. *Mechanisms of carcinogenesis in risk identification*. IARC, 1992.
73. Stewart BW. Role of DNA repair in carcinogenesis. In: Vainio H, Magee PN, MacGregor DB, MacMichael AJ, eds. *Mechanisms of carcinogenesis in risk identification*. IARC, 1992.
74. McClellan RO. Risk assessment and biological mechanisms: lessons learned, future opportunities. *Toxicology* 1995;102:239–258.
75. Dybing E, Huitfeldt HS. Species differences in carcinogen metabolism and interspecies extrapolation. In: Vainio H, Magee PN, MacGregor DB, MacMichael AJ, eds. *Mechanisms of carcinogenesis in risk identification*. IARC, 1992.
76. Green T. Species differences in carcinogenicity: the role of metabolism in human risk evaluation. *Teratog Carcinog Mutagen* 1990;10:103–113.
77. Conolly RB. Cancer and non-cancer risk assessment: not so different if you consider mechanisms. *Toxicology* 1995;102:179–188.
78. Goddard MJ, Krewski D. The future of mechanistic research in risk assessment: where are we going and can we get there from here? *Toxicology* 1995;102:53–70.
79. Perera F, Mayer J, Santella RM, et al. Biological markers for risk assessment for environmental carcinogens. *Environ Health Perspect* 1991;90:247–254.
80. Rosenkranz HS. Structure-activity relationships for carcinogens with different modes of action. In: Vainio H, Magee PN, MacGregor DB, MacMichael AJ, eds. *Mechanisms of carcinogenesis in risk identification*. IARC, 1992.
81. Luster MI, Pait DG, Portier C, et al. Qualitative and quantitative models to aid in risk assessment for immunotoxicology. *Toxicol Lett* 1992;64/65:71–78.
82. Kinlen LJ. Immunosuppression and cancer. In: Vainio H, Magee PN, MacGregor DB, MacMichael AJ, eds. *Mechanisms of carcinogenesis in risk identification*. IARC, 1992.
83. Balls M. *In vitro* methods in regulatory toxicology: the crucial significance of validation. *Arch Toxicol Suppl* 1995;17:155–162.
84. Zbinden G. The concept of multispecies testing in industrial toxicology. *Regul Toxicol Pharmacol* 1993;17:85–94.
85. Walum E, Forsman B, Stagh T. Scientific, ethical and legal aspects of the acceptance of *in vitro* methods in regulatory toxicology. *Arch Toxicol Suppl* 1995;17:163–169.

SECTION

II

Prevention, Regulatory, Safety, and Legal Issues

CHAPTER 7

Laws and Regulations Regarding Hazardous Materials

Linda M. Micale and Paul D. Phillips

U.S. environmental laws and regulations that control hazardous exposures and toxic substances date to 1906 (Table 7-1). Since the 1970s, the federal government has enacted a host of environmental laws to address the nation's concern over pollution and its uncertain effects on health and well-being. These laws emerged after images of toxic pollutants, combustible or decaying waterways, and hazy skies were printed, broadcast, and became visible to average citizens in their own communities. The U.S. Congress passed legislation to curb air pollution, water pollution, solid and hazardous-waste, and the cleanup of hazardous-waste sites (Table 7-2). The laws sought to encourage the development of procedures for monitoring, recordkeeping and reporting, improving management, applying technology to reduce pollution, and defining which hazardous materials would be subject to each law.

In the intervening years, the numbers of regulated hazardous materials in environmental statutes has evolved from a handful in each law to hundreds covered by a single law alone. The terms used to describe these materials varies from law to law. In the Clean Air Act (CAA), for example, facilities must concern themselves with regulated air pollutants, hazardous air pollutants (HAPs), criteria pollutants, and "112(r) chemicals." The Comprehensive Environmental Response, Compensation and Liability Act (CERCLA), commonly known as *Superfund*, brought the term *hazardous substances* to the forefront. In 1986, Title III of the Superfund Amendments and Reauthorization Act (SARA) added *extremely hazardous substances*. The same law carried its own list of "toxic chemicals" that would be subject to special reporting provisions. The Resource Conservation and Recovery Act (RCRA) defines *solid wastes*, *hazardous-wastes*, and *recyclable materials*, among other terms. These laws brought new language to commerce and industry as well as swirling lists of materials that must be individually assessed, managed, or reported to achieve the national goal of reducing pollution and waste.

An overview is presented of the objectives of eight federal environmental laws and the hazardous materials, chemicals, or substances they target. The laws and their related programs are covered roughly in the order that Congress enacted them in the modern era of environmental cleanup, chemical management, and pollution control:

- CAA; 1970, as amended
- Federal Water Pollution Control Act or Clean Water Act (CWA; 1972, as amended)
- Federal Insecticide, Fungicide, and Rodenticide Act (FIFRA; 1972, as amended)
- Safe Drinking Water Act (SDWA; 1974, as amended)
- RCRA; 1976, as amended
- Toxic Substances Control Act (TSCA; 1976, as amended)
- CERCLA; 1980, as amended
- Emergency Planning and Community Right-to-Know Act (EPCRA or SARA Title III; 1986)

This chapter summarizes information on why these materials are regulated and gives references on where individual lists can be found.

LAW VERSUS REGULATION

A federal law, enacted by Congress, describes the intent of legislators and the purpose of the law. The law describes its application, defines major terms and phrases used, prescribes enforcement provisions, and sets deadlines for the promulgation of regulations by the U.S. Environmental Protection Agency (EPA). The law is published in the *United States Code* (*USC*). It also can be accessed through other resources, including EPA's Web site at http://www.epa.gov. *Titles* and *Sections* refer to the law. In turn, EPA develops rules to implement the intent of Congress. Proposed rules or regulations are published first in the *Federal Register* (*FR*), a daily chronicle of federal actions and notices. Once finalized, these regulations are "codified" in the *Code of Federal Regulations* (*CFR*). They include definitions and descriptions of rule applicability, thresholds for triggering certain requirements, and management practices or operating requirements. Regulations also include permitting, notification, and registration requirements, as well as written documents required for compliance demonstrations and data gathering. The term *Parts* refers to the rule. In addition to the *FR* and *CFR*, rules can be reviewed on EPA's Web site.

CLEAN AIR ACT

Legal citation:	42 *USC* §§ 7401 *et seq.*
Regulations:	*CFR* 50–99

TABLE 7-1. Federal laws related to exposures to toxic substances

Legislation	Administering agency	Regulated products
Food, Drug and Cosmetics Act (1906, 1938, amended 1958, 1960, 1962, 1968)	FDA	Food, drugs, cosmetics, food additives, color additives, new drugs, animal and feed additives, and medical devices
Federal Insecticide, Fungicide and Rodenticide Act (1948, amended 1972, 1975, 1978)	EPA	Pesticides
Dangerous Cargo Act (1952)	DOT, USCG	Water shipment of toxic materials
Atomic Energy Act (1954)	NRC	Radioactive substances
Federal Hazardous Substances Act (1960, amended 1981)	CPSC	Toxic household products
Poultry Products Inspection Act (1968)	USDA	Food, feed, color additives, and pesticide residues
Occupational Safety and Health Act (1970)	OSHA, NIOSH	Workplace toxic chemicals
Poison Prevention Packaging Act (1970, amended 1981)	CPSC	Packaging of hazardous household products
Clean Air Act (1970, amended 1974, 1977)	EPA	Air pollutants
Hazardous Materials Transportation Act (1972)	DOT	Transport of hazardous materials
Clean Water Act (formerly Federal Water Control Act) (1972, amended 1977, 1978)	EPA	Water pollutants
Marine Protection, Research and Sanctuaries Act (1972)	EPA	Ocean dumping
Consumer Product Safety Act (1972, amended 1981)	CPSC	Hazardous consumer products
Lead-Based Paint Poison Prevention Act (1973, amended 1976)	CPSC, HEW (HHS), HUD	Use of lead paint in federally assisted housing
Safe Drinking Water Act (1974, amended 1977)	EPA	Drinking water contaminants
Resource Conservation and Recovery Act (1976)	EPA	Solid waste, including hazardous-wastes
Toxic Substances Control Act (1976)	EPA	Hazardous chemicals not covered by other laws, includes premarket review
Federal Mine Safety and Health Act (1977)	DOL, NIOSH	Toxic substances in coal and other mines
Superfund Amendments and Reauthorization Act (1986); Comprehensive Environmental Response, Compensation, and Liability Act (1981)	EPA	Hazardous substances, pollutants and contaminants at waste sites

CPSC, U.S. Consumer Product Safety Commission; DOL, U.S. Department of Labor; DOT, U.S. Department of Transportation; EPA, U.S. Environmental Protection Agency; FDA, U.S. Food and Drug Administration; HEW, U.S. Department of Health, Education, and Welfare; HHS, U.S. Department of Health and Human Services; HUD, U.S. Department of Housing and Urban Development; NIOSH, National Institute for Occupational Safety and Health; NRC, Nuclear Regulatory Commission; OSHA, Occupational Safety and Health Administration; USCG, U.S. Coast Guard; USDA, U.S. Department of Agriculture.

List of National Ambient Air Quality Standards (NAAQS) for "criteria pollutants:"	40 *CFR* 50.4–50.12
Reference test methods for measuring pollutants:	Appendices A–K to Part 50
List of air toxics (HAPs):	40 *CFR* 61 and Section 112(b) of the act
List of regulated substances:	40 *CFR* 68.130
List of ozone-depleting chemicals (ODCs):	40 *CFR* 82, Appendices A, B, and F
Acid rain hotline:	(202) 233-9620
Asbestos abatement ombudsman:	(800) 368-5888
Ozone protection and stratospheric ozone information hotline:	(800) 296-1996

Like most federal environmental laws, today's CAA has evolved over 30 years. Initially enacted in 1963, it is considered the nation's first true environmental law (1–3). The purpose of the law is to control and reduce sources of air pollutants that affect human health. Early versions of the law focused on a limited number of regulated air pollutants, including six pollutants covered by national standards and eight HAPs. With the Clean Air Act Amendments (CAAA) in 1990, Congress and EPA have significantly augmented or enhanced air quality programs and added the litany of regulated pollutants noted previously. These include an expansion of the list of HAPs to 189 chemicals and the addition of the list of substances regulated under the Accidental Release Prevention Program.

Key elements of the CAA and its 1990 amendments related to regulated pollutants are

1. NAAQS, which regulate six "criteria pollutants" (Title I)—carbon monoxide (CO), lead, nitrogen oxides (NOx), sulfur dioxide (SO_2), ozone (ground-level rather than stratospheric), and particulate matter (PM).
2. State Implementation Plans (SIPs), which must be developed and approved by EPA to ensure state compliance with NAAQS (40 *CFR* 51 and 52). Under the CAAA, areas in "nonattainment" for ozone, for example, must demonstrate reductions in volatile organic compounds by 3% annually (1). The SIP also implements the Visibility Protection Program, aimed at eradicating any visibility impairment from human sources in designated "Class I" areas such as national parks.
3. New Source Performance Standards (NSPS), which involve the listing of 61 specific "source categories" or large industrial processes that must meet specific air quality or technology requirements on construction (40 *CFR* 60). NSPS regulates criteria pollutants and seven other contaminants through its controls on these source categories (see Regulated Air Pollutants).
4. New Source Review and Prevention of Significant Deterioration programs, which also affect construction of defined "major" sources or "major modifications" that have the potential to adversely affect compliance with NAAQS. Permits are issued under these programs after a lengthy planning and review process to ascertain the nature and extent of air quality impacts from proposed activities. The Prevention of Significant Deterioration Program also requires best available control technology to be applied to address criteria pollutants.
5. The Mobile Sources Program in Title II, which includes vehicle standards to reduce hydrocarbon and NOx emissions from these sources, and reformulated or "clean alternative fuels."
6. The Air Toxics Program in Title I, Section 112, involving listed HAPs and National Emissions Standards for Hazardous Air Pollutants, known as NESHAPs.

TABLE 7-2. Summary of environmental health laws and regulations

Act and year enacted	Authority, enforcement, and purpose
Clean Air Act (CAA), 1963	The U.S. Environmental Protection Agency (EPA) is charged with regulation of air pollutants from stationary and mobile sources. The CAA was passed in 1963 but had few enforcement provisions. The 1970 amendments established National Ambient Air Quality Standards (NAAQS) to protect public health and welfare. The 1970 and 1977 amendments provided the legal authority and enforcement required. States were given the responsibility to attain and maintain the standards set forth. Each state was required to submit provisions that set specific emissions limitations, known as *New Source Performance Standards* (NSPS). In 1977, EPA set National Emission Standards for Hazardous Air Pollutants (NES-HAPs) designed to set the standards for and regulate new as well as existing sources of designated hazardous air pollutants. The act prohibits the use of dispersion techniques or intermittent control devices for the control of air emissions. It regulates vehicles that travel highways. EPA insures compliance of automobile manufacturers for control of vehicle emissions and regulates the amount of lead and additives in gasoline.
Clean Water Act (CWA), 1972	Begun as the Federal Water Pollution Control Act in 1948. It was revised in 1972 to introduce technology forcing effluent standards to make waters fishable and swimmable. The CWA has as its purpose to provide federal assistance for construction of publicly owned sewage treatment plants, to regulate the discharge of pollutants from point sources, and to regulate spills of hazardous-waste and oil. The 1972 amendment established standards (National Pollutant Discharge Elimination System, NPDES) for regulating direct discharge of pollutants into water in interstate as well as intrastate waterways. There were two deadlines for polluters: 1977 and a more stringent 1983 date. A 1977 amendment extended the 1977 deadline for industrial polluters if certain requirements were being met and extended the deadline for publicly owned treatment companies if noncompliance was the result of construction delays or lack of federal funding. Also, cost considerations regarding the best available versus the best conventional technology to use to comply with standards was included. The CWA requires EPA to set standards for the direct discharge of toxic pollutants into waterways, for pretreatment of waste that is discharged by a private company into publicly owned waste treatment facilities, and standards that regulate thermal pollution such as is caused by power plants. A federal permit system was established to enforce water quality standards and effluent standards. Discharge without a permit or in violation of a permit could bring about sanctions.
Safe Drinking Water Act (SDWA), 1974	SDWA provides for maximum contaminant levels in piped drinking water used for human consumption. Identified pollutants are: lead, arsenic, mercury, cadmium, barium, chromium, selenium, silver, nitrates, coliform bacteria, fluoride, turbidity, lindane, endrin, methoxychlor, trihalomethanes, toxaphene, radionuclides, 2,4-dichlorophenoxyacetic acid, and 2,4,5-trichlorophenoxyacetic acid. The SDWA is designed to protect human health from contaminated drinking water. Secondarily it is designed to protect the public by specifying the taste, color, odor, and other conditions of water for human consumption. Under the SDWA, individual states have the authority of regulation as well as enforcement. EPA reserves the right to compel compliance through federal court if necessary. It also has emergency powers to take whatever necessary action to protect the public from contaminants that have entered a water system if EPA finds that state authorities have not acted in a timely manner to relieve the threat to the public. Additionally, EPA can use what is termed *Suggested No Adverse Response Levels*, or SNARLs, to help guide regional EPA offices and states in setting levels of selected water contaminants. SNARLs are used as guidelines in determining imminent threats to human health.
Federal Insecticide, Fungicide, and Rodenticide Act (FIFRA), 1947	FIFRA, amended in 1972, 1975, and 1978, regulates the production, use, and distribution of pesticides. Since 1970, EPA has had the authority to regulate pesticides. Pesticide regulation first occurred in 1910 under the authority of the Insecticide Act. This act protected the consumer against mislabeling and ineffective products. A pesticide is defined under FIFRA as any substance or mixture of substances that is intended for preventing, destroying, repelling, or mitigating any pest, and any substance or mixture intended for use as a plant regulator, defoliant, or desiccant. These include insecticides, fungicides, herbicides, desiccants, defoliants, nematocides, and rodenticides. FIFRA requires the registration of all pesticides with EPA. Pesticides are classified as general use or restricted use. Restricted use pesticides can only be applied by licensed applicators. Along with the FDA, FIFRA establishes pesticide tolerance levels for agricultural products and foods. EPA can force removal or discontinuation of a pesticide that is in violation of the act. Individual states have the right, responsibility, and authority to regulate pesticides under FIFRA. EPA can always override a state if a state is not or cannot enforce the regulations.
Resource Conservation and Recovery Act (RCRA), 1976	RCRA regulates the generation and disposal of hazardous-waste. This is distinct from regulating an environmental medium such as air or water. RCRA grew out of amendments to the Solid Waste Act, 1965. RCRA gives a broad definition to the term *solid waste* and actually defines *hazardous-waste* in terms of a waste or combination of wastes that may cause or contribute to an increase in mortality or illness or pose a present or potential hazard to human or environmental health. RCRA targets waste that is transported, stored, treated, or disposed of improperly. RCRA is a means to regulate the management of hazardous-waste from generation to disposal. EPA was required by RCRA to identify and list hazardous materials. To do so, RCRA provides a tracking system for the generators of hazardous-wastes. Generators must keep records of their wastes. They are ultimately liable for the proper transport, storage, treatment, and disposal of these wastes.
Comprehensive Environmental Response, Compensation, and Liability Act (CERCLA), 1980	Commonly referred to as *Superfund*, CERCLA was the result of federal legislation directed at compensation for cleanup of hazardous-waste sites. CERCLA was designed to expedite remediation and reimbursement for cleanup activities. The act created a fund to pay for cleanup and remediation after the release of a hazardous substance that presents a public health threat. The Superfund consists of $1.6 billion financed over a 5-year period by fees levied on petroleum (87.5%) with the remainder generated by tax revenue (12.5%). The concept of a "release" is central to CERCLA. A release of a hazardous material does not include occupational exposures, exhaust emissions, release of radioactive material from a nuclear accident, or the normal application of pesticides. Governmental response is limited to 6 months or a sum of $1 million in expenses, whichever comes first. Mandatory reporting is required for a release of any reportable amounts of hazardous materials. Fines exist if reporting does not occur.
Toxic Substances Control Act (TSCA), 1976	TSCA regulates hazardous chemicals currently in existence and prevents chemicals from entering the market that may have an unreasonable risk to health or the environment. TSCA is directed at the inherent toxicity of the chemical. The act mandates that EPA maintain and publish a listing of chemicals manufactured or processed in the United States. Manufacturers are required to report to EPA data concerning uses, amounts produced, by-products, number of exposed workers, and adverse effects of a chemical on the health of humans and the environment. Manufacturers and processors of new chemicals are required to give EPA a 90-day notice prior to manufacturing or use. This notice, which is made available to the public, must include data concerning health and environmental consequences. EPA can require testing of chemicals. It has the authority to prohibit use, production, processing, distribution, or disposal of a chemical. Labeling and proper recordkeeping are required.
Emergency Planning and Community Right-to-Know Act (EPCRA: 40 *CFR* 350–374), 1986	Referred to as *Title III of the Superfund Amendments and Reauthorization Act* (SARA). Enacted in response to chemical disasters. Three levels of chemical hazards are identified: hazardous chemicals, extremely hazardous substances, and toxic chemicals. Requires facilities to determine if extremely hazardous substances on site exceed threshold planning quantities (TPQs) and, if so, to work with Local Emergency Planning Committees (LEPCs) to assist in planning to prevent chemical releases. The LEPCs must prepare comprehensive emergency plans identifying risk-related facilities, designating a community emergency coordinator, and have equipment and methods to respond to emergencies. A list of Material Safety Data Sheets for hazardous chemicals and extremely hazardous substances exceeding TPQs is required as part of Community Right-to-Know provisions of EPCRA. Section 312 of EPCRA requires facilities to submit Tier 1/Tier 2 reports identifying quantities, storage location, and container types of hazardous materials. Section 313 requires Toxic Chemical Release Inventory Reporting on an "R" form to be filed annually covering emission, on- and off-site disposal, accidental releases, wastewater discharges, and recycling activity of the facilities.

7. The Air Toxics Program, which also involves the application of Maximum Achievable Control Technology (MACT) for "source categories" that emit HAPs and for control of individual HAPs. The statutory goal for this program is to reduce emissions of 189 air toxics by 75% over 10 years (1).
8. The Accidental Release Prevention Program in Title III, which has separate lists of "regulated substances" that require risk management planning by certain regulatory deadlines because they are especially toxic, explosive, or flammable.
9. The Acid Rain Program in Title IV, which addresses control of SO_2 and NOx to stem acid deposition. Large utilities are the current focus. Acid rain provisions in the CAAA require the removal of 12.5 million tons of SO_2 and NOx from utility sources—a 50% reduction from 1980 levels—by 2000 (Section 401 of the act).
10. The comprehensive Operating Permits Program in Title V, which requires new, existing, and modified stationary sources (facilities) to estimate potential emissions of "regulated air pollutants" to determine whether they will be regulated as "major" or "minor" sources. A litany of federal, state, and local applicable requirements also must be evaluated during this process. A facility seeking a 5-year permit must certify its compliance with these requirements, including an annual emissions cap.
11. Stratospheric Ozone Protection, Title VI, which requires phaseouts for listed "Class I" and "Class II" ozone-depleting chemicals in general accordance with international initiatives documented in the *Montreal Protocol*. The CAAA bans the production of Class I substances (excluding methyl chloroform) by 2000 and all Class II substances by 2030.
12. Enforcement Provisions in Title VII include civil and criminal penalties and compliance programs.

National Ambient Air Quality Standards for Criteria Pollutants

Historically, the NAAQS have focused on six "big hitter" pollutants. The CAA included primary, "health-based" and secondary "welfare-based" standards for six criteria pollutants listed in 40 *CFR* 50:

- CO
- NOx
- Lead (Pb)
- SO_2
- O_3 [related to pollution from volatile organic compounds (VOCs) and NOx]
- Particulates (PM_{10} = particulates with diameter of 10 μm or smaller)

VOCs involve a regulatory definition in Part 51.100(s) rather than a list of chemicals.

Geographic areas that do not achieve these standards are considered to be in various stages of nonattainment. Before the passage of the 1990 CAAA, nonattainment areas above 120 parts per million (ppm) concentrations had 3 to 5 years to improve air quality. Despite their limited coverage, these programs had some success in the years before the CAAA completely changed the face of air quality management and compliance. For example, one source reported that

- Nationwide, particulate emissions were reduced by 30% between 1970 and 1980.
- SO_2 levels from fossil fuel combustion and industry were cut by almost 25% in the same decade.
- The average number of days that cities reported "unhealthful" or "very unhealthful" air quality was reduced.

In 1990, at the time of the CAAA, one source estimated that

- 96 U.S. cities were nonattainment for ozone
- 41 cities were nonattainment for CO
- 70 cities were nonattainment for particulates

Motor vehicles were still the single largest source of ozone pollution (contributing an estimated 50%) and CO (approximately 90%) in the country.

Under the revised program, each pollutant is designated specific time frames for improvements based on the "severity" of the problem (2). Classifications are based on specific concentrations of the criteria pollutants. SIPs identify how attainment will be achieved by each state. For example, the deadline for attainment of ozone NAAQS in ozone nonattainment areas was or is by November 15 of

- 1993 for marginal nonattainment (3 years)
- 1996 for moderate nonattainment (6 years)
- 1999 for serious nonattainment (9 years)
- 2005 for severe nonattainment (15 years)
- 2010 for extreme nonattainment (20 years)

Current data on nonattainment areas can be found by region at EPA's Web site (http://www.epa.gov/region09/air).

Revised Standards for Ozone and Particulate Matter

The CAA requires EPA to review NAAQS every 5 years. The standards are to be updated if the agency finds that it is necessary to "protect public health with an adequate margin of safety." EPA states that it must consider only the public health, and not the costs of compliance, when setting these standards. Cost considerations are to be addressed during the implementation phase.

The last thorough review of the ozone standard was in 1978. Particulate matter was last reviewed in 1999 (Air Quality Criteria for Particulate Matter, http://www.epa.gov/ncea/partmatt.htm, October 1999). The EPA has embarked on a scientific review of peer-reviewed studies on these pollutants, set up an independent advisory body, and held more than 125 hours of public discussion. For ozone alone, EPA estimated that 3,000 new studies had been published on the health and environmental effects of ozone since the 1980s. A large body of evidence was cited to determine that

- "Longer-term exposures at levels below the existing standard were found to cause significant health effects, including asthma attacks, breathing and respiratory problems, loss of lung function, and possible long-term damage and lowered immunity to disease."
- "Exposures to particles smaller than those regulated by the EPA can lodge in the lungs and cause premature deaths and respiratory problems" (http://www.epa.gov, July 17, 1996 and http://www.epa.gov/ncea/partmatt.htm, October 1999).

Consequently, EPA set a new 8-hour standard for ozone at 0.08 ppm to protect the public against longer exposure periods. This is the "health-based" or "primary" standard. The old "secondary" or "welfare-based" standard is replaced with the primary standard for protection of the environment, national parks, forests, and so forth. The 0.12-ppm, 1-hour standard is in place until an area presents 3 years of data showing compliance with the standard. The standard is remaining in place, in part, to facilitate a smoother transition to the new requirements (http://www.epa.gov; EPA Fact Sheet, July 17, 1997, Office of Air & Radiation, Office of Air Quality Planning & Standards, "EPA's Revised Ozone Standard").

EPA augmented its PM standard with a new $PM_{2.5}$ for particles 2.5 μm or smaller. The standard is 15 micrograms per cubic meter (μg/m^3) and a new 24-hour $PM_{2.5}$ standard at 65 μg/m^3. The current PM_{10} standard for 50 $\mu g/m^3$ is being retained and the 24-hour standard was revised to express a "1 expected exceedance over three years" form. The secondary standards are being revised to be the same as the primary standards. EPA also is issuing new rules to monitor PM, particularly in light of the new network required to measure $PM_{2.5}$ (http://www.epa.gov, EPA Fact Sheet, July 17, 1997, Office of Air & Radiation, Office of Air Quality Planning & Standards, "EPA's Revised Particulate Matter Standard," and also http://www.epa.gov/ncea/partmatt.htm, October 1999).

According to EPA, the new NAAQS "will prevent approximately

- 15,000 premature deaths
- 350,000 cases of aggravated asthma
- 1 million cases of significantly decreased lung function in children." (http://www.epa.gov, August 1997)

The debate raged in 1996 and 1997 over the scientific basis for listing these standards, because the costs of compliance are perceived by the regulated community to be enormous. EPA estimates that 57,000 comments were received. The March 1997 issue of *EM*, a magazine of the Air & Waste Management Association, featured a vigorous open forum about the validity of the scientific review undertaken by EPA and the acceptability of health risks under the previous standards.

At a minimum, the list of nonattainment areas covered is expected to expand significantly with the advent of these standards. EPA's implementation package for ozone will involve transitional classifications through which areas can comply partially with requirements until 2004, with compliance determinations as late as 2007. On the PM side, the key question is identifying cost-effective pollution controls to meet the new standards. EPA will complete an additional study before new nonattainment areas are added.

Hazardous Air Pollutants

In the 1970s, the structure of the HAP program took shape, but only eight pollutants were initially regulated: radon, beryllium, mercury, vinyl chloride, radionuclides, benzene, asbestos, and inorganic arsenic (40 *CFR* 61).

The list increased in the CAAA under Section 112(b) to 189 chemicals. It includes both organics and metals. EPA's administrator was given authority to periodically review and revise the list "by rule, adding pollutants which present, or may present, through inhalation or other routes of exposure, a threat of adverse human health effects (including, but not limited to, substances which are known to be, or may reasonably be anticipated to be carcinogenic, mutagenic, teratogenic, neurotoxic, which cause reproductive dysfunction, or which are acutely or chronically toxic) or adverse environmental effects whether through ambient concentrations, bioaccumulation, deposition, or otherwise, but not including releases subject to regulation under subsection (r) [Accidental Release Prevention] as a result of emissions to the air. No air pollutant which is listed under section 108(a) [NAAQS] may be added to the list under this section" and "no substance, practice, process or activity regulated under Title VI (ODCs) of this act shall be subject to regulation under this section solely due to its adverse effects on the environment." A 1989 EPA study estimated that 2.7 billion lb of HAPs were released to the air by major manufacturers in 1987 (1).

The thresholds for major source regulation of these chemicals is the potential to emit actual emissions from a stationary source that equal or exceed 10 tons per year of a single pollutant or 25 tons per year in aggregate. Major sources of HAPs that are subject to MACT represent

- The average emission limitation achieved by the best-performing 12% of the existing sources (see also lowest achievable emission rate in Section 171 of the act) prevailing at 30 or more sources, or
- The average emission limitation achieved by the best-performing five sources in categories with less than 30 sources [Section 112(d)].

MACT currently is determined on a case-by-case basis for most HAPs that are not part of source categories [Section 112(g)]. Most HAPs are regulated by the EPA's Hazardous Organic NESHAP, which applies to the synthetic organic chemical manufacturing industry (Final Rule Controlling Air Toxic Emissions from Synthetic Organic Chemical Manufacturing Industry, http://www.epa.gov/reg3artd/hazpollut/fshon.htm, March 1, 1994) (4).

In addition to listing specific chemicals, the CAAA identifies "source categories" that represent 90% of the stationary source emissions of the 30 HAPs that present the greatest threat to public health in the largest number of urban areas [Section 112(c)]. EPA designates source categories for regulation under 40 *CFR* 63. Source categories include halogenated solvent cleaning, synthetic organic chemical manufacturing, secondary lead melting, and magnetic tape manufacturing, among others. MACT rules developed to date are defined for these sources at that citation.

Ozone-Depleting Chemicals

EPA lists these chemicals in concert with the guidelines of the *Montreal Protocols* of 1987 and 1990. The CAAA provided phase-out dates, depending on the damaging effects of the chemicals. Class I substances—chlorofluorocarbons (CFCs), Halon, and tetrachloride—were set to be banned in 2000. A 2-year delay was granted for the Class I substance methyl chloroform. Class II chemicals are to be phased out by 2030. These substances include hydrochlorofluorocarbons, which are considered less dangerous to the stratosphere than CFCs because of the addition of hydrogen molecules. In addition to the phaseouts, the program contains a series of production and consumption controls that include tradable allowances. Uses of unsafe alternatives are prohibited. EPA is required to establish a list of safe substitutes for these products. Since the early 1990s, components of this program also have included

- A national recapture and recycling program
- Safe disposal of controlled substances
- Mandatory labeling
- A ban on "nonessential" CFC products

Some exceptions are noted in the law for "essential uses." These include applications involving medical devices and aviation safety testing (2).

Chemicals Regulated under the Accidental Release Prevention Program [Section 112(r)]

The Accidental Release Prevention Program includes 100 "regulated substances" initially based on the list of "extremely hazardous substances" in EPCRA. It ties closely to the provisions for process safety management in the Occupational Safety and Health Act for "highly hazardous chemicals." It involves the establishment of an independent Chemical Safety and Hazard Identification Board subject to presidential review. EPA's initial list included

- 77 acutely toxic substances, with a threshold quantity of 500 to 20,000 lb
- 63 flammable gases and volatile flammable liquids, with a threshold quantity of 10,000 lb
- Division 1.1 high explosive substances as listed by the U.S. Department of Transportation in 49 *CFR* 172.1, with a threshold quantity of 5,000 lb

The list is meant to identify substances that, "in the event of an accidental release, are known to cause or may be reasonably expected to cause death, injury, or serious adverse effects to human health and the environment" (5). EPA considered the severity of health effects, the likelihood of a release (i.e., "the accident history of a substance") and the potential magnitude of human exposure. Details on listing rationale is provided in the *FR* that proposed changes to the initial list and threshold quantities (6). Volatile substances were chosen because they are likely to become airborne and impact the public. Highly flammable gases and liquids and high explosives were listed because "vapor cloud explosions and blast waves from detonations have caused injuries to the public and damage to the environment" (7).

Facilities with listed substances that exceed threshold quantities are subject to a variety of provisions, including hazard assessment, compliance audits, training, emergency response, and risk management planning. The program is tiered so that sources most at risk are subject to more intensive requirements. The compliance deadline was June 21, 1999.

Regulated Air Pollutants

The Operating Permits Program in Title 5 involves "regulated air pollutants." But no single list of these pollutants were contained in EPA's regulations. Regulated air pollutants, based on regulatory provisions, encompass (4)

1. Criteria pollutants for which NAAQS is established
2. Pollutants regulated under the NSPS program:
   - VOCs
   - NOx
   - Dioxin/furan [Part 60.53(a)]
   - Fluorides
   - Hydrogen chloride
   - Hydrogen sulfide (H_2S)
   - Sulfuric acid mist
   - Total reduced sulfur
   - Reduced sulfur compounds
   - Total suspended particulates
3. Class I and Class II substances under Title VI (ODCs)
4. Pollutants for which a NESHAP is established and lists HAPs [Section 112 and 112(b)]
5. Section 112(r) pollutants (61 *FR* 31668) on final promulgation of the list

CLEAN WATER ACT

Legal citation:	33 *USC* §§ 1251 *et seq.*
Regulations:	40 *CFR* 100–141 (water programs), 400–471 (effluent guidelines and standards)
List of priority pollutants:	Appendix A to Section 126 of the act
List of federally promulgated water quality standards:	40 *CFR* 131, Subpart D
List of toxic pollutants:	Section 307(a) of the act; 40 *CFR* 423, Appendix A
List of categorical industries:	40 *CFR* 405–471
National small (wastewater) flows information hotline:	(800) 624-8301

Water quality contamination and protection are covered at length in another part of this volume; abbreviated information is provided in this chapter to address regulated pollutants.

The jurisdiction of the CWA is extensive, applicable to all "navigable waters" of the United States, an area broadly defined by the federal government. The original goal of the CWA was to make all surface waters fishable and swimmable by 1983, with zero discharges to these waters by 1985 (33 *USC* § 1251). Although these goals were not met, measurable and visible water quality improvements were observed (8).

Key elements of the CWA related to regulation of substances with potentially adverse effects on waters of the United States are

1. Provisions for development of surface water quality standards form one of the foundations of the act. Standards are established through designation of uses for water bodies, including full body contact, incidental human contact, domestic water source, aquatic life and wildlife, and so forth. The act requires states to identify waters within their boundaries and adopt numeric and narrative water quality standards that protect designated uses. States must review these standards every 3 years, at a minimum, a process known as the *triennial review* (33 *USC* § 1313 and 40 *CFR* 131.20).
2. EPA has authority to review the standards and require changes. If a state fails to make the changes in 90 days, EPA can set standards for that state (40 *CFR* 131, Subpart D).
3. When toxic pollutants are a concern, states must adopt a numeric standard sufficient to protect designated uses (Section 307 of the act, 40 *CFR* 423, Appendix A).
4. National Pollutant Discharge Elimination System (NPDES) permits are required for "point sources" of pollution that discharge to a water of the United States (40 *CFR* 122 and Section 402 of the act).
5. A key condition of the NPDES permit is the effluent limitations applicable to the specific discharge and its pollutants. Waste stream analyses are necessary to determine the components of a discharge so that controls are appropriate and ensure compliance with the limitations. Effluent limitations are based on three criteria (9):
   - Level of best available technology or best conventional technology
   - Meeting a water quality parameter in the receiving waters
   - Minimizing toxicity of the discharge (40 *CFR* 400–471)
6. Sources that discharge to a publicly owned treatment works do not typically require a NPDES permit. Instead a pretreatment or wastewater discharge permit is required from the local treatment facility. The publicly owned treatment works, in turn, must manage discharges from multiple sources to comply with permit conditions, including water quality standards. Pretreatment requirements include prohibited discharges identified in 40 *CFR* 403.5, such as
   - Pollutants that create a fire or explosion hazard
   - Discharges with a pH lower than 5.0 unless the works is designed to accommodate them
   - Petroleum oil and other mineral products that will impede pass-through
   - Pollutants resulting in toxic gases
7. The CWA's storm water programs for permitting, management, and pollution prevention planning were installed through amendments to the act. They extend the NPDES program to covered discharges and facilities [Section 402(p) of the act].
8. Delegated authority for regional water quality planning appears in Section 208 and 40 *CFR* 130. This authority directed states to develop "area-wide" plans to address

sources of "non-point" pollution. Land-use planning and regional waste treatment planning were emphasized.

9. Other provisions of the CWA include permit requirements for dredge and fill operations, called *Section 404 permits*; rules to address spills of oil or hazardous substances (including spill prevention, control, and countermeasure plans) that later became a cornerstone of CERCLA; and a construction grants program to assist municipalities with development of sewage treatment plants.
10. Enforcement provisions appear in Section 309, and citizen suits are addressed in Section 505 of the act.

Definition of Pollutant

The definition of *pollutant* in Section 502 of the CWA includes dredged soil; solid waste; incinerator residue; sewage; garbage; sludge; munitions; chemical wastes; biological materials; radioactive materials; heat; wrecked or discarded equipment; rock; sand; cellar dirt; and industrial, municipal, and agricultural waste discharged into water. Conventional pollutants subject to water quality standards include biological oxygen demand, pH, fecal coliform, suspended solids, and oil and grease (Section 316 of the act).

Toxic Pollutants and Priority Pollutants

EPA has listed 126 toxic pollutants in 40 *CFR* 423, Appendix A, because they can cause death, illness, mutations, behavioral abnormalities, or physiological malfunctions in living organisms (33 *USC* § 1362). The agency also has published criteria documents that identify the scientific basis for setting water quality standards and recommending a range of reasonable standards for certain uses.

The Natural Resources Defense Council sued EPA because its early toxics programs were alleged to be inadequate to meet the intent of the CWA. A consent decree was issued in the late 1980s to require a program that regulated 65 categories of priority pollutants (including the toxic pollutants) by 34 industry categories, called "categorical sources" (Appendix A to Section 126). One source estimated that more than 70% of U.S. industries were affected by this requirement (9). The regulation of these pollutants and industrial "categories" is addressed through CWA effluent limitations and the NPDES permit program.

FEDERAL INSECTICIDE, FUNGICIDE, AND RODENTICIDE ACT

Legal citation:	7 *USC* §§ 135 *et seq.*
Regulations:	40 *CFR* 150–189
List of registered pesticides:	http://www.epa.gov
National Pesticides Telecommunications Network:	(800) 858-7378
Pesticide Information Network:	(703) 305-5919 (via modem)

Congress enacted the first version of FIFRA in 1947 to require that pesticides used in interstate commerce be registered with the U.S. Department of Agriculture (10). The primary thrust of this law was to ensure the effectiveness of pesticide products, although a limited recognition of their potential harm to human health and animals was also present in the law. In 1970, pesticide regulation was transferred from the Agriculture Department to EPA. FIFRA was amended numerous times in the 1970s and 1980s to provide EPA with more authority over pesticides. The issue of residual pesticide concentrations in food recently has been elevated to a major policy initiative under the Food, Drug and Cosmetics Act (21 *USC* § 346a *et seq.*). Much debate has occurred over the effectiveness of FIFRA in addressing hazards from pesticides versus their benefits to national commerce and agricultural production.

The law and its regulations do not provide specific lists but do define *pesticide*, *rodenticide*, *fungicide*, and *insecticide*. Like many substances found in individual federal environmental laws, pesticides are regulated to some degree through other programs (10):

- Food, Drug and Cosmetics Act, noted above, and through the monitoring of residues in food.
- CAA, as HAPs.
- CWA, under discharge permit requirements in Section 301, as "toxic substances" under Section 307, and through "non-point" sources of pollution that result in discharges to waterways (Section 208).
- RCRA through hazardous-waste listing (40 *CFR* 261) for controlling waste from pesticide manufacturing and use. However, proper land application of a registered pesticide is exempted from RCRA regulation.
- Occupational Safety and Health Administration (OSHA), for the protection of agricultural workers during application of pesticides.

Key elements of this law related to regulated hazardous materials are

1. Pesticide registration procedures for nearly all new pesticide products used in the United States, including full disclosure of the formula; a proposed label describing its proper use; and a complete discussion of tests proving the effectiveness of the product.
2. Experimental use permits for pesticides undergoing registration to obtain the information necessary for EPA review.
3. EPA approval of a specific pesticide formulation, once registration information is evaluated, including the criterion that it will not cause "unreasonable adverse effects on the environment" [Section 2(bb)] when used in accordance with standard practice.
4. Provisions for "suspension," an immediate ban for imminent hazards, or cancellation of pesticide registrations based on scientific review of a "substantial question of safety."
5. Classification of "general" and "restricted" categories of pesticide products. Restricted products are available for use only to "certified applicators." The pesticide label indicates that a product is restricted and must be applied "under the direct supervision of a Certified Applicator."
6. A certification program, which has been the subject of much scrutiny and concern about its integrity, to train and certify applicators.
7. Penalties for use of restricted pesticides in violation of the label.

Regulations in 40 *CFR* involve proper management, storage, and use of pesticides. Special handling is required, but the regulations often involve "recommendations" rather than strict measures. Label restrictions, for example, require special protection for products but the rules recommend storage in dry, well-ventilated buildings or covered areas where fire protection is provided. Identification signs are recommended for all rooms and buildings to advise of the contents of the pesticides. These rules are distinct from other parts of 40 *CFR*, which typically define requirements for management of regulated substances.

SAFE DRINKING WATER ACT

Legal citation:	42 *USC* §§ 300 *et seq.*

Regulations:	40 *CFR* 141–149
List of chemicals subject to drinking water standards [maximum contaminant levels (MCLs)]:	40 *CFR* 141–143
SDWA hotline:	(800) 426-4791

The original purpose of the SDWA was to enable EPA to set standards or treatment methods for waterborne "contaminants" that could adversely affect human health and ensure that drinking water quality, treatment, and distribution systems would be monitored for safety. The 1974 act was amended in 1986 in part to expedite the standard-setting process, set up a program to monitor specific unregulated contaminants, require disinfection for all "public water systems" (including groundwater systems), and develop corrosion control programs to diminish introduction of lead and copper residues from pipes into water supplies.

Ten elements of the SDWA are

1. Regulation of "public water systems" that routinely provide drinking water for human consumption, have at least 15 service connections, and serve at least 25 persons [Section 1401(4) of the act]. Water for human consumption also applies to bathing, cooking, dishwashing, and maintaining oral hygiene.
2. Public water supplies are subdivided into three categories: "community," "non-community," and "non-transient, non-community." Community systems serve at least 25 year-round residents. Non-community systems are all others that meet the public water system criteria (40 *CFR* 141.2), such as restaurants and gas stations. Non-transient, non-community systems serve at least 25 persons over a 6-month period. The rationale for the distinction is to develop standards that address continued consumption of water from a system. One source estimates that 60,000 community water systems and 200,000 non-transient, non-community systems exist in the United States (11). Public water systems must meet drinking water standards.
3. Section 1401 of the act requires EPA to establish national primary water regulations and national secondary water regulations. Both sets of regulations are based on MCLs for regulated pollutants. Primary standards are enforceable, apply to public water systems, and are based on MCL goals aimed at preventing adverse impact to human health. MCL goals, by contrast, are not enforceable. Secondary standards also apply to public water systems but are based instead on aesthetic characteristics of the water as a product, such as taste, odor, and appearance. The standard-setting process is lengthy and subject to much scientific review and debate.
4. The MCL means the "maximum permissible level of a contaminant in water which is delivered to the free-flowing outlet of the ultimate user of public water systems . . ." [Section 300(f)(3) of the act]. Before 1986, less than 20 MCLs had been set by EPA. Approximately 76 were set by the early 1990s. EPA was required to set 25 new MCLs every 3 years, beginning in 1991, an enormous effort with significant implications for suppliers (40 *CFR* 141 and 143). MCLs are critically linked to RCRA corrective action, CERCLA cleanup criteria, RCRA land disposal restrictions, and solid waste disposal requirements, among other environmental rules.
5. If EPA determines that it is not economically or technically feasible to set a level, a treatment method may be established as an MCL instead [Section 1412(7)(A)].
6. The National Primary Drinking Water Standards also involve EPA's identification of methods to monitor for MCLs (Section 1400 and 1401) and rigorous recordkeeping on the part of the supplier to ensure compliance with the MCLs (Section 1445 of the act).
7. Public water systems can obtain a variance from EPA if it cannot meet the MCL, even after application of best available treatment technologies, caused by the inherent characteristics of the water supply. The variance must not result in unreasonable risk to consumers and the supplier must ultimately comply with the MCL (Section 1415).
8. EPA's enforcement provisions include mandatory notification to customers and the agency for violations of standards and other requirements of the act (Section 1414). Customers are notified through local newspapers no more than 14 days after the violation. Acute risks from violations must be reported to local radio and television stations within 72 hours (40 *CFR* 141.32).
9. The SDWA also encompasses an Underground Injection Control Program to protect drinking water supplies from contamination by subsurface disposal of wastes into wells [40 *CFR* 144.31(a)]. EPA has defined five classes of well systems, ranging from wells with wastes injected below the lowermost source of drinking water to wells where wastes are injected above or into drinking water sources. The fifth class covers everything that may have been missed by the other categories. One source places EPA's estimate for wells covered by the program at 400,000 (11).
10. Programs to protect wellhead and sole-source aquifers were added to the SDWA through the 1986 amendments. Wellhead protection involves inventories of potential source of contamination with a plan to protect the supply from these concerns (Section 1428). The sole-source aquifer program is rather limited in that it provides for designation of such aquifers, involves federal assistance in developing protection plans, and prohibits expenditure of federal dollars on activities that could result in contamination of the aquifer (Section 1424).

RESOURCE CONSERVATION AND RECOVERY ACT

Legal citation:	42 *USC* §§ 6901 *et seq*.
Regulations:	40 *CFR* 240–259 (solid wastes), 260–272 (hazardous-wastes), 273 (universal wastes), 279 (used oil), 280–282 [underground storage tanks (USTs)]
Hazardous-wastes lists and characteristics:	40 *CFR* 261
EPA hotline:	(800) 424-9346
Pollution prevention information clearinghouse:	(202) 260-1023

The generation and disposal of hazardous-wastes represent a critical subset of the broader topic of hazardous materials toxicology. The manufacture, use, processing, or accidental release of hazardous materials may result in wastes that are considered hazardous under RCRA. Passed in 1976, this federal law and its regulations seek to reduce public health risks and environmental impacts by controlling hazardous-wastes from the time they are generated to the time of their disposal. A common phrase used to describe RCRA's approach is a "cradle-to-grave" system of managing hazardous-wastes.

Key elements of RCRA related to regulated wastes are

1. Hazardous-waste Identification Program (40 *CFR* 261 and 60 *FR* 66344), which lists and characterizes mixtures and recycled materials. The rules provide criteria for exemptions for wastes that are not "hazardous" under RCRA but that may be managed through another law, for example, the CWA. The program also provides criteria for the lengthy process of

"delisting" a hazardous-waste (40 *CFR* 260.22) if a generator can demonstrate that the waste is not hazardous based on the reasons for which it was listed in Appendix IX of Part 261.

2. The Dec. 15, 1996 hazardous-waste identification rule for process wastes (40 *CFR* 260) and for contaminated media, which provides an alternative to delisting by identifying numeric parameters for listed wastes below which they are not considered hazardous. The rationale behind the agency's proposals is that these wastes are "low-risk." Using the sampling and analysis procedures in the rule, the waste could "exit" the Subtitle C Program, assuming concentration thresholds were not exceeded and the waste exhibited no hazardous-waste characteristics. The final rule for process wastes is anticipated in 2001; the final rule for dye and pigment industries was issued on July 23, 1999 (40 *CFR* 148261) (12).
3. Notification of hazardous-waste activities is required under RCRA Section 3010(a) for any person who manages a hazardous-waste. Notification must be filed with EPA within 90 days after a rule says that the waste one generates is hazardous. EPA has a standard form for this purpose.
4. Standards for generators of hazardous-wastes (40 *CFR* 262), which involve waste characterization, proper on-site handling and storage, proper shipping through the use of a uniform hazardous-waste manifest, and recordkeeping and reporting requirements. The rules provide tiered requirements for large-quantity, small-quantity, and conditionally exempt small-quantity generators. Standards involve management requirements rather than numeric limits.
5. Standards for transporters of hazardous-wastes (40 *CFR* 263) whether by air, rail, highway, or water, which also include proper handling, manifest requirements, and spill response.
6. Standards for treatment, storage, and disposal facilities (TSDFs; 40 *CFR* 264, 265), which are extensive, including general facility standards, RCRA permitting, and standards for specific types of facilities such as surface impoundments and landfills. Many facilities take stock of their activities to avoid this level of RCRA regulation.
7. The RCRA permitting program for TSDFs (40 *CFR* 280), which results in voluminous narrative and data that essentially describe the approved manner in which a TSDF will be operated to prevent or address releases of hazardous-wastes during operations. The permit also includes a detailed closure plan for removal or containment of all hazardous-wastes so that a release will be prevented. Permits are issued for 10 years and may require several years to obtain. Prior to issuance of a permit, the TSDF is subject to interim standards in 40 *CFR* 265.
8. The Land Disposal Ban Program (40 *CFR* 278), which radically changed the nation's approach to disposal by requiring treatment to specific standards before land disposal of wastes containing leachable liquids. Land disposal includes use of landfills, injection wells, surface impoundments, waste piles, and other similar units. EPA listed wastes that would be subject to the ban in "thirds" to phase-in standard-setting activities for hazardous-wastes and to allow generators and TSDFs to identify suitable technologies for compliance. This program is a complex and significant result of the 1984 amendments to RCRA entitled the "Hazardous and Solid Waste Amendments."
9. RCRA's USTs provisions (40 *CFR* 280), which involve "regulated petroleum substances" and the proper management, configuration, and removal of USTs to prevent or address releases to the environment.
10. RCRA includes used oil as a non-hazardous-waste in 40 *CFR* Part 279, with emphasis on proper storage and handling before recycling or other disposition.
11. The Universal Waste Program was recently added by EPA to address widely generated waste streams that were not managed as hazardous-wastes but were determined to have potential effects on human health and the environment because of the volumes of material involved:
    - Waste batteries, including lead-acid batteries that are for reclamation under Part 266
    - Recalled pesticides or stocks of unused pesticides that will be discarded
    - Mercury thermostats

    If any of these wastes exhibits hazardous-waste characteristics, they must be managed as hazardous, rather than universal, wastes.

    The rule provides proper waste management standards for small-quantity and larger-quantity "handlers" of universal wastes: storage, labeling and marking, accumulation time limits, spill response, and off-site shipping and disposal (40 *CFR* 279).
12. Corrective action provisions under RCRA typically address facilities in operation that have caused a release of hazardous-wastes within and beyond the facility boundary (Section 3004). This authority is very similar to that found under CERCLA.
13. Enforcement provisions, including EPA inspections, citizen suits, imminent hazard actions, and civil and criminal penalties, also are included in RCRA, Sections 3007, 3008, 7002, and 7003.

Hazardous-wastes are so designated owing to the physical, biological, or chemical characteristics they present as risks to the public or environment. Short-term health risks associated with hazardous-wastes include immediate effects from inhalation, ingestion, or skin absorption (5). Environmental impacts include risks of fire, explosion, production of noxious gases, and polluted discharges to land or surface waters. Long-term health risks associated with chronic exposure to low doses of hazardous-wastes include central nervous system problems, cancer, and birth defects (12). These health risks may be tied to long-term environmental impacts. Hazardous-wastes improperly disposed of on land may accumulate in and contaminate subsurface soils; soil contaminants may ultimately migrate to drinking water supplies (13).

Characterizing Solid Wastes and Hazardous-Wastes

RCRA requires that waste generators must be able to "characterize" their wastes in accordance with the definitions provided in 40 *CFR* Part 261. When characterizing wastes, facility operators first must determine whether the material they generate is indeed a "waste" by EPA definition. A waste is a material that has served its original intended use and is discarded, intended to be abandoned, recycled or "inherently waste-like." EPA does not consider materials that can be reused directly as wastes (14).

Facility operators then must determine whether the waste they generate is "solid waste." According to the regulations, solid wastes may be liquid, contained gaseous, semisolid, or solid. The category covers almost all wastes, including hazardous-wastes and municipal garbage. Some materials are excluded from the definition of solid waste and from RCRA regulations. These include point sources of pollution regulated under the CWA, irrigation return flow, domestic sewage, and *in situ* mining wastes, among others (Part 261.4). Although they are not regulated by RCRA, these wastes may still be "hazardous" from a chemical, physical, or biological perspective. Beyond these and other exclusions identified in the regulations, two types of materials clearly are not solid waste: products or intermediary products of a manufacturing or mining process, and materials other than garbage, refuse, or sludge that are always used (15).

Once identified as a solid waste, facilities must determine whether their wastes are hazardous by RCRA definition. As noted above, hazardous-wastes are a subset of solid wastes and are addressed by the Subtitle C portion of RCRA. Hazardous-wastes may be specifically listed within the regulations or exhibit at least one of four characteristics outlined by EPA. The waste may be a mixture of hazardous and solid waste, with some exceptions. Exclusions from RCRA hazardous-wastes currently include household wastes, agricultural wastes used as fertilizers, mining overburden, and oil and natural gas exploration drilling waste, among others (40 *CFR* 261.4). Although many recycling activities are exempt from RCRA Subtitle C, wastes that exhibit a hazardous-waste characteristic when they are recycled are subject to hazardous-waste regulations.

EPA's basis for defining listed and characteristic hazardous-wastes is their toxicity. The *CFR* (Part 261.10) explains that characteristic hazardous-wastes were identified as those which

- Cause or significantly contribute to mortality or irreversible illness
- Pose a substantial present or potential hazard to human health or the environment during waste management

40 *CFR* Part 261.11 indicates that listed hazardous-wastes may also

- Be fatal to humans in low doses or meet specific lethal dose criteria in animals
- Contain certain toxic constituents listed in the regulations (Subpart B, Appendix VIII), unless specific circumstances are reviewed by EPA with the finding that substantial risk is not present

Listed Hazardous-Wastes (40 *CFR* Part 261.30)

EPA has established four waste lists. The "F" list contains wastes from nonspecific sources. The list is broadly used by industry because it includes spent solvents such as toluene and methylene chloride. The "K" list contains hazardous-wastes from specific sources such as petroleum refining or the production of pigments and certain chemicals. The "U" list identifies discarded commercial chemical products and all off-specification containers and spill residues of the products. The "P" list parallels the "U" list by identifying "acutely" hazardous, discarded commercial chemical products. Listed wastes that will be recycled, reused, or reclaimed must adhere to applicable hazardous-waste regulations before these activities. Several hundred hazardous-wastes are currently listed in the regulations at the reference given above. EPA has authority to list additional wastes based on toxicity factors.

Mixtures of listed hazardous-waste and solid waste are regulated as hazardous unless they can be successfully "delisted" through a comprehensive testing and reporting process. The process is intended to demonstrate that the specific waste stream in question is not hazardous by EPA definition. EPA publishes industry proposals to delist wastes in the *FR* and allows for public comment before making a final decision. Successfully delisted wastes and the facility that was granted the petition are identified in Appendix IX at 40 *CFR* 261.

Characteristic Hazardous-Wastes (40 *CFR* Part 261.21)

In addition to listed wastes, RCRA allows EPA to identify hazardous-wastes by characteristics that make them harmful to human health or the environment. There are four characteristics, each with specific definitions:

- *Ignitability*: most common definition is the flash point below 140°F
- *Corrosivity*: most commonly a pH equal to or less than 2 or equal to or greater than 12.5
- *Reactivity*: extremely unstable, tends to react violently or explode during management
- *Toxicity*: specific standards for certain metals, volatile organics, and pesticides based on a test that extracts these constituents from a waste. The method assumes a dilution factor that corresponds to the constituent concentration necessary to leach from a municipal solid waste landfill to ground water.

Mixtures of characteristic and solid wastes are hazardous only if the entire mixture exhibits one of the four characteristics.

Recyclable Materials

The rules on recycling currently are rather complex. Some materials are solid wastes when recycled, some are hazardous-wastes, others are neither. Part 261.2 states that materials are intended as solid wastes if they are "used in a manner constituting disposal," burned for energy recovery, "inherently waste-like," reclaimed, or "accumulated speculatively." Materials that are solid wastes when they are recycled include those

- Used as an ingredient in an industrial process to make a product but are not reclaimed first
- Used or re-used as substitutes for a commercial product
- Returned to the original process without first being reclaimed

Part 261.6 identifies requirements for "recyclable materials" that are hazardous-wastes, such as hazardous-waste fuels and used oil, that exhibit a hazardous-waste characteristic before recycling. Except for those materials identified above, recyclable materials are hazardous and must be managed according to RCRA Subtitle C rules before recycling. Some facilities have requested that EPA simplify these criteria on what is and is not hazardous to reduce potential cost barriers to recycling.

TOXIC SUBSTANCES CONTROL ACT

Legal citation:	15 *USC* §§ 2601 *et seq.*
Regulations:	40 *CFR* 700–799
The TSCA inventory:	40 *CFR* 710.4
List of health and safety studies:	40 *CFR* 716.120
National Lead Information Center hotline:	(800) LEADFYI and (800) 424-LEAD
National Radon hotline:	(800) SOS-RADON
TSCA Assistance Information Service:	(202) 554-1404

TSCA was enacted in 1976 to "fill the cracks" left by other environmental laws (16). It gives EPA broad authority to regulate production, use, distribution, and disposal of "chemical substances." TSCA also addresses the need for manufacturers to supply data on the environmental and health effects of the chemicals and mixtures they produce. The key goal of TSCA is to identify and document risks associated with new products before they are distributed commercially and prevent those with "unreasonable risks" or "imminent hazards" from being introduced (16). It is a statute with enormous implications for commerce and public health.

TSCA's main components include

1. Premanufacture notice (PMN) of new chemical substances must occur 90 days before their commercial production and introduction into the marketplace (Section 5 of the act). Significant new uses of existing chemicals must be described to EPA under TSCA rules as well.
2. Testing may be required by EPA for chemicals that may present a significant risk or that are produced in substantial quantities and result in substantial human or environmental exposure (Section 4). Congress created the Interagency Testing Committee to recommend to the EPA administrator which substances should be prioritized for testing. Testing is triggered by either risks or potential for widespread exposure.
3. EPA has authority to limit or prohibit the manufacture, use, distribution, and disposal of existing chemicals (Section 6). This authority is particularly critical if submitted information was inadequate to determine risks to the public, or a new use or product presents an "unreasonable" risk (16). EPA has 90 days from the date of receipt of the PMN to review it and decide on the need for regulatory action.
4. The TSCA "inventory," the cornerstone of the law, is a list of chemical substances manufactured or processed for commercial use in the United States. EPA must maintain this list as a result of Section 8. Chemicals not listed require a PMN. More than 60,000 substances appear on the inventory (16,17). Production information must be updated by importers and manufacturers every 4 years (40 *CFR* 710).
5. Health and safety study reporting provides EPA with access to changing information on health and safety studies related to the substances (Section 8). The list of these studies is found at 40 *CFR* 716.120. Chemicals subject to specific reporting requirements are listed in the rules at 40 *CFR* 704 and 712.
6. Substantial risk notification is required under Section 8(e) when manufacturers, processors, or distributors learn of such risks associated with a substance, usually related to its toxicity, mutagenic or teratogenic effects. *Substantial risk* is not defined in TSCA.
7. EPA requires significant adverse reaction recording for reports of actual or suspected adverse reactions from the use of a chemical or mixture. EPA can review these records on request [15 *USC* § 2607(c)]. Commonly known health effects, or those that appear on the product's label, need not be recorded under this provision.
8. Export notice requirements are included in the act to allow EPA to inform foreign governments of shipments of chemical substances to their countries (Section 12). Conversely, import certifications are included so chemical substances brought into the United States comply with TSCA (Section 13).
9. Chemical-specific regulations in TSCA address six substances: asbestos, CFCs, dioxins, metal working fluids, hexavalent chromium, and polychlorinated biphenyls (PCBs) (40 *CFR* 761, 762, and 749).
10. Enforcement provisions involve EPA inspections (Section 11), imminent hazard authority" (16,17), civil and criminal penalties for violations (Section 16). It is illegal to commercially use, distribute, or manufacture a substance without first meeting TSCA requirements. Private citizens can bring suit under TSCA after notifying EPA. They can petition the EPA administrator to revise rules under the act (Section 20 of the act and 40 *CFR* 702).

Chemical Substances

Under TSCA, the term *chemical substance* means "any organic or inorganic substance of a particular molecular identity, including any combination of such substances occurring in whole or in part as a result of a chemical reaction or occurring in nature, and any chemical element or uncombined radical." The TSCA inventory includes five volumes of reportable chemical substances that meet the foregoing definition and were manufactured, processed, or imported for commercial use in the United States between January 1, 1975, and the first publication of the inventory on June 1, 1979. The law excludes the following materials from the TSCA inventory (40 *CFR* 710):

- Any mixture of a chemical substance
- Chemical substances manufactured for research and development [Section 8(b)]
- Any pesticide when manufactured, processed, or distributed in commerce for use as a pesticide
- Tobacco or any tobacco product, but not including any derivative products
- Any source material, special nuclear material, or by-product material
- Any pistol, firearm, revolver, shells, and cartridges
- Any food, food additive, drug, cosmetic, or device manufactured or processed for these uses
- Articles with no change in composition in end use
- Impurities "unintentionally" present in another chemical substance
- By-products without specific commercial intent
- Chemicals produced from incidental reactions
- "Non-isolated intermediates," which may be partially or totally consumed during manufacture

To provide a context for some of its authority, a number of terms are described in the regulations. For example, *significant adverse reactions* of human health include, but may be broader than

- Long-lasting or irreversible damage, such as cancer or birth defects
- Partial or complete impairment of bodily functions, such as reproductive disorders, neurologic disorders, or blood disorders
- An impairment of normal activities experienced by all or most of the persons exposed at one time
- An impairment of normal activities experienced each time an individual is exposed (40 *CFR* 717.12)

"Significant adverse reactions" of the environment include

- Gradual or sudden changes in the composition of animal life or plant life, including fungal or microbial organisms, in an area
- Abnormal number of deaths of organisms (such as fish kills)
- Reduction of the reproductive success or the vigor of a species
- Reduction in agricultural productivity, whether crops or livestock
- Alterations in the behavior or distribution of a species
- Long-lasting or irreversible contamination of components of the physical environment, especially in the case of groundwater and surface water and soil resources that have limited self-cleansing capability (40 *CFR* 717.12).

The terms *substantial risk* and *unreasonable risk* are not defined in TSCA. The legislative history indicates that such risks are somewhat subjective and involve "balancing the probability that harm will occur and the magnitude and severity of that harm against the effect of proposed regulatory action on the availability to society of the benefits of the substance or mixture" [H.R. Rep. No. 13,441, 94th Cong., 2d Sess. 13–14 (1976)].

An *imminently hazardous chemical substance or mixture* is defined in the act as one that presents "an imminent and unreasonable risk of serious or widespread injury to health or the environment . . . before a final rule . . . can protect against such risk" [15 *USC* § 2606 (f)]. As noted previously, TSCA gives EPA the authority to begin judicial proceedings to seize such substances. Relief under this authority includes "risk notification to purchasers, risk notification to the public, recall, and replacement or repurchase of the imminently hazardous substance" (16). EPA must act within 180 days when information suggests that a chemical substance poses a significant risk of human cancer, gene mutations, or birth defects.

Polychlorinated Biphenyls

In addition to the general requirements for chemical substances, TSCA contains regulations for the safe handling and disposal of PCB substances. Concentration thresholds for management of PCBs vary depending on the type of item (40 *CFR* 761). Items include PCB transformers, electrical equipment, and light ballasts, among others, containing mineral oil dielectric fluids. The regulations were written, in large part, to address Congress' presumption of unreasonable risk to humans, animals, and the environment [Section 6(e)]. EPA regulations require manufacturing, processing, and distribution of PCBs in a "totally enclosed manner" to prevent unreasonable risks. Standard warning labels are prescribed, as well as storage, recordkeeping, manifesting, and reporting requirements. TSCA regulations also define a spill cleanup policy for releases of PCB-containing materials greater than 50 ppm (40 *CFR* 761.120–135). Regulations regarding disposal of PCBs are strict; any release of 50 ppm or more is prohibited. PCB disposal typically involves destruction through incineration, although a variety of disposal standards appear in the regulations.

The act was also amended to add titles for

- Regulation of asbestos hazards (Title II, the Asbestos Hazard and Emergency Response Act)
- Regulation of indoor radon hazards (Title III, The Indoor Radon Abatement Act)
- Regulation of exposure to lead-based paint (Title IV, Lead-Based Paint Exposure Reduction Act)

COMPREHENSIVE ENVIRONMENTAL RESPONSE, COMPENSATION, AND LIABILITY ACT

Legal citation:	42 *USC* §§ 9601 *et seq.*
Regulations:	40 *CFR* 300–311
List of hazardous substances and reportable quantities (RQs):	40 *CFR* 302.4
National Response Center (NRC) for Reportable Releases:	(800) 424-8802
EPA hotline:	(800) 424-9346

CERCLA, better known as *Superfund*, was enacted in 1980 to create a national program for responding to releases of "hazardous substances." The act gives EPA the authority and funding to investigate and take remedial action at abandoned waste sites and to regulate the cleanup of accidental spills or releases of hazardous substances to the environment. CERCLA was amended by SARA of 1986, which added major provisions, such as selection of cleanup standards, cost recovery settlements, civil penalties, the hazard ranking system, and citizen suits provisions. Most guidance related to CERCLA is found in the statute and in case law, records of decisions, and agency guidance documents rather than in EPA regulations.

To a certain extent, CERCLA embraces other environmental laws that were in existence at the time, but handled a specific type of medium or problem. CERCLA provides authority for cleanup of releases in any medium, whether air, water, land, or subsurface. CERCLA is the main trigger behind the Phase I Environmental Site Assessment process required by lenders, buyers, or sellers seeking to characterize the condition of sites involved in a real estate transaction. The process is critical to limiting the liability of these entities by demonstrating what is known or in place at a site at the time of a transaction. It has resulted in a massive shift in national commitment to pollution control and prevention.

Recognized problems with CERCLA include

- The high emphasis on identification of liability that may defer and prolong cleanup.
- The difficulty in determining acceptable levels of risk that may lead to inconsistent cleanups.
- EPA's slow approval rate of emerging cleanup technologies, in part to ensure that the technology is effective, but in part due to bureaucracy.
- EPA's slow-moving bureaucracy makes it difficult to apply innovative solutions.
- The difficulty in communicating risks and allaying public concerns about uncertainties associated with cleanup protract the process to balance the need for health assurance versus the unfeasibility of a zero-risk cleanup.
- The disuse of real estate involved in CERCLA cleanups after the site has been cleared by EPA.

To respond to some of these difficulties, EPA and several states have launched initiatives to streamline cleanup balanced by the statutory mandate to remain protective of human health and the environment. For example, the "Brownfields Program" is aimed at redeveloping idle or abandoned sites where real or perceived environmental contamination makes it difficult to do so. EPA's Office of Solid Waste and Emergency Response states its "Brownfields Mission" as "empowering States, communities and other stakeholders in economic development to work together in a timely manner to prevent, assess, safely clean up, and sustainably reuse brownfields" (http://www.epa.gov/swerosps/bf/mission.htm, August 1997). EPA also has established a Reinvention for Innovative Technologies Program to increase incentives for development and use of potentially beneficial new technologies and remove that barrier to innovation. In August 1997, Reinvention for Innovative Technologies was supporting 40 projects to change this critical framework within EPA jurisdiction.

Key elements of CERCLA related to regulated materials are

1. The National Contingency Plan, or the National Oil and Hazardous Substances Pollution Contingency Plan (Section 105 of the act), which provides guidelines for federal response actions to hazardous substances releases. The plan states that
   - Remedial action alternatives must be cost-effective.
   - Alternatives must be effective in protecting public health, welfare, and the environment.
   - The remedy must be technically feasible.
   - The effects of the remedy on the surrounding environment also must be considered. Actions may be short term to address releases or threats requiring expedited response or longer term when the situation is not immediately life threatening (Section 106).
2. The list of Hazardous Substances and Reportable Quantities (Section 102 of the act) is a compendium of lists primarily from other federal programs existing at the time the law was enacted (40 *CFR* 302.4). CERCLA requires incident reporting to the NRC for releases of any substance on the list, beyond the workplace, which exceeds its RQ (in pounds).

3. EPA requires that certain persons must notify the agency of the existence of sites where hazardous-wastes from industries, businesses, governments, hospitals, and other sources were stored, treated, or disposed of and are still present [Section 103(c)].
4. The decision about how, where, and when to use the Superfund (Section 111 of the act) is defined through the site discovery process, preliminary assessments and site inspections, and the use of the Hazard Ranking System to identify candidates for the National Priorities List [(NPL); Section 105]. Site discovery can involve the Section 103(c) notification, citizen referral, and release notifications to the NRC. The Comprehensive Emergency Response Compensation and Liability Information System (CERCLIS) database contains information on these potential and NPL sites (http://www.epa.gov/enviro/html/cerclis/cerclis_overview.html).
5. Section 118 of the act gives a high priority for protection of drinking water supplies.
6. The Remedial Investigation, Feasibility Study, and Remediation processes involve a thorough evaluation to gather data that determine the nature and extent of site contamination, establish the criteria for cleanup, identify alternatives for cleanup, and provide technical and cost analyses of these alternatives. A remedial design is selected through a Record of Decision for the site, which is a public document that describes how cleanup will occur.
7. Strict, joint, and several liability for responsible parties makes CERCLA provisions difficult to evade, but also has had the unintended effect of seriously delaying cleanups and causing much money to be spent in litigation (Section 107 of the act).
8. Cost-recovery provisions in Section 122 allow EPA to seek out and hold parties responsible for remedial investigations and cleanup. The act also allows the EPA to enter into settlements with responsible parties for cleanup costs. Responsible parties who refuse to pay may be sued for as much as three times the cost of cleanup.
9. Federal facilities are addressed in Section 120 of CERCLA to ensure that the rules encompass these vast areas where contamination has occurred.
10. Development of cleanup standards for a site is addressed in Section 121, including the selection of a remedial action, the degree of cleanup, state involvement, and permits and enforcement. Standards must be "adequate to protect human health and the environment." This criterion is defined primarily through risk assessment procedures that meet all federal applicable, relevant, and appropriate requirements.

Wastes Excluded from Notification Requirements in Section 103(c)

Wastes excluded from EPA notification include

- Solid waste that is not regulated as hazardous-waste under RCRA
- Household waste, including garbage, trash, and septic tank wastes
- Solid waste generated and returned to the soil as fertilizers through agricultural practice and livestock production
- Mining overburden returned to the mine site
- Drilling fluids, produced waters, and wastes associated with crude oil and gas development
- Cement kiln dust waste (unless regulated as a hazardous-waste under RCRA)
- Natural gas and petroleum (unless specifically regulated as a hazardous-waste under RCRA)

Hazardous Substances

A *hazardous substance* is any material that poses a threat to public health or the environment. As noted above, CERCLA encompasses lists and designated substances found in other laws, in part, to address pollution that may have occurred before their enactment. Section 101 of CERCLA states that *hazardous substances* means

- Any substance designated according to Section 311(b)(2)(A) of the CWA (33 *USC* § 1321)
- Any element, compound, mixture, solution, or substance designated pursuant to Section 102 of this act (list of hazardous substances and reportable quantities)
- Any hazardous-waste having the characteristics identified under or listed pursuant to Section 3001 of the Solid Waste Disposal Act (RCRA; 42 *USC* § 6921)
- Any toxic pollutant listed under Section 307(a) of the CWA
- Any hazardous air pollutant listed under Section 112 of the CAA (42 *USC* § 7412)
- Any imminently hazardous chemical substance or mixture with respect to which the EPA has taken action under Section 7 of TSCA (15 *USC* § 2606)

Typical hazardous substances are materials that are toxic, corrosive, ignitable, explosive, or chemically reactive. An RQ, a quantity (in pounds) designated for listed hazardous substances, triggers notification of the NRC within 24 hours so that the need for remedial action can be evaluated. Federally permitted releases defined in Section 101 of the act are excluded.

The EPA Web site provides 1994 and 1995 data on the progress of site remediation at NPL sites under the CERCLA program:

Remediation status	No. of sites (1994)	No. of sites (1995)
Remedial action not begun	98	90
Study under way	263	213
Remedy selected	74	82
Remedial design under way	211	169
Construction under way	430	472
Construction completions	278	346

Of the 1,372 NPL sites listed in 1995, construction of the remedial alternative was under way or completed at 59% of the sites (http://www.epa.gov). A 1997 report from the General Accounting Office found that over the 1986–1996 period, it took longer to place sites on the NPL and to clean them up:

- Placing a site on the NPL "rose from four to more than nine years."
- Cleanup rose from about "two years to almost eleven years over the same time period"(18).

EMERGENCY PLANNING AND COMMUNITY RIGHT-TO-KNOW ACT

Legal citation:	42 *USC* § 11001 *et seq.*
Regulations:	40 *CFR* 350–374
List of extremely hazardous substances:	40 *CFR* 355, Appendix B
List of toxic chemicals:	40 *CFR* 372.65(a)
Summary reference:	*EPA's Title III List of Lists*, Document No. EPA 560/4-92-011
EPA hotline:	(800) 535-0202

EPCRA was signed into law in 1986 as Title III of SARA (19). It is widely described as a law enacted in response to the Bhopal, India, chemical disaster a few years before. Lawmakers saw that the U.S. population was at risk from similar accidents and recognized a serious need to close the gap through prevention activities. This law brought with it three new hazardous material categories: (a) "hazardous chemicals," (b) "extremely hazardous substances," and (c) "toxic chemicals." It also triggered a massive effort among industries and government to identify and quantify chemical products in storage, in the manufacturing process, or otherwise used for the purpose of preventing and swiftly addressing potentially large environmental releases.

Key elements of EPCRA related to the management of regulated hazardous materials include

1. The Emergency Planning and Notification provisions (Sections 301–303), which required facilities to determine whether amounts of extremely hazardous substances on site exceeded threshold planning quantities. If so, the facility is required to send an emergency coordinator to work with the Local Emergency Planning Committee (LEPC), authorized by the State Emergency Response Commission (SERC), to assist in planning to avert environmental disasters. LEPCs must prepare comprehensive emergency response plans that comprise a list of information that includes the identification of all risk-related facilities, designation of a community emergency coordinator, and descriptions of methods and equipment to be used to address emergency scenarios.
2. Immediate Notification of Releases of Extremely Hazardous Substances (Section 304), which is required if a release of a listed hazardous or extremely hazardous substance occurs in an amount over an RQ that is not otherwise permitted by law. The LEPC and the SERC must be notified under EPCRA. This notification does not relieve a facility from incident notification requirements found in other federal, state, or local laws. For example, EPCRA cross-references CERCLA notification requirements to the NRC [40 *CFR* 255.40(b)].
3. A list of Material Safety Data Sheets (MSDSs) for hazardous chemicals and extremely hazardous substances exceeding listed thresholds, which is required by the LEPC and the SERC as part of EPCRA's Community Right-to-Know Reporting provisions (Section 311). The deadline for initial reporting was 1990; new facilities or covered new chemicals must be accounted for within 3 months.
4. Section 312 of the act, which requires covered facilities to submit Tier One and Tier Two reports that identify quantities, storage locations, and container types. Mixtures must be evaluated for the presence of hazardous chemicals and extremely hazardous substances. Tier Two reports are submitted annually in March; the Tier One is filed on an initial basis only (40 *CFR* 370.20). The report excludes articles and chemicals present as a solid in a manufactured item to the extent that exposure does not occur in normal use.
5. Toxic Chemical Release Inventory Reporting (Section 313), which focuses on certain types of industrial facilities (Standard Industrial Classification codes 20–39) that manufacture, process, or otherwise use listed toxic chemicals over regulatory thresholds. The annual Toxics Release Inventory (TRI), also called the "Form R" report, is filed annually in July and covers the breadth of emissions, treated wastewater discharges, on-site and off-site disposal, accidental releases, and recycling activities (40 *CFR* 372). EPCRA's effect was so widespread that EPA requires suppliers of products that contain Form R reportable chemicals to notify their customers. This is usually performed through the Material Data Safety Sheets (40 *CFR* 372.45). Provisions for protecting legitimate Trade Secrets are included in EPCRA at 40 *CFR* 350.5.
6. Enforcement authority and civil and criminal penalties, which are addressed in Sections 325 and 326 of the act.

A striking result of this law was that information compiled through EPCRA's reporting requirements was much more accessible to the general public though local libraries and local emergency planning commissions. EPCRA specified that the public be able to obtain these data during working hours. Perhaps no environmental law, other than CERCLA, had more initial impact in preventing pollution than EPCRA when it was enacted. The TRI, for example, provided citizens with data for a "top ten" list no industry wanted to be on. The TRI, or "Form R" report presented numbers related to discharges, emissions, releases, and land disposal with no explanation of what efforts had been under way to mitigate these numbers. Many companies went to great lengths to ensure that the next year's report showed obvious reductions.

Extremely Hazardous Substances

Extremely hazardous substances are listed in the Appendices at 40 *CFR* 355. The list is an extension of the hazardous substances list compiled under CERCLA. As noted above, it invokes several responsibilities for facilities: evaluation of facility quantities for planning purposes, assessment of releases greater than RQ for immediate emergency notification, and reporting on Tier One and Tier Two forms (items 1 through 4, above).

Hazardous Chemicals

EPCRA borrows from OSHA when it uses the term *hazardous chemicals* (40 *CFR* 370.20 and 29 *CFR* 1910.1200) to cover a broad spectrum of possible materials that would need to be addressed in a community-based emergency response plan. A *hazardous chemical* is defined to mean any element, chemical, or compound that is a physical or health hazard. Typically, this is interpreted as any chemical that requires an MSDS. Neither OSHA nor EPCRA provides a specific list of hazardous chemicals. EPCRA's threshold for reporting a hazardous chemical to the LEPC is amounts equal to or greater than 10,000 lb (item 3, above). In reporting, EPCRA offers the option of submitting MSDSs or listing the chemicals by common name and identifying its associated hazard category. Each of these categories correlates to related OSHA hazard categories (18):

- Immediate or acute health hazard, corresponding to OSHA's "highly toxic," "toxic," "corrosive," "irritant," and "sensitizer" health hazard categories
- Delayed or chronic health hazard, related to OSHA's definition for *carcinogen*
- Fire hazard, corresponding to the physical categories "flammable," "oxidizer," "combustible liquid," and "pyrophoric" under OSHA
- Sudden release of pressure hazard, relating to OSHA's "compressed gas" and "explosive" categories
- Reactive hazard, based on OSHA's "organic peroxide," "unstable reactive," and "water reactive"

Regarding the EPCRA requirements, facilities may inadvertently overlook this ongoing reporting requirement for hazardous chemicals once the original list has been submitted. As noted above, the requirement involves continued reporting of new chemicals over the thresholds within 3 months. If the LEPC asks for an MSDS, it must be submitted regardless of the quantity stored or used on site (40 *CFR* 370.30). As noted above, hazardous chemicals are also reported on the Tier One and Tier Two forms if regulatory criteria are met (item 4, above).

Toxic Chemicals

Toxic chemicals are listed by EPA strictly for the purpose of the TRI Form R reporting each July 1 (item 5, above, 40 *CFR* 372.65). The source of this list was a combination of chemical lists developed by New Jersey and Maryland for their own toxic release reporting and planning laws. The list of toxic chemicals nearly doubled in 1995 when 648 chemicals and chemical categories were listed. Most recently, EPA proposed to add "dioxin" and "dioxin-like" compounds to the toxic chemicals list (62 *FR* 24887-24896, May 7, 1997). Several of these compounds encompass PCBs (19).

EPA has developed information summaries and fact sheets on more than 200 TRI chemicals to describe how the public might be exposed and how exposure might affect them and the environment. The sheets are based in large part on New Jersey's Hazardous Substance Fact Sheet Program. This information can be accessed online through the TRIFACTS database, a subset of the National Library of Medicine's TOXNET system.

In determining the applicability of the TRI report, it is critical that a facility evaluate the definitions of *manufacture*, *process*, and *otherwise used* in relation to the listed toxic chemicals on site (40 *CFR* 372.3). Thresholds for reporting apply under each category: 25,000 lb for manufactured and processed, 10,000 lb for chemicals otherwise used. Once reporting thresholds are met, the facility must quantify the ways these chemicals are "released" by a facility. The term *release* includes virtually all planned and unplanned methods of treatment and disposition.

An Alternate Form R reporting rule is available for facilities that generate less than 500 lb per year of reportable chemicals as wastes, counting all possible discharges and releases. A new threshold of 1,000,000 lb applies for these facilities, and a two-page certification form is used rather than the detailed Form R. This alternative was provided to streamline regulatory reporting for those facilities that have been successful in waste minimization efforts since the enactment of EPCRA.

The breadth of Form R reporting under EPCRA is expected to be expanded in other ways by adding types of facilities that are subject to reporting, such as metal mining, coal mining, electric utilities, commercial hazardous-waste treatment facilities, and others. EPA promulgated a final rule on this issue in May 1997 with an effective date of December 31, 1997—in time for the 1998 Form R reporting cycle (62 *FR* 23834).

SUMMARY

The history of U.S. environmental regulation is traced to public response to a general fouling of the environment. The federal government's approach to pollution control and prevention has relied heavily on the identification and listing of hazardous materials in laws and regulations. The eight environmental acts reviewed mandate regulatory control over the vast majority of environmental hazards affecting health and the environment in America. The future of U.S. regulatory action is predicted to be more conscious of cost-benefit analyses and outcomes research to prove health benefits. Other nations witnessing the success of U.S. environmentalism have begun to develop their equivalent laws and regulations.

REFERENCES

1. Commerce Clearing House Editorial Staff. Clean air act, law and explanation. Chicago: Commerce Clearinghouse, Inc. 1990.
2. Brownell WF. Clean air act. In: *Environmental law handbook*, 14th ed. Rockville, MD: Government Institutes, 1997:72–108.
3. Tobin RJ. Revising the clean air act: legislative failure and administrative success. In: Vig NJ, Kraft ME, eds. *Environmental policy in the 1980s*. Washington: CQ Press, 1984:227.
4. List of regulated air pollutants (as of April 1993). In: *CAA guidance, EPA's policy and interpretations*. Issue 1. New York: Elsevier Science, Inc., 1995:175–183.
5. Goldman BA, Hulme JA, Johnson C. Hazardous waste management: reducing the risk. Washington: Island Press, 1986.
6. Paigen B, Goldman LR, Higland JH, Magnant MM, Steegman AT Jr. Prevalence of health problems in children living near Love Canal. *Hazardous Waste and Hazardous Materials* 1985;2(1):23–44.
7. Proposed Rule. *Federal Register* 1996 Apr 15; 61(73):16598.
8. Ingram HM, Mann DE. Preserving the clean water act: the appearance of environmental victory. In: Vig NJ, Kraft ME, eds. *Environmental policy in the 1980s*. Washington: CQ Press, 1984:252.
9. Gallagher LM. Clean water act. In: *Environmental law handbook*, 14th ed. Rockville, MD: Government Institutes, 1997:109–160.
10. Miller ML. Pesticides. In: *Environmental law handbook*, 14th ed. Rockville, MD: Government Institutes, 1997:284–327.
11. Williams SE. Safe drinking water act. In: *Environmental law handbook*, 14th ed. Rockville, MD: Government Institutes, 1997: 196–225.
12. HWIR to be promulgated sometime next century. *The Hazardous Waste Consultant* 1997;15(4).
13. Krag BL. Hazardous wastes and their management. *Hazardous Waste and Hazardous Materials* 1985;2(3):251–308.
14. Buchanan MW. Recycling issues. In: *The resource conservation and recovery act (RCRA): the teenage years*. Scottsdale, AZ: State Bar of Arizona, 1989.
15. Case DR. Resource conservation and recover act. In: *Environmental law handbook*, 14th ed. Rockville, MD: Government Institutes, 1997:328–359.
16. Phillips PD, Hofstetter DL. The toxic substances control act. In: Sullivan JB Jr, Krieger GR, eds. *Hazardous materials toxicology, clinical principles of environmental health*. Baltimore: Williams & Wilkins, 1992.
17. Landfair, SW. Toxic substances control act. In: *Environmental law handbook*, 14th ed. Rockville, MD: Government Institutes, 1997:328–359.
18. CERCLA cleanups progressing slower than program goals. *The Hazardous Waste Consultant* 1997;15(4).
19. Halblieb, WT. Emergency planning and community right-to-know act. In: *Environmental law handbook*, 14th ed. Rockville, MD: Government Institutes, 1997:481–509.

CHAPTER 8

Medical Surveillance and Medical Screening for Toxic Exposure

Gary R. Krieger, Caryl S. Brailsford, Marci Balge, and Myron C. Harrison

The ultimate goal of medical surveillance is primary prevention. Comprehending the concept of medical surveillance depends on a clear understanding of the distinction between surveillance and screening (Table 8-1). *Medical surveillance* is defined as "ongoing scrutiny, generally using methods distinguished by their practicability, uniformity, and frequently their rapidity, rather than by complete accuracy. Its main purpose is to detect changes in trend or distribution in order to initiate investigative or control measures" (1).

The purpose of surveillance is the elimination of exposures that cause disease. To accomplish this, it is not sufficient to merely identify adverse health outcomes in individuals. There must also be a means to link these outcomes back to work exposures to analyze the plausibility of causation. Surveillance also depends on the ability to define groups of individuals who have similar work histories, thereby facilitating the detection of unusual distributions of disease.

TABLE 8-1. Medical surveillance versus medical screening

Medical surveillance	Medical screening
Purpose is to identify opportunities for primary prevention (i.e., elimination of exposure opportunities)	Purpose is secondary prevention (i.e., early identification of clinical disease in order to intervene)
Ideally is very broad, varied, practical, rapid, and highly sensitive in order to not miss a problem in the work environment; often sacrifices accuracy	Ideally is highly accurate in order to minimize the harm that occurs to individuals from false-positives and false-negatives
Focused on populations of similarly exposed individuals; analysis of aggregate data is important	Focused on the individual clinical interaction; analysis of aggregate data is not necessary
Rarely accomplished in industry	Very common in industry; millions of examinations performed annually

Medical screening has a different purpose than medical surveillance. It focuses on the individual for the purpose of secondary prevention (i.e., the early detection and treatment of disease) (2). The benefit of medical screening—either in early detection of disease or in the provision of reassurance—is to the individual. High predictive value is critical when counseling individuals. Applying medical tests of little or no proven value to asymptomatic populations with low prevalence of disease is questionable and costly. An unfortunate reality of most screening programs is that the false-positives greatly outnumber the true positives. False-negatives are also a significant issue in that they provide false reassurance to both an individual and the company.

Medical surveillance programs are designed to systematically collect and analyze health information on workers exposed to hazardous materials. Components of a medical surveillance program include

- Biological monitoring
- Protocols for testing
- Determination of health hazards, exposures, and job-related risks
- Tracking systems
- Specific job descriptions, job duties, and job requirements
- Exposure monitoring system

The end results of this surveillance are used to take both preventive and ongoing action in the workplace. To be effective, a medical surveillance program must meet all appropriate regulatory requirements and must be managed in a cost-effective and businesslike fashion. Program goals include the following (3):

- Establish epidemiologic surveys with the purpose of determining the frequency or natural history of a particular condition.
- Protect the health of the public (e.g., from communicable diseases).
- Produce data that would meet regulatory and internal company exposure monitoring requirements. Regulatory exposure standards are not always available for all substances. Thus, many large companies have developed exposure standards for their internal use; however, most industrial-based medical surveillance programs are regulatory driven.

To manage a successful program, internal evaluation criteria must be established. These criteria are based on several key issues:

- The type of organization establishing the program (e.g., industrial, medical group practice)
- The program administrators (e.g., funded versus internal vendor service)
- Income source
- Internal audits
- The employees in the surveillance program

Within a program, the specific goals of the various managers and customers may not be the same. For example, the managers may view cost control within a context of minimum regulatory compliance as the primary goal, whereas the worker's perspective of the program may focus on the desire to have maximum medical testing regardless of cost or effectiveness. Given this clear dichotomy, it is essential for the physician to balance these perspectives when developing overall program goals, objectives, and outcomes. Table 8-1 presents an example of specific program elements in the evaluation process. By using this model, it is possible—based on past efforts—to determine the direction of future program activities.

Surveillance does not occur unless a link is made between a health outcome and the work environment. Cohort mortality studies can be a form of surveillance if there is enough information available to link outcomes to specific work environments and if there are historical records that document the exposures and work practices in these environments. Other effective forms of surveillance include the willingness of many physicians, nurses, and industrial hygienists to pursue specific worker reports or a "sentinel event" by doing job inspections. These practices create an immediate link between health outcomes and the work environment. But these efforts are reactive and dependent on the interest and commitment of the particular professional and willingness of the company to cooperate.

Systematic, documented programs designed to periodically link outcomes (reports, diagnoses, and test results) to specific work environments are infrequent. Given all of the exposure assessment activity and all of the clinical examinations that occur annually in industry, this statement may seem puzzling. But the truth is that these two activities generally operate independent of each other. One reason is that most industry activity in the safety, health, and environmental areas is compliance driven, and Occupational Safety and Health Administration (OSHA) regulations do not require genuine surveillance activities.

Another reason for the rarity of surveillance programs is that they are very difficult to achieve technically. Classifying employees with similar jobs into exposure groups at a point in time is difficult. Subsequently tracking and documenting exposure group changes for an employee caused by either new work assignments or process alterations is even more challenging. Furthermore, there are no practical, widely available tools for analyses of group data. Methods that employ the rigor of formal epidemiology studies are too slow and too expensive to serve as surveillance systems.

HUMAN EXPOSURE STANDARDS

Since September 1988, OSHA has indicated support for generic regulations in the areas of exposure monitoring and medical surveillance (4,5). If these proposed rule changes occur, they would have the effect of setting general examination requirements for all chemical exposures.

Unlike current requirements, the proposed generic requirements would have a broader scope:

- Initial exposure monitoring of workers will be required of employers.
- The frequency of follow-up monitoring will be specified.

- The placement of air-sampling techniques in terms of personal and environmental monitoring will be specified.
- Procedures will be developed for employee observance of ambient sampling.
- Medical surveillance will be required for all employees exposed to one-half the exposure limit.
- The fact that employees will not be charged for the examinations will be emphasized.

Currently, OSHA regulations listed in 29 *CFR* 1910.120 require employers to implement medical surveillance programs in the following situations (6):

- Implement programs for employees who may be exposed to hazardous substances or health hazards at or above the permissible exposure limits (PELs) for 30 days or more per year.
- In the absence of PELs, medical surveillance should be established for those employees working at limits above the published exposure levels for a given substance.
- Employees who wear a respirator for 30 days or more per year must be examined.
- HAZMAT (hazardous material) employees, defined as employees who are designated to plug, patch, or temporarily control leaks from containers that hold hazardous substances, must be examined.
- All employees who are injured as a result of overexposure from an emergency incident involving hazardous substances must be examined.

The large number of potentially hazardous materials and the frequency of their use virtually ensures that people will be exposed to hazardous substances at some time and to some degree.

Exposure refers to any contact of an organism with a chemical or physical agent. For the majority of the health effects, there is a general correlation between the amount of a toxic substance absorbed and the production of a response. This dose-response relationship implies that for many materials, there are levels of exposure that can be tolerated without adverse health effects. Thus, it is important to accurately assess the magnitude, frequency, duration, and route of exposure. This exposure assessment generates a series of standards or limits that are considered safe for each material encountered.

Exposure limits vary from country to country, depending on the original data source. The United States, Western Europe, and Australia generally use health impairment data, whereas Russian scientists frequently focus on neurophysiologic changes in experimental animals. In addition, the safety factors applied to a data source can widely vary because of technical and socioeconomic factors. In the United States, exposure limits are statutory requirements, whereas in some countries, exposure limits are included in labor agreements.

In the United States, one of the first groups to develop specific exposure guidelines was the American Conference of Government Industrial Hygienists (ACGIH). In 1941, ACGIH suggested maximum allowable concentrations for use in industry. A list of maximum allowable concentrations was compiled by ACGIH and published in 1946. In the early 1960s, ACGIH revised their recommendations and renamed them *threshold limit values* (*TLVs*). TLVs are a registered trademark of the ACGIH and refer to the concept that there is a threshold dose or concentration of air contaminants in the working environment below which there are no adverse effects. Broadly, a TLV refers to an airborne concentration and workplace condition under which it is believed that nearly all workers may be repeatedly exposed day after day without adverse effects. TLVs were formulated for use in the normal industrial workplace, not as general environmental or community standards. The notion of a TLV is not easily transferable to the situation found at chemical spills or at complex hazardous-waste sites, because TLVs are not risk-based calculations based on Environmental Protection Agency exposures and toxicity factors.

The ACGIH system has been widely disseminated and is extremely influential both in the United States and internationally.

Compliance with regulations does not ensure corporate liability protection. The National Institute of Occupational Safety and Health (NIOSH) developed recommendations for medical surveillance covering more than 400 chemicals. These recommendations differ from OSHA PELs for more than 100 chemicals. It is quite common to discover that an exposure level is well below OSHA requirements but above NIOSH recommendations. In this situation, it may be prudent to monitor these exposures as part of the overall medical surveillance program; however, the OSHA PELs are the legally binding standards.

OCCUPATIONAL SAFETY AND HEALTH ADMINISTRATION REQUIREMENTS RELATING TO SPECIFIC HAZARDOUS EXPOSURES

There are exposures to specific chemical hazards and hazardous environments that have legally mandated OSHA examination requirements. In most cases, it is the responsibility of the employer to provide the physician with a copy of the relevant OSHA standard when requesting medical surveillance for their workers; however, physicians must also independently be aware of OSHA examination requirements. The OSHA standards will require that specific history, physical examination, and biological testing be performed at strict intervals, and the standards will affect medical management of abnormal findings.

OSHA has specific medical surveillance requirements for hazardous chemicals, exposures, and environments (7,8). Some states, such as California, also have their own state OSHA-equivalent regulatory system. States may enact more stringent, but not less stringent, occupational standards. Physicians should therefore be familiar with current OSHA standards from their state OSHA equivalent. Copies of federal standards may be obtained from the U.S. Department of Labor through the U.S. Government Printing Office. These standards are periodically updated, and new standards are added. Up-to-date OSHA medical surveillance and biological exposure indices can be found at www.osha-slc.gov/SLTC/medicalsurveillance/index.html.

NIOSH is charged with providing guidance to OSHA for use in regulations. Many hazardous chemicals and environments have been evaluated by NIOSH that have suggested medical surveillance protocols. These protocols are not legally required until promulgated by OSHA, but they generally provide standards for good medical practice. Guidance is also provided by the American National Standards Institute, which provides protocols for generally accepted medical surveillance. OSHA standards are frequently based on American National Standards Institute standards for physical hazards, such as laser exposures. Other sources include the ACGIH, which also lists biological exposure indexes (BEIs). BEIs are useful suggestions for medical surveillance and medical monitoring. The guidelines cover only a small number of chemicals and typically are much more specific than the OSHA equivalent.

In addition to requiring special history and physical examinations and tests, some standards require the administration of legally mandated questionnaires: asbestos, cotton dust, cadmium, and formaldehyde (6–12).

The use of personal protective equipment does not negate the need for following medical surveillance requirements. The need for participation in a medical surveillance program is determined by exposure type and exposure. It is the responsibility of the employer to supply the examining physician with information about actual or anticipated environmental exposure levels and duration and types of personal protective equipment used. Most standards also require that the current examining physician be provided with the names and addresses of previous examiners to allow for obtaining old records and comparison of lab and other test results and health status.

The legal examination requirements are specific to the anticipated toxicity of the exposure and are less complete than the standard of care for hazardous materials examinations. The examination requirements are usually organ or toxicity specific. Some latitude is given to the examining physician for determining types of testing required. For example, many standards require the use of respiratory protective equipment. The regulatory guidance for respiratory protection clearance does not require obtaining spirometry or testing of any type other than a history and physical directed toward the respiratory tract (*CFR* 1910.0134). Most physicians would recommend spirometry as an additional method of determining an individual's capability for using personal protective equipment; however, spirometry is not legally required by OSHA. Guidance from other agencies, such as NIOSH (13,14), also recommend spirometry as a method of evaluating fitness for respirator use.

Conversely, many standards require the use of specific tests at specific frequencies. Some of these tests are uncommon outside of occupational exposures that may well be anachronistic because of poor sensitivity and specificity. For example, arsenic workers (*CFR* 1910.1018) and coke oven workers (*CFR* 1910.1029) are required to submit sputum for cytology at regular intervals.

There are also legal requirements for the qualifications of test administrators. Most standards (especially asbestos and cotton dust) require that persons administering spirometry be trained and certified by NIOSH. Likewise, calibrations of the testing equipment must be performed at specified (usually daily) intervals.

Chest x-rays must be evaluated by specially trained examiners using standardized guidelines. Classification is either done according to the International Labor Organization, such as coke oven workers and arsenic workers, or evaluated by B-readers (asbestos), specially trained physicians who rate chest x-rays based on specialized ranking standards.

Most OSHA standards require that the employer be provided with reports of the employee's capability to perform work in the proposed hazardous environment. Any medical symptoms reported by the employee relating to the exposure should be included in the written opinion. If an individual has a medical condition that puts him or her at increased risk from the occupational exposure, restrictions relating to this condition must be included in the medical opinion. Confidentiality must also be protected if the medical condition is personal and not related to the exposure. The results of laboratory and other testing generally must also be provided to the employer. Depending on the standard, employers are required to maintain employee monitoring results and medical records for 30 years. In case the business is terminated, records can be sent to OSHA for retention.

SPECIFIC PROGRAMS UNDER THE OCCUPATIONAL SAFETY AND HEALTH ADMINISTRATION

Asbestos (*CFR* 1910.1000, *CFR* 1926.1101)

Asbestos is covered under two standards, one for general industry (*CFR* 1910.1000) and one for construction industry (*CFR* 1926.1101). The medical surveillance requirements are similar. Examinations are required before assignment, annually, and at termination of employment. The examination requires a medical and work history. There is a legally mandated history questionnaire included in the standard, which should be administered to the employee. There are two versions of the history questionnaire, the annual and the initial. The physical examination requires evaluation of the respiratory, cardiac, and gastrointestinal tract. Pulmonary function testing is required annually. Chest x-ray is required as a baseline, then periodically, based on number of years of exposure and smoking status (Table 8-2).

TABLE 8-2. Asbestos chest x-ray guidelines

Years since first exposure	Age of employee		
	15–35	36–45	46+
0–10	Every 5 y	Every 5 y	Every 5 y
10+	Every 5 y	Every 2 y	Every 1 y

As with other standards, the physician should be provided with a copy of the standard, a description of the affected employee's duties and anticipated exposure level, a description of personal protective equipment used, and the location of any previous medical testing. The physician must provide the employer with a written opinion of whether the employee has any detected medical conditions that would put him or her at increased risk of health impairment from exposure to asbestos and any recommended limitations on the employee relating to use of personal protective equipment. The written statement to the employer must include a statement that the employee has been informed by the physician of any medical conditions present that may have been caused by asbestos exposure. The employee must be notified by the physician of the increased risk of lung cancer attributable to the combined effects of smoking and asbestos exposure.

Cadmium (*CFR* 1910.1027, *CFR* 1296.1127)

The general requirements of the cadmium standard are similar to other standards. The laboratory monitoring and medical removal protocols are based on combinations of three laboratory results: urinary β-2 microglobulin standardized to grams of creatinine (μg/g-Cr), blood cadmium in micrograms cadmium per liter whole blood (μg Cd/L), and urinary cadmium in micrograms per gram of creatinine (μg/g-Cr).

For the initial monitoring, if urine cadmium (CdU) is less than 3 μg/g-Cr, β-2 microglobulin is less than 300 μg/g-Cr, or the blood Cd is less than 5 μg/L, the employer shall provide the minimum level of medical surveillance, which includes second examination 1 year after the initial examination, then at least biennially thereafter and annual laboratory screening. Annual laboratory screening includes the three tests described above.

If the results of monitoring show CdU is greater than 3 μg/g-Cr, β-2 microglobulin is greater than 300 μg/g-Cr, or the blood Cd greater than 5 μg/L, the employer shall

1. Notify the employee and reassess the employee's work practices and personal hygiene.
2. Reevaluate the employee's respirator use, if any, and respiratory protection program.
3. Review the hygiene facilities.
4. Reevaluate engineering exposure controls.
5. Assess employee's smoking status.
6. Correct any deficiencies within 90 days.
7. Provide a full medical examination to the employee within 90 days.

If the physician determines that medical removal is not necessary, the laboratory testing should be repeated semiannually and the medical examination annually until the CdU is less than 3 mg/g-Cr, β-2 microglobulin is less than 300 mg/g-Cr, and the blood Cd is less than 5 mg/L. Once levels are below these thresholds, then the minimum medical surveillance may be performed.

If the biomonitoring results show CdU is greater than 15 μg/g-Cr, the level of cadmium in blood (CdB) is greater than 15 μg/L, or the β-2 microglobulin level is greater than 1,500 μg/g-Cr, the employer shall provide a medical examination within 90 days (which includes repeat biomonitoring) and should reevaluate the employee's work and hygiene practices. The physician should provide a written medical opinion regarding whether medical removal is indicated. If an employee's β-2 microglobulin urinary levels are greater than 1,500 μg/g-Cr, for mandatory medical removal to be required either the employee's CdU level must also be greater than 3 μg/L of whole blood. If the employee is not medically removed from exposure, biomonitoring should reoccur quarterly and medical evaluations should be repeated semiannually until the levels reach CdU less than 3 mg/g-Cr, β-2 microglobulin less than 300 mg/g-Cr, and blood Cd less than 5 mg/L. At that time, the employer may provide the minimum level of medical surveillance, which includes second examination 1 year after the initial examination, with repeat medical examinations at least biennially thereafter and annual laboratory screening.

In 1999, the requirements for medical removal became more stringent. If both the initial biomonitoring results and the laboratory results at the time of medical evaluation show a CdU level higher than 7 mg/g-Cr, or the level of CdB is greater than 10 mg/L, or the β-2 microglobulin level is greater than 750 mg/g-Cr—*and* either the Cd level is greater than 3 mg/g-Cr or the CdB level is greater than 5 mg/L—then medical removal is required.

Cotton Dust (*CFR* 1910.1043)

The cotton dust standard is similar in format to other standards. It has specific testing requirements regarding timing and frequency of spirometry. Spirometry must be performed on the first day of the work week, after at least 35 hours with no exposure to cotton dust. The test should be repeated between 4 and 10 hours of the start of the shift, no more than 1 hour after the end of exposure. The testing must be performed annually when employees are exposed at or above the exposure action level (AL), which varies for different processes: for employees exposed at or below the AL, for all employees who work only with cotton dust from washed cotton, and for all employees in cottonseed processing and waste processing operations. Medical surveillance must include, at a minimum, the cotton dust standardized questionnaire, Schilling byssinosis grade, and spirometry.

Medical surveillance should be provided every 6 months for employees with abnormal spirometry. *Abnormal* is defined as an FEV_1 (forced expiratory volume in 1 second) greater than 80% of predicted, but with an FEV_1 decrement of 5% or 200 mL on first working day of testing; or FEV_1 less than 80% of predicted; or when the physician determines that any significant change in questionnaire results, pulmonary function results, or other diagnostic tests has occurred.

Pulmonary function results that are less than 60% of the predicted value should result in referral to a specialist for more detailed evaluation.

Lead (*CFR* 1910.1025, *CFR* 1926.62)

Lead is covered by two standards (15,16), one for the construction industry (*CFR* 1926.62), another for general industry (*CFR* 1910.1025). The examinations are similar, but the level for medical removal and the frequency of examinations and blood lead monitoring are different. The employer should notify the physician as to which standard applies to the employees requiring medical surveillance. General industry lead standards apply to workers working with lead in all industries except agriculture and construction and includes manufacturing of materials using lead; foundries; lead production facilities; lead battery manufacturing; electronics; and processes in which lead is handled, ground, or otherwise used in manufacturing. The construction industry is defined as "construction, alteration and/or repair, including painting and decoration." Workers performing remediation of lead contamination and transport of lead-contaminated materials and construction maintenance workers are included in the construction industry standard. Exposure assessment is necessary in both construction and general industries. The results of environmental testing should be provided to the examining physician.

The general industry standard requires medical surveillance for all employees exposed to airborne lead concentrations at or above the AL of 30 mg/m^3, averaged over an 8-hour day for more than 30 days per year, regardless of whether respiratory protection is used. Medical surveillance includes biological monitoring and medical examinations. Biological monitoring includes blood lead level (BLL) and zinc protoporphyrin (ZPP) level testing. The BLL and ZPP testing must occur at least every 6 months for all employees covered under the standard whose BLLs are less than 40 mg/dL and every 2 months for BLLs greater than 40 mg/dL. Medical removal from lead exposure must occur with a BLL greater than 50 mg/dL averaged over the previous 6 months or a single BLL greater than 60 mg/dL. If medical removal occurs, BLL monitoring should occur at least monthly.

The medical examination portion of the medical surveillance program for general industry must occur at least annually for workers whose BLL exceeds 40 mg/dL at any time during the previous year. Medical examinations should also occur before assignment; when the employee develops signs of lead-related health problems, including infertility; when failure of personal protective equipment occurs; and with medical removal.

The medical examination must include the following:

- A detailed work history and medical history with particular attention to past lead exposure (both occupational and nonoccupational); personal habits, especially smoking; and past gastrointestinal, hematologic, renal cardiovascular, reproductive, and neurologic problems.
- A thorough physical examination with attention to teeth, gums, and hematologic, gastrointestinal, renal, cardiovascular, and neurologic systems; pulmonary status must be included if respiratory protection is to be used.
- Blood pressure.
- Blood testing to include BLL, hemoglobin, hematocrit, red cell indices, examination of peripheral smear morphology, ZPP, blood urea nitrogen, serum creatinine, and a routine urinalysis with microscopic evaluation.

The lead standard is unique in that it requires a second physician opinion be provided to the employee, at the employee's request, if the employer selects the initial evaluating physician. A method of resolving disputes occurring between the two physicians is contained within the standard. The examining physician must provide the employee and employer with a written medical opinion regarding whether any detected medical conditions exist that would place the employee at increased medical risk as a result of exposure to lead. The details and diagnoses of these medical conditions must remain confidential and should not be reported to the employer unless the medical conditions are a direct result of employment. The report must include clearance to use personal protective equipment, if indicated. BLLs must also be reported to the employer and employee. The employee must be notified of any medical conditions discovered during the medical examination.

The construction industry standard is very similar to the general industry standard. The difference is primarily in the requirements for BLL testing and the frequency of BLL testing. Initial medical surveillance is required for workers exposed for any 1 day at or above the AL (30 mg/m^3).

Initial medical surveillance includes BLL and ZPP testing. A full medical surveillance program must be instituted if exposure occurs for more than 30 days per year at or above the AL. Full medical surveillance includes BLL and ZPP levels at least every 2 months for the first 6 months of the program, then every 6 months thereafter. Any employee who has a BLL greater than 40 mg/dL must have BLL and ZPP testing performed every 2 months until BLL is less than 40 mg/dL on two consecutive tests. Medical removal must occur when BLL exceeds 50 mg/dL. If a BLL exceeds the medical removal level of 50 mg/dL, repeat testing is required within 2 weeks.

Medical examinations are required at least annually for workers for whom any BLL obtained during the previous year equals or exceeds 40 mg/dL. Workers removed from exposure must be provided with a medical examination. Workers reporting any signs and symptoms of lead-related health problems must be provided with a medical examination as described above in the general industry standard (29 *CFR* 1910). The content of the examination, reporting requirements of the examination, and provision for multiple physician review is the same for both standards.

Medical removal under both lead standards requires a BLL less than 40 mg/dL before the worker may return to a lead-exposed environment. If medical removal occurs, the employee must be provided with the same earnings, benefits, employee rights, and seniority as if performing the same lead-exposed job, as long as the employee cooperates with ongoing medical surveillance and testing during medical removal. If medical removal occurs, the employer may remove the employee from exposure to lead, provide special protective equipment, or place limitations on the employee consistent with the medical findings or recommendations of any of the examining physicians.

1,3-Butadiene (29 *CFR* 1910.1051)

The butadiene standard (17) was recently released. It requires a reduction in allowable exposure and adds medical surveillance requirements where exposure occurs. Medical surveillance mandates an annual medical screening for (a) all employees exposed at or above the action level for 30 days or more, (b) employees exposed 10 to 29 days at or above the PEL or short-term exposure level, (c) employees who have had exposures at or above the PEL or short-term exposure level for 309 or more days per year for 10 or more years, (d) employees who have had exposure at or above the AL for 60 or more days per year for 10 or more years, (e) employees exposed above 10 ppm on 30 or more days within the past year, and (f) employees exposed to butadiene in an emergency situation (within 48 hours). The employer is required to aggregate medical surveillance data to explore whether the health of the worker group is adversely affected by exposure.

The annual medical evaluation will include a standardized questionnaire to elicit symptoms relating to the hematologic system. It specifically looks for signs or symptoms of leukemia or blood abnormality or reproductive abnormalities. A complete blood count (CBC) with platelets and white blood cell differential is required. Comparison with the individual's own prior laboratory results is required, and variations from an individual's usual results should be considered abnormal, even if within the normal range. Abnormal results, including both variations from the individual's normal and abnormalities outside of the laboratory normal range, should be repeated within 6 weeks. Medical removal should occur when clinically significant abnormalities in the CBC occur.

The physical examination should occur before assignment and be repeated every 3 years. The examination can be directed to the hematopoietic system: lymph nodes, spleen, and liver. Physical examinations are to be provided to workers identified by the screening questionnaire and CBC and to those with concerns about reproductive and developmental toxicity.

Physical examinations are also to be provided to workers after acute, significant exposure and should be directed to the respiratory system, eyes, sinuses, skin, nervous system, and other affected systems. CBC must be obtained within 48 hours and repeated at 1, 2, and 3 months.

EMPLOYEE SELECTION FOR MEDICAL SURVEILLANCE

Companies are constantly faced with a dilemma regarding whom to actually include in their medical surveillance program. There are many employers who are involved with projects that require fieldwork in areas in which the exposures are not well characterized and in which the industrial hygiene database is incomplete. In addition, many employees with episodic exposures are in positions that involve contact with hazardous materials for fewer than 30 days per year. For example, supervisors and project managers go to hazardous job sites but rarely do any actual fieldwork and have significantly decreased opportunity for exposures. Also, some employers hire temporary employees for large jobs that last fewer than 30 working days. Thus, a variety of scenarios can occur that create confusion for employers in determining whether an employee belongs in a medical surveillance program.

There are several ways to approach this issue (3,18). One approach is to survey everyone in the company. The overall program is established with a preventive medicine focus, and exposure-specific protocols are provided for employees who perform hazardous materials work. A second possibility for defining participants is to include all employees, regardless of exposure length, who may at some point in the year perform work involving hazardous materials. A third and more job-specific way of selection is to include employees only on a project-by-project basis; however, there are operational problems associated with this method. Many jobs have quick starts that leave minimum time for performing an adequate baseline examination. Thus, employees can be sent to the field without appropriate medical evaluation and clearance.

In general, the current OSHA regulations direct the frequency of medical surveillance examinations for hazardous materials (19):

- Depending on the prior job assignment and the potential of exposure to toxic substances
- At least once every 12 months unless the examining physician believes a longer interval (every 2 years) is appropriate
- Discretionary initiation by the examining physician for more frequent examination intervals
- At termination of employment or reassignment of job duties or location
- As soon as an employee states that he or she has concerns related to signs and symptoms indicating overexposure to hazardous substances

In addition, if an unprotected employee has been exposed in an emergency situation, then an examination is required.

To facilitate the examination process, there is a standard set of information that ideally should be available to the physician or nurse:

- The OSHA standards and surveillance requirements related to the hazardous substance
- The employee's job description, with emphasis on specific duties that may generate exposure
- Any exposure history and industrial hygiene monitoring data
- Use of personal protective equipment data from OSHA 1910.134 (20)
- Data from prior examinations

Review of Occupational Safety and Health Administration Standards

Occupational health professionals in industry generally understand that systematic, proactive medical surveillance is a rare activity. This reality includes the medical examination programs that are mandated by OSHA. A review of the medical evaluations mandated by OSHA found 21 standards that contain some requirement for medical evaluation or testing (2). Each standard was scored in terms of three characteristics: overall quality control, medical screening usefulness, and medical surveillance use. The score for medical screening use was based on an assessment of the elements most necessary to assure the generation of information useful to the delivery of clinical services. The medical surveillance score assessed elements necessary to assure evaluation of aggregate or sentinel data and the application of these data to prevention. The mean medical screening score for the standards was 52%. The medical surveillance use score was 31%. The author concluded that very few OSHA standards have added features to the traditional packaging of clinical medical services, which might make them more powerful as surveillance tools. The situation may be improving, as evidenced by the 1996 OSHA Butadiene Standard, which is the first OSHA standard to include a requirement for the analysis of aggregate data.

HEALTH CARE PROVIDER SELECTION

Generally, the choice of physician(s) providing the medical surveillance examination is directed by the company. In many cases, the company's human resources manager is responsible for the selection of services. There are specific criteria for physician selection recommended by the American Industrial Hygiene Association (21):

- The physician should be board certified in occupational medicine. If a board-certified physician is not available, either a board-eligible physician or a physician with experience and training in occupational medicine should be selected.
- In the absence of a board-certified physician in occupational medicine, it is recommended that the examining physician provide employee medical records to a board-certified physician for review.
- The American Industrial Hygiene Association also recommends verifying state licensure, reviewing resumés, and performing a standard general employment interview and background check.

EXAMINATION CONTENT

OSHA's regulations state that the medical examination should include a medical and work history. Special emphasis is placed on possible symptoms related to the handling of hazardous substances, as well as overall fitness for duty. *Fitness for duty* includes the ability to wear personal protective equipment at any level as well as fitness for exposure to other hazards that may be expected at the work site. For example, because of temperature extremes, an individual may be medically fit to work as a driller in Level B in Colorado in January but not able to do the same work in Phoenix, Arizona, in July.

Unlike the general surveillance recommendations for most categories of workers, OSHA has specific rules for hazardous-waste workers. The *Federal Register* of March 6, 1989, outlines the final rule related to 29 *CFR* 1910: Hazardous-waste Operations and Emergency Response (19). The section on medical surveillance includes specific provisions for baseline, periodic, and exit medical examinations. The overall content of the examination is determined by the examining physician. After the examination and testing are complete, a formal written summary is required.

The physician's written opinion is specifically directed to include the following:

- Recommended limitations or restrictions for the specific job duties
- Results of the medical examination and tests conducted
- Statement that the employee has been informed of the examination results and of any conditions that require follow-up

In addition, the written medical information sent to the employer should not reveal specific findings that are not work related.

RECORD KEEPING

According to *CFR* 1910.120, medical records of the medical surveillance program should be retained for a period of 30 years past the employee's termination date.

When an employee requests access to a record, the employer is responsible for assuring that access is provided within 15 days of the request by the employee or the employee's designated representative. The designated representative should have written consent from the employee for access to the record. Upon receiving a request for medical records, the company physician may recommend that the employee (a) consult with the examining physician to review the records, (b) accept a summary of the record in lieu of the entire record, or (c) recommend that the record be released only to a physician or other designated representative. If the physician believes that direct employee access to information contained in the records regarding a specific diagnosis of terminal illness or psychiatric condition could be detrimental to the employee's health, the employer may inform the employee that access will be provided to a designated representative with written consent. A physician maintaining the records may delete from the record identities of family members, personal friends, or fellow employees who have provided confidential information relative to the employee's health status.

Employers must provide the OSHA representative with immediate access to medical and exposure records on request. Rules regarding OSHA access to records are covered in *CFR* 1910.20.

CLINIC SELECTION FOR MEDICAL SURVEILLANCE

The choice of examining physician and clinic has become highly competitive. Hospitals, clinics, and emergency departments compete for this source of revenue. There are several variables that a company should consider in its selection criteria: location, proximity to the company, cost, local reputation among employees, access, turnaround time for results, ease of scheduling in a timely manner, physician specialties and certifications, and ability to comply with contractual arrangements established with laboratories.

Access and timely turnaround of examination results are critical. Ideally, an applicant is not placed in a position until the presence or absence of work restrictions has been medically determined. The physician performing the examination should have job descriptions and physical and psychological job requirements for each position, so an appropriate decision can be made regarding work restrictions specific to a position.

Aside from logistic criteria, there are other equally important considerations:

- Availability of ancillary services [Are electrocardiographic (ECG), pulmonary, x-ray, audiology, and laboratory services readily available? If an employee has to schedule appointments with several different services before the examination, it can become very time consuming and cumbersome.]
- Turnaround time for receipt of laboratory results
- Certification of technicians performing ancillary testing, specifically pulmonary functions and audiometrics
- Clinic personnel's knowledge of OSHA regulations pertaining to medical surveillance, medical record storage, and release of information
- Ease of scheduling examinations and meeting time constraints

CONSULTING MEDICAL DIRECTOR

Employers without in-house medical departments generally select a physician consultant for the management of the medical surveillance program. This individual should be board certified or eligible in occupational medicine and should perform the following tasks:

- Oversee the selection of clinics and medical providers.
- Provide quality assurance and quality control by reviewing all examination results and, when necessary, consulting with the physician who performed the examination.
- Collaborate with industrial hygienists, safety professionals, and occupational health nurses in developing policies and protocols for the medical surveillance program.
- Serve as a resource in toxicology.
- Conduct epidemiologic studies as indicated.

EXAMINATION CATEGORIES

There are five categories of examinations:

- The *post-offer* examination is designed to determine the need for medical accommodation after a particular job has been offered by the employer.
- The *baseline* examination is conducted before work with hazardous materials or conditions; this examination establishes initial testing levels and determines the presence or absence of work restrictions for a particular position.
- The *periodic/annual* examination is conducted on an annual basis beginning 1 year after the baseline examination to monitor ongoing health status and determine the presence or absence of work restrictions.
- The *exit* examination is conducted when an employee terminates employment from a position requiring work involving hazardous materials or conditions.
- The *special* examination is conducted to determine possible health effects related to a specific exposure or event. *Fitness-to-work* examinations are also considered special examinations.

Baseline Examinations

If an applicant or employee has received an exit examination from his former employer within 6 months, the results can be obtained, reviewed for completeness and appropriateness, and used as the baseline for the current employer. If components are missing, only those missing should be ordered.

Components of a baseline examination include the following:

- Complete health history
- Physical examination
- Visual examination, with and without glasses
- ECG; 12-lead resting ECG
- Chest x-ray, posteroanterior view
- Audiometric testing to include 500, 1,000, 2,000, 4,000, 6,000, and 8,000 Hz
- A complete and thorough health history

A wide variety of questionnaires have been developed and are currently in use at many occupational medicine clinics. Because of the importance of vision with respect to job efficiency and safety, a detailed vision examination measuring visual acuity for near and distance, visual fields, color discrimination, and depth perception should be included.

Periodic/Annual Examinations

The components of an annual examination should be consistent with age, medical history, and job-related activities during the past year. Periodic examinations are usually done for employees with ongoing work activities involving hazards or exposures, but they are also useful in the monitoring of individuals with previous exposures to substances that can have long latency periods.

Special Examinations

These examinations are generally done to evaluate the effects of a specific hazardous material or general overexposure situation (e.g., fire, smoke exposure). Special examinations are also conducted to obtain biological exposure samples before and after shift. Fitness-to-work examinations are frequently obtained for employees reentering the workplace after absences that were due to nonwork-related medical problems.

SPIROMETRY

Routinely assessing pulmonary function with simple spirometry has become common practice in occupational medicine. When used in conjunction with the health history, physical examination, and chest x-ray results, spirometry results can identify preexisting pulmonary disease.

OSHA currently requires spirometry for employee exposure to asbestos, coke oven emissions, and cotton dust. NIOSH recommends spirometry for airborne substances including beryllium, cadmium, chlorine, formaldehyde, nitrogen dioxide, silica, sulfur dioxide, toluene diisocyanate, and wood dust.

There are several problems associated with spirometry:

- Inadequate training of personnel conducting the tests
- Technically deficient spirometers
- Lack of standardization of test methodology
- Lack of physician knowledge in interpreting test results

In 1978, the American Thoracic Society published standardization for spirometry (22). The society recently updated its recommendations (23). Spirometers do not need to perform all tests, but the ones they do perform should meet the specifications for that test (24).

MONITORING PROTOCOLS

Two essential elements in the management of medical surveillance programs are the accurate evaluation of monitoring results and the development of monitoring protocols that are appropriate to the actual exposures encountered in the workplace.

Unlike employees in a stable manufacturing environment, hazardous-waste workers encounter potential exposures to a variety of unidentified substances. Ambient monitoring and sampling data are generally not available before the initiation of work. Because of these unknown factors, these workers rely heavily on the use of personal protective equipment.

Biological monitoring includes measurement of appropriate determinants in biological specimens collected from the worker. BEIs are reference values intended as guidelines for the evaluation of potential health hazards (25). BEIs represent levels most likely to be seen in healthy workers exposed to chemicals to the same extent as workers with inhalation exposures to the TLV–time-weighted average. BEIs apply to 8-hour exposures, 5 days per week, and are not intended for use as a measure of adverse effects or for diagnosis of occupationally related illnesses. Using human data, the BEI is based either on the relationship between intensity of exposure and biological levels of the determinant or on the relationship between biological levels and health effects. Biological monitoring, which is complementary to air monitoring, should be conducted when it can (a) enhance or substantiate air monitoring, (b) test the efficacy of preplacement examinations, (c) determine the potential for absorption, or (d) detect nonoccupational exposure.

BEI offers a more direct measure of the exposure intensity, but there are multiple confounding factors:

- Physiologic and health status of the employee: body build, diet, sex, age, medication
- Exposure sources: intensity of the physical workload and fluctuations of exposure intensity and skin exposure
- Environmental sources: community and home air pollutants, water, and food contaminants
- Lifestyle variations: smoking, alcohol, personal hygiene
- Methodologic sources involving specimen collection, storage, and analyses

Urine, exhaled air, and blood specimens are used as biological specimens. Quantitative collection of urine during a specific time period can be difficult because of the variability of urine output and concentration. Quality control over individual collection of a 24-hour urine specimen can also be difficult when employees are working in remote job sites.

In evaluation of exhaled air, there are rapid changes of the concentration with time; in addition, the concentration is changing during expiration. Therefore, it is important to specify whether alveolar (end-exhaled air) or mixed-exhaled air is indicated. Workers with altered pulmonary function may not be suitable for exposure monitoring by exhaled air, because it has been demonstrated that differences in metabolism can result in as much as 100% variation.

In the analysis of data based on blood specimens, several factors should be considered. The plasma-erythrocyte ratio and the distribution of determinants among blood constituents can affect the outcome measurements. Unless indicated, the BEIs for volatile chemicals relate to venous blood, not capillary blood. A list of the current adopted biological exposure indices is available from ACGIH (25).

Drugs can also affect the accuracy of biological exposure indices because they alter the efficiency of specific metabolic pathways. Therefore, a careful medication history is critical (26).

LIVER FUNCTION STUDIES

Chronic alcohol consumption induces the hepatic metabolism of many chemicals. Studies have shown that blood ethanol levels between 5 and 15 mmol/L increase the internal exposure time and the concentration of toluene and styrene at TLVs. Exposure to chemicals can also increase the sensitivity to the effects of alcohol. Many possible mechanisms exist in which alcohol can modify the disposition and kinetics of workplace chemicals. It is therefore essential in evaluating laboratory results during medical surveillance examinations to pay particular attention to the overall liver enzyme abnormalities. It is not uncommon to find mild transient abnormalities of liver function. Before conclusions are drawn, the tests should be serially repeated, and confounders such as alcohol, illness, and exercise should be controlled.

TRACKING

There are a variety of computer software systems available for managing a medical surveillance program. Medical clinics tend to focus on systems that store data while emphasizing tracking functions, such as examination frequency and due dates. A well-integrated program offers the ability to track frequency, results, and the movement of an employee from one plant/location to another. This is important to prevent examination duplication and unnecessary testing.

IMPLEMENTATION OF A PHYSICAL EXAMINATION PROGRAM

Communication between the employer and physician regarding expectations is essential in implementing a successful medical surveillance program. Agreement on communication, protocols, and pricing is essential.

The physical examination is usually scheduled by the employee or the company's health and safety representative. To ensure efficiency, several steps should be followed.

When the examination is scheduled, all appropriate ancillary services should be completed within the same time. Thus, the entire examination is completed in a relatively short time period, and the physician has all results at the time of the physical.

IMPROVING MEDICAL SURVEILLANCE PROGRAMS

A medical surveillance program should be described in a written document, and it should be accessible to any employee or other interested party. This document should explicitly describe the purpose of the testing and the reasons for inclusion of specific groups of employees. It should also address the management of positive screening results in the individual participant, including who will pay for the costs of further evaluation. It should describe methods for the periodic reporting of results to employees and management.

With few exceptions, medical surveillance should be driven by results of exposure assessments (qualitative and quantitative) performed or overseen by industrial hygiene professionals.

In other words, medical surveillance should be targeted to groups who are shown to have significantly high risk. The resources involved in medical surveillance are valuable and should not be wasted on groups of employees who are not at risk. It is also true that the medical practitioner and the company that he or she represents will feel less uneasy about harmful outcomes that inevitably accompany screening if the participants were genuinely at increased risk of disease.

Medical surveillance programs need to be directed and coordinated by appropriately trained and credentialed health professionals. Medical surveillance is a highly complex activity that mixes issues of bioethics, scientific knowledge, medical procedures, data analysis, medical confidentiality, priority setting, and the need for professional judgment (27). The professionals who accept the responsibility must thoroughly understand both the benefits and pitfalls of medical testing. Additionally, they must recognize that they have a fiduciary obligation to the participants, and they must be willing to be accountable for negative outcomes. Ultimately, medical surveillance programs will be judged not only by regulation or company policy, but also by the ethical and legal standards of medical practice.

There should be a concerted effort to increase the specificity of screening tests of biological function by pushing them upstream in the natural history of a disease (Fig. 8-1).

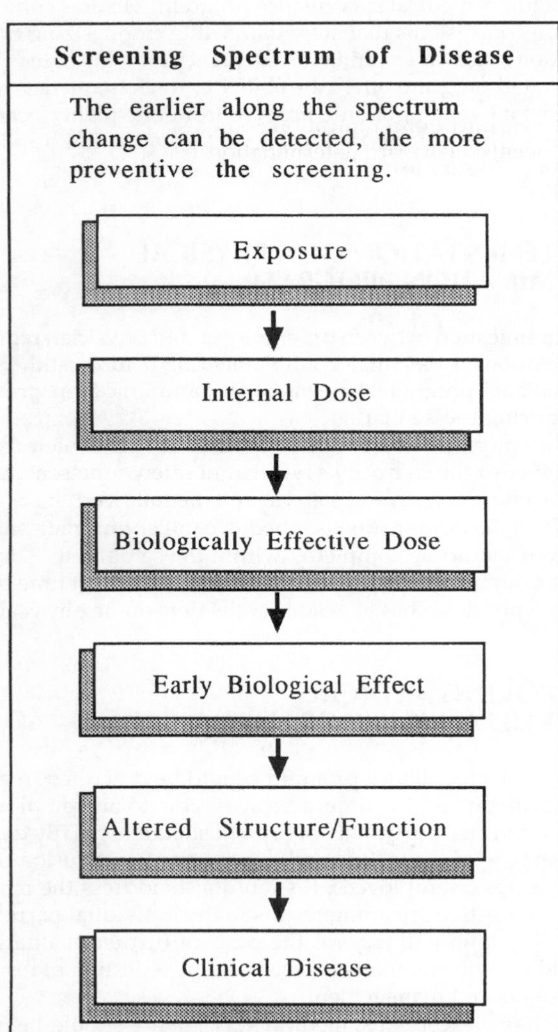

Figure 8-1. Screening spectrum of disease.

As a general rule, the farther along the spectrum that people can be initially screened, the more accurate and ethically defensible the exercise becomes. This concept argues strongly for increased activity in the broad area of biological monitoring. Health professionals should look for opportunities to increase the use of available biological monitoring technologies and decrease the use of nonspecific physical examination procedures. This includes educating the companies for which they work about the need to develop accurate biological monitoring tests for the materials they produce and use. This is part of overall product stewardship.

It should be recognized that any employee's decision to participate in a medical surveillance program must be fully informed and voluntary and should be preceded by a sufficient understanding of both the benefits and liabilities. Some thoughtful observers believe that participants in medical surveillance should sign informed consent forms (28).

SUMMARY AND CONCLUSIONS

Medical surveillance is a critical cornerstone of any occupational medicine program. Successful programs combine state-of-the-art science with high levels of managerial control. As OSHA moves toward a generic surveillance examination, the need for well-designed and managed programs will increase.

REFERENCES

1. Last JM. *A dictionary of epidemiology.* New York: Oxford University Press, 1983.
2. Silverstein M. Analysis of medical screening and surveillance in 21 occupational safety and health administration standards: support for a generic medical surveillance standard. *Am J Ind Med* 1994;26:283–295.
3. Ducatman AM. Medical surveillance programs (postgraduate seminar). Boston: American Occupational Medicine Conference, May 1989.
4. Code of Federal Regulations: 29 *CFR* 1910.120. Washington: US Government Printing Office; 1988.
5. Gochfield M, Favata EA. Hazardous waste workers. *Occup Med* 1990;5(1): 151–155.
6. Code of Federal Regulations: 29 *CFR* 1910.120. Washington: US Government Printing Office; 1988:82–89.
7. Code of Federal Regulations: 29 *CFR* 1910. Washington: US Government Printing Office; 1995.
8. Code of Federal Regulations: 29 *CFR* 1926. Washington: US Government Printing Office; 1995.
9. Code of Federal Regulations: 29 *CFR* 1910.1001. Washington: US Government Printing Office; 1995.
10. Code of Federal Regulations: 29 *CFR* 1910.1043. Washington: US Government Printing Office; 1995.
11. Code of Federal Regulations: 29 *CFR* 1910.1000. Washington: US Government Printing Office; 1995.
12. Code of Federal Regulations: 29 *CFR* 1910.1048. Washington: US Government Printing Office; 1995.
13. NIOSH Spirometry Workbook, Division of Training and Manpower Development, US Department of Health and Human Resources. Public Health Service, Centers for Disease Control, National Institute for Occupational Safety and Health; 1980:6–9.
14. *NIOSH spirometry training guide.* Washington: National Institute of Occupational Safety and Health, Division of Respiratory Disease Studies, 1997.
15. Code of Federal Regulations: 29 *CFR* 1926.62. Washington: US Government Printing Office; 1995.
16. Code of Federal Regulations: 29 *CFR* 1910.1025. Washington: US Government Printing Office; 1995.
17. Code of Federal Regulations: 29 *CFR* 1910.1051. Washington: US Government Printing Office; 10/24/1996.
18. Rempel D, ed. Medical surveillance in the workplace: overview. *Occup Med* 1990;5(3):435–438.
19. *Screening and surveillance: a guide to OSHA standards.* Washington: US Department of Labor, Occupational Safety and Health Administration, 2000.
20. Code of Federal Regulations: *CFR* 1910.134. Washington: US Government Printing Office; 1988:360.
21. American Independent Hygiene Association. Proposed criteria for the selection of appropriate medical resources to perform medical surveillance for employees engaged in hazardous waste operations. Joint AIHA and ACGIH Hazardous Waste Committee. *J Am Ind Hyg Assoc* 1989;50(12):A820–872.

22. George RB, et al. American Thoracic Society Respiratory Care Committee—position papers. *ATS News* 1978;4:6.
23. Gardner RM. Standardization of spirometry; a summary of recommendations from the American Thoracic Society: the 1987 update. *Ann Intern Med* 1988;108:217–220.
24. Horvath EP Jr. Manual of spirometry in occupational medicine. Cincinnati: National Institute for Occupational Safety and Health, Division of Training and Manpower Development, 1981.
25. American Conference of Governmental Industrial Hygienists. Threshold limit values and biological exposure indices. Cincinnati: American Conference of Governmental Industrial Hygienists; 1999.
26. Thomas V, Pierce F-B, Thomas J. Biological monitoring V: dermal absorption. *Appl Ind Hyg* 1989;4(8):F14–F21.
27. Shickle D, Chadwick R. The ethics of screening: is "screeningitis" an incurable disease? *J Med Ethics* 1994;20:12–18.
28. Rothstein MA. Legal concerns in worker notification and the use of biomarkers in medical surveillance. In: Mendelsohn ML, Peeters JP, Normandy MJ, eds. *Biomarkers and occupational health: progress and perspectives*. Washington: Joseph Henry Press, 1995:37–47.

CHAPTER 9

Hazard Communication and Material Safety Data Sheets

John G. Danby

The Hazard Communication Standard, 29 Code of Federal Regulations (*CFR*) 1910.1200(a) states, "The purpose of this section (of 29 *CFR*) is to ensure that the hazards of all chemicals produced or imported are evaluated, and that information concerning their hazards is transmitted to employers and employees."

An additional purpose of this standard was to provide a program that was consistent throughout the United States. The Occupational Safety and Health Administration (OSHA) regulation specifically preempted states, cities, towns, or other political subdivisions of a state from adopting or enforcing their own different forms of hazard communication programs. The only exemption to this preemption was for states with federally approved OSHA programs. These state programs would be required to submit their hazard communication program to OSHA for approval before their adoption. In effect, this allowed OSHA to approve a state's hazard communication program to ensure consistency between the states and within the federal system.

OSHA published its original Hazard Communication Standard on November 23, 1983. The standard directed chemical manufacturers or importers to assess the hazards of chemicals they manufacture or import and to provide this information to those companies in the manufacturing sector, SIC Codes 20 through 39, that used the product. The companies were then required to transmit this information to their employees through the use of a comprehensive hazard communication program. This program involves the use of container labeling and other forms of warning, material safety data sheets, and employee training.

On August 24, 1987, OSHA's revised Hazard Communication Standard was promulgated, requiring nonmanufacturing employers—including agriculture, forestry, fishing, mining, construction, wholesale and retail trade, finance, insurance, real estate, and service groups—to provide their employees with hazard communication programs similar to those required in the manufacturing sector. Because of legal challenges by the construction industry, the revised Hazard Communication Standard did not become effective for this industry until February 15, 1989.

Another revision to the Hazard Communication Standard was promulgated on February 9, 1994 (1). This rule modified and clarified many issues regarding labeling, the written hazard communication program, material safety data sheets (MSDSs), and the duties of manufacturers, importers, and distributors to provide MSDSs to employees.

Manufacturing laboratories are only required to comply with limited aspects of the standard. Labels must remain on the chemical containers and not be defaced; MSDSs received from the distributor must be maintained and accessible to the employees; and employees must be informed of the chemical hazards and trained in the proper methods of handling these materials. For nonmanufacturing labs, the Hazard Communication Standard is preempted by the Occupational Exposure to Hazardous Chemicals in Laboratories Standard, which incorporates many aspects of the Hazard Communication Standard. The standard covers a wide variety of chemicals that could cause adverse health effects. Examples of health hazards include carcinogens, irritants, sensitizers, corrosives, and specific organ system toxicants. The appendix gives OSHA-detailed definitions of each physical and health hazard.

There are many materials that are not included under this standard. Examples include (a) hazardous-wastes regulated by the U.S. Environmental Protection Agency under the Resource Conservation and Recovery Act and the Comprehensive Environmental Response, Compensation and Liability Act; (b) tobacco and tobacco products; (c) wood or wood products (except wood dust); (d) manufactured items that meet specific criteria under the standard; and (e) food, drugs, or cosmetics intended for personal consumption by employees.

The Hazard Communication Standard consists of five major components: (a) hazard determination, (b) MSDSs, (c) labels and other forms of warning, (d) a written hazard communication program, and (e) employee information and training.

HAZARD DETERMINATION

Chemical manufacturers and importers must evaluate their materials and determine whether they are considered hazardous. Employers may rely on the hazard evaluations conducted by the chemical manufacturers or importers, or they may choose to perform their own hazard evaluations on the chemicals used in their businesses. In general, because of both the cost and the technical skills required to perform a hazard determination, the majority of employers rely on the evaluations of the manufacturers or importers.

At a minimum, all chemicals listed in the Occupational Safety and Health Administration Regulations, 29 *CFR* Part 1910, Subpart Z, Toxic and Hazardous Substances, or in the *Threshold Limit Values for Chemical Substances and Physical Agents* published by the American Conference of Governmental Industrial Hygienists (ACGIH, latest edition) must be considered as hazardous. In addition, the following sources must be reviewed to determine whether a chemical is carcinogenic or potentially carcinogenic:

- National Toxicology Program *Annual Report on Carcinogens* (latest edition)
- International Agency for Research on Cancer *Monographs* (latest edition)
- 29 *CFR* 1910, Subpart Z, Toxic and Hazardous Substances, Occupational Safety and Health Administration

However, all available scientific data on carcinogenicity must be evaluated when making a determination of carcinogenicity; one must go beyond the three references listed above.

Mixtures of chemicals involve several complex issues compared with single component materials when attempting to determine the mixture's hazards; however, this does not relieve the manufacturer or importer from performing a hazard determination on a chemical mixture. Initially, a mixture can be tested as a whole to determine its physical and health hazards. For example, a given mixture could be submitted to a toxicology testing laboratory for health hazard evaluation. The same material could also be submitted to a chemical laboratory for determination of its physical properties. Generally, it is extremely time-consuming and costly to evaluate a chemical mixture for potential health hazards; fortunately, many chemicals may be evaluated using an alternative procedure. As an example, if the mixture is not tested as a whole, the mixture is considered to have the health hazards exhibited by those components comprising 1% or more, by weight or volume, of the mixture. If one of the components is a carcinogenic hazard, the mixture is considered a carcinogen if the carcinogenic component is present in concentrations of 0.1% or more. Finally, if the employer has evidence that a given component present in the mixture in concentrations less than 1% (or less than 0.1% for carcinogens) could reasonably be expected to be released in concentrations that would exceed an established OSHA permissible exposure limit (PEL) or an ACGIH threshold limit value (TLV), the mixture is assumed to pose a health hazard.

The evaluation procedures used by the chemical manufacturer, importer, or employer must be documented in writing and should describe the health and physical hazards that were evaluated for the chemical. The written procedures need only describe the general process used to perform the evaluations and are not required to describe in detail the procedures used for individual chemicals. However, some companies have described their specific hazard determination procedures in order to better document the evaluation process. This strategy has proven useful when the health hazard determination was challenged by a regulatory agency. It could also be used to limit future product liabilities.

The Hazard Communication Standard requires additional information that should be provided in the evaluation procedures:

- The person(s) responsible for the evaluation process
- The information sources to be used
- The criteria to be used to evaluate the studies or sources, e.g., statistical significance, number of positive results, whether conducted according to commonly accepted scientific principles
- A plan for reviewing and updating the hazard evaluations and MSDSs.

MATERIAL SAFETY DATA SHEETS

An MSDS is defined in the OSHA Hazard Communication Standard as "...written or printed material concerning a hazardous chemical...." This form of information transfer was intended to be a cornerstone of an employer's hazard communication program in that the MSDS details the types of hazards associated with that material and the proper methods of protecting personnel from these hazards. A properly prepared MSDS should provide employers and employees sufficient information so that the product can be used in a safe manner.

The exact form or layout of the MSDS was not specified in the Hazard Communication Standard; however, in 1985, OSHA released its concept of a generic MSDS form (Fig. 9-1). An MSDS must be written in English and contain, at a minimum, this information: identity of the compound, chemical and common names, exposure limits, physical and chemical characteristics, physical hazards, health hazard data, carcinogenic potential, routes of entry, methods for controlling employee exposure, and precautions for safe handling and use.

Identity of the Compound

The identity of the material specified on the MSDS should be identical to the label on the materials container. In some cases, this identity could be a product name (e.g., Product XYZ) or it could be a very specific chemical name (e.g., ethylene glycol monomethyl ether).

Chemical and Common Names

If the material is composed of a single chemical, the MSDS must list its chemical and common names. In many cases, the chemical's unique Chemical Abstract Service identification number is also included. If the material is a mixture, the MSDS must identify each component contributing to a known hazard by its chemical and common name, but the exact percentage of each component is not required to be listed. Those mixtures that have not been tested as a whole to determine the specific hazard must list those components considered to be health hazards (see the previous section, Hazard Determination) by comprising more than 1% of the materials or more than 0.1% for those components considered to exhibit carcinogenic potential. Those components of a mixture that are considered physical hazards must also be listed by their chemical and common names when the mixture has not been tested as a whole.

Exposure Limits

OSHA PELs, ACGIH TLVs, National Institute for Occupational Safety and Health recommended exposure limits, or other employee exposure limits recommended by the manufacturer, importer, or employer should be included for each component listed by chemical and common name. If the mixture has been tested as a whole and a recommended exposure limit determined, this value should also be listed. It should be noted that this form of exposure limit technically is not considered a TLV, as these terms are trademarks of the ACGIH.

Physical and Chemical Characteristics

Certain physical and chemical characteristics assist in evaluating the potential hazards posed by the material. Boiling point and vapor pressure are important in determining the ease with which a liquid will evaporate. Generally, liquids with low boiling points and high vapor pressures evaporate quickly. For example, acetone quickly evaporates; it has a boiling point at 133°F (56°C) and a vapor pressure of 226.3 mm Hg at 25°C. In contrast, malathion has a boiling point at 156°C at 0.7 mm Hg and a vapor pressure of 0.00004 mm Hg at 20°C; it slowly evaporates. If the material is a flammable liquid, an increased fire hazard may result. An inhalation exposure could occur as a result of the evaporation of a toxic liquid.

Vapor density is another important physical characteristic typically listed on an MSDS. Vapor densities less than 1.0 indicate that a gas or vapor is lighter than air and tends to rise; in contrast, a gas or vapor with a vapor pressure higher than 1.0 tends to concentrate in low areas and creates potential health or physical hazards (e.g., oxygen deficiency or a flammable environment).

Appearance and odor of the material are other characteristics commonly included on the MSDS. It is important to remember that odor should not be relied on to determine potential exposure or overexposures to a material, as the minimum odor detection concentration can be well above the OSHA PEL or the ACGIH TLV. Two other important physical and chemical characteristics are water solubility and specific gravity. These parameters are useful in the determination of proper spill and fire

Material Safety Data Sheet
May be used to comply with
OSHA's Hazard Communication Standard,
29 CFR 1910.1200. Standard must be
consulted for specific requirements.

U.S. Department of Labor
Occupational Safety and Health Administration
(Non-Mandatory Form)
Form Approved
OMB No. 1218-0072

IDENTITY *(As Used on Label and List)*	Note: *Blank spaces are not permitted. If any item is not applicable, or no information is available, the space must be marked to indicate that.*

Section I

Manufacturer's Name	Emergency Telephone Number
Address *(Number, Street, City, State, and ZIP Code)*	Telephone Number for Information
	Date Prepared
	Signature of Preparer *(optional)*

Section II — Hazardous Ingredients/Identity Information

Hazardous Components (Specific Chemical Identity; Common Name(s))	OSHA PEL	ACGIH TLV	Other Limits Recommended	% *(optional)*

Section III — Physical/Chemical Characteristics

Boiling Point		Specific Gravity (H_2O = 1)	
Vapor Pressure (mm Hg.)		Melting Point	
Vapor Density (AIR = 1)		Evaporation Rate (Butyl Acetate = 1)	
Solubility in Water			
Appearance and Odor			

Section IV — Fire and Explosion Hazard Data

Flash Point (Method Used)	Flammable Limits	LEL	UEL
Extinguishing Media			
Special Fire Fighting Procedures			
Unusual Fire and Explosion Hazards			

(Reproduce locally) OSHA 174, Sept. 1985

Figure 9-1. Generic material safety data sheet. ACGIH, American Conference of Governmental Hygienists; IARC, International Agency for Research on Cancer; NTP, National Toxicology Program; OSHA, Occupational Safety and Health Administration; PEL, permissible exposure limit; TLV, threshold limit value. *(continued)*

Section V — Reactivity Data

Stability	Unstable		Conditions to Avoid
	Stable		

Incompatibility (*Materials to Avoid*)

Hazardous Decomposition or Byproducts

Hazardous Polymerization	May Occur		Conditions to Avoid
	Will Not Occur		

Section VI — Health Hazard Data

Route(s) of Entry: Inhalation? Skin? Ingestion?

Health Hazards (*Acute and Chronic*)

Carcinogenicity: NTP? IARC Monographs? OSHA Regulated?

Signs and Symptoms of Exposure

Medical Conditions
Generally Aggravated by Exposure

Emergency and First Aid Procedures

Section VII — Precautions for Safe Handling and Use

Steps to Be Taken in Case Material Is Released or Spilled

Waste Disposal Method

Precautions to Be Taken in Handling and Storing

Other Precautions

Section VIII — Control Measures

Respiratory Protection (*Specify Type*)

Ventilation	Local Exhaust	Special
	Mechanical (*General*)	Other

Protective Gloves	Eye Protection

Other Protective Clothing or Equipment

Work/Hygienic Practices

Page 2

★ U.S.G.P.O.: 1986-491-529/45775

Figure 9-1. *(continued)*

control methods. For example, a material's specific gravity determines whether a material will float on water (e.g., specific gravity less than 1.0) or if it will sink in water (e.g., specific gravity greater than 1.0).

Physical Hazards

Fire and reactivity are physical hazards of a material. The fire-related characteristics listed on the MSDS would include (a) *flash point,* the minimum temperature at which a liquid gives off sufficient flammable vapors to ignite in the presence of an ignition source, and (b) *lower flammable limit* (*LFL*) and *upper flammable limit* (*UFL*), which indicate the ability of a material to pose a fire hazard. The LFL is the lowest concentration of the material in air that will produce a fire when an ignition source is present, whereas the UFL is the highest concentration of the material in air that will produce a fire when an ignition source is present. The concentration of material in air between the LFL and UFL is considered the *flammable range* and defines where a fire can be initiated or sustained, provided sufficient fuel and oxygen are present. Below the LFL, the mixture is too lean to burn; above the UFL, the mixture is too rich to burn.

Other information that may be contained in this section of the MSDS includes (a) fire-extinguishing media, such as water, foam, or dry chemical; (b) special fire-fighting procedures, such as use of self-contained breathing apparatus or other special forms of personal protective equipment; and (c) unusual fire and explosion hazards exhibited by the material when involved in a fire (e.g., the potential production of phosgene and hydrogen chloride in fires involving carbon tetrachloride or other chlorinated solvents).

Reactivity refers to a material's tendency to undergo chemical reactions with a subsequent release of energy. Information typically provided in an MSDS related to this hazard includes stability, chemical incompatibilities, hazardous decomposition products, or hazardous polymerization. For example, mercury fulminate is an unstable material that is explosive when dry. This would be noted on the MSDS under Conditions to Avoid. When potassium cyanide comes in contact with a strong acid, such as sulfuric acid, the resulting reaction can release toxic hydrogen cyanide gas. This type of reactivity hazard would be included under the heading of Incompatibility.

Health Hazard Data, Carcinogenic Potential, and Routes of Entry

This section of the MSDS informs the reader about the type of health hazard associated with exposure to the material. Typically, the three primary routes of exposure in an industrial setting are inhalation, ingestion, and dermal. To ensure that proper personal protective equipment or other forms of control measures are used, it is important for employees and employers to know the routes by which a material could enter the body.

Acute and chronic health hazards associated with exposure to a chemical will be listed on the MSDS, as will a material's carcinogenic potential. If a material is listed in the National Toxicology Program, in the International Agency for Research on Cancer *Monographs,* or by OSHA as a carcinogen, this must be noted in the MSDS. As required by the standard, additional information must be included to assist physicians or other emergency medical personnel in determining whether a person has been, or may be, seriously injured from exposure to the material. This information includes signs and symptoms of exposure, medical conditions that could be aggravated by exposure, and emergency and first aid procedures.

Methods for Controlling Employee Exposure

After reviewing the hazard data, a logical regimen of measures is recommended to reduce employee exposure levels to the material. Control measures could include general dilution or local exhaust ventilation, proper work or personal hygiene practices, the use of personal protective equipment, or a combination of all these measures. If personal protective equipment is to be used, the specific type of protective equipment should be listed on the MSDS. For example, if an employee is exposed to airborne dusts containing lead, then a half-face or full-face respirator with a high-efficiency particulate air filter cartridge may be specified. In some cases, a supplied air respirator may be specified in the MSDS. The specific types of glove material, eye protection, and other types of personal protective equipment may also be included in this category. Work or hygienic practices that might be recommended include washing hands before eating, drinking, or smoking; not smoking in the area; and not using high-pressure air to clean work surfaces.

This portion of the MSDS must be evaluated very closely by the employer or employee, as the contents may be of limited use. For example, when describing the type of gloves to use, the MSDS might state "Use impermeable gloves" or "Use of gloves recommended" rather than specifying a particular glove material, such as butyl rubber, Viton, or polyvinyl chloride. Liability concerns may cause a chemical manufacturer or importer to recommend the use of a supplied air respirator when an air-purifying respirator would be adequate.

Precautions for Safe Handling and Use

Information required in this section details four areas: (a) the proper methods of handling and storing the materials, (b) measures needed to properly handle the material in the event of a release or spill, (c) disposal of the waste materials following a cleanup, and (d) other special precautions recommended by the importer, distributor, or employer preparing the MSDS. Disposal requirements can significantly vary from state to state and within given municipalities; therefore, information in this section may be of limited use. Thus, a typical recommendation on an MSDS would be "Dispose of in accordance with federal, state, or local regulations."

Other Requirements for MSDSs

The MSDS must list the name and address of the manufacturer, importer, or employer who prepared the MSDS. In addition, an emergency telephone number must be included so that employers or emergency medical personnel can obtain additional information on the material. The date of the latest preparation or revision of the MSDS must also be included.

All portions of the MSDS must be filled out; no blanks are permitted on the MSDS. If relevant information concerning some aspect of the material required on the MSDS could not be ascertained, then "N/A" or another designation must be indicated.

Occasionally, new information concerning a chemical becomes available. When this occurs, the chemical manufacturer, importer, or employer must then revise the MSDS within 3 months to reflect this change. Manufacturers and importers must supply the employer with the revised MSDS with the first shipment of the material after the revised MSDS is prepared.

Although there are many obvious advantages to a well-prepared MSDS, there are several problems associated with the current system. For example, there is no required or specified format for an MSDS, only types of information required to be included in the MSDS. This may increase the difficulty of identifying desired information. In addition, the technical nature of this document may increase the potential of its misrepresentation by personnel unfamiliar with its terminology.

Some of the issues associated with MSDSs were addressed by the American National Standards Institute, Inc. (ANSI) in the *National Standard for Hazardous Industrial Chemicals: Material Safety Data Sheets: Preparation* (2). This consensus standard, ANSI Z400.1-1993, issued in 1993, expands the MSDS to 16 sections and emphasizes "completeness, clarity, and format consistency." The foreword to the standard notes that "there are several items in the American National Standard that have not been a part of MSDSs in the past. The principal items are the headings and order of the sections, the emergency overview, and sections 11 through 16." The sections included in the ANSI MSDS include the following:

1. Chemical Product and Company Identification
2. Composition, Information on Ingredients
3. Hazards Identification
4. First Aid Measures
5. Fire-Fighting Measures
6. Accidental Release Measures
7. Handling and Storage
8. Exposure Controls, Personal Protection
9. Physical and Chemical Properties
10. Stability and Reactivity
11. Toxicologic Information
12. Ecological Information
13. Disposal Considerations
14. Transport Information
15. Regulatory Information
16. Other Information

Many MSDS preparers now use the ANSI MSDS format on a regular basis.

Another difficulty related to MSDSs is that they are typically written only in English. Many employees in the United States are recent immigrants from non–English-speaking areas of the world, such as Southeast Asia and Central or South America. This type of employee may understand or speak limited English and subsequently may not comprehend the technical portions of the MSDS. Therefore, training in these alternative languages and use of effective (multilingual) container labeling is essential to ensure that non–English-speaking employees comprehend the chemical's hazards.

One aspect related to the MSDS program that may create a serious difficulty, especially under emergency conditions, is a provision of the standard that allows a chemical manufacturer, importer, or employer to designate a product a *trade secret*. Under this designation, the specific chemical name is not required to be included on the MSDS, provided the MSDS contains information regarding the specific properties and hazards associated with the material. In the case of medical emergencies, the standard does contain an additional provision permitting physicians and nurses to request the specific identity of a hazardous chemical; this information must be immediately provided by the chemical manufacturer, importer, or employer. Under nonemergency situations, the specific chemical identity may be requested in writing by physicians, industrial hygienists, toxicologists, or other health personnel to assist them in the determination of toxicity. If the information is provided, a strict confidentiality agreement can be required by the manufacturer or importer. In difficult situations, OSHA can be contacted to resolve release-of-information issues.

LABELS AND OTHER FORMS OF WARNING

An integral portion of a facility's overall hazard communication program is the use of labels or other forms of warnings on chemical containers. Compliance with this portion of the Hazard Communication Standard is divided between those individuals who manufacture and distribute the chemicals and those who use the chemicals in the workplace. The following are chemical containers that do not require labeling by this standard:

- Pesticides regulated by the Federal Insecticide, Fungicide, and Rodenticide Act, which are labeled in accordance with those regulations
- Foods, food additives, color additives, drugs, cosmetics, or medical or veterinary devices, regulated by the Food, Drug, and Cosmetic Act, which are labeled in accordance with those regulations
- Distilled spirits, wines, or malt beverages (beer) intended for nonindustrial use regulated by the Federal Alcohol Administration Act, which are labeled in accordance with those regulations
- Consumer products regulated by the Consumer Product Safety Act, which are labeled in accordance with those regulations.

Chemical Manufacturers and Distributors

Chemical manufacturers, importers, or distributors of chemicals covered by the Hazard Communication Standard must label each chemical container (e.g., 55-gallon barrel, 1-gallon bottle) with its identity, appropriate hazard warnings, and the name and address of the manufacturer or other responsible party. If the chemical is regulated by OSHA within 29 *CFR* 1910.1001 through 29 *CFR* 1910.1052 as a carcinogen (e.g., asbestos, arsenic, vinyl chloride), the container must be labeled with the appropriate hazard warning as required by the applicable standard. Warnings of other hazards posed by these materials should also be listed on the label.

Employers and the Workplace

Employers are required to ensure chemical containers used in their workplaces are properly labeled. If a container arrives from the chemical manufacturer or distributor with an appropriate label affixed to it [e.g., identity of the hazardous chemical(s) and appropriate hazard warnings], the employer is not required to add labeling. If the employer wants to place additional warning information on the container, he or she may do so, provided he or she does not remove, deface, or make illegible the original hazard label. The hazard warning can be of any type that conveys the special physical and health hazards, including target organ effects of the chemical. Words, pictures, symbols, or combinations of these can be used.

One alternative hazard warning system commonly used in industry to label containers is the Hazardous Material Identification System (HMIS) devised by the National Paint and Coatings Association (3). This system provides information concerning a material's health, flammability, and reactivity hazards, as well as the proper types of personal protective equipment to be used while handling this material. The severity of each hazard is denoted using a numeric rating system, with a scale of 0 to 4. A rating of 0 indicates a minimum hazard, whereas 4 denotes a severe hazard. Table 9-1 summarizes HMIS ratings.

The HMIS and its variation also identify the types of personal protective equipment that should be used by personnel when handling a given material. Figure 9-2 is a facsimile of an HMIS label that could be used on a chemical container. For example, a facility could state that the use of safety glasses and gloves is required by employees, which would be indicated on the HMIS under Personal

TABLE 9-1. Summary of the Hazardous Material Identification System ratings

Health hazard rating		
0	Minimal hazard	No significant risk to health.
1	Slight hazard	Irritation or minor reversible injury possible.
2	Moderate hazard	Temporary or minor injury may occur.
3	Serious hazard	Major injury likely unless prompt action is taken and medical treatment is given.
4	Severe hazard	Life-threatening, major, or permanent damage may result from single or repeated exposures.
Flammability hazard rating		
0	Minimum hazard	Materials that are normally stable and will not burn unless heated.
1	Slight hazard	Materials that must be preheated before ignition will occur; flammable liquids in this category will have flash points (the lowest temperature at which ignition will occur) at or above 200°F (93.3°C) (NFPA Class IIIB).
2	Moderate hazard	Material that must be moderately heated before ignition will occur, including flammable liquids with flash points at or above 100°F (37.7°C) and below 200°F (93.3°C) (NFPA Class II and Class IIIA).
3	Serious hazard	Materials capable of ignition under almost all normal temperature conditions, including flammable liquids with flash points below 73°F (22.8°C) and boiling points above 100°F (37.7°C), as well as liquids with flash points between 73°F (22.8°C) and 100°F (37.7°C) (NFPA Class 1B and 1C).
4	Severe hazard	Very flammable gases or very volatile flammable liquids with flash points below 73°F (22.8°C) and boiling points below 100°F (37.7°C) (NFPA Class 1A).
Reactivity hazard rating		
0	Minimum hazard	Materials that are normally stable, even under fire conditions, and will not react with water.
1	Slight hazard	Materials that are normally stable but can become unstable at high temperatures and pressures; these materials may react with water, but they will not release energy violently.
2	Moderate hazard	Materials that, in themselves, are normally unstable and will readily undergo violent chemical change but will not detonate; these materials may also react violently with water.
3	Serious hazard	Materials that are capable of detonation or explosive reaction but require a strong initiating source or must be heated under confinement before initiation, or materials that react explosively with water.
4	Severe hazard	Materials that are readily capable of detonation or explosive decomposition at normal temperatures and pressures.

Protective Equipment Required as *A*. The use of gloves and full-face respirator with organic vapor cartridges could be labeled as *B*.

For employees to use the HMIS properly, wall posters summarizing the hazard information and personal protective equipment designations should be placed within the work areas for easy reference. Wallet cards are also available for distribution to employees. An adequate training program explaining the system is also required (see Employee Information and Training later in this chapter).

Another example of an alternative hazard warning system is the National Fire Protection Association (NFPA) 704 System (4). This system was designed to provide basic information primarily for fire-fighting personnel during fire emergencies. It uses a diamond-shaped figure divided into four sections (Fig. 9-3). Each section has a numeric rating of 0 through 4 to depict the chemical's health hazard (blue diamond), flammable hazard (red diamond), and stability hazard (yellow diamond) (e.g., water reactive, radioactive, oxidizers, or etiologic agents). The general explanation of the numeric ratings for the health hazard portion of the symbol is given in Table 9-2.

Although the NFPA 704 system is very useful for properly trained fire-fighting personnel, it may be very confusing and could lead to misinterpretations. For untrained personnel, the system provides minimal information regarding the material's

HEALTH HAZARD RATING ________

FLAMMABILITY
HAZARD RATING ________

REACTIVITY
HAZARD RATING ________

PERSONAL PROTECTIVE
EQUIPMENT REQUIRED ________

____

Figure 9-2. Hazardous Materials Identification System (HMIS)–type label. With permission from *National Paint and Coatings Association's HMIS Hazardous Materials Identification System's Revised Raw Materials Rating Manual.*

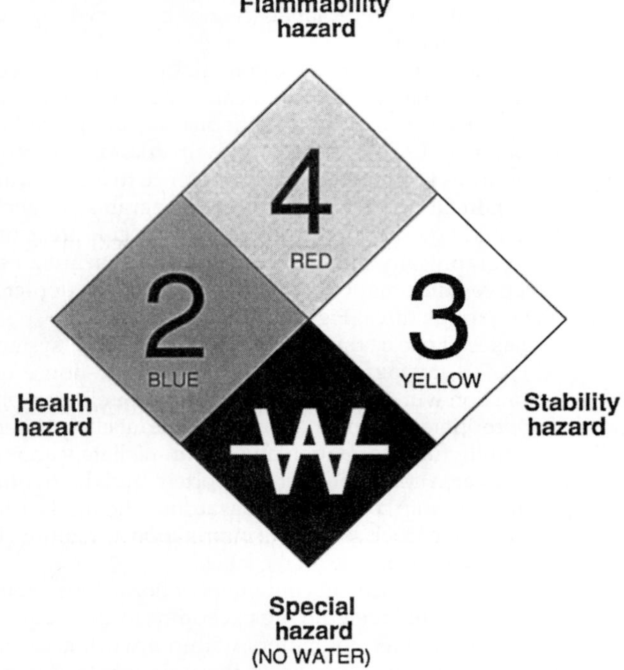

Figure 9-3. National Fire Protection Association 704 hazard warning symbol.

TABLE 9-2. Explanation of numeric ratings for the health hazard portion of symbols

	Identification of health hazard (color code: BLUE)	Identification of flammability (color code: RED)	Identification of reactivity (stability) (color code: YELLOW)
Signal	**Type of possible injury**	**Susceptibility of materials to burning**	**Susceptibility to release of energy**
4	Materials that on very short exposure could cause death or major residual injury even if prompt medical treatment was given	Materials that will rapidly or completely vaporize at atmospheric pressure and normal ambient temperature or that are readily dispersed in air and will burn readily	Materials that in themselves are readily capable of detonation or of explosive decomposition or reaction at normal temperatures and pressures
3	Materials that on short exposure could cause serious temporary or residual injury even if prompt medical treatment was given	Liquids and solids that can be ignited under almost all ambient temperature conditions	Materials that in themselves are capable of detonation or explosive reaction but require a strong initiating source, or that must be heated under confinement before initiation, or that react explosively with water
2	Materials that on intense or continued exposure could cause temporary incapacitation or possible residual injury unless prompt medical treatment is given	Materials that must be moderately heated or exposed to relatively high ambient temperatures before ignition can occur	Materials that in themselves are normally unstable and readily undergo violent chemical change but do not detonate; also, materials that may react violently with water or may form potentially explosive mixtures with water
1	Materials that on exposure would cause irritation but only minor residual injury, even if no treatment is given	Materials that must be preheated before ignition can occur	Materials that in themselves are normally stable, but that can become unstable at elevated temperatures and pressures, or that may react with water with some release of energy, but not violently
0	Materials that on exposure under fire conditions would offer no hazard beyond that of ordinary combustion material	Materials that will not burn	Materials that in themselves are normally stable, even under fire exposure conditions, and that are not reactive with water

hazards and must be used in conjunction with the OSHA labeling requirements.

To assist employees in better understanding the NFPA 704 system, signs could be posted in the work areas that describe what each number means from a health, flammability, and stability hazard viewpoint. Although acceptable for use on chemical containers used in the workplace, the NFPA 704 system could be mistaken for shipping labels required by the Department of Transportation because of the similarity in the labels' designs. Therefore, the NFPA labels cannot be placed on containers during shipment.

One other method that relates potentially harmful effects from contact with a hazardous chemical is the use of pictorial depictions (Fig. 9-4). These pictorial depictions are placed on chemical containers used in Germany, Switzerland, and other European countries to provide a quick reference to a chemical's hazard(s) (5,6). In addition to using these pictograms on labels, pictograms could be used on signs posted in specific areas of a workplace to graphically remind workers of the hazards. Personal protective equipment can also be adequately depicted through the use of pictures (Fig. 9-5).

OSHA makes it clear that such alternative label systems (HMIS, NFPA 704, pictograms) are for employer in-house use only in conjunction with an effective hazard communication program and appropriate training that describes the labeling system. Additional amplifying information must be immediately accessible in each work area. Manufacturers, importers, and distributors are not permitted to ship containers of hazardous chemicals using any of the alternative labels; complete information as required by the standard must be available on the label.

As previously discussed, all containers of hazardous chemicals must be properly labeled. One exception to this requirement concerns stationary containers within a work area that have similar contents and hazards. In these circumstances, it is sufficient to place signs or placards that display the hazard information in the area of the containers. Standard operating procedures, process sheets, batch or blend tickets, or similar written materials can be posted on stationary containers in lieu of labels if they provide the required information that would otherwise be on a label. Written materials must be readily available to the employees in their work area throughout each work shift. Pipes and piping systems are not required to be labeled, although this generally is a good practice to follow, as doing so provides quick information in the event of a leak or a break in the piping system.

The only other exception to the labeling requirement is for portable containers that have materials transferred into them from labeled containers and are intended for the immediate use of the employee who makes the transfer. Caution should be used under these conditions. It is very easy to visualize empty, portable, nonlabeled containers left on a workbench by one employee and picked up by another employee to use for a different chemical. Combining of incompatible materials could occur, resulting in serious injuries to unsuspecting employees. Thus, in order to standardize operations and reduce potential labeling problems, it may be more prudent to label all containers.

EMPLOYEE INFORMATION AND TRAINING

The Hazard Communication Standard requires that all employers provide each potentially exposed employee with certain information and training. This training should cover both normal work assignments and the accidental exposures from spills or leaking containers. Training must be hazard specific. For example, if the information and training program initially covered flammable hazards and the employee will now be exposed to a corrosive hazard, additional specific information and training related to corrosive hazards must be provided.

Each affected employee must be informed of the following:

Figure 9-4. Chemical hazards pictorial descriptions. Modified with permission after refs. 5 and 6.

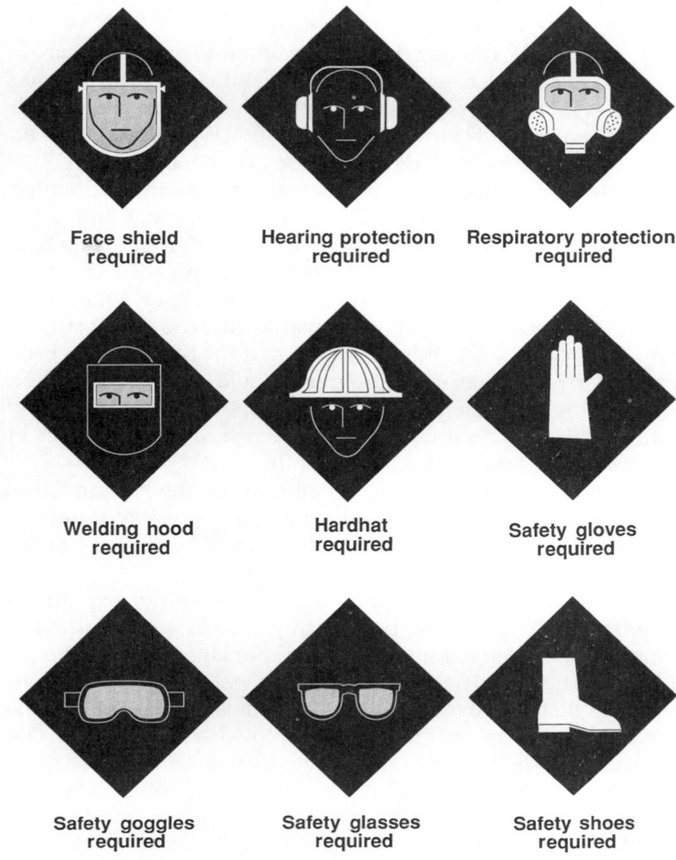

Figure 9-5. Personal protective equipment pictorial descriptions. Modified with permission after refs. 5 and 6.

- The existence of the Hazard Communication Standard and what the standard requires of the employer
- The operations within the facility where hazardous substances are present and employee exposure could occur
- The location(s) within the facility where the written hazard communication program, the written procedures used for the hazard evaluation determinations, the lists of hazardous chemicals used in the facility, and the copies of MSDSs for the hazardous chemicals are maintained

One of the most important aspects of the training is the hazard recognition and specificity. For example, if the facility uses materials that only exhibit the hazards of flammability and corrosiveness, the employees should be trained only in those hazards; discussion of the other types of hazards that would not be encountered at the facility is not required. Training can be done by individual chemical or by categories of hazards. If only a small number of different chemicals are used in the facility, the training may be more meaningful if each chemical is discussed individually. If there are a large number of chemicals or if the types of chemicals change on a regular basis, the training program may be based on general hazard categories. When training is based on general hazard categories, it is essential that the discussion groups the facility's chemicals into their respective hazard categories.

The format of the training program has been left to the discretion of the employer. It can involve the use of videotapes, classroom lectures, slides, movies, hands-on training, or combinations of these.

The correct interpretation of MSDSs and container labels is essential for the employee's knowledge and understanding of the hazards with which he or she works. Because much of this information may be very technical in nature, the training program must present the information in a manner that is easy to comprehend. This also may involve the use of a multimedia presentation of the material. For example, the explanation of flash point and LFLs and UFLs may be presented with a demonstration followed by a discussion of these physical properties.

Employee training must include methods—such as color or odor—that can be used to detect the presence of a chemical that could create a hazard in the workplace. Monitoring systems used by the employer to determine employee exposures, including personal monitoring or continuous monitoring instruments, should also be discussed in the training sessions.

Other aspects of the training would include the means by which employees can be protected from the chemical hazards. This could include a discussion of ventilation controls presently used at the facility to reduce the hazard potential, a discussion of the proper work practices that employees can use to reduce their exposure, or a discussion of the use of any personal protective equipment used by the employees (e.g., gloves, respirators, or safety glasses). If emergency equipment is located in the facility—such as emergency showers or eyewashes, fire blankets, or fire extinguishers—this equipment should also be included in the discussion of protective equipment.

Other specific training that may be required involves nonroutine operations, such as reactor vessel cleaning, work on charged piping systems, and cleanup of spills or other releases of hazardous substances. This form of work situation typically exposes an employee to more hazards than those experienced during normal day-to-day operations. This may require more detailed training in the use of personal protective equipment, simulated hands-on demonstrations, or more detailed information on hazard assessment and preventive measures to prevent accidents.

Finally, it is important for the employees to know where copies of the MSDSs are retained in the facility and the means by which they can access this information. If the MSDSs have been computerized, the training program should include instruction on how to access the MSDS information on the computer system. Again, MSDSs must be readily accessed by employees in each work area during each work shift.

In addition to training facility employees, the Hazard Communication Standard requires the training of on-site contractors and temporary employees. The training must be consistent with the requirements for permanent employees.

The Hazard Communication Standard does not require the use of formal pre- and posttesting means to monitor the employee's understanding of the presented materials. However, because the standard is performance oriented, it is recommended that employers use some mechanism to ensure that the training program provided the employees with appropriate information and the employer with adequate feedback.

Although the standard does not require training records, many employers do keep this type of record. These records document that the employee actually received the training. An attendance sheet signed daily by each employee attending a training course should be used, and a copy should be placed in each of the attending employee's personnel files. The data and content of the training course should also be a part of the attendance record.

WRITTEN HAZARD COMMUNICATION PROGRAM

The employer's written hazard communication program is a document that describes how the employer complies with the requirements of the Hazard Communication Standard. Many nonspecific or generic plans have been developed by consultants, trade organizations, and other groups to provide an "easy" method of complying with the standard's requirements; however, it is essential that at least the following six specific items are discussed:

- Hazardous substance list
- Labels and other forms of warning
- Material safety data sheets
- Employee information and training
- Hazards of nonroutine tasks
- On-site contractors

Thus, generic plans must still be facility specific.

OSHA's 1994 revision of the standard includes a new Appendix E, Guidelines for Employer Compliance, which provides information designed to aid the employer in developing and implementing an effective program.

Hazardous Substance List

A list of each hazardous substance used within the facility must be generated and maintained in an orderly manner. Smaller facilities generally are aware of the materials used in their processes, and the generation of the hazardous substance list should not be too difficult; however, large, complex manufacturing facilities may have a more difficult time generating the initial list. The use of departmental questionnaires, facility walk-throughs, and reviews of purchasing department records may facilitate this record-keeping requirement.

The facility's hazardous substance list should include four areas of information: (a) the product name of each material; (b) the common name used by the employees; (c) the manufacturer of the material; and (d) for larger facilities, the departments or areas within the facility where the material is used.

In addition to the master list maintained for the entire facility, smaller lists arranged in alphabetical order should be maintained for each department or work area within the facility. Whenever a new product is introduced into a department, the department's list and the facility's master list could then be amended.

The Hazard Communication Standard requires that the method used to determine the hazard(s) posed by a material or chemical used in the workplace be described. Obviously, before the effective development of a hazardous substance list for a facility, the employer must have this procedure in place. If the employer decides to use the manufacturer's or importer's determination, this should be so stated in the written plan. If the employer's decision is to evaluate the material him- or herself, the specific procedures used for the evaluation should be outlined or described. Regardless of which method is used to perform the hazard determination, the responsible person should be identified.

Labels and Other Forms of Warning

This section of the facility's written hazard communication program describes the methods used to label containers of hazardous substances properly. If the employer uses only those containers of materials as provided by the manufacturer or supplier, the employer can rely on the labels provided by those entities. If, however, the employer provides additional or alternative labeling, then the system must be described. If alternative methods of labeling are used in the facility (batch tickets or warning signs posted in work areas), written descriptions must be provided. A copy of each alternative method should be included in this section of the written plan.

Clearly, chemical hazard information changes; therefore, a system must be initiated by the employer for review and update of the hazard warnings and information on container labels. Manufacturers, distributors, and employers are responsible for revising labels within 3 months of becoming aware of new significant information regarding a chemical's hazards. The written plan should also include a designation of the person(s) responsible for ensuring labeling of in-plant containers and shipping containers and for reviewing and updating hazard labels.

Material Safety Data Sheets

As one of the cornerstones of an effective hazard communication program, the dissemination of information contained in the MSDS is critical. Information required in the written plan includes the following:

- How the MSDSs are maintained in the facility (e.g., The MSDSs are maintained in the supervisor's office of each work station in a notebook that can be accessed by employees during each work shift; or the MSDSs are transferred to the facility's computer system and employees have access to a computer terminal during their work shift.)

- Procedures required if an MSDS is not received with the initial shipment of a hazardous substance (e.g., The supplier and manufacturer of the hazardous substance will be sent a letter stating that an MSDS was not received and the employer is now formally requesting an MSDS for that material; this letter would be followed by a registered letter within 1 month if an MSDS has still not been received.)
- Description of alternative methods used in the workplace other than MSDSs [e.g., use of written standard operating procedures or an MSDS that covers groups of chemicals used in a specific manufacturing process (these methods must also be available to employees at all times, and the written plan should address this requirement)]
- A written procedure for updating an MSDS if the employer prepares his or her own MSDSs (e.g., Available hazard data will be reviewed and evaluated, and on the positive determination of new and significant information, the MSDS will be changed within 30 days.)
- The name of the person(s) responsible for obtaining and maintaining MSDSs

EMPLOYEE INFORMATION AND TRAINING

This section of the written hazard communication program discusses the means by which the facility will provide its employees with the following:

- The identity of chemical workplace hazards
- Schedule of training and retraining
- An outline of the training program
- Location of the written hazard communication plan
- The person(s) responsible for conducting the training program

Hazards of Nonroutine Tasks

Some tasks at a facility may not be done on a routine basis and may present their own specific hazards. For example, cleaning or repair of a Freon degreasing tank may pose an asphyxiation hazard if personnel are required to enter the tank. The written hazard communication plan must address these nonroutine tasks in a systematic fashion.

CONCLUSION AND SUMMARY

The OSHA Hazard Communication Standard provides for a systematic transfer of information from manufacturers of chemicals to the users of these materials. Through the use of MSDSs, training sessions, and written hazard communication programs, employers and employees are made aware of the safety and health hazards associated with the materials used in the workplace and the methods to protect against those hazards. Proper use and implementation of a facility's hazard communication program should assist in the reduction of chemically related occupational injuries and illnesses.

REFERENCES

1. US Department of Labor, Occupational Safety and Health Administration. Hazard communication—final rule. Washington: Occupational Safety and Health Administration, 1994;59:FR 6126–6184.
2. American National Standards Institute, Inc. American national standard for hazardous industrial chemicals—material safety data sheets—preparation. New York: American National Standards Institute; 1993:v.
3. National Plant and Coatings Association. Hazardous materials identification system's revised raw materials rating manual: fall. Washington: National Plant and Coatings Association; 1984:RM/8.
4. National Fire Protection Association. Fire protection guide on hazardous materials, NFPA 704, standard system for the identification of the fire hazards of materials, 9th ed. Quincy: National Fire Protection Association, 1986;704.5–704.8.
5. Toxler R. *Wegleitung durch die arbeitssicherheit*. Luzer: Eidgenossiche Koordinations Kommission fur Arbeitssicherheit, 1987:303–309.
6. Kuhn R, Birett K. *Merkblatter gefahrliche Arbutstoffe*, vol 5. Landsberg/Lech: Ecomed, 1980:Warnsybole, 27.

APPENDIX 9-1
Hazardous Definitions and Terms

A. Physical Hazards

Combustible liquid means any liquid having a flash point at or above 100°F (37.8°C) but below 200°F (93.3°C), except any mixture having components with flash points of 200°F (93.3°C) or higher, the total volume of which makes up 99% or more of the total volume of the mixture.

Common name means any designation or identification—such as code name, code number, trade name, brand name, or generic name—used to identify a chemical other than by its chemical name.

Compressed gas means

(i) A gas or mixture of gases having, in a container, an absolute pressure exceeding 40 psi at 70°F (21.2°C); or

(ii) A gas or mixture of gases having, in a container, an absolute pressure exceeding 104 psi at 130°F (54.4°C), regardless of the pressure at 70°F (21.1°C); or

(iii) A liquid having a vapor pressure exceeding 40 psi at 100°F (37.8°C) as determined by the American Society for Testing Materials D-323-72.

Explosive means a chemical that causes a sudden, almost instantaneous release of pressure, gas, and heat when subjected to sudden shock, pressure, or high temperature.

Flammable means a chemical that falls into one of the following categories:

(i) *Aerosol, flammable* means an aerosol that, when tested by the method described in 16 *CFR* 1500.45, yields a flame projection exceeding 18 inches at full valve opening or a flashback (a flame extending back to the valve) at any degree of valve opening.

(ii) *Gas, flammable* means:

(a) A gas that, at ambient temperature and pressure, forms a flammable mixture with air at a concentration of 13% by volume or less; or

(b) A gas that, at ambient temperature and pressure, forms a range of flammable mixtures with air wider than 12% by volume, regardless of the lower limit.

(iii) *Liquid, flammable* means any liquid having a flash point below 100°F (37.8°C), except any mixture having components with flash points of 100°F (37.8°C) or higher, the total of which make up 99% or more of the total volume of the mixture.

(iv) *Solid, flammable* means a solid, other than a blasting agent or explosive as defined in 190.109(a), that is liable to cause fire through friction, absorption of moisture, spontaneous chemical change, or retained heat from manufacturing or processing, or that can be ignited readily and, when ignited, burns so vigorously and persistently as to create a serious hazard. A chemical shall be considered to be a flammable solid if, when tested by the method described in 16 *CFR* 1500.44, it ignites and burns with a self-sustained flame at a rate greater than one-tenth of an inch per second along its major axis.

Organic peroxide means an organic compound that contains the bivalent -O-O-structure and that may be considered to be a structural derivative of hydrogen peroxide when one or both of the hydrogen atoms has been replaced by an organic radical.

Oxidizer means a chemical other than a blasting agent or explosive as defined in 1910.109(a) that initiates or promotes combustion in other materials, thereby causing fire either of itself or through the release of oxygen or other gases.

Physical hazard means a chemical for which there is scientifically valid evidence that it is a combustible liquid, a compressed gas, an explosive, a flammable, an organic peroxide, an oxidizer, a pyrophoric, an unstable (reactive), or a water reactive.

Pyrophoric means a chemical that will ignite spontaneously in air at a temperature of 130°F (54.4°C) or below.

Unstable (reactive) means a chemical that, in its pure state, or as produced or transported, will vigorously polymerize, decompose, or condense, or will become self-reactive under conditions of shocks, pressure, or temperature.

Water reactive means a chemical that reacts with water to release a gas that is either flammable or presents a health hazard.

The chemical manufacturer, importer, or employer evaluating chemicals shall treat the following sources as establishing that the chemicals listed in them are hazardous:

(i) 29 *CFR* Part 1910, Subpart Z, Toxic and Hazardous Substances, Occupational Safety and Health Administration; or

(ii) *Threshold Limit Values for Chemical Substances and Physical Agents in the Work Environment*, American Conference of Governmental Industrial Hygienists (latest edition).

B. Health Hazards

i. *Carcinogen*: A chemical is considered to be a carcinogen if
   (a) It has been evaluated by IARC and found to be a carcinogen or potential carcinogen; or,
   (b) It is listed as a carcinogen or potential carcinogen in the *Annual Report on Carcinogens* published by the National Toxicology Program (latest edition); or,
   (c) It is regulated by the Occupational Safety and Health Administration as a carcinogen.

ii. *Corrosive*: A chemical that causes visible destruction of, or irreversible alterations in, living tissue by chemical action at the site of contact. For example, a chemical is considered to be corrosive if, when tested on the intact skin of albino rabbits by the method described by the U.S. Department of Transportation in Appendix A to 49 *CFR* Part 173, it destroys or changes irreversibly the structure of the tissue at the site of contact after an exposure period of 4 hours. This term shall not refer to action on inanimate surfaces.

iii. *Highly toxic*: A chemical falling within any of the following categories:
   (a) A chemical that has a median lethal dose (LD_{50}) of 50 mg or less per kg of body weight when administered orally to albino rats weighing between 200 and 300 grams each.
   (b) A chemical that has a median lethal dose (LD_{50}) of 200 mg or less per kg of body weight when administered by continuous contact for 24 hours (or less if death occurs within 24 hours) with the bare skin of albino rabbits weighing between 2 and 3 kg each.
   (c) A chemical that has a median lethal concentration (LD_{50}) in air of 200 parts per million by volume or less of gas or vapor, or 2 mg per L or less of mist, fume, or dust, when administered by continuous inhalation for 1 hour (or less if death occurs within 1 hour) to albino rats weighing between 200 and 300 grams each.

iv. *Irritant*: A chemical that is not corrosive but that causes a reversible inflammatory effect on living tissue by chemical action at the site of contact. A chemical is a skin irritant if, when tested on the intact skin of albino rabbits by the methods of 16 *CFR* 1500.41 for 4 hours of exposure or by other appropriate techniques, it results in an empirical score of five or more. A chemical is an eye irritant if so determined under the procedure listed in 16 *CFR* 1500.42 or other appropriate techniques.

v. *Sensitizer*: A chemical that causes a substantial proportion of exposed people or animals to develop an allergic reaction in normal tissue after repeated exposure to the chemical.

vi. *Toxic*: A chemical falling within any of the following categories:
   (a) A chemical that has a median lethal dose (LD_{50}) of more than 50 mg per kg but not more than 500 mg per kg of body weight when administered orally to albino rats weighing between 200 and 300 grams each.
   (b) A chemical that has a median lethal dose (LD_{50}) of more than 200 mg per kg but not more than 1,000 mg per kg of body weight when administered by continuous contact for 24 hours (or less if death occurs within 24 hours) with the bare skin of albino rabbits weighing between 2 and 3 kg each.
   (c) A chemical that has a median lethal concentration (LD_{50}) in air of more than 200 parts per million but not more than 2,000 parts per million by volume of gas or vapor, or more than 2 mg per L but not more than 20 mg per L of mist, fume, or dust, when administered by continuous inhalation for 1 hour (or less if death occurs within 1 hour) to albino rats weighing between 200 and 300 grams each.

vii. *Target-organ effects*: The following is a target-organ categorization of effects that may occur, including examples of signs, symptoms, and chemicals that have been associated with these effects. These examples are presented to illustrate the range and diversity of effects and hazards found in the workplace as well as the broad scope employers must consider in this area, but they are not intended to be all inclusive.
   (a) *Hepatotoxins*: Chemicals that produce liver damage. Signs and symptoms: jaundice, liver enlargement. Chemicals: carbon tetrachloride, nitrosamines
   (b) *Nephrotoxins*: Chemicals that produce kidney damage. Signs and symptoms: edema, proteinuria. Chemicals: halogenated hydrocarbons, uranium
   (c) *Neurotoxins*: Chemicals that produce their primary toxic effects on the nervous system. Signs and symptoms: narcosis, behavorial changes, decrease in motor functions. Chemicals: mercury, carbon disulfide
   (d) Agents that act on blood or the hematopoietic system: decrease hemoglobin function, deprive the body tissues of oxygen. Signs and symptoms: cyanosis, loss of consciousness. Chemicals: carbon monoxide. cyanides
   (e) Agents that damage the lung: chemicals that irritate or damage the pulmonary tissue. Signs and symptoms: Cough, tightness in chest, shortness of breath. Chemicals: Silica, asbestos

(f) *Reproductive toxins*: Chemicals that affect the reproductive capabilities, including chromosomal damage (mutations) and effects on fetuses (teratogenesis). Signs and symptoms: birth defects, sterility. Chemicals: lead, dichlorobromopropane
(g) *Cutaneous hazards*: Chemicals that affect the dermal layer of the body. Signs and symptoms: defatting of the skin, rashes, irritation. Chemicals: ketones, chlorinated compounds
(h) *Eye hazards*: Chemicals that affect the eye or visual capacity. Signs and symptoms: conjunctivitis, corneal damage. Chemicals: organic solvents, acids

Adapted with permission from 29 *CFR* 1200.

CHAPTER 10

Environmental Contamination and Minority Communities

Miguel C. Fernández and Herbert H. Ortega

As is the case with many social and political conflicts, environmental health issues in U.S. minority communities are determined in large part by basic economic disparities and historical discriminatory practices in housing, education, employment opportunities, health care access and availability, legal representation, and voting rights (1,2). More affluent communities are able to wield greater influence and power through community organizations and political representation because of established social, political, and economic advantages. Their communities are able to exclude proximal development of enterprises or projects that carry environmental risk such as waste incinerators, dumps, and handling of radioactive minerals and waste.

In general, more affluent communities develop in areas away from toxic-waste sites and industrial pollutants and thus insulate themselves from most forms of environmental contamination. In some wealthy urban core enclaves, smog, primarily from vehicle emissions, may be unavoidable. Overall, however, the wealthy can afford homes at a comfortable distance from the urban core and other economically depressed areas in peripheral urban quadrants. In areas where city or groundwater is considered contaminated, the affluent are able to afford water purification systems or bottled water. These trends may seem obvious, but have been poorly studied.

Historical, social, and economic discrimination, based primarily on ethnicity and physical appearance, has led to varying degrees of poverty among some ethnic minority groups. Poverty and social stressors play a role with regard to disease engenderment and susceptibility, and has led to the creation of the terms *environmental racism* and *environmental inequity*, or conversely *environmental equity*, *eco-justice*, and *environmental justice* (2,3). Each term carries its own degree of sociopolitical interpretation, but *environmental justice* seems to be the most enduring.

Health care access and poverty have been associated with racial and ethnic discrimination. Health services research indicates that minority groups and the poor have a higher risk for occupational illnesses (4). In a landmark study, the U.S. Department of Health and Human Services' 1985 "Report of the Secretary's Task Force on Black and Minority Health" linked discrimination, race, and ethnicity with disease (5).

NATIVE PEOPLES AND RADIOACTIVE CONTAMINATION

In 1946, the 167 inhabitants of the Bikini atoll of the Marshall Islands in the Pacific Ocean were moved to accommodate nuclear weapons testing under the Operation Crossroads program. Although the Bikinians were given a cursory explanation of what was to occur, the regional native populace was not aware of the massive destruction and contamination that would follow. The Marshall Islands became the primary thermonuclear testing area for the United States in the 1940s and 1950s, continuing there through 1958, including the first hydrogen bomb detonation in 1954, code-named BRAVO. Several atolls and islands in the area were damaged and contaminated by the detonations and their subsequent fallout containing cesium-137 (^{137}Cs).

Beyond the acute effects of exposure to nuclear fallout, other associated medical effects described among the chronically exposed population of the region include the induction of one case of fatal acute myeloid leukemia and a large number of thyroid tumors (benign and malignant) in addition to hypothyroidism in adults and children, and two cases of cretinism (6). At approximately the same time, and related in large part to the development of nuclear weapons, Native Americans of the Colorado Plateau faced a similarly insidious situation. Mines had been opened at the turn of the century on Navajo (Dineh), Acoma Pueblo, and Laguna Pueblo lands to produce steel-hardening vanadium. Vanadium, uranium, and uranium's natural decay product, radium, are found together as the mineral carnotite. Radium became highly valued in Europe and the United States as a cytotoxic antitumor agent until a number of gruesome deaths in the watch-dial painting industry linked it to the development of leukemia and bone tumors. Uranium oxide found an early use in pottery glazes and iridescent glass, owing to its bright yellow color. The value of uranium-235 (^{235}U) developed as a source of energy for the production of nuclear fission reactions. Most of these mines overwhelmingly employed Navajo labor (7).

The potential adverse health effects of acute and chronic exposure to radioactive substances was well known to the scientific community by mid-century. Despite this knowledge, the underground uranium mines notoriously lacked adequate ventilation or methods to contain radioactive waste and contamination. Consequently, workers developed illness related to mining operations such as silicosis and other forms of pulmonary fibrosis. It has since been determined that Native American miners have more nonmalignant respiratory disease from underground uranium mining, and less disease from smoking, than other U.S. miners studied (8).

Breathing radon progeny elements, which occur as natural decay products of uranium, had been linked in early studies of European pitchblende miners who had a 75% death rate from lung cancers. This link has been supported by later studies (9). Mine workers in the United States in general come from poor and rural populations.

Occupational disease related to mining is not confined to Native Americans or other minority groups (10). However, in the retrospective cohort mortality study, despite lower smoking rates, Navajo miners from the Colorado Plateau have shown several-fold elevated standardized mortality ratios for lung cancer (3.3), tuberculosis (2.6), and pneumoconioses and other respiratory diseases (2.6) 23 years after their last exposure to radon progeny (11). In testimony given to a U.S. Senate subcommittee in 1990, the National Institute for Occupational Safety and Health's chief statistician, Dr. Robert Hornung, reported that of 4,146 uranium miners studied, more than 350 had died from lung cancer (approximately 1 in 12), five times the rate for the general population (12).

The Radiation Exposure Compensation Act was enacted by Congress in 1990 after more than 20 years of intermittent hearings and committee activities, finally leading to a recognition of the harmful effects of mining activities and exposure to atomic weapon detonations (7).

The problem of radiation exposure related to mining is widespread and not limited to the miners themselves. Nearly 1,200 mines were dug on the Navajo reservation. Some open-pit mines have filled with water and become watering holes for animals. In addition, after numerous milling sites were established to convert the crude uranium ore into yellowcake, leftover tailings from the conversion process resulted in environmental contamination. Millions of tons of open tailings piles, containing the water-soluble radium-226 and other radioactive components, are scattered in 24 states. On the Navajo reservation and other nearby communities, tailings piles have been located near the center of town, potentially exposing children playing near them. Windblown dust has contaminated groundwater, irrigation water, and cattle water supplies with other such waste products as arsenic, lead, nitrate, selenium, and uranium. Despite the Uranium Mill Tailings Radiation Control Act passed by Congress in 1978, cleanup continues (7).

PESTICIDES AND FARM WORKERS

The modern environmental movement developed rapidly after the publication of biologist Rachel Carson's haunting 1962 book *Silent Spring*. The main thrust of this movement centered on the effects of pesticides on wildlife and humans (13). Few focused on the effects that widespread use of pesticides had on millions of farm workers. It would be more than a decade later when a small number of studies would explore unequal exposure risks among different social groups (2).

In the early 1960s, California farm worker Cesar Chavez organized the mostly Mexican, Mexican-American, and Filipino laborers to form the National Farm Workers Association (later the United Farm Workers of America). Chavez began the first minority-engendered popular movement organized in large part around environmental issues. Although primarily a labor movement, the newly unionized farm workers strongly protested the spraying of pesticides over workers and crops, and brought national attention to this occupational hazard and potential public health problem. In response to this risk, the first union contracts signed by Chavez in 1970 specifically banned the use of DDT, aldrin, and dieldrin, several years before the U.S. government ban on these pesticides (13). In addition to the established population of farm workers, under the postwar Bracero program (1942–1964), impoverished Mexicans lacking English fluency and education were brought to the United States to provide an inexpensive labor force. Agricultural workers, particularly migrants, are excluded from many key laws and regulations concerning labor practices and protections. Lacking economic, sociopolitical, educational, and legal resources, the agricultural workers represent a vulnerable population (13).

Migrant farm workers and their families, the majority of whom are of Mexican ancestry in the United States, are considered to have a disproportionately increased risk of adverse health effects related to pesticides; yet, they have often been excluded from pesticide health effect studies (14,15). Migrant workers and their families often live on, or are adjacent to, fields and orchards where pesticide applications occur. Families, including small children, often work together in contaminated farm fields. Skin and respiratory exposures occur from direct contact with contaminated crops, soil, and airborne pesticides, leading to increased total body burdens (15,16).

Beyond the ongoing research into toxic effects of acute pesticide exposure and carcinogenicity, interest has been raised with regard to neuropsychological, neurobehavioral, reproductive, developmental, respiratory, and immunologic health-related problems (17). Malnutrition and other chronic diseases that occur at higher frequencies in lower socioeconomic groups may increase susceptibility to pesticide toxicities (15).

AFRICAN-AMERICAN AND LATINO COMMUNITIES

By the 1980s, hundreds of community groups had organized around issues of differential exposure to environmental risks (Fig. 10-1). In 1982, North Carolina's impoverished Warren County community, largely African American, gained national attention by protesting a proposed hazardous-waste site to dump soil contaminated with polychlorinated biphenyls in a landfill that would be 10 ft above the water table (18). Then, in 1983, the U.S. General Accounting Office (GAO) published a study of southeastern U.S. communities surrounding four large commercial hazardous-waste landfills. The GAO found that three of four sites were located in predominantly African-American communities (19). Bullard, also in 1983, showed that in Houston, 21 of 25 solid-waste facilities were located in its African-American communities (20).

In 1987, a landmark study by the United Church of Christ's Commission for Racial Justice described the extent of inequitable environmental risks and the consequences for those who are victims of polluted environments (21). Their study revealed that race was the most significant variable associated with the location of hazardous-waste sites, even after controlling for urban and regional differences in socioeconomic status. The greatest number of commercial hazardous-waste facilities were located in communities with the highest proportions of racial and ethnic minorities. Another important finding was that the average minority population in communities with one commercial hazardous-waste facility was twice the average minority percentage in communities without such facilities (21).

The United Church of Christ report also showed that three out of every five African and Hispanic Americans lived in communities with one or more toxic-waste sites. More than 15 million African Americans, more than 8 million Hispanics, and approximately one-half of all Asian/Pacific Islanders and Native Americans were living in communities with one or more abandoned or uncontrolled hazardous-waste sites (21).

Studies since then have shown a relationship between race or ethnicity and the location or attempted location of hazardous-waste sites. This relationship appears to be independent of social class. Additionally, other studies have shown that race or ethnicity and income are associated risk factors for a variety of environmental exposures and susceptibility (2).

Countering this picture of environmental racism, a GAO report in 1995 showed that neither minorities nor low-income people were overrepresented in any consistent manner within a 1-mile radius of municipal landfills (22). However, this conclusion only referred to municipal solid-waste facilities (i.e., city dumps) and compared groups overall at the national level. It did not examine variations on the regional level, and population densities were not taken into account. The relationship between an arbitrary 1-mile radius and effects on the local water supply or air quality within a

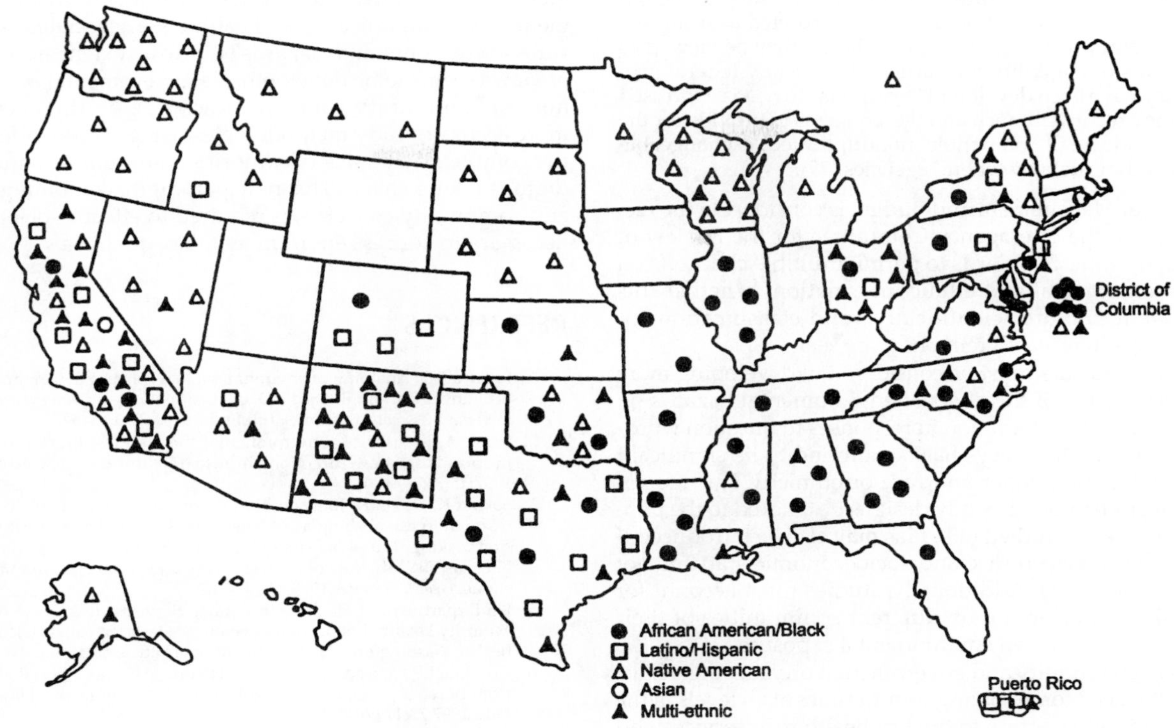

Figure 10-1. Location of grassroots environmental justice groups by race or ethnicity. (With permission from ref. 1.)

larger area was not specified. The report only cited existing sites and did not address, for example, the numerous attempts by hazardous-waste disposal firms to locate waste facilities on Native American lands and other impoverished communities (23).

Aside from the siting of hazardous-waste sites, minorities and the poor face a concentration of toxin-producing industries within their communities. One obvious reason for the disproportionate siting of potentially hazardous industries and waste sites is that land and labor costs tend to be less in many of these communities. Another explanation is the dire need for employment and a perception by business and community leaders that impoverished minorities prefer to have jobs, even those that expose themselves and their communities to hazardous conditions. The location of these industries has been termed *LULU*, for *l*ocally *u*ndesirable *l*and *u*se. After one LULU has taken hold within a community, there seems to be a decreased barrier to establishing subsequent LULUs. This phenomenon of concentrated industrialization may contribute greatly to the exposure of a community to multiple potential toxins (24).

Lead exposure, particularly in children, has been a particular concern of poor communities living close to industries. Long-term negative health impacts include neurobehavioral and hematopoietic abnormalities in children and hypertension in adults. Children living in substandard housing, especially those with poor nutritional status, are particularly at risk for lead toxicity. Sources of lead exposure in children include paint chips, contaminated soil and air from industry, and, in some communities, ceramic glazes and cosmetics. Repeated studies have shown that the poor, particularly African-American and Latino children, are disproportionately exposed to toxic levels of lead (25).

The health effects of industrial pollutants on a particular population can be difficult to assess owing to multiple confounding variables. These variables include nutritional status, health status, age, genetic susceptibility, degrees and quality of exposure (i.e., route, dose, duration, repetitive, additive, synergistic), or exposure to complex mixtures of toxins, latency, prior exposure to other toxins, the quality and accuracy of methods used to determine the degree of exposure, and the ability of testing to detect subtle health effects (3).

CHALLENGES IN RESEARCH, DATA COLLECTION, AND INTERPRETATION

With the growing concern that minority and economically disadvantaged communities bear a disproportionate share of the risks of environmental pollutant exposure, funding additional research has been proposed to help address the environmental health issues discussed (3,26). The challenge of designing studies that involve comparisons of ethnically and culturally diverse groups demands a critical assessment of how these groups are defined and how individuals may self-identify. In the scientific community, little thought has been given to the basic presumptions of what constitutes a race, a concept that has been criticized as inaccurate (27).

Racial and ethnic classifications are just one of many complexities that arise in research bias. One of the difficulties in classifying people into racial and ethnic categories is that the U.S. population as a whole is becoming increasingly multiethnic, with a growing number of individuals having parents of more than one ancestry (28). In scientific literature, most researchers have used a government standard as defined by the 1977 U.S. Office of Management and Budget Statistical Directive 15, which recognizes four racial groups (American Indian or Alaskan Native, Asian or Pacific Islander, black, and white) and one ethnic category (Hispanic):

> This directive provides standard classifications for record keeping, collection, and presentation of data on race and ethnicity in

federal program administrative reporting and statistical activities. These classifications should not be interpreted as being scientific or anthropologic in nature, nor should they be viewed as determinants of eligibility for participation in any federal program. They have been developed in response to needs expressed by both the executive branch and the Congress to provide for the collection and use of compatible, nonduplicated, exchangeable racial and ethnic data by federal agencies (29).

The Office of Management and Budget is considering the recommendation of the Interagency Committee for the Review of the Racial and Ethnic Standards to permit multiple checkoffs on forms that solicit racial and ethnic information. Whether this will translate into more scientifically valid classifications of minority groups in research remains to be seen.

Several other factors must be considered in developing more accurate assessments of the effect of environmental hazards on minority communities. Variation in responses to question wording in health research surveys has been found to be significant and is dependent on gender and race or ethnicity. It is recommended that epidemiologic study designs be tailored to the population groups being studied (30). Bias may also be introduced if the relationship between race and socioeconomic status is not taken into account (31). Additionally, studies must account for the variability of perception by different communities of their estimated risk from a given environmental exposure (24).

Leaders in community and governmental organizations have recognized the need for involving communities at all levels in the pursuit of improving access to quality health care services and performing research that addresses environmental inequalities (3,32–34). In recognition of this need, several governmental agendas have been prepared. The Environmental Justice Act, passed by Congress in 1992, and the presidential Executive Order 12898 (1994) are examples of federal actions directed specifically at these needs. The U.S. Environmental Protection Agency's Environmental Equity Workgroup and the Department of Health and Human Service's Subcommittee on Environmental Justice, Environmental Health Policy Committee, are examples of strategic plans developed in accordance with these federal actions (35). Grants addressing environmental equity issues have become available as a result of such plans (36,37).

Creating new strategies to address environmental equity problems involves development and encouragement of scientists and other researchers from minority and economically disadvantaged backgrounds. As an example of an increased awareness of this need, some epidemiologists are recognizing the relative underrepresentation of minority professionals within their field and formulating plans to address them (38).

Many community activists express dichotomous viewpoints from those expressed by scientists. The community perspective generally tends to the belief that the goals of research should go beyond a given that sufficient evidence of environmental racism exists. The community activists believe that the focus of research should be on participation of affected communities, and on the recognition, prevention, and remediation of existing inequities and injustices based on race and income that have not been adequately addressed by government and industry. Among other concerns, they challenge the Environmental Protection Agency, when making permit decisions, to consider the aggregate risk to communities already saturated with toxin-producing industries (23).

SUMMARY

The prevailing scientific position is that of viewing research goals focused primarily on nonconfrontational, "value-free methods of identification, assessment, comparison, management and communication of health risks associated with exposures to environmental hazards" (3). To an extent, a convergence of views seems to be developing as governmental agencies take note of community concerns. Recognizing the necessity for more accurate study methodologies using an expanded view of the complex dynamics of minority communities, a new paradigm is taking shape. This new paradigm, combining scientific and community concerns, is required to effect a societal change necessary to address environmental inequalities.

REFERENCES

1. Bullard RD. Anatomy of environmental racism and the environmental justice movement. In: Bullard RD, ed. *Confronting environmental racism: voices from the grassroots*. Boston: South End Press, 1993:15–39.
2. Szasz A, Meuser M. Environmental inequalities: literature review and proposals for new directions in research and theory. *Current Sociology* 1997;45(3):99–120.
3. Sexton K, Olden K, Johnson BL. Environmental justice: the central role of research in establishing a credible scientific foundation for informed decision making. *Toxicol Ind Health* 1993;9(5):685–727.
4. Nickens HW. The role of race/ethnicity and social class in minority health status. *Health Serv Res* 1995;30:151–162.
5. US Department of Health and Human Services, Task Force on Black and Minority Health. Report of the secretary's task force on black and minority health. Washington: US Department of Health and Human Services; 1986.
6. Cronkite EP, Conrad RA, Bond VP. Historical events associated with fallout from Bravo Shot: Operation Castle and 25 years of medical findings. *Health Phys* 1997;73(1):176–186.
7. Eichstaedt PH. *If you poison us: uranium and Native Americans*. Santa Fe: Red Crane Books, 1994:47–65, 123–126, 127–149.
8. Mapel DW, Coutlas DB, James DS, et al. Ethnic differences in the prevalences of nonmalignant respiratory disease among uranium miners. *Am J Public Health* 1997;87(5):833–838.
9. Harley N, Samet JM, Cross FT, et al. Contribution of radon and radon daughters to respiratory cancer. *Environ Health Perspect* 1986;70:17–21.
10. Roscoe RJ. An update of mortality from all causes among white uranium miners from the Colorado Plateau Study Group. *Am J Ind Med* 1997;31(2):211–222.
11. Roscoe RJ, Deddens JA, Salvan A, Schnoor TM. Mortality among Navajo uranium miners. *Am J Public Health* 1995;85(4):535–540.
12. Impacts of past uranium mining practices, 1990: hearing on 101–0683 before the Subcommittee on Mineral Resources Development and Production of the Senate Committee on Energy and Natural Resources, 101st Cong, 2nd Sess (1990) (testimony of RW Hornung).
13. Moses M. Farm workers and pesticides. In: Bullard RD, ed. *Confronting environmental racism: voices from the grassroots*. Boston: South End Press, 1993:161–178.
14. Mines R, Gabbard S, Boccalandro B. *Findings from the National Agricultural Workers Survey (NAMS): a demographic and employment profile of perishable crop workers*. Washington: US Department of Labor, Office of Program Economics; 1990. Research report no. 1.
15. Fleming LA, Herzstein JA. Emerging issues in pesticide health studies. *Occup Med: State of the Art Reviews* 1997;12(2):387–397.
16. Moses M, Johnson ES, Anger WK, et al. Environmental equity and pesticide exposure. *Toxicol Ind Health* 1993;9(5):913–959.
17. Sever LE, Arbuckle TE, Sweeney A. Reproductive and developmental effects of occupational pesticide exposure: the epidemiologic evidence. *Occup Med: State of the Art Reviews* 1997;12(2):305–325.
18. Lee C. Toxic waste and race in the United States. In: Bryant B, Mohai P, eds. *Race and incidence of environmental hazards: a time for discourse*. Boulder: Westview Press, 1992:10–27.
19. US General Accounting Office. Siting of hazardous-waste landfills and their correlation with racial and economic status of surrounding communities. Washington: US Government Printing Office; 1983. Publication GAO/RCED–83–168.
20. Bullard RD. Solid waste sites and the black Houston community. *Sociological Inquiry* 1983;53(spring):273–288.
21. United Church of Christ, Commission for Racial Justice. Toxic waste and race in the United States: national report on the racial and socioeconomic characteristics of communities with hazardous waste sites. New York: Public Data Access, 1987.
22. US General Accounting Office. Hazardous and non-hazardous waste: demographics of people living near waste facilities. Washington: US Government Printing Office; 1995; GAO/RCED–95–84.
23. Bullard RD. Conclusion: environmentalism with justice. In: Bullard RD, ed. *Confronting environmental racism: voices from the grassroots*. Boston: South End Press, 1993:195–206.
24. Benson L. Environmental health in minority communities. In: Brooks SM, Bochfeld M, Herzstein J, Jackson RJ, Schenker MF, eds. *Environmental medicine*. St. Louis: Mosby–Year Book, 1995:412–415.

25. Kurin D, Therrell BL, Patterson P. Demographic risk factors associated with elevated lead levels in Texas children covered by Medicaid. *Environ Health Perspect* 1997;105(1):66–68.
26. Anderson YB, Coulberson SL, Phelps J. Overview of the EPA/NIEHS/ATSDR workshop, equity in environmental health: research issues and needs. *Toxicol Ind Health* 1993;9(5):679–683.
27. Williams DR. Race and health: basic questions, emerging directions. *Ann Epidemiol* 1997;7:322–333.
28. Lott JT. Policy purposes of race and ethnicity: an assessment of federal racial and ethnic categories. *Ethn Dis* 1993;3(3)(summer):221–228.
29. Office of Management and Budget. Race and ethnic standards for federal statistics and administrative reporting. Washington: Office of Federal Statistical Policy and Standards, US Department of Commerce; 1978. Directive no. 15.
30. Warnecke RB, Johnson TP, Chavez N, et al. Improving question wording in surveys of culturally diverse populations. *Ann Epidemiol* 1997;7:334–342.
31. Herman AA. Toward a conceptualization of race and epidemiologic research. *Ethn Dis* 1996;6(5)(winter/spring):7–20.
32. Nickens HW. A compelling research agenda. *Ann Intern Med* 1996;215:237–239.
33. Bullard RD, Wright BH. Environmental justice for all: community perspectives on health and research needs. *Toxicol Ind Health* 1993;9(5):821–842.
34. Anonymous. Stronger voice for environmental justice advocates? *Environmental Science & Technology* 1995;29(1):22A.
35. Subcommittee on Environmental Justice, Environmental Health Policy Committee, US Department of Health and Human Services. Strategic elements for environmental justice. *Environ Health Perspect* 1995;103(9):796–800.
36. Anonymous. Toxic waste research. *Environ Health Perspect* 1993;101:474.
37. Anonymous. Colleges get environmental justice grants. *Environmental Science & Technology* 1995;29(11):491A.
38. St. George DM, Schoenbach VJ, Reynolds GH, et al. Recruitment of minority students to US epidemiology degree programs. *Ann Epidemiol* 1997;7:304–310.

CHAPTER 11
Personal Protection and Hazardous Materials

Richard L. Urie

Protection of employees from hazardous materials consists of three broad areas:

1. Administrative controls
2. Engineering controls
3. Personal protective equipment

Administrative controls consist of managerial efforts to reduce risks of accidents or toxic exposures through planning, training, employee rotation on job sites, changes in processes, and product substitution. These managerial efforts include the development of standard operating procedures along with emergency response plans. The development of environmental and medical surveillance programs may be part of policy and procedures.

Engineering controls are measures that are planned and constructed for the purpose of reducing accidents and/or chemical and physical hazards. Engineering controls may be implemented at the source of the hazard, along the exposure path (such as with a pipeline), or at the operator or receiver of the hazardous substance. Examples include the use of exhaust ventilation, dust suppressants to control fugitive dust emissions, radiation shielding, and the installation of physical protective guards over machinery.

Personal protective equipment (PPE) includes a wide variety of items worn by an individual to prevent injury or exposure. Generally, administrative and engineering controls are used to prevent exposure of personnel to hazardous materials. However, direct personnel response to a hazardous materials site is frequently required to conduct environmental sampling, clean up spills, or respond to accidents and injuries. For these instances, protective equipment is required. Such equipment must offer respiratory, ocular, and dermal protection from chemical or physical hazards. Proper protection is important for two reasons:

1. Because of the nature of most hazardous materials incidents and hazardous-waste site investigations, the use of PPE is often the only feasible means of preventing or reducing chemically related exposures.
2. The misuse of PPE may directly or indirectly contribute to accidents, chemical or radiologic exposures, dermal injury, burns, heat stress, and related impairments.

RESPIRATORY PROTECTION

Respiratory protective devices come in a wide variety of configurations, materials, sizes, and intended applications. The selection, use, and maintenance of respirators are complex subjects requiring extensive training and experience. Yet workers are often assigned respirators without consideration given to medical clearance, respirator fit testing, job-specific selection criteria, or adequate maintenance of the equipment. The large number of Occupational Safety and Health Administration (OSHA) citations issued for inadequate respirator programs attests to this frequent violation.

Respirators of each class require an apparatus or framework that serves toisolate the wearer from contaminated air. Such apparatus may be provided in the form of a tight-fitting face piece, a snorkel-like mouthpiece, or a loose-fitting cover such as a hood, suit, hard hat assembly, or blouse.

Examples of tight-fitting face pieces include the quarter-mask that covers the mouth and nose (Fig. 11-1), the half-mask that fits over the nose and under the chin (Fig. 11-2), and the full face mask that covers the face from the hairline to below the chin (Fig. 11-3). These face pieces are generally constructed of neoprene, silicone, or molded rubber. Full face respirators provide limited eye protection against impact and chemical contact.

Mouthpiece respirators are inserted into the mouth in the same fashion as a snorkel (Fig. 11-4). Respirators of this type may include attached nose pinchers to prevent entry of air through the nostrils. Mouthpiece respirators are seldom used for purposes other than emergency escape contingencies.

Loose-fitting respirators typically cover at least the face and a portion of the head and may include full body suits. Some are built into a hard hat and face shield assembly (Fig. 11-5), thereby providing limited protection against impact or chemical contact.

The type of face piece, cover, or mouthpiece determines the degree of protection provided against barrier breakthrough. *Barrier breakthrough* is the passage of contaminated air through a

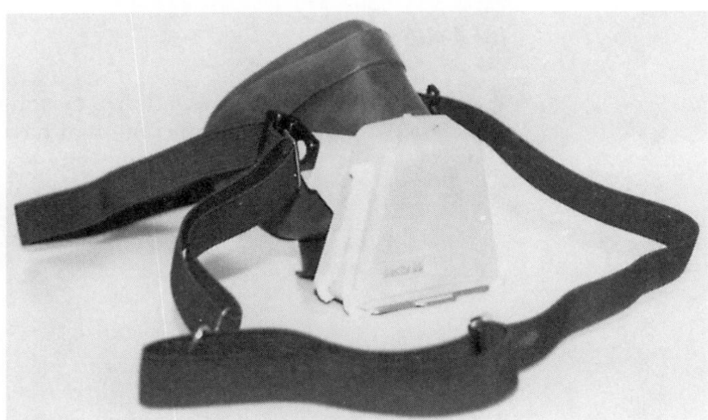

Figure 11-1. Quarter-mask respirator.

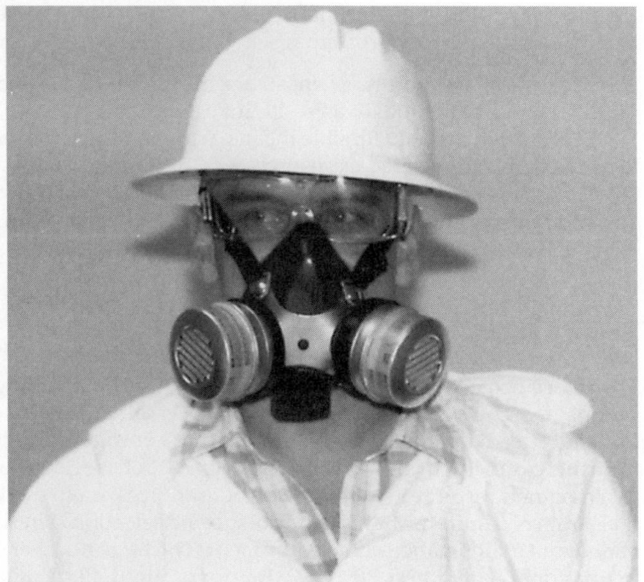

Figure 11-2. Half-mask respirator.

breach in the respirator-to-face seal. This level of sealing or barrier protection in conjunction with the efficiency of the air-purifying element or air-supplied system determines the overall protection factor for the protective device.

The National Institute of Occupational Safety and Health (NIOSH) has assigned protection factors to various representative respiratory protection ensembles, as indicated in Tables 11-1 and 11-2. The protection factor is the ratio of the concentration of the contaminant present in the ambient atmosphere to the concentration within the face piece of the respirator. NIOSH describes the application of the protection factor as follows: "The maximum specified use concentration for a respirator is generally determined by multiplying the exposure limit for the contaminant by the protection factor assigned to a specific class of respirators" (1).

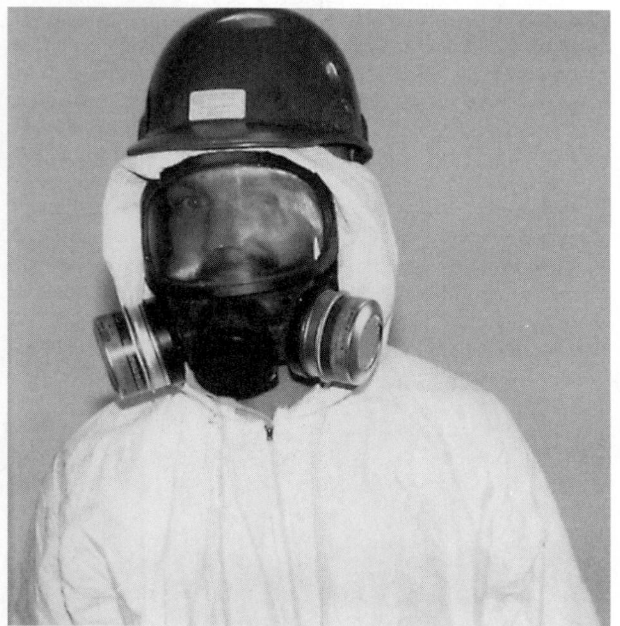

Figure 11-3. Full face respirator.

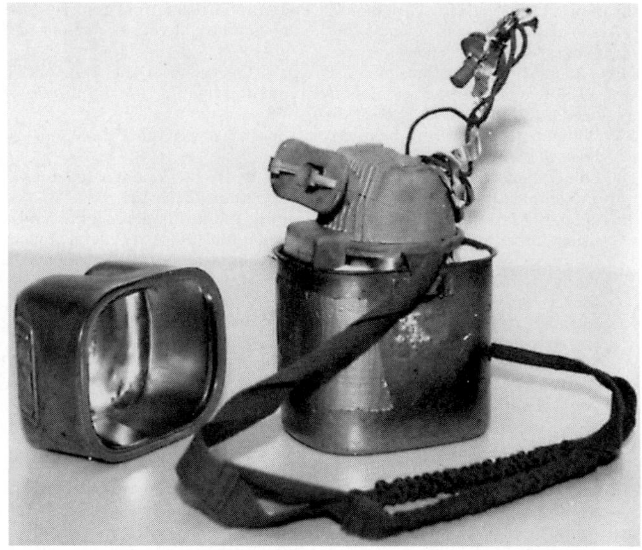

Figure 11-4. Mouthpiece respirator.

The respirators on the market may be broadly classified as the following types:

1. Air-purifying respirator
2. Supplied air respirator
3. Self-contained breathing apparatus

Air-Purifying Respirators

These incorporate any one of the apparatuses previously discussed with a particulate filter, gas or vapor removal element, or a combination particulate and gas or vapor removal system. Respirators within this class may be powered by a portable battery-driven blower (e.g., powered air-purifying respirator), or operated under the negative pressure generated by inhalation (e.g., negative pressure air-purifying element).

Particulate filtering respirators use a fibrous material that traps dusts, mists, and fumes. Some filters are impregnated with a resin base and are electrostatically charged to enhance the filtration efficiency. However, conditions such as high humidity or exposure to oily mists may result in the loss of this electrostatic charge.

Filters can be either standard configuration, offering moderate particulate arresting efficiencies, or approved as high efficiency particulate air filters (HEPA filters). HEPA filters typically consist of a larger cartridge or canister as opposed to the relatively flat disk-like standard filter element (Fig. 11-6). The standard filter has an approximate efficiency of 80% to 90% against 0.6-μm particles; the HEPA element has a tested efficiency of 99.9% against 0.3-μm particles. Both classes of filters develop increased efficiency as the particle load within the filter increases with use. Conversely, as the openings within the filter media become smaller, breathing resistance increases. Filters of both types are typically used until such a time as breathing becomes difficult due to this resistance. However, the policy of filter reuse should not be followed in situations involving the filtration of radioactive particles that may emit ionizing radiation other than alpha particles.

One-piece disposable dust respirators are also available. However, they are seldom used for applications other than those involving nuisance dusts due to poor filtration efficiency and inadequate face-sealing properties (Fig. 11-7).

Gas and vapor cartridges or canisters are engineered to collect toxic or irritating gases or chemically convert gases to safe material (Fig. 11-8). The purification device contains a granulated high

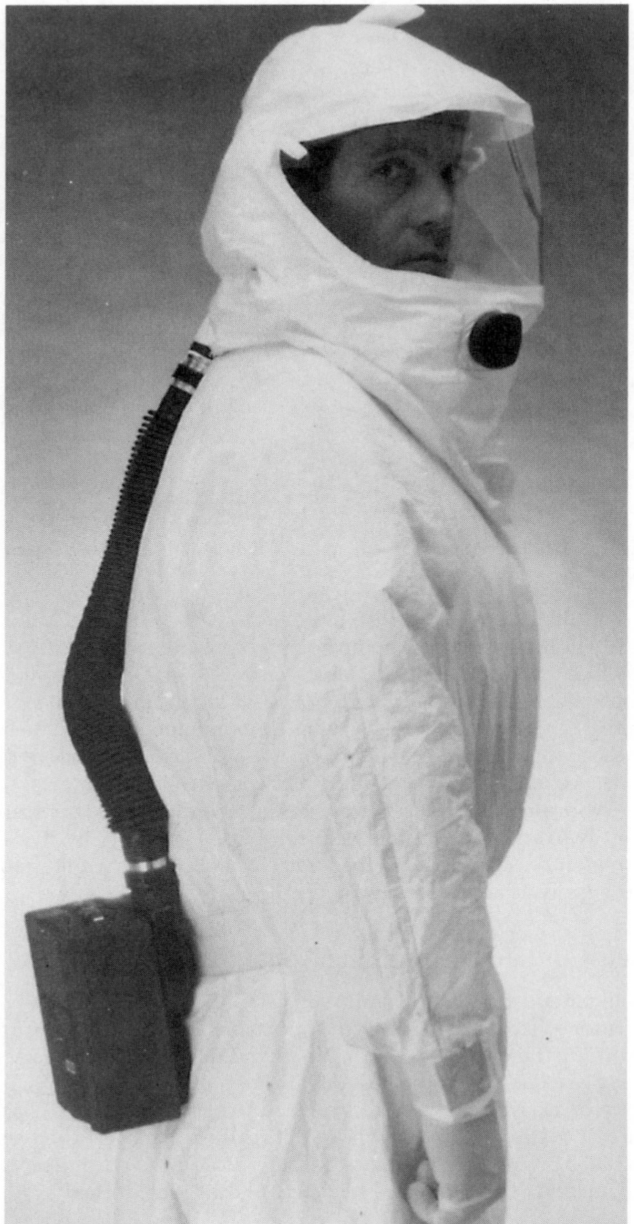

Figure 11-5. Mine Safety Appliances powered air-purifying respirator. Total assembly.

TABLE 11-1. Assigned protection factor classifications of respirators for protection against particulate exposures[a]

Assigned protection factor	Type of respirator
5	Single-use or quarter-mask respirator
10	Any air-purifying half-mask respirator, including disposable equipped with any type of particulate filter except single use[b,c]
	Any air-purifying full face piece respirator equipped with any type of particulate filter[d]
	Any supplied air respirator equipped with half-mask and operated in a demand (negative pressure) mode[b]
25	Any powered air-purifying respirator equipped with a hood or helmet and any type of particulate filter[e]
	Any supplied air respirator equipped with a hood or helmet and operated in a continuous flow mode[e]
50	Any air-purifying full face piece respirator equipped with a high efficiency filter[b]
	Any powered air-purifying respirator equipped with a tight-fitting face piece and a high efficiency filter[e]
	Any supplied air respirator equipped with a full face piece and operated in a demand (negative pressure) mode[b]
	Any supplied air respirator equipped with a tight-fitting face piece and operated in a continuous flow mode[d]
	Any self-contained respirator equipped with a full face piece and operated in a demand (negative pressure) mode[b]
1,000	Any supplied air respirator equipped with a half-mask and operated in a pressure demand or other positive-pressure mode[b]
2,000	Any supplied air respirator equipped with a full face piece and operated in a pressure demand or other positive-pressure mode[b]
10,000	Any self-contained respirator equipped with a full face piece and operated in a pressure demand or other positive-pressure mode[b]
	Any supplied air respirator equipped with a full face piece operated in a pressure demand or other positive-pressure mode in combination with an auxiliary self-contained breathing apparatus operated in a pressure demand or other positive-pressure mode[b]

[a]Only high-efficiency filters are permitted for protection against particulates having exposure limits less than 0.05 mg/m^3.
[b]The assigned protection factors (APFs) were determined by Los Alamos National Laboratories by conducting quantitative fit testing on a panel of human volunteers.
[c]An APF of 10 can be assigned to disposable particulate respirators if they have been properly fitted using a quantitative fit test.
[d]The APF was based on consideration of efficiency of dust, fume, and mist filters. From ref. 1, with permission.
[e]The APFs were based on workplace protection factor data or laboratory data more recently reported than the Los Alamos National Laboratories data.

surface-area media referred to as *sorbent*. Sorbent interacts with the gas molecules through adsorption, absorption, chemisorption, or catalytic chemical reactivity. The most commonly used sorbent media is activated carbon that alone is an effective adsorbent for some organic vapors or gases. Activated carbon may also be impregnated with chemical substances to enhance the adsorption action for other specific gases. Examples include iodine-impregnated activated carbon for use against mercury vapor and metallic oxide–impregnated carbon that collects acid gases. Other agents used as adsorbents include silica gel and activated alumina. Absorbents that rely on chemical interactions can include alkaline sorbents used to neutralize acid gases. Sorbents can also use catalysts to speed up the conversion of toxic gases to relatively nontoxic products. The "self-rescuer" respirators carried by underground mine workers use a catalyst called *hopcalite*, which converts carbon monoxide to carbon dioxide.

Combination cartridges and canisters are available and consist of multiple elements for various gases or for gases and particulates. Cartridges and canisters are labeled and color coded for their intended use. Table 11-3 depicts the color code system established by American National Standard, K.13.1. All U.S. manufacturers of respirators conform to this color code system; however, cartridges, filters, and canisters are not interchangeable with different brands of respiratory devices, despite the uniform color code.

Supplied Air Respirators

Supplied air respirators consist of a source of respirable air that is supplied to the wearer's face or headpiece. They are defined as type A, B, or C:

TABLE 11-2. Assigned protection factor classifications of respirators for protection against gas and vapor exposures

Assigned protection factor[a]	Type of respirator
10	Any air-purifying half-mask respirator (including disposable) equipped with appropriate gas and vapor cartridges[b]
	Any supplied air respirator equipped with a half-mask and operated in a demand (negative pressure) mode[b]
25	Any powered air-purifying respirator with a loose-fitting hood or helmet[c]
	Any supplied air respirator equipped with a hood or helmet and operated in a continuous flow mode[c]
50	Any air-purifying full face piece respirator equipped with appropriate gas and vapor cartridges or gas mask (canister respirator)[b]
	Any powered air-purifying respirator equipped with a tight-fitting face piece and appropriate gas and vapor cartridges or canisters[c]
	Any supplied air respirator equipped with a full face piece and operated in a demand (negative pressure) mode[b]
	Any supplied air respirator equipped with a tight-fitting face piece operated in a continuous flow mode[c]
	Any self-contained respirator equipped with a full face piece and operated in a demand (negative pressure) mode[b]
1,000	Any supplied air respirator equipped with a half-mask and operated in a pressure demand or other positive-pressure mode[b]
2,000	Any supplied air respirator equipped with a full face piece and operated in a pressure demand or other positive-pressure mode[b]
10,000	Any self-contained respirator equipped with a full face piece and operated in a pressure demand or other positive-pressure mode[b]
	Any supplied air respirator equipped with a full face piece operated in a pressure demand or other positive-pressure mode in combination with an auxiliary self-contained breathing apparatus operated in a pressure demand or other positive-pressure mode[b]

[a]The assigned protection factor (APF) for a given class of air-purifying respirators may be further reduced by considering the maximum use concentrations for each type of gas and vapor air-purifying element.
[b]The APFs were determined by Los Alamos National Laboratories by conducting quantitative fit testing on a panel of human volunteers.
[c]The APFs were based on workplace protection factor data or laboratory data more recently reported than the Los Alamos National Laboratories data.
From ref. 1, with permission.

Type A: Consists of a tight-fitting face piece attached to a large-diameter hose supplied with fresh air from a mechanical blower. The blower may be motor driven or hand operated.

Type B: Respirators also consist of a tight-fitting face piece attached to a large-diameter hose with low breathing resistance. Air is drawn through the hose by the force of inhalation only.

Type C: Respirators consist of a tight- or loose-fitting face or head assembly, a high-pressure air line not to exceed 300 ft, couplings, regulators, control valves, and a supply of breathing air typically from compressed air cylinders or an approved compressor (Fig. 11-9).

Breathing air used for any respirator system must meet the requirements for type 1 gaseous air (grade D or higher quality) set forth by the Compressed Gas Association (Table 11-4).

Type C respirators may be further classified with respect to the air flow and pressurization of air in the face piece. They may be supplied with (a) continuous air flow, (b) air flow that is delivered on inhalation only ("demand"), or (c) constant pressurization of the mask with additional air flow on inhalation ("pressure-demand").

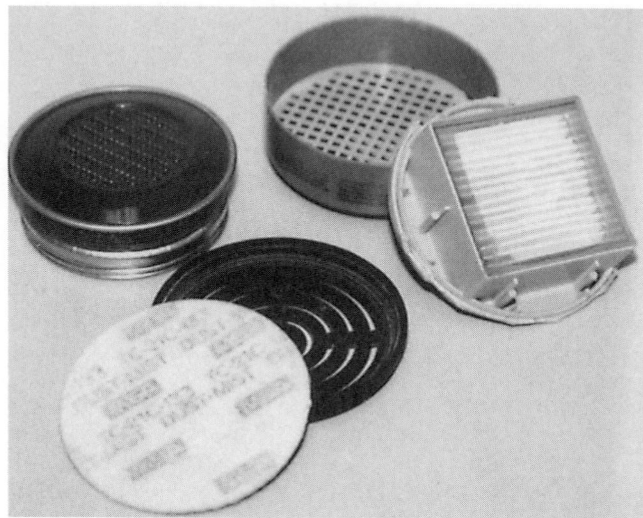

Figure 11-6. Filter pad, high efficiency particulate air filters cartridge and canister.

The continuous flow system provides constant pressurization of the face piece but requires a large volume of air. Demand systems conserve the air supply, but do not provide constant positive pressure, thereby potentially allowing contaminants into the mask if the face-to-face piece seal is broken. Pressure-demand systems provide a constant positive pressure and conservation of air.

Work on hazardous-waste sites or chemical incident scenes that warrant supplied air respirator use typically involve the type C pressure-demand system with an auxiliary emergency air supply attached to the wearer.

Self-Contained Breathing Apparatus

Self-contained breathing apparatuses (SCBAs) are individual respirator systems consisting of a portable air or oxygen supply worn by the user (Fig. 11-10). No physical link to a stationary air supply exists, as in the case of supplied air respirators. SCBAs may be classified as *closed circuit* or *open circuit* systems. Closed circuit systems, also known as "rebreathers," recycle the user's exhaled breath after removing carbon dioxide and adding oxygen as needed. The gases are recycled within a contained system,

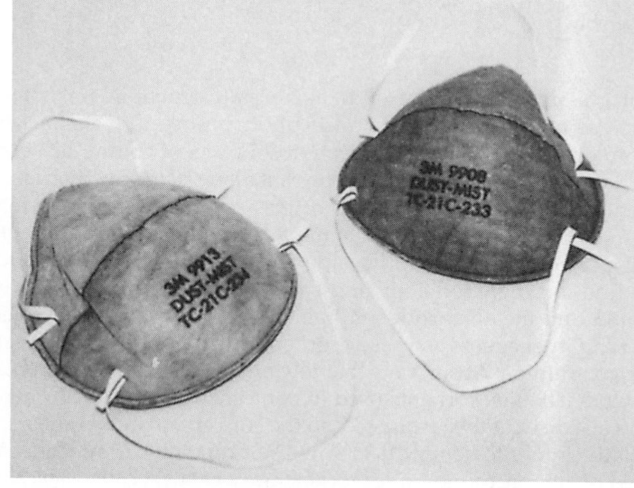

Figure 11-7. Disposable dust respirators.

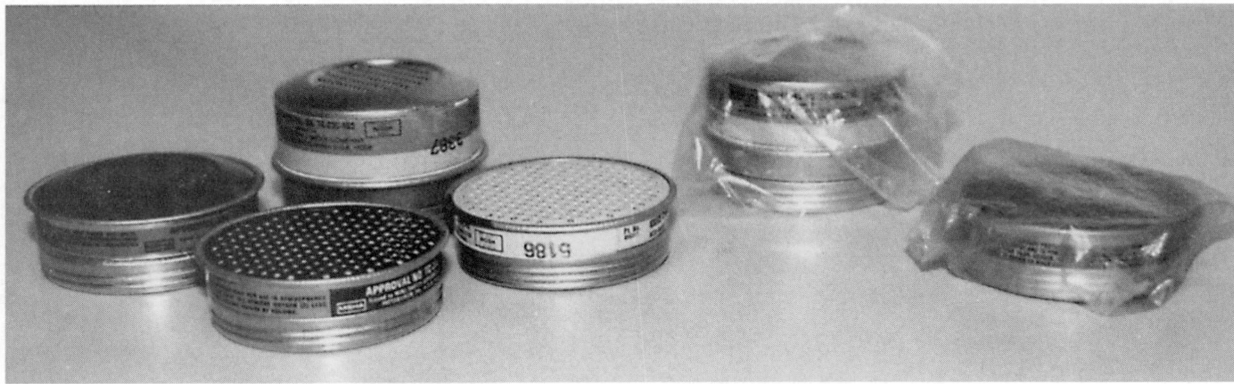

Figure 11-8. Single element and combination cartridges.

except in the event of excess pressurization, in which case air is vented out the relief valve. Closed circuit SCBAs that provide up to 4 hours of use per charge are available. The two basic types of rebreathers use either a cylinder of compressed oxygen or a solid oxygen–generating substance such as potassium superoxide. Rebreathers have limited use at hazardous-waste sites or chemical spill sites due to the high expense of the units and the danger of flammability associated with oxygen-enriched systems (2).

Open circuit SCBAs exhaust the exhaled air to the atmosphere, rather than recycling it. They typically consist of a 30- or 60-minute supply of compressed grade D air worn on the back of the user and a tight-fitting face piece (see Fig. 11-10). As with type C respirators, these SCBAs may use either a demand or pressure-demand regulator system. The complete system typically weighs 30 to 38 lb. Open circuit SCBAs are available with an optional valve stem that allows the attachment of an airline from a stationary source of air (Fig. 11-11). This feature allows the option of creating a type C respirator with a 30- or 60-minute escape bottle.

TABLE 11-3. Atmospheric contaminants to be protected against

Contaminants	Colors assigned[a]
Acid gases	White
Hydrocyanic acid gas	White with 1/2-in. green stripe completely around the canister near the bottom
Chlorine gas	White with 1/2-in. yellow stripe completely around the canister near the bottom
Organic vapors	Black
Ammonia gas	Green
Acid gases and ammonia gas	Green with 1/2-in. white stripe completely around the canister near the bottom
Carbon monoxide	Blue
Acid gases and organic vapors	Yellow
Hydrocyanic acid gas and chloropicrin vapor	Yellow with 1/2-in. blue stripe completely around the canister near the bottom
Acid gases, organic vapors, and ammonia gases	Brown
Radioactive materials, excepting tritium and noble gases	Purple (magenta)
Particulates (dusts, fumes, mists, fogs, or smokes) in combination with any of the above gases or vapors	Canister color for contaminant, as designated above, with 1/2-in. gray stripe completely around the canister near the top
All of the above atmospheric contaminants	Red with 1/2-in. gray stripe completely around the canister near the top

[a]Gray shall not be assigned as the main color for a canister designed to remove acids or vapors.

Note: Orange shall be used as a complete body or stripe color to represent gases not included in this table. The user should refer to the canister label to determine the degree of protection the canister affords.

[Secs. 4(b)(2), 6(b), and 8(c), 84 Stat. 1592, 1593, 1596, 29 *U.S.C.* 653, 655, 657; Secretary of Labor's Order No. 8-76 (41 FR 25059); 29 *CFR* Part 1911 (39 FR 23502, June 27, 1974, as amended at 43 FR 49748, Oct. 24, 1978)

From ref. 2, with permission.

CHEMICAL PROTECTIVE CLOTHING

Chemical protective clothing (CPC) is a broad class of garments worn to protect the wearer against contaminant-related injury

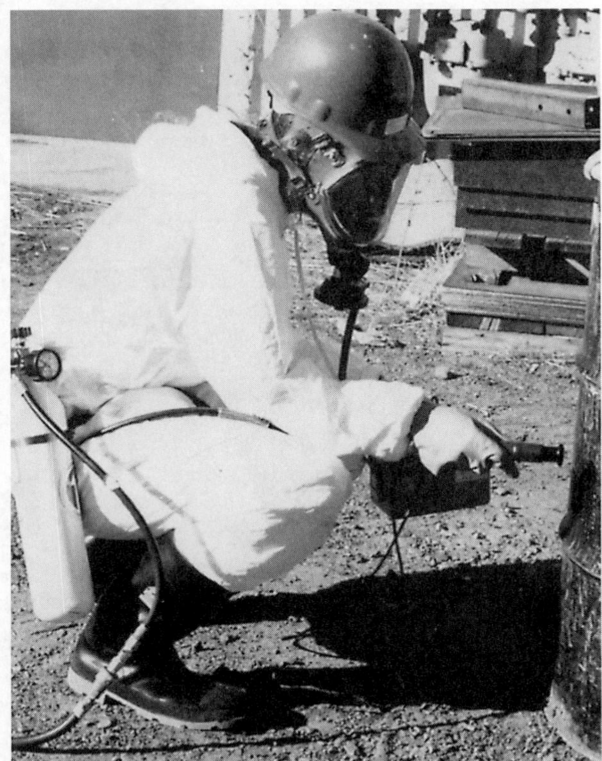

Figure 11-9. Supplied air system.

TABLE 11-4. Characteristics of grade D and better breathing air

Limiting characteristics	Grades					
	D	E	F	G	H	I
% O_2 (v/v) Balance predominantly N^2V	atm. 19.5–23.5[a]	atm. 19.5–23.5	atm. 19.5–23.5	atm. 19.5–23.5	atm. 19.5–23.5	atm. 19.5–23.5
Water	*b*	*b*	*b*	*b*	*b*	1°–10.4°F
Hydrocarbons (condensed) in mg/m^3 of gas at normal temperature[c]	5	5	—	—	—	—
CO	20	10	5	5	5	1
Odor	*d*	*d*	*d*	*d*	*d*	*d*
CO_2	1,000	500	500	500	0.5	—
Gaseous hydrocarbons (e.g., methane)	—	—	25	15	10	0.5
Nitrogen dioxide	—	—	—	2.5	0.5	0.1
Nitrous oxide	—	—	—	—	—	0.1
Sulfur dioxide	—	—	—	2.5	1	0.1
Halogenated solvents	—	—	—	10	1	0.1
Acetylene	—	—	—	—	—	0.05

[a]The term "atm" (atmospheric) denotes the normal oxygen content of atmospheric air; numbers indicate oxygen limits for synthesized air.
[b]The water content of compressed air required for a particular grade can vary from saturated to dry depending upon the intended use. If a specific water limit is required, it should be specified as a limiting dewpoint (expressed in temperature °F at one atmosphere absolute pressure) or concentration in ppm (v/v).
[c]No limits are given for condensed hydrocarbons beyond grade E as gaseous hydrocarbon limits could not be met if condensed hydrocarbons were present.
[d]Adapted from Compressed Gas Association, Inc., Air Specification G-7.1
From ref. 2, with permission.

or as a means of controlling the spread of the contaminant. The term *chemical* protective clothing is somewhat misleading, as it typically includes garments worn in situations involving infectious or radiologic waste as well as chemicals. Hazardous material incidents in which CPC is needed include exposure to any of the following: toxic gases, asphyxiants, corrosive liquids, flammable vapors, solvent vapors, explosives, and carcinogens.

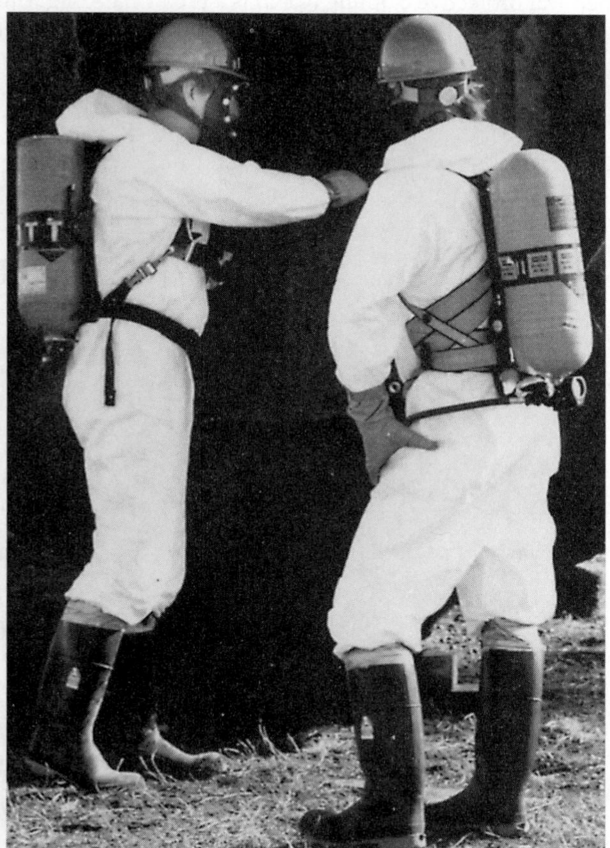

Figure 11-10. Self-contained breathing apparatus.

Clearly, no universal ensemble appropriate to all situations exists. Such factors as garment flammability, chemical resistance, strength, degree of vapor sealing, heat transfer, cost, and so forth dictate the need for a wide variety of garment materials and designs. A few representative styles and materials are discussed to introduce some of the most commonly used CPC ensembles.

Fully Encapsulating Suits

One-piece garments that provide chemical protection for the entire body exist (see Fig. 11-11). They represent the most extensive degree of PPE skin protection available. The suit also protects the enclosed breathing apparatus from chemical degradation and excessive decontamination requirements. Most reusable encapsulating suits are made of butyl rubber, Viton, Teflon, or a combination of these. The suits may have integral boots and gloves made of neoprene, polyvinylchloride, or other natural or synthetic materials. The face shield may be made of glass or acrylate compounds. Disposable encapsulating suits that are manufactured from a variety of polymer-covered fibrous materials are also available. Encapsulating suits are used in conjunction with SCBAs and a type C air-line respirator.

Nonencapsulating Suits

Nonencapsulating suits consist of one or two pieces. One-piece hooded coveralls are generally the suit of choice; however, a hooded jacket worn with a pair of pants or bib overalls is also an option. Usually, when these suits are worn in the field, seams, gaps, and connection points are tape sealed (3). Nonencapsulating suits are often purchased with the intent of disposing of the garment after a day of field use.

Aprons, Boots, Boot Covers, and Gloves

Aprons are also used as a means of partial skin protection for such activities as chemical sampling and packaging. Aprons

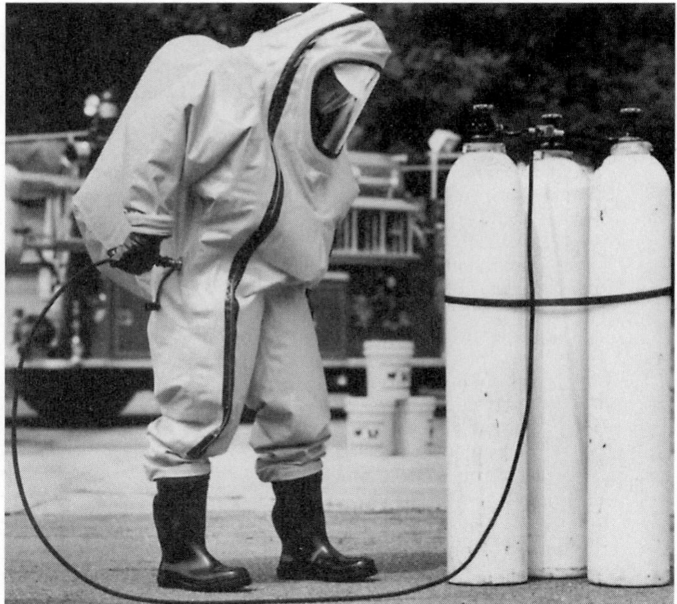

Figure 11-11. Fully encapsulating suit with self-contained breathing apparatus in a level A hazardous materials operation. User is changing the self-contained breathing apparatus air bottle with air from the stationary bottle.

may cover only the chest and abdomen or extend the full length of the chest to the feet and include full sleeves.

Boots, boot covers, and gloves are a necessary addition to most ensembles, as the hands and feet are the most likely portion of the body to come in contact with contaminants.

Barrier creams are available that, when applied directly to the skin, offer temporary protection against some chemical products. Barrier creams are more appropriate for use in controlled industrial settings than in hazardous material situations. Such creams may be used to help prevent the dermal absorption of chlorinated solvents.

Specialized Protective Equipment

Specialized protective equipment and accessories are available for applications other than chemical/skin contact and include such items as flame-resistant suits, flotation gear, antiradiation suits, blast fragmentation suits, and cooling accessories.

Flame-resistant suits: Consist of aluminized encapsulating suits, fire fighter's bunker coats, or one-piece nonencapsulating suits (Fig. 11-12) such as the Nomex coverall. Garments of this nature are sometimes worn in conjunction with chemical protective clothing that alone offers little protection against a flashback.

Antiradiation suits: Designed to prevent ingestion, inhalation, or spread of radiation-bearing particles. They offer little protection against the effects of electromagnetic radiation exposure.

Blast and fragmentation suits: Used when handling explosive materials. However, no gear exists that adequately protects against the impact of more than a minute quantity of explosive material at distances less than approximately 20 ft.

Cooling devices: Due to the potential for heat stress associated with chemical protective clothing, cooling accessories are sometimes incorporated into the protective ensemble. These accessories consist of three basic types: (a) evaporation cooling garments involving the circulation of cool, dry air; (b) water and ice jackets using conductive cooling properties; and (c) garments containing battery-powered pumps and tubes that circulate cool liquid across the chest and back.

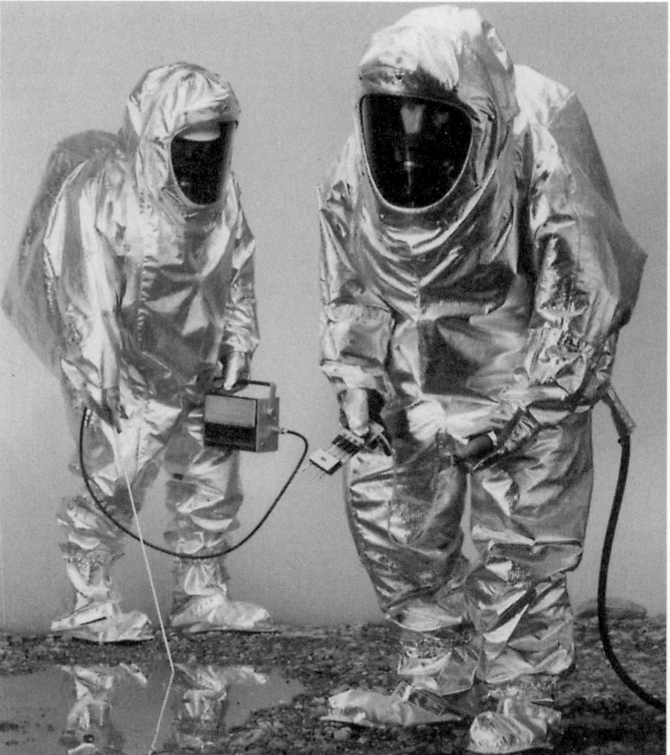

Figure 11-12. Flame-resistant suits.

The overall effectiveness of these devices on hazardous-waste sites is limited owing to the added weight, bulk, and maintenance requirements. Other protective gear commonly used on hazardous-waste sites includes hard hats and goggles or face shields.

Levels of Hazardous Material Protection

The U.S. Environmental Protection Agency (EPA) has established distinct combinations of respirators and chemical protective garments for use in certain hazardous materials situations. These classes or "levels of protection" are referred to as *A*, *B*, *C*, and *D*.

Level A: Represents the maximum degree of skin and respiratory protection offered by a combination of a supplied air respirator and an encapsulating suit

Level B: Consists of a supplied air respirator and a nonencapsulating garment

Level C: Involves a moderate degree of respiratory protection and skin protection through the use of an air-purifying respirator and a nonencapsulating garment

Level D: Consists of standard work clothes—no respirator and no chemical protectivegarment

The specific EPA ensembles for levels A through D are presented in Table 11-5. Many companies and agencies have adopted the terminology of the EPA.

REGULATIONS AND CERTIFICATIONS IMPACTING ON PERSONAL PROTECTIVE EQUIPMENT USE

Respiratory protective devices must be tested and certified by the NIOSH and the Mine Safety and Health Administration

TABLE 11-5. Protective equipment selection guide[a]

Level of protection	Equipment	Protection provided	Should be used when	Limiting criteria
A	Recommended Pressure-demand, full face piece SCBA or pressure-demand supplied air respirator with escape SCBA Fully encapsulating, chemical-resistant suit Inner chemical-resistant gloves Chemical-resistant safety boots and shoes Two-way radio communications Optional Cooling unit Coveralls Long cotton underwear Hard hat Disposable gloves and boot covers	The highest available level of respiratory, skin, and eye protection.	The chemical substance has been identified and requires the highest level of protection for skin, eyes, and the respiratory system based on either Measured (or potential for) high concentration of atmospheric vapors, gases, or particulates or Site operations and work functions involving a high potential for splash, immersion, or exposure to unexpected vapors, gases, or particulates of materials that are harmful to skin or capable of being absorbed through the intact skin. Substances with a high degree of hazard to the skin are known or suspected to be present, and skin contact is possible. Operations must be conducted in confined, poorly ventilated areas until the absence of conditions requiring level A protection is determined.	Fully encapsulating suit material must be compatible with the substances involved.
B	Recommended Pressure-demand, full face piece SCBA or pressure-demand supplied air respirator with escape SCBA Chemical-resistant clothing (overalls and long-sleeved jacket; hooded, one- or two-piece chemical splash suit; disposable chemical-resistant one-piece suit) Inner and outer chemical-resistant gloves Chemical-resistant safety boots or shoes Hard hat Two-way radio communications Optional Coveralls Disposable boot covers Face shield Long cotton underwear	The same level of respiratory protection but less skin protection than level A. It is the minimum level recommended for initial site entries until the hazards have been further identified.	The type and atmospheric concentration of substances have been identified and require a high level of respiratory protection, but less skin protection. This involves atmospheres: With IDLH concentrations of specific substances that do not represent a severe skin hazard or That do not meet the criteria for use of air-purifying respirators. Atmosphere contains less than 19.5% oxygen. Presence of incompletely identified vapors or gases is indicated by direct-reading organic vapor detection instrument, but vapors and gases are not suspected of containing high levels of chemicals harmful to skin or capable of being absorbed through the intact skin.	Use only when the vapor or gases present are not suspected of containing high concentrations of chemicals that are harmful to skin or capable of being absorbed through the intact skin. Use only when it is highly unlikely that the work being done will generate either high concentrations of vapors, gases, or particulates or splashes of material that will affect exposed skin.
C	Recommended Full face piece, air-purifying, canister-equipped respirator Chemical-resistant clothing (overalls and long-sleeved jacket; hooded, one- or two-piece chemical splash suit; disposable chemical-resistant one-piece suit) Inner and outer chemical-resistant gloves Chemical resistant safety boots or shoes Hard hat Two-way radio communications Optional Coveralls Disposable boot covers Face shield Escape mask Long cotton underwear	The same level of skin protection as level B, but a lower level of respiratory protection.	The atmospheric contaminants, liquid splashes, or other direct contact will not adversely affect any exposed skin. The types of air contaminants have been identified, concentrations measured, and a canister is available that can remove the contaminant. All criteria for the use of air-purifying respirators are met.	Atmospheric concentration of chemicals must not exceed IDLH levels. The atmosphere must contain at least 19.5% oxygen.

(continued)

TABLE 11-5. *(continued)*

Level of protection	Equipment	Protection provided	Should be used when	Limiting criteria
D	Recommended Coveralls Safety boots or shoes Safety glasses or chemical splash goggles Hard hats Optional Gloves Escape mask Face shield	No respiratory protection. Minimal skin protection.	The atmosphere contains no known hazard. Work functions preclude splashes, immersion, or the potential for unexpected inhalation of or contact with hazardous levels of any chemicals.	This level should not be worn in the Exclusion Zone. The atmosphere must contain at least 19.5% oxygen.

IDLH, immediately dangerous to life or health; SCBA, self-contained breathing apparatus.
[a]Based on EPA protective ensembles.
From ref. 13, with permission.

(MSHA). NIOSH and MSHA performance requirements are stipulated in Title 30, Code of Federal Regulations, part II.

Users of respirators must meet a variety of requirements established by the appropriate agency in authority, such as OSHA, MSHA, and the Nuclear Regulatory Commission. The OSHA requirements are representative of other agency requirements and incorporate the American National Standards Institute (ANSI) standard Z88.2-1969, "Practices for Respiratory Protection"; 49 *CFR* Part 173, "Shipping of Compressed Gas Cylinders"; ANSI standard 248.1-1954, "Marking of Compressed Gas Cylinders"; and Compressed Air Standard G-7.1-1966.

The major requirements of the OSHA 29 *CFR* 1910.134 Respiratory Protection Standard are

1. Standard operating procedures governing the selection and use of respirators shall be in writing.
2. Respirators shall be selected on the basis of hazards to which the worker is exposed.
3. The user shall be instructed and trained in the proper use of respirators and their limitations.
4. Where practicable, the respirators should be assigned to individual workers for their exclusive use.
5. Respirators shall be regularly cleaned and disinfected. Those issued for the exclusive use of one worker should be cleaned after each day's use, or more often if necessary. Those used by more than one worker shall be thoroughly cleaned and disinfected after each use.
6. Respirators shall be stored in a convenient, clean, and sanitary location.
7. Respirators used routinely shall be inspected during cleaning. Worn or deteriorated parts shall be replaced. Respirators for emergency use, such as self-contained devices, shall be thoroughly inspected at least once a month and after each use.
8. Appropriate surveillance of work area conditions and degree of employee exposure or stress shall be maintained.
9. There shall be regular inspection and evaluation to determine the continued effectiveness of the program.
10. Persons should not be assigned to tasks requiring use of respirators unless it has been determined that they are physically able to perform the work and use the equipment. A physician shall determine what health and physical conditions are pertinent. The respirator user's medical status should be reviewed periodically (e.g., annually).
11. Approved or accepted respirators shall be used when they are available. The respirator furnished shall provide adequate respiratory protection against the particular hazard for which it is designed in accordance with standards established by competent authorities. The U.S. Department of Interior, Bureau of Mines, and the U.S. Department of Agriculture are recognized as such authorities. Although respirators listed by the U.S. Department of Agriculture continue to be acceptable for protection against specified pesticides, the U.S. Department of the Interior, Bureau of Mines, is the agency now responsible for testing and approving pesticide respirators.

OSHA also prohibits facial hair on respirator users due to data indicating poor respirator-to-face sealing. Contact lenses are also prohibited. Individuals dependent on the use of corrective lenses need special respirator spectacle kits.

Respirator filters and cartridges must meet certain test criteria as defined by MSHA in 30 *CFR* Part II. Particulate filters are tested against silica dust, lead fume, silica mist, and dioctylphthalate. Chemical cartridges are tested with the agents listed in Table 11-6.

Other standards that define respirator selection and use under specific circumstances are in effect. Examples include OSHA standards for asbestos, lead, and arsenic exposure. Due to the complex integration of various agency standards, an organization such as NIOSH should be consulted for clarification.

Unlike respirators, protective garments are not stringently regulated. Although a variety of recommended tests and manufacturing guidelines are available, few have been incorporated into regulatory standards. Many of the more established manufacturers have adopted guidelines from the American Society of Testing and Materials, ANSI, and the National Fire Protection Association regarding permeability and breakthrough testing, sizing, and garment flammability, respectively (4,5).

Protective accessories, including eye and face protection, head protection, and foot protection, are well addressed by agencies such as OSHA. OSHA regulations incorporate ANSI standard 287.1-1968, "Occupational and Educational Eye and Face Protection"; ANSI standard 289.1-1969, "Safety Requirements for Industrial Head Protection"; and ANSI standard 241.1-1967, "Men's Safety-Toe Footwear."

SELECTION OF PERSONAL PROTECTIVE EQUIPMENT

Much has been written on this complex subject and is too extensive to consolidate in this text. However, detailed decision trees and selection guides are available, including two NIOSH publications:

1. "Respirator Decision Logic," publication 87-108

TABLE 11-6. Chemical cartridges and their testing agents

Cartridge	Test atmosphere
Ammonia	Ammonia
Acid gas	Sulfur dioxide, chlorine, hydrochloric acid
Methylamine	Methylamine
Organic vapors	Carbon tetrachloride
Pesticides	Silica dust, lead fume, dioctylphthalate
Carbon monoxide	Carbon monoxide

2. "Personal Protective Equipment for Hazardous Material Incidents: A Selection Guide," publication 84-114.

Some of the major respirator selection criteria to be evaluated include the following:

- Level of oxygen in the atmosphere
- Toxicity of contaminant, including conditions immediately dangerous to life and health and permissible exposure limits
- Sealing efficiency of mask
- Sorption efficiency of cartridge media for the specific contaminant of concern
- Odor or irritant threshold of contaminant
- Concentration of contaminant
- Service life of respirator
- Conditions of use (i.e., fire, humidity)

The selection of chemical protective clothing is based on a variety of scientific data and judgment. Criteria such as permeation and breakthrough are good indicators of chemical resistance. However, stitching, sizing, dexterity, and general durability must be closely inspected for a given brand. The manufacturing process should also be evaluated. For example, two gloves of the same material and thickness may have different degrees of protection if one is latex-dipped and one is solvent- or cement-dipped, the difference being that solvent dipping involves multiple dipping or layering, whereas latex dipping is a single-dip process (6). It has been speculated that the single dip may result in a higher rate of imperfections.

Protective suits, aprons, boots, and gloves are manufactured by different methods and in a wide variety of materials, thicknesses, and configurations. All of these variables must be considered when selecting a chemical protective garment for a given application. One major set of parameters to be assessed is the breakthrough time and permeation rate of a chemical or group of chemicals for the material used to construct the garments. *Breakthrough* is defined as the differential time from initial contact of the outside surface of the CPC with a chemical to the first detection of the chemical on the inside surface (4,6). Permeation rate is a numeral expression that indicates the amount of a chemical that passed through a given area of clothing per unit time. It is important to note that these data are based on laboratory conditions. Use in the presence of increased heat increases the movement of the chemicals through the garment. In addition, the data pertain to the material only; seams, zippers, and face shields may not offer the same degree of chemical resistance as the material itself. Breakthrough and permeation data for several materials are available from manufacturers of disposable chemical protective garments [e.g., Tyvek (Dupont)].

Combining the various criteria for selecting respirators and protective clothing results in some variation of the EPA "levels of protection." The basic advantages and limitations of each level are also provided (see Table 11-5).

Many qualifiers should be evaluated before assigning an initial level of protection. However, some general examples are presented based on my experience:

Level A operations: Includes work with concentrated corrosives, such as a chlorine cylinder leak or an anhydrous ammonia line repair; handling of highly toxic materials, such as military chemical agents or highly infectious microorganisms; and entry into unknown chemical or infectious waste releases.

Level B operations: Includes confined space entry situations in which oxygen concentration may be below 19.5% and toxic products are present; work involving volatile carcinogens, such as hydrazine; and products irritating to the skin that exceed an immediately dangerous-to-life-and-health value, such as a 200 parts per million vapor concentration of hydrofluoric acid.

Level C operations: Includes some low-level uranium tailings cleanup, lead dust exposure, low to moderate asbestos sampling, and low-level exposure to solvent vapors.

Level D operations: Operations conducted in the support area of a hazardous waste operation, equipment mobilization, and noninvasive geophysical surveys.

PROBLEMS ASSOCIATED WITH PERSONAL PROTECTIVE EQUIPMENT USE

Although the various forms of eye, skin, and respiratory protection described in this chapter can be critical elements of a safety program, they also present some health concerns related to physical fitness of workers, heat stress, and exposure to multiple chemicals.

Heat stress is a common concern among users of impermeable garments when temperatures exceed 75°F (23.9°C) and the physical labor demand is high. The added weight of an SCBA and confinement within a full face mask add to the workload, heat retainment, and loss of evaporative cooling. The end result may be a 35% loss of cooling, an additional 40 lb of carrying weight, and an environment within the suit equal to 100% humidity. Some suits cannot be worn for more than 15 minutes above 80°F (26.7°C) (15). Therefore, measures must be taken to restrict the wearing time of impermeable garments to temperature-dependent work and rest regimes (7,8). In addition, workers should be encouraged to replace lost fluids throughout the day, avoid alcoholic beverages, monitor body temperature or heart rate, and schedule heavy work for cooler parts of the day. Workers new to a warm work environment should be acclimated over a week-long period, beginning with a 50% workload that is progressively increased by approximately 10% each day (9,10).

Signs and symptoms of heat-related illness and loss of thermoregulatory control should be monitored and include headache, disturbances in gait, tachycardia, dizziness, skin that is warm or hot to the touch with little sweating, rapid respirations, and altered mental status. Supervisors of hazardous materials workers should be aware of these warning signs and intervene immediately if they become apparent. Emergency medical response is required to prevent serious illness or death. Workers in level A protective gear may not be easily observed until they have serious signs and symptoms.

Dermatoses may result from the moisture and abrasion caused by some protective garments. Respirator masks that are disinfected but inadequately rinsed can result in severe skin irritation caused by residual chemicals. Suits and masks may be worn for hours at a time before being removed. Any dirt, disinfectant, or moisture trapped within the face piece seal remains in contact with the skin under pressure. Workers must be advised of the importance of PPE cleaning, disinfection, and rinsing.

The use of SCBAs and air-line respirators has been related to complaints of headaches and upper airway irritation. Some drying of the mucous membranes can be expected. This is a result of the removal of water vapor from the compressed air, which prevents corrosion within the regulator systems (11). Some symptoms of irritation may be related to the pressure placed on the temples by the respirator straps or the constant flow of cool air across the face and eyes.

The negative pressure requirements, exhalation residence, and dead air space of air-purifying respirators may result in such physiologic changes as increased alveolar carbon dioxide tension, decreased oxygen uptake, and an increased oxygen debt (12). The end result of such reactions may be fatigue, dyspnea, and headache. This may contraindicate the use of negative pressure air-purifying respirators at high altitudes, during heavy exertion, or for workers with significant respiratory impairments.

Restricted vision and reduced dexterity associated with PPE use may increase the possibility of falls, vehicular accidents, and other conventional safety concerns. Workers should be advised to work in pairs (i.e., the buddy system), and take additional time, if needed, to complete field tasks in high-risk areas. Mobile equipment operators must be particularly watchful of workers near their operations, as hearing may also be compromised by hoods, shrouds, or masks.

Permeability of level A garments are typically studied only with single chemicals and not mixtures. NIOSH has stated that the permeation parameters of single chemicals cannot be relied on to determine the permeability of mixtures (10).

SUMMARY

Of the three forms of employee protection, administrative controls, engineering controls, and personal protective equipment, the latter is the least desirable, but often the most applicable to situations involving hazardous materials work. Proper selection of PPE begins with a thorough knowledge of the equipment and the contaminants. Users of PPE must be properly trained in its use, fitted, and examined by a physician before being qualified for field duty. Some equipment, such as respirators and flotation gear, must meet certain agency approvals. Improper use of PPE may result in a variety of hazardous conditions, including chemical or radiologic exposure due to inadequate protection, heat stress, dermatoses, fatigue, and general discomfort.

REFERENCES

1. Bollinger NJ, Schutz RH. National Institute of Occupational Safety and Health guide to industrial respiratory protection. Washington: US Department of Health and Human Services, September 1987; National Institute of Occupational Safety and Health publication no. 87-116.
2. Ronk R, White MK, Linn H. Personal protective equipment for hazardous materials incidents: a selection guide. Washington: US Department of Health and Human Services, October 1984. National Institute of Occupational Safety and Health publication no. 84-114.
3. US Environmental Protection Agency. Hazardous materials incident response operations—training manual. Washington: US Environmental Protection Agency, 1982:3–4.
4. Schwope AD, Costas PP, Jackson JO, Weitzman DJ. Guidelines for the selection of chemical protective clothing: field guide. Vol. l. Cincinnati: American Conference of Governmental Industrial Hygienists, 1983.
5. Mine Safety Appliances Company. Chempruf II total-encapsulating suit instruction manual, publication 481127. Pittsburgh: Mine Safety Appliances Company, nd.
6. Siebe North. North hand protection: permeation resistance guide, publication IH-200. Charleston, SC: Siebe North, 1984.
7. Raven PB, Dodson A, Davis TO. Stresses involved in wearing PVC supplied air suits: a review. *Am Ind Hyg Assoc J* 1979;40:592–599.
8. Levine SP, Martin WF. *Protecting personnel at hazardous waste sites*. Stoneham, MA: Butterworth Publishers, 1985.
9. US Public Health Service. NIOSH recommended standard for occupational exposure to hot environments. Washington: National Institute of Occupational Safety and Health, 1977; National Institute of Occupational Safety and Health publication no. 757-009/26.
10. Moran, J. Personal protective equipment, Hazmat, Hazwaste, Hazchem and Lady SARA. *Appl Ind Hyg* 1989;4(2):F7–F9.
11. International Fire Service Training Association. *Self-contained breathing apparatus*. Tulsa, OK: Fire Protection Publications, Oklahoma State University, 1982.
12. Raven PB, Dodson AT, Davis TO. The physiological consequences of wearing industrial respirators: a review. *Am Ind Hyg Assoc J* 1979;40:517–534.
13. *Occupational safety and health guidance manual for hazardous waste site activities*. Washington: National Institute for Occupational Safety and Health, 1985.

CHAPTER 12
Recognition of Hazardous Materials

William V. Gustin

When incidents involving hazardous materials occur, a team of specially trained, hazardous-material technicians usually responds to control and mitigate the situation. But it is usually the first responder (i.e., the first arriving police, fire, or emergency medical service unit) that must quickly and accurately determine the presence of hazardous materials, identify the products involved, ascertain the degree of risk, and determine means necessary to protect themselves and the public. Often, the safe and successful outcome of a hazardous material incident depends on the action taken by first responders during the first few critical minutes after their arrival on the scene.

FIRST RESPONDER

Approach and Initial Action at a Hazardous-Materials Incident

Emergency response personnel are conditioned to rapidly intervene at emergencies to save lives and property. A quick response, rapid fire control, and prompt patient care are desirable qualities in any responder. But the mind-set of emergency personnel (to rush in and mitigate the situation) can put them at unnecessary risk at a hazardous-materials incident. Known or potential hazardous-materials incidents require a more thorough and cautious assessment of conditions before the scene can be safely approached, victims rescued, and materials identified.

The difference between successfully handling a hazardous-materials incident and becoming part of the problem depends largely on an awareness of the presence of hazardous and toxic materials. Labeling and documentation systems are, at best, tools to assist in product hazard identification. No marking system is designed to identify all hazardous materials before they can do harm to emergency response personnel. Markings are just one of many possible indicators of the presence of hazards that should be identified, understood, and heeded. Markings and labels are often of no use to first responders if they do not suspect the presence of hazardous materials. Information is key to safe and effective mitigation of a hazardous-material emergency. The first responder to arrive can gather critical information to assist other emergency personnel and prevent further injury or contaminations. But responding agencies should not wait to obtain information until units arrive on the scene; conditions may rapidly deteriorate before they arrive. Police or fire dispatchers and 911 operators should begin the process of gathering pertinent information from the parties reporting the incident and then transmit it to responding units. The following information helps first-arriving units to safely approach the scene and begin operations, as well as assists later-arriving specialists with mitigation:

- Exact address and name of involved person(s)
- Names and types of materials involved, spelled out if possible
- Types and numbers of containers involved
- Status of product (i.e., spilled, leaking, or burning)
- Visible placards, labels, and four-digit United Nations (UN) identification numbers
- Whether the product was being off-loaded, mixed, or transferred
- Physical state of hazard (i.e., solid, liquid, or gas)
- Quantity of material released, spilled, or burning
- Number of victims
- Status of victims
- Exposure status of victims (i.e., dermal or inhalational)
- Special hazards (i.e., biological, radioactive, or explosive)

First responders can use various sources or clues to detect the presence of hazardous materials and determine the products involved. They should know how to safely approach a hazardous-materials incident to identify materials and determine their hazards while minimizing risk of exposure and contamination or adding a source of ignition.

Many hazardous materials behave in ways that can give notice of their presence to first responders. However, almost all of this behavior occurs after these materials have exited their containers or have been exposed to fire. Therefore, strange odors, vapor clouds, or noxious fumes are as much a signal to withdraw to a safe distance as they are a cause for further investigation. Emergency personnel should never intentionally expose themselves to odors or close-in views of product release. They must be observant and respond appropriately to any of the following conditions:

- Foul, unusual, or noxious odors. Some materials, such as hydrogen sulfide, paralyze the olfactory senses after a few whiffs.
- A vapor cloud caused by the refrigeration effect of a liquefied gas, such as propane, or a cryogenic liquid, such as liquid oxygen, boiling into a gas as they leave their containers (Fig. 12-1).
- Fumes, possibly from a spilled corrosive material, such as concentrated nitric acid, which emits brownish fumes.
- Irritation to the eyes, nose, and throat. Leaking chlorine or anhydrous ammonia can cause slight discomfort 1 minute and overwhelm or kill the next as the wind direction shifts and blows concentrated fumes toward emergency responders and bystanders.
- Unusually intense or large fires for the size of the building, vehicle, or container involved may be the only clue that hazardous materials are involved (Fig. 12-2).
- Fires that do not subside, or actually intensify, on application of water.

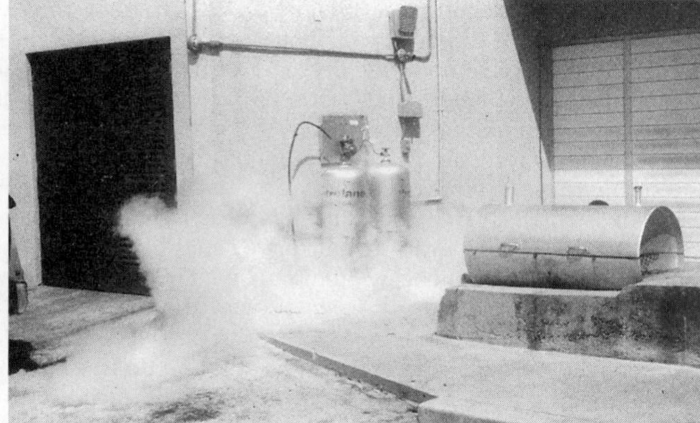

Figure 12-1. Vapor cloud caused by refrigeration effect of liquid propane. A dangerous situation of a leak involving a gas under pressure.

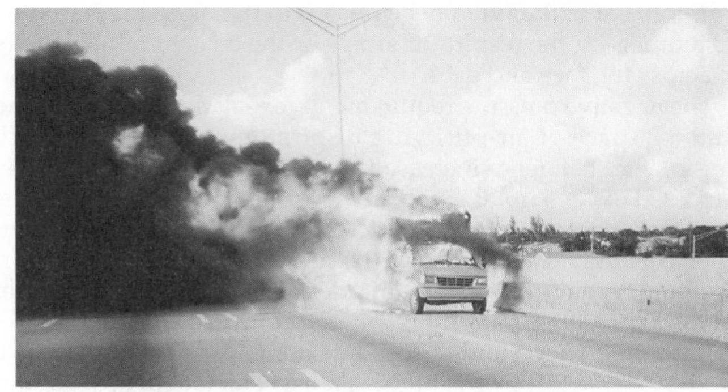

Figure 12-2. Intense fire in truck containing hazardous flammable paint and lacquer was the only clue that hazardous materials were involved.

- Loud, jet-like noise or jets of flame indicative of containers venting or relief devices operating to relieve rising internal pressures.
- Explosions.

Sometimes, emergency personnel are at the greatest risk when danger is not readily apparent. This is often the case with hazardous materials when police, fire, or emergency medical personnel have unknowingly exposed themselves to toxic, flammable, or explosive products. Loss of life involving hazardous materials has occurred when firefighters, who are generally well versed in hazard recognition and procedures, were unsure of a hazards presence and approached an incident as if it were a routine operation. Emergency rescue personnel must use extreme caution when approaching a person down for unknown reasons in a transportation or industrial setting, or they could become victims themselves of an unknown toxic material (Table 12-1).

Approaching the Scene

Wind direction and speed should be ascertained en route or at least at a great distance from the immediate scene. Wind direction has a great bearing on the direction of approach and positioning of responding units. Even the slightest breeze can be detected by discharging a small amount of chemical extinguishing agent into the air from a fire extinguisher. The following guidelines allow for a safe approach to a known or suspected hazardous materials scene:

- Approach the scene from upwind and uphill.

TABLE 12-1. Do's and don'ts for first responders

Do's of first responders
Do assess the situation and use best judgment.
Do park upwind, upgrade, pointing away from site and at a safe distance.
Do consult current *North American Emergency Response Guidebook*.
Do confirm that local authorities have been notified of the incident and that hazardous materials may be involved.
Don'ts of first responders
Do not drive through or walk through spilled materials.
Do not allow equipment to become contaminated.
Do not attempt rescue unless trained and properly equipped with appropriate personal protective equipment.
Do not become exposed by entering a contaminated area.
Do not attempt to recover shipping papers, manifests, or bills of lading unless adequately protected.

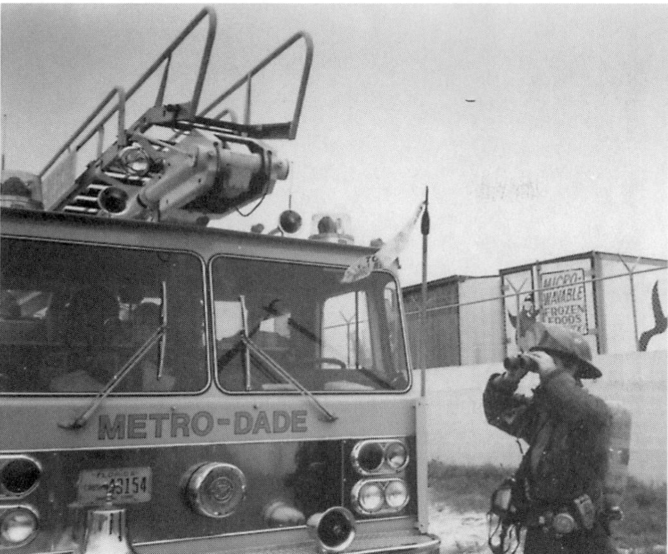

Figure 12-3. Fire department personnel assessing a hazardous scene with binoculars at a safe distance. Note wind sock showing correct position for personnel to be in (upwind).

- Stop at a safe distance and observe conditions (with binoculars, if necessary) before approaching the immediate scene (Fig. 12-3).
- Position the vehicle so that it is heading away from the scene in case sudden retreat is necessary.
- Approach the scene, on foot, with extreme caution. A vehicle's catalytic converter operates at a minimum of 1,200°F, a sufficient temperature to ignite all flammables.
- Approach the scene with a minimum number of personnel to conduct the initial assessment. Keep other responding units staged at a safe distance outside the hazard area.
- Use protective equipment. Obviously, units not equipped with protective clothing and self-contained breathing apparatuses are not able to safely intervene in an incident to the extent that a properly protected unit can.

Initial Action after Arriving at Scene

A decision to withdraw and wait for more qualified responders is based on conditions, level of protective equipment required, and collective level of expertise of those on the scene. Understand limitations of personnel at the scene. The safest and most prudent action for first responders may be to do nothing except to evacuate the area and isolate the scene. Direct involvement in an incident should be preceded by the question: Would the outcome of this incident be any different if we did nothing? With these points in mind, responding personnel should protect themselves and others by adhering to the following:

- Isolate the scene and deny entry to bystanders, unprotected responders, and responders who do not have a definite mission in the hazard area.
- Control traffic without the use of flares. Do not add another source of ignition.
- Eliminate sources of ignition, but do not start vehicles or operate electrical switch-gear in the hazard area.
- Post a wind sock and plan for a sudden change in wind direction. A small flag or a piece of police line taped on an antenna or post does the job (see Fig. 12-3).
- Plan for sudden ignition of spilled or leaking materials. Assign standby positions on dry chemical fire extinguishers and foam hose lines.
- Do not walk or drive through spilled material or enter a vapor cloud.
- Perform rescues only at an acceptable level of risk to rescuers and with realistic chances for success.
- Attempt to identify the materials involved through placards, markings, labels, shipping papers, and information received from a driver or plant personnel.

Dangers of Confined Spaces

Emergency medical personnel face a very dangerous and often insidious situation when they are called on to rescue a person found unconscious in a confined space. A *confined space* is defined as an enclosure with a restricted means of entry and exit that is not normally occupied but can be entered temporarily for maintenance, repair, cargo moving, and so on.

Many case histories exist of rescuers who themselves became victims when they succumbed to the effects of a toxic or oxygen-deficient atmosphere in a confined space. Rescuers should suspect oxygen deficiency and protect themselves from toxic or flammable gases within confined spaces. The removal of an unconscious or incoherent patient from a confined space requires special training, breathing apparatus, and devices to detect and monitor the presence of toxic or flammable gases. Confined spaces that can be immediately dangerous to life and health include

1. Interior of tanks, vats, bins, or silos (Fig. 12-4)
2. Inside boilers and industrial ovens
3. The hold of a ship contaminated with carbon monoxide, spilled chemicals, or leaking refrigerant gases
4. Cargo trailers and boxcars contaminated with leaking chemicals or fumigated with pesticides
5. Refrigerated trucks and rail cars filled with oxygen-excluding refrigerant gases
6. Below-grade utility holes, cable vaults, and sewers that are oxygen deficient and toxic from organic decomposition

Symptoms of Chemical Exposure

Emergency medical personnel with prior knowledge of an occupancy or mode of transport involved with hazardous materials are more likely to interpret any unusual signs exhibited by a patient as signs of possible exposure to hazardous chemicals. Immediate measures must be taken to protect rescuers from exposure, determine the material involved, and decon-

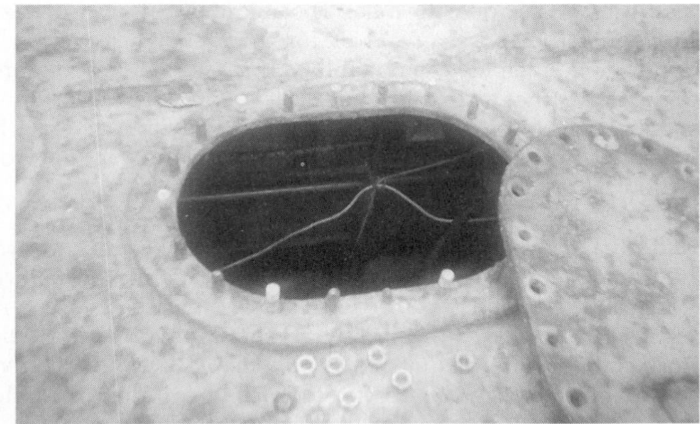

Figure 12-4. Confined space that could be O_2 deficient.

taminate the patient before admission to a hospital emergency department (1).

IDENTIFYING POTENTIALLY HAZARDOUS SITES

Marking and labels are just two of many indicators of the presence of hazardous materials. But it would be foolish to determine the strategy at a hazardous-materials incident solely on the information provided by a sign or label. Markings, labeling, and documentation regulations have limitations. National Fire Academy courses on hazardous materials detail several clues or indicators for detecting the presence of hazardous materials that first responders should look for before they intervene in an incident (2):

1. Prior knowledge of an occupancy, processes, reactions, and contents of the site or business
2. Facility inventory documents and Material Safety Data Sheets (MSDSs)
3. Placards and labels
4. Shipping papers
5. Container markings and colors
6. Shape and design of container
7. Other indications (i.e., visual, odors)

Occupancy and Location

When the subject of hazardous materials is discussed, many emergency response personnel tend to conjure up thoughts of exotic chemicals with long, multisyllabic names. Actually, the vast majority of hazardous-materials incidents involves common hydrocarbon gas and liquid fuels, solvents, and corrosives. The garage in a typical American home is replete with a variety of chemical hazards: gasoline, solvents, pesticides, propane cylinders, acids, and oxidizing swimming pool chemicals. Multiplying the contents of the average home by 10,000 gives some indication of the inventory of potential hazards in stock at a local hardware store or home improvement center.

The degree of danger to which emergency response personnel are exposed is often in inverse proportion to the amount of knowledge they have of the presence of hazardous materials at a particular occupancy. To illustrate the point, consider the clandestine drug laboratory. The operation dangerously and illegally stores, uses, and disposes of toxic, flammable, and corrosive substances, often in the garage or basement of a house in a quiet residential neighborhood. Each designer drug requires different chemicals for its production. A typical illegal laboratory uses large quantities of acetone, ether, and hydrochloric acid in the manufacturing or refining process and often disposes of these volatile materials down the toilet. The unknown presence of hazardous materials poses great risk for emergency responders if they do not anticipate the possibility. If emergency responders are not aware that hazardous materials are present, they cannot protect themselves. Expect large amounts of hazardous materials and chemicals to be found where they are involved in production, storage, use, and transportation.

PRODUCTION

Sites that manufacture or process hazardous materials are likely candidates for hazardous materials releases and emergencies. Production of hazardous materials involves ingredients, catalysts, intermediate compounds, and byproducts that may be more dangerous than the finished product. In some respects, however, an incident at a facility that is known to produce hazardous materials may be less dangerous for emergency personnel than at a site where the presence of hazardous materials is unknown. For example, firefighters and medics responding to a report of a fire or unconscious person at the Apex Chemical Company would naturally suspect that hazardous materials could be involved and approach the incident from its onset as a hazardous-material emergency. Additionally, plant personnel, familiar with their products and processes, may be available or can be summoned to the facility to offer technical information on hazards and advice on how to mitigate the situation. A word of caution, however: Information provided by employees or management of facilities must be considered with cautious skepticism and should be verified because it may be incomplete or inaccurate. Experience teaches that plant personnel have a tendency to understate the hazards of their products.

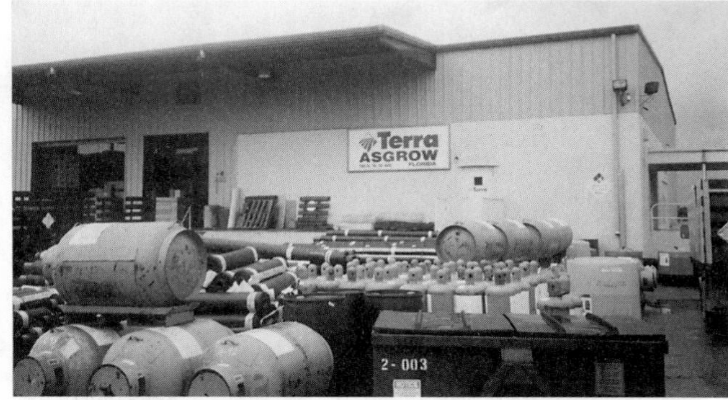

Figure 12-5. Agricultural chemical warehouse showing methylbromide tanks outside with flammable substances and insecticides inside.

STORAGE

Examples of storage facilities include bulk plants and tank farms containing petrochemicals; chemical distributors storing corrosives, oxidizers, flammable solvents, pressurized gases, and insecticides; and bonded warehouses storing large inventories of liquor (Fig. 12-5).

Many warehouses store large quantities of flammable, poisonous, and corrosive liquids in one of the most common yet potentially dangerous containers: the 55-gallon drum (Fig. 12-6). The widespread use and familiar presence of drum storage should not lull public and corporate safety personnel into a sense of complacency. Fifty-five–gallon drums have caused or contributed to many hazardous-materials spills, fires, and explosions because of

1. Their vulnerability to puncture and release of contents by accidental penetration by a forklift or other mechanical damage. Tests conducted with drums filled with 55 gallons of water revealed that a punctured drum spills its contents over 1,200 square feet of level surface.
2. The absence of pressure relief devices. When drums are exposed to heat, rising internal pressures have no way to escape. Drums give no clear and reliable indication of an impending explosion, which results from excessive pressure and the failure of the container.

USE

Facilities that use chemicals in manufacturing, processes, or reactions have the potential for a hazardous release or other accident. This grouping refers to handling of hazardous materials on a consumable basis. Listed below are sites where I have responded to hazardous-material emergencies:

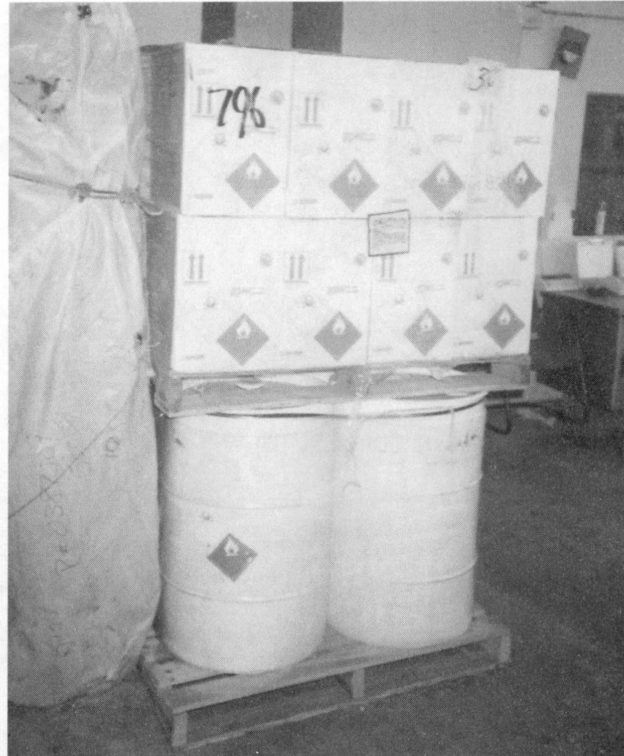

Figure 12-6. Storage of flammable, toxic material with 55-gallon drums. These drums are one of the most common yet potentially dangerous containers if punctured or exposed to fire.

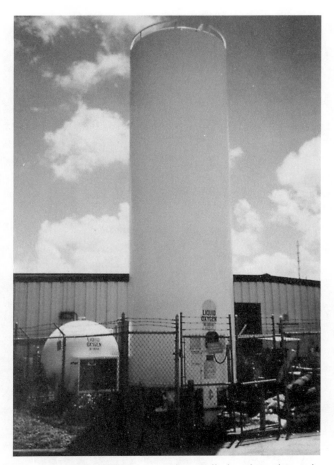

Figure 12-8. Liquid oxygen storage tank typically found near hospitals.

1. Home: Improper mixing of cleaning agents or drain cleaners producing toxic fumes; fires resulting from contamination of oxidizing swimming pool chemicals; explosion of 20-lb propane cylinder.
2. Office: A blueprint duplication machine leaking toxic fumes of anhydrous ammonia.
3. Farm: Pesticides, oxidizers, and anhydrous ammonia (Fig. 12-7).
4. Schools: Old, unstable chemicals (e.g., ether) found in chemistry laboratories.
5. Health care: Infectious wastes, anesthetic gases, compressed gases, cryogenic oxygen, and ethylene oxide sterilizing gas (Figs. 12-8 and 12-9).

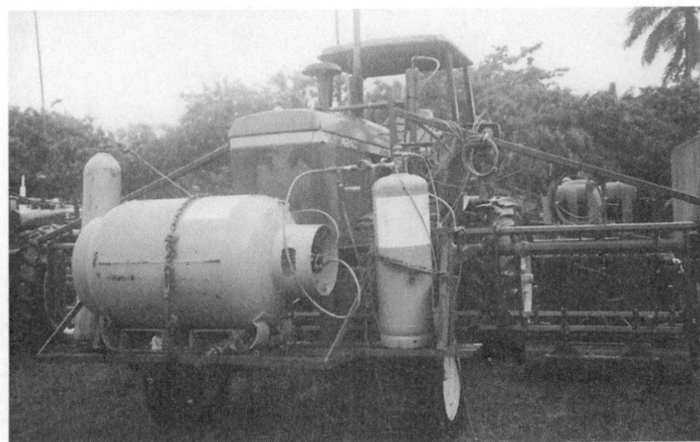

Figure 12-7. Tractor rigged with cylinders of methylbromide/chloropicrin for soil fumigation.

6. Swimming pools and water treatment plants using chlorine gas and strong oxidizing chemicals.
7. Industry: Relatively safe products, such as plastics and fiberglass boats, require large quantities of toxic, reactive, and flammable ingredients and catalysts in their manufacture (Fig. 12-10).
8. Auto repair: Fires involving flammable paints and solvents. Automotive repair shops have at least one set of oxygen and acetylene cylinders for welding and cutting (Fig. 12-11).
9. Cold storage warehouses: Leaks of anhydrous ammonia refrigerant gas.
10. Construction: Blasting for excavation involves blasting agents, such as ammonium nitrate, fuel-oil mixture, and explosive-detonating devices (Fig. 12-12).

PREVENTIVE MEASURES

The best way to deal with hazardous materials in production, storage, and use is before an incident occurs. Progressive emergency medical service, fire, and rescue services prepare for incidents at fixed facilities by

- Conducting preplan surveys and inspections
- Developing preincident plans with plant personnel and all responding agencies
- Developing a system for quick retrieval of MSDSs for each site and ensuring that facilities place their MSDSs in an easily accessible location
- Requiring by local law that facilities use a marking system for fixed installations (Fig. 12-13)

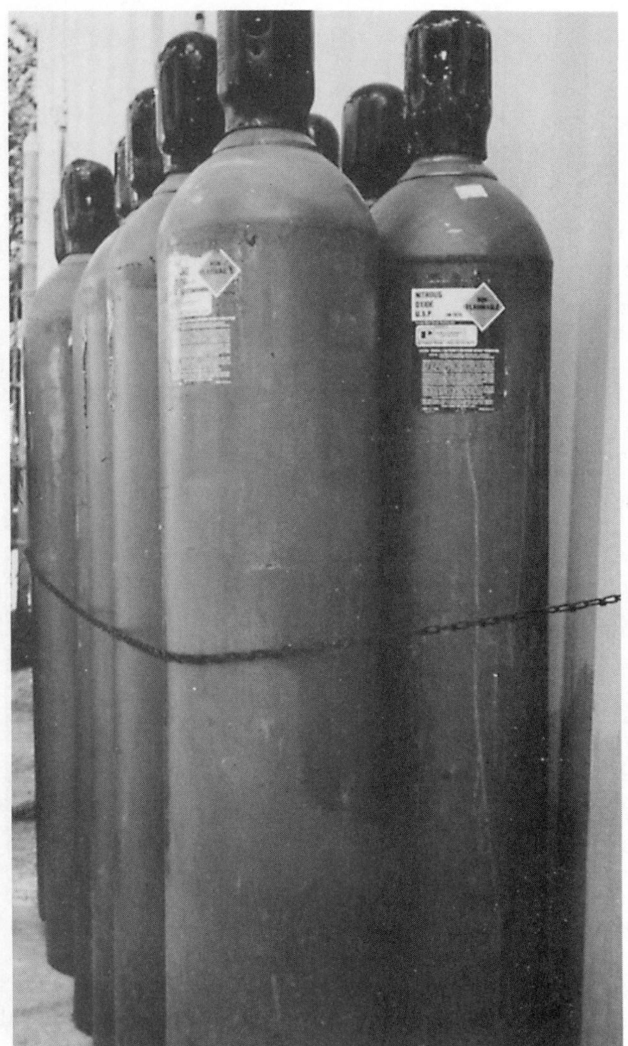

Figure 12-9. Compressed gas cylinders of nitrous oxide.

TRANSPORTATION

Industrialized countries, such as the United States, depend heavily on thousands of chemicals and materials with hazardous properties that are transported each day from producer to user, and, ultimately, to a waste-disposal facility. All but a very

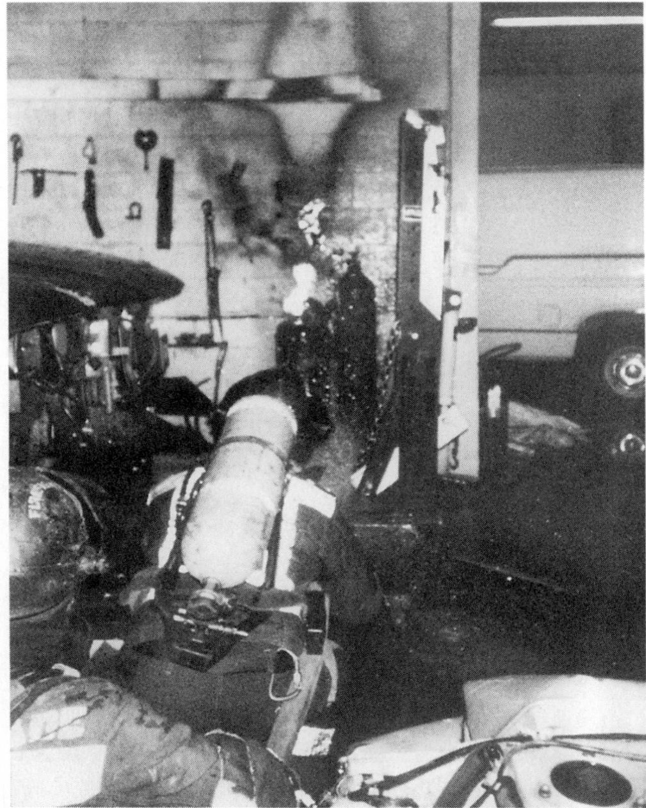

Figure 12-11. Firefighters apply stream of water to cool burning acetylene cylinder; a common hazard in auto repair shops.

few of these shipments reach their destination safely and without incident. This is partly because of regulations governing the transportation of hazardous materials.

In the United States, hazardous materials are defined, classified, and regulated by the U.S. Department of Transportation (DOT). The laws for transporting hazardous materials, which DOT administers and enforces, are detailed in Title 49 of the *Code of Federal Regulations* (49 *CFR*). Forty-nine *CFR* sections specify the types and quantities of substances that can be transported and requirements for packaging containers and transport vehicles. Additional sections list requirements for identifying hazardous materials in transit and providing emergency information to

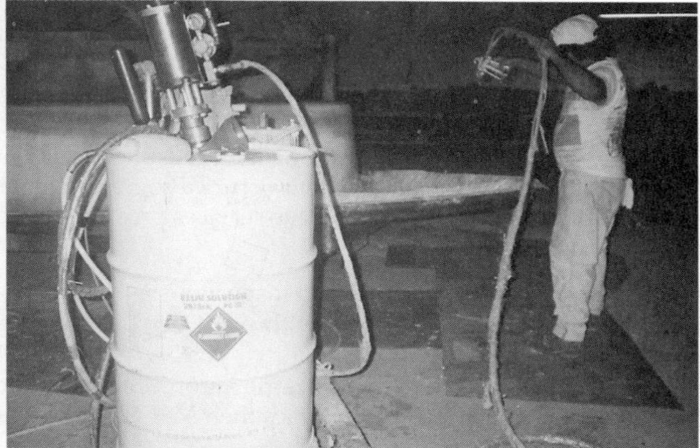

Figure 12-10. Fiberglass boat manufacturing dispensing flammable polyester resin from 55-gallon drum.

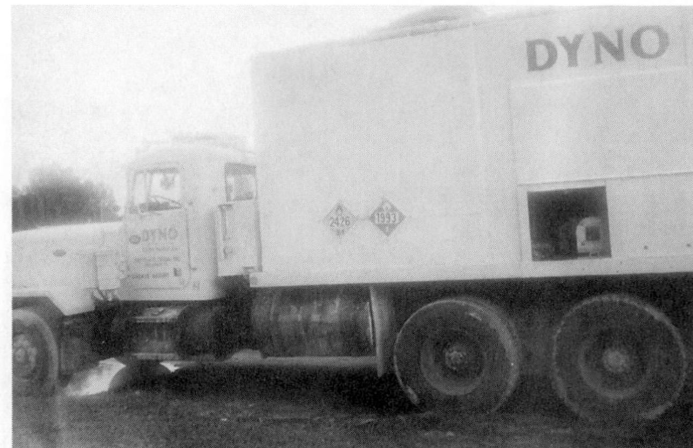

Figure 12-12. Truck dispenses mixture of ammonium nitrate and fuel oil blasting agents.

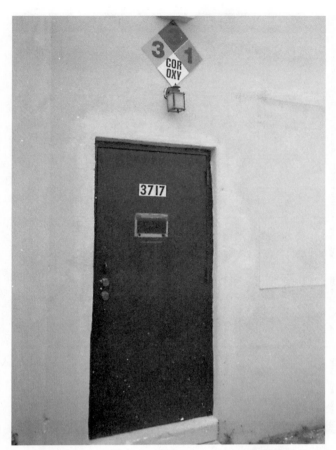

Figure 12-13. The presence of the National Fire Protection Association (NFPA) warning placard above the door indicates the presence of corrosive and oxidizing materials. The placard indicates that the building contains materials that are extremely dangerous to health, ignite at normal temperatures, or are unstable if heated.

assist response personnel in recognizing hazards and taking proper action to protect themselves and the public.

DEFINITIONS OF HAZARDOUS MATERIAL

DOT defines *hazardous material* as a substance or material, including a hazardous substance, hazardous waste, marine pollutant, or elevated-temperature material, that has been determined by the secretary of transportation to be capable of posing an unreasonable risk to health, safety, and property when transported in commerce, and that has been so designated. The U.S. Environmental Protection Agency (EPA), in conjunction with DOT, regulates the transportation of hazardous wastes and hazardous substances that could adversely affect the environment.

Regulations for international shipments of dangerous goods (hazardous materials) are developed by the UN. For example, international transport of hazardous materials by vessel must comply with standards written by the International Maritime Organization, an agency of the UN. DOT has revised its regulations for domestic shipments to bring them closer in line with UN standards. These changes are intended to simplify requirements and facilitate commerce and shipping in a global economy.

TRANSPORTATION OF HAZARDOUS MATERIALS

Transportation emergencies involving hazardous materials often are more dangerous than those at fixed facilities. The materials involved may be unknown. Warning signs may not be present or they may be obscured by rollover, smoke, or debris. The driver may be killed or incapacitated and unable to provide information. Additionally, the force of collision or rollover may cause incompatible substances to leak and react with each other, creating hazards that are worse than if each material was released separately.

Hazardous materials are transported by five basic modes: (a) roadway, (b) rail, (c) water, (d) air, or (e) pipeline. Emergency medical personnel should be prepared for the possibility of a patient being exposed and contaminated by a hazardous substance any time accidents involve railroad lines and rail yards, trucking and freight terminals, river and oceangoing vessels, or waterfront warehouses.

Shippers and emergency responders should recognize and understand hazardous material markings, labels, placards, and documentation. Emergency response personnel must be aware of the limitations of the placard and labeling system. They must attempt to verify data on product identification, hazards, and protection by seeking more than one source of information.

HAZARD CLASSIFICATION AND IDENTIFICATION NUMBERS

The UN and DOT assign hazardous materials to classes according to their primary, or most significant, hazard. Most of these hazard classes are further divided into divisions that have numerical decimal values (Fig. 12-14). Pressurized gases, for example, are in hazard class No. 2. This class is further broken down into division 2.1-flammable gas, 2.2-nonflammable nontoxic gas, and 2.3-toxic gases.

Hazardous materials also are assigned a four-digit identification number that must appear on shipping papers and packaging.

The hazard class of dangerous goods is indicated either by its class (or division) number or name. For a placard corresponding to the primary hazard class of a material, the hazard class or division number must be displayed in the lower corner of the placard. However, no hazard class or division number may be displayed on a placard representing the subsidiary hazard of a material. For other than Class 7 or the OXYGEN placard, text indicating a hazard (for example, "CORROSIVE") is not required. Text is shown only in the U.S. The hazard class or division number must appear on the shipping document after each shipping name.

Class 1 - Explosives
- Division 1.1 Explosives with a mass explosion hazard
- Division 1.2 Explosives with a projection hazard
- Division 1.3 Explosives with predominantly a fire hazard
- Division 1.4 Explosives with no significant blast hazard
- Division 1.5 Very insensitive explosives; blasting agents
- Division 1.6 Extremely insensitive detonating articles

Class 2 - Gases
- Division 2.1 Flammable gases
- Division 2.2 Non-flammable, non-toxic* compressed gases
- Division 2.3 Gases toxic* by inhalation
- Division 2.4 Corrosive gases (Canada)

Class 3 - Flammable liquids (and Combustible liquids [U.S.])

Class 4 - Flammable solids; Spontaneously combustible materials; and Dangerous when wet materials
- Division 4.1 Flammable solids
- Division 4.2 Spontaneously combustible materials
- Division 4.3 Dangerous when wet materials

Class 5 - Oxidizers and Organic peroxides
- Division 5.1 Oxidizers
- Division 5.2 Organic peroxides

Class 6 - Toxic* materials and Infectious substances
- Division 6.1 Toxic* materials
- Division 6.2 Infectious substances

Class 7 - Radioactive materials

Class 8 - Corrosive materials

Class 9 - Miscellaneous dangerous goods
- Division 9.1 Miscellaneous dangerous goods (Canada)
- Division 9.2 Environmentally hazardous substances (Canada)
- Division 9.3 Dangerous wastes (Canada)

Figure 12-14. Hazard classification system from the *North American Emergency Response Guidebook*. *The words *poison* or *poisonous* are synonymous with the word *toxic*.

U.S. Department of Transportation
Research and Special Programs Administration

DOT CHART 10

Hazardous Materials Marking, Labeling & Placarding Guide

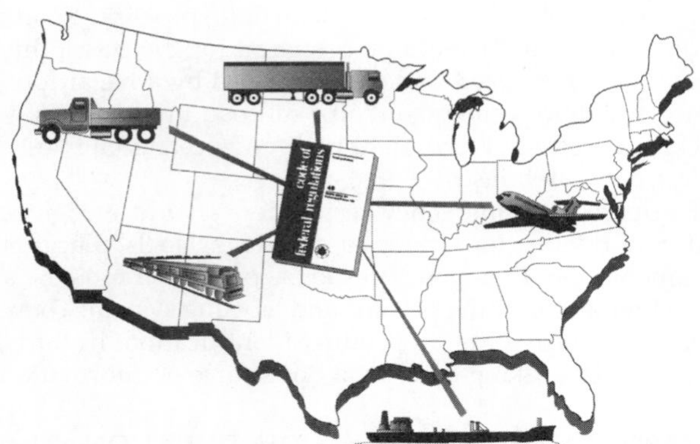

Refer to 49 CFR, Part 172:

Marking - Subpart D

Labeling - Subpart E

Placarding - Subpart F

Emergency Response - Subpart G

NOTE: **This document is for general guidance only and must not be used to determine compliance with 49 CFR, Parts 100-199.**

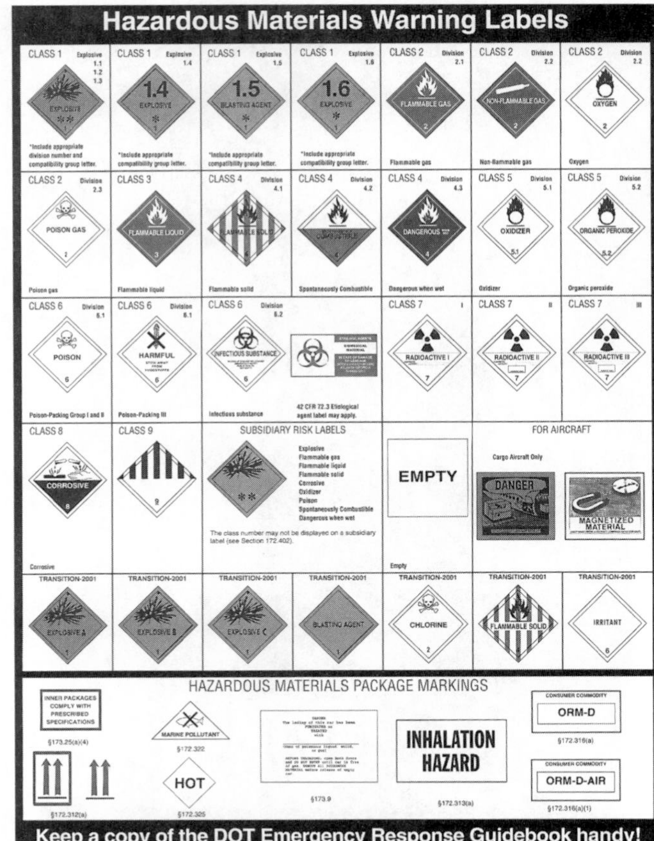

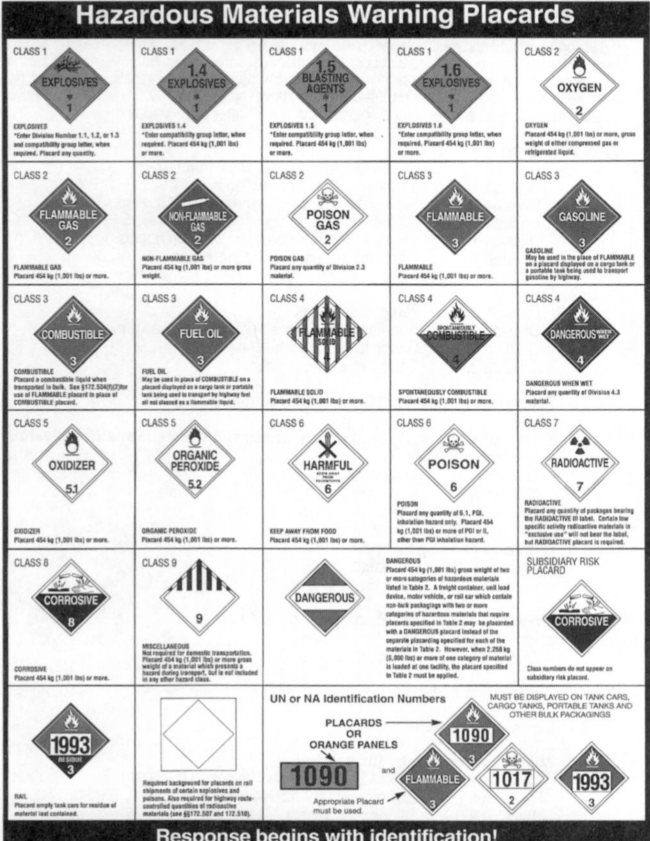

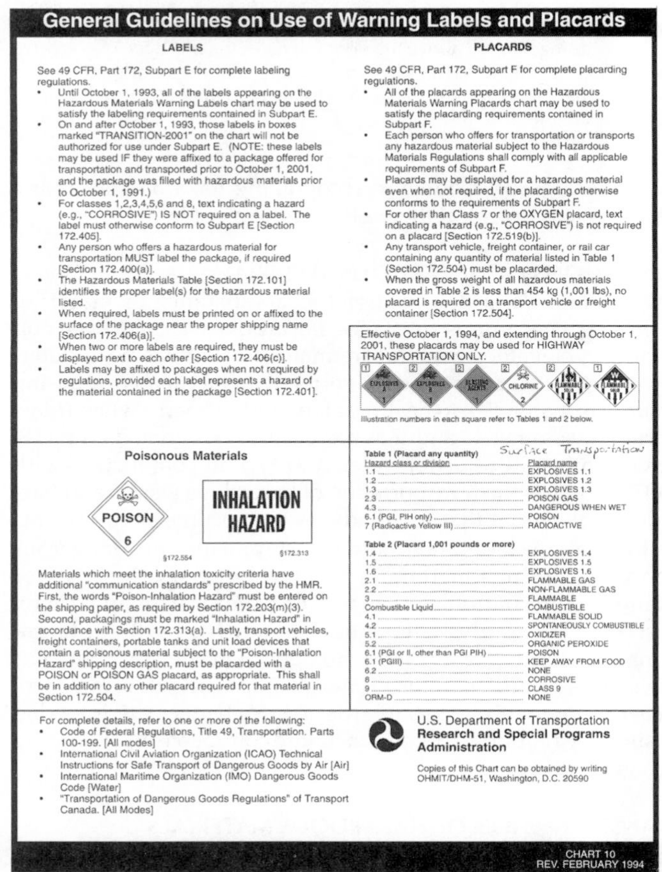

General Guidelines on Use of Warning Labels and Placards

LABELS

See 49 CFR, Part 172, Subpart E for complete labeling regulations.

- Until October 1, 1993, all of the labels appearing on the Hazardous Materials Warning Labels chart may be used to satisfy the labeling requirements contained in Subpart E.
- On and after October 1, 1993, those labels in boxes marked "TRANSITION-2001" on the chart will not be authorized for use under Subpart E. (NOTE: these labels may be used IF they were affixed to a package offered for transportation and transported prior to October 1, 2001, and the package was filled with hazardous materials prior to October 1, 1991.)
- For classes 1,2,3,4,5,6 and 8, text indicating a hazard (e.g., "CORROSIVE") IS NOT required on a label. The label must otherwise conform to Subpart E [Section 172.405].
- Any person who offers a hazardous material for transportation MUST label the package, if required [Section 172.400(a)].
- The Hazardous Materials Table [Section 172.101] identifies the proper label(s) for the hazardous material listed.
- When required, labels must be printed on or affixed to the surface of the package near the proper shipping name [Section 172.406(a)].
- When two or more labels are required, they must be displayed next to each other [Section 172.406(c)].
- Labels may be affixed to packages when not required by regulations, provided each label represents a hazard of the material contained in the package [Section 172.401].

PLACARDS

See 49 CFR, Part 172, Subpart F for complete placarding regulations.

- All of the placards appearing on the Hazardous Materials Warning Placards chart may be used to satisfy the placarding requirements contained in Subpart F.
- Each person who offers for transportation or transports any hazardous material subject to the Hazardous Materials Regulations shall comply with all applicable requirements of Subpart F.
- Placards may be displayed for a hazardous material even when not required, if the placarding otherwise conforms to the requirements of Subpart F.
- For other than Class 7 or the OXYGEN placard, text indicating a hazard (e.g., "CORROSIVE") is not required on a placard [Section 172.519(b)].
- Any transport vehicle, freight container, or rail car containing any quantity of material listed in Table 1 (Section 172.504) must be placarded.
- When the gross weight of all hazardous materials covered in Table 2 is less than 454 kg (1,001 lbs), no placard is required on a transport vehicle or freight container [Section 172.504].

Effective October 1, 1994, and extending through October 1, 2001, these placards may be used for HIGHWAY TRANSPORTATION ONLY.

Illustration numbers in each square refer to Tables 1 and 2 below.

Poisonous Materials

Materials which meet the inhalation toxicity criteria have additional "communication standards" prescribed by the HMR. First, the words "Poison-Inhalation Hazard" must be entered on the shipping paper, as required by Section 172.203(m)(3). Second, packagings must be marked "Inhalation Hazard" in accordance with Section 172.313(a). Lastly, transport vehicles, freight containers, portable tanks and unit load devices that contain a poisonous material subject to the "Poison-Inhalation Hazard" shipping description, must be placarded with a POISON or POISON GAS placard, as appropriate. This shall be in addition to any other placard required for that material in Section 172.504.

Table 1 (Placard any quantity) Surface Transportation

Hazard class or division	Placard name
1.1	EXPLOSIVES 1.1
1.2	EXPLOSIVES 1.2
1.3	EXPLOSIVES 1.3
2.3	POISON GAS
4.3	DANGEROUS WHEN WET
6.1 (PGI, PIH only)	POISON
7 (Radioactive Yellow III)	RADIOACTIVE

Table 2 (Placard 1,001 pounds or more)

Hazard class or division	Placard name
1.4	EXPLOSIVES 1.4
1.5	EXPLOSIVES 1.5
1.6	EXPLOSIVES 1.6
2.1	FLAMMABLE GAS
2.2	NON-FLAMMABLE GAS
3	FLAMMABLE
Combustible Liquid	COMBUSTIBLE
4.1	FLAMMABLE SOLID
4.2	SPONTANEOUSLY COMBUSTIBLE
5.1	OXIDIZER
5.2	ORGANIC PEROXIDE
6.1 (PGI or II, other than PGI PIH)	POISON
6.1 (PGIII)	KEEP AWAY FROM FOOD
6.2	NONE
8	CORROSIVE
9	CLASS 9
ORM-D	NONE

For complete details, refer to one or more of the following:

- Code of Federal Regulations, Title 49, Transportation. Parts 100-199. [All modes]
- International Civil Aviation Organization (ICAO) Technical Instructions for Safe Transport of Dangerous Goods by Air [Air]
- International Maritime Organization (IMO) Dangerous Goods Code [Water]
- "Transportation of Dangerous Goods Regulations" of Transport Canada. [All Modes]

U.S. Department of Transportation
Research and Special Programs Administration

Copies of this Chart can be obtained by writing OHMIT/DHM-51, Washington, D.C. 20590

CHART 10
REV. FEBRUARY 1994

Figure 12-15. U.S. Department of Transportation (DOT) chart of hazardous materials marking, labeling, and placarding.

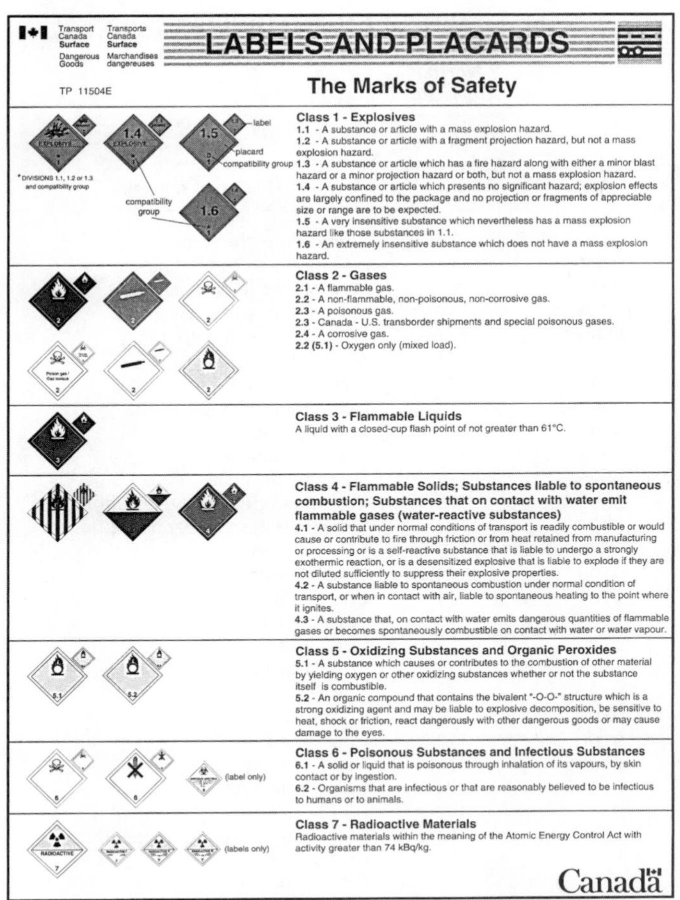

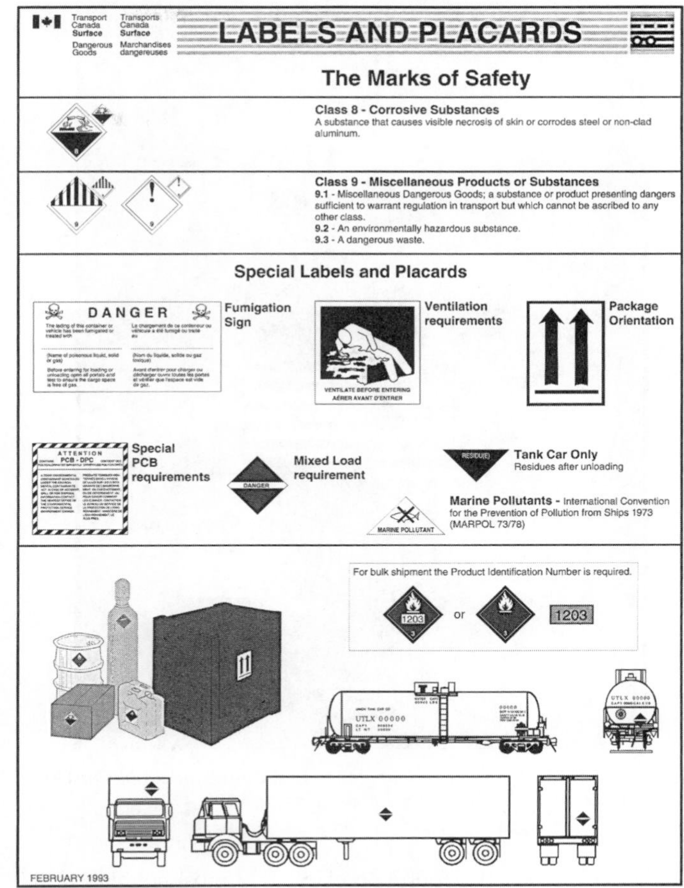

Figure 12-16. Canadian labels and placards.

Identification numbers for certain products may be required to be displayed on or beside placards on bulk-transport containers, such as tank vehicles and portable tanks (Figs. 12-15 through 12-17). An identification number with the prefix *UN* is authorized for international shipments. A number with the prefix *NA* (North America) means that the product is not recognized for international shipments, except between the United States and Canada.

The name of a hazardous material can be determined by referencing the product's identification number in the *North American Emergency Response Guidebook* (3). Developed jointly by the governments of Canada, the United States, and Mexico, the guidebook is intended to aid first responders in quickly identifying a product, determining its specific or generic hazards, and protecting themselves and the public during the initial response phases of a transportation incident. The guidebook may be of somewhat lesser value in application at fixed facility locations (Fig. 12-18). The publication contains two listings of chemicals, one indexed alphabetically and one in numerical order according to the UN/NA identification numbers of the chemicals (Table 12-2).

Each product is assigned a number for one of 62 guides that provide preliminary information on hazards, isolation, protective clothing, evacuation, initial action in case of fire or spill, and first aid (Fig. 12-19).

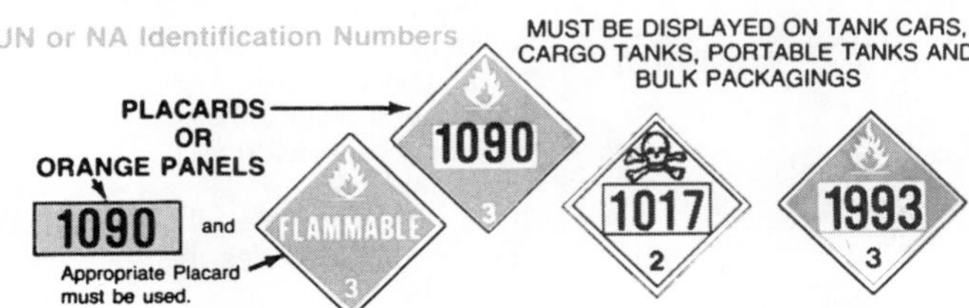

Figure 12-17. United Nations UN)/North American (NA) identification number.

PLACARDS

Placards are diamond-shaped signs displayed on the sides and ends of a truck, trailer, shipping container, or rail car. They indicate the presence of hazardous materials in a shipment and, with some notable exceptions, generally identify the type or nature of the hazard. Placards provide information in a number of ways (Figs. 12-20 through 12-22):

- Shape: A distinctive diamond shape "square on point," measuring 10.75 in.
- Colored background: Emergency responders should study placards to associate their colors with hazard classes. Color is definitely the first distinguishing characteristic of a placard to be visible. Color may be the only clue to identify a hazard if other features of a placard cannot be seen because of distance, damage, smoke, or vapor cloud (Fig. 12-23).
- Symbol in the top corner: These symbols graphically describe the hazard of a material. For example, a skull and crossbones would indicate a toxic hazard. It would be displayed on the top corner of placards for poisons.

Symbols are located in the top corner of placards and labels (Fig. 12-24). Text in English that indicates the hazard (e.g., "Flammable

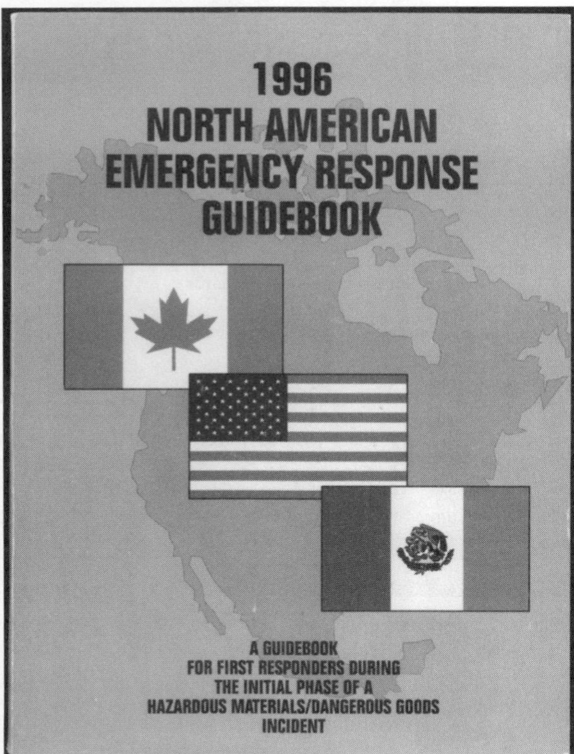

Figure 12-18. *North American Emergency Response Guidebook* (NAERG) for first responders to a hazardous-materials site, 1996.

Gas" or "Corrosive") is found on placards of most nonbulk shipments within the United States. Other than "Radioactive" or "Oxygen" placards, DOT does not require text. It is not likely to be found on Canadian or other international placards.

UNITED NATIONS AND NORTH AMERICAN IDENTIFICATION NUMBERS

UN or NA identification numbers are found on or beside placards for shipments of hazardous materials in bulk. Bulk packaging includes containers or transport vehicles in which hazardous materials are loaded with no intermediate form of containment that have a capacity greater than 450 L (119 gallon) for liquids, a maximum net weight greater than 400 kg (822 lb), and a water capacity greater than 454 kg (1,000 lb) for a gas. Beside a standard placard, the four-digit identification number is displayed in an orange rectangle (Figs. 12-21 and 12-25). Placards also can be written in other languages, such as Spanish, yet the international symbols provide a clear warning (Fig. 12-26). Hazard classes 1 to 9 and their divisions also are displayed in the lower corner of labels and placards.

CONTAINER MARKINGS AND LABELS

Packaging for hazardous materials must bear the proper shipping name of its contents and UN/NA identification number. Combination packages (e.g., a cardboard carton containing plastic jugs of a liquid, hazardous material) must display orientation arrows (Fig. 12-27). Packaging, containers, and transport vehicles destined for shipment by vessel must display a marine pollutant mark if their contents meet criteria for marine pollutants.

Information found on packages containing pesticides and other chemicals used on the farm, lawn, and garden can be very valuable in identifying their ingredients and determining the type and degree of hazard they present. The words *caution*, *warning*, and *dan-*

TABLE 12-2. Hazard names

Identification No.	*North American Emergency Response Guidebook* No.	Name of material
9086	143	Ammonium chromate
9087	171	Ammonium citrate, dibasic
9088	154	Ammonium fluoborate
9089	171	Ammonium sulfamate
9089	171	Ammonium sulphamate
9090	171	Ammonium sulfite
9090	171	Ammonium sulphite
9091	171	Ammonium tartrate
9094	153	Benzoic acid
9095	171	*n*-Butyl phthalate
9096	171	Calcium chromate
9097	171	Calcium dodecylbenzenesulfonate
9097	171	Calcium dodecylbenzenesulphonate
9100	171	Chromic sulfate
9100	171	Chromic sulphate
9101	171	Chromic acetate
9102	171	Chromous chloride
9103	171	Cobaltous bromide
9104	171	Cobaltous formate
9105	171	Cobaltous sulfamate
9105	171	Cobaltous sulphamate
9106	171	Cupric acetate
9109	171	Cupric sulfate
9109	171	Cupric sulphate
9110	171	Cupric sulfate, ammoniated
9110	171	Cupric sulphate, ammoniated
9111	171	Cupric tartrate
9117	171	Ethylenediaminetetraacetic acid
9118	171	Ethylenediaminetetraacetic acid
9119	171	Ferric ammonium citrate
9119	171	Ferric ammonium oxalate
9120	171	Ferric fluoride
9121	171	Ferric sulfate
9121	171	Ferric sulphate
9122	171	Ferrous ammonium sulfate
9122	171	Ferrous ammonium sulphate
9125	171	Ferrous sulfate
9125	171	Ferrous sulphate
9126	171	Fumaric acid
9127	171	Isopropanolamine dodecylbenzene-sulfonate
9127	171	Isopropanolamine dodecylbenzene-sulphonate
9134	171	Lithium chromate
9137	171	Naphthenic acid
9138	171	Nickel ammonium sulfate
9138	171	Nickel ammonium sulphate
9139	171	Nickel chloride
9140	154	Nickel hydroxide
9141	154	Nickel sulfate
9141	154	Nickel sulphate
9142	171	Potassium chromate
9145	171	Sodium chromate
9146	171	Sodium dodecylbenzenesulfonate (branched chain)
9146	171	Sodium dodecylbenzenesulphonate (branched chain)
9147	171	Sodium phosphate, dibasic
9148	171	Sodium phosphate, tribasic
9149	171	Strontium chromate
9151	171	Triethanolamine dodecylbenzenesulfonate
9151	171	Triethanolamine dodecylbenzene-sulphonate

From ref. 3, with permission.

NAERG96 **Flammable Solids - Toxic and/or Corrosive** **GUIDE 134**

EMERGENCY RESPONSE

FIRE

Small Fires

- Dry chemical, CO_2, water spray or alcohol-resistant foam.

Large Fires

- Water spray, fog or alcohol-resistant foam.
- Move containers from fire area if you can do it without risk.
- Do not use straight streams.
- Do not get water inside containers.
- Dike fire control water for later disposal; do not scatter the material.

Fire involving Tanks or Car/Trailer Loads

- Fight fire from maximum distance or use unmanned hose holders or monitor nozzles.
- Cool containers with flooding quantities of water until well after fire is out.
- Withdraw immediately in case of rising sound from venting safety devices or discoloration of tank.
- ALWAYS stay away from the ends of tanks.

SPILL OR LEAK

- Fully encapsulating, vapor protective clothing should be worn for spills and leaks with no fire.
- ELIMINATE all ignition sources (no smoking, flares, sparks or flames in immediate area).
- Stop leak if you can do it without risk.
- Do not touch damaged containers or spilled material unless wearing appropriate protective clothing.
- Prevent entry into waterways, sewers, basements or confined areas.
- Use clean non-sparking tools to collect material and place it into loosely covered plastic containers for later disposal.

FIRST AID

- Move victim to fresh air. • Call emergency medical care.
- Apply artificial respiration if victim is not breathing.
- **Do not use mouth-to-mouth method if victim ingested or inhaled the substance; induce artificial respiration with the aid of a pocket mask equipped with a one-way valve or other proper respiratory medical device.**
- Administer oxygen if breathing is difficult.
- Remove and isolate contaminated clothing and shoes.
- In case of contact with substance, immediately flush skin or eyes with running water for at least 20 minutes.
- For minor skin contact, avoid spreading material on unaffected skin.
- Keep victim warm and quiet.
- Effects of exposure (inhalation, ingestion or skin contact) to substance may be delayed.
- Ensure that medical personnel are aware of the material(s) involved, and take precautions to protect themselves.

Figure 12-19. Guide page from *North American Emergency Response Guidebook* shows typical information about hazards.

ger in the precautionary statements indicate the relative degree of toxicity. *Caution* indicates a relatively low toxic hazard, *warning* indicates moderate toxicity, and *danger* indicates a substance with a high level of toxicity (Fig. 12-28). Packages of pesticides and agricultural chemicals also display information for first-aid treatment and emergency phone numbers through which physicians and emergency responders can obtain additional information on the product. In addition to a list of ingredients found on the labels, all pesticides and agricultural chemicals sold in the United States display an EPA registration number that can assist emergency response personnel, poison control centers, and physicians in accurately identifying the product.

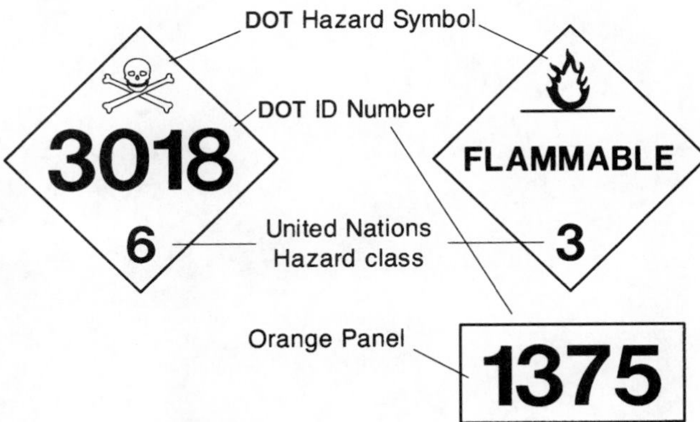

Figure 12-20. Components of a vehicle placard. DOT, Department of Transportation.

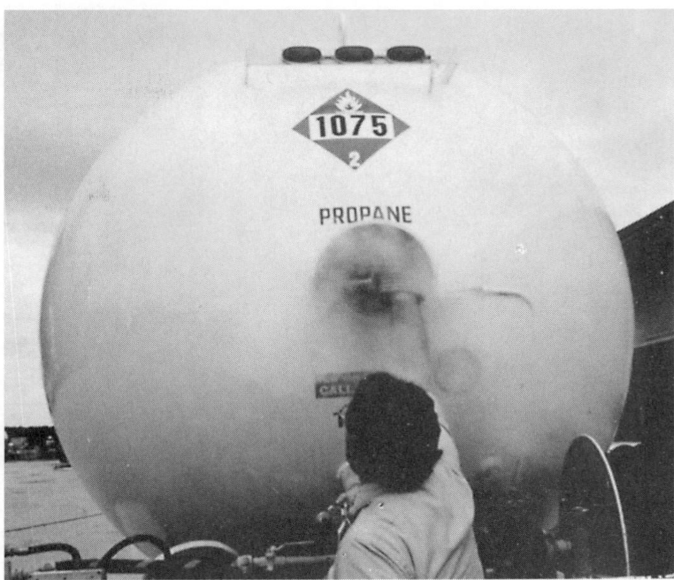

Figure 12-21. Placard on pressurized propane tank has United Nations/North American identification number 1075 in the center. Note the U.S. Department of Transportation symbol for flammable gas at the top.

LABELS

Hazardous-material labels are 4-in. versions of placards that are attached to packages and nonbulk containers (e.g., 55-gallon drums). The labels display the same colors and figures as placards do. They must appear on packages next to the proper shipping name and UN/NA identification number. Labels on compressed gas cylinders may be attached with a tag because of the irregular shape of the containers (Fig. 12-29). Although text is often found on labels used for domestic shipments, (e.g., "Corrosive"), it is not required on labels for hazard classes 1, 2, 3, 4, 5, 6, and 8. It is not likely to be found on labels from other countries.

REQUIREMENTS FOR LABELS AND PLACARDS

First responders must not assess the degree of hazard or attempt to identify specific hazardous materials solely on the current DOT

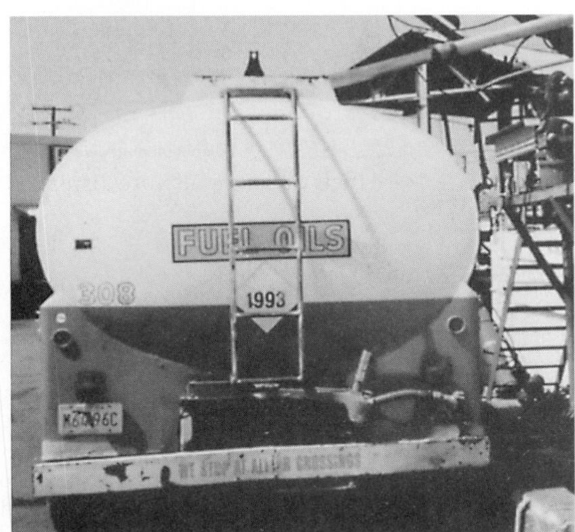

Figure 12-22. Flammable liquid placard with red background bleached by sunlight shows the United Nations/North American identification numbering on tanker trucks.

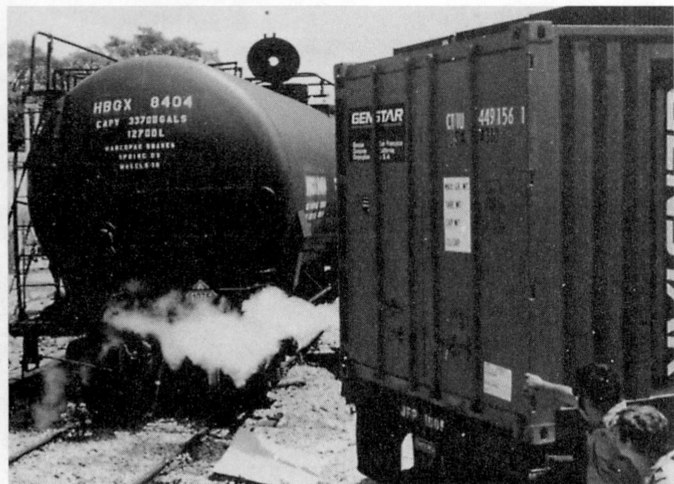

Figure 12-23. Placard partially obscured by vapor cloud.

placard and labeling system. A study of 49 *CFR* reveals that not every hazardous material is placarded or labeled every time, on every container, and in every mode of transport. But seven hazard classes and divisions of material require a placard for any quantity:

Hazard class/division	Placard name
1.1	Explosives 1.1
1.2	Explosives 1.2
1.3	Explosives 1.3
2.3	Poison gas
4.3	Dangerous when wet
6.1	Poison: Inhalation hazard

UN ID Number	DOT Symbol	Hazard Class
1		Explosives
2		Gases
3		Flammable liquids
4		Flammable solids Spontaneously combustible materials Materials dangerous when wet
5		Oxidizers Organic peroxides
6		Poisonous materials
		Biohazard
7		Radioactive materials
8		Corrosives
9		Other regulated materials

Figure 12-24. U.S. Department of Transportation (DOT) hazard symbols describing hazard class in terms of the nature of the hazard and the United Nations (UN) identification number.

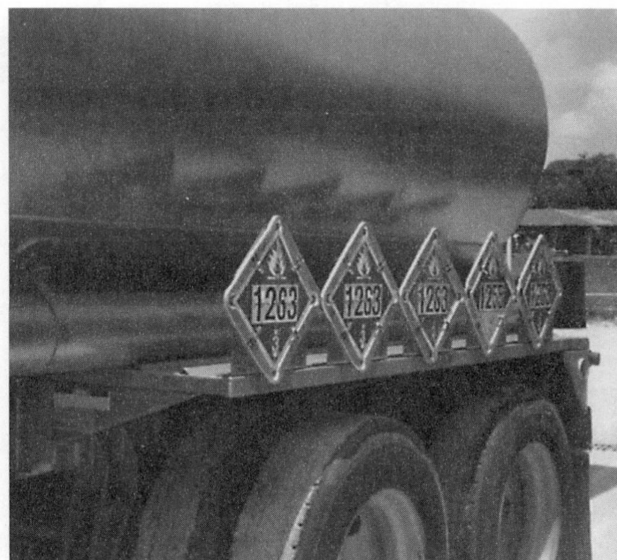

Figure 12-25. A liquid tanker capable of transporting five separate liquids due to compartmentalization. Each liquid requires a separate placard.

All other materials require a placard only when 454 kg (1,001 lb) is transported. As a result, emergency personnel may approach an overturned or burning truck with no outward indication that it is carrying 1,000 lb of flammable, poisonous, corrosive, or oxidizing materials. DOT also does not require placards or labels on combustible liquids shipped in nonbulk packaging or small containers, such as lighter fluid, regardless of their quantity.

SUBSIDIARY RISK LABELS AND PLACARDS

Materials may present more than one hazard. For example, a toxic insecticide also may be a flammable liquid. Corrosive materials that present a threat to the skin also may be toxic if its vapors are inhaled. If a material meets the criteria for more than one hazard, the additional or subsidiary hazards should be indicated after the primary hazard on the shipping papers. Subsidiary hazards must be indicated by an additional label on packages. For

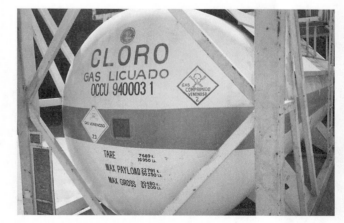

Figure 12-26. Intermodal tank containing chlorine, United Nations No. 1017. Note placard in Spanish.

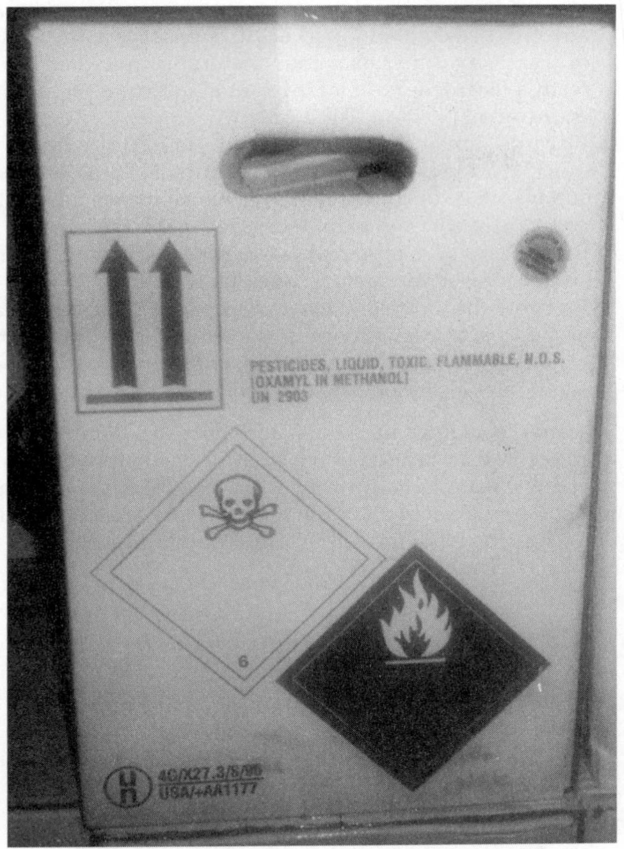

Figure 12-27. Pesticide packaging bearing United Nations/North American identification number with orientation arrows showing poison label with subsidiary flammable label.

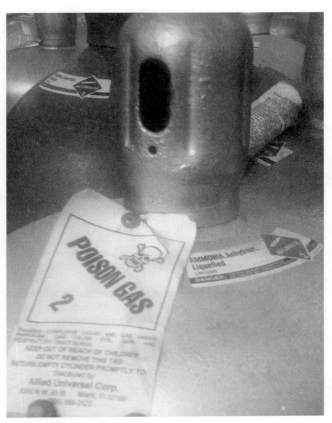

Figure 12-29. Anhydrous ammonia cylinder displays tag indicating poison gas for international shipment.

PRECAUTIONARY STATEMENTS
HAZARDS TO HUMANS & DOMESTIC ANIMALS

DANGER: Causes irreversible eye damage. Do not get in eyes. Wear goggles or face shield when handling concentrate. Harmful if swallowed or inhaled. Avoid contact with skin or clothing. Avoid breathing spray mist. Wash thoroughly after handling. Do not graze animals around treated trees or feed foliage or fruit to animals. **FIRST AID:** In case of eye contact, flush eyes immediately with fresh water for at least 15 minutes and see a doctor. If on Skin – Wash with plenty of soap and water. If Swallowed – Give water or milk to drink and telephone for medical advice. **DO NOT** make person vomit unless directed to do so by medical personnel. If medical advice cannot be obtained, then take person and product container to the nearest medical emergency treatment center or hospital. **Note to Physicians:** Emergency Information call 1-800-454-2333. **ENVIRONMENTAL HAZARDS:** Do not apply directly to water. Do not contaminate water by cleaning of equipment or disposal of wastes. **PHYSICAL OR CHEMICAL HAZARDS: FLAMMABLE.** Keep away from heat and open flame.

NOTICE: Buyer assumes all responsibility for safety and use not in accordance with directions.

Figure 12-28. Pesticide container label indicating "Danger" level of toxicity.

certain substances, a second placard on vehicles and shipping containers may be required. A material that is classified as having a subsidiary risk of toxicity by inhalation would be labeled and placarded "Poison" or "Poison Gas" in addition to being labeled and placarded for its primary hazard. Labels and placards indicating subsidiary hazards must appear next to the label or placard indicating the primary hazard but must not display a hazard class number in the lower corner (see Fig. 12-27).

MIXED SHIPMENTS

Regulations from DOT allow shipments of mixed loads of materials from different hazard classes to be placarded "Dangerous" instead of displaying two or more placards for the individual products being shipped (Fig. 12-30). But there are limits to when a "Dangerous" placard can be used. The seven classes and divisions of materials that require a placard at any quantity always take precedence. If 2,260 kg (5,000 lb) or more of one category of material is loaded at one facility, the placard specific to the hazard class must be used. First responders encountering a vehicle or container displaying the "Dangerous" placard should expect a mixed bag of goods and should examine the shipping papers to determine the exact materials involved.

LIMITATIONS OF PLACARDS AND LABELS AS AN IDENTIFICATION SYSTEM

The current DOT identification system has weaknesses. However, it was never intended to be an all-inclusive system for identifying every hazardous material in transit. The following is a summary of the weaknesses and limitations of the placard and label system:

1. Placard and label regulations apply only to materials in transit and may not be present at fixed facilities.

DANGEROUS
Placard 454 kg (1,001 lbs) gross weight of two or more categories of hazardous materials listed in Table 2. A freight container, unit load device, motor vehicle, or rail car which contain non-bulk packagings with two or more categories of hazardous materials that require placards specified in Table 2 may be placarded with a DANGEROUS placard instead of the separate placarding specified for each of the materials in Table 2. However, when 2,268 kg (5,000 lbs) or more of one category of material is loaded at one facility, the placard specified in Table 2 must be applied.

Figure 12-30. Explanation of dangerous placard for mixed loads.

2. Placards and labels indicate only the most significant hazards of a material, but not all of them. Gasoline, for example, is placarded only as a flammable liquid even though inhalation of gasoline vapors can cause dizziness, impaired mental acuity, and chemical pneumonia.
3. Materials have to meet narrow criteria to be placed in a specific hazard class. For example, DOT criteria classify anhydrous ammonia as a nonflammable gas because of its high upper explosive limit. But ammonia has fueled some deadly, devastating explosions after accumulating in a confined space.
4. Most mixed loads qualify for the "Dangerous" placard, which provides no outward indication of the hazards of the contents.
5. Shipments of most hazardous materials (except the seven mentioned previously in Requirements for Labels and Placards) do not require placards for less than 454 kg (1,001 lb). Nine hundred pounds of flammable liquids in a burning truck can be an unrecognized, life-threatening hazard for an unsuspecting first responder.
6. Labels are very small. The vehicle must be opened to observe them, and they are required on only one side of a package. This makes a label impossible to read if it is in the wrong position or blocked by other packages, as in a loaded semitrailer.
7. Narrowly written requirements based on container size may allow a substantial amount of flammable liquid to be unlabeled because it is in small containers (e.g., aerosol cans).

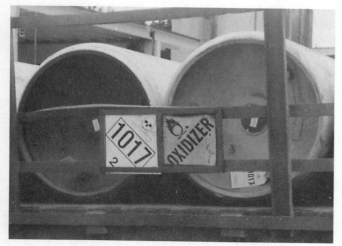

Figure 12-31. This truck is transporting 1-ton chlorine gas containers (United Nations No. 1017, Gas Class 2) and calcium hypochlorite (oxidizer). Note incorrect position of placards.

8. Hazardous-material shipments often are labeled and placarded incorrectly. Some surveys reveal that as many as 50% of trucks hauling hazardous materials are either incorrectly placarded, not placarded at all, or have placards in an incorrect position (Fig. 12-31).
9. Placards deteriorate from weather. Rain, dirt, and snow quickly obliterate cardboard placards. Several weeks of sun bleach colors out of placards, which makes them difficult to identify from a distance (see Fig. 12-22).
10. Placards can be obscured by darkness, rollover, debris, smoke, fire, or vapor cloud (see Fig. 12-23).
11. Probably the most significant weakness of labels and placards is that a responder must get dangerously close to the container or vehicle to read them. Often, if emergency personnel are close enough to read a placard, they are too close!

Placards, container markings, and shipping papers cannot give an accurate indication of what happens when two or more incompatible materials are mixed or come into contact with each other. The result can be the formation of more toxic or reactive materials, such as the mixture of aluminum phosphide and an acid, which releases phosphine gas.

MAKING THE MOST OF AN IMPERFECT SYSTEM

Placards and labels can be a very useful tool for hazard identification if emergency responders follow these guidelines:

1. Memorize the symbols and, more important, the colors of all placards and labels.
2. Practice sighting placards on trucks and trains. Look up the UN/NA identification number on vehicles and containers and find the material in the *North American Emergency Response Guidebook.*
3. Use binoculars to observe placards at a safe distance (see Fig. 12-3).

Shipping Papers

Transportation of hazardous materials must be documented on shipping papers that accompany a shipment to its destination. Shipping papers may be known by different names, depending on the mode of transportation. Because current regulations do not require placarding on most shipments of hazardous materials less than 454 kg (1,001 lb), shipping papers are the first clue of the presence of dangerous materials. Placards and labels provide only general information of the most significant hazards. They usually do not identify specific products. Shipping papers can help fill the void of information about the precise identification of materials, their quantity, specific hazards, and emergency action (Fig. 12-32).

Shipping papers must provide the following information:

1. Quantity and specific type of packaging. Examples: three drums, six boxes, one pail, three skids.
2. Proper shipping name.
3. Hazard class. If a material has a subsidiary risk, the secondary-class name and number follow the primary-hazard class. As examples, silicon tetrafluoride: Class 2.3, Poison gas (8); or silicon tetraflouride: Class 2.3, Poison gas (Corrosive). This would indicate that the product is in the primary-hazard class 2.3, poison gas, with a subsidiary hazard class 8, corrosive.
4. UN/NA identification number.
5. Packing group number. Classes 3, 4, 5, 6, 8, and 9 each have an assigned packing group (PG) that appears on the shipping

SHIPPING DOCUMENTS (PAPERS)*

The shipping document provides vital information when responding to a hazardous materials/dangerous goods** incident. The shipping document contains information needed to identify the materials involved. Use this information to initiate protective actions for your own safety and the safety of the public. The shipping document contains the proper shipping name (see blue-bordered pages), the hazard class or division of the material(s), ID number (see yellow-bordered pages), and, where appropriate, the Packing Group. In addition, there must be information available that describes the hazards of the material which can be used in the mitigation of an incident. The information must be entered on or be with the shipping document. This requirement may be satisfied by attaching a guide from the NAERG96 to the shipping document, or by having the entire guidebook available for ready reference. Shipping documents are required for most dangerous goods in transportation. Shipping documents are kept in

- the cab of the motor vehicle,
- the possession of the train crew member,
- a holder on the bridge of a vessel, or
- an aircraft pilot's possession.

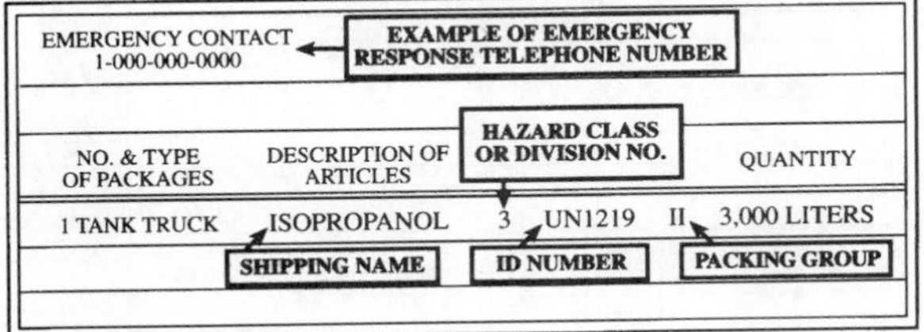

Figure 12-32. Inside cover of *North American Emergency Response Guidebook* shows shipping document.

papers. These groups are based on the level of danger presented by the materials. The PG classification numbers are

- PG I: Great danger
- PG II: Moderate danger
- PG III: Minor danger

6. Total weight.
7. Signature of the shipper certifying that the hazardous materials have been properly prepared for transportation in compliance with regulations.
8. Emergency response phone contact. This must be a phone contact that can provide information in the event of a spill, fire, or accident, such as CHEMTREC 1-800-424-9300.

Materials in divisions 2.3 (Poisonous gas) and 6.1 (Poison) may be toxic by inhalation. The regulations describe criteria for this classification that depends on the lethal concentration that kills 50% of test animals (LC_{50}) for the gas and LC_{50} and volatility for a 6.1 material. The words *inhalation hazard* must be part of the description on the shipping papers.

When a hazardous material is listed on a shipping paper along with nonhazardous goods, the hazardous materials must be

1. Entered first
2. Entered in a different color that clearly contrasts with the printing for nonhazardous entries
3. Identified by the entry of X or RQ (reportable quantity of hazardous substance, as regulated by EPA) in the hazardous material (HM) column, located to the left of the proper shipping name

COMPLIANCE WITH SHIPPING REGULATIONS

DOT and UN regulations governing the transport of hazardous materials often are confusing, virtually impossible to enforce, and constantly being revised. Consequently, vast differences exist between written regulations and their application in the field. As a practical matter, compliance with regulations governing the transport of hazardous materials depends largely on the competency and honesty of shippers and whether they accurately declare goods as hazardous materials.

Consider this scenario: A large resort in the Caribbean receives most of its supplies by ship from the United States. Its agent in Miami, Florida, purchases the supplies locally and loads them into 40-foot shipping containers that are taken by truck to a cargo vessel berthed on the Miami River. One shipment, consisting of several hundred pounds of oxidizing swimming pool chemicals, pesticides, propane, and acetylene cylinders, is loaded into one container with several bags of rice and flour. This load is clearly in violation of international marine shipping regulations: Flammables cannot be shipped in the same container with oxidizers. Poisons cannot be shipped with foodstuffs. This unscrupulous shipper identifies the entire load with some vague description as hotel supplies or household goods on the shipping paper. As much as the captain of the ship transporting the container technically has the responsibility to inspect and verify the contents of the container, it is impossible to open and examine each piece of freight in every container. Additionally, no one outside of U.S. Customs or the coast guard wants to break the seal that the shipper placed on the doors of the container and then incur the liability for goods that are reported missing. Imagine the danger and difficulties that the ship's crew, coast guard, and local fire department face when smoke or fumes begin issuing from the container.

Terra

GF36P DELIVERY TICKET BILL OF LADING 004972
MAIL TO:

SHIP TO: CUSTOMER ACCT #:
DELIVERY DATE:
SHIP VIA:

WAREHOUSE: HOMESTEAD-ORNAMENTAL SALESMAN:

QUANTITY ORDERED SHIPPED | PRODUCT DESCRIPTION PACKAGE DESC EPA #/LOT | SL CUST | SO # PO# | GROSS WT PRODUCT#

BIPYRIDILIUM PESTICIDES, LIQUID, TOXIC (CONTAINS PARAQUAT), 6.1, UN3016, PG II ERG GUIDE 55 OR ERG GUIDE 151
2.000 ________ *GRAMOXONE EXTRA 2-1/2 GAL 00 005268 50
5.000 GALLON 2.5 GALLONS 10182-280 63477422

CHLOROPICRIN AND METHYL BROMIDE MIXTURES, 2,3, UN1581,

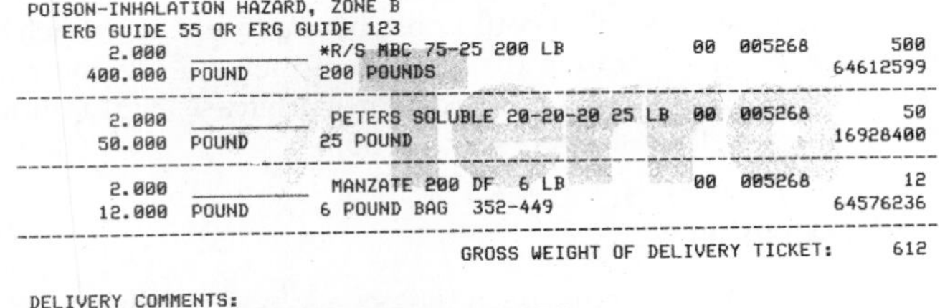

POISON-INHALATION HAZARD, ZONE B
ERG GUIDE 55 OR ERG GUIDE 123
2.000 ________ *R/S MBC 75-25 200 LB 00 005268 500
400.000 POUND 200 POUNDS 64612599

2.000 ________ PETERS SOLUBLE 20-20-20 25 LB 00 005268 50
50.000 POUND 25 POUND 16928400

2.000 ________ MANZATE 200 DF 6 LB 00 005268 12
12.000 POUND 6 POUND BAG 352-449 64576236

GROSS WEIGHT OF DELIVERY TICKET: 612

DELIVERY COMMENTS:
THIS IS NOT A TRUE ORDER FOR INFORMATION ONLY

*FOR RESALE ONLY

THIS IS TO CERTIFY THAT THE ABOVE NAMED MATERIALS ARE PROPERLY CLASSIFIED, DESCRIBED, PACKAGED, MARKED AND LABELED, AND ARE IN PROPER CONDITION FOR TRANSPORTATION, ACCORDING TO THE APPLICABLE REGULATIONS OF THE DEPARTMENT OF TRANSPORTATION.
SHIPPER SIGNATURE ________________ DATE ________

Figure 12-33. Bill of lading for truck delivery. Note *North American Emergency Response Guidebook* (*ERG Guide*) No. 55 on document as reference for hazmat response team in case of spill.

```
10/25/96                  Train Consist * FINAL *                      Page     1
13:48:40                                                               RSMTPFR

                CARS IN THIS TRAIN ARE COUNTED FROM FRONT TO REAR

---------------------------------------------------------------------------------
Originating Station 0366    Destination Station 0007     Train ID 0208
Conductor                   Engineer                  Trainman
Date 10/25/96  Time 13:00   Time Crew on Duty 12:30
---------------------------------------------------------------------------------

    ----Equip----                                       -----Destination----- Left-at
Seq Init Number    LE KD  Commodity   Consignee    Patron            Station Station

    FEC      431    O  D  LOCOS,ELEC .                                   0007    0007

    FEC      437    O  D  LOCOS,ELEC .                                   0007    0007

  1 CSXT 502734     E  A  **EMPTY**   JEFFERSON SM CSXT           JAC 0007    0007

  2 CSXT 130305     E  A  **EMPTY**   JEFFERSON SM CSXT           JAC 0007    0007

  3 TILX 300822     E  T  PETROLEUM   TEXACO       CSXT           JAC 0007    0007
     ***************************
     *                         *
     ***************************
     EMERGENCY CONTACT:
       8004249300
                                               1 Tank
                                               RESIDUE: LAST CONTAINED
                                               LIQUEFIED PETROLEUM GAS
                                               2.1
                                               UN1075
                                               HAZMAT STCC=4905752
                                               ****************************************
                                               ******************** END OF HAZMAT DATA

     TO/CONSIGNEE                              FROM/SHIPPER
     TEXACO                                    NATIONAL PROPANE
     NORCO                  LA                 MIAMI                  FL

  4 SOEX    3400    E  T  PETROLEUM   SHELL OIL CO CSXT           JAC 0007    0007
     ***************************
     *                         *
     ***************************
     EMERGENCY CONTACT:
       800-424-9300-0000
                                               1 Tank
                                               RESIDUE: LAST CONTAINED
                                               LIQUEFIED PETROLEUM GAS
                                               2.1
                                               UN1075
                                               HAZMAT STCC=4905752
                                               ****************************************
                                               ******************** END OF HAZMAT DATA

     TO/CONSIGNEE                              FROM/SHIPPER
     SHELL OIL COMPANY                         SYNERGY GAS
     MCELROY                LA                 MEDLEY                 FL
```

Figure 12-34. Train consist. Note that third and fourth cars from locomotive contain residues of liquid propane gas.

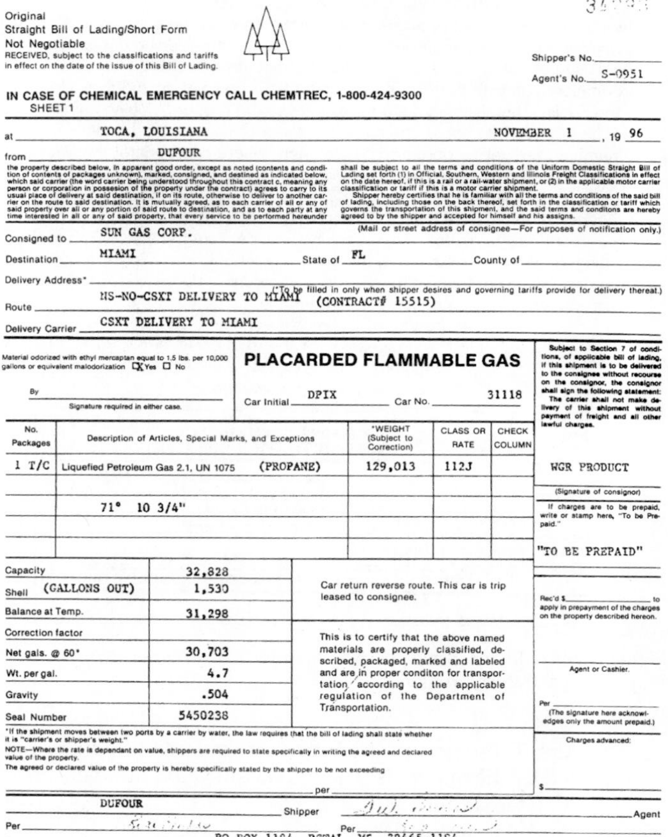

Original
Straight Bill of Lading/Short Form
Not Negotiable
RECEIVED, subject to the classifications and tariffs in effect on the date of the issue of this Bill of Lading.

Shipper's No. ______
Agent's No. S-0951

IN CASE OF CHEMICAL EMERGENCY CALL CHEMTREC, 1-800-424-9300
SHEET 1

at TOCA, LOUISIANA NOVEMBER 1, 19 96
from DUFOUR

the property described below, in apparent good order, except as noted (contents and condition of contents of packages unknown), marked, consigned, and destined as indicated below, which said carrier (the word carrier being understood throughout this contract c, meaning any person or corporation in possesion of the property under the contract) agrees to carry to its usual place of delivery at said destination, if on its route, otherwise to deliver to another carrier on the route to said destination. It is mutually agreed, as to each carrier of all or any of said property over all or any portion of said route to destination, and as to each party at any time interested in all or any of said property, that every service to be performed hereunder shall be subject to all the terms and conditions of the Uniform Domestic Straight Bill of Lading set forth (1) in Official, Southern, Western and Illinois Freight Classifications in effect on the date hereof, if this is a rail or a rail-water shipment, or (2) in the applicable motor carrier classification or tariff if this is a motor carrier shipment.
Shipper hereby certifies that he is familiar with all the terms and conditions of the said bill of lading, including those on the back thereof, set forth in the classification or tariff which governs the transportation of this shipment, and the said terms and conditons are hereby agreed to by the shipper and accepted for himself and his assigns.

Consigned to SUN GAS CORP. (Mail or street address of consignee—For purposes of notification only.)
Destination MIAMI State of FL County of ______
Delivery Address* ______ (*To be filled in only when shipper desires and governing tariffs provide for delivery thereat.)
Route NS-NO-CSXT DELIVERY TO MIAMI (CONTRACT# 15515)
Delivery Carrier CSXT DELIVERY TO MIAMI

Material odorized with ethyl mercaptan equal to 1.5 lbs. per 10,000 gallons or equivalent malodorization ☒ Yes ☐ No
By ______
Signature required in either case.

PLACARDED FLAMMABLE GAS
Car Initial DPIX Car No. 31118

Subject to Section 7 of conditions, of applicable bill of lading, if this shipment is to be delivered to the consignee without recourse on the consignor, the consignor shall sign the following statement:
The carrier shall not make delivery of this shipment without payment of freight and all other lawful charges.
WGR PRODUCT
(Signature of consignor)

No. Packages	Description of Articles, Special Marks, and Exceptions	*WEIGHT (Subject to Correction)	CLASS OR RATE	CHECK COLUMN
1 T/C	Liquefied Petroleum Gas 2.1, UN 1075 (PROPANE)	129,013	112J	
	71° 10 3/4"			

If charges are to be prepaid, write or stamp here, "To be Prepaid."
"TO BE PREPAID"

Capacity	32,828
Shell (GALLONS OUT)	1,530
Balance at Temp.	31,298
Correction factor	
Net gals. @ 60°	30,703
Wt. per gal.	4.7
Gravity	.504
Seal Number	5450238

Car return reverse route. This car is trip leased to consignee.

This is to certify that the above named materials are properly classified, described, packaged, marked and labeled and are in proper conditon for transportation according to the applicable regulation of the Department of Transportation.

Rec'd $ ______ to apply in prepayment of the charges on the property described hereon.
Agent or Cashier.
Per ______
(The signature here acknowledges only the amount prepaid.)
Charges advanced:
$ ______

*If the shipment moves between two ports by a carrier by water, the law requires that the bill of lading shall state whether it is "carrier's or shipper's weight."
NOTE—Where the rate is dependant on value, shippers are required to state specifically in writing the agreed and declared value of the property.
The agreed or declared value of the property is hereby specifically stated by the shipper to be not exceeding ______ per ______

DUFOUR Shipper ______ Agent
Per ______ Per ______
Permanent postoffice address of shipper PO BOX 1184 PETAL MS 39465-1184

NGL-103

Figure 12-35. Bill of lading.

Locating Shipping Papers

Shipping papers should be located and examined as soon as a close approach to an incident can be accomplished safely. A close approach to the scene may be impossible for the first responders because of fire, explosion, toxic fumes, and lack of proper protective equipment.

Truck Transport

Truck drivers hold the shipping papers, or bill of lading, for truck shipments. They may be stored in a holder, which is mounted to the inside of the door on the driver's side of the vehicle. When attempts to locate the bill of lading beside the driver are unsuccessful, it could possibly be found: (a) attached to packages in the trailer, (b) on the engine cover in the cab, (c) on the dashboard, (d) in the driver's briefcase, or (e) under the mattress in the "sleeper" (Fig. 12-33).

Rail Transport

Rail shipping papers must be in the possession of the train crew. If the train has a caboose, they would be in the possession of the conductor at the end of the train. The papers are found in the engine for trains without cabooses. The train crew should furnish two types of shipping papers. The first is the train consist or wheel report. This computer printout lists all the cars as they appear in the train beginning with the lead engine, a general description of each car's contents (e.g., merchandise, compressed gas), and whether the car is carrying a hazardous material. The consist is valuable in a derailment situation for piecing together cars and their contents when several have left the track (Fig. 12-34). The second document is the waybill or bill of lading for individual rail cars (Fig. 12-35). The waybill provides all required information. It also must mention the residue of the last hazardous product carried in any empty tank cars (Fig. 12-36). Content

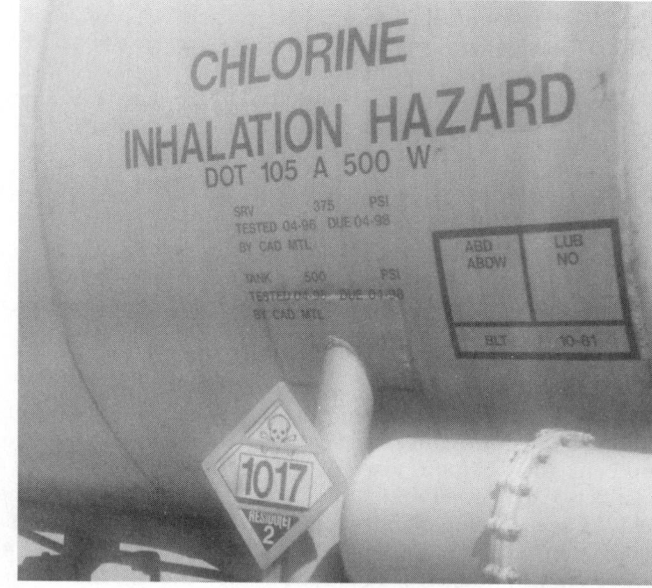

Figure 12-36. "Empty" chlorine tank car with residue placard.

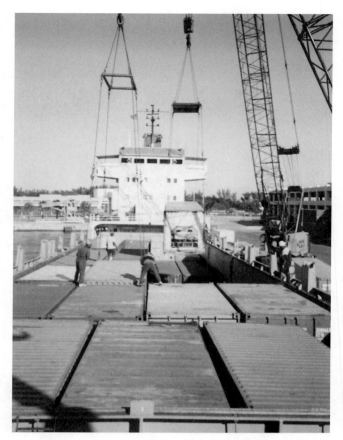

Figure 12-37. Loading of shipping containers. Note confined space.

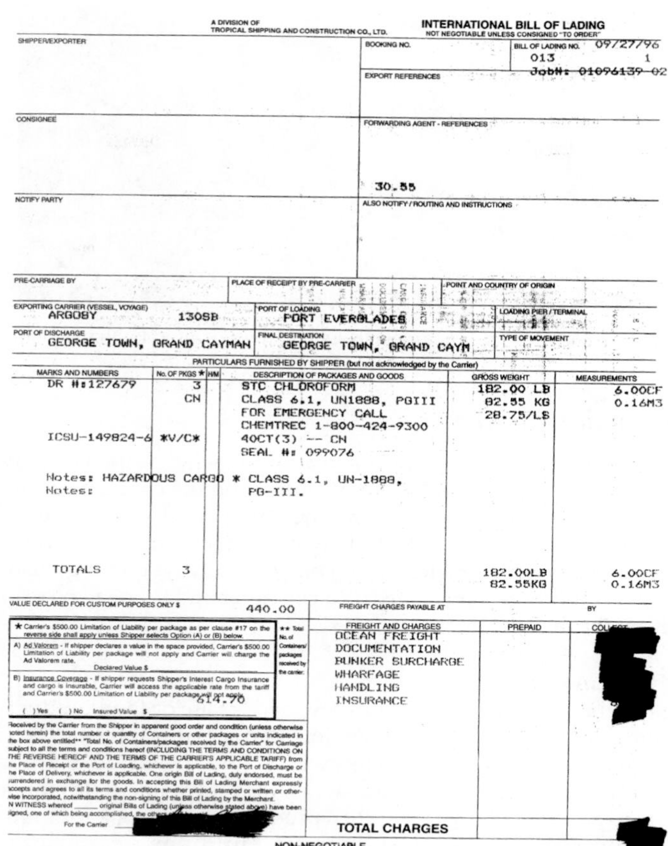

A DIVISION OF TROPICAL SHIPPING AND CONSTRUCTION CO., LTD.

INTERNATIONAL BILL OF LADING

NOT NEGOTIABLE UNLESS CONSIGNED "TO ORDER"

SHIPPER/EXPORTER

BOOKING NO.

BILL OF LADING NO. 09727796 013 1

~~JobH: 01096139-02~~

EXPORT REFERENCES

CONSIGNEE

FORWARDING AGENT - REFERENCES

30.55

NOTIFY PARTY

ALSO NOTIFY / ROUTING AND INSTRUCTIONS

PRE-CARRIAGE BY	PLACE OF RECEIPT BY PRE-CARRIER	POINT AND COUNTRY OF ORIGIN
EXPORTING CARRIER (VESSEL, VOYAGE) ARGOBY 130SB	PORT OF LOADING PORT EVERGLADES	LOADING PIER / TERMINAL
PORT OF DISCHARGE GEORGE TOWN, GRAND CAYMAN	FINAL DESTINATION GEORGE TOWN, GRAND CAYM	TYPE OF MOVEMENT

PARTICULARS FURNISHED BY SHIPPER (but not acknowledged by the Carrier)

MARKS AND NUMBERS	No. OF PKGS *	HM	DESCRIPTION OF PACKAGES AND GOODS	GROSS WEIGHT	MEASUREMENTS
DR #:127679	3 CN		STC CHLOROFORM CLASS 6.1, UN1888, PGIII FOR EMERGENCY CALL CHEMTREC 1-800-424-9300	182.00 LB 82.55 KG 28.75/L$	6.00CF 0.16M3
ICSU-149824-6	*V/C*		40CT(3) -- CN SEAL #: 099076		
Notes: HAZARDOUS CARGO * CLASS 6.1, UN-1888, PG-III. Notes:					
TOTALS	3			182.00LB 82.55KG	6.00CF 0.16M3

VALUE DECLARED FOR CUSTOM PURPOSES ONLY $ 440.00

FREIGHT CHARGES PAYABLE AT BY

* Carrier's $500.00 Limitation of Liability per package as per clause #17 on the reverse side shall apply unless Shipper selects Option (A) or (B) below.

A) Ad Valorem - If shipper declares a value in the space provided, Carrier's $500.00 Limitation of Liability per package will not apply and Carrier will charge the Ad Valorem rate. Declared Value $

B) Insurance Coverage - If shipper requests Shipper's Interest Cargo Insurance and cargo is insurable, Carrier will access the applicable rate from the tariff and Carrier's $500.00 Limitation of Liability per package will not apply. 614.70

( ) Yes ( ) No Insured Value $

** Total No. of Containers/packages received by the carrier.

FREIGHT AND CHARGES	PREPAID	COLLECT
OCEAN FREIGHT		
DOCUMENTATION		
BUNKER SURCHARGE		
WHARFAGE		
HANDLING		
INSURANCE		
TOTAL CHARGES		

Received by the Carrier from the Shipper in apparent good order and condition (unless otherwise noted herein) the total number or quantity of Containers or other packages or units indicated in the box above entitled** "Total No. of Containers/packages received by the Carrier" for Carriage subject to all the terms and conditions hereof (INCLUDING THE TERMS AND CONDITIONS ON THE REVERSE HEREOF AND THE TERMS OF THE CARRIER'S APPLICABLE TARIFF) from the Place of Receipt or the Port of Loading, whichever is applicable, to the Port of Discharge or the Place of Delivery, whichever is applicable. One origin Bill of Lading, duly endorsed, must be surrendered in exchange for the goods. In accepting this Bill of Lading Merchant expressly accepts and agrees to all its terms and conditions whether printed, stamped or written or otherwise incorporated, notwithstanding the non-signing of this Bill of Lading by the Merchant. IN WITNESS whereof ______ original Bills of Lading (unless otherwise stated above) have been signed, one of which being accomplished, the other

For the Carrier

NON-NEGOTIABLE

Figure 12-39. International bill of lading for shipment by vessel.

and hazard information can be obtained from the yard master for incidents in a railroad yard.

Air Shipments

Airbills on each piece of the shipment must be in the possession of the pilot in the cockpit and are usually in the pilot's briefcase.

Water Shipments

Shipping containers may carry hazardous materials. Placarding and labeling depend on the competency and honesty of shippers to provide appropriate and accurate information (Figs. 12-37 and 12-38). A dangerous cargo manifest must be on the vessel in a designated holder on the bridge or in the wheelhouse (Fig. 12-39). Barges have a dangerous cargo manifest located in the pilot house of the tugboat. Unmanned barges keep the manifest in a pipe or cylinder holder near the warning sign indicating hazardous cargo.

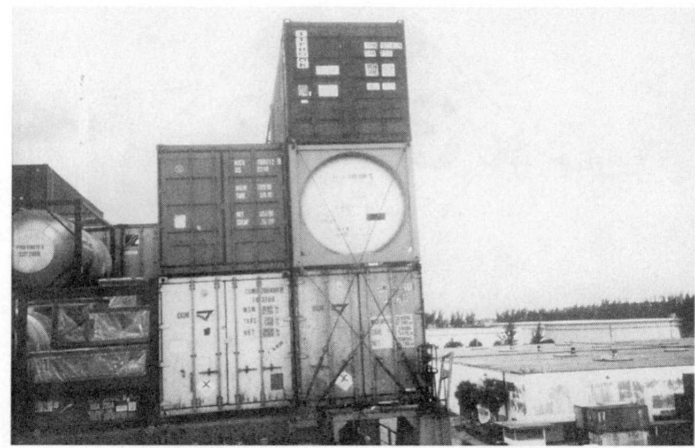

Figure 12-38. Containers on ship. Note "flammable" placard.

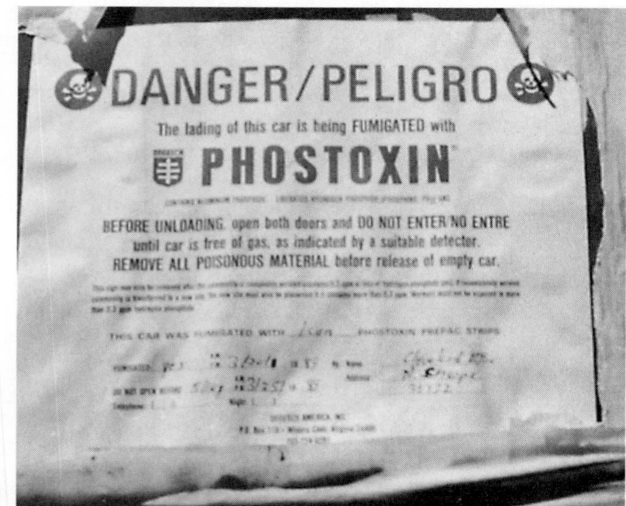

Figure 12-40. Fumigation notice indicates the potential for a confined space toxic hazard. With permission from National Fire Protection Association.

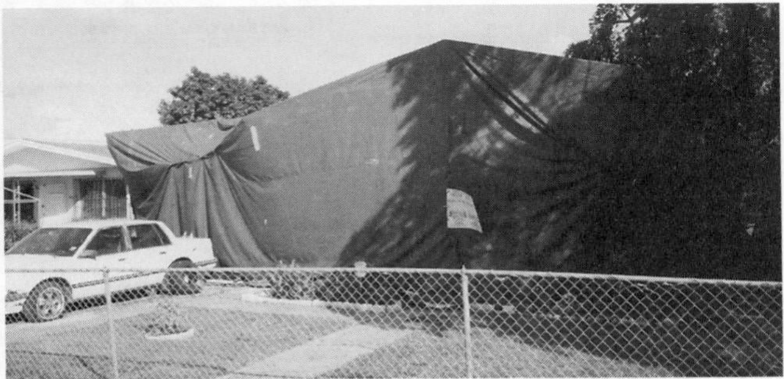

Figure 12-41. Tented structure with sulfuryl fluoride used for fumigation.

Container Markings

Containers used in transport and at fixed facilities often display the name of the owner or manufacturer and the product within. Obviously, a container bearing the name and logo of Amoco, Texaco, Dow, or Union Carbide would indicate a possible presence of hazardous materials. A company's name and logo usually are the largest markings on a container and thus can be read from the farthest distance.

FUMIGATION

Sites that store, process, or purvey food, grain, or food products often undergo pesticide fumigation. Rail cars transporting foodstuffs are routinely fumigated with a toxic pesticide, such as phostoxin or methyl bromide, when they are loaded. Responders to an incident involving such products should look for fumigation notices posted at doors to buildings or transport containers (Figs. 12-40 through 12-42). Tented buildings would give immediate indication of a building undergoing fumigation. A light smoke or vapor should give rise to suspicion of pesticide fumigation. Soil fumigation may use a combination of toxic materials (see Fig. 12-7).

RAIL CARS

Some rail cars are designed or set aside by the owner to transport only one commodity. These cars generally have the name of the product stenciled on the rail car. DOT regulations require more than 40 hazardous products to have their names stenciled in 4-in. letters on the sides of the rail car. These products include anhydrous ammonia, chlorine, hydrocyanic acid, liquefied hydrogen, liquefied petroleum gas, nitric acid, and phosphorous. Note the "residue" placard in the rail car for chlorine transport (see Fig. 12-36).

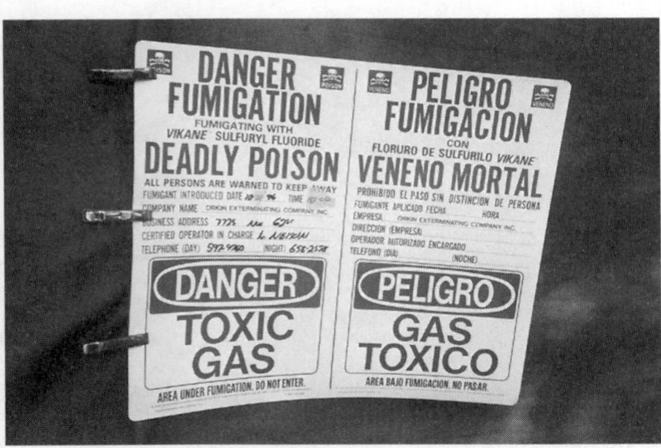

Figure 12-42. Sign required by law to be at fumigation site.

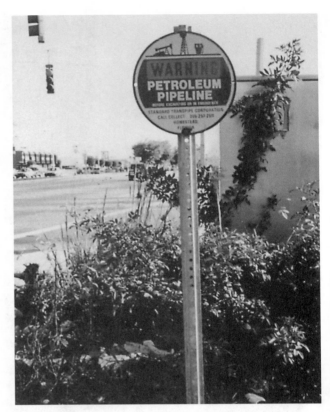

Figure 12-43. High-pressure liquid fuel transmission line. Marker posts such as this one are usually found where the pipeline crosses highways, railways, and waterways.

PIPELINE HAZARDS

Pipelines, including high-pressure transmission pipelines containing natural gas and other petroleum fuels, transfer products across sections of the country. Transmission pipelines operate at an extremely high rate of flow; consequently, a leak or break usually results in a significant release of product before sensing equipment can initiate closing of valves and shutdown of pipes (Fig. 12-43).

National Fire Protection Association 704 System

The 704 system, developed by the National Fire Protection Association, is used at fixed facilities, such as storage or industrial

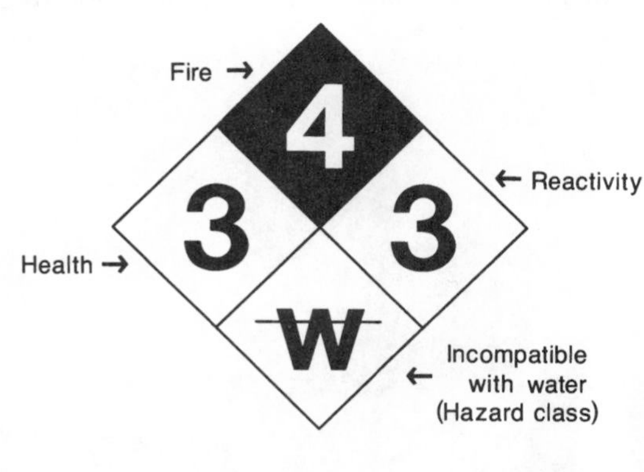

Figure 12-44. Components of a National Fire Protection Association 704 System signage.

sites, to indicate the presence of hazardous materials and their relative degree of hazard. The system uses a diamond, which is divided into quadrants of smaller diamonds. Each diamond quadrant addresses a different hazard category (Fig. 12-44):

- The blue diamond in the 9 o'clock position identifies "Health Hazard."
- The red diamond in the 12 o'clock position identifies "Flammability Hazard."
- The yellow diamond in the 3 o'clock position identifies the reactivity or instability of a material.
- The white diamond in the 6 o'clock position provides information on special hazards of a material. This quadrant may contain a symbol, such as that indicating radioactive materials, or letters, such as that indicating water-reactive, or "OXY" for oxidizer.
- The relative hazards of health, flammability, and reactivity of a product are rated by a number from zero (0), indicating no special hazard, to four (4), indicating severe hazard (Fig. 12-45).

The 704 system is nationally recognized but not mandated by federal law. Many industries voluntarily post 704 diamonds at their facilities in cooperation with their local fire department. Many local governments require the use of the system.

The 704 system provides a simple arrangement of readily recognizable colors, numbers, and symbols that gives the first responder an idea of the general hazards of a material at a glance. But it does not identify the specific product involved and is not used in transportation. The presence of such a warning at a building site indicates that hazardous materials are present (see Fig. 12-13).

CONTAINER SHAPE AND DESIGN

Some hazardous materials require specialized containment that has a specific shape, which can give a clue to the identity of its contents. Determining whether a hazardous material is present or not based on container design alone would be dangerously inadequate. New and different container designs are being produced to meet the needs of changing regulations and technology. Years ago, pressurized-gas rail tanker cars used to be identified by their white color, rounded ends, and dome arrangement. Now DOT regulations require that the cars be retrofitted with thermal insulation that is sprayed on or under a metal jacket. Today, pressurized gas cars may very well be black

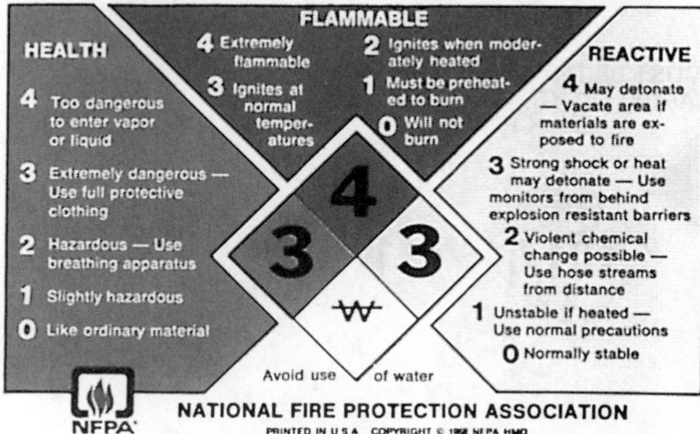
EMERGENCY GUIDE FOR HAZARDOUS MATERIALS
FLAMMABLE
HEALTH
4 Too dangerous to enter vapor or liquid
3 Extremely dangerous — Use full protective clothing
2 Hazardous — Use breathing apparatus
1 Slightly hazardous
0 Like ordinary material
4 Extremely flammable
3 Ignites at normal temperatures
2 Ignites when moderately heated
1 Must be preheated to burn
0 Will not burn
REACTIVE
4 May detonate — Vacate area if materials are exposed to fire
3 Strong shock or heat may detonate — Use monitors from behind explosion resistant barriers
2 Violent chemical change possible — Use hose streams from distance
1 Unstable if heated — Use normal precautions
0 Normally stable
4
3
3
Avoid use of water
NFPA
NATIONAL FIRE PROTECTION ASSOCIATION

Figure 12-45. National Fire Protection Association 704 signing system shows shape, color coding, and symbol indicating presence and degree of hazard and hazardous materials at fixed facilities. Copyright 1985, National Fire Protection Association, Quincy, MA 02269.

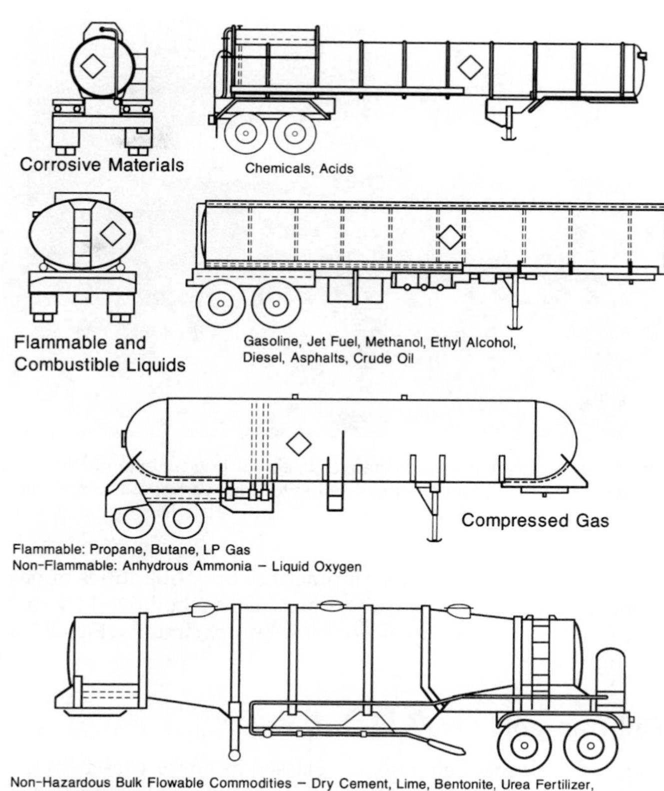

Figure 12-46. Basic shapes of truck trailers that transport hazardous materials.

with squared-off ends. Hazardous materials in small containers up to and including the 55-gallon drums are transported in general cargo trailers and stored in unmarked warehouses that give no clue to their presence.

All limitations aside, container shape and design can give the first responder a clue to the presence of hazardous materials at a distance, which can make the task of product identification safer. What follows is a brief overview of container-product relationships.

Trucks

The trucking industry uses different types of vehicles (other than general cargo trailers that are used to ship hazardous car-

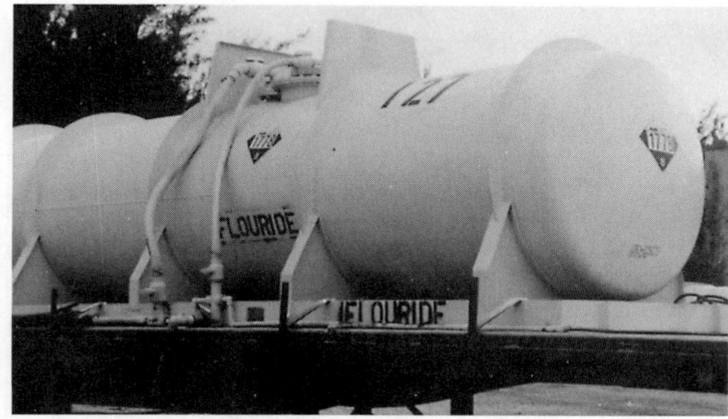
FLOURIDE

Figure 12-47. Specialized transport container for fluoride. Note reinforcing ribs and protection for valves at the top. This is typical for a tank that contains a corrosive.

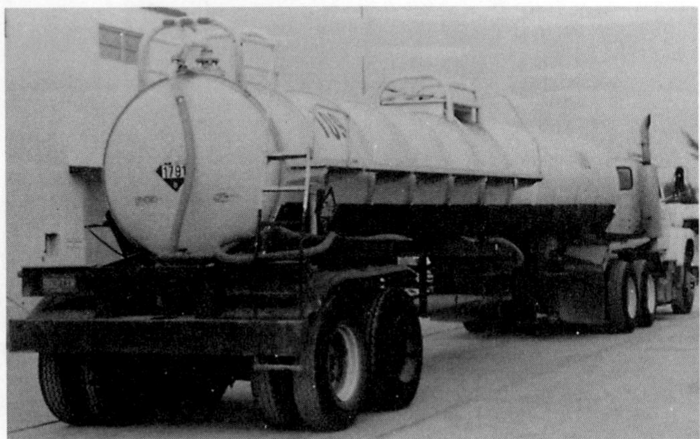

Figure 12-48. Corrosive liquid tanker distinguished by external ribs and relatively small tank container in relation to truck carriage. These features indicate a heavy liquid.

gos in small containers) for shipment of bulk quantities of hazardous materials. These trailers are easily recognized by their shape and may consist of one or more compartments (Figs. 12-46 through 12-48).

Rail Transport

Railroad tank cars generally are classed as either pressurized or nonpressurized. Pressurized tank cars carry a variety of hazardous liquids and pressurized gases. Some of the most common include chlorine, propane, butane, and anhydrous ammonia. They are recognized by a protective dome on the top of the car, which houses all the valves, gauging fixtures, and relief devices, and by the absence of any valves or piping under the car (Fig. 12-49).

Nonpressurized cars carry flammable, poisonous, and corrosive liquids and a variety of nonhazardous products. These cars have a variety of valves, pipe outlets, and relief devices along the top of the car and usually have outlets at the bottom (Fig. 12-50). Nonpressurized cars carrying corrosive materials generally can be identified by a black band around the tank at the outlets to protect the tank from spills when loading or off-loading acids or alkalis.

Small Cylinders

The compressed gas industry has a suggested standard for color coding cylinders to indicate their contents:

Oxygen cylinders: Green

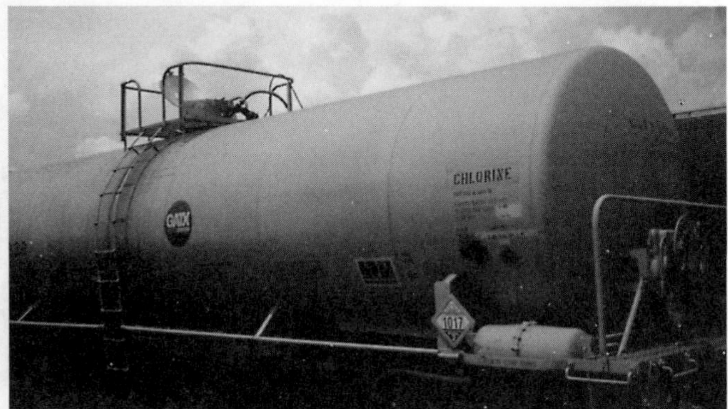

Figure 12-49. Profile of a pressurized tank car carrying chlorine. Note the dome on top that contains all outlets.

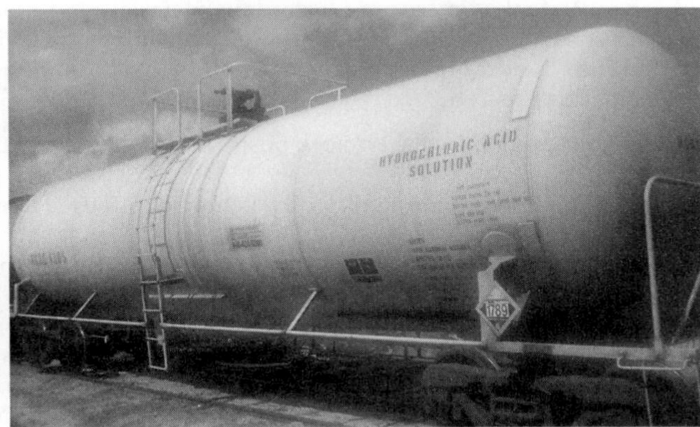

Figure 12-50. Nonpressurized tank car with valves and outlets at both top and bottom of car.

Helium cylinders: Brown
Nitrous oxide cylinders: Blue

This color-code system is a suggested standard and not required by law. Emergency response personnel should check for the extent of voluntary compliance in their jurisdiction.

Incidents involving liquid propane (LP) gas cylinders are on the rise. As with 55-gallon drums, the hazards of small LP cylinders are taken lightly or ignored because the containers are so common. An exploding 20-lb propane cylinder used to fuel barbecue grills creates a fireball, ground flash, shock wave, and flying metal tank fragments. First responders must anticipate their presence in homes, LP-powered vehicles, or even gas-powered floor-scrubbing machines. Their presence may be hidden but must be expected at accidents or fires involving snack trucks, mobile homes, and recreational vehicles (Fig. 12-51).

CONCLUSION

It can be very frustrating for emergency personnel who are used to rushing into an incident to do nothing but await the arrival of more qualified responders. The degree of risk to be taken must be commensurate with the amount to be gained by any act on the scene. Detecting the presence of hazardous materials is the

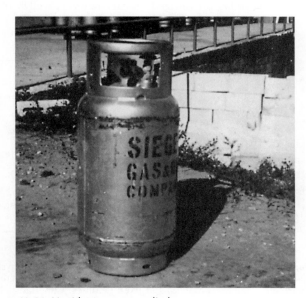

Figure 12-51. Liquid propane gas cylinder.

EMERGENCY RESPONSE TELEPHONE NUMBERS

CANADA

1. **CANUTEC**
   613-996-6666
   (Collect calls are accepted)

UNITED STATES

1. **CHEMTREC®**
   1-800-424-9300
   (Toll-free in the U.S. and Canada)
   703-527-3887 For calls originating elsewhere
   (Collect calls are accepted)

   or

2. **CHEM-TEL, INC.**
   1-800-255-3924
   (Toll-free in the U.S. and Canada)
   813-979-0626 For calls originating elsewhere
   (Collect calls are accepted)

3. **MILITARY SHIPMENTS**
   703-697-0218 - Explosives/ammunition incidents
   (Collect calls are accepted)
   1-800-851-8061 - All other dangerous goods incidents

MEXICO

1. **SETIQ**
   91-800-00-214 in the Mexican Republic
   For calls originating in Mexico City and the Metropolitan Area
   575-0838, 575-0842 or 559-1588
   For calls originating elsewhere, call
   0-11-52-5-575-0838 or 0-11-52-5-575-0842

2. **CECOM**
   91-800-00-413 in the Mexican Republic
   For calls originating in Mexico City and the Metropolitan Area
   550-1496, 550-1552, 550-1485, or 550-4885
   FAX 616-5560 or 616-5561
   For calls originating elsewhere, call
   0-11-52-5-550-1496, 0-11-52-5-550-1552, 0-11-52-5-550-1485, or 0-11-52-5-550-4885

Figure 12-52. Back cover, inside, of *North American Emergency Response Guidebook* with emergency phone numbers.

goal, but not at the expense of exposure or contamination of personnel. Emergency response telephone numbers in North America (the United States, Canada, and Mexico) are available for assisting emergency responders (Fig. 12-52).

REFERENCES

1. Bronstein A, Currance P. *Emergency care for hazardous materials exposure*. St. Louis: Mosby, 1988.
2. National Fire Academy. Hazardous materials incident analysis, student manual. Emmitsburg, MD: National Fire Academy, National Emergency Training Center, 1985.
3. US Department of Transportation. North American Emergency Response Guidebook. Mexico: US Department of Transportation, Transport Canada, Secretariat of Communications and Transportation, 1996.

CHAPTER 13

Radiation and Radioactive Emergencies

James M. Woolfenden and John B. Sullivan, Jr.

Since the discovery of x-rays in 1895 and radioactive decay in 1896, many sources of ionizing radiation have been developed for medical and industrial use. Nuclear power now provides a significant part of the energy needs of the United States and other countries. Nuclear medicine uses radioactive isotopes for diagnostic studies as well as treatment of diseases such as hyperthyroidism and thyroid cancer. Radioactive tracers have contributed to fundamental discoveries throughout the life sciences, from physiology to molecular biology to genetics. Virtually all new drugs are developed using radiolabeled forms to study pharmacokinetics and biodistribution. Radioactive isotopes have a wide variety of industrial and commercial applications, from smoke detectors to well logging. Use of x-rays is not confined to medicine, and industrial radiography is widely used for tasks such as testing the integrity of welded joints.

All applications of radiation and radioactive isotopes have potential for accidents and exposure to excessive levels of radiation. Exposure to high doses of radiation can have serious health consequences, although the risks attributed to lower levels of exposure are the subject of ongoing debate. The world was reminded of the dangers of radioactive hazards from the Chernobyl nuclear power plant explosion in 1986. Since this disaster, scientists worldwide have been studying the continuing health effects on nearby populations.

FUNDAMENTALS OF RADIATION AND RADIOACTIVITY

The term *radioactivity* refers to atoms with unstable nuclei that decay with the emission of particles or electromagnetic radiation. There are many technical terms to be familiar with regarding radiation and radioactivity (Table 13-1). Four modes of radioactive decay exist. *Alpha decay* involves emission of a helium nucleus, or alpha particle, that consists of two protons and two neutrons. *Beta decay* involves emission of a negatively charged electron, or beta particle ($\beta-$), from the nucleus. *Positron decay* is associated with emission of a positively charged electron, or positron ($\beta+$). The positron is the antiparticle of the electron, and when a positron encounters an electron, the two annihilate, with emission of two photons that travel in opposite directions. (Detection of both photons is the basis of positron emission tomography.) *Electron capture,* as the name implies, involves capture of an inner-shell electron by the nucleus, and the electron combines with a proton to form a neutron.

In each of these four modes of decay, the number of protons in the nucleus changes, and so the new nucleus (referred to as the *daughter*) represents a different element. In another mode of decay, called *isomeric transition,* the nucleus emits a gamma ray but no particles, and so the daughter is the same element as the parent.

When radiation interacts with matter, including tissue, it deposits energy. The energy transfer results in ionization or excitation, in which orbital electrons in the target atoms are ejected or disturbed by the incoming radiation, causing molecular damage and disrupting normal functioning of cells. Adaptive and repair processes are also induced by radiation exposure, and these may counteract much of the damage at low exposure levels.

Charged particles are more efficient at depositing energy in tissue than are gamma rays or x-rays, and the greater the mass of the particle, the greater the energy deposited. The electron mass is about 1/1,800 of the mass of a proton, and so electrons produce less ionization in tissue than protons. The energy deposited per unit distance traversed in tissue is known as *linear energy transfer* (LET), expressed in kiloelectron volts per micrometer. For example, a 5-MeV alpha particle has an LET in tissue of approximately 100 keV/mm, compared with 16 keV/mm for a 2-MeV proton and 0.25 keV/mm for a 1-MeV electron (1). Alpha particles lose energy so rapidly that they travel only

TABLE 13-1. Definitions

Absorbed dose: The amount absorbed per unit mass of irradiated material when ionizing radiation passes through the matter. The units of measurement of absorbed dose are the rad and the gray.
Activity: The number of nuclear transformations occurring in a given quantity of material per unit time.
Alpha particle: A particle with a positive charge made up of two neutrons and two protons emitted by certain radioactive materials. It is the least penetrating of the three types of emitted radiation and can be stopped by a sheet of paper.
Beta particle: An elementary particle emitted from a nucleus during radioactive decay. It has a single electrical charge and a mass 1/1,837 of a proton. A negatively charged beta particle is identical to an electron; a positively charged beta particle is a positron.
Curie: The unit of activity of nuclear transformation per unit time. One curie equals 3.7×10^{10} nuclear transformations per second.
Daughter and daughter product: A nuclide formed by radioactive decay of another nuclide, the product of which may be stable or unstable.
Effective half-life: Time required for a radionuclide contained in a biological system to reduce its activity by one-half as a combined result of radioactive decay and biological elimination.
Electron capture: The unit of exposure to x-rays and gamma rays. Capture of an inner-shell electron by a nucleus when the electron combines with a proton to form a neutron.
Gamma rays: High-energy, nuclear in origin, short-wavelength electromagnetic radiation that is very penetrating.
Ionizing radiation: Any radiation displacing electrons from atoms or molecules, thus producing ions.
Isotopes: One of two or more atoms with the same atomic number but with different atomic weights. The nuclei of isotopes have the same number of protons but a different number of neutrons.
Neutron: An uncharged elementary particle with a mass slightly greater than that of a proton. A free neutron is unstable and decays with a half-life of 13 minutes into an electron, proton, and neutrino.
Physical half-life: The time required for a radioactive substance to lose one-half of its activity by decay.
Positron decay: Emission of positively charged electron (β+).
Proton: An elementary particle with a single positive charge and a mass 1,837 times that of an electron.
Rad: Absorbed dose of radiation deposited per unit mass of tissue.
Radioactivity: Spontaneous release of particles or electromagnetic radiation from atoms with unstable nuclei.
Radionuclide: A radioactive form of an element.
Rem: The special unit of dose equivalent.
Roentgen (R): Amount of radiation that produces a given amount of ionization in a given volume of air.
X-ray: A penetrating form of electromagnetic radiation that is nonnuclear in origin, emitted when the inner orbital electrons of an excited atom return to their normal state or when a metal target is bombarded with high-speed electrons.

very short distances in air, however, and they require a kinetic energy of at least 7.5 MeV to penetrate intact skin (1). Alpha particles are usually not a significant radiation hazard unless they are inhaled, ingested, or deposited in open wounds. The distance traveled by beta particles in tissue also depends on their kinetic energy, with typical distances ranging from less than 1 mm up to 1 to 2 cm.

Neutrons are uncharged and do not interact readily with tissues and, therefore, are much more penetrating than charged particles. Neutrons are absorbed by nuclei of atoms in the absorbing material, such as tissue, and may produce a variety of particles and nuclear fragments depending on the neutron energy. Nuclear absorption of neutrons may induce radioactivity, a process referred to as *neutron activation*.

Radionuclides that decay by isomeric transition and electron capture do not emit any particles from the nucleus and, in general, deliver lower tissue radiation doses than radionuclides that decay by emission of beta particles. Tc-99m, the radionuclide used most commonly (in a variety of chemical forms) for nuclear medicine imaging, decays by isomeric transition; most of the other imaging radionuclides decay by electron capture. Although such radionuclides do not emit particles from the nucleus, they may emit orbital electrons that contribute to the radiation dose that they deliver. The biological effects of these relatively low-energy electrons depend on their intracellular localization and, in particular, whether they are in close proximity to DNA (2).

Gamma rays are photons that arise from the nucleus. They are much less efficient at depositing energy in tissue than charged particles, but they can travel much greater distances than particles. The basic considerations for reducing exposure to gamma rays and x-rays are time, distance, and shielding. If work in a radiation field is required, it should be planned ahead of time to minimize the duration of exposure. Increasing distance from a radiation source can be very effective in reducing dose, because the radiation exposure from a point source decreases as the inverse square of the distance. Lead and other high-atomic-number materials can be used to shield gamma rays and x-rays; the thickness required depends on the gamma-ray energy. Lead is generally not an appropriate shield for a pure beta emitter; if the lead is close enough to the source, the beta particles produce x-rays when they strike the lead. Usually just distance from the source is adequate for protection from beta emitters because the beta particles have limited range in air. If shielding is required, then low-atomic-number materials, such as lucite, are preferable to lead.

RADIONUCLIDES

Radioactive forms of elements are termed *radionuclides* (Table 13-2). Radionuclides are commonly used throughout many industries and medical facilities. The risk of injury to tissues from incorporation of the various radionuclides varies and is a function of the following: (a) specific activity, (b) dose, (c) half-life, (d) biological elimination, (e) target-organ concentration, and (f) route of exposure and absorption. The disintegration time (half-life) and the type of radiation emitted vary with the species and are critical features of radionuclide toxicity. The toxicity of a radionuclide to a particular tissue is a function of the type of radiation emitted, the half-life of the radiation, and biological elimination of the element. Biological elimination and the actual half-life combine to create an *effective half-life* of elimination. The site of greatest injury from a radionuclide occurs within the tissue (critical organ) that concentrates the radionuclide (see Table 13-2). The route of exposure influences toxicity. Inhalation can present a different order of toxicity as compared with ingestion or wound contamination.

The decay of radionuclides follows an exponential equation: $A = A_0e^{-\lambda t}$, where A is the activity at time t, A_0 is the starting activity at time t_0, e is the natural logarithm base, λ is the decay constant of the radionuclide, and t is the elapsed time from t_0. This equation is very useful for calculating the amount of a radionuclide deposited at an earlier time or the amount that remains at a later time. $A = A_0/2$ at the physical half-life of the radionuclide. Because $\lambda = 0.693/t_{1/2}$, where $t_{1/2}$ is the physical half-life of the radionuclide, the equation can also be expressed as $A = A_0e^{-0.693t/t_{1/2}}$. Because $e^{-0.693} = 1/2$, the equation can be further simplified as $A = A_0(0.5)^{t/t_{1/2}}$. This last form can be used on pocket calculators that lack natural logarithms.

Even when a radionuclide is retained in the body, its activity decreases according to the decay equation. Most internally deposited radionuclides are excreted to some extent, however, and body clearance is often expressed in terms of the biological

TABLE 13-2. Radionuclides

Radionuclides	Radiation type	Physical $T_{1/2}$	Effective $T_{1/2}$	Organ
Americium 241	Alpha, gamma	458 y	139 y	Bone
Americium 243	Alpha, gamma, daughters	7,950 y	195 y	Bone
Arsenic 74	Beta, gamma	18 d	17 d	Total body
Arsenic 77	Beta, gamma, daughters	39 h	24 h	Total body
Barium 140	Beta, gamma, daughters	13 d	11 d	Bone
Cadmium 109	Gamma, daughters	453 d	140 d	Liver
Calcium 45	Beta	165 d	162 d	Bone
Calcium 47	Beta, gamma, daughters	4.5 d	4.5 d	Bone
Californium 252	Gamma, alpha, neutron, daughter	2.6 y	2.2 y	Bone
Carbon 14	Beta	5,730 y	12 d	Total body
Cerium 141	Beta, gamma, daughters	32 d	30 d	Liver
Cerium 144	Beta, gamma, daughters	284 d	280 d	Bone
Cesium 137	Beta, gamma, daughters	30 y	70 d	Total body
Chromium 51	Gamma	28 d	27 d	Total body
Cobalt 57	Gamma	270 d	9 d	Total body
Cobalt 58	Beta, gamma	71 d	8 d	Total body
Cobalt 60	Beta, gamma	5.3 y	10 d	Total body
Curium 242	Alpha, neutron, gamma	163 d	155 d	Liver
Curium 243	Alpha, gamma	32 y	27.5 d	Liver
Curium 244	Alpha, neutron, gamma	17.6 y	16.7 y	Liver
Europium 152	Beta, gamma, daughters	13 y	3 y	Kidney
Europium 154	Beta, gamma	16 y	3 y	Bone
Europium 155	Beta, gamma	2 y	1.3 y	Kidney
Fluorine 18	Beta, gamma	2 h	2 h	Total body
Gallium 72	Beta, gamma	14 h	12 h	Liver
Gold 198	Beta, gamma	2.7 d	2.6 d	Total body
Indium 114m	Beta, gamma, daughters	49 d	27 d	Kidney, spleen
Iodine 125	Beta, gamma	60 d	42 d	Thyroid
Iodine 131	Beta, gamma, daughters	8 d	8 d	Thyroid
Iron 55	Gamma	2.6 y	1 yr	Spleen
Iron 59	Beta, gamma	46 d	42 d	Spleen
Lead 210	Beta, gamma, daughters	20 y	1.3 y	Kidney
Mercury 197	Gamma	2.7 d	2.3 d	Kidney
Mercury 203	Beta, gamma	46 d	11 d	Kidney
Molybdenum 99	Beta, gamma, daughters	2.8 d	1.5 d	Kidney
Neptunium 237	Alpha, gamma, daughters	2 million y	200 y	Bone
Neptunium 239	Beta, gamma	2.3 d	2.3 d	Gastrointestinal tract
Phosphorus 32	Beta	14 d	14 d	Bone
Plutonium 238	Alpha, gamma	88 y	63 y	Bone
Plutonium 239	Alpha, gamma	24,000 y	197 y	Bone
Polonium 210	Alpha	138 d	46 d	Spleen
Potassium 42	Beta, gamma	12 h	12 h	Total body
Promethium 147	Beta	2.6 y	1.6 y	Bone
Promethium 149	Beta, gamma	2.2 d	2.2 d	Bone
Radium 224	Alpha, gamma, daughters	3.6 d	3.6 d	Bone
Radium 226	Alpha, gamma, daughters	1,600 y	44 y	Bone
Rubidium 86	Beta, gamma	19 d	13.2 d	Total body
Ruthenium 106	Beta, daughters	368 d	2.5 d	Kidney
Scandium 46	Beta, gamma	84 d	40 d	Liver
Silver 110m	Beta, gamma, daughters	255 d	5 d	Total body
Sodium 22	Beta, gamma	950 d	11 d	Total body
Sodium 24	Beta, gamma	15 h	14 h	Total body
Strontium 85	Gamma	65 d	65 d	Total body
Strontium 90	Beta, daughters	28 y	15 y	Bone
Sulfur 35	Beta	88 d	44 d	Testis
Technetium 99m	Gamma	6 h	5 h	Total body
Technetium 99	Beta	200,000 y	20 d	Kidney
Thorium 230	Alpha, gamma	80,000 y	200 y	Bone
Thorium 232	Alpha, gamma, daughters	1.4×10^{10} y	200 y	Bone
Thorium (natural)	Alpha, beta, gamma	—	200 y	Bone
Tritium (^3H)	Beta	12 y	12 d	Total body
Uranium 235	Alpha, gamma, daughters	7.1×10^8 y	15 d	Kidney
Uranium 238	Alpha, gamma, daughters	4.5×10^9 y	15 d	Kidney
Uranium (natural)	Alpha, beta, gamma	4.5×10^9 y	15 d	Kidney
Yttrium 90	Beta	64 h	64 h	Bone
Zinc 65	Beta (+), gamma	245 d	194 d	Total body
Zirconium 95	Beta, gamma, daughter	66 d	56 d	Total body

$T_{1/2}$, half-life.
Adapted from National Council on Radiation and Protection Measurements, Report No. 65. *Management of persons accidentally contaminated with radionuclides.* Washington, DC: National Council on Radiation and Protection Measurements, 1979.

half-life, even though the clearance may not be well represented by a single exponential equation. The biological half-life is simply the time at which half of the radionuclide has been excreted from the body (ignoring physical decay). The combined effect of physical decay and biological excretion is often expressed in terms of the effective half-life. The relationship between physical, biological, and effective half-life is as follows: $1/T_p + 1/T_b = 1/T_{eff}$. The effective half-life is used in radiation dose calculations.

The unit of exposure to x-rays and gamma rays is the roentgen (R), which is the amount of radiation that produces a given amount of ionization in a given volume of air. For biological systems, exposure is usually expressed as a rate of ionization per unit time, such as R per hour. Radiation dose is expressed in terms of the absorbed dose, which is defined as energy deposited per unit mass of tissue. The units of absorbed dose are ergs per gram or joules per kilogram, although absorbed dose is more commonly given in rad (100 erg/g) or gray (Gy; 1 Gy = 1 J/kg = 100 rad = 10^4 erg/g). Because the effectiveness of different types of radiation varies with LET in causing biological effects, the absorbed dose may be modified by a quality factor to take these differences into account. The quality factor is dimensionless, and so the modified absorbed dose still has units of erg/g or J/kg; the modified units are the roentgen equivalent man (rem) and the sievert (Sv).

Environmental Radiation Exposure

All life on earth is exposed to environmental radiation and has adapted to its presence. The main sources of naturally occurring environmental radiation are cosmic rays, radionuclides in the earth, radionuclides in the body, and radon and its decay products in air. The average effective dose equivalent (a sum of weighted absorbed doses in tissues times a quality factor) to the U.S. population is about 300 mrem (3 mSv) per year (3). This figure is the sum of about 28 mrem from cosmic rays, 28 mrem from terrestrial radionuclides, 40 mrem from radionuclides in the body, and 200 mrem from inhaled radon decay products. There are considerable local variations in background radiation that are caused by differences in naturally occurring radionuclides in the soil as well as by altitude. For example, cosmic-ray exposure approximately doubles with every 2,000 m of altitude (3).

Human-made sources add another 60 mrem to the average effective dose equivalent of the U.S. population. Of this total, 50 mrem is attributable to medical diagnosis and 10 mrem to consumer products (4). Radioactive fallout from nuclear weapons testing is now an insignificant source of radiation exposure, as it results in less than 1 mrem per year (4).

Occupational exposure adds still further to selected groups of the population. It is estimated that aircraft crew members receive 100 to 200 mrem exposure annually from cosmic radiation compared with 24 mrem exposure at sea level (3,5). Mean annual occupational doses for industrial radiographers are 430 mrem; for health care workers who receive occupational exposure, the figure is less than 200 mrem (5). The regulatory limit for whole-body occupational exposure of adults in the United States is 5 rem (5,000 mrem) per year; for the general public it is one-tenth of that value.

In assessing the significance of exposure to low levels of radiation, it is important to remember that an exposure represents an increment in exposure, not a new event. Exposures to radiation levels similar to those present in the environment are not likely to be associated with detectable biological changes.

Radiation Exposure and Contamination

The two best-known examples of radiation emergencies are use of nuclear weapons and disasters at nuclear power plants. The two differ fundamentally in potential for casualties and radiation-associated injury. At Hiroshima, conservative estimates for deaths after the atomic blast are 45,000 immediately and 19,000 over the next 4 months; at Nagasaki, the estimates are 22,000 immediately and 17,000 over the next 4 months (6). Many of the deaths were caused by the blast, flash burns, and trauma, and it is not possible to know for sure what fraction died directly or indirectly from radiation. The Chernobyl nuclear reactor accident in 1986 resulted in 28 radiation-associated deaths (7). The accident at the Three Mile Island nuclear power plant in 1979 resulted in no injury or death, and radiation exposure to plant workers and the general public was insignificant (8).

Radiation accidents can occur at any point in the nuclear fuel cycle, from mining and milling through final use and disposal, but such accidents and injuries have been rare (8). (The increased incidence of lung cancer in uranium miners falls outside the category of radiation accident.) Based on reports of accidental radiation exposures (9,10), radiation injuries are much more likely to be encountered in other circumstances. An important cause of radiation injury is inadvertent exposure of industrial radiographers to gamma-ray sources. Such sources are housed in a shielded container and are extended out of the container during radiography. Exposures and injury occur when the source fails to retract into the container or becomes detached, or when the operator loses track of whether the source is in the extended or retracted position.

Another important cause of radiation exposure and injury is lost or discarded sealed sources that are found by members of the public who are unaware of the contents. The sources may be handled or carried in pockets for extended periods, and they may result in serious injury or death. The most common sealed sources in these accidents are iridium 192, cesium 137, and cobalt 60. Physical properties of these radionuclides are listed in Table 13-3. In one such accident, pellets of ^{60}Co from a teletherapy machine were scattered in a junkyard where metal from the machine was being recycled, and some of the pellets were left in a pickup truck used for deliveries. Radiation doses to workers in the junkyard, estimated from cytogenetic studies, ranged up to nearly 200 rad acute dose and 1,500 rad protracted dose. Some hot spots in the junkyard had exposure rates up to 600 R/hour (11).

Uncommon causes of inadvertent radiation exposure and injury include whole-body irradiation from sealed-source irradiators and irradiation of a portion of the body from accelerator beams (9). Such accidents have occurred when safety interlocks have been malfunctioning or have been turned off. Incidents of inappropriately high radiation doses to patients resulting in fatalities have occurred from teletherapy machines and from brachytherapy sources (12).

TABLE 13-3. Properties of common sealed-source radionuclides

Radionuclide	Half-life	Decay mode	Emissions
Cobalt 60	5.21 y	β–	β– E_{max} 314 keV; γ 1.173, 1.333 MeV
Cesium 137	30.0 y	β–	β– E_{max} 1.18 MeV; γ 661 keV
Iridium 192	73.8 d	β–, EC	β– E_{max} 670 keV; γ 296–612 keV

β–, beta; EC, electron capture; E_{max}, maximum energy; eV, electron volt; γ, gamma ray.
Data from Browne E, Firestone RB. *Table of radioactive isotopes.* New York: Wiley-Interscience, 1986; and Lederer CM, Hollander JM, Perlman I. *Table of radioactive isotopes,* 6th ed. New York: Wiley, 1967.

TABLE 13-4. Properties of selected radionuclides in nuclear medicine and life sciences

Radionuclide	Half-life	Decay mode	Main emissions	Use
Carbon 14	5,730 y	β–	β– E_{max} 156 keV	Research
Fluorine 18	1.83 h	β+	β+ E_{max} 635 keV; g 511 keV	Imaging
Gallium 67	3.26 d	EC	γ 93–396 keV	Imaging
Iodine 123	13.2 h	EC	γ 159 keV	Imaging
Iodine 125	60.1 d	EC	γ and x-rays 27–35 keV	Research, RIA
Iodine 131	8.04 d	β–	β– E_{max} 606 keV, g 364 keV	Imaging, therapy
Indium 111	2.81 d	EC	γ 171, 245 keV	Imaging
Phosphorus 32	14.3 d	β–	β– E_{max} 1.71 MeV	Research, therapy
Samarium 153	1.95 d	β–	β– E_{max} 800 keV, g 103 keV	Therapy
Strontium 89	50.6 d	β–	β– E_{max} 1.46 MeV	Therapy
Sulfur 35	87.5 d	β–	β– E_{max} 167 keV	Research
Technetium 99m	6.01 h	IT	γ 140 keV	Imaging
Thallium 201	3.05 d	EC	x-ray 69–80 keV; g 135, 167 keV	Imaging
Tritium	12.3 y	β–	β– E_{max} 18.6 keV	Research, other[a]
Xenon 133	5.25 d	β–	β– E_{max} 346 keV, g 81 keV	Imaging

β–, beta; β+, positron; EC, electron capture; E_{max}, maximum energy; eV, electron volt; γ, gamma ray; IT, isomeric transition; RIA, radioimmunoassay.
[a]Other uses of tritium (H-3) include self-luminous signs and dials.
Physical data from Browne E, Firestone RB. *Table of radioactive isotopes.* New York: Wiley-Interscience, 1986; and Lederer CM, Hollander JM, Perlman I. *Table of radioactive isotopes*, 6th ed. New York: Wiley, 1967.

Unsealed radionuclide sources may be involved in several different accident scenarios. Laboratory accidents can result in exposure to many different radionuclides, although the ones most commonly used in life sciences and pharmaceutical laboratories are iodine 131, iodine 125, phosphorus 32, carbon 14, tritium, and sulfur 35. Transportation accidents involving vehicles or aircraft carrying radionuclides for research or clinical nuclear medicine may result in radiation exposure, although radiation injury in such circumstances had not been reported in the United States as of 1990 (13). Properties of radionuclides commonly used in nuclear medicine and in life sciences research are given in Table 13-4.

In determining the appropriate treatment a patient requires and the nature of the precautions taken by those personnel involved in the medical care, the modality of exposure must be considered: (a) irradiation, (b) external contamination, or (c) internal contamination or incorporation.

In the first situation—irradiation—the patient has been subjected to gamma or x-rays. In these cases, the patient has been exposed to radiation but is not radioactive and, therefore, poses no risk to medical personnel. The patient has already sustained whatever injury is going to occur, and it manifests itself over time. Of interest, one exception exists to the rule that an irradiated victim poses no hazard: the patient who has been exposed to high-dose neutron radiation. In these extremely rare cases, the patient may, in fact, become radioactive.

The second situation—external contamination—involves external, surface contamination of the patient. In these cases, decontamination must occur while protecting medical personnel and equipment from exposure. Monitoring of the patient and the decontamination effort must be performed using appropriate radiation detection devices.

The third situation—internal contamination or incorporation—occurs by inhalation, ingestion, or deposition of material into an open wound. This route of exposure is of particular concern because of the potential for internal irradiation and the permanent incorporation of the radioactive material in the molecules of cells. Usually, the effects of an internal contamination accident, such as radionuclide intake, manifest themselves over a period of years, except in cases of massive exposure. In these cases, urgent removal is indicated with possible utilization of chelating agents.

Planning for Radiation Emergencies

No substitute exists for a well-thought-out plan for radiologic emergencies that has been tested in simulated emergency situations. Parts of the plan are elements of the broader disaster plan for the institution, but certain considerations exist that are specific to the possible presence of radioactive contamination. These considerations do not apply to individuals who have been irradiated by sealed sources, accelerators, or teletherapy machines. These individuals are not radioactive and do not pose any radiologic threat to emergency personnel.

An area in or adjacent to the emergency department for decontamination of patients should be identified. It should be possible to restrict access to the area. There should be no through traffic, so that contamination is not spread elsewhere in the department. Isolation clothing and booties should be used by those working in the area, and the isolation clothing should not be worn out of the area. Because contaminated individuals may have sustained trauma, the area should be suitable for providing trauma services as well. A decontamination table should be in the room; ideally, it should be possible to collect the wash water from the table. A cabinet with necessary supplies should be in the restricted area. Suggested supplies are listed in Table 13-5.

An impoundment area should be designated near the emergency department. Emergency transport vehicles may have been contaminated during transport, and they need to be surveyed before they are released. Emergency transport personnel may also need to be surveyed.

Personnel responsibilities should be spelled out in the emergency plan. The emergency response team should include an individual knowledgeable about radioactive materials and radiation safety. An experienced technician or professional should perform the radiation surveys, including surveys of the medical staff before they leave the restricted area. A security officer should be designated to control access to the restricted area. Because radiation accidents arouse great public curiosity, a public information spokesperson should be designated.

Radiation Survey Instruments

Geiger-Müller (G-M) survey meters are inexpensive and widely available, and they are usually the instrument of choice

TABLE 13-5. Supplies for radioactive emergencies and decontamination

Radiation-monitoring equipment
- Geiger-Müller survey meter
- Ionization chamber survey meter
- Pocket dosimeters and charger
- Film badges and thermoluminescence dosimeters
- Batteries for Geiger-Müller survey meter

General protective equipment
- Plastic sheeting for floor
- Duct tape
- Masking tape, 2-inch
- Masking tape, 1-inch
- Polyethylene bags, large
- Polyethylene bags, small
- Scrub suits
- Disposable protective suits
- Disposable shoe covers
- Goggles
- Half-face filtered respirators
- Dust and mist respirators, disposable
- Surgical masks
- Surgical gloves, sterile
- Examination gloves, nonsterile
- Neoprene industrial gloves
- Coveralls (contaminated clothing exchange)

Decontamination equipment
- Scissors, heavy duty
- Large plastic basin
- Large plastic containers for wash water
- Wash bottle
- Liquid soap
- Prep sponges
- Surgical hand brushes
- Disposable towels
- Absorbent cotton balls
- Forceps for sponges
- Sterile gauze 4″ × 4″ pads
- Sterile gauze 1″ × 1″ pads
- Cotton-tipped applicators
- Plastic containers for used sponges and pads
- Remote handling tongs, large
- Remote handling tongs, small
- Sterile suture sets
- Sterile irrigation fluid
- Irrigation syringe
- Hair clipper
- Nail clipper

Bioassay equipment
- Alcohol wipes
- Vacutainer holder and tubes (Becton, Dickinson, Franklin Lakes, NJ)
- Sterile culture swabs
- Sterile urine sample container
- Plastic urine container, large, nonsterile
- Wide-mouth plastic sample containers and lids

Area control equipment
- Signs, *Radiation area*
- Warning rope, yellow and magenta
- Barrier tape
- Identification badges
- Access log book

Miscellaneous
- Felt marker pens
- Ballpoint pens
- Tags, with wire, for bag labeling
- Peel-off stickers for container labeling
- Tape *Radioactive* for labeling samples and bags
- Sealable plastic bags, assorted sizes
- Flashlight and batteries
- Notebook pads

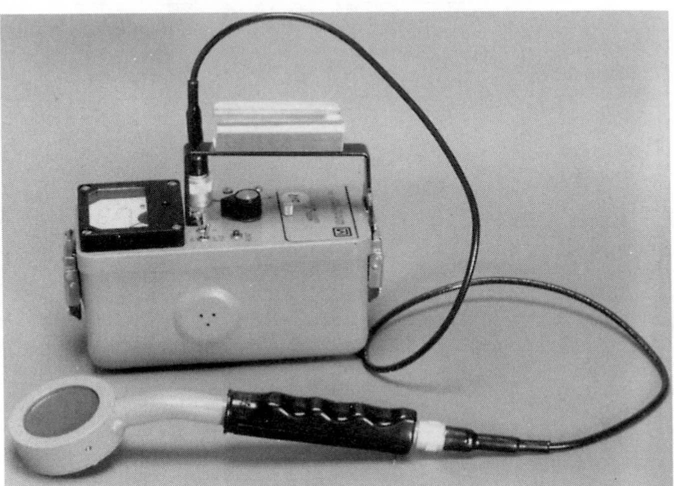

Figure 13-1. Geiger-Müller survey meter.

for detecting contamination and monitoring decontamination efforts (Fig. 13-1). Most G-M detectors are battery powered. Batteries should be tested before use; a test setting exists on the survey meter for this purpose. Most G-M detectors have a section with a protective covering over a thin window of mica or mylar that permits particles and low-energy photons to be detected when the window covering is opened. Beta particles must have a kinetic energy of approximately 30 keV to pass through the window, however, so typical G-M detectors do not detect tritium, which has a maximum beta particle energy of 18.6 keV.

A G-M detector is best used as a qualitative indicator that radiation is present in excess of natural background. It should not be used to estimate radiation exposure or dose rates. The counting efficiency for x-rays and gamma rays is quite low, typically 1% or less. G-M detectors provide no information on energy of detected radiation, although comparison of readings with the window open and closed can be used to distinguish between beta and gamma rays. G-M detectors may become paralyzed by high radiation levels, and in this circumstance, they indicate either no increase in counts or a count rate much lower than actually present. Detector paralysis can be checked by moving the detector much farther from the source and seeing if a paradoxical increase occurs in count rate.

If high radiation levels are anticipated, then an ionization chamber is preferable to a G-M detector. Ionization detectors can be used to measure radiation exposure rate and to estimate dose rate, but they are less sensitive than G-M detectors. Scintillation detectors are much more sensitive than either G-M detectors or ionization detectors in detecting low-level contamination and are able to determine gamma-ray energy, but they are more expensive and not as widely available.

Direct-reading pocket dosimeters, a type of ionization chamber, are needed for monitoring radiation exposure of staff during decontamination and emergency care (Fig. 13-2). A charger is needed to reset the dosimeters. The advantage of these devices is the immediate reading of cumulative exposure since the last resetting, but they do not provide a permanent record of exposure. Film badges and thermoluminescence detectors provide more accurate radiation exposure data than pocket dosimeters, and they result in a permanent record, but the results are not immediately available.

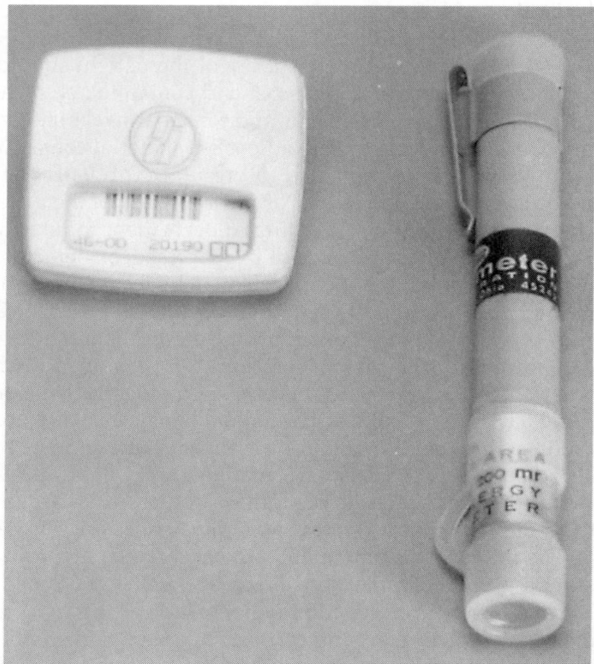

Figure 13-2. Personal dosimeters worn by staff.

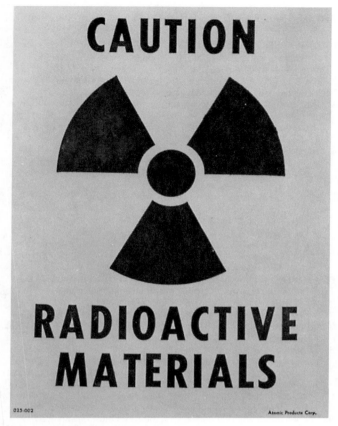

Figure 13-3. Radioactive hazard warning sign.

MANAGEMENT OF RADIATION ACCIDENTS

Prehospital Management

At the scene of a radiation accident, a number of tasks must be accomplished rapidly. The site must be secured, a command post set up upwind of the site, and a contamination/decontamination perimeter established. The number of personnel inside the contaminated sector should be limited to the minimum necessary to evacuate victims and accomplish necessary tasks. Contaminated clothes and objects should be left inside the control line. The nature of the exposure should be ascertained (irradiation versus radioactive contamination), and a determination of whether the exposure is continuing should be made. If, in fact, the exposure is continuing, emergency personnel must ensure their own safety before attempting to rescue any victims. If the radiation source cannot be isolated or shielded, allowable exposure times for rescuers must be calculated before entering the contaminated site.

The immediate priority for any victim of a radiation accident, whether in the prehospital setting or the emergency department, is to address any life threats that may exist not from radiation but from concomitant injury. The combination of associated injuries and radioactive contamination requires expert management to prevent incorporation. Although rescuers and emergency personnel should take appropriate steps to avoid personal contamination, lifesaving interventions should never be delayed. Protective clothing, such as shoe covers, gowns, coveralls, masks, and gloves, may be donned to prevent skin contamination.

As soon as is practical, the radiation victim should be moved away from the contaminated site to the control line. Proper signs should be in place to warn of the hazards (Fig. 13-3). At this control site, a survey can be performed using a G-M survey meter to determine the extent of contamination. If the meter indicates the presence of radioactivity, all clothing and valuables should be removed from the victim, bagged, and labeled. This step may reduce the contamination by as much as 70%. All metal objects should be identified and saved for possible neutron activation analysis, which can aid estimates of the radiation dose received. It should be remembered that unless associated serious injuries exist, there is really no reason to rush to the hospital. Whenever possible, the victim should be washed at the site. Most of the threat of contaminating others is removed when the clothing is gone and the victim has showered. The victim should then be wrapped in a sheet, to decrease the possibility of spreading any remaining contaminated material, and moved to the ambulance for transport. The rescuers should remove the victim's outer clothing. The interior of the ambulance can be covered or draped to minimize contamination, and transporting personnel should wear protective clothing, gloves, and masks during the transport.

Emergency Department Management

Emergency medical care of injured individuals takes precedence over decontamination, and lifesaving care should never be deferred for assessment of radiologic injuries or contamination. The hospital is usually notified of possible contamination before a victim arrives, however, and activation of the radiologic emergency plan should permit medical assessment and decontamination to proceed (Table 13-6). If a radiologic accident involves multiple individuals, it may be more practical to triage at the scene and initially transport only those who are injured. If individuals are contaminated at a site with decontamination facilities, it may be preferable to decontaminate uninjured individuals on site (14). Some individuals may not be contaminated. Also, exposures to sealed sources are not associated with contamination (unless a sealed source has been opened).

The nature of the accident or radiologic exposure should be determined at the earliest possible time so the hospital's radiation disaster plan can be activated. Some individuals know exactly the radionuclide and activity involved, such as in a lab-

TABLE 13-6. Emergency department and staff preparation

1. Remove all patients and pregnant women from the arrival zone of the ambulance, the entrance into the emergency department, and the route of all contaminated patients.
2. The route from the ambulance arrival zone to the decontamination room is covered with polyethylene plastic secured to the floor with tape.
3. The arrival route and entryway for patients are demarcated with rope or *radioactive*-labeled ribbon. Proper *radioactive* signs are in place. This area remains as such until cleared by radiation safety officers or the health physicists in charge.
4. The decontamination room is marked with proper signs. The floors and walls are covered with polyethylene plastic sheeting secured by tape. A demarcation line of bright, clearly identifiable tape separates clean from unclean areas on entrance to the decontamination room. Ventilation to the room is turned off and ventilation ducts covered with appropriate filters or plastic. The room must be self-contained. Electrical switches and handles of doors and equipment should be covered with tape.
5. A designated radiation safety officer maintains watch at the entrance of the decontamination room to monitor all personnel, equipment, and samples leaving the room.
6. A designated nurse or technical assistant is on standby outside the decontamination room to pass in supplies to the medical team in the room. This person does not enter the decontamination room.
7. All equipment in the room is essential to the care and decontamination of the patient and must remain in the room until cleared by radiation therapy.
8. Protective garments are donned by the decontamination team. Two pairs of gloves should be worn. The inner gloves are removed as the last pieces of protective equipment as the person exits the room post-decontamination. The minimum protection includes surgical scrub wear, pants and shirt, cap, masks, shoe covers, surgical gown with sleeves taped, two pairs of gloves, and eye protection.
9. All personnel entering and leaving the room must be surveyed for radiation safety for contamination. Contaminated items and clothing must remain in the room.

oratory accident. It may be possible from the history to determine the likelihood of external or internal contamination and to make an early assessment of radiologic risk.

EXTERNAL CONTAMINATION AND DECONTAMINATION

One room should be designated as the decontamination room and prepared for the victim. Nonessential equipment should be removed, the ventilation system turned off, and coverings placed on the floor and all door handles, cabinet handles, drawer handles, and light switches. Entry to and exit from the room must be controlled to prevent the spread of contamination. Optimally, the room selected should be close to the ambulance entrance to minimize exposure, and the route from the ambulance entrance to the designated room should be covered with paper and sheets. A decontamination table should be available where the victim can be washed and the effluent collected for disposal. If the effluent can be directly flushed into ordinary drains and diluted with large amounts of water, then no risk exists in allowing the contaminated fluid to be disposed of in this fashion.

Once the patient arrives at the hospital, he or she should be transferred to a hospital stretcher, and the transporting vehicle secured until it can be surveyed and declared free of contamination. Ambulance personnel should be monitored for contamination and, if positive, should remove all clothing, shower, and then be checked again. All hospital personnel involved in evaluating and treating victims should wear protective clothing, including gowns, gloves, masks, caps, and shoe covers and utilize film badges or dosimeters to monitor their exposure.

Evaluation and decontamination of the patient may proceed once all immediate life-threatening problems have been addressed. A careful, complete survey of the patient should be performed by the radiation physicist and contaminated areas of the body documented. Nasal, oral, and ear canal swabs should be obtained and sent for analysis. Radioactive material contaminating wounds, ingested, or inhaled can result in irradiation of tissues throughout the body as well as incorporation of the material into biochemical reactions, resulting in permanent radioactivity. Treatment of contaminated wounds by surgical debridement may be necessary if wounds cannot be adequately decontaminated.

Decontamination of any open wound is the first priority. If an open wound is found to be contaminated, decorporation treatment should be started. Also, decorporation should be instituted for inhaled or ingested radioactive material. Thus, identification of the type and nature of the radioactive contaminant is crucial. Copious irrigation of the wounds with normal saline usually removes some of the radioactive material. If oral contamination is found, ingestion is presumed, and aspiration of stomach contents by nasogastric tube is indicated. If the aspirate is contaminated, gastric lavage follows. The finding of contamination in nasal swabs is considered presumptive proof of inhalation of radioactive material.

Dermal absorption of radionuclides and radioactivity is of primary concern in planning for the management of patients. Absorption is a passive process determined by the nature of the radionuclide, the physical condition of the skin, the extent of contamination, the solubility of the contaminant, and the chemical nature of the radionuclide. The horny layer of the skin is the most important barrier to penetration. Mechanical damage to the skin substantially increases absorption. Injury from acids and alkalis can either facilitate or, in some cases, inhibit percutaneous absorption. Dilute acid burns facilitate the dermal penetration of plutonium.

The initial evaluation of external contamination should include gamma, beta, and alpha monitoring. Experience in monitoring for beta emitters and alpha emitters is essential. An inexperienced person using this sophisticated equipment can miss beta-emitting contamination, and beta burns to the skin can occur if this contamination remains in contact too long.

Once the patient is medically stabilized, and if the initial survey indicates contamination, decontamination should begin (Table 13-7). Clothing should be removed—preferably by cutting and folding back on itself to minimize further spread of contamination—and placed in a plastic bag. Intact skin is an effective barrier, and skin contamination can usually be removed by routine washing with soap and water. Contaminated wounds may be cleaned gently with a surgical sponge and irrigation. Skin decontamination should continue until no further decrease in activity occurs, no significant contamination remains, or further decontamination is more harmful than helpful (14). The use of a soft brush or soft sponge is recommended to prevent abrading the skin. Attention should be paid to the hair, nails, and web spaces of toes and fingers. The wash solution should be collected in a containment vessel, and the decontamination team adequately garbed in protective clothing. Between decontamination procedures, the skin should be dried and monitored for effectiveness of the decontamination. If contaminant remains, this process should be repeated until background levels are demonstrated by monitoring. The use of 5% sodium hypochlorite (household bleach) has been recommended for more persistent contamination. A problem with sodium hypochlorite is that a weakly acidic solution tends to make plutonium soluble and could increase risk of percutaneous absorption.

Once these procedures are performed, the patient is moved to a clean stretcher and then resurveyed. Hair that cannot be decontaminated should be removed by clipping and saved by

TABLE 13-7. Management and decontamination of patients

1. The physician in charge directs medical care and decontamination of the patients.
2. Radiation safety officer monitors patient front and back on arrival. Contaminated areas are recorded by nurse on patient cards or tags.
3. Patient's clothes are removed and sealed in plastic bag, containing proper patient identification.
4. Routine cotton swab samples are obtained of mouth, eye conjunctivae and mucosa, nasal mucosa, and ear canals and placed in sample containers marked with the patient's identification. Other samples are obtained as needed, such as of wound sites and all skin contaminated areas. Samples are given to radiation safety officer for proper storage.
5. Radiation safety officer monitors all decontamination personnel and biological samples obtained during management and decontamination.
6. Medical assessment identifies medical needs of the patient. Patients with contaminated open wounds have priority.
7. Contaminated wounds:
   A. If decorporation treatment with diethylenetriamine pentaacetic acid is indicated, begin as soon as possible.
   B. Open wounds are washed with normal saline for 3 to 5 minutes and remonitored for contamination level. This step is repeated if contamination persists.
   C. Persisting contamination of open wounds despite repeated saline washings can be managed with a 3% hydrogen peroxide wash.
   D. Contaminated tissue not being successfully removed by repeated washings may require surgical debridement. Surgical debridement may be necessary if the radionuclide is toxic, has a long half-life, and is not removed by appropriate decontamination methods.
   E. Save and label all tissue removed and place in appropriate specimen containers for storage by radiation safety.
   F. Cover all decontaminated wounds with sterile dressing and protect them from other areas of the skin that may be undergoing decontamination.
8. Contaminated eyes, ears, mouth, nose:
   A. Irrigate eyes with water or saline. Do not allow cross-contamination to the other eye during irrigation.
   B. Irrigate ears with warm saline or a 50:50 mixture of warm saline with 3% hydrogen peroxide using a bulb syringe. Monitor decontamination process, and repeat irrigation as needed. Do not allow irrigation solution to flow into patient's mouth, eyes, or wounds.
   C. Irrigate nose with saline using a bulb syringe. Have suction available, and do not allow patient to swallow irrigant. Monitor irrigant for radioactivity during the process.
   D. Have patient irrigate mouth without swallowing the water. Insert nasogastric tube into stomach and monitor contents of stomach for radioactivity. If gastrointestinal contents are contaminated, then lavage stomach until clear and begin decorporation with diethylenetriamine pentaacetic acid.
   E. Monitor level of decontamination and repeat irrigations as needed.
9. External contamination:
   A. Decontamination of the skin should begin with mild washing and gentle scrubbing using a detergent and water. A soft sponge or soft brush should be used to avoid skin abrasions. Monitor skin and washing fluid for radioactivity and repeat washing three to four times to remove residual contaminant.
   B. For persisting levels of contamination, use a mixture of 50:50 cornmeal and powdered detergent (Tide, Procter & Gamble, Cincinnati) mixed in water to form a paste. Gently scrub the skin with this mildly abrasive material using soft sponges.
   C. For persisting contamination, a 5% sodium hypochlorite solution (household bleach) can be used either at full strength over most areas or diluted 1:4 (bleach:water) over areas such as the face and neck.
   D. Citric acid 3% can be applied to the areas and rinsed off with water.
   E. For persistent contamination, and in extreme cases only, the application of 4% potassium permanganate followed by a 4% sodium bisulfite rinse may be tried. Potassium permanganate is an oxidizer and stains the skin as well as removes the outer layer of the skin.
   F. All skin areas, front and back, should be decontaminated until radiation safety agrees that the process is successful.
   G. Washings are collected in a containment vessel.
   H. Avoid splashing decontamination fluid, and do not allow washings to contaminate eyes, mouth, other mucous membranes, or wounds of the patient.
   I. Contaminated hair is washed with water and soap, then rinsed and monitored. Repeat as necessary. Hair may have to be cut. Do not shave hair because of risk of cutting skin.
10. Patients may be removed from the decontamination room after radiation safety indicates that the level of contamination is safe. The patient should be dried. All materials should remain in the decontamination room. Wounds can be closed as needed after decontamination. Monitoring of patients and personnel is performed before anyone is allowed to leave the room.
11. Entire body of patient is monitored by radiation safety before leaving room.
12. All previously sampled areas should be resampled and labeled as *postdecontamination* with time and patient identification.
13. New polyethylene floor covering is laid out from the patient to the door of the decontamination room, and a clean stretcher is brought into the room. The patient is placed on the stretcher by a clean team and removed from the room. The process is monitored by radiation safety.
14. Decontamination team exit:
   A. The team may be rotated in and out, depending on the level of contamination. This is guided by radiation safety.
   B. An exiting team member goes to the designated clean line at the door of the room. All protective clothing is placed in a predesignated drop zone or placed in a predesignated container. Outer gloves are removed first. Personnel monitors are then given to a radiation safety officer. Remove tape from sleeves and trouser cuffs. Remove outer surgical gown, then shirt and pants. Shoe covers are removed one at a time. Radiation safety monitors the first shoe and if clean, the person can step over the line into the clean area and remove the second shoe cover. The inner gloves are then removed after the person is over the clean line and dropped into the designated area.
   C. The team member then showers and is remonitored by the radiation safety officer for any contamination.

radiation safety. Shaving is to be avoided, because small breaks in the skin may be produced.

After triage and patient assessment, samples of body fluids should be obtained for analysis. Blood is sent for a complete blood count, differential, and platelet count. It is essential that samples be drawn as early as possible to determine a baseline leukocyte count and to type lymphocytes for possible marrow transplantation later in the patient's course. Absolute lymphocyte count of more than 1,500 cells/mm^3 48 hours after exposure indicates minimum exposure, whereas fewer than 1,000 lymphocytes at 24 hours or 500 at 48 hours indicates a severe radiation exposure. Serum electrolytes and a chromosome analysis are also performed on blood specimens. Urine and fecal samples are collected daily; however, initial samples that are negative for contamination may be misleading. Several days may be needed before an accurate assessment can be made.

Possible inhalation or ingestion of radionuclides resulting in internal contamination can be assessed quickly by counting swabs of the nares and mouth, but negative swab counts do not exclude internal contamination. All excreta should be collected, labeled by time and date, and saved for later counting and assessment of internal contamination. Such specimens are very helpful in estimating internal radiation dose. If any significant amount of contamination is thought to have been ingested, gastric lavage may be useful.

When decontamination of the patient has been completed, the patient should be moved to a clean stretcher for removal to another room. At this time the medical staff must remove surgical attire, gloves, and booties and be monitored before they leave the decontamination area. Any contamination on the medical staff must be removed before they leave the area.

Care should be taken in all of the G-M detector surveys to make sure that unintended radiation sources are not contributing to the counts. Such sources might include internal contamination in the patient, contaminated clothing in a bag nearby, or contamination on the surface of the survey probe itself. It is advisable to cover the G-M probe with a plastic bag so that the probe itself does not become contaminated.

Patients Who Have Received Diagnostic or Therapeutic Radionuclides

Several circumstances exist in which patients who have recently received diagnostic or therapeutic radionuclides may cause concern regarding radioactive contamination and its consequences. Such patients may be involved in accidents, they may die of disease or trauma, or they may be incontinent and contaminate the local environment. In each of these circumstances, the potential for diagnostic radiopharmaceuticals to produce a significant radiologic hazard is virtually nil, although any contamination should be contained and removed.

Patients who have received therapeutic doses of radionuclides may cause some radiation exposure of others. Patients who have been treated with pure beta emitters, such as ^{32}P sodium phosphate for polycythemia vera or strontium 89 chloride for intractable bone pain from skeletal metastases, do not usually require any special precautions because the beta particles are completely absorbed by body tissues; minor exposure to the hands of others might occur during surgery, autopsy, or embalming. Patients treated with high doses of ^{131}I sodium iodide for thyroid cancer, on the other hand, emit enough gamma rays so that radiation precautions are required. ^{131}I emits both beta particles, which deliver most of the therapeutic radiation dose, and gamma rays. Federal and state regulations require that patients receiving high doses of ^{131}I be confined, however, so encounters with such patients in an emergency department are unlikely.

Acute Radiation Injury and Biological Effects

The signs and symptoms of acute radiation exposure are affected by radiation dose, dose rate, and area of the body affected. Acute radiation syndrome assumes whole-body exposure; similar manifestations may be seen after exposure of large areas of the head, thorax, and abdomen (15). The acute radiation syndrome usually occurs with doses higher than 100 rad (1 Gy) (16). When radiation passes through cells (irradiation), molecules are bombarded with energy, causing atoms to become excited and bonds to break. This leads to the formation of ions (thus, the term *ionizing radiation*) and charged fragments called *radicals*, which cause further damage and alterations in function when they interact with other cellular components. The most radiosensitive tissues are generally those with high cellular turnover, including the hematopoietic, gastrointestinal, and reproductive systems. The exception to this rule is the lymphocyte, which, although it has a slow turnover rate, is very radiosensitive.

TABLE 13-8. Acute total-body radiation exposure dose physiologic response

Dose in rads	Medical effects
20–100	Alterations in number of circulating white blood cells and some chromosomal changes
100–200	Nausea and vomiting along with reduction in circulating white blood cells
200–400	Severe reduction in circulating white blood cells, nausea and vomiting, hair loss, increased chance of infection, some deaths
600–1,000	50% death rate in 30 days, bone marrow suppression, sterility, diarrhea, erythema, and loss of skin cells
1,000–2,000	Destruction of intestinal mucosa, diarrhea, death in 2 weeks
2,000–3,500	Vascular collapse, cerebral anoxia, death within 48 hours

Irradiation by high-energy gamma rays produces tissue damage but does not cause contamination unless source material was actually contacted. Irradiation may be localized or total-body irradiation. If total-body irradiation has occurred, then the patient may experience the onset of the radiation syndrome. The significance and extent of the irradiation injury can be determined by the time of onset of gastrointestinal symptoms (nausea, anorexia, vomiting) after exposure. The biological effects of radiation may become manifest within hours, days, or several weeks, or may take years or even decades to become evident. Those symptoms that occur rapidly are called *acute radiation syndrome,* whereas those that occur years later are *long-term effects* (Table 13-8). Total-body radiation exposure has been characterized as sublethal (less than 200 rads), potentially lethal (200 to 1,000 rads), or supralethal (greater than 1,000 rads). The acute syndrome is divided into four phases: prodrome, latent, manifest illness, and recovery.

Prodrome is an initial toxic period characterized by nausea, vomiting, intestinal cramps, diarrhea, salivation, and dehydration. Fatigue, apathy, fever, and hypotension may also be noted. This phase usually occurs with exposure greater than 100 rads and always with doses greater than 400 rads. Onset of symptoms occurs within 2 hours if doses exceed 600 rads; symptoms may begin in 2 to 6 hours at doses less than 400 rads. As a general rule, the faster the prodrome occurs, particularly vomiting, the greater the dose received. If vomiting occurs within 1 to 5 hours, the patient has received a significant dose of radiation; if it starts within 1 hour, the patient has probably received a near-lethal dose; and if vomiting begins within minutes, the patient has likely been exposed to lethal amounts.

The *latent period* is a period of well-being after the prodrome symptoms resolve, but it is dose related and may not be present in high-level exposure. This period may last days to weeks.

Manifest illness results from the injury sustained by susceptible organ systems. The hematopoietic system is exquisitely sensitive, and the result is pancytopenia. The usual sequence of changes is lymphocytopenia, granulocytopenia, thrombocytopenia, and, finally, decreased erythrocytes. Lymphocytes may disappear within 24 hours of exposure. Granulocytes often disappear within several days and platelets in 1 to 2 weeks. As a result, the patient is at extreme risk for infection or bleeding diathesis. Damage to the gastrointestinal tract may lead to profound electrolyte disturbances and dehydration. Death usually occurs within 2 weeks if the dose of radiation exceeded 1,000 rads, and within 2 days if the exposure was greater than 2,000 rads.

Long-term effects of radiation may result from a single, acute exposure or from prolonged, chronic exposure. The biological effects include increased incidence of various types of cancer, shortening of life span, sterility, and cataracts.

The prodromal period is associated with transitory symptoms beginning 1 to 6 hours after exposure. Symptoms may include anorexia, nausea, vomiting at lower absorbed doses, and fatigue, diarrhea, fever, and headache at higher doses (16). The latent period extends from the end of the prodromal phase to the onset of symptoms associated with hematologic, gastrointestinal, cardiovascular, and neurologic abnormalities. With doses less than 400 rad (4 Gy), the symptom-free latent period may extend for 1 to 3 weeks.

The hematologic syndrome is associated with radiation doses in the range of 150 to 600 rad (1.5 to 6 Gy). The basic pathogenesis is pancytopenia resulting from myelosuppression. Anemia is less prominent than leukopenia because of the longer life of circulating red cells. Lymphocytes are extremely radiosensitive, and lymphocyte reactivity may drop in less than 1 hour after exposure. Lymphocyte counts and cytogenetic changes can be used to estimate radiation dose down to a lower limit of approximately 20 rad (0.2 Gy) (11). Loss of granulocytes and lymphocytes results in immunosuppression. The main complications of the hematologic syndrome are infection resulting from leukopenia and bleeding caused by thrombocytopenia.

The gastrointestinal syndrome develops at doses of about 600 rad (6 Gy). Time to onset is related to dose, with onset in about 1 week at lower doses and 2 to 3 days at much higher doses (15). The severity of diarrhea increases with higher radiation doses. The syndrome results from mitotic arrest of stem cells in the crypts of the small intestine, so that when the outer cells are normally sloughed over a period of 48 to 72 hours, they are not replaced. Fluid and electrolyte loss occurs from the denuded epithelium, and bacteria normally present in the intestine cause infection and sepsis.

Radiation doses more than 1,500 rad (15 Gy) may cause hypotension, vascular damage, and cerebral edema, but only limited human data exist on doses in this range. These doses are almost invariably fatal (16).

Treatment of Acute Radiation Syndrome

Life-supporting measures and emergency treatment should take precedence over specific treatment for radiation injury. Treatment of trauma and burns may need to be combined with decontamination when the patient has been stabilized. Biological samples obtained at the outset may be helpful in assessing radiation dose and prognosis. A complete blood count provides baseline granulocyte, lymphocyte, and platelet levels; a sample of blood should be saved for possible lymphocyte cytogenetic analysis. Urine and feces can be used to test for the presence and magnitude of internal contamination. A sperm count may be helpful in assessing radiation dose, and the baseline sample can be obtained as long as several weeks after exposure (17).

Treatment of the hematologic syndrome is similar to treatment of complications of cytotoxic chemotherapy or immunosuppression. It is possible that colony-stimulating factors may be helpful in stimulating marrow recovery, although data in radiation-injury patients are limited (15). Use of bone marrow transplantation in radiation accident victims is controversial. If radiation doses exceed 1,500 rad (15 Gy), death from gastrointestinal or other nonhematologic causes is virtually certain, and so marrow transplantation is futile. A number of complicating factors exist in attempted bone-marrow transplantation in radiation-accident victims, and it is not clear that any of the previous transplantation attempts have been beneficial (15).

Treatment of the gastrointestinal syndrome centers on fluid and electrolyte replacement and therapy for sepsis and endotoxemia. There have been relatively few cases of the gastrointestinal syndrome from radiation accidents. Ten patients at Chernobyl were thought to have the syndrome, and all died within 3 weeks (16).

Treatment of Internal Contamination

Initial decontamination should help to minimize internal deposition of radionuclides. If radionuclides are present in the gastrointestinal tract, gastric lavage and purgatives may reduce absorption. If radioiodine has been absorbed or ingested, stable potassium iodide can partially block thyroid uptake if given orally within a few hours of the accident. Potassium iodide blocks reuptake of radioiodine by the thyroid, so it should generally be started, even if the time elapsed from the accident is more than a few hours, and continued for 1 to 2 weeks after initial exposure to ^{131}I.

Expert help and guidance should be sought before attempting to mobilize and remove internally deposited radionuclides. Fluids and diuretics may be helpful in promoting urinary excretion of some radionuclides. It may be useful to calculate the expected radiation dose from the deposited radionuclides to see if mobilization is advisable and whether the benefit outweighs the risks. Chelating agents, such as diethylenetriamine pentaacetic acid (DTPA), may be useful for transuranic and rare earth elements. Stable isotopes can be administered to dilute and competitively inhibit binding of the corresponding radioisotopes.

Also termed *incorporation,* internal contamination results from the inhalation, ingestion, or wound contamination of a radioactive material or radionuclide. The radioactive material thus has the opportunity to become incorporated into the body and irradiate internal tissues. This situation is a serious medical emergency. Some radionuclides can become permanently incorporated into the biological molecules of the body. Methods to decorporate these radioactive materials should be carried out according to a standard protocol. Patients who are judged to have high probability of internal contamination should undergo treatment as rapidly as possible to minimize incorporation of the radioactive substance. Treatment modalities revolve around enhanced elimination or excretion and reduction of absorption; however, specific therapy depends on identification of the radioactive contaminant involved.

If gastrointestinal contamination is likely, the first procedure utilized is gastric lavage. The stomach is washed with large amounts of water to remove as much material as possible. The aspirate should be tested for contamination and lavage continued until the fluid return is free of radioactivity. Purgatives may be utilized to increase the rapidity with which the radioactive material traverses the bowel. In addition, certain cathartics, such as magnesium sulfate, may produce insoluble salts with some radionuclides and further limit absorption. Barium- and aluminum-containing antacids are used for strontium ingestion and act to decrease uptake by forming insoluble salts.

Pulmonary lavage may be used for inhalation of radioactive material that is not soluble. This decontamination technique is performed under general anesthesia and involves the use of a double-lumen endotracheal tube so the two lungs can be isolated from each other and lavaged independently to remove deposited material.

Blocking agents may be administered to reduce uptake by saturating metabolic pathways with stable or nonradioactive compounds. For example, radioiodine can be competitively blocked by giving potassium iodine. Stable forms of strontium can be used to reduce uptake of radioactive strontium. The same is true for radioactive forms of calcium, zinc, and potassium.

Prompt and proper handling of contaminated wounds is especially important to prevent further incorporation of radioactive material. Surveying the wound with the radiation detector indicates whether the site is contaminated; sampling of wound tissue, exudate, any foreign bodies, and wound irrigation solution should be accomplished. Elimination can be enhanced by the use of chelating agents, which bind target compounds and then are excreted by the kidney. Multivalent radioisotopes in the actinide series (transuranic elements plutonium, neptunium, and americium) as well as rare earths have been effectively chelated using DTPA. Other metal chelators, such as calcium disodium ethylenediaminetetraacetic acid (calcium versenate), dimercaprol (BAL), dimercaptosuccinic acid, dimercaptosulfonate, penicillamine, and deferoxamine, can be used for the appropriate metals. Calcium disodium ethylenediaminetetraacetic acid can be used for transuranium metals, but DTPA is much more effective. Dimercaptosuccinic acid and dimercaptosulfonate, analogues of BAL, are newer chelators and are superior to other chelators for removing many metals, including cadmium, chromium, mercury, lead, arsenic, and copper. The use of combined chelators DTPA and BAL has been successful in removing cadmium in animal models.

Although human data on the use of DTPA are limited, its administration is recommended as soon as possible within the first few hours to be effective. DTPA is available from the Radiation Emergency Assistance Center/Training Site (REAC/TS) in Oak Ridge, Tennessee [telephone number (865) 576-3131]. Decorporation with chelating agents should be started as soon as possible in patients with contaminated wounds. Patients with residual contamination from skin break or foreign bodies may also benefit from pharmacologic therapy. Treatment depends on the chemical properties of the particular radioisotope involved and should be done in conjunction with advice from a nuclear medicine physician or radiation medicine specialist. DTPA chelates multivalent radionuclides that can then be renally excreted. The calcium and zinc salts of DTPA are approved for human use. CaDTPA is 10 times more effective than ZnDTPA for increasing renal excretion of actinide radionuclides within the first few hours of exposure. ZnDTPA is equally efficacious after the first 1 or 2 days of exposure.

In an acute exposure, 1 g of CaDTPA diluted in 250 mL of dextrose 5% in water should be infused over 60 to 90 minutes. The dose may be repeated daily for 5 days. For immediate field administration, an aerosol inhalation treatment can be accomplished by placing the entire contents of a vial in a nebulizer. ZnDTPA appears to be less toxic than CaDTPA, but because of its lower efficacy should not be the first drug of choice. CaDPTA should be continued at a once-daily dose of 1 g intravenously. During this time, blood samples, total-body and chest counts, 24-hour urine collections, and stool samples should be collected and monitored for radioactivity to determine need for further chelation. If further chelation is required beyond 5 days, then ZnDTPA should be substituted for more prolonged therapy. A DTPA administration protocol and consent form is available from REAC/TS.

A nuclear medicine specialist should be consulted as soon as possible in cases of incorporation or if it is suspected to have occurred.

Radiation Emergency Assistance Center/Training Site

Specialized assistance in medical management of radiation accidents is available from REAC/TS. The program supports the U.S. Department of Energy, World Health Organization, and International Atomic Energy Agency in medical management of radiation accidents. It is based at the Oak Ridge Institute for Science and Technology in Tennessee and offers 24-hour emergency response. Further details about REAC/TS and its services may be obtained at the program's Web site (http://www.orau.gov/reacts/).

SUMMARY

Radiation is a part of our environment. Radiation accidents are infrequent, but health care facilities should be prepared to deal with them. The nature of the radiation accident, the presence of radioactive contamination, and the estimated radiation dose determine the appropriate action.

REFERENCES

1. Mettler FA Jr, Upton AC. *Medical effects of ionizing radiation*, 2nd ed. Philadelphia: WB Saunders, 1995.
2. Adelstein SJ, Kassis AI. Radiobiology. In: Wagner HN Jr, Szabo Z, Buchanan JW, eds. *Principles of nuclear medicine*, 2nd ed. Philadelphia: WB Saunders, 1995.
3. National Council on Radiation Protection and Measurements. Exposure of the population in the United States and Canada from natural background radiation. Bethesda, MD: National Council on Radiation Protection and Measurements, 1987 [NCRP report no 94].
4. National Council on Radiation Protection and Measurements. Ionizing radiation exposure of the population of the United States. Bethesda, MD: National Council on Radiation Protection and Measurements, 1987 [NCRP report no 93].
5. National Council on Radiation Protection and Measurements. Exposure of the U.S. population from occupational radiation. Bethesda, MD: National Council on Radiation Protection and Measurements, 1989 [NCRP report no 101].
6. Kondo S. *Health effects of low-level radiation*. Madison, WI: Medical Physics Publishing, 1993.
7. Royal HD. The Three Mile Island and Chernobyl reactor accidents. In: Mettler FA Jr, Kelsey CA, Ricks RC, eds. *Medical management of radiation accidents*. Boca Raton, FL: CRC Press, 1990.
8. Eisenbud M. *Environmental radioactivity from natural, industrial, and military sources*, 3rd ed. Orlando, FL: Academic Press, 1987.
9. Hübner KF, Fry SA. *The medical basis for radiation accident preparedness*. New York: Elsevier/North Holland, 1980.
10. Mettler FA Jr, Kelsey CA, Ricks RC, eds. *Medical management of radiation accidents*. Boca Raton, FL: CRC Press, 1990.
11. Littlefield LG, Joiner EE, Hübner KF. Cytogenetic techniques in biological dosimetry: overview and example of dose estimation in ten persons exposed to gamma radiation in the 1984 Mexican ^{60}Co accident. In: Mettler FA Jr, Kelsey CA, Ricks RC, eds. Medical management of radiation accidents. Boca Raton, FL: CRC Press, 1990.
12. Mettler FA Jr, Ricks RC. Historical aspects of radiation accidents. In: Mettler FA Jr, Kelsey CA, Ricks RC, eds. *Medical management of radiation accidents*. Boca Raton, FL: CRC Press, 1990.
13. Jefferson RM. Transporting radioactive materials and possible radiological consequences from accidents as might be seen by medical institutions. In: Mettler FA Jr, Kelsey CA, Ricks RC, eds. *Medical management of radiation accidents*. Boca Raton, FL: CRC Press, 1990.
14. Rosenberg R, Mettler FA Jr. Emergency room management of radiation accidents. In Mettler FA Jr, Kelsey CA, Ricks RC, eds. *Medical management of radiation accidents*. Boca Raton, FL: CRC Press, 1990.
15. Saenger EL, Silberstein EB. Radiation accidents. In: Wagner HN Jr, Szabo Z, Buchanan JW, eds. *Principles of nuclear medicine*, 2nd ed. Philadelphia: WB Saunders, 1995.
16. Mettler FA Jr. Effects of whole-body irradiation. In: Mettler FA Jr, Kelsey CA, Ricks RC, eds. *Medical management of radiation accidents*. Boca Raton, FL: CRC Press, 1990.
17. Saenger EL. Evaluation of extent of injury. In: Mettler FA Jr, Kelsey CA, Ricks RC, eds. *Medical management of radiation accidents*. Boca Raton, FL: CRC Press, 1990.

CHAPTER 14

United States–Mexico Environmental Health Issues

Miguel C. Fernández and Herbert H. Ortega

The uniqueness of the U.S.-Mexico border makes it difficult to draw parallels with political borders elsewhere. It is an unusual region, in which an important industrialized country meets a developing one, characterized by a collage of two worlds containing peoples who represent extremes of affluence and poverty, education and illiteracy, technology and folk medicine, and urban teaching hospitals and rural clinics. Portraying a reversal of expected norms, the incidence of developing world diseases, such as tuberculosis, parasitoses, and diarrheal diseases, is rising north of the border. Communities south of the border are beset by the increased incidence of cardiovascular diseases and other chronic illnesses, which may be related to a number of factors, including increasing rates of tobacco use and exposure to environmental pollutants (1).

On both sides of the border, the consequences of major economic inequities create a third world setting. Consequently, environmental health issues cannot be approached independent of the context of the economic, political, social, and cultural factors that characterize and determine the quality of life on the border. The intense daily interaction between the people, industry, and commerce of both countries is a testimony of mutual dependence. The border catalyzes and plays out binational tensions derived from major issues, such as immigration and border patrolling, drug trafficking, commerce and economic development, health, energy and water resources and use, environmental pollution, interdiction, and national security. The consequences of the 1993 North American Free Trade Agreement (NAFTA) between the United States, Canada, and Mexico has dynamically increased international contacts and cultural and economic exchanges that may be expected to cause sweeping positive and negative changes in both countries (2).

GEOGRAPHY AND POPULATION

From east to west, the border consists of ten states: Texas, New Mexico, Arizona, and California in the United States, and Tamaulipas, Nuevo Leon, Coahuila, Chihuahua, Sonora, and Baja California del Norte Mexico in Mexico. The border stretches approximately 3,200 kilometers (2,000 miles) across the continent, from the Gulf of Mexico cities of Brownsville, Texas, and Matamoros, Tamaulipas, in the east to San Diego, California, and Tijuana, Baja California del Norte, on the Pacific coast (Fig. 14-1). The elevation ranges from 1,397 meters above sea level at Ciudad Juarez, Chihuahua, to 84 meters below sea level in some regions of Baja California Norte (3).

Together, the 1990 U.S. and Mexico censuses showed a population of 65,222,233 in the ten border states, with 79% of that number living on the U.S. side. Most of the people on the border live in fourteen pairs of cities. The population living in the 23 U.S. counties and the 39 Mexican *municipios* (municipalities) that touch the international line was 9,089,508. At the county level, 57% of the border population resided on the U.S. side. If the growth rate remains stable, the estimated population-doubling time for the U.S. border counties is 47 years, but only 9 years for the *municipios* (4).

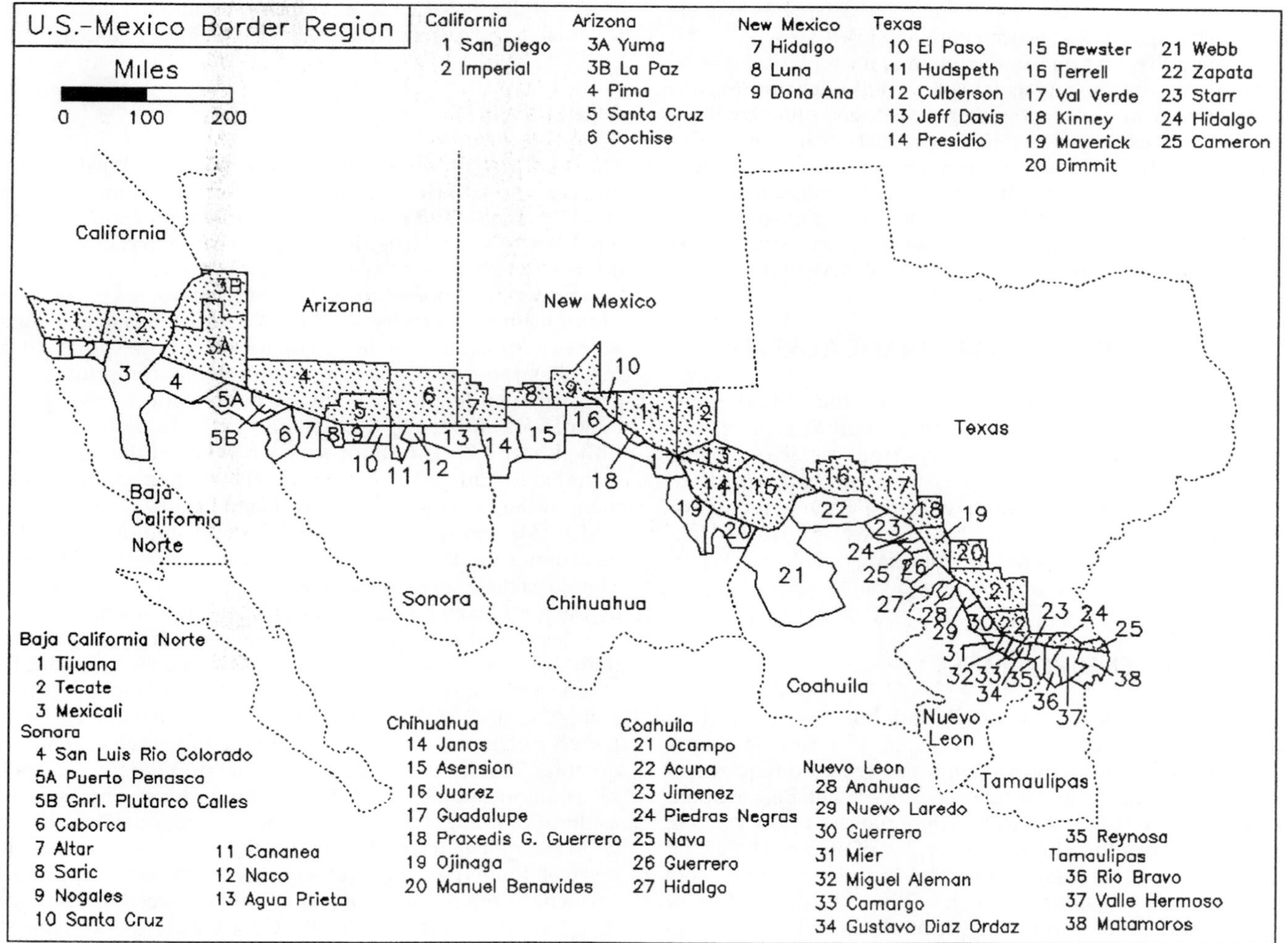

Figure 14-1. U.S.-Mexico border region.

THE ECONOMY AND THE *MAQUILA* INDUSTRY

Mexico's principal economic policy, from 1940 to 1960, was import substitution. This practice, principally oriented toward internal markets, needs foreign investment. The growing profits leaving the country increased the negative balance of payments until it became a chronic problem. The situation worsened during the 1970s and 1980s as oil prices plunged, the peso devalued in 1982, and the external debt increased. Industrial growth that was based on import substitution came to a standstill. Whereas Mexico needed an economic reorientation based on employment, the United States needed to lower production costs.

In 1965, American tariff laws and Mexican legislation established the National Border Program to foster the *maquiladora*, or twin plant industries. *Maquiladoras* are foreign-owned border industrial plants with special tariff benefits. They began as a U.S. initiative, but soon countries like Brazil, Germany, and Japan realized the advantages of production close to the U.S. market, and on a modest scale established their own plants in Mexico. The program entered an important growth phase during the early 1980s, which has not abated. Initially, the National Border Program required plants to locate along the border. However, *maquila* industrial parks can now be found throughout the country. *Maquilas* have become the second largest source of foreign exchange for Mexico, second only to proceeds from oil. Gross production at the end of August 1996 was U.S. $21.4 billion, which represents an increase of 29% from the same period in 1995. Women once comprised as much as 85% of the workforce but now make up less than 60% of it. As of August 1996, there were 2,355 plants in operation, employing 730,777 Mexican nationals (5).

Twin plants have become one solution to unemployment in an unstable economy. Premanufactured products brought into Mexico for assembly because of the low cost of labor and other corollary benefits are then exported as a finished product or component. The *maquiladora* enterprise, however, has not represented a permanent capital investment for Mexico. It currently uses minimum national supply sources (approximately 2%) and results in little transfer of technologic expertise. Evidence exists that these two situations are slowly beginning to change, in part because of NAFTA (6).

THE NORTH AMERICAN FREE TRADE AGREEMENT

The NAFTA between Canada, Mexico, and the United States came into effect in 1993. Labor unions, religious groups, and nongovernment environmental groups from Mexico, Canada, the United States, and elsewhere pressured the U.S. Congress to mesh environmental agreements with the trade agreements. This eventually happened. Thus, NAFTA has become the catalyst for a broad array of discussions, programs, and projects pertaining to environmental health internationally.

THE BORDER ENVIRONMENT

The accelerated urbanization of Mexican border cities such as Nuevo Laredo, Ciudad Juarez, Nogales, and Tijuana occurs without a corresponding growth in infrastructure required to prevent environmental and human endangerment. Because both governments recognize the health consequences of unclean air, water, and soil resulting from the interplay of personal behavior, industry practices, and environmental factors, measures were established on both sides for the handling and disposition of industrial, agricultural, and domestic products and waste. However, underfunded regulatory enforcement and administrative processes have been ineffective in achieving adequate compliance. These problems are compounded by a relatively very young, undereducated, and impoverished workforce. Consequently, government, business, and residents are faced with the formidable challenge to create and maintain a workable and comprehensive program of environmental hygiene (3).

Improvements in water availability, sanitation, and control of effluents have been slow despite efforts by the Mexican government to provide each family with an adequate water supply. In the established urban areas of the border states, as many as 87% of housing units have tap water. Families without access to running water share 200-liter plastic or metal drums, which often are contaminated and release toxic substances. As water storage tanks, these serve as breeding grounds for pathogen vectors (primarily mosquitos), parasites, and other infectious agents (2).

The U.S. border states have a better water supply and better delivery systems, but a trend toward substandard housing indicates that water supply problems are not exclusive to Mexico. Unincorporated settlements on both sides of the border, termed *colonias*, have not been annexed by local towns and cities. Hence, the *colonias* lack the tax base necessary to support sewers, running water, and electricity. Outhouses, septic tanks, or surface waste commonly drain into well water, causing a water supply that is unfit for human consumption (7).

Some chemicals that are banned in the United States, primarily pesticides, are used in Mexican agriculture. These substances and their persistent residues first affect Mexican farmworkers and then those who consume contaminated produce in the United States and elsewhere. Both countries contribute to the contaminations as legal and illegal pesticides find their way into the underground water table and rivers that cross the international boundary (2).

AGREEMENTS

The border is an area of confused jurisdiction. Weak enforcement of regulations offers ample opportunities for those who choose to ignore and abuse them. Clandestine export of hazardous wastes—including, for example, mercury, cyanide and arsenic compounds, polychlorinated biphenyls, asbestos, and various hydrocarbons—from the United States is a prime example of criminal activity with ecologically disastrous consequences (8). American laws governing these exports do not include strong sanctions against those who dump toxic waste across the border. Mexico fares no better, with excessive numbers of laws and poorly funded agencies that make enforcement difficult (2). Efforts to improve conditions on the border have included initiatives in the areas of education, housing, employment, water, sewage, environment, and health.

The Agreement for the Protection and Improvement of the Environment in the border region between the United States and Mexico, better known as the *La Paz Agreement*, was signed in 1983 by the presidents of both countries. In the agreement, the border was designated as extending 100 kilometers north and south, and numerous norms for environmental cooperation were established.

The International Boundary and Water Commission (IBWC), along with its Mexican counterpart, *la Comisión Internacional de Limites y Aguas*, has been an important and successful bilateral organization on the U.S.-Mexico border. Its charge includes the distribution, supply, and quality of the water resources, as well as the addressing of issues pertaining to groundwater (9). It is a good example of what a bilateral program can accomplish when it is well funded (through respective State Department budgets) and when both countries are equals in every respect. Its longevity is its best testimonial. The IBWC turned 110 years old in 1999.

In 1991, *Project Consenso* (consensus) was assembled. Participants were nongovernment border residents with an interest in alerting people to border health and environmental issues. They identified six categories of urgent concern: health promotion/ disease prevention, primary health care, maternal and child health, substance abuse, environmental health, and occupational health. The specific recommendations for the environmental health category were the following (10):

- Assure proper disposal of hazardous waste generated by the *maquila* industries.
- Establish a binational entity empowered to address and improve health and environmental needs along the U.S.-Mexico border.
- Increase potable water and establish additional sewage disposal facilities along the border.
- Prevent food contamination by pesticides.
- Decrease environmentally related disease conditions.
- Identify and reduce pollution sources affecting water quality in the Rio Grande river.
- Quantify the level of contaminants in the environment and initiate abatement efforts as necessary.

The occupational health category centered on the *maquila* industry and specifically recommended the following (10):

- Design and implementation of preventive programs dealing with hygiene and safety in the workplace
- Initiation of studies focusing on occupational health and safety to provide epidemiologic databases
- Establishment of joint training and exchange programs for regulatory agencies
- Increase in the cooperation and coordination between environmental and occupational health agencies

The Integrated Environmental Plan for the U.S.-Mexico border area (which borrowed concepts from *Project Consenso*), known as the *Border Plan*, was adopted in February 1992. This effort was the environmental parallel track to NAFTA. The four principal objectives of the Border Plan are the following (11):

- Cooperative efforts to strengthen the enforcement of environmental laws relating to polluting activities
- Increases in investments for pollution control efforts
- Cooperative efforts to increase the understanding of pollution problems confronting citizens in the border region
- Cooperative efforts in environmental education and training

Border Program XXI is a binational initiative (12). The program, which also borrowed concepts from *Project Consenso*, proposes to charge federal agencies with border environmental responsibility for the sustainable protection of health, environment, and natural resources. The strategy includes public participation, decentralization of environmental management from federal to local governments, and strengthening of local infrastructures by increasing resources and communication. The goal of this program is to achieve sustained development, which by definition must include improvement in other economic and social conditions on both sides of the border. The 5-year goals of Border Program XXI are to (12)

- Improve the capacity of the state, local, and indigenous environment and health services to evaluate the relationship between human health and the environment through surveillance, monitoring, and research
- Improve the capacity of the state, local, and indigenous environment and health services in order to deliver programs in environmental health, prevention, and education
- Augment the participation of other participants on the border (such as individuals, community organizations, occupational groups) in environmental health initiatives
- Improve the opportunities for training of environment and health personnel
- Strengthen public consciousness and increase the understanding of the problems regarding environmental health through information and educational opportunities

U.S. federal agencies assigned primary responsibilities for Border Program XXI are the Environmental Protection Agency (EPA), the Department of Health and Human Services, the IBWC, and the Departments of the Interior and Agriculture. Adjunct U.S. government organizations include the Agency for International Development and the Departments of State, Justice, and Energy. Primary Mexican federal agencies assigned are the Secretariat of Social Development (Sedesol); the Secretariat of Environment, Natural Resources, and Fishing (Semarnap); and the Secretariat of Health. Supporting Mexican agencies include the Secretariat of Foreign Relations, the Secretariat of Transportation and Communications, the Department of Energy, and the National Institute of Statistics (12).

The Intersectorial Coordinating Committee (ICC) was formally created by the Department of Health and Human Services and the EPA in 1995 to promote activities related to environmental health. The ICC is made up of federal and state environmental and health professionals and includes participation by the Pan American Health Organization and its Mexican counterpart on this project, the Secretariat of Health. The ICC defined *environmental health* as "human health exposed to the effects of chemical, physical and biological agents in the community, at the work place and at home" (13).

Other organizations active in border environmental health projects are the U.S.-Mexico Border Health Association, the U.S. Centers for Disease Control and Prevention, and the Agency for Toxic Substance and Disease Registry (2).

Mexico and the United States created the U.S.-Mexico Border Environmental Cooperation Agreement to assist in funding the improvement of border conditions. In turn, the agreement established two organizations: the Border Environment Cooperation Commission, aimed to facilitate building infrastructure, and the North American Development Bank (NADBank) to supplement other funding sources. NADBank is to be funded by the World Bank, the Inter-American Development Bank, and by the respective governments. It is estimated that of the projected U.S. $20 billion needed, NADBank will generate about $8 billion (14).

CLINICAL CONSIDERATIONS

Border environmental health issues are receiving more attention. *Maquila* and agricultural activities generate or use a wide range of substances that represent considerable dangers to the environment, workers, and other regional inhabitants.

Lead and Other Metals

Lead is considered dangerous primarily because of its potentially detrimental impact on the developing nervous system and intellect of children. Lead exposure is common in Mexico. Sources implicated so far include auto emissions, lead smelter emissions, lead-based glazes and ceramics, folk remedies, and canned food and beverages (15). As of 1991, nearly 90% of gasoline sold in Mexico was leaded (16). Companion cities along the border share a common atmosphere polluted by vehicle emissions resulting from the combustion of gasoline refined in Mexico. Higher concentrations of air lead were found to be the strongest factor associated with whole blood lead (BPb) levels exceeding 15 μg/dL in children in Mexico City (17).

One of the most well-known examples of lead poisoning in a border community was studied in the early 1970s in El Paso,

Texas. Landrigan et al. (18) found that 53% of the children ages 1 through 9 years living within 1.6 kilometers of a lead-emitting smelter had BPb levels of at least 40 μg/dL. They were found to be exposed to high levels of lead in dust and air. Lead exposure from paint, water, food, and pottery was also found to occur, but each was relatively less significant. Lead levels declined dramatically after the smelter was shut down (18). Calderon-Salinas et al. (19) compared two groups of children living near a lead smelter in the Mexican border state of Coahuila. In the group of children living closest to the smelter, they found more clinically significant impairment of neuromuscular conduction velocity and motor coordination, a decreased intelligence quotient unrelated to socio-economic status, and more general symptoms, including colic, headache, paresthesia, myalgia, and dizziness (19).

Lead-based glazes and ceramics are commonly used in Mexico and in the border region and have been associated with increased BPb in Mexico City and several border *colonias*. In Mexico City, the major predictors of BPb exceeding 10 μg/dL were the use of lead-glazed ceramics in food preparation, exposure to airborne lead, and the lead content of the dirt from children's hands (20). In a longitudinal study of 603 children in a Mexico City suburb ages 12 to 59 months, higher BPb levels were found in those living in households using lead-glazed pottery and in those who habitually chew colored pencils (21). A cohort study comparing pregnant women in Mexico City of high versus low socioeconomic status also showed increased BPb levels in those who use lead-glazed pottery (generally poorer women) (22). Although lead is known to be a ubiquitous health hazard in the urban environment, it also affects community health in rural areas. Needleman et al. showed that the use of lead-glazed ceramics was the most important determinant of BPb levels in rural Mexican communities (23).

Air contamination occurs with a number of other metals besides lead. Arsenic is abundant in the natural environment but may be increased with industrialization without pollution controls. In Texas, five of twenty areas found to have the highest 24-hour levels of ambient air arsenic were located along the Texas-Mexico border region (24). Air arsenic levels had increased over time and remained high for more than 2 years after significant emission source reductions (24).

Folk Remedies

Home remedies have also been implicated as a cause of lead and mercury poisoning in Mexican communities on both sides of the border. One implicated lead poisoning source is an orange powder stomach ailment remedy known variably as *azarcon* or *greta* (25,26). Mercurous chloride from a Mexican-produced beauty cream (Crema de Belleza-Manning) has been associated with several cases of mercury poisoning along the border (27). These and other folk remedies are easily obtained south of the border without a prescription and are easily brought northward (28). As recently as 1994, *azarcon* or *greta* was still to be found in Mexican herbal stores north of the border in cities such as Phoenix.

Gases, Fumes, and Other Air Contaminants

In addition to the contamination of air by metals from vehicles and some industries, the population of arid border cities share the irritating effects of other emissions, such as organic solvents, dust particles from a number of sources, and poisonous gases and fumes. Sulfur dioxide, carbon monoxide, and ozone from vehicle emissions and elevated ambient measures of particulate matter are pollutants found in higher quantities in border city regions. Results of binational environmental health studies have shown particulate ambient air levels higher than the U.S. federal primary standards long before the *maquiladora* industrialization phenomenon (29).

Open burning and unpaved streets are cited as the principal sources of suspended particulate matter in the Ciudad Juarez-El Paso area (30). This area has been cited for having air quality below the EPA standards for particulates, ozone, and carbon monoxide (31). These pollutants have been strongly associated with symptom exacerbations of asthma and emphysema. Even children with mild asthma are shown to be affected by high ambient levels of particulates and ozone (32). Indoor air quality is an issue in poorer border households, which often use traditional wood stoves for heating and cooking. Home use of these types of domestic stoves has been shown to have a causal role in chronic bronchitis and chronic airflow obstruction (33).

Blood carboxyhemoglobin levels have been shown to be elevated in border customs agents as they work among vehicles crossing at border stations (34). This situation would seem to have significance for only a relatively small group of workers. However, border inspectors are not the only people being exposed to high air levels of CO at the border stations. Many workers from both sides make cross-border commutes daily and may wait for up to several hours to cross while hundreds of vehicles are idling and spewing CO and other toxic fumes. Additionally, one finds hundreds of vendors, as well as beggars with young children and infants, mingling between the idling vehicles. After adding these various groups together, one can surmise that thousands may be exposed daily to high air levels of CO at an undetermined, yet probably significant, cumulative cost to their health.

Water Contamination

Water supplies in border communities are dangerously contaminated in a number of ways. One primary concern is the illegal but common practice of dumping hazardous wastes into bodies of water directly, into the soil, and into municipal sewage systems. Aquifers are shared across the border, and thus contamination on one side affects both sides. Sanchez published the results of a transborder water-quality monitoring program covering the Arizona and Sonora cities both known as Nogales (35). It was shown that municipal water supplies were fairly safe. However, well water trucked into poor communities that lack running water contained volatile organic chemicals and nitrates. Trichloroethane, tetrachloroethylene, trichloroethylene, dichloroethylene, and dichloroethane were found in levels exceeding the Mexican safety standard in three wells sampled twice at 4 months apart (35). The clinical significance of acute and chronic exposure to these compounds in these communities has yet to be determined.

In addition to unsafe water sources in these arid communities, those people in the *colonias* who lack running water may resort to storing water in unsafe containers, particularly discarded industrial chemical barrels (7). Depending on what chemical was originally stored in a particular barrel, a casual rinsing may not be sufficient to ensure that water stored in this way is free of chemical residues.

Dumping raw industrial sewage–containing metals may affect the health of border residents as well as those remotely located from the region. Examples of this problem in coastal waters have been shown by measurements of elevated levels of metals found in shrimp off the northwest Pacific coast of Mexico and in oysters found off the northeast coast in the Gulf of Mexico (36,37). These and other aquatic sources of nutrition may lead to increased total body burdens of metals.

Although industrial wastewater contamination is very important, the paramount water-related health problem remains enteric infections. The persistently higher rates of infant mortality on the Mexican side of the border are directly the result of diarrheal disease that is a consequence of the consumption of water contaminated by human and animal waste (38). In

El Paso County, Texas, nearly 18% of wells tested in 1992 were contaminated by fecal coliforms, and more contained other pathogenic bacteria (39). Because of the common and very shallow aquifer there, groundwater may be contaminated by pathogenic bacteria and viruses across the border. Fewer than 20% of the people of the *colonias* have access to sewer or wastewater treatment, and as many as 40% have no municipal water (39). Nearly all wells sampled in Ciudad Juarez, directly across the border from El Paso, were fecally contaminated, according to a 1987 study reported by Cech and Essman. Their study serves as an excellent review and summary of the multitude of border water supply contamination problems through 1992 (40).

Sewer line breaks are common in Mexican communities along the border. In Nogales, Sonora, the population growth has outgrown the capacity of the municipal sewage lines. Nogales is unique in that it actually has a sewage treatment facility, a binational plant serving both sides of the border since the late 1950s that was expanded in 1991. However, deficiencies in operations, maintenance, and expansion of the system have led to capacity overload. Because sewer lines often run parallel to washes, raw effluent from breaks in sewage lines lead to direct contamination of the groundwater, streams, and rivers, leaving them with high concentrations of coliform bacteria and industrial waste (35). Other Mexican border cities dump untreated sewage directly into the ground and water. Given these conditions, it is not surprising that amebiasis, hepatitis A, *Salmonella typhi* infections, and shigellosis are much more common in the border communities, particularly in the *colonias*, because the lack of sewers and sewage treatment plants allows for a continuous recycling of infectious agents (40).

Infectious Diseases

In addition to those diseases acquired from the consumption of contaminated water supplies, infectious diseases are common in the border communities. They include respiratory infections; brucellosis attributed to the consumption of unpasteurized goat cheese; sexually transmitted diseases, including acquired immunodeficiency syndrome; rabies from wild dogs, bats, and coyotes; and tuberculosis. Water stored in open containers and drums allows the proliferation of the *Aedes aegypti* mosquito, the vector responsible for transmitting Dengue fever to humans (41).

Pesticides, Fumigants, and Other Agricultural Exposures

Many of the communities close to the border work in agriculturally related businesses. Certain sectors of this group of people are exposed to a wide variety of hazardous conditions. Trauma ranks highly in agricultural area morbidity and mortality. Prolonged sun exposure is common. Windswept and tractor-raised soil, airborne plant fibers, harvested grain dust, and farm vehicular emissions exposure are important with regard to respiratory illnesses (42). Occasionally, deaths of unsuspecting stowaway train passengers have occurred because of riding in fumigated railroad boxcars carrying fresh produce along the border (43).

In Mexico, restrictions on the production, import, and use of persistent organochlorine pesticides, mostly DDT, toxaphene, and benzene hexachloride, have been limited (44). In fact, the legal production and use of DDT is still allowed under Mexican law for use in public health campaigns. As recently as 1982, Mexico was producing an estimated 5,700 tons per year (44). Despite a growing awareness of the long-term adverse environmental and health effects of widespread use of organochlorine, underfunding of research and a lack of enforcement of regulatory restrictions has remained the norm (44). Political pressure beginning in the 1970s culminated in the creation of *la Comisión Intersecretarial para el Control del Proceso y Uso de Plaguicidas, Fertilizantes y Sustancias Tóxicas* (Interministerial Commission for the Control of the Process and Use of Pesticides, Fertilizers, and Toxic Substances) and a shift to the production of organophosphorous and carbamate insecticides (44).

Farmers, farmworkers, and their children are commonly exposed to pesticides through agricultural work environments. Given the number of workers exposed and the number and absolute quantity of chemicals used, relatively few studies of the effects on this population exist. However, evidence exists that persons exposed to either organochlorine or organophosphate pesticides may exhibit clinically significant toxicities. For example, a study of lactating women in a northern Mexican town confirmed previous studies performed elsewhere that showed that dichlorodiphenyl dichloroethene (1,1-bis[*p*-chlorophenyl]-2,2-dichloroethylene), the major excretory product in workers exposed to DDT, may affect a woman's ability to lactate. This is especially important in border communities with contaminated water supplies, in which those most at risk for enteric-related morbidity and mortality are newly weaned children, the youngest being most at risk (45).

Organophosphates and carbamates are well known to cause severe acute cholinergic syndromes and delayed neurotoxicity. Some evidence suggests associations between organophosphate pesticides and some cancers, aplastic anemia, spontaneous abortion, and stillbirth. Parental agricultural occupations are associated with male worker infertility and Ewing's bone sarcoma in children of male farmworkers. Finally, a number of congenital birth defects have been related to exposure to agricultural chemicals during preconception, including neural tube defects, facial clefts, and renal agenesis (46).

Mexico shifted from the production and widespread use of organochlorine pesticides to organophosphates beginning in the 1970s. In essence, a tradeoff was made between the gradual restriction on the use of environmentally persistent organochlorine and the use of relatively nonpersistent organophosphates. This shift created more acute clinical problems, especially for workers involved in their production, distribution, mixing, and application, as well as for those in the fields, in addition to those potential chronic effects as described above (44).

Neural Tube Defects

A great deal of controversy was generated by reports of neural tube defects (NTDs) along the Texas-Mexico border since the early 1990s. A cluster of cases in Brownsville, Texas, led to much publicity in the popular press about environmental pollution from Matamoros, the Mexican city across the border (47,48). Most cases were found to be in babies born to mothers living in poverty and in close proximity to the severely polluted waters of the Rio Grande (*Río Bravo* in Mexico). Studies have focused on this industrial-agricultural area and the questions regarding the etiology of these defects. Industrial solvent vapors from the *maquiladoras* and pesticide residues are evident in and around the Río. Paternal exposure to solvents and pesticides has been suggested as being associated with the development of NTDs (49).

Other exposures and occupations associated with NTDs are organic solvents, anesthetic gases (maternal exposure), mercury (paternal exposures), ionizing radiation (both maternal and paternal exposures), food and beverage processing, nurses, painters, and farmers/farmworkers (49). Additionally, suggested environmental associations are vinyl chloride, water nitrates, hazardous-waste sites involving solvents or metals, water-borne pathogens, and water disinfection by-products (48). NTDs are more common among Mexican than Anglo populations in North America. In one study, periconceptional use of folate-containing multivitamins seemed to be protective against NTDs in Anglo women but not California Latinas (50).

Maquiladoras

Workers in the *maquiladoras* are exposed to many chemicals, some of them carcinogenic. Items of particular concern include metals, fumes, corrosives, acetates, epoxy resins, pentachlorophenol, trichlorophenol, trichloroethylene, and other organic solvents and vapors. Additionally, workers are subjected to long work shifts; repetitive motion tasks; poor lighting, ventilation, and sanitation; and temperature stress. Surveys on the health of *maquiladora* workers have been difficult to perform and interpret. Surveys are dependent on self-reporting by the economically vulnerable workers, who may be reluctant to report negative information. Although their lives may be improved economically and socially in the short term, exposure to some chemicals may have long-term effects that may not become evident for many more years (51).

Reported occupational symptoms and diagnoses include dermatitis, nausea, headaches, visual disturbances, mouth and throat irritation, respiratory hypersensitivities, renal disease, increased rates of spontaneous abortion, growth and development problems in the children of solvent-exposed workers, nervousness and irritability, and various musculoskeletal ailments (51). In a survey, more than 60% of 497 *maquiladora* workers perceived health-related risks associated with working conditions (52).

A 1990 study of 480 women confirmed earlier studies that have shown that compared with women working in the service industry, women working in *maquiladoras* delivered significantly lower birthweight babies. Specifically, reduced birthweight was associated with work in the electronics and garment industries, which make up the vast majority of *maquiladora* jobs (53).

Although much concern has been placed on workplace exposure, the *colonias* serve as the homes for many of the workers. Moure-Eraso et al. surveyed Mexican community leaders and *maquiladora* workers in the towns of Matamoros and Reynosa, Tamaulipas. The majority of community leaders felt the *maquiladoras* brought few positive developments. They voiced serious concerns regarding overextended infrastructures, reports of community illness related to toxic wastes found in *colonias*, and environmental deterioration in general (54).

SUMMARY

The border between Mexico and the United States involves historically complex issues that cross many disciplines. The large economic disparity between the countries gives Mexico a strong incentive to make de facto concessions, including those with large negative environmental impact, in exchange for economic and political gains from welcoming U.S. industries within its borders in the form of the *maquiladoras*. The capital net gain by the United States can be measured in terms of lower labor, infrastructure, and environmental protection costs. Thus, perceived mutual gains are economy driven and are at the expense of the public health and the environment shared by both countries along the border and beyond.

The economic drive has led to rapid development of U.S. industry along the Mexican side of the border. Many of these industries use and generate diverse groups of natural and synthesized substances that are a cause for toxicologic and environmental health concerns in the region. Creating solutions to these problems requires further development of international cooperative agreements, and collaborations and exchanges in the educational, economic, and scientific research realms. Unfortunately, political and economic considerations could continue to hamper these types of development. To move beyond these roadblocks, we need to focus on the border as a shared environment. We must realize that borders are dictated by social, economic, and political conceptions, but that toxicology and the environment are oblivious to these borders.

REFERENCES

1. Soberón G, Frenk J, Sepúlveda J. The health care reform in Mexico: before and after the 1985 earthquakes. *Am J Public Health* 1986;76:673–680.
2. Ortega HH. *Present trends and future possibilities of health along the United States–Mexico border states*. Washington: Pan American Health Organization, 1992:13–17.
3. National Center for Environmental Health, Centers for Disease Control and Prevention. Interagency strategy to address environmental health issues along the U.S.–Mexico border. Atlanta: Centers for Disease Control and Prevention, 1996.
4. Ortega H. United States–Mexico border: vital statistics review. El Paso, TX: The InterAmerica Institute for Border Health, 1995:9–12.
5. Federal Reserve Bank of Dallas, El Paso Branch. The Maquiladora Industry in Historical Perspective (Parts I and II). *Business Frontier*. Issues 3 and 4, 1998.
6. Profile of the maquila industry in the state of Chihuahua. Regional information system of economic development of Ciudad Juarez, 1996:14–17.
7. Jones D. Trouble on the border: international health problems merge at the Rio Grande [Editorial]. *Tex Med* 1989;85:28–33.
8. Ponciano G, Moreno R, Espinosa RM, et al. Situación actual en México. La zona fronteriza México–Estados Unidos. In: Rivero Serrano O, Ponciano Rodríguez G, Gonález Martínez S, eds. *Los residuos peligrosos en México*. México City: Universidad Nacional Autónoma de México, 1996.
9. Sepulveda C, Utton A. *The US-Mexico border region: anticipating resource needs and issues to the year 2000*. El Paso, TX: Texas Western Press, 1984:353–364.
10. Pan American Health Organization. *Project consenso*. Washington, 1991:5–27.
11. Atkeson. The Mexican-U.S. border environmental plan. *J Envt & Dev* 1992: 143–147.
12. Secretariat of Health of Mexico, Environmental Health Division. Border XXI program: draft document. Mexico City: Mexican Social Security Institute, 1996:I–18.
13. Secretariat of Health of Mexico, Environmental Health Division. Border XXI program: draft document. Mexico City: Mexican Social Security Institute, 1996:III–21.
14. Houseman R. Reconciling trade and environment: lessons from the North American Free Trade Agreement. Washington: Center For Environmental Law, 1994.
15. Romieu I, Palazuelos E, Meneses F, Hernández–Avila M. Vehicular traffic as a determinant of blood lead levels in children: a pilot study in Mexico City. *Arch Environ Health* 1992;47:246–249.
16. Driscoll W, Mushak P, Garfias J, Rothenberg SJ. Mexico's experience. *Environ Sci Technol* 1992;26:1702–1705.
17. Olaiz G, Fortoul TI, Rojas R, et al. Risk factors for high levels of lead in blood of school children in Mexico City. *Arch Environ Health* 1996;51:122–126.
18. Landrigan PJ, Gehlbach SH, Rosenblum BF, et al. Epidemic lead absorption near an ore smelter: the role of particulate lead. *N Engl J Med* 1975;292:123–129.
19. Calderón-Salinas JV, Valdez-Anaya B, Mazuniga-Charles, Albores-Medina A. Lead exposure in a population of Mexican children. *Hum Exp Toxicol* 1996;15:305–311.
20. Romieu I, Carreon T, Lopez L, et al. Environmental lead exposure and blood lead levels in children of Mexico City. *Environ Health Perspect* 1995;103(11): 1036–1040.
21. López-Carrillo L, Torres-Sánchez L, Garrido F, et al. Prevalence and determinants of lead intoxication in Mexican children of low socioeconomic status. *Environ Health Perspect* 1996;104:1208–1211.
22. Farias P, Borja-Aburto VH, Rios C, et al. Blood lead levels in pregnant women of high and low socioeconomic status in Mexico City. *Environ Health Perspect* 1996;104:1070–1082.
23. Needleman HL, Schell A, Bellinger DC, et al. The long term effects of exposure to low doses of lead in childhood: an 11 year follow-up report. *N Engl J Med* 1990;322:83–88.
24. Shields J. Ambient air arsenic levels along the Texas-Mexico border [Abstract]. *J Air Waste Manag Assoc* 1991;41:827–831.
25. Flattery R, Gambatese R, Schlag L, et al. Lead poisoning associated with use of traditional ethnic remedies: California, 1991 through 1992. *Ethn Dis* 1994;4:95–97.
26. Snyder DC, Mohle-Boetani JC, Palla B, Fentersheib M. Development of a population-specific risk assessment to predict elevated blood lead levels in Santa Clara County, California. *Pediatrics* 1995;96:643–648.
27. Mercury poisoning associated with beauty cream—Texas, New Mexico, and California, 1995–1996. *MMWR Morb Mortal Wkly Rep* 1996;45:400–403.
28. Casner PR, Guerra LG. Purchasing prescription medication in Mexico without a prescription—the experience at the border. *West J Med* 1992;156:512–516.

29. Davila GH. Joint air pollution sampling program in twin cities on the U.S.-Mexico border. *Bull Pan Am Health Organ* 1976;10:241–246.
30. Applegate HG, Bath CR, Brannon JT. Binational emissions trading in an international air shed: the case of El Paso, Texas and Ciudad Juarez. *J Borderland Stud* 1989;4:1–25.
31. EPA lists areas failing to meet ozone or carbon monoxide standards. *EPA Environ News* 1988 May;3:1–8.
32. Romieu I, Meneses F, Ruiz S, et al. Effects of air pollution on the respiratory health of asthmatic children living in Mexico City. *Am J Resp Crit Care Med* 1996;154:300–307.
33. Perez-Padilla R, Regalado J, Vedal S, et al. Exposure to biomass smoke and chronic airway disease in Mexican women: a case-control study. *Am J Resp Crit Care Med* 1996;154:701–706.
34. Cohen SI, Dorion G, Goldsmith JR, Permutt S. Carbon monoxide uptake by inspectors at a United States–Mexico border station. *Arch Environ Health* 1971;22:47–54.
35. Sanchez RA. Water quality problems in Nogales, Sonora. *Environ Health Perspect* 1995;103[Suppl 1]:93–97.
36. Paez-Osuna F, Tron-Mayen L. Distribution of heavy metals in tissues of the shrimp *Penaeus californiensis* from the northwest coast of Mexico. *Bull Environ Contam Toxicol* 1995;55:209–215.
37. Vazquez FG, Sharma VK, Alexander VH, Frausto CA. Metals in some lagoons of Mexico. *Environ Health Perspect* 1995;103[Suppl 1]:33–34.
38. Simonelli JM. Defective modernization and health in Mexico. *Soc Sci Med* 1987;24:23–36.
39. Mroz RC Jr., Pillai SD. Bacterial populations in the groundwater on the US-Mexico border in El Paso County, Texas. *South Med J* 1994;87:1214–1217.
40. Cech I, Essman A. Water sanitation practices on the Texas-Mexico border: implications for physicians on both sides. *South Med J* 1992;85:1054–1064.
41. Warner DC. Health issues at the U.S.-Mexican border. *JAMA* 1991;265:242–247.
42. Weiss JA. The U.S./Mexico border health concerns and implications for nursing. *Nurs Health Care* 1992;13:418–424.
43. Deaths associated with exposure to fumigants in railroad cars—United States. *MMWR Morb Mortal Wkly Rep* 1994;43:489–491.
44. Albert LA. Persistent pesticides in Mexico. *Rev Environ Contam Toxicol* 1996;147:1–44.
45. Gladen BC, Rogan WJ. DDE and shortened duration of lactation in a northern Mexican town. *Am J Public Health* 1995;85:504–508.
46. Metzger R, Delgado JL, Herrell R. Environmental health and Hispanic children. *Environ Health Perspect* 1995;103[Suppl 6]:25–32.
47. Suro R. Rash of infant brain defects disturbs border city. *New York Times* 1992; May 31.
48. Krieger GR. The investigation of a cluster of neural tube defects in Cameron County, Texas. *Occup Environ Med* 1992;6:89–92.
49. Sever L. Looking for causes of neural tube defects: Where does the environment fit in? *Environ Health Perspect* 1995;103[Suppl 6]:165–171.
50. Harris JA, Shaw GM. Neural tube defects—why are rates high among populations of Mexican descent? *Environ Health Perspect* 1995;103[Suppl 6]:163–164.
51. Hovell MF, Sipan C, Hofstetter CR, et al. Occupational health risks for Mexican women: the case of the maquiladora along the Mexican–United States border. *Int J Health Serv* 1988;18:617–627.
52. Balcazar H, Denman C, Lara F. Factors associated with work-related accidents and sickness among maquiladora workers: the case of Nogales, Sonora, Mexico. *Int J Health Serv* 1995;25:489–502.
53. Eskenazi B, Guendelman S, Elkin EP. A preliminary study of reproductive outcomes of female maquiladora workers in Tijuana, Mexico. *Am J Ind Med* 1994;24:667–676.
54. Moure-Eraso R, Wilcox M, Punnett L, et al. Back to the future: sweatshop conditions on the Mexico–U.S. border. I. Community health impact of maquiladora industrial activity. *Am J Ind Med* 1994;25:311–324.

SECTION

III

The Individual and Organ Systems

CHAPTER 15

Clinical Dermatotoxicology

John B. Sullivan, Jr., Robert J. Levine, Jerry L. Bangert, Howard Maibach, and Philip Hewitt

STRUCTURE AND FUNCTION OF SKIN

The skin is the body's largest organ. The skin of an adult weighs 3 to 4 kg, constitutes as much as 7% of body weight, and measures approximately 2 m^2 (1). The skin serves as a protective barrier against harmful substances, is involved in thermoregulation, is a sensory organ, and has immune system functions. Skin consists of three layers: the epidermis, dermis, and subcutaneous fat (Fig. 15-1).

Epidermis

The epidermis provides physical protection for the skin and a major barrier against chemicals. The epidermis consists of four zones or layers extending from the dermis to the skin surface: the basal layer, the spinous cell layer, the granular layer, and the cornified layer (*stratum corneum*), which is the outermost area of the skin (Fig. 15-2). A major function of the epidermis involves production of the outer cornified protective layer of the skin. Most of the barrier function of the skin is found in the stratum corneum.

The basal cell layer of the epidermis consists of cuboid or columnar cells from one to three cell layers in thickness. The basal cell layer is the proliferative area of the epidermis. Basal cells have large oval nuclei and basophilic cytoplasm and replace cells lost from the epidermal surface. The epidermis turns over every 12 to 14 days (1). In addition, the cell transit time of the stratum corneum is another 14 days. The basal cell layer contains distinct populations of cells, including melanocytes. The undersurface of the epidermis undulates, which forms projections called *rete ridges* that separate dermal papillae.

Cells within the spinous layer include keratinocytes, which are polygonal in shape and have spiny projections known as *desmosomes*. Langerhans' cells and dendritic cells are scattered throughout the spinous layer. These cells have a function in immune reactions. Langerhans' cells serve as antigen-presenting cells to T cells.

The granular layer is composed of keratinocytes, which contain keratohyalin granules. This layer is two to three cell layers in thickness and is between the spinous and cornified layers. Lamellar bodies that are found in the granular layer keratinocytes are involved in the cornification process. A protein called *filaggrin*, which is a component of keratohyalin granules, causes keratin filament aggregation. Formation of keratin is a major function of epidermal keratinocytes.

The cornified layer, or the stratum corneum, is composed of flat polyhedral cells called *corneocytes* that have lost their nuclei and cytoplasmic organelles. Stratum corneum is the thinnest over the eyelids and genitalia, and thickest on palms and soles.

Nails

The nail unit consists of the nail plate and surrounding tissue (1). Nail plates are cornified cells that insert proximally and laterally into skin grooves known as the *proximal* and *lateral* skin folds. Nail plates consist of the same four layers as the epidermis. The cuticle is the cornified area of the ventral part of the proximal nail fold, extending 1 to 2 mm over the nail plate. The matrix of the nail unit contains cells that multiply to form the cornified nail plate. The lunula, a crescent-shaped zone distal to the proximal nail fold, marks the distal extension of the nail matrix. Beneath the nail plate lies the nail bed, which is rich in vascularity and arteriovenous shunts. Nail blood supply comes from two arterial arches branching from digital arteries. Fingernails grow 0.1 mm per day. Toenails grow 0.03 to 0.05 mm per day. A narrow zone of skin at the distal end of the nail bed, the hyponychium, merges with the skin at the tip of the digit.

Dermis

The dermis supports the epidermis with its connective tissue matrix. The dermis consists of connective tissues such as collagen, elastic tissues, and ground substance. These tissues help protect against trauma and mechanically support the epidermis. Within the dermis are blood vessels, lymphatics, nerves, hair follicles, sebaceous glands, apocrine glands, and eccrine glands. Collagen is the major structural component of the dermis. Ground substance is amorphous material filling spaces between the cellular components of the dermis and is composed of plasma proteins, water, electrolytes, and mucopolysaccharides.

An important component of the ground substance is fibronectin, high-molecular-weight glycoproteins. Fibronectins attach fibroblasts, macrophages, and keratinocytes to cell membranes, basement membranes, collagen, and fibrin. Fibronectin also has chemotactic properties and attracts fibrocytes and monocytes and endothelial cells (1).

The dermis is rich in vasculature, nerves, and specialized sensory receptors. Arteries arising from areas of subcutaneous fat form plexus, from which capillaries supply dermal papillae. Veins return blood to subcutaneous vessels. The rate of return of blood aids in thermoregulation. The dermal microvascular unit is associated with mast cells, T lymphocytes, and fibroblasts. The glomus is a

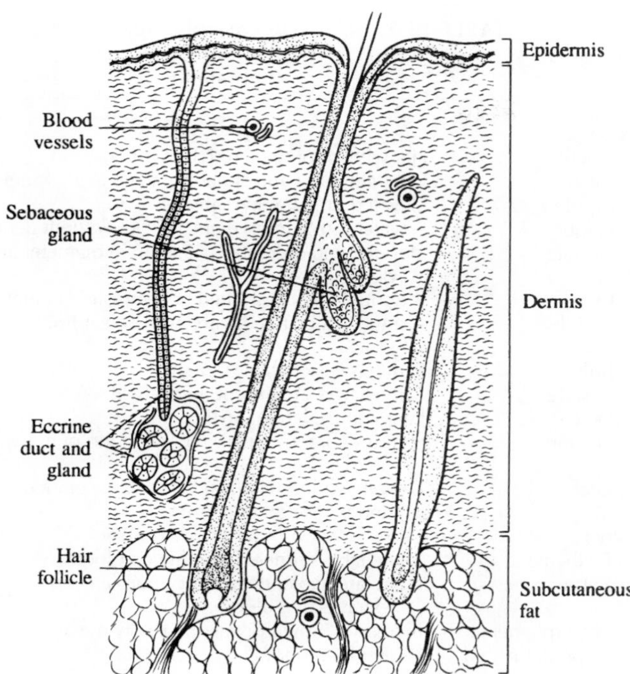

Figure 15-1. Layers of the skin. (Reprinted with permission from Arndt K, LeBoit P, Robinson J, Wintroub B. *Cutaneous medicine and surgery,* vol. I. Philadelphia: WB Saunders, 1996;4.)

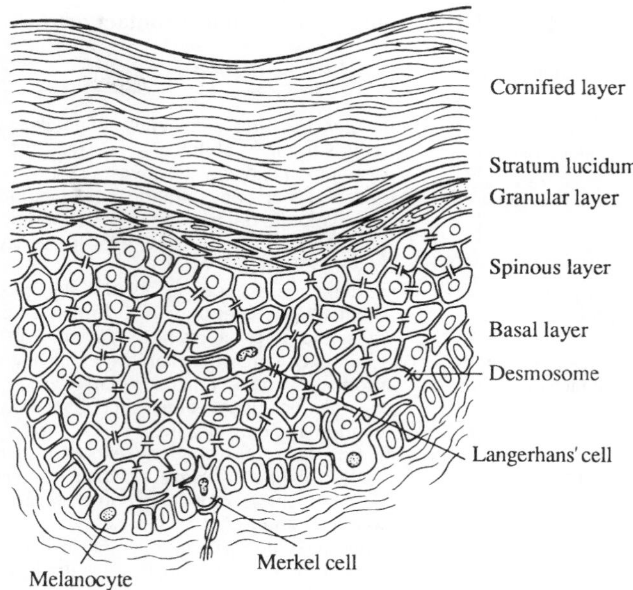

Figure 15-2. Epidermis structure. (Reprinted with permission from Arndt K, LeBoit P, Robinson J, Wintroub B. *Cutaneous medicine and surgery,* vol. I. Philadelphia: WB Saunders, 1996;6.)

specialized arterial venous shunt in the pads and nail beds of the fingers and toes and also on the skin of the ears and parts of the central face. The epidermal-dermal junction, also known as the *basement membrane zone,* separates the dermis from the epidermis.

Sensory Organs

The skin possesses a variety of specialized sensory receptors: temperature, pressure, pain, and touch. These sensory receptors are either free or encapsulated. The free nerve endings consist of single nerve fibers, whereas the encapsulated nerve fibers are elaborate and contain different kinds of cells and nerve endings. The free nerve endings can be myelinated or unmyelinated and are found forming networks in the dermis, especially around hair follicles (1).

Encapsulated neuroreceptors include Meissner's corpuscles, Ruffini corpuscles, Pacini corpuscles, and mucocutaneous corpuscles. Pacini corpuscles are located in the dermis and subcutaneous tissue and function as pressure receptors. Meissner's corpuscles are found in the center of palms and soles, lips, eyelids, external genitalia, and nipples and are mechanoreceptors. Ruffini corpuscles are found mainly in the soles in the lower part of the dermis and subcutaneous fat and are similar to Meissner's corpuscles. Mucocutaneous corpuscles are in the papillary dermis or submucosa of conjunctiva, tongue, gingiva, perianal area, and external genitalia (1).

Free nerve endings are myelinated or unmyelinated in the papillary dermis. Merkel cells are specialized free nerves attached to cells and are thought to be touch receptors. Merkel cells are found in skin and oral mucosa (1). Free nerve endings form complexes around hair follicles.

Dermal Glands

Glandular structures within the skin include eccrine glands, apocrine glands, and sebaceous glands. Eccrine glands are sweat glands and are found abundantly in the skin's surface, with highest concentration in the palms, soles, and axillary regions. These sweat glands produce a hypotonic solution and assist in thermoregulatory mechanisms.

Apocrine glands are found primarily in the axillary region, anogenital region, external auditory canal (cerumen glands), and eyelids (glands of Moll). Apocrine glands are not involved in thermoregulation and are not sweat glands. These glands are thought to function as scent glands and produce a viscous white odorous substance.

Sebaceous glands are found on all parts of the body except palms and soles, and they open directly onto the surface of the skin. They empty also into the outer portion of hair follicles. Hair follicles are responsible for hair growth on the skin and scalp areas. Sebaceous glands produce an oil called *sebum*—a mixture of triglycerides, phospholipids, and cholesterol—which helps lubricate and protect the skin.

CLINICAL DERMATOTOXICOLOGY

Dermatotoxicology can be categorized into the clinical areas of acute contact dermatitis, irritant contact dermatitis, allergic contact dermatitis, contact urticaria, phototoxicity and photosensitivity reactions, systemic toxicity from percutaneous absorption of chemicals, disorders of the nails, hair loss or alopecia, chemical burns, and ulceration.

Clinical Approach to Dermatotoxicity

The clinical approach to dermal lesions should proceed with a medical history and an examination of anatomic areas involved (Table 15-1).

SKIN LESION TERMS

Describing dermal lesions is the first step in diagnosis of a dermatitis. Dermal lesions have three basic morphologic features:

- Color
- Appearance and shape
- Surface change

TABLE 15-1. Clinical evaluation of chemical contact dermatitis

Step	Consider
Identify the chemical characteristics	Molecular structure, allergenicity, chemical nature, irritancy, ability to vaporize, skin penetration capacity, reactivity
Define the exposure	Dose depends on concentration, site of exposure, volume, duration on the skin, and penetrability of the compound; exposures may be multiple, acute, or chronic
Define preexisting problems	Physical trauma, skin drying, abraded skin, prior dermatitis, hobbies or work that might cause other exposures, atopic history, prior exposure
Identify environmental factors	Low humidity increases irritability, cool weather produces stronger reactions than warmer weather, occlusion of the skin enhances penetration and may also increase irritation
Identify airborne routes	Evaluate areas more commonly exposed, such as face, hands, and arms; chemicals and particulates can become lodged in sweat areas and in clothing
Note anatomic site differences	Skin permeability varies in different sites and is greater in the thinner areas; the palm is the thickest area, the face and upper back are thinnest
Note age factors	Skin irritation develops more easily in babies and children younger than age 8 years; skin problems are common in the elderly

TABLE 15-2. Skin lesion morphology

	Appearance
Lesion	
Macule	Flat with color (e.g., red, brown)
Patch	Flat with color and surface change (e.g., scale)
Papule	Elevated <0.5 cm in diameter
Plaque	Elevated >0.5 cm in diameter, but without depth
Nodule	Elevated and indurated, >0.5 cm in diameter and depth
Cyst	A nodule filled with fluid or semisolid content
Vesicle	A small blister, filled with visible clear fluid, <0.5 cm
Bullae	Same as vesicle but >0.5 cm
Pustule	Same as vesicle except fluid is yellow
Wheal	Edematous plaque (hive)
Erosion	Shallow sore from partial denudation of the epidermis
Ulcer	Deeper wound with loss of all of the epidermis and part or all of dermis
Colors	
Erythema	Blanchable redness from dilated blood vessels
Purpura	Nonblanchable, deep red or purple color from extravasated blood
Hyperpigmented	Increased brown pigment, usually melanin
Hypopigmented	Whiter than normal
Surface change	
Crust	Dried serum or blood on surface of skin (scab)
Scale	White or whitish flakes on surface of skin from thickened stratum corneum
Lichenification	Thickened skin with accentuated surface markings

Adapted from Lookingbill D. Principles of diagnosis. In: Callen J, ed. *Principles of diagnosis in current practice of dermatology.* Philadelphia: Current Medicine, 1995. With permission from Current Medicine.

Eczema is a generic term for inflammatory conditions of the skin typically manifested by vesiculation, erythema, edema, papules, and crusting. *Rashes* are inflammatory processes that involve blood vessels and the dermis. There is no vasculature in the epidermis. A rash without a surface change is solely dermal. Erythema is discerned from purpural changes because erythematous changes blanch on pressure. Purpurae are due to blood extravasation into the dermis. Surface changes may show crusting, scaling, lichenification, or fissuring. The skin may show erosion as in ulceration or be edematous (wheal). The lesion's morphology can vary from flat (macule) to elevated (papule, plaque, nodule) to fluid filled (vesicle, bullae, cyst).

MEDICAL HISTORY

Along with describing the morphologic features and location of the lesions, the medical evaluation should include the following questions.

What is the patient's environmental exposure or occupation? Defining exposure is essential, and understanding the actual tasks and job a worker performs is important to understanding exposure. Job titles do not always indicate exactly what the worker does on a daily basis. Therefore, relying on a job title may not provide correct information regarding exposures.

What anatomic area is involved? Because most occupational skin disease is contact dermatitis, generally the area where the chemical makes contact with the skin is where the lesion begins. Spread of the offending irritant or allergen can occur to other sites from the point of contact. The eyelids and face are typical secondary sites of spread from the hands. It should be noted if the dermatitis is symmetric, unilateral, or bilateral.

Is there a preexisting problem? Clinicians must differentiate a dermatitis that may have been preexisting versus one that occurred away from the worksite. What hobbies does the individual partake in away from work? Could there be multiple exposures of different agents?

What are the signs and symptoms? Contact irritant dermatitis tends to burn or sting. Contact allergic dermatitis itches. An acute allergic contact dermatitis has a polymorphic eruption with erythema, clusters of papules, vesiculation, edema, exudation, and crusting. An irritant contact dermatitis starts with burning and stinging and scaliness, with later development of vesicular or papular eruption. Discerning the two is frequently difficult without patch testing. The dermatitis should be described in terms of its location and clinical appearance (Table 15-2).

Are protective clothing and personal protective devices used? Gloves and other protective devices may not provide complete protection. Gloves can tear and be penetrated by chemicals, depending on the nature of the glove. Are chemically resistant gloves used? Chemically resistant gloves made of nitrile rubber are much more protective than latex gloves. Also, gloves can act as occlusive barriers to increase the chance of dermatitis if chemicals come in contact with the skin under the glove.

Is there trauma to the skin? Mechanical trauma to the skin can result in enhanced chemical penetration. Chronic trauma may also produce dermatitis and fissuring of the skin.

Are other people affected at work? If other people are affected, then an airborne allergenic or irritative chemical might be a cause.

TABLE 15-3. Irritant dermatitis versus allergic dermatitis clinical differentiation

Allergic dermatitis	Irritant contact dermatitis
Delayed onset	Acute onset
Itching	Stinging, burning
Vesicles	History of contact with known irritant
Erythroderma	Negative patch tests to relevant allergens
History of contact with known allergen	Localized to the site of contact; airborne contact irritants usually affect hands, face, and eyelids
(+) Patch test to relevant allergen	(–) Patch test for allergy

Does the rash improve when the person is away from work and worsen when the person returns to work? The answer to this question helps determine whether the rash is work related. However, the clinician must be sure that the individual has not come into contact with other chemicals from hobbies or other sources that could exacerbate or produce the dermatitis. Additionally, the role of stress must be evaluated in this context, as the patient may have a stress-exacerbated dermatitis that is not related to a work exposure.

The clinician should explore the occurrence of previous rashes and dermatitis. Allergies and medication use should be probed. Clinicians should inquire about any family history of atopic disease and history of other dermal lesions, such as psoriasis. General health and review of systems may reveal predisposing factors for dermatitis or other medical disorders. Dermatitis might be caused by medications and not an environmental exposure.

PHYSICAL EXAMINATION

Physical examination should take note of the anatomic location and the clinical patterns of the rash. Most occupational contact dermatitis affects the hands. If the individual has no protective devices and the hands are not affected, then the contact might be airborne. Airborne contact dermatitis may affect any area of the body. Exposed skin areas and areas affected by sweat are usually involved the most; these include the neck, eyelids, face, chest, and upper back. Allergic contact dermatitis can be generalized and involve systemic manifestations, such as angioedema, urticaria, and systemic reactions.

IRRITANT CONTACT DERMATITIS VERSUS ALLERGIC DERMATITIS

It is difficult to separate an irritant contact dermatitis from allergic or endogenously induced dermatitis (Table 15-3). Involvement of the popliteal fossae and the antecubital fossae tends to be endogenous or allergic contact dermatitis. Pattern of rash alone cannot rule in or rule out contact versus endogenous dermatitis, and competent dermatologic consultation is required (2,3).

Patch testing is the best method to discern between irritant and allergic dermatitis and should be undertaken by dermatologists proficient with this method of diagnosis.

Acute Contact Dermatitis

This is an acute reaction of the skin induced by a single exposure or multiple exposures to toxic substances. Such a toxic reaction is caused by dermal contact with obviously hazardous substances, such as acids, alkalis, solvents, and highly irritant and necrosing chemicals (Table 15-4). Injury to the skin ranges from erythema to burns, ulceration, or eczema.

TABLE 15-4. Agents causing acute toxic contact dermatitis and burns

Acetic acid	Barium hydroxide
Acrylic acid	Calcium carbonate
Acrolein	Calcium hydroxide
Benzoic acid	Calcium oxide
Boric acid	Hydrazine
Bromoacetic acid	Lithium hydroxide
Chloroacetic acids	Potassium hydroxide
Chlorosulfuric acid	Sodium carbonate
Fluorophosphoric acid	Sodium hydroxide
Fluorosilicic acid	Sodium metasilicate
Fluorosulfonic acid	Acrylonitrile
Formic acid	Antinomy trioxide
Fumaric acid	Acrylates
Hydrobromic acid	Methacrylates
Hydrochloric acid	Chromates
Hydrofluoric acid	Chromic acid
Lactic acid	Epichlorohydrin
Nitric acid	Epoxy reactive diluents
Perchloric acid	Formaldehyde
Peroxyacetic acid	Isocyanates
Phosphonic acids	Methylene chloride
Phosphoric acids	Peroxides
Phthalic acids	Benzoyl
Picric acid	Cumene
Propionic acid	Cyclohexanone
Salicylic acid	Methyl ethyl ketone
Sulfonic acids	Potassium
Sulfuric acid	Sodium
Tartaric acid	Lithium
Toluene sulfonic acid	Tetrahydronaphthalene
Tungstic acid	Phenolic compounds
Quaternary ammonium compounds	Phenol
Tributylin oxide	Phthalic anhydrides
Amines	Pentafluorophenol
Ammonia	

Adapted from Kanerva L, Mjorkner B, Estlander T, Jolanki R, Tarvainen K. Plastic materials: occupational exposures: skin irritance and its prevention. In: Van der Valk P, Maibach H, eds. *The irritant contact dermatitis syndrome*. Boca Raton, FL: CRC Press, 1996; and Bruze M, Freger S. Chemical skin burns. In: Van der Valk P, Maibach H, eds. *The irritant contact dermatitis syndrome*. Boca Raton, FL: CRC Press, 1996. With permission from CRC Press.

Irritant Contact Dermatitis

Irritant dermatitis constitutes 90% of occupationally related dermatitis (2–4). The clinician's challenge is to distinguish contact dermatitis from allergic dermatitis (see Table 15-3). Contact dermatitis from a chemical can appear as an acute onset, be delayed 12 to 24 hours, or can develop slowly over weeks or months. Clinical characteristics vary, depending on the onset. Certain clinical features suggest etiologies (Table 15-5).

Acute onset contact dermatitis from chemicals usually appears as an erythematous reaction of the skin with or without vesicles, bullae, edema, or erythematous vesiculopapular lesions. Delayed contact dermatitis usually appears as vesicles, papules, or erythema. Dermatitis that develops after trauma may appear as lichenification, scaling, or erythematous areas with papules and pustules.

Chronic dermatitis may cause fissuring, lichenification, dryness, and scaling of the skin. Delayed contact dermatitis appears as inflammation that is usually not visible for 8 to 24 hours after the exposure (2–4). The clinical course after that period of time resembles that of acute irritant contact dermatitis.

Many contact irritants are airborne. These include volatile organic chemicals, ammonia, acid alkalies, cleaning products,

TABLE 15-5. Lesions and possible etiology of irritant contact dermatitis

Lesions	Etiologies
Ulcerations	Strong acids, especially chromic, hydrofluoric, nitric, hydrochloric, sulfuric
	Strong alkalis, especially calcium oxide, sodium hydroxide, potassium hydroxide, ammonium hydroxide, calcium hydroxide, sodium metasilicate, sodium silicate, potassium cyanide, trisodium phosphate
	Salts, especially arsenic trioxide, dichromates
	Solvents, especially acrylonitrile, carbon bisulfide
	Gases, especially ethylene oxide, acrylonitrile
Folliculitis and acneiform lesions	Arsenic trioxide
	Glass fibers
	Oils and greases
	Tar
	Asphalt
	Chlorinated naphthalenes
	Polyhalogenated biphenyls and others
Milia	Occlusive clothing and dressing
	Adhesive tape
	Ultraviolet
	Infrared
	Aluminum chloride
Pigmentary alterations	Hyperpigmentation
	Any irritant or allergen, especially phototoxic agents such as psoralens, tar, asphalt, phototoxic plant
	Metals, such as inorganic arsenic (systemically), silver, gold, bismuth, mercury
	Radiation: ultraviolet, infrared, microwave, ionizing
	Hypopigmentation
	p-tert-Amylphenol
	p-tert-Butylphenol
	Hydroquinone
	Monobenzyl ethyl of hydroquinone
	Monomethyl ether of hydroquinone
	p-tert-Catechol
	p-Cresol
	3-Hydroxyanisole
	Butylated hydroxyanisole
	1-tert-Butyl-3,4-catechol
	1-Isopropyl-3,4-catechol
	4-Hydroxypropriophenone
Alopecia	Chloroprene, thallium, bismuth, borax, arsenic, barium
Urticaria	Numerous chemicals, cosmetics, animal products, foods, plants, textile, woods
Granulomas	Keratin
	Silica
	Beryllium
	Talc
	Cotton fibers
	Bacteria
	Fungi
	Parasites and parasite parts

Adapted from Harvell J, Lammintausta K, Maibach H. Irritant contact dermatitis. In: Guin J, ed. *Practical contact dermatitis: a handbook for the practitioner.* New York: McGraw-Hill, 1995; 11.

epoxy resins, metals, particulates, metal oxides, silicates, carbonless copy paper, and sawdust (2–4).

Diagnosis tends to be a process of exclusion, even though irritant contact dermatitis is more common than allergic contact dermatitis. Diagnostic evaluation should consider history of atopy; occupation; exposures; type of chemicals that could be contacted; whether the chemical irritants could be trapped in clothes, gloves, or areas of sweat; the anatomic region; distribution of the dermatitis; the presence of preexisting dermatoses; and skin that would be less resistant to the irritants, such as skin that has suffered mechanical trauma (2–4).

Airborne contact irritants or allergens commonly affect the eyelids. Contamination of a person's fingers with chemicals can allow spreading to other areas of the body, such as the face and eyelids. Contact dermatitis is the most common dermatitis of the eyelid and is frequently caused by cosmetics, chemical vapors, soaps, or hair products (2–4).

Cumulative Irritant Dermatitis

Cumulative irritant dermatitis is probably the most common type of irritant contact dermatitis. This manifestation occurs from repetitive chemical exposure causing recurrent symptoms. The condition can develop after days, weeks, or years of exposure (2–4).

Irritant dermatitis can develop after acute skin trauma and presents as erythema, vesicles, scaling, and papules. Irritant dermatitis may also appear as pustular acneiform lesions. Pustular and acneiform irritant dermatitis has been known to develop after exposure to metals, oils, greases, tars, asphalts, and naphthalenes. Some individuals exposed to chemicals experience subjective irritation or itching of the skin without visible inflammation.

The areas of skin most commonly affected by chemicals should be examined: eyelids, hands, neck, and face. The thick stratum corneum of the palms usually prevents reactions in this location. Irritants can lodge in clothing and produce dermatitis, most commonly on the thighs, upper back, axillary areas, and feet.

The histopathology of chronic irritant dermatitis differs from acute contact dermatitis (Figs. 15-3 and 15-4).

DERMAL GRANULOMA FORMATION

Dermal granulomas are a type of irritant contact dermatitis. Granulomas are due to the response of macrophages to foreign body injection into cutaneous tissues. They may be accompanied by giant cell formation histologically. Granuloma formation in the skin is commonly due to tissue injections of metal or metallic parts. The following agents can cause dermal granulomatous disease (4):

- Beryllium
- Silica
- Talc

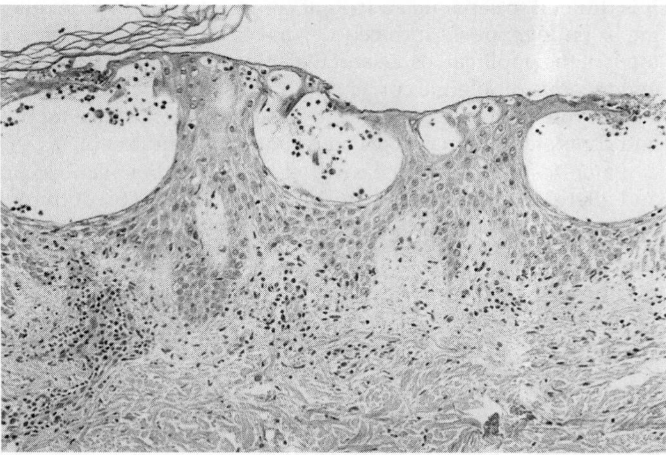

Figure 15-3. Acute contact dermatitis histopathology.

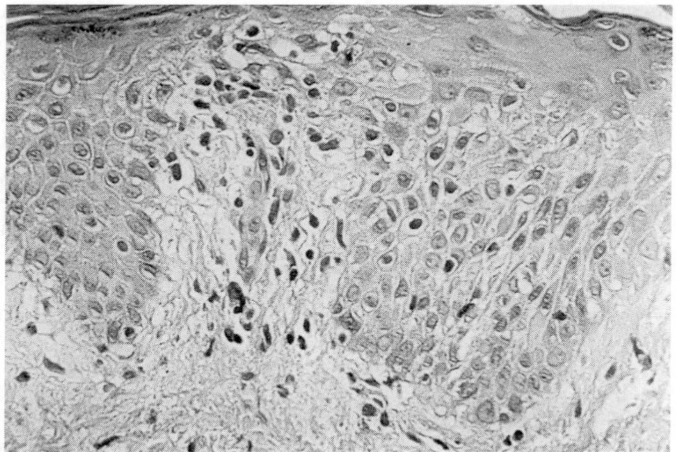

Figure 15-4. Chronic irritant dermatitis histopathology.

- Cotton fibers
- Biological and infectious agents
- Powders

DERMAL ULCERATIONS

Corrosive substances, such as alkalies and acids, can produce ulcerative skin lesions. Ulcerations occur because of the direct corrosive and necrotizing effect of chemicals on dermal tissues. Trauma to the skin increases the risk of ulceration when an individual is exposed to chemicals. Depending on the chemical involved, further systemic absorption may occur, producing systemic toxicity, such as in the case with chromic acid, arsenic, and epichlorhydrin. Otherwise, treatment of dermal ulcerations from most chemicals is localized and symptomatic, with emphasis directed toward dressing changes and prevention of infection.

LEUKODERMA

Chemical injuries, burns, and repetitive trauma to the skin can produce depigmentation known as *leukoderma*, which cannot easily be distinguished from vitiligo. Hands and forearms are most affected, usually in a symmetric fashion. Leukoderma can also appear in sites distal from direct contact from the chemical and be associated with alopecia. Loss of pigment may take between 4 weeks and 6 months after exposures. Chemicals that are associated with leukoderma include the following (2–4):

- Phenol
- Alkyl phenols
- Catechol
- *p*-Phenylenediamine
- Hydroquinone
- Monobenzylether of hydroquinone
- *p*-tert-Butylphenol
- *p*-tert-Butylcatechol
- Monomethylether of hydroquinone
- *p*-tert-Amyl phenol
- *p*-Cresol
- *p*-Aminophenol
- *p*-Octylphenol
- *p*-Nonyl phenol
- Mercaptoamines

Occupational exposure situations associated with skin depigmentation include photographic chemicals; germicides; disinfectants; detergents; deodorants; inks; and the manufacturing of paints, plastics, synthetic rubber, and insecticides.

Leukoderma is a result of structural changes to the melanocytes in the skin. There is no effective treatment outside of avoiding contact with the chemicals and use of appropriate barrier devices and barrier creams.

MELANODERMA

Melanoderma is a hyperpigmentation of the skin caused by chemical injury, thermal burns, and chronic skin trauma. Melanoderma can be caused by coal tar pitch, coal tar, asphalt, creosote, and other coal tar derivatives (2–4).

TREATMENT OF IRRITANT CONTACT DERMATITIS

Preventive measures are the most successful in preserving healthy skin and preventing contact dermatitis. Contact dermatitis is mostly a chronic eczematous process, and topical therapy must be directed at rehydrating the skin. Nonirritating fatty substances hydrate the skin and help restore barrier function. Topical therapy should contain low percentages of drying agents (2–4).

Topical corticosteroids can decrease inflammation. However, steroids also make the epidermis thinner and vulnerable to trauma. Consequently, more chemicals may be absorbed through skin if contact is not terminated. In cases in which the skin is dry or fissured, a moisturizer should be applied and steroids avoided. Dermatologic consultation should be obtained as necessary. In cases that cannot be adequately controlled by prevention, barrier creams and personal protective devices should be provided.

Protective gloves can help prevent contact dermatitis and are made of a variety of synthetic rubber materials. Specialized gloves and industrial gloves usually are thicker and can protect against chemical penetration. Synthetic rubber materials include nitrile, chloroprene, butyl rubber, fluoro rubber, and styrene-butadiene rubber. A disadvantage of gloves is irritation from sweating from their occlusive influence on the skin surface. Also, prolonged glove wearing can exacerbate a preexisting dermatitis. Contact urticaria dermatitis can be caused by latex rubber gloves (3).

LYMPHOMATOID CONTACT DERMATITIS

Cases are reported of plaquelike, infiltrated lesions from contact dermatitis that are histologically similar to mycosis fungoides or lymphoma (5–7). This lesion was first described as due to contact with an allergen in the striker surface of a matchbox. Other cases describe recurrent and progressive erythematous patchy dermatitis with flares of erythema.

Pathology of the lesions shows lymphocytic dermal reticulosis and chronic epithelial response (5–7). The clinical condition is chronic, and patch tests are positive with unrelated allergens. The condition may represent a transitional lymphoproliferative premalignant state.

The association of photosensitivity and lymphomalike histopathologic lesions has been reported. Clinically, these cases show generalized, persistent, photosensitive dermal reactions with skin thickening and edema. Tissue histology shows lichenoid infiltrates resembling mycosis fungoides and granulomatous infiltrates of the dermis. Lymphomatoid dermatitis has been reported from nickel contact with a thick lymphohistocyte infiltrate occupying most of the dermis (7). The cellular infiltrate consisted of CD-3 and CD-4 cells.

COMMON SUBSTANCES THAT CAUSE CONTACT DERMATITIS

Numerous commonly available chemicals cause contact dermatitis and are components of products used daily (2–4).

Antiseptics and Disinfectants

Antiseptics are applied to skin or other tissue to kill bacteria and viruses. Disinfectants are used on nonliving or inanimate objects, such as countertops and floors. Some health care–use disinfectants contain compounds advertised to kill human immunodeficiency virus-1. Medical facility disinfectant/cleaners contain alkaline corrosives, cationic and anionic detergents, and ethylenediaminetetraacetic acid (EDTA), which are sensitizers. Hospital disinfectants, germicidals, and deodorants can contain phenylphenol, quaternary ammonium chloride, EDTA, and cationic detergents (octyldecyldimethyl ammonium chloride, dioctyldimethyl ammonium chloride, didecyldimethyl ammonium chloride, *n*-alkyldimethylbenzyl ammonium chloride). Disinfectants must be effective on organic material and nondestructive to the surface they contact. Some disinfectants are applied to the skin for antiseptic activity.

Quaternary ammonium compounds are contact irritants found in deodorants, hair products, antistatic compounds, softeners, and common cleaners/disinfectants. Quaternary ammonium compounds are surface-active agents (surfactants) with a positive charge (2–4). They include the following:

- Benzalkonium chloride
- Cetylpyridinium chloride
- Cetalkonium chloride
- Cetyldimethylethylammonium bromide
- Cetrimonium bromide

Benzalkonium chloride (Zephiran chloride) is used as a skin disinfectant and for treatment of superficial dermal wounds, abrasions, and superficial infections. Its antibacterial activity is limited to gram-positive organisms and a few gram-negative organisms. It is a rare sensitizer. Delqualinium chloride, another quaternary ammonium compound, is a contact irritant and sensitizer. It has caused ulcers of the skin in some instances (2).

Alcohols are used as antiseptics in many products. Alcohols are divided into (a) primary, secondary, or tertiary alcohols; (b) by the number of hydroxyl groups; and (c) by whether their carbon chain is open or closed. The hydroxyl groups in alcohol contribute a degree of polarity. The lower the molecular weight, the more easily the alcohol dissolves in water (methanol, ethanol, and propanol). Alcohols are used as antiseptics because they denature proteins. As such, they are effective antibacterial agents. Isopropyl alcohol is used as an antiseptic in a 70% solution.

Alcohols have drying effects on the skin. Alcohol, such as isopropanol, can be absorbed through the skin and cause clinical toxicity. The irritancy of many commercial products is related to their alcohol content.

Aldehydes are irritants and sensitizers used in disinfectants for medical instruments. The most common cold-sterilizing aldehyde in use is glutaraldehyde. Aldehydes act by alkylating microbe DNA and RNA. Glutaraldehyde vapors cause eye and throat irritation, cough, shortness of breath, and dermatitis.

Formaldehyde is a contact irritant and a skin sensitizer. When used as a disinfectant, it is usually in a low concentration of 2%. Many cleaning agents, soaps, and disinfectants contain formaldehyde releasers (Table 15-6), which may cause irritation or sensitization.

Povidone-iodine (Betadine) solution is an iodoform with less irritancy than weak iodine solutions. Povidone-iodine is available in solutions ranging from 0.01% to 10.00% (2–4).

Irritant chlorine compounds in disinfectants include chlorites and chloramine. Sodium hypochlorite is an oxidizing agent and combines with water and organic material to release free chlorine gas, which is able to denature protein. Chloramine is a strong irritant and releases chlorine on contact with organic material. Chloramine is found in toilet bowl cleaners, bathtub cleaners, and floor cleaners.

Cleaning Agents, Detergents, and Soaps

Cleaning agents and detergents are common causes of contact dermatitis. Detergents are divided into anionic, cationic, amphoteric, and nonionic (Table 15-7). Detergents contain surfactants, which act to decrease the surface tension between two unmixable phases. Surfactants lower surface tension because their molecu-

TABLE 15-6. Formaldehyde releasers in common products

Formaldehyde releaser	Product
Benzylhemiformal	Cleaning agents Polishes
Bioban CS-1246	Cutting fluids
Nitrobutyl morfoline	Cutting fluids
Bromonitrodioxane	General cleaners Dishwashing liquids Automotive cleaners
Bromonitropropanediol	Automotive cleaners Dishwashing liquid Disinfectants General cleaners
Chloroallylhexaminium chloride	Cleaning agents Coloring agents Paints and lacquers Polishes Shampoo Hair care products Soap and skin care products
Diazolidinyl urea	Soap and skin care products
Dimethylol urea	Cleaning agents Cutting fluids
DMDM hydantoin	Shampoo, hair care products Soap and skin care products
Dimethoxymethane	Cleaning agents
Formaldehyde	Cleaning agents Coloring agents Curing agents Cutting fluids Paints Lacquers Polishes Shampoo Hair products Soap Skin care products Surface active agents Toilet cleaners
Hexamethylenetetramine	Cleaning agents
Imidazolidinyl urea	Shampoo and hair care products
N-methylolchloroacetamide	Coloring agents
N-methylolethanolamine	Paints and lacquers
Trihydroxyethylhexahydro *s*-triazine	Disinfectants
Paraformaldehyde	Disinfectants Descaling agents

TABLE 15-7. Types of detergents

Anionic
- Alkyl carboxylate (soap)
- Alkyl sulfate
- Alkyl benzene sulfonate
- Secondary alkyl sulfonate
- Alkyl poly-ethoxy sulfate
- Alkyl poly-ethoxy sulfosuccinate
- Alkyl sulfo acetate
- Fatty acid isethionate
- Protein fatty acid condensation products

Cationic
- Alkyl quaternary ammonium chloride
- Alkyldimethylbenzyl ammonium chloride
- Octyldecyldimethyl ammonium chloride
- Dioctyldimethyl ammonium chloride
- Didecyldimethyl ammonium chloride

Amphoteric
- Alkyl glycinate
- Alkyl amino propionate
- Alkyl amino betaine

Nonionic
- Alkyl poly-ethoxylate
- Alkyl phenol poly-ethoxylate
- Alkylic acid amino poly-ethoxylate

Adapted from Typker R. Detergents and cleansers. In: Van der Valk P, Maibach H, eds. *The irritant contact dermatitis syndrome.* Boca Raton, FL: CRC Press, 1996. With permission from CRC Press.

lar structure has a hydrophilic and hydrophobic part. Detergents and cleaners have other components that facilitate soil removal, emulsifying, and surface wetting (2–4).

Surfactants are soaps of fatty acids in their true form and are made from alkali action on fatty acids. Fatty acids contained in soaps include lauric, palmitic, oleic, stearic, and myristic acids. Early surfactants were carboxylates. More modern surfactants are versatile, with properties adjusted by the hydrophobic and hydrophilic groups (2–4).

Soaps, cleaning agents, and detergents consist of numerous additives and compounds that serve to act as surface-active agents or surfactants, which facilitate removal of dirt, grime, and soil. Soaps and detergents generically contain the following ingredients: surfactants, alkalies, builders, perfumes, dyes, pigments, fatting agents, corrosion inhibitors, whiteners, suds-controlling agents, enzymes, abrasives, and solvents (2–4).

Cleaning agents cause significant episodes of contact dermatitis and are one of the leading causes of contact dermatitis.

Soap solutions generally have alkaline pHs. Constant contact of the skin to alkaline pH soaps can cause irritation of the skin, increase the pH of the skin, and allow other chemicals to penetrate the skin, predisposing to infection. Ethylenediaminetetraacetic acid is an allergen found in some soap solutions, disinfectants, and cleaning products (2–4).

Detergents and cleaning agents can damage the stratum corneum and impair the barrier function of the dermis. Detergents may contain other toxic chemicals, as well as sensitizers. Detergents and cleaners can cause clinical reactions, from wrinkling of the skin to erythema and fissure formation.

Anionic detergents have a negatively charged group in addition to the lipophilic noncharged group. Cationic detergents have a positively charged group with a lipophilic group. Depending on pH, amphoteric detergents can take on either cationic or anionic properties. Nonionic detergents do not dissociate into ions in solution.

Cationic detergents have weaker cleansing power than anionic detergents. Ethoxy groups present in detergents help to determine solubility in water or lipids. High content of ethoxy groups increases water solubility. Low content of ethoxy groups increases fat solubility.

Anionic detergents tend to be highly irritating. Cleaning agents can contain many other components besides cationic, anionic, amphoteric, and nonionic chemical components. Cleaning agents with disinfectants may contain quaternary ammonium chlorides, formaldehyde or formaldehyde releasers, alcohols, and silicates, as well as alkaline substances, such as sodium hydroxide or sodium carbonate.

FIBERGLASS

Fiberglass is made of silicon dioxide. Glass fibers cause intense irritation when glass particles smaller than 3.5 microns in diameter embed in the skin. The dermatitis is irritant and pruritic.

Fiberglass dermatitis has a rapid onset with intense itching. Dermatitis usually occurs on exposed areas of skin. Scratching can transfer the glass spicules to other areas. Fiberglass dermatitis is more common in humid, warm conditions. Glass spicules may be seen under the microscope after skin scraping. The skin should be scrubbed with a sponge. Adhesive tape has been used to help remove the glass particles.

ORGANIC SOLVENTS

Hydrocarbon solvents are used for their ability to distribute between water and lipids to dissolve other compounds. The extent of this action is determined by the lipophilicity of the solvent. Aromatic solvents and chlorinated aliphatic solvents are more lipophilic. Alcohols tend to be more hydrophilic.

Solvents are estimated to cause as many as 20% of cases of occupational dermatitis (2–4). The percutaneous penetrating ability of the solvent determines the extent of dermal injury produced. Poorly absorbed solvents tend to cause more skin damage than those that are rapidly absorbed. Those solvents that are readily absorbed may cause systemic toxicity.

Solvents cause dermatitis by dissolving the protective oil layer on the skin. Solvents dissolve and dissipate surface lipids of the stratum corneum, increasing their absorption and the penetration of other compounds. Solvents can also damage the stratum corneum.

The irritant properties of solvents are ranked as follows: aromatic > aliphatic > chlorinated > turpentine > alcohols > esters > ketones (2). Dermal exposure to solvents can cause clinical signs and symptoms of erythema, dryness, fissuring, and eczema. Solvents can also involve other areas of the body as a result of vapor contact. More extensive burn lesions of the skin can occur from organic solvents, such as methylene chloride and gasoline, in close contact with the skin.

Ninety percent of occupational dermatoses are contact dermatitis, with solvents being implicated as a major source. Solvent irritancy varies according to the compound's percutaneous absorption, the irritating nature of the chemical, and the contact time with skin. Also, skin irritation decreases as the range of boiling point for the organic solvents increases. Therefore, organic solvents with lower-boiling-point ranges are more irritating than higher-boiling-point solvents. Clinically, solvents cause contact dermatitis with folliculitis, hyperpigmentation, and hyperkeratotic responses. Also, contact dermatitis and irritancy of solvents is enhanced by occlusive equipment, such as gloves or clothes, in addition to a prolonged contact. Organic solvents can produce burns on prolonged contact with the skin (2–4).

Solvents have a defatting action on dermal lipids, which can cause water loss from the skin. This defatting produces a whitening and drying of the skin after contact. Solvents can also cause drying, cracking, and fissuring of skin, which can result in a lymphangitis that is hard to distinguish from an infection.

Loss of barrier function is caused by damage to the stratum corneum and can result in increase of dermal absorption of solvents. Examples include isopropanol, propanol, ethanol, acetone, and chloroform, which cause dehydration through loss of water from the skin. Propylene glycol causes irritation that is due to drying and deoiling of the skin barrier.

Solvents also cause allergic contact dermatitis by either forming a neohapten in the skin or causing contact dermatitis that injures the skin and allows other allergens in an occupational environment to cause sensitization (2–4).

ALIPHATIC HYDROCARBONS

These are commonly found in kerosene, Stoddard solvent, gasoline, and individually in paints and lacquers. Lower-boiling-point aliphatics have greater defatting action and, therefore, potential to cause dermatitis. Clinical manifestations include inflammation, folliculitis, acneiform dermatitis, and hyperpigmentation (2–4).

AROMATIC SOLVENTS

In general, solvents with benzene ring resonating structures are greater irritants than aliphatic compounds. In addition to their defatting capacity, they can cause dermal burns. Benzene causes dermal erythema, skin drying, scaling, vesiculation, and dermal burns on prolonged contact (2–4).

Toluene—a component of gasoline, paints, adhesives, and lacquers—produces contact irritant dermatitis. Xylenes (*p*-xylene, *o*-xylene, *m*-xylene) are irritants to the eyes, skin, and respiratory tract. Xylenes defat the skin and cause contact dermatitis. Ethylbenzene is a skin and eye irritant and is probably the most irritating of the benzene compounds. Styrene causes defatting and dermatitis (2–4).

HALOGENATED SOLVENTS

The halogenated solvents cause contact dermatitis and, in cases of prolonged skin contact, burns. TCE, a degreasing solvent, can cause blistering on prolonged contact, dryness of skin, irritancy, exfoliative dermatitis, or scarlatiniform dermatitis. Perchloroethylene dermal lesions range from erythema to blistering. Distal pulp of the fingers and nails may become painful and swollen when workers use TCE or perchloroethylene without protective gloves.

PESTICIDES

Pesticides are classified as fungicides, herbicides, insecticides, and rodenticides. Hexachlorocyclohexane (lindane) and pyrethrums are common sensitizers. Pentachlorophenol and chlorophenols are irritants and sensitizers (2–4). Most pesticide dermal reactions are irritant in nature.

Chlorophenoxy Compounds and Chloroanilines

Eczema and chloracne are associated with 2,4,5-trichlorophenoxyacetic acid and 2,4-dichlorophenoxyacetic acid. Chloracne is also associated with dichloroaniline herbicides and urea herbicides, such as diuron and linuron. Chloracne is difficult to discern from acne vulgaris. Porphyria cutanea tarda has been reported in association with hexachlorobenzene and diazinon. Porphyria cases may have blistering skin lesions on sun exposure.

Organophosphates

Sensitizers include malathion, parathion, naled, dichlorvos, and plondrel. Dermatitis is also reported from dermal exposure to carbaryl, a carbamate.

Fungicides

Sensitizers include thiocarbamates, thirams, ziram, phenylmercuric acetate, tetrachloroisophthalonitrile, benomyl, captan, diflolantan, dithiocarbamates, chlorothalonil, atrazine, triazoles, and triazines.

Dermatitis caused by fungicides is commonly reported. Thiocarbamates are a group of fungicides with chemical structure similar to disulfiram. Ethylene thiourea is a carcinogenic metabolite of ethylene bisdithiocarbamates and is a skin sensitizer. Maneb and Zineb are other thiocarbamates. Maneb contains manganese and Zineb contains zinc. Both are sensitizers.

Benomyl is a carbamate fungicide, is an allergen, and causes allergic dermatitis in nursery workers. Captan is used on fruit as a powder and is a sensitizer. Chlorothalonil is used on ornamental flowers and fruit and causes allergic dermatitis. Erythema dyschromicum perstans is associated with chlorothalonil in banana plantation workers.

Ethoxyquin is used on apples and pears and can cause allergic dermatitis.

Herbicides

Paraquat and diquat are irritants and cause irritant bulbous dermatitis and damage to fingernails. Propachlor is a reported irritant and sensitizer. Paraquat and diquat are bipiridyl herbicides that cause dermal injury by corrosive action and irritation. Severe contact dermatitis can occur from both agents. Damage to the fingernails from hand exposure occurs. Transfer of the herbicides to other skin areas from the hands can cause spreading dermatitis.

Glyphosate is an isopropylamine chemical structure. Concentrated solutions can cause dermal irritation.

Pyrethrums and Pyrethroids

Allergic contact dermatitis occurs with paresthesia of the involved areas. Pyrethrum is an extract from chrysanthemum flowers and contains sesquiterpene lactones that are potent sensitizers. Synthetic pyrethrins can cause dermal irritancy and paresthesia.

Algicides

Organic polyamines are sensitizers. Acrolein is a strong irritant and may cause burns. Dinitrochlorobenzene is a strong sensitizer. Mercaptobenzothiazole is a weak sensitizer. Tributylin is an irritant and is a phototoxic compound.

Fumigants

Methylbromide causes skin burns and contact dermatitis. It is absorbed through the skin, is a potent neurotoxin, and has caused death by this route of absorption. Metam sodium (Vapam) produces carbon disulfide, methylamine, and H_2S and causes dermatitis.

ALLERGIC CONTACT DERMATITIS

Allergic contact dermatitis involves approximately 30% of all occupational skin disorders. Lesions begin with erythema and proceed to eczema with multiple morphologic features: clusters of papules, vesicles, edema, weeping, exudation, and crusting. Intense itching is a hallmark (Fig. 15-5). Allergic contact dermatitis is a type IV delayed hypersensitivity reaction. An initial encounter can sensitize the skin through direct contact, and a subsequent encounter with an antigen can result in clinical features.

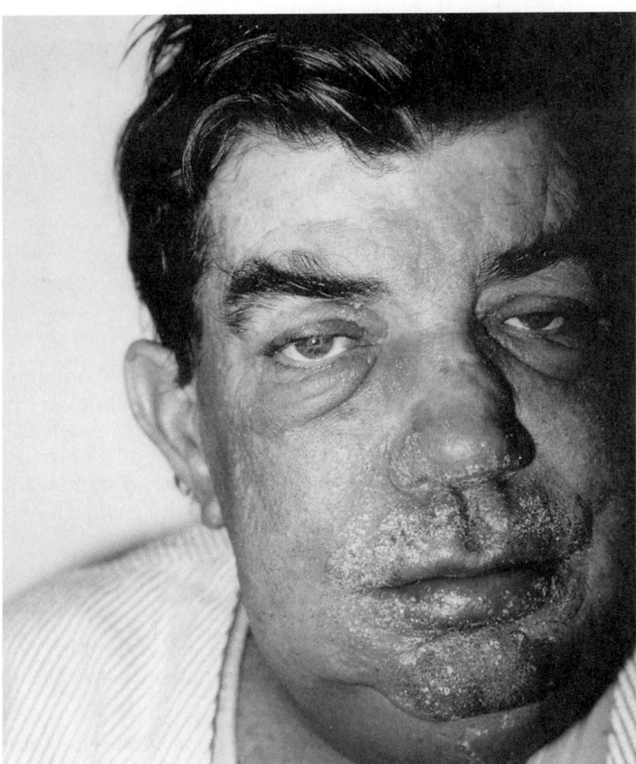

Figure 15-5. Allergic contact dermatitis.

A mononuclear cell infiltrate appears at the site of the lesion in 6 to 8 hours, peaking at approximately 12 hours after reexposure.

The clinical appearance is similar to contact dermatitis. If palms and soles are involved, vesicles might be seen. Sensitized individuals may also show other reactions, such as urticaria or erythema multiforme. Scaliness, drying of skin, and fissures may occur in the postacute phase. Common contact allergens are listed in Table 15-8.

TABLE 15-8. Contact allergens

Epoxy resins	Cellulose ester plastics
Phenol-formaldehyde plastics	Azobenzene dyes
Acrylic acids	*p*-tert-Butylphenol
Polyester plastic	Ethylene glycol
Ammonia	Monoethyl ether acetate
Naphthylamines	*P*-aminophenol sulfate
Paraphenylenediamine	Ammonium thioglycolate
Mercaptobenzothiazole phenols	Glyceryl
Dibutyl phthalates	Monothioglycolate
Diethyl phthalates	*P*-toluene diamine sulfate
Dioctyl phthalates	Triethanolamine
Ethylene diamine	Ethanolamine
Diethylene triamine	Dibromodicyanobutane
Triethylene tetraamine	Soybean oil
Ethylenediamine	Kojic acid (5-hydroxy-2-hydroxymethyl-4-pryene)
Tetraacidic acid	Carbonless copy paper
Bisphenol	Polyethylene glycol
Epichlorhydrin	Butylhydroxytoluene
Aliphatic polyamines	Diethyltoluamide
Polycarboxylic acids	Nickel
Dicarboxylic acid anhydrides	Chromium
Amine epoxy hardeners	Platinum
Formaldehyde	Rhodium
Toluene sulfonamide-formaldehyde resin	Sodium silicate
Latex	Xylene
Ammonium persulfate	Wood
Aminophenol	Vinyl pyridine
Resorcinol	Terpinylacetate
Cresol	Oleylamide
Alkyl phenols	Aminothiazole
Acrylate and methacrylates	Castor bean pomace
Acrylamide	Lindane
Acrylonitrile	Sodium sulfide
Acrylate monomers	Sulfur dioxide
Methacrylate compounds	Curing agents and accelerators

Immune Function of the Skin

The skin has immunologic functions carried out by Langerhans' cells. Also included in the dermis are macrophages and mast cells. Langerhans' cells are antigen-presenting cells and express the major histocompatibility complex class II. They also express CD1A receptors, complement receptors, and receptors for the Fc portion of immunoglobulin (Ig) G and IgE antibodies. Langerhans' cells present antigens to T lymphocytes as the initiating event in dermal allergic contact hypersensitivity and delayed-type hypersensitivity.

The keratinocytes in the skin also have a role in cell-mediated immune function. They secrete a variety of cytokines and growth factors that play a role in modulating immunity and inflammation in the skin. Keratinocytes produce prostaglandin E_2, which is a down-regulator of the inflammatory responses.

Formation of Contact Allergens

Contact allergens are low-molecular weight substances that penetrate through the epidermis and reach deeper tissues of the skin. The first step in allergic contact hypersensitivity involves the conjugation of the chemical with cutaneous cellular proteins to form a complete antigen. This complete antigen is taken up by the Langerhans' cells, which process it and then express the antigen on the surface of their cells in a complex with the major histocompatibility complex class II receptor. The Langerhans' cells then migrate to lymph nodes and present the antigen to T cells. This results in clonal expansion of lymphocytes, which migrate to the site of the antigen to create the inflammatory and immune response.

The histopathology of allergic contact dermatitis has three subdivisions: acute, subacute, and chronic. The histopathologic features of these three vary in terms of spongiosis (intercellular edema) severity and inflammatory infiltration. Subacute allergic contact dermatitis has less intercellular edema than acute allergic contact dermatitis, and in chronic allergic contact dermatitis, spongiosis or edema is modest.

Cross-Sensitization

Cross-sensitization can occur after exposure to an antigen that is recognized by the immune system. Consequently, exposure to structurally similar chemicals can cause a recurrence of the disease manifestation. A common sensitizing agent in cosmetics, paraphenylenediamine, can cross-react with many related substances in other products.

Allergic Contact Dermatitis and Systemic Symptoms

Severe allergic contact dermatitis may be associated with systemic manifestations. Such clinical signs and symptoms include

- Headache
- Fever
- Anorexia
- Nausea

- Fatigue
- Paresthesias of lesion sites
- Diarrhea
- Respiratory symptoms
- Anaphylaxis
- Immune-complex reactions with vasculitis and nephritis
- Angioedema
- Lymphangitis
- Lymphedema

CONTACT URTICARIA

Contact urticaria is the wheal and flare reaction caused by chemical agents that are allergenic or are primary urticariogenic agents. There are four types of contact urticarias: (a) nonallergenic, (b) immune-mediated or allergic, (c) a combination of allergic and nonallergic, and (d) a combination of allergic eczematous and urticarial (8).

Nonimmune-mediated urticaria does not require previous sensitization of the skin, whereas allergic-mediated urticaria requires sensitization. A mixture of allergic and nonallergic mechanisms may also occur.

The nonimmune-mediated urticarial reaction is the most common form of contact urticarial reactions and is probably related to releases of vasoactive substances by a non-antibody–mediated release mechanism. Chemical agents producing nonallergenic contact urticaria include benzoic acid, sorbic acid, cinnamic acid, cinnamic aldehyde, sodium benzoate, and acetic acid. Benzoic acid, sorbic acid, cinnamic acid, and cinnamic aldehyde are the strongest of these agents (8).

Dimethyl sulfoxide is a promoter of cutaneous absorption of chemicals and can cause erythema and nonallergenic contact urticaria. Sorbic acid is a natural preservative and may also be found in creams and ointments that may cause iridemia or itching. Benzoic acid is also a preservative for food products and can cause both nonallergenic contact urticaria and systemic type I hypersensitivity reactions that are IgE mediated (8). Cinnamic acid is a flavoring ingredient that can produce contact urticaria. Cinnamic aldehyde, present in cinnamon and used as a flavoring agent, may cause erythema, itching, and nonallergenic contact urticaria.

Balsam of Peru contains aromatic substances that cause nonallergic and allergic contact urticaria. Allergic contact urticaria is probably caused by immune mechanisms that require IgE and also by IgG and IgM through activation of the complement pathway.

Many different foods have been reported to cause allergic contact urticaria, such as potatoes, fish, eggs, milk, flour, and lettuce. Contact urticaria is known to occur from metals such as nickel, rhodium, and platinum (2–4). The following are criteria for diagnosing allergic contact urticaria:

- History of previous exposure to an allergen without the provocation of symptoms
- Degree of chemical reaction and sensitivity reaction that increases with ongoing recurring exposures
- Low number of affected exposed persons
- Possible nonspecific elevation of serum IgE
- More common in atopic individuals
- Positive skin testing with suspected agent

PATCH TESTING

Patch testing is used to help determine the existence of a delayed hypersensitivity dermatitis or contact allergic dermatitis. Suspicion of an allergic contact dermatitis is an indication for patch testing (2–4,8). Patch testing should involve a low enough level of sensitizing agent to avoid a false-positive result. A false-positive result is an irritant reaction with a similar clinical appearance to an allergic dermatitis. If the sensitizer in the patch test is too low, a false-negative reaction may result. This patch testing must balance the dose of the sensitizing agent. Patch testing variables include

- Concentration of sensitizer
- Dose
- Technique
- Occlusion time
- Variation in skin absorption of sensitizer

Patch testing kits and systems are supplied by commercial vendors with premeasured allergens. With 3,000 known allergens, it is impossible to test for all sensitizers. Fortunately, 20 to 30 allergens account for most cases of allergic contact dermatitis. Most patch testing kits group those allergens into standardized testing kits. International patch testing specialty groups have set standards for testing (Table 15-9).

Technique of Patch Testing

Patch testing involves appropriate testing and then interpretation of the results. The technique and mechanics of patch testing include (9)

- *Application of the allergen in a vehicle or medium.* The vehicle should not be irritating or sensitizing. It should be inert

TABLE 15-9. The American standard patch test series

Test preparation
Benzocaine
Mercaptobenzothiazole
Colophony
p-Phenylenediamine
Imidazolidinyl urea (Germall 115)
Cinnamic aldehyde
Lanolin alcohol (wool wax alcohols)
Carba mix (carba rubber mix)
1,3-Diphenylguanidine
Zinc diethyldithiocarbamate
Zinc dibutyldithiocarbamate
Neomycin sulfate
Thiuram mix (thiuram rubber mix)
Tetraethylthiuram disulfide
Tetramethylthiuram monosulfide
Tetramethylthiuram disulfide
Dipentamethylenethiuram disulfide
Formaldehyde (contains methanol)
Ethylenediamine dihydrochloride
Epoxy resin
Quaternium-15 [*N*-(3-chloroallyl)-hexaminium chloride]
p-tert-Butylphenol formaldehyde resin
Mercapto mix (mercapto rubber mix)
N-Cyclohexyl-*s*-benzothiazole-sulfonamide
2,2-Benzothiazyl disulfide
Morpholinylmercaptobenzothiazole
Black rubber (*p*-phenylenediamine) mix
N-Phenyl-*N*'cyclohexyl-*p*-phenylenediamine
N-Isopropyl-*N*'phenyl-*p*-phenylenediamine
N-*N*'-Diphenyl-*p*-phenylenediamine
Potassium dichromate
Balsam of Peru
Nickel sulfate (anhydrous)

From Guin J. *Practical contact dermatitis: a handbook for the practitioner.* New York: McGraw-Hill, 1995;50. With permission from McGraw-Hill.

and nonreactive with the allergen. Common vehicle media include water, ethanol, petrolatum, olive oil, methylethyl ketone, and acetone. Control tests with the vehicle are important, because some can be irritants and give a false-positive test.

- *Adhesive.* Tapes or adhesives are used to ensure adequate occlusion against the skin. A too-tight occlusion may cause an irritant reaction.
- *Marking of the test area.* To be able to identify the test area, it must be marked; otherwise, patch test reactions cannot be reliably identified. Skin markers enable correct reading of patch tests.
- *Occlusion time.* Sensitizers in the patch test vehicle migrate into the epidermis. Patch test occlusion times are standardized to 48 hours. Any change from the standard time can affect the test.

Reading Patch Test Results

Interpreting patch test results requires great skill and experience. The patch test strip is removed after 48 hours, but some reactions show up as late as 72 hours after the test is applied (9). A single reading at 48 hours may miss 30% of contact allergies (9). If only one reading is done, it should be on day 3 or 4 (9). Reading at 48 hours alone will miss reactions and is not recommended.

The contact allergen dose may produce varying dermal reactions. In a very sensitive individual, a high allergen dose may produce vesiculation and bullae, whereas a smaller dose may only result in erythema. Patch testing is interpreted as follows (9):

- Negative reaction: nothing
- Doubtful reaction: erythema only
- Weak reaction: erythema, no vesiculation, papules, infiltration
- Strong reaction: erythema proceeding to vesicular eruption with edema
- Extreme reaction: bullae or ulceration
- Irritant reaction

Irritant reactions from skin testing are usually manifested as erythema. Patch testing can be repeated to rule in or out an offending allergen. Irritant reactions can manifest in different clinical morphologies, from erythema to eczematous reactions. Patients may also be positive to more than one test.

It is difficult to discern between allergic and irritant reactions. Atopic individuals are also more prone to irritant reactions (9). Plus, many sensitizing agents are also irritants. False-positive and false-negative reaction interpretation requires an experienced dermatologist.

METAL IMMUNOLOGY AND DERMAL TOXICITY

Many metals and compounds of metals have immunogenic properties (Table 15-10). For metals or any other chemical to activate an immune process, the metal or chemical must first penetrate the stratum corneum and act as a hapten by reacting with proteins in the skin. This forms a complete allergen or antigen, which can then be taken up by macrophages or the Langerhans' cells for antigen presentation to T lymphocytes to set up a sensitization process.

Many metals and compounds of metals are dermal sensitizers and cause allergic contact dermatitis. Nickel and platinum are well known to cause immediate type I hypersensitivity with urticaria and type IV delayed hypersensitivity. In some cases, the immunogenic metal, such as beryllium, can form granulomas. Zirconium and beryllium are granulomatogenic metals. Histologically, the lesion contains monocytes, epithelioid cells, and giant cells (2–4).

Common Dermal Problems from Metals

BERYLLIUM

Beryl ore is not hazardous to skin, but beryllium compounds are extremely hazardous to the skin and pulmonary systems. Compounds can cause dermal ulceration, contact dermatitis, granulomatous lesions, and contact sensitization.

ARSENIC

Arsenic compounds and arsenic metal dust causes contact dermatitis with erythema and pruritus. Vesicular and papular lesions may appear with pustular folliculitis. Organic arsenic compounds have been reported to be allergens. Other dermal lesions caused by arsenic include hyperkeratosis, melanosis, and skin ulceration and carcinoma.

CHROMIUM

Chromium exists in oxidation states from Cr^{-2} to Cr^{+6}. Trivalent Cr^{+3} and hexavalent Cr^{+6} forms are toxic; the remaining valences are unstable. Cr^{+3} is the most common form used in industry. Hexavalent forms are the most toxic systemically and dermally. Hexavalent forms, such as in chromic acid, cause dermal ulceration, burns, and necrosis. Hexavalent forms are allergens and can induce sensitization. The classic chromium skin lesion is an ulcer. Ulceration is increased when chromate compounds—such as chromic acid, potassium chromates, or sodium chromates—contact wet skin surfaces. This is why nasal septal tissue is commonly affected. Chromium ulcers are common over joints of the hand and where skin breaks happen on the skin surface. The lesions are small, painless, and appear "punched out." They heal slowly and leave scars. Allergic contact dermatitis to chromium is eczematous in clinical appearance.

Chromium dermatitis can become chronic despite removal from contact. Chromium ulcers can be prevented by decontaminating the skin with water and a solution of 10% ascorbic acid, which reduces Cr^{+6} to Cr^{+3}.

COBALT

Cobalt is a commonly occurring metal present in paints, varnishes, inks, feed additives, alloys, ceramics, electronics, pigments, and some hair dyes. Cobalt causes allergic contact dermatitis. Cobalt and nickel sensitivity occur together in many instances, because the two metals are found naturally together. Individuals with a positive patch test to nickel are likely to be positive to cobalt. When used in tattoo pigments, susceptible individuals may develop granulomatous reactions.

GOLD

Gold in element form is stable and nonreactive. Gold in ores may be contaminated with other metals. Hydrocyanic acid is used during extraction procedures and is highly irritating to skin. Gold chloride is a sensitizer. Most gold dermatitis is due to jewelry and is probably related to gold chloride. Gold sodium thiosulfate also causes dermatitis.

NICKEL

Nickel is probably the most common cause of metal contact dermatitis, especially from jewelry. Nickel dermatitis clinically is widespread, chronic, and persistent, justifying the term *metastatic eczema*. Nickel dermatitis starts locally with intense itching. Scratching causes spread to other sites. The palm is frequently involved. Nickel dermatitis can be chronic and severe.

ZIRCONIUM

Zirconium produces hypersensitivity and granulomatous skin disease. Granulomas occur after contact with zirconium salts.

TABLE 15-10. Dermal immunology and toxicity of metals

Metal	Dermal action	Dermal immunology	Dermal toxicology
Beryllium	Preferentially binds to epidermal proteins. Highly reactive with protein. Retained in tissue. Interferes with normal phagocyte action. Can cause ulcers.	Produces a complete antigen by reacting with dermal protein. Delayed hypersensitivity. Granuloma formation cell-mediated hypersensitivity. Sensitization is permanent.	Salts are very corrosive and irritating to skin, allowing significant absorption to occur. Toxic to any tissue it contacts. Can exist as (+) or (–) ions, depending on pH of environment.
Mercury	All forms of Hg are absorbed dermally. Organic Hg is most readily absorbed. Reacts with protein –SH groups. Taken up selectively by Langerhans' cells.	Moderate sensitizer causes delayed and immediate hypersensitivity reactions. Allergic contact dermatitis.	Occurs in three forms: elemental, organic, inorganic. All types can cause allergic reactions. Hypersensitivity symptoms improve on chelation.
Indium	Poor or no human skin absorption because of indium's precipitation at physiologic pH.	Indium trichloride is a contact allergen in animals.	No toxicity skin reports in humans.
Silver	Reacts with dermal proteins—sulfhydryl, carboxyl, or imidazole groups. Denatures protein. Penetration of skin results in argyria or hyperpigmentation. Does not deposit in epidermis. Deposits around sweat glands, basement membrane, and connective tissue.	Isolated cases of immediate (type I) hypersensitivity and delayed (type IV) contact dermatitis.	No toxic activity to skin reported outside of hyperpigmentation.
Aluminum	Aluminum salts penetrate skin and inhibit eccrine sweat glands. Aluminum chlorohydrate used in antiperspirants. Precipitates hydroxide gels in sweat glands.	Weak allergen, occasional allergic contact sensitization.	Skin irritation.
Arsenic	Trivalent form binds to sulfhydryl groups on protein. Skin absorption occurs. Accumulates in skin, hair, and nails.	Increased incidence of skin tumors and cutaneous malignant melanoma. Skin sensitizers causing eczematous and follicular dermatitis. Irritant dermatitis.	Trivalent form is most toxic. Dermal hyperkeratosis, melanosis, and precancerous dermatitis (Bowman's disease). Skin ulceration. Skin irritation.
Gold	Stable and nonreactive monovalent gold binds with sulfhydryl groups on proteins. Accumulates in hair, nails, and skin.	Allergic stomatitis from dental work. Contact dermatitis. Gold chloride is a sensitizer. Gold cyanide solutions are suspected sensitizers.	Exfoliative dermatitis. Mucous membrane dermatitis. Chrysiasis-bluish color of skin on exposure to ultraviolet light. Gold chloride is a strong irritant that damages and penetrates skin.
Cadmium	Dermal absorption is not significant although it can be absorbed through damaged skin. Concentrates in hair.	Inconclusive proof that Cd is a sensitizer.	Highly toxic metal to kidneys and lungs. Cadmium sulfide used in tattooing causes ultraviolet light reactions in skin.
Cobalt	Poor skin absorption.	Cobalt compounds are allergenic and photoallergenic. Anaphylactoid reactions have occurred from inhaled dust.	Irritant dermatitis from salts.
Chromium	Hexavalent (Cr^{+6}) is readily absorbed via skin. Chromium adheres to skin and is retained for as long as 3 weeks following a single contact. Cr^{+3} and Cr^{+6} penetrate skin; Cr^{+3} forms complexes with dermal and epidermal tissues. Cr^{+6} does not complex with proteins.	Hexavalent forms are sensitizers. Metallic Cr is nonimmunogenic. Chromate salts are potent allergens—they have delayed-type sensitivity and cause systemic reaction. Cr^{+3} can cause antibody formation with +RAST test (IgE mediated).	Hexavalent forms are most toxic. Primary irritants and corrosive to skin. Burns, ulceration with systemic renal toxicity. Chromium ulcers (punched-out lesions). Nasal septum perforation.
Copper	Binds to –SH groups of protein. Cu compounds are absorbed via skin and appear in sweat, nails, hair, skin, blood, and urine. Cu(II) penetrates intact skin.	Hypersensitivity is uncommon but is reported to cause immediate (type I) and delayed (type IV) hypersensitivity skin reactions. Eczematous and urticarial reactions.	Contact stomatitis. Copper sulfate is corrosive and an irritant.
Iron	Affinity for nucleophiles. Skin absorption reported only for chelated form of iron.	Rare cases of allergic contact dermatitis.	None reported.
Molybdenum	Can accumulate in skin following systemic absorption bound to collagen.	Metal dust exposure can cause IgE type of sensitization. $MoCl_5$ is a potent contact sensitizer.	Dermatitis eczema.
Nickel	Affinity for keratin. Absorbed via skin and binds to epidermal tissue. Occlusion increases skin penetration tenfold. Epidermis serves as nickel reservoir and is bound to carboxyl groups. Eliminated in sweat.	All of nickel compounds can cause allergenicity: contact dermatitis, delayed contact dermatitis, antibody-mediated IgE urticaria, and asthma from skin exposure. Most common cause of allergic contact dermatitis in females.	Contact dermatitis.
Lead	Combines with –SH groups, nitrogen, and oxygen. Complexes with anionic ligands in proteins. Skin absorption is insignificant.	Rare allergic reactions.	Lead acetate may be absorbed in toxic amounts. No direct skin toxicity.
Antimony	Hard, brilliant metal. Antimony trioxide is used in paints, pigments, ceramics, and for flame-proofing of paper and textiles.	Not an allergen.	Skin irritants. Pruritic, erythematous papules. Lichenoid dermatitis.

Granulomas caused by soluble salts tend to disappear in a few months. Those caused by insoluble zirconium salts persist for years. Zirconium is used in alloys, surgical implants, paints, ceramics, and varnishes. Common zirconium compounds are zirconium acetate, zirconium hydroxide, zirconium oxide, zirconium oxychloride, zirconium potassium fluoride, zirconium sulfate, and zirconium tetrafluoride.

Cosmetics

Cosmetic skin care products and hair products are leading causes of contact and allergic dermatitis (2–4,8). Hand dermatitis among hairdressers is frequent. Ingredients responsible for most cosmetic-related allergies are the following:

- Fragrances
- Preservatives
- Antioxidants
- Hair colors
- Nail lacquer resins, acrylates, methacrylates, cyanoacrylates
- Lanolin
- Permanent waving agents
- Sunscreens

Cosmetics are regulated by the Food, Drug, and Cosmetic Act. Most dermatitis problems related to cosmetics are caused by those products that remain on the skin versus those that are rinsed off. Common allergens in hair products include the following (2–5):

- Phenylenediamine
- Fragrances (cinnamic alcohol, musk ambrette, balsam of Peru, isoeugenol)
- Quaternium-15
- Glyceryl thioglycolate
- Thioglycolic acid
- MEA-thioglycolate
- Sodium persulfate
- Ammonium thioglycolate
- Glycerylmonothioglycolate
- Monoethanolamine
- Triethanolamine
- Benzoin
- Propylene glycol
- Formaldehyde
- Lanolin
- Pyrogallol
- Resorcinol
- Toluene-2,4-diamine
- *p*-Toluenediamine sulfate
- *N*-phenyl-*p*-phenylene-diamine
- 2-bromo-2-nitropropane-1,3-diol
- Toluene sulfonamide/formaldehyde resin
- Imidazolidinyl urea
- Parabens
- Ammonium persulfate
- Aminophenols

Cosmeticians, manicurists, and individuals who are exposed to methacrylates, acrylates, and cyanoacrylates risk allergic reactions from products that include initiators and stabilizers.

Many case descriptions exist of allergic reactions of the hands and fingers to methacrylate and methacrylate monomers. In addition to allergic contact dermatitis, nail dystrophy, paronychia, and permanent nail loss and onycholysis can occur. Dermatitis caused by methyl methacrylate can result in persistent paresthesias lasting months. Acrylates and methacrylates readily penetrate latex, rubber gloves, and polyvinyl gloves. Acrylates and methacrylates are also used in dental materials. Hair coloring agents contain potent allergens and sensitizers. Phenylenediamine is a primary ingredient in hair coloring and is oxidized by hydrogen peroxide in the process and coupled with the hair shaft. This produces the permanent coloring of hair. Hair dyes are common causes of contact dermatitis and sensitization. Cross-sensitization and reaction to other dyes and compounds can occur once an individual is sensitized to an allergen.

Plastics and Synthetic Resins

Plastics are large chains of long molecules made from small molecules called *monomers* that are linked together. The longer-chain molecules are called *polymers*. *Polymerization* is the cross-linking of the monomers to form polymers.

Plastics are classified as *thermoplastic* or *thermosetting*. Thermoplastics contain polymers that are side by side and can take different shapes when heated. Thermosetting plastics are long polymeric chains joined together, cross-linked by smaller molecules. Turning thermoplastics into thermosetting plastics is called *curing*. Unlike thermoplastics, heating thermosetting plastics does not change their shape. Polymerization of plastics is caused by the addition of curing agents, stabilizers, plasticizers, and catalysts. The components of plastics and resins—such as monomers, stabilizers, plasticizers, and curing agents—are known to cause allergic and irritant dermatitis.

Some plastics rarely, if ever, cause dermatitis, such as polypropylene, polyurethane, Teflon, polyvinylchloride, and silicones. Many additives, however, are potent sensitizers, such as phthalates. Synthetic resins that are cured or in the solid state and are fully polymerized rarely cause dermatitis. The finished product is usually free of irritating agents and allergens. Cutting, grinding, and sawing of polymerized resin materials can release particles and potentially some monomers that may be responsible for causing contact dermatitis and respiratory problems. The more common causes of synthetic resins that produce dermatitis include acrylic nails, uncured acrylic dentures, epoxy resins, formaldehyde resins, and toluene sulfonamide resins.

Epoxy Resins

Epoxy resin systems consist of two basic components: a resin monomer and a curing or hardening agent. These two components are mixed just before use. Curing or polymerization is an exothermic reaction.

The majority of epoxy resins used are made from epichlorohydrin and bisphenol A, both of which can cause dermal lesions. Epichlorohydrin causes contact dermatitis and skin ulceration. High-molecular-weight epoxy resins are solids, and those of low molecular weight are generally liquids. Allergic dermatitis is rare with resins of molecular weight of 1,000 and higher.

Epoxy resins are thermosetting, and curing agents or hardeners are used in their formation. There are three kinds of hardeners: tertiary amines, acid anhydrides, and polyamines, which are added to the mixture to induce a curing or polymerization. The pH of the amines is between 13 and 14, and they are potent skin irritants. Reactive diluents are added to reduce plastic viscosity. These reactive diluents are glycidyl ethers or esters, and they are allergens. They include the following:

- Glycidyl ethers
- Glycidyl esters
- 1,4-butanediol diglycidyl ether
- *N*-butyl glycidyl ether

- *O*-cresyl glycidyl ether
- Butyl diglycidyl ether
- Phenyl glycidyl ether
- 1,6-hexanediol diglycidyl ether

There are alternative epoxy systems to the epichlorohydrin-bisphenol A complex. The contact dermatitis caused by epoxy resins is generally from the resin and not the diluent or the curing agent. Epoxy resins can remain incompletely cured for several days but are generally considered nonallergenic when they are cured. The clinical pattern of dermatitis from epoxy resins generally begins on the fingers and then spreads to the face and eyelids. This is generally caused by direct contact and not by vapor spread.

Phenol-Formaldehyde Resins

This resin mixture is produced when phenol is mixed with an aldehyde in the presence of an alkaline catalyst. The phenols include cresols, phenol, xylenols, *p*-tert-butylphenol or phenylphenol, and bisphenol or resorcinol. Formaldehyde, urea, furfural, and melamine are commonly used aldehydes. Contact dermatitis can occur from formaldehyde, phenol, or furfural, which are sensitizing agents. Formaldehyde is both a sensitizing agent and an irritant. *P*-tert-Butylphenol can cause depigmentation of the skin.

Acrylics

Acrylics are another important group of plastic resins that cause dermatitis (Table 15-11). Acrylic plastic systems include acrylates and methacrylates, which undergo polymerization to form plastics like plexiglass. The addition of methyl groups to the acrylate acrylic monomer decreases allergenicity. Diacrylic monomers and triacrylic monomers are potent sensitizers. Dimethacrylate and trimethacrylate monomers are weaker sensitizers. Monoacrylates are moderate irritants. Irritant reactions increase with increasing numbers of acrylic double bonds and the presence of hydrophilic groups.

Acrylates are used in nail products, hair products, cosmetics, medical device adhesion, and plastics. Acrylic resin systems consist of the following components:

- A *prepolymer*, which is a monomer or multifunctional acrylate ester, such as ethyl acrylate or methylmethacrylate
- An *inhibitor* to prevent premature polymerization, such as hydroquinone
- An *initiator* to trigger polymerization, such as *N,N*-dimethyl-*p*-toluidine or benzoyl peroxide

Some acrylate resin systems use ultraviolet light as an initiator of polymerization. An acrylate resin system typical for bone cement includes methylmethacrylate monomers, hydroquinone, and *N,N*-dimethyl-*p*-toluidine contained in 1 ampul and is a sweet-smelling liquid. The other component is a powder mixture of polymethyl methacrylate polymer with a copolymer of methyl methacrylate-styrene. The powder and liquid are mixed, which creates an exothermic reaction that forms a soft, pliable mass. This hardens into cement in a few minutes. Epoxy systems contain reactive diluents and hardeners that can cause contact dermatitis.

Dermatitis caused by resin systems usually appears on the fingertips and hands. In the case of dental resins, allergic stomatitis is reported. Eczema and nail onycholysis occurs from hand contact. Dermatitis can be spread to other areas, such as the eyelids. Raynaud's syndrome is reported after chronic contact (9). Also, persistent paresthesias—lasting months—may occur after dermatitis from acrylic resins. Patch testing confirms the existence of allergy.

TABLE 15-11. Acrylic compound sensitizers

Acrylamide
Acrylated epoxy resin
Acrylated polyester
Acrylonitrile
Butanediol diacrylate
Butyl acrylate
n-Butyl acrylate
tert-Butyl acrylate
Butyl emthacrylate
Diethylene glycol dimethacrylate
Dipentaerythritol monohydroxypentaacrylate
Ethyl acrylate
2-Ethylbutyl acrylate
2-Ethylhexyl acrylate
Ethyl methacrylate
Glycidyl acrylate
1,6-Hexanediol diacrylate
Hexahydro-1,3,5-triacrylol-*s*-triazine
2-Hydroxyethyl methacrylate
1-Hydroxypropyl methacrylate
Methyl methacrylate
N-methylol acrylamide
N,N'-Methylene*bis* (acrylamide)
n-tert-Butyl maleamic acid
Pentaerythritol triacrylate
Tetraethylene glycol dimethacrylate
Trimethylolpropane triacrylate

Adapted from Rietschel R, Fowler J. Plastic (synthetic resin) dermatitis. In: *Fisher's contact dermatitis,* 4th ed. Baltimore: Williams & Wilkins, 1995:651. Permission from Williams & Wilkins.

Polyurethanes

Isocyanates are the monomers or prepolymer bases of polyurethanes and have the general formula $R - (N = C - O)n$. Common isocyanates include toluene diisocyanate, 4,4'-diphenylmethane diisocyanate, and 1,6-hexamethylene diisocyanate. Isocyanates are contact sensitizers and may produce eczematous eruptions at the point of exposure. Toluene diisocyanate can be airborne and is also a cause of occupational asthma. Liquid isocyanate monomers produce an inflammatory skin reaction on contact. Isocyanate resin systems use amine catalysts, which are potent sensitizers.

CHEMICAL PHOTOTOXICITY AND PHOTOSENSITIVITY REACTIONS

Photosensitivity and phototoxicity are skin disorders—termed *photodermatoses*—that require the dual presence of a photosensitizing chemical and appropriate radiation, usually in the ultraviolet range, to produce a lesion. Chemically induced photosensitivity is categorized as either a phototoxic reaction or a photoallergic reaction.

Phototoxicity

Phototoxicity-induced dermatitis is a result of chemically induced reactivity of the skin to ultraviolet light and occurs by a nonimmunologic mechanism. Phototoxic reactions are directly related to the toxin—that is, the response of the skin is related to the dose of the chemical and the dose of the radiation of appropriate wavelength.

The basis of phototoxic reactions is the light-absorbing nature of the molecule or chemical involved. The molecular structure of the chemical becomes excited by the spectrum of energy that it absorbs and dissipates its energy in a very short period of existence. During this energy dissipation, photochemical reactions occur, with resulting photo by-products that induce toxic responses in the skin. These by-products can induce photo adducts with DNA, as exemplified by psoralens. Ultraviolet light and ultraviolet A, B, and C absorption spectrum bands are all involved (2–4,8–10).

Most phototoxic reactions result in a first-degree sunburn reaction, although other reactions can occur, depending on the photosensitizing chemical. Clinical features consist of immediate irritating and burning sensation with erythema, swelling of the skin, and urticaria. Delayed erythema and edema can occur hours or days later. Blistering occurs in more severe reactions. Hyperpigmentation may occur as a consequence of the reaction. In some cases, hyperpigmentation may be the only consequence of the phototoxic reaction. On biopsy of lesions, epidermal edema (spongiosis) with necrotic keratinocytes may be seen.

Phototoxic reactions are limited to the areas of skin exposed to light. Phototoxic drugs taken systemically may cause other reactions, including damage to the fingernails called *photoonycholysis*, papular skin reactions, severe localized edema, and periorbital edema. The degree of phototoxicity is influenced by natural pigmentation of the skin. Light-skinned individuals experience greater photosensitivity than dark-skinned individuals. Also, the vehicle in which a phototoxic chemical is applied to the skin affects the reaction. Increased humidity also amplifies a phototoxic reaction. Common phototoxic substances include the following (2–4,8–10):

- Sulfonamides
- Phenothiazines
- Sulfonylureas
- Tetracyclines (mainly doxycycline and minocycline)
- Psoralen
- 8-Methoxy psoralen
- 4,5,8-Trimethyl psoralen
- Creosote
- Coal tar
- Anthracene
- Acridine
- Amyl-ortho-dimethylaminobenzoic acid
- Pyrene
- Anthraquinone rivanol
- Phenanthrene
- Benzo(a)pyrene
- Acriflavine
- Angelica
- Figs
- Pyridine
- Parsnip
- Parsley
- Celery
- Lime
- Methylene blue
- Dispense blue 35
- Rose bengal
- Eosin stain

Coal tar vapors can expose roofers to chemicals that can produce phototoxic reactions as well as phototoxic keratoconjunctivitis. Corneal ulceration can progress from this lesion. Coal tar products, including creosote, are phototoxic.

Psoralens are derivatives of plants and are phototoxic chemicals. Several plant species contain phototoxins. *Phytophoto dermatitis* is the term applied to phototoxic reactions caused by contact with plants containing phototoxic chemicals. Supermarket clerks and baggers have developed papular dermatitis confined to the upper extremities from exposure to celery contaminated with a fungal parasite. Carrots and limes are also a cause of phytophotodermatitis. Lesions can spread into bullae, leaving residual hyperpigmentation. Plants of the chrysanthemum family contain alpha-terthienyl, which is a phototoxic chemical. Mangos and ornamental oranges are also phototoxic agents.

Photoallergy

Photoallergic reactions are immune mediated and occur in individuals who have been sensitized by exposure to the photosensitizing substance simultaneously exposed to appropriate radiation. Photoallergy is much less common than phototoxicity. Except for the role of ultraviolet radiation in the conversion of a hapten into a complete allergen, photoallergy is similar to allergic contact dermatitis. The ultraviolet radiation induces a more potent allergen in the molecule as a basis for further hapten formation (2–4,8–10).

After the sensitization, reexposure to the photoallergen induces a delayed hypersensitivity reaction. Clinical features of photoallergic reactions are characterized by sun-induced eczematous reactions or lichenoid papules. The reaction usually occurs within 24 to 48 hours after combined exposure to sunlight and the photoallergen. Clinical presentation is an eczematous reaction similar to allergic contact dermatitis. Pigmentation changes and thickening of the involved area of skin may also occur. Histologic biopsies show epidermal spongiosis and dermal infiltration of lymphocytes and histiocytes. Exposure to sunlight through clothing can also evoke photoallergic dermatitis. The most serious complication of photoallergy is the development of a persistent light reaction, which is characterized by extreme photosensitivity. Many agents that cause photoallergy are in consumer products, such as cosmetics, drugs, soap, shampoos, sunscreens, and fragrances. These agents include the following:

- Chlorpromazine
- Promethazine
- Para-aminobenzoic acid (PABA) and PABA esters in sunscreens
- Sulfonylureas
- Thioureas
- Thiazides
- Digalloyltrioleate
- Trioleate
- Plants of the chrysanthemum family
- Chromium
- Lichens
- Diphenylhydramine
- 4,6-Dichlorophynolphenol
- Sulfanilamide
- Hexachlorophene
- Bithionol
- Hexa chloropane
- Dichlorophen
- Fenticlor
- Tribromosalicylanilide
- Fenticlor
- Dibenzoylmethanes
- Halogenated salicylanilides
- Triclosan
- Quinoxaline
- 1,4-Di-*N*-oxide
- Musk
- 6-Methylcouramine

TABLE 15-12. Differentiation of photoallergy from phototoxicity

Reaction characteristics	Phototoxicity	Photoallergy
First exposure reaction	Yes	No
Time of onset	Minutes to hours	24–48 hours
Dermal lesion	Sunburn	Eczematous morphology
Biopsy	Epidermal spongiosis with necrotic keratinocytes	Epidermal spongiosis with dermal infiltration of lymphocytes and histiocytes
Ultraviolet light spectrum	Ultraviolet-A	Ultraviolet-A
Diagnosis	History and clinical features	Photopatch test

- Benzophenones
- Cinnamates
- Sandalwood oil
- Thiourea

Differentiation of Photoallergy from Phototoxicity

Both photoallergy and phototoxicity require the presence of a photosensitizing agent and appropriate ultraviolet radiation. Diagnosis is based on the morphology of the lesion, time of onset, and positive photopatch testing in the case of photoallergy (Table 15-12).

NAIL DISORDERS

Nail disorders can be due to local injury, systemic diseases, or infection. They may be congenital or hereditary (11). Physical examination should note nail pattern changes: thickening, thinning, pitting, ridging, discoloration, separation of nail from nail bed (onycholysis), complete shedding of nail, subungual hyperkeratosis, inflammation, and a combination of nail lesion with hand or other skin area dermatitis.

Fungal infection (onychomycosis) is a common problem, especially of toenails, due to chronic moisture and occlusion from shoes. Organisms frequently involved include *Trichophyton*, *Aspergillus*, *Cephalosporium*, and *Fusarium*. *Candida* infection occurs in immune deficiency. Clinically, the nail can present with onycholysis, nail-bed hyperkeratosis, and yellow-brown discoloration.

Paronychia is an infection of the nail folds. It is usually bacterial but may be fungal. Swelling, redness, and pain are present. Purulent material may accumulate.

Onycholysis, or separation of the nail plate from the nail bed, occurs from chemical exposure, trauma, and chronic exposure to moisture. Physical examination can help discern a local reaction from a systemic one. Local reactions involve either upper or lower nails separately. Systemic drug reactions involve both. Onycholysis can occur from contact exposure to acrylates/methacrylates and cyanoacrylate nail glues (11).

Drug reactions involving the nail plate may be local or systemic. Photoonycholysis is induced by tetracyclines combined with exposure to sunlight. Cancer chemotherapeutics produce nail changes with pigmentation alterations (11).

Contact dermatitis of the nail area occurs with erythema, scaling, and vesicle formation. Cosmetics can cause nail contact dermatitis, especially acrylate monomers used in artificial nails. Secondary *Pseudomonas* and yeast infections may accompany acrylate or cyanoacrylate onycholysis (11). Table 15-13 lists causes of discolored nails.

TABLE 15-13. Discolored nails

Leukonychia (white nails)
- Arsenic
- Paraquat
- Thallium
- Butchers
- Salt plant workers
- Rust removers
- Silver workers
- Textile workers

Yellow nails
- Phenylenediamine
- Epoxies
- Methylene dianiline
- Diquat
- Dinitrosalicylic acid
- Dinitrobenzene
- Dinitrotoluene
- Trinitrotoluene
- Pesticide workers
- Flower handlers
- Dinitro-*o*-cresol

Blue nails
- Aluminum anodizers
- Oxalic acid
- Radiator workers
- Auto mechanics
- Dye makers
- Electroplaters
- Ink makers
- Metal cleaners
- Photographers
- Paint removers

Black nails
- Hydrochloric acid
- Gunsmiths
- Vintners (red wine)
- Woodworkers (ebony)

Brown nails
- Cobblers
- Cigar makers
- Coffee bean workers
- Photographers
- Road pavers
- Roof tarrers
- Shoeshiners
- Walnut pickers
- Varnish
- Gold potassium cyanide

Green nails
- Dishwashers
- Bartenders
- Electricians
- Fruit handlers
- Laundry workers
- Metallurgists
- Restaurant workers
- Sugar factory workers

Adapted from Table 9-2 in Baran R. Occupational nail disorders. In: Adams R, ed. *Occupational skin disease,* 2nd ed. Philadelphia: WB Saunders, 1990:162. With permission from WB Saunders.

Ionizing radiation causes nail-loss radiodermatitis with early signs of longitudinal ridging and brittleness (11). Nails become dull, then opaque, and atrophy, with black spots appearing. Nail changes of radiodermatitis may not develop for months after the exposure. Microwaves have also been reported to damage nails without causing pain (11).

Chemical hazards to the nails can produce allergic dermatitis in the periungual skin areas. Nails can be weakened by chemical contact with acids, alkalis, and chlorine compounds. Hydrofluoric acid is especially harmful to fingertip tissue and nail beds. Nail discoloration can occur as a result. Koilonychia (spear nails) can occur in cement workers and in auto mechanics with contact dermatitis.

Nails can be softened by detergents, motor oils, and solvents. Gold potassium cyanide causes a purple-brown discoloration (11). Turpentine is a sensitizer that can cause periungual eczema with hyperkeratosis. Nonoxynol 6, a nonionic emulsifier found in waterless hand cleaners, has caused transverse nail dystrophy (11).

CHEMICAL-INDUCED ALOPECIA

Alopecia includes hair loss, involution, miniaturization, or increased hair fragility. Alopecia is divided into scarring and nonscarring. Scarring alopecia is permanent because of loss of hair follicles. Chemicals and drugs may produce alopecia (Table 15-14).

Hair growth consists of asynchronous cycles of generation and loss. Hair has a cycle consisting of three phases (10):

1. *Anagen*: Production of mature hair. Hair grows at a rate of 0.35 mm per day. The anagen phase lasts 2 to 6 years.
2. *Catagen*: Follicular cells stop their division and the hair root shrinks. This phase lasts for days to a few weeks.

TABLE 15-14. Chemicals and drugs associated with alopecia

Accutane	Melphalan
Androgens	Mepesulfate
Arsenic	Mephenasin
Auranofin	Methotrexate
Barium	Methyldopa
Bismuth	Methylsergide
Borax	Metoprolol
Carbimazole	Mitomycin
Chloroprene	Mitoxantrone
Chloroquine	Monobenzone
Cimetidine	Nicotinyl alcohol
Clofibrate	Nitrofurantoin
Clonazepam	Oral contraceptives
Colchicine	Para-aminosalicylic acid
Cyclophosphamide	Propanol
Dacarbazine	Quinacrine
Danazol	Radiotherapy
Doxorubicin	Salicylates
Ethambutol	Thallium
Ethionamide	Thiouracil
Etoposide	Trichlormethiazide
Etretinate	Trimethadione
Gold	Triparanol
Heparin	Valproic acid
Ifosfamide	Vinblastine
Indomethacin	Vincristine
Interferon-α	Vindesine
Isotretinoin	Vitamin A
Levodopa	5-Fluorouracil
Lithium	6-Mercaptopurine

Hair Loss (MEDITEXT Medical Management). In: Hall AH, Rumack BH, eds. TOMES System. (V93 edition.) Englewood, CO: Micromedix. Reprinted with permission from Micromedix, Inc.

3. *Telogen*: A resting phase in which the hair shafts shed and the hair bulb lies dormant in the follicle. This is the shedding phase of hair and lasts for 2 to 4 months.

The cycles of hair growth occur randomly around various sites in the body. In the scalp region, 85% to 95% of the follicles are in anagen phase, and 5% to 15% are in the telogen phase. For the eyebrows, the telogen phase lasts approximately 9 months, whereas the anagen phase lasts 10 weeks (10). Areas of the skin with a high percentage of anagen activity (rapidly dividing cells) are affected more by chemical and drug injury. Telogen areas tend to be more resistant.

Chemicals causing hair loss usually do so by precipitating the telogen phase or are toxic to the anagen phase and the hair root when combed or plucked. Anagen hair has its root in an elongated translucent sheath of living cells from the hair follicle. Telogen hair has a spheric, nonpigmented bulb.

Alopecia may be spotty or diffuse, or excessive hair shedding may be noted. Chemical- or drug-induced alopecia can be difficult to diagnose. Anagen hair also may fracture, leaving the bulb behind in the hair follicle. Chronic systemic lupus erythematosus is the most common cause of inflammatory alopecia (11).

CHEMICAL BURNS AND INJURY

Although most thermal burns share common management approaches, chemical burns are distinguished by their broad range of pathophysiologic processes. Unlike thermal sources of burns, chemicals may continue to injure tissue for several days unless neutralized or removed. Chemical burns are usually occupation related and account for only 2% to 4% of burn admissions (12,13).

The extent of burn caused by chemical agents is a function of several factors, including the quantity and concentration of the agent, the duration of contact, the depth of penetration, the specific agent involved, and the anatomy involved. Some studies have also suggested a possible genetic susceptibility to injury by certain agents. Underlying state of health and age are two other relevant factors.

The use of the term *burn* to describe injury by these chemicals is a bit of a misnomer, because tissue destruction by thermal activity is not the primary mechanism of injury. Different classes of agents may destroy tissue proteins by oxidation, reduction, vesicant activity, desiccation, metabolic inhibition, or protoplasmic poisoning. Oxidizing agents denature tissue proteins and are oxidized themselves during this process. The oxidized agent is frequently cytotoxic and causes further cell damage. Protoplasmic poisons form salts with cellular proteins as their method of action. Desiccants act to dehydrate cells, often producing exothermy in the process. Vesicants induce the release of tissue amines after a chain of physiologic reactions. Acids with pH less than 2 often produce coagulation necrosis on dermal contact. Alkalis with pH greater than 11.5 can produce extensive tissue injury through liquefaction necrosis (12,13). Because liquefaction necrosis can cause a loosening of the tissue planes that allows for deeper penetration of the offending agent, alkali burns tend to cause more tissue destruction than acid burns.

Skin Injury from Hazardous Materials

The stratum corneum constitutes the principal anatomic barrier against penetration by exogenous chemicals. For example, the buffering action of lactic acid, amines, and weak bases present in this layer affords some protection against alkaline substances. The remainder of perceptible skin thickness is a loose matrix composed of dermal connective tissue consisting of fibrous proteins (collagen, elastin, reticulin) imbedded in a proteinaceous ground substance. By attacking and destroying the various proteins and lipoproteins present in the epidermis and dermis, hazardous chemicals cause local tissue destruction and penetrate into the more vascular tissue layers from which systemic absorption and deeper tissue damage may occur.

Burns and Tissue Chemical Injury

Chemical burns may be considered a special form of irritant contact dermatitis, in which substantial skin necrosis and inflammation may result from one-time exposure to a chemical substance. For example, exposure to formaldehyde may result in first-degree burns, or a sensitization dermatitis may occur in previously exposed persons. The dermatitis may be characterized by an eczematous vesicular reaction, which occurs suddenly with eruptions on the eyelids, feet, neck, scrotum, and arms. Urticaria has been reported as well.

Clearly, the inherent caustic or corrosive chemical properties of an agent influence the extent of injury. However, other physical properties—such as molecular size, weight, polarity, and ionization—also have an impact on the ability of a substance to penetrate the protective skin barrier and promote injury. In general, larger molecular weight substances, when ionized, are poor penetrants and are less likely to cause injury. The concentration of the chemical and the duration and frequency of exposures play an important role in tissue injury. Cutaneous injury is less likely to occur with lower concentrations, shorter exposures, and less frequent contact. Also, skin becomes more permeable and less of a protective barrier as the temperature rises, which directly increases the irritant potential of toxic substances. If the skin surface is injured or otherwise compromised, chemical irritation is also more likely to develop.

The anatomic skin site influences the extent of injury because of the relative differences in thickness of the protective epidermal layers in different parts of the body. In general, the eyelids, face, and genital skin have the thinnest protective barriers and are therefore the most susceptible to chemical irritation. Finally, there have been several studies to determine the impact of genetics and race on host susceptibility to injury. These studies have not demonstrated conclusive evidence that susceptibility is influenced by these factors.

ALKALI DERMAL INJURIES

The inorganic alkalis include sodium, potassium, lithium, barium, and calcium hydroxides, as well as the silicates of these metals. These compounds are used extensively in home and industry, in such products as washing powders, drain cleaners, and paint removers. Another household source of alkaline toxicity are button batteries, which are often misplaced by children in the nose, ear, or mouth. Anhydrous sodium hydroxide may cause severe injury to tissues based on its ability to saponify lipids, denature proteins and collagen, and dehydrate tissues and cells.

The alkalis often produce a brown, friable, gelatinous eschar in the areas of skin contact, referred to as *liquefaction necrosis*. The initial injury with alkalis is typically not as fulminant as those caused by acids. Ultimate tissue destruction, however, is often more profound with alkali exposure. As with other chemicals that "burn," the concentration of the alkali and duration of exposure are critical determinants of the degree of tissue injury. Skin biopsies from human subjects having 1-*N*-sodium hydroxide applied to their arms for an average of 80 minutes showed progressive inflammatory changes resulting in the total destruction of the epidermis within 60 minutes.

Management of alkali dermal injury should begin in the prehospital setting with removal of the patient from the source of exposure. All clothing and footwear contaminated with the alkali should be removed and irrigation of the burn areas initiated. Supportive therapy including oxygen and intravenous fluids should be used as needed. On arrival in the emergency department, irrigation and supportive therapy should continue while a thorough evaluation of dermal injury and systemic toxicity is performed.

In addition to injury from skin contact, alkalis may also cause injury through ocular exposure, inhalation, and ingestion. Ocular injury may be very severe, including disintegration and sloughing of the conjunctival and corneal epithelium, corneal opacification, and ultimately blindness. With the advent of automobile air bags, cases of alkali keratitis have recently been reported in association with air-bag deployment (14). Treatment for ocular exposures should begin in the prehospital setting with irrigation, using large amounts of water. These patients should be brought immediately to an emergency department, in which irrigation should continue until corneal pH returns to normal. An urgent referral to an ophthalmologist should be made on all cases with significant exposures.

Inhalation injuries that are due to alkalies may be life-threatening. Respiratory injury may range from mild irritation of the mucous membranes to significant injuries of respiratory tissues causing pneumonitis and pulmonary edema. Severe tissue hypoxia and shock may occur. Prehospital treatment for inhalation injuries from these agents should include removal from the exposure area, oxygen therapy, and maintenance of airway and blood pressure. Subsequent emergency department care should include continued maintenance of supportive therapy, with specific attention to the degree of systemic injury. Ingestion of these agents may cause extensive injuries to oral, esophageal, and intestinal mucosa. Patients may present with severe oral, chest, and abdominal pain, with hematemesis and bloody diarrhea. Esophageal or intestinal perforation may result in mediastinitis, peritonitis, shock, and subsequent cardiovascular collapse (15). The estimated fatal dose in adults is 5 g. Gastric lavage or emesis is contraindicated. Initial therapy should involve dilution of the alkali with milk or water as well as airway support and fluid resuscitation when appropriate (Fig. 15-6).

1. 2R (solid) + $2H_2O$---2R + 2OH−(aqueous) + H_2 (gas)

2. 2R + (aqueous) + 2OH−(aqueous) ---2ROH (aqueous)

NET REACTION

2R (solid) + $2H_2O$---2ROH (aqueous) + H_2 (gas)

(where R represents either metallic sodium or potassium)

Figure 15-6. Reaction of water and metallic sodium or potassium.

Cement burns represent another common alkali burn seen in emergency departments. Many of the commercial cements in use today are a combination of tri- and dicalcium silicates with varying amounts of alumina, tricalcium aluminate, and iron oxide. When cement becomes wet, sodium, potassium, and calcium hydroxides are formed, and the pH of the cement rises above 12. Wet cement often comes in contact with workers' skin through work clothes or footwear, which provide a partial barrier to these substances. The resultant burn is typically discovered hours after the initial contact. The same principles of management as for alkali burns should be used.

CHROMIC ACID BURNS

Chromic acid is commonly used during the electroplating process. Of the three valences of chromium (Cr^{+2}, Cr^{+3}, and Cr^{+6}), the hexavalent form is the most toxic because of its ability to freely cross cell membranes. Most tissue damage is caused by the change of valence (Cr^{+6} to Cr^{+3}) that occurs in the presence of protein. Chromic acid is a strong desiccant, and the readily absorbed hexavalent ionic form causes remote organ injury. Chromic acid is commonly used in combination with sulfuric acid at elevated temperatures in the electroplating process, enhancing its toxicity (16).

Relatively minor exposures of chromic acid cause immediate skin damage, permitting rapid absorption of the toxic chromium ion in the absence of prompt decontamination. If an explosion is part of the injury process, total body exposure may be quite large and include contamination of the mucosa. Full-thickness burns covering as little as 1% of the body surface area may lead to irreversible acute tubular necrosis secondary to acute chromium intoxication. The mortality rate is high if the burned area exceeds approximately 10% of the body surface area.

Presenting symptoms of someone exposed to chromic acid include localized pain of the involved skin surfaces, with subsequent diarrhea, gastrointestinal bleeding, hemolysis, hepatic injury, and renal damage. Severe poisoning follows the ingestion of as little as 1 to 2 g of compounds containing hexavalent chromium ion. The lethal dose is approximately 6 g.

Treatment is directed at immediate, copious irrigation of all exposed areas. If irrigation cannot be achieved within seconds to minutes, full thickness burns and cutaneous absorption of the chromium ion will result. A variety of compounds have been recommended for limiting the toxic effects of the hexavalent chromium ion, including dressings of sodium thiosulfate, sodium citrate, 10% vitamin C gel to convert Cr^{+6} to Cr^{+3}, lactate, and sodium metabisulfite. Recommended systemic antidotes include sodium thiosulfate, dimercaprol, calcium disodium ethylenediaminetetraacetic acid, and *n*-acetyl-cysteine. Some have advocated a prompt, deep, tangential incision of all contaminated tissues to prevent systemic ion penetration. All these approaches must be regarded as experimental.

ELEMENTAL METALS

The elemental metals, such as sodium and potassium, have several industrial applications, including use as coolants in nuclear reactors, as polymerization catalysts in the manufacture of tetraethyl lead, and in the production of photoelectric cells. Injuries caused by the elemental metals may be particularly devastating as a result of the production of both chemical and thermal burns (17). On reaction with water in tissues, these elements are explosive and form hydroxides, which cause significant tissue destruction. As a result, the usual therapy of copious water irrigation is not appropriate.

As with other chemicals that "burn," any contaminated clothing or footwear should be rapidly removed, as should any obvious metal particles in tissue. The burn area should be covered with oil (mineral oil or common cooking oils) to prevent further chemical reaction. Any burning metal in tissue should be extinguished by an extinguisher containing sodium chloride, sodium carbonate, or a graphite base.

After the initial therapy in the prehospital setting, the patient should be rapidly transported to an appropriate emergency department, in which further wound debridement and metal extraction can be performed. Any extracted sodium or potassium particles should be placed for disposal in isopropyl alcohol and tert-butyl alcohol, respectively. After excision of all metal particles, treatment is the same as for traditional alkali burns.

WHITE PHOSPHORUS

White phosphorus is an incendiary used in modern weaponry, as well as in the manufacture of various insecticides, fertilizers, and rodent poisons. It is a translucent, solid substance with a garlic-like odor, which, on exposure to air, may fume or flame spontaneously.

White phosphorus is an oxidizing agent that is highly toxic to skin, causing both thermal and chemical burns. Much has been learned about burns caused by this agent from the study of wartime injuries. As a general rule, exposures to this agent cause second- and third-degree burns to the contact area. This substance continues to oxidize and injure tissue until debrided, completely oxidized, or neutralized by tissue. Particles of this agent are often driven deeply into tissue layers, making neutralization very difficult (18).

Treatment of dermal injuries caused by white phosphorus should begin in the prehospital setting and include copious irrigation, removal of visible particles from the wound, and removal of all garments and footwear contaminated with the substance. Any particles removed from tissue should be placed under water and disposed of to prevent spontaneous combustion with air. In the emergency department setting, more extensive debridement should be performed. Irrigation with copper sulfate solution is often helpful in identifying occult white phosphorus particles in the wound by causing a characteristic black color change. After the identification process is completed, it is very important to fully irrigate the wound to remove all residual copper sulfate to prevent systemic copper toxicity (19). Perhaps a safer method of detecting white phosphorous is the use of the Wood's lamp, which causes phosphorous to fluoresce under ultraviolet light (20). White phosphorus rarely causes systemic toxicity via percutaneous absorption or inhalation. Ingestions of this substance do occur, and a dose of 1 mg per kg is considered potentially lethal (21). Systemic ingestions are associated with fatty degeneration of the liver and with the signs and symptoms of acute liver failure.

ORGANIC ACIDS (PHENOLS, CRESOLS, CREYSILIC ACIDS)

Organic acids are characterized by the presence of a benzene ring with one or more substituted hydroxyl groups. These compounds are used in the pharmaceutical industry and as deodorant sanitizers and home disinfectants. Organic acids are highly corrosive to skin and mucous membranes and may cause serious systemic effects after percutaneous absorption.

Phenol is a white crystalline solid at room temperature. In liquid form, it is known as *carbolic acid*. Phenol is extremely corrosive to skin surfaces, causing third-degree chemical burns (22). Eye contact may cause severe damage to the cornea, resulting in blindness (23). Phenol is effectively absorbed by inhalation, skin exposure, or ingestions. Systemic toxicity begins with central nervous system stimulation, which can lead to hyperreflexia and convulsions, followed by depression of the central nervous system (leading to respiratory depression) and a direct negative effect on the myocardium (24). Hepatotoxicity, renal failure, and methemoglobinemia can also be life-threatening (24). Approximately 50% of all reported burns and intoxications with phenol have resulted in fatalities (25). Because diluting phenol with water may paradoxically increase tissue penetration, water irrigation is not uniformly recommended, unless a high-density shower is available. Instead, phenol is more soluble in polyethylene glycol, which can be used more effectively to remove phenol from the skin (26). If polyethylene glycol is not available, intense water irrigation should be performed until it can be obtained.

Pentafluorophenol causes dermal burns and erythema. Treatment is similar to phenols, because the fluorides are tightly bound to the benzene ring structure. When confronted with a case of an emergency skin burn, one of the authors (Sullivan) elected to treat with irrigation and calcium gluconate gel because of a lack of toxicity data on the compound. The outcome was good, probably because the fluoride is tightly bound to the aromatic ring.

Cresol is an organic acid with toxicity similar to phenol. Cresol causes significant dermal injury by its denaturing effect on tissue proteins, leading to inflammation and necrosis of epidermal and dermal tissues. Repeated skin contact with low concentrations may cause tawny discoloration of the skin and chronic inflammatory changes. Cresol may be absorbed systemically after chronic dermal exposure, resulting in some cases of central nervous system, liver, and kidney injury.

Appropriate management of dermal injuries from these agents should begin in the prehospital setting. Removal from the source of the agent is standard, as is removal of all contaminated clothing and footwear. Copious irrigation is performed on all affected areas. Supportive measures, such as oxygen therapy and fluid resuscitation, are initiated as needed. Emergency department evaluation includes a careful assessment of extent of injury and a careful search for systemic toxicity.

INORGANIC ACIDS

Sulfuric acid, hydrochloric acid, and nitric acid are inorganic acids that are highly corrosive to tissues. These agents injure tissues primarily by dehydration and heat production, resulting in protein denaturation and cellular death.

Sulfuric acid, also known as *sodium bisulfate*, has a variety of home and industrial uses. On contact with skin, a hard eschar forms with deep ulceration into the underlying tissues. Extensive destruction of tissue occurs, and considerable heat is released during this reaction. This process of injury is sometimes referred to as *coagulation necrosis*. Ingestions from this substance are rare because of its caustic nature, but may cause shock, glottic and laryngeal injury, asphyxia, and even intestinal perforation.

Injuries caused by hydrochloric and nitric acids are similar to those of sulfuric acid. The burning process is more indolent than that of sulfuric acid, producing deeper, more extensive ulcers.

Therapy for these agents includes removal of all contaminated garments and footwear and copious irrigation with water of all affected areas. Because concentrated sulfuric acid produces extreme heat when combined with water, it is helpful to neutralize this substance with soap or lime water before lavage. If there is any evidence of systemic toxicity, appropriate supportive care is initiated. In the emergency department, appropriate management of burns from these agents often requires debridement and prolonged irrigation to prevent further tissue injury. Because of the highly corrosive nature of these acids, it is critical to quickly neutralize or remove them from tissues. In addition to the danger of injury from oral and skin contact, certain acids, such as nitric acid, are highly toxic if inhaled. Inhalation of the substance may cause severe respiratory irritation with associated burns of the mucous membranes. After severe exposures, pulmonary edema may develop rapidly but generally does so after a latent period of 5 to 72 hours. Systemic symptoms include dizziness, headache, nausea, weakness, chest tightness, dyspnea, and frothy sputum production. Complete recovery may occur after days to weeks or longer. In severe exposures, death that is due to anoxia may occur within a few hours of exposure.

Chronic inhalations of lower concentration may lead to erosion of teeth, inflammatory and ulcerative changes in the mouth, chronic bronchial irritation with cough, and chronic dyspnea. Patients exposed to the inorganic acid fumes should be removed from the exposure area immediately and given airway and hemodynamic support as needed. Victims should be brought immediately to an emergency facility for definitive care and evaluation.

HYDROFLUORIC ACID

Hydrofluoric acid is the inorganic acid of elemental fluorine. It is a colorless, fuming liquid or gas with an irritating, pungent odor that has multiple industrial and home uses, including glass etching, rust removal, and cleansing.

The compound is highly corrosive and produces a characteristic injury to skin by two different mechanisms. First, there is tissue destruction through the operation of free hydrogen ions. Second, more extensive injury is caused by penetration of fluoride ions deep into tissues. As with other chemicals that "burn," the extent of injury is dependent on surface area involved, concentration of the acid, and duration of exposure (27).

Hydrofluoric acid burns are characterized by a blanched appearance of the skin with persistent pain, edema, and necrosis (28,29). When the concentration of acid is less than 20%, pain and erythema may occur after a latent period of as long as 24 hours. Concentrations between 20% and 50% cause burns that are often apparent within 1 hour. Burns associated with hydrofluoric acid concentrations higher than 50% cause immediate tissue damage on contact with resultant severe pain, swelling, and necrosis of tissue (30). With more extensive burns, fluoride ions may penetrate into the deeper tissues, in which they can complex with available bivalent cations, such as calcium and magnesium, to form insoluble fluoride salts. This interaction has several deleterious effects on cellular function, including disruption of membrane function and impairment of cellular metabolism, which ultimately results in extensive tissue necrosis and cellular death (31,32).

Patients with hydrofluoric acid burns classically present with pain at the site of contact. The pain is often described as excruciating and may seem out of proportion to the surface area involved. Despite therapy, cellular injury may progress, with vesiculation and eventual necrosis appearing at the contact site. In very serious exposures, fluoride ions may actually penetrate to underlying bone and cause marked demineralization (see Chapter 64).

ALDEHYDES

Aldehydes are chemical compounds that can be reduced to an alcohol or oxidized to an acid. A large number of aldehydes are capable of dermal injury and include formaldehyde, acrolein, and glutaraldehyde. These compounds are used in a variety of settings, including the production of chemicals, the production of food products, plastics production, the textile industry, and the leather industry. Most aldehydes are highly volatile and tend to cause eye and mucous membrane irritation.

Formaldehyde is well known as an irritant to eyes and mucous membranes. Skin contact with formaldehyde has a variety of dermal effects, including irritation, allergic contact dermatitis, and urticaria. Formaldehyde is a frequent cause of allergic contact dermatitis in the industrial and health care setting. Minor epidemics of allergic contact dermatitis have been described among health care workers who handle equipment immersed in formaldehyde solutions. Because of its ubiquity in our environment, humans can come into frequent contact with low concentrations of formaldehyde sufficient to provoke responses in those with allergic contact sensitization (33). These diverse sources include components of plastics, glues, antifungal disinfectants, preservatives, paper, fabrics, leather, coal and wood smoke, fixatives for histology, and photographic materials. Formaldehyde is a skin irritant and a skin sensitizer. The best treatment is to avoid contact by the use of protective wear, including gloves.

Acrolein is a highly volatile aldehyde, which in liquid form causes severe skin irritation. Exposure should be treated with copious irrigation; exposures are rarely serious.

Glutaraldehyde is a strong mucous membrane irritant. Occasional contact with skin can cause an allergic response leading to contact dermatitis. Sensitization to glutaraldehyde occurs much less frequently than to formaldehyde, and cross-reactivity with formaldehyde-sensitive individuals does not appear to occur. Exposure should be treated with irrigation, and repeated exposure should be avoided to prevent sensitization.

EPOXY RESINS

Epoxy resin systems contain resins, hardeners, and reactive diluents. Other compounds, such as tar, glass, dyes, and other plastics, are occasionally added to the system. Epoxy resins have a wide range of applications and are increasingly used as a glue for metal, rubber, plastics, and ceramics and for repair work in a variety of areas including concrete, electrical insulation, metals, and floor coverings.

The primary dermal effect of epoxy resin systems is allergic contact dermatitis. More than 90% of those with the contact allergy are sensitized specifically to the resin. The allergic dermatitis is usually evident in localized areas of the hands and forearms, but it occasionally appears on the face and neck (34).

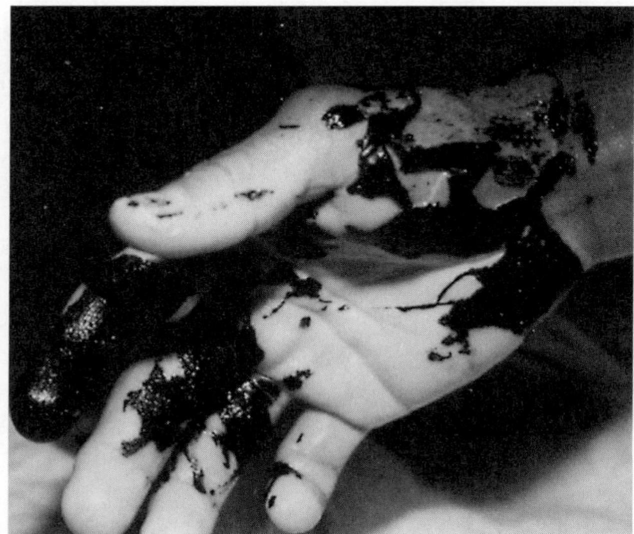

Figure 15-7. Hot tar burns to the hand.

The treatment of epoxy dermatitis is to avoid ongoing contact. This occasionally necessitates discontinuing of job activity and retraining. Prevention is the best cure.

HOT TAR

Asphalt tar, used in surfacing, is a product of the residues of coal tar. It is heated to approximately 450°F to maintain its liquid form for application. On contact with skin, it cools rapidly, but its retained heat is usually sufficient to produce first- and second-degree burns (Fig. 15-7). Burns that are due to hot tar present a difficult management problem because of the difficulty of removing the hot tar without inflicting further injury to the underlying injured skin (35).

Traditional approaches to tar burn injuries have included cooling of the tar with irrigation or ice pack applications followed by debridement. However, there has been a shift to the use of emulsifying agents, which are readily available and can avoid the secondary injury inflicted by the debridement procedure. The compound polyoxyethylene sorbitan has been found to have excellent lipophilic and hydrophilic properties, making it an excellent emulsifier of tar that can be washed off with water (Fig. 15-8). This compound is found in Neosporin cream, Neosporin ointment, and Tween 80. Liquid Tween 80 is deemed to be preferable to Neosporin cream, because it is more water soluble and easily washable, and emulsification is more rapid (36). However, Neosporin is generally more readily available and is perfectly adequate. There are anecdotal reports of the use of mayonnaise as a reportedly highly effective emulsifier.

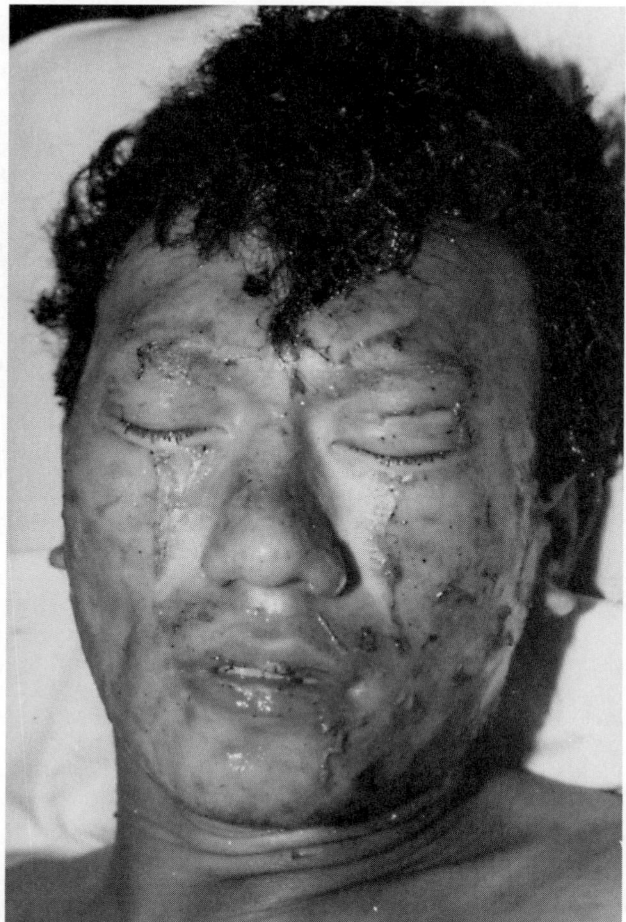

Figure 15-8. Hot tar burns to the face after removal with polyoxyethylene sorbitan.

ORGANIC SOLVENTS

Hydrocarbons are derivatives of petroleum distillation, the major classes of which include straight-chain saturated and unsaturated aliphatic, cyclic, and halogenated hydrocarbons.

Hydrocarbons are directly irritating to the epidermal tissue and as a consequence of their high lipid solubility may cause dissolution of fatty tissues and penetration of cell membranes (37). Various forms of cutaneous injury may occur, including contact dermatitis, eczematoid eruption, burns, and epidermal necrosis. In order of decreasing dermal toxicity are the short-chain aliphatics, aromatics, and chlorinated solvents (Table 15-15). As with other dermal toxins, the depth of injury appears directly related to the duration of exposure and concentration of the specific agent. Prolonged contact with gasoline and other short-chain hydrocarbons has traditionally been felt to cause only partial-thickness burns, but reports of full-thickness injury dispel this notion (38). Significant cutaneous absorption of gasoline and other hydrocarbons is felt to be uncommon (39).

Therapy for hydrocarbon dermal injury involves removal from the source of exposure, removal of contaminated clothing and footwear, and irrigation with copious amounts of water or saline to the exposed areas. General supportive care should be administered on an individual basis, depending on the severity of the exposure and the agent involved.

ALIPHATIC ALCOHOLS AND GLYCOLS

The aliphatic alcohols are hydrocarbon compounds that contain one substituted hydroxyl group. The glycols are alcohols with two substituted hydroxyl groups. Like other hydrocarbons, they are excellent solvents that cause minimal toxicity when associated with routine exposures.

Methyl alcohol, also known as *methanol* or *wood alcohol*, is a colorless, volatile liquid used as a solvent in the production of paints, dyes, cements, and inks. Toxicity from this agent usually occurs after inhalation, although serious injury and death have

TABLE 15-15. Agents associated with dermal injury

Agent	Application	Mechanism of injury	Therapy
Alkalis	Cement, sugar reagents, drain cleaners, paint removers	Saponify lipids Denature proteins Dehydrate tissues	Water or saline irrigation
Chromic acid	Electroplating Metal cleanser	Oxidizing effects Systemic absorption	Water or saline irrigation, $CaNa_2$ EDTA, dimercaprol for systemic toxicity
Elemental metals	Nuclear coolants Polymerization catalysts	Corrosive Thermal	Wound débridement; excision of all metal particles
White phosphorus	Insecticides Fertilizers Weapons	Corrosive	Water or saline irrigation, copper sulfate irrigation, wound debridement
Phenols Cresols	Pharmaceuticals Deodorants Disinfectants	Corrosive	Polyethylene glycol, water or saline irrigation
Inorganic acid (sulfuric, nitric, hydrochloric)	Glass industry Car batteries Metal cleansing	Corrosive Thermal	Water or saline irrigation
Hydrofluoric acid	Glass etching Rust removal Home cleaner	Corrosive Protoplasmic poison	Water or saline irrigation, subcutaneous or intraarterial calcium
Aldehydes	Plastic, leather, food production	Oxidizers	Water or saline irrigation
Epoxy resins	Floor coverings Glue Electrical insulators	Irritant contact dermatitis	Avoid contact, cortisone ointment
Hot tar	Road surfacing	Thermal	Emulsifying agents (Neosporin and Tween 80), then saline or water irrigation
Organic solvents	Solvents Fuels Pharmaceutical	Mild corrosive	Water or saline irrigation
Aliphatic alcohols and glycols	Paint, dye, antifreeze, heat exchangers	Mild corrosive	Water or saline irrigation
Sodium hypochlorite	Bleaches, disinfectants, water purifiers	Corrosive Oxidizer	Water or saline irrigation

EDTA, ethylenediaminetetraacetic acid.

occurred from ingestions and percutaneous absorption. Methyl alcohol causes dermal injury similar to other hydrocarbons, the most common being a chronic fissured dermatitis. Systemic toxicity is usually associated with metabolic acidosis and visual disturbances secondary to optic nerve injury. Central nervous system effects include headaches, vertigo, unsteady gait, and inebriation. An ingestion of as little as 15 mL has caused death. The metabolic products of formic acid and formaldehyde are the responsible toxic agents.

Ethylene glycol is used in hydraulic fluids, antifreeze, and heat exchangers. It causes dermal toxicity similar to other hydrocarbons, and significant percutaneous absorption may occur. Inhalation at room temperature is unlikely because of its low vapor pressure. The estimated lethal dose for adults is 100 mL, and in cases of fatal ingestions, coma, respiratory failure, kidney failure, and death may ensue within 72 hours.

Management strategies for dermal injuries secondary to these agents are similar to those outlined for other hydrocarbons.

SODIUM HYPOCHLORITE

This agent is used in disinfectants, bleaches, deodorizers, and water purifiers. As an oxidizing agent, sodium hypochlorite is very corrosive to tissues. The toxicity of sodium hypochlorite is related to available chlorine in solutions containing this substance. Solutions containing less than 6% available chlorine usually cause significant injury to tissues in large volumes only; concentrations of available chlorine higher than 15% can cause significant skin injury in much smaller volumes and after shorter exposures.

Contact with diluted solutions may cause mild irritation of the skin. However, more concentrated solutions may bleach the skin and cause pain, erythema, blistering, and skin necrosis. Sensitization dermatitis may occur in previously exposed individuals.

Initial treatment for these burns includes removal of contaminated clothing and footwear and irrigation of the affected area with soap or mild detergent and large amounts of water. Patients should be promptly transferred for definitive emergency department care. In addition to its dermal toxicity, sodium hypochlorite may also cause injury from ocular exposure, inhalation, or ingestion. Ocular toxicity is dependent on the concentration of available chlorine, with predictable corneal injury occurring on exposure to concentrations higher than 15%.

PHYSICAL AGENTS CAUSING DERMAL INJURY

High-Pressure Injuries

Many chemical agents are being used in relatively high-pressure devices that develop pounds-per-square-inch pressures of 1,500 or greater. Injuries from such devices are extremely hazardous for several reasons. As in other chemical burns, there is exposure to a substance that can cause substantial tissue injury. In addition, the chemical may be injected much more deeply into tissues, making removal or neutralization very difficult. Because of the high-pressure injection and deep tissue penetration, it is very easy to underestimate the severity of injury.

The most common substance injected is grease, typically delivered into the nondominant hand (40,41). Paint, paint solvent, hydraulic fluid, diesel fuel, water, and air are also commonly injected (42,43). The site of entry, the chemical characteristics of the injected material, the velocity of injection, and the duration of exposure all contribute to the extent of injury (44). Paint solvent is generally regarded as the most destructive, because its low viscosity allows extensive spread into soft tissue and also causes direct tissue necrosis because of its corrosive properties (45). The acute phase of these injuries is often characterized by a localized compartment syndrome (44).

Common errors in the management of these injuries include administration of local anesthetic, local exploration of the wound, and application of a tourniquet (44). Generally recommended management of these injuries includes tetanus prophylaxis, elevation and splinting of the injured limb, administration of broad spectrum antibiotics, and, most important, emergency surgical consultation for the decompression, debridement, and deep structure repair that define the definitive treatment for these injuries (44).

Microwave Injuries

Industrial and home use of microwave energy devices has become prevalent. Microwaves are defined as nonionizing high-frequency electromagnetic radiation and are positioned on the high-frequency long-wavelength portion of the electromagnetic spectrum. Although microwave appliances are for the most part quite safe, there are clear hazards associated with their use.

The deleterious effects of microwave radiation on the human body are due largely to heat production and subsequent thermal injury. The amount of heat generated is a function of the power output of the microwave device, distance of the tissue from the source, type of tissue involved, and duration of exposure. Significant dermal injuries secondary to microwave exposure are relatively rare and generally involve the upper extremity. Exposures as brief as 2 to 3 seconds may cause significant injury, with the occurrence of erythema, pain, blistering, and tissue necrosis. In some instances, the skin may demonstrate only minimal signs of injury, whereas underlying muscle, nerves, and blood vessels may be significantly damaged. Sensory nerves are particularly vulnerable to microwave energy. Cases of persistent neuritis and even compressive neuropathy have been reported after these exposures. Occasionally, burns of the oral mucosa and esophagus have occurred secondary to overheating of food products, particularly by children not familiar with the proper use of these devices.

Much still needs to be learned about injuries resulting from microwave exposure. An emphasis on preventive measures limiting the risk of these devices needs to be an ongoing focus of regulatory and health agencies.

Tissue injury resulting from microwave exposure should be managed by standard wound-care techniques. The thermal injury is generally localized to the areas of exposure without propagation along tissue planes or the creation of exit-type wounds. Adequate exposure and debridement of injured tissue, as well as close observation for potential complications, remains the cornerstone of good therapy.

MANAGEMENT SUMMARY

The treatment of dermal injuries from hazardous materials should be approached from the perspective of optimizing local wound care and appropriately evaluating the need for systemic supportive therapy. Emergency treatment is directed at elimination of the offending agent and the accurate diagnosis of extent of injury. Removal of the toxin generally requires dilution, neutralization, and debridement of the wound (see Table 15-15). Additionally, measures to promote systemic detoxification and facilitation of excretion of the offending agent are necessary for certain compounds. Supportive care typically includes adequate fluid resuscitation and ventilatory support.

The rapid removal of contaminated garments and footwear and the initial dilution of the agent should begin in the prehospital setting. The initial irrigation may require gallons of water or saline over a period of several hours. Dilution has many salutary effects, including reduction of the concentration of the offending chemical agent and removal of the agent from the contact surface. These effects greatly decrease the rate of chemical reaction and help to restore wound pH levels toward the normal range. It is universally accepted that early intervention is critical in preventing full-thickness injury. Thus, it is essential that the irrigation process be started in the prehospital setting.

The neutralization process, whether by water or tissue exposure, usually causes an exothermic reaction that has the potential for further thermal injury. However, this effect may be minimized by continuous irrigation. Certain chemical burns, such as those caused by hydrofluoric acid, may require more specific interventions.

Two issues are of critical importance when confronted with chemical burns and planning a management strategy. First, it is essential not to underestimate the extent of the initial injury. Second, tissue penetration and subsequent injury may continue for several days. Thus, early definitive evaluation and treatment by experienced personnel afford the best chance for minimizing morbidity and mortality.

Dermal injuries from physical agents, such as microwaves and high-pressure tissue injectors, although uncommon, require familiarity with their effects for appropriate management.

REFERENCES

1. White C, Bigby M. What is normal skin? In: Arndt K, Laboit P, Robinson J, Wintroub B, eds. *Cutaneous medicine and surgery: an integrated program in dermatology*, vol 1. Philadelphia: WB Saunders, 1996.
2. Rietschel R, Fowler J. *Fisher's contact dermatitis*, 4th ed. Baltimore: Williams & Wilkins, 1995.
3. Van der Valk P, Maibach H. *The irritant contact dermatitis syndrome*. Boca Raton, FL: CRC Press, 1996.
4. Adams R. *Occupational skin disease*, 2nd ed. Philadelphia: WB Saunders, 1990.
5. Orbanega J, Diez L, Lozano L, Salazar C. Lymphomatoid contact dermatitis. *Contact Dermatitis* 1976;2:139.
6. Ecker R, Winkelmann R. Lymphomatoid contact dermatitis. *Contact Dermatitis* 1981;7:84.
7. Danese P, Bertzzoni M. Lymphomatoid contact dermatitis due to nickel. *Contact Dermatitis* 1995;33:268.
8. Fisher A. Contact urticaria due to occupational exposures. In: Adams R, ed. Occupational skin disease. Philadelphia: WB Saunders, 1990.
9. Guin J. *Practical contact dermatitis*. New York: McGraw-Hill, 1995.
10. Marzulli F, Maibach H. *Dermatotoxicology*. New York: Hemisphere Publishing Corporation, 1987.
11. Norton L. *Dermatology*, 3rd ed. Moschella S, Hurley H, eds. Philadelphia: WB Saunders, 1992.
12. Lutterman A, Curreri PW. Chemical burn injury. In: Boswick JA, ed. *The art and science of burn care*. Aspen, CO: Aspen Publishers, 1987:233.
13. Sykes RA, Mani MM, Heibert JM. Chemical burns: retrospective review [Review]. *J Burn Care Rehabil* 1986;7:343.
14. Swanson-Biearman B, Mrvos R, Dean BS, et al. Airbags: lifesaving with toxic potential. *Am J Emerg Med* 1993;11(1):38.
15. Lecgaard T. Corrosive injuries of the esophagus. *J Laryngol Otol* 1945;60:389.
16. Wang AW, Davis JWL, Sirvant SUU, et al. Chromic acid burns in acute chromium poisoning. *Burns* 1985;11:181.
17. Clare RA. Chemical burns secondary to elemental metal exposure. *Am J Emerg Med* 1988;6:355.

18. Konjoyan TR. White phosphorus burns: case report and literature review. *Mil Med* 1983;148:881.
19. Chuttani HK, Gupta PS, Gulati S, et al. Acute copper sulfate poisoning. *Am J Med* 1965;39:849.
20. US Department of Defense, North Atlantic Treaty Organization. Emergency war surgery. Washington: US Government Printing Office, 1975.
21. Summerlin WT, Adler AI, Moncrief JA. White phosphorus burns and massive hemolysis. *J Trauma* 1967;7:476.
22. Abraham AJ. A case of carbolic acid gangrene of the thumb. *Br J Plast Surg* 1972;25:282.
23. Freidenwald JS, Hughes WF, Herman H. Acid burns of the eye. *Arch Ophthalmol* 1946;35:98.
24. Pardoe R, Minami RT, Sato M, et al. Phenol burns. *Burns* 1976;3:29.
25. Horch R, Spilker G, Stork GB. Phenol burns and intoxications. *Burns* 1994;20(1):45.
26. Mozingo DW, Smith AA, McManus WF, et al. Chemical burns. *J Trauma* 1988;28(5):642.
27. Derelanko MJ. Acute dermal toxicity of dilute hydrofluoric acid. *J Toxicol—Cut Ocular Toxicol* 1985;4:73.
28. Craig RDP. Hydrofluoric acid burns of the hands. *Br J Plast Surg* 1964;17:53.
29. Dibbell DG, Iverson RE, Jones W, et al. Hydrofluoric acid burns of the hand. *J Bone Joint Surg* 1970;52(A):931.
30. Iverson RE, Laub DR, Madison MS. Hydrofluoric acid burns. *Plast Reconstr Surg* 1971;48:107.
31. Burke WJ, Hoegg UR, Phillips RE. Systemic fluoride poisoning resulting from a fluoride skin burn. *J Occup Med* 1973;15:39.
32. Tepperman PB. Fatality due to acute systemic fluoride poisoning following hydrofluoric acid skin burn. *J Occup Med* 1980;22:691.
33. Committee on Aldehydes. Formaldehyde and other aldehydes. Washington: National Academy Press, 1981.
34. Fregert S. Contact dermatitis from epoxy resin systems. In: Benneter HM, ed. *Occupational and industrial dermatology.* Chicago: Year Book Medical Publishers, 1987.
35. Demling RH, Buerstatte WR, Perea A. Management of hot tar burns. *J Trauma* 1980;20:242.
36. Bose B, Tredjet T. Treatment of hot tar burns. *CMAJ* 1982;127:21.
37. Hunter GA. Chemical burns of the skin after contact with petrol. *Br J Plast Surg* 1968;21:337.
38. Walsh WA, Scarpa FJ, Brown RS, et al. Gasoline immersion burn. *N Engl J Med* 1974;291:830.
39. Ainsworth RW. Petrol vapour poisoning. *BMJ* 1960;5185:1547.
40. Schoo MJ, Scott FA, Boswick JA Jr. High pressure injection injuries of the hand. *J Trauma* 1980;20:229–239.
41. Harter BT Jr, Harter KC. High pressure injection injuries. *Hand Clin* 1986;2:547.
42. Walker WA, Burns RP, Adams J Jr. High pressure water injury: case report. *J Trauma* 1989;29:258.
43. Welmer JB Jr., Pack LL. High pressure water-gun injuries to the extremities. *J Bone Joint Surg* 1988;70-A(8):1221.
44. Fialkou JA, Freiberg A. High pressure injection injuries: an overview. *Emer Med* 1991;9:367.
45. Serio CA, Smith JS, Graham WP. High pressure injection injuries of the hand: a review. *Am Surg* 1989;55(12):714.

CHAPTER 16
Clinical Pulmonary Toxicology

Lee S. Newman

RESPIRATORY TRACT ANATOMY

Deposition and retention of airborne substances is dictated in part by the anatomy of the respiratory tract. A useful, albeit simplified, approach divides the respiratory tract into three major regions: (a) nasopharyngeal, (b) tracheobronchial, and (c) pulmonary (Fig. 16-1). These subdivisions of the respiratory tract are somewhat arbitrary. Although toxic agents may tend to affect one area more than others, the effects of inhaled agents are commonly detected in varying degrees throughout the respiratory tract. Furthermore, the respiratory tract is more than a series of interconnected tubes. More than 40 types of specialized cells are found in the respiratory tract, and they vary in their susceptibility to inhalational injury.

Nasopharynx

The nasopharynx begins at the anterior nares where air enters the nose in an upward direction and passes horizontally backward to join the pharynx. To do so it must negotiate two 90-degree bends before lining up with the pharyngo-laryngeal-tracheal path to the lungs. These bends in airflow with inspiration form the first barrier to the inhalation of airborne toxicants. The air turbulence created by the turbinates causes the larger particles (those in the 5- to 10-mg range) to be impacted and trapped in mucosa lined by highly vascular, mucous epithelium (see Fig. 16-1). The larynx lies in series with the nasopharynx, trachea, and conducting airways. Therefore, laryngeal injury may result if the causative agent can successfully negotiate the nasopharynx.

Conducting Airways

On passing through the larynx, air enters the trachea where airway dimension is relatively more fixed. The trachea, bronchi, and bronchioles serve as the conducting airways. As the conduit to the gas exchange components of the lungs, these airways are the second major line of defense against inhaled toxicants. The conducting airways are lined by ciliated epithelium. Mucus-secreting cells, goblet cells, brush cells, Clara cells, and a number of other rare cell types produce a thin mucus layer. The cilia on the surface of the airways rhythmically beat to remove particles from the deeper recesses of the lung along the mucociliary escalator. Transport rates along the mucociliary escalator in the trachea and large bronchi can be as rapid as 1 to 4 cm per minute. Mucociliary transport is a major mechanism for clearing inhaled particles from the conducting airways and hence serves as a major method of pulmonary detoxification.

The intrapulmonary airways can be subdivided into three major categories: (a) cartilaginous bronchi, (b) membranous or respiratory bronchioles, and (c) gas exchange ducts and sacs. The upper airway plus the cartilaginous bronchi are responsible for most of the airways resistance and so-called dead space measured by physiologic methods.

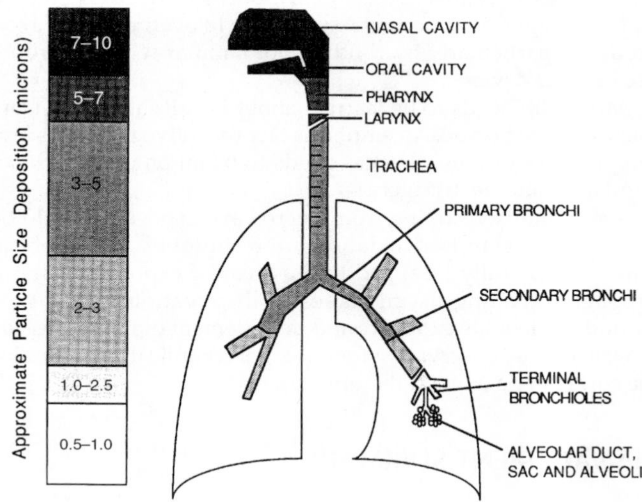

Figure 16-1. Schematic illustration of respiratory tract anatomy and approximate pattern of particle deposition.

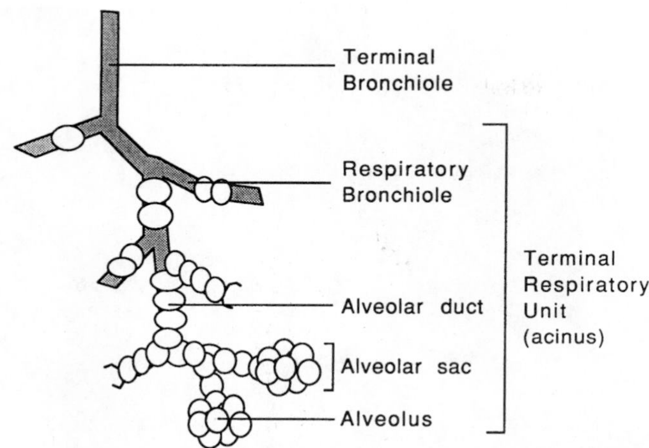

Figure 16-2. Gas exchange occurs starting at the level of the respiratory bronchiole. The terminal respiratory unit (or acinus) is composed of a respiratory bronchiole and the distal alveolar ducts, sacs, and alveoli.

Respiratory bronchioles are 0.5-mm-wide tubes that are short, numerous, and highly distensible. Respiratory bronchioles are lined by some ciliated epithelium and cuboidal epithelium, which flatten into alveolar epithelium as the bronchioles open into the gas exchange portions of the lung. They extend into the alveolar ducts and alveolar sacs, which are thin-walled tubes that serve as conducting airways and in gas exchange. The sacs are clusters of several alveoli that terminate in one or more alveoli branching from alveolar ducts.

Pulmonary Parenchyma

The alveoli themselves are thin pouches that open at one end into either an alveolar sac, an alveolar duct, or directly onto a respiratory bronchiole. Discrete fingers of several hundred alveoli sacs and ducts are referred to as *terminal respiratory units* (Fig. 16-2).

Gas exchange occurs principally in the alveoli. The barrier to gas exchange consists of three main layers: (a) the alveolar epithelium, (b) a thin interstitial space, and (c) the capillary endothelium (Fig. 16-3). The alveolar epithelium is composed principally of two cell types. Type I alveolar cells form thin sheets of cytoplasm to facilitate gas exchange. Type II alveolar cells are cuboidal and covered with microvilli with cytoplasm rich in lamellar bodies. These are intracellular storage sites for the surfactant that help maintain the pulmonary surface area. Type III alveolar cells are extremely rare but are also found lining the alveoli. Alveolar macrophages in the alveoli ingest foreign particles and play a key role in triggering inflammatory and immunologic reactions in the lung. They contain many lysosomes filled with digestive enzymes, especially acid hydrolases. The macrophages can transverse the alveolar unit via the airway, lymphatics, or pulmonary blood vessels.

The interstitial space normally consists of a few elastic fibers, collagen fibrils, and fibroblasts, among other cell types. Distortion of this space by fibrosis or inflammatory cell infiltration can produce devastating alterations in the gas exchange capabilities of the lung.

Pathologic processes that affect any part of the terminal respiratory unit—epithelium, interstitium, or vascular endothelium—can produce profound alterations in gas exchange. Denudation of epithelium may alter surface tension and produce intraalveolar exudation of cells and edema, interstitial fibrosis may alter gas diffusion properties, and blood flow changes may lead to ventilation-perfusion mismatching, among other physiologic effects.

Pulmonary Circulation and Lymphatics

The pulmonary blood vessels parallel the airways. The bronchial (systemic) circulation provides for the metabolic needs of the airways as far distal as the terminal bronchioles. This bronchial circulation is composed of arteries branching from the aorta or intercostals, sending branches to the trachea and esophagus along the path of the mainstem bronchi and pulmonary vessels to the deep lung and to the visceral pleura. Bronchial capillaries interdigitate in the bronchial submucosa. Venous blood returns from the trachea and cartilaginous bronchi into bronchial veins draining into the azygous or hemiazygous. In the deeper lung, the bronchial blood anastomoses with pulmonary venules, returning to the left side of the heart in venous admixture.

The pulmonary arteries are responsible for carrying oxygen-poor blood to the lung's gas exchange units. They enter the lungs at the hilum adjacent to the main bronchi and travel in parallel with the branches as each airway generation subdivides to the level of the respiratory bronchiole. Venous return similarly parallels bronchi and pulmonary arteries but at some slight distance away from the airways. In the region of gas exchange, the pulmonary arteries branch out to supply each discrete terminal respiratory unit. The pulmonary veins drain parts of several such terminal respiratory units. This pulmonary vascular bed is extremely dynamic. The arteries are as distensible as veins in other parts of the body.

The capillary network is an extremely high-volume bed where blood slows to allow gas exchange through the tripartite alveolar wall. Capillary networks cross several alveoli and then merge into venules.

The lungs have extensive lymphatics that help maintain the homeostasis of the lung both in terms of volume shifts and defense mechanisms. Although most inhaled toxic compounds are carried up the airways by the mucociliary escalator, some are cleared via the lymphatics. The lymphatics can be divided into (a) capillaries, located in the connective tissue but not in the alveolar walls, and (b) collecting lymphatics, which are recognized by their smooth muscle cells and valves and carry lymph from the periphery of the lung to hilar lymph nodes. Anatomically, there are interconnected superficial and deep plexuses. The two carry lymph to the hilum or to regional lymph nodes found around the major bronchi and trachea. Lymph ultimately flows into the right lymphatic duct or into the thoracic duct. Patches of lymphoid tissue are also found along the tracheobronchial tree, and such bronchus-associated lymphoid tissue serves an important role in immune responses to antigen stimulation.

RESPIRATORY TRACT PHYSIOLOGY

A clinically relevant way to think about respiratory physiology is in terms of (a) ventilation, (b) gas exchange, and (c) nonventilatory functions. This section discusses these aspects by placing the physiology in context with tests of pulmonary function.

Ventilation

Ventilation is the action of moving air through the nasopharynx and tracheobronchial tree into terminal respiratory units where gas exchange can occur. The ability to ventilate is dependent on mechanical factors such as the ability of the thoracic cage to

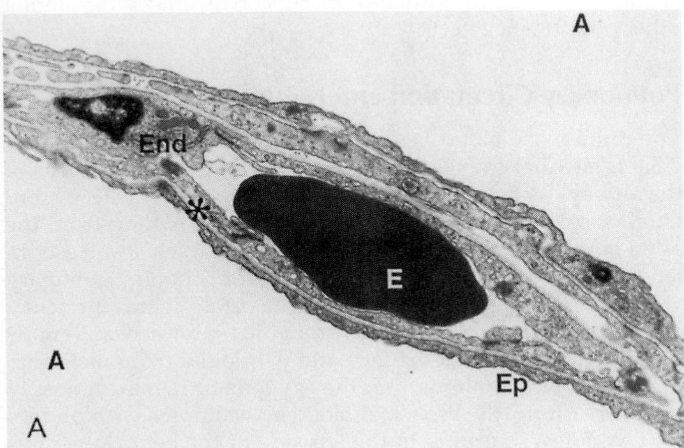

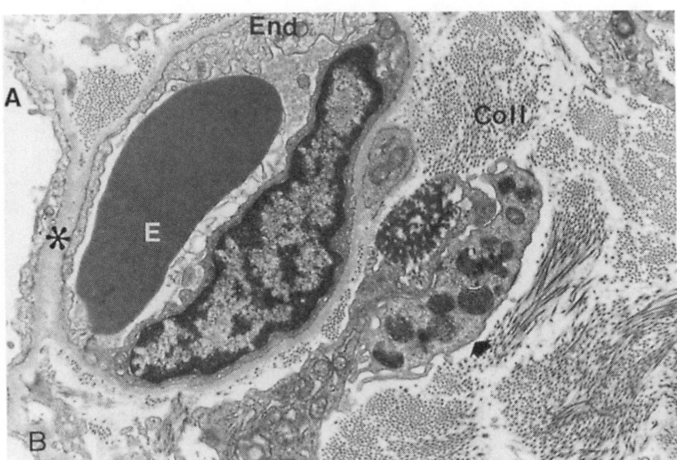

Figure 16-3. A: Electron micrograph (12,000× original magnification) of alveolar wall from normal lung. Alveolar air space (*A*) is separated from the alveolar capillary by attenuated epithelium (*Ep*) and basal lamina (*). An endothelial cell (*End*) containing an erythrocyte (*E*) completes the gas exchange unit. (Photomicrograph by Sheryl Campbell.) **B:** In comparison with the normal alveolar wall in **(A)**, marked alterations can be seen in this gas exchange unit from a patient with pulmonary fibrosis. The alveolar space (*A*) at far left abuts an alveolar epithelial cell with thickened basal lamina (*) separating it from the capillary endothelium (*End*). An erythrocyte (*E*) is contained within the capillary. Marked collagen deposition (*Coll*) can be seen to distort the alveolar capillary unit. Arrow indicates a mast cell in the fibrotic interstitium (12,000× original magnification). (Photomicrograph by Jan Henson.)

enlarge and the diaphragm to move downward during inspiration. It is also dependent on the elastic properties of the lung, which includes passive recoil of the lung during expiration.

Pathologic processes in the respiratory system may affect ventilation in one of several ways:

1. Mechanical or structural: Conditions that alter neuromuscular function, coordination, or that prevent full expansion of the lung (e.g., distortion of the thoracic cage, pain, obesity) can limit the ability to fully inspire, thereby reducing ventilation. Such problems may be recognized on pulmonary function tests as a restrictive pattern of low lung volumes.
2. Airways: Alterations of the airways either owing to acute injury and edema (e.g., alkali or acid burns) or chronic bronchial wall inflammation (e.g., chronic bronchitis from cigarette smoking or asthma from inhalation of sensitizing chemicals) slows the rate at which air is expired. These abnormalities are recognized on pulmonary function tests as an obstructive pattern.
3. Elasticity: Alterations in the compliance properties of the lungs greatly affect ventilation. Increasing stiffness, as seen in fibrotic lung disease, is associated with low lung volumes and an inability to increase volumes on demand. Airflow itself may be normal; however, the total volume of inspired air is restricted. Alternately, decreasing stiffness, as seen in emphysema, is associated with airflow obstruction.

Any of these alterations may be associated with abnormalities in gas exchange.

MEASUREMENT OF AIRFLOW AND LUNG VOLUMES

Appreciation of how inhalational exposures affect pulmonary performance requires an understanding of the lung capacities, volumes, and airflow as illustrated in Figure 16-4 and summarized in Table 16-1.

Lung Volumes and Capacities. The amount of air that can be exchanged in and out of the lung with maximum inspiratory and expiratory effort is referred to as the *vital capacity* (VC). Even with the most complete expiration possible, the lung never completely collapses but retains a small volume referred to as the *residual volume* (RV). The sum of the VC plus the RV is the *total lung capacity* (TLC). Under normal resting conditions, the amount of air that we breathe in and out of our lungs represents only a part of the VC. This normal amount of air exchange is the *tidal volume* (TV). The air that is left in the lungs at the end of the tidal breath is the functional residual capacity. When exertion places greater demands on the body, normal individuals can improve ventilation and thereby improve gas exchange in two ways: by increasing lung volume and by increasing respiratory rate.

Lung volumes can be greatly altered by certain pathologic conditions induced by inhaled toxicants, as illustrated in Figure 16-5. For example, the lung volumes and capacities can become exceedingly large due to air trapping, as is seen in asthma and chronic obstructive lung disease with emphysema. In such cases, the TLC increases, but a disproportionately greater increase occurs in the RV and functional residual

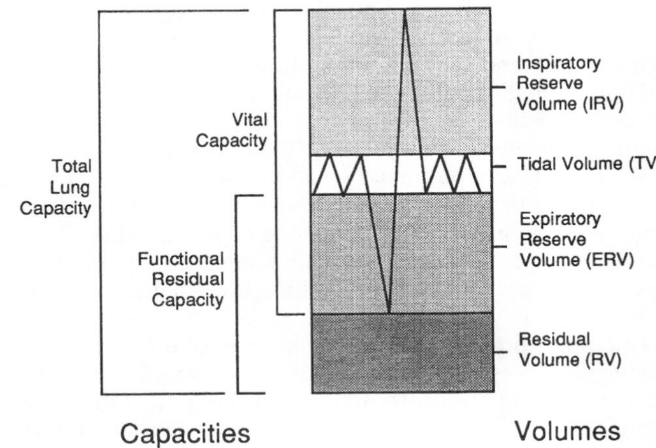

Figure 16-4. Lung volumes and capacities.

TABLE 16-1. Principal measurements of lung physiology

Measure	Common abbreviation	Significance
Airflow		
Forced expiratory volume at 1 second	FEV_1	Most common measure of airflow obstruction; estimates amount of air forced from lungs in 1 second of effort; see FEV_1/FVC ratio.
Forced expiratory volume at 1 second/forced vital capacity	FEV_1/FVC ratio	To understand the relevance of FEV_1, it must be considered in ratio to the total amount of expirable air (see FVC). High or normal ratio suggests no airflow obstruction; low ratio indicates reduced airflow compared to total amount of air expirable.
Forced expiratory flow, 25% to 75%	$FEF_{25\%-75\%}$	Reflects airflow in smaller conducting airways by measuring amount of expired air in middle half of expiratory effort. Low in obstructive disease.
Specific conductance	S_{gaw}	Sensitive measure of the ability of airways to conduct air; used in more sophisticated lung function laboratories, especially in detecting response to bronchodilators and in inhalation challenge testing.
Airway resistance	R_{aw}	Inverse of conductance; measures resistance to airflow.
Peak expiratory flow rate	PEFR	Often measured by use of handheld peak flow meter; provides an estimate of the degree of airflow limitation without use of spirometer; helps patients estimate severity of asthma exacerbation.
Provocative concentration 20%	PC_{20}	The concentration of an inhaled bronchoconstricting agent that is sufficient to reduce FEV_1 by 20%; used to measure the effect of histamine or methacholine in reducing airflow, aiding asthma diagnosis.
Lung volumes		
Forced vital capacity	FVC	Best estimate of the amount of air that can be exchanged in a single breath. Does not include residual volume left in lungs at end of expiration. Low FVC suggests either restriction or implies air trapping, with air left in lungs at end of expiration (see FEV_1/FVC ratio).
Total lung capacity	TLC	Sum of all lung volumes; measures total size of the lungs, including residual left at the end of expiration.
Thoracic gas volume	TGV	Comparable to the functional residual capacity (FRC); measured by body plethysmography ("body box").
Functional residual capacity	FRC	Amount of air expirable if one blows out the "extra" volume of air left in the lungs at the end of a normal breath (tidal volume) down to residual capacity; low in restriction and obesity.
Residual volume	RV	Amount of air left in lungs after all possible volume has been expired; high in obstructive lung diseases that cause air trapping (e.g., asthma and emphysema); low in restrictive lung disease.
Gas exchange		
Diffusing capacity for carbon monoxide	DLCO	Estimates ability of gases to transfer in and out of lungs by tracing CO; reflects mismatch in ventilation and perfusion, diffusion block; high in asthma, congestive heart failure; low in interstitial lung disease and in emphysema.
Diffusing capacity for carbon monoxide, corrected for alveolar volume	DLCO/VA	Corrects DLCO for amount of air volume, thus reflecting the degree of gas exchange in those parts of the lungs in which air is being exchanged.
Alveolar-arterial oxygen difference (alveolar-arterial gradient)	$PAO_2 - PaO_2$ (A-a) gradient	Calculated from arterial blood gases, this composite number estimates the amount of O_2 and CO_2 in alveoli compared to partial pressures in the arteries. Increased $PAO_2 - PaO_2$ indicates gas exchange abnormalities.
Exercise capacity		
Oxygen consumption at maximum exercise	O_2max	Reliable measure of the amount of oxygen consumed, hence the amount of work performed when the patient is exercising; used to estimate impairment caused by cardiovascular and respiratory disease.

capacity. Conversely, conditions that produce an increase in lung stiffness (elastic recoil), such as the granulomatous diseases and interstitial fibrosis, cause the TLC and other volumes and capacities to decrease. The net effect is a decrease in the amount of air exchanged in and out of the alveoli. Under such circumstances, the body must rely less on recruitment of lung volume to meet the needs for improving ventilation and increasing gas exchange.

To investigate diseases that may have affected lung volume, it is necessary to perform pulmonary function tests that include the actual measurement of lung volumes, usually by the helium dilution method or the body plethysmograph.

Simple spirometry cannot be used to measure most lung volumes and capacities. Spirometry principally gives information about airflow, with the exception of measuring the VC. But as can be seen in Figure 16-5, VC cannot be used alone to distinguish between restrictive disease and air trapping. It only gives a hint of the source of the abnormality.

Airflow. Airflow limitation is a common consequence of many inhalational injuries. Here, the simple spirometer is the single most useful tool to generate a picture of the dynamics of air movement out of the lung. Specifically, the tool allows measurement of how much air has been moved over what period, which translates into airflow rates. By convention, the expiratory volume forced out of the lungs in 1 second (FEV_1) is the focus. But airflow limitation can also occur during other parts of expiration, as measured by the forced expiratory flow in the middle half of expiration ($FEF_{25\%-75\%}$). To make the most out of the FEV_1, it should always be examined in relation to the total amount of air that was expired during the test, the forced VC (FVC). The FEV_1/FVC ratio allows the determination not only if airflow is decreased but also whether the decrease is owing to a parallel decrease in the total amount of air in the lung, or is a true obstruction of airflow.

By performing spirometry before and after the use of a bronchodilator it is possible to detect whether airflow obstruction is fixed or whether there is an element of reversibility suggesting underlying bronchospasm and reactive airways disease (asthma).

Exercise Physiology and Ventilation. Because ventilation is a dynamic process, the simple assessment of resting lung volumes and resting airflow frequently does not give a complete picture of the severity of an insult to the respiratory system. Exercise studies help to assess what ventilatory reserve the pulmonary system has after inhalational injury, and the degree to which overall exercise capacity is impaired.

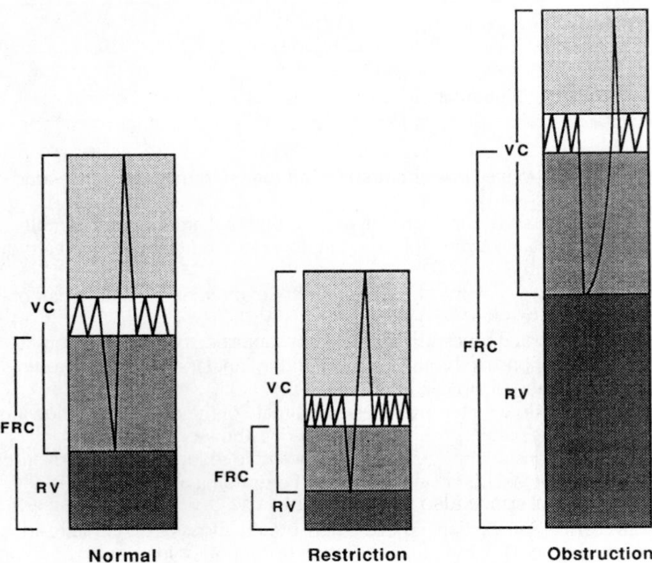

Figure 16-5. Lung volumes and capacities in normal individuals and in restrictive and obstructive lung disease. FRC, functional residual capacity; RV, residual volume; VC, vital capacity.

To maximize ventilation, an individual has two options: (a) increase respiratory rate and (b) increase the amount of air exchanged with each breath. Both increase when normal individuals exercise. A normal individual can triple or quadruple his or her TV with exercise. But some patients with interstitial lung disease have normal resting lung volumes but fail to recruit additional respiratory units during exercise, leading to dyspnea, high respiratory rate, and possibly even gas exchange problems.

A second type of ventilatory abnormality detected by exercise studies but which is not always obvious on resting studies is referred to as *exercise-induced bronchospasm*. Individuals with reactive airways disease develop nonspecific airways hyperreactivity, meaning that even if one specific toxic agent caused the asthma, bronchospasm can be triggered by a number of other irritants. Exercise itself can provoke bronchospasm, which can be detected by measuring airflow before and after exercise.

Gas Exchange

Gas exchange occurs along the entire alveolar surface, with oxygen moving by diffusion from the alveolar side into the blood and carbon dioxide diffusing from the blood into the alveolus, as illustrated in Figure 16-5. The gases must diffuse across the pulmonary epithelial cell, across the basement membrane, through the interstitial space, through the basement membrane underlying the endothelial cells, and through the capillary endothelium. Oxygen must then exchange through the plasma and across the membrane of red blood cells to combine with hemoglobin to form oxyhemoglobin.

Alterations in diffusion of gases can occur due to pathologic changes in any of these layers. The classic example is thickening of the interstitial space as seen in pulmonary fibrosis, or replacement of the normally attenuated alveolar epithelial cells by cuboidal-shaped cells as seen in diffuse alveolar epithelial damage from chemical inhalation. Gas exchange abnormalities may also occur due to alterations in the matching between ventilation and perfusion, as seen in emphysema, in which large regions of lung may be perfused but not adequately ventilated.

The major measurable physiologic effects of impaired gas exchange include (a) abnormal ventilation owing to increased respiratory rate and attempts to increase TV; (b) hypoxemia at rest and with exercise; and (c) exercise limitation, related to an early switch to anaerobic metabolism and subsequent lactic acidosis. These abnormalities can occur in association with lung diseases that produce restrictive, obstructive, or mixed patterns on pulmonary function testing. For example, both interstitial fibrosis and emphysema can cause gas exchange abnormalities.

DIFFUSING CAPACITY

In estimating the extent of gas exchange abnormalities, clinicians rely on several tests, including the use of carbon monoxide diffusing capacity. To estimate the diffusing capacity of the lung, one must know the amount of gas that is diffusing across the barrier in some unit of time. One must also know the mean difference in the partial pressures of the gas between the alveolus and the capillary. The calculation of the actual mean difference in partial pressures for oxygen between alveolus and capillary is difficult, because the partial pressures vary across the course of the capillary. In contrast, carbon monoxide has such high affinity for hemoglobin that the mean gradient is easier to estimate. This is the main reason that carbon monoxide is typically used to assess diffusing capacity of the lungs for carbon monoxide (DLCO). The single-breath technique, although easier to perform than the multiple-breath (steady-state) technique, is performed under conditions of breath holding and therefore may not be as accurate a reflection of a true diffusion abnormality. When abnormal, the DLCO is helpful, but it is a relatively late and insensitive indicator of gas exchange abnormalities in some disease states.

ARTERIAL BLOOD GAS ANALYSIS

To obtain an overall estimate of gas exchange, most clinical laboratories perform arterial blood gas analysis. The resting arterial blood gas provides information about the partial pressure of gases (oxygen and carbon dioxide) dissolved in the blood and can be used to estimate the alveolar-arterial difference in partial pressure of oxygen. In normal persons this alveolar-arterial (A-a) gradient is usually between 2 and 17 mm Hg at room air, but widens in pathologic states that affect gas exchange.

Patients can have normal resting arterial blood gases and still have significant gas exchange abnormalities. For this reason, the estimation of gas exchange during exercise can become especially important. If abnormalities in gas exchange are not evident during exercise, then a clinically significant gas exchange problem does not exist. Whether performed on a cycle ergometer or on a treadmill, the information obtained about an individual's pulmonary impairment and gas exchange abnormalities is invaluable. If the study is performed correctly, it is one of the most sensitive indicators of underlying respiratory disease. Such studies provide information about the level of exercise that an individual can maximally tolerate, and how much of the exercise limitation is related to gas exchange or ventilatory or cardiovascular disorders. Although time-consuming and expensive, exercise tests play an important role in the long-term assessment and follow-up of patients with toxicologic lung injury.

Nonventilatory Functions of the Lung

Aside from ventilation and gas exchange, the respiratory system has several other important functions. These include the production and secretion of hormones and mediators, biotransformation of chemical compounds, and removal of vasoactive agents from the blood stream. Examples of the ability of the lungs to metabolize foreign chemicals include the handling of basic amines. Enzymes exist in the lung capable of transforming substances such as aromatic polycyclic hydrocarbons. However, compared to other organs such as the liver, the lung plays a small role in the biotransformation of drugs and toxic chemicals. It must be remembered, however, that the lung is capable of selective uptake of some compounds and of the metabolic activation of certain compounds, such as paraquat, into agents that produce pulmonary toxicity. With regard to removal of vasoactive agents, the classic example is the conversion of the polypeptide angiotensin I into angiotensin II as the enzyme passes through the lung. The converting enzyme is found in pulmonary capillary cells. Major inactivation of 5-hydroxytryptamine also occurs in the lung. A number of prostaglandins are inactivated or removed from circulation in the lung.

DEPOSITION AND CLEARANCE OF INHALED SUBSTANCES

Toxic materials in inhaled air come in basically two forms: (a) gases and (b) aerosols. Aerosols are droplets of liquid or are particles suspended in gas.

The site of deposition for inhaled gases is largely determined by the solubility of the gas in the aqueous layer of the respiratory mucosa. Gases that are extremely water soluble, such as ammonia and sulfur dioxide, are deposited and removed predominantly by the upper respiratory tract. Thus, they exert their main toxic effects on the upper airways and only damage the peripheral air spaces when inhaled in high concentrations. Alternatively, gases that are of low water solubility, such as oxides of nitrogen and phosgene, may predominantly injure the pulmonary parenchyma. The less soluble the gas, the greater the potential for damage at the level of the terminal respiratory unit.

Many factors influence the deposition of particulate matter. These factors include (a) the characteristics of the aerosol itself, (b) the anatomy of the respiratory tract, and (c) the breathing pattern of the individual. The size of the particle is usually the predominant factor affecting deposition, although particle density and shape also contribute to the pattern seen. The majority of particles larger than approximately 10 μm in diameter are successfully filtered out by the nasopharynx. Particles in the range of 0.5 to 3.0 μm are deposited predominantly in distal airways and alveoli. Evidence suggests that particles smaller than approximately 0.5 μm in diameter behave much like gases do. Although it was believed that such small particles were mainly exhaled without significant deposition, studies indicate that so-called submicron particles may be significant contributors to lung injury at the level of the respiratory bronchioles and alveoli (see Fig. 16-1).

Another major determinant of how inhaled agents affect the respiratory tract pertains to the types of lung cells found at the deposition site. Cells vary in their susceptibility to toxic agents. For example, not only are the upper airway and tracheobronchial tree the sites of deposition of sulfur dioxide, but smooth muscle cells located there appear to be especially susceptible to toxic injury.

Clearance of particles is also of great importance in determining the toxic effects of inhaled agents. *Particle clearance* can refer to elimination of particles from the body or to their translocation to other organs after their initial deposition in the respiratory tract. In general, highly water-soluble particles and gases are absorbed through the epithelial layer into the blood stream near where they have been deposited. The clearance of insoluble particles is dependent on where they impact. If they are deposited in the nasopharynx and tracheobronchial tree, where there is ciliated epithelium and a layer of mucus, then most of the particles are transported up the mucociliary escalator where they are swallowed or expectorated. At the alveolar level, where there is no ciliated epithelium, the defense against foreign matter is largely in the hands of alveolar macrophages. These alveolar macrophages phagocytose particles, destroy microorganisms, and may then migrate up the tracheobronchial tree or into the lymphatics. Some particles engulfed by the macrophages are not successfully digested, and may cause cell lysis. The fate of such particles is less certain. Some of the dead macrophages and associated particles are presumably removed by tracheobronchial clearance. Some are retained and become part of an ongoing pulmonary inflammatory reaction. The death of alveolar macrophages and the subsequent liberation of cellular products may, in fact, trigger a number of pathologic responses, including fibrosis, emphysema, and granuloma formation. Neutrophils also play an important role in the handling of particles in the lung, especially after the inflammatory reaction has commenced. And some foreign particles in the alveolar space also may pass into the pulmonary lymphatics or eventually dissolve and diffuse into the capillary blood.

ASSESSMENT OF PULMONARY TOXICITY

Occupational and Environmental Exposure Assessment

HISTORY

One of the first steps in the evaluation of an individual with suspected pulmonary injury from a toxic exposure is to determine the exposure. Sometimes it is easy (e.g., when a worker gets sprayed in the face with ammonia and promptly develops respiratory symptoms). But more often it is not a trivial task. It requires a careful environmental and occupational history. When the disease onset is delayed or the suspected exposure is complex, the physician must generate a database that includes the jobs that the individual has had and the types of exposures that he or she may have experienced on those jobs. The simplest and most systematic way of approaching the occupational history is to generate a chronological list of all jobs. One can then elaborate on each of those jobs by asking specific questions about the exposures encountered. This can be a time-consuming task, but such detective work is often rewarding.

It is also important to obtain information about non–work-related exposures, including medications, pets, hobbies, and smoking habits. For example, a patient was diagnosed with occupational asthma owing to the inhalation of toluene diisocyanate as part of an automotive spray paint. He left his job, but continued to be exposed by doing spray painting in his garage as a hobby. Part-time dental technicians may work out of basement shops producing amalgams that contain beryllium that can induce chronic granulomatous disease. Weekend welders run some risk of developing metal fume fever that their clinician might erroneously call "the flu." Secondary or passive exposure to toxic substances can occur if carried home by family members. This occurred historically with asbestos fibers on the clothes of asbestos workers, causing asbestosis and cancer in family members. Smoking history should always be obtained. Cigarette smoke can sometimes cause the same symptoms as those seen with other exposures and can have additive or multiplicative effects when combined with toxicants.

MATERIAL SAFETY DATA SHEETS

Sometimes it is apparent that there is a hazard in the workplace that has caused pulmonary symptoms, but additional informa-

TABLE 16-2. Identifying occupational and environmental causes of lung disease

- Occupational history
  - Chronologic job list
  - Potential exposures from each job
- Environmental history
  - Dwelling location, heating and ventilation, furnishings, fabrics
  - Chemicals: insecticides, herbicides, cleaning agents
  - Hobbies and associated exposures
  - Pets
  - Habits: smoking, illicit drugs
  - Other inhabitants and their exposures
- Biological monitoring
  - Medical examination
  - Lung tissue analysis for mineral content
  - Arterial blood gas analysis (e.g., carboxyhemoglobin)
  - Immunologic testing
- Worksite or home evaluation
  - Material Safety Data Sheet review for evidence of pulmonary irritants or sensitizers
  - Discuss job exposures with plant foreman, supervisor, or health and safety personnel
  - Review industrial hygiene data if available from company or from federal agency investigations
  - Conduct walkthrough investigation
  - Survey workforce and perform atmospheric analyses if indicated by walkthrough findings

tion is needed to help pinpoint the specific cause. Some investigative options are listed in Table 16-2. Workers frequently do not know all of the chemicals they come in contact with and cannot fully assess the associated risks. Material Safety Data Sheets (MSDSs) form a crucial link between the exposures and the diagnosis. MSDSs are required by law to be present and available in the workplace. MSDSs should be routinely reviewed when patients present with possible work-related symptoms for indirect evidence of exposure to sensitizers and pulmonary irritants.

ONSITE INVESTIGATION

In the occupational medicine clinic setting, one further step in linking a patient's disease and his or her workplace involves onsite investigation. Walkthroughs of a plant can usually be arranged with the plant manager and commonly provide insights unobtainable in the doctor's examining room. In our own practice, we work as a team with industrial hygienists. When needed, it is possible to do onsite atmosphere analysis and obtain information on the health of other workers. The clinician should inquire if any federal agencies have investigated the workplace.

DETECTION OF MINERALS IN THE LUNG

Analysis of the dust content of tissue specimens can serve as another way of confirming exposure. If a large piece of material, such as an entire lobe of lung or at least several grams of lung tissue can be obtained, the tissue can be treated chemically or washed to remove organic material. Mineral content of the remaining inorganic matter is then analyzed. The inorganic particles can be measured for size and number and their mineral content determined. Most of these methods destroy the tissue and therefore do not allow observation of how the dust burden correlates with anatomy and pathology. Numerous methodologic and standardization problems with digested tissue analysis for mineral and fiber content exist. These include potential sampling error and variability in digestion techniques, fiber extraction, counting, and analysis methods.

Alternatively, tissue can be sectioned for light microscopy, for scanning, or for transmission electron microscopy. Microscopy methods, although subject to significant sampling errors owing to the very small amount of tissue being studied, can yield a great deal of information about particle size, composition, and crystalline structure. Microscopy potentially gives critical information about the relationship of particle to pathology, but provides a relatively poor estimate of the amount of mineral present.

Light Microscopy. The light microscope detects only large particles that can be either identified by their polarization characteristics or staining properties. Some crystalline minerals, such as talc and silica, are birefringent when examined under polarized light. Carbonaceous dusts, such as graphite, carbon particles, and coal dust, are readily seen using routine histologic staining methods, especially as they are ingested by alveolar macrophages. Asbestos bodies (ferruginous bodies) can be seen on routine hematoxylin- and eosin-stained sections, but are better seen using iron stains (e.g., Prussian blue) due to their ferritin coating. The light microscope only detects particles larger than approximately 0.5 μm in size.

Electron Microscopy. The transmission electron microscope allows the pathologist to see the shadows of electron-dense materials as the electron beam is passed through the tissue specimen. The scanning electron microscope generates a three-dimensional image as the electron beam reflects off the surface of the tissue. These methods can be linked with an electron probe, crystallographic diffraction methods, and x-ray energy spectrometry to give more specific information about the actual mineral contact of the particles being observed. However, these analyses are expensive, time-consuming, and subject to sampling error. Also, certain lightweight minerals are poorly detected.

Clinical Examination

The patient's symptoms should be carefully reviewed with at least three goals in mind: (a) identifying the level of the respiratory tract that has been affected (e.g., nasopharynx versus bronchial tree); (b) assessing the timing of onset, latency, and severity of the illness; and (c) guiding further diagnostic testing. Details of the signs and symptoms produced by various toxic injuries to the respiratory system are described in subsequent chapters.

The physical examination may provide a few crucial clues. Patients with asbestosis or other pneumoconioses may have dry rales heard at the lung bases on inspiration. The patient with occupational asthma may have wheezing heard on auscultation; however, given the reversible nature of reactive airways disease, there may be clinical examinations that are completely normal. An individual who has developed acute mucosal injury caused by an alkali or acid burn may have stridor. However, none of these clinical findings is pathognomonic for a specific toxic insult.

Chest Imaging

RADIOGRAPHY

The chest radiograph is one of the cornerstones in the assessment of toxic injuries to the respiratory tract. Although evidence of obstructive lung disease can be found on chest radiograph,

TABLE 16-3. Common radiographic findings in occupational and environmental lung disease

Radiographic finding	Disease
Diffuse infiltrates, interstitial pattern (nodular, reticular, reticulonodular)	Aluminum lung (Shaver's disease)
	Asbestosis
	Bronchiolitis obliterans
	Chronic beryllium disease
	Chronic brucellosis
	Coalworker's pneumoconiosis
	Drug-induced disease (e.g., bleomycin, methotrexate, gold, busulfan)
	Extrinsic allergic alveolitis (hypersensitivity pneumonitis)
	Fuller's earth
	Hard-metal disease (cobalt)
	Histoplasmosis
	Kaolinosis (china clay)
	Mixed dust fibrosis
	Oxygen toxicity
	Paraquat poisoning
	Pneumoconiosis caused by radiopaque dusts (siderosis, silver, stannosis, baritosis, antimony, rare-earth pneumoconiosis, titanium, zirconium, chromite)
	Radiation pneumonitis
	Silo filler's disease (oxides of nitrogen) (late phase)
	Talcosis
	Thesaurosis (hair spray)
	Vineyard sprayer's lung (copper sulfate)
	Zinc chloride
Diffuse infiltrates, acinar/alveolar pattern (including pulmonary edema)	Acetaldehyde
	Acrolein (acrylic aldehyde)
	Acute aspiration (water, alcohol, kerosene)
	Acute cadmium poisoning
	Acute beryllium disease
	Acute silicoproteinosis
	Adult respiratory distress syndrome
	Ammonia
	Burns
	Chlorine
	Cobalt
	Fire smoke
	Hydrocarbon pneumonitis
	Hydrogen chloride
	Hydrogen fluoride
	Hydrogen sulfide
	Hydrogen phosphide (phosphine)
	Hydrogen selenide
	Lithium hydride
	Manganese
	Mercury vapors
	Methyl bromide
	Nickel carbonyl
	Organophosphates
	Oxides of nitrogen (silo filler's disease)
	Ozone
	Paraquat poisoning
	Phosgene
	Polymer fume fever
	Selenium
	Sulfur dioxide
	Titanium tetrachloride
	Toluene diisocyanate
	Trimellitic anhydride lung disease/anemia
	Zinc chloride
Diffuse infiltrates, "mixed" acinar and reticulonodular pattern	Chronic beryllium disease
	Drug-induced disease (methotrexate, bleomycin)
	Extrinsic allergic alveolitis (hypersensitivity pneumonitis)
	Pulmonary edema (many causes)
Segmental consolidation	Occupational infections (including brucellosis, tularemia, anthrax)
	Psittacosis-ornithosis
	Vanadium (heavy exposure)
Cystic or cavitary lesions	Coalworker's pneumoconiosis, complicated (large opacities)
	Caplan's nodules
	Coccidioidomycosis
	Cystic bronchiectasis
	Histoplasmosis
	Silicosis, complicated (large opacities)
	Silicotuberculosis
Solitary or multiple pulmonary nodules	Coalworker's pneumoconiosis
	Progressive massive fibrosis
	Caplan's necrobiotic nodules
	Complicated (large opacities)
	Cryptococcosis
	Histoplasmosis
	Occupational or environmental lung malignancies
	Silicosis
	Complicated (large opacities)
	Rheumatoid silicotic nodules
Hyperinflation	Chronic obstructive lung disease
	Emphysema (tobacco exposure, possible cadmium)
	Occupational asthma (many causes)
Hilar and mediastinal lymphadenopathy	Chronic beryllium disease
	Mushroom workers' lung (rare in other extrinsic allergic alveolitis)
	Occupational infections (including brucellosis, tularemia, histoplasmosis, coccidioidomycosis)
	Silicosis
Mediastinal widening	Aluminum lung (Shaver's disease)
	Anthrax
Pleural effusions	Asbestos exposure
	Asbestosis
	Mesothelioma
Pleural plaques	Asbestos exposure
	Chronic beryllium disease
	Diatomaceous earth lung (free silica)
	Extrinsic allergic alveolitis (chronic)

the greater application pertains to toxic injuries that produce interstitial infiltrates, such as the pneumoconioses. Table 16-3 lists the common radiographic findings in occupational and environmental lung diseases. Classically, one looks at (a) the shape of opacities (e.g., irregular versus rounded); (b) the size of opacities; (c) profusion (the number of opacities per unit lung); (d) the extent and location of the infiltrates (e.g., upper lobe versus lower lobe predominance); and (e) presence of ancillary findings such as pleural plaques, adenopathy, pulmonary hypertension, cardiac enlargement, and Kerley's lines. These five main observations form the basis of a formal reading system known as the International Labor Organization (ILO) 1980 Classification of Radiographs of the Pneumoconioses. Although designed for the systematic recording of radiographic changes caused by inhalation of mineral dusts, the principles can be applied in reading films from any of the diffuse interstitial diseases listed in Table 16-3.

By this classification, small opacities (smaller than 10 mm in diameter) are described as rounded as seen in diseases such as silicosis, or irregular as seen in asbestosis. The letters *p*, *q*, and *r* are used to subdivide rounded opacities according to size—up to 1.5 mm, 1.5 to 3.0 mm, and 3.0 to 10.0 mm, respectively. Similarly, the letters *s*, *t*, and *u* describe the predominant sizes of small irregular opacities. In the classification system, each radiograph's opacities are classified according to the most common and next most common shape and size. For example, s/t indicates that the majority of opacities are size s, and the second most common size is t. Profusion, the number of small rounded or small irregular opacities per lung zone, is divided into four main categories from 0 through 3, and these are further divided along a 12-point scale ranging from 0/− to 3/+. To score the extent of involvement, each lung is arbitrarily divided into three zones by horizontal imaginary lines one-third and two-thirds of the distance between the apex of the lung and the dome of the diaphragm.

The ILO classification also systematically describes large opacities (larger than 10 mm) as well as pleural plaques and other abnormalities. A set of standard ILO reference films are routinely used by readers in judging the shape, size, and profusion of opacities on a given chest radiograph.

The opacity's shape (round versus irregular) is of limited use. Most interstitial lung diseases can present with a range of opacities from pure round to reticular nodular to pure linear or irregular. Even in simple silicosis—the classic example of rounded opacities—the opacities can assume a more reticular appearance on the chest radiograph, depending on factors such as dust burden and duration of illness.

Distribution of diffuse infiltrates may be of slightly greater predictive value, although again there are many exceptions. Opacities are found throughout the lungs in most interstitial lung diseases. However, in a number of toxicant-induced diseases there is a lower-lung predominance. Examples include nitrofurantoin-induced disease, metallic mercury embolism, interstitial pulmonary edema, pulmonary fibrosis, asbestosis, and talcosis. Relatively few of the diffuse interstitial lung diseases show an upper-lung field predominance, with two notable exceptions from the standpoint of toxic inhalation: silicosis and chronic beryllium disease.

Hilar adenopathy, with or without eggshell calcifications, is seen in silicosis as well as in some cases of coal workers' pneumoconiosis and, occasionally, in chronic beryllium disease.

A pattern of acute pulmonary edema in a patient without trauma or heart disease raises the spectra of chemical exposure. The typical pattern is that of diffuse fluffy alveolar infiltrates but with a normal heart size. Drugs that can cause a noncardiogenic pulmonary edema pattern include amphotericin B, aspirin, hydrochlorothiazide, lidocaine, major tranquilizers, opiates, sedatives, and sympathomimetic agents. Alveolar hemorrhage is often indistinguishable from the pulmonary edema pattern on chest radiograph. This can result from a number of exposures, including agents such as D-penicillamine and trimellitic anhydride.

The limitations of the chest radiograph should be acknowledged. First, the chest radiograph often correlates poorly with the clinical activity of interstitial lung diseases. For example, the chest radiograph may be markedly abnormal in coal workers who have normal pulmonary function. A number of inhaled dusts may produce benign pneumoconioses. When dusts are radiodense, they produce radiographic changes, but with little or no pathologic or physiologic abnormality on further investigation. Conversely, some patients with significant pulmonary embarrassment have normal-appearing chest radiographs. Radiographically inapparent clinical illness can occur in patients with farmers' lung or other hypersensitivity pneumonitides, beryllium disease, and asbestosis.

A second major limitation of the chest radiograph is its lack of specificity. Many types of injuries produce similar radiographic changes. This lack of specificity prevents heavy reliance on the chest radiograph in differential diagnosis of chest disease. For example, although it is classically taught that silicosis produces small, rounded opacities predominantly in the upper- and mid-lung fields, there are many cases described in which the disease may have lower lobe predominance with a more reticular appearance on chest radiograph. Asbestosis is classically credited with producing small, irregular opacities in the lower-lung fields; however, this disease can produce mid- and upper-lung field predominant disease. Even the presence of pleural plaques, which many occupational medicine physicians equate with asbestos exposure, has limited specificity. Many pulmonary diseases (related or unrelated to toxicologic insult) exist that can produce bilateral pleural disease, including silicosis, diatomaceous earth pneumoconiosis, and chronic beryllium disease. Previous chest surgery or chest trauma may also confound the assessment of pleural disease. However, in the proper clinical context, presence of plaques and infiltrates in an asbestos-exposed individual may be sufficient to diagnose asbestosis.

GALLIUM SCINTIGRAPHY

^{67}Gallium imaging has been applied in the examination of inflammatory lung disease, but has relatively limited proven application. The limitations of this nuclear medicine technique are based on (a) its lack of specificity and (b) the fact that the examination takes a long time to perform, with useful data obtainable at the earliest 18 to 24 hours after injection of the ^{67}Gallium tracer. In principle, the gallium acts by binding to transferrin. In inflammatory lesions, such as malignancies; infections; and chronic inflammation, such as granulomatous disease, the gallium is transferred from transferrin to local iron-binding proteins such as lactoferrin. These proteins are found on the surface of macrophages or in the granules of leukocytes. The net effect is localization of ^{67}Gallium at sites of cellular inflammation.

In practice, gallium scanning has limited use. It may be applied when routine radiographic procedures have been unrevealing, but the clinical scenario still suggests that there is an active pulmonary process. Under such circumstances, a positive gallium scan may help the clinician decide to proceed with more invasive and specific tests, such as lung biopsy.

COMPUTED TOMOGRAPHY

Computed tomography (CT) has become an indispensable tool for imaging the chest. It provides information not only about the pulmonary parenchyma but also about the mediastinum, pleura, and chest wall. Improvements in resolution, in particular the advent of thin-section, high-resolution CT scanning, allows visualization of even minute and subtle interstitial lung abnormalities. In some cases, the CT scan's level of detection is far superior to that of the conventional chest radiograph. With it, subtle plaques and effusions are visualized from asbestos, conglomerate masses from silicosis, and even small cavities from silicotuberculosis that would otherwise evade early detection. With high-resolution CT scans, it is easy to diagnose bronchiectasis and spot radiographically inapparent interstitial infiltrates that may be less apparent on chest radiographs. CT scans have also demonstrated great sensitivity in imaging the upper respiratory tract, including the sinuses, posterior pharynx, and tracheobronchial tree.

The role of CT scanning in comparison to the use of magnetic resonance imaging has yet to be fully explored in relation to the respiratory tract. At its current level of development, magnetic resonance imaging has no advantages over CT of the lungs, mediastinum, and hilar regions.

Physiologic Assessment

Pulmonary function tests provide clues to the type of toxicologic insult to the respiratory tract. The specific measurements relied

TABLE 16-4. Examples of physiologic abnormalities in occupational and environmental lung disease

- Airflow limitation (obstruction)
  - Without bronchodilator response
    - Bronchiectasis (e.g., ammonia)
    - Chronic bronchitis (e.g., irritant dusts and fumes, coal dust, tobacco smoke)
    - Chronic obstructive lung disease (e.g., tobacco smoke)
    - Emphysema (e.g., tobacco smoke, possibly cadmium, nitrogen dioxide)
    - Upper airway obstruction (e.g., tracheal stenosis after chemical burn to airway; laryngeal malignancy caused by asbestos)
    - Vocal cord dysfunction (irritant-induced)
  - With bronchodilator response
    - Reactive airway disease (asthma) (see Table 16-5)
    - Reactive airways disease syndrome (e.g., high-dose, single exposure to airways irritants)
  - Restrictive physiology
    - Bronchiolitis obliterans (e.g., oxides of nitrogen, sulfur dioxide)
    - Chronic beryllium disease
    - Chronic extrinsic allergic alveolitis (e.g., avian proteins, fungal spores)
    - Hard-metal disease (giant cell pneumonitis caused by cobalt)
    - Interstitial fibrosis (e.g., methotrexate, nitrofurantoin, oxygen toxicity)
    - Pneumoconioses (e.g., asbestosis, silicosis)
    - Talcosis
    - Pleural disease (e.g., mesothelioma, diffuse pleural thickening)
  - Mixed disorder (obstructive plus restrictive physiology)
    - Asbestosis
    - Bronchiolitis obliterans
    - Chronic beryllium disease
    - Extrinsic allergic alveolitis
    - Silicosis
    - Tobacco smoke plus toxicant exposure

on in pulmonary physiologic assessment are summarized in Table 16-1. Table 16-4 lists the common physiologic findings in a number of occupational and environmental lung diseases. But, by and large, the main value of pulmonary function tests and exercise physiology studies lies more in the assessment of degree of impairment and response to treatment than in diagnosis.

The clinician must be aware of the limitations of each test. Spirometry and measurements of lung volumes are greatly influenced by factors such as (a) patient effort and understanding of the testing procedure, (b) skill of the technician performing the testing, (c) the equipment and testing methods being used, (d) standardization and quality control of the equipment used in physiologic assessment, and (e) variation in definition of physiologic abnormalities by various interpreters of pulmonary function tests.

SPIROMETRY

Simple spirometry is commonly used in industry and in clinical practice as a screening test. However, even with NIOSH-certified spirometry technicians, a great deal of mediocre data are still being generated. Even with good quality spirometry, simple spirometry only gives the clinician a few key pieces of information: (a) low FEV_1/FVC ratio indicates airflow obstruction; (b) low flows during the middle half of expiration (the $FEF_{25\%-75\%}$) also help indicate airflow limitation; (c) improvement in FEV_1/FVC after bronchodilators indicates reversible airflow obstruction; (d) serial decrements in FEV_1/FVC ratio on annual examinations is a useful indicator of disease progression; (e) used pre- and postexposure, FEV_1/FVC can help to define the cause of airflow obstruction; and (f) low FVC may imply restrictive physiology but cannot and should not be relied on as the sole indicator of lung volume status.

In addition to relying on the numbers themselves, clinicians should review the shape of the curves produced as air flows in and out of the lungs. Such flow volume loops can provide important clues to upper airway obstruction. For example, premature truncation or flattening of the inspiratory portion of the loop can be seen in patients with vocal cord dysfunction, a condition linked to irritant exposures that mimics asthma.

Normal spirometry does not exclude the possibility of significant, impairing lung disease. It does not give sufficient information about lung volumes, gas exchange, or response to specific triggers of asthma. Furthermore, a single set of normal spirometry values does not exclude possible asthma. Because airflow limitation can be completely reversible, serial measurements may be required.

A frequently encountered scenario is one in which an individual has inhaled a suspected toxic agent and presents with symptoms of shortness of breath, chest tightness, or wheezing. Spirometry is normal, with no bronchodilator response. The clinician might conclude erroneously that there is nothing physiologically wrong with the individual, on the basis of a single clinical interview. However, when evaluated during a time of significant symptoms, the patient's pulmonary function tests may show a dramatic airflow limitation. If the spirometry is still normal, but symptoms persist, several options are available for ruling out occult asthma. These include

1. Nonspecific inhalation challenge testing, using methacholine or histamine as the challenge substance. Individuals with airways hyperreactivity develop transient bronchospasm and a concomitant drop in airflow on inhaling these compounds.
2. Peak flow meter recording. Measurements of peak flow can be conveniently performed by the individual during symptomatic and asymptomatic periods. If significant variation in peak flows is recorded by the patient, this serves as a clue to airways hyperreactivity. Furthermore, if used correctly, peak flows can help identify specific patterns of hyperreactivity.
3. Airways resistance and conductance measurement. An increasing number of clinical pulmonary physiology laboratories have the capacity to detect airflow limitation both by flow measurements and by directly measuring airways resistance and airways specific conductance. The principle is simple: High airways resistance and low conductance imply narrowing of the conducting airways. The advantage of measuring specific conductance and airways resistance is that these tests are often more sensitive than FEV_1 in detecting airflow abnormalities. They are also more effort-independent than other measures of airflow. Like measures of airflow, they can be performed both pre- and postbronchodilator.

LUNG VOLUME ASSESSMENT

Measurement of the lung compartments (volumes and capacities) is generally made by one of several methods, including helium dilution, nitrogen washout, and body plethysmography. The latter is by far the faster method. It is more expensive but only slightly more difficult to perform compared with inert gas methods. Some patients are unable to use the "body box" due to claustrophobia, obesity, or skeletal deformity. Again, the quality of results is dependent on patient understanding, effort, and technician skill. When assessing for the presence of either air trapping or restrictive lung disease, one of these methods should be used to generate an accurate picture of lung volumes. As in spirometry, normal lung volumes alone do not fully exclude the possibility of significant underlying lung disease.

A common scenario in which lung volumes are normal but fail to identify serious underlying toxicologic injury is seen with interstitial lung diseases such as pneumoconioses. A patient with asbestosis may have normal lung volumes, leading the clinician to conclude erroneously that this individual is unimpaired. However, individuals with pneumoconioses or other interstitial lung diseases may have normal lung volumes but severe derangement of gas exchange. When the clinical suspicion is high, the workup should not stop with lung volumes but include tests designed to examine abnormalities of gas exchange.

GAS EXCHANGE

The ultimate task of the respiratory system is to regulate oxygen and carbon dioxide tension in the blood. As such, tests that measure abnormalities in gas exchange are critical to the assessment of respiratory damage. Gas exchange is evaluated clinically using the DLCO, and arterial blood gas determinations at rest and during exercise. The DLCO provides a relatively good approximation of gas exchange abnormalities caused by ventilation-perfusion mismatching, venous admixture (shunting), and barriers to diffusion of gases. But it does not separate among these causes. Simply put, the diffusing capacity is a measure of the ability of the respiratory system to conduct air from alveolus to capillary blood. The test is performed by either a single-breath or steady-state technique. The latter is preferred because breath-holding creates artificial conditions in which to measure diffusion and also may be more difficult for patients with lung disease. A number of theoretical considerations must be taken into account in such testing, including the hemoglobin, alveolar volume, and temperature. DLCO has limited sensitivity, and should not be singularly relied on in the estimation of pulmonary gas exchange.

A resting room air arterial blood gas can be extremely useful and sometimes is the only clue to abnormal gas exchange, even in the face of normal lung volumes and normal diffusing capacity. From the blood gas, one should examine not only the absolute partial pressures of oxygen and carbon dioxide, but also calculate the A-a gradient. This A-a gradient for PO_2 is an estimation of the differential passage of oxygen and carbon dioxide between the alveolus and the arterial blood. It is an indirect equivalent of DLCO, but can be abnormal even when DLCO is not. Exercise physiology testing can be done with either continuous measurement of oxygen saturation by oximetry or by the use of an indwelling arterial catheter for the serial sampling of arterial blood gases. The latter is more invasive but gives more accurate and reliable information. When oximetry is used, blood gases should be drawn at rest and at peak exercise to confirm the correlation between PO_2 and oximetry. A maximal exercise study provides invaluable information about a patient's exercise capacity and about the degree of gas exchange abnormality. Normal individuals increase ventilation and improve oxygenation. Patients with interstitial lung disease suboptimally increase ventilation and desaturate during exercise. This test provides a wealth of practical information and is often more sensitive than DLCO.

Endoscopy

Flexible fiberoptic scopes have had an important impact on the evaluation of the upper and lower respiratory tracts. Rhinoscopy is extremely useful in helping to examine alterations in the region of first-line defense against inhaled toxicants. Direct laryngoscopy permits careful examination of the nasopharynx, including the larynx and proximal trachea. This can prove very useful when faced with suspected acute chemical burns, possible vocal cord dysfunction in which the vocal cords adduct during inspiration, or in assessing for chronic scarring of the upper respiratory tract.

The fiberoptic bronchoscope allows inspection of the airway from the level of the posterior pharynx through four or five generations of bronchi and to obtain samples of lung tissue for histologic examination. Sometimes simple visual inspection of the airway can help clarify a confusing clinical picture. The small pieces of bronchial and parenchymal tissue obtainable with a biopsy forceps are often sufficient to make outpatient diagnoses of lung disease. For example, there is an extremely high yield on transbronchial biopsy for the diagnosis of granulomatous diseases such as beryllium disease and extrinsic allergic alveolitis (hypersensitivity pneumonitis).

Bronchoalveolar lavage, a technique in which aliquots of normal saline are instilled and suctioned from a small segment of peripheral lung, is still principally a research tool, with a few important exceptions. Examination and immunologic testing of the cells from lavage has helped to identify a number of inhalational injuries, including beryllium disease and extrinsic allergic alveolitis. In these diseases, there is a marked increase in lavage lymphocytes, whereas a normal lavage contains mainly macrophages. Good correlation exists between the high lymphocyte counts and the underlying granulomatous pathology. Furthermore, testing of cells obtained from lavage for their immunologic reactivity allows the clinician to make a specific diagnosis of beryllium disease. With these few exceptions, bronchoalveolar lavage still has relatively limited clinical application in the evaluation of pulmonary toxic insults.

Immunologic Evaluation of Pulmonary Toxicity

An emerging area of intense research and new clinical application is the immunologic assessment of inhaled toxicant effects. Some offending agents have nonspecific inflammatory effects on cell populations. Others are either (a) immunosuppressants, causing defects in normal immune regulation, or (b) act as antigens, causing specific hypersensitivity immune responses both within the lung and systemically. Normally, the local immune system can handle the routine barrage to which the lung is subjected. But the response can go awry, producing harmful effects such as granuloma formation, pulmonary fibrosis, and bronchial hyperreactivity. This topic has been well reviewed elsewhere and is discussed only briefly here. The main applications of immunology in assessment of occupational and environmental lung disease fall into several areas: (a) occupational asthma, (b) extrinsic allergic alveolitis (hypersensitivity pneumonitis), (c) pneumoconioses, and (d) occupational diseases caused by metal sensitization.

Most of the industrial agents that cause occupational asthma have known or suspected allergic properties, although occupationally and environmentally triggered asthma often occurs via multiple inflammatory, irritant, and pharmacologic mechanisms. Although immunologic tests of hypersensitivity may help pinpoint a putative allergen, they generally do not prove causation, short of bronchoprovocation testing.

High-molecular-weight compounds, such as those found in plant dusts, enzymes, animal dander, and urine, can produce allergic bronchoconstriction by producing specific immunoglobulin E (IgE) and sometimes specific IgG antibodies. Therefore, it is sometimes possible to use skin prick and patch testing, precipitins testing, radioallergosorbent tests (RAST), or enzyme-linked immunosorbent assays (ELISAs) to detect responses to these agents. Examples of clinical application of such immunologic tools include the use of latex skin tests, RAST inhibition, and ELISA to detect latex hypersensitivity and asthma. Low-molecular-weight compounds, such as the anhydrides, plicatic acid, isocyanates, and metal salts, may serve as protein-bound haptens, inducing both humoral or cellular immune responses. Immunologic meth-

TABLE 16-5. Examples of occupational and environmental causes of asthma

Agent source	Population at risk
Animal products	
Laboratory animals	Laboratory workers
Sea squirt fluid	Oyster/pearl gatherers
Avian proteins	Bird fanciers
Insects	
Locusts	Laboratory workers
Mites	Grain, flour mill workers, bakers
Moths, butterflies	Environmental exposure
Fungi	
Alternaria species	Bakers
Aspergillus species	Bakers
Cladosporium spores	Farm workers
Mushroom spores	Mushroom cultivation
Grains, flour, plants	
Wheat	Millers
Grain	Farm workers, grain handlers
Flour	Bakers
Castor beans	Farmers, gardeners
Gum acacia	Printers
Tobacco dust	Cigarette factory workers
Spices	Spice factory workers
Coffee beans	Exposure to green and roasted beans
Western red cedar	Workers, miller, joiners, carpenters
Oak	Millers
Cocabolla	Wood finishers
Redwood	Carpenters
Cotton, hemp, sisal, flax, and possible bacterial contaminants, endotoxin (part of clinical spectrum of *Byssinosis*)	Textile manufacturing, carders, sorters, weavers
Metals	
Chromates	Chrome plating and polishing
Platinum salts	Platinum refining
Nickel sulfate	Nickel plating
Nickel carbonyl	Chemist
Vanadium and vanadium pentoxide	Boiler cleaners
Cobalt	Tungsten carbide grinding
Stainless steel	Welders (chromium and nickel exposure)
Chemicals	
Fluorine	Aluminum potroom workers
Formalin	Laboratory workers, resin molding, hospital personnel
Ethanolamines	Aluminum cable soldering
Paraphenylenediamine	Fur dyers
Ethylene diamine	Rubber, shellac workers
Isocyanates Toluene diisocyanate, hexamethylene diisocyanate, diphenylmethane diisocyanate, naphthalene diisocyanate	Isocyanate manufacturing, plastics, factory workers, polyurethane foam manufacturing, automobile painters, printers, rubber workers, chemists, laminators, boat construction, tinners, insulators
Phthalic anhydride	Paint manufacturing, plastics molding
Trimellitic anhydride	Chemical workers
Colophony (pine resin)	Electronics soldering
Polyvinyl chloride fumes	Meat wrappers
Dyes	Dye manufacturing, hairdressers
Drugs	
Methyl dopa	Pharmaceutical manufacturing
Penicillins	Pharmaceutical manufacturing
Psyllium	Pharmaceutical manufacturing
Tetracycline	Pharmaceutical manufacturing
Sulfathiazole	Pharmaceutical manufacturing
Chloramines	Pharmaceutical manufacturing
Enzymes	
Trypsin	Plastics manufacturing
Pancreatic extract	Manufacturing, parents of children with cystic fibrosis
Bacillus subtilis	Detergent manufacturing

ods available for evaluating occupational asthma have been thoroughly reviewed elsewhere. The demonstration of specific antibodies indicates sensitization but may also be found in persons who have no asthma or allergic symptoms. Furthermore, some patients with allergen-induced asthma may be negative on immunologic tests, due to factors such as time since last exposure and methodologic flaws in assays. Therefore, results of immunologic tests must always be taken in the full clinical context. Major causes of occupational asthma are listed in Table 16-5.

Extrinsic allergic alveolitis is an immunologically mediated hypersensitivity reaction that occurs after exposure to a variety of organic dusts. Examples include farmers' lung disease, involving an immune response to one or more bacterial or fungal antigens found in moldy hay; pigeon breeders' disease; bagassosis; and humidifier fever, among others. A partial list of causes of extrinsic allergic alveolitis is found in Table 16-6. In the clinical setting of this hypersensitivity reaction, precipitins tests can help identify new antigens. They can also be used to confirm the clinical suspicion of hypersensitivity. However, because of the high rate of positive precipitin in asymptomatic-exposed subjects as well as the variability of precipitin responses over time and the lack of a truly exhaustive battery of test antigens, precipitins testing should only be considered an adjunct to diagnosis. A positive precipitins test can support the clinical diagnosis of extrinsic allergic alveolitis but should not be relied on to either solely include or exclude this diagnosis.

With regard to the pneumoconioses, specifically coal workers' pneumoconiosis, silicosis, and asbestosis, a number of immunologic abnormalities in blood and in bronchoalveolar lavage has been identified. None of these has any specific diagnostic or prognostic value in the clinical setting at this time. Clearly, immune regulation itself is altered in these disease states as evidenced by the increased risk of mycobacterial infection and connective tissue disease in individuals with pneumoconioses.

Occupational lung diseases caused by sensitizing metals have served as the paradigm for interstitial lung disease involving cell-mediated immune responses. Perhaps the single best application of these principles has been in the detection of chronic beryllium disease, in which immunologic evaluation using the beryllium lymphocyte proliferation test has become the key to the diagnosis and medical screening of exposed workers. Testing for cellular immunity has been preliminarily described in other metal-induced diseases, such as aluminum-induced granulomatosis, as well as for titanium, chromium, nickel, gold, and zirconium.

OCCUPATIONAL AND ENVIRONMENTAL LUNG DISORDERS

The list of agents that can induce lung injury is legion, ranging from minor irritants to carcinogens. Damage varies from reversible upper airway inflammation to permanent airway bronchoconstriction and from reversible hypersensitivity reactions to irreparable fibrosis. Table 16-7 outlines the principal types of pulmonary responses to toxic insults.

TABLE 16-6. Examples of agents causing extrinsic allergic alveolitis (hypersensitivity pneumonitis)

Agent	Source	Disease
Amoebae		
Naegleria gruberi	Humidifier water	Humidifier lung
Acanthamoeba spp.	Humidifier water	Humidifier lung
Animal proteins		
Bovine, porcine	Pituitary snuff	Snuff taker's lung
Murine	Rat, mouse urine	
Avian proteins		
Pigeon serum protein	Pigeon droppings	Pigeon breeder's disease
Parrot serum protein	Parrot droppings	Budgerigar fancier's disease
Chicken proteins	Chicken products	Feather plucker's lung
Bacterial		
Bacillus spp.	Humidifier water	Humidifier lung
	Wood dust	
	Detergent (enzyme)	
Chemicals		
Isocyanates	Chemical manufacturing	—
Trimellitic anhydride	Chemical manufacturing	—
Fungi		
Alternaria spp.	Moldy wood pulp	Pulp worker's disease
Aspergillus spp.	Moldy malt, barley	Malt worker's lung
	Moldy hay	Farmer's lung
Graphium spp.	Moldy redwood dust	Sequoiosis
Penicillium spp.	Cheese mold	Cheese washer's lung
	Humidifier water	Humidifier lung
	Moldy cork	Suberosis
Insects		
Wheat weevil	Grain contamination	Miller's lung
Plant products		
Ramin	Sawdust, coffee dust, dried grass	Sequoiosis, coffee worker's lung, thatched roof disease
Thermophylic actinomycetes		
Micropolyspora faeni	Moldy hay	Farmer's lung
	Mushroom waste	Mushroom worker's lung
Thermoactinomyces sacchari	Bagasse	Bagassosis
Thermoactinomyces vulgaris	Moldy hay	Farmer's lung
	Mushroom waste	Mushroom worker's lung

The remainder of this chapter focuses on several common classes of injurious agents and clinical presentations of respiratory disorders produced by inhaled toxicants, providing a diagnostic approach to such problems.

Clinical Approach to Suspected Toxicant-Induced Asthma

The diagnosis of asthma related to pulmonary toxicants is a two-part process. First, one must confirm the presence of airways hyperreactivity. Second, one must establish an association between the asthma and the suspected causative agent. Figure 16-6 illustrates an approach to the diagnosis of toxicant-induced asthma.

TABLE 16-7. Examples of agents that produce acute respiratory tract injury

Irritant gases, high solubility
- Acetaldehyde (CH_3CHO)
- Acrolein (acrylic aldehyde) (CH_2:CHCHO)
- Ammonia (NH_3)
- Hydrogen chloride (HCl)
- Sulfur dioxide (SO_2)

Irritant gases, intermediate to low solubility
- Chlorine (Cl_2)
- Nitrogen oxides (NO_x)
- Ozone (O_3)
- Phosgene (carbonyl chloride) ($COCl_2$)

Asphyxiants
- Carbon monoxide (CO)
- Hydrogen cyanide (HCN)
- Hydrogen sulfide (H_2S)

Systemic toxicants
- Metal oxides (metal fume fever)
- Tetrafluorethylene resin pyrolysis products (polymer fume fever)

Patients with environmental or occupational causes of asthma generally present as any asthmatic patient does. Symptoms may include chest tightness, episodic shortness of breath, and, sometimes, wheezing. Not infrequently the patient may present only with cough. At this point, it is incumbent on the clinician to take a careful occupational environmental history. The symptoms may or may not have coincided with doing particular jobs at work or in a hobby. Other exposed individuals might have similar complaints. The patient may make the association between his or her symptoms and a particular exposure if the provocative agent induces an immediate pattern of hyperreactivity. But frequently the temporal relationship is missed because many substances can cause a late asthmatic response without any evidence of immediate airways hyperreactivity. In those individuals, the symptoms of cough, wheezing, shortness of breath, or chest tightness may only occur after work or even during sleep. In such cases, inquiry about weekend and holiday improvement and relapses on returning to work may yield important clues.

As illustrated in Figure 16-6, once the suspicion of reactive airways disease has been raised, the clinician must confirm the diagnosis of asthma. The examination may or may not reveal obvious wheezing and airflow limitation on forced expiration. Pulmonary function tests that confirm the presence of airflow limitation with improvement after bronchodilator are sufficient to make the diagnosis of asthma. But some patients with occupationally induced asthma have normal lung function at the time of presentation. In such individuals, it is best to proceed with nonspecific bronchoprovocation testing with methacholine or histamine inhalation.

Having thus demonstrated the presence of hyperreactive airways, it is then necessary to obtain objective evidence that the asthma is related to a specific agent in the environment. In some cases, this is helped greatly by reviewing MSDSs. These may reveal the presence of a known sensitizer or pulmonary irritant. But more often than not it will not be possible to pinpoint the specific agent without a great deal of additional testing. Even then this exercise is often futile. Several ways in which a more specific diagnosis can be made include (a) skin and serologic tests, (b) pulmonary function tests at the time of exposure, and (c) specific bronchoprovocation tests.

Immunologic tests are one indirect method for making a causal link of exposure to illness. Skin and serologic tests are useful usually only if the particular agent in question is an allergen and if the

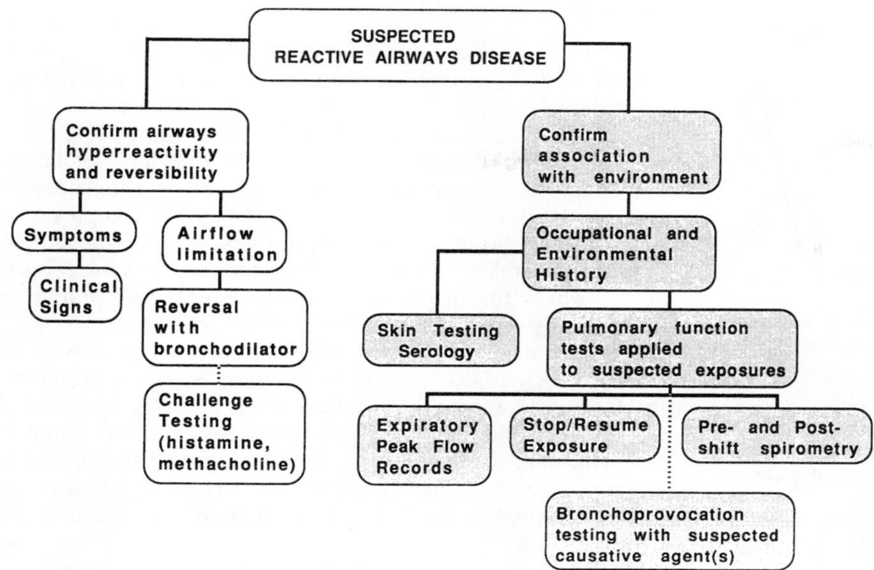

Figure 16-6. Clinical approach to the evaluation of suspected reactive airways disease (asthma) related to environmental or occupational exposure. Dotted lines indicate tests less commonly used in clinical evaluation (see text for explanation).

specific allergen has been well characterized. When the agent causes the individual to mount specific antibodies, skin-prick and skin-patch testing, RAST, or ELISA testing may be successful. But negative immunologic testing does not exclude the diagnosis.

Several methods of pulmonary function testing are used to obtain more compelling evidence of environmentally related asthma. Peak flow measurements are particularly useful if the individual is continuing to have frequent exposure. In our practice, individuals are asked to make peak flow readings using a peak flow meter approximately six times a day, including measurements in and out of the environment in question. Such records preferably should be kept for 2 or more weeks, while in and out of exposure. If the workplace is suspected, peak flows are used during periods on and off work, preferably including weekends off and at least 1 to 2 weeks completely off. Figure 16-7 shows a typical pattern of peak flows in an individual with work-related asthma. Drawbacks to peak expiratory flow recordings exist. Some individuals only have intermittent exposure, and hence, intermittent symptoms. The symptoms may last not simply minutes but up to days after a single exposure. If an individual's asthma is poorly reversible, removal from exposure might not lead to demonstrable improvement in peak flows. Concurrent treatment, such as with corticosteroids or cromolyn sodium, may confound results. Variation in the patient's technique and accuracy of record keeping may, in some individuals, be additional drawbacks. In conscientious patients, however, peak flows can be invaluable in helping to identify asthma triggers.

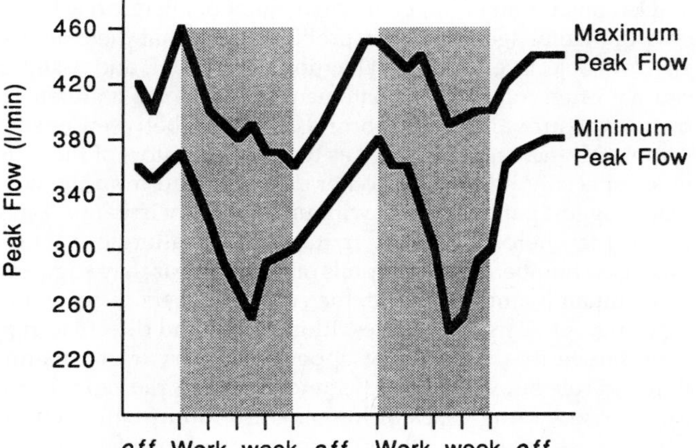

Figure 16-7. Work-related patterns of airflow obstruction can be documented using an peak expiratory flow meter. One such work-related pattern is shown in which there is progressive decline in peak flow across the workweek with weekend recovery of lung function.

Another method of demonstrating the environment link to asthma involves the measurement of lung function before and after exposure. In the occupational setting, for example, preshift and postshift spirometry can be performed. This can be time-consuming and requires onsite spirometry, as airways hyperreactivity may reverse very quickly after removal from exposure. However, documentation of a 20% fall in FEV_1 over the work shift and a progressive drop in lung function across the course of the workweek can be compelling. Pre- and postshift spirometry does not necessarily provide clues to the specific agent in question, but can rule in or rule out workplace triggers in general. Again, this technique may miss late asthmatic responses that may occur hours after exposure.

A third pulmonary function method of assessing for an association between the environment and asthma is to remove the individual from exposures and monitor symptoms, medications, and spirometry until he or she is stable. Then the patient is "rechallenged" to the environment in question, and reassessed for changes in symptoms, medication use, and pulmonary function.

In rare instances, it may be necessary to perform specific bronchoprovocation tests with suspected agents and placebo control. The indiscriminate use of such challenge tests is strongly discouraged, however. They are potentially dangerous as well as time-consuming and costly. They should be performed by experienced personnel in a clinical setting in which patients can be carefully monitored for precipitous, severe reactions. The clinician must be prepared to handle severe reactions that can occur immediately or 8 to 24 hours after the challenge.

One form of bronchoprovocation is the simple challenge in which the individual is asked to simulate his or her normal activity, such as pouring dust or removing and snapping latex gloves. Pulmonary function testing is performed before, during, and after exposure. More sophisticated methods use whole-body exposure chambers with accurate real-time measurement of the exposure level. This technology is crucial in challenges that involve highly toxic chemicals, such as isocyanates.

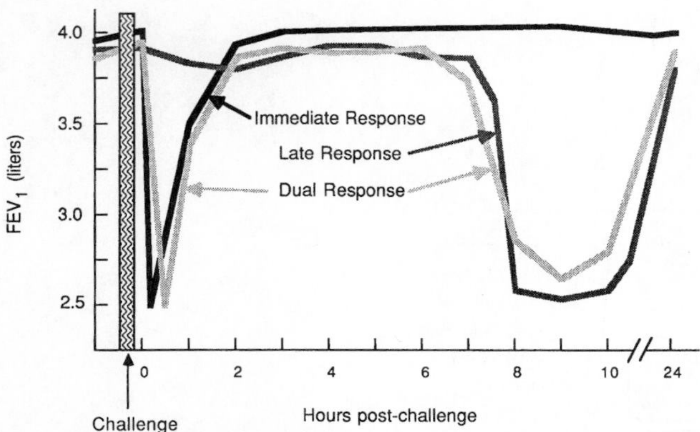

Figure 16-8. Three common patterns of airways hyperreactivity in response to inhaled agents are (a) immediate airflow obstruction, (b) late occurrence of airflow obstruction, and (c) dual pattern with both an immediate and delayed response.

After challenge, the individual is monitored carefully for development of one of the three patterns of asthmatic reactions: immediate, late, or dual responses, as shown in Figure 16-8.

Challenge testing should be reserved for (a) the research setting, to study previously unrecognized causes of asthma, and (b) rare occasions when the patient may otherwise refuse to believe that the causative agent is causing his or her asthma and refuse to leave exposure. Challenge testing has been advocated for use for medical-legal purposes; however, this is rarely in and of itself a sufficiently good reason to perform potentially dangerous provocation testing.

Physicians are often taught that environmental causes of asthma can be expected to resolve with removal from exposure. However, this is not always the case. More than one-half of individuals who have developed asthma from compounds as diverse as isocyanates and plicatic acid from Western red cedar remain symptomatic and have persistent bronchial hyperreactivity for years after cessation of exposure. Some patients with environmentally induced asthma improve after removal from exposure but do not recover completely. Prognosis is linked to the duration of exposure, severity of airflow limitation at the time of diagnosis, and the specific causative agent, among other factors.

Reactive Airways Disease Syndrome

Asthma is typically thought of as requiring a period of chronic antigen or irritant exposure before the development of clinical symptoms and signs. However, it is now clear that individuals can develop the signs, symptoms, physiology, and pathology of reactive airways disease (asthma) after a single, high-level accidental exposure to irritating gases, fumes, or smoke, including chlorine and ammonia. The symptoms commonly occur within several hours of the initial exposure and resolve within several weeks, but some individuals develop persistent airways hyperreactivity.

The message is clear: Airways hyperreactivity can be induced by a single, high-level exposure to irritants. This should be borne in mind at the time that patients present with acute accidental overexposures. For example, even if an individual with an acute inhalational injury has been successfully treated and released from the hospital, early pulmonary function assessment should be performed to exclude the possibility of persistent airways hyperreactivity.

Acute Inhalational Injury

Many mists, gases, and fumes can produce acute respiratory tract injury, as outlined in Table 16-7. Mechanisms include (a) irritant, (b) asphyxiant, and (c) systemic toxicity.

The site of action is in part dependent on extent of exposure and solubility of the gas or size and structure of the particulate. Sometimes the specific agent is clearly identified, as in chemical tank accidents. But sometimes the agent may be a complex mixture of combustion and pyrolysis products, as occurs in welding or in smoke-inhalation injuries. Often, the onset of symptoms is acute, as in sulfur dioxide and ammonia exposures, but may be delayed, as seen with nitrogen oxides and phosgene.

The irritant gases induce cellular injury in the airway by (a) forming acids (e.g., hydrogen chloride, sulfur dioxide); (b) depositing alkalis that produce deep, smoldering mucosal injury (e.g., ammonia); and (c) releasing oxygen-free radicals (e.g., chlorine, ozone). The outcomes range from reversible conjunctival and upper airway irritation to airway hyperreactivity, laryngospasm, bronchiolitis obliterans, pulmonary edema, and death.

Asphyxiants interfere with the normal delivery of oxygen. Some do this by (a) blocking oxygen binding to hemoglobin, as seen with nitrogen dioxide and carbon monoxide; (b) blocking oxidative phosphorylation, as seen with hydrogen sulfide; or (c) displacing oxygen, as seen with carbon dioxide, methane, and helium.

Metal oxide fumes, such as zinc, magnesium, and copper, or heated polymers, such as Teflon fluorocarbons, can induce flulike symptoms of fever, chills, chest pain, cough, and arthralgias, with negative chest radiographs. The mechanisms underlying polymer and metal fume fever are obscure. Neither is associated with prolonged symptomatology or permanent respiratory dysfunction.

The clinical approach to these acutely injurious agents is dependent on the specific chemical and its mechanism of injury.

Upper Airway Inflammation

Numerous agents can potentially injure the upper respiratory tract—our first line of defense. Symptoms are often immediate and obvious to the patient: burning sensation in the nose and throat, watery nasal discharge, epistaxis, hoarseness, sore throat, and cough that may be present acutely and even develop into chronic bronchitis. Any or all of these symptoms may occur, depending on the nature of the specific agent inhaled and its pattern of airway deposition.

Demonstration of upper airway irritant or allergic reactions to environmental agents is often problematic in that there are usually few objective findings. Diagnosis is clinical, and assigning cause is often conjectural. Abatement of symptoms with removal from exposure and a temporal association between onset of symptoms and exposure serve as the best indicators of the causal link, especially if MSDSs or other data obtained from the workplace suggest patient contact with upper airway irritants. A nasal smear may help to identify irritant versus allergic reactions. Increased numbers of neutrophils on nasal smear may suggest an acute inflammatory response. Increased numbers of eosinophils may suggest allergic etiologies. Rhinoscopy and direct laryngoscopy can verify the degree of upper respiratory tract inflammation and rule out vocal cord dysfunction. Sinus radiographs may assist in assessing cases of longer duration in which chronic sinusitis has occurred with or without secondary infection.

When cough is the predominant symptom, it is critical that cough-variant asthma and vocal cord dysfunction be excluded by performing pulmonary function tests and even methacholine or histamine challenge, sometimes preceded or followed by

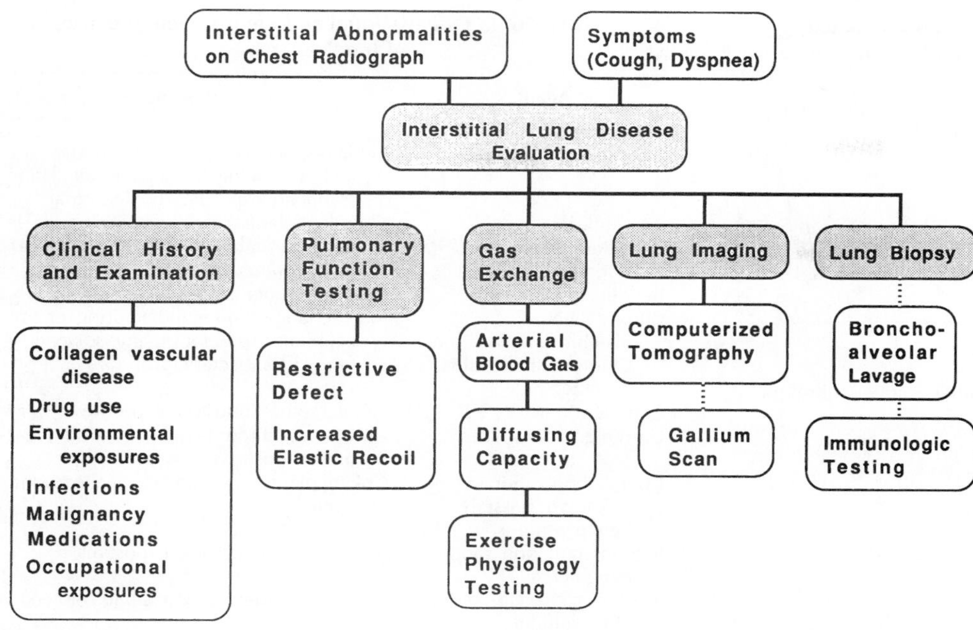

Figure 16-9. Clinical approach to the diagnosis of interstitial lung disease caused by environmental or occupational agents. Dotted lines indicate tests that are less commonly used but that may be useful in specific circumstances, as discussed in the text.

direct laryngoscopy. Industrial bronchitis is defined as persistent cough owing to an occupational exposure with no other apparent cause for cough. It usually occurs in the absence of airways hyperreactivity. In some cases of industrial bronchitis, we have proceeded to fiberoptic bronchoscopy to confirm and document the extent of the bronchial inflammation. But in most cases of upper respiratory inflammation from environmental agents, these more invasive tests are not performed. The cornerstone of treatment is removal from exposure. Symptomatic measures, such as inhaled, insufflated, or oral corticosteroids, or cromolyn sodium may be prescribed empirically.

Most cases of environmentally induced rhinitis, sinusitis, and tracheobronchitis resolve without significant long-term sequelae, unless there is concomitant airways hyperreactivity or deep lung injury. Another exception is in the case of chemical "burns" of either an acute or smoldering type as is seen with hydrochloric, nitric, or hydrofluoric acids. If severe injury occurs, secondary problems, such as bronchiectasis, tracheal stenosis, or laryngeal dysfunction, may result.

Assessment of Environmental Causes of Interstitial Lung Disease

Interstitial lung diseases represent a large portion of what pulmonologists see, secondary to inhaled toxic agents. There are two common presentations. In one scenario, the patient obtains a routine chest radiograph that shows increased interstitial markings. This may occur as part of an annual physical, on a routine preoperative radiograph, or perhaps as part of an asbestos-worker screening. Alternatively, the patient may present with unexplained symptoms of cough, dyspnea on exertion, and shortness of breath. Once suspected, the clinical evaluation of interstitial lung disease should have four goals: (a) to obtain sufficient information to make a firm diagnosis of the type of interstitial disease, (b) to determine the causative agent, (c) to assess the severity of impairment from the disease, and (d) to determine a treatment plan.

Most pulmonologists start with the chest radiograph. It may provide important insights. Clues include the presence of associated findings, such as adenopathy, which might be suggestive of sarcoidosis or beryllium disease; pleural plaques, which, if the history is compatible, may be sufficient to confirm asbestos exposure, cavitary lesions suggesting tuberculosis, along with silicosis. More often than not, however, the findings on chest radiograph are not sufficiently specific to allow the clinician to forego the further diagnostic evaluation outlined in Figure 16-9.

The workup begins with a careful history, focusing on causes of interstitial disease, including medications; drug abuse; heart disease; malignancy; collagen vascular disease; fungal, viral, or bacterial infection; and occupational and environmental exposures. Table 16-8 lists some of the recognized environmental and occupational causes of the interstitial lung diseases. These are subdivided into those producing a principal pattern of (a) interstitial fibrosis, (b) granuloma formation, (c) bronchiolitis obliterans, (d) pulmonary edema, and (e) other, such as respiratory bronchiolitis and giant cell pneumonitis. Chronicity of symptoms and any temporal association of exposure to organic and inorganic agents may greatly help focus the diagnostic workup.

More often than not, additional testing, including lung biopsy, is required to make a firm diagnosis. Transbronchial lung biopsy has proved extremely useful in diagnosis of granulomatous lung diseases. But because it is less accurate and less sensitive in the diagnosis of bronchiolitis obliterans and fibrosing lung disease, such cases may require open lung biopsies.

In certain instances, lung biopsy can be completely avoided; examples include asbestosis. If an individual has a history of asbestos exposure, a typically long latency between first exposure and development of interstitial infiltrates, slow disease progression, and a typical x-ray pattern with irregular opacities and pleural plaques, further workup is probably unnecessary. This is sufficient information to make a presumptive diagnosis without proceeding to bronchoscopy or open lung biopsy. Similar principles apply to the noninvasive diagnosis of silicosis and coal workers' pneumoconiosis. But if the clinical picture is not fully compatible with the physiologic and radiographic presentations of these diseases, biopsy is needed to rule out other interstitial lung diseases.

A second example is the individual with clinical symptoms of acute extrinsic allergic alveolitis (hypersensitivity pneumonitis) in whom there is a readily identifiable etiologic agent—such as being a bird fancier or having pitched moldy hay. Such individuals can be given the clinical diagnosis of hypersensitivity pneumonitis, even without serum precipitins testing. Rather

TABLE 16-8. Common pathologic changes associated with occupational and environmental causes of interstitial lung disease

Diffuse interstitial fibrosis (usual interstitial pneumonitis, desquamative interstitial pneumonitis, fibrotic nodules)
- Aluminum
- Asbestos
- Beryllium (end stage)
- Chronic extrinsic allergic alveolitis from fungal spores, avian proteins, isocyanates (see Table 16-6)
- Chronic pulmonary edema (numerous causes, see Table 16-3)
- Coal dust
- Cobalt
- Copper
- Diatomaceous earth
- Drugs (e.g., bleomycin, busulphan, cyclophosphamide, nitrofurantoin)
- Ionizing radiation
- Kaolin (china clay)
- Mercury fumes
- Mixed dust fibrosis
- Nickel
- Oil mists (lipoid pneumonia)
- Paraquat
- Silica
- Talc

Granulomatous and mononuclear cell infiltration (hypersensitivity and foreign body reactions)
- Aluminum
- Asbestos
- Beryllium
- *Blastomyces dermatides* (North American blastomycosis)
- *Brucella abortis* (chronic infection)
- Coal dust
- Cobalt
- *Coccidioides immitis*
- Copper (vineyard sprayer's lung)
- Drugs (e.g., methotrexate, gold)
- Extrinsic allergic alveolitis (see Table 16-6)
- *Histoplasma capsulatum*
- Oil mist (lipoid pneumonia)
- Polyvinyl chloride dust
- Silicotuberculosis
- Talc

Bronchiolitis obliterans
- Ammonia
- Cadmium oxide
- Chlorine
- Chloropicrin
- Hydrogen fluoride
- Hydrogen sulfide
- Methyl sulfate
- Oxygen toxicity
- Oxides of nitrogen
- Ozone
- Phosgene
- Sulfur dioxide
- Trichloroethylene

Other
- Giant cell pneumonitis caused by cobalt (hard metal disease)

than proceeding immediately to additional diagnostic procedures such as lung biopsy, such patients can be treated by removing them from exposure and sometimes administering a short course of oral corticosteroids. If the clinical diagnosis was correct, one can anticipate a prompt reversal of symptoms, signs, pulmonary function, and x-ray abnormalities. If, however, the symptoms have been more chronic, the clinical diagnosis may be less clear and lead ultimately to biopsy.

Bronchoalveolar lavage at the time of transbronchial lung biopsy may lend additional specificity to the diagnosis of interstitial lung disease in the case of extrinsic allergic alveolitis, chronic beryllium disease, hard metal disease due to cobalt, and asbestosis. In fact, in some countries, asbestos fibers in bronchoalveolar lavage are counted and used as an indication of underlying asbestosis.

TABLE 16-9. Occupational and environmental causes of lung cancer

Agent	Sources of exposure
Asbestos	Insulators, brake repair, textile industry, asbestos mining, heating and ventilation, secondary exposures, nonindustrial
Acrylonitrile	Chemical plants
Arsenates, arsenites, arsenic trioxide	Smelting, pesticide manufacturing, vineyard workers
Beryllium	Beryllium processing
Chloroethers Bis-chloromethyl ether Chloromethyl methyl ether	Ion-exchange resin manufacturing, chemical plants (used for organic solvents, fungicides, bactericides)
Cadmium	Smelter, other industrial exposures
Chromium, chromates	Chromium, chromite ore extraction, pigment industry
Coal carbonization (agent unknown, possibly benzpyrene)	Coking plants, gas workers, steel carbonization
Ionizing radiation, radon daughters	Miners, potential home exposures
Mustard gas (bis[β-chloroethyl]sulfide)	Chemical warfare (workers and soldiers)
Nickel dust, fume	Nickel smelting, refining, calcining, nickel carbonyl processes
Silica	Mining, tunneling, stone cutting
Tobacco smoke	Cigarette, cigar, pipe smoking
Vinyl chloride	Polymer industry

Environmentally Induced Lung Cancer

The demonstration of respiratory tract malignancy secondary to toxic exposures is complicated by a number of factors. Tobacco smoke is the overwhelming respiratory carcinogen and confounds many studies of other suspected carcinogens. In some instances, there is an additive or multiplicative risk when smoking is added to a cocarcinogen such as asbestos or ionizing radiation.

Much of what we know about carcinogens is predicated on animal studies that may or may not be pertinent to man and on epidemiologic studies of cancer incidence in industrial cohorts in which appropriate matching of control groups is sometimes a problem. This is a major topic that is beyond the scope of this chapter and has been well reviewed elsewhere.

Table 16-9 lists the major known and suspected causes of occupational lung cancer.

IRRITANT-ASSOCIATED VOCAL CORD DYSFUNCTION

Irritant-associated vocal cord dysfunction (IVCD) is a newly recognized clinical entity often misdiagnosed as asthma. Cases of IVCD are being reported secondary to an occupational or environmental exposure. Clinical criteria for irritant versus nonirritant vocal cord dysfunction have been established (Table 16-10) (16). Vocal cord dysfunction is a disorder of the larynx in which the vocal cords adduct inappropriately during an inspiration or expiration. The criteria for diagnosis for IVCD are demonstrated by laryngoscopy, and diagnosis is based on the presence of vocal cord adduction during inspiration with a posterior chink or adduction during early expiration with a posterior chink (1). Signs and symptoms of IVCD are listed in Table 16-11. Types of

TABLE 16-10. Clinical criteria for vocal cord dysfunction

IVCD
- Documented absence of preceding VCD or laryngeal disease
- Onset of symptoms after a single specific exposure or accident
- Exposure to an irritating gas, smoke, fume, vapor, mist, or dust
- Onset of symptoms within 24 hours after exposure
- Symptoms of wheezing, stridor, dyspnea, cough, or throat tightness
- Abnormal direct laryngoscopy for vocal cord dysfunction either in the asymptomatic state, during symptoms, or with a provocative study
- Exclusion of other types of significant vocal cord disease

Non–irritant-induced VCD
- Symptoms of wheezing, stridor, dyspnea, cough, or throat tightness
- Abnormal direct laryngoscopy for vocal cord dysfunction either in the asymptomatic state, during symptoms, or with a provocative study
- Exclusion of other types of significant vocal cord disease
- Absence of onset of symptoms after a single specific exposure or accident

IVCD, irritant-associated vocal cord dysfunction; VCD, vocal cord dysfunction.
From ref. 16, with permission.

the exposures are ammonia, flux fumes, cleaning chemicals, odors, smoke, organic solvents, machine fluid, and ceiling tile dust. The abnormality can occur in inspiration, expiration, or in both phases of the respiratory cycle. Patients with IVCD express a significant increase in chest complaints.

Vocal cord dysfunction often mimics asthma, and, therefore, it is important to consider the diagnosis of IVCD in symptomatic patients after irritant exposures to distinguish it from reactive airways dysfunction. The pathogenesis of IVCD is not known, but direct inflammation caused by irritants is suggested. A statistically significant difference in spirometry between IVCD groups and vocal cord dysfunction groups from other causes exists. Normal airflow in a dyspneic and wheezing patient should raise the index of suspicion for vocal cord dysfunction–mimicking asthma. The flow-volume loop can provide additional clues to the diagnosis of vocal cord dysfunction. Vocal cord dysfunction subjects undergoing methacholine challenge show a fall in the mid-inspiratory flow at 50% of the VC.

Vocal cord dysfunction may be associated with symptoms of panic, depression, and anxiety. Psychopathology can also occur. Chronic symptoms of sinusitis, rhinitis, and voice changes occur and can exacerbate vocal cord dysfunction. The frequency of gastroesophageal reflux disease is higher in IVCD than other causes of vocal cord dysfunction (2,3). The irritation caused by reflux of gastric acid onto the vocal cords may also have a role in the pathogenesis of irritant vocal cord dysfunction. Gastric acid reflux produces distinct symptoms of hoarseness, persistent nonproductive cough, a sensation of pressure deep in the throat, and a continual need to clear the throat. Many of these symptoms overlap with vocal cord dysfunction. The association of gastroesophageal reflux disease with respiratory conditions is appreciated, although its association with vocal cord dysfunction should be further investigated.

TABLE 16-11. Vocal cord dysfunction–associated symptoms

Symptom	IVCD	VCD	*P* Value
Wheeze	9/11 (82)	26/33 (79)	.83
Cough	11/11 (100)	31/33 (94)	.40
Shortness of breath	11/11 (100)	30/33 (91)	.30
Choking or throat tightness	9/10 (90)	22/26 (85)	.68
Chest pain or chest tightness	6/6 (100)	17/30 (57)	.04
Stridor	4/6 (67)	6/8 (75)	.73
Gastroesophageal reflux	7/10 (70)	19/32 (59)	.55
Voice changes	11/11 (100)	14/16 (88)	.22
Dysphagia	5/9 (56)	8/30 (27)	.44
Rhinosinusitis	8/11 (73)	30/33 (91)	.13

IVCD, irritant-associated vocal cord dysfunction; VCD, vocal cord dysfunction.
Note: Expressed as number of patients reporting symptom/number of patients for whom the symptom was adequately recorded, percentage in parentheses.
From ref. 16, with permission.

The differentiation and correct diagnosis of vocal cord dysfunction are important because therapy for vocal cord dysfunction is different from that for asthma or reactive airways disease syndrome, and patients may benefit greatly from speech therapy to retrain muscles that cause laryngeal dysfunction. Vocal cord dysfunction does not benefit from inhaled corticosteroids, bronchodilators, or leukotriene inhibitors.

SUGGESTED READING

1. American Medical Association. *Guides to the evaluation of permanent impairment*. Chicago: American Medical Association, 1993.
2. American Thoracic Society. Guidelines for the evaluation of impairment/disability in patients with asthma. *Am Rev Respir Dis* 1993;147:1056.
3. Breeze R, Turk M. Cellular structure, function, and organization in the lower respiratory tract. *Environ Health Perspect* 1984;55:3.
4. Chan-Yeung M, Malo J-L. Occupational asthma. *N Engl J Med* 1995; 33:107.
5. Cherniack RM. *Pulmonary function testing*. Philadelphia: WB Saunders, 1977.
6. Cone JE. Occupational lung cancer. In: Rosenstock L, ed. *Occup Med: State of the Art Reviews*. Philadelphia: Hanley and Belfus, 1987.
7. Harber P, Schenker MB, Balmes JR. *Occupational and environmental respiratory disease*. St. Louis: Mosby–Year Book, 1996:3.
8. Kennedy SM. Acquired airway hyperresponsiveness from non-immunogenic irritant exposure. In: Beckett WS, Bascome R, eds. *Occup Med: State of the Art Reviews*. Philadelphia: Hanley and Belfus, 1992:7287.
9. National Research Council. *Biologic markers in immunotoxicology*. Washington: National Academy Press, 1992.
10. National Research Council. Subcommittee on Pulmonary Toxicology Committee on biologic markers. *Biologic markers in pulmonary toxicology*. Washington: National Academy Press, 1989:105.
11. Newman L, Storey E, Kreiss K. Immunologic evaluation of occupational lung disease. In: Rosenstock L, ed. *Occup Med: State of the Art Reviews*. Philadelphia: Hanley and Belfus, 1987:345.
12. Newman LS. Occupational illness. *N Engl J Med* 1995;333:1128.
13. Schwartz DA. Acute inhalational injury. In: Rosenstock L, ed. *Occup Med: State of the Art Reviews*. Philadelphia: Hanley and Belfus, 1987:2297.
14. Schwarz MI, King TE Jr., eds. *Interstitial lung disease*, 2nd ed. St. Louis: Mosby–Year Book, 1993:1.
15. Wasserman K, Hansen JE, Sue DY, Whipp BJ. *Principles of exercise testing and interpretation*. Philadelphia: Lea & Febiger, 1987:32.

REFERENCES

1. Perkner J, Fennelly KP, Balkissoon R, et al. Irritant associated vocal cord dysfunction. *J Occup Environ Med* 1998;40(2):136.
2. Rontal E, Rontal M, Jacob HJ, Rolnick MI. Vocal cord dysfunction—an industrial health hazard. *Ann Otol Rhinol Laryngol* 1979;88(Pt 1):818.
3. Newman K, Mason U, Schmaling K. Clinical features of vocal cord dysfunction. *Am J Respir Crit Care Med* 1985;152:1382.

CHAPTER 17
Acute Pulmonary Injury

John R. Balmes

The widespread use in modern society of materials potentially hazardous to the respiratory tract makes inhalational injury a relatively common occurrence. Short-term exposure to high concentrations of noxious gases, fumes, or mists is generally because of industrial or transportation accidents. The resultant inhalation injury from such high-intensity exposures can result in severe impairment or death. The most common cause of inhalation injury called into poison control centers is the improper mixing of household cleaning products containing bleach and acid that leads to the generation of hydrochloric acid. Although inhalation injury because of household cleaning exposures is usually mild, persistent symptoms can occur (1). Pulmonary insufficiency caused by smoke inhalation probably accounts for more fire-related deaths than any other cause, and the components of smoke most toxic to the lungs are gases produced by the pyrolysis of synthetic materials. Many smoke and toxic inhalation–related deaths occur at the scene, but a large number of patients with inhalation injuries die after hospitalization. Early recognition of inhalation injury in fire, industrial, and environmental accident victims could well result in increased survival and decreased long-term disability.

DETERMINANTS OF TOXICITY

The effects of inhalational exposure to toxic materials can range from transient, mild irritation of the mucous membranes of the upper airway to fatal adult respiratory distress syndrome (ARDS). The anatomic site of injury in the respiratory tract depends on what is inhaled. The site of deposition of an inhaled gas is determined primarily by its water solubility, but also by the duration of exposure and the minute ventilation of the victim. Because of the efficient scrubbing mechanism of the moist surfaces of the nose and throat, the concentration of an inhaled water-soluble gas such as formaldehyde is greatly reduced by the time it reaches the trachea. In contrast, a relatively water-insoluble gas such as phosgene is not well absorbed by the upper airways and, thus, may penetrate to the alveoli. During vigorous exertion, the oral breathing necessary to meet increased ventilatory demands decreases the contact time between the moist upper airway surfaces and the inhaled gas such that a significant concentration of even a very water-soluble gas may reach the distal lung. Another mechanism by which water-soluble toxic chemicals may penetrate more deeply into the respiratory tract is adsorption onto inhaled particulate matter, such as in smoke.

The site of deposition of an aerosol, whether it consists of solid or liquid particles, is determined primarily by particle size. Particles larger than 10 μm in diameter mostly deposit in the nose, oropharynx, and larynx, whereas particles smaller than 3 μm tend to deposit in terminal lung units. Particles between 0.5 and 10.0 μm in diameter also are deposited in the conducting airways. Particle size is not the only determinant of the toxic effect of inhaled particles. For example, acid aerosols are neutralized to some extent by the ammonia generated by oral bacteria, and smaller acid droplets, despite their greater ability to penetrate to the distal lung, are more completely neutralized than larger droplets (2).

The toxicity of an inhaled material also is dependent on the varying susceptibility of different populations of respiratory tract cells to the effects of the material. Although ozone is a relatively water-insoluble gas and, thus, penetrates well into the distal lung, cells of the conducting airways clearly can be injured by inhalation of this gas. The underlying health of the exposed individual can be an important determinant of toxicity. Inhaled sulfur dioxide, which is largely absorbed onto the mucous membrane of the nose and throat because of its water solubility, causes bronchospasm in asthmatic individuals at relatively low concentrations.

MECHANISMS OF TOXICITY

The mechanisms by which inhaled materials can produce toxic effects include the following (Table 17-1): (a) simple asphyxiation owing to replacement of atmospheric oxygen by other gases such as methane or nitrogen, (b) tissue asphyxia owing to pulmonary absorption of agents capable of interfering with oxygen transport or poisoning cellular respiratory enzymes such as carbon monoxide or cyanide, (c) nonrespiratory effects owing to pulmonary absorption of agents such as lead or hydrocarbon solvents, (d) excessive stimulation of physiologic responses by agents inhaled in concentrations below those required to cause morphologic evidence of injury, and (e) direct cellular injury. This chapter focuses only on the emergency medical management of pulmonary injury owing to inhaled materials (i.e., toxic effects caused by the last two mechanisms previously listed).

Cough, mucus secretion, bronchoconstriction, and, perhaps, even airway edema are normal physiologic responses to the inhalation of noxious materials. Afferent nerves in the airways that trigger the cough reflex can be stimulated directly by inhaled irritants or indirectly through the release of mediators such as histamine or prostaglandins (3). Although the cough response is generally protective, prolonged or excessive stimulation of this response by inhaled materials can be a cause of significant morbidity in susceptible individuals. Inhalation of concentrations of irritants that cause little effect in most people may induce incapacitating cough in individuals with preexisting airway hyperresponsiveness caused by asthma or viral upper respiratory infections. Stimulation of mucus secretion from submucosal glands and goblet cells by inhaled materials is another protective response of the airways that also can lead to significant morbidity (4). Hypertrophy of submucosal glands and goblet cell hyperplasia have been demonstrated in rats and dogs after repeated exposures to sulfur dioxide (5,6). So-called benign mucus hypersecretion or industrial bronchitis is common among individuals occupationally exposed to relatively low levels of irritant dusts, gases, fumes, or mists. Whether workers with mucus hypersecretion are at increased risk for the development of chronic airflow obstruction is a matter of debate, but considerable data are available to support such a position (7,8).

Bronchoconstriction is probably a normal response to the inhalation of noxious materials; it serves to protect the pulmonary parenchyma from excessive exposure. Whereas some inhaled materials, such as ozone, only cause bronchoconstriction at concentrations that also are associated with direct epithelial injury, other materials, such as cigarette smoke and sulfur dioxide, appear to induce bronchoconstriction at concentrations well below those required to produce morphologic evidence of injury (9).

TABLE 17-1. Toxicity from inhaled materials

Mechanism	Examples
Simple asphyxia	Nitrogen, methane (replacement of atmospheric oxygen)
Tissue asphyxia	Carbon monoxide, cyanide, hydrogen sulfide
Nonrespiratory effects owing to pulmonary absorption	Hydrocarbon solvents, lead
Excessive stimulation of physiologic responses	Formaldehyde, sulfur dioxide
Direct cellular injury	Ammonia, chlorine, nitrogen dioxide, phosgene

Airway edema is certainly a feature of direct epithelial injury owing to inhaled materials. However, airway edema also may be produced by stimulation of an axonal reflex in airway afferent nerves by exposure to relatively low concentrations of an inhaled irritant (10). Low-molecular-weight peptides, known as *tachykinins*, are released from stimulated airway afferent nerves. These peptides cause vasodilatation and increased vascular permeability of submucosal vessels (11). Inhaled cigarette smoke, formaldehyde, and toluene diisocyanate have been shown to produce tachykinin-mediated airway edema.

Direct injury of the airway mucosa occurs when cytotoxic materials are inhaled at sufficiently high concentrations. Epithelial cell injury and death give rise to a number of effects that impact on a patient's respiratory status. Mucociliary clearance is markedly decreased, the normally tight intercellular junctions become porous (allowing the penetration of foreign material, including bacteria), and sloughing of dead epithelial cells may cause mechanical obstruction of airway lumina. In addition, the release of a variety of cytokines and mediators by injured cells of the airway mucosa leads to local inflammation, edema, and constriction of airway smooth muscle. Thus, direct epithelial injury from higher concentrations of an inhaled toxic material amplifies the stimulation of physiologic responses that occurs at lower concentrations.

Although much is known about the mechanisms of acute airway injury caused by the inhalation of toxic materials, little is known about the possible long-term sequelae of such acute injury. It is clear that most persons who develop acute chemical bronchitis recover completely within a period of weeks, presumably due to the regeneration of a normal airway mucosa. However, a small percentage of persons may develop persistent airway hyperresponsiveness and, even clinically, significant asthma after a single, high-intensity exposure to certain toxic materials. The risk factors for the development of this syndrome, which has been termed *reactive airways dysfunction syndrome* (RADS) (12), are unknown, although cigarette smoking is suspected of being one such factor. The observation that many workers who develop toluene diisocyanate–induced occupational asthma have been exposed repeatedly to high concentrations of the material during accidental spills may be relevant to the development of an asthma-like syndrome after single massive exposures to isocyanates and other agents (13).

Inhaled water-insoluble gases and small particles tend to penetrate to terminal lung units where they can cause injury to epithelial cells of the terminal and respiratory bronchioles and of the alveoli, pulmonary capillary endothelial cells, and alveolar macrophages. Water-soluble gases can cause such pulmonary parenchymal injury if inhaled in sufficiently high concentrations. Type I alveolar epithelial cells are particularly susceptible to injury, presumably due to their high surface area to volume ratio. Pulmonary parenchymal injury is characterized by diffuse bronchiolar obstruction owing to edema and infiltration by inflammatory cells of bronchiolar walls, and by alveolar flooding (pulmonary edema) owing to increased permeability of both layers of the alveolar-capillary membrane. In addition, injury to alveolar macrophages may play a role in the frequent development of superimposed bacterial infection with chemical pneumonitis.

The delayed onset of symptoms and clinical findings that often occur with chemical pneumonitis may be a result of injury to the alveolar-capillary membrane from inflammatory cells, such as polymorphonuclear leukocytes, recruited to the lungs, rather than from a direct effect of the inhaled material. Although most persons appear to recover remarkably well from even severe chemical pneumonitis if they can be adequately supported through the acute phase of their illness, a small percentage develop progressive inflammation and obliteration of distal airways (i.e., bronchiolitis obliterans) that can be responsible for considerable impairment.

SITE OF INJURY

Upper Airways

The nose, pharynx, and larynx are exposed to the highest concentrations of an inhaled gas and, thus, frequently bear the brunt of the injury (Table 17-2). In particular, water-soluble gases such as ammonia and chlorine are more likely to cause laryngeal edema and resultant upper airway obstruction than pulmonary parenchymal injury. Such gases are capable of producing severe mucous membrane ulceration, hemorrhage, and edema. Although such physical evidence of chemical injury may be present early, it may take several hours for sufficient edema to develop to produce hoarseness and stridor. Chemical injury of the face, mouth, and throat may increase upper airway secretions and impair the ability to clear lower airway secretions. Generally, the greater the chemical injury of the upper airways, the greater the likelihood of concomitant chemical injury of the lower airways.

Lower Airways

Breath holding and laryngospasm in response to irritation of the airways are protective mechanisms that occur in the conscious victim of a toxic inhalation. These mechanisms are not operative in the unconscious victim, however, so that more severe injury to the lower airways (and pulmonary parenchyma) is likely to be present in such a setting.

Inhalation of many toxic materials produces a severe tracheobronchitis (see Table 17-2). Cilia become paralyzed, and the clearance of mucus and inhaled particles is reduced (14). Toxic chemicals adsorbed onto the surfaces of inhaled particles have a greater opportunity to cause airway mucosal injury. Pathologic examination of tissue from fire victims who experienced chemical injury to the respiratory tract has shown carbonaceous material (i.e., soot) with adsorbed toxic chemicals to be firmly adherent to the tracheobronchial mucosa (15).

A few hours after a severe chemical inhalation injury, one finds extensive but mild mucosal edema and scattered submu-

TABLE 17-2. Effects of irritant gas inhalation

Site of injury	Effects
Mucous membranes of the eyes, nose, and oropharynx	Erythema Edema Ulcerations and hemorrhage Burns
Upper airways	Mucosal inflammation and burns Laryngeal obstruction
Lower airways	Tracheobronchitis Impairment of mucociliary clearance Bronchorrhea Mucosal sloughing Bronchoconstriction Airway edema Atelectasis
Pulmonary parenchyma	Pulmonary edema/adult respiratory distress syndrome Impaired bacterial clearance/pneumonia
Systemic effects (hydrogen fluoride)	Hypocalcemia, hypomagnesemia Methemoglobinemia (nitrogen dioxide)

cosal hemorrhage without ulceration. The victim may have minimum clinical signs or symptoms at this point. Later (8 to 48 hours postinhalation), progressive edema develops. A mucopurulent membrane subsequently develops on the mucosal surface. Bronchorrhea also may occur. At 48 to 72 hours postinhalation, if the injury is severe enough, sloughing of the tracheobronchial mucosa begins, yielding what has been described as a pseudomembranous tracheobronchitis (15). In this stage, expectoration of bronchial casts may be observed.

Even when direct injury to the lower airways is not severe, the stimulation of irritant receptors in the large airways may cause bronchoconstriction. When this effect is coupled with the peribronchial edema that occurs with more severe injury, significant airways obstruction is likely to develop. When sloughing of bronchial mucosa is also present, occlusion of central airways may cause significant atelectasis as well.

Pulmonary Parenchyma

Although less common than injury to the airways, chemical injury at the alveolar level owing to the inhalation of toxic materials involves damage to epithelial and endothelial membranes, resulting in increased permeability-induced edema (see Table 17-2). The injury may range from mild interstitial edema to progressive pulmonary insufficiency. Severe chemical pneumonitis caused by toxic inhalation can be considered a form of ARDS.

Experimental animal evidence confirms that increased pulmonary microvascular permeability to high-molecular-weight compounds is a feature of chemical pneumonitis (16,17). Although the mechanism by which the increased permeability develops has not been completely defined, it is clear that alveolar flooding may occur even when pulmonary capillary hydrostatic pressure is normal. Because many victims of inhalation injury also have severe cutaneous burns and thus require large volumes of fluid replacement, management of such patients can be difficult. In addition, some evidence exists that cutaneous burns, even in the absence of inhalation injury, may induce increased pulmonary capillary permeability (18).

Studies in dogs have demonstrated an immediate reduction in pulmonary surfactant after toxic inhalation (19). This reduction may explain the early development of peripheral atelectasis in many victims of inhalation injury. Loss of surfactant also may play a role in the increased alveolar-capillary membrane permeability that characterizes chemical pneumonitis.

When the pulmonary parenchyma becomes edematous due to toxic inhalation injury, as in the other forms of ARDS, lung compliance decreases, the alveolar-arterial oxygen difference increases (caused by shunting of blood away from damaged areas), and pulmonary vascular resistance increases.

The onset of pulmonary edema may be immediate if the injury is severe, although in most cases it is delayed 24 to 48 hours and may occur as late as 1 week postinhalation. Several investigators have found little evidence of pulmonary edema in animals that died shortly after smoke inhalation (20–22). Respiratory failure associated with radiographic infiltrates with an onset more than 1 week postinhalation is likely owing to sepsis and bacterial pneumonia.

DIAGNOSIS

Due to the delayed onset of many of its clinical features, the early diagnosis of inhalation injury often proves difficult. Certain findings should lead one to suspect the presence of inhalation injury in a fire or environmental accident victim, including facial burns, inflamed nares, sputum production, and wheezing (Table 17-3). Victims of fires or explosions in enclosed spaces, where synthetic materials were burned or where irritating materials were released, should be suspected of having experienced inhalation injury. Because of the likelihood of increased exposure in the unconscious victim, neurologic status at the scene is an important determinant of the severity of lung injury. Firefighters and emergency medical technicians at the scene can often provide information as to how and where the victims were found.

TABLE 17-3. Action criteria for toxic inhalation injury

- Criteria for transportation to the hospital
  - Burned in an enclosed space
  - Burning of synthetic material
  - Altered mental status
  - Facial burns
  - Chest pain
  - Older than 60 years
- Criteria for admission to the hospital
  - Altered mental status
  - Any respiratory symptoms (i.e., cough, chest tightness, dyspnea)
  - Hoarseness, wheezing
  - History of ischemic heart disease or chronic obstructive pulmonary disease
  - Elevated carboxyhemoglobin (>20%)
- Criteria for admission to intensive care unit
  - Depressed consciousness
  - Abnormal arterial blood gases
  - Abnormal electrocardiogram
  - Hoarseness, wheezing
  - Decreased peak expiratory flow rates or abnormal spirometry
- Criteria for intubation
  - Depressed consciousness
  - Severe laryngeal obstruction
  - Respiratory insufficiency by arterial blood gas measurement

Any fire or explosion victim with actual or suspected altered consciousness should be assumed to have carbon monoxide intoxication. The possibility of cyanide and hydrogen sulfide intoxication should be considered as well. Dizziness, headache, chest pain, nausea, and vomiting should suggest intoxication with a systemic poison capable of causing tissue asphyxia.

Chest radiographic and arterial blood gas values are often normal in the immediate postinhalation period and cannot be relied on to clear a victim for discharge from an emergency room. A low oxyhemoglobin saturation in the face of a normal PaO_2 should alert one to the likelihood of carbon monoxide intoxication. Simple spirometry or peak expiratory flow rate measurements to detect early airway obstruction are often quite useful.

Carboxyhemoglobin saturation should be obtained in all fire or explosion victims. Elevated carboxyhemoglobin levels have been shown to correlate relatively well with the presence of smoke inhalation injury (23) and concomitant elevated cyanide levels (24). Significant metabolic acidosis should also alert one to the possibility of cyanide or hydrogen sulfide intoxication.

Direct laryngoscopy or fiberoptic bronchoscopy has been advocated by some authors to be performed routinely in the setting of a significant inhalation injury. If laryngeal edema is present, these authors recommend prophylactic endotracheal intubation. Some degree of laryngeal edema is common, however, and most patients improve spontaneously and do not require intubation. Only a small percentage of victims with facial, nasal, and oropharyngeal burns (thermal or chemical) go on to develop life-threatening upper airway obstruction, and it is difficult to predict which patients are likely to have such an outcome. I advocate careful clinical monitoring of fire and toxic inhalation victims, preferably in an intensive care setting, rather than routine laryngoscopy or bronchoscopy. These procedures can be quite uncomfortable when the mucosal surfaces of the nose, throat, and airways are inflamed.

If bronchoscopy is performed, evidence of inhalation injury includes erythema, edema, ulceration, and hemorrhage of the airway mucosa (25). If particulate material was inhaled, then its presence on the airway mucosa also may be seen. The presence of endobronchial polyps has been noted on occasion in patients with severe inhalation injury (26). It has been speculated that these polyps are the large airway correlates of the bronchiolitis obliterans that can develop in small airways after inhalation injury.

The results of early ventilation-perfusion lung scanning of victims of toxic inhalation injury have been used to predict subsequent respiratory complications (25). Flow-volume loops have been used to diagnose upper airway obstruction and as a more sensitive detector of early lower airways obstruction than simple spirometry or peak expiratory flow rates (27–29). Measurement of diffusing capacity has been suggested as a sensitive indicator of pulmonary parenchymal injury (26). Alveolar epithelial permeability by calculation of lung clearance of inhaled radiolabeled tracers has been used to quantitate the degree of lung injury in patients with ARDS and has been used experimentally in animals to characterize inhalation injury (30). However, practical considerations of availability and patient ability to perform limit the clinical applicability of these more "sensitive" tests.

TREATMENT

Treatment at the scene of a fire or explosion should assume significant exposure to carbon monoxide and, thus, high flow (10 to 15 L per minute) oxygen via face mask should be administered to most victims (see Table 17-3). Administration of high concentrations of oxygen may cause persons with chronic obstructive pulmonary disease who chronically retain carbon dioxide to stop breathing. Thus, victims must be carefully observed during fire and explosion scene triage and transportation to the hospital. If a victim requires ventilatory support, 100% oxygen should be administered by positive pressure during transportation. Particular attention should be paid to profuse secretions in unconscious victims.

Fire, explosion, or environmental accident victims older than 40 years and those with frequent extrasystoles or tachycardia should be monitored via telemetry en route to the hospital. Because seizures may occur as a result of hypoxemia or systemic intoxication with carbon monoxide, cyanide, or hydrogen sulfide, one must be prepared for this complication.

Any victim at the scene observed to have evidence of inhalation injury should be taken to a hospital emergency room for evaluation. At the hospital, the initial history should include a concerted effort to determine the types of materials burned or inhaled and the intensity of exposure. The oral and nasal mucosal membranes should be examined for injury, and concurrent skin burns, even if relatively slight, should not be overlooked. Because of the potential for central nervous system effects from toxic chemical inhalation, a mental status evaluation should always be performed, even in fully ambulatory victims.

All fire or toxic inhalation victims with mental status abnormalities should be hospitalized for at least 24 hours of observation, even if they are otherwise without symptoms or signs. Asymptomatic fire victims with a high probability of smoke inhalation injury (i.e., those with facial, nasal, or oral burns; those with significantly elevated carboxyhemoglobin levels; and those with histories of exposure to toxic fumes or in confined spaces) also should be observed for at least 24 hours. The following parameters should be monitored: vital signs, including respiratory rate; central nervous system status; degree of airway obstruction (serial spirometry or peak expiratory flow rate measurements are better than the stethoscope); arterial blood gases; chest radiograph; and electrocardiogram and cardiac monitoring in patients older than 40 years with chest pain or with irregular heart rates.

Supportive treatment of victims with evidence of inhalation injury at the time of admission should include: (a) maintenance of an adequate airway, (b) removal of mucus and debris from the tracheobronchial tree, (c) reversal of airflow obstruction, and (d) correction of hypoxemia.

Early intubation may be critical to prevent rapid asphyxia caused by upper airway obstruction. A victim of a toxic inhalation with stridor; hoarseness; or severe facial, nasal, and oral injuries should be closely monitored with arterial blood gases for respiratory insufficiency and intubated if necessary. Tracheostomy is rarely required initially and should not be done through burn tissue because of the substantial risk of infection in the wound and in the airway.

The severe tracheobronchitis that develops in many patients with inhalation injury requires vigorous bronchial hygiene measures. Adequate hydration, deep inspiratory maneuvers, postural drainage, and chest physical therapy may help promote drainage of mucous plugs and secretions. Frequent suctioning of intubated patients with smoke inhalation injury is a way to debride the airways of the adherent soot that may contain irritant and corrosive chemicals. Some authors have advocated the use of fiberoptic bronchoscopy as a treatment and a diagnostic modality in the management of smoke inhalation injury to facilitate the removal of adherent soot by lavage (31).

Bronchospasm should be treated with the usual agents as if for acute asthma, except that corticosteroids should be avoided if possible. Corticosteroids may reduce lung bacterial clearance (32), and sustained use may increase the risk of opportunistic infection (33).

Hypoxemia can usually be corrected by the administration of oxygen when not complicated by carbon monoxide intoxication. Hypoxemia not corrected by bronchial hygiene measures, bronchodilators, and supplemental oxygen suggests the presence of severe pulmonary parenchymal injury.

Supportive care of patients with severe parenchymal injury that is evolving into ARDS is critical. Mechanical ventilation with positive end-expiratory pressure is usually required to correct hypoxemia with sufficiently low concentrations of supplemental oxygen to avoid oxygen toxicity. Monitoring of pulmonary hemodynamics, cardiac output, and blood gases must supplement the use of formulas in the determination of intravenous fluid replacement in the patient with severe cutaneous burns to avoid exacerbation of alveolar flooding.

Use of corticosteroids in the treatment of toxic inhalation injury remains controversial. Whereas some authors have advocated prophylactic corticosteroid therapy to reduce parenchymal inflammation and subsequent fibrosis (34), others have noted increased infectious complications with their use (33,35). In an animal model of acrolein-induced inhalation injury, the administration of methylprednisolone 30 minutes after exposure reduced mortality but was not associated with amelioration of histologic evidence of lung damage (36). The methylprednisolone-treated animals had improved survival despite showing more pulmonary vascular congestion than was seen in the control animals. This study confirmed earlier observations and suggests a possible role for steroids in the management of inhalation injury. However, because of the apparent increased risk of pneumonia associated with administration of steroids in patients with inhalation injury, their routine use cannot be recommended. Furthermore, two clinical trials have shown either no benefit or increased mortality in steroid-treated patients (37,38).

Pneumonia is the most common late complication in patients with inhalation injury. It can result from either aspiration of microorganisms or hematogenous dissemination from contaminated wounds. Because fever and leukocytosis may be present after inhalation injury in the absence of infection, repeated examination of Gram's stain sputum is necessary, and cultures should be obtained if the flora changes. Prophylactic use of antibiotics has not been demonstrated to be of benefit in patients with inhalation injury (33).

PROGNOSIS

The mortality rate from smoke inhalation injury without concomitant severe burns ranges from 5% to 10%. However, with severe cutaneous burns, the mortality rate increases to 49% to 80% (20). The cause of this high mortality for combined injury remains unclear. It is likely that the risk of developing ARDS in these patients is determined by the degree of damage to the alveolar epithelium from toxic gas inhalation and damage to the pulmonary capillary endothelium secondary to sepsis or inflammatory response-related complement activation and platelet and leukocyte aggregation (17,18). Severely burned patients with inhalation injury often require large volumes of fluid replacement. The inability of these patients' more permeable alveolar-capillary membranes to handle the replaced fluid also may contribute to the high mortality. In a review of more than 1,000 consecutive burn patients, 35% had inhalation injury, and of the patients with inhalation injury, 38% developed pneumonia (39). Inhalation injury alone increased mortality by a maximum of 20%, and pneumonia alone by a maximum of 40%; when both were present, the maximum mortality approached 60%.

Age is a major risk factor for mortality from inhalation injury (40–42). The physiologic stress of inhalation injury is probably less tolerated in older persons, who are more likely to have a preexisting cardiopulmonary disorder. An analysis of hospitalized burn patients who were older than 60 years found the following: (a) the cause of death frequently was pneumonia in patients who died but did not have burns over a large surface area; (b) once pneumonia developed, death was almost an invariable outcome; and (c) the mean fluid requirement to maintain adequate vital signs was less for survivors than for those who died (40). An aging cardiovascular system burdened with increased alveolar-capillary permeability owing to inhalation injury and to severe cutaneous burns is easily pushed into pulmonary edema, which compromises gas exchange and can lead to pneumonia. Patients with inhalation injury are already at increased risk for pneumonia by virtue of their bronchorrhea and impaired respiratory defense mechanisms. Pneumonia is poorly tolerated by elderly patients, even in the absence of inhalation injury.

In addition to severity of concomitant cutaneous burns and age, the presence of facial burns (even when the total body surface area burned is small) and elevated carboxyhemoglobin levels (greater than 15% saturation) also have been associated with high rates of inhalation injury and mortality (23,43).

Because it is difficult to assemble and to study a cohort of patients with inhalation injury that is of sufficient size, few data exist on long-term follow-up of such patients. One study did systematically characterize the pulmonary function of fire victims immediately after injury, and sequentially during treatment and recovery (44). The results of this study confirmed that the incidence of respiratory complications in fire victims is related to the severity of cutaneous burns and the presence or absence of smoke inhalation. Smoke inhalation caused severe airway obstruction in most patients by 9 hours after exposure. Patients with cutaneous burns tended to develop a significant restrictive ventilatory defect over the first several days that correlated with the surface area of the burns, whether or not the chest was burned, fluid was retained, and the colloid osmotic pressure was reduced. As expected, the combination of surface burns and smoke inhalation was associated with the greatest deterioration in pulmonary function. Although most parameters of pulmonary function gradually improved over the 5 months after injury, still some evidence existed of mild airway obstruction in those subjects who had sustained smoke inhalation.

EVALUATION OF LESS SEVERE INHALATION INJURY

One who carefully evaluates ambulatory patients who have sustained milder degrees of inhalation injury can successfully identify and diagnose sequelae in most cases. The following four areas of approach are recommended: (a) careful medical and exposure history, (b) thorough physical examination, (c) appropriate imaging studies, and (d) pulmonary function testing.

History

A detailed history of the patient's complaints and environmental and occupational exposures is essential. Hazardous material or fire department incident reports should be reviewed if pertinent and available. Work practices should be extensively explored with attention to types and duration of exposures, whether appropriate environmental controls are present, and if respiratory protective gear is used. Material Safety Data Sheets should be reviewed, if available. These documents profile the important health, safety, and toxicologic properties of the product's ingredients and, under federal law, are to be furnished by the employer to the worker and his or her health care provider on request. If available, actual industrial hygiene data on the level of exposure and the agent to which the patient was exposed should be obtained. The history should include the condition of the patient's home, any hobbies, and social habits, because exposures contributing to or causing the respiratory tract injury may be discovered.

Physical Examination

Inhalation injury does not present with specific clinical findings. It is difficult to distinguish chemical bronchitis from infectious bronchitis or irritant-induced asthma from other types of asthmas. Only in the context of the exposure history can the correct diagnosis be made. A physician suspecting the presence of inhalation injury should, nonetheless, perform a complete physical examination rather than focus narrowly on findings suggested by the exposure history. Relevant nonexposure-related disease may otherwise be missed.

The physical examination may be helpful if abnormal, but it is, in general, insensitive for detection of mild respiratory tract injury. The vital signs and the level of respiratory distress, if any, should be assessed. The presence of cyanosis and finger clubbing should be noted. Examination of the skin and eyes can yield signs of irritation and inflammation. Oropharyngeal and nasal areas should be inspected for inflammation, ulcers, and polyps. The presence of wheezing and rhonchi is evidence of airways disease, and crackles are suggestive of the presence of parenchymal disease. Examination of the cardiovascular system for evidence of left ventricular failure is important when crackles are heard. The presence of isolated right ventricular failure suggests the possibility of cor pulmonale as a result of chronic severe lung disease with hypoxemia.

Imaging Studies

A chest radiograph should be part of the workup when inhalation injury is suspected. However, normal radiographic findings do not exclude significant damage to the lung. Immediately after toxic inhalational injury, the chest radiograph is frequently normal. On the other hand, dramatically abnormal chest radiographs can be seen in individuals without significant lung injury who are exposed chronically to iron oxide or tin oxide. Abnormalities on the chest radiograph do not necessarily correlate with the degree of pulmonary impairment or disability. These are better assessed by pulmonary function testing and arterial blood gas determination.

Computed tomography (CT) is a radiographic technique that scans axial cross-sections and produces tomographic slices of the organ scanned. Conventional CT of the chest is better able to detect abnormalities of the pleura and the mediastinal structures than plain chest radiography, in large part because it is more sensitive to differences in density. However, conventional CT scanning adds little to chest radiography for evaluation of the lung parenchyma. High-resolution CT scanning (HRCT) incorporates thin collimation (1 to 2 mm as opposed to 10 mm in conventional CT), with high spatial-frequency reconstruction algorithms that sharpen interfaces between adjacent structures. Multiple studies suggest that HRCT is more sensitive than either conventional CT or chest radiography for assessing the presence, character, and severity of diffuse lung processes such as emphysema and interstitial fibrosis (45,46). Two potential sequelae of toxic inhalation injury that are often more focal—bronchiectasis and bronchiolitis obliterans—are also best imaged by HRCT (47,48).

Pulmonary Function Testing

Pulmonary function testing is used to detect and quantitate abnormal lung function. Measurement of lung volumes and diffusing capacity, gas exchange analysis, and exercise testing should be performed in a well-equipped pulmonary function laboratory, but spirometry can and should be done in most evaluating centers. Performance requirements for spirometers are described in a 1995 American Thoracic Society (ATS) statement (49).

The most valuable of all pulmonary function parameters are those obtained from spirometry, namely forced expiratory volume in 1 second (FEV_1), forced vital capacity (FVC), and the FEV_1/FVC ratio. These parameters provide the best method of detecting the presence and severity of airway obstruction as well as the most reliable assessment of overall respiratory impairment. The forced expiratory flow from 25% to 75% of vital capacity and the shape of the expiratory flow-volume curve are more sensitive indicators of mild airway obstruction. A simple portable spirometer can be used to obtain the necessary measurements. Lack of patient cooperation, poor testing methods, and unreliable equipment can produce misleading results. The 1995 ATS statement contains criteria for the performance of spirometry. Results of spirometry can be compared to predicted values from reference populations (adjusted for age, height, and gender) and expressed as a percentage of the predicted value (50). The presence of obstructive, restrictive, or mixed ventilatory impairment can then be determined from the comparison of observed values with predicted values. Because the commonly used reference populations consist entirely of white people, there can be problems using predicted values to evaluate patients of different ethnic backgrounds. Typically, a 10% to 15% lowering of the predicted value is done to correct for the generally smaller lungs of these patients.

Another commonly used single-breath test that reflects the degree of airway obstruction is the peak expiratory flow rate. Portable instruments, such as the mini-Wright peak flow meter, can be used for its measurement. The major limitation of the peak expiratory flow rate is that patient self-recording of measurements is usually done and, thus, a considerable potential for recording error exists. Despite this limitation, the test is useful in detecting changes in airway obstruction over time. Serial peak flow measurements are especially valuable in the diagnosis of asthma (51).

Because FVC can be reduced due to disease processes that either restrict airflow into or obstruct airflow from the lungs, differentiation of restrictive from obstructive processes often requires measurement of static lung volumes [i.e., total lung capacity (TLC), functional residual capacity, and residual volume]. These lung volumes are measured by inert gas dilution or body plethysmography (52). Restrictive lung diseases cause a reduction in TLC and other lung volumes, whereas obstructive diseases may result in hyperinflation and air trapping (i.e., increased TLC and residual volume/TLC ratio).

The diffusing capacity of the lung for carbon monoxide (DLCO) is a test of gas exchange in which the amount of inhaled carbon monoxide absorbed per unit time is measured (53). The DLCO is closely correlated with the capacity of the lungs to absorb oxygen. A reduced DLCO is a nonspecific finding; obstructive, restrictive, or vascular diseases can all cause reductions. Nevertheless, the DLCO is often used in combination with other clinical evidence to support a specific diagnosis or to assess respiratory impairment.

Nonspecific bronchoprovocation testing is useful in the diagnosis of asthma (54). Pulmonary function responses to inhaled histamine and methacholine are relatively easy to measure and give an indication of the presence and degree of nonspecific hyperresponsiveness of the airways. A measure of airway obstruction, such as FEV_1, is obtained repeatedly after progressively increasing doses of histamine or methacholine to generate a dose-response curve. The test is usually terminated after a 20% fall in FEV_1. Patients with asthma typically respond with such a change in lung function after a relatively low cumulative dose of methacholine. Nonspecific challenge testing with methacholine is relatively inexpensive and can be performed on an outpatient basis.

MANAGEMENT OF LESS SEVERE INHALATION INJURY

Symptoms of respiratory irritation may be treated with bronchodilators and cough suppressants as needed. Corticosteroids, either systemic or inhaled, are thought by some people to have a salutary effect on the resolution of airway inflammation, although no data from controlled trials exist to support their use. Prompt diagnosis and treatment of secondary infection are essential. Follow-up of inhalation injury should be early and frequent until progression toward recovery is evident.

CHRONIC SEQUELAE

The paucity of data regarding follow-up of fire victims leads one to turn to studies of firefighters with repeated occupational inhalation of smoke. It is clear that routine fire fighting is associated with acute decrements in pulmonary function (55,56) and increased airway responsiveness (56,57). The persistence of these decrements in some firefighters (56,58) and the apparent increased prevalence of airway hyperresponsiveness among firefighters (59) suggest that inhalation of toxic combustion products may lead to chronic airway inflammation and remodeling. Of course, the relationship between the effects of recurrent occupational exposure of firefighters and the effects of single massive toxic gas exposures is problematic.

Data are collected in follow-up of victims of massive exposure to chlorine (60,61) and sulfur dioxide (62) that tend to show a progressive decline in pulmonary function for the first 6 months after exposure. Beyond this point, usually either a lack of further deterioration or even a gradual improvement exists in pulmonary function. However, a persistent restrictive ventilatory impairment and increased airway responsiveness may be present years after inhalation injury in a small minority of patients (61,62).

Anecdotal reports of victims who developed chronic sequelae such as bronchiolitis obliterans, bronchiectasis, and lung parenchymal fibrosis have existed for some time (63,64). Recovery from bronchiolitis obliterans may be aided by a course of corticosteroid treatment. Persistence of airway hyperresponsiveness and an asthma-like syndrome (i.e., irritant-induced asthma) have been anecdotally reported (12,65,66). Irritant-induced asthma occurs without a latent period after substantial exposure to an irritating dust, mist, vapor, or fume. RADS is an irritant-induced asthma caused by a short-term, high-intensity exposure (12).

Irritant-induced asthma involves persistent nonspecific airway hyperresponsiveness but not specific responsiveness to an etiologic agent. Although no doubt exists that irritant-induced asthma can be caused by a single, intense exposure (i.e., RADS), it appears that lower-level exposure over a longer duration of time (months to years) can also cause the disease (66). Whereas the mechanisms by which airway inflammation occurs in irritant-induced asthma are not well understood, neurogenic pathways may be involved. The axonal reflex involving C-fiber stimulation and the release of neuropeptides have been implicated in models of irritant-induced airway hyperresponsiveness (67). With high-level irritant exposure, direct chemical injury can lead to an inflammatory response. Because respiratory symptoms resolve within weeks to several months in most individuals who develop airway inflammation after a toxic inhalation (i.e., chemical bronchitis), an important unanswered question is what causes this response to persist in the small number of individuals who develop irritant-induced asthma. Cigarette smoking and a preexisting tendency to develop wheezing are two risk factors that have been identified for persistent asthma-like symptoms after inhalation injury (1).

Management of irritant-induced asthma does not differ from that of other types of asthmas (51). The cornerstone of asthma management is prevention of acute exacerbations by avoidance of exposure to asthma triggers and antiinflammatory therapy. Acute asthma attacks requiring emergency management should be treated with supplemental oxygen, beta-agonists, corticosteroids, and, if infection is suspected, antibiotics. Hospitalization should be considered in the more severe cases because of the potential for respiratory failure. If irritant-induced asthma is caused by recurrent occupational exposures, the use of personal protective equipment may lower exposures to levels that do not induce bronchospasm. Workers who are able to continue in their jobs should have regular follow-up visits, including monitoring of their lung function and nonspecific airway responsiveness. In addition to reduction or elimination of exposure to the causative agent, workers with irritant-induced asthma should also avoid exposure to other materials and processes that generate irritating dusts, mists, vapors, and so forth. Cessation of smoking and avoidance of exposure to environmental tobacco smoke are also essential.

IMPAIRMENT AND DISABILITY ASSESSMENT

Physicians may be called on to assess their patients' respiratory impairment and to make judgments about disability based on these assessments. *Impairment* refers to a loss of function, and *disability* refers to a decreased ability to perform work as a consequence of this loss of function. An impairment and disability evaluation typically involves the following questions:

1. Has the patient's condition reached a point of maximal medical improvement or is substantial improvement likely with further treatment?
2. What is the degree of impairment, if any?
3. Does the impairment prevent the patient from performing his or her usual and customary job, or any job?
4. Should the patient be precluded from specific duties (e.g., from tasks that involve exposure to respiratory tract irritants)?
5. Does a need for future medical treatment exist?
6. What is the long-term prognosis?
7. Does the patient require vocational rehabilitation?

Although some of the state worker's compensation systems require the use of specific rating schemes, the most widely recognized impairment classification scheme is that of the American Medical Association (AMA) (68). The AMA scheme involves four classes of impairment—none, mild (10% to 25%), moderate (26% to 50%), and severe (51% to 100%). This classification is based on the results of spirometry, DLCO, and maximal oxygen consumption during exercise. The presence of hypoxemia (i.e., a resting PaO_2 less than 55 mm Hg) is rated as a severe impairment. Exercise testing is recommended when dyspnea seems out of proportion to the results of the resting pulmonary function tests. The AMA classification scheme is best applied to rating impairment from chronic lung diseases that cause relatively stable dysfunction.

Asthma is a dynamic disease that does not generally result in a static level of impairment. Therefore, a different approach to the evaluation of impairment in patients with asthma than that of the AMA guidelines is required. The ATS proposed an impairment rating scheme for asthma that used the following criteria: degree of postbronchodilator airway obstruction by spirometry, measurement of airway responsiveness, and medication requirements (69). Assessment of impairment and disability should be done only after optimization of therapy and whenever the worker's condition changes substantially, whether for better or worse.

SPECIFIC EXAMPLES OF IRRITANT GASES

Ammonia

Ammonia (NH_3) is a highly irritating, highly water-soluble gas that is colorless but has a distinctive odor. It is used extensively as a refrigerant and in the manufacture of plastics, explosives, fertilizers, and pharmaceuticals. Accidental industrial exposure to ammonia usually occurs after rupture of a tank or pipeline (70–72). Transportation accidents have resulted in large-scale environmental exposures to ammonia gas (73).

Because ammonia is highly water soluble, it can cause extensive damage to mucous membranes of the eyes, nose, oropharynx, larynx, and tracheobronchial tree. Ammonia and water combine to form ammonium hydroxide that dissociates to ammonium (NH_4^+) and hydroxyl (OH^-) ions. The latter cause a severe alkaline burn characterized by liquefaction necrosis. In addition, ammonia gas releases heat as it dissolves and is, thus, capable of causing thermal injury (74).

Exposure to high concentrations of ammonia produces severe burns of the cornea and upper airway. Death may result from acute laryngeal edema (70,71,74). Diffuse tracheobronchitis with severe bronchoconstriction and bronchorrhea is a common feature of ammonia inhalation. Mild cases present with inflamed mucous membranes and a normal chest examination. Moderate cases present with wheezing, rhonchi, productive cough, and burns of the cornea, nose, and mouth. Severe cases present in respiratory distress, with blood-tinged sputum, stridor, pulmonary edema, and burns of the upper airway. Severity of inhalation injury relates to the concentration of the gas and the duration of exposure.

Victims of ammonia exposure require prompt decontamination of eyes and skin as well as aggressive airway management. Because ammonia tends to cause more airway than parenchymal injury, chest radiographic findings correlate poorly with degree of inspiratory distress. Signs of improvement are generally apparent within 48–72 hours of admission, and most patients recover without significant residual impairment. However, anecdotal reports of bronchiectasis and bronchiolitis obliterans exist (72,73). One case of severe ammonia inhalation injury requiring intubation and mechanical ventilatory support during the acute phase was reported to have been followed by a persistent asthma-like syndrome and airway hyperresponsiveness (75).

Chlorine

Chlorine is an irritant gas that is somewhat less water soluble than ammonia. It is used widely as a bleaching agent, as a disinfectant, and in the manufacture of many chemicals, plastics, and resins. Chlorine is often transported and stored under pressure in pipes, trucks, or tanks, and exposure occurs during industrial or transportation accidents (60,76); as a result of mixing chlorine bleach with an acid cleaner (77); or during cylinder changes at swimming pools (78). Chlorine toxicity appears to be mediated by the evolution of hydrogen chloride on contact with moist mucous membranes and by the generation of free radicals at the cellular level (79). The oxidant effect of chlorine is thought to be the explanation for the fact that it is approximately 20 times more toxic to the respiratory tract than hydrogen chloride alone.

Because chlorine is less water soluble than ammonia, inhalation injury caused by chlorine is characterized by relatively less upper airway and more parenchymal injury than that caused by ammonia. Still, chlorine exposure does cause significant local irritation to mucous membranes. Substernal, burning chest pain and paroxysmal cough are frequent features of chlorine inhalation injury. Headache is also a common complaint. High-intensity exposure can lead to respiratory distress and pulmonary edema. Chest radiographic findings tend to lag somewhat behind the course of the clinical presentation. Pulmonary function tends to be abnormal after chlorine exposure, even if pulmonary edema is not clinically evident (60,76). Typically, airway obstruction and significant air trapping are found in the immediate postexposure period (60). Over time, pulmonary function tends to improve, although some persons may be left with a residual restrictive ventilatory impairment with increased lung elastic recoil and airway hyperresponsiveness (61).

Nitrogen Dioxide

Nitrogen dioxide (NO_2) is a relatively water-insoluble gas that is reddish brown in color. It is encountered in grain storage silos (80), welding (81), combustion of fuels or nitrogen-containing materials (82), production and use of nitrate explosives (81), and handling of rocket fuel oxidizers (83). Because nitrogen dioxide is relatively insoluble in water, little absorption by, and irritation of, the mucous membranes of the eyes, nose, and throat exists. Thus, persons inhaling even high concentrations of nitrogen dioxide may not become immediately aware of their exposure. Again, because of its lack of water solubility, inhaled nitrogen dioxide penetrates well to the pulmonary parenchyma, where it causes oxidant injury to terminal bronchioles and to endothelial and epithelial layers of the alveolar-capillary membrane (84–87).

The onset of respiratory symptoms after inhalation of nitrogen dioxide is typically delayed for several hours to up to 30 hours. Cough, dyspnea, fever, and leukocytosis are common clinical features of nitrogen dioxide inhalation injury. As with chlorine, chest radiographs may be normal on clinical presentation but usually progress to show evidence of pulmonary edema. Most victims of nitrogen dioxide inhalation who can be adequately supported throughout the initial acute injury recover completely, but a few patients go on to develop a late phase of illness 2 to 6 weeks later. This late phase is characterized by progressive dyspnea, fever, and patchy infiltrates on chest radiographs (88). The mechanism of the late phase of nitrogen dioxide inhalation injury is not understood. Anecdotal reports suggest that treatment with corticosteroids may be beneficial, although no data from controlled clinical trials are available (80,81,83,89,90). Bronchiolitis obliterans has been described after nitrogen dioxide inhalation injury, but it is not clear that all cases with late phase illness are caused by bronchiolitis (91). The likelihood of developing late phase illness does not appear to be related to the severity of the initial illness.

Inhalation of nitrogen dioxide also may lead to the generation of methemoglobin (92,93), which can complicate hypoxemia caused by pulmonary injury, by adding an impairment of oxygen transport to extrapulmonary tissues.

REFERENCES

1. Blanc P, Galbo M, Hiatt P, Olson KR. Morbidity following acute irritant inhalation in a population-based study. *JAMA* 1991;266:664–669.
2. Larson TV, Covert DS, Frank R, Charlson RJ. Ammonia in the human airways: neutralization of inspired acid sulfate aerosols. *Science* 1977;197:161–163.
3. Coleridge HM, Coleridge JCG, Ginzel KN, Baker DG, Banzett RB, Morrison MA. Stimulation of "irritant" receptors and afferent C-fibers in the lung by prostaglandins. *Nature* 1976;264:451–452.
4. Nadel JA. Regulation of bronchial secretions. In: Newball HH, ed. *Immunopharmacology of the lung*. New York: Marcel Dekker Inc, 1983:109–139.
5. Reid L. An experimental study of hypersecretion of mucus in the bronchial tree. *Br J Exp Pathol* 1963;44:437–445.
6. Scanlon PD, Seltzer J, Ingram RH, Reid L, Drazen JM. Chronic exposure to sulfur dioxide: physiologic and histologic evaluation of dog exposure to 50 or 15 ppm. *Am Rev Respir Dis* 1987;135:831–839.
7. Becklake MR. Chronic airflow limitation: its relationship to work in dusty occupations. *Chest* 1985;88:608–617.
8. Kennedy SM. Agents causing chronic airflow obstruction. In: Harber P, Schenker M, Balmes J, eds. *Occupational and environmental respiratory disease*. St. Louis: Mosby–Year Book, 1996:433–449.
9. Nadel JA, Salem H, Tamplin B, Tokiwa G. Mechanism of bronchoconstriction during inhalation of sulfur dioxide. *J Appl Physiol* 1965;20:164–167.
10. Lundberg JM, Saria A. Capsaicin-induced desensitization of the airway mucosa to cigarette smoke, mechanical and chemical irritants. *Nature* 1983;302:251–253.
11. Lundberg JM, Brodin E, Saria A. Effects and distribution of vagal capsaicin sensitive neurons with special reference to the trachea and lungs. *Acta Physiol Scand* 1983;119:243–252.
12. Brooks SM, Weiss MA, Bernstein IL. Reactive airways dysfunction syndrome (RADS): persistent asthma syndrome after high level irritant exposure. *Chest* 1985;88:376–384.
13. Moller DR, Brooks SM, McKay RT, Cassedy K, Kopp S, Bernstein IL. Chronic asthma due to toluene diisocyanate. *Chest* 1986;90:494–499.
14. Loke J, Paul E, Virgulto JA, Smith GJW. Rabbit lung after acute smoke inhalation: cellular response and scanning electron microscopy. *Arch Surg* 1984;199:956–959.

15. Chu C-S. New concepts of pulmonary burn injury. *J Trauma* 1981;21:958–961.
16. Rowland RRR, Yamaguchi K, Santibanez AS, Kodama KT, Ness VT, Grubbs DE. Smoke inhalation model for lung permeability studies. *J Trauma* 1986;26:153–156.
17. Till GO, Johnson KJ, Kunkel R, Ward PA. Intravascular activation of complement and acute lung injury. *J Clin Invest* 1982;69:1126–1135.
18. Till GO, Beauchalp C, Menapace D, et al. Oxygen radical dependent lung damage following thermal injury on rat skin. *J Trauma* 1983;23:269–277.
19. Nieman GF, Clark WR Jr, Wax SD, Webb WR. The effect of smoke inhalation on pulmonary surfactant. *Ann Surg* 1980;191:171–181.
20. Zawacki BE, Jung RC, Joyce J, Rincon E. Smoke, burns, and the natural history of inhalation injury in fire victims: a correlation of experimental and clinical data. *Ann Surg* 1977;185:100–110.
21. Stephenson SF, Esrig BC, Polk HC, Fulton RL. The pathophysiology of smoke inhalation injury. *Ann Surg* 1975;182:652–660.
22. Dressler DP, Skornik WA, Kupersmith S. Corticosteroid treatment of experimental smoke inhalation. *Ann Surg* 1976;183:46–52.
23. Zikria BA, Budd DC, Floch F, Ferrer JM. What is clinical smoke poisoning. *Ann Surg* 1975;181:151–156.
24. Clark CJ, Campbell D, Reid WH. Blood carboxyhemoglobin and cyanide levels in fire survivors. *Lancet* 1981;1:1332–1335.
25. Hunt JL, Agec RN, Pruitt BA Jr. Fiberoptic bronchoscopy in acute inhalation injury. *J Trauma* 1975;15:641–649.
26. Williams DO, Vanecko RM, Glassroth J. Endobronchial polyposis following smoke inhalation. *Chest* 1983;84:774–776.
27. Moylan JA, Wilmore DW, Mouton DE, Pruitt BA. Early diagnosis of inhalation injury using 133 xenon lung scan. *Ann Surg* 1972;176:477–484.
28. Petroff PA, Hander EW, Clayton WH, Pruitt BA. Pulmonary function studies after smoke inhalation. *Am J Surg* 1976;132:346–351.
29. Haponik EF, Meyers DA, Munster AM, et al. Acute upper airway injury in burn patients: serial changes of flow-volume curves and nasopharyngoscopy. *Am Rev Respir Dis* 1987;135:360–366.
30. Mason GR, Effros RM, Uszler JM, Mena I. Small solute clearance from the lungs of patients with cardiogenic and noncardiogenic pulmonary edema. *Chest* 1985;88:327–334.
31. Clark CJ, Reid WH, Telfer ABM, Campbell D. Respiratory injury in the burned patient: the role of flexible bronchoscopy. *Anaesthesia* 1983;38:35–39.
32. Skornik WA, Dressier DP. The effects of short-term steroid therapy in lung bacterial clearance and survival in rats. *Ann Surg* 1974;179:415–421.
33. Levine BA, Petroff PA, Slade CL, Pruitt BA. Prospective trials of dexamethasone and aerosolized gentamicin in the treatment of inhalation injury in the burned patient. *J Trauma* 1978;18:188–193.
34. Welch GW, Lull RJ, Petroff PA, Hander EW, McLeod CG, Clayton WH. The use of steroids in inhalation injury. *Surg Gynecol Obstet* 1977;145:539–544.
35. Moylan JA, Chan C. Inhalation injury—an increasing problem. *Ann Surg* 1978;188:34–37.
36. Beeley JM, Crow J, Jones JG, Minty B, Lynch RD, Pryce DP. Mortality and lung histopathology after inhalation lung injury: the effect of corticosteroids. *Am Rev Respir Dis* 1986;133:191–196.
37. Moylan JA. Diagnostic techniques and steroids. *J Trauma* 1979;19[suppl]: 917.
38. Shirani KZ, Moylan JA, Pruitt BA. Diagnosis and treatment of inhalation injury in burn patients. In: Loke J, ed. *Pathophysiology and treatment of inhalation injuries*. New York: Marcel Dekker Inc, 1988:239–280.
39. Shirani KZ, Pruitt BA, Mason AD. The influence of inhalation injury and pneumonia on burn mortality. *Ann Surg* 1987;205:82–87.
40. Anous M, Heimbach DM. Causes of death and predictors in burned patients more than 60 years of age. *J Trauma* 1986;26:135–139.
41. Thompson PB, Herndon DN, Traber DL, et al. Effect on mortality of inhalation injury. *J Trauma* 1986;26:163–165.
42. Clark CJ, Reid WH, Gilmour WH, Campbell D. Mortality probability in victims of fire trauma: revised equation to include inhalation injury. *BMJ* 1986;1:1303–1305.
43. Wroblewski DA, Bower GC. The significance of facial burns in acute smoke inhalation. *Crit Care Med* 1979;7:335–338.
44. Whitener DR, Whitener LM, Robertson KJ, Baxter CR, Pierce AK. Pulmonary function measurements in patients with thermal injury and smoke inhalation. *Am Rev Respir Dis* 1980;122:731–739.
45. Grenier P, Valeyre D, Cluzel P, Brauner MW, Lenoir S, Chastang C. Chronic diffuse interstitial lung disease: diagnostic value of chest radiography and high-resolution CT. *Radiology* 1991;179:123–132.
46. Murata K, Kahn A, Herman PG. Pulmonary parenchymal disease: evaluation with high resolution CT. *Radiology* 1989;170:629–635.
47. Munro NC, Cooke JC, Currie DC, Strickland B, Cole PJ. Comparison of thin section computed tomography with bronchography for identifying bronchiectatic segments in patients with chronic sputum production. *Thorax* 1990;45:135–139.
48. Morrish WF, Herman SJ, Weisbrod GL, Chamberlain DW. Bronchiolitis obliterans after lung transplantation: findings at chest radiography and high-resolution CT. *Radiology* 1991;179:487–490.
49. American Thoracic Society. Standardization of spirometry: 1994 update. *Am Rev Respir Dis* 1995;152:1107–1136.
50. American Thoracic Society. Lung function testing: selection of reference values and interpretative strategies. *Am Rev Respir Dis* 1991;144:1202–1218.
51. National Asthma Education Program. *Guidelines for the diagnosis and management of asthma*. Bethesda, MD: National Institutes of Health, 1991:17–25.
52. Ries AL. Measurement of lung volumes. *Clin Chest Med* 1989;10:177–186.
53. American Thoracic Society. Single breath carbon monoxide diffusing capacity (transfer factor): recommendations for a standard technique. *Am Rev Respir Dis* 1987;136:1299–1307.
54. Sterk PJ, Fabbri LM, Quanjer PH, et al. Airway responsiveness: standardized challenge testing with pharmacological, physical and sensitizing stimuli in adults. *Eur Respir J* 1993;6[suppl 16]:53–83.
55. Musk AW, Smith JT, Peters JM, McLaughlin E. Pulmonary function in firefighters: acute changes in ventilatory capacity and their correlates. *Br J Ind Med* 1979;36:29–34.
56. Sheppard D, Distefano S, Morse L, Becker CE. Acute effects of routine firefighting on lung function. *Am J Ind Med* 1986;9:333–340.
57. Sherman CB, Barnhart S, Miller MF, et al. Firefighting acutely increases airway responsiveness. *Am Rev Respir Dis* 1989;140:185–190.
58. Loke J, Farmer W, Matthay RA, Putnam CE, Smith GJW. Acute and chronic effects of firefighting on pulmonary function. *Chest* 1980;77:369–373.
59. Niederman MS, Abrams C, Virgulto JA, et al. Increase in bronchial reactivity of firefighters with normal lung function. *Am Rev Respir Dis* 1981;123:488–491.
60. Charan NB, Lakshinarayan S, Myers CG, Smith DD. Effects of accidental chlorine inhalation on pulmonary function. *West J Med* 1985;143:333–336.
61. Schwartz DA, Smith DD, Lakshinarayan S. The pulmonary sequelae associated with accidental inhalation of chlorine gas. *Chest* 1990;97:820–825.
62. Harkonen H, Nordman H, Korhonen O, Winblad I. Long-term effects of exposure to sulfur dioxide. *Am Rev Respir Dis* 1983;128:890–893.
63. Donnellan WI, Poticha SM, Hallinger PM. Management and complications of severe pulmonary burn. *JAMA* 1965;194:1323–1325.
64. Perez-Guerra F, Walsh RE, Sagel SS. Bronchiolitis obliterans and tracheal stenosis: late complications of inhalation burn. *JAMA* 1971;218:1568–1570.
65. Boulet L-P. Increases in airway responsiveness following acute exposure to respiratory irritants. *Chest* 1988;94:476–481.
66. Tarlo SM, Broder I. Irritant-induced occupational asthma. *Chest* 1989;96: 297–300.
67. Thompson JE, Scypinski LA, Gordon T, Sheppard D. Tachykinins mediate the acute increase in airway responsiveness caused by toluene diisocyanate in guinea pigs. *Am Rev Respir Dis* 1987;136:43–49.
68. American Medical Association. *Guides to the evaluation of permanent impairment*, 4th ed. Chicago: American Medical Association, 1993:153–167.
69. American Thoracic Society. Guidelines for the evaluation of impairment/disability in patients with asthma. *Am Rev Respir Dis* 1993;147:1056–1061.
70. Close LG, Catlin FI, Cohn AM. Acute and chronic effects of ammonia burns of the respiratory tract. *Arch Otolaryngol* 1980;106:151–158.
71. Walton M. Industrial ammonia gassing. *Br J Ind Med* 1973;30:78–86.
72. Sobonya R. Fatal anhydrous ammonia inhalation. *Hum Pathol* 1977;8:293–299.
73. Kass I, Zamal N, Dobry CA, Holzer M. Bronchiectasis following ammonia burns of the respiratory tract. *Chest* 1972;62:282–285.
74. O'Kane GJ. Inhalation of ammonia vapor. *Anaesthesia* 1983;38:1208–1213.
75. Flury KE, Dines DE, Rodarte JR, Rodgers R. Airway obstruction due to inhalation of ammonia. *Mayo Clin Proc* 1983;58:389–393.
76. Weill H, George R, Schwartz M, Ziskind M. Late evaluation of pulmonary function after acute exposure to chlorine gas. *Am Rev Respir Dis* 1969;99:374–379.
77. Murphy DMF, Fairman RP, Lapp NL, Morgan WKC. Severe airway disease due to inhalation of fumes from cleaning agents. *Chest* 1976;69:372–376.
78. Decker WJ, Koch HF. Chlorine poisoning at a swimming pool: an overlooked hazard. *Clin Toxicol* 1978;13:377–381.
79. Adelson L, Kaufman J. Fatal chlorine poisoning: report of two cases with clinicopathologic correlation. *Am J Clin Pathol* 1971;56:430–442.
80. Lowery T, Shuman LM. Silo filler's disease—a syndrome caused by nitrogen dioxide. *JAMA* 1956;162:153–160.
81. Jones GR, Proudfoot AT, Hall JI. Pulmonary effects of acute exposure to nitrous fumes. *Thorax* 1973;28:61–65.
82. Nichols BH. The clinical effects of inhalation of nitrogen dioxide. *AJR Am J Roentgenol* 1930;23:516–520.
83. Yockey CC, Eden BM, Byrd RB. The McConnell missile accident: clinical spectrum of nitrogen dioxide exposure. *JAMA* 1980;244:1221–1223.
84. Guidotti TL. Toxic inhalation of nitrogen dioxide: morphologic and functional changes. *Exp Mol Pathol* 1980;33:90–103.
85. Sherwin RP, Richters V. Lung capillary permeability—nitrogen dioxide exposure and leakage of tritiated serum. *Arch Intern Med* 1971;128:61–68.
86. Pickrell JA, Hahn FF, Rebar AH, et al. Pulmonary effects of exposure to 20 ppm NO_2. *Chest* 1981;80:50S–52S.
87. DeNicola DB, Rebar AH, Henderson RF. Early indicators of lung damage: biochemical and cytological response to NO_2 inhalation. *Toxicol Appl Pharmacol* 1981;60:301–312.
88. Becklake MR, Goldman KI, Boxman AR, Freed C. The long-term effects of exposure to nitrous fumes. *Am Rev Tuber* 1957;76:398–409.
89. Horvath EP, do Pico GA, Barbee RA, Dickie HA. Nitrogen dioxide induced pulmonary disease. *J Occup Med* 1978;20:103–110.
90. Ramirez J, Dowell AR. Silo filler's disease: nitrogen dioxide induced lung injury—long-term follow-up and review of the literature. *Ann Intern Med* 1971;74:569–576.
91. Milne JEH. Nitrogen dioxide inhalation and bronchiolitis obliterans. *J Occup Med* 1969;11:538–547.
92. Clutton-Brock J. Two cases of poisoning by contamination of nitrous oxide with higher oxides of nitrogen during anesthesia. *Br J Anaesth* 1967;39:388–392.
93. Prys-Roberts C. Principles of treatment of poisoning by higher oxides of nitrogen. *Br J Anaesth* 1967;39:432–438.

CHAPTER 18
Clinical Hepatotoxicity

Caryl S. Brailsford, Samir M. Douidar, and Wayne R. Snodgrass

The liver, as the main organ responsible for the metabolism of xenobiotics, is particularly susceptible to injury from drugs and environmental toxins (1). A wide variety of substances that induce liver toxicity are recognized. These include natural hepatotoxins, such as products of plants (fungal or bacterial metabolites) and minerals (2); products of the chemical or pharmaceutical industry (3); or industrial by-products and waste materials that, by polluting the environment, may gain access to humans (4,5) (Table 18-1). Chemical-induced hepatic injury follows three general patterns: cytotoxic injury causing hepatocellular necrosis, cholestatic injury, or mixed hepatocellular and cholestatic injury. Cytotoxic injury involves liver parenchyma and produces necrosis, fatty change, and cirrhosis. Cholestatic injury can result in interference with bile secretion and in jaundice. Often, liver injury is a mixture of both (6,7). Carcinoma can also be a manifestation of chemical-induced hepatic injury.

Drug- and chemical-induced liver disease may be so clinically subtle that estimates of incidence are influenced by the method used to identify cases. Laboratory screening of all persons at risk most certainly detects liver injury more often than reliance on clinical symptoms or signs. However, this approach may be overly sensitive, and positive results may or may not be indicative of significant hepatotoxicity. On the other hand, routine tests may not be sensitive enough to detect other drug-induced liver disease (e.g., chronic methotrexate therapy) or toxic exposure–related liver disease (e.g., angiosarcoma that is due to vinyl chloride). Also, in some cases, these toxicities may appear gradually, after several months or years of exposure, making detection difficult. Testing either by laboratory methods or imaging techniques may not be able to discriminate between occupationally induced hepatotoxicity and hepatotoxicity caused by nonindustrial exposures or health problems.

Medical screening and surveillance for hepatotoxicity that is due to environmental and occupational chemical exposure have become important for documenting workers' health and safety. Hepatic injury can be acute, subacute, or chronic. Fortunately, because of improved industrial hygiene monitoring of the most serious hepatotoxins, acute hepatotoxicity is rare. It is now more likely that hepatotoxicity will manifest as subacute and chronic hepatic injury. However, current laboratory methods of detecting hepatic damage remain best at detecting acute hepatotoxicity. Subacute or chronic hepatic disease is much more difficult to screen for, because the methods used may not detect the damage done or may be overly sensitive, leading to unnecessary detection of false-positive results (8) or, more importantly, may miss true subacute or chronic disease (high false-negatives). Screening and surveillance programs must be structured with this in mind.

Mechanisms of liver toxicity include the following (7):

- Lipid peroxidation
- Reactive oxygen species formation
- Covalent binding to liver protein
- Glutathione depletion
- Peroxisome proliferation
- Interference with protein synthesis
- Plasma membrane damage

TABLE 18-1. Chemical classes of hepatotoxic agents

A. Inorganic agents
  - Metals and metalloids: antimony, arsenic, beryllium, bismuth, boron, cadmium, chromium, cobalt, copper, iron, lead, manganese, mercury, gold, phosphorus, selenium, tellurium, thallium, zinc
  - Hydrazine derivatives
  - Iodides

B. Organic agents
  - Natural
    - Plant toxins: albitocin, cycasin, icterogenin, indospicine, lanthana, ngaione, nutmeg, pyrrolidizine, safrole, tannic acid
    - Mycotoxins: aflatoxins, cyclochlorotine, ethanol, luteoskyrins, ochratoxins, rubratoxins, sterigmatocystins, and other antibiotics
    - Bacterial toxins: exotoxins (*Corynebacterium diphtheria, Clostridium botulinum, Streptococcus hemolyticus*), endotoxins, ethionine
  - Synthetic
    - Nonmedicinal
      - Haloalkanes and halolefins
      - Nitroalkanes
      - Organic amines
      - Azo compounds
      - Phenol and derivatives
      - Various other organic compounds
    - Medicinal agents
      - Antibiotics: chloramphenicol, erythromycin estolate, erythromycin ethyl succinate, penicillins, cephalosporins, novobiocin, rifampicin, tetracyclines, sulfonamides, nitrofurans, clindamycin, spectinomycin, sulfones, and quinolones
      - Antifungal agents: amphotericin, 5-fluorocytosine, griseofulvin, ketoconazole, and saramycetin
      - Antimetazoal and antiprotozoal agents: emetine, amodiaquine, carbarsone, 8-hydroxyquinolines, metronidazole, thiabendazole, hycanthone, and mepacrine
      - Antituberculous agents: cycloserine, isoniazid, rifampicin, *p*-aminosalicylic acid, and ethionamide
      - Antiviral agents: cytarabine, idoxuridine, vidarabine, and xenylamine
      - Endocrine agents: antithyroid drugs, oral hypoglycemics, and steroids (e.g., oral contraceptives, anabolic C-17, glucocorticoids, and tamoxifen)
      - Anesthetic agents: halothane, methoxyflurane, ether, chloroform, nitrous oxide, and cyclopropane
      - Psychotropic agents: phenothiazines, thioxanthenes, butyrophenones, benzodiazepines, monoamine oxidase inhibitors, and tricyclic antidepressants
      - Anticonvulsants: phenytoin, phenobarbital, valproic acid, and mephenytoin
      - Analgesics and nonsteroidal antiinflammatory drugs: acetaminophen, salicylates, indomethacin, diflunisal, ibuprofen, sulindac, phenylbutazone, naproxen, and fenoprofen
      - Cardiovascular agents: anticoagulants, antiarrhythmics (e.g., quinidine, procainamide, verapamil, and nifedipine), antihypertensives (e.g., hydralazine, methyldopa, and captopril), diuretic agents, antianginal agents, and antihyperlipidemic agents
      - Antineoplastic agents
      - Miscellaneous drugs: colchicine, allopurinol, cimetidine, disulfiram, vitamin A, iodide ion, thorotrast, ranitidine, British anti-Lewisite penicillamine, dantrolene, zoxazolamine, and others

Modified from Zimmerman HJ. *The adverse effects of drugs and other chemicals on the liver.* New York: Appleton-Century-Crofts, 1978:4.

ANATOMY AND PHYSIOLOGY

Because of its anatomy and physiology, the liver is uniquely sensitive to xenobiotic damage. The liver receives blood from two sources. The portal system brings venous blood from the gut. The liver also receives arterial blood from the hepatic artery. In

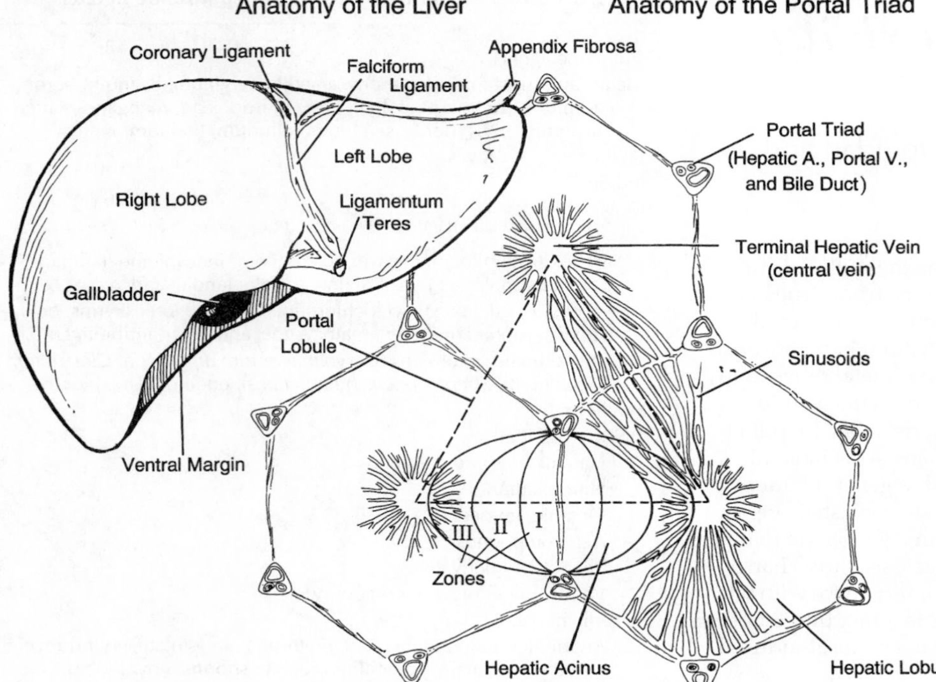

Figure 18-1. Functional acinus zones. Zone I: periportal zone. Highest concentration of O_2, nutrients, hormones, and unmetabolized xenobiotics. Also has high concentration of glycogen synthesis enzymes and mitochondria. Zone II: intermediate zone. Zone III: Receives blood with lower O_2 tension. Less active in glycogen and protein synthesis. More active in glycogen storage and fat formation. Contains high concentration of enzymes for chemical biotransformation, cytochrome P-450 system.

addition, lymphatics from the gut travel to the liver. Toxins that are ingested, inhaled, then swallowed, or produced by gut bacteria enter the liver through portal blood. Inhaled gases and dermally absorbed toxicants enter the liver through the arterial system via the hepatic artery. The liver receives approximately 25% of the cardiac output. Of the total hepatic blood flow, 25% is arterial from the hepatic artery, and 75% is venous from the portal veins (and thus deoxygenated).

The hepatic artery and portal vein branch together with the lymphatics and sympathetic nerves to form the portal triad. The bile-collecting system forms the last constituent of the portal triad. The blood travels from the portal triad through the hepatic sinusoids and is collected in the terminal hepatic vein. The endothelium has wide fenestrations in the sinusoids, and the hepatocytes have microvilli, which increase surface area to absorb materials from the plasma. After percolating through the sinusoids, blood is collected into the terminal hepatic vein, where it rejoins the systemic circulation (9).

The functional unit of the liver is the acinus. The area around the portal triad is called *zone I*, or the *periportal area*. The area surrounding the portal vein is called *zone III*, or the *peripheral* or *centrilobular area*. *Zone II* is intermediate between zones I and III (10). Older descriptions of hepatic microanatomy were based on nonfunctional histologic patterns, whereas the zonal description of the acinus is based on the physiologic microstructure as described by Rappaport (10) (Fig. 18-1).

The blood in zone I contains the highest concentration of oxygen, nutrients, hormones, and unmetabolized xenobiotics. Zone I cells have a higher concentration of glycogen synthesis enzymes, as well as a high concentration of mitochondria involved in the Krebs cycle. More protein synthesis also occurs in zone I (10).

Zone III cells receive blood with a lower oxygen tension and are less active in glycogen and protein synthesis. However, the glucose/glycogen systems can vary in concentrations between zone I and zone III, depending on nutritional status and other factors (11). Zone III is more active in glycogen storage and fat formation (10). Most important to toxicology is the high concentration of enzyme systems for biotransformation in zone III. Most notable is the cytochrome P-450 system, also called the *mixed function oxidase system* (*MFO*) (12). Associated enzymes, such as nicotinamide adenine phosphate dehydrogenase cytochrome c-reductase are also highest in zone III. MFO and nicotinamide adenine phosphate dehydrogenase cytochrome c-reductase, are formed in and located on the endoplasmic reticulum (10). Agents that induce cytochrome P-450 function also increase the smooth endoplasmic reticulum in zone III cells (13).

HEPATIC CELL METABOLISM OF XENOBIOTICS

Many organic xenobiotic agents are lipid soluble. To be excreted in the urine, they must be made more polar or water soluble. A molecule can be made more polar by oxidation or hydrolysis. It can be made more polar by attaching another molecule that can facilitate excretion into the bile or kidney. The liver adds both types of groups to accomplish this excretion.

These reactions are divided into two sequential sets of reactions: phase I and phase II. Phase I reactions make a compound more polar by oxidation, reduction, or hydrolysis (14). Phase II reactions modify components—generally by conjugation reactions—to make a compound more excretable and, in some cases, to make a product less toxic (15). The hepatic toxicity of many xenobiotics is due to phase I (or sometimes phase II) biotransformation (16). The metabolism of a toxic chemical can have three outcomes: It can become less toxic; it can be metabolized to a more toxic intermediate, which is subsequently detoxified; or it can be bioactivated to a more toxic metabolite, which can cause cellular damage (Fig. 18-2).

Phase I reactions occur predominantly in the hepatic smooth endoplasmic reticulum of zone III but are not limited to that location. The major reaction types and substrates are:

- *Flavin-containing monooxygenase*: oxidation of tertiary and secondary amines, hydrazines, thioamides, thiols, disulfides, amino thiols, imines, and aryl amines

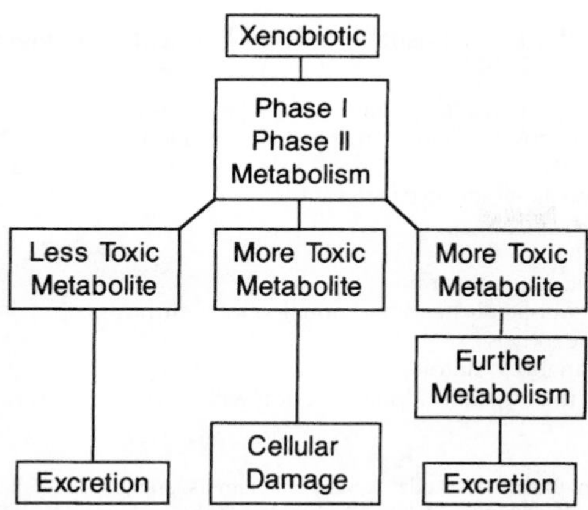

Figure 18-2. Possible outcomes of xenobiotic metabolism.

- *Epoxide hydrolase*: hydrates, arene oxides, and aliphatic epoxides
- *Esterases and amidases*: hydrolytic cleavage of esters, amides, and thioesters
- *Alcohol, aldehyde, ketone oxidation, and reduction systems*: oxidation, dehydrogenation, or reduction of alcohols, aldehydes, and ketones
- *MFO (P-450)*: hydroxylation of aliphatic and aromatic structures; epoxidation of alkenes; oxidative deamination of aliphatic structures with a primary amino group; oxidative dealkylation of a carbon group attached to an O, N, S atom; oxidation of sulfur and nitrogen or desulfurization of sulfur-containing organic compounds; and oxidative dehalogenation of halogenated compounds
- *Microsomal (P-450)-mediated reductions*: azo and aromatic nitro compounds and reductive dehalogenations

Phase I reactions biotransform many chemicals. The xenobiotic is biotransformed to a more reactive molecule by this metabolism, and then a more chemically stable—and more or less toxic—molecule can be formed. For example, a possibly more toxic, reactive, electrophilic molecule can be formed, which can then alkylate proteins, DNA, or lipids. Free radicals can also be formed; these very active molecules participate in a self-propagating chain reaction of free-radical transfer in the cell. Free radicals can cause peroxidation of lipid structures in the cell, inactive proteins, and DNA (17). Phase I reactions can be induced, causing a much greater capacity for metabolism through phase I reactions. Phenobarbital and 3-methyl-cholanthrene are notable inducers of phase I metabolism (18). If a toxic metabolite is created by phase I metabolism, then coadministration of an inducer will increase the production of toxic metabolites.

Phase II reactions occur both in the endoplasmic reticulum and in the cytosol. They require energy, usually adenosine triphosphate, and add functional groups, which increase molecular weight (17). In many cases, they inactivate toxic intermediates formed in phase I reactions (14). Most also require cofactors. Major phase II reactions are the following:

- *Glucuronidation*: adds glucuronic acid to a wide variety of functional groups, including aliphatic and aromatic alcohols, carboxyl acids, primary and secondary aromatic and aliphatic amines, and free sulfhydryl groups; promotes excretion of the substrate by liver and kidney organic acid transport systems
- *Sulfotransferase*: transfers inorganic sulfate to hydroxyl groups, commonly aliphatic alcohols and phenols [Cysteine, required as a sulfur source, can be rate limiting. Sulfate conjugates are renally excreted (17).]
- N-*Acetyl transferases*: acetylates arylamines, hydrazines, hydrazides, sulfonamides, and primary aliphatic amines; the rate of acetylation can be genetically variable (17)
- *Amino acid conjugation*: acts on groups containing a carboxylic acid group, most commonly glycine, glutamine, and serine [Concentrations of these amino acids can affect the rate of conjugation (17).]
- *Glutathione* S-*transferase*: important phase II enzyme that can detoxify highly reactive intermediates; acts on electrophilic intermediates and is a cofactor for glutathione peroxidase, which inactivates lipid peroxidation (14)

MORPHOLOGIC PATTERNS OF HEPATIC INJURY

Phase I and phase II reactions can contribute to the biotransformation of hazardous chemicals. These products of biotransformation are often the agents that ultimately cause hepatocellular damage. Regardless of the etiology of hepatocellular damage, the liver can only make a few pathologic responses. Hepatic injury from any source can manifest as steatosis, necrosis, cholestasis, fibrosis/cirrhosis, or cancer. The main types of morphologic changes in the liver produced by chemicals, drugs, and other agents are listed in Table 18-2.

Steatosis

Steatosis, or fatty liver, often is an early sign of hepatotoxicity. It is associated with a decrease in the concentration of plasma lipids and plasma lipoproteins as demonstrated by studies with

TABLE 18-2. Morphologic types of drug-induced liver diseases

Type	Examples
Zonal necrosis	Acetaminophen, carbon tetrachloride
Nonspecific hepatitis	Aspirin, oxacillin
Viral hepatitis-like lesion	Isoniazid, methyldopa, halothane
Chronic active hepatitis	Methyldopa, dantrolene, isoniazid, propylthiouracil, sulfonamides, papaverine, clometacin
Cholestasis	
Hepatocanalicular	Chlorpromazine, erythromycin estolate, organic arsenicals
Canalicular	Estrogens, anabolic steroids
Fatty liver	
Large globules	Ethanol, corticosteroids
Small droplets	Tetracycline, valproic acid
Vascular lesions	
Hepatic vein thrombosis	Oral contraceptives
Venoocclusive disease	Certain antineoplastic agents
Peliosis hepatis	Anabolic steroids
Noncirrhotic portal hypertension	Vinyl chloride
Cirrhosis	Ethanol, methotrexate, chronic hepatitis-inducing drugs except glucocorticoids
Tumors	
Adenoma	Oral contraceptives, androgens
Focal nodular hyperplasia	Oral contraceptives
Carcinoma	Oral contraceptives, thorotrast, vinyl chloride, anabolic steroids
Angiosarcoma	Thorotrast, vinyl chloride, arsenic, copper sulfate

From Ockner RK. Drug-induced liver disease. In: Zakim D, Boyer T, eds. *Hepatology: a textbook of liver disease.* Philadelphia: WB Saunders, 1982:693, with permission.

carbon tetrachloride. Carbon tetrachloride can interfere with the synthesis of the protein for triglyceride export from the liver. A similar mechanism likely is involved in other fatty liver damage (19). Other suspected occupationally occurring causes of steatosis include chlorinated and aromatic hydrocarbons, hydrazine derivatives, pesticides, and phosphorus (20).

Necrosis

Carbon tetrachloride has been extensively used to demonstrate possible mechanisms of hepatocellular necrosis. It seems likely that the final irreversible step in necrosis is disruption of calcium homeostasis. Calcium ions influx as a result of damage to the plasma membrane and other vital cell structures. This influx of calcium ions inactivates mitochondria, inhibits enzymes, and denatures structural proteins (21).

The cellular mechanism resulting in the disruption of calcium homeostasis is unclear. Studies on carbon tetrachloride demonstrate that inhibition of protein synthesis occurs before calcium homeostasis disruption via damage to ribosomes by carbon tetrachloride metabolites. Lipid peroxidation in the endoplasmic reticulum, which is involved with both calcium ion and triglyceride excretion, occurs in carbon tetrachloride–induced necrosis (17). How this explains necrosis for other hepatotoxins is unclear, but a similar mechanism is likely.

Cholestasis

Cholestasis is poorly understood but can be due to bile flow alterations, bile permeability, or dysfunction of microfilaments involved in bile transport (22). This may be caused by membrane damage or immune damage caused by a chemical or its metabolite. It can acutely be detected by elevations of serum bilirubin and alkaline phosphatase. In the case of chemically induced cholestatic liver disease, more common causes, such as obstructive cholestasis, must be ruled out. Histologically, bile plugs in the canaliculi may be observed, or an exudative reaction of the portal tracts may occur. Mild hepatocellular necrosis may also be observed (23). Occupationally occurring compounds associated with cholestasis include methylenediamine, toluene diisocyanate, and paraquat (20).

Fibrosis and Cirrhosis

Fibrosis and cirrhosis are the end result of ongoing hepatic injury. Septate of collagen are deposited throughout the liver, leading to distortion of the hepatic circulation. It is the disruption of circulation that leads to portal hypertension and the clinical syndrome associated with end-stage liver disease. It is associated most commonly with hepatitis and chronic ethanol use and has been observed in chronic carbon tetrachloride exposure (24). The mechanism is not clear, but increased collagen proline synthesis has been observed (20). Early fibrosis has also been demonstrated after exposure to organic solvents, such as trichloroethylene and 1,1,1-trichloroethane (25,26). Other compounds associated with cirrhosis include arsenicals, pesticides, dimethylnitrosamine, and hydrocarbons (20).

Hepatic Carcinogenesis

Hepatic carcinogenesis has been demonstrated for a number of naturally occurring and industrially produced chemicals. For many agents, the exact mechanism of tumor production has not been determined. Carcinogenesis involves a two-step process of induction followed by a long latent period, during which neoplasm develops. A promoter is required during this latent period to produce a cancer. Most chemical carcinogens act as initiators by causing structural damage to DNA (27). Several human hepatic carcinogens have been identified (Table 18-3). Some are industrially produced chemicals, but many are naturally occurring biological agents.

TABLE 18-3. Suspected liver chemical carcinogens

Aflatoxin (*Aspergillus flavus* and *Aspergillus parasiticus*)
Other mycotoxins (fumonisin, sterigmatocystin, luteoskyrin, cyclochlorotine)
Plant alkaloids
Pyrrolizidine alkaloids: cycasin, safrole
Nitrosamines
Nitrosamides
Heterocyclic aromatic amines
Ethanol (alcoholic cirrhosis and nonalcoholic cirrhosis)
Oral contraceptives
Androgen-anabolic steroids
Thorotrast (ThO_2)—emits alpha radiation with a half-life of 1.4×10^{10} yr
Azo dyes

Adapted from Okuda K, Okuda H. Malignant tumors: primary liver cell carcinoma. In: Bircher J, Benhamou J, McIntyre N, Rizzetto M, Rodes J, eds. *Oxford textbook of clinical hepatology*, vol. 2, 2nd ed. Oxford: Oxford Medical Publications, 1999:1491; Degunier Y, Turlin B. Other causes of hepatocellular carcinoma. In: Okuda K, Tabor E, eds. *Liver cancer.* New York: Churchill Livingstone, 1997:97.

Occupationally induced liver carcinoma is well described for angiosarcoma of the liver (28). Arsenicals and dimethylnitrosamine are also associated with hepatocellular carcinoma (20).

CLASSIFICATION OF HEPATOTOXINS AND MECHANISMS OF TOXICITY

Hepatotoxins are classified into two main categories: predictable (intrinsic) and unpredictable (idiosyncratic) (29). Predictable hepatotoxicity is usually dose related, can be produced in experimental animals, and usually affects a particular region of the hepatic lobule. Unpredictable or idiosyncratic hepatotoxicity occurs in unusually susceptible persons, cannot be reproduced in experimental animals, and is usually in a diffuse form (Fig. 18-3).

Intrinsic Hepatotoxins

The mechanism by which intrinsic, predictable hepatotoxins and their metabolic products induce hepatic injury falls into two main categories: direct and indirect (24,30). Direct hepatotoxins act by a physicochemical destruction of hepatocyte membranes through

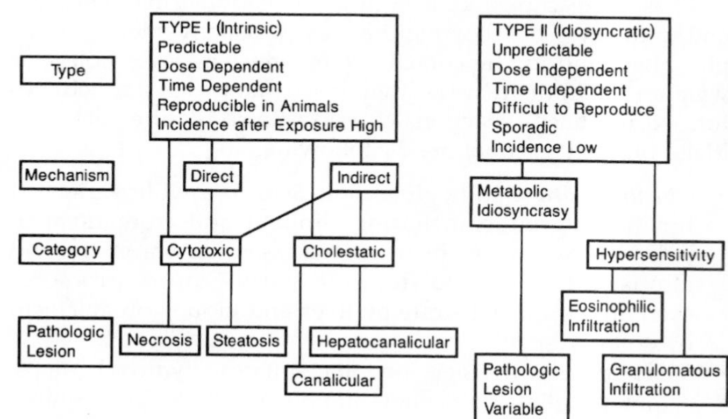

Figure 18-3. Classification of pathologic lesions produced by hepatotoxins.

peroxidation with free radicals or activated oxygen formation. This membrane injury is the first step in direct hepatotoxicity, which ends in either cell necrosis or steatosis. Few intrinsic hepatotoxins produce injury by a direct mechanism; examples are carbon tetrachloride (CCl_4), several other halogenated hydrocarbons, acetaminophen, and yellow phosphorus (22,31,32).

Most intrinsic hepatotoxins produce injury by indirect mechanisms. This injury results from a binding of the toxic agent or its products to cell membranes or molecules, which leads to distortion of physiologic or biochemical pathways essential for cell integrity. This binding may be covalent (e.g., acetaminophen and bromobenzene) or noncovalent (e.g., phalloidin) (33–35). Covalent binding appears to be the most important form of indirect hepatotoxicity. Protection against the toxic effects of covalent binding is provided by glutathione, which itself binds covalently to the reactive electrophilic metabolites of toxic agents (e.g., acetaminophen), converting them to nontoxic products that are readily excreted (36). Also, glutathione serves to reduce peroxides and so provides protection against the peroxidation by activated oxygen (32,37).

The hepatotoxic damage produced by indirect hepatotoxins may by either cytotoxic (expressed as steatosis or necrosis) or cholestatic (expressed as arrested bile flow).

Cytotoxic indirect hepatotoxins cause hepatic injury by interfering with metabolic pathways essential for parenchymal cell integrity. The biochemical and physiologic lesions induced by these agents lead to steatosis, necrosis, or both. Examples of agents that produce steatosis are tetracyclines (38), L-asparaginase (39), methotrexate (40), aflatoxin (24), and puromycin (41). Agents that cause necrosis include bromobenzene (42), 6-mercaptopurine (43), urethane (44), and thioacetamide (24). Some agents produce both steatosis and necrosis, such as toxins of amanita phalloides and tannic acid (24).

Ethanol can be classified as an indirect hepatotoxin. It leads to fatty metamorphosis by a number of adverse effects on hepatocyte metabolism (45). It also can lead to necrosis, perhaps by the effects of acetaldehyde (46) or by increasing oxygen requirements of hepatocytes (47). Ethanol also potentiates the hepatotoxic effects of a number of known toxic agents through induction of the MFO system and consequent enhancement of biotransformation of these agents to toxic metabolites (48,49). Of special clinical importance is the enhancement of the hepatotoxic effects of chlorinated hydrocarbons (50) and acetaminophen (51) by ethanol. Many cytotoxic indirect hepatotoxins are hepatocarcinogens, which likely happens through alkylation or arylation of DNA (52).

Cholestatic indirect hepatotoxins, on the other hand, produce jaundice or impaired liver function by selective interference with hepatic mechanisms of excretion into the bile canaliculi, by injury to bile ducts, or by inhibition of hepatocellular uptake from the blood of substances destined for biliary excretion (24). Cholestatic indirect hepatotoxins of clinical significance include methyltestosterone and some C-17 alkylated anabolic steroids, such as ethinyl estrogen and progesterone derivatives used as oral contraceptives (43,53,54). The effect of these agents is dose related but modified by the individual susceptibility of the recipient. As an example, oral contraceptives are likely to produce jaundice in women who have had the benign cholestatic jaundice of pregnancy, a syndrome with a genetic basis (55). Most agents causing cholestatic disease are drugs rather than industrial or chemical hazardous materials (24).

The mechanism for the impaired function induced by these anabolic, progestational, and estrogenic steroids is unknown. There is evidence that indicates a precise structural requirement to induce injury, namely an alkyl group at C-17. Testosterone, which lacks this type of substituent, does not lead to impaired function, whereas methyl testosterone with the C-17 methyl group does (24).

There are several agents that produce cholestasis by selectively damaging the ductal system. 4,4-Diaminodiphenylmethane, a plastics hardener, led to an epidemic of cholestatic jaundice in England as a result of its presence as a contaminant of flour (56). A similar lesion has been reported in Spain as the result of ingestion of rapeseed oil contaminated with aniline (57). Paraquat poisoning also can produce ductal destruction (58). 5-Fluorouridine given by infusion through the hepatic artery in the treatment of metastatic carcinoma of the liver leads to an injury of the biliary tree resembling sclerosing cholangitis (59). Mycotoxins such as sporidesmin mainly cause ductal injury in some species (60).

Idiosyncratic Unpredictable Hepatotoxins

Many drugs unpredictably produce hepatic injury in a small proportion of recipients. Two mechanisms of idiosyncratic hepatic injury have been recognized: hypersensitivity and metabolic aberration.

Hypersensitivity-related hepatic injury develops after a relatively fixed sensitization period of 1 to 5 weeks and recurs promptly on readministration of the agent. It tends to be accompanied by systemic (fever, rash, eosinophilia) and histologic (eosinophil-rich or granulomatous inflammatory infiltrate in the liver) evidence of hypersensitivity. These hallmarks of hypersensitivity, especially when supported by a recurrence of the syndrome in response to a challenge dose, permit the inference that the hepatic injury is due to drug allergy and that the drug or a metabolite has acted as a hapten.

Lack of these hallmarks of hypersensitivity suggests that the idiosyncrasy may be the result of a metabolic aberration rather than of hypersensitivity. This is strongly supported by the observations of Spielberg and coworkers (61), who found that patients who had sustained hepatic injury in a hypersensitivity-type reaction to phenytoin had an apparent defect in converting the active metabolite (arene oxide) to the inactive dihydrodiol. The active metabolite probably acts as a hapten or may be cytotoxic.

Even among the agents that appear to produce hepatic injury related to hypersensitivity, there appear to be several categories. The circumstantial evidence for the role of hypersensitivity is most strongly suggestive for those drugs that produce hepatic injury only in association with systemic features suggestive of an allergic response, such as phenytoin (62). The role of hypersensitivity is somewhat less clear for drugs such as chlorpromazine, erythromycin estolate, and halothane, which produce hepatic injury that may or may not be accompanied by systemic features suggestive of drug allergy (53). On the other hand, drugs that cause systemic hypersensitivity do not necessarily cause hepatic injury, such as penicillin and procainamide (63). Furthermore, there are drugs that produce hepatic injury without clinical features of hypersensitivity. Some of these respond promptly to a challenge dose [e.g., ticrynafen-associated hepatic injury (64)], whereas others do not (e.g., isoniazid and valproic acid).

It has been hypothesized that hypersensitivity leads to hepatic injury only when the respective drug has some intrinsic hepatotoxic potential. Those reactions that do not resemble serum sickness but are provoked by a challenge dose may be the result of hypersensitivity, but by a different immunologic mechanism (3). Hypersensitivity and metabolic idiosyncratic reactions can also occur in occupationally induced liver injury (65).

FACTORS AFFECTING HEPATOTOXICITY

A variety of factors can influence both hepatic metabolism and hepatotoxicity of toxic chemicals, usually via modification of MFO or other phase I reaction. In many cases, induction of P-450

MFO system can lead to the increased production of a toxic metabolite by favoring a biotransformation pathway, which leads to that toxic product. The most notable inducer is ethanol, but other factors influence metabolism and toxicity as well.

MFO function can be modified in a number of ways. It can be induced by drugs like phenobarbital, but many xenobiotics also produce P-450 enzyme system induction. Histologically, proliferation of the hepatic smooth endoplasmic reticulum occurs, predominantly in zone III when MFO induction occurs. Inducers of MFO include synthetic steroids, ethanol, 1,1,1-trichloroethane, polyhalogenated aromatics including DDT, polychlorinated or brominated biphenyls, tetrachlorodibenzodioxin (66), aldrin, hexachlorobenzene lindane, and chlordane (17). The P-450 system can be induced by cigarette smoking and consumption of charcoal-broiled foods (18).

The MFO system can be inhibited in a variety of ways as well. The activity of the MFO system can influence how a compound is metabolized, thus influencing the type of intermediate produced, and therefore modifying the toxicity produced. Other factors that influence the P-450 MFO systems are the following:

- *Nutritional state*: Calcium, copper, iron, magnesium, and zinc deficiencies decrease MFO activities. Vitamin deficiencies (ascorbic acid, tocopherol, and B-complex) decrease MFO function, as does starvation. Low-protein diets increase the toxicity of some xenobiotics.
- *Age*: Newborn and fetal animals are less able to biotransform xenobiotics by MFO. Old age increases toxicity of some agents; however, this may be due to factors other than the MFO system (i.e., decreased blood flow, uptake, or renal excretion).
- *Genetic factors*: Multiple isozymes of MFO system exist, and the distribution of these can be genetically influenced (17,18). This will determine biotransformation products by favoring some reactions. Some phase II enzyme systems, such as acetylases, are also genetically variable (16). There are also some differences between species regarding distribution of types of P-450 isozymes, which must be considered when extrapolating from animal data (18).
- *Gender*: Gender influences proportions of MFO isozymes in rats. This has not been reproduced in humans (17,18).
- *Physical activity and smoking cigarettes*: These also influence the MFO system.

The ingestion of ethanol increases the toxicity of carbon tetrachloride and trichloroethylene (67). Ethanol and trichloroethylene are both metabolized by alcohol dehydrogenase, and concurrent administration of both competitively inhibit each other's metabolism and prolong the half-life of both agents (68). Methylene chloride toxicity was increased when chronically administered with ethanol for 5 days. However, when ethanol and methylene chloride were administered at high dose for 1 day, the toxic effects were antagonized (69). Chloroform toxicity likewise is increased by coadministration with ethanol. Manganese and mercury toxicity may also be increased by ethanol (70). Blood concentrations of xylene, styrene, toluene, and trichloroethylene are all increased with concurrent ethanol administration (71).

Several toxins inhibit ethanol metabolism similar to the drug disulfiram. Disulfiramlike reactions are caused by the buildup of the metabolite acetaldehyde, which causes tachycardia, flushing, and throbbing headache, and can lead to cardiovascular collapse. Hepatic alcohol dehydrogenase is inhibited by some amides, pesticidal dithiocarbamates, thirams, carbamates, cyanamides, nitroglycerol, and some oximes (72), as do carbon disulfide and dimethylformamide (Table 18-4) (73). Solvents also influence the metabolism of other solvents. In most cases, the long-term effects of the altered metabolism by ethanol and solvent mixtures are unknown. However, ethanol may potentiate the angiosarcoma rate from vinyl chloride exposure (72).

TABLE 18-4. Chemical: ethanol metabolic interactions

Disulfiram reactions	Enhancement of solvent hepatotoxicity
Amides	Halogenated hydrocarbons
Dimethyl formamide	Carbon tetrachloride
	Trichloroethylene
Oximes	Methylene chloride
N-Butyraldoxime	
Cyclohexanone oxime	
Methyl ethyl ketoxime	Metals
Acetaldoxime	Manganese
Isobutyladoxime	Mercury
Thirams	Vinyl chloride
Disulfiram	Xylene
Carbamates	
Pyrazole	Styrene
Ziram	Toluene
Manam	
Sulfonureas	Carbon disulfide
Nitroglycerol	
Cyanamide	
Calcium cyanamide	
N-Butyramide	
Isobutyramide	
Trichloroethylene	
Carbon disulfide	

From Hills BW, Venable HL. The interaction of ethyl alcohol and industrial chemicals. *Am J Ind Med* 1982;3:321–333; Dossing M. Metabolic interactions between organic solvents and other chemicals. In: Riihimaki V, Ulfvarson U, eds. *Safety and health aspects of organic solvents.* New York: Alan R. Liss, 1986:97–105.

NONOCCUPATIONAL EXPOSURE TO HEPATOTOXINS

Not all hepatotoxicity is caused by industrial exposure or medication administration. Hepatotoxins that may be encountered in the home include chemical toxins (e.g., CCl_4, yellow phosphorus, copper salts), botanical agents (e.g., mycotoxins), and large overdoses of ordinarily safe drugs (e.g., acetaminophen, ferrous salts, salicylates) (Table 18-5).

Poisonous mushrooms are still an important cause of acute hepatic necrosis injury (60,74). Food contaminated with aflatoxins has been implicated in the causation of acute hepatic disease as well as in etiology of hepatic carcinoma (61,62,75,76). Pyrrolidine alkaloid toxicity has been reported as a cause of hepatic disease in the United States and other parts of the world. Some items obtained in "natural food" stores and some health remedies sold in pharmacies in the southwestern region of the United States have been reported to contain pyrrolidine alkaloids (63,77). Exposure to these hepatotoxins can confuse evaluation of liver disease from industrially produced chemicals or occupational exposures to hepatotoxic agents.

Widely employed insecticides include a number of chlorinated aromatic hydrocarbons, some of which are hepatotoxic in large doses. Exposure of humans to these agents may be through contaminated food, occupational exposure, or accidental ingestion. Long-term storage in human tissues of DDT and other insecticides and their metabolites has been demonstrated (64,78). Nevertheless, there is no significant evidence of hepatic injury from sustained occupational exposure to the chlorinated insecticides (21). Accidental ingestion of large amounts of DDT

TABLE 18-5. Routes of exposure to hepatotoxic agents

- Toxicologic
  - Occupational
    - Routine exposure to toxic agents
    - Accidental exposure
  - Domestic
    - Accidental or suicidal exposure
    - Ingestions of toxic contaminant food
    - Exposure to euphoric toxic agents as a form of drug abuse
    - Autogenic (synthesis in gastrointestinal tract of nitrosamines, ethionine, lithocholate)
  - Environmental
    - Pollution, food, or water; pesticides, industrial pollution
    - Pollution of atmosphere (hypothetical hepatotoxic hazard)
    - Natural hepatotoxins
- Pharmaceutical
  - Iatrogenic
  - Self-medication (drug overdose)

From Zimmerman HJ. *Hepatotoxicity: the adverse effects of drugs and other chemicals on the liver.* New York: Appleton-Century-Crofts, 1978:4, with permission.

(approximately 6 g) (65,79) and of paraquat (approximately 20 g) (66,80), however, has led to rare instances of centrilobular hepatic necrosis, which has been fatal. Paraquat also has been reported to lead to destruction of intrahepatic bile ducts and cholestasis (53). In general, overt acute hepatic injury is a rare consequence of occupational exposure to toxic chemicals today.

IMPORTANT INDUSTRIALLY OCCURRING HEPATOTOXINS

To a large degree, the rate of overt, acute hepatotoxicity that is due to industrial agents has decreased as a result of the identification of a few agents that have been eliminated or hygienically controlled at the worksite. These agents include carbon disulfide, chloroform trichloroethylene, trichloroethane, toluene, halothane, and solvent mixtures (67,81). Other possible hepatotoxic agents, including metallic and inorganic compounds, have also been described (21). Agents that have been reported to cause occupationally induced hepatotoxicity in humans are included in Table 18-6.

Carbon tetrachloride and chloroform are accepted hepatotoxins. Carbon tetrachloride is metabolized to a free radical and interrupts protein synthesis, leading to steatosis and necrosis (21). A cross-sectional study of hepatic function in England showed that workers exposed to carbon tetrachloride showed significant differences between exposed workers and control subjects in alkaline phosphatase and gamma-glutamyl transferase levels; however, no clinical disease was shown. Three-year follow-up showed that the liver enzyme changes were stable (82). Chloroform acts by a different metabolite but causes steatosis and zone III necrosis (67).

Perchlorethylene is commonly used in dry-cleaning processes. Mild to moderate hepatic parenchymal changes were noted on ultrasound in 69% of dry-cleaning workers and were noted in only 39% in a comparison group of laundry workers. Elevations of alanine aminotransferase (ALT) of as much as 1.5 times compared with control subjects were noted in only 29% of the dry-cleaning workers. This suggests both hepatotoxicity of perchlorethylene and a lack of sensitivity of liver enzyme testing in detecting hepatotoxicity (83).

Trichloroethylene hepatotoxicity was demonstrated by intentional solvent sniffing. Elevations of ALT and aspartate aminotransferase (AST) have occurred. Liver biopsy demonstrated centrilobular fibrosis with repeated exposures. Cardiac and neurologic effects were also noted (68,84). A case report of industrial trichloroethylene exposure resulting in liver enzyme elevation without cholestasis with atypical lymphocytosis, eosinophilia, and erythematous, peeling skin rash with reoccurrence with reexposure suggests a possible sensitization or idiosyncratic reaction to trichloroethylene or one of its metabolites (85). In a study of screening tests for trichloroethylene, induced hepatotoxic effects have not been able to correlate abnormalities with exposure when controlled for age and alcohol use (86).

1,1,1-Trichloroethane (a similar halogenated hydrocarbon to carbon tetrachloride and trichloroethylene) has been noted to cause acute hepatotoxicity in rare instances (69,70,87,88). Liver biopsy after 1,1,1-trichloroethane overexposure has demonstrated eosinophilic infiltration in periportal cells and cholestasis. On electron microscopy, proliferation of peroxisomes and smooth endoplasmic reticulum occurred. This case also had symptoms consistent with hypersensitivity, namely fever and urticaria (71,72). Cirrhosis has also been described after recurrent episodes of exposure to trichloroethylene and 1,1,1-trichloroethane (73,74). However, a matched-pair study was unable to demonstrate the effect of low-level exposure to trichloroethylene on liver function laboratory tests (75,89).

Methylene chloride is a suspected hepatotoxin. A study of workers chronically exposed to relatively high levels of methylene chloride did not show any clinically significant difference in control workers and exposed worker workers for AST, ALT, or total bilirubin (90).

Toluene has been demonstrated to cause mild pericentral fatty change with an elevation of ALT/AST ratio from occupational exposure in a print shop (76,91). Other investigations have not found associations of liver enzyme abnormalities and hepatotoxicity with toluene exposure (77–79,92–94).

Dichloropropanol is associated with submassive hepatic necrosis after acute overexposure in two individuals with the same exposure. Follow-up investigation in an animal model using 1,3-dichloro-2-propanol showed similar results, suggesting that this is the active compound in dichloropropanol hepatotoxicity (95).

Solvent mixture exposure is often more common than isolated solvent exposure. Solvent mixtures have been investigated in the literature with conflicting results. Car painters using solvent mixtures of toluene, xylene, butyl acetate, and white spirit—plus other alcohols and ketones—showed no statistically significant elevation in liver function tests when compared with controls (80,96). House painters exposed to white spirit (which is a combination of aromatic and aliphatic hydrocarbons), paints and lacquers, xylene, petroleum spirits, toluene, methyl ethyl ketone, and occasional use of industrial alcohols demonstrated elevated aminotransferases. Biopsy results included significant steatosis with focal necrosis, enlarged portal tracts, and fibrosis (81,97).

Another study of solvent mixture exposure involving a mixture of isopropyl alcohol, toluene, methyl ethyl ketone, and ethyl acetate suggested that the sole cause of toxicity was due only to the toluene component of the mixture. There also appeared to be no interaction between the components of the solvent mixture to cause increased toxicity over the toxicity of the toluene alone (98).

Other studies of solvent mixtures in paint workers showed elevations in workers compared with control subjects but, when controlled for alcohol consumption and age, any differences between exposed and control groups were eliminated (99). This suggests that alcohol consumption was an important factor in occupational hepatotoxicity. Concurrent use of two or more hepatotoxic agents may cause potentiation of hepatotoxicity of one or both agents (100). Another study of house painters sug-

TABLE 18-6. Select occupational hepatotoxins

A. Aliphatic hydrocarbons
1. Alicyclic hydrocarbons, e.g., cyclopropane
2. *n*-Heptane
3. Turpentine

B. Alcohols
4. Allyl alcohol
5. Ethyl alcohol
6. Ethylene chlorohydrin
7. Methyl alcohol
8. Ethylene glycol ethers and derivatives

C. Ethers and epoxy compounds
9. Dioxane
10. Epichlorohydrin
11. Ethylene oxide
12. Ethyl ether

D. Acetates
13. Methyl, ethyl, *N*-propyl, isopropyl, *N*-butyl, and amyl
14. Ethyl silicate

E. Carboxylic acids and anhydrides
15. Phthalic anhydride

F. Aliphatic halogenated hydrocarbons
16. Carbon tetrachloride
17. Chloroform
18. Chloroprene
19. Dibromochloropropane
20. 1,2-Dibromoethane
21. 1,2-Dichloroethane
22. Ethylene dibromide
23. Ethylene dichloride
24. Methyl bromide
25. Methyl chloride
26. Methylene chloride
27. Propylene dichloride
28. Tetrachloroethane/tetrabromo
29. Tetrachloroethylene
30. 1,1,1-Tetrachloroethane
31. 1,1,2-Tetrachloroethane
32. Trichloroethylene
33. Vinyl chloride

G. Aliphatic amines
34. Ethanolamines
35. Ethylene diamine

H. Cyanides and nitriles
36. Acetonitrile
37. Acrylonitrile
38. Hydrogen cyanide

I. Aromatic hydrocarbons
39. Benzene
40. Diphenyl
41. Naphthalene
42. Styrene/ethyl benzene
43. Toluene
44. Xylene

J. Phenols and phenolic compounds
45. Cresol
46. Phenol

K. Aromatic halogenated hydrocarbons
47. Benzyl chloride
48. Chlorodiphenyls and derivatives
49. Chlorinated benzenes
50. Chlorinated naphthalenes
51. Polychlorinated biphenyls
52. Polybrominated biphenyls

L. Aromatic amines
53. 2-Acetylamino-fluorene
54. 3,3-Dichlorobenzidine and its salts
55. 4-Dimethylaminoazobenzene

M. Nitrocompounds
56. Dinitrobenzene
57. Dinitrophenol
58. Dinitrotoluene
59. Nitrobenzene
60. Nitroparaffins
61. Nitrophenol
62. Picric acid
63. Tetryl
64. Nitromethane
65. Trinitrotoluene
66. 2-Nitropropane

N. Miscellaneous organic nitrogen compounds
67. Dimethylnitrosamine
68. *N,N*-Dimethylformamide
69. Ethylenediamine
70. Hydrazine and derivatives
71. Methylene dianiline
72. *N*-Nitrosodimethylamine
73. Pyridine
74. *N,N*-Dimethylacetamide

O. Miscellaneous organic chemicals
75. β-Propiolactone
76. Carbon disulfide
77. Dimethyl sulfate
78. Mercaptans
79. Tetramethylthiuram disulfide

P. Halogens
80. Bromide/hydrogen bromides

Q. Metallic compounds
81. Arsenic
82. Arsine
83. Beryllium
84. Bismuth and compounds
85. Boron and compounds (excluding the hydrides)
86. Boron hydrides
87. Cadmium and compounds
88. Carbonyls (metal)
89. Chromium and its compounds
90. Copper
91. Germanium
92. Iron
93. Naphthol
94. Nickel and compounds
95. Phosphine
96. Phosphorus and compounds (excluding phosphine)
97. Pyrogallol
98. Selenium and compounds
99. Stibine
100. Thallium and compounds
101. Thorium dioxide (Thorotrast)
102. Tin and compounds
103. Uranium and components

R. Pesticides
104. Bipyridyls
105. Thallium sulfate
106. Kepone

S. Physical hazards
107. Ionizing radiation
108. Vibration, whole body

Adapted from World Health Organization. *Early detection of occupational disease.* Geneva: World Health Organization, 1986; Davidson CS. Guidelines for hepatotoxicity due to drugs and chemicals. *NIH Publication No. 79-313.* Washington: Department of Health, Education, and Welfare, 1979.

gests that the interaction between solvent exposures and other medicinal and nonoccupational hepatotoxins is important in elevations of liver enzyme levels, more so than simply exposure to solvents. However, history of heavy exposure to organic solvents was also associated with changes in liver enzyme levels, even when recent exposure to solvents was minimal (101). This study also suggests that the interaction between exposure to both occupational and personal hepatotoxic agents (medications or alcohol) may have been important in the causation of hepatotoxicity.

These studies suggest that there may be some interactions between the components of solvent mixtures to cause cotoxicity, but in other circumstances, one component of the mixture (such as toluene) may dominate the toxicity. Investigations also suggest that ethanol consumption may dominate the toxicity of solvent exposures or may potentiate the toxicity of the solvent mixture, perhaps by induction of liver enzymes.

Carbon disulfide has caused fatty degeneration and hemorrhages of the liver in animals (102). It causes liver enlargement and periacinar degeneration and can inhibit drug-metabolizing enzymes (103).

Dimethylacetamide is a potential hepatotoxin. A case report of accidental overexposure to dimethylacetamide and ethylenediamine resulted in toxic hepatitis, rhabdomyolysis, esophagitis, conjunctivitis, skin burns, and hallucinations with delirium (104). Dimethylacetamide is suspected to be a hepatotoxin after chronic exposure. A large epidemiologic study of workers in an acrylic fiber plant did not show any correlation between exposure levels and liver chemistry tests (105,106).

Many other agents are suspected carcinogens (see Table 18-3). Most notable is vinyl chloride, which causes angiosarcoma.

CLINICAL EVALUATION OF HEPATOTOXICITY

Detection of hepatotoxicity caused by hazardous chemicals can be difficult. Investigation of acute liver injury is fairly routine clinically. Initial evaluation is usually done by measurement of liver enzyme levels. The assessment of chronic hepatotoxicity is less common and more difficult. Hepatotoxicity from occupational exposure is nonspecific (except in the case of vinyl chloride or methylene dianiline), and it is difficult to discriminate from many other causes of hepatotoxicity (107), especially by laboratory methods. Most of the tests for hepatotoxicity evaluation were developed to detect acute, severe liver damage.

This section first discusses the evaluation of acute hepatotoxicity. Screening for chronic hepatotoxicity is then addressed, with the application of tests commonly used in acute hepatic function evaluation as applied to chronic or subacute liver damage.

Acute Hepatic Toxicity

Because chemical- or drug-induced liver disease may present initially with quite nonspecific symptoms (e.g., fever or virallike syndrome), a thorough and careful history regarding medication, alcohol intake, drug or chemical abuse, exposure to chemicals, and type of occupation is essential. Occupational and environmental toxic exposures can produce acute toxicity (see Table 18-6). Medical history of other diseases, particularly those involving the liver, should be explored. Personal and family history of allergy or hypersensitivity to food, medication, or chemicals is important in idiosyncratic-mediated hepatitis.

When a patient presents with clinical or laboratory findings suggestive of impaired liver function, other diagnostic possibilities, which are not always easily distinguishable from chemical-induced liver injury, should be considered. These may include viral hepatitis (A, B, C, and others), systemic bacterial, fungal, rickettsial or parasitic diseases, postoperative intrahepatic cholestasis, choledocholithiasis and/or acute pancreatitis, bile duct injury, congestive heart failure, cancer, and deterioration of preexisting liver disease. This broad differential diagnosis, together with the fact that the hepatotoxic potentials of most newly introduced agents are not known, makes it necessary for the clinician to remain constantly alert to the possibility that a seemingly nonspecific, unfavorable turn of events or change in liver function may represent chemical-induced liver injury.

The chemical and biochemical manifestations of chemical- or drug-induced hepatic disease reflect the histologic pattern of injury. Hepatocellular injury with necrosis usually resembles viral hepatitis in both clinical and laboratory findings. This type of injury is associated with malaise, nausea, and vomiting followed by jaundice. High levels of aminotransferase enzymes (AST, ALT) and depressed levels of plasma coagulation factors are characteristic findings. The most useful clinical clues to severity of necrosis are the prothrombin time and serum bilirubin concentration (108,109).

Diffuse parenchymal degeneration with little necrosis, as in salicylate-induced hepatic injury, can lead to a syndrome resembling anicteric hepatitis (110). Toxic steatosis of the microvesicular type, as in tetracycline-induced hepatic injury, may lead to a syndrome resembling the fatty liver of pregnancy and Reye's syndrome (111) in its clinical, histologic, and biochemical features.

Cholestatic hepatic injury is clinically manifested by jaundice and pruritus. Laboratory findings include moderate elevations of aminotransferases, alkaline phosphatase, bilirubin, and cholesterol. The two types of cholestatic jaundice in humans (hepatocanalicular and canalicular) differ in their biochemical findings as they differ in their histologic findings. Levels of alkaline phosphatase are elevated more than threefold, and cholesterol values are increased in hepatocanalicular (e.g., chlorpromazine-induced) but not in canalicular (e.g., methyltestosterone-induced) hepatotoxicity (24). Fever, rash, and eosinophilia are usually associated with the hypersensitivity type of drug-induced hepatic injury. The pseudomononucleosis or serum sickness–like syndrome of fever, rash, lymphadenopathy, and lymphocytosis with atypical lymphocytes in the blood is a characteristic hypersensitivity reaction to a number of drugs (e.g., phenytoin, sulfonamides, aminosalicylic acid) (24,53). Renal injury may occur as a result of nephrotoxic metabolites (methoxyflurane) (112) or as a manifestation of generalized hypersensitivity (53).

Toxic porphyria may be associated with several forms of hepatic injury. Hexachlorobenzene liver toxicity is associated with a form of porphyria resembling porphyria cutanea tarda (113). Griseofulvin-induced hepatic injury also may be accompanied by a similar defect in porphyria metabolism (114). Most cases of porphyria cutanea tarda are associated with alcoholism and alcoholic liver disease (115).

Several well-known hepatotoxins tend to present clinically in three distinct phases: (a) immediate, severe gastrointestinal or neurologic manifestations; (b) an asymptomatic period of relative well-being; (c) a phase of overt hepatic injury that often includes renal failure. This sequence is characteristic of poisoning due to CCl_4 (116), yellow phosphorus (117), and hepatotoxic mushrooms (118).

Detecting Subacute and Chronic Hepatotoxicity

Acute hepatotoxicity is usually easy to recognize clinically by laboratory means, particularly after large doses of toxic agents. Acute, occupationally induced hepatic injury has decreased because of control of certain hazardous agents and is comparatively uncommon (20). Hepatic damage, however, is not limited to acute toxicity but includes subacute and chronic toxicity (24).

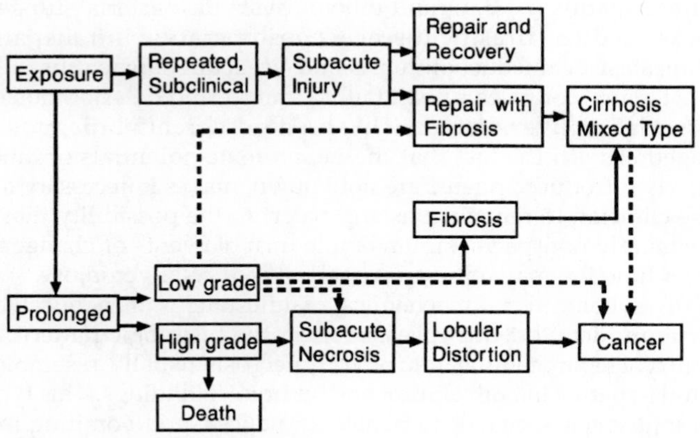

Figure 18-4. Possible outcomes of chronic hepatotoxin exposure. (Modified from Tamburro CH, Liss GM. Tests for hepatotoxicity: usefulness in screening workers. *J Occup Med* 1986;28:1034–1044.)

Figure 18-4 demonstrates how the dose and administration interval can have a profound effect on eventual outcome.

It is also evident why different tests are appropriate to detect the various outcomes of exposure to toxic agents. Vinyl chloride is an example of a hepatotoxin that causes damage from low-level chronic exposure at doses below which acute toxicity is seen. Angiosarcoma and nonmalignant hepatocellular damage due to vinyl chloride are difficult to detect by current methods. Indeed, vinyl chloride has served as a model for developing surveillance methods for subacute and chronic hepatic damage from hazardous industrial chemicals (119). Through screening and surveillance, hepatotoxicity can be minimized and, it is hoped, prevented.

An effective surveillance program for hepatotoxicity, as in all screening programs, needs to follow basic principles. It must be selective and tailored to the population at risk. It must detect disease before damage is evident. Treatment should be available for the condition. (In the case of occupational hepatotoxicity, eliminating or minimizing exposure is usually the only treatment.) The test itself must be valid and reliable. The risks and costs of the test should not outweigh the benefits. Finally, adequate follow-up is necessary (120).

In this discussion of medical surveillance and laboratory testing methods, it must be remembered that occupational and medical history remain the best tools for detecting chronic or subacute hepatotoxicity (121,122).

HEPATOTOXICITY TESTING

Subclinical hepatic damage is more difficult to detect than acute hepatotoxicity. In terms of liver function tests, it is difficult to know what represents normal and abnormal in an asymptomatic population. Indeed, liver enzyme testing in an asymptomatic population results in 2.5% to 10.0% abnormal values (123). In many cases, abnormalities in standard liver enzyme batteries reflect hepatotoxicity from ethanol, acute illness, or other transient, nonoccupational fluctuations. It may also be that the pathogenesis of subacute or chronic hepatic injury is different from acute hepatotoxicity. In this case, tests designed to detect acute hepatotoxicity may be difficult to interpret. In an industrial setting, the goal is to identify latent hepatotoxicity to prevent irreversible future liver damage.

Enzyme Levels

Hepatic enzymes are the most commonly obtained tests of liver function. ALT and AST are often obtained as paired indicators of hepatocellular damage. They reflect changes in cellular permeability rather than cellular function and can be indicators of cellular necrosis. A variety of conditions—including nutritional state, infection, and alcohol use—can influence these levels (123). AST and ALT can also be found in heart, muscle, and lung (24). Obesity elevates levels of AST/ALT. ALT is elevated to a somewhat greater degree in obesity (124).

Ratios of AST/ALT have been used to aid in diagnosis of liver injury. An elevated AST/ALT ratio has been associated with alcoholic liver disease (123). An elevation of the ALT/AST ratio of higher than 1.6 has been associated with pericentral fatty change that is due to toluene (125).

Gamma glutamic acid transferase (GGT) is a sensitive indicator of liver injury and is specific to the liver. Elevation of GGT is associated with ethanol consumption and has a high false-positive rate (123). Lactate dehydrogenase likewise can be elevated with liver damage but is not specific for the liver, because it is present in heart, muscle, lungs, and a variety of disease states (24).

Serum enzyme levels represent loss of hepatocyte cellular integrity and are accurate indicators of acute hepatic disease. They do not represent the metabolic function of the liver (53). In subacute or chronic hepatic injury, liver enzymes may only transiently elevate and then return to normal. Also, diminished functioning parenchyma is often not reflected by serum enzymes; indeed, in end-stage liver disease, falling enzyme levels may reflect worsening disease as a result of loss of hepatic parenchyma. Overall, serum enzyme levels have lacked sensitivity for detecting early liver injury (119).

Usually accompanying hepatic enzyme testing are one or two tests that measure cholestatic functioning. Alkaline phosphatase (AP) and serum bilirubin (direct and indirect) are the most common tests for this. AP can also be present in bone and elevated with bone disease or damage. However, if bone disease is excluded, AP can be a very specific test of liver and biliary function (123). Bilirubin can be elevated in as much as 5% of a population. This can be due to a congenital and benign disorder called *Gilbert's disease*. Usually, bilirubin elevation reflects late changes of biliary injury or acute infection, so it is often not helpful in detecting damage from hazardous chemicals. 5'-Nucleotidase (5'NT) is specific to biliary tract disease. It has been used in evaluation of clinical disease, but not in screening for liver disease (123).

Functional Tests

Tests of actual liver function, rather than levels of circulating liver enzymes, are also useful. Clearance tests have been proposed as being more sensitive and specific for detecting the functional ability of the liver (126).

The investigation of liver disease by laboratory tests involves a variety of hepatic functions (127):

- Uptake, conjugation, and excretion of anionic compounds
  - Total serum bilirubin (direct and indirect)
  - Urinary bilirubin and urobilinogen
  - Bile acids
- Hepatocellular damage
  - Aspartate aminotransferase (AST) (glutamic oxaloacetic transaminase)
  - Alanine aminotransferase (ALT) (glutamic pyruvate transaminase)
  - Glutathione-*S*-transferase (GST)
  - Lactate dehydrogenase and LD5 isoenzyme
  - Serum ferritin
  - Vitamin B_{12}
- Bile flow obstruction
  - Alkaline phosphatase

  - γ-Glutamyltransferase
  - 5'-Nucleotidase
  - Leucine aminopeptidase
  - Lp-X
  - Secretory component and IgA
- Synthetic function
  - Serum albumin
  - Prealbumin
  - Cholinesterase
  - Prothrombin time
  - Partial thromboplastin time
  - Serum proteins
  - Lecithin cholesterol acyltransferase

Testing the functional ability of the liver has been demonstrated to identify early, subclinical disease. In the case of vinyl chloride, indocyanine green clearance (128) and serum bile acids (119) have detected early hepatic damage. Several other functional tests are currently possible. They include the aminopyrine breath test, antipyrine, caffeine, and phenacetin clearances. Serum bile acids and ionic dye clearances are also used.

The aminopyrine breath test is used to assess the functional reserve of end-stage liver failure. Aminopyrine is oxidized by the MFO system and then demethylated. By radiolabeling aminopyrine and checking for expired $^{14}CO_2$, an indication of hepatic function is obtained. Due to the use of radiolabel, lack of data in an asymptomatic population, and uncertainties about interpretation of results, this is a difficult examination to use for detecting subacute or chronic hepatic disease caused by toxic chemicals (124). The test requires physical rest for 2 hours after administration of aminopyrine until sample collection. Measuring sequential radiolabel excretion rates during the 2 hours of study has enabled some authors to quantitate changes in microsomal enzyme function before and after exposure to inducers of the microsomal system. It is most useful for quantitating prognosis in known liver disease (128).

Antipyrine is a widely used index of microsomal enzyme activity. It is well absorbed from the gastrointestinal tract. It is oxidized in phase I metabolism (MFO) to five metabolites, which are conjugated in phase II and excreted. Antipyrine is eliminated in a linear fashion over time and is also distributed in total body water; therefore, samples of urine or saliva can be used to determine the clearance of antipyrine, giving an indication of microsomal function (127).

The test is limited because of its multiple metabolic pathways, any of which could be inhibited or turned on, making total clearance more complex than at first glance (123). It is best used for comparison of individuals rather than for screening populations. It also cannot be repeatedly used, because it is an inducer of its own metabolism. Its advantages are that it is noninvasive and simple to administer.

Other tests of P-450 (MFO) function are under study. These include caffeine and phenacetin breath tests (123). Also under study are *d*-galactose elimination capacity and 6-hydroxycortisol excretion. The advantage to the latter two methods is that both measure the metabolism of endogenous substances.

A Polish study of acetaminophen clearance in workers exposed to polyvinyl chloride showed a correlation between accelerated acetaminophen clearance and exposure. There was no corresponding change in paracetamol clearance or liver enzyme levels with exposure to polyvinyl chloride (129). If this test is validated in other studies, it may be a useful screening tool.

Measurements of anionic dye clearances also have been used to detect subclinical liver disease. Bromosulfobromophthalene clearance has been discarded because of its toxicity. Indocyanine green (ICG) has been studied, and at certain doses it shows great sensitivity to chemical-induced liver injury. It also shows dose-response correlation with vinyl chloride and vinyl monomer exposure, a known hepatocarcinogen and hepatotoxin (123).

Measurement of serum bile acids does not require administration of exogenous compounds. A single measure of fasting conjugated cholic acid (CCA) and cholylglycine can indicate the hepatic excretory function in a fashion similar to the way serum creatinine measurements indicate the excretory function of the kidney (123). CCA and cholylglycine are similar in sensitivity to GGT in detecting chemical-induced liver injury. CCA and AP are most specific for liver disease and correlate with portal tract changes in vinyl monomer disease. Serum bile acids correlate with ICG clearance in vinyl chloride liver disease. Serum bile acids may also be more sensitive to styrene-induced hepatotoxicity (120,130).

Liver disease from chronic toxic exposure tends to demonstrate more fibrosis and evidence of chronic injury. Acute hepatotoxicity is more likely to show a cytotoxic response, as seen in alcoholic, drug-related, and infectious acute hepatitis. This may explain why functional tests, such as bilirubin and bile salt levels, may correlate better with chronic or subacute hepatotoxicity, whereas serum enzyme levels are more useful in acute or nonchemically induced hepatic injury (119).

Methods of detecting genetic damage by electrophilic compounds are also being investigated. Measurements of RNase (ribonuclease activity) suggesting high DNA turnover and urinary thioether levels and alpha esterase levels have correlated with exposure to styrene and benzidine. Correlation between these measures of exposure was stronger than other measures of liver enzymes or measurements of specific metabolites (131). Many new tests for levels of DNA adducts and DNA synthesis are being developed. These may ultimately lead to better methods of detecting chronic or precarcinogenic liver toxicity from occupational exposures.

Hepatic Synthesis Tests

The liver is responsible for production of many circulatory proteins. Most commonly tested are serum albumin, prothrombin time, cholesterol, amino acids, and carrier protein molecules such as transferrin. All are insensitive tests for screening for early liver toxicity. Prothrombin time, for example, indicates clotting factor deficiency. It is commonly used as a measure of severe acute hepatotoxicity because of the short half-life of the clotting-factor activity measured. It is also useful in monitoring end-stage liver failure. It, like other tests for hepatic synthesis, is insensitive to mild or early liver injury. The liver has vast synthetic reserve, and only with extensive parenchymal loss will diminished tests of synthetic function be abnormal (123).

Structural Studies

Physical examination is a highly specific study, but it has low sensitivity for evaluating early liver damage, because hepatomegaly is a late effect of hepatotoxicity. Multiple radiologic studies—including computerized tomography, magnetic resonance imaging, isotope studies, and ultrasound studies—have not been helpful in screening an industrial population for hepatic injury. As many as 12% false-positives and 35% to 40% false-negatives have been demonstrated when using these methods in an industrial population (123).

Liver biopsy is highly sensitive and specific. It is obviously not indicated for screening purposes because of the risk of the procedure to an asymptomatic person. It is indicated for persistent abnormalities detected on screening evaluations, particularly when exposure to a possible hepatotoxin has occurred (123). Other etiologies for abnormal screening studies, such as viral infections and therapeutic drugs, should be ruled out before undertaking liver biopsy. Other indications for biopsy include unexplained hepatomegaly or splenomegaly, cholestasis of uncertain cause, suspected systemic or infiltrative disease, and suspected primary or metastatic liver tumor (132). In addition, liver biopsy results are difficult to interpret, because the liver is limited in the types of pathologies it can demonstrate (see Table 18-2).

PROTOCOL FOR SCREENING FOR HEPATOTOXICITY IN A POPULATION EXPOSED TO HAZARDOUS CHEMICALS

Current testing methods for hepatotoxicity are not easily applied to screening programs. As many as 30% of asymptomatic workers subjected to a standard battery of serum liver chemistries had results in excess of laboratory control subjects (133). Indeed, because elevated liver chemistries are so common, many physicians ignore abnormal liver chemistries, unless they are greater than twice normal (124). This may lead to misdiagnosis and continuing indolent hepatic injury. Tests of low specificity are often used for screening. This is responsible for much of the difficulty, because as tests of low specificity, they lead to high false-positive results. The low sensitivity of other testing methods leads to high false-negative results, particularly in a population with low disease prevalence. In addition, the range of normal for a laboratory is usually set to include 95% of the population it tests. Often a hospital laboratory is called on to test people with other illnesses and known hepatic disease. The range of normal for this group may be different from the range of normal in an occupational group.

The risks of screening are also important to consider. If liver chemistries are passed as normal when they may represent early toxicity, a worker may be returned to a dangerous environment. If abnormal results are obtained on a nonspecific test, a worker may be removed unnecessarily from a worksite and be subjected to expensive, unnecessary, and sometimes risky evaluations or procedures.

These problems can be minimized by using the following guidelines:

- Set normal levels for the population being screened. Setting the upper limit of normal to the 95th percentile with respect to the screened population has been shown to decrease the false-positive results without increasing false-negatives (133). A sample size of 150 to 250 gives adequate accuracy (134).
- Use a wider range of normal if performing multiple tests. Multiple tests done on an individual increases the chance that an isolated false-positive result will occur. If it is necessary to test using a panel of examinations, setting the normal range to include the 99th percentile decreases false-positives (134).
- Screen with tests of high specificity first. Using a battery of tests of varying sensitivity and specificity increases false-positive results (123).
- Follow tests of high specificity with tests of higher sensitivity to correctly identify true-positives (123).
- Follow up positive results with more extensive diagnostic evaluations, as the chance of a false-positive is minimized (123).

One study used a sequence of alkaline phosphatase or serum bile acids as specific initial screens. The positives were followed with GGT or ICG tests. Positives in both the screen and subsequent testing require evaluation by a specialist as well as liver biopsy (Table 18-7). This sequence decreased false-positive occurrence and did not increase false-negative occurrence (123). Further validation of this method is warranted before it can be recommended as a standard procedure.

TABLE 18-7. Health monitoring in a hepatotoxic environment

Initial employee screening

Goal: Rule out preexisting liver disease that would put employee at increased risk.

1. Medical history with specific questions about ethanol use, hepatitis, and previous liver disease.
2. Occupational history including previous worksite exposure and home or hobby exposures to hepatotoxins.
3. Medical examination directed toward the hepatobiliary system to detect hepatic enlargement or signs of chronic hepatic disease.
4. Urinalysis for urobilinogen and bile pigments.
5. Serum enzymes aspartate aminotransferase or γ glutamic acid transferase.
6. Serum bilirubin or alkaline phosphatase.
7. Follow-up or repeat abnormal examinations.

Periodic surveillance

Goals: (a) Rule out nonoccupational liver disease; (b) detect hepatic damage from hepatotoxic environment.

1. Same protocol as initial screening.
2. Tests more specific followed by test more sensitive to hepatic injury caused by the hepatotoxic agent. In the case of vinyl chloride, fasting bile salts followed by indocyanine green clearance or γ glutamic acid transferase.
3. Follow up abnormal values with further diagnostic tests.
4. Refer persistently abnormal screening studies or abnormal secondary studies to a specialist for consideration of biopsy and further diagnostic workup.
5. Remove worker with abnormal screening tests from hepatotoxic environment until definitive diagnosis made. Follow abnormal tests after exposure ceases.

Adapted from Tamburro CH, Liss GM. Tests for hepatotoxicity: usefulness in screening workers. *J Occup Med* 1986;28:1034–1044; Davidson CS, Leevy CM, Chamberlayne EC, eds. Guidelines for detection of hepatotoxicity due to drugs and chemicals. *NIH Publication No. 79-313*. Washington: Department of Health, Education, and Welfare, 1979; World Health Organization. *Early detection of occupational diseases*. Geneva: World Health Organization, 1986.

Finally, workers assigned to a known or likely hepatotoxic environment should have adequate preplacement screening to rule out factors that would put them at increased risk. In this instance, it is wise to rule out preexisting damage to the liver from hepatitis, alcohol, or other causes. For this purpose, standard tests of hepatic disease, such as enzyme levels and bile products, are appropriate. An approach to medical surveillance of workers in a hepatotoxic environment is provided in Table 18-7.

EVALUATION OF THE INDIVIDUAL WITH ABNORMAL LIVER FUNCTION TEST RESULTS

The above discussion, while relevant, does not give much guidance for management of the individual who is asymptomatic and working in a low-risk environment who is noted on examination to have elevation of one or more standard liver function enzymes, especially if in-house normal values have not been established. There are three factors for consideration. First, is the abnormality representative of liver pathology? Minor elevation (less than 10% greater than the upper limit of normal) of a single liver enzyme is not likely to represent significant liver pathology (135,136). In this case, no further evaluation or work restriction is needed.

The following questions need to be answered next: Is there liver pathology present? Can it be determined to be work related or not? If liver pathology is suggested by the liver function test abnormalities, the most common causes of nonoccupational liver enzyme abnormalities should be ruled out. Because ethanol use is a most common cause of abnormal liver function tests, the tests should be repeated after a period of abstinence. The medical history should be reviewed for any evidence of medication use that may cause liver function abnormalities. If medically feasible, all medications should also be discontinued before retest of liver function tests. Additional laboratory tests to rule out other causes of liver damage, especially hepatitis B and C, should be obtained, especially if the liver function abnormalities persist after abstinence from ethanol. If no other etiology for the liver function abnormalities can be found, careful investigation of the work environment occupational and medical history is warranted. This will assist in determining if there is any exposure that may be related to the liver enzyme abnormalities.

Finally, once persistent liver function abnormalities have been documented, work restrictions are indicated in cases in which workers are exposed to agents with clearly documented hepatotoxicity. It is less clear what to do with workers whose primary exposure is to hazardous materials when the hepatotoxicity is not well documented in humans or only documented in animals, when the exposure is only intermittent or very low dose, or when there is only the potential for exposure to materials that are possibly hepatotoxic.

One method of addressing this problem is to conduct a "study" with a population of one—that is, with the individual in question. The individual can be sequentially tested in various exposure circumstances in an attempt to correlate exposure with liver function abnormalities. Initially, weekly liver function tests can be obtained away from any exposure, then work assignments can be switched on a monthly basis. A worker could then be assigned to an environment where the potential hepatotoxin(s) were present for a 4-week period of time, then reassigned to a workplace where no potential for exposure to hepatotoxins exists. This cycle could be repeated several times until a pattern of change was noted (137). Because this is a "clinical trial," appropriate consent must be obtained before initiating the investigation. There are also other limitations to this type of investigation. It does not ensure that ongoing, subclinical hepatotoxicity is not occurring. It is possible that the liver enzyme tests are not sensitive enough to reliably detect ongoing hepatotoxicity for the hepatotoxin in question, and the hepatotoxicity may be missed.

SUMMARY

Hepatotoxicity continues to be a consequence of exposure to toxic chemicals. It is uniquely sensitive to their effects because of physiologic and anatomic factors that distribute absorbed chemicals to the liver. The liver metabolizes chemicals to facilitate excretion, but, in some cases, this biotransformation creates a more reactive or toxic compound, which can produce hepatocellular damage insult to another organ.

Damage done to the liver can manifest in several forms, depending on the dose and frequency of exposures as well as on the severity of the toxin. A single high dose of a chemical or small dose of an extremely toxic chemical can cause acute hepatitis and cytotoxic damage, which can lead to death.

Chronic exposure or frequent, subacute exposure to hepatotoxic chemicals can produce more indolent hepatic disease. This may ultimately lead to fibrosis, scarring, and parenchymal loss. It may also induce or promote carcinogenesis.

Detection of acute hepatotoxicity is achievable with methods of testing commonly used today. In most cases, these methods were developed for detecting acute liver disease and end-stage liver failure. The challenge for the future is detecting chronic and subacute hepatic damage from toxic chemicals. In this way, liver disease from toxic chemicals in use today can be prevented.

REFERENCES

1. Zimmerman HJ. Hepatotoxic effects of oncotherapeutic agents. *Prog Liver Dis* 1986;8:621.
2. Kraybill HR. The toxicology and epidemiology of natural hepatotoxin exposure. *Isr J Med Sci* 1974;10:416.
3. Zimmerman HJ, Maddrey WC. Toxic and drug-induced hepatitis. In: Schiff L, Schiff ER, eds. *Diseases of the liver*, 6th ed. Philadelphia: JB Lippincott Co, 1987:591.
4. Anonymous. Drinking water: another source of carcinogens. *Science* 1974;186:809.
5. Ridder WE, Oehma FW. Nitrates as an environmental, animal and human hazard. *Clin Toxicol* 1974;7:145.
6. Rouiller CH. Experimental toxic injury of the liver. In: Rouiller CH, ed. *The liver*. New York: Academic Press, 1964:335.
7. Schaffner F, Raisfeld IH. Drugs and the liver: a review of metabolism and adverse reactions. *Adv Intern Med* 1969;15:221.
8. Tamburro CH, Liss GM. Tests for hepatotoxicity: usefulness in screening workers. *J Occup Med* 1986;28:1034.
9. Campra JL, Reynolds TB. The hepatic circulation. In: Arias IM, Jakoby WB, Popper H, et al., eds. *The liver: biology and pathobiology*, 2nd ed. New York: Raven Press, 1988:911.
10. Rappaport AM. Physioanatomical basis of toxic liver injury. In: Farber E, Fisher MM, eds. *Toxic injury of the liver*. New York: Marcel Dekker Inc, 1979:1.
11. Gumucio JJ, Chianale J. Liver cell heterogeneity and liver function. In: Arias IM, Jakoby WB, Popper H, et al., eds. *The liver: biology and pathobiology*, 2nd ed. New York: Raven Press, 1988:931.
12. Caldwell J. Biological implications of xenobiotic metabolism. In: Arias IM, Jacoby WB, Popper H, et al., eds. *The liver: biology and pathobiology*, 2nd ed. New York: Raven Press, 1988:355.
13. Nickels J. Effects of organic solvents on liver cell morphology. In: Riihimaki V, Ufvarson U. *Safety and health aspects of organic solvents*. New York: Alan R. Liss, 1986:115.
14. Jakoby WB. Detoxication: conjugation and hydrolysis. In: Arias IM, Jacoby WB, Popper H, et al., eds. *The liver: biology and pathobiology*, 2nd ed. New York: Raven Press, 1988:375.
15. Ziegler DM. Detoxication: oxidation and reduction. In: Arias IM, Jacoby WB, Popper H, et al., eds. *The liver: biology and pathobiology*, 2nd ed. New York: Raven Press, 1988:363.
16. Anders MW. Bioactivation mechanisms and hepatocellular damage. In: Arias IM, Jacoby WB, Popper H, et al., eds. *The liver: biology and pathobiology*, 2nd ed. New York: Raven Press, 1988:389.
17. Sipes IG, Gandolfi AJ. Biotransformation of toxicants. In: Klaassen CD, Amdur MO, Doull J, eds. *Casarett and Doull's toxicology: the basic science of poisons*, 3rd ed. New York: Macmillan, 1986:64.
18. Watkins PB. Role of cytochrome P450 in drug metabolism and hepatotoxicity. *Semin Liver Dis* 1990 Nov;10(4):235.
19. Dianzani MU. Reactions of the liver to injury, fatty liver. In: Farber E, Fisher MM, eds. *Toxic injury of the liver, part A*. New York: Marcel Dekker Inc, 1979:281.
20. Dossing M, Skinhoj P. Occupational liver injury: present state of knowledge and future perspective. *Int Arch Occup Environ Health* 1985;56(1):1.
21. Farber JL. Reaction of the liver to injury, necrosis. In: Farber Fisher MM, eds. *Toxic injury of the liver, part A*. New York: Marcel Dekker, Inc, 1979:281.
22. Plaa GL. Toxic responses of the liver. In: Klaassen CD, Amdur MO, Doull J, eds. *Casarett and Doull's toxicology: the basic science of poisons*, 3rd ed. New York: Macmillan, 1986:286.
23. Kaplowitz N, Aw TY, Simon FR, Stoltz A. Drug-induced hepatoxicity. *Ann Intern Med* 1986 Jun;104(6):826.
24. Zimmerman HJ. *Hepatotoxicity: the adverse effects of drugs and other chemicals on the liver*. New York: Appleton-Century-Crofts, 1978.
25. Thiele DL, Eigenbrodt EH, Ware AJ. Cirrhosis after repeated trichloroethylene and 1,1,1-trichloroethane exposure. *Gastroenterology* 1982;83:926.
26. Baerg RD, Kimberg DV. Centrilobular hepatic necrosis and acute renal failure in solvent sniffers. *Ann Intern Med* 1970;73:713.
27. Williams GM, Weisburger JH. Chemical carcinogens. In: Klaassen CD, Amdur MO, Doull J, eds. *Toxicology: the basic science of poisons*, 3rd ed. New York: Macmillan, 1986:99.
28. Dossing M, Skinhoj P. Occupational liver disease. *Int Arch Occup Environ* Health 1985;56:1.
29. Popper H. Drug-induced hepatic injury. In: Gall EA, Mostofi FK, eds. *The liver*. Baltimore: Williams & Wilkins, 1973:182.
30. Farber JL, Gerson RJ. Mechanisms of cell injury with hepatotoxic chemicals. *Pharmacol Rev* 1984;36:71s.
31. Recknagel RO. A new direction in the study of carbon tetrachloride hepatotoxicity. *Life Sci* 1983;33:401.
32. Nelao SD. Mechanisms of the formation and disposition of reactive metabolites that can cause acute liver injury. *Drug Metab Rev* 1995;27(1,2):147.
33. Mitchell JR, Jollow DJ. Metabolic activation of drugs to toxic substances. *Gastroenterology* 1975;68:392.
34. Mitchell JR, Nelson SD, Thorgeirsson SS, et al. Metabolic activation: biochemical basis for many drug-induced liver injuries. *Prog Liver Dis* 1976;5:259.
35. Kroker R, Hegner D. Solubilization of phalloidin binding sites from rat liver hepatocytes and plasma membranes by trypsin. *Naunyn Schmiedebergs Arch Pharmacol* 1973;279:339.

36. Mitchell JR, Thorgeirsson SS, Potter WZ, et al. Acetaminophen-induced hepatic injury: protective role of glutathione in man and rationale for therapy. *Clin Pharmacol Ther* 1974;16:676.
37. Aw TY, Hanna P, Petrini J, et al. Hepatic drug metabolism and drug-induced liver injury. In: Gitnick G, ed. *Current hepatology*, vol 5. New York: John Wiley and Sons, 1985:113.
38. Schenker S. Pathogenesis of tetracycline-induced fatty liver. In: Gerog W, Sickinger K, eds. *Drugs and the liver*. Stuttgart: FK Schattauer-Verlag, 1975:269.
39. Pratt CB, Johnson WW. Duration and severity of fatty metamorphosis of the liver following L-asparaginase therapy. *Cancer* 1971;28:361.
40. Dahl MGC, Scheuer PJ. Methotrexate hepatotoxicity in psoriasis. Comparison of different dose regimens. *BMJ* 1972;1:654.
41. Farber E. Biochemical pathology. *Annu Rev Pharmacol Toxicol* 1971;11:71.
42. Reid WD, Christie B, Krishina G, et al. Bromobenzene metabolism and hepatic necrosis. *Pharmacology* 1971;6:41.
43. Einhorn M, Davidson I. Hepatotoxicity of mercaptopurine. *JAMA* 1964; 188:802.
44. Weiss DL, De Los Santos R. Urethane-induced hepatic failure in man. *Am J Med* 1960;28:476.
45. Leiber CS. Alcohol and the liver: transition from adaptation to tissue injury. In: Khanna JM, Israel Y, Kalant H, eds. *Alcoholic liver pathology*. Ontario: Addiction Research Foundation, 1975:171.
46. Farber E. Some fundamental aspects of liver injury. In: Khanna JM, Israel Y, Kalant H, eds. *Alcoholic liver pathology*. Ontario: Addiction Research Foundation, 1975:289.
47. Videla L. Increased oxidative capacity in the liver following ethanol administration. In: Khanna JM, Israel Y, Kalant H, eds. *Alcoholic liver pathology*. Ontario: Addiction Research Foundation, 1975:331.
48. Zimmerman HJ. Effects of alcohol on other hepatotoxins. *Alcohol Clin Exp Res* 1986;10:3.
49. Strubelt O. Alcohol potentiation of liver injury. *Fund Appl Toxicol* 1978;4:144.
50. Plaa GL. Toxic responses of the liver. In: Doull J, Klaassen CD, Amdur MO, eds. *Casarett and Doull's toxicology: the basic science of poisons*, 2nd ed. New York: Macmillan, 1980:206.
51. Soto C, Lieber CS. Increased hepatotoxicity of acetaminophen after chronic ethanol consumption in the rat. *Gastroenterology* 1981;80:140.
52. Miller EC, Miller JA. Hepatocarcinogenesis by chemicals. *Prog Liver Dis* 1976;5:699.
53. Zimmerman HJ. Clinical and laboratory manifestations of hepatotoxicity. *Ann N Y Acad Sci* 1963;104:954.
54. Metreau JM, Dhumeaux D, Berthelot D, et al. Oral contraceptives and the liver. *Digestion* 1972;7:318.
55. Holzbach RT, Sanders JH. Recurrent intrahepatic cholestasis of pregnancy: observations on pathogenesis. *JAMA* 1965;193:542.
56. Kopelman H, Scheuer PJ, Williams R, et al. The liver lesion of the Epping jaundice. *Q J Med* 1966;35:553.
57. Solis-Herruzo JA, Castellano G, Colina F, et al. Hepatic injury in the toxic epidemic syndrome caused by ingestion of adulterated cooking oil (Spain 1981). *Hepatology* 1984;4:131.
58. Mullick FG, Ishak KG, Mahabir R, et al. Hepatic injury associated with paraquat toxicity in humans. *Liver* 1981;1:209.
59. Hohn D, Melnick J, Stagg R, et al. Biliary sclerosis in patients receiving hepatic arterial infusions of floxyuridine. *J Clin Oncol* 1985;3:98.
60. Slater TF, Strauli UD, Sawyer B, et al. Sporidesmin poisoning in the rat. *Res Vet Sci* 1964;5:540.
61. Spielberg SP, Gordon GB, Blake DA, et al. Predisposition to phenytoin hepatotoxicity assessed in vitro. *N Engl J Med* 1981;305:722.
62. Lee TJ, Carney CN, Lapis JL, et al. Diphenylhydantoin-induced hepatic necrosis. *Gastroenterology* 1976;70:422.
63. Davies GE, Holmes JE. Drug-induced immunological effects on the liver. *Br J Anaesth* 1972;44:941.
64. Zimmerman HJ, Lewis JH, Ishak KG, et al. Ticrynafen-associated hepatic injury: analysis of 340 cases. *Hepatology* 1984;4:315.
65. Bond GR. Hepatitis, rash and eosinophilia following trichloroethylene exposure: a case report and speculation on mechanistic similarity to halothane induced hepatitis. *J Toxicol Clin Toxicol* 1996;34(4):461.
66. Reynolds ES, Moslen MT. Liver and biliary tree. In: Mottet NK, ed. *Environmental pathology*. New York: Oxford University Press, 1985:248.
67. Cornish HH, Adefuin J. Ethanol potentiation of halogenated aliphatic solvent toxicity. *Am Ind Hyg Assoc J* 1966;57.
68. Muller G, Spassowski M, Henschler D. Metabolism of trichloroethylene in man. *Arch Toxicol* 1975;33:173.
69. Balmer MF, Smith FA, Leach LJ, Yuile CL. Effects in the liver of methylene chloride inhaled alone and with ethyl alcohol. *Am Ind Hyg Assoc J* 1976;345.
70. Hills BW, Venable HL. The interaction of ethyl alcohol and industrial chemicals. *Am J Ind Med* 1982;3:321.
71. Dossing M. Metabolic interactions between organic solvents and other chemicals. In: Riihimaki V, Ulfvarson U, eds. Safety and health aspects of organic solvents. New York: Alan R. Liss, 1986:97.
72. Rueff B, Benhamou JP. Acute hepatic necrosis and fulminant hepatic failure. *Gut* 1973;14:805.
73. Krishnamachari KAVR, Bhat RV, Nagarajan V, et al. Hepatitis due to aflatoxicosis: an outbreak in Western India. *Lancet* 1975;1:1061.
74. Wagon GN. Aflatoxins and their relationship to hepatocellular carcinoma. In: Okuda K, Peters RL, eds. *Hepatocellular carcinoma*. New York: John Wiley and Sons, 1976:25.
75. Ridker PM, Ohkuma S, McDermott WV, et al. Hepatic veno-occlusive disease associated with the consumption of pyrrolizidine-containing dietary supplements. *Gastroenterology* 1985;88:1050.
76. Bick M. Chlorinated hydrocarbon residues in human body fat. *Med J Aust* 1969;1:1127.
77. Smith NJ. Death following accidental ingestion of DDT: experimental studies. *JAMA* 1948;136:469.
78. Bullivant CM. Accidental poisoning by paraquat: report of two cases in man. *BMJ* 1966;1:1272.
79. Klockars M. Solvents and the liver. In: Riihimaki V, Ufvarson U, eds. *Safety and health aspects of organic solvents*. New York: Alan R. Liss, 1986:139.
80. Tomenson JA, Baron CE, O'Sullivan JJ, Edwards JC, et al. Hepatic function in workers occupationally exposed to carbon tetrachloride. *Occup Environ Med* 1995;52(8):508.
81. Brodkin CA, Danielle W, Checoway H, Echeverria D, et al. Hepatic ultrasonic changes in workers exposed to perchlorethylene. *Occup Environ Med* 1995;52(10):679.
82. Baerg RD, Kimberg DV. Centrilobular hepatic necrosis and acute renal failure in "solvent sniffers." *Ann Intern Med* 1970;73:713.
83. Lee TJ, Carney CN, Lapis JL, et al. Diphenylhydantoin-induced hepatic necrosis. *Gastroenterology* 1976;70:422.
84. Rasmussen K, Brogren CH, Sabroe S. Subclinical affection of liver and kidney function and solvent exposure. *Int Arch Occup Environ Health* 1993;64(6):445.
85. Stewart RD, Andrews JT. Acute intoxication with methylchloroform. *JAMA* 1966;195:904.
86. Nathan AW, Towsland PA. Goodpastures syndrome and trichloroethane intoxication. *Br J Clin Pharmacol* 1979;8:284.
87. Halevy J, Pitlik S, Rosenfeld J. 1,1,1-trichloroethane intoxication: a case report with transient liver and renal damage: review of the literature. *Clin Toxicol* 1980;16:467.
88. Thiele DL, Eigenbrodt EH, Ware AJ. Cirrhosis after repeated trichloroethylene and 1,1,1-trichloroethane exposure. *Gastroenterology* 1982;83:926.
89. Kramer CG, Ott GM, Fulkerson JE, Hicks N, Imbus HR. Health of workers exposed to 1,1,1-trichloroethane: a matched-pair study. *Arch Environ Health* 1978;33:331.
90. Soden KJ. An evaluation of chronic methylene chloride exposure. *J Occup Med* 1993 Mar;35(3):282.
91. Guzelian P, Mills S, Fallon HJ. Liver structure and function in print workers exposed to toluene. *J Occup Med* 1988;30:791.
92. Tahti H, Karkkainen S, Pyykko K, Rintala E, Kataja M, Vapaatalo H. Chronic occupational exposure to toluene. *Int Arch Occup Environ Health* 1981;48:61.
93. Brugnone F, Perbellini L. Toluene coma and liver function. *Scand J Work Environ Health* 1985;11:55.
94. Brugnone F, Perbellini L. Toluene coma and liver function. *Scand J Work Environ Health* 1985;11:55.
95. Haratake J, Furuta A, Iwasa T, Wakasugi C, Imazu K. Submassive hepatic necrosis induced by dichloropropanol. *Liver* 1993;13(3):123.
96. Kurppa K, Husman K. Car painters' exposure to a mixture of organic solvents. *Scand J Work Environ Health* 1982;8:137.
97. Dossing M, Arlien-Soborg P, Petersen LM, Ranek L. Liver damage associated with occupational exposure to organic solvents in house painters. *Eur J Clin Invest* 1983;13:151.
98. Ukai H, Takada S, Inui S, Imai Y, et al. Occupational exposure to solvent mixtures: effects on health and metabolism. *Occup Environ Med* 1994;51(8):523.
99. Rees D, Soderlund N, Cronje R, Song E, Kielkowski D, Myers J. Solvent exposure, alcohol consumption and liver injury in workers manufacturing paint. *Scand J Work Environ Health* 1993;19(4):236.
100. Dossing M, Skinhoj P. Occupational liver injury: present state of knowledge and future perspective. *Int Arch Occup Environ Health* 1985;56(1):1.
101. Lundbeerg I, Nise G, Hedenborg G, Hogberg M, Vesterberg O. Liver function tests and urinary albumin in house painters with previous heavy exposure to organic solvents. *Occup Environ Med* 1994 May;51(5):347.
102. Magos L, Butler WH. Effect of phenobarbitone and starvation on hepatotoxicity in rats exposed to disulfide vapor. *Br J Ind Med* 1972;29:95.
103. Bond EJ, DeMatteis F. Biochemical changes in rat liver after administration of carbon disulphide, with particular reference to microsomal changes. *Biochem Pharmacol* 1969;18:2531–2549.
104. Marino G, Anastopoulos H, Woolf AD. Toxicity associated with severe inhalational and dermal exposure to dimethylacetamide and 1,2 ethanediamine. *J Occup Med* 1994;35(6):637.
105. Spies GJ, Rhyne RH Jr, Evans RA, et al. Monitoring acrylic fiber workers for liver toxicity and exposure to dimethylacetamide. 2. Serum clinical chemistry results of dimethylacetamide-exposed workers. *J Occup Environ Med* 1995;37(9):1102.
106. Spies GJ, Rhyne RH Jr, Evans RA, et al. Monitoring acrylic fiber workers for liver toxicity and exposure to dimethylacetamide. 1. Assessing exposure to dimethylacetamide by air and biological monitoring. *J Occup Environ Med* 1995;37(9):1093.
107. Dossing M. Occupational toxic liver damage. *J Hepatol* 1986;3:131.
108. Clark R, Borirak-Chanyavat V, Davidson AR, et al. Hepatic damage and death from overdose of paracetamol. *Lancet* 1973;i:66.
109. Ritt DJ, Whelan G, Werner DJ, et al. Acute hepatic necrosis with stupor or coma: an analysis of thirty-one patients. *Medicine* 1969;48:151.
110. Zimmerman HJ. Aspirin-induced hepatic injury. *Ann Intern Med* 1974;80:103.
111. Hoyumpa AM, Jr, Greene HL, Dunn GD, et al. Fatty liver: biochemical and clinical considerations. *Am J Dig Dis* 1975;20:1142–1170.

112. Elkington SG, Goffinet JA, Conn HO, et al. Renal and hepatic injury associated with methoxyflurane anesthesia. *Ann Intern Med* 1968;69:1229.
113. Schmid R. Cutaneous porphyria in Turkey. *N Engl J Med* 1960;263:397.
114. Hurst EW, Paget GE. Protoporphyrin, cirrhosis and hepatomata in the livers of mice given griseofulvin. *Br J Dermatol* 1963;75:105.
115. Lundvall O. Alcohol and porphyria cutanea tarda. In: Engel A, Larsson T, eds. *Alcoholic cirrhosis and other toxic hepatopathies.* Stockholm: Nordiska Bokhandelns Forlag, 1970:356.
116. Jennings RB. Fatal fulminant acute carbon tetrachloride poisoning. *Arch Pathol* 1955;59:269.
117. Rodriguez-Iturbe B. Acute yellow phosphorus poisoning. *N Engl J Med* 1971;284:157.
118. Harrison DC, Coggins CH, Welland FH, et al. Mushroom poisoning in five patients. *Am J Med* 1965;38:787.
119. Liss GM, Greenberg RA, Tamburro CH. Use of serum bile acids in the identification of vinyl chloride hepatotoxicity. *Am J Med* 1985;78:68.
120. Levy BS, Halperin WE. Screening for occupational disease. In: Levy BS, Wegman DH, eds. *Occupational health: recognizing and preventing work-related disease.* Boston: Little, Brown and Company, 1988:75.
121. Davidson CS, Leevy CM, Chamberlayne EC, eds. *Guidelines for detection of hepatotoxicity due to drugs and chemicals.* Washington: Department of Health Education and Welfare, 1979. [NIH publication no 79313].
122. World Health Organization. *Early detection of occupational diseases.* Geneva: World Health Organization, 1986.
123. Tamburro CH, Liss GM. Tests for hepatotoxicity: usefulness in screening workers. *J Occup Med* 1986;28:1034.
124. Hodgson MJ, Van Thiel DH, Lauschus K, Karpf M. Liver injury tests in hazardous waste workers: the role of obesity. *J Occup Med* 1989;31:238.
125. Guzelian P, Mills S, Fallon HJ. Liver structure and function in print workers exposed to toluene. *J Occup Med* 1988;30:791.
126. Brody DH, Leichter L. Clearance tests of liver function. *Med Clin North Am* 1979;63:621.
127. Rosalki S, McIntyre N. Biochemical investigations in the management of liver disease. In: Bircher J, Benhamou J, McIntyre N, Rizzetto M, Rodes J, eds. *Oxford textbook of clinical hepatology,* vol. 2, 2nd ed. Oxford: Oxford Medical Publications, 1999:503.
128. Tamburro CH, Greenberg RA. Effectiveness of federally required medical laboratory screening in the detection of chemical liver injury. *Environ Health Perspect* 1981;41:117.
129. Smilgin Z, Drozdzik M, Gawronska-Szkarz B, Wojcocki J, et al. Pharmacokinetics of acetaminophen in individuals occupationally exposed to polyvinyl chloride modified with plasticizers (in Polish). *Med Pr* 1993;44(5):423.
130. Edling C, Tagesson C. Raised serum bile acid concentrations after occupational exposure to styrene: a possible sign of hepatotoxicity? *Br J Ind Med* 1984;41:257.
131. El Gazzar RM, Adbel Hamid H, Shamy MY. Biologic monitoring of exposure to electrophilic compounds. *J Environ Pathol Toxicol Oncol* 1994;13(1):19.
132. Isselbacher KJ, LaMont JT. Diagnostic procedures in liver disease. In: Petersdorf RG, Adams RD, et al., eds. *Harrison's principles of internal medicine,* 10th ed. New York: McGraw-Hill, 1983.
133. Wright C, Rivera JC, Baetz JH. Liver function testing in a working population: three strategies to reduce false-positive results. *J Occup Med* 1988;30:693.
134. Reed AJ, Henry RJ, Mason WB. Influence of statistical method used on the resulting estimate of the normal range. *Clin Chem* 1971;17:275.
135. Wright C, Rivera JC, Baetz JH. Liver function testing in a working population: strategies to reduce false positive results. *J Occup Med* 1988;30:693.
136. Herip DS. Recommendations for the investigation of abnormal hepatic function in asymptomatic workers. *Am J Ind Med* 1992;21:331.
137. Anonymous. What restrictions regarding work duties or exposures are appropriate when liver function abnormalities (especially elevated enzymes) are noted? *J Occup Med* 1993;35(11):1082.

CHAPTER 19

Clinical Neurotoxicology and Neurobehavioral Toxicology

Christopher M. Filley and James P. Kelly

An understanding of neurotoxicology depends on a working knowledge of the nervous system and its potential for toxic injury (Table 19-1). The CNS is comprised of the brain and spinal cord. The PNS is divided into the somatic and autonomic nervous systems. The autonomic nervous system is subdivided into sympathetic and parasympathetic.

TABLE 19-1. Major components of central nervous system and peripheral nervous system

Central nervous system
- Brain
- Spinal cord
- Optic nerves (cranial nerve II)

Peripheral nervous system
- Somatic division
  - Cranial nerves (except optic nerves)
  - Spinal nerves
  - Dorsal root ganglia
  - Peripheral nerves
    - Motor—neuromuscular junction
    - Sensory—special receptors
- Autonomic division
  - Parasympathetic—cranial and sacral nerves and ganglia
  - Sympathetic

The neuron is the basic functional element of the nervous system, and consists of the cell body, multiple branching dendrites, and a single axon (Fig. 19-1). The cell body contains the neuronal nucleus and other organelles that are involved with cellular metabolism, whereas the dendrites and axons are responsible for signal reception and transmission, respectively. Many axons of the CNS and PNS are invested with an insulating sheath of myelin that is approximately 70% lipid and 30% protein. Myelin is laid down by glial cells known as *oligodendrocytes* in the CNS

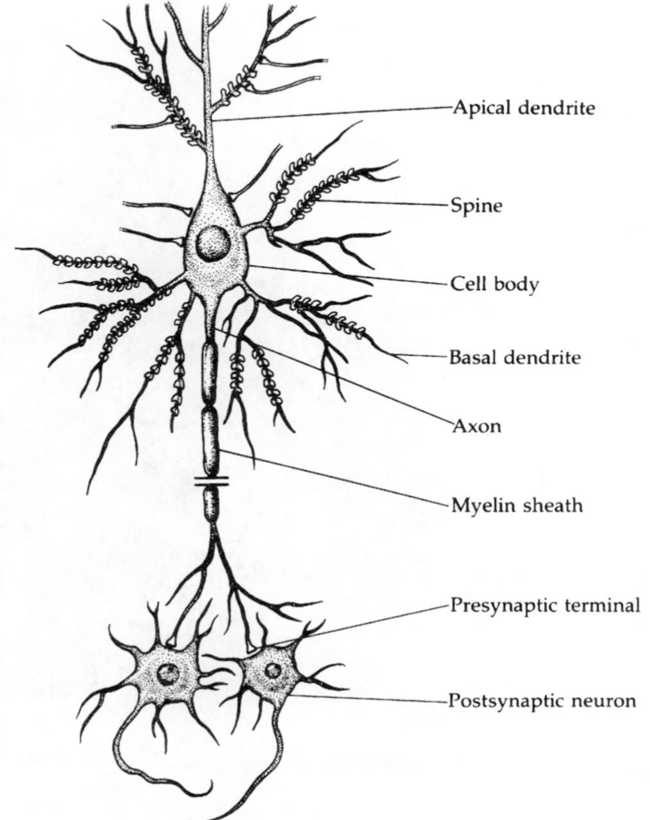

Figure 19-1. Nerve cell. (Reprinted with permission from Martin J. *Neuroanatomy.* New York: Elsevier, 1989.)

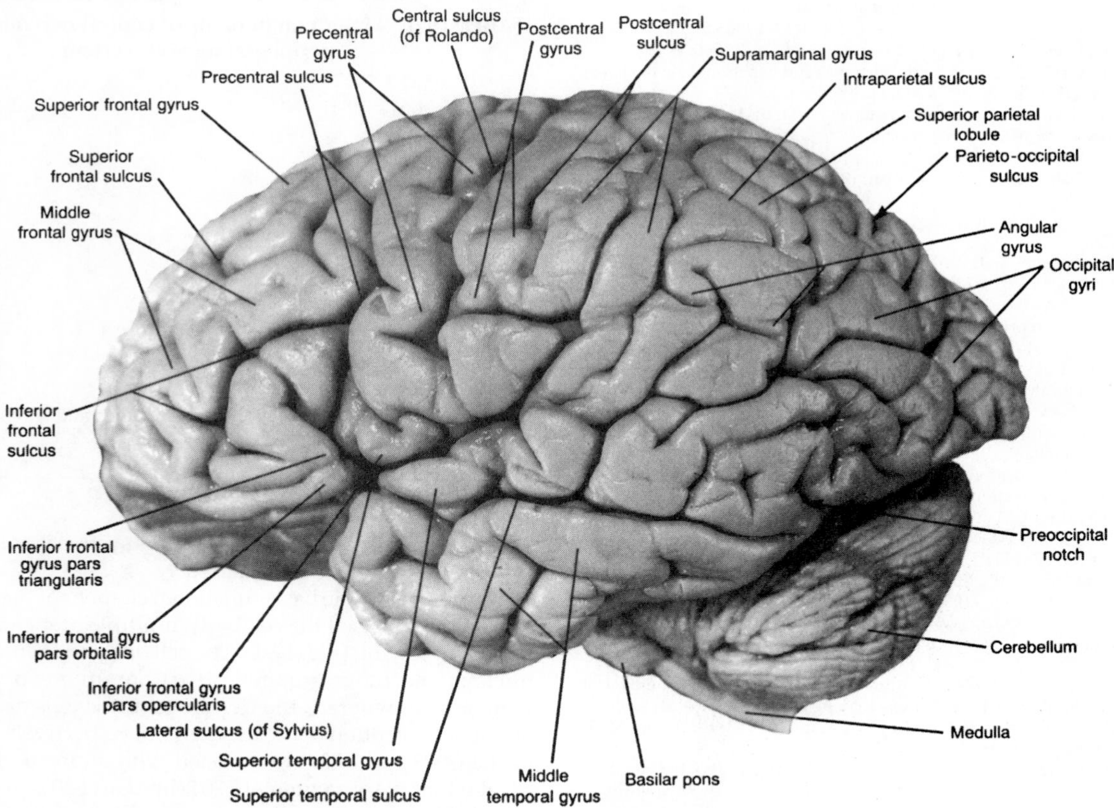

Figure 19-2. Lateral view of left cerebral hemisphere. (Reprinted with permission from Bhatnagar S, Andy O. *Neuroscience for the study of communicative disorders*. Baltimore: Williams & Wilkins, 1995.)

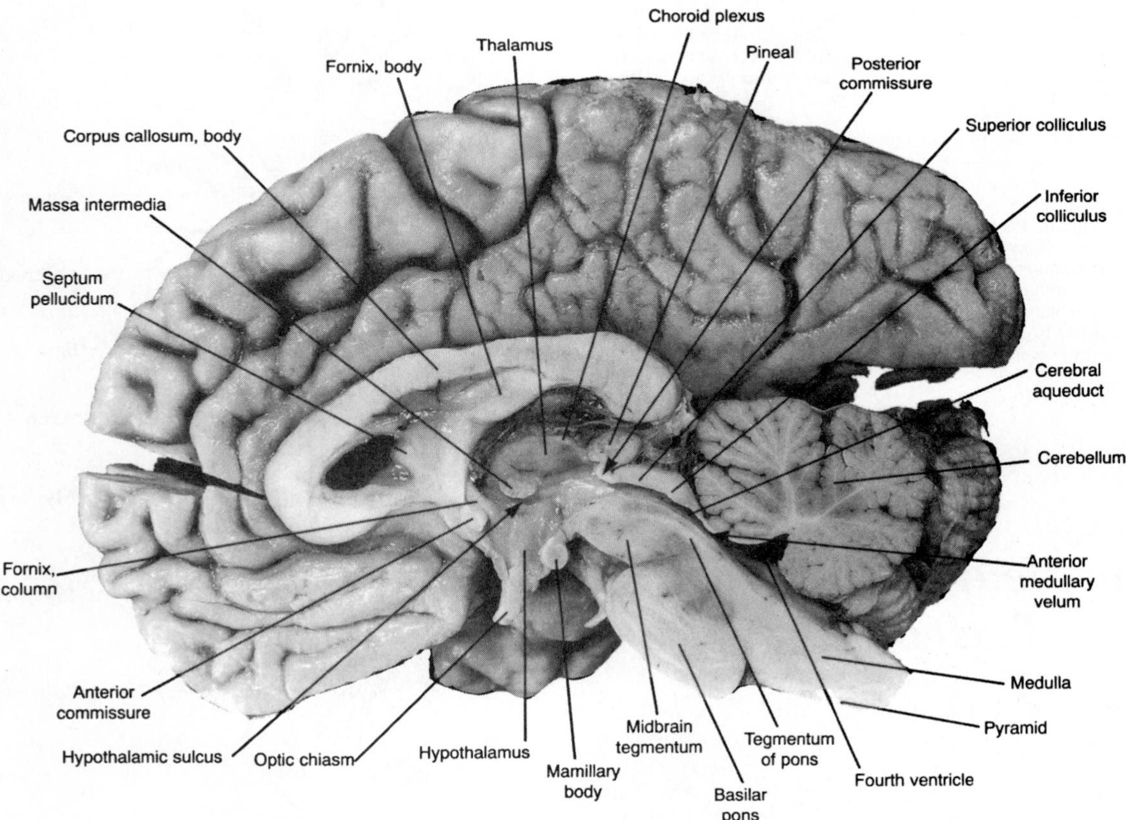

Figure 19-3. Midsagittal surface of diencephalon, second brain stem. (Reprinted with permission from Bhatnagar S, Andy O. *Neuroscience for the study of communicative disorders*. Baltimore: Williams & Wilkins, 1995.)

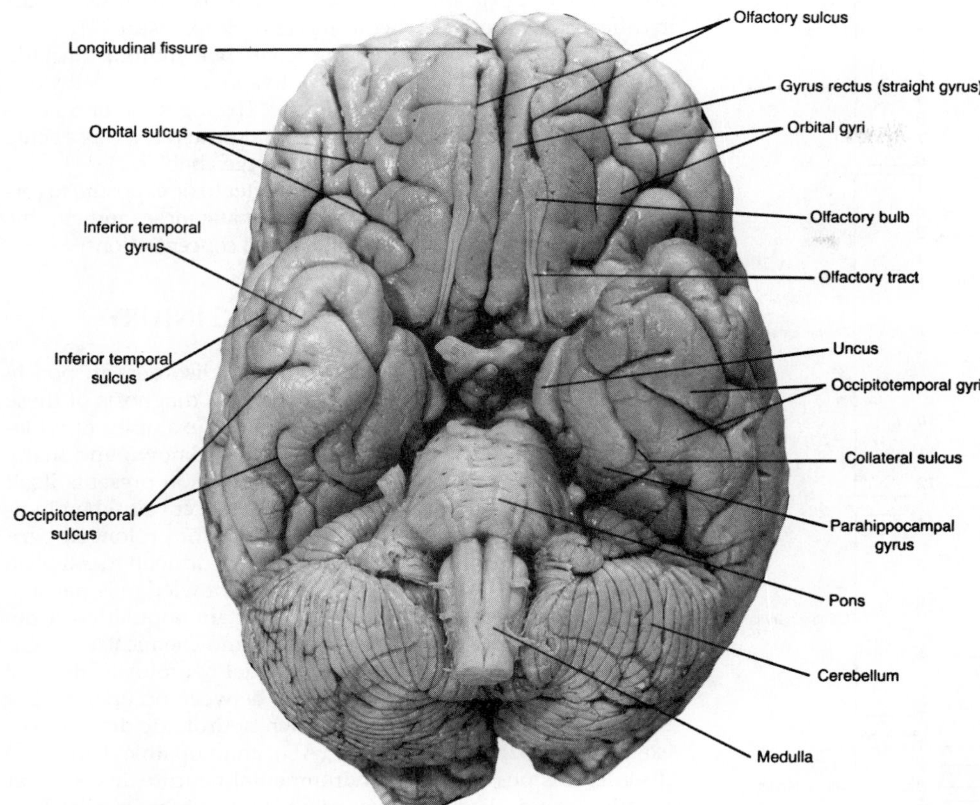

Figure 19-4. Ventral surface of cerebral hemisphere. (Reprinted with permission from Bhatnagar S, Andy O. *Neuroscience for the study of communicative disorders.* Baltimore: Williams & Wilkins, 1995.)

and Schwann cells in the PNS. Other types of CNS glial cells are astrocytes, which maintain a stable environment for neurons, and phagocytic cells called *microglia*.

The brain consists of the cerebrum, the brainstem, and the cerebellum (Fig. 19-2). The cerebrum contains the paired cerebral hemispheres, in which gray matter and white are easily distinguishable grossly. The gray matter includes the cerebral cortex on the outer surface of the brain, and the basal ganglia and diencephalon (thalamus and hypothalamus) deep within the hemispheres (Fig. 19-3). The white matter is made up of numerous myelinated tracts within and between the hemispheres that serve to connect cortical and subcortical gray matter structures.

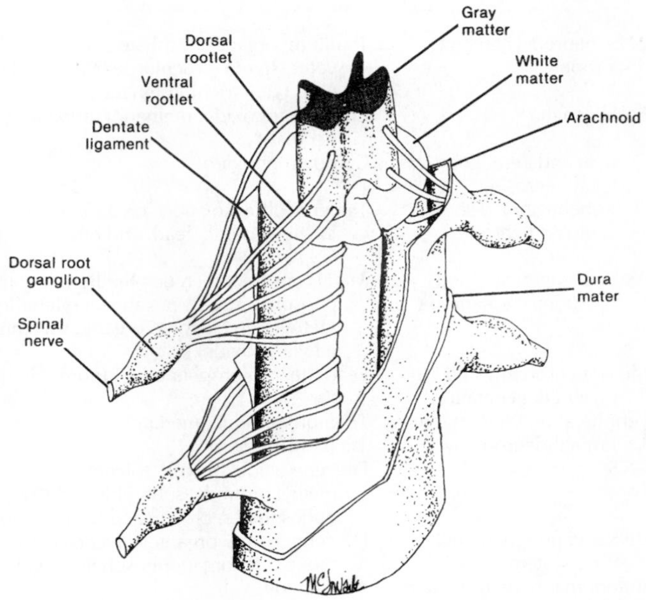

The ventral surface of the cerebral hemispheres reveals olfactory bulb and tracts, cerebellum, medulla, pons, and better views of the temporal lobe external anatomy (Fig. 19-4).

The spinal cord is a cylinder surrounded by pia mater. A dural sac is lined on the inside with the arachnoid membrane enclosing cerebrospinal fluid that occupies the subarachnoid space (Fig. 19-5). Denticulate ligaments anchor the spinal cord to the dura. Spinal nerves are connected to the spinal cord in pairs: eight cervical, 12 thoracic, five lumbar, five sacral, and one coccygeal (Fig. 19-6). Each spinal nerve has dorsal and ventral roots forming continuous rows along the spinal cord.

The response of the nervous system to toxic substances depends to a large extent on the function of the blood–brain barrier and its relatives, the blood–nerve and blood–cerebrospinal fluid (CSF) barriers (1,2). These barriers protect the CNS and PNS from bloodborne toxins that may damage other organs. The blood–brain barrier is effective in this regard because of (a) the presence of capillary endothelial cells that are invested with glial (astrocytic) processes, (b) tight junctions between the endothelial cells, and (c) a basement membrane between the endothelial cells and the astrocytic processes (1,2).

Figure 19-5. Spinal cord, meninges, and spinal nerves. (Reprinted with permission from Nulte J. *The human brain*, 2nd ed. St. Louis: CV Mosby Company, 1988.)

NEUROTOXICOLOGY

The nervous system enjoys relative protection from toxic insults. However, compounds that are nonpolar and lipid soluble—such as general anesthetics, analgesics, and organic solvents—

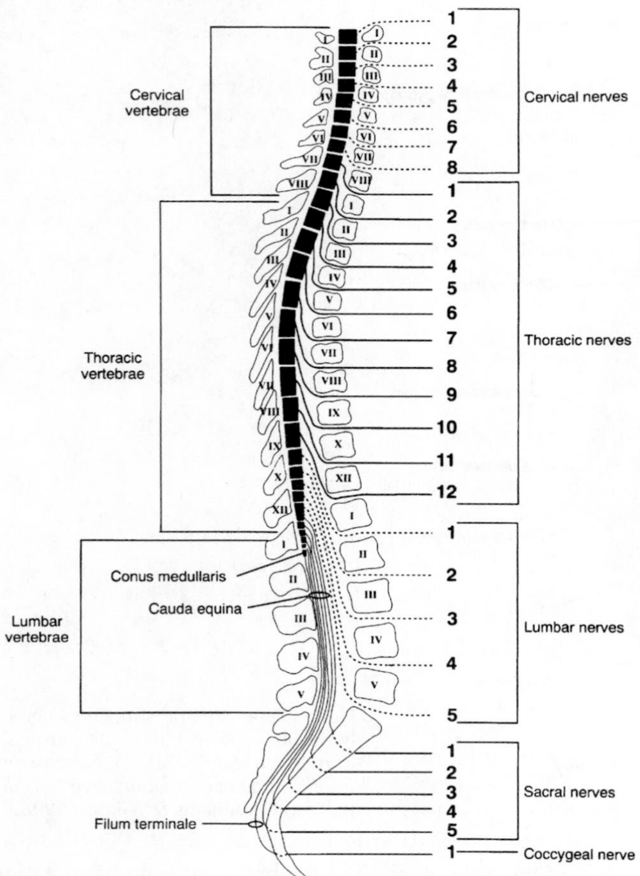

Figure 19-6. Spinal nerves in relation to vertebrae. (Reprinted with permission from Bhatnagar S, Andy O. *Neuroscience for the study of communicative disorders.* Baltimore: Williams & Wilkins, 1995.)

readily cross the blood–brain barrier. Moreover, age differences may influence the vulnerability of the nervous system to toxins; lead toxicity, for example, may cause acute or chronic encephalopathy in children because the blood–brain barrier is not yet fully developed, but rarely does so in adults.

Once the toxin has entered the nervous system, harmful sequelae may be caused by effects on the cell body, dendrites, axon, myelin, glial cells, or blood vessels. In clinical terms, toxic effects may manifest as neurobehavioral syndromes, seizures, movement disorders, cerebellar ataxia, cranial nerve disorders, and peripheral neuropathy (motor, sensory, or mixed) (3).

The route of exposure for neurotoxic chemicals varies considerably, but the three major ones are the lungs via inhalation, the gastrointestinal (GI) tract via ingestion, and the skin via absorption. Many chemicals can be absorbed through more than one route. Solvents and gases are best absorbed through the lungs, and metals through the GI tract; pesticides are well absorbed through the skin and the GI tract.

In general, two types of neurotoxicities may occur: acute and chronic. Acute neurotoxicity typically causes a physiologic or biochemical change in the nervous system that involves no structural change. The effect is usually rapidly reversible after withdrawal of the toxin, although exceptions to this rule are known; carbon monoxide, for example, may cause permanent structural brain injury and clinical sequelae after a single exposure.

Chronic exposures are more often associated with structural changes in the nervous system. These changes are due either to long-standing metabolic derangements that damage nervous tissue or to hypoxia and ischemia. A single toxin may also result in different syndromes in acute and chronic exposure (4).

Examples of neurotoxins causing acute CNS syndromes include high concentrations of organic solvent vapors such as methylene chloride, trichloroethylene, and toluene. The ingestion of concentrated hydrogen peroxide solutions (3% or greater) can cause acute cerebral infarction due to formation of oxygen bubbles.

Chronic CNS syndromes may occur after toxic exposure to certain metals, such as lead, mercury, and manganese, and chronic exposure to some organic solvents at high concentrations.

EPIDEMIOLOGY OF NEUROTOXIC INJURY

The incidence and prevalence of neurotoxic disorders are poorly known. The main reason is the difficulty in diagnosis of these syndromes. Data are mostly available from examples of widespread exposure in which the toxin is well known and many individuals are heavily exposed. This situation presents itself when accidental environmental exposures occur or when individuals abuse a substance at high levels or for prolonged periods. Low-level exposure, in contrast, is very difficult to establish as a cause of neurotoxicity. This lack of knowledge is particularly regrettable because of the risk to certain populations from exposure to a wide variety of pollutants and chemicals.

One approach to determining potential neurotoxic effects of chemicals is to search for associations between occupational or environmental exposures and known neurologic disease. For example, in Alzheimer's disease (AD), an idiopathic dementing disease, it is possible that environmental neurotoxins, such as aluminum and silicon, may contribute to the pathogenesis; these elements are found within neuritic plaques that are the neuropathologic hallmarks of the disease. However, the data implicating aluminum in AD are contradictory, and these elements are not likely to play an important role in the pathogenesis of the dis-

TABLE 19-2. Common neurotoxins affecting the central nervous system and peripheral nervous system

Target	Neurotoxins
CNS, neurons, cerebral atrophy	Thallium, organophosphates, organic solvents (styrene, trichloroethylene, toluene, 1,1,1-trichloroethane)
Basal ganglia	Carbon monoxide, methanol (putamen necrosis)
Cortical and cerebellar focal necrosis	Carbon monoxide
Neurobehavioral disorders, acute and chronic	Toluene, other solvents, organometallics, ethylene oxide, lead, and other metals, CS_2
Axon degeneration and sensorimotor neuropathy	Metals (arsenic, mercury, thallium, organophosphates, CS_2, hexane, acrylamide, methyl butyl ketone, organic solvents, ethylene oxide)
Motor neuropathy and myelin degeneration	Lead, hexachlorophene, tellurium, triethyl tin
Peripheral nervous system	Thallium, arsenic, mercury
Trigeminal neuropathy	Trichloroethylene
CNS	Ethylene oxide, organic solvents, metals, methyl bromide, sulfurylfluoride, organophosphates, chlorinated hydrocarbons
CNS and peripheral nervous system	Ethylene, oxide, organic solvents, carbon monoxide, organophosphates, lead
Autonomic nervous system	Acrylamide

CNS, central nervous system.

ease (5). Other studies have found no association of AD with any of eight occupational categories, ranging from factory worker to professional (6), further suggesting that environmental substances may not contribute to the etiology. Epidemiologic studies have merit, but they must often rely on indirect means of determining the neurotoxicity of a given substance.

The most important chemical classes with respect to occupational and environmental toxicity include organic solvents, metals, pesticides, and gases (Table 19-2).

DIAGNOSIS OF NEUROTOXIC SYNDROMES

The diagnosis of neurotoxic disorders is not difficult in the uncommon case of epidemic exposure or with a well-described syndrome. More common and challenging are individuals with neurologic symptoms in whom exposure to chemicals is unclear or poorly documented (7). It is appropriate in this setting to consider the possibility of a naturally occurring neurologic or nonneurologic disorder that could provide a more convincing explanation for the patient's complaints. Although some cases remain obscure even after extensive evaluation, the intelligent use of the history, neurologic examination, and diagnostic tests can significantly improve the accuracy of diagnosis (Table 19-3).

History

The foundation of the clinical neurotoxicologic evaluation is the history (4). Key elements include a detailed account of known or suspected toxic agents, the nature and duration of exposure, and the response to removal from presumed toxic exposure. In general, neurotoxic illness develops at the time of exposure or shortly thereafter and improves or resolves with removal of the toxin (4). Adherence to these principles often promptly settles a vexing clinical issue.

TABLE 19-3. Diagnostic approach to neurotoxicology

- History
  - Neurologic examination
    - Factual evidence sought regarding suspected exposure
    - Documentation of premorbid level of functioning
    - Preexisting neurologic or psychiatric disorders
    - Occupational and social history
    - Family history
  - Laboratory tests
    - Analysis for toxins (or metabolites) in blood, urine, hair, and nails as appropriate
    - Liver and kidney functions
    - Thyroid functions
    - Vitamin B_{12}
    - Serology
    - EMG and nerve conduction studies
    - Erythrocyte sedimentation rate
    - Spinal fluid analysis
  - Neuropsychological consultation
    - Thorough battery of cognitive and emotional tests
    - Comparison with prior level of functioning or test data when available
  - Special tests
    - Magnetic resonance imaging (MRI)
    - Computed tomography (CT)
    - Single photon emission computed tomography (SPECT)
    - Positron emission tomography (PET)
    - Evoked potentials

EMG, electromyelogram.

Other medical or neurologic problems, such as diabetes, that might contribute to the presentation should be pursued. The use of medications and alcohol or other drug use should be carefully documented. In patients with neurobehavioral impairment, it is often necessary to corroborate or obtain historic information from others who can provide it, such as family, friends, coworkers, and health professionals in the workplace.

Occupational history-taking is often neglected. The details elicited may serve to establish that neurotoxic exposure has or has not occurred (8,9):

1. Where do you work and how long have you been employed?
2. What type of service or product is produced?
3. Describe specifically what you do while working.
4. What materials, chemicals, or process do you work with?
5. Are the materials vapors, liquids, or solids?
6. Do you have skin contact with the materials?
7. Do you inhale or breathe any vapors?
8. Do you use protective equipment such as gloves, respirators, barrier creams, or clothing?
9. Were you given training and instruction on proper use, maintenance, and cleaning of protective equipment?
10. What are the conditions of your work area with regard to ventilation and drainage?
11. Is there a temporal relationship between your symptoms and your workplace?
12. What happens to your symptoms before beginning work? During work? After leaving work? On weekends or prolonged times away from work?
13. Do others at work have similar problems?

Neurologic Examination

A complete neurologic examination should evaluate the mental status, cranial nerves, motor system, coordination, gait, and reflexes (Table 19-4). Special attention should be directed to the areas of patient concern. Cognitive loss, for example, focuses the examination on the mental status, and distal paresthesias point to the peripheral nerves. Because toxic effects on the nervous system are typically diffuse, signs of involvement are nonfocal (4). The examination of a patient with neurotoxic disease may in fact suggest a metabolic, nutritional, degenerative, or demyelinating disease (4). If these etiologies are excluded, a toxic cause becomes more likely. Thus, a symmetric peripheral neuropathy may be quite helpful, whereas spastic hemiplegia should prompt a search for an alternative diagnosis. The same principle is true of neurobehavioral disorders; signs of acute confusion or dementia are typical of neurotoxic disorders whereas evidence of aphasia is not.

Neurotoxic agents affect the nervous system in a diffuse fashion and usually bilaterally and symmetrically. Also, toxins can produce multiorgan signs and symptoms resulting in different syndromes. Different exposure levels (acute or low-level), chronic exposures, and doses can also produce different symptomatology.

Laboratory Tests

The use of toxicologic testing depends on the particular agent involved and whether an established assay exists. Toxic substances or their metabolites can sometimes be detected in blood or urine. In many situations, these tests are of limited usefulness because of the time that has elapsed between the presumed exposure and neurologic evaluation (4).

TABLE 19-4. Summary of the clinical neurologic examination

I. Tests for cerebral function
 A. General cerebral function:
  1. General behavior and affect: Note eccentricities, mannerisms, disarray of dress, gestures. Is the patient cooperative? Note attitude and affect.
  2. Level of consciousness: Orientation to time, person, and place. Is the person conversant? Level of concentration.
  3. Intellectual performance: Level of intellect for education and background. Capacity for calculation, abstract reasoning.
  4. Emotional status: Tension, anxiety, hostility, depression, euphoria, inappropriateness.
  5. Thought content: Note preoccupations, delusions, illusions, hallucinations, excessive thought processes, or repetitions.
  6. Short-term memory: Retention of digits, repetition of series of numbers.
  7. Long-term memory: Can be tested for in taking a history.
 B. Specific cerebral functions
  1. Cortical sensory interpretation: An abnormality between peripheral sensory receptors and the cortex might compromise transmission of basic sensory information: tactile identification of shapes (stereognosis), recognition of numbers traced on skin (graphesthesia), two-point discrimination on the skin.
  2. Cortical motor integration: To carry out a skilled act, the person must be able to understand what is desired and the instruction. The inability to carry out purposeful or skilled acts in the absence of motor paralysis is called *apraxia*.
  3. Language: Characteristics of conversational speech and ability to comprehend spoken language, competency in repetition, naming, reading, and writing. Comprehension of spoken language, word finding, word listing, reading out loud.

II. Tests for the cranial nerves
 A. Olfactory: Tested by common smells with patient's eyes closed. Disorders of smell can occur from head trauma, sinusitis, upper respiratory infection, nasal obstruction, toxins, and medications.
 B. Optic: Visual acuity testing, visual field testing for visual impairment. Optic pathways are retina, optic nerves, nerve tracts, lateral geniculate body, geniculocalcarine tract, and occipital lobe.
 C. Oculomotor, IV trochlear, VI abducens: Tested as a unit because all supply muscles for eye movement. Cranial nerve (CN) III supplies muscles that cause pupillary constriction and elevate eyelids. Check range of extraocular movements in all directions. Difficulty with eye movement up, down, or medially involves CN III. Ptosis of eyelid and pupil dilation involves CN III. CN IV involves looking down with lateral motion of eye. Check for double vision and nystagmus. Pupillary reflexes are accommodation, constriction, consensual.
 D. Trigeminal: Facial sensation bilaterally, corneal reflex, masseter and temporal muscles, muscles of mastication, and sensation to mucosa of nose and mouth.
 E. Facial: Test wrinkling of forehead, frown, smile, raising eyebrows, and strength of closed eyelids. Sensory portion tested by sugar or salt on periphery of tongue. CN VII maintains facial symmetry. Paresis in lower face indicates involvement of supranuclear fibers supplying facial nerve. Paralysis of whole face involves motor nucleus or peripheral portion of CN VII. Motor nucleus is located in caudal portion of pons.
 F. Acoustic: Divided into cochlear nerve and vestibular nerve. Hearing can be checked with watch and tuning fork for lateralization and air and bone conductivity.
 G. Glossopharyngeal, X. Vagus: Tested together. Swallowing is mediated by vagus nerve. Gag reflux is mediated by CN IX. CN IX nucleus is in medulla. Motor and autonomic nuclei of CN X is in medulla.
 H. Accessory: Test strength of trapezius muscle while shoulders are shrugged against resistance. Test sternocleidomastoid strength.
 I. Hypoglossal: Test strength of the tongue while protruded. Move tongue side to side. Nucleus of CN XII is in medulla.

III. Tests for cerebellar function and coordination: Finger-to-nose testing for each hand, rapid alternating movements—feet tapping, pronating, and supinating hand on thigh while sitting, heel-to-toe walking, heel-to-shin test, Romberg's test, gait.

IV. Tests for the motor system
 A. Muscle size: Check for size and shape. Note any atrophy. Check hand muscles for wasting. Check for fasciculations or tremor. Fasciculations may indicate lower motor neuron wasting.
 B. Muscle tone: Check resistance to passive movement, check for spasticity, rigidity, and flaccidity.
 C. Involuntary movements: Note dystonic movements, jerky motions, choreiform movements, myoclonic contractions, tics, or tremors. Involuntary movements suggest extrapyramidal pathway involvement.
 D. Muscle strength: Compare strength of corresponding muscles on each side. Weakness indicates a lesion anywhere in the pathway from peripheral nerves, neuromuscular junction, muscles themselves, pyramidal tract in cerebrum, brainstem, and spinal cord.

V. Tests for the sensory system
 A. Primary forms of sensation
  1. Superficial tactile sensation (cotton test)
  2. Superficial pain (pinprick)
  3. Sensitivity to temperature (hot and cold)
  4. Vibration (tuning fork)
  5. Deep pressure pain
  6. Motion and position
 B. Cortical and discriminatory forms of sensation—requires interpretation by cerebral cortex: Two-point discrimination, point localization, stereognosis, texture discrimination, graphesthesia, and extinction phenomenon.

VI. Tests for reflex status
 A. Deep reflexes
  1. Biceps (cervical nerves 5 and 6)
  2. Brachioradialis (cervical nerves 5 and 6)
  3. Triceps (cervical nerves 6, 7, 8)
  4. Patellar (lumbar nerves 2, 3, 4)
  5. Achilles (sacral nerves 1, 2)
  6. Ankle clonus
 B. Superficial reflexes
  1. Abdominal
  2. Plantar
  3. Gluteal (cremasteric)
 C. Pathologic reflexes
  1. Babinski's
  2. Chaddock
  3. Oppenheim
  4. Gordon

TABLE 19-5. Neuroimaging pathology of select toxins

Toxin	Procedure	Neuropathology
Manganese	MRI, CT	Radiodensities in the basal ganglia areas
Methanol	CT	Putamen, globus pallidus lesions
Toluene	MRI	Cerebral atrophy, cerebellar atrophy, brain atrophy, increased periventricular white matter signal intensity, loss of differentiation of gray and white matter
Hydrogen peroxide	MRI, CT	Ischemic changes, cerebral infarction
Organic solvents	CT	Cerebral atrophy
Carbon monoxide	CT, MRI	Basal ganglia lesions, particularly globus pallidus, white matter lesions

CT, computed tomography; MRI, magnetic resonance imaging.

Standard screening blood tests are often indicated when other neurologic diseases are suspected; a chemistry survey, complete blood cell count, erythrocyte sedimentation rate, thyroid function tests, vitamin B_{12} and folate levels, serologic test for syphilis, and human immunodeficiency virus test may all be helpful.

Spinal fluid studies for inflammatory or infectious disorders can be performed if clinical suspicion is high.

Special Diagnostic Tests

Neurology has a variety of diagnostic methods that can prove helpful in diagnosis of neurotoxic disorders. Whereas none of these can provide a definitive answer in most cases, the information gained is often useful in supporting a clinical impression. The three categories of special tests are neuroimaging, clinical neurophysiology studies, and neuropsychological testing.

NEUROIMAGING

Computed tomography (CT) and then magnetic resonance imaging (MRI) have rapidly evolved to provide excellent structural imaging of the brain. Despite these advances, most CT and MRI scans are normal or show nonspecific cerebral volume loss in neurotoxic disorders because the injury is at a microscopic level that is below the resolution of the technology. Exceptions to this rule occur, however, as in the examples of carbon monoxide (10), methanol (11), toluene, and manganese (12) (Table 19-5). Functional imaging studies, including single photon emission computed tomography (SPECT), positron emission tomography (PET), and functional MRI have not yet been widely applied to neurotoxicology.

Neuroimaging evaluates anatomic or structural changes in the CNS by either CT scan or by MRI. Functional evaluation of the CNS is performed by PET, SPECT, and MRS.

CT scanning allows visualization of the brain and spinal cord in submillimeter detail; however, lack of metabolic information and specificity significantly reduces the use of CT scanning for neurotoxicology. CT scanning has been used to detect cerebral atrophy after toxic organic solvent exposure.

MRI allows imaging and visualization of abnormalities of the white matter of the brain, metabolic disorders, traumatic disorders, and inflammatory and degenerative disorders. MRI scanning has been used in detection of radiodense manganese concentrations in the basal ganglia areas of the brain (Fig. 19-7). As MRI and CT scanning become more widely used in evaluating neurotoxic disorders, more information regarding their usefulness is forthcoming.

PET scanning allows noninvasive measurement of metabolic activity, blood flow, and neurotransmission. Tracer molecules are tagged with a positron emitting radioisotope and injected systemically. Many radial isotopes are available. Most commonly used, however, are oxygen-labeled water for cerebral blood flow, fluorine-labeled fluorodeoxyglucose for glucose metabolism, and fluorine-labeled fluorodopa for dopamine receptor mapping. PET scanning is useful in evaluation of Par-

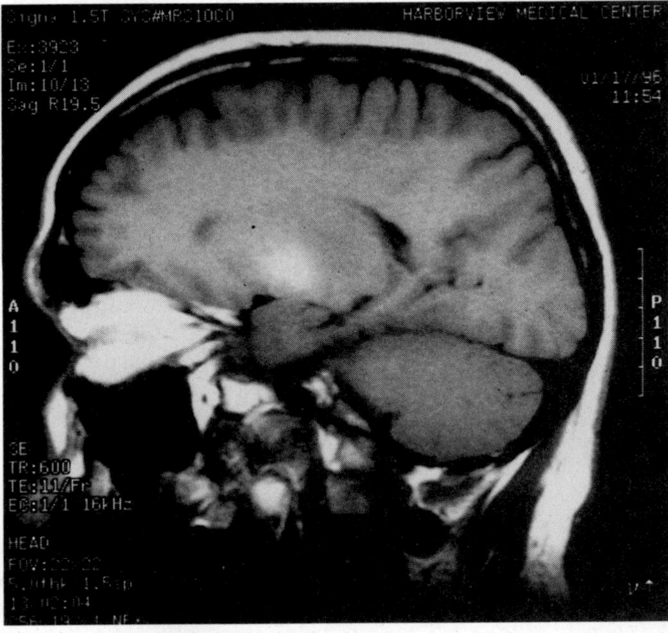

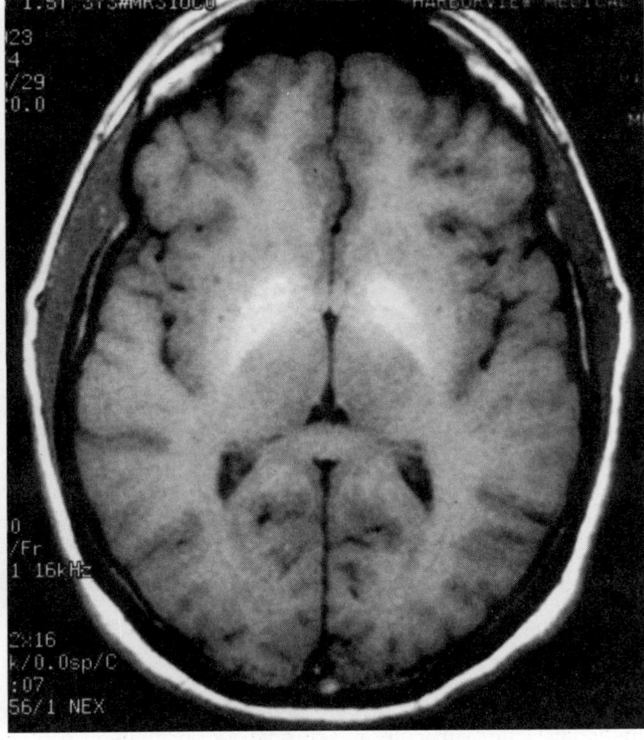

Figure 19-7. A: MRI scan showing deposition of manganese in area of the basal ganglia (*bright oval area*). **B:** MRI scan showing deposition of manganese (*bright area*) in the basal ganglia area. Courtesy of Jeff Burgess, M.D.

kinson's disease (PD), movement disorders, dementias, brain tumors, cerebral asemia, and schizophrenia. PET scanning has not been widely applied to neurotoxicology.

SPECT scanning is sometimes used in place of PET scanning. SPECT allows regional cerebral metabolism and neurotransmitter receptor imaging to be studied. SPECT has been used in evaluating AD and dementias. It is also used in brain injury from trauma. MRS allows detection of brain injury metabolites and allows for detection of subtler abnormalities than does MRI.

NEUROPHYSIOLOGY STUDIES

Clinical neurophysiology studies include nerve conduction velocities (NCVs), electromyography (EMG), electroencephalography (EEG), and evoked potentials (EPs). These tests allow a functional assessment of various regions in the CNS and PNS.

Electromyography and Nerve Conduction Velocities. EMGs and NCVs are used to document a distal axonal neuropathy, typically seen in neurotoxic disorders (13). However, a normal NCV or EMG study does not rule out toxic neuropathy because even a minority of normal conducting fibers can produce a normal electrical pattern (13). Changes indicating demyelination of peripheral nerves are unlikely to be toxin induced. EMGs and NCVs can also be used to diagnose other causes of peripheral nerve dysfunction such as entrapment syndromes (carpal tunnel) or mononeuropathy multiplex. Nerve conduction studies and EMG can detect subclinical abnormalities caused by peripheral neurotoxins.

EMG involves a needle examination. Nerve conduction studies are recordings of the amplitude and conduction philosophy of sensory nerve action potentials or compound muscle action potentials after nerve stimulation. EMG and NCV studies are used to determine the severity of a peripheral nerve disorder and sometimes can diagnose the underlying pathology. A properly conducted EMG and NCV study can determine the involvement of sensory or motor fibers and whether changes are axonal degeneration or demyelination:

Segmental demyelination
- Destruction of myelin sheath
- Axon may be spread
- Results in decreased nerve condition velocity
- Recovery may be complete

Axonal degeneration
- Entire neuron may be involved
- Distal axonal degeneration (distal axonopathy)
- Myelin sheath degeneration may occur
- Nerve conduction velocity is normal early, but amplitude of action potential may be decreased
- Distal muscle denervation
- Recovery is slow and may be incomplete

Peripheral neuropathies generally involve axonal degeneration as demonstrated in Fig. 19-8.

Usually, large fibers are preferentially affected; therefore, sensory nerve action potentials may be reduced in amplitude or may be absent altogether. Involvement of motor fibers and distal muscle groups and distal extremity muscle groups causes a reduced compound muscle action potential. Conduction velocity studies reflect size of the nerve, the nerve myelin content, the nodal and internodal links, resistance of the axon, and the temperature of the nerve. Myelin sheath lesions result in dramatic reductions of conduction velocity whereas axonal loss may be associated with borderline low conduction velocity abnormalities.

EMG is sensitive for axonal degeneration and abnormal EMG may be the first finding in subclinical neuropathies. EMG can also differentiate acute, subacute, and chronic peripheral neuropathies.

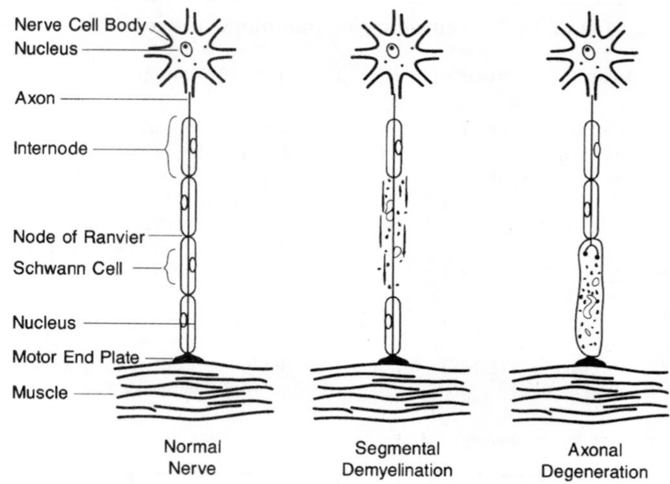

Figure 19-8. Pathologic features of toxic neuropathies.

EMG and NCV data must be compared to population normative values to determine if the EMG and NCV are abnormal in a tested individual.

Evoked Potentials. Three basic EPs are used in clinical neurology to test the integrity of sensory CNS pathways from receptor to cortex: Visual evoked potentials (VEPs), auditory evoked potentials (AEPs), and somatosensory evoked potentials.

EPs can generate reliable information about the integrity of sensory pathways from the periphery to the cortex. VEPs, AEPs, and somatosensory evoked potentials may all be performed. Although abnormalities of AEPs have been found in persons heavily exposed to toluene (12), the usefulness of EPs in detecting low-level or occupational exposure remains uncertain.

Electroencephalogram. EEGs are basically not very useful as a neurologic diagnostic technique for toxic disorders. An EEG's value for neurotoxicity detection and determination is limited.

The EEG has long been a useful test for seizure disorders and metabolic-toxic disorders, but its use in many instances of suspected toxic disorder is limited because findings are nonspecific and may relate to other causes of brain dysfunction (14).

Neuropsychological Studies. In many cases of neurobehavioral impairment, the need for quantified evaluation dictates that formal neuropsychological testing be performed. This provides a useful extension of the mental status examination, but standardization of this assessment is difficult (15) because of the wide variety of neuropsychological tests in common use (16). Table 19-6 provides a list of tests often used in neurobehavioral toxicology along with the cognitive and emotional domains they are designed to assess. Whereas the procedures of neuropsychology offer helpful information, they usually cannot lead to an unequivocal diagnosis, and clinical judgment in light of all the available information is the best final arbiter. This uncertainty applies especially to computerized testing (17) that has been proposed as a means of evaluating large numbers of individuals in the field and in epidemiologic studies.

Neuropsychological studies assess subtle brain dysfunctions caused by neurotoxic substances. It also assesses the functional integrity of the CNS. Besides being frequently used, neuropsychological studies also have generated disagreement and some controversy. Patients suspected of a neurotoxicity should be evaluated within the larger scope of educational background, preexisting psychological problems, sociologic data, and demo-

TABLE 19-6. Neuropsychological tests

Attention and concentration
  Paced Auditory Serial Attention Test
  Digit Span
Memory
  Wechsler Memory Scale
  Benton Visual Retention
Psychomotor performance
  Finger tapping
  Grip strength
  Santa Ana Dexterity Test
Sensation and perception
  Tactual Performance Test
  Seashore Rhythm Test
  Speech Sounds Perception Test
  Reitan-Klove Sensory Perceptual Examination
Sequencing, planning, and efficiency
  Trail Making Tests A and B
  Digit Symbol Test (subtest of Wechsler Adult Intelligence Scale—Revised)
Abstraction and cognitive flexibility
  Halstead Category Test
  Wisconsin Card Sorting Test
  Stroop Color-Work Interference Test
Language skills
  Reitan Indiana Aphasia Screen Test
  Boston Diagnostic Aphasia Examination
Personality and emotional state
  Minnesota Multiphasic Personality Inventory
  Taylor Manifest Anxiety Scale
Intelligence and academic skills
  Wechsler Adult Intelligence Scale—Revised
  Wechsler Intelligence Scale for Children—Revised
  Peabody Individual Achievement Test

graphic data that influence the outcome of the testing. Neuropsychological testing is an adjunct to proper diagnostic approaches, including a logical examination, ancillary testing, and neuroimaging. Neuropsychological testing for neurotoxicity should take a comprehensive approach examining cognitive, affective, and neurobehavioral functions.

The World Health Organization (WHO) and the National Institute of Occupational Safety and Health (NIOSH) have provided a battery of neuropsychological testing that they term a "core" battery of tests selected for their sensitivity to neurotoxic effects as well as providing a comprehensive neuropsychological survey. The WHO and NIOSH battery includes the following tests (15):

- Aiming
- Simple Reaction Time
- Santa Ana Dexterity Test
- Digital Symbol Test
- Benton Visual Retention Test
- Digit Span
- Profile of Mood States

CLINICAL SYNDROMES OF NEUROTOXICOLOGY

Neurotoxic disorders can affect any area of the nervous system, and produce a variety of clinical syndromes: central and peripheral neuropathies, cranial nerve neuropathies, neurobehavioral disorders, seizures, movement disorders, cerebellar disorders, acute confusional states, and dementia. Toxic causes are multiple.

Neurotoxicity of Organic Solvents

Organic solvents can be absorbed by inhalation, ingestion, and percutaneous absorption. Toxicity from organic solvents can be acute or chronic. In general, acute toxicity from organic solvents produces diffuse central neurologic manifestations. However, some solvents may cause more focal neurotoxic presentations such as the peripheral neuropathy induced by hexane and methyl butyl ketone (2-hexanone) after chronic exposure.

Neurotoxicity from organic solvent is divided into PNS and CNS syndromes. High-level exposure to organic solvents can induce an acute encephalopathy. Long-term exposure may result in irreversible neurotoxicity. Toluene is an example of a solvent that can produce severe CNS damage on high-level inhalation characterized by ataxia and focal CNS damage.

High concentration inhalation exposure is most common in two situations: inhalational abuse of a solvent and confined space exposure. Intentional inhalational exposure of solvents can result in a person's being exposed acutely to concentrations varying from 100- to 1,000-fold higher than occupational permissible exposure levels. Such intentional abuse results in an acute CNS syndrome and acute encephalopathy.

Confined space exposure in occupational settings can result in solvent vapor exposure that is immediately dangerous to life and health. Acute intoxication of an organic solvent can range from feelings of euphoria, dizziness, lightheadedness, and ataxia to loss of consciousness, seizures, and death.

Acute intoxication with toluene produces euphoria, ataxia, headache, paresthesias, and depressed reflexes. Exposure to high concentrations produces acute confusional states. Persistent neurotoxicity after high-dose toluene exposure includes cognitive disorders, cerebellar ataxia, optic neuropathy, hearing loss, and other multifocal CNS defects. Brainstem dysfunction and corticospinal lesion signs also occur. Chronic toluene inhalation also can produce diffuse brain white matter pathology that can be seen on MRI.

SOLVENT SYNDROME

The "solvent syndrome" is a controversial topic and many studies of the topic have been criticized. The syndrome is thought to be induced by a chronic exposure to organic solvents that results in personality changes, memory loss, fatigue, depression, and a psychoorganic syndrome.

One problem involving solvent exposure and the occupational environmental arena is that, generally, mixtures of solvents are involved instead of one single solvent, and dealing with mixtures can be complicated. Standardization of a diagnostic approach to the solvent syndrome or the psychoorganic syndrome has been attempted by WHO and summarized by Rosenberg (18):

Type 1: Symptoms only. Complaints of nonspecific symptoms; completely reversible if exposure discontinued; equivalent to "neurasthenic syndrome."

Type 2A: Sustained personality or mood change. Same as type 1, but symptoms are not reversible.

Type 2B: Impairment in intellectual function. Symptoms are accompanied by objective evidence of impairment on neuropsychological tests; "minor neurologic signs" may be seen and may not be reversible, synonymous with "psychoorganic syndrome" and "mild dementia."

Type 3: Dementia. Marked global deterioration in intellectual function; neurologic signs evident, poorly reversible, if at all, but is generally nonprogressive once exposure has ceased.

This classification ranges from complaints of nonspecific symptoms that are reversible with discontinuation of exposure, to changes in personality and mood, impairment of intellectual function, and dementia. Many studies on the psychoorganic syndrome or the solvent syndrome are lacking in terms of methodology, and diagnosis of chronic toxic encephalopathy differs greatly. The solvent syndrome has been reported in a variety of workers and in a variety of industries with these reports focusing on neuropsychological studies, EEG changes, vestibular function, EMG and nerve conduction testing, VEPs, cerebral blood flow, and CT scan.

In summary, it is unclear whether cerebral atrophy differs between the control groups and those who are said to have a solvent syndrome. The medical literature is in disagreement over low-level solvent exposure resulting in psychoorganic syndrome or the solvent syndrome. The data point to the fact that below recognized permissible exposure limits, the solvent syndrome does not occur.

Seizures

A seizure is a paroxysmal and excessive discharge of cerebral neurons. A seizure disorder, or epilepsy, is a condition of recurrent unprovoked seizures, and implies that an epileptogenic brain lesion is present. Thus, a single seizure or flurry of seizures does not necessarily imply that a seizure disorder exists. This distinction is important in neurotoxicology because many neurotoxins can cause seizures during periods of acute intoxication, but it is exceedingly rare for toxin exposure to be the cause of a seizure disorder (19). Seizures can be classified as follows (19):

I. Generalized, symmetric, and bilateral
  A. Tonic-clonic
    1. Clonic
    2. Tonic
    3. Aclonic
  B. Myoclonic
  C. Absence
II. Partial seizures
  A. Simple partial (unimpaired consciousness)
    1. Motor
    2. Sensory
    3. Autonomic
  B. Complex partial (impaired consciousness)
  C. Partial with secondary generalization

A wide variety of solvents, metals, pesticides, and gases can cause acute seizures, and the severity of the episode generally parallels the degree of exposure (Table 19-7). Withdrawal of the offending agent typically leads to resolution of the problem without recurrence.

TABLE 19-7. Toxins associated with seizures

Solvents	Hydrogen sulfide
Methanol	Carbon monoxide
Ethylene glycol	Pesticides and insecticides
Carbon tetrachloride	Organophosphates
Benzene	Carbamates
Chlorobenzene	Strychnine
Dioxane	Picrotoxin
Nitromethane	Methylbromide
2-Naphthol	Sulfuryl fluoride
Metals	Ethylene oxide
Arsenic	Aldrin
Lead	Dieldrin
Thallium	Lindane
Mercury	Toxaphene
Antimony	Endrin
Aluminum	Chlordane
Reducing agents	Isobenzan
Monomethylhydrazine	Endosulfan
Decaborane	Pyrethrins
Pentaborane	Pyrethroids
Chemical asphyxiants	Nicotine
Hydrogen cyanide	

Movement Disorders

The term *movement disorders* refers to motor dysfunction related not to weakness but to abnormalities of muscle tone, voluntary movement, and posture. Movement disorders encompass involuntary movements such as tremor, dystonia, chorea, athetosis, dyskinesia, myoclonus, and ballismus, but for purposes of neurotoxicology, the most common syndrome is parkinsonism. Toxins associated with movement disorders are

Parkinsonism
- Carbon disulfide
- Manganese
- Carbon monoxide
- Hydrogen cyanide
- Carbon disulfide
- 1-Methyl-4-phenyl-1,2,3,6-tetrahydropyridine (MPTP)
- Carbon tetrachloride

Ataxia, tremor, myoclonus
- Hydrazine
- Phosphine
- Methyl mercury
- Chlordecone
- Acrylamide
- Methylbromide

In keeping with the classic features of PD, the degenerative disease from which the name of this syndrome is derived, parkinsonism manifests as resting tremor, bradykinesia, and rigidity. Parkinsonism has been observed after exposure to manganese (20), carbon monoxide (21), carbon disulfide (22), carbon tetrachloride (23), methanol (24), cyanide (25), and MPTP (26). MPTP is particularly intriguing because it produces a clinical syndrome very similar to PD and involves selective damage to the substantia nigra that also mimics the pathology of PD (27). MPTP produced acute parkinsonism in individuals who thought they were injecting an analog of meperidine intravenously for abuse purposes.

Cerebellar Ataxia

Disorders of coordination are typically caused by cerebellar dysfunction. Solvents are especially likely to cause cerebellar ataxia, and heavy toluene exposure is associated with ataxia and cerebellar white matter damage (28). Mercury (29), the pesticide chlordecone (30), and the fumigant gas methyl bromide (31) also can lead to cerebellar dysfunction.

Cranial Neuropathy

Unlike the peripheral nerves, the cranial nerves are rarely the target of neurotoxic assault. Probably the best-known toxic syndrome of the cranial nerves is trigeminal neuropathy related to trichloroethylene (TCE) exposure (32). More than 3.5 million individuals are exposed to TCE (18), and it was once used as an anesthetic agent. Cranial neuropathies after TCE general anesthesia were noted. TCE splash or high vapor exposures have produced trigeminal neuropathy and weakness in the facial nerve and optic nerve. Attempts to reproduce trigeminal neurotoxicity with pure TCE have been unsuccessful, indicating that TCE breakdown products, such as dichloracetylene, are the most likely causative agent (18).

TABLE 19-8. Toxins associated with peripheral neuropathy

Arsenic
Lead
Mercury
Thallium
Organo-tin compounds (trimethyl tin)
Carbon disulfide
Chronic ethanol ingestion
Ethylene oxide
n-Hexane
Trichloroethylene
Methylhexane
Methylbromide
Styrene
Methyl-*n*-butyl ketone
Acrylamide
Organic solvent mixtures
Dimethylaminopropionitrile
Delayed neuropathy of organophosphates

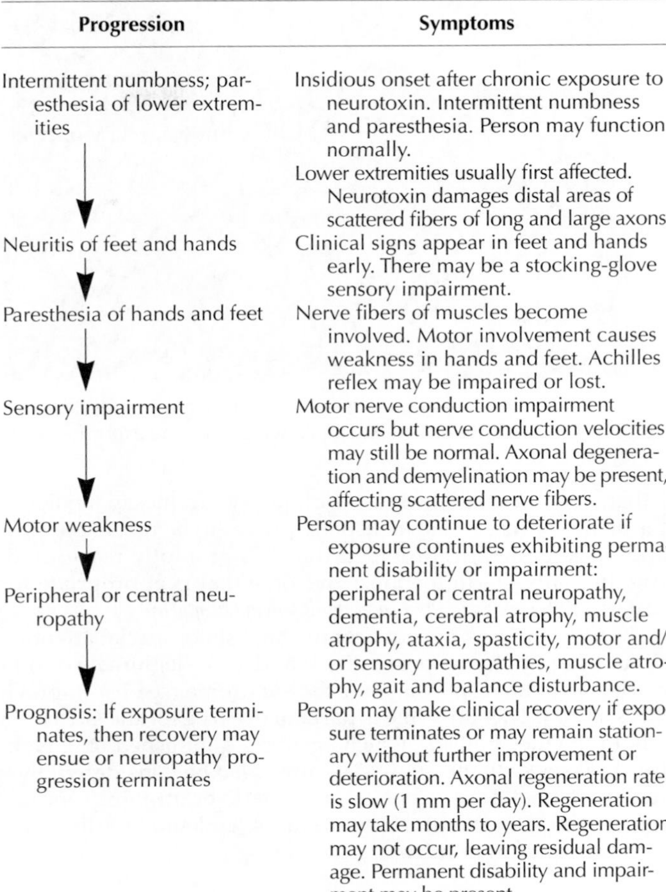

TABLE 19-9. Clinical progression of toxic neuropathy

Progression	Symptoms
Intermittent numbness; paresthesia of lower extremities	Insidious onset after chronic exposure to neurotoxin. Intermittent numbness and paresthesia. Person may function normally. Lower extremities usually first affected. Neurotoxin damages distal areas of scattered fibers of long and large axons.
Neuritis of feet and hands	Clinical signs appear in feet and hands early. There may be a stocking-glove sensory impairment.
Paresthesia of hands and feet	Nerve fibers of muscles become involved. Motor involvement causes weakness in hands and feet. Achilles reflex may be impaired or lost.
Sensory impairment	Motor nerve conduction impairment occurs but nerve conduction velocities may still be normal. Axonal degeneration and demyelination may be present, affecting scattered nerve fibers.
Motor weakness	Person may continue to deteriorate if exposure continues exhibiting permanent disability or impairment:
Peripheral or central neuropathy	peripheral or central neuropathy, dementia, cerebral atrophy, muscle atrophy, ataxia, spasticity, motor and/or sensory neuropathies, muscle atrophy, gait and balance disturbance.
Prognosis: If exposure terminates, then recovery may ensue or neuropathy progression terminates	Person may make clinical recovery if exposure terminates or may remain stationary without further improvement or deterioration. Axonal regeneration rate is slow (1 mm per day). Regeneration may take months to years. Regeneration may not occur, leaving residual damage. Permanent disability and impairment may be present.

Peripheral Neuropathy

Neurotoxic disease is an important source of occupational neurologic disorders. One must be aware that there are many other causes of peripheral neuropathy, including alcohol abuse, diabetes mellitus, and medications in common use, such as vincristine (33), cisplatin (34), and podophyllin (35). Many environmental and occupational substances can also cause neuropathy (Table 19-8). Some well-known peripheral neurotoxins include the solvents *n*-hexane (36) and methyl-*n*-butyl-ketone (37); the metals lead (38), mercury (39), arsenic (40), and thallium (41); the organophosphate pesticides (42); and the gases carbon disulfide (43) and ethylene oxide (44).

Symptoms typically start insidiously and include numbness and paresthesias of feet and hands, and progress to involve distal weakness (Table 19-9). Autonomic features are rare, but pain may be prominent. Gait disorder and muscle atrophy may develop after prolonged exposure. Toxic neuropathy is usually axonal in nature, and may involve large fibers (with prominent vibratory sense impairment) or small fibers (with pain and temperature impairment). Withdrawal of the toxin can often lead to recovery, with axonal regeneration at a rate of approximately 1 mm per day.

A patient may interpret numbness as loss of sensation, tingling, or weakness. Most peripheral neuropathies from toxic causes are symmetric with distal nerve involvement. Clinical findings usually demonstrate sensory loss early on, and motor and sensory deficits as the neuropathy progresses. Cranial nerve function and CNS function are usually normal. Motor involvement typically shows decreased muscle tone and weakness that are usually symmetric and more commonly seen in the lower extremities. Motor weakness usually involves toe extensors (extensor digitorum brevis), foot dorsiflexors (anterior tibialis), and the extensor muscles in the hands (hypothenar or dorsal interossei) (18). Reflexes may be hypoactive or absent. The Achilles reflex may be impaired or absent in long nerve neuropathies. Gait problems may be related to neurosensory impairment, but ataxia is usually absent. Rapid alternating movements are intact. A tremor may be seen with large fiber neuropathy (18). Also, impaired vibratory sensation may occur distally, but is normal more proximally. Small-fiber involvement causes loss of pinpoint pain discrimination with a stocking-glove distribution. Hot and cold sensation may also be impaired if small fibers are involved. Two-point discrimination and stereognosis are not selectively impaired relative to any sensory loss.

An axonal neuropathy pattern can be seen on electrophysiologic examination. Conduction velocities reflect nerve size, myelin content, axonal resistance, nodal and internodal lengths, and nerve temperature (18). Myelin sheath lesions reflect a dramatic loss in NCVs (Fig. 19-9). Axonal loss of large fibers may cause a borderline loss in NCVs. EMG is a sensitive indicator of axonal degeneration and may show abnormalities early in the course of a peripheral neuropathy. EMG also helps to define the chronicity of a lesion (18).

Neurobehavioral Syndromes

Two major syndromes can occur after neurotoxic exposure: acute confusional state (45) and dementia (46). These are two of the most familiar neurobehavioral syndromes and each has a wide range of potential etiologies (47). Most toxic agents can, in fact, produce either syndrome depending on the degree and duration of exposure (46). Table 19-10 lists toxic chemicals associated with neurobehavioral dysfunction.

The clinician's task is first to identify the syndrome and then to pursue its specific diagnosis in a systematic fashion. The possibility of drug abuse often demands consideration in this process (48), and even prescription medications can play a role.

ACUTE CONFUSIONAL STATE

Acute confusional state is a rapidly evolving disorder of arousal and attention that can take the form of agitation and autonomic overactivity (delirium), or, more commonly, somnolence and

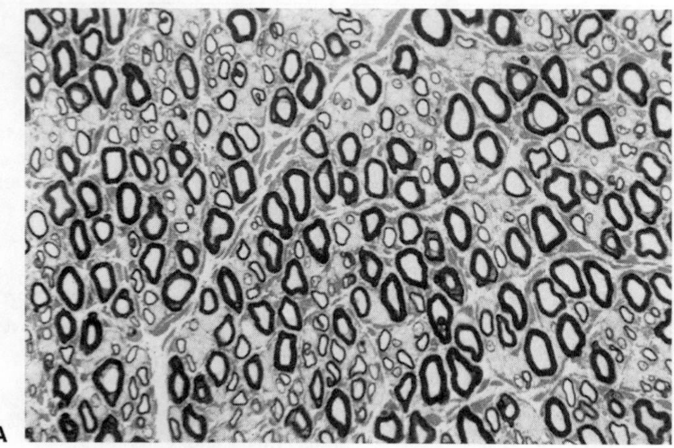

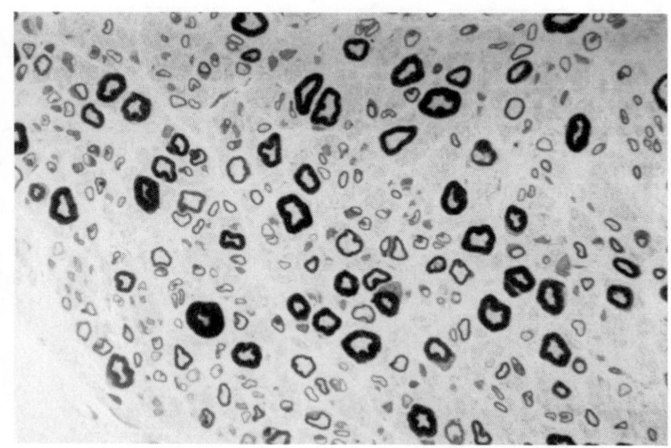

Figure 19-9. A: Normal sural nerve. **B:** Abnormal sural nerve biopsy showing loss of myelin sheath and degeneration following *n*-hexane exposure.

lethargy (45). One of the most common syndromes in medicine, the acute confusional state usually proves to be reversible with appropriate therapy, provided that it is promptly recognized. An alternative term for this syndrome that is appropriate for neurotoxicologists is *toxic-metabolic encephalopathy.*

In the diagnosis of acute confusional state, special attention should be paid to the possibility that drugs—legitimate or otherwise—can be responsible for the syndrome (see list in previous section). This principle is particularly true for the elderly, in whom the metabolism of such agents is diminished (49). Nontoxic causes of acute confusion must also be considered. Systemic metabolic disturbances, traumatic brain injury, stroke, infectious and inflammatory diseases, and seizure disorders may cause a similar picture.

DEMENTIA

Dementia is an acquired and persistent impairment of neurobehavioral function that generally spares attention but affects cognitive and emotional competence (46). This impairment is sufficient to interfere with normal social and occupational function. Because it most often affects older people, dementia is a syndrome with steadily increasing importance in our aging society, but younger individuals may also be affected. In advanced countries, AD is by far the most common of the dementias, accounting for more than one-half the cases that are diagnosed (50). The ominous nature of the syndrome, which in most cases is irreversible, understandably results in a growing concern on the part of people exposed to potentially neurotoxic substances.

TABLE 19-10. Toxic chemicals associated with neurobehavioral dysfunction

Toluene	Lead
Styrene	Mercury
Xylene	Arsenic
Methanol	Manganese
Trichloroethylene	Thallium
Perchloroethylene	Aluminum
Carbon disulfide	Organophosphates
n-Hexane	Organochlorines
Ethylene glycol	Paraquat
Carbon tetrachloride	Carbon monoxide
Methylene chloride	Nitrous oxide

Some individuals, in fact, are found to have AD or another dementia when a neurotoxic disorder is first suspected.

The list of potential neurotoxins causing dementia is long, although it is often unclear whether a given substance has been definitely proven to be culpable. Substances known to cause dementia include lead, carbon monoxide, and toluene. These are discussed in some detail to illustrate important principles of this syndrome.

Lead poisoning or plumbism has been known since antiquity. Lead encephalopathy typically affects children. In adults, a predominantly motor neuropathy is more common. The vulnerability of children to lead has been shown in children who ingest lead paint from older buildings, so-called pica (51), and in a case of gasoline sniffing that resulted in irreversible encephalopathy attributable to tetraethyl lead intoxication (52). Lead encephalopathy can also result from ingestion of "moonshine" whiskey contaminated with lead (53). Diagnosis can be established by blood testing for lead, and chelation therapy with dimercaptosuccinic acid, ethylenediaminetetraacetic acid, or penicillamine can be helpful in acute poisoning; persistent dementia may result, however, despite treatment (53).

Exposure to carbon monoxide can occur from suicide attempts or poorly ventilated areas in which motorized machinery is active (54). Neurobehavioral effects can range from mild confusion to coma and death. Because of its high affinity for hemoglobin, carbon monoxide deprives the brain of normal oxygen delivery, and neuropathologic changes mimic those seen with anemic anoxia: neuronal loss in the hippocampus, laminar necrosis in the cortex, and degeneration in the basal ganglia. Carboxyhemoglobin levels more than 30% are associated with cognitive changes; these may take the form of a cortical dementia with amnesia, aphasia, apraxia, and agnosia (55). A delayed dementia may also occur after several days of early recovery, and is thought to be owing to cerebral demyelination (56). Treatment of carbon monoxide poisoning involves removal from the source and the use of hyperbaric oxygen.

The dementia of toluene abuse has become better understood. This disorder is particularly instructive, and serves as an example of a toxic neurobehavioral syndrome with well-defined neuropathology. Toluene is a widely used solvent and a major constituent of commercially available spray paints. When toluene vapor is inhaled, acute exposure can induce euphoria, and toluene has become an inexpensive and easily obtained drug of abuse. Prolonged heavy exposure has been shown to cause central neurotoxicity, of which dementia is the most prominent feature (27). Individuals so affected have abnormalities in the cerebral white matter on MRI scans (12), and these changes appear to result from solvent-induced leukoencephalopathy in the brain (57). The severity of the dementia correlates with the degree of white matter involvement on MRI (58), and this disorder is an example of a white matter dementia (59).

More uncertainty surrounds the problem of low-level exposure to toluene and other solvents in the workplace. As is often the case in neurotoxicology, occupational exposures are difficult to link with clinical syndromes. An extensive literature has appeared in Scandinavian countries regarding the purported neurobehavioral effects of low-level solvent exposure (7). The psychoorganic syndrome (7) or the "painter's syndrome" (7,60) refers to a syndrome of fatigue, irritability, depression, and memory loss in workers exposed to solvents (60). Initial reports implicating neurobehavioral toxicity have been questioned by later studies that suggest no association between exposure and symptoms (61). The role of alcohol in causing these symptoms was not clearly excluded (62). Studies have often been confused by the possibility of psychiatric factors that could also explain some or all of these complaints (63).

A final area of concern is the appearance of two syndromes related to American military involvement. The first is the possible neurotoxicity of the defoliant Agent Orange that was widely used in the Vietnam War, and the second is the so-called Gulf War syndrome. Both of these issues have generated much controversy because of the large number of individuals potentially involved who may be eligible for governmental compensation.

Between 1962 and 1971, more than 11 million gallons of the herbicide Agent Orange were sprayed over South Vietnam (64). A by-product of Agent Orange was dioxin, which was implicated in causing birth defects and cancer (64), and public concern led to major studies examining the possible health effects of herbicides used in Vietnam. Although hampered by methodologic problems, these studies concluded that no association of herbicides and clinical neurologic disorders (neurobehavioral or otherwise) could be established, and that no strong biological plausibility for such associations was suggested (64).

The war in the Persian Gulf was waged in 1990 and 1991. Since then, reports have appeared describing many veterans who have a variety of nonspecific symptoms: attention and memory impairment, depression, insomnia, headaches, vertigo, joint and muscle pain, paresthesias, and fatigue (65). These complaints are more prevalent in military personnel who participated in this war than in those who were not deployed in the Persian Gulf (66), and these symptoms have been postulated to result from exposure to cholinesterase-inhibiting chemicals, such as organophosphate compounds and pyridostigmine bromide (67). Moreover, neuropsychological abnormalities compatible with exposure to these chemicals have been documented in a small sample of Gulf War veterans (68). Despite the suggestion, however, that exposure to chemical warfare agents may be responsible, no direct evidence exists of a culpable agent in this syndrome (69).

REFERENCES

1. Lewis AJ. Functions of supporting cells. In: Lewis AJ, ed. *Mechanisms of neurological disease*. Boston: Little, Brown and Company, 1976:77.
2. Norton S. Toxic responses of the central nervous system. In: Klassen CD, Amdur MO, Doull J, eds. *Casarett and Doull's toxicology: the basic science of poisons*. New York: Macmillan, 1986:359.
3. Anger WK, Johnson BL. Chemicals affecting behavior. In: O'Donoghue JL, ed. *Neurotoxicity of industrial and commercial chemicals*. Boca Raton, FL: CRC Press, 1985:51.
4. Schaumburg HH, Spencer PS. Recognizing neurotoxic disease. *Neurology* 1987;37:276.
5. Blass JP. Pathophysiology of the Alzheimer's syndrome. *Neurology* 1993;43[Suppl 4]:S25.
6. Amaducci LA, Fratiglioni L, Rocca WA, et al. Risk factors for clinically diagnosed Alzheimer's disease: a case-control study of an Italian population. *Neurology* 1988;36:922.
7. Flodin U, Edling C, Axelson O. Clinical studies of psycho-organic syndrome among workers with exposure to solvents. *Am J Ind Med* 1984;5:287.
8. Lee WR, McCallum RI. The occupational history. In: Raffle PAB, Lee WR, McCallum RI, Murray R, eds. *Hunter's diseases of occupation*. Boston: Little, Brown and Co., 1987:229.
9. Imbus HR. Clinical aspects of occupational medicine. In: Zenz C, ed. *Occupational medicine*. Chicago: Year Book Medical Publishers, 1988:107.
10. Klawans HL, Stein RW, Tanner CM, Goetz CG. A pure parkinsonian syndrome following acute carbon monoxide intoxication. *Arch Neurol* 1982;39:302.
11. Rubinstein D, Escott E, Kelly JP. Methanol intoxication with putaminal and white matter necrosis: MRI and CT findings. *Am J Neuroradiol* 1995;16:1492.
12. Rosenberg NL, Spitz MC, Filley CM, Davis KA, Schaumburg HH. Central nervous system effects of chronic toluene abuse—clinical, brainstem evoked response and magnetic resonance imaging studies. *Neurotoxicol Teratol* 1988;10:489.
13. Schaumburg HH, Spencer PS. Toxic neuropathies. *Neurology* 1979;29:429.
14. Seppalainen AM. Neurophysiological findings among workers exposed to organic solvents. *Acta Neurol Scand* 1982;66[Suppl 92]:109.
15. Hartman DE. *Neuropsychological toxicology*. New York: Pergamon Press, 1988.
16. Lezak MD. *Neuropsychological assessment*, 3rd ed. New York: Oxford University Press, 1995.
17. Agnew J, Schwartz BS, Bolla KI, Ford DP, Bleecker ML. Comparison of computerized and examiner-administered neurobehavioral testing techniques. *J Occup Med* 1991;33:1156.
18. Rosenberg NL. Neurotoxicity of organic solvents. In: Rosenberg NL. *Occupational and environmental neurology*. Boston: Butterworth–Heinemann, 1995.
19. Gulevich SJ, Lewin E, Rosenberg NL. Paroxysmal disorders and occupational neurology. In: Rosenberg NL, ed. *Occupational and environmental neurology*. Boston: Butterworth–Heinemann, 1995:129.
20. Mena I, Marin O, Fuenzalida S, Cotzias GC. Chronic manganese poisoning—clinical picture and manganese turnover. *Neurology* 1967;17:128.
21. Ringel SP, Klawans HL. Carbon monoxide-induced parkinsonism. *J Neurol Sci* 1972;16:245.
22. Peters HA, Levine RL, Matthews CG, Sauter SL, Rankin JH. Carbon disulfide-induced neuropsychiatric changes in grain storage workers. *Am J Ind Med* 1982;3:373.
23. Melamed E, Lavy S. Parkinsonism associated with chronic inhalation of carbon tetrachloride. *Lancet* 1977;1(8019):1015.
24. Guggenheim MA, Couch JR, Weinberg W. Motor dysfunction as a permanent complication of methanol ingestion. Presentation of a case with beneficial response to levodopa treatment. *Arch Neurol* 1971;24:550.
25. Rosenberg NL, Myers JA, Martin WRW. Cyanide-induced parkinsonism: clinical, MRI, 6-fluorodopa PET studies. *Neurology* 1989;39:142.
26. Langston JW, Ballard P, Tetrud JW, Irwin I. Chronic parkinsonism in humans due to a product of meperidine-analog synthesis. *Science* 1983;219:979.
27. Davis GC, Williams AC, Markey SP. Chronic parkinsonism secondary to intravenous injection of meperidine analogs. *Psychiatry Res* 1979;1:249.
28. Hormes JT, Filley CM, Rosenberg NL. Neurologic sequelae of chronic solvent vapor abuse. *Neurology* 1986;36:698.
29. Albers JW, Kallenbach LR, Fine LJ, et al. Neurological abnormalities associated with remote occupational mercury exposure. *Ann Neurol* 1988;24:651.
30. Taylor JW, Selhorst JB, Houff SA, Martinez AJ. Chlordecone intoxication in man, I: clinical observations. *Neurology* 1978;28:626.
31. Moses H, Klawans HL. Bromide intoxication. In: Vinken PJ, Bruyn GW, eds. *Handbook of clinical neurology: intoxications of the nervous system*. Part 1, vol. 36. Amsterdam: North Holland, 1979:291.
32. Feldman RG. Trichloroethylene. In: Vinken PJ, Bruyn GW, eds. *Handbook of clinical neurology: intoxications of the nervous system*. Part 1, vol. 36. Amsterdam: North Holland, 1979:457.
33. Casey EB, Jellife AM, Le Quesne M, Millett YL. Vincristine neuropathy: clinical and electrophysiological observations. *Brain* 1973;96:69.
34. Roelofs RI, Hrushesky W, Rogin J, Rosenberg L. Peripheral sensory neuropathy and cisplatin chemotherapy. *Neurology* 1984;34:934.
35. Filley CM, Graff-Radford NR, Lacy JR, Heitner M, Earnest MP. Neurologic manifestations of podophyllin toxicity. *Neurology* 1982;32:308.
36. Herskowitz A, Ishii N, Schaumburg HH. *N*-hexane neuropathy: a syndrome occurring as a result of industrial exposure. *N Engl J Med* 1971;285:82.
37. Allen N, Mendell JR, Billmaier DJ, et al. Toxic polyneuropathy due to methyl-*n*-butyl ketone: an industrial outbreak. *Arch Neurol* 1975;32:209.
38. Feldman RG, Hayes MK, Younes R, et al. Lead neuropathy in adults and children. *Arch Neurol* 1977;34:481.
39. Albers JW, Kallenbach LR, Fine LJ, et al. Neurological abnormalities associated with remote occupational mercury exposure. *Ann Neurol* 1988;24:651.
40. Heyman A, Pfeiffer JB, Willett RW, et al. Peripheral neuropathy caused by arsenic intoxication. *N Engl J Med* 1956:254:401.
41. Anderson O. Clinical evidence and therapeutic indications in neurotoxicology, exemplified by thallotoxicosis. *Acta Neurol Scand Suppl* 1984;70:185.
42. Gutmann L, Besser R. Organophosphate intoxication: pharmacologic, neurophysiologic, clinical, and therapeutic implications. *Semin Neurol* 1990;10:46.
43. Aaserud O, Hommeren OJ, Tvedt B, et al. Carbon disulfide exposure and neurotoxic sequelae among viscose rayon workers. *Am J Ind Med* 1990;18:25.
44. Gross JA, Haas ML, Swift TR. Ethylene oxide neurotoxicity: report of four cases and review of the literature. *Neurology* 1979;29:978.
45. Strub RL, Black FW. *Neurobehavioral disorders: a clinical approach*. Philadelphia: F. A. Davis, 1988:107.

46. Cummings JL, Benson DF. *Dementia: a clinical approach*, 2nd ed. Boston: Butterworth–Heinemann, 1992.
47. Filley CM. *Neurobehavioral anatomy.* Niwot, CO: University Press of Colorado, 1995.
48. Brust JCM. *Neurological aspects of substance abuse.* Boston: Butterworth–Heinemann, 1993.
49. Meredith LA, Filley CM. Acute confusional state. In: Jahnigen DW, Schrier RW, eds. *Geriatric medicine.* Cambridge, MA: Blackwell Science, 1996:283.
50. Filley CM. Alzheimer's disease: it's irreversible but not untreatable. *Geriatrics* 1995;50:18.
51. Albert JJ, Breault HJ, Friend WK, et al. Prevention, diagnosis, and treatment of lead poisoning in children. *Pediatrics* 1969;44:291.
52. Valpey R, Sumi SM, Copass MK, Goble GJ. Acute and chronic progressive encephalopathy due to gasoline sniffing. *Neurology* 1978;28:507.
53. Whitfield CL, Ch'ien LT, Whitehead JD. Lead encephalopathy in adults. *Am J Med* 1972;52:289.
54. Gilbert GJ, Glaser GH. Neurologic manifestations of chronic carbon monoxide poisoning. *N Engl J Med* 1969;261:1217.
55. Winter P, Miller J. Carbon monoxide poisoning. *JAMA* 1976;236:1502–1504.
56. Plum F, Posner JB, Hain RF. Delayed neurological deterioration after anoxia. *Arch Intern Med* 1962;110:18.
57. Rosenberg NL, Kleinschmidt-DeMasters BK, Davis KA, Dreisbach J, Hormes JT, Filley CM. Toluene abuse causes diffuse central nervous system white matter changes. *Ann Neurol* 1988;23:611.
58. Filley CM, Heaton RK, Rosenberg NL. White matter dementia in chronic toluene abuse. *Neurology* 1990;40:532.
59. Filley CM, Franklin GM, Heaton RK, Rosenberg NL. White matter dementia: clinical disorders and implications. *Neuropsychiatry Neuropsychol Behav Neurol* 1989;1:239.
60. Arlien-Soberg P, Bruhn P, Glydensted C, Melgaard B. Chronic painters' syndrome: chronic toxic encephalopathy in house painters. *Acta Neurol Scand* 1979;60:149.
61. Gade E, Mortenson EL, Bruhn P. Chronic painter's syndrome: a reanalysis of psychological test data in a group of diagnosed cases, based on comparisons with matched controls. *Acta Neurol Scand* 1988;77:293.
62. Juntunen J, Matikainen E, Antii-Poika M, Souranta H, Valle M. Nervous system effects of long-term occupational exposure to toluene. *Acta Neurol Scand* 1985;72:512.
63. Filley CM. Neurobehavioral disorders in workers. In: Rosenberg NL. *Occupational and environmental neurology.* Boston: Butterworth–Heinemann, 1995:115.
64. Goetz CG, Bolla KI, Rogers SM. Neurologic health outcomes and Agent Orange: Institute of Medicine report. *Neurology* 1994;44:801.
65. Haley RW, Kurt TL, Hom J. Is there a Gulf War syndrome? Searching for syndromes by factor analysis of symptoms. *JAMA* 1997;277:215.
66. Iowa Persian Gulf study group. Self-reported illness and health status among Gulf War veterans: a population-based study. *JAMA* 1997;277:238.
67. Haley RW, Kurt TL. Self-reported exposure to neurotoxic chemical combinations in the Gulf War: a cross-sectional epidemiologic study. *JAMA* 1997;277:231.
68. Haley RW, Hom J, Roland PS, et al. Evaluation of neurologic function in Gulf War veterans: a blinded case-control study. *JAMA* 1997;277:223.
69. Landrigan PJ. Illness in Gulf War veterans: causes and consequences. *JAMA* 1997;277:259.

CHAPTER 20
Clinical Cardiac Toxicology

Neal L. Benowitz

Approximately 50% of deaths in the United States result from heart disease or stroke. Although many cardiovascular deaths may be accounted for by the known risk factors of hypertension, diabetes, cigarette smoking, hyperlipidemia, and genetic factors, many other cardiovascular deaths are not explained by these risk factors. Exposure to toxic chemicals—both in the workplace and in the general environment—may be responsible for a significant number of cases of cardiovascular disease.

Toxins can affect the cardiovascular system at a variety of sites (Table 20-1). The heart may be injured by ischemia (atheromatous or nonatheromatous coronary artery disease), asphyxia, direct myocardial injury, or disturbances in electric impulse formation or conduction. Blood vessels can be affected diffusely, by systemic vasoconstriction (resulting in hypertension) or by focal obstruction (arterial occlusive disease). This chapter discusses toxic cardiovascular disease from the perspective of types of injuries, with discussion of the epidemiology, mechanisms of toxicity, and clinical features for specific toxins within each class of injury. The scope of the chapter is limited to industrial and environmental chemicals. Medications, food poisoning, and plant poisoning, although important causes of acute cardiovascular disease, are not discussed. The reader is referred elsewhere for detailed discussion of cardiovascular complications of drug intoxication (1).

TABLE 20-1. Chemical toxins and cardiovascular disease

Atherosclerotic ischemic heart disease
Carbon disulfide (1)[a]
Carbon monoxide (3)
Combustion products (3)
Environmental tobacco smoke (2)
Arsenic (3)
Nonatheromatous ischemic heart disease
Organic nitrates (1)
Myocardial asphyxiants
Carbon monoxide (1)
Cyanide (1)
Hydrogen sulfide (1)
Direct myocardial injury
Cobalt (2)
Arsenic (1)
Arsine (1)
Lead (3)
Antimony (2)
Organic solvents (3)
Arrhythmias
Halogenated hydrocarbons (1)
Organophosphates (1)
Antimony (2)
Arsenic (1)
Arsine (1)
Hypertension
Lead (2)
Cadmium (3)
Carbon disulfide (3)
Arsenic (2)
Peripheral arterial occlusive disease
Arsenic (2)
Lead (2)
Carbon disulfide (2)

[a]Probability of causation: 1, definite; 2, probable; 3, possible.
Adapted from ref. 2, with permission.

CAUSATION OF CHEMICAL-INDUCED CARDIOVASCULAR DISEASE

Cardiovascular disease is common in all industrialized countries, and causation of such disease by chemical exposures is often difficult to establish. Occasionally, massive exposures to carbon monoxide or cyanide produce acute injury and clear causation. More commonly, cardiovascular disease is seen in the context of low-dose, repeated exposure. It is difficult to establish the cause of cardiovascular disease for several reasons:

- Cardiovascular disease is common, even in the absence of toxic exposures. Thus, in the typical workplace, many workers have cardiovascular disease, and it is difficult to spot clusters or epidemics.
- There is often nothing specific, either clinically or pathologically, to establish toxic cardiovascular disease. If present,

other risk factors are usually assumed to be the cause of cardiovascular disease.

- It is rarely possible to document high tissue levels of suspected toxicants.
- It is difficult to establish the level of exposure of a worker to industrial chemicals over the many years it may take to develop cardiovascular disease.
- Cardiovascular toxicants are likely to interact with other risk factors or preexisting disease in causing or manifesting cardiovascular disease.

For the most part, our ideas about causation of toxic cardiovascular disease are based on epidemiologic studies. Establishing causation through such studies is difficult because of the generally small increases in relative risk and potential confounding with cardiovascular risk factors, including lifestyle and diet. In only a few cases has it been shown that removing a person or a population from a toxic exposure reduces the risk of cardiovascular disease.

Epidemiologic studies on chemical-induced cardiovascular disease must be viewed considering these limitations. The epidemiologic literature on chemical factors in causing cardiovascular disease has been comprehensively reviewed elsewhere (2). An attempt was made in that review to evaluate the methodological quality of studies that support causation for particular toxins. Based on the number of studies, the number of subjects studied, and the quality of the research design, the probability of causation by chemical risk factors was judged as summarized in Table 20-1. Selected epidemiologic studies or specific toxic exposures will be mentioned in the section on cardiovascular diseases caused by specific chemicals.

CARDIOVASCULAR DISEASES CAUSED BY SPECIFIC CHEMICALS OR TOXINS

Atherosclerotic Vascular Disease

There is substantial evidence for accelerated development of atherosclerotic coronary artery disease after exposure to carbon disulfide, combustion products, and arsenic. Nitroglycerin and carbon monoxide have also been associated with an increased incidence of coronary heart disease.

CARBON DISULFIDE

Epidemiology. Chronic exposure to carbon disulfide is well documented to increase mortality from ischemic heart disease. Research has primarily been conducted on viscose rayon workers. A 2.5-fold excess in mortality from coronary heart disease in workers exposed to carbon disulfide was first reported in 1968 (3). Subsequently, a prospective study from Finland demonstrated a 5.6-fold relative increase in coronary heart disease mortality and a threefold increased risk of first nonfatal myocardial infarction in carbon disulfide–exposed workers (4). Interventions that reduce carbon disulfide exposure have been shown to reduce the risk of cardiovascular disease to control levels (5). This observation—along with findings of another recent study showing that ischemic heart disease mortality was increased with increasing exposure in the previous 2 years, whereas the increased risk did not persist in workers who had left the industry (6)—suggests that carbon disulfide may also produce an acute reversible effect on the cardiovascular system. Of note, two recent studies of the relationship between carbon disulfide exposure to risk factors for coronary heart disease, performed in viscose rayon workers under modern threshold-limit value (TLV) standards, report conflicting results. A U.S. study of 165 workers with an average 8-hour exposure ranging from 0.6 to 11.8 ppm showed a significant positive relationship between low-density lipoprotein cholesterol and diastolic blood pressure with carbon disulfide exposure (7). A German study of 247 workers with exposures ranging from less than 0.2 to 65.7 ppm (median, 4.0) found no relationship between carbon disulfide exposure and blood pressure, blood lipids, blood glucose, or fibrinolytic activity (8). Thus, it is unclear whether the TLV of 10 ppm is adequate to prevent cardiovascular risk.

Exposure. Carbon disulfide is primarily used as a solvent in the manufacturing of viscose rayon but is also used as a solvent for rubber, fats, oils, resins, and the synthesis of other chemicals. Inhalation of the vapors is the major route of exposure, although carbon disulfide can also be absorbed through the skin.

Exposure to levels of 2,000 ppm carbon disulfide results in narcosis; 1,000 ppm has been associated with severe neuropsychiatric disturbance; 300 to 400 ppm produces mild poisoning after several hours. The concentration of carbon disulfide in workers with increased coronary heart disease who have been exposed is reported at 20 to 60 ppm. The current TLV is 10 ppm.

Mechanisms of Toxicity and Pathophysiology. Carbon disulfide–induced cardiovascular disease has been clearly demonstrated, and several likely mechanisms have been described. Carbon disulfide reacts with amines or amino acids in the body to form dithiocarbamates, which in turn form complex trace metals (particularly copper and zinc) and chemically react with certain enzymatic cofactors such as pyridoxine (9,10). The chelation of metals that are cofactors for enzymes, as well as direct inactivation by carbon disulfide, results in inhibition of many enzyme systems (including dopamine β-hydroxylase). Carbon disulfide may interfere with normal inhibition of elastase activity, resulting in excess elastase activity with disruption of blood vessel walls and formation of aneurysms. Carbon disulfide has also been proposed to decrease fibrolytic activity with a resultant enhancement of thrombosis.

Inhibition of enzymatic processes is thought to produce a number of metabolic disturbances—including abnormalities of lipid metabolism and thyroid function—that can lead to hypercholesterolemia and hypothyroidism (9,11). Inhibition of dopamine β-hydroxylase, an enzyme that converts dopamine to norepinephrine, may be responsible for hypertension as well as for some of the neuropsychiatric features of carbon disulfide intoxication. Inhibition of aldehyde dehydrogenase may result in a disulfiram-like reaction to alcohol, with flushing and hypotension.

Accelerated atherosclerotic vascular disease may occur as a consequence of carbon disulfide effects on blood pressure, lipids, thyroid function, glucose tolerance, and fibrolytic activity. The risks of carbon disulfide exposure remained after adjusting for hypertension and serum cholesterol, indicating that carbon disulfide may have other toxic effects on the cardiovascular system (12).

The resultant pathology includes atherosclerotic vascular disease involving the coronary, cerebral, and peripheral arteries. Renal vascular hypertension has also been reported. Microaneurysms and atrophic changes of the retina are seen in the eyes of workers chronically exposed to excessive amounts of carbon disulfide (13).

Clinical Features. Acute intoxication may produce symptoms and signs of encephalopathy or polyneuropathy, including fatigue, headaches, dizziness, disorientation, paresthesias, psychoses, and delirium. After chronic exposure, patients may present with hypertension or manifestations of atherosclerotic vascular disease, such as angina or myocardial infarction. It is noteworthy that the typical patient demonstrates one or more of the known risk factors for coronary artery disease, and only from an occupational history will the role of carbon disulfide be suspected. Work in rayon or rubber manufacturing, chemical manufacturing, or chemistry laboratories should prompt further inquiry into possible exposure to carbon disulfide.

An early sign of chronic carbon disulfide poisoning on physical examination is abnormal ocular microcirculation, characterized by microaneurysms and hemorrhages resembling those of diabetic retinopathy.

Laboratory findings may include a decrease in serum thyroxine levels and an increase in serum cholesterol levels, particularly those of the very-low-density β-lipoproteins. Carbon disulfide concentration in blood can be measured by gas chromatography–mass spectrometry (14), although the assay is not available for routine monitoring. In one group of 42 workers occupationally exposed to carbon disulfide, the mean free and acid labile carbon disulfide concentrations were 261 and 9,482 ng per L, respectively. In contrast, the carbon disulfide concentrations in individuals taking disulfiram (200 mg per day) for treatment of alcoholism were many-fold higher—mean free and acid labile carbon disulfide, 897 and 40,084 ng per L, respectively. The urinary excretion of 2-thiothiazolidine-4-carboxylic acid, a conjugation product of carbon disulfide and glutathione, is proportional to exposure as measured by ambient air monitoring and may be a more practical measure of occupational exposure (15).

Other diagnostic studies that may be of use include fluorescein angiography of the retinal blood vessels, which may show delayed filling of retinal arteries as an early sign of vascular disease. The electrocardiogram (ECG) sometimes shows evidence of ischemia or previous myocardial infarction. The presence of coronary artery disease may be confirmed by exercise stress testing and coronary angiography.

The vascular findings in patients with chronic carbon disulfide poisoning are similar to those seen in any patient with atherosclerotic vascular disease. The most specific finding is an abnormal ocular microcirculation in the absence of diabetes. The diagnosis is based on the clinical picture of premature vascular disease and history of exposure to excessive levels of carbon disulfide for more than 5 to 10 years.

COMBUSTION PRODUCTS (INCLUDING ENVIRONMENTAL TOBACCO SMOKE)

Combustion of organic materials produces a complex mixture of particulates and gases that include polycyclic aromatic hydrocarbons, nitrosamines, aldehydes, hydrogen cyanide, nitrogen oxides, carbon monoxide, and, depending on the source, certain trace metals, including cadmium, arsenic, and lead. The fact that exposure to combustion products can cause atherosclerotic heart and vascular disease has been suggested by the strong association between cigarette smoking and atherosclerotic vascular disease. Although the mechanism of disease is unknown, carbon monoxide, polycyclic aromatic hydrocarbons, and, in cigarette smokers, nicotine and certain glycoproteins have been suspected as contributing to the process.

Epidemiology. Acute carbon monoxide poisoning can cause myocardial injury or aggravate underlying vascular disease. High-level chronic exposures [carboxyhemoglobin (HbCO), 20% to 30%] have been reported to produce a several-fold increase in the incidence of coronary artery disease in tatami mat makers in Northern Japan (16). These workers heated their buildings with charcoal braziers while tightly sealing windows and doors to conserve heat during cold winter weather.

It has been suggested that chronic carbon monoxide exposure at levels more relevant to occupational exposure (HbCO, 5% to 15%) places workers at increased risk of coronary artery disease. This observation is based on studies of carbon monoxide in animals (which have had conflicting results) and the association between HbCO level and coronary artery disease risk in cigarette smokers (17,18). The latter is difficult to interpret, because carbon monoxide exposure is strongly associated with exposure to other toxic substances in cigarette smoke. Epidemiologic studies of carbon monoxide exposure in humans report conflicting results. One study reported a dose-related association between carbon monoxide exposure and angina symptoms, but not ECG abnormalities, in foundry workers (19). One study found excess mortality from atherosclerotic heart disease in New York City tunnel officers (exposed to carbon monoxide from auto exhaust) with a standardized mortality ratio of 1.35 (95% confidence intervals of 1.09 to 1.68) (20). No relationship between duration of exposure and risk of disease was found; however, the excess risk did appear to decline after improvements in ventilation of the tunnels, and did decline after workers were no longer exposed. On the other hand, other studies in firefighters and foundry workers found no association between the level of carbon monoxide exposure and coronary heart disease risk (2). Thus, the relationship between chronic carbon monoxide and atherosclerotic vascular disease remains uncertain.

Significant excess mortality for ischemic heart disease has been reported in chimney sweeps, aluminum reduction workers, tar distillation workers, and gas workers who are exposed to combustion tar (21–26). A role for polycyclic aromatic hydrocarbons has been suggested.

Exposure to environmental tobacco smoke has been of considerable concern, particularly in regard to the risk of lung cancer, respiratory infection in children, and abnormal pulmonary function (27). Evidence also exists, however, that environmental tobacco smoke may increase the risk of coronary artery disease. A number of studies have been reported, nearly all of which have found an increased relative risk for ischemic heart disease among nonsmokers married to smokers compared with nonsmokers married to nonsmokers (28,29). The overall relative risk is small (on average 1.3), but, considering the large number of people exposed, it may account for a significant number of cases of ischemic heart disease.

The biological plausibility of a relative risk of 1.3 for passive smokers compared with a risk of 2 for active smokers has been questioned. However, the relative risk of smoking is based on comparisons with groups of nonsmokers, which includes passive smokers who appear to have a higher risk of ischemic heart disease than nonexposed nonsmokers. As a result, the relative risk of coronary artery disease in smokers may have been underestimated.

Exposure. Exposure to combustion products is primarily by inhalation. Exposure to carbon monoxide may occur whenever combustion engines or other types of combustion are present, such as in foundries and in fire fighting. Carbon monoxide poisoning may also occur with the use of faulty furnaces or heaters. Typical workplace exposure results in HbCO concentrations of 2% to 8%, whereas cigarette smokers commonly have concentrations of 5% to 15%. Studies of environmental tobacco smoke exposure using levels of cotinine (a metabolite of nicotine) in the blood and urine indicate that environmental tobacco smoke exposure may result in an intake equivalent to one-fourth to one cigarette per day (30,31). It is noteworthy, however, that the composition of sidestream smoke that is released into the environment is different from that of mainstream smoke that is inhaled by the smoker because of differences in heat of combustion and oxygen concentrations at the burning end. Consequently, compared with mainstream smoke, the concentrations of some toxic chemicals—including polycyclic aromatic hydrocarbons, nitrosamines, and formaldehyde—in sidestream smoke are substantially enhanced over those of nicotine. In addition, with aging of environmental tobacco smoke, nicotine vaporizes, and nicotine concentrations in the air decline more quickly than particulate concentrations. For these reasons, measurement of nicotine-based markers in nonsmokers to derive cigarette-equivalents of exposure underestimate the exposure to other toxic constituents of tobacco smoke.

Mechanisms of Toxicity. Carbon monoxide might contribute to atherosclerosis by altering lipid metabolism, increasing the permeation of lipids into blood vessel walls, and enhancing platelet aggregation. High levels of carbon monoxide exposure accelerate atherosclerosis in hypercholesterolemic animals. Carbon monoxide could contribute to angina pectoris/ischemic heart disease mortality by aggravating coronary ischemia and by reducing the amount of oxygen carried by and released from hemoglobin. The effects of carbon monoxide on patients with preexisting coronary artery disease is discussed in detail in the section Myocardial Asphyxiants.

The possible role of polycyclic aromatic hydrocarbons in accelerating atherogenesis is suggested by a hypothesis that the atherosclerotic plaque may derive from single smooth muscle cells that have been mutated (32,33). Chemical carcinogens, such as the polycyclic aromatic hydrocarbons, are known to cause mutations in various types of cells. High levels of exposure to benzo[*a*]pyrene or other polycyclic aromatic hydrocarbons enhance the development of atherosclerotic lesions in some experimental animals.

Clinical Features. A history of exposure to combustion engines, fire, or foundry work in association with atherosclerotic vascular disease should suggest the possible role of carbon monoxide or other combustion products. Patients may present with any manifestation of atherosclerotic vascular disease, including angina pectoris, myocardial infarction, occlusive peripheral vascular disease, or sudden death. The risk of death from ischemic heart disease declines after cessation of exposure in cigarette smokers and similarly seems to decline with cessation of some occupational exposures, such as in tunnel officers (20). Laboratory studies may show increased concentrations of HbCO at the end of work, but levels will be back to normal within 24 to 36 hours of the last exposure. Elevation of hemoglobin concentrations is commonly seen in cigarette smokers and has been reported in some, but not all, studies of chronic carbon monoxide exposure.

ARSENIC

Epidemiology. Three epidemiologic studies have reported positive (although of small magnitude) associations between arsenic exposure (arsenic trioxide) and cardiovascular disease in copper smelter workers (34,35). One of these, a case-control study, reported dose-related increases in ischemic heart disease risk, with a standardized mortality ratio of 2.8 for ischemic heart disease among the more heavily exposed workers (36). High levels of arsenic in drinking water, particularly in areas of southwestern Taiwan, where high arsenic-containing artesian well water is consumed, have also been associated with a dose-related increase in mortality from ischemic heart disease (37).

Exposure. Occupational toxicity has been of concern primarily in workers in smelters, where ore containing large amounts of arsenic is processed. Arsenical insecticides have been used in vineyards, and chronic arsenic poisoning has been reported in vintners. Exposure may be by inhalation of contaminated dusts or plant debris or may be by ingestion of contaminated foods (especially wine or beer). The major exposure to arsenic in large populations is by drinking arsenic-containing well water.

Clinical Features. The clinical features are those of atherosclerotic vascular disease, as discussed in the section Atherosclerotic Vascular Disease. Excessive exposure to arsenic in drinking water has also been associated with an increased prevalence of hypertension, an important factor for ischemic heart disease (38). Specific signs and symptoms of chronic arsenic poisoning—gastrointestinal disturbances, dermatitis or hyperpigmentation of the skin, and peripheral neuropathy—should be sought, but one does not usually find these with chronic low-level exposures.

Nonatheromatous Ischemic Heart Disease

Ischemic heart disease may result from coronary vasospasm in the absence of atherosclerosis. Occupational exposure to nitrates, particularly nitroglycerin and ethylene glycol dinitrate, have been associated with such toxicity.

ORGANIC NITRATES

Epidemiology. In the 1950s, epidemics of chest pain and sudden death in munitions workers were observed. These events typically occurred 36 to 72 hours after withdrawal from exposure to organic nitrates and were felt to be part of a nitrate withdrawal syndrome (39,40). Initial reports described workers with ischemic heart disease symptoms in the absence of or with only minimal atherosclerotic coronary artery disease. Subsequent epidemiologic studies have confirmed the association with a relative risk of 2.5 for cardiovascular mortality in workers exposed for 20 or more years (40). Epidemiologic studies have suggested that nitrate exposure might contribute to accelerated atherosclerosis as well (41). Sulfide-ore miners in Finland have been reported to have a significantly excess mortality from ischemic heart disease, which might be attributable to nitroglycerin exposure while working with dynamite (42). In this study, it is unclear whether the ischemic heart disease was atheromatous or nonatheromatous, or both.

Exposure. Nitroglycerin and nitroglycol (ethylene glycol dinitrate) exposures occur in the munitions and explosives industries and among construction workers who handle dynamite. Dynamite is composed of approximately 60% organic nitrates, 25% blasting oil, and 10% dinitrotoluene, with a small amount of nitrocellulose and fillers. Blasting oil is 80% nitroglycol and 20% nitroglycerin and is the source of the volatile nitrates. Exposures tend to be greatest during explosive-mixing and cartridge-filling operations. Nitrates are highly volatile and are readily absorbed through the skin and lungs. Nitrates can permeate the wrapping material of dynamite sticks, so workers who handle dynamite should be advised to wear cotton gloves. Natural rubber gloves should not be used, because they become permeated with nitrates, and the gloves may enhance cutaneous nitrate absorption.

With current automated processes in explosives manufacturing, direct handling of nitrates by employees is minimized. However, levels of nitrates in the workplace environment must be controlled by adequate ventilation and by air conditioning during periods of hot weather. The current Occupational Safety and Health Administration exposure limit is 0.2 ppm for nitroglycerin, but even at lower levels (0.02 ppm or above) personal protective gear is recommended to avoid headache. Although there are no readily available biochemical measures to detect excessive nitrate exposure, findings of progressively decreasing blood pressure and increasing heart rate during the workday are suggestive of excessive exposure. Monitoring for these signs in employees may help prevent adverse effects of exposure to nitrates.

Blood concentrations of nitroglycerin have been measured in the workplace during production of gunpowder (43). Plasma concentrations of nitroglycerin in workers in the roll mill area were as high as 98.1 nmol per L (median) as compared with 5.7 nmol per L after taking 1.0 mg nitroglycerin sublingually. Thus occupational exposures produce many-fold greater blood levels of nitroglycerin than does nitroglycerin in therapeutic doses.

Mechanisms and Pathogenesis. The occurrence of the nitrate withdrawal syndrome requires prolonged exposure to nitrates or nitrites. Initially, workers experience the vasodilatory effects of nitrates, including flushing, headaches, and palpitations. These reactions tend to diminish over time, particularly over the course of the work week. With prolonged exposure, usually a year or longer, symptoms of nitrate withdrawal develop. The pathogenesis is thought to involve adaptation of physiologic systems to the vascular actions of nitrates. Nitrates directly dilate blood vessels, including those of the coronary circulation. With prolonged exposure, compensatory vasoconstriction—believed to be mediated by sympathetic neural responses—and activation of the renin-angiotensin system develops. If exposure to nitrates is stopped, compensatory vasoconstriction becomes unopposed, and coronary vasospasm with angina, myocardial infarction, or sudden death may result. Chest pain occurring during nitrate withdrawal has been termed *Monday morning angina*, because it typically occurs 2 or 3 days after the last day of nitrate exposure. Mechanisms by which nitrates may promote atherosclerotic vascular disease are unknown.

Clinical Features. Workers exposed to excessive levels of nitrates typically experience headaches and may demonstrate hypotension, tachycardia, and warm, flushed skin. With continued exposure, these symptoms and signs become less prominent. After 1 to 2 days without exposure to nitrates (generally occurring on weekends), signs of acute coronary ischemia—ranging from angina at rest to myocardial infarction or sudden death—may occur (40,44).

During episodes of pain, the ECG shows evidence of ischemia: either ST segment elevation or depression, with or without T-wave abnormalities. At other times, the ECG may be perfectly normal. Typical findings of myocardial infarction on ECG are an elevation of serum concentrations of the MB isoenzyme of creatine phosphokinase. Results of exercise stress testing and coronary angiography when the patient is asymptomatic may be normal.

Treatment of myocardial ischemia that is due to nitrate withdrawal should include the administration of cardiac nitrates (e.g., nitroglycerin or isosorbide dinitrate) and calcium blockers. Case reports indicate that ischemic symptoms may recur—indicating a persistent tendency to coronary spasm—for weeks or months (45,46). Therefore, long-term cardiac nitrate or calcium block therapy may be needed. The worker should be removed from sources of organic nitrate exposure.

OTHER CHEMICAL EXPOSURES

Acute myocardial infarction in the absence of coronary artery disease has occurred after acute exposures to solvents, presumably as a result of arrhythmias, and after acute intoxication with myocardial asphyxiants.

Myocardial Asphyxiants

Acute intoxication with asphyxiant chemicals can produce myocardial as well as generalized tissue injury. Such chemicals include carbon monoxide, cyanide, and hydrogen sulfide. Acute myocardial necrosis, including papillary muscle necrosis and pulmonary edema, have been observed (47,48). Severe intoxication with altered levels of consciousness would be expected to accompany asphyxia severe enough to produce myocardial injury.

CARBON MONOXIDE

Exposure. The major problem from asphyxiants occurs from carbon monoxide exposure in patients with preexisting coronary artery disease. Sources of exposure to carbon monoxide were described in the section Combustion Products (Including Environmental Tobacco Smoke). Levels of carbon monoxide should be monitored if there are sources of combustion such as combustion engines or furnaces in the workplace. The current 8-hour TLV is 25 ppm, which at the end of an 8-hour workday results in a HbCO concentration of 3% to 4%. This concentration is tolerated well by healthy individuals but not by people with cardiovascular or chronic lung disease. Workplace monitoring is easily done with a portable carbon monoxide meter. Biological monitoring of workers involves measuring either the HbCO concentration in blood or the level of expired carbon monoxide, which is directly proportionate to the HbCO concentration. Elevated carbon monoxide levels should be anticipated in cigarette smokers.

Mechanisms and Pathogenesis. The pathogenesis of carbon monoxide poisoning occurs as a result of the high affinity of carbon monoxide for hemoglobin. The affinity of carbon monoxide for hemoglobin is more than 200 times that of oxygen. Binding of carbon monoxide and hemoglobin to form HbCO reduces delivery of oxygen to body tissues, because the oxygen-carrying capacity of hemoglobin is decreased and because less oxygen is released to tissues at any given oxygen tension (i.e., there is a shift in the oxygen dissociation curve). Thus, a HbCO concentration of 20% represents a greater reduction in oxygen delivery than a 20% reduction in erythrocyte count. Other heme-containing proteins (e.g., myoglobin, cytochrome oxidase, and cytochrome P-450) bind 10% to 15% of the total body carbon monoxide, but the medical significance of their binding at usual levels of exposure to carbon monoxide is unsettled.

In healthy individuals exposed to carbon monoxide, the decrease in delivery of oxygen to tissues causes the cardiac output and coronary blood flow to increase to meet the metabolic demands of the heart. Although these compensatory responses allow healthy individuals to perform at normal work levels, their maximum exercise capacity is decreased. If, on the other hand, compensatory responses are limited, as in patients with coronary artery disease, carbon monoxide exposure may cause angina or myocardial infarction.

Clinical Features. Reduced exercise thresholds for the development of angina have been reported when HbCO concentrations are as low as 2.0% (49,50). Carbon monoxide decreases the ventricular fibrillation threshold in experimental animals and may do the same in humans (51). Severe carbon monoxide poisoning may cause acute myocardial infarction or sudden death, particularly in people with underlying coronary heart disease (52,53).

In patients with angina pectoris, peripheral arterial occlusive disease, or chronic obstructive lung disease, low levels of carbon monoxide (blood HbCO, 4% or less) reduce exercise capacity to the point of angina, claudication, or dyspnea, respectively (49,50,54,55). Low-level carbon monoxide exposure may reduce maximum exercise capacity even in healthy workers (56).

Symptoms of carbon monoxide poisoning include headache (at HbCO concentrations as low as 10%) and nausea, dizziness, fatigue, and dimmed vision at higher concentrations.

The only specific laboratory finding is elevation of HbCO concentration. When arterial blood gases are measured, the arterial oxygen tension is usually normal or slightly reduced, whereas the venous partial pressure of oxygen (PO_2) and oxygen content are substantially reduced. Respiratory alkalosis that is due to hyperventilation is commonly observed in mild to moderate poisonings, whereas respiratory failure may complicate the severest poisonings. When there is marked tissue hypoxia, lactic acidosis develops.

Carbon monoxide is eliminated from the body by respiration, and the rate of elimination depends on ventilation, pulmonary blood flow, and inspired oxygen concentration. The half-life of carbon monoxide in a sedentary adult breathing air is 4 to 5 hours. The half-life can be reduced to 80 minutes by giving 100% oxygen by face mask, or it can be reduced to 25 minutes by giving hyperbaric oxygen (3 atmospheres) in a hyperbaric chamber.

Direct Myocardial Injury

Several chemicals are of concern as potential causes of myocardial injury.

COBALT

Epidemiology. Concern with cobalt has arisen from epidemics of cardiomyopathy first seen in the 1960s in drinkers of beer containing cobalt added to stabilize the foam (57,58). The mortality rate in people affected with cobalt-induced cardiomyopathy was as high as 50% in some series. Evidence for the importance of cobalt as an industrial cardiac toxin is becoming stronger. A study of tungsten carbide workers exposed to cobalt-containing dust found no overt systolic left ventricular dysfunction as tested by radionuclide ventriculography (59). However, a weak but statistically significant inverse correlation existed between resting left ventricular ejection fraction and duration of exposure, supporting a possible role for cobalt in causing myocardial disease. Workers with abnormal chest x-rays, presumably the result of metal-induced interstitial lung fibrosis ("hard metal" pneumoconiosis), did show a reduced right ventricular ejection fraction, felt to be an early stage of cor pulmonale. Although no other convincing epidemiologic evidence indicates that cobalt is a risk factor for cardiovascular disease, there are several case reports of cardiomyopathy in cobalt-exposed workers, including cases in which high levels of cobalt in the heart were measured at autopsy or in explanted hearts (60–62).

Exposure. Cobalt is used along with tungsten carbide in the production of metal alloys used especially in the manufacturing of drills and bits. Exposure is primarily to cobalt powder and dust. Cobalt-60 is used medicinally for radiotherapy. Human exposure can be assessed by measuring urinary cobalt concentrations.

Pathophysiology. Cobalt depresses oxygen uptake by mitochondria of the heart and interferes with energy metabolism in a manner biochemically similar to the effects of thiamine deficiency (63). Cobalt appears to exert its effects by binding to sulfhydryl groups of α-lipoic acid and preventing oxidation of α-ketoglutarate and pyruvate to succinyl coenzyme A (CoA) and acetyl CoA, respectively, in the citric acid cycle. Because cobalt-exposed beer drinkers, but not individuals receiving high doses of cobalt for medical therapeutic reasons, develop cardiomyopathy, it has been speculated that cobalt, excessive alcohol consumption, malnutrition, or a combination of these act synergistically to produce myocardial injury. Most affected people have been heavy drinkers for many years, but the cardiomyopathy itself appeared within 1 year of the time that cobalt was added to the beer. The pathology in those who have died from cobalt-induced cardiomyopathy included myocardial necrosis with thrombi in the heart and major blood vessels. Cobalt produces a dose-dependent cardiomyopathy in several animal species (62). Cardiomyopathy develops more rapidly in animals with lower exposure to cobalt in the presence of a protein-deficient or thiamine-deficient diet.

Clinical Features. The clinical picture is that of a congestive cardiomyopathy with low cardiac output, venous congestion, pericardial effusion, and polycythemia. The ECG typically shows low voltage, ST segment depression, T-wave inversions, and, in some cases, Q-waves suggestive of myocardial infarction.

ARSENIC/ARSINE

Subacute arsenic poisoning caused by ingestion of arsenic-contaminated beer has been associated with cardiomyopathy and cardiac failure. In one epidemic in Manchester, England, 6,000 people were affected, which included 70 deaths (64). Arsenic poisoning can cause electrographic abnormalities including ST- and T-wave changes and QT-interval prolongation. Case reports indicate that arsenic poisoning can cause ventricular arrhythmias of the torsades de pointes type (65,66). Little is known of the mechanism of arsenic-induced myocardial injury.

Arsine gas causes red blood cell hemolysis and, in some cases, death from cardiac failure. Massive hemolysis, which may persist for several days, produces hyperkalemia, which can result in cardiac arrest. ECG manifestations of acute arsine poisoning include high, peaked T-waves; conduction disturbances; various degrees of heart block; and asystole (67). Arsine may also directly affect the myocardium, causing a greater magnitude of cardiac failure than would be expected from the degree of anemia.

LEAD

The major cardiovascular concern for lead is its association with hypertension. Lead poisoning has also been associated with myocarditis and ECG abnormalities in children (68,69). Case reports of myocarditis manifested as sinus bradycardia, ventricular ectopy, and diffuse ST-T wave changes on ECG have been reported, as well as sinus bradycardia with or without first-degree atrioventricular block in lead-exposed workers (70,71). In rats, chronic exposure to lead produces degeneration of myofibrils with impairment of electric and contractile function (71–73).

ANTIMONY

The therapeutic use of antimonial compounds for treatment of parasitic infections produces ECG abnormalities—primarily T-wave changes and QT-interval prolongation—and has caused sudden death in some patients. An epidemic of sudden death and ECG abnormalities in workers exposed to antimony trisulfide in one factory has been described (74). When use of antimony was stopped, no further deaths occurred, although ECG abnormalities persisted in some of the exposed individuals. Studies in animals confirm that chronic exposure to antimony can produce myocardial injury (74), although the mechanism has not been elucidated. One cohort study of Hispanic men working in a Texas antimony smelter found no significant increase in cardiovascular mortality (75). Although not an expected occupational hazard, acute oral ingestion of antimony potassium tartrate (tartar emetic), used to treat schistosomiasis japonicum, may produce respiratory failure, cardiogenic shock, and death (76).

ORGANIC SOLVENTS

The major cardiovascular concern with solvent exposure is cardiac arrhythmias. However, several reports of myocardial failure in solvent-exposed individuals have been published (77–81). Dilated cardiomyopathy with severe cardiac failure developed in several people who were occupationally exposed to solvents (toluene or 1,1,1-trichloroethylene). In two of these cases, biopsy evidence of myocarditis was present, and in one case there was no evidence of myocarditis at autopsy. One man developed an acute toxic myocarditis while painting in an unventilated room with a methyl cellulose–based paint. Another man, who had been exposed to a toluene-based glue for 3 years as a furniture upholsterer, developed acute myocarditis associated with hepatic necrosis and renal failure. Although these case reports raise concern about myocardial toxicity caused by excessive solvent exposure, the possibility of coincidental viral myocarditis must also be considered.

Arrhythmias

Arrhythmias are a common complication of ischemic heart disease and congestive cardiomyopathy but also may be precipitated by chemical exposures, particularly to halogenated hydrocarbons.

HALOGENATED HYDROCARBONS

Epidemiology. Numerous cases of cardiac arrhythmias or sudden death (presumably because of arrhythmias) in people abusing solvents or occupationally exposed to high levels of organic solvents or fluorocarbons have been described (82–85). Epidemiologic studies in general have not supported an overall increase in cardiovascular mortality in solvent-exposed workers, other than that with carbon disulfide (86). The primary cardiovascular risk from solvents appears to occur during acute intoxication. A study of hospital pathology residents showed an association between exposure to Freon 22 and palpitations and arrhythmias as documented by ambulatory ECG monitoring (87). In a study of ten healthy firefighters experimentally exposed to 1,000 ppm bromochlorodifluormethane (halon 1211, a fire-extinguishing agent) during treadmill exercise, complex ectopy (ventricular couplets and/or idioventricular rhythm) occurred in two subjects with halon and none with placebo exposure (88). Concentrations of 1,000 ppm or higher of halon are encountered in the environment when halon is used to extinguish a fire. However, two studies of ambulatory ECGs in refrigerator repairmen exposed to fluorocarbons found no relationship between exposure and arrhythmias (89,90).

Exposure. Exposure to solvents is widespread in industrial settings such as dry cleaning, degreasing, painting, and chemical manufacturing. Fluorocarbons are used extensively as refrigerants and propellants in a wide variety of products. Solvent abuse—including sniffing of glue, spray paints, shoe polish, and typewriter correction fluid—most commonly occurs among adolescents and young adults. A variety of hydrocarbons have been implicated in sudden deaths. These include toluene, 1,1,1-trichloroethane, benzene, and fluorocarbons (Freon). Assessment of exposure is most easily done by making workplace air measurements, although concentrations of some hydrocarbons may be measured in the expired air or in the blood of intoxicated patients.

Pathogenesis. Halogenated hydrocarbons have complex effects on the heart. At low levels of exposure, solvents sensitize the heart to effects of catecholamines. Experimental studies have shown that the dose of epinephrine required to produce ventricular tachycardia or fibrillation is reduced after solvents are inhaled (91). Catecholamine release is induced by euphoria and excitement because of the central nervous system effects of the solvents and also by exercise. Sensitization of the myocardium to effects of catecholamines and enhanced catecholamine release, in combination with asphyxia and hypoxia, is believed to be the cause of the arrhythmias, which can result in sudden death. At higher levels of exposure, solvents may depress sinus node activity and thereby cause sinus bradycardia or arrest. Solvents may also depress atrioventricular nodal conduction and cause atrioventricular block. Bradyarrhythmias may then predispose to escape ventricular arrhythmias or, in cases of more severe intoxication, to asystole. The arrhythmogenic action of solvents may be enhanced by alcohol or caffeine (92,93).

The cardiac pathology in death cases is usually unremarkable, consistent with a sudden arrhythmic death, although acute myocardial infarction secondary to solvent intoxication has also been described. The finding of a fatty liver suggests chronic exposure to high levels of solvents or to ethanol.

Clinical Features and Treatment. The presence of symptoms of acute hydrocarbon exposure preceding the onset of arrhythmias or collapse should be ascertained. Symptoms of intoxication with hydrocarbon solvents or fluorocarbon propellants include dizziness, lightheadedness, headaches, nausea, drowsiness, lethargy, palpitations, and syncope. Physical examination may reveal ataxia, nystagmus, or slurred speech. The heart rate and blood pressure are usually normal, except at the time of arrhythmias, when a rapid or irregular heartbeat is present and may be accompanied by hypotension.

Convulsions, coma, or cardiac arrest may occur after severe intoxication. Workers who have heart disease or chronic lung disease with hypoxemia may be more susceptible to the arrhythmogenic actions of solvents. Arrhythmias induced by solvents or propellants are expected to occur only at work, while the worker is exposed to these agents. Arrhythmias may include premature atrial or ventricular contractions, atrial fibrillation, ventricular tachycardia or fibrillation, and asystole.

Solvent-exposed workers who report palpitations, dizzy spells, or syncopal episodes should be evaluated by 24-hour ambulatory ECG monitoring, including while at work. Workers with heart disease—especially those with chronic arrhythmias—should be advised to avoid exposure to potentially arrhythmogenic chemicals.

Because arrhythmias from hydrocarbons are related to the sensitization of the heart to the actions of catecholamines, the use of β-adrenergic–blocking drugs is most rational in treating solvent-induced arrhythmias. For workers who experience episodic arrhythmias in the workplace, the worker should be removed from the exposure or advised to use protective respiratory equipment. If a worker collapses and resuscitation is required, the use of epinephrine or other sympathomimetic drugs should be avoided if possible, because these agents may precipitate further arrhythmias.

ORGANOPHOSPHATES

Epidemiology. Acute intoxication with organophosphates and carbamate insecticides can produce diverse cardiovascular disturbances, including hypotension, sinus tachycardia, sinus bradycardia, varying degrees of heart block, prolonged Q-T interval, ventricular premature beats, and ventricular tachycardia, often of the torsades de pointes type (94,95). In one series, 41% of patients with severe organophosphate poisoning had one or more cardiac arrhythmias (94). Chronic exposure to organophosphates and carbamate insecticides has been associated with an increased prevalence of ECG abnormalities (96), although the significance of these abnormalities with respect to clinical cardiovascular disease is unknown.

Exposure. Organophosphate and carbamate insecticides are widely used in agriculture. They can be applied to crops by aerial spraying or by hand. Agricultural workers may therefore absorb insecticide by inhalation of mist or via cutaneous absorption. Continuing exposure may occur from contact with contaminated clothing or hair. The presence of some of the organophosphates may be measured in the blood or gastric fluid. Some organophosphates, such as parathion, have metabolites that may also be measured in the urine.

Pathophysiology. Organophosphates and carbamates inhibit acetylcholinesterase. The result is accumulation of acetylcholine at cholinergic synapses and myoneural junctions. The cardiovascular effects may vary over the time course of organophosphate poisoning. Early in acute poisoning, acetylcholine stimulates nicotinic receptors at sympathetic ganglia and causes tachycardia and mild hypertension. Later, when acetylcholine acts at muscarinic receptors or blocks ganglionic transmission by hyperpolarization, it causes bradycardia and hypotension. As a consequence of autonomic imbalance and asynchronous repolarization of different parts of the heart, there may be Q-T interval prolongation, and polymorphous ventricular tachycardia (torsades de pointes) has been reported (95).

The excess of acetylcholine at the myoneural junctions initially causes muscle paralysis, including paralysis of the diaphragm, which results in respiratory arrest. Other consequences are described with clinical findings below. As organophosphates act on autonomic neurotransmission, there are no specific pathologic findings.

Clinical Findings and Treatment. Typical symptoms of mild organophosphate and carbamate poisoning include weakness, headache, sweating, nausea, vomiting, abdominal cramps, and diarrhea. Moderate poisoning may be associated with chest discomfort, dyspnea, inability to walk, and blurred vision. Physical signs are those of cholinergic excess and include small pupils, diaphoresis, salivation, lacrimation, an increase in bronchial secretions (which may resemble pulmonary edema), and muscle fasciculations. Adult respiratory distress syndrome has also been reported (97).

Early cardiovascular manifestations include tachycardia and hypertension. Later, there may be bradycardia and hypotension. There is sometimes frank muscular weakness or, in severe poisoning, paralysis accompanied by respiratory failure, convulsions, or coma.

The failure of usual doses of atropine—a competitive antagonist of acetylcholine at muscarinic receptors—to reverse cholinergic signs strongly supports the diagnosis of organophosphate or carbamate poisoning.

The diagnosis is confirmed by the finding of a markedly depressed level of cholinesterase in red blood cells. Depression below 50% of normal is usually seen in patients with symptoms, and depression to less than 10% of normal is usually seen in patients with severe poisoning. Plasma cholinesterase activity is usually depressed also, but this correlates less well with clinical manifestations. Arterial blood gases may show carbon dioxide retention, hypoxia, or both.

Delayed repolarization with delayed Q-T interval prolongation on the ECG and episodes of ventricular tachycardia may be seen for as long as 5 to 7 days after acute intoxication (95). The ECG also commonly shows nonspecific ST- and T-wave changes.

In addition to ventricular tachycardia and fibrillation, a number of other arrhythmias have been seen during organophosphate or carbamate insecticide poisoning. These include sinus bradycardia; atrioventricular junctional bradycardia; atrioventricular dissociation; and varying degrees of heart block, including complete heart block, as well as systole (98,99). The chest x-ray may resemble pulmonary edema.

The differential diagnosis of signs and symptoms of cholinergic excess includes treatment with cholinesterase inhibitors, such as pyridostigmine, for myasthenia gravis. Small pupils may also be seen following ingestion of narcotics, clonidine, phenothiazine, sedative drugs, and α-adrenergic–blocking drugs, and in patients with pontine brain infarction or hemorrhage.

General treatment measures include decontamination (removal of clothing and thorough cleaning of skin and hair), support of respiration (including mechanical ventilation for respiratory failure), and support of circulation. Specific measures include the use of pralidoxime to reverse muscular paralysis and other manifestations of excess acetylcholine, and the use of atropine to reverse bronchorrhea and bradycardia.

Intensive cardiac and respiratory monitoring of patients for several days after exposure is recommended, with particular attention to the possible late development of arrhythmias or respiratory failure. Heart block and polymorphous ventricular tachycardia with a prolonged Q-T interval are optimally treated by cardiac pacing. The use of antiarrhythmic drugs (e.g., quinidine, procainamide, and disopyramide) that depress conduction and calcium channel blockers should be avoided.

OTHER CHEMICALS

Antimony has been associated with ECG abnormalities and an increased risk of sudden death, presumably because of arrhythmias (74). Acute arsenic poisoning can cause ECG abnormalities; recurrent ventricular tachycardia of the torsades de pointes type has been described (65,66). Arsine exposure production disturbance includes various degrees of heart block and asystole, probably related in part to hyperkalemia resulting from hemolysis (67).

Hypertension

As chronic hypertension is a major risk factor for premature atherosclerotic coronary vascular disease and stroke, the possibility that occupational and environmental factors can induce or aggravate hypertension is of concern. Evidence exists that nonchemical factors, such as work stress and noise, may increase the prevalence of hypertension, but this section focuses on chemical factors, for which there is also evidence.

LEAD

Epidemiology. Epidemiologic studies suggest that low-level lead exposure can chronically elevate blood pressure (100,101). Such exposures can occur in the workplace or from other environmental sources. Several studies in large unselected populations have reported a positive relationship between lead concentration and systolic blood pressure (102,103). The National Health and Nutrition Examination Survey study in the United States found an average 5-mm Hg rise per 15 μg per dL blood lead concentration increment (102). Over the range of commonly observed blood lead concentrations (0.8 to 35 μg per dL), a blood pressure elevation of 10 to 15 mm Hg would be predicted. A case-control study comparing 135 hypertensive patients and a similar number of age- and sex-matched normotensive controls supports the relationship between blood lead and diastolic blood pressure, and suggested even a greater quantitative contribution of lead to blood pressure elevation (104). Several mortality studies of lead-exposed workers have reported significant associations between blood pressure, the risk of cerebrovascular disease, and the extent of lead exposure, although not all studies have confirmed that relationship (2,100,101).

It is noteworthy that chronic lead exposure increases the risk of chronic renal disease. Chronic renal disease may be contributed to by and may cause or aggravate hypertension. Several workplace epidemiologic studies have found increased mortality from chronic renal disease in lead-exposed workers (105).

Exposure. Environmental sources of lead include inhalation of automobile exhaust from gasoline containing alkyl lead additives, from ingestion of dust contaminated with lead paint, and from drinking water that had passed through lead piping. Occupational exposures to lead-containing dust or fumes occur in lead smelters; foundries; and industries, such as battery manufacturing, construction work, demolition, and vehicle radiator repair, where lead compounds are used.

Lead exposure can be assessed by measuring blood lead concentration. The average blood lead concentration in adults in the United States not exposed to lead is approximately 10 μg per dL (102). The normal range is up to approximately 35 μg per dL. Even within this range, there is evidence of an increase in blood pressure with increasing concentrations of lead (102,106). Workplace exposures may result in levels that are much higher. Lead concentrations above 40 to 50 μg per dL are considered to be excessive. Erythrocyte protoporphyrin concentration, a biochemical test that correlates with blood lead concentration, begins to increase at blood lead levels of 25 to 30 μg per dL.

Pathophysiology. Low-level chronic lead exposure increases blood pressure in animals (100,101). The major hemodynamic effect appears to be increased vascular resistance. Lead may increase vascular resistance by increasing plasma renin activity; by increasing responsiveness of vascular smooth muscle to the pressor effects of endogenous vasoconstrictors, such as norepinephrine or angiotensin II; and/or by direct contraction of vascular smooth muscle. The importance of increased plasma renin has been questioned, because angiotensin II levels are not correspondingly increased, suggesting that lead may also inhibit angiotensin-converting enzyme. Furthermore, in people chronically exposed to lead, plasma renin activity is normal or low. Increased vascular tone and reactivity may result from increased intracellular calcium. Lead exposure increases calcium levels in various tissues, possibly as a result of inhibition of sodium potassium–adenosine triphosphatase (ATPase) and effects on calmodulin-mediated calcium transport.

Clinical Features. The clinical features of lead-induced hypertension are similar to those from hypertension of any cause. Other features of lead intoxication at low levels include slowed nerve conduction, impaired biosynthesis of hemoglobin (related to inhibition of δ-aminolevulinic acid and ferrochelatase) with an increase in erythrocyte protoporphyrin concentration, and hyperuricemia (due to increased tubular reabsorption of uric acid). At higher lead levels, evidence of frank toxicity—including anemia, peripheral neuropathy, and renal failure—is seen. Even in the general population, an inverse relationship exists between blood lead concentration and creatinine clearance, although there is still a question as to whether low-level lead exposure impairs renal function or whether impaired renal function leads to retention of lead (107).

CADMIUM

In animal studies, low-level cadmium exposure elevates blood pressure (108). Many epidemiologic human studies on hypertension and cardiovascular disease have examined the relationship to cadmium, and the results are generally inconclusive (2,109). Those studies reporting positive associations tend to be more methodologically flawed. Overall, the evidence that exposure to cadmium in the workplace increases the risk of hypertension or cardiac vascular disease is unconvincing.

OTHER CHEMICALS

Carbon disulfide exposure may be associated with hypertension, possibly mediated by inhibition of dopamine β-hydroxylase. Some data indicate that long-term arsenic exposure via drinking water is associated with a dose-related increase in the prevalence of hypertension (38). Exposure to organic solvents during pregnancy has been reported to increase the risk of hypertension and of preeclampsia (i.e., hypertension with edema and proteinuria) (110). In a case-referent study of 90 exposed American women, relative risks of 3.0 (95% confidence interval, 0.9 to 9.9) and 3.9 (95% confidence interval, 2.5 to 5.4) for hypertension and preeclampsia, respectively, were observed. Of note, the level of exposure to solvents was moderate, in most cases barely exceeding one-third of the TLV. This study is provocative but requires replication with a large number of patients. A provocative but difficult-to-explain report describes two men with acute accidental intense exposure to Freon (in one case, Freon 22 and Freon 12; in the other, Freon 113), followed by new onset of persistent hypertension (111). In one case, labile hypertension persisted, whereas in the other case, hypertension resolved after 16 months. It was speculated that Freon that was lipid soluble was gradually released from adipose over time, producing long-lasting effects, although the mechanism for hypertensive action was not identified.

Peripheral Arterial Occlusive Disease

Chronic high-level exposure to carbon disulfide, arsenic, and lead are associated with an increased prevalence of peripheral vascular disease. Arterial disease with dry gangrene of the lower extremities that is due to chronic arsenic poisoning, called *Blackfoot disease*, has been endemic in diverse areas of the world, such as Taiwan, Chile, and Mexico, where arsenic levels in drinking water are high (38,112,113). Typically, Blackfoot disease is of insidious onset with numbness and coldness of the extremities as initial symptoms, followed by localized ulceration and subsequently gangrenous changes. The name of the disease comes from the black coloration of the dry gangrene. Spontaneous amputation may ensue, or surgical amputation may be required. The pathology of Blackfoot disease includes thickening and fibrinoid necrosis of subcutaneous arterioles. The pathophysiology of chemically induced peripheral vascular disease, with the possible exception of carbon disulfide, is unknown. Worldwide, cigarette smoking is the major risk factor for peripheral vascular disease. Once a person has peripheral arterial occlusive disease with intermittent claudication, exposure to carbon monoxide, even at low levels, significantly reduces exercise tolerance (54).

MANAGEMENT SUMMARY

A number of chemicals have been implicated in the causation of cardiovascular disease. Although there has been considerable scientific investigation, there are still many unanswered questions about causation for chemicals that have been discussed. A survey of the probability for causation for various chemicals is presented in Table 20-1. A problem in the evaluation of any particular patient is that cardiovascular disease is very common in the general population, and the clinical manifestations are generally nonspecific, so causality for a specific toxic exposure is difficult to establish.

However, the data reviewed in this chapter may be of use in occupational and environmental medicine in several ways:

- Knowledge of the potential cardiovascular toxins and associated diseases makes it possible for health care personnel to intelligently monitor exposed workers for early evidence of cardiovascular disease. An example of this is the use of funduscopy to assess early cardiovascular toxicity from carbon disulfide.

- Knowledge of interactions between chemical toxins and medical diseases provides a basis for health care personnel to advise workers about safe workplace exposures. For example, a patient with angina pectoris should be advised not to work on a job in which he or she is exposed to significant levels of carbon monoxide.
- Knowledge of cardiovascular toxicology allows for more rational preemployment screening. Patients with underlying cardiovascular disease should not be placed in workplaces in which they are exposed to chemicals that may aggravate their diseases.
- Specific epidemiologic data have been used to improve workplace conditions and decrease occupation-related cardiovascular disease. For example, control of carbon disulfide exposure has reduced the incidence of ischemic heart disease in viscose rayon workers (5). Reduction of nitrate exposure in explosives manufacturing has reduced the incidence of sudden death in those workers. Similar controls are indicated for other known toxic exposures, including environmental tobacco smoke.

REFERENCES

1. Benowitz NL, Goldschlager N. Cardiac disturbances in the toxicologic patient. In: Haddad LM, Winchester JF, eds. *Clinical management of poisoning and drug overdose*, 2nd ed. Philadelphia: WB Saunders, 1990.
2. Kristensen TS. Cardiovascular diseases and the work environment: a critical review of the epidemiologic literature on chemical factors. *Scand J Work Environ Health* 1989;15:245–264.
3. Tiller JR, Schilling RSF, Morris JN. Occupational toxic factor in mortality from coronary heart disease. *BMJ* 1968;4:407–411.
4. Hernberg S, Partanen T, Nordman CH, Sumari P. Coronary heart disease among workers exposed to carbon disulphide. *Br J Ind Med* 1970;27:313–325.
5. Nurminen M, Hernberg S. Effects of intervention on the cardiovascular mortality of workers exposed to carbon disulphide: a 15-year follow-up. *Br J Ind Med* 1985;42:32–35.
6. Sweetnam PM, Taylor SWC, Elwood PC. Exposure to carbon disulphide and ischaemic heart disease in a viscose rayon factory. *Br J Ind Med* 1987;44:220–227.
7. Egeland GM, Burkhart GA, Schnorr TM, Hornung RW, Fajen JM, Lee ST. Effects of exposure to carbon disulphide on low density lipoprotein cholesterol concentration and diastolic blood pressure. *Br J Ind Med* 1992;49:287–293.
8. Drexler H, Ulm K, Hubmann M, Hardt R, et al. Carbon disulphide. III. Risk factors for coronary heart diseases in workers in the viscose industry. *Int Arch Occup Environ Health* 1995;67:243–252.
9. Tolonen M. Vascular effects of carbon disulfide: a review. *Scand J Work Environ Health* 1975;1:63–77.
10. Coppock RW, Buck WB. Toxicology of carbon disulfide: a review. *Vet Hum Toxicol* 1981;23:331–336.
11. Cavalleri A. Serum thyroxine in the early diagnosis of carbon disulfide poisoning. *Arch Environ Health* 1975;30:85–87.
12. Nurminen M, Mutanen P, Tolonen M, Hernberg S. Quantitated effects of carbon disulfide exposure, elevated blood pressure, and aging on coronary mortality. *Am J Epidemiol* 1982;115:107–118.
13. Karai I, Sugimoto K, Goto S. A fluorescein angiographic study on carbon disulfide retinopathy among workers in viscose rayon factories. *Int Arch Occup Environ Health* 1983;53:91–99.
14. Brugnone F, Maranelli G, Zotti S, eds. Blood concentration of carbon disulphide in "normal" subjects and in alcoholic subjects treated with disulfiram. *Br J Ind Med* 1992;49:658–663.
15. Riihimaki V, Kivisto H, Peltonen K, Helpio E, Altio A. Assessment of exposure to carbon disulfide in viscose production workers from urinary 2-thiothiazolidine-4–carboxylic acid determinations. *Am J Ind Med* 1992;22:85–97.
16 Goldsmith JR. Carbon monoxide research: recent and remote. *Arch Environ Health* 1970;21:118–120.
17. Weir FW, Fabiano VL. Reevaluation of the role of carbon monoxide in production as aggravation of cardiovascular disease processes. *J Occup Med* 1982;24:519–525.
18. Wald N, Howard S, Smith PG, Kjeldsen K. Association between atherosclerotic diseases and carboxyhaemoglobin levels in tobacco smokers. *BMJ* 1973;1:761–765.
19. Hernberg S, Karava R, Koskela RS, Luoma K. Angina pectoris, ECG findings and blood pressure of foundry workers in relation to carbon monoxide exposure. *Scand J Work Environ Health* 1976;2[Suppl 1]:54–63.
20. Stern FB, Halperin WE, Hornung RW, Ringenburg VL, McCammon CS. Heart disease mortality among bridge and tunnel officers exposed to carbon monoxide. *Am J Epidemiol* 1988;182:1276–1288.
21. Theriault GP, Tremblay CG, Armstrong BG. Risk of ischemic heart disease among primary aluminum production workers. *Am J Ind Med* 1988;13:659–666.
22. Hansen ES. Mortality from cancer and ischemic heart disease in Danish chimney sweeps; a five-year followup. *Am J Epidemiol* 1983;177:160–164.
23. Ronnenberg A. Mortality and cancer morbidity in workers from an aluminium smelter with prebaked carbon anodes—part III: mortality from circulatory and respiratory diseases. *Occup Environ Med* 1995;52:255–261.
24. McLaren WM, Hurley JF. Mortality of tar distillation workers. *Scand J Work Environ Health* 1987;13:404–411.
25. Gustavsson P, Reuterwall C. Mortality and incidence of cancer among Swedish gas workers. *Br J Ind Med* 1990;47:169–174.
26. Evanoff BA, Gustavsson P, Hogstedt C. Mortality and incidence of cancer in a cohort of Swedish chimney sweeps: an extended followup study. *Br J Ind Med* 1993;50:450–459.
27. US Environmental Protection Agency, Office of Health and Environmental Assessment, Office of Air and Radiation. *Respiratory health effects of passive smoking: lung cancer and other disorders.* Washington: US Environmental Protection Agency, Office of Health and Environmental Assessment, Office of Research and Development, 1992.
28. Glantz SA, Parmley WW. Passive smoking and heart disease. *JAMA* 1995;273:1047–1053.
29. Kawachi I, Graham A, Colditz GA. A prospective study of passive smoking and coronary heart disease. *Circulation* 1997;95:2374–2379.
30. Benowitz NL. Cotinine as a biomarker of environmental tobacco smoke exposure. *Epidemiol Rev* 1996;18:188–204.
31. US Surgeon General. The health consequences of involuntary smoking. Rockville, MD: US Department of Health and Human Services, 1986.
32. Bond JA, Gown AM, Yang HL, Benditt EP, Juchau MR. Further investigations of the capacity of polynuclear aromatic hydrocarbons to elicit atherosclerotic lesions. *J Toxicol Environ Health* 1981;7:327–335.
33. Penn A, Snyder C. Arteriosclerotic plaque development is promoted by polynuclear aromatic hydrocarbons. *Carcinogenesis* 1988;9:2285–2189.
34. Pinto SS, Enterline PE, Henderson V, Varner MO. Mortality experience in relation to a measured arsenic trioxide exposure. *Environ Health Perspect* 1977;19:127–130.
35. Lee-Feldstein A. Arsenic and respiratory cancer in humans: follow-up of copper smelter employees in Montana. *J Natl Cancer Inst* 1983;70:601–609.
36. Axelson O, Dahlgren E, Jansson CD, Rehnlund SO. Arsenic exposure and mortality: a case-referent study from a Swedish copper smelter. *Br J Ind Med* 1978;35:8–15.
37. Wu MM, Kuo TL, Huang YH, Chen CJ. Dose-response relationship between arsenic concentration in well water and mortality from cancers and vascular diseases. *Am J Epidemiol* 1989;130:1123–1132.
38. Chen CJ, Hsueh YM, Lai MS, et al. Increased prevalance of hypertension and long-term arsenic exposure. *Hypertension* 1995;25:53–60.
39. Morton WE. Occupational habituation to aliphatic nitrates and the withdrawal hazards of coronary disease and hypertension. *J Occup Med* 1977;19:197–200.
40. Lange RI, Reid MS, Tresch DD, Keelan MH, Bernhard VM, Coolidge G. Nonatheromatous ischemic heart disease following withdrawal from chronic industrial nitroglycerin exposure. *Circulation* 1972;46:666–678.
41. Levine RJ, Andjelkovich DA, Kersteter SL, et al. Heart disease in workers exposed to dinitrotoluene. *J Occup Med* 1986;28:811–816.
42. Ahlman K, Koskela RS, Kuikka P, Koponen M, Annanmaki M. Mortality among sulfide ore miners. *Am J Ind Med* 1991,19:603–617.
43. Gjesdal K, Bille S, Bredesen JE, et al. Exposure to glyceryl trinitrate during gun powder production: plasma glyceryl trinitrate concentration, elimination kinetics, and discomfort among production workers. *Br J Ind Med* 1985;42:27–31.
44. Amnon B-D. Cardiac arrest in an explosives factory due to withdrawal from nitroglycerin exposure. *Am J Ind Med* 1989;15:719–722.
45. Klock JC. Nonocclusive coronary disease after chronic exposure to nitrates: evidence for physiologic nitrate dependence. *Am Heart J* 1975;89:510–513.
46. Przybojewski JZ, Heyns MH. Acute coronary vasospasm secondary to industrial nitroglycerin withdrawal: a case presentation and review. *S Afr Med J* 1983;63:158–165.
47. Corya BC, Black MJ, McHenry PL. Echocardiographic findings after acute carbon monoxide poisoning. *Br Heart J* 1976;38:712.
48. Middleton GD, Ashby DW, Clark F. Delayed and long-lasting electrocardiographic changes in carbon-monoxide poisoning. *Lancet* 1961;1:12.
49. Allred EN, Bleecker ER, Chaitman BR, et al. Short-term effects of carbon monoxide exposure on the exercise performance of subjects with coronary artery disease. *N Engl J Med* 1989;321:1426–1432.
50. Allred EN, Bleecker ER, Chitman BR. Effects of carbon monoxide on myocardial ischemia. *Environ Health Perspect* 1991;91:89–132.
51. Aronow WS, Stemmes EA, Zweig S. Carbon monoxide and ventricular fibrillation threshold in normal dogs. *Arch Environ Health* 1979;34:184–186.
52. Atkins EH, Baker EL. Exacerbation of coronary artery disease by occupational carbon monoxide exposure: a report of two fatalities and a review of the literature. *Am J Ind Med* 1985;7:73–79.
53. Scharf SM, Thames MD, Sargent RK. Transmural myocardial infarction after exposure to carbon monoxide in coronary artery disease: report of a case. *N Engl J Med* 1974;15:409.
54. Aronow WS, Stemmer EA, Isbell MW. Effect of carbon monoxide exposure on intermittent claudication. *Circulation* 1974;49:415–417.
55. Calvery PMA, Leggett RJ. Carbon monoxide and exercise tolerance in chronic bronchitis and emphysema. *BMJ* 1981;283:878.
56. Horvath SM, Raven PB, Dahms TE, et al. Maximum aerobic capacity at different levels of carboxyhemoglobin. *J Appl Physiol* 1975;38:300–303.

57. Bonenfant JL, Miller G, Roy PE. Quebec beer-drinkers' cardiomyopathy: pathological studies. *Can Med Assoc J* 1967;97:910–916.
58. Kesteloot H, Roeland J, Willems J, Claes JH, Joosens JV. An enquiry into the role of cobalt in the heart disease of chronic beer drinkers. *Circulation* 1968;37:854–864.
59. Horowitz SF, Fischbein A, Matza D, et al. Evaluation of right and left ventricular function in hard metal workers. *Br J Ind Med* 1988;45:742–746.
60. Barborik M, Dusek J. Cardiomyopathy accompanying industrial cobalt exposure. *Br Heart J* 1972;34:113–116.
61. Kennedy A, Dornan JD, King R. Fatal myocardial disease associated with industrial exposure to cobalt. *Lancet* 1981;1:412–414.
62. Jarvis JQ, Hammond E, Meier R, Robinson C. Cobalt cardiomyopathy. *J Occup Med* 1992,34:620–626.
63. Alexander CS. Cobalt and the heart. *Ann Intern Med* 1969;70:411–413.
64. National Research Council. Biologic effects of arsenic on man. In: *Arsenic*. Washington: National Academy of Sciences, 1977:173–191.
65. Goldsmith S, From AHL. Arsenic-induced atypical ventricular tachycardia. *N Engl J Med* 1980;303:1096–1098.
66. Beckman KJ, Bauman JL, Pimental PA, Garrard C, Hariman RJ. Arsenic-induced torsade de pointes. *Crit Care Med* 1991;19:290–292.
67. Josephson CJ, Pinto SS, Petronella SJ. Arsine: electrocardiographic changes produced in acute human poisoning. *Arch Ind Hyg* 1951;4:43–52.
68. Kline TS. Myocardial changes in lead poisoning. *Am J Dis Child* 1960;99:48.
69. Silver W, Rodriguez-Torres R. Electrocardiographic study in children with lead poisoning. *Pediatrics* 1968;41:1124–1127.
70. Read JI, Williams JP. Lead myocarditis: report of a case. *Am Heart J* 1952;44:797–802.
71. Myerson RM, Eisenhauler JH. Atrioventricular conduction defects in lead poisoning. *Am J Cardiol* 1963;11:409–412.
72. Asokan SK. Experimental lead cardiomyopathy: myocardial structural changes in rats given small amounts of lead. *J Lab Clin Med* 1974;84:20–25.
73. Williams BJ, Hejtmancik MR, Abreu M. Cardiac effects of lead. *Fed Proc* 1983;42:2989–2993.
74. Brieger H, Semisch CW, Stasney J, Piatnek DA. Industrial antimony poisoning. *Ind Med Surg* 1954;23:521–523.
75. Schnorr TM, Stenland K, Thun MJ, Rinsky RA. Mortality in a cohort of antimony smelter workers. *Am J Ind Med* 1995;27:759–770.
76. Lauwers LF, Roelants A, Rosseel PM, Heyndickx B, Baute L. Oral antimony intoxications in man. *Critical Care Med* 1990;18:324–326.
77. Mee AS, Wright PL. Congestive (dilated) cardiomyopathy in association with solvent abuse. *J R Soc Med* 1980;73:671–672.
78. Weissberg PL, Green ID. Methyl-cellulose paint possibly causing heart failure. *BMJ* 1979;1114.
79. McLeod AA, Marjot R, Monaghan MJ, Hugh-Jones P, Jackson G. Chronic cardiac toxicity after inhalation of 1,1,1-trichloroethane. *BMJ* 1987;294:728–729.
80. Wiseman MN, Banim S. "Glue sniffer's" heart? *BMJ* 1987;294:739.
81. Knight AT, Pawsey CGK, Aroney RS, Lawrence JR, Jones BJ, Newland RC. Upholsterers' glue associated with myocarditis, hepatitis, acute renal failure and lymphoma. *Med J Aust* 1991;154:360–362.
82. Bass M. Sudden sniffing death. *JAMA* 1970;212:2075–2079.
83. Kleinfeld M, Tabershaw IR. Trichloroethylene toxicity: report of five fatal cases. *Arch Ind Hyg Occup Med* 1954;10:134–141.
84. Wright MF, Strobl DJ. 1,1,1-Trichloroethane cardiac toxicity: report of a case. *J Am Osteopath Assoc* 1984;84:285–288.
85. May DC, Blotzer MJ. A report of occupational deaths attributed to fluorocarbon-113. *Arch Environ Health* 1984;39:352–354.
86. Wilcosky TC, Simonsen NR. Solvent exposure and cardiovascular disease. *Am J Ind Med* 1991;19:569–586.
87. Speizer FE, Wegman DH, Ramirez A. Palpitation rates associated with fluorocarbon exposure in a hospital setting. *N Engl J Med* 1975;292:624–626.
88. Kaufman JD, Morgan MS, Marks ML, Greene HL, Rosenstock L. A study of the cardiac effects of bromochlorodifluoromethane (halon 1211) exposure during exercise. *Am J Ind Med* 1992;21:223–233.
89. Antti-Poika N, Heikkila J, Saarinen L. Cardiac arrhythmias during occupational exposure to fluorinated hydrocarbons. *Br J Ind Med* 1990;47:138–140.
90. Edling C, Ohlson C-G, Ljungkvist G, Oliv A, Soderholm B. Cardiac arrhythmia in refrigerator repairmen exposed to fluorocarbons. *Br J Ind Med* 1990;47:207–212.
91. Kobayashi S, Hutchenon DE, Regan J. Cardiopulmonary toxicity of tetrachloroethylene. *J Toxicol Environ Health* 1982;10:23–30.
92. White JF, Carlson GP. Epinephrine-induced cardiac arrythmias in rabbits exposed to trichloroethylene: potentiation by caffeine. *Fund Appl Toxicol* 1982;2:125–129.
93. White JF, Carlson GP. Epinephrine-induced cardiac arrythmias in rabbits exposed to trichloroethylene: potentiation by ethanol. *Toxicol Appl Pharmacol* 1981;60:466–471.
94. Finkelstein Y, Kushnir A, Raikhlin-Eisenkraft B, Taitelman U. Antidotal therapy of severe acute organophosphate poisoning: a multihospital study. *Neurotoxicol Teratol* 1989;11:593–596.
95. Ludomirsky A, Klein HO, Sarelli P, et al. Q-T prolongation and polymorphous ("torsade de pointes") ventricular arrhythmias associated with organophosphorous insecticide poisoning. *Am J Cardiol* 1982;49:1654–1658.
96. Saiyed HN, Sadhu HG, Bhatnagar VK, Dewan A, Venkaiah K, Kashyap SK. Cardiac toxicity following short-term exposure to methoxyl in spraymen and rabbits. *Hum Experi Toxicol* 1992;11:93–97.
97. Kass R, Kochar G, Lippman M. Adult respiratory distress syndrome from organophosphate poisoning. *Am J Emerg Med* 1991;9:32–33.
98. Kiss Z, Fazekas T. Arrythmias in organophosphate poisonings. *Acta Cardiol* 1979;34:323–330.
99. O'Malley MA, McCurdy SA. Subacute poisoning with phosalone, an organophosphate insecticide. *West J Med* 1990;153:619–624.
100. Sharp DS, Becker CE, Smith AH. Chronic low-level lead exposure: its role in the pathogenesis of hypertension. *Med Toxicol* 1987;2:210–232.
101. Schwartz J. Lead, blood pressure, and cardiovascular disease in men. *Environ Health* 1995;50:31–37.
102. Pirkle JL, Schwartz J, Landis JR, Harlan WR. The relationship between blood lead levels and blood pressure and its cardiovascular risk implication. *Am J Epidemiol* 1985;121:246–258.
103. Menditto A, Morisi G, Spagnolo A, Menotti A, NFR Study Group. Association of blood lead to blood pressure in men aged 55 to 75 years: effect of selected social and biochemical confounders. *Environ Health Perspect* 1994;102[Suppl 9]:107–111.
104. Beevers DG, Erskine E, Robertson M, et al. Blood lead and hypertension. *Lancet* 1976;1:1–3.
105. Landrigan PJ. Toxicity of lead at low dose. *Br J Ind Med* 1989;46:593–596.
106. Wolf C, Wallnofer A, Waldhor T, Vutuc C, Meisinger V, Rudiger HW. Effect of lead on blood pressure in occupationally nonexposed men. *Am J Ind Med* 1995;27:897–903.
107. Staessen JA, Lauwerys RR, Buchet JP, et al. Impairment of renal function with increasing blood lead concentrations in the general population. *JAMA* 1992;327:151–156.
108. Schroeder HA. Cadmium, chromium, and cardiovascular disease. *Circulation* 1967;35:570–582.
109. Staessen J, Amery A, Bernard A, et al. Blood pressure, the prevalence of cardiovascular diseases, and exposure to cadmium: a population study. *Am J Epidemiol* 1991;134:257–267.
110. Eskenaza B, Bracken MB, Holford TR, Grady J. Exposure to organic solvents and hypertensive disorders of pregnancy. *Am J Ind Med* 1988;14:177–188.
111. Voge VM. Secondary arterial hypertension linked to freon exposure. *South Med J* 1996;89:516–518.
112. Chen CJ, Wu MM, Lee SS, Wong JD, Cheng SH, Wu HY. Atherogenicity and carcinogenicity of high-arsenic artesian well water: multiple risk factors and related malignant neoplasmas of blackfoot disease. *Arteriosclerosis* 1988;8:452–460.
113. Tseng WP. Blackfoot disease in Taiwan: a 30-year followup study. *Angiology* 1989;40:547–557.

CHAPTER 21
Clinical Ocular Toxicology

Robert J. Noecker

ANATOMY AND PHYSIOLOGY OF THE EYE

The eye and visual system are susceptible to injury from many different hazards in the environment. Chemicals, heat, electromagnetic radiation, and ionizing radiation all have potential adverse effects on the function of the eye and vision. It is important to be aware of the unique problems that each of these environmental agents presents.

Anatomy of the Eye

The eye is located in the orbit, which is a bony structure consisting of seven cranial bones. Six extraocular muscles are responsible for moving the globe. There are four recti muscles: the superior, inferior, medial, and lateral rectus. There are also the superior oblique and inferior oblique muscles. The eyelids protect the anterior surface of the eye. The skin that covers the eyelids is the thinnest in the body, and there is no subcutaneous fat present. The protractor muscle of the eye, which causes the eyelid to close, is the orbicularis oculi muscle, which is innervated by the seventh cranial nerve. The retractor muscles, which include the levator (innervated by cranial nerve III) and Müller's muscle (innervated by the sympathetic system). The tarsus is a firm, dense connective tissue plate located at the margin of the eyelids, which contains meibomian glands and eyelashes (Figs. 21-1 through 21-3).

The inside surface of the eyelids and the surface of the globe are lined with the conjunctiva. The conjunctiva is nonkeratinized squamous epithelium, which contains mucin-secreting goblet cells. The sclera is a tough, white outer shell, which helps maintain the shape of the globe and protect the inner contents. The cornea is the clear, centrally located tissue responsible for focusing light into the posterior pole. The cornea consists of five layers, including epithelium, Bowman's layer, stroma, Descemet's membrane, and the endothelium. The anterior chamber is located behind the cornea, and this is the space through which aqueous humor circulates before exiting the eye. Trabecular meshwork, the drain through which the aqueous humor flows out of the eye, is located at the junction between the cornea and the iris. The iris is the colored portion of the eye responsible for increasing or decreasing the amount of light allowed into the eye via the dilator and sphincter muscles. Attached to the lens and iris is the ciliary body. The ciliary body produces aqueous humor, which maintains pressure in the eye and changes the shape of the lens. The lens of the eye is located directly behind the pupil and changes its shape to focus light. The vitreous is a jelly-like substance that forms the bulk of the posterior chamber and is optically clear. The retina lines the posterior four-fifths of the eye, and its nutrition is supplied by the underlying choroid and pigment epithelium. The nerve fiber layer of the retina coalesces to form the optic nerve.

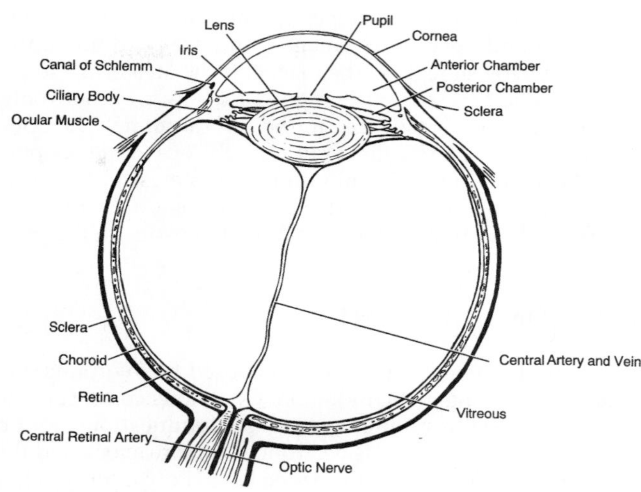

Figure 21-2. Anatomy of the internal eye.

Physiology of the Eye

The surface of the eye is covered with a tear film. The three components to the tear film are the outer lipid layer, produced by the meibomian glands; the middle aqueous layer, produced by the lacrimal glands; and the inner mucous layer, produced by goblet cells on the conjunctiva. The function of the tear film is to provide a smooth optical surface with the air. It is a medium through which debris is removed and through which oxygen is supplied to the cornea. The tear film also contains numerous antimicrobial agents, which inhibit infections and lubricates the cornea, eyelids and conjunctiva, and presenting desiccation of these surfaces. The central cornea is approximately 0.5 mm thick and is the main refractive element of the eye. The cornea aqueous interface produces 40 to 45 diopters of focusing power. The epithelium of the cornea is hydrophobic and prevents excess water from entering the corneal stroma. The endothelium of the cornea is a single layer of cells, which acts to pump water out of the cornea back into the aqueous humor. The cornea needs to be partially dehydrated to remain clear and function effectively.

The aqueous humor is for the most part located in the anterior chamber. It is produced by the nonpigmented inner epithelial cells of the ciliary body. It originates from behind the iris, goes through the pupil into the anterior chamber, and out through the trabecular meshwork and canal of Schlemm. The canal of Schlemm is a large venous channel that drains the aqueous into venous channels of the sclera. The iris acts as a filter to light coming into the posterior pole of the eye. The dilator muscle is innervated by the sympathetic system, and the sphincter muscle is innervated by the parasympathetic system.

The lens is the weaker of the two refractive surfaces, and is responsible for approximately 10 to 12 diopters of focusing power. It is a biconvex in structure and is held in place by zonules, which are attached to the ciliary muscle. During accommodation, there are changes in the lens thickness so that light is focused more anteriorly in the eye. The ciliary muscle contracts, causing relaxation of zonule fibers, resulting in increased thickness of the lens with accommodation. Presbyopia is a condition that occurs with aging, and is owing to increasing lens stiffness, which limits the amount of shape change the lens can undergo. Furthermore, as cataracts develop with aging, less light passes through the lens.

The vitreous occupies four-fifths of the volume of the globe, taking up approximately 4 mL. It is 99% water, with the major component being hyaluronic acid. It provides a passageway of metabolites to be utilized by the lens, ciliary body, and retina. The retina produces signals from light stimulation, which are then carried by the optic nerve to the occipital cortex. The rods and cones are the photoreceptors, which are responsible for collecting the light input. Rods provide more of the vision in dim lighting and

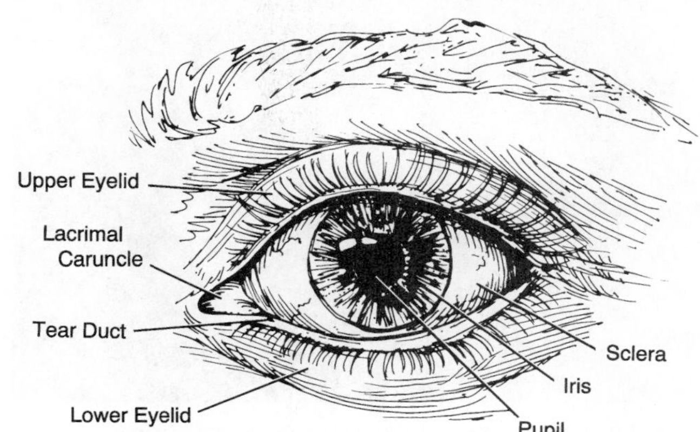

Figure 21-1. Anatomy of the external eye.

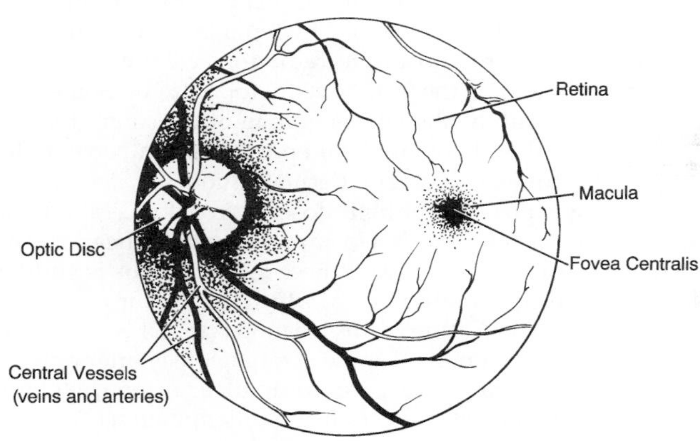

Figure 21-3. Anatomy of the retina.

are more predominantly in the peripheral retina. Cones provide color vision and very sharp images, and are predominantly located in the foveal region. The macula is the area of the retina that gives the best and sharpest vision. It is made up of cones only, and takes up a very small area in the central retina. The optic nerve ganglion cells carry the input from the eye to the occipital cortex. Approximately 120 million neurons exist in the optic nerve. The number of neurons decrease with age, and are lost at an accelerated rate due to glaucoma or high pressure in the eye.

RADIATION AND LIGHT

Humans are becoming increasingly exposed to environmental sources of electromagnetic radiation. Of serious concern is the potential damage from microwaves, communications, radon gas levels, x-rays, radiation leaks from nuclear reactors, and the progressive deterioration of the ozone layer. Public concern has mainly focused on the potential carcinogenic effects; however, radiation can cause other noncarcinogenic yet very damaging effects on the eye. In the electromagnetic spectrum, radiant energy is categorized according to wavelength frequency or photon energies. Radiation of wavelength 10 nm or less is classified as ionizing radiation (1).

Radiation can affect any structure of the eye, including the cornea, conjunctiva, lens, retina, and optic nerve. The damage from radiation exposure is usually slowly progressive and delayed in onset. Typically, it becomes evident months to years after the exposure. The main mechanism of decreased vision in patients is increased permeability of the blood vessels, especially in the retina and optic nerve.

At the cellular level, ionizing radiation has two effects. The first is on individual cells, causing death or functional alterations, and the second is an indirect effect of vascular damage. The direct injury may cause an arrest in mitosis. The vascular changes include early swelling of the vessels with degeneration of the intima and endothelial cells. Clinically, the early changes are seen as vascular dilatation or engorgement, hemorrhage, vascular tortuosity, and hyperemia of the tissue. Most of these changes develop 3 to 5 weeks after the injury, but severe sequelae can be seen in the tissues 1 to 2 years after the exposure.

EXTERNAL DISEASE

Radiation affects the eye in two ways. One effect develops within a few weeks after exposure and another response occurs between months to years after exposure. A large amount of radiation in a short period may cause a corneal flash burn, with few serious or permanent consequences. A smaller concentration over a longer period may cause cumulative effects to the lens and retina. The early reactions are similar to those produced by ultraviolet (UV) light, conjunctival hyperemia, and conjunctival inflammation. After exposure to radiation, there is very little active inflammation in the form of cellular infiltrates. Some scarring can occur with hyaline degeneration of the connective tissue. The corneal and conjunctival epithelia often become dry and show keratinization and epidermalization.

With long exposure and high doses, corneal ulceration and necrosis may develop with accompanying opacification and vascularization. The severest of these late reactions is sudden widespread necrosis of the cornea, which may occur years after exposure. The main feature of this reaction is that the whole area exposed to radiation may ulcerate spontaneously after appearing normal for years. A large chronic ulcer often develops, which is accompanied by infection and inflammation (2). Often, this late reaction is accompanied by glaucoma, massive intraocular hemorrhage, and inflammation.

Radiation may also cause keratitis and dry eye by killing the goblet cells of the conjunctiva, thus reducing the wettability of the ocular surface. This in turn causes chronic problems and exposure keratopathy secondary to inadequate surface lubrication.

The ocular surface may be further compromised by drying due to a relative insufficiency of tears. One study of children who were relocated from Chernobyl to Israel documented significantly decreased tear production in the population that was exposed to the most radiation from the nuclear power plant. Of the children studied, 18% had blepharoconjunctivitis and 15% had significantly decreased tear production. Typically, reduced tear production is usually associated with older age groups and is unusual in children. The relatively high rate of blepharoconjunctivitis has also been associated with dry eyes. Although it is not known if the changes in tear production are transient or permanent, the effect of decreased tear production was present 7 years after the exposure and may result in significant morbidity over time (3).

LENS

The lens is the most sensitive structure to ionizing radiation in the adult eye. The basic mechanism for cataractogenesis or opacification of the lens is damage to the DNA of cell membranes by free radical formation and oxidative reactions. The damage tends to be cumulative and is dose-related.

Histopathologic studies of human lenses exposed to long-term, low-dose radiation showed alterations in the anterior epithelial cells, germinal epithelial cells, and equatorial cortical fibers (4,5). Radiation first affects the nuclei of cells and mitosis, which line the preequatorial zone of the lens epithelium (6). Radiation causes mitosis to be inhibited for a short time, but later it recommences. The distorted cells form and migrate to the posterior pole in the axial region where they produce a subcapsular opacification.

With larger doses of radiation, all of the epithelial cells may be harmed with no normal fibers forming, and hence the entire lens may become opaque. In humans, the earliest cataractous changes are discreet dots in the cortex near the posterior pole. These opacified areas later spread, producing a disc-shaped cataractous lesion. Later, a central opacity occupies the region of the posterior cortex (Fig. 21-4).

Most of the complications from radiation exposure occur between approximately 3,000 and 4,000 rad with external beam radiation. However, the minimum cataractogenic dose has been estimated to be 500 rad but may be as low as 200 rad. Merriam suggested that some people develop cataracts after receiving 200 rad in a single exposure or 550 rad over 3 months (7). Studies have shown that a single large dose is more cataractogenic than several

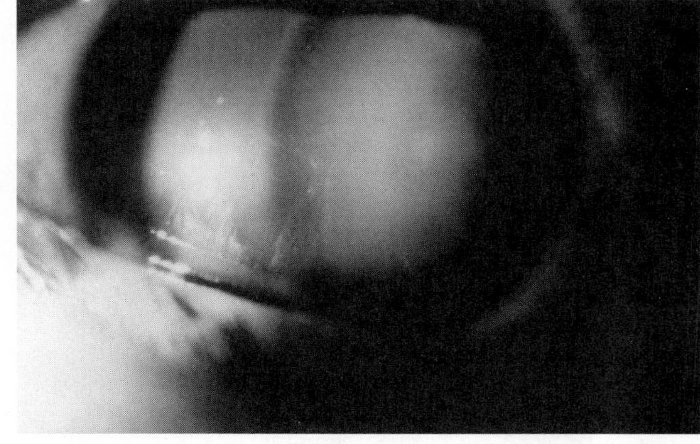

Figure 21-4. Cataract after radiation exposure. Nuclear sclerotic and posterior subcapsular cataractous changes in the lens of this eye are apparent 1 year after external beam radiation exposure.

small doses. Ionizing radiation may cause cataracts in the lens even when the rest of the eye may appear normal. In the past, workers were not aware of the lens changes caused by ionizing radiation because of the long waiting period before the clinical opacities developed. The younger the person, the more susceptible the lens is to radiation injury and the shorter the latency period. The larger the dose, the shorter the latency period.

No medical therapeutic modality is available for the treatment or prevention of radiation cataracts. The only surgical therapy is removal of the cataractous lens. Therefore, exposure to radiation should be minimized by shielding and avoidance of inadvertent dosing.

RETINA

Radiation retinopathy is a delayed onset, slowly progressive occlusive vasculopathy. It may lead to capillary nonperfusion, large vessel occlusion, vascular incompetence, and neovascularization, which in turn leads to loss of visual function (8). The vaso-occlusive process is often slow and unrelentingly progressive (9).

Clinically, the signs that are seen in radiation retinopathy are identical to those seen in diabetic retinopathy (Fig. 21-5A). To differentiate between the two, a history of radiation exposure must be elicited. Macular edema is often the earliest finding and is frequently the cause of decreased vision in people with radiation retinopathy (10). The next most common changes in order of frequency are microaneurysms, intraretinal hemorrhages, hard exudates, nerve fiber layer infarcts, and capillary nonperfusion. Characteristic findings, such as microaneurysms or telangiectasias, are seen earlier in the course of the disease. Cotton wool spots are seen transiently, with large areas of capillary nonperfusion seen later. Retinal hemorrhages and exudates may occur at any time. Later, extensive retinovascular occlusion may lead to neovascularization. Widespread neovascularization may be seen in the retina, optic nerve, and iris, which may in turn lead to vitreous hemorrhage and neovascular glaucoma. Later in the course of the disease, retinal pigment epithelial atrophy is seen, giving the fundus a salt-and-pepper appearance (11).

In the largest series of patients followed after irradiation for choroidal melanomas with proton beam therapy, 89% developed some manifestation of radiation retinopathy. Retinal neovascularization was relatively rare, seen in only 6% of cases (12). The threshold for radiation retinopathy depends both on the total dose delivered and the daily fraction size. In general, the incidence of tissue damage increases with greater total dosage. Most reports indicate that at least 30 to 35 Gy to the head are needed before retinopathy can be expected (13,14). However, retinal vascular changes have been seen after as little as 11 Gy of external beam radiation (15,16).

Histopathologic studies have shown that retinal vessel endothelial cell damage leads to vascular occlusion. The thickening of the arteriolar walls is due to deposition of fibrillar and hyaline material. Human studies have shown ganglion cell loss, intraretinal exudates, and cystic changes of the outer plexiform layers. The rods and cones are relatively resistant to radiation damage (17).

The diagnosis of radiation retinopathy should be considered if there is any history of radiation exposure for any reason. Fluorescein angiography findings consistently demonstrate areas of capillary nonperfusion; without these findings it is difficult to make the diagnosis of radiation retinopathy (11) (Fig. 21-5B).

Treatment of radiation retinopathy is difficult. When the vision loss is owing to ischemic maculopathy secondary to capillary nonperfusion, there is no treatment available. However, cystoid macular edema may be helped by laser grid therapy. Panretinal photocoagulation is beneficial in reducing the neovascularization of the optic nerve and retina, and may prevent progression of neovascular glaucoma (10). Pars plana vitrectomy has been performed to treat nonclearing vitreous hemorrhages, with improvement in visual function.

In conclusion, radiation retinopathy is a delayed onset progressive disease that often leads to vision loss from central macular capillary nonperfusion. In later stages, vision loss may result from vitreous hemorrhage, neovascular glaucoma, or retinal detachment. Although the retinopathy is progressive, regression has been seen in some cases. Three conditions appear to exacerbate the retinopathy. Patients with preexisting microangiopathy have worse disease. Patients with preexisting diabetic retinopathy have more changes at lower doses (11). Those patients with exposure to chemotherapeutic agents, such as fluorouracil, appear predisposed to and have a lower threshold for development of radiation retinopathy, even if therapy is not concurrent (18).

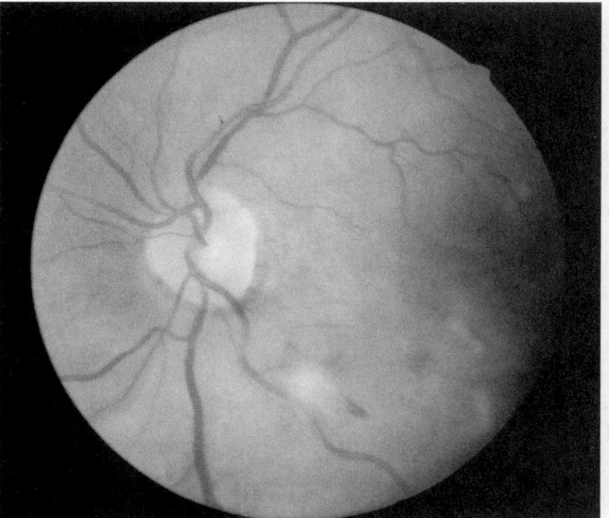

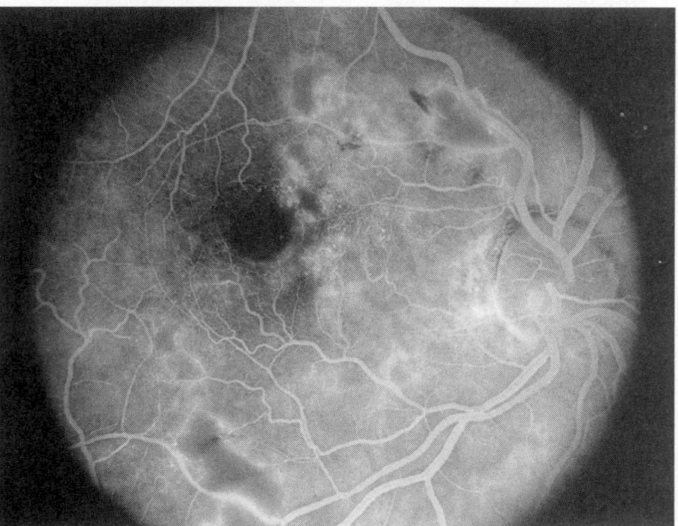

Figure 21-5. A: Radiation retinopathy. The retina of a patient 1 year after being exposed to external beam radiation. This photograph demonstrates intraretinal hemorrhages and telangiectasias. Cotton wool spots are also evident, which indicate retinal ischemia. **B:** Fluorescein of same patient demonstrating areas of capillary nonperfusion, microaneurysms, and hemorrhages.

OPTIC NERVE

Optic neuropathy may occur in conjunction with radiation retinopathy or alone. Optic nerve damage from radiation may first be manifested by optic nerve edema. Often, surrounding hemorrhages, cotton wool spots, and exudates occur. Eventually the edema resolves, and the optic nerves become atrophic. One study that followed 335 patients who had received proton beam radiation showed that optic disc pallor was the most common lesion seen in 63% of cases at 5 years. Disc edema was seen in approximately one-third of cases. The least common finding was neovascularization of the disc, which was present in only 7% of cases at 5 years. The optic nerve changes were more prominent when the disc received higher radiation levels (70 Gy). Older patients tended to have more optic nerve hemorrhages than nerve layer infarcts (12).

One histopathologic study examined the optic nerve of a patient who had received 6,000 rad of radiation. The eye was removed 18 months after the radiation exposure because of intractable glaucoma (19). The sensory retina showed absence of ganglion cells. The optic nerve showed areas of necrosis with round cell infiltrates and vessels, with the changes seen in retinal vessels with radiation retinopathy.

Clinically, vision usually begins to decrease months to years after exposure. The earliest changes may be diffuse decrease in visual sensitivity, followed by central scotomas and, potentially, loss of all vision.

Sunlight and Ultraviolet Radiation

In the electromagnetic spectrum, the UV spectrum is located just below the visible spectrum of light. For convenience and based on biological effects, the spectrum is subdivided into UV-C (200 to 290 nm), UV-B (290 to 320 nm), and UV-A (320 to 400 nm). The wavelengths 200 to 300 nm are absorbed by the cornea. The 300 to 400 nm wavelengths are transmitted through the cornea and are absorbed by the lens (20).

EXTERNAL DISEASE

Superficial keratitis is caused by radiation with a peak at 288 nm, in which longer wavelengths above 310 nm are believed to be harmless. Experimental studies have shown that UV damage can be seen in epithelial cells within 24 hours of exposure. The damage is represented by increased membrane permeability (21). After exposure to a large amount of UV light, intense and painful inflammation occurs, with conjunctival inflammation and keratopathy of the cornea occurring several hours later. This inflammation usually lasts for several days, and is analogous to an acute, blistering sunburn. This photokeratitis is frequently seen as a welder's flash, caused by momentary exposure to UV-C during arc welding. Photokeratitis has also been reported in association with defective glass envelopes surrounding mercury vapor lamps and also accounts for 59% of all injuries associated with tanning booths (22). This condition is also seen as snow blindness, which is usually encountered when the UV ray's reflectivity is extremely high, such as during spring skiing. At high altitudes, UV with the sunlight is more intense than at sea level because of less atmospheric absorption. Usually, no permanent damage occurs, but the eye may remain photophobic for some time.

Depending on the intensity and duration of the radiation, the corneal epithelial cells may die or be stimulated to active proliferation. In the cornea, acute injuries produce nuclear fragmentation similar to that after exposure to mustard gas. Long-term exposure to the cornea and conjunctiva results in damage not only to the epithelium but also in the subepithelial connective tissue. The subepithelial tissues exhibit fragmentation of collagen, and elastoid degeneration results.

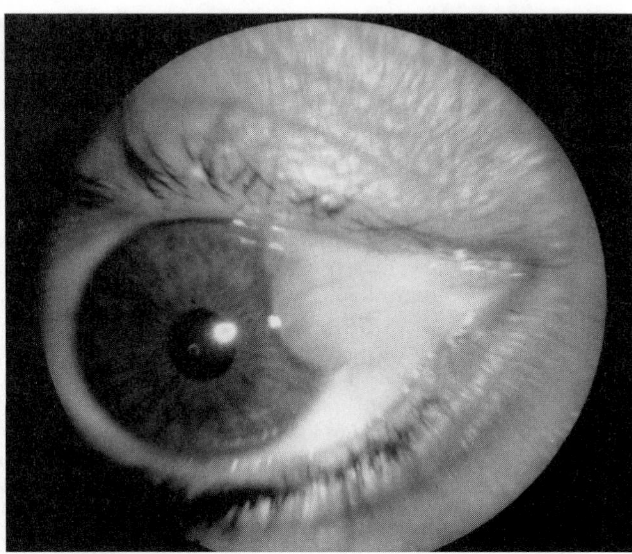

Figure 21-6. Pterygium. Pterygium has grown onto the cornea and is growing toward the visual axis.

Pingueculae and pterygia may occur from chronic exposure to UV light (23). Pingueculae are localized, yellowish, fleshy lesions that appear on the conjunctival surface near the limbus, usually in the interpalpebral fissure. Histologically, the epithelium may be normal or hyperkeratotic, and the substantia propria shows actinic degeneration. The prevalence of pingueculae increases with age and is usually clinically insignificant.

Pterygia are similar in appearance but involve the peripheral cornea as well. These lesions are highly vascular compared to pingueculae (Fig. 21-6). Like pingueculae, histologically pterygia are comprised of degenerating collagen fibers and elastoid fibers. Pterygia occur more commonly in tropical or sunny areas versus more temperate climates and have been clearly associated with exposure to UV light. They are more common in people aged 20 to 40 years who work outdoors (24).

Clinically, pterygia can cause irritation and discomfort. More seriously, they can grow across the cornea, causing astigmatism and decreased vision. In this case, the pterygia should be removed surgically. A relatively high recurrence rate is associated with pterygia.

Climatic droplet keratopathy is a spheroidal degeneration of the superficial corneal stroma. This is characterized by yellow, oily-appearing droplets in Bowman's layer. The degeneration is thought to be caused by changes in the serum proteins that normally diffuse through the cornea. Many studies have shown the relationship between UV exposure and disease prevalence and severity (25,26). Spheroidal degeneration can lead to a significant decrease in vision due to clouding of the cornea and is a major cause of blindness in some parts of the world (27).

CATARACTS

The evidence of whether UV light is cataractogenic from usual daily doses is mainly statistical based on cataract incidence in different regions. Some epidemiologic studies suggest that UV-B exposure is an important risk factor for the development of cataracts. One study showed a very clear dose-response effect between exposure to UV-B and cortical cataracts (28). In another study, cumulative exposure of UV-B was associated with increased incidence of posterior subcapsular cataracts (29). Based on this evidence, it is recommended that adequate protection be used to minimize chronic exposure.

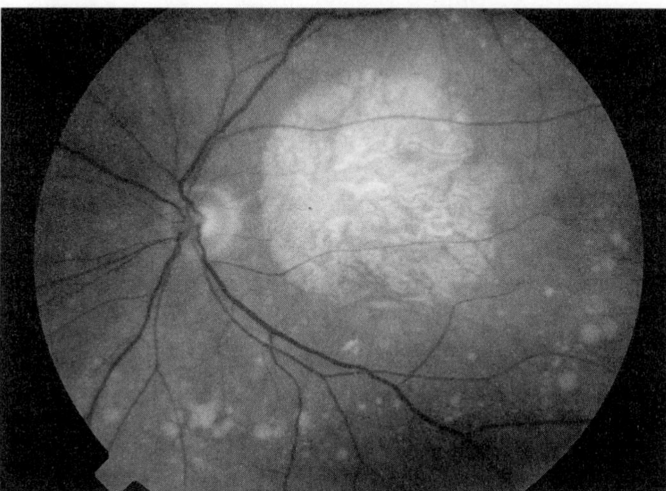

Figure 21-7. Macular degeneration. The retina pigment epithelium has become atrophic, resulting in degeneration of the retina in the macular region.

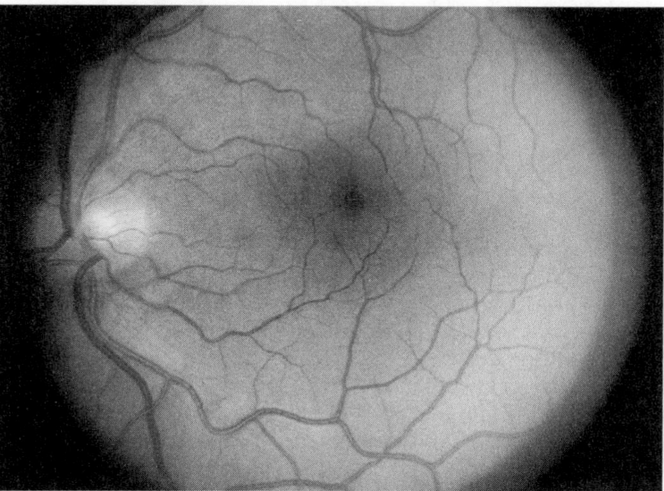

Figure 21-8. Retinal solar burn. Retina of the right eye of a patient who gazed at a solar eclipse in southern Arizona. The characteristic retinal change is present in the macula.

Retina

MACULAR DEGENERATION

Much less is known about the role of chronic UV exposure in macular degeneration (Fig. 21-7). The primary reason macular degeneration was first linked to UV light exposure was the clinical observation in a large series of patients with macular degeneration. Van der Hoeve found that macular degeneration was much less common in patients who had significant cataracts, and he thought that patients with their lenses intact were offered some protection from the UV and blue light (30). Experimentally, the histologic changes induced by cumulative photochemical injury are similar to those seen in macular degeneration in people. Some investigators have shown that macular degeneration is associated with light iris and hair color. It has been suggested that the lighter pigmentation may reflect a lower level of melanin and, thus, less protection against photooxidative damage because of the direct absorption of light. The aging lens becomes increasingly brown and acts as a blue light filter to protect the retina from shorter wavelengths. However, with the removal of the crystalline lens after cataract surgery, many patients lose this shortwave protection.

Taylor showed, in a study of Chesapeake Bay watermen, high levels of exposure to blue or visible light may have caused ocular damage, especially later in life, and may be related to development of macular degeneration (23). The Beaver Dam Eye Study also suggested that exposure to sunlight may be associated with macular degeneration but that longitudinal studies are needed (31).

ACUTE SOLAR EXPOSURE

Solar retinopathy is a condition in which both visible and infrared sunlight is concentrated on the macular area of the retina. The mechanism of injury is thought to be a photochemical reaction that results from the retina being heated with prolonged gazing at the sun, especially with a dilated pupil (32). Solar retinopathy is usually bilateral and associated with visual dazzling and scotoma, or blind spot. Initially, minimal changes in the retina occur, but, within 24 hours, several yellow-whitish spots may develop (Fig. 21-8). After several weeks, lesions and edema disappear, and a perifoveal defect in the pigment epithelium may remain. Postinjury visual acuity may be normal but is often reduced while final visual acuity usually ranges from 20/20 to 20/40 (33).

One report by Rothkoff documented a 16-year-old student who was using welder's glasses and had a visual acuity of 20/80 after gazing at a solar eclipse. Six months later, the patient's visual acuity was 20/60 with a central scotoma. Another 16-year-old student, viewing the eclipse through old exposed film, had developed bilateral macular edema and macular exudates with visual acuity of 20/200 in the right eye and 20/80 in the left eye. After six months, the patient's visual acuity improved to 20/30 in each eye with normal-appearing maculas (34).

VISIBLE LIGHT TOXICITY

Retinal light toxicity has been shown to occur at low thresholds for blue light. Experimental studies in monkeys showed that there was a permanent loss of blue cone sensitivity and that the effect was cumulative. Ham showed that light toxicity depends on the wavelength or color (35). Damage increases rapidly with the transition from green to blue to violet. Sperling showed that long wavelengths produce mostly thermal lesions, whereas short wavelengths in the visible spectrum produce mainly photochemical lesions (36). Moderate photochemical lesions are repairable with time.

PROTECTION FROM ULTRAVIOLET LIGHT AND SUNLIGHT

Strong reason exists to believe that there are significantly higher levels of UV radiation exposure because of the changes in the earth's atmosphere (37). Protection of the eyes from UV radiation has become a multi-million-dollar industry, which has spurred the development of UV-absorbing spectacles, sunglasses, intraocular lenses, and contact lenses.

Even "cheap" sunglasses absorb most of the UV-B radiation. The ability of a lens to filter UV light is largely a function of the chromophores embedded in the plastic material, and the chromophores have little or no effect on the color or darkness of the lens. Therefore, the color or darkness of a lens gives no indication of the UV-light-absorbing characteristics, and even clear spectacle lenses have significant UV-absorbing properties.

Although it is true that there is no definite proof that wearing UV-protecting sunglasses prevents macular degeneration and cataracts, there is a growing amount of evidence that suggests that light exposure does play a role in these disease processes. Therefore, young, lightly pigmented people who live in hot climates should wear sunglasses. People who have had cataract surgery with a nonabsorbing intraocular lens should also wear sunglasses, as should patients treated with photosensitizing drugs and patients who have malabsorption syndromes. Sunglasses would augment their natural defenses of pupillary reflexes, squinting, blinking, and eyebrow shadowing (33,38).

Laser Light

Lasers are being used more and more in the work environment. They are used clinically in medicine every day and in retail scanning devices. They are being used in industrial work settings more and more, and are used in the military as sighting devices and weapons.

A significant risk of photic retinopathy from laser scatter exists. Usually, during the operation of the laser, the operator is protected through filters. However, subtle blue-green defects have been documented in the long-term laser operators. Color contrast defects have been detected and have been thought to be secondary to chronic exposure to argon blue-green light (39,40). Industrial accidents happen most often when operators have removed their safety glasses and the laser is inadvertently turned on. Treatment is aimed at using adequate protection and avoiding exposure.

Microwaves

Microwave radiation is at the low end of the electromagnetic spectrum and extends from 1 mm to 2 m. It is being used in many applications (e.g., microwave ovens, radar, satellite communications, and insect-control devices). Microwaves are very common in the work environment. The energy levels are much less than those required to break chemical bonds. Therefore, microwaves are a nonionizing form of energy in which the only molecular effects are vibrational or rotational. The only biological effect is thermal.

Microwave-induced posterior subcapsular cataracts may occur when the subject is given high, repeated doses. The potential for lens damage in small, chronic doses is unclear (6). Experimental evidence of the ocular effects of microwaves has been demonstrated in rabbits and dogs. Most of the experiments were performed in the UHF (ultrahigh frequency) range. Even in the UHF range, most ocular effects have been confined to the adnexa (e.g., thermal injury to the lids) and conjunctiva (e.g., anterior segment keratitis, iritis). It is also possible for microwaves to cause cataracts, but only at dose levels so high as to cause hypothermic brain death. There have been scattered and isolated reports in medical literature implicating that microwaves are the cause of cataracts in humans. None of these cases is fully documented, and the cause-and-effect relationship is conjectural. For human exposure to microwaves, there has never been a documented case of ocular damage. Furthermore, it does not appear that there ever could be such a case (6).

Heat and Infrared Injuries

EXTERNAL DISEASE

Most conjunctival injuries caused by exposure to cold air, flames, or hot fluids also affect the eyelids and corneas (41). The extent of the tissue destruction varies with the initial temperature and the nature of the causative agent, as well as the duration of the contact with the conjunctiva. Minor thermal injuries may only damage the conjunctival epithelium and cause loss of the epithelial cells. More severe injuries, especially those caused by hot foreign bodies, may affect the underlying stroma and may cause coagulation necrosis followed by scarring, and in severe cases, symblepharon. The conjunctiva is less likely to have ischemia because it is protected by the eyelid skin. Freezing of the eyelid or periorbital skin (frostbite) results in solidification of the dermal and epidermal cells with accompanying vasoconstriction.

Corneal burns after exposure to heat are usually less severe than chemical burns. Flash burns usually produce some mild epithelial injury followed by uncomplicated healing. Prolonged exposure to heat may result in degeneration of corneal stroma collagen. Exposure to cold temperature for short durations rarely causes significant injury to the stroma or posterior cornea.

LENS

Exfoliation of the lens capsule is a syndrome originally described by Elshnig in 1922. It was seen in glass blowers who worked with tanks of molten glass at temperatures of 1,500°C. These tanks gave off thermal radiation rich in infrared rays. The resultant injury involved capsular peeling and frequent posterior subcapsular cataract after several decades of exposure. This occupational thermal injury has been virtually eliminated by use of protective goggles (42).

In humans, heat cataract is rare, although it has been seen for many years in glass blowers and steel puddlers. An opacity in the posterior cortex has been noted. Often, a cobweb-like opacity occurs in the outer layers of the posterior cortex, which later develops into a saucer-shaped disc. Eventually the entire lens may become involved (43).

Electric Shock

Lens opacification may follow electric shock, especially if the contact area involves the head. Initially, there is anterior subcapsular vacuolization that, in turn, may become an anterior subcapsular cataract. In the severest cases, the opacities may form within a few days (44). One 33-year-old man was studied after an electric burn of 15,000 volts on the forehead. The man developed bilateral cataracts, and electron microscopic studies showed anterior subcapsular epithelial proliferation seen in other forms of subcapsular cataracts (44).

Electricity may also affect other parts of the eye. The passage of high-voltage electric current through the body causes effects seen in individuals similar to those seen in lightning strikes. The retinal changes include retinal edema and hemorrhages, macular edema, and macular hole (45). The effect of passage of electric current and the resistance of the tissue leads to changes in the vessels and other tissues. No treatment is usually necessary, and, after a time, the retinal edema usually subsides. Macular holes require surgery to be repaired.

Cathode Ray Tubes or Video Display Terminals

The U.S. Food and Drug Administration Bureau of Radiologic Health has evaluated visual display terminals (VDTs) and televisions for hazards of ionizing radiation and found that all commercial models, when properly encased, emitted far less radiation than permitted by applicable standards (46). No ophthalmic disease has been identified with the use of cathode ray displays (47).

Color vision changes have been documented in approximately 10% of VDT users (48). Color vision changes caused by VDTs may last for several hours. Affected individuals may report that small light-colored objects appear tinted when viewed against a dark background. Also, the color of the tint is complementary to that of the VDT. Color vision testing by pseudoisochromatic plates shortly after use is often abnormal in these subjects but returns to normal after several hours (49). Those workers who are troubled by the complementary chromatopsia or those who work in jobs in which color vision is critical, such as color-processing laboratories or dye and paint industries, may prevent the chromatopsia by switching to an achromatic or trichromatic VDT (48,49).

In addition, problems with glare, poor contrast, and improper angulation motion may cause problems for any user. Users of VDTs need to have accurate current refractions and presbyopic spectacles for aid in using these units. Extended use of VDTs may cause ocular and physical discomfort, fatigue, and frustration.

CHEMICALS

Heavy Metals

COPPER

Copper-containing metal foreign bodies in the eye and brass, bronze, and aluminum alloys containing copper present serious problems because of the toxic effect on the eye. The characteristic reaction to copper and its alloys is a purulent exudation and collection of inflammatory cells around the foreign body (Fig. 21-9). In the external eye, a purulent inflammatory reaction is provoked, and this may lead to expulsion of the particle. In the anterior chamber, a fibrinous anterior uveitis may result around the foreign body and soon cover it. When the foreign body is completely embedded in the lens, it causes the least amount of inflammatory reaction but may cause a blue-green discoloration.

Copper-containing intraocular foreign bodies or systemic increases in serum copper may lead to deposition of copper into the lens capsule. The lens opacity has a characteristic "sunflower" configuration, with an anterior central disc occupying the pupillary area and radiating petals on the posterior surface of the iris (50). Microscopic studies of the lens have demonstrated granular copper deposits within the anterior posterior lens capsule, mostly in the polar regions. The combined deposition of copper in the cornea and lens can result in reduced visual acuity and distortion of color vision. Penicillamine may be administered with subsequent reduction in the deposition of the copper.

The effects of copper are most serious when they are embedded in the posterior pole of the eye in the vitreous or retina. A purulent exudative reaction develops around the foreign body with the intensity being related to the percentage of copper in the foreign body. Usually, widespread inflammatory and degenerative changes in the retina and vitreous result. The vitreous may cloud and then shrink, leading to a retinal detachment. If the retina does remain in place, the toxic reaction of the dissolved copper may soon poison the retina, causing degeneration of the retina and retinal pigment epithelium. Glaucoma rarely results from retained intraocular copper foreign bodies. In comparison with some other intraocular foreign bodies that may not necessarily need to be removed, every effort should be made to remove a copper-containing foreign body (51).

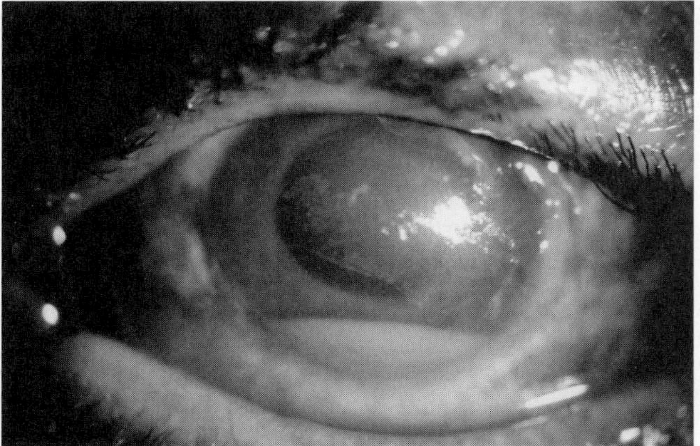

Figure 21-9. Hypopyon and corneal abrasion status after intraocular copper foreign body. The copper has caused inflammation manifested by the layered white cells (hypopyon).

IRON

Iron and iron compounds can have a variety of toxic actions on the eye. Impregnation of eye tissues with iron, such as that which may come from a foreign body, is known as siderosis. Small iron-containing foreign bodies may become lodged in the cornea, and, if they are retained for days to weeks, may break down and deposit iron within the epithelium, Bowman's layer, and the anterior stroma. These may appear clinically as a brownish or rust-colored ring surrounding the foreign body that may persist for months after the removal. Histologically, there is localized siderosis with metallic particles lying within the damaged stromal lamellae in macrophages and stromal keratocytes. The extent of the siderosis is influenced by the site of a foreign body. Although cornea and scleral foreign bodies may have local effects, the particle in the anterior chamber may be diffused away by the aqueous humor. Foreign bodies in the lens tend to have localized effects.

The most widespread effects tend to be owing to iron particles in the posterior pole. The iris is often changed in color early and may remain so years after the foreign body is removed. However, in other cases it has been reported that the iris color may return to normal. The activity of the pupil is often affected, resulting in poor accommodation and reaction to light. Although good visual acuity may result for a long time in the presence of intraocular iron, the retina may be severely injured and eventually destroyed by the toxic action of the iron. Even though the media may remain clear, there is a gradual decrease in visual acuity, ultimately leading to blindness. Glaucoma occurs in some cases of ocular siderosis, but the incidence is uncertain (52).

Intraocular iron foreign bodies can be diagnosed by plane films and computed tomography scans. The most efficacious treatment is attempted removal of the intraocular iron, especially with a magnet.

Rust rings that result in the cornea may be initially removed. However, there is often residual rust that may be removed later. Treatment with ophthalmic ointment has been shown to hasten the disappearance of rust rings and result in easy removal, up to days to weeks after the initial injury (52).

SILVER

Silver may be deposited in the cornea as a result of prolonged environmental exposure (i.e., industrial silver polishing or engraving after topical application of silver-containing eyedrops or ingestion of solutions that contain silver) (53). The deposits appear to be inert and cause no visual functional deficit. Clinically, there is a gray-brown discoloration of the conjunctiva and of Descemet's membrane. This is visible at the slit lamp as a diffuse granular brown pigmentation. After prolonged ingestion of silver-containing solutions, silver can be seen deposited within the vascular endothelium, Bruch's membrane, and the lens capsule (54).

GOLD

Gold can accumulate in the cornea and conjunctiva after prolonged systemic ingestion. In most cases, there is no inflammation or visual disturbance. The gold disappears within 3 to 5 months after ingestion is discontinued. Rarely, superficial corneal ulceration or opacification may occur in association with inflammation to adjust the hypersensitivity or toxicity of gold. A more common asymptomatic condition is characterized by the presence of glittering granules throughout the corneal stroma, which are more numerous in the deeper layers (55).

MERCURY

Mercury that gains entry to the aqueous from external sources accumulates in the lens capsule basement membrane, as do silver and gold (56). Pigmentation of the anterior lens capsule has been observed in patients who work with mercury in the manufacture of thermometers, in the felt hat industry, and in patients who work with mercury zinc amalgams in the battery industry (56,57). The reports of mercury toxicity on the retina and optic nerve are rare, and those that have been presented do not demonstrate a causative relationship. Awareness of the problem and enforcement of preventive measures have reduced exposure to inorganic materials.

LEAD

Ocular complications may occur in only 1% to 2% of cases of systemic lead poisoning. Usually, the manifestations are delayed and occur several months after the chronic exposure. The retinal changes include hemorrhages and posterior pole vascular sheathing and shiny dots in the macula associated with optic nerve edema. There may be true optic neuritis and involvement of any portion of the optic tract, radiations, or visual cortex. Treatment involves removing as much of the lead as soon as possible from the circulatory system with ethylenediaminetetraacetic acid, dimercaprol, or penicillamine. Iodides have also been used to withdraw blood from the bone to allow excretion of the metal.

Other Chemicals: Delayed Injuries

CHANGES IN REFRACTION

Many side effects of drugs or toxic action of chemicals may disrupt the ability of the eye to accommodate or change its focus in a normal manner. These disturbances may be divided into weakness or paralysis of accommodation, acute transient myopia, or cataract formation.

The weakness or paralysis of accommodation is by far the most common interference caused by drugs that have anticholinergic properties. Besides anticholinergic drugs, ganglion-blocking agents may block parasympathetic innervation of the ciliary muscle at the ciliary ganglion. Botulinum toxin may interfere with accommodation and cause mydriasis, through interference and release of the acetocholine from the parasympathetic nerve endings (58).

A second group of substances may cause myopia or nearsightedness combined with miosis or a small pupil. These substances act by causing contraction of the ciliary muscle and the iris sphincter muscle. Once again, the most common agents are the anticholinesterase agents, miotics such as pilocarpine, muscarine, physostigmine, and organophosphate insecticides (58).

CATARACTS

Only six or seven substances have been shown to produce cataracts in human beings. On the other hand, more than 50 substances have been shown to cause cataracts in animals. The group of drugs that have antimitotic actions similar to those produced by radiation have the biggest effect. These drugs include busulfan, dibromomannitol, dimethylaminostyrocliniline, iodoacetate, nitrogen mustards, tetramine, and triaziquone.

Other opacity-inducing agents and anticholinesterase drugs, such as isofluorphate, demecarium, or echothiophate, may cause increased lens opacity with vacuolization below the anterior lens epithelium and capsule. Other substances, such as naphthalene, may also cause these changes. A mechanism of these cataracts is thought to be osmotic swelling brought about by a breakdown of the lens pump leak system (58).

TABLE 21-1. Common environmental substances associated with optic nerve dysfunction

Amyl acetate	Lead
Benzene	Methyl acetate
Carbon dioxide	Methylene blue
Carbon disulfide	Methyl chloride
Carbon tetrachloride	Nitrobenzene
Cyanide	Pentachlorophenol
DDT	Styrene
Dieldrin	Tetraethyl lead
Dinitrobenzene	Thallium
Dinitrotoluene	Tobacco smoke
Ethylene glycol	Trichloroethylene

RETINAL DAMAGE

Retinal edema has been associated with a variety of drugs in humans, including cyanide, glue sniffing, and methanol. Retinal hemorrhages may be seen with toxicity of a number of agents. Poisoning with lead, licorice, triethyl, tin, and vitamin A have been associated with elevated intracranial pressure and vascular congestion. Only a few substances are noteworthy on the list of retinotoxic substances for humans. On this list are corticline, copper, iodate, iron, oxygen, piperidylchlorophenodiazine, and thioridazine (58).

OPTIC NEURITIS

Optic neuritis is caused by a variety of substances. Clinically, optic neuritis is seen as optic nerve disc edema with hyperemia. There may be surrounding vascular congestion of the retina. The list of substances that may cause toxic neuropathies is found in Table 21-1.

METHANOL

Optic neuropathy is usually seen in alcoholic individuals who have accidentally or intentionally consumed methanol (Fig. 21-10). Methanol can be toxic in small amounts, and poisoning can occur with ingestion of less than half an ounce. The clinical picture has been established from a collection of reported cases. Nausea, inebriation, headache, dyspnea, vomiting, abdominal pain, and then bilateral visual impairment occur. Vision loss is typically profound, and there is usually pupillary dilatation. Usually, optic nerve edema extends into the peripapillary retina. Optic atrophy usually develops after 1 or 2 months. Treatment for this problem includes correction of the acidoses, hemodialysis, and administration of ethanol to interfere with the metabolism. Vision loss in methanol intoxication is usually much worse than that seen in other optic neuropathies. The optic nerve edema that is seen is exceptional for this group of disorders. Few patients may show improvement, but relapses are also common. The prognosis is generally very poor with methanol toxicity.

CHEMICAL INJURIES

Accidental splashing or squirting of substances into the eyes is the most common of toxic eye injuries. Chemicals can be divided into three categories: (a) caustic, (b) solvent, and (c) detergent. Of these, the caustic injuries are the most dangerous and cause the most damage to the eye. Solvent injuries may cause ocular discomfort and pain and may result in loss of some or all of the corneal epithelium, but, as a general rule, these chemicals do not damage the underlying corneal stroma. Most

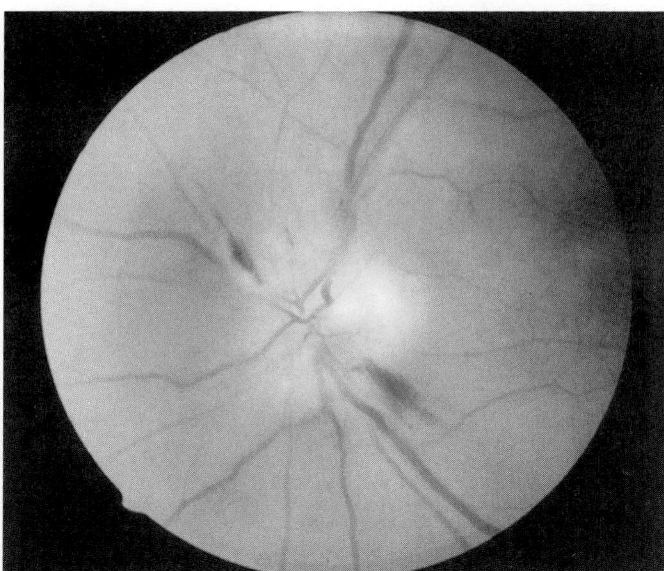

Figure 21-10. Optic nerve edema. Right eye of patient who ingested methanol and experienced severe vision loss. Note blurred optic disc margins and associated flame hemorrhages in the nerve fiber layer of the retina.

of these substances have no alkaline or acidic properties and are used for dissolvent properties. The prolonged irrigations that are necessary for acid or alkali burns are not necessary. The long-term prognosis is usually good with solvents, and there tend to be no long-term sequelae.

Injuries to the eye with detergents or surfactants are more complex. Most household and industrial-use detergents rarely cause serious injuries in human eyes. Some surfactants have been demonstrated to have a delayed effect on the cornea, however, with resultant corneal edema hours after exposure. In addition, some surfactants, such as the polyoxyethylene glycol ethers, may have an anesthetic property that may lead to delay in irrigation treatment. Toxic degeneration has been caused by accidental irrigation of the conjunctiva and cornea with presurgical skin antiseptic solutions (59). Solutions containing chlorhexidine, isopropyl alcohol, and detergents have been observed to produce conjunctival hyperemia chemosis, as well as corneal exchanges that range from diffuse punctate keratitis to stromal edema and almost total loss of endothelium.

Acid corneal burns tend to be nonprogressive, with little tendency to be chronic. Penetration of the acid is limited by the buffering reaction of the tissues, and the lesions are sharply delineated. Healing is usually rapid, but the epithelial reattachment may be delayed. In a study by Hirst, the original basement membrane remained in place, but the secretion of a new basement membrane and epithelial adhesion was delayed for up to 8 weeks (60). The most commonly encountered acid injuries include those caused by sulfuric, hydrochloric, acetic, and nitrous acids. The most common etiology of injury is from battery explosions. Compared to alkali injury, penetration is limited, and permanent impairment usually does not result unless additional damage from foreign bodies or thermal injuries exists. Usually, no long-term treatment is necessary once the surface has reepithelialized.

The most important alkali agents causing chemical injuries to the eye include ammonia, lye, potassium hydroxide, magnesium hydroxide, and lime. Of these, ammonia and lye tend to produce the most serious injuries. Lime, most frequently encountered in the form of plaster, is the most commonly encountered alkali injury; however, it tends to be the least severe.

Deep perilimbal alkali burns can cause scarring of the episcleral aqueous outflow channels, resulting in secondary glaucoma. Burns may produce corneal opacification, symblepharon, conjunctival shrinkage, trichiasis, and xerophthalmia (43) (Fig. 21-11A). In severe alkali burns, the lens rapidly becomes cataractous, and the iris and ciliary body may become necrotic, resulting in decreased aqueous production and eventual phthisis. Even in mild cases, associated inflammation persists until the injury is healed. Immediately after application of alkali, the epithelial cells die and the stroma becomes denatured. For a period of up to 2 weeks, the damaged area remains in a relatively acellular state. After this period, there is stromal infiltration by polymorphonuclear leukocytes and fibroblasts with neovascularization extending in from the periphery. Collagenase is produced by the adjacent epithelium, and corneal ulcers may develop central to the cellular infiltrate where the collagenase levels are the highest (61).

The parameters that are followed in the first week after injury include corneal reepithelialization, corneal clarity, intraocular pressure, anterior chamber inflammation, and lens clarity. The two most important factors in early treatment concern control of the ocular surface and intraocular inflammation. If too much inflammation exists, epithelial cells will not migrate and defects

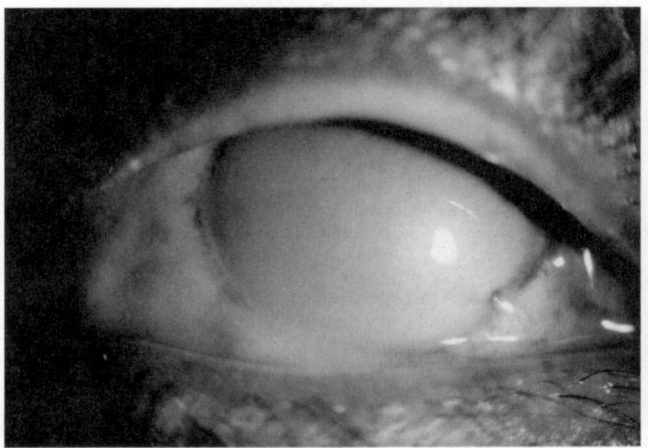

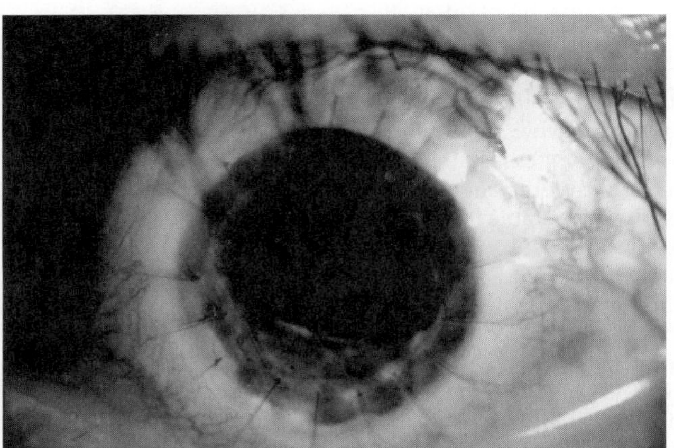

Figure 21-11. A: Alkali burn to cornea in a 47-year-old man splashed in eye while cleaning stove in a restaurant with lye. Despite immediate medical therapy, alkali burn resulted in a total opacification of cornea with limbal ischemia and chronic inflammation. **B:** Same patient. Status after corneal transplant and Molteno tube to control intraocular pressure.

will not heal. In addition, there is increased risk of vascularization of the corneal surface.

In the second and third weeks after injury, the corneal and conjunctival epithelium and keratocytes continue to proliferate in an effort to restore structural and functional normal surfaces. In severe cases, the reepithelialization is delayed or does not occur. In this phase, proteolytic digestion may occur excessively in the stroma, causing corneal thinning and potential perforation of the eye.

Several weeks to months after injury, the corneas are examined for recovery of sensation and for the presence of surface epithelial defects. Lubrication is extremely important in this phase as normal function and structure begins returning to the ocular surface. In cases in which damage is more widespread, corneal reepithelialization must occur from the conjunctival epithelium. This reepithelialization is very slow and may not occur in some individuals. The patients are at risk for severe vascularization, scarring, and opacification of the corneal surface with goblet cell mucin deficiency or persistent epithelial erosions (62).

THERAPY

Therapy in the first week after the injury is aimed at promoting epithelial wound healing. Prompt reepithelialization is associated with successful stromal repair processes. Slower reepithelialization may result in persistent problems. The mainstay of therapy is tear substitutes. In young people, there may be adequate tear protection and tear substitutes may not be necessary. If a delay in reepithelialization occurs, however, tear supplementation can be beneficial. In these patients, preservative-free tears and ointments should be used to avoid further toxicity to the epithelium. Punctal occlusion may be a beneficial adjunct to tear substitutes, particularly in those patients with preexisting dry-eye disorders. Topical antibiotics in the form of ointment or drops are used to prevent bacterial infection. Cycloplegics, such as atropine, are often helpful for treating inflammation and increasing patient comfort.

If epithelial defects persist into the second week, occlusive therapy in the form of tarsorrhaphy (sewing the eyelids closed), bandaged contact lens, or collagen shield may be necessary to protect the corneal surface. Contrary to popular belief, corticosteroids do not have an adverse effect on the rate of epithelial wound healing, and the intensive use of topical corticosteroids in the early phases may increase epithelial recovery (63). Corticosteroids increase the risk of bacterial superinfection, and therefore prophylactic antibiotics must be used in conjunction with them. After 10 to 14 days, corticosteroid use becomes potentially hazardous, and it should be tapered off, especially in corneas in which reepithelialization has not occurred yet.

Other agents, such as ascorbate, have been shown to aid in the reformation of collagen. Also, citrate is a calcium chelator that is effective in reducing corneal ulceration and perforation after alkali burns.

In the worst cases, in which perforation is a risk, the use of a tissue adhesive, specifically isobutyl cyanoacrylate (Histoacryl), is usually preferable to emergency corneal transplant. The tissue adhesives prevent further ulceration, and they support stromal repair and neovascularization. However, tissue adhesives do induce vascularization and complicate subsequent surgical procedures to improve vision (62).

REHABILITATION

Long-term treatment of chemical injuries involves maximizing function and restoration of vision, usually through a corneal transplant (Fig. 21-11B). To achieve success, there must be normal blinking, eyelid contour, and the absence of any corneal exposure. In addition, there must be a sufficient tear film layer, to which a new cornea may adapt. Also, epithelial stem cells must be present for the cornea transplant, and there must not be any active ulceration, inflammation, or uncontrolled glaucoma.

Preparatory procedures for corneal transplant include lysing conjunctival adhesions and eliminating eyelid dysfunction. Secondary glaucoma must be controlled with medication, filtration surgery, or laser cyclophotocoagulation. Corneal stem cells lost from disease or injury should be replaced. If the injury is monocular, then autotransplantation can be done from the uninjured eye. With bilateral injury, homologous tissue may be an option.

The process of visual rehabilitation is usually delayed for 1 to 2 years to allow a quiet, stable eye to develop (62).

REFERENCES

1. Larman S. Radiant. Energy and the eye. In: *Functional ophthalmology*. New York: Macmillan, 1980.
2. Spencer WH. *Ophthalmic pathology: an atlas and textbook*, 4th ed. American Academy of Ophthalmology, 1996:157–325.
3. Gamus D, Weschler Z, Greenberg S, Romano A. Decreased tear secretion in Chernobyl children: external eye disorders in children subjected to long-term low-dose radiation. In: Sullivan DA, ed. *Lacrimal gland tear film in dry eye syndromes*. New York: Plenum Press, 1994:513.
4. Haze BP, Fisher RF. Influence of a prolonged period of low dosage x-rays on the optic and ultrastructural appearance of cataract on the human lens. *Br J Ophthalmol* 1979;63:457–464.
5. Richards RD, Riley EF, Leinfelder PJ. Lens changes following x-ray radiation of a single and multiple quadrant. *Am J Ophthalmol* 1956;42:44–50.
6. Lipman RM, Tripathi BJ, Tripathi RC. Cataracts induced by microwave and ionizing radiation. *Surv Ophthalmol* 1988;33:200.
7. Merriam GRJ, Focht EF. A clinical study of radiation cataracts and their relationship to dose. *AJR Am J Roentgenol* 1957;77:759–785.
8. Maguire AM, Schaschat AB. Radiation retinopathy. In: Roian SJ, ed. *Retina*, 2nd ed. St. Louis: Mosby, 1994.
9. Amoaku WMK, Archer DB. Fluorescein angiographic features, natural course and treatment of radiation retinopathy. *Eye* 1990;4:657–667.
10. Chandhuri PR, Austin DJ, Rosenthal AR. Treatment of radiation retinopathy. *Br J Ophthalmol* 1981;65:623–625.
11. Brown GC, Shields JA, Sanborn G, Augsberger JJ, Sevino PJ, Schatz NJ. Radiation retinopathy. *Ophthalmology* 1982;89:1494–1501.
12. Guyer DR, Mukai S, Eagan KM, et al. Radiation maculopathy following proton beam irradiation for choroidal melanoma. *Ophthalmology* 1992;99:1278–1285.
13. Merriam GR, Jr., Szechter A, Focht EF. The effects of ionizing radiation on the eye. *Front Radiat Ther Oncol* 1972;6:346–385.
14. Nakissa N, Ruben P, Strohl R, Keys H. Ocular and orbital complications following radiation therapy of perinasal sinus malignancies: a review of literature. *Cancer* 1983;51:980–986.
15. Perrers-Taylor M, Brinkley D, Reynolds T. Choroido-retinal damage as a complication of radiotherapy. *Acta Radiol Ther Phys Biol* 1965;3:431–440.
16. Elsas T, Thorud E, Jetne V, Conradi IS. Retinopathy after low dose irradiation for an intracranial tumor of the frontal lobe. *Acta Ophthalmol Scand* 1988;66:65–68.
17. Saornil MA, Eagan KM, Gragoudas ES, et al. Histopathology of uveal melanomas treated with proton beam irradiation: a comparison study. *Arch Ophthalmol* 1992;110:1112–1118.
18. Chacko DC. Considerations in the diagnosis of radiation injury. *JAMA* 1981;245:1255–1258.
19. Ross HS, Rosenberg S, Friedman AH. Delayed radiation necrosis of the optic nerve. *Am J Ophthalmol* 1973;76:683–686.
20. Hamill MB. Corneal injury. In: Kruchmer J, ed. *Cornea*. St. Louis: Mosby, 1996.
21. Clarke SM, Doughty MJ, Cullen AP. Acute effects of ultraviolet B radiation on the corneal surface of the pigmented rabbit. A study by scanning electron microscopy. *Acta Ophthalmol* 1990;68:639–650.
22. Injuries associated with ultraviolet tanning devices: Wisconsin. *MMWR Morb Mortal Wkly Rep* 1989;38:333.
23. Taylor HR, West S, Munos B, et al. The long-term effects of visible light on the eye. *Arch Ophthalmol* 1992;110:99–104.
24. Hill JC, Maske R. Pathogenesis of pterygia. *Eye* 1989;3:218–226.
25. Norn M, Franck C. Long-term changes in the outer part of the eye in welders: prevalence of spheroidal generation pingueculae, pterygium, and corneal cicatrices. *Acta Ophthalmol* 1991;69:382–386.
26. Norn MS. Spheroid generation pingueculae and pterygium among Arabs in the Red Sea territory (Jordan). *Acta Ophthalmol* 1982;60:949–954.
27. Rodgers FC. Clinical findings, course and the progress of Bietti's corneal degeneration in the dahlak ions. *Brit J Ophthalmol* 1973;57:657–664.
28. Hiller R, Sperduto RD, Ederer F. Epidemiological associations with nuclear, cortical, and posterior subcapsular cataracts. *Am J Epidemiol* 1986;124:916.
29. Bochow TW, West SK, Azar A, et al. Ultraviolet light exposure and the risk of posterior subcapsular cataracts. *Arch Ophthalmol* 1989;107:369.
30. Van der Hoeve J. Eye lesions produced by light rich in ultraviolet rays: senile cataract, senile degeneration of the macula. *Am J Ophthalmol* 1920;3:178–194.
31. Cruickshanks KJ, Klein R, Klein BEK. Sunlight and age-related macular degeneration: the Beaver Dam Eye Study. *Arch Ophthalmol* 1993;111:514–518.

32. White TJ, Mainster MA, Wilson PW, Tipps JH. Choreoretinal temperature increases from solar observation. *Bull Math Biophys* 1971;33:1–17.
33. Mainster MA, Kahn JA. Photic retinal injury. In: Roian SJ, ed. *Retina*. St. Louis: Mosby, 1994:1767–1781.
34. Rothkoff L, Kushelevsky A, Blumenthal M. Solar retinopathy: visual prognosis in 20 cases. *Isr J Med Sci* 1978;14:238–243.
35. Ham WT, Jr., Mueller HA, Ruffolo JJ Jr, et al. Sensitivity of the retina to radiation damage as a function of wavelength. *Photochem Photobiol* 1979;29:735–743.
36. Lanum J. The damaging effect of light on the retina: empirical findings, theoretical and practical implications. *Surv Ophthalmol* 1978;22:221–249.
37. Farmer CB, Toon GC, Schaper W, et. al. Stratospheric trace gases in Spring 1986 Antarctic atmosphere. *Nature* 1987;329:126.
38. Sliney DH. Eye protective techniques for bright light. *Ophthalmology* 1983;90:937–944.
39. Arden GB, Berninger T, Hogg CR, Perry S. A survey of color discrimination in German ophthalmologists: changes associated with the use of lasers and operating microscopes. *Ophthalmology* 1991;98:567–575.
40. Berninger TA, Canning CR, Gundez K, Strong N, Arden GB. Using argon laser blue light reduces ophthalmologist's color contrast sensitivity. *Arch Ophthalmol* 1989;107:1453–1459.
41. Linhart RW. Burns of the eyes and eyelids. *Ann Ophthalmol* 1988;10:999–1000.
42. Eshnig A. Ablösung der Zonulalamelle bei Glasbläsern. *Klin Monatsbl Augenheilkd* 1922;69:732–734.
43. Folberg R, Spencer WH, ed. *Ophthalmic pathology atlas and textbook*, 4th ed. American Academy of Ophthalmology, 1996:38.
44. Fraunfelder FT, Hannah C. Electric cataracts. I. Sequential changes, unusual and prognostic findings. *Arch Ophthalmol* 1972;87:179–183.
45. Campo RV, Lewis RS. Lightning induced macular hole. *Am J Ophthalmol* 1984;97:792–794.
46. U.S. Department of Health and Human Services, Food and Drug Administration. An evaluation of radiation emission from video display terminals: radiological health. Washington: U.S. Department of Health and Human Services, Food and Drug Administration, 1981.
47. Panel on impact of video viewing on vision of workers: executive summary. In: *Video displays, work and vision*. Washington: National Academy Press, 1983:1–4.
48. Greenwald MJ, Greenwald SJ, Blake R. Long-lasting visual after effect from viewing a computer video display. *New Engl J Med* 1983;309:315.
49. Kajn JA, Fitts J, Psaltis P, Ide CH. Prolonged complimentary chromatopsia in users of video display terminals [letter]. *Am J Ophthalmol* 1985;99:736–737.
50. Tso MOM, Fine BS, Thorpe HE. Kayser-Fleischer ring and associated cataract and Wilson's disease. *Am J Ophthalmol* 1975;79:479–488.
51. Grant WM. *Toxicology of the eye*, 2nd ed. Springfield, IL: Charles C Thomas Publisher, 1974:312–320.
52. Grant WM. *Toxicology of the eye*, 2nd ed. Springfield, IL: Charles C Thomas Publisher, 1974:594–605.
53. Spencer WH, Garron LK, Contreras F, et al. Endogenous and exogenous ocular and systemic silver deposition. *Trans Ophthalmol Soc UK* 1980;100:171–178.
54. Grant WM. *Toxicology of the eye*, 2nd ed. Springfield, IL: Charles C Thomas Publisher, 1974:913–918.
55. Roberts WH, Wolter JR. Ocular chrysiasis. *Arch Ophthalmol* 1956;56:48–52.
56. Kark RAP, Poskanzer DC, Bullock JO, et. al. Mercury poisoning and its treatment with *N* acetyl-D, L-penicillamine. *New Engl J Med* 1971;285:10.
57. Rosen E. Mercurialentis. *Am J Ophthalmol* 1950;33:1287–1288.
58. Grant WM. *Toxicology of the eye*, 2nd ed. Springfield, IL: Charles C Thomas Publisher, 1974:22–47.
59. Macrae SM, Brown B, Edelhauser HF. The corneal toxicity of presurgical skin antiseptics. *Am J Ophthalmol* 1984;97:221–232.
60. Hirst LW. Corneal epithelial regeneration and adhesions following acid injuries in the rhesus monkey. *Invest Ophthalmol Vis Sci* 1982;23:764–773.
61. Brown SI, Weller CA, Akiya S. Pathogenesis of ulcers of alkali-burned cornea. *Arch Ophthalmol* 1970;83:205–208.
62. Pfister RR, Pfister BL. Alkali-injuries of the eye. In: Krachner E, ed. *Cornea*. St. Louis: Mosby, 1997:1443–1452.
63. Ho PC, Elliot JH. Kinetics of corneal epithelial regeneration: II. Epidermal growth factor and topical corticosteroids. *Invest Ophthalmol Vis Sci* 1975;14:630.

CHAPTER 22
Clinical Renal Toxicology

Alfred M. Bernard

The unusual susceptibility of the kidney to toxic injury mainly stems from its function of regulating the volume and composition of body fluids. The two organs weigh approximately 300 g in humans and receive 25% of the cardiac output. This blood flow is distributed to the nephrons, which constitutes the functional and morphologic unit of the kidney (10^6 nephrons per kidney). Each nephron is composed of a vascular part, the glomerulus, followed by an epithelial part, the tubule, which is divided into several segments, as illustrated in Figure 22-1.

The glomerulus functions as a charge and size-selective filter, efficiently retaining in the vascular compartment blood cells and proteins with a molecular weight higher than 40,000 (i.e., most plasma proteins) and allowing the passage of small molecules, including the waste products of the organism. In humans, approximately 20% (i.e., 180 L per day) of the renal plasma flow is filtered by the glomeruli. From this copious filtrate, the tubule then recovers water, sodium chloride, and numerous other solutes. If this procedure is highly effective in removing toxic waste products, it implies, however, various physiologic processes that may concentrate toxic chemicals in some regions of the nephron or the interstitium.

Because most of the transport systems are localized in the proximal tubule, that part of the nephron is the most frequent target of nephrotoxic chemicals. In addition, because of its high energy and substrate requirements, the proximal tubule is also very sensitive to ischemia.

The loop of Henle enables the kidney to concentrate urine by a countercurrent mechanism. Substances like urea, which are not reabsorbed by the proximal tubule, progressively concentrate in the loop of Henle and can reach high concentrations in the deep medulla or the papilla (e.g., analgesics).

Sodium chloride and water can be further reabsorbed by the distal tubule and the collecting duct, the latter under the influence of antidiuretic hormone. These two segments can also acidify urine through the secretion of H^+ and NH_4^+ (1).

EPIDEMIOLOGY

A substantial proportion of the human population is exposed to potentially nephrotoxic chemicals as a result of drug treatment, living or working in a contaminated environment, and accidental or intentional poisonings (2). The exact contribution of these various sources of exposure to the occurrence of acute or chronic nephropathies is largely unknown.

For the occupational exposure only, it is estimated that in the United States nearly 4 million workers are potentially exposed to nephrotoxic chemicals (3).

The annual incidence of acute renal failure is approximately 2 per 100,000. According to some authors (4,5), up to 20% of the cases of acute renal failure might be ascribed to a toxic injury, mostly by drugs.

With respect to chronic renal failure, available data concern only the analgesic abuse nephropathy, which could be responsible for approximately 3% of end-stage renal failure cases in Europe. In some countries (Switzerland, Belgium), up to 20% of patients on renal dialysis have been analgesics abusers. It must be stressed, however, that approximately 50% of the cases of chronic renal failure are of uncertain etiology (6).

It is thus possible that some widespread occupational or environmental pollutants (e.g., heavy metals, solvents, mycotoxins) or drugs other than analgesics (e.g., antibiotics, lithium) are involved in the development of chronic renal failure. Several observations tend to support this hypothesis: (a) the well-documented occurrence of renal effects in subjects occupationally or environmentally exposed to nephrotoxicants such as lead or cadmium (7–11), (b) the excess of mortality from renal diseases in cohorts of workers with previous exposure to these two heavy metals, and (c) the demonstration that subclinical renal effects caused by the occupational exposure to cadmium are the

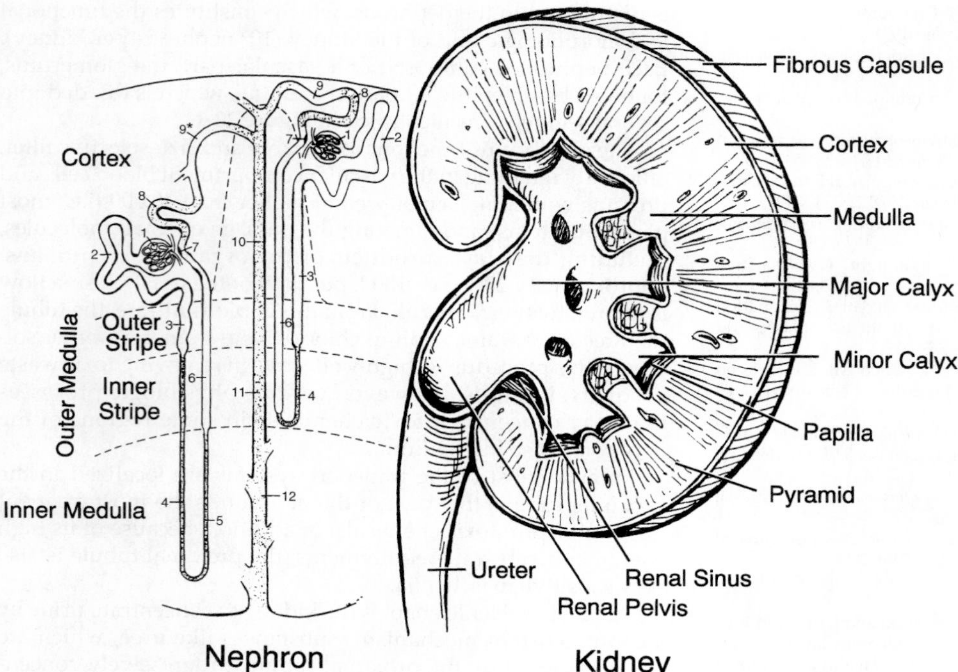

Figure 22-1. 1, Renal corpuscle, including Bowman's capsule and the glomerulus (glomerular tuft); 2, Proximal convoluted tubule (S1 and S2); 3, Proximal straight tubule (S3); 4, Descending thin limb; 5, Ascending thin limb; 6, Distal straight tubule (thick ascending limb); 7, Macula densa located within the final portion of the thick ascending limb; 8, Distal convoluted tubule; 9, Connecting tubule; 9*, Connecting tubule of the juxtaglomerular nephron that forms an arcade; 10, Cortical collecting duct; 11, Outer medullary collecting duct; 12, Inner medullary collecting duct. (From ref. 2, with permission.)

forerunner signs of an accelerated and irreversible decline of the renal function (12).

ROUTES OF EXPOSURE AND ABSORPTION

The types of exposures to nephrotoxic chemicals may be domestic, occupational, environmental, therapeutic, or intentional. Heavy metals and solvents are widely used in industry. Solvents are also components of a number of chemical products such as paints, cleaning agents, glues, paint strippers, and pesticides used by the general population.

The routes of entry of nephrotoxins may be inhalation, ingestion, or skin contact. In industry, inhalation represents the major route of exposure to metal fumes or dusts. Some ingestion of dusts may also occur either by the swallowing of inhaled particles cleared from the lungs or as a result of bad hygiene habits (e.g., smoking at the workplace or eating with contaminated hands). Inhalation is also the main route by which workers absorb solvents, although in some circumstances skin absorption may be very important (e.g., in cleaning or degreasing operations). For the general population, metals are usually absorbed via contaminated foods or drinks, whereas hydrocarbons may be absorbed by inhalation, skin contact, and accidental or deliberate ingestion. Children may ingest high amounts of heavy metals through pica or mouthing when playing on contaminated surfaces (e.g., in the vicinity of a smelter, in old houses with crumbling lead-based paints).

NEPHROTOXINS

Chemicals can affect the renal function or structures through a direct toxic action or through various systemic effects, such as intravascular hemolysis, rhabdomyolysis, or cardiac failure. Only those chemicals producing specific effects on the kidney are considered here. The types of renal effects may vary from subclinical enzymuria or proteinuria to acute tubular necrosis or chronic renal failure, depending on the conditions of exposure (dose and duration) and the toxicologic properties of the chemical.

Table 22-1 lists occupational or environmental toxins that may cause acute or chronic renal diseases in humans. The list of drugs with possible side effects on the kidney is still longer, including more than 300 compounds (13). The nephrotoxic effects caused by chemicals to which humans can be exposed in the environment or at the workplace are briefly described.

Metals and Inorganic Chemicals

LEAD

Lead has been a very common cause of acute or chronic renal failure in the past. Acute tubular necrosis has been described after accidental or intentional absorption of high doses of lead. Cases of chronic renal failure have been reported in adults who had ingested high amounts of leaded paints during childhood and in workers with a long history of occupational exposure. In the chronically exposed adult, lead nephropathy occurs as a progressive tubulointerstitial nephritis characterized by the absence of proteinuria or albuminuria in its early phase, which presently can only be detected by the measurement of the glomerular filtration rate (14). Studies that have applied a wide battery of renal effect markers have failed to identify a test for the early diagnosis of incipient lead nephropathy (15). The accumulation of lead in kidneys, particularly in the proximal tubules, can be associated with the presence of intranuclear inclusion bodies formed by protein lead complexes (Fig. 22-2). These intranuclear bodies, however, usually disappear with the progression of the renal disease. Lead nephropathy may be associated with heme synthesis disturbances, gout, and hypertension.

Lead stored in tissues can be mobilized and eliminated in urine by the administration of chelators [e.g., Na_2Ca ethylenediaminetetraacetic acid (EDTA) or dimercaptosuccinic acid]. A urinary excretion of lead higher than 800 µg per 24 hours after the intravenous injection of 0.5 g Na_2Ca EDTA is an indication of an excessive lead body burden.

CADMIUM

Chronic exposure to cadmium in the workplace or general environment may give rise to a progressive form of tubulointerstitial

TABLE 22-1. Examples of industrial chemicals that have been associated with acute or chronic renal damage in humans

Metals
- Arsenic
- Bismuth
- Chromium
- Cadmium
- Copper
- Germanium
- Gold
- Lithium
- Mercury
- Platinum
- Silver
- Thallium
- Uranium

Hydrocarbons
- Carbon tetrachloride
- 1,2-Dichloromethane
- Trichloroethylene
- Chloroform
- Toluene
- Styrene
- Methanol
- Ethylene glycol
- Diethylene glycol
- Ethylene glycol ethers
- Hexachloro-1,3-butadiene
- Dichloracetylene
- Carbon disulfide
- Dioxane
- Perchlorethylene
- Trichloroethane

Mixtures of hydrocarbons
- Gasoline, automobile exhaust, degreasing solvents, paints, paint solvents and thinners, glues, glue solvent vapors, hairdressing solvents and sprays, pesticide solvents

Miscellaneous
- Silica and silicon compounds
- Paraquat ochratoxin A
- Aristolochic acid

nephritis resulting from the accumulation of the metal in the renal cortex, especially in the proximal tubules. Epidemiologic studies conducted in occupationally exposed workers or in inhabitants of cadmium-polluted areas in Japan have documented the constellation of renal effects of cadmium, which consist of an increased urinary excretion of various tubular antigens, enzymes, or plasma-derived proteins (16,17). The thresholds of urinary cadmium (an indicator of the body burden) associated with their occurrence range from less than 2 µg per g creatinine (i.e., the upper limit of normal for nonoccupationally exposed populations) for the onset of some biochemical effects up to 10 µg per g creatinine, the level associated with the development of the classical tubular proteinuria (increased urinary excretion of β_2-microglobulin and retinol-binding protein) (18). So far, only effects associated with the latter threshold are known to be irreversible from a certain threshold (above 1,000 µg per g creatinine) and to predict an accelerated decline of the renal function with age (19). The concentration of cadmium in the renal cortex—the so-called critical concentration—corresponding to the threshold of 10 µg per g creatinine is estimated at 180 parts per million (17). The half-life of cadmium in kidneys exceeds 15 years in humans. No efficient chelation therapy is available for chronic cadmium poisoning. Na_2Ca EDTA has been successfully used in cases of acute poisoning.

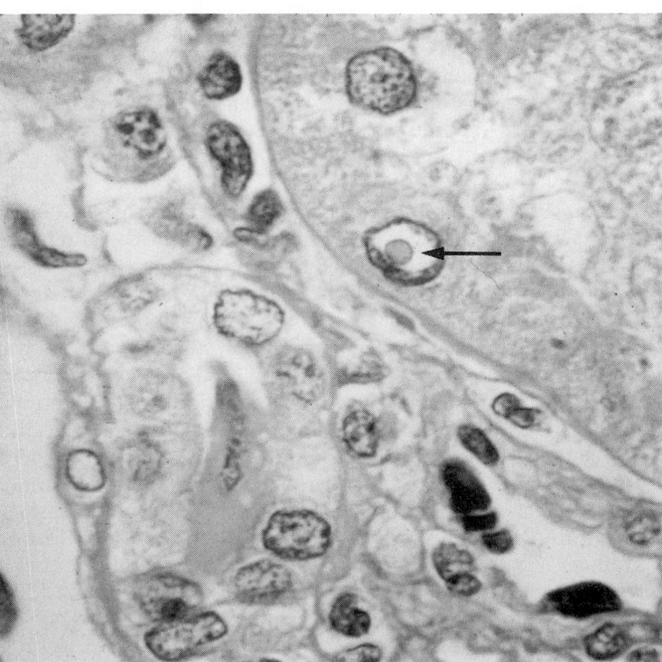

Figure 22-2. Lead inclusions in nucleus of tubular cells of kidney in the case of lead poisoning. (Masson's Trichrome ×1,120.)

MERCURY

Acute exposure to certain inorganic or organic forms of mercury can cause an acute tubular necrosis and renal failure. It has been known for a long time that patients treated with mercurial compounds can develop a glomerulonephritis usually associated with proteinuria and occasionally with nephrotic syndrome. Cases of glomerulonephritis have also been reported after the chronic exposure to high levels of mercury vapor in industry (20). At lower levels of exposure, mercury vapors or salts can cause various subclinical renal disturbances such as an increased urinary excretion of enzymes or of high-molecular-weight plasma proteins (21). Some evidence exists that in industrial workers these early effects may be irreversible.

The concentration of mercury in urine from which these manifestations of nephrotoxicity may occur is estimated at 50 µg per g creatinine (21). Various chelating agents can be used in cases of acute or chronic mercury poisoning (dimercaprol, D-penicillamine, or dimercaptosuccinic acid).

SILICA

An association between exposure to silica and silicon-containing compounds and chronic nephropathy has been suspected for many years. Several cases of rapidly progressive glomerulonephritis without significant immune deposits have been reported in workers exposed to silica. Cross-sectional studies on workers exposed to crystalline silica and animal studies support the hypothesis of a nephrotoxic action of silica (22). It has been also suggested that exposure to silicon-containing compounds (e.g., in grain dust) might play a role in the etiology of Wegener's granulomatosis.

CHROMIUM

The acute tubular toxicity of chromate and dichromate salts in animals is well documented, and cases of renal tubular necrosis have been described in humans after acute poisoning. Slight signs of tubular dysfunction, such as low-molecular-weight proteinuria or enzymuria, have been reported in workers chronically exposed to hexavalent chromium. Some studies have suggested a threshold approximately 15 µg per g creatinine for the appearance of these tubular effects (23). In the environment, even in areas in which soil is highly contaminated by chromium, the risk of renal effects can be considered as negligible in view of the amount of metal (mostly trivalent) likely to be absorbed by ingestion or inhalation.

OTHER INORGANIC COMPOUNDS

Acute arsenic poisoning may cause tubular necrosis. Acute or severe chronic poisoning is usually treated with the chelating agent 2,3-dimercaprol. Inhalation of arsine may also produce an acute tubular necrosis as a result of intravascular hemolysis. Germanium is a semimetal increasingly used in the electronic industry. In Japan, cases of renal failure have been reported in subjects who had consumed large amounts of germanium (50–250 mg per day, normal intake being approximately 1 mg) over a period of 4 to 18 months. Renal biopsy showed degeneration of the renal tubules with little involvement of the glomeruli. Uranium salts can produce acute tubular injury and tubular necrosis in animals and humans. Chronic effects, except a slight elevation of β_2-microglobulin excretion in uranium mill workers, have not been reported. Bismuth administration results in the formation in tubular cells of nuclear inclusion bodies comparable to those observed with lead. It is unknown whether it can result in a chronic nephropathy (24).

Organic Chemicals

A number of solvents used in industry or home products (e.g., halogenated hydrocarbons, ethylene glycol, petroleum distillates, and toluene) are direct tubular toxins. Acute exposure to these solvents by inhalation or ingestion can produce tubular effects that, depending on the dose and the solvents, vary from a mild proteinuria or enzymuria to an acute tubular necrosis (25). For instance, glue, paint, or toluene sniffing may cause various signs of tubular dysfunction consistent with Fanconi's syndrome (e.g., aminoaciduria, glucosuria, tubular-type proteinuria, and renal tubular acidosis). Several case reports and case-control studies suggest that subacute or chronic exposure to hydrocarbons may lead to various types of glomerulonephritis, particularly anti-glomerular basement membrane (GBM) antibody-mediated diseases (Fig. 22-3) such as Goodpasture's syndrome (26). The latter is a rapidly progressive glomerulonephritis characterized by recurrent lung hemorrhages and by the presence of antibodies directed against the GBM. A number of hydrocarbon mixtures and specific chemicals, such as organic solvents, automobile exhausts, hairdressing solvents, gasoline, glues, trichloroethane, or tetrachloroethane, have been associated with these anti-GBM diseases. Evidence for a genetic disposition (HLA-DR2) and an influence of tobacco smoking has been reported (27). The hypothesis of a nephrotoxic risk associated with chronic exposure to organic solvents is further supported by a series of cross-sectional studies showing subclinical tubular and tubular lesions in workers exposed to various specific hydrocarbons (e.g., toluene, perchlorethylene, or styrene) or mixtures of hydrocarbons (e.g., emissions of petroleum refinery or refueling stations). Depending on the type of solvent, organs other than the kidney may be damaged [e.g., the liver (halogenated hydrocarbons) and the central nervous system]. Paraquat, a dipyridilium herbicide, is a tubular toxin that can produce acute renal failure.

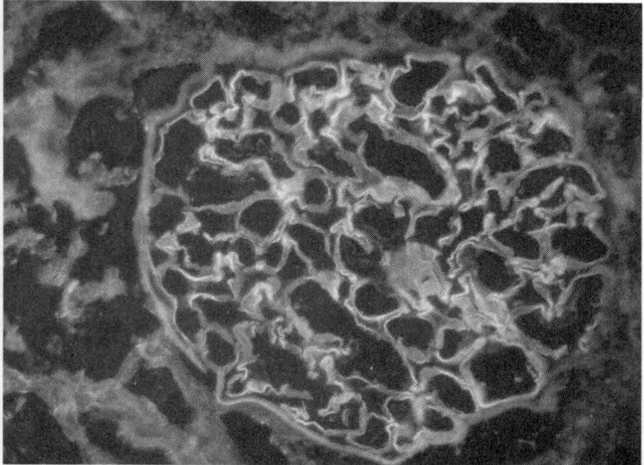

Figure 22-3. Linear immunoglobulin G deposits along the glomerular capillary wall from a patient who developed an antiglomerular basement membrane disease after acute exposure to solvents (×280).

Natural Nephrotoxins

Several mycotoxins are nephrotoxic after acute or chronic administration. Citrinin and ochratoxin A are products of *Aspergillus* that can be found in a variety of cereal grains. These compounds can cause proteinuria, oliguria, and even renal failure and death (28). Fumonisins produced by the *Fusarium* species are commonly found on corn and corn products and have been found to produce nephrotoxicity in rats. Cases of tubulointerstitial nephritis with renal failure have been reported after the consumption of certain mushrooms such as *Cortinarius orellanus* and *Cortinarius preciosissimus*, and *Amanita phalloides* (hepatorenal failure). A rapidly progressive renal disease leading to renal failure has been described in Belgium after the consumption of a slimming regimen based on Chinese herbs (29). Aristolochic acid, a nephrotoxic and genotoxic substance produced by *Aristolochia*, is the suspected agent of the disease. Several natural nephrotoxins (e.g., ochratoxin A, aristolochic acid, and silica) have also been implicated in the etiology of a nephropathy endemic to the Balkan area (Balkan endemic nephropathy).

MECHANISMS OF NEPHROTOXICITY

The mechanisms leading to nephrotoxicity may be biochemical, immunologic, or hemodynamic.

Biochemical Mechanisms

Biochemical mechanisms are numerous and reviews are available (16). With respect to tubular lesions, the mechanisms frequently follow the same pattern: entry of the chemical into the tubular cell via the luminal or basolateral site by an active or passive transport system; accumulation of the chemical in one or several cellular compartments (lysosomes for aminoglycosides, cytoplasm for cadmium); and binding of the chemical or its metabolites to target macromolecules (e.g., membrane components, cytoskeleton, and enzymes). Nephrotoxicity usually develops in a dose-dependent fashion from a certain concentration in the tubular cell (the so-called critical concentration) (30). Figure 22-4 depicts the mechanism of tubular toxicity of cadmium, one of the most hazardous nephrotoxicants in the environment. After absorption, cadmium is taken up by the liver where a liver Cd,Zn-metallothionein is synthesized. Once released into the circulation, the Cd,Zn-metallothionein complex is rapidly cleared from plasma by glomerular filtration to be taken up by the proximal tubule cells via an absorptive endocytosis mechanism. It is likely that part of circulating cadmium bound to albumin enters tubular cell via the same pathway. In the lysosomal compartment, the Zn^{2+} and Cd^{2+} ions are released from metallothionein, and the apo-metallothionein is degraded

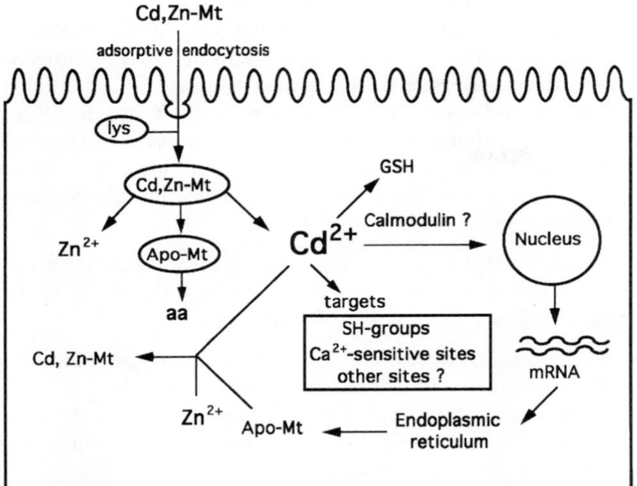

Figure 22-4. Mechanism of cadmium nephrotoxicity. mRNA, messenger RNA; Mt, metallothionein; lys, lysosome.

by proteases. Two protective mechanisms then intervene to neutralize the free cadmium ion: The first is the binding of the metal ion to intracellular reduced glutathione (GSH), and the second, which intervenes after 1 or 2 hours, is the sequestration of the ion by the newly synthesized renal metallothionein. It is assumed that kidney damage occurs when these two mechanisms are saturated, which allows the free cadmium ion to interact with different molecular targets such as sulfhydryl groups of the skeleton tubulin or of metalloenzymes, and calcium-sensitive sites such as calmodulin, cytoskeleton actin, or calcium-dependent endonucleases (activation of apoptosis). Cadmium exerts its toxicity mainly on the S1 and S2 segments with an early manifestation of increased leakage of brush border enzymes or antigens in urine, and a decreased endocytotic uptake of proteins. No evidence of free radical involvement exists.

The tubular toxicity of inorganic mercury presents several similarities with that of cadmium because mercury bound to sulfhydryl groups of filtered proteins (e.g., metallothionein whose synthesis is stimulated by mercury) is also taken up by the proximal tubular cells via an absorptive endocytosis mechanism. Part of the circulating mercury probably also enters the tubular cell by amino acids, dipeptide, or organic anion transporters located at the luminal/basolateral site. The S3 segment of the tubule is the initial site of injury but, as the dose increases, the S2 and S3 segments are progressively damaged. Early markers of inorganic mercury tubular toxicity include brush border antigens, enzymes, or proteinuria. At higher doses, inorganic mercury produces a decrease of glomerular filtration rate (GFR), which may lead to acute renal failure. Mercury has a very high affinity for sulfhydryl groups, and this interaction, when involving sensitive sites (e.g., enzymes, cytoskeleton proteins, membrane proteins), probably plays an important role in the cellular toxicity of mercury.

For most organic nephrotoxins, the binding to cellular targets requires the activation of the substance into electrophilic metabolites. Some compounds are activated by the P-450–dependent monooxygenases. An example is chloroform, which transforms into trichloroethanol before giving rise to phosgene, which can react with target macromolecules. In the case of a halogenated alkenes (trichloroethylene, hexachloro-1,3-butadiene) the formation of GSH conjugates is an important step in the development of nephrotoxicity. The GSH conjugates or their derivatives, the cysteine conjugates, can be transported to the kidney where, after hydrolysis by β-lyase, they release the ultimate nephrotoxic species. Reactive oxygen species are involved in the nephrotoxicity of some compounds (e.g., cephaloridine, puromycin aminonucleoside) (31).

Immunologic Mechanisms

Immune-type nephritis may result from two basic processes: (a) the deposition of circulating immune complexes in the glomerular structures (granular deposits by immunofluorescence) or (b) the in situ formation of immune complexes between a circulating antibody and glomerular antigens or antigens "planted" in the glomerulus. In the latter case, the immunofluorescence pattern appears linear or granular, depending on the distribution of the antigens. Immune complexes formed or deposited in renal structures may cause tissue lesions in a sequence of events involving, namely, the activation of the complement, the recruitment of leukocytes, and the release by the latter of proteases, reactive oxygen species, prostaglandins, and various inflammatory mediators (e.g., cytokines, growth factors) (32).

Immunologic mechanisms of nephrotoxicity may lead to a glomerulonephritis (e.g., membranous glomerulonephritis induced by gold salts, mercurials, or D-penicillamine) or an acute interstitial nephritis (penicillin derivatives). The exact mechanisms by which chemicals trigger the hypersensitivity reaction are usually unknown. The chemical might in some cases behave as a hapten (e.g., methicillin), modify a self-antigen, or else release into the circulation normally hidden tissue antigens. In the gold-, D-penicillamine-, or mercury-induced glomerulonephritis, the immune reaction might be the consequence of a polyclonal activation. The gold- and D-penicillamine-induced membranous glomerulonephritis are more frequently observed in patients with the HLA-DR4 or -DR3 antigen, respectively (12).

Hemodynamic Mechanisms

Hemodynamic alterations are frequently involved in the initiation or progression of toxic nephropathies.

In acute tubular injury, the renal function can be impaired by casts and cell debris obstructing the tubular lumen, by a back flow of glomerular filtrate across disrupted tubular epithelium, or by vasoconstricting substances such as thromboxane, endothelin, or the renin-angiotensin system. Nonsteroidal antiinflammatory drugs inhibit the synthesis of prostaglandins and may precipitate renal failure in subjects with circulatory impairment. Once the glomerular filtration rate has been reduced to approximately 30% of normal as a result of toxic injury or renal disease, the evolution to end-stage renal failure becomes unavoidable, probably because remnant nephrons are progressively destroyed by the compensatory increase in the single nephron glomerular filtration rate (elevation of glomerular pressure and flow) (33).

Necrosis and Apoptosis

Cell death may occur through necrosis or apoptosis. These two forms of cell deaths are distinct in both their mechanisms and implications. Necrotic death is the outcome of a cascade of events that leads to major alterations of the cell membranae permeability. A number of cellular targets and events have been identified to play a role in necrotic cell death: altered cell volume and ion homeostasis by changes in cell membrane permeability, activation of calcium-dependent proteinases and phospholipases, disruption of cytoskeleton and cell polarity, mitochondrial dysfunction, rupture of lysosomes and release of lysosomal enzymes. As opposed to necrotic death, apoptotic cell death is a process whereby a cell is activated by various signals to undergo a programmed process of self-induced death. It is a normal and widespread phenomenon in morphogenesis and cell development processes that necessitate cell deletion. Fragmentation of genomic DNA is an early and irreversible event that commits the cell to die and that is triggered by Ca^{2+}-activated endonucleases. Data suggest that apoptosis could be involved in the nephrotoxicity of compounds like cadmium, mercury, or aminoglycosides. The kinetics of intracellular calcium could be critical in determining the type of cell death: An abrupt and marked increase would lead to necrosis whereas a small and progressive rise would orient the cell to die by apoptosis.

Response of Kidney to Tissue Injury

After nephrotoxic insult, paracrine or autocrine mechanisms are activated to release several mediators that participate in tissue regeneration at different sites of the nephron or kidney. These factors include epidermal growth factor (GF), insulin-like GFs, platelet-derived GF, fibroblast GF, hepatocyte GF, and transforming GFs alpha and beta. Adequate repair leads to reepithelization and functional recovery, whereas inadequate repair can result in fibrosis and irreversible dysfunction. An increased DNA synthesis is the manifestation of tissue repair after renal injury.

Tubulointerstitial inflammation is an important consequence of chronic renal parenchyma injury that may lead to renal fibrosis and loss of renal function whether the primary injury occurs in the tubular, interstitial, glomerular, or vascular compartment. Humoral factors released from infiltrating and residential cells stimulate kidney cells and especially fibroblasts to produce extracellular matrix molecules such as collagen. Transforming growth factor B1, which can stimulate synthesis of extracellular matrix while down-regulating matrix metalloproteinases, is presently considered as one of the key mediators promoting renal fibrosis (34).

An irreversible loss of renal nephrons entails a compensatory hypertrophy in remnant nephrons to maintain renal function. This compensatory response is particularly remarkable at the glomerular level. The GFR of remnant nephrons can increase by more than 50% as a result of increases in glomerular plasma flow rate and glomerular hydrostatic pressure. These compensatory mechanisms, however, may progressively damage the glomerular capillary wall and lead to mesangial thickening due to local deposition of filtered macromolecules. These mechanisms are believed to be important factors in the development of glomerulosclerosis.

In some cases, chronic injury to the kidney may lead to kidney hyperplasia, metaplasia, and cancer. In animals, various hydrocarbons (e.g., unleaded gasoline, D-limonene, 1,4-dichlorobenzene, tetrachloroethylene) have been shown to produce renal tumors. The tumorigenicity of these hydrocarbons is, however, secondary to the alpha$_{2U}$-globulin nephropathy that is specific to the male rate (31). Cases of renal cancer have been reported in humans after high exposure to lead and some solvents (i.e., perchloroethylene).

DIAGNOSIS

The main clinical manifestations that may reflect renal injury are

- Hematuria, which denotes the presence of blood in urine and damage to the glomerular capillary wall.
- Proteinuria (greater than 0.5 g per 24 hours). A proteinuria higher than 3.5 g per 24 hours is characteristic of the nephrotic syndrome. The proteinuria may be of glomerular type composed mainly of high-molecular-weight proteins (i.e., with a molecular weight greater than 40,000) or of tubular type with a predominance of low-molecular-weight proteins (molecular weight less than 40,000). The latter usually results from proximal tubule injury, whereas the former is indicative of a loss of the glomerular barrier selectivity.
- Oliguria (urine output of less than 600 mL per day).
- Azotemia (i.e., the elevation of the serum concentration of small molecules such as urea, creatinine, or low-molecular-weight proteins such as β_2-microglobulin).
- Generalized edema, which in the absence of cardiac failure or cirrhosis is characteristic of the nephrotic syndrome (hypoalbuminemia).
- Hypertension, which may develop as a consequence of glomerulosclerosis.

These manifestations often occur in groups or syndromes. The main clinical syndromes that may be induced by acute or chronic exposure to nephrotoxins are

- Acute renal failure, which is the acute suppression of the renal function with azotemia and often oliguria.
- Chronic renal failure, which is the permanent loss of renal function with azotemia, acidosis, anemia, hypertension, and various other disturbances.
- Tubulointerstitial nephritis (chronic or acute) with various signs of tubular dysfunction (e.g., tubular-type proteinuria, urine acidification and concentration deficits, and salt wastings).
- Nephrotic syndrome, characterized by heavy proteinuria (greater than 35 g per 24 hours), hypoproteinemia, edema, hyperlipidemia, and hyperlipiduria. Nephrotic syndrome can be owing to several types of glomerulonephritis (e.g., membranous and minimal change).
- Rapidly progressive glomerulonephritis, a syndrome with hematuria and oliguria leading to renal failure within weeks (e.g., Goodpasture's syndrome).

The diagnosis of specific types of nephropathies rests on various clinical tests or investigations such as urine analysis and microscopy; estimation of the GFR on the basis of serum creatinine or urea, or of the clearance of creatinine, inulin, or labeled compounds; assessment of the tubular function (e.g., urine concentration and acidification ability and phosphate clearance); radiographic and radioisotopic investigations; and examination of renal biopsies by immunofluorescence, light, or electron microscopy.

Hygiene improvements in modern factories have considerably decreased the risk of acute or rapidly progressive renal diseases of occupational origin. The nephrotoxic action of industrial chemicals manifests essentially through various biological renal anomalies such as proteinuria or enzymuria. These renal effects, which are detectable only by the use of sensitive screening tests might, however, reflect in some cases an incipient renal disease.

The diagnosis of a toxic nephropathy rests essentially on the patient history. It consists of questioning to determine whether the patient has or could have absorbed high doses of nephrotoxins either in the preceding hours or days for a nephropathy of acute onset or during his or her lifetime for a long-standing renal disease. This search must be conducted by considering all possible sources of exposure: diseases or affections requiring prolonged treatment with potentially nephrotoxic drugs such as antibiotics or analgesics, including exposure in the home or work environment to nephrotoxic chemicals such as solvents or heavy metals; ingestion of contaminated food or drinks (e.g., by heavy metals or ethylene glycol); exposure to environmental pollutants (e.g., lead for children); drug addiction (e.g., glue sniffing); and use of nontraditional medicines such as herbal preparations. The possibility of synergisms between chemicals should not be overlooked, and one must be aware that the absorption of relatively low doses of a nephrotoxin may in some predisposed individuals cause severe renal damage. For instance, a moderate exposure to carbon tetrachloride vapors may produce an acute hepatorenal failure in subjects taking barbiturates (35).

Toxic nephropathies can be differentiated from other types of renal diseases on the basis of clinical or biochemical signs that are highly suggestive of a certain type of intoxication (e.g., heme synthesis deficits in cases of chronic lead poisoning, neurologic and hepatic symptoms for acute inhalation of halogenated hydrocarbons, or central nervous system disturbances in cases of chronic poisoning by mercury).

The diagnosis of a toxic nephropathy is also greatly facilitated if the suspected chemical is found in high concentrations in biological materials such as urine, blood, tissue biopsy, or gastric fluid. The maximum time that can elapse between the exposure and the sample collection for a reliable estimation of the absorbed dose depends on the kinetics of the chemicals in the analyzed compartment. It may range from a few hours for rapidly eliminated toxins up to years for cumulative toxins such as lead or cadmium (36). A definitive diagnosis of a toxic nephropathy can be made only after having excluded all other possible causes such as infections, systemic disorders with renal involvements (e.g., diabetes, hypertension, amyloidosis, vasculitis, gout, and metabolic diseases), hereditary nephritis, and malignancy.

SCREENING TESTS FOR NEPHROTOXICITY

At the present time, most clinicians rely on the use of serum creatinine for an indirect assessment of renal function. Although this test has the advantage of being simple, it is not sufficiently sensitive to be used for a screening purposes. Because of its nonlinear relationship with the GFR, serum creatinine rises significantly only when the GFR has been decreased by 30% to 50%. Serum β_2-microglobulin has been reported to be more sensitive than serum creatinine, but this marker cannot be recommended as a reliable GFR indicator because false-positive results can be observed in a number of lymphoproliferative disorders. Serum cystatin C, although equally as sensitive as β_2-microglobulin, appears as a more specific indicator of the GFR (37).

A direct estimate of the GFR based on the clearance of endogenous creatinine, inulin, or labeled compounds permits a more sensitive assessment of the renal function, but such tests are not suitable for routine or large-scale screening of populations at risk. Furthermore, these tests fail to detect early renal effects because of the extensive reserve of the kidneys, which masks the toxic injury until a considerable amount of renal parenchyma (up to 50%) is irreversibly lost. The prevention of renal diseases caused by occupational or environmental nephrotoxins requires the use of more sensitive tests capable of detecting renal effects at a stage when they are still reversible, or at least not so advanced as to trigger a progressive renal disease. The following tests are presently the most sensitive for that purpose (Tables 22-2, 22-3) (38).

Proteinuria

An increased urinary output of proteins is frequently an early and sensitive indicator of renal damage. Determination of the total protein excretion as a screening test for nephrotoxicity in populations at risk has long been abandoned in favor of more sensitive tests measuring specific urinary proteins with appropriate immunoassay. In practice, one usually recommends the determination in urine of at least two plasma-derived proteins, a high-molecular-weight protein such as albumin for the early detection of glomerular barrier defect, and a low-molecular-weight protein such as retinol-binding protein for the early screening of proximal tubule damage (39). In women, the assay of urinary Clara cell protein allows detection of very subtle defects in proximal tubule dysfunction that pass completely unseen with other microproteins (Fig. 22-5) (40). The simultaneous determination of a high- and low-molecular-weight protein allows detection of proteinuria of glomerular, tubular, or mixed origin. In the absence of an increase in low-molecular-weight proteins, a high-molecular-weight proteinuria can be interpreted as the result of an increased permeability of the glomerular filter owing to a loss of glomerular polyanion (loss of charge-permselectivity); structural alterations of the glomerular basement membrane (e.g., increased pore size or appearance of a nonrestrictive shunt); or hemodynamic changes (decreased GFR, increased glomerular hydrostatic pressure). A low-molecular-weight proteinuria, by contrast, can result from a decreased tubular uptake of proteins, a saturation of the tubular transport mechanisms, or a competitive inhibition of protein uptake by exogenous (e.g., aminoglycosides) or endogenous (albumin) compounds. In the absence of renal insufficiency (GFR greater than 60 mL per minute) and of a massive proteinuria (albuminuria less than 1 g

TABLE 22-2. Biomarkers of nephrotoxicity

Biological specimen	Biomarkers
Serum	
Markers of the GFR	Creatinine, β_2-microglobulin
Markers of the GBM integrity	Anti-GBM antibodies, laminin
Urine	
Plasma proteins of high molecular weight	Albumin, transferrin
Renal-derived low-molecular-weight proteins	β_2-Microglobulin, retinol-binding protein, α_1-microglobulin, α-amylase, Tamm-fall protein (loop of Henle)
Antigens	Fibronectin, mainin, brush border antigens

GBM, glomerular basement membrane; GFR, glomerular filtration rate.

TABLE 22-3. Normal levels of some markers of nephrotoxicity

Markers	Normal levels	Remarks
Serum (mg/L)		
Markers of the GFR		
Creatinine	<13	Influence of meat consumption.
β_2-Microglobulin	<2.4	Influence of immunoproliferative disorders.
Cystatin	<2	—
Urine (mg/g creatinine)	—	—
Glomerular markers		
Albumin	<20	More sensitive than albumin but less stable in urine.
Transferrin	<0.8	—
Tubular markers		
β_2-Microglobulin	<0.3	Unstable at urinary pH ≤5.6 GFR >60 mL/min. GFR >60 mL/min.
Retinol-binding protein	<0.3	Possible influence of increased glomerular permeability.
α_1-Microglobulin	<20	Useful in women only. More sensitive than other microproteins.
Clara cell protein	<0.03	Stable at 4°C for months. Isoenzyme B more specific of cell damage.
B-*N*-acetyl-D-glucosaminidase (μg/g creatinine)	<2	—

GFR, glomerular filtration rate.
Note: For all protein markers, repeated freezing-thawing cycles should be avoided. The samples must be stored frozen if the analysis cannot be carried out within 2 to 3 weeks.

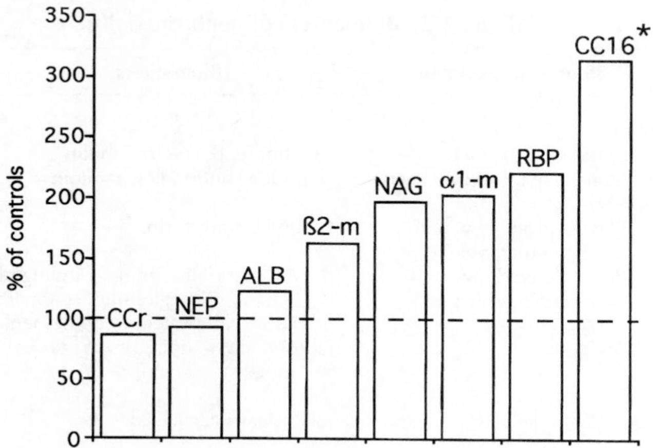

Figure 22-5. Urinary excretion of proteins and tubular enzymes in a group of 27 women who had followed a slimming regimen based on Chinese herbs and who had normal renal function (serum creatinine less than 13 mg/L). The geometric [arithmetic for creatinine clearance (CCr)] means of values are shown in percentage of that found in an age-matched control group of 31 healthy women. α_1-m, α_1-microglobulin; ALB, albumin; β_2-m, β_2-microglobulin; CC16, Clara cell protein; NAG, B-*N*-acetylglucosaminidase; NEP, neutral endopeptidase; RBP, retinol binding protein. *Significantly different from controls. (Adapted from ref. 41.)

per g creatinine), an increased excretion of low-molecular-weight proteins such as retinol-binding protein can be undoubtedly ascribed to a decreased tubular transport capacity by absorptive endocytosis. In the case of retinol-binding protein or β_2-microglobulin, because the fractional excretion of these low-molecular-weight proteins is approximately 0.03%, the percent loss of the tubular reabsorptive capacity can be roughly estimated by dividing the relative increase of the urinary output by 30.

Enzymuria

Injury to the kidney and particularly to the proximal tubule can be detected by measuring the urinary activity of kidney-derived enzymes. Of all the urinary enzymes that have been proposed as the nephrotoxicity index, so far the lysosomal enzyme β-*N*-D-glucosaminidase (NAG) has proven to be one of the most valuable. Advantages of this enzyme include its stability in urine, its high molecular weight (excluding a plasmatic origin), and its high activity in the kidney. The diagnostic value of NAG can be further enhanced by measuring the two isoenzymes of NAG, which consist mainly of the A isoenzyme (functional form released by exocytosis) and the B isoenzyme (lesional form released with fragments of cell membranes).

Urinary Excretion of Renal Antigens

Destruction of renal tissue can also be detected by measuring in urine kidney components that, when they are quantitated by immunochemical methods, are referred to as *renal antigens*. Renal antigens that have been proposed as urinary markers of nephrotoxicity include ligandin, carbonic anhydrase, alanine aminopeptidase, adenosine deaminase-binding protein, and intestinal alkaline phosphatase for the proximal tubule; fibronectin for the glomerulus; and Tamm-Horsfall glycoprotein for the thick ascending limb of the loop of Henle. It is possible that renal antigens, like kidney-derived enzymes, are mainly markers of the acute phase of renal tissue destruction and may be less appropriate than assays relying on plasma protein excretion for detecting chronic phases of renal diseases. A cautious interpretation of the urinary excretion of a renal antigen of any nature or function is also warranted by the fact that the amount released in urine depends on both the extent of renal damage as well as the antigen store of the kidney. As this was demonstrated with Tamm-Horsfall glycoprotein and with the neutral endopeptidase 24.11, the urinary excretion of renal antigen decreases when the renal mass is reduced (positive correlation with the GFR) so that one change (increased leakage due to tubular injury) can be masked by another (decreased production and secretion accompanying the renal mass reduction) (41).

These various markers of nephrotoxicity can be measured on a 24-hour urine sample or on a spot (ideally midstream) urine sample provided a correction is made for diuresis on the basis of urinary density or creatinine. Sampling time is usually not critical except for markers that are unstable in urine (e.g., β_2-microglobulin) for which first-morning samples should be avoided. Because the urinary excretion rate of some markers (e.g., low-molecular-weight proteins) may be to some extent influenced by the diuresis, it is therefore advisable to avoid extreme variations in the urinary flow. This is especially true when the results are corrected for the urinary concentration of creatinine, which at extreme values (e.g., less than 0.3 and greater than 3.0 g per L) is no more linearly related to the diuresis.

Numerous epidemiologic studies have successfully used these markers to identify potentially nephrotoxic industrial chemicals or to establish dose response/effect relationships (42). The tests that have proven the most useful in these studies are those measuring the urinary excretion of specific plasma proteins (e.g., retinol-binding protein and albumin).

In a health surveillance program, it is also useful to examine the urine with a classic reagent strip, a test that is simple to perform and that can detect urinary anomalies such as glucosuria or hematuria. The microscopic examination of urine may be a useful additional test, but it is usually not applicable during routine monitoring of populations. It is important to stress that none of the previously described screening tests has an *ex officio* unfavorable prognosis. In some situations, they may merely reflect physiologic changes that do not necessarily imply a loss of functional or structural integrity of the renal tissue (e.g., orthostatic, febrile, or exercise proteinuria), whereas in other situations, they may reveal transient and reversible renal effects. This frequently applies to the acute tubulotoxic effects, not accompanied by a decline of GFR, which may be observed in a number of situations such as short treatment with antibiotics, surgery, or acute poisonings. By contrast, when markers of nephrotoxicity become increasingly abnormal over months or years, they may suggest the development of a progressive and irreversible nephropathy with a less favorable prognosis.

UROTHELIUM

The function of the lower urinary tract is to transport urine from the renal pelvis through the ureters to the bladder where it is stored until eliminated via the urethra. The lower urinary tract consists thus of the renal pelvis, ureters, bladder, and urethra. A transitional epithelium referred to as *urothelium* lines these different areas (43). The bladder is usually the most sensitive area to toxic injury, probably because of longer exposure to toxicants. Although the bladder may be the site of nonneoplastic lesions causing inflammation and hyperplasia, the most significant toxic response is neoplasia. Aromatic amine (benzidine, β-naphthylamine, 4-aminobiphenyl) have been known for a long time to produce bladder cancer in humans. The mechanism of carcinogenesis involves the excretion of an unstable *N*-glucuronide, which, on hydrolysis in the bladder, releases an ultimate carcinogen reacting with the bladder epithelium. Subjects with the slow acetylator phenotype in whom glucuronoconjugation is more active are at higher risk of developing bladder cancer. Another activation mechanism is via the prostaglandin synthesis pathway, which is particularly active in the bladder epithelium. Urothelial cancers have been reported in women who had consumed Chinese herbs contaminated with aristolochic acid (44). Urinary cytology is the most appropriate method for the early detection of this cancer.

REFERENCES

1. Leaf A, Cortran RS. *Renal pathophysiology,* 3rd ed. Oxford: Oxford University Press, 1985.
2. The Renal Commission of the International Union of Physiological Sciences. A standard nomenclature for structures of the kidney. *Kidney Int* 1988;33:1–7.
3. Landrigan PJ, Goyer RA, Clarkson TW, et al. The work-relatedness of renal diseases. *Arch Environ Health* 1984;39:225–230.
4. Anderson RJ, Linas SL, Berns AS, et al. Non-oliguric acute renal failure. *N Engl J Med* 1977;296:1134–1138.
5. Hou SH, Bushinsky DA, Wish JB, Cohen JJ, Harrington JT. Hospital acquired renal insufficiency: a prospective study. *Am J Med* 1983;74:243–248.
6. Gregg JH, Elseveirs MM, DeBroe ME, Bach PH. Epidemiology and mechanistic basis of analgesic-associated nephropathy. *Toxicol Lett* 1989;46:141–151.
7. Wedeen RP. Occupational renal disease. *Am J Kidney Dis* 1984;4:241–257.
8. Buchet JP, Lauwerys R, Roels H, et al. Renal effects of cadmium body burden of the general population. *Lancet* 1990;336:699–702.
9. Staessen JA, Lauwerys R, Geert I, Roels H, Vyncke G, Amery A. Renal function and historical environmental pollution from zinc smelters. *Lancet* 1994;343:1523–1527.
10. Bernard A, Vyskocil A, Roels H, Kriz J, Kodl M, Lauwerys R. Renal effects in children living in the vicinity of a lead smelter. *Environ Res* 1995;68:91–95.
11. Verberk M, Willems T, Verplancke A, DeWolf F. Environmental lead and renal effects in children. *Arch Environ Health* 1996;51:83–87.
12. Roels H, Lauwerys R, Buchet JP, Bernard AM, Vos A, Oversteyns M. Health significance of cadmium-induced renal dysfunction: a five-year follow-up. *Br J Ind Med* 1989;46:755–764.
13. Hamel JD, Biour M, Cheymol G. Nephrotoxicite medicamenteuse. Fichier bibliographique des atteintes renales et des medicaments responsables: "nephrotox." *Therapie* 1988;43:211–217.
14. Bennett WM. Lead nephropathy. *Kidney Int* 1985;28:212–220.
15. Cardenas A, Roels H, Barbon R, et al. Markers of early renal changes induced by industrial pollutants II: application to workers exposed to lead. *Brit J Ind Med* 1993;50:28–36.
16. Bernard A, Lauwerys R. Effects of cadmium exposure in man. In: Foulkes ED, ed. *Cadmium toxicology, handbook of experimental pharmacology.* New York: Springer-Verlag, 1986:136–177.
17. Bernard A, Roels H, Cardenas A, Buchet JP, Lauwerys R. Cadmium and health: the Belgian experience. *IARC Sci Publ* 1992;108:15–33.
18. Roels H, Bernard AM, Cardenas A, et al. Markers of early renal changes induced by industrial pollutants III: application to workers exposed to cadmium. *Brit J Ind Med* 1993;50:37–48.
19. Bernard A. Biomarkers in the surveillance of workers exposed to cadmium. *Int J Occup Med Environ Health* 1996;2:S33–S36.
20. Druet P. Contribution of immunological reactions to nephrotoxicity. *Toxicol Lett* 1989;46:55–64.
21. Cardenas A, Roels H, Barbon R, et al. Markers of early renal changes induced by industrial pollutants I: application to workers exposed to mercury vapor. *Brit J Ind Med* 1993;50:17–27.
22. Hotz P, Lorenzo J, Fuentes E, Cortes G, Lauwerys R, Bernard A. Subclinical signs of kidney dysfunction after short exposure to silica in the absence of silicosis. *Nephron* 1995;70:438–442.
23. Franchini I, Mutti A. Selected toxicological aspects of chromium (VI) compounds. *Sci Total Environ* 1988;71:379–387.
24. IPCS CEC. *Principles and methods for the assessment of nephrotoxicity associated with exposure to chemicals.* Geneva: World Health Organization, 1991. Environmental Health Criteria 119.
25. Lauwerys R, Bernard A, Viau C, Buchet JP. Kidney disorders and hematotoxicity from organic solvent exposure. *Scand J Work Environ Health* 1985;11(Suppl 1):84–90.
26. Churchill DN, Fine A, Gault MH. Association between hydrocarbon exposure and glomerulonephritis: an appraisal of the evidence. *Nephron* 1983;33:166–172.
27. Bombassei GJ, Kaplan AE. The association between hydrocarbon exposure and antiglomerular basement antibody-mediated diseases (Goodpasture's syndrome). *Am J Ind Med* 1992;21:141–153.
28. De Paolo N, Guarnieri A, Loi F, Sacchi G, Mangioratti AM, De Paolo M. Acute renal failure from inhalation of mycotoxins. *Nephron* 1993;64:621–625.
29. Vanherweghem JL, Depierreux M, Tielemans C, et al. Rapidly progressive interstitial renal fibrosis in young women: association with slimming regimen including Chinese herbs. *Lancet* 1993;341:387–391.
30. Ford SM, Hook JB. Biochemical mechanisms of toxic nephropathies. *Semin Nephrol* 1984;f:88–106.
31. Goldstein RS, Schnellmann RG. The toxic responses of the kidney. In: Klaassen CD, ed. *Casarett & Doull's toxicology, the basic science of poisons.* New York: McGraw-Hill, 1996:417–442.
32. Schreiber BD, Groggel GC. Immunological mechanisms in renal diseases. In: Goldstein RS, ed. *Mechanisms of injury in renal diseases and toxicity.* Boca Raton, FL: CRC Press, 1994:247–265.
33. Brenner BM, Meyer TW, Hostetter TH. Dietary protein intake and the progressive nature of kidney diseases: the role of hemodynamically mediated glomerular injury in the pathogenesis of progressive glomerulosclerosis in aging, renal ablation and intrinsic renal disease. *N Engl J Med* 1982;307:652–659.
34. Roderman HP, Binder A, Burger A, Guven N, Lofler H, Bamberg M. The underlying cellular mechanism of fibrosis. *Kidney Int* 1996;49:S32–S36.
35. Mahieu P, Geubel A, Rahier J, Scailteur V, Dieryck JP, Lauwerys R. Potentiation of carbon tetrachloride hepato-nephrotoxicity by phenobarbital in man. *Int J Clin Pharmacol Res* 1983;3:427–430.
36. Bernard A. Biokinetics and stability aspects of biomarkers: recommendations for application in population studies. *Toxicol Lett* 1995;101:65–71.
37. Nilsson-Ehle P, Grubb A. New markers for the determination of GFR: iohexol clearance and cystatin C serum concentration. *Kidney Int* 1994;46:S17–S19.
38. Lauwerys R, Bernard A. Preclinical detection of nephrotoxicity: description of the tests and appraisal of their health significance. *Toxicol Lett* 1989;46:13–29.
39. Bernard A, Thielemans N, Lauwerys R. Urinary protein 1 or Clara cell protein: a new sensitive marker of proximal tubular dysfunction. *Kidney Int* 1994;46:S34–S37.
40. Bernard A, Lauwerys R. Proteinuria: changes and mechanisms in toxic nephropathies. *Crit Rev Toxicol* 1991;21:373–405.
41. Nortier J, Deschodt-Lanckman M, Simon S, et al. Proximal tubular injury in Chinese herbs nephropathy: monitoring by neutral endopeptidase enzymuria. *Kidney Int* 1997;1:288–293.
42. Bernard A, Lauwerys R. Epidemiological application of early markers of nephrotoxicity. *Toxicol Lett* 1989;46:293–306.
43. Alden C, Frith C. Urinary system. In: Haschek WM, Rousseaux CG, eds. *Handbook of toxicologic pathology.* San Diego, CA: Academic Press, 1991:315–387.
44. Cosyns JP, Jadoul M, Squifflet JP, Van Cangh PJ, van Ypersele de Strihou C. Urothelial malignancy in nephropathy due to Chinese herbs. *Lancet* 1994;344:188.

CHAPTER 23
Teratogenesis and Reproductive Toxicology

Michael A. McGuigan and Benoit Bailey

Human reproduction involves a complex, integrated series of neurophysiologic events. Toxins may adversely affect successful reproduction at any level, from sexual maturation and function of the individual in question to the growth, development, and reproductive capacity of the offspring (Table 23-1). The complexity of the entire reproductive process makes it particularly susceptible to toxic injury. Adding to the difficulties in understanding *reproductive toxicity* is that adverse consequences may result from a toxic insult to the mother, the father, or the fetus. To begin to understand reproductive toxicology, it is necessary to be familiar with both the female and male reproductive systems as well as fetal growth and development.

Women

The female reproductive organ system consists of four anatomic components, the functions of which are regulated by steroids and hormones secreted from the pituitary gland and the ovaries.

The ovaries are two almond-shaped organs located on either side of the uterus. Physiologically, the ovaries are responsible for steroid and hormone secretion and for oogenesis, the production of female gametes (ova or oocytes).

The fallopian tubes (or oviducts) are tubular structures that connect the surface of each ovary with the uterine lumen. The fallopian tubes have two functions: They are the conduits by which the ovulated ovum (or oocyte) is transported to the uterus, and they are the location in which fertilization of the ovum occurs.

The uterus, located in the pelvic cavity, is a pear-shaped organ with thick walls and a single central lumen. Anatomically, it is

TABLE 23-1. Scope of reproductive toxicology

Preconception
Sexual maturation
Libido
Genetic structure
Gamete formation
Gamete transport
Conception
Fertilization
Implantation
Placentation
Fetal loss
Pregnancy
Embryo development
Embryo teratogenicity
Embryo fetotoxicity
Fetal maturation
Birth
Delivery
Neonatal transition
Lactation
Growth and development
Altered reproduction of offspring
Impaired intellectual function
Transplacental carcinogenesis

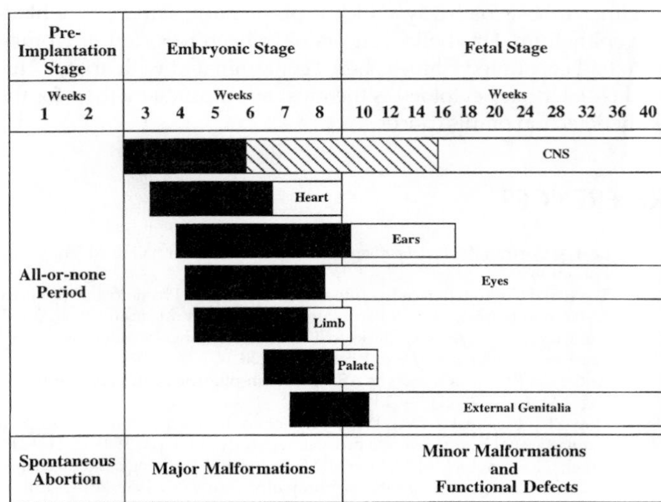

Figure 23-1. Time frame of susceptibility to teratogens for different organs. The number of weeks represents the time postconception; for gestational age, 2 weeks should be added if the menstrual cycle is regular and of 28 days. Solid bars denote higher susceptibility. Hatched bars denote intermediate susceptibility. Empty bars denote lower susceptibility. CNS, central nervous system. (Modified from Sadler TW. *Langman's medical embryology,* 6th ed. Baltimore: Williams & Wilkins, 1990;130.)

divided into four regions (fundus, corpus, isthmus, and cervix) and is composed of three layers: the endometrium (the lining in which the fertilized ovum implants and grows, and in which the placenta develops and attaches), the myometrium (the muscular tissue responsible for the expulsion of the fetus), and the peritoneum.

The vagina is a fibromuscular tube that connects the lower part of the uterine cervix with the outside environment.

Men

The male reproductive organ system consists of three anatomic components, the functions of which are regulated by steroids and hormones secreted from the pituitary gland and the testes.

The testes are two ovoid structures located in the scrotal sac. Physiologically, the testes are responsible for steroid and hormone secretion and for spermatogenesis, the production of male gametes (spermatozoa).

The epididymis is a convoluted tubular structure that connects each testis with the vas deferens (the tube that carries the spermatozoa to the prostatic urethra). The function of the epididymis is to provide an environment conducive to the maturation of the spermatozoa.

The urethra is divided into two sections: the prostatic and the penile urethra. The urethra is the conduit between the vas deferens and the outside environment.

Fetus

Conception occurs within the fallopian tube, and the fertilized ovum is transported to the uterus, in which implantation occurs and placentation begins. The period between conception and implantation is known as the *preimplantation stage* and takes approximately 2 weeks. During that period, the fertilized ovum is not usually susceptible to teratogenic insults, because it is relatively isolated from the maternal circulation. If major abnormalities or critical loss of cells occurs during this period, the embryo is usually spontaneously aborted early enough so that the pregnancy is rarely identified. Because of that, the preimplantation stage has become known as the *all-or-none period* (1). Therefore, any exposure to 2 weeks after conception—or, if the menstrual cycle is regular and of 28 days, to 4 weeks of gestational age—is unlikely to be responsible for congenital malformations.

Once implantation into the uterine lining is established, the embryonic stage is begun and lasts for approximately 6 weeks. It is during this period that susceptibility to toxins is high and major morphologic abnormalities occur (Fig. 23-1) (2). After the embryonic stage, the fetus grows and develops for the balance of the gestation. During this period, the susceptibility of developing organ systems to toxic injury varies. Each organ system has a critical time frame during which it is particularly susceptible to the development of morphologic abnormalities. Organogenesis is largely limited to the first trimester, but genital development continues until near term, and central nervous system development continues throughout the gestation and into the postnatal period.

EPIDEMIOLOGY OF TOXIC INJURY

Reproductive toxicology is the study of the adverse effects of environmental agents on the process of human reproduction. The incidence and prevalence of reproductive disorders caused by toxic injury depend on the particular outcome that is measured and the methods of the data collection. All information must always be compared with the normal background rates of fetal loss and spontaneous malformations.

Measured outcomes related to reproductive toxicity include

- Fertility
- Fecundity
- Malformation

Fertility measures the ability of a woman to conceive or become pregnant. True fertility measures only preimplantation events and does not distinguish between toxic injuries that occurred to the male or to the female reproductive system.

Fecundity is the ability to bear liveborn offspring and measures overall reproductive function. It does not distinguish between male and female toxic insults or normal and abnormal births, nor does it identify infants that are born prematurely or die shortly after birth. Term gestation is a reflection of a

TABLE 23-2. Probabilities of spontaneous abortion

Time from ovulation	Probability of fetal death in gestation interval (%)	Cumulative risk after missed menstrual period (%)
1–6 days	54.6	—
7–13 days	24.7	—
14–20 days	8.2	8.2
3–5 weeks	7.6	15.8
6–9 weeks	6.5	22.3
10–13 weeks	4.4	26.7
14–17 weeks	1.3	28.0
18–21 weeks	0.8	28.8
22–25 weeks	0.3	29.1
26–29 weeks	0.3	29.4
30–33 weeks	0.3	29.7
34–37 weeks	0.3	30.0
38+ weeks	0.7	30.7

Modified from Kline J, Stein Z. Very early pregnancy. In: Dixon RL, ed. *Reproductive toxicology.* New York: Raven Press, 1985;259.

TABLE 23-3. Causes of malformations in humans

Cause	Percentage
Unknown	65%–70%
Genetic defects	20%
Drugs/environmental chemicals	4%–6%
Chromosomal abnormalities	3%–5%
Maternal infections	2%–3%
Maternal metabolic imbalances	1%–2%
Maternal reactions	< 1%

Modified from Wilson JG. Teratogenic effects of environmental chemicals. *Fed Proc* 1977;36:1699.

woman's ability to carry the fetus to term (38–40 weeks of gestation) and measures postimplantation events.

Fertility and fecundity (the so-called reproductive rates) are not accurate ways of measuring the teratogenic potential of a substance. First of all, it is not always easy to diagnose an early pregnancy or to establish when conception occurred. Groups of women who are being studied prospectively may be more aware of pregnancies. The identification of fetal loss depends on the accurate diagnosis of pregnancy, and any suspected increases in fetal loss rates may be within the normal background of spontaneous postconceptual loss rate, estimated to range from 20% to 56% (3–5). The calculated estimates of the likelihood of spontaneous abortion at any given period of gestation are presented in Table 23-2. Also, as shown in Table 23-2, most of the spontaneous abortions occurred before the woman missed her menstrual period, and thus, the vast majority of them go unrecognized. The causes of spontaneous abortions are heterogeneous, made up of chromosomally abnormal fetuses (30% to 50%) and chromosomally normal conceptions (6).

A third commonly measured outcome is malformations. Malformations may be observable at birth (congenital) or may not be noticed until much later. The specific malformation is traditionally anatomic or structural in nature, but malformations may also include physiologic (metabolic) or behavioral (psychological) abnormalities. Despite human malformations being a common occurrence, difficulty arises in defining what is a major and what is a minor malformation, because the most accepted definition of *major malformation* is rather vague: any anomaly that has an adverse effect on either the function or the social acceptability of the individual (7). However, it is generally accepted that the general rates of major and minor malformations are 1% to 3% and 15% of all live births, respectively. Those risks are called *baseline risks* and should not be expected to be lower. As an example, major malformations would include neural tube defects and most congenital heart disease, whereas minor malformations would include abnormalities of hand creases, ears, and skin color. Although the incidences of some malformations are well established, the etiologies are not. In fact, for the majority of malformations, the cause is unknown (8) (Table 23-3).

Establishing the particular outcome to be monitored is difficult when trying to assess reproductive toxicity. The results of an acute exposure might not be expressed until weeks, months, or even years later. For example, the timing of the spermatogenic cycle may delay the expression of a toxic effect on spermatocytes until the cells have matured into spermatozoa and been ejaculated, a process that takes months. Toxic effects may also occur after long-term low-level exposure, especially if the toxic molecular insults are cumulative. Such effects could hasten menopause or alter sexual performance and behavior (9).

DATA COLLECTION METHODS

A number of different types of study methods are used to collect data regarding the association of environmental and occupational exposure to adverse reproductive consequences (10). Correlative studies of groups of subjects compare (or correlate) the frequencies of occurrence of a particular disorder among different at-risk groups with the levels of exposure of these groups to the toxin in question. Results suggesting that an exposure is teratogenic are those demonstrating that the particular defect or malformation is more common in those groups with higher degrees of exposure.

Case reports of adverse consequences of an exposure often serve as the initial basis for implicating specific compounds. These reports are common but are not initially helpful unless the results are rare or unique (e.g., thalidomide). The hypotheses generated by case reports need to be tested systematically before they can be regarded as conclusive.

Retrospective studies of individuals compare cases of a disorder with controls, with respect to the extent of exposure to possible toxins. These studies are also known as *case-control studies*, a very common type of report in which controls are selected to match the subjects. When an exposure is recalled more often by parents of children with defects than by control subjects, the results are considered suggestive that the exposure was teratogenic. Because these studies rely on individual recall, they are subject to a considerable amount of bias.

Prospective studies of individuals compare those exposed to a possible toxin with those who were not exposed (or who were exposed to a greater or lesser degree) with respect to the frequency of an adverse reproductive effect. These studies are also known as *cohort studies*, in which the identified exposed and control groups are studied over a period of time. Results suggesting that an exposure was teratogenic occur when the defects were found to be especially common in infants whose parents were known to have been exposed. These studies are also subject to bias, although less so, and they are incapable of detecting rare outcomes in most situations because of the large sample size needed.

Intervention studies try to establish the frequency with which a disorder occurs in a control group (exposed to a possible toxin) compared with a group in which action has been taken to prevent or reduce exposure to the same toxin. If malformations occur less commonly after intervention, then the results suggest that exposure is teratogenic.

TABLE 23-4. Agents reported to affect female reproductive capacity

Antineoplastic agents
 Alkylating agents, antimetabolites
Environmental agents
 Carbon monoxide; electromagnetic field; hypoxia; alpha, beta, and gamma radiation; x-rays
Food additives and contaminants
 Cyclohexylamine, diethylstilbestrol, dimethylnitrosamines, monosodium glutamate, nitrofuran, nitrosamines, sodium nitrite
Fungicides/fumigants/sterilants
 Benomyl, dibromochloropropane, ethylene oxide, ethylene thiourea, hexachlorobenzene, thiram
Industrial chemicals
 Acrylonitrile, aniline, benzene, benzo[a]pyrene, caprolactam, carbon disulfide, carbon tetrachloride, chloroform, chloroprene, cyanides, di-*n*-butylphthalate, DNT, ethanol, formaldehyde, formamides, glycol ethers, hexane, methylene chloride, polychlorinated biphenyls, styrene, tetrachloroethylene, toluene, trichloroethylene, vinyl chloride, xylene
Infections
 Cytomegalovirus, parvovirus B-19, rubella virus, toxoplasmosis, varicella-zoster virus
Metals and trace elements
 Arsenic, boron, cadmium, chromium, copper, lead, manganese, mercury, molybdenum, nickel, selenium, thallium
Personal habits
 Caffeine, cocaine, ethanol, heroin, marijuana, nicotine
Pesticides
 Acrolein, aldrin, carbaryl, chlordane, chlordecone, cyanazine, DDT, dichloran, dieldrin, ethylene oxide, hexachlorobenzene, lindane, methoxychlor, mirex, paration, toxaphene, 2, 4-D, 2, 4, 5-T
Steroids
 Natural and synthetic androgens, antiandrogens, estrogen, antiestrogen, progestins
Therapeutic agents
 Angiotensin-converting enzyme inhibitors, anesthetic gases/vapors, anticonvulsants, etretinate, isotretinoin, levodopa, lithium, monoamine oxidase inhibitors, opioids, phenothiazines, quinacrine, reserpine, selective serotonin reuptake inhibitors, sympathomimetic amines, tetracyclines, thalidomide, tricylic antidepressants, warfarin

Modified from Dixon RL. Toxic responses of the reproductive system. In: Klaassen CD, Amdur MO, Doull J, eds. *Casarett and Doull's toxicology: the basic science of poisons,* 4th ed. New York: MacMillan, 1995;566.

TABLE 23-5. Agents reported to affect male reproductive capacity

Antineoplastic agents
 Alkylating agents, antimetabolites, antitumor antibiotics
Environmental agents
 Deuterium oxide; heat; hypoxia; light; alpha, beta, and gamma radiation; x-rays
Food additives and contaminants
 Aflatoxins, cyclamate, diethystilbestrol, dimethylnitrosamines, gossypol, metanil yellow, monosodium glutamate, nitrofuran derivatives
Fungicides/fumigants/sterilants
 Apholate, captin, carbendazim, dibromochloropropane, epichlorohydrin, ethylene oxide, ethylene dibromide, thiocarbamates, triphenyltin
Industrial chemicals
 Acrylonitrile, aniline, benzene, benzo[a]pyrene, caprolactam, carbon disulfide, carbon tetrachloride, chloroform, chlorpropene, dioxin, dimethylbenzanthracene, di-*n*-butylphthalate, dithiocarbamates, DNT, epichlorohydrin, formamides, glycidyl ethers, glycol ethers, hexafluoroacetone, hexane, methylene chloride, polybrominated biphenyls, polychlorinated biphenyls, styrene, tetrachloroethylene, thiophene, toluene, trichloroethylene, vinyl chloride, xylene
Infections
 Mumps virus
Metals and trace elements
 Aluminum, boranes, boron, cadmium, chromium, gold, lead, manganese, mercury, molybdenum, nickel, uranium
Personal habits
 Caffeine, cocaine, ethanol, heroin, marijuana, nicotine
Pesticides
 Aldrin, carbaryl, chlordane, chlordecone, DDT, dichloran, dichlorvos, dieldrin, dinoseb, diquat, hexamethylphosphoramide, lindane, methoxychlor, paraquat, 2, 4-D, 2, 4, 5-T
Steroids
 Natural and synthetic androgens, antiandrogens, estrogen, antiestrogen, progestins
Therapeutic agents
 Aldactone, amphotericin B, anesthetic gases/vapors, bretylium, chloroquine, chlorpropamide, cimetidine, clonidine, colchicine, guanethidine, levodopa, methyldopa, monoamine oxidase inhibitors, nitrofurans, opioids, phenacetin, phenothiazines, phenytoin, quinacrine, quinine, reserpine, selective serotonin reuptake inhibitors, tricyclic antidepressants, thiazides

Modified from Dixon RL. Toxic responses of the reproductive system. In: Klaassen CD, Amdur MO, Doull J, eds. *Casarett and Doull's toxicology: the basic science of poisons,* 4th ed. New York: Macmillan, 1995;566.

Randomized trials are those in which subjects are exposed to a potential toxin at random. These studies are generally not subject to much bias but are almost never available in the field of reproductive toxicology.

The discovery of the teratogenicity of many chemicals and the suspicions and allegations directed against others have fostered the view that the chief causes of congenital malformations are environmental or workplace chemicals (11). This view is not correct (see Table 23-3). The identification of substances that have potentially deleterious effects of human reproduction is difficult. Although a great deal of work has been done in animals, little has been established with respect to the dangers of industrial chemicals on human reproduction. Factors that make it difficult and problematic to extrapolate from animal data to humans include genetic susceptibility; intrinsic sensitivity of the developing tissues to the particular toxin; and interspecies variability in pharmacokinetic processes (including metabolism), which affects the magnitude and duration of exposure relative to the developmental stage (and metabolic capabilities) of the fetus (12).

It is clear from animal experiments and human epidemiologic studies that many industrial chemicals have the potential to be reproductive toxins. An estimate is that more than 2,800 chemicals have been tested for teratogenicity, and approximately 62% are not teratogenic (11). As more substances are tested and the sophistication of the evaluation process improves, more substances will be added to the reproductive toxicity list. Some of the substances that are believed to have adverse reproductive effects in humans are presented in Tables 23-4 and 23-5.

ROUTES OF EXPOSURE AND ABSORPTION

For the worker, the routes of exposure and absorption for most industrial chemicals are inhalation and dermal. However, environmental exposure could also occur by other routes, including oral or irradiation. Generally, once the substance has been absorbed, it will be distributed throughout the mother's body.

Pregnancy alters a number of pharmacokinetic parameters that modify the distribution and renal excretion of toxins (Fig. 23-2). Also, the activities of maternal phase I and II metabolic pathways are modified compared with the nonpregnant state. The results for substances studied to date are higher clearance rates during pregnancy. This suggests that a given exposure will

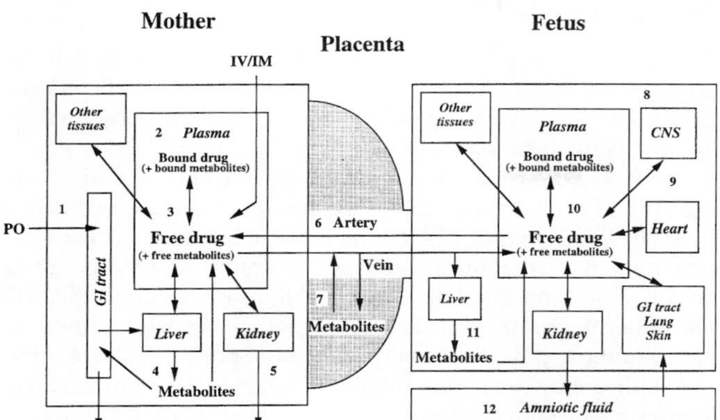

Figure 23-2. Maternal–placental–fetal pharmacokinetic relationships. 1, altered maternal absorption; 2, increased maternal plasma volume; 3, increased maternal unbound drug fraction; 4, altered hepatic clearance; 5, increased maternal renal blood flow and GFR; 6, maternal–fetal blood pH differences; 7, possible placental metabolism; 8, undeveloped fetal blood–brain barrier; 9, preferential fetal circulation to the heart and brain; 10, increased fetal unbound drug fraction; 11, immature fetal liver enzyme activity; 12, large peripheral fetal compartment; CNS, central nervous system; GI, gastrointestinal; IM, intramuscular; IV, intravenous; PO, by mouth.

result in comparatively lower blood levels in a pregnant woman than in a nonpregnant woman. Toxic substances may also be metabolized by the placenta or may cross the placenta unchanged. Once the toxic substance reaches the fetal circulation, it is distributed throughout the body of the fetus.

The capabilities of fetal hepatic metabolism are limited and variable (13). Smooth endoplasmic reticulum appears at approximately 40 to 60 days of gestation. By midgestation, fetal phase I reactions function at 20% to 40% of adult values but vary considerably, depending on which isoenzymes are involved. Fetal phase II reaction activities are variable; glucuronidation capabilities are low, but enzyme systems for sulfate, glycine, and glutathione conjugation exist. The major pathways and maternal-fetal interrelationships are depicted in Figure 23-2. The variability of the fetotoxic effects resulting from this distribution depends on the timing of the exposure (see Fig. 23-1): Not only are different organ systems forming at different times and rates, but the activities of the fetal enzyme systems that may make a substance more or less toxic are also changing throughout the gestational period. A well-known example of this is the risk associated with acetaminophen overdose in pregnancy (14). Because the fetal metabolic capacity increases during pregnancy, an acetaminophen overdose that would cause no fetal effect in the first trimester could cause fetal death if it occurs during the third trimester (14).

Breast milk may also serve as a source of xenobiotic chemicals in the broad sense of reproductive toxicology. Such things as metals (mercury, lead), halogenated hydrocarbons [tetrachloroethylene, polybrominated biphenyls, polychlorinated biphenyls (PCBs)], and pesticides (DDT residues, dieldrin, heptachlor epoxide) may be transferred to the infant in significant quantities (15).

BASIC TOXICITY MECHANISMS

The reviews of published reports of reproductive toxicity document that slightly less than one-half of the reports deal with male and the rest with female reproduction (16,17). Approximately 45% of the reports on female reproduction are concerned with toxicity to the embryo/fetus or placenta, which results in spontaneous abortion or pregnancy toxicity; 40% of the reports focus on the hypothalamic-pituitary-ovarian-uterine axis (18).

The condition that must be met for a teratogenic agent to act is that a susceptible organism must come in contact with the required amount of an appropriate toxin at a vulnerable period in development. The basic mechanism of action of a toxin is the interruption of normal reproductive function. To accomplish this, the toxin must be absorbed and distributed within the body. Once at its target site, the toxin must exert some measurable effect (19). Understanding the ways in which teratogenesis can be induced and the mechanisms through which chemicals act may allow the anticipation of risk to the fetus and a more accurate extrapolation from controlled animal data to random human exposures:

- *Mutations* consist of a change in the sequence of nucleotides on the DNA molecule. The altered DNA code is responsible for the generation of abnormal cell proteins. Examples of substances that cause mutations include ionizing radiation, some cancer chemotherapy agents (alkylating agents), and some carcinogens.
- *Chromosome mechanisms* include breaks or nondisjunction (failure to separate properly). Chromosomal abnormalities occur normally with increasing maternal age but also result from viral infections and irradiation.
- *Mitosis* consists of a complex of various processes by which two daughter cells normally receive identical complements of chromosomes. Many cancer chemotherapy agents (e.g., cytosine arabinoside, colchicine, vincristine) interfere in mitosis.
- *Nucleic acid integrity or function* can be adversely affected by toxins. Improperly functioning nucleic acids result in abnormal production of cellular proteins and, thus, malfunction of the cell. Examples of substances that interfere in nucleic acid function include cancer chemotherapy agents (e.g., 6-mercaptopurine, actinomycin D, 5-fluorouracil) and antibiotics (e.g., lincomycin, streptomycin).
- *Biosynthesis precursors or substrates* may be used incorrectly if specific substances are deficient in the fetus because of maternal dietary deficiency or failure of absorption through the maternal gut, or if the toxin interferes with placental transport of essential fetal nutrients.
- *Energy sources* within the cells may be inhibited and lead to teratogenesis or fetal death. For example, dinitrophenol or cyanide may interfere with the cellular electron transport system.
- *Alteration in enzyme function* by toxins may result in teratogenesis (e.g., hydroxyurea, folic acid antagonists) or in mutagenesis due to inhibition of the enzymes that repair damaged DNA. In reproductive toxicology, this basic approach is made more complex because the process may involve an adult (female or male) only, or an adult female and a developing fetus separated by a metabolically active placenta. Thus, damage to the fetus may arise from the toxin's effects on the mother, on the placenta, or on the fetus itself.

Although the exact etiology and mechanism of teratogenesis for the largest group of congenital anomalies are listed as unknown, the probable causes include polygenic mechanisms (involvement of multiple genes), multifactorial mechanisms (interaction between the genes and one or more exogenous agents), synergistic interaction of toxins, and spontaneous errors of development. Once the toxin has exerted its effects, it is metabolized (usually a process of detoxification) and excreted. The final step is that of repair of damage (20).

Substances that have been reported to cause ovarian toxicity after occupational exposure act directly or indirectly. Indirect-acting toxins are substances that either change the physiologic control mechanisms of the organism or are metabolized (activated) to form molecules that then act in a direct fashion. Examples of indirect-acting toxins include natural or synthetic sex steroids (e.g., androgens, oral contraceptives), which compete with endogenous sex hormones; pesticides, which interact with estrogen receptors (e.g., organochlorine and organophosphate insecticides) or alter the rate of steroid production or clearance (e.g., DDT, PCBs); and metals (e.g., lead, mercury), which alter endogenous hormonal control (21). Other examples of indirect-acting toxins are those that affect the hepatic metabolism of gonadal hormones in the neonatal period (e.g., tetrachlorodibenzo-*p*-dioxin, PCBs, chlordane) (22). PCBs alter the hepatic metabolism of gonadal hormones and, therefore, have the potential to alter the reproductive characteristics of the affected individual. PCBs administered to neonatal rats exerted long-lasting effects on hepatic function (23), resulting in altered circulating levels of gonadal hormones. These data suggest that prenatal exposure to PCBs may result in compromised fertility later in life as a result of altered function, not only in the genital organ system but also in extragenital organs (e.g., liver) (22).

Direct-acting toxins may be structurally similar to a normal endogenous compound (e.g., diethylstilbestrol) or be chemically reactive (e.g., alkylating agents, cadmium) (21). Other examples of direct-acting toxins include such compounds as cyclophosphamide, dibromochloropropane, and the polycyclic aromatic hydrocarbons. For other substances—such as carbon disulfide and organic compounds (e.g., hydrocarbons)—the mechanism of action is not clear (18).

SPECIFIC REPRODUCTIVE TOXINS

To put the above theories into perspective, it is useful to review the existing data on specific compounds.

Mercury Compounds

Mercury compounds are uniformly teratogenic in animals, but this has not been the case in humans. Organic mercury crosses the placenta more easily than elemental mercury. Elemental mercury crosses the placenta more readily than inorganic mercury (24). Mercuric chloride has been associated with abortion, but transplacental transfer of inorganic mercury has not been associated with congenital anomalies (16).

Elemental mercury is absorbed by inhalation and may cause menstrual disturbances (16). Elemental mercury has been found in increased concentrations in the placenta and fetal tissues of dental workers (25). However, theses workers do not appear to be at increased risk of spontaneous abortion or bearing offspring with malformations or neurologic sequelae (26,27).

Methyl mercury has been associated with a syndrome produced by the dietary ingestion of various forms of methyl mercury originally described in a fishing village of Japan, Minamata Bay. The syndrome has been known as the *Minamata disease*. Sources of the methyl mercury included chemically polluted fish in Minamata Bay, but other outbreaks have linked Minamata disease with contaminated flour or pork and fungicide-treated grain.

Methyl mercury causes extensive damage to the fetal brain, with neural degeneration and glial proliferation occurring throughout the cerebral and cerebellar cortices (28). The clinical characteristics and the severity of the fetal disorder are related to the age of fetal exposure—namely, the second or third trimester. Although some of the effects of fetal methyl mercury exposure are recognizable at birth, others may not be identified until several months later. The manifestations of fetal exposure consist primarily of cerebral palsy (spasticity, hypotonia), mental retardation, microcephaly, abnormal eye movements (nystagmus, strabismus), and abnormal dentition (11). Absence of ingested-dose data has precluded establishing a dose-response relationship for fetal damage.

Polychlorinated Biphenyls

PCBs are a group of more than 100 chemicals with different degrees of toxicity. Commercial formulations of PCBs are usually mixtures of PCB isomers with contamination by the more toxic dibenzofurans.

PCBs are considered to be nonteratogenic in most animal studies (16). In humans, maternal ingestion of cooking oil containing 1,000 to 1,500 ppm of PCBs (which was contaminated with large amounts of dibenzofurans) during the first trimester has resulted in congenital abnormalities. Reported findings included stillbirths, intrauterine growth retardation, exophthalmos, dark brown skin discoloration, gingival hyperplasia, and spotted calcifications of the skull. Follow-up of the children revealed that the growth disturbances resolved over a few years but that the children tended to be apathetic and listless, with soft neurologic signs (29,30). PCBs are transferred through breast milk, and this may be a significant source for infants of mothers exposed to these compounds.

Long-term environmental exposure to PCBs has been studied in pregnant women eating contaminated fish from Lake Michigan (31). Overall, it appears that PCB-exposed children were at greater risk of fetal and postnatal growth deficit and had lower full-scale and verbal IQ in infancy, which was still present at age 11 years (32,33). The significance of this in other populations is not known.

Lead

Lead is a known teratogen in animals, but its ability to induce major physical malformations in a human fetus has not been established. However, lead has been known to be a human reproductive hazard for more than a century. It was even used as an abortifacient.

Lead begins to cross the placenta as early as 12 to 14 weeks of gestation. As maternal exposure continues, lead accumulates in fetal tissues so that fetal concentrations tend to rise throughout the balance of the pregnancy. The potential for cumulative toxicity is of special concern.

Among the major effects associated with maternal lead exposure are a higher incidence of spontaneous abortion, preterm births, and perinatal mortality (34). Reports also exist of poorer neurobehavioral performance in the children of women with blood lead levels higher than 10 mg per dL (0.5 mmol per L) (35). Although these results were never confirmed, it appears wise to suggest to women to wait until their lead levels are less than 10 mg/dL before becoming pregnant.

Paternal lead exposure has been claimed to be associated with adverse fetal effects, but it is not clear whether this is due to direct lead effects on sperm (chromosomal aberrations or abnormal sperm number, shape, or activity) or to maternal exposure to the lead dust brought home by her spouse.

Cases of fetal lead exposure need to be followed carefully. The newborns of such pregnancies need to be evaluated at birth for biochemical evidence of lead poisoning (levels of blood lead). Because lead is transferred in breast milk, periodic biochemical screening should be carried out through infancy. As the children grow and develop, they should be screened periodically for subtle neurologic deficits.

Organic Solvents

Organic solvents generally have the potential to be reproductive hazards under the appropriate laboratory circumstances. In humans, several studies suggest that organic solvents are associated with an increased risk of spontaneous abortion, although these claims have not always been confirmed (36). This is not surprising because of the complexity and diversity of possible exposure in the workplace. However, it appears that this is true in workers of semiconductor manufacturing exposed to ethylene glycol ethers (37).

Although organic solvents are considered to be teratogenic in experimental animals, exposure during human pregnancy has been associated only sporadically with a number of congenital anomalies, including sacral agenesis, central nervous system malformations, and cleft lip (11). These studies are suggestive, but suffer from significant methodologic problems. Other studies suggest that exposure to organic solvents is related to decreased libido, impotence, sperm abnormalities, menstrual irregularities, decreased fertility, preterm births, low birth weights, and neonatal problems.

None of the claimed associations concerning the induction of birth defects by industrial solvents has been convincing (11), although some probably increased the risk of spontaneous abortion. However, because of their potential to induce adverse reproductive effects in animals, caution should be used in exposing women of childbearing age to this class of chemicals in the workplace. Minimizing exposure includes adequate ventilation and appropriate protection clothing and devices.

Cancer Chemotherapy Agents

Cancer chemotherapy agents have teratogenic potential in the human when exposure occurs early in pregnancy. Proven teratogens include alkylating agents (busulfan, chlorambucil, cyclophosphamide, mechlorethamine) and antimetabolites (aminopterin, azaserine, azathioprine, azauridine, cytarabine, 5-fluorouracil, methotrexate) (11). Women who receive chemotherapeutic agents for the treatment of cancer have a significant risk of bearing malformed infants, ranging from 1 to 10 to 1 to 50, depending on the agent and the exposure. Exposure to these drugs has been associated with spontaneous abortion, stillbirth, and neonatal mortality. The types of malformations attributed to cancer chemotherapy agents include multiple anomalies, as well as defects in the central nervous system, skull and face, kidney and ureter, and the extremities and digits (11). On the other hand, no evidence exists that women treated for cancer before conception are at increased risk of adverse reproductive outcomes. However, nurses who had miscarriages were 2.6 times more likely to have been exposed occupationally to these drugs than nurses who bore live children (38). Also, increased rates of chromosomal abnormalities have been found in the nurses who were chronically exposed to these drugs (38).

No evidence exists that paternal exposure to cancer chemotherapy agents before or around the time of conception carries an increased teratogenic risk. Although the numbers in the study group were small, the incidence of birth defects in children fathered by 27 men treated for testicular cancer did not differ from that in the general population (39). Temporary infertility is often observed after treatment with cancer chemotherapy agents because of azoospermia.

Ionizing Radiation

Ionizing radiation exposure in dosages less than 10 rads (100 mGy) is not associated with any increase in congenital malformations. In the dose range of 10 to 15 rads (100 to 150 mGy), there may be a barely discernible increase, but this is uncertain. With dosages higher than 15 rads (150 mGy), there is a two- to threefold increase in the incidence of major malformations (40). The classic effects of high doses of radiation include embryonic or fetal death, congenital anomalies (microcephaly, eye malformations, genital and skeletal malformations), mental retardation, and intrauterine growth retardation. These findings may occur after an acute exposure of more than 50 rad (500 mGy) (40).

Preconception radiation may cause reduction or obliteration of gamete (ova or spermatozoa) production and a decrease in the production of ovarian hormones (41). The sensitivity of the ovary appears to be greater in older women (41). Preconception radiation has not been demonstrated to lead to significant genetic hazards or subsequent fetal malformations in children. A study of a limited number of women who had been exposed to high levels of radiation before conception demonstrated normal offspring (42). Radiotherapy may cause temporary or permanent amenorrhea, depending on the dose and age of the woman. It may be advisable for patients receiving more than 25 rads (250 mGy) to the gonads to wait for several months before conceiving (40).

Maternal radiation exposure has been associated with an increase in childhood leukemia in the offspring; this observation has not been confirmed in another study (43,44). However, paternal exposure to x-ray in the latter was associated with an increased risk of leukemia (44). Also, an increase in chromosomally abnormal abortuses has been reported from fathers who were occupationally exposed to x-rays (45). Overall, the risk associated with a fetal exposure of 0.5 rem (5 mSv) has been estimated to be none for spontaneous abortion, major malformation, and severe mental retardation, but has been estimated to add 166 cases of childhood leukemias by age 10 years by 1 million pregnancies (46).

Women of childbearing age working regularly with radiation must be monitored if there is a reasonable possibility of receiving more than a quarter of their maximum quarterly recommended limit of 1.25 rem (12.5 mSv). The National Council on Radiation Protection and Measurements recommends that the maximum permissible dose equivalent to the embryo and fetus from occupational exposures of the pregnant woman should be 0.5 rem (5 mSv) during the entire pregnancy (47). The Nuclear Regulatory Commission suggests that women who are or expect to become pregnant and whose fetus could receive 0.5 rem (5 mSv) or more before birth should seek ways to reduce their exposure within their present job or delay having children until they change job locations. This recommendation does not address the potential risk of increased carcinogenesis, for which safe level of exposure is not known at this time.

Cadmium

Cadmium has quite a variable teratogenic potential in the laboratory. This seems to depend on the particular salt used, as well as the species of animal, the gestational exposure time, and the route of administration (11). These factors make it highly problematic to extrapolate from animal experiments to human occupational exposures. Based on animal data, the mechanism of cadmium teratogenesis appears to be through carbonic anhydrase inhibition. In addition, cadmium is concentrated in the placenta, and placenta malfunction has been noted.

In humans, the picture is less convincing. Reports of cadmium-induced testicular damage, impaired reproduction, and teratogenicity appear to be confined to high-level exposure in animals (48). No fetal damage has been reported in women with Itai-Itai disease, a syndrome associated with high cadmium exposure (49). Other than an association of infants with lower birth weights with material occupational exposure to cadmium (50), cadmium does not appear to have any causal relationship to the induction of birth defects.

Video Display Terminals

Video display terminals (VDTs) have been used more and more frequently, not only at work but also at home. Previous adverse pregnancy outcomes reported in women exposed to VDTs included spontaneous abortion, prematurity, and birth defects

(51). However, earlier reports were faulted for selection and recall bias (52). Current data do not support any relation between exposure to VDTs and adverse pregnancy outcome (53). Because of the high number of women exposed, it is normal to find a certain number of spontaneous abortions and malformations that, so far, have not conclusively been shown to be higher than the baseline risk (54).

VDTs use cathode ray vacuum tubes similar to those used in televisions, and therefore can be a potential source of ionizing and nonionizing radiation. Ionizing radiation emission has been shown to be severalfold lower than the permitted level of 0.5 rem during pregnancy. The effect of nonionizing radiation—the electromagnetic field—is controversial in general and is for pregnancy as well. Because the strength of the electromagnetic field decreases with distance and the strongest fields are emitted from the rear, sitting 18 to 24 inches (50 cm) in front of the screen is quite effective in limiting the exposure and decreasing any risk (55).

DIAGNOSTIC STRATEGIES: DEFINING TOXIC EXPOSURE

All substances are poisons; there is none which is not a poison. The right dose differentiates a poison and a remedy.

Paracelsus (1493–1541)

Diagnostic strategies for the evaluation of reproductive risks and defining what constitutes a toxic exposure must be based on a consideration that no chemical is completely safe under all circumstances. An important aspect of the diagnosis is establishing the degree of exposure. A dose-response relationship must be rationally applied to the particular individual. However, reliable use of a dose-response curve is difficult (56). It is likely that the dose-response relationship is different for each chemical and physical agent, and the characteristics of the curve depend on the gestational timing of the exposure and the reproductive outcome (response) observed. To improve reliability, more than one outcome should be followed, such as fertility, fetal loss, and malformation rates.

History

The past exposure of the woman provides the background against which the risks of the occupational exposure must be interpreted. Important aspects of the general history include the patient's age and her race or ethnic background. The last two personal items are important because certain races or ethnic groups may have a predilection for the development of certain inherited abnormalities (e.g., neural tube defects). These data must be known to counsel accurately. If the woman is pregnant, information must be gathered about the types of birth control methods used, whether any ovulatory drugs were used, when her last menstrual period was, and what her estimated date of delivery is. In addition, prepregnancy and current weights must be documented. Because certain chronic disease conditions or their treatment are associated with an increased risk to the fetus, questions must be asked about the existence of heart disease, hypertension, renal disease, diabetes mellitus, thyroid disease, epilepsy, and cancer. Intercurrent acute disease states (e.g., infections) and therapy need to be documented. Rubella, toxoplasmosis, and cytomegalovirus infections have been associated with congenital malformations. Also, details of the patient's dietary history should be explored, including such things as caffeine intake or special diets.

Signs and Symptoms

Reasons for concern about reproductive toxicity vary considerably, and these reasons dictate the approach to the case. First, a worker may ask for information about toxic substances before he or she starts working in a particular area. In this case, no search for symptoms is required. Second, a worker may be concerned about an exposure and want information on his or her personal reproductive risk. In this type of case, the details of the exposure and any symptoms need to be obtained. All symptoms associated with the exposure should be carefully documented, along with their sequence of development, intensity, duration, and treatment. Even those symptoms that might be attributed to other causes (e.g., nausea and vomiting from morning sickness) should be recorded. Any symptoms reported by coworkers should be noted as well. Third, a couple may present with infertility and question the role of toxic exposures. For these cases, the physiologic causes should be explored in an appropriate setting by a qualified individual. Toxicologic causes must be included as part of the evaluation. Fourth, parents may be asking for information to make a retrospective causal judgment regarding existing malformations in their child.

Cofactors

Consideration must be given to the confounding secondary exposures and nonoccupational substances to which the woman may be exposed. Information must be obtained regarding the use of ethanol, tobacco, and illicit drugs. Exposure to heat (hot tubs, saunas) and radiation must be asked about. Hobbies (e.g., lead or solvents from painting or ceramics), gardening (e.g., fertilizers, pesticides), or home renovations (e.g., paint removers, solvents, lead dust) may expose a pregnant woman to potentially toxic chemicals. One report claimed that 28% of a small study population had household exposure to chemicals during their pregnancies, primarily to paints, solvents, oven cleaners, hair dyes, and laboratory chemicals (57).

Partner History

If the patient is a pregnant woman, similar information must be obtained concerning her partner: his age, race, or ethnic background; occupation; history of disease; use of medications; and use of ethanol, tobacco, and drugs of abuse. Mumps infection in an adult male may be associated with reduced fertility.

The retrospective evaluation of potentially toxic exposures is difficult, because recall bias is a significant problem. Individuals with reproductive failures are much more likely to recall exposures than couples with successful outcomes. The establishment of the time of an exposure relative to the pregnancy depends on the method used for establishing when conception occurred. The most commonly used method, recollection, is notoriously inaccurate. The critical periods of fetal organ development make accurate timing very important in trying to determine the type of malformations that might be expected.

Definition and Identification of Exposure

Of primary importance are the identification of the chemicals in question and the extent of the exposure. Chemicals may be identified by the appropriate Material Safety Data Sheet. However, this may not be accurate or complete enough. A detailed description of the work performed by the patient should be obtained, including the frequency and duration of exposures and the types of protection used (e.g., ventilation system, respirator, protective clothing). Using job descriptions may be helpful in determining types of potential exposures. Documentation of the extent of the exposure in industrial settings is often lacking, and almost everyone has had multiple episodes of exposures to more than one substance. Certain occupations of the mother (e.g., those involving exposure to anesthetic gases, cancer chemotherapy agents, ethylene oxide, ethylene glycol ethers) have been associated with an increase in spontaneous abortion rates (7,37).

A wide range of measures are available to estimate the degree of exposure or dose of a toxic substance, including estimates of emissions, limited monitoring information, direct monitoring of ambient conditions, analysis of concentrations present in blood or other body tissues, and identification of biological markers of exposure. These data are not often available. In some cases, the best information available is that the worker was exposed or not exposed. This type of classification is not optimal, because it reduces the probability of identifying changes in response occurring with exposure and may limit the ability to recognize the effects of exposure. The best measure of exposure is the actual measured level of the toxin (preferably in biological fluids or in the environment). Even with accurate exposure data, undependable results may occur if the appropriate reproductive outcome (e.g., malformations or spontaneous abortions) is not recorded. A reasonable approach to categorizing exposure is to group the exposures into rational biologically appropriate categories (however they are defined). Whatever measure of exposure is used, it is critically important to consider the measured outcome in terms of the gestational timing of the exposure (56).

Family Medical History

Certain disease states tend to run in families and may not necessarily be present in each generation. For this reason, questions should be asked about the presence of the following diseases in members of the paternal and maternal extended families: heart disease, hypertension, renal disease, diabetes mellitus, thyroid disease, epilepsy, and cancer. It is particularly important to establish the presence or absence of genetic diseases or malformations in the extended family. Common major malformations that tend to be familial include anencephaly, spina bifida, club foot, cleft lip or palate, and congenital dislocation of the hip (58).

Physical Examination

The physical examination of the pregnant woman exposed to a toxic substance should be complete and thorough. The examination should include a thorough evaluation of the fetus, including its movements, heart rate, and size.

Tests

Biological markers can provide accurate estimates of the human dose and uptake of hazardous chemicals. With respect to reproductive effects, biological markers might be sought in semen, vaginal fluid, breast milk, and urine (9), but these types of tests are not widely available. The values obtained from biological and environmental monitoring are useful for helping to establish the dose or quantity of a chemical to which a woman was exposed. Biological or environmental values that are considered as normal, safe, or acceptable for a worker cannot be assumed to be normal, safe, or acceptable for the fetus.

Potentially useful measures of male reproductive toxicity include body weight, testicular size and weight, semen analysis (including sperm count, motility, and morphology), and endocrine function (levels of luteinizing hormone, follicle-stimulating hormone, testosterone, and gonadotropin-releasing hormone).

TABLE 23-6. Methods used for prenatal diagnosis

- Maternal serum markers
  - α-Fetoprotein
  - DNA testing
- Visualization of the fetus
  - Noninvasive
    - Ultrasonography
    - Radiography
  - Invasive
    - Fetoscopy
    - Fetography
    - Amniography
- Analysis of fetal tissues
  - Amniocentesis
  - Chorionic villus sampling
  - Fetoscopy
    - Fetal blood sampling
    - Fetal skin biopsy
    - Fetal liver biopsy

Measurements of female reproductive toxicity include body weight, endocrine function (levels of cyclicity of gonadotropin-releasing hormone, luteinizing hormone, follicle-stimulating hormone, prolactin, chorionic gonadotropin, estrogen, and progesterone), and evaluation of cervical mucus and cytology/histology.

Prenatal Testing

A number of tests are potentially useful for making a prenatal diagnosis of congenital disorders (Table 23-6). The procedure that is used depends on the type of defect being sought. Ultrasound is the procedure of choice for the visualization of fetal body parts. Examples of the disorders that may be diagnosed by ultrasonography in the second trimester are presented in Table 23-7.

Radiographic studies have been used to evaluate the fetus. Plain radiography provides information about fetal skeletal ossification and may be useful in diagnosing some forms of bone dysplasias. Fetography and amniography use the introduction of a contrast material into the amniotic cavity. These techniques are

TABLE 23-7. Disorders that may be diagnosed by ultrasonography

- General conditions
  - Hydrops
  - Oligohydramnios/polyhydramnios
- Central nervous system
  - Anencephaly
  - Encephalocele
  - Meningomyelocele
  - Hydrocephalus
- Chest
  - Congenital heart disease
  - Diaphragmatic hernia
  - Pulmonary hypoplasia
- Abdomen/gastrointestinal
  - Esophageal/duodenal atresia
  - Gastroschisis
  - Omphalocele
- Renal/genitourinary
  - Cystic kidney
  - Renal agenesis
  - Hydronephrosis
- Skeletal
  - Digital anomalies
  - Limb reduction deformities
  - Skeletal dysplasias

used to visualize the contour of the fetal body and, because some of the contrast material is swallowed by the fetus, the outline of the fetal gastrointestinal tract. Radiographic techniques have, for the most part, been replaced by ultrasonography because of the risks associated with exposure to ionizing radiation and with the introduction of a catheter into the amniotic cavity.

Fetoscopy and amniocentesis are also invasive techniques. Fetoscopy is used to visualize fetal body parts and to obtain fetal tissue samples (e.g., blood, skin, liver) for analysis. Amniocentesis is used to obtain amniotic fluid for cell and biochemical analysis. All of the above invasive procedures carry the risks of inducing spontaneous abortion, amnionitis, blood loss, and Rh isoimmunization.

Chorionic villus sampling is a safe and effective technique for the early prenatal diagnosis of cytogenetic abnormalities (59). The primary advantage to this technique is that it can be done substantially earlier than amniocentesis.

Moreover, maternal blood testing can also be useful in prenatal diagnosis. α-Fetoprotein measured in maternal serum can serve as a marker for several fetal anomalies, including neural tube defects. Also, DNA testing can be done to detect if the mother or father has a specific mutation for certain diseases.

Work Environment Monitoring

Continuous monitoring or surveillance of adverse consequences, another method for identifying reproductive hazards in the workplace, can serve many purposes (60). Reproductive defects monitoring systems can be used to monitor newborns and identify as quickly as possible an increase in the prevalence of specific malformations or groups of malformations. Surveillance systems also may be used to identify cases (infants born with a specific type of birth defect) for a case-control study. If the defect in question is a relatively rare one, without a registry system, it may be difficult to identify a large enough number of cases to make study worthwhile, especially if one does not want to trace cases too far back in time and risk jeopardizing the quality of the retrospectively collected information. Reproduction monitoring systems also can be used to look at the outcome of deliveries of a specific cohort of women (identified by occupation, degree of exposure, or other characteristics). To be useful, this type of service needs to be coupled with a registry of all births (to give a denominator) and include such data as the number of births in the area, the maternal age distribution, and birth weight and gestational age of the infants. The last function of a monitoring system is to compare trends in overall malformation rates in the general population with the trends in specific exposure populations.

DIAGNOSTIC STRATEGY SUMMARY

- *Gather* accurate patient and exposure information.
- *Establish* the patient's intervention options.
- *Collect* available literature information regarding pertinent human and animal exposures.
- *Evaluate* the patient and literature data for medical and statistical quality. Review the data critically.
- *Estimate* the risk based on the nature, extent, and timing of the exposure.
- *Compare* the estimated risk realistically to baseline risks.
- *Weigh* the benefits of exposure versus the estimated risks of exposure.
- *Determine* the present condition of the fetus.
- *Ask* for expert help, if needed.
- *Help* the patient make a realistic decision.
- *Support* the patient's choices.
- *Follow* and document the patient's course and the outcome of the pregnancy. Follow-up may continue as the newborn infant grows and develops.

MANAGEMENT SUMMARY

The evaluation of the reproductive risks to women and men from environmental and occupational exposure to chemicals or physical agents is a complex and emotional issue. Unfortunately, the knowledge of the reproductive toxicity of those agents in humans is often incomplete or nonexistent. Although many chemicals are potentially reproductive toxins, many are not. Similarly, some malformations are caused by toxins, but most are not. Suspicions are justified, but it is not wise to present suspicions and beliefs as facts. Be specific about dangers, but do not condemn all drugs and chemicals as fetotoxic.

REFERENCES

1. Fabro S. On predicting environmentally-induced human reproductive hazards: an overview and histological perspective. *Fund Appl Toxicol* 1985;5: 609–614.
2. Sadler TW. *Langman's medical embryology,* 7th ed. Baltimore: Williams & Wilkins, 1995;133.
3. Edmonds DK, Lindsay KS, Miller JF, et al. Early embryonic mortality in women. *Fertil Steril* 1982;38:447–453.
4. French FE, Bierman JM. Probabilities of fetal mortality. *Public Health Rep* 1962;77:835–847.
5. Whittaker PG, Taylor A, Lind T. Unsuspected pregnancy loss in healthy women. *Lancet* 1983;1:1126–1127.
6. Kline JK. Maternal occupation: effects on spontaneous abortions and malformations. *Occup Med* 1986;1:381–403.
7. Marden PM, Smith DW, McDonald MJ. Congenital anomalies in the newborn infants including minor variations. *J Pediatr* 1964;64:357–371.
8. Wilson JG. Teratogenic effects of environmental chemicals. *Fed Proc* 1977;36:1698–1703.
9. Dixon RL, Nadolney CH. Assessing risk of reproductive dysfunction associated with chemical exposure. In: Dixon RL, ed. *Reproductive toxicology.* New York: Raven Press, 1985:329–339.
10. Leck I. Teratogenic risks of disease and therapy. *Contrib Epidemiol Biostat* 1979;1:23–43.
11. Schardein JL. *Chemically induced birth defects.* New York: Marcel Dekker Inc, 1985.
12. Nau H. Species differences in pharmacokinetics and drug teratogenesis. *Environ Health Perspect* 1986;70:113–129.
13. Manson JM. Teratogens. In: Klaassen CD, Amdur MO, Doull J, eds. *Casarett and Doull's toxicology. The basic science of poisons.* 3rd ed. New York: Macmillan, 1986:195–220.
14. Tenenbein M. Poisoning in pregnancy. In: Koren G, ed. *Maternal–fetal toxicology.* New York: Marcel Dekker Inc, 1994:226–231.
15. Wolff MS. Occupationally derived chemicals in breast milk. In: Mattison DR, ed. *Reproductive toxicology.* New York: Alan R. Liss, 1983:259–281.
16. Barlow SM, Sullivan FM. *Reproductive hazards of industrial chemicals.* New York: Academic Press, 1982.
17. Pruett JG, Winslow SG. Health effects of environmental chemicals on the adult human reproductive system. A selected bibliography with abstracts, 1963–1981. Federation of American Societies for Experimental Biology (FASEB) Special Publication NLM/TIRC-82/1. Bethesda, MD: Federation of American Societies for Experimental Biology.
18. Mattison DP. Clinical manifestations of ovarian toxicity. In: Dixon RL, ed. *Reproductive toxicology.* New York: Raven Press, 1985:109–130.
19. Wilson JG. Current status of teratology. In: Wilson JG, Fraser FC, eds. *Handbook of teratology,* vol 1. New York: Plenum Press, 1977:47–73.
20. Steinberger E, Lloyd JA. Chemicals affecting the development of reproductive capacity. In: Dixon RL, ed. *Reproductive toxicology.* New York: Raven Press, 1985:1–20.
21. Mattison DP. Effects of biologically foreign compounds on reproduction. In: Abdul-Harim RW, ed. *Drugs during pregnancy.* Philadelphia: George F. Stickley, 1981:101–125.
22. McLachlan JA, Newbold RR, Korach JC, et al. Transplacental toxicology: prenatal factors influencing postnatal fertility. In: Kimmel CA, Buelke-Sam J, eds. *Developmental toxicology.* New York: Raven Press, 1981:212–232.
23. Lucier GW, McLachlan JA, Davis GJ. Transplacental toxicology of the polychlorinated and polybrominated biphenyls. In: Mahlum DD, Sikov MR, Hackett PC, Andrew FD, eds. *Developmental toxicology of energy-related pollutants.* Washington: Technical Information Center, US Department of Energy; 1978:188–203.

24. Berlin M, Jua J, Logdberg B, Warfvinge K. Prenatal exposure to mercury vapor: effects on brain development. *Fund Appl Toxicol* 1992;19:324–326.
25. Wannag A, Skajaerasen J. Mercury accumulation in placenta and fetal membranes: a study of dental workers and their babies. *Environ Physiol Biochem* 1975;5:348–352.
26. Brodsky JB, Cohen EN, Whitcher C, Brown BW, Wu ML. Occupationnal exposure to mercury in dentistry and pregnancy outcome. *J Am Dent Assoc* 1985;111:779–780.
27. Ericson A, Kallen B. Pregnancy outcome in women working as dentists, dental assistants or dental technicians. *Int Arch Occup Environ Health* 1989;61:329–333.
28. Matsumoto H, Koya G, Takeuchi T. Fetal Minamata disease. *J Neuropathol Exp Neurol* 1965;24:563–574.
29. Harada M. Intrauterine poisoning. Clinical and epidemiological studies and significance of the problem. *Bull Inst Const Med Kumamato Univ* 1976;25[Suppl]:1–60.
30. Yamashita F. Clinical features of polychlorobiphenyls (PCB)-induced fetopathy. *Paediatrician* 1977;6:20–27.
31. Fein GG, Jacobson JL, Jacobson SW, Schwartz PM, Dowler JK. Prenatal exposure to polychlorinated biphenyls: effect on birth size and gestational age. *J Pediatr* 1984;105:315–319.
32. Jacobson JL, Jacobson SW, Humphrey HEB. Effects of in utero exposure to polychlorinated biphenyls and related contaminants on cognitive functioning in young children. *J Pediatr* 1990;116:38–45.
33. Jacobson JL, Jacobson SW. Intellectual impairment in children exposed to polychlorinated biphenyls in utero. *N Engl J Med* 1996;335:783–789.
34. Rom WN. Effects of lead on the female and reproduction: a review. *Mt Sinai J Med* 1976;43:542–552.
35. Bellinger D, Leviton A, Waternaux C, et al. Longitudinal analyses of prenatal lead exposure and early cognitive development. *N Engl J Med* 1987;316:1037–1043.
36. Bentur Y, Koren G. The common occupational exposures encountered by pregnant women In: Koren G, ed. *Maternal–fetal toxicology.* New York: Marcel Dekker Inc, 1994:428–433.
37. Correa A, Gray RH, Cohen R, et al. Ethylene glycol ethers and risks of spontaneous abortion and subfertility. *Am J Epidemiol* 1996;143:707–717.
38. Selevan SG, Lindbohm M-L, Hornung RW, Hemminki K. A study of occupational exposure to antineoplastic drugs and fetal loss in nurses. *N Engl J Med* 1985;313:1173–1178.
39. Senturia YD, Peckham CS, Peckham MJ. Children fathered by men treated for testicular cancer. *Lancet* 1985;2:766–769.
40. Brent RL. The effect of embryonic and fetal exposure to x-ray microwaves, and ultrasound. *Clin Perinatol* 1986;13:615–648.
41. Mettler FA, Moseley RD. *Medical effects of ionizing radiation*. Orlando, FL: Grune & Stratton, 1985:126–191.
42. Horning SJ, Hoppe RT, Kaplan HS, Rosenberg SA. Female reproductive potential after treatment for Hodgkin's disease. *N Engl J Med* 1981;304:1377–1382.
43. Diamond EL, Schmerler H, Lilienfeld AM. The relationship of intrauterine radiation to subsequent mortality and development of leukemia in children: a prospective study. *Am J Epidemiol* 1973;97:283–313.
44. Shu XO, Reaman GH, Lampkin B, et al. Association of paternal diagnostic x-ray exposure with risk of infant leukemia. *Cancer Epidemiol Biomarkers Prev* 1994;3:645–653.
45. Boue J, Boue A, Lazar P. Retrospective and prospective epidemiological studies of 1500 karyotyped spontaneous abortions. *Teratology* 1975;12:11–26.
46. Stewart A, Webb D, Hewitt D. A survey of childhood malignancies. *BMJ* 1958;1:1495–1508.
47. Review of NCRP radiation dose limit for embryo and fetus in occupationally exposed women: recommendations of the National Council on Radiation, Protection and Measurement. Washington: National Council on Radiation, Protection and Measurement, 1977 [Publ no 53].
48. Webb M. Cadmium. *Br Med Bull* 1975;31:246–250.
49. Thueraut J, Schaller KH, Engelhardt E, Gossler K. The cadmium content of the human placenta. *Int Arch Occup Environ Health* 1975;36:19–27.
50. Sullivan FM, Barlow SM. Congenital malformations and other reproductive hazards from environmental chemicals. *Proc R Soc Lond* 1979;205:91–110.
51. Bentur Y. Ionizing and nonionizing radiation in pregnancy. In: Koren G, ed. *Maternal–fetal toxicology.* New York: Marcel Dekker Inc, 1994:553–555.
52. McDonald AD, Chesy NM, Delrome C, McDonald JC. Visual display units and pregnancy: evidence from the Montreal survey. *J Occup Med* 1986;28:1226–1231.
53. Schnorr TM, Grajewski B, Hornung R, et al. Video display terminals and the risk of spontaneous abortions. *N Engl J Med* 1991;324:727–733.
54. Marcus M. Epidemiologic studies of video display terminals and pregnancy outcome. *Reprod Toxicol* 1990;4:51–56.
55. Paul M. Video display terminals. In: Paul M, ed. *Occupational and environmental reproductive hazards*. Baltimore: Williams & Wilkins, 1993:190–200.
56. Selevan SG, Lemasters GK. The dose-response fallacy in human reproductive studies of toxic exposures. *J Occup Med* 1987;29:451–454.
57. Hill RM, Craig JP, Chaney MD, et al. Utilization of over-the-counter drugs during pregnancy. *Clin Obstet Gynecol* 1977;20:381–394.
58. Fraser FO. The epidemiology of the common major malformations as related to environmental monitoring. In: Hook EB, Janerich DT, Poter IH, eds. *Monitoring birth defects and environment: the problem of surveillance*. New York: Academic Press, 1971:85–96.
59. Rhoads GG, Jackson LG, Schlesselman SE, et al. The safety and efficacy of chorionic villus sampling for early prenatal diagnosis of cytogenetic abnormalities. *N Engl J Med* 1989;320:609–617.
60. Kallen B, Hay S, Klingberg M. Birth defects monitoring systems. Accomplishments and goals. In: Kalter H, ed. *Issues and reviews in teratology*, vol 2. New York: Plenum Press, 1984:1–21.

CHAPTER 24

Carcinogenesis, Mutagenesis, and Genotoxicity

Thomas J. Mason, Chodaesessie Wellesley-Cole Morgan, and John B. Sullivan, Jr.

In 1775, Percival Pott described the occurrence of scrotal cancer in a subpopulation of his male patients who were chimney sweeps (1). The fact that these sweeps had been occupationally exposed to soot led Dr. Pott to conclude that exposure to soot was associated with the development of scrotal cancer in this defined population. In the 200-plus ensuing years, a number of substances have been associated with carcinogens in animals and humans. Based on studies by the International Agency for Research on Cancer (IARC), at least 24 substances are strongly associated with the occurrence of cancer in humans (2). A summary is presented in Table 24-1.

Industrial processes strongly associated with carcinogenesis, even though the causative agent is not always clearly identified, include manufacturers of amines (bladder cancer), chromate (lung cancer), cadmium (prostate cancer), hematite mining (lung cancer), nickel (nasal cavity and lung cancer), and the rubber industry (lung cancer). The IARC monographs have evaluated 860 agents, mixtures, and exposures, of which 78 are carcinogenic to humans, 63 are probably carcinogenic to humans, and 235 are possibly carcinogenic to humans (see Table 24-1).

Occupational exposures associated with a technological process and medical treatments that are known to be carcinogens are listed in Table 24-2 (3). The substances listed in the table have been evaluated by scientists from the National Toxicology Program and other U.S. federal agencies as part of a hazard identification program. Substances that are known to be carcinogenic are defined as those substances for which there is sufficient evidence of carcinogenicity from studies in humans that indicates a causal relationship to the agent, substance, or mixture and human cancer. This publication (3) was updated in 2000. Several agents, substances, or mixtures have been added to the list as "known to be a human carcinogen," and multiple other chemicals have been added as "reasonably anticipated to be a human carcinogen" (http://ehis.niehs.nih.gov/roc/toc9.html).

CRITERIA FOR CHEMICAL CARCINOGENESIS

A *chemical carcinogen* is an agent that increases the occurrence of cancer compared with untreated controls when administered to animals. This definition is based on an increased relative rate of cancer—that is, the absolute risk of a cancer in the population is irrelevant. Four types of increased neoplastic responses are accepted as evidence of carcinogenesis: (a) increased incidence of "naturally" occurring tumors, (b) development of new types of cancers, (c) a new multiplicity of cancers, and (d) a decrease in median time to tumor. These criteria tend to blur the distinction between initiation and promotion of cancers but are useful and conservative.

A wide variety of chemicals can produce one or more of these responses. Although these agents fall into several broad classes, the chemical structures and modes of action are diverse. In some cases, the term *promoter* or *enhancer* may be more appropriate than *carcinogen*. In any case, the varying mechanisms of expo-

TABLE 24-1. Some chemicals and processes carcinogenic to humans as determined by the International Agency for Research on Cancer

Aflatoxins	Estrogen replacement therapy
Aluminum production	Estrogen, nonsteroidal[a]
4-Aminobiphenyl	Estrogen, steroidal
Analgesic mixtures containing phenacetin	Furniture and cabinet working
Arsenic and arsenic compounds[a]	Hematite mining, underground, with exposure to radon
Asbestos	Iron and steel founding
Auramine, manufacture of	Isopropyl alcohol manufacture, strong-acid process
Azathioprine	Magenta, manufacture of
Benzene	Melphalan
Benzidine	8-Methodxypsoralen (Methoxsalen) plus ultraviolet radiation
Betel quid with tobacco	Mineral oils, untreated and mildly treated
N,N-Bis(2-chloroethyl)-2-naphthylamine (chlornaphazine)	MOPP (combined therapy with nitrogen mustard, vincristine, procarbazine, and prednisone) and other combined chemotherapy including alkylating
Bis(chloromethyl)ether and chloromethyl methyl ether (technical grade)	Mustard gas (sulfur mustard)
Boot and shoe manufacture and repair	2-Naphthylamine
1,3-Butanediol dimethanesulfonate (Myleran)	Nickel and nickel compounds[a]
Chlorambucil	Oral contraceptives, combined
1-(2-Chloroethyl)-3-(4-methylcyclohexyl)-1-nitrosourea	Oral contraceptives, sequential
Chromium compounds, hexavalent[b]	Rubber industry
Coal gasification	Shale oils
Coal-tar pitches	Soots
Coal tars	Talc containing asbestiform fibers
Coke production	Tobacco products, smokeless
Cyclophosphamide	Tobacco smoke
Diethylstilbestrol	Treosulfan
Erionite	Vinyl chloride

[a]Applies to the group of chemicals or process used and not necessarily to all individual chemicals.
[b]These agents have a protective effect against cancers of the ovary and endometrium.
Adapted from ref. 2, with permission.

sure that these different agents imply point to the need for specialized risk analysis and management.

Mechanisms of Action

The primary site of action of many chemical carcinogens is DNA. Current investigations focus on these nucleotides—to which these carcinogens bind—and the type of binding or adduct formation. Many details have been elucidated, such as the action of methylnitrosourea in producing carbonium ions and their binding to guanine. In humans, no direct evidence exists that DNA adducts—other than those covalently bound—can cause cancer. However, in bacteria, even intercalated binding of some chemicals is mutagenic, leading to the suspicion that covalent binding may not be required in other species.

The evidence in favor of DNA's being the critical target of carcinogens can be summarized as follows:

- Most cancers display some chromosomal abnormalities.
- Most cancers display abnormal gene expression.
- Many cancers display activated oncogenes.
- Neoplasia is self-propagating—that is, cancer is inherited at the cellular level.
- Some genetic alterations predispose to cancer.
- Carcinogens can be shown to react covalently with DNA.
- Defective DNA repair predisposes to cancer.

TABLE 24-2. Substances/groups of substances, occupational exposures associated with a technological process, and medical treatments that are known to be carcinogenic

Aflatoxins
Alcoholic beverage consumption
4-Aminobiphenyl
Analgesic mixtures containing phenacetin
Arsenic and certain arsenic compounds
Asbestos
Azathioprine
Benzene
Benzidine
Bis (chloromethyl) ether and technical-grade chloromethyl methyl ether
1,3-Butadiene
1,4-Butanediol dimethyl sulfonate (Myleran)
Cadmium and cadmium compounds
Chlorambucil
1-(2-Chloroethyl)-3-(4-methylcyclohexyl)-1-nitrosourea
Chromium and hexavalent compounds
Coke oven emissions
Conjugated estrogens
Cyclophosphamide
Cyclosporin A
Diethylstilbestrol
Dyes that metabolize to benzidine
  Direct black 38
  Direct blue 6
Environmental tobacco smoke
Erionite
Ethylene oxide
Melphalan
Methoxsalen with ultraviolet A therapy
Mustard gas
2-Naphthylamine
Radon
Silica, crystalline
  Quartz
  Cristobalite
  Triclyme
Smokeless tobacco
Solar radiation and exposure to sunlamps or sunbeds
Soots
Strong inorganic acid mists containing sulfuric acid
Tamoxifen
Tars and mineral oils
Thiotepa
Tobacco smoking
Thorium dioxide
Vinyl chloride
Soots, tars, and mineral oils

Adapted from the Ninth Report on Carcinogens. U.S. Department of Health and Human Services, Public Health Service, National Toxicology Program, 2000.

Many carcinogens are activated by host metabolism. These reactive species bind covalently to DNA and other macromolecules. However, enzyme repair systems can replace damaged sections of DNA, allowing the cell to recover. If cellular reproduction occurs in the presence of DNA damage, point mutations, transpositions, and other genetic alterations can occur. It is also plausible that binding and alteration of proteins that regulate gene expression can transform cells. Reproduction of damaged or transformed cells may produce preneoplastic lesions, some perhaps clinically evident.

The different chemical classes of carcinogens typified in Figure 24-1 do not have common structural features. However, they have been shown to have common metabolic characteristics and tendencies to form reactants of a specific type. Much of the work demonstrating these pathways was accomplished by J. A. and E. C. Miller (4–6). During hepatocarcinogenesis, azo dyes were shown

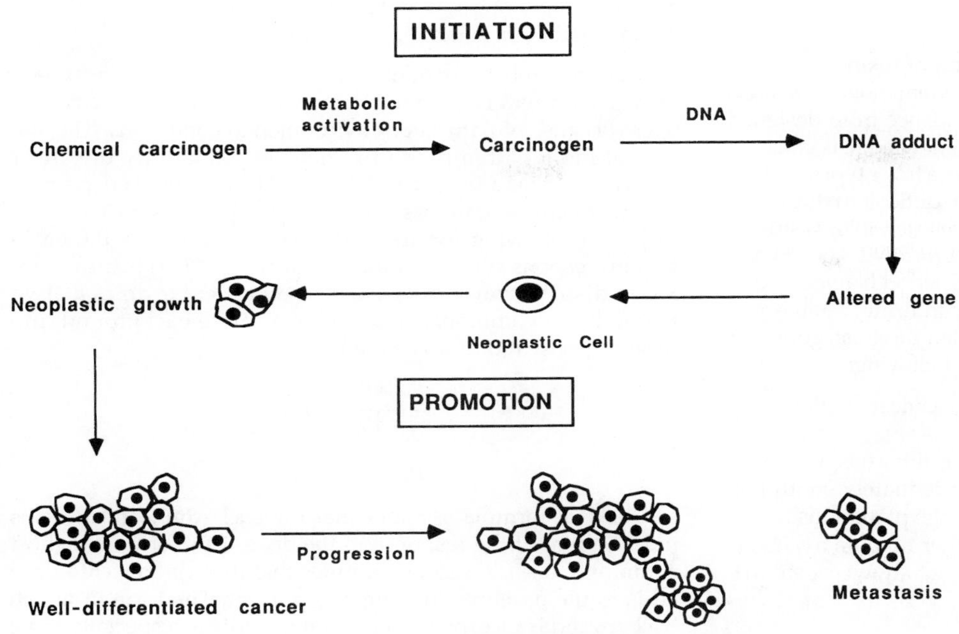

Figure 24-1. Carcinogenesis steps.

to become covalently bound to liver proteins (4). Similarly, benzo[1]pyrene became covalently bound to proteins in the skin of mice (5). Similar results were obtained in studies of other chemical carcinogens. The common metabolic pathway for the structurally dissimilar compounds appears to be conversion to electrophils (electron-deficient molecules), which then covalently bind to a variety of biological macromolecules, most notably DNA.

In addition, for the electrophilic reactants, studies also suggest that free radicals are produced during metabolism (7). They carry no net change but do have an unpaired electron. The evidence in favor of this pathway is strengthened by observations that antioxidants, which inhibit free radical formation, can diminish the activity of some carcinogens (8).

These mechanistic explanations are satisfying for several reasons. They demonstrate why metabolism of carcinogens is necessary for activation. Species differences in metabolism undoubtedly exist, which is consistent with other experimental evidence indicating that some carcinogens are species specific. Also, the genetic mode of action of most carcinogens may explain the long lead time between exposure to toxins and the appearance of cancer. However, not all carcinogens are activated by metabolism. A few—for example, some chemotherapeutic drugs—do not require activation. Examples of carcinogens needing no direct activation are β-propiolactone, nitrogen mustard, and bis(chloromethyl)ether. Furthermore, there appear to be epigenetic and other mechanisms by which some other carcinogens act. These include the cytotoxic agents mentioned, plastics, hormones, and immune suppressants (2,3).

Cancer Initiation

The previous section emphasized the latency period between the application of a carcinogen and the ultimate appearance of the tumor. This delay is not due solely, or even principally, to the growth of neoplastic cells from micro- to macroscopic size. Instead, it is explained by the need for a second developmental stage in carcinogenesis for many chemicals. Such a latency period, with the same implication, is also seen for cancers induced by viruses and ionizing radiation.

Rous and Kidd (9) use the term *initiation* to describe the application of tar to a rabbit's ear, which could then be made to produce a tumor by wounding. Initiation alone is not sufficient to produce neoplasia in most cases, and host and environmental factors may provide the subsequent requirements. Many chemical carcinogens can provide requirements for both stages.

The process of pure initiation has the following characteristics:

- Irreversibility
- Cumulative effects of repeated exposures to initiator
- No morphologic changes in initiated cells
- Dependency on metabolism and the cell cycle
- No threshold dose or maximum response to the initiator

Cancer Promotion

Promotion is the process by which initiated cells complete the neoplastic transformation. In many cases, promotion requires the presence of an additional substance (promoter), which, by itself, may not be carcinogenic. The promoting agent probably alters gene expression with the subsequent manifestation of neoplasia in initiated cells. Promoters are often hormones, drugs, or plant products that react with cell membrane, nuclear, or cytoplastic receptors.

Most chemical carcinogens are both initiators and promoters (complete carcinogens) (see Fig. 24-1). A few are pure initiators, especially at low doses, with promotion becoming manifest at higher doses. However, promoters cannot initiate a cancer but may transform neoplasms that were initiated by other environmental exposures or chance events.

Promotion is characterized by the following:

- Reversibility and nonadditivity
- Morphologic changes in cells and gross appearance of neoplasia
- Noninitiation
- Modulation by environmental and lifestyle factors
- Threshold and maximal response

A number of environmental factors are likely to be tumor promoters. In fact, human neoplasia may represent the effects of environmental and dietary promotion more than initiation. Environmental promoting agents probably include dietary fat, cigarette smoke, asbestos, halogenated hydrocarbons, and alcohol, as well as estrogens.

HUMAN CARCINOGENESIS

Inferences regarding the carcinogenic action of toxins in human populations have come from two sources: epidemiologic investigations in small exposed populations and evidence from designed experiments in animals in which sufficient knowledge is obtained to draw conclusions across species lines. These latter types of studies are particularly important; it is extremely difficult to draw firm conclusions regarding carcinogenesis from epidemiologic studies alone because of recall bias regarding exposure, low-level and otherwise unknown exposures, and a long lag period between exposure and outcome. Because of the difficulty in firmly establishing carcinogenicity in humans, IARC has adopted three categories for the strength of such evidence. These are the following:

- Sufficient evidence indicating human cancer is definitely caused by exposure
- Limited evidence indicating that causality has not been proved because these studies have inadequately controlled confounders, bias, chance, or alternative explanations
- Inadequate evidence, which means either no data available, weak epidemiologic data, or studies that showed convincingly no evidence of carcinogenicity

There are large numbers of epidemiologic studies that demonstrate convincing carcinogenicity for lifestyle factors and dietary exposures in humans. These include alcohol, smoking, and aflatoxin.

Aflatoxin is associated primarily with liver cancer; high concentrations of this substance are found in the diet of some individuals in Africa and East Asia. In fact, the dose of aflatoxin ingested by certain individuals greatly exceeds the dose that has been proven carcinogenic in laboratory animals.

No discussion of chemical carcinogenesis in humans would be complete without mention of the leading human carcinogen: cigarette smoke. Current epidemiologic estimates indicate that approximately 90% of the lung cancer cases in the United States are a direct consequence of tobacco smoking. Considering the attributable risk of tobacco smoking in bladder cancer and gastrointestinal tract cancer, as many as 30% of the cancer deaths in the United States are a consequence of exposure to cigarette smoke.

A number of occupations are associated with higher incidence of cancer in humans. Most of these are listed in Tables 24-1 and 24-2. In many cases, the precise mechanism by which cancers are produced is not known. For example, although considerable evidence exists that exposure to asbestos is carcinogenic, the exact mechanism is unknown. Fiberglass has been shown to be carcinogenic in rodents through an unknown mechanism, but it does not pose a detectable increased risk for humans.

Many of the manufacturing processes listed in Tables 24-1 and 24-2 involve exposure to a variety of chemicals, such as dyes, benzene, cadmium, and pesticides. However, some industrial processes seem not to involve known carcinogens, indicating unknown mechanisms of action or interaction. The attributable risk that is due to occupational exposure for cancer deaths in the United States is under some dispute. Although estimates have been as high as 20%, it is more realistic to conclude that approximately 5% of cancer deaths in the United States can be attributed to occupational exposure.

Dose-Response Models

The primary quantitative issues in dose-response modeling are the following:

- The mathematic form of the dose-response function
- The incorporation of "background" in the model
- The number of doses and animals per dose tested
- The method of estimation of model parameters

That the probability of observing cancers of a specific type is greater than zero is quite likely, even in the absence of a carcinogen, because of natural or environmental conditions. The statistical model attempts to predict the probability of cancer occurrence, p, as a function of dose, d. The observed effects may include death, weight loss, and number of tumors.

In the following formulas, we assume that P_0 is the background response or probability of cancer and $F(d)$ is the cumulative distribution of responses at a particular dose, d. Two methods are commonly used to incorporate background into dose-response models. These are:

$$\frac{Pd - P_0}{1 - P_0} = F(d)$$

$$Pd = F(d + d_0)$$

The first formula assumes that the background response is independent of the response to the dose. This formula is most commonly used. A second assumes that the administered dose adds to the baseline dose already present. The form in which background is incorporated is often not critical, especially if the model is linear at low doses.

Two general categories of models are used for low-dose extrapolation. These are termed *tolerance* and *mechanistic* models. Tolerance models are not derived from biological explanations of dose response and are mainly statistically motivated. Commonly used tolerance models are the log-probit and log-logistic models. In contrast, mechanistic models are derived from theories about carcinogenesis that give rise to quantitative probabilities of cancer incidence. Common mechanistic models are the one-hit, gamma multihit, multistage, and Weibull models. Mechanistic models, for obvious reasons, are generally preferred over tolerance models. Several commonly used carcinogenic risk models are shown in Table 24-3.

The log-probit mode was first used in bioassay and was adopted in risk assessment primarily for convenience. The log-logistic model has a sigmoid curve very similar to the probit, because of the similarity between the logit and normal probability distributions. However, at low doses, the logistic model is more conservative. Because of its shape at low doses, the one-hit model was very conservative. In many instances, it does not provide a reasonable model for low-dose extrapolation in spite of its simplicity (10). The gamma model is intuitively appealing because of

TABLE 24-3. Commonly used models for assessing risk from chemical carcinogens

Model	Mathematical form
Log-probit	$F(d) = \Phi[(\log(d) - \mu)/\sigma]$ $= \Phi[a + b \log(d)]$ where $a = \frac{-\mu}{\sigma}$, $b = \frac{1}{\sigma}$, and $\Phi(\cdot)$ is the cumulative normal distribution function.
Log-logistic	$F(d) = 1/([1 + e^{a - b\log(d)}]b > 0)$
One-hit	$F(d) = 1 - e^{\lambda d}$
Gamma	$F(d) = 1 - e^{-(a_1 + b_1 d)(a_2 + b_2 d)}$
Multihit	$F(d) = 1 - e^{-\lambda_0 - \lambda_1 d - \ldots - \lambda_k d^k}$, $\lambda_i \geq 0$
Weibull	$F(d) = 1 - e^{-bd^k}$

the assumptions underlying its derivation (11), but its practical implementation is difficult for computational reasons. The multistage model has the same mathematic form as the one-hit model, with a polynomial in the exponent. It has been widely used. The Weibull model behaves similarly to the gamma, especially at low doses, and is a special case of multistage model.

Estimation Procedures

Estimation procedures for the parameters of the dose-response function are similar in concept for all the models. They usually follow methods to obtain maximum likelihood estimates of the parameters. Simply stated, these procedures generate values for the parameters that were most likely to have produced the observed data if the model was correct. In some instances, mathematic transformation of the models can be used with alternative estimation procedures (e.g., weighted least squares) to produce estimates with the same or similar desirable properties as maximum likelihood estimates.

After estimation of model parameters, low-dose extrapolation is generally straightforward. Two techniques for extrapolation have been advocated: (a) direct mathematic extrapolation to low doses based on estimated parameters and (b) linear extrapolation back to the estimated background response from the lowest dose modeled, regardless of the dose-response model. The linear extrapolation technique has been discussed by Gaylor and Kodell (1980) (12). Linear extrapolation resembles the one-hit model, which is linear at low doses.

A major endpoint of these analyses is the estimation of a virtually safe dose (VSD). This is a dose at which there is a small effect above control, usually in the range of 10^{-5} to 10^{-8}. Because the VSD is outside the range of experimentally obtained data, its estimation is subject to many nuances and difficulties.

Because of the relatively small number of data on which model parameter estimates are based, there is often little difference between models in the observed range. However, when the incidence over background is small, as with VSD of 10^{-5} or less, the results can be quite different. In general, the predicted dose is smallest for the one-hit and multistage models and largest for the gamma multihit and log-probit models. Typically, the Weibull and log-logistic models are intermediate. This is a rough guideline and is not infallible for all data sets.

Other Considerations in Quantitative Risk Assessment

Other major issues in carcinogenic risk assessment are time-to-event analyses and pharmacokinetics. Time-to-event analyses attempt to model the incidence of tumors as a function of the interval between exposure and appearance of the cancer. Recall that shortening of median time to tumor is an indication of chemical carcinogenesis. In a commonly used form, the probability of observing a tumor at time, t, and dose, d, is given by the equation:

$$P(d,t) = 1 - e^{-g(d)H(t)}$$

for which $H(t)$ is the cumulative hazard and $g(d)$ is the dose function. The dose function, g, can be taken to be a polynomial. In a lifetime study, $H = 1$, and the model becomes equivalent to the multistage model.

Pharmacokinetic considerations become important because of a possible nonlinear relationship between administered dose and effective dose. Based on Michaelis-Menten kinetics, the effective and administered doses are related by:

$$E = \frac{aA}{(b + A)}$$

for which E is the effective dose and A is the administered dose. More complicated relationships between these two quantities are biologically plausible. However, the quantity and quality of data do not frequently support such modeling efforts.

In practice, pharmacokinetic information is frequently used to extrapolate across animal species—that is, from rodent to human. This information can be used to correct for different routes of exposure, for example. In general, there are no widely accepted principles for using data in this way.

In summary, chemical carcinogens are substances that increase the occurrence of cancer in humans. These substances act primarily by binding covalently to DNA. In many instances, this initiation must be accompanied by a second step (promotion), which can be produced by environmental or dietary substances, continued exposure to the carcinogen, or other factors. Many chemical substances are both initiators and promoters. Extensive studies and reviews by IARC have determined that a sizable number of chemicals and processes are convincingly associated with human carcinogenesis. An even larger number of additional substances are suspected of being carcinogenic, but less convincingly so.

For the toxicologist, it is important to assess quantitatively the risk associated with specific chemical carcinogens or other suspected carcinogens. The mathematic and statistical techniques for doing so represent a compromise between analytic rigor and sufficient experimental data. Risk-assessment studies are typically performed at doses much higher than those experienced in an environmental setting. Mathematic techniques are used to extrapolate the results of such experiments back to the low levels of environmental exposure. Estimation of a "safe dose" also depends on assumptions about background incidence of the cancers being observed.

BIOMARKERS

From 1987 to the present, researchers have been developing interest in the role and use of biological markers or biomarkers in epidemiologic research. A *biological marker* can be defined as a biological indicator of exposure, effects of exposure, early disease, or of susceptibility to any of these (13). It is thought that the use of biomarkers may help researchers to enhance exposure assessment, gain insight into disease mechanisms, and become more knowledgeable about acquired and inherited susceptibility (14). One of the goals of molecular epidemiologists is to prevent disease by using biological markers to identify risks before clinical onset to allow for effective interventions (15). Major contributions have been made to the field of biomarkers and molecular biology. A brief review of these contributions to the field is presented.

To evaluate markers of internal dose and biologically effective dose (BED) of carcinogens, Perera et al. (16) conducted a pilot study to compare three complementary markers of BED of carcinogens by taking a variety of measurements on blood samples from 22 smokers and 24 nonsmokers. The BED is the amount of activated carcinogen interacting with critical cellular targets (16). The researchers investigated the relationships between each individual marker and cotinine, a highly specific biochemical marker of internal dose of active and passive cigarette smoke, and made comparisons among the three individual markers. The biological markers measured were polycyclic aromatic hydrocarbon (PAH)–DNA adducts, 4-Amino biphenyl-Hb adducts, and sister chromatid exchanges (SCEs). Benzo[a]pyrene (B[a]P) is a PAH that is found in the workplace, urban air, and drinking water (17). It is a constituent of main and sidestream cigarette smoke and a carcinogen that contributes to lung cancer in smokers and nonsmokers. 4-Amino biphenyl-Hb is a carcinogen and mutagen also found in main and sidestream cigarette smoke; it is also present in azo dyes and is a constituent in ambient air pollution. SCEs indicate chromosomal damage and are biomarkers of dose and cellular response to occupational and environmental exposure. Methods to quantify the BED would enhance the epidemiology of human carcinogenesis and improve risk extrapolation between species (16). A population of smokers was used in this study because measures of external exposure to cigarette smoke could be estimated.

B[a]P and PAH have been linked with increased risk of lung cancer in smokers and nonsmokers (18) and in occupational groups, such as foundry workers (19). Perera et al. (20) conducted a detailed occupational study among Finnish foundry workers with the intent of validating PAH-DNA adducts as markers of the BED. This population had a well-characterized occupational exposure to PAHs, and their smoking status was known. Methods to quantify the BED would enhance the epidemiology of human carcinogenesis and improve risk extrapolation between species (20). DNA adducts were found to be significantly related to B[a]P exposure. The study supported the feasibility of monitoring adduct formation in a population occupationally exposed to carcinogens.

Harris et al. (21) reviewed the literature and concluded that the primary goal of biochemical and molecular biology was to identify individuals at an increased risk of cancer before clinical manifestation of these conditions. This area of cancer research would combine epidemiologic and laboratory techniques by which biochemical and molecular epidemiologists would be able to predict disease risk in individuals rather than in populations.

Hulka and Wilcosky (22) identified issues relevant to and the rationale for the use of biological markers in epidemiologic research. The researchers intimated that the most important limitation in many epidemiologic studies was the inadequacy of accurate methods for measuring quantifying exposure variables, especially in the area of environmental epidemiology. The researchers concluded that biological markers had the potential to improve the accuracy of exposure measures and increase the validity of the results.

Schulte (23) analyzed the medical and epidemiologic literature to examine methods used for assessing genetic factors in occupational disease studies. It was found that genetic variables had often been excluded from multivariate models for evaluating disease risk factors because of the inadequacy of data collected by survey questionnaires. The researchers concluded that the role of genetics in occupational disease should be clarified to have a better understanding of the occurrence of disease. This knowledge could be used to develop appropriate intervention programs.

In another review of the literature, Schulte (24) noted that a great opportunity existed for the use of biological markers for epidemiologic research in the future. The use of biological markers in epidemiologic studies would allow for the quantification of exposure variables. However, important considerations in the use of the markers would have to be taken into account. These include how the marker is to be used in the study, the type of marker, confounding factors, sensitivity, specificity, predictive value, ethical and legal implications, and interpretation and communication of results.

Schulte and Singal (25) critically analyzed the notification and communication techniques that had been followed in notifying participants in field studies performed by National Institute for Occupational Safety and Health investigators. The evaluation was undertaken to recommend communication methods that would reduce the likelihood of misleading study participants and give meaningful interpretation to results. An example of the problems that can arise when communication of test results to study participants is unclear occurred during a pilot cytogenetic study in 1980 in the Love Canal area in Niagara Falls, New York (26). Some residents of this area were informed by the investigators that they had abnormally high numbers of chromosomal aberrations, and the study results indicated an increased risk of cancer and adverse reproductive outcomes. It was not made clear to the study participants that the prevalence of these abnormalities among the study participants was what would have been expected in the general population (26).

Environmental pollution in the highly industrialized region of Silesia in Poland has been associated with increased risk of cancer and adverse reproductive outcomes. Perera et al. (27) used a variety of biological markers to measure molecular and genetic damage in peripheral blood samples from residents from the town of Gliwice in the province of Katowice in Silesia and from residents living in Biala Podlaska, a rural, less polluted area in northeastern Poland. Results showed that environmental exposure was associated with significant increases in PAH-DNA and aromatic-DNA adducts, SCEs, and chromosomal aberrations. The researchers found that the aromatic-DNA adducts were significantly correlated with chromosomal mutation, providing a molecular link between environmental exposure and genetic alteration relevant to cancer.

Carcinogen-DNA adducts and somatic gene mutation at the hypoxanthine guanine phosphoribosyl transferase locus were evaluated in a study by Perera et al. (28), in peripheral leukocytes of workers in an iron foundry exposed to low levels of B[a]P and other PAHs. The levels of the biomarkers PAH-DNA, aromatic-DNA, and hypoxanthine guanine phosphoribosyl transferase mutation increased with exposure among the 64 workers sampled. However, the markers showed differential response to the change in exposure, depending on the individual lifetime of each biomarker. These results support a molecular link between the PAHs and somatic gene mutation and indicate the need to consider the individual lifetime of each particular biomarker.

Perera (29), in a review, reported that molecular epidemiologic research provides evidence that environmental factors are contributors to human cancer and that the risk factors can be modified by genetic susceptibility to exogenous exposures. Molecular epidemiologic studies have suggested that certain defined populations—such as very young children, those with predisposing genetic traits or nutritional deficits, and certain ethnic groups—may be more likely to have a greater risk from specific exposures than other members of the population. To have effective intervention strategies, it is important that risk assessments include data on individual variability to exposure and susceptibility.

A paper by Hulka and Margolin (30) highlighted methodologic problems related to the use of biological markers in epidemiologic research. A number of issues—including sources of misclassification, confounding, and study designs to reduce the bias—were discussed, as well as sample size estimates and validation of biomarkers. Despite the problems and the fact that the concept of using biomarkers in epidemiologic research is still relatively new, these markers could help to increase knowledge about health and disease among defined populations.

Numerous risk factors have been identified for breast cancer. Some of the risk factors are related to steroid hormones, gender, early menarche, late menopause, obesity in postmenopausal women, parity, and late age of first pregnancy. Hulka et al. (31) reviewed highlights of some of the biomarkers relevant to studies of breast cancer and precursor lesions with emphasis on those that could be hormonally induced or altered. Their conclusion was that biomarkers for breast cancer pathogenesis need to be better defined, and the risks associated with environmental exposure need to be better evaluated.

Harris et al. (32) investigated the role played by six families of activated protooncogenes in human lung cancer. Experiments on human bronchial epithelial cells *in vitro* indicated that the tumor suppressor genes play a dominant role in lung carcinogenesis. In 1991, Harris (33) reviewed the literature on the role of mutations in cancer-related genes in human and animal models. The p53 tumor suppressor gene was implicated in the majority of human cancers, and analysis of the p53 mutational spectrum in human cancer has provided evidence that both exogenous and endogenous causes of mutation contribute to human carcinogenesis. Harris (34) also observed that carcinogenesis is a multistage process involving activation of protooncogenes and inactivation of tumor suppressor genes, such as the p53 tumor suppressor gene, which is mutated in approximately 50% of almost all cancer types. These p53 mutations can help to identify particular carcinogens and define the biochemical mechanisms responsible for genetic lesions in DNA that cause human cancer. p53 Mutations can also act as a molecular dosimeter of carcinogenic exposure, thereby providing information about the molecular epidemiology of human cancer risk. A better understanding of molecular carcinogenesis and molecular epidemiology should help to improve public health decisions concerning cancer hazards.

Schulte (35) noted that occupational diseases were being assessed at the cellular and molecular level using biological markers with a greater degree of analytic sensitivity to describe events in the continuum from first exposure to clinical disease. There has been an increase in sensitivity in measuring exposures from parts per million, units of the order of 10^{-6}, to measures of dose (DNA adducts) in picomoles or femtomoles, units of the order of 10^{-12} or 10^{-15} (20). The increase in sensitivity has to be tempered with the knowledge that many factors can and do alter the appearance of biological markers. For example, not all workers with similar exposures develop diseases or markers indicative of the exposure (35). It is, therefore, of paramount importance to take into account the variation among individuals when interpreting these data. The use of biological markers in occupational health research also has clinical, legal, and ethical implications that need to be considered. Schulte (35) concluded that information from workers themselves would still be of critical importance. However, the information gleaned could be further enhanced by the effective use of markers. Schulte (36) noted that the markers could then be used to reduce misclassification of exposure, provide better interpretation of exposure-disease associations (exposure assessment is one of the weakest aspects of epidemiology), or be used in support of developing cancer intervention programs. Schulte (37) stressed that a strategy for realizing the potential of newly developed biological markers to enhance epidemiologic research was needed. This strategy could include the development of programs to encourage interdisciplinary collaboration and train molecular epidemiologists.

Biomarkers could be potentially useful when there is well-defined epidemiologic evidence of an exposure-disease association. Once the relationship has been established and replicated, it could eventually be feasible to look for the marker of exposure and thereby indicate the possible risk for developing a specific disease. When epidemiologic evidence is inconclusive about an exposure-disease relationship, biomarkers could be used to assess whether the exposure-disease relationship truly exists. Finally, when epidemiologic methods do not conclusively establish exposure-disease associations, assessment of biomarkers in a known-to-be-exposed population may contribute information concerning the risk of disease in a target population (38).

Rothman (39) noted that certain issues must be recognized when using biological markers to assess genetic susceptibility. He cautioned that exposure assessment should be given as much importance as biomarker measurement, and cases with a wide range of exposure patterns should be studied to facilitate the development and testing of hypotheses. Rothman also observed that epidemiologic studies evaluating genetic susceptibility are subject to a number of biases, including misclassification and confounding. This fact needs to be taken into account when designing studies. Finally, Rothman advocates the importance of demonstrating the biological plausibility of an observed interaction among measures of exposure, risk for disease, and genetically associated susceptibility.

The list of known carcinogens to human beings has not remained constant since 1987 (2,3). Instead, a marked improvement in ascertainment of exposure and of the response of the individual to the exposure has taken place, as well as in improved characterization of the individual. With the development of molecular epidemiology, it is sometimes possible to ascertain the dose of exposure received by the individual, observe that there are differences in individual responses to the dose, and examine individual characteristics even more closely. It is possible to medically monitor certain defined populations with regard to risk assessment, and with this ability has arisen the legal, ethical, and societal implications of such surveillance.

Shields and Harris (40) concluded that "the assessment of cancer risk in an individual and on a molecular level is currently not possible because no single genetic factor is sufficiently predictive." It is likely to change, though.

FEMALE BREAST CANCER AND ENVIRONMENTAL EXPOSURE(S)

The risk of development of breast cancer after involuntary environmental exposure to organochlorine pesticides is used here to illustrate the strengths, weaknesses, and controversy that have arisen from using biological markers to ascertain exposure dose.

King and Schottenfeld (41) argued that although increased mammography screening could have explained the increase in breast cancer incidence rates in United States during the mid-1980s, it was possible that differences in the distribution of risk factors could also have accounted for part of the increase in incidence rates during this period. These differences could have included age at menarche, age at birth of the first child, estrogen replacement therapy, and exposure to environmental organochlorines.

Wolff et al. (42) reported that even though breast cancer had been associated with endogenous hormone exposure, more attention was being focused on the environmental exposures that could be responsible for a proportion of breast cancer incidence. A number of chemicals, including pesticides and PAHs, have been shown to induce breast cancer in rodents. These results could serve as leads to studies in humans. Wolff et al. also reported that age when exposure takes place is important, and this claim has been strongly supported by data on cigarette smoking (42). It has been demonstrated that mammary tissue is more susceptible to carcinogens at certain periods of breast development.

Dunnick et al. (43) reported that breast cancer incidence rates among populations change as people migrate from one part of the world to another. This indicated that environmental exposures may contribute to the disease. Carroll (44) reported that migrant studies have shown that breast cancer incidence and mortality increase among people who move from countries with low-fat diets to those with high-fat diets. This observation indicates that geographical differences in breast cancer could be due to environmental factors in addition to genetic factors. Dunnick et al. also reported that the halogenated hydrocarbons and aromatic nitro compounds were included in a class of chemicals identified as causing mammary gland cancer in rodents in studies by the National Toxicology Program (43).

Velentgas and Daling reviewed the literature on risk factors for breast cancer in general and compared risks for younger premenopausal women with older postmenopausal women (45). Ethnicity, parity, and large body size have been associated with increased risk for younger premenopausal women, but not for older, postmenopausal women. Kelsey and Hom-Ross (46) reported that when comparing breast cancer incidence rates throughout the world, rates were highest in the North American and Northern European countries, intermediate in Southern and Eastern European and in South American countries, and lowest in African and Asian countries. The authors noted that investigation into the cause of increasing incidence rates of breast cancer in developing countries would help to understand the epidemiology of breast cancer.

Hoffman (47) reported that it had been postulated that exposure to organochlorines increases the development of breast cancer. Ahlborg et al. (48) also state that from experimental studies, evidence exists that certain organochlorine compounds may cause estrogenic effects, whereas others cause antiestrogenic effects.

Wolff et al. (49) analyzed sera from stored blood specimens of participants enrolled in the New York Women's Health Studies between 1985 and 1991. In this population of New York City women, breast cancer was strongly associated with DDE in the serum. Falck et al. (50) reported that the etiology of human breast cancer is unknown, and because risk factors such as menstrual, reproductive, and family histories account for fewer than 50% of all the cases, it is thought that the environmental halogenated hydrocarbons acting either as cocarcinogens or promoters could be involved in breast cancer research.

Djordjevic et al. (51) developed a method based on supercritical fluid extraction, column chromatography on neutral alumina, and gas chromatography with electron capture detection for the assessment of organochlorinated pesticide and polychlorinated biphenyl residues in adipose tissues. It is a quantitative method allowing for the analyses of organochlorinated compounds in specimens as small as 50 µg. Chlorinated pesticides have been quantified in drinking water, polluted air, tobacco, tobacco smoke, and in several food items (52). DDT and DDE are xenoestrogens that are known to influence estrogen-responsive tissues. Therefore, it has been hypothesized that these organochlorinated compounds contribute to the risk of breast cancer. Djordjevic et al. (53) devised a study to determine the levels of organochlorinated compounds to which cigarette smokers in the United States had been exposed. A significant correlation had been found by Mussalo-Rauhamaa et al. (54) between DDT content of human adipose tissue and smoking. The study indicated that between the late 1940s and the mid-1970s, the amounts of organochlorinated compounds deposited in adipose breast tissue of U.S. women were influenced by their personal cigarette smoking habits.

Davis (55) reviewed existing toxicologic and epidemiologic data to evaluate the role of naturally occurring carcinogens and anticarcinogens in the cause and prevention of human cancer. Davis concluded that well-designed studies using common mixtures in foods should be tested for carcinogenicity in human tissue cultures and in other animals. Such studies should examine whether the action of synthetic organic carcinogens could be inhibited by naturally occurring anticarcinogens. Skolnick and Cannon-Albright (56) reviewed the methodology in genetic analysis of predisposition to breast cancer. Familial aggregations of breast cancer susceptibility have been shown to be linked to chromosome 17q and mutations in the p53 tumor suppressor gene, as well as to familial groups exhibiting genetic susceptibility that is not due to either of the previous conditions. Skolnick and Cannon-Albright (56) concluded that these findings would help in future understanding of breast cancer predisposition at the molecular level.

Eby et al. (57) noted that epidemiologic studies have shown that families linked to *BRCA1*, the breast cancer–susceptibility gene, were more likely to have early onset of breast cancer or to have breast and ovarian cancer in the family. Different degrees of risk for breast cancer exist, depending on whether the woman affected is a first-degree relative. The problem with such an observation is that the nature of the underlying risk factor(s) is obscured, and it is impossible to tell whether the factors are due to genetics, environmental exposure, or a mixture of the two. Tumor-suppressor genes have also been implicated in hereditary cancers (58).

Weber et al. (59) wrote that because of the identification of *BRCA1* and the localization of *BRCA2*, it is imperative to assess breast cancer intervention strategies for women at risk of developing breast cancer. This is important, because there is a paucity of data on the efficacy of chemopreventive agents, and there is potential for psychosocial harm, family disruption, loss of medical insurance, and livelihood when testing for genetic susceptibility to any disease. Participants and their families need to be protected by law from some of these risks, but they also need to be counseled and made aware of the implications of informed consent before being tested for genetic susceptibility to breast cancer.

No consensus of opinion exists in epidemiologic research literature on the direction of an association between smoking and the risk of breast cancer. Ambrosone et al. (60) initiated a study that considered genetic variability and susceptibility to carcinogens in cigarette smoke. The authors hypothesized that polymorphisms in *N*-acetyl transferase (NAT) and NAT2 could result in decreased capacity to detoxify the carcinogenic aromatic amines in cigarette smoke. This could lead to an increase in susceptibility to breast cancer. The acetylator polymorphism is included in studies of cancer epidemiology, because the enzyme acts on carcinogens in compounds such as cigarette smoke (61). People who have defective acetylator enzymes are referred to as *slow acetylators* (62). The results of the study by Ambrosone et al. (60) indicated that smoking appeared to increase the risk of breast cancer among postmenopausal women who were slow acetylators. The study population consisted of pre- and postmenopausal white women in New York. Fifty-five percent of the women studied were slow acetylators, and among these, women who had begun to smoke at an early age appeared to be at an increased risk for breast cancer. These results need to be confirmed by research using additional well-designed epidemiologic studies. The data from this study suggest that some types of breast cancer could be prevented in the white female population of the United States if smoking is averted, especially from an early age.

Sondik (63) presented a paper that described the differences in incidence and mortality for breast cancer among ethnic groups in the United States. African-American and white women younger than 50 years of age have approximately the same incidence rates; however, African-American women have higher mortality rates. Elledge et al. (64) reported that breast cancer, which is a heterogeneous disease, appeared to be more aggressive in African-American women because of biological differences, such as genetic susceptibility to certain environmental exposures, hormonal levels, or interaction between both factors. Taioli et al. (65) examined the role of *CYP1A1* polymorphisms as potential molecular markers of breast cancer susceptibility in white and African-American women, because estrogens have been implicated in the initiation and promotion of breast cancer. Taioli et al. reported that a polymorphism in the *CYP1A1* gene, which is involved in estrogen metabolism, is significantly associated with breast cancer in African-American women but not in white women. Davis et al. (66) reviewed the literature on the role of estrogens and xenoestrogens in the induction of breast cancer.

Experimental evidence indicates that compounds such as the chlorinated organocompounds, polycyclic aromatic hydrocarbons, and some pharmaceutical drugs affect estrogen production and thereby function as xenoestrogens (see Chapter 27). Some xenoestrogens have been experimentally shown to induce mammary carcinogenesis. Davis et al. hypothesized that changes in exposure to xenoestrogenic substances could account for some trends in breast cancer and provide an opportunity for investigation into primary prevention strategies (66). If it can be intimated that xenoestrogens play a role in breast cancer carcinogenesis, then reducing exposure to these compounds could be viewed as a means of primary prevention of this disease. Silbergeld and Davis (67) wrote that if xenoestrogens affect pathways of hormonal metabolism, then the appropriate biomarkers of exposure may be identified and characterized.

Bradlow et al. (68) described the mechanism by which xenoestrogens could affect the development of breast cancer. Estradiol metabolism involves hydroxylation of the steroid at one of two mutually exclusive sites: C2 and C16β. This reaction results in the formation of 2-hydroxyestrone (2-OHE1) metabolite, which is weakly antiestrogenic, nongenotoxic, and inhibits breast cell proliferation (68), and also in the formation of 16β-hydroxyestrone (16β-OHE1), which is tumorigenic, genotoxic, and enhances breast cell growth (68). 16β-OHE1, a product of this metabolism, is thought to enhance breast cell growth. The authors suggest that 16β-hydroxylation is a biological marker for breast cancer risk and may act as an initiator in breast cancer. This study measured the amount of estradiol metabolized via the two pathways in the presence of a number of substances, including indole-3-carbinol and a variety of chlorinated pesticides. The chlorinated pesticides increased the ratio of 16β-OHE1 to 2-OHE1 metabolites, whereas indole-3-carbinol reduced the level of this ratio to below levels that occurred in unexposed control cells. The authors concluded that substances that increase the ratio of 16β-OHE1 to 2-OHE1 should be identified as potential breast carcinogens. It may be possible to efficiently measure assays of this ratio in women, thereby identifying women at a higher risk for breast cancer and putting in place preventive nutritional strategies and interventions.

Wolff et al. (49) found that higher serum levels of organochlorines are associated with a fourfold increase in breast cancer. Savitz (69) noted that estradiol metabolism appeared to differ among white, African-American, and Asian women. Other researchers have confirmed that among breast cancer cases, African-American and white women have higher organochlorine levels and 2 to 3 times more breast cancer than Asian women. Taioli et al. (70) reported that a polymorphism in the *CYP1A1* gene, which is involved in estrogen metabolism, is significantly associated with breast cancer in African-American women but not in white women. Taioli et al. (70) presented data that indicated that African-American women had higher 16β-OHE1 to 2-OHE1 urinary metabolite ratios than white women. Bradlow et al. (68) and Davis et al. (66) suggested that the observed differences in this ratio between the two ethnic groups could be caused by genetic factors, diet, physical activity, or environmental exposure to substances, such as dioxins and organochlorine pesticides. Taioli et al. (70) indicated that a study is being planned to investigate in detail the differences in the estrogen metabolite ratio between white and African-American women. If these results are confirmed, biomarkers for identifying groups of women at high risk for developing breast cancer for whom preventive strategies would be the most beneficial could be developed.

Michnovicz et al. (71) noted that cigarette smoking in women induced an increase in estradiol 2-hydroxylation, which led to a corresponding decrease in the competing pathway involving 16β-hydroxylation. The authors concluded that further investigation into the mechanisms of the reaction could lead to the development of strategies to reduce the risk of hormone-dependent tumors, such as breast cancer. Michnovicz and Bradlow (72) reported that an increase or decrease in estradiol 2-hydroxylation can be achieved in a number of ways; however, estradiol 16β-hydroxylation cannot be altered easily. The authors suggest that this knowledge could be used to design interventions for diseases with either too little or too much estrogen.

Michnovicz and Bradlow (73) investigated the effects of indole-3-carbinol—a compound obtained from cruciferous vegetables, such as cabbage and broccoli—on human beings. It was found that indole-3-carbinol altered the endogenous estrogen metabolism. This conclusion was drawn from the evidence of increased excretion of 2-OHE1 metabolites in urine samples. The results indicate that dietary intervention could reduce the risk of some types of cancers. Jellinck et al. (74) further found that dietary indoles induced increased synthesis in the competing pathways of 2- and 16β-hydroxylation. This mechanism reduces the levels of 16β-hydroxylation, which are able to form stable covalent adducts with estrogen receptors, thereby interfering in the mechanism of mammary carcinogenesis.

Liehr (75) reviewed the mechanism of mammary carcinogenesis, which emphasized tumor initiation by metabolic activation of estrogens in combination with cell transformation and growth stimulated by estrogen receptor–mediated processes. Estrogen receptors are almost undetectable in normal epithelial tissue, so it is believed unlikely that tumor initiation by metabolic activation of estrogens alone is the only contribution of estrogens to tumor development in the mammary gland (75). It was also found that in animal models, synthetic estrogens with extremely potent hormonal activity have been identified that were found to be weakly tumorigenic (76). It was concluded that hormonal potency and carcinogenic activity are separate characteristics of estrogens and are not inherently linked. It was also concluded that hormonal activity of estrogens was a necessary but not sufficient cause for tumor induction to occur (75).

Liehr (75) also reviewed the hormonal potency of catecholestrogen metabolites and their potential for inducing DNA damage during estrogen-induced tumorigenesis. The prevention of breast cancer initiation by interfering in the metabolic activation of estrogens is believed possible (75). A prevention strategy had been studied in the hamster kidney model (76). Ascorbic acid is thought to have inhibited kidney carcinogenesis by interfering in the metabolism of estrogen. Liehr intimated that ascorbic acid and vitamin C could play a role in the prevention of breast cancer and that the role of diet in the prevention of breast cancer had been indicated in other epidemiologic studies (56).

If specific biomarkers that identify the extent of biologically available exposure could be validated, then the ability to predict which women would be at highest risk for breast cancer will be greatly enhanced. However, many ethical problems are involved in pursuing this course of action. Weber et al. (59) have reviewed the potential risks of testing for genetic susceptibility. Lin (62) wrote that lawmakers are investigating methods of ensuring safe and ethical use of tests for *BRCA1* gene mutators. If a familial risk for breast cancer exists, Eby et al. (57) argue that this observation does not clarify the true nature of the underlying risk factors, which could be genetic or otherwise. Malkin and Friend (58) warned that the ethical and psychosocial implications of being able to use biomarkers should be considered before embarking on this line of investigation. Wolff (77) has intimated that damage to genetic material is not necessarily associated with disease. Therefore, researchers must understand the behavior of the marker that they are trying to quantify, why it is to be quantified, what the marker actually measures, what the result means, and how it should be communicated to a study participant. Schulte and Singal (25) reported that biomarkers should only be used in epidemiologic studies when validation studies—including measurements of sensitivity, specificity, and positive and negative predictive values—have been completed. In conclusion, biomarkers must be thoroughly evaluated through methodologic research before they are incorporated into epidemiologic studies (78,79). Selected contributions to this area of research are summarized in chronologic sequence in Table 24-4.

TABLE 24-4. Selected contributions to biomarker research

Year	Primary author	Study subjects [nos.] and exposures	Biological materials	Markers of exposure (E), response (R), susceptibility (S)	Known/suspected carcinogens	Target organ/system	Impact on future research
1987	Harris et al. (21)	Women and men occupationally exposed to PAHs	Cells and tissues, blood sera	PAH-DNA adducts (E)	Polycyclic aromatic hydrocarbons	Lung	Indicated primary goal of biochemical and molecular epidemiology is to predict disease in high-risk individuals instead of populations and to do this before onset of clinically manifest disease
1987	Perera et al. (16)	Female [12] and male [10] smokers, female [12] and male [12] nonsmokers	Blood samples	PAH-DNA adducts (E), 4-ABP-Hb adducts (E), sister chromatid exchanges (E, R)	B[a]P, 4-ABP	Lung	Markers needed to detect and quantify exposure to carcinogens resulting from environmental exposures
1988	Perera et al. (20)	Volunteer female and male workers in Finnish iron foundry occupationally exposed to PAHs [35] and their unexposed controls [10]	Blood samples	Aromatic DNA adducts (E)	Occupational exposure to PAHs	Leukocytes	Postlabeling assays need to be incorporated into studies of exposure to known or suspect carcinogens
1992	Perera et al. (27)	Residents of region of Poland exposed to environmental pollution	Blood samples	PAH-DNA and aromatic adducts (E), chromosomal aberrations (E), sister chromatid exchanges (E, R), doubling in frequency of *ras* oncogene overexpression (E)	Carcinogens in environmental air pollution	Associated with increased risk of cancer and adverse reproductive outcomes	Molecular link between environmental exposure and genetic alteration pertaining to cancer and reproductive risk
1994	Perera et al. (28)	Female [13] and male [51] foundry workers exposed to B[a]P and other PAHs	Leukocytes	PAH-DNA adducts (E), aromatic DNA (E), hypoxanthine guanine, phosphoribosyl, transferase mutation (E)	B[a]P and other PAHs	Leukocytes, lymphocytes	Suggests a molecular link between somatic gene mutation and exposure to PAHs
1995	Bradlow et al. (68)	Effect of organochlorine pesticides on estradiol metabolism	Urine	1 β-Hydroxylation (E)	—	Breast	Ratio of 16β-hydroxyestrone to 2 hydroxyestrone may provide a marker for breast cancer risk
1995	Taioli et al. (65)	51 women with breast cancer [21 African-American, 30 white] and 269 female controls [86 African-American, 183 white]	Blood samples	Polymorphism in *CYP1A1* gene, which is involved in estrogen metabolism (E, S)	—	Breast	Elevated frequency of the homozygous MspI polymorphism among African-American women with breast cancer
1996	Taioli et al. (70)	White [15] and African-American [18] women ages 18–73 years	Urine	16β-OHE½-OHE1, urinary metabolite ratio (E)	—	Breast	Ratio higher among African-American women than white women

ABP, amino biphenyl; B[a]P, benzo[a]pyrene; PAH, polycyclic aromatic hydrocarbon.
From refs. 85–87, with permission.

CAUTIONARY NOTE

A *sentinel health event* can be defined as a rare disease appearing in an unlikely place at an unusual time, a disability, or an untimely death, the occurrence of which should serve as a warning signal (80). Occurrence of a sentinel health event is an indication that an individual has had contact with a hazardous environmental exposure and that some action (an investigation or analysis) should be taken by the authorities. Hepatic angiosarcoma (HAS) in humans was first associated with exposure to polyvinyl chloride in Louisville, Kentucky, in a vinyl chloride polymerization plant (81). Early in 1974, a plant physician reported several cases of the rare disease to the authorities (82). This disease was so rare in humans that a single case was sufficient to be recognized as a sentinel health event. Ten cases of HAS were eventually reported from the same plant (81). Epidemiologic studies at that plant and other polyvinyl chloride polymerization plants identified vinyl chloride monomer as the causative agent. Experimental studies in early 1974 confirmed vinyl chloride monomer as a hepatic carcinogen capable of producing HAS and other tumors (82).

Breast cancer among women does not fit the usual definition of a sentinel health event. It is not a rare occurrence when compared with the preceding example. The disease has many previously identified and likely subsequently to be identified risk factors, some of which may be modifiable. It is in this latter context that breast cancer among females may be viewed as a "clarion disease," because its multifactorial etiology with defined population differences in exposure, response, and susceptibility has served as a call to action in the scientific pursuit of an improved understanding of carcinogenesis, mutagenesis, and genotoxicity.

An area of specific interest has been that of assessing the role that environmental chemicals might play in the synergistic activation of estrogen receptor (83). Findings by Arnold et al. (83) stimulated considerable interest and scientific debate. However, their report has been formally withdrawn (84). Thus, this cautionary note is offered for our readers' consideration. We must continue our scientific pursuits as they relate to chemical and environmental carcinogenesis, with the commitment to replication and verification exemplified by these investigators (83,84).

REFERENCES

1. Pott, P. *Chirurgical observations relative to the cataract, the polypus of the nose, the cancer of the scrotum, the different kinds of rupture, and the mortification of the toes and feet*. London: Hawkes, Clarke, and Collins, 1775.
2. IARC. Overall evaluations of carcinogenicity to humans as evaluated in IARC Monographs volumes 1 to 77. http://193.51.164.11/monoeval/crthall.html, 2000.
3. Ninth Report on Carcinogens. U.S. Department of Health and Human Services, Public Health Service, National Toxicology Program, 2000.
4. Miller EC, Miller JA. The presence and significance of bound amino azo dyes in the livers of rats fed *p*-dimethylaminoazobenzene. *Cancer Res* 1947;7:468.
5. Miller EC. Studies on the formation of protein-bound derivatives of 3,4-benzopyrene in the epidermal fraction of mouse skin. *Cancer Res* 1951;11:100.
6. Miller JA, Cramer JW, Miller EC. The n- and ring-hydroxylation of 2-acetylaminofluorene during carcinogenesis in the rat. *Cancer Res* 1960;20:950.
7. Nagta C, Kodama M, Ioki Y, Kimura T. Free radicals produced from chemical carcinogens and their significance in carcinogenesis. In: Floyd RA, ed. *Free radicals and cancer.* New York: Marcel Dekker Inc, 1982:1.
8. Wattenberg LW. Inhibition of chemical carcinogenesis. *J Natl Cancer Inst* 1978;60:11.
9. Rous P, Kidd JG. Conditional neoplasms and subthreshold neoplastic states. *J Exp Med* 1941;73:365.
10. Food Safety Council. Quantitative risk assessment. proposed system for food safety assessment. Washington: Food Safety Council, 1980b:137–160.
11. Rai K, van Ryzin J. Risk assessment of toxic environmental substances using a generalized multi-hit dose response model. In: Breslow NE, Whittemore AS. *Energy and health.* Philadelphia: Society for Industrial and Applied Mathematics, 1979:99–117.
12. Gaylor DW, Kodell RL. Linear interpolation algorithm for low dose risk assessment of toxic substances. *J Environ Pathol Toxicol* 1980;4:305–312.
13. National Research Council. Biological environmental health research. *Environ Health Perspect* 1987;74:1–191.
14. Rothman N, Stewart WF, Schulte PA. Incorporating biomarkers into cancer epidemiology: a matrix of biomarker and study design categories. *Cancer Epidemiol Biomarkers Prev* 1995;4(4):301–311.
15. Perera FP, Weinstein IB. Molecular epidemiology and carcinogen DNA adduct detection. New approaches to studies of human cancer causation. *J Chronic Dis* 1982;3:581–600.
16. Perera FP, Santella RM, Brenner D, et al. DNA adducts, protein adducts and sister chromatid exchange in cigarette smokers and nonsmokers. *J Natl Cancer Inst* 1987;79(3):449–456.
17. International Agency on Research for Cancer. Polynuclear aromatic compounds. Chemical, environmental and experimental data. *IARC Monogr Eval Carcinog Risk Chemicals in Humans* 1983;32(Pt 1):1–453.
18. International Agency on Research for Cancer. Tobacco smoking. *IARC Monogr Eval Carcinog Risks Chem Hum* 1986;38:35–394.
19. International Agency on Research for Cancer. Polynuclear aromatic hydrocarbons. *IARC Monogr Eval Carcinog Risk Chem Hum* 1984;34(Pt 3).
20. Perera FP, Hemmonshi K, Yaina TL, Brenner D, Kelly G, Santella RM. Detection of polycyclic hydrocarbon DNA adducts in white blood cells of foundry workers. *Cancer Res* 1988;48(8):2288–2291.
21. Harris CC, Weston A, Wiley JC, Trivers GE, Mann DL. Biochemical and molecular epidemiology of human cancers, indicators of carcinogen exposure, DNA damage and genetic predisposition. *Environ Health Perspect* 1987;75:109–119.
22. Hulka BS, Wilcosky T. Biological markers in epidemiologic research. *Arch Environ Health* 1988;43:83–89.
23. Schulte PA. Simultaneous assessment of genetic and occupational risk factors. *J Occup Med* 1987;29:884–891.
24. Schulte PA. Methodologic issues the use of biologic markers in epidemiologic research. *Am J Epidemiol* 1987;126:1006–1016.
25. Schulte PA, Singal M. Interpretation and communication of the results of medical field investigations. *J Occup Med* 1988;31:589–594.
26. Wolff S. Love Canal revisited. *JAMA* 1984;251:1464.
27. Perera FP, Hemminki K, Gryzbowska L, et al. Molecular and genetic damage in humans from environmental pollution in Poland. *Nature* 1992;360:256–258.
28. Perera FP, Orchey C, Santella R, et al. Carcinogen-DNA adducts and gene mutation in foundry workers with low-level exposure to polycyclic aromatic hydrocarbons. *Carcinogenesis* 1994;15:2905–2910.
29. Perera FP. Molecular epidemiology insights into cancer susceptibility risk assessment and prevention. *J Natl Cancer Inst* 1996;88:496–509.
30. Hulka BS, Margolin BH. Methodological issues in epidemiologic studies using biomarkers. *Am J Epidemiol* 1992;135:200–209.
31. Hulka BS, Liu ET, Liniger RA. Steroid hormones and the risk of breast cancer. *Cancer* 1994;74[Suppl 3]:1111–1124.
32. Harris CC, Reddel R, Pfeifer A, et al. Role of oncogenes and tumor suppressor genes in human lung carcinogenesis. *IARC Sci Publ* 1991a;105:294–304.
33. Harris CC. Molecular basis of multi-stage carcinogenesis. *Princess Takamatsu Symp* 1991b;22:3–19.
34. Harris CC. Deichmann lecture. *p53* tumor suppression gene: at the crossroads of molecular carcinogenesis, molecular epidemiology and cancer risk assessment. *Toxicol Lett* 1995;82,83:1–7.
35. Schulte PA. Contribution of biological markers to occupational health. *Am J Ind Med* 1991;20:435–446.
36. Schulte PA. Biomarkers in epidemiology: scientific issues and ethical implications. *Environ Health Perspect* 1992;98:143–147.
37. Schulte PA. Use of biological markers in occupational health research and practice. *J Toxicol Environ Health* 1993;40:359–366.
38. Schulte PA. Opportunities for the development and use of biomarkers. *Toxicol Lett* 1995;77:25–29.
39. Rothman N. Genetic susceptibility biomarkers in studies of occupational and environmental cancer: methodologic issues. *Toxicol Lett* 1995;77:221–225.
40. Shields PJ, Harris CC. Molecular epidemiology and the genetics of environmental cancer. *JAMA* 1991;266:681–687.
41. King SE, Schottenfeld D. The "epidemic" of breast cancer in the US—determining factors. *Oncology* 1996;10:453–462. [Discussion 462, 464, 470–472]
42. Wolff MS, Collman GW, Barnett JC, Huff J. Breast cancer and environmental risk factors: epidemiological and experimental findings. *Ann Rev Pharmacol Toxicol* 1996;36:573–596.
43. Dunnick JK, Elwell MR, Huff J, Barrett JC. Chemically induced mammary gland cancer in the National Toxicology Program's carcinogenesis bioassay. *Carcinogenesis* 1995;16:173–179.
44. Carroll KK. Dietary fat and breast cancer. *Lipids* 1992;27:793–797.
45. Velentgas P, Daling JR. Risk factors for breast cancer in younger women. *J Natl Cancer Inst Monogr* 1996;(16):15–24.
46. Kelsey JL, Hom-Ross PL. Breast cancer: magnitude of the problem and descriptive epidemiology. *Epidemiol Rev* 1993;15:7–16.
47. Hoffman W. Organochlorine compounds: risk of non-Hodgkin's lymphoma and breast cancer? *Arch Environ Health* 1996;51:189–192.
48. Ahlborg US, Lipworth L, Titus-Ernstoff L, et al. Organochlorine compounds in relation to breast cancer, endometrial cancer, and endometriosis: an assessment of biological and epidemiological evidence. *Crit Rev Toxicol* 1995;25:463–531.
49. Wolff MS, Toniolo PS, Lee EW, Rivera M, Dubon N. Blood levels of organochlorine residues and risk of breast cancer. *J Natl Cancer Inst* 1993;85:648–652.
50. Falck F, Ricci A Jr, Wolff MS, Godbold J, Dechers P. Pesticides and polychlorinated biphenyl residues in human breast lipids and their relation to breast cancer. *Arch Environ Health* 1992;47:163–166.

51. Djordjevic MV, Hoffman D, Fan J, Prokopczyk B, Citron ML, Stellman SD. Assessment of chlorinated pesticides and polychlorinated biphenyls in adipose breast tissue using a supercritical fluid extraction method. *Carcinogenesis* 1994;15:2581–2585.
52. International Agency for Research on Cancer. DDT and associated compounds. *IARC Monogr Eval Carcinog Risk Hum* 1991;53:179–249.
53. Djordjevic MC, Fan J, Hoffman D. Assessment of chlorinated residues in cigarette tobacco based on supercritical fluid extraction and GE-ECD. *Carcinogenesis* 1995;16:2627–2632.
54. Mussalo-Rauhamaa H, Pyysalo H, Moilanen R. Influence of diet and other factors. *J Toxicol Environ Health* 1984;13:689–704.
55. Davis DL. Natural anti-carcinogens, carcinogens, and changing patterns in cancer: some speculation. *Environ Res* 1989;50:322–340.
56. Skolnick MH, Cannon-Albright LA. Genetic predisposition to breast cancer. *Cancer* 1992;70[Suppl 6]:1747–1754.
57. Eby N, Chang-Claude J, Bishop DT. Familial risk and genetic susceptibility for breast cancer. *Cancer Causes Control* 1994;5:458–470.
58. Malkin D, Friend SH. Screening for susceptibility in children. *Curr Opin Pediatr* 1994;5:46–51.
59. Weber BL, Giusti RM, Liu ET. Developing strategies for intervention and prevention in hereditary breast cancer. *J Natl Cancer Inst Monogr* 1995;17:99–102.
60. Ambrosone CB, Freudenheim JL, Graham S, et al. Cigarette smoking, *N*-acetyltransferase 2 genetic polymorphisms, and breast cancer risk. *JAMA* 1996;276:1494–1501.
61. International Agency for Research on Cancer, World Health Organization. Chemistry and analysis of tobacco smoke in tobacco smoking. *IARC Monogr Eval Carcinog Risk Chem Hum* 1996;38:83–126.
62. Lin HJ. Smokers and breast cancer: "chemical individuality" and cancer predisposition. *JAMA* 1996;27b:1511–1512.
63. Sondik EJ. Breast cancer trends: incidence, mortality and survival. *Cancer* 1994;74[Suppl 3]:995–999.
64. Elledge RM, Clark GM, Chamness GC, Osborne CK. Tumor biologic factors and breast cancer prognosis among white, Hispanic, and black women in the United States. *J Natl Cancer Inst* 1994;86:705–712.
65. Taioli E, Trachman J, Chen X, Toniolo P, Garte SJ. A CYP1A1 restriction fragment length polymorphism is associated with breast cancer in African-American women. *Cancer Res* 1995;55:3757–3758.
66. Davis DL, Bradlow HL, Wolff M, Woodruff T, Hoel DA, Anton-Culver H. Medical hypothesis: xeno-estrogens as preventable causes of breast cancer. *Environ Health Perspect* 1993;101:372–377.
67. Silbergeld EK, Davis DL. Role of biomarkers in identifying and understanding environmentally induced disease. *Clin Chem* 1994;40(Pt 2):1363–1367.
68. Bradlow HL, Davis DL, Lin A, Sepkovic DW, Tiwan R. Effects of pesticides on the ratio of 16 alpha/2-hydroxyestrone: a biologic marker of breast cancer risk. *Environ Health Perspect* 1995;103[Suppl 7]:147–150.
69. Savitz DA. Breast cancer and serum organochlorines: a prospective study among white, black, and Asian women. *J Natl Cancer Inst* 1994;86:1256.
70. Taioli E, Garte SJ, Trachman J, et al. Ethnic differences in estrogen metabolism in healthy women. *J Natl Cancer Inst* 1996;86:617.
71. Michnovicz JJ, Hershcopf RJ, Naganuma H, Bradlow HL, Fishman J. Increased 2-hydroxylation of estradiol as a possible mechanism for the anti-estrogenic effect of cigarette smoking. *N Engl J Med* 1986;315:1305–1309.
72. Michnovicz JJ, Bradlow HL. Dietary and pharmacological control of estradiol metabolism in humans. *Ann N Y Acad Sci* 1990;595:291–299.
73. Michnovicz JJ, Bradlow HL. Altered estrogen metabolism and excretion in human beings following consumption of indole-3-carbinol. *Nutr Cancer* 1991;16:59–66.
74. Jellinck PH, Forhort PA, Riddick DS, Okey AB, Michnovizc JJ, Bradlow HL. Ah receptor bonding properties of indole carbinols and induction of hepatic estradiol hydroxylation. *Biochem Pharmacol* 1993;45:1129–1136.
75. Liehr JG. Dual role of estrogens as hormones and procarcinogens: tumor initiation by metabolic activation of estrogens. *Eur J Cancer Prev* 1997;6(1):3–10.
76. Liehr JG, Wheeler WJ. Inhibition of estrogen-reduced renal carcinogen in Syrian hamsters by vitamin C. *Cancer Res* 1983:43:4638–4644.
77. Wolff S. Problems and prospects in the utilization of cytogenetics to estimate exposure at toxic chemical waste dumps. *Environ Health Perspect* 1985;48:25–27.
78. Nauman CH, Griffith J, Blancato JN, Aldrich TE. Biomarkers in environmental epidemiology. In: Cooke C, ed. *Environmental epidemiology and risk assessment*. New York: Van Nostrand Reinhold 1993;152–181.
79. Schulte PA, Perera FP, eds. *Molecular epidemiology: principles and practices*. San Diego, CA: Academic Press Inc, 1993.
80. Rothwell CJ, Hamilton CB, Leaverton PE. Identification of sentinel health events as indicators of environmental contamination. *Environ Health Perspect* 1991;94:261–263.
81. Falk H. Vinyl chloride induced hepatic angiosarcoma. *Princess Takamatsu Symp* 1987;18:39–46.
82. Dannaher CL, Tamburro CH, Yam LT. Occupational carcinogenesis: the Louisville exposure with vinyl chloride–associated hepatic angiosarcoma. *Am J Med* 1981;70:279–287.
83. Arnold SF, Klotz DM, Collins BM, Vonier PM, Guillette LJ Jr, McLachlan JA. Synergistic activation of estrogen receptor with combinations of environmental chemicals. *Science* 1986;272:1489–1492.
84. McLachlan JA. Synergistic effect of environmental estrogens: report withdrawn. *Science* 1997;277:462–463.
85. Šrám RJ. Effect of glutathione s-transferase M1 polymorphisms on biomarkers of exposure and effects. *Environ Health Perspect* 1998;106(Suppl 1):231–239.
86. Bearer CF. Biomarkers in pediatric environmental health: a cross-cutting issue. *Environ Health Perspect* 1998;106(Suppl 3):813–816.
87. Autrup H, Daneshvar B, Dragsted L, et al. Biomarkers for exposure to ambient air pollution: comparison of carcinogen-DNA adduct levels with other exposure markers and markers for oxidative stress. *Environ Health Perspect* 1999;107:233–238.

CHAPTER 25
Clinical Immunotoxicology and Allergy

John B. Sullivan, Jr., Bradford O. Brooks, and William J. Meggs

The immune apparatus is an intricate homeostatic system that plays a crucial role in striking a delicate balance between health and disease. Immunity is maintained via a series of complex, highly regulated, multicellular, and physiologic mechanisms designed to accomplish a singular goal: to differentiate *self* from *nonself*. Nonspecific (innate) and specific (adaptive) mechanisms are deployed through a network of blood and lymphatic vessels and lymphoid organs. *Immunotoxicity* is defined as the adverse effect of an inappropriate immune response, induced directly or indirectly, by a xenobiotic (pharmacologic agents, environmental and occupational contaminants, or biologicals) or physical agent. This adverse effect is generally immunosuppression or immunostimulation (Fig. 25-1).

Immunity is divided into nonspecific and specific immunity. Nonspecific immune defense mechanisms include (1) mechanical

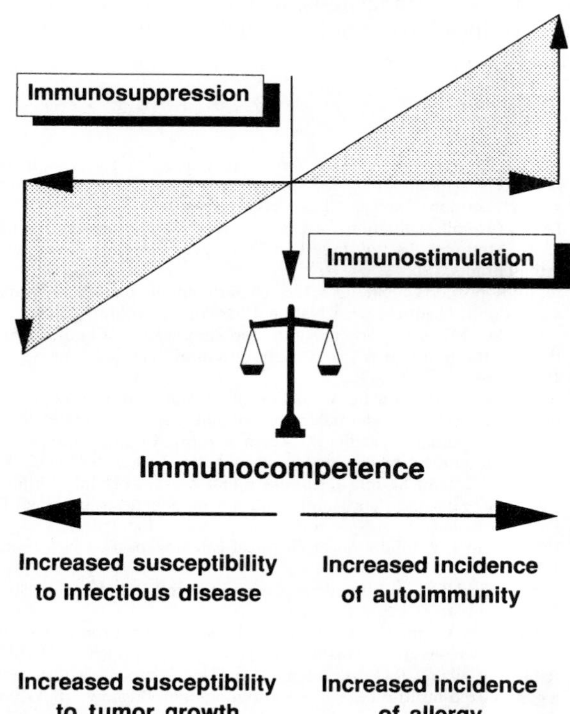

Figure 25-1. Immunocompetence.

constraints, such as epithelial and mucosal barriers and associated lymphoid tissue that maintain the physical/chemical barrier found in the skin and mucous membranes; (2) natural killer cells, macrophages, and polymorphonuclear cells that mediate nonspecific immune responses and inflammation; and (3) secreted chemical products and humoral mediators of protection.

In healthy individuals, nonspecific resistance is always operative, and is incapable of distinguishing between self and nonself. It cannot increase response intensity on reexposure. Nonspecific resistance mechanisms have evolved to respond quickly to a broad spectrum of hazards, relying on specific immune mechanisms for backup.

Unlike nonspecific immunity, specific immune mechanisms are silent until evoked by a specific agent. Although much remains to be discovered and mechanistically defined, seven distinguishing characteristics of the immune system are responsible for its unique effectiveness:

1. *Specificity*: Resistance to disease was known to be specific long before our current understanding of the immune system. Immune reactions can discriminate between even closely related molecules (1).
2. *Collaboration*: The nature of cell-cell and cell-cytokine (humoral cell product) collaboration in antibody formation and cell-mediated responses has been described in detail (2). Collaboration of lymphocytes with cell products such as antibody or cytokines and nonlymphoid cells allows for an optimized, maximally effective immune response.
3. *Clonal expansion*: Although millions of functional immune cells—sessile or in circulation—are ready to participate in an immune response, only a few cells are capable of recognizing a specific antigen at any one time. After antigen-specific recognition, these selected cells immediately progress into a blastogenic phase, cloning themselves. This expansion allows for an amplified and effective immune response.
4. *Differentiation*: Lymphocytes, when activated by antigen recognition, begin to synthesize new RNA, get larger, and secrete proteins, such as lymphokines and antibodies. These proteins account for the majority of phenomena typically associated with immunity. A subset of these differentiated cells develop into long-lived memory cells.
5. *Mobility*: The cells and effector molecules of specific and nonspecific resistance mechanisms must disseminate throughout the body to be effective. The mobility of these elements also accounts for local immune interactions, which often result in systemic effects.
6. *Memory*: Once an antigen (molecule not recognized as self) has elicited an immune response, specific elements of the immune apparatus are forever changed. Usually, future encounters with the same antigen result in an augmented response (positive memory). In other cases, a second encounter with the same antigen results in a diminished response or acquired tolerance (negative memory). Together, specificity and memory are criteria used to distinguish between immunologic and nonimmunologic responses.
7. *Regulation*: The time of onset, intensity, humoral/cellular participants, and duration of an effective immune response must be carefully controlled. Most responses of the immune system represent a balance between up-regulatory and down-regulatory circuits. Many of the known immunopathologic disease processes are thought to result from defects in immune regulation.

Specific immunity is subdivided into humoral and cellular limbs (Fig. 25-2). In the humoral limb, B lymphocytes are the pivotal cell, whereas in the cellular limb, T lymphocytes are the central participant. Originating from the bone marrow, B lymphocytes mature into plasma cells that produce immunoglobulins, which bind antigens through variable region combining sites. Antibody produced by mature B lymphocytes can only recognize a single antigenic specificity. Diversity in antibody specificity results from somatic recombination of genes affecting different regions of the immunoglobulin molecule. After antibody binding of antigen, antigen-antibody complexes are cleared with the help of complement and macrophages.

In contrast to antibody, T lymphocytes recognize small antigenic sequences of amino acids, but only when they are presented by the gene products of the major histocompatibility complex (MHC). T lymphocytes recognize antigen only when presented in the context of self-MHC; this phenomenon is referred to as *MHC restriction*. T cells are often found to recognize antigenic determinants deep within the interior of antigens that are not freely accessible on the surface. This feat is caused by the processing performed by antigen-presenting cells (APCs), with subsequent presentation of degraded antigen in conjunction with self-MHC to the T cells.

ANATOMIC COMPONENTS OF THE IMMUNE SYSTEM

The human body has two types of immune defenses—*innate* and *adaptive*—that work together to provide defense against adverse challenges. Innate immunity is nonspecific and is present from birth in all individuals (Table 25-1). Two broad mechanisms of innate immunity are inflammation and phagocytosis. Innate immunity is the first defense against external challenging agents by nonspecific mechanisms that do not discriminate. Innate immunity consists of the skin barrier, mucous membranes, lysozymes and other defense mechanisms of the mucosal surfaces of the body, acidity of the stomach, tears from the eyes, cilia motion and mucous barrier of the respiratory tract, skin lactic acid, and saturated fatty acids. Adaptive immunity, on the other hand, is acquired and developed after an individual is specifically challenged.

Lymphoid organs are divided in two broad categories based on their function: (a) primary lymphoid organs and (b) secondary lymphoid organs (Table 25-2, Fig. 25-3). Primary lymphoid organs are the sites of antigen-independent differentiation of lymphocytes. They are areas in which cells are protected from interaction with antigen, so they can mature and be released into the general circulation, then migrate to secondary lymphoid organs. The primary lymphoid organs are more centralized:

- Bone marrow
- Fetal liver
- Thymus

Secondary lymphoid organs are more peripheral. They are sites of antigen-dependent activation in which differentiation of the immune cells occurs:

- Spleen
- Lymph nodes
- Mucosal-associated lymphoid tissue (MALT) and bronchial-associated lymphoid tissue (BALT)

Secondary lymphoid organs located throughout the body trap antigens and provide a network for lymphocyte and antigen interactions and the immune response. Another organized response of the immune system is the reticuloendothelial system. This system is located in secondary lymphoid organs and forms a network through which lymphatic fluid and blood pass.

The bone marrow, the site of blood cell production, contains pluripotent stem cells that can develop into either lymphoid or

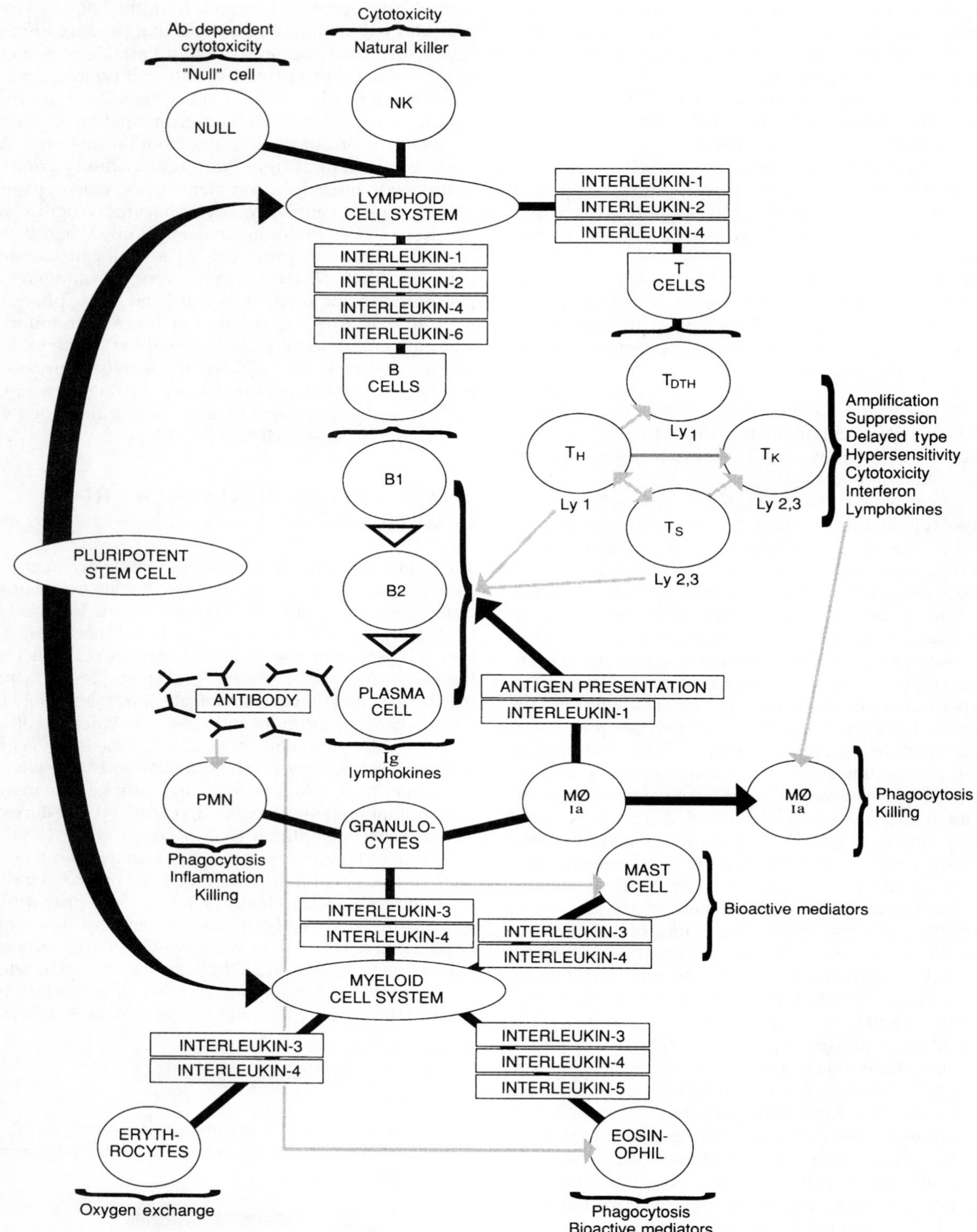

Figure 25-2. The immune system.

myeloid lines. The bone marrow also serves as a secondary lymphoid organ.

Thymus

The thymus is a primary lymphoid organ. Fetal lymphocytes migrate to the thymus, which is located in the anterior mediastinum. The thymus reaches maximum size in puberty, then atrophies. This process is called *thymic involution* and is accelerated by corticosteroids. The thymus is divided into lobules separated by connective tissue. Each lobule has an outer cortex and an inner medulla (Fig. 25-4). Pre–T lymphocytes migrate from the bone marrow and enter the thymic cortex. As they mature, they enter the medulla, in which they further mature. T cells in the outer cor-

TABLE 25-1. Components of the nonspecific immune response

Mucosal barrier epithelial cells
Polymorphonuclear leukocytes
Eosinophils
Mast cells
Basophils
Platelets
Mononuclear phagocyte system
Mucosal defenses
Complement system
Acute-phase reactants
Inflammation
Enzymes
Vasoactive amines
Phagocytosis

tex are immature and divide frequently. More mature T cells are found in the inner medulla areas. After maturation, these T cells move into the circulatory system and lymphatic system.

Thymosin is a thymic hormone that acts on T cells at different stages of development. Thymopoietin also helps induce T-cell maturation. Other serum thymic factors produce expression of clusters of deviation (CD) markers on lymphocyte cell membranes.

Lymph Nodes

Lymph nodes are secondary lymphoid organs in which antigen-dependent immune responses occur. All secondary lymphoid organs have similar characteristics anatomically (see Fig. 25-4). Each has a special port of entry and discrete areas to which the B lymphocytes and T lymphocytes migrate. Each has a tissue architecture, allows trapping of antigens, and allows a proficient lymphocyte antigen interaction.

Lymph nodes are encapsulated and are located throughout the body. Lymph nodes are composed of an outer cortex and an inner medulla. The cortex contains follicles to which B cells migrate and a paracortical area to which T cells migrate. Follicles are classified as primary or secondary. Primary follicles are aggregates of small B lymphocytes. On stimulation, a primary lymph node follicle transforms into a secondary follicle.

The secondary follicle contains a germinal center with small and large lymphocytes, blast cells, macrophages, and dendritic cells. The outer zone of the germinal center contains small lymphocytes.

The paracortex area is a mixture of lymphocytes and contains a predominant number of small T lymphocytes with APCs. The medulla contains sinuses and cords that contain plasma cells and larger lymphocytes.

Lymph nodes are generally located at the junctions of lymphatic vessels around the body. The lymph nodes drain and filter fluid. They consist of a series of sinusoids. These sinusoids are located throughout the lymph nodes that the lymph fluid first travels through; the lymph fluid then leaves by efferent lymphatic vessels entering back into the venous system by the thoracic duct. Antigens that enter lymph nodes in the lymphatic circulation are

TABLE 25-2. Primary and secondary lymphoid organs

Primary lymphoid organs	Secondary lymphoid organs
Thymus	Spleen
Bursa of fabricius (avian)	Lymph nodes
Fetal liver (mammal)	Gut-associated lymphoid tissue
Adult bone marrow	

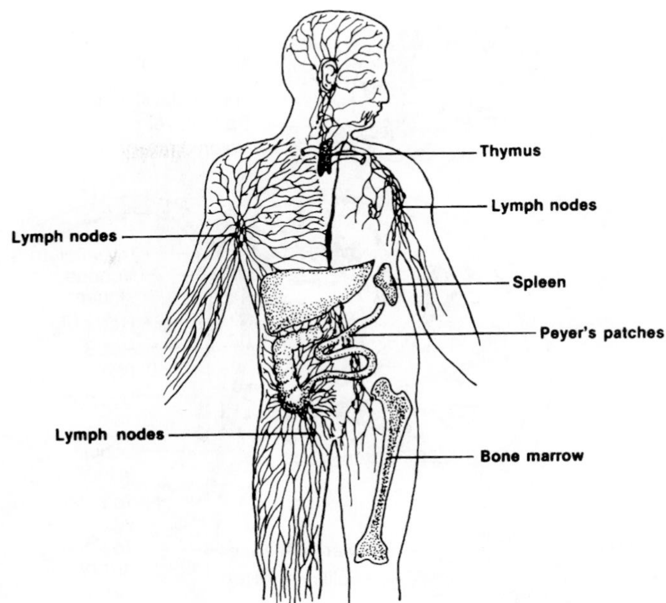

Figure 25-3. Primary and secondary lymphoid organs. (Courtesy of the Agency for Toxic Substances Disease Registry, Office of Technology Assessment, 1991.)

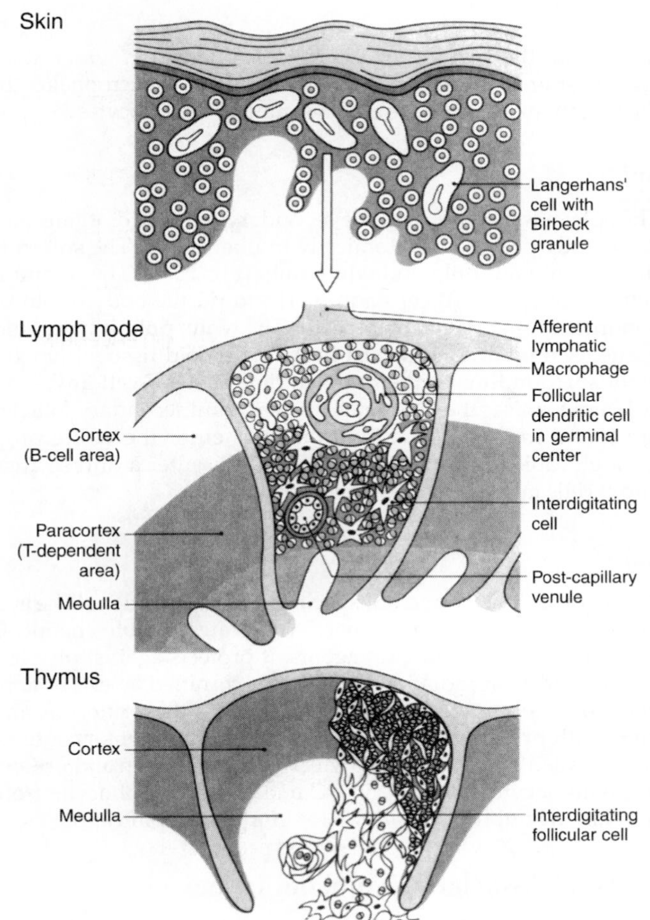

Figure 25-4. Lymphoid organs: skin, lymph nodes, thymus. (From Roitt I, Brostoff J, Male D. *Immunology.* St. Louis: C.V. Mosby/Gower Publishing Co, 1985.)

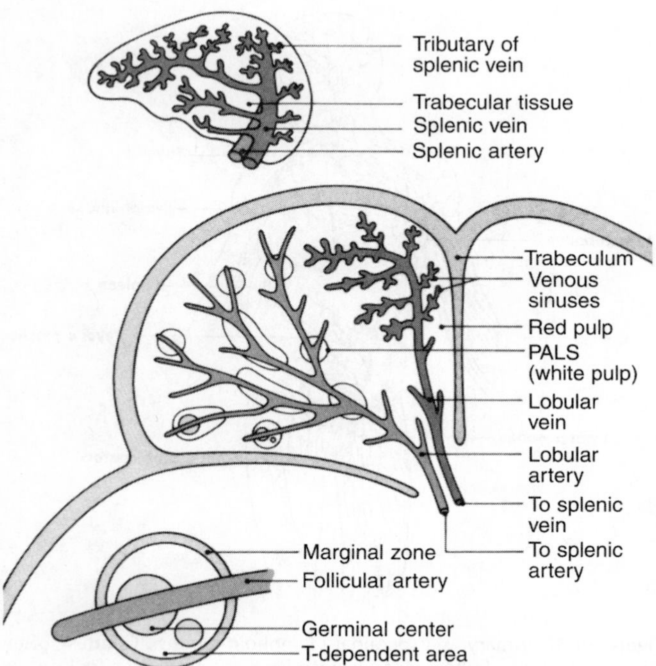

Figure 25-5. Spleen. PALS, periarteriolar lymphocyte sheath. (From Roitt I, Brostoff J, Male D. *Immunology.* St. Louis: C.V. Mosby/Gower Publishing Co, 1985.)

trapped in the lymph node–meshed network, in which they encounter immune cells and can be engulfed by macrophages. In the lymph nodes, antigens are presented to lymphocytes.

Spleen

The spleen is the largest of the secondary lymphoid organs and is specially designed anatomically to filter blood. The spleen is divided into red pulp and white pulp (Fig. 25-5). The red pulp consists of red blood cells and works to rid the body of old or abnormally shaped red blood cells. The white pulp is lymphoid tissue. Central arterioles exist in the lymphoid tissue. Immediately surrounding the central arteriole is the T-cell area, and adjacent to this is the B-cell area. Primary and secondary follicles are found in the spleen. Lymphocytes enter the white pulp through capillaries. The T cells and B cells enter a diffuse area, and B cells migrate to the follicles.

Skin

The skin has specific and nonspecific immune functions. The epidermis forms a mechanical barrier to water-soluble chemicals and physical and biological agents. It protects against physical trauma and solar radiation by its upper cornified layer. For antigens to be recognized, they must penetrate the epidermis and bind with proteins to form a neohapten. The dermis contains APCs, called *Langerhans' cells,* which process antigen and present it to lymphocytes (see Fig. 25-4). Circulation of lymphocytes from the skin to lymph nodes allows for immune amplification.

Mucosal-Associated Lymphoid Tissues

MALTs are located in submucosal areas of the gastrointestinal, respiratory, and urogenital tracts. (The respiratory lymphoid tissue is also referred to separately as BALT.) Because these mucosal surfaces interact with the environment, they are important in host resistance and immune response. Areas of MALT can be organized into follicles similar to germinal centers in secondary lymphoid organs. An example of such an area is the Peyer's patches located in the gastrointestinal tract. The Langerhans' cells of the skin are also a component of MALT.

FUNCTIONAL COMPONENTS OF THE HUMAN IMMUNE SYSTEM: HUMORAL AND CELLULAR

Adaptive immunity comes into play when the innate defense systems are unable to defend against the foreign substance or invading organism. The adaptive immune system has two major arms: humeral-mediated immunity (HMI) and cellular-mediated immunity (CMI).

Humoral-Mediated Immunity

Antibodies are the main component of HMI and are proteins produced by B cells that are present in bodily secretions and plasma.

Antibody response can be described as primary and secondary. A primary response is elicited when an antigen is introduced to the immune system for the first time. During the primary response, there is a latent phase in which there is no detectable circulating antibody. This latent phase lasts between 5 and 7 days. After the latent phase, there is a gradual rise and then decline of the antibody titer that is associated with decreased antibody production and clearance of antibody from the system. The first immunoglobulin class to appear in a primary antibody response is immunoglobulin M (IgM). This is followed by the production of IgG. Reexposure to the same antigen causes a secondary antibody response that has a shorter latent phase, with IgG being the predominant immunoglobulin produced at a higher titer, and the antibody response is more persistent for a longer period. This is called the *anamnestic response.*

Antibodies have two physiochemically functional areas (Fig. 25-6). The F(ab) portion binds to antigen; the F(c) portion establishes antibody class—IgG, IgM, IgE, IgA, and IgD. Antibodies are found as components of serum proteins in the gamma (γ) and beta (β) regions as isolated by protein electrophoresis. The binding of antibody to antigen forms an immune complex.

IgG is found in the γ region. IgA migrates to γ and β regions. IgM migrates to γ, β, and α-2 regions. IgD and IgE electrophoretically isolate to the β region.

Antibodies consist of two heavy chains and two light chains held together by disulfide bonds (see Fig. 25-6). Each heavy and

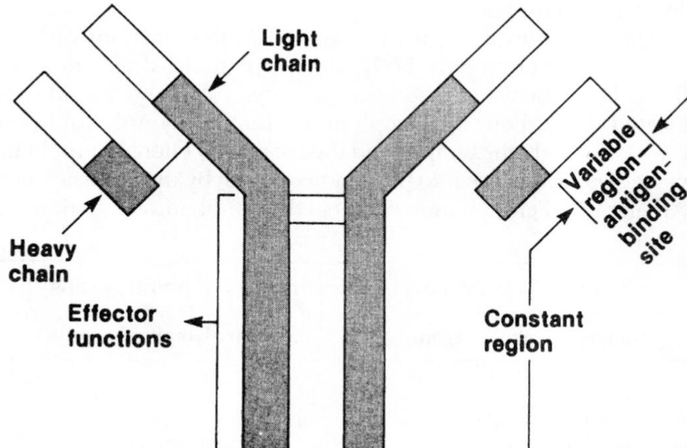

Figure 25-6. Antibody structure. (Courtesy of the Agency for Toxic Substances Disease Registry, Office of Technology Assessment, 1991.)

TABLE 25-3. Immunoglobulin G monomers

Immunoglobulin	T ½	Serum concentration	Molecular weight
IgG_1	21 days	10 mg/mL	150
IgG_2	21 days	5 mg/mL	150
IgG_3	7 days	1 mg/mL	170
IgG	21 days	0.5 mg/mL	150

light chain contains variable domains and constant domains with diverse amino acids. The variable region of antibody defines its unique ability to bind to antigen. Variable regions of immunoglobulins are encoded by gene combinations.

Papain enzymatically splits immunoglobulins at their hinge region into three fragments: two F(ab)s and one F(c). F(ab) is derived from the term *f*ragment *a*ntigen *b*inding. F(ab)s consist of the whole light chain with variable regions and part of the constant domain of the heavy chain.

The F(c) fragment crystallizes (fragment crystallizable). The F(c) portion of immunoglobulins binds to F(c) receptors on immune cells.

Pepsin activity on immunoglobulins cleaves the protein into two fragments: the $F(ab)_2$ fragment, held together by disulfide bonds, and the remainder of F(c) fragments of heavy chains not held together.

There are two types of light chains: kappa (κ) and lambda (λ). For any given immunoglobulin, only one type of chain is present, either kappa or lambda, but not both. Each immunoglobulin class has a unique heavy chain that defines its nature: IgG = gamma (γ) chains; IgM = mu (μ) chains; IgA = alpha (α) chains; IgD = delta (δ) chains; and IgE = epsilon (ε) chains.

Following are the major classes of antibodies.

IGG

IgG is the predominant antibody synthesized in the secondary antibody response. It is a specific antitoxin antibody. IgG is the only antibody that crosses the placenta. Its half-life equals 23 days. IgG activates the classical complement pathway. It has four subclasses (IgG_1, IgG_2, IgG_3, IgG_4). Each IgG is a monomer with varying serum half-lives (Table 25-3).

IGM

IgM is made up of five basic units (pentamer) held together by a J piece, a glycoprotein that attaches to heavy chains by a disulfide bond. IgM is consequently a large molecule. IgM is the antibody of first response to an antigen and is present in primary and secondary immune response. IgM is commonly found in B-cell surfaces and activates the classical complement pathway. Its serum half-life is 5 days with a serum concentration of 2 mg per mL. Its molecular weight is 900.

IGE

The plasma concentration of IgE is the lowest of all the antibodies. IgE is a monomer and is also termed *reagin*. IgE is responsible for type I (allergic) hypersensitivity reactions. The F(c) portion of IgE binds to mast cell receptors. Bridging of IgE molecules by antigen results in release of vasoactive mediators of allergy. IgE receptors are found also on eosinophils. Its serum concentration is 0.0001 mg per mL, and its half-life is 3 days.

IGA

IgA exists in two forms: secretory and serum. Serum IgA concentration is 3 mg per mL, and 0.5 mg per mL for IgAs has a half-life of 7 days. The function of serum IgA is antigen clearance and immune regulation.

Secretory IgA is found in biological secretions of mucosal areas of the body: nasal, gastrointestinal, respiratory, saliva, tears, prostate fluid, and vaginal secretions. Secretory IgA is a formation of two IgA molecules (dimer), attached by a J-chain glycoprotein plus the secretory component.

Secretory and serum IgAs are controlled by different mechanisms. Plasma cells release IgA dimers, which then bind to the secretory component located on epithelial cell membranes. The IgA-S complex is taken up by the epithelial cell and transported to the mucosal fluids on the surface of tissue. At this point, the secretory component may be cleaved off the IgA dimer. Secretory IgA is resistant to proteolysis.

The function of secretory IgA is basically first-line defense at mucosal barrier surfaces. IgA-S assists in destruction of pathogens via antibody-dependent cell-mediated cytotoxicity.

IGD

The serum concentration of IgD is less than 1% of total serum immunoglobulins (0.3 mg per mL). IgD has a half-life of 2 to 3 days. The exact function of IgD is unknown, but it has activity to insulin, penicillin, nuclear antigens, and thyroid antigen. It is found on the surface of B cells.

Cellular-Mediated Immunity

Immune system cells are derived from a pluripotent stem cell that follows two broad cell lines: myeloid and lymphoid (Fig. 25-7). Myeloid cells develop into monocytes, macrophages, and granulocytes. Lymphoid cells are T cells, B cells, and granular lymphocytes. Myeloid cell lines are responsible for nonspecific innate immunity and circulate in the peripheral blood and tissues of the body. The cellular immune system is also classified according to broad cell types and functions (Tables 25-4, 25-5): primary effector cells, APCs, and accessory cells.

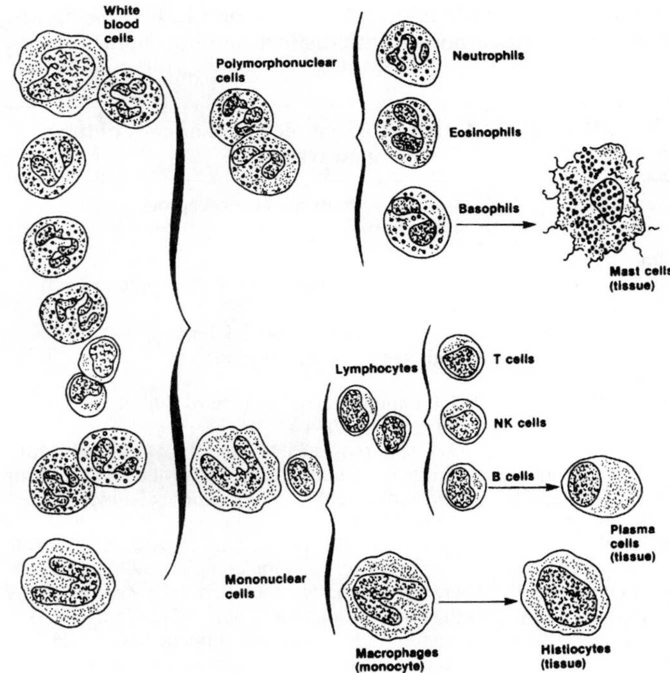

Figure 25-7. White blood cells differentiating into lymphoid and myeloid cell lines. NK, natural killer. (Courtesy of the Agency for Toxic Substances Disease Registry, Office of Technology Assessment, 1991.)

TABLE 25-4. Major cell classes of the immune system

- Primary effector cells
  - B lymphocytes
  - T lymphocytes
  - Natural killer cells
- Antigen-presenting cells
  - B lymphocytes
  - Macrophages/monocytes
  - Follicular dendritic cells
  - Interdigitating dendritic cells
  - Langerhans' cells
  - Endothelial cells
- Accessory cells
  - Neutrophils
  - Basophils and mast cells
  - Eosinophils
  - Platelets

National Research Council. *Biologic markers in immunotoxicology.* National Research Council, Commission on Life Sciences, Board on Environmental Studies and Toxicology, Committee on Biologic Markers, Subcommittee on Immunotoxicology. Washington: National Academy Press, 1992.

MONOCYTES AND MACROPHAGES

Monocytes make up 4% to 10% of nucleated cells in the blood with a diameter of 12 to 16 μm. The cells have a horseshoe-shaped nucleus with neutrophilic granules. Monocytes that migrate into tissue become tissue macrophages. Macrophages are larger than monocytes, with more prominent granules. Macrophages perform two vital functions for the immune system: (a) phagocytosis of particulate matter, and (b) presentation of an antigen to a T cell. Antigen presentation to T cells by macrophages begins the T-cell–dependent immune process that activates other T cells and B cells to respond specifically to an antigen. Macrophages have surface receptors on their cells, including the MHC, receptors for complement, and F(c) receptors for immunoglobulins.

GRANULOCYTES

Granulocytes include neutrophils, eosinophils, and basophils. Each of these has granules with distinct staining characteristics.

TABLE 25-5. Activity/surface receptors of cells of the immune system

Cells	Activity/surface receptors
Granulocytes	
Neutrophils	Inflammation, phagocytosis, F(c) receptor, CO11b, CD35
Eosinophils	Allergic response, helminth killing
Basophils	Allergic reactions, IgE receptor
Lymphocytes	
T cells	Cellular immunity, helper/cytotoxic MHC Class II, CD2, CD3, CD4
B cells	Suppressor activity, MHC class II, CD2, CD3, CD8
Large granulocytic lymphocytes	Antibody formation, F(c) receptor MHC class I, complement receptor, natural killer cell function CD2, CD16
Macrophages/monocytes	Antigen-presenting cells, phagocytosis, MHC class II receptor, F(c) receptor, complement receptor
Mast cells	Allergic reaction, degranulation, IgE receptors
Langerhans' cells	Antigen-presenting cell in skin, MHC class II, CD1
Dendritic cells	Antigen-presenting cell in lymphatic tissue, MHC class II, CD1

MHC, major histocompatibility complex.

Mature granulocytes have a diameter of 10 to 15 microns and contain a multilobulated nucleus. Neutrophils form 70% of nucleated cells in the blood and contain granules that store the enzymes myeloperoxidase, hydrolase, and muramidase. Neutrophils also perform phagocytosis and have receptors for complement and F(c) receptors for immunoglobulin.

EOSINOPHILS

Eosinophils form 2% to 5% of the circulating leukocytes in the blood and generally increase in response to an allergic situation. They contain yellow to red granules when stained with Wright's stain. This property of high affinity for eosin dye helped to originally name the cell type.

Eosinophils are bilobed and approximate the size of neutrophils. They contain four types of granules: crystalloid core granules, primary granules, small granules containing arylsulfatase and other enzymes, and tubulovesicles. Eosinophils originate from the bone marrow, and their differentiation is promoted by cytokines and granulocyte-macrophage-colony–stimulating factor.

Eosinophils have receptors for IgG, IgA, and IgE. They also have membrane receptors for complement components and cytokines. Granules of eosinophils contain lysosomal hydrolases, cationic proteins, a neurotoxin, peroxidase enzyme, and major basic protein, which is toxic to helminth parasites and tumor cells. The neurotoxin was named so because it produces cerebrocerebellar dysfunction in rabbits. Eosinophil peroxidase, along with hydrogen peroxide, kills helminth parasites and protozoa.

Eosinophils also produce cytokines. Their granules contain mediators to assist in regulating the IgE-mediated response. Such mediators as histaminase help inactivate the IgE-mediated allergic response.

BASOPHILS AND MAST CELLS

Basophils and mast cells share similar features. Basophils are large cells with coarse granules that stain a deep blue with basophilic dyes. The granules of basophils contain histamine and other vasoactive amines. They have surface receptors for IgE only and not for other antibodies. On the crosslinking of two IgE antibodies, the granules release their contents and produce allergic reactions. Basophils form as much as 0.5% of the circulating leukocytes in the blood.

Mast cells and basophils contain granules and are major sources of histamine and other chemical mediators. They are derived from pluripotent stem cells in the bone marrow. Both cell types express cell membrane receptors that bind the F(c) portion of IgE.

Basophils generally have a segmented nucleus that contains dense nuclear chromatin and oval cytoplasmic granules. Mast cells are round or elongated morphologically and have a nonsegmented nucleus or, occasionally, a bilobed nucleus.

Mast cells are distributed throughout connective tissue, lying adjacent to blood vessels, near nerves, and just under epithelial surfaces near the external environment, such as the respiratory system and skin. Unlike basophils, mast cells do not circulate in the blood.

Mast cells and basophils have potent mediators stored in their granules, such as histamine, serine proteases, proteoglycans, and carboxypeptidase A. Other bioactive mediators are synthesized when the cells are activated by IgE or products of arachidonic acid oxidation or platelet-activating factor. Cytokines are stored in mast cell and basophil granules and are synthesized on cell activation.

LYMPHOCYTES

Lymphocytes make up 20% to 30% of peripheral white cells and are classified according to their size. Small lymphocytes have a diameter of 8 to 10 μm and high nuclear-to-cytoplasm ratios. They lack cytoplasmic granules. Small lymphocytes are subdivided into T cells and B cells, based on their function. A third type of lymphocyte is a large granular lymphocyte with a diameter of as much as 16 μm and a small nuclear to cytoplasmic ratio. Whereas the small lymphocytes lack granules, the large granular lymphocytes contain granules.

B Lymphocytes (B Cells). B lymphocytes make up 5% to 15% of circulating lymphocytes and have receptors that express immunoglobulins. B cells also have immunoglobulin F(c) receptors (CD-16), complement receptors, and the MHC receptors. Other glycoprotein cell markers present on B cells identified by monoclonal antibodies include CD-19, CD-20, and CD-21 receptors.

B cells can be antigen independent or antigen dependent. Antigen-independent B cells do not express immunoglobulins. Antigen-dependent B cells undergo proliferation, activation, and differentiation into plasma cells that secrete specific immunoglobulins. These activated cells do not express MHC, CD-19, CD-20, or CD-21 receptors found on other B lymphocytes.

T Lymphocytes. Eighty percent of circulating lymphocytes are T cells that are either effectors or regulators. Effector T cells perform the function of cytolysis of cells infected by viruses or tumor cells and produce lymphokines. The regulator function of T cells increases or suppresses other lymphocytes. T cells also express cell-surface markers. Helper T cells express the CD-4 marker, and suppressor T cells express the CD-8 marker. All circulating T cells express CD-3 markers and the CD-2 marker. T cells that express the CD-4 marker are also called *T-helper (Th) cells* (Table 25-6).

T cells differentiate in the fetal liver or bone marrow, then migrate to the thymus, which then provides a further environment for maturation. While in the thymus, these cells are known as *thymocytes*. Along the cortex of the thymus, T cells develop CD-2 and CD-3 receptor expressions on their cell-surface. Further maturation allows for the development of CD-4 and CD-8 molecules on the cell membrane. Maturing T lymphocytes express four CD molecules: CD-2, CD-3, CD-4, and CD-8 (Fig. 25-8). As the immature T cell migrates into the medullary area of the thymus, the CD-4 or the CD-8 receptor is lost, thus differentiating the cell as a helper cell (T_h) with CD-4 marker or a suppressor cell (T_s) with a CD-8 marker.

TABLE 25-6. Major functions of T cells

Abbreviation	Function
T_D	T cells responsible for delayed-type hypersensitivity. After reacting with antigen, T_D cells release cytokines that can kill target cells *in vitro* (cytotoxins) and activate macrophages, inducing inflammation.
T_H	T-helper cells assist in humoral immunity, i.e., antibody production. They are required if a B cell is to produce antibody. One characteristic feature of T-helper cells is a surface marker called *CD4*.
T_K	Often referred to as *killer T cells*, or *cytotoxic lymphocytes*, this subclass of T cells, after being specifically sensitized, directly interacts with target cells to kill them *in vitro*. They are distinguished from natural killer cells by the requirement for sensitization and cell-surface markers.
T_S	T cells that serve to control immune responses by producing factors that can act on both B cells and T_H cells. T-suppressor cells can be distinguished from T-helper cells because they exhibit a signature molecule referred to as *CD8*.

Courtesy of the National Research Council. *Biologic markers in immunotoxicology.* National Research Council, Commission on Life Sciences, Board on Environmental Studies and Toxicology, Committee on Biologic Markers, Subcommittee on Immunotoxicology. Washington: National Academy Press, 1992.

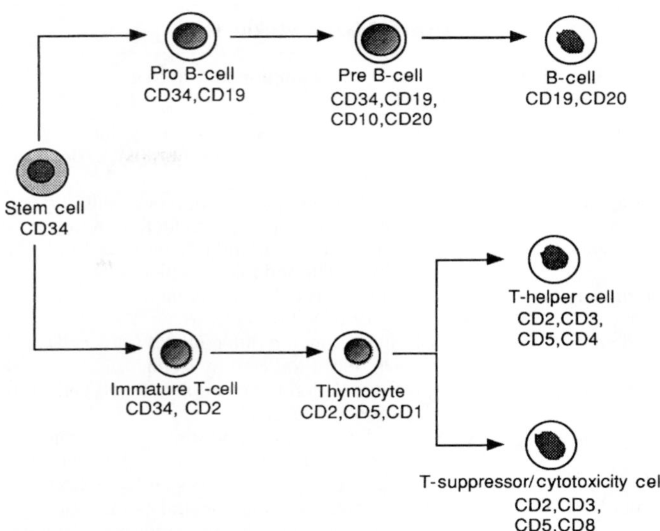

Figure 25-8. Clusters of differentiation (CDs) of T cells.

T-Cell Helpers and T-Cell Suppressors. T-cell helpers, or T_h cells, promote activation of B cells and T-suppressor cells, or T_s cells will down-regulate B-cell activity. T cells can be divided into T-cell subsets based on membrane surface glycoproteins, CD-4 and CD-8. CD-4 cells are referred to as T_h cells and are divided into the subsets of T_h-1 and T_h-2, based on the cytokines that they release.

CD-8 positive cells are either cytotoxic lymphocytes (T_c cells) or T_s cells. T_h and T_s cells regulate cell-mediated immune response and the specific functions of B cells and cytotoxic lymphocytes. The T_h cells form a special feature of memory. When stimulated by antigen, the T_h cells secrete cytokines, which induce activated B cells and T cells to become memory cells.

LARGE GRANULOCYTIC LYMPHOCYTES

Large granulocytic lymphocytes contain cytoplasmic granules. Some of these are natural killer (NK) cells. NK cells have CD-2, CD-16, and CD-56 cell-surface markers. NK cells attack and lyse tumor cells, cells infected by viruses, and allogeneic transplant cells without need of antibody or complement. NK cells also participate in antibody-dependent cell-mediated cytolysis.

ANTIGEN-PRESENTING CELLS

APCs initiate specific immune response by presenting antigens to T cells or B cells. Macrophages, dendritic cells, and Langerhans' cells are APCs. Langerhans' cells are present in the dermis and epidermis and play a key role in immune surveillance. Dendritic cells are long filamentous cells present in lymphoid organs. Mast cells are the other APCs; they are located in connective tissue throughout the body. Mast cells contain IgE receptors. Basophils and mast cells contain similar granular enzyme content and vasoactive mediators.

CYTOKINES

Cytokines are protein molecules that transmit messages between cells. Cytokines regulate cell growth and cell differentiation. Four major groups of cytokines are mediators of immune function (Table 25-7):

- Colony-stimulating factors (CSFs)
- Interferons (IFNs)
- Tumor necrosis factors (TNFs)
- Interleukins (ILs)

TABLE 25-7. Cytokines

Cytokine	Function and source
Interleukin-1	Inflammation, fever, immunoregulation. Produced by monocytes, fibroblasts, dendritic cells.
Interleukin-2	Activation and proliferation of T cells and B cells, macrophage production of tumor necrosis factor and interferon-α. Produced by T cells and natural killer cells.
Interleukin-3	Functions as colony-stimulating factor and is produced by T cells.
Interleukin-4	Proliferation and differentiation of T cells and B cells. Produced by T cells.
Interleukin-5	Differentiation of eosinophils and B cells. Produced by T cells.
Interleukin-6	Cell differentiation and stimulates production of acute-phase reactants by the liver. Produced by macrophages and lymphocytes.
Tumor necrosis factor-α	Stimulates inflammation and cytotoxicity. Produced by lymphocytes and macrophages.
Tumor necrosis factor-β	Stimulates inflammation and cell killing. Produced by lymphocytes and macrophages.
Interferon-α	Antiviral activity. Produced by leukocytes.
Interferon-β	Antiviral activity. Produced by fibroblasts.
Interferon-γ	Immune regulation and antiviral activity. Produced by T cells and natural killer cells.
Granulocyte-macrophage colony-stimulating factor	Produced by macrophages and causes proliferation of granulocytes and monocytes.
Granulocytic colony-stimulating factor	Produced by macrophages and fibroblasts and causes proliferation of granulocyte colonies.
Macrophage colony-stimulating factor	Produced by activated T cells, B cells, and fibroblasts and causes monocyte colony proliferation.

Colony-Stimulating Factors. CSFs cause the proliferation and differentiation of immature bone marrow cells. Granulocytic CSF stimulates growth of mature granulocytes. Macrophage CSF stimulates monocyte macrophage colonies. Granulocyte-macrophage CSF stimulates formation of granulocytes, monocytes, and macrophages.

Interferons. IFNs are glycoproteins produced in response to viral infections, immune stimulation, or chemical stimuli. Three types exist: IFN alpha, IFN beta, and IFN gamma (IFNα, IFNβ, and IFNγ). IFNα is produced by leukocytes, IFNβ is produced by fibroblasts, and IFNγ is produced by T cells. IFNα and IFNβ are active against viral replication, interfering with viral RNA. IFN also helps present cells to cytotoxic T cells and activated NK cells to help destroy these virus-infected cells. IFNγ activates macrophages and increases the expression of MHC class 1/class 2 molecules on activated macrophages. It also activates NK cells and activates B cells to secrete antibody.

Tumor Necrosis Factors. There are two TNFs, alpha and beta. TNF-α is produced by macrophages, monocytes, lymphocytes, and NK cells in response to bacterial components; viruses, tumor cells, and bacterial toxins; the complement component C5A; and fungal and parasitic toxins. TNF-β, also known as *lymphotoxin*, is produced by CD-4 and CD-8 cells after they are exposed to antigen. TNF-γ is cytotoxic for certain selected cells.

Interleukins. ILs are produced by leukocytes (IL-1, IL-2, IL-3, IL-4, IL-5, IL-6, IL-10, and IL-12). IL-1 is produced by macrophages and fibroblasts, and it serves as an initiator molecule for inflammation responses. IL-1 activates T cells and causes T cells to release other lymphokines. It helps provide for B-cell proliferation and acts on the bone marrow to produce CSF. IL-1 also activates and increases the number of T cells and B cells and activates NK cells. IL-1 induces fever and the synthesis of acute-phase proteins by the liver. It also produces differentiation of hematopoietic precursors and activates cells to produce and release other cytokines and mediators of inflammation. It supports and helps amplify the specific immune responses.

IL-2 is produced by CD-4 lymphocytes that are stimulated. IL-2 causes proliferation of activated T and B cells and increases production of NK cells.

Activated T cells produce IL-2, which induces proliferation of antigen-activated T cells and enhances NK-cell activity. Activated T cells also produce B-cell growth factor, IL-4, and IL-6, which stimulate proliferation and differentiation into antibody-secreting cells. Macrophage inhibition factor and macrophage activating factor are products of activated T cells and activate macrophage function. Two cytokines produced by macrophages are IL-1 and TNF. IL-1 stimulates IL-2 expression.

IL-3 is a glycoprotein produced by activated T cells. It serves as a growth factor for hematopoietic precursors.

IL-4 is a glycoprotein produced by activated T cells. It helps in the proliferation of T cells, B cells, and NK cells, and in the suppression of T-cell production of IFNs and TNFs.

IL-5 is produced by activated T cells. It stimulates B cells to produce antibody.

IL-6, produced by activated T and B cells, monocytes, and fibroblasts, has a short half-life and may regulate hematopoiesis, acute-phase protein production, and antibody production.

IL-10 and -12 inhibit IFNγ production, antigen presentation, and macrophage production of IL-1. IL-12 acts in just the opposite way of IL-10—it activates macrophages and NK cells and increases IFNγ production.

Antigen Processing

B cells and T cells both recognize antigens, but by different mechanisms. The B-cell antigen receptor is a surface immunoglobulin made up of a heavy chain and light chain. Each B-cell clone has one type of immunoglobulin on its surface and can bind directly to antigens through this surface immunoglobulin. T cells, on the other hand, recognize antigen that has been processed by APCs. The binding of a T cell to an APC is controlled by MHC. MHC can be class 1 or class 2. The number of APCs that can interact with T_h cells is limited and includes macrophages, dendritic cells, Langerhans' cells, and B lymphocytes. These cells contain a large number of surface MHC class 2 molecules. All nucleated cells have MHC class 1 proteins on their surface.

The delivery and processing of antigen to either CD-4 lymphocytes or CD-8 lymphocytes are different. The presentation to CD-4 lymphocytes requires antigen to be taken up by the APC and broken down into fragments. These fragments are then combined with the MHC class 2 receptor, and the peptide-MHC complex is transported to the surface of the APC for recognition by the T_h cell. For CD-8 cells, antigen is broken down and complexed with MHC class 1 molecules and is then exported to the cell-surface for presentation to T_s cells.

Antibody response to the majority of antigens requires T_h cells, and these antigens are known as T-dependent antigens. They are usually complex structures and protein in nature. T-independent antigens can activate B cells without T-cell assistance. These independent antigens are usually large molecules.

T-CELL ACTIVATION

On stimulation by antigen T_h cells, an activation process called blast transformation occurs. This blastogenic transformation amplifies the number of functional T_h cells. Direct contact between the original T_h cell and antigen is necessary for T-cell activation. The APC contains not only the antigen but also the MHC class 2 receptor on its surface, and the T cell must recognize both this and the antigen. This is called MHC restriction, and it allows the interacting cells to recognize that they are from the same host or from genetically similar individuals. The T-cell receptor consists of the MHC receptor and the CD-3 glycoprotein. Recognition of the antigen on the APC and the MHC class 2 molecules present on the APC surface is accomplished by the T-cell receptor on the T_h cell.

Activation of an effector T cell requires antigenic stimulation, IL-1, and IL-2. T_h cells undergo blastogenic transformation on stimulation with antigen contained on APCs. The T cells must recognize both the antigen and the MHC class II molecule on the APC surface to undergo blastogenesis. During contact, the APC can receive signals from the release of IL-1 from the T_h cell. IL-1 promotes IL-2 receptor expression and synthesis by the T cells. T cells sensitized by the antigen and stimulated by IL-1 express IL-2 receptors. In the presence of IL-2, the effector T cell undergoes blastogenic transformation and differentiation into a T cell that is cytotoxic or cytokine producing.

CYTOTOXIC T_C-CELL ACTIVATION

T_c cells are cytotoxic T cells and are capable of destroying cells without antibody. On contact with foreign cells, the T_c cell releases substances that kill the target cell. The T cells can repeat killing activity. IL-2 is a cytokine released by the T_h cells that activates the T_c cell for it to become a cytotoxic cell.

B-CELL ACTIVATION

A *hapten* is a substance of low molecular weight that is not capable of causing an immune response unless it is bound to a larger macromolecular structure. Activation of B cells requires binding of immunoglobulin receptors to an antigen. IL-2, IL-4, IL-6, and IL-10 are cytokines required for B-cell proliferation. These cytokines arise from macrophages in a T-cell–independent immune response and from T_h cells in a T-cell–dependent response.

NATURAL KILLER CELL ACTIVATION

NK cells are large lymphocytes with cytoplasmic granules that can kill cells infected by viruses, can kill cancer cells, and do not require previous sensitization by antigen. NK cells do not have T-cell or B-cell markers. They do have F(c) receptors on their cell-surface, and their activity is modulated by cytokines.

ANTIBODY-DEPENDENT CELL-MEDIATED CYTOLYSIS

The killing, or lysing, of antibody-coated target cells by cells with cytolytic activity is known as *antibody-dependent cell-mediated cytolysis*. The antibody involved is IgG.

Complement System

The complement system is a component of nonspecific immunity and involves fourteen separate components involving two separate pathways of activation: the classical pathway and the alternate pathway.

The components of the complement system act and interact in a cascading sequence. The alternate pathway and the classical pathway are divided into three mechanisms: recognition, activation, and membrane attack.

The consequences of complement activation include the following:

- Amplification of the classical and alternative pathway components to enhance the activation of other complement components.
- Release of anaphylatoxins, which are cleavage products of C4, C3, and C5 complement components and cause the release of active peptides C4A, C3A, and C5A—the anaphylatoxins that mediate inflammation and induced release of histamine from basophils and mast cells. Anaphylatoxins also increase vascular permeability and cause smooth muscle contraction.
- Immune adherence, which involves covalent bonding between complement components and soluble immune complexes or particles. A portion of the complement component that does not adhere is exposed and available for binding to other cell receptors, monocytes, B lymphocytes, erythrocytes, or mast cells.
- Opsonization, the enhancement of phagocytosis by polymorphonuclear leukocytes or monocytes.
- Chemotaxis, which results from the cleavage of C5, from either the classical or alternative pathway. C5 convertase produces C5A, a potent chemotactic factor and anaphylatoxin. C5A causes migration of inflammatory cells, including neutrophils and monocytes.
- Kinin activation by the complement system, which results in smooth muscle contraction, mucous secretion, pain, and increased vascular permeability.
- Lysis, which is the destruction of cells and the lytic function of complement. Lysis is necessary for host defense against some bacterial infections.

ACUTE-PHASE REACTANTS

Acute-phase reactants are a component of nonspecific immunity and are synthesized by chemical proteins by the liver in response to inflammation. Acute-phase responses include fever, which occurs after inflammation caused by infectious or noninfectious states. Fever is caused by IL-1. Acute-phase reactants include C-reactive protein, haptoglobin, fibrinogen, α-1 antitrypsin, ceruloplasmin, and α-2 macroglobulin.

IMMUNOCOMPETENCE AND IMMUNOTOXICOLOGY

In concert with lymphoid organs, specific and nonspecific cellular and humoral factors maintain immunocompetence, a state of functional immunity that provides effective resistance to infectious agents and neoplastic cells. Rapid, mobile, and specific responses of the immune system may be manifested locally or systemically, reversibly or irreversibly, acutely or chronically. There is ample evidence that the immune apparatus can be the target for toxic effects caused by a wide variety of environmental (3–13), occupational (11,14–22), and pharmaceutic agents or drugs (23–30) at one or more points in the immune system.

Immunotoxicology is the subdiscipline of toxicology that views the immune system as a potential target organ of toxicity. Immunotoxicity can be expressed as:

- Immunosuppressive responses
- Immunostimulatory responses (hypersensitivity and allergy)
- Autoimmunity

Immunotoxicology attempts to predict, detect, characterize mechanistically, quantify, and interpret the adverse human consequences of direct and indirect alterations of the immune system that occur as a result of various agents. If immunocompetence represents an optimally balanced immune response, then profound immunosuppression or overt hypersensitivity represents the extremes of inappropriate and ineffective immune responsiveness.

Historically, early efforts in immunotoxicology were devoted to the following:

- Demonstrating that the immune system can be the target organ for toxin-induced alterations

- Documenting hypersensitivity, autoimmunity, and immunosuppression as the predominant sequelae of immunotoxin exposures
- Development of rodent-based, standardized batteries of tests to detect systemic immunotoxicity (31,32)
- Refinements of immunotoxicity testing to enhance its use in risk-assessment algorithms (33,34)
- Development of effective diagnostic protocols for the detection of clinical immunotoxicity

As immunotoxicology matures as a scientific endeavor, additional effort will be needed to further characterize significant issues, such as the immunologic fragility of the fetus and other susceptible subpopulations, reversibility of immunotoxicity, genetic control of immunotoxic responses, identification of reliable biomarkers of immunotoxicologic relevance, and the relevance of local/regional immunotoxic responses in contrast to systemic responses.

Although immunotoxicology has become a vital subdiscipline of toxicology, it is important to note that immunotoxic effects are influenced by factors common to basic toxicology (Table 25-8).

Immunosuppression

Some of the most forceful demonstrations of the importance of an intact immune system are seen in experiments of nature. Included in this category are the known human and animal genetic/congenital abnormalities of the immune system (35). Pathogenic states of decreased immune responsiveness are documented in these well-characterized primary immunodeficiencies (36). However, until the acquired immune deficiency syndrome (AIDS) (37) epidemic, chronic immunosuppressive defects were considered rare. The clinical sequelae of immunosuppression can range from significant and life-threatening to laboratory curiosities (36–48).

Immunosuppression is a decrease in immune function measured as an effect on cellular, humoral, or nonspecific immune parameters. In general, primary immune responses are susceptible to suppression, whereas secondary (anamnestic) immune responses are refractory. Therefore, drug- or chemically induced immunosuppression is dependent not only on the characteristics of the xenobiotic, but also on the timing of exposure relative to the generation of an immune response. In addition to gross effects, subtle immunosuppression may occur through the triggering of apoptosis (49–52), differentiation (53), MHC product expression or restriction (54–56), and delays in IgM to IgG antibody production shift in plasma cells (57). Furthermore, studies indicate that certain chemicals may exert an indirect immunologic effect via stress responses (58,59). The clinical relevance of these subtle changes is difficult to assess. Ongoing studies involving patients exposed to heavy metals (22,60), polybrominated biphenyls (61–63), polychlorinated biphenyls (22,50,64), certain pesticides (22,65–70), and drugs of abuse (28,29,71) reveal that immunosuppressive effects of xenobiotics can be significant and persistent. It should be noted that the immune system is a multifaceted network that maintains a level of functional reserve, and therefore a toxic effect on a particular cell or circuit may not necessarily lead to a detectable clinical manifestation. The likely clinical sequelae of immunosuppression are increased rates of infectious diseases and neoplasia.

TABLE 25-8. Factors influencing immunotoxicity

Characteristics of the immunotoxic agent
Structure of chemical
Physical characteristics
Presence/level of contaminants or other chemicals in mixture
Stability of chemical/chemical mixture
Bioavailability of chemical/chemical mixture
Characteristics of exposure scenario
Route of exposure
Concentration/volume of exposure
Frequency of exposure
Duration of exposure
Characteristics of individual
Genetic makeup of individual
Immunologic status of individual
Hormonal status of individual
Nutritional status of individual
Preexisting disease or organ pathology in individual
Pregnancy status of individual
Age, sex, and weight of individual
Concurrent lifestyle attributes of individual

IMMUNOSUPPRESSION AND INFECTIOUS DISEASE

Opportunistic infections are common in immunocompromised hosts (38,40,72–77). Recurrent opportunistic infections are often harbingers of an underlying immunodeficiency (75,78,79). Exposure to immunosuppressive chemicals and drugs has resulted in decreased host resistance (79). More ominous is the finding that exposure to common air pollutants, such as ozone, nitric oxide, and sulfur dioxide, increases host susceptibility to infection (80). Multiple mechanisms are deployed by the immune apparatus to neutralize and eradicate different infectious agents; innate and specific immune responses can be required, depending on the pathogen encountered. The clearance of extracellular microbial pathogens requires the interaction of pathogen-specific antibody with leukocytes and complement. The clearance of intracellular microbes involves primarily cell-mediated immune mechanisms. Toxigenic infections, which typically result from the production of toxins by certain bacteria, require the production of specific antibody for neutralization. Antitoxin antibodies prevent binding of the toxin to specific receptors, thus preventing their deleterious effects. Based on the knowledge of immunity to microbes, groups of infectious agents can be linked to broad classifications of immune alterations (Table 25-9) and can be an indication of the underlying immune defect in patients.

In addition to their clinical significance as sequelae of human immunosuppression, infectious agents, used as probes, are effective tools for studying potential immunotoxins (81). Numerous infectious disease models have been used to screen xenobiotics for immunotoxic potential in animal-based host-resistance assessments: cytomegalovirus (82), influenza virus (83), herpes simplex virus (84), *Listeria monocytogenes* (85), *Streptococcus pneumoniae* (86), *Trypanosoma musculi* (87), *Plasmodium yoelii* and *berghei* (88), and *Trichinella spiralis* (89). Each of these infectious agents requires a complex recital of the immune system's repertoire for its successful elimination. In predictive immunotoxicity testing, the elegance of the host-resistance models arises from their ability to test functionally several circuits of the immune apparatus during a single experiment.

IMMUNOSUPPRESSION AND CANCER

The interaction between tumor cells and the host immune system is complex, involving innate and adaptive resistance mechanisms. Human antisera and monoclonal antibodies reactive with autologous tumors have been isolated. Nevertheless, a strong antibody response to tumor antigens has not been correlated with effective host resistance to tumors. Cytotoxic T lymphocytes and nonspecific NK cells are thought to play pivotal roles in limiting tumor growth and metastasis (90). In addition, the macrophage plays a dual role, functioning nonspecifically as a phagocytic effector or specifically through lymphokine activation in acquired immune responses (91).

TABLE 25-9. Infectious agents associated with immune alterations

B-lymphocyte defects	T-lymphocyte defects	Granulocyte defects
Virus		
Hepatitis B	Rubeola	
Echovirus	Varicella	
Epstein-Barr		
Cytomegalovirus		
Herpes simplex		
Poxvirus		
Bacteria		
Pseudomonas spp.	*Mycobacterium* spp.	*Staphylococcus* spp.
Hemophilus spp.	*Listeria* spp.	*Klebsiella* spp.
Streptococcus spp.	*Legionella* spp.	*Nocardia* spp.
Meningococcus spp.	*Salmonella* spp.	
Neisseria spp.		
Yeast and fungi		
Candida spp.	*Candida* spp.	
Histoplasma spp.	*Aspergillus* spp.	
Cryptococcus spp.		
Parasite		
Giardia lamblia	*Pneumocystis carinii*	
Pneumocystis carinii	*Toxoplasma gondii*	
	Entamoeba histolytica	
	Cryptosporidium spp.	

Several lines of evidence implicate immunosuppression with an increased incidence of cancer. First, from the onset of the AIDS epidemic in the early 1980s, several neoplastic diseases have been associated with this condition. Kaposi's sarcoma, systemic non-Hodgkin's lymphoma, primary central nervous system lymphoma, and invasive cervical cancer may affect as many as 40% of AIDS patients in some stage of their illness (39,92). Second, there is a growing literature describing an increase in cancer incidence after immunosuppression associated with organ transplantation (93–98). Third, review of the relationship between the degree of immunosuppression and malignancy in patients on immunosuppressive drugs provides further convincing evidence of the importance of intact immunity in resistance to cancer (99).

These findings are concordant with a popular theory that the immune system, particularly elements responsible for CMI, is responsible for anticancer reconnaissance or immune surveillance (100). This hypothesis is based on two premises: (a) that neoplastic and normal cells generally have different antigenic portraits, and (b) that the immune system responds to the antigenically modified (nonself) cells in essentially the same way it responds to infectious agents. Most, if not all, carcinogens are mutagens that may cause mutations leading to the expression of tumor-specific antigens. It is hypothesized that the immunogenicity of a tumor is directly proportional to the dose of the carcinogen responsible for its induction. This hypothesis would explain the usually low or absent immunogenicity of "spontaneous" tumors induced by undetectable levels of environmental carcinogens.

When studied in well-defined experimental models, tumors can be remarkably effective probes for the study of relevant immunotoxic effects of chemicals and drugs (81). *In vivo* tumor-resistance models can be implemented using either transplantable (101) or virus-induced (102) tumors that have been characterized as to their behavior in specific inbred strains of rodents. Endpoints for *in vivo* assays of tumor resistance include mean survival time, mean time to tumor rejection, response to secondary tumor challenge, and quantitation of metastases or tumor size. *In vivo* tumor-resistance assays are sensitive and well adapted to the screening of potentially immunotoxic compounds for immunosuppressive activity (32,101). Using PYB6 sarcoma (nonmetastatic), B16F10 melanoma (metastatic), and murine sarcoma virus tumor-resistance models, accumulating evidence indicates that exposure to immunotoxicants can diminish innate and adaptive immune responses to tumors (103). In addition, either innate (NK cells) or adaptive (cytotoxic T cells) tumor-resistance mechanisms can be studied *in vitro*. As with most *in vitro* assays, these techniques have the advantage of refined control, manipulation of variables, the ability to use either human- or animal-derived cell systems, and significantly reduced time requirements (days). The practical combination of *in vivo* and *in vitro* tumor-resistance analyses provides sensitive endpoints for detecting biologically relevant immunotoxicity. It should be noted that, like host-resistance models using infectious agents, the sensitivity of *in vivo* tumor-resistance assays results from the recital of multiple mechanisms that control the *in vivo* immune response. To date, no single *in vitro* assay system can sufficiently address the multiple parameters exercised in the *in vivo* host-resistance models.

Alterations of immune responsiveness caused by xenobiotic exposures are demonstrable in humans and animals. Furthermore, xenobiotic-induced immunosuppression can lead to increased susceptibility to infectious disease, cancer, or both. However, it should be noted that, contrary to popular public perception, evidence directly implicating environmental or industrial chemicals in the suppression of human immune responses is considerably less robust than the evidence linking such agents to allergy and hypersensitivity reactions (11).

Hypersensitivity

Despite evidence that certain controlled hypersensitivity reactions can be beneficial (e.g., IgE response to parasites), most manifestations of hypersensitivity are adverse. Hypersensitivity disorders are the most prominent form of immunotoxicity recognized in humans. Hypersensitivity is best portrayed as an exaggerated response to an antigenic stimulus, commonly distinguished by a reduced threshold to antigen. Regardless of their type, all hypersensitivity reactions are induced by recall antigens in or on a host who has previously effected an immune response to the antigen. It is estimated that more than 40 million Americans suffer from some form of hypersensitivity disease (104), and approximately 9% of all patients seeking medical care do so for treatment of hypersensitivity disorders. Immunopathology can be antibody mediated, cell mediated, or a combination.

In addition to being the most predominant form of immunotoxicity, hypersensitivity disorders are certainly the most problematic form. Allergic disorders tend to be more individualized than most other forms of toxicity. Exposure conditions that elicit an allergic response in certain individuals may have no effect on others similarly exposed. Clearly, genetic predisposition plays a role in hypersensitivity disorders (104,105). Because hypersensitivity disorders can be elicited by a diversity of antigens and occur in or on numerous organ systems of the body, they arise in what appears to be a bewildering array. Although the Gell and Coombs' classification of immunopathology (Table 25-10) allows some insight into the mechanisms that underlie hypersensitivity disorders, it is particularly important to realize that more than one of these mechanisms can operate simultaneously in an individual.

One characteristic common to all types of hypersensitivity reactions is the necessity of prior exposure to elicit a reaction. In the case of types I, II, and III, prior exposure to antigen leads to the production of specific antibody, IgE, IgM, or IgG. In the case of type IV, prior exposure to antigen leads to the generation of memory T lymphocytes. Most potentially allergenic chemical agents are low molecular weight and may act as haptens. The type of hypersensitivity an agent elicits in a susceptible host

TABLE 25-10. Gell and Coombs' classification of immunopathology

Type	Hypersensitivity reactions	Cells	Immunoglobulin	Complement activation	Examples
I	IgE mediated. Most cells bind IgE by their R(c) receptors. On antigen encounter, IgE is cross-linked, inducing mast-cell degranulation with release of mediators.	Mast cells Basophils	IgE	No	Anaphylaxis Asthma Allergic rhinitis
II	Antibody-dependent cytotoxicity. Antibody directed against antigens on a person's own cells or tissues. Interaction with complement pathway and effector cells cause damage to cells or tissues. Antibodies interact with complement (Clq) and effector cells via their F(c) receptors. The antibody serves as a bridge between antigen and effector cells.		IgG IgM	Yes	Transfusion reactions Hemolytic disease of newborn Host-versus-graft reaction Goodpasture's syndrome
III	Immune complex disease. Immune complexes are deposited in tissues, complement is activated, and polymorphonuclear leukocytes are attracted to the area, causing inflammation and tissue damage.		IgG	Yes	Serum sickness Farmer's lung disease
IV	Delayed hypersensitivity (48–72 hours). Antigen-sensitized T cells release lymphokines after secondary contact with the same antigen. Lymphokines induce an inflammatory response that activates mast cells to release mediators.	T cells Macrophage	IgM	Yes	Tuberculosis skin test Granulomatous disease Contact allergic dermatitis

depends on its route of exposure and the nature of the host constituent with which it interacts (Table 25-11).

Although the majority of our understanding of hypersensitivity has been derived from study of immune responses to natural antigens such as pollens, house dust, or danders, it is now apparent that occupational and environmental exposures to chemicals and other xenobiotics is an important and growing cause of hypersensitivity disorders (106). It is important to note that most threshold limit values are quantitatively determined by irritant or toxic effects rather than by their sensitizing effects (107). Workers can become sensitized to chemicals well below the allowable threshold limit (107).

CLINICAL HYPERSENSITIVITY AND ALLERGY

Terms used to describe hypersensitivity reactions and allergic reactions include the following:

- *Anaphylaxis*: This term was introduced in 1902 to indicate adverse reactions to horse serum injected for therapy of infectious disease. The term suggests a reaction that is the opposite of prophylaxis. In the context of immunotoxicology, anaphylaxis has taken on the implication of an acute reaction involving immunologic and inflammatory mechanisms.

TABLE 25-11. Immune interactions in hypersensitivity

Host constituent	Immune interaction	Hypersensitivity
Protein	Antibody (IgE or IgG) Response to hapten Sensitization of mast cells	Asthma or allergic rhinitis
	Antibody (IgM or IgG) response Ag-Ab complex formation Complement activation	Hypersensitivity pneumonitis
Cell	Antibody (IgG) response to Ag-altered host cell	Autoimmune hemolytic anemia
	T-lymphocyte response to Ag-altered host cell	Contact dermatitis

Ig, immunoglobulin.

- *Atopy*: This term was introduced in the 1920s to describe a multiplicity of curious reactions then thought to be unique to humans. This word is derived from the Greek word *atopia*, meaning strangeness. Those curious reactions are now known to be allergies. In the context of immunotoxicology, atopy implies a constitutional or hereditary tendency to develop chronic hypersensitivity states, such as hay fever or asthma, especially to antigens that provoke no adverse reactions in so-called normal subjects.
- *Allergy*: This term was introduced in 1906 to indicate altered reactivity as a result of a previous exposure. The term *allergy* is often used to describe either atopic or anaphylactic reactions (104,108–112).

The most clinically relevant hypersensitivity reactions encountered with chemical hazards are: (a) immediate hypersensitivity, (b) immune complex reactions, (c) delayed hypersensitivity, (d) antibody-dependent cytotoxicity, and (e) pseudoallergic reactions.

IMMEDIATE HYPERSENSITIVITY REACTIONS (TYPE I)

Hypersensitivity reactions are beneficial expressions of the immune response that cause inflammation damage directed against antigens. Occasionally, in some circumstances, the hypersensitivity response causes disease. Type I, or immediate hypersensitivity, occurs when IgE antibody response is directed against antigens that are typically considered innocuous. Type I or IgE-mediated hypersensitivity reactions are characterized by allergic reactions immediately after contact with an antigen. Such reactions include anaphylaxis, allergic rhinitis, allergic dermatitis, and asthma. Type I reactions are dependent on specific triggering of IgE-sensitized mast cells by an antigen, with a resulting release of pharmacologically active mediators of inflammation. Such reactions include asthma, eczema, hay fever, urticaria, and anaphylaxis.

Asthma and allergic rhinitis are the most common forms of immediate hypersensitivity (81). These diseases are produced as the result of a two-step inflammatory reaction initiated by mediators that are released by reaction of multivalent antigen with mast cells and basophils passively sensitized with cytophilic antibody on the surface. Effector cells release an arsenal of biologically active substances including histamine, heparin, serotonin, and arachidonic acid (Fig. 25-9). The early phase is characterized by

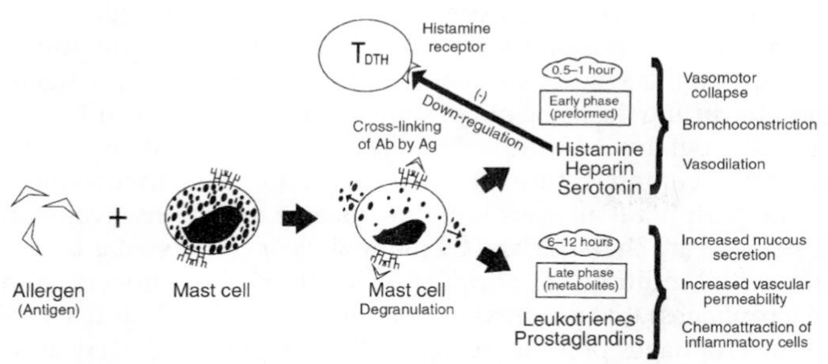

Figure 25-9. Mechanisms of early- and late-onset type I hypersensitivity.

two events. The first is smooth muscle contraction or dilatation of arterioles, mediated by histamine via H_2 receptors, typified by a wheal-and-flare skin reaction. The second is immediate smooth muscle contraction in pulmonary bronchi, resulting in bronchospasm and asthma. The late phase of immediate hypersensitivity is characterized by painful, indurated skin lesions on the one hand or compromised airway flow rate on the other. Late-phase reactions are mediated by leukotrienes and prostaglandins, which are cellular metabolites of arachidonic acid.

Evidence suggests that histamine also is capable of switching off—or down-regulating—delayed hypersensitivity responses by interaction with histamine receptors on T lymphocytes, which participate in these reactions (82).

Contact with an allergen or an antigen results in development of IgE antibody response, usually to a local event, at the site of the allergen's entry into the body. This is typically a mucosal surface, the skin, or some local lymph node. Antigen is presented to the B cells with the help of T cells, which stimulate B cells to produce the IgE antibody. Because it is locally produced, IgE first sensitizes local mast cells and then enters the general circulation, binding to receptors on circulating basophils and tissue-fixed mast cells throughout the body.

This ability to bind to mast cells and basophils is a major characteristic of the IgE antibody. The serum half-life of IgE is 2.5 days, but mast cells remain sensitized for as long as 12 weeks. A wheal-and-flare reaction of the skin is typical of the response to an individual whose sensitizers rechallenge with an antigen. The skin-sensitizing ability of IgE resides in the F(c) portion.

Allergic diseases usually are associated with elevated serum IgE concentrations. However, a normal IgE concentration does not exclude atopy. Studies dating from the 1920s indicate that parents who have allergic manifestations have a higher proportion of children who have allergic manifestations than parents who are not allergic. With two allergic parents in the family, there is a 50% chance the children may have an allergy. With one allergic parent, the chances are still approximately 30%. Thus, genetics plays a role in allergy.

When IgE binds to the F(c) receptors on mast cells and basophils, degranulation and release of vasoactive inflammatory mediators are triggered by crosslinking of the IgE molecules with antigen. In addition to mast cells and basophils, other cells have F(c) receptors for IgE antibodies: T cells, B cells, monocytes, alveolar macrophages, eosinophils, and platelets. Monocytes with F(c)-IgE receptors are increased in circulation in cases of atopic eczema. Eosinophils and platelets also have F(c) receptors for IgE and participate in cytotoxicity against parasites. The breakdown products of complement activation called *anaphylatoxins* (C3A and C5A) affect neutrophils, platelets, and macrophages.

Mucosal mast cells require T cells for maturation. Lymphokines from stimulated lymphocytes can release histamine from basophils in addition to that released by IgE combination with antigen. Such a histamine-releasing factor may be involved with amplifying delayed hypersensitivity and regulating type I reactions.

Release of mediators from mast cells and basophils involves an influx of calcium ions first. This is followed by the release of preformed mediators, the chief ones being histamines. After this is the synthesis of new mediators from arachidonic acid leading to the production of prostaglandins and leukotrienes. The release of mediators has an immediate direct effect on tissues, causing edema, bronchoconstriction, and hypersecretion, leading to asthma and the other allergic reactions.

Stimulation of β receptors increases the intracellular level of cyclic adenosine monophosphate. Drugs that block β receptors decrease intracellular levels of cyclic adenosine monophosphate and place individuals at risk for more severe allergic reactions.

IgE plays a beneficial role in parasitic infections. If IgA does not stop the penetration of the gut mucosa by a parasite, contact with IgE-sensitized mast cells causes a reaction that attracts eosinophils and neutrophils needed for local defense. IgE plays a major role in the defense against parasitic infections.

Multiple factors influence human capacity to mount an immediate hypersensitivity response. Included are genetic makeup; dose, duration, and route of exposure to allergen; antigen type; age; and lifestyle or habit. Of these factors, the most important is genetic makeup. Data suggest that the atopic state exhibits a defect in T-lymphocyte (T-suppressor) function (82,83). Even animal models of sensitization demonstrate high and low responder strains (82). In addition, exposure to soluble, high-molecular-weight antigens—including peptides, proteins, glycoproteins, and polysaccharides—tend to select for type I reactions (72). However, when combined with host carrier proteins, even low-molecular-weight haptens can become complete antigens and elicit an immediate hypersensitivity response. Furthermore, characteristics of the chemicals or other xenobiotics that sensitize an individual may not necessarily be the same as those that elicit an allergic response (58,72). It is the atopic worker who is most likely to suffer an allergic response to chemicals in the workplace.

TYPE II HYPERSENSITIVITY (ANTIBODY-DEPENDENT CYTOTOXICITY)

This form of hypersensitivity involves antibody directed against surface or tissue antigen (Table 25-10). Complement is involved, and its activation, along with effector cells, brings about tissue damage to those cells and tissues that contain the cell-surface antigen. Antibodies interact with complement C1Q and the effector cells by the F(c) regions. The antibody, therefore, acts like a bridge between the antigen and the effector cells, thus denoting the antibody-dependent cytoxicity reaction.

Clinical manifestations of type II reactions include transfusion reactions, hemolytic disease of the newborn, autoimmune hemolytic anemias, drug-induced reactions to blood components, acute graft rejection, and glomerular basement membrane (GBM) damage, such as Goodpasture's syndrome, which involves pulmonary hemorrhage and nephritis. Myasthenia gravis is an extreme muscular weakness associated with antibodies to the acetylcholine receptor present on surface of muscle membranes.

Activation of the complement system results in binding of activated C3 to target cells and antigens, which opsonizes the target tissue or cells for the effector cells, such as neutrophils. Chemotaxis attracts effector cells to the site of type II hypersensitivity reactions. C5A is particularly important in this action. C5A is split by C5 convertases from C5, a component of complement. When antibody binds to antigens on the target cell membrane, it activates the first component of the complement pathway, C1. This activates the classical pathway depositing C3B and C4B2B3B on the target cell. C3B acts as an opsonin for cells with appropriate receptors. C5 convertases activate lytic pathway, causing membrane damage by the complement component C5-C9 complex.

Goodpasture's syndrome is an example of cross-reactivity of lung basement membrane with GBM. Goodpasture's syndrome is associated with organic solvent exposure. The syndrome consists of pulmonary hemorrhage and nephritis with immune complex deposition.

TYPE III HYPERSENSITIVITY REACTION (IMMUNE COMPLEX DISEASE)

Immune complexes occur when antibody contacts antigen and the antigen is effectively removed by cells of the immune system (see Table 25-10). However, this type of reaction can go awry and lead to hypersensitivity reaction of type III variety, also called *immune complex disease*. Clinical syndromes that are type III–mediated include serum sickness and autoimmunity diseases.

Three broad groups of immune complex formation diseases exist: (a) persistent infections presenting microbial antigens, resulting in complex formation; (b) autoimmunity with the presence of a self-antigen, resulting in clinical diseases such as nephritis, arthritis, and dermatitis; and (c) extrinsic environmental causes, such as environmental antigens, which can damage tissue.

Persistent infections, such as endocarditis, viral hepatitis, or those caused by parasites that produce weak antibody response, can lead to chronic immune complex formation. Autoimmunity is the production of autoantibodies to self-antigens leading to immune complex formation. Systemic lupus erythematosus (SLE) is an example. Extrinsic environmental causes usually form at a surface contact area, such as the lungs or skin, with an environmental agent. They result in immune complex diseases such as farmer's lung or allergic alveolitis. The antibodies induced by these antigens are primarily IgG rather than IgE.

The immune complexes trigger inflammatory processes and can interact with the complement system, leading to generation of C3A and C5A. Vasoactive amines are released from mast cells and basophils, and chemotaxis of other inflammatory cells occurs. Immune complexes may react with platelets through F(c) receptors. Polymorphonuclear leukocytes attempt phagocytosis of the complex and release lysosomal enzymes, causing further tissue damage.

Serum sickness is an example of circulating immune complexes that are deposited in the tissues, leading to inflammatory syndrome, such as glomerular nephritis and arthritis. Serum sickness is also known as *antigen excess disease*.

The Arthus reaction is a localized reaction in and around the walls of small blood vessels in the skin. The Arthus reaction occurs after repeated immunization with a development of high levels of precipitating IgG antibody. Edema, hemorrhage, and erythema can develop at the site of the repeated injection within 4 to 10 hours after the injection. Antigen antibody and complement are deposited in the vessel wall, followed by neutrophil infiltration and the intravascular clumping of platelets. Platelet reactions can lead to vascular occlusion and necrosis in severe cases.

Immune complexes are normally removed by the mononuclear phagocyte system in the liver, spleen, and lungs. However, smaller complexes can circulate for longer periods of time, whereas larger complexes are usually rapidly removed.

Immune complex deposition is more probable in sites in which high blood pressure and turbulence are present. Such sites are glomerular capillaries and the lungs, walls of arteries, vessel bifurcation, and choroid plexus of the ciliary body of the eye.

Mounting evidence exists that injury to tissue caused by antigen-antibody complexes is more common than initially supposed (84–87).

Hypersensitivity pneumonitis includes a group of respiratory diseases caused by inhalation of organic dusts and chemicals. After exposure, patients experience dyspnea, fever, cough, and malaise (86). Symptoms start 4 to 6 hours after exposure to the causative antigen and may last for 12 to 24 hours. Chest roentgenograms during the acute phase show interstitial edema and, occasionally, patchy infiltrates (86). Hypersensitivity pneumonitis exhibits common features: (a) There is predominant involvement of the peripheral airways without systemic organ involvement; (b) lesions are characterized by mononuclear cell, alveolar filling, interstitial infiltrates (T-suppressor/cytotoxic lymphocytes and macrophages) that progress to granulomas; (c) T cells and alveolar macrophages present are markedly activated; and (d) disease is associated with high levels of precipitating antibody against offending particulate antigens, with bronchial washes showing elevated levels of IgG, IgA, IgM, and T-cell lymphokines.

TYPE IV HYPERSENSITIVITY REACTIONS OR DELAYED HYPERSENSITIVITY REACTION

Delayed-type hypersensitivity (DTH) reaction requires a time period to develop. Unlike other forms of hypersensitivity, it cannot be transferred from one animal to another by serum, but can be transferred by lymphocytes bearing surface phenotypes. T cells are necessary for producing the delayed response and are referred to as NK cells, which have become sensitized to the particular antigen by a previous encounter. Examples of delayed hypersensitivity reactions include granulomatous diseases and the positive reaction to a tuberculin skin test. Granulomatous hypersensitivity reactions are generally the more serious type of type IV reaction. Allergic contact dermatitis characterized by eczema is another example.

Granulomatous hypersensitivity involving T-cell–mediated immunity results from the persistent presence of some agent within a macrophage that it is unable to destroy. Immunologic granuloma formation occurs with certain metals, such as beryllium and zirconium, and from nonantigenic stimuli, such as talc.

The epithelioid cell is the characteristic cell of granulomatous hypersensitivity diseases and is seen on electron microscopy as a large flattened cell with an increased amount of endoplasmic reticulum. Another type of cell seen in this reaction is the multinucleated giant cell. Giant cells have nuclei distributed around the periphery and contain little endoplasmic reticulum.

A granulomatous hypersensitivity reaction requires as long as 4 weeks for the reaction time and histologically contains epithelioid cells or giant cells, macrophages, fibrosis, and necrosis. A number of chronic infectious diseases manifest delayed hypersensitivity, such as mycobacteria, protozoa, and fungi, which produce tuberculosis, leprosy, leishmaniasis, listeriosis, deep fungal infections, and helminthic infections. These diseases present with chronic antigenic stimulation.

DTH reactions usually occur 24 hours or more after interaction of soluble antigen with previously sensitized, antigen-specific T lymphocytes. The histologic hallmark of this reaction is a mononuclear cell infiltrate containing lymphocytes, monocytes, and basophils. Pathology is mediated by lymphokines, such as IFN-γ, which activates monocytes/macrophages and causes them to secrete enzymes and other pharmacologically active mediators that induce tissue damage. A classical example of DTH is the allergic contact dermatitis induced by contact with poison ivy. Plant catechols, such as urushiol and toxicodendrol, are the causative allergens in this disorder.

PSEUDOALLERGIC REACTIONS

The intersection of immunotoxicity and hypersensitivity is often complex. Multiple etiologies and mechanisms may induce similar signs and symptoms. An example of this complexity is the reactive airway type of disorder, which can be induced by irritant, toxic, or immunologic mechanisms (113–115). Circumstances in which patients may present symptoms characteristic of immune-mediated hypersensitivities range from skin rashes to anaphylaxis, in which it is impossible to establish that any immune mechanism is involved. The molecular basis of such phenomena is not understood completely. Certain chemicals and other xenobiotics have the ability to bypass the regular two-stage mast-cell triggering process and act directly to cause degranulation (114–116). Mechanisms by which this may occur include (a) direct cytolysis of the mast cell (cytotoxicity), (b) direct, noncytolytic mast-cell degranulation not involving immune mechanisms (114,115), and (c) direct chemical interaction with complement to form anaphylatoxic complement subcomponents (114,115).

CHEMICALLY INDUCED HYPERSENSITIVITY

Some chemicals can cause respiratory or dermal hypersensitivity, inducing asthma or contact dermatitis.

The precise mechanisms responsible for hypersensitivity to low-molecular-weight chemicals are hypothesized to be that certain low-molecular-weight chemicals can act as haptens and bind to protein carriers (e.g., self-proteins or MHC molecule), leading to an immune response directed against the hapten:carrier complex. A number of factors are known to influence either in the induction or elicitation phases of hypersensitivity (Table 25-12): (a) genetic predisposition; (b) preexisting disease or dysfunction; (c) inherent sensitizing potential of the chemical; (d) route of exposure during sensitization; (e) concentration, duration, and frequency of exposure; and (f) other lifestyle factors. Dermal and respiratory routes of exposure are the predominant portals for occupational and environmental agents.

Skin Immune System

The skin is a major organ of defense. Its first line of defense, the physical/chemical barrier, results from the physiochemical properties of the cornified layer of the epidermis. This layer serves as a barrier to water-soluble compounds, photons of sunlight, mechanical trauma, and invasion by microbial agents. However, allergens and antigens are often able to penetrate the outermost layer of the epidermis, necessitating a second line of defense, the immune system.

The immune network of the skin is thought to be compartmentalized and is often referred to as the *skin immune system* (117). Compartmentalized immune networks are dependent on constant recirculation of lymphoid cells to increase the random chance of antigen-specific lymphocytes interacting with APCs. After interaction with antigen-bearing Langerhans' cells (skin APC), recirculation of lymphocytes from the skin to draining lymph nodes and other lymphoid organs allows for amplification of the immune response by directing effector cells to the site of antigen deposition. A functioning skin immune system not only protects against skin infections that are due to viral, fungal, or bacterial agents, but also plays a pivotal role in immune surveillance against skin tumors.

TABLE 25-12. Mechanisms responsible for chemically induced hypersensitivity

Chemical and/or metabolites are directly antigenic by themselves.
Chemicals or metabolites may haptenize with serum proteins to form new immunogens and autoantigens.
Chemicals or metabolites covalently bind to macromolecules present in the target organ areas of the lung, gastrointestinal tract, or skin.
Chemicals directly affect the immune system with activation of T-cell lymphocytes, activation of B-cell lines, and an increase in helper to suppressor T-cell ratio.
Autoantigens are released following tissue damage by chemical exposures.
There are shared antigen determinants between the chemical and tissue of the organism.

Examples of skin diseases in which chemical hypersensitivity plays a role include the following:

- *Allergic contact dermatitis*: A T-lymphocyte–mediated, DTH response. The resulting inflammatory reaction is usually localized at the site of antigen deposition in the skin. DTH responses can be elicited months after the initial (priming) exposure, with the local cellular infiltrate predominantly being mononuclear cells. Unresolved inflammatory responses at the site of antigen deposition result in thickening, fissuring, and lichenification of the skin (108).
- *Urticaria/hives*: Mediated through an antigen-specific IgE antibody and mast-cell collaboration, resulting in release of pharmacologically active mast-cell factors. These mast-cell factors induce a localized increase in vascular permeability, resulting in erythema and edema of the dermis, and often resulting in intense itching, tingling, or burning. Contact urticaria occurs through dermal contact with the chemical allergen (109).

DIAGNOSIS OF DERMAL HYPERSENSITIVITY

Clinical diagnosis of chemically induced dermal hypersensitivities involves the following elements: (a) careful clinical, occupational, and recreational histories; (b) epicutaneous (patch) testing; (c) cutaneous (prick or intradermal injection) tests; (d) provocation tests, when deemed appropriate (118–123); and (e) biopsy of a lesion.

Respiratory Immune System

The respiratory tract is protected by innate and adaptive immune mechanisms. Innate immunity is provided by epithelial cells, the mucociliary escalator, nonspecific phagocytes, NK cells, and lysozymes. Adaptive immunity is provided to the respiratory tract through an extensive lymphoid apparatus comprised of B and T lymphocytes, alveolar macrophages, and other antigen-presenting cells. Histologically, lymphoid tissue can be observed throughout the respiratory tract, from the nasopharynx to alveoli.

Regional lymph nodes receiving lymphatic drainage from most of the lungs are located at the level of the trachea and major bronchi (tracheobronchial and hilar lymph nodes). In addition to these typical lymph nodes, the respiratory tract contains lymphoid nodules comprised of follicular structures, but lacking capsules. These lymphoid elements—BALT—occur in the walls of the bronchi. BALT is distributed at strategic intersections between arteries and bronchus epithelium. Lymphocytes and phagocytes are distributed throughout the submucosa and lamina propria in close proximity to blood and lymphatic vessels. Bronchioles contain discrete aggregates of lymphoid tissue juxtaposed with specialized lymphoepithelium. These unique structures allow intimate communication between respiratory epithelium, lymphatic tissue, and blood vessels, and it is likely that filtration and subsequent transport of antigenic material to the immune apparatus occurs at this location.

Chemical respiratory allergy is an immune-mediated reaction in the respiratory tract resulting in numerous conditions, such as asthma (104,110,124–127), hypersensitivity pneumonitis (104,111,112,128–131), and rhinitis (104,127,132,133). Sensitization is thought to occur via inhalation exposure to appropriate antigens, but dermal exposures may also contribute to the induction of pulmonary hypersensitivities. Respiratory reactions in individuals previously sensitized are usually elicited by inhalation of recall antigen. Allergic responses to chemicals in the respiratory

TABLE 25-13. Examples of occupational respiratory allergens

	Chemicals	Metal fumes	Medications
Asthma	Acid anhydrides Aminoethyl ethanolamine Azodicarbonamide Colophony Cutting oils Cyanoacrylate esters Fluoride Formaldehyde Glutaraldehyde Hexamethylene diisocyanate Paraphenylene diamine Plicatic acid Reactive organic dyes Toluene diisocyanate	Chromium Cobalt Nickel Platinum Vanadium Welding flux	Amprolium HC Cimetidine Penicillins Piperazine Spiramycin Sulfonamide Tetracycline
	Chemicals	**Microbial antigens**	
Hypersensitivity pneumonitis	Copper sulfate Diphenylmethane diisocyanate Hexamethylene diisocyanate Pyrethrum Sodium diazobenzene sulfate Toluene diisocyanate Trimellitic anhydride	*Alternaria* spp. *Aspergillus* spp. *Aureobasidium pullans* *Cladosporium* spp. *Faenia rectivirgula* *Graphium* spp. *Merulius lacrymans* *Naegleria gruberi* *Penicillium* spp. *Thermoactinomyces* spp. *Trichosporon cutaneum*	

tract are often associated with type I immunopathology, but types II, III, and IV mechanisms can also be involved (Table 25-13).

ASTHMA

Asthma is a complex inflammatory disease characterized by airway obstruction that is reversible (but not completely so in some individuals), either spontaneously or with treatment, and increased airway responsiveness to a variety of stimuli. Allergy is often associated with asthma in childhood, but many adults with asthma do not appear to be sensitized to specific allergens. The risk of developing asthma has a genetic component; children with asthmatic parents are at increased risk for developing the disease themselves. The histologic hallmarks of asthma are infiltration of inflammatory cells, especially eosinophils; edema; and loss of respiratory epithelial integrity. Individuals with asthma typically develop acute episodes characterized by respiratory symptoms (e.g., dyspnea, cough, wheezing) and airflow obstruction.

HYPERSENSITIVITY PNEUMONITIS

Hypersensitivity pneumonitis results from repeated inhalation of organic dust, low-molecular-weight chemicals, or chemicals. This classification of respiratory hypersensitivity constitutes a spectrum of granulomatous, interstitial and bronchiolar, and alveolar lung diseases. Initially considered a rare disease, advances in diagnosis demonstrate that the disease is more common than earlier thought (112). The histologic hallmark of hypersensitivity pneumonitis includes an interstitial mononuclear cell infiltrate and the presence of activated lymphocytes in bronchoalveolar lavage fluid. Pathogenesis of hypersensitivity pneumonitis involves (a) repeated antigen exposure, (b) immunologic sensitization of the host to specific antigens, and (c) immune-mediated damage to the lung.

DIAGNOSIS OF RESPIRATORY HYPERSENSITIVITY

Clinical history, including familial and occupational findings, and the frequent coexistence of rhinitis or sinusitis are key factors in diagnosis of respiratory hypersensitivities. Spirometry should be performed before and after beta-agonist bronchodilator administration to identify reversible airflow limitation. If spirometry shows no airflow limitation and asthma is suspected, a methacholine or histamine challenge test should be administered to identify nonspecific airway hyperresponsiveness. Because of the complexity of most respiratory hypersensitivities, other tests may also be indicated, including complete blood cell count, chest radiography, sputum/nasal secretion cytology, complete pulmonary function testing, sinus radiography, and tests to identify gastroesophageal reflux.

Predictive Testing for Respiratory Hypersensitivity

Respiratory hypersensitivity to chemicals is a growing public concern. Although the number of chemicals known to cause respiratory hypersensitivities is limited, predictive testing is essential for the development of occupational and environmental health protection. Approaches used to predict chemicals with respiratory sensitization potential include structure-activity studies, assessment of *in vitro* binding of reactive chemicals to proteins, and *in vivo* exposure characterizations including serology, histopathology, and pulmonary function.

AUTOIMMUNITY

How does the immune system respond to foreign antigens without responding to self? Thanks to the early work of Bretscher and Cohn (134) and others, we know that two signals are required to activate lymphocytes. Signal 1 is the binding of lymphocyte receptors with antigen, whereas signal 2 is engendered by *costimulatory molecules* (135–137). Costimulatory signals can emanate from microbial constituents, from lymphokines such as IL-1 and IL-2, or from a variety of extracellular matrix proteins, subsequently named *adhesion pro-*

teins. Costimulatory adhesion proteins have been demonstrated on APCs, B lymphocytes, T lymphocytes, and activated endothelial cells. Paradoxically, recognition and response to nonself is MHC restricted (requires recognition of self). Binding of antigen (signal 1) in the absence of a costimulatory signal (signal 2) down-regulates the immune response into a specific state of unresponsiveness, clonal anergy (138). The importance of down-regulation of lymphocytes in avoiding autoimmunization should be obvious. However, the converse up-regulation of lymphocytes, especially the activation of antiself lymphocytes by costimulatory molecules, can result in a destructive cycle of immunopathology.

For any given autoimmune disease, no specific gene, no specific environmental agent, and no specific perturbation of the immune apparatus, in and of itself, causes this disorder. Rather, a concentration of obligatory MHC and non-MHC genes interacts with environmental agents and inherent anomalies of a specific target organ to trigger and maintain an autoimmune response. Interestingly, the capacity to produce autoantibodies is an inherent property of the normal immune apparatus. B-cell–derived autoantibodies and autoreactive T cells are commonly found in persons not otherwise demonstrating an autoimmune disease. These innocuous natural autoantibodies are present in small amounts and only as low-affinity antibodies in normal sera. Autoimmunity becomes a pathologic event (e.g., autoimmune disease) with the production of large amounts of certain kinds of IgM autoantibodies or specific high-affinity IgG autoantibodies. High-affinity IgG autoantibodies require autoreactive T cells and are likely to be derived from an antigen-driven response.

The overwhelming problem in autoimmune disease lies not in the existence of autoantibody or autoreactive T cells, but rather in the complex interactions of genes, immune factors, and environmental agents that drive autoimmunization into a profound deviation from the normal: a self-destructive immune response. Germline/phenotypic variations and defects in T-lymphocyte maturation are hypothesized to contribute to impaired immune regulation, setting the stage for later development of autoimmune disease (Table 25-14).

With many autoimmune diseases, the preponderance of women who have the disease is intriguing. Often, this same phenomenon is observed in animal models of autoimmune diseases (139). It has been shown that sex hormones can modify immune responses. Orchidectomy amplifies immune responses, and women typically produce higher antibody titers after antigen challenge than men (140). How female sex hormones alter immune responses is largely unknown. A direct effect on lymphocytes or macrophages, or both, has been postulated (140), and estrogens are known to have complex effects on T-cell maturation (138).

Despite an incomplete understanding of the complex interaction of genes, hormones, and environmental agents associated with autoimmune disease, it is obvious that failure to effectively regulate autoimmunity can result in clinically important consequences (141–151). Just as self-recognition is essential to the immune system, uncontrolled self-reaction is perilous. The weight of evidence from numerous studies indicates that numerous environmental agents may be implicated in the induction or maintenance of autoimmune disease. Evidence exists to support infectious agents (150,152–157), therapeutic agents (147,158–160), and chemicals (12,17,22,145,158–162) as etiologic agents in the induction of autoimmunity. Because chemicals influence lymphocyte activation, antibody synthesis, production of cytokines, and other cellular interactions, it is not surprising that they may also induce autoimmune responses and autoimmune disease.

Autoimmune disorders induced by chemicals can be either tissue specific (e.g., myasthenia gravis and thyroiditis) or systemic (e.g., SLE). Drugs such as hydralazine, procainamide, and methyldopa are frequently implicated in the induction of autoimmunity (138,158–160). Other agents, such as mercuric chloride (158,161), gold salts (158), dieldrin (163), and methylcholanthrene (164), have also been implicated in the induction of autoimmune disease.

TABLE 25-14. Autoimmune disease

Syndrome	Associated antigens (Ags)
Antibody-mediated pathology	
Systemic lupus erythematosus	Double- or single-stranded DNA
Autoimmune granulocytopenia	Nuclear and cytoplasmic Ags
Autoimmune thrombocytopenia	Granulocytes
Goodpasture's syndrome	Thrombocytes
Myasthenia gravis	Glomerular basement membrane
Pernicious anemia	Acetylcholine receptors
Autoimmune thyroiditis	Intrinsic factors
Autoimmune endocrinopathies	Thyroglobulin
Autoimmune hemolytic anemia	Selected hormones
Pemphigus	Erythrocytes
Immune granulocytopenia	Intracellular epidermal Ags
Immune thrombocytopenia	Xenobiotics bound to self-Ags
Serum sickness	Xenobiotics bound to self-Ags
Anaphylaxis	Xenobiotics bound to self-Ags
Immune hemolytic anemia	Xenobiotics bound to self-Ags
Cell-mediated pathology	
Experimental allergic encephalomyelitis	T-cell specificity for basic protein of myelin
Experimental arthritis	T-cell specific for *Mycobacterium* tuberculosis and synovial tissue
Contact dermatitis	Xenobiotics bound to self-Ags

Xenobiotics may elicit an autoimmune response via at least four different hypothesized mechanisms:

1. *Direct effects on the immune system*: Xenobiotics or their metabolites may directly alter lymphocytes and macrophages. These effects may be manifested as reductions in T-cell suppressor activity or polyclonal activation of B cells (165,166). Direct evidence of methyldopa interference with T-cell suppressor activity in human autoimmune hemolytic anemia has been elucidated (167). Procainamide has also been demonstrated to disrupt immune regulation by inhibiting cyclic adenosine monophosphate generation and stimulating T-cell helper functions (168). Metals such as mercury are reported to stimulate polyclonal B-lymphocyte stimulation (158).
2. *Release or expression of autoantigens*: Xenobiotics may disrupt and release tissue antigens into the general circulation, a qualitative effect. Alternatively, chemical agents may induce a quantitative increase in autoantigens present normally in the circulation. This mechanism may explain autoimmune responses after chronic exposure to metals such as mercury or gold (158).
3. *Altered-self*: Xenobiotics may interact with autoantigens in such a manner as to no longer be recognized as self. Interactions with chemicals may either expose "hidden" antigenic determinants or induce the production of new autoantigens. Hydralazine is thought to induce autoimmune responses via this mechanism by its ability to complex with deoxyribonucleoprotein.
4. *Molecular mimicry*: Increasing evidence shows that certain infectious agents may contain antigenic determinants that closely resemble host heat-shock proteins (169–171). Interestingly, SLE patients demonstrate an enhanced expression of a heat-shock-protein gene by circulating mononuclear

cells (172). Theory would suggest—but no evidence supports—that possible shared antigenic determinants exist between xenobiotics and autoantigens. In fact, autoantibodies induced by procainamide, methyldopa, penicillamine, and hydralazine do not cross-react with these drugs.

The weight of evidence accumulated to date demonstrates that autoimmunity, as well as autoimmune disease, can be induced by chronic exposure to common xenobiotics. Studies from humans and animals reveal that autoimmune phenomena are induced by a complex interaction of genes, hormones, and environmental factors. Although therapeutic drugs are the most common xenobiotics implicated in autoimmune disease, individuals charged with the prevention, diagnosis, and treatment of autoimmune disease should be aware of the potential role that other chemicals may play in the development of these disorders.

PREDICTIVE IMMUNOTOXICITY TESTING

As the importance of the immune system becomes better elucidated, more attention is being placed on protecting it—and, if possible, manipulating it—therapeutically. Humans are often subjected to unavoidable exposures to many potentially hazardous environmental and occupational agents. These potential hazards—occurring as undesirable consequences of inadequately tested technologies, increases in population and pollution, and emerging infectious diseases—have become a worldwide concern. The interaction of xenobiotics with various circuits of the immune apparatus has therefore become an area of notable scientific and clinical concern. Fueled by this concern, demand has grown for the capability to predict potential immunotoxicity before human exposure.

Immune responses are numerous and varied, producing markers that can be used to predict environmental exposures, develop dose-response relationships, and facilitate assessment of risk associated with low-level exposures. These markers include quantitative alterations in total immunoglobulins, antigen-specific antibodies, and immune-cell populations. Quantitative and qualitative changes in functional responses to biological and chemical antigens, mitogens, vaccines, infectious agents, and neoplastic cell lines also are used as markers of immunotoxicity. These biomarkers of immunotoxicity can be grouped into three main categories:

- *Markers of exposure* can be xenobiotics or their metabolites. This marker can also be the product of interaction between the xenobiotic and a target cell or biomolecule. Immune system biomarkers indicating exposure are xenobiotic-specific antibodies or cellular responses.
- *Markers of effect* are measurable cellular, biochemical, or molecular alterations within an organism that can be recognized as either being established or having potential adverse health effects. Immune-system biomarkers of effect include alterations in the cells or biochemistry, resulting in impairment of the immune system and immune-mediated pathology manifested in tissues outside of the immune apparatus.
- *Markers of susceptibility* are factors known to alter immune responsiveness, resulting in differences between populations and individuals and within individuals over time. The three most important factors are genetics, age-related alterations, and neuropsychological factors (173). Examples of immune system biomarkers of susceptibility include certain genes or gene products associated with increased susceptibility to certain immune-mediated diseases (allergy, autoimmunity), pregnancy (estrogen-induced immunosuppression, placental antigen-induced immune responses), age-related immune variations (decline in thymic hormone levels), and the immunologic fragility of the developing fetus.

Using sensitive methods that measure changes in these biomarkers of immunotoxicity, predictive immunotoxicity testing is performed to determine (a) the potential adverse immune alterations induced by occupational or environmental agents, or (b) the potential adverse or beneficial immunomodulatory effects of pharmaceutics.

The International Seminar on the Immunological System as a Target Organ for Toxicity has recommended that "a chemical substance should be considered immunotoxic when undesired events of the chemical are 1) a direct and/or indirect action of the xenobiotic (and/or biotransformation product) on the immune system; or, 2) an immunologically based host response to the compound and/or its metabolites, or host antigens are modified by the compound or its metabolites" (174).

Historically, predictive immunotoxicity testing has been performed using laboratory animals, particularly rodents. No single immune function test can accurately predict immunotoxicity; the structural and functional complexity of the immune apparatus requires that multiple parameters be scrutinized for a comprehensive assessment. Immunotoxicology and its sister discipline, clinical immunology, use sensitive batteries of descriptive and functional assays to determine the immunologic status of individuals. Exposures, challenges, and measurements are implemented using *in vivo* and *in vitro* methods (175). It should be noted that application of modern immunologic methods, in concert with traditional toxicologic studies, have demonstrated a very effective partnership, resulting in a burgeoning immunotoxicology literature. Standard toxicology endpoints, such as organ weights, cellularity, and cell-subpopulation dynamics, can and do serve as important cornerstones in assessing immune injury. However, a fortuitous feature of the immune system is the ability of its cells to be removed from the body and retain their function *in vitro*. This unique feature has allowed the development of numerous immunotoxicology methods that can yield a realistic analysis of both immune parameters (biomarkers of immunotoxicity) and functional (host resistance) aspects of the immune system (Table 25-15).

TABLE 25-15. Examples of immune (biomarker) and host-resistance assays

Immune (biomarker) assays
Thymus/body weight ratio
Spleen/body weight ratio
Complete blood cell count with differential cell counts
Cell-surface marker expression (qualitative and quantitative)
Total immunoglobulin and IgG, IgM, IgA, and IgG titers
Delayed-type hypersensitivity responses against keyhole limpet hemocyanin
Autoantibody titers
Spleen cellularity (nucleated cells)
IgM (primary response) and IgG (secondary response) plaque-forming cells to sheep erythrocytes
T-cell mitogenic responses to concanavalin A
B-cell mitogenic responses to lipopolysaccharide
Mixed-leukocyte response against allogeneic leukocytes
Natural killer–cell activity against tumor lines (YAC-1 tumor cells)
Host-resistance assays
Lung tumor burden after injection with B16F10 melanoma cells
Tumor growth after subcutaneous implantation of PYB6 tumor cells
Parasitemia after infection with *Trypanosoma musculi*
Parasitemia after infection with *Plasmodium yoelii*
Parasitemia after infection with *Trichinella spiralis*
Morbidity after challenge with influenza virus
Morbidity after challenge with *Streptomyces monocytogenes*
Morbidity after challenge with *Listeria monocytogenes*

For detailed protocols for these assays, please refer to Burleson GR, Dean JH, and Munson AE, eds. *Methods in immunotoxicology.* New York: Wiley-Liss, 1995.

TABLE 25-16. Two-tier immunotoxicity panel

Parameters	Procedures
Tier I (screen)	
Immunopathology	Hematology: Complete blood workup and differential count
	Weights: Body, spleen, thymus, kidney, liver, and lungs
	Cellularity: Spleen
	Histology: Spleen, thymus, lymph nodes
Humoral-mediated immunity	Enumeration of IgM antibody plaque-forming cells to T-dependent and T-independent antigens and lipopolysaccharide mitogen response
Cell-mediated immunity	Con A mitogen response and mixed-leukocyte response
Nonspecific immunity	Natural killer–cell activity (spleen)
Tier II (mechanism)	
Immunopathology	Quantitation of splenic B- and T-cell numbers
Humoral-mediated immunity	Enumeration of IgG antibody plaque-forming cells to T-dependent Ags
Cell-mediated immunity	Cytotoxic T-lymphocyte function and delayed hypersensitivity responses
Nonspecific immunity	Enumeration of peritoneal macrophages and analysis of their phagocytic capacity
Host-resistance models (endpoints)	Syngeneic tumor models: PyB6 sarcoma (tumor incidence), B16F10 melanoma (lung burden)
	Bacterial models: *Listeria monocytogenes* (mortality), *Streptococcus* spp. (mortality)
	Parasite models: *Trypanosoma musculi* (parasitemia), *Plasmodium yoelii* (parasitemia)
	Virus models: Influenza (mortality)

Numerous detailed methodologies for the assessment of chemically induced immunotoxicity are available (81). Typically, these methods are grouped into tiered batteries of tests. We present a two-tiered battery of tests for the screening of immunotoxicity (Table 25-16) that differs only slightly from that recommended by the National Toxicology Program (NTP), National Institute of Environmental Health Sciences (32). Our modifications include the use of T-independent antigen probes (176), in addition to T-dependent antigens (tier I) and the substitution of a *Trypanosoma musculi* host-resistance model (87) for *Plasmodium yoelii* (tier II). These modifications are included because of the increased sensitivity they add to each of their respective tiers.

The remainder of the two tiers is essentially the same as that of the NTP testing regimen. Tier I assays are limited and are positioned to readily detect potent immunotoxicants. Tier I tests are presumably less effective in detecting weak immunotoxicants. Nevertheless, no compound has been identified that can affect a tier II assay without also exhibiting an effect in some tier I assessment (34,177). Tier II tests are intended to confirm the immunotoxicity of xenobiotics identified in tier I and further elucidate possible cellular and molecular mechanisms of immunotoxic activity for those xenobiotics (32). Predictive immunotoxicity testing has elucidated an interesting array of immunotoxins (11,13,16,19,21,22,24,28,51,59,60,64–66,68–71,162,178–228).

Another approach that holds great promise for predictive immunotoxicity testing is the use of human peripheral blood cells. Using these cells to detect the adverse effects of environmental exposures is relevant in that immune cells circulate through the body, making contact with all the major organ systems; control numerous host defense mechanisms; and can metabolically alter many xenobiotics. Because of the ready access to human peripheral blood cells, immunotoxicology represents a unique scientific arena in which *in vivo* immunology can be carefully examined using minimally invasive techniques.

Using mononuclear cells recovered from healthy human blood donors, hypersensitivity reactions, autoimmune responses, and immunosuppression induced by chemical agents can be assessed *in vitro* using human cells cultured in the presence of xenobiotics or examined directly after a potential *in vivo* exposure has occurred. Data derived from *in vivo* exposures can be used to confirm or refute the validity of data derived from *in vitro* methods.

The powerful combination of human- and animal-based predictive immunotoxicity assessments provides a sound basis for further study of the immune system as a target organ for toxic chemicals. Future efforts will be devoted to cataloging the testing results for several hundred compounds for use in assessing the efficacy of various test combinations. Further refinement of cellular and molecular biomarkers of immunotoxicity will also be necessary to resolve the economic and laboratory limitations inherent in predicting chemical immunotoxins.

RISK ASSESSMENT AND IMMUNOTOXICOLOGY

Although the adoption of a battery of tests to evaluate immunotoxicity has advanced our knowledge of xenobiotic-induced damage to the immune system in the regulatory context, it is important not only to identify, quantify, and predict adverse alterations in the immune system, but also to determine the toxicologic significance of such information. It is economically impossible to completely test for immunotoxic effects associated with all of the chemicals released into the environment. Therefore, methods to more accurately predict risk to the immune system must be developed using limited but critical immunotoxicity data sets. The flurry of activity and intense controversy associated with risk assessment and its use in regulatory decisions can be viewed as a vectored dilemma, driven by competing—sometimes antagonistic—forces. Concerns of industry that costs of complying with environmental regulations are excessive given the weak scientific basis for many risk assessments, concerns of environmentalists that risk-assessment practices and policies do not adequately protect human and environmental health, and the public's lack of confidence in regulatory decision making all contribute to an adversarial atmosphere.

Risk assessment for chemical agents focused on estimating the incidence of cancer from chronic or lifetime exposures to a chemical agent at some unit dose. However, increasing demand exists for risk estimates using noncancer endpoints, such as reproductive, nervous, and immune system disorders. Whether establishing cancer or noncancer endpoints, some similarities exist; both necessitate calculations that incorporate assumptions and uncertainties (229–231). As defined by the National Academy of Sciences (232), risk assessment comprises four steps. These steps—as well as their applicability to immunotoxicology data—are summarized as the following:

1. *Hazard identification* attempts to determine whether a specific xenobiotic can cause adverse health effects. This step involves a qualitative evaluation of animal and human data to determine the potential hazard of a xenobiotic. Important considerations in hazard identification include dose, route, and duration of exposure in the test species. When attempting to identify immunotoxic hazards, it is generally assumed that alterations in immune function, lymphoid organ histology, or host resistance to infectious agents or neoplasia could potentially evolve into adverse effects.
2. *Dose-response assessment* attempts to determine the relationship between xenobiotic dose and incidence of adverse effects in humans. For noncancer toxicity, a no-observable-adverse-effect level (NOAEL) is established

for a chosen adverse response. This value is obtained from either a dose-response curve or estimated from the lowest-observable-adverse-effect level. Once a NOAEL has been established, safety factors are typically applied to allow for uncertainties in interspecies variations, irreversibility versus reversibility, and chronic versus acute exposures. Application of dose-response assessment to immunotoxicology data remains difficult. Although the NOAEL is heavily dependent on the sensitivity of an assay, the presence or absence of an immunotoxic effect is dependent on statistically significant alterations occurring in a multiplicity of tests, each with different sensitivities. Furthermore, it has been shown that immune tests often show interdependence with one another (177). Before conducting a dose-response assessment, it may be necessary to rank tests or combinations of tests in order of sensitivity and interdependence.

3. *Exposure assessment* attempts to determine what exposures are currently experienced or anticipated under different conditions in defined populations. This element of risk assessment is performed parallel to hazard identification and dose-response assessment. Exposure assessment is dependent on field measurements, estimates based on job/task/time matrices, or biological/clinical effects to determine a quantitative description of exposure linked to a specific population. Again, application of this risk-assessment tool to immunotoxicology data is difficult. Unfortunately, even seemingly reliable exposure surrogates, such as body burdens of a specific xenobiotic, may not be robust in that they seldom establish concentrations at or in a specific immunologic target organ, tissue, or cell.
4. *Risk characterization* is an aggregation of the previous three steps and attempts to estimate the incidence of an adverse effect in a given population and potential health problems that might reasonably be expected to accompany such an effect.

The two-tiered NTP battery of tests has been used to examine an ever-increasing array of compounds by the National Institute of Environmental Health Sciences and other institutions (32). The database generated by testing more than 50 compounds in both tiers of the NTP battery has been examined in an attempt to improve the accuracy and efficiency of screening chemicals for immunotoxicity and to select those tests that predict immune-mediated diseases (34,177,233). Comparing the result of each immune test with the overall result of the compound tested, the sensitivity, specificity, and concordance (combination of sensitivity and specificity) of each test were determined. Identification of immune parameter tests (biomarkers) that could accurately predict altered host resistance was emphasized. The results of this insightful analysis revealed that (a) as few as two selected assays (lymphocyte enumeration and T-dependent antibody responses) can successfully predict immunotoxicity in mice; (b) an excellent correlation exists between alterations in immune response assays and altered host resistance; (c) no single immune test studied could predict altered host resistance; (d) based on a cyclophosphamide data set, most immune function–host resistance relationships were linear rather than linear-quadratic (threshold) models; and (e) using the same cyclophosphamide data set, it was possible to model the quantitative relationship between immune-function tests and host-resistance tests.

Obviously, additional analyses using other chemical/immune test data sets and animal species are necessary before risk assessments for immunotoxic endpoints will be common. However, results demonstrate that it may be possible to determine the immunotoxic risk of a chemical based on the results of immune (biomarker) tests instead of the more laborious and expensive host-resistance assays.

DEVELOPMENTAL IMMUNOTOXICITY

Although ample evidence exists that the immune system can be adversely altered by xenobiotics, the consequences of these alterations on the developing (fetal) immune system are not well characterized. Lifelong capacity for immunocompetence is determined early in development, during prenatal and early postnatal development. In fetal development, lymphoid precursors first appear in the blood islands of the yolk sac, later move to the liver, and finally reside in the bone marrow (234). At birth, and throughout most of life, the primary lymphocyte-producing organs are the bone marrow and thymus. Injury during prenatal development of the immune system may be initially subtle; xenobiotic-induced alterations in immunocompetence may not be recognized clinically until long after exposure. In rodent-based models, *in utero* treatment with any of a diverse array of immunotoxicants induces more significant and persistent alterations of subsequent postnatal immune responses than similar exposures in adults (3,235).

Many of the predictive methods used to assess immune function in adult humans and animals (e.g., NTP, tier I and II assays) are not readily adaptable to the developmental model (e.g., plaque-forming cell assays, cell-mediated immunoassays, etc.). However, certain immune tests (e.g., cell-surface marker expression) are readily applied to developmental models. Furthermore, studies demonstrate that fetal thymus and liver immune cells are qualitatively and quantitatively altered after immunotoxin exposure (236). Alterations of fetal liver and fetal thymocyte cell-surface antigen expression have also been demonstrated after *in utero* immunotoxin exposure (237). Additional studies in the NZB/NZW mouse model of SLE suggest that exposure to environmental endocrine-disrupting chemicals—which bind to estrogen receptors and thus mimic the action of estradiol—may affect the fetus and alter the subsequent course of autoimmune disease in adults (238). Full characterization of the sensitivity, specificity, and reproducibility of these tests in the unique context of the developing immune apparatus is lacking. Before immunotoxicity assessments can be included in routine developmental toxicity studies, biomarkers of developmental immunotoxicity must be identified and validated.

CLINICAL IMMUNOTOXICOLOGY

Clinical immunotoxicology is concerned with the adverse effects of foreign substances on the immune system of humans. Immunotoxicity is not the same as immunomodulation, unless it results in adverse health effects. Immune alterations that result in harmful responses in the host are considered immunotoxic.

Three broad categories of immunopathology can occur from adverse alteration of the immune system's response:

- Immunosuppression (enhanced susceptibility to infections or cancer)
- Hypersensitivity reactions (type I, type II, type III, type IV)
- Autoimmunity

Immunomodulation can result in immune-system-function changes, such as immunoglobulin production and numbers of cells. But immunotoxicology includes both *harmful change* to the immune system and *adverse effects* to the host. Two broad mechanisms of immunologic responses exist:

- Antigen-specific responses
- Innate, or nonantigen, specific immunity

Antigen-specific responses require primary exposure to an antigen that induces a specific response, such as antigen-specific immunoglobulins or T-cell receptors on lymphocytes. On subsequent contact with the antigen, an enhanced response occurs because of immunologic memory. Nonantigen-specific immunity involves inflammatory effectors, which are activated by nonantigen mechanisms. Examples include NK cells, macrophages, platelet activation, complement activation, and acute-phase reactants.

Immunotoxicity versus Immune Alteration

The immune system is complex, and an amplified response to foreign antigens and haptens is normal. The immune system communicates in a bidirectional manner with the brain and responds to stressors, both acute and chronic. This psychoneuroendocrine connection can be activated by different stressors: physical, environmental, chemical, and psychological. Activation of the hypothalamic-pituitary-adrenal axis increases circulating catecholamines, which may produce immune-system responses, both in quantity and quality, with an increase in NK-cell numbers, increase in CD-8–bearing T-cell lymphocytes, decreased level of NK-cell activity, and depressed lymphocyte response to mitogens.

These immune changes are not a result of toxicity but are a response related to adaptation or maladaptation to stressors. Lymphocytes have membrane receptors for catecholamines, and NK cells are highest in catecholamine-receptor concentration. CD-4–bearing T cells have the lowest number of catecholamine receptors. CD-8 cells are midway between. Research also shows that peripheral cytokine release by activated T cells can influence the brain. Astrocytes in the brain modulate immune responses, and glial cells have cytokine receptors. Inflammation is known to induce CNS responses of anorexia, lethargy, and depression. Activation of macrophages in the inflammatory process releases IL-1, which may induce further cytokine production by the brain. Mast cells are located in close proximity to neurons in the CNS and peripheral nervous system, so chemicals that activate macrophages may induce neuroimmune responses. Production of cytokines peripherally may activate production of CNS cytokines, which may explain the neurobehavioral symptoms experienced by patients with chronic inflammation.

Functional activation of the immune system is demonstrated in situations of stress, particularly chronic stress. Family members caring for Alzheimer patients exhibit functional immune changes. Subjects under stress also show suppression of immune-cell function, such as lymphocyte response to mitogens and an associated increase in antibodies to Epstein-Barr IgG titers. In evaluating patients, these physiologically responsive immune alterations should not be confused with immunopathology.

Polychlorinated and Polybrominated Hydrocarbons

Polyhalogenated aromatic compounds include polychlorinated dibenzo-*p*-dioxins, polychlorinated dibenzofurans, polychlorinated biphenyls (PCBs), and polybrominated biphenyls (PBBs). PCBs were produced in the United States as a mixture of 209 congeners of PCBs. After reports of animal and human toxicity, the production of PCBs in the United States was suspended in 1977. Approximately one-half of the PCBs produced between 1966 and 1974 were used in electrical transformers.

PCBs are inert and are resistant to environmental degradation; therefore, they tend to accumulate in the environment. Human exposure occurs via inhalation or ingestion. The high lipid solubility of these compounds allows them to accumulate up the food chain. Toxic effects of PCBs include chloracne, ocular irritation, arthritis, gastrointestinal symptoms, and hepatotoxicity.

Herbicides, such as 2,4-D (2,4-dichlorophenoxyacetic acid) and 2,4-T (2,4,5-trichlorophenoxyacetic acid), have been contaminated with dibenzo-*p*-dioxins or, more specifically, TCDD 2,3,7,8-tetrachlorodibenzo-*p*-dioxin (239). The toxicity of polychlorinated hydrocarbons is mediated through binding to the arylhydrocarbon receptor (AhR) in cells. The AhR is an intracellular protein that mediates the induction of enzymes such as arylhydrocarbonhydroxylase and 7-ethoxyresorufin-*o*-deethylase (239). Tissues containing this AhR protein are targets for polyhalogenated aromatic chemical toxicity.

PCBs are immunotoxic in various animal species, and as persistent environmental contaminants, they form an important class of compounds of concern. Thymic atrophy occurs in PCB-treated animals, as do alterations in immunity after exposure. PCBs affect humoral and CMI in animal models (240). In humans accidentally exposed to PCB, decreases in the total number of T lymphocytes have been demonstrated, along with decreases in the percentage of peripheral T lymphocytes and concentrations of IgM and IgA. PCBs have also been found to affect polymorphonuclear (PMN) leukocyte function *in vitro*. These effects do not appear to be related to the arylhydrocarbon receptor. Aroclor 1242 stimulates PMN production of superoxide anion (O^{2-}). It appears that exposure to PCBs enhances the respiratory burst *in vitro* of PMNs. Aroclor 1242 also stimulates degranulation in PMNs.

In experimental animal studies, TCDD was the most toxic member of a class of polychlorinated dibenzo compounds. It is a potent carcinogen and promoter of carcinogenesis and affects the developing immune system of animals. However, human toxicity has been difficult to determine.

Humans accidentally exposed from 1977 were retrospectively studied. One Michigan study concluded that 18 of 45 people exposed to PBBs used throughout the state in 1973 and 1974 showed a statistically significant decrease in the absolute number of T cells, as well as decreased mitogenic responses to T-cell mitogens. No change in the absolute number of B cells was evident, but lymphocytes showed decreased mitogenic responses to a B-cell mitogen. A persistent increase in NK cells was also present in these same subjects; this increase remained 5 years later (241). It appears that PBB exposure resulted in a persistent increase in NK cells. However, the exposed population has not been affected by an unusual number of infectious diseases or cancers.

One of the most intensely studied PCB compounds is TCDD, a contaminant of the herbicide 2,4,5-trichlorphenoxyacetic acid (2,4,5-T). The incident in Michigan involving the contamination of dairy cattle feed with PBBs highlighted the concern over these compounds (242). Local farmers and Michigan residents who consumed these contaminated dairy products were found to have PBBs in the plasma. Immunologic investigations demonstrated that 34% of farm residents and 59% of PBB-manufacturing workers had a reduction in T-lymphocyte numbers (243). B-cell and T-cell lymphocyte blastogenesis was reduced in exposed farmers and workers as compared with controls. In the Michigan population overall, T cells and B cells were normal as compared with controls (243).

In a Taiwan incident, 2,000 people were exposed to rice oil contaminated with PCBs. Immunologic changes showed a depression in the percentage of total T cells and active T cells 1 year after exposure. Three years later, there was a partial recovery and an increase in the CD-8 T cells (244). No increase in infectious diseases was associated with this immune change.

In humans, the immunologic health effects of PCBs have been difficult to demonstrate. Chloracne, a recognized dermatologic effect of PCB exposure, is probably the best described toxicity of the compounds with hepatotoxicity. Although animal studies have proven the carcinogenicity of PCBs, no conclusive evidence shows that exposure to PCBs results in an increased incidence of cancer in humans. Small, short-term epidemiologic studies of capacitor manufacturing workers exposed to PCBs have not indicated an increased incidence of cancer (245). Other epidemiologic studies have also failed to demonstrate an increased incidence in cancer rates of exposed humans (246–248). The delayed immune response in 30 patients from the Taiwan incident was studied and compared with the response with 50 controls (249). The study found that dermal lesions appeared to correlate with whole-blood PCB concentrations. The study also demonstrated decreases in IgM and IgA, but no effect on IgG. In addition, there was a decrease in the percentage of T lymphocytes and T-lymphocyte helper cells, as well as a suppression of delayed hypersensitivity to antigens.

Health effects from long-term exposure to TCDD have been reported after spills or contaminations that resulted in human exposure. In 1971, sludge oil contaminated with TCDD was sprayed on dirt roads at various sites in eastern Missouri (250). Twelve years later, in 1983, one of the nine residential sites in which TCDD spraying had occurred became the focus of investigation. The area chosen had TCDD concentrations in surrounding soil ranging from 39 to 1,100 ppb. The mobile homes in the area had inside dust concentrations higher than 1 ppb. The study included 155 exposed individuals. No increase in the number of medical symptoms above the control population was documented in the study, nor were there any incidences of chloracne or increased incidences of cancer. No increased incidences of spontaneous abortions, reproductive problems, or congenital malformations were detected. Basic liver function tests of all exposed individuals were normal. However, subclinical hepatotoxicity was suggested by some of the assays, particularly higher mean urinary uroporphyrin concentrations in exposed persons and correlation of serum levels of five liver enzymes (aspartate aminotransferase, alanine aminotransferase, γ-glutamyltranspeptidase, alkaline phosphatase, and alanine aminopeptidase) with years of residence at the contaminated site. Immunologic evaluation of the exposed individuals revealed an elevated incidence of anergy and relative anergy compared with controls. T-cell-surface marker analyses demonstrated statistically significant decreases in percentages of T-CD3, T-CD4, and T-CD11 cells in exposed groups. The number of non–T lymphocytes in peripheral blood samples was elevated in the exposed group. No significant difference in T-lymphocyte proliferative response to mitogen stimulation or cytotoxic T-cell activity was present in either of the groups.

Overall, the exposed group had a nonstatistically significant increased frequency of abnormal T-cell subsets as well as a nonstatistically significant abnormality in T-cell function (250). The presence of *in vitro* immune alterations in the exposed population, with the absence of overt clinical signs and symptoms of immune deficiency, points to a subclinical immunotoxicity from TCDD after prolonged exposure.

Another study on individuals exposed to TCDD for 10 years who lived or worked near contaminated areas in Missouri showed no difference in the study population as compared with the control group in delayed hypersensitivity, T-cell subsets, and cytotoxic T-cell proliferation assays (251). A separate study reported health effects of TCDD in children after an environmental accident near Seveso, Italy, in 1976 (252). The exposed children totaled approximately 1,500 and ranged in age from 6 to 10 years. Immunologic parameters were not studied, but liver function tests showed alterations in alanine aminotransferase and γ-glutamyltransferase.

An immunologic investigation of 55 transformer repairmen with high adipose concentrations of PCBs has been reported (245). These workers were predominantly exposed to Aroclor 1260 and some to Aroclor 1242. Physical examinations, as well as immunologic evaluations, were performed. Delayed hypersensitivity, evaluated with an intradermal injection of mumps and trichophytin antigens, was no different than in the nonexposed controls. No incidence of chloracne was reported in this study.

Although animal studies have supported the immunotoxicity of PCBs, human studies to date have been questionable in terms of immunopathology and subsequent adverse health effects.

Metals

Metals have immune consequences after systemic and dermal exposure. Immunotoxic metals include arsenic, lead, mercury, cadmium, chromium, nickel, beryllium, indium, silver, gold, cobalt, molybdenum, platinum, and zirconium.

Exposure to inorganic lead, mercury, and cadmium is associated with glomerulonephritis secondary to GBM deposition of anti-GBM antibodies (253–255). Clinical manifestations include proteinuria and nephrotic syndrome. Metal-induced glomerulonephritis does not appear to be dose related. An immune glomerulonephritis may occur in as many as 10% of patients receiving gold salt therapy for rheumatoid arthritis (255).

Cadmium is reported to produce renal tubular lesions as well as glomerulonephritis (255). Animal studies have demonstrated IgG glomerular deposits in the basement membrane, as well as antibodies directed against GBM glycoproteins after chronic cadmium exposure. Cadmium has been shown to suppress antibody formation in animals and has been epidemiologically linked to respiratory cancer (256).

Although lead can reduce host resistance to infection and interfere with reproductive functions, lead-induced immunotoxicity in humans has not been well documented. One study, which examined the effect of lead on 12 children documented to have measurable blood lead concentrations, did not demonstrate any significant effect on major immunoglobulin concentrations, total complement, C3 component of complement, or the antigenic response to tetanus toxoid (257,258).

Metals can produce dermal and respiratory problems, ranging from rashes to occupationally induced asthma. Chromium, beryllium, and platinum are particularly potent sensitizing metals and produce a variety of hypersensitivity pulmonary diseases and dermal lesions after human exposure. Hexavalent chromium compounds can produce corrosive and irritating effects after dermal exposure, which consists of skin ulceration, dermatitis, and nasal septum ulceration. Chromium, a shiny white metal, is nontoxic in the elemental state. Chromium salts, trioxides, and chromic acid are strong irritants and oxidants that can produce immune-mediated glomerulonephritis (255). Chronic inhalation of chromium dust can produce asthma and reactive airway disease.

Beryllium can cause pulmonary disease in microgram amounts. Controlling environmental air concentrations of beryllium has been demonstrated to control acute pulmonary disease in workers; however, chronic pulmonary disease is not dose related, and minute exposures can be a definite risk factor. Beryllium in all forms can cause human disease, usually via inhalation. Acute beryllium inhalation can cause tracheobronchitis and necrosis of the mucous membranes of the tracheobronchial area, as well as conjunctivitis and rashes. Berylliosis may be delayed for several years postexposure. Chronic beryllium disease is characterized by granulomatous lesions in the lungs, skin, spleen, liver, lymph nodes, and kidneys. Acute exposure to beryllium dusts can produce inflammatory pneumonitis. Immunotoxicity from beryllium exposure is thought to occur through an antibody-mediated sensitization process (121,122). A specific lymphocyte transformation test is available to test humans for sensitivity to beryllium. Nodular granulomatous, noncaseating lesions have been documented in workers with inhalational beryllium exposure. Direct skin contact with beryllium can cause hypersensitivity dermatitis.

Beryllium is a potent sensitizing metal that can produce pulmonary and dermal disease via immunologic mechanisms not fully understood. Epidemiologic data also suggest an association between beryllium and lung cancer.

Nickel and nickel compounds (nickel, nickel carbonyl, nickel sulfate, nickel hydroxide, and nickel carbonate) can induce dermal and pulmonary disease. Nickel is associated with lung and nasal cancer in exposed human populations. Workers who chronically inhale high concentrations of nickel dust may develop asthma. In addition, high environmental nickel exposure can cause nasal septum necrosis. Nickel carbonyl, a potent toxin, the toxicity of which can be delayed hours after exposure, can produce a severe, delayed pulmonary distress syndrome consisting of pneumonitis and cerebral edema. Nickel carbonyl is metabolized in the body to Ni^{2+} and carbon monoxide (259). Nickel carbonyl is an animal teratogen. Nickel is also a cause of allergic contact dermatitis. It has been reported to be a stimulus for lymphocyte blastogenesis transformation in human lymphocytes and has been shown to bind directly to lymphocyte cell-surface membranes.

Chronic exposure to manganous compounds can result in increased pulmonary infections and neurologic effects similar to parkinsonism (259). Manganese dioxide inhalational exposure can reduce host defense mechanisms of the lungs and result in pulmonary inflammation and impairment of pulmonary macrophages (259).

Chronic arsenic toxicity can produce hematologic effects with resulting disturbance of erythropoiesis, thrombocytopenia, granulocytopenia, and other blood dyscrasias. Lymphatic cancers and leukemia have been associated with chronic arsenic exposure. Arsenic-related dermatologic lesions include eczematous dermatitis, follicular dermatitis, and hyperkeratosis. Arsenic is also associated with basal cell and squamous cell skin cancers. Arsenic-related increased incidence of respiratory cancers has been reported in epidemiologic studies of smelter workers (260,261).

Selenium is a unique metal in that it may enhance the immune response. This immune enhancement has been demonstrated in animal models.

It is of interest to note that the metals that are considered to be primary irritants and human sensitizers are also those associated with human carcinogenesis (262).

The skin is an important route of exposure to metals, resulting in allergies and contact dermatitis. Subclinical lead effects on the immune system also have been studied (263). Fifty-four volunteers underwent immune system testing; this included one group of volunteers with blood lead concentrations of 25 µg per dL or higher (the high-lead group) and another with amine blood lead concentration of 4.6 µg per dL (the low-lead group). In the high-lead group, there were reductions in the percentage and absolute number of circulating T cells of the CD3 variety of surface markers and T_h cells (CD4) compared with lesser reductions in the low-lead group. There was also a significant reduction in the CD4-CD8 ratio in the high-lead group caused by a decrease in CD4 marker cells without an increase in the CD8 cells. Reduction in phytohemagglutinin (PHA) mytogenic response was present in the high-lead group, with a lesser impairment in the low-lead group. This study indicates an immunotoxic effect on T lymphocytes and T_h cells at blood lead concentrations of 25 µg per dL and possibly higher. Reduced neutrophil function has also been found in lead-exposed workers with low-lead concentrations.

Allergic reactions of the skin to lead or lead salts are rare and have only been seen in chronic lead intoxication. Lead acetate, which has been used to darken hair cosmetically, has not been shown to be an allergen.

Arsenicals can cause immediate and delayed contact allergy and anaphylactoid reactions. Arsenic has also been associated with cell-mediated contact dermatitis.

Mercury reduces mytogenic responses in a dose-dependent fashion in *in vitro* studies of human peripheral blood cells (264). This effect was monocyte dependent. Removing the monocytes actually enhanced mitogenicity. Nickel and chromium can induce contact dermatitis, IgE-mediated asthma, and urticaria. Chromium metals are inducers of immediate and delayed contact dermatitis. Inhalation of chromate fumes is associated with occupational asthma.

Nickel is a skin sensitizer producing contact dermatitis of the delayed variety in antibody-mediated immediate-type urticaria and asthma. Exposures dermally or by inhalation or ingestion can produce these allergic manifestations. Nickel is one of the most common causes of allergic contact dermatitis.

Platinum salts are sensitizers and are highly allergenic. Reactions to platinum salts include allergic conjunctivitis, rhinitis, asthma, urticaria, and allergic contact sensitization.

Tin has been shown to be a contact sensitizer; this has been confirmed by human patch tests. However, few adverse effects are reported from skin contact.

Zirconium can induce granulomatous hypersensitivity reactions after repeated skin exposure. Zirconium compounds can cause closure of the sweat duct as a result of protein precipitation. Zirconium complexes have been used commercially in deodorants and antiperspirants. The allergic reaction is of the delayed variety.

Studies on lead in relationship to the immune system have been conflicting. Some studies have shown depressed serum immunoglobulins, whereas others using occupationally exposed individuals with nonoccupationally controlled populations have shown no changes or no differences in the immunoglobulin level. Other studies have shown that children with lead levels ranging from 22 to 42 µg per dL showed higher frequencies of abnormal serum IgM and secretory IgA values than children from low-lead comparison groups, with levels ranging from 11 to 24 µg per dL (265). Many of the studies investigating pediatric exposures to lead have reported complement deficiencies. Because the complement system activation involves a highly organized cascade that generates immune and inflammatory responses to tissue invasion, particularly from bacteria, deficiencies may predispose individuals to infections. Other studies have correlated lead exposures in autoimmune renal disease (266). In this study, 21 of 57 workers undergoing renal function tests had excessive body burdens of lead with impaired renal function. Glomerular membrane studies for immunofluorescence were obtained from 7 of 15 workers diagnosed as having lead-induced nephropathy. In 5 of the 7, granular deposition of IgG with C3 in 2 of them was detected. In one other sample, IgM was present in glomerular capillaries. Others showed linear immunoglobulin deposition along the basement membrane of either IgG or IgG plus complement.

Effective neutrophil chemotaxis in respiratory burst activity for superoxide anions is reported in workers occupationally exposed to lead who had a mean blood lead concentration of 41 µg per dL compared with a healthy unexposed control population with a blood lead level less than 10 µg per dL (266).

An increase in T-suppressor cell activity has been reported in occupational exposures (267). However, despite all the studies, there remains much uncertainty about lead and its cause-and-effect relationship with immunotoxicity. Lead may be an immune modulator, but overt toxicity does not appear to be the cause.

Reviews of immunotoxic effects of metals indicate that at high concentration, metals exert immunosuppressive activity, but at low concentrations, immunoenhancement may be seen.

Pesticides and Insecticides

Defined immunotoxicity of pesticides in humans is limited to a few studies. However, animal studies have demonstrated wide-ranging immunologic dysfunctions, including atrophy of lymphoid tissues as well as CMI and HMI immunosuppression induced by a variety of pesticides. Prenatal exposure of mice to chlordane has resulted in depressed CMI.

Bioaccumulation of chlorinated pesticides in adipose tissue of humans is documented by fat biopsy. These pesticides can be detected in serum as well as adipose tissue in a range of parts-per-million concentrations. DDT and its metabolite, DDE, are detected in adipose tissue and serum of nonexposed individuals because of bioaccumulation up through the food chain. Other pesticides found in adipose and serum of the general population include benzene hexachloride and its isomers, lindane, chlordane, heptachlor, heptachlor epoxide, and dieldrin. These organochlorine pesticides can be assayed for in adipose tissue as well as serum. Their presence in the general population creates a confounding factor. The presence of these pesticides and their metabolites in adipose tissue and serum at low parts per million and parts per billion does not appear to constitute an immunologic health risk in terms of altered host defense in the general population. Again, their presence indicates exposure and not disease.

Contact dermatitis from pesticide exposure is probably the most commonly recognized adverse consequence from dermal exposure to organophosphates, fungicides, fumigants, and pyrethroid compounds. Autoimmunity in humans exposed to pesticides has been suggested but is lacking. Studies of human leukocyte functions *in vitro* have demonstrated alterations after pesticide exposure (268). Cultures of human lymphocytes undergoing PHA mitogen blastogenic stimulation in the presence of pesticides demonstrated inhibition (268). In this study, carbamates inhibited lymphocyte PHA stimulation by 10%, organophosphates by 11% to 18%, and organochlorine pesticides (BHC, endrin, DDT) by 11% to 17%. Lymphocyte stimulation in response to PHA, as well as rosette formation of sheep red blood cells when exposed to human lymphocytes, are characteristics of T lymphocytes. DDT was a potent inhibitor of *in vitro* human erythrocyte rosette formation. In the same study, DDT did not alter neutrophil chemotaxis. However, methyl parathion and benzyl benzoate did inhibit PMN chemotaxis (268).

Studies with lindane have shown inhibiting effects on human lymphocyte PHA mitogenesis. Lindane was found to alter T-lymphocyte membrane-associated events leading to mitogen activation by PHA (269). Other studies have shown defects in chemotaxis, nitro blue tetrazolium (NBT) reduction by phagocytes, and phagocytosis in occupationally exposed workers (270). In addition, the incidence of infectious episodes was higher in these workers (271). In contrast, children exposed to DDT did not show alteration in antibody titers to diphtheria immunization (272).

Defined immunotoxic effects of insecticides in humans are lacking. Immediate hypersensitivity reactions and contact hypersensitivity reactions are probably the most common immunotoxic effects of pesticides reported. It is also important to remember that pesticides may be mixtures of compounds and not pure, and it may be the vehicle that the pesticide is dissolved in that is actually toxic. In terms of overall host defense mechanisms, no evidence suggests that pesticides reduce host defense ability to fight infections or cancer.

Studies show changes in T-cell subsets and immune functions with depression of lymphocyte mitogen-induced stimulation with respect to pentachlorophenol. However, prolonged exposure of humans to pentachlorophenol did not show significant changes in T-cell subsets of CD-3, CD-4, CD-8, or CD-4/CD-8 ratios or an effect on immunoglobulins or complement (273). The study did show a significant depression of PHA mitogen-induced lymphocyte blastogenesis, but only at high concentrations of exposure. Also, a small study of 12 workers exposed to chloropyrofos with multiple objective symptoms also failed to show significant immune alterations and lymphocyte subsets, except for a decrease in CD-4 marker T lymphocytes and an increase in CD-26 lymphocyte, a marker of activated T lymphocytes (274). Such studies have lacked adequate controls and been few in number.

Organochlorine pesticides have been studied extensively for their toxic effects in mammals, plants, insects, and humans. These organochlorine pesticides mainly include aldrin, endrin, and dieldrin, as well as DDT, chlordane, heptachlor, and lindane. Aldrin is metabolized to dieldrin in soil by mammals, plants, insects, bioconcentrates, and adipose tissue. Endrin forms an epoxide called isodrin and does not accumulate in adipose tissue. Whereas immunotoxic effects of these compounds are seen quite readily in mice, in which they decrease the resistance to infections, these effects do not occur in human exposure (275). Data relating to chlordane immunotoxicity are controversial (276), whereas animal studies adequately demonstrate the effect of chlordane on the developing immune system, showing a profound deficit in contact hypersensitivity response to allergens. This contact hypersensitivity deficit, however, is not shown to be a T-cell deficit (275). Prenatal exposure of other animals to chlordane also shows effects on pluripotent colony-forming units and the granulocyte macrophage colony-forming unit stem-cell populations.

Allergic and Hypersensitivity Pulmonary Disease

Allergic-mediated asthma and nonallergic-mediated asthma have been documented to occur from chemicals, vegetable matter, exotoxins, and proteins. Repeated exposure to the offending agent can produce sensitization. Once an IgE-mediated problem occurs, an exposure to minute amounts can precipitate inflammation, edema, and bronchospasm.

Sensitizing environmental contaminants and chemicals act as haptens by combining with proteins present in mucosal surfaces or to albumin and other serum proteins. After repeated exposure, IgE antibodies directed against this hapten complex can form.

Occupationally related immunologic lung disease may present as asthma, hypersensitivity pneumonitis, or granulomatous or fibrotic lung disease. Reactive hypersensitivity of the airways that is nonimmunologically mediated can also be a result of exposure to chemicals. Stimulation of subepithelial vagal receptors by chemicals inhaled as vapors, aerosols, or dusts can induce this clinical syndrome of hyperreactive airways. Many common chemicals and respiratory irritants can produce reactive airway clinical problems by nonimmune mechanisms.

Allergenic metals can cause pulmonary disease and asthma. Fifteen metals have the properties of both allergenicity and carcinogenicity. Arsenic, beryllium, chromium, and nickel are accepted as animal and human carcinogens as well as potent sensitizing agents.

Trimellitic anhydride, a component of resin-curing agents, toluene diisocyanate, methylene diphenyl diisocyanate, and phthalatic anhydrides (plasticizers) are well-known precipitators of allergic asthma. Trimellitic anhydride may produce an asthmatic syndrome, an irritant syndrome, and a hypersensitivity pneumonitis syndrome.

The biotechnology industry is an occupational source of exposure to a variety of proteins, peptides, and chemicals that can result in IgE-mediated asthma. This includes enzymes such as papain, pepsin, alkaline phosphatase, glucosoxidase, peroxidase, ribonuclease; acrylamide monomers and aliphatic amines; and chemicals used to haptenize drugs to albumin molecules, such as carbodiamides, toluene diisocyanate, glutaraldehyde, and phenylenediamine.

Nickel sulfate exposure has been demonstrated to cause a positive inhalational challenge test as well as antibody formation. Platinum workers can experience not only pulmonary sensitization with development of specific IgE and asthma, but also conjunctivitis and rhinitis.

Formaldehyde exposure is widespread because of its presence in multiple commonly used products, including fabrics, wood products, particle board, and carpets. Formaldehyde is a direct upper-airway and respiratory irritant.

Hypersensitivity pneumonitis can be acute or chronic. The acute form of chemically induced hypersensitivity pneumonitis presents with fever, chills, nonproductive cough, chest pain, and dyspnea and usually resolves in 24 hours. Chronic pneumonitis from an immunologic etiology may occur after a chronic or subchronic exposure to low concentrations of chemicals. Fever, cough, fatigue, weight loss, and shortness of breath are the clinical manifestations. Permanent pulmonary fibrosis can occur.

A one-time exposure or multiple inhalational exposures to certain irritant chemicals can result in reactive airway disease manifested by chronic cough, bronchospasm, chest tightness, and shortness of breath on reexposure to the same or other irritating chemicals. Chemicals that produce irritant effects on the airways do so via nonimmune mechanisms.

Fibrotic pulmonary disease associated with immunologic abnormalities can occur as a result of the chronic inhalation of dusts and human-made fibrogenic materials, including asbestos, mica, graphite, silica, and beryllium. The release of lysosomal enzymes from macrophages occurs as a result of the phagocytosis of these human-made fibers.

Patients with silicosis have been found to have elevated circulating immune complexes, including antinuclear antibody and rheumatoid factor (277). No direct correlation between severity of disease and the presence of immune complexes is documented. In addition, patients with silicosis have documented increased immunoglobulins with increased secretory IgA.

Asbestos-related lung disease has immunologic features. Asbestos fibers activate classical and alternate complement pathways. Activity of NK cells and antibody-dependent cellular cytotoxicity (K cells) has been demonstrated to be depressed in patients with asbestosis (277–279). In addition, asbestosis is associated with a decrease in the number of T cells, increased immune complexes, and increased serum immunoglobulin concentrations (280).

CLINICAL SPECTRUM OF IMMUNE-RELATED RESPIRATORY DISEASE

The spectrum of respiratory disease described in humans exposed to inhaled toxins includes asthma, hypersensitivity pneumonitis, pulmonary fibrosis, and pulmonary infiltrates with eosinophilia. More than 200 chemicals are known to cause respiratory hypersensitivity (281). Low-molecular-weight chemicals bind to proteins to form neohaptens, thus exposing the immune system to new epitopes, which can elicit immune responses. These low-molecular-weight chemicals include isocyanates, acid and hydrides, wood dust, and metals. Occupational asthma can be divided into immunologic causes and nonimmunologic causes. Immunologic mechanisms are induced through IgE-mediated hypersensitivity responses, antigen antibody complex responses, complement activation, and cell-mediated responses. Nonimmunologic asthma is induced by damage to bronchial epithelial tissue, which allows inflammation to occur, and stimulation of vagal afferent nerves beneath the epithelium, which can result in bronchial constriction of nonspecific hyperresponsiveness of the airways. Release of substance P, neurokinin A, and other tachykinins results in increased airway responsiveness. Also, the inhibition of neutral endopeptidase that is responsible for tachykinin degradation furthers the hyperresponsive effects of chemicals. Toluene diisocyanate causes release of tachykinins, interferes with neutral endopeptidase, and stimulates local release of substance P and calcitonin-generated–related peptide from nerve endings in the lungs. This neurogenic inflammation induces bronchoconstriction and inflammation in a nonimmune manner (282).

Plicatic acid in the western red cedar can activate the classic or alternate complement pathways, causing production of anaphylatoxins, which can activate mast cells to release bioactive mediators and produce respiratory responses (283).

Acid anhydrides are constituents of resins such as phthalic anhydride, maleic anhydride, and trimellitic acid anhydride. Acid anhydrides are used in paints, varnishes, and plastics, and as curing agents in adhesive coatings and sealant materials. Acid anhydrides can produce adverse reactions in humans through direct effects of skin, mucous membrane, lungs, nose, and through hypersensitivity reactions. These hypersensitivity reactions of acid anhydrides can be IgE-mediated cytotoxic, immune-complex, or cell-mediated mechanisms (284). Trimellitic anhydride can induce antibody responses of IgA, IgG, and IgM. IgE-mediated reactions are also demonstrated against anhydride-protein conjugated haptens. A late respiratory systemic syndrome resembling a hypersensitivity pneumonitis can begin 4 to 12 hours after trimellitic anhydride exposure and is associated with productive cough, fever, chills, arthralgias, and myalgias (285). Acid anhydrides include phthalic anhydride, hemic anhydride, trimellitic anhydride, hexahydrophthalic anhydride, and tetrachlorophthalic anhydride.

Isocyanates are common chemicals causing occupationally related respiratory disease. Isocyanates are mucous membrane irritants: irritants to the eyes, nose, and throat. Isocyanate respiratory disease includes asthma, hypersensitivity pneumonitis, and bronchiolitis obliterans. The immune lesion involves the conjugation of isocyanates to proteins forming neohaptens recognized by the immune system. Isocyanates induce immune responses and neurogenic inflammation effects in the pulmonary system. Isocyanates can produce IgE-mediated immune responses as well as IgG- and IgM-specific antibodies.

The clinical picture may present as early asthmatic reactions, late asthmatic reactions, or dual asthmatic reactions. Early asthmatic reactions are seen most frequently with higher-molecular-weight compounds. Delayed or late asthmatic reactions are more frequently seen in low-molecular-weight chemical-induced asthma, and dual asthmatic reactions are frequently seen in IgE-mediated asthma. Late asthmatic responses occur 4 to 12 hours after exposure to the chemical and are associated with inflammatory influx and inflammation of the airways. Bronchial hypersensitivity usually precedes this inflammation.

Isocyanate-induced asthma is associated with late asthmatic responses that occur 4 to 12 hours after exposure and are preceded by an inflammatory cell influx into the respiratory tissues. Persistent bronchial hyperactivity is also present, and the initiation of the inflammatory stage preceding the asthmatic response could be the result of either an immunologic response or a direct toxic response on the epithelial cell lining and the alveolar macrophages. The inflammatory cascade occurring after exposure results in pathologic changes, airway edema, smooth muscle hypertrophy, and collagen deposition. Bronchial hyperactivity can persist for long periods of time after a worker is removed from exposure to isocyanates.

Fumes or dust of metallic salts can cause chemical pneumonitis, bronchitis, adult respiratory distress syndrome, and pulmonary hypersensitivity. Pulmonary reactions produced by metallic salts can be immunologic and nonimmunologic. Nickel, platinum, cobalt, and chromium are metal salts that produce respiratory disease and asthma by immunologic mechanisms. Other metal salts, such as zinc, cadmium, aluminum, and vanadium pentoxide, can produce pulmonary disease and asthma by nonimmune mechanisms. Metal fume fever is a well-recognized pulmonary pneumonitis produced by metal oxide fume inhalations producing symptoms 4 to 12 hours after exposure that may last as long as 2 days with coughing, shortness of breath, myalgia, and fever.

ORGANIC DUST TOXIC SYNDROME

Organic dust toxic syndrome (ODTS) is an acute febrile reaction to organic dust and is distinct from hypersensitivity pneumonitis. It is a noninfectious febrile response associated with chills, myalgia, cough, dyspnea, headache, nausea, and malaise, which occur after a high exposure to organic dust. Although ODTS shares some clinical features with hypersensitivity pneumonitis, including increased neutrophils in the bronchoalveolar lavage, it is a different disease (286). In ODTS, there is a paucity of or no infiltrates on chest x-ray. Severe hypoxemia does not occur, and prior sensitization to antigens is not required. No sequelae of recurrent attacks appears to result in pulmonary fibrosis.

Acute hypersensitivity pneumonitis is characterized by restrictive airway disease and a reduced diffusing capacity for carbon monoxide and hypoxemia. Also, hypersensitivity pneumonitis can be a recurring disease and can result in chronic dyspnea on exertion, cough, and other pathology. Farmer's lung disease is a hypersensitivity disease with immunologic mechanisms; it has been recognized since the eighteenth century.

It has been assumed for years that any case of febrile illness after organic dust exposure was a hypersensitivity pneumonitis; however, this is not the case. Influenzalike syndromes after organic dust exposure are probably ODTS as opposed to an immunologically mediated pulmonary pneumonitis.

ODTS can be seen in individuals who are exposed to high dust concentrations in agricultural and nonagricultural environments. The etiology of ODTS includes endotoxin and maybe β-1,3 glucans from fungus. Levels of respirable endotoxin are quite high in agricultural settings. Endotoxin is known to produce fever and malaise and pulmonary injury. There are generally no sequelae of ODTS as compared with pulmonary hypersensitivity diseases, and there is no evidence of an immune reaction occurring with ODTS.

Contact Allergic Dermatitis

Dermatitis caused by chemical exposure can be immunologic or nonimmunologic. Contact dermatitis secondary to irritant and sensitizing chemicals is a commonly recognized occupational injury. Exposures occur by direct contact with chemicals in vapor phase, liquids, or solids or by systemic exposure via inhalation.

Rashes may appear in a variety of areas, including exposed surfaces of the neck, arms, legs, face, and hands, and nonexposed areas as well. Frequently, chemicals or fibrogenic materials, such as fiberglass, accumulate in work clothes and are in chronic contact with the skin. Soluble chemicals in a vapor phase may dissolve in the sweat present on skin surfaces. Clinical symptoms of airborne dermal irritants are itching, burning sensation, and ocular irritation. The clinical presentation of dermatitis varies from eczema to erythema, urticarial lesions, papillary lesions, or vesicular lesions. Dermatitis is subdivided into allergic contact dermatitis, nonimmunologic urticarial rash, phototoxic contact dermatitis, photoallergic contact dermatitis, irritant contact dermatitis, and acne venenata. The more commonly recognized contact urticarial rashes are to formaldehyde and nickel. Nickel dermatitis can occur either by direct dermal exposure or via systemic exposure. Patients with sensitivity to nickel may develop chronic eczema.

Contact dermatitis from corrosive chemicals, such as cement, range from erythema and burns to ulceration. Carbonless paper is recognized as a source of irritancy and allergic reactions, including dermal and pulmonary irritation (287).

Making a diagnosis of contact dermal allergy can be difficult, because many chemicals produce dermatitis via irritant nonimmunologic methods. Patch testing and biopsy are methods to discern the two lesions.

Respiratory Immune Effects and Air Pollutants

The respiratory system has nonspecific immune mechanisms that protect against disease. However, air pollutants can compromise these protective mechanisms, leading to increased risk of illness. Macrophages responsible for removing or neutralizing particles that invade the lungs are found in interstitial tissues of the alveoli or free in the alveolar luminal surface. The effectiveness and efficiency of the phagocytosis and lysis functions by pulmonary macrophages dictate the ultimate level of pulmonary protection. Any chemical or particulate matter that interferes with either the absolute macrophage number or basic functions can produce pulmonary susceptibility to damage. Macrophage elimination of particulates involves the following (288):

- Chemotaxis
- Opsonization by complement and antibody
- Attachment of particle to phagocyte
- Phagocytosis of particle
- Formation of primary lysosome
- Fusion with secondary lysosome
- Destruction of particle

Interruption of normal pulmonary host defense can occur if any one of these phagocytosis events is interfered with by a pollutant. A variety of environmental pollutants stimulate increased numbers of macrophages in the pulmonary environment. These include lead oxide (PbO), nickel chloride ($NiCl_2$), nickel oxide (NiO), cadmium chloride ($CdCl_2$), carbon monoxide, quartz crystals, tobacco smoke, and a variety of environmental dusts (288).

Some environmental contaminants—such as silica, chrysotile asbestos, cadmium, acrolein, manganese dioxide, some lead oxides, and antimony—reduce the absolute number of free pulmonary macrophages (288). Acute exposure of macrophages to ozone (O_3) or nitrogen dioxide (NO_2) can decrease phagocytic activity and ability (288,289). Other chemicals directly impairing phagocytic functions include nickel chloride ($NiCl_2$), cadmium, nickel, copper, mercury, zinc, platinum, vanadium oxides (V_2O_5), and cadmium oxide (CdO).

Shape, size, chemical composition, and surface area of inhaled particles help to determine macrophage dysfunction. The ultimate fate of the macrophage that ingests particles entering the respiratory system depends on whether the cell can destroy the particle or whether the particle destroys the cell. If the macrophage is killed, the toxin is then released into the lung environment to promote further damage. In some situations, the macrophage viability is affected, but cell lysis does not occur.

IFN production by macrophages is depressed after exposure to ozone, automobile exhaust, and NO_2 (288). Alteration of macrophage lysosomal enzymes and release of these enzymes, as well as other biologically active substances, is promoted by certain environmental contaminants, including release of prostaglandins, collagenase, elastase, plasminogen-activating factor, and lytic enzymes. Asbestos and silica particles stimulate the release of lysosomal enzymes, which subsequently elicit inflammatory processes with tissue destruction and fibrosis of the lungs. Macrophage contents are then released to repeat the cycle (288,289).

Air pollution is a risk factor for respiratory infection, and air pollutants have an effect on the increasing susceptibility to allergic and infectious diseases. Ozone (O_3), nitrogen dioxide (NO_2), and sulfur dioxide (SO_2) have been extensively studied, and epidemiologic studies now indicate relationships between these air pollutants and respiratory infections. Respiratory tract infections are more prevalent in children living in areas highly polluted with SO_2 emissions. Children have more frequent colds, cough, and bronchitis when air pollution alerts occur (290). Similar effects have not been found for nitrogen dioxide. Studies indoors did not find a correlation between NO_2 generated by cooking and respiratory illness in infants younger than 2 years of age (291). Other studies, however, indicate an increased incidence of respiratory illness in children in homes with gas stoves, and a 15-ppb increase in household nitrogen dioxide exposure was associated with an increase of 20% in the incidence of lower-respiratory-tract symptoms in children (292,293). Other studies have shown associations between NO_2 exposure indoors and an increased incidence of respiratory symptoms and croup in children younger than 2 years of age (294). Still others have shown that exposure to photochemical pollutants that contain a predominance of ozone is associated with a 50% increase in the duration of episodes of coughing, phlegm production, and sore throat (295).

These studies, among others, indicate that air pollutants indoors and outdoors can have immunosuppressive effects on the respiratory system, leading to increased incidence of infections and inflammation. These same pollutants are thought to have serious effects on exacerbation of existing respiratory disease, such as asthma and bronchitis. Air pollutants—including particulates, ozone, nitrogen dioxide, and sulfur dioxide—appear to enhance asthmatic disease and exacerbate asthmatic disease and reactive airways. Air pollutants themselves promote nonspecific airway hyperreactivity and cause decrements in pulmonary function.

Concern has arisen about the decreased resistance to infections (bacterial and viral) and the effect on enhancing allergic responses from these pollutants. Studies have shown that air pollutants modulate immune responses in the lungs, increasing susceptibility to bacterial infections in laboratory rodents (290). Also, suppression of phagocytic activity appears to play a key role in this immune-modulating effect. Animal models studied for decreased resistance to bacterial infection have shown enhanced mortality after exposure to concentrations of ozone as low as 0.1 ppm and 0.01 ppm of phosgene (290). Investigations demonstrate that alveolar macrophages function is impaired after ozone exposure in animal models as well as in humans (296). Nitrogen dioxide exposure also suppresses alveolar macrophage function in animal models and in humans (297–300). In conclusion, exposure to atmospheric pollutant gases increases susceptibility due to bacterial infections in rodent models. Most directly, they suppress the activity of alveolar macrophages. Also, we know that ozone suppresses alveolar macrophage function in humans, and it impairs the phagocytic activity of macrophages.

Showing the impaired resistance to viral infections in animal models has been more difficult, as opposed to the ease with which increased bacterial infections have been shown. This is important, because most of the infections in young children and many in adults are virally induced. Human clinical studies have not been any more successful than the laboratory animal studies in demonstrating increased susceptibility to viral infections.

It may be that the studies that have been performed are examining symptoms that are related to enhanced inflammation or allergic responses in the respiratory system. It also may be that although virus replication may not be enhanced by pollutant exposure, an enhanced inflammatory response does occur, and this enhanced inflammatory response to the virus may be modulated by the atmospheric pollutant exposure. Animals infected with influenza virus showed an increased airway hyperresponsiveness to methacholine after exposure to ozone. When infection and exposure were combined, the hyperreactive effect was increased. Thus, pollutants may exacerbate hyperreactive and asthmaticlike responses that are a result of respiratory infections (301).

Only a few studies have linked exposure to atmospheric pollutants and increased allergic responsiveness in humans. One study reported that an exposure to 0.12 ppm of ozone increased bronchial responsiveness to antigen in some individuals (302). Other investigators have reported changes in pulmonary immune functions involving exposure to ozone. These changes include modulation of T lymphocytes, modulation of bronchus-associated lymphoid tissue, elevation of specific antibody (IgE antibody in some cases), and suppression of delayed T-cell hypersensitivity. The discovery that there are two distinct populations of CD-4 (T_h) cells, T_h-1 and T_h-2, has helped understanding of these modulations. T_h cell type 1 produces IL-2 and γ-IFN, the engine behind delayed T-cell hypersensitivity reactions and IgG production, whereas T_h-2 cells produce IL-4, which stimulates IgE production, the key to immediate hypersensitivity type I reactions. It is important to note that these two populations of cells are also antagonistic to each other and influence the types of immune responses that develop. Thus, atmospheric pollutants may enhance some antibody responses, suppress delayed hypersensitivity responses, and modulate T-cell activity as a result of the disturbance of balance between these two T-cell helper-cell populations. Apparently, such a disturbance of the balance favors a type I reaction versus a type IV hypersensitivity reaction.

TOBACCO SMOKE

Tobacco smoke has been demonstrated to have a profound health risk on the respiratory system as well as the kidney, bladder, pancreas, and digestive tract. It is a known carcinogen. Also, long exposure to tobacco smoke is associated with a high frequency of respiratory diseases. Smokers have an increased incidence of influenza and other respiratory tract infections. Tobacco smoke impairs granulocyte chemotaxis, increases leukocyte numbers, increases the release of elastase and superoxide from lung macrophages, and stimulates degranulation of basophils (303). In animal models, tobacco smoke depresses lymphocyte blastogenesis, decreases antibody production, and decreases the level of respiratory lymphoid tissue. Exposure to passive tobacco smoke is thought to increase the susceptibility of children to respiratory infections. Tobacco smoke contains more than 4,000 different chemicals that are toxic or carcinogenic, or both (304).

Sidestream tobacco smoke is a source of environmental indoor contamination, and the chemical contents are different from mainstream smoke inhaled into a person's lungs. The particulate phase of tobacco smoke contains a majority of genotoxic and carcinogenic substances. Nitrosamines are inducers of benign and malignant tumors in the respiratory tracts of laboratory animals (303). Tobacco smoking is a significant risk factor for acute respiratory illnesses and chronic obstructive pulmonary disease. Tobacco smoke induces changes in alveolar macrophages by increasing their number three- to fivefold. Evidence shows that alveolar macrophages from tobacco smokers produce more oxygen radicals and products of myeloperoxidase activity (305). Tobacco smoke also causes many other functional alterations in alveolar macrophages, including depressed response to antigens and increased chemotactic responses. Thus, alveolar macrophages in smokers are constantly in a heightened activated state compared with nonsmokers.

Macrophages accumulate in the alveoli and respiratory bronchiole of smokers and, because of their ability to secrete biologically active substances, can play a role in pathogenesis of pulmonary disease. The increased release of radicals and elastase may contribute to connective tissue damage. Tobacco smoke also increases recruitment of neutrophils and macrophages from the peripheral blood into the lungs. Agreement exists that tobacco smoking decreases serum immunoglobulin concentrations, including decreased concentrations of IgG, IgA, and IgM. Levels of IgE, however, are significantly higher in smokers than in nonsmokers.

Tobacco smoke also induces leukocytosis and an increase in lymphocytes. Decreases in CD-4/CD-8 ratios have also been noted. Some investigators have reported an increase in the percentage of CD-4 T cells over time in smokers, whereas others have found a significant increase in total T cells along with an increase in the CD-4/CD-8 ratio (306). Decreased mitogen responses to PHA are found in older chronic male smokers. Other investigators have shown that NK-cell activity in the peripheral blood was significantly lower in smokers compared with nonsmokers. Differences may exist in the genetic background of the population studied on the NK-cell activity.

CLINICAL IMMUNOLOGIC TESTING

The components of immune system testing are basically determining whether both cell-mediated and humoral-mediated arms are intact.

- Quantitation and characterization of serum immunoglobulins through protein electrophoresis
- Immunofixation electrophoresis to detect monoclonal immunoglobulins in serum, urine, or cerebrospinal fluid
- Immunoassays for specific immunoglobulins
- Complement assays
- Evaluation of lymphocyte numbers and functions
- Evaluation of lymphocyte subsets (CD membrane markers)
- Evaluation of lymphocyte mitogenesis
- Skin tests for delayed hypersensitivity
- Detection and quantitation of autobodies
- Neutrophil functioning

Protein Electrophoresis and Immunoglobulin Quantitation

Immunoglobulin quantitation and protein electrophoresis provide direct information concerning the absence of an immunoglobulin class or the presence of a monoclonal or polyclonal gammopathy. The three major immunoglobulins quantitated are IgG, IgM, and IgA. IgE can be measured if allergies are part of the clinical syndrome; however, IgE may or may not be elevated. The detection of antigen-specific IgE and IgG requires more sophisticated testing, such as by enzyme-linked immunosorbent assays. Hypogammaglobulinemias are usually the result of a secondary immune deficiency. The most frequent immunoglobulin deficiency is IgA, and in 50% of these cases, the patient is clinically asymptomatic. Secretory IgA is a mucosal barrier defense mechanism, and its assay is separate from the measurement of regular IgA. Examination of the protein electrophoretic pattern can quickly indicate whether a patient has normal concentrations of immunoglobulins, hypogammaglobulinemia, or a dysgammaglobulinemia.

IgG is the most prevalent immunoglobulin class, ranging in the serum from 5 to 15 g per L. IgM serum concentrations range from 0.4 to 2 g per L, and IgA ranges from 0.5 to 4 g per L. Immunoassays include enzyme-linked immunoassays, radioimmunoassays, precipitin immunoassays using radial immunodiffusion, fluorescent immunoassays, and chemiluminescent immunoassays.

Skin Test for Delayed Hypersensitivity

Skin tests for delayed hypersensitivity can be performed using common antigens such as *Trichophyton*, *Candida albicans*, purified protein derivative, and mumps antigen. An erythematous dermal reaction and induration greater than 10 mm in diameter at 24, 48, or 72 hours after intradermal injection of 0.1 mL of the antigen into the volar surface of the forearm indicates that a complex series of cell-mediated events occurred: The antigen was recognized by lymphocytes and appropriately processed, helper/inducer T cells were activated, lymphokines were secreted, and recruitment of nonsensitized lymphocytes to the antigen deposition area occurred. Development of a positive skin test is dependent on previous antigen exposure. A positive skin test result for delayed hypersensitivity indicates a normally functioning cell-mediated immune system, and 95% of the normal population will react to three out of five skin tests. Standardization of skin test antigens has been a problem, and lack of standardized reagents may complicate the skin test. This should be checked before applying any skin tests. Also, a negative result may indicate an improperly administered test and not an immune defect. A positive delayed hypersensitivity skin test indicates an intact and normally functioning cell-mediated immune system.

Autoantibody Assays

Measurement of autoantibodies can be useful in diagnosing connective tissue diseases. The commonly measured autoantibodies are antibodies against nuclei, smooth muscle, DNA, and thyroid tissue. Autoimmune diseases and chronic inflammatory states may be misdiagnosed as an immunotoxicity from xenobiotics. Antinuclear antibodies (ANA) can be present in healthy individuals, in persons with rheumatic and nonrheumatic disease, in family members of persons with autoimmune disease, and in the elderly (307). The finding of low-titer autoantibodies in an individual is of little significance in making a diagnosis of an immune dysfunction. Approximately 35% of healthy people will have a positive ANA titer if their serum is checked at dilutions less than 1:10, and 4% will be positive at dilutions higher than 1:10 (308). Approximately 38% of persons older than 60 years of age will be positive for ANA (308).

Normally, humans have antibodies against common antigens to which everyone is exposed. These antibodies occur as a normal response and can be quantitated: isohemagglutinins, antistreptolysin-O, and antibodies to measles, mumps, polio, and tetanus toxoid immunizations (308). The primary and secondary immune response to an antigen can be determined in some situations. Evaluation of the primary immune response requires an antigen to which the person has never been exposed. This can produce some problems and introduce risk to the patient. The secondary immune response is easier to evaluate and can be as easy as administration of tetanus toxoid and measuring antibody titers. However, the primary immune response is usually the most sensitive to immunosuppressants.

Complement Function

The complement system consists of approximately 30 cascading and interacting proteins circulating in the blood. The complement system is divided functionally into the classical pathway and the alternate pathway, both of which lead to the cleavage of C3. Activation of the classical pathway requires IgG or IgM antibody combined with antigen. The alternate pathway can be activated by IgA and polysaccharides with repeating structure. The membrane attack complex of complement consists of C5-C9, which becomes activated as the terminal functioning unit of complement.

The clinical evaluation of the complement system involves the following:

- Total hemolytic complement in serum (CH_{50})
- Complement component assays
- Measurement of immune complexes

CH_{50} measures overall complement function by assaying the amount of diluted serum necessary to produce 50% hemolysis of a standard amount of red blood cells coated with antibody. CH_{50} varies per laboratory and evaluates the functional integrity of the complement system.

Complement system function can be screened for by quantifying C3 (alternate complement pathway), C4 (classical pathway), and CH_{50} (total complement). The measurement of CH_{50} is more useful for monitoring immune complex diseases such as glomerulonephritis or SLE. Deficiencies in selected complement components can present with different disease patterns. Indications for assaying complement function are repeated infections by pyogenic bacteria, systemic bacterial infections, or suspected autoimmune disease. Some of the clinical syndromes associated with inappropriate activation of complement include recurring angioedema, chronic urticaria, palpable purpura, arthralgias, cutaneous vasculitides, unexplained fever, nephritis, and arthritides (309).

Reduced serum concentration of the C4 is a sensitive indicator of a low-level activation of the complement system. C3 usually has a high serum concentration, and its measurement provides information about the alternate complement pathway. A normal C4 with a low concentration of C3 indicates alternate pathway activation of the complement system (310). Low C3, C4, and CH_{50} is associated with classical pathway activation. Normal C3 and C4 with a low CH_{50} suggests a deficiency of one of the other complement components.

Activation of the complement system and the presence of autoantibodies indicates immune complex diseases and autoimmunity. Positive results for immune complexes, the presence of certain autoantibodies, and complement system activation should encourage the clinician to search for end-organ pathology in specific organ systems involved in the clinical syndrome. Negative results in the immune complex assays for complement and autoantibodies are helpful in ruling out a humoral-mediated cause of clinical defense.

TABLE 25-17. Cluster designation markers

Cluster designation	Location
CD1a (T6, OKT6, Leu6)	Found on cortical thymocytes, Langerhans' cells
CD2 (T11, OKT11, Leu5)	Found on T cells and natural killer-cell subset, designated as LFA-2
CD3 (T3, OKT3, Leu4)	Found on T cells, multichain receptor associated with the T-cell antigen receptor
CD4 (T4, OKT4, Leu3)	Found on T-cell subset and low-density monocytes, cytoadhesion receptor for MHC class II binding, receptor for human immunodeficiency virus
CD5 (T1, OKT1, Leu5)	Found on T cells, a B-cell subset, and B-cell CLL
CD7 (3A1, OLT16, Leu9)	Found on thymocytes, most T cells, most natural killer cells, platelets, some myeloid leukemia cells
CD8 (T8, OKT8, Leu2)	Found on T-cell subset and in low density on natural killer cells, cytoadhesion receptor for MHC class I binding
CD10 (J5, OKB cALLa, CALLA)	Found on pre-B cells, neutrophils, common acute leukemia cells of childhood
CD11a (BD11A)	Found on leukocytes, α chain of LFA-2, binds to CD18
CD11b (Mo1, OKM1, Leu15)	Found on T-cell subset, natural killer cells, monocytes, granulocytes, β chain of complement receptor 3 (CR3, C3b), binds to CD18
CD11c (ROS65, LeuM5)	Found on T-cell subset, natural killer cells, monocytes, granulocytes, β chain of complement receptor 4 (CDR4), binds to CD18
CD13 (My7, OKM13, LeuM7)	Found on monocytes and neutrophils
CD14 (Mo2, OKM14, LeuM3)	Found on monocytes
CD16 (Leu11)	Found on T-cell subset, natural killer cells, granulocytes, F(c) receptor for IgG [F(c)γRIII]
CD18	Found on leukocytes, β chain bound to CD11a, CD11b, or CD11c (α chain)
CD19 (B4, OKB22, Leu12)	Found on B cells and pre-B cells
CD20 (B1, Leu16)	Found on B cells, pre-B cells, pro-B cells
CD21 (B2, OKB7, anti-CD2)	Found on B cells, complement receptor 2 (CR2, C3d), EBV receptor
CD22 (B3, OKB22, Leu14)	Found on B cells and hairy leukemia cells
CD23 (Leu20)	Found on activated B cells, T cells, eosinophils, low-density F(c) IgE receptor [F(c)γRII]
CD25 (IL2T1, OKT26a, IL2R)	Found on activated T cells, B cells, monocytes, low-affinity interleukin-2 receptor α chain, p55, Tac
CD28 (Leu28)	T-cell subset, activated B cells, costimulatory receptor for T-cell activation
CD29 (4B4)	Found on leukocytes and platelets, adhesion receptor
CD33 (My9, LeuM9)	Found on myeloid progenitors
CD34 (HPCA-1)	Found on hematopoietic progenitors
CD38 (T10, Leu17)	Found on activated T cells, plasma cells, thymocytes
CD40	B cells, monocyte/macrophage, dendritic cells
CD4OL (gp39)	Found on activated T cells
CD45 (KC56, HLE)	Found on leukocytes
CD45RA (2H4, Leu18)	Found on T-cell subsets, most B cells and natural killer cells; isoform of CD45 appears to identify naive CD4 T cells
CD45RO (BD45RO, UCHL-1)	Found on T-cell subsets, isoform of CD45 appears to identify memory CD4 T cells
CD56 (NKH-1, Leu19)	Found on natural killer cells, T-cell subset
CD57 (Leu7, HNK-1)	Found on natural killer-cell subset, T-cell subset
CD69	Found on activated T cells, activated B cells, activated natural killer cells, and macrophages
CD71	Found on activated T cells and activated B cells, proliferating cells, transferrin receptor
CD95 (APO-1, Fas antigen)	Activated T cells, B cells, natural killer cells, thymocytes, receptor for apoptosis signal
CD117 (c-kit, stem-cell factor receptor)	Hematopoietic stem-cell subset, mast cell
CD122	T cells, B cells, natural killer cells, β chain of the interleukin 2 receptor

CLL, chronic lymphocytic leukemia; EBV, Epstein-Barr virus; Ig, immunoglobulin; MHC, major histocompatibility complex.
Adapted from Fleisher TA, Tomar RH. Diagnostic laboratory immunology. *JAMA* 1997;278(22):1825, with permission.

Immune Cell Assays

Any significant decrease in the number of T lymphocytes results in a lymphopenia in peripheral blood smears, because they make up approximately 75% to 85% of the peripheral blood lymphocyte population. Determination of the number of T cells in peripheral blood is also performed by using the sheep erythrocyte rosette formation method. Another method for enumerating T cells involves the use of fluorescent-labeled monoclonal antibodies directed against mature T cells.

The development of monoclonal antibodies against markers on cell surfaces of lymphocytes and flow cytometry allows for classification and enumeration of cells. Cellular assays of T-cell subsets are used to monitor quantitative and qualitative changes in the immune system. Cellular assessment includes a complete blood count and differential, enumeration of T cells and B cells, and cell classification according to surface markers. Monoclonal antibodies have been developed against CD on cell surfaces. In 1982, the nomenclature of monoclonal antibodies for cell differentiation was standardized, giving CD to antigenic epitopes on cell surfaces.

Flow cytometry provided a second technology to characterize and enumerate blood cells. Flow cytometry provides a means of counting lymphocytes labeled with monoclonal antibodies, which allows automated counting of lymphocytes and lymphocyte subsets. Flow cytometry measures the light scatter of cells as they pass through a laser beam. Cells enter the instrumentation flow cell and pass through the laser beam one by one, using a process called *laminar flow*. If the cell has an attached monoclonal antibody, a fluorescent dye on the monoclonal antibody will be excited by the laser beam and emit light that is detected by a photomultiplier tube.

Lymphocytes express CD markers as shown in Figure 25-8 and Table 25-17. Similar CD clusters can be found on different cells. Cells expressing CD-3 and CD-4 markers are helper/inducer phenotypes. Those expressing CD-3 and CD-8 are suppressor/cytotoxic phenotypes. Although CD-4 differentiation receptors are found on Th cells, CD-4 is also found on monocytes. It is important to exclude monocytes from the lymphocyte count during flow cytometry analysis; otherwise, the CD-4 count may be erroneously elevated. Monoclonal antibodies are also used for B-cell analysis. CD-19 and CD-20 markers identify B lymphocytes. NK cells, monocytes, and granulocytes are also defined by monoclonal antibodies.

Lymphocyte Mitogenesis

Lymphocyte transformation can be tested by three separate mitogens that stimulate blastogenesis of lymphocytes. The most commonly used mitogens are PHA, concanavalin-A, pokeweed mitogen, and staphylococcal protein A. PHA and concanavalin-A stimulate T cells. Pokeweed mitogen stimulates T cells and B lymphocytes, and staphylococcal protein A stimulates B cells. Lymphocytes exposed to these mitogens normally undergo blastogenesis. The incorporation of tritiated thymidine added to the assay indicates blastogenesis, because dividing cells incorporate the radiolabel into their DNA of dividing cells.

Cell-Mediated Cytotoxicity

Cell-mediated cytotoxicity can also be tested. The effector cell that is being analyzed must correspond to the target cell selected. In testing NK activity, the target cells must be sensitive to the NK killing. Most cell-mediated cytotoxicity assays are designed using cells labeled with radioactive chromium (Cr^{51}). The release of the radioisotope is proportional to the extent of cell killing in the assay.

Phagocyte Functioning

Defects in CMI may be recognized by clinical symptoms of infections associated with common CMI functions: killing of intracellular pathogens, delayed hypersensitivity reactions to recognized antigens, tumor-cell rejection, contact dermatitis, and tissue injury from autoimmunity. Defects usually present as an increase in infections with agents such as viruses, intercellular pathogens, and fungi.

For proper functioning of the immune system, especially the HMI, the participation of nonimmune cells and complement is critical to effectively protect the host against infectious agents. The complement system and phagocytes must function normally for antibody to provide host defense. Phagocytes are divided into neutrophils and macrophages (monocytes). A complete evaluation of phagocyte functions includes the following tests:

- Neutrophil count in peripheral blood
- NBT reduction
- Chemotaxis
- Phagocytosis
- Killing ability

However, not all of these tests are needed in screening for abnormalities. The absolute neutrophil count should be obtained by Wright's stain of a peripheral blood smear. This may reveal any neutrophil morphologic abnormalities. A PMN count lower than 1,000 per mm^3 is associated with an increased risk of infection. Neutropenia has many etiologies, including infections, drugs, and heredity. Neutropenia that is drug or chemical induced may be caused by peripheral PMN destruction from an autoimmunity or to depression of granulocyte formation in the bone marrow.

Critical functions of neutrophils are chemotaxis, phagocytosis, and killing of ingested microbial agents. Interference with any one of these functions can produce clinical disease. Ingestion and oxidative killing functions of neutrophils can be measured using the NBT reduction test. It is a limited test and is most useful for the diagnosis of chronic granulomatous disease. Another test of phagocytosis is the elicitation of chemiluminescence measured by scintillation counter.

Neutrophil function can be assayed by testing with the NBT test. This test measures a respiratory burst of the neutrophils producing superoxide anions. Neutrophils reduce the NBT dye to formazan, which appears as dark blue grains in the cytoplasm. Patients with chronic granulomatous disease lack the ability to reduce NBT. Patients with dysfunction of neutrophils generally have recurring bacterial diseases. Chemotaxis can also be measured using stimulants such as informal-l methionyl-l leucyl-phenylalanine, which tests the migration of neutrophils compared with normal controls.

Immune Activation

Measurement of immune activation generally includes a complete blood cell count, differential immunoglobulin concentrations, and complement levels. The general signs and symptoms of immune activation include lymphadenopathy, fever, and lethargy. Cytokines are generally in low concentration in the blood and have very short half-lives. The most common cytokine measurement is IL-2, which induces proliferation and maturation of T cells. IL-2 is assayed using an enzyme immunoassay technique.

CLINICAL ALLERGY

The allergic diseases are a group of disorders that are triggered by exposure to antigens to which an individual produces IgE antibody. *Atopy* refers to the state of producing IgE antibody to environmental antigens. An *atopic* individual manufactures IgE antibody to one or more environmental substances. Atopy can be a familial trait, particularly with regard to certain antigens. An allergic reaction requires several components. An individual must manufacture IgE antibody to a substance, be exposed to the substance, and have an organ or organ system that reacts adversely to the exposure. To understand this last point, consider an inhalation exposure to ragweed pollen of a group of individuals that are allergic to ragweed pollen. Some individuals will respond to the challenge with rhinitis but not asthma, some will develop an asthma attack but not rhinitis, and some will develop both asthma and rhinitis. A few individuals will develop urticaria from a pollen exposure, and some individuals will remain asymptomatic.

An allergic reaction requires an initial exposure, which triggers the production of IgE antibody to the antigen. On subsequent exposures, antigen molecules cross-link IgE antibodies bound to mast cells and basophils, triggering basophil and mast-cell degranulation and the extrusion of cell granules and preformed mediators into the extracellular space. These mediators include the vasoactive amine histamine and chemotactic factors for neutrophils and eosinophils.

Other mediators, such as the arachidonic acid metabolites of the leukotriene and prostaglandin classes, are manufactured after antigen stimulation of the mast cell.

Chemotactic factors attract neutrophils and eosinophils to the area of stimulation. The eosinophil is a white blood cell that migrates into tissues and releases major basic protein, eosinophil cation protein, and eosinophil protein-X (311). The eosinophil is prominent in the defense against parasites, but these proteins can also damage host tissues, as observed in the hypereosinophil syndrome (312).

Neutrophils migrate into the area of mast-cell degranulation and secrete factors that degranulate mast cells, leading to a recurrence of symptoms approximately 4 to 8 hours after the initial allergy attack. *Late-phase reactions* is the term given for these delayed reactions, which can occur in the airway, skin, and in systemic anaphylaxis. Corticosteroids and cromolyn can ablate late-phase reactions, but β adrenergic agents, such as albuterol, are ineffective in preventing late-phase reactions.

Specific IgE antibody is produced by plasma cells and binds avidly to receptors on the surfaces of mast cells and basophils. Mast cells reside in tissues in close proximity to blood vessels and nerves, whereas basophils are found circulating in the blood and can migrate into tissues. The initiation process involves the presentation of antigen to T lymphocytes by macrophages, which then induce B lymphocytes to differentiate into plasma cells.

Allergic diseases can be triggered by nonimmunologic stimuli. Cold dry air, exercise, chemical irritants, and emotional stress have been identified as triggers of asthma attacks. Some substances can directly degranulate mast cells or basophils, and reactions to these substances are termed *anaphylactoid reactions*. The term *anaphylactic reactions* is reserved for immunologically mediated reactions. Examples of substances that degranulate mast cells directly that are of clinical significance include iodinated radiocontrast media and opioids at high doses (313).

The mechanism by which low-molecular-weight irritants trigger allergic symptoms has been the subject of intense investigation. There are chemical irritant receptors called *chemoreceptors* on the surface of sensory nerve c-fibers in the skin, airway, and gut. When chemical irritants bind to these receptors, substance P and other mediators of inflammation are released. In addition, the binding of irritants to the chemoreceptors triggers a nerve impulse that travels to the central nervous system (314,315).

Human challenge studies have verified that environmental tobacco smoke can induce asthma (316) and rhinitis (317) in susceptible individuals, presumably through neurogenic inflammation. Perfumes have also been demonstrated to induce asthma in asthma patients with a history of sensitivity to perfumes (318).

A relationship exists between neurogenic inflammation and immunogenic inflammation in that human skin mast cells contain receptors for substance P (319). When substance P binds to mast cells, the mast cells degranulate and release mast-cell mediators. Further sensory nerve C-fibers have surface receptors for histamine. The binding of histamine to the nerve fibers triggers substance P release, and a nerve impulse is transmitted to the CNS (320).

Reactions most commonly occur at the site of inoculation with antigen or chemical irritant. For example, asthma and rhinitis most commonly result from inhalation exposures, whereas ingestions generally lead to gastrointestinal symptoms. Sometimes, the site of response is switched (321). Examples include systemic anaphylaxis to ingestions of food and drugs, in which there is a rapid development of signs and symptoms in many organ systems. Food allergy can result in asthma, urticaria, systemic anaphylaxis, and laryngeal edema. Site switching is believed to take place in the CNS. The response to the sensory nerve signal from the site of inoculation is rerouted to another peripheral location, leading to substance P release at the other location. The phenomenon of site switching has been termed *neurogenic switching* (321).

It has been shown in animal studies that systemic anaphylaxis can be blocked by ablating nerve pathways, even though histamine release still occurs at the inoculation site (322,323). Hence, systemic anaphylaxis occurs because the initial inoculation triggers a nerve impulse that travels to the CNS. Nerve impulses then travel throughout the body, and substance P is released, which triggers mast-cell degranulation and multiorgan system involvement.

A remarkable increase over the last few decades of the twentieth century occurred in the prevalence, incidence, and death rate from asthma in industrialized countries. A number of studies have documented this increase, and prevalence rates have increased in the range of 20% to 40% per decade. Examples include a National Institutes of Health Statistics study of children and adolescents that found a 23% increase in the prevalence of asthma from 3.1% in 1970 to 3.8% in 1978 to 1980 (324). A special child health study found a 39% increase in the prevalence of asthma from 3.2% in 1981 to 4.3% in 1988 (325). A study of young adult, nonsmoking Michigan Medicaid recipients found a 40% increase in the prevalence of asthma, from 2.0% in 1981 to 2.8% in 1988 (326). An increase of 54% in the incidence of asthma was seen from 1964 to 1983, with the largest increases in incidence rates for children and adolescents (327). Asthma hospitalizations among children rose at a rate of 4.5% a year from 1974 to 1983 (328). Mortality from asthma increased 6.2% per year during the 1980s after declining 7.8% per year during the 1970s (329). Similar increases have been observed in other allergic diseases, although data are limited. There was an approximately 100% increase in asthma, rhinitis, and eczema in Swedish schoolchildren from 1979 to 1991 (330). Large increases in both asthma and allergic rhinitis were observed in young Italian men from 1983 until 1993 to 1995 (331).

Hypotheses to explain this remarkable increase in allergic diseases include the proposal that there is an epidemic of asthma-inducing viral illnesses. Viral infections can induce asthma and may play a role in the epidemic (332). Many observers believe that the effects of environmental toxins are responsible. Two mechanisms by which toxic exposures may lead to allergic diseases are

- Toxic exposures that may induce antibody production against previously benign substances. Toxins that operate in this manner are called *environmental adjuvants.*
- Toxic exposures that may induce end-organ sensitivity to allergic and other stimuli—that is, a toxic exposure may convert a normal lung to an asthmatic lung, etc.

An *adjuvant* is a substance that enhances the development of immunity to other substances. Adjuvants produce different types of immune responses that are specific for the adjuvant. Alum induces IgE antibody to a coinjected protein. Freund's complete adjuvant, which is an oil immersion of mycobacterial antigens, induces cellular immunity to a coinjected protein. Chemicals that induce immune responses to other substances in the environment are *environmental adjuvants*. Environmental contamination with adjuvants has been suggested as a cause of the increasing prevalence of respiratory allergy in industrialized countries. Substances known to induce IgE-antibody production to concomitantly administered substances in experimental models include diesel exhaust particles, sulfur dioxide, nitrogen dioxide, and ozone (333–336).

The polyaromatic hydrocarbons in diesel exhaust particles enhance the production of IgE antibodies by B cells *in vitro* (337) and enhance the *in vivo* IgE production in the human upper airway (338). *In vivo* nasal challenge with diesel exhaust particles has been shown to increase cytokine production in the human upper airway (339). Diesel exhaust particles may play a role in the worldwide increase in allergic respiratory disease.

RADS has been defined as an asthmalike illness induced by a single high-dose irritant exposure. The asthmatic condition persists and becomes chronic (340). High-dose exposures associated with the induction of asthma include acetic acid (341), ammonia (342), chlorine (343), ethylene oxide (344), sulfur dioxide (345), glacial acetic acid (346), smoke (340), dust (340), and toluene diisocyanate (347). In addition to asthma attacks, patients with RADS report constitutional symptoms associated with previously tolerated chemical exposures, so that RADS overlaps with chemical sensitivity (348–350). Endobronchial biopsies of patients with RADS has revealed chronic inflammation with lymphocytic infiltrates (343).

An upper airway analogue of RADS, the reactive upper-airway dysfunction syndrome (RUDS), has been described. RUDS refers to the induction of chronic rhinitis after an irritant exposure, and these individuals have a persistent intolerance to chemical irritants (348). Nasal biopsy findings in patients with RUDS include proliferation of peripheral nerve fibers, basement membrane thickening, chronic inflammation with lymphocytic infiltrates, and gaps in tight junctions (349). A mechanism for the persistent inflammation and reactivity to chemicals is suggested by these findings (350).

EXPOSURE RESPONSE VERSUS IMMUNOTOXICITY

Exposure to a chemical with a subsequent immune response must not be confused with immunotoxicity. A normal immune response involves the following:

1. Encounter of lymphocyte with antigen
2. Antigen recognition by the immune system
3. Activation of lymphocytes
4. Amplification of the immune response
5. Immune discrimination between self and nonself
6. Regulation and control over the immune response

In the process of deciding toxic causation, the clinician must account for the difference between exposure and actual disease, which may result from end-organ damage or altered immune status. An example of this is the presence of antibodies to the conjugate of formaldehyde and human serum albumin. The presence of such IgG and IgM antibodies has been demonstrated in some individuals exposed to formaldehyde. The presence of these antibody titers means that haptenization of human serum proteins has occurred and that an immune response recognized the new immunogen. The presence of specific circulating IgG and IgM antibodies to formaldehyde–human serum albumin haptens demonstrates that exposure to formaldehyde can result in immune system stimulation to a neoantigen. However, the clinician must be careful not to interpret this normal immune relapse as disease.

REFERENCES

1. Chase M. Specificity of serological reactions: Landsteiner centennial. *Ann N Y Acad Sci* 1970;169:9–10.
2. Paul W. *Fundamental immunology*, 3rd ed. New York: Raven Press, 1993:1–1490.
3. Holladay SD, Smith BJ. Alterations in murine fetal thymus and liver hematopoietic cell populations following developmental exposure to 7,12-dimethylbenz[a]anthracene. *Environ Res* 1995;68:106–113.
4. Botham PA. Are pesticides immunotoxic? *Adverse Drug React Acute Poison Rev* 1990;9:91–101.
5. Ullrich SE. Potential for immunotoxicity due to environmental exposure to ultraviolet radiation. *Hum Exp Toxicol* 1995;14:89–91.
6. Burmester GR. Lessons from Lyme arthritis. *Clin Exp Rheumatol* 1993;11(Suppl 8):S23–S27.
7. Friedman SM, Tumang JR, Crow MK. Microbial superantigens as etiopathogenic agents in autoimmunity. *Rheum Dis Clin North Am* 1993;19:207–222.
8. Hanson CD, Smialowicz RJ. Evaluation of the effect of low-level 2,3,7,8-tetrachlorodibenzo-*p*-dioxin exposure on cell mediated immunity. *Toxicology* 1994;88:213–224.
9. Harris JP, Keithley EM. Inner ear inflammation and round window otosclerosis. *Am J Otol* 1993;14:109–112.
10. Holmdahl R, Malmstrom V, Vuorio E. Autoimmune recognition of cartilage collagens. *Ann Med* 1993;25:251–264.
11. Luster MI, Rosenthal GJ. Chemical agents and the immune response. *Environ Health Perspect* 1993;100:219–226.
12. Yoshida S, Gershwin ME. Autoimmunity and selected environmental factors of disease induction. *Semin Arthritis Rheum* 1993;22:399–419.
13. Sharma RP. Immunotoxicity of mycotoxins. *J Dairy Sci* 1993;76:892–897.
14. Harper N, Steinberg M, Safe S. Immunotoxicity of a reconstituted polynuclear aromatic hydrocarbon mixture in B6C3F1 mice. *Toxicology* 1996;109:31–38.
15. Kusaka Y. Occupational diseases caused by exposure to sensitizing metals. *Sangyo Igaku* 1993;35:75–87.
16. Descotes J. Immunotoxicology of cadmium. *IARC Sci Publ* 1992;385–390.
17. van den Tweel JG. Immunotoxiciteit en pathogeniteit van stoffen. *Ned Tijdschr Geneeskd* 1992;136:1949–1951.
18. Claassen E. Immunotoxicologie; nieuwe ontwikkelingen en perspectieven. *Ned Tijdschr Geneeskd* 1991;135:879–885.
19. Karol MH, Jin RZ. Mechanisms of immunotoxicity to isocyanates. *Chem Res Toxicol* 1991;4:503–509.
20. Verdier F, Virat M, Schweinfurth H, Descotes J. Immunotoxicity of bis(tri-*n*-butyltin) oxide in the rat. *J Toxicol Environ Health* 1991;32:307–317.
21. Zaidi SI, Raisuddin S, Singh KP, et al. Acrylamide induced immunosuppression in rats and its modulation by 6-MFA, an interferon inducer. *Immunopharmacol Immunotoxicol* 1994;16:247–260.
22. Krzystyniak K, Tryphonas H, Fournier M. Approaches to the evaluation of chemical-induced immunotoxicity. *Environ Health Perspect* 1995;103(Suppl 9):17–22.
23. Nagayama Y, Ohta K, Tsuruta M, et al. Exacerbation of thyroid autoimmunity by interferon alpha treatment in patients with chronic viral hepatitis: our studies and review of the literature. *Endocr J* 1994;41:565–572.
24. Jeong TC, Matulka RA, Jordan SD, Yang KH, Holsapple MP. Role of metabolism in cocaine-induced immunosuppression in splenocyte cultures from B6C3F1 female mice. *Immunopharmacology* 1995;29:37–46.
25. Schuurman HJ, Kuper CF, Vos JG. Histopathology of the immune system as a tool to assess immunotoxicity. *Toxicology* 1994;86:187–212.
26. Descotes J. Immunotoxicology of immunomodulators. *Dev Biol Stand* 1992;77:99–102.
27. Fornasiero MC, Ferrari M, Gnocchi P, Trizio D, Isetta AM. Immunodepressive activity of FCE 23762 on humoral and cell-mediated immune responses in normal mice: comparison with doxorubicin. *Agents Actions* 1992;37:311–318.
28. Pirozhkov SV, Watson RR, Chen GJ. Ethanol enhances immunosuppression induced by cocaine. *Alcohol* 1992;9:489–494.
29. Chang MP, Norman DC. Immunotoxicity of alcohol in young and old mice. II. Impaired T cell proliferation and T cell-dependent antibody responses of young and old mice fed ethanol-containing liquid diet. *Mech Ageing Dev* 1991;57:175–186.

30. Misra RR, Bloom SE. Roles of dosage, pharmacokinetics, and cellular sensitivity to damage in the selective toxicity of cyclophosphamide towards B and T cells in development. *Toxicology* 1991;66:239–256.
31. Luster MI, Germolec DR, Rosenthal GJ. Immunotoxicology: review of current status. *Ann Allergy* 1990;64:427–432.
32. Luster MI, Munson AE, Thomas PT, et al. Development of a testing battery to assess chemical-induced immunotoxicity: National Toxicology Program's guidelines for immunotoxicity evaluation in mice. *Fundam Appl Toxicol* 1988;10:2–19.
33. Luster MI, Pait DG, Portier C, et al. Qualitative and quantitative experimental models to aid in risk assessment for immunotoxicology. *Toxicol Lett* 1992;64–65:71–78.
34. Luster MI, Portier C, Pait DG, et al. Risk assessment in immunotoxicology. I. Sensitivity and predictability of immune tests. *Fundam Appl Toxicol* 1992;18:200–210.
35. Huber J, Zegers B, Schuurman H. Pathology of congenital immunodeficiencies. *Semin Diagn Pathol* 1992;9:31–62.
36. Buckley R. Primary immunodeficiencies. In: Paul W, ed. *Fundamental immunology,* 3rd ed. New York: Raven Press, 1993:1353–1374.
37. Rosenberg Z, Fauci AS. Immunology of HIV infection. In: Paul W, ed. *Fundamental immunology,* 3rd ed. New York: Raven Press, 1993:1375–1398.
38. Purtillo D, Linder J, Seemayer J. Inherited and acquired immunodeficiency disorders. In: Covin B, Bhan A, McCluskey R, eds. *Diagnostic immunopathology.* New York: Raven Press, 1988:121–150.
39. Geh JI, Spittle MF. Oncological problems in AIDS—a review of the clinical features and management. *Ann Acad Med Singapore* 1996;25:380–391.
40. Arribas JR, Storch GA, Clifford DB, Tselis AC. Cytomegalovirus encephalitis. *Ann Intern Med* 1996;125:577–587.
41. Miralles ES, Nunez M, De Las Heras ME, Perez B, Moreno R, Ledo A. Pityriasis rubra pilaris and human immunodeficiency virus infection. *Br J Dermatol* 1995;133:990–993.
42. Sanchez Munoz-Torrero JF, Yniguez TR, Garcia-Onieva E, et al. Nocardiosis en enfermos con infeccion por virus de la inmunodeficiencia humana en España. *Rev Clin Esp* 1995;195:468–472.
43. Moss PJ, Read RC, Kudesia G, McKendrick MW. Prolonged cryptosporidiosis during primary HIV infection. *J Infect* 1995;30:51–53.
44. Ali NJ, Kessel D, Miller RF. Bronchopulmonary infection with *Pseudomonas aeruginosa* in patients infected with human immunodeficiency virus. *Genitourin Med* 1995;71:73–77.
45. Ognibene FP, Shelhamer JH, Hoffman GS, et al. *Pneumocystis carinii* pneumonia: a major complication of immunosuppressive therapy in patients with Wegener's granulomatosis. *Am J Respir Crit Care Med* 1995;151:795–799.
46. Greenspan JS. Periodontal complications of HIV infection. *Compendium* 1994;(Suppl 18):S694–S698, S714–S717 [Quiz].
47. Straus WL, Ostroff SM, Jernigan DB, et al. Clinical and epidemiologic characteristics of *Mycobacterium haemophilum,* an emerging pathogen in immunocompromised patients. *Ann Intern Med* 1994;120:118–125.
48. Domer JE, Garner RE. Immunomodulation in response to *Candida. Immunol Ser* 1989;47:293–317.
49. Rhile MJ, Nagarkatti M, Nagarkatti PS. Role of Fas apoptosis and MHC genes in 2,3,7,8-tetrachlorodibenzo-*p*-dioxin (TCDD)-induced immunotoxicity of T cells. *Toxicology* 1996;110:153–167.
50. Batt AM, Ferrari L. Manifestations of chemically induced liver damage. *Clin Chem* 1995;41:1882–1887.
51. Raffray M, Cohen GM. Thymocyte apoptosis as a mechanism for tributyltin-induced thymic atrophy in vivo. *Arch Toxicol* 1993;67:231–236.
52. Raffray M, McCarthy D, Snowden RT, Cohen GM. Apoptosis as a mechanism of tributyltin cytotoxicity to thymocytes: relationship of apoptotic markers to biochemical and cellular effects. *Toxicol Appl Pharmacol* 1993;119:122–130.
53. Burchiel S, Hadley W, Barton S, Fincher R, Laure L, Dean J. Persistent suppression of humoral immunity produced by 7,12-dimethylbenz(a)anthracene (DMBA) in B6CF1 mice: correlation with changes in spleen cell surface markers detected by flow cytometry. *Int J Immunopharmacol* 1988;10:369–376.
54. Katz D. Genetic control of cell-cell interactions. *Pharmacol Rev* 1982;34:51–62.
55. Hanse T, Carreno B, Sachs D. The major histocompatibility complex. In: Paul W, ed. *Fundamental immunology,* 3rd ed. New York: Raven Press, 1993:577–628.
56. Germain R. Antigen processing and presentation. In: Paul W, ed. *Fundamental immunology,* 3rd ed. New York: Raven Press, 1993:629–676.
57. Teal J, Abraham K. The regulation of antibody class expression. *Immunol Today* 1987;8:122–126.
58. Wilder RL. Neuroendocrine-immune system interactions and autoimmunity. *Annu Rev Immunol* 1995;13:307–338.
59. Pruett SB, Ensley DK, Crittenden PL. The role of chemical-induced stress responses in immunosuppression: a review of quantitative associations and cause-effect relationships between chemical-induced stress responses and immunosuppression. *J Toxicol Environ Health* 1993;39:163–192.
60. Fugere N, Brousseau P, Krzystyniak K, Coderre D, Fournier M. Heavy metal-specific inhibition of phagocytosis and different in vitro sensitivity of heterogeneous coelomocytes from *Lumbricus terrestris* (Oligochaeta). *Toxicology* 1996;109:157–166.
61. Damstra T, Jurgelski W, Jr., Posner HS, et al. Toxicity of polybrominated biphenyls (PBBs) in domestic and laboratory animals. *Environ Health Perspect* 1982;44:175–188.
62. Amos HE. Inadvertent immunosuppression as a health hazard. *Br J Clin Pract* 1986;40:336–340.
63. Fries GF. The PBB episode in Michigan: an overall appraisal. *Crit Rev Toxicol* 1985;16:105–156.
64. Tryphonas H. Immunotoxicity of PCBs (Aroclors) in relation to Great Lakes. *Environ Health Perspect* 1995;103(Suppl 9):35–46.
65. Vial T, Nicolas B, Descotes J. Clinical immunotoxicity of pesticides. *J Toxicol Environ Health* 1996;48:215–229.
66. Thomas PT. Pesticide-induced immunotoxicity: are Great Lakes residents at risk? *Environ Health Perspect* 1995;103(Suppl 9):55–61.
67. Keil DE, Padgett EL, Barnes DB, Pruett SB. Role of decomposition products in sodium methyldithiocarbamate-induced immunotoxicity. *J Toxicol Environ Health* 1996;47:479–492.
68. Institoris L, Siroki O, Desi I. Immunotoxicity study of repeated small doses of dimethoate and methylparathion administered to rats over three generations. *Hum Exp Toxicol* 1995;14:879–883.
69. Bernier J, Girard D, Krzystyniak K, et al. Immunotoxicity of aminocarb. III. Exposure route–dependent immunomodulation by aminocarb in mice. *Toxicology* 1995;99:135–146.
70. Rodgers K. The immunotoxicity of pesticides in rodents. *Hum Exp Toxicol* 1995;14:111–113.
71. Pirozhkov SV, Watson RR, Chen GJ. Ethanol enhances immunosuppression induced by cocaine. *Alcohol Alcohol Suppl* 1993;2:75–82.
72. Buckley R. Immunodeficiency diseases. *JAMA* 1987;258:2841–2850.
73. Duggan JM, Goldstein SJ, Chenoweth CE, Kauffman CA, Bradley SF. *Achromobacter xylosoxidans* bacteremia: report of four cases and review of the literature. *Clin Infect Dis* 1996;23:569–576.
74. Moss RL, Musemeche CA, Kosloske AM. Necrotizing fasciitis in children: prompt recognition and aggressive therapy improve survival. *J Pediatr Surg* 1996;31:1142–1146.
75. Harril WC, Stewart MG, Lee AG, Cernoch P. Chronic rhinocerebral mucormycosis. *Laryngoscope* 1996;106:1292–1297.
76. Guay DR. Nontuberculous mycobacterial infections. *Ann Pharmacother* 1996;30:819–830.
77. Berna JD, Garcia-Medina V, Cano A, Guirao J, Lafuente A, Garcia-Orenes MC. Neumonia por *Rhodococcus equi* en pacientes infectados por el HIV: presentacion de 2 casos y revision de la literatura. *Enferm Infecc Microbiol Clin* 1996;14:177–180.
78. Heinz T, Perfect J, Schell W, Ritter E, Ruff G, Serafin D. Soft-tissue fungal infections: surgical management of 12 immunocompromised patients. *Plast Reconstr Surg* 1996;97:1391–1399.
79. Bradley G, Morahan P. Approaches to assessing host resistance. *Environ Health Perspect* 1982;43:61–69.
80. Brooks B. *Understanding indoor air quality,* 1st ed. Boca Raton, FL: CRC Press, 1992:1–189.
81. Burleson GR, Dean JH, Munson AE. *Methods in immunotoxicology.* New York: Wiley-Liss, 1995.
82. Garssen J, Van der Vliet H, De Klerk A, et al. A rat cytomegalovirus infection model as a tool for immunotoxicity testing. *Eur J Pharmacol* 1995;292:223–231.
83. Lebrec H, Burleson GR. Influenza virus host resistance models in mice and rats: utilization for immune function assessment and immunotoxicology. *Toxicology* 1994;91:179–188.
84. Bradley SG, Morahan PS. Approaches to assessing host resistance. *Environ Health Perspect* 1982;43:61–69.
85. Bradley G. Listerial host resistance model. In: Burleson G, Dean J, Munson A, eds. *Methods in immunotoxicology,* 1st ed. New York: Wiley-Liss, 1995:169–180.
86. Bradley G. *Streptococcus* host resistance model. In: Burleson G, Dean J, Munson A, eds. *Methods in immunotoxicology,* 1st ed. New York: Wiley-Liss, 1995.
87. Brooks B, Sullivan J. Immunotoxicology. In: Sullivan J, Krieger G, eds. *Hazardous materials toxicology: clinical principles of environmental health,* 1st ed. Baltimore: Williams & Wilkins, 1992:190–214.
88. Luebke R. Assessment of host resistance to infection with rodent malaria. In: Burleson G, Dean J, Munson A, eds. *Methods in immunotoxicology,* 1st ed. New York: Wiley-Liss, 1995:221–242.
89. van Loveren H, Luebke R, Vos J. Assessment of immunotoxicity with the parasitic infection model *Trichinella spiralis.* In: Burleson G, Dean J, Munson A, eds. *Methods in immunotoxicology,* 1st ed. New York: Wiley-Liss, 1995:243–276.
90. Brittenden J, Heys D, Ross J, Eremin O. Natural killer cells and cancer. *Cancer* 1996;77:1226–1243.
91. Keever-Taylor C, Witt P, Truitt R, Ramanujam S, Borden E, Ritch P. Hematologic and immunologic evaluation of recombinant human interleukin-6 in patients with advanced malignant disease: evidence for monocyte activation. *J Immunother* 1996;19:231–243.
92. Wang CY, Schroeter AL, Su WP. Acquired immunodeficiency syndrome–related Kaposi's sarcoma. *Mayo Clin Proc* 1995;70:869–879.
93. Buchsel PC, Leum EW, Randolph SR. Delayed complications of bone marrow transplantation: an update. *Oncol Nurs Forum* 1996;23:1267–1291.
94. Goldstein DJ, Austin JH, Zuech N, et al. Carcinoma of the lung after heart transplantation. *Transplantation* 1996;62:772–775.
95. Tan-Shalaby J, Tempero M. Malignancies after liver transplantation: a comparative review. *Semin Liver Dis* 1995;15:156–164.
96. Yellin SA, Weiss MH, Kraus DH, Papadopoulos EB. Tonsil lymphoma presenting as tonsillitis after bone marrow transplantation. *Otolaryngol Head Neck Surg* 1995;112:544–548.
97. Melosky B, Karim M, Chui A, et al. Lymphoproliferative disorders after renal transplantation in patients receiving triple or quadruple immunosuppression. *J Am Soc Nephrol* 1992;2:S290–S294.

98. Herreros J, Florez S, Echevarria JR, Fernandez AL, Pardo Mindan FJ. Enfermedad linfoproliferativa y cancer en el enfermo trasplantado. *Rev Esp Cardiol* 1995;48(Suppl 7):129–134.
99. Oliver RT, Nouri AM. T cell immune response to cancer in humans and its relevance for immunodiagnosis and therapy. *Cancer Surv* 1992;13:173–204.
100. Kripke ML. Immunoregulation of carcinogenesis: past, present, and future. *J Natl Cancer Inst* 1988;80:722–727.
101. Dean J, Luster M, Boorman GA, Leubke R, Lauer LD. Application of tumor, bacterial, and parasite susceptibility assays to study immune alterations induced by environmental chemicals. *Environ Health Perspect* 1982;43:81–88.
102. Hinton DM. Immunotoxicity testing applied to direct food and colour additives: US FDA "Redbook II" guidelines. *Hum Exp Toxicol* 1995;14:143–145.
103. Murray MJ, Kerkvliet NI, Ward EC, Dean J. Models for the evaluation of tumor resistance following chemical or drug exposure. In: Dean J, Luster M, Munson A, Amos H, eds. *Immunotoxicology and immunopharmacology,* 1st ed. New York: Raven Press, 1985:113–122.
104. Plaut M, Zimmerman E. Allergy and mechanisms of hypersensitivity. In: Paul W, ed. *Fundamental immunology.* New York: Raven Press, 1993:1399–1425.
105. Garssen J, Vandebriel J, Kimber I, van Loveren H. Hypersensitivity reactions: definitions, basic mechanisms, and localizations. In: Vos J, Younes M, Smith E, eds. *Allergic hypersensitivities induced by chemicals: recommendations for prevention.* Boca Raton, FL: World Health Organization/CRC Press, 1996:19–58.
106. Vos J, Younes M, Smith E, eds. *Allergic hypersensitivities induced by chemicals: recommendations for prevention.* Boca Raton, FL: World Health Organization/ CRC Press, 1996:1–348.
107. Salvaggio J. Overview of occupational immunologic lung disease. *J Allergy Clin Immunol* 1982;70:5–10.
108. Sheretz E, Storrs F. Contact dermatitis. In: Rosenstock L, Cullen MR, eds. *Textbook of clinical occupational and environmental medicine.* Philadelphia: WB Saunders, 1994:514–529.
109. Hjorth N. The allergens. In: Maibach H, ed. *Occupational and industrial dermatology,* 2nd ed. Chicago: Year Book Medical Publishers, 1987:22–27.
110. Balmes J. Asthma. In: Harber P, Schenker M, Balmes J, eds. *Occupational and environmental respiratory disease.* St. Louis: Mosby–Year Book, 1996:189–202.
111. Murphy D, Morgan K, Seaton A. Hypersensitivity pneumonitis. In: Morgan W, Seaton A, eds. *Occupational lung diseases.* Philadelphia: WB Saunders, 1995:525–567.
112. Rose C. Hypersensitivity pneumonitis. In: Harber P, Schenker M, Balmes J, eds. *Occupational and environmental respiratory disease.* St. Louis: Mosby–Year Book, 1996:201–215.
113. Kaliner M, Eggleston P, Matthews K. Asthma and rhinitis. *JAMA* 1987;258:2851–2873.
114. Stanworth D. Mechanisms of hypersensitivity. In: Gibson G, Hubbard R, Parke D, eds. *Immunotoxicology.* New York: Academic Press, 1983:71–86.
115. Stanworth D. Current concepts of hypersensitivity. In: Dean J, Luster M, Munson A, Amos H, eds. *Immunotoxicology and immunopharmacology,* 1st ed. New York: Raven Press, 1985:91–98.
116. Sell S. *Immunology, immunopathology, and immunity.* New York: Elsevier Science, 1987:1–507.
117. Bos J, Das P, Kapsenberg M. The skin immune system (SIS). In: Bos J, ed. *Skin immune system (SIS).* Boca Raton, FL: CRC Press, 1990:3–8.
118. Ring J. Diagnosis and treatment of hypersensitivity reactions of the skin. In: Vos J, Younes M, Smith E, eds. *Allergic hypersensitivities induced by chemicals,* 1st ed. Boca Raton, FL: CRC Press, 1996:225–236.
119. Hannuksela M. Tests for immediate hypersensitivity. In: Maibach H, ed. *Occupational and industrial dermatology,* 2nd ed. Chicago: Year Book Medical Publishers, 1987:168–178.
120. Fischer T, Maibach H. Patch testing in allergic contact dermatitis, an update. In: Maibach H, ed. *Occupational and industrial dermatology,* 2nd ed. Chicago: Year Book Medical Publishers, 1987:190–210.
121. Mauer T. Predictive testing for skin allergy. In: Vos J, Younes M, Smith E, eds. *Allergic hypersensitivities induced by chemicals,* 1st ed. Boca Raton, FL: CRC Press, 1996:237–260.
122. Magnusson B, Kligman A. The identification of contact allergens by animal assay: the guinea pig maximization test. *Journal Invest Dermatol* 1969;52:268–276.
123. Buehler E. Delayed contact hypersensitivity in the guinea pig. *Arch Dermatol* 1965;91:171–177.
124. Chan-Yeung M. Asthma. In: Rosenstock L, Cullen MR, eds. *Textbook of clinical occupational and environmental medicine.* Philadelphia: WB Saunders, 1994:197–209.
125. Malo J, Cartier A. Occupational asthma. In: Harber P, Schenker M, Balmes J, eds. *Occupational and environmental respiratory disease.* St. Louis: Mosby–Year Book, 1996:420–432.
126. Seaton A. Occupational asthma. In: Morgan W, Seaton A, eds. *Occupational lung diseases,* 3rd ed. Philadelphia: WB Saunders, 1995:457–483.
127. Peterson B, Saxon A. Global increases in allergic respiratory disease: the possible role of diesel exhaust particles. *Ann Allergy Asthma Immunol* 1996;77:263–268, 269–270 [Quiz].
128. Paky A, Knoblauch A. Staubbelastung, staubbedingte Lungenkrankheiten und Atemschutzmassnahmen in der Landwirtschaft. *Schweiz Med Wochenschr* 1995;125:458–466.
129. Laurent K, De Jonghe M, Flemale A, Kimbimbi P, Defrance P, Gillard C. Un nouveau cas de pneumopathie d'hypersensibilité á la Salazopyrine? *Rev Pneumol Clin* 1985;41:340–343.
130. Reynolds HY. Hypersensitivity pneumonitis: correlation of cellular and immunologic changes with clinical phases of disease. *Lung* 1988;166:189–208.
131. Perez Arellano JL, Sanchez Sanchez R, Pastor Encinas I, Losa Garcia JE, Garcia Martin MJ, Gonzalez Villaron L. Pathogenesis of hypersensitivity pneumonitis. *Allergol Immunopathol (Madr)* 1989;17:225–232.
132. Wardlaw AJ. Air pollution and allergic disease. Report of a working party of the British Society for Allergy and Clinical Immunology. *Clin Exp Allergy* 1995;25(Suppl 3):6–8.
133. Eccles R. Rhinitis as a mechanism of respiratory defense. *Eur Arch Otorhinolaryngol Suppl* 1995;1:S2–S7.
134. Bretscher P, Cohn M. A theory of self-nonself discrimination. *Science* 1970;163:1042–1049.
135. Guerder S, Flavell RA. Costimulation in tolerance and autoimmunity. *Int Rev Immunol* 1995;13:135–146.
136. Perrin PJ, Scott D, June CH, Racke MK. B7-mediated costimulation can either provoke or prevent clinical manifestations of experimental allergic encephalomyelitis. *Immunol Res* 1995;14:189–199.
137. Ostrand-Rosenberg S, Baskar S, Patterson N, Clements VK. Expression of MHC Class II and B7-1 and B7-2 costimulatory molecules accompanies tumor rejection and reduces the metastatic potential of tumor cells. *Tissue Antigens* 1996;47:414–421.
138. Schwartz R. Autoimmunity and autoimmune diseases. In: Paul W, ed. *Fundamental immunology,* 3rd ed. New York: Raven Press, 1993:1033–1087.
139. Talal N. Autoimmunity and sex revisited. *Clin Immunol Immunopathol* 1989;53:355–357.
140. Ahmed S, Penhale W, Talal N. Sex hormones, immune responses, and autoimmune diseases. *Am J Pathol* 1985;12:531–551.
141. Bach J. Organ-specific autoimmunity. *Immunol Today* 1995;16:353–355.
142. Black CM. Scleroderma and fasciitis in children. Curr Opin Rheumatol 1995;7:442–448.
143. Strassburg CP, Manns MP. Autoimmune hepatitis versus viral hepatitis C. *Liver* 1995;15:225–232.
144. Yung RL, Johnson KJ, Richardson BC. New concepts in the pathogenesis of drug-induced lupus. *Lab Invest* 1995;73:746–759.
145. Bigazzi PE. Autoimmunity and heavy metals. *Lupus* 1994;3:449–453.
146. Hayashi Y, Haneji N, Hamano H. Pathogenesis of Sjögren's syndrome-like autoimmune lesions in MRL/lpr mice. *Pathol Int* 1994;44:559–568.
147. Lorber M, Gershwin ME, Shoenfeld Y. The coexistence of systemic lupus erythematosus with other autoimmune diseases: the kaleidoscope of autoimmunity. *Semin Arthritis Rheum* 1994;24:105–113.
148. Sakata S. Autoimmunity against thyroid hormones. *Crit Rev Immunol* 1994;14:157–191.
149. Carnaud C, Bach JF. Cellular basis of T-cell autoreactivity in autoimmune diseases. *Immunol Res* 1993;12:131–148.
150. ter Meulen V, Liebert UG. Measles virus–induced autoimmune reactions against brain antigen. *Intervirology* 1993;35:86–94.
151. Weetman AP. Extrathyroidal complications of Graves' disease. *Q J Med* 1993;86:473–477.
152. Tomer Y, Davies TF. Infections and autoimmune endocrine disease. *Baillieres Clin Endocrinol Metab* 1995;9:47–70.
153. Fohlman J, Friman G. Is juvenile diabetes a viral disease? *Ann Med* 1993;25:569–574.
154. Rasmussen HB, Perron H, Clausen J. Do endogenous retroviruses have etiological implications in inflammatory and degenerative nervous system diseases? *Acta Neurol Scand* 1993;88:190–198.
155. Wright P, Murray RM. Schizophrenia: prenatal influenza and autoimmunity. *Ann Med* 1993;25:497–502.
156. Tomer Y, Davies TF. Infection, thyroid disease, and autoimmunity. *Endocrin Rev* 1993;14:107–120.
157. Kirch DG. Infection and autoimmunity as etiologic factors in schizophrenia: a review and reappraisal. *Schizophr Bull* 1993;19:355–370.
158. Pelletier L, Castedo M, Bellon B, Druet P. Mercury and autoimmunity. In: Dean J, Luster M, Munson A, Kimber I, eds. *Immunotoxicology and immunopharmacology,* 2nd ed. New York: Raven Press, 1994:539–552.
159. Condemi J. The autoimmune diseases. *JAMA* 1987;258:2920–2929.
160. Smith H, Steinberg A. Autoimmunity—a perspective. In: Paul W, Fathman G, Metzger H, eds. *Annual review of immunology.* Palo Alto, CA: Annual Reviews, 1983:175–210.
161. Bigazzi P. Autoimmunity induced by chemicals. *J Toxicol Clin Toxicol* 1988;26:125–156.
162. Descotes J, Nicolas B, Vial T. Assessment of immunotoxic effects in humans. *Clin Chem* 1995;41:1870–1873.
163. Hamilton H, Morgan D, Simmons A. A pesticide (dieldrin)-induced immunohemolytic anemia. *Environ Res* 1978;17:155–164.
164. Bigazzi P. Mechanisms of chemical induced autoimmunity. In: Dean J, Luster M, Munson A, Amos H, eds. *Immunotoxicology and immunopharmacology,* 1st ed. New York: Raven Press, 1985:277–290.
165. Theofilopoulos A. The basis of autoimmunity: Part I—Mechanisms of aberrant self-recognition. *Immunol Today* 1995;16:91–97.
166. Theofilopoulos A. The basis of autoimmunity: Part II—Genetic predisposition. *Immunol Today* 1995;16:150–158.
167. Kirtland H, Mohler D, Horowitz D. Methyldopa inhibition of suppressor lymphocyte function: a proposed cause of autoimmune hemolytic anemia. *N Engl J Med* 1980;302:825–832.
168. Miller K, Salem K. Immune regulatory abnormalities produced by procainamide. *Am J Med* 1982;73:487–492.

169. Dhillon V, Latchman D, Isenberg D. Heat shock proteins and systemic lupus erythematosus. *Lupus* 1991;1:3–8.
170. van Eden W. Heat shock proteins as immunogenic bacterial antigens with the potential to induce and regulate autoimmune arthritis. *Immunol Rev* 1991;121:5–28.
171. van Eden W, Holoshitz J, Nevo Z, Frenkel A, Klajman A, Cohen I. Arthritis induced by a t-lymphocyte clone that responds to *Mycobacterium tuberculosis* and to cartilage proteoglycans. *Proc Natl Acad Sci U S A* 1982;82:5117–5120.
172. Deguchi Y, Kishimoto S. Enhanced expression of the heat shock protein gene in peripheral blood mononuclear cells of patients with active systemic lupus erythematosus. *Ann Rheum Dis* 1990;49:893–895.
173. Subcommittee on Immunotoxicology. Biologic markers in immunotoxicology. Washington: National Academy Press, 1992:1–206.
174. Bennet E, Mercier M. Preface. In: Berlin A, Dean J, Draper M, Smith E, Spreafico R, eds. *Immunotoxicology.* Boston: Martinus Nijhoff Publishers, 1987.
175. Munson A, LeVier D. Experimental design in immunotoxicology. In: Burleson G, Dean J, Munson A, eds. *Methods in immunotoxicology.* New York: John Wiley and Sons, 1993.
176. Brooks B, Neuman E, Reed N. Differential recovery of antibody production potential after sublethal whole-body irradiation in mice. *J Leukoc Biol* 1986;40:335–345.
177. Luster MI, Portier C, Pait DG, et al. Risk assessment in immunotoxicology. II. Relationships between immune and host resistance tests. *Fundam Appl Toxicol* 1993;21:71–82.
178. Descotes J, Nicolas B, Pham E, Vial T. Sentinel screening for human immunotoxicity. *Arch Toxicol Suppl* 1996;18:29–33.
179. Kerkvliet NI. Immunological effects of chlorinated dibenzo-*p*-dioxins. *Environ Health Perspect* 1995;103(Suppl 9):47–53.
180. Bernier J, Brousseau P, Krzystyniak K, Tryphonas H, Fournier M. Immunotoxicity of heavy metals in relation to Great Lakes. *Environ Health Perspect* 1995;103(Suppl 9):23–34.
181. Ban M, Hettich D, Cavelier C. Use of Mishell-Dutton culture for the detection of the immunosuppressive effect of iron-containing compounds. *Toxicol Lett* 1995;81:183–188.
182. Lawrence BP, Leid M, Kerkvliet NI. Distribution and behavior of the Ah receptor in murine T lymphocytes. *Toxicol Appl Pharmacol* 1996;138:275–284.
183. Urso P, Majekodunmi MJ, Cobb JR, et al. Zidovudine as an immunomodulatory agent. *Cell Mol Biol* 1995;41(Suppl 1):S103–S112.
184. Moszczynski P, Moszczynski P Jr. Ekspozycja na rtec a zdrowie populacji. I. Immunotoskycznosc rteci. *Med Pr* 1995;46:385–393.
185. Harper N, Connor K, Steinberg M, Safe S. Immunosuppressive activity of polychlorinated biphenyl mixtures and congeners: nonadditive (antagonistic) interactions. *Fundam Appl Toxicol* 1995;27:131–139.
186. Soderberg LS, Barnett JB. Possible mechanisms of immunotoxicity following in vivo exposure to the inhalant, isobutyl nitrite. *Adv Exp Med Biol* 1995;373:189–192.
187. Chiappelli F, Kung MA, Villanueva P, Lee P, Frost P, Prieto N. Immunotoxicity of cocaethylene. *Immunopharmacol Immunotoxicol* 1995;17:399–417.
188. Zelikoff JT, Bowser D, Squibb KS, Frenkel K. Immunotoxicity of low level cadmium exposure in fish: an alternative animal model for immunotoxicological studies. *J Toxicol Environ Health* 1995;45:235–248.
189. Schlumpf M, Parmar R, Butikofer EE, et al. Delayed developmental neuro- and immunotoxicity of benzodiazepines. *Arch Toxicol Suppl* 1995;17:261–287.
190. Zheng YT, Zhang WF, Ben KL, Wang JH. In vitro immunotoxicity and cytotoxicity of trichosanthin against human normal immunocytes and leukemia-lymphoma cells. *Immunopharmacol Immunotoxicol* 1995;17:69–79.
191. Rice CD, Banes MM, Ardelt TC. Immunotoxicity in channel catfish, *Ictalurus punctatus*, following acute exposure to tributyltin. *Arch Environ Contam Toxicol* 1995;28:464–470.
192. Williams WC, Riddle MM, Copeland CB, Andrews DL, Smialowicz RJ. Immunological effects of 2-methoxyethanol administered dermally or orally to Fischer 344 rats. *Toxicology* 1995;98:215–223.
193. van Loveren H, Steerenberg PA, Vos JG. Early detection of immunotoxicity: from animal studies to human biomonitoring. *Toxicol Lett* 1995;77:73–80.
194. McKallip RJ, Nagarkatti M, Nagarkatti PS. Immunotoxicity of AZT: inhibitory effect on thymocyte differentiation and peripheral T cell responsiveness to gp120 of human immunodeficiency virus. *Toxicol Appl Pharmacol* 1995;131:53–62.
195. Narasimhan TR, Craig A, Arellano L, et al. Relative sensitivities of 2,3,7,8-tetrachlorodibenzo-*p*-dioxin-induced Cyp1a-1 and Cyp1a-2 gene expression and immunotoxicity in female B6C3F1 mice. *Fundam Appl Toxicol* 1994;23:598–607.
196. van Loveren H, Gianotten N, Hendriksen CF, Schuurman HJ, van der Laan JW. Assessment of immunotoxicity of buprenorphine. *Lab Anim* 1994;28:355–363.
197. Neubert R, Golor G, Helge H, Neubert D. Risk assessment for possible effects of 2,3,7,8-tetrachlorodibenzo-*p*-dioxin (TCDD) and related substances on components and functions of the immune system. *Exp Clin Immunogenet* 1994;11:163–171.
198. Tryphonas H. Immunotoxicity of polychlorinated biphenyls: present status and future considerations. *Exp Clin Immunogenet* 1994;11:149–162.
199. Rice CD, Merchant RE, Jeong TC, Karras JB, Holsapple MP. The effects of acute exposure to 2,3,7,8-tetrachlorodibenzo-*p*-dioxin on glioma-specific cytotoxic T-cell activity in Fischer 344 rats. *Toxicology* 1995;95:177–185.
200. Burns LA, Bradley SG, White KL, et al. Immunotoxicity of 2,4-diaminotoluene in female B6C3F1 mice. *Drug Chem Toxicol* 1994;17:401–436.
201. Burns LA, White KL, Jr., McCay JA, et al. Immunotoxicity of mono-nitrotoluenes in female B6C3F1 mice: II. Meta-nitrotoluene. *Drug Chem Toxicol* 1994;17:359–399.
202. Burns LA, Bradley SG, White KL Jr, et al. Immunotoxicity of nitrobenzene in female B6C3F1 mice. *Drug Chem Toxicol* 1994;17:271–315.
203. Bradley SG, White KL Jr, McCay JA, et al. Immunotoxicity of 180 day exposure to polydimethylsiloxane (silicone) fluid, gel and elastomer and polyurethane disks in female B6C3F1 mice. *Drug Chem Toxicol* 1994;17:221–269.
204. Yoshida SH, Teuber SS, German JB, Gershwin ME. Immunotoxicity of silicone: implications of oxidant balance towards adjuvant activity. *Food Chem Toxicol* 1994;32:1089–1100.
205. Davis DA, Archuleta MM, Born JL, Knize MG, Felton JS, Burchiel SW. Inhibition of humoral immunity and mitogen responsiveness of lymphoid cells following oral administration of the heterocyclic food mutagen 2-amino-1-methyl-6-phenylimidazo[4,5-b]pyridine (PhIP) to B6C3F1 mice. *Fundam Appl Toxicol* 1994;23:81–86.
206. Zelikoff JT, Sisco MP, Yang Z, Cohen MD, Schlesinger RB. Immunotoxicity of sulfuric acid aerosol: effects on pulmonary macrophage effector and functional activities critical for maintaining host resistance against infectious diseases. *Toxicology* 1994;92:269–286.
207. Messiha FS. Developmental toxicity of cesium in the mouse. *Gen Pharmacol* 1994;25:395–400.
208. Houben GF, Penninks AH. Immunotoxicity of the colour additive caramel colour III; a review on complicated issues in the safety evaluation of a food additive. *Toxicology* 1994;91:289–302.
209. Cohen MD, Yang Z, Zelikoff JT. Immunotoxicity of particulate lead: in vitro exposure alters pulmonary macrophage tumor necrosis factor production and activity. *J Toxicol Environ Health* 1994;42:377–392.
210. Gaworski CL, Vollmuth TA, Dozier MM, Heck JD, Dunn LT, Ratajczak HV, Thomas PT. An immunotoxicity assessment of food flavouring ingredients. *Food Chem Toxicol* 1994;32:409–415.
211. Basketter DA, Bremmer JN, Kammuller ME, et al. The identification of chemicals with sensitizing or immunosuppressive properties in routine toxicology. *Food Chem Toxicol* 1994;32:289–296.
212. Zelikoff JT, Smialowicz R, Bigazzi PE, Goyer RA, Lawrence DA, Maibach HI, Gardner D. Immunomodulation by metals. *Fundam Appl Toxicol* 1994;22:1–7.
213. Soderberg LS, Barnett JB. Inhaled isobutyl nitrite compromises T-dependent, but not T-independent, antibody induction. *Int J Immunopharmacol* 1993;15:821–827.
214. Arnold DL, Bryce F, Karpinski K, et al. Toxicological consequences of Aroclor 1254 ingestion by female rhesus (*Macaca mulatta*) monkeys. Part 1B. Prebreeding phase: clinical and analytical laboratory findings. *Food Chem Toxicol* 1993;31:811–824.
215. De Krey GK, Baecher-Steppan L, Deyo JA, Smith B, Kerkvliet NI. Polychlorinated biphenyl-induced immune suppression: castration, but not adrenalectomy or RU 38486 treatment, partially restores the suppressed cytotoxic T lymphocyte response to alloantigen. *J Pharmacol Exp Ther* 1993;267:308–315.
216. Furuhama K, Benson RW, Knowles BJ, Roberts DW. Immunotoxicity of cephalosporins in mice. *Chemotherapy* 1993;39:278–285.
217. Kaminski NE, Stevens WD. The role of metabolism in carbon tetrachloride-mediated immunosuppression. In vitro studies. *Toxicology* 1992;75:175–188.
218. Harvey RB, Elissalde MH, Kubena LF, Weaver EA, Corrier DE, Clement BA. Immunotoxicity of ochratoxin A to growing gilts. *Am J Vet Res* 1992;53:1966–1970.
219. Hajoui O, Flipo D, Mansour S, Fournier M, Krzystyniak K. Immunotoxicity of subchronic versus chronic exposure to aldicarb in mice. *Int J Immunopharmacol* 1992;14:1203–1211.
220. Barnett JB, Gandy J, Wilbourn D, Theus SA. Comparison of the immunotoxicity of propanil and its metabolite, 3,4-dichloroaniline, in C57Bl/6 mice. *Fundam Appl Toxicol* 1992;18:628–631.
221. Shenker BJ, Rooney C, Vitale L, Shapiro IM. Immunotoxic effects of mercuric compounds on human lymphocytes and monocytes. I. Suppression of T-cell activation. *Immunopharmacol Immunotoxicol* 1992;14:539–553.
222. Oyama Y, Chikahisa L, Tomiyoshi F, Hayashi H. Cytotoxic action of triphenyltin on mouse thymocytes: a flow-cytometric study using fluorescent dyes for membrane potential and intracellular Ca^{2+}. *Jpn J Pharmacol* 1991;57:419–424.
223. Hatori Y, Sharma RP, Warren RP. Resistance of C57Bl/6 mice to immunosuppressive effects of aflatoxin B1 and relationship with neuroendocrine mechanisms. *Immunopharmacology* 1991;22:127–136.
224. Davis D, Safe S. Halogenated aryl hydrocarbon-induced suppression of the in vitro plaque-forming cell response to sheep red blood cells is not dependent on the Ah receptor. *Immunopharmacology* 1991;21:183–190.
225. Smialowicz RJ, Simmons JE, Luebke RW, Allis JW. Immunotoxicologic assessment of subacute exposure of rats to carbon tetrachloride with comparison to hepatotoxicity and nephrotoxicity. *Fundam Appl Toxicol* 1991;17:186–196.
226. Nair BS, Erickson JR, Pillai R, Estrada A, Watson RR. Immunotoxicity of poly-drug use: abnormalities in the active and high-affinity CD2 antigen (E-rosette receptor) bearing T-lymphocytes. *Toxicol Lett* 1991;57:339–345.
227. Smialowicz RJ, Riddle MM, Luebke RW, et al. Immunotoxicity of 2-methoxyethanol following oral administration in Fischer 344 rats. *Toxicol Appl Pharmacol* 1991;109:494–506.
228. Blank JA, Joiner RL, Houchens DP, Dill GS, Hobson DW. Comparative immunotoxicity of 2,2′-dichlorodiethyl sulfide and cyclophosphamide:

evaluation of L1210 tumor cell resistance, cell-mediated immunity, and humoral immunity. *Int J Immunopharmacol* 1991;13:251–257.
229. Fan A, Howd R, Davis B. Risk assessment of environmental chemicals. *Annu Rev Pharmacol Toxicol* 1995;35:341–368.
230. Fielder RJ. Risk assessment of chemicals: general principles (and how these relate to immunotoxicity). *Hum Exp Toxicol* 1995;14:150.
231. Faustman E, Omenn G. Risk assessment. In: Klassen C, ed. *Toxicology—the basic science of poisons*, 5th ed. New York: McGraw-Hill, 1995:75–88.
232. National Research Council (US) Committee on the Institutional Means for Risk Assessment in the Federal Government. Managing the process. Washington: National Academy Press, 1983.
233. Luster M, Portier C, Pait D, Rosenthal G, Germolec D. Immunotoxicology and risk assessment. In: Burleson G, Dean J, Munson A, eds. *Methods in immunotoxicology.* New York: Wiley-Liss, 1996:51–68.
234. Osmond D. The ontogeny and organization of the lymphoid system. *J Invest Dermatol* 1985;85:2s–9s.
235. Holladay S, Luster M. Developmental immunotoxicity. In: Kimmel C, Buelke-Sam J, eds. *Developmental toxicity,* 2nd ed. New York: Raven, 1994:93–118.
236. Holladay S, Smith B. Fetal hematopoietic alterations after maternal exposure to benzo[a]pyrene: a cytometric evaluation. *J Toxicol Environ Health* 1994;42:259–273.
237. Holladay S, Luster M. Alterations in fetal thymic and liver hematopoietic cells as indicators of exposure to developmental immunotoxicants. *Environ Health Perspect* 1996;104:809–813.
238. Walker S, Keisler L, Caldwell C, Kier A, vom Saal F. Effects of altered prenatal hormonal environment on expression of autoimmune disease in nzb/nzw mice. *Environ Health Perspect* 1996;104:815–821.
239. Kafafi S, et al. Environmental binding of polychlorinated biphenyls to the arylhydrocarbon receptor. *Environ Health Perspect* 1993;101:422–428.
240. Ganey P, Sirois JE, Denison M, Robinson JP, Roth RA. Neutrophil function after exposure to polychlorinated biphenyls in vitro. *Environ Health Perspect* 1993;101:430–434.
241. Burrell R. Immunotoxic reactions in the agricultural environment. *Ann Agric Environ Med* 1995;2:11–20.
242. Bekesi JG, Holland JF, Anderson HA, et al. Lymphocyte function of Michigan dairy farmers exposed to polybrominated biphenyl. *Science* 1978;199:1207–1209.
243. Descotes J. Biphenyls: 1. Polybrominated biphenyls. In: Descotes J, ed. *Immunotoxicology of drugs and chemicals.* Amsterdam: Elsevier Science, 1986:342.
244. Lu YC, Wu YC. Clinical findings and immunologic abnormalities in Yu-Cheng patients. *Environ Health Perspect* 1985;59:17–29.
245. Emmett EA, Maroni M, Schmith JM, Levin BK, Jefferys J. Studies of transformer repair workers exposed to PCBs: I. Study design, PCB concentrations, questionnaire, and clinical examination results. *Am J Ind Med* 1988;13:415–427.
246. Evans RG, Webb KB, Knutsen AP, et al. A medical follow-up of the health effects of long-term exposure to 2,3,7,8-tetrachlorodibenzeno-*p*-dioxin. *Arch Environ Health* 1988;43:273–278.
247. Stehr-Green PA, Burse VW, Welty E. Human exposure to polychlorinated biphenyls at toxic waste sites: investigations in the United States. *Arch Environ Health* 1988;43:420–424.
248. Brown DP. Mortality of workers exposed to polychlorinated biphenyls—an update. *Arch Environ Health* 1987;42:333–339.
249. Kimbrough RD. Human health effects of polychlorinated biphenyls (PCBs) and polybrominated biphenyls (PBBs). *Annu Rev Pharmacol Toxicol* 1987;27:87–111.
250. Hoffman RE, Stehr-Green PA, Webb KB, et al. Health effects of long-term exposure to 2,3,7,8-tetrachlorodibenzeno-*p*-dioxin. *JAMA* 1986;255:2031–2038.
251. Webb K, Evans RK, Stehr P, Ayres SM. Pilot study on health effects of environmental 2,3,7,8-TCDD in Missouri. *Am J Ind Med* 1987;11:685–691.
252. Mocarelli P, Marocchi A, Brambilla P, Gerthoux P, Young DS, Mantel N. Clinical laboratory manifestations of exposure to dioxin in children. A six-year study of the effects of an environmental disaster near Seveso, Italy. *JAMA* 1986;256:2687–2695.
253. Koller LD. Review/commentary: immunotoxicology of heavy metals. *Int J Immunopharmacol* 1980;2:269–279.
254. Koller LD. Effects of environmental contaminants on the immune system. *Adv Vet Sci Comp Med* 1979;23:267–295.
255. Druet P, Bernard A, Hirsch F, et al. Immunologically mediated glormerulonephritis induced by heavy metals. *Arch Toxicol* 1982;50:187–194.
256. Koller LD, Exon JH, Roan JG. Antibody suppression by cadmium. *Arch Environ Health* 1975;30:598–601.
257. Reigart JR, Graber CD. Evaluation of the humoral immune response of children with low level lead exposure. *Bull Environ Contam Toxicol* 1976;16:112–117.
258. Sachs HK. Intercurrent infection in lead poisoning. *Am J Dis Child* 1978;132:315–316.
259. Smith TJ, Blough S. Chromium, manganese, nickel, and other elements. In: Rom WN, ed. *Environmental and occupational medicine.* Boston: Little, Brown and Co, 1983:491–510.
260. Enterline PE, March GM. Cancer among workers exposed to arsenic and other substances in a copper smelter. *Am J Epidemiol* 1982;116:895–911.
261. Pershagen G. Lung cancer mortality among men living near an arsenic-emitting smelter. *Am J Epidemiol* 1985;122:684–694.
262. Eisenbud M. Carcinogenicity and allergenicity. *Science* 1987:1613.
263. Fischbein A, Tsang P, Luo J, Bekesi J. The immune system is target for subclinical lead-related toxicity. *Br J Ind Med* 1993;50:185–186.
264. Shenker B, Rooney C, Vitale L. Immunotoxic effects of mercuric compounds on human lymphocytes and monocytes—suppression of T-cell activation. *Immunopharmacol Immunotoxicol* 1992;14:539–553.
265. Wagnerova M, Wagner V, Madlo Z, et al. Seasonal variations in the level of immunoglobulins and serum proteins of children differing by exposure to airborne lead. *J Hyg Epidemiol Microbiol Immunonol* 1986;30:127–138.
266. McCabe M. Mechanisms and consequences of immunomodulation by lead. In: Dean J, Lester M, Munson A, Kimber I, eds. *Immunotoxicology and immunopharmacology,* 2nd ed. New York: Raven Press, 1994.
267. Vorella P, Giardino A. Lead and cadmium at very low doses affects in vitro immune responses of human leukocytes. *Environ Res* 1991;55:165–177.
268. Lee TP, Moscati R, Parks BH. Effects of pesticides on human leukocyte functions. *Res Commun Chem Pathol Pharmacol* 1979;23:597–609.
269. Roux F, Treich I, Brun C, Desoize B, Fournier E. Effect of lindane on human lymphocyte responses to phytohemagglutinin. *Biochem Pharmacol* 1979;28:2419–2426.
270. Descotes J. Biphenyls: 1. Polybrominated biphenyls. In: Descotes J, ed. *Immunotoxicology of drugs and chemicals.* Amsterdam: Elsevier Science, 1986:314–332.
271. Hermanowicz A, Nawarska Z, Borys D. The neutrophil function and infectious disease in workers occupationally exposed to organochlorine insecticides. *Int Arch Occup Environ Health* 1982;50:329.
272. Costa M, Schvartsman S. Antibody titers and blood levels of DDT after diphtheric immunization in children. *Acta Pharm Toxicol* 1977;41:249.
273. Colosio C, Maroni M, Barcellini W, et al. Toxicological and immune findings in workers exposed to pentachlorophenol (PCP). *Arch Environ Health* 1993;48:81–88.
274. Thrasher J, Madison R, Broughton A. Immunologic abnormalities in humans exposed to chloropyrofos: preliminary observations. *Arch Environ Health* 1993;48:89–93.
275. Barnett J, Rodgers K. Pesticides. In: Dean J, Luster M, Munson A, Kimber I, eds. *Immunotoxicology and immunopharmacology,* 2nd ed. New York: Raven Press, 1994.
276. McConnachie P, Zahalsky A. Immune alterations in humans exposed to the termidicide technical chlordane. *Arch Environ Health* 1992;47:295–301.
277. Doll NJ, Stankus RP, Highes J, et al. Immune complexes and autoantibodies in silicosis. *J Allergy Clin Immunol* 1981;68:281–285.
278. Kubota M, Kagamimori S, Yokoyama K, Okada A. Reduced killer cell activity of lymphocytes from patients with asbestosis. *Br J Ind Med* 1985;42:276–280.
279. Barbers RG, Oishi J. Effects of in vitro asbestos exposure on natural killer and antibody-dependent cellular cytotoxicity. *Environ Res* 1987;43:217–226.
280. Grammer LC. Occupational immunologic lung disease. In: Patterson R, ed. *Allergic diseases diagnosis and management.* Philadelphia: JB Lippincott Co, 1985:691–708.
281. Berstein D. Occupational asthma. *Clin Allergy* 1992;76:917–934.
282. Sheppard D, Thompson J, Scypinski L, et al. Toluene diisocyanate increases airway responsiveness to substance P and decreases airway neutral endopeptidase. *J Clin Invest* 1988;81:1111–1115.
283. Chan-Yeung M. Immunologic and nonimmunologic mechanisms in asthma due to western red cedar. *J Allergy Clin Immunol* 1982;70:32–37.
284. Bernstein J, Bernstein L. Clinical aspects of respiratory hypersensitivity to chemicals. In: Dean J, Luster M, Munson A, Kimber I, eds. *Immunotoxicology and immunopharmacology,* 2nd ed. New York: Raven Press, 1994.
285. Zeiss C, Wolkonsky P, Pruzansky J, Patterson R. Clinical and immunologic evaluation of trimellitic anhydride workers in multiple industrial settings. *J Allergy Clin Immunol* 1982;70:15–18.
286. Essen S, Robins R, Thompson A, Rennard S. Organic dust toxic syndrome: an acute febrile reaction to organic dust exposure distinct from hypersensitivity pneumonitis. *Clin Toxicol* 1990;28:389–420.
287. LaMarte FP, Merchant JA, Casale TB. Acute systemic reactions to carbonless paper associated with histamine release. *JAMA* 1988;260:242–243.
288. Gardner DE. Alterations in macrophage functions by environmental chemicals. *Environ Health Perspect* 1984;55:343–358.
289. Descotes J. *Immunotoxicology of drugs and chemicals.* Amsterdam: Elsevier Science, 1986:359–362.
290. Selgrade M, Gilmour M. In: Dean J, Luster M, Munson A, Kimber I, eds. *Immunotoxicology and immunopharmacology,* 2nd ed. New York: Raven Press, 1994.
291. Samet J, Lambert W, Skipper B, et al. Nitrogen dioxide and respiratory illness in infants. *Am Rev Respir Dis* 1993;148:1258–1265.
292. Speizer F, Ferris B, Bishop Y, et al. Respiratory disease rates and pulmonary function in children associated with NO_2 exposure. *Am Rev Respir Dis* 1980;121:3–10.
293. Neas L, Dockery D, Ware J, et al. Association of indoor nitrogen dioxide with respiratory symptoms and pulmonary function in children. *Am J Epidemiol* 1991;134:204–218.
294. Schwartz J, Spix C, Wichmann H, Malin E. Air pollution and acute respiratory illness in five German communities. *Environ Res* 1991;56:1–14.
295. Schwartz J. Air pollution and the duration of acute respiratory symptoms. *Arch Environ Health* 1992;47:116–122.
296. Devlin R, McDonnell R, Mann R, et al. Exposure of humans to ambient levels of ozone for 6.6 hours causes cellular and biochemical changes in the lung. *Am J Respir Cell Mol Biol* 1991;4:72–81.

297. Suzuki T, Akita S, Kanoh T, et al. Decreased phagocytosis and superoxide anion production in alveolar macrophages of rats exposed to nitrogen dioxide. *Arch Environ Contam Toxicol* 1986;15:733–739.
298. Hoof T, Man R, Kuper C, Appelman L. Comparitive sensitivity of histopathology and specific lung parameters in the detection of lung injury. *J Appl Toxicol* 1988;8:59–65.
299. Devlin R, Horstman D, Becker S. Inflammatory response in humans exposed to 2.0 ppm NO_2. *Am Rev Respir Dis* 1992;145:A456.
300. Gilmour M, Park P, Doefler D, Selgrade M. Factors which influence the suppression of pulmonary antibacterial defenses in mice exposed to ozone. *Exp Lung Res* 1993;19:299–314.
301. Zoratti E, Busse W. The role of respiratory infections in airway responsiveness and the pathogenesis of asthma. *Immunol Allergy Clin North Am* 1990;10:449–461.
302. Molfino N, Wright S, Katz I, et al. Effects of low concentrations of ozone on inhaled allergen responses in asthmatic subjects. *Lancet* 1991;338:199–203.
303. Sopori M, Goud N, Kaplan A. Effects of tobacco smoke on the immune system. In: Dean J, Luster M, Munson A, Kimber I, eds. *Immunotoxicology and immunopharmacology,* 2nd ed. New York: Raven Press, 1994.
304. Stedman R. The chemical composition of tobacco and tobacco smoke. *Chem Rev* 1968;68:153–207.
305. Hoidal J, Fox R, LeMarbe P, et al. Altered oxidated metabolic responses in vitro of alveolar macrophages from asymptomatic cigarette smokers. *Am Rev Respir Dis* 1981;23:85–87.
306. Hughes D, Haslam P, Townsend P, et al. Numerical and functional alteration in circulatory lymphocytes in cigarette smokers. *Clin Exper Immunol* 1985;61:459–466.
307. Condemi JJ. The autoimmune diseases. *JAMA* 1987;258:2920–2929.
308. DeShazo RD, Lopez M, Salvaggio JE. Use and interpretation of diagnostic immunologic laboratory tests. *JAMA* 1987;258:3011–3031.
309. Rosenfeld SI. Interpretation of complement and immune complex assays. In: Grieco MH, Meriny DK, eds. *Immunodiagnosis for clinicians: interpretation of immunoassays*. Chicago: Year Book Medical Publishers, 1983:161–187.
310. Katz P. Clinical and laboratory evaluation of the immune system. *Med Clin North Am* 1985;69:453–464.
311. Gleich GG, Adolphson CR. The eosinophilic leukocyte structure and function. *Adv Immunol* 1986;39:137–253.
312. Straetmans N, Ferrant A, Martiat P, Sokai G, Michaux JL. Hypereosinophilia syndrome: apropos of 2 cases and literature review. *Acta Belgica* 1992;47:90–99.
313. Lieberman P. Anaphylactoid reactions to radiocontrast material. *Clin Rev Allergy* 1991;9:319–338.
314. Nadel JA. Neutral endopeptidase modulates neurogenic inflammation. *Eur Respir J* 1991;4:745–754.
315. Nielsen GD: Mechanisms of activation of the sensory irritant receptor by airborne chemicals. *Crit Rev Toxicol* 1991;21:183–208.
316. Danuser B, Weber A, Hartmann AL, et al. Effects of bronchoprovocation challenge test with cigarette sidestream smoke on sensitive and healthy adults. *Chest* 1993;103:353–358.
317. Willes SR, Fitzgerald TK, Bascom R. Nasal inhalation challenge studies with sidestream tobacco smoke. *Arch Environ Health* 1992;47:223–230.
318. Shim C, Williams MH Jr. Effect of odors in asthma. *Am J Med* 1986;80:18–22.
319. Church MK, el-Lati S, Caulfield JP. Neuropeptide-induced secretion from human skin mast cells. *Int Arch Allergy Appl Immunol* 1991;94:310.
320. Cavagnaro J, Lewis RM. Bidirectional regulatory circuit between the immune and neuroendocrine systems. *Year Immunol* 1989;4:241–252.
321. Meggs WJ. Neurogenic switching: a hypothesis for a mechanism for shifting the site of inflammation in allergy and chemical sensitivity. *Environ Health Perspect* 1995;103:54–56.
322. Leslie CA, Mathe AA. Modification of guinea pig lung anaphylaxis by central nervous system (CNS) pertubations. *J Allergy Clin Immunol* 1989;83:94–101.
323. Levy RM, Rose JE, Johnson JS. Effect of vagotomy on anaphylaxis in rat. *Clin Exp Immunol* 1976;24:96–101.
324. Evans R, Mullaly DI, Wilson RW, Gergen PJ. National trends in the morbidity and mortality of asthma in the U.S. *Chest* 1987;91:65S–74S.
325. Weitzman M, Gortmaker SL, Sobol MA, et al. Recent trends in the prevalence and severity of childhood asthma. *JAMA* 1992;268:2673–2677.
326. Gertsman BB, Bosco LA, Tomita DK, et al. Prevalence and treatment of asthma in the Michigan Medicaid patient population younger than 45 years, 1980-1986. *J Allergy Clin Immunol* 1989;83:1032–1039.
327. Yunginger JW, Reed CE, O'Connell EJ, et al. A community-based study of the epidemiology of asthma: incidence rates, 1964–1983. *Am Rev Respir Dis* 1992;146:888–894.
328. Gergen PF, Weiss KB. Changing patterns of asthma hospitalization among children: 1979 to 1987. *JAMA* 1990;264:1688–1692.
329. Weiss KB, Wagener DK. Changing patterns of asthma mortality: identifying target populations at high risk. *JAMA* 1990;264:1683–1687.
330. Aberg N, Hesselmar B, Aberg B, Eriksson B. Increase of asthma, allergic rhinitis and eczema in Swedish schoolchildren between 1979 and 1991. *Clin Exp Allergy* 1995;25:815–819.
331. Ciprandi G, Vizzaccaro A, Cirillo I, et al. Increase of asthma and allergic rhinitis prevalence in young Italian men. *Int Arch Allergy Immunol* 1996;111:278–283.
332. Kava T. Acute respiratory infection, influenza vaccination and airway reactivity in asthma. *Eur J Respir Dis* 1987;150:1–38.
333. Matsumura Y. The effects of ozone, nitrogen dioxide, and sulfur dioxide on the experimentally induced allergic respiratory disorder in guinea pigs. I. The effects of sensitization with albumin through the airway. *Am Rev Respir Dis* 1970;102:430–437.
334. Matsumura Y. The effects of ozone, nitrogen dioxide, and sulfur dioxide on the experimentally induced allergic respiratory disorder in guinea pigs. II. The effects of ozone on the absorption and the retention of antigen in the lung. *Am Rev Respir Dis* 1970;102:438–443.
335. Matsumura Y. The effects of ozone, nitrogen dioxide, and sulfur dioxide on the experimentally induced allergic respiratory disorder in guinea pigs. III. The effect on the recurrence of dyspnea attacks. *Am Rev Respir Dis* 1970;102:444–447.
336. Biagini RE, Moorman WJ, Lewis TR, et al. Ozone enhancement of platinum asthma in a primate model. *Am Rev Respir Dis* 1986;134:719–725.
337. Takenaka H, Zhang K, Diaz-Sanchez D, Tsien A, Saxon A. Enhanced IgE production results from exposure to the aromatic hydrocarbons from diesel exhaust: direct effects on B-cell IgE production. *J Allergy Clin Immunol* 1995;95:103–115.
338. Diaz-Sanchez D, Dotson AR, Takenaka H, Saxon A. Diesel exhaust particdles induce local IgE production in vivo and alter the pattern of IgE messenger RNA isoforms. *J Clin Invest* 1994;94:1417–1425.
339. Diaz-Sanchez D, Tsien A, Casillas A, Dotson AR, Saxon A. Enhanced nasal cytokine production in human beings after in vivo challenge with diesel exhaust particles. *J Allergy Clin Immunol* 1996;98:114–123.
340. Brooks SM, Weiss MA, Bernstein IL. Reactive airways dysfunction syndrome (RADS): persistent asthma syndrome after high level irritant exposure. *Chest* 1985;88:376–384.
341. Rajan KG, Davies BH. Reversible airways obstruction and interstitial pneumonitis due to acetic acid. *Br J Ind Med* 1989;46:67–68.
342. Flury KE, Ames DE, Rodarte JR, et al. Airway obstruction due to inhalation of ammonia. *Mayo Clin Proc* 1983;58:389–393.
343. Gautrin D, Boulet L-P, Boutet M, et al. Is reactive airways dysfunction syndrome a variant of occupational asthma? *J Allergy Clin Immunol* 1994;93:12–22.
344. Deschamps D, Rosenberg N, Soler P, et al. Persistent asthma after accidental exposure to ethylene oxide. *Br J Ind Med* 1992;49:523–525.
345. Charan NB, Myers CG, Lakshminarayan S, et al. Pulmonary injuries associated with acute sulfur dioxide inhalation. *Am Rev Respir Dis* 1979;119:555–560.
346. Kern DG. Outbreak of the reactive airways dysfunction syndrome after a spill of glacial acetic acid. *Am Rev Respir Dis* 1991;144:1058–1064.
347. Luo JC, Nelsen KG, Fischbein A. Persistent reactive airways dysfunction syndrome after exposure to toluene diisocyanate. *Br J Ind Med* 1990;47:239–241.
348. Meggs WJ, Cleveland CH Jr. Rhinolaryngoscopic examination of patients with the multiple chemical sensitivity syndrome. *Arch Environ Health* 1993;48:14–18.
349. Meggs WJ, Elsheik T, Metzger WJ, et al. Nasal pathology and ultrastructure in patients with chronic airway inflammation (RADS and RUDS) following an irritant exposure. *J Toxicol Clin Toxicol* 1996;34:383–396.
350. Meggs WJ. Hypothesis for the induction and propogation of chemical sensitivity based on biopsy studies. *Environ Health Perspect* 1997;105(Suppl 2):473–481.

CHAPTER 26

Clinical Rheumatologic Diseases

Bridget T. Walsh and David E. Yocum

ENVIRONMENTAL FACTORS AND RHEUMATOLOGIC/AUTOIMMUNE DISEASE

The underlying etiology of most autoimmune or connective tissue diseases has been the source of much research and debate. As more and more is known about autoimmune disease, it is clear that genetics and environmental or external factors share in the development of disease, but the exact amount each contributes remains unclear. Immunotoxicologic studies have provided evidence that chronic exposure to certain chemicals can directly affect the immune system *in vitro*: some in an immune-suppressive manner, some in an immune-potentiating manner (1–5). The induction of autoantibodies by acute and chronic exposure to chemicals represents an immune-potentiated effect. Several mechanisms have been proposed for the induction of an autoimmune response by toxic chemical exposures,

tion of an autoimmune response by toxic chemical exposures, including stimulation of T and B lymphocytes, inhibition of T-suppressor cells, chemical cross-reactivity with self-antigens, chemicals forming haptens with serum proteins to form new immunogens, and changes in cytokine production (2,6,7). An autoimmune response in animals, measured by the production of autoantibodies, does not equate with autoimmune disease. Although many chemicals in humans (especially low molecular weight) are known to induce autoantibody production [drugs (8–10), formaldehyde (2,3), pesticides and hydrocarbons (1,2), and some heavy metals (10–12)], the leap from this to actual disease induction is much less substantiated, especially because most autoimmune diseases are difficult to diagnose or trace to specific causes.

Progressive systemic sclerosis (PSS, or scleroderma), Goodpasture's syndrome, and drug-induced lupus are three autoimmune diseases with the clearest associations with certain environmental/chemical factors. Other autoimmune diseases may be triggered by certain chemicals, but there is a paucity of evidence demonstrating clear associations (Table 26-1).

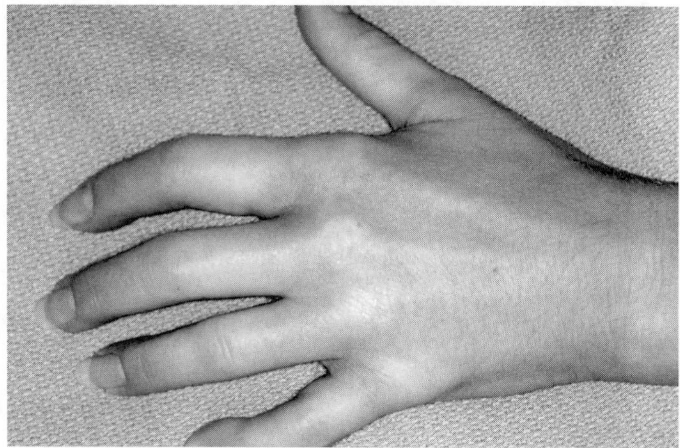

Figure 26-1. Hand of idiopathic scleroderma. (Courtesy of Mike Maricic, M.D.)

Progressive Systemic Sclerosis

PSS, or scleroderma, is an uncommon autoimmune disease affecting multiple organ systems. The prevalence of scleroderma is reported to range between 4 and 290 cases per 1,000,000 individuals in the population (13,14). The characteristic pathologic findings include a predominant mononuclear cell infiltrate in tissues associated with a proliferative vasculopathy (microangiopathic and occlusive microvascular changes), which results in tissue atrophy and fibrosis. Clinical manifestations include cutaneous tissue swelling in the early phases and severe, tight, bound-down skin as the disease progresses (Fig. 26-1). After the skin, the most common systemic-organ problems include gastrointestinal (esophageal dysmotility, reflux, intestinal malabsorption, and colonic wide-mouth diverticula), pulmonary (interstitial lung disease, pulmonary hypertension, and pleural effusions), cardiac (pericardial or vascular proliferation), renal (proliferative vasculopathy resulting in hypertension, proteinuria, and renal failure), and musculoskeletal (acute myositis, chronic myopathy, acroosteolysis, and a seronegative nonerosive polyarthritis and joint contractures) problems. Acroosteolysis (lytic/resorptive changes at the distal phalanges) is fairly distinctive, as seen in Figure 26-2. Raynaud's phenomenon, a vasospastic condition triggered by cold exposure resulting in pain and color changes (paleness, cyanosis, and often erythema on rewarming), is a common syndrome that often predates scleroderma (Fig. 26-3).

TABLE 26-1. Chemicals associated with autoimmune diseases

Hydrocarbons
- Goodpasture's syndrome
- Scleroderma
- ? SLE

Silica/mining
- Scleroderma
- RA

Aromatic amines and hydrazines
- Drug-induced lupus
- ? SLE

Heavy metals
- Glomerulonephritis
- Gout (lead exposure)

Implants
- Bovine collagen
  - Dermatomyositis/polymyositis
- Silicone
  - Fibromyalgia
  - ? Scleroderma, RA, SLE, dermatomyositis, polymyositis
- Paraffin
  - Scleroderma

?, weak association; SLE, systemic lupus erythematosus; RA, rheumatoid arthritis.

Scleroderma has the clearest evidence linking it to occupational and toxic chemical exposures (Table 26-2). The strongest associations include silica exposure and vinyl chloride. Trichloroethylene (TCE), perchloroethylene (PCE), epoxy resins, other organic solvents, and certain drugs have less convincing associations. Denatured rapeseed oil and L-tryptophan have been associated with clear sclerodermalike changes.

Silica/Silicone

Silica exposure has been clearly linked with the development of scleroderma, especially in miners with silica pulmonary disease

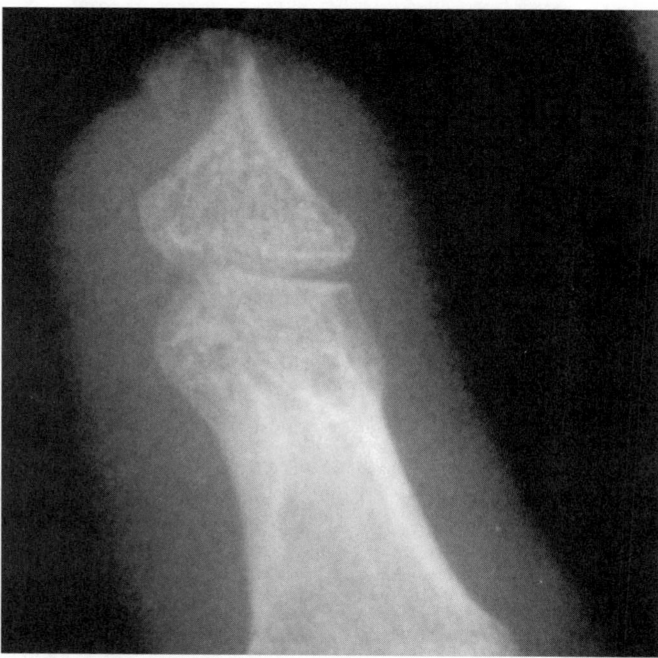

Figure 26-2. Photograph of x-ray showing acroosteolysis. (Courtesy of Mike Maricic, M.D.)

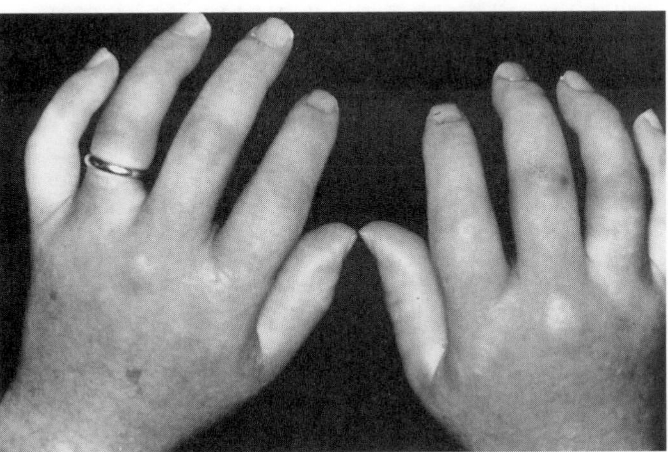

Figure 26-3. Raynaud's phenomenon. (Courtesy of Mike Maricic, M.D.)

(15–19). Erasmus (15) reported on 17 gold miners who developed scleroderma in a population of 40,013 miners. This was almost twice the rate found when they examined those with scleroderma or reviewed medical records of those admitted to a local hospital over a 5-year period (n = 10) with scleroderma out of 50,000 admissions (only one with gold-mining exposure). He noted the high prevalence in men (100%) of miner-associated scleroderma compared with those in the hospital setting without exposure (all women, more consistent with idiopathic PSS). Haustein and Ziegler (16) reported a relative risk of 25 for developing scleroderma after exposure to silica and a relative risk of more than 100 in those who had frank silicosis (a restrictive pulmonary disease associated with silica exposure). One series of 66 males with scleroderma found that almost one-half (26 men) had worked in the coal mines primarily. Of these, 14 reported dyspnea and cough, 8 of whom had radiographic changes of silicosis. Raynaud's phenomenon was seen in 15 of the 26 individuals with silica exposure (17). The study concluded that the clinical presentation of PSS was similar in the environmentally exposed group and the idiopathic scleroderma group. Sanchez-Roman et al. (20) investigated 50 individuals working in a scouring-powder production plant and found 32 individuals (64%) with an autoimmune-related disease or clinical manifestations supporting an autoimmune process: 8 with criteria for systemic lupus erythematosus (SLE) or overlap with scleroderma, 5 with scleroderma, and 6 with Sjögren's syndrome (an autoimmune disease with lymphocytic infiltration in glandular tissue).

TABLE 26-2. Chemical agents associated with scleroderma

Agent	Occupation/ exposure	Strength of association
Silica	Mining: gold, coal	Strong:
Dust	Stone masons	RR = 25 for exposure
Silicone polymers	Scouring powders	RR = 100 for individuals with pulmonary disease
Silicone polymers	Silicone breast implants	Weak: Case reports and case series; case control studies show no increased risk
Chemicals		
Solvents: aromatic hydrocarbons	Toluene, benzene, xylene Mixtures	Moderate to strong association: Case reports, case series
Aliphatic hydrocarbons, chlorinated	(Poly) Vinyl chloride TCE PCE	Case reports/case series and case control studies
Other (plastics, vapors)	Epoxy resins Metaphenylenediamine Naphtha-*n*-hexane Urea formaldehyde	Case reports
Drugs		Mild association:
	Bleomycin	Case reports, small case series
	Carbidopa	
	L-5-hydroxytryptophan	Case report, biological plausibility
	Pentazocine	Case series
	Appetite suppression	Case reports
	Cocaine	Case reports
Miscellaneous		Moderate to strong association:
Toxic oil, Spain	Denatured rapeseed oil	Case reports and case series
L-Tryptophan	1'-ethylidenedis [tryptophan]; weak association	Case control studies

RR, relative risk; TCE, trichloroethylene; PCE, perchloroethylene.

SILICONE BREAST IMPLANTS AND PROGRESSIVE SYSTEMIC SCLEROSIS

Much debate has taken place concerning the role of silicone breast implants as a cause of PSS or other autoimmune diseases. Silicones are a class of polymers built from alternating atoms of silicon and oxygen. They are developed from the quartz rock (silica or SiO_2) (20) and are composed of 25% to 33% silica (21). The most ubiquitous silicone, developed in the 1930s, is polydimethylsiloxane (PDMS), with variable length chains of the Si—O—Si— moiety, in which methyl groups are attached off each side of the Si atom. By varying the length of the number of cross-links between chains, the physical form can be changed (gel, liquid, or solid elastomer), and it can come close to replicating the weight and consistency of human tissue (22). The most widely used application of PDMS is for medical implants, test tube linings, and disposable syringes. It is estimated that insulin-dependent diabetics inject 25,000 to 50,000 microdroplets (25–50 g) of PDMS over a lifetime (21,22).

Although silicone is chemically inert, questions about its biological activity exist. Only a few case reports and small series have linked PSS to the use of silicone, although there have been many animal-study (23) reports of local tissue inflammatory reactions to silicone, including that used for total joint replacements without the development of PSS. Several reports have associated acute pulmonary toxicity with the injection of silicone into breast tissue and thigh tissue of transsexual men (24) without the development of PSS. Numerous published case reports and small case series suggest a relationship of silicone breast implants to connective tissue diseases in general (rheumatoid arthritis [RA], fibromyalgia, undifferentiated connective tissue disease [CTD]) and PSS specifically (25–28). However, more objective, well-conducted population-based studies have not shown a clear relationship and actually suggest a possible protective effect.

Sanchez-Guerrero and colleagues found a total of 293 individuals reporting some type of connective tissue disease related to their silicone gel-filled breast implants (out of the millions of women who have had implants). Thirty-eight of these individuals had definable PSS, although they had more rapid development of disease, including pulmonary manifestations, than idiopathic PSS. The majority of the remaining individuals in their review had vague undefinable musculoskeletal symptoms, and a minority had other connective tissue diseases (21). Hochberg et al. (29) conducted a case-control study of 837 women with scleroderma and

2,507 race-matched female controls and found the adjusted odds ratio associating scleroderma with silicone breast implants to be 1.11 [95% confidence interval (CI), 0.55 to 2.24], suggesting no significant increase in scleroderma in those with implants. In a retrospective population-based medical record review in Olmstead County, Minnesota, Gabriel et al. (30) examined silicone breast implants in 749 cases and 1,498 connective tissue disease controls. None of the cases and one of the controls were identified as having PSS. The overall relative risk of developing a defined connective tissue disease was 1.06 (95% CI, 0.34 to 2.98) (27). Sanchez-Guerrero et al. (31) looked at women followed in the Nurses Health Study (n = 87,501), identifying those with silicone breast implants and those with reported connective tissue diseases. Five hundred sixteen were confirmed as having definite connective tissue disease, and 1,183 as having silicone breast implants of various types. Only three of the silicone breast implant individuals had a definable connective tissue disease (RA). No silicone breast implant individuals were found to have PSS. They concluded that the age-adjusted relative risk of having a definable connective tissue disease in women with silicone breast implants is 0.6 (95% CI, 0.2 to 2.0), suggesting a protective effect.

SILICONE BREAST IMPLANTS AND AUTOIMMUNE RESPONSE

The data do not support silicone breast implantation as a risk of developing scleroderma (as they do inhaled forms of silica) or any other true autoimmune disease. However, the question of silicone as an immunogenic stimulant remains. Silicone breast implants have been known to leak, and several studies have documented inflammatory reactions with particles of silicone in the surrounding tissues (32) and lymphatics (33). The presence of autoantibodies to BB' polypeptide, which is a rare autoantibody found primarily in connective tissue diseases, has been found in individuals with implanted silicone devices (24). Additionally, specific antibodies to implanted silicone have been documented in some individuals with various types of silicone devices, including silicone breast implants (34). Kossovsky et al. looked at anti–silicone surface-associated antigen antibodies (anti-SSAAs) in individuals with silicone breast implants with rheumatologic-like diseases (n = 310), those with silicone breast implants without rheumatologic diseases (n = 11), and those without silicone breast implants who had rheumatologic disease (n = 88: 50 with RA, 19 with SLE, 19 with PSS). They looked at several surface-silicone antigens [including fibronectin-associated antigen (anti-SSAA [fn]); fibrinogen-associated antigen (anti-SSAA [fbgn]); myelin basic protein (anti-SSAA [my]); and insulin, Collagen I and Collagen III (anti-SSA [in]) (Col1, Col3), respectively] and found higher rates of anti-SSAAs in symptomatic silicone breast implant individuals compared with all other groups ($p < .05$).

Several other autoantibodies have been found in individuals with silicone breast implants (26), suggesting an immunologic response to the silicone implants. Lewy and Ezrailson (35) tested 3,380 individuals with silicone breast implants for antinuclear antibodies, gamma globulins, and other autoantibodies and found 22% with antinuclear antibodies (ANAs) in titers of 1:40 or greater (compared with 5% of the general public when tested). A direct relationship was found between the rate of ANA positivity and the duration of implant, regardless of age. Using historical controls, they calculated a relative risk of 4.4 for having a positive ANA in the presence of silicone breast implants ($p < .001$). Silverman et al. (36) reported on 3,184 individuals with symptomatic silicone breast implants and found 59.6% with ANA titer of 1:40 or greater (using a Hep 2 assay), 35.2% with titer of 1:80 or greater, and 17.6% with a titer of 1:160 or greater. This was comparable to only 3% positive ANA for asymptomatic silicone breast implant individuals (n = 37) and 5% for healthy controls (n = 40). Only fibromyalgia controls had similar autoantibody production (ANA 1:80 or greater, 28%, n = 200). Bridges et al. had similar results (37). Claman and Robertson (38) looked at the rate of positive ANA titers in two groups (above 1:80 in one group and 1:256 in another), both comparing only healthy, asymptomatic individuals who had silicone breast implants to healthy controls. They found a positive ANA in 27% of the asymptomatic silicone breast implants compared with only 3% of the controls. No difference was found when controlling for age or type of implant. No mention was made about the length of time the implant had been in place.

Several other autoantibodies were found, including double-stranded DNA, thyroglobulin, myelin basic protein antibodies, smooth muscle, antiparietal cells, anti–glomerular membrane antibodies, rheumatoid factor, and Sjögren's antibodies (anti-SSA and anti-SSB), the highest titers of which were found in symptomatic silicone breast implant patients (35–37). Low complement levels were found as well (20.4% with a low C3 level and 10.5% with a low C4 level), suggesting some ongoing immune complex process (36).

Interestingly, autoantibodies specific to idiopathic scleroderma [i.e., anti-topoisomerase (SCL70)] have not been found in as many cases of silicone breast implant individuals compared with idiopathic scleroderma (13% compared with 20% to 40%, respectively) (39). Silicone breast implant individuals had more anticentromere antibody than idiopathic scleroderma (40% versus 10%). This antibody is seen more commonly in a related condition called the *CREST syndrome* (calcinosis, Raynaud, esophageal dysmotility, sclerodactyly, and telangiectasia). Bridges et al. (25) demonstrated similar findings.

Although these studies certainly suggest an immunologic reaction to the silicone, considerable controversy remains over whether they truly cause disease. Investigators are looking into the characteristics of silicone in implants to see if differences may be significant. Some data suggest the composition of the silicone implant and the molecular weight of the complex have a lot to do with reactivity (21). Investigating the genetics of those who have developed diseases may also give insight into susceptibility.

Vinyl Chloride

Vinyl chloride (CH_2=CHCl) is a gaseous material used to make the solid plastic material polyvinyl chloride by a process called *polymerization*. The first reported cases of disease related to exposure of vinyl chloride were in 1963 (40), which described Raynaud's phenomenon in 6% of the 168 individuals exposed to vinyl chloride. The study additionally described sclerodermalike skin changes in 3.6% of those examined. Since then, numerous reports have related vinyl chloride exposure to disease. Cordier et al. (41), Harris and Adams (42), and others (43–47) have described the process of acroosteolysis, Raynaud's phenomenon, and sclerodermalike changes in individuals exposed to vinyl chloride; thus came the term *occupational acroosteolysis*. Wilson et al. found 5 of 31 cases of vinyl chloride exposure with acroosteolysis out of 3,000 workers in a vinyl chloride industrial plant (48). An additional 25 cases were reported by Dinman et al. in their review of more than 5,000 workers in plants across the United States and Canada who developed sclerodermalike skin changes, osteolysis, and Raynaud's phenomenon (49). Histologic findings are similar in idiopathic and occupational sclerodermatous diseases. Fewer vascular changes occur with occupational acroosteolysis (43,45,50), although the type of acroosteolysis appears to be different (less distal tuft resorption with vinyl chloride) (50). Table 26-3 outlines differences between idiopathic vinyl chloride–associated and silica-associated scleroderma.

Other manifestations of occupational acroosteolysis syndrome have been described in varying frequency. These include fatigue, a few cases of pulmonary or gastrointestinal involvement, signif-

TABLE 26-3. Occupational scleroderma compared with idiopathic scleroderma

Characteristic	Idiopathic PSS	Occupational acroosteolysis (vinyl chloride)	Silica
Skin changes			
Edematous early	++	++	++
Bound-down late	++++	+++	+++
Histologic changes			No data
Thickened dermis	+++	+++	
Thickened collagen fibers	+++	+++	
Increased fragmented elastic fibers	?	+++	
Nodules	–	++	
Vasculopathy	+++	–	
Lymphocytic infiltration	±	++	
Raynaud's phenomenon	+++	+++	+++
Musculoskeletal:			
Osteolysis	+++	++++ (acroosteolysis)	++
Digital pitting/ulcers	+++	–	+
Joint contractures	++++	++	++
Sacroiliitis	–	++	No data
Arthralgia/arthritis/myalgia	+++	+++	+
Pulmonary involvement	+++	+	++++
Gastrointestinal	+++	+	+
Hepatic	–	+++	No data
Renal	+++	+	+
Serologic			
ANAs	+++	++	+
Antitopoisomerase	+++	No data	No data
Anticentromere	+	No data	No data
Genetic association			
HLA-DR5	++	++	
HLA-DR3	++	+++ (more severe disease)	No data
HLA-B8	++	++ (more severe disease)	

+, present; –, absent; ++ to ++++, increasing positive; ±. equivocal; ?, weak association; ANAs, antinuclear antibodies; HLA, human leukocyte antigen, PSS, progressive systemic sclerosis.

icant hepatic changes, erosive and sclerotic changes in the sacroiliac joint, erosions of the calcaneus, tendon contractures, and thrombocytopenia (44). Interestingly, little involvement of the renal system has been reported with occupational acroosteolysis compared with that typically found with idiopathic PSS.

Evidence suggests that the type of vinyl chloride exposure and the length of exposure influence the development of this disease (48). Dinman et al. noted that all but one of the 25 individuals in their series had been involved in cleaning the vats in which the polymerization process was performed (49). Length of exposure was studied by Lilis et al. (46), who surveyed 267 individuals and examined 87 former workers of a polyvinyl chloride plant. Of these individuals, 83% had 2 or more years of exposure. Besides the significant hepatic effects of chronic exposure (hepatomegaly, esophageal varices, fibrosis of the liver capsule, thrombocytopenia, and hemangiosarcoma) and pulmonary effects noted in a few (fibrotic changes in those inhaling polyvinyl chloride dust and one report of granulomatous reaction), they found classic Raynaud's in 5.6% of the total individuals exposed. Those with exposures of more than 20 years had twice the rate of Raynaud's phenomenon, and 53% of those with abnormal chest radiographs had Raynaud's phenomenon. Pseudoclubbing was noted in 8.7% of the total and in 17.3% of those with more than 20 years of exposure. This persisted even after cessation of exposure. More than 26% of those examined had sclerodermatous changes of the fingers, hands, and forearms, with some cases involving the face. No cases of linear scleroderma were seen. Eight percent of individuals reported pain in the small joints of the fingers, although none had documented synovitis and, as reported, no evidence of sacroiliitis was present (44). Lilis estimated the prevalence of acroosteolysis with vinyl chloride exposure to be approximately 1.7% of workers, certainly a much higher rate than idiopathic PSS (46).

Not all individuals exposed to the chemical develop disease, raising the question of whether other factors (e.g., genetics) may be involved. Black et al. (51,52) investigated the genetic susceptibility to vinyl chloride–induced sclerodermalike syndrome. In one study (51), they found 16 of 44 individuals with vinyl chloride disease to be human leukocyte antigen (HLA)–DR5 positive, compared with only 22 of 148 controls (p <.05). They also determined that the individuals with more severe vinyl chloride disease had higher rates of possessing the HLA-DR3 and B8 alleles (p = .004). They compared the individuals with vinyl chloride disease with 50 individuals with classic idiopathic scleroderma and found similar HLA associations (i.e., DR5, DR3, and B8 were present in both groups). The most significant association was with those individuals with severe vinyl chloride disease. Unfortunately, no significant association of the anti-Scl-70 (topoisomerase) was typically associated with scleroderma, nor the anticentromere antibodies (typically seen with a related syndrome of CREST) in individuals with vinyl chloride disease (51,52).

Because thrombocytopenia had been seen in so many individuals, Ward et al. (53) investigated possible immunologic mechanisms in the pathogenesis of polyvinyl chloride disease by looking at 58 individuals who had worked at a polyvinyl chloride plant and were referred to a local hospital. They divided patients according to the amount of disability that they had and demonstrated circulating immune complexes (by the presence of mixed cryoglobulins, depressed values of C3 and C4), which correlated with the severity of disease. They also showed positive antinuclear antibodies (titers of 1:20 to 1:50), a reduction in T-cell population with a slight increase in B-cell population (most prominent in the most severely affected group), and biopsies of the skin, muscle, lung, and vascular endothelium showing aggregates of immunoglobulin G (IgG), C3, C4, and fibrin deposition.

That the exposure of vinyl chloride, specifically cleaning of the autoclave vats, increases one's risk of developing occupational acroosteolysis (of which scleroderma and Raynaud's phenomenon are prominent features) would appear fairly clear. It may be that the presence of HLA-DL5 increases one's susceptibility to this exposure. Given the presence of thrombocytopenia and immune complex deposition, it is likely that an immunologic process is related to the pathophysiology of this disease.

Organic Solvents

Organic solvents, both aromatic and aliphatic hydrocarbons (especially chlorinated ones), have been implicated as etiologic factors in the development of scleroderma. Walder (54) noted seven individuals with scleroderma, six of whom had contact with various types of organic solvents, including toluene and chemicals used for dry cleaning (benzene or white spirits). Five additional cases of solvent-associated illness were presented in 1981, with the addition of dieselene to the list (55).

Besides the aromatic hydrocarbon solvents, chlorinated hydrocarbons have also been implicated, primarily in case reports and small case series. TCE ($CHCl{=}ClCl_2$) is a degreasing solvent chemically related to vinyl chloride. Exposure to TCE has been associated with fatigue, weakness, irritability, hepatitis, cardiac conduction abnormalities, depression, and neuropathies, depending on the extent and the type of exposure. Additionally, because TCE is in a vaporized form and is often absorbed in the pulmonary vasculature, it can produce pulmonary symptomatology, including pulmonary edema. Several reports of TCE exposure and development of a sclerodermalike illness exist (56–58). Saihan et al. (56) reported the first case of Raynaud's, scleroderma, peripheral neuropathy, and lymphadenopathy in a middle-aged man exposed to TCE while working in the Royal Navy and helicopter factory. Unfortunately, the individual had also been a heavy drinker and had been on allopurinol, so it is difficult to separate which clinical features might be related to the exposure versus his habits.

PCE ($CCl_2=CCl_2$) is a chlorinated solvent, often used in the dry cleaning industry. It is felt to be relatively nontoxic unless associated with chronic exposure, when it can be associated with hepatic toxicity and neurologic effects (59). Sparrow reported on a 19-year-old man who worked in a dry cleaning factory and was exposed to PCE during cleaning of the drums, which contained PCE used for dry cleaning. He was also exposed to fumes. He developed Raynaud's phenomenon, weakness, early scleroderma changes in his hands, serologic evidence of hepatitis, and impotence (59). Laboratory findings showed a very high ANA (1:10,240) and a muscle biopsy demonstrating lymphocytic infiltrate. He did not have acroosteolysis or sacroiliitis, and there is some question of an underlying autoimmune process, because he had a history of alopecia and vitiligo. Sparrow also reviewed nine cases of chronic PCE exposure reported with development of Raynaud's phenomenon, myalgias, hepatotoxicity, and fatigue (59).

Other solvents have also been implicated. Yamakage and Ishikawa reported ten individuals with a localized scleroderma (morphea) and Raynaud's phenomenon who had various exposures to organic solvents, some of which were vapors and some direct contact (the specific solvents were not listed) (60). To determine the causative relationship, they injected solvents into the peritoneum of ddY strains of mice and found sclerotic changes in skin biopsy specimens. This was most pronounced when aliphatic hydrocarbons were injected (60). Czirjak reported on 8 of 21 individuals with PSS who had various chemical exposures, including naphtha, crude solvents, and polyethylene (58), and Owens and Medsger reported on two individuals with PSS exposed to metaphenylenediamine (61). Amines, such as epoxy resins [specifically cyclohexamine (bis[4-amino-3-methyl-cyclohexyl] methane)], have been indicated in the development of scleroderma as well (62).

The possibility that an amine might result in sclerodermatous skin changes has been the source of much interest. Several researchers have investigated skin accumulation of tryptophan-derived biological amines found in scleroderma patients, and Stachow et al. demonstrated the harmful effects these amines have on blood vessels and sympathetic nerve endings, speculating that deficiencies in the oxidation of amines (and tryptophan-derived amines specifically) were the potential etiologic factors (60,63–65). Interestingly, the intermediate products of vinyl chloride are similar to epoxy resins and may tie in the relationship as an etiologic reason for the sclerodermalike changes seen with this agent.

Considerable interest has developed in looking at the association of tryptophan metabolism and the relationship to idiopathic scleroderma and other of the chemical-induced sclerodermalike syndromes. Sternberg and colleagues (66) reported a drug-associated sclerodermalike illness when a patient was treated with L-5 hydroxytryptophan and carbidopa for intention myoclonus. They reported increased levels of kynurenine in the plasma, which remained elevated after the drugs were withdrawn. The levels went even higher on drug rechallenge. They speculated that there was a defect in the enzyme capsule that catabolizes kynurenine. They further investigated 15 patients with idiopathic scleroderma and found seven of them to have elevated levels of plasma kynurenine. They concluded that scleroderma, both idiopathic and sclerodermalike disorders, may be associated with high plasma serotonin levels (the recorded physiologic results of the two drugs, carbidopa and hydroxytryptophan) and elevated plasma levels of kynurenine. These findings are further supported by the discovery of L-tryptophan–induced eosinophilia-myalgia syndrome.

Eosinophilia-Myalgia Syndrome

The eosinophilia-myalgia syndrome was initially identified in the early fall of 1989 in New Mexico and Minnesota, where three patients were reported to have developed eosinophilia with severe myalgia after taking L-tryptophan. By the summer of 1990, more than 1,500 cases had been reported, including 26 deaths (67). The syndrome was characterized by incapacitating muscle aches, eosinophilia with counts higher than 2,000 per μL, fever, weakness, dysesthesias, dyspnea on exertion, arthralgias, rash, and other vaguer symptomatology (68,69). Two case-control studies (70,71) subsequently confirmed an association with L-tryptophan, leading to a ban on sales in the United States. It was determined that in almost all cases, the source of L-tryptophan could be traced to a single Japanese manufacturer (67). The search for the exact chemical contaminate was undertaken. Belongia and colleagues (71) suggested that the contamination came during the fermentation process of *Bacillus amyloliquesaciens* when a different strain was used in the fermentation process, along with a decrease in the amount of powdered carbon in the purification process. The Centers for Disease Control and Prevention also investigated the potential etiologic agent within the L-tryptophan and examined indol-containing compounds, β-carbolines, and vasotracin, all of which have been identified within certain peaks (e.g., peak 97) when high-performance liquid chromatography was used. The changes in the fermentation and purification process appeared to result in a specific new amino acid called *1'-ethylidenedis [tryptophan]*, which is distinct from L-tryptophan. Specifically, this new amino acid duplicates the L-tryptophan moiety in a mirror image and attaches via a carbon chain (67,72).

L-Tryptophan is degraded in the liver and metabolized to serotonin, a neurotransmitter, which has been used to treat sleep disorders and depression (71). Silver et al. (73) have investigated the degradation products of L-tryptophan in the eosinophilia-myalgia syndrome and found increased levels of metabolites, including quinolinic acid and kynurenine. The kynurenine pathway may be involved in a variety of inflammatory triggers, such as IL-2, interferon gamma, and possibly secondary to indoleamine-2,3,-dioxygenase from the macrophage. It has also been speculated that individuals with eosinophilia-myalgia syndrome may have an abnormal production of 3-methylindole or similar toxic substances that may be involved during the breakdown of L-tryptophan in the gut (67). Sternberg and colleagues (66) hypothesized that the sclerodermalike skin changes may result from two factors, one being a defect in an enzyme resulting in elevated kynurenine levels or increased blood serotonin levels. With the association of sclerodermalike skin changes and exposures to L-tryptophan or epoxy resins (a biogenic amine), the possibility of a tie-in relating these disorders to tryptophan, serotonin, and kynurenine metabolic systems needs to be more fully investigated.

Toxic Oil Syndrome

During the early summer of 1981 in the industrial section of Madrid, Spain, an epidemic of fever, acute respiratory distress, abdominal pain, pruritic skin rash, myalgia, hepatosplenomegaly, neurologic abnormalities, cardiac conduction defects, and eosinophilia was reported (74). After intensive searching, the epidemic was traced to the use of rapeseed oil for cooking, which had been denatured with aniline (colorizing agent) and contained acetanilide. It was being sold door to door in Spain with no labeling or safety information. Because the syndrome differed from the typical expected reaction to aniline or acetanilide intoxication, further investigation was undertaken, which revealed an association to oleoanilide, which is formed when a fatty acid reacts with acetanilide (74).

Approximately 20,000 individuals were affected after ingestion of the oil, some with repeated exposure. More than 350 deaths have been reported in association with the ingestion. Some individuals developed a more chronic disease manifested by arthralgias, arthritis, muscle atrophy, sclerodermalike skin changes, and Raynaud's phenomenon (75). The clinical syndrome is similar to scleroderma in the following ways: initial edematous skin with gradual bound-down skin and contractures around the joints, Raynaud's phenomenon, dysphagia, alopecia, hypertension, and sicca symptoms. Alonso-Ruiz et al. (76) also examined laboratory abnormalities in 32 of these individuals noting eosinophilia (600 to 11,102 eos per μL) in 28; elevated lactate dehydrogenase (which persisted for more than 36 months) in 33%; a low-positive ANA (titer, 1:40) in three individuals; and no individuals with rheumatoid factor, abnormal complements, or immunoglobulins. However, no real autoimmune disease was found.

Although the eosinophilia-myalgia syndrome and toxic oil syndrome are clinically similar to idiopathic PSS, they have only a few histologic features that are truly comparable. The most prominent similarity is the perivascular inflammatory response with a resultant microangiopathy. Idiopathic PSS typically has very little inflammatory infiltrates in the tissue, unlike the significant inflammatory cells in both of the other processes. Idiopathic PSS has a significant increase in fine collagen fibrils, followed by atrophic changes with thinning of the dermis and loss of rete pegs and dermal appendages (65,67,77) and very little eosinophilia, unlike eosinophilia-myalgia or toxic oil syndrome.

Drugs Inducing Sclerodermalike Illness

Numerous drugs have been implicated in causing a sclerodermalike illness. Bleomycin has been associated with skin changes but no other manifestation of scleroderma and improves or resolves on discontinuation of the medication (78–80). Injections of pentazocine, a nonnarcotic analgesic agent, were found to cause cutaneous changes consistent with scleroderma in 17 individuals (81). Histologic features were similar to idiopathic PSS, with the exception of panniculitis, fat necrosis, and granulomatous inflammation found in these individuals, not typically seen in scleroderma. Appetite suppressants have also been implicated in several reports (82–84). Methysergide, chemically similar in structure to serotonin, has been reported to cause cardiac and pulmonary fibrosis similar to that seen in PSS without skin manifestations (85).

AUTOIMMUNE GLOMERULONEPHRITIS

Goodpasture's Disease (Antiglomerular Basement Membrane Antibody)

Goodpasture's disease is an autoimmune disease characterized by pulmonary hemorrhage, glomerulonephritis, and autoantibodies to basement membrane of the glomerulus in the kidney and alveoli in the lung [antiglomerular basement antibody (anti-GBM)]. The disease is named after Ernest Goodpasture, who first described the hemoptysis and glomerulonephritis in a young man.

Hydrocarbons have been implicated in many of the cases of Goodpasture's syndrome (86–95), along with pesticides (96) and glue sniffing (97), although the majority of reports are case reports or case series. Sprecace first reported on this relationship in three of six individuals with pulmonary hemorrhage who had a prior exposure to hydrocarbons (86); one had glomerular involvement. Beirne and Brennan (87) reported on five patients with pulmonary hemorrhage and glomerulonephritis and one with nephritis alone, all with anti-GBM antibodies being detected. All had prior exposure to hydrocarbons (two to degreasing solvents, three to paint solvents, one to hair sprays, and one to jet propulsion fuel) (98). Other chemicals have been implicated. D'Apice et al. (94) reported on 18-year-old female twins who developed pulmonary hemorrhage and glomerulonephritis, one after exposure to gasoline and one after exposure to turpentine. Whitworth et al. reported on a 20-year-old woman exposed to dry cleaning solvents who developed pulmonary hemorrhage and glomerulonephritis (93). Bonzel et al. reported on a 16-year-old woman (99), and Rees et al. (100) reported on six individuals, with anti-GBM antibodies detected in the serum who were exposed to glue sniffing, various solvents, or chemical fumes. No data were mentioned regarding pulmonary or renal disease. Bernis et al. (101) reported on a 19-year-old female hairdresser who developed anti-GBM antibody glomerulonephritis. Withdrawal of the permanent wave solution from her job description resulted in remission of the disease. This may support a causative relationship.

Several case-control studies support these observations. Bell et al. did a case-control study of 50 individuals with biopsy-proven proliferative glomerulonephritis and 100 age-, sex-, and social class–matched controls. Significantly more cases were found with "solvent" exposure compared with controls (102). In these studies, they divided exposure into heavy exposure (house painting, industrial spray painting, carpet cleaning, floor covering cleaning, glue sniffing) with moderate exposure (non-occupational household painting) and slight exposure (outdoor painting, handling of petrol fluids, and hobby gluing). In addition, they assigned each exposure an intensity factor and estimated the number of exposure hours, coming up with a solvent exposure score. Cases had averaged 13,186 ± 3,716 solvent exposure score compared with controls of more than 3,030 ± 1,152 solvent exposures ($p < .01$). Ravnskov et al. (98) looked at 50 individuals with biopsy-proven glomerulonephritis and 100 matched controls. Fifty percent of individuals with glomerulonephritis reported solvent exposure compared with only 20% of controls. Daniell et al. (92) reviewed nine case-control studies, specifically looking at the association between solvent exposure and the development of glomerulonephritis. An odds ratio was reported that could be calculated in six of the studies, yielding a 2.8- to 8.9-fold increased risk for developing glomerulonephritis in those exposed to solvents. In several of the studies, there appears to be a dose-response relationship.

This causative relationship of hydrocarbons to the development of anti-GBM antibody disease has been supported *in vitro* using animal studies (87,103–105). Evidence suggests that hydrocarbons damage the basement membrane, thereby damaging the alveoli and glomerular type IV collagen, resulting in exposure of the antigen on the basement membrane (87,90,103). Cigarette smoking has been implicated as a potential etiologic contributor to the development of anti-GBM–mediated pulmonary hemorrhage (106), although the interaction between smoking and hydrocarbons was not specifically investigated. Of 47 patients with glomerulonephritis, 37 were smokers. Ten individuals did not smoke, and only two of those developed pulmonary hemorrhage. It is speculated that smoking also injures the basement membrane collagen, exposing the antigen.

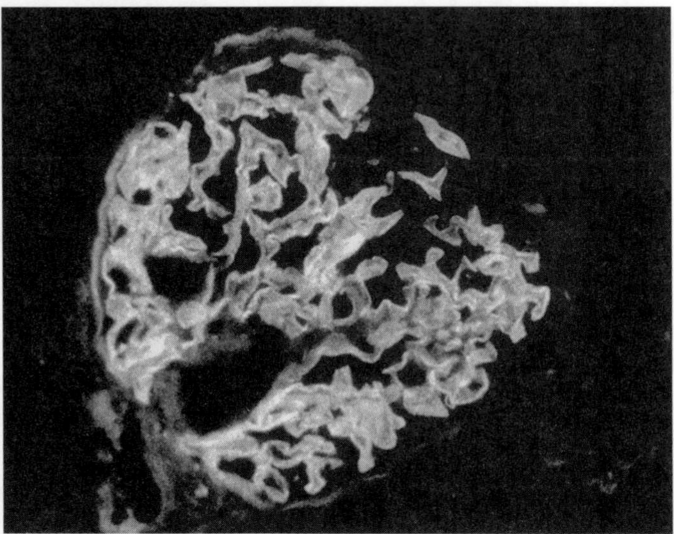

Figure 26-4. Renal biopsy from Goodpasture's syndrome. (Courtesy of Ellinor Angel, M.D.)

At our institution, five patients with Goodpasture's syndrome were hospitalized between 1991 and 1999. Only one mentioned an association with hydrocarbon exposure. He was a 34-year-old man presenting with pulmonary hemorrhage and glomerulonephritis who admitted to significant hydrocarbon exposure (generator exhaust) in his job. His chest radiograph demonstrated bilateral interstitial infiltrates, he had a positive anti-GBM, negative C-ANCA and P-ANCA, and his renal biopsy demonstrated glomerulonephritis with immunofluorescence stain revealing linear deposits of IgG consistent with Goodpasture's syndrome (Fig. 26-4). This patient had a 15 pack-year history of smoking.

Toxin exposure does not explain all cases of Goodpasture's syndrome, and thousands of individuals have been exposed to gasoline fumes and solvents who have not developed disease (only approximately 500 cases of Goodpasture's have been reported), suggesting that a genetic predisposition may contribute to an individual's risk. Rees and colleagues (100) have demonstrated a strong association with HLA-DR2 antigen in people with solvent exposure, which has also been demonstrated by other investigators.

Other Immunologically Mediated Glomerulonephritis Syndromes

Gold salts used for the treatment of RA have been implicated in the development of glomerulonephritis associated with an immune complex deposition process and are thought to be encountered in approximately 1% to 10% of RA patients treated with gold (107). This may in part be related to genetic susceptibility, as noted by Wooley et al. (108), who demonstrated an increased frequency of DRw3 in RA patients developing immune complex glomerulonephritis. Mercury has been implicated as a cause of glomerulonephritis and membranous glomerulopathy in various strains of mice (109), as well as proteinuria and nephrotic syndrome in humans (110). An immune complex–mediated process does appear involved in this; some have demonstrated mineral deposits and granular IgG deposits along various similar structures. D-Penicillamine, a chelating agent used in Wilson's disease and RA, has been shown to cause glomerulonephritis in an immunologically mediated mechanism (110). Cadmium in chronic exposure has also been shown to cause glomerulonephritis (107,111).

Systemic Lupus Erythematosus

SLE is a relatively rare (prevalence rate, 10–50 per 100,000) multisystem disease with an underlying pathogenesis that is related to several immunologic abnormalities (B-cell hyperactivity, autoimmunity with autoantibody production, and defective down-regulation of immune responses) coupled with immune complex deposition and inflammatory reactions leading to tissue damage. The resultant clinical manifestations are often diverse, differing between patients and within a given patient over time. Exacerbations and remissions of SLE are common. Individuals with more mild lupus typically have skin, musculoskeletal, and mucosal abnormalities in addition to constitutional symptoms (fatigue, myalgias, and headaches). More severe involvement occurs in approximately 30% to 40%, including renal disease, pleuritic and pericardial disease, hematologic abnormalities, and neurologic involvement. Fortunately, with the availability of corticosteroids and cytotoxics, individuals with severe disease can now be controlled so that the 5-year mortality is well above 90%.

Epidemiologic studies suggest that prevalence rates differ depending on sex (preponderance of 10:1 in women to men) (112), ethnicity (African-American women with rates above 200 per 100,000, and both female and male Hispanics with 94 per 100,000) (113–115), and genetic factors (C4 null allele and 21-hydroxylase allele) (116,117). External factors, such as infection, sunlight, and even dietary factors (e.g., the amino acid L-canavanine, found in alfalfa sprouts), have been associated with lupus-like symptoms in monkeys (112,118–122) and flares of human SLE (120). Chemical factors are suggested as a stimulus for the development of this autoimmune disease; however, investigations have failed to show conclusively an association. Before reviewing the data suggesting an association between chemicals and SLE, it is useful to look at drug-induced lupus, a related condition that may serve as a comparable model.

Drug-Induced Lupus

Drug-induced lupus (DIL) syndrome comes the closest to supporting an association between chemicals and autoimmune disease. DIL is a disorder that is clinically similar to SLE (skin rashes, musculoskeletal manifestations, serositis, constitutional symptoms, and autoantibody production); however, it is typically not associated with the severe manifestations of renal or central nervous system involvement. Additionally, DIL affects men to the same degree as women and usually resolves on withdrawal of the drug.

DIL was first described in 1945 in a patient on sulfadiazine (123). Since that time, more than 70 medications and drugs have been implicated. Procainamide, hydralazine, various anticonvulsants, psychiatric medications, and antituberculous medication are the most convincingly implicated drugs (124,125) and seem to have the chemical structure related to aromatic amines or substituted hydrazines (126–129). Procainamide is associated with the development of antinuclear antibodies in close to 90% of the individuals, oftentimes without the development of any clinical symptomatology.

The chemical agents associated with DIL are not only found in medications. Hydrazines, for example, are found in pesticides, herbicides, preservatives, plastic products, mushrooms, and tobacco; aromatic amines are found in hair dyes, food dyes, and related products (124,129,130). Permanent hair dyes (especially those that darken hair) contain aromatic amines that can be absorbed through the scalp (125) and have been implicated in the development of lupuslike diseases in animals. Freni-Titulaer et al., for example, looked at 23 individuals with SLE (along with 21 subjects with other connective tissue diseases and 88 age-, sex-,

TABLE 26-4. Definite and probable systemic lupus erythematosus cases

Sex	Age	Diagnosis date[a]	Highest ANA titer[a]	Highest DS DNA titer	Symptom or organ system	Years of residence in Nogales, AZ
Diagnosis: Definite SLE cases (four or more ACR criteria)						
F	36	1990	1:320	1:256	R, S, CNS	16
F	50	12/91	1:1,280	1:800	CNS, P, A, H	47
F	35	1988	1:5,120	1:2,560	M, A	6
F	43	3/89	1:320	0	S, M, P	27
F	37	1987	1:5,120	1:2,390	S, CNS, M, P, A	37
F	43	1990	1:2,560	1:431	P, OU	NA
F	51	1989	1:1,280	157	A, P, S	50
F	47	1985	1:640	Negative	S, M, P, A	31
F	48	1970s	"Strong +"[b]	0	A, S, H, P	31
F	53	1992	1:640	NA	S, H, M	32
F	24	1979	1:40	NA	R, S, M, OU	NA
F	44	1969	1:640	Negative	R, M, P, A	21
F	42	6/94	1:80	Negative	S, M, P, A	8
F	27	1991	1:5,120	1:10	S, M, P, A	NA
F	21	12/89	1:40,960	1:1,280	H, A	13
F	32	4/94	NA	NA	A, R, P, S	NA
F	48	1972	"Strong +"	NA	M, R, A, LE prep	16
F	48	1992	1:160	0	S, M, P, A	41
F	49	1971	1:80	0	S, M, P, A	33
Diagnosis: Probable SLE cases (three SLE criteria)						
F	45	3/94	1:40	NA	OU, P, A	33
F	35	3/94	0	0	S, A, OU	NA
F	46	3/94	1:2,560	1:627	S	28
F	46	1981	1:1,280	1:320	A	14
F	53	3/94	1:160	0	P, A	51
F	71	3/94	1:2,560	0	S, A	30
F	44	4/94	1:20	Negative	S, A, P	NA

A, arthritis; ACR, American College of Rheumatology; ANA, antinuclear antibodies; CNS, central nervous system; DS DNA, double-stranded DNA; F, female; H, hematologic; LE prep, lupus erythematosus prep; M, malar; NA, not available; OU, oral ulcer; P, photosensitivity; R, renal; S, serositis; SLE, systemic lupus erythematosus.
[a]Date of diagnosis and highest ANA based on best medical record documentation.
[b]"Strong +" = indicates quote from medical record.

and race-matched controls). Hair-dye use was the clearest risk factor, with an odds ratio (risk ratio) of 7.1 (95% CI, 1.9 to 26.9) for developing SLE. Using darkening agents raised one's risk more than lightening agents (130). Additionally, Hochberg et al. (131) found prior hair-dye use in 74 patients studied. This association has been called into question by two other investigators: Sanchez-Guerrero and colleagues looked at 106,390 participants in the Nurse's Health Study, ranging in ages from 30 to 55 years (132). They were questioned about such things as disease, medical history, habits, medications, and family history and were studied for more than 10 years. They found that the use of hair dye and SLE had a relative risk of 0.96 (95% CI, 0.63 to 1.47), despite hair-dye use for as many as 15 years. Petri and Allbritton looked at 218 of the lupus cohort patients at Johns Hopkins, compared them with 178 first-degree or second-degree relatives and 186 best friends, and found no difference in the use of hair dyes (133).

The exact reason why certain individuals develop this autoimmune response to medication and others do not has been the topic of much research. Reidenberg and others have hypothesized that such individuals are slow acetylators (134,135); however, this could not be confirmed by Baer et al. (136).

Chemicals in the Development of Systemic Lupus Erythematosus

Aliphatic hydrocarbons have been implicated in the development of autoantibody production and SLE-like symptoms, but convincing evidence as an etiologic agent of SLE is lacking. Kilburn and Warshaw (137) investigated individuals in south Tucson, where TCE—used for cleaning airplanes—allegedly percolated into groundwater supplies and was found in toxic levels in ground wells [ranging from 6 to more than 500 ppb; the Environmental Protection Agency (EPA) accepted level is less than 5 ppb]. They measured ANA production (by fluorescence ANA) and looked for the symptoms of lupus (definite diagnosis being confirmed in 10 cases), using a control population living in Phoenix, outside the contamination area. They found that women in the exposed area were 2.3 times more likely to have positive ANAs (titer 1:80 or higher) and had significantly more lupuslike symptoms than in the control area. No significant difference was evident in men. Although there has been some criticism of the methodology (138), the finding of significantly greater autoantibodies in certain areas of exposure compared with areas without the exposure is certainly disturbing. Criticism of these data has come from individuals who were supported by the industry implicated in the pollution of the groundwater, raising questions of bias.

Broughten and Thrasher (139) have also recorded significantly higher autoantibodies in individuals exposed to TCE compared with controls (91% versus 21%, respectively); after withdrawal of the exposure, the number with positive antibodies decreased to 41%. Unfortunately, no specifics regarding the number of individuals or the type of exposure were included.

We have investigated a reported cluster of SLE along the Mexican-American border in the small town of Nogales, Arizona (population 19,000, 90% Hispanic). Seventy-six individuals and their medical records were examined, and ANA and anti–double-stranded DNA testing was done (113). Nineteen individuals were determined to have definite and seven to have

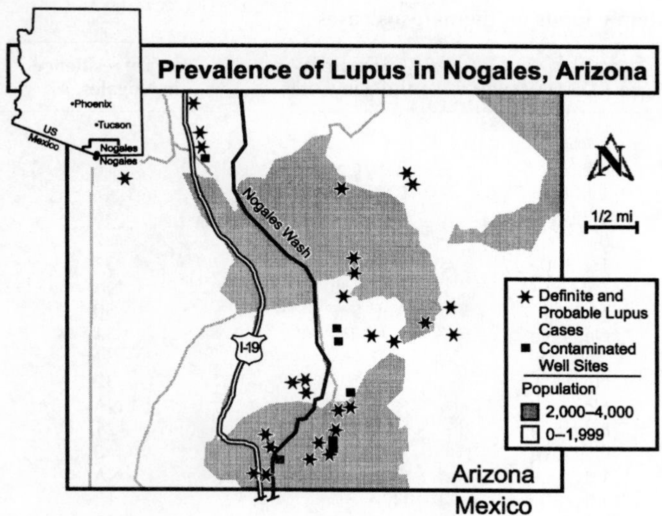

Figure 26-5. Map of Nogales, Arizona, with plotted cases and toxic wells.

probable SLE based on American College of Rheumatology (ACR 1984) criteria. This translated to a prevalence rate of 94 per 100,000, which is significantly higher than the highest rate recorded for the continental United States. Table 26-4 demonstrates the demographic, serologic, and disease manifestations data for this group of individuals. When plotting individual cases on the map of Nogales, it became apparent that the vast majority (more than 80%) lived within 3.5 miles of the Mexican-American border and within 1 mile of either side of the riverbed called the *Nogales Wash* (Fig. 26-5). The significance of this distribution resides in the town's concern for environmental toxins that have been demonstrated in this same area. The Arizona Department of Environmental Quality (ADEQ) has sampled air concentrations of particulate matter measuring 10 µm (PM_{10}) periodically since 1985 and has found that these concentrations violated standards on multiple occasions (140). They revealed chemicals such as chlorinated organic compounds, neoprene, exhaust fumes, and cooking oils in significant quantities (141). Groundwater-quality testing by the Earth Technology Corp. for the ADEQ revealed the presence of several volatile organic compounds (VOCs). TCE, 1,1,1-trichloroethane (1,1,1-TCE), digromochloromethene, tetrachloromethylene, bromoform, chloroform, 1,1-dichloroethane, and *trans*-1-2-dichloroethylene were documented as being above recommended EPA levels in the groundwater and well sampling along the Nogales Wash (ADEQ, 1990) (142).

This clustering of patients in close proximity to areas of environmentally exposed air and water led to a second phase of the investigation. Because all of the cases were Mexican-American, there was a question of whether the excess prevalence rate was more ethnically related or was a true environmentally related process. This phase was a population-based cross-sectional survey using a validated lupus screening questionnaire (143), followed by ANA testing and use of a comparison town, Patagonia, which was out of the air and watershed area of Nogales. Two nested case-control studies were also conducted, using three controls per case; however, the numbers were too small to detect any differences. Nogales was divided into 141 neighborhood blocks, each with 30 to 50 households (a total population of approximately 20,000), and sampling was done randomly. Case families and cases from the initial phase were excluded from this phase. For the purpose of analysis, Nogales was divided into three zones of concern for environmental exposures: low, moderate, and high concern based on communities reporting.

A total of 757 individuals completed the interview process, and 206 individuals gave biological specimens. No differences were evident between Nogales and the control community in terms of reporting lupuslike symptoms. Differences in the level of ANA titers were, however, found between Nogales and the control community, and also within Nogales, stratified on the geographic areas of concern for toxic exposure. ANA titers of 1:160 or higher were seen in areas of moderate to high concern for environmental exposures compared with areas of low concern ($p = .05$) (Table 26-5). Even when controlling for female gender and Hispanic race, this relationship held true with a relative risk of 6 (CI, 0.8 to 47; $p = .05$). The fact that the ANA stratified according to areas of geographic concern rather than being randomly distributed in this town certainly supports evidence from prior investigators suggesting that chemicals can induce autoantibody production. A paucity of evidence exists, however, linking the chemicals to development of actual disease, and there is concern for the subjective way areas of geographic concern for environmental exposure were determined. Whether chemicals just induce the autoantibodies without having specific disease-potentiating effects, whether the autoantibody itself has disease-modifying or inciting capability, or whether the chemical itself can cause the lupuslike illness and the ANA is just a marker remain to be seen.

DERMATOMYOSITIS AND POLYMYOSITIS

Dermatomyositis and polymyositis are uncommon inflammatory myopathic processes with an annual incidence rate of approximately 5.0 to 8.9 per 1,000,000 (144). The underlying etiology of these diseases has been investigated in many series. Only rare reports have been made of chemical exposures being implicated as an etiologic factor in dermatomyositis and polymyositis.

TABLE 26-5. Antinuclear antibody titers of 1:160 or more by community-defined areas of concern score (female respondents)

	Concern for environmental toxicity		Low concern 1		Moderate concern 2		High concern 3	
ANA titer	N	%	N	%	N	%	N	%
Less than 1:160	41	97.6	15	100.0	34	89.5	26	89.7
1:160 or more	1	2.4	0	0.0	4	10.5	3	10.3

ANA, antinuclear antibody titer.
Relative risk: 6.0; confidence interval: 0.8, 47.0; $p = .05$.
From ref. 113, with permission.

Cukier et al. (144) reported on eight patients with dermatomyositis and an additional patient with polymyositis who had received bovine collagen dermal implants in the 1980s and developed the syndrome an average of 6.4 months after the injection. They calculated the standardized incidence ratio of 5.05 (95% CI, 2.31 to 9.59, p <.0001) for dermatomyositis and polymyositis in collagen-treated patients, compared with the general population and a standardized incidence ratio of 18.8 (CI, 8.1 to 37.0, p <.0001) for dermatomyositis specifically. Type I and type III bovine collagen had been used for injection. Other authors have reported dermatomyositis in association with bovine collagen injections and silicone breast implants (145). Castro and Krull (146) reported one patient with dermatomyositis in 7,000 collagen-treated patients on the basis of responses from 316 dermatologists who had used collagen bovine implants. An additional 14 patients had suffered from arthritis and arthralgias. Other scattered reports exist of patients with autoimmune polyarthritis after injection (147). DeLustro and colleagues (148) reported on eight patients that had rheumatologic conditions after bovine injections, including RA (three patients), dermatomyositis (two patients), polymyositis (one patient), and two with other autoimmune diseases (two of the patients reported by DeLustro were included in Cukier's group of patients).

Ciguatera toxin has been implicated in polymyositis in three cases (149,150). All individuals had ingested tropical fish and developed an acute illness manifest with arthralgias, myalgias, pruritus, peripheral neuropathies, abdominal pain, and diarrhea. Polymyositis developed 6 months after exposure in one individual and years later in the other two (6 years and 11 years), raising the question of true association. However, given that dermatomyositis and polymyositis are rare conditions, as is Ciguatera poisoning (annual incidence estimated to be 1 in 2,000 per year) (151), this is a possible association.

RHEUMATOID ARTHRITIS

Rheumatoid arthritis (RA) is a chronic systemic inflammatory disorder characterized by inflammation and erosion involving synovial joints. It is associated with rheumatoid nodules, neuropathies, vasculitis, lymphadenopathy, and splenomegaly, and in the majority of cases, a positive rheumatoid factor. It is seen worldwide and has a prevalence ranging from 0.3% to 1.5% of the population.

RA is actually a New World disease. Archeologic remains of bones with erosive changes similar to what would be expected in RA date back only to the 1700s in Europe, Africa, and the Middle East. Remains of Native Americans in North America, however, found in archeologic digs in northern Alabama, have demonstrated changes consistent with RA dating back thousands of years (152). Given that travel from Europe to the Americas increased in the 17th century, many speculate that an environmental agent had a great deal to do with the development of this disease in Europe at this time. The most likely agents are suspected to be infectious (i.e., viral or bacterial).

Chemical toxins and occupational exposures have been investigated with a suggested link to mining. Klockars et al. (153) demonstrated a relative risk of 5 for granite miners in RA with an increased incidence of RA of 1.7 per 1,000, compared with the expected incidence rate of 0.5 per 1,000. Interestingly, in this series, most of the RA individuals did not have silicosis (153). Sluis-Cremer et al. (154) reported on gold miners with relative risk (odds ratio) of 3.79 (CI, 1.72 to 8.39) for those with silicosis, but not associated with simple dust exposure. Miall et al. (155) reported on an increased rate of RA in coal miners who had massive pulmonary fibrosis. This syndrome, when accompanied by rheumatoid nodules and arthritis, is called *Caplan's syndrome*. Overall, however, coal miners did not have an increased rate of RA compared to nonminers in the same area, making it only speculative that coal mining was the etiologic factor. Silica exposure resulting in silicosis was implicated as an etiologic factor in the increased rate of RA in pyrite miners in Italy; however, as reviewed by Silman and Hochberg, the study had several epidemiologic flaws that make drawing conclusions risky (13).

Other than these instances, in which mining has been associated with increased rates of RA, no other convincing reports show that environmental or occupational exposure raises one's risk of developing the disease.

Summary

Autoimmune disease has been thought to be genetically driven, but data suggest that genetics primarily confer susceptibility to an infectious or environmental agent(s). Given the rarity of many of the autoimmune diseases, the unpredictable penetrance and ultimately the exposure to such an agent make population studies and strong conclusions difficult. Finally, the human immune system has evolved to a point at which certain cell populations (e.g., TH and TH2), which were fixed and able to be cloned in animals, can now shift in response to things such as stress or coexistent infections. Therefore, proving that an environmental agent is causative may prove difficult.

SIGNIFICANCE OF AUTOANTIBODIES

The term *horror autotoxicus* was the term for the situation in which the immune system could turn against the host, leading to severe tissue damage. Although transient responses to damaged self-tissues do occur, normal individuals do not mount sustained adaptive immune responses to their own antigens. Although self-tolerance is the general rule, in certain disease states, sustained immune responses to self-tissues occur, and these responses can result in severe tissue damage. By definition, autoimmune diseases are largely those in which autoantibodies are found. The first autoantibodies thoroughly studied—the antibodies of acquired hemolytic anemias—required little extensive investigation (156). These antibodies bound to red cells, thus sensitizing them to lysis by complement or to phagocytosis by the reticuloendothelial system. They typically caused the clinical diseases in which they were found, and therefore direct correlation exists between the autoantibodies and disease.

However, with the discovery of autoantibodies, such as rheumatoid factor and ANA, no such clear role is apparent between these and the diseases in which they occur. A great deal of research has been devoted to establishing the potential pathogenetic pathways between these antibodies and the diseases, such as RA and SLE, in which they occur. Most autoimmune diseases arise spontaneously—that is, we do not understand the events in which the immune response is initiated to self-antigens. Some strong associations have been made between certain infections and the onset of autoimmune diseases (157,158). These later observations suggest that infectious agents may play a critical role in this process. In experimental animals, autoimmune diseases can be induced by mixing tissue extracts with strong adjuvants containing bacteria and injecting them into genetically susceptible animals (159,160). These animals then develop a specific adaptive immune response to self-antigens and, ultimately, autoimmune diseases. However, such associations have not been clear in human disease. Therefore, it is important not only to identify autoantibodies in certain autoimmune diseases, but also to demonstrate the pathways of pathogenicity of the autoantibodies. With environmental factors,

TABLE 26-6. HLA genotype and susceptibility to autoimmune disease

Disease	HLA allele	Relative risk
Rheumatoid arthritis	DR4	4.2
Systemic lupus erythematosus	DR3	5.8
Pemphigus vulgaris	DR4	14.4
Insulin-dependent diabetes	DR3 and DR4	3.2
Graves' disease	DR3	3.7
Myasthenia gravis	DR3	2.5
Hashimoto's thyroiditis	DR5	3.2
Multiple sclerosis	DR2	4.8
Goodpasture's syndrome	DR2	15.9
Acute anterior uveitis	B27	10.04
Ankylosing spondylitis	B27	87.4

HLA, human leukocyte antigen.

such as chemicals or other substances, defining a pathogenetic relationship is even more difficult. Often, syndromes of fatigue, myalgias, and arthralgias have been associated with certain exposures. However, it has been very difficult to demonstrate consistent autoantibodies and so far impossible to associate these autoantibodies with clear-cut disease.

Genetic Role

Susceptibility to most autoimmune diseases, and thus the development of autoantibodies, shows a significant genetic component (Table 26-6) (161). In fact, familial associations are common. To date, the only consistent genetic marker for susceptibilities to autoimmune disease has been the major histocompatibility complex (MHC) genotype. Many human autoimmune diseases show HLA-linked disease associations, and these associations appear to grow stronger as the ability to HLA genotype becomes more accurate. For example, RA was associated with certain MHC class II genes—DW4, DW14, DW15, DW16, DW1—depending on ethnicity (161). However, with further and more specific analysis, it has been found that a stretch of amino acids in residues 67 through 74 was common to all 5 HLA genes and termed the *HLA DR beta 1 epitope* (DRB1) (162). Susceptibility and severity are now associated not only with having this gene, but also with whether one has a single or double copy of the gene. So-called "double-dose patients" have not only severe RA but also more severe systemic disease. Such patients are more likely to be positive for the autoantibody rheumatoid factor. Most diseases have been associated with MHC class II alleles, but in some cases, susceptibility is linked to MHC class I alleles.

It makes sense that autoimmune responses and diseases would be associated with the MHC genotype. Autoimmune responses involve T cells, and the ability of T cells to respond to a particular antigen—self or nonself—depends on the MHC genotype. Unfortunately, models depicting how particular MHC genotypes determine susceptibility to autoimmune disease and thus the development of autoantibodies have not been proven. Although attractive, models suggesting that allelic differences of the MHC molecule are more able to bind autoantigens to autoreactive T cells—thus determining autoimmune disease—remain hypothetical.

Criteria for Pathogenicity

Antibodies exert their effects by a variety of mechanisms, including aggregation, stimulation, opsonization, complement fixation, and indirect sensitization of a target site to other enzymatic action. Although the affinity and valence of the antibody are probably important and influence their pathogenetic role, it is probably the epitope or the site to which the antibody is directed that is the most critical of all. To establish pathogenicity, one must be able to describe how the antibody's combining with its antigen results in damage, and the resultant lesion should be similar to that one seen in the true autoimmune disease. In the actual autoimmune disease, one should find antibody and antigen in the site of tissue damage. In addition, one would like to see a correlation between autoantibody levels and disease activity.

To be associated with an autoimmune disease, an autoantibody should be found in higher concentrations and more frequently in affected versus unaffected individuals. In other words, the antibody should be specific for the disease, and the antibody titer should be associated with the severity of the disease.

Pathogenetic Autoantibodies

The following are groups of diseases in which autoantibodies have been found at the site of the disease process and in which their concentration has been associated with disease severity.

MYASTHENIA GRAVIS

Myasthenia gravis is a disease characterized by weakness and fatigability of skeletal muscles. It has been strongly associated with autoantibodies to the acetylcholine receptor (AChR) (163). Animal models demonstrate that, when certain animals are injected or immunized with the receptor and produce antireceptor antibodies, they develop symptoms resembling myasthenia gravis (164). In humans, antibodies to the receptor are detected in as many as 90% of individuals and are absent in healthy controls. Treatments directed at the immune system, such as immunosuppressive drugs, result in clinical improvement and are associated with a lowering in the level of the autoantibody (165). Although the association between autoantibodies to the AChR receptor appears directly pathogenic, no direct evidence exists for pathogenicity of the human AChR by adoptive transfer.

PEMPHIGUS

Pemphigus is a skin disease characterized by blistering, not only of the skin but also of the mucous membranes. Autoantibodies that bind to the surface of the epidermal cells are found in pemphigus and appear to play a major role in its induction (166). Immunohistology of the skin demonstrates immunoglobulin bound to the epidermal cell surface in nearly all patients with pemphigus. In addition, the level of antiepidermal antibodies correlates with disease activity, and removal of these antibodies leads to clinical improvement. Passive transfer of these antibodies to neonatal mice reproduces the human disease clinically, histologically, and immunologically (167). Finally, children of mothers with pemphigus may have transient disease because of maternal antibodies (168). These results strongly support the role of such autoantibodies in the pathogenicity of this disease.

Associated Autoantibodies

Whereas the previous examples demonstrate strong association with autoantibody titer and disease activity, as well as a high prevalence of the antibodies in affected individuals, other autoantibodies in human diseases demonstrate strong associations with the autoimmune disease, but true pathogenetic correlations have not been made (Table 26-7). Autoantibodies in Graves' disease are directed against the thyroid-stimulating hormone receptor, and they actually mimic the action of the pituitary hormone (169). Although the autoantibodies in this

TABLE 26-7. Autoantibodies and disease association

Disease	Autoantibodies to:
Graves' disease	Thyroid-stimulating hormone receptor
Rheumatoid arthritis	Immunoglobulin
Systemic lupus erythematosus	DNA, histones, ribosomes, others
Multiple sclerosis	Myelin basic protein
Diabetes mellitus, insulin dependent	Unknown B-cell antigen
Polyarteritis nodosa	Hepatitis B surface antigen
Goodpasture's syndrome	Basement membrane
Antiphospholipid syndrome	Cardiolipin and lupus anticoagulant
Primary biliary cirrhosis	Mitochondria
Myositis	Aminoacyt + RNA synthetase
Wegener's vasculitis	Serine protease (C-ANCA)

disease are associated strongly, they have also been found in many cases of closely related goitrous conditions.

In some patients with repeated episodes of thrombosis, recurrent fetal loss, and thrombocytopenia, antiphospholipid antibodies have been identified and described as the *antiphospholipid syndrome* (170). These autoantibodies include antibodies against cardiolipin, as well as the so-called lupus anticoagulant. The main feature of the antiphospholipid syndrome, thrombosis, may occur in nearly any blood vessel and may be associated with thrombocytopenia, transverse myolitis, and chorea. These antibodies are also associated with recurrent abortions, fetal death, and retardation of intrauterine growth. However, although the frequency of these autoantibodies is greater in lupus patients, autoantibodies can be found in healthy populations in whom disease is not present. Thus, evidence shows that there may be an association with these autoantibodies and clinical manifestation. However, this association is far from clear.

Autoantibodies to nuclear material (ANA) and systems are seen in a variety of individuals, including 5% of the healthy population. However, the titers are higher, primarily in those patients who suffer from SLE (171). In addition, many of these individuals may have low complement levels, and in certain cases, this may be associated with active flares of disease. However, it is not clear that these autoantibodies are clearly pathogenetic. Evidence—such as the lack of effect of plasmapheresis in which these antibodies are removed—on the outcome of SLE or severe nephritis suggests the role is far from clear.

Normal Autoantibodies

It appears that many autoantibodies may serve normal important functions in the body. Although typically high in RA, rheumatoid factor has also been found in healthy individuals at low levels (172). Some data would suggest that rheumatoid factor may function as a regulatory antibody in the normal situation. In addition, autoantibodies against T-cell receptors have been found in high levels in SLE as well as in RA and in aging individuals (173). However, they have also been found in healthy individuals and in preparations of intravenous gamma globulin, although at lower levels. Therefore, such "normal" autoantibodies may represent important regulatory mechanisms in normal immune functioning.

Finally, certain viruses and other adjuvants may nonspecifically stimulate the immune system, resulting in high levels of circulating immunoglobulin (hypergammaglobulinemia) (174). If one would measure a specific antibody, it might appear high, but in relationship to the overall high levels of immunoglobulin, this would not be the case. Therefore, one has to be extremely careful in measuring autoantibodies in these situations. Such situations occur regularly in SLE and RA.

Autoantibodies may represent the actual pathogenetic agent of certain diseases: the secondary consequences of tissue damage or chronic inflammation or just the harmless footprints of an etiologic agent. Establishing a pathogenetic role for autoantibodies requires not only their presence, but also that they appear at the location of the presumptive target antigen and that their levels are associated with disease activity. A majority, if not all, of infected individuals should have autoantibodies present. Finally, it should be shown that passive transfer of the antibodies is capable of inducing disease in animals and that removal of the autoantibodies from the affected individual results in disease amelioration. One must be extremely careful in attributing a disease association or pathogenetic role to autoantibodies. For example, although ANAs may identify patients with SLE, they may also be found in a significant proportion of healthy individuals, and although some patients with SLE have disease activity strongly associated with levels of certain autoantibodies, many patients have no such association. It could be extremely harmful if one were to identify a presumptive autoantibody as being pathogenetic for a disease process and treating it as such. Such autoantibodies may actually represent the immune response's attempt to correct the disease process, and removal of these autoantibodies would result in disease worsening.

REFERENCES

1. Vojdani A, Ghoneum M, Brautbar N. Immune alteration associated with exposure to toxic chemicals. *Toxicol Ind Health* 1992;8:239–254.
2. Bigazzi PE. Autoimmunity induced by chemicals. *Clin Toxicol* 1988;26:125–156.
3. Thrasher JD, Broughton A, Madison R. Immune activation and autoantibodies in humans with long term inhalation exposure to formaldehyde. *Arch Environ Health* 1990;45:217–223.
4. Levin A, Byers V. Environmental illness: a disorder of immune regulation. *Occup Med* 1987;2(4):669–681.
5. Trizio D, Basletter DA, Botham PA, et al. Identification of immunotoxic effects of chemicals and assessment of their relevance to man. *Food and Chem Toxicol* 1988;26(6):527–539.
6. Amos HE, Park BK. Understanding immunotoxic drug reactions. In: Dean J, et al., eds. *Immunotoxicology and immunopharmacology.* New York: Raven Press, 1985:207–229.
7. Brooks B, Sullivan JB. Immunotoxicology. In: Sullivan JB, Krieger GR, eds. *Hazardous materials toxicology: clinical principles of environmental health.* Baltimore: Williams & Wilkins, 1992.
8. Bluestein HG, Redelman D, Zvaifler N. Procainamide-lymphocyte reactions. *Arthritis Rheum* 1981;24:1019–1023.
9. Mongey A. The potential role of environmental agents in systemic lupus erythematosus and associated disorders. In: Wallace DJ, Hahn BH, eds. *Dubois' lupus erythematosus*, 4th ed. Philadelphia: Lea & Febiger, 1993:37–63.
10. Hahn BH. An overview of the pathogenesis of systemic lupus erythematosus. In: Wallace DJ, Hahn BH eds. *Dubois' lupus erythematosus*, 4th ed. Philadelphia: Lea & Febiger, 1993:65–70.
11. Bigazzi PE. Autoimmunity and heavy metals. *Lupus* 1994;3:449–453.
12. Cardenas A, Roels H, Bernard AM, et al. Markers of early renal changes induced by industrial pollutants. I. Application to workers exposed to mercury vapour. *Br J Ind Med* 1993;7:294–296.
13. Silman AJ, Hochberg MC. *Epidemiology of the rheumatic diseases.* New York: Oxford University Press, 1993:192–219.
14. Smith EA, LeRoy EC. Systemic sclerosis. In: Klippel JH, Dieppe PA, eds. *Rheumatology.* St. Louis: Mosby–Year Book, 1998: Chapter 7.
15. Erasmus LD. Scleroderma in gold-miners on the Witwatersrand with particular reference to pulmonary manifestations. *South Africa J Lab Clin Med* 1957;3:209–231.
16. Haustein UF, Ziegler V. Environmentally induced systemic sclerosis–like disorders. *Int J Dermatol* 1985;24:147–151.
17. Rodnan GP, Benedek TG, Medsger TA, Cammarata RJ. The association of progressive systemic sclerosis (scleroderma) with coal miners' pneumoconiosis and other forms of silicosis. *Ann Int Med* 1967;66:323–334.
18. Steenland K, Goldsmith D. Silica exposure and autoimmune diseases. *Am Ind Med* 1995;28:603–608.
19. Balaan M, Banks D. Silicosis. In: Rom W, ed. *Environmental and occupational medicine.* Boston: Little, Brown and Company, 1992:345–358.
20. Sanchez-Roman J, Wichmann I, Salaberri J, Varela JM, Nunez-Roldam A. Multiple clinical and biologic autoimmune manifestations in 50 workers after occupational exposure to silica. *Ann Rheum Dis* 1993;52:534–538.

21. Sanchez–Guerrero J, Schur PH, Sergent JC, Liang MH. Silicone breast implants. *Clin Immunol Epidemiol Studies* 1994;37:158–168.
22. Cook R, Harrison MC, Levier RR. The breast implant controversy. *Arthritis Rheum* 1994;37:153–157.
23. Kossovsky N, Heggers JP, Robson MC. Experimental demonstration of the immunogenicity of silicone-protein complexes. *J Biomed Mater Res* 1987;21:1125–1133.
24. Chastre J, Basset F, Viau F, et al. Acute pneumonitis after subcutaneous injections of silicone in transsexual men. *N Engl J Med* 1983;308:764–767.
25. Bridges AJ, Conley C, Wang G, Burns D, Vasey F. A clinical and immunologic evaluation of women with silicone breast implants and symptoms of rheumatic disease. *Ann Intern Med* 1993;118:929–936.
26. Cuellar ML, Gluck O, Molina JF, Gutierrez S, Garcia C, Espinoza R. Silicone breast implant–associated musculoskeletal manifestations. *Clin Rheum* 1995;14:667–672.
27. Kumagai Y, Shiokawa Y, Medsger TA, Rodnan GP. Clinical spectrum of connective tissue disease after cosmetic surgery. *Arthritis Rheum* 1984;27:1–12.
28. Kaiser W, Biesenbach G, Stuby U, Grafinger P, Zazgornik J. Human adjuvant disease: remission of silicone induced autoimmune disease after explantation of breast augmentation. *Ann Rheum Dis* 1990;49:937–938.
29. Hochberg MC, Perlmutter DL, Medsger TA, et al. Lack of association between augmentation mammoplasty and systemic sclerosis (scleroderma). *Arthritis Rheum* 1996;39:1125–1131.
30. Gabriel SE, O'Fallon WM, Kurland LT, et al. Risk of connective tissue diseases and other disorders after breast implantation. *N Engl J Med* 1994;24:1697–1702.
31. Sanchez-Guerrero J, Graham AC, Karlson EW, et al. Silicone breast implants and the risk of connective tissue disease and symptoms. *N Engl J Med* 1995;332:1666–1670.
32. Kasturi KN, Hatakeyama A, Spiera H, Bona CA. Antifibrillarin autoantibodies present in systemic sclerosis and other connective tissue diseases interact with similar epitopes. *J Exp Med* 1995;181:1027–1036.
33. Truong LD, Cartwright J, Goodman MD, Woznicki D. Silicone lymphoidenopathy associated with augmentation mammoplasty: morphologic features of nine cases. *Am J Surg Pathol* 1988;12:484–491.
34. Kossovsky N, Conway D, Kossowsky R, Petrovich D. Novel anti–silicone surface–associated antigen antibodies (anti-SSAA(x)) may help differentiate symptomatic patients with silicone breast implants from patients with classical rheumatic diseases. *Curr Top Microbiol Immunol* 1996;210:327–336.
35. Lewy RI, Ezrailson E. Laboratory studies in breast implant patients: ANA positivity, gammaglobulin levels, and other autoantibodies. *Curr Top Microbiol Immunol* 1996;210:337–353.
36. Silverman S, Gluck O, Silver D, et al. The prevalence of autoantibodies in symptomatic and asymptomatic patients with breast implants and patients with fibromyalgia. *Curr Top Microbiol Immunol* 1996;210:317–322.
37. Bridges AJ, Anderson JD, Burns DE, Kemple K, Kaplan JD, Lorden T. Autoantibodies in patients with silicone implants. *Curr Top Microbiol Immunol* 1996;210:277–282.
38. Claman HN, Robertson AD. Antinuclear antibodies in apparently healthy women with breast implants. *Curr Top Microbiol Immunol* 1996;210:265–268.
39. Sanchez-Guerrero J, Schur PH, Sergent JS, Liang MH. Silicone breast implant and rheumatic disease. *Arthritis Rheum* 1994;37:156–168.
40. Sucin I, Drejman I, Valaskai M. Study of disease caused by vinyl chloride. *Med Lav* 1967;58:261–271. Cited in: Markowitz SS, McDonald CJ, Fethiere W, Kerzner MS. Occupational acro-osteolysis. *Arch Dermatol* 1967;106:219–223.
41. Cordier JM, Fievez C, Lefeure MT, Seurin A. Acroosteolyses et lesions cutanoes associeces chez duez ouvriers affects on nettoyege d'autoclaves. *Cahiers Med Travail* 1996;4:14. Cited in: Dodson VN, Dinman BD, Whitehouse WM, Nasr ANM, Magnuson HJ. Occupational acro-osteolysis. *Arch Envion Health* 1971;22:83–91.
42. Harris DK, Adams WGF. Acro-osteolysis occurring in men engaged in the polymerization of vinyl chloride. *BMJ* 1967;3:712–714.
43. Markowitz SS, McDonald CJ, Fethiere W, Kerzner MS. Occupational acro-osteolysis. *Arch Dermatol* 1972;106:219–223.
44. Dodson VN, Dinman BD, Whitehouse WM, Nasr ANM, Magnuson HJ. Occupational acro-osteolysis. *Arch Environ Health* 1971;22:83–91.
45. Veltman G, Lange CE, Juhe S, Stein G, Bachner U. Clinical manifestations and course of vinyl chloride disease. *Ann N Y Acad Sci* 1975;246:6–17.
46. Lilis R, Anderson H, Nicholson WJ, Daum S, Fischbein AS, Selikoff IJ. Prevalence of disease among vinyl chloride and polyvinyl chloride workers. *Ann N Y Acad Sci* 1975;246:22–41.
47. Gama C, Meira JBB. Occupational acro-osteolysis. *J Bone Joint Surg Am* 1978;60A:86–90.
48. Wilson RH, McCormick WE, Tatum CF, Cheech JL. Occupational acroosteolysis: report of 31 cases. *JAMA* 1967;201:577–581.
49. Dinman BD, Cook WA, Whitehouse WM, et al. Occupational acroosteolysis in an epidemiological study. *Arch Environ Health* 1971;22:61–73.
50. Meyerson LB, Meier GC. Cutaneous lesions in acro-osteolysis. *Arch Dermatol* 1972;106:224–227.
51. Black C, Pereira S, McWhirter A, Welsh K, Laurent R. Genetic susceptibility to scleroderma-like syndrome in symptomatic and asymptomatic workers exposed to vinyl chloride. *J Rheum* 1986;13:1059–1062.
52. Black CM, Welsh KI, Walker AE, et al. Genetic susceptibility to scleroderma-like syndrome induced by vinyl chloride. *Lancet* 1983;1:53–55.
53. Ward AM, Udnoon S, Watkins J, Walker AE, Darke CS. Immunological mechanisms in the pathogenesis of vinyl chloride disease. *BMJ* 1976;1:936–938.
54. Walder B. Solvents and scleroderma [Letter]. *Lancet* 1965;2:436–437.
55. Walder BK. Do solvents cause scleroderma? *Int J Dermatol* 1983;22:157–158.
56. Saihan EM, Burton JL, Heaton KW. A new syndrome with pigmentation, scleroderma, gynaecomastia, Raynaud's phenomenon and peripheral neuropathy. *Br J Dermatol* 1978;99:437–440.
57. Lockey JE, Kelly CR, Cannon GW, Colby TV, Aldrich V, Livingston GK. Progressive systemic sclerosis associated with exposure to trichloroethylene. *J Occup Med* 1987;29:493–496.
58. Czirjak L, Danko K, Schlammadinger J, Suranyi P, Tamasi L, Szegedi GY. Progressive systemic sclerosis occurring in patients exposed to chemicals. *Int J Dermatol* 1987;26:374–378.
59. Sparrow GP. A connective tissue disorder similar to vinyl chloride disease in a patient exposed to perchlorethylene. *Clin Exp Dermatol* 1977;2:17–22.
60. Yamakage A, Ishikawa H. Generalized morphea-like scleroderma occurring in people exposed to organic solvents. *Dermatologica* 1982;165:186–193.
61. Owens GR, Medsger TA. Systemic sclerosis secondary to occupational exposure. *Am J Med* 1988;85:114–116.
62. Yamakage A, Ishikawa H, Saito Y, Hattori A. Occupational scleroderma-like disorder occurring in men engaged in the polymerization of epoxy resins. *Dermatologica* 1980;161:33–44.
63. Stachow A, Jablonska S, Skiendzielewska A. 5-Hydroxytryptamine and tryptamine pathways in scleroderma. *Br J Dermatol* 1977;97:147–154.
64. Stachow A, Jablonska S, Skiendzielewska A. Biogenic amines derived from tryptophan in systemic and cutaneous scleroderma. *Acta Derm Venerol* 1979;59:1–5.
65. Brunjes S, Arterberry JD, Shankel S, Johns VJ. Decreased oxidative deamination of catecholamines associated with clinical scleroderma. *Arthritis Rheum* 1964;7:138–152.
66. Sternberg EM, Van Woert MH, Young SN, et al. Development of a scleroderma-like illness during therapy with L-5-hydroxytryptophan and carbidopa. *N Engl J Med* 1980;303:782–787.
67. Hertzman PA, Falk H, Kilbourne EM, Page S, Shulman LE. The eosinophilia-myalgia syndrome: the Los Alamos conference. *J Rheum* 1991;18:867–873.
68. Martin RW, Duffy J, Engel AG, et al. The clinical spectrum of the eosinophilia-myalgia syndrome associated with L-tryptophan ingestion. *Ann Int Med* 1990;113:124–134.
69. Hertzman PA, Blevins WL, Mayer J, Greenfield B, Ting M, Gleich GJ. Association of the eosinophilia-myalgia syndrome with the ingestion of tryptophan. *N Engl J Med* 1990;322:869–873.
70. Eidson M, Philen RM, Sewell CM, Voorhees R, Kilbourne EM. L-Tryptophan and eosinophilia-myalgia syndrome in New Mexico. *Lancet* 1990;335:645–648.
71. Belongia EA, Hedberg CW, Gleigh GJ, et al. An investigation of the cause of the eosinophilia-myalgia syndrome associated with tryptophan use. *N Engl J Med* 1990;323:357–365.
72. Anonymous. Eosinophilia-myalgia syndrome—New Mexico. *MMWR Morb Mortal Wkly Rep* 1989;38:765–767.
73. Silver RM, Heyes MP, Maize JC, Quearry B, Vionnet-Fuasset M, Sternberg EM. Scleroderma, fasciitis, and eosinophilia associated with the ingestion of tryptophan. *N Engl J Med* 1990;322:874–881.
74. Tabuenca JM. Toxic-allergic syndrome caused by ingestion of rapeseed oil denatured with aniline. *Lancet* 1981;2:567–568.
75. Mateo IM, Izquierdo M, Fernandez-Dapica MP, Navas J, Cabello A, Gomez-Reino JJ. Toxic epidemic syndrome: musculoskeletal manifestations. *J Rheum* 1984;11:3:333–338.
76. Alonso-Ruiz A, Zea-Mendoza AC, Salazar-Vallinas JM, Rocamora-Ripoll A, Beltran-Gutierrez J. Toxic oil syndrome: a syndrome with features overlapping those of various forms of scleroderma. *Semin Arthritis Rheum* 1986;15:200–212.
77. LeRoy EC. Scleroderma (systemic sclerosis). In: Kelly WA, Harris ED, Ruddy S, Sledge CB, eds. *Textbook of rheumatology.* Philadelphia: WB Saunders, 1985:1183–1201.
78. Kerr LD, Spiera H. Scleroderma in association with the use of bleomycin: a report of 3 cases. *J Rheumatol* 1992;19:294–296.
79. Cohen IS, Mosher MB, O'Keefe EJ, Klaus SN, De Conti RC. Cutaneous toxicity of bleomycin therapy. *Arch Dermatol* 1973;107:553–555.
80. Finch WR, Rodnan GP, Buckingham RB, Prince RK, Winkelstein A. Bleomycin-induced scleroderma. *J Rhuem* 1980;7:651–659.
81. Palestine RF, Millns JL, Spigel GT, Schroeter AL. Skin manifestations of pentazocine abuse. *Am Acad Dermatol* 1980;2:47–55.
82. Tomlinson IW, Jayson MIV. Systemic sclerosis after therapy with appetite suppressants. *J Rheum* 1984;11:254.
83. Aeschlimann A, De Truchis P, Kahn MF. Scleroderma after therapy with appetite suppressants. *Scand J Rheum* 1990;19:87–90.
84. Trozak DJ, Gould NM. Cocaine abuse and connective tissue disease. *J Am Acad Dermatol* 1984;10:525.
85. Graham JR. Cardiac and pulmonary fibrosis during methysergide therapy for headache. *Am J Med Sci* 1967;254(1):1–12.
86. Sprecace GA. Idiopathic pulmonary hemosiderosis. *Am Rev Respir Dis* 1963;88:330–336.
87. Beirne GJ, Brennan JT. Glomerulonephritis associated with hydrocarbon solvents. *Arch Environ Health* 1972;25:365–369.
88. Keogh AM, Ibels LS, Allen DH, Isbister JP, Kennedy MC. Exacerbation of Goodpasture's syndrome after inadvertent exposure to hydrocarbon fumes. *BMJ* 1983;288:188.
89. Kleinknecht D, Morel-Maroger L, Callard P, Adhemar J, Mahieu P. Antiglomerular basement membrane nephritis after solvent exposure. *Arch Intern Med* 1980;140:230–232.

90. Bombassei GJ, Kaplan AA. The association between hydrocarbon exposure and anti-glomerular basement membrane antibody-mediated disease (Goodpasture's syndrome). *Am J Ind Med* 1992;21:141–153.
91. Von Scheele C, Althoff P, Kempi V, Schelin U. Nephrotic syndrome due to subacute glomerulonephritis—association with hydrocarbon exposure? *Acta Med Scand* 1976;200:427–429.
92. Daniell WE, Couser WG, Rosenstock L. Occupational solvent exposure and glomerulonephritis. *JAMA* 1988;259:2280–2283.
93. Whitworth JA, Lawrence JR, Meadows R. Goodpasture's syndrome. *Aust N Z J Med* 1974;4:167–177.
94. D'Apice AJF, Kincaid-Smith P, Becker GJ. Goodpasture's syndrome in identical twins. *Ann Intern Med* 1978;88:61–62.
95. Ravnskov U. Acute glomerulonephritis and exposure to organic solvents in father and daughter. *Acta Med Scand* 1979;205:581–582.
96. Polla B, Pirson Y, Cosyns JP, Van Ypersele De Strihou C. Toxic anti-GBM glomerulonephritis. *Clin Nephrol* 1983;19:45–47.
97. Nathan AW, Toseland PA. Goodpasture's syndrome and trichloroethane intoxication. *Br J Clin Pharmacol* 1979;8:284–286.
98. Ravnskov U, Forsberg B, Skerfving S. Glomerulonephritis and exposure to organic solvents. *Acta Med Scand* 1979;205:575–579.
99. Bonzel KE, Muller-Wiefel DE, Ruder H, Wingen AM, Waldherr R, Weber M. Anti-glomerular basement membrane antibody-mediated glomerulonephritis due to glue sniffing. *Eur J Pediatr* 1987;146:296–300.
100. Rees AJ, Lockwood CM, Peters DK Nephritis due to autoantibodies to GBM. In: Kincaid-Smith P, D'Apice AJF, Atkins RC, eds. *Progress in glomerulonephritis*. New York: John Wiley and Sons, 1979:347–366.
101. Bernis P, Hamels J, Quoidbach A, Mahieu PH, Bouvy P. Remission of Goodpasture's syndrome after withdrawal of an unusual toxic. *Clin Nephrol* 1985;23:6:312–317.
102. Bell GM, Gordon ACH, Lee P, et al. Proliferative glomerulonephritis and exposure to organic solvents. *Nephron* 1985;40:161–165.
103. Yamamoto T, Wilson CB. Binding of anti-basement membrane antibody to alveolar basement membrane after intrtracheal gasoline instillation in rabbits. *Am J Pathol* 1987;126:497–505.
104. Klavis G, Drommer W. Goodpasture syndrome and Benzineinwirkung. *Arch Toxicol* 1969;26:40–55.
105. Harman JW. Chronic glomerulonephritis and the nephrotic syndrome induced in rats with N,N'-diacetylbenzidine. *J Pathol* 1970;104:119–128.
106. Donaghy M, Rees AJ. Cigarette smoking and lung hemorrhage in glomerulonephritis caused by antibodies to glomerular basement membrane. *Lancet* 1983;2:1390–1392.
107. Druet P, Bernard A, Hirsch F, et al. Immunologically mediated glomerulonephritis induced by heavy metals. *Arch Toxicol* 1982;50:187–194.
108. Wooley PH, Griffin J, Panayi GS, Batchelor JR, Welsh KI, Gibson TJ. HLA-DR antigens and toxic reactions to sodium aurothiomalate and D-penicillamine in patients with rheumatoid arthritis. *N Engl J Med* 1980;303:300–302.
109. Guery JC, Druet E, Glotz D, Hirsch F, Mandet C, De Heer E, Druet P. Specificity and cross-reactive idiotypes of anti-glomerular basement membrane autoantibodies in $HgCl_2$-induced autoimmune glomerulonephritis. *Eur J Immunol* 1990;20:93–100.
110. Jaffe IA. Penicillamine. In: Kelly WA, Harris ED, Ruddy S, Sledge CB, eds. *Textbook of rheumatology*. Philadelphia: WB Saunders, 1993:760–765.
111. Joshi BC, Dwivedi C, Powell A, Holscher M. Immune complex nephritis in rats induced by long-term oral exposure to cadmium. *J Comp Pathol* 1981;91:11–15.
112. Hochberg MC. The epidemiology of systemic lupus erythematosus. In: Wallace DJ, Hahn BH, eds. *Dubois' lupus erythematosus*, 4th ed. Philadelphia: Lea & Febiger, 1993:49–57.
113. Clark LC, Giuliano A, Walsh BJ, et al. The Santa Cruz community health survey. December, 1994.
114. Siegel M, Holley HL, Lee SL. Epidemiologic studies on systemic lupus erythematosus: comparative data for New York City and Jefferson County, Alabama. *Arthritis Rheum* 1970;13:802–811.
115. Fessel WJ. Systemic lupus erythematosus in the community. *Arch Int Med* 1974;134:1027–1035.
116. Howard PE, Hochberg MC, Bias WB, Arnett FC Jr, McLean RH. Relationship between C4 null gene, HLA D region antigens and genetic susceptibility to systemic lupus erythematosus in caucasians and black americans. *Am J Med* 1986;88:187–192.
117. Schur PH, Marcus-Bagley D, Awdeh Z, Yunis EJ, Alper CA. The effect of ethnicity on major histocompatibility complex complement allotypes and extended haplotypes in patients with systemic lupus erythematosus. *Arthritis Rheum* 1990;33:985–992.
118. Malinow MR, Bardana EJ, Goodnight SH. Pancytopenia during ingestion of alfalfa seeds. *Lancet* 1981;8220:615.
119. Bardana EJ, Malinow MR, Houghton DC, et al. Diet-induced systemic lupus erythematosus (SLE) in primates. *Am J Kidney Dis* 1982;1:345–352.
120. Roberts JL, Hayashi JA. Exacerbation of SLE associated with alfalfa ingestion. *N Engl J Med* 1983;308:1361.
121. Alcocer-Varela J, Iglesias A, Llorente L, Alarcon-Segovia D. Effects of L-canavanine on T cells may explain the induction of systemic lupus erythematosus by alfalfa. *Arthritis Rheum* 1985;28:52–57.
122. Malinow MR, Bardana EJ, McLaughlin P. Systemic lupus erythematosus-like syndrome in monkeys fed alfalfa sprouts: role of nonprotein amino acid. *Science* 1982;216:415–417.
123. Hoffman BJ. Sensitivity to sulfadiazine resembling acute disseminated lupus erythematosus. *Arch Dermatol Syphil* 1945;51:190–192.
124. Hess EV. Environmental lupus syndromes. *Br J Rheum* 1995;34:597–601.
125. Reidenberg MM. The chemical induction of systemic lupus erythematosus and lupus-like illnesses. *Arthritis Rheum* 1981;24:1004–1008.
126. Stratton MA Drug-induced systemic lupus erythematosus. *Clin Pharmacol* 1985;4:657.
127. Hess E. Drug-related lupus. *N Engl J Med* 1988;318:1460.
128. Solinger AM. Drug-related lupus: clinical and etiologic considerations. *Rheum Dis Clin North Am* 1988;14:187.
129. Reidenberg MM, Durant PJ, Harris RA, De Boccardo G, Lahita R, Stenzel KH. Lupus erythematosus–like disease due to hydrazine. *Am J Med* 1983;75:365–370.
130. Freni-Titulaer LWJ, Kelley DB, Grow AG, McKinley TW, Arnett FC, Hochberg MC. Connective tissue disease in southeastern Georgia: a case-control study of etiologic factors. *Am J Epidemiol* 1989;130:404–409.
131. Hochberg MC, Kaslow RA Risk factors for the development of systemic lupus erythematosus: a case control study. *Clin Res* 1983;31:732A.
132. Sanchez-Guerrero J, Karlson EW, Colditz GA, Hunter DJ, Speizer FE, Liang MH. Hairdye use and the risk of developing systemic lupus erythematosus. *Arthritis Rheum* 1996;39:657–662.
133. Petri M, Allbritton J. Hair product use in systemic lupus erythematosus: a case-controlled study. *Arthritis Rheum* 1992;35:625–629.
134. Reidenberg MM. Aromatic amines and the pathogenesis of lupus erythematosus. *Am J Med* 1983;75:1037–1042.
135. Perry HM, Tan EM, Carmody S, Sakamoto A. Relationship of acetyl transferase activity to antinuclear antibodies and toxic symptoms in hypertensive patients treated with hydralazine. *J Lab Clin Med* 1970;76:114–125.
136. Baer AN, Woosley RL, Pincus T. Further evidence for the lack of association between acetylator phenotype and systemic lupus erythematosus. *Arthritis Rheum* 1986;29:508–514.
137. Kilburn KH, Warshaw RH. Prevalence of symptoms of systemic lupus erythematosus (SLE) and of fluorescent antinuclear antibodies associated with chronic exposure to trichloroethylene and other chemicals in well water. *Environ Res* 1992;57:1–9.
138. Wallace DJ, Quismorio FP Jr. The elusive search for geographic clusters of systemic lupus erythematosus. Critical review. *Arthritis Rheum* 1995;38:1564–1567.
139. Broughton A, Thrasher JD. *Chemical exposures: low levels and high stakes*. New York: Van Nostrand Reinhold, 1991.
140. Meuzelaar HLC. University of Utah, Center for Micro Analysis and Reaction Chemistry [Letter], Dec. 15, 1992.
141. Zurick P. Testimony before the United States House of Representatives Subcommitee on Regulation, Business Opportunities and Energy. Feb. 21, 1992.
142. Water Quality Assurance Revolving Fund Phase 1 Report, Nogales Wash Study Area Task Assignment E-3, Nogales, Arizona. Report prepared for the Arizona Department of Environmental Quality by Earth Technology Corporation, March 1990.
143. Liang MH, Meenan RF, Cathcart ES, Schur PH. A screening strategy for studies in systemic lupus erythematosus: series design. *Arthritis Rheum* 1980;23:153.
144. Cukier J, Beauchamp RA, Spindler JS, Spindler S, Lorenzo C, Trentham DE. Association between bovine collagen dermal implants and a dermatomyositis or a polymyositis-like syndrome. *Ann Intern Med* 1993;118:920–928.
145. Love LA, Weiner SR, Vasey FB, et al. Clinical and immunologic features of women who develop myositis after silicone implants. *Arthritis Rheum* 1995;68:S46.
146. Castro FF, Krull EA. Injectable collagen implant—update. *J Am Acad Derm* 1983;9:889–893.
147. Jarrett MP, Roguska-Kyts J. Collagen induced arthritis in humans. *Arthritis Rheum* 1982;25:1024–1025.
148. DeLustro F, Fries J, Kang S, Kaye R, Reichlin. Immunity to injectable collagen and autoimmune disease: a summary of current understanding. *J Dermatol Surg Oncol* 1988;14:57–65.
149. Stommel EW, Parsonnet J, Jenkyn LR. Polymyositis after ciguatera toxin exposure. *Arch Neurol* 1991;48:847–877.
150. Stommel EW, Jenkyn LR, Parsonnet J. Another case of polymyositis after ciguatera toxin exposure. *Arch Neurol* 1993;50:571.
151. Lawrence DN, Enriquez MB, Lumish RM, Msceo A. Ciguatera fish poisoning in Miami. *JAMA* 1980;224:254–258.
152. Rothchild BM, Turner KR, DeLuca MA. Symmetrical erosive peripheral polyarthritis in the late archaic period of Alabama. *Science* 1988;241:1498–1501.
153. Klockars M, Koskela R-S, Jarvinen E, Kolari PJ, Rossi A. Silica exposure and rheumatoid arthritis: a follow up study of granite workers 1940–81. *BMJ* 1987;294:997–1000.
154. Sluis-Cremer GK, Hessel PA, Hnizdo E, Churchill AR. Relationship between silicosis and rheumatoid arthritis. *Thorax* 1986;41:596–601.
155. Miall WE, Ball J, Kellgren JH. Prevalence of rheumatoid arthritis in urban and rural populations in South Wales. *Ann Rheum Dis* 1958;17:264–272.
156. Naparstek Y, Plotz DH. The role of autoantibodies in autoimmune disease. *Annu Rev Immunol* 1993;11:79–104.
157. Kaufman DL, Erlander MG, Clare-Salzler M, Atkinson MA, Maclaren NK, Tobin AJ. Autoimmunity to two forms of glutamate decarboxylase in insulin-dependent diabetes mellitus. *J Clin Invest* 1992;89:283–292.

158. Kaplan MH, Svec KH. Immunologic relation of streptococcal and tissue antigens. III. Presence in human sera of streptococcal antibody cross-reactive with heart tissue, association with streptococcal infection, rheumatic fever, and glomerulonephritis. *J Exp Med* 1964;119:651–665.
159. Kakimoto K, Katsuki M, Hirofuji T, Iwata H, Koga T. Isolation of T-cell line capable of protecting mice against collagen-induced arthritis. *J Immunol* 1988;140:78–83.
160. Brostoff SW, Mason DW. Experimental allergic encephalomyelitis in successful treatment in vivo with a monoclonal antibody that recognizes T-helper cells. *J Immunol* 1984;133:1938–1942.
161. Nepom GT, Nepon B. The major histocompatibility complex. In: Klippel JH, Dieppe PA, eds. *Rheumatology.* St. Louis: Mosby-Year Book, 1998: Chapter 12.
162. Seyfried CE, Mickelson E, Hansen JA, Nepom GT. A specific nucleotide sequence defines a functional T cell recognition epitope shared by diverse HLA-DR specificities. *Hum Immunol* 1988;21:289–299.
163. Schonbeck S, Chrestel S, Hohlfeld R. Myasthenia gravis: prototype of the anti-receptor autoimmune diseases. *Int Rev Neurobiol* 1990;32:175–200.
164. Patrick J, Lindstrom J. Autoimmune response to acetylcholine receptor. *Science* 1973;180:871–872.
165. Kuks JB, Gusterhuis HJ, Limburg PC. Anti-acetylcholine receptor antibodies decrease after thymectomy in patients with myasthenia gravis: clinical correlations. *J Auto Immun* 1991;4:197–211.
166. Grando SA, Drannik GN, Glukhenky BT, et al. Clinical and laboratory evaluation of hemocarboadsorption in autoimmune bullous dermatoses. *Int J Artif Organs* 1990;13:181–188.
167. Rock B, Labib RS, Diaz LA. Monovalent fab immunoglobulin fragments from endemic pemphigus foliaceus autoantibodies reproduce the human disease in neonatal bal 1c mice. *J Clin Invest* 1990;85:296–299.
168. Anhalt GJ, Diaz LA. In vivo studies of antibody dependent acantholysis. *Immuno Ser* 1989;46:291–316.
169. Burman KD, Baker JR Jr. Immune mechanisms in Graves' disease. *Endocrinol Rev* 1985;6:183–232.
170. McNeil HP, Chesterman CN, Krilis SA. Immunology and clinical importance of antiphospholipid antibodies. *Adv Immunol* 1991;49:193–280.
171. Weinstein A, Bordwell B, Stone B, Tibbe HSC, Rothfield NF. Antibodies to native DNA and serum complement (C3) levels. Application to diagnosis and classification of systemic lupus erythematosus. *Am J Med* 1983;74:206–216.
172. Schrohenloher RE, Bridges SL Jr, Koopman WJ. Rheumatoid factor. In: WJ Koopman, ed. *Arthritis and allied conditions: a textbook of rheumatology,* 13th ed. Philadelphia: Williams & Wilkins, 1996:1109–1130.
173. Marcholonis JJ, Schluter SF, Wang E, et al. Synthetic autoantigens of immunoglobulins and T-cell receptors: their recognition in aging, infection and autoimmunity. *Proc Soc Exp Biol Med* 1994;207:129–147.
174. Braun J, Stiehm ER. The B-lymphocyte system. In: Stiehm ER, ed. *Immunologic disorders in infants and children,* 4th ed. Philadelphia: WB Saunders, 1996:35–74.

CHAPTER 27

Endocrine-Disrupting Chemicals

Janet E. Kester

It has long been recognized that various xenobiotics (naturally occurring and synthetic compounds that interact with an organism but do not occur in the normal metabolic pathways of that organism) (1) may exert profound influences on the vertebrate endocrine system, including the adrenals, hypothalamic-hypophyseal axis, pancreas, pineal gland, thyroid gland, and sex organs. There has been significantly increased scientific, regulatory, and public interest in and concern about the potential effects of exposure to these "endocrine disruptors"—environmental agents that influence the complex and interdependent function of endocrine systems, particularly reproductive systems, in humans and wildlife. This concern stems from a series of reports in the popular and scientific press that "xenoestrogens," xenobiotics with specifically estrogenlike effects, may play a role in reportedly increased rates of breast cancer and endometriosis in women, testicular and prostate cancers and reduced semen quality in men, and abnormal sexual development in both sexes (2–9). In addition, observations of wildlife with deformed genitalia, sterility, aberrant mating behavior, and other physical and behavioral abnormalities have been linked to exposure to xenoestrogens (10–13).

Books such as *Our Stolen Future* (14) and associated articles in the popular press have promoted the unproved hypothesis that xenoestrogens and other endocrine disruptors may exert these effects by blocking, mimicking, or otherwise interfering with the activities of natural hormones, causing adverse effects at the level of the organism, its progeny, and subpopulations of organisms. In June 1996, Arnold et al. (15) of Tulane University reported that mixtures of some weakly estrogenic chemicals (e.g., the pesticides endosulfan, dieldrin, chlordane, and toxaphene) and hydroxylated polychlorinated biphenyls (PCBs) were up to 1,600 times more active than single compounds in a simple yeast estrogen system containing human estrogen receptor and an estrogen-sensitive reporter gene. This widely publicized finding of synergy appeared to offer a mechanism by which the low environmental concentrations of these chemicals might cause profound adverse effects. As such, it played a significant role in prompting mandates in the 1996 Food Quality Protection Act and the Safe Drinking Water Act requiring the U.S. Environmental Protection Agency (EPA) to develop a screening and testing strategy for chemicals possessing endocrine-disrupting activity within 2 years, despite lack of knowledge regarding (a) the identity, potency, and mechanisms of action of chemicals that might interfere with endocrine system functions and (b) the magnitude or even existence of any resultant human or ecological health problems. The legislation cites the Federal Insecticide, Fungicide, and Rodenticide Act and the Toxic Substances Control Act (TSCA) as the two statutes under which the EPA implements an endocrine screening and testing strategy, and also provides supplementary order authority to require testing (16).

However, by November 1996, laboratories at Texas A&M University, Duke University, the National Institute of Environmental Health Sciences, the Chemical Industry Institute of Toxicology, and Zeneca had tried but failed to reproduce the findings of Arnold et al. (17,18). The Tulane group was also unable to confirm its previous results, and has officially retracted them, stating that "despite the enthusiasm it [the publication] generated, it is clear that any conclusions drawn from this paper must be suspended until such time, if ever, the data can be substantiated" (19). However, the legislative imperative to identify endocrine disruptors and its 2-year timetable remain.

The EPA has established the Endocrine Disruptor Screening and Testing Advisory Committee (EDSTAC) to carry out the congressional mandate. EDSTAC's commission is to recommend a strategy for identifying chemical substances or mixtures in the 70,000 chemicals in the TSCA inventory that could cause any kind of endocrine disruption in either humans or ecological receptors. Not surprisingly, research efforts to examine endocrine disruption abound. The White House's Committee on Environment and Natural Resources' endocrine disruptors working group has identified 394 endocrine disruptor projects funded by 14 federal agencies. The National Institute of Environmental Health Sciences topped the list with 93 studies, the National Cancer Institute had 59, and EPA had 51. Of these, 272 projects (69%) focused on human health, 70 (18%) on ecology, and only 52 (13%) on exposure. By topic, 178 studies looked at reproduction and development, 97 at carcinogenesis, 83 at neurologic effects, 37 at immunologic questions, and 98 at other issues.

Although the issue of endocrine disruptors in the environment increasingly includes agents that may act on androgenic, thyroid, pituitary, and other endocrine systems, the greatest scrutiny to date has been focused on compounds thought to exert estrogenic (agonist) and antiestrogenic (antagonist) effects. The purpose of this chapter is therefore to provide a concise overview of available information on potential effects of environmental xenoestrogens and antiestrogens on human health. Given the rate of publication in this field, this review must be understood to be a snapshot of the state of knowledge at the time of writing.

A WIDE VARIETY OF ENVIRONMENTAL COMPOUNDS EXHIBIT ESTROGENIC AND ANTIESTROGENIC ACTIVITY

EPA defines an environmental endocrine disruptor as "an exogenous agent that interferes with the synthesis, secretion, transport, binding, action, or elimination of natural hormones in the body that are responsible for the maintenance of homeostasis, reproduction, development, and/or behavior" (20). These compounds may mimic, enhance (an agonist), or inhibit (an antagonist) the action of endogenous hormones. As noted by Neubert (21), it is critical to distinguish between qualitative findings that "may be interesting from a scientific point of view, but may have no significance at all for the situation of relevant human exposures." It is thus of especial importance in defining such chemicals from a public and environmental health standpoint that (a) the effect must be manifested at the level of the intact organism, and (b) the effect must be adverse. Thus, Ashby et al. (22) have suggested that an endocrine-disrupting chemical be defined as "an agent that can induce adverse health effects in an intact organism, consequent to disruption of the organism's endocrine system. Specifically, the activity of a chemical in any of the available *in vitro* assays does not define it as an endocrine disruptor. . . ." This point is reinforced by Neubert (21), who emphasizes that "especially when considering the relevance of *in vitro* data, it must be proven that a possible effect also occurs under realistic *in vivo* conditions."

As discussed in this chapter, potential xenoestrogens and antiestrogens include not only synthetic industrial chemicals, but also a wide variety of natural products (Table 27-1). Natural xenoestrogens and antiestrogens include not only phytoestrogens manufactured by plants and mycoestrogens manufactured by fungi, but also polycyclic aromatic hydrocarbons (PAHs), which are naturally occurring products of combustion. Synthetic xenoestrogens and antiestrogens include pharmaceuticals [e.g., tamoxifen and diethylstilbestrol (DES)] and industrial chemicals (e.g., organochlorine pesticides, plasticizers, and detergents) and by-products (e.g., dioxins and furans). It is important to note that, as indicated in Table 27-1, several of the organochlorine compounds implicated as estrogen agonists or antagonists have been banned from use in the United States for decades. In addition, environmental regulations regarding the use and disposal of chemicals have resulted in significantly lower emissions of most industrial compounds and associated by-products. As a result, the concentrations of even persistent chemicals have been generally declining in the environment and in biotic tissues (23–25).

TABLE 27-1. Environmental compounds exhibiting estrogenic and antiestrogenic properties

Compound	Use and source	Estrogenic (+) or antiestrogenic (–) activity
Synthetic chemicals		
o,p'-DDT and its major metabolite, DDE (dichlorodiphenyldichloroethylene)	Insecticide for tobacco and cotton; most uses in the United States prohibited since 1973, but manufacturing for export is permitted.	+
Kepone (decachlorooctahydro-1,3,4-metheno-2H-cyclobuta(cd)pentalene-2-one)	Insecticide for food and nonfood crops, used in household roach traps. No longer produced commercially in the United States.	+
Methoxychlor (2,2-bis(*p*-methoxyphenol)-1,1,1-trichloroethane)	Insecticide against a wide range of pests, including houseflies and mosquitoes, cockroaches, chiggers, and various arthropods commonly found on field crops, vegetables, fruits, stored grain, livestock, and domestic pets.	+
Dieldrin	Insecticide; all uses canceled.	+
Endosulfan	Insecticide for more than 60 food and nonfood crops, especially tobacco, cotton, fruits, lettuce, and tomatoes.	+
Toxaphene (technical chlorinated camphene)	Insecticide for food and nonfood crops; control of livestock ectoparasites. All uses have been banned since 1990.	+
Polychlorinated biphenyls (PCBs)	Dielectric and heat-exchange fluids; manufacture discontinued in the United States in 1976.	+
Hydroxylated PCBs	Metabolic products of PCBs.	±
2,3,7,8-Tetrachlorodibenzo-*p*-dioxin (TCDD) and related compounds	Unwanted by-products in synthesis of chemicals derived from chlorophenols and chlorobenzenes.	–
Phthalate esters	Plasticizers used in the production of polymeric materials such as polyvinyl chloride; produced in extremely large volumes.	+
Bisphenol-A	Used in manufacture of polycarbonate-derived products.	+
Phenol red	pH indicator used in cell culture media.	+
Alkyl phenols	Used for preparation of polyethoxylates in detergents.	+
Naturally occurring chemicals		
Polycyclic aromatic hydrocarbons	Ubiquitous products of combustion.	–
Indole-3-carbinol and related compounds	A major component of cruciferous vegetables such as brussels sprouts and cauliflower.	±
Isoflavonoids and coumestans	Plant compounds with a flavonoid backbone; especially abundant in legumes.	±
Lignans	Synthesized by the action of intestinal microflora on dietary precursors.	±
Zearalenone and related compounds	Mycotoxin.	+

See text for references.

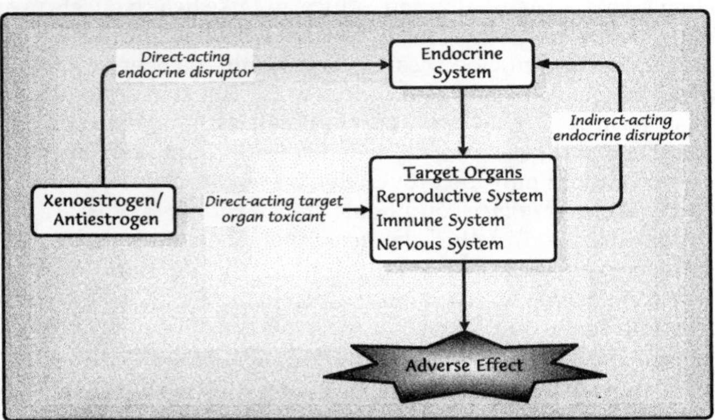

Figure 27-1. Direct and indirect modes of action of xenoestrogens and antiestrogens. (From ref. 26, with permission.)

POSSIBLE MECHANISMS OF ACTION OF XENOESTROGENIC AND ANTIESTROGENIC COMPOUNDS

It must be emphasized that the effects exerted by xenoestrogenic compounds (as well as endogenous hormones) are dependent on and vary with experimental system, dose or concentration, body burden, timing, and duration and timing of exposure. Effects may be reversible or irreversible, of delayed or immediate onset, and of short or long duration. Many components of the endocrine system are functionally interlinked with each other and with other organ systems. The endocrine system is subject to servoregulation via a number of hypothalamo-hypophyseal–target organ feedback loops, and interacts importantly with the immune system. As such, there are many possible target organ sites at which a xenoestrogen could disrupt normal function, any combination of which could be mechanistically involved in the estrogenic or antiestrogenic activity.

Adverse (or therapeutic) effects can arise from either primary (direct) or secondary (indirect) effects on endocrine function (21,26). A direct-acting endocrine disruptor affects the endocrine organ first, resulting in secondary toxicity in other organ systems, whereas an indirect-acting endocrine disruptor affects some other target organ first, influencing the endocrine system to cause indirect effects on other organ systems secondarily. These relationships are shown in Figure 27-1. Effects could occur as a consequence of altered (a) hormone concentration (i.e., hormone synthesis or breakdown, storage and release, transport and clearance), (b) interaction with the hormone receptor (i.e., binding and dissociation kinetics, agonistic versus antagonistic effects), (c) receptor concentration, and (d) hormone-receptor complex interactions with DNA (Fig. 27-2).

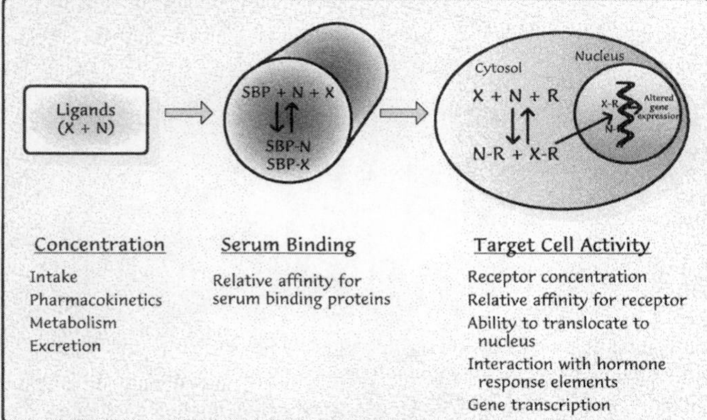

Figure 27-2. Possible loci of xenoestrogen/antiestrogen action. N, endogenous ligand; R, estrogen receptor; SBP, serum binding protein; X, xenoestrogen/antiestrogen.

ENVIRONMENTAL COMPOUNDS WITH ESTROGENIC EFFECTS

A wide range of synthetic chemicals has been shown to exert estrogenic and antiestrogenic effects in various systems (3,4,27) (see Table 27-1). Estrogenic effects are generally attributed to the ability of xenoestrogens to bind, albeit relatively weakly, to the cytosolic estrogen receptor and initiate estrogenic effects on gene expression.

Synthetic Xenoestrogens

The estrogenic potential of organochlorine pesticides, including methoxychlor, DDT and its major metabolite (DDE), and kepone was first reported in the 1960s and 1970s (28–30). The organochlorine pesticides endosulfan, toxaphene, and dieldrin have been reported to exhibit estrogenic activity in MCF-7 human breast cancer cells (31). Other chemicals shown to elicit estrogenic responses in various systems include polychlorinated and polybrominated biphenyls [PCBs and polybromated biphenyls (PBBs)] and hydroxylated PCBs (32–38), phthalate esters (39,40), alkylphenols (41–43), phenol red (44), and bisphenol-A (45) (see Table 27-1).

Natural Xenoestrogens

Many plants produce endocrine-modulating chemicals that are thought to have evolved as part of an astonishingly diverse and effective armamentarium in their phylogenetic war against the kingdom Animalia. A survey of the literature identified 149 "phytoestrogens," nonsteroidal compounds that have structural homology to steroidal estrogens and may behave as either estrogen agonists or antagonists. Two major classes of phytoestrogens exist: isoflavonoids and lignans (see Table 27-1). Although isoflavonoids are formed in a wide variety of edible plants, including dozens that are common components of the human diet (Table 27-2), the lignans are mainly synthesized by the action of intestinal microflora on dietary precursors. In addition, various mycotoxins that are present in the human diet, including zearalenone and related compounds, have demonstrated estrogenicity (46–49).

TABLE 27-2. Common edible plants with estrogenic effects

Barley	Field bean	Plum
Cabbage	Garlic	Pomegranate
Carob	Ginseng	Potato
Carrot	Grapefruit	Rhubarb
Celery	Green pea	Rice
Chick pea	Hops	Safflower
Cinnamon	Kidney bean	Sage
Cloves	Lime	Sesame seed
Coconut	Liquorice	Soybean
Coffee bean	Olive	Sugar beet
Common oat	Parsley	Sunflower
Corn	Parsnip	Wheat
Cumin	Peanut	Wild cherry
Fennel	Pineapple	Wild ginger

The estrogenic effects of flavonoids were first noted in the 1940s, when reproductive disorders in Australian ewes were linked to their consumption of the legume *Trifolium subterraneum*, a species of clover (reviewed in ref. 50). The isoflavonoid phytoestrogens are heterocyclic phenols that are structurally similar to estrogens. They include several structural classes with a common flavonoid backbone: flavones, flavanones, flavonols, isoflavones, and related condensation products (e.g., coumestrol). The four most common isoflavones are formononetin, daidzein, genistein, and biochanin A, which is metabolized to genistein. Formononetin may be metabolized to daidzein, which is further metabolized to equol (a more potent phytoestrogen) and O-desmethylangolensin. Isoflavonoids, which are consumed daily in gram quantities, are especially abundant in legumes (46). Soybeans, the third largest crop in the United States, have received particular attention as sources of phytoestrogens in the human diet. Soybeans contain significant levels of genistein (1,107 mg per kg dry weight) and daidzein (846 mg per kg dry weight) (50). Approximately 80% of the vegetable oil consumed in the United States is from soybeans, with an estimated annual per capita consumption rate of 65 lb per year. In addition, the majority of infant formulas contain soy solids and proteins (50).

The lignans enterolactone and enterodiol were first identified in human urine. These compounds are actually the products of intestinal microbial metabolism of secoisolariciresinol and matairesinol, substances found in whole grains, fibers, flax seeds, fruits, and vegetables. Products of lignan and isoflavone metabolism may be either excreted or absorbed. If absorbed, they may be conjugated with glucuronic acid or sulfate in the liver. The conjugated products may then be either excreted via bile or urine, or deconjugated by intestinal bacteria and absorbed again in a process of enterohepatic recirculation.

ENVIRONMENTAL COMPOUNDS WITH ANTIESTROGENIC EFFECTS

Natural and synthetic chemicals have also been shown to exhibit antiestrogenic activity (see Table 27-1).

Phytoestrogens

Isoflavonoids that bind to the estrogen receptor have also been characterized as antiestrogenic, depending on relative concentration, experimental system, and endpoint. Thus, although isoflavonoids such as luteolin and quercetin antagonized estrogenic responses in the rat uterus and inhibited breast, ovarian, pancreatic, and colon cancer cell proliferation *in vitro* and estrogen-independent mammary tumor growth in mice (51–55), coumestrol, genistein, and zearalenone were found not to be antiestrogenic in transfected HeLa human breast cancer cells (56). The weakly estrogenic isoflavonoid naringenin also exhibited antiestrogenic activity in rats cotreated with estradiol (57). Markaverich et al. characterized coumestrol as an "atypical estrogen" in a paper examining its effects on estrogen receptor function and uterine growth in ovariectomized rats (58). These results illustrate the difficulty of making general statements about the nature and magnitude of effects of these chemicals.

Aryl Hydrocarbon Receptor Agonists

The most potent member of a large family of related chemicals (including polyhalogenated dibenzofurans and some biphenyls) that exert their characteristic effects via binding to the aryl hydrocarbon (Ah) receptor, a member of the steroid hormone receptor superfamily of gene regulatory proteins, is 2,3,7,8-tetrachlorodibenzo-*p*-dioxin (TCDD) (59,60). Ah receptor agonists such as TCDD have exhibited a broad spectrum of antiestrogenic activity in rodent and cell models, including several human breast and other cancer cell lines (61–73). Hydroxylated PCBs, which are estrogenic in some systems, have been shown to have antiestrogenic effects in breast cancer cell lines (74,75). The PAHs and indole-3-carbinol (a major component of cruciferous vegetables such as brussels sprouts and cauliflower) and related compounds also bind to the Ah receptor and exhibit antiestrogenic effects (57,70,76–80).

As with their other effects, Ah receptor binding plays a central role in the antiestrogenic effects exerted by these compounds (70,73,77). A study showed that the antiestrogenic effects exerted by Ah receptor agonists are caused by direct interference of the Ah receptor-ligand complex with binding of the estrogen receptor-ligand complex to genomic estrogen response elements (72).

STRUCTURE-ACTIVITY RELATIONSHIPS

The universe of xenoestrogenic compounds is diverse in structure and potency (81). In addition, the magnitude and nature of effects depend on dose, experimental system, and exposure regime. Therefore, considerable difficulty exists in attempting to reconcile chemical structure with estrogenic (or antiestrogenic) potency (82). For example, the structure-activity relationships (SARs) for estrogenicity and antiestrogenicity for hydroxylated PCBs are shown to be complex and response-specific (74). No SAR can be identified for alkyl polychlorinated dibenzofurans (83). Thus, although useful SARs among discrete chemical series acting by the same mechanism may be discernible in specific systems for specific effects (84), it is unlikely that any general SARs capable of encompassing all categories of endocrine disruptors may be developed (85).

REPORTED EFFECTS OF XENOESTROGENS ON REPRODUCTIVE SYSTEMS

Hormonal influences are essential for normal function at multiple stages of mammalian development, from prenatal until late postnatal life (Fig. 27-3). The processes involved and the effects elicited are characteristic of the particular life stage. In general, the developing organism may be especially sensitive to xenoestrogens; many of the differentiations that occur during the fetal and perinatal period, if perturbed, cannot be compensated for in later life (21).

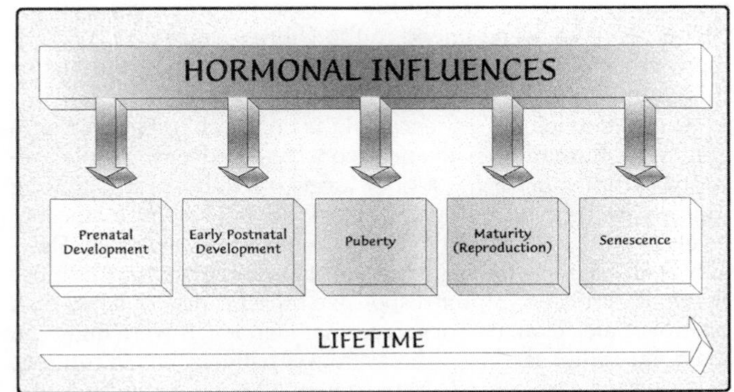

Figure 27-3. Developmental stages at which hormonal influences are essential. (From ref. 21, with permission.)

Female Reproductive System

The reproductive process is orchestrated by sequential hormonal actions in parents and developing young. Thus, significant disturbance of hormonal balance in females may jeopardize the reproductive health of the mother and the developmental and reproductive integrity of her offspring, male and female. A variety of chemicals have been shown to disrupt female reproductive function in experimental animals. Observed effects include abnormal sexual differentiation, ovarian function, fertilization, implantation, and pregnancy. However, with the exception of endometriosis and vaginal and breast cancer, environmental endocrine disruptors have not been implicated as causative agents for serious effects on human female reproduction.

VAGINAL CANCER

The only xenoestrogen for which a causal relationship has been demonstrated is DES, a synthetic estrogen used widely in the United States between the 1940s and 1970 to prevent miscarriage. Administration of the drug before the eighteenth week of pregnancy has been associated with vaginal clear cell adenocarcinoma and other disorders of the reproductive tract (e.g., vaginal adenosis, cervical erosion, and pseudopolyps) in female children (86). Many of the same structural and developmental abnormalities also have been observed in laboratory animals treated with DES (27).

BREAST CANCER

Breast cancer is the second leading cause of cancer deaths in women after lung cancer. The incidence of this disease appears to have increased approximately 1% annually since the 1940s after correcting for improved detection (87), although death rates for breast cancer (and all other cancers except lung) are decreasing in the United States (88,89). A wide variety of risk factors has been associated with human breast cancer, including genetics; age at menarche, menopause, and first birth; diet; socioeconomic status; height; weight; exposure to environmental radiation; and cumulative estrogen exposure (90–93). However, the mechanisms of mammary gland carcinogenesis and the precise roles played in its etiology by chemical carcinogens, radiation, viruses, lifestyle factors, oncogenes, tumor suppressor genes, and exposure to estrogens have yet to be elucidated.

The hypothesized causal role for organochlorine xenoestrogens in breast cancer is based primarily on the results of case-control studies demonstrating correlation between tissue concentrations of certain pesticides (e.g., DDT and related metabolites) and PCBs in cancer patients (4,6,8,91,94,95). Because of their lipophilicity and resistance to metabolism, many of these compounds tend to accumulate in human adipose tissue and are excreted in milk (96–98). Blood levels of these compounds represent highly stable markers of exposure (99,100). However, a number of these chemicals have been banned in the United States and levels of them in the environment and in tissues have been declining in this country (see Table 27-1).

The epidemiologic evidence linking organochlorine xenoestrogens with human breast cancer consists of several small case-control studies reporting higher levels of DDE or PCBs among cancer patients than controls. Wolff et al. (6) linked breast cancer to levels of DDT and related metabolites in serum or tumors. Dewailly et al. (95) reported higher levels of DDE in mammary adipose tissue of estrogen receptor-responsive breast cancer patients than controls. Falck et al. (94) observed that PCB levels were higher in mammary adipose tissue in breast cancer patients than in controls, and a nested case-control study showed that women with serum PBB levels of 2 to 4 parts per billion had a higher estimated risk for breast cancer than women with less than 2 parts per billion (91). However, the hypothesized linkage between organochlorine compounds and human breast cancer is questionable on several grounds (101–103). First, other studies show that levels of these chemicals are not elevated in breast cancer patients relative to controls. A comparison of DDE and PCB levels in mammary adipose tissue from Scandinavian breast cancer patients versus controls showed no significant differences (104). In a nested case-control study designed to evaluate organochlorine levels in patients long before breast cancer diagnosis, adjusting for other known risk factors for breast cancer and stratified across racial and ethnic subpopulations, Krieger et al. (105) concluded that the data do not support the hypothesis that exposure to DDE and PCBs increases risk of breast cancer. The results of a European case-control study with 264 case patients and 341 controls also did not support the hypothesis that DDE increases risk of breast cancer in postmenopausal women in Europe (106). Hunter et al. (107) compared the blood levels of DDE and PCBs in 240 women with breast cancer and matched controls from the Nurses' Health Study. Their results indicated no evidence of a positive association between high levels of plasma DDE or PCBs and a risk of breast cancer (107).

Second, the levels of DDE observed in blood samples collected in 1989 to 1990 for the study of Hunter et al. (107) were similar to those measured in samples obtained between 1985 and 1991 for the study of Wolff et al. (6). However, the median concentrations in samples taken in the late 1960s (before the 1972 ban of DDT) were six times higher (105). This finding is consistent with the continuing decline in DDE levels in the environment and suggests that even the higher levels of DDE present when DDT was used are not related to cancer. This suggestion is reinforced by the findings that no increased risk of breast cancer exists in either women who are occupationally exposed to relatively high levels of PCB (108,109) or women in Mexico, where DDT is still being used, whose mean serum levels of DDE were much higher than those currently prevailing in the United States.

Third, the available data are not compatible with the theory that exposure to DDT and other organochlorines *in utero* or during early childhood constitutes a significant risk factor, as the postmenopausal women who have accounted for most of the increase in the incidence of breast cancer were already adults when these compounds were most widely used in the 1940s and 1950s.

Fourth, the organochlorines are weakly estrogenic compounds, and their contribution to total dietary estrogen equivalents (0.0000025%) is dwarfed by that of phytoestrogens (101). Finally, in three epidemiologic reviews of breast cancer incidence and the possible role of organochlorine chemicals in its etiology, the weight of evidence for an association between organochlorines and human breast cancer was found not compelling (110–112). Robbins et al. (113) concluded that the relatively high incidence of breast cancer in the San Francisco Bay area can be accounted for by known risk factors, including reproductive history and alcohol consumption. Thus, the weight of available evidence does not support a causal role for xenoestrogens in human breast cancer (20,26,102,103).

ENDOMETRIOSIS

Endometriosis is a reproductive and immunologic disease of unknown etiology that often causes infertility. It is characterized by aberrant location of uterine endometrial cells (114). Results of a single study with seven rhesus monkeys suggested a dose-response relationship between dioxin exposure and the development of endometriosis (115). However, a reproductive toxicology study in rhesus monkeys concluded that the incidence and severity of endometriosis lesions was not related to the ingestion of the PCB mixture Aroclor 1254, which contains dioxin-like congeners (15). In addition, no statistically significant correlations between disease status and serum levels of 22 of the most common dioxin, furan, and PCB congeners were found in a clinical comparison of 15 patients with varying severity of endometriosis versus an equal number of age- and location-matched controls. Thus, evidence supporting the hypothesis that dioxin and PCBs are causally related to endometriosis in either humans or monkeys is lacking.

Male Reproductive Effects

Reports that human sperm counts and semen quality are declining have attracted much media and scientific attention, providing a strong impetus for the interest in endocrine disruptors. The actual starting point was papers published in the early 1980s suggesting that donor semen parameters had changed over time (116) and that the fertility of Danish men had declined between 1952 and 1972 (117). However, it was not until the 1992 reports of Brake and Krause (118) and Carlsen et al. (2) that real alarm arose. Carlsen et al. (2) reviewed 61 scientific papers published between 1938 and 1990 and performed a metaanalysis of mean sperm density data on nearly 15,000 men. This analysis revealed what the authors termed a "highly significant" decrease in mean sperm count, from 113 million per mL in 1940 to 66 million per mL in 1990. A simple linear regression analysis of the data showed that, at the calculated rate of decline, all males would have a zero sperm count by 2020. These results appeared to be generally corroborated by other European studies (119–121). Carlsen et al. (2) also linked the declining semen quality with a twofold rise in incidence of testicular cancer over this period, and suggested that a common explanation for the two phenomena might be that estrogens or estrogen-like compounds could be damaging testicular function. Sharpe (122) and Sharpe and Skakkebaek (5) proposed that xenoestrogens are involved in the decline of sperm counts as well as other male reproductive disorders, including prostate cancer, hypospadias, cryptorchidism, and decreased fertility. They also speculated that similar effects on the male fetus, during a vulnerable stage of its development, may be induced by maternal exposure to xenoestrogenic chemicals. Unlike the proposed link between xenoestrogens and breast cancer this contention is not based on observations of increased levels of xenoestrogens in males; rather, it is premised on observations of reproductive system abnormalities in male offspring of women treated with DES during pregnancy. In support of this hypothesis, Sharpe et al. (123) reported a 5% to 15% decrease in testis size and sperm production in male rats whose mothers received low doses of 4-octylphenol and butyl benzyl phthalate during gestation and lactation.

Although biologically plausible and intensely interesting to the news media, this theory has several significant shortcomings. First, other prior (124,125) and subsequent studies (126–128) have shown no decline in semen quality. Second, and of great importance, several other workers have reached quite different conclusions from the study of Carlsen et al. (2) data. Using the same data set, Bromwich et al. (129) pointed out that a change in the lower reference value for normal sperm concentration could have changed donor selection criteria such that men with lower sperm concentrations would have been excluded from earlier studies but included later on. Olsen et al. (130) noted that the individual variability in sperm concentration exceeded the year-to-year changes. Application of different mathematic models to describe the data resulted in very different interpretations (including increased sperm counts) with as good or better correlation (131). The reanalysis of the Carlsen et al. data by Fisch and Goluboff (132) and Fisch et al. (133) revealed marked regional variations in mean sperm concentrations. These authors suggested that the observed variability may be a significant confounding factor in data interpretation. Sherins (134) pointed out that the lack of control for abstinence time before sample collection could be a significant confounding factor.

Third, Ekbom et al. (135) have reported an inverse correlation between decreasing levels of DDE in human milk in Finland and Denmark and rising testicular cancer rates. In addition, although DDE levels in milk in these countries are similar, the age-specific testicular cancer incidence rate is approximately 25 per 100,000 in Denmark but only 5 per 100,000 in Finland (136). Thus, there appears to be no dose-response relationship between estimates of tissue concentration and adverse effects on the male reproductive system.

Fourth, the effects of butyl benzyl phthalate on rat testis size and sperm production observed by Sharpe et al. (123) could not be reproduced by Ashby et al. (137) in a larger follow-up experiment. As noted by Ashby and colleagues (16,138,139), this discrepancy underlines the difficulties inherent in attempting to control and interpret the subtle results of complex endocrine toxicity studies.

Finally, as previously mentioned, the abnormalities observed in male offspring born to women who received high doses of DES during pregnancy in the 1950s, including epididymal cysts, hypoplastic testes, and microphallus (140), have been cited as a major basis for assuming that xenoestrogens are adversely affecting male sexual development and reproductive capacity. Furthermore, the average sperm concentration in DES-exposed men was significantly lower than that in controls. These effects, which appear to be related to reduced testis size, have been replicated in animals (123,139). Despite these anomalies, however, a follow-up study of the DES-exposed men reported no change in fertility compared to controls, based on time to pregnancy (140,141), and no reports have indicated an increase in reproductive tract cancers in them (20).

COMPARATIVE POTENCY OF AND RELATIVE EXPOSURE TO NATURAL AND SYNTHETIC XENOESTROGENS

With regard to the human health significance of existing levels of exposure to environmental xenoestrogens, Neubert (21) makes the important point that "meaningful for humans is only a *quantitative* risk assessment, taking the extent of possible human exposures and the biological potency of the substance into account." Safe (101) examined the hypothesis that dietary xenoestrogens may play a significant role in human reproductive disorders using an estrogen-equivalency factor approach to estimate the relative contribution of synthetic chemicals and naturally occurring phytoestrogens to total estrogenic activity in the human diet. In this approach, the estrogen equivalents (EQs) in any mixture are assumed to be equal to the sum of the product of the concentration of individual compounds (*ECs*) times their potency (*EP*) relative to estradiol:

$$\text{Total EQ}\left[\frac{\mu\text{g}}{\text{day}}\right] = \sum([EC_{1-n}] \times EP_{1-n})$$

Winter (142) estimated a total dietary intake of estrogenic pesticides based on the U.S. Food and Drug Administration's total diet study of approximately 2.5 µg per day for the maximally exposed group (adolescent males aged 14 to 16 years). The average estimated daily intake of all flavonoids in food products was 1,045 mg per day (46). The potencies of xenoestrogens and phytoestrogens relative to that of estradiol were estimated as 0.000001 and 0.0001, respectively, based on *in vitro* study results (101). As shown in Table 27-3, the estimated daily estrogen equivalents derived from phytoestrogens is 104.5 µg per day,

TABLE 27-3. Estimated estrogen equivalents associated with phyto- and xenoestrogenic dietary components and hormonal therapies

Estrogenic compound	Daily intake rate (mg per day)	Relative estrogenic potency	Estrogen equivalents (μg per day)
Flavonoids in foods	1,045,000	0.0001	104.5
Estrogenic pesticides	2.5	0.000001	0.0000025
Birth control pill	—	—	16,675
Postmenopausal therapy	—	—	3,350

Modified from ref. 101, with permission.

whereas that derived from pesticides is only 0.0000025 μg per day (a factor of almost 42 million times lower). Estrogen intakes for various hormonal drug therapies (47) are provided for reference (101). The estrogen equivalents associated with postmenopausal estrogen therapy and birth control pills exceed that of estrogenic pesticides by factors of approximately 1.3 billion and 6.7 billion, respectively (see Table 27-3).

Safe's conclusions have been confirmed by Zava et al. (143), who evaluated the relative estrogen receptor-binding affinity of various endogenous and xenoestrogenic and antiestrogenic compounds in MCF-7 human breast cancer cells, and estimated the approximate concentrations of various endogenous and xenoestrogens in human serum (Table 27-4). These investigators estimated that the phytoestrogen concentration after consumption of a soy meal would be at least 100 times the reported serum concentrations of organochlorine pesticides. Because the phytoestrogens bind to the estrogen receptor with approximately 10-fold greater affinity, the binding of organochlorines such as DDT to the estrogen receptor would be reduced by approximately 1,000-fold (143). Thus, Zava et al. concurred that the high relative concentrations of phytoestrogens are likely to significantly reduce the binding of other weak xenoestrogens to the estrogen receptor (143). However, they also noted that significant differences in the metabolism and pharmacokinetics of phytoestrogens and organochlorines may tend to increase the relative biological impact of the latter.

TABLE 27-4. Approximate concentrations of endogenous estrogens, xenoestrogens, and antiestrogens in human serum

Compound	Relative estrogen receptor-binding affinity	Estimated concentration in human serum (nM)
Natural		
Estradiol	100	0.2–1.0
Therapeutic compounds		
Tamoxifen	0.1	100–1,000
4-Hydroxytamoxifen	1.0	10–100
Plant- and fungus-derived compounds		
Genistein	0.1	0–3,000
Equol	0.1	<100
Quercetin	0.001	<200
Organochlorines		
o,p′-DDT	0.012	2
o,p-DDE (dichlorodiphenyldichloroethylene)	0.006	60
PCB-126	0	4–20
PCB-153	0	0.2–10.0

PCB, polychlorinated biphenyl.
Modified from ref. 172, with permission.

XENOESTROGENS AND ANTIESTROGENS AS ANTICANCER AGENTS

Although much of the public concern about environmental chemicals, including endocrine disruptors, is related to fear that they are a significant cause of human cancer, a large body of data indicates that some xenoestrogens and antiestrogens under certain conditions are actually protective against cancer. Therefore, effective design of studies to evaluate endocrine-disrupting potential and management of associated risks require that these effects also be carefully examined and their mechanisms elucidated.

Synthetic Compounds

TCDD is a well-known antiestrogen (101). Although considered the most potent known carcinogen in some animal species, it is also known to exert anticarcinogenic effects (144). For example, TCDD decreased the formation of mammary and uterine tumors in Sprague-Dawley rats after long-term feeding (145), and inhibited growth of mammary tumors induced by 7,12-dimethylbenzanthracene in the same rat strain (146). TCDD also inhibited estradiol-dependent postconfluent growth of MCF-7 and T47D human breast cancer cells (67,147). Weekly administration of TCDD in mice bearing MCF-7 tumor xenografts resulted in transient tumor growth suppression (67). Pretreatment with PCBs protected rats against liver cancer induced by hepatocarcinogens (148). In addition, PCBs, PBBs, and TCDD all inhibited skin tumor initiation by PAHs (149–152).

Human epidemiologic studies also reveal evidence of anticarcinogenic effects. In a 10-year follow-up of populations exposed to TCDD after a trichlorophenol plant accident near Seveso, Italy, Bertazzi et al. (153) reported that breast cancer incidence was below expectations in the most contaminated areas and that a clear deficit for endometrial cancer was observed in the less contaminated areas. An update of this continuing study found 4 out of 159 possible associations between estimated TCDD exposure and cancer incidence to be statistically significant but no increase for all-cancer mortality or major specific sites (154). Based on a comparison of observations in human epidemiologic studies and the Kociba et al. (145) lifetime rat study, Kayajanian (155) concluded that TCDD is a net anticarcinogen in humans and that dioxin exposure provides substantial prophylactic benefits to many of those destined to develop cancer, even after the cancer has been initiated. Much more work is needed to elucidate the complex interactions of this potent chemical with biological systems. Given the foregoing, it is clear that researchers investigating toxicological mechanisms and regulators attempting to manage risks associated with human exposure must be mindful of the potential for different, even opposite, effects under different circumstances and tailor interventions to effects reasonably expected to occur under relevant human exposure conditions.

Natural Compounds

The natural, plant-derived phytoestrogens have been used medicinally for thousands of years. As discussed earlier in this chapter, the phytoestrogenic isoflavonoids and lignans may exert weak estrogenic and antiestrogenic effects. Isoflavonoids and lignans bind to the estrogen receptor and induce estrogenic or antiestrogenic responses (143,156,157). They have been shown to inhibit the aromatase enzyme that converts androstenedione to estrone (158–161). They also possess antioxidant properties and have been shown to influence not only sex hormone metabolism and activity, but also protein synthesis, intracellular enzymes, growth factor action, malignant cell proliferation, differentiation, and angiogenesis (50,162).

TABLE 27-5. Some studies suggesting possible anti–breast cancer effects of isoflavonoids and lignans in humans

Compound or food	Species or cell type	Effect or result
Diet	Human	Low urinary excretion of phytoestrogens in women with breast cancer
Soy food	Human	High phytoestrogen intake associated with low risk
Soybean chips	Rat	Inhibition of mammary tumor growth
Flax seed	Rat	Protective against breast cancer
Flax seed	Rat	Inhibition of promotional phase
Heated soybean protein isolate	Rat	Inhibition of tumor progression
Genistein	Rat	Suppression of mammary tumor formation
Genistein, biochanin A	MCF-7 and other human breast cancer cells	Competition with estradiol
Daidzein	ZR-75-1 human breast cancer cells	Growth inhibition
Enterolactone	MCF-7 human breast cancer cells	Inhibition of proliferation in the presence of estradiol
Thirteen isoflavonoids, flavonoids, and lignans	MCF-7 human breast cancer cells	Biphasic effects on DNA synthesis
	MDA-MB-231 estrogen-independent human breast cancer cells	Inhibition of DNA synthesis

Modified from ref. 50, with permission.

These properties suggest a role for these natural compounds as anticancer agents, a role that is supported by epidemiologic studies demonstrating that Asian populations, who typically consume a diet that is very rich in the phytoestrogens genistein and daidzein, exhibit a significantly lower rate of hormone-dependent cancers and a much lower incidence of hormone-associated health problems, such as osteoporosis and menopausal symptoms, than do Westerners (16,50,163). For example, breast cancer patients or individuals at high risk for breast cancer typically excrete low amounts of lignans and isoflavonoids (164,165), whereas people in areas with low incidence of hormone-dependent cancers have relatively high levels (165–169). Furthermore, hormone-dependent cancer rates in Asian immigrants to Western countries rise when they assume the typical Western diet (163), suggesting that dietary and not physiologic differences are responsible. *In vitro* studies have shown that phytoestrogens stimulate proliferation of cancer cells in the absence of endogenous estrogens, but inhibit the growth of the same cells in the presence of estradiol (170–172). In addition, the effects of synthetic xenoestrogens and antiestrogens would be expected to be blocked by the comparatively much higher levels of phytoestrogens in the diet (101,102,143). A summary of results suggesting a possible protective role against breast cancer is presented in Table 27-5.

CONCLUSIONS AND FUTURE DIRECTIONS

The wide publication and aggressive promotion of speculative assertions regarding the relationship between environmental chemicals, including endocrine disruptors, and human and ecological health problems has fueled widespread public concern. Public concern has, in turn, spurred establishment by the U.S. government of an ambitious 2-year schedule for development of a screening and testing strategy for chemicals among the 70,000 in the TSCA inventory that may possess endocrine-disrupting activity. Even a cursory review of the burgeoning literature on the often conflicting effects of endocrine disruptors on *in vitro* and *in vivo* systems reveals the daunting complexity of this task. In terms of potential cost, it is instructive to note that the National Toxicology Program has spent hundreds of millions of dollars to investigate the rodent carcinogenicity of only approximately 400 chemicals.

In considering the empirical basis for all this activity, it is important to note that although several etiologic links between heavy exposure to xenobiotics and adverse impacts on wildlife have been confirmed (10–13), available data have, as yet, revealed but one causal relationship between a xenoestrogen and human cancer: the synthetic estrogen DES and vaginal cancer (22,26). Kavlock et al. (26) conducted a comprehensive review of data adduced during an EPA-sponsored workshop held in April 1995 to identify data gaps and establish research priorities related to the principal human health effects tentatively associated with endocrine disruptors: cancer, reproductive toxicity, neurotoxicity, and immunotoxicity. They concluded that no clear relationships exist between any of these effects (some of which, like the alleged decline in human semen quality, remain equivocal) and exposure to xenobiotics (Table 27-6). Ashby et al. (22) further evaluated the database in accordance with Hill's criteria for distinguishing between epidemiologic association and causation (173). This analysis also indicated only tentative associations between human exposure to xenobiotics and health effects (Table 27-7). At the same time, it is clear that dietary and lifestyle habits play an important role in modulating the health effects of greatest concern.

Given the concomitant existence of strong public and regulatory pressure to act and the absence of compelling evidence linking xenoestrogens and antiestrogens (or other endocrine-disrupting chemicals) with adverse human health effects, Ashby et al. (137)

TABLE 27-6. Conclusions and recommendations regarding the association of adverse human health effects with endocrine-disrupting chemicals

Possible human endocrine toxicity	Conclusion and recommendation
Breast cancer	Conflicting data regarding the etiologic roles of DDT, DDE, and PCBs
Ovarian and testicular cancer	No evidence that endocrine-disrupting chemicals are a risk factor
Reduced semen quality and sperm counts	The reality of the effect has not been established
Reproductive deficits	First priority: hypotheses generated from field observations must be tested
Neurologic deficits	First priority: studies to define the biological effects most likely to occur
Immunologic deficits	First priority: studies to determine if there has been an increase in cases of immune dysfunction

DDE, dichlorodiphenyldichloroethylene; PCBs, polychlorinated biphenyls.
Modified from ref. 22, with permission.

TABLE 27-7. Application of Hill's criteria for epidemiologic causation to chemical endocrine toxicities in humans

Hill's criteria for establishing causation	Chemical endocrine toxicities in humans
Strength of evidence	– (except diethylstilbestrol)
Consistency of evidence	–
Specificity of effect	–
Temporality of effect	–
Dose responsiveness of effect	–
Plausibility of effect	+
Coherence with existing knowledge	+
Experimental evidence (in rodents)	?
Analogy (structure activity)	?

–, no toxicity; +, toxicity; ?, unknown.
Modified from ref. 22, with permission.

have identified three interdependent needs that must be addressed individually: (a) confirm the uncertain human and wildlife health effects, (b) evaluate the extent to which endocrine-disrupting chemicals are implicated in these effects, and (c) distinguish effects associated with accidental massive exposures from those expected under general ambient conditions. Progress depends on broad agreement regarding what adverse responses are of concern and development of reliable and practical assays for their detection or prediction. A significant concern is ensuring that the mounting pressure for action does not result in the testing of chemicals merely for the sake of testing, without clear reference to their potential to cause adverse effects under realistic exposure conditions. Because of the immense variability in chemical structure among endocrine-disrupting chemicals, SARs are unlikely to provide a useful screening mechanism in the near future. Accordingly, a rigorously validated *in vitro* test battery that is predictive of significant effects *in vivo* must be developed to assist in screening. This, in turn, requires (a) clear definition of significant adverse effects (as opposed to non-toxic adaptive responses) in animal models whose responses are shown to correspond to those of the receptors of concern (i.e., humans, wildlife) under environmentally realistic exposure conditions (as opposed to the relatively massive dosing typical of toxicologic studies) and (b) identification of positive control chemicals for reference within the assay. If the necessarily gradual and deliberate development of such a rational scientific process is short-circuited by arbitrary time constraints and public misconceptions about sources of risk, results are liable, like those obtained to date, to be inflammatory without being interpretable.

REFERENCES

1. Hodgson E, Mailman RB, Chambers JE. *Dictionary of toxicology.* New York: Van Nostrand Reinhold Company, 1988.
2. Carlsen E, Giwercman A, Keiding N, Skakkebaek NE. Evidence for the decreasing quality of semen during the past 50 years. *BMJ* 1992;305:609–613.
3. Colborn T, vom Saal FS, Soto AM. Developmental effects of endocrine-disrupting chemicals in wildlife and humans. *Environ Health Perspect* 1993;101:378–384.
4. Davis DL, Bradlow HL, Wolff M, Woodruff T, Hoel DG, Anton-Culver H. Medical hypothesis: xenoestrogens as preventable causes of breast cancer. *Environ Health Perspect* 1993;101(5):372–377.
5. Sharpe RM, Skakkebaek NE. Are oestrogens involved in falling sperm counts and disorders of the male reproductive tract? *Lancet* 1993;341:1392–1395.
6. Wolff MS, Toniolo PG, Leel EW, Rivera M, Dubin N. Blood levels of organochlorine residues and risk of breast cancer. *J Natl Cancer Inst* 1993;85:648–652.
7. Birnbaum LS. Endocrine effects of prenatal exposure to PCBs, dioxins, and other xenobiotics: implications for policy and future research. *Environ Health Perspect* 1994;102:676–679.
8. Davis DL, Bradlow HL. Can environmental estrogens cause breast cancer? *Sci Am* 1995;273:166–171.
9. Kelce RW, Stone RC, Laws CS, Gray EL, Kemppainen AJ, Wilson ME. Persistent DDT metabolite *p,p'*-DDE is a potent androgen receptor antagonist. *Nature* 1995;373:581–585.
10. LeBlanc GA. Are environmental sentinels signaling? *Environ Health Perspect* 1995;103:888–890.
11. Rolland R, Gilbertson M, Colborn T. Environmentally induced alterations in development: a focus on wildlife. *Environ Health Perspect* 1995;103:162–167.
12. LeBlanc GA, Bain LJ. Chronic toxicity of environmental contaminants: sentinels and biomarkers. *Environ Health Perspect* 1997;105[Suppl 1]:65–80.
13. Semenza JC, Tolbert PE, Rubin CH, Guillette LJ Jr, Jackson RJ. Reproductive toxins and alligator abnormalities at Lake Apopka, Florida. *Environ Health Perspect* 1997;105:1030–1032.
14. Colborn T, Dumanoski D, Myers JP. *Our stolen future: are we threatening our fertility, intelligence, and survival? A scientific detective story.* New York: Dutton Books, 1996.
15. Arnold SF, Klotz DM, Collins BM, Vonier PM, Guillette LJ Jr, McLachlan JA. Synergistic activation of estrogen receptor with combinations of environmental chemicals. *Science* 1996;272:1489–1492.
16. Ashby J, Elliott BM. Reproducibility of endocrine disruption data. *Regul Toxicol Pharmacol* 1997a;26:94–95.
17. Gaido KW, McDonnell DP, Korach KS, Safe SH. Estrogenic activity of chemical mixtures: Is there synergism? *CIIT Activities* 1997;17:1–7.
18. Ramamoorthy K, Wang F, Chen I-C, et al. Estrogenic activity of a dieldrin/toxaphene mixture in the mouse uterus, MCF-7 human breast cancer cells, and yeast-based estrogen receptor assays: no apparent synergism. *Endocrinology* 1997;188:1520–1527.
19. McLachlan JA. Synergistic effect of environmental estrogens: report withdrawn. *Science* 1997;277:459–463.
20. US Environmental Protection Agency. Special report on environmental endocrine disruption: an effects assessment and analysis. Washington: Office of Research and Development, 1997, EPA/630/R-96/012.
21. Neubert D. Vulnerability of the endocrine system to xenobiotic influence. *Regul Toxicol Pharmacol* 1997;26:9–29.
22. Ashby J, Harris CA, Lefevre PA, Odum J, Routledge EJ, Sumpter J. Synergism between synthetic estrogens? *Nature* 1997b;385:494.
23. Robinson PE, Mack GA, Remmers J, Levy R, Mohadjer L. Trends of PCB, hexachlorobenzene, and benzene hexachloride levels in the adipose tissue of the U.S. population. *Chemosphere* 1990;53:175–192.
24. Giesy JP, Ludwig JP, Tillitt DE. Deformities of birds in the Great Lakes region: assigning causality. *Environ Sci Technol* 1994;28:128A–135A.
25. Wolff MS. Pesticides—how research has succeeded and failed in informing policy: DDT and the link with breast cancer. *Environ Health Perspect* 1995; 103[Suppl 6]:87–91.
26. Kavlock RJ, Daston GP, DeRosa C, et al. Research needs for the risk assessment of health and environmental effects of endocrine disruptors: a report of the U.S. EPA-sponsored workshop. *Environ Health Perspect* 1996;104[Suppl 4]:715–740.
27. McLachlan JA. Functional toxicology: a new approach to detect biologically active xenobiotics. *Environ Health Perspect* 1993;101:386–387.
28. Tullner WW. Uterotrophic action of the insecticide methoxychlor. *Science* 1961;133:647–648.
29. Bitman J, Cecil HC, Harris SJ, Fries GF. Estrogenic activity of o,p'-DDT in the mammalian uterus and avian oviduct. *Science* 1968;162:371–372.
30. Hammond B, Katzenellenbogen BS, Krauthammer N, McConnell J. Estrogenic activity of the insecticide chlordecone (Kepone) and interaction with uterine estrogen receptor. *Proc Natl Acad Sci U S A* 1979;76:6641–6645.
31. Soto AM, Chung KL, Sonnenschein C. The pesticides endosulfan, toxaphene, and dieldrin have estrogenic effects on human estrogen-sensitive cells. *Environ Health Perspect* 1994;102:380–383.
32. Bitman J, Cecil HC, Harris SJ. Biological effects of polychlorinated biphenyls in rats and quail. *Environ Health Perspect* 1972;145–149.
33. Ecobichon DJ, MacKenzie DO. The uterotropic activity of commercial and isomerically pure chlorobiphenyls in the rat. *Res Commun Chem Pathol Pharmacol* 1974;9:85–95.
34. Korach KS, Sarver P, Chae K, McLachlan JA, McKinney JD. Estrogen receptor-binding activity of polychlorinated hydroxybiphenyls: conformationally restricted structural probes. *Mol Pharmacol* 1988;33:120–126.
35. Jansen HT, Cooke PS, Porcelli J, Liu TC, Hansen LG. Estrogenic and antiestrogenic actions of PCBs in the female rat: *in vitro* and *in vivo* studies. *Reprod Toxicol* 1993;7:237–248.
36. McKinney JD, Waller CL. Polychlorinated biphenyls as hormonally active structural analogues. *Environ Health Perspect* 1994;102:290–297.
37. Soontornchat S, Li M-H, Cooke PS, Hansen LG. Toxicokinetic and toxicodynamic influences on endocrine disruption by polychlorinated biphenyls. *Environ Health Perspect* 1994;102:568–571.
38. Waller CL, Minor DL, McKinney JD. Using three-dimensional quantitative structure-activity relationships to examine estrogen receptor binding affinities of polychlorinated hydroxybiphenyls. *Environ Health Perspect* 1995; 103:702–707.
39. Jobling S, Reynolds T, White R, Parker MG, Sumpter JP. A variety of environmentally persistent chemicals, including some phthalate plasticizers, are weakly estrogenic. *Environ Health Perspect* 1995;103(6):582–587.
40. Harris CA, Henttu P, Parker MG, Sumpter JP. The estrogenic activity of phthalate esters *in vitro*. *Environ Health Perspect* 1997;105:802–811.
41. Soto AM, Justicia H, Wray JW, Sonnenschein C. p-Nonyl-phenol: an estrogenic xenobiotic released from "modified" polystyrene. *Environ Health Perspect* 1991;92:167–173.

42. Jobling S, Sumpter JP. Detergent components in sewage effluent are weakly estrogenic to fish: an *in vitro* study using rainbow trout (*Oncorhynchus mykiss*) hepatocytes. *Aquat Toxicol* 1993;27:361–372.
43. White R, Jobling S, Hoare SA, Sumpter JP, Parker MG. Environmentally persistent alkylphenolic compounds are estrogenic. *Endocrinology* 1993;135:175–182.
44. Berthois Y, Katzenellenbogen JA, Katzenellenbogen BS. Phenol red in tissue culture media is a weak estrogen: implications concerning the study of estrogen-responsive cells in culture. *Proc Natl Acad Sci U S A* 1986;83:2496–2500.
45. Krishnan AV, Stathis P, Permuth SF, Tokes L. Bisphenol-A: an estrogenic substance is released from polycarbonate flasks during autoclaving. *Endocrinology* 1993;132:2279–2286.
46. Kuhnau J. The flavonoids. A class of semi-essential food components: their role in human nutrition. *World Rev Nutr Diet* 1976;24:117118–117191.
47. Verdeal K, Ryan DS. Naturally occurring estrogens in plant foodstuffs—a review. *J Food Protection* 1979;42:577–583.
48. Whitten PL, Naftolin F. Dietary estrogens: a biologically active background for estrogen action. In: Hochberg RB, Naftolin F, eds. *The new biology of steroid hormones*. New York: Raven Press, 1991:155–167.
49. Miksicek RJ. Commonly occurring plant flavonoids have estrogenic activity. *Mol Endocrinology* 1993;44:37–43.
50. Adlercreutz H. Phytoestrogens: epidemiology and a possible role in cancer protection. *Environ Health Perspect* 1995;103[Suppl 7]:103–112.
51. Markaverich BM, Roberts RR, Alejandro MA, Johnson GA, Middleditch BS, Clark JH. Bioflavonoid interaction with rat uterine type II binding sites and cell growth inhibition. *J Steroid Biochem* 1988;30:71–78.
52. Carbone A, Ranelletti FO, Rinelli A, et al. Type II estrogen receptor in the papillary cystic tumor of the pancreas. *Am J Cancer Res* 1989;92:572–576.
53. Piantelli M, Ricci R, Larocca LM, et al. Type II estrogen binding sites in human colorectal carcinoma. *J Clin Pathol* 1990;43:1004–1006.
54. Scambia G, Ranelletti FO, Benedetti Panici P, et al. Inhibitory effects of quercetin on OVCA 433 cells and the presence of type II oestrogen binding sites in primary ovarian tumors and cultured cells. *Br J Cancer* 1989;62:942–946.
55. Scambia G, Ranelletti FO, Benedetti Panici P, et al. Quercetin inhibits the growth of multidrug-resistant estrogen-receptor negative MCF-7 human breast cancer cell line expressing type II estrogen-binding sites. *Cancer Chemother Pharmacol* 1991;28:255–258.
56. Mäkelä S, Davis VL, Tally WC, et al. Dietary estrogens act through estrogen receptor-mediated processes and show no antiestrogenicity in cultured breast cancer cells. *Environ Health Perspect* 1994;102:572–578.
57. Ruh MF, Zacharewski T, Connor K, Howell J, Chen I, Safe S. Naringenin: a weakly estrogenic bioflavonoid that exhibits antiestrogenic activity. *Biochem Pharmacol* 1995;50:1485–1493.
58. Markaverich BM, Webb B, Densmore CL, Gregory RR. Effects of coumestrol on estrogen receptor function and uterine growth in ovariectomized rats. *Environ Health Perspect* 1995;103:574–581.
59. Landers JP, Bunce NJ. The Ah receptor and the mechanism of dioxin toxicity. *Biochem J* 1991;276:273–287.
60. Safe S, Krishnan V. Cellular and molecular biology of aryl hydrocarbon (Ah) receptor-mediated gene expression. *Arch Toxicol Suppl* 1995;17:99–115.
61. Krishnan V, Porter W, Santostefano M, Wang X, Safe S. Molecular mechanism of inhibition of estrogen-induced cathepsin D gene expression by 2,3,7,8-tetrachlorodibenzo-*p*-dioxin (TCDD) in MCF-7 cells. *Mol Cell Biol* 1995;15:6710–6719.
62. Astroff B, Rowlands C, Dickerson R, Safe S. 2,3,7,8-Tetrachlorodibenzo-*p*-dioxin inhibition of 17J-estradiol-induced increases in rat uterine EGF receptor binding activity and gene expression. *Mol Cell Endocrinol* 1990;72:247–252.
63. Astroff B, Safe S. 2,3,7,8-Tetrachlorodibenzo-*p*-dioxin as an antiestrogen: effect on rat uterine peroxidase activity. *Biochem Pharmacol* 1990;39:485–488.
64. Biegel L, Safe S. Effects of 2,3,7,8-tetrachlorodibenzo-*p*-dioxin (TCDD) on cell growth and the secretion of the estrogen-induced 34-, 52-, and 160-kDa proteins in human breast cancer cells. *J Steroid Biochem Mol Biol* 1990;37:725–732.
65. Safe S, Astroff B, Harris M, et al. 2,3,7,8-Tetrachlorodibenzo-*p*-dioxin (TCDD) and related compounds as antiestrogens: characterization and mechanism of action. *Pharmacol Toxicol* 1991;69:400–409.
66. DeVito MJ, Thomas T, Martin E, Umbreit TH, Gallo MA. Antiestrogenic action of 2,3,7,8-tetrachlorodibenzo-*p*-dioxin: tissue-specific regulation of estrogen receptor in CD1 mice. *Toxicol Appl Pharmacol* 1992;113:284–292.
67. Gierthy JF, Bennett JA, Bradley LM, Cutler DS. Correlation of *in vitro* and *in vivo* growth suppression of MCF-7 human breast cancer by 2,3,7,8-tetrachlorodibenzo-*p*-dioxin. *Cancer Res* 1993;53:3149–3153.
68. Krishnan V, Safe S. Polychlorinated biphenyls (PCBs), dibenzo-*p*-dioxins, (PCDDs) and dibenzofurans (PCDFs) as antiestrogens in MCF-7 human breast cancer cells: quantitative structure-activity relationships. *Toxicol Appl Pharmacol* 1993;120:55–61.
69. Rowlands C, Krishnan V, Wang X, et al. Characterization of the aryl hydrocarbon receptor and aryl hydrocarbon responsiveness in human ovarian carcinoma cell lines. *Cancer Res* 1993;53:1802–1807.
70. Harper N, Wang X, Liu H, Safe S. Inhibition of estrogen-induced progesterone receptor in MCF-7 human breast cancer cells by aryl hydrocarbon (Ah) receptor agonists. *Mol Cell Endocrinol* 1994;104:47–55.
71. Zacharewski T, Bondy K, McDonell P, Wu ZF. Antiestrogenic effects of 2,3,7,8-tetrachlorodibenzo-*p*-dioxin on 17J-estradiol-induced pS2 expression. *Cancer Res* 1994;54:2707–2713.
72. Kharat I, Saatcioglu F. Antiestrogenic effects of 2,3,7,8-tetrachlorodibenzo-*p*-dioxin are mediated by direct transcriptional interference with the liganded estrogen receptor. Cross-talk between aryl hydrocarbon- and estrogen-mediated signaling. *J Biol Chem* 1996;271:10533–10537.
73. Nodland KI, Wormke M, Safe S. Inhibition of estrogen-induced activity by 2,3,7,8-tetrachlorodibenzo-*p*-dioxin (TCDD) in the MCF-7 human breast cancer and other cell lines transfected with vitellogenin A2 promoter constructs. *Arch Biochem Biophys* 1997;338:67–72.
74. Connor K, Ramamoorthy K, Moore M, et al. Hydroxylated polychlorinated biphenyls (PCBs) as estrogens and antiestrogens: structure-activity relationships. *Toxicol Appl Pharmacol* 1997;145:111–123.
75. Moore M, Mustain M, Daniel K, et al. Antiestrogenic activity of hydroxylated polychlorinated biphenyl congeners identified in human serum. *Toxicol Appl Pharmacol* 1997;142:160–168.
76. Bjeldanes L, Kim J-Y, Grose K, Bartholomew J, Bradfield C. Aromatic hydrocarbon responsiveness—receptor agonists generated from indole-3-carbinol *in vitro* and *in vivo*: comparisons with 2,3,7,8-tetrachlorodibenzo-*p*- dioxin. *Proc Natl Acad Sci U S A* 1991;88:9543–9547.
77. Chaloupka K, Krishnan V, Safe S. Polynuclear aromatic hydrocarbon carcinogens as antiestrogens in MCF-7 human breast cancer cells: role of the Ah receptor. *Carcinogenesis* 1992;13:2223–2239.
78. Liu H, Wormke M, Safe S, Bjeldanes LF. Indole[3,2-b]carbazole: a dietary-derived factor that exhibits both antiestrogenic and estrogenic activity. *J Natl Cancer Inst* 1994;86:1758–1765.
79. Tiwari RK, Guo L, Bradlow HL, Telang NT, Osborne MP. Selective responsiveness of breast cancer cells to indole-3-carbinol, a chemopreventative agent. *J Natl Cancer Inst* 1994;86:126–131.
80. Chen I, Safe S, Bjeldanes L. Indole-3-carbinol and diindolylmethane as aryl hydrocarbon (Ah) receptor agonists and antagonists in T47D human breast cancer cells. *Biochem Pharmacol* 1996;51:1069–1076.
81. Lucier GW. Dose-response relationships for endocrine disruptors: what we know and what we don't know. *Regul Toxicol Pharmacol* 1997;26:34–35.
82. Katzenellenbogen JA. The structural pervasiveness of estrogenic activity. *Environ Health Perspect* 1995;103[Suppl 7]:99–101.
83. Sun G, Safe S. Antiestrogenic activities of alternate-substituted polychlorinated dibenzofurans in MCF-7 human breast cancer cells. *Cancer Chemother Pharmacol* 1997;40:239–244.
84. Tong W, Perkins R, Strelitz R, et al. Quantitative structure-activity relationships (QSARs) for estrogen binding to the estrogen receptor: predictions across species. *Environ Health Perspect* 1997;105:1116–1124.
85. Ashby J, Houthoff E, Kennedy SJ, et al. The challenge posed by endocrine disrupting chemicals. *Environ Health Perspect* 1997;105(2):164–169.
86. Poskanzer D, Herbst A. Epidemiology of vaginal adenosis and adenocarcinoma associated with exposure to stilbestrol *in utero*. *Cancer* 1977;39:1892–1895.
87. Feuer EJ, Wun L-M. How much of the recent rise in breast cancer can be explained by increases in mammography utilization? A dynamic population model approach. *Am J Epidemiol* 1992;136:1423–1436.
88. Peto R, Lopez AD, Boreham J, Thun M, Heath C Jr. *Mortality from smoking in developed countries 1950–2000*. Oxford, UK: Oxford University Press, 1994.
89. Ames BN, Gold LS. The causes and prevention of cancer: gaining perspective. *Environ Health Perspect* 1997;105[Suppl 4]:865–873.
90. Harris JR, Lippman ME, Veronesi U, Willett W. Breast cancer (first of three parts). *N Engl J Med* 1992;327(5):319–328.
91. Henderson AK, Rosen D, Miller GL, et al. Breast cancer among women exposed to polybrominated biphenyls. *Epidemiology* 1995;6(5):554–546.
92. Hunter DJ, Willett WC. Diet, body size, and breast cancer. *Epidemiol Rev* 1993;15:110–132.
93. Hulka BS, Liu ET, Lininger RA. Steroid hormones and risk of breast cancer. *Cancer* 1994;74:1111–1124.
94. Falck F, Ricci A, Wolff MS, Godbold J, Deckers P. Pesticides and polychlorinated biphenyl residues in human breast lipids and their relation to breast cancer. *Arch Environ Health* 1992;47:143–146.
95. Dewailly E, Dodin S, Verreault R, et al. High organochlorine body burden in women with estrogen receptor-positive breast cancer. *J Natl Cancer Inst* 1994;86:232–234.
96. Rogan WJ, Gladen BC, McKinney JD, et al. Polychlorinated biphenyls (PCBs) and dichlorodiphenyl dichloroethane (DDE) in human milk: effects of maternal factors and previous lactation. *Am J Public Health* 1986;76:172–177.
97. Rogan WJ, Gladen BC, McKinney JD, et al. Polychlorinated biphenyls (PCBs) and dichlorodiphenyl dichloroethane (DDE) in human milk; effects on growth, morbidity, and duration of lactation. *Am J Public Health* 1987;77:1294–1297.
98. Savage EP, Keefe TJ, Tessari JD, et al. National study of chlorinated hydrocarbon insecticide residues in human milk, USA. I. Geographic distribution of dieldrin, heptachlor, heptachlor epoxide, chlordane, oxychlordane, and mirex. *Am J Epidemiol* 1981;113:413–422.
99. Gammon MD, Wolff MS, Neugut AI, et al. Treatment for breast cancer and blood levels of chlorinated hydrocarbons. *Cancer Epidemiol Biomarkers Prev* 1996;5:467–471.
100. Gammon MD, Wolff MS, Neugut AI, et al. Temporal variation in chlorinated hydrocarbons in healthy women. *Cancer Epidemiol Biomarkers Prev* 1997;6: 327–332.
101. Safe SH. Environmental and dietary estrogens and human health: Is there a problem? *Environ Health Perspect* 1995;103:346–351.
102. Safe SH. Is there an association between exposure to environmental estrogens and breast cancer? *Environ Health Perspect* 1997a;105[Suppl 3]:675–678.
103. Safe SH. Xenoestrogens and breast cancer. *New Engl J Med* 1997b;337:1303–1304.
104. Unger M, Kiaer H, Blichert-Toft M, Olsen J, Clausen J. Organochlorine compounds in human breast fat from deceased with and without breast cancer

and in biopsy material from newly diagnosed patients undergoing breast surgery. *Environ Res* 1984;34:24–28.

105. Krieger N, Wolff MS, Hiatt RA, Rivera M, Vogelman J, Orentreich N. Breast cancer and serum organochlorines: a prospective study among white, black, and Asian women. *J Natl Cancer Inst* 1994;86:589–599.
106. van't Veer P, Lobbezoo IE, Martin-Moreno JM, et al. DDT (dicophane) and postmenopausal breast cancer in Europe: case-control study. *BMJ* 1997;315:81–85.
107. Hunter DJ, Hankinson SE, Laden F, et al. Plasma organochlorine levels and the risk of breast cancer. *New Engl J Med* 1997;337:1253–1258.
108. Brown DP. Mortality of workers exposed to polychlorinated biphenyls—an update. *Arch Environ Health* 1987;42:333–339.
109. Adami HO, Lipworth L, Titusernstoff L, et al. Organochlorine compounds and estrogen-related cancers in women. *Cancer Causes Control* 1995;6:551–566.
110. Key T, Reeves G. Organochlorines in the environment and breast cancer. *BMJ* 1994;308:1520–1521.
111. Houghton DL, Ritter L. Organochlorine residues and risk of breast cancer. *J Am Coll Toxicol* 1995;14:71–89.
112. Ahlborg UG, Lipworth L, Titusernstoff L, et al. Organochlorine compounds in relation to breast cancer, endometrial cancer, and endometriosis: an assessment of the biological and epidemiological evidence. *Crit Rev Toxicol* 1995;25:463–531.
113. Robbins AS, Bresciani S, Kelsey JL. Regional differences in known risk factors and the higher incidence of breast cancer in San Francisco. *J Natl Cancer Inst* 1997;89:960–965.
114. Olive DL, Schwartz LB. Endometriosis. *N Engl J Med* 1993;328:1759–1769.
115. Rier SE, Martin DC, Bowman RE, Dmowski WP, Becker JL. Endometriosis in Rhesus monkeys (*Macaca mulatta*) following chronic exposure to 2,3,7,8-tetrachlorodibenzo-*p*-dioxin. *Fund Appl Toxicol* 1993;21:433–441.
116. Leto S, Fresnilli FJ. Changing parameters of donor semen. *Fertil Steril* 1981;36:766–770.
117. Bostofee E, Serup J, Rebbe H. Has the fertility of Danish men declined through the years in terms of semen quality? *Int J Fertil* 1983;28:91–95.
118. Brake A, Krause W. Decreasing quality of semen. *BMJ* 1992;305:1498.
119. Auger J, Kunstmann JM, Czyglik F, Jouannet P. Decline in semen quality among fertile men in Paris during the past 20 years [see comments]. *New Engl J Med* 1995;332:281–285.
120. Irvine S, Cawood E, Richardson D, MacDonald E, Aitken J. Evidence of deteriorating semen quality in the United Kingdom: birth cohort study in 577 men in Scotland over 11 years [see comments]. *BMJ* 1996;312:467–471.
121. Van Waeleghem K, DeClercq N, Vermeulen L, Schoonjans F, Comhaire F. Deterioration of sperm quality in young healthy Belgian men. *Hum Reprod* 1996;11:325–329.
122. Sharpe RM. Declining sperm counts in men—is there an endocrine cause? *J Endocrinol* 1993;136:357–360.
123. Sharpe RM, Fisher JS, Millar MM, Jobling S, Sumpter JP. Gestational and lactational exposure of rats to xenoestrogens results in reduced testicular size and sperm production. *Environ Health Perspect* 1995;103:1136–1143.
124. Smith KD, Steinberger E. What is oligospermia? In: Troen P, Nankin HR, eds. *The testis in normal and infertile men*. New York: Raven Press, 1977:489–503.
125. MacLeod J, Wang Y. Male fertility potential in terms of semen quality: a review of the past, a study of the present. *Fertil Steril* 1979;31:103–116.
126. Suominen J, Vierula M. Semen quality of Finnish men. *BMJ* 1993;306:1579.
127. Paulsen CA, Berman NG, Wang C. Data from men in the greater Seattle area reveal no downward trend in semen quality: further evidence that deterioration of semen quality is not geographically uniform. *Fertil Steril* 1996;65:1015–1020.
128. Bujan L, Mansat A, Pontonnier F, Mieusset R. Time series analysis of sperm concentration in fertile men in Toulouse, France, between 1977 and 1992. *BMJ* 1996;312:471–472.
129. Bromwich P, Cohen J, Stewart I, Walker A. Decline in sperm counts: an artefact of changed reference range of "normal?" *BMJ* 1994;309:19–22.
130. Olsen GW, Ross CE, Bodner KM, Lipschultz LI. Sperm decline—real or artifact? A reply of the authors. *Fertil Steril* 1996;65:451–453.
131. Olsen GW, Bodner KM, Ramlow JM, Ross CE, Lipschultz LI. Have sperm counts been reduced 50 percent in 50 years? A statistical model revisited. *Fertil Steril* 1995;63:887–893.
132. Fisch H, Goluboff ET, Olson JH, Feldshuh J, Broder SJ, Barad DH. Semen analyses in 1,283 men from the United States over a 25-year period: no decline in quality [see comments]. *Fertil Steril* 1996;65:1009–1014.
133. Fisch H, Goluboff ET. Geographic variations in sperm counts: a potential cause of bias in studies of semen quality. *Fertil Steril* 1996;65:1044–1046.
134. Sherins RJ. Are semen quality and male fertility changing? *N Engl J Med* 1995;332:327–328.
135. Ekbom A, Wicklund-Glynn A, Adami HO. DDT and testicular cancer. *Nature* 1996;347:553–554.
136. Adami HO, Bergstrom R, Mohner M, et al. Testicular cancer in nine northern European countries. *Int J Cancer* 1994;59:33–38.
137. Ashby J, Odum J, Tinwell H, Lefevre PA. Assessing the risks of adverse endocrine-mediated effects: Where to from here? *Regul Toxicol Pharmacol* 1997e;26:80–93.
138. Ashby J, Lefevre PA, Odum J, et al. Failure to confirm estrogenic activity for benzoic acid and clofibrate: implications for lists of endocrine-disrupting agents. *Regul Toxicol Pharmacol* 1997d;26:96–101.
139. Ashby J, Tinwell H, Lefevre PA, et al. Normal sexual development of rats exposed to butyl benzyl phthalate from conception to weaning. *Regul Toxicol Pharmacol* 1997;26:102–188.
140. Wilcox AJ, Baird DD, Weinberg CR, Hornsby PP, Herbst AL. Fertility in men exposed prenatally to diethylstilbestrol. *New Engl J Med* 1995;332:1411–1416.
141. Leary FJ, Resseguie LJ, Kurland LT, O'Brien PC, Emslander RF, Noller KL. Males exposed *in utero* to diethylstilbestrol. *JAMA* 1984;252:2894–2989.
142. Winter CK. Dietary pesticide risk assessment. *Rev Environ Contam Toxicol* 1992;127:23–67.
143. Zava DT, Blen M, Duwe G. Estrogenic activity of natural and synthetic estrogens in human breast cancer cells in culture. *Environ Health Perspect* 1997;105[Suppl 3]:637–645.
144. US Environmental Protection Agency. Health assessment document for 2,3,7,8-tetrachlorodibenzo-*p*-dioxin (TCDD) and related compounds, volumes I–III. Washington: EPA, 1994.
145. Kociba RJ, Keyes DG, Beger JE, et al. Results of a 2-year chronic toxicity and oncogenicity study of 2,3,7,8-tetrachlorodibenzo-*p*-dioxin (TCDD) in rats. *Toxicol Appl Pharmacol* 1978;46:279–303.
146. Holcomb M, Safe S. Inhibition of 7,12-dimethylbenzanthracene-induced rat mammary tumor growth by 2,3,7,8-tetrachlorodibenzo-*p*-dioxin. *Cancer Lett* 1994;82:43–47.
147. Fernandez P, Safe S. Growth inhibitory and antimitogenic activity of 2,3,7,8-tetrachlorodibenzo-*p*-dioxin (TCDD) in T47D human breast cancer cells. *Toxicol Lett* 1992;61:185–197.
148. Makiura S, Aoe H, Sugihara S, Hirao K, Arai M, Ito N. Inhibitory effect of polychlorinated biphenyl on liver tumorigenesis in rats treated with 3'-methyl-4-dimethylaminoazobenzene, *N*-2-fluorenyl-acetamide and diethylnitrosamine. *J Natl Cancer Inst* 1974;53:1253–1257.
149. Berry DL, Slaga TJ, DiGiovanni J, Juchau MR. Studies with chlorinated dibenzo-*p*-dioxins, polybrominated biphenyls, and polychlorinated biphenyls in a two-stage system of mouse skin tumorigenesis: potent anticarcinogenic effects. *Ann N Y Acad Sci* 1979;320:405–414.
150. Cohen GM, Bracken WM, Iyer RP, Berry DL, Selkirk JK, Slaga TJ. Anticarcinogenic effects of 2,3,7,8-tetrachlorodibenzo-*p*-dioxin on benzo(a)pyrene and 7,12-dimethylbenz(a)anthracene tumor initiation and its relationship to DNA binding. *Cancer Res* 1979;39:4027–4033.
151. DiGiovanni J, Berry DL, Juchau MR, Slaga TJ. 2,3,7,8-Tetrachlorodibenzo-*p*-dioxin: potent anticarcinogenic activity in CD-1 mice. *Biochem Biophys Res Commun* 1979;86:577–584.
152. DiGiovanni J, Berry DL, Gleason GL, Kishore GS, Slaga TJ. Time-dependent inhibition by 2,3,7,8-tetrachlorodibenzo-*p*-dioxin of skin tumorigenesis with polycyclic hydrocarbons. *Cancer Res* 1980;40:1580–1587.
153. Bertazzi A, Pesatori AC, Consonni D, Tironi A, Landi MT, Zocchetti C. Cancer incidence in a population accidentally exposed to 2,3,7,8-tetrachlorodibenzo-para-dioxin. *Epidemiology* 1993;4:398–406.
154. Bertazzi PA, Zocchetti C, Guercilena S, et al. Dioxin exposure and cancer risk: a 15-year mortality study after the "Seveso accident." *Epidemiology* 1997;8:646–652.
155. Kayajanian G. Dioxin is a promoter blocker, a promoter, and a net anticarcinogen. *Regul Toxicol Pharmacol* 1997;26:134–137.
156. Martin PM, Horwitz KB, Ruyan DS, McGuire WL. Phytoestrogen interaction with estrogen receptors in human breast cancer cells. *Endocrinology* 1978;103:1860–1867.
157. Eckert RL, Katzenellenbogen BS. Effects of estrogens and antiestrogens on estrogen receptor dynamics and the induction of progesterone receptor in MCF7 human breast cancer cells. *Cancer Res* 1982;42:139–144.
158. Kellis JT Jr., Vickery LE. Inhibition of human estrogen synthetase (aromatase) by flavones. *Science* 1984;225:1032–1034.
159. Adlercreutz H, Bannwart C, Wähälä K, et al. Inhibition of human aromatase by mammalian lignans and isoflavonoid phytoestrogens. *J Steroid Biochem Mol Biol* 1993;44:147–153.
160. Campbell DR, Kurzer MS. Flavonoid inhibition of aromatase enzyme activity in human preadipocytes. *J Steroid Biochem Mol Biol* 1993;46:381–388.
161. Wang C, Mäkelä T, Hase T, Adlercreutz H, Kurzer MS. Lignans and isoflavonoids inhibit aromatase enzyme in human preadipocytes. *J Steroid Biochem Mol Biol* 1994;50:205–212.
162. Knight DC, Eden JA. A review of the clinical effects of phytoestrogens. *Obstet Gynecol* 1996;87:897–904.
163. Adlercreutz CH, Goldin BR, Gorbach SL, et al. Soybean phytoestrogen intake and cancer risk. *J Nutr* 1995;125[Suppl 3]:757S–770S.
164. Adlercreutz H, Fotsis T, Heikkinen R, et al. Excretion of the lignans enterolactone and enterodiol and of equol in omnivorous and vegetarian women and in women with breast cancer. *Lancet* 1982;2:1295–1299.
165. Adlercreutz H, Höckerstedt K, Bannwart C, Hämäläinen E, Fotsis T, Bloigu S. Association between dietary fiber, urinary excretion of lignans and isoflavonic phytoestrogens, and plasma non-protein bound sex hormones in relation to breast cancer. In: Bresciani F, King RTB, Lippman ME, Raynaud JP, eds. *Progress in cancer research and therapy.* Volume 35: hormones and cancer. New York: Raven Press, 1988:409–412.
166. Adlercreutz H, Fotsis T, Bannwart C, et al. Determination of urinary lignans and phytoestrogen metabolites, potential antiestrogens and anticarcinogens, in urine of women on various habitual diets. *J Steroid Biochem* 1986;25:791–797.
167. Adlercreutz H, Höckerstedt K, Bannwart C, et al. Effect of dietary components, including lignans and phytoestrogens, on enterohepatic circulation and liver metabolism of estrogens, and on sex hormone binding globulin (SHBG). *J Steroid Biochem* 1987;27:1135–1144.

168. Adlercreutz H, Honjo H, Higashi A, et al. Urinary excretion of lignans and isoflavonoid phytoestrogens in Japanese men and women consuming traditional Japanese diet. *Am J Clin Nutr* 1991;54:1093–1100.
169. Adlercreutz H, Hämäläinen E, Gorbach S, Goldin B. Dietary phyto-oestrogens and the menopause in Japan. *Lancet* 1992;339:1233.
170. Mousavi Y, Adlercreutz H. Enterolactone and estradiol inhibit each other's proliferative effect on MCF-7 breast cancer cells in culture. *J Steroid Biochem Mol Biol* 1992;41:615–619.
171. Wang C, Kurzer MS. Phytoestrogen concentration determines effects on DNA synthesis in human breast cancer cells. *Nutr Cancer* 1997;28:236–247.
172. Zava DT, Duwe G. Estrogenic and antiproliferative properties of genistein and other flavonoids in human breast cancer cells *in vitro*. *Nutr Cancer* 1997; 27:31–40.
173. Hill AB. The environment and disease: association or causation? *Proc R Soc Med* 1965;59:295–300.

CHAPTER 28
Clinical Hematotoxicology

John B. Sullivan, Jr., Janet S. Weiss, and Gary R. Krieger

The hematopoietic system consists of blood, bone marrow, vasculature, and various organs, such as the spleen and lymph nodes. Bone marrow provides the microenvironment that induces stem cell differentiation into blood cell lines. Cytokines are proteins that are essential to the production and behavior of hematopoietic cells, that control stem cell replication, clonal selection, maturation rate, and growth inhibition, and that are involved with other interleukins and interferons as biological response modifiers (1). Blood cells consist of the circulating cellular elements of white blood cells (WBCs), red blood cells (RBCs), and platelets.

ANATOMIC AND CELLULAR FEATURES OF THE HEMATOPOIETIC SYSTEM

Bone Marrow

The bone marrow stroma consists of a matrix of interlaced strands of fibroblasts and endothelial cells. Embedded in this meshwork are closely packed nests or clusters of hematopoietic cells admixed with adipose tissue. Immediately adjacent to this network are vascular sinusoids, which provide access for mature cells to migrate into the general circulation. Colonies of erythroid, myeloid, and lymphoid cells and megakaryocytes proliferate from stem cells (Fig. 28-1). The process of hematopoiesis allows a small number of stem cells to produce progressively more mature progenitor cells, which in turn generate mature blood cells. The most primitive stem cell is the pluripotential stem cell, which has the capacity to generate progenitor cells in all blood cell lineages. Cellular progenitors divide, and each generation doubles the number of its predecessor generation. The cell line sequentially advances along the developmental continuum, differentiating and maturing into the terminal forms: the reticulocytes, polymorphonuclear cells, and lymphocytes. Clonal units remain clustered in closely packed colonies, and the degree of maturation can be evaluated by examining the marrow.

Hematopoiesis occurs within a microenvironment of the bone marrow located in the medullary cavity of bone. The process of *commitment* describes a transition from pluripotent stem cells to progenitor cells. Progenitor cell areas within bone marrow consist of cells with the capacity to differentiate along one cell lineage. This process involves acquiring specific growth factor receptors and losing other growth factor receptors. Progenitor cells are functionally defined by their capacity to form colonies in *in vitro* assays. The proliferation, differentiation, and survival of these immature cells are sustained by a family of glycoproteins, hematopoietic growth factor, or colony-stimulating factors. Growth factors are produced by the endothelial cells.

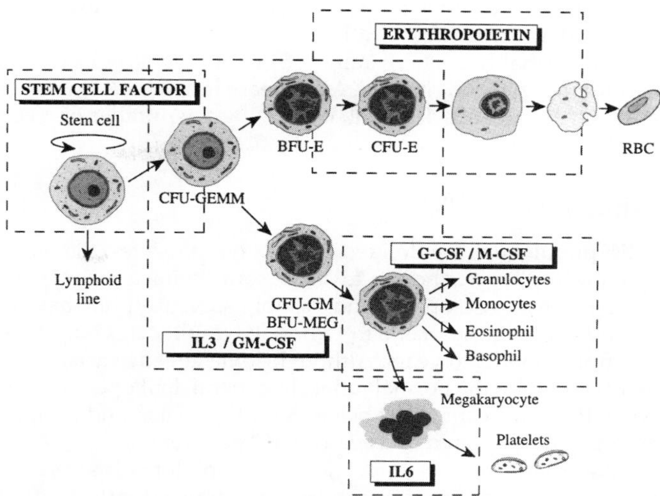

Figure 28-1. Marrow cell differentiation and proliferation. BFU-E, burst-forming unit, erythroid; BFU-MEG, burst–forming unit, megakaryocyte; CFU-E, colony-forming unit, erythroid; CFU-GEMM, colony–forming unit, granulocyte erythrocyte monocyte megakaryocyte; CFU-GM, colony-forming unit, granulocyte macrophage; CSF, colony stimulating factor; GM-CFU, granulocyte-macrophage colony-forming unit; IL, interleukin; RBC, red blood cell. (Reprinted with permission from Hillman R, Ault K. *Hematology in clinical practice.* New York: McGraw-Hill, 1995.)

Adults use approximately 50% of the available medullary bone cavities and have hematopoietically active marrow in the proximal epiphyses of the long bones, skull, vertebrae, pelvis, ribs, and sternum. In myelodysplastic conditions, hematopoiesis extends into additional bony areas and to extramedullary sites, such as the liver and spleen.

Pluripotent stem cells retain the capacity for self-renewal and maintain hematopoiesis by clonal proliferation. Approximately 75% of the hematopoietic cells in the marrow are of myeloid lineage, 25% are erythroid, and fewer than 1% are megakaryocytic.

Red Blood Cells

Erythrocytes contain hemoglobin, a protein that reversibly binds and transports oxygen. The oxygen-transporting site of the heme group is a Fe^{2+} ion on the porphyrin ring. Hemoglobin consists of four porphyrins, so that at full saturation four oxygen molecules bind to the hemoglobin protein. The release of the first oxygen facilitates the release of the second, and the release of the second oxygen facilitates the release of the third. The fourth oxygen usually is not released from the protein. Human RBCs enter the circulation at the reticulocyte stage, after final generation of the normoblast has extruded its nucleus. The reticulocyte continues to synthesize hemoglobin until its supply of messenger RNA is exhausted, and then it decreases slightly in size and becomes a mature erythrocyte. RBCs have an average life span of 120 days in circulation.

Erythropoietin, a glycoprotein produced by the kidney, is the primary regulator of RBC production. Hypoxia, hemolysis, and bleeding cause a rapid increase in serum concentrations of erythropoietin. The marrow responds by increasing erythroid precursors, increasing mitoses, shortening transit time, increasing hemoglobin synthesis, and increasing the uptake of iron.

The marrow becomes hypercellular with an increase in the erythroid–to–myeloid cell ratio.

The normal hematocrit ranges from 36% to 48% in women and from 40% to 52% in men. An increase in total RBC mass acts as a negative feedback signal, decreasing the number of recognizable erythroid precursors in the marrow.

White Blood Cells

WBC populations are divided into the lymphocytes, the monocyte-macrophages, and the myeloid series, which includes the granulocytes, eosinophils, and basophils. Neutrophils have an intravascular life span of 6 to 12 hours; lymphocytes may circulate from months to years. Although some genetic variability is associated with the normal range, in general, leukopenia occurs when the WBC count falls below 3×10^9 per liter, and lymphocytosis occurs when it exceeds 10×10^9 per liter.

Monocytopenia, eosinopenia, and basophilopenia are seen in bone marrow failure syndromes that adversely affect all cell lines or selectively affect granulocytes. Eosinopenia often is caused by redistribution of these cells from the vascular space into tissues and is incited by severe infections, burns, neoplasms, and severe traumatic injuries.

Lymphocytes are involved in cellular and humoral immunity. Mononuclear cells spend very little time in the circulating blood. They differentiate further into macrophages, which ingest waste and debris and kill invading pathogens. They also participate in the immune response by consuming antigenic material and presenting it to a T cell, which then becomes activated. T and B lymphocytes replicate in the lymph nodes, spleen, and tonsils, as well as in the bone marrow. The normal range in the peripheral blood is 2 to 4×10^9 per liter. Seventy percent are B lymphocytes, and 20% are T lymphocytes. Lymphopenia may cause a number of clinical problems, depending on the degree to which cellular and humoral immunity are impaired and on which lymphocyte subsets are affected.

Fluctuations in leukocytes are proportionally greater than in the RBC population. A number of physiologic and environmental conditions have been reported to cause transient changes that may exceed the normal range.

Platelets

Platelets are anuclear cells derived from bone marrow megakaryocytes. Platelets are formed when the cytoplasm of a mature megakaryocyte fractures into small fragments. The average megakaryocyte can generate 1,000 to 2,000 platelets. Normal platelet numbers range from 140,000 to 440,000 per cubic millimeter. Platelets function primarily in hemostasis and thrombosis. They adhere to irregular and injured surfaces and then secrete prostaglandins and adenine diphosphate, initiate the coagulation cascade, aggregate, fuse, and retract, forming a thrombus. The average life span of a platelet is 7 to 10 days before removal by the reticuloendothelial system.

ERYTHROCYTE DISORDERS

Anemias

Anemia is a reduction in the body's RBC mass. The RBC mass is regulated within limits by a feedback loop via erythropoietin and involves a response of the renal peritubular cells to tissue oxygen content. RBCs circulate in the peripheral circulation for 90 to 120 days. Each day, 0.8% of the body's RBC pool must be replaced by erythrocytes released from bone marrow. The spleen is the major site of aged RBC removal. Anemia, which is a deficiency in RBC mass and hemoglobin content, occurs when normal RBC production and destruction are upset. It can be caused by primary bone marrow factors or by increased peripheral loss of erythrocytes.

Anemia represents a general index of health or illness, and its diagnosis requires a systematic approach (Table 28-1) (2). The general diagnostic approach entails examination of a peripheral blood smear and RBC indices: hematocrit, hemoglobin, RBC count, mean corpuscular volume (MCV), mean corpuscular hemoglobin, and mean corpuscular hemoglobin concentration. In addition, the WBC count, platelet count, reticulocyte count, and a stool smear for occult blood should be obtained.

Anemias can be classified broadly as *hyporegenerative* or *hyperregenerative* (2). Anemia of blood loss or hemolytic destruction peripherally leads to increased erythropoietin secretion and reticulocytosis (more than 0.5% to 2.0%). The increased concentration of circulating reticulocytes compensates for peripheral RBC deficits, assuming that the bone marrow is intact and functioning normally. The absence of reticulocytosis in the face of anemia indicates that RBC production is impaired. Thus, the reticulocyte

TABLE 28-1. Laboratory tests useful for diagnosing anemia

Initial assessment
- RBC number: RBCs, hemoglobin, hematocrit
- RBC indices: mean cell volume, mean cell hemoglobin, mean cell hemoglobin concentration, RBC distribution width
- WBC count, WBC differential
- Platelet count
- Blood film morphology: cell size, symmetry (anisocytosis, poikilocytosis, polychromasia)
- Reticulocyte count
- Stool examination for occult blood

Hypoproliferative anemia, aplastic anemia
- Serum ferritin
- Serum iron and total iron-binding capacity
- Marrow examination
- Marrow aspirate: erythroid-myeloid ratio, cell morphology and maturation, iron stain
- Marrow biopsy: cellularity, morphology
- Cytogenetics (bone marrow)
- Monoclonal antibody assays (bone marrow)
- Special stains (trichrome, silver stain for reticulin, peroxidase, esterase, periodic acid–Schiff): bone marrow
- Marrow incubation assay
- Blood lead
- Peripheral blood lymphocyte incubation assay
- Viral studies (e.g., hepatitis, human immunodeficiency virus, Epstein-Barr virus)

Hemolytic anemia
- Serum haptoglobin
- Coombs' test
- Cold agglutinin titer
- Serum and urine hemosiderin
- Serum unconjugated bilirubin
- Serum lactate dehydrogenase
- Osmotic fragility
- Incubated autohemolysis test
- Glucose-6-phosphate dehydrogenase screen
- Methemoglobin level
- Hemoglobin electrophoresis

Maturation disorders
- Free erythrocyte or zinc protoporphyrin
- Serum B_{12} level
- Serum and RBC folate level
- Hemoglobin electrophoresis

RBC, red blood cell; WBC, white blood cell.

TABLE 28-2. Selected causes of anemia

Microcytic anemia	Acute and chronic leukemias
Iron deficiency	Infiltration of the marrow by carcinoma
Anemia of chronic disease	Granulomas
Thalassemias	Human immunodeficiency virus
Aluminum toxicity	Macrocytic anemia
Thyrotoxicosis	Cobalamin and folate deficiencies
Hereditary sideroblastic anemia	Alcoholism
Lead poisoning	Drugs, especially those that interfere with DNA synthesis
Normocytic anemia	Nitrous oxide (occupational exposure, abuse)
Iron deficiency	Arsenic poisoning
Anemia of chronic disease	Liver disease
Renal failure	Marrow aplasia
Liver disease	Myelodysplasia
Lead poisoning	Myelofibrosis
Hemolytic anemias	Sideroblastic anemia
Endocrine disorders (hypothyroidism, hypopituitarism, primary adrenal insufficiency, thyrotoxicosis, hyperparathyroidism)	Acute myeloblastic leukemia
Marrow aplasia	Multiple myeloma
Myelodysplasia	Lymphoma
Myelofibrosis	Hypothyroidism

Adapted with permission from Lee GR, Foerster J, Lukens J, Wintrobe MM, eds. *Wintrobe's clinical hematology,* 10th ed. Philadelphia: Lippincott Williams & Wilkins, 1999.

count helps to isolate quickly the etiology of anemia: either peripheral RBC loss or destruction or abnormal marrow sources.

The size of RBCs also helps to classify anemias: normal MCV values are 80 to 95 fL, and MCVs that exceed this range are classified as *macrocytic anemias*. The MCV is a useful screen for assisting in the diagnosis of anemias. *Microcytic anemias* are associated with deficits in hemoglobin synthesis (iron deficiency, chronic disease, thalassemia). Macrocytic anemias (MCV greater than 115 fL) are commonly due to folate or vitamin B_{12} deficiency. Liver disease and inherited abnormalities in purine-pyrimidine metabolism can cause macrocytic anemia (2). The mean corpuscular hemoglobin and mean corpuscular hemoglobin concentration do not provide any further information beyond the MCV for categorizing anemias. Table 28-2 lists causes of anemia.

Examination of the peripheral blood smear is crucial in differentiating the causes of anemia. Anemia due to hyporegenerative processes requires bone marrow examination. Most patients with anemia do not require a bone marrow biopsy, as less invasive testing readily identifies the etiology. For example, anemia accompanied by leukopenia or thrombocytopenia suggests a primary or secondary disorder of the bone marrow, a megaloblastic process, or hypersplenism. If examination of the peripheral smear shows hypersegmented neutrophils accompanying macrocytic erythrocytes, megaloblastic anemia is suggested. Further assessment of workplace exposures to folate-inhibiting chemicals and testing of vitamin B_{12} and folate levels would be indicated.

The absolute reticulocyte count is helpful when distinguishing hypoproduction from shortened RBC survival. If an adequate compensatory response—reflected by an increased reticulocyte count—is seen, a bone marrow examination may not be required. In some anemias, hypoproduction occurs in conjunction with shortened RBC survival: The anemias of chronic disease, iron deficiency, vitamin B_{12} deficiency, folate deficiency, and β-thalassemia major are included in this list.

Patients who present with pancytopenia or bicytopenia (decreases in two cell lines) should have aspirate and bone marrow biopsies.

RBC morphologic features on the peripheral blood smear provide valuable clues to the diagnosis of anemia. Hypochromia and microcytosis suggest iron deficiency, thalassemia, sideroblastic anemia, and anemia of chronic disease. Coarse basophilic stippling of RBCs suggests lead intoxication and thalassemia. Macroovalocytes are seen in cobalamin and folate deficiencies, but they can also be found in acute arsenic poisoning, myelodysplasia, myelofibrosis, and hemolytic anemia. Teardrop cells and nucleated RBCs are indicative of myelofibrosis or functional or anatomic asplenia but can also occur in immune hemolysis, megaloblastic anemia, thalassemia major, and extensive metastatic cancer to bone. Microspherocytes suggest immune hemolysis, hereditary spherocytosis, microangiopathic anemia, and hypophosphatemia. Sickle cells suggest hemoglobinopathy (hemoglobins SS, SC, S-thalassemia, and C_{Harlem}).

RBC fragments (schistocytes) indicate microangiopathic or traumatic hemolysis and are seen occasionally in cases of iron deficiency or megaloblastic anemia and in patients having cancer chemotherapy. Target cells are present in hemoglobinopathies (C, SC, SS), thalassemias, liver disease, iron deficiency, and after splenectomy. They are also common artifacts. Elliptocytes are seen in hereditary elliptocytosis, iron deficiency, myelofibrosis, and megaloblastic anemias. Burr cells (echinocytes) are seen in renal failure and pyruvate kinase deficiency. Spur cells (acanthocytes) are characteristic of liver disease and abetalipoproteinemia. Polychromatophilic RBCs and increased reticulocytosis suggest intense marrow stimulation after hemorrhage, hypoxia, splenectomy, or hemolysis. Rouleaux (RBCs stacked like coins) suggest myeloma and macroglobulinemia, and agglutinated RBCs suggest cold agglutinin disease.

The peripheral smear in aplastic anemia reveals pancytopenia. RBC morphology is normochromic and normocytic without membrane defects. No abnormal (leukemic) cells or nucleated RBCs are seen.

Examination of the bone marrow is a definitive diagnostic tool for distinguishing hypoproliferative processes from conditions that accelerate peripheral destruction (hyporegenerative versus hyperregenerative). Hypoproliferative processes diminish cellular elements. When a single cell line is affected, an obvious shift takes place in the ratio between myeloid and erythroid precursors, and few of the more mature erythroid cells are present. At its most extreme, in aplastic anemia, the bone marrow consists of fat, fibrous tissue, and lymphocytes with little evidence of regeneration. Cellular elements are reduced to 25% or less. Mature lymphocytes are the predominant cellular element. In some instances, the marrow is actually hypercellular but shows severe dyserythropoiesis. Erythroid colonies are in disarray, and nuclear maturity and the cytoplasm are dyssynchronous. The normoblast has a finely stippled appearance rather than the coarser clefts usually seen at this stage, and the cytoplasm retains its basophilia as the cell matures. The latter finding is also common in vitamin B_{12}-, folate-, and iron-deficiency conditions.

Megaloblastic anemias have enlarged, abnormal-appearing normoblasts (macroblasts in the marrow) and show characteristic changes in the myeloid line, including giant metamyelocytes and hypersegmented neutrophils. Dyserythropoiesis may extend to the megakaryocytes as well.

Ringed sideroblasts are found in sideroblastic anemias as a result of lead poisoning, chronic alcohol consumption, or treatment with isoniazid, cycloserine, chloramphenicol, lincomycin, or penicillamine. In sideroblasts, a ring of iron granules is arranged around the nucleus. The defect involves the mitochondria, and iron builds up at the site of heme synthesis (3).

When increased peripheral destruction has occurred, as in the hemolytic processes, the marrow often is hyperplastic, with a substantial increase in the erythroid-myeloid ratio. The rate of maturation is compressed, and the orthochromatic normoblast is released earlier than it would be if there were not an increased demand for RBCs.

The methemoglobin level and complete blood count should be obtained if methemoglobinemia is suspected. The level of hypoxia should be assessed clinically and biochemically. The peripheral blood smear may show reticulocytosis and RBCs that appear irregularly fragmented. Assaying for glucose-6-phosphate dehydrogenase (G6PD) deficiency is appropriate but cannot be performed when an individual presents after an acute episode. Young RBCs generally contain normal levels of the enzyme and, during an acute hemolytic episode, the older RBCs are destroyed, leaving only younger cells. Consequently, the best time to screen is before exposure or 1 to 2 months after hemolysis has resolved.

Occult blood loss, the most common cause of anemia, must be excluded. Disruption of vascular integrity may be subtle or overt and requires thorough assessment. Coagulation abnormalities may contribute to occult blood loss. Some drugs that may promote blood loss as a result of disruption of coagulation include aspirin, alcohol, nonsteroidal antiinflammatory drugs, corticosteroids, and anticoagulants.

Hemolytic Anemia and Methemoglobinemia

Increased RBC destruction is termed *hemolysis*. A common mechanism of hemolysis is the oxidation and then denaturation of hemoglobin, which precipitates within the RBC, alters the surface, and causes leakage and, ultimately, hemolysis. The precipitated globin chains (Heinz bodies) are removed by macrophages in the liver and spleen. The RBC is unable to reform into a smooth sphere, so it continues along in circulation with a piece missing. These irregularly shaped RBCs may be seen on the usual peripheral smear, whereas Heinz bodies can be visualized only with a special preparation, a supravital stain. Tables 28-3 and 28-4 list selected agents that may cause hemolytic anemia and methemoglobinemia.

TABLE 28-3. Drugs, chemicals, and processes that cause hemolytic anemia

Alcoholism
Apiole
Arsine (AsH_3)
Bee sting
Benzene
Chlorates (ClO_3^-)
Copper
Glycerol (intravenous)
Hemodialysis
Hornet sting
Intravenous alimentation without phosphorus supplementation
Ionizing radiation
Lead
Mephenesin
Methylene chloride
Mitomycin C
Nonoxidant chemicals
Prolonged antacid ingestion
Propylthiouracil
Pyrogallic acid
Snake venoms (cobras, vipers, Australian king brown snake)
Spider venoms (*Loxosceles reclusa* and *Loxosceles laeta*)
Stibine (SbH_3)
Thermal burns
Trimellitic anhydride
Water
Zinc ethylene–bis–dithiocarbamate (zineb)

TABLE 28-4. Selected methemoglobin-generating agents

Aromatic (cyclic) compounds
- Acetanilid
- Aminophenol
- Ammonium nitrate
- Aniline[a]
- Bromoaniline
- Chloronitrobenzene
- Cresol[a]
- Dinitrophenol
- Dinitrotoluene
- Hydroquinone
- Naphthalene[a]
- Naphthyl amines
- Nitrates
- Nitroaniline
- Nitrobenzene[a]
- Nitrofurantoin[a]
- Nitroglycerin
- Nitrophenol
- Phenacetin[a]
- Phenazopyridium
- Phenol[a]
- Phenylhydrazine
- Phenylsemicarbazide[a]
- Resorcin[a]
- Salicylates[a]
- Sulfonamides[a]
- Sulfones (Dapsone)[a]
- Toluidine
- Trinitrotoluene

Bromates
Chlorates
Hematin
Hydroxylamine
Hyperbaric oxygen
Methylene blue (in infants)
Nitrates
Pentachlorophenol

[a]May cause hemolysis at high dose, even in the setting of apparently normal red blood cell counts.

Hemoglobin is unique in that it has the ability to bind with oxygen without being oxidized. This ability is attributable to the fact that the iron on the heme moiety is continuously shuttled from Fe^{3+} to Fe^{2+} via enzymatic reduction by the anaerobic Embden-Meyerhof pathway. RBCs have an extensive number of protective antioxidant and redox mechanisms, including the glutathione system, reduced nicotinamide adenine dinucleotide phosphate, reduced nicotinamide adenine dinucleotide, superoxide dismutase, catalase, and membrane-associated vitamins E and C. Various chemicals increase the rate of heme oxidation 100- to 1,000-fold, overwhelming these mechanisms. Methemoglobin and denaturation of hemoglobin occur when hemoglobin oxidation exceeds the normal reducing capacity of the system. Methemoglobin is potentially reversible, but sulfhemoglobin and Heinz bodies are irreversible. Chemicals either may act as oxidizing agents directly or may interact with oxygen to form free radicals or peroxides. Unless such chemicals are detoxified by the glutathione-dependent reduction system, cellular damage—methemoglobinemia, sulfhemoglobinemia, or hemolytic anemia—ensues. Why exposure to oxidants produces methemoglobin in some individuals, sulfhemoglobin in others, and hemolytic anemia in yet others is unclear.

Some of these oxidant compounds are powerful enough to overcome even normal-appearing erythrocytes and produce methemoglobinemia and Heinz body hemolytic anemia. Although some diversity is present in their chemical composition and structure, many possess an arylamine nucleus or are aniline derivatives.

Methemoglobin is unable to transport oxygen. It increases the oxygen affinity of the remaining heme groups in the tetramer, shifting the oxygen dissociation curve to the left and thereby reducing oxygen delivery to the tissues (4).

Environmental exposures that cause methemoglobinemia and oxidative hemolysis disproportionately affect infants. Infants' increased susceptibility can be explained thus: Until the age of 6 months, infants have lower levels of the soluble reduced form of nicotinamide adenine dinucleotide cytochrome-b_5 reductase as compared with adults. Other contributions include a relatively higher consumption of foodstuffs and liquids from the gastrointestinal tract because of the higher metabolic demands of infants and a higher surface to volume ratio for substances absorbed through the skin. Although infants are more susceptible, all age groups are at risk if exposure is sufficient.

Well water contaminated with excessive amounts of fertilizer containing nitrates is an environmental source of methemoglobinemia. Poisonings, sometimes fatal, have been reported in infants given well water high in nitrates or fed formula reconstituted with water containing nitrates (5). Nitrates are converted by gastrointestinal tract bacteria into nitrites, which are the active agents. Water-soluble vitamin K analogs given to infants and aniline dyes used as marker inks on diapers have also caused fatalities (6). Other common situations involving nitrates include consumption of foodstuffs high in nitrates (sausages, preserved meats), spinach that has been left out for some time before cooking, or foods accidentally contaminated with nitrates (7). Recreational use of butyl and amyl nitrate; topical application of bismuth subnitrate, ammonium, potassium, and silver nitrate to burns; and ingestion of room deodorizers containing butyl nitrite have caused methemoglobinemia.

The aromatic nitro and amino compounds, nitrates, chlorates, and metals can cause occupational and environmentally related hemolytic anemias via excessive skin absorption. Phenol, cresol, and pentachlorophenol are frequently encountered industrial chemicals that may cause hemolysis via oxidation. Nitrous gases generated by arc welding and by stored grains (silo-filler gas), as well as potassium chlorate and other chlorate salts used in pesticides and herbicides, can cause methemoglobinemia and hemolysis via oxidation mechanisms (8–14).

Sulfhemoglobinemia is formed when a sulfur atom substitutes for an oxygen on one or more of the porphyrin rings. It produces cyanosis at approximately 0.5 g per dL, methemoglobinemia at 2 g per dL, and reduced hemoglobin at 5 g per dL (15).

Signs and symptoms of methemoglobinemia are greater than the comparable decrease in the amount of RBC mass, because oxidized heme increases the affinity of the remaining oxygen-binding sites on the molecule. In contrast, despite often intense cyanosis, sulfhemoglobinemia is rarely symptomatic, because the sulfonated site decreases the affinity of the remaining oxygen-binding sites, facilitating rather than impairing tissue oxygenation. The most common agents associated with sulfhemoglobinemia are acetanilid, phenacetin, and the sulfonamides. Rarely, sulfhemoglobinemia is associated with hemolysis due to Heinz body formation.

Direct-acting agents are those that can oxidize hemoglobin *in vivo* as well as *in vitro*. These include the nitrites, nitrates, chlorates, and quinones. Indirect-acting agents include other aromatic amino and nitro compounds, such as the aniline dyes, acetanilid, phenacetin, sulfonamides, and phenazopyridine.

Individuals deficient in G6PD or other components of the hexose monophosphate shunt are particularly sensitive to the hemolytic effect of oxidant compounds. These deficiencies often involve genetic polymorphisms of enzymes of the hexose monophosphate pathway and glutathione. The gene *G6PD* is found on the X chromosome and is inherited as an X-linked trait. Variants of *G6PD* are found with differing frequency in different populations, affecting more than 130 million people worldwide. Most of these polymorphisms produce no symptoms until challenged with oxidants. Some variants, such as Mediterranean and Canton, exert very low enzyme activity, and individuals with such variants develop severe intravascular hemolysis when challenged by fava beans or by oxidant drugs. Chicago and Oklahoma are two variants that induce chronic extravascular hemolysis that is exacerbated by oxidants.

Hemolysis caused by oxidants in G6PD deficiency is dose-dependent. Hemolysis can occur in G6PD-deficient individuals at lower levels of exposure than would affect people with normal RBCs. G6PD activity falls exponentially with the age of the RBC, and young RBCs often have near-normal activity. Older RBCs are generally adversely affected by oxidants. Oxidant stress is generated also by infection, lowering the threshold at which those with G6PD deficiency produce methemoglobinemia or hemolysis in response to an oxidant.

Chlorate salts and chloramines (formed by combining chlorine with ammonia) can cause methemoglobinemia and hemolysis that is unresponsive to methylene blue.

Some metals may cause hemolytic anemia. Cytolytic metals can bind to sulfhydryl groups and can have a high affinity for the thiol groups present on the surfaces of RBCs and on cysteine residues on hemoglobin. Binding of the metals causes increased membrane permeability and leads to hemolysis. Inorganic arsenic (arsenic trioxide and arsenic pentoxide) causes RBC hemolysis in animal studies and in human ingestions. Copper may cause intravascular hemolysis and methemoglobinemia. People who experience accidental or suicidal ingestion of copper sulfate have presented with these findings. Hemolysis may also occur after hemodialysis with water contaminated by copper pipes. Copper accumulates within RBCs and causes hemolysis by inactivating enzymes of the pentose phosphate and glycolytic pathways and disrupting membrane integrity.

Lead shortens RBC survival and may cause hemolysis. Severe acute hemolysis is rare but may be seen with very high exposures, such as those produced by power sanding and use of a blow torch on leaded paint surfaces. Lead-induced hemolysis may be caused by inhibition of pyrimidine 5' nucleotidase.

Inhalational exposure to arsine and stibine gases may cause intravascular hemolysis. These gases are colorless, nonirritating, and highly toxic and are produced when acids react with metallic arsenic and antimony, respectively. The most common exposures occur during the refining and processing of metals that contain metallic arsenic and antimony as impurities. Arsine exposures may also occur during galvanizing, soldering, etching, and lead plating. Arsine is used in the semiconductor industry as well. Adverse effects generally appear 2 to 24 hours after exposure, and presentation may be dramatic, with near-fatal outcomes (16). Symptoms from severe, acute exposure consist of abdominal pain, nausea, vomiting, and passage of dark-red urine. Findings include jaundice, anemia, reticulocytosis, leukocytosis, and RBC hemolysis. Hemolytic anemia has been reported also after exposure to zinc ethylene–bis-dithiocarbamate (zineb), a fungicide (17).

Immune hemolysis involves destruction of RBCs by antibodies directed against antigens that are either present in the RBC membrane or adsorbed onto the RBC surface. Drugs (and polypeptides) that elicit immunoglobulin G or anticomplement antibodies induce primarily extravascular hemolysis. Bacterial polysaccharide antigens elicit immunoglobulin M antibodies that may lead to intravascular hemolysis. Although immune hemolysis is a common cause of drug-induced disease, it is not usually associated with industrial exposures, with the exception of exposure to trimellitic anhydride.

Erythrocytosis

The RBC mass (erythrocytes) is maintained within narrow limits and does not vary more than 10% among people of the same age and gender. Erythrocytes lost daily via senescence are replaced by new erythrocytes as long as nutrients remain adequate. Erythrocyte production is regulated by erythropoietin, produced by peritubular interstitial fibroblasts in the inner renal cortex. This same peritubular site contains a heme protein that functions as an oxygen sensor to upregulate erythropoietin messenger RNA transcription via nucleoproteins called *hypoxia-inducible factors* that interact with an enhancer in the 3' region of the erythropoietin gene (18). Anemia or hypoxia increases erythropoietin production by increasing the number of producing cells. Erythropoietin is produced also by liver fibroblasts and hepatocytes. The plasma concentrations of erythropoietin range from 4 to 26 mU per milliliter. Chronic, low-level exposure to carbon monoxide and oxidants may cause a compensatory erythrocytosis. Polycythemia has also been noted after chronic phosphorus exposure in the match industry (19), although it is possible that this finding was caused by liver damage.

Generally, the modest degree of polycythemia that accompanies chronic hypoxemia from any of these agents is asymptomatic and does not lead to the problems seen in polycythemia rubra vera, a neoplastic disease that causes a much greater increase in RBC mass. Findings are typical of the underlying process.

Acquired Porphyrias

The porphyrias arise as a result of defective heme biosynthesis and buildup of heme precursors. Primary (hereditary) and secondary (due to chemical exposures) porphyrias have been described. The buildup of heme functions to inhibit δ-aminolevulinic acid synthetase, creating a negative feedback loop. The critical rate-limiting step is the synthesis of δ-aminolevulinic acid from glycine and succinyl coenzyme A.

The urine-soluble heme precursors—δ-aminolevulinic acid and porphobilinogen—are toxic to nervous tissue and cause symptoms of psychiatric disturbances, sensorimotor neuropathy, and autonomic dysfunction (abdominal colic, constipation). The urine-insoluble precursors—uroporphyrin III, coproporphyrin III, and protoporphyrin IX—fluoresce in the skin when exposed to sunlight, particularly the 400-nm wavelength. These precursors cause cutaneous photosensitivity. Their effects include blistering of the skin, scarring, and deformity with hypertrichosis. The teeth often are discolored and deformed. Occasionally, RBC hemolysis is observed as well. The toxic porphyrias associated with chemical exposure are similar to the inherited disorder porphyria cutanea tarda. Clinical manifestations are similar, with adverse effects seen in skin and liver, accompanied by deranged heme synthesis.

The first reported outbreak of acquired porphyria occurred in Turkey between 1956 and 1961 and involved more than 4,000 people (21). Symptoms developed approximately 6 months after people ingested wheat treated with the fungicide hexachlorobenzene. The wheat was intended for planting but instead was ground into flour and consumed. Adults and children of both genders were affected. Presenting findings included cutaneous photosensitivity, blistering and hyperpigmentation of the skin, hypertrichosis, weakness, and hepatomegaly. Marked porphyrinuria was seen, and the urine often was colored red or brown. The overall mortality rate was 10%. Breast-fed infants younger than age 2 whose mothers were affected had a 95% mortality rate.

Follow-up studies of the originally exposed population indicated that porphyrinuria persisted in some individuals throughout the ensuing 25 years (21). Hyperpigmentation was found in 71% of those originally exposed, and 47% had hypertrichosis. Residual scarring of sun-exposed skin was found in 87%. Additional findings included perioral scarring, small hands, arthritis, short stature, weakness, paresthesias, and myotonia. Fifty-six samples of breast milk obtained from affected mothers showed an average of 0.51 parts per million (ppm) hexachlorobenzene, as compared with 0.07 ppm in samples from unaffected mothers.

The mechanism by which hexachlorobenzene produces porphyria remains unclear. Animal studies suggest that the porphyrinogenic compounds interfere with recognition of the inhibitory signal generated by heme (22). Thus, δ-aminolevulinic acid synthetase activity continues to generate porphyrins. Other theories suggest that porphyrinogenic compounds induce the enzyme either by acting on the electron transport chain, which stimulates the production of succinyl coenzyme A, or by depressing intracellular adenosine triphosphate levels.

TABLE 28-5. Selected chemicals associated with acquired porphyria

Aluminum
Disinfectants
2-Benzyl-4,6-dichlorophenol
o-Benzyl-*p*-chlorophenol
Fungicide: hexachlorobenzene
Herbicides
2,3,7,8-Tetrachlorodibenzo-*p*-dioxin
2,4-Dichlorophenol
2,4,5-Trichlorophenol
Lead
Vinyl chloride

Iron seems to play a permissive rather than a causative role in the porphyrias and may provide a clue to the susceptibility of some individuals and not others to the porphyrinogenic properties of some of the polychlorinated compounds. In a porcine and a human liver model (23), iron overload inhibited uroporphyrinogen III cosynthase activity, enhanced total porphyrin production, and increased uroproporphyrin I. In rats treated with hexachlorobenzene, iron overload caused decreased production of liver heme, cytochrome P-450, and cytochrome b_5, and an absence of uroporphyrinogen decarboxylase activity. In addition, mice were protected from the porphyrinogenic effect of 2,3,7,8-tetrachlorodibenzo-*p*-dioxin when made iron-deficient by phlebotomy, as compared with controls.

The dramatic presentation of acquired porphyria seen in this and other epidemics as a result of ingestion of contaminated foodstuffs has not been observed after exposure to the other agents listed in Table 28-5. Two studies of populations whose occupation was the manufacture of herbicides and who were exposed to 2,4-dichlorophenol and 2,4,5-trichlorophenol found a high percentage of workers with chloracne, hyperpigmentation, hirsutism, and skin fragility (24,25). Many workers demonstrated increased excretion of porphyrins (uroporphyrin and coproporphyrin). In one of the manufacturing plants, a follow-up study conducted 6 years later, during which time industrial exposures had decreased, found no residual symptoms of porphyria and only one worker who had persistent uroporphyrinuria. The authors also postulated that the true porphyrinogenic agent may have been 2,3,7,8-tetrachlorodibenzo-*p*-dioxin and that a change in manufacturing practices had eliminated this contaminant (23).

Mild porphyria cutanea tarda has been observed in some hemodialysis patients, many of whom are aluminum-overloaded from aluminum contaminants present in dialysis fluid. Plasma and urine uroporphyrins are increased, whereas coproporphyrins are decreased. Aluminum has been shown to inhibit some heme synthetic enzymes.

Studies of vinyl chloride workers revealed that in patients who had cirrhosis of the liver, esophageal varices, splenomegaly, Raynaud's phenomenon, sclerodermalike skin changes, acroosteolysis, and thrombocytopenia, urinary levels of coproporphyrin were significantly elevated (26).

At blood levels of approximately 40 μg per dL, lead interferes with heme synthesis by inhibiting δ-aminolevulinic acid dehydrase, which increases urinary porphobilinogen. Lead also interferes with heme synthesis by blocking ferrochelatase, which interferes with the incorporation of iron into protoporphyrin IX and depresses coproporphyrinogen oxidase activity. Symptoms of lead poisoning, especially at levels higher than 60 μg per dL, include abdominal pain, constipation, and vomiting. At even higher levels, paresthesias, diarrhea, neuropsychiatric signs, and seizures are similar to those seen in acute intermittent porphyria.

Diagnosis of acquired porphyrias requires a high index of suspicion, as presenting symptoms often are vague and appear to be multisystemic in origin. The history should explore the onset, character, nature, and duration of symptoms. A thorough evaluation of occupational exposures to suspected porphyrinogenic compounds is indicated. In addition, a detailed family history should be obtained in which related familial and genetic diseases are noted, because the inherited hepatic porphyrias are transmitted as autosomal dominant traits with variable expressivity (3). Symptoms of the familial form generally begin between the ages of 40 and 60 years and may be precipitated by estrogens or known hepatotoxic drugs. Sporadic cases of porphyria cutanea tarda also occur. They probably are the most commonly diagnosed cases of hepatic porphyria and are associated with alcoholic liver disease and contraceptive steroids.

Laboratory results include increased urinary excretion of uroporphyrin and coproporphyrin, without an increase in porphyrin precursors (δ-aminolevulinic acid and porphobilinogen). Anemia is uncommon, as are other abnormalities of the peripheral blood. Additional tests may include biological monitoring, depending on the suspected agent. Measurement of other porphyrin precursors may help to distinguish between porphyria cutanea tarda and the other hepatic porphyrias.

APLASTIC ANEMIA AND BONE MARROW SUPPRESSION

The incidence of aplastic anemia ranges between two and six cases per 1 million population (27). Aplastic anemia is diagnosed by the presence of pancytopenia and hypocellular bone marrow. Individuals with aplastic anemia usually seek medical help owing to their symptoms, which result from low blood cell counts. The patient may report easy bruising and gum bleeding as common symptoms due to thrombocytopenia or fever and bleeding secondary to pancytopenia. All blood cellular elements can be depressed, or a decrease in a single element may be dominant clinically. Heavy menstrual flows may occur in young women. In most cases of aplastic anemia, peripheral blood counts are uniformly depressed, and the peripheral blood smear shows a paucity of platelets and leukocytes with normal RBC morphology. Toxic granulations may be present in neutrophils.

Bone marrow examination is the primary basis for the diagnosis of peripheral pancytopenia and aplastic anemia. Both the bone marrow aspirate and the biopsy must be examined in suspected cases. In aplastic anemia, total marrow cellularity is low, but residual lymphocytosis may be noted. Hemophagocytosis or macrophage ingestion of RBCs frequently is present.

Aplastic anemia can be acquired or inherited. Acquired forms may be due to immune-mediated mechanisms or direct damage to DNA in stem cells or progenitor cells (or both). The International Aplastic Anemia and Agranulocytosis Study is the largest and most comprehensive study of the epidemiology of bone marrow failure (27). Most causes of aplastic anemia remain unknown. However, certain drugs, chemicals, and viruses, and irradiation are known to be causative of or associated with aplastic anemia (Table 28-6). The proposed mechanisms of marrow production defects from acquired xenobiotics are as follows:

- *Direct cytotoxicity*: destruction of the hematopoietic stem cells or progenitor cells
- *DNA mutations*: interference with progenitor cells' ability to replicate or differentiate
- *Immunologic mechanisms*: suppression of hematopoiesis or an imbalance of production or concentration of stimulatory or inhibitory growth factors in the bone marrow microenvironment caused by T lymphocytes

Ionizing radiation is a well-known cause of bone marrow failure secondary to DNA injury. Radiation can produce not only aplastic anemia but also myelodysplasia and leukemia. Stem cells and progenitor cells are damaged by irradiation. Mortality from bone marrow toxicity is a function of the marrow's ability to tolerate both depletion of its cells that are actively pro-

TABLE 28-6. Chemical and physical agents associated with the development of pancytopenia and marrow hypoplasia

Agents that cause marrow hypoplasia in a dose-dependent manner
- Chemotherapeutic agents
  - Alkylating agents: busulfan, melphalan, cyclophosphamide
  - Antibiotics: daunorubicin, doxorubicin hydrochloride (adriamycin)
  - Antimetabolites: antifolic compounds, purine or pyrimidine analogs, etoposide
  - Antimitotic agents: colchicine, vincristine, vinblastine
- Arsine
- Benzene
- Cymene
- Dichlorovinyl cysteine
- Estrogens
- Inorganic arsenic
- Ionizing radiation: x-rays, radioactive isotopes, nuclear fallout
- Trinitrotoluene

Other agents associated with marrow injury (low probability)
- Arsenic
- Bismuth
- Colloidal silver
- Dinitrophenol
- Gold salts
- Hair dyes
- Insecticides: chlorophenothane (DDT), parathion, chlordane, pentachlorophenol
- Medicinal agents
- Analgesic and antiinflammatory drugs: acetylsalicylic acid, diclofenac, fenbufen, fenoprofen, gold compounds, indomethacin, naproxen, phenylbutazone, piroxicam, sulindac
- Angiotensin-converting enzyme inhibitor antihypertensives: captopril, enalapril, lisinopril
- Antiarrhythmic drugs: amiodarone, tocainide
- Anticonvulsants: carbamazepine, ethosuximide, felbamate, phenacemide, phenobarbital
- Antidiabetic drugs: carbutamide, chlorpropamide, tolbutamide
- Antihistamines: cimetidine, ranitidine, tripelennamine
- Antimicrobial agents: amphotericin B, chloramphenicol, chlortetracycline, methicillin, organic arsenicals, oxytetracycline, penicillin, quinacrine, streptomycin, sulfamethoxypyridazine, sulfisoxazole, sulfonamides
- Antithyroid drugs: methimazole, methylthiouracil, propylthiouracil
- Azidothymidine (AZT)
- Carbonic anhydrase inhibitors: acetazolamide, mesalazine, methazolamide
- D-Penicillamine
- Sedatives and hypnotic agents: chlordiazepoxide, chlorpromazine, meprobamate, mepazine, methyprylon, promazine
- Thiocyanate

Mercury

Solvents: carbon tetrachloride, glycol ethers, mixed solvent exposure

Toxigenic fungus (present on moldy grain)

Adapted from ref. 33 and Williams DM, Pancytopenia, aplastic anemia, and pure red cell aplasia. In: Lee GR, Foerster J, Lukens J, Wintrobe MM, eds. *Wintrobe's clinical hematology*, vol 1, 9th ed. Philadelphia: Lea & Febiger, 1993:915.

ducing neutrophils and platelets and direct damage to the stem cell. Bone marrow hypoplasia occurs with radiation doses in excess of 1.5 to 2.0 Gy. Lethal exposure in animals begins at approximately 4 Gy, and whole-body exposures of 10 to 50 GY in humans generally are incompatible with survival (27).

Aplastic anemia and myelodysplasia sometimes are confused. Myelodysplasia is usually a disease of the elderly, whereas aplastic anemia is primarily a disease of the young. Also, in myelodysplasia, patients are generally asymptomatic at presentation, and their blood counts tend to be less severely depressed than those of aplastic anemia patients. Peripheral blood smears from myelodysplasia patients can show more striking abnormalities than those from aplastic anemia patients, with erythrocyte anisocytosis, giant platelets, and hypogranulated or hyposegmented polymorphonuclear leukocytes. Also, bizarre nuclear morphology of leukocytes and granulocytes may occur in myelodysplasia. The bone marrow in myelodysplasia is normally cellular or hypercellular, but a hypocellular variant has been described (27).

Some drugs, chemicals, and viral infections cause aplastic anemia through immune mechanisms (27,28). However, although several drugs and chemicals are cited as causes of bone marrow failure and aplastic anemia, clear etiologic relationships have been established in only a few cases. Benzene is the chemical that is most convincingly linked to aplastic anemia by both clinical and epidemiologic studies. Benzene causes aplastic anemia in a dose-related manner and requires exposure to high levels (29,30). Also, metabolites of benzene have been shown to be the true etiologic agents of bone marrow–induced toxicity to stem cells and progenitor cells (31). The risk of producing benzene-related aplastic anemia in the 1- to 10-ppm chronic exposure range is estimated to be as high as 1 per 100,000 to as low as 1 per 1 million (30). Large population studies demonstrate that inhalational exposure to high benzene concentrations over a chronic period are required to produce aplastic anemia. One study of 74,828 benzene-exposed Chinese workers showed a significant excess of aplastic anemia (9 cases, or an incidence of 1.2 per 10,000 population) and myelodysplasia cases, as compared with 35,805 unexposed controls, in whom no cases were found (32). The average benzene exposure was 16.7 ppm.

Agents that are bone marrow–toxic may selectively affect the erythroid precursors (pure RBC aplasia) or all three cell lines (33). The cellular progenitors, the stromal microenvironment, or both may be affected. The earliest hematopoietic stem cells are most vulnerable to injury; thus, when chemical injury occurs, hypoplasia of all three cell lines is more common than RBC aplasia. In addition to chemical and physical agents, viruses and immune diseases can cause aplastic anemia. Associated viruses include Epstein-Barr virus, hepatitis (non-A, non-B, non-C, and non-G), parvovirus, and the human immunodeficiency virus (33). Immune processes also are associated with aplastic anemia and include eosinophilic fasciitis, hypoimmunoglobulinemia, thymoma and thymic carcinoma, graft-versus-host disease, systemic lupus erythematosus (SLE), pregnancy, and paroxysmal nocturnal hemoglobinuria (27,34). Altered immunity involving cytokines such as interferon-γ with T-lymphocyte activation has been associated with aplastic anemia (27).

Chemical and physical agents may also interfere with the biosynthetic steps necessary for DNA synthesis (35). The most common mechanism is interference with the incorporation of purine or pyrimidine bases. A chemical—typically an electrophilic compound or intermediary metabolite—binds to the DNA base, causing substitution of an incorrect base pair or sterically hindering replication and blocking DNA strand duplication. Examples of such chemicals are antineoplastic drugs. Disrupting the microtubules of the mitotic spindle interferes with separation of chromosomes and inhibits DNA synthesis. Colchicine, periwinkle, and taxol act in this way.

The topoisomerase II–directed epipodophyllotoxins (etoposide and teniposide) cause DNA damage via the intranuclear enzyme topoisomerase II and stabilize the DNA–topoisomerase II covalent linkage (36). The DNA-intercalating anthracyclines also inhibit topoisomerase II. These agents increase the frequency of chromosomal translocations, which are cytotoxic and leukemogenic. Translocations on chromosome 11 are especially important, as they frequently involve the mixed lineage or myeloid leukemia gene found at 11q23. Benzene metabolites *p*-benzoquinone and hydroquinone inhibit human DNA topoisomerase II (37).

Drugs and chemical agents may interfere with RNA formation. In addition, the translation and transcription processes needed for protein synthesis are a third mechanism that disrupts DNA synthesis (35). Such antibiotics as doxorubicin (Adriamycin) and daunorubicin are examples.

Another way in which a chemical may interfere with cell production is to interfere with the incorporation of vitamin B_{12}, folate, or iron. Examples of agents that act in this way include nitrous oxide (in cases of occupational exposure or abuse), anticonvulsant drugs, methotrexate, isoniazid, and cycloserine. Hypersegmented neutrophils in the peripheral blood are present in addition to the RBC findings, indicating that these agents adversely affect more than one cell line.

Other chemicals and drugs are suspected to cause bone marrow toxicity on an idiosyncratic basis. Their effects may be because of a metabolite that is formed by a secondary pathway and is appreciable in only a minority of individuals, by immunologic sensitization, or by mechanisms not elucidated. Most of these agents have been identified on the basis of individual case reports published in the medical literature (in the American Medical Association Adverse Reactions Registry or to the Food and Drug Administration) or collected by the International Agranulocytosis and Aplastic Anemia Study (38).

Immunologic mechanisms in aplastic anemia have been implicated in decreased production and increased destruction of cellular elements (33). In such cases, the marrow often contains increased numbers of mature lymphocytes and plasma cells. Aplastic anemia shares characteristics with other autoimmune disorders characterized by T-cell–mediated tissue and organ-specific pathology. Common immune events include cytotoxic T-cell activation, cytokine production, and specific target tissue immunopathology. Support for the immune etiology comes from studies that showed that blood cells and marrow samples from patients with aplastic anemia suppressed *in vitro* hematopoietic colony formation by progenitor cells and the removal of T cells improved colony formation *in vitro* (39). The soluble inhibitory factors were found to be IFN-γ and tumor necrosis factor-α, which suppressed proliferation of early and late hematopoietic progenitor and stem cells (40). A marrow incubation assay using the parent compound and its metabolites may assist in ascertaining the causative agent, but a negative assay does not completely exonerate the agent in question.

Drugs and chemicals may form bone marrow–toxic metabolites via activation by cytochrome P-450 monooxygenases and the epoxide hydrolases, which produce electrophilic intermediaries, which in turn can react with and damage macromolecules. Often, toxicity is caused by a minor metabolic pathway that may become significantly active only when major pathways have been saturated or require induction by specific compounds. Some metabolic pathways demonstrate genetic variability (genetic enzyme polymorphism) (38). Four examples of metabolizing enzymes that have been associated with bone marrow injury are (i) aryl hydrocarbon hydroxylase, (ii) epoxide hydrolase, (iii) *S*-methylation, and (iv) *N*-acetylation.

Aryl hydrocarbon hydroxylase is induced by aromatic hydrocarbons. Experimentally, animals that contain an aryl hydrocarbon gene variant that is poorly responsive to induction develop aplastic anemia when exposed to benzo[a]pyrene, benzene, and other aromatics. They can be protected from marrow failure when pretreated by chemicals that induce P-450 microsomal oxidases, such as phenobarbital, or by agents that inhibit P-450 metabolism, such as *a*-naphthoflavone. The basis on which a P-450 enzyme inducer confers protection to the marrow is the first-pass detoxification effect of the liver and intestine. These organs have a vastly greater capacity to metabolize the compound, leaving fewer unaltered hydrocarbon molecules available to reach the marrow.

Another category of substrate-specific enzymes is the epoxide hydrolases, which convert epoxides to phenols. Intrinsic activity and inducibility vary widely among individuals and ethnic groups. Epoxide hydroxylase activity can be measured indirectly by incubating a susceptible patient's lymphocytes with drug intermediates formed by rat hepatic microsomes. The lymphocytes demonstrate the effect of the toxic intermediates and act as a source of epoxide hydroxylase. An example of a drug the effect of which is mediated by this enzyme is phenytoin. Phenytoin-induced aplastic anemia, hepatotoxicity, and birth defects may be detected by lymphocyte incubation assays.

Methylation is an important metabolic pathway for many drugs, some of which may cause myelosuppression. Thiopurine methyltransferase catalyzes the *S*-methylation of the antimetabolites 6-mercaptopurine, 6-thioguanine, and azathioprine. Thiopurine methyltransferase activity is high in 89%, medium in 11%, and absent in 0.03% of the population. When the individuals in whom activity is absent are given doses of azathioprine or 6-mercaptopurine, they accumulate intracellular 6-thioguanine, a purine analog that can be incorporated into DNA. Elevated levels of 6-thioguanine and low or absent enzyme levels were noted in patients with thiopurine- and azathioprine-induced myelosuppression.

Acetylation is another metabolic pathway with polymorphic activity. Fast acetylation is more common among certain ethnic groups (Asians) than others (whites). Acetylation is associated with drug-induced lupus erythematosus, bladder cancer (slow), isoniazid treatment failure against tuberculosis (fast), and sulfonamide toxicity (slow). Sulfa is shunted from the acetylation pathway to the P-450 pathway, generating increased amounts of toxic metabolites such as hydroxylamine. *N*-acetylation is also a major pathway for procainamide metabolism, and slow acetylation is associated with the development of antinuclear antibodies and an SLE-like syndrome.

ALTERATIONS IN SPECIFIC CELL LINES

Agranulocytosis

Agranulocytosis is a syndrome marked by sudden onset and associated with fever, chills, malaise, pharyngitis, mouth ulcers, and cervical lymphadenopathy. Peripheral blood smears show a deficiency in granulocytes, but other leukocytes may also be decreased. Leukocyte counts are usually fewer than 500 cells per µL (41). The absolute number of monocytes and lymphocytes may be decreased or normal. Erythrocyte and platelet counts remain normal. The bone marrow aspirate shows normal erythropoiesis and megakaryocyte production, but myelopoiesis is markedly reduced, with a block at the promyelocyte stage (41). Drugs and chemicals associated with agranulocytosis are listed in Table 28-7. Drugs are implicated in the majority of cases of agranulocytosis (42). Agranulocytosis can result in septicemia, and death due to sepsis may occur. Use of any suspected drug or exposure to a suspected chemical should be discontinued. Spontaneous regeneration occurs within 5 to 9 days in most cases when the causative agent is withdrawn (41).

Leukopenia, as compared to agranulocytosis, is defined as a WBC count of fewer than 4,000 cells per µL. Some chemical agents and certain drugs may reduce the number of WBCs by decreasing production in the bone marrow or increasing peripheral destruction. Some of these agents, if given in sufficient doses, produce neutropenia in a predictable fashion. Production and destruction defects may be immunologically mediated or may be caused by the generation of toxic metabolites. Although some of these pathways have been elucidated, many have not and can be described only as an inherent sensitivity to the chemical or one of its metabolites.

Neutropenia is the most common cause of leukopenia. *Neutropenia* is defined as a neutrophilic granulocyte count of fewer than 1,500 cells per µL. The propensity to infection depends on the severity of neutropenia and underlying disease processes. Patients with neutropenia secondary to bone marrow failure or chemotherapy are at great risk for bacterial infection. Although modest neutropenia of 1,000 to 1,500 cells per µL has little propensity to infection, the affected person may manifest fever and can be managed as an outpatient if not being treated with chemotherapeutic agents or affected with bone marrow failure. Neutropenia ranging from 500 to 1,000 cells per µL does carry a risk of infection. Patients with severe neutropenia (fewer than 500 cells per µL; agranulocytosis) have a high propensity to infection but may not show clinical signs of infection. Neutropenia can be secondary to decreased granulocyte production, a shift of peripheral granulocytes to tissues, margination, or increased peripheral destruction. A large number of chemicals may cause mild, nonprogressive neutropenias that readily return to normal after cessation of exposure to such chemicals.

Ionizing radiation exposure may give rise to lymphopenia. Relatively low exposures are able to lyse lymphocytes and, at higher levels, radiation injures progenitor cells. The most common presentation of chronic toxic exposure to benzene is lymphocytopenia, which often precedes anemia and thrombocytopenia. Therapeutic agents include the alkylating agents, immunosuppressive agents, and antithymocyte globin, which may cause primary marrow damage and inhibit replication of more mature lymphoid elements. Endogenous and administered steroids cause lymphopenia by transiently shifting lymphocytes away from the peripheral blood compartment. Additional causes of lymphopenia include viral, bacterial, and granulomatous infections and antibody-mediated lymphocyte destruction (42).

The bone marrow in chemically induced neutropenia is often hypocellular and exhibits maturation arrest. Mature myeloid elements—myelocytes, metamyelocytes, and polymorphonuclear leukocytes, which are the cells most commonly found in the normal marrow—are absent, whereas earlier granulocytic precursors are preserved.

In immunogenic agranulocytosis, mature lymphocytes and plasma cells, which are not normally found in the marrow, may be present and are believed to produce immunoglobulins. When drug-related antibody is directed at mature neutrophils, the bone marrow may be hypercellular, with a disproportionate increase in myeloid colonies, and all stages of maturation are evident (42).

Leukocytosis

Various host and environmental factors influence the peripheral blood leukocyte count (43). Cigarette smoking, male gender, white race, and increased total body adiposity are associated with an increased peripheral leukocyte count, whereas alcohol ingestion, increasing height and age are inversely related to leukocyte count (43). Heat and intense solar radiation (both sunlight and ultraviolet light) can cause leukocytosis. Acute anoxia, as a result of anemia or hypoxia, causes neutrophilic leukocyto-

TABLE 28-7. Agents associated with agranulocytosis and neutropenia

Chemical exposures
- Antimony
- Arsenic
- Benzene (lymphopenia)
- DDT
- Dinitrophenol
- Gold salts
- Thioglycolic acid (cold wave)

Medicinal agents
- Allopurinol
- Analgesics, sedative and antiinflammatory agents
  - Acetylsalicylic acid
  - Aminopyrine
  - Antipyrine
  - Carbamazepine
  - Colchicine
  - Dipyrone
  - Fenoprofen
  - Ibuprofen
  - Indomethacin
  - Oxyphenbutazone
  - Phenacetin
  - Phenylbutazone
  - Tolmetin
- Antiarrhythmics
  - Procainamide
  - Propranolol
  - Quinidine
- Anticonvulsants
  - Barbiturates
  - Carbamazepine
  - Diphenylhydantoin
  - Ethosuximide
  - Mephenytoin
  - Methylphenylhydantoin
  - Phenytoin
  - Phethenylate
  - Trimethadione
  - Trimethyloxazolidine
- Antihistamines (H_1 and H_2 blockers)
  - Chlorpheniramine
  - Cimetidine
  - Methapheniline
  - Ranitidine
  - Thenaldine
  - Tripelennamine
- Antihypertensives
  - Captopril
  - Enalapril
  - Hydralazine
  - Methyldopa
  - Propranolol
  - Rauwolfia
- Antimalarials
  - Dapsone
  - Hydroxychloroquine
  - Pyrimethamine
  - Quinine
- Antimicrobial agents
  - *p*-Aminobenzoic acid
  - Ampicillin
  - Augmentin
  - Carbenicillin
  - Cephalexin
  - Cephalothin
  - Chloramphenicol
  - Clindamycin
  - Cloxacillin
  - Doxycycline
  - Gentamicin
  - Griseofulvin
  - Isoniazid
  - Isonicotinic acid hydrazine
  - Levamisole
  - Lincomycin
  - Methicillin
  - Metronidazole
  - Nafcillin
  - Nitrofurantoin
  - Norfloxacin
  - Novobiocin
  - Oxacillin
  - Penicillin
  - Rifampin
  - Ristocetin
  - Streptomycin
  - Thiosemicarbazone
  - Vancomycin
- Antithyroid drugs
  - Carbimazole
  - Methimazole
  - Methylthiouracil
  - Propylthiouracil
  - Thiouracil
- Bumetanide
- Cinchophen
- Diethazine
- Drugs associated with antileukocyte antibodies
  - Aminopyrine
  - Ampicillin
  - Chlorpromazine
  - Chlorpropamide
  - Clozapine
  - Dicloxacillin
  - Lidocaine
  - Methimazole
  - Nafcillin
  - Phenytoin
  - Procainamide
  - Propylthiouracil
  - Sulfasalazine
- Ethacrynic acid
- Levamisole
- Mercurial diuretics
- Organic arsenicals
- Penicillamine
- Phenindione
- Phenothiazines and other tranquilizers
  - Butyrophenones
  - Chlorpromazine
  - Clozapine
  - Desipramine
  - Diazepam
  - Haloperidol
  - Imipramine
  - Loxapine
  - Mepazine
  - Meprobamate
  - Molindone
  - Prochlorperazine
  - Promazine
  - Thioridazine
  - Thiothixene
- Plasmochin
- Sulfonamides, antibacterial
  - Succinyl sulfathiazole
  - Sulfadiazine
  - Sulfadiazine silver
  - Sulfaguanidine
  - Sulfanilamide
  - Sulfasalazine
  - Sulfisoxazole
  - Trimethoprim-sulfamethoxazole
- Sulfonamides, nonantibacterial
  - Acetazolamide
  - Carbutamide
  - Chlorothiazide
  - Chlorpropamide
  - Chlorthalidone
  - Hydrochlorothiazide
  - Tolbutamide

Adapted with permission from Lee GR, Foerster J, Lukens J, Wintrobe MM, eds. *Wintrobe's clinical hematology*, vol 1, 9th ed. Philadelphia: Lea & Febiger, 1993:1593; and Handin R, Lux S, Stossel T. *Blood: principles and practice*. Philadelphia: JB Lippincott Co, 1995:524.

sis, even in the absence of an adrenal surge. Acclimatization to high altitudes causes a transient neutrophilia, which then is replaced by a relative lymphocytosis and eosinophilia. Endogenous histamine release that is caused by allergic reactions may also cause a transient neutrophilia.

Strenuous exercise regularly causes neutrophilia and, occasionally, lymphocytosis. Generally, this is due to a shift of leukocytes from the marginal pool to the circulation, and counts return to normal within a few hours. Convulsive seizures, both endogenous and electrically induced, are associated with neutrophilia in a manner similar to the neutrophilia induced by strenuous exercise.

Epinephrine injection produces neutrophilia that peaks and returns to normal rapidly, generally within an hour. Adrenal steroid effects cause transient surges in neutrophils and rapid declines in T and B lymphocytes. These effects probably are responsible for diurnal fluctuations and the leukocytosis reported during exertion, attacks of paroxysmal tachycardia, pain, nausea, and vomiting (in the absence of infection). Administration of cortisone increases blood levels of 17-hydroxycorticosteroids, which cause a transient neutrophilia followed by a more protracted and dose-dependent eosinopenia and lymphopenia.

Some chemicals may produce leukocytosis. Poisoning by lead, especially at levels sufficiently high to produce lead colic, may cause elevated leukocyte counts. Acute poisoning by iron, ethylene glycol, potassium chlorate, digitalis, camphor, antipyrine, acetanilid, phenacetin, quinidine, pyrogallol, turpentine,

TABLE 28-8. Chemical agents associated with thrombocytopenia

Agents that suppress platelet production
- Chemicals that produce generalized bone marrow suppression (see Table 28-6)
- Chemicals that selectively suppress megakaryocytes
  - Chlorothiazide
  - Estrogen
  - Ethanol
  - Tolbutamide

Agents that directly damage platelets
- Bleomycin
- Protamine sulfate
- Ristocetin

Agents associated with antiplatelet antibodies
- Acetaminophen
- Allyl isopropyl carbamide and congeners
- *p*-Aminosalicylic acid
- Cephalothin
- Diazepam
- Diphenylhydantoin
- Gold salts
- Heparin
- Methicillin
- Methyldopa
- Novobiocin
- Penicillin
- Quinidine
- Quinine
- Rifampin
- Stibophen
- Sulfisoxazole

Agents whose mechanism is unknown (presumably immunologic but lacking definitive evidence of antibody formation)
- Acetazolamide
- Allopurinol
- Alprenolol
- Aminopyrine
- Amiodarone
- Ampicillin
- Amrinone
- Antazoline
- Aspirin
- Barbiturates
- Bismuth
- Butalbital
- Carbamazepine
- Carbutamide
- Cephalexin
- Chlordiazepoxide
- Chloroquine
- Chlorothiazide
- Chlorpheniramine
- Chlorpromazine
- Chlorpropamide
- Chlorthalidone
- Cimetidine
- Clinoril
- Clonazepam
- Clopamide
- Codeine
- Colloidal silver
- Copper sulfate
- Clotrimazole
- DDT
- Desipramine
- Dextroamphetamine sulfate
- Diazoxide
- Digitalis
- Digitoxin
- Digoxin
- Dinitrophenol
- Disulfiram
- L-Dopa
- Ergot
- Erythromycin
- Ethyl allyl acetylurea
- Ethylchlorovinyl
- 5-Ethylphenylhydantoin
- Fenoprofen
- Furosemide
- Gentamicin
- Glymidine
- Heroin
- Hexopropynate
- Hydroxychloroquine
- Hydroxyquinolone
- Imipramine
- Indomethacin
- Insecticides
- Iopanoic acid
- Isoniazid
- Lidocaine
- Lincomycin
- Meperidine
- Meprobamate
- Mercurial diuretics
- Minoxidil
- Morphine
- Nitrofurantoin
- Nitroglycerin
- Nitroprusside
- Organic arsenicals
- Organic hair dyes
- Oxyphenbutazone
- Oxytetracycline
- Paramethadione
- Penicillamine
- Pentamidine
- Phenacetin
- Phenobarbital
- Phenylbutazone
- Phenytoin
- Phthalazinol
- Potassium iodide
- Prednisone
- Primidone
- Procainamide
- Prochlorperazine
- Promethazine
- Propylthiouracil
- Pyrazinamide
- Reserpine
- Sodium salicylate
- Spironolactone
- Streptomycin
- Sulfadiazine
- Sulfadimetine
- Sulfamerazine
- Sulfamethazine
- Sulfamethoxazole
- Sulfamethoxypyridazine
- Sulfathiazole
- Tetracycline
- Tetraethyl ammonium
- Thioguanine
- Thiouracil
- Thiourea
- Tobramycin
- Tolbutamide
- Toluene diisocyanate
- Trimethadione
- Trimethoprim
- Turpentine
- Valproate
- Vinyl chloride

Adapted from Bithell TC. Thrombocytopenia caused by immunologic platelet destruction: idiopathic thrombocytopenic purpura (ITP), drug-induced thrombocytopenia, and miscellaneous forms. In: Lee GR, Foerster J, Lukens J, Wintrobe MM, eds. *Wintrobe's clinical hematology,* vol 2, 9th ed. Philadelphia: Lea & Febiger, 1993:1329–1355.

benzene, and arsphenamine causes a transient leukocytosis. Any agent responsible for tissue necrosis can cause increases and decreases in leukocytes, especially neutrophils. Envenomation by reptiles, insects, and jellyfish also may cause a transient neutrophilia because of endogenous release of histamine and adrenal steroids. Chronic inorganic mercury exposure may produce leukocytosis, and therapeutic treatment with corticosteroids and lithium chloride may produce neutrophilia.

Clues to the diagnosis of leukocytosis may be provided by examination of the peripheral smear. Toxic granulations in the neutrophils suggest an infectious etiology, often accompanied by increased numbers of neutrophils with bilobed nuclei (bands) containing Döhle's bodies. Polylobated neutrophils suggest a megaloblastic process. Large numbers of primitive or bizarre-appearing cells suggest an acute leukemia.

Eosinophilia is associated with allergic sensitization, parasitism, and other medical conditions of unknown etiology, such as eosinophilic fasciitis. A contaminant in the manufacture of the amino acid L-tryptophan caused a disorder characterized by eosinophilia, severe generalized myalgia, fever, polyneuropathy, swelling, and induration of the skin.

Thrombocytopenia

Thrombocytopenia is characterized by a reduced number of platelets in the circulating blood. It is the most common cause of abnormal bleeding. Thrombocytopenia results from three processes: (i) deficient platelet production in the bone marrow, (ii) accelerated platelet destruction, and (iii) abnormal distribution or pooling of the platelets. Of these, increased platelet destruction is the most common etiology and generally leads to compensatory stimulation of thrombopoiesis. When destruction exceeds the marrow's ability to increase platelet production, thrombocytopenia develops. The peripheral blood smear and the marrow contain diagnostic clues.

Causes of Thrombocytopenia

Causes of thrombocytopenia include chemical and physical agents that produce accelerated platelet destruction through immunologic mechanisms or primary marrow injury (Table 28-8). Agents that cause bone marrow suppression also produce thrombocytopenia. Platelets often are the last cell type to return to normal levels after toxic insult, and, in some patients, thrombocytopenia persists indefinitely. Other disorders that suppress or reduce megakaryocytes include aplastic anemia, acute and chronic leukemias, myelodysplastic syndromes (MDSs), myelophthisic processes (metastatic carcinomas, histiocytosis, some viruses, myelofibrosis, and osteopetrosis), congenital megakaryocytic hypoplasia, and Fanconi's anemia.

Ineffective thrombopoiesis may be caused by excessive ethanol consumption, deficiencies of vitamin B_{12} or folic acid, severe iron-deficiency anemia, paroxysmal nocturnal hemoglobinuria, and some hereditary syndromes. Deficient thrombopoietin may also cause decreased production of platelets. Some drugs, such as chlorothiazide, may suppress thrombopoiesis and induce platelet antibodies. Mild asymptomatic thrombocytopenia may be seen in as many as 25% of people on chlorothiazide therapy. This agent may also cause thrombocytopenia in the neonate if taken by the mother during pregnancy. Megakaryocyte production is impaired in the neonate, whereas mothers rarely are found to be thrombocytopenic.

Accelerated platelet destruction often is caused by immunologic mechanisms. For many of these drug- or chemical-induced thrombocytopenias, no antibody can be identified, and the mechanism is presumed to be immunologic. Antibodies that may damage platelets are associated also with idiopathic thrombocytopenia purpura, hemolytic anemias, SLE, lymphoreticular disorders, the acquired immunodeficiency syndrome, and hypothyroidism (44). Other immunologic processes that may cause a transient thrombocytopenia include vaccinations, anaphylaxis, and allergic reactions to insect bites and foods (44). Additional causes of increased platelet destruction are diffuse intravascular coagulation, tumors, infectious diseases, microangiopathic processes, and splenic sequestration.

Thrombocytopenia has been reported from exposures to benzene, cresol, naphthalene, and several insecticides, including DDT, lethane, pyrethrin, dieldrin, 2,2-dichlorovinyldimethylphosphate, chlordane, and γ-benzene hexachloride (45–49). The mechanism appears to be marrow toxicity, as megakaryocytes were reported to be reduced (45–49). Two agents associated with immunologically mediated thrombocytopenia are toluene diisocyanate and turpentine (45,46). Two cases of symptomatic thrombocytopenia occurred after acute, high exposures to toluene diisocyanate that induced bronchospasm. Subsequently, the platelet count in each of these patients dropped to 6,000 and $30,000 \times 10^9$ per liter. Turpentine also is reported to have caused symptomatic thrombocytopenia after exposure (46). On bone marrow examination in this case, megakaryocytes were plentiful, peripheral platelet destruction was increased, and thrombocytopenia resolved with steroid treatment.

Vinyl chloride has been reported to cause thrombocytopenia in workers who have developed vinyl chloride–induced hepatic fibrosis with esophageal varices and splenomegaly (47). The thrombocytopenia was likely due to splenic sequestration.

Abnormal bleeding may be caused by interference with platelet function. Environmental exposures to DDT (via its metabolite pp'DDE) and polychlorinated biphenyls (Arochlor 1242) are associated with coagulation defects by inhibiting platelet cyclooxygenase, which interferes with aggregation (48,49). Drugs that interfere with platelet function are listed in Table 28-9.

TABLE 28-9. Agents that interfere with platelet function

Antihistamines (H_1)
Aspirin
Caffeine
Cephalothin
Clofibrate
Corticosteroids
Dextrans
Dipyridamole
Ethanol
Fenoprofen
Furosemide
Ibuprofen
Indomethacin
Naproxen
Nonsteroidal antiinflammatory agents
Penicillins
Phenothiazine
Phentolamine
Piroxicam
Procaine
Propranolol
Snake venoms (vipers and crotalids)
Tricyclic antidepressants

Significant bleeding is unusual with platelet counts higher than 50,000 and usually does not become evident until platelet counts fall to fewer than 20,000. An enlarged spleen suggests platelet sequestration. Petechiae, pallor, and fever suggest aplasia or leukemia.

BONE MARROW

Increased peripheral destruction usually causes a compensatory proliferation in megakaryocytes in bone marrow. When platelet production is directly suppressed, megakaryocytes in the marrow are reduced in number or appear abnormal (i.e., hypoplastic and small, with a small rim of cytoplasm). When ineffective thrombopoiesis occurs, the total number of megakaryocytes in the marrow increases, but the cytoplasm does not increase in volume. The number of platelets produced per megakaryocyte is diminished, and the megakaryocytic nucleus appears to be hyperlobulated.

HEMATOPOIETIC MALIGNANCIES

Leukemias, lymphomas, multiple myeloma, and myelodysplasia are clonal diseases that arise from primitive precursor cells. When exposed to a specific causative chemical agent or radiation, cells in the marrow may be damaged. However, only a single cell initiates a clone that continues to expand, giving rise to a malignant process.

Some clonal diseases start at the level of the pluripotential stem cell. Other neoplasms, such as acute myeloblastic leukemia or the lymphocytic leukemias, are descendants from a committed cellular progenitor that is further along the granulocytic or lymphocytic pathway. Table 28-10 provides an overview of the hematopoietic malignancies, organized by probable cell of origin, a nomenclature established by a French-American-British (FAB) cooperative group (50,51).

As with most cancers, no single factor is responsible for the development of leukemia. It is likely that most leukemias arise

TABLE 28-10. Classification of neoplastic diseases of the hematopoietic system

I. Neoplasms of stem cell origin
  A. Without maturation: chronic myelogenous leukemia in myeloblastic phase (Philadelphia chromosome bcr/abl translocation present)
    1. Myeloid differentiation predominant
    2. Lymphoid differentiation predominant
  B. With maturation: chronic myelogenous leukemia
  C. Mixed lymphoid-myeloid differentiation (FAB M0, M1, L1, L2)
II. Neoplasms of multipotential stem cell origin
  A. Myelodysplastic syndromes
    1. Refractory anemia
    2. Refractory anemia with ring sideroblasts
    3. Refractory anemia with excess blasts
    4. Chronic myelomonocytic leukemia
    5. Refractory anemia with excess blasts in transformation
  B. Chronic myeloproliferative disorders
    1. Polycythemia rubra vera
    2. Thrombocythemia
    3. Myelofibrosis not associated with acute myelogenous leukemia
III. Neoplasms that originate in myeloid-committed precursors
  A. Acute myeloid leukemia
    1. (FAB) M0: Myeloblastic leukemia with minimal differentiation
    2. (FAB) M1: Myeloblastic leukemia without maturation
    3. (FAB) M2: Myeloblastic leukemia with maturation
    4. (FAB) M3: Promyelocytic leukemia
    5. (FAB) M4: Myelomonocytic leukemia
    6. (FAB) M5: Monocytoid leukemia
    7. (FAB) M6: Erythroleukemia
    8. (FAB) M7: Megakaryoblastic leukemia
IV. Neoplasms of lymphoid-committed precursors
  A. Immature phenotype: acute lymphoblastic leukemia (FAB L1 and L2)
  B. Intermediate or mature phenotype: non-Hodgkin's lymphoma
  C. Mature lymphocytic phenotype
    1. Prolymphocytic leukemia
    2. Chronic lymphocytic leukemia
    3. Hairy-cell leukemia
  D. Plasmacytoid phenotype (multiple myeloma)
V. Neoplasms of controversial (possibly lymphoid) origin: Hodgkin's disease

FAB, French-American-British cooperative group (Groupe Française de Morphologique Hematologique).
Kinney MC, Lukens JN. Classification and differentiation of the acute leukemias. In: Lee GR, Foerster J, Lukens J, et al., eds. *Wintrobe's clinical hematology,* vol 1, 10th ed. Baltimore: Williams & Wilkins, 1999:2209–2240; and Stock W, Thirman MJ. Pathobiology of acute myeloid leukemia. In: Hoffman R, Benz E, Shattil S, et al., eds. *Hematology: basic principles and practice,* 3rd ed. New York: Churchill Livingstone, 1999:979–999.

from the interaction of host susceptibility and one or more chemical or physical agents. On the molecular level, leukemogenic agents appear to act by damaging DNA in critical areas or interfering with cell signaling. Evidence is mounting that suggests that the critical step in this process is inhibition of the activity of a suppressor gene or activation of an oncogene.

Tumor Suppressor Gene Inhibition and Oncogene Activation

A malignant transformation involves somatic and heritable changes in some genes that control normal cell growth and cell development (52). The affected genes are of two types: oncogenes, which induce oncogenic growth, and tumor suppressor genes, which negatively regulate cell growth. Many oncogenes were discovered because of their presence in retroviruses that induced animal tumors. In hematologic neoplasms, inappropriate activation of oncogenes—either from transcription errors or structural rearrangements—often occurs and is believed to be fundamental to neoplastic transformation. Loss of genetic material, especially involving chromosomes 5, 7, and Y, are observed in acute nonlymphocytic leukemia (ANLL) and in MDSs and may result in inactivation of tumor suppressor genes located in specific regions on these chromosomes (53). Genetic alterations are found in cases of acute myelogenous leukemia (AML). Genetic alterations that are specific to AML include loss of the long arms of chromosomes 5, 7, and 20, which occurs in therapy-related AML and AML associated with prior MDS. Chromosomal alterations may be balanced or unbalanced, and recurrent gain or loss of chromosomes and structural rearrangements may be evident. In one study of 354 patients, a gain of chromosome 8 was the most frequent abnormality seen in AML (13%), loss of chromosome 7 was the second most frequent change (9%), and loss of chromosome 5 was seen in 6% (54).

Environmental associations with AML have been reported. A retrospective study of 52 patients with *de novo* AML who were exposed to various chemicals demonstrated a 75% rate of clonal chromosomal abnormalities as compared with 32% of a control group (55). Seventy-nine percent of the chromosomally abnormal cases had at least one of four specific abnormalities: –5/del(5q), –7/del(7q), +8, or +21. Other studies have reported on the association among smoking, irradiation, exposure to solvents and hair dyes, and specific cytogenetic abnormalities and *ras* oncogene activation in patients with AML or acute lymphoblastic leukemia (56).

Studies of secondary leukemias—those that clearly followed treatment with radiotherapy and alkylating agents, as well as those following chemical exposures—show that a large percentage have abnormal karyotypes. A high percentage of patients with therapy-related leukemias have abnormal chromosomes (50). In one study, 93% of patients (252 of 270) had abnormal chromosomes (50). These abnormalities involved loss of chromosome 5 following unbalanced translocation, del(5q), loss of chromosome 5, loss of chromosome 7, del(7q), and loss of 7q as a result of unbalanced translocation of 7q22. Overall, 43% of patients had a loss of 5q, and 51% had a loss of 7q. The most common aberration was del(5q).

Karyotypic abnormalities include structural aberrations: deletions, unbalanced translocations, isochromosomes, and ring chromosomes. Of particular interest are translocations. One, which is present in more than 90% of chronic myelogenous leukemias (CMLs), is the Philadelphia chromosome, which is a balanced translocation between chromosomes 9 and 22 that causes fusion of gene sites coding for the breakpoint cluster region (bcr) and the avian blastic leukemia (abl) proteins. The protooncogene c-*sis* is very similar to the simian sarcoma virus oncogene. A related fusion protein is seen in approximately one-third of patients with acute lymphoblastic leukemia. The bcr/abl fusion protein acts to disrupt transcription control by increasing tyrosine kinase activity. This occurs via an interaction between the *ras* oncogene and p21 (57–59). Acute promyelocytic leukemia (FAB M3) often shows a translocation [15,17] that alters the promyelocytic leukemia and retinoic acid receptor-α gene sites (60). Fusion proteins also are produced by this translocation and are similar to proteins that may transform cells into malignancy by fusing onto protooncogenes and altering transcription.

Genetic alterations in the *ras* oncogenes are the most common molecular abnormalities found in the ANLLs and MDSs. The N, K, and H *ras* oncogenes encode membrane-bound G-proteins, which are components of the intracellular signal transduction pathways controlling mitogenesis and differentiation (61). In one report, a disproportionate number of AML patients with mutations in *ras* had been employed for 5 or more years in work involving exposure to benzene, as compared with AML patients who did not have *ras* mutations (odds ratio, 9.1) (62). Taylor et al.

(62) noted that *ras* mutations were present also in one worker who did not have disease. Mutations in the *myc* protooncogenes (L, N, and c) have been implicated in human hematopoietic malignancies, including AML. These mutations encode nuclear phosphoproteins, which are believed to participate in the control of cell proliferation and differentiation. The relationship between c-*myc* mutations and chemical exposure has not been elucidated.

Environmental Leukemogenic Agents

BENZENE

Some studies suggest that people who pursue certain occupations are at increased risk of developing hematolymphatic malignancies. Any chemical capable of inducing bone marrow damage must be assumed to be a potential leukemogen. Two known environmental leukemogenic agents are ionizing radiation and benzene. People exposed to ionizing radiation from nuclear fallout or treatment with x-rays for benign and malignant disease and those who work on nuclear submarines have exhibited excess mortality from leukemia.

Industries in which workers are chronically exposed to benzene have demonstrated an increased incidence of AML among their workers (32,63–69). In addition, chronic high-level inhalational benzene exposure has been shown to be linked to bone marrow suppression, aplastic anemia, pancytopenia, lymphopenia, leukocytopenia, and anemia of the macrocytic variety (32,63–69).

Epidemiologic studies show that of the leukemia subtypes, only AML incidence is elevated significantly in association with benzene exposure. In a large cohort study of cancer among 74,828 benzene-exposed workers, the incidence of AML alone was found to be significantly elevated (66). Although this cohort study also identified cases of CML and ALL, these were nonsignificant excesses. In addition, the same large cohort study found a significant excess of cases of aplastic anemia (n = 9) and MDS (66).

Research indicates that individuals vary in their susceptibility to benzene hematotoxicity, possibly due to interindividual variation in metabolic activation and benzene detoxification. Benzene is metabolized to benzene oxide by the enzyme CYP2E1, which then spontaneously forms phenol, which is metabolized to hydroquinone (70). The hydroquinone and its related hydroxymetabolites are converted by myeloperoxidase in the bone marrow to benzoquinones, potent genotoxic and hemotoxic compounds. These hematotoxic metabolites also can be converted back to less toxic compounds by NQO1 enzymes (70). One study examined whether high CYP2E1 enzyme activity and low NQO1 enzyme activity would increase an individual's susceptibility to benzene toxicity (70). The study involved a retrospective cohort of 11,177 benzene-exposed workers in China. Of these workers, benzene poisoning was diagnosed in 103. Three of these subjects developed hematologic malignancies—one ANLL, one MDS, and one non-Hodgkin's lymphoma. Within 4 to 14 years after the diagnosis of benzene toxicity, seven subjects in the study in whom benzene poisoning was not found were diagnosed with hematologic malignancy—three non-Hodgkin's lymphoma, two ANLL, one CML, one multiple myeloma, and one MDS. Benzene poisoning was associated with a 71-fold risk for ANLL or MDS. Results showed that benzene poisoning cases were associated with the $NQO1^{609}$ C→T mutation and a rapid fractional secretion of chlorozoxazone, thus documenting that interindividual variation in a metabolic process in humans is associated with increased risk of benzene hematotoxicity (70).

Studies of patients with occupational exposure to benzene show a pattern of cytogenetic aberrations involving chromosome 5 or 7 (or both) and trisomy 8 (71). Another study demonstrated that hydroquinone induces a specific chromosome loss found in secondary MDS and AML (72). AML and its subtypes (mainly M1, M2, M4, or M6) are the most frequent hematologic malignancies associated with chronic benzene exposure and alkylating agents (73). The metabolites of benzene are clastogenic, causing micronuclei and aneuploidy and disrupting microtubular assembly, which interferes with spindle formation during mitosis (72,74). Hydroquinone, a major benzene metabolite, has been demonstrated to cause genetic alterations of chromosomes 5 and 7 that are associated with early events in benzene-induced AML (72).

Cancer is believed to be an evolutionary process in which multiple events involving independent genetic alterations along with environmental factors contribute to the development of malignant phenotype. Leukemia is a multistep process, and such a model for benzene-induced AML has been proposed involving progressive dysplastic changes accompanied by a pattern of clonal cytogenetic abnormalities in hematopoietic target cells (74). This model involves altered proliferation accompanied by genetic damage that leads to progressive selection and gives rise to the evolution of a leukemic hematopoietic progenitor cell clone. Frequently, cases of ANLL are preceded by pancytopenia or myelodysplasia.

Studies of benzene-related leukemias suggest similarities to leukemias that occur after treatment with cancer chemotherapeutic agents: the so-called secondary leukemias (75). In such cases, the risk of secondary MDS or ANLL is increased ten- to 105-fold over that of the general population. Factors that seem to increase risk are abnormalities of cellular immunity and treatment with alkylating agents, topoisomerase II inhibitors, and total or partial body irradiation (73,75–77). Similarities between secondary and benzene-related leukemias include an increased incidence of mutant *ras* oncogene activity, an increased incidence of deletions and translocations (often involving chromosomes 5 and 7), and a poorer prognosis (78,79).

Some researchers report that *p*-benzoquinone and hydroquinone, reactive metabolites of benzene, inhibit topoisomerase II activity (37,80). Topoisomerase II is an endonuclease required for replication, recombination, chromosome segregation, and chromosome structure. However, the pattern of chromosome aberrations typically associated with inhibition of topoisomerase II has not been observed in occupationally exposed populations (72). In a study of a Chinese cohort occupationally exposed to benzene, increases in cytogenetic aberrations were noted (81). The study showed that exposure to benzene was associated with a marked increase in the loss and long-arm deletions of chromosomes 5 and 7 [–5, –7, del(5sq), and del(7sq)] in lymphocytes of workers (81). Particularly interesting was the finding of a partial deletion of the long arm of chromosome 5 (–5q), which has been found by others in increased frequency in series of patients who have an MDS or AML (82). An increase in glycophorin A mutations was observed also in this group of workers heavily exposed to benzene (70).

1,3-BUTADIENE

Workers exposed to 1,3-butadiene are reported to be at increased risk for lymphohematopoietic cancers (69,83). The standard mortality ratio (SMR) in one cohort of 2,795 men equaled 191 for lymphosarcoma, 113 for leukemia, and 152 for other lymphatic tissue malignancies among the 1,222 deaths identified (83). Ward et al. (84) studied 364 men in three butadiene plants, noting an SMR of 577 for lymphosarcoma and reticulosarcoma and a non–statistically significant increase in stomach cancer among the 185 deaths observed overall in the study cohort (84,85). Another study included 15,649 men in eight styrene-butadiene rubber plants (86), in which 3,976 deaths occurred: The leukemia SMR was 194 for hourly workers who had been employed 10 or more years in the industry and whose disease was diagnosed 20 or more years after their date of hire. The study found that the SMR equaled 251 for workers in polymerization, 265 for maintenance laborers, and 431 for laboratory personnel—three labor divisions in which workers potentially experienced higher exposure to butadiene or styrene monomer. Macaluso et al. (87) studied a cohort of 16,610 subjects employed at six styrene-butadiene rubber-manufacturing plants. Among these workers, the risk of leukemia rose to 4.5 in their highest exposure category, which was defined as 80 ppm-years or more.

Complicating factors in 1,3-butadiene studies are multiple exposures to other chemicals used in the styrene-butadiene rubber-production process and potential confounding agents [dithiocarbamates (DTCs)] that are employed in the rubber industry. DTCs represent a class of thiono-sulfur-containing compounds used as accelerators in the vulcanization of rubber. The hematotoxicity of DTCs has been associated with the risk of developing leukemia in styrene-butadiene rubber production (88).

Overall, the regulatory and scientific categorization of 1,3-butadiene has been fraught with controversy. In 1998, the U.S. Environmental Protection Agency's Science Advisory Board held 2 days of open hearings on 1,3-butadiene toxicology. After extensive discussion and review, the board did not upgrade 1,3-butadiene to a group A known human carcinogen. In contrast, on the basis of the same epidemiologic and toxicologic database, the U.S. National Toxicology Program, in its ninth report on carcinogens released in the spring of 2000, upgraded the status of 1,3-butadiene to "known to be a human carcinogen" (89). Finally, in a series of studies similar to the Chinese benzene research, Hayes et al. (90) were unable to show specific genotoxic effects at the chromosomal or genetic levels related to 2-ppm exposure levels in Chinese butadiene polymer–production workers.

Myelofibrosis

The MDSs are a group of five related chronic diseases of stem cells in which marrow fibrosis and ineffective extramedullary hematopoiesis occur in the liver and spleen. A high percentage of MDSs transform into acute leukemias. Occupational exposure to benzene and ionizing radiation and treatment with cytotoxic drugs are known causes, but the vast majority of cases are of unknown etiology. The megakaryocyte mass in marrow is increased, liberating large amounts of platelet-derived growth factor and transforming growth factor–β, interleukin-1, and tumor necrosis factor–α, agents known to cause fibrosis.

Many patients with myelofibrosis are asymptomatic, but some report fatigue, weight loss, weakness, symptoms of splenomegaly and hepatomegaly (abdominal fullness, early satiety), bone pain, and easy bruising. Physical findings include splenomegaly, hepatomegaly, bruising, petechiae, and adenopathy. Signs of portal hypertension may exist. Fever, edema, pallor, extramedullary masses, Sweet's syndrome (neutrophilic dermatosis), and effusions containing hematopoietic cells also are seen. Men are disproportionately affected, and the typical age at diagnosis is older than 60 years. A detailed occupational and exposure history is necessary to determine whether work situations existed in which the patient may have been exposed to myelotoxicants or products contaminated with them.

Examination of the peripheral blood shows teardrop cells, circulating normoblasts, evidence of hemolysis, reticulocytosis, leukocytosis with immature elements, circulating megakaryocytes or their fragments, and hypersegmented or hyposegmented polymorphonuclear leukocytes. Platelets often are increased but may be decreased or normal. The bone marrow in myelofibrosis often cannot be aspirated. A moderate to marked increase in reticulin and collagen is detectable. Megakaryocytosis often is present. Patchy hypercellularity with mild maturational abnormalities is common. Cytogenetic abnormalities are significant, often with bizarre metaphases and fragmented chromosomes. Generally, all three cell lines are affected. Alterations in chromosomes 5, 7, 8, 9, and 20 are found in more than 50% of some case series. Monoclonal and polyclonal cell populations have been described (91,92). Immunologic tests often are positive, including antinuclear antibodies, RBC antibodies, and immune complexes. As MDS evolves, a significant increase occurs in the percentage of CD34 cells among all myeloid cells (92).

Nonneoplastic conditions that may cause marrow fibrosis include immune diseases (SLE, polyarteritis nodosa), tuberculosis, rickets, histiocytosis, sarcoidosis, and sickle cell anemia.

MEDICAL SURVEILLANCE FOR HEMATOLOGIC INJURY

Blood counts alone are a poor predictor of early hematopoietic toxicity of either an acute or chronic nature. This is so because of the variability in the healthy population, as reflected in the broad ranges cited as normal and the diversity of benign conditions that may increase or decrease cellular parameters. Published studies of occupational cohorts comment on the lack of sensitivity, specificity, and predictive value of blood count determinations (93,94). Complete blood count surveillance of petrochemical manufacturing workers is an ineffective tool in identifying leukemia or preleukemic states.

Nonetheless, much of the WBC count variability is due to neutrophils, which respond to a wide range of physiologic and nonoccupational stressors. Eliminating the neutrophil component diminishes the variability of the total WBC count substantially. Studies suggest that absolute lymphocyte counts may be useful to identify workers who may be experiencing hematotoxicity from occupational exposures (66). Studies have identified exposure-response correlations between airborne benzene dose or exposure and decreases in lymphocyte counts (69). One study, which used two independent determinations of benzene exposures—organic vapor passive dosimetry and measurement of urinary metabolites (muconic acid, phenol, catechol, and hydroquinone conjugates)—found that the mean absolute lymphocyte count fell 16% in the group of workers exposed to 7.6 ppm benzene as compared with unexposed controls and fell 31% in the group of workers exposed to 31 ppm as compared with controls (66). A second study on a rubber hydrochloride cohort showed similar findings even at maximum exposure levels of 1.4 ppm daily (68).

The MCV may be used to monitor chemical exposures that are associated with microcytic or megaloblastic changes. One can screen also for chemicals that are associated with increased RBC destruction, because a compensatory reticulocytosis will be reflected in a modest increase in MCV that can be confirmed by a reticulocyte count.

Studies on workers exposed to benzene suggest that MCV may be useful when evaluating hematotoxicity (66), with one study suggesting that statistically significant changes are observed even at median exposures of 1.4 ppm (68). An even more sensitive but nonspecific parameter that may be used to assess the RBCs quantitatively is the RBC distribution width. This measurement, which is the coefficient of variation of the MCV, evaluates the size distribution of the RBCs. Alterations in this measurement can be seen before changes in MCV are appreciated.

RBC and WBC counts exhibit less intraindividual than interindividual variation. Medical surveillance programs may take advantage of this by performing baseline studies on each worker and comparing yearly changes. The variance drops substantially. More than a 10% to 20% change in hematocrit or 50% alteration in MCV or absolute lymphocyte count suggests an adverse effect. These variances should, of course, be correlated with environmental sampling and integrated with biological monitoring results.

Examination of the peripheral smear is an inexpensive, relatively sensitive tool for evaluating early changes in RBC and WBC morphology and, in conjunction with the parameters noted previously, can be of some value. It has not been the subject of rigorous study in the context of occupational surveillance.

Increasingly, enzyme polymorphisms are being identified that may predict individual sensitivities or susceptibilities. Critical enzyme systems are those involved with metabolism and detoxification of potentially hematotoxic agents, such as those that are involved with production of energy and transfer of oxygen. Prescreening for some of these enzyme polymorphisms may be indicated when target chemicals are likely to be encountered in the work environment. Candidates include polymorphisms in aryl hydrocarbon hydroxylase, glutathione synthetase, *S*-methylation, epoxide hydrolase, G6PD, and methemoglobin reductase.

A gradation in risk between cases of hematopoietic disease and controls may be due to genetic polymorphisms. One study measured CYP2E1 and NQO1 variants, determining that subjects with both variant CYP2E1 (as measured by fast chloroxazone excretion) and two copies of variant NQO1 (with C→T mutation) had a 7.6-fold increased risk of benzene toxicity as compared with those who had wild-type enzymes (94a).

Another study measured glutathione-*S*-transferase isoenzyme polymorphisms and showed that the lymphocytes from GST-M1–negative individuals had a higher number of sister chromatid exchanges (SCEs) when incubated with butadiene epoxides than did the lymphocytes of GST-M1–positive donors and that GST-T1–negative donors had a higher number of SCEs when incubated with butadiene monoepoxide than did GST-T1–positive donors (95). This study indicates that susceptibility to the effects of 1,3-butadiene is modulated by these enzyme variants.

Molecular biomarkers can be examined for peripheral blood lymphocytes. Genetic alterations are common in leukemias, suggesting that cytogenetics may prove fruitful in predicting increased risk for neoplastic disease. A number of studies performed in diverse occupational settings have explored the potential for using DNA adducts, SCEs, abnormalities in reporter genes (*hprt*), glycophorin A oncogenes (*p53* and *ras*), and fixed translocations (96). DNA adducts are specific but transient and are excellent markers of exposure but not of effect. SCEs also are short-lived. Studies evaluating stable or persistent DNA changes offer intriguing possibilities for evaluating effects and predicting risk.

Studies in benzene-exposed workers provide compelling evidence that persistent cytogenetic changes are sensitive indicators of early biological effect that may have prognostic significance. The structural aberrations, particularly deletions and translocations, have been examined in cross-sectional cohort studies as well as in case-control studies. These studies potentially provide support for risk stratification on the basis of abnormalities in cytogenetic markers (97–101).

Other studies underscore the utility of examining persistent cytogenetic aberrations and continuing follow-up for long periods. Hagmar et al. (102) cytogenetically studied 1,982 subjects, with follow-up from 1970 to 1990, and noted that risk of cancer increased with the number of chromosomal aberrations.

Bonassi et al. (103) studied 871 hospital workers exposed to ionizing radiation and found that chromosomal aberrations closely tracked radiation exposure.

Studies using fluorescent *in situ* hybridization and chromosome probes offer a relatively rapid and sensitive method by which to assess cytogenetic abnormalities quantitatively in peripheral lymphocytes. Prospective studies, however, have yet to be reported. The predictive value of these surveillance tools is under study, so it is too soon to recommend their use for routine surveillance.

G6PD and methemoglobin-reductase variants predict increased susceptibility to methemoglobin-forming agents. Polymorphisms in P-450 isotopes, *N*-acetyl transferase, and glutathione synthetase reflect individual differences in the metabolism of xenobiotics. Assessment of genotypic and phenotypic enzymatic polymorphisms can be performed by standardized techniques that are available from reference laboratories.

DNA adducts are specific but transient and are excellent markers of exposure but not of effect. SCEs are useful as nonspecific markers but are short-lived. Those studies evaluating stable or persistent DNA changes offer possibilities for evaluating effects and predicting risk.

DNA repair efficiency has been studied in benzene- and butadiene-exposed workers (104). The rationale for this test stems from the hypothesis that some environmental toxicants induce genetic damage by disrupting the normal DNA repair enzymes, so that somatic mutations, once formed, are more likely to persist. The assay challenges lymphocytes from exposed workers with a clastogenic agent (ionizing radiation or bleomycin), then measures mutational foci that persist after cell replication. Preliminary studies appear promising.

More prospective studies are needed to determine the predictive value and true utility of these surveillance tools. Increasingly, cytogenetic markers, gene polymorphisms, and mutational events are being incorporated into epidemiologic tools, and their incorporation into routine medical surveillance may be forthcoming (103).

REFERENCES

1. Roath S, Laver J, Lawman J, Gross S. Biologic control mechanisms. In: Gross S, Roath S, eds. *Hematology: a problem-oriented approach*. Baltimore: Williams & Wilkins, 1996.
2. Schnall SF, Berliner N, Duffy TP, Benz EJ. Approach to the adult and child with anemia. In: Hoffman R, Benz E, Shattil S, et al., eds. *Hematology: basic principles and practice*, 3rd ed. New York: Churchill Livingstone, 2000.
3. Wiley JS, Moore MR. Heme biosynthesis and its disorders: porphyrias and sideroblastic anemias. In: Hoffman R, Benz E, Shattil S, et al., eds. *Hematology: basic principles and practice*, 3rd ed. New York: Churchill Livingstone, 2000.
4. Mansouri A. Review: methemoglobinemia. *Am J Med Sci* 1985;289:200–209.
5. Fan AM, Steinberg VE. Health implications of nitrate and nitrite in drinking water: an update on methemoglobinemia occurrence and reproductive and developmental toxicity. *Regul Toxicol Pharmacol* 1996;23(1, part 1):35.
6. Fisch RO, Berglund EB, Bridge AG, et al. Methemoglobinemia in a hospital nursery. *JAMA* 1963;185:760.
7. Singley TL. Secondary methemoglobinemia due to the adulteration of fish with sodium nitrite. *Ann Intern Med* 1962;57:800.
8. Djerassi LS, Vitany L. Hemolytic episode of G6PD deficient workers exposed to TNT. *Br J Ind Med* 1975;32:54.
9. Gannon PF, Sherwood Burge P, Hewlett C, Tee RD. Haemolytic anemia in a case of occupational asthma due to maleic anhydride. *Br J Ind Med* 1992;49:142.
10. Minami H, Katsumata M, Tomoda A. Methemoglobinemia with oxidized hemoglobins and modified hemoglobins found in bloods of workers handling aromatic compounds and in those of a man who drank cresol solution. *Biomed Biochem Acta* 1990;49:S327.
11. Hassan AB, Seligmann H, Bassan HM. Intravascular hemolysis induced by pentachlorophenol. *BMJ* 1985;291:21.
12. Romeo L, Apostoli P, Kovacic M, Martini S, Brugnone F. Acute arsine intoxication as a consequence of metal burnishing operations. *Am J Ind Med* 1997;32:211.
13. Adams KF, Johnson G Jr, Hornowski KE, Lineberger TH. The effect of copper on erythrocyte deformability: a possible mechanism of hemolysis in acute copper intoxication. *Biochim Biophys Acta* 1979;550:279.
14. Fairbanks VF. Copper sulfate induced hemolytic anemia. *Arch Intern Med* 1967;120:428.
15. Curry S. Methemoglobinemia. *Ann Emerg Med* 1982;11:214–221.
16. Klimecki WT, Carter DE. Arsine toxicity: chemical and mechanistic implications. *J Toxicol Environ Health* 1995;46(4):399.
17. Pinkhas J. Sulfhemoglobinemia and acute hemolytic anemia with Heinz bodies following contact with a fungicide—zinc ethylene bis-dithiocarbamate—in a subject with G6PD deficiency and hypocatalasemia. *Blood* 1963;21:484.
18. Koury ST, Koury MJ, Bondurant MC, et al. Quantitation of erythropoietin-producing cells in kidneys of mice by in situ hybridization: correlation with hematocrit, renal erythropoietin MRNA, and serum erythropoietin concentration. *Blood* 1989;74:645–651.
19. LeBeau MM, Albain KS, Larson RA, et al. Clinical and cytogenetic correlation in 63 patients with therapy-related myelodysplastic syndromes and acute nonlymphocytic leukemia: further evidence for characteristic abnormalities of chromosomes nos. 5 and 7. *J Clin Oncol* 1986;4:325–345.
20. Cam C, Nigogosyan G. Acquired porphyria cutanea tarda due to hexachlorobenzene: report of 348 cases due to the fungicide. *JAMA* 1963;183:88.

21. Peters H, Cripps D, Gocmen A, et al. Turkish epidemic hexachlorobenzene porphyria: a 30-year study. *Ann N Y Acad Sci* 1987;514:183.
22. Gocmen A, Peters HA, Cripps DJ, et al. Hexachlorobenzene episode in Turkey. *Biomed Environ Sci* 1989;2:36.
23. Calvert GM, et al. Evaluation of porphyria cutanea tarda in US workers exposed to 2,4,7,8-tetrachlorodibenzo-*p*-dioxin. *Am J Ind Med* 1994;25:559.
24. Sterling TD, Arundel AV. Health effects of phenoxy herbicides. A review. *Scand J Work Environ Health* 1986;12:161.
25. Kauppinen T, Kogevinas M, Johnson E, et al. Chemical exposure in manufacture of phenoxy herbicides and chlorophenols and in spraying of phenoxy herbicides. *Am J Ind Med* 1993;23:903.
26. Pirastu R, Comba P, Reggiani A, Foa B, Masena A, Maltoni C. Mortality from liver disease among Italian vinyl chloride monomer–polyvinyl chloride manufacturers. *Am J Ind Med* 1990;17:155.
27. Young NS, Maciejewski JP. Aplastic anemia. *Hematology: basic principles and practice*, 3rd ed. New York: Churchill Livingstone, 1999.
28. Kaufman DW, Kelly J, Jurgelm J, et al. Drugs in the etiology of agranulocytosis and aplastic anemia. *Eur J Haematol Suppl* 1996;60:23.
29. Aksoy M. Hematotoxicity and carcinogenicity of benzene. *Environ Health Perspect* 1989;82:193–197.
30. Smith M. Overview of benzene-induced aplastic anemia. *Eur J Haematol Suppl* 1996;57:107–110.
31. Ross D. Metabolic basis of benzene toxicity. *Eur J Haematol* 1996;57(Suppl): 111–118.
32. Yin S, Hayes R, Linet M, et al. A cohort study of cancer among benzene exposed workers in China: overall results. *Am J Ind Med* 1996;29:227–235.
33. Young NS, Maciejewski JP. Aplastic anemia. In: Hoffman R, Benz E, Shattil S, et al., eds. *Hematology: basic principles and practice,* 3rd ed. New York: Churchill Livingstone, 1999.
34. Wallace D, Hahn B. *Dubois' lupus erythematosus*, 5th ed. Baltimore: Williams & Wilkins, 1997.
35. LeBeau MM, Larson RA. Cytogenetics and neoplasia. In: Hoffman R, Benz E, Shattil S, et al., eds. *Hematology: basic principles and practice,* 3rd ed. New York: Churchill Livingstone, 1999.
36. Wang JC. DNA topoisomerases. *Annu Rev Biochem* 1996;65:635–692.
37. Hutt AM, Kalf GF. Inhibition of human DNA topoisomerase II by hydroquinone and *p*-benzoquinone: reactive metabolites of benzene. *Environ Health Perspect* 1996;(Suppl 6):1265.
38. Kaufman DW, Kell JP, Levy M, Shapiro S. *The drug etiology of agranulocytosis and aplastic anemia.* New York: Oxford University Press, 1991.
39. Kagan WA, Ascensao JA, Pahwa RN, et al. Aplastic anemia: presence in human bone marrow cells that suppress myelopoiesis. *Proc Natl Acad Sci U S A* 1976;73:2890–2894.
40. Selleri C, Maciejewski JP, Sato T, Young NS. Interferon-γ constitutively expressed in the stromal microenvironment of human marrow cultures mediates potent hematopoietic inhibition. *Blood* 1996;87:4149–4157.
41. Munker R, Hiller E, Paquette R. *Modern hematology: biology and clinical management.* Totowa, NJ: Humana Press, 2000:97–104.
42. Curnutte JT, Coates TD. Disorders of phagocyte function and number. In: Hoffman R, Benz E, Shattil S, et al., eds. *Hematology: basic principles and practice,* 3rd ed. New York: Churchill Livingstone, 1999.
43. Schwartz J, Weiss S. Host and environmental factors influencing the peripheral blood leukocyte count. *Am J Epidemiol* 1991;134(12):1402–1409.
44. Levine SP. Thrombocytopenia caused by immunologic platelet destruction. In: Lee GR, Foerster J, Lukens J, et al, eds. *Wintrobe's clinical hematology,* vol. 1, 10th ed. Baltimore: Williams & Wilkins, 1999;1583–1611.
45. Jennings GH, Gower ND. Thrombocytopenic purpura in toluene di-isocyanate workers. *Lancet* 1963;1:406.
46. Wahlberg P, Nyman D. Turpentine and thrombocytopenic purpura. *Lancet* 1969;2:215.
47. Micu D, Mihailescu E, Vilau C, Tarpa A, Chircu V, Zgoanta C. The value of some cytochemical investigations of the leukocytes and platelets in estimating the effects of occupational exposure to benzene, vinyl chloride and carbon disulfide. *Med Interne* 1985;23:115.
48. Lundholm CE, Bartonek M. A study of the effects of pp'DDE and other related chlorinated hydrocarbons on the inhibition of platelet aggregation. *Arch Toxicol* 1991;65:570.
49. Raulf M, Konig W. In vitro effects of polychlorinated biphenyls on human platelets. *Immunology* 1991;72:287.
50. Kinney MC, Lukens JN. Classification and differentiation of the acute leukemias. In: Lee GR, Foerster J, Lukens J, et al, eds. *Wintrobe's clinical hematology,* vol. 1, 10th ed. Baltimore: Williams & Wilkins, 1999;2209–2240.
51. Stock W, Thirman MJ. Pathobiology of acute myeloid leukemia. In: Hoffman R, Benz E, Shattil S, et al., eds. *Hematology: basic principles and practice,* 3rd ed. New York: Churchill Livingstone, 1999:979–999.
52. Rosenberg N, Krontiris TG. The molecular basis of neoplasia. In: Hoffman R, Benz E, Shattil S, et al., eds. *Hematology: basic principles and practice,* 3rd ed. New York: Churchill Livingstone, 1999:870–885.
53. Mitelman F, Brandt L, Nilsson P. Relation among occupational exposure to potential mutagenic/carcinogenic agents, clinical findings and bone marrow chromosomes in acute nonlymphocytic leukemia. *Blood* 1978;52:1229.
54. Pedersen-Bjergaard H, Rowley JD. The balanced and the unbalanced chromosome aberrations of acute myeloid leukemia may develop in different ways and may contribute differently to malignant transformation. *Blood* 1994;83:2982.
55. Mitelman F, Nilsson PG, Brandt L, et al. Chromosome pattern, occupation and clinical features in patients with acute nonlymphocytic leukemia. *Cancer Genet Cytogenet* 1981;4:197–214.
56. Taylor JA, Sandler DP, Bloomfield CD, et al. *Ras* oncogene activation and occupational exposures in acute myeloid leukemia. *J Natl Cancer Inst* 1992;84:1626.
57. Kurzrock R, Shtalrid M, Romero P, et al. A novel c-abl protein product in Philadelphia-positive acute lymphoblastic leukemia. *Nature* 1987;325:631–635.
58. Hermans A, Heisterkamp N, von Linden M, et al. Unique fusion of *bcr* and *c-abl* genes in Philadelphia chromosome–positive acute lymphoblastic leukemia. *Cell* 1987;51:33–40.
59. Daley G, McLaughlin J, Witte O, et al. The CML-specific P210 bcr/abl protein, unlike v-abl, does not transform NJH/3T3 fibroblasts. *Science* 1987;237:532–535.
60. Larson RA, Kondo K, Vardiman J, et al. Evidence for a 15:17 translocation in every patient with acute promyelocytic leukemia. *Am J Med* 1984;76:827–841.
61. Rubnitz JE, Look AT. Pathobiology of acute lymphoblastic leukemia. In: Hoffman R, Benz E, Shattil S, et al., eds. *Hematology: basic principles and practice,* 3rd ed. New York: Churchill Livingstone, 1999:1052–1069.
62. Taylor C, Hughes DC, Zappone E, et al. A screen for *ras* mutations in individuals at risk of secondary leukemia due to occupational exposure to petrochemicals. *Leuk Res* 1995;19(5):299.
63. Yin SN, Li GL, Tain FD, et al. A retrospective cohort study of leukemia and other cancers in benzene workers. *Environ Health Perspect* 1989;82:207–213.
64. Austin H, Delzell E, Cole P. Benzene and leukemia: a review of the literature and a risk assessment. *Am J Epidemiol* 1988;127(3):419–439.
65. Brett S, Rodricks J, Chinchilli V. Review and update of leukemia risk potentially associated with occupational exposure to benzene. *Environ Health Perspect* 1989;82:267–281.
66. Rothman N, Li G, Dosemeci M, et al. Hematotoxicity among Chinese workers heavily exposed to benzene. *Am J Ind Med* 1996;29:236–246.
67. Linet MS, Yin SN, Travis LB, et al. Clinical features of hematopoietic malignancies and related disorders among benzene-exposed workers in China. *Environ Health Perspect* 1996;104(Suppl 6):1353.
68. Collins JJ, Conner B, Friedlander BR, et al. A study of the hematologic effects of chronic low-level exposure to benzene. *J Occup Med* 1991;33(5):619–626.
69. Ward E, Hornung R, Morris J, et al. Risk of low red or white blood cell count related to estimated benzene exposure in a rubber worker cohort (1940–1975). *Am J Ind Med* 1996;29:247.
70. Rothman N, Smith M, Hayes R, et al. Benzene poisoning, a risk factor for hematological malignancy, is associated with the NQO1609 C→T mutation and rapid fractional excretion of chlorzoxazone. *Cancer Res* 1997;57:2839–2842.
71. Narod SA, Dube ID. Occupational history and involvement of chromosomes 5 and 7 in acute nonlymphocytic leukemia cancer. *Cancer Genet Cytogenet* 1989;38:261–269.
72. Stillman WS, Varella-Garcia M, Irons RD. The benzene metabolite, hydroquinone, induces dose-dependent hypoploidy in a human cell line. *Leukemia* 1997;11:1540–1545.
73. Levine EG, Bloomfield CD. Leukemias and myelodysplastic syndromes secondary to drug, radiation and environmental exposure. *Semin Oncol* 1992;19:47–84.
74. Irons RD, Stillman WS. Impact of benzene metabolites on differentiation of bone marrow progenitor cells. *Environ Health Perspect* 1996;104(Suppl 6):1247–1250.
75. Smith MA, McCaffrey RP, Karp JE. The secondary leukemias: challenges and research directions. *J Natl Cancer Inst* 1996;88:407–418.
76. Pedersen-Bjergaard J, Phillip P. Balanced translocations involving chromosome bands 11q23 and 21q22 are highly characteristic of myelodysplasia and leukemia following therapy with cytostatic agents targeting at DNA–topoisomerase II. *Blood* 1991;78:1147–1148.
77. Smith M, Rubenstein L, Ungerleider R. Therapy related acute myeloid leukemia following treatment with epipodophyllotoxins: estimating the risks. *Med Pediatr Oncol* 1994;23(2):86–98.
78. Heim S, Mitelman F. Cytogenetic analysis in the diagnosis of acute leukemia. *Cancer* 1992;70(Suppl 6):1701–1709.
79. Pedersen-Bjergaard J, Pedersen M, Roulston D, Philip P. Different genetic pathways in leukemogenesis for patients presenting with therapy related myelodysplasia and therapy related acute myeloid leukemia. *Blood* 1995;86(9):3542–3552.
80. Chen HW, Eastmond DA. Topoisomerase inhibition by phenolic metabolites: a potential mechanism for benzene's clastogenic effects. *Carcinogenesis* 1995;16:2301–2307.
81. Zhang L, Rothman R, Wang Y, et al. Increased aneusomy and long arm deletion of chromosomes 5 and 7 in lymphocytes of Chinese workers exposed to benzene. *Carcinogenesis* 1998;19(11):1955–1961.
82. Smith MT, Zhang L. Biomarkers of leukemia risk: benzene as a model. *Environ Health Perspect* 1998;106(Suppl 4):937–946.
83. Divine BJ, Hartman CM. Mortality update of butadiene production workers. *Toxicology* 1996;113(1–3):169.
84. Ward EM, Fajen JM, Ruder AM, et al. Mortality study of workers employed in 1,3-butadiene production units identified from a large chemical workers cohort. *Toxicology* 1996;113:157–168.
85. Ward EM, Fajen JM, Ruder AM, et al. Mortality study of workers in 1,3-butadiene production units identified from a chemical workers cohort. *Environ Health Perspect* 1995;103:598–603.
86. Delzell E, Sathiakumar N, Hovinga M, et al. A follow-up study of synthetic rubber workers. *Toxicology* 1996;113:182–189.

87. Macaluso M, Larson R, Delaell E, et al. Leukemia and cumulative exposure to butadiene, styrene and benzene among workers in the synthetic rubber industry. *Toxicology* 1996;113(1–3):190.
88. Irons RO, Pyatt DW. Dithiocarbamates as potential confounders in butadiene epidemiology. *Carcinogenesis* 1998;19(4):539–542.
89. Ninth report on carcinogens. Washington: US Department of Health and Human Services, Public Health Service, National Toxicology Program, 2000.
90. Hayes RB, Zhang L, Yin L, et al. Genotoxic markers among butadiene polymer workers in China. *Carcinogenesis* 2000;21(1):55–62.
91. Noel P, Tefferi A, Pierre R, et al. Karyotypic analysis in primary myelodysplastic syndromes. *Blood Rev* 1993;7:10–18.
92. Span LFR, Dar SE, Shetty V, et al. Apparent expansion of CD34+ cells during the evolution of myelodysplastic syndromes to acute myeloid leukemia. *Leukemia* 1998;12:1685–1695.
93. Cowles MF, Bennett JM, Ross CE. Medical surveillance for leukemia at a petrochemical manufacturing complex: four year summary. *J Occup Med* 1991;33(7):808–812.
94. Tsai SP, Dowd CM, Cowles SR, Ross CE. Morbidity patterns among employees at a petroleum refinery. *J Occup Med* 1991;33(10):1076–1080.
94a. Rothman N, Smith MT, Hayes RB, et al. Benzene poisoning, a risk factor for hematological malignancy, is associated with the NQO1 609C $\rightarrow$ T mutation and rapid fractional excretion of chlorzoxazone. *Cancer Res* 1997;57:2839–2842.
95. Wiencke JK, Pemble S, Keterer B, Kelsey KT. Gene deletion of glutathione *S*-transferase theta: correlation with induced genetic damage and potential role in endogenous mutagenesis. *Cancer Epidemiol Biomarkers Prev* 1995;4(3):253–259.
96. Srám RJ, Binková, B. Molecular epidemiology studies on occupational and environmental exposure to mutagens and carcinogens, 1997–1999. *Environ Health Perspect* 2000;108[Suppl 1]:57–70.
97. Stillman WS, Varella-Garcia M, Irons RD. The benzene metabolite, hydroquinone, selectively induces 5q31– and –7 in human CD34+CD19– bone marrow cells. *Exp Hematol* 2000;28:169–176.
98. Smith MT, Zhang L, Jeng M, et al. Hydroquinone, a benzene metabolite, increases the level of aneusomy of chromosomes 7 and 8 in human CD34-positive blood progenitor cells. *Carcinogenesis* 2000;21:1485–1490.
99. Masuba V, Rozgaj R, Sentiga K. Cytogenetic changes in subjects occupationally exposed to benzene. *Chemosphere* 2000;40:301–310.
100. Zhang L, Rothman N, Wang Y, et al. Increased aneusomy and long arm deletion of chromosomes 5 and 7 in the lymphocytes of Chinese workers exposed to benzene. *Carcinogenesis* 1998;19:195–1961.
101. Zhang L, Wang Y, Shang N, Smith MT. Benzene metabolites induce the loss and long arm deletion of chromosomes 5 and 7 in human lymphocytes. *Leuk Res* 1998;22:105–113.
102. Hagmar L, Brogger A, Hansteen IL, et al. Cancer risk in humans predicted by increased levels of chromosomal aberrations in lymphocytes: Nordic study group on the health risk of chromosome damage. *Cancer Res* 1994;54(11):2919–2922.
103. Bonassi S, Abbondandolo A, Camurri L, et al. Are chromosome aberrations in circulating lymphocytes predictive of future cancer onset in humans? Preliminary results of an Italian cohort study. *Cancer Genet Cytogenet* 1995;79(2):133–135.
104. Hallberg LN, el Zein R, Grossman L, Au WW. Measurement of DNA repair deficiency in workers exposed to benzene. *Environ Health Perspect* 1996;104(Suppl 3):529–534.

CHAPTER 29

Olfactory and Nasal Toxicology

John B. Sullivan, Jr.

OLFACTION AND COMMON CHEMICAL SENSES

The ability to detect airborne chemicals is dependent on two sensory mechanisms located in the nasal passages: olfaction and the common chemical senses (CCS). Evolution has relegated odor detection in humans to a minor function in survival, food gathering, and most daily living activities. Humans depend much more on senses of sight and hearing for protection against danger and daily living. However, there are episodes in which loss of smell can lead to extreme consequences.

Individuals with olfactory disorders can be hazards to themselves and others working in occupations in which odor detection of vapors is a necessary part of safety. More than 2 million Americans have some kind of sensory dysfunction of olfaction or taste, and approximately 200,000 people visit physicians each year for taste and smell disorders (1).

The common chemical senses are comprised of branches of the trigeminal (V) cranial nerve. Together, the olfactory nerves and CCS form an early warning system to detect airborne chemicals.

At least 120 different chemicals, more than 60 drugs, and numerous medical conditions can cause olfactory dysfunction (Tables 29-1 through 29-3). Of the majority of etiologies of smell and taste dysfunction, only 5% of these are caused by toxic exposures. Most are caused by head injury, upper respiratory tract infection, and disease.

TABLE 29-1. Toxic substances associated with olfactory dysfunction in humans

Toxic substances
Acetaldehyde
Acetic acid
Acetone
Acetonitrile
Acetophenone
Acid chlorides
Benzaldehyde
Benzene
Benzylic acid
Butyl acetate
Butylene glycol
Carbon tetrachloride
Chloroform
Chloromethanes
Dimethylsulfate
Ethyl acetate
Ethyl ether
Formaldehyde
Furfural
Halogenated organic compounds
Iodoform
Isocyanates
Menthol
Nitro compounds
Organic fluorine compounds
Pentachlorophenol
Phenylenediamine
Selenium compounds
Sulfur compounds
Tetrachloroethane
Trichloroethane
Trichloroethylene
Xylene
Metals and metallic compounds
Aluminum fumes
Arsenic
Arsenite
Asphalt
Cadmium
Cement dust
Chromium compounds
Copper
Copper fumes
Cotton dust
Dust and particulates
Flax
Flour
Lime
Manganese
Mercury
Nickel
Nickel hydroxide
Osmium
Potash
Potassium sulfide
Silica
Silver nitrate
Strontium sulfate
Tetroxide
Tin fumes
Wood dust
Zinc
Zinc fumes
Other hazards
Ammonia
Bromine
Carbon disulfide
Carbon monoxide
Chlorine
Coal tar vapors
Flue gas
Fluorides
Hydrogen chloride
Hydrogen fluoride
Hydrazine
Nitric acid
Nitrogen dioxide
Phosgene
Selenium dioxide
Sewer gas
Sulfur dioxide
Sulfuric acid

Adapted from ref. 1, with permission.

Terms applied to olfactory and taste dysfunctions are listed in Table 29-4. *Anosmia* is the term used to describe a complete loss of smell. *Hyposmia* indicates a diminished sense of smell. *Hyperosmia* is an enhanced sensitivity to odors. *Dysosmia* is a distortion in perception of odors, and *parosmia* is a distortion in perception caused by environmental factors and stimuli. *Cacosmia* is the term applied to odor intolerance problems produced from environmental chemicals that results in symptoms of illness. *Dysgeusia* is a distortion in taste perception, and *ageusia* is a complete loss of taste.

Chemoreceptors of the olfactory system can detect and discriminate among thousands of distinct odors. Odors alert individuals to potentially very dangerous situations. Examples include the detection of hydrogen sulfide at concentrations much lower than would be harmful. In the vast majority of cases, humans detect odors at a threshold much below irritancy levels or a concentration that would produce physical damage to the airways.

Otolaryngologists are increasingly concerned about environmental pollutants and their potential to damage olfaction and chemoreception. The olfactory system is similar to the immune system in the numbers of genes related to it. There may be more than 1,000 olfactory receptor genes (1).

Anatomy and Physiology of Olfaction

The human olfactory epithelium is a 1- to 2-cm square area of neuroepithelium located high in the nasal cavity (Fig. 29-1). For molecules to reach the olfactory nerves, they must first dissolve in the aqueous medium of mucus that coats the olfactory epithelium. When chemicals penetrate this aqueous barrier, they interact first with primary olfactory neurons (PON). The cells of the olfaction and taste are the only sensory cells that are replaced throughout the life span, and PONs, if damaged, can regenerate from basal cells. Axons of PONs are grouped into bundles of 50 to 100 and surrounded by Schwann's cell sheath. PONs are unmyelinated and send a single unbranched dendrite to the surface of the epithelium terminating in the olfactory knob (1,2).

Cilia extend from each dendrite into the mucous layer covering the olfactory neuroepithelium (Fig. 29-2). The cilia of the primary olfactory neurons form a very dense, compact area covering the neuroepithelium. PONs synapse with a second olfactory in the olfactory via an excitatory amino acid neurotransmitter.

The aqueous mucous lining of the neuroepithelium contains odorant-binding proteins. Hundreds of olfactory receptor proteins respond to tens of thousands of different odors. The olfactory neurosensory mechanism is capable of detecting odors of newly synthesized chemicals and distinguishing them from chemicals that have not yet been synthesized, emphasizing the olfactory system's ability to respond to environmental stimuli in a manner similar to the immune system. This amplification of response allows odor detection of mere molecules. Each protein receptor must be able to produce a unique pattern of response so that the central nervous system is able to distinguish even newly synthesized chemicals (1,2).

In contrast to humans, animals have a much larger area of neurosensory epithelium. Supporting cells in the epithelial layer mechanically isolate the primary olfactory neuron cell bodies from the environment, forming tight junctions between the dendrites and the supporting cells, which provides a barrier to chemical molecules in the environment.

Bowman's glands, located at the basement membrane structure of the olfactory epithelial structure, secrete a mucous cover for the epithelium. These glands are sympathetically and parasympathetically mediated. The covering of the neuroepithelium with mucous creates a specialized environment critical for odor detection. It allows the ciliated portion of the primary olfactory neurons to function by providing proper ionic and osmotic environments. Disruption of this mucous layer by chemicals, infection, or trauma can be associated with smell disorders. Bowman's glands are responsible for maintaining this important mucous layer that allows olfactory action potentials to be generated. The mucous layer also allows molecules of chemicals to be trapped from the air into this aqueous environment.

Because primary olfactory neurons maintain a contact with the environment outside of the brain, there is a potential that toxins can be transferred directly from the outside air into the brain and central nervous system (2). The olfactory mucous layer also provides immune and defense mechanisms, including immunoglobulin A, secreted by Bowman's glands, as well as the microbial proteins lactoferrin and lysozyme. Other defense mechanisms of the mucous layer include metabolic enzymes, including P-450, cytochrome enzymes that play a role in the metabolism of toxins that reach olfactory receptors (1,2).

TABLE 29-2. Diseases associated with smell disorders

Infections and inflammation	Tumors
Glossitis	Intracranial
Oral mycosis	Intranasal
Parotitis	Sinus
Rhinitis	Submandibular gland
Sinusitis	Anatomic
Viral URI	Nasal obstruction
Endocrine	Polyposis
Adrenal insufficiency	Gastrointestinal
Diabetes mellitus	Chronic liver disease
Hyperthyroidism	Cirrhosis
Hypothyroidism	Crohn's disease
Kallmann's syndrome (hypogonadotrophic hypogonadism)	Hepatitis
Pseudohypoparathyroidism	Congenital
Neurologic	Cleft palate
AIDS dementia	Familial
Alzheimer's disease	Kallmann's syndrome (hypogonadotrophic hypogonadism)
Craniofacial trauma	Turner's syndrome
Epilepsy	Others
Guillain-Barré syndrome	Cystic fibrosis
Huntington's disease	Ethmoidectomy
Korsakoff's psychosis	Giant cell arteritis
Meningioma	High altitude syndrome
Migraine headaches	Pregnancy
Multiple sclerosis	Radiotherapy
Parkinson's disease	Sarcoidosis
Temporal lobe epilepsy	Sjögren's syndrome
Nutritional	Tonsillectomy
Alcoholism	Uremia
Pellagra	Xerostomia
Pernicious anemia	

AIDS, acquired immunodeficiency syndrome; URI, upper respiratory infection.
Adapted from ref. 9, with permission.

Evidence exists for specific olfactory receptor proteins as the first step in the creation of odorant sensation. G-proteins serve as messenger proteins. A stereospecificity of chemical odorants exists so the olfactory system can detect different odors of stereoisomer pairs of molecules (1,2).

Olfactory cilia contain membrane-associated GTP-binding proteins (guanosine triphosphate) (G proteins). When odorant molecules bind to olfactory receptors, they activate G proteins, which then activate adenylate cyclase to generate cyclic AMP as a second messenger, resulting in a membrane potential and action potential. The stages of olfaction represent steps of amplification that provide increased sensitivity to detect odorants. Continuous odorant stimulation can cause olfactory fatigue, or desensitization. This may be caused by rapid reduction in C-AMP or cyclic-GMP levels (1,2).

Disorders of Olfaction

Olfactory function problems can be divided into two broad areas: (a) high-level toxic exposures that damage the neuroepithelium and (b) odor perception problems that produce cacosmia or parosmia. Exposure to numerous chemicals at a high enough concentration can cause olfactory epithelial damage.

Approximately 5% of patients with a head injury have associated olfactory loss, most involving a frontal or occipital injury

TABLE 29-3. Medications associated with disturbances of taste or smell

Medication	Disturbance of taste or smell	Medication	Disturbance of taste or smell
Opiates	Smell depression	Methylthiouracil	T and smell loss
Azelastine	Bitter, metallic dysgeusia, altered T	Thiamazole	T loss
Cefamandole	"Bad T"	Allopurinol	Metallic dysgeusia
Doxycycline	Anosmia, parosmia	Auranofin	Altered T, metallic dysgeusia
Lincomycin	T disorder	Penicillamine	T loss, metallic dysgeusia
Procaine penicillin	Metallic dysgeusia	Amiloride	Decreased T for salt, decreased salt T
Metronidazole HCl	Metallic dysgeusia	Amrinone	Hypogeusia, dysosmia
Sulfasalazine	DT	Beta-blockers	Anosmia
Tetracycline	Metallic dysgeusia	Bretylium	Enhances salt T
Amphotericin B	DT	Captopril	Increased T, DT, and RT parosmia
Griseofulvin	DT	Diltiazem	Hypogeusia, hyposmia
Ethambutol	Metallic dysgeusia	Dipyridamole	"Bizarre" T and parosmia
Metronidazole	T disorder	Enalapril	Parosmia: metallic, sweet, salt dysgeusias, T loss
Scopolamine (SQ)	Impaired odor detection		
Phenindione	T disorder	Nifedipine	T and smell distortions
Tegretol	Hypogeusia, "bad T" to alcohol, ageusia	Nitroglycerin (transdermal)	Ageusia
		Spironolactone	T loss
Biguanide	Metallic dysgeusia	Dextroamphetamine	Decreased olfactory acuity, increased sucrose threshold, decreased bitter threshold
Acetyl sulfosalicylic acid	T disorder		
Phenylbutazone	Ageusia, hypogeusia	Chlorhexidine	DT, persistent aftertaste, T loss, salt T loss
Cholestyramine	T abnormality	Hexetidine	Altered T
Clofibrate	Decreased T sensitivity	Sodium lauryl sulfate	DT
5-fluorouracil	Alterations in bitter and sour sensitivity, increased sweet sensitivity	Acetazolamide	Bitter dysgeusia
		Isotretinoin	Citric acid ageusia, hyposmia
Adriamycin/methotrexate	Altered T	Baclofen	Ageusia, hypogeusia
Azathioprine	DT	Acetyl-beta-methyl-choline HCl	Decreased DT for smell
Bleomycin	T loss	Acetylcholine HCl	Decreased DT for smell
Cisplatin	Ageusia	Cocaine, tetracaine	Anosmia, olfactory loss
Methotrexate	Sour and metallic dysgeusia, ageusia	Menthol	Decreased DT for smell
Levodopa	DT	Strychnine	Decreased DT for smell
Lithium carbonate	Unpleasant T, metallic dysgeusia	Zinc sulfate	Anosmia, hyposmia, parosmia
Carbimazole	T and smell loss	Chlormezanone	Ageusia
Methimazole	T and smell loss	Zopiclone	T perversion

DT, disturbance taste; RT, reduced taste; T, taste.
Adapted from ref. 9, with permission.

(3). Craniofacial injury can result in a shearing effect of the olfactory filaments at the point at which they pass through the cribriform plate (4). One patient evaluated was a plumber who sustained a frontal inferior contusion documented on magnetic resonance imaging (MRI) from a fall. Afterwards, he developed anosmia. This individual used welding equipment in his business and could not detect the odor of acetylene, which placed him and others at risk, nor could he detect other flammable gases while welding. This is an example of how anosmia can cause serious health threats and lead to serious accidents.

The second most common cause of smell disorders is a viral infection or upper respiratory tract infection. Many patients describe olfactory dysfunctions after resolutions of colds or flu.

TABLE 29-4. Terms describing taste and smell dysfunction

Term	Taste and smell dysfunction
Anosmia	Complete loss of smell
Hyposmia	Decreased sense of smell
Hyperosmia	Increased odor sensitivity
Dysosmia	Distortion in odor perception
Ageusia	Loss of taste
Hypogeusia	Decreased taste sensitivity
Hypergeusia	Enhanced taste sensitivity
Dysgeusia	Distortion in taste perception

Olfactory diminution occurs as one ages but usually is not significant until well into the 70s. Loss of taste is relatively rare but may follow loss of smell. Because smell and taste are closely related, individuals with olfactory dysfunction may also present with taste dysfunction, when in reality taste is intact. Taste qualities are salty, sour, sweet, and bitter, and it is important to test individuals to determine whether they actually have a taste deficit. Olfactory dysfunction secondary to toxic exposures gener-

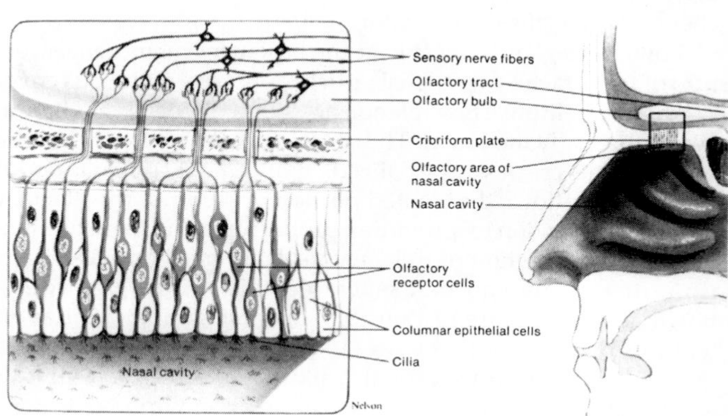

Figure 29-1. Olfactory neuroepithelium and anatomic location in nasal cavity. (Reprinted from Hole J Jr. *Human anatomy and physiology,* 2nd ed. Dubuque, IA: WC Brown Co, 1981, with permission.)

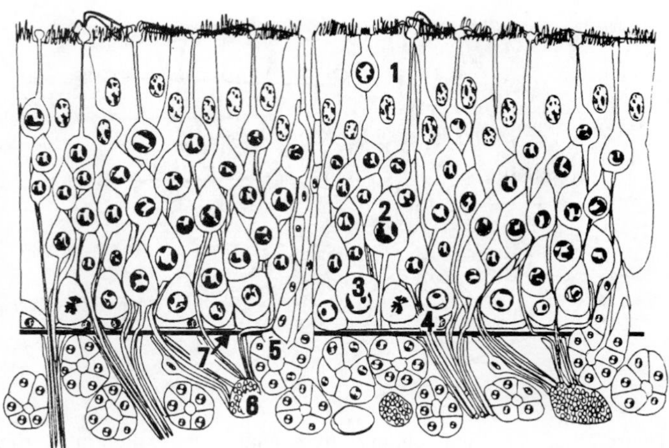

Figure 29-2. Layers of olfactory epithelium. 1, sustentacular cell; 2, mature receptor neuron; 3, globose basal cell; 4, pyramidal basal cell; 5, Bowman's gland; 6, olfactory nerve bundle; 7, basement membrane. (Reprinted from ref. 1, with permission.)

ally involves a sudden exposure and a high concentration rather than chronic low-grade exposures.

A history of chronic sinusitis, allergic rhinitis, nasal symptomatology, upper respiratory tract infections, and head traumas is important to ascertain when differentiating toxic exposure etiologies from other etiologies (5). It is also important to review medication, because more than 60 medications have been known to alter smell and taste (see Table 29-2) (1–7).

Olfactory loss has been reported in association with many diseases, such as diabetes, Parkinson's disease, alcoholism, Usher's syndrome, hypothyroidism, neurodegenerative disease, and renal failure (6–9) (see Table 29-3). Also, radiation to the head and neck can cause taste and smell dysfunction.

Toxic compounds can also affect the function of the olfactory system indirectly by causing inflammation of the nasal passages, leading to swelling around olfactory receptors. Exposure to such airborne hazards as ozone, sulfur dioxide, nitrogen dioxide, and formaldehyde has caused changes in olfactory thresholds. Studies involving toluene and xylene show a shift in the detection threshold after exposure to toluene xylene or a mixture of the two (6–9).

When olfactory cells are damaged by inhaled toxins, self-repair requires approximately 30 days (1). Sometimes it may take much longer for olfactory function to return, depending on the specific anatomic structures that are damaged. Also, exposure to a toxic hazard during an upper respiratory tract infection can result in greater damage than either alone (1).

Olfactory dysfunction has been reported after high exposure to cadmium, methyl mercury, toluene diisocyanate, manganese, sulfur dioxide, acrylates, methacrylates, ammonia, and organic solvent compounds (10–17).

Clinical Evaluation of Olfactory Dysfunction

The main points of clinical evaluation include history, physical examination, chemosensory tests, radiological evaluation with MRIs, or computed tomography (CT) scanning of the head and sinuses (1,3). Referral to an otolaryngologist is important to differentiate a conductive from sensorineural etiology. Rhinolaryngoscopy can evaluate for the presence of inflammation or rhinitis, and helps differentiate allergic versus nonallergic disease, or vasomotor rhinitis. Evaluation should rule out infections, polyps, toxic exposures, medications, cancers, and other sources of inflammation (see Tables 29-1 through 29-3).

Nasal endoscopy allows for accurate diagnoses and can detect pathologic changes that could prevent chemical odor molecules from reaching the olfactory neuroepithelium (18). Histories of exposure, occupational work history, and hobbies should be explored. History of head trauma and other diseases and dental work should be explored. Neurodegenerative processes should be ruled out. Olfactory loss secondary to sinus and nasal pathology should be ruled out. Biopsy of neuroepithelium has been used.

Chemosensory testing should be conducted by experts to discern conductive from neurosensory losses. The Smell Identification Test (Sensonics, Inc., Haddon Heights, NJ) is a chemosensory testing system that is self-administered. The test has a normative database of 4,000 men and women ranging in ages from 4 to 99 years. The Smell Identification Test has found use in clinical screening for a variety of diseases that have olfactory dysfunction as a component: Parkinson's disease, Usher's syndrome, temporal lobe epilepsy, chemical exposure, Down's syndrome, cystic fibrosis, and alcoholism. The test is particularly sensitive to frontal lobe dysfunction (19).

Radiologic evaluation includes CT scanning of the paranasal sinuses looking for soft tissue and bony changes and ruling out obstructive lesions, fractures, and other pathology of bones and soft tissue. CT scanning is the definitive test to rule out bone and soft tissue lesions and conductive losses (1,2). Other diseases, such as lupus and sarcoidoses, have been associated with smell and taste disorders in rare cases (1,2).

Toxic Exposures and Olfactory Dysfunction

Humans breathe 10,000 to 20,000 L of air per day, mainly through their noses. Thus, the olfactory system comes into contact with many varieties of concentrations of chemicals. As an example, the indoor air of multiple modern environments of public buildings and offices contains between 50 and 350 different volatile organic chemicals, usually at very low concentrations that generally do not stimulate odor perceptions (see Chapter 53). Approximately 5% of cases of smell disorder are related to toxic exposures. The olfactory system, including the mucous surface, secretes IgA and contains antimicrobial proteins and P-450 enzymes as a part of a defense mechanism against toxic chemicals and inhaled pathogens (20).

Cadmium exposure is a well-recognized toxin that causes anosmia in humans. Chronic exposure is required. Also, in cadmium-exposed individuals, proteinuria was associated with the presence of anosmia (12,17). Individual β-2-microglobulin in the urine also is associated with hyposmia. Organic mercury exposure can cause olfactory dysfunction (11). Exposure to irritant corrosive gases, SO_2, and ammonia at high concentration has also caused olfactory dysfunction. Anosmia has occurred after long-term exposure to solvents. Acrylates and methacrylates have shown some diminished impairment or some mild impairment (13).

Most of the data on olfactory toxicity are derived from animal models and from clinical and anecdotal case reports. Mechanisms of study through neuroepithelial biopsy should be performed only by those who are experts in the procedure (21).

Olfactory-Limbic Connections

Olfactory connections track into the rhinencephalon, one of the most ancient parts of the brain, and interconnect extensively with structures in the limbic system.

Each olfactory bulb sends projections to the olfactory cortex and to limbic structures: amygdala, periamygdaloid cortex, thalamus, nucleus of the lateral olfactory tract, locus coeruleus, and raphe nuclei. Increased odor sensitivity is termed *hyperosmia*, whereas odor distortion is termed *dysosmia*. Odor sensitivity and odor distortion are sometimes referred to as *cacosmia*, which generally refers to reactions to odors that have no adverse effect on other individuals and cannot be explained by biological models. Cacosmic individuals express somatic and neuropsychiatric symptom amplification on detection of low-level environmental odors (22–24). However, individuals with odor sensitivity have been diagnosed with posttraumatic stress disorder, panic disorder, somatoform disorder, and recurrent major depression when their true problem may not be psychiatric.

The limbic system is the portion of the brain most sensitive to chemical stimuli and is responsible for human emotions and reaction to threats.

Because the limbic system controls emotions, reactions to threat, and "fight or flight" responses, its extensive interconnections with the olfactory system might theoretically explain why some people express odor intolerance to some chemicals. Olfactory nerve fibers connect to functional and anatomic areas of the limbic system, such as the hippocampus, amygdala, and hypothalamus. These areas are involved with arousal, rage, apathy, emotions, and recent memory. Amygdala functions include fear, rage, indifference to surroundings, drowsiness, increase in the pituitary-adrenocortic activity, changes in blood pressure, increased gastrointestinal motility, changes in respiration, and pupillary reactions. The hypothalamus regulates the autonomic nervous system and sends out autonomic discharges that produce physical expressions of emotions: rapid heart rate, gastrointestinal disturbance, elevation of blood pressure, increased sweating, flushing of the skin, dry mouth, and dry skin. Olfactory sensitivity can be induced in animals (25).

Another phenomenon that could be involved in producing an altered sense of smell is called *response facilitation*. The olfactory-limbic system is especially susceptible to habituation-facilitation phenomena. Odors can stimulate either habituation or a facilitation response. If the odor is mild and pleasant, no objection exists and habituation occurs. The individual ignores the stimulus. If the odor is offensive and strong, facilitation can occur and odor threshold response is lowered. This mechanism is a variant of kindling, in which individuals are sensitized to low levels of environmental odors not perceived by others.

These hypotheses could help explain strange symptoms and the sensitivity of some individuals to odors that others believe are trivial nuisances. However, none has been demonstrated to be operative in human studies.

NASAL CAVITY RESPONSE TO CHEMICALS

Three types of epithelia reside in the nasal cavity: squamous, secretory ciliated, and olfactory. Entering the nasal cavity, air first comes into contact with squamous epithelium. This cell type transitions into a transitional cell type with microvilli: columnar epithelium (respiratory type) begins at the anterior portion of turbinates (Fig. 29-3). This area contains serous submucosal cells and mucus-secreting goblet cells, and is highly vascularized.

The nasal epithelium humidifies and warms inspired air. Expired air passes over the nasal mucosa, which has just transferred warmth to inhaled air. Expired air traveling over the cooler mucosa causes water to condense, thus recycling moisture.

Common Chemical Senses and Airborne Irritants

A major function of the nasal cavity involves sensing of airborne irritants by the trigeminal nerve endings (cranial nerve V) that make up our common chemical senses. Stimulation of the trigeminal nerve endings by airborne irritants causes reflex inhibition of breathing, reduced heart rate, and elevated blood pressure, presumably to protect deeper airways from chemical injury.

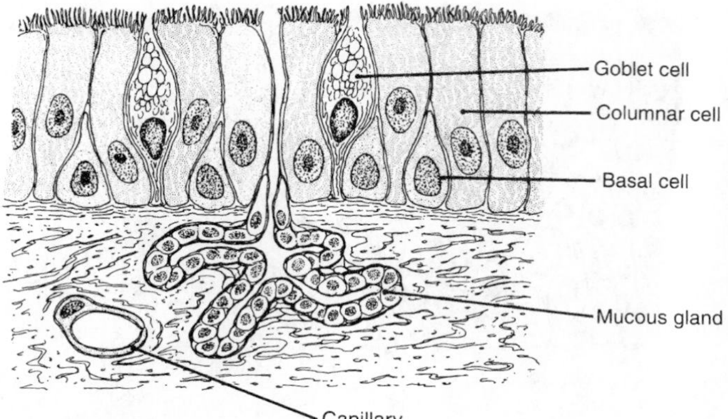

Figure 29-3. Nasal epithelium of the columnar type. (Reprinted from Donald J, Gluckman J, Rice D. *The sinuses*. New York: Raven Press, 1995, with permission.)

The trigeminal nerve, the fifth cranial nerve, is divided into three afferent branches (Fig. 29-4): the ophthalmic branch, the maxillary branch, and the mandibular branch. The ophthalmic branch innervates the interior part of the nose (ethmoidal nerve), the conjunctiva of the eye, the cornea, and the iris. The maxillary branch innervates the posterior and inferior areas through the pterygopalatine nerve and the infraorbital nerve. The mandibular branch innervates the tongue and the mouth. The trigeminal branches contain myelinated as well as unmyelinated fibers and contain high amounts of substance P, a potent neuropeptide that causes inflammation.

In addition to these nerves, the nasal passages have other defensive mechanisms against airborne hazards. For instance, the nasal cavity can secrete antibodies and proteins that act against inhaled microbial pathogens. The nasal passages also contain certain enzymes that can detoxify inhaled chemicals. Therefore, the nasal passages serve as part of the organism's detoxification response.

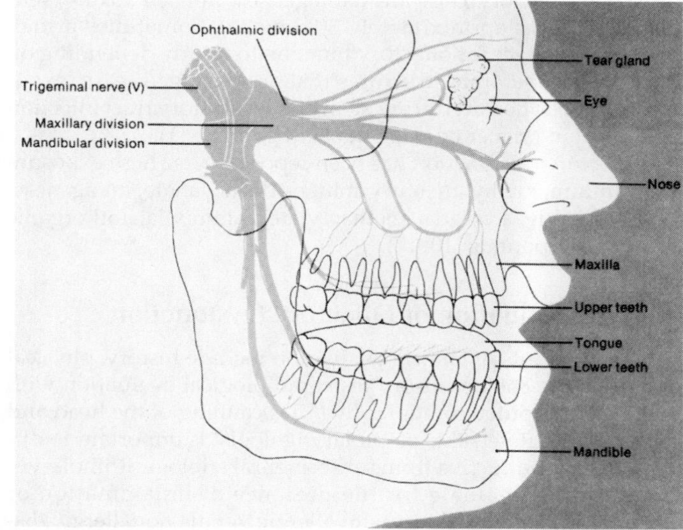

Figure 29-4. Branches of the trigeminal nerve innervating the nasal cavity. (Reprinted with permission from Hole J Jr. *Human anatomy and physiology*, 2nd ed. Dubuque, IA: WC Brown Co, 1981, with permission.)

Lesions to the nasal mucosa by airborne chemicals can be erosion, ulceration, inflammation, hypertrophy, exudative, altered mucociliary function, or squamous metaplasia (26).

Nasal sinus disease can affect olfactory function. Nasal and sinus disease is associated with olfactory dysfunction in up to 27% of patients presenting with olfactory loss (1).

Many threshold limit values (TLVs) have been established based on nasal irritancy (26).

Exposure to sensory irritants in air promotes a burning and painful sensation in the nasal passages, head, and cornea caused by stimulation of trigeminal nerve endings. Such sensory irritation is important to help protect against occupational and environmental exposures. Activation of the trigeminal nerve endings in the nasal passages depends on the chemical nature of the material. Trigeminal nerves can also be activated by physical irritants, such as dust, particulates, and biologicals.

Trigeminal nerves in the nose are also sensitive to pressure changes, mechanical changes, and chemical activation. Airborne chemicals can induce activation or stimulation of unmyelinated and myelinated trigeminal fibers. The compound capsaicin has a high effect on unmyelinated C-fibers of the trigeminal nerve. Stimulation of C-fibers releases substance P, which induces a neurogenic inflammatory response. Substance P antagonists can prevent this response. Because irritation reactions are mediated through receptor processes, a desensitization, as well as a sensitization, process can occur (27,28).

The trigeminal nerve contains other neuropeptides besides substance P, which belong to the tachykinin group: neurokinin A and calcitonin gene–related peptide. Another neuropeptide is the atrial natriuretic factor, which may be involved in pain mechanisms. Activation of C-fibers induces an outpouring of neuropeptides, which can result in neurogenic inflammation. The signs and symptoms of neurogenic inflammation are sneezing, nasal stuffiness, rhinorrhea, facial pain, eye irritation, watery eyes, headache, sinus congestion, cough, throat irritation, and wheezing. Substance P can also be found in the lungs, and its presence and release are probably related to production of inflammation in asthma on sensory irritation of chemical irritants (27,28).

Neurogenic inflammation is different from inflammation produced by prostaglandins. Substance P causes vasodilation and increased vascular permeability. Substance P is a potent releaser of mediators from mass cells and causes a depolarizing effect on trigeminal neurons. Therefore, it can increase the effect of other agonists. Substance P sensory efferent nerves have axon reflexes to the parasympathetic cholinergic neurons and the sphenopalatine ganglion, in which substance P activates cholinergic neurons causing nasal secretion.

Release of tachykinins from airway sensory nerves causes bronchial constriction, vasodilation, plasma exudation, mucus secretion, and inflammation, resulting in cough, shortness of breath, and wheezing, and other signs and symptoms of neurogenic inflammation. Airway epithelial damage by airborne chemicals can result in exposure of afferent nerve endings to subsequently inhaled irritants.

The effects of tachykinins can be amplified further by the loss of the neuropeptide degrading enzyme neutral endopeptidase, from epithelial cells. Tachykinins can produce effects by activating specific receptors localized to smooth muscles of all airways from the trachea to the smaller bronchioles. Substance P appears to be the most potent activator of these receptors. Viral infections can deactivate neutral endopeptidase in the airway epithelium, resulting in a hyperresponsiveness of the airways or reactive airways dysfunction. On exposure to other substances (i.e., noxious irritants in the air), the airways can become hyperresponsive, producing asthma, cough, chest tightness, and shortness of breath (27–29).

Many chemicals and particulates are irritants that stimulate sensory nerve endings, releasing substance P and other neuropeptides to produce inflammation. When the level of neutral endopeptidase enzyme is decreased or inhibited by respiratory viral infection by chronic inflammation, the neurogenic inflammatory responses can be amplified or exaggerated. This mechanism is postulated to play a role in irritant-induced reactive airways. Neutral endopeptidase modulates responses of neurogenic inflammation by degrading neurokinins. Anything that decreases neutral endopeptidase activity exaggerates neurogenic inflammatory responses (27–29).

The nasal cavity also has metabolic capabilities, which, on a g-per-g basis, are higher than that of the liver. Nasal tissue contains P-450 enzyme systems. Metabolic activation can give rise to high concentration of reactive metabolites at sensory receptor sites in the nose (26).

Irritancy versus Odor Threshold

For alkyl compounds, irritancy potency increases with carbon length. However, the lower the carbon number, the higher the vapor pressure; therefore, lower carbon number alkyl compounds such as *n*-propylacetate and 1-propanol can achieve higher concentrations in the nasal cavity to trigger reactions by the common chemical senses (27). Irritation produced by these highly volatile organics occurs at concentrations around their odor threshold. Otherwise, for more potent chemical irritants that are not as volatile, the irritancy threshold far exceeds odor thresholds.

The irritation threshold decreases with increasing carbon length for alcohols, ketones, acetates, and alkylbenzenes (27).

Water solubility plays a role in irritancy and odor detection. Layer molecules that are less water soluble may tend to dissolve less rapidly in the water-mucoid lining covering the nasal epithelium or olfactory epithelium. Reactive chemicals that can break disulfide bonds, oxidize thiol groups, or undergo acid-base reactions are known to be irritants (27). Low-level volatile organic chemicals (VOCs) can be additive and produce irritation at concentrations far lower than individual threshold limit values.

For halogenated benzenes and halogenated alkylbenzenes, the irritancy potency depends on their ability to dissolve in nasal mucus and reach receptors. The more hydrophobic the compound, the less it dissolves. The sensory irritation capacity of ketones and ethers increases with increasing lipophilicity.

Research has also shown that for some airborne chemicals, a reaction occurs at the receptor site. There are sensory irritants that chemically attack nucleophilic groups in the nasal neuroreceptor. Benzylidene malonitrile is such a compound. Sensory irritation receptors contain thiol groups, which can chemically react with some airborne irritants.

In summary, the sensory receptors in the nasal passages can be activated by one physical adsorption, as demonstrated by alkanes, alkylbenzenes, alcohols, ketones, and ethers, in which the receptor is activated by a benzene binding site. The alcohols activate the receptor by a hydrogen bond. Another mechanism or reaction is chemical reactions by more potent substances that chemically react with receptors instead of physically binding with the receptor. This reaction involves breakage of a disulfide bond in the receptor at a thiol group, which is how sulfur dioxide activates the receptor. Other substances activate the receptor by chemical reaction with a nucleil filate group. Formaldehyde, acrolein, and chlorobenzylidine malonitrile react with thiol groups in the receptors. Chlorine and ozone may actually oxidize the thiol group and activate the receptor (28,29).

The assay developed to measure common chemical sense irritancy has been the reflex depression of the respiratory rate in mice. The concentration of the compound that leads to a 50% depression of respiratory rate (RD-50) forms the basis to assess irritancy potency of chemicals. The RD-50 correlates with the TLVs recommended by the American Conference of Governmental Industrial Hygienists in approximately 40 compounds. This correlation validates these TLVs (26,29).

SUMMARY

Odors and irritation are complex subjects. The neurosensory mechanisms of olfaction and common chemical senses provide protection against noxious airborne chemicals. Activation and amplification of these neurosensory mechanisms could explain symptoms experienced by people exposed to airborne irritants and odors.

The olfactory and nasal epithelium can be damaged by numerous chemicals. They also have a tremendous detoxification capacity, which helps protect humans against noxious substances.

REFERENCES

1. Seiden A. *Taste and smell disorders*. New York: Thieme Medical Publishers, 1997.
2. Doty R, ed. *Handbook of olfaction and gustation*. New York: Marcel Dekker Inc, 1995.
3. Duncan H, Seiden A, Paik S, Smith D. Differences among patients with smell impairment resulting from head trauma, nasal disease, or prior upper respiratory infection. *Chem Senses* 1991;16:517.
4. Duncan H, Seiden A. Long-term follow-up of olfactory loss secondary to head trauma and upper respiratory tract infection. *Arch Otolaryngol Head Neck Surg* 1995;121:1183–1187.
5. Apter A, Mott A, Cain W, et al. Olfactory loss and allergic rhinitis. *J Allergy Clin Immunol* 1992;90:670–680.
6. Schiffman S. Drugs influencing taste and smell perception. In: Getchell T, Doty R, Bratoshuk L, Snow J, eds. *Smell and taste in health and disease*. New York: Raven Press, 1991.
7. Schiffman S. Taste and smell and disease. *N Engl J Med* 1993;308:1337–1343.
8. Deemes D, Doty R, Settle R. Smell and taste disorder, a study of 750 patients from the University of Pennsylvania Smell and Taste Center. *Arch Otolaryngol Head Neck Surg* 1991;117:519.
9. Mott A, Leopold D. Disorder in taste and smell update in otolaryngology I. *Med Clin North Am* 1991;75(6):1321–1346.
10. Amoore J. Effect of chemical exposure on olfactories in humans. In: Barrow C, ed. *Toxicology of the nasal passages*. Washington: Hemisphere Publishing, 1986.
11. Furuta S, Nishimoto K, Egawa M, et al. Olfactory dysfunction in patients with Minamata disease. *Am J Rhinol* 1994;8:259–263.
12. Rose C, Heywood P, Costanzo R. Olfactory impairment after chronic occupational cadmium exposure. *J Occup Environ Med* 1992;34:600–605.
13. Schwartz B, Doty R, Monroe C, et al. Olfactory function in chemical workers exposed to acrylate and methacrylate vapors. *Am J Public Health* 1989;79:613–618.
14. Hotz P, Tschopp A, Soderstrom D, et al. Smell or taste disturbances, neurological symptoms and hydrocarbon exposures. *Int Arch Occup Environ Health* 1992;63:525–530.
15. Sandmark B, Broms I, Lofgren L, Ohlson C. Olfactory function in painters exposed to organic solvents. *Scand J Work Environ Health* 1989;15:60–63.
16. Emmett E. Parosmia and hyposmia induced by solvent exposure. *Br J Indust Med* 1976;33:196–198.
17. Potts C. Cadmium proteinuria: the health of battery workers exposed to cadmium oxide dust. *Ann Occup Hyg* 1965;8:55–61.
18. Lanza D, Moran D, Doty R, et al. Endoscopic human olfactory biopsy technique: a preliminary report. *Laryngoscope* 1993;103:815–819.
19. Doty R, Shaman P, Dann M. Development of the University of Pennsylvania Smell Identification Test—a standardized microencapsulated test of olfactory function. *Physiol Behav* 1984;32:489–502.
20. Mellert T, Getchel M, Sparks L, Getchel T. Characterization of the immune barrier in human olfactory mucosa. *Otolaryngol Head Neck Surg* 1992;106:181–188.
21. Lovell M, Jafek B, Moran D, et al. Biopsy of human olfactory mucosa: an instrument and a technique. *Arch Otolaryngol Head Neck Surg* 1982;108:247–249.
22. Bell I, Miller C, Schwartz G. An olfactory-limbic model of multiple chemical sensitivity syndrome: possible relationships to kindling and affective spectrum disorders. *Biol Psychiatry* 1992;32:218–242.
23. Rossi J. Sensitization induced by kindling and kindling-related phenomena as a model for multiple chemical sensitivity. *Toxicology* 1996;III:87–100.
24. Bell I, Miller C, et al. Neuropsychiatric and somatic characteristics of young adults with and without self-reported chemical odor intolerance and chemical sensitivity. *Arch Environ Health* 1996;51(1):9–21.
25. Wang H, Wysocki C, Golbe G. Induction of olfactory receptor sensitivity in mice. *Science* 1993;260:998–1000.
26. Barrow C. *Toxicology of the nasal passages*. New York: McGraw-Hill, 1984.
27. Cain W, Cometto-Muniz J. Irritation and odor as indicators of indoor pollution. *Occup Med State of the Art Reviews* 1995;10(1):133–145.
28. Damgard G. Mechanisms of activation of the sensory irritant receptor by airborne chemicals. *Toxicology* 1991;21(3):183–208.
29. Cometto-Muniz J, Cain W. Thresholds for odor and nasal pungency. *Physiol Behav* 1990;48:719–725.

CHAPTER 30

Neuropsychological Evaluation of Toxic Exposures

Lidia Artiola i Fortuny

Neuropsychological investigation is recognized as the most sensitive way to examine the possibility of brain dysfunction and is considered by some to be a first-line diagnostic tool in the assessment of toxic exposure (1). The advantages of neuropsychological assessment are numerous. Neuropsychological procedures are noninvasive and are therefore safe, reliable, replicable, easily transportable, and relatively cost-effective (1), despite their time-intensive nature. The neuropsychological examination's degree of sensitivity can allow detection of neurotoxicity before more objective neurologic symptoms emerge (2). However, although neuropsychological procedures are highly sensitive to cognitive changes that can occur secondary to exposure to toxic substances, they do not possess high levels of specificity; that is, the results of the neuropsychological examination can alert the clinician to the possible presence of brain dysfunction, but they alone do not provide definitive information as to what may be causing the dysfunction.

The greatest challenge to the neuropsychologist, when faced with psychometric abnormalities in exposed individuals, is to distinguish between the potential effects of toxic agents and other possible causes of dysfunction. Clinical diagnosis in cases of neurotoxin exposure necessitates the integration of information gathered from the patient's mental health and medical history, record review, clinical observation, testing, and collateral sources, as well as information from other fields (i.e., toxicology, neurology, neuroradiology, and neurophysiology).

In this chapter, the various aspects of the neuropsychological examination of adults with suspected toxic exposure are examined. A brief outline of areas of behavior and cognition that have been documented to be vulnerable to the possible effects of neurotoxins is provided. Variables known to have potentially profound effects on the neuropsychological profile are addressed. These variables are independent from alleged exposure, but their effects can be similar to those commonly reported in toxic exposure. Finally, an outline of procedures is suggested for use with neuropsychological referrals.

Psychometric measurement of populations exposed to toxic substances began in the 1970s in Scandinavia (3). Since then, the use of behavioral tests has expanded significantly (4), with a great deal of activity in the area of neuropsychological assessment for the detection of adverse effects of various substances on the central nervous system, and a number of investigators have compiled these findings into books (1,5,6). Researchers have also been active in the development of neuropsychological batteries (7–10). In response to the need for normative information, a number of investigators have focused on normative data collection (4,9). The work of Anger and his colleagues (4) addressed the need for standardized test batteries and attempted to identify nervous system effects of chemical exposures in human populations worldwide.

In the United States, the University of Pittsburgh group (9) has collected appropriate age-scaled norms from blue-collar workers, delineated the factor structure of a test battery, and examined the interrelationships among test scores and certain demographic variables on test data.

Exposure to toxic substances commonly found in the workplace or in the environment is known to potentially cause neuropsychological disturbances. A body of literature exists on the various deficits documented over the years for these substances. Attention, memory and learning, visuospatial, psychomotor, and sensory and motor impairment, as well as a number of neurobehavioral alterations, have been documented after exposure to organic solvent mixtures (11–17), organophosphates (18–21), metals (e.g., lead, mercury, arsenic) (22–26), carbon monoxide (moderate and severe exposure) (27,28), and ethylene oxide (29).

Despite positive findings of cognitive impairment in exposed individuals, the literature is by no means in agreement. For example, it is not possible to conclude that all workers with organic solvent exposure show evidence of dysfunction. In fact, most epidemiologic studies of workers exposed to solvents at or below threshold limit values (TLVs) have failed to demonstrate the presence of cognitive deficits (30–33) or consistent effects of organic solvents on neurobehavioral function (34). Neither is it possible to conclude that documented deficits are permanent or remain stable in all individuals. Morrow and her coworkers (35) found that the presence of certain risk factors, a peak exposure and psychological distress, was detrimental for long-term neuropsychological outcome in workers with solvent exposure, raising the issue of vulnerability.

Although the evidence from industrial exposure is inconclusive in regard to the effects of many potential neurotoxins on cognition and neurobehavior, available evidence does point to significant and widespread cognitive effects and possible structural changes in the brain with chronic solvent abuse (36–40).

Individual cases of dementia attributable to exposure to neurotoxins are certainly seen clinically. Hartman (1) reported on the disastrous effects of 13 to 14 years of chronic exposure to neurotoxic solvents on a man in his 50s whose job was to clean a spray paint booth. This clinician has seen several printers from Mexico with 20 to 30 years of exposure to lead, and significant body burdens of lead (2 to 4 years after cessation of exposure), whose neuropsychological profiles were of generalized cognitive dilapidation. However, extreme cases notwithstanding, for most individuals with documentable neuropsychological deficits, these tend to be mild to moderate in severity and are usually limited to measures of learning, abstract reasoning, visuospatial abilities, psychomotor speed, and reaction time.

Most referral questions in cases of possible neurotoxin exposure revolve around diagnostic issues. The referral source is usually interested in knowing whether the patient's complaints can be directly attributed to toxic exposure or to any other factor, including, but not exclusively, an unrelated neurologic process, psychiatric illness, or malingering. The referral source may also ask for guidance as to management or treatment planning if problems are documented during the examination. For the neuropsychologist to be able to provide cogent answers regarding the nature of the patient's complaints and symptoms, the following is required: appropriate training and experience on the part of the clinician (1,41), access to background information on the patient, behavioral observation of the patient, and neuropsychological testing.

EFFECTS OF DEMOGRAPHIC VARIABLES

The effects of education on tests of cognitive ability are profound and well documented in the cross-cultural and educational literature (42). Clinical neuropsychology has long recognized the profound negative effects of increasing age and low education on test performance (41,43). More specifically these effects are documented in the body of research that addresses toxic encephalopathy (9,44). Anger and his associates (4) found such negative effects on their battery when it was administered to subjects in Latin America with extremely low levels of education. Italian researchers also found low levels of education to be an important moderator variable (45). South African investigators (44,46) stressed that, when applied to non-Western subjects, results of neuropsychological tests that have been well standardized in Western countries may be misleading unless validity issues have been addressed. The pervasive effects of formal schooling on neuropsychological performance must be stressed, as they are present even in areas of behavior that would seem to be free of the influences of formalized learning. Indeed, education has been found to affect performance in simple and complex motor tasks (47,48).

In the English-speaking industrialized world, the neuropsychological examination takes place within the framework of normative comparison standards. For adults, the norm for many measurable psychological functions is a score that represents the average or median performance of a population (41) possessing certain characteristics. Normative standards can be based on age, educational level (usually number of years of formal education), or both. Some normative standards are also stratified by gender. Raw test scores are usually converted into scaled scores for the purpose of comparison with the standardization sample. Many clinicians use the range of plus or minus one standard deviation from the mean to imply "normality" (43) during neuropsychological assessment of an individual possessing the demographic characteristics of the normative sample. Scores below that level are "outside of the normal range" and are therefore assigned the label "impaired." Rating of severity depends on how much the score deviates from the expected mean.

Clinical neuropsychology as practiced in the English-speaking industrialized world has made important strides through the collection of massive databases of normative information. However, toxic exposure is a worldwide phenomenon and, hence, is likely to touch individuals from an array of different cultural and linguistic backgrounds (4,45,46).

Although neuropsychological test norms may be accepted as gold standards in the United States, England, and Australia, it cannot be assumed that the same procedures and their normative information are applicable to other populations. Administration of a neuropsychological procedure that is well established in the United States, and use of U. S. mainstream norms on a subject with little or no formal education, is likely to lead to invalid, uninterpretable results. The neuropsychologist who wishes to embark in test administration to individuals whose demographic characteristics are not those of the sample used to norm the procedures has to proceed with a great deal of caution. Within the North American context, it should be stressed that a significant number of neurotoxicologic referrals are likely to be individuals who have immigrated to the United States for economic reasons, who have little in the way of formal schooling in their own country, and who have nonexistent or marginal command of the English language. Such individuals should not be assessed with instruments and normed on individuals with mainstream demographic characteristics. It goes without saying that the patient's fluent command of the language is a requirement for the clinician wishing to undertake such evaluations, as is an in-depth knowledge of the patient's background and culture of origin. The clinician has to resort to historic and anecdotal information much more heavily than he or she would with a mainstream referral, as tests normed for individuals with these demographic characteristics are not widely available. Use of interpreters is a questionable practice to be used only after it has become clear that referral to a qualified native speaker of the patient's language is impossible.

The need for standardization of neuropsychological test batteries for use with occupational populations exposed to chemicals in developing countries is well recognized, and projects are ongoing to meet this need, with some promising cross-cultural results (4,46). Despite intense activity in the area of neuropsychological neurotoxicology, no widely accepted battery of tests exists that can be used in the clinic for individuals with very low levels of education and whose knowledge of the English language is poor.

EFFECTS OF PSYCHIATRIC VARIABLES

Evaluation of a toxic exposure suspected of causing neurobehavioral effects necessitates inclusion of a psychological assessment. Psychiatric symptoms are frequently identified in assessment of possible toxic encephalopathy and may range from minor fluctuations of mood to severe disturbance meeting diagnostic criteria for psychiatric illness, such as panic disorder (49), posttraumatic stress disorder (50,51), and psychosis (52). Mood changes are commonly reported by exposed workers, with subjective complaints of fatigue, irritability, and poor anger control (53,54). A number of studies from Scandinavia have reported adverse effects of solvents, including fatigue, irritability, alcohol intolerance, and depression (16,55,56). Nevertheless, a U.S. study (23,57) failed to demonstrate an association with chronic low-level solvent exposure, reporting only a small effect on one of the symptoms (depression). Another study (58) found no solvent-related increase in psychiatric symptoms in painters and solvent-exposed populations in the United Kingdom. The importance of documenting present emotional state and previous personality, family, social, and work stressors is underscored. Effects of preexisting mental illness, fear of brain damage (1,59), and the possibility of mass psychogenic illness (1) should be considered.

The issue of whether significant psychological disturbance without evidence of neurologic deficit in the aftermath of toxic exposure is attributable to neuropathologic or functional causes is unresolved. Nevertheless, in neurotoxicologic assessment, as in assessment of other possible causes of brain damage, neuropsychological abnormalities have to be interpreted in the light of reported or documented psychological problems. Also, documentation of psychological status clarifies the task of referral for intervention and management.

Exposed patients frequently complain of a variety of somatic symptoms. For example, pain is reported frequently. This is not surprising, given the high prevalence of chronic pain of any origin in the general population—one-third of Americans, according to Bonica (60). Pain is rarely attributable to exposure, but depression and anxiety are frequent concomitants of pain (61), and it is suggested that pain amplifies depression (62). A pain syndrome can trigger a downward spiral in which the patient loses contact with sources of positive reinforcement, such as coworkers and the positive self-esteem that comes from being productive (62). This can lead to depression with loss of energy and decreased ability to interact with others. Social contact that does take place becomes organized around pain complaints. Secondary gain may be a factor, inasmuch as the individual is able to avoid unwanted responsibilities. It can also become a factor when the possibility of financial gain appears (62).

Many symptoms and complaints by individuals who have been exposed to potentially toxic substances are common in a number of other, unrelated disease states, psychiatric illnesses, or in situations involving substance abuse. A number of these complaints have very high base rates in the normal population (e.g., anxiety, depression, headaches, back pain, fatigue, concern about health, irritability, restlessness, memory problems), and even higher in individuals who are in litigation for reasons other than toxic exposure (63).

NEUROPSYCHOLOGICAL EXAMINATION

The neuropsychological examination of the patient with possible neurotoxic exposure should ideally proceed within the framework of a multidisciplinary team including a medical toxicologist, a neurologist, and a neurophysiologist. Background information on the patient is necessary and includes school, military, medical, and employment records, as well as exposure records from industrial hygienists, engineers, and the like. This information assists in the diagnostic process. For the neuropsychologist working on a clinical referral, however, all of the mechanisms are rarely in place. Nevertheless, it is still the obligation of the neuropsychologist to obtain as much information, enlisting the help of the patient and referral sources to obtain records, as possible to ascertain that no crucial piece of information is overlooked.

Review of Relevant Documentation

Review of developmental, school, and past medical records, as well as the occupational and mental health history, is a crucial part of the examination. Past medical and mental health information should be obtained directly from the patient and from records and other collateral sources of information. Detailed information on the duration and intensity of neurotoxin exposure can be obtained through records and directly from the patient, either through structured interview or through a questionnaire. Information on the possibility of a peak exposure should be obtained. Estimating severity of toxic exposure can be an arduous task, as evaluation of deficits generally occurs after exposure has ceased, at a time when the body burden of suspected toxic substances is no longer elevated.

Interview and Behavioral Observations

A detailed interview of the patient, with collection of demographic and social information, deserves a great deal of attention. In this context, the following historical aspects of the patient should be reviewed: family composition during childhood; marital history; academic history, including investigation into the possibility of a learning disability; medical history, including past substance abuse; military history; legal history, including encounters with the law; family history of genetic, psychiatric, or neurologic illness; and detailed occupational and recreational history. Information on present life circumstances and current medical status, including use of prescription medication and substance abuse, should be elicited from the patient. Eliciting a list of present complaints from the patient in writing (dictated if the patient is unable to write) gives a better idea of the problems that are most troubling to the patient. Asking the patient to check a list of complaints can also be useful, particularly to compare the results of this with spontaneous generation. However, symptom checklists can elicit literally masses of complaints from patients who are very focused on issues of somatization. Checklists also may provide individuals who wish to appear sicker than they are with the opportunity of overreporting symptoms. A history of evolution of symptoms should be carefully elicited.

Direct observation of the patient, including how he or she moves about and responds to the examiner and to others in the examination process, his or her stamina and expressions of self, on what he or she focuses, to what he or she attends, how feelings are expressed, how guarded he or she is, and his or her level of self-disclosure, may provide valuable clues to the patient's emotional status, social adaptation, and language competence on spontaneous speech.

Indirect reports on the patient's behavior through the technician's observations during testing, such as level of effort and cooperation, stamina, requests for breaks, and any unusual behaviors, can be useful ways to learn more about the patient.

An interview with at least one collateral source of information (preferably someone who lives with the patient and has known him or her pre- and postexposure) regarding the patient's premorbid versus present status, ability to interact with the family and proceed in day-to-day living activities, and progression of symptoms can give the clinician a better sense of the changes (or lack thereof) that the patient may have experienced.

Cognitive Measurement

Depending on what neurotoxin is involved, at what exposure levels, and for what period of time the exposure occurred, the difficulties that may arise from toxic exposure can range from frank generalized cognitive dilapidation (i.e., dementia) to subtle, frequently difficult to substantiate, cognitive complaints. Test selection must reflect consideration of all of the possibilities.

In most cases of assessment of possible toxic encephalopathy, to provide a profile of abilities and deficits, and to address diagnostic issues, it is appropriate to select neuropsychological tests that assess a variety of functions. It is important to sample those cognitive areas reported to have been affected by toxic exposure and those that have not.

Measurement of possible deficit presupposes that there is some sort of standard against which the patient is measured. Results obtained are scored and compared to published normative data based on expected ranges of results stratified by age, education, and, for some procedures, gender.

A list of tests is proposed for examination of possible toxic encephalopathy (Table 30-1). This list is by no means intended to be comprehensive. Neither is the list meant as a battery, but as possible procedures that have generally been validated in research and clinical settings on patients with known brain damage. Some of the procedures overlap with others in the behavior they sample. Most of the tests suggested have a track record in the field of neuropsychology and are generally recognized as valid and reliable. Clinicians wishing to use alternative testing procedures have a number of possible choices and may wish to consult compendia of neuropsychological test procedures.

Selection of Test Procedures

An initial review of records and an interview of the patient, including information on the patient's level of orientation to person, time, place, and situation, guide the clinician as to choice of test procedures. In cases of extremely low levels of functioning (i.e., dementing-type condition), the clinician may have to resort to a brief mental status examination of the patient using such instruments as the Mini-Mental Status Examination (64), the Alzheimer's Disease Assessment Scale (65), or the Mattis Dementia Rating Scale (66). Results on these screening procedures give a glimpse into the patient's general cognitive status and shed some light on the patient's ability to undergo a more complex examination. For the majority of toxic exposure referrals, the examination (i.e., patient contact) is a reasonably lengthy undertaking. A general consensus exists on the areas that necessitate specific attention during the neuropsychological examination of the individual exposed to toxic substances.

The pros and cons of fixed batteries versus flexible neuropsychological batteries are well documented (41,67). The Halstead-Reitan Battery (HRB) and the Luria-Nebraska Neuropsychological Battery (LNNB) are the most commonly used batteries in the field of neuropsychology. However, relatively little neurotoxicology research has been undertaken with either of these batteries. They possess relatively poor focus on memory, a clear limitation in an area in which difficulties, when present, are with new learning. If used, both batteries should be supplemented with some memory tasks. Most research in neurotoxicology has used flexible batteries (1). Most of these batteries have been assembled using preexisting procedures with a track record in the area of mental measurement. The WHO Neurobehavioral Core Test Battery (NCTB) (68) was intended as a brief set of tests with emphasis on international use. Norms were collected for 2,300 control subjects in three different continents (4). The Neurobehavioral Evaluation System (NES) (69), a computerized battery, has been validated in different parts of the world (70). The Pittsburgh Occupational Exposures Test (POET) (9) includes a commonly used set of tests and is intended for clinical and research use. Whether the clinician uses an existing battery or whether a set of tests is chosen to address the specific referral question, care should be taken that the procedures sample an array of cognitive domains.

ASSESSMENT OF ATTENTION AND CONCENTRATION

In the real world, ability to attend to the environment is a prerequisite for efficient behavior. No universally accepted definition of attention exists, although there appears to be general agreement in the field of neuropsychology that (a) attention is a system in which processing occurs in a series of sequential stages within different brain systems, and (b) attention has a limited capacity that varies between individuals and within the same person depending on the time and situation (41). Also, general agreement exists on the fragility of attention. This aspect of behavior can be affected by any type of brain damage, but it is also susceptible to emotional factors, general medical condition, and adverse environmental influences. Similarly, during the neuropsychological evaluation, the patient's ability to attend to the information presented has a profound impact on his or her ultimate success in completing the tasks. This ability can be affected by a variety of environmental or internal factors. Attention and concentration tasks clearly possess components that can be identified as executive, language, visuospatial, or visuomotor in nature. Nevertheless, a number of tasks hold special interest for their attention components (see Table 30-1). Neuropsychology has a number of procedures designed to assess various aspects of attention, including vigilance, short-term storage capacity, tracking, sequencing, scanning, and rate of information processing. Attention cannot be measured in isolation.

ASSESSMENT OF INTELLECTUAL FUNCTION

Assessment of the current level of intellectual functioning is an important part of the assessment of toxic encephalopathy. In the English-speaking world, and in many areas of the industrialized non–English-speaking world, administration of the Wechsler Intelligence Scales (WAIS, WAIS-R) is clearly the most thorough, if somewhat time-consuming, avenue available. The importance of administering lies in the fact that IQ generally correlates with neuropsychological test performance and control of IQ is, therefore, important. Additionally, whereas a number of the subtests of the WAIS are very resilient to the effects of brain dysfunction (i.e., Information, Vocabulary, and Picture Completion), others appear to be sensitive to the effects of subclinical toxic exposure (i.e., Digit Symbol, Block Design, Similarities, and Digit Span) (1). However, use of the WAIS with individuals whose demographic characteristics, particularly level of educational attainment and

TABLE 30-1. Names and types of tests for neuropsychological evaluation

Name of test	Type of test	Reference
Mini-Mental Status Examination	Index of cognitive function	64
Alzheimer's Disease Assessment Scale	Index of cognitive function	65
Mattis Dementia Rating Scale	Index of cognitive function	66
Digit Span Wechsler Intelligence Scales-R	Short-term memory	74
Digit Symbol Wechsler Intelligence Scales-R	Psychomotor speed	74
Symbol-Digit Modalities (Smith)	Psychomotor speed	75
Paced Auditory Serial Addition Test	Information processing, sustained attention	76,77,78
WAIS-R	Intellectual function (IQ)	74
Progressive Matrices	Reasoning (visual)	79,80,81
National Adult Reading Test	Estimate of premorbid intellectual ability	82,83
Wide Range Achievement Test-III	Reading, spelling, math	84
Peabody Individual Achievement Test-R	Scholastic abilities	85
Wisconsin Card Sorting Test	Abstraction, mental flexibility	86,87
Category Test	Concept formation	88,89
Stroop Color-Word Test	Shifting perceptual set	90
Controlled Oral Word Association	Verbal organization	91
Thurstone Written Fluency	Verbal organization	92
Token Test	Syntactic comprehension	93
Boston Naming Test	Confrontation naming	94
Aphasia Screening Test	Language screening	95,96
Hooper Visual Organization Test	Visual organization	97
Rey-Osterreith Figure (Copy)	Constructional praxis	98,99
Embedded Figures	Visual search	100
Wechsler Memory Scale-Revised	Verbal and visual learning	101
Memory Assessment Scales	Verbal and visual learning	102
California Verbal Learning Test	Verbal learning and memory	103
Rey Auditory Verbal Learning Test	Verbal learning and memory	104
Story Memory Test	Prose learning and memory	43
Figure Memory Test	Visual learning and memory	43
Rey-Osterreith Figure (Delayed Recall)	Visual learning and memory	98,99
Grooved Pegboard	Manual dexterity	105,106
Finger Tapping Test	Motor speed	95
Grip Strength	Motor strength	89
Beck Depression Inventory	Depression self-report	107
Beck Anxiety Inventory	Anxiety self-report	108
Symptom Checklist 90-R	Symptom self-report	109
Minnesota Multiphasic Personality Inventory II	Personality assessment, self-report	110
Personality Assessment Inventory	Personality assessment, self-report	111
Profile of Mood States	Mood self-assessment	112
15-Item Memory Test	Cooperation	113
Dot Counting Test	Cooperation	98
Forced Choice Test	Cooperation	114
Portland Digit Recognition Test	Cooperation	115

WAIS-R, Wechsler Adult Intelligence Scale, revised.

language, are different from those of the standardization sample is likely to yield invalid, meaningless results.

Estimation of previous level of intellectual ability is frequently desirable and can be roughly achieved through administration of the North American Adult Reading Test (NAART) (71). Indeed, reading of phonetically irregular words is thought to be a good predictor of premorbid mental ability.

SCHOLASTIC ACHIEVEMENT

The assessment of verbal and mathematic academic skills is considered an important part of the examination, as these areas are also likely to reflect, to an important degree, the patient's level of premorbid functioning. Poor spelling or writing can be an indicator of low scholastic achievement, but also of a developmental language deficit, a dyslexic deficit, or an acquired deficit. Comparison of present results with scholastic records, if available, can provide unique insights to the patient's abilities.

ASSESSMENT OF EXECUTIVE FUNCTIONING

Executive functions are those abilities that permit an individual to successfully engage in independent behavior. They include such aspects of behavior as initiation, planning, volition, self-monitoring and self-regulation, purposive action, judgment, abstracting, generalizing from particulars, decision making, and modifying behavior in response to a changing environment. These functions differ from cognitive functions in that they address how, whether, and under what circumstances an individual goes about doing something, whereas cognitive functions address what and how much people know or can do (41). Executive function assessment is one of the most challenging aspects of the neuropsychological examination, as its measurement remains elusive. However, executive dysfunction can exert a profound effect on the patient's ability to operate efficiently and in a self-motivated manner.

Executive dysfunction has been documented as a sequela of solvent inhalation (5). However, at the present time only a limited set exists of well-established neuropsychological procedures that allow the subject to demonstrate his or her ability to abstract from particulars, choose among alternatives, and make decisions regarding the most efficient way to complete a task. The assessment of executive functions, then, is not only achieved through the administration of tests (see Table 30-1), but also through careful observation of the subject during interview and testing, and through interview of significant others.

ASSESSMENT OF LANGUAGE

Although language is rarely disrupted in toxic encephalopathy, it is important to address it during the examination of possible toxic encephalopathy, as patterns of deficits in language tests can signal the presence of an aphasic disorder (and hence the possibility of another neuropathologic process), a developmental language disorder, or even lack of cooperation on the subject's part. Extensive assessment of language functions, such as administration of a full aphasia battery, is generally unnecessary. However, some brief screening procedures are recommended (see Table 30-1).

ASSESSMENT OF VISUOSPATIAL AND CONSTRUCTIONAL FUNCTIONS

Our ability to perceive the world around us dictates how well we can function in it. Visual perception is an exceedingly complex array of functions, including basic perception of color and form, complex visual arrays, motion, and perception of oneself. With the exception of Embedded Figures (45) and tests of color perception (72), perceptual tests requiring no manipulation of the test material have received little attention in the neuropsychological assessment of toxic exposure. Most tests involving visual perception contain attention, spatial orientation, language, memory, and constructional components (e.g., Block Design, Object Assembly, Digit Symbol subtests of the WAIS, Trail Making Test, and drawing tests). Intact executive functions are also frequently a prerequisite for correct performance of the tests (e.g., Rey-Osterreith Figure). Given the complexity and interconnection of functions involved in performance of these tasks, and given that impairment in any of the areas can impact successful completion of the task, it is good practice to observe subject behavior carefully during testing and to observe the quality of the work product. Abnormalities in a variety of visuospatial tests and in tests with visuospatial components have been found after toxic exposure (e.g., immediate visual reproduction, as well as delayed visual reproduction, embedded figures, and mental rotations) (45,73).

ASSESSMENT OF MEMORY AND LEARNING

What we call *memory* is a complex system through which organisms encode, retain, recall, and recognize information or material to which they have previously been exposed. Some aspects of memory are much more susceptible to disruption owing to brain damage than others. The pattern of complaints reported by the patient and significant others during the interview can begin to give the clinician some idea as to where the problem may lie. Neuropsychology possesses a vast array of memory assessment procedures (see Table 30-1). The neuropsychological examination of the exposed subject should include procedures that sample initial registration of information (immediate recall), rate of learning (learning curve), spontaneous recall of information after a delay (delayed free recall), and recognition of information previously learned. Sampling of these aspects of memory in the visual and verbal modalities is advisable, as patterns of results can provide useful diagnostic information. Knowledge about remote life events (via history taking) and about information acquired long ago (i.e., lexical stock, general information) is a critical part of the examination, as these aspects of cognition are unlikely to be affected by exposure to neurotoxins. Careful examination of the pattern of results obtained in these tests is crucial to the diagnostic accuracy. Indeed, for example, impaired immediate recall of information is a common symptom in early forms of progressive dementing illness. However, it is also commonly seen in depression. Failure to address delayed recall or recognition may lead to a flawed diagnostic impression.

ASSESSMENT OF MOTOR SPEED AND DEXTERITY

Motor speed and dexterity deficits are often seen in toxic encephalopathy. A number of simple procedures are available (see Table 30-1). All are timed tests and involve an apparatus with a counting or strength measurement device.

PSYCHOLOGICAL ASSESSMENT

A number of tests of personality and emotional status are available. The effects of deficits may manifest through response endorsement or indirectly through patterns of responses, suggestive of attempts to mask deficits, or, conversely, attempts at symptom magnification. Caution must be exercised that the patient's level of reading permits understanding of the task.

ASSESSMENT OF DECEPTION AND MALINGERING

The possibility of exaggeration of symptomatology, or even frank malingering, deserves our attention when assessing individuals with possible toxic encephalopathy. The possibility of secondary gain can and does affect the results of neuropsychological tests, and may influence the willingness of the individual to give a forthright history of complaints. Exaggeration of deficits can be owing to a psychogenic disturbance, deliberate distortion, or a combination of both. The problem is further complicated by the fact that symptom amplification may coexist with genuine neurologic compromise.

Neuropsychological referrals for assessment of a possible toxic encephalopathy frequently occur within a context in which the patient may stand to gain from being impaired (worker compensation, disability determination, or personal injury). The first line of assessment of malingering lies in careful recording of history. Guardedness around social circumstances that might explain some of the complaints or around the possibility of a preexisting medical or mental health history should alert the clinician as to the possibility of malingering. Inconsistent results between the present and past examination, discrepancies within the present examination, and a pattern of results that is inconsistent with known neurotoxic syndromes should also raise questions.

A number of tests have been used to distinguish between genuine neurologically based injury and simulated deficits (see Table 30-1). Most of these tests are psychometrically simple tasks requiring immediate recall of information. For example, the 15-Item Memory Test asks the subject to reproduce overlearned strings of numbers, letters, and simple geometric designs.

Symptom Validity Testing is intended to measure faked deficits in memory or sensory functions. It involves the presentation of stimuli in which perception or recognition is affirmed or denied by the examinee. The tests are made to appear quite difficult when, in fact, they are very easy, if not trivial. In fact, the tasks are so easy that even significantly neurologically impaired persons should perform them satisfactorily. The subject's performance on a large number of test items is compared with expected levels based on the binomial probability distribution.

INTERPRETATION OF RESULTS

Once all data have been collected, the diagnosis of toxic encephalopathy can only be made if the evidence points to toxic exposure as the primary etiology, and alternative explanations for the patient's symptoms and other causes have been ruled out. Special attention should be paid to avoiding such interpretation errors as confirmatory bias, overgeneralization, over- and underinterpretation, and underuse of base rates (41).

Before the clinician embarks on careful pattern analysis and integration of results with historical, medical, and toxicologic information, it is important to verify that the patient's performance was effortful and valid. Guardedness, defensiveness, and vagueness of responses during the interview should alert the clinician to the possibility of deception. Important levels of emotional distress during the examination can cause the patient to put forth varying levels of effort and lead to unreliable results. In cases in which the patient has undergone prior neuropsychological examination, a comparison of present to past performance can give excellent clues as to the stability of symptoms, complaints, and neuropsychological test scores. Inconsistent findings should be carefully examined, as they may be indicative of fluctuating effort or significant emotional interference. Departures from expected levels of performance in tests designed to assess malingering indicate a purposeful attempt to manipulate results. When performance defies statistical rules for malingering, the neuropsychologist has to conclude that the patient's level of cooperation was not sufficient to generate valid or reliable results. The only conclusion that can be derived from the examination at that point is that the true nature of the patient's neuropsychological problems is not known. It should be noted that sophisticated subjects can frequently see through these relatively simple tests, so that detection of malingering in such individuals can be more challenging, requiring careful examination of history and data analysis for inconsistencies. When the clinician possesses reasonable certainty regarding the validity of the results obtained (i.e., that the results are a good representation of the patient's current level of functioning), analysis of available information can proceed.

It is not good clinical practice to automatically link test abnormalities to the effects of neurotoxins. Hartman (1) remarks that the clinician has the obligation to make a comprehensive effort to determine whether significant exposure occurred. Complaints, symptoms, and neuropsychological data should make sense from a toxicologic standpoint. Is the substance that the patient was exposed to known to be toxic under the conditions of exposure that were documented for the patient? In this respect, efforts should be directed toward investigating the temporal relationship between the complaints or symptoms and the exposure. Similarly, complaints that appear for the first time only years after termination of exposure (and coinciding with initiation of legal proceedings) should be highly suspect.

Evidence of generalized cognitive dilapidation on testing and real-life level of functioning should incite investigation into the possibility of a progressive dementing illness, unrelated to exposure, particularly if the documented exposure is not deemed likely to be sufficient to have caused dementia.

Neuropsychological results that show a clear pattern of lateralization should alert the clinician to the possibility of a neurologic event affecting only one hemisphere. A complaint of difficulty reading may well precede the exposure and be linked to a developmental learning disability. School records can be very helpful here.

Complaints, symptoms, and data should also make sense with respect to what is known about consistency of neuropsychological deficits in testing. For example, a patient who cannot repeat more than two digits backward is unlikely to be able to learn a list of 16 words. Test results should make sense in light of the patient's level of function in real life. For instance, extremely low scores in language tests in a patient who demonstrates no language problems during spontaneous speech, understands instructions, and lives independently should clearly be scrutinized as to the possibility of symptom magnification. In general, scores that fall "off the scales" should lead to careful scrutiny of motivational factors.

Documentation of progression is an important part of the diagnostic process. Indeed, the literature reflects that symptoms tend to stabilize, improve, or disappear after removal from alleged exposure. Appearance of symptomatology for the first time after exposure has ceased should alert the clinician to the possibility of an unrelated factor at play. Intensification of cognitive symptomatology after cessation of exposure has been reported, but it is unclear whether this is owing to exposure itself or to the effects of possible moderator variables, such as ability to return to work, or psychological distress (9).

In summary, neuropsychological data should be interpreted within the context of the examination, direct observation, and examination of other existing information. Test scores alone may be summary statements about observed behavior, but they are based on one narrowly defined aspect of behavior. Neuropsychology has a very prominent role in the assessment of toxicity in the central nervous system. However, in the complex area of neurotoxicology, the clinician's acquaintance with the limitations of qualitative and quantitative data and familiarity with the art of avoiding common interpretation errors determines the ultimate value of his or her contribution.

REFERENCES

1. Hartman DE. *Neuropsychological toxicology: identification and assessment of human neurotoxic syndromes*, 2nd ed. New York: Plenum Press, 1995.
2. Gamberale F, Kjellberg A. Behavioral performance assessment as a biological control of occupational exposure to neurotoxic substances. In: Gilioli R, Cassitto MG, Foa V, eds. *Neurobehavioral methods in occupational health: proceedings of the International Symposium on Neurobehavioral Methods in Occupational Health (State of the Art and Emerging Trends)—Como and Milan, Italy, June 23-26, 1982*. Oxford, UK: Pergamon Press, 1983:111–121.
3. Hänninen H. Psychological tests in the diagnosis of carbon disulfide poisoning. *Work Environ Health* 1966;2:16–20.
4. Anger WK, Cassitto MG, Liang Y, et al. Comparison of performance from three continents on the WHO-recommended neurobehavioral core test battery. *Environ Res* 1993;62:125–147.
5. Arlien-Søborg P. *Solvent neurotoxicity*. Boca Raton, FL: CRC Press, 1992.
6. Johnson BL, Baker EL, Giglioli R, et al, eds. *Prevention of neurotoxic illness on working populations*. New York: Wiley, 1987.
7. Baker EL, Feldman RG, White RF, Harley JP, Dinse GE, Berkey CS. Monitoring neurotoxins in industry: development of a neurobehavioral test battery. *J Occup Med* 1983;25(2):125–130.
8. Baker EL, Letz R, Fidler A. A computer-administered neurobehavioral evaluation system for occupational and environmental epidemiology: rationale, methodology and pilot study results. *J Occup Med* 1985;27:206–212.
9. Ryan CM, Morrow LA, Bromet EJ, Parkinson DK. Assessment of neuropsychological dysfunction in the workplace: normative data from the Pittsburgh Occupational Exposures Test Battery. *J Clin Exp Neuropsychol* 1987;9:665–679.

10. Bowler RM, Mergler D, Huel G, Garrison R, Cone J. Neuropsychological impairment among former microelectronics workers. *Neurotoxicology* 1991; 12:87–104.
11. Lindström K. Behavioral changes after long-term exposure to organic solvents and their mixtures. *Scand J Work Environ Health* 1981;7[Suppl 4]:48–53.
12. Linz DH, deGarmo PL, Morton WE, Weins AN, Coull BM, Maricle RA. Organic solvent-induced encephalopathy in industrial patients. *J Occup Med* 1986;28:119–125.
13. Allison WM, Jerrom DWA. Glue sniffing: a pilot study of cognitive effects of long-term use. *Int J Addict* 1984;19:453–458.
14. Ryan CM, Morrow LA, Hodgson M. Cacosmia and neurobehavioral dysfunction associated with occupational exposure to mixtures of organic solvents. *Am J Psychiatry* 1988;145:1442–1445.
15. Morrow LA, Robin N, Hodgson MJ. Assessment of attention and memory efficiency in persons with solvent neurotoxicity. *Neuropsychologia* 1992;10:911–922.
16. Arlien-Soborg P, Bruhn P, Gyldensted C, Paulson OB. Chronic painter's syndrome: toxic encephalopathy in house painters. *Acta Neurol Scand* 1979;60:149–156.
17. Troster AI, Ruff RM. Neuropsychological sequelae of exposure to the chlorinated hydrocarbon solvents trichloroethylene and trichloroethane. *Arch Clin Neuropsychol* 1990;5:31–47.
18. Korsak RJ, Sato MM. Effects of chronic organophosphate pesticide exposure on the central nervous system. *Clin Toxicol* 1977;11:83–95.
19. Levin HS, Rodnitzky RL. Behavioral aspects of organophosphorous pesticides in man. *Clin Toxicol* 1976;9:391.
20. Levin HS, Rodnitzky RL, Mick DL. Anxiety associated with exposure to organophosphate compounds. *Archives Gen Psychiatry* 1976;33:225–228.
21. Kaplan JG, Kessler J, Rosenberg N, Pack D, Schaumburg HH. Sensory neuropathy associated with Dursban (chlorpyrifos) exposure. *Neurology* 1993;43(11):2193–2196.
22. Bleecker ML, Bolla-Wilson K. *Neuropsychological impairment following inorganic arsenic exposure: unmasking a memory disorder. Neurobehavioral methods in occupational health*. Copenhagen: World Health Organization, 1985;3:172–176.
23. Bleecker ML, Bolla KI, Agnew J, Schwartz BS, Ford DP. Dose-related subclinical neuropsychological effects of chronic exposure to low levels of organic solvents. *Am J Ind Med* 1991;19:715–728.
24. Bolter JF, Stanczik DF, Long CJ. Neuropsychological consequences of acute, high level, gasoline inhalation. *Clin Neuropsychol* 1983;5:47.
25. Hänninen H. Behavioral effects of occupational exposure to mercury and lead. *Acta Neurol Scand* 1982;66[Suppl 92]:167–175.
26. Uzzell B, Oler J. Chronic low-level mercury exposure and neuropsychological functioning. *J Clin Exp Neuropsychol* 1986;8:581–593.
27. Lishman WA. *Organic psychiatry*, 2nd ed. Oxford: Blackwell Scientific, 1987.
28. Jackson DL, Menges H. Accidental carbon monoxide poisoning. *JAMA* 1980;243:772–774.
29. Klees JE, Lash A, Bowler RM, Shore M, Becker CE. Neuropsychologic "impairment" in a cohort of hospital workers chronically exposed to ethylene oxide. *J Toxicol Clin Toxicol* 1990;28(1):21–28.
30. Bromet E, Parkinson D, Cohen S. Health effects of long-term solvent exposure in blue-collar women. *Am J Ind Med* 1990;17:661–676.
31. Cherry N, Hutchins H, Pace T, Waldron HA. Neurobehavioral effects of repeated occupational exposure to toluene and paint solvents. *Br J Ind Med* 1985;42:291–300.
32. Cherry N, Gautrin D. Neurotoxic effects of styrene: further evidence. *Br J Ind Med* 1990;47:29–37.
33. Maizlish NA, Langolf GD, Whitehead LW, et al. Behavioral evaluation of workers exposed to mixtures of organic solvents. *Br J Ind Med* 1985;42:579–590.
34. Kishi R, Harabuchi I, Katakura Y, Ikeda T, Miyake H. Neurobehavioral effects of chronic occupational exposure to organic solvents among Japanese industrial painters. *Environ Res* 1993;62:303–313.
35. Morrow LA, Ryan CM, Hodgson MJ, Robin N. Risk factors associated with persistence of neuropsychological deficits on persons with organic solvent exposure. *J Occup Med* 1990;32:444–450.
36. Filley CM, Heaton RK, Rosenberg NL. White matter dementia in chronic toluene abuse. *Neurology* 1990;40:532–534.
37. Rosenberg NL, Spitz MC, Filley CM, Davis KA, Schaumberg HH. Central nervous system effects of chronic toluene abuse-clinical, brainstem evoked response and magnetic resonance imaging studies. *Neurotoxicol Teratol* 1988;10:489–495.
38. Rosenberg NL, Kleinschmidt-DeMasters BK, Davis KA, Dreisbach JN, Hormes JT, Filley CM. Toluene abuse causes diffuse central nervous system white matter changes. *Ann Neurol* 1988;23:611–614.
39. Grigsby J, Rosenberg NL, Dreisbach JN, Busenbark D, Grigsby P. Chronic toluene abuse produces neuropsychological deficits. *Arch Clin Neuropsychol* 1993;8:229–230.
40. Tsushima WT, Towne WS. Effects of paint sniffing on neuropsychological test performance. *J Abnorm Psychol* 1977;86(4):402–407.
41. Lezak M. *Neuropsychological assessment*, 3rd ed. New York: Oxford University Press, 1995.
42. Rogoff B, Chavajay P. What's become of research on the cultural basis of cognitive development? *Am Psychol* 1995;50:859–877.
43. Heaton RK, Grant I, Matthews CG. Comprehensive norms for an Expanded Halstead-Reitan Battery: demographic corrections, research findings, and clinical applications. Odessa, FL: Psychological Assessment Resources, 1991.
44. Colvin M, Myers J, Nell V, Cronje R. A cross-sectional survey of neurobehavioral effects of chronic solvent exposure on workers in a paint manufacturing plant. *Environ Res* 1993;63:122–132.
45. Camerino D, Cassitto MG, Giliori R. Prevalence of abnormal neurobehavioral scores in populations exposed to different industrial chemicals. Institute of Occupational Health, University of Milan. *Environ Res* 1993;61:251–257.
46. Nell V, Myers J, Colvin M, Rees D. Neuropsychological assessment of organic solvent effects in South Africa: test selection, adaptation, scoring, and validation issues. Health Psychology Unit, University of South Africa. *Environ Res* 1993;63:301–318.
47. Bornstein RA. Normative data on selected neuropsychological measures from a nonclinical sample. *J Clin Psychol* 1985;41:651–659.
48. Warner MH, Ernst J, Townes BD. Relationships between IQ and neuropsychological measures in neuropsychiatric populations: within-laboratory and cross-cultural replications using WAIS and WAIS-R. *J Clin Exp Neuropsychol* 1987;9:545–562.
49. Dager SR, Holland JP, Cowley DS, Dunner DL. Panic disorder precipitated by exposure to organic solvents in the work place. *Am J Psychiatry* 1987;144:1056–1058.
50. Schottenfeld RS, Cullen MR. Recognition of occupation-induced post-traumatic stress disorders. *J Occup Med* 1986;28:365–369.
51. Morrow LA, Ryan CM, Goldstein G, Hodgson MJ. A distinct pattern of personality disturbance following exposure to mixtures of organic solvents. *J Occup Med* 1989;31:74–746.
52. Goldblum D, Chouinard G. Schizophrenia psychosis associated with chronic industrial toluene exposure: case report. *J Clin Psychiatry* 1985;46:350–351.
53. Baker EL, Letz RE, Eisen RE. Neurobehavioral effects in solvents in construction painters. *J Occup Med* 1988;30:116–123.
54. Morrow LA, Ryan CM, Hodgson MJ, Robin N. Alterations in cognitive and psychological functioning after organic solvent exposure. *J Occup Med* 1990;32:440–450.
55. Hane M, Axelson O, Blume J, Hogstedt C, Sundell L, Ydreborg B. Psychological function changes among house painters. *Scand J Work Environ Health* 1977;3:91–99.
56. Struwe G, Wennberg A. Psychologic and neurological symptoms in workers occupationally exposed to organic solvents. *Acta Psychiatr Scand* 1983;[Suppl 303]:68–80.
57. Bolla KI, Schwartz BS, Agnew J. Subclinical neuropsychiatric effects of chronic low level solvent exposure in U.S. paint manufacturers. *J Occup Med* 1990;32:8.
58. Spurgeon A, Gray CN, Sims J, et al. Neurobehavioral effects of long-term occupational exposure to organic solvents: two comparable studies. *Am J Ind Med* 1992;22:325–335.
59. Schottenfeld RS. Psychiatric manifestations of occupational toxic exposure. *Res Staff Physic* 1984;30:54PC–62PC.
60. Bonica JJ. Evolution and current status of pain programs. *J Pain Symptom Manage* 1990;5:368–374.
61. Blumer D, Heilbronn M. Chronic pains as a variant of depressive disease: the pain prone disorder. *J Nerv Ment Dis* 1982;170:381–406.
62. Brose WG, Spiegel D. Neuropsychiatric aspects of pain management. In: Yudofsky ST, Hales RE, eds. *The American Psychiatric Press textbook of neuropsychiatry*, 2nd ed. Washington: American Psychiatric Press, 1992.
63. Lees-Haley PR, Brown RS. Neuropsychological complaint base rates of 170 personal injury claimants. *Arch Clin Neuropsychol* 1993;8:203–209.
64. Folstein MF, Folstein SE, McHugh P. Mini-mental state: a practical method for grading the cognitive state of outpatients for the clinician. *J Psychiatr Res* 1975;12:189–198.
65. Rosen WG, Mohs RC, Davis KL, Longitudinal changes: cognitive, behavioral, and affective patterns in Alzheimer's disease. In: Poon LW, ed. *Handbook for clinical memory assessment of older adults*. Washington: American Psychiatric Association, 1986.
66. Mattis S. *Dementia Rating Scale (DRS)*. Odessa, FL: Psychological Assessment Resources, 1988.
67. Franzen MD. *Reliability and validity in neuropsychological assessment*. New York: Plenum Publishing, 1989.
68. Baker EL, Letz R. Neurobehavioral testing in monitoring hazardous workplace exposures. *J Occup Med* 1986;28:987–990.
69. Baker EL, Letz RE, Fidler AT. A computer-administered neurobehavioral evaluation system for occupational and environmental epidemiology. *J Occup Med* 1985;27:206–212.
70. Letz R. The Neurobehavioral Evaluation System: an international effort. In: Johnson BL, ed. *Advances in neurobehavioral toxicology: applications in environmental and occupational health*. Chelsea, MI: Lewis Publishers, 1990.
71. Spreen O, Strauss E. *A compendium of neuropsychological tests: administration, norms, and commentary*. New York: Oxford University Press, 1991.
72. Mergler D, Bowler R, Cone J. Color vision loss among disabled workers with neuropsychological impairment. *Neurotoxicol Teratol* 1990;12:669–672.
73. Estrin WJ, Bowler RM, Lash A, et al. Neurotoxicological evaluation of hospital sterilizer workers exposed to ethylene oxide. *Clin Toxicol* 1990;28(1):1–20.

74. Wechsler D. *Manual for the WAIS-R*. New York: Psychological Corporation, 1981.
75. Smith A. *Symbol Digit Modalities Test-Revised*. Los Angeles: Western Psychological Services, 1992.
76. Gronwall D. Paced auditory serial-addition task: a measure of recovery from concussion. *Percept Mot Skills* 1977;44:367–373.
77. Gronwall D, Sampson H. *The psychological effects of concussion*. Auckland, NZ: Auckland University Press, 1974.
78. Gronwall D, Wrightson P. Delayed recovery of intellectual function after minor head injury. *Lancet* 1974;2:605–609.
79. Raven JC. *Progressive matrices: a perceptual test of intelligence*. London: HK Lewis, 1938.
80. Raven JC. *Colored progressive matrices sets A, Ab, B*. London: HK Lewis, 1947.
81. Raven JC. *Advance progressive matrices sets I and II*. London: HK Lewis, 1965.
82. Nelson HE. *National Adult Reading Test (NART): test manual*. Windsor, UK: NFER Nelson, 1982.
83. Nelson HE, O'Connell A. Dementia: the estimation of pre-morbid intelligence levels using the new adult reading test. *Cortex* 1978;14:234–244.
84. Wilkinson G. *The Wide Range Achievement Test—1993 edition*. Wilmington, DL: Jastak Associates, 1993.
85. Markwardt FC. *Peabody Individual Achievement Test—revised*. Circle Pines, MN: American Guidance Service, 1989.
86. Berg EA. A simple objective technique for measuring flexibility in thinking. *J Gen Psychol* 1948;39:15–22.
87. Grant DA, Berg EA. A behavioral analysis of degree of impairment and ease of shifting to new responses in a Weilg-type sorting problem. *J Exp Psychol* 1948;39:404–411.
88. Halstead WC. *Brain and intelligence*. Chicago: University of Chicago Press, 1947.
89. Reitan RM, Davidson LA. *Clinical neuropsychology: current status and applications*. Washington: VH Winston, 1974.
90. Stroop JR. Studies of interference in serial verbal reaction. *J Exp Psychol* 1935;18:643–662.
91. Benton A, Hamsher K de S. *Multilingual aphasia examination*, 2nd ed. Iowa City, IA: AJA Associates, Inc., 1989.
92. Thurstone LL, Thurstone TG. *Primary Mental Abilities—revised*. Chicago: Science Research Associates, 1962.
93. De Renzi E, Faglioni P. Normative data and screening power of a shortened version of the Token Test. *Cortex* 1978;14:41–49.
94. Kaplan EF, Goodglass H, Weintraub S. *The Boston Naming Test*, 2nd ed. Philadelphia: Lea & Febiger, 1983.
95. Reitan RM. Manual for administration of neuropsychological test batteries for adults and children. Indianapolis University Medical Center, unpublished data, 1969.
96. Halstead WC, Wepmann JM. The Halstead-Wepman Aphasia Screening Test. *J Speech Hear Disorders* 1959;14:9–15.
97. Hooper HE. *The Hooper Visual Organization Test: manual*. Beverly Hills, CA: Western Psychological Services, 1958.
98. Rey A. L'examen psychologique dans les cas d'encéphalopathie traumatique. *Archives de Psychologie* 1941;28:286–340.
99. Osterrieth PA. Le test de copie d'une figure complexe: contribution a l'etude de la perception et de la memoire. *Archives de Psychologie* 1944;30:286–356.
100. Spreen O, Benton AL. *Embedded Figures Test*. Victoria, BC: University of Victoria, Neuropsychology Laboratory, 1959.
101. Wechsler D. *Wechsler Memory Scale—revised*. New York: The Psychological Corp., 1987.
102. Williams JM. Cognitive Behavior Rating Scale. Odessa, FL: Psychological Assessment Resources, 1991.
103. Delis DC, Kramer JH, Kaplan E, Ober BA. *The California Verbal Learning Test—research edition*. San Antonio: The Psychological Corporation, 1987.
104. Taylor EM. *Psychological appraisal of children with cerebral deficits*. Cambridge: Harvard University Press, 1959.
105. Kløve H. Clinical neuropsychology. In: Forster FM, ed. *The medical clinics of North America*. New York: Saunders, 1963.
106. Matthews CG, Kløve H. *Instruction manual for the Adult Neuropsychology Test Battery*. Madison, WI: University of Wisconsin Medical School, 1964.
107. Beck AT, Beck RW. Screening depressed patients in family practice. *Postgrad Med* 1972;52:81–85.
108. Beck A. *Beck Anxiety Inventory*. San Antonio: The Psychological Corporation, 1987.
109. Derogatis L. *SCL-90-R administration, scoring, and procedures manual-II*. Towson, MD: Clinical Psychometric Research, 1977.
110. Butcher JN, Dahlstrom WG, Graham JR, et al. *MMPI-2: Minnesota Multiphasic Personality Inventory-2. Manual for administration and scoring*. Minneapolis: University of Minnesota Press, 1989.
111. Maurey LC. *Personality Assessment Inventory Manual*. Odessa, FL: Psychological Assessment Resources Inc., 1991.
112. McNair DM, Lorr M, Droppleman LF. *EDITS manual for the profile of mood states*. San Diego, CA: Educational and Industrial Service, 1981.
113. Rey A. *L'Examen clinique en psychologie*. Paris: University of France Press, 1964.
114. Hiscock M, Hiscock C. Refining the forced-choice method for the detection of malingering. *J Clin Exp Neuropsychol* 1989;11:967–974.
115. Binder, LM. Assessment of malingering after mild head trauma with the Portland Digit Recognition Test. *J Clin Exp Neuropsychol* 1993;15:170–182.

CHAPTER 31
Psychological Sequelae of Hazardous Materials Exposures

Iris R. Bell, Carol M. Baldwin, and Richard S. Schottenfeld

The psychological sequelae of chemical and hazardous materials exposures result from the interaction of biological, psychological, and sociocultural factors within a community or individual. Such sequelae derive in part from the physiologic effects of the agent and in part from the perceived short-term and long-term effects and risks from a given exposure. Individual differences in vulnerability to these effects emerge from genetic, social, cultural, and personality-related variables.

Neuropsychiatric symptoms, including weakness, fatigue, malaise, anxiety, depressed or irritable mood, difficulty concentrating, distractibility, and memory impairment, are commonly experienced after acute or chronic exposure to a wide range of noxious and toxic substances. These symptoms can result from the direct toxic effects of exposure on the central nervous system, from psychological or emotional reactions to exposure, or from a combination of both. Preexisting symptoms may also be exacerbated by and mistakenly attributed to exposure. Owing to the fact that neuropsychiatric symptoms may lead to considerable disability regardless of etiology, accurate and early diagnosis and institution of appropriate therapeutic interventions are essential (1).

First, it is crucial to recognize that the direct, toxic effects of an exposure can cause psychiatric and behavioral symptoms and syndromes. In many fields of medicine, a common but erroneous assumption is that the cause must be psychogenic because the resulting manifestations are psychiatric in nature. On the contrary, the brain is a complex biological system that controls behavior (2). Exposures to many chemical substances can cause central and peripheral nervous system dysfunction, even without obvious structural changes. With the newer diagnostic tools for functional testing, such as functional magnetic resonance imaging, positron emission tomography (PET), single photon emission computerized tomography (SPECT), evoked potentials, and quantitative electroencephalography, the ability to understand the biological mediation of many neuropsychiatric conditions related to toxic exposures is likely to expand rapidly in the near future.

Second, an important cautionary note is that although *hysteria* and some of its modern derivative terms, such as *somatoform disorder*, are frequent diagnoses of exclusion when organic etiologies are not readily found, classic studies on mixed clinical populations have shown that a large proportion of patients who receive such diagnoses are subsequently diagnosed with specific medical conditions (3,4). In controversial conditions, such as chronic fatigue syndrome (which shares the symptom of low-level chemical intolerance with multiple chemical sensitivity), some research has demonstrated that the determination of "medically explained" as opposed to "medically unexplained" symptoms relies heavily on the biases of the evaluator rather than on objective data (5). Controlled studies have shown that even patients with documented neurologic lesions also exhibit some symptoms usually considered "hysterical" in clinical practice (6).

Consequently, symptoms after exposure to known or suspected neurotoxins, including heavy metals, pesticides, and organic solvents, often pose a diagnostic challenge. The diagnosis of a toxic syndrome is facilitated when exposures exceed established thresholds for biological effects and symptoms follow classic patterns for intoxication. It is in the area of chronic persistent disability after recovery from an acute exposure that the issue of organic versus psychogenic factors becomes especially problematic.

PEAK EXPOSURES AND DISTRESS

Several studies have shown that, in the case of solvents (7) and pesticides (8), a history of an acute "peak exposure" event may be a better predictor of chronic neuropsychological and cognitive sequelae than is cumulative exposure *per se*. A *peak exposure* is defined as a discrete time-limited event involving toxic or subtoxic levels of a hazardous agent and requiring acute medical treatment (e.g., in a hospital emergency room) (7). Even in situations of definite central nervous system toxicity, however, psychological and emotional reactions may play a part in the persistence of symptoms and may complicate recovery and exacerbate disability. For example, the study of peak exposures to solvents found that high levels of emotional distress at the time of the original exposure are also a risk factor for persistent neuropsychological deficits and disability (7).

POSTTRAUMATIC STRESS DISORDER

Conversely, in the absence of definite neurotoxicity, or after low-level exposure, symptoms can result from psychological and emotional reactions secondary to the fact that an exposure occurred. Toxic exposure events may initiate acute (lasting less than 3 months) and chronic (lasting longer than 3 months) posttraumatic stress disorder (PTSD). PTSD is a disabling psychiatric diagnosis in which a traumatic event (e.g., a life-threatening toxic spill) initiates a syndrome involving persistent reexperiencing of the original event, persistent avoidance of trauma-related stimuli and numbing of overall responsiveness, and persistent psychophysiologic arousal (9). Individuals with PTSD have high rates of comorbid psychiatric problems, such as major depression, dysthymia, generalized anxiety disorder, obsessive-compulsive disorder, and mania, as well as substance abuse (10).

Vulnerability to developing PTSD derives in part from characteristics of the affected individual (10). These include poorer socioeconomic status in childhood, preexisting psychiatric problems, reported childhood abuse, being female (in mid-30s to 50 years old), and degree of social support after the event. PTSD vulnerability also derives in part from the characteristics of the traumatic event. Such characteristics include the experience of physical injury and physical proximity to the perceived danger during the event.

Notably, some chronic effects of toxic exposures and the symptoms of PTSD may share endogenous mechanisms. For example, solvent-exposed workers with and without histories of traumatic events have psychological profiles that overlap those of prisoners of war with PTSD more than they do those of chronic medical patients (11). In other words, it is possible that exposures to certain chemicals may activate some of the same psychophysiologic processes that underlie PTSD, even without an associated traumatic event. Neural sensitization is one proposed mechanism for the development of enhanced reactivity to environmental agents (12,13) and to psychological trauma (14). In sensitization, certain susceptible neuronal pathways develop a persistent change in their degree of responsiveness to stimuli (i.e., not only pharmacologic agents, but also psychological and physical stressors). In fact, pharmacologic agents and stress can cross-sensitize (13).

These considerations make it extremely difficult and perhaps clinically unrealistic to try to distinguish definitively between toxic and psychological sequelae of some exposures. Consistent with this ambiguity, a study of symptom clusters in persons living near two Superfund sites found that almost two times as many of those with the highest cumulative exposure had five or more neurologic symptoms in comparison with those with the lowest cumulative exposure (15). Cumulative exposure was calculated on the basis of distance from the sites and length of time exposed to various amounts of chemicals at the sites. Most of the neurologic symptoms were nonspecific, however, and could occur in medical and psychiatric conditions such as PTSD.

Consequently, the differential diagnosis of neuropsychiatric symptoms includes (a) organic mental disorders; (b) psychological or emotional reactions secondary to exposure and resulting illness; and (c) preexisting or concomitant psychiatric disorders (including psychological or emotional reactions to life problems or stressors unrelated to exposure and problematic alcohol or other substance use). These diagnoses are not mutually exclusive. Symptoms may reflect a combination of disorders, and complete differentiation of organic from nonorganic disorders is not always possible. Adjustment disorders with anxious or depressed mood after toxic exposures, for example, may be difficult to differentiate from organic affective disorders resulting from direct toxic effects on the central nervous system; both may be present in the same individual. Preexisting psychiatric disorders or coexisting stressors (e.g., family or economic problems) can also make it difficult to sort out the relative contributions of toxic central nervous system effects and psychological or emotional reactions to exposure.

Accurate diagnosis of neuropsychiatric syndromes associated with exposure depends on (a) a detailed history of exposure and chronology of symptoms; (b) knowledge of the possible neurotoxic effects of exposure; (c) psychiatric evaluation, including a thorough psychosocial history, history of drug and alcohol use, and neurologic and mental status examination; (d) awareness of the client's cultural background or beliefs regarding psychological symptoms and psychologically based interventions; and often (e) results of special tests, including neuropsychological testing, electroencephalogram, and diagnostic imaging.

Treatment must include helping the exposed person and others in his or her environment gain an understanding of the etiology and significance of the neuropsychiatric symptoms. In addition, a realistic view of the prognosis for immediate and long-term symptom relief underlies effective preventive interventions and treatments. Cognitive and behavioral treatments are often useful in bringing about symptomatic relief regardless of the specific diagnosis and etiology. However, when members undergo a toxic exposure, these primarily dominant culture–based treatments may need modifications geared to a given ethnic minority and to the individual's degree of acculturation.

A BIOPSYCHOSOCIAL MODEL OF POSTEXPOSURE ILLNESS

The likelihood that neuropsychiatric symptoms follow an acute or chronic exposure depends on environmental and host factors.

Environmental factors are exposure-related or psychosocial-related. Exposure-related factors include (a) neurotoxicity of the chemical or material, (b) dose or concentration of chemical or material, and (c) exposure duration (acute, subacute, chronic). Psychosocial-related factors include (a) speed and efficiency of recognition, evaluation, and resolution of problematic exposure, (b) shared belief system concerning the danger of the exposure that develops among those exposed, (c) shared belief system concerning the danger of the exposure that exists within the community, and (d) intensity of preexposure and postexposure social strife and community divisiveness.

Host factors include (a) the biological sensitivity or susceptibility of the exposed person to the toxic effects of exposure and (b) the psychological makeup of the exposed person. The latter includes the tendency of the individual to somatize anxiety (i.e., to interpret the dangers or significance of the exposure, the person's interpretive set) and the individual's coping skills, social support system, psychological defenses, and underlying psychological vulnerability (16,17).

INCIDENCE OF NEUROPSYCHIATRIC SYMPTOMS AFTER ACUTE AND CHRONIC EXPOSURE

Baseline rates of occurrence of many neuropsychiatric symptoms in the general adult population are quite high, making it difficult to assess whether symptoms resulted from toxic exposure. A National Center for Health Statistics national survey found that 78% of Americans reported being bothered by at least one of 12 common symptoms, such as headache, palpitations, or dizziness (18). Studies of college students show similarly high rates of reported symptoms (19).

Another estimate of population baseline rates of neuropsychiatric symptoms comes from reported prevalence of symptoms in control or referent groups used in studies of the neuropsychiatric effects of exposure. Symptoms of fatigue, for example, were reported by 72% of locomotive engineers and assistants used as case controls in a study of neuropsychiatric symptoms associated with solvent exposure in car painters, 80% of control subjects reported being irritable sometimes or frequently, 70% reported difficulties with concentration and sleep, 44% reported mood lability, and 37% reported being bothered by heart pounding (20). Between one and five chronic neurobehavioral symptoms (including fatigue, sleep disturbances, irritability, lack of concentration, memory problems, instability of mood, headache, decreased libido or potency, and diminished alcohol tolerance) were reported by 56% of paper mill workers and urban farm dwellers used as controls in a study of neurobehavioral changes in shipyard painters exposed to solvents (21).

Despite high baseline rates of neuropsychiatric symptoms in the community, several controlled studies have documented excess rates of neuropsychiatric symptoms after a variety of exposure conditions. Twelve days after exposure to a chemical cloud of malathion, for example, exposed seamen who were compared with seamen on a vessel that was not exposed to the chemical cloud reported significantly more symptoms of headache, dizziness, and fainting (73% versus 24%), visual disturbances (41% versus 10%), nasal or pharyngeal irritation (59% versus 19%), and appetite or taste loss (43% versus 5%). Many of the symptoms reported by exposed seamen were consistent with the acute effects of exposure to malathion, but information about the exposure was limited and did not entirely explain the occurrence of symptoms on the basis of the direct toxic effects of the chemical. The more knowledgeable workers were about the effects of malathion exposure, the less likely they were to suffer psychological distress (22). Thirty percent of 20,000 persons evaluated for the effects of ingestion of toxic cooking oil in Spain required psychiatric evaluation because of anxious, depressive, or phobic psychological reactions. Neuropsychological testing failed to document evidence of organic brain damage resulting from the toxic effects of the cooking oil. Their psychiatric disorders were classified as adjustment disorders (23).

Evaluations of workers involved in the Three Mile Island (TMI) nuclear power plant accident and of workers with long-term occupational exposure to asbestos provide the clearest indication of the incidence of psychiatric symptoms after exposures that are not directly toxic to the central nervous system. Compared with control subjects working at a second nuclear power plant, TMI workers experienced significantly more angry reactions (40% versus 29% among supervisors and 51% versus 31% among nonsupervisors), worry (27% versus 6% and 30% versus 8%), and somatic symptoms (26% versus 12% and 29% versus 17%). Distress levels were in the high normal range, did not appear to interfere significantly with functioning, and declined over the 6 months after the accident (24). Similarly, insulation workers who were at significantly increased risk for asbestosis or lung cancer as a result of high-level asbestos exposure also experienced more somatic symptoms, alcohol abuse, and diminished mental health functioning at times of stress compared with postal worker control subjects (25).

CLINICAL ISSUES IN ORGANIC MENTAL DISORDERS: NEUROPSYCHIATRIC SYNDROMES ASSOCIATED WITH SPECIFIC NEUROTOXINS

Specific syndromes of neurotoxic and neurobehavioral dysfunction are recognized consequences of toxic exposure to specific chemicals. These exposures can result in pronounced psychiatric manifestations (26,27).

Erethism, or the syndrome of organic mental disturbances seen in chronic inorganic mercury poisoning, is characterized by irritability, difficulty concentrating, and insomnia. Affected persons often suffer from overwhelming tiredness, extreme timidity, shyness, embarrassment, discouragement, and apathy. Memory loss and cognitive impairments usually accompany the disorder. Hallucinations and seizures may also occur. Although psychiatric symptoms may be the earliest manifestation of intoxication, gingivitis, dermatitis, and tremor are also characteristic features of inorganic mercury exposure (28).

Although severe intoxication with inorganic lead has long been recognized as a cause of encephalopathy in adults, the subtler effects of lower-level intoxications in adults have been elucidated only in the past decade (29). Severe depression, anxiety, sleep disorders, irritability, fatigue, difficulties in concentration, and memory loss can all be a result of intoxication with inorganic lead. Because not all lead-intoxicated patients with depression or other psychiatric symptoms suffer from other classic features of intoxication, such as anemia, colic, or peripheral neuropathies, a history of exposure to inorganic lead is the most important clue to the diagnosis. Depressive symptoms may be severe enough to meet criteria for a major depression, but the disorder is best characterized as an organic affective disorder, which places proper emphasis on the etiologic significance of intoxication with inorganic lead (29,30). Exposure to other metals may also lead to severe neuropsychiatric symptoms.

A manic syndrome is associated with manganese intoxication ("manganese madness"); the syndrome is characterized by emotional lability, increased motor activity, auditory hallucinations, irritability, nervousness, and compulsive behavior. The manic syndrome may precede other signs and symptoms of intoxication. A parkinsonian syndrome secondary to manganese toxicity consists of muscular weakness and rigidity, impaired speech and gait, and loss of facial expression; usually only appears after the onset of psychiatric symptoms; and is irreversible (31). Severe anxiety, fears of dying, and neurasthenia (or severe weakness) caused by intoxication with organic tin compounds are usually accompanied by signs of encephalopathy (severe headache, alterations in consciousness, delirium, and seizures). Chronic intoxication with bromides historically has resulted from medicinal use of bromides but not from environmental or occupational exposure; depression, hallucinosis, and schizophreniform psychosis can be seen in the absence of other signs of intoxication (32).

Intoxication with arsenic, thallium, bismuth, inorganic tin, aluminum, gold, and zinc usually produce widespread systemic signs in addition to central nervous system disturbances, making the diagnosis of an organic mental disorder readily apparent (33–35). Toxic exposure to methyl bromide used as a fumigant can result in psychosis, suicidal ideation, and homicidal thoughts.

PSYCHOLOGICAL EFFECTS OF EXPOSURE

Fear is a feeling of alarm, apprehension, disquiet, or trepidation caused by danger, whereas *anxiety* is defined as a similar state of uneasiness, distress, or dread lacking an unambiguous cause or specific threat (36). Fear and anxiety are commonly accompanied by symptoms of motor tension (trembling, twitching, feeling shaky; muscle tension, aches, soreness; restlessness; easy fatigability), autonomic hyperactivity (shortness of breath; palpitations or tachycardia; sweating or cold, clammy hands; dry mouth; dizziness or lightheadedness; nausea, diarrhea, or abdominal distress; flushes or chills; frequent urination; trouble swallowing or "lump in the throat"), and increased vigilance and scanning (feeling keyed up or on edge; exaggerated startle response; difficulty concentrating or losing train of thought; trouble falling or staying asleep; irritability) (9,37). The symptoms of fear or anxiety are identical to the chronic neuropsychiatric symptoms that are often experienced after many toxic exposures. No one would doubt that fear could account for the occurrence of these symptoms immediately after a life-threatening event or an acute, frightening toxic exposure. There has been considerable controversy, however, about whether these symptoms could develop in individuals exposed to lesser degrees of trauma or could persist in individuals for prolonged periods after traumatic events in the absence of preexisting personality or anxiety disorders.

Research on PTSDs has provided the most compelling evidence for the widespread persistence of severe anxiety symptoms in persons exposed to traumatic circumstances, regardless of predisposing personality vulnerability. The diagnostic hallmarks of a classic PTSD include persistent reexperiencing of the traumatic event, avoidance of stimuli associated with the trauma, or generalized numbing of responsiveness, and severe symptoms of anxiety (9). Reexperiencing the traumatic event occurs in the form of recurrent recollections or dreams or reenactments of the trauma. Avoidance is characterized by efforts to avoid thoughts, feelings, activities, or situations associated with the trauma or by psychogenic amnesia regarding aspects of the trauma.

Studies of Vietnam veterans indicate that, even 15 years after the end of the war, 15% of those who served in Vietnam were still suffering from PTSD. Lifetime rates of PTSD approached 50% of Vietnam veterans. Higher rates of PTSD were found in those with the most extensive combat experience, and combat experience opposed to any precombat variables accounted for the greatest amount of variability in the development of PTSD (38). Combat veterans of World War II reported similarly high rates of symptoms of depression, anxiety, tension, irritability, startle reactions, impairment of memory, and obsession with thoughts of wartime experiences (39). High rates of PTSD have also been reported in survivors of disasters (e.g., concentration camps or rape). Traumatic experiences can worsen preexisting conditions as well. For example, chronic fatigue syndrome patients living in a county heavily impacted by Hurricane Andrew experienced greater illness burden and more physical symptoms than did chronic fatigue syndrome patients living in less affected areas of southern Florida (40).

On the basis of these studies, there can be little doubt that severe traumatic events, including potentially life-threatening toxic exposures, can cause long-lasting and severe psychiatric impairment regardless of preexisting personality vulnerability or underlying psychiatric disorder. Also, evidence exists suggesting that less severe traumas can also lead to symptoms. Horowitz, for example, conducted an experimental study demonstrating that healthy volunteers experienced greater fear responses after watching a short film depicting bodily injury compared with control subjects watching a neutral film, an erotic film, or a film depicting separation. The occurrence of intrusive and repetitive thoughts correlated significantly with exposure to a stressful film (41).

PSYCHOLOGICAL EFFECTS MEDIATED BY COGNITIVE APPRAISAL OF DANGER AND COPING ABILITIES

The psychological consequences of a traumatic experience, including acute or chronic exposure to toxic or noxious substances, depend to a considerable degree on the exposed person's cognitive appraisal of the severity or danger of the experience. Relatively minor or even entirely nontoxic exposures may be interpreted as life-threatening and subsequently may lead to severe psychological sequelae. Alternatively, extremely dangerous exposures may go unnoticed or unrecognized by those exposed and lead to no psychological reactions. Uncertainty over short- and long-term risks from an exposure is a major psychological factor in the adverse outcomes of exposed persons.

Factors affecting the cognitive appraisal of severity of an exposure include (a) the nature and severity of symptoms produced by the exposure; (b) the exposed person's previous experience with similar symptoms and illness; (c) the exposed person's knowledge, expectations, and beliefs about the dangers and potential consequences of exposure; (d) the type, quality, and credibility of information presented to the person about the exposure (17,42,43); and (e) the credibility and referent power of the individual or organization presenting the information. Repeated exposures, for example, may become increasingly frightening if they are experienced as unavoidable and believed likely to lead to cumulative effects. Exposures in environments known to contain highly toxic substances are interpreted differently than identical exposures in environments known to contain nontoxic substances. Based on a combination of these factors, identical symptoms may be interpreted as indicative of entirely benign or extremely malignant conditions. The former interpretive set may evoke little or no anxiety, whereas the latter may evoke considerable anxiety and a cascade of anxiety-related symptoms that amplify the symptom complex.

Social and cultural factors may also play a role. That is, in surveys, white men perceive the lowest degree of risk from a wide range of potential environmental hazards compared to white women or minority men and women (44). Investigators have postulated that these differences in perception relate in part to the higher sense of control and perceived power over their environment that white men typically experience, as compared with white women or members of minority groups. In reality, society has chosen to place many toxic hazard sites close to the residential areas of persons of lower socioeconomic status, many of whom are from disadvantaged ethnic and racial minority backgrounds. Minorities may also have jobs that place them in higher-exposure work situations (45). Apart from exposures, even with good knowledge of risks, belief systems can affect whether individuals engage in self-protective behaviors (16). For example, a large proportion of pesticide-exposed immigrant farm workers (60%) do not consistently use self-protective methods. Studies have shown that it is the perception of having no control over the consequences of the environmental exposure, more than fear of pesticides, belief about amount of exposure, or perception of the effectiveness of the protective behavior, that most influences the workers' decision not to use self-protective strategies during work.

The effectiveness of the exposed person's coping skills and psychological defenses and the adequacy and timeliness of community response also affect the severity of psychological sequelae to traumatic experiences or toxic exposure. Denial of the significance of exposure can function to ward off what would otherwise be intolerable levels of anxiety. The ability to modulate anxiety by focusing on current activities or future benign outcomes rather than on malignant possibilities may also lessen the severity of adverse psychological effects. Difficulties coping with or responding sensitively to emotions that frequently follow traumatic experiences, such as fear, helplessness, anger, guilt, shame, and loss, may complicate the psychological sequelae. Reassurance in the form of accurate information provided by credible experts and acknowledgment by those responsible for the damage caused, combined with empathic, informed support from family and friends, can lessen anxiety after an exposure (17). Misleading or inaccurate information, refusal by those in charge to accept responsibility, or exaggerated concern of family and friends, however, can exacerbate psychological reactions.

The potential impact of psychological distress from an exposure to a toxic or hazardous agent on medical outcomes is substantial. For instance, individuals living near TMI nuclear power plant or those living near a toxic landfill exhibited not only increased global psychological and subjective somatic distress, but also elevations in blood pressure and stress hormone levels (46). Similarly, residents of a Northern California town exposed to a spill of a toxic pesticide, metam sodium, had higher blood pressure and less fluctuation of cortisol levels than controls from an unexposed location (47). The long-term risks of hypertension include increased risk of cardiovascular and cerebrovascular diseases as well as of late-life dementias (48).

DEPRESSIVE REACTIONS

Although anxiety is the most common psychological reaction to exposure, significant depression may also result. In addition to depressed mood, depressive states are characterized by diminished interest or pleasure in activities; feelings of hopelessness, helplessness, worthlessness, or guilt; psychomotor agitation or retardation; fatigue; indecisiveness or difficulties concentrating; vegetative symptoms (disturbances of appetite, libido, sleep); and suicidal ideation (9).

Depression may result from a loss of bodily functioning or health caused by exposure (depression associated with chronic illness caused by exposure) or from an anticipated or threatened loss of health (depression associated with violation of a person's sense of invulnerability and intactness). Depression may also result from the exposed person's inability or failure to live up to his or her own ideals in response to exposure; for example, becoming frightened or running away from an exposure scene may be experienced as an act of cowardice and lead to loss of self-esteem. Depressive reactions are usually transient but may become persistent if not managed appropriately. Of note, a community survey of 13 Alaska communities one year after the *Exxon Valdez* oil spill found increased risk for depression, generalized anxiety disorder, and PTSD in the highly exposed as compared with the unexposed group (45). In community evaluations, it is also possible to control for the concomitantly elevated psychological distress in determining the effects of exposure to a hazardous substance on physical health (15).

Notably, a study of solvent-exposed workers found that, although they had clinically elevated scores on standardized measures of emotional distress, including depression, they did not differ from unexposed controls in self-concept, perceived daily hassles and uplifts, or belief in ability to control their environment (49). The relatively intact self-concept and locus of control in these persons suggests that their depression may have resulted more from the effects of the solvents themselves on the brain than from poor coping capacity within the exposed persons. Thus, although the affective phenomenology may be indistinguishable at first glance, thorough clinical evaluation may permit some degree of differentiation in cases of depression and other psychological disturbances related more to the toxic exposure itself from those related more to intrapsychic vulnerabilities.

CONVERSION REACTIONS

The term *conversion reactions* refers to transformations and attempted resolutions of psychological conflict into alterations or loss of physical functioning that suggest physical disorder (9,50,51). Classic conversion symptoms include paralysis, aphonia, seizures, uncoordination, blindness, tunnel vision, anosmia, anesthesia, and paresthesia. Conversion reactions often develop suddenly during extremely stressful circumstances, such as combat, life-threatening accidents, and environmental or occupational toxic exposures. Symptoms usually achieve some primary gain for the exposed person (e.g., paralysis of a limb prevents the person from acting on aggressive and angry feelings) and may also result in secondary gain (e.g., the symptom results in evacuation from a dangerous situation or provision of outside support from others). In clinical practice within industrialized countries, conversion reactions are less common than adjustment disorders, PTSD, and anxiety and depressive disorders. Vulnerability to conversion reactions is higher in rural populations, those with lower socioeconomic status, and those with a limited capacity for comprehending psychological concepts. Rates of conversion reactions are highest in developing countries. In such locales, it is essential to take the cultural health beliefs and practices into account in delineating the possible role of stress versus toxic exposures in the clinical presentation (16).

PREEXISTING OR CONCOMITANT PSYCHIATRIC DISORDERS

The Epidemiologic Catchment Area survey documented a high prevalence of anxiety disorders, depression, and drug and alcohol use disorders in the general population. The Epidemiologic Catchment Area survey documented lifetime prevalence rates of alcohol abuse or dependence in adults of between 11% and 16%; drug abuse and dependence affected between 5% and 6%; major depression was experienced by approximately 5%; panic disorder affected 1.4%; and somatization disorder affected 0.1% (52). In the *Diagnostic and Statistical Manual IV* used for psychiatric diagnosis (9), substance-related disorders involve substance use (dependence, abuse) as well as substance-induced (intoxication, withdrawal, delirium, dementia, amnestic disorder, psychotic disorder, mood disorder, anxiety disorder, sexual dysfunction, sleep disorder) conditions from a drug of abuse, a medication, or a toxin. Substance use disorders, which are the most common psychiatric disorders experienced by the general adult population, may lead to symptoms or prolonged disability after a toxic exposure that are mistakenly attributed to exposure. A careful history of drug and alcohol use, obtained in a nonjudgmental manner, often helps lead to the diagnosis. Affirmative responses to the questions Have you tried to cut down on drinking? Have you been annoyed by criticism about your drinking? Have you felt guilty about your alcohol use? or modifications of these questions for other drugs indicate possible alcohol or drug problems (53).

Although somatization disorder is quite rare in the general population, symptoms of the disorder may also be mistakenly attributed to toxic exposure. Somatization disorder is characterized by a history of recurrent and multiple somatic symptoms, of several years' duration, for which medical attention has been sought, or from which everyday functioning is impaired, but that are not owing to any physical disorder (9). The disorder begins before age 30 years and has a chronic, fluctuating course. In the United States, women receive somatization disorder diagnoses more often than men, but cultural factors may lead to a different gender ratio in other countries, such as Greece or Puerto Rico. Predominant symptoms over the long-term course of somatization disorder include pain symptoms in at least four different sites (e.g., head, abdomen, back, joints), at least two gastrointestinal symptoms other than pain (e.g., nausea, bloating, diarrhea, multiple food intolerances), at least one sexual dysfunction symptom other than pain (e.g., sexual indifference, irregular menses), and at least one pseudoneurologic symptom (e.g., conversion symptoms or amnesia).

An accurate chronology of symptoms and exposure usually establishes a history of somatization disorder before exposure. The biological bases of the symptoms in somatization disorder are poorly understood at this time, but they constitute a relatively stable cluster of symptoms over time (54). Somatization disorder, like PTSD, is associated with high rates of childhood abuse and other, comorbid psychiatric disorders. In contrast, individuals with good health and work histories earlier in life may first develop somatizationlike clinical pictures after a toxic exposure in their 30s or later. As in other psychiatric disorders that begin after the usual age of onset (e.g., later-onset depression), it is essential to rule out organic causes. No studies have yet addressed the parallel issue of organicity, perhaps caused by toxic substances in some cases (55), in the differential diagnosis of late-onset somatization disorder.

Errors in attribution of symptoms to exposure are not usually the result of deliberate falsification. Symptoms of preexisting psychiatric disorders, including PTSD, may become more pronounced or noticeable after toxic exposures or other traumatic environmental events, and thus come to be associated with the exposure. In addition, a natural tendency exists to search for a specific, discernible cause of symptoms, such as a toxic exposure, rather than to view the symptoms as part of an underlying psychiatric disorder.

SOLVENT SYNDROMES

Although extensive literature exists describing an association between chronic, relatively low-level exposure to organic solvents and solvent mixtures and neuropsychiatric symptoms and disability, controversy exists in the United States about the significance of the deficits reported or the specific etiologic role of repeated exposure to organic solvents.

Spencer and Schaumburg reviewed the scientific criteria for human neurotoxicity and the evidence suggesting that specific solvents and solvent mixtures are neurotoxic (56). Five solvents met scientific criteria for proven human neurotoxicity. Central nervous system effects (impaired intellectual functioning and psychomotor deficits), as well as evidence of subclinical peripheral neuropathy, have been demonstrated after chronic exposure to carbon disulfide at levels previously believed to be safe (10–30 ppm, with brief periods of up to 100 ppm). Deliberate, repeated inhalation of toluene for its euphorigenic effect can lead to early emotional and neuropsychological changes, including anxiety, irritability, mood swings, and forgetfulness. Tremor, nystagmus, slurred speech, hearing impairment, and ataxic gait occur later in the course of repeated exposures. Hexane and ketones produce primarily peripheral neuropathies in the absence of cognitive or emotional changes. Acute intoxication with trichloroethylene and perchloroethylene may cause reversible sensory and motor cranial neuropathies, most often of the trigeminal nerve (57). Chronic, low-level exposure to trichloroethylene has also been reported to cause neuropsychological and emotional changes, but studies have reported contradictory results. Chronic exposure to other solvents or solvent mixtures has also been reported to result in central nervous system toxicity (26,27,58).

The neuropsychological deficits most commonly reported after chronic solvent exposure include short-term memory deficits, impaired visuomotor performance, and slowed reaction time (20,21,59–71). The abnormal findings on neuropsychological testing are partially explainable on the basis of attention and concentration difficulties under increased cognitive load and are consistent with an organic affective disorder or other organic mental disorders associated with chronic solvent exposure, as well as a primary psychiatric disturbance. Neuropsychological deficits have been reported to persist for more than 2 years after cessation of exposure, suggesting that the deficits may be irreversible (66,72). Notably, although the solvent-exposed workers' somatic symptoms lessen over time, their objective dysfunction on neuropsychological testing largely persists (66). Thus, chronic preoccupation with physical symptomatology is unlikely to account in full for the cognitive difficulties. Heavy concomitant alcohol use in solvent-exposed workers may act synergistically with the solvents to produce the more severe neuropsychological impairments (68).

Studies have shown that solvent-exposed workers have a significantly greater slowing of the latency of the P300 wave in their auditory evoked potential, an objective measure of attention deficits, than either chronic schizophrenics or normal controls (73). Increased duration of solvent exposure correlates with longer P300 latencies. In contrast, lower P300 amplitude of the evoked potential correlates with a greater degree of psychological disturbance (74). Furthermore, SPECT and PET brain scans of neurotoxin-exposed workers, most of whom exhibit neuropsychological deficits, suggest diffuse brain dysfunction rather than gross structural changes, especially in the temporal lobes, frontal lobes, basal ganglia, and thalamus (64). Hence, carefully selected, sensitive tests of neurologic function, in combination with detailed clinical assessment, may help in confirming the diagnosis (26,75).

In many Scandinavian countries, disability is accepted and compensation awarded for neurotoxicity after repeated exposure to paint, lacquers, and solvent mixtures. A uniform nomenclature for solvent-related neuropsychiatric symptoms has been proposed (76). When cognitive or neurobehavioral deficits are present, a diagnosis of toxic encephalopathy is warranted. In the absence of demonstrable deficits in psychomotor, perceptual, or cognitive function, a mood disturbance associated with chronic solvent exposure characterized by symptoms of depression, irritability, and loss of interest in activities is best considered an organic affective disorder (77).

Three cases of panic disorder have also been reported to have been precipitated by occupational exposure to organic solvents (78). Panic disorder is characterized by the sudden emergence of feelings of intense fear in situations that usually do not cause anxiety. Cognitive, autonomic, and motor symptoms of anxiety are also present during an episode of panic. In all cases, panic attacks were initially experienced only at work after acute exposure to organic solvent mixtures; episodes recurred repeatedly at work after subsequent exposures and eventually were experienced spontaneously outside of the workplace. One patient had a prior history of panic attacks during adolescence. Two patients experienced panic attacks in response to a diagnostic challenge with sodium lactate. All three patients responded to pharmacologic interventions. The authors suggested that sensitization or a limbic kindling mechanism might account for the disorder (78,79). A subsequent study found that panic patients who have symptoms of limbic system dysfunction, such as depersonalization or derealization, exhibit more divergent quantitative electroencephalogram responses to odors than do panic patients without limbic symptoms or normal controls (80). Although more research is needed, history, together with selected tests of neurologic function, may assist in differentiating solvent-induced organic subtypes from other psychiatric disorders of unknown etiology (73,74).

APPROACH TO DIAGNOSIS

Psychiatric disorder or emotional disturbance should be suspected especially in the following circumstances: (a) when recovery appears to be delayed longer than was originally anticipated based on the severity of exposure and resulting impairment; (b) when neuropsychiatric symptoms predominate, especially in the absence of detectable neurologic impairment; and (c) after any severe, life-threatening traumatic situation.

Relatively brief screening instruments can be useful in assessing the likelihood of a psychiatric disorder complicating recovery after toxic exposure. The Beck Depression Inventory (BDI-II) is a 21-item, self-administered questionnaire that can be completed in 5 minutes. Elevated scores on the BDI suggest depression (81). The Symptom Checklist-90 (SCL-90-revised) is a 90-item, self-administered questionnaire that can be used to assess general psychiatric severity, anxiety, depression, interpersonal sensitivity, obsessive-compulsiveness, paranoia, psychoticism, and somatization (82). Elevated BDI or SCL-90 scores should be followed by complete psychiatric evaluation.

In the psychiatric evaluation, diagnosis is facilitated by obtaining a complete and accurate history and chronology of symptoms and of the disabling effects of illness. The evaluation needs to include a thorough review of the person's current and past life situation (family relationships and relationships with coworkers, supervisors, or other persons involved in the exposure), prior history of psychiatric disorders, history of somatization, and drug and alcohol use history. The meaning and significance of the exposure to the person, as well as the person's coping skills and characteristic psychological defenses, should also be assessed. A complete mental status examination is also essential. Auditory, visual, and chemosensory evoked response potentials may add valuable adjunctive information in an evaluation (73,74,83).

Neuropsychological testing can also be useful to assess impairment resulting from exposure (26,70,71), but the interpretation of test results is not always straightforward. Age-adjusted population norms are not available for many of the most commonly used neuropsychological tests. Preexposure test results are rarely available for comparison, so that the determination of exposure-related neuropsychological impairment requires estimation of preexposure functioning. School performance or scores on grade school or high school achievement tests often provide the best basis for estimating preexposure functioning. Considerable variability in cognitive and intellectual functioning in different domains (e.g., verbal abilities, visual-spatial ability) is common in the general population. Although suggestive of impairment, intratest scatter on subscales of the Wechsler Intelligence Scales test is not definitive. When evidence exists of overall good preexposure functioning, consistent, onset impairment in one area of functioning known to be affected by the toxic substance strongly supports the likelihood of exposure-related central nervous system toxicity.

PREVENTION AND TREATMENT OF POSTEXPOSURE PSYCHIATRIC DISORDERS

The initial response to a toxic exposure of emergency personnel (e.g., firefighters, emergency medical technicians, and emergency physicians) and the subsequent response of workplace survivors, employers, and persons with expertise brought in to evaluate the exposure (e.g., toxicologists, industrial hygienists, occupational and environmental physicians, counseling and community psychologists) are of critical importance in preventing severe psychological and emotional sequelae.

During the process of evacuation, reassurance and attempts to maintain some sense of calm are in order. In the days after the discovery of exposure or evacuation, accurate information about dangers of exposure should be presented in a straightforward, clear fashion by knowledgeable persons who are viewed as credible experts by those who have been exposed. Information should be presented accurately and in a way that does not overwhelm a person's defenses (i.e., denial may be quite useful for some people when nothing can be done to prevent toxic consequences after an exposure); others function better only after they have fully reviewed all of the potential sequelae of exposure. Because acute stress may diminish the exposed person's ability to comprehend fully elaborate information, it is important to make sure that those who have been exposed and others in their community develop an accurate understanding of the information presented.

To ensure that information is accurately and completely comprehended, presentation of information may need to be repeated over a period of days or weeks. Distribution of clearly written information, with references to the scientific literature, may also be useful. Persons exposed to toxic or potentially toxic substances, as well as their family members, often need an opportunity to ask questions about the potential dangers of the exposure and to discuss their personal risk of present or future damage with scientific experts. Those individuals responsible for providing information need to take sufficient time to discover what misperceptions, if any, those who were exposed may have and to address these misperceptions. The process is complicated when scientific information about the dangers is limited or nonexistent (17,55).

When human error or design problems have led to exposure, psychological sequelae can be minimized if those persons in charge of ensuring safety (e.g., employers, in the case of occupational exposures) accept responsibility and attempt to rectify problems. Regardless of who is "at fault," an employer's acknowledgment that an exposure has occurred and expression of sincere interest in the recovery of those exposed and in preventing future recurrences can create a climate that fosters healing. Research has shown that the public's perception of risk is often more important than quantitative risk assessment information (17). Some investigators have proposed that acceptability of an environmental risk depends on a set of issues, including voluntariness of exposure, controllability of the consequences, distribution of the consequences in time and space, context of probability assessment, context of accident evaluation, combination of accident probability and seriousness, knowledge about the risky activity, condition of the individual, social factors, and confidence in the experts and regulators (17,84).

Especially after severe, potentially life-threatening exposures, early referral for psychiatric evaluation and assistance may be critical in lessening the psychological impact of the exposure. Culturally relevant psychotherapy and intervention can help exposed persons resolve psychological conflicts aroused by the exposure. Working through feelings of anger and blame about the exposure, guilt, loss, or vulnerability can ameliorate symptoms associated with emotional disturbance and facilitate recovery. If present, mistaken attribution of preexisting psychiatric symptoms can be confronted gently in the context of a supportive psychotherapy. Mental health professionals using cognitive and behavioral techniques, as well as community-based health promotors in underserved neighborhoods comprised of primarily ethnic minorities, also may be helpful in facilitating successful return to full functioning of traumatized persons. Finally, psychopharmacological treatments may also be useful to treat symptoms of posttraumatic stress disorders, anxiety disorders, or depression occurring in the aftermath of exposure.

REFERENCES

1. Wells KB, Stewart A, Hays RD, et al. The functioning and well-being of depressed patients. *JAMA* 1989;262:914–919.
2. Frazer A, Molinoff P, Winokur A, eds. *Biological bases of brain function and disease*. New York: Raven Press, 1994.
3. Hall RCW, Popkin MK, Devaul RA, et al. Physical illness presenting as psychiatric disease. *Arch Gen Psychiatry* 1978;35:1315–1320.
4. Slater EO, Glithero E. A follow-up of patients diagnosed as suffering from "hysteria." *J Psychosom Res* 1965;9:9–13.
5. Johnson SK, DeLuca J, Natelson BH. Assessing somatization disorder in the chronic fatigue syndrome. *Psychosom Med* 1996;58:50–57.
6. Gould R, Miller BL, Goldberg MA, Benson DF. The validity of hysterical signs and symptoms. *J Nerv Ment Dis* 1986;174:593–597.
7. Morrow LA, Ryan CM, Hodgson MJ, Robin N. Risk factors associated with persistence of neuropsychological deficits in persons with organic solvent exposure *J Nerv Ment Dis* 1991;179:540–545.
8. Rosenstock L, Keifer M, Daniell WE, et al. Chronic central nervous system effects of acute organophosphate pesticide intoxication. *Lancet* 1991;338:223–227.
9. American Psychiatric Association. *Diagnostic and statistical manual of mental disorders*, 4th ed., revised. Washington: American Psychiatric Association, 1994.
10. Fairbank JA, Schlenger WE, Saigh PA, Davidson JRT. An epidemiologic profile of posttraumatic stress disorder. Prevalence, comorbidity, and risk factors. In: Friedman MJ, Charney DS, Deutch AY, eds. *Neurobiological and clinical consequences of stress: from normal adaptation to PTSD*. Philadelphia: Lippincott–Raven, 1995:415–427.
11. Morrow LA, Ryan CM, Goldstein G, Hodgson M. A distinct pattern of personality disturbance following exposure to mixtures of organic solvents. *J Occup Med* 1989;31:743–746.
12. Bell IR. Neuropsychiatric aspects of sensitivity to low level chemicals: a neural sensitization model. *Toxicol Indust Health* 1994;10:277–312.
13. Antelman SM. Time-dependent sensitization as the cornerstone for a new approach to pharmacotherapy: drugs as foreign/stressful stimuli. *Drug Devel Res* 1988;14:1–30.
14. Yehuda R, Antelman SM. Criteria for rationally evaluating animal models of posttraumatic stress disorder. *Biol Psychiatry* 1993;33:479–486.
15. Dayal H, Gupta S, Trieff N, et al. Symptom clusters in a community with chronic exposure to chemicals in two Superfund sites. *Arch Environ Health* 1995;50:108–111.
16. Vaughan E. Individual and cultural differences in adaptation to environmental risks. *Am Psychologist* 1993;48:673–680.
17. Wandersman AH, Hallman WK. Are people acting irrationally? Understanding public concerns about environmental threats. *Am Psychologist* 1993;48:681–686.
18. National Center for Health Statistics. *Selected symptoms of psychological distress*. Public Health Services. Washington: US GPO, 1970. Series 11, no. 37.
19. Pennebaker J, Skelton J. Psychological parameters of physical symptoms. *J Pers Soc Psychol* 1978;4:213.
20. Husman K. Symptoms of car painters with long-term exposure to a mixture of organic solvents. *Scand J Work Environ Health* 1980;6:19–32.
21. Valciukas JA, Lilis R, Singer RM, et al. Neurobehavioral changes among shipyard painters exposed to solvents. *Arch Environ Health* 1985;40:47–52.
22. Markowitz JS, Gutterman EM, Link BG. Self-reported physical and psychological effects following a malathion pesticide incident. *J Occup Med* 1986;28:377–383.
23. Loper-Ibor JJ, Soria J, Canas F. Psychopathological aspects of the toxic oil syndrome catastrophe. *Br J Psychiatry* 1985;147:352–365.
24. Kasl SV, Chisholm RF, Eskenazi B. The impact of the accident at Three Mile Island on the behavior and well-being of nuclear workers. Part II: job tension, psychophysiological symptoms, and indices of distress. *Am J Public Health* 1981;71:484–495.
25. Lebovits AH, Byrne M, Bernstein J, Strain JJ. Chronic occupational exposure to asbestos: more than medical effects? *J Occup Med* 1988;30:49–54.
26. Hartman DE. *Neuropsychological toxicology: identification and assessment of human neurotoxic syndromes*, 2nd ed. New York: Plenum Publishing, 1995.
27. Isaacson RL, Jensen KF, eds. *The vulnerable brain and environmental risks*. Vol 3. *Toxins in air and water*. New York: Plenum Publishing, 1994.
28. Kark RAP. Clinical and neurochemical aspects of inorganic mercury intoxication. In: Vinken PJ, Bruyn GW, eds. *Handbook of clinical neurology*. Amsterdam: North Holland, 1979.
29. Cullen MR, Robins JM, Eskenazi B. Adult inorganic lead intoxication: presentation of 31 new cases and a review of recent advances in the literature. *Medicine* 1983;62:221–247.
30. Schottenfeld RS, Cullen MR. Organic affective illness associated with lead intoxication. *Am J Psychiatry* 1984;141:1423–1425.
31. Mena I. Manganese poisoning. In: Vinken PJ, Bruyn GW, eds. *Handbook of clinical neurology*. Amsterdam: North Holland, 1979.
32. Moses H, Klawans HL. Bromide intoxication. In: Vinken PJ, Bruyn GW, eds. *Handbook of clinical neurology*. Amsterdam: North Holland, 1979.
33. Foncin JF, Gruner JE. Tin neurotoxicity. In: Vinken PJ, Bruyn GW, eds. *Handbook of clinical neurology*. Amsterdam: North Holland, 1979.
34. Chhuttani PN, Chopra JS. Arsenic poisoning. In: Vinken PJ, Bruyn GW, eds. *Handbook of clinical neurology*. Amsterdam: North Holland, 1979.
35. Goetz CG, Klawans HL. Neurologic aspects of other metals. In: Vinken PJ, Bruyn GW, eds. *Handbook of clinical neurology*. Amsterdam: North Holland, 1979.
36. Morris W, ed. *The American heritage dictionary of the English language*. Boston: Houghton Mifflin, 1981.
37. Yates FE, Marsh DJ, Moran JW. The adrenal cortex. In: Mountcastle VB, ed. *Medical physiology*. St. Louis: CV Mosby, 1974.
38. Scrignar CB. *Posttraumatic stress disorder: diagnosis, treatment, and legal issues*. New York: Praeger Publishers, 1988.
39. Hocking F. Extreme environmental stress and its significance for psychopathology. *Am J Psychother* 1970;24:4–26.
40. Lutgendorf SK, Antoni MH, Ironson G, et al. Physical symptoms of chronic fatigue syndrome are exacerbated by the stress of Hurricane Andrew. *Psychosom Med* 1995;57:310–323.
41. Horowitz MJ. *Stress response syndromes*. New York: Jacob Aronsen, 1976.
42. Lazarus RS, Averill JR, Opton EM. The psychology of coping: issues of research and assessment. In: Coelho G, Hamburg DA, Adams JE, eds. *Coping and adaptation*. New York: Basic Books, 1974:249–315.
43. Schottenfeld RS. Workers with multiple chemical sensitivities: a psychiatric approach to diagnosis and treatment. *Occup Med State Art Rev* 1987;2:739–753.
44. Flynn J, Slovic P, Mertz CK. Gender, race, and perception of environmental health risks. *Risk Anal* 1994;14:1101–1108.
45. Palinkas LA, Russell J, Downs MA, Petterson JS. Ethnic differences in stress, coping, and depressive symptoms after the *Exxon Valdez* oil spill. *J Nerv Ment Dis* 1992;180:287–295.
46. Baum A, Fleming I. Implications of psychological research on stress and technological accidents. *Am Psychologist* 1993;48:665–672.
47. Bowler R, Mergler D, Huel G, Cone JE. Aftermath of a chemical spill: psychological and physiological sequelae. *Neurotoxicology* 1994;15:723–729.
48. Skeeog I, Lernfelt B, Landahl S, et al. Fifteen-year longitudinal study of blood pressure and dementia. *Lancet* 1996;347:1141–1145.
49. Morrow LA, Kamis H, Hodgson MJ. Psychiatric symptomatology in persons with organic solvent exposure. *J Consult Clin Psychol* 1993;61:171–174.
50. Laplanche J, Pontalis JB. *The language of psychoanalysis*. Nicholson-Smith D, trans. New York: WW Norton, 1973.
51. Lazare A. Current concepts in psychiatry: conversion symptoms. *N Engl J Med* 1981;305:745–748.
52. Robins LN, Helzer JE, Weissman MM, et al. Lifetime prevalence of specific psychiatric disorders in three sites. *Arch Gen Psychiatry* 1984;41:949–958.
53. Mayfield D, McLeod G, Hall P. The CAGE questionnaire; validation of a new alcoholism screening instrument. *Am J Psychiatry* 1980;131:1121–1128.
54. Bell IR. Somatization disorder: health care costs in the decade of the brain. *Biol Psychiatry* 1994;35:81–83.
55. Bowler RM, Mergler D, Rauch SS, Bowler RP. Stability of psychological impairment: two year follow-up of former microelectronics workers' affective and personality disturbance. *Women Health* 1992;18:27–48.
56. Spencer PS, Schaumburg HH. Organic solvent neurotoxicity—facts and research needs. *Scand J Work Environ Health* 1985;1[Suppl 11]:53–60.
57. Cavanagh JB, Buxton PH. Trichloroethylene cranial neuropathy: is it really a toxic neuropathy or does it activate latent herpes virus? *J Neurol Neurosurg Psychiatry* 1989;52:297–303.
58. Office of Technology Assessment. *Neurotoxicity: identifying and controlling poisons of the nervous system*. New York: Van Nostrand, 1990.
59. Orbaek P, Risberg J, Rosen I, et al. Effects of long-term exposure to solvents in the paint industry. *Scand J Work Environ Health* 1985;11[Suppl 2]:1–28.
60. Larsen F, Leira HL. Organic brain syndrome and long-term exposure to toluene: a clinical, psychiatric study of vocationally active printing workers. *J Occup Med* 1988;30:875–878.
61. Gyntelberg F, Vesterhauge S, Fog P, et al. Acquired intolerance to organic solvents and results of vestibular testing. *Am J Ind Med* 1986;9:363–370.
62. Rasmussen K, Jeppesen HJ, Sabroe S. Solvent-induced chronic toxic encephalopathy. *Am J Ind Med* 1993;23:779–792.
63. Iregren A, Gamberale F. Human behavioral toxicology. Central nervous effects of low-dose exposure to neurotoxic substances in the work environment. *Scand J Work Environ Health* 1990;16[Suppl]:17–25.
64. Callender TJ, Morrow L, Subramanian K, Duhon D, Ristovv M. Three-dimensional brain metabolic imaging in patients with toxic encephalopathy. *Environ Res* 1993;60:295–319.
65. Flodin U, Edling C, Axelson O. Clinical studies of psycho-organic syndromes among workers with exposure to solvents. *Am J Ind Med* 1984;5:287–295.
66. Orbaek P, Lindgren M. Prospective clinical and psychometric investigation of patients with chronic toxic encephalopathy induced by solvents. *Scand J Work Environ Health* 1988;14:37–44.
67. Gregersen P, Angelso B, Nielsen TE, et al. Neurotoxic effects of organic solvents in exposed workers: an occupational, neuropsychological, and neurological investigation. *Am J Ind Med* 1984;5:201–225.
68. Cherry N, Labreche FP, McDonald JC. Organic brain damage and occupational solvent exposure. *Br J Ind Med* 1992;49:776–781.
69. Kraut A, Lilis R, Marcus M, et al. Neurotoxic effects of solvent exposure on sewage treatment workers. *Arch Environ Health* 1988;43:263–268.
70. Oberg RGE, Udesen H, Thomsen AM, et al. Psychogenic behavioral impairments in patients exposed to neurotoxins. Neuropsychological assessment in differential diagnosis. In: *WHO. WHO environmental health series, docu-*

ment 3. Neurobehavioral methods in occupational and environmental health. Copenhagen: WHO, 1985:130–135.

71. Morrow LA, Robin N, Hodgson MJ, Kamis H. Assessment of attention and memory efficiency in persons with solvent neurotoxicity. *Neuropsychologia* 1992;30:911–922.
72. Bruhn P, Arlien-Soborg P, Gyldensted C, Christensen EL. Prognosis in chronic toxic encephalopathy—a two-year follow-up study in 26 house painters with occupational encephalopathy. *Acta Neurol Scand* 1981;64:259–272.
73. Morrow LA, Steinhauer SR, Hodgson MJ. Delay in P300 latency in patients with organic solvent exposure. *Arch Neurol* 1992;49:315–320.
74. Morrow LA, Steinhauer SR, Condray R. Differential associations of P300 amplitude and latency with cognitive and psychiatric function in solvent-exposed adults. *J Neuropsych Clin Neurosci* 1996;8:446–449.
75. Amler RW, Anger WK, Seyemore OJ, eds. *Adult Environmental Neurobehavioral Test Battery.* Atlanta: US Department of Health and Human Services, Public Health Service, Agency for Toxic Substances and Disease Registry, 1995.
76. Arlien-Soborg P, Hansen L, Ladefoged O, Simonsen L. Report on a conference on organic solvents and the nervous system. *Neurotoxicol Teratol* 1992;14:81–82.
77. Baker EL. Organic solvent neurotoxicity. *Ann Rev Health* 1988;9:223–239.
78. Dager SR, Holland JP, Cowley DS, Dunner DL. Panic disorder precipitated by exposure to organic solvents in the work place. *Am J Psychiatry* 1987;144:1056–1058.
79. Bell IR, Miller CS, Schwartz GE. An olfactory-limbic model of multiple chemical sensitivity syndrome: possible relationship to kindling and affective spectrum disorders. *Biol Psychiatry* 1992;32:218–242.
80. Locatelli M, Bellodi L, Perna G, Scarone S. EEG power modifications in panic disorder during a temporolimbic activation task: relationships with temporal lobe clinical symptomatology. *J Neuropsychiatry Clin Neurosci* 1993;5:409–414.
81. Beck AT, Steer RA, Brown GK. *Beck Depression Inventory II.* San Antonio: The Psychological Corp., 1996.
82. Derogatis L. *SCL-90-R administration, scoring, and procedures manual, II.* Towson, MD: Clinical Psychometric Research, 1983.
83. Otto DA, Hudnell HK. The use of visual and chemosensory evoked potentials in environmental and occupational health. *Environ Res* 1993;62:159–171.
84. Vlek C, Stallen P. Rational and personal aspects of risk. *Acta Psychologia* 1980;45:273–300.

CHAPTER 32

Low-Level Chemical Sensitivity and Chemical Intolerance

John B. Sullivan, Jr., Iris R. Bell, and William J. Meggs

Multiple chemical sensitivity (MCS) is a controversial subject that has provoked a major schism among health care professionals. Legal and regulatory committees are similarly divided with passionate advocates on both sides of the controversy.

Most individuals seen in clinical settings who claim MCS profess that they have experienced some initial acute environmental exposure and experience recurring symptoms triggered by subsequent low-level exposures (Table 32-1). Symptoms are subjective and confusing: fatigue, pain, headache, memory problems, feelings of rage or apathy, irritability, dizziness, anxieties, myalgias, and various other somatic complaints. Those claiming MCS express a range of illness from infrequent nuisance symptoms to disability. Such claims are confounding because such low levels of environmental chemicals generally have no adverse biological effect on the majority of others exposed.

MCS and the practice of clinical ecology have been discounted by professional organizations, including the American Academy of Allergy and Immunology in 1986, the California Medical Association Scientific Task Force on Clinical Ecology in 1986, American College of Physicians in 1989, the American College of Occupational and Environmental Medicine in 1991, and the Subcommittee on Immunotoxicology of the National

TABLE 32-1. Symptoms and conditions reported to be associated with low-level chemical exposures

Respiratory system	Neurologic system
Rhinitis	Headache
Sinusitis	Mental confusion
Asthma	Difficulty with concentration
Nasal congestion	Seizures
Sneezing	Coma
Sinus headaches	Tinnitus
Eyes	Syncope
Conjunctivitis	Depression
Blurred vision/tearing	Anxiety
Gastrointestinal system	Psychosis
Irritable bowel syndrome	Musculoskeletal system
Nausea	Myalgias
Vomiting	Myositis
Diarrhea	Arthralgias
Abdominal cramping	Arthritis
Bloating	

Research Council, and the American Academy of Clinical Toxicology in 1995. Furthermore, the Centers for Disease Control and Prevention does not recognize MCS because it lacks case definition and objective diagnostic criteria. Adding to the confusion, the Americans with Disabilities Act includes MCS as a disability. The U.S. Department of Housing and Urban Development also established disability status for MCS in 1992.

The philosophical gap between traditional clinicians versus those who accept MCS as a disease remains profound. As a unique disease, however, MCS has little scientific support to date. No studies have shown prospectively a causal role for any proposed mechanism for MCS, psychogenic or toxigenic in nature (1). In fact, labeling patients as having MCS can place them at a disadvantage in seeking health care from many medical practitioners. The debate swirling around MCS remains acrimonious, with little middle ground. But the problem seems to be growing. It is time for a balanced approach to MCS that explores hypothetical models and theories that can be tested.

The National Research Council, Agency for Toxic Substances and Diseases Registry, National Institute of Environmental Health, and U.S. Environmental Protection Agency have sponsored or cosponsored conferences to advance the scientific consideration of these issues.

This chapter explores hypotheses that could assist in explaining the polysymptomatic condition known as *MCS*. No model has been confirmed as an operative mechanism for those claiming to have or diagnosed as having MCS or chemical intolerance, but the hypothetical models do serve as a rational starting point for discussion and testing of this vexing problem.

DEFINING TERMS: MULTIPLE CHEMICAL SENSITIVITY, CHEMICAL INTOLERANCE, AND CACOSMIA

Debate swirls around definitions of MCS (2). Confusion results because MCS is sometimes used interchangeably with other terms such as *chemical sensitivity* (*CS*), *chemical intolerance* (*CI*), or *cacosmia*. Cullen has provided a definition for MCS that is useful for research purposes (3). Although controversial as a valid medical diagnosis, a definition of MCS helps test hypotheses and differentiate these complaints from other validated medical disorders. The term *MCS* is used in this chapter to describe a broad spectrum of patients claiming illness consistent with the Cullen definition: "An acquired disorder characterized by recurrent symptoms, referable to multiple organ systems, occurring in response to demonstrable exposure to many chemically unrelated compounds at doses far below those established in the general population to cause biologically harmful effects. No single widely accepted test of physiologic function can be shown to correlate with symptoms."

Further confusion arises because of the interchangeable use of terms that apply to different conditions of odor perception dysfunction and perceived CI. The terms *CI*, *cacosmia*, and *CS* are used interchangeably to the point of confusion in the medical literature. Those claiming CI may or may not meet Cullen's definition of MCS. The reader should be wary of the casual misapplication of terms without appropriate definition when evaluating research articles published on MCS or CS. Only recently have validated self-report questionnaires become available to assist in determining the numbers of chemicals that patients identify as triggering agents. One is a 122-item comprehensive scale and the other a five-item screening index (4,5). Scores on a four-item survey to assess the number of lifestyle changes reported because of CS have correlated with degree of rated disability (6). Such tools offer a replicable way to compare subject populations across studies. But no single currently validated questionnaire captures the full Cullen criteria or any other definition of MCS.

Cacosmia refers to distorted odor perception with an increased sensitivity to odors (7). Odor sensitivity is a commonly expressed symptom in MCS patients. The literature defines various dysfunctions of olfaction: *Hyperosmia* indicates increased sensitivity to some or all odorants. *Dysosmia* describes a distortion in the perception of a smell. It can occur as an unpleasant odor when no odor is present. *Parosmia* describes a distorted perception in response to a particular odor stimulus (7). The term *cacosmia*, however, is frequently used instead of hyperosmia, dysosmia, or parosmia.

Other investigators refer to illness from low-level chemicals as *CS* or *CI*. In this chapter, *CS* and *CI* refer to these as a core symptom characteristic of MCS, not the complete symptomatic presentation of these patients.

Clinicians and researchers continue to struggle with MCS's lack of an accepted case definition to guide rational decision making. Despite the controversy over the nature of the condition, its cause and treatment, proponents and skeptics of MCS generally agree that patients who express symptoms are experiencing some kind of health problem.

OVERLAPPING SYNDROMES WITH MULTIPLE CHEMICAL SENSITIVITY

Some of the symptoms expressed by those claiming MCS and forms of CI overlap other syndromes, some of which are controversial and/or unsubstantiated (8):

- Sick building syndrome (SBS)
- Chronic fatigue syndrome (CFS) and fibromyalgia (FM)
- Gulf War syndrome
- Solvent syndrome

Sick Building Syndrome

The World Health Organization described SBS in 1983 as an illness associated with low-level indoor air contaminants from a variety of difficult-to-define sources. SBS is complex. It is linked to chemical, physical, biological, and psychosocial factors. Symptoms of SBS can be vague and subjective. They involve multiple organ systems but many are related to respiratory irritation. Symptoms described include headache, fatigue, neurobehavioral disturbances, respiratory irritation, wheezing, coughing, eye burning, and symptoms of mucous membrane irritancy. Irritancy symptoms, inflammation, and neurocognitive symptoms are documented to occur in human-controlled studies with mixtures of volatile chemicals at levels found in common indoor environments at airborne concentrations less than Occupational Safety and Health Administration permissible exposure standards or threshold limit values for any one individual chemical (9–13). In some cases, individuals have claimed onset of MCS symptoms from an episode of poor indoor air quality after new carpet installation (14,15).

Although illness caused by low-level indoor pollutants has been controversial in the past, research has demonstrated the onset of symptoms in humans at low levels of total volatile organic chemicals.

Chronic Fatigue Syndrome and Fibromyalgia

CFS, another polysymptomatic condition characterized by overwhelming and disabling fatigue, overlaps MCS symptoms because fatigue is often a feature of those claiming MCS (16). From 46% to 67% of those diagnosed with CFS also report some form of vague CI (17). CFS patients (as defined by the Centers for Disease Control and Prevention) also have higher rates of depression and anxiety than normal controls (18). CFS appears to have some overlapping symptoms that are claimed by MCS patients.

FM, which often overlaps CFS, is a chronic, debilitating, non-articular rheumatic disease of unknown etiology. FM involves chronic, diffuse musculoskeletal pain at multiple tender points. Up to 55% of FM patients also meet specific criteria for MCS (19).

Gulf War Syndrome

Gulf War syndrome is a recent, controversial, and likely heterogeneous, problem of chronic unexplained illness reported by some American and British military personnel who served in the Gulf War of 1991. These military personnel claim to have been exposed to immunizations to germ warfare agents, petroleum products, insect repellents, pesticides, corrosion-resistant paints, depleted uranium, antidotes for chemical warfare agents, and, perhaps, chemical weapons from enemy attacks or "friendly fire" destruction of nerve gas arsenals. No published, large-scale studies of Gulf War veterans have addressed the prevalence of CI or MCS. A pilot survey study of randomly selected veterans enrolled for any reason as outpatients at a southwestern U.S. Veterans Administration medical center (not necessarily on the Gulf War Registry) found that 86% of 14 Gulf War veterans claiming acquired chronic illness on a global health rating reported considering themselves to be "especially sensitive to certain chemicals." This rate was much higher than the 30% of ten healthy Gulf War veterans and 30% of ten healthy Gulf-era (nondeployed) veteran control groups who endorsed the same question (20). Federally sponsored researchers on Gulf War illnesses report that many Gulf veterans exhibit the same qualitative symptom patterns seen in civilians with CFS, FM, and MCS, but only a small subset of chronically ill veterans to date meet strict criteria for these disorders (21,22). It is unknown whether wartime chemical exposures *per se* initiated the current conditions.

Solvent Syndrome

The *solvent syndrome*, as the term is commonly used, is a controversial diagnosis applied to individuals who report forgetfulness, difficulty concentrating, depression, irritability, incoordination, and cognitive dysfunction, including loss of reading abilities. Some individuals occupationally exposed to solvents report cacosmia, with previously innocuous odors producing symptoms of headache and nausea in as many as 60% of this population (23). Controlled human clinical studies (not epidemiologic) of organic-solvent-exposed workers matched for age, educational level, and intelligence showed cognitive impairments, particularly of memory and concentration, when evaluated by standardized neuropsychometric tests (24). Cacosmia accounted for a significant portion of the variance in the cognitive findings (23,24). Still, solvent syndrome remains unsubstantiated as a distinct medical diagnosis.

PSYCHIATRIC AND MEDICAL COMORBIDITY

Many individuals claiming MCS date their illness from a specific chemical exposure or to an environment such as remodeling or installation of new carpeting, moving into a new house, industrial exposures, or a chemical spill (Table 32-2). But in one controlled comparison of MCS and CFS, 40% of patients claiming MCS symptoms in an occupational medicine clinic did not recall a specific exposure associated with the onset of their illness. They were indistinguishable in terms of their present symptoms from those who did recall some inciting event (18). Such a finding, if replicable and validated, provides some support for Cullen's definition of MCS, but raises the need for an accepted case definition of patients without an identifiable initiating chemical exposure to cover a broader spectrum of patients (1).

The same study that used the Cullen case definition to define MCS subjects showed less psychiatric disturbance in case definition MCS subjects compared to those who did not report an initiating chemical exposure event. Standardized measures of psychiatric and neuropsychological function also did not differentiate subjects reporting sensitivities to chemicals from those with CFS. Of great interest, 74% of the case definition MCS patients did not meet criteria for any current psychiatric disorder (18). However, those reporting no initiating event relating to claimed CS had a 69% rate of current and lifetime psychiatric disorders.

Table 32-3 summarizes selected MCS studies and their potential methodology and design flaws. One review criticized studies that had reached the conclusion that MCS was of primarily psychogenic origin (25). This review revealed serious study design problems judged to be prominent in nine of ten of the published articles on MCS that claimed a psychogenic basis. As stated in the review: "The reporting of multiple organ symptoms in the absence of obvious pathophysiologic signs or positive findings on standard laboratory tests is not evidence of psychogenic causation" (25). Others have made a similar point in a review of the scientific evidence involving MCS—that is, the cross-sectional designs of past studies do not prove psychogenic causality (1).

The reader should be cautioned that further research on overlapping syndromes and MCS is required to validate these previous studies before final conclusions can be drawn. In many case series, peer-reviewed research and population surveys published regarding MCS can be faulted for design and method errors. However, the body of peer-reviewed, replicated research on the subject is growing.

Although psychiatric comorbidity is increased in patients claiming MCS as a broad group, especially depression, anxiety, and somatization disorders (see Table 32-3), a subset of patients have no identified past or current history of such diagnoses, especially those meeting Cullen's MCS case definition (6,26,27). Many patients claiming MCS actually have other diagnosable medical conditions such as rhinitis, dermatitis, asthma, migraine headache, arthritis, irritable bowel syndrome, stress-induced symptoms, and comorbid psychological problems. No studies have presented medical-record-confirmed data with objective, confirmatory, laboratory test data on medical comorbidity in MCS patients. Using an epidemiologic survey approach without medical record confirmation, one study of 28 self-identified MCS patients recruited via patient-support newsletters gave increased histories of reported physician-diagnosed rhinitis, chronic bronchitis, migraine, irritable bowel, arthritis, CFS, hypoadrenocortical function, candidiasis, ovarian cysts, chronic pelvic pain, and menstrual disorders, as well as depression, anxiety, and panic disorders, compared with 17 healthy, community-recruited persons with the symptom of multiple CIs and with 20 normals (27). In that survey study, the MCS patients reported significantly increased rates of physician-diagnosed family histories of rhinitis (MCS: 46%; healthy CI: 24%; normal: 10%, $p = .02$) and diabetes mellitus (MCS: 57%; health CI: 35%; normal: 15%, $p = .01$).

A population-based epidemiologic study of county government employees and kin in southern Arizona (n = 181; 113 households) replicated the personal history finding of increased, self-reported medical attention for bronchitis (as well as asthma and pneumonia), this time in chemically intolerant nonpatients (28). Similar to the preceding MCS survey, this study found a trend toward more maternal histories of diabetes mellitus among the 22.6% of persons with increased CI (rating three of five chemicals as triggering moderate to severe illness, but not necessarily MCS) compared with the 31.5% of persons with no CI at all (rating zero of five chemicals as triggering agents) [i.e., 24% versus

TABLE 32-2. Examples of chemicals associated with multiple chemical sensitivity

Products of combustion
- Environmental tobacco smoke
- Exhaust fumes from diesel and gasoline engines
- Fumes from gas cook stoves
- Furnace fumes
- Fumes from charcoal lighter fluid

Organic solvents
- Fresh paint
- Printing ink
- Turpentine
- Glues and adhesives
- Pesticide diluents

Cleaning products
- Bleach
- Ammonia
- Disinfectants
- Detergents, particularly those with fragrance

Materials that emit gas into indoor air
- Synthetic carpets
- Carpet mats
- Carpet adhesives
- Synthetic materials in furniture
- Wall board and particle board
- Synthetic draperies
- Fumes from office machines
- Fumes from office materials, such as carbonless copy paper and correction fluid

Pesticides
- Organochlorine pesticides
- Organophosphate pesticides
- Pyrethrums and pyrethroids
- Xylene and other pesticide solvents

Chemicals in foods
- Preservatives, including sulfites
- Additives
- Pesticide residues
- Naturally occurring food chemicals

Products containing fragrances
- Perfumes
- Deodorants
- Shampoos
- After-shave lotions
- Detergents
- Sunscreen and sun-tanning products

8% of the respective group maternal diabetes histories (p <.10)]. Notably, the relative risk for heart problems in the individuals with high levels of self-reported CI was markedly elevated at 7.05 compared with the nonchemically intolerant controls (p <.05).

Potentially consistent with the increased risk of cardiovascular disease in chemically intolerant individuals, one laboratory study found that the waking supine blood pressures of 12 healthy community elderly individuals with higher ratings of CI on the five-item screening index were significantly higher than those of 13 healthy elderly persons with lower ratings of CI (5). Such findings suggest that the physiologic and genetic traits of chemically intolerant persons may differ from those of normals but do not address the question of cause-effect relationships to environmental factors such as chemicals or nonspecific stressors. These findings require replication in larger samples. The relevance of such data to Cullen-defined MCS patients or other similarly chronically ill populations is unexamined.

DISABILITY ISSUES AS CONFOUNDING FACTORS IN MULTIPLE CHEMICAL SENSITIVITY STUDIES

Those claiming MCS complain of acute flares of symptoms that they say interfere with their daily living activities and lead to

TABLE 32-3. Summary of key findings from controlled studies in multiple chemical sensitivity (MCS) patients

Study	Design (between or within subjects)	Baseline or with chemical exposure	Key findings in MCS patients	Comments
Doty et al. 1988	Between	Chemical exposure	Normal olfactory detection thresholds Increased nasal resistances, respiration rates, Beck Depression scores Most had food sensitivities MCS women showed less heart rate decrease after methyl ethyl ketone than did normal women MCS women showed less nasal resistance after phenyl ethyl alcohol	MCS with psychiatric histories screened out of study Randomized exposures blinded to visual cues but not odor
Black et al. 1990	Between	Baseline	Increased rates of current or past depression/anxiety/somatoform disorders	Healthy community controls only Cases from support groups/flyers, psychiatric and occupational medical clinics
Simon et al. 1990	Between	Baseline	Increased history of anxiety/depressive disorders Increased history of medically unexplained symptoms	Limited to aerospace plastics workers with compensation claims
Simon et al. 1993	Between	Baseline	Immunologic and neuropsychological results not different from chronic pain controls Increased current anxiety/depressive disorders Somatization diagnoses in 25% No psychological diagnosis in 56%	Immunologic laboratory found unreliable with split samples Inclusion criteria required central nervous system symptoms
Staudenmayer and Selner 1990	Between	Baseline	EEG spectral patterns similar to those of mixed psychiatric patients	Psychiatric patient controls not screened for chemical sensitivity
Staudenmayer et al. 1993	Within	Chemical exposure	No reliable response pattern	Use of masking odor could produce active placebo Outcome measures not sensitive (dichotomous, mainly subjective)
Buchwald and Garrity 1994	Between	Baseline	30% met criteria for chronic fatigue syndrome Less postexertional fatigue than in chronic fatigue or fibromyalgia groups Averaged 23.3 medical provider visits per year	Symptom questionnaire-based
Bell et al. 1995	Between	Baseline	Increased food intolerance and lower alcohol use than in healthy chemical intolerant or normals Increased rhinitis, bronchitis, migraine, irritable bowel, arthritis, ovarian cysts, menstrual dysfunction, psychiatric diagnoses Increased family histories of rhinitis and diabetes mellitus	Cases recruited by newsletter Questionnaire-based
Fiedler et al. 1996	Between	Baseline	No current psychiatric diagnosis in 74% Highest rate of false alarms on Continuous Visual Memory Test	Cases recruited from occupational medicine clinic Chemically sensitive without identifiable chemical initiating event had highest rate of psychiatric diagnoses
Hummel et al. 1996	Within	Chemical exposure	Room air shortened chemosensory event-related potential latencies (EEG CSERP) relative to 2-propanol exposure Ability after 2-propanol compared with after room air challenge 20% of patients had increased symptoms after room air challenge	Double-blind without masking odor [used olfactory threshold concentrations; ability to detect odor = at chance (50%)] Room air and 2-propanol delivered from plastic containers—potential for active placebo

CSERP, chemosensory event-related potential latencies; EEG, electroencephalographic.
Note: Additional findings on (a) chemically intolerant individuals without MCS diagnoses versus controls (5,6,9,10,15,24–28,30,32,34,35,69,81) and (b) MCS patient studies without controls (7,80,98–101,106,108,110) are discussed in the text.

marked changes in their lifestyle (6). Patients expressing mild symptoms usually remain employed and lead normal lives, though most make choices for their home environment. Their only intervention outside of the home may be to request that a coworker not wear particular perfumes or fragrances or to request no smoking sections in restaurants. At the other extreme are patients who express disabling symptoms, think they are unable to work, and have highly restricted social lives.

Because of the nature of MCS complaints, individuals claiming MCS as an illness are embroiled in litigation and worker's compensation claims that may bias their involvement in research. As a result, occupational medicine physicians and medical toxicologists may see a skewed sample of the patients (i.e., a disproportionate number of MCS patients seeking legal decisions related to their health status).

It is necessary to distinguish the possible contributing factors in the disability claims from motivating factors in health-care-seeking behavior and from possible etiological factors in the self-reported CI. For example, one study demonstrated that FM patients recruited from a tertiary referral clinic had significantly more lifetime psychiatric diagnoses than did nonpatient controls who also met FM diagnostic criteria but were recruited from the community without a history of obtaining medical attention for their symptoms in the past 10 years (29). These authors concluded that the increased comorbid psychiatric diagnoses in many FM studies may relate more to the variable of who seeks health care than to the illness itself. If this finding extends at least to the 55% of the FM population with MCS, clinicians and researchers must use great caution in generalizing their observations of comorbid psychiatric or any other problems in MCS patients to the larger population of chemically intolerant persons outside their specific setting and recruitment procedures (19).

Many published studies on MCS contain design and method flaws, so they must be carefully scrutinized. One such flaw is the bias of secondary gain involving disability claims or litigation (30). This limitation can occur when CI as a complaint in a clinical practice is used to recruit MCS subjects without a proper control group that contains a comparable number of disabled patients without CS. As an example of a more appropriate approach to considering the nature of CS or intolerance independent of disability or litigation issues, one investigation that recruited female subjects for a low-level CI study involving electroencephalographic evaluation excluded subjects if they were involved in pending worker's compensation or chemical injury–related litigation (31). These subjects also were thoroughly screened with batteries of health questionnaires, medical history, physical examination, and psychological measures (31).

The Cullen definition of MCS, as opposed to other verifiable inflammatory and irritancy reactions to irritant chemicals, requires that the person express sensitivity to more than one chemical and that symptoms involve more than one organ system. The multiorgan symptoms expressed tend to involve cognitive complaints such as concentration, memory problems, fatigue, musculoskeletal pain, and headache (1,6,32).

Although clinicians have focused mainly on trying to understand the subjectively enhanced reactivity to environmental chemicals in MCS patients, individuals who have self-identified CI for research purposes, as opposed to litigation, also report adverse effects from common foods, prescription drugs, and alcohol (1,6,16,18,20,23,24,26,27,32). This type of pervasive difficulty with the environment could have an extensive impact on quality of life for affected individuals. No published outcomes studies have yet systematically examined this issue of the subjective effects of MCS or CS or of specific treatments on patient satisfaction with their health and social, emotional, and professional role functioning.

PREVALENCE AND DEMOGRAPHICS

Claims of MCS have been reported among industrial workers and white-collar workers, male and female. Women tend to report more MCS symptoms and CI than men (clinical populations are up to 80% female) (1,6,16,26,27,32). Studies suggest that patients with MCS as defined by Cullen are in their 30s to 40s at diagnosis and have above-average educational backgrounds. Epidemiologic studies show that 15% to 30% of the general population reports mild-to-moderate CIs or forms of chemical sensitivities. Between 4% and 6% indicate a physician diagnosis of MCS or daily symptoms they ascribe to low-level chemical exposure (33–35). Similar constitutional and somatic complaints are high in the general population background and thus confound research unless accounted for in study design. Specific populations with higher prevalence of self-reported MCS symptoms include a 60% rate in solvent-exposed workers, rates of 46% to 67% for chronic fatigue and FM patients, and an 86% rate in Persian Gulf War veterans claiming chronic illness (17–20,23,24).

Subsets of Multiple Chemical Sensitivity

Reports reviewed indicate that two subgroups of individuals claiming low-level CS might exist: those who can identify an initiating chemical exposure (which is referred to as *MCS* because it satisfies the Cullen case definition) and those who cannot (which is termed *CS*) (18,26). These two subsets also appear to differ in psychiatric comorbidity and in cognitive performance in studies. The MCS group had fewer psychiatric diagnoses and poorer performance on a visual memory test than did the CS group (18,28,36–43).

Similarly, ten nonpatient, community-recruited, middle-aged individuals with CS and lifestyle changes because of their symptoms also differed in polysomnographic sleep patterns, cognitive test performance disturbances, and heart rate reactivity from the eight subjects with CS who denied such changes and from the 12 normals (28,36–43). In the cognitive area, the CS with lifestyle changes exhibited certain problems in performing a continuous visual memory test, an ability regulated more by the frontal brain regions (44) similar to those reported previously in the Cullen definition MCS patients (18). In contrast, the CS patients without lifestyle changes performed like normals on the visual memory test but did the worse, even with practice, on a visuospatial divided attention test, an ability regulated more by temporal-parietal brain regions (45). The divided attention test finding is a replication and extension of a similar observation in elderly patients with CI but no lifestyle changes from a separate study (37). None of the subjects in the community-recruited or elderly studies were involved in chemical-related disability or other litigation claims. However, the community-based studies did not differentiate subjects on the basis of presence or absence of an identifiable chemical initiator. Thus, the comparability of subject samples between studies is uncertain. Nevertheless, the data suggest the testable hypothesis that the brain regions most affected in MCS and some CS patients with lifestyle changes (i.e., frontal) may differ from those most affected in CS without lifestyle changes (i.e., temporoparietal). Further research is needed to determine if patterns of neurophysiologic findings reliably distinguish different subpopulation persons with CS.

In summary, the limited evidence to date suggests that subtypes of individuals might exist that express potentially distinct characteristics that could be overlooked by labeling them all as having a single condition termed MCS. Presence or absence of an initiating chemical exposure history, of comorbid psychiatric conditions, or of concomitant lifestyle changes are among the subtyping possible approaches for MCS and CS.

TWO-STEP HYPOTHESIS OF CAUSATION: INITIATION AND TRIGGERING

A hypothetical two-step process is proposed for the onset of MCS as defined by Cullen: initiation (or sensitization) followed by triggering (or elicitation) of symptoms (46). Different chemicals and different doses can be theorized to contribute to each step of this hypothetical process, but the initiation exposure subjectively is reported to be a higher exposure level than the later eliciting doses by history.

Initiation may involve a smaller number of specific substances, often listed in the categories of solvents or pesticides, but at higher initial doses than those later required to elicit an adverse reaction (16). Triggering or elicitation of response is reported to involve a broader array of environmental agents at lower doses than those involved for the initiation step. This hypothetical process is diagrammed in Figure 32-1.

However, this model does not explain symptoms in those 40% of patients in one study who did not experience a high-level exposure (18). But those not reporting an initiating chemical event tend to have the highest rate of psychiatric comorbidity compared to Cullen case-definition MCS patients (18).

One way of understanding the origins of CS without an initiating chemical is to consider that early life stress could itself have been the initiating event, with low-level chemicals as the current eliciting agents (34). Both MCS patients and community-recruited persons with CS rate their earlier lives as more stressful than do normal controls (27,34). This model is consistent with numerous animal studies showing neurobehavioral cross-sensitization between stress and certain pharmacologic substances (47,48).

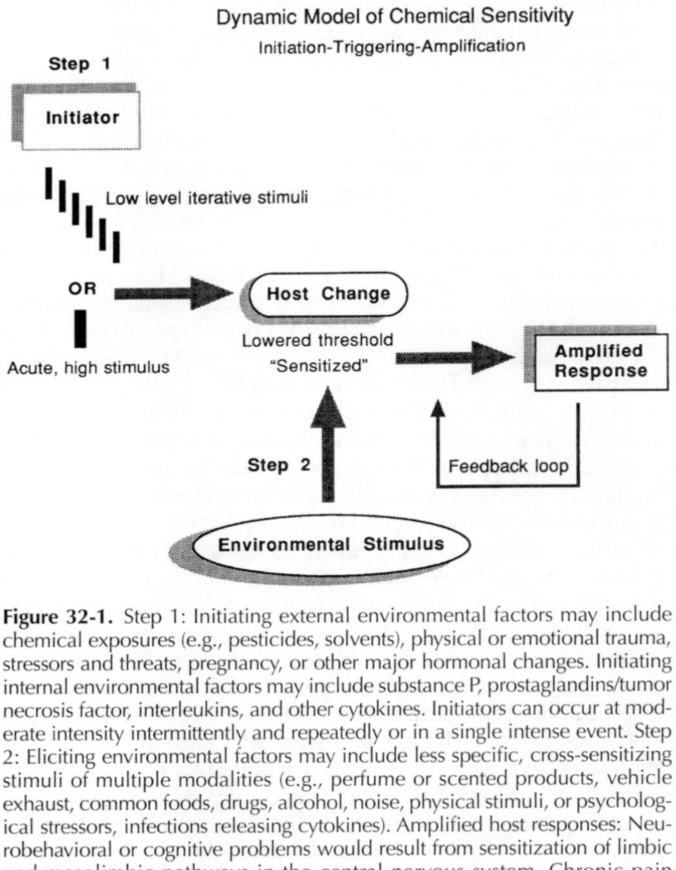

Figure 32-1. Step 1: Initiating external environmental factors may include chemical exposures (e.g., pesticides, solvents), physical or emotional trauma, stressors and threats, pregnancy, or other major hormonal changes. Initiating internal environmental factors may include substance P, prostaglandins/tumor necrosis factor, interleukins, and other cytokines. Initiators can occur at moderate intensity intermittently and repeatedly or in a single intense event. Step 2: Eliciting environmental factors may include less specific, cross-sensitizing stimuli of multiple modalities (e.g., perfume or scented products, vehicle exhaust, common foods, drugs, alcohol, noise, physical stimuli, or psychological stressors, infections releasing cytokines). Amplified host responses: Neurobehavioral or cognitive problems would result from sensitization of limbic and mesolimbic pathways in the central nervous system. Chronic pain response would result from sensitization of peripheral sites and of central nervous system pain pathways (e.g., dorsal horn spinal neurons, cingulum). Maladaptive response to cycling stressors would result in physical, behavioral, and psychological signs and symptoms: difficulty sleeping, somatic complaints, depression, irritability, difficulty concentrating, lethargy, anxiety.

The corollary from the initiation-triggering hypothesis is that enhanced responsiveness is related specifically to the activation of the same systems the initiating stimulus altered. Data consistent with this theory include

1. *Olfactory sensory ability* (e.g., demonstration of heightened ability of MCS patients to discriminate a series of different chemical odors in the laboratory after exposure to a widely used solvent, 2-propanol, as compared with exposure to room air alone) (41)
2. *Stress hormone output* [e.g., overall elevation and lability in levels of the physiologic stress hormone, plasma beta-endorphin, after ingestion of different foods (milk or soy beverage) in chemically intolerant elderly patients versus normal controls (the authors acknowledge that either nonspecific stress or specific foods could have accounted for the findings)] (42)
3. *Amplification of physiologic responses with repetition of a given factor over time* (e.g., evidence from different studies of amplification rather than habituation in chemically intolerant individuals of their autonomic or electroencephalographic responses to a given laboratory procedure over time) (28,31,38,42,43,49)

Thus, neither the initiating nor the eliciting stimulus has to be a specific chemical exposure. Rather, the susceptible host may be capable of amplified responses to stimuli of various classes: chemicals, foods, drugs, noise, physical stress, cognitive stress, or psychological stress.

Furthermore, synergism between different environmental factors may play a role in MCS such as they do in SBS where temperature and volatile organic compound load can interact to initiate symptoms (11). Examples of such synergisms might be chemicals and stress, or chemicals and noise, or chemicals and foods. Among young adult college students, for example, those with personal and family medical or psychiatric history profiles similar to MCS patients rate themselves higher in frequency of illness from low-level chemicals and in noise sensitivity compared to peers without increased sensitivity (50). In a survey of 490 young adults, those who rated themselves high in illness from chemicals and foods had the highest rates of irritable bowel, premenstrual tension syndrome, illness from small amounts of alcohol, depression, and anxiety compared to peers who rated themselves as being low in both classes of sensitivity (51).

A different, more general model of toxin-induced loss of tolerance is also postulated (52). That is, a given chemical exposure event initiates a loss of tolerance in the host, by a variety of as yet undetermined mechanisms. Subsequent exposures to chemicals, foods, and drugs then elicit an enhanced response. If true, toxin-induced loss of tolerance could underlie a class of disorders rather than simply a single diagnostic entity.

One investigation examined olfactory and trigeminal neurosensory systems in a double-blind fashion using MCS patients who met the Cullen case definition (41). A total of 23 participants, 13 women, and ten men, were involved based on a thorough medical history. All 23 were evaluated by an otolaryngologist who performed a physical examination for upper airway disease, otoneurological disease, or audiological disturbances. In this study, patients related the onset of their symptoms to a variety of chemical exposures (e.g., permethrins, solvents, and formaldehyde). A detailed history ruled out upper respiratory tract disease. The study included reproducible, quantifiable measurements such as discrimination of odorants, acoustic rhinometry, and chemosensory event-related potentials. The study concluded that changes in chemosensory event-related potential latencies indicated an alteration in the processing of olfactory and trigeminal stimuli in MCS subjects who met the case definition. It was postulated that this change could account for the increased susceptibility of MCS patients to environmental chemicals. A criticism of this study, as noted by the investigators, is that comparison groups of healthy age- and sex-matched controls are required before definitive conclusions can be drawn.

Initiating (sensitizing) and triggering (eliciting of symptoms) steps are an established mechanism for other disease processes, for example, (a) allergic asthma and allergic rhinitis via the immune system and (b) airway inflammation caused by inhaled xenobiotics initiating hyperresponsive airways and asthma through nonimmune mechanisms (39–41). In the nonimmune model, it is postulated that an irritant exposure may disrupt intercellular tight junctions between bronchoepithelial cells and cause desquamation of the respiratory epithelium with exposure of afferent nerve fibers (53–55). If the initial exposure damages the respiratory epithelium, the threshold for subsequent low-level chemical exposures to induce inflammation by interacting with sensory nerve c-fibers is reduced, resulting in reactive airways. Chemical exposures at levels that did not induce inflammation before the exposure could now induce inflammation, which in turn could propagate further respiratory epithelium damage. Also in support of the nonimmune mechanism is the release of inflammatory mediators by nonspecific defense cells such as macrophages caused by irritant chemicals.

Proposed Models

Various hypothetical models consistent with an initiation-triggering concept have been proposed to theorize why MCS individuals could experience the symptoms they express. These models are divided into four general themes:

1. Direct biological effects of chemicals on the body (neural sensitization, neurogenic inflammation, porphyria, immune dysregulation)
2. Psychosomatic effects of chemicals as perceived, but nonbiological, stressors on the body, with biological mediation of resultant physiologic changes (nonimmunologically mediated stress responses, psychoneuroimmunologic changes, classic conditioning)
3. Misattribution of symptoms of psychiatric disorders to chemicals rather than to psychological state [depression, anxiety, or panic disorder, somatization disorder, posttraumatic stress disorder (PTSD)]
4. Delusions (false beliefs of psychotic proportions) of chemically caused symptoms (delusional disorder)

No single, let alone replicated, study exists in the peer-reviewed literature that proves any of these models to a definitive degree. For the current discussion, the first two themes are focused on as the most promising. These themes implicitly assume that the patient's symptoms are valid, subjective experiences requiring a biological explanation. Symptoms are by definition not imaginary. They must have some mechanism in the body by which they occur, including "psychiatric" symptoms (56).

It is crucial to remember that correlation is not proof of causation. Finding a specific immune system disturbance or a metabolic anomaly provides no more direct proof that the finding causes MCS symptoms than does finding a specific psychiatric diagnosis or a high level of psychological stress. It is well established that certain drugs (e.g., reserpine and propranolol) and environmental chemicals (e.g., cholinesterase-inhibiting organophosphate pesticides) can cause depressogenic neurochemical changes in the brain. A diagnosis of a condition such as major depression cannot by itself rule out a drug or an environmental chemical, as opposed to a psychogenic etiology, for the psychological state. But environmental chemicals may or may not play a causal role in MCS depressions. No study as yet has addressed that question.

Any finding in MCS must not only be replicated in independent laboratories, but also ultimately tested for the presence or absence of a causal, facilitative, or permissive role in the production of patients' symptoms. Studies in which psychiatric histories were directly assessed have never reported a dramatic excess of psychoses or delusions in MCS or persons with CS. Consequently, the last model theme is not further addressed here.

Direct Biological Models

NEURAL SENSITIZATION AND KINDLING

At the basis for the sensitization model is the concept of *dynamic diseases*. *Dynamic processes* refer to an amplified response to low-level iterative stimuli using feedback or regulatory loops (57). Asthma and seizures are examples of dynamic diseases in which a small stimulus results in amplified clinical responses. An initiation-triggering mechanism is at the core of such a dynamic process and several of the proposed models involving direct biological effects of chemicals (see Fig. 32-1).

The plausibility of an initiation-triggering model is supported by basic science literature on neurally based, nonimmunologic sensitization of the central and peripheral nervous systems (47,58–62). Neural sensitization is the progressive amplification of a given response by the passage of time after a single intense stimulus or over repeated intermittent reexposures to the same initiating stimulus. Pathways in the brain most susceptible to sensitization in animal research include the olfactory system, limbic system, and mesolimbic system.

Neural sensitization can occur in the central nervous system (CNS) from repeated, intermittent exposure to moderate levels or even to a single high-intensity exposure level of agents that have activating or sedating effects. Stimuli of diverse classes also can cross-sensitize. A nondrug stressor can initiate sensitization, which is later elicited by a stimulant drug (e.g., amphetamine) in the form of a heightened locomotor behavioral response (48). A psychological stressor can initiate sensitization, which is later elicited by a neuroleptic drug (haloperidol) in the form of a prolonged period of catalepsy (63–65). Repeated low-level formaldehyde exposures [measured at 1.43 ± 0.14 parts per million (ppm) on day 1 and at 0.633 ± 0.012 ppm on day 10 of the study] can initiate sensitization of vertical locomotor activity, which is later elicited by a stimulant drug (e.g., cocaine) (66). The phenomenon of neural sensitization might help to explain a role for environmental initiators and triggering of different chemical classes.

In addition to formaldehyde cross-sensitization with cocaine, animal studies using other chemicals have demonstrated neurobehavioral sensitization. For example, repeated toluene exposures at levels within occupational limit standards (80 ppm over 4 weeks, 5 days per week for 6 hours per day) initiates sensitization in animals (67). The result is subsequent enhancement, not of the spontaneous or resting status of the sensitized animals, but rather of the psychomotor response to administration of the dopamine agonist drug apomorphine. Evidence of the sensitized state requires an eliciting stimulus, in this case a drug. Moreover, these sensitized animals exhibit impairment in spatial learning and memory function long after clearance of the toluene and its metabolites from the body (68). Dopamine receptor changes persisting after the end of the toluene exposures have been implicated in the latter findings.

In another study, both toluene and mint odors initiated sensitized electroencephalographic (EEG) beta activity responses in animals with electrodes implanted in the limbic system of the brain, a highly sensitizable region with strong neuroanatomic and neurophysiologic links to olfactory pathways (69). Sensitization of the limbic structure of the amygdala can result in an extreme and special case of the process (i.e., kindling). Kindling is a permanent neurophysiologic phenomenon in which repeated lower-level electrical or chemical stimuli applied daily for 10 to 14 days can eventually elicit tonic-clonic seizures in animals at doses that elicited no behavioral response on the first exposure. For instance, repeated exposures to the pesticide lindane initiate persistent changes in sensitized behavior and electrophysiologic responses in the limbic system of rats receiving oral doses (70). Other pesticides facilitate the acquisition of electrical kindling of the amygdala as well (70).

These preclinical data suggest the hypothesis that it may be difficult to find differences between MCS patients and controls in a single-session study. The preferred experimental design may be repeated sessions involving some type of initiating and eliciting stimulus, if sensitization is indeed relevant to the MCS process at all. Most studies have found few significant objective differences between MCS patients and controls at rest on single-session clinical testing (1).

No studies have yet tested the neural sensitization model in MCS patients (71). Several small-sample (e.g., 8 to 12 subjects per group) studies have demonstrated statistically significant sensitization of specific quantitative EEG (qEEG) frequency bands in community-recruited persons with multiple CIs.*

Determination of the qEEG frequencies in these studies was completely automated via the processing of the electronically recorded raw EEG signal by a commercial fast Fourier transform software program and thus not susceptible to experimenter bias.

The data demonstrate that certain chemically intolerant persons without disability or litigation biases are more sensitizable than are control groups. Increased alpha activity is also a marker of neural sensitization to repeated stimulant drug exposures in animals (74), and solvent-exposed workers exhibit increases in alpha and delta activity after work (75). The only published single-session qEEG study of MCS patients (76) produced ambiguous results. They failed to screen their control groups (psychiatric patients and normals) for CS and did not control for group differences in drug exposures that could alter EEG. It is unknown if MCS patients show EEG sensitization findings in properly controlled research. The clinical significance of the sensitized responses also is unknown.

The theory that neural sensitization plays a role in response amplification of MCS patients may explain several observations. First, neural sensitization is a leading model for the development of drug craving and addiction (77). Despite their own documented intolerance of alcohol and other drugs reported in MCS, a subset of individuals who report CS have increased rates of family histories of drug (50) or alcohol abuse problems compared with normals (78). In view of the findings of an increased prevalence of somatization disorder in MCS, it is notable that familial and genetic research has shown that male offspring of alcoholics have increased rates of alcoholism and sociopathy. Female offspring of alcoholics have increased rates of somatization disorder (79). The biology of somatization as a possible variant of addiction-related genetics is largely unexplored at this point (80). But these elevated rates of family drug addiction and alcohol abuse might also indicate psychosocial factors in the health problems.

Many claiming MCS show not only adverse reactions to certain environmental agents, but also addictive-like patterns of craving and ingestion of foods such as wheat, corn, milk, sugar, and caffeine (46,81). More chemically sensitive college students score higher than do nonchemically sensitive college students on a scale measuring carbohydrate craving (50). Unlike adverse chemical reactions, which are often more immediate in onset, the negative phase of food reactions with unpleasant symptoms is delayed in many cases. But non-MCS patients have similar addictive cravings.

Animals that sensitize best to amphetamine show elevated rates of spontaneous sucrose ingestion before drug exposure, consistent with the possibility of shared mechanisms between the spectrum of symptoms in MCS and those in drug addiction (82). Formaldehyde cross-sensitizes with the stimulant drug cocaine over time in an animal model studied as an approach to drug craving and addiction (47). It has been hypothesized that MCS patients may be genetically addiction-prone, but their primary addictive substances may be foods rather than drugs (34).

Second, neural sensitization is also a leading model for the development of PTSD and recurrent depression (68,83). Investigators have found increased rates of histories of childhood abuse in patients professing MCS and in others with CI (40,78,84). Such abuse histories are often increased in patients with PTSD, major depression, and somatization disorder (85–87). Leading psychiatric investigators have proposed that the intense stress of the abuse could have initiated irreversible changes in brain function, including prior sensitization of limbic and mesolimbic pathways. If so, these considerations might explain the reported increase in comorbid psychiatric disorders in some samples of MCS and CS patients. In this case, neither psychiatric disorders nor MCS would cause each other, but rather, simply share a common initiating factor.

Third, the sensitization model is consistent with the fact that women complain of CI and sensitivity more than men. Female animals sensitize to drugs and stress more readily than do male animals (47). Castration of adult males modifies their vulnerability to sensitization closer to that of females (88). Removal of ovaries in females affects sensitizability more in the young than in adults. These findings indicate that a high estrogen-to-progesterone ratio favors development of sensitization (89). It could be postulated that testosterone in men may protect against sensitization, but an increased estrogen to progesterone ratio in women may facilitate it. Prospective studies assessing baseline and postsurgical degrees of CS and laboratory chemical qEEG sensitizability in patients undergoing therapeutic castration or complete hysterectomy could help test the role of hormonal status in the sensitization hypothesis for human subjects.

Fourth, in a previously sensitized individual, under certain circumstances, sufficient eliciting stimuli might be the perceived threat of chemical exposure or odors that mobilize the stress response, even without an actual exposure. Evidence exists that animals sensitize to injections of saline (presumably to the stress of the procedure) compared with untreated controls (90). This type of placebo reactivity in MCS during chemical testing protocols is reported but without normal comparison groups (41,91).

However, in criticism, these studies omitted the necessary design (i.e., they did not use a parallel group as opposed to crossover of conditions within the same individuals). Proper design for controlled studies of this type of sensitization precludes the use of active and placebo treatments in the same person, even on different days (71). It is essential to compare separate no-treatment, placebo-treatment, and active-treatment groups over time by randomly assigning different but comparable patients and controls to complete each of the different conditions for the duration of their participation (i.e., a parallel group design). Otherwise, the risk of carryover effects from prior exposures to either placebo or active agents might obscure the ability to demonstrate the presence of persistent sensitization, if any occurs (92).

XENOBIOTIC-INDUCED INFLAMMATION MODEL, INCLUDING NEUROGENIC INFLAMMATION

Although the neural sensitization model may partly explain amplified somatic symptoms and neurobehavioral problems in

*Studies demonstrated increased alpha activity at multiple sites by week 3 compared with week 1 in response to 2-second sniffs of propylene glycol and peppermint but not vanilla odor in CS women, a pattern different from that of sexually abused women without CS (who increased alpha to most exposures, including sham) and normals (who did not increase alpha over the three sessions) (72); increased frontal alpha activity from session one to session two a week later and at rest before chemical exposure sessions in CS women, although depressed women without CS and normals showed decreased alpha (31); and increased central-posterior delta during 1-minute inhalation of 10^{-1} vol/vol diluted musk odor in CS adults without lifestyle changes versus CS adults with lifestyle changes and normals (73).

MCS patients, it does not account for some of the other symptoms expressed by those claiming MCS, such as headache, eye irritation, chest tightness, respiratory complaints, nasal irritancy, and congestion, myalgias, and fatigue. It is postulated that inflammation might play a role in the generation of some of these symptoms, particularly those that suggest an irritation-based etiology. As an example, studies in which chemically intolerant individuals are recruited revealed complaints such as sinus problems, nasal problems, eye and skin problems, allergies, bronchitis, and other respiratory complaints that could have inflammation or irritancy as their basis (18,31,93). Complaints of irritancy and respiratory symptoms are frequently mixed in with other complaints that lack a clear inflammatory basis for their explanation: dizziness, fatigue, depression, irritability, and light-headedness. This has led some to theorize that inflammation, especially neurogenic, nonimmunologic types, may play a role in the generation of some, but not all, of the symptoms expressed by MCS patients (94).

Supporting the theory are anecdotal reports of chronic fatigue in reported clinical cases exposed to fungal contamination indoors (95). Fungal cell walls contain 1,3-β-glucans, polyglucose compounds that incite airway inflammation when inhaled and are found in airborne sampling (96). Also, some indoor fungal contaminants release volatile organic chemicals that cause nonimmunoglobulin E (IgE)–mediated histamine release from human bronchoalveolar lavage cells (97). The same effect was obtained from low-molecular-weight alcohols. Although these studies are not evidence of a link between chemical exposure and the fatigue claimed by MCS patients, they do provide indirect evidence that exposure to proinflammatory volatile chemicals can be associated with cytokine mediator release and reports of fatigue in patients. Further studies of low-level volatile organic chemical exposure indoors frequently list fatigue as a symptom expressed by those experiencing illness from poor indoor air quality (10,11,98).

Some xenobiotics may be immunosuppressive and decrease specific cytokines. One study examined the effect on human basophils and lymphocytes of subjects produced by permethrin (99). Subjects were atopic, normal controls and a permethrin-exposed nonatopic group. Permethrin concentrations in indoor house dust for the chemically exposed group claiming neurologic symptoms varied between 100 and 700 μg per kg. This group also had higher permethrin metabolites in their urine compared to nondetectable for nonatopic controls and the non-exposed atopic subjects. The aim of the study was to examine the *in vitro* effects of permethrin (commonly used indoors as a termiticide) on human lymphocytes and basophils, and to measure interleukin-4 (IL-4) and interferon-α (IFN-α) production and histamine release patterns. The results indicated that permethrin induced a significant inhibition of phytohemagglutinin-stimulated lymphocyte proliferation that was greater for atopic subjects. The cytokine response was more sensitive in atopics. IFN-α and IL-4 levels were reduced in a dose-dependent fashion in all groups, as was lymphocyte proliferation. Histamine release was no different among the three groups. The authors speculate that these results could indicate that permethrin induces immunosuppression, especially in atopics after indoor use. Because IL-4 is involved in lymphocyte transformation to B-cell production of IgE, these authors speculate that lymphocyte function may be damaged by permethrin. This study can be criticized for its small numbers of subjects. Further duplication of results is necessary in a larger population before conclusions can be made.

Inflammation and cytokine release are recognized events caused by xenobiotics (100). Research reveals the role played by inflammation and cytokines in the CNS, particularly acting on the hypothalamic-pituitary-adrenal (HPA) axis to increase circulating catecholamines and glucocorticosteroids (101,102). The concept of a form of toxic inflammation is derived from reports of respiratory inflammation (termed *toxic pneumonitis*) induced by chemicals and organic dusts, mainly seen in agricultural environments (103).

Whether cytokines are involved in patients claiming MCS remains speculative, unproved, and a topic for further research. But the connection between inflammation cytokines and the CNS is substantiated. Inflammatory processes involving peripheral tissues cause the release of cytokines that further act to produce a cascade of inflammatory events (101). Interleukin-1 (IL-1), a cytokine released by T-cell lymphocytes in inflammatory processes, activates the HPA axis along with central and peripheral catecholamine pathways (104,105). One of the more defined functional loops involving cytokines, the CNS, and immune function involves IL-1. IL-1 increases corticotropin-releasing factors in the CNS, which increases output of catecholamines and corticosteroids (105). As opposed to IL-1, IL-2 does not alter corticosteroid levels, but instead increases adrenergic and dopaminergic turnover (101,105). IL-6 increases the turnover of serotonergic and dopamine systems without altering noradrenergic systems (101,105). The effect of increased circulating catecholamines and corticosteroids would be to inhibit immune activation, thus reducing IL-1 levels. Therefore, excessive circulating IL-1 levels would tend to inhibit its own production and reduce its concentration (105).

Of interest are animal studies showing that IL-1 given systemically or into cerebral ventricles produces fever and sleep (106,107). In humans, interferons and IL-2 share common features of inducing fatigue, weakness, lethargy, and confusion (108). One study showed sedative effects of IL-2 in a rat model consistent with being mediated at the locus ceruleus level of the brain via stimulation of opiate receptors (109). It is reported also that IFN-α binds to opiate receptors in the human brain and produces endorphinlike effects that can be prevented or reversed with naloxone (110,111). Studies support that cytokines induce anorexia, lethargy, and fever in animals and humans. If cytokines produced peripherally can induce cytokine production in the CNS, such a mechanism of inflammatory mediator release might theoretically explain some of the neurobehavioral symptoms frequently complained of by MCS patients, such as fatigue, lassitude, and confusion, assuming that they might have elevated cytokine levels. Alterations in responsivity of cytokine receptor numbers or affinities may also contribute to enhanced cytokine responses (112).

Controlled studies have not demonstrated that those claiming MCS have abnormally elevated cytokines. Some studies show the opposite. One such study comparing immunologic functions in patients claiming MCS with normal controls showed no difference in IL-2 concentrations between cases and controls, but did show significantly lower levels of IL-1 generated by cultured monocytes in the cases versus controls (113). But this study's potential design flaws include not meeting Cullen's case definition of MCS, inconsistency in timing the measurement of IL-1 levels, and inconsistency between split sample findings from the same commercial laboratory. If IL-1 levels were found to be reduced in case definition MCS patients, this might indicate activation of the regulatory feedback loop described (105). This is a hypothesis for further study.

Another form of inflammation involves the trigeminal nerve endings in the upper airways and nasal passages. This is termed *neurogenic inflammation* and is generated by chemical irritants (114). The nasal passage is innervated by fibers of the trigeminal nerves, which form the common chemical senses. Trigeminal nerve ends are scattered throughout the nasal passages and surface of the eyes. The common chemical senses respond to airborne irritants and chemical with signs and symptoms of pain, irritancy, and inflammation (114,115). Human susceptibility to an inflammatory reaction from low-level indoor contaminants, both allergenic and nonallergenic, probably has a genetic predisposition (115). A growing body of research on chronic pain has focused on neural sensitization to mediators of the initial response to injury. Neurogenic inflammation is a testable model for end-organ dysfunction that could account for chronic pain and inflammation at multiple sites, without immunologic mediation.

Controlled human studies on mixtures of low-level volatile organic solvents (below Occupational Safety and Health Administration–recognized permissible exposure limits of any one chemical) indicate that inflammation, pungency, and irritation probably play primary roles in symptoms, and atopic subjects report more SBS-like symptoms from newly painted indoor surfaces: eye irritation, nose irritation, throat irritation, and facial irritation and fatigue in 50% of subjects (98).

Exogenous stimuli, such as chemicals, can activate chemosensitive c-fiber afferent nerves that release neuropeptides such as substance P. They cause inflammation both at the site and locations in the body different from that of the initiating stimulus. For example, results of one study show that neural elements are present in synovial tissue and that neurogenic inflammation may play a role in the arthralgia and inflammation of rheumatoid arthritis (116). Although such findings do not necessarily explain joint pains expressed by some MCS patients, at least there is a basis for the role of neurogenic, inflammation-inducing pain at sites other than the upper and lower airways. The c-fibers also send neural signals to the CNS that can activate autonomic nervous system responses and initiate sensitization of CNS neurons involved in pain perception (117–120).

Some patients claiming MCS and other chemically intolerant individuals report symptoms such as migraine headache, rhinitis, sinusitis, and asthma that have an inflammatory or irritancy basis. Neurogenic inflammation could conceivably contribute to some of these symptoms. Headache of migraine nature is attributed to neurogenic inflammation. Notably, substance P analogues and certain interleukins (which modulate inflammation) can also initiate sensitization (78,120,121).

Furthermore, exposure of cultured rat sensory neurons to the cytokine tumor necrosis factor-α (TNF-α) can sensitize neuronal electrophysiologic responsivity to subsequent chemostimulation from the c-fiber stimulant, capsaicin (122). TNF-α levels and receptors also have been shown to be altered in patients with CFS, a condition in which some MCS symptoms overlap (112).

In an individual susceptible to neural sensitization, chronic activation of inflammatory events might initiate a chain of events in the periphery leading to both peripheral sensory nerve and sensitization by neuropeptides and cytokines. In this case, the immediate sensitizing agent would be endogenous mediators rather than environmental chemicals, yet the external inciting event is a chemical that activates the pathway. Some support for such a theory is derived from the fact that macrophages cross from the periphery into the CNS where they secrete cytokines that affect immune activities and lymphocyte responses to mitogens (123,124). Also, astrocytes in the CNS modulate immune responses and have been discovered to be antigen-presenting cells (125–128).

Another metabolic marker of inflammation is neopterin. Elevated levels occur in inflammatory diseases such as autoimmunity and vasculitis (129,130). Neopterin plays a role in neurotransmission, vasodilation, platelet aggregation inhibition, antiproliferative action of cytokines, and reduction of oxidative stress (129–131). It is generated in the synthesis of biopterins, a folate-dependent biosynthetic pathway affecting neurotransmitter synthesis and release, and nitric oxide synthesis (131). Human monocytes and macrophages can produce tetrahydrobiopterin in response to cytokines, such as IFN-α, which leads to accumulation of neopterin (132). Higher levels of serum neopterin, a nonspecific marker of monocyte/macrophage activation and inflammation, correlated with higher scores for somatization, limbic system somatic symptoms, and fatigue in community-recruited chemically intolerant women with lifestyle changes, but not in depressed controls without CS (78). Researchers performing the assays were blind to the group membership of the subjects. But this exploratory study is limited because it involved only a small number of patients, and the findings are correlational. They must be considered preliminary and inconclusive. Further studies on larger samples using MCS patients and other control groups are needed to validate these results, both at resting baseline and after repeated chemical exposures.

Mast cells located in the periphery around neurons in the CNS release vasoactive inflammatory mediators. The brain may thus be a target for inflammatory chemical mediators. Whereas inflammatory diseases of tissues peripheral to the CNS can cause fatigue, anorexia, lethargy, fever, and depression, is it possible that inflammatory mediators released in the CNS may cause such symptoms? This remains to be proven. Animal models demonstrate that intraperitoneal injections of the cytokine IL-1 induces CNS proinflammatory cytokine protein markers in the brain (133). Consequently, peripherally produced cytokines might theoretically act locally to induce cytokines in the CNS that result in neurobehavioral symptoms (133). Such a mechanism could theoretically explain some of the neurobehavioral symptoms experienced by those with well-recognized, chronic inflammatory diseases and some of the neurobehavioral symptoms in MCS patients if inflammation indeed actually plays a role.

In summary, the inflammation model as a hypothetical basis to explain some of the symptoms expressed by MCS patients is attractive. It also has drawbacks. Studies are lacking that demonstrate inflammation as an operative mechanism in MCS patients. MCS patients do not appear to be experiencing the chronic debilitating effects of inflammation seen in well-known autoimmune diseases. More research is needed before conclusions can be made.

PORPHYRIA

Another theory is that MCS might involve inborn or acquired metabolic errors (i.e., enzyme abnormalities) that enhance susceptibility to the effects of exogenous chemicals. These would include defects in liver detoxification enzymes and variants of porphyria, a set of diseases related to disturbed heme metabolism (134,135). Ziem and McTamney reported finding unusually high rates of disorders of porphyrin metabolism on assays done at the Mayo Medical Laboratories in a case series of 14 MCS patients (136). The nature of the abnormalities did not overlap those characteristic of the congenital porphyrias. No published study has replicated and extended these findings under blind conditions in MCS patients, compared with control groups without CS. Disorders of heme metabolism, which can cause neurologic, behavioral, and gastrointestinal manifestations, remain an incompletely evaluated hypothesis for some cases of MCS.

DIRECT CHEMICAL TOXICITY CAUSING IMMUNE DYSREGULATION

One of the widely debated issues is whether immunotoxicity plays a role in the production of MCS symptoms. The immune system is the most well-recognized system capable of producing amplified reactivity (fulfilling the dynamic model hypothesis), and much research has been performed on immunotoxicity of xenobiotics. No evidence for classic, atopic IgE elevations in MCS has been found. MCS patients have not been shown to have evidence of decreased cancer surveillance or increased opportunistic infections—hallmarks of immune system dysfunction.

Immunologic findings reported in claimed cases of MCS include increased immunoglobulin levels, antichemical antibodies, autoantibodies, activated lymphocytes, altered T-cell subsets, changes in natural killer cell (NK) numbers and activity, and depressed T-cell response to mitogen stimulation (137,138). In the only systematically designed study, patients claiming CS and musculoskeletal patient controls did not differ in the variables previously reported in those case series (113). These other studies were criticized as being flawed by subsequently released evidence that the commercial laboratory used for many case series reportedly yielded reliability close to chance rates on a small number of split samples (139).

Anecdotal instances exist in which immune function tests repeated on MCS patients in different laboratories are normal. No persuasive evidence exists of an immunotoxic abnormality in MCS patients. The possibility that chemical exposures induce immune dysfunction in subsets of MCS patients with certain characteristics or with specific comorbid diagnoses remains to be proven.

The use of heterogeneous patient samples may have contributed to the difficulty in replicating previously reported clinical findings. Studies of function in both the immune and nervous systems require careful control over the state of the individual at the time of testing, as well as attention to circadian rhythm influences to avoid confounding factors. A starting point may be to evaluate the effects of chemical, drug, and food exposures on MCS patients with disorders having known immune system mediation. Until standardized clinical protocols are established, the clinical usefulness of ascribing immunologic dysfunction to MCS patients or of recommending specific immune tests as part of a clinical evaluation for a given individual is unproved.

A viable alternative hypothesis for immunologic alterations in some MCS patients is the biological effects of stress on the immune system.

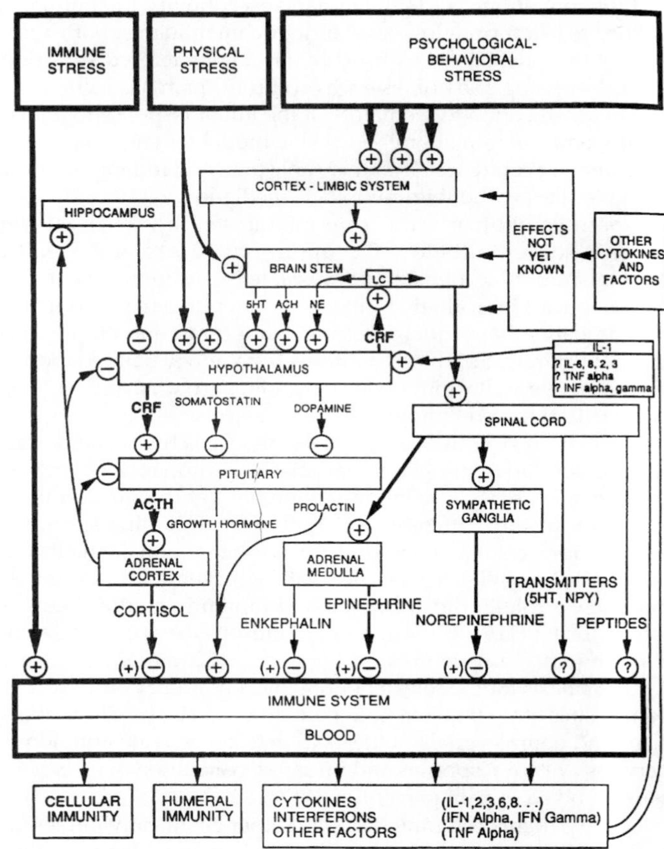

Figure 32-2. Schematic representation of the pathways involved in the neuroendocrine response to stress and its effect on the immune system. The anatomic and functional interrelationships (stimulatory or inhibitory) of the different neuroendocrine components involved in the stress response are illustrated. ACH, acetylcholine; ACTH, adrenocorticotropic hormone; CRF, corticotropin-releasing factor; IFN, interferon; IL, interleukin; NE, norepinephrine; NPY, neuropeptide Y; 5-HT, serotonin; LC, locus ceruleus; TNF, tumor necrosis factor; –, mild stimulation; ?, unknown.

Psychosomatic Effects of Chemicals, with Biological Mediation

STRESS AND THE IMMUNE SYSTEM

For both symptom production and for any observed immune system changes, the chronic effects of stress are another hypothesis in and of itself or in addition to other mechanisms for some MCS cases. Research validates the following (105,140): (a) stress activates areas of the brain that are linked to the immune system and the endocrine system; (b) stress activates the HPA axis and the sympathetic nervous system, releasing epinephrine and norepinephrine; (c) immune cells have receptors on their surfaces for catecholamines, and glucocorticoids respond to stressful activation, altering numbers and functions of certain immune cells; and (d) blocking of the catecholamine binding to these receptors prevents stressful episodes from altering immune system function.

When individuals are exposed to stressful stimuli, the HPA axis can be activated. HPA activation increases the excretion of corticosteroids and catecholamines. Glucocorticoids are released from the adrenal gland in response to adrenocorticotropic hormone (ACTH) release from the pituitary gland. ACTH release from the pituitary gland is caused by corticotropin-releasing hormone (CRH) release from the hypothalamus. Lymphocyte function may be influenced by ACTH and CRH because lymphocytes have receptors for both of these neuroendocrine chemicals on their surface in addition to receptors for catecholamines.

Other receptors found on lymphocytes include those for opioid compounds. Endogenous opioid peptides are endorphins, enkephalins, and dynorphins. Studies have shown that elevation of these opioid compounds can alter functions of immune cells of lymphocytes and macrophages (141,142). One study did show elevated and labile levels of plasma beta endorphin in elderly patients with CS but no lifestyle changes (42). No studies have examined endogenous opioids in MCS patients.

Understanding health stressors that could produce immune system alterations deserves much more research. Factors that assist an individual in coping with the stressors also can modify a person's response to stress. Such factors include nutrition, physical exercise, and stress reduction.

Stress from any source (i.e., chemical, physical, or psychological) can have effects on the immune system through neuroendocrine responses of the CNS and HPA axis (Fig. 32-2) (105,143–146). Although stress responses can cause release of endogenous opioids, cortisol, and catecholamines that may alter the humoral and cellular immune system, this immune response is not direct, chemically induced immunotoxicity as claimed by some. Rather, it is a physiologic response of the immune system to various types of chronic stressors.

Studies show that stress can elevate numbers of T cells and B cells, impair responsiveness of lymphocytes to mitogens, decrease CD4/CD8 (T-helper/T-suppressor) ratios, increase NK populations, and decrease NK cell activity (147–152). Individuals treated with β-adrenergic antagonist drugs, such as propranolol, show inhibition of immune alterations after stressful episodes (140). After a stressor—psychological or chemical—there is a complex feedback cascade involving the brain that activates neural stress pathways. This causes functional activation of immune cells that secrete cytokines and influence the CNS (153).

In animal models, exposure to chemicals evokes expression of brain biomarkers indicative of a neuronal excitation response to stress (70,154–157). The primary response to stress actually serves to augment immune function. But as stress becomes overwhelming, chronic immune functions can be altered and suppressed.

Mood and anxiety disorders and other psychiatric conditions are sometimes associated with changes in the immune system. It is reported that there is a linear relationship between severity of depression and immune compromise, including a marked reduction in the response to mitogens by lymphocytes, reduced NK activity, and alteration of immune cell numbers—primarily an increase in CD8 T-cell lymphocytes (158).

Marital discord, bereavement, and other such stressors are associated with immunosuppression and higher antibody titers to Epstein-Barr virus, lower NK activity, and reduced lymphocyte response to mitogens (148,149,159,160). The chronic stress of providing care to family members with debilitating disease shows decreases in CD4 T cells, lower helper to suppressor cell ratios, and increased antibody titers to Epstein-Barr virus (159,160). Bereavement, depression, and anxiety activate neuroendocrine functions that reduce NK activity and reduce T-cell numbers with CD4 markers.

Research has shown that moderate exercise modulates the effects of chronic diseases and has positive effects on immune function (161). Relaxation methods also positively modulate the immune system through stress reduction (148).

Individuals under stress show higher titers of Epstein-Barr viral capsid antigen IgG. Negative moods also depress mitogen stimulation of lymphocytes. Studies show that stressors increase the number of CD8 marker T cells and CD16/56 cells (NK cells), decrease mitogen response, and increase numbers of B cells (CD19) within 5 minutes of the stressor (105,143–145). These immune changes can persist for hours.

Chronic stressors probably increase susceptibility to common viral respiratory infections in humans and more serious infections in animals (105,143,161,162). Also, chronic stress acts opposite of acute stress in producing immune function changes. Chronic stress reduces NK cell numbers and activity. Acute stress elevates NK cell numbers and activity. Acute stress elevates lymphocyte subsets. In contrast, chronic stress decreases lymphocyte mitogen responsiveness. The stress-induced, increased NK cell activity is blocked by propranolol (140).

The phenomenon of acute reactions or triggering of symptoms when rechallenged with a chemical stressor has been observed in animals. It was termed the *generalized adaptation syndrome* by Selye in his 1950 book, *Stress*. The term *generalized* was introduced because he was able to show that chemicals and other stressors also lead to a maladaptive response.

In summary, the available data do not currently support a direct immunotoxic role of chemicals in the mediation of MCS. Instead, some immune alterations and activation could result from multiple stressors (physical or psychological) and may be reversible. Odors and activation of inflammation by low-level chemical exposure might also serve as such stressors. No research has directly tested any of these proposed cause-effect relationships.

Chronic stress and associated somatic, behavioral, and psychological responses outlast their initiating cause with symptoms persisting for long periods. Chronic stress also is associated with a loss of personal control over one's health. Providing patients with personal control over their health can thus be beneficial (163). But assigning a victim status to MCS patients or stripping them of their personal control could exacerbate chronic stress (e.g., by rendering controversial diagnoses that the patients may perceive as untreatable and inescapable). Efforts to increase patients' sense of control over their health should have positive health effects, especially if an environmental chemical etiology is demonstrable.

STRESS AND THE BRAIN

Exposures to chemicals may evoke expression of brain biomarkers indicative of a neuronal excitation response to stress. Pyrethroid insecticides administered intraperitoneally in animal models evoke c-Fos and c-Jun protein biomarkers in brain neurons in the thalamus, hypothalamus, hippocampus, and cortex to varying degrees (154). c-Fos and c-Jun proteins are transcription factors encoded by rapidly inducible proto-oncogenes (155,156). Such markers indicate changes in neuron activity and programming. c-Fos expression in homogenates is demonstrated after the application of lindane. The expression of c-Fos and c-Jun biomarkers reflects an intense and lasting neuronal excitation. Such brain markers appear in the cells of the brain that are functionally activated by stressors of all varieties. With the use of c-Fos and c-Jun markers, scientists can study areas of the brain that are activated by adverse stimuli (157).

Animals studied using conditioned stressors (stressors that produce fear or anxiety without pain or without some kind of insult) show activation of areas in the hypothalamus that contain CRH. Other areas activated in the studies included the amygdala, the basal ganglia, and thalamic nuclei (154–157). The areas of the brain activated by stressors (physical, chemical, or psychological) are associated with the HPA, and the sympathetic nervous system. If a similar activation of stress areas in the brain of MCS patients occurs, then subsequent activation of the sympathetic nervous system might explain some of their symptoms, such as anxiety or difficulty concentrating. Preliminary data indicate that mood and stress *per se* are not sufficient to account for poorer neuropsychological test performance, at least in chronically ill Gulf War veterans (164).

Some MCS patients claim that odors incite their symptoms. At issue is how different chemicals at low levels can give rise to qualitatively different odor experiences. Olfactory bulbs track into the limbic system of the brain, interconnecting extensively with limbic structures (Fig. 32-3 A,B,C). No researchers have been able to show any differences between MCS patients and normals in their objective olfactory sensory abilities (49,165,166). But the limbic system is sensitive to chemical stimuli and controls emotions, reactions to threat, and fight-or-flight responses.

Olfactory fibers connect with functional and anatomic areas of the limbic system such as the amygdala, hippocampus, and hypothalamus. These areas are involved with apathy, rage, emotions, and recent memory. Amygdala functions include fear, rage, indifference to surroundings, drowsiness, and increased pituitary-adrenocortical activity, blood pressure changes, gastrointestinal motility, respiratory rate changes, and pupillary reactions. The hypothalamus regulates the autonomic nervous system. Along with sensitization of the olfactory system, the presence of interconnecting olfactory-limbic neural circuits could possibly account for amplified responses to odors. The circuits may explain some symptoms experienced by MCS patients as defined by Cullen. Such neuroanatomic and neurophysiologic connections could also account for odor perception problems, or cacosmia, experienced by other individuals.

PSYCHONEUROIMMUNOLOGY

Stress can result in complex neuroendocrine and immune alterations. The bidirectional neuroendocrine and immune connections with the brain have been established as a component of the stress response (102). In one direction, cytokines can activate neuropathways. In the other direction, the brain can implement

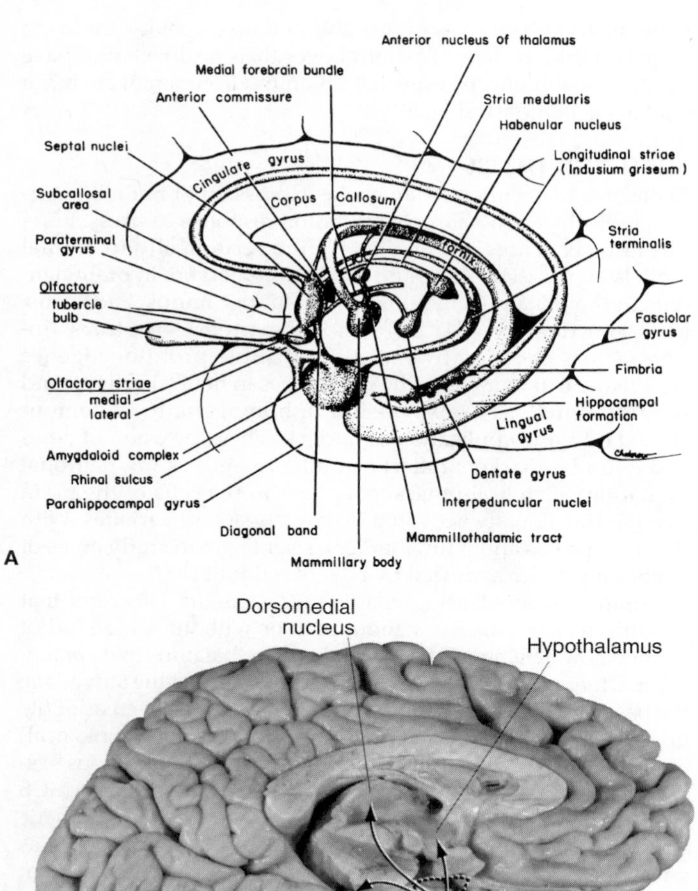

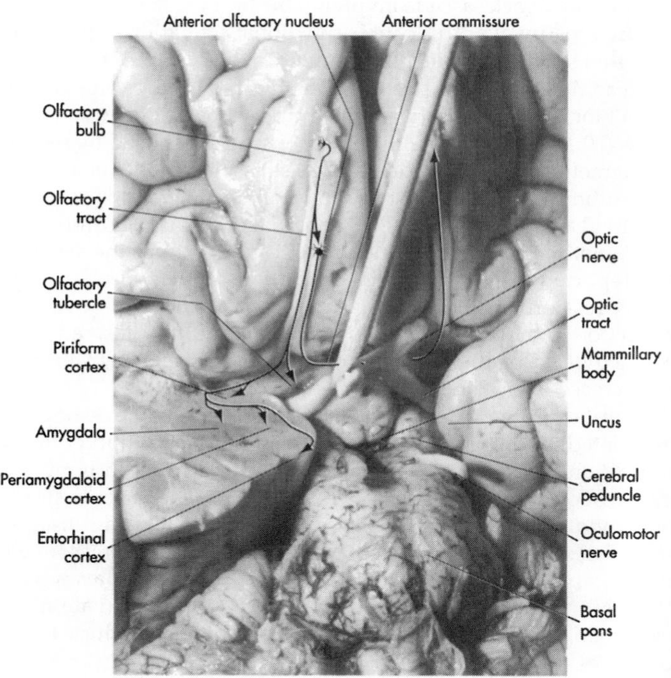

Figure 32-3. **A:** Limbic lobe—olfactory connections. **B,C:** Neuroanatomic structures showing the relationship of olfactory bulb to the limbic system.

changes in immune function. The interplay can become multidimensional. For example, in one experiment, researchers used IFN-α, which causes increased NK activity, as a means to study an unconditioned stimulus in an animal model. The administration of the IFN-α was paired with an initially neutral odor. When the odor alone was presented, the same immune alteration occurred without administration of the interferon (104,167). This study shows an olfactory-HPA link and demonstrates the capacity of conditioned odor effects to alter the immune system through activating the HPA axis. The relevance of this research to MCS is hypothetical and untested.

Cells of the immune system communicate with other cells of the immune system through cytokines. Lymphocytes have receptors on their cell surfaces for glucocorticoid steroids and catecholamines generated by the HPA neuroendocrine connections after cytokine excitation or stressful stimuli (168). NK cells have the highest number of catecholamine receptors. CD4 lymphocytes have the lowest number. CD8 lymphocytes and B cells are intermediate between the NKs and the CD4 lymphocytes with regard to catecholamine receptors. Macrophages have a high number of receptors for catecholamines.

The CD4 population of lymphocytes, known as *helper/inducer T cells*, are distinguished by two subpopulations, TH-1 and TH-2. When CD4 T cells are activated, they produce cytokines. The pattern of these cytokines determines the type of immune response. T-cell clones develop into TH-1 or TH-2 subtypes based on their cytokine profile influence. Generation of the TH-2 subtype is influenced by high IL-4 and IL-5. TH-1 subtype depends on high IL-2 and IFN-α. TH-1 cells promote cellular immune reactions and the TH-2 population promotes antibody production by B cells with IL-4 stimulation. An increase in the functional activity of TH-1 populations suppresses the TH-2 cell population and vice versa.

One effect of stress on the immune system is a decrease in cellular immune function and an increase in antibody production (143,147,169,170). This could result from suppression of the TH-1 population, which would then result in enhancement of TH-2 functions. Stress can produce alterations in the function of the immune system because the neuroendocrine-immune interconnections are both anatomic and chemical (105,147,169,170). The sympathetic nervous system also is involved in stress-induced immune alterations in animals and in humans. Activation of the sympathetic nervous system releases epinephrine and norepinephrine that can cause quantitative and qualitative changes in peripheral blood lymphocytes such as an increase in NK cells, increase in T-cell lymphocytes bearing the CD8 membrane receptor, and a decrease in mitogenesis of lymphocytes.

Acute stress and chronic stress have different actions on immunity and health in humans and animals (105,162,169–171). Individuals who have been studied under situations of chronic stress, such as after the death of a spouse or when caring for family members with Alzheimer's disease, demonstrate functional alteration of the immune system (148,149,159,160). Stress also predisposes individuals to increased susceptibility to viral infections and higher titers of latent Epstein-Barr virus (148,149,160,162).

Studies have shown that students subjected to stress show suppression of immune-cell function and an associated increase in antibodies to the Epstein-Barr virus, in particular, titers of Epstein-Barr viral capsid antigen IgG (149). NK cells, which have the highest number of adrenergic receptors, are the cell population with the largest increase subsequent to a stressful event. But NK activity and lymphocyte response to mitogens are suppressed in episodes of stress (149,150).

Acute or chronic stress produces health problems if maladapted to by those experiencing it. The health effects of stress reactions, particularly chronic stress, are divided into somatic, behavioral, and psychological. Symptoms expressed by MCS patients frequently overlap those produced by stress: anxiety, lethargy, irritability, bodily aches, and difficulty concentrating. Activation of the HPA stress mechanism by fear of exposures or threat may explain some MCS symptoms or some flares of symptoms under certain circumstances. As an analogy from the field of neurology, patients with documented epileptic disorders can experience bona fide seizures and pseudoseizures at different times.

The possibility of chemically elicited and stress-elicited MCS symptoms in the same patient is untested. If MCS shares hormonal features of PTSD, CFS, or FM, related data in those conditions indicate that patients may show a reduction rather than an elevation in 24-hour urinary free cortisol output. They also may show hypersuppression rather than loss of suppression of serum cortisol by a low-dose steroid exposure (i.e., opposite to the HPA axis pattern of major depression) (172–174).

In summary, stressful events can elicit neuroendocrine responses that can alter the immune system. Such stressful events might play a significant role in some MCS patients as primary or secondary factors in clinical course.

CLASSICAL CONDITIONING

A plausible psychophysiologic hypothesis that merits consideration is that of classical conditioning (175,176). In this model, the pairing of a biologically active stimulus [an unconditioned stimulus (UCS)] with an initially neutral, biologically inactive stimulus (e.g., CS) can result in the later ability of the CS alone to elicit conditioned responses that are the same or opposite to the unconditioned responses (UCRs) caused by the UCS. Like sensitization, conditioning is a type of psychobiological learning. The UCS in MCS would be a chemical exposure, with the CS a low-level odor with no inherent biological activity or physical surroundings of a specific building or location (176). Generalization of the CS would help account for the spread of sensitivities in MCS from the initiating chemical to multiple other substances.

The degree to which conditioning explains elements of MCS in certain patients can be tested. One limitation of this model is that the symptoms elicited by a CS should be those induced by the UCS or their opposite (if compensatory mechanisms are involved). The initiating chemical exposure in MCS is often either unknown or subtoxic in level. Even MCS patients with an identifiable initiating exposure have multiple symptoms that are not characteristic of any specific toxicologic syndrome. It is not clear how the UCR to a particular chemical could serve as the basis for a conditional response such as the polysystem symptoms of MCS. In chemically sensitive patients with no identifiable, initiating, toxic-chemical exposure, the nature of the UCS and UCR would be even more difficult to determine.

One form of neural sensitization has a conditioned component, termed *context-dependent* (92). The sensitized response develops in a particular setting paired with the administration of the exogenous agent. It later appears only in the same setting. Administration of the agent in a different setting does not elicit the sensitized response. This scenario might approximate SBS more than it would MCS. Although some have suggested that sensitization is simply a form of conditioning, some animal studies have demonstrated that the context-dependent, conditioned component can be extinguished (eliminated) while retaining the sensitized (amplified) reactivity component to a given drug (92,177). It is possible to establish context-independent sensitization in which varying the site within which the substance is originally administered allows subsequent elicitation of hyperactivity in any environment (178). This context-independent scenario may best approximate MCS, in which flares are claimed to occur in any setting.

Misattribution of the Symptoms from Psychiatric Disorders

Many clinical samples of MCS or CS patients have increased rates of lifetime or current psychiatric disorders, especially major depression, anxiety disorders, and somatization disorder. Some observers have concluded that all of the symptoms in MCS patients reduce to misattribution of symptoms from their diagnosable psychiatric disorders (179,180).

But somatization disorder is a diagnosis rendered without objective criteria, based on the lack of medical explanation for symptoms. Two different research groups have said it is the opinion of the observer whether a given controversial diagnosis (e.g., CFS or FM) is an acceptable medical explanation for symptoms (181,182). It is a subjective process on the clinician's or researcher's part that determines whether patients meet criteria for a label of somatization disorder.

No published studies have tested MCS patients with and without psychiatric problems under controlled conditions for differences in reactivity to active versus sham chemical exposures. The only published challenge study in MCS patients used strong odors, such as peppermint, as placebos and masking odors to cover the active odors. It did not control for possible sensitization to either active or placebo exposures in the same patients over time (91), thereby rendering the placebo potentially active (69,178).

Some studies that have linked MCS with purely psychogenic origins have been criticized as having serious design and method faults (25). Models of neural sensitization and neurogenic inflammation offer rational starting points for study of MCS mechanisms. But they do not rule out a role for maladaptive stress responses, dysfunctional coping responses, secondary phobic or avoidant behaviors, personality disorders, malingering, or other psychogenic processes as primary causation or complicating factors in MCS patients.

No MCS studies have demonstrated that scores on scales of psychological distress account for a large portion of the variance in the self-reported CS. In a sample of 643 healthy college students, multiple regression analyses did not demonstrate that depression, anxiety, or repression accounted for any of the variance in CI index scores (183). Even if psychological distress turns out to explain some of the variance in CS of MCS patients, it would not apply in those cases with past but not current histories of psychiatric conditions. No strong evidence exists that supports psychological distress as a sufficient explanation for CS in clinic or nonclinic samples.

A growing body of research in psychiatry and neurosciences does implicate neurobiological dysfunction in the mediation of symptoms in the major psychiatric disorders, even those initiated by psychological trauma (56,184–187). For instance, studies suggest that severe life stress plays its largest role in the initiation phase of PTSD or in a person's first episode, rather than later episodes, of major depression (83). Individuals differ in their susceptibility to developing chronic PTSD. Thereafter, mild stress or no stress at all is associated with recurrences or flares of symptoms. Combat veterans with PTSD also show greater opioid-mediated, naloxone-inhibited analgesia to a standardized heat stimulus on reexposure to trauma-relevant stimuli than do matched combat veteran controls without PTSD (188). These findings have prompted psychiatrists to conclude that an endogenous amplifying process followed the original insult. That process then induced persistent changes in brain function that allowed elicitation of symptoms by factors far different from the initiating trauma (189).

As an example, although the original psychological stress may not have involved noise, heightened startle to sudden environmental noise is a hallmark symptom of PTSD. Everyday minor hassles not necessarily similar to the original trauma can elicit flares of PTSD to a degree previously seen only with much more intense earlier events.

In brief, MCS and PTSD have parallels, especially in that affected individuals have amplified reactivity to certain environmental stimuli, but the current triggering stimuli are not necessarily the same as those that initiated the process. But these two conditions differ in the following important respects: (a) MCS patients have low rates of substance use or abuse (unless food cravings are considered); (b) PTSD patients have increased rates of alcohol and drug problems; and (c) MCS patients exhibit increased difficulty with certain spatial or visual attention and memory tasks, whereas PTSD patients show increased difficulty with verbal memory (18,25,37,39,40,190,191). The latter findings suggest that opposite sides of the brain may play greater roles in the neurobehavioral symptomatology of MCS and PTSD (right hemisphere in MCS and left hemisphere in PTSD).

Consistent with this possibility, opposite patterns of resting EEG alpha asymmetry over the frontal regions of the brain are seen in chemically intolerant (more alpha on right) versus depressed (more alpha on left) women, even though both groups have comparably high rates of prior abuse histories and current levels of depression (31,40). Participants in this study were middle-aged women who reported illness from the odor of common chemicals, depressed persons without such odor intolerance, and normal controls. The subjects completed a set of psychological scales and underwent two separate qEEG recording laboratory settings spaced a week apart at the same time of day for each subject. qEEG spectral analysis was automated and performed by a research assistant blind to the study hypotheses. The data indicated that those expressing CI, as defined in the study, differed significantly from depressed subjects and normal controls in qEEG alpha patterns at resting baseline. Subjects were excluded who were involved in any litigation or worker's compensation claims that could pose secondary bias. Medication use also was accounted for in the study. As the authors noted, these findings require replication, more rigorous controls, and extension to larger samples, including MCS patients, before final conclusions can be drawn.

Psychiatric diagnoses are descriptive labels for clusters of symptoms. As such, they can provide only directions for research on possible mechanisms. Some patients claiming MCS symptoms may be explained solely on a psychogenic basis. Others cannot (24). Problems such as childhood abuse or panic disorder, which have been found in elevated rates in MCS patients, have mediating biological processes, including electrophysiological data showing limbic system dysfunction of the type postulated to occur via neural sensitization (87,116). Even panic patients in remission show evidence for stress-reactive cardiovascular response amplification that could be a manifestation of neural sensitization (151,152).

Controlled studies have demonstrated neurochemical dysfunction (e.g., vulnerability to depletion of precursors of mood-regulatory neurotransmitters) and EEG changes (e.g., lateral asymmetry) in persons with depression, the most common comorbid psychiatric diagnosis in MCS patients (192,193). Behavioral interventions help in numerous other medical (e.g., cancer, heart disease, diabetes mellitus, asthma) and psychiatric (e.g., obsessive-compulsive disorder, schizophrenia) conditions without proving a psychogenic etiology for any of them. As would be expected, clinicians have also reported that behavioral interventions are beneficial in MCS (84,91,194).

CURRENT CLINICAL ISSUES INVOLVING CHEMICAL SENSITIVITY

Much of the controversy surrounding MCS stems not only from skepticism that low-level chemicals could cause such illness, but that some physicians who care for MCS patients often use purportedly unproved therapies (195). Much of the medical literature on MCS has limited data on both sides of this debate. The literature has delineated specific editorial opinions of various authors and organizations concerning the nature of the clinical problem or treatment approaches of physicians who specialize in managing MCS patients. Many of the therapies recommended for MCS patients are unproved and remain controversial. These therapies range from avoidance of eliciting agents, use of intradermal or sublingual dilutions of offending agents to neutralize symptoms, and sauna detoxification, to treatment for presumptive infectious disease comorbidities, immune system supports, nutritional supplements, psychotropic and anticonvulsant (e.g., gabapentin) drugs, and various alternative or complementary medicine techniques (196). However, neither appropriate epidemiological or health outcomes nor controlled trials of most of these approaches have been published in the peer-reviewed literature.

A summary of 305 MCS patients' self-ratings of the helpfulness or harmfulness of many different treatments was published in a 1996 patient newsletter (*Chronic Fatigue Immunodeficiency Syndrome Chronicle*) (197). The scientific validity of such a survey can be criticized, but it does provide clues to how those who describe themselves as having MCS feel about therapies. For example, 93% of the respondents considered chemical avoidance practices to be a "major" or "enormous" help (n = 304 tried). Only 41% had a similar rating for antifungal, anti-*Candida* therapies (n = 234 tried), 34% for intravenous vitamin C infusions (n = 110 tried), and 18% (n = 50 tried) for fluoxetine. By far, the treatments most often identified as 'harmful' were antidepressant drugs [including tricyclic and serotonin reuptake inhibitors and the newer agent bupropion (a catecholaminergic drug), with adverse ratings ranging from 52% to 67% of respondents]. This informal survey outlines the beliefs of a sample of MCS patients, 41% of whom reported CFS and 28% FM diagnoses. The findings suggest that this sample of MCS patients did not have globally positive beliefs about all nonconventional therapies. Many held negative views of the conventional medications usually prescribed for their psychiatric comorbid conditions. It should be noted that avoidance success could mean that (a) chemicals were a direct cause of their problem or (b) the increased sense of self-efficacy from implementing an avoidance program helped, independent of whether chemicals were a biological factor in the etiology.

Such findings create a quandary for clinicians who treat patients claiming MCS. Most of these patients find that avoidance techniques are beneficial, but some practitioners recommend extreme forms of isolation. Critics express concern over extreme social isolation and the financial costs of overzealous and costly environment changes. The following rational approaches are recommended:

1. Establish a healthy and clean home or work environment that meets the ventilation standards of the American Society of Heating, Refrigerating and Air-Conditioning Engineers. This reduces existing volatile chemicals to concentrations that the vast majority of people can tolerate. Identify and eliminate sources of odors. Install appropriate air filtration to clean and filter entering air.
2. Reduce chronic stress, if identified, with appropriate intervention.
3. Within reason, avoid situations in which odors or chemicals may cause problems. This may be difficult, but anecdotally it may help. It also is a logical extension of inferential causation reasoning that if an exposure to an odor or chemical is perceived to be the basis of symptoms, then avoidance may be of benefit, regardless of the mechanisms by which the exposure might be triggering symptoms.
4. Nonsedating antihistamines, if tolerated, may help prevent irritant upper airway effects of chemicals on the mucous membranes, such as nonallergic rhinitis. The use of antihistamines for nonallergic rhinitis has support (198). Appropriate precautions to patients for adverse effects and drug interactions are important.
5. Those claiming MCS can be considered to be individuals who may have lost a key aspect of control over their health and lifestyle. A general program of health promotion, stress reduction, nutrition, and moderate exercise is beneficial. Exercise has antidepressant, antianxiety, and mood-enhancing effects that are all positive for those claiming MCS or not (199). This enables the individual to regain a controlling feature over his or her general health. Such personal control consists of an individual's beliefs about how well he or she can bring about good events and avoid bad events (163,200).

Although these recommendations can only theoretically be said to benefit MCS cases, they do have support for their positive health benefits.

If a physician decides to provide longitudinal care for an individual claiming MCS, the establishment of a trusting relationship between the patient and an empathetic health care provider is essential. Such a relationship facilitates joint decisions about integrating reasonable diagnosis and treatment and avoiding therapies with no proven benefit. This approach may serve to improve the sense of control a patient experiences. Studies in behavioral medicine have demonstrated that increased sense of control has beneficial effects on psychological and medical outcomes in many different illnesses. Treatment of any identified comorbid psychiatric disorders by proven psychotherapies or tolerated medications is important.

To dismiss a patient from care asserting MCS to be purely psychiatric risks communicating a harmful negative attitude. Such rejecting behaviors of the physician can make the patient feel devalued with problems that the doctor considers to be imaginary or trivial. However, a common bias in U.S. society is that psychiatric disorders are less important and treatable than medical diagnoses. On the other extreme, labeling a patient with unsubstantiated diagnoses for which there is no effective treatment may be harmful and exacerbate chronic stress. An open patient-physician communication and an open mind are essential for any physician willing to be involved with these cases. Despite the lack of medical science to explain CS, many positive benefits can be derived by practicing the art of medicine in the care of these patients.

CONCLUSION

Research is needed to test the different models proposed for the vexing problem referred to as *MCS*. The eventual explanation may involve integration of several models. Research is advancing to a point at which scientifically replicable methods are beginning to elucidate some intriguing mechanisms underlying the phenomenon. The debate over MCS should not continue along dualistic, argumentative lines (i.e., toxigenic versus psychogenic). As with psychiatric conditions and other illnesses, biological and psychosocial factors could contribute to the basis of the problem. Only well-designed research studies can demonstrate if this is the case. Research models for MCS must account for the clinical phenomenology and have rigorous evidence, or they must be abandoned in favor of others that have scientific validation.

REFERENCES

1. Fiedler N, Kipen H. Chemical sensitivity: the scientific literature. *Environ Health Perspect* 1997;105[Suppl 2]:409–415.
2. Nethercott JR, Davidoff LL, Curbow B, Abbey H. Multiple chemical sensitivities syndrome: toward a working case definition. *Arch Environ Health* 1993;48:19–26.
3. Cullen MR. The worker with multiple chemical sensitivities: an overview. In: Cullen MR, ed. *Occup Med State of the Art Reviews*. Philadelphia: Hanley and Belfus, 1987:655–662.
4. Kipen HM, Hallman W, Kelly-McNeil K, Fiedler N. Measuring chemical sensitivity prevalence: a questionnaire for population studies. *Am J Public Health* 1995;85:574–577.
5. Szarek MJ, Bell IR, Schwartz GE. Validation of a brief screening measure of environmental chemical sensitivity: the chemical odor intolerance index. *J Environ Psychol* 1997;17(4):345–351.
6. Simon GE, Katon WJ, Sparks PJ. Allergic to life: psychological factors in environmental illness. *Am J Psychiatry* 1990;147:901–906.
7. Duncan H, Smith D. Clinical disorders of olfaction. In: Doty R, ed. *Handbook of olfaction and gustation*. New York: Marcel Dekker Inc, 1998.
8. Sparks PJ, ed. *Occupational medicine: state of the art reviews*. Philadelphia: Hanley and Belfus, 2000:497–675.
9. Molhave L. Controlled experiments for studies of the sick building syndrome. *Ann N Y Acad Sci* 1992;641:46–55.
10. Kjaergaard S, Molhave L, Pedersen O. Human reactions to a mixture of indoor air volatile organic compounds. *Atmospheric Environ* 1991;25A(8): 1417–1426.
11. Molhave L, Liu Z, Jorgensen A, Pederson L, Kjaergaard S. Sensory and physiological effects on humans of combined exposures to air temperatures and volatile organic compounds. *Indoor Air* 1993;3:155–169.
12. Holcomb L, Seabrook B. Indoor concentrations of volatile organic compounds: implications for comfort, health and regulation: review. *Indoor Environ* 1995;4:7–26.
13. Molhave L. Volatile organic compounds, indoor air quality and health. *Indoor Air* 1991;4:357–376.
14. Hirzy JW, Morison R. Carpet/4-pehnylcyclohexene toxicity: the EPA headquarters case. In: Garrick BJ, Gekler WS, eds. *The analysis, communication, and perception of risk*. New York: Plenum Publishing, 1991:51–61.
15. Welch LS, Sokas R. Development of multiple chemical sensitivity after an outbreak of sick building syndrome. *Toxicol Ind Health* 1992;8:47–50.
16. Miller CS, Mitzel HC. Chemical sensitivity attributed to pesticide exposure versus remodeling. *Arch Environ Health* 1995;50:119–129.
17. Buchwald D, Garrity D. Comparison of patients with chronic fatigue syndrome, fibromyalgia, and multiple chemical sensitivities. *Arch Intern Med* 1994;154:2049–2053.
18. Fiedler N, Kipen HM, DeLuca J, Kelly-McNeil K, Natelson B. A controlled comparison of multiple chemical sensitivities and chronic fatigue syndrome. *Psychosom Med* 1996;58:38–49.
19. Slotkoff AT, Radulovic DA, Clauw DJ. The relationship between fibromyalgia and the multiple chemical sensitivity syndrome. *Scand J Rheumatol* 1997;26:364–367.
20. Bell IR, Warg-Damiani L, Baldwin CM, Walsh ME, Schwartz GE. Self-reported chemical sensitivity and wartime chemical exposures in Gulf War veterans with and without decreased global health ratings. *Mil Med* 1998;163:725–732.
21. Clauw D, Kin T, Barbey J. Physiologic abnormalities in fibromyalgia, chronic fatigue syndrome, and Gulf War illness. Presentation at the Conference on Federally Sponsored Gulf War Veterans' Illnesses Research Conference. Washington: June 1998.
22. Proctor SP, White RF, Wolfe J. Summary of environmental interview data from Persian Gulf War (PGW) veterans. Presentation at the Conference on Federally Sponsored Gulf War Veterans' Illnesses Research Conference. Washington: June 1998.

23. Ryan CM, Morrow LA, Hodgson M. Cacosmia and neurobehavioral dysfunction associated with occupational exposure to mixtures of organic solvents. *Am J Psychiatry* 1988;145:1442–1445.
24. Morrow LA, Ryan CM, Hodgson MJ, Robin N. Alterations in cognitive and psychological functioning after organic solvent exposure. *J Occup Med* 1990;32:444–450.
25. Davidoff AL, Fogarty L. Psychogenic origins of multiple chemical sensitivities syndrome: a critical review of the research literature. *Arch Environ Health* 1994;49:316–325.
26. Simon GE, Daniell W, Stockbridge H, Claypoole K, Rosenstock L. Immunologic, psychological, and neuropsychological factors in multiple chemical sensitivity: a controlled study. *Ann Intern Med* 1993;19(2):97–103.
27. Bell IR, Peterson JM, Schwartz GE. Medical histories and psychological profiles of middle-aged women with and without self-reported illness from environmental chemicals. *J Clin Psychiatry* 1995;56:151–160.
28. Baldwin CM, Bell IR. Increased cardiopulmonary disease risk in a community-based sample with chemical odor intolerance: implications for women's health and health care utilization. *Arch Environ Health* 1998;53:347–353.
29. Aaron LA, Bradley LA, Alarcon GS, et al. Psychiatric diagnoses in patients with fibromyalgia are related to health care-seeking behavior rather than to illness. *Arthritis Rheum* 1996;39:436–445.
30. Terr AI. Environmental illness: a clinical review of 50 cases. *Arch Intern Med* 1986;146:145–149.
31. Bell IR, Schwartz GE, Baldwin CM, Hardin EE, Kline JP. Differential resting EEG alpha patterns in women with environmental chemical intolerance, depressives, and normals. *Biol Psychiatry* 1998;43:376–388.
32. Sparks PJ, Daniell W, Black DW, et al. Multiple chemical sensitivity syndrome: a clinical perspective. I. Case definition, theories of pathogenesis, and research needs. *J Occup Med* 1994;36:718–730.
33. Bell IR, Baldwin CM, Schwartz GE. Illness from low levels of environmental chemicals: relevance to chronic fatigue syndrome and fibromyalgia. *Am J Med* 1998;105:745–825.
34. Bell IR, Schwartz GE, Amend D, Peterson JM, Stini WA. Sensitization to early life stress and response to chemical odors in older adults. *Biol Psychiatry* 1994;35:857–863.
35. Meggs WJ, Dunn KA, Bloch RM, Goodman PE, Davidoff AL. Prevalence and nature of allergy and chemical sensitivity in a general population. *Arch Environ Health* 1996;51:275–282.
36. Bell IR, Bootzin RR, Ritenbaugh C, et al. A polysomnographic study of sleep disturbance in community elderly with self-reported environmental chemical odor intolerance. *Biol Psychiatry* 1996;40:123–133.
37. Bell IR, Wyatt JK, Bootzin RR, Schwartz GE. Slowed reaction time performance on a divided attention task in elderly with environmental chemical odor intolerance. *Int J Neurosci* 1995;84:127–134.
38. Bell IR, Schwartz GE, Bootzin RR, Wyatt JK. Time-dependent sensitization of heart rate and blood pressure over multiple laboratory sessions in elderly individuals with chemical odor intolerance. *Arch Environ Health* 1997;52:6–17.
39. Bell IR, Szarek MJ, Dicenso DR, Baldwin CM, Schwartz GE, Bootzin RR. Patterns of waking EEG spectral power in chemically intolerant individuals during repeated chemical exposures. *Int J Neurosci* 1999;97:41–59.
40. Bell IR, Baldwin CM, Russek LG, Schwartz GE, Hardin EE. Early life stress, negative paternal relationships, and chemical odor intolerance in middle-aged women: support for a neural sensitization model. *J Womens Health* 1998;7:1135–1147.
41. Hummel T, Roscher S, Jaumann MP, Kobal G. Intranasal chemoreception in patients with multiple chemical sensitivities: a double-blind investigation. *Regul Toxicol Pharmacol* 1996;24:S79–S86.
42. Bell IR, Bootzin RR, Davis T, Hau V, Ritenbaugh C, Johnson KA, Schwartz GE. Time-dependent sensitization of plasma beta-endorphin in community elderly with self-reported environmental chemical odor intolerance. *Biol Psychiatry* 1996;40:134–143.
43. Morrow LA, Steinhauer SR. Alterations in heart rate and pupillary response in persons with organic solvent exposure. *Biol Psychiatry* 1995;37:721–730.
44. Retzlaff PD, Morris GL. Event-related potentials during the Continuous Visual Memory Test. *J Clin Psychol* 1996;52:43–47.
45. Fink GR, Halligan PW, Marshall JC, Frith CD, Frackowiak RSJ, Dolan RJ. Where in the brain does visual attention select the forest and the trees? *Nature* 1996;382:626–628.
46. Ashford NA, Miller CS. *Chemical exposures, low levels and high stakes,* 2nd ed. New York: Van Nostrand–Reinhold, 1998.
47. Antelman SM. Time-dependent sensitization in animals: a possible model of multiple chemical sensitivity in humans. *Toxicol Indust Health* 1994;10:335–342.
48. Antelman SM, Eichler AJ, Black CA, Kocan D. Interchangeability of stress and amphetamine in sensitization. *Science* 1980;207:329–331.
49. Doty RL, Deems DA, Frye RE, Pelberg R, Shapiro A. Olfactory sensitivity, nasal resistance, and autonomic function in patients with multiple chemical sensitivities. *Arch Otolaryngol Head Neck Surg* 1988;114:1422–1427.
50. Bell IR, Hardin E, Baldwin CM, Schwartz GE. Increased limbic system symptomatology and sensitizability of young adults with chemical and noise sensitivities. *Environ Res* 1995;70:84–97.
51. Bell IR, Schwartz GE, Peterson JM, Amend D. Symptom and personality profiles of young adults from a college student population with self-reported illness from foods and chemicals. *J Am Coll Nutr* 1993;12:693–702.
52. Miller CM. Toxicant-induced loss of tolerance—an emerging theory of disease? *Environ Health Perspect* 1997;105[Suppl 2]:445–453.
53. Lemanske R, Busse W. Asthma. *JAMA* 1997;278(22):1855–1873.
54. Farley J. Inhaled toxicants and airway hyperresponsiveness. *Ann Rev Pharmacol Toxicol* 1992;32:67–88.
55. Barnes P. Neurogenic inflammation and asthma. *J Asthma* 1992;29(3):165–180.
56. Kandel ER. A new intellectual framework for psychiatry. *Am J Psychiatry* 1998;155:457–469.
57. May R. The chaotic rhythms of life. In: Hall N, ed. *Exploring chaos—a guide to the new science of disorder.* New York: Norton, 1993.
58. Bell IR, Miller CS, Schwartz GE. An olfactory-limbic model of multiple chemical sensitivity syndrome: possible relationship to kindling and affective spectrum disorders. *Biol Psychiatry* 1992;32:218–242.
59. Bell IR. Neuropsychiatric aspects of sensitivity to low level chemicals: a neural sensitization model. *Toxicol Indust Health* 1994;10:277–312.
60. Kalivas PW, Sorg BA, Hooks MS. The pharmacology and neural circuitry of sensitization to psychostimulants. *Behav Pharmacol* 1993;4:315–334.
61. Sorg BA, Prasad BM. Potential role of stress and sensitization in the development and expression of multiple chemical sensitivity. *Environ Health Perspect* 1997;105[Suppl 2]:467–471.
62. Antelman SM. Time-dependent sensitization as the cornerstone for a new approach to pharmacotherapy: drugs as foreign/stressful stimuli. *Drug Devel Res* 1988;14:1–30.
63. Antelman SM, Caggiula AR, Knopf S, Kocan DJ, Edwards DJ. Amphetamine or haloperidol 2 weeks earlier antagonized the plasma corticosterone response to amphetamine: evidence for the stressful/foreign nature of drugs. *Psychopharmacology* 1992;107:331–336.
64. Sorg BA, Willis JR, Nowatka TC, Ulibarri C, See RE, Westberg HH. A proposed animal neurosensitization model for multiple chemical sensitivity in studies with formalin. *Toxicology* 1996;111:135–145.
65. Antelman SM, Kocan D, Knopf S, Edwards DJ, Caggiula AR. One brief exposure to a psychological stressor induces long-lasting, time-dependent sensitization of both the cataleptic and neurochemical responses to haloperidol. *Life Sci* 1992;51:261–266.
66. Sorg BA, Willis JR, See RE, Hopkins B, Westberg HH. Repeated low-level formaldehyde exposure produces cross-sensitization to cocaine: possible relevance to chemical sensitivity in humans. *Neuropsychopharmacology* 1998;18:385–394.
67. vonEuler G, Ogren S, Eneroth P, Fuxe K, Gustafsson J. Persistent effects of 80 ppm toluene on dopamine-regulated locomotor activity and prolactin secretion in the male rat. *Neurotoxicology* 1994;15:621–624.
68. vonEuler G, Ogren SO, Li XM, Fuxe K, Gustafsson JA. Persistent effects of subchronic toluene exposure on spatial learning and memory, dopamine-mediated locomotor activity and dopamine D2 agonist binding in the rat. *Toxicology* 1993;77:223–232.
69. Kay LM. Support for the kindling hypothesis in multiple chemical sensitivity syndrome (MCSS) induction. Presentation at the 26th Annual Meeting of the Society for Neuroscience. Washington: November, 1996.
70. Gilbert ME. Repeated exposure to lindane leads to behavioral sensitization and facilitates electrical kindling. *Neurotoxicol Teratatol* 1995;17:131–141.
71. Bell IR, Rossi J, Gilbert M. Testing the neural sensitization and kindling hypothesis for illness from low levels of environmental chemicals: working group report. *Environ Health Perspect* 1997;105[Suppl 2]:539–547.
72. Fernandez M. EEG measures of subjects with idiopathic chemical sensitivity: a test of the sensitization model. Ph.D. diss., University of Arizona, 1998.
73. Bell IR, Szarek MFJ, Dicenso DR, Baldwin CM, Schwartz GE, Bootzin RR. Patterns of waking EEG spectral power in chemically intolerant individuals during repeated chemical exposures. *Int J Neurosci* 1999;97:41–59.
74. Ferger B, Stahl D, Kuschinsky K. Effects of cocaine on the EEG power spectrum of rats are significantly altered after its repeated administration. Do they reflect sensitization phenomena? *Naunyn Schmiedebergs Arch Pharmacol* 1996;353:545–551.
75. Muttray A, Lang J, Mayer-Popken O, et al. Acute changes in the EEG of workers exposed to mixtures of organic solvents. *Int J Occup Med Environ Health* 1995;8:131–137.
76. Staudenmayer H, Selner JC. Neuropsychophysiology during relaxation in generalized, universal "allergic" reactivity to the environment: a comparison study. *J Psychosom Res* 1990;34:259–270.
77. Robinson TE, Berridge KC. The neural basis of drug craving: an incentive-sensitization theory of addiction. *Brain Res Rev* 1993;18:247–291.
78. Bell IR, Patarca R, Baldwin CM, Klimas NG, Schwartz GE, Hardin EE. Serum neopterin and somatization in women with chemical intolerance, depressives, and normals. *Neuropsychobiology* 1998;38:13–18.
79. Hill SY, Smith TR. Evidence for genetic mediation of alcoholism in women. *J Substance Abuse* 1991;3:159–174.
80. Bell IR. Somatization disorder: health care costs in the decade of the brain. *Biol Psychiatry* 1994;35:81–83.
81. Parker SL, Leznoff A, Sussman GL, Tarlo S, Krondl M. Characteristics of patients with food-related complaints. *J Allergy Clin Immunol* 1990;86:503–511.
82. Sills TL, Vaccarino FJ. Individual differences in sugar intake predict the locomotor response to acute and repeated amphetamine administration. *Psychopharmacology* 1994;116:1–8.
83. Post RM. Transduction of psychosocial stress into the neurobiology of recurrent affective disorder. *Am J Psychiatry* 1992;149:999–1010.
84. Staudenmayer H, Selner ME, Selner JC. Adult sequelae of childhood abuse presenting as environmental illness. *Ann Allergy* 1993;71:538–546.
85. Bremner JD, Southwick SM, Johnson DR, Yehuda R, Charney DS. Childhood physical abuse and combat-related posttraumatic stress disorder in Vietnam veterans. *Am J Psychiatry* 1993;150:235–239.

86. Morrison J. Childhood sexual histories of women with somatization disorder. *Am J Psychiatry* 1989;146:239–241.
87. Teicher MH, Glod CA, Surrey J, Swett C. Early childhood abuse and limbic system ratings in adult psychiatric outpatients. *J Neuropsychiatry Clin Neurosci* 1993;5:301–306.
88. Robinson TE, Becker JB, Presty SK. Long-term facilitation of amphetamine-induced rotational behavior and striatal dopamine release produced by a single exposure to amphetamine: sex differences. *Brain Res* 1982;253:231–241.
89. Peris J, Decambre N, Coleman-Hardee ML, Simkins JW. Estradiol enhances behavioral sensitization to cocaine and amphetamine-stimulated striatal [3H] dopamine release. *Brain Res* 1991;566:255–264.
90. Jodogne C, Marinelli M, LeMoal M, Piazza PV. Animals predisposed to develop amphetamine self-administration show higher susceptibility to develop contextual conditioning of both amphetamine-induced hyperlocomotion and sensitization. *Brain Res* 1994;657:236–244.
91. Staudenmayer H, Selner JC, Buhr MP. Double-blind provocation chamber challenges in 20 patients presenting with Multiple Chemical Sensitivity. *Reg Toxicol Pharmacol* 1993;44–53.
92. Bell IR, Schwartz GE, Baldwin CM, Hardin EE, Klimas N, Kline JP, Patarca R, Song ZY. Individual differences in neural sensitization and the role of context in illness from low level environmental chemical exposures. *Environ Health Perspect* 1997;105[Suppl 2]:457–466.
93. Bell I, Miller C, Schwartz C, et al. Neuropsychiatric and somatic characteristics of nondisabled young adults with cacosmia. *Arch Environ Health* 1996;51:9–21.
94. Meggs WJ. Hypothesis for induction and propagation of chemical sensitivity based on biopsy studies. *Environ Health Perspect* 1997;105[Suppl 2]:473–478.
95. Auger P, Gourdeau P, Miller D. Clinical experience with patients suffering from a chronic fatigue-like syndrome and repeated upper respiratory infections in relation to airborne molds. *Am J Ind Med* 1994;25:41–42.
96. Fogelmark B, Rylander R, Sjostrand M. Pulmonary inflammation induced by repeated inhalation of beta(1,3)-D-glucan and endotoxin. *Int J Exp Pathol* 1994;75:85–90.
97. Larsen F, Clementsen P, Hansen M, et al. Volatile organic compounds from the indoor mold *Trichoderma viride* cause histamine release from human bronchoalveolar cells. *Inflamm Res* 1998;47[Suppl 1]:55–84.
98. Wieslander G, Norback D, Nordstrom K, Walinder R, Venge P. Nasal and ocular symptoms, tear film stability, and biomarkers in nasal lava in relation to building-dampness and building design in hospitals. *Int Arch Occup Environ Health* 1999;72:451–461.
99. Diel F, Detscher M, Borck H, et al. Effects of permethrin on human basophils and lymphocytes in vitro. *Inflamm Res* 1998;47[Suppl 1]:511–512.
100. Schook L, Laskin D, eds. *Xenobiotics and inflammation*. New York: Academic Press, 1994.
101. Whal S, Brandes M. Inflammatory cytokines: an overview. In: Schook L, Laskin D, eds. *Xenobiotics and inflammation*. New York: Academic Press, 1994.
102. Smith T, Hewson A. Neuroendocrine-induced immune modulation and autoimmunity. In: Kresina T, ed. *Immune modulating agents*. New York: Marcel Dekker Inc, 1998.
103. Rylander R. Organic dusts and lung disease: the role of inflammation. Review Articles. *Ann Agric Environ Med* 1994;1:7–10.
104. Banks W, Castin A, Gutierrez E. Interleukin-1 alpha in blood has direct access to cortico brain cells. *Neurosci Lett* 1993;163:41.
105. Heninger G. Neuroimmunology of stress. In: Friedman MJ, Charney DS, Deutch AY, eds. *Neurobiological and clinical consequences of stress: from normal adaptation to PTSD*. Philadelphia: Lippincott–Raven Publishers, 1995.
106. Dinarello C. Multiple biological properties of recombinant human interleukin-1 (beta). *Immunobiology* 1986;172:301–315.
107. Krueger J, Walter C, Dinarello C, et al. Sleep-promoting effects of endogenous pyrogen (interleukin-1). *Am J Physiology* 1984;246:R994–R999.
108. Fent K, Zbinden G. Toxicity of interferon and interleukin. *Trends Pharmacol Sci* 1987;8:1001–1005.
109. Sarro G, Masuda Y, Ascioti C, Audino M, Nistico G. Behavioral and ECoG spectrum changes induced by intracerebral infusion of interferons and interleukin 2 in rats are antagonized by naloxone. *Neuropharmacology* 1990;29(2):167–179.
110. Blalock J, Smith E. Human leukocyte interferon (HuIFN-alpha): potent endorphin-like opioid activity. *Biochem Biophys Res Commun* 1981b;101:472–278.
111. Blalock J, Stanton J. Common pathways of interferon and hormonal action. *Nature* 1980;283:406–408.
112. Patarca R, Klimas NG, Garcia MN, et al. Deregulated expression of soluble immune mediator receptors in a subset of patients with chronic fatigue syndrome: cross-sectional categorization of patients by immune status. *J Chronic Fatigue Syndrome* 1995;1:81–96.
113. Simon G, Daniell W, Stockbridge H, Claypoole K, Rosenstock L. Immunologic, psychological and neuropsychological factors in multiple chemical sensitivity. *Ann Intern Med* 1993;19(2):97–103.
114. Nielsen G. Mechanisms of activation of the sensory irritant receptor by airborne chemicals. *Crit Rev Toxicol* 1991;21(3):183–208.
115. Bascom R, Ksavanathan, Swift D. Human susceptibility to indoor contaminants. *Occup Med* 1995;10(1):119–132.
116. Gronblad M, Konttinen Y, Korkala O, et al. Neuropeptides in synovium of patients with rheumatoid arthritis and osteoarthritis. *J Rheum* 1988;15(1):1807–1810.
117. Coderre TJ, Katz J, Vaccarino AL, Melzack R. Contribution of central neuroplasticity to pathological pain: review of clinical and experimental evidence. *Pain* 1993;52:259–285.
118. Vaccarino AL, Melzack R. Temporal processes of formalin pain: differential role of the cingulum bundle, fornix pathway, and medial bulboreticular formation. *Pain* 1992;49:257–271.
119. Gracely RH, Lynch SA, Bennett GJ. Painful neuropathy: altered central processing maintained dynamically by peripheral input. *Pain* 1992;51:175–194.
120. Kalivas PW, Stewart J. Dopamine transmission in the initiation and expression of drug- and stress-induced sensitization of motor activity. *Brain Res Rev* 1991;16:223–244.
121. Denicoff KD, Kurkin TM, Lotze MT, et al. The neuroendocrine effects of interleukin-2 treatment. *J Clin Endocrinol Metab* 1989;69:402–410.
122. Nicol GD, Lopshire JC, Pafford CM. Tumor necrosis factor enhances the capsaicin sensitivity of rat sensory neurons. *J Neurosci* 1997;17:975–982.
123. Lotan M, Schwartz M. Cross talk between the immune system and the nervous system in response to injury—implications for regeneration. *FASEB J* 1994;8:1026.
124. Black P. Central nervous system immune system interactions: psychoneuroendocrinology of stress and its immune consequences. *Antimicrob Agents Chemother* 1994;3:1.
125. Smith T, DeGirolami U, Hickey W. Neuropathology of immunosuppression. *Brain Pathol* 1992;2:183.
126. Montgomery D. Astrocytes—form, functions and roles in disease. *Vet Pathol* 1994;31:145.
127. Graber M, Streit W. Microglia—immune network in the CNS. *Brain Pathol* 1990;1:2.
128. Otero G, Merrill J. Cytokine receptors on glial cells. *Glia* 1994;11:117.
129. Fuchs D, Weiss G, Wachter HI. Neopterin, biochemistry, and clinical use as a marker for cellular immune reactions. *Int Arch Allergy Immunol* 1993;101:1–6.
130. Nassonov E, Sasonov M, Beketova T, Semenkova I, Wachter H, Fuchs D. Serum neopterin concentrations in Wegener's granulomatosis correlate with vasculitis activity. *Clin Exp Rheum* 1995;13:353–356.
131. Patarca R, Bell IR, Fletcher MA. Pteridines and neuroimmune function and pathology. *J Chronic Fatigue Syndrome* 1997;3:69–86.
132. Werner-Felmayer G, Werner ERR, Fuchs D, Hausen A, Eibnegger G, Wachter H. Neopterin formation and tryptophan degradation by a human myelomonocytic cell line (THP-1) upon cytokine treatment. *Cancer Res* 1990;50:2863–2867.
133. Johnson R, Dantzer R, Kelley K. Neurobehavioral toxicity of cytokines. *Neurotoxicology* 1996;17(3–4):943(abst).
134. Calabrese EJ. Biochemical individuality: the next generation. *Reg Toxicol Pharmacol* 1996;24:S58–S67.
135. Ellefson RD, Ford RE. The porphyrias: characteristics and laboratory tests. *Reg Toxicol Pharmacol* 1996;24:S119–S125.
136. Ziem G, McTamney J. Profile of patients with chemical injury and sensitivity. *Environ Health Perspect* 1997;105[Suppl 2]:417–436.
137. Thrasher JD, Broughton A, Madison R. Immune activation and autoantibodies in humans with long-term inhalation exposure to formaldehyde. *Arch Environ Health* 1990;45:217–223.
138. Thrasher JD, Wojdani A, Cheung G, Heuser G. Evidence for formaldehyde antibodies and altered cellular immunity in subjects exposed to formaldehyde in mobile homes. *Arch Environ Health* 1987;42:347–350.
139. Simon GE. Questions and answers #3. *Toxicol Ind Health* 1994;4/5:523–535.
140. Bachen E, Manuck S, Cohen S, et al. Adrenergic blockade ameliorates cellular immune responses to mental stress in humans. *Psychosom Med* 1995;57:366–372.
141. Shabit Y. Stress induced immune modulation in animals: opiates and endogenous opioid peptides. In: Ader R, Felten D, Cohen N, eds. *Psychoneuroimmunology.* New York: Academic Press, 1991.
142. Sibinga N, Goldstein A. Opioid peptides and opioid receptors and cells of the immune system. *Ann Rev Immunol* 1988;6:219–249.
143. Kicolt-Glaser J, Glaser R. Psychoneuroimmunology and health consequences: data and shared mechanisms. *Psychosom Med* 1995;57:269–274.
144. Herbert T, Cohen S, Marsland A, Bachen E, et al. Cardiovascular reactivity and the course of immune response to an acute psychological stressor. *Psychosom Med* 1994;56:337–344.
145. O'Leary A. Stress, emotion, and human immune function. *Psychol Bull* 1990;108(3):363–382.
146. Zakowski S, McAllister C, Deal M, Baum A. Stress, reactivity, and immune function in healthy men. *Health Psychol* 1992;11(4):223–232.
147. Kusnecov A, Rabin B. Stressor induced alterations of immune function—mechanisms and issues. *Int Arch Allergy Immunol* 1994;105:107.
148. Esterling B, Antoni M, Kumar M. Emotional repression, stress disclosure responses and Epstein-Barr viral capsid antigen titers. *Psychosom Med* 1990;52:392–410.
149. Kicolt-Glaser J, Speicher C, Holliday J, Glaser R. Stress and the transformation of lymphocytes by Epstein-Barr virus. *J Behav Med* 1984;7:1.
150. Khan M, Sansoni P, Silverman E, et al. Beta adrenergic receptors on human suppressor, helper, and cytolytic lymphocytes. *Biochem Pharmacol* 1986;35:1137.
151. Weilburg JB, Schacter S, Worth J, et al. EEG abnormalities in patients with atypical panic attacks. *J Clin Psychiatry* 1995;56:358–362.
152. Leyton M, Belanger C, Martial J, et al. Cardiovascular, neuroendocrine, and monoaminergic responses to psychological stressors: possible differences between remitted panic disorder patients and healthy controls. *Biol Psychiatry* 1996;40:353–360.
153. Black P. Central nervous system immune system interactions: psychoneuroendocrinology of stress and its immune consequences. *Antimicrob Agents Chemother* 1994;36:1.

154. Hassouna I, Wickert H, El-Elaimy I, Zimmermann M, Herdegen T. Systemic application of pyrethroid insecticides evokes differential expression of c-Fos and c-Jun in rat brain. *Neurotoxicology* 1996;17(2):415–432.
155. Hoffman G, Smith M, Berbalis J. c-Fos and related immediate early gene products as markers of activity in neuroendocrine systems. *Front Neuroendocrinol* 1993;14:173.
156. Rabin B, Pezzone M, Kusnecov A, Hoffman G. Identification of stressor activated areas in the central nervous system. *Methods Neurosci* 1995;24:185.
157. Pezzone M, Lee W, Hoffman G, et al. Activation of brain stem catecholaminergic neurons by condition and uncondition aversive stimuli as revealed by c-fos immunoreactivity. *Brain Res* 1993;608:310.
158. Marazziti D, Ambrogi F, Vanacore R, et al. Immune cell imbalance in major depressive and panic disorders. *Neuropsychobiology* 1992;26:23–26.
159. Kiecolt-Glazer J, Glaser R, Shuttleworth E, et al. Chronic stress and immunity in family care givers of Alzheimer's disease victims. *Psychosom Med* 1987;49:523–535.
160. McKinnon W, Weisse C, Reynolds C, et al. Chronic stress, leukocyte subpopulations and humoral response to latent viruses. *Health Psychol* 1989;8:389–402.
161. Irwin M, Mascovich A, Gillin C, et al. Partial sleep deprivation reduces natural killer cell activity in humans. *Psychosom Med* 1994;56:493–498.
162. Bachen E, Marsland A, Manuck S, Cohen S. Psychological stress and immune competence. In: Kresina T, ed. *Immune modulating agents.* New York: Marcel Dekker Inc, 1998:145–159.
163. Peterson C, Stunkard A. Personal control and health promotion. *Soc Sci Med* 1989;28(8):819–828.
164. White RF, Krengel M, Proctor S, et al. Neuropsychological findings among Persian Gulf War veterans. Presentation at the Federally Sponsored Gulf War Veterans' Illnesses Research Conference. Washington: June 1998.
165. Reference deleted by author.
166. Kurtz D, White T, Belknap E. Perceived odor intensity and hedonics in subjects with multiple chemical sensitivity. *Chem Senses* 1993;18:584.
167. Hiramoto R, Ghanta V, Solvason B, et al. Identification of specific pathways of communication between the CNS and NK cell system. *Life Sci* 1993;53:527.
168. Madden K, Felten D. Experimental basis for neural-immune interactions. *Physiol Rev* 1995;75:77.
169. Levy J, Bell K, Lachar B, Fernandez F. Psychoneuroimmunology. In: Rolak L, Harati Y, eds. *Neuroimmunology for the clinician.* Boston: Butterworth–Heinemann, 1996:35–55.
170. Kort W. The effect of chronic stress on the immune system. *Adv Neuroimmunol* 1994;4:1–11.
171. Martins T, Aguas A. Stress modulates acute inflammation triggered by mycobacteria in autoimmunity-prone and normal mice. *Inflamm Res* 1995;44:393–399.
172. Demitrack MA, Dale JK, Straus SE. Evidence for impaired activation of the hypothalamic-pituitary-adrenal axis in patients with chronic fatigue syndrome. *J Clin Endocrinol Metab* 1991;73:1224–1234.
173. Crofford LJ, Pillemer SR, Kalogeras KT. Hypothalamic-pituitary-adrenal axis perturbations in patients with fibromyalgia. *Arthritis Rheum* 1994;37:1583–1592.
174. Yehuda R, Teicher MH, Trestman RL, Levengood RA, Siever LJ. Cortisol regulation in posttraumatic stress disorder and major depression: a chronobiological analysis. *Biol Psychiatry* 1996;40:79–88.
175. Bolla-Wilson K, Wilson RJ, Bleecker ML. Conditioning of physical symptoms after neurotoxic exposure. *J Occup Med* 1988;30:684–686.
176. Siegel S, Kreutzer R. Pavlovian conditioning and multiple chemical sensitivity. *Environ Health Perspect* 1997;105[Suppl 2]:521–526.
177. Stewart J, Vezina P. Extinction procedures abolish conditioned stimulus control but spare sensitized responding to amphetamine. *Behav Pharmacol* 1991;2:65–71.
178. Post RM, Weiss SRB, Pert A. The role of context and conditioning in behavioral sensitization to cocaine. *Psychopharmacol Bull* 23:425–429 (1987).
179. Terr AI. Multiple chemical sensitivities [Editorial]. *Ann Intern Med* 1993;119:163–164.
180. Gots RE. Multiple chemical sensitivities—public policy. *Clin Toxicol* 1995;33:111–113.
181. Johnson SK, DeLuca J, Natelson BH. Assessing somatization disorder in the chronic fatigue syndrome. *Psychosom Med* 1996;58:50–57.
182. Hudson JI, Geldenberg DL, Pope HG, Keck P, Schlesinger L. Comorbidity of fibromyalgia with medical and psychiatric disorders. *Am J Med* 1992;92:363–367.
183. Bell IR, Schwartz GE, Peterson JM, Amend D. Self-reported illness from chemical odors in young adults without clinical syndromes or occupational exposures. *Arch Environ Health* 1993;48:6–13.
184. Charney DS, Deutch AY, Krystal JH, Southwick SM, Davis M. Psychobiologic mechanisms of posttraumatic stress disorder. *Arch Gen Psychiatry* 1993;50:294–305.
185. Gabbard GO, Goodwin FK. Integrating biological and psychosocial perspectives. In: Dickstein LJ, Riba MB, Oldham JM, eds. *Review of psychiatry,* vol 15. Washington: American Psychiatric Press, 1996:527–548.
186. Perna G, Barbini B, Cocchi S, Bertani A, Gasperini M. 35% CO_2 challenge in panic and mood disorders. *J Affect Disord* 1995;33:189–194.
187. Pitman RK, van der Kolk BA, Orr SP, Greenberg MS. Naloxone-reversible analgesic response to combat-related stimuli in posttraumatic stress disorder. *Arch Gen Psychiatry* 1990;47:541–544.
188. van der Kolk BA, Greenberg MS, Orr SP, Pitman RK. Endogenous opioids, stress induced analgesia, and posttraumatic stress disorder. *Psychopharmacol Bull* 1989;25:417–421.
189. Yehuda R, Antelman SM. Criteria for rationally evaluating animal models of posttraumatic stress disorder. *Biol Psychiatry* 1993;33:479–486.
190. Miller NS, Stimmel B, eds. *Comorbidity of addictive and psychiatric disorders.* New York: Haworth Press, 1993.
191. Shalev A, Bleich A, Ursano RJ. Posttraumatic stress disorder: somatic comorbidity and effort tolerance. *Psychosomatics* 1990;31:197–203.
192. Heninger GR, Delgado PL, Charney DS. The revised monoamine theory of depression: a modulatory role for monoamines, based on new findings from monoamine depletion experiments in humans. *Pharmacopsychiatry* 1996;29:2–11.
193. Davidson RJ. EEG measures of cerebral asymmetry: conceptual and methodological issues. *Int J Neurosci* 1988;39:71–89.
194. Staudenmayer H. Clinical consequences of the EI/MCS "diagnosis": two paths. *Reg Toxicol Pharmacol* 1996;24:S96–S110.
195. American Medical Association, Council on Scientific Affairs. Clinical ecology. *JAMA* 1992;268:3465–3467.
196. Sparks PJ, Daniell W, Black DW, et al. Multiple chemical sensitivity syndrome: a clinical perspective. II. Evaluation, diagnostic testing, treatment, and social considerations. *J Occup Med* 1994;36:731–737.
197. LeRoy J, Davis TH, Jason LA. Treatment efficacy: a survey of 305 MCS patients. *The CFIDS Chronicle* Winter 1996;52–53.
198. Wihl J, Peterson B, Peterson L, et al. Effect of the nonsedative H-1 receptor antagonist astemizole in perennial allergic and nonallergic rhinitis. *J Allergy Clin Immunol* 1985;75(6):720–727.
199. Byrne A, Byrne D. The effect of exercise on depression, anxiety and other mood states: a review. *J Psychosom Res* 1993;37(6):565–574.
200. Futterman A, Kemeny M, Shapiro D, Fahey J. Immunological and physiological changes associated with induced positive and negative mood. *Psychosom Med* 1994;56:499–511.

SECTION

IV

Environmental Health Hazards of Business, Industry, Sites, and Locations

CHAPTER 33

Semiconductor Manufacturing Hazards

Michael L. Fischman

Electronics is projected to be the world's largest industry in terms of revenue. Semiconductor integrated circuits, known as *chips*, underpin the entire electronics industry. Worldwide sales of semiconductor devices are approximately $132 billion, with U.S. companies accounting for approximately 40% of the revenue (1).

The number of people directly involved in semiconductor manufacturing is surprisingly small. U.S. Department of Labor figures for 1995 place total employment in the industry in the United States at approximately 235,000, with five states (i.e., California, Texas, Oregon, Massachusetts, and New York, in descending order) accounting for nearly 60% of employment (2). Probably no more than 45,000 people, however, work in clean rooms directly handling the product. The remaining total are employed in a variety of engineering, non–clean room manufacturing, support, sales, and administrative functions. From a health perspective, this small group of clean room workers requires much more attention because of the large number of chemical and physical hazards associated with clean room operations.

Potential health risks in semiconductor manufacturing occur from the manufacture of substrate through the completed chip. Three broad areas of concern for occupational exposures are the following:

1. The clean room environment
2. The manufacturing process and tools
3. Selected chemicals used

The complex nature of this highly competitive industry and rapid changes in technology and materials pose obstacles to the delineation of health risks. Knowledge of manufacturing processes and controls, coupled with an understanding of the inherent toxicology of the chemicals used, enables a health professional to make informed assessments of health risks in the semiconductor industry.

CLEAN ROOM

Electronic device fabrication occurs in an environment that demands unusual accommodations by workers. Many of the work-related health problems observable among semiconductor workers are directly attributable to the clean room environment rather than to any of the process chemicals.

Semiconductor wafers are processed in clean rooms that are designed to minimize deposition of airborne particles onto the product. Federal Standard 209-D defines environmental classes of such rooms; the most frequently used parameter is the maximum number of particles of diameter 0.5 μm or greater per cubic foot of air (0.028 m^3). For example, a class 10,000 clean room is defined as having no more than 10,000 0.5-μm particles per cubic foot of air. A similar count in normal ambient air would typically exceed 500,000 particles per cubic foot. As circuit geometries shrink, manufacturers concentrate on progressively smaller particles, in addition to maintaining lower particle concentrations. Production clean rooms that average much less than one particle equaling or exceeding 0.1 μm diameter per cubic foot are not uncommon and are expected to be the norm.

It is difficult to understand the potential health hazards in clean rooms without understanding the techniques used to create particle-free environments. Essentially, three configurations or generations of semiconductor clean rooms exist (3):

Mixed-flow rooms usually combined with vertical-laminar-flow workstations
Mixed-flow rooms arranged into aisles and core areas
Vertical-laminar-flow clean rooms

Clean Room Design and Evolution

The original controlled environments in semiconductor manufacturing were relatively airtight rooms kept under positive pressure, in which air was continuously filtered to remove particles. Filtered air entered through vents in the ceiling and exited through vents placed in side walls near the floor. Airflow in these rooms (often termed *mixed-flow*) was random and turbulent; therefore, particles remained suspended for long periods of time. Many air changes (one air change amounts to replacing the equivalent of the volume of air contained in the room) were required before all particles were flushed from the room.

The next generation of clean rooms provided specially designed clean workstations used in combination with these mixed-flow clean rooms (Fig. 33-1). These freestanding stations provide a small workspace in which filtered air flows in parallel lines (*laminar flow*). Laminar flow is extremely efficient at removing particles from the air. The stations also use high-efficiency particulate air (HEPA) filters to capture particles. HEPA filters, whether they are in freestanding hoods or in the ceiling of the clean room, effectively remove all particles larger than 0.05 μm in diameter.

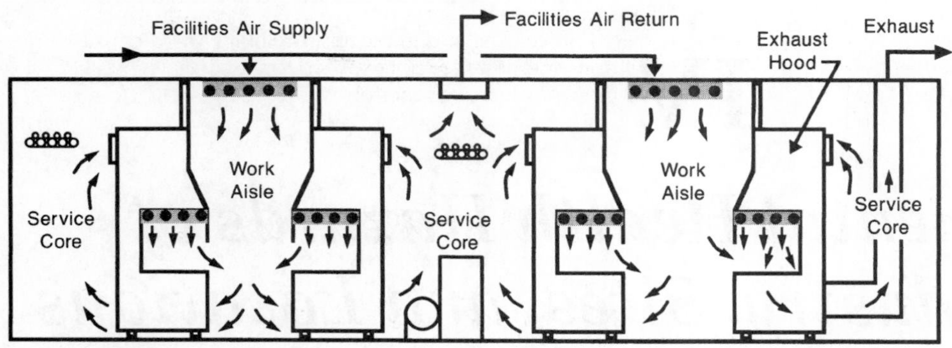

Figure 33-1. Older clean room with clean workstations.

Clean room workstations were a decided improvement for the product but not necessarily for the worker. Although they appear similar to ventilation hoods used in a chemical laboratory, they are not intended to protect the worker (i.e., to pull air inward and upward away from the worker). In fact, some air is always being pushed out the front of the hoods toward the worker's breathing zone (Fig. 33-2). This ventilation technique used in clean room workstations protects the product under the hood from any particles in the room, but can expose the worker to vapors or other air contaminants being generated in the workstation. HEPA filters are ineffective at removing gases or vapors. If vapors are generated, protection of the worker requires the addition of a separate externally vented exhaust system at each workstation. These types of clean room configurations are only seen in older facilities that have not been upgraded.

The next step in the evolution of clean rooms was to arrange workstations adjacent to one another to form aisles. In this arrangement, the rear of the workstation faced a service core in which all the tool equipment, wet chemicals, and gas distribution lines and facilities were located. Partitions filled the space between the top of the hoods and the ceiling to physically separate the work aisles from the core areas (Fig. 33-3).

The workstation's hood air intakes are in the core areas. The air is pulled into the back of the workstation hood, and then it goes up to the top of the hood where a fan pushes it down through a HEPA filter. The air spills over the work surface and out into the work aisle. Approximately 85% of the airflow into the work aisles comes through these hoods. The remaining air is supplied through HEPA filters in the ceiling of the clean room.

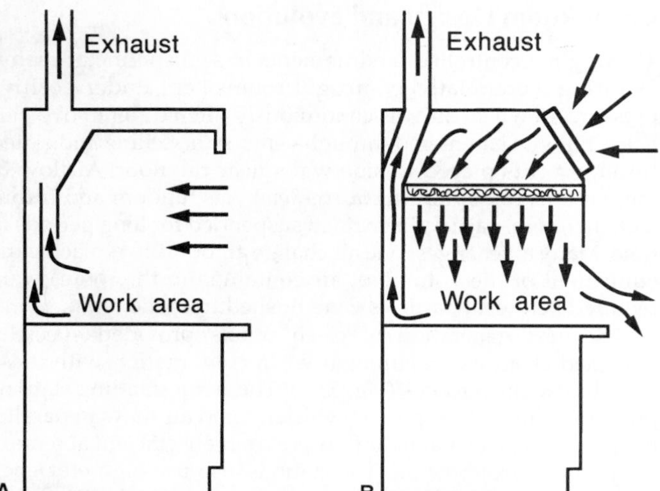

Figure 33-2. Airflow in traditional ventilation hoods (A) and in semiconductor clean room hoods (B).

The air entering through the ceiling is conditioned air, the temperature and humidity of which have been adjusted within prescribed parameters. Air exits the work aisles through vents in the side walls to the core areas. Part of the air in the cores returns via air plenums to the facility ventilation system, but most returns directly to the clean room via the workstation hoods.

Airflow remains relatively turbulent in this configuration, although other features yield a significantly cleaner environment for the product. The design focuses all freshly filtered air at the work aisle while return air is channeled through the service core. This results in a high air change rate of 250 to 300 air changes per hour in the work aisle, combining air recirculated through the hoods and facilitating ventilation. Consequently, this system is able to achieve airborne particle levels much lower than those found in standard mixed-flow clean rooms. Many of these rooms achieve better than class 100 in the work aisles.

Because the bulk of the air entering the clean room is recirculated from the core areas, workers can be exposed to any contaminants released in the core area. Among these contaminants are any gas leaks from uncontrolled lines or cylinders, oil mists from pumps and tools, vapors from wet chemical spills, and air from work aisles that communicate with the same core. Additionally, the equipment in some core areas generates large heat loads that are circulated directly into the work aisles. This sometimes results in individual aisles that are uncomfortably warm.

The state of the art in clean room ventilation is the vertical-laminar-flow (VLF) clean room. Air above the ceiling pressurizes a plenum that is comprised of HEPA filters. The air flows straight down through the room to exit through perforations in a raised floor. In some facilities, air is captured in a plenum under the floor and is returned through ducts to the ceiling plenum. Other VLF facilities direct the air exiting the perforated floor through the service core (also termed *service bay* or *service chase*), from which it returns to the ceiling plenum. Although this airflow pattern provides protection for the product, it also yields additional protection to workers from gas and vapor leaks in the service cores. Straight laminar flow prevents eddying of air currents, and particles are effectively contained within the area in which they

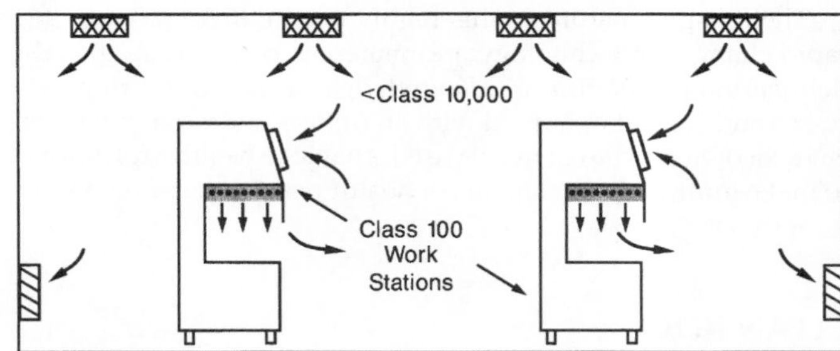

Figure 33-3. Work aisle and core area type 1 configuration of clean room.

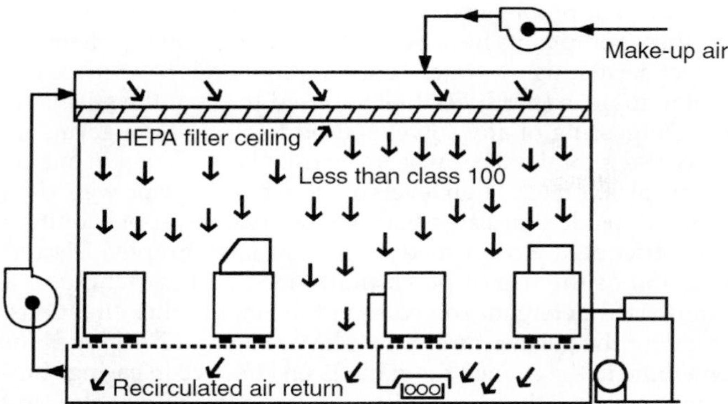

Figure 33-4. Vertical-laminar-flow room. HEPA, high-efficiency particulate air.

are generated. Air moves down through the room like a giant piston, quickly driving all particles through the floor (Fig. 33-4). In VLF clean rooms, the entire volume of air in the room is recirculated and refiltered 9 to 10 times per minute, or approximately every 6 seconds. Better than class 1 environments can be achieved. Thus, a typical fabrication (fab) facility is divided into production bays and maintenance (service) chases. Laminar airflow is provided through the entire ceiling of each production bay and is returned through a perforated raised floor in the bay to the maintenance chase, from which it flows back into the interstitial plenum above the ceiling to be recirculated through HEPA filters before returning to the production bay. Noticeably absent in the VLF environment are the individual workstation hoods that are integral to mixed-flow clean rooms. Tool exhaust systems are the same as those in other semiconductor clean rooms.

The VLF clean room is a marked improvement for product yield and for diminishing worker exposure to chemicals. Even in this environment, it must be remembered that low concentrations of vapors or other airborne chemicals, not captured by local exhaust systems, escape from wet tools, from which they are quickly distributed and diluted into the entire volume of the clean room. In contrast, gas contamination of the clean room environment generally requires a significant tool failure or other accident. Health professionals faced with specific employee complaints or with more general questions of long-term safety should to take the time to understand the details of any clean room ventilation scheme. Clean rooms are not generic and are no longer exclusive to the semiconductor industry. The aerospace, medical products, ceramics, chemical, biotechnology, and pharmaceutical industries have included clean rooms in many of their processes.

Protection of Workers from Airborne Contaminants

To protect workers from uncontrolled releases, process tools and process lines delivering chemicals are enclosed and externally vented through an exhaust system. If inadvertent leaks occur, they are readily swept out of the work area. *Wet stations* with open baths of chemicals can generate mists or vapors during normal processing. Exhaust ventilation is provided as slotted exhaust around the perimeter of each sink, as well as slots to the rear, both of which remove contaminated air. It is necessary to provide a fine balance between the laminar airflow and exhaust to prevent the product from being contaminated, as well as to prevent emissions from escaping from the front of the wet station toward the worker.

Many dry plasma processes mix chemicals and gases, some of which are highly toxic, in low-pressure closed reactor chambers that are exhausted through vacuum pumps to a scrubber or other treatment device before release to the atmosphere. During normal processing and in the absence of an accident or tool malfunction, operators are not exposed to the gases or exhaust products of these enclosed reactions. Tool maintenance personnel, as discussed throughout subsequent sections, have greater opportunity for exposure when chambers are opened.

Air Exchange in Clean Rooms

Constant loss of air from the clean room circulation occurs through the tool exhausts. These losses are replaced with outside air, causing a continual dilution of clean room air. Any makeup air must be conditioned and adds a new particle load that must be filtered. Facilities engineers prefer to minimize this burden, but because of losses through tool exhausts, they have no choice but to continually add fresh air. The volume of makeup air can be considerable. For instance, a single wet station can exhaust approximately 1,500 to 2,000 cubic feet of air per minute (42 to 56 m^3), and a chemical vapor deposition tool or dry etch reactor approximately 650 cubic feet per minute (18.2 m^3). A good rule of thumb is that 10% of the total clean room volume is being removed (and replaced by outside air) per hour. In the case of a particularly noxious odor or irritating vapor, building engineers can purge the entire clean room volume much more rapidly.

Clean Room Health Problems

Semiconductor clean rooms can be described as hot, dry, and windy. Process optimization requires close control of the temperature, which is maintained at approximately 68° to 75°F. Humidity is maintained constant from 15% to 50% to protect wafers from condensation of water droplets. This warm, relatively dry air is moving constantly at 80 to 100 linear feet per minute. These three conditions, especially the rapid air movement, dehydrate the stratum corneum of the skin and the mucous membranes.

SKIN PROBLEMS IN THE SEMICONDUCTOR CLEAN ROOM

Rycroft has written on the importance of "low-humidity occupational dermatoses" that can manifest as either pruritus, urticaria, or eczema (4,5). Workers with recurrent, intractable dermatoses that rarely receive a specific etiologic diagnosis occasionally demand a medical transfer out of the clean room.

Health professionals faced with dermatitis from the clean room too often pursue a chemical irritant or putative allergen, when the problem can often be easily ameliorated by maintaining hydration of the stratum corneum. Prevention is the best strategy. Some skin problems can be avoided by offering a selection of clean room approved moisturizing creams or lotions in the change areas. The possibility that the formulation of a specific cream may further aggravate the problem should be remembered. An added benefit of skin hydration is decreased shedding of dry skin particles into the processing environment.

SENSITIZATION

It is likely that dehydrated, microfissured skin is at increased risk of irritation or sensitization. Health professionals sometimes attempt patch testing to try to rule out the possibility of chemical allergy. However, this diagnostic technique is imperfect and only occasionally yields useful information (6,7). This is especially true when testing with unknown compounds or compounds for which clinical experience in testing is limited.

UPPER RESPIRATORY PROBLEMS

Other problems besides dermatoses are directly attributable to the warm, dry environment. Complaints of mucous membrane dryness of the eye, nose, and throat are relatively common. Recurrent epistaxis, sinusitis, and laryngitis are problems that occur in a very small percentage of workers. Often, dryness can be controlled by encouraging and facilitating regular intake of water, sometimes supplemented by the use of over-the-counter nasal sprays.

ASTHMA

Asthmatics sometimes find that the clean room air worsens their symptoms, perhaps because of drying of the airways. An alternative, but generally less likely explanation (assuming properly functioning exhaust systems), is that low levels of airborne chemicals are aggravating or precipitating bronchospasm. For allergic asthmatics, an anecdotal suggestion is that their asthma may improve in the clean room, reflecting reduced exposure to environmental aeroallergens. In any case, no need exists for preplacement restrictions for asthmatics.

EYE PROBLEMS

The semidesert conditions of the semiconductor clean room can also contribute to eye problems. Some workers complain of constantly irritated eyes, but usually this can be ameliorated by the use of over-the-counter eyedrops to moisturize the conjunctivae. Individuals with problems such as a chronic corneal ulcer or chronic or recurring conjunctivitis often fare poorly and may have to be transferred.

Contact lens use had historically not been permitted in clean rooms. The reason had been the fear that contact lenses might contribute to a chemical injury of the eye. Prohibition of contact lens use in clean rooms, as in industry as a whole, is an outdated policy that is based on unsubstantiated rumors and fears. In fact, experimental and anecdotal evidence exists that contact lenses provide some protection against either chemical or mechanical insult (8,9). Obviously, contact lenses by themselves do not serve as adequate protection against either form of injury. Appropriate eye protection must be worn with or without contact lenses.

Contact lenses may be troublesome for some clean room workers because of the dry air, not because of the intermittent presence of chemicals in the environment. Workers requiring visual correction should be allowed to choose between spectacles and contact lenses.

Garments

Clean room garments provide protection of wafers from people. These garments are worn generally over a worker's own clothes to prevent shedding of contaminant particles. Skin flakes, hair follicles, dust on clothes, cosmetics, and skin bacteria are all frequent sources of contamination. Dressed in his or her own clothes, a person sitting and working sheds from 500,000 to 1,000,000 particles per minute (10). When walking, the number increases to 5,000,000 to 10,000,000 particles per minute. Clean room garments keep most of these particles out of the manufacturing environment.

The suits are designed and woven to minimize fraying and shedding of particles or fibers. Gore-Tex (polytetrafluoroethylene) laminate is sometimes used. Disposable Tyvek (spunbound olefin) suits are commonly worn by visitors.

Many garments also incorporate a small percentage of conductive carbon filaments (approximately 1% by weight) that dissipate static electricity. High-density, very large scale integrated circuits can be damaged by voltages as low as 20 V—several orders of magnitude less than the charge that can be generated from a clean room worker.

Clean room suits are laundered and repaired at special facilities that maintain a class 100 environment. Workers often attribute skin problems to garment laundering, and, occasionally, these complaints have been substantiated. One epidemic of contact dermatitis was traced back to high levels of residual tetrachlorethylene (perchlorethylene) used to clean the garments (11). Outgassing of any solvents used to clean these garments before use is minimal because the garments are sealed in impermeable plastic bags. High levels of tetrachlorethylene were documented inside the sealed bags using organic vapor monitors and subsequently confirmed by gas chromatography. Discontinuation of the use of perchlorethylene and switching to a water-based detergent solved the problem. In other situations, removing the garment from the plastic bag and hanging it for some time in the change room has been effective in easing complaints, apparently by permitting outgassing of dry cleaning solvents before garment wear.

Switching to a detergent is not a sure solution. Another clean room was afflicted with an epidemic of dermatitis that was eventually attributed to the alkalinity of residual detergent. This problem was solved when an additional rinse cycle was added to the cleaning procedure. In a semiconductor facility in Europe, an epidemic (i.e., five cases of facial dermatitis) was traced to high residual levels of the laundering chemical—in this case, peroxyacetic acid. Again, the problem was solved with the addition of another rinse cycle.

The possibility of irritation from residual cleaning chemicals trapped in clean room garments is a consideration that should be explored very early in the investigation of dermatitis. Health personnel should be especially suspicious of this possibility if the dermatitis is most noticeable on the skin that is in contact with seams on the garment. These seams are usually areas in which the material is folded over and stitched, making an efficient trap for residual laundering agents.

THERMAL ASPECTS OF CLEAN ROOM GARMENTS

Clean room garments can also cause thermal discomfort, because they represent an additional layer of relatively nonporous clothing in an environment that is already warm. No ability exists to open or shed clothing based on personal comfort. The perception of overheating is not unusual in areas near open diffusion furnaces. True hyperthermic syndromes have not been documented.

Fortunately, little physical labor is required of operators in the semiconductor clean room so that workers are not generating a significant internal heat load. An exception occurs in the maintenance of tools, which occasionally can be strenuous.

Hot flashes that accompany menopause can be quite intolerable in the clean room garment. Tight, misfitted garments also can contribute to overheating in the clean rooms. The need to protect the product must be balanced against worker comfort. It is not feasible to create a perfect barrier between the worker and the product.

HEADGEAR

In most instances, headgear has been a fabric hood designed to cover the head, mouth, and sometimes nose, leaving an exposed area for the eyes. In some situations, goggles have been added to this uniform. A fairly frequent phenomenon with entry into the clean room is the aggravation of facial acne. The problem is usually attributed to irritation from rubbing of the hoods. Work around clean room furnaces can cause sweating and aggravate acne. Acne might seem trivial in an industry replete with potential chemical catastrophes, but it is an issue of concern to affected employees. The acne typically responds to more aggressive conventional treatment. Very rarely, the only solution is medical transfer.

Bubble hoods or helmets that completely enclose the head and face have been introduced to some fabrication areas, typically those attempting to maintain very low particle counts. These hoods or helmets require a portable, powered blower to draw air into them. Exhausted air passes through a small HEPA filter, preventing the escape of contaminants and particles from the worker into the clean room. These hoods or helmets are not respirators; they are used to protect the product from particles. Self-contained breathing apparatuses have also been used in some situations. Any of these initiatives to further enclose the worker may make it more difficult for some workers to adapt. Some workers have complained of head or neck discomfort or skin problems in association with use of these hoods or helmets.

GLOVES

Latex or polyvinyl chloride gloves with no powder are usually part of the clean room uniform. Other synthetics, such as neoprene, nylon, and polyurethane, are sometimes used. Many workers find that their hands perspire in the gloves. Because the gloves are impermeable to water, they can be quite uncomfortable. A small percentage of workers cannot work in clean rooms because of their inability to wear these gloves without developing dermatitis. Most frequently, these difficulties are caused by an occlusive aggravation of a preexisting eczema or other latent dermatitis, caused by moisture, heat, friction, and occlusion. Workers with significant histories of eczema, including atopic, dyshidrotic, and irritant contact eczema involving the hands, psoriasis, lichen planus of the hands, or with chronic paronychia often do not fare well in occlusive gloves. Wearing cotton or nylon underliners under the occlusive gloves sometimes ameliorates a dermatitis. Good hand hygiene, use of nonirritating soaps, use of moisturizers, and more frequent glove changes may also help. Occasionally, employees may develop an allergic contact dermatitis to a glove additive or accelerator, detectable on patch testing. Despite the increased attention to latex protein allergies in settings in which these gloves are regularly worn, such as health care institutions, latex allergy appears to be a very uncommon problem in the semiconductor industry, perhaps because of the use of high-quality, nonpowdered latex gloves. When problems caused by delayed or immediate hypersensitivity to glove materials occur, substitution is often difficult because of the demanding microcontamination (particle) control requirements to qualify new materials.

All the garment items discussed thus far are worn for the protection of the product, and offer little or no protection from chemicals in the work environment. With some processes, additional personal protective equipment must be worn.

Illumination

Yellow or amber light is provided in lithography areas of semiconductor manufacturing facilities. Some employees in this area complain about the yellow or amber light. The selective filtration of light is necessary to exclude ultraviolet radiation and the lower end of the visible spectrum, as semiconductor photoresists used in the lithography process are sensitive in the 300- to 400-nm spectrum. The complaints are nonspecific, but many workers state that they find the lighting depressing. No documented adverse health effects (physical or psychological) exist from exposure to this unnatural light.

Lighting that is unnecessarily bright can aggravate the perception of heat in the clean rooms. Fifty foot-candles of illumination (4.6 lux) are adequate for almost all clean room operations, but higher levels are frequently encountered. Lowering the level of illumination from 80 to 50 foot-candles (7.4 to 4.6 lux) in one clean room aisle markedly decreased employee complaints of overheating.

Noise

VLF clean rooms can be noisy because of the large ventilation systems and the tool noise. Measurements of 70 to 75 dB are common noise levels, but higher readings are occasionally documented. These noise levels pose no potential damage to hearing and are below any threshold for other extraauditory effects of noise. Nonetheless, visitors are surprised at the difficulty in carrying on conversation in these environments. The garment hoods or helmets covering ears and mouth contribute to this difficulty. Some workers with hearing impairment find the environment very difficult. Completely deaf workers tend to have no problems. Even in the absence of the opportunity to read lips, they usually have developed effective alternative systems of communication.

Ionization of Air

Air filtration removes ions and therefore increases the accumulation of static electricity on surfaces (including wafers). The dryness of the clean room makes control of static electricity all the more difficult. Some semiconductor manufacturers intentionally add ions to the clean room to lessen the possibility of product damage from electrical static discharge.

Speculation about whether the lack of negative ions in air can cause adverse health effects is a recurring topic, for which no scientific support exists. Of more concern is the fact that ionization systems (static eliminators) used in clean rooms can generate ozone. Health professionals should be aware of this possibility and the possible respiratory effects. Instances have occurred in which entire semiconductor fabrication buildings have been evacuated and temporarily closed because of high ozone levels. In one case, six fabrication workers presented simultaneously with symptoms of irritation of eyes and throats, headache, and shortness of breath. Exact ozone levels were not documented but were well in excess of the threshold limit value (TLV) of 0.1 parts per million (ppm). The building was temporarily closed, the ion generators were eliminated, and the problem did not recur.

Another device used by some manufacturers to lessen electrical static discharge is a sealed polonium 210 source that emits alpha particles. These are sometimes placed at every workstation. They can present a health hazard if the source is broken and workers either inhale or ingest polonium particles.

Problems of Shift Work

Building and equipment overhead contributes a little more than 50% to the cost of a completed chip. Chemicals and supplies are approximately 40% of the cost, and labor is no more than 10%. Semiconductor manufacturers are therefore pressured to minimize equipment purchases and operate around the clock. The health effects of unusual shifts are not unique to this industry. Any health professional working in this industry should become knowledgeable about the physiologic and social aspects of this difficult subject. Particularly difficult to solve are work-life issues that often present initially as medical problems.

Psychological Problems

Clean room environments are notable for emotional sterility and dehumanized surroundings. Walls and furniture are usually gray or white metal or plastic. The ambient lighting in some areas is a pale yellow or amber color. Windows are rare and usually look out on equally uninteresting production areas or hallways. No change occurs in temperature or humidity, regardless of time of year. Airflow is even and constant, and the ventilation systems create a persistent mechanical noise. Generally, no music is allowed.

Everyone in the semiconductor clean room is dressed in identical garments that conceal any individual identity. Personal features, such as jewelry or makeup, are not visible. In some settings, name tags are viewed as a potential source of contamination and are not used. It is difficult to see facial expressions because of the hoods that cover the mouth and forehead, although the newer helmets with blowers allow the whole face to be seen. Nevertheless, perhaps as a testament to our social natures, workers learn to recognize one another based on those limited features that are visible. No private workspaces, desks, or space that a worker can own or individualize exist. Limited areas for sitting exist.

Fewer particles are generated if human activity is inhibited. Rules or guidelines that discourage assembling in groups, rapid movement, or frequent entry and exit are common. In some organizations, employees are told to avoid excessive talking and to avoid humming, singing, and laughing, because all of these activities release contaminants from the mouth into the clean room. Movements are limited to those that are absolutely essential to the job. Rapid movements, such as twitching or gesturing or clapping hands, are avoided. Unfortunately, many of these rules are unrealistic. It is usual to see small groups of workers talking and laughing while they wait for processes to finish. The benefit to morale and, ultimately, productivity of this communal behavior probably outweighs the losses incurred from additional particle generation.

The typical work of semiconductor fabrication can be repetitive and monotonous. Basically, the job of many operators is to carry wafers to a tool, load them, and log the job number into a keyboard. The tool is connected to a central computer from which it receives detailed instructions on the parameters of the process. A separate group of process engineers monitors the product and makes all the decisions about changes in the process. Tools are extremely complex, and often routine maintenance is done by a small group of technicians. However, some manufacturers have begun to involve operators in significant maintenance activities, thus blurring the distinction between operators and technicians and presumably increasing the challenges and opportunities for operators.

With many tasks, the largest part of the job is simply waiting for a tool to finish a process step so that the wafers can be moved to the next tool. It has been estimated that a semiconductor clean room operator typically spends approximately 10% of the shift actively working and the remainder waiting. Some jobs are exceptions to this generalization. Photoexposure tool work and inspection of wafers with microscopes are two examples in which the work is continuous.

Workers may have very little sense of ownership of the final product because of the great number of processing steps (often more than 500). The importance of one's contribution to these microscopic devices is difficult to appreciate. Little sense of craftsmanship exists. To some extent, this notion may be countered by the sharing of statistics regarding yield and productivity, management recognition of contributions, and more participative team and group management.

The potential for dissatisfaction with or even alienation from one's work, sometimes resulting from the organizational, job design, and environmental factors, is certainly not unique to the semiconductor industry. However, from the perspective of a health professional, it may affect the reporting of complaints, discomfort, and injuries, and may increase the anxiety associated with exposures and health hazards.

PHYSICAL ISOLATION OF THE CLEAN ROOM

Because of the special garments and, in some cases, the need for multiple clothes changes, clean room ingress and egress are difficult and time-consuming. Other company personnel seldom enter. Management offices are outside the manufacturing floor because of the high cost of clean room space. Clean rooms that are currently under construction offer increased barriers to access; as many as three separate clothes changes are required before entry.

PSYCHOLOGICAL EFFECTS OF THE ENVIRONMENT

To what extent the unnatural environment, the physical isolation, and the unstimulating work content affect mood, psychology, or motivation is unstudied. Some observers have speculated that the semiconductor clean room operator is more likely to be depressed because of this environment. No data exist to support this idea. Health professionals who work in the industry state that clean room workers as a group seem to be no more afflicted with psychological problems than other manufacturing groups. In any case, it is important not to forget the unique and alien features of this environment. A few specific syndromes deserve discussion in the context of semiconductor clean rooms.

PHOBIAS

A variety of phobias can be aggravated by the environment and cause a small number of workers to be medically removed from clean rooms. Claustrophobia and chemophobia are the two most common. Either the physical environment or the restrictive headgear can precipitate the former. Phobias often manifest as classic panic attacks within hours or days of entry into this environment. It is not always easy for health professionals to distinguish between discontent and a true phobia, especially in cases that are slow to manifest. Psychiatric or psychological referral is important if this diagnosis is entertained. In some cases, desensitization therapy successfully treats the problem (12–14).

MULTIPLE CHEMICAL SENSITIVITIES

A proposed and controversial syndrome termed *multiple chemical sensitivities* refers to the occurrence of recurrent diverse symptoms involving multiple organ systems (e.g., variably central nervous system, gastrointestinal tract, skin, respiratory tract), reportedly occurring when the individual is exposed at very low levels to multiple chemically unrelated compounds (15). It seems unlikely that these symptoms, typically without any objective, conventionally accepted physical or laboratory findings, truly constitute a specific disorder. Patients with the condition have been found to have a high prevalence of psychiatric disorders, including depression and somatoform or somatization disorders, and no demonstrable evidence of any immunologic disorders (16).

Complaints suggestive of multiple chemical sensitivities are not commonly reported by semiconductor workers, but, given the not infrequent odors of chemicals reported in clean rooms, it is likely that such individuals have difficulty tolerating clean room work. Should they occur, these complaints should be addressed promptly by occupational health professionals. Although it is naïve to believe that the complaints are never exaggerated for the purpose of achieving a job transfer or a disability settlement, it is best to avoid such a judgment in any individual case. A percentage of these patients, particularly soon after onset of symptoms, benefit from reassurance, including review of data indicating lack of significant exposure and measures to prevent exposures, and psychiatric diagnosis and treatment. Any other approach is likely to steer the patient into the care of clinical ecologists or environmental medicine doctors who often inflict serious additional psychological and financial harm on these people (17).

MASS PSYCHOGENIC ILLNESS

Chemical odors are not uncommon in clean room settings. The combination of these odors with work that is often inherently monotonous, and the tendency to be isolated from management, makes a natural setting for mass psychogenic illness (MPI). The electronics industry has been particularly susceptible to this phenomenon (18,19).

MPI is suspected when an epidemic of symptoms occurs in individual members of a group of people, without any objective medical findings or any identifiable environmental explanation. MPI is not a clinical diagnosis; it is a sociologic phenomenon describing the collective behavior of a group of people (20).

The words *psychogenic* and *illness* imply that psychopathology is present in the affected individuals. Quite the opposite, the response, although not conscious, is a natural, healthy coping reaction to a stressful work situation perceived to be unresolvable.

The specific response of the occupational health team and line management to one of these episodes varies greatly from situation to situation. The best and quickest resolution is obtained if qualified occupational health professionals are directing the investigation.

Discussion of MPI is not meant to imply that every unexplained epidemic of symptoms in the clean room falls into this category. MPI should not be automatically invoked merely because of the absence of other explanations (20). A variety of symptoms (e.g., reflex nausea, headaches, and mucous membrane irritation) may occur as a direct result of unpleasant odors and concern about one's environment (21). Episodes of symptom occurrence that resemble indoor air quality problems, related to such factors as airflow, odor dispersion, temperature, and humidity, in office buildings have occurred in semiconductor manufacturing facilities. Many episodes of mass symptoms rightfully remain unexplained.

PROCESSES AND TOOLS USED IN SEMICONDUCTOR MANUFACTURING

Semiconductor manufacturing is divided into three groups of processes:

1. Substrate manufacture (making the wafer)
2. Device fabrication (making microelectronic devices, such as the transistors on the wafer)
3. Device interconnection (wiring together the devices to form a circuit)

In actual production of an integrated circuit, the substrate wafer passes through each process many times.

Substrate Manufacture

Integrated circuits are fashioned onto the surface of thin silicon wafers that typically vary from 3.25 to 8.00 and 12.00 in. in diameter (82.5 to 300.0 mm). Silicon is the basic substrate used to make more than 95% of wafers. The manufacture of the wafer or substrate does not take place in wafer fab facilities. It occurs in a few specialized independent facilities that then supply wafers to semiconductor manufacturers.

Raw silicon dioxide (quartz) is first reduced to silicon by melting in a carbon arc furnace at more than 1,900°C. This metallurgic-grade silicon is ground to a powder, heated, and exposed to high-purity hydrogen chloride gas, producing trichlorosilane ($SiCl_3H$). Trichlorosilane is reduced to very pure silicon by reacting it with hydrogen at a high temperature. This electronic-grade silicon has less than 1 part per billion of impurities. The ability to later create microscopic devices by selectively contaminating the silicon depends on starting with a pure substrate. As little as 1 ppm impurity in silicon can profoundly alter its electrical properties.

CRYSTAL PULLERS

Almost all crystal growth is done by the Czochralski method. The *crystal puller* tools are large tools in which a quartzite (i.e., noncrystalline silica) crucible holds molten silicon (1,420°C) heated by radiofrequency (RF) energy. A starter or seed crystal of silicon is placed onto the end of a rod and dipped into the melt. The rod is pulled out slowly and rotated while the molten silicon crucible is turned in the opposite direction. Silicon atoms attach to the rod, and the crystal grows in size.

The melt is usually selectively contaminated or *doped* with a few grams of boron powder to create silicon with a desired number of electron-deficient areas called *holes*. Phosphorus or arsenic is used to dope the melt if an area with a surplus of electrons is desired. The dopant comes in premeasured vials that present little opportunity for exposure.

Crystal growth occurs in an argon atmosphere to prevent oxidation of the silicon crystal and the introduction of impurities from air. Energy to heat the melt is supplied by RF heaters. Magnetic confinement of the melt using large external magnets (1,000 to 5,000 G, 0.1 to 0.5 T) is being used experimentally to lessen convective flow in the melt. This technique results in a structurally more uniform ingot. Finished ingots are usually approximately 2 ft long (61 cm) and weigh approximately 200 lb (90 km).

The ingot is removed from the reactor by using mechanical hoists, and the crucible is discarded. The graphite susceptor that holds the quartzite crucible should be vacuumed and then wiped with methanol or isopropyl alcohol. The debris on the susceptor is primarily silicon dioxide (SiO_2) and silicon carbide in large flakes and pieces that pose no inhalation hazard.

MACHINING OPERATIONS

The tools used in milling, grinding, and notching of the ingot, as well as slicing and lapping of the wafers, are standard metal machining tools. The hazards are primarily those of mechanical trauma, machining oils, and noise. Before machining, the ingot is attached to an aluminum or graphite key with an epoxy resin. It is then ground to a uniform-diameter cylinder. A small notch is machined lengthwise onto the ingot to assist in later positioning of wafers, resulting in one flat edge on each wafer. Wafers are sliced from the ingot at specific angles to ensure the desired crystal orientation on the processing surface. Internal diameter diamond saws are used in this operation. X-ray crystallography is used to position the ingots. Further edge contouring is done to complete the milling operations. Silicon dust from these operations has no special toxicity, but is generally kept well below nuisance standards by using wet processes.

LAPPING

Lapping is done to achieve flatness and parallelism on both sides of the wafers. State-of-the-art processing technologies require wafers with 1 nm or less variation in the elevations on the surface of the wafer. Most lapping operations use slurries of either alumina or silicon carbide. The machines enclose the wafers, and pressures are adjusted automatically.

ACID ETCH

After the machining operations, the wafer surface is chemically etched in *silicon etch*, a mixture of nitric, acetic, and hydrofluoric acids. This is followed by an etch with chromic acid and hydrofluoric acid. Filling the baths and handling the wafers require standard precautions to protect skin and eyes. The ventilation hood over a wet station in these non–clean room settings is a standard hood that pulls air away from the worker. Complaints about acid aerosols are rare to nonexistent at these well-ventilated workstations.

POLISHING

Before polishing, the wafers are usually preannealed in furnaces in an atmosphere of nitrogen and hydrogen chloride. To polish wafers, a table holding an abrasive pad rotates while the plates holding the wafers are pressed against it. The wafers are bathed in a slurry of colloidal silica and potassium hydroxide at a pH of approximately 11. The polishing is accomplished by a chemical-mechanical reaction rather than mechanical friction alone. A colloid of SiO_2 and silicon hydroxide (SiOH) forms between the silica particles and the wafer surface, and pulls SiO_2 off the wafer. The process is well enclosed so that exposure to the highly alkaline solution is not a concern while the machines are running. After polishing, class one lasers are used to scribe an identification number on each wafer.

CLEANING

The last step in wafer preparation is removing the silica colloid in a mixture of HCl-H_2O_2 or H_2SO_4-H_2O_2, followed by rinsing in deionized water. These are standard wet station operations, with good ventilation. Some manufacturers have substituted less corrosive solutions with which to clean the wafers, such as 5% sodium hypochlorite, because some workers developed irritation of eyes and upper airway. A tendency exists in the industry to move away from any chlorine-containing solutions because of contamination problems with chloride ions in later processing. Organic surfactants, such as ethoxylated amines, are being introduced as substitutes. A final wafer-cleaning step uses ammonium hydroxide solution.

GALLIUM ARSENIDE WAFERS

Although the overwhelming majority of wafers continues to be silicon, some special applications (e.g., generally optoelectronics, military hardware, or very high-speed semiconductors) warrant the use of gallium arsenide (GaAs). The primary advantage of GaAs compared with silicon is that electrons move 5 to 6 times faster in GaAs. Unfortunately, GaAs wafer manufacture is much more hazardous than the manufacture of silicon wafers and, therefore, requires more stringent industrial hygiene controls than has been customary with silicon.

Polycrystalline GaAs material is formed by reacting elemental arsenic and elemental gallium inside a sealed tube at high temperatures. Workers are potentially exposed to arsenic when preparing the reaction vessel and removing products. The greatest potential exposure occurs with milling. The polycrystalline GaAs is milled to remove oxides. The ends are sawed off, and the entire chunk is sandblasted. Air levels of arsenic ranging from 540 to 1,500 μg per m^3 have been measured in these areas (22).

Single crystal GaAs ingots are manufactured from the polycrystalline product by several different methods. The first is a liquid-encapsulated Czochralski technique similar to the crystal pulling of silicon ingots. The main difference is that the surface of the melted GaAs is covered with a layer of molten boron oxide that prevents the loss of vaporized gallium at the high temperatures needed to melt arsenic. The process is enclosed and offers no hazard while in operation. Cleaning a GaAs crystal puller is an extremely hazardous procedure. The graphite susceptor is first vacuumed and the surfaces are wiped with isopropyl alcohol. Personal sampling done by the National Institute of Occupational Safety and Health (NIOSH) has documented average exposures in excess of 1,000 μg per m^3 of air during these cleaning operations (22). Self-contained breathing apparatuses under positive pressure or an air-supplied respirator must be used to provide adequate protection. Access to the room during cleaning procedures should be highly restricted, and frequent area sampling is necessary to identify potential air contamination.

The other method used to manufacture GaAs ingots is the horizontal Bridgeman technique. Elemental arsenic is loaded into one end of a horizontal quartz ampule, and liquid gallium is loaded into a small boat in the other end. A seed crystal of GaAs is placed into the ampule to provide the initial structure for the growth, then heated and cooled. After cooling, the ampule is broken and discarded and the ingot removed. Sampling data have demonstrated that this process is inherently cleaner than the crystal puller method, but the exposure potential is still well in excess of accepted standards (22).

Subsequent machining operations are similar to those used with silicon ingots, but the GaAs dust must be treated as inorganic arsenic dust. Sampling data in these areas has shown them to be cleaner than some other parts of GaAs processing, but still in excess of the NIOSH's Recommended Exposure Level (REL) of 10 μg per m^3 (22).

OTHER ELEMENTS IN COLUMNS THREE AND FIVE OF THE PERIODIC TABLE USED FOR ELECTRONIC DEVICE FABRICATION

GaAs is the only material that has gained acceptance in the microelectronics industry as a substitute for silicon substrate. Six of the ten elements in columns three and five of the periodic table (III and V) lend themselves to electronic device fabrication: aluminum, gallium, indium, phosphorous, arsenic, and antimony. The other four elements are not generally used, because their atomic size precludes easy combination. Boron and nitrogen are too small, and thallium and bismuth are too large. Exotic binary, tertiary, and quaternary combinations of III and V materials are common in research labs and pilot operations. It is likely that some of these materials ultimately will enter into production. With them come more advanced growth techniques, such as molecular beam epitaxy and metalloorganic chemical vapor deposition. Unfortunately, investigation of the toxicology of the exotic metalloorganic chemicals used in these processes is in an embryonic stage.

SUMMARY OF WAFER MANUFACTURE

The manufacture of substrate wafers, including all of the steps discussed in this section, takes place before the receipt of the wafer by the semiconductor manufacturer. With the exception of gallium arsenide, wafer manufacture is relatively safe. Chemical use is less intensive than other parts of semiconductor manufacturing, and control engineering is better understood because the processes are not in the clean room environment.

Overview of Device Fabrication

The fabrication of microscopic electronic devices onto the surface of the wafers presents tremendous challenges for health and safety professionals. Device fabrication entails the large majority of all the chemical hazards encountered in semiconductor manufacturing. Wafers are the basic parts that are handled and reprocessed in a wafer fabrication process. Eventually, each wafer is cut into a hundred or more individual integrated circuits (i.e., chips). Transistors, diodes, resistors, and capacitors are the electronic components fabricated onto each wafer. This is accomplished by creating areas of altered electrical conductivity within the high-purity silicon substrate. Unadulterated silicon is a poor conductor of electricity because the four electrons in the outer shell are shared equally with contiguous silicon atoms, creating stable bonds. Addition to the silicon of materials, such as arsenic and phosphorus, that have an excess of electrons in their outer shell creates an electron-rich area. These areas are known as *n*, or *negative*, areas. Similarly, addition of materials (most commonly boron) that are deficient in electrons in their outer shell creates an area that is electron poor, known as a *p*, or *positive*, area. The interface between p and n areas is called the *p-n junction*. The ability to control the flow of electricity across p-n junctions was the fundamental discovery that is the basis of all microelectronic circuits. Doping of microscopic areas of the substrate is achieved through the technologies of ion implantation, diffusion, and chemical vapor deposition.

LITHOGRAPHY

Lithography means "writing in stone." In this case, the stone is a layer of SiO_2 created on the surface of the silicon substrate by oxidation. Patterns can be written into the SiO_2 by applying a protective layer (i.e., a *resist*) to selected areas of the SiO_2 surface and subsequently destroying the unprotected SiO_2 with a chemical etchant, such as a strong acid. In essence, the engineers are sculpting a bas-relief impression in the SiO_2 by means of a chemical attack rather than hammer and chisel. Destroying this protective layer of SiO_2 exposes the underlying silicon substrate to enable implantation with a dopant, such as arsenic.

After the implantation of a dopant into the substrate, the resist is stripped away from the remaining SiO_2 layer. The remaining SiO_2 can be completely removed or left as a base for a subsequent step in the process. Many processing steps (more than 500 in some complicated logic circuits) are required to manufacture a single microscopic device. Fortunately, many devices (up to 10 billion in memory applications) are created simultaneously on each wafer, and, in some steps, several hundred wafers are processed simultaneously. Figure 33-5 is a schematic representation of the basic steps in manufacturing microelectronic devices.

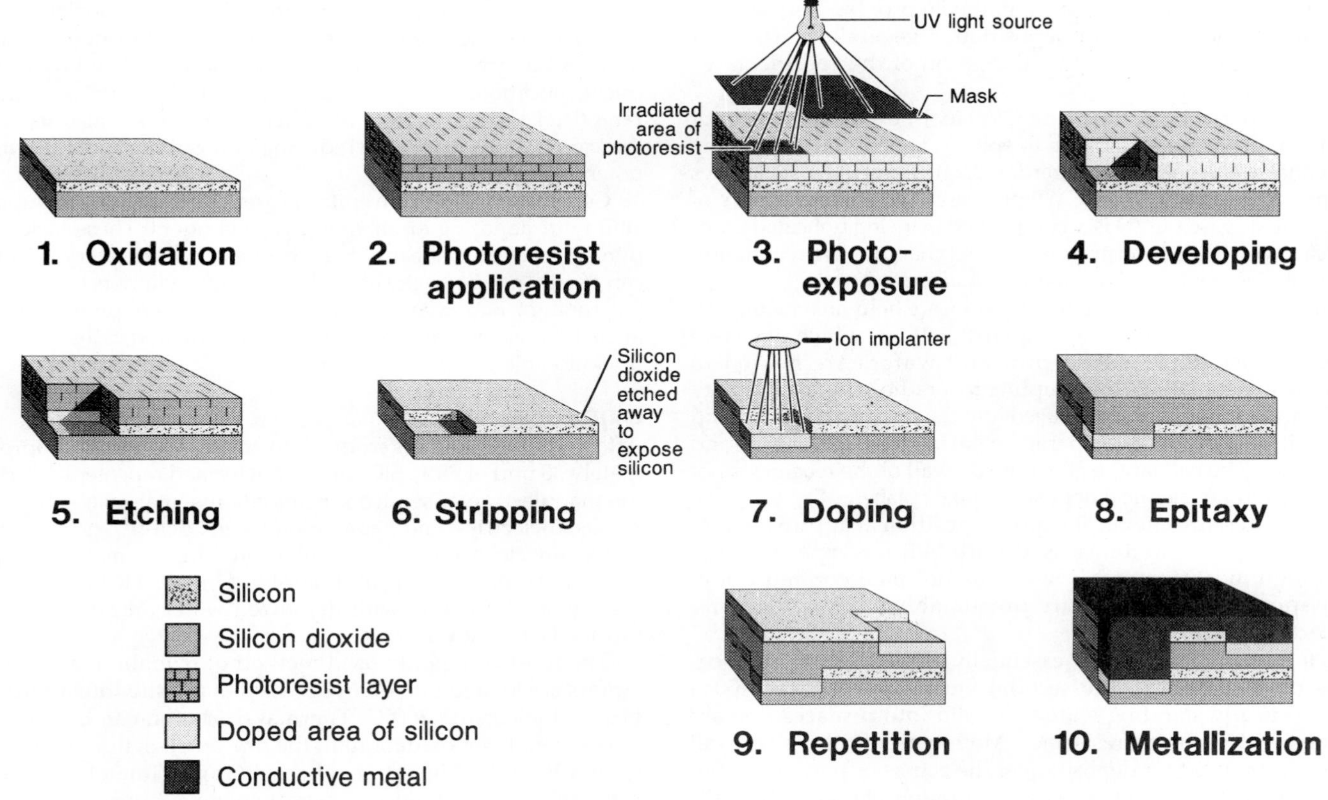

Figure 33-5. Schematic of manufacture of semiconductor devices.

1. *Oxidation*: The first step is to form a thin layer of chemically resistant silicon oxide over the surface of the silicon wafer. Sometimes, this is preceded by an epitaxial layer of silicon on silicon.
2. *Photoresist application*: The silicon dioxide layer is located with a thin protective layer called a *photoresist*.
3. *Photoexposure*: The coated wafer is exposed to ultraviolet radiation through a mask that allows light to strike only parts of the photoresist surface. Masks determine the patterns or circuits in the photoresist. With a typical positive photoresist, the areas struck by light undergo a chemical reaction that makes the photoresist more soluble in an alkaline solution.
4. *Developing*: The developer is an alkaline solution that removes the areas of the photoresist that were exposed to ultraviolet light. The silicon dioxide under removed areas of photoresist is now protected and can be attacked by etching. The underdeveloped or remaining photoresist is hardened by baking to a surface much like the enamel on an automobile.
5. *Etching*: The unprotected silicon dioxide is etched away either by hydrofluoric acid (i.e., wet etching) or by ionized gases (i.e., dry etching). The photoresist layer protects the silicon dioxide that engineers do not wish to remove.
6. *Stripping*: The remaining photoresist has served its purpose, and is now removed or stripped off the wafer surface using highly caustic wet chemicals (i.e., wet stripping) or by ionized O_2 (i.e., dry stripping or ashing).
7. *Doping*: Areas, in which the silicon dioxide layer has been removed to reveal silicon, now exist on the wafer. This silicon can be contaminated or doped with atoms, such as arsenic, to change its electrical conductivity. Altering conductivity in selected areas of the silicon is the essence of creating microelectronic devices, such as transistors and diodes. The doping is accomplished by either ion implantation or diffusion.
8. *Chemical vapor deposition*: Another layer of silicon (i.e., epitaxy) or of another compound (e.g., silicon nitride) is now applied to the wafer, thereby burying the area of silicon that was altered or doped.
9. *Repetition*: Subsequent oxidations, resist layers, exposures, etching, and doping create additional areas of either increased or decreased electrical conductivity relative to the substrate silicon.
10. *Metallization*: The last step is to wire together the devices to create electronic circuits. This is done by depositing patterns of metal by the same photolithographic technique used to create devices.

THIN FILMS—CHEMICAL VAPOR DEPOSITION

A variety of processes are used to deposit a layer of a material on the wafer in the thin films area, most of which involve chemical vapor deposition (CVD). Epitaxy, a type of chemical vapor deposition and a method of growing more silicon on the wafer surface, is often the first production step on the surface of the wafer. *Epitaxy* is the process of growing a thin elemental crystal layer on top of an identical substrate crystal. The main advantage of epitaxy is that a lightly doped layer of epitaxial silicon can be grown on top of a heavily doped silicon substrate, thus creating a sharp transition of electrical properties between the two layers. This junction can serve as an effective insulating layer between the epilayer and substrate. This prevents currents from flowing via substrate between adjacent devices formed in the epilayer. Silicon on silicon is the most common epitaxial process. The thickness of the epitaxial layer is usually 5 to 10 μm. Almost all epitaxial processes are accomplished by chemical vapor deposition. A general discussion of CVD processes precedes the discussion of the specific gases used in silicon epitaxy.

It is important to understand CVD tools, used in a number of thin film processes in addition to epitaxy, to appreciate the many potential health and safety hazards (23,24). Use of these techniques is increasing rapidly, and CVD processes are intensive users of highly toxic gases. CVD is accomplished by using unheated gases to react with heated substrate in a closed chamber. Two configurations of these tools are common, *cold wall* and *hot wall*.

In cold wall reactors, 10 to 50 wafers are held on a metal susceptor that is lowered into a quartz bell jar, which is subsequently sealed. The susceptor and wafers are heated to approximately 1,100°C by coupling to a radio frequency energy source. Gases are then introduced into the reaction chamber, and deposit only on high-temperature surfaces on the wafers and susceptor. The bell jar (i.e., the outside wall of the reactor) is not heated, and no chemical deposition takes place.

Low-pressure chemical vapor deposition at approximately 50 mm Hg is sometimes used with bell jar–type reactors, although more commonly with the hot wall configuration. Low-pressure chambers are presumably safer in that any leaks are inward.

Hot wall reactors are essentially typical stack furnaces (described in the Oxidation section). Quartz boats holding 100 to 200 vertically standing wafers are slid into furnaces that are heated with electrical resistance. More typically, these hot wall reactors are used for deposition of dielectrics or polysilicon but are sometimes found in epitaxial applications. Because the walls of the reactor are hot in these furnaces, they react with introduced gases just as the boat and wafers do. Deposited material is cleaned from the inside of the chamber by introducing hydrogen chloride (HCl) gas at high temperatures.

Increasingly, low-pressure vacuums are used in CVD processes. Somewhat surprisingly, low-pressure techniques are potentially more dangerous than atmospheric depositions. The reason is that the concentration of gases used is much higher. In atmospheric epitaxial growth, the silicon might be doped with arsine (AsH_3) gas in the parts per million range of concentration. Low-pressure chemical vapor deposition epitaxy requires AsH_3 gas in at least 2% concentration.

Low-pressure depositions pose additional hazards to tool maintenance personnel. Exhaust gases can dissolve into the vacuum pump oil, which makes handling this material hazardous, although many factories are now using oil-free pumps (25). Many of the gases used in CVD processes react with air to form solids. Small leaks cause particles to form within incoming gas lines or exhaust lines. Eventually, this can lead to plugged lines and ruptures. Maintenance of these lines can be hazardous, as some of the deposited waste products explode on exposure to air. Maintenance personnel should be disciplined about eye protection when working on CVD exhaust systems.

Electrical shock is another hazard of CVD tools that require voltages as high as 10,000 V. In fact, the presence of very high voltages is true of most semiconductor manufacturing tools. Safety professionals in the semiconductor industry often identify the risk of electrocution as their greatest single concern, making electrical safety training and practices extremely important.

GASES USED IN EPITAXY AND CHEMICAL VAPOR DEPOSITION

Epitaxy, a CVD process used to grow a thin layer of silicon, uses a great diversity of potentially very toxic gases. Typically, in a silicon deposition, HCl gas is used first to etch the wafers. Gases such as silane (SiH_4), dichlorosilane ($SiCl_2H_2$), and trichlorosilane ($SiCl_3H$) are used to deposit silicon. Light doping of the new crystal growth is common and is accomplished by introducing additional gases such as AsH_3, phosphine (PH_3), or diborane (B_2H_6) to the reactor chamber. Hydrogen is also used in these operations to create a reducing atmosphere and presents a potential explosion hazard.

Generally, operators in epitaxial areas do not have the responsibility of handling or changing gas cylinders. These tasks are done by special gas teams. State-of-the-art gas delivery systems can greatly minimize the hazard by moving cylinders to a distant gas room or pad. Many semiconductor workers prefer epitaxy areas because no wet processes are present, and, consequently, no noticeable vapors are present.

OXIDATION

After epitaxy, a wafer is oxidized to create a thin layer (approximately 30 nm) of SiO_2. SiO_2 layers are formed repeatedly during the manufacture of semiconductor circuits, mainly as diffusion masks, dielectrics, and passivation layers. Before oxidation, the wafers are cleaned of all particulate and organic matter in typical wet stations with a solution of H_2O-H_2O_2-HCl at approximately 80°C. Rinsing with deionized water and drying with nitrogen gas follows.

The most commonly used method of oxidation is thermal. Wafers are loaded into quartz boats that are slid into a furnace heated to 900° to 1,200°C. Thermal oxidation can be divided into dry and wet oxidation. In the dry process, thin oxides are grown in an O_2-HCl atmosphere at approximately 1 atm of pressure. Dry oxidation processes create extremely corrosive exhaust because of the presence of HCl. Except in the instance of a system failure, operators have no potential for exposure to these gases.

Thicker oxides require higher pressures and the use of steam (wet oxidation). Wet oxidation is accomplished by reacting H_2 with O_2 in the furnace chamber. Hydrogen is used with extreme care because of its potential for explosion. The furnaces must be maintained at or above the autoignition temperature of H_2. Leaks from furnaces are also a concern. Unless the concentration of H_2 in the air is kept below 4%, a danger of explosion exists. Area monitors for any H_2 gas leak are very prominent in clean room areas that use hydrogen. Because the specific gravity of hydrogen is only 0.07, hydrogen sensors in other industries are typically placed at the ceiling. Clean room ventilation schemes make this strategy inadequate in the semiconductor industry (26).

Chemical vapor deposition is sometimes used to deposit SiO_2. This process is done by reacting silane with oxygen, and it gives a better-quality oxide. The process temperatures are much lower than those used in typical wet and dry oxidations.

DIELECTRIC FILM DEPOSITION

Dielectric layers are electrical insulators used to separate conducting metals or provide protection from the environment. Commonly used layers are polycrystalline silicon, silicon nitride, polyimide, and silicon dioxide. The method of deposition is most commonly physical vapor deposition. However, chemical vapor deposition with its attendant-controlled use of toxic and flammable gases is used increasingly, as smaller products require more level depositions.

Undoped SiO_2 is used as an insulating layer between multilevel metallizations and is usually sputtered onto the wafer. Often, a tool is used to do a series of sputter depositions with each followed by an etch cycle to try to level or *planarize* the surface of the wafer. The etch cycle is accomplished with an ionized chlorinated hydrocarbon gas.

PASSIVATION

Silicon nitride (Si_3N_4) is often used as a final passivating or protective layer for silicon devices because it is highly impermeable to the diffusion of water or sodium from the environment. This CVD process uses two hazardous gases, silane and ammonia. Another final passivating layer that is sometimes deposited is *p-glass*. This is a layer of SiO_2 doped with phosphorus to make it more pliant and less likely to crack during the sawing and separation of chips. The source of the phosphorus is PH_3 gas.

FURNACES

Furnaces are used not only for oxidation, but also for diffusion, annealing, and some CVD processes. Furnaces are long cylindrical tubes that have historically been configured in a horizontal four-stack. Six- to eight-foot-long (1.8- to 2.4-m) quartzware boats are loaded with wafers and slid into the furnaces. Technologies are using vertical diffusion furnaces that have become necessary as wafer size has increased and greater contamination control is required. Open-atmosphere furnaces are the usual configuration for horizontal and vertical furnaces. Loading and unloading are usually highly mechanized, although some older horizontal installations required the workers to push and pull the boats with glass rods. Most commonly, microprocessor-controlled cantilevers handle the quartzware boats. The need to eliminate manual handling of the wafers is driven by process requirements but also lessens human exposure to heat, thermal burns, and exhaust from the furnaces. Heating of the furnace is done with electrical resistance. Most processes occur at either atmospheric pressure or slightly elevated pressures. In newer installations, vertical furnaces are better enclosed and are mechanically loaded, significantly reducing the potential for worker exposure to heat and physical stressors, compared with the traditional horizontal furnace.

Gases are introduced into the reaction chamber of the furnace after the load door is locked. The gas cylinders supplying these gases are stored in well-ventilated gas cabinets, typically located at a remote gas pad, and delivered to the furnace through double contained lines to prevent leakage. All systems have overrides that purge the furnace with inert gas whenever process conditions exceed preset limits. The source and load ends of the furnaces have local exhaust systems.

In the older horizontal furnaces, worker exposures to toxic exhaust can occur when they open the diffusion furnaces, if the furnaces have been inadequately purged, which is unlikely, or from offgassing of the wafers (27,28). The automated process used with vertical furnaces has eliminated this possibility.

One persistent problem in horizontal furnace areas is that the temperature can be much higher than is typically found in other parts of the semiconductor clean room. Even if the air temperature is not excessive, the infrared radiation from the furnaces can make these areas very uncomfortable for some workers. Facial dermatitis, most commonly acne, can be aggravated by chronic sweating caused by the heat in these areas. Workers in marginal physical condition may also have difficulty in these areas.

Another potential hazard of furnaces is cleaning the quartzware tubes that slide into the furnaces. One method of cleaning the tubes is dipping them into large baths of highly concentrated hydrofluoric acid outside the fabrication area. In newer-generation clean rooms, the tubes are cleaned in automated tube washers with appropriate rinse cycles. Workers performing these duties are potentially exposed to hydrofluoric acid burns and inhalation of acid aerosols if ventilation and enclosure integrity are not maintained. Bulk delivery of hydrofluoric acid has also reduced the incidents of spills and splashes.

Ceramic fiber insulation has replaced asbestos insulation in almost all furnaces. Whenever the operating temperatures are higher than 1,000°C, a potential exists for exposure to free silica. Studies have demonstrated that the aluminosilicate fiber devitrifies at approximately 1,000°C to form crystobalite. Release of crystobalite into the air under actual maintenance procedures has been documented (29). Personnel involved in these maintenance operations should take precautions against inhalation of free silica.

Photolithography

PHOTORESIST APPLICATION

After the creation of an SiO_2 layer, the wafer is covered with a photoresist. Although photoresists comprise a very small proportion of the total chemical usage in semiconductor manufacturing, many workers handle these chemicals and are potentially exposed via inhalation and skin absorption.

WAFER TRACKS

The basic tool for application of photoresist is called a *wafer track* or *spin coater*. Unlike most semiconductor manufacturing tools, the wafer processing portions of wafer tracks sit out in the clean room process bay. The operator loads a cassette of wafers into one end of these machines. Individual wafers are moved on air tracks or cantilevered arms to a wafer priming area in which, most commonly, hexamethyldisilazane (HMDS) is dispensed to promote adhesion of the resist. HMDS readily hydrolyzes in air to release ammonia, adding to the odor potential of this process if it is not well contained and ventilated. The wafer then moves to a photoresist apply station or spin cup. The entire surface of a wafer is covered with a resist solution by dispensing a measured volume of resist onto the center of a rapidly spinning wafer. The spinning wafer is contained inside a cup that captures spattered photoresist. The cup is under exhaust ventilation to remove vapors arising from the photoresist solvents.

The wafer is then carried automatically through small ovens or hotplates that bake a wafer at approximately 80° to 90°C. This is the *softbake* or *prebake* process, which causes 80% to 90% of the resist solvent to vaporize. With older or poorly maintained tools, this heating step can be a source of significant vapor releases. In newer tools, the softbake ovens are purged with nitrogen, and exhaust ventilation and oven seals have been improved to carry away the solvent vapors. Even new, well-designed tools need constant cleaning of the exhaust tubes that become clogged with photoresist polymers. In older tools, resist canisters were stored under the tool and became a potential source of solvent vapors caused by frequent spills. However, in newer tools, they have been moved to specially designed dispensing cabinets in the maintenance chase that are ventilated. The steel canisters have also been replaced by one-time-use, disposable plastic containers supplied directly by the resist manufacturer, thereby eliminating another potential source for spill or vapor release.

Environmental sampling at wafer tracks invariably yields results that are under all published exposure standards (27,30). These data have not been wholly successful in addressing worker perceptions. Workers seem to dislike these tools more than any others in the semiconductor clean room. Odors are common, and concerns have been generated by the prior presence of ethylene glycol ethers in almost all photoresist formulations.

Wafer track tools are also used to apply materials that are not photoresists. Other polymers, such as polysulfone and polyimides, are applied as dielectric layers usually in the metallization stage of manufacture. Operators generally make no distinction between photoresists and dielectrics, and anything applied at a wafer track is known as a *resist*. The dielectric polymers use different solvents—primarily *n*-methylpyrrolidone (NMP), but perhaps dichloromethane, dimethylformamide, and dimethylacetamide in some settings.

PHOTOEXPOSURE

Exposure tools, also known as *aligners*, *steppers*, *scanners*, or *projection tools*, use a variety of methods to expose photoresist to ultraviolet (UV) radiation that has passed through a mask. The UV source is an intense mercury arc lamp (approximately 1,500 kW). Although most of the radiation given off by the lamps is greater than 350 nm in wavelength, significant amounts are also below 315 nm. Leakage of UV radiation during operation or exposure during maintenance, although not likely, can cause serious acute and chronic damage to skin, cornea, and the retina. Photoexposure may cause anxiety about the hazards of UV radiation among some operators. Monitoring with a UV actinic radiometer may be helpful in reassuring the operators.

Another potential exposure of the optical exposure process is to ozone, generated by the strong electrical fields surrounding the mercury arc lamps. Levels in excess of published exposure standards have been documented around inadequately ventilated photoexposure tools, although tool heat exhaust and general fab ventilation typically are expected to minimize the potential for significant exposures.

The mercury arc lamps are a potential source of mercury exposure. These lamps eventually fail, burst, and release vaporized mercury (approximately 2 mg) into the clean room environment. Depending on the volume of the room and the rate of dilution of the air, an inhalation exposure could occur. No such overexposures have ever been documented; presumably, the rate of general ventilation and local exhaust in this area would minimize the potential for exposure. Routinely changing bulbs after a defined number of hours of operation prevents this possibility.

Photoexposure tools are somewhat unusual in the clean room in that they demand long periods of sitting in static postures. This can generate a variety of musculoskeletal complaints. The work also entails prolonged use of microscopes and video display terminals (VDTs), and can be a source of eyestrain or fatigue.

DEVELOPING

Developing of the exposed photoresist, similar to film developing, is accomplished with the use of strong bases, such as NaOH, KOH, or tetramethylammonium hydroxide, with a pH of approximately 13. The hazards to skin and eye are easily appreciated, and proper protective equipment is crucial. Alkaline burns are a special hazard to the cornea. Even small splashes into the eye require immediate and copious irrigation followed by prompt referral to an ophthalmologist, whether symptoms are present. Developing is typically conducted on a spinner track similar to the resist dispense track, in which a small amount of developer is applied to the surface of the wafer. Storage of development chemicals is also enclosed and ventilated with similar controls to prevent leaks, splashes, and spills.

WET STATIONS

Wafers are repeatedly cleaned, etched, and stripped in wet chemical baths. Wet stations are used for cleaning in diffusion and some resist-stripping operations, as well as in wet-etch processes. A typical wet station or wet bench consists of a number of process tanks, chemical recirculators, filters, rinse tanks, a wafer dryer, exhaust system, and, in most cases, automatic chemical dispensing systems. Very often, the baths are heated by electrical immersion heaters. The use of scrubbing, ultrasonics, megasonics, and acoustics is sometimes added. Robots to handle the wafers have been introduced to most of these operations, especially in the VLF type of clean rooms. Mixed-flow design rooms with individual hoods, although rarely seen, generally do not have enough space under the hoods to allow robotic tools. Automated handling of cassettes and chemicals is safer than manual techniques, but most accidents at wet stations have occurred when workers were manually draining and refilling the baths. New-generation clean rooms have largely eliminated this hazard by the use of bulk chemical delivery systems plumbed into the wet stations.

A wide variety of inorganic acids and organic solvents are used at wet stations. Table 33-1 lists some of the chemicals that are found in wet baths in semiconductor manufacturing. Proper personal protective gear must be used, including full-coverage aprons with arms, appropriate gloves, and eye and face protection. The potential hazards at wet stations are so readily apparent that compliance is generally not an issue.

Possible inhalation hazards at wet stations are more difficult to define. Sporadically and unpredictably, a noticeable amount of chemical vapor is expelled transiently into the worker's breathing zone. This problem is identified primarily at stations in which highly irritant chemicals with good warning properties are used. The typical complaints are odors, eye irritation, or throat irritation. Environmental or personal sampling invariably yields numbers that are well within published short-term exposure limit and time-weighted standards. Some of these sampling data have been published (27). The potential for this transient spike exposure can be reduced by following strict work practice controls and ensuring a good balance between laminar airflow and the wet station local exhaust.

WET STATION EXHAUST SYSTEMS

Perimeter and subsink exhaust systems exist at wet stations in clean rooms to carry away vapors and aerosols. These exhausts

TABLE 33-1. Chemicals commonly found at wet stations

Alkalis
Ammonium hydroxide
Potassium hydroxide
Sodium hydroxide
Acids
Acetic acid
Hydrochloric acid
Hydrofluoric acid
Nitric acid
Perchloric acid
Sulfuric acid
Chromic acid
Other
Ammonium fluoride
Hydrogen peroxide
Methanol
Isopropyl alcohol
Sodium peroxide
Acetone
Xylene
N-Methyl pyrrolidone

must be balanced against positive airflow of the laminar air provided at the front of each station. Ventilation balance is not a static phenomenon. Any time an additional tool is added to an exhaust system, the exhaust on adjacent tools may be diminished, affecting control of hazards. Likewise, any change in laminar airflow in the clean room affects capture capabilities of a wet station. To reduce this potential, it is imperative that impacts to changes in exhaust and laminar airflow be understood and monitored.

Spills or overflows of acids or solvents into a subsink can be pulled into tool exhaust systems. Nonvolatile chemicals can stay suspended in the exhaust system indefinitely. Eventually, a saturation point is reached and the chemicals start to come out of the exhaust system, although not necessarily from the points through which they entered. This phenomenon can be an interesting source of odors and exposures in the clean room, which is very difficult to investigate.

FIRE HAZARD AT WET STATIONS

Fires at wet stations previously were relatively frequent events but are not common now. These fires usually occurred when the baths were drained without turning off the heater and were later refilled, igniting the chemicals. In some cases, the electrical immersion heater ignites the bench, which is often constructed of polypropylene. An electrical immersion heater has a surface temperature of approximately 180°F (82°C) in ambient water and 1,300°F (704°C) in ambient air. A variety of over-temperature monitors and liquid level controls are available to reduce the chance of accidental ignition. Even when installed, these monitors frequently fail or are ignored by operators. More than one-half of the insurance losses encountered in the semiconductor industry were caused by fire (31). In 1977, an entire semiconductor facility in Scotland was lost to a fire that began at a wet bench. Controls and automation in newer wet stations appear to have reduced the risk of fire.

Fire suppression techniques that are adequate in most industrial settings fail to be effective in the VLF clean room. Laminar flow moves air downward through the floor, whereas heat-activated sprinklers are naturally placed in the ceiling. In a demonstration study performed in a mock clean room, it took 35 minutes before a conventional fire system detected a wet station fire (31). The trend in the industry is to install Halon 1301 extinguishing systems at each wet station, although this material is now being replaced by another Halon that is not an ozone-depleting substance. New fire codes, specific to the semiconductor industry, state that fire protection systems must be placed directly on the wet station. These codes also address construction of semiconductor fab facilities, as well as the handling, storage, and use of the chemicals (32–34).

HARDBAKE

After the removal of the undeveloped photoresist in a wet station, a thermal baking process hardens the remaining photoresist to a finish much like the enamel on an automobile. The photoresist is now ready to protect the underlying SiO_2 from an etchant chemical attack. The hardbake process occurs in well-enclosed and well-ventilated ovens.

Etching

SiO_2 that is not protected by resist is removed in the etching process to uncover silicon and enable subsequent doping. Etching is accomplished either by submersion of the wafer in an acid bath or by an enclosed *dry etch*, which uses ionized gases.

ACIDS USED IN WET ETCHING

Wet etches historically have been manual processes, although in more advanced clean rooms, robots move baskets of wafers in and out of the baths. In wet etching, the acids most frequently used are hydrofluoric acid (HF), HCl, sulfuric acid (H_2SO_4), nitric acid (HNO_3), and chromic acid (CrO_3). Dermal hazards are usually very well controlled. Poorly engineered stations can expose workers to significant concentrations of acid aerosols that are irritating to the upper and lower respiratory tract.

DRY ETCHING

Dry etching has supplanted wet etching because of shrinking geometries on the surface of wafers. Wet etching is difficult to control, because it etches in all directions. Dry etching uses ionized gases in closed reactors with most processes carried out at pressures lower than 1 mm Hg (0.01 atm). At least a dozen different methods of dry etching exist, but the best known are plasma etching and reactive ion etching (RIE) (35). The only difference between the two is that in RIE the wafers are situated on the anode, whereas in plasma systems they are on the cathode plate. RIE systems achieve better directional etching action. In either system, activated fluorine-based or chlorine-based etchants are created by exposing a gas to an RF field through the electrodes in a chamber. The most popular gases are hexafluoroethane (C_2F_6), sulfur hexafluoride (SF_6), chlorine (Cl_2), nitrogen trifluoride (NF_3), and trifluoromethane (CHF_3), with lesser use of boron trichloride (BCl_3), HCl, bromine (Br_2), carbon tetrafluoride (CF_4), carbon tetrachloride (CCl_4), and boron trifluoride (BF_3). A number of other compounds, at least 200 gaseous etchants, most of which are chlorine or fluorine based, have been investigated (36,37). The reactive species etch physically and chemically. The by-product of the etching process is usually a halogenated compound of the material being etched. These products are removed continuously by vacuum pumps. Etch chambers are closed systems, and the potential for exposure to the gases and by-products contained within them is extremely remote. If a chamber is inadvertently opened prematurely, emissions of by-products into the fab area are possible. If vacuum pump exhaust lines plug and leak, a potential for release of by-products also exists. Some of the reactor effluents are highly toxic. They are trapped in either pump oil or liquid nitrogen, and, unless handled appropriately, present a potential hazard to workers who must maintain the pumps (38). Many controls are in place to eliminate this risk. Most modern pumps do not use oil. An automatic shutdown mechanism is typically built into the vacuum pump, such that if an exhaust line leaks or plugs, the pressure change is detected and the pump is shut down.

REACTIVE ION ETCHING OF METALS

As with device formation, dry etching of deposited aluminum is increasingly preferred to wet etching, because smaller geometries can be achieved. The tools and potential means of exposure do not differ from the etching of silicon. Because of the high reactivity of metals with ambient O_2 and H_2O, plasma etching of metals often involves more emphasis on etching oxides of the metal rather than the metal itself. Chlorocarbon and fluorocarbon gases, rather than pure halogens, are typically used to etch metal films because they are more effective in reducing the metal oxides. Examples of gases used in metal etching are CCl_4 with BCl_3, $SiCl_4$, $C_2Cl_2F_4$, and $CClF_3$.

The exhaust products are a halogenated compound of whatever metal is used for interconnection. Because nitrogen is used as a carrier gas for the reactive halogenated gases, by-products of the reactions can incorporate nitrogen atoms. Hydrogen cyanide is commonly measured at levels of 1 to 2 ppm on opening reactors that are used to dry etch aluminum; in addition, cyanogen chloride has also been detected in excess of the TLV ceiling (39). These gases have been detected only in aluminum-etch chemistries.

DRY ETCHING OF GALLIUM ARSENIDE

As GaAs wafers become more widely used, maintenance of dry etching tools becomes more hazardous. It has been demonstrated that large amounts of arsenic accumulate in the cartridge filters, nitrogen traps, and pump oil (40).

RADIOFREQUENCY RADIATION EMISSIONS IN DRY ETCHING

The charged gas plasmas are created with RF energy, and these tools sometimes leak electrical and magnetic energy. In 1983, 23 plasma etching units from four different facilities were monitored by NIOSH for release of RF energy. Five of the 23 units emitted electrical field energies above American Conference of Governmental Industrial Hygienists (ACGIH) standards, and three emitted magnetic fields above ACGIH standards (27). Measurements were done 10 cm from the units. Because workers generally are not standing near the units when the units are in operation, the actual potential for significant exposure is greatly diminished. Nonetheless, frequent monitoring of the tools for RF emission is warranted. Exposure to less than the published ACGIH standards prevents thermal injuries. Tools are maintained in such a way as to minimize leakage well below the standards, in part because the RF leaks interfere with robotic equipment in the process area.

INCREASED POTENTIAL FOR RADIOFREQUENCY EXPOSURE

Evaporators and sputterers are among other tools, besides etchers and plasma tools, that use RF energy. The potential for exposure to RF energy is increasing rapidly. Many of the tools used in semiconductor manufacturing use wavelengths that are particularly well absorbed by human tissue (13.56 MHz). Careful maintenance and regular monitoring of tools eliminate the possibility of exposure.

STRIPPING THE RESIST

After etching of unprotected SiO_2, the resist has served its purpose and must be removed from the protected SiO_2. *Ashing* or *dry stripping* is usually the first step. Tools used in this step are essentially the same as dry etch tools. Wafers are placed in a chamber that is pumped down to approximately 2 mm Hg. Oxygen is introduced and subjected to microwave energy, typically at 2.45 GHz, that creates oxygen radicals. These radicals react with resist to oxidize it to water, carbon monoxide, and carbon dioxide that are pumped away.

The primary reason for the initial introduction of dry stripping was to reduce chemical consumption and disposal problems. However, other process changes now mandate the use of dry stripping. During dry etch, the top surface of the photoresist mask becomes fluorinated or chlorinated, which renders it insoluble to most wet chemistries. Resist that has been exposed to ion implantation is also hardened and difficult to remove with wet processes alone. Therefore, an ashing step is used to remove the top layer of the resist, or the *skin* as it is sometimes called. After this top layer of resist is removed, wet or dry processes can be used to strip the remaining resist.

Another approach that has been used to strip resist is to use a combination of UV radiation and ozone at atmospheric pressure (41). This process is not widely used. Because this process occurs at ambient pressures, rather than in a vacuum, increased potential exists for exposure of workers to the reactant gases.

WET STRIPPING

Very corrosive chemicals based on formulations developed in the metal paint industries are used in wet stripping. These processes occur at typical wet stations, in which cassettes of wafers are dunked into baths. In the past, hot solvent processes (90° to 120°C) had been used, and ultrasound energy was added to increase the penetration. Wet stripping uses NMP and organic acids at room temperatures in wet stations.

Previous strippers typically contained a primary solvent, a cosolvent, an activator (penetrant), and a surface wetting agent. Historically, the most popular primary solvent for the diazonaphthoquinone/novolak (DQN) photoresist system had been dichloromethane, but this has largely been replaced by NMP. In the past, phenol, tetrachloroethylene, *o*-dichlorobenzene, and *p*-toluene sulfonic acid, H_2O_2-H_2SO_4, Cr_2O_3-H_2SO_4, and an ammonia solution of hydrogen peroxide had been used in mixtures as strippers with DQN.

FUTURE OF WET STRIPPING OPERATIONS

Because wet stripping is considerably more hazardous than dry stripping and is less controllable from a process perspective, it is natural to question why wet stripping is still used. The reason is that photoresist is typically contaminated with metal ions that do not volatilize during the ashing or dry stripping process. These ions are left on the surface of the wafer and are driven into the wafer during subsequent processing. The metal ions can short microscopic circuits. Wet stripping is much more effective at removing metal ions from the surface of the wafer. Until photoresists are free of metal contamination, wet stripping stations remain part of the clean room environment.

Doping

Doping of the substrate to create n and p regions is achieved either by thermal diffusion or ion implantation. The latter is a more advanced technique that is necessary for smaller geometries. It also has considerably more potential for hazardous exposures than does diffusion.

DIFFUSION

Diffusion is based on the fact that, at 1,000°C, impurities diffuse into and through the silicon substrate. Because the dopants move much more slowly through SiO_2, a protective layer of that material allows selective doping.

The first step is called *predeposition* and coats the wafer with the dopant material. Wafers are placed into quartz tubes that are pushed into a typical stack furnace to heat the wafers. The dopant source may be a powdered form of the desired dopant or in the form of a dummy wafer. Liquid sources can also be used by bubbling an inert carrier gas, such as phosphorus oxychloride, through a liquid form of the dopant.

The wafers are then heat treated by putting them into a second furnace at higher temperatures (approximately 1,300°C) to drive in the dopant. This step occurs in an oxidizing atmosphere that forms a thin layer of quartz over the freshly doped silicon.

The source cabinets in which the dopants are supplied are ventilated to an exhaust system. Scavenger boxes enclose the loading worker end of the furnaces and are also exhausted. All reported sampling data taken while the furnaces are operating have been either undetectable or below published standards (27).

ION IMPLANTATION

Ion implantation is a critical technology in modern semiconductor manufacturing. A controllable quantity of almost any element can be mingled with the host material, in this case the silicon substrate (42). Ion implantation tools generate a beam of dopant ions by boiling them from a heated filament. The ions are accelerated in electrical fields and directed against a gaseous form of the element to be introduced. AsH_3, PH_3, and B_2H_6 are common dopant gases. Collision with the high-velocity electrons strips away the dopant's electrons to create a plasma. An electrical field pulls the plasma from the chamber. Magnets are used to deflect the ion beam at precise angles, causing heavier or lighter ions to be selected out of the focused beam. This results in a highly purified beam of dopant ions that impact the substrate surface. The entire process occurs in a vacuum of 10^{-6} mm Hg (10^{-8} atm) or less. The vacuums are created by either oil diffusion or cryogenic pumps backed by a mechanical roughing pump.

Operator interaction with the tools is ordinarily limited to loading and unloading a cassette of wafers and entering the job number into a keyboard. Nonetheless, potential health hazards for operators exist. These hazards include catastrophic gas leakage (highly unlikely), ionizing radiation (slight possibility of exposure), and fumes, such as arsenic trioxide, from newly implanted wafers. The use of solid sources, such as arsenic or phosphorus, eliminates the potential for catastrophic releases. The development of vacuum delivery systems for dopants, in which the hydride is adsorbed onto a solid sorbent in a cylinder below atmospheric pressure, also dramatically minimizes this potential, in that a leak would cause air to move into the cylinder. Great efforts are taken in the semiconductor industry to ensure against exposure to the toxic gases used in implantation.

All implanters use high voltages to accelerate the charged particles of the ion beam. The energy of accelerated electrons created by this process is high enough to generate x-rays. Much of the ion implanter is lined with lead shielding to protect personnel, but leaks can occur if the equipment is not well maintained or monitored. Film badges are not adequate for identifying exposures from implanters, because most emissions are in the form of narrow beams from cracks and holes in the cabinet. It is unlikely that the film badge, whether worn by personnel or placed on the implanter, is in the line of a leak. X-ray surveys should be done with a Geiger-Müller counter after major preventive maintenance activities to ensure that ionizing radiation is not leaking (43). Actual doses can be quantified with an ion chamber.

A study performed by NIOSH in 1985 demonstrated small amounts of inorganic arsenic being emitted from implanted wafers up to 3.5 hours after removal from the tool (28). A survey of ion implantation operations in three semiconductor facilities documented routine worker exposure to levels of airborne dopants below ACGIH or Occupational Safety and Health Administration (OSHA) standards. Area sampling demonstrated the potential for more worrisome exposures (44). A separate study confirmed the presence of low levels of the airborne contaminant at these tools (43). The maximum exposure was quite low, 0.04 µg per m^3. In both studies, surfaces in the implanter areas were contaminated with arsenic, but at very low levels. PH_3 has also been documented as a gas leaking from wafers implanted with phosphorus, even though the source was solid phosphorus. Barring unusual circumstances, employee exposures by this route are expected to be negligible.

Workers who maintain or repair the implanters have the same potential exposures described for operators, plus additional hazards. Significant levels of arsenic have been documented in pump oils, to which maintenance workers are potentially exposed. Contact with the oil theoretically could enhance the absorption of toxic material contained within it, such as arsenic, through the skin. Inhalation of toxins contained in the oil mists is a theoretical concern, but of doubtful actual significance.

Cleaning the tool parts, especially beam line components, provides another opportunity for exposure to arsenic for maintenance personnel. Although AsH_3 and PH_3 have been detected from samples taken inside cryopumps, employee exposures from maintenance activities have not been documented. A strong odor of garlic (similar to AsH_3 or PH_3) often occurs when beam lines and pumps are opened, and sometimes forces building evacuations. Sampling, even in the presence of the odors, has yet to document the presence of AsH_3 or PH_3. The cause of these odors has not yet been determined. Work practice controls have been successful in preventing escape of these odors.

Bead blasters are used to clean the implanter parts after they have been removed from the tool. Typically, the bead blasters, which are enclosed and exhausted, are housed in dedicated maintenance areas outside the clean room. Handling of parts and cleaning of the bead blasters present other hazards that require personal protection. Wet slurry blasters are inherently safer than dry blasters and have been adopted by some companies. The industry is also looking at the use of CO_2 pellet cleaning, which could lead to a further reduction in waste and employee exposure potential.

Several components inside the implanter operate at very high voltages, up to 100,000 V. Use of grounding hooks before any contact with these tools is essential, even if the tool is not operating. Ordinarily, it is not possible to get into implanters without turning off the power. Some maintenance and fine-tuning require technicians to adjust these tools with parts charged to high voltage.

Any worker who changes gas cylinders of toxic or corrosive gases is at risk of a catastrophic accident and should perform all gas source changes in a self-contained breathing apparatus under positive pressure. Solid sources (usually vaporizers of elemental arsenic or phosphorus) are changed and loaded almost daily for each tool and present potential for exposure to inorganic arsenic dust. At a minimum, this work should be done under a ventilation hood with appropriate personal protective equipment. Some companies require glove boxes for solid source changes.

ANNEALING

Implantation damages the surface of the wafer. Slowly heating the wafer returns it to its original condition and incorporates the dopant atoms into the silicon crystal lattice. Annealing is done in stack furnaces at approximately 800°C.

Occasionally, high-energy lasers, electron beams, or flash lamps are used to anneal surfaces, because they minimize the diffusion of dopant that occurs with prolonged heating. Rapid thermal annealing with lasers can cut the heating time to less than 10^{-7} seconds.

Device Interconnection (Metallization)

Interconnection of completed semiconductor devices is accomplished by depositing patterns of metal (*wiring*) onto the surface of the chip. The width of these wires varies from 0.5 to 5.0 µm in products. The patterns are created by the use of photolithography. Most modern integrated circuits require at least three levels of metallization, with each separated by an insulating layer.

Metallization processes are presently less of a health and safety challenge than device formation processes, because of the absence of ion implanters and the less frequent use of chemical vapor deposition tools. These two types of tools are the heaviest users of hazardous gases. Metallization relies on inherently safer physical vapor-depositing methods.

PHYSICAL VAPOR DEPOSITION OF METALS

Deposition of metals has traditionally been accomplished by two physical vapor deposition methods, either evaporation or sputtering. Aluminum is the most commonly used metal for connecting devices. Other commonly deposited metals are chromium, nickel, gold, silver, titanium, tungsten, platinum, and silicon. Combinations such as copper-chrome-gold and lead-tin are frequently used.

EVAPORATION

Evaporation uses a two-chambered tool. The wafers are loaded onto a dome and placed into the upper chamber. A solid slug of the metal that is to be evaporated and deposited is placed in a lower chamber. No reactive gases are used at these tools. The metal is evaporated by RF, thermal, or electron beam heating, and the vapors deposit on wafers in the chamber above. All the reactions occur in a vacuum, and operator exposure to the metals in a vaporized state is not a consideration.

CLEANING OF EVAPORATORS

Exposure to metallic dust can occur with cleaning of the tools. Between runs, the operator sometimes vacuums the reaction chamber for any loose flakes or particles of metal. After a certain number of runs, the inside of the tool is taken out and cleaned in a bead blaster. Parts of the tool that cannot be removed are mechanically scrubbed with wire pads or brushes. Exposure levels to the metal deposited in the tool are extremely high during these cleaning procedures. For instance, personal sampling on a worker cleaning a lead-tin evaporator documented a 90-minute mean airborne lead level in excess of 1,200 μg per cubic meter. Appropriate respirators are one solution to this problem. A preferable solution is to substitute chemical cleaning methods for the mechanical methods.

SPUTTERING

Sputtering is done by bombarding the target metal with argon ions in a vacuum to release metal ions from the surface of the target. These atoms condense on the substrate to form a film. Sputtering processes are used to deposit semiconductors and dielectrics as well as metals. Sputtering is carried out at relatively high pressures, 10^{-2} mm Hg (10^{-4} atm). RF or direct current power sources are used to create the ionized argon. As with evaporation tools, exposure to metals can occur with cleaning.

Exposure to RF energy is a possibility at sputterer tools. These emissions are generally the result of incorrect placement of shielding after maintenance procedures.

CHEMICAL VAPOR DEPOSITION OF METALS

Continued reduction of device and interconnection dimensions cause the current evaporation and sputtering of metals to be obsolete. CVD metal systems allow better contouring, as well as better control of composition of binary or tertiary metal systems. Metal silicides are already used in some circuits as first-layer metallizations. A typical reaction is to combine tungsten hexafluoride gas with silane to deposit tungsten silicide. Silane is often used in 100% concentrations to ensure the desired composition of the silicide deposition. Metal hydrides, halides, and carbonyls, as well as an infinite variety of organometallics, are also used to accomplish CVD of metals. As these processes become more prevalent in the production environment, they present a major challenge to health and safety professionals, in part because of the paucity of toxicologic information on these materials.

LIFT OFF

Photoresists are traditionally used in device photolithography to assist in a subtractive or etching process. In metallization processes, they are often used to deposit a solid onto the substrate, an additive process. In one technique, the metal is deposited, then covered with a patterned resist, and subsequently etched. In another technique, the resist is used to *lift off* deposited metal. This is done by evaporating a metal onto a surface that is partially protected by an already patterned and developed resist. The wafer is then placed in a solvent that causes swelling of the resist. As the resist swells, it lifts the overlaid metal away from the surface of the wafer and allows it to be washed away. Metal that was deposited onto the substrate is left behind. Lift off stations are much like wet stripping stations in terms of the chemicals used. The solvent is generally heated, which adds to the potential for exposure to vapors. Worker complaints about eye and throat irritation are frequent. Fires are not uncommon.

SILYATION

Etching deposited metals requires a more aggressive chemical attack than etching of SiO_2. Consequently, the resists need to be tougher. Silyation is frequently performed to harden a photoresist before it is subjected to etching. *Silyation* is a process of introducing silicon atoms into the surface of the organic resist. The process can be accomplished with either wet or dry procedures. Most commonly, a wet bath using either HMDS or silazone in xylene is used.

OTHER ACTIVITIES AND HAZARDS

Inspection and Microscopes. Much of the work done in clean rooms is inspection of the wafers through microscopes or, increasingly, by looking at VDTs. Either tends to involve long hours in static postures. Too often, the workstations and tools are not well fitted to the particular individual. Generalized aches and pains are a frequent complaint as a result of this work. Workers with neck problems seem to have special difficulty. Eyestrain and fatigue are also reported with these tools. Complaints associated with microscopic work are among the most frequently reported of all problems in semiconductor clean rooms.

Microscopes pose another interesting hazard: the potential for spread of infectious eye disease. Management and health personnel should be careful that no worker with conjunctivitis works with microscopes. The most dramatic example of this potential problem occurred in 1987 among microscope users at a microelectronics assembly facility (45). An epidemic of conjunctivitis eventually affected 196 of 350 workers and caused a 5-day shutdown of the plant. This episode cost the manufacturer more than $600,000. Another epidemic of ocular infections in a class 100 semiconductor facility has been reported (46). The likely pathogen in both epidemics was thought to be an adenovirus. Simple hygiene measures, such as handwashing and use of isopropyl alcohol wipes on the oculars between uses, are adequate to prevent transmission of infection. UV lamps are used in some facilities to sterilize the ocular pieces, but they are not entirely effective against viruses. Some workers have solved the problem of dirty oculars by carrying a set of eyepieces in and out of the clean room.

Musculoskeletal Trauma in Semiconductor Manufacturing. Aside from the sequelae of inspection work or other tasks requiring prolonged sitting, the semiconductor clean room is relatively free of musculoskeletal stressors. Heavy physical labor is nearly nonexistent. Highly repetitive tasks, which are often associated with other parts of the microelectronics industry, are infrequent. OSHA logs from the industry show that sprains and strains are the most frequently reported incidents (47), although many companies have experienced increased rates of cumulative trauma disorders, consistent with the experience in other industries.

Video Display Terminals (VDTs). VDTs are very common in inspection areas. It is not unusual to see a worker using three or four terminals simultaneously at some inspection stations. All of the usual ergonomic considerations with VDT use are as important in the clean room as they are elsewhere (48,49).

One possible outcome of VDT use is especially interesting in the clean room environment. Reports of outbreaks of facial dermatitis among VDT users have been published (50,51). These rashes usually appear within hours to days after the use of the VDT. Typically, the patient complains of a prickly sensation and eventually develops a facial erythema. It has been proposed that the electrostatic field between the VDT and the operator can cause increased deposition of irritant particles on the face of the user. This is an unproved hypothesis, but, given the presence of low concentrations of airborne chemicals and the prevalence of static electricity in semiconductor clean rooms, it should be kept in mind. The problem of VDTs and facial dermatitis has usually been solved by raising the ambient humidity, a solution that is not available in the semiconductor environment.

Chip Separation, Assembly, and Testing

Most wafers are put through an automated furnace called a *reflow oven*. This finely controlled warming of the wafers causes the terminal pads that are usually a lead-tin alloy to soften and reshape into more rounded contours. These are well-ventilated tools that present no hazard to operators, except for the use of hydrogen in the ovens to prevent oxidation, and there is always a potential for explosion with hydrogen. Concern has been raised about reflow ovens when the substrate is gallium arsenide rather than silicon because of the potential to generate AsH_3.

Testing of the circuits is done by automated tools before the wafers are cut into individual chips (die). Almost always, a number of defective chips exists on any wafer.

Operators then mount wafers onto an adhesive tape that is in a frame. Diamond wheels on a wafer saw are used to cut the wafer into individual integrated circuits. The remaining parts of the procedure are almost entirely automated, including alignment, cutting, cleaning, and selection of good chips. No hazards for operators exist in these operations, except for ergonomic stressors of prolonged microscope use.

The chips are then packaged individually or into modules by a wide variety of techniques. Epoxy adhesives and encapsulants are often used in attaching the die and sealing the package containing the die. Little potential for contact exists with the epoxy compounds, which are not applied manually. A small amount of solvent, such as isopropyl alcohol and NMP, is used for cleaning. Curing ovens, reflow ovens, and burn-in ovens, all of which are typically vented, occasionally are the sources of odors, but not demonstrated exposures of concern. Although lead is used, significant exposures to airborne lead typically do not occur. After the packages are complete, they are marked, either with lasers or ink. At that point, the completed devices are tested using an array of different electrical equipment. Operations in these assembly and test facilities are not chemically intensive, in contrast to wafer fab facilities.

Mask Making

Mask making is an integral part of the manufacture of semiconductors and uses many of the same techniques as the manufacture of devices. Masks are used in photoexposure tools to determine the patterns of UV light imaged onto a photoresist. Masks are simpler in that only one layer of patterned material is necessary. The process begins with a quartz blank, onto which a thin layer of chrome is deposited by an evaporation process. A layer of polymethylmethacrylate (PMMA) or a derivative is deposited over the chrome as a resist. PMMA is a positive, one-component resist. Electron-beam radiation is used to cause scissions of the polymer backbone. The scissioned PMMA polymer has a lower molecular weight and is more amenable to removal by a ketone solvent developer.

ELECTRON-BEAM TOOLS

An electron beam is used to expose the PMMA resist, which is an example of radiolithography rather than photolithography. Narrow electron beams are used to directly write a pattern of exposure onto the PMMA resist without an intervening mask. The desired pattern is generated from digital data written by circuit engineers and stored electronically. As electron beams cannot exist outside a vacuum, no potential exists for human exposure to this radiation. The beams are focused onto the masks by magnets.

Outgassing of the exposed resist generates a variety of simple hydrocarbons and other organics, including CO, CO_2, and aldehydes. These are removed from the vacuum by high-speed exhaust so that internal tool surfaces do not become contaminated.

ETCHING CHROME

Etching of the chrome is done most commonly by wet acid. Newer process requirements are going to force the introduction of more accurate dry etches. One option is plasma etching, which is already widely used in the photolithographic process. Another process, called *ion-milling*, in which argon is ionized and bombarded against the target, is used to etch in some mask-making facilities. No chemical reaction takes place in this process; the argon atoms mechanically sputter against the target.

The plates are cleaned in acid baths and with mechanical brushing. Defects in the chrome pattern on the reticle larger than 1 μm in size can be repaired by depositing additional metal, usually molybdenum. This is accomplished by heating small areas with a laser and then using chemical vapor deposition to deposit metal on the heated areas. Extra metal can be ablated by the same laser tool.

Lasers in Semiconductor Manufacturing

Lasers are used widely in semiconductor manufacturing. Die separation, trimming, annealing, scribing, mask repair, alignment of wafers, and etching endpoint detection are just a few uses. Visible light lasers offer a hazard, but a well-defined hazard. Rigorous compliance with published American National Standards Institute standards helps to avoid any injuries. The only fail-safe way to control lasers is to engineer a way to eliminate the possibility of exposure. Experience has shown that a system that depends on personal protection (e.g., goggles) fails regularly. Incidents of retinal burns may be underreported (52), although they appear to be uncommon in the presence of a good laser safety program, including training.

SUMMARY OF SEMICONDUCTOR MANUFACTURING

The basic processes that should be understood are crystal growth, machining of wafers, CVD processes, including epitaxy, oxidation, photoresist application, exposure, development, wet and dry etching, wet and dry stripping, doping by either diffusion or implantation, and metallization. A reasonable generalization about state-of-the-art facilities is that operators are very seldom exposed to the chemicals they use. Tool maintenance and setup personnel are at greater risk. The specific chemicals and work practices in any particular setting are highly variable, and it is incumbent on a health professional to take the time to understand each situation before making statements on the presence or absence of health risk. Professionals associated with this industry have invariably commented on the rapid pace of change in tools and materials and on the fact that adequate toxicologic assessment of chemicals almost never precedes their introduction into manufacturing settings. The pace of change is quickening under the pressure of severe economic competition. A typical schedule of new technology introduction from research through development and pilot lines into full-scale manufacturing was approximately 6 to 8 years. The executives who manage microelectronic businesses are now demanding that this schedule be compressed into a 2- or 3-year time frame. Engineers are not typically evaluated or rewarded on their ability to appreciate or understand new or unusual health hazards. This task is the responsibility of health and safety professionals. Unfortunately, the opportunities for these professionals to be involved before new processes arrive at the manufacturing floor are sometimes being diminished by the quickening pace of technologic change. On the other hand, in some organizations, the health and safety professionals have become an integral part of the process development team, such that potential health issues can be identified and resolved before the actual introduction of the new technology.

SELECTED TOXIC HAZARDS

Any large semiconductor facility uses several thousand chemicals. An attempt to review the toxicology of all these materials is doomed to be superficial and of little value. Instead, some issues that are particularly topical in the industry are discussed:

1. Solvent use in photolithography
2. Arsenic
3. Gases
4. Photoresists
5. Hydrofluoric acid
6. Waste products of dry etching

Solvent Use in Photolithography

Until the early to mid-1990s, ethylene glycol ethers were used extensively as major components of photoresist solvent systems in the semiconductor industry. Since then, in part because of reproductive health concerns raised by animal studies and industry epidemiologic studies discussed in the following section, these solvents have been replaced by other solvents, primarily ethyl lactate and propylene glycol monomethyl ether acetate (PGMEA). Because of their historical significance in the industry, it is important to briefly review their use and toxicologic properties. In the years before substitution, the primary ethylene glycol ether used in photoresist formulations was 2-ethoxyethanol acetate. Some companies used diethylene glycol dimethyl ether, commonly known as *diglyme*. A particularly useful characteristic of the glycol ethers is that they are completely miscible with water as well as with most organic solvents, so that they serve as ideal coupling agents in many solvent systems (53). From a health perspective, they have other valuable features: They are nonflammable, noncarcinogenic, and nonmutagenic.

The OSHA standards were adopted from ACGIH in 1971 and are based on long-recognized acute toxic effects of glycol ethers on the kidney, liver, hematopoietic system, and central nervous system. Reproductive and developmental hazards that became evident in subsequent animal tests, beginning with a report by Nagano in 1979 (54), were not known when the OSHA limits were established. Table 33-2 lists recommended standards.

ETHYLENE GLYCOL ETHERS

Regulatory History and Scientific Developments for the Ethylene Glycol Ethers. The following discussion traces the history of regulatory thinking about the glycol ethers, as well as the state of knowledge about their toxicology. Reproductive and developmental effects are the focus, as these outcomes are driving regulatory thinking. On May 2, 1983, NIOSH published a Current Intelligence Bulletin on the glycol ethers (55). At that time, NIOSH did not recommend a specific exposure standard. Rather, they stated that 2-methoxyethanol and 2-ethoxyethanol had the potential to cause reproductive damage in male and female workers and that exposure should be limited as much as possible. NIOSH recommended that OSHA reassess the standards.

On January 24, 1984, the U.S. Environmental Protection Agency published an advance notice of proposed rulemaking, stating its intent to establish stricter standards for the glycol ethers. Completed animal studies had been brought to the EPA's attention. On May 20, 1986, the EPA, in accordance with the Toxic Substances Control Act, referred the responsibility of determining an appropriate standard to OSHA. In the interim, the EPA published a risk assessment on the glycol ethers. Their recommended exposure limits are shown in Table 33-2.

ACGIH lowered its TLVs for the four chemicals in 1985, based on animal studies that demonstrated reproductive and developmental toxicity. Those TLVs have remained unchanged and are shown in Table 33-2. On April 2, 1987, OSHA published an advance notification to establish health and safety standards for 2-methoxyethanol (2-ME), 2-ethoxyethanol (2-EE), and their respective acetates, 2-methoxyethanol acetate (2-MEA) and 2-ethoxyethanol acetate (2-EEA) (56). In its Criteria Document, NIOSH issued RELs of 0.1 ppm for 2-ME and 2-MEA, and 0.5 ppm for 2-EE and 2-EEA. These are very close to the EPA recommendations of 1984 (see Table 33-2). The NIOSH document also strongly encouraged implementation of biological monitoring for the metabolites of glycol ethers, whenever time-weighted average

TABLE 33-2. Recommended exposure standards for glycol ethers (in ppm)

Name	OSHA PEL, 1991; draft standard, 1993	Current ACGIH threshold limit value, 1997	U.S. EPA recommended exposure limit, 1984	NIOSH Crit Doc, 1991
Methoxyethanol (CH_3-O-CH_2-CH_2-OH)	25/(0.1)	5	0.03	0.1
2-Methoxyethanol acetate (CH_3-O-CH_2-CH_2-COOH)	25/(0.1)	5	0.03	0.1
2-Ethoxyethanol (CH_3-CH_2-O-CH_2-CH_2-OH)	200/(0.5)	5	0.5	0.5
2-Ethoxyethanol acetate (CH_3-CH_2-O-CH_2-CH_2-COOH)	100/(0.5)	5	0.5	0.5

ACGIH, American Conference of Governmental Industrial Hygienists; EPA, Environmental Protection Agency; NIOSH, National Institute for Occupational Safety and Health; OSHA, Occupational Safety and Health Administration; PEL, permissible exposure limit.
Note: All standards include a skin notation.

(TWA) exposures exceed one-half of the REL or dermal contact occurs, in recognition of the large contribution of skin absorption.

Animal outcomes, manifesting as fetal death or resorptions, were observed at inhalation levels for 2-ME as low as 10 ppm in rabbits and 50 ppm in rats (57). The no-observed-effect level (NOEL) for fetal resorption in these studies was 3 ppm in rabbits and 10 ppm in rats. Other fetal effects, such as skeletal and soft-tissue lesions, were observed at higher levels of exposure.

Testicular damage was observed in rats and rabbits after inhalation exposures of 2-ME (58). The NOEL was 30 ppm in the rabbit. In the rat, inhalation exposures produced similar testicular damage with a NOEL of 100 ppm.

In rabbits, fetal skeletal abnormalities were observed in inhalation studies with 2-ME at 175 ppm (59). Inhalation studies with 2-ME in rats also produced skeletal defects as well as decreased birth weight (60). The NOEL in both studies was 50 ppm. 2-EE has been shown to produce similar fetal toxicity in dermal studies (61). Maternal or paternal exposures to 2-EE both result in neurotoxic effects in offspring manifested as impaired neuromuscular ability (62).

A 2-EEA inhalation study used New Zealand White rabbits and Fischer 344 rats exposed to vapor on gestational days 6 through 18 at concentrations of 0, 50, 100, 200, and 300 ppm for 6 hours a day. Both species showed developmental toxicity and teratogenicity at levels of 100 to 300 ppm. At 50 ppm, both species were free of effect (63). Testicular damage was observed in rabbits after exposure of 2-EE with a NOEL of 100 ppm (64).

Many other bioassays have been reported, but the ones mentioned are representative of the findings. A complete catalogue of studies can be found in the NIOSH Criteria Document (65). The number of studies and consistency of results are highly persuasive.

Epidemiologic Evidence. The epidemiologic data available specifically on glycol ethers are meager and poorly controlled. Three studies pertain to male reproduction. A study of men exposed to 2-EE demonstrated a decrease in average sperm count when compared with control subjects. The airborne levels of 2-EE were measured as nondetectable up to 33.8 ppm (66). A study in a glycol ether production facility found decreased testicular size in exposed men, but no decrease in sperm counts or other sperm abnormalities (67).

A study of shipyard painters exposed to 2-ME at a mean concentration of 2.6 mg per m^3 (1.2 ppm) and 2-EE at a mean concentration of 9.9 mg per m^3 (2.6 ppm) found an increased prevalence of oligospermia and azoospermia (68). The results, when controlled for smoking, also demonstrated an increased odds ratio for lower sperm count per ejaculation. It is important to note that these exposure levels are well within current OSHA and ACGIH standards. Biological monitoring for metabolites of 2-ME and 2-EE was positive.

Metabolism of Ethylene Glycol Ethers. Three general concepts in glycol ether toxicology emerge from pharmacokinetic data (53,69–71). The first is the biological activation of ethylene glycol ethers by liver-dependent alcohol dehydrogenase (ADH) to an alkoxyacetic acid metabolite that is the actual toxin. Glycol ethers with a secondary alcohol group, such as the common isomers of propylene glycol ethers, do not serve as substrates for ADH. Instead, they are metabolized by cytochrome P-450–dependent O-demethylation, and subsequently biotransformed to carbon dioxide. No toxic metabolite is formed.

The second concept is that a mole of a glycol ether is toxicologically equivalent to a mole of its acetate. The glycol ether acetates are rapidly converted to the corresponding glycol ethers by esterases present in the mucosa, liver, kidneys, lungs, and blood.

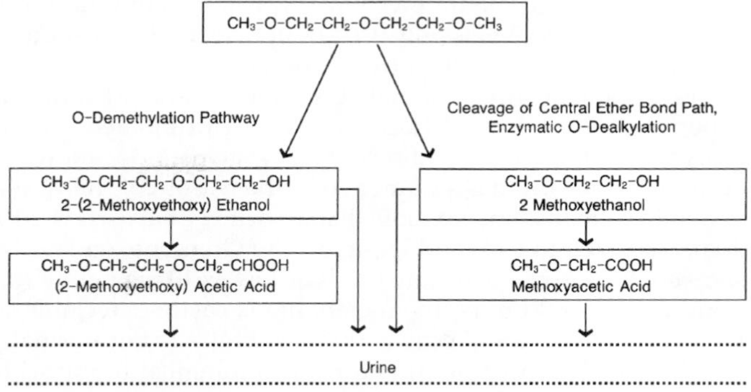

Figure 33-6. Metabolism of diethylene glycol dimethyl ether.

Subsequent biotransformation to an alkoxyacetic acid occurs as in Figure 33-5. The third important concept is that an inverse relationship exists between the length of the substituted alkyl group and reproductive toxicity. 2-ME is more toxic than 2-EE that is, in turn, more toxic than 2-butoxyethanol.

Of note, studies have revealed that the likely first step in the metabolism of diethylene glycol dimethyl ether (diglyme) is the hydrolysis of the ether bond, yielding at least one molecule of 2-methoxyethanol. Metabolism studies in rats and mice have demonstrated that diglyme is, as was suspected, biotransformed in part to yield 2-ME, and ultimately the toxic metabolite 2-MAA (72) (Fig. 33-6). Bioassays demonstrate that all the adverse effects seen with 2-ME occur at similar exposure levels of diglyme (73–76).

Mechanism of Toxicity for Ethylene Glycol Ethers. The mechanism by which glycol ethers cause reproductive toxicity is not known. Studies at the Chemical Industry Institute of Toxicology suggest that interference with DNA or RNA synthesis may be involved (77,78). One hypothesis is that alkoxyacetic acids interfere with the availability of one-carbon units for incorporation into purine and pyrimidine bases, thereby affecting the formation of nucleic acids. At a time of rapid cellular proliferation, such as embryogenesis, a limitation in the availability of these precursors presumably could be highly damaging.

Skin Absorption of Ethylene Glycol Ethers. *In vitro* studies using the skin of beagle dogs demonstrated that 2-EEA is absorbed at a rate of 2.3 mg per cm^2 per hour (79). *In vitro* studies of isolated human skin show absorption rates of 2.8 mg per cm^2 per hour for 2-ME and 0.9 mg per cm^2 per hour for 2-EE (80). The area of a human hand is approximately 650 cm^2. Therefore, immersion of a hand in 2-ME could result in the absorption of 400 mg in 15 minutes. This is equivalent to exposure to 10 ppm in the air for 8 hours. Just 10 seconds of hand immersion causes absorption of an amount of 2-ME equivalent to 8 hours of exposure at the NIOSH draft REL of 0.1 ppm. Of course, proper work practices with photoresist preparations does not result in hand immersion or prolonged unprotected skin contact.

Biological Monitoring. Because the glycol ethers are rapidly absorbed through the skin, environmental sampling of airborne concentrations is an incomplete assessment of total exposure, unless the potential for skin exposure can be completely excluded. Fortunately, analytical techniques exist to determine the levels of alkoxyacetic acid metabolites of 2-ME and 2-EE in the urine (81,82).

Groeseneken has performed experiments on human volunteers to determine the rate of pulmonary absorption of 2-EE and subsequent excretion of metabolite (83). A steady state was reached almost immediately, and respiratory elimination of unmetabolized 2-EE was only 0.4% of uptake. Ethoxyacetic acid (EAA) was observed in the urine during exposure and up to 42 hours after exposure. The half-life of absorbed 2-EE in this experiment was 10 to 12 hours. Only 23% of inhaled 2-EE is recovered as EAA. Conjugation of EAA to glycerine is known to occur in animals, and is assumed to be the reason for this observation in humans. It is possible that a portion of absorbed 2-EE is metabolized to CO_2 and expired. The Groeseneken studies showed that even at exposure levels as low as 10 mg per m^3 (2.8 ppm) of air for 4 hours, the metabolite is easily detectable 18 hours after exposure. Because the metabolite is not normally present in human urine, this form of biological monitoring could serve as a qualitative indicator of exposure.

A field application of this technology studied five women exposed to a combined concentration of 4 ppm of 2-EE and 2-EEA in a silk-screening process (84). All were wearing gloves. The urinary excretion of EAA showed a clear increase over the week, and EAA was still detectable 12 days after exposure ceased. The half-life of EAA excretion was estimated to be 1 to 2 days. A correlation coefficient of 0.92 was found between average exposure over the week and the EAA excretion at the end of the week.

It is premature to state that a quantitative correlation can be made between the amounts of alkoxyacetic acids found in the urine and absorption of glycol ethers. Most trials have shown great intraindividual variability between the amount of alkoxyacetic acids excreted, given the same absorption. The variation was as much as tenfold in one study (85). Among factors that have been demonstrated to affect the excretion of the toxic metabolite of a glycol ether are metabolic induction by xenobiotics, metabolic inhibition by xenobiotics, and dose-dependent pharmacokinetics. This deficiency in the data should not discourage the use of biological monitoring. Although the amount of metabolite in the urine may not be linearly correlated to the absorbed dose of glycol ether, it is likely to be closely correlated to the concentration of toxic metabolite being presented to target organs.

Environmental Exposure Data. A few published reports exist of sampling data for glycol ether exposure within the semiconductor industry. The EPA contracted a report on glycol ether exposure data in a variety of industries (56). The data showed that most large industries had exposures of less than the 0.03 ppm level for 2-ME and 1 ppm for 2-EE. The exceptions were the trade industries involved in surface coating applications and the use of inks. The former category includes the microelectronics industry. It is important to remember that these data address only exposure via inhalation, and that any skin absorption is additional.

The Semiconductor Industry Association conducted an industry-wide survey of industrial hygiene air sampling data during 1984 to 1985 to describe typical levels of exposure to the ethylene glycol ethers. Seven member companies provided a total of 277 samples. In 1982, NIOSH had done similar sampling in the semiconductor industry and generated 92 data points. The data from these two studies were published together in 1989 (30). The mean concentration in air of personal samples of 2-EE was 0.55 ppm, just slightly higher than the NIOSH draft REL of 0.5 ppm. A total of 24 area samples was collected, and the arithmetic mean was 0.99 ppm. The results for 2-EEA were lower with a mean of 0.05 ppm, although the mean of short-term samples (15 minutes or less) was 2.82 ppm. Area samples were also low at 0.05 ppm. Geometric means, statistical measures that better fit the distribution of occupational exposure data, were even lower for 2-EEA at 0.02, 0.09, and 0.01 ppm, respectively. For purposes of the statistical analysis, data points that were less than the limit of detection were assumed to equal the limit of detection, a conservative approach that would tend to overestimate the actual mean exposure levels.

Qualitative Risk Assessments of Glycol Ethers. The EPA risk assessment of 1984 calculated the margins of safety—defined as the NOEL in the most sensitive species divided by the estimated human exposure level. The NOELs for testicular toxicity were 30 ppm for 2-ME and 100 ppm for 2-EE. For developmental toxicity, the NOELs were 3 ppm for 2-ME and 50 ppm for 2-EE. The NOEL for each acetate was assumed to be the same as its parent compound.

An exposure level with a 100-fold margin of safety is considered unlikely to produce adverse effects in humans. This safety factor is often explained as tenfold for differences between humans and test species, and another tenfold for protection of hypersusceptible subgroups in the human population. The EPA estimated that between 206,000 and 350,000 workers in the U.S. workforce are exposed to the four ethylene glycol ethers at levels exceeding the 100-fold margin of safety. The EPA recommended adoption of acceptable exposure levels of 0.03 ppm for 2-ME and 2-MEA, and 0.5 ppm for 2-EE and 2-EEA.

Another qualitative risk assessment was published in 1988 (86). This work was done under contract to the Semiconductor Industry Association. The assessment's author chose to use a safety factor of 10 rather than the more traditionally accepted factor of 100. Given the consistency of glycol ether bioassay results among different species, this may be a reasonable decision. The assessment's author also chose to reject the Dow Chemical study of 1982 that had demonstrated a NOEL of 3 for developmental effects in rabbits (57). No other study has shown a NOEL this low. The result of these two choices was to conclude that the current ACGIH TLVs of 5 ppm offer adequate margins of safety for reproductive and developmental effects. Based on this analysis and the environmental monitoring data, the assessment's author concluded that workers in the semiconductor industry would not be expected to experience reproductive or developmental effects from glycol ether use, so long as inhalation exposures remained controlled to or below these levels and dermal contact was avoided.

SUBSTITUTES FOR GLYCOL ETHERS IN PHOTORESISTS

Manufacturers and users of photoresists have taken efforts to eliminate ethylene glycol ethers from their products and processes. Four commonly explored substitutes are propylene glycol monomethyl ether acetate (PM acetate, PGMEA), ethyl-3-ethoxypropionate, ethyl lactate, and 4-butyrolactone (71). The acute toxicity of the possible substitutes as established by median lethal dose value is apparently low (71). Furthermore, they seem to be free of chronic toxicity, including reproductive and developmental effects, except at very high exposure levels. The most commonly used substitutes, PGMEA and ethyl lactate, appear to represent significant improvements to the ethylene glycol ethers from a health perspective.

Ethyl lactate is a colorless liquid with a characteristic odor and a vapor pressure at 30°C of 5 mm Hg. Its toxicologic properties resemble those of ethyl acetate, which is low in toxicity and is also an ethyl ester of a low-molecular-weight carboxylic acid. Ethyl lactate produced no skin irritation or sensitization in human subjects patch tested with a concentration of 8% in petrolatum. It has a high median lethal dose orally, greater than 5 gm per kg in rats and 2.5 gm per kg in mice. It is irritating in the rabbit eye and, like ethyl acetate, is a central nervous system depressant at very high concentrations in animals (87). It can probably be absorbed through the skin, as well as via inhalation. It is converted in nasal mucous membranes and in the skin to ethyl alcohol and lactic acid; presumably, hydrolysis of the ester linkage occurs in other tissues as well, leading to these products. It did not have mutagenic activity in bacteria. Ethyl lactate is used in a variety of commercial products, present in the following concentrations: soap—usual 0.01%, max 0.2%; perfume—usual 0.1%, max 0.8%. It is used in some nail polish removers in concentrations from 10% to 50%. It is approved by the U.S. Food and Drug Administration for food use. It is present naturally in apples, citrus fruits, pineapple, peas, sauerkraut, vinegar, bread, beer, grape brandy, rum, whisky, cider, sherry, wine, and cocoa, among other foods. It is volatilized from a variety of beverages and foods (detectable by headspace collection and analysis), including vinegar, soy sauce, wine, and beer (87). Although longer-term health effects from this material have not been studied in animals, its relatively low volatility, conversion to well-studied compounds (lactic acid and ethanol), and its presence in relatively high concentrations naturally in foods suggest that it is unlikely to pose significant health risks through controlled use in semiconductor manufacturing.

Propylene glycol monomethyl ether acetate (PM acetate, PGMEA) possesses essentially identical toxicity to propylene glycol monomethyl ether (PGME), to which it is hydrolyzed. It is a colorless liquid with a relatively high vapor pressure of 3.8 mm Hg at 20°C (71). Its vapors are a mild upper respiratory irritant. It possesses low acute toxicity in humans and experimental animals, much lower than the comparable ethylene glycol ethers. It is absorbed through the skin. Unlike ethylene glycol ethers, it is not metabolized to an alkoxyacetic acid derivative, presumably because it is a secondary rather than a primary alcohol. Extensive testing in laboratory animals demonstrates that it is not a reproductive or developmental toxin, except perhaps at very high maternally toxic doses. This lack of developmental toxicity contrasts sharply with that of the ethylene glycol ethers, which are selective developmental toxins. It is thought that these differences reflect the different metabolic pathways (88,89). Of note, the other isomer of PGMEA, the β (beta) isomer, which is a primary alcohol and can be a contaminant of PGMEA, is metabolized to 2-methoxypropionic acid and is a selective fetal toxin (89). Consequently, it is important to confirm that this isomer constitutes a very small percentage (less than 1%) of the supplied PGMEA, because the reassuring toxicology data on PGMEA derive from a commercially available product with less than 1% of the contaminant.

OTHER SOLVENTS AND CHEMICALS USED IN PHOTOLITHOGRAPHY

Ethyl-3-ethoxypropionate (EEP) has been used as a less-flammable substitute for acetone in edge bead removal, to remove accumulated spun-on photoresist from the edge of the wafer. It appears to be of low toxicity, but relatively few data on its toxicity exist. By analogy to related esters, such as vinyl propionate and ethyl acetate, it is probably a mild upper respiratory tract irritant. Several studies have been conducted in rats and rabbits, which demonstrate that it is of low toxicity. No health effects have been observed at concentrations below 250 ppm. Concentrations of approximately 1,000 ppm for 90 days caused decreased activity and reduced body weight gain in rats. Concentrations of 500 ppm for 90 days caused decreased weight gain, but no health effects were seen at 250 ppm. In other studies, EEP did not cause teratogenic effects (i.e., birth defects in offspring of pregnant animals) at exposure levels as high as 1,000 ppm. It may cause slight reduction in fetal growth but only at concentrations (500 to 1,000 ppm) high enough to cause observable toxicity in the maternal animal (71). A study of the metabolism of EEP in rats found no evidence that this material was metabolized to an alkoxypropionic acid derivative, which might raise concerns of toxicity similar to that of the ethylene glycol ethers (90). Although the toxicologic data for this compound do not suggest a concern, its use in practice has triggered odor complaints from employees and nearby community residents, because of its very low odor threshold and unpleasant odor. These complaints have created an impetus for a further substitute.

NMP is a colorless liquid with a mild amine odor and a low vapor pressure, 0.334 mm Hg at 25°C. It is used as a photoresist stripper primarily, as well as in polyimide photoresists. It is of low acute toxicity with oral median lethal doses in laboratory animals of approximately 4 to 7 gm per kg body weight. It is well absorbed through the skin and can cause irritant contact dermatitis (91,92). It does not appear to be a selective developmental toxin in laboratory animals from oral or dermal exposures (91). Some controversy exists on this point, with EPA scientists interpreting a two-generation rat dietary study as showing effects such as decreased male fertility, female fecundity, reduced litter size, and reduced body weight at a dose of 50 mg per kg lowest observed adverse effect level (LOAEL), with a parental no observed adverse effect level (NOAEL) of 160 mg per kg (93). However, other scientists have reported a problem with experimental design, based on the strain of rats used, raising questions about the validity of these findings and prompting a replication of this study. Very high and naturally unachievable air concentrations of NMP (150 and 165 ppm) resulted in an increase in preimplantation losses, decreased fetal body weight, and a delay in neurobehavior development in the offspring of exposed rats, without observable maternal toxicity (94,95). Although the overall reproductive and developmental toxicology database on NMP is largely reassuring, these uncertainties suggest a need to minimize any potential for exposure. Neither inhalation, because of the very low vapor pressure of NMP, nor oral exposures are likely in the workplace. Confirming this, a detailed industrial hygiene survey of operations using NMP by one large semiconductor manufacturer found that 88% of 169 samples fell below the limit of detection, with the remaining detectable samples falling well below 1 ppm. Avoidance of exposure thus primarily requires attention to avoiding unprotected skin contact, through the use of face shields, and chemically resistant gloves and aprons during chemical handling or maintenance activities.

HMDS is in the chemical class of silazanes, which are silicon compounds containing nitrogen. HMDS is a colorless, transparent liquid that smells like ammonia. In addition to its use in the semiconductor industry as a surface-active agent spun onto wafers in photolithography, HMDS is used in organic synthesis in the chemical and pharmaceutical industry. HMDS undergoes rapid hydrolysis in the presence of atmospheric moisture, to liberate one molecule of ammonia and one molecule of hexamethyldisiloxane per molecule of HMDS (96). When HMDS undergoes thermal decomposition in the presence of oxygen (at high temperatures more than approximately 300°F), formaldehyde may be released. HMDS shares this property with other compounds containing a silicon atom bound to a methyl group. Formaldehyde is not released at the much lower temperatures (200°F or less) maintained in the bake ovens on coaters. A study in rats found reduced activity, ataxia, dyspnea, sedation, and loss of the righting reflex at HMDS exposures of 5,600 mg per m^3. The LC_{50} for an unspecified time interval was 10,300 mg per m^3. Bleeding into the lungs was the only pathologic abnormality detected in those animals that died. Comparative studies using ammonium hydroxide solution (ammonia), instead of HMDS, indicated that most of the toxicologic effects of HMDS were consistent with those associated with acute exposure to ammonia at very high concentrations (96). One study of HMDS and other compounds conducted in the United States in 1975 examined the ability of HMDS to induce benign lung tumors (i.e., adenomas) in mice. Exposure was by intraperitoneal injection at levels close to the maximally tolerated dose. No excess of benign lung tumors existed in the HMDS-exposed animals compared to the control groups (97). HMDS is a skin and eye irritant with direct contact (98). Hexamethyldisiloxane, formed during atmospheric hydrolysis, is a respiratory tract irritant, as is ammonia, obviously. Animal evidence exists that hexamethyldisiloxane causes central nervous system depression with comparably high air concentrations, suggesting that it may be the proximate cause of the central nervous system depression noted with HMDS. Most short-term tests for genotoxicity or mutagenicity with hexamethyldisiloxane have been negative. It is used in some cosmetics. Hexamethyldisiloxane has a relatively high vapor pressure, 42 mm Hg at 25°C (99). In sum, HMDS appears to be a respiratory irritant and central nervous system depressant with very high concentration exposures, which would never be encountered in a wafer fab. It is possible that low levels of ammonia released by hydrolysis could lead to mild transient eye or mucous membrane irritation, although local exhaust on coaters should prevent this.

Arsenic

The acute effects of exposure to inorganic arsenic are well characterized (100,101). Realistically, exposures in the semiconductor industry are extremely unlikely to be sufficient to cause acute symptoms. Concern about exposure in semiconductor manufacturing is driven by the chronic health effects—primarily cancer and, to a lesser degree, concern about possible effects on the fetus. Documented chronic health effects in occupationally exposed populations include lung cancer, perforation of the nasal septum, laryngitis, pharyngitis, bronchitis, peripheral neuropathy, and encephalopathy. Cutaneous manifestations have been seen in individuals exposed to arsenic in drinking water and drugs, but not in occupationally exposed groups. These clinical findings have included hyperkeratosis of the palms and skin cancer. The possibility of fetal toxicity in humans is not widely discussed, but some animal studies suggest a teratogenic effect (102,103).

Arsenic used in silicon-based fabs currently is typically AsH_3, alkylated arsines, or solid source elemental arsenic, although some older processes used trivalent and pentavalent arsenic compounds. Some organizations have eliminated the use of AsH_3 or developed new delivery systems that contain lower volumes of AsH_3 at subatmospheric pressures (not compressed). A detailed industrial hygiene investigation of ion implant activities, in which solid source elemental arsenic served as the only arsenic source, revealed extremely low airborne arsenic concentrations during maintenance activities. With two different types of implanters, the geometric means of TWA samples for 46 and 27 samples were 8% and 5% of the permissible exposure limit (10 µg per m^3), respectively. Cleaning of equipment in the fab for one type of implanter, such as cleaning the source housing and scraping the beam line, was associated with higher levels than cleaning in the arsenic parts clean shop. The addition of supplemental local exhaust in the fab led to further reduced airborne concentrations. With 23 measurements, sampling for AsH_3 was below the limit of detection. Subsequent chemical and solubility testing of the residue from these implanters strongly suggested that the arsenic remained in an elemental form (rather than an oxide or compound of arsenic) (104). Furthermore, concurrent pre- and postshift urinary monitoring for inorganic arsenic and its metabolites, and air sampling during maintenance operations on implanters, demonstrated an inability of biomonitoring to detect arsenic exposure (*personal communication*). This finding was not surprising, given the relationship between TWA exposure to arsenic and urine concentrations of inorganic arsenic and its metabolites. The background urinary concentration, which varies with arsenic in drinking water and diet, is expected to be less than 10 to 20 µg per L in the United States. At a TWA exposure of 2 µg per m^3, urinary arsenic concentration does not exceed this background level (105). Given air concentrations lower than this, even during maintenance activities and the use of personal protective equipment, it is unlikely that one could detect an increment in urinary arsenic from these activities. If the residue is insoluble elemental arsenic, which appears to be the case, absorption of arsenic into the body and subsequent urinary excretion does not occur.

A study of airborne arsenic and hair arsenic levels in maintenance workers in a silicon wafer fab using 15% AsH_3 in implanters found three of 12 short-term (not TWA) breathing zone samples greater than the detection limit, ranging from 2 to 15 µg per m^3. Hair arsenic levels did not clearly distinguish maintenance workers from the control group in this population (106).

Excess risk of lung cancer from arsenic has been demonstrated in workers exposed to arsenic in smelters, including copper smelters, insecticide manufacturing, and mining. Heavily exposed workers in epidemiologic studies had been exposed to arsenic concentrations from 200 to more than 50,000 µg per m^3. Low exposure groups generally ranged from 10 to 500 µg per m^3. The groups with the lowest cumulative exposures in these studies typically had 1 to 10 mg per m^3 per year of exposure; in many of the studies, the risk of lung cancer in these low-exposure groups was not distinguishable from that in the control group. Especially when considering the noncontinuous nature of exposures and the use of respiratory protective equipment, exposures in ion implanter maintenance workers likely are three or four orders of magnitude below levels in these studies that conferred a clear excess of lung cancer. Admittedly, epidemiology has problems in detecting risks at very low exposures. In addition, some epidemiologic studies have suggested a supralinear dose-response curve (i.e., a proportionately greater effect at lower doses, which are still much higher than doses in the semiconductor industry) (107). Other epidemiologic studies at low doses (e.g., from arsenic in drinking water) have demonstrated a sublinear dose-response relationship (108). Studies on the genotoxicity of arsenic, including the induction of chromosomal aberrations and the potentiation of the effect of mutagens, generally demonstrate a sublinear or threshold dose-response relationship, probably because of an indirect genetic effect. These data, suggesting a threshold, provide further support for the notion that the very low levels of exposure in the semiconductor industry are unlikely to lead to lung cancer or other adverse effects (108). Nevertheless, efforts to minimize arsenic exposure, through engineering controls, local exhaust ventilation, training in good work practices, and use of respiratory protective equipment, are clearly warranted for this group of semiconductor workers.

GALLIUM ARSENIDE

In October 1987, NIOSH issued an alert about potential health hazards of GaAs (109). It is important to understand that this alert is based entirely on the known adverse health effects of exposure to inorganic arsenic.

A number of experiments have demonstrated that GaAs dissociates in the lung or gut of mammals to gallium and arsenic, with the latter behaving metabolically as any other inorganic arsenic species (110–112). NIOSH has recommended that GaAs be handled in accordance with the 1975 NIOSH recommendation for inorganic arsenic (113). The NIOSH recommendation is that GaAs be controlled to not exceed 2 µg per m^3 of air as a 15-minute ceiling. OSHA has a less-restrictive standard for inorganic arsenic that includes a permissible exposure limit (PEL) (TWA of 8 hours) of 10 µg per m^3 (114).

ROLE OF BIOLOGICAL MONITORING FOR INORGANIC ARSENIC

Biological monitoring for arsenic can, in some circumstances, be a useful complement to airborne environmental sampling in ensuring worker safety. Biological monitoring of total and inorganic arsenic excretion is available to supplement the usual air sampling and wipe samples. Some understanding of the metabolism of arsenic is necessary to properly interpret these tests.

Arsenic from dietary sources (primarily seafood) is in the form of either arsenobetaine, arsenocholine, or trimethylarsenic acid. These forms of arsenic are referred to as *organic* arsenic and have not been associated with any adverse health outcomes.

Exposure to inorganic arsenic occurs in a variety of environmental and industrial settings. Natural drinking water sources, anthropogenic environmental contamination from mine wastes, and seaweed are examples. The latter poses a problem when monitoring Japanese workers but is generally not a consideration for American workers (115). Inorganic arsenic can be inhaled or ingested in many possible forms. It is excreted in one of three forms: arsenic cations, monomethylarsonic acid, or dimethylarsinic (cacodylic) acid. Only inorganic arsenic can cause the well-documented acute and chronic adverse health effects of arsenic.

Measurement of total arsenic in urine measures the organic and inorganic forms. This test is widely available and is what many surveillance programs have relied on for evidence of absorption. Workers are generally asked to refrain from consuming seafood for 5 days before giving the urine sample. Health practitioners faced with a high result invariably repeat the test after delivering more adamant dietary instructions to the worker. The repeat test is usually normal, and a tendency exists to pursue the problem no further. The abnormal result is ascribed to diet, but the reality is that a normal repeat urine does not definitively indicate that the initial high number was not caused by a transient workplace exposure. Potentially correctable engineering problems or breaches in safe work practices could be overlooked.

A solution to this dilemma exists. It is possible to measure the inorganic component of the total arsenic excreted in urine (116,117). Until late 1989, this test (often termed *fractionation* or *speciation* of arsenic) was not readily available commercially. Small amounts of inorganic arsenic are absorbed from seafood. For this reason, even if total arsenic is not being determined, it is important to continue to emphasize the usual dietary restrictions before routine screening. Any urine inorganic arsenic level in excess of 25 μg per L should be pursued very aggressively to find sources of exposure, although it may reflect nonoccupational sources.

Although some arsenic is accumulated in the body—primarily in hair, skin, nails, and the lungs—most is excreted into the urine quite rapidly (101,118). Annual samples donated on arbitrary dates, such as birthdays, are not likely to detect intermittent absorption. Attempts should be made to collect samples soon after potential exposures. Workers should be encouraged to present for monitoring whenever they suspect an exposure may have occurred.

Because of the very low levels of airborne arsenic in modern silicon wafer fabs, it is unlikely that urinary biomonitoring is able to detect increments in exposure. Thus, a study of gallium arsenide workers with mean TWA exposures approximately two times the PEL of 10 μg per m^3 was unable to detect changes in arsenic concentration postshift or differences from the control group (115). These levels are substantially higher than levels documented in silicon-based fabs using optimal control technologies. Along these lines, since its inception, a prior program of urinary inorganic arsenic testing at one large semiconductor manufacturer over several years never detected elevated urinary arsenic levels in any employee tested, including implanter maintenance staff (*personal communication*). A decision to implement a urinary biomonitoring program for arsenic should take into consideration the arsenic species present (AsH_3, elemental arsenic, trivalent or pentavalent arsenic, gallium arsenide), the adequacy of industrial hygiene controls, and the results of air monitoring during maintenance operations. Similarly, hair arsenic testing, which theoretically can detect arsenic absorption over a longer time interval, is unlikely to be useful in this setting because of the very low levels of exposure and the additional problem of external contamination of hair, which cannot be distinguished from internal absorption and deposition in hair.

OTHER MEDICAL SURVEILLANCE FOR ARSENIC

In addition to biological monitoring for inorganic arsenic absorption, few other medical surveillance measures are productive. Taking a good history to try to elicit any concerns about the workplace or arsenic exposures is certainly useful. Given the proper environmental control of arsenic, examination components, such as the neurologic or skin examination that might be useful with higher exposures, are unlikely to yield relevant findings. The remainder of the typical physical examination is unlikely to be worthwhile. No laboratory work, except the biological monitoring already discussed, is specific enough to be of value. Of course, if environmental monitoring results exceed the OSHA action level, which is unlikely, then a company is legally obligated to conform to the arsenic standard, which unfortunately includes a number of insensitive and nonspecific screening tests (114).

GALLIUM OXIDE TOXICITY

Because experiments have shown that gallium is not absorbed from either the lung or the gut, there has been little concern about the systemic effects of gallium in gallium arsenide operations. One paper raises concerns about local pulmonary toxicity (119). Significant pulmonary pathology in rats was caused by inhalation of gallium oxide particles at a high dose, 23 mg per m^3. The exposure was 4 weeks in duration, at which time alveolar proteinosis was seen. By 6 to 12 months postexposure, the lesions progressed to fibrosis. The paper's authors stated that the cytotoxic, inflammatory, and fibrotic responses were equal to or greater than those observed with quartz particles. In the future, exposure to gallium may be regulated as more than a nuisance dust. In the meantime, employers should take prudent steps to minimize inhalation of gallium or its compounds, although constraints on airborne particles in the fab would clearly prevent exposures at the level studied experimentally.

Gases

Every semiconductor manufacturer must develop a strategy for the safe handling of gases, because the use of toxic, hazardous, and corrosive gases entails a potential for sudden release into the work environment that could lead to serious injury, other health effects, or property damage. The first step in safe gas handling is to identify every gas used and the potential of each to cause injury or illness. With a clear understanding of the gases and their inherent hazards, it is possible to decide which gases can be brought into work areas by cylinder, which require a more expensive system of gas lines with remote storage, and which may benefit from substitution. Available state-of-the-art control systems for toxic and hazardous gases, including double contained gas lines, sensitive monitoring and alarm systems, automatic gas shut-off systems, and appropriate work practices and personal protective equipment, prevent any routine exposure to these gases and should be able to preclude accidental releases and exposures. Currently, most toxic, hazardous, and corrosive gases are supplied via specially contained gas lines from a remote gas pad.

SILANE AND CHLORINATED DERIVATIVES

Silane gas is used extensively in semiconductor manufacturing for the deposition of thin dielectric films. Silane presents a significant health hazard because of its potential to detonate. Until the early 1980s, the conventional wisdom was that silane, although pyrophoric, could not explode. A series of experiments established that under certain conditions, generally with high volume leaks into stagnant air, silane could accumulate and subsequently detonate (120). Manufacturers of monitoring equipment report that 15 to 20 ppm leaks of silane in semiconductor fabrication areas and around gas cabinets are found routinely (37). One of the major problems of handling silane is that it does not always immediately ignite on contact with air. Small leaks can produce sizable quantities of silane and air mixtures that have subsequently detonated (121).

As an explosive, 1 lb of silane (0.45 km) is equivalent to 6 lb (2.7 km) of TNT. A typical 9-by-52-in. (23-by-132-cm) cylinder of silane contains 5,000 g or just more than 14 lb (6.4 km) of silane, which is equivalent to 84 lb (38.2 km) of TNT. An unfortunate demonstration of silane's explosive potential occurred in March 1988. A single cylinder of silane that had been contaminated with nitrous oxide exploded and killed three people. The explosion occurred at an analytical laboratory after the cylinder had been removed from a semiconductor facility because of the contamination problem.

No catastrophic detonations of silane have been reported in the semiconductor industry, although in 1988 a silane gas leak at a semiconductor facility in California ignited and caused four injuries and a plant evacuation. Serious burns to a technician, after a cylinder leak in gas cabinets on a gas pad, with accumulation and then ignition of silane, have been reported.

ACGIH has a rather curious TLV of 5 ppm for silane (122). This level was adopted in 1983 and replaced a TLV of 0.5 ppm that had been in effect since 1974. The rationale for either concentration is unclear, but is probably a response to the inhalation toxicity of other metallic hydrides. Acute toxicity testing in laboratory animals has shown no toxicity in rats up to 1,400 ppm for 6 hours (122). Four-hour inhalation studies established the LC_{50} in rats and mice, respectively, at 4,000 and 9,600 ppm (123). In any case, the threat of silane is not pulmonary or systemic toxicity via inhalation, but rather the danger of fire or detonation.

Dichlorosilane, trichlorosilane, and silicon tetrachloride are also used extensively in the semiconductor industry. Dichlorosilane (SiH_2Cl_2, DCS) appears to form hydrochloric acid and small particles containing silicon and chlorine on contact with water vapor in air. The LC_{50} in male mice for a 4-hour exposure was 144 ppm, whereas a 2-hour exposure to 64 ppm resulted in wheezing and histopathologic changes in the nose and trachea. Exposure to 32 ppm 6 hours per day for 2 and 4 weeks also resulted in wheezing and more pronounced histopathologic changes in the nose and trachea, including squamous metaplasia (124). Trichlorosilane ($SiHCl_3$, TCS) and silicon tetrachloride ($SiCl_4$) are liquids with low boiling points and sharp, unpleasant odors that are severe irritants to the eye and respiratory tract. Similar to DCS, both compounds yield hydrochloric acid and other silicon-containing compounds on exposure to water, water vapor, or moist mucous membranes (125,126). After a spill of silicon tetrachloride at a chemical plant, most individuals developed mild eye and upper respiratory irritation, but six individuals who were involved in the clean-up developed a variety of transient symptoms, including cough, wheezing, burning throat, lacrimation, and rhinorrhea. Chest x-rays and pulmonary function studies revealed no abnormalities attributable to the exposure (127).

ARSINE

AsH_3 is a highly toxic gas. Thus, at 250 ppm, AsH_3 is said to be lethal to humans instantly, or with exposure for 30 minutes, variably. Lower levels of exposure, in the 10- to 50-ppm range, for longer intervals may cause hemolytic anemia and ultimately lead to death. The principal pathologic effect is hemolysis leading to a severe anemia and hypoxemia. Renal failure also occurs either from direct nephrotoxicity of AsH_3 or from hemoglobinuria. Hydration, dialysis, and general support are the mainstays of therapy. Exchange transfusion is recommended as the treatment for severe hemolysis. Recognizing that the resources, including the units of blood, required to treat a massive AsH_3 intoxication are substantial, particularly if it involved several individuals, prevention of releases and exposure is critical.

How likely is a significant AsH_3 release in the semiconductor industry? AsH_3 has not caused a death in the semiconductor industry, although in 1988 a graduate student who was changing an AsH_3 cylinder in a laboratory on an ion implantation tool was killed by a gas leak. Multiple deaths have been caused by AsH_3 in other industries. Given its high acute toxicity, relatively small releases of AsH_3 could lead to toxicologically important concentrations in nearby areas, although the rapidity of air changes in the fab would tend to rapidly dilute the gas. Rigorous control systems, including monitors, alarms, containment, use of small cylinders, and local exhaust, and work practices have presumably lowered the risk of a significant release substantially. Nevertheless, concerns about AsH_3 hazards have prompted some semiconductor manufacturers to eliminate or minimize its use.

SUBSTITUTION FOR ARSINE

Several semiconductor manufacturers have been able to completely eliminate AsH_3 from their processes by using elemental arsenic in implantation tools and alkylated arsine in epitaxy. Elemental arsenic is a solid and is relatively easy to work with safely under a ventilation hood or in a glove box. Alkylated arsines are liquids, therefore, the potential for catastrophe is minimal. They are also less toxic than the hydride. The introduction of subatmospheric cylinders, containing small volumes of AsH_3 adsorbed to carbon, should significantly reduce the risk of AsH_3 release. AsH_3 is released from the cylinder only when exposed to a higher vacuum inside the tool after desorption from carbon, eliminating the potential for releases to the work environment should a leak occur.

PHOSPHINE

PH_3 is a severe pulmonary irritant at high concentrations, with 4-hour LC_{50} values reported in the literature as low as 11 ppm in rats. Symptoms in humans include nausea, vomiting, cough, chest tightness, and headache, with dyspnea and chest pressure in more severe exposures. The most common cause of death in human exposures has been pulmonary edema (128). With 6-hour exposures to 10 ppm PH_3 for 4 days in mice, evidence for mild liver and kidney damage exists, histologically and on clinical chemistry tests. Similar exposures, 5 days per week for 2 weeks, to 5 ppm caused no evidence of tissue injury but slight increases in blood urea nitrogen (BUN) in male mice; no effects were observed at 2.5 ppm (128).

As a result of a report of increased chromosomal aberrations in lymphocytes from fumigant applicators exposed to PH_3 (generated from metal phosphides), the genotoxicity of PH_3 has been evaluated in several additional studies. Exposures of rats and mice to PH_3 at concentrations up to 5 ppm for 6 hours per day for 9 days did not lead to measurable evidence of genotoxicity using several assays, including measurement of sister chromatid exchange, chromosomal aberrations, and micronuclei (129). Other investigators found evidence for weak genotoxicity in mice, with an increase in the frequency of micronuclei after 13 weeks of exposure to PH_3 at 4.5 ppm, whereas a number of other assays revealed no genotoxic effect (130). A study of fumigators in Australia revealed no evidence of increases in micronuclei in lymphocytes or in urine mutagenicity using a bacterial mutation (Ames) assay, despite measured exposures as high as 2.4 ppm over 1 hour (6 of 23 exposures were more than 0.5 ppm, although 14 of 23 exposures were below the limit of detection). A higher number, although not statistically significant, of fumigators with mild liver enzyme elevations existed as compared to the controls (131). Based on industrial hygiene data and the controls in place during use of PH_3 in semiconductor manufacturing, exposures of semiconductor workers to PH_3 are unlikely and certainly below those for fumigant applicators.

DIBORANE

B_2H_6 is a pulmonary irritant, causing symptoms in humans of chest tightness, cough, dyspnea, and wheezing with acute exposures. In animal experiments, it causes pulmonary edema with acute exposures (132). Although other hydrides of boron (i.e., pentaborane, decaborane) are known central neurotoxins and some older reports of neurotoxicity caused by B_2H_6 exist, literature does not suggest that B_2H_6 is a neurotoxin (133). In male mice, the 4-hour LC_{50} was 31.5 ppm. Exposure to 5 ppm for 6 hours per day, 5 days per week, for 2 weeks led to significant increases in lung weight, as did a single 2-hour exposure to 15 ppm. Pathologically, changes with acute exposure to 15 ppm included diffuse bronchiolitis, congestion, and pulmonary edema, whereas subacute exposure over 2 weeks to 5 ppm led to perivascular inflammation and pulmonary congestion; no changes were noted in the brain or other organs (133). Significant changes in several bronchoalveolar lavage parameters occurred with a single 4-hour exposure in rats to 1 ppm B_2H_6, with more pronounced changes at 10 ppm (132). A study in male mice defined a NOEL of 1 ppm for an 8-hour exposure; subtle effects of peribronchiolar inflammation at 0.2 ppm for a 2-week subacute exposure precluded the identification of a NOEL for longer duration exposures (134).

OTHER GASES AND LOW BOILING POINT LIQUIDS

Some gases or low boiling point liquids used in different semiconductor processes, such as metal etching and diffusion, have the property of hydrolyzing in air to yield hydrochloric or hydrofluoric acid, thereby resulting in the potential for respiratory irritation. Boron trichloride (BCl_3) and phosphorus oxychloride ($POCl_3$) hydrolyze to yield hydrochloric acid (and phosphoric acid, in the case of $POCl_3$), whereas boron trifluoride and tungsten hexafluoride yield hydrogen fluoride (135–138). Nitrogen trifluoride (NF_3) has been shown to be a methemoglobin-former at high concentrations in animals (139).

GAS DELIVERY SYSTEMS FOR HIGHLY TOXIC GASES

State-of-the-art gas handling systems for highly toxic gases, such as AsH_3, isolate all cylinders in remote gas rooms. The use of cylinders with critical orifices or excess flow valves reduces the risk of a sudden large-volume release of gas. Some gas systems deliver gas to the processing area by coaxial (double-walled) lines. In some situations, the inside or delivery line containing toxic gas is pressurized to 20 to 30 lb per square inch (psi) (1.4 to 2.0 atm), whereas the annular or outside line is pressurized to approximately 100 psi (6.8 atm) with nitrogen. When a defect occurs in the delivery line, the leak is inward from the annular space. The pressure in that space is monitored, and a pressure drop causes a regulator to shut off the source of the toxic gas, as well as alarming operators of the gas system. Another promising delivery system, already described, stores the hydride adsorbed onto a solid in a cylinder maintained at subatmospheric pressures. Leaks in the cylinder do not allow leakage of the hydride from the cylinder; instead air moves into the cylinder.

Unfortunately, gas is not currently piped into ion implanters. These tools use a very high voltage chamber (approximately 100,000 V). It is, therefore, not possible to safely connect to metal gas lines. Cylinders of gas (typically AsH_3, PH_3, or B_2H_6) are placed into the tool. The industry is experimenting with sections of glass ceramic delivery line to hopefully allow gas to be delivered from outside lines.

Some highly corrosive etching gases have very low vapor pressure and, therefore, must be brought to the tool in cylinders. An example is tungsten hexafluoride, which has a very low vapor pressure.

SAFE GASES

Highly toxic gases, such as AsH_3, or explosive gases, such as silane, receive the most focus in the semiconductor industry. Inert gases, such as argon and nitrogen, receive less attention, although these safe gases are used in tremendous quantities. Unlike either silane or AsH_3, inert gases have caused deaths in the industry.

Four cases of oxygen-deficient syncope in 1 year at a single semiconductor facility illustrate the ever-present danger of these gases (*personal communication*). In two of the cases, workers succumbed after entering rooms with wafer storage cabinets that maintained an internal atmosphere of nitrogen at slight positive pressure, to protect product from ingress of particles. If a cabinet leaks slightly and is not maintaining positive pressure, the temporary solution is to turn up the flow of gas. This increases flow of nitrogen into the room, and, at some point in a small room, it replaces enough of the oxygen to present an asphyxiation hazard.

The other two cases occurred in a partially enclosed area at the end of an aisle in a clean room (*personal communication*). Process engineers introduced a nitrogen drying step to the end of a wet station without installing an exhaust for the nitrogen. It was assumed that the air changes and dilution in the clean room would be adequate to protect workers. The problem was identified when the second of two workers experienced syncope at the tool. The first episode had initially been attributed to the fact that the worker was dieting to lose weight. In each of these four cases, the worker was a healthy individual, with no permanent harm. The outcomes might have been more serious in an individual with coronary artery disease.

Two lessons may be learned from these incidents. First, no gas is so safe that engineers can simply depend on environmental dilution to protect workers. Second, any case of syncope in an industry in which gases or vapors are present needs a thorough workplace investigation by health professionals.

Photoresists

No reported incidents exist of harm from photoresists as they are used in semiconductor manufacturing, although a basis for some health concerns does exist. Clearly, the greatest concern about photoresists had been the potential for reproductive and developmental toxicity because of the high content of glycol ether solvents.

CHEMISTRY OF PHOTORESISTS

Photoresists are chemical mixtures that can be altered by exposure to electromagnetic energy, such as ultraviolet radiation, E beams, or x-rays. The radiation is passed through a mask, exposing only a desired pattern on the surface of a layer of photoresist. If the photoresist is a *negative photoresist*, the area exposed to light is hardened and becomes less soluble. If a *positive photoresist* is used, the exposed area becomes weakened and is more easily removed by a solvent during development. The pattern of photoresist left behind after development allows selective exposure of the underlying material to other processes, such as etching or ion implantation.

NEGATIVE PHOTORESISTS

Most negative resists become insoluble through some type of radiation-induced cross-linking. The first resist used to fabricate solid-state devices was a negative resist based on cyclized 1,4-poly(*cis*-isoprene) that becomes cross-linked on exposure. Typically, the cyclized rubber matrix was sensitized with a bis(aryl azide) photosensitive cross-linking agent. The use of a negative photoresist in photolithography is severely limited by the fact that the cyclized rubber polymers require organic solvent developers that cause image distortion because of swelling of the photoresist. It is unlikely that health professionals encounter negative resists in semiconductor manufacturing, although negative resists may be used to fabricate larger-scale components in the electronics industry.

POSITIVE PHOTORESISTS

The mechanism of positive resist action involves either chain-scission or a polarity change in the polymer. Photoresists based on the latter mechanism are the most widely used for semiconductor manufacturing because they possess high resolution and excellent resistance to dry etching processes. DQN resists, discussed later, are typically polarity change positive resists.

CHAIN SCISSION RESISTS

The classic positive chain-scission resist is PMMA. It is a widely used electron beam photoresist in some steps of semiconductor manufacturing and in mask manufacturing. The acrylic monomer (methyl methacrylate, MMA) is a potent sensitizer and causes paresthesias of the fingertips (i.e., with direct skin contact on the fingertips). Sensitization to MMA has occurred in medical professionals who use it to cement a variety of prostheses. No problems have been observed with the use of PMMA in semiconductor manufacturing, probably because of an absence of contamination with the monomer and more easily controlled work practices. The typical developer for PMMA is a combination of methyl isobutyl ketone and isopropyl alcohol. A great number of substituted methacrylates have been experimented with to try to improve the sensitivity of PMMAs to radiation and their resistance to dry etching.

Another class of positive chain-scission resists is the poly(olefin sulfones). The polymers are alternating copolymers of an olefin and sulfur dioxide. The weak carbon-sulfur (C—S) bond is cleaved on irradiation. These types of resists are typically used in mask making.

DIAZONAPHTHOQUINONE-NOVOLAK PHOTORESISTS

DQN resists are typical of the polarity change positive resists. They operate via a dissolution-inhibition mechanism. The major component is an alkali-soluble resin (novolak) that is rendered insoluble in aqueous alkaline solutions through incorporation of a hydrophobic material (a diazonaphthoquinone). On irradiation, this photoactive hydrophobic material may either be removed or converted to an alkali-soluble species, thereby allowing selective removal of the irradiated portion of the resist by an alkaline developer.

The DQN photoresist system is the most widely used in semiconductor manufacturing. This system is discussed in detail to give a sense of potential exposures in photolithography. The overall formulation of a typical DQN resist is shown in Table 33-3.

TABLE 33-3. Typical formulation of a diazonaphthoquinone/novolak photoresist

Novolak resin	8 g
Diazonaphthoquinone	2 g
Glycol ether	20 g
Butyl acetate	2 g
Xylene	2 g
Additives	Trace
Hexamethyldisilazane	
Organic acids	
Phthalic anhydride	
Silanes	
Imidazoles	

NOVOLAK RESIN

The resin, polymer, or plastic used to form a protective layer over the wafer is a *novolak*, a phenol-formaldehyde resin. An important feature of the resin is its insolubility in alkaline solutions. Variations on the solubility of the novolak resin are made by adding other alkyl groups to the aryl ring of the phenol monomer before polymerization. A typical resin is formed by the condensation of formaldehyde and a substituted phenol, such as meta-cresol.

As a high-molecular-weight polymer, the novolak resin is without significant health hazard. Small amounts of formaldehyde and substituted phenols contaminate the finished resin and, therefore, are also present in the final photoresist formulation. It is possible that these monomers are partially vaporized in the softbake process, although the more likely exposure occurs through skin contact with the liquid photoresist (Fig. 33-7).

Formaldehyde presents a theoretical concern because it can be a dermal sensitizing agent. However, significant airborne release or concentrations of formaldehyde are highly unlikely and have not been observed with the conventional use, in photolithography areas, of photoresist formulations containing low levels of free formaldehyde. Formaldehyde's ability to produce dermal sensitization after contact and experience with phenol-formaldehyde resins in other industries have demonstrated the potential for contact dermatitis. Irritant contact dermatitis has been reported, but most reports document allergic contact dermatitis. Besides formaldehyde, 14 other contact sensitizers have been recognized in resins based on phenol and formaldehyde (140). Para-tertiary-butyl-phenol has been the most widely documented.

DIAZONAPHTHOQUINONE

The sensitizer or photoactive element of the DQN system is diazonaphthoquinone (DQ). Novolak resins are rendered insoluble in alkaline solutions by the addition of 10% to 20% by weight of DQ. Several hundred variations of DQ have been patented. DQ is often in the form of a diester or triester of sulfonic acid (Fig. 33-8).

TRIHYDROXYBENZOPHENONE

Trihydroxybenzophenone (THBP) is used by many photoresist manufacturers to create diesters and triesters of the diazonaph-

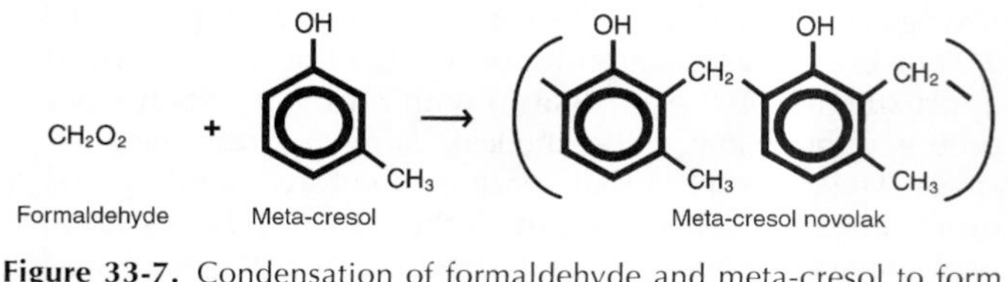

Figure 33-7. Condensation of formaldehyde and meta-cresol to form novolak resin.

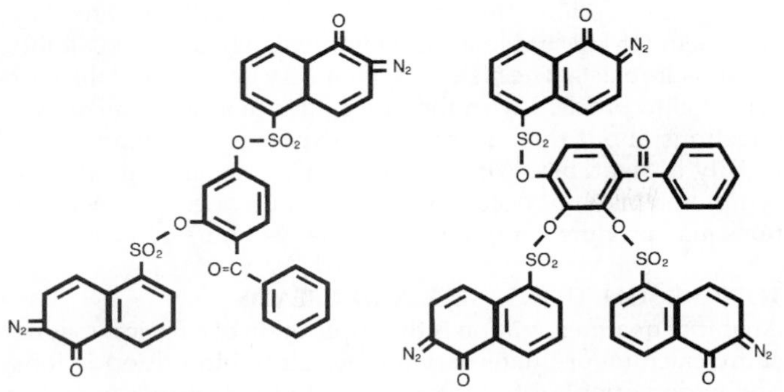

Figure 33-8. Diester and triester of diazonaphthoquinone.

thoquinones. A small amount of THBP always contaminates the most fastidiously prepared DQ esters. At least one manufacturer adds THBP to its photoresist formulations in significant amounts to improve the sensitivity of the resist. The interest in this chemical resides in the fact that it was found to be genotoxic in two tests *in vitro*. Mutation and chromosomal aberrations were observed using Chinese hamster ovary cells (141). Subsequent *in vitro* tests of THBP were negative. No animal studies have been performed.

The THBP results are not surprising. All photoactivators and sensitizers used in photoresists are, by their nature, expected to be biologically active. Very little testing has been done, except for bacterial mutation (Ames) assays and a few *in vitro* tests for genotoxicity. Surprisingly, when photoactivators or sensitizers are tested, they are in their inactivated state. An interesting test that has not been done with these materials is to paint them onto the skin of animals and then expose the molecules to UV radiation. This would mimic an exposure scenario that may occur to workers when they leave the clean room environment and are exposed to sunlight. A related compound, benzophenone, is used widely in topical sunscreens to absorb UV-A and UV-C radiation and can be a contact sensitizer.

Epidemiologic data from the printing industry may be pertinent to the semiconductor industry. The printing industry uses the same basic process of combining polymers with photosensitive chemicals and exposure to UV radiation to produce an image as the semiconductor industry uses. However, it uses different specific chemicals in an environment that is generally much less well controlled from an industrial hygiene perspective. Several reports have suggested an excess of malignant melanoma among workers in the printing industry (142,143), including a cohort study (144). The authors in the latter study suggested that hydroquinone may be the cause for the observed increased risk, based on retrospective exposure assessment and its ability to cause depigmentation and changes in melanocytes with skin contact.

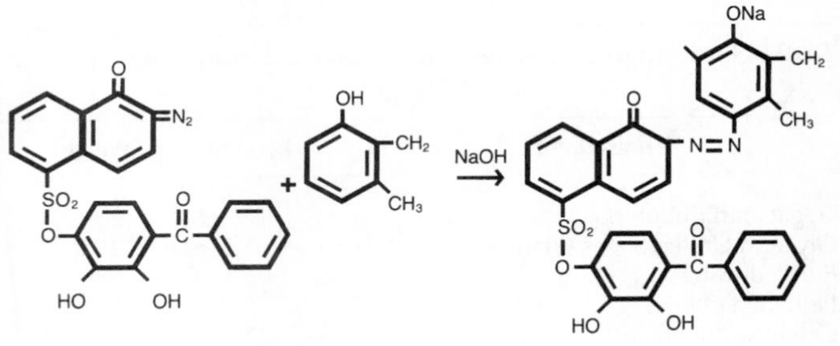

Figure 33-9. Diazonium-azo coupling reaction.

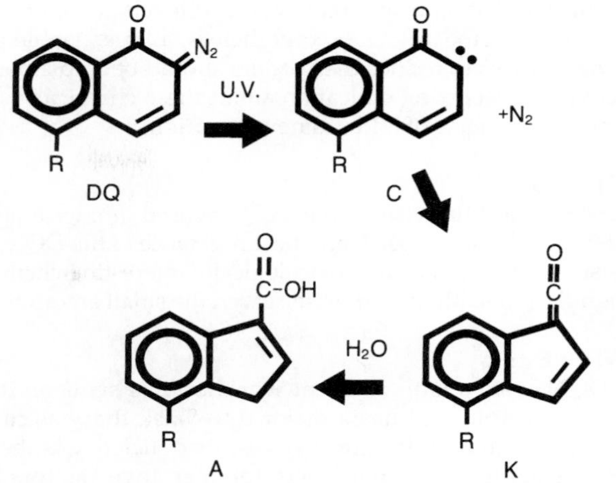

Figure 33-10. Rearrangement of diazonaphthoquinone on exposure to ultraviolet radiation.

COUPLING OF DIAZONAPHTHOQUINONE PHOTOINITIATOR TO THE NOVOLAK POLYMER

Before exposure to light, the DQ ester acts to inhibit the dissolution of the novolak resin. This inhibition is thought to involve a diazonium-azo coupling reaction promoted by immersion in an alkaline developer (Fig. 33-9).

TOXICITY OF AZO COMPOUNDS

Azo compounds are synthetic compounds not found in nature. They consist of two aromatic rings joined by an azo (—N=N—) bond. They are chromophores and have been widely used as dyes in the past. Dyes, such as Direct Blue 6, Direct Black 38, and Direct Brown 95, possess multiple azo bonds and are very potent carcinogens in laboratory animals (145). Their toxicity is thought to be dependent on biotransformation to benzidine. It is unlikely that the transient azo-coupled diazonium compounds in Figure 33-9 could be similarly metabolized to benzidine.

EXPOSURE OF DIAZONAPHTHOQUINONE TO ULTRAVIOLET RADIATION

After exposure to UV light, the DQ inhibitor no longer functions. The exposed DQ is rearranged first to a carbene, then to a ketene, and finally to an indene acid complexed to the novolak resin. This makes the novolak resin more hydrophilic and more soluble (Fig. 33-10).

HEALTH HAZARDS OF DIAZONAPHTHOQUINONES

The health hazards of DQs are not known. Their structure is similar to potent antibiotics and cancer chemotherapeutic agents, suggesting biological activity. Some data about similar compounds are available. 9,10-Anthraquinone shows evidence of carcinogenic activity when fed to mice and is also a potent skin sensitizer. Hydroquinone is mutagenic, is a well-known skin sensitizer, has been shown to cause respiratory sensitization in humans (146), and, as already noted, has been postulated as a cause for the observed increased risk for melanoma in printers. Its use in the photography industry has shown it to be a skin-bleaching agent (147).

DIAZONAPHTHOQUINONE-NOVOLAK SOLVENTS

A large part of the typical DQN formulation is the solvent carrier combination of *n*-butyl acetate (NBA), xylene, and a glycol ether. The first two are a constant source of troublesome odors in the typical clean room environment. NBA has an odor threshold of less than 1 ppm. The TLV of 150 ppm often becomes a moot point to the workers. Xylene is another chemical with a very low odor threshold and no apparent hazard at levels encountered in the semiconductor industry. Nonetheless, all reasonable engineering controls to reduce these odors should be implemented. Effective and recurring education about these chemicals is also an important means of addressing perceptions.

ADDITIVES

A variety of additives (see Table 33-3) are used in trace amounts to alter the adhesion, speed, and heat resistance of the DQN photoresists. Although they are toxicologically interesting chemicals, no significant health hazard exists, given the small amounts.

NEWER RESISTS

The DQN system is the current workhorse of semiconductor photolithography but has a major drawback that has caused investigators to look for alternatives. Its deficiency is the low thermal stability of the hardened polymer. Investigators have experimented with other phenolic polymers to try to find resists that are stable beyond 120°C. The candidates include poly(*p*-hydroxystyrene), poly(*p*-hydroxy-α-methylstyrene), and *N*-(*p*-hydroxyphenyl)maleimide. Organosilicon polymers are being used extensively in research laboratories as a photoresist, especially in multilevel resist systems.

Poly(dimethylglutarimide) is used as a deep UV resist in production settings. Many new resists are being explored for use with excimer laser radiation, which allows finer resolution than that obtainable with current UV sources. A large class exists of inorganic resists, such as germanium-selenium (Ge-Se) and arsenic trisulfide, that would, if used, introduce toxic metals into photoresist formulations. X-ray lithography, the introduction of which seems imminent, may require other types of photoresists. Accompanying each new resist polymer are different photoinitiators, different solvent formulations, and different developers. It is the responsibility of a health professional to read with skepticism the material data safety sheets that invariably accompany photoresists. The lack of adverse health effects on these sheets often merely reflects the lack of toxicity testing on the compound. All photoresist materials should be handled with very fastidious work practices and controls.

Hydrofluoric Acid

The special dangers of delayed and continuing HF burns are widely appreciated in the microelectronics industry. However, most burns are treated by medical personnel outside the industry, who, barring specific outreach and training efforts by industry health and safety professionals, may not be familiar with the unique medical management required for HF burns. HF burns are often undertreated in emergency departments and private physicians' offices, unless the physicians are trained in appropriate treatment.

INITIAL TREATMENT

The initial treatment of any HF burn is to remove the HF from the skin by irrigation with water for at least 10 to 15 minutes. Instead of a gentle stream, the irrigation should be done forcefully enough to accomplish this purpose. Showers or hoses are the ideal methods. A water tap at a sink suffices for smaller burns. No work area that uses HF should be allowed to operate without these options immediately nearby. Workers should clearly understand the importance of immediate irrigation. Unfortunately, in their haste to transport burned victims to a medical facility, coworkers sometimes forego the crucial initial step of irrigation, allowing more prolonged contact with and deeper penetration of fluoride ions.

Clothes saturated with HF are sometimes a source of continuing exposure. Especially in the instance of a splash, it is best to remove and dispose of all clothing. Clothing that has absorbed HF can cause serious burns to anyone who handles it carelessly. Treatment for HF should proceed immediately if any possibility of exposure exists. The history is often very unclear, and the wise course is to proceed with therapy rather than to agonize over questions about the nature of the exposure that may not be readily answerable. With HF concentrations as high as 50%, symptoms may not occur for up to 8 hours. Lesser concentrations may produce symptoms only after 24 hours.

TOPICAL SOLUTIONS, GELS, AND CREAMS

An initial treatment option is the application of a topical magnesium, calcium, or quaternary amine salt to bind fluoride ions. The wide variety of favorites attests to the fact that none has clearly established efficacy over the others. Magnesium sulfate solution, magnesium oxide paste, calcium gluconate gel, benzethonium chloride (Hyamine), and benzalkonium chloride (Zephiran) are among the treatments that have been used, and they continue to be recommended by many sources.

The best-controlled animal study to date concluded that calcium gluconate is the most effective topical treatment (148). Zephiran, magnesium ointment, and aloe gel did not alter the histopathologic progression of the HF burn. However, some authors have questioned the relevance of animal models to the typical human exposure, and use of the quaternary amine and magnesium compounds still remains reasonable (149,150).

Calcium gluconate as a 2.5% gel can be made (see list of ingredients in Table 33-4). The tragacanth is initially weighed, then wet with glycerin and mixed in a blender. Warm water (600 mL) is then added to the blender to solubilize the initial mixture. The liquefied phenol is added next. This is followed by the calcium gluconate 10% solution, and the concoction is then thoroughly mixed. Afterward, it can be stored in tubes for application. Calcium gluconate gel is also available from some pharmaceutical suppliers.

INJECTION OF TISSUE WITH CALCIUM IONS

HF is highly soluble in biological membranes and, therefore, behaves differently from other acids, such as HCl and H_2SO_4, whose immediate corrosive and thermal effects occur immediately and on the most proximate tissue. HF can absorb deeply and insidiously into tissue before dissociating and releasing highly destructive fluoride ions. The quickest and surest way to bind fluoride ions and halt tissue destruction and symptoms is to inject the afflicted dermal and subcutaneous tissue with calcium ions. This is done with calcium gluconate, usually a 5% solution. A rule of thumb is to use 0.5 mL for each centimeter squared of burned skin. A 27- or 30-gauge needle is used with multiple injection sites. No need exists to use anesthesia before infiltration with calcium gluconate. As with most subcutaneous injections, the pain is a function of pressure and tissue distension and can be minimized by injecting slowly. Relief of pain from the burn provides a good indicator to judge the adequacy of treatment and the necessity of further injections.

TABLE 33-4. Ingredients needed to make calcium gluconate as a 2.5% gel

Ingredient	Percent	Weight
Tragacanth ribbon no. 1	2	20 g
Glycerin United States Pharmacopeia	2.5	25 g
Purified water	68	680 mL
Liquefied phenol	0.13	1.3 mL
Calcium gluconate 10%	27.4	250 mL

Calcium gluconate injections are clearly indicated when severe pain persists after adequate topical treatment or with apparent severe burns on presentation. Delay in the initiation of irrigation and topical treatment and recognition that the HF was more concentrated (particularly if well above 20%) provide additional impetus to consider injections. When faced with a likely HF burn that fails to respond promptly to topical treatment, the physician is in the fortunate situation in which appropriate therapy may be highly efficacious, and in almost no instance is the injection harmful. Granted, injections must be done with reasonable care into small spaces, such as digits, but this is not a significant contraindication.

Occasionally, the physician is faced with a hard indurated HF burn of a finger into which calcium gluconate injection is neither wise nor possible. This situation may be best treated with intraarterial 10% calcium gluconate infusion. More aggressive use of percutaneous calcium gluconate injections into early HF burns would in many instances prevent progression to induration and tissue destruction.

RISK OF HYPERCALCEMIA FROM INJECTIONS

Also, the remote possibility exists of causing hypercalcemia with the injections. If large volumes of calcium gluconate are being injected (greater than 20 mL of 5% solution), it is prudent to monitor the serum calcium before further injections. In a crisis situation in which larger volumes are indicated, a rhythm strip can be monitored for indications of either hypercalcemia or hypocalcemia.

LATE TREATMENT

A late presentation, often after several days, of a probable HF burn is not uncommon. Calcium gluconate injections have caused rapid and dramatic amelioration of signs and symptoms as late as 5 days after the burn. If any reason exists to think that the tissue is still reacting to fluoride ion, then it is not too late to inject calcium gluconate. Except in the case of fingers or toes, it is always possible to inject around and under the most indurated HF burn. Repeat injections, at an interval of 4 to 6 hours or a day later, are also perfectly reasonable if clinical signs and symptoms indicate continued tissue destruction.

CALCIUM CHLORIDE CONTRAINDICATED

It is important to mention that calcium chloride cannot be used for dermal or subcutaneous injections. This drug causes severe irritation and necrosis of tissue. Disastrous incidents have occurred in which calcium chloride was mistakenly substituted for calcium gluconate to treat HF burns.

HYDROFLUORIC ACID BURNS OF THE EYE

Splashes of HF into the eye should be irrigated copiously. Introduction of any other chemicals besides water into the eye should be done with caution. Anecdotal evidence exists from several case reports suggesting benefit from the irrigation of the eye with roughly 500 mL of 1% calcium gluconate solution (149). Quaternary ammonium compounds and calcium chloride should not be used for eye irrigation. Individuals with an eye splash of HF should be referred for immediate ophthalmologic consultation after irrigation.

METABOLIC DISORDERS OF HYDROFLUORIC ACID

Death from systemic fluorosis is a rare, but documented, sequela of topical HF burns (151,152). One fatality followed an HF burn of only 2.5% of the body surface area (152). All deaths have involved profound hypocalcemia with subsequent arrhythmias and cardiac arrest. The mechanism of this hypocalcemia is probably the removal of free calcium ions via the formation of CaF_2.

Patients with significant burns should receive cardiac monitoring and intermittent serum calcium determination for 6 to 8 hours postexposure. If metabolic problems develop, they manifest within that period of time. The QT interval is very sensitive to hypocalcemia, and a lengthened QT interval is usually the first sign of hypocalcemia secondary to HF exposure (153). This can occur as quickly as 25 to 30 minutes postexposure. Classic physical findings, such as carpopedal spasm, Chvostek's sign, or Trousseau's sign, are often absent even when hypocalcemia, a prolonged QT interval, and bradycardia are present. Treatment is slow intravenous infusion of calcium gluconate diluted in intravenous fluids, and stopping the absorption of fluoride. The latter consists of removal of all clothing, irrigation, topical calcium gluconate treatment, and infiltration of the burn area with calcium gluconate.

SURGICAL EXCISION

Surgical excision of severely HF-burned tissue is an option that has been used not only to remove necrotic tissue but also to remove an ongoing source of fluoride ion absorption. The most dramatic case report describes a worker who experienced a 5% body surface HF burn and who developed severe hypocalcemia and cardiac arrhythmias. This problem could not be corrected despite large doses of intravenous calcium replacement and appropriate wound therapy, including infiltration of calcium gluconate. The situation was brought under control only when the burned skin on the forearm was surgically removed (153).

INTRAARTERIAL CALCIUM INFUSION

Several articles have been published on the treatment of HF burns with an intraarterial calcium infusion (154,155). This approach has proven to be efficacious in situations in which local infiltration was not possible, but logistically, it is difficult to perform, and complications of the procedure have occurred. Only physicians who can manage any complications should undertake this treatment. It is not an outpatient procedure.

INHALATION EXPOSURE TO HYDROFLUORIC ACID

As inhalation of HF can result in respiratory tract irritation, including potentially pulmonary edema, the patient exposed to hydrogen fluoride gas or experiencing significant facial burns should be monitored for respiratory symptoms. Supportive treatment, including oxygen administration, is appropriate. Anecdotal evidence exists of a beneficial effect from the administration of a nebulized mist containing 2.5% to 3% calcium gluconate (149). Monitoring for systemic effects of HF absorption is also necessary, with appropriate calcium gluconate administration, if indicated.

PREVENTION AND BETTER TREATMENT

The most important strategy for working with HF remains primary prevention, and the semiconductor industry has been quite aggressive in eliminating these burns. Equipment design, increased worker education, better personal protective equipment, and the change to dry etching have all contributed to this progress. Local medical facilities and emergency department personnel may need periodic review of appropriate evaluation and management.

Waste Products of Dry Etching

A multitude of complex organic compounds is produced during the process of dry etching, particularly during metal etching using chlorine-containing source gases. More than 600 different chemicals have been detected in residues in the chambers of plasma etchers. Less volatile materials tend to settle in these residues, whereas more volatile materials may be removed in the vacuum exhaust and may deposit in lines or in vacuum pump oil.

These waste products are generated by chemical reactions of the process gases with organic photoresist polymers and chemicals. Classes of chemicals generated with common representative chemicals in these classes include aromatic compounds (e.g., hexachlorobenzene), aliphatic compounds (e.g., hexachloroethane, tetrachloroethylene, hexachlorobutadiene), cycloalkanes (e.g., hexachlorocyclopentadiene), heterocyclic compounds (e.g., pentachloropyridine), and nitriles (e.g., trichloroacrylonitrile, pentachloropropionitrile) (156,157). Many of these materials have never been the subject of toxicologic study, although some are known to be mutagenic (e.g., hexachlorobutadiene). In addition to organic chemicals, several metals and metallic compounds (e.g., aluminum, aluminum trichloride, boron trichloride, iron, titanium), hydrochloric acid, hydrogen cyanide, and cyanogen chloride have been identified in the residue (39,156,158).

Several studies have now demonstrated that these waste products are capable of causing adverse effects *in vitro* and *in vivo* in animals. Waste samples removed from the chamber caused unscheduled DNA synthesis in mouse hepatocytes in culture, and mutation in bacterial DNA repair assays and other bacterial assays, but were not clastogenic as indicated by tests for chromosomal aberrations (156). Subchronic administration of waste oil from a vacuum pump to Wistar rats in high doses caused liver enlargement and histologic changes in the liver. Assays for micronuclei demonstrated increased frequencies in Wistar rats given the waste oil by gavage *in vivo*, supported by positive findings in a bacterial mutation (Ames) assay, although positive findings using uncontaminated vacuum pump oil in these assays complicate the interpretation of the findings (158). A presented but unpublished report reportedly found higher rates of micronuclei in lymphocytes of workers engaged in maintenance and cleaning operations (158). In another study using solid waste products in a gas pipeline from a metal etcher, the authors found statistically significant increased postimplantation fetal losses, decreased fetal body weight, and increased malformations (cleft palates) in mice fed the material by gavage in large amounts (up to 750 mg per kg per day) (157).

The precise health significance of these findings is difficult to discern, in that, during normal operations, there should be little or no exposure to waste products from dry etching operations. The extent of exposure leading to effects in these animal bioassays was much greater than could be postulated for a semiconductor worker. The low volatility of most of these organic compounds would largely prevent inhalation exposure, although some volatile materials may be present in vacuum lines and pump oil. The reported findings in maintenance workers, if confirmed, certainly warrant concern. The greatest potential for exposure to these materials would be during maintenance and cleaning of chambers, lines, and pumps, in which dermal and perhaps inhalation exposures could occur. Given the potential for serious chronic adverse health effects, attempts to maintain exposure and absorption as close to zero as possible are warranted. Availability of appropriate engineering controls and personal protective equipment (including air line or comparable respirators and protective gloves and clothing) and use of meticulous work practices are certainly prudent and indicated for this small group of maintenance workers.

HEALTH ISSUES AND CONCERNS IN THE SEMICONDUCTOR INDUSTRY

Reproductive Health Concerns

As an attempt to evaluate concerns raised by a number of women working in a digital equipment corporation wafer fab who had experienced spontaneous abortions, a group of researchers from the University of Massachusetts conducted a small reproductive epidemiology study, the results of which were published in 1988 (69). This case-control study demonstrated a doubling of the odds ratio for spontaneous abortion among clean room–exposed women. The scientific quality and size of the study were not adequate to allow definitive statements about the risks of work in clean rooms, but presented the hypothesis that clean room work could be associated with adverse reproductive outcomes.

In response to this, two additional studies have been conducted, one by researchers at the University of California (UC) Davis involving a number of semiconductor manufacturers and sponsored by the Semiconductor Industry Association, and the second by researchers at Johns Hopkins University sponsored by IBM (159,160). Both studies included two components to study reproductive outcomes, a historical and a prospective component.

The historical component in the UC Davis study identified 904 eligible pregnancies and 113 spontaneous abortions (SABs) from a sample of 7,269 female employees from 14 companies. The relative risk (RR) for SABs in fab workers, after adjustment for confounding factors, was 1.43 (95% CI = 0.95 to 2.09). Similar adjusted RRs were statistically significantly elevated for the photolithography (1.67, 95% CI = 1.17 to 2.62) and etching (2.08, 95% CI = 1.04 to 2.55) subgroups, but not the furnace (1.07, 95% CI = 0.57 to 1.93) and thin film/ion implant (1.38, 95% CI = 0.70 to 2.53) subgroups (159,161). Exposure to photoresist chemicals, including ethylene-based glycol ethers (EGEs), was associated with increased risk for SABs with a dose-response relationship. Exposure to fluoride in etch areas (as part of buffered oxide etch) was also associated with increased risk for SABs, but no dose-response relationship existed. Together, these materials accounted for the observed excess risk in fab employees, such that no excess risk existed in workers not working around these materials (RR = 0.98). Self-reported stress in fab workers was also associated with an elevated RR for SABs (RR = 2.18). Studies of individuals working around cleaning solvents (e.g., acetone, isopropyl alcohol, and methanol), dopants (e.g., arsenic, phosphorus, boron, or antimony), and extremely low-frequency magnetic fields and RF did not suggest any increased risk for SABs (159,162).

Similarly, the IBM retrospective study identified 1,174 pregnancies among women employed at two sites. The investigators found a similar overall adjusted RR of 1.4 (95% CI = 0.9 to 1.9), comparing clean room workers to women working outside the clean room. Interestingly, the risk of SABs was nearly identical in clean room and nonmanufacturing workers, with both of these groups having significantly higher RRs of similar magnitude compared to the other manufacturing group. They also found a statistically significantly increased adjusted RR for SABs in women working in areas involving high potential exposure to EGE-based photoresist (2.8, 95% CI = 1.4 to 5.6), with a lower risk for those less intensively exposed (1.4, 95% CI = 0.8 to 2.6). They did not specifically study exposure and outcomes among fluoride-exposed workers, although miscarriage rates were not elevated in the broad process group of develop and etch, which included the etch area. They found no effect of paternal clean room exposure on the risk of SABs in the wives of these workers (160).

The UC Davis prospective study assessed reproductive outcomes in 403 women using daily diaries and assays of urinary hormones, allowing detection of clinically recognized and subclinical SABs. The authors found an adjusted risk ratio for SAB of 1.25 (95% CI = 0.63 to 1.76), reflecting a total of 52 detected conceptions in the fab and nonfab populations. Although limited by a small sample size, a nonsignificant association existed between the potential for EGE exposure and SABs, but no similar association for fluorides was observed (163). The prospective component of the Johns Hopkins study identified 92 pregnancies, of which 32 were subclinical. The study identified a nonsignificant excess of SABs in clean room employees compared to the other two non–clean room groups (adjusted OR 1.3, 95% CI = 0.9 to 2.0), as well as a nonsignificant excess of SABs in women working around EGEs compared to these control groups (RR 1.5, 95% CI = 0.8 to 2.9) (160).

Analyses from the prospective component of the UC Davis study suggested reduced per cycle probability of conception (i.e., fecundability) when adjusted for confounders in the fab population compared to the nonfab population, but results from the prospective and cross-sectional components did not suggest reduced fertility in fab workers. A similar nonsignificant reduction in fecundability was observed in clean room workers in the prospective component of the Johns Hopkins study.

The most consistent result from these two large studies is the finding of an increased risk of SABs among women working around photoresists and EGEs. The authors of the studies acknowledge the inability to specifically implicate EGEs, because they are consistently used in mixtures with other chemicals. The implication of an EGE effect stems largely from the extensive literature supporting adverse reproductive and developmental effects of EGEs in laboratory animals, along with little evidence supporting such effects from the other chemicals used concurrently. The findings of exposure and risk assessment studies relying on the low measured air concentrations of EGEs in the semiconductor industry tend to belie a role for EGEs (30). These risk assessments, however, do not consider several factors that might reduce their applicability to the clean room worker population—the potential role for dermal exposures, the potential occurrence and effect of transient high airborne concentrations of EGEs, or a potential greater susceptibility of humans to EGE effects compared with animals. The contradictory findings of risk assessment methods and epidemiologic approaches, both grounded in industrial hygiene methods, are worrisome and leave uncertainty as to the role of EGEs in the induction of SABs in fab workers, which cannot be scientifically resolved.

The finding regarding fluoride exposure in workers exposed to buffered oxide etch was not seen in the Johns Hopkins study and is less biologically plausible, in the absence of compelling animal data suggesting adverse reproductive effects of fluoride with low-level exposures. Furthermore, unlike with EGEs, no dose-response relationship was observed between exposure measures and SABs. After the release of the UC Davis study, one large semiconductor manufacturer conducted a detailed industrial hygiene assessment of multiple etch wet stations at several different fabs involving multiple air samples for acids, alkalis, and solvents, including 12 samples for ammonium fluoride and 32 samples for HF. Averaging of all of the full-shift results, which were largely below the limit of detection, amounted to less than 2.1% of the TLVs. Ammonium fluoride and HF results, all below the limit of detection, averaged less than 0.41% and less than 1.3% of the respective TLVs (*personal communication*). These results are far below levels implicated in animal studies as possibly causing reproductive toxicity. Consequently, the role of etch fluoride in inducing SABs in this industry remains in considerable doubt, despite the epidemiologic findings.

The response of semiconductor manufacturers to these studies has generally included extensive communication with workers regarding the findings, a reduction and then elimination of use of implicated ethylene glycol ethers (*personal communication*), an effort to better characterize and control exposures that might impact reproductive outcomes, and the reinforcement or development of policies to permit accommodations for pregnant employees who have concerns about their work area. In the face of uncertainty regarding specific risks, many companies permit transfers out of the clean room for pregnant employees or women contemplating pregnancy. At the same time, policies to require transfer or exclude pregnant women have not been adopted, as they are neither scientifically indicated nor legally acceptable. The limited ability of epidemiologic studies to establish causal associations with specific chemical exposures, particularly in a setting with use of multiple chemicals present at low or nondetectable levels, suggests a need for such a multifaceted approach to deal with these concerns. Efforts to eliminate use and prevent new introduction of chemicals with documented adverse reproductive effects are clearly prudent.

Concerns Regarding Carcinogens and Cancer

A limited number of known carcinogens are used in semiconductor manufacturing. As discussed, arsenic, specifically including trivalent and pentavalent compounds of arsenic, is a known human lung and skin carcinogen. No epidemiologic or toxicologic data exist relating to elemental arsenic, but its insolubility would presumably limit its biological availability and potential for carcinogenicity. Properly managed, there should be no exposure to arsenic for semiconductor manufacturing employees, with the possible exception intermittently of ion implant maintenance workers. Use of rigorous engineering controls and work practices and appropriate respiratory protective equipment should result in no significant increment in arsenic exposures in this group relative to background environmental exposures in the general population.

Several other agents, sulfuric acid, chromic acid, silica, and nickel, identical or related to agents known or suspected to be carcinogenic to humans in other settings with high-level exposures, are used in the semiconductor industry. According to the International Agency for Research on Cancer (IARC), sufficient evidence exists that occupational exposures to strong inorganic acid mists containing sulfuric acid are carcinogenic to humans. Epidemiologic evidence for the association between this exposure and the development of lung and laryngeal cancer was derived from studies in industries involved in steel pickling and electroplating, in which airborne concentrations often have exceeded 0.5 mg per m^3 (164). Several factors, including effects of high-concentration exposures on lung defense mechanisms, on the ability to neutralize hydrogen ion, and on cell injury and proliferation, as well as the epidemiologic data, suggest the existence of a threshold for sulfuric acid carcinogenicity (165). In any case, exposures to acid aerosols of sulfuric acid and sulfates are ubiquitous in the general population, because of ambient air pollution. In contrast, barring unusual circumstances, mists of sulfuric acid and other acids are not generated in the semiconductor industry because of the way in which acids are handled in wet stations and the need to minimize airborne particles. Use of bulk chemical delivery systems and extensive local exhaust ventilation systems on wet stations minimizes the potential for exposure to sulfuric acid. Confirming this, industrial hygiene monitoring for sulfuric acid for manual and automated wet stations at four fabs of one large manufacturer revealed no measurements above the limit of detection. For the 27 of 30 samples, in which sampling technique and duration permitted a low limit of detection, the results were nondetectable, with the highest limit of detection being 0.063 mg per m^3 (*personal communication*). Exposures sufficient to raise concerns about carcinogenicity do not appear to occur in the semiconductor industry.

Chromic acid, a hexavalent chromium compound, is used to a limited degree in wet stations. Epidemiologic data from cohorts of chromium platers and chromium pigment workers are sufficient, according to IARC, to conclude that hexavalent chromium compounds are carcinogenic to humans, primarily causing lung cancer. Chromic acid, a highly soluble hexavalent chromium compound, has not been clearly implicated; the sparingly soluble compounds, such as zinc chromate, are most implicated, as opposed to insoluble and highly soluble compounds (166). With controls similar to those for sulfuric acid, airborne exposure levels for chromic acid were consistently nondetectable in the wet station study discussed (*personal communication*). Although silica dust may be encountered during some semiconductor processes, it is rarely airborne, at very low air concentrations, and is almost exclusively amorphous (noncrystalline) silica. Whereas IARC believes that limited evidence exists for the carcinogenicity of crystalline silica in humans (lung cancer) and sufficient animal evidence exists, making crystalline silica a probable human carcinogen, inadequate evidence exists for the carcinogenicity of amorphous silica in humans and experimental animals (167). Like aluminum, nickel is occasionally deposited as a metallic layer on wafers. IARC considers that sufficient evidence exists indicating human carcinogenicity for nickel and nickel compounds, primarily from studies of nickel refineries in which excesses of lung and sinonasal cancer were observed. The precise nickel compounds implicated remain unclear, although nickel sulfides and oxides are most often implicated and metallic nickel has not been clearly implicated (168). Because nickel is deposited in sealed chambers, the potential for exposure to any nickel compounds is limited, perhaps during maintenance and cleaning operations.

In addition, some of the noted waste products of dry etching have demonstrated sufficient (S) or limited (L) evidence for carcinogenicity in animals, according to IARC: hexachlorobenzene (S), hexachlorobutadiene (L), and tetrachloroethylene (S). Other waste products are chemically related to suspect carcinogens, such as acrylonitrile (S) (169).

Close analysis of the use of these agents in semiconductor manufacturing suggests very limited potential for exposure, largely because of the use of rigorous engineering controls and appropriate personal protective equipment. Although there is some uncertainty about the existence of threshold doses below which no effect occurs for carcinogens, it seems unlikely that these intermittent exposures, which would be very low concentrations if they occur at all, would confer any increased risk of cancer. For some of these agents, exposures from work would not likely result in a significant increment in total exposure above general environmental exposures.

In March 1996, several newspapers reported on a lawsuit filed by former employees at an IBM semiconductor fab against a number of chemical manufacturers, alleging a connection between workplace exposures and cancers they had developed (170). On April 18, 1997, the NBC-TV news program *Dateline* contained a segment dealing with alleged health risks, including cancer, from the use of chemicals at this IBM semiconductor manufacturing plant in New York State. Because information regarding these cases has not appeared in the medical literature, precise information about the types of cancers and the nature, duration, and intensity of exposures for these former workers has not been available. Limited information suggests that these former employees had several different types of cancers, including testicular, brain, colon, and cervical cancer and lymphoma, suggesting that a cluster of like cancers did not exist. Critical information to permit a scientific assessment, such as clustering of cases in time or space (i.e., work areas) and time from initial employment to development of cancer (i.e., potential induction-latency intervals), is either not available or not suggestive of a workplace causation. The types of cancers do not conform to what one might expect, based on the chemicals with carcinogenic properties used in the industry as discussed (i.e., lung cancer). Certainly, it is appropriate to gather additional information about these individuals and the areas in which they worked. However, the allegations in the lawsuit alone cannot provide scientific evidence of an increased risk of cancer associated with work in the semiconductor industry.

A single published study exists of cancer incidence and mortality in the semiconductor industry, based on a population of approximately 1,800 workers at an English semiconductor fab. The study is limited because of the relatively short duration of follow-up since first employment and small size of the study population. Forty-six cancer deaths occurred [standard mortality ratio (SMR) 79], with no statistically significant excesses of any type of cancer. For respiratory cancers, 12 deaths occurred when 11.9 were expected. An initial small excess of melanoma cases did not persist in the follow-up of the cohort through 1988 (171).

Given undetectable to very low exposures to a limited number of carcinogens, little scientific basis exists to suspect excesses of cancer in semiconductor workers. Chemicals that have been implicated as causes of human occupational cancers invariably were identified as such in industries with high, uncontrolled exposures, although to some degree this reflects limitations in the sensitivity of epidemiologic methods. A number of obstacles exist to the conduct of a meaningful epidemiologic study of cancer in the semiconductor industry. Unlike most industries, in which one or two predominant chemical exposures exist, a multitude exists of potential low-level exposures in the semiconductor industry. Moreover, the frequent changes in processes and chemicals, typically over several years or less, mean that workers do not experience a consistent and limited set of exposures over a working lifetime, as they do in most industries. These changes would markedly complicate the exposure assessment and exposure subcohort identification portions of a study. More so than in other industries, it is likely that the findings of any present-day cancer study, which would reflect exposure 15 to 20 years previously, would not be useful in identifying current high-risk areas, as the processes theoretically underlying any identified excesses of cancer would no longer be in use. Moreover, the number of workers with potential for exposure, primarily equipment maintenance workers, would represent a small subset of fab employees, limiting the power of any study. Even if it were possible to overcome these obstacles, it is unlikely that conventional epidemiologic approaches would be able to detect increased risks for cancer in potentially exposed semiconductor workers because of the limited sensitivity in detecting small excess risks that might be associated with very low, intermittent exposures. As with reproductive health concerns, an approach that avoids the use or introduction of known or suspected carcinogens, combined with strict controls to preclude exposure for those agents that are used, would appear to provide the best protection to workers.

Occupational Illnesses in the Semiconductor Industry

Worker's compensation data from the California Bureau of Labor Statistics and Research (BLSR), presented in a review of health hazards in the microelectronics industry, suggest a higher frequency of occupational illnesses, as a percentage of all work-loss injuries, among semiconductor workers in California compared with workers in all California manufacturing industries (e.g., 16.5% versus 6.9%, respectively) in 1989. Of these occupational illnesses leading to work loss, a higher percentage of illnesses was because of systemic poisonings (i.e., illness caused by toxic materials) in this industry (6.7%) compared again with general industry (1.1%) (172). Unfortunately, these aggregate data do not permit an understanding of the precise nature and severity of the occupational illnesses and systemic poisonings, with the exception that they were sufficiently severe to lead to work loss. This finding of relatively frequent occupational illnesses caused by systemic poisoning contrasts with the results of a small published study assessing the reliability of the recording of injuries and illnesses in a number of companies in this industry. Of the 16 occupational illnesses among the 101 reportable cases, 14 were skin conditions and 2 were cumulative trauma (173). Data from one large semiconductor manufacturing company indicate that more than 80% of reportable occupational illnesses fit within one of these two categories, cumulative trauma or dermatitis, with less than 1% caused by systemic poisonings (*personal communication*). From a different perspective, extensive literature searches in a number of occupational medicine and toxicology databases failed to identify published case reports of significant systemic illness stemming from chemical exposures in the semiconductor industry. It is difficult to reconcile the differences in reported illnesses between these data sources. Because of the peculiarities of the OSHA reporting system, a case becomes an illness because it stems from a noninstantaneous exposure, not because it conforms to a conventional biological definition of illness (173). A case can be correctly reported as an occupational illness caused by systemic poisoning, even if a brief but noninstantaneous exposure occurred to chemicals leading to minor transient symptoms with or without objective findings. Obviously, it would be desirable to avoid all chemical exposures and symptoms therefrom. A more detailed review of the records from which the aggregate BLSR data are derived might permit a better understanding of the nature and severity, or lack thereof, of the reported cases. However, the interpretation of the significance of the BLSR data alone must be cautious, in the absence of other corroborating evidence indicating frequent or serious illnesses caused by chemical exposure in this industry.

Review and Approval of Chemical Use and Introduction

Given the obvious limitations of most material safety data sheets, a key element of a health and safety program in the semiconductor industry is a chemical review program. Appropriately trained staff, typically an industrial hygienist, working with a toxicologist and an occupational physician, review the toxicologic properties of new chemicals proposed for use before their introduction. Typically, this process entails literature searches in relevant databases (e.g., TOXLINE, NIOSHTIC, Registry of Toxic Effects of Chemical Substances, and Hazardous Substances Data Bank) and review of toxicologic literature on a particular chemical. In addition to acute health hazards, one must consider information regarding genotoxicity, carcinogenicity, and reproductive and developmental toxicity. Physical and chemical properties of the chemical (e.g., physical form, vapor pressure, odor, and reactivity) also need to be considered, as do the proposed use and controls for the material (e.g., enclosure and local exhaust ventilation) From this information, it is possible to assess the likelihood that the use of this chemical under these circumstances might pose a hazard to the worker.

Development of criteria with which to classify chemicals is helpful. For potential developmental toxins, for example, one can classify agents with regard to the strength of scientific evidence for adverse effects from animal experiments and with regard to evidence for selective effects on the fetus with no maternal toxicity. For carcinogens, use of a scheme similar to that used by IARC is helpful, with category 1 agents being carcinogenic to humans and category 2A agents being probably carcinogenic to humans. One can also classify with regard to potency and dose-response considerations. With these categories, one can set *a priori* guidelines with regard to the hurdles required for approval or the controls required for use. One constraint using this process occurs when few or no toxicologic data exist on the compound from which to make an assessment. In this case, barring evidence to indicate no exposure potential or the safety of closely related materials, it is prudent to insist on very tight controls to prevent exposure. It seems appropriate for the semiconductor manufacturer to apply pressure on the chemical manufacturer to conduct appropriate toxicologic studies in these situations.

With these programs and categories, it is possible to rationally compare alternative processes and chemicals from a health hazard perspective, not only against one another but also against the existing chemicals. This approach permits a commitment to continuous improvement, making process changes that not only improve manufacturing but also reduce potential health hazards. This process occasionally forces the health and safety professional to deny approval for the use of a particular chemical, although more often the approval is granted with conditions on use and controls. Close involvement with process research and development staff can permit the abandonment of a problematic chemical early, before there has been a significant investment into its introduction and use. The program must be enforceable (e.g., controls over chemical purchasing and management support). Because new toxicologic information becomes available periodically on existing chemicals, it is important to create a mechanism to identify relevant information and, if indicated, to make changes in the use or controls on these materials. It is difficult to quantify the benefits from such programs, measuring problems that might have happened, but they intuitively make considerable sense in this industry characterized by continuous change.

REFERENCES

1. World Semiconductor Trade Statistics. *Blue Book*. WSTS/Semiconductor Industry Association, 1996.
2. Department of Labor, Bureau of Labor Statistics. Washington: US Department of Labor, 1997.
3. Rapa A. Clean rooms for VLSI manufacturing. IBM technical report [Tr 22.2497]. East Fishkill, NY: IBM General Technology Division, 1983.
4. Rycroft RCG. Low humidity and microtrauma. *Am J Ind Med* 1985;8:371–373.
5. Rycroft RCG. Low humidity occupational dermatoses. In: Gardner AW, ed. *Current approaches to occupational health*, 3rd ed. Boston: Wright, 1987.
6. Fischer T, Maibach HI. Patch testing in allergic contact dermatitis: an update. In: Maibach HI, ed. *Occupational and industrial dermatology*, 2nd ed. Chicago: Year Book Medical Publishers, 1987;22:190–210.
7. Shama SK. Monitoring and updating patch test allergens used in the United States. The Occupational and Environmental Medicine (OEM) Report. Boston: OEM Health Information, 1989:6792.
8. Nilsson SEG, Anderson L. The use of contact lenses in environments with organic solvents, acids, or alkalies. *Acta Ophthalmol* 1982;60:599–608.
9. Randolph SA, Zavon MR. Guidelines for contact lens use in industry. *J Occup Med* 1987;29:237–242.
10. Pogge BH. Metals and semi-metals in the semiconductor device technologies. In: Clarkson TW, ed. *Biological monitoring of toxic metals*. New York: Plenum Publishing, 1988.
11. Redmond SF, Schappert KR. Occupational dermatitis associated with garments. *J Occup Med* 1987;29:243–244.
12. Dager SR, Holland JP, Cowley DS, et al. Panic disorder precipitated by exposure to organic solvents in the work place. *Am J Psychiatry* 1987;144:1056–1058.
13. Klein DF, Zitrin CM, Woerner MG, Ross DC. Treatment of phobias. II. Behavior therapy and supportive psychotherapy: are there any specific ingredients? *Arch Gen Psychiatry* 1983;40:139–145.
14. Tearnan BH, Goetsch V, Adams HE. Modification of disease phobia using a multifaceted exposure program. *J Behav Ther Exp Psychiatry* 1985;16:57–61.
15. Cullen MR. Workers with multiple chemical sensitivities. *Occup Med* 1987;2:655–806.
16. Simon G, et al. Immunologic, psychological, and neuropsychological factors in multiple chemical sensitivity: a controlled study. *Ann Intern Med* 1993;119(2):97–103.
17. Terr Al. Clinical ecology. *Ann Intern Med* 1989;111:168–178.
18. Boxer PA. Occupational mass psychogenic illness. *J Occup Med* 1985;27:867–872.
19. Olkinuora M. Psychogenic epidemics and work. *Scand J Work Environ Health* 1984;10:501–504.
20. Colligan MJ. Mass psychogenic illness: some clarification and perspectives. *J Occup Med* 1981;23:635–638.

21. Shusterman D, Lipscomb J, Neutra R, Satin K. Symptom prevalence and odor–worry interaction near hazardous waste sites. *Environ Health Perspect* 1991;94:25–30.
22. Lenihan KL, Sheehy JW, Jones JH. Assessment of exposures in gallium arsenide processing: a case study. In: American Conference of Governmental Industrial Hygienists. *Hazard assessment control technology in semiconductor manufacturing*. Chelsea, MI: Lewis Publishers, 1989.
23. Hammond ML. Safety in chemical vapor deposition. *Solid State Technol* 1989;(Dec):104–109.
24. Rhoades BJ, et al. Safety and environmental control systems used in chemical vapor deposition (CVD) reactors at AT&T Microelectronics, Reading, Pennsylvania. In: American Conference of Governmental Industrial Hygienists. *Hazard assessment and control technology in semiconductor manufacturing*. Chelsea, MI: Lewis Publishers, 1989.
25. Bachmann P, Berges HP. Safety aspects of oil sealed rotary vane vacuum pumps in CVD applications. *Solid State Technol* 1986;(July):83–87.
26. Schaeffer J. Hydrogen monitoring throughout the semiconductor manufacturing facility. *Semiconductor Safety Assoc J* 1988;(Sept).
27. Jones JH. Exposure and control assessment of semiconductor manufacturing. *Proc Am Inst Phys Conf U S A* 1988;166:44–53.
28. Ungers LJ, Jones JH, McIntyre AJ, et al. Release of arsenic from semiconductor wafers. *Am Ind Hyg Assoc J* 1985;46:416–420.
29. Holroyd D, Rea MS, Young J, Briggs G. Health related aspects of the devitrification of aluminosilicate refractory fibers during use as a high temperature furnace insulant. *Ann Occup Hyg* 1988;3:171–178.
30. Paustenbach DJ. Risk assessment methodologies for developmental and reproductive toxicants: a study of the glycol ethers. In: Paustenbach D, ed. *The risk assessment of environmental hazards*. New York: John Wiley and Sons, 1989:725–768.
31. Singer PH. Wet bench fire suppression. *Semiconductor Int* 1987;(Sept):154–157.
32. Uniform building code. Chapter 9, Group H, Division 6; 1988.
33. Uniform fire code. Article 80; 1987. [Companion document—the toxic gas model ordinance; 1988].
34. Uniform fire code. Article 51; 1987.
35. Singer PH. Dry etching of SiO_2 and Si_3N_4. *Semiconductor Int* 1986;(May):98-103.
36. Moreau WM. *Semiconductor lithography*. New York: Plenum Publishing, 1988.
37. Mucha A. The gases of plasma etching: silicon based technology. *Solid State Technol* 1985;(March):123–127.
38. Ohlson J. Dry etch chemical safety. *Solid State Technol* 1986;(July):69–73.
39. Mueller MR, Kunesh RF. Safety and health implications of dry chemical etching. In: American Conference of Governmental Industrial Hygienists. *Hazard assessment and control technology in semiconductor manufacturing*. Chelsea, MI: Lewis Publishers, 1989.
40. Ruuskanen J, et al. Gallium arsenide etchers: beware of the pump oil. *Semiconductor Int* 1988;(June):88–90.
41. Skidmore K. Use the right plasma to strip away resist. *Semiconductor Int* 1988;(Aug):54-59.
42. Picraux ST, Percy PS. Ion implantation of surfaces. *Sci Am* 1985;237:102–113.
43. Baldwin DG, King BW, Scarpace LP. Ion implanters: chemical and radiation safety. *Solid State Technol* 1988;(Jan):99–105.
44. Ungers LJ, Jones JH. Industrial hygiene and control technology assessment of ion implantation operations. *Am Ind Hyg Assoc J* 1986;47:607–614.
45. Doyle L, Gallagher K, Heath BS, Patterson WB. An outbreak of infectious conjunctivitis spread by microscopes. *J Occup Med* 1989;31:758–762.
46. Paul M, Himmelstein J, Weinstein S, et al. Ocular infections and the industrial use of microscopes. *J Occup Med* 1989;31:763-766.
47. McCurdy SA. Occupational injury and illness in the semiconductor manufacturing industry. *Am J Ind Med* 1989;15:499–510.
48. Marriott MD, Stuchly MA. Health aspects of work with visual display terminals. *J Occup Med* 1986;28:833–848.
49. Rose L. Workplace video display terminals and visual fatigue. *J Occup Med* 1987;29:321–324.
50. Rycroft RJG, Calnan CD. Facial rashes among video display unit operators. In: Pearce, BG ed. *Health hazards of VDTs*. New York: John Wiley and Sons, 1984.
51. Tjonn HH. Report of facial rashes among VDU operators in Norway. In: Pearce BG, ed. *Health hazards of VDTs*. New York: John Wiley and Sons, 1984.
52. Fthenakis VM. Hazards from radiofrequency and laser equipment in the manufacture of a-SI photovoltaic cells. Brookhaven National Laboratory; 1985:15.
53. Hattis D, Berg R. Pharmacokinetics of ethoxyethanol in humans. MIT Center for Technology, Policy and Industrial Development. February 1988. [Report no 88-1].
54. Nagano K, et al. Embryotoxic effects of ethylene glycol monomethyl ether in mice. *Toxicology* 1981;20:335.
55. National Institute of Occupational Safety and Health. Current intelligence bulletin 39: glycol ethers. Cincinnati: US Department of Health and Human Services, 1983. [DHHS Pub 83-112].
56. US Department of Labor, Occupational Safety and Health Administration. ANPR for health and safety standards: occupational exposure to 2-methoxyethanol, 2-ethoxyethanol and their acetates. *Federal Register* 1987;52:10585–10593.
57. Hanley TR, Yano BL, Nitschke KD, John JA, et al. Comparison of the teratogenic potential of inhaled ethylene glycol monomethyl ether in rats, mice and rabbits. *Toxicol Appl Pharmacol* 1984;75:409–422.
58. Miller RR, Ayers JA, Young JT, McKenna MJ, et al. Ethylene glycol monomethyl ether. I. Subchronic vapor inhalation study with rats and rabbits. *Fund Appl Toxicol* 1983;3:49–54.
59. Tinson DJ. Ethylene glycol monomethyl ether: inhalation teratogenicity study in rabbits. Submitted to Environmental Protection Agency by ICI Center Toxicology Laboratory; 1983 April 21.
60. Tinson DJ. Ethylene glycol monomethyl ether: inhalation teratogenicity study in rats. Submitted to Environmental Protection Agency by ICI Center Toxicology Laboratory; 1983 April 14.
61. Niemeier RW, Smith RJ, Hardin ED, et al. Teratogenicity of 2-ethoxyethanol by dermal application. *Drug Chem Toxicol* 1982;5:277–294.
62. Nelson BK. Ethoxyethanol behavioral teratology in rats. *Neurotoxicology* 1981;2:231–247.
63. Tyl RW, Pritts IM, France AK, Fisher LC, Tyler TR. Developmental toxicity evaluation of inhaled 2-ethoxyethanol acetate in Fischer 344 rats and New Zealand white rabbits. *Fund Appl Toxicol* 1988;10:20–39.
64. Terrill JB. A 13-week inhalation study of ethylene glycol monomethyl ether in the rabbit. Report 82-7589 to the Chemical Manufacturers Association; 1983.
65. National Institute of Occupational Safety and Health. Criteria for a recommended standard occupational exposure to ethylene glycol monomethyl ether, ethylene glycol monoethyl ether, and their acetates. Cincinnati: US Department of Health and Human Services/NIOSH, 1991.
66. Ratcliffe JM, Schrader SM, Clapp DE, et al. Semen quality in workers exposed to 2-ethoxyethanol. *Br J Ind Med* 1989;46:399–406.
67. Cook RR, Bodner KM, Kolesar RC, et al. A cross-sectional study of ethylene glycol monomethyl ether process employees. *Arch Environ Health* 1982;37:346.
68. Welch LS, Schrader SM, Turner TW, Cullen MR, et al. Effects of exposure to ethylene glycol ethers on shipyard painters. II. Male reproduction. *Am J Ind Med* 1988;14:509–526.
69. Pastides H, et al. Spontaneous abortion and general illness symptoms among semiconductor manufacturers. *J Occup Med* 1988;30:543.
70. Snyder R, Andrews LS. Toxic effects of solvents and vapors. In: Klaassen CD, Doull J, Amdur MO, eds. *Casarett and Doull's toxicology: the basic science of poisons*, 5th ed. New York: McGraw-Hill, 1996;24:737–771.
71. Boggs A. A comparative risk assessment of casting solvents for positive photoresist. *Appl Ind Hyg* 1989;4:81–87.
72. Cheever KL, Richards DE, Weigel WW, et al. Metabolism of bis(2-methoxyethyl) ether in the adult male rat: evaluation of the principal metabolite as a testicular toxicant. *Toxicol Appl Pharmacol* 1988;94:150–159.
73. Teratogenicity study of diglyme in the rat. Submitted to Environmental Protection Agency under Toxic Substance Control Act. [DuPont HLR 515–87].
74. Subchronic inhalation toxicity study with diglyme. Submitted to Environmental Protection Agency under Toxic Substance Control Act. [DuPont HLR 129–88].
75. Subchronic inhalation toxicity study with diglyme. Submitted to Environmental Protection Agency under Toxic Substance Control Act. [DuPont HLR 562–88].
76. Price CJ, Kimmell CA, George JD, Marr MC. The developmental toxicity of diethylene glycol dimethyl ether in mice. *Fund Appl Toxicol* 1987;8:115–126.
77. Stedman DB, Welch F. Inhibition of DNA synthesis in mouse whole embryo culture by 2-methoxyacetic acid and attenuation of the effects by sample physiological compounds. *Toxicol Lett* 1989;45:111–117.
78. Mebus CA, Welsch F. The possible role of one-carbon moieties in 2-methoxyethanol and 2-methoxyacetic acid–induced developmental toxicity. *Toxicol Appl Pharmacol* 1989;99:98–109.
79. Guest D, Hamilton ML, Deisinger PJ, Divincenzo GD, et al. Pulmonary and percutaneous absorption of 2-propoxyethyl acetate and 2-ethoxyethyl acetate in beagle dogs. *Environ Health Perspect* 1984;57:177–183.
80. Dugard PH, Walker M, Mawdsley SJ, Scott RC, et al. Absorption of some glycol ethers through human skin in vitro. *Environ Health Perspect* 1984;57:193–197.
81. Groeseneken D, VanVelm E, Veulemans H, Masschelein R. Gas chromatographic determinations of methoxyacetic and ethoxyacetic acids in urine. *Br J Ind Med* 1986;43:62–65.
82. Smallwood AW, Debord KE, Lowry LK. Analyses of ethylene glycol monoalkyl ethers and their proposed metabolites in blood and urine. *Environ Health Perspect* 57:249–253.
83. Groeseneken D, Veulemans H, Masschelein R. Urinary excretion of ethoxyacetic acid after experimental human exposure to ethylene glycol monoethyl ether. *Br J Ind Med* 1986;43:615–619.
84. Veulemans H, Groeseneken D, Masschelein R, et al. Field study of the urinary excretion of ethoxyacetic acid during related daily exposure to the ethyl ether of ethylene glycol and ethyl ether of ethylene glycol acetate. *Scand J Work Environ Health* 1987;13:239–242.
85. Johanson G, Kronborg H, Naslund PH, et al. Toxicokinetics of inhaled 2-butoxyethanol (ethylene glycol monobutyl ether) in man. *Scand J Work Environ Health* 1986;12:594–602.
86. Paustenbach DJ. Assessment of the developmental risks resulting from occupational exposure to select glycol ethers within the semiconductor industry. *J Toxicol Environ Health* 1988;23:29–37.
87. US National Library of Medicine. Ethyl lactate. Hazardous Substances Data Bank 1996. Available at http://toxnet.nlm.nih.gov.
88. US National Library of Medicine. 1-methoxy-2-hydroxypropane (PGME). Hazardous Substances Data Bank 1996. Available at http://toxnet.nlm.nih.gov.
89. Merkle J, Klimisch HJ, Jäckh R. Prenatal toxicity of 2-methoxypropylacetate-1 in rats and rabbits. *Fund Appl Toxicol* 1987;8:71–79.
90. Deisinger PJ, Boatman RJ, Guest D. The metabolism and disposition of ethyl 3-ethoxypropionate in the rat. *Xenobiotica* 1990;20:989–997.

91. US National Library of Medicine. 1-methyl-2-pyrrolidone (NMP). Hazardous Substances Data Bank 1996.
92. Leira HL, et al. Irritant cutaneous reactions to *n*-methyl-2-pyrrolidone (NMP). *Contact Dermatitis* 1992;27:148–150.
93. US Environmental Protection Agency. Lifecycle analysis and pollution prevention assessment for *n*-methylpyrrolidone (NMP) in paint stripping. Washington: EPA; 1993.
94. Hass U, Lund S, Elsner J. Effects of prenatal exposure to *n*-methylpyrrolidone on postnatal development and behavior in rats. *Neurotoxicol Teratol* 1994;16:241–249.
95. Hass U, Jakobsen B, Lund SP. Developmental toxicity of inhaled *n*-methylpyrrolidone in the rat. *Pharmacol Toxicol* 1995;76:406–409.
96. Stark F. Toxicity studies on TX-85 (hexamethyldisilazane). Dow Corning Corporation. Washington: US Environmental Protection Agency, 1992. TSCA Section 8(e) [Notification 8EH6-0192-2068].
97. Stoner G, Weisburger E, Shimkin M. Brief communication: tumor response in strain A mice exposed to silylating compounds used for gas-liquid chromatography. *J Natl Cancer Inst* 1975;54:495–497.
98. Myers RC, Ballantyne B. Acute toxicologic evaluation of hexamethyldisilazane. *J Am Coll Toxicol* 1993;12:576.
99. US National Library of Medicine. Hexamethyldisiloxane. Hazardous Substances Data Bank 1996. Available at http://toxnet.nlm.nih.gov.
100. Fowler BA, ed. *Biological and environmental effects of arsenic*. Amsterdam: Elsevier, 1983.
101. Finkel AJ. Arsenic. In: Hamilton A, Hardy HL, Finkel AJ, eds. *Hamilton and Hardy's industrial toxicology*, 4th ed. Littleton, MA: PSG Publishing, 1983.
102. Beaudoin AR. Teratogenicity of sodium arsenate in rats. *Teratology* 1974;10:153–158.
103. Hood RD, Thacker GT, Patterson BL. Effects in the mouse and rat of prenatal exposure to arsenic. *Environ Health Perspect* 1977;19:219–222.
104. Kosnett M. Unpublished study. San Francisco: Center for Occupational and Environmental Health, University of California, San Francisco, 1991.
105. Lauwerys R, Hoet P. Arsenic. In: Lauwerys R, Hoet P, eds. *Industrial chemical exposure: guidelines for biological monitoring*. Boca Raton, FL: Lewis Publishers, 1993:21–28.
106. De Peyster A, Silvers J. Arsenic levels in hair of workers in a semiconductor fabrication facility. *Am Ind Hyg Assoc J* 1995;56:377–383.
107. Hertz-Picciotto I, Smith AH. Observations on the dose-response curve for arsenic exposure and lung cancer. *Scand J Work Environ Health* 1993;19:217–226.
108. Rudel R, Slayton T, Beck B. Implications of arsenic genotoxicity for dose response of carcinogenic effects. *Reg Toxicol Pharmacol* 1996;23:87–105.
109. National Institutes of Occupational Safety and Health. Health alert: request for assistance in reducing the potential risk of developing cancer from exposure to gallium arsenide in the microelectronics industry. Cincinnati: Department of Health and Human Services (NIOSH), 1987. [Publication no 88-100].
110. Rosner MH, Carter DE. Metabolism and excretion of gallium arsenide and arsenic oxides by hamsters following intratracheal instillation. *Fund Appl Toxicol* 1987;9:730–737.
111. Webb DR, Wilson SE, Carter DE. Pulmonary clearance and toxicity of respirable gallium arsenide particulates intratracheally instilled in rats. *Am Ind Hyg Assoc J* 987;48:660–667.
112. Webb DR, Wilson SE, Carter DE. Comparative pulmonary toxicity of gallium arsenide, gallium oxide, or arsenic oxide intratracheally instilled into rats. *Toxicol Appl Pharmacol* 1986;82:405–416.
113. National Institute of Occupational Safety and Health. Criteria for a recommended standard: occupational exposure to inorganic arsenic. Cincinnati: National Institute of Safety and Health, 1975.
114. Occupational Safety and Health Administration. Standard on arsenic. Washington: Office of the Federal Register, National Archives and Records Service, General Services Administration [29 CFR1910.1018].
115. Yamauchi H, Takahashi K, Mashiko M, Yamamura Y. Biological monitoring of arsenic exposure of gallium arsenide and inorganic arsenic exposed workers by determination of inorganic arsenic and its metabolites in urine and hair. *Am Ind Hyg Assoc J* 1989;50:606–612.
116. Foa V, et al. The speciation of the chemical forms of arsenic in the biological monitoring of exposure to inorganic arsenic. *Sci Total Environ* 1984;34:241–259.
117. Norin H, Vahter M. A rapid method for the selective analysis of total urinary metabolites of inorganic arsenic. *Scand J Work Environ Health* 1981;7:38–44.
118. Vahter ME. Arsenic. In: Clarkson TW, et al. *Biological monitoring of toxic metals*. New York, NY: Plenum Publishing, 1988.
119. Wolff RK, Henderson RF, Edison AF, et al. Toxicity of gallium oxide particles following a 4-week inhalation exposure. *Appl Toxicol* 1988;8(3):191–199.
120. Balboni HA, Ziemer EJ. *Study of silane self-ignition and explosion potential*. Essex Junction, VT: IBM General Technical Division, 1979.
121. Ring MA. Silane-O_2 explosions, their characteristics and their control. *Proc Am Inst Phys Conf U S A* 1988;166:175–182.
122. American Conference of Governmental Industrial Hygienists. *Documentation of the threshold limit values and biological exposure indices*, 6th ed. Cincinnati: American Conference of Governmental Industrial Hygienists, 1991.
123. Stokinger HE. The halogens and the nonmetals boron and silicon. In: Clayton GD, Clayton FE, eds. *Patty's industrial hygiene and toxicology*, 3rd rev. Vol 2B. New York: John Wiley and Sons, 1981.
124. Nakashima H, et al. Acute and subacute inhalation toxicity of dichlorosilane in male ICR mice. *Arch Toxicol* 1996;70:218–223.
125. US National Library of Medicine. Trichlorosilane. Hazardous Substances Data Bank 1997. Available at http://toxnet.nlm.nih.gov.
126. US National Library of Medicine. Silicon tetrachloride. Hazardous Substances Data Bank 1997. Available at http://toxnet.nlm.nih.gov.
127. Kizer KW, Garb LG, Hine CH. Health effects of silicon tetrachloride. Report of an urban accident. *J Occup Med* 1984;26:33–36.
128. Morgan D, et al. Inhalation toxicity of phosphine for Fischer 344 rats and B6C3F1 mice. *Inhal Toxicol* 1995;7:225–238.
129. Kligerman A, et al. Cytogenetic and germ cell effects of phosphine inhalation by rodents. II. Subacute exposures to rats and mice. *Environ Mol Mutagen* 1994;24:301–306.
130. Barbosa A, et al. Determination of genotoxic and other effects in mice following short term repeated-dose and subchronic inhalation exposure to phosphine. *Environ Mol Mutagen* 1994;24:81–88.
131. Barbosa A, Bonin A. Evaluation of phosphine genotoxicity at occupational levels of exposure in New South Wales, Australia. *Occup Environ Med* 1994;51:700–705.
132. Nomiyama T. Inhalation toxicity of diborane in rats assessed by bronchoalveolar lavage examination. *Arch Toxicol* 1995;70:43–50.
133. Uemura T, et al. Acute and subacute inhalation toxicity of diborane in male ICR mice. *Arch Toxicol* 1995;69:397–404.
134. Nomiyama T, et al. No-observed-effect level of diborane on the respiratory organs of male mice in acute and subacute inhalation experiments. *Sangyo Eiseigaku Zasshi* 1995;37:157–160.
135. US National Library of Medicine. Boron trichloride. Hazardous Substances Data Bank 1997. Available at http://toxnet.nlm.nih.gov.
136. US National Library of Medicine. Phosphorus oxychloride. Hazardous Substances Data Bank 1997. Available at http://toxnet.nlm.nih.gov.
137. US National Library of Medicine. Boron trifluoride. Hazardous Substances Data Bank 1997. Available at http://toxnet.nlm.nih.gov.
138. Canadian Centre for Occupational Health and Safety. Tungsten hexafluoride. MSDS database 1993.
139. US National Library of Medicine. Nitrogen trifluoride. Hazardous Substances Data Bank 1996. Available at http://toxnet.nlm.nih.gov.
140. Bruze M. Contact dermatitis from phenol-formaldehyde resins. In: Maibach HI, ed. *Occupational and industrial dermatology*, 2nd ed. Chicago: Year Book Medical Publishers, 1987.
141. Toxic Substance Control Act. [TSCA 8e/report HQ-0484-0510].
142. Dubrow R. Malignant melanoma in the printing industry. *Am J Ind Med* 1986;10:119–126.
143. McLaughlin JK, Malker HS, Blot WJ, et al. Malignant melanoma in the printing industry. *Am J Ind Med* 1988;13:301–304.
144. Nielsen H, Henriksen L, Olsen JH. Malignant melanoma among lithographers. *Scand J Work Environ Health* 1996;22:108–111.
145. National Institute of Safety and Health. Current intelligence bulletin: benzidine derived dyes. 1978 [DHEW pub 78-148] no 24.
146. Choudat D, Neukirch F, Brochard P, et al. Allergy and occupational exposure to hydroquinone and to methionine. *Br J Ind Med* 1988;45:376–380.
147. National Institute of Safety and Health. A recommended standard for occupational exposure to hydroquinone. 1978 [DHEW pub 78-115].
148. Bracken W, et al. Comparative effectiveness of topical treatments for hydrofluoric acid burns. *J Occup Med* 1985;27:733–739.
149. Upfal M, Doyle C. Medical management of hydrofluoric acid exposure. *J Occup Med* 1990;32:726–731.
150. Dunn BJ, MacKinnon MA, Knowlden NF, et al. Topical treatment for hydrofluoric acid dermal burns: further assessment of efficacy using an experimental pig model. *J Occup Environ Med* 1996;38(5):507–514.
151. Mullet T, Zoeller T, Bingham H, et al. Fatal hydrofluoric acid cutaneous exposure with refractory ventricular fibrillation. *J Burn Care Rehab* 1987;8:216–219.
152. Tepperman PB. Fatality due to acute systemic fluoride poisoning following a hydrofluoric acid skin burn. *J Occup Med* 1980;22:691–692.
153. Buckingham FM. Surgery: a radical approach to severe hydrofluoric acid bums: a case report. *J Occup Med* 1988;30:873–874.
154. Vance MV, Curry SC, Kunkel DB, et al. Digital hydrofluoric acid burns: treatment with intraarterial calcium infusion. *Ann Emerg Med* 1986;15:890–896.
155. Velbart J. Arterial perfusion for hydrofluoric acid burns. *Hum Toxicol* 1983;2:233–238.
156. Braun R, Huttner E, Merten H, Raabe F. Genotoxicity studies in semiconductor industry. 1. In vitro mutagenicity and genotoxicity studies of waste samples resulting from plasma etching. *J Toxicol Environ Health* 1993;39:309–322.
157. Schmidt R, Scheufler H, Bauer S, Wolff L, Pelzing M, Herzschuh R. Toxicological investigations in the semiconductor industry. III. Studies on prenatal toxicity caused by waste products from aluminum plasma etching processes. *Toxicol Ind Health* 1995;11:49–61.
158. Bauer S, Wolff I, Werner N, Schmidt R, Blume R, Pelzing M. Toxicological investigations in the semiconductor industry. IV. Studies on the subchronic oral toxicity and genotoxicity of vacuum pump oils contaminated by waste products from aluminum plasma etching processes. *Toxicol Ind Health* 1995;11:523–541.
159. Schenker M, et al. Association of spontaneous abortion and other reproductive effects with work in the semiconductor industry. *Am J Ind Med* 1995;28:639–659.
160. Gray RH, Corn M, Cohen R, et al. Final report: the Johns Hopkins University retrospective and prospective studies of reproductive health among IBM employees in semiconductor manufacturing. Baltimore: The Johns Hopkins University Press, 1993.

161. Beaumont JJ, Swan SH, Hammond SK, et al. Historical cohort investigation of spontaneous abortion in the Semiconductor Health Study: epidemiologic methods and analyses of risk in fabrication overall and in fabrication work groups. *Am J Ind Med* 1995;28:735–750.
162. Swan SH, Beaumont JJ, Hammond SK, et al. Historical cohort study of spontaneous abortion among fabrication workers in the semiconductor health study: agent-level analysis. *Am J Ind Med* 1995;28:751–769.
163. Eskenazi B, Gold EB, Lasley BL, et al. Prospective monitoring of early fetal loss and clinical spontaneous abortion among female semiconductor workers. *Am J Ind Med* 1995;28:833–846.
164. International Agency for Research on Cancer. Occupational exposures to mists and vapours from sulfuric acid and other strong inorganic acids. *IARC Monogr Eval Carcinog Risks Chem Hum* 1992;54:103–106.
165. Schlesinger R. Effects of inhaled acids on respiratory tract defense mechanisms. *Environ Health Perspect* 1985;63:25–38.
166. International Agency for Research on Cancer. Chromium and chromium compounds. *IARC Monogr Eval Carcinog Risks Hum Suppl* 1987;7:165–168.
167. International Agency for Research on Cancer. Silica. *IARC Monogr Eval Carcinog Risks Hum Suppl* 1987;7:341–343.
168. International Agency for Research on Cancer. Nickel and nickel compounds. *IARC Monogr Eval Carcinog Risks Hum Suppl* 1987;7:264–269.
169. International Agency for Research on Cancer. Table 1. Degrees of evidence for carcinogenicity in humans and in experimental animals. *IARC Monogr Eval Carcinog Risks Hum Suppl* 1987;7:56–74.
170. Glaberson W. Ailing chip workers cite chemicals, not chance. *New York Times* 1996 March 28.
171. Sorahan T, Pope DJ, McKiernan MJ. Cancer incidence and cancer mortality in a cohort of semiconductor workers: an update. *Br J Ind Med* 1992;49:215–216.
172. LaDou J, Rohm T. Occupational hazards in the microelectronics industry. In: Rom W, ed. *Environmental and occupational medicine*, 2nd ed. Boston: Little, Brown and Company, 1992:1051–1062.
173. McCurdy S, Schenker M, Samuels S. Reporting of occupational injury and illness in the semiconductor manufacturing industry. *Am J Public Health* 1991;81:85–89.

CHAPTER 34

Plastic Manufacturing

Richard Lewis and John B. Sullivan, Jr.

Articles made from plastics are ubiquitous in industrialized societies and are found in appliances, automobiles, toys, home furnishings, clothing, insulation, food and beverage containers, and countless other applications. Advances in plastics technology have resulted in the development of materials with properties that equal or exceed those of metal, wood, and glass. Plastics can be formed into sheets, coatings, or laminates or molded into virtually any shape or size. Plastic materials may have equal strength, durability, and impact resistance compared with some metals but are much lighter, a distinct advantage in the transportation industry. The synthetic nature of these materials allows the industry to readily adapt products to current needs. With different combinations of polymers and additives, the production of materials with unique properties and applications is seemingly limitless.

As the plastics industry has grown, the major focus has been on the chemical and mechanical properties of the materials as they relate to specific applications. The presumption has been that high-molecular-weight polymers are biologically inert. As the industrial and medical experience with these compounds has grown, so has the recognition of a variety of potential health hazards. In the industrial medical setting, health providers need to be familiar with the basic materials and processes of this industry to recognize adverse health effects in this ever-expanding and changing industry.

Plastics are divided into two main classes: (a) thermoplastics, which can be repeatedly softened and reshaped with the application of heat or pressure; and (b) thermoset plastics, which undergo a chemical reaction during processing that results in permanent cross-linking. Table 34-1 lists the major thermoplastic and thermoset polymers in use.

TABLE 34-1. Thermal degradation products of some plastics

Polymer	Degradation product(s)	Hazard
Polyethylene	Carbon monoxide	S
Polyvinyl chloride	Vinyl chloride	S, C
	HCl, phosgene	I, R
	Dioxins, furans	C
Polystyrene	Styrene	S
	Benzene	S, C
Fluoropolymers	Carbonyl fluoride	I, R
	Perfluoroisobutylene	I, R
	Hydrofluoric acid	I, R
Polyurethane	Aldehydes, ammonia	I, R
	Cyanide	S
	Isocyanates	I, R
	Nitrogen dioxide	R
Phenolic	Formaldehyde	I, R, S
	Aldehydes, ammonia	I, R
	Cyanide	S
	Nitrogen dioxide	R

C, carcinogen; I, mucous membrane irritant; R, respiratory irritant; S, systemic toxin.

Thermoplastic compounds have the characteristic that their shape can be altered by heating and then cooling. During heating, the distances between the macromolecules increase with the decrease in Van der Waals forces. During the cooling process, the distances decrease with a subsequent increase in Van der Waals forces. The newly shaped plastic thus retains the new position. Thermoplastics may be recycled and reused. Thermoset plastics cannot be altered once formed, because the macromolecules undergo a chemical reaction during formation. This thermoset linkage usually involves more than two functional chemical groups, which are cross-links between the chains (1).

RESIN MANUFACTURE

Resins are the basic building blocks of plastic and synthetic rubber materials. The raw materials for the production of polymers are derived primarily from crude oil and natural gas, and the growth of the plastics industry is dependent on the availability of these resources. The chemicals that serve as intermediates or monomers are obtained by crude oil distillation followed by catalytic cracking and reformation. Other chemical reactions, such as the addition of halogens, may take place before polymerization (2).

Polymerization reactions occur in closed systems under controlled conditions. Chain reaction polymerization is initiated when a catalyst reacts with a substrate material, forming a free radical from a double bond. Chain growth results when additional monomeric units are added to the growing polymer chain, until there is either deliberate or spontaneous termination. In step reaction polymerization, two different chemicals react with the elimination of small molecules.

Before polymeric resins are used in the fabrication or manufacture of plastic products, a variety of additives and fillers may be added in the process of compounding. These include colorants, plasticizers, biocides, antioxidants, flame retardants, and fillers. The intimate mixing of polymer and additives requires heavy machinery, including ball mills, high-speed propeller mixers, kneading machines, and Banbury mixers or extruders. The compounded polymers may be supplied as sheets or formed into pellets, beads, or powders.

PLASTIC PROCESSING

The plastic processing industry converts a resin into finished products. Granules and powders may be compounded with additives before processing, and workers in these operations may have exposures similar to those of the resin manufacturers. Thermoset and partially polymerized materials may be supplied in solid or liquid form, and workers handling these materials may have exposure to unreacted intermediates and additives.

Plastic material processing requires that the resin be converted to a soft, malleable state through the application of heat or pressure followed by mechanical constriction to mold the material to the desired form and then cool it. Two of the primary processes used in the manufacture of plastic products are blow molding and injection molding. In blow molding, a hollow tube of heated plastic is formed, usually by extrusion, and placed in a mold with the desired final shape. The tube is filled with air under high pressure, which expands the plastic into the mold cavity. The air is exhausted and the finished part ejected. This process can be used to form small bottles or 55-gallon drums. Injection molding uses high pressures to convert thermoplastic materials into articles with complex shapes. Pellets or granules are heated in a barrel, and the melted plastic is injected into a cooled metal mold by a helical screw. The parts are held under pressure until cool, then removed from the mold and trimmed. In compression molding, heat and pressure are applied to resin granules within a mold, forcing the material to conform to the mold shape. In transfer molding, thermoset materials are heated in a cavity and then transferred into a separate mold using a plunger. Extrusion forces a continuous flow of heated plastic through a die of the desired shape and is used for production of piping, tubing, gutters, and sheets. Calendering uses heated rollers to form sheets and coatings. Thermoforming and vacuum forming use pressure and suction, respectively, to conform heated sheet plastic to a mold.

Finishing processes include the use of paints, adhesives, and solvents, as in many other manufacturing industries. Molded items often need to be trimmed by hand before packaging and shipping. Scrap thermoplastic materials are usually recycled after grinding.

HEALTH HAZARDS

Most of the polymerization processes take place in closed systems, and the health hazards of resin manufacture are similar to those of the petrochemical industry (1–4). Workers may have exposure to vapors and dusts containing chemical intermediates, polymers, and additives during loading, mixing, pelletizing, and maintenance operations. Proper storage and handling of chemicals and additives are mandatory. Reactions must be carefully controlled to avoid chemical release or explosion. Dry mixing and pelletizing operations may generate high concentrations of airborne dusts of combustible plastic materials, presenting an explosion hazard.

Plastic processing equipment operates using high temperatures and pressures and needs to be equipped with proper guards and safety rails to avoid serious burns, amputations, and crush injuries. The overheating of plastic materials during processing, cleaning, and maintenance operations may expose workers to the thermal decomposition products of the polymer materials. Finishing operations may expose workers to a variety of other chemical compounds, such as solvents and adhesives. In addition, cutting of plastics may result in repetitive motion injuries, such as tendinitis, sprains, and carpal tunnel syndrome.

COMBUSTION PRODUCT HAZARDS

Thermoplastic materials must be heated during processing. The temperatures required to achieve proper fluidity vary with the composition of the polymer and the additives. Overheating of plastics results in thermal decomposition and the release of oligomers, monomers, and other combustion products. The composition of the mixture of gases and vapors that are evolved is complex and is dependent not only on the chemical constituents of the polymer, but also on the temperature. At lower temperatures (300° to 400°F), combustion is incomplete, releasing larger, more complex molecules, whereas at higher temperatures (higher than 1,600°F), complete combustion and oxidation produce low-molecular-weight gases. Workers may be exposed to the thermal decomposition products of plastics through accidental overheating during processing or during cleanout and maintenance operations. In addition, the burning of plastic materials during fires may present a health hazard to firefighters and the public.

The main combustion hazards that have been identified for the major classes of plastic materials are listed in Table 34-1. New thermal degradation products will be identified as research in this area proceeds. Although combustion hazards are primarily respiratory irritants (hydrochloric acid, aldehydes), significant pulmonary injury from nitrogen oxides and phosgene, as well as systemic poisoning from CO and cyanides, may occur. The long-term health effects of exposure to combustion products of plastics are unknown.

POLYETHYLENE AND POLYPROPYLENE

High- and low-density polyethylene resins account for almost one-third of the plastics produced in the United States. More than 100 different brands of polyethylene are available.

Polyethylene is produced by the polymerization of ethylene in either continuous-flow or tubular reactors. Polyethylene is formed from a polymerization reaction of alkenes and conjugated dienes. Ethylene heated under pressure with oxygen produces a high-molecular-weight compound, polyethylene, made up of many ethylene subunits:

$$nCH_2 = CH_2 \xrightarrow[\text{Heat pressure}]{O_2} (-CH_2-CH_2-)n$$

This type of polymerization, the end-to-end addition of monomers, is termed *addition polymerization*. The other type of polymerization—in which monomers are combined and in the process a molecule is lost—is termed *condensation polymerization*.

Polypropylene is characterized by resistance to heat and chemical corrosion. Propylene polymerization can occur in three different arrangements. All the methyl groups can be on one side of an extended chain (isotactic), methyl groups can alternate from side to side (syndiotactic), or methyl groups can alternate on each side of the chain randomly (atactic). Isotactic polypropylene is crystalline and forms strong fibers with a high melting point. Atactic polypropylene is a soft, elastic, pliable material. Polymerization of polypropylene generally occurs in a slurry with a hydrocarbon solvent diluent. Production of both plastics uses organometallic catalysts. Solvent vapors are evaporated off during drying and grinding. Liquid polymer is then cooled and formed into pellets.

High-density polyethylene is used to form containers ranging from fuel tanks to milk bottles. Low-density polyethylene has higher clarity and is used for films, coatings, shrink wrap, and food packaging. Polypropylene is used in containers, including medical syringes, as well as automotive components.

Both ethylene and propylene are asphyxiant gases. Several of the organometallic catalysts used are potent respiratory and skin irritants. Occupational asthma has also been reported due to both agents (1). The thermal decomposition products of polyethylene and polypropylene include carbon dioxide as well as formaldehyde and acrolein, both respiratory irritants. Preliminary research suggesting that workers exposed to polypropylene were at excess risk for developing colorectal cancer was not supported by subsequent investigations (2).

Ethylene and propylene should be stored properly in well-ventilated areas. Workers should not enter reaction vessels without using proper air-supplied respirators. Care should be taken to avoid overheating or burning these polymers to prevent the formation of aldehydes and other decomposition products.

POLYVINYL CHLORIDE

Polyvinyl chloride (PVC) is a versatile plastic used widely in diverse applications. This product is produced by polymerization of vinyl chloride monomer, a gas at room temperature:

$$nCH_2 = \underset{\displaystyle Cl}{CH} \xrightarrow{\text{Peroxides}} (-CH_2-\underset{\displaystyle Cl}{CH}-)n$$

Polymerization reactions take place in pressure vessels using a process in which vinyl chloride is suspended in water using a colloid with a peroxide catalyst. Residual monomer is removed from the vessels, and the slurry is dried, then pelletized.

PVC is used widely in pipe, wire, and cable coatings for its strength and corrosion resistance. Diverse other uses range from floor tile and records to medical tubing and intravenous solution bags. PVC plastics commonly include plasticizers to increase flexibility. The major class of plasticizers are the phthalate esters, such as di(2-ethylhexyl) phthalate and dioctyl phthalate.

From 1927 until 1970, there was extensive exposure to unreacted vinyl chloride monomer in chemical plants producing PVC resin (Fig. 34-1). In the early years of production, air levels of vinyl chloride routinely exceeded 1,000 ppm, at times resulting in very high exposure. While entering and cleaning reactor vessels (or "polys"), workers at times were overcome by narcotic concentrations of vinyl chloride (15,000 to 20,000 ppm).

In the mid-1970s, the toxicity and carcinogenicity of vinyl chloride monomer were recognized after the identification and reporting of a cluster of cases of angiosarcoma of the liver in workers at a PVC production plant in Louisville, Kentucky. The marked excess of this extremely rare tumor also occurred at several other PVC production plants around the world. The association of exposure to vinyl chloride monomer and angiosarcoma of the liver and hepatic carcinoma has subsequently been confirmed in several epidemiologic investigations (3–7).

Several other effects related to vinyl chloride exposure have been reported. The hand-cleaning of reactors in the late 1960s caused a condition termed *acroosteolysis*, a combination of Raynaud's phenomenon and lytic lesions of the distal phalanges (8). This condition was reversible with the use of proper hand protection. Subacute liver injury with fibrosis has also occurred with repeated heavy exposure. The primary target area of injury appears to be the endothelial cells in the hepatic sinusoids (9). Exposure to PVC dust has been associated with the development of a pneumoconiosis, and vinyl chloride monomer and PVC dust have been associated with development of a sclerodermalike syndrome in case reports (10).

In the United States and European countries, worker exposure to vinyl chloride has been reduced significantly, from 100 ppm to 200 ppm in the early 1970s to less than 5 ppm since the promulgation of the Occupational Safety and Health Administration (OSHA) standard in 1974. In other parts of the world, high levels of exposure to vinyl chloride monomer may have continued well into the 1980s. With this reduction in exposure, the risk of developing subacute liver injury appears to be minimal. The risk for developing angiosarcoma and possibly other malignancies (brain tumors, leukemia) remains uncertain. Workers who were first exposed before 1970 appear to remain at risk, with latencies as long as 50 years being reported. A register of angiosarcoma cases is maintained by the Association of Plastics Manufacturers of Europe.

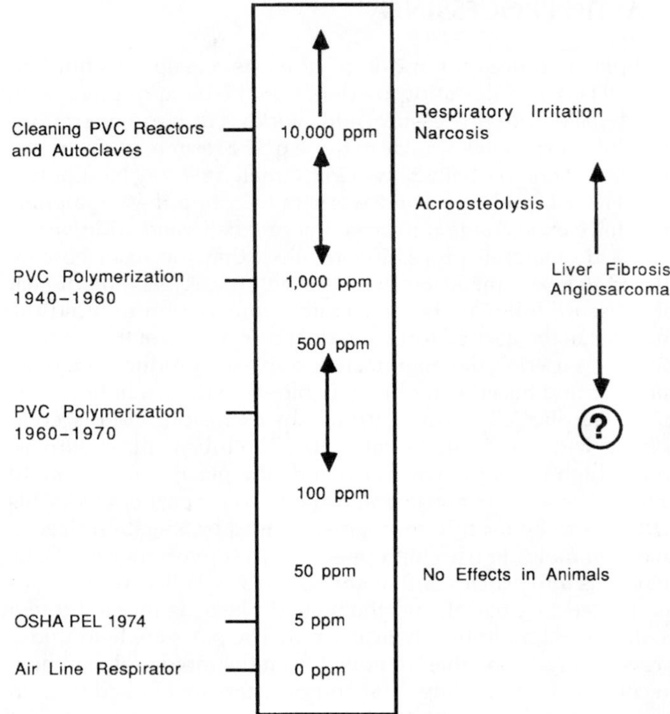

Figure 34-1. Vinyl chloride exposure and health effects at various times and under different conditions. OSHA, Occupational Safety and Health Administration; PEL, permissible exposure limit; PVC, polyvinyl chloride.

The risk of exposure to unreacted vinyl chloride monomer is much less in the processing of PVC resins into finished products. There has been limited evidence that exposure to PVC dust during grinding and other fabrication operations may result in the development of a pneumoconiosis in some workers, accompanied by a slight reduction in pulmonary function. The plasticizer di(2-ethylhexyl)phthalate is also hepatotoxic and is an animal carcinogen as well (11). The thermal decomposition products of PVC include hydrochloric acid and phosgene, both respiratory irritants. Other thermal decomposition products are polychlorodibenzodioxins and polychlorodibenzofurans.

It appears that the marked reduction in exposure to vinyl chloride has been effective in preventing workers from developing the significant health problems of the past. Care should be taken to prevent accidental overexposure to vinyl chloride during PVC production through the use of proper respiratory protection. Workers should also avoid exposure to PVC dust generated during grinding, drying, or cleaning operations. Medical surveillance under the OSHA standard required annual examinations of workers exposed to vinyl chloride, including liver enzymes. Assessment of lung function is also recommended. Any workers exposed to high levels of vinyl chloride monomer should be aware that they may be at risk for the development of liver cancer throughout their lives.

Unfortunately, routine tests have been inadequate in detecting angiosarcoma of the liver, most cases presenting clinically with advanced disease. Elevations of serum bile acids and hyaluronic acid have been reported in workers with histologically proven vinyl chloride–induced liver damage and may be better tools for surveillance of currently exposed workers (9). An elevation of van Willebrand factor has also been reported in individuals diagnosed with angiosarcoma, and levels have been used to track disease progression (12). Vinyl chloride–induced mutations in the p53 (13) and the *k-ras* genes (14) have been identified through identification of altered serum proteins, and these show promise in identifying excessive exposure as well as disease risk.

POLYSTYRENE

Styrene-based polymers rank third in production behind polyethylene and PVC. In addition to polystyrene plastics, other styrene polymers are used in the manufacture of synthetic rubber. Polystyrene resins are produced by a bulk polymerization process. A bead polymerization process in suspension is used to produce polystyrene foams (Fig. 34-2). Copolymerization of 1,3-butadiene with styrene produces styrene-butadiene rubber.

Polystyrene packaging materials are used widely for food products such as egg cartons, plates, cups, and disposable food containers. Copolymers of styrene with acrylonitrile are much more durable and used in machine housings, battery casings, and automotive components.

There is potential exposure to unreacted styrene monomer during resin production, particularly during mixing, loading, and maintenance operations. Styrene monomer may also be released if styrene polymers are heated. Styrene is used as a cross-linking agent in reinforced plastics used in boat building (see Polyesters, below).

At high concentrations (higher than 100 ppm), styrene is a respiratory and mucous membrane irritant. Skin contact may result in the development of primary irritant dermatitis. The manifestations of overexposure to styrene include lightheadedness, dizziness, and uncoordination. Limited clinical investigations of workers with long-term exposure to styrene have suggested subtle central and peripheral nervous system injury as well as possible liver damage (15). Styrene is mutagenic and has been associated with the induction of chromosomal aberrations in humans, although human epidemiologic studies have not shown a definitive cancer risk (16).

Acrylonitrile ($CH_2 = CH - CN$) is an explosive, flammable liquid used in manufacturing acrylic fibers and as an intermediate in pesticide manufacturing. Acrylonitrile (vinyl cyanide) vapor is also a potent eye, mucous membrane, and skin irritant and may also cause symptoms of headache, fatigue, and nausea. Acrylonitrile may act as a chemical asphyxiant similar to hydrogen cyanide, and acute poisoning should be managed with amyl nitrate or sodium thiosulfate. Acrylonitrile has been regulated as a carcinogen in the United States, although epidemiologic studies have not consistently shown excesses of lung, colon, or prostatic cancers (17).

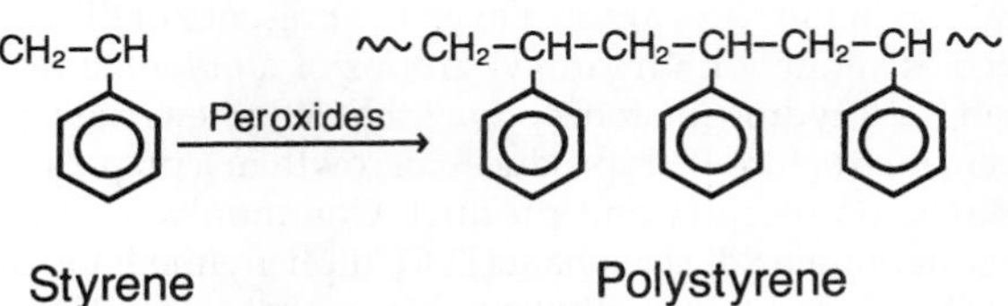

Figure 34-2. Styrene; polystyrene.

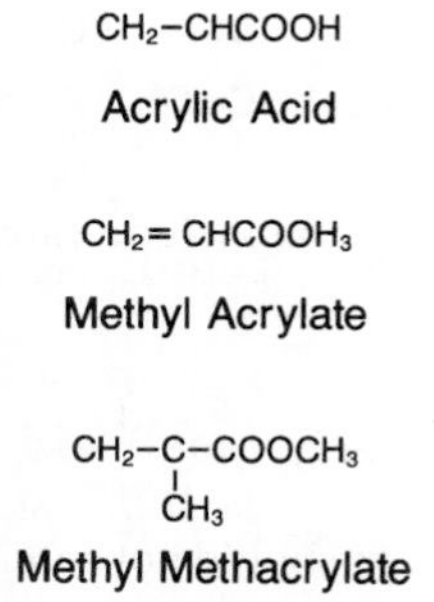

CH_2–CHCOOH

Acrylic Acid

CH_2= CHCOOH$_3$

Methyl Acrylate

CH_2–C(–CH_3)–COOCH$_3$

Methyl Methacrylate

Figure 34-3. Acrylic acid; methyl acrylate; methyl methacrylate.

The main measures in protecting the health of workers involved in the production of styrene polymers is control of exposure to styrene and acrylonitrile. Styrene polymers are generally inert, although free monomers may be released during combustion. Biological monitoring of worker exposure to styrene involves the measurement of urine metabolites (phenylglyoxylic acid and mandelic acid) or styrene in blood or exhaled air.

ACRYLICS

Acrylic materials are formed from acrylic acid and methyl acrylate (Fig. 34-3). Acrylates have a resilience and clarity that have led to extensive use in coatings, lights, windows, and face shields. Most are polymers of methyl methacrylate formed through bulk polymerization with peroxide catalysts (Fig. 34-4). Resins are supplied in sheets, pellets, or syrups.

The methacrylates are upper respiratory and mucous membrane irritants, but skin sensitization may occur leading to allergic contact dermatitis (18). Other symptoms reported after overexposure to methyl methacrylate include headache, fatigue, and irritability.

Prevention of skin sensitization is best achieved through limiting skin contact. Patch testing confirms the diagnosis. Further work with acrylics should be avoided in sensitive individuals.

FLUOROPOLYMERS AND CHLOROPOLYMERS

Fluoropolymers or chloropolymers comprise a small but growing class of materials that combine resistance with low friction (Fig. 34-5). In addition to nonstick cookware, fluoropolymers are

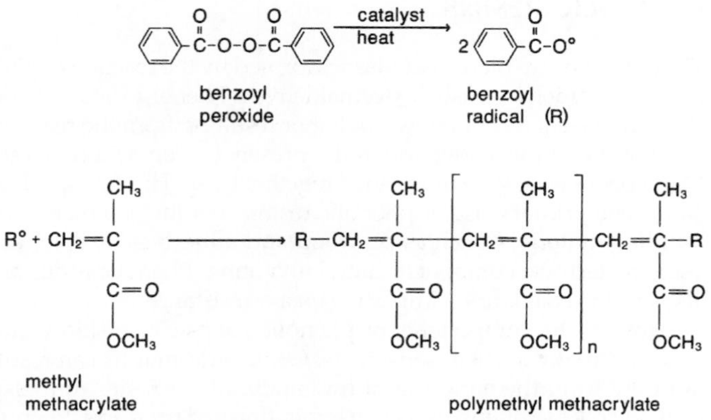

benzoyl peroxide —catalyst, heat→ 2 benzoyl radical (R)

R° + CH_2=C(CH_3)(C=O)(OCH_3) → R–CH_2=C(CH_3)(C=O)(OCH_3)–[CH_2=C(CH_3)(C=O)(OCH_3)]$_n$–CH_2=C(CH_3)(C=O)(OCH_3)–R

methyl methacrylate — polymethyl methacrylate

Figure 34-4. Polymethyl methacrylate.

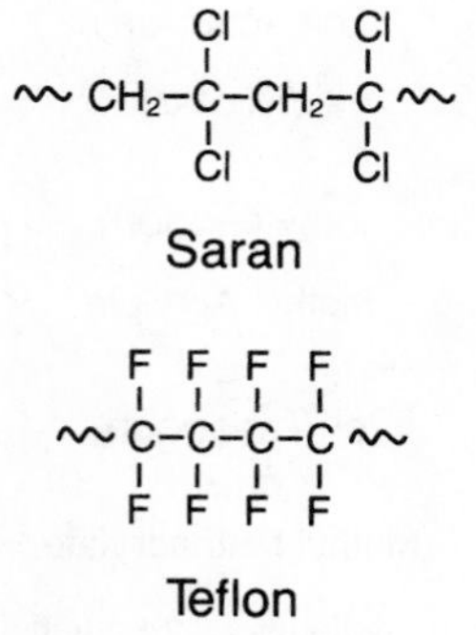

Saran

Teflon

Figure 34-5. Fluoro- and chloropolymers.

used to form sheaths and coatings for wire and cable. A large number of different fluoropolymer resins exist, most produced using hydrogen fluoride in combination with various aliphatic and chlorinated hydrocarbons. The high viscosity of fluoropolymers requires the use of high pressure and high temperature during processing.

During resin production, a variety of fluorinated and chlorinated hydrocarbons may be employed. Many of these are used more commonly as industrial refrigerants and solvents. The main hazard of these materials is the induction of solvent narcosis with overexposure. Hydrogen fluoride is a potent respiratory irritant, potentially causing delayed pulmonary edema (19). Hydrofluoric acid may also be used; it is an agent notorious for causing extensive necrotic skin burns. Immediate treatment of any symptomatic hydrofluoric acid is critical; calcium gluconate creams and injections are effective in anecdotal reports.

Polymer fume fever is a condition ascribed to the inhalation of the thermal decomposition of polytetrafluoroethylene $(-CF_2 = CF_2-)n$. After exposure to the overheated polymer, symptoms of fever, chills, cough, and dyspnea develop over several hours, resolving spontaneously in a few days. Smoking cigarettes coated with the polymer has also caused this syndrome. Although this has generally been a benign, self-limited condition, there are a few reports of individuals developing chronic pulmonary impairment (20).

Prevention of illness and injury in fluoropolymer production requires careful recognition of the toxicity of the materials used in production. High-temperature processing operations require use of local exhaust ventilation to limit exposure to thermal decomposition products. Respiratory protection must be worn if molds or equipment are heated during cleaning. Good housekeeping practices and restriction of smoking in work areas prevents inadvertent development of polymer fume fever.

PHENOLIC RESINS

The phenolics are thermoset plastics formed by the reaction of phenol and an aldehyde, usually formaldehyde. Phenol-formaldehyde resins represent a well-known polymer resulting from the reaction of phenol and formaldehyde in the presence of an acid or alkali. Many phenol rings are thus joined together by $-CH^2-$ groups (Fig. 34-6). The primary use of phenolic resins is in the production of building materials, such as plywood and adhesives. Resoles are used in electrical components and laminating. Phenolic resins are also used to coat fabrics, imparting crease resistance.

Most of the components of phenolic resins cause skin irritation, and many are skin sensitizers. Contact dermatitis can result not only from the handling of raw materials or resins, but also from the release of uncured resins from finished products. Phenol, formaldehyde, and hexamethylene tetramine are also respiratory

Phenol + HCHO Formaldehyde → (H_2SO_4 or NaOH) Hydroxymethylphenol → (Heat) Phenol-Formaldehyde Resin

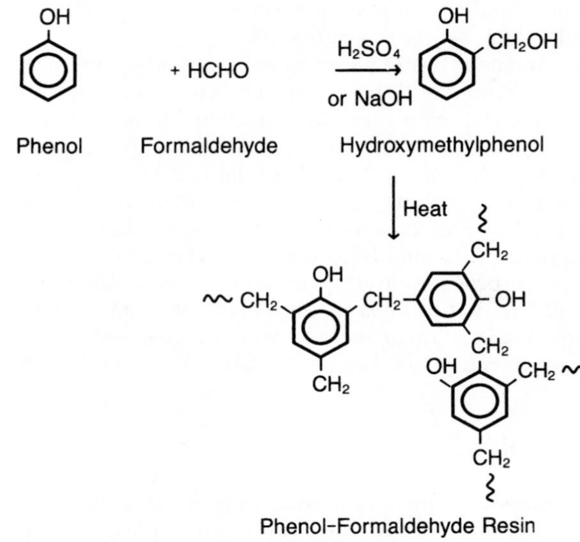

Figure 34-6. Phenol-formaldehyde resin.

and mucous membrane irritants. Phenol may be absorbed through the skin, with overexposure causing fatigue, weight loss, and liver injury. Operations that generate dust—such as grinding of phenolic materials—have been reported to cause pulmonary impairment and x-ray changes consistent with a pneumoconiosis. Thermal decomposition products of phenolic polymers include phenol, formaldehyde, acrolein, and carbon monoxide.

As with acrylics, avoidance of skin contact through proper material handling is essential in the prevention of dermatitis and sensitization. Proper respiratory protection should be worn when handling resin powders and during grinding operations.

POLYURETHANES AND URETHANES

Polyurethanes are used widely in furnishings and construction in the form of flexible and rigid foams. These complex cellular polymers are formed by a reaction of an isocyanate with an alcohol group from a polyol, polyester, or polyether (9). The foams are formed in a one-shot process, with the addition of an organometallic catalyst and a blowing agent (water or a chlorofluorocarbon). The liquid polymer is poured on a moving conveyor and heat-cured into slabs.

Urethanes are prepared from an isocyanate or polyisocyanate prepolymer. Isocyanates are chemicals that contain the NCO group. Polyisocyanates usually contain three or more NCO groups. The basic unit of polyurethane materials is a monomer. Monomers are made to react with each other by an exchange of atoms. A stepwise reaction of monomers is the basis of how diisocyanates are used to make longer chains of polyurethane. The propagation reaction using the monomer-starting material can occur either by the use of radicals or the use of a chemical that transfers a hydrogen atom. Usually, a polyol compound is used to transfer the hydrogen atom needed to the isocyanate. This chemical reaction saturates the double bond between the nitrogen and the carbon in the NCO group. Given the presence of diisocyanate molecules, along with hydroxyl groups of a polyol, a repeating exchange of hydrogen atoms occurs that lengthens the repeating molecular structure. This produces a growth in a prepolymer to a large macromolecular end product. Commonly used diisocyanates are toluene diisocyanate (TDI), diphenylmethane diisocyanate (MDI), and hexamethylene diisocyanate (Fig. 34-7). These compounds react with the dipolyfunctional hydroxy group, such

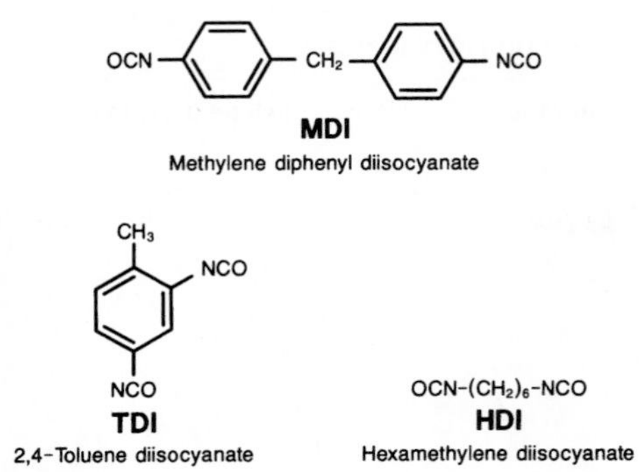

Figure 34-7. Toluene diisocyanate; methylene diphenyl diisocyanate; hexamethylene diisocyanate.

as is present on polyol compounds, to form polyurethanes (9,10). Polyurethanes are used as foams and as surface coating in the form of adhesives and sealants. The typical polyol compound is a trihydroxy resin or polyglycol, which reacts with the diisocyanate to form a prepolymer. The polymerization reaction is exothermic. The heat that evolves helps cure and set the foam. Because of this exothermic reaction, some diisocyanate may volatilize and escape into the atmosphere of the environment. Other curing agents used in polyurethane manufacturing include amines and esters (Table 34-2).

Diisocyanates are the most commonly recognized isocyanates, with TDI being the most commonly used commercial diisocyanate. Two isomers are available: 2,4-TDI and 2,6-TDI. Other commonly used isocyanates include hexamethylene diisocyanate, naphthalene diisocyanate, and para-tolyl monoisocyanate (Table 34-3). After proper curing, the foams and polyurethanes that have been shaped usually contain no free diisocyanate compounds.

Occupations with the potential of having exposure to isocyanate products include diisocyanate workers, polyurethane manufacturing workers, upholstery workers, spray painters, coating workers, plastic film makers, plastic molders, and rubber workers (21).

Decrement of pulmonary functions and asthma are known consequences of pulmonary exposure to diisocyanate compounds (10,12,13). Human toxicology from diisocyanates is a result of dermal and inhalation contact with the chemical in a liquid or aerosolized form. Dermal contact can be direct or indirect via contact with vapors. Inhalational exposure is via vapor phase of the material or through inhalation of aerosolized material during spraying. Volatility of the isocyanate directly influences toxicity (9,10,12,13).

MDI and polyether polyol are frequently used in the formation of urethane foams. The polyol is used to react with the MDI to form a prepolymer, polymethylene polyphenylisocyanate (PAPI) (Fig. 34-8). MDI is manufactured from the condensation of aniline and formaldehyde to form methylene dianiline. This is then reacted with phosgene to form MDI. PAPI is a thick amber gel with little or no volatility and very low toxicity (9).

Exposure hazard of isocyanates is directly related to volatility and molecular weight. Isocyanates with low volatility and larger molecular weight, such as MDI and PAPI, are much less toxic than highly volatile, low-molecular-weight isocyanates, such as TDI or methyl isocyanate (MIC) (9). The vapor pressures of MDI and PAPI are significantly less in comparison to the vapor pressure of TDI. Because vapor pressure is directly related to inhalation potential, the pulmonary exposure to PAPI and MDI is less than TDI and would occur only if the material were heated to vaporization or aerosolized (Table 34-4).

Because the isocyanates with higher molecular weight and lower volatility are less toxic, health effects and exposure hazards from polyisocyanates tend to be much less. The low-molecular-weight and highly volatile MIC and TDI are dermal and pulmonary irritants and can produce severe pulmonary damage in concentrated forms (10,12–14). The higher-molecular-weight and less volatile MDI and PAPI are much less toxic than TDI and MIC. The dermal toxicity of MDI and PAPI is limited to mild irritation and requires direct contact.

The respiratory system is the main target organ for isocyanate toxicity (21–28) and occurs via particle formation or vaporization of the isocyanates. This volatilization can occur with increasing temperatures. Reasonable estimations of the respiratory exposure hazard from isocyanates is based on molecular weight, volatility, ambient temperatures, and the airborne concentration reaching the breathing zone of the individual. If the breathing zone concentration is more than 0.5 ppm, then pulmonary toxicity is more likely (13). The higher the dose and the longer the exposure, the sooner respiratory symptoms develop. Usually, with an exposure exceeding 0.5 ppm, symptoms may begin within a few hours (13). Traditionally, these symptoms consist of

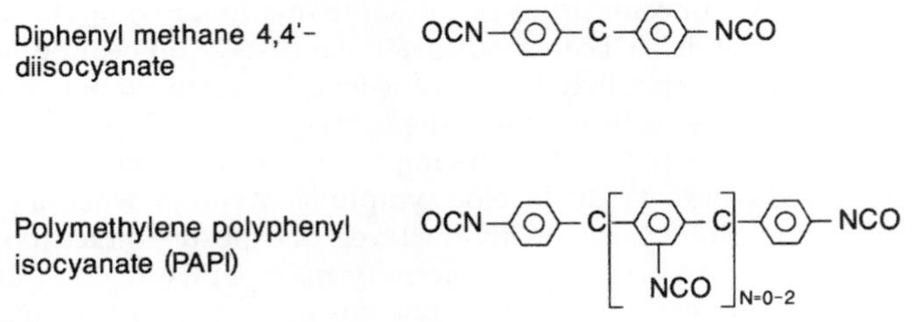

TABLE 34-2. Isocyanate curing agents

Trihydroxyl resin (castor oil)
Polyglycol (dipropylene glycol)
Aromatic amino polyol
Trichlorofluoromethane
Silicone oil
Phosphate esters
Tetramethyl butane diamine
Tetramethyl propane diamine
Diethanolamine
Tetramethylguanidine
Triethylene diamine
Triethylamine
Dimethylethanolamine
Diethylethanolamine
Dichlorobenzidine
Dianisidine
Tolidine
4,4-Methylene-bis(2-chloroamiline)

TABLE 34-3. Common isocyanates

Toluene diisocyanate (TDI)
Hexamethylene diisocyanate (HDI)
Methylene diphenyl diisocyanate (MDI)
Naphthalene diisocyanate (NDI)
Polymethylene polyphenyl isocyanate (PAPI)
Para-tolyl monisocyanate (PTI)
Dicyclohexyl methane-4,4-diisocyanate (DMDJ)
Triphenyl methane-4,4',4''-triisocyanate
Isophorone diisocyanate (IPDI)

Figure 34-8. Polymethylene polyphenyl isocyanate.

TABLE 34-4. Comparison of physical features of certain isocyanates

	Toluene diisocyanate	Methylene diphenyl diisocyanate	Polymethylene polyphenyl isocyanate
Molecular weight	174.4	250.3	400
Appearance	Clear to yellow liquid	White solid	Dark amber viscous liquid
Vapor pressures (mm Hg)			
50°F (10°C)	0.02	0.00006	0.00024
77°F (25°C)	0.05	0.00014	0.00006
100°F (37.7°C)	0.10	0.00031	0.00016
Relative vapor pressures (mm Hg)			
50°F (10°C)	898	1.5	1.0
77°F (25°C)	834	1.5	1.0
100°F (37.7°C)	612	1.5	1.0

cough, pleuritis, wheezing, and chest tightness. If concentrations are high enough, pulmonary edema and hemorrhagic alveolitis may occur. This type of exposure results in pulmonary pathology evident within 4 to 8 hours postexposure. The allergic manifestation of isocyanate exposure in terms of asthma does not occur until reexposure.

Previous human exposures in the medical literature to either TDI or MDI have been in the monomeric form. The main form of MDI used industrially is in the prepolymeric form (polymeric-MDI) or PAPI (see Fig. 34-8). This material is a mixture of bifunctional monomers (45% to 55%), with the remainder being three- and four-ring homologues having three or four NCO groups per molecule. Most of the industrial hygiene work on human exposure standards to isocyanates and diisocyanates has been confined to the monomer form, and not to prepolymers. Ample clinical and experimental evidence shows that TDI and MDI monomers produce dermal and pulmonary disease in the form of allergic contact dermatitis, pulmonary hypersensitivity, pneumonitis, and asthma (14–18). The medical literature further reflects that MDI monomers and polymers have an impressive safety record in industrial exposures, even though direct chronic and long-term exposures are associated with decrements in forced expiratory volume (FEV_1; greater than 1 second), forced vital capacity, and diffusion capacity. However, given adequate safety controls, MDI workers do not demonstrate FEV_1 decrements (28).

OSHA recommends an exposure standard for TDI and MDI of 0.005 ppm for a time-weighted average. A ceiling value of 0.02 ppm is also recommended for TDI. A ceiling limit cannot be violated at any time. Exposure limits exist only for diisocyanates. Exposure limits for the prepolymeric forms of diisocyanates, such as PAPI, do not exist, because their volatility is so low and toxicity hazard is minimal.

In general, isocyanates are irritants to the skin, cause contact and allergic dermatitis, and are irritants to the mucous membranes. Concentrated forms of the more volatile isocyanates, such as TDI and MIC, can produce chemical bronchitis and acute asthma at room temperatures in addition to inflammatory changes in the airways. Sensitization to isocyanates in an occupational setting can result in an asthma recurrence or reexposure to even low concentrations of the same or similar compound. The less volatile MDI can produce similar disease on heating.

There is evidence that the exposure level is an important factor in respiratory sensitization and the subsequent development of occupational asthma—thus the importance of prevention (28). Sensitized workers may develop symptoms of cough, wheezing, and chest tightness, even with low levels of exposure on reexposure. Chronic airway hyperreactivity may persist even after removal from exposure. Other concerns in the production and handling of polyurethanes include exposure to chlorinated and fluorinated solvents during batch preparation and curing. Many of the catalysts used are also potent irritants. Thermal decomposition products of polyurethanes—including free isocyanates, hydrogen cyanide, and carbon monoxide—are very hazardous.

Material handling and process ventilation are the key steps in preventing exposures during manufacturing. Proper eye, skin, and respiratory protection is critical in preventing overexposure to isocyanates. Periodic medical surveillance for possible respiratory or skin effects helps to ensure the adequacy of these measures in limiting exposure.

AMINO RESINS

The amino resins are thermoset materials used primarily in adhesives, coatings, and insulating materials. These are formed by a reaction of formaldehyde with an amino group from either urea or melamine (Fig. 34-9). The controlled polymerization reaction occurs in the presence of an acid catalyst and heat, with the evolution of water and formaldehyde. Amino resins are supplied as liquids, air-dried solids, or powders.

Exposure to formaldehyde is the main health hazard in the production and use of the amino resins. Formaldehyde is a respiratory and mucous membrane irritant, but may also cause nonspecific symptoms of headache and fatigue. Formaldehyde is also an animal carcinogen and is suspected of being a human carcinogen. The release of formaldehyde from finished products, such as plywood and urea-formaldehyde insulation, may contribute to air-quality problems in new buildings. Urea-formaldehyde insulation was banned from home use in 1982. Thermal decomposition products include carbon monoxide, formaldehyde, ammonia, and cyanide.

Proper ventilation is important in reducing formaldehyde levels in virtually any use of amino resins. Skin contact should also be avoided to prevent skin irritation or cutaneous sensitization.

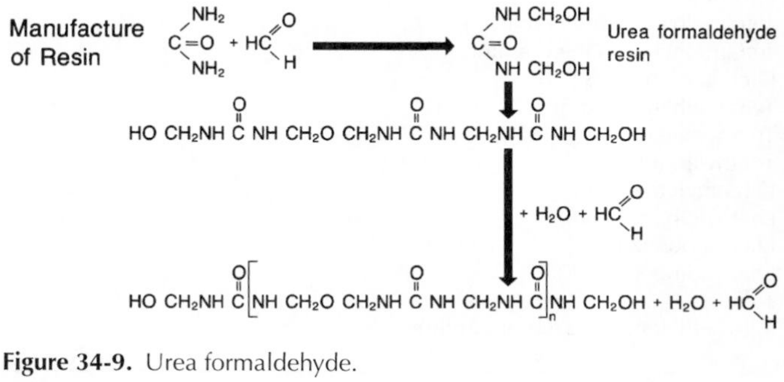

Manufacture of Resin

Urea formaldehyde resin

Figure 34-9. Urea formaldehyde.

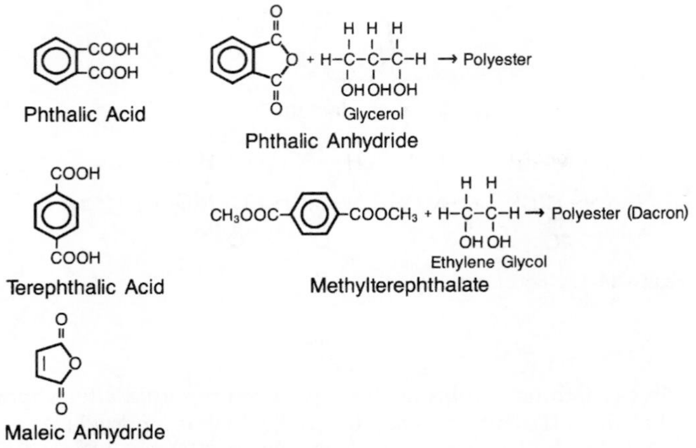

Phthalic Acid

Phthalic Anhydride + Glycerol → Polyester

Terephthalic Acid

Methylterephthalate + Ethylene Glycol → Polyester (Dacron)

Maleic Anhydride

Figure 34-10. Dibasic acids and polyester formation.

POLYESTERS

The basic building components of polyesters are dibasic carboxylic acids (phthalic acids) and anhydrides (Fig. 34-10). Carboxylic acids react with alcohols to form esters. Polyesters are formed when carboxylic acids react with compounds containing more than one –OH group. Polyesters include saturated resins, polyethylene terephthalate, and polybutylene terephthalate, used in containers, coatings, and fabrics. These are formed through a polycondensation reaction of an acid (dimethyl terephthalate) and an alcohol (ethylene glycol or 1,4-butanediol) (Fig. 34-11).

Unsaturated polyesters are formed from dibasic acids (phthalic or maleic anhydride) and glycol. Styrene is used as a cross-linking agent, and a filler such as fiberglass is also added. The unsaturated polyesters are used in boat hulls, paneling, shower stalls, and automotive bodies. These may be molded or applied by spraying or by hand.

Polyesters do not cause dermatologic or respiratory irritation or sensitization, although their basic building components can. The major hazard in the application of unsaturated polyesters as reinforced plastics is exposure to styrene vapor, particularly during spraying. These operations require the use of proper ventilation and respiratory protection.

EPOXY RESINS

Epoxy resins are formed by the reaction of epichlorhydrin (C_3H_5OCl) and a diglycidyl ether ($C_6H_{10}O_3$) of the bisphenol-A type. Epoxies are used primarily for protective coatings and laminates for metals, woods, and other plastics. Other uses include adhesives and bonding agents, flooring, and reinforced plastics for electrical and tooling applications.

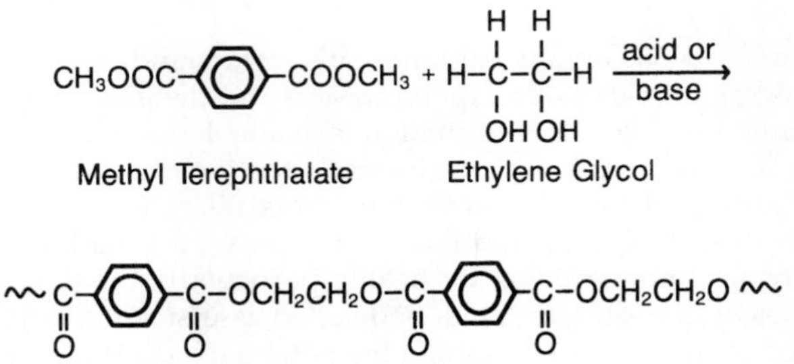

$$CH_3OOC-C_6H_4-COOCH_3 + HOCH_2CH_2OH \xrightarrow{\text{acid or base}}$$

Methyl Terephthalate Ethylene Glycol

$$\sim C(=O)-C_6H_4-C(=O)-OCH_2CH_2O-C(=O)-C_6H_4-C(=O)-OCH_2CH_2O \sim$$

Figure 34-11. Polyester.

Epoxy resin

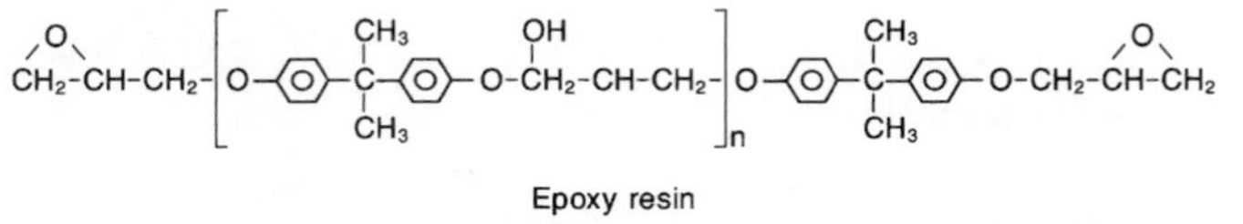

when n = 0, molecular weight = 340
n = 1, molecular weight = 624
n = 2, molecular weight = 908
n = 3, molecular weight = 1,192

Figure 34-12. Molecular formula of epoxy resin.

The main health hazard of exposure to epoxies is allergic dermal or respiratory sensitization, usually to low-molecular-weight oligomers of the cured resin (molecular weight = 340) (29,30). Contact allergies to epoxy resins usually develop after months of exposure. The majority of cases are caused by contact with the 340-molecular-weight oligomer (Fig. 34-12) (29). The epoxy system consists of a resin, a curing agent (hardener), and a reactive compound.

Epoxy resins are used as glues, floor coverings, and paints and coatings. Epoxy resins vary in molecular weight. A low-molecular-weight resin is less than 1,000 and is a liquid. High-molecular-weight resins are greater than 1,000 and are typically solids. Resins are made up of oligomers with differing molecular weights. The primary sensitizing oligomer in bisphenol-A resins has a molecular weight of 340 (22). Oligomers of molecular weight 624 are less sensitizing, and those of molecular weight 908 are not sensitizing.

Hardeners are curing agents. They are usually amines, such as aliphatic polyamines (diethylenetetramine, triethylenetetramine, trimethylhexamethylenediamine), and are potent sensitizing agents (Fig. 34-13) (22). Sometimes, cycloaliphatic polyamines are used as curing agents. Hardeners include aliphatic and cycloaliphatic amines, which are strong irritants, as well as sensitizers. Amine-curing chemicals are dermal and pulmonary sensitizers. The lower-molecular-weight aliphatic amines have greater volatility and a much greater chance to contact skin and the airway. Epoxy reactive diluents are also strong sensitizers (Fig. 34-14). Diglycidyl ether is a liquid used as a diluent for epoxy resins and causes ocular, respiratory, and skin irritation. Exposure of the liquid to skin can produce severe damage.

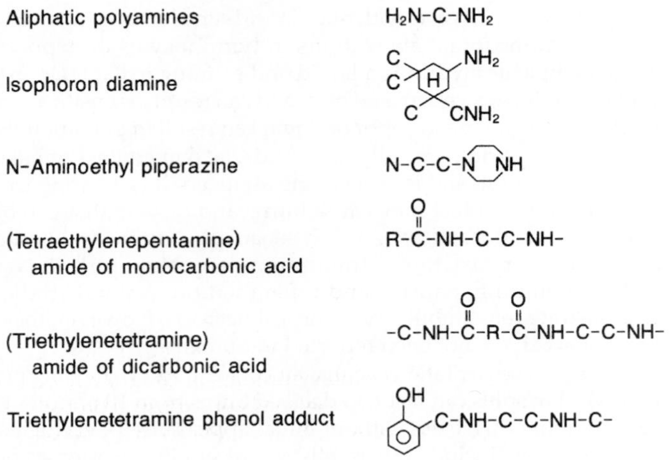

Aliphatic polyamines	$H_2N-C-NH_2$
Isophoron diamine	(cyclohexane ring with C, C, C, NH_2, CNH_2)
N-Aminoethyl piperazine	N-C-C-N NH (piperazine)
(Tetraethylenepentamine) amide of monocarbonic acid	R-C(=O)-NH-C-C-NH-
(Triethylenetetramine) amide of dicarbonic acid	-C-NH-C(=O)-R-C(=O)-NH-C-C-NH-
Triethylenetetramine phenol adduct	(phenol, OH)-C-NH-C-C-NH-C-

Figure 34-13. Epoxy resin hardeners.

Diglycidyl ether of diphenylol propane

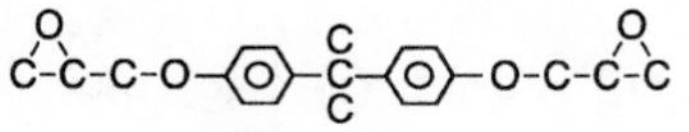

Glycidaldehyde

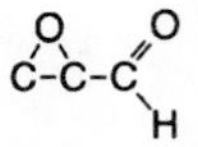

Glycidol

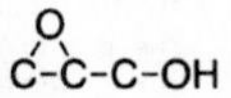

Isooctyl glycidyl ether

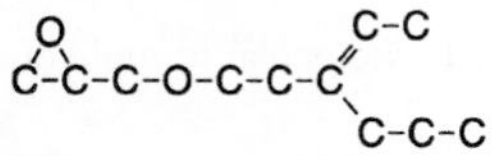

Cresyl glycidyl ether

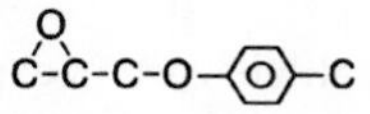

1,2-Epoxydodecane

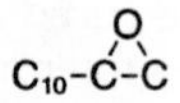

Monoglycidyl ester of a synthetic fatty acid

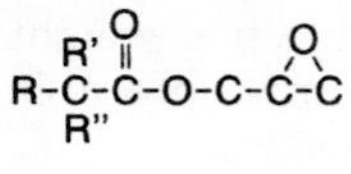

Monoglycidyl ether of isomeric alcohols

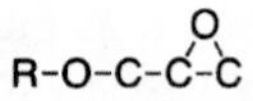

Diglycidyl ether of butanediol

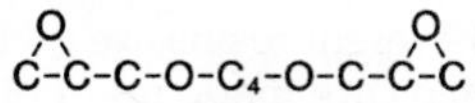

Diglycidyl ether of neopentylglycol

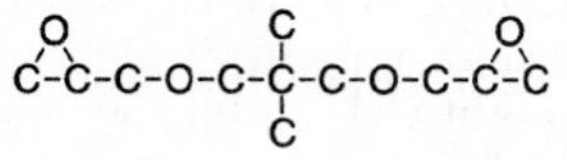

Figure 34-14. Epoxy reactive diluents.

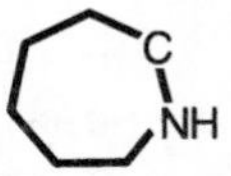

EPICHLORHYDRIN

Epichlorhydrin (C_3H_5ClO) is a highly reactive and flammable curing agent. It is used in the manufacturing of epoxy resins, glycol, plasticizers, dye stuffs, lubricants, adhesives, pharmaceuticals, and oil emulsification products. Epichlorhydrin is a solvent for resins, gums, cellulose, esters, paints, and lacquers. It is also used as a stabilizer in chlorine-containing products like rubber, solvents, and pesticides.

Epichlorhydrin is a colorless liquid with a chloroformlike odor. Its vapor density is 1.7 (air = 1.0). The compound is released into the environment through its use in various processes and industries. Epichlorhydrin is biodegradable, and bioaccumulation is negligible (31).

Epichlorhydrin reacts with nucleic acids and has been shown to induce chromosomal aberrations in lymphocytes of exposed workers. Epichlorhydrin is a liquid and a strong irritant. Dermal contact produces a vesiculated burn and can result in sensitization. Pulmonary exposure to vapor or liquid can result in pneumonitis.

Epichlorhydrin is rapidly absorbed via skin contact, inhalation, or ingestion, and is quickly metabolized. It is a strong irritant, and skin contact may cause burns and blisters that can be delayed. Epichlorhydrin is a skin sensitizer. Vapors and liquid are pulmonary irritants. Inhalation can cause pulmonary edema, vomiting, nausea, and inflammation. Animal studies demonstrate renal tubular and cortical necrosis. However, these renal effects have not been reported in humans (31).

Eye and nasal irritation occur at air concentrations of 76 mg per m^3 (31). Skin spills can result in delayed burns from 10 minutes to several hours (31), even without initial appearance of erythema. Dermal lesions include burns, blisters, ulceration, erosions, and sensitization. Epichlorhydrin penetrates leather and rubber gloves. Asthma and bronchitis have been reported after vapor inhalation (31). Fatty degeneration of the liver is reported (31).

Caprolactam

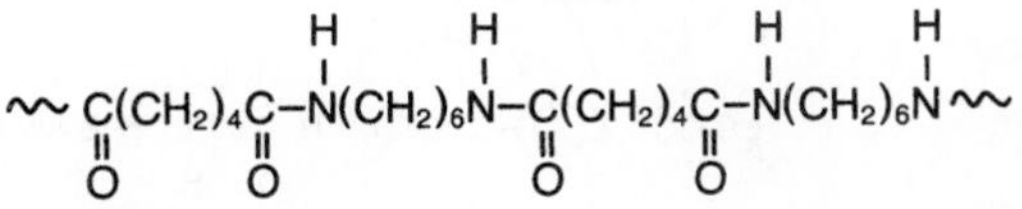

Figure 34-15. Polyamide (nylon).

Epichlorhydrin-air mixtures of 3.8% to 21% epichlorhydrin per volume of air are explosive at temperatures higher than 34° C and can be ignited by hot surface contact or flame at a distance because of the chemical's vapor density. Contact of epichlorhydrin with strong bases, acids, zinc, aluminum, metal chlorides, alcohols, trichloroethylene, isopropylamine, and oxidizing agents can cause fires or explosions. Burning epichlorhydrin produces a mist of hydrogen chloride, phosgene, and CO. The chemical may rapidly polymerize if its container is in a fire and explodes. It should be stored in a cool, dry room. The permissible exposure limit equals 10 mg per m^3, the threshold limit value/time-weighted average equals 10 mg per m^3, and the short-term exposure limit equals 20 mg per m^3.

NYLON

Nylon polymers are polyamides formed by either the polymerization of a lactam (caprolactam) (Fig. 34-15) or the reaction of an amine and a dibasic acid. A major use of nylon is in the production of fibers and filaments for textiles and furnishings. Molded compounds are used in automotives, housewares, and appliances. The raw materials are respiratory and skin irritants. Most reductions take place in closed systems. Nylon compounds are a rare cause of allergic sensitization.

CELLULOSICS

Cellulosics are formed by the chemical modification of naturally occurring polymers from wood and cotton. They are used for films, sheeting, tools, and personal items (brushes, pens). Exposure to organic raw wood and cotton fibers may cause allergic respiratory problems. A major hazard with the use of cellulose nitrate films is the formation of high levels of nitrogen oxides with thermal decomposition.

ADDITIVES

More than 500 organic and inorganic compounds are added to plastic materials to alter their physical and chemical properties. Limited toxicologic information is available on many of these compounds, requiring continuing attention to worker health. Additives include plasticizers, colorants, fillers, foaming agents, asbestos, stabilizers, and flame retardants. Past work practices may also influence worker health, particularly the past use of asbestos and silica as fillers. A detailed assessment of additives used is critical in determining the potential hazard of a specific operation.

REFERENCES

1. Gannon PF, Burge PS, Benfield GF. Occupational asthma due to polyethylene shrink wrapping (paper wrapper's asthma). *Thorax* 1992;47:759.
2. Langast H, Tomenson J, Stringer DA. Polypropylene production and colorectal cancer: a review of the epidemiologic evidence. *Occup Med (Oxf)* 1995;45:69.
3. Apfeldorf R, Infante PF. Review of epidemiologic study results of vinyl chloride-related compounds. *Environ Health Perspect* 1981;41:221–235.
4. International Agency for Research on Cancer. IARC monographs on the evaluation of the carcinogenic risk of chemicals to humans: some monomers, plastics and synthetic elastomers, and acrolein. *IARC Monogr Eval Carcinog Risk Chem Hum* 1979;19:1–513.
5. Doll R. Effects of exposure to vinyl chloride: an assessment of the evidence. *Scand J Work Environ Health* 1988;14:61.
6. Wong O, Whorton MD, Foliart DE, Ragland D. An industry-wide epidemiologic study of vinyl chloride workers, 1942–82. *Am J Ind Med* 1991;20:317–334.
7. Laplanche A, Clavel-Chapelon F, Contassot JC, Lanouziere C. Exposure to vinyl chloride monomer: results of a cohort study after a seven year follow up: the French VCM Group. *Br J Ind Med* 1992;49:134–137.
8. Dodson V, Dinman B, Whitehouse WM, Nasr AN, Magnuson HJ. Occupational acroosteolysis III: a clinical study. *Arch Environ Health* 1971;22:83–91.
9. Liss GM, Greenberg RA, Tamburro CH. Use of bile acids in the identification of vinyl chloride hepatotoxicity. *Am J Med* 1985;78:68.
10. Studnicka MJ, Menzinger G, Drlicek M, Maruna H, Neumann MG. Pneumoconiosis and systemic sclerosis following 10 years of exposure to polyvinyl chloride dust. *Thorax* 1995;50:583–585, 589.
11. Garberg P, Hogberg J, Lundberg I, Lundberg P. NIOH and NIOSH basis for an occupational health standard: Di92-ethylhexylphthalate (DEHP). Cincinnati: National Institute for Occupational Safety and Health, 1990. [DHHS publication no 90-110].
12. Froment O, Marion MJ, Lepot D, Contassot JC, Trepo C. Immunoquantitation of von Willebrand factor (factor VIII–related antigen) in vinyl chloride exposed workers. *Cancer Lett* 1992;61:201–206.
13. Trivers GE, Cawley HL, DeBenedetti VM, et al. Anti-p53 antibodies in sera of workers occupationally exposed to vinyl chloride. *J Natl Cancer Inst* 1995;87:1400–1407.
14. DeVivo I, Marion MJ, Smith SJ, Carney WP, Brandt-Rauf PW. Mutant c-Kiras p21 protein in chemical carcinogenesis in humans exposed to vinyl chloride. *Cancer Causes Control* 1994;5:273–278.
15. Cherry N, Gautrin D. Neurotoxic effects of styrene: further evidence. *Br J Ind Med* 1990;47:29–37.
16. Wong O, Trent LS, Whorton MD. An updated cohort mortality study of workers exposed to styrene in the reinforced plastics and composite industry. *Occup Environ Med* 1994;51(6):386–396.
17. Swaen GM, Bloemen LJN, Twisk J, Scheffers T, Slangen JJM, Sturmans F, Mortality of workers exposed to acrylonitrile. *J Occup Med* 1992;34:801–809.
18. Kiec-Swierczynska MK. Occupational allergic contact dermatitis due to acrylates in Lodz. *Contact Dermatitis* 1996;34(6):419–422.
19. National Institute for Occupational Safety and Health. *Criteria for a recommended standard: occupational exposure to decomposition products of fluorocarbon polymers*. Cincinnati: Department of Health, Education and Welfare (NIOSH), 1977.
20. Shusterman DJ. Polymer fume fever and other fluorocarbon pyrolysis-related syndromes. *Occup Med* 1993;8:519–531.
21. Musk AW, Peters JM, Wegman DH. Isocyanates and respiratory disease: current status. *Am J Ind Med* 1988;13:331–349.
22. Fuortes LJ, Kiken S, Makowsky M. An outbreak of naphthalene di-isocyanate-induced asthma in a plastics factory. *Arch Environ Health* 1995;50:337–340.
23. Rando RJ, Abdel-Kader H, Hughes J, Hammad YY. Toluene diisocyanate exposure in the flexible polyurethane foam industry. *Am Ind Hyg Assoc J* 1987;48:580–585.
24. Simpson C, Garabrant D, Torrey S, Robbins T, Franzblau A. Hypersensitivity pneumonitis-like reaction and occupational asthma associated with 1,3-bis(isocyanatomethyl) cyclohexane prepolymer. *Am J Ind Med* 1996;30:48–55.
25. Banks DE, Butcher BT, Salvaggio JE. Isocyanate-induced respiratory disease. *Ann Allergy* 1986;57:389–396.
26. Mapp CE, Vecchio LD, Boschetto P, Fabbri LM. Combined asthma and alveolitis due to diphenylmethane diisocyanate (MDI) with demonstration of no crossed respiratory reactivity to toluene diisocyanate (TDI). *Ann Allergy* 1985;54:424–429.
27. Olsen GW, Shellenberger R, Bodner KM, et al. An epidemiologic investigation of forced expiratory volume at 1 second and respiratory symptoms among employees of a toluene diisocyanate production plant. *J Occup Med* 1989;31:664–667.
28. Musk AW, Peters JM, Berstein L. Absence of respiratory effects in subjects exposed to low concentrations of TDI and MDI: a reevaluation. *J Occup Med* 1985;27:917–920.
29. Jolanki R, Tarvainen K, Tatar T, et al. Occupational dermatoses from exposure to epoxy resin compounds in a ski factory. *Contact Dermatitis* 1996;34:390–396.
30. Fregert S. Contact dermatitis from epoxy resin systems. In: Maibach H, ed. *Occupational and industrial dermatology*, 2nd ed. Chicago: Year Book Medical Publishers, 1987.
31. *Epichlorhydrin—environmental health criteria 33*. Geneva: World Health Organization, 1984.

SUGGESTED READING

Jarvisalo J, Pfaffli P, Vaino H, eds. *Industrial hazards of plastics and synthetic elastomers*. New York: Alan R. Liss, 1984.

Malten KE. Problems in the production and processing of plastics. In: Maibach H, ed. *Occupational & industrial dermatology*, 2nd ed. Chicago: Year Book Medical Publishers, 1987.

Radian Corporation. *Polymer manufacturing*. Park Ridge, NJ: Radian Corporation, 1986.

Tosti A, Guerra L, Vincenzi C, Pelua AM. Occupational skin hazards from synthetic plastics. *Toxicol Ind Health* 1993;9:493–502.

Vainio H, Pfaffli P, Zitting A. Chemical hazards in the plastics industry. *J Toxicol Environ Health* 1980;6:259–266.

CHAPTER 35
Tire and Rubber Manufacturing Industry

John B. Sullivan, Jr., Mark D. Van Ert, and Richard Lewis

RUBBER INDUSTRY HAZARDS

The production of rubber products involves a mixture of complex chemicals to which workers may be exposed. In addition to the multiple chemicals used in rubber production, there are many by-product chemicals produced by the various processes and reactions.

It was in the early part of the nineteenth century that the rubber industry began in the United States. The vulcanization process discovered by Charles Goodyear in 1839 (using sulfur and heat to cross-link natural rubber molecules), as well as the use of additives to improve processing, led to a demand for rubber products that exceeded supplies. By the end of the nineteenth century, rubber plants were being exported from Brazil to plantations in southeast Asia, Sri Lanka, Indonesia, Liberia, and Zaire. These countries remain the primary producers of natural rubber today.

The growth of the petrochemical industry and advances in polymer technology, coupled with shortages of natural rubber during World War II, led to the creation of the synthetic rubber industry in the 1940s.

Finished rubber products consistj of basic elastomers plus a multitude of chemical additives. The increasing demand for natural and synthetic rubber has resulted in an increase in the production of processing chemicals. Today, the demand for synthetic rubber is outpacing the demand for natural rubber. The fastest growing demand will be for ethylene-propylenediene rubber. Demand for styrene-butadiene synthetic rubber (SBR) and SBR-latex is less (1).

Four types of synthetic rubbers have become widely used since 1950: SBR, butyl rubber, nitrile rubber, and polychloroprene. Other synthetic rubbers are polysulfide, polyurethane, and ethylene-propylenediene. SBR is used mainly in tire production and is the most commonly used rubber in the world (1).

In concert with the steady growth in output of the various rubber products, the output of rubber-processing chemicals is expected to continue to increase. These chemicals impart the desirable characteristics for the final rubber product. Tire manufacturing remains the leading consumer of nearly one-half of all natural and synthetic rubber produced annually. This industry employs more than one-half million workers in nearly 400 plants around the world. A single tire may require the use of several hundred raw materials. Workers' exposures may vary, not only with different jobs within a plant, but also with changes in production techniques and material use over time. Many changes have occurred in the industry over the years with regard to the kinds of chemicals used as well as the processes used to manufacture rubber (2).

Natural rubber is obtained from plants, especially the *Hevea braziliensis* tree, native to the Amazon region of South America. Preliminary processing involves filtering to remove dirt and debris and coagulation with formic and acetic acids. The rubber is then rolled into sheets, cut, and cured with either smoke or sodium bisulfite bleach, then formed into bales for shipping (3).

The production of natural rubber shares many of the occupational health hazards of other agricultural industries. These include use of sharp cutting implements, exposure to pesticides (including sodium arsenite), and risk of tropical diseases in endemic areas. The acids and caustics used in processing are potential respiratory and skin irritants. Increasing use of processing equipment requires careful attention to safety practices to prevent worker injuries.

The basic ingredient of synthetic rubber is polymeric material (elastomer) similar to plastic resin. Rubber in its crude state is lacking in strength and resiliency. Cross-linking using sulfur or sulfur donors during the vulcanization process creates a durable, pliable, thermoset material.

The manufacturing of synthetic rubber involves the use of large volumes of raw materials. Polymerization of rubber ingredients takes place in enclosed vessels. Leaks from these vessels and maintenance operations, such as the cleaning of reaction vessels and maintenance of distribution pipes, were major sources of exposure before implementation of proper venting and respiratory protection measures.

cis-1,4-Polyisoprene is the basic natural rubber. The synthetic SBR is produced through an emulsion polymerization reaction of aqueous styrene and gaseous butadiene. Unreacted monomers are recycled. The latex polymer is coagulated with sulfuric acid and dried before shipping. Other chemicals may be added—such as carbon black, antioxidants, and curing agents—depending on the intended end use of the product (2).

Overexposure to unreacted styrene monomer can result in central nervous system effects of giddiness, loss of coordination, and possible liver damage. Worker exposure to 1,3-butadiene can result in mucous membrane and respiratory irritation at high concentrations; it is also a suspected human carcinogen.

Neoprene (polychloroprene) combines the mechanical properties of natural rubber with increased resistance to aging, oils, and chemicals. Neoprene is used in belts, hoses, footwear, gloves, and low-voltage insulation. Chloroprene (2-chloro-1,3-butadiene) is flammable, and exposure to high concentrations of unreacted monomers as well as partially polymerized intermediates may produce narcosis, respiratory and skin irritation, alopecia, and liver and kidney damage.

Other synthetic rubbers include butyl (isobutylene-isoprene polymers), nitrile (NBR) copolymers of acrylonitrile and butadiene, and polyurethane. Acrylonitrile is a respiratory and mucous membrane irritant, and overexposure can produce cyanide poisoning. Acrylonitrile is a suspected human carcinogen (2).

INDUSTRY PROCESS AND REACTIONS

The rubber industry work environment is quite diverse with respect to physical and chemical exposures. Hundreds of different chemicals are used as rubber additives in the process of manufacturing rubber products (2). These chemicals are grouped into various functional categories:

- Elastomers (natural or synthetic)
- Fillers
- Antidegradents
- Vulcanizing agents
- Solvents
- Accelerators
- Activators
- Retarders
- Reinforcing agents
- Pigments and dyes
- Antitack agents
- Bonding agents
- Miscellaneous chemicals

The major reinforcement and filler materials are carbon black and amorphous silica, although asbestos-containing materials have been used. Vulcanizing agents include sulfur, zinc oxide, stearic acid, and other sulfide and sulfur compounds. Thiurams, thiocarbamates, and various amine and aldehyde compounds are used as accelerators to increase the rate of rubber curing. Other additives include activators (soaps and fatty acids), extenders (mineral oils), plasticizers (phthalates), antioxidants (amines, quinones), and pigments.

The basic production stages in the manufacturing of rubber tires and tubes are presented in Figure 35-1 and summarized in this chapter. Descriptions for each of these processes are as follows (Table 35-1):

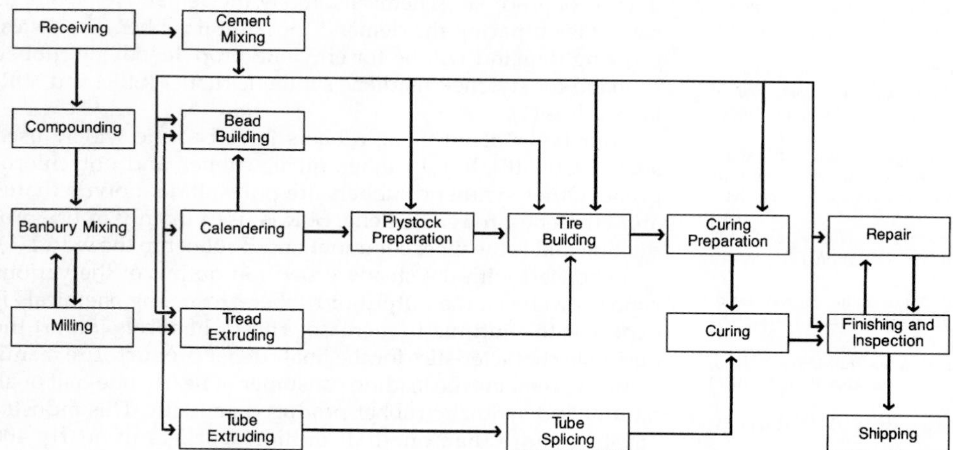

Figure 35-1. Production stages in manufacturing of tires and tubes. (Adapted from ref. 13, with permission.)

TABLE 35-1. Summary description of major work areas (occupational title groups)

1. *Shipping and receiving*: Receiving unloads and stores all incoming ingredients that go into making the final products, e.g., carbon black, pigments, rubber, etc. Shipping stores and loads the final products (e.g., tires) into trucks or boxcars.
2. *Compounding and mixing, cutting and milling*: Cement mixing—raw ingredients (rubber, fillers, oils, pigments) are weighed and mixed together in a Banbury mixer. Environmental exposure to particulates (e.g., carbon black, accelerators, antioxidants, talc) is high. Cements are solvents such as paraffin HC (e.g., hexane), aromatic hydrocarbons (e.g., toluene, xylene), chlorinated HC (e.g., CCl_4, trichloroethylene), and ketones (e.g., methyl ethyl ketone).
3. *Mill-mixing*: Service to batch preparation—mill-mixing is a largely superseded mixing process. Service jobs are for the compounding and mixing operations. Environmental exposures are similar to compounding and mixing.
4. *Milling*: Rubber mix from Banbury is processed further under heat and pressure, until rubber is in a soft, plastic state. This is probably the first work area where there is substantial exposure to reaction products.
5. *Calender, plystock handling*: The rubber stock from the mill is rolled out into a sheet of controlled thickness, usually covering a fabric. The calender stock (plystock) is then cut and spliced for use in building the ply of the tire. There is some exposure to reaction products and solvents.
6. *Tuber (extrusion), tread cementing*: Rubber stock from a mill is forced through a die forming a tread or tube. The tread is cut in appropriate lengths and cemented with solvents on the cut end so as to be tacky.
7. *Tire building, bead building*: Beads are rubber-and-fabric-covered wire that in a finished tire rest on the rim of the wheel. The treads, beads, and plystock are used to build the tire. The major exposures are to solvents.
8. *Green tire inspection, paint and line*: The green (uncured) tire is inspected and repaired and sprayed with solvents or lined with talc so it will not stick in the curing mold. Solvents—and in some cases, talc—are the major environmental exposures.
9. *Tube and flap building, valves*: The tube from the extruder is cut and valves attached. The inside of the tube is coated with talc and then cured, buffed, and sprayed with solvent to make it tacky.
10. *Curing*: The green uncured product (tire, tube) is cured under heat and pressure. The major environmental exposure is to reaction products, and, in tube curing, to talc.
11. *Inspection, finishing, repair*: The cured product is inspected (repaired if necessary) and made ready for shipping (finishing). Environmental exposures are in repairing (solvents, rubber dust).
12. *Maintenance*: This job group includes mechanics, pipefitters, electricians, welders, painters, and carpenters.
13. *Mechanical and special products*: A variety of products and jobs are included in this group, most of them similar to machine shop types of exposures.
14. *Reclaim operations*: Scrap vulcanized rubber products are shredded, ground up, and devulcanized. By the application of heat and chemicals, the rubber compound is restored to its original plastic state. Exposures are to particulates and chemicals.
15. *Synthetic plant*: This is essentially a chemical plant making elastomers that approximate one or more of the properties of natural rubber. SBR is the most important synthetic rubber. Others include neoprene, nitrile, ethylene-propylene-diene, etc. Exposures are to the gases or liquids that are the ingredients for the particular synthetic rubber being made.
16. *Janitoring, trucking, power plant, etc.*: This is a miscellaneous group with a variety of different jobs and exposures.

SBR, styrene-butadiene rubber.
Adapted from ref. 15, with permission.

- Raw material handling, compounding, and mixing
- Milling
- Extruding and calendering
- Component assembly and building
- Curing or vulcanizing
- Inspection, repair, and finishing
- Storage and dispatch

Raw Materials Handling

The initial step in product fabrication involves weighing and mixing (compounding) various additives with either natural or synthetic rubber. The manual weighing and filling of hoppers results in generation of dust. Additives may be in the form of powders, flakes, or pellets and are supplied in bags or drums.

Carbon black and occasionally zinc oxide arrive in bulk form, either in tankers or metal containers. Antioxidant and other oils are usually received in 55-gallon drums or tank cars. Exposure to dusts or vapors may occur during the handling of these raw materials. Compounding and mixing of materials may be a dusty process, especially when clinical agents stored in open drums and bags are weighed and transferred for mixing in the Banbury units (2).

Raw rubber and other additives are usually fed into a mixer or Banbury unit by conveyor or manual process. These components are mixed together under pressure between the rotors and against the walls of the chamber. The chamber is usually water cooled to reduce heat. However, in some operations, the chamber may be steam heated to reduce the viscosity of the mixture. Retarders, antidegradents, processing oils, reinforcing agents, and fillers are often added to the raw rubber stock at this stage (2).

Milling

The mixer drops its batch of mixed rubber directly onto the rollers of a discharge mill, in which further mixing takes place. This mixture is then cooled to between 65° and 80°C and often transferred to other mills for further processing. Local exhaust ventilation is frequently used to collect fumes and vapors that arise from the process. Workers may be exposed to vapors, aerosols from the hot rubber, and dust from incompletely mixed additives or other compounding agents added on mix mills.

Rubber comes off the mill in a continuous sheet, which is fed by a conveyor to a dip that prevents the rubber from sticking together. Mineral dust (talc and soapstone) slurries are commonly used as antisticking agents. The newly dipped or detackified rubber sheet is dried, folded, placed on pallets, and—in the case of the first-stage rubber—stored. After this stage, rubber is ready for fabrication to the components from which a tire is built.

Rubber stock is heated and remilled to obtain softness and plasticity for further processing. Time and temperature of the milling process govern the chemical reactions within the batch, thus determining the properties of the finished material. During the formation of rubber sheets, the uncured rubber is coated with an antitack agent to reduce sticking. Talc (either in a dry or slurry form) was used extensively for this purpose but has now been replaced by the use of amorphous silica and liquid soaps. The rubber stock is cooled in dip tanks, generating steam.

All of these operations result in potential exposure to reaction products from heated but unvulcanized rubber stock. In addition, there is potential exposure to dust, such as talc or soapstone from the antitack agents.

Extruding and Calendering

The tread and sidewall of a tire are produced by an extrusion process. In the manufacture of tread for tires, the milled rubber sheet is extruded through a die corresponding to specific tread dimensions and weight. It is then cut into specified lengths, and the ends are joined manually or automatically with cement at a tire-building station.

Rubber sheet may also be formed into plystock by calendering. Steel cord and fabrics (nylon, rayon, polyesters, and fiberglass) may be pretreated using a phenol-formaldehyde solution to improve adhesion.

The tread and sidewalls of a tire can be manufactured separately or in the same operation. The tread-sidewall extruder laminates the two types of strips to form a tire tread and sidewalls. Strips are bonded by heat and pressure generated by a rotating extruder screw. The tread and sidewall may also be formed separately in similar types of production lines. Extrusion temperatures are in the range of 80°C and may result in volatilization of constituents that are applied earlier in the mixing of the rubber. The extruder operator may also be exposed to volatile organic compounds used at the tread-end cement station or other nearby operations. After extrusion, the tread is sometimes cooled in a water bath and dipped in a solvent bath. Solvents typically used in this phase of tire building include naphtha, heptane, hexane, isopropanol, and toluene. The continuous rubber tread is then cut into specified lengths and the tread ends tackified. Tackification usually involves applying a cement containing dissolved rubber and solvents (naphtha and toluene) on the tread ends. Local exhaust ventilation may be available to control solvent vapor exposure.

Calendering is the operation that produces plies and belts, which form the body of the tire and give it strength and stability. Plies and belts are composed of rubber reinforcements of fabric, steel wire, or glass fiber. Plies, belts, and liners are made of a calender, a multiple roll mill that produces stock of carefully controlled thickness. A rolled fabric, normally rayon or some other synthetic fiber, is spliced either by adhesive or a high-speed sewing machine onto the end of a previously processed roll. This continuous sheet of fabric is then dipped under controlled tension into a tank containing latex. Solutions of formaldehyde, caustic soda, and resorcinol—or other synthetic adhesive combinations—may be added to the latex at this point. After dipping, the fabric travels past either rotating meter bars or vacuum suction lines and then through a drying oven to remove excess solvent. The latex-dipped fabric is then passed through a calendering machine, which impregnates it with rubber. Temperature during the calendering operation is 70° to 80°C. Potential toxins emitted from this process are similar in character to those from milling or extrusion.

Tire Building and Component Assembly

Rubber tires represent combinations of many different rubber components. Tires are assembled on a drum combining ply stock, beads, sidewalls, and other components. The surface of the components may be treated with solvent, primarily naphtha, during the tire-building process. Many rubber products, such as hoses, are already formed into their final shape before curing. Tires are sprayed with a mold-release agent and placed into steel molds to impart the final shape and surface characteristics during the curing process.

Passenger car tires are built as cylinders on a collapsible rotating drum. First, the inner liner is wrapped around the drum followed by a variable number of rubber impregnated fabric plies. Next, the edges of the fabric and inner liner are wrapped around the bead assemblies. Then, pressure is applied manually or automatically from the tread center out to the bead to expel air trapped between the assembled components. Belts made of fabric, steel, or glass fiber are laid onto the cord, and finally the tread and sidewall components are wrapped around the assembled components and bonded. Organic solvents, such as naphtha, heptane, hexane, isopropanol, methanol, and toluene, may be used during the building to tackify the rubberized components. Potential sources of human exposure at such stations occur during solvent application and the handling of green (uncured) tire components.

Curing or Vulcanizing

Before curing, the assembled unvulcanized part is inspected and repaired if necessary. The tire is then placed in a ventilated booth, in which it is sprayed on the inside with lubricants and on the outside with release agents, which prevent the tire from sticking to the mold after curing. Either organic-based lubricants or water-based suspensions of silicone solids may be used for outside sprays. Solvent-based lubricants may contain naphtha, hexane, heptane, isopropanol, and toluene. Evaporation of these solvents can contribute to human exposure.

The tire is then molded and vulcanized in a curing press. In this process, the tire is shaped, the tread design created, and chemical cross-linking of the rubber product triggered, allowing the tire to hold its shape. Curing usually takes 20 to 60 minutes at a temperature of 100° to 200°C. All freshly molded tires release substantial volumes of curing fumes into the work area and continue to do so as they are transported—usually by conveyor—to the finishing and storage areas.

Finishing and Inspection

After vulcanization, tires are inspected for faults and may undergo further processing, such as grinding, trimming, repair, painting, and assembly. Potential occupational health hazards in the refinishing operations involve exposure to rubber dust, particularly from trimming, fumes from grinding, and solvent vapors from cleaning, patching, and painting of blemishes.

Storage

Final rubber products can degas a variety of chemicals and chemical by-products during storage, although concentrations are minimal compared with those generated during the cure operation.

CHEMICAL COMPOUNDS USED IN RUBBER COMPOUNDING

Types of Rubber Compounds

A multitude of chemical agents are used to produce the final rubber product. Elastomers, the basic polymers used in rubber manufacturing, are divided into three functional classes:

- General purpose
- Solvent resistant
- Heat resistant

General-purpose elastomers are the SBR type, butyl, natural rubber, and polybutadiene (Fig. 35-2). Chemical- and solvent-resistant elastomers are nitrile, polyurethanes, and polychloro-

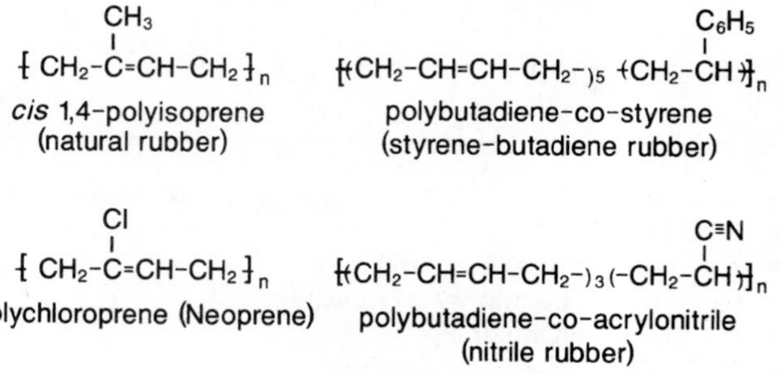

$$\{CH_2-\overset{CH_3}{\overset{|}{C}}=CH-CH_2\}_n$$

cis 1,4-polyisoprene (natural rubber)

$$\{(CH_2-CH=CH-CH_2-)_5\ (CH_2-\overset{C_6H_5}{\overset{|}{CH}})\}_n$$

polybutadiene-co-styrene (styrene-butadiene rubber)

$$\{CH_2-\overset{Cl}{\overset{|}{C}}=CH-CH_2\}_n$$

polychloroprene (Neoprene)

$$\{(CH_2-CH=CH-CH_2-)_3(-CH_2-\overset{C\equiv N}{\overset{|}{CH}})\}_n$$

polybutadiene-co-acrylonitrile (nitrile rubber)

Figure 35-2. Rubber compounds classified by chemical structures. (From ref. 2, with permission.)

TABLE 35-2. Types of synthetic rubbers

Styrene-butadiene rubber (SBR): The major synthetic rubber produced. Makes up 40% of the world's production. Weaker than natural rubber but ages more slowly.
Butyl rubber: Low permeability for air and gases. Used for inner tubes.
Nitrile rubber: Abrasion resistant. Resistant to penetration by chemicals, water, and oils.
Polyisoprene: Used mainly as a blending component with other rubbers. Synthetic polyisoprene rubber contains a high percentage of cisisoprene.
Polychloroprene: Known as neoprene. Flame resistant and wears longer than SBR. Possesses resistance to oil, solvent, and water penetration. Used mainly in the transportation industry and for sealants, cables, coatings, and adhesives.
Ethylene-propylene: Possesses resistance to ozone, sunlight, weather, and aging.
Silicone rubber: Resists degradation in temperature extremes. Used in aerospace industry and medical-surgical field.
Polyurethane: Used for coatings, insulation, packaging, and in automotive industry.
Polysulfide: Resistant to solvents and used in sealants in construction and building.
Chlorosulfonated polyethylene rubber: Used in cable covering.
Polyacrylic rubber: Plastic rubber that resists oils and aging. Used as seals and gaskets.
Fluoroelastomers: High thermal stability. Used in aerospace industry.
Thermoplastic elastomers: Melt at high temperatures and resolidify on cooling without loss of elastic property.

Adapted from ref. 2, with permission.

prene (neoprene). Heat-resistant examples are silicone, polyethylene, and polyacrylates. Today, SBR is the major synthetic rubber produced. It makes up approximately 40% of the world production and is the primary component of tires. Examples of synthetic rubber and their properties are shown in Table 35-2.

Vulcanizing Agents

Vulcanizing agents are necessary to induce cross-linking of rubber elastomers during the process of rubber manufacturing. The most common vulcanizing agent in general-purpose use is sulfur, in which cross-links and cyclic structures are formed (2). Other common sulfur donors used are morpholine, dithiocarbamates, dithiophosphates, and tetraethylthiuram disulfide and tetramethylthiuram disulfide.

Other agents used in the vulcanization process are benzoyl peroxide, dicumyl peroxide, aromatic nitrogen compounds, dioximes, phenols, diisocyanates, and dinitroso compounds (3). Silicone rubber, which is fully saturated, cannot be vulcanized with sulfur. Instead, peroxides are necessary to achieve cross-linking by formation of free radicals on the polymer chain (2).

Accelerators

The reaction between sulfur donors and rubber is very slow, and to speed the process a group of chemicals termed *accelerators* is used (Table 35-3).

Accelerators function at curing temperatures of 140° to 200°C. Accelerators can be classified by their chemical structure, their rate of vulcanization, and their sulfur demand. Less active accelerators require large amounts of sulfur donors, whereas more active ones require a smaller quantity.

Slow accelerators are amines and thiourea derivatives. Moderately fast accelerators are sulfonamides, 1,3-diphenylguanidine, and mercaptobenzothiazole (MBT). Very fast accelerators are thiurams, dithiocarbamates, and thiophosphates (Figs. 35-3 through 35-6).

TABLE 35-3. Common rubber accelerators

- Thiurams
  - Tetramethylthiuram disulfide (TMTD)
  - Tetraethylthiuram disulfide (TETD)
  - Dipentamethylenethiuram disulfide (PTD)
  - Tetramethylthiuram monosulfide (TMTM)
- Mercapto group
  - 2-Mercaptobenzothiazole (MBT)
  - Cyclohexylbenzothiazolesulfenamide (CBS)
  - Dibenzothiazoledisulfide (MBTS)
  - Morpholinomercaptobenzothiazole (MMBT)
- PPD group
  - Phenylcyclohexyl-PPD (CPPD)
  - Isopropylphenyl-PPD
  - Isopropylaminodiphenylamine (IPPD)
  - Diphenyl-PPD (DPPD)
  - Diaminodiphenylmethane (DDM)
- Naphthyl group
  - Phenyl-β-naphthylamine (PBN)
  - Sym-Di-β-naphthyl-PPD (DBNPD)
- Carbamates
  - Zinc diethlydithiocarbamate (ZDC)
  - Zinc dibutyldithiocarbamate (ZBC)
- Miscellaneous
  - 1,3-Diphenylguanidine (DPG)
  - Dithiodiomorpholine (DOD)
  - Monobenzyl ether of hydroquinone
  - Butyraldehyde-aniline
  - Ethylene thiourea

Adapted from ref. 3, with permission.

The variety of chemical structures ranges from primary, secondary, and tertiary amines; aldehydes; thiophosphates; dithiocarbamates; xanthates; sulfonamides; guanidines; thioureas; and benzothiazoles. The need for better accelerators has led to development of a benzothiazole class of chemicals, particularly 2-MBT, which accounts for 90% of the accelerators in use (2,3). Reacting MBT with amines led to the production of sulfonamide accelerators. Cure rate and scorch safety (scorching devalues a product) are also important factors to consider in the choice of accelerators (2).

Studies have demonstrated that nitrosamines—suspected human carcinogens—are released when compounded rubber is heated, as occurs in milling, calendering, and curing operations.

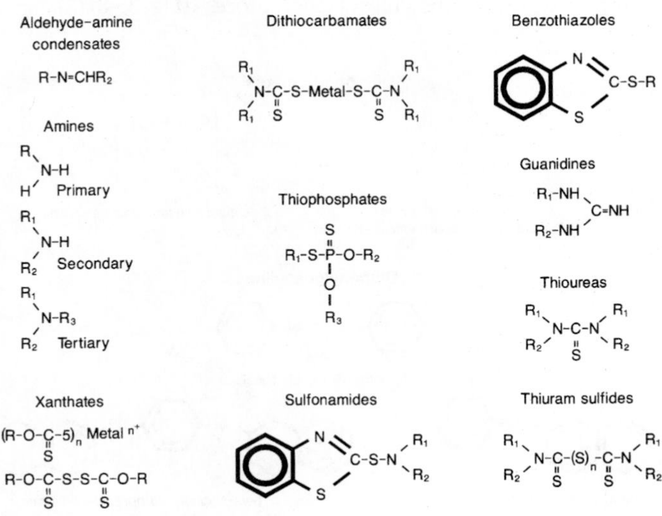

Figure 35-3. Accelerator types classified by chemical structure. (From ref. 2, with permission.)

Tetraethylthiuram disulfide (TETD)
Tetraethylthiuram monosulfide (TMTM)
Dipentamethylenethiuram disulfide (PTD)
N-Phenylcyclohexyl-p-phenylenediamine (CPPD)
Diphenyl-p-phenylenediamine (DPPD)
Isopropylphenyl-p-phenylenediamine (IPPD)
Diethylthiourea

Figure 35-4. Thiurams. (Adapted from ref. 3, with permission.)

Nitrosamines are also present as contaminants in accelerator chemicals (Table 35-4; Fig. 35-7). The highest air concentrations of nitrosamines have been measured in curing areas. Changes in rubber formulations have helped to reduce or even eliminate these by-products. Nitrosamines are the result of the use of amines, which are nitrosated by nitrogen oxides in the manufacturing process.

Activators

Activators are used to make accelerators more effective and speed the process of vulcanization. Activators are usually inorganic compounds and metal oxides such as zinc oxide, lead oxide, magnesium oxide, and sodium carbamate. Organic acids, such as stearic acid or lauric acid, are used to solubilize the metal oxides in the rubber mixture (2). The most common activator is zinc oxide.

Retarders

Retarders are mainly organic acids, anhydrides, and phthalimides; they delay the action of an accelerator. They are sometimes used to slow the vulcanization process. Also, accelerated rubber may cure prematurely, and retarders slow this process. Commonly used retarders are *N*-nitrosodiphenylamine, cyclohexylthiophthalimide, and a sulfonamide (2). Cyclohexylthiophthalimide degrades to phthalimide during the vulcanization process (Fig. 35-8) (2).

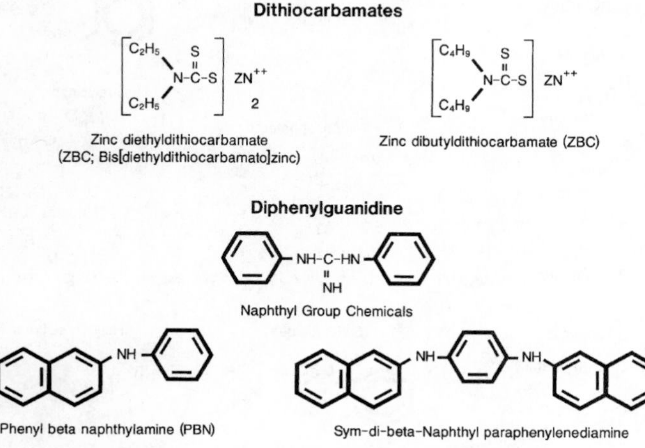

Figure 35-5. Dithiocarbamates and diphenylguanidine. (Adapted from ref. 3, with permission.)

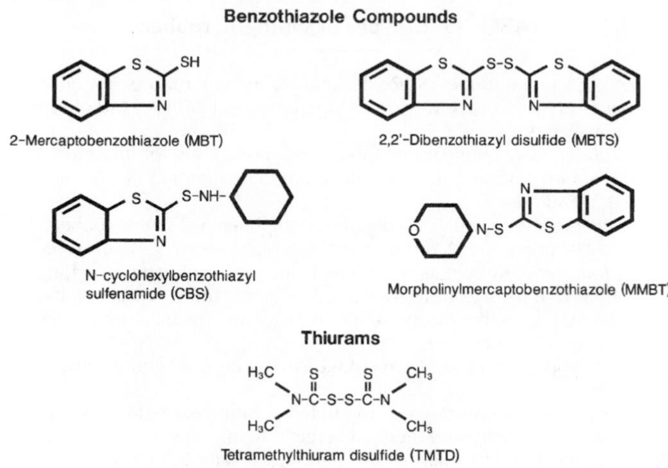

Figure 35-6. Benzothiazole compounds and thiurams. (Adapted from ref. 3, with permission.)

Antidegradants and Antioxidants

Because rubber deteriorates with aging by oxidation, antidegradants are usually incorporated in the final rubber products to prevent or slow oxidation processes. Oxidation can produce cross-linking of butadiene molecules, resulting in stiffness of rubber products. Antioxidants prevent the polymer chain from degrading. Naphthylamine antioxidants were associated with bladder cancer and have been withdrawn from use. Current antioxidants include phenols, thioesters, and amines. Commonly used antioxidants are diphenylamines and dihydroquinolines. *p*-Phenylenediamine is useful in preventing degradation because of ozone. Antioxidants with phenolic structures fall into five classes: (a) phenols with varying side groups, (b) bisphenols with side groups, (c) thiobisphenols, (d) polyphenols, and (e) polyhydroxyphenols (3).

Processing Aids

Processing aids are used to make uncured rubber malleable and more easily mixed, extruded, or calendered. In the early years of rubber manufacturing, pine tars were used for this purpose, but they have been replaced by naphthenic and aromatic mineral oils (2). Aromatic processing oils are widespread in the rubber industry. Many rubber formulations contain as much as 20% or more of aromatic mineral oil, with large amounts of polycyclic aromatic hydrocarbons (PAH) present in these oils. Mercaptan derivatives, thiophenols, or MBT may also be used to help soften rubber.

TABLE 35-4. Nitrosamine contamination in commercial rubber chemicals

Accelerator	Nitrosamine present
N-pentamethylene dithiocarbamate, piperidine salt	*N*-Nitrosopiperidine
Tetramethylthiuram disulfide	*N*-Nitrosodimethylamine
Tetraethylthiuram disulfide	*N*-Nitrosodiethylamine
Zinc pentamethylene dithiocarbamate	*N*-Nitrosopiperidine
Zinc dibutyldithiocarbamate	*N*-Nitrosodibutylamine
Zinc diethyldithiocarbamate	*N*-Nitrosodiethylamine
Morpholine derivatives	*N*-Nitrosomorpholine

Adapted from ref. 18, with permission.

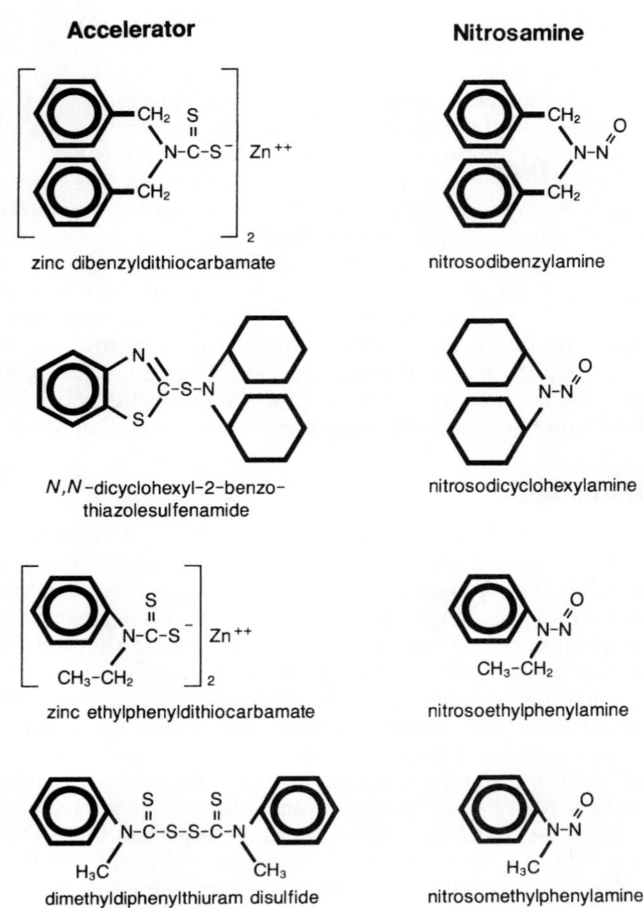

Figure 35-7. Accelerators and corresponding nonvolatile nitrosamines. (Adapted from ref. 2, with permission.)

Reinforcing Agents

Reinforcing agents are very important ingredients in rubber technology and add tensile strength and abrasion resistance to vulcanized rubber (2). The most important reinforcing agents are carbon black and amorphous silicas. Channel black became the carbon black most popular in rubber after 1942. Soon after this, the channel blacks were replaced by furnace blacks. Furnace blacks are manufactured from oil and contain PAHs.

Miscellaneous Agents

A variety of other agents used in the manufacture of rubber products are silicones, fluorinated hydrocarbons, polyethylene glycols, bonding agents, antitack agents, and a variety of organic solvents, including aliphatic hydrocarbons, acetones, 1,1,1-trichloroethane, methyl ethyl ketone, methylene chloride, trichloroethylene, toluene, xylene, tetrahydrofuran, and dimethylformamide. Benzene, employed in the very early history of rubber manufacture, was replaced in the early 1940s with naphtha-type solvents. Flame retardants are added when heat resistance is a required property.

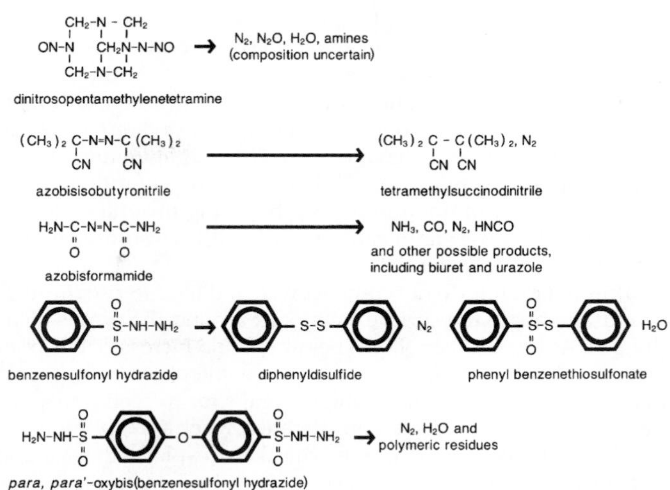

Figure 35-9. Blowing agents and their routes of decomposition. (Adapted from ref. 2, with permission.)

These include clay fillers, ammonium phosphates, magnesium hydroxide, aluminum hydroxide, antimony oxide, chlorinated paraffins, and brominated aromatics, which increase the heat resistance of rubber (3).

Blowing agents are used to produce foam rubber by decomposing at curing temperature to produce gas (Fig. 35-9) (2). Other additive groups are pigments, bonding agents(isocyanates, *p*-dinitrosobenzene, resorcinol-hexamethylenetetramine), antitack agents (mica and talc), and mold release agents (silicones, fluorinated hydrocarbons, polyethylene glycols) (2).

GENERAL HEALTH HAZARDS OF THE RUBBER INDUSTRY

The environmental impacts associated with the disposal of tires is quite substantial and frequently overlooked because of the obvious importance of worker exposure issues. Nevertheless, disposal and potential recycle issues are a major concern to this industry. The most important human health and environmental problem surrounding the treatment, storage, and disposal of tires is associated with their large-scale combustion hazard. The potential and actual impacts of tire fires have been well documented in the United States. The U.S. Environmental Protection Agency (EPA) has published monitoring data from 22 actual tire fire emergencies (4). Previously, the EPA had published detailed characterization data from emission of burning scrap tires in a controlled test experiment (5,6,7). Similar data have been published in standard well-known environmental journals (8,9).

In the United States, tire fires are a relatively common occurrence. More than 240 million vehicle tires are discarded annually in the United States. Less than 25% of this total are reprocessed. Therefore, more than 170 million scrap tires are discarded in landfills, aboveground stock piles, or illegal dumps. Federal legislation has been introduced to address this problem. Proposed legislation has been directed toward reducing the number of

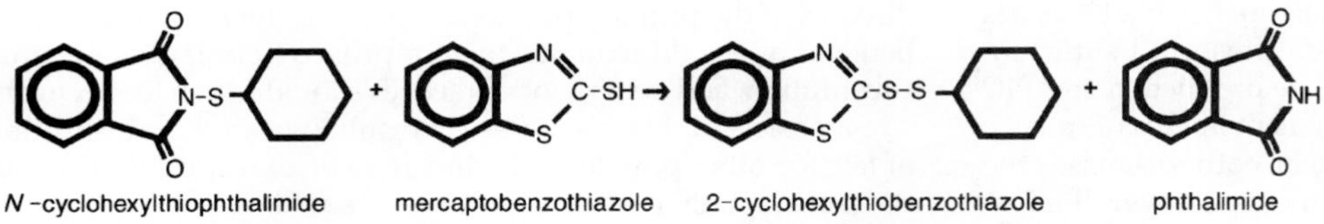

N-cyclohexylthiophthalimide + mercaptobenzothiazole → 2-cyclohexylthiobenzothiazole + phthalimide

Figure 35-8. Decomposition of the retarder *N*-cyclohexylthiophthalimide during vulcanization. (Adapted from ref. 2, with permission.)

tires permitted in a given location (less than 2,500) and their state of intactness. The latter refers to the need to shred intact tires to below specific size levels.

Tire fires are most commonly associated with arson, although lightning strikes are also a recognized ignition source, as are spontaneous outbreaks that are caused by a combination of heat and vibration. Tire piles are well-known sources of rodent infestations and are common mosquito breeding grounds. Hence, large tire piles pose significant public health risks unreliable to their combination potential.

Tires in landfills do not compact well and tend to rise through a landfill mass to the surface as the dirt around the tires is compressed. As the number of tires below ground increases, this phenomenon tends to be accentuated. The geometry of aboveground piles is such that there are numerous gaps for oxygen transport. This mechanism is a crucial consideration when a tire pile ignites.

The mechanism of tire fires is critical and explains the extreme difficulty in extinguishing these fires. Once ignited, tires produce approximately 18,000 BTUs per second of heat energy, compared with approximately 6,000 BTUs per second for a traditional class A fuel fire. The tires produce tremendous quantities of oil, which also contributes to the fire's persistence. The high heat output severely complicates fire fighting attempts because of the difficulty of working near this extreme thermal source.

Although water may be trapped around and inside disposed tires, this water does not mitigate the inherent fire risk. Water alone has almost always been insufficient to extinguish class A tire fires. Water has strong surface tension and spontaneously rolls off most fuels and rubber surfaces. Therefore, the water moves away too rapidly from the heat to absorb the available heat capacity. Furthermore, extensive water use is associated with substantial environmental impacts because of surface water runoff and subsequent groundwater contamination. Although water alone is insufficient to extinguish the tire fire, it temporarily lowers fire temperatures and increases emissions of particulate and other products of incomplete combustion (PIC).

Water's utility as a tire fire extinguishing material has been enhanced by the use of foams that act by decreasing surface tension. This surface tension reduction allows the water to sheet out, covering the tire surface and penetrating deeper into the fire. This mechanism is different than the use of blanketing foams, which act by a pure oxygen deprivation mechanism. Unfortunately, these types of applied foam blankets are easy to disturb, and their ability to deal with large fires appears to be poor.

Traditionally, the use of sand and large earth-moving equipment has been the mainstay of firefighters with large tire fires. The sand acts as an oxygen deprivation agent and also has the benefit of soaking up some of the produced oil. The earth-moving equipment is used to apply the sand and reconfigure the tire pile into a more favorable geometry.

Toxicologically, tire fires produce tremendous quantities of (a) particulates; (b) heavy metals, particularly zinc and lead; (c) emission of organics, including benzene, toluene, and styrene; (d) volatile PIC; (e) PAHs; and (f) dioxins and furans. Levels of benzene greater than 1 ppm in air have been measured within 300 miles of tire fires. One large tire fire in Hagerstown, Maryland, produced 200,000 gallons (800,000 L) of oil. This oil is itself combustible but frequently is not burned. The water prevents the oil from igniting but does not extinguish the overall fire. In this particular situation, the oil becomes a major source of surface- and groundwater pollution. Hence, if adequate firefighting materials are not available, it is better to let the fire burn at high temperatures until sufficient resources can be used. Otherwise, particulate production and PIC are enhanced without meaningful improvement in fire control.

The ineffective use of water or foams, or both, decreases the overall fire burn rate but paradoxically increases overall emission. As the temperature of the fire is temporarily lowered, the rubber binds to the cord material. This new material is more difficult to combust at the new, but temporary, lower temperature. The rubber material can be pyrolyzed, which produces volatiles and other PICs, but it does not fully combust. Therefore, overall toxicity and pollution are enhanced rather than mitigated.

As in many other manufacturing industries, noise remains a major concern in the rubber industry. The extensive use of mixing and milling equipment, extruders, calenders, conveyers, and hydraulic tools in the tire industry results in noise levels exceeding 85 dB throughout most operations. Other physical hazards include risk of thermal and chemical burns and heat stress. Besides trauma, dermal and pulmonary exposures from chemicals are common hazard sources. Health hazards are also peculiar to certain sites and processes in the rubber industry because of the variety of chemicals, processes, and reactions that occur.

Dermatitis

Many rubber additives are capable of producing dermatitis (3). Because natural rubber is not considered a contact allergen, people who develop dermatitis after contact with natural rubber products are reacting to persistent additives (3). Rubber additives can produce dermatitis even from cured products by migrating to the surface of the product over time.

A number of accelerators and other compounds used in the rubber industry—including thiurams; amines; guanidines; disulfides; and certain thiazoles, such as MBT—are skin sensitizers causing contact and allergic contact dermatitis in rubber workers. Many of the common rubber sensitizers are included in patch test batteries used by dermatologists and allergists. Cross-reactivity to similar substances may occur, and sensitized individuals generally need to be removed from further exposure to avoid worsening of their condition.

Irritant dermatitis may be precipitated or aggravated by contact with solvents, caustics, and acids. Treatment with topical steroids and emollients is usually effective. Minimizing skin contact with these substances is the best means of prevention. Phenols and hydroquinones can cause focal hypopigmentation (leukoderma).

Respiratory Disease

Several studies have demonstrated an excess of respiratory symptoms and pulmonary function abnormalities in rubber workers. Studies have documented that asthma, chronic lung changes, respiratory problems, and bronchitis have been prevalent in the rubber industry, particularly in dusty areas such as compounding and mixing (10). Findings consistent with mucous hypersecretion and mild airway obstruction have been reported in workers exposed to carbon black, additives, talc, and curing fumes (10). Symptoms reported by these workers have included cough and sputum production, frequent upper respiratory infections, and episodes of bronchitis. Spirometry has shown decrements in flow rates with preservation of lung volumes. In general, the effects of smoking and workplace exposures appear to be additive.

The long-term impact of exposures in the rubber industry on respiratory status is uncertain. Radiographic evidence of pulmonary fibrosis has been reported only rarely in rubber workers and has been related to specific materials and work practices. Mortality studies have not shown excess mortality from these respiratory diseases. If the primary pulmonary insult is the inhalation of particulates and mild irritants, then improved ventilation, material substitution, and better work practices should lessen these effects.

Silicosis and talcosis have also resulted from the substitution of talc for other powder. Talc dust may be of respirable size and contain crystalline silica and fibrous tremolite.

Workers exposed to curing fumes may have a higher prevalence of chronic bronchitis. Respiratory morbidity is related to the intensity and length of exposure to these fumes (10,11). Other studies have shown that employment in the curing departments is associated with shortness of breath, chest tightness, wheezing, and changes in respiratory function tests (10–12).

Chronic lung diseases, such as pneumoconiosis, pulmonary fibrosis, bronchitis, and emphysema, can occur in workers overexposed chemically to carbon black as well as to dusts and particulates (13).

Because of the multitude of chemicals that are either used or formed in the manufacture of rubber products, and the observation that workers are frequently exposed to mixtures of chemical agents, it is often difficult to pinpoint a specific chemical in the etiology of disease. General mortality patterns among rubber industry workers have been investigated in relation to the overall industry as well as to the specific jobs or tasks (14,15).

MEDICAL SURVEILLANCE AND PREVENTION

Health surveillance programs for rubber workers should include periodic audiometry and spirometry. If possible, the information should be standardized to allow assessment of the effectiveness of controls in high-risk areas. Physical examinations should focus on the respiratory system as well as the skin. Despite the many uncertainties regarding the true cancer risks in the rubber industry, screening for gastrointestinal cancer should be considered. This is relatively common in the general population, and early detection can markedly improve outcome, particularly for cancer of the colon.

Reduction in the release of air contaminants into the work environment through the use of proper ventilation and substitution of less toxic materials presents a continuing challenge for the rubber industry. Given the potential risks of respiratory disease and cancer in this industry and that smoking tends to potentiate the effects of some chemicals, workplace smoking restriction policies and smoking cessation programs may be extremely beneficial for rubber workers.

TABLE 35-5. Exposure situation for *N*-nitrosamines in the rubber industry

Job description	Chemical	Concentration in the air (μg/m³)
Raw material handling, weighing, mixing	Nitrosodimethylamine	0.2–0.9
	Nitrosomorpholine	0.1–2.0
Milling, extruding, calendering	Nitrosodimethylamine	0.1–2.0
	Nitrosomorpholine	0.1–9.0
Assembly and building	Nitrosodimethylamine	0.1–1.0
	Nitrosomorpholine	0.5–3.0
Curing or vulcanizing	Nitrosodimethylamine	0.1–2.0
	Nitrosodimethylamine	15–130
	Nitrosodimethylamine	1.0–4.5
	Nitrosomorpholine	0.1–17.0
	Nitrosodimethylamine	1–40
	Nitrosodiethylamine	0.1–5.0
	Nitrosomorpholine	0.1–3.0
	Nitrosodimethylamine	40–90
	Nitrosomorpholine	120–380
	Nitrosodimethylamine	500–1,060
	Nitrosomorpholine	200–4,700
	Nitrosodimethylamine	1
	Nitrosodiethylamine	5
	Nitrosopiperidine	0.3
	Nitrosomorpholine	0.1
	Nitrosodimethylamine	1.0–3.5
	Nitrosomorpholine	3–9
	Nitrosodimethylamine	0.2–3.5
	Nitrosodimethylamine	1
	Nitrosodiethylamine	3
Inspection and finishing	Nitrosodimethylamine	0.1–1.5
	Nitrosodiethylamine	0.1–20.0
	Nitrosodimethylamine	1–10
Storage and dispatch	Nitrosodimethylamine	0.2–10.0
	Nitrosodimethylamine	1–19
	Nitrosomorpholine	0.3–17.0
	Nitrosodimethylamine	0.2–1.0

Adapted from Spiegelhalder B. Carcinogens in the workroom air in the rubber industry. *Scand J Work Environ Health* 1983;9(2):15–25.

HEALTH HAZARDS BY AREAS

Raw Material Handling, Weighing, and Mixing Areas

Raw material handling, weighing, and mixing exposes the worker to particulate matter (13). In some rubber manufacturing plants, the majority of particulate exposure consists of carbon black, whereas in others, talc and compounding agents may be significant. Cross-contamination of other areas may also occur as a result of ventilation patterns, although the magnitude of such exposures is relatively much less (13).

Mill operators can also be exposed to incompletely mixed compounds from the Banbury mixers and from compounding materials added during mix milling. Talc exposures were common owing to the use of this compound as a detackifier for stored rubber sheets (2,13).

In cement mixing, workers may be exposed to solvents used to prepare cements for use in extrusion, calendering, tire building, repair, and other operations. These solvent mixtures, which often include the addition of dissolved rubber solids, are prepared in the cement house.

Component Assembly and Tire Building

Various organic solvents, including petroleum naphthas, often are used in specific tire-manufacturing operations (2,14). These include tuber or tread-end cementing, bead building, tire building, and spray booth (doper) operations for green (uncured) tires.

Although petroleum naphtha is a common component of many of the solvents applied to green tire components, other solvents including toluene (tread-end cementing) and *N*-hexane (bead building) are also used (14). Because petroleum naphthas may contain small amounts of aromatics such as toluene, benzene, and xylene, proper evaluation of worker exposure should include monitoring for these chemicals as well.

Repair of cured tires sometimes requires the use of solvents to preclean flawed areas of the tire before application of solvent-rich rubber repair material. Mixtures of toluene and naphtha and other petroleum solvents may be used in such preparations.

Curing or Vulcanization

Before curing, rubber products, including green tires, are frequently sprayed with a solvent-based lubricant in spray booth (doping) operations. This process generates solvent vapors. The subsequent cure cycle generates condensed volatiles, vapors, gases, and reaction products (2,15,16). The curing fume itself consists of a complex array of organic compounds, including nitrosamines, which arise from the actual cure of the tires (2,12,15,17). Nitrosamines—which have been found in curing as well as milling, extrusion, and calendering—include *N*-nitrosodibutylamine, *N*-nitrosodimethylamine (NDMA), *N*-nitrosodiphenylamine, *N*-

TABLE 35-6. Summary of vapor in air concentrations of solvent components from selected work areas

Work area component	Chemical	Range (ppm)
Cement mixing	Pentane	0.91–61.20
	Hexane	0.83–98.50
	Heptane	0.39–90.70
	Octane	0.16–7.64
	Benzene	0.18–16.50
	Toluene	0.37–19.30
	Xylene	0.02–1.50
	Isopropanol	0.01–28.50
Tire building	Pentane	0.29–5.45
	Hexane	0.3–135
	Heptane	0.06–12.20
	Octane	0.19–1.79
	Benzene	0.09–1.52
	Toluene	0.13–3.29
	Xylene	0.01–1.38
	Isopropanol	0.07–6.83
Final inspection	Pentane	0.04–0.82
	Hexane	0.59–6.40
	Heptane	0.09–0.81
	Octane	0.02–0.27
	Benzene	0.01–0.19
	Toluene	0.03–0.64
	Xylene	0.02–0.54
	Isopropanol	0.08–0.44
Warehouse	Pentane	0.03–0.56
	Hexane	0.02–0.45
	Heptane	0.07–0.19
	Octane	0.02–0.21
	Benzene	0.01–0.48
	Toluene	0.01–0.37
	Xylene	0.03–0.51

Adapted from Van Ert M, et al. Worker exposures to chemical agents in the manufacture of rubber tires: solvent vapor studies. *Am Ind Hyg Assoc J* 1980;41:212–219.

nitrosomorpholine (NMOR), *N*-nitrosopiperidine T, and *N*-nitrosopyrrolidine (Table 35-5) (17–19).

Final Inspection and Repair and Finishing Area

Inspection may involve the handling of hot cured rubber products. As a result, workers other than those in curing may be exposed to condensed volatiles, vapors, and gases, although in much lower levels. In final inspection, repair activities may require the use of solvent-based rubber products leading to employee exposure to these vapors (Table 35-6) (14).

Storage and Dispatch Area

Stored rubber products release or degas low concentrations of solvent vapors that were used in the manufacturing process, as well as other less volatile products (see Table 35-6) (14).

CARCINOGENIC AND MUTAGENIC PROPERTIES OF CHEMICALS

Commonly used accelerators and curing agents (thiuram compounds including tetramethylthiuram disulfide, tetraethylthiuram disulfide, and tetramethylthiuram monosulfide) have been demonstrated to be carcinogenic in animal studies (2).

Solvents used in the rubber industry include petroleum naphthas, toluene, hexane, isopropyl alcohol, trichloroethylene, 1,1,1-trichloroethane, and methylene chloride. Occupational studies suggest some evidence of increased carcinogenesis secondary to solvent exposure (20).

Small amounts of monomers such as acrylonitrile, butadiene, chloroprene, ethylene, propylene, styrene, vinyl acetate, vinyl chloride, and vinylidene chloride remain in solid rubber polymer and could be released into the work environment, but probably at concentrations lower than existing standards. Most of these monomers have not been known to bind directly with cellular macromolecules, but their metabolites might do so (2,16). Sufficient evidence exists to implicate acrylonitrile as a suspected human carcinogen based on animal studies (2,16). Vinyl chloride is a confirmed human carcinogen (2). There is limited animal evidence of the carcinogenicity of styrene (2,16).

Epichlorohydrin is also used in the manufacture of elastomers. It can react directly with macromolecules and serum proteins. Epichlorohydrin is a mutagenic chemical and is also carcinogenic in mice and rats (2,16). No adequate epidemiologic observations are in the literature as to its carcinogenicity in humans.

Talc, widely used as an antitacking agent, is mainly associated with respiratory disease. However, some talcs may contain asbestos fibers and fibrous tremolite.

Carbon blacks contain variable amounts of compounds, some of which have not been identified. The most probable carcinogenic hazard of carbon black is associated with benzene-extractable chemicals, consisting mainly of aromatic hydrocarbons and sulfur compounds (21–23). Among these chemicals are benz(a)anthracene, benzo(a)pyrene, and indenopyrene, which are known carcinogens. Chrysene has been described as a tumor-initiating agent, and nitro derivatives of polycyclic hydrocarbons have also been found in extracts of commercial carbon black (21–23). Data indicate that the known carcinogens present in carbon blacks are strongly absorbed but can be eluted by biological fluids (21–23). A 1962 study reported that the polycyclic hydrocarbons, including benzopyrene, present in the furnace and channel blacks were not eluted by human blood, plasma, or gastric juice (22).

Cancer of the bladder has long been recognized as a problem within the rubber industry and has been associated with specific aromatic hydrocarbons. The cause was probably an organic antioxidant added to the rubber mixture—β-naphthylamine—although subsequent concern has focused on α-naphthylamine, benzidine, and 4-aminobiphenyl (xenylamine). Bladder cancer has been associated with three occupational title groups in the rubber industry—receiving and shipping, compounding and mixing, and milling—although the number of bladder cases is small. Reactive metabolic intermediates from aromatic amines and their interaction with cellular macromolecules have been extensively reviewed (2,16,24,25). The carcinogenic or genotoxic activity of aromatic amines and amides is dependent on metabolic activation or *N*-hydroxylation to hydroxylamines. Naphthylamine-acetaldehyde was introduced as an antioxidant in the rubber industry in 1928. It was associated with an increase in incidence of bladder cancer. 4-Aminobiphenyl, benzidene, and β- or 2-naphthylamine are known to be carcinogenic for humans. Their use was discontinued in the early years of the industry. Phenyl β-naphthylamine was used as an antioxidant. Research indicated that phenyl β-naphthylamine is metabolized by the body to β-naphthylamine. There is sufficient evidence for the carcinogenicity of simpler amines—2,4-diaminotoluene and 2-chloroaniline—in experimental animals.

Phthalate Esters

Phthalate esters are plasticizers used in numerous plastic products, including rubber tires. Consequently, they are widely distributed. The two most common plasticizers are diethylhexylphthalate and di-*n*-butylphthalate. Phthalate esters are not known to be acutely toxic. They contaminate soil and water in wide-ranging areas of the United States. Diethylhexylphthalate and di-*n*-butylphthalate are considered weak animal carcinogens.

Curing Fumes and Other Curing Emissions

During the vulcanization process, fumes and vapors are emitted into the air because of volatilization of rubber ingredients. No experimental data are available concerning the long-term toxicity of curing fumes. Curing fumes from the tire vulcanization process contain a number of chemicals and chemical by-products (2,11,12,15,16). These products are dependent on the temperature, the type or composition of the rubber, and the presence or absence of oxygen. Increased incidence of lung cancer in workers who are in the curing area has been demonstrated in various epidemiologic studies (15,26–27). Many airborne nitrosamines are formed during rubber processing and are found in the work atmosphere (2,17–19,28). No direct evidence yet exists that nitrosamines cause cancer in humans.

Polycyclic Aromatic Hydrocarbons

PAHs are fused benzene ring compounds present in crude oil and generated by burning organic materials. PAHs are found in aromatic oils, which are extensively used in the rubber industry as plasticizers and softeners. A tire may contain as much as 20% aromatic and paraffinic oils (2). These aromatic oils may contain large amounts of PAHs, some of which contain concentrations of carcinogens. Benzo(a)pyrene is a well-known PAH carcinogen (2,21–23).

PAHs in rubber factory atmospheres include

- Fluoranthene
- Pyrene
- Benzo(a)fluorene
- Benz(a)anthracene
- Chrysene
- Benzo(b)fluoranthene
- Benzo(a)pyrene
- Dibenz(a,j)anthracene
- Dibenz(a,h)anthracene
- Indenopyrene
- Benzo(g,h,i)perylene
- Anthanthrene
- Perylene

PAHs are potent skin carcinogens in animal models. Normally, in the rubber industry, humans do not frequently come into direct contact with these aromatic oils. However, uncured rubber, with which workers have much contact, contains large amounts of these oils. Thus, PAH transfer to the skin may be facilitated. Carbon black also contains PAHs. Fortunately, only small amounts of PAHs are released into biological fluids by carbon black because of its high absorption feature. Solvent extract of carbon black is carcinogenic, but carbon black itself is not.

PAHs are undoubtedly released during the heating of rubber, but studies have not demonstrated this to be a significant problem in the industry in relation to existing airborne concentrations.

PAHs are metabolized by the P-450 mixed oxidase enzyme system in the liver to carcinogenic compounds. DNA binding studies have shown that several benzo(a)pyrene metabolites bind covalently to DNA.

Mineral oils, such as coal tar oils, petroleum, and other tar products, are widely used in the rubber industry as extenders. The use of mineral oils has increased considerably over the years because they are cheap and impart desirable properties to the finished rubber. These oils contain relatively large quantities of

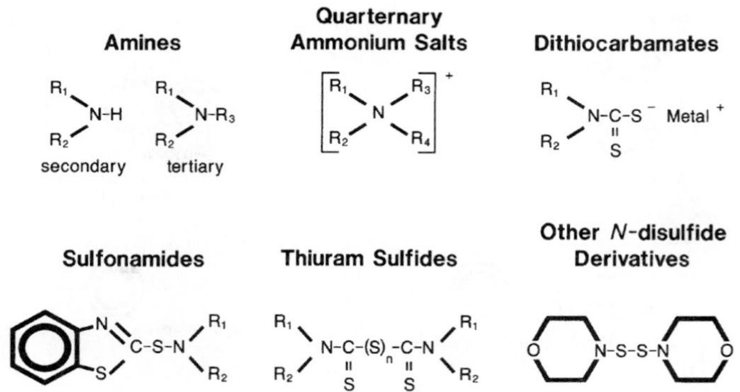

Figure 35-10. Groups of chemicals that can be converted to *N*-nitrosamines. (Adapted from ref. 18, with permission.)

PAHs. PAHs also may be formed when the tars and mineral oils are heated. These mineral oils and tar products vary in composition. They all, however, may induce carcinogenic effects in mammals, including humans. This carcinogenic effect may be due to the presence of the PAHs.

Nitroso Compounds and Nitrosamines

Very little information is available on the health effects of chemical by-products generated during rubber processing. During vulcanization, air is excluded, and the mold contains a reducing atmosphere. Products that can be formed during vulcanization and released from the surface of the rubber include amines and organic sulfides derived from accelerators (Fig. 35-10). There are many reports of these chemicals breaking down at curing temperatures. Because the maximum temperature of the vulcanization or curing of rubber is approximately 240°C, pyrolysis does not normally occur (2). On removal from the mold, the rubber can undergo oxidating reactions in which peroxy-substituted amines and acids can be formed, such as NMOR, NDMA, and *N*-nitrosopyrrolidine (see Table 35-5) (2,24,28). These compounds, demonstrated to be carcinogenic in a number of animal models, have been identified in the extrusion, milling, calendering, curing, and cooling (postcuring) areas of tire factories (15,17–19). The discovery of such compounds in the air of specific areas of tire plants has led to control measures such as improved ventilation and compound substitutions to reduce or eliminate these agents from the workplace environment.

N-Nitroso compounds are produced by acid-catalyzed reactions of nitrites with certain nitrogen-containing amine compounds (24). Nitroso compounds are divided into nitrosamines and nitrosamides. Most of these have been demonstrated to be potent carcinogens. The antidegradant process and curing process involves amines, nitrosamines, and quinolines, which are suspected carcinogens. Possibly, these compounds are precarcinogens that require metabolic activation by the body to become carcinogens (24).

NMOR, a known animal carcinogen, has been quantitated in rubber industry factory air sampling (17). Also, small amounts of another carcinogen, NDMA, have been identified. NDMA was found as an indoor air pollutant at concentrations ranging from 0.07 to 0.14 µg per m^3. NMOR was also found in the rubber factory as an impurity in morpholine and in the cross-linking accelerator bismorpholinecarbamylsulfenamide. NMOR was found at all sites sampled in the rubber industries surveyed, including milling, extrusion, calendering, and curing. The lowest level was in the finishing area and the highest levels in the extruding areas (17).

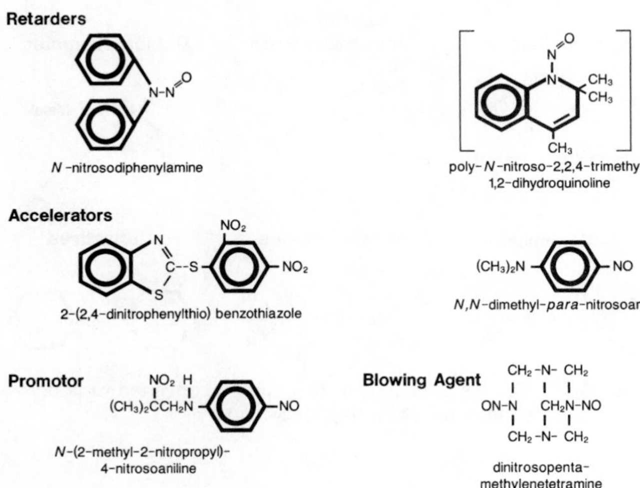

Figure 35-11. Nitro and nitroso compounds used in the rubber industry that can act as precursors of nitrogen oxides. (Adapted from ref. 18, with permission.)

Chemicals containing nitro or nitroso groups can serve as nitrosating agents (18). These chemicals can thermally decompose in hot processes to form nitrogen oxide and directly nitrosate amines contained in rubber (Fig. 35-11) (18). Nitrogen oxides can also be formed as by-products of internal combustion processes secondary to machine use.

Nitrosamines have been reported in numerous worksite air samples in the United States and Germany in breathing zone samples (18). These nitrosamines included NDMA, NMOR, *N*-nitrosobutylamine, *N*-nitrosopiperidine, and *N*-nitrosopyrrolidine. The nitrosatable precursor of each of these compounds is used in the rubber industry, with the exception of *N*-nitrosopyrrolidine.

In addition to the nitrosation of secondary amines, reactions involving tertiary amines or amine derivatives occur in aqueous systems and solid systems, as well as in the gaseous phase. The following two nitrosation reactions are possible:

- Nitrosatable compounds dissolved or dispersed in latex solution can be nitrosated during the production of latex articles. Nitrogen oxide from the air has been proposed as the nitrosating agent in this case. Atmospheric levels of nitrogen oxides can be complemented by other combustion processes, such as open flames and other pollutant sources (17,18,24).
- Chemicals that contain nitro or nitroso groups are potential nitrostating agents, as some of these chemicals may decompose thermally during processing of the rubber to form nitrogen oxides. Direct nitrosation of specific compounds contained in solid rubber is therefore possible. Animal studies have demonstrated that airborne concentrations of nitrosamines, similar to those found in the rubber industry, can induce cancers of the lung, kidney, and liver (18).

The rubber industry as a whole has several hundred different chemicals involved in the manufacture of various rubber products. The choice of chemicals used in different stages of the processing of the rubber varies from company to company, and even within the different departments and factories within the same company.

RUBBER INDUSTRY AND CANCER

Studies of rubber workers in the United States and other countries have demonstrated that the death rate due to all cancers appears lower than in the general population. But a detailed review of the mortality experience of these cohorts has shown excesses for specific causes of death (26–40). Among U.S. rubber workers, excess malignancies of the lung, lymphatic system, and hematopoietic system—particularly lymphatic leukemia—have been associated with certain jobs in the rubber industry (26–40). Stomach cancers have been associated with jobs in the production line, including compounding and mixing, milling, and extrusion. Lung cancer has been associated with curing jobs in certain rubber industries (26–40).

Establishing causation of these health outcomes with many of the materials and chemicals that occur in the work atmosphere in the rubber industry has been difficult because of the diverse and changing nature of exposures within the rubber industry, the multiple exposures experienced by many workers because of job mobility over a working lifetime, and the lack of historical industrial hygiene data. Most epidemiologic studies of cancer and other diseases in rubber workers have not always been exposure specific, or they have used job descriptions as a substitute for exposure estimates. Consequently, there is sometimes considerable difficulty in identifying etiologic factors in cancer and other disease causation (29). This process is confounded by the need to estimate exposures that occurred several decades ago in relation to cancer occurring more recently. Evidence of human carcinogenicity to either a single chemical or a complex mixture of chemicals in the rubber industry has been derived from the following types of studies (29):

- Reports on individual cancer patients who have a history of exposure to the suspected carcinogen
- Descriptive epidemiologic studies in which the incidence of cancer in human populations is found to vary with exposure to the agent or agents in question
- Analytic epidemiologic evidence—such as case-control or cohort studies—in which individual exposure to the agents is found to be associated with an increased risk of cancer

The first two study types provide only suggestive evidence of causation. The third one, an analytic epidemiologic study, provides better insight if there is no identified bias, error in the design of the study, or confounding factors.

The rubber industry has gone through many evolutionary changes involved with technology and chemicals. To try to define a typical rubber manufacturing operation is difficult in terms of either the process, end product, or environmental controls. Multiple processes in the rubber industry can be associated with different exposure hazards. The variables that arise include variations in production and control technology, variations in process requirements, and variations in work practice (2,15,29).

Assessing exposures of rubber workers is also rather difficult for the following reasons (2,29):

- An individual experiences a large variety of exposures from the multiple chemicals used in a given job and cross-contamination from adjacent work areas.
- Several hundred chemicals, including some complex solvent mixtures, are used in the rubber industry.
- Few workers in the industry remain in the same job during the entire period of their employment, although job mobility for these workers may be minimal. However, they may work at many different jobs over the course of their employment, making it very difficult to track their exposure history.
- Cancer excesses that occur in the industry may have resulted from chemical exposures that occurred within or outside the industry many years before clinical diagnosis of the disease.
- Industrial processes can result in the formation of new materials as by-products of those processes.

Excess mortality from various cancers has been reported in rubber workers, and the International Agency for Research on Cancer has classified specific exposures in the rubber industry as potentially carcinogenic in humans (2). Despite changes in manufacturing materials, operations, work conditions, and worker mobility, epidemiologic investigations have identified excesses of several different cancers in rubber workers, depending on the study population and time frame of interest. Although in some instances specific causes have been suggested, specific factors contributing to cancer excess in rubber workers remain uncertain.

The first cancer identified in rubber workers was an excess in bladder cancer in Great Britain. The cancer excess in workers studied was ultimately attributed to the use of aromatic amines, primarily β-naphthylamine, as an accelerator. The use of this chemical was discontinued by 1950, and excess bladder cancer has not been identified in subsequent studies.

Studies have also shown certain rubber workers to be at an increased risk for developing leukemia (39). Excess has been found in other studies, including a risk of lymphocytic leukemia with exposure to solvents other than benzene (26–40). Limited studies of workers producing SBR have also suggested an excess of leukemia risk (39).

Although rubber workers overall have not been found to be at an increased risk for developing lung cancer, excess lung cancer has been identified in a variety of rubber worker subpopulations. Lung cancer has been associated with exposure to compounding, mixing and milling, and curing fume exposure, but these studies are inconsistent (26–39). Smoking, interactions of smoking with other exposures in the industry, and chance clustering (given the extensive investigation of this industry) all remain possible explanations for the findings related to lung cancer to date.

Most epidemiologic studies of the rubber industry are retrospective follow-up studies of cohorts of rubber workers or case-control studies of people with cancer. Typically, the rate of occurrence or death, or both, from cancer is compared with the rates in a control population. This control may be the general population.

Frequently, in follow-up studies, the rate of death in the study population is less than that in the general population. This difference is termed the *healthy worker effect*. This selection bias occurs because only relatively healthy people enter the employment force, but it usually applies less to cancer than to other causes of death.

In occupational cohort studies, the standardized mortality ratio (SMR) is commonly used. The SMR is the number of deaths observed in a group divided by the number expected in the same group. The quotient is multiplied by 100. The expected numbers, which are customarily based on the mortality experience of the general population, are usually standardized for age and calendar time. In case-control studies, disease rates are not computed because of the small size of the population studied.

The main studies of the rubber industry in the United States consist of those from the Harvard School of Public Health and the University of North Carolina (2,26). Data in the Harvard study included 13,571 male production workers (26). These people were working at a plant on or after January 1, 1940, and worked at least 5 years at the plant between that time and June 1971. They were studied from January 1940 through June 1974. During that period, 980 deaths from cancer were observed; 1,046 were expected. In the second phase of the study, cancer morbidity between 1964 and 1974 was examined by a review of the area tumor registry. The rates of cancer were measured among workers in specific areas of the rubber plant. Lung cancer excesses were noted in the tire-curing area in people who had worked there for at least 5 years, tire-molding people who had worked there for at least 5 years, and in the fuel cell de-icer manufacturing area. In the tire-curing area, there were 31 cases of cancer with 14.1 cases expected; in the fuel cell de-icer area, there were 46 cases of cancer with 29.1 expected (26).

University of North Carolina Studies

In the studies from the University of North Carolina (UNC), 6,678 production workers were studied, and 351 cancer deaths occurred during a 9-year follow-up; 336.9 deaths were expected, based on the U.S. male age and race-specific rate (2,28,29).

McMichael et al. in 1976 detailed job histories of seven specific cancer case groups in this industry (15,40). They found that respiratory cancer excess was found in the following areas: receiving and shipping, compounding and mixing, milling, extrusion, tubing, and reclaim.

Excess mortality from lung cancer was found in one United Kingdom study; an excess of lung cancer was found among workers in many occupations in the tire industry and nontire sectors. Excess cases of lung cancer in U.S. studies were associated with work in compounding and mixing, extrusion, tire curing, and rubber reclaim (2,15,26,32,33,40).

Two populations were defined in the UNC study. The first population consisted of 6,678 men who were alive on January 1, 1964, and had worked for at least 10 years in a large Akron, Ohio, tire plant (40). This population was studied for 9 years, starting from 1964. Overall results of the study demonstrated cancers of other organ systems without excess lung cancer. A parallel study of 1,339 men in a second tire factory in Akron showed essentially the same, with no evidence of increased lung cancer rates (15,40). A case-control study conducted on 61 cases of lung cancer and 61 matched control subjects demonstrated a strong correlation between the rubber curing process and lung cancer. Twenty-five percent of the cases were exposed to curing agents versus 15% of control subjects (15,40).

The second UNC study was conducted on 8,418 white male production workers from 1964 to 1973. Again, lung cancer was not a prominent disease among the cancers observed.

Harvard School of Public Health Studies

This study defined a population of 13,570 white male workers employed in an Akron plant from 1940 to 1971 (2,26). All members of the study had worked for at least 5 years. The number of overall cancer deaths was less than the general population. Bladder cancer appeared in excess. A subsequent cancer study was carried out in this particular plant showing correlations between type of job and excess cancers. The results of this study demonstrated an excess of lung cancer in the curing, molding, and fuel cell area of the plant (32). The mortality of 13,571 white, male rubber employees was studied from 1940 through 1974 as part of the Harvard study. An excess of lung cancer in the tire curing area (observed, 20; expected, 12.4) was identified. In addition, the curing workers had a higher incidence of chronic bronchitis. Of the curing workers with at least 10 years' experience, 25% had chronic obstructive lung disease. Smoking did not account for the difference between the curing versus the control group in terms of increased respiratory disease.

Results of a 5-year analysis from 1967 to 1971 of 40,807 British rubber workers demonstrated an overall 19% increase in the incidence of cancer (34). There was also excess lung cancer in the tire manufacturing area (34).

Smoking habits were not accounted for in this large study; however, the SMR for other smoking and urban-related disease was approximately the same in all sectors. This suggests that smoking is not a primary cause for the excess lung cancer seen in this study (34).

The risk of neoplasms in general was higher for the tire industry as compared with the cable-making industry. No evidence was found to suggest this excess might be due to smoking habits. The death rates for smoking-related causes—in particular, for chronic obstructive lung disease and bronchitis—in the tire industry is approximately the same for the cable-making industry (34). The first prospective study to report on excess lung cancer deaths in the rubber industry was by Mancuso (29).

British Rubber Manufacturer Association/ Birmingham University Study

The British Rubber Manufacturer Association (BRMA) initiated a retrospective study that covered 33,815 men who worked in the rubber industry from 1946 to 1960. Thirteen factories were included: eight tire and five general rubber products. The study population worked for a minimum of 1 year and was divided into three cohorts (28):

- Cohort 1, January 1946 to December 1950
- Cohort 2, January 1951 to December 1955
- Cohort 3, January 1956 to December 1960

The study looked at all causes of death, not just cancer, and was extended until 1975. The final report focused only on cancer cases in the industry.

The initial study analyzed deaths from cancer by studying only members of the population who survived for a minimum for 10 years past beginning employment. This removed all cases of cancer deaths that occurred close to the point of entry into employment. Using this refined 10-year latency technique, an excess of cancer was observed (28).

The lung cancer mortality was analyzed in terms of occupational groups in the rubber industry. The results of this analysis suggested that certain occupations in the rubber industry were associated with higher-than-expected mortality rates for respiratory cancer (28).

Excess lung cancer has been associated with work in the curing, inspection, and mixing areas of the rubber industry in general, as demonstrated by a number of studies. In the BRMA study, the individual environmental exposure of workers was considered to be important in delineation of carcinogenesis. These work environments were identified by obtaining detailed occupational histories as well as job descriptions from workers. For each chemical exposure, the fraction of the subgroup reported to have some exposure to that chemical was recorded and generated data that indicated excess lung cancer with exposure to curing vapors.

A case-control study was conducted with four control subjects being chosen for each case of lung cancer. These control subjects were matched for age, factory, cohort, and duration of service. No single environmental area stands out as a cause of lung cancer; however, curing vapors (vulcanizing) were highlighted.

Extended British Rubber Manufacturer Association Study

Reported in 1982, the extended BRMA study followed the original study population through December 31, 1975, allowing another 5 years of analysis. This study excluded all those workers who died in the 10 years after the beginning of their employment. This restraint reduced the study population from 36,695 participants to 33,815 and removed the healthy worker effect influence (28). The overall results for cancer deaths in the population showed increased SMRs for all cancer types, excess lung cancer, excess leukemia, and excess stomach cancer (28). Lung cancer excess seen in the previous study was reconfirmed by this extended study data. The extended study also confirmed suspected information regarding occupational site and the excess lung cancer cases. In addition, the results were worse for general rubber goods than for tire industries alone.

The general rubber goods and tire manufacturing rubber industries show excess lung cancer rates in the curing, tire-building, and inspection and finishing areas of the workplace.

CONCLUSION

The rubber industry employs hundreds of chemicals in a variety of processes, and reactions leading to potentially hazardous exposures can occur in multiple environments. Decomposition products from chemical reactions may account for many unknown exposures to potential carcinogens at various sites with excess of lung cancer, leukemia, and lymphomas having been described in certain occupational groups. As a result, control of exposures is an important preventive health issue.

REFERENCES

1. Greek BF. Rubber chemicals face more demanding market. *Chem Eng News* 1989;25–54.
2. International Agency for Research on Cancer. The rubber industry. *IARC Monogr Eval Carcinog Risk Chem Hum* 1982;28:1–486.
3. Feinman SE. Sensitivity to rubber chemicals. *J Toxicol Cutan Ocul Toxicol* 1987;6:117–153.
4. US Environmental Protection Agency, Office of Air Quality Planning and Standards. *Final report: analysis of the ambient monitoring data in the vicinity of open tire fires*. Research Triangle Park, NC: Environmental Protection Agency, 1993.
5. Ryan JV, Acurex Corporation. *Characterization of emissions from the simulated open burning of scrap tires*. Washington: US Environmental Protection Agency, 1989. [EPA-600/2-89-054].
6. US Environmental Protection Agency, Control Technology Center for the Office of Air Quality Planning and Standards. *Burning tires for fuel and tire pyrolysis: air implications*. Research Triangle Park, NC: US Environmental Protection Agency, 1991.
7. DeMarini DM, Lemieux PM. *Mutagenicity of emissions from the simulated open burning of scrap rubber tires*. Washington: US Environmental Protection Agency, 1992. [EPA-600/R-92-127]
8. Levendis A, Atal A, Carlson J, Dunayevskiy Y, Vouros P. Comparative study on the combustion and emissions of waste tyre crumb and pulverized coal. *Environ Sci Technol* 1996;30:2742–2754.
9. Teng H, Chyang C, Shang S, Ho J. Characterization of waste tire incineration in prototype vortexing fluidized bed combustor. *J Air Waste Manage Assoc* 1997;47:49–57.
10. Weeks JL, Peters JM, Monson RR. Screening for occupational health hazards in the rubber industry. Part I. *Am J Ind Med* 1981;2:125–141.
11. Weeks JL, Peters JM, Monson RR. Screening for occupational health hazards in the rubber industry. Part II: health hazards in the curing department. *Am J Ind Med* 1981;2:143–151.
12. Fraser DA, Rappaport S. Health aspects of the curing of synthetic rubbers. *Environ Health Prospect* 1976;17:45–53.
13. Williams TM, Harris RL, Arp EW, Symons MJ, Van Ert MD. Worker exposure to chemical agents in the manufacture of rubber tires and tubes: particulates. *Am Ind Hyg Assoc J* 1980;41:204–211.
14. Delzell E, Monson RR. Mortality among rubber workers: IV. General mortality patterns. *J Occup Med* 1981;23:850–856.
15. McMichael AJ, Spirtas R, Gamble JF, Tousey PM. Mortality among rubber workers: relationship to specific jobs. *J Occup Med* 1976;18:178–185.
16. Fishbein L. Core problems in chemical industries: additives used in the plastics, polymer, and rubber industries. In: Stich HF, ed. *Carcinogens and mutagens in the environment*. Boca Raton, FL: CRC Press, 1982.
17 Fajen JM, Carson GA, Rounbehler DP, et al. *N*-Nitrosamines in the rubber and tire industry. *Science* 1979;205:1262–1264.
18. Spiegelhalder B. Carcinogens in the workroom air in the rubber industry. *Scand J Work Environ Health* 1983;9:15–25.
19. Nutt A. Rubber work and cancer: past, present and perspectives. *Scand J Work Environ Health* 1983;9[Suppl 2]:49–57.
20. Wilcosky TC, Checkoway H, Marshall EG, Tyroler HA. Cancer mortality and solvent exposures in the rubber industry. *Am Ind Hyg Assoc J* 1984;45:809–811.
21. Nutt A. Measurement of some potentially hazardous materials in the atmosphere of rubber factories. *Environ Health Perspect* 1976;17:117–123.
22. Neal J, Thornton M, Nau CA. Polycyclic hydrocarbon elution from carbon black or rubber products. *Arch Environ Health* 1962;4:46–54.

23. Locati G, Fantuzzi A, Consonni G, Li Gotti I, Bonomi G. Identification of polycyclic aromatic hydrocarbons in carbon black with reference to cancerogenic risk in tire production. *Am Ind Hyg Assoc J* 1979;40:644–652.
24. Mirvish SS. Formation of *N*-nitroso compounds: chemistry, kinetics and in vivo occurrence. *Toxicol Appl Pharmacol* 1975;31:325–351.
25. Dipple A, Michejda CJ, Weisburger EK. Metabolism of chemical carcinogens. *Pharmacol Ther* 1985;27:265–296.
26. Monson RR, Fine LJ. Cancer mortality and morbidity among rubber workers. *J Natl Cancer Inst* 1978;61:1047–1053.
27. McMichael AJ, Andjelkovic DA, Tyroler HA. Cancer mortality among rubber workers: an epidemiologic study. *Ann N Y Acad Sci* 1976;271:125–137.
28. Parkes HG, Veys CA, Waterhouse JAH, Peters A. Cancer mortality in the British rubber industry. *Br J Ind Med* 1982;39:209–220.
29. Mancuso TF. Problems and perspective in epidemiological study of occupational health hazards in the rubber industry. *Environ Health Perspect* 1976; 17:21–30.
30. Delzell E, Manson R. Mortality among rubber workers: III. Cause-specific mortality, 1940–1978. *J Occup Med* 1981;23:677–684.
31. Delzell E, Monson RR. Mortality among rubber workers: VII. Aerospace workers. *Am J Ind Med* 1984;6:265–271.
32. Delzell E, Monson RR. Mortality among rubber workers: X. Reclaim workers. *Am J Ind Med* 1985;7:307–313.
33. Delzell E, Louik C, Lewis J, Monson RR. Mortality and cancer morbidity among workers in the rubber tire industry. *Am J Ind Med* 1981;2:209–216.
34. Fox AJ, Lindars DC, Owen R. A survey of occupational cancer in the rubber and cablemaking industries: results of five-year analysis, 1967–1971. *Br J Ind Med* 1974;31:140–151.
35. Kilpikari I. Mortality among male rubber workers in Finland. *Arch Environ Health* 1982;37:295–298.
36. Delzell E, Andjelkovich D, Tyroler HA. A case-control study of employment experience and lung cancer among rubber workers. *Am J Ind Med* 1982; 3:393–404.
37. Norseth T, Andersen A, Giltvedt J. Cancer incidence in the rubber industry in Norway. *Scand J Work Environ Health* 1983;9:69–71.
38. Meinhardt TJ, Lemen RA, Crandall MS, Young RJ. Environmental epidemiologic investigation of the styrene-butadiene rubber industry: mortality patterns with discussion of the hematopoietic and lymphatic malignancies. *Scand J Work Environ Health* 1982;8:250–259.
39. Matanoski GM, Santos-Burgoa C, Schwartz L. Mortality of a cohort of workers in the styrene-butadiene polymer manufacturing industry (1943–1982). *Environ Health Perspect* 1990;86:107–117.
40. McMichael AJ, Spirtas R, Kupper LC. An epidemiologic study of mortality within a cohort of rubber workers, 1964–1972. *J Occup Med* 1976;18:178–185.

CHAPTER 36
Automobile Airbag Hazards

J. Michael Hitt

Although the inclusion of automobile airbags in motor vehicles was federally mandated in the 1990s, the concept and research date to the 1960s. Concern for the effectiveness and safety of the device was originally tested by placing a baboon in a cockpit of a simulated aircraft crashing at 120 miles per hour. Research on the safety of the device has continued since that time.

There is no question that airbags perform the function for which they were designed: to protect the driver in moderate- to high-speed frontal crashes. Studies demonstrate that driver fatalities in airbag-equipped cars were reduced by 24% in frontal crashes relative to comparable cars equipped only with manual belts (1). In 1991, nonpedestrian motor vehicle crashes claimed 36,500 lives, with the total cost of all fatal motor vehicle accidents estimated to be $96.1 billion, excluding the inestimable human loss. Uninjured survivors of fatal crashes were three times more likely to have been restrained. Only 28.9% of fatalities were restrained by either seat belts or airbags or both. I would conservatively estimate that 4,000 lives are saved annually in the United States specifically as a result of the presence and deployment of airbags.

The Federal Motor Vehicle Safety Standard Number 208, *Occupant Crash Protection*, requires that all passenger cars manufactured after September 1, 1989, be equipped with automatic crash protection. This requirement has generally been met by providing airbags on all new passenger vehicles since that time. This has opened up a new field of applied toxicology. Thousands of airbag deployments now occur every year. Most generate no toxicologic concern; however, some individuals have reported physical and metabolic injury as the result of these deployments. The popular press has been keenly interested in the subject, as is evidenced by a quotation found in the newspaper *USA Today*: "At least 32 children and 20 adults have been killed by the explosive force of air bags in the USA since mid-1990" (2).

Thousands of workers in the United States and other countries are involved in the production of automobile airbags. Airbag-related industrial injuries occur every year, and some years' fatalities are the direct result of the manufacturing process.

The body of knowledge of the toxicologic effects of automobile airbags and their components on both workers and consumers is rapidly growing. It is increasingly becoming a fascinating topic to physicians, environmental health experts, regulators, lawmakers, and attorneys.

This product will eventually be in the possession of 80% of adult Americans. As with any common product containing chemicals, questions as to potential toxic effects have been and continue to be raised.

The deployment of the airbag requires a controlled rapid generation of gas within centimeters of the driver's face. In newer vehicles, the same scenario is true for the passenger. This results in the release of the products of combustion and creates a unique and potentially hazardous situation within the confines of the passenger compartment. Previously, automotive reactions of this nature had been isolated to the engine compartment and, in the case of the internal combustion engine, shielded by massive metal blocks. The airbag, however, aims a high-speed chemical reaction of similar intensity directly at the automobile occupant. Instead of massive steel shielding, the airbag offers only the protection of a cloth bag, fiber screens, and a thin metal inflator body. The engineering required to protect humans from this protective device is substantial and impressive. The record largely bears out the fruits of the scientific work that went into its development.

AUTOMOBILE AIRBAG MODULE

Figure 36-1 demonstrates the major components of a driver's side automobile airbag module. A passenger side airbag is similar. This system operates by placing the module in the center of the steering wheel. The back side of the inflator is attached to the steering wheel, and the opposite side, facing the driver, contains the airbag, housed within a plastic container and cover. The module is connected to crash sensors at the front, sides, and possibly the passenger compartment of the vehicle (Fig. 36-2). The sensor, which typically consists of an accelerometer, will detect an extremely rapid deceleration and send an electric current to activate the inflator.

The inflator is the heart of the driver's side system. It consists of a lightweight, stainless steel, or aluminum housing, which contains a stack of gas-generating disks or pellets composed primarily of sodium azide and an oxidizer (Fig. 36-3). The gas-generating material is housed within a combustion chamber. The inflator walls are permeated by holes or ports, which allow gas to escape. These holes are screened by a final filter, which serves to cool the gases and protect the airbag itself from particles that might burn or rupture. The entire inflator sits within the circular opening of the airbag. The bag is woven of soft, porous fabric, allowing rapid inflation and deflation.

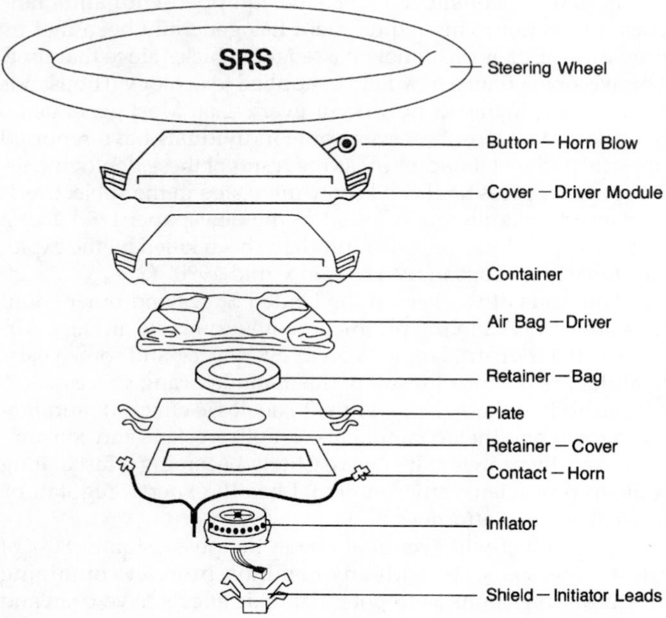

Figure 36-1. Major components of a driver's side supplemental restraint system (SRS), automobile airbag module. (Reprinted with permission by TRW Safety System, Mesa, Arizona.)

Combustion occurs when an electronically activated squib ignites the enhancer (booster) charge, which ignites the main charge placed within the material.

Beginning in 1996, some automobile models were delivered with a simpler deployment system containing less toxic materials. These vehicles contain azide-free generators, allowing for a module that is lighter than previous airbag modules. Hybrid systems and a pyrotechnic heater are also being used. The hybrid systems, however, use the best qualities of both systems: A small, nontoxic propellant charge breaks open the seal on the gas canister, and the high-pressure contents rapidly flow out. Some hybrid systems generate little heat, allowing for a lighter-weight airbag and virtually no chance of vehicle occupant burns. As an adjunct to these systems, new sensing mechanisms (Fig. 36-4) are being developed to further protect vehicle occupants (3).

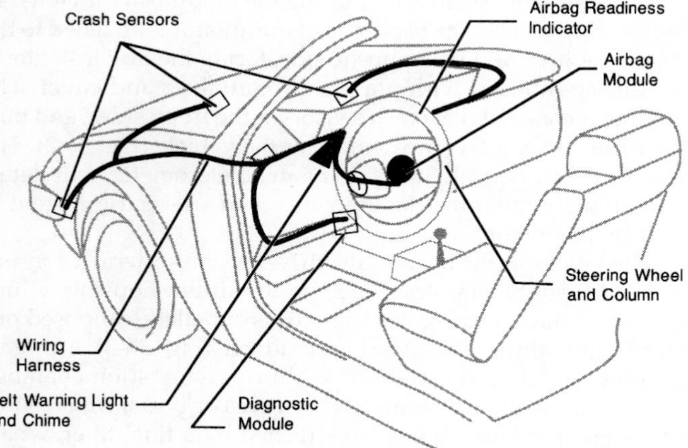

Figure 36-2. Operation of an automobile airbag module. At extremely rapid deceleration, the sensor will signal, causing an electrical current to activate the inflator. (Reprinted with permission by TRW Safety System, Mesa, Arizona.)

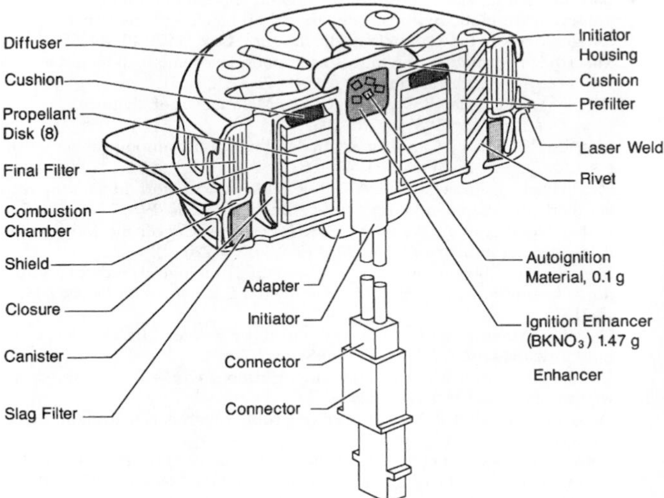

Figure 36-3. Driver inflator component of an automobile airbag module. (Reprinted with permission by TRW Safety System, Mesa, Arizona.)

CHEMICAL CONSTITUENTS AND TOXICITY

Table 36-1 illustrates some of the typical components of airbags, along with the associated toxicologic effects. Components vary by manufacturer. Most airbags contain sodium azide (N_3Na) salt. This is the major functional component and the one with

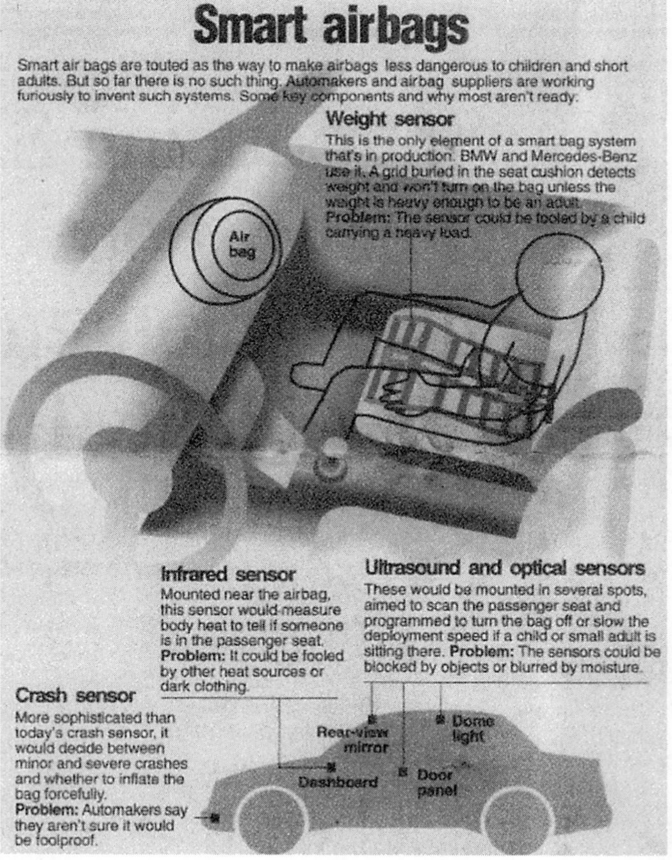

Figure 36-4. Smart air bags. (Used with permission by *USA TODAY.* Copyright 1996.)

TABLE 36-1. Chemical hazards of airbag industry

Agent	Use	Exposure	Hazard
Sodium azide salt	Propellant and source of detonation	Ingestion of salt or inhalation of hydrazoic acid	May affect cardiovascular, neurologic, and pulmonary systems and blood. Blocks cytochrome oxidase and mitochondrial phosphorylation. Can cause hypotension, syncope, headache, muscular weakness, seizures, metabolic acidosis, pulmonary edema, methemoglobinemia, angina, cardiac dysrhythmias, cyanosis.
Ceramic fibers	Filter assembly	Inhalation, dermal, ingestion	Irritant to skin and mucous membrane. Nausea, vomiting, and diarrhea may occur following fiber ingestion.
Boron	Enhancer present as boron potassium nitrate	Dermal, inhalation	Irritant to eyes and mucous membranes in aerosolized form
Potassium nitrate	Enhancer assembly	Dermal, ingestion	Dermatitis, methemoglobinemia, vasodilator, hypotension, syncope, angina
Nitrocellulose	Enhancer assembly	Inhalation, dermal, ingestion	None
Molybdenum disulfide	Oxidizer	Inhalation, dermal	Fatty degeneration of liver

the greatest potential for toxicity. Sodium azide is the primary constituent that reacts to produce the nitrogen gas.

Boron and potassium nitrate are commonly used as the primary ignition material. Nitrocellulose and other materials may be used as enhancers or as an autoignition material. Together, they ignite the propellant, initiating the chemical reaction that ultimately leads to inflation and off-gassing of combustion products. Other chemical components frequently present are sulfur, molybdenum disulfide, iron oxide, or silicon dioxide. The products of combustion are present in gaseous and particulate form. Tables 36-2 and 36-3 summarize the chemical products present from the deployment of a driver's airbag using a sodium azide–based gas-generating agent.

The principal chemical component of the entire system—and certainly the major toxic raw material—is sodium azide, which makes up the bulk of the gas-generating disks. These disks are securely contained in a metal housing, leaving little potential for toxic exposure in the context of their use in automobiles. As noted in Tables 36-2 and 36-3, the products of combustion in a normal airbag deployment are safe and well below the American Conference of Governmental Industrial Hygienists limits of exposure.

TABLE 36-2. Analysis of typical atmosphere in vehicle after airbag deployment for one type of inflator

Component	Range of typical concentrations (ppm)	ACGIH TLVs-STEL (ppm)
Carbon dioxide	<500–2,170[a]	30,000
Hydrogen	100–408	N/A[b]
Carbon monoxide	<5.0–60.3	400
Ammonia	<2.0	35
Hydrogen sulfide	<1.0–2.3	15
Nitric oxide	<5.0	125
Nitrogen dioxide	<5.0	5
Benzene	<0.10–0.45	50

ACGIH, American Conference of Governmental Industrial Hygienists; STEL, short-term exposure limits, 1991–1992; TLVs, threshold limit values.
Tested in a 100-cubic-foot chamber. Analysis excludes N_2O_2 and water vapor, which will remain close to predeployment levels.
[a]< indicates that the numerical value following it is the lower limit of detection for that species and that the actual level present is less than this value.
[b]Not applicable for one-time exposure, or chemical species is an ACGIH unlisted substance.
Automotive Safety Products. Driver air bag technical data sheet, revision 3. Ogden, UT: Morton International, Inc., July 29, 1996. Used with permission.

In other settings, such as laboratories and manufacturing plants, sodium azide toxicity can occur from inhalation of azide gas (hydrazoic acid), which is released through hydrolysis in aqueous solutions of the azide salt or from ingestion of the sodium azide salt. Respiratory toxicity can involve respiratory failure and pulmonary edema. Methemoglobinemia can occur as a result of oxidation of hemoglobin similar to nitrites.

Clinical signs and symptoms of toxicity are dose dependent. Ingestions of 40 mg and less have produced headache. Doses of up to 60 mg have resulted in syncope and hypotension. Doses of 80 to 150 mg have resulted in angina, dyspnea, tachycardia, nausea, vomiting, diarrhea, and headache (4). A fatal ingestion can be as little as 1 to 2 g (5).

Sodium azide has caused at least seven fatalities after ingestion (6). It is a chemical of highly acute toxicity with an unknown mechanism of action. It has some chemical properties and biological effects similar to cyanide, but its lethality is not because of inhibition of cytochrome oxidase. A clinical picture similar to cyanide intoxication may occur in large doses with metabolic acidosis, severe hypotension unresponsive to fluids, and vaso-

TABLE 36-3. Analysis of solid particulate levels in typical vehicle atmosphere after airbag deployment for one type of inflator

Category	Range of typical concentrations (mg/m^3)	ACGIH TLVs-STEL (mg/m^3)
Total particulate	24.2–92.2	N/A[a]
Respirable particulate	21.9–86.2	N/A
Sodium[b]	4.73–29.80	N/A
Acetate	2.05–3.70	N/A
Potassium	<0.10–1.23	N/A
Nitrate	0.23–0.72	N/A
Nitrite	<0.100–0.327	N/A
Sulfate	<0.10–0.14	N/A
Lead	<0.040–0.043	0.75
Sodium azide	<0.0031–0.0044	0.29 (ceiling limit)

ACGIH, American Conference of Governmental Industrial Hygienists; STEL, short-term exposure limits, 1991–1992; TLVs, threshold limit values.
Tested in a 100-cubic-foot chamber. Chemical analysis provided of respirable particulate fraction.
[a]Not applicable for one-time exposure, or chemical species is an ACGIH unlisted substance.
[b]Some of the sodium may be present as sodium hydroxide, which has a TLV ceiling limit of 2 mg/m^3.
Automotive Safety Products. Driver air bag technical data sheet, revision 3. Ogden, UT: Morton International, Inc., July 29, 1996. Used with permission.

constrictors and seizures. In unknown ingestions, sodium azide poisoning may be mistaken for cyanide poisoning. Possibly, its toxicity is due to its metabolic conversion to nitric acid (6).

Sodium azide is a common preservative for laboratory reagents and is widely used in the explosives industry. Sodium azide is a white crystal. The pK_a of sodium azide is 4.8, so in acidic fluids such as gastric juice, a large amount of hydrazoic acid HN_3 will be present (7).

In the industrial setting, the two most common routes of exposure are inhalation and skin absorption. Sodium azide is easily absorbed through the skin, and this can create a significant exposure for workers and consumers who might tamper with or otherwise come in contact with the salt (8). Low-level exposure over long periods of time is likely to produce diarrhea and a mild lowering of blood pressure. More acute low-level exposure may also produce hypotension, as in the case of nine dialysis patients who suddenly developed low blood pressures within 30 minutes of receiving dialysis from a system using glycerine-preserved ultrafilters that had not been rinsed before use (9). Sodium azide shares certain cardiovascular effects with nitrites, and human deaths from it appear to be due to cardiovascular collapse (10). One such case, involving an accidental ingestion of approximately 1 g of sodium azide, resulted in acute myocardial infarction in a 29-year-old individual. This progressed to cardiomyopathy and death within 48 hours (11).

Sodium azide has been studied as an antihypertensive drug in human clinical trials. It appears to be an effective pharmaceutical agent with no adverse effects noted in 25 years of study, when dosages were kept below 0.75 mg per day. This dose is significant, because it represents the approximate daily dose of an industrial worker working one shift at the ceiling exposure limit of 0.3 mg per m^3 (12). For this reason, mild depression of blood pressure may be expected in sodium azide workers. Anecdotal reports cite a greater hypotensive effect in hypertensive workers as compared to normotensive workers. There have been no reports of rebound hypertension on weekends or vacations. In animal studies, however, toxic doses of azide have resulted in centrally mediated *hypertension*, tachycardia, cardiac arrhythmia, respiratory depression, seizures, and death (13). Hypertension after sodium azide ingestion has also been demonstrated in humans, as in the case of a 30-year-old who intentionally ingested 15 to 20 g of the substance and who later died from a combination of acidosis, respiratory depression, and ventricular fibrillation (14).

Diarrhea appears to be a common symptom of sodium azide workers. Nausea, vomiting, and abdominal pain have also been noted (12).

Sodium azide is not listed as a carcinogen, although it is a known plant mutagen. Some conflicting animal studies have been performed with no clear evidence of animal mutagenicity (15). There is no evidence of teratogenic effects in humans. Only one study has demonstrated any teratogenic effects. This experiment was performed on pregnant golden hamsters by subcutaneously implanting osmotic minipumps containing 400 mg per mL of sodium azide over 7 to 9 days, delivering a total dose of 6×10^{-2} mmol per kg per hour. This dose produced obvious toxicity in the animal but also resulted in an increased incidence of gross malformations in the form of encephaloceles and caused resorptions of embryos (16).

The neurotoxicity of sodium azide is significant. In animal studies, chronic administration of sodium azide induced progressive movement disorders and central nervous system necrosis (17). Striatal necrosis has been experimentally induced in rats via sodium azide injections (18). Cerebellar cortical degeneration has been demonstrated by injecting monkeys with a single dose of sodium azide, ranging from 8 to 13 mg per kg. Most of the animals demonstrated, at a minimum, transient ataxia, with most having more persistent ataxia. All symptomatic monkeys demonstrated cerebellar changes (19).

Sodium azide exposure on a chronic basis produces behavioral changes in animals and has been considered to be a model for some aspects of Alzheimer's disease (20).

From a practical perspective, the components of airbag modules offer little potential for toxicity. The public is at little risk from any of the chemicals, because the chemicals are sealed in metal and not easily accessible for tampering. The public's principal risk of exposure is when an airbag is deployed; however, the thermal degradation destroys the module's chemical components and yields principally nitrogen gas with traces of other gases and particulates (see Tables 36-2, 36-3).

The other chemicals contained in airbags do offer potential for toxicity during the manufacturing and repair process and possibly, under certain conditions, during and after the deployment of the airbag. One of these hazards is ceramic fiber. The ceramic fiber used in the module consists of vitreous luminosilicate fibers. These fibers are used as components of the filter assemblies. No known chronic health effects occur in humans from long-term exposure to ceramic fibers. Ceramic fibers have been injected into the peritoneal cavity of laboratory animals, as well as into the pleural cavity, and tumors have been produced. This is not a unique effect, and similar results have been detected in various fibrous materials.

Several studies have suggested a low order of potential of inducing pulmonary tumors in animals, whereas others have contradicted this. The International Agency of Research on Cancer classified fibrous glass wool, mineral wool, and ceramic fiber as group 2B carcinogens. Group 2B agents are possibly carcinogenic to humans (21).

Ceramic fibers also are irritating to skin and mucosal membranes. Ingestion may cause gastrointestinal disturbances, such as irritation, nausea, vomiting, and diarrhea.

The enhancer assembly contains powdered ignition and enhancer material, commonly consisting of boron potassium nitrate, nitrocellulose, and 2.4-dinitrotoluene. Boron potassium nitrate has toxic properties similar to any nitrate and also is mildly irritating to mucous membranes. Environmental monitoring in the enhancer assembly operation has demonstrated that exposure to all propellant dusts and particles is well below Occupational Safety and Health Administration standards. Heavy exposures to processes involving potassium nitrates can cause dermatitis and dermal burns, and chronic exposure to low levels can cause chronic coronary vessel dilation. This coronary artery dilation can be a problem during worker furlough, on weekends, and during holidays, because the possibility of reflex constriction or spasm of the coronary vessels may occur. However, this only happens in long-term, heavy exposures.

Ingested nitrates can be converted by enzymatic activity to nitrites, which can cause methemoglobinemia. Nitrites can also be converted by the body into nitrosamines. Several members of this class of compounds have been identified as carcinogens or potential carcinogens. Boron itself is relatively nontoxic and is a mild irritant.

2,4-Dinitrotoluene, which is used by a minority of airbag manufacturers, is toxic by inhalation and ingestion. It is a mucous membrane irritant and may cause methemoglobinemia. In animals, central nervous system, reproductive, and bone marrow abnormalities have been noted. 2,4-Dinitrotoluene is an animal carcinogen. Tests for mutagenic activity of this compound are ambiguous.

In industry, the principal effects are mucous membrane and skin irritation, but in large exposures, cyanosis, weakness, and shortness of breath are common findings. Workers occasionally have nonspecific symptoms such as nausea, headache, confusion, incoordination, loss of consciousness, cough, and joint pain. Interestingly, the compound appears to permeate the skin to a significant extent. Workers with preexisting central or peripheral nervous system, lung, or reproductive disorders may have increased susceptibility to 2,4-dinitrotoluene exposure. The International Agency of Research on Cancer, Occupational Safety and Health Administration, and the National Toxicology Program have not rated 2,4-dinitrotoluene as a carcinogen. Nitrocellulose is not known to have harmful toxic effects in humans (22).

Cupric oxide, also rarely used by modern airbag manufacturers, is occasionally a component of the airbag inflator module. This chemical has a low inherent toxicity, but exposure to copper-containing material may cause ulceration and perforation of the nasal septum over time. Sensitization to copper also occurs in the rarely reported cases of dermatitis associated with copper.

As airbags become more common, the scrapping of cars is a potential source for exposure to all the chemical components of the module (23). Reassuringly, azides are quickly detoxified by bacteria and fungi and in fact are commonly used in the agriculture industry and in fungicides, herbicides, and nematodicides. More concern is present for the rapid release of gas during scrapping operations, tampering, and repair. Azide toxicity, however, should not be a problem in these circumstances.

POSTDEPLOYMENT VEHICLE OCCUPANT INJURY AND TOXICITY

The medical literature has become replete with anecdotal reports of orthopedic, ocular, and cardiothoracic injuries and deaths associated with airbag deployment. These have even occurred at speeds as low as 15 miles per hour. Such injuries occur because of the physical force of the inflating airbag, which at its maximum speed travels between 50 and 200 mph (24). The Transport Department of Canada has undertaken a study that appears to indicate that airbags cause, rather than preclude, morbidity in crashes that occur at the lower end of the collision severity spectrum, when the occupant is wearing a seat belt. The seat belt alone would have been expected to protect the occupant. Their conclusion is that the airbag deployment threshold is set too low, at least for belted occupants (25).

One of the most common groups of physical injuries are those that damage the eyes, orbits, and facial structure of the vehicle occupant. There is a considerable variation in the type of injury reported, but some individuals have been blinded by the impact of the bag (26). One detailed study of ten level 1 trauma center patients who had incurred substantial lower extremity trauma in vehicles equipped with airbags concluded that airbags do not prevent injuries to the lower extremity (27).

Perhaps the most troubling data about airbag morbidity and mortality are the reports of injury and death, including decapitation, that occur when infants and small children encounter a deployed airbag. Warnings have been issued regarding children riding in the front seats of passenger airbag–equipped vehicles (28). Considerable testing is now being performed regarding this issue. Simulated crashes and full-blown crash tests using baboons in various positions and unembalmed human cadavers are being undertaken to explore this issue further.

Of more relevance to the field of toxicology are the potential chemical hazards to automobile occupants that can be encountered after activation or deflation of an airbag. Similar hazards may be encountered by paramedical personnel responding to an accident. Exposure to irritating gas on deflation of an airbag can occur. The airbag is inflated with nitrogen, which is produced when approximately 80 g total of sodium azide is detonated. Byproducts of detonation of sodium azide include sodium hydroxide and nitrogen (see Tables 36-2, 36-3). These gases and particles have been demonstrated to be within the recommended guidelines for human exposures, but no guidelines exist for particle exposures of this magnitude (150 to 220 mg per m^3). Powder residue can produce ocular and nasal irritation. On detonation of the sodium azide, nitrogen gas inflates the bag. Nitrogen gas is also vented to the sides of the steering column toward the driver's feet. The nitrogen gas is warmed by the explosion, sometimes to temperatures high enough to physically burn the occupant's extremities or face (29).

Additionally, an alkaline powder will be present around the driver's compartment. This powder can produce injuries that are most commonly manifested as chemical keratitis and other eye burns (30). The powder consists of talc and sodium hydroxide. It has been suggested that all occupants who have been passengers in a vehicle in which an airbag has deployed undergo thorough skin irrigation to decrease the potential for dermal irritation or burns (29).

Those occupants with lung disease, particularly asthmatics, may be more prone to aggravation of their preexisting disease. Significant asthmatic reactions have occurred in some asthmatic individuals after airbag deployment. One study placed 24 patients with histories of asthma in the rear seats of vehicles equipped with airbags. The airbags were deployed, and the subjects remained in the vehicle with no outside ventilation for 20 minutes or until they perceived or demonstrated signs of chest tightness and bronchoconstriction. Ten of the individuals demonstrated clinically significant bronchoconstrictive episodes (31).

In rare instances, the airbag may not properly or completely inflate. In the only case of this occurring to my knowledge, the effects on the occupant of the vehicle were difficult to delineate and confirm. This case—in which I had personal involvement—was one in which a previously healthy 27-year-old woman remained in the passenger compartment for approximately 10 minutes after the apparently faulty deployment of the airbag. She reported seeing a "snakelike" device emerge from the steering column some 30 seconds after the crash. The vehicle interior filled with a grayish smoke, and a grayish powder residue was propelled into the passenger compartment. She relates a momentary loss of consciousness with an essentially normal checkup at her physician later the same day. A skin burn was noted and treated. A minor cough ensued, and progressively, over months, the individual developed cognitive difficulties and intolerance of many types of normal household chemical exposures. Neuropsychological testing revealed motor and cognitive slowing, balance difficulties, and problems with immediate recall of information. A magnetic resonance imaging scan of the brain was negative, and single-photon-emission computed tomography scans demonstrated temporal lobe asymmetry, mild diminution of global cerebral perfusion, left temporal hypoperfusion, and bilateral orbitofrontal hypoperfusion.

WORKER PROTECTION

Clearly the most hazardous component of the airbag manufacturing industry is that of fire or explosion. Automobile airbags are much more than channeled rapid chemical reactions attached to cloth bags. They represent a vast amount of engineering effort, stress analysis, and finite element analysis. Despite the superb engineering used by this industry, the potential for explosion throughout the manufacturing process is inevitably present. Raw materials must be ground to appropriate size, mixed with other chemical constituents, pressed into appropriate form, and packaged with other components. All of these parts of the process have some inherent risk associated with them. Workers need to be isolated from the most hazardous parts of the process. These components (principally grinding, pressing, and blending) can be done by automated equipment behind reinforced concrete walls and monitored by closed-circuit television.

The dust generated from the grinding and pressing process is a potential health hazard, both from inhalation and skin exposure. Workers cleaning and servicing equipment, as well as working around the grinding process, should have dermal protection with appropriate garments. The appropriate respiratory protective device is also required. Worker protection is required until the disk is sealed into the canister.

Employees who cut or manipulate the ceramic fiber may be exposed to airborne fiber components and should wear respiratory protection or perform such work in appropriately hooded work stations. Air flows should be adjusted so that the fiber products are not released into the environment at levels exceeding the threshold limit value.

Care should be taken to electrically ground the entire manufacturing process from start to finish. This precaution, however, may not be totally necessary, because the sodium azide propellant is not very static sensitive. Ignition of sodium azide requires 250 times the Department of Defense standard for electrostatic discharge sensitivity. No fire or explosive accident involving sodium azide–based propellant has been clearly linked to electrostatic discharge. Nonetheless, explosions and fatalities do occur in airbag manufacturing plants.

MEDICAL MONITORING

Not all workers in the manufacture of airbags need to be medically monitored. Only those employees whose jobs require the use of respirators—that is, those directly involved in the manufacture, grinding, pressing, and to a lesser extent, the packaging of the explosive components—require monitoring. The only additional job classification personnel that would require such monitoring would be those working around ceramic fiber. The current industry standard would dictate that all of the above classifications of employees need to have periodic respirator examinations.

The American National Standard for Respiratory Protection-Respirator Use specifies that any employee who is required to wear a respirator in the course of his or her duties must be appropriately medically monitored. Industrial hygienists and safety engineers must establish the type of respirator indicated for the particular components being used. The physician will then classify each employee as class I, II, or III. Class I individuals have no restrictions on respirator use. Class II individuals have some restrictions. Class III individuals are restricted from respirator use. The physician must perform a medical evaluation, stressing cardiac, pulmonary, auditory, and psychological factors. The employee must be examined for facial deformities, adequate hearing, tympanic membrane ruptures, adequate respiratory and cardiovascular function, endocrine disorders, neurologic disorders, and psychological conditions.

Assessment is necessary of any medications that the employee may be taking, including legal and illegal drugs and alcohol. Generally, the physician will want to perform spirometry and may occasionally require an exercise stress test, depending on the type of respirator used and the conditions under which the use occurs, as well as the employee's physical condition. These examinations may be repeated as often as the physician feels necessary, but generally this type of examination is not required any more frequently than every 5 years in those younger than age 35 years, with exams every 2 years in those age 35 to 45 years, and annually thereafter. More frequent examinations may be necessary for employees who smoke, have known lung disease, or have cardiac disease. Examination on termination is usually advisable, as well as on return from prolonged absences or disability (21a).

Workers who have potential skin or inhalation exposure to sodium azide should have periodic blood pressure screening. Hypertensive individuals should be identified, and their blood pressure should be monitored weekly. Other individuals not found to be hypertensive initially should be monitored weekly for 4 weeks until a baseline is obtained, then every 2 to 4 weeks thereafter. Monitoring is for the purpose of identifying hypotension, which may or may not be symptomatic in individuals exposed to sodium azide.

Individuals with heart disease or who are at high risk for heart disease should be restricted from working with sodium azide and potassium nitrate. Both of these chemicals potentially could exacerbate preexisting cardiac conditions.

Preplacement physicals should be performed on all workers in these areas to identify cardiac, pulmonary, dermatologic, neurologic, and any other medical conditions that might place a worker at increased risk in this environment.

As with any plant environment, periodic audiograms should be performed in any areas identified as noisy or borderline noisy. Noise-level monitoring in a work environment should be routinely performed as good industrial hygiene and safety practice dictates.

CUMULATIVE TRAUMA DISORDERS

In this era of prevalence and concern for cumulative trauma disorders, no discussion of any manufacturing process would be complete without some mention of this problem. The automobile airbag industry, like most industries, involves some jobs that require repetitive use of the upper extremities. Most of the positions within the automobile airbag industry are automated, so that repetitive use of the hands and wrists is minimal. One area of concern, however, is a very traditional function—that of sewing. In some plants, the airbags themselves are hand sewn by workers sitting or standing at an industrial sewing machine. This work usually involves repeated ulnar and radial deviation of the hands throughout an 8-hour day. There is also some flexion and prolonged gripping in this process. Individuals with histories of carpal tunnel syndrome; tendinitis; or neck, shoulder, and elbow problems should be restricted from duty in this area. Individuals who become symptomatic with any of these problems while working in the sewing area should be taken off work or transferred, at least temporarily, to a different function within the plant. The module assembly operation also has ergonomic implications, considering the repetitive use of the hands and arms.

SUMMARY

The automobile airbag industry is a uniquely new manufacturing process using several potentially hazardous chemicals (see Table 36-1). As the deployment of airbags progresses under federal mandate, this industry will grow, and new work-related and non–work-related medical conditions will most probably be identified. There are considerable concerns as to the safety of airbag deployment for children riding in the front seat of vehicles. There are also a number of other injuries and fatalities caused by airbag deployment. Occasional mild toxicologic problems occur after deployment in rare cases. Overall, the automobile airbag saves a great many more lives than it costs, even though definable morbidity and mortality are associated with its use. New versions and designs of the classic airbag may significantly decrease some of the problems associated with it.

REFERENCES

1. Lund AK, Ferguson SA. Driver fatalities in 1985–1993 cars with airbags. *J Trauma* 1995;38:469–475.
2. Canada joins search for solutions. *USA Today* 1996;15(73):2B.
3. Wanted: smart air bags. *USA Today* 1996;15(73):1B.
4. Lott AL. Material safety data sheet—airbag inflators/module. In: *TRW safety systems*. Mesa, AZ: 1989.
5. Klein-Schwartz W, Gorman RL, Oderda GM, Massaro BP, Kurt TL, Garriott JC. Three fatal sodium azide poisonings. *Med Toxicol Adverse Drug Exp* 1989;4:219–227.
6. Smith RP, Louis CA, Kruszyna R, Kruszyna H. Acute neurotoxicity of sodium azide and nitric oxide. *Fundam Appl Toxicol* 1991;17:120–127.
7. Abrams A, El-Mallakh JL, Meyer R. Suicidal sodium azide ingestion. *Ann Emerg Med* 1987;16:1378–1380.
8. Layne RD. Sodium azide exposure from canisters used to inflate safety air bags. Washington: Occupational Safety and Health Administration, 1989.
9. Gordon SM, Drachman J, Bland LA, Reid MH, Favero M, Jarvis WR. Epidemic hypotension in a dialysis center caused by sodium azide. *Kidney Int* 1990;37:110–115.
10. Smith RP, Wilcox DE. Toxicology of selected nitric oxide-donating xenobiotics, with particular reference to azide. *Crit Rev Toxicol* 1994;24:355–377.
11. Judge KW, Ward NE. Fatal azide-induced cardiomyopathy presenting as acute myocardial infarction. *Am J Cardiol* 1989;64:830–831.
12. Sodium azide. Material safety data sheets; 1989. [EXP 0064/88D].
13. Kaplita PV, Borison HL, McCarthy LE, Smith RP. Peripheral and central actions of sodium azide on circulatory and respiratory homeostasis in anesthetized cats. *J Pharmacol Exp Ther* 1984;231:189–196.
14. Abrams A, El-Mallakh JL, Meyer R. Suicidal sodium azide ingestion. *Ann Emerg Med* 1987;16:1378–1380.
15. Fung VA, Huff J, Weisburger EK, Hoel DG. Predictive strategies for selecting 379 NCI/NTP chemicals evaluated for carcinogenic potential: scientific and public health impact. *Fundam Appl Toxicol* 1993;20:413–436.
16. Sana TR, Ferm VH, Smith RP. Sodium azide (NaN_3) has weak teratogenic effects in the golden hamster. *Toxicology* 1990;10:124.
17. O'Donoghue JL. Carbon monoxide, inorganic nitrogenous compounds, and phosphorus. In: O'Donoghue JL, ed. *Neurotoxicity of industrial and commercial chemicals*, vol 1. Boca Raton, FL: CRC Press, 1985:193–203.
18. Miyoshi K. Experimental striatal necrosis induced by sodium azide. *Acta Neuropathol (Berl)* 1967;9:199–216.
19. Mettler FA, Sax DS. Cerebellar cortical degeneration due to acute azide poisoning. *Brain* 1972;95:505–516.
20. Bennett MC, Rose GM. Chronic sodium azide treatment impairs learning of the Morris water maze task. *Behav Neural Biol* 1992;58:72–75.
21. Fiberfax Material safety data sheets. The Carborundum Company—Fibers Division; 1980. [MSDS no AVP/B07-2].

21a. American National Standards Institute. American national standard for respiratory protection—respirator use—physical qualifications for personnel. New York, NY: ANSI, 1984.

22. Single base smokeless powder. Material safety data sheets. Exbro Chemical Products Company; 1988.
23. Pietz JF. Problem considerations of using sodium azide in the air cushion restraint system. In: *Talley industries of Arizona*. Mesa, AZ: 1978. [Report no 11988].
24. Schreck RM, Rouhana SW, Santrock J, et al. Physical and chemical characterization of airbag effluents. *J Trauma* 1995;38:528–532.
25. Dalmotas DJ, et al. Airbag deployments: the Canadian experience. *J Trauma* 1995;38:476–481.
26. Onwuzuruigbo CJ, Fulda GJ, Larned D, Hailstone D, et al. Traumatic blindness after airbag deployment: bilateral lenticular dislocation. *J Trauma* 1996;40:314–316.
27. Burgess AR, Dischinger PC, O'Quinn TD, Schmidhauser CB. Lower extremity injuries in drivers of airbag-equipped automobiles: clinical and crash reconstruction correlations. *J Trauma* 1995;38:509–516.
28. From the Centers for Disease Control and Prevention. Air-bag–associated fatal injuries to infants and children riding in front passenger seats—United States. *JAMA* 1995;22:1752–1753.
29. Swanson-Biearman B, Mrvos R, Dean BS, Krenzelok EP. Air bags: lifesaving with toxic potential? *Am J Emerg Med* 1993;11:38–39.
30. Smally AJ, Binzer A, Dolin S, Viano D. Alkaline chemical keratitis: eye injury from airbags. *Ann Emerg Med* 1992;21:1400–1402.
31. Gross KB, Haidar AH, Basha MA, et al. Acute pulmonary response of asthmatics to aerosols and gases generated by airbag deployment. *Am J Respir Crit Care Med* 1994;150:408–414.

CHAPTER 37
Aerospace Industry Exposure Hazards

Bradley Y. Dennis

Aerospace manufacturing and repair present numerous potential hazardous exposures. Many workers and employers are unaware of these health risks.

This chapter deals primarily with advanced composites and solvents but also covers other common chemical hazards found in the aerospace industry. Specific health and safety information concerning several chemicals is provided. It also is important to consider basic health and safety issues. Hazardous exposure may occur through oral ingestion, dermal contact, or inhalation. Because the industrial setting does not lend itself to frequent oral ingestion, data from skin contact and inhalation studies are more relevant than readily available information on the oral toxicity of a compound.

Regardless of a substance's hazard or toxicity, careful steps should be taken when handling any chemical to minimize individual exposure. If chemicals are handled correctly, even the most toxic substances pose little hazard to the worker.

Material-safety data sheets furnished by a supplier are helpful. Control measures also are available to ensure a safe work environment on an individual basis. For instance, administrative controls are provisions made by a company's management to control hazards. They include material handling, training, isolation of operations (lunch areas separated from work areas), personal protective equipment, personal hygiene (hand washing before eating, drinking, and smoking), warning labels, housekeeping, work practices for chemical storage and transportation, and emergency instructions. Engineering controls, such as closed-system processing and effective ventilation, should provide, as nearly as possible, complete containment of dusts, fumes, and vapors from hazardous materials. When general ventilation is not sufficient to control airborne exposures, engineering controls, such as local exhaust ventilation at the emission source, should be provided and supplemented by personal protective equipment, when necessary.

Workers should not be exposed to airborne contaminants in excess of threshold limit values set by the American Conference of Governmental Industrial Hygienists or the Occupational Safety and Health Administration (OSHA) permissible exposure limits. Air monitoring of personal breathing zones should be considered to establish baseline exposure levels, with periodic assessments in areas where toxic chemicals are processed, unusual odors exist, or heavier than normal visible contamination appears.

ADVANCED COMPOSITES

A composite is a material made from several components. An early example of a composite is reinforced concrete, in which a reinforcement is embedded in a type of matrix. A composite is expected to have mechanical properties superior to those of its components. The 1950s saw the modern era of composite materials begin with the introduction of metal alloys, fiberglass, and plastics. Lightweight materials with increased strength, stiffness, and resistance to high temperatures were not introduced until the more recent development of carbon and graphite fiber composites. Since the early 1980s, use of carbon and graphite composites has increased significantly in sports equipment, industrial machinery, medical prostheses, and, especially, the aerospace industry.

Advanced composites consist of carbon or graphite fibers bound in a resin matrix, which provides the insulation and physical-resistance properties of composites. The resin matrix that binds the fibers may consist of different substances such as epoxy, polyester, polyacetal, polyethylene, and polystyrene. The most commonly used resin is epoxy, which is usually derived from diglycidyl ether of bisphenol A (DGBA) or from a non-bisphenol A epoxy such as 4-glycidiloxy-*N*,*N*-diglycidilaniline. Epoxy resins are reacted with curing agents to solidify the epoxy and convert it to a thermoset plastic.

The primary concerns in the production, machining, and maintenance of advanced composites involve the release of low-molecular-weight and high-vapor-pressure compounds. These compounds include solvents, reactive diluents, epoxies, and hardeners released during preimpregnation or evaporation from the stored preimpregnation material. In addition, inhalation of carbon fibers and dust can occur during grinding and cutting. Dermal exposure with potential skin sensitization or contact dermatitis and local eye and skin irritation are possible.

TOXICOLOGIC PROPERTIES OF COMPOSITES

Epoxy Resins

Propylene and chlorine react to form epichlorohydrin, which is mixed with bisphenol A, a backbone chemical formed from acetone and phenol. Epichlorohydrin and bisphenol A form a glycidyl group, which is reacted with hardeners or curing agents (normally amines) to produce epoxy resin for preimpregnating fibers (Fig. 37-1). The term *epoxy* is applied to compounds containing one or more oxirane rings. The term *prepreg* defines sheets of pyrolized carbon fibers impregnated with a liquid binder, such as epoxy resin, then reacted with a curing agent to solidify the epoxy, convert it to a thermoset plastic, and mold into a desired shape. Approximately 30% to 45% of prepreg is resin, and 1% to 10% is solvent.

Almost all bisphenol A–based epoxy resins contain less than 1 part per million (ppm) residual epichlorohydrin. The Chemical Abstracts Service notes a threshold limit value, permissible-exposure limit, and time-weighted average of 2 ppm and carries a "skin" notation. Care should be taken with any resin containing epichlorohydrin because the International Agency for Research on Cancer (IARC) has classified it as a probable human carcinogen (group 2A) based on animal data (1), and the National Toxicology Program (NTP) has classified it as a substance anticipated to be carcinogenic (2). The IARC has decided that insufficient data exist to classify DGBA as a potential carcinogen (3).

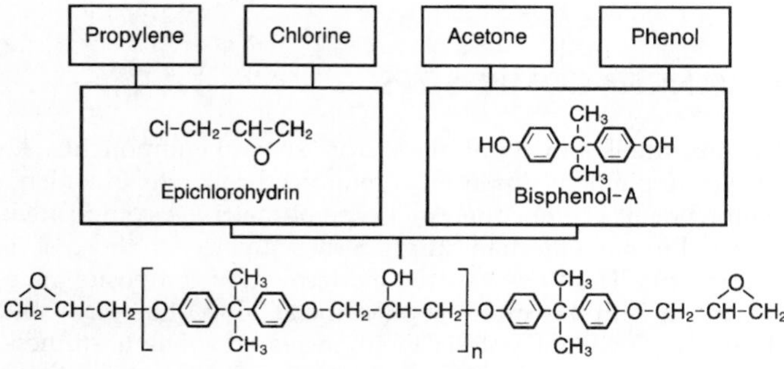

Figure 37-1. Manufacturing process for bis A-based epoxy resins.

Epoxy resins formed from bisphenol A and epichlorohydrin have a low order of acute toxicity and cause only slight to moderate skin irritation. Rarely, individuals develop a skin sensitivity. Chronic dermal application of DGBA on mice did not cause skin cancer, nor did it cause any hematologic or clinical chemistry changes (4–6). Bisphenol F epoxy resins cause minor skin and eye irritation and are thought to be toxicologically similar to bisphenol A resins.

Cycloaliphatic epoxy resins have an irritant effect on the skin and mucous membranes but most are not considered mutagenic. Neither NTP, IARC, nor OSHA considers them carcinogenic. However, animal studies indicate a possible carcinogenic effect for certain cycloaliphatic epoxy resins. Precautionary measures should be followed carefully when handling these products. Cycloaliphatic glycidyl ethers and esters irritate the skin and mucous membranes and may have a sensitizing effect. Neopentylglycol diglycidyl ether has been reported to cause skin tumors with chronic exposure to shaved mice skin (7).

Polyurethane Resins

Polyurethane resins consist of isocyanates and polyols. Most commercial isocyanates are highly toxic through skin absorption with systemic toxicity or skin and lung sensitization. Proper ventilation is a necessity because of the high inhalation toxicity. Respiratory sensitization has also been described for some isocyanate exposure.

Toluene diisocyanate (TDI) has a threshold limit value, time-weighted average (TLV-TWA) of 0.005 ppm and a TLV–short-term exposure limit (TLV-STEL) of 0.02 ppm. Permissible exposure limits (PELs) are set at the same levels. Because TDI has no odor-warning characteristics, it is hazardous in vapor or liquid forms and causes skin and respiratory sensitization. Some cross-reactivity may occur with other isocyanates. Once sensitization occurs, even a few hundredths of a ppm causes recurrent allergic reaction. TDI is a strong skin and eye irritant. Prolonged contact with skin causes burns. Exposure to high vapor concentrations may cause pulmonary edema.

TDI has been classified as possibly carcinogenic by IARC (group 2B), based on animal but no human data (8). This classification has been criticized for its poorly conducted oral intubation route of administration, high test doses used, and lack of characterization of the test substance in the body. A study using an inhalation administration did not confirm the earlier NTP study findings (9).

Polyols include polyether and polyester and are used for cross-linking isocyanate compounds. They provide no health hazard other than the occasional presence of unreacted ethylene oxide in some polyols used in poorly ventilated work areas.

Phenolic and Amino Resins

Phenol-, urea-, and melamine-formaldehyde resins have a low toxicity potential. However, contact with the phenol-formaldehyde resin in the uncured state should be avoided because of potential phenol absorption through the skin. Small amounts of formaldehyde and phenol also may be given off during the curing process, which requires good ventilation.

The current TLV-TWA for formaldehyde is 1 ppm, with a STEL of 2 ppm. The permissible exposure limit TWA (PEL-TWA) for formaldehyde is 1 ppm, with a STEL of 2 ppm. Formaldehyde is a strong skin sensitizer and an eye, skin, and respiratory irritant (10). Formaldehyde is an animal carcinogen but study results are inconclusive in humans.

Bismaleimide Resins

Bismaleimide resins (polyimides) have not been studied extensively. Prolonged or repeated skin contact has been reported to cause irritation or sensitization, and dust may cause eye, nose, and throat irritation.

Thermoplastics

Other than the styrene group of thermoplastics (polystyrene), these compounds are not considered harmful to humans. Most cause no toxic effects by ingestion, skin contact, or inhalation. The styrene monomer is of concern because its vapors can cause eye irritation, and liquid exposure causes eye, skin, and mucous membrane irritation. Central nervous system (CNS), liver, and kidney effects also have been reported (11). Styrene sickness, a syndrome characterized by drowsiness, dizziness, nausea, and headache, has been reported in workers exposed to 200 to 700 ppm styrene (11). The styrene monomer has been labeled "possibly carcinogenic to humans" by IARC based on limited animal studies (12).

Hardeners and Curing Agents

Aromatic amine hardeners are slightly irritating to skin and mucous membranes. Inhalation has been shown to cause damage to internal organs, such as the liver, and may form methemoglobin to decrease the blood's oxygen-transporting ability. Methylene dianiline, 4,4-methylene dianiline (MDA) has a TLV-TWA of 0.1 ppm with a recommended PEL of 0.01 ppm. Chronic exposure is capable of causing liver damage in humans after oral or dermal exposure (11,13). NTP has classified MDA to be a carcinogen, but no confirmed reports exist of MDA-related cancer in humans.

The manufacturer's prepregging and "B-staging" operations usually markedly decrease any free MDA that may be present in an amine-cured, epoxy resin system. Although no free MDA is likely to be detected in cured laminates, it is recommended that a high-efficiency particulate air-filtered, ventilated, hand tool be considered for cutting and trimming MDA-containing prepregs instead of stripping and peeling by hand. 4,4-Sulfonyl dianiline (Dapsone, DDS) has no established workplace standards. No history or evidence exists of human carcinogenicity with this substance (14).

Aliphatic and cycloaliphatic amine hardeners are strong bases and should be considered severe irritants or corrosives. Some also are sensitizers. Polyaminoamide hardeners have a slightly irritating effect on skin but may cause sensitization. Amide hardeners are only slight irritants. Anhydride curing agents are severe eye irritants and strong skin irritants. Good ventilation is necessary for work areas where these curing agents are used.

Solvents

Preparation of composite materials requires the use of solvents at numerous stages; during the manufacture of the basic resin and fibers, while impregnating reinforcements, and in tool- and work-area cleanup. Skin contact with most organic solvents results in drying, defatting, and dermatitis. Because some solvents are absorbed through the skin, an additional potential hazard exists when other materials are dissolved and carried through the skin with the solvent. For instance, although it should never be allowed, solvents are occasionally used to remove sticky epoxy resins from the skin, which may facilitate the penetration of epoxy resin into the body (10,15).

Inhalation of solvent vapors may cause delayed pulmonary edema, respiratory irritation, and CNS depression with narcosis, incoordination, dizziness, unconsciousness, and even death.

Ketone Solvents

Acetone has a TLV and PEL-TWA of 750 ppm and a TLV and a PEL-STEL of 1,000 ppm. Inhalation may cause mucous membrane irritation, nausea, and headache. Skin contact can cause defatting and dermatitis. Systemic injury probably does not occur with skin absorption but repeated exposure to high levels of acetone may cause CNS depression.

Methyl ethyl ketone (MEK) has TLV- and PEL-TWAs of 200 ppm and TLV and PEL-STELs of 300 ppm. MEK causes nose, throat, and eye irritation above 200 ppm (11). A recognizable odor is noted at the TLV for MEK, but few serious health effects have been reported at this level (11). Minor embryo- and fetotoxic effects have been observed in female rats exposed to MEK levels greater than 1,000 ppm (16).

Chlorinated Solvents

Exposure to very high concentrations of halogenated hydrocarbon solvents have been reported to cause CNS depression and cardiac muscle sensitization. Animal studies have demonstrated liver and kidney changes with chronic exposure. Two separate case-control studies have suggested a possible association of chlorinated organic solvents used in de-icer and fuel cell manufacturing with excess lung cancer (17,18).

Methylene chloride (dichloromethane) has a TLV-TWA of 50 ppm. OSHA has established a PEL of 500 ppm with an acceptable ceiling concentration of 1,000 ppm. Exposure to methylene chloride vapors well above the TLV may cause CNS depression but use at or below the TLV has caused no adverse health effects (11). Liquid methylene chloride may cause eye and skin irritation, and high concentrations of vapors may cause respiratory irritation. Methylene chloride is metabolized to carbon monoxide, forming carboxyhemoglobin, thus decreasing the body's ability to carry oxygen to the tissues. Studies have shown that methylene chloride causes cancer in animals. NTP has concluded that methylene chloride is carcinogenic in rodents, based on inhalation studies (19). Methylene chloride appears to be a genotoxic carcinogen, exerting its effect through direct chemical interaction between itself or one of its metabolic products and genetic structures of the cell (20).

New toxicokinetic studies, which reduce reliance on animal experiments and provide a more systematic approach to hazard evaluation, have found that the conventional research approach overestimates the human risk from methylene chloride by a factor of 100. Because of the discrepancy between the toxicokinetic approach and conventional risk assessment, the U.S. Environmental Protection Agency (EPA) has reconsidered its rule making for methylene chloride.

1,1,1-Trichloroethane (methylchloroform) has TLV- and PEL-TWAs of 350 ppm. The TLV and PEL-STELs are 450 ppm. Trichloroethane generally is less toxic than methylene chloride, and exposure of humans to 500 ppm for 7 hours per day for 5 days showed no evidence of abnormal clinical findings (11). Severe overexposure can cause CNS depression, which may lead to respiratory arrest. But rapid and complete recovery usually follows if the victim is alive when removed from exposure (21). Overexposure also is reported to cause fat deposits and necrosis in the liver and occasional kidney damage (22). Alcohol should be avoided before, during, and after trichloroethane exposure because both are metabolized by the liver. This solvent is not teratogenic and carcinogenicity and mutagenicity testing has proven inconclusive (23).

Other solvents include dimethylformamide (DMF) and *N*-methylpyrrolidone (NMP). DMF has a TLV- and PEL-TWA of 10 ppm (skin). It is irritating to the eyes, skin, and mucous membranes. Overexposure may cause nausea, abdominal pain, loss of appetite, and possible liver damage (11). IARC has classified DMF as possibly carcinogenic to humans (group 2B), based on controversial studies linking DMF to the development of testicular cancer (24,25). NMP has a TWA of 100 ppm (vapor). It can cause dermatitis with blistering, edema, and erythema with prolonged or repeated contact. It is not a skin sensitizer. Vapor contact may cause eye irritation (26). No teratogenicity has been noted in animal studies.

REINFORCING MATERIALS

Reinforcement materials are added to the resin matrix of advanced composites to provide strength to the cured material. Once the composite is produced, exposure is limited to that encountered during drilling, grinding, and sanding operations.

Dusts generated during such operations should be controlled by nuisance dust standards. Based on chemical and morphologic studies showing high chemical stability of composites, and the fact that most secondary products from machining composites are particulate rather than fibrous, it is more important to consider the size and shape of the particles than the resin chemical or fabric composition (27).

The difference between total and respirable dust should be considered. Particles smaller than 3.5 μm in diameter can reach deeper areas of the lung. Particles larger than 10 μm in diameter cannot reach the deep lung tissues. These particles are not considered respirable. Dusts with a mean aerodynamic diameter of 3.5 μm or less are considered respirable (28).

Carbon and Graphite Fibers

Carbon fibers can be made from any carbonaceous, fibrous raw material that pyrolyzes to a char and leaves a high carbon residue. Early carbon fibers were made from rayon but are now made from polyacrylonitrile or petroleum pitch. The precursor is heated to 1,200°C to produce a carbon fiber and 2,200° to 2,700°C to produce a graphite fiber. These carbon-based fibers provide the strength of composites, as graphite fibers are 1.5 to 2.0 times stronger than steel.

The TLV-TWA for synthetic forms of graphite has been established at 10 mg per m^3. Natural graphite is to be controlled to 2.5 mg per m^3 (respirable dust), but proposals are being considered to specify 10 mg per m^3 for all forms of graphite, natural and synthetic. No established limits have been set for carbon fibers, although the U.S. Navy has established a limit of 3 carbon fibers per cm^3. As a minimum, the OSHA nuisance dust standard of 10 mg per m^3 total dust, 5 mg per m^3 respirable fraction, should not be exceeded. The size of carbon fibers produced by machining of composites is considered too large to be damaging to the respiratory system, but it does cause mechanical abrasion and irritation of the skin and eyes (29). Allergic or sensitizing reactions are not reported to occur when handling unsized carbon or graphite fibers (30,31).

Animal studies found no tumors or scar tissue in the lungs of guinea pigs after significant exposure to carbon fibers (32). The EPA found insufficient data to classify the carcinogenic potential of carbon fibers (33).

Aramid fiber (Kevlar) is another type of reinforcing material. DuPont has established an acceptable exposure limit of 5 respirable fibers per cm^3. Aramid fiber is not a sensitizer and shows only occasional mild irritation of skin. Animal inhalation studies show little evidence of lung damage. The EPA found insufficient data to classify aramid fibers as a possible human carcinogen (34).

Fiberglass is a type of human-made fiber that is supplied in two basic forms: textile (continuous filament) fibers and wool-type fibers used in insulation. The TLV-TWA for fiberglass dust is 10 mg per m^3. OSHA has not established a PEL, but a TWA of 15 mg per m^3 of total dust and 5 mg per m^3 of respirable fraction is presently used. The National Institute of Occupational Safety and Health is pursuing a standard level of 3 fibers per cm^3.

The continuous filament fibers used in composite reinforcement differ from the wool-type in that all textile fibers are greater than 6 μm in diameter and thus are nonrespirable (35). The glass fibers may break into shorter lengths, but their diameter will not permit them into the deep lung areas. Fiberglass itself causes only mechanical irritation of the eyes, nose, and throat, but skin sensitization may occur from the uncured resins and hardeners used to manufacture the reinforced laminate. Human and animal studies have failed to demonstrate a cancer risk, and the IARC has categorized continuous filament fiberglass as not classifiable for human carcinogenicity. Fiberglass wool was classified as a possible human carcinogen by IARC, based on animal studies using nonnatural routes of exposure such as injection or implantation (35).

Ceramic fibers are another reinforcement material with no specific TLV or OSHA PEL. Ceramic fibers may cause temporary local skin or respiratory irritation. No studies are available on the health effects from exposure to ceramic fibers in humans.

Composite Hazard Controls

Proper ventilation systems are most important in controlling potential composite hazards. Dilution ventilation, such as open hangars, are probably inadequate. Paint booths are often inadequate because the filters become saturated quickly by the dust concentration generated. In addition, makeup air volumes are often too small. Aerospace manufacturers traditionally have a metallic background, and older facilities have ventilation systems designed for metallic rather than chemical use.

Composite machining should be performed, when possible, in shops dedicated to this operation. A two-room format should be considered with lay-up operations performed in a room ventilated for solvents. A separate room should be used for machining of composites where full body coveralls (preferably disposable), side-shield safety glasses, and gloves provide skin protection.

Local exhaust ventilation should be used to remove composite particulates. An exhaust hood designed for air flow to be drawn from under a sanding operation is preferable. A direct tool attachment with high-velocity, low-volume exhaust, or plastic bags designed to fit around or near the tool in use also are acceptable.

Dust masks are adequate respiratory protection for most operations. The National Institute for Occupational Safety and Health respirator selection guide should be consulted for airborne concentrations above acceptable exposure levels. When very small composite particulates in the 0.5- to 1.0-μm range are generated, the use of high-efficiency, particulate air filters should be considered. A high-efficiency vacuum system is a very helpful general housekeeping tool for eliminating significant proportions of dust and fibers. Compressed air should not be used to blow dust off workers. Hand washing should be mandated, and hands, arms, and face should be thoroughly washed before eating.

Repair Material Toxicity

Composite repair materials include polymers, such as adhesives and prepregs, and aerosol coatings. Repairs may take place in the manufacturing facility, in depots, or in the field. The potential routes of exposure are the same as those for composite fabrication and include skin contact, inhalation, and ingestion.

Polymers

Polymeric materials may be staged into three categories. The A stage is an early stage in the preparation of thermosetting resins in which the material is still soluble in certain liquids and fusible. Monomeric reactants are present, and health concern is highest in this stage, especially for two-part, room temperature adhesives. The B stage is an intermediate stage in the reaction of thermoset resins in which the material swells and softens in contact with liquids and softens when heated but may not dissolve or fuse. B-stage materials are partially polymerized into long chain molecules and are less chemically reactive. Health concern is moderate in this stage, which includes epoxy and condensation polyimide prepregs and most film and foam adhesives. The C stage is the final, fully cured state of composites and adhesives. No chemical reactivity exists, and the health concern is for dust from machining and sanding.

More than 90% of polymeric materials used are epoxy. They include a glycidyl ether family, mild pulmonary and eye irritation from dusts and vapors, and potential for sensitization with exposure to uncured resin. Epoxy paste adhesive is 100% resin and has a similar chemistry to the epoxy prepregs and adhesives. It is important to keep in mind that mixing paste adhesives in batches greater than 1 lb may result in an exothermic reaction in the container, thus releasing toxic gases.

Polyimide polymer materials also include prepregs, film adhesives, and paste adhesives. These materials also are occasionally used in high-tech, advanced-composite repair work. The condensation polyimide prepreg has a low toxicity in B stage, but mild irritation and dark staining of the skin may occur. Polyimide film adhesive (B stage) may cause moderate skin and eye irritation. The presence of xylene may act as a pulmonary irritant, and silica may cause lung injury. Polyimide paste adhesive (A stage) contains MDA, which may cause liver damage. Silica and xylene are also found in the paste adhesive, as well as ethanol, which acts as a CNS depressant.

The skin route of entry for the polymeric repair materials is of concern only in the A and B stages. It is prevented by using nonpermeable gloves and shop coats that can be cleaned frequently. Protective clothing is especially important during the lay-up of prepregs or adhesive mixing operations. Inhalation occurs with the low volatility of B-stage polymers, the higher volatility of A-stage products, and C-stage dust from machining and sanding operations. Proper ventilation or outdoor work help prevent inhalation toxicity. Manufacturing and depot areas must have ventilation systems suited to chemical, not metal, operations. All polymers should be cured under vacuum bags with a carbon filter on an exhaust hose. Respirators should be worn to prevent dust inhalation. Ingestion has a very low probability of occurring.

Coating Repairs

Coatings are applied as respirable aerosols, usually within paint booths or paint hangars. They are more toxic than polymer materials because they contain lead in topcoats, chromium (Cr^{+6}) in primers and topcoats, methylene chloride in solvents, diisocyanates in urethane topcoats, and MDA in a few topcoats. Coatings may enter the body more easily than polymer materials and protective clothing is less effective.

Plating: Surface Preparation Operations

Potential exposures in plating include cadmium, chromium, and nickel. Plasma spraying can cause a potential exposure to chromium. A high risk of ground water contamination exists from repeated spills in plating operations. Risk assessment may be required for cadmium and chromium.

Paint Strippers

Paint strippers are potentially exposed to several solvents such as dioxane, methylene chloride, ethylene dichloride, phenol, toluene, xylene, and trichloroethylene. All depainting operations should be performed in paint booths, using catch basins to eliminate the potential for sewer runoff. Exposure to methylene chloride may require a risk assessment performance.

Controlled Chemicals

States such as California are beginning to develop strict laws to control certain chemical exposures. California has adopted Proposition 65, the Safe Drinking Water and Toxic Enforcement Act of 1986 which controls known or suspected carcinogenic air contaminants. Because so many aerospace manufacturers are located in California, a list of controlled chemicals and their typical use is provided (36) (Table 37-1).

Administrative controls to ensure employee education in proper maintenance and cleanup methods and correct use of personal protective equipment and respirators are important. Material Safety Data Sheets should be made available to personnel.

TABLE 37-1. Controlled chemicals

Chemical	Prop. 65	Typical use
Acetaldehyde	X	Solvent-structural adhesives
Acrylamide		Adhesives
Acrylonitrile	X	Acrylic and elastomers
Allyl chloride		Resin for varnish/plastic/adhesive
Benzene	X	Solvent-phenol prepregs
Benzidene	X	Stiffening agent-rubber
1,3-Butadiene	X	Synthetic elastomers
Cadmium	X	CD plating-ceramics
Chlorobenzene		Solvent-methylene diisocyanate
Chloroform	X	Laboratory solvent
Chromium (hexavalent)	X	Paints-plating
Dichlorobenzidene		Cure agent-urethanes
Diethanolamine		Cutting oils-detergent for emulsion paints
Dioxane		Lacquers/paints/strippers
Epichlorohydrin	X	Epoxy prepregs-resins
Ethylene dichloride		Paint strippers
Formaldehyde	X	Phenol prepregs
Lead	X	Paints
Maleic anhydride		Polyester resins
Methylene chloride	X	Solvent-paints
4-4'-Methylene dianiline	X	Polyamide prepregs
Nickel		Plating-paints
Phenol		Phenolic prepregs
Propylene oxide		Polyols for urethane foams
Titanium oxide		White pigment in paints
Toluene		Solvent-paints
Trichloroethylene		Solvent-paints
Xylene		Solvent-paints
Urethane	X	Elastomers-paints

Data from South Coast Air Quality Management District in Los Angeles, with permission.

REFERENCES

1. International Agency for Research on Cancer. Overall evaluations of carcinogenicity: an updating of IARC monographs volumes 1 to 42. *IARC Monogr Eval Carcinog Risks Hum Suppl* 1987;7.
2. National Toxicology Program. Fourth annual report on carcinogens: summary. Washington: US Department of Health and Human Services, Public Health Service, 1985. [NTP 85-002].
3. International Agency for Research on Cancer. Vol 47. Organic solvents, some resin monomers, some pigments, and occupational exposures in the painting trades. Lyon, France: WHO, International Agency for Research on Cancer, 1989.
4. Holland JM, et al. *Chronic dermal toxicity of epoxy resins. I. Skin carcinogenic potency and general toxicity.* Oak Ridge, TN: Oak Ridge National Laboratory, 1981. [ORNL 5762 special].
5. Holland JM, et al. *Test of carcinogenicity in mouse skin: methylenedianiline, gamma-glycidyloxytrimethyloxysilane, gamma-aminopropyltriethoxysilane and a mixture of m-phenylenediamine, methylenedianiline and diglycidylether of bisphenol-A.* Oak Ridge, TN: Oak Ridge National Laboratory, 1987. [ORNL/TM-10472].
6. Zakova N, Zak F, Froehlich E, Hess R. Evaluation of skin carcinogenicity of technical 2,2-bis-(*p*-glycidyloxyphenyl)-propane in CF1 mice. *Food Chem Toxicol* 1985;23:1081–1089.
7. US Environmental Protection Agency 8EHQ-0481-0397 and 8EHQ-0481-0397S. In: Preliminary evaluations of initial TSCA section 8(e) substantial risk notifications; February 1, 1980 to December 31, 1982. EPA 560/2-83-001. Environmental Protection Agency, 1983.
8. International Agency for Research on Cancer. Some chemicals used in plastics and elastomers. *IARC Monogr Eval Carcinog Risk Hum* 1986;39.
9. Loeser E. Long-term toxicity and carcinogenicity studies with 2,4/2,6-toluene diisocyanate (80/20) in rats and mice. *Toxcol Lett* 1983;15:71–81.
10. Greenblatt M. Formaldehyde toxicology: a review of recent developments. *Proc Int Cong Role Formaldehyde Biol Syst* 1987;2:53–59.
11. American Conference of Governmental Industrial Hygienists. *Documentation of the threshold limit values and biological exposure indices*, 5th ed. Cincinnati: American Conference of Governmental Industrial Hygienists, 1988.
12. International Agency for Research on Cancer. Overall evaluations of carcinogenicity: an updating of IARC monographs volumes 1 to 42. *IARC Monogr Eval Carcinog Risk Hum Suppl* 1987;7.
13. Kopelman H, Robertson MH, Sanders PG, Ash I. The Epping jaundice. *BMJ* 1966;1:514–516.
14. Mandell GL, Sande MA. Antimicrobial agents (continued): drugs used in the chemotherapy of tuberculosis and leprosy. In: Gilman AG, Goodman LS, Gilman A, eds. *Goodman and Gilman's the pharmacological basis of therapeutics*, 8th ed. New York: Macmillan, 1990.
15. Clayton GD, Clayton FE. *Patti's industrial hygiene and toxicology*, 3rd rev ed. New York: John Wiley and Sons, 1981:2141–2159; 2217–2232.
16. Deacon MM, Pilny MD, John JA, et al. Embryo- and fetotoxicity of inhaled methyl ethyl ketone in rats. *Toxicol Appl Pharmacol* 1981;59:620–622.
17. Delzell E, Andjelkovich D, Tyroler HA. A case control study of employment experience and lung cancer among rubber workers. *Am J Ind Med* 1982;3:393–404.
18. Manson RR, Fine LJ. Cancer mortality and morbidity among rubber workers. *J Natl Cancer Inst* 1978;61:1047–1053.
19. National Toxicology Program. Toxicology and carcinogenesis studies of dichloromethane (methylene chloride) in F344/N rats and B6C3F1 mice (inhalation studies). Technical report 306. Washington: National Toxicology Program, 1986. [CAS no 75-09-2].
20. Clewell HJ, Andersen ME, MacNaughton MG, Stuart BO. Toxicokinetics: an analytical tool for assessing chemical hazards to man. *Aviat Space Environ Med* 1988;A125–A131.
21. Gosselin RE, Smith RP, Hodge HC, Braddock JE. *Clinical toxicology of commercial products*, 5th ed. Baltimore: Williams & Wilkins, 1984.
22. Prendergast JA, Jones RA, Jenkins LJ Jr, Siegel J. Effects on experimental animals of long-term inhalation of trichloroethylene, carbon tetrachloride, 1,1,1-trichloroethane, dichlorodifluoromethane, and 1,1-dichloroethylene. *Toxicol Appl Pharmacol* 1967;10:270–289.
23. US Environmental Protection Agency. Draft criteria document for 1,1,1-trichloroethane. NTIS Doc. No. PB84-199520. 1984.
24. Chen JL, Kennedy GL. Dimethylformamide and testicular cancer. *Lancet* 1988;1(8575–8576):55.
25. Levin SM, Baker DB, Landrigan PJ, et al. Testicular cancer in leather tanners exposed to dimethylformamide. *Lancet* 1987;8568:1153.
26. GAF Chemicals Corporation. *GAF Material Safety Data Sheet: M-pyrol.* Wayne, NJ: Gaf Chemicals Corporation, 1986.
27. Boatman ES, Covert D, Kalman D, Luchtel D, Omenn GS, et al. Physical morphological and chemical studies of dusts derived from the machining of composite-epoxy materials. *Environ Res* 1988;45:242–255.
28. American Conference of Governmental Industrial Hygienists. *TLVs. Threshold limit values and biological exposure indices for 1990–1991.* Cincinnati: American Conference of Governmental Industrial Hygienists, 1990–91.
29. Kowalska M. Carbon fiber reinforced epoxy prepregs and composites—health risk aspects. *SAMPE: Journal of Advanced Materials* 1982;(Jan):13–19.
30. Reference deleted by author.
31. Zumwalde RD, et al. *Carbon/graphite fibers: environmental exposures and potential health implications.* Cincinnati: National Institute of Safety and Health, Division of Surveillance, Hazard Evaluation and Field Studies, 1980.
32. Holt PF, Home M. Dust from carbon fibre. *Environ Res* 1978;17:276–283.
33. Vu V. *Health hazard assessment of nonasbestos fibers*, final draft. Washington: US Environmental Protection Agency, Health and Environmental Review Division, Office of Toxic Substances, 1988.
34. Zahr GE. DuPont comments: health hazard assessment of nonasbestos fibers (final draft). OPTS 62036E (Appended to letter from Zahr to SACMA, August 19, 1988).
35. International Agency for Research on Cancer. Man-made mineral fibres and radon. *IARC Monogr Eval Carcinog Risks Hum* 1988;43.
36. Morris VL. Repair material toxicity: a presentation to workshop on composites—Northrop Corp., B-2 Division-Materials and Processes, Los Angeles, California, March 23, 1989.

CHAPTER 38
Hazards of Biotechnology

Alan M. Ducatman, Cheryl S. Barbanel, and Daniel F. Liberman

Biotechnology is defined as the application of biological systems to technical and industrial processes. This implies the integration of a variety of biological sciences with chemical and process engineering in a way that optimizes the biological system (1). That biotechnology can play an important role in any industrial biological process or any process in which a biological catalyst can replace a chemical one (2) was clearly illustrated in the Office of Technology Assessment report (3) that examined potential industrial applications in the pharmaceutical, animal and plant, agricultural, specialty chemical, food additive, commodity chemical energy, bioelectronics, and environmental sectors. Some scientific developments with industrial applications in biotechnology are protein engineering, genetic engineering, transgenic animal development, and site-specific mutagenesis.

APPLIED MICROBIOLOGY OVERVIEW

From the beginning of recorded history, the microbe has been used by humans. *Applied microbiology* has been defined as the use of microorganisms to produce useful products for the benefit of mankind. For centuries, yeasts, molds, and bacteria were used to preserve meats, fruits, and vegetables and to enhance the quality of life with products including beverages, cheeses, bread, foods, and vinegar. Pasteur's investigation of the underlying mechanisms of these processes had a remarkable impact on the advancement of science. As a result, not only was microbiology viewed as a distinct discipline, but the development of vaccines and the concepts of hygiene, which underscore modern medicine, were advanced as well. The use of microorganisms by the Buchners led to the discovery that cell-free yeast extracts could convert sucrose to ethanol, thus giving rise to the discipline of biochemistry (4). The discoveries of penicillin and streptomycin and their subsequent commercial success marked the start of the antibiotic era. Microorganisms not only produce antibiotics, but are also used as tools in basic research and are one of the driving forces responsible for the remarkable advances in the fields of molecular genetics and molecular biology. These advances were a part of a continuous series of major developments and discoveries—for example, the development of efficient industrial processes for the manufacture of vitamins, plant growth factors, enzymes, amino acids, flavorings, polysaccharide, and single-cell protein for animal and human consumption (4).

The use of living organisms or their components in industrial processes is desirable, because microorganisms naturally produce countless substances during their lifetime. Fermentation using yeast to produce bread and beer—or bacteria and fungi to produce yogurt, cheese, sausage, soya, and sake—has been carried out for centuries. Vitamins (1930s), antibiotics (1940s), enzymes, hybrid plants (foods), and amino acids are all important products of biotechnology. Scientific discoveries in the 1940s, 1950s, and 1960s set the stages for the first successful DNA cloning experiments in 1972 (5). A number of industries have been created out of the use of microorganisms as natural factories. The cultivation of populations of cells that are selected as the best producers of certain gene products under conditions designed to enhance their abilities has resulted in a multimillion-dollar industry (see reference 6 for an extensive review). The cornerstone that forms the foundation of this industry can be traced to three characteristics of the microorganisms: the tremendous variety of reactions that microorganisms can carry out; the ability to adapt to various environments, thus allowing growth on readily available carbon and nitrogen sources in successively larger volumes; and the ability to grow and attain high rates of metabolism and biosynthesis.

Applied microbiologists have been successful in exploiting these characteristics, and the knowledge accumulated as a result of their efforts has revolutionized the fermentation industry. The emergence of genetic engineering techniques has allowed us to produce an ever-increasing number and variety of gene products in bacterial and cell cultures. We are able to exploit an organism's ability to produce primary and secondary metabolites for commercial purposes. The only limitations appear to be the availability of an isolated gene and an appropriate expression system to produce it. Table 38-1 (7) lists a selection of scientific disciplines using applied molecular genetics.

Biotechnology is the application of biological systems to basic and applied technical and industrial processes. Although these processes vary substantially in their details, they all share a common feature: They are all based on the use of microorganism or cell to serve as a catalyst in the conversion of substrate to product. A concern that is common to all applications is the need to maintain aseptic conditions. This is because most products are made by a pure culture (a population of cells derived from a single strain or clone). To avoid contamination, all phases of the process must be carefully evaluated and monitored.

TABLE 38-1. A selection of scientific disciplines using applied molecular genetics

Agricultural science	Medicine
Anthropology	Epidemiology
Archeology	Diagnosis
Biochemistry	Treatment
Cell biology	Gene therapy
Receptor biology	Vaccine development
Environmental science	Organ transplantation
Ecology	Immunology
Environmental biology	Microbiology
Enzymology	Taxonomy
Evolutionary biology	Metabolism
Genetics	Paleontology
Microbial genetics	Polymer science: biopolymers
Human, animal, plant genetics	Systematics, taxonomy
Population genetics	
Pharmacogenetics	

Adapted from Jackson DA. DNA: template for an economic revolution. *Ann N Y Acad Sci* 1995;758:356–365.

COMMON FEATURES OF BIOTECHNOLOGY PROCESSES

Although each technical process is associated with its own unique starting material (bacteria, fungi, yeast, plant or animal cell, or enzyme), technical manipulation (cell or enzyme immobilization, bacterial or cell genetic engineering, cell fusion), processes (continuous or batch fermentation), and scale (small to very large), certain common features or stages lend themselves to a more general discussion.

Biotechnologic activity involves the following:

- Isolation and preservation of the organism or cell that is to serve as the biocatalyst or the source of the biocatalyst of interest
- Preparation of the biocatalyst
- Process scale-up for the biocatalyst or large-scale growth of the organism
- Separation of the desired product
- Purification of the product

CULTURE PRESERVATION

Organisms to be preserved are usually cultivated in small volumes (less than 100 mL), and the resultant suspension is distributed in 1-mL aliquots into tubes containing a cryopreservative. These tubes are sealed and usually stored at ultralow temperatures until needed. Alternatively, samples are freeze-dried and stored under ambient conditions. Even though the volume of cell suspension or the number of organisms in the starting sample is small, the biology of the organism (e.g., pathogen or saprophyte, mechanism of pathogenicity, virulence, host range, type of illness) should be understood before work begins. Appropriate procedures and practices that protect the worker and the biological material from gross contamination should be clearly defined.

PREPARATION OF THE BIOCATALYST

Organisms to be preserved are usually cultivated in small volumes (less than 100 mL), and the resultant mixture is transferred in quantities of as much as 1 mL into small tubes with a cryopreservative. These tubes are sealed and stored in or above liquid nitrogen in a low-temperature freezer (–80°C) or in a standard freezer (–20°C) (8). Alternatively, samples can be lyophilized (freeze-dried) and stored between room temperature and 0°C (8,9). These samples serve as the starting material for all future cultivations. Each sealed tube may contain a few micrograms (dry weight) of microorganism. The number of organisms per tube may vary from 1×10^8 for yeast and molds to 1×10^{10} for bacteria (10). Appropriate work practices in an appropriate biological safety cabinet should protect the worker and the biological system from gross contamination. When a lyophilizer is used, care should be taken to prevent the vacuum lines from being contaminated. The insertion of a suitable filter or trap is usually sufficient. All lines, tubing, or glass connectors that come in contact with the primary vessel or tube should be decontaminated by chemical disinfection, followed by extensive washing to remove residual disinfectant or by steam sterilization before reuse. Inoculum preparation is typically from a viable preserved stock culture. This may involve stepwise transfer into successively larger culture vessels to develop the final seed culture for large-scale fermentation. The next stage is to provide the required number and quality of organisms or enzymes to initiate a larger-scale cultivation or process.

CELLS

A tube of preserved material is opened, and its contents are transferred into a flask or bottle containing an appropriate volume of a sterile nutrient solution. The culture is capped or closed with a filter or plug, which permits the passage of gases but not of organisms. The culture is then maintained at an appropriate growth temperature, dependent on the organism involved, until satisfactory growth is achieved. It is then used to seed a similar but larger vessel. This flask is maintained at the appropriate temperature and is often placed on an automatic shaker, roller, or stirrer to increase gaseous interchange across the liquid-air interface (8). After a suitable growth period, the culture is transferred to a sterile container from which it is further transferred into a larger culture vessel (bioreactor).

To this point, it is frequently necessary to limit the amount of growth at each of these amplification phases to prevent the medium from becoming too acidic or alkaline, which might result in a cessation of growth or even kill the organism. Once the seed culture has been transferred to the culture vessel, these restrictions no longer apply. Typically, there may be a few grams (dry weight) of organism at this point, which means that the increase in the number of organisms present is on the order of 10^3 to 10^4 (10).

ENZYMES

If the biocatalyst is a purified enzyme, then sufficient enzyme must be isolated from the producing organisms. The preparation of the starting inoculum would be similar to that described in the section Preparation of the Biocatalyst.

When a sufficient number of organisms are attained, the enzyme is isolated and attached to a suitable carrier. By definition, *immobilization* is the conversion of enzymes from a water-soluble, mobile state to a water-insoluble, immobile state (11).

All plastic or glassware that comes in contact with the organism should be decontaminated or disposed of promptly after use and not allowed to accumulate. Unattended vessels (e.g., bottles, flasks, plates) containing medium (or even a residual film of medium) can support the growth of saprophytes, which may result in unnecessary contamination of the system. Keep in mind that many of these environmental organisms are spore formers and therefore are capable of extensive contamination.

If pathogens are to be used, precautions to prevent accidental breakage of flasks during shaking are necessary. All glassware should be examined before use; any item that is chipped or cracked should not be used.

When a dry air shaker or a shaker platform is used with pathogens (especially for organisms known to be respiratory tract pathogens), the unit should be enclosed in a chamber that operates under a negative pressure, and the exhaust air should be cleaned by filtration. If a vessel should break or a cotton plug or stopper come off, then any aerosol that might be generated would be trapped in the filter.

If such an accident does occur, then personnel who are suitably trained, clothed, and provided with appropriate respiratory protection should remove the undamaged vessels, clean up the debris, and decontaminate the shaker and chamber surfaces appropriately (see reference 12 for a listing of appropriate disinfectants and decontaminants and procedures for their use).

SCALE-UP OF THE PROCESS

To maximize the yield of a desired product, microorganisms are grown in bioreactors under rigorously controlled conditions. Often the final process is preceded by growth in successively larger vessels—for example, 20 L, 200 L, and 2,000 L (13), usually constructed of stainless steel.

There are three basic fermenter-bioreactor designs: (a) small, portable units that are filled with medium and sterilized in an autoclave; (b) portable units that are sterilized in an autoclave and filled aseptically with sterile medium; and (c) fixed units that are sterilized in place (13–15). In a batch process, most of the constituents of the medium are combined with the biological catalyst at the start. The process vessel is sterilized before the medium is introduced. Depending on the scale of operation, the starting materials are added by means of tubes and pipes (13,15). In the vessel, the catalyst and constituents of the medium are mixed by a rotating control shaft that carries several impeller rotor blades. As the biological conversion proceeds, any additional nutrients needed can be added via additional tubes and lines. This requires that conditions in the reaction vessel be monitored during the conversion and that sensors be inserted through the vessel wall at various locations. A vessel for a continuous process is similar, except that nutrient is continuously added and the products of the reaction are continuously removed (13).

In either the batch or continuous mode of operation, the design of fermentation equipment and facilities is central to the containment strategy for biological control. The term *biological control* is used because both the worker and the integrity of the culture must be protected. To avoid contamination of the culture, all materials that come in contact with it—as well as the medium constituents—must be sterilized. Air should be filtered through a deep bed of glass wool or by special high-efficiency particulate air filters. Reactor vessels, pipelines, and other surfaces with which the medium comes in contact are steam sterilized. The mechanical system must be designed and operated so that the opportunities for contaminants to enter—or for organisms to escape—are eliminated or minimized. Maintaining the integrity of various entry and exit points in the system is both crucial and often difficult. The potential for human error and mechanical failure is great, and culture contamination unfortunately does occur.

Massive contamination is usually caused by mistakes, whereas slight contamination that develops gradually is frequently caused by inadequate sterilization. If the contamination is chronic, the whole system should be given a detailed critical inspection. In the initial installation and during contamination review, care must be taken to ensure that all piping and fittings are welded properly and that the use of connecting fittings is minimized (13,14). Dead spaces, crevices, and nondraining portions of lines should be avoided. Sterile and nonsterile segments of the system should be separated by steam blocks. Valves should be examined for dead spots or crevices before being installed.

In dealing with pathogens, exhaust gases must be either filter sterilized or incinerated to remove or destroy any organisms suspended in them. An effluent stream with a high moisture content reduces high-efficiency particulate air (HEPA) filtration efficiency, and in the event of a "foam out," it will reduce containment efficacy. In such a situation, hydrophobic prefilters in conjunction with a catch basin or tank to collect condensate or foam should be included in the design.

Agitator seals must be examined for leaks. The possibility that leaks can occur is not trivial. The recommendation for top-mounted agitation for large-scale processes involving recombinant DNA organisms is an attempt to reduce the impact of a seal malfunction (16). If the impeller shaft is located at the bottom, then a seal leak can result in the vessel's contents contaminating the motor, the floor, etc. If the system is located at the top, then the extent of contamination is reduced substantially. Three types of seals (packed seal, lip or oil seal, and mechanical seal) are commonly used (14,15). The current trend in design of contained fermenter is toward double mechanical seals.

Sampling ports must also be considered as possible routes of contamination. Samples should be taken via a closed system to avoid the generation of aerosols (16). Flush-mounted valves that eliminate dead spaces should be used where possible. Piston and ball valves can be designed to include a steam block, in which the sample flows from the vessel to the sample port when the valve is open, and steam flows back through the valve toward the sample port and the vessel when the valve is closed. Butterfly valves are also very popular. Ports must be provided for probes to monitor the progress of the fermentation. Probes that can be sterilized along with the reaction vessel should be used. It is important to avoid crevices on the ports and to incorporate both internal and external seals in the design of probe ports.

Large-scale growth of the organism in a bioreactor (fermentation) under controlled conditions maximizes the yield of the desired product. The design of the bioreactor used is dependent on the organism being grown and the degree of containment and asepsis required. The large-scale growth phase may be carried out in bioreactors ranging from open-pan vessels to highly enclosed systems. To facilitate gaseous exchange and to ensure transport of nutrients and waste products, the culture may require agitation by mechanical stirring or by aeration (15).

RECOVERING THE PRODUCT

The specific method of product recovery and purification depends on the properties of the product, such as its location (intracellular, dissolved in medium, or both) and its stability to heat and chemical disinfectants (reagents used in the extraction and purification may inactivate the product). Yeasts and fungi are usually harvested by continuous filtration, whereas bacteria, viruses, and cells are routinely harvested by centrifugation. Recovery on the order of 100 kg of wet cell material from 1,000 L of culture is possible (10,14).

Separation and subsequent processing always involve the breaking of air-liquid interfaces and therefore results in the release of aerosols. If the biocatalyst is a pathogen, it is desirable to inactivate the organism first. This can be accomplished by "in place" sterilization within the reactor vessel (batch sterilization). Alternatively, the reactor contents can be sterilized by being passed through a heat exchanger (continuous-flow sterilization) (16). Either method is acceptable if the product of interest is stable under the conditions of sterilization.

If the product is heat labile, then it is necessary to consider chemical inactivation of the organism. This requires that the product be unaffected by the disinfectant selected. In the event that the product is not stable, then it must be separated from the cells before further processing. Such bulk processing must be performed under closed conditions to minimize personnel and environmental exposures (13).

The vessel contents must be delivered to the separation tank, filtration column, or centrifuge by a series of lines, the integrity of which should be examined in the same fashion as that of the vessel itself. The columns and centrifuge should be a closed system (primary containment) or placed in a chamber or room that is specifically designed to control the spread of aerosols (secondary containment). Such rooms or chambers are maintained under negative pressure (more air is exhausted than supplied) to prevent dissemination of organisms to neighboring areas or to the environment (16).

PROCESSING THE PRODUCT

Subsequent processing methods vary widely and depend on the purpose of the fermentation. In some cases, the whole culture may be used without separation of cells. Separated microorganisms may be used without further processing beyond drying, such as the yeasts, fungi, and bacteria used as single-cell proteins (13). In other instances, the cells may be subjected to some form of chemical or physical disruption to release the desired product (14).

Cells may be disrupted by nonmechanical methods—such as osmotic shock, or enzymatic or chemical lysis—or by mechanical methods. Because of difficulties in scaling up the former procedures, mechanical methods are more popular on the industrial scale. Two types of mechanical disrupters are widely used: high-pressure homogenizers and high-speed agitator mills. Because both have the potential for generating aerosols, the system design must ensure either that any aerosol generated be retained within the unit itself or—as mentioned above for filtration systems and centrifuges—that the unit be placed within a suitable chamber or room that provides the necessary aerosol control.

Often it is essential to protect the product from contamination. In this case, efforts must be directed toward keeping external organisms out rather than keeping process organisms in. This requires facilities and equipment that are operated under positive pressure conditions. Containment facilities then are transformed into barrier facilities (17). In such circumstances, it is essential that any pathogenic organism used as the biocatalyst be inactivated before processing to avoid personnel exposures.

BIOHAZARDS OF BIOTECHNOLOGY PROCESSES

The biotechnology processes may include the isolation of growth medium components, viable and nonviable organisms, and suspended solids. Most reported health problems are associated with downstream processes (18). In particular, cell separation and disruption processes have the potential to generate substantial aerosols (19). The extraction of intracellular enzymes involves handling large quantities of cell debris and places the greatest demands on biosafety (20). Centrifuges and rotary vacuum filters are also capable of creating contaminated aerosols. Disruption processes such as homogenization and bead-milling sonication may generate aerosols, both of the organism and its components. Purification processes such as ultrafiltration, chromatography, and dialysis are less likely to generate aerosols. Aerosol generation could, however, occur in the event of failures in seals or piping. Exposure may also occur during activities such as filling bags, vials, or other containers (18). With many biological products, the risk of allergic reaction is greatest after the product is more concentrated during purification and packaging (21). The degree of risk may be influenced by the product formulation—whether solid, powder, or liquid form. Effluent from the process may be an additional source of exposure for workers and may have a significant influence on the environment at the point of discharge (19). Table 38-2 lists the biohazard potential of biotechnology processes.

Who Is at Risk?

Biotechnologists are scientists drawn from a variety of disciplines. These disciplines include biochemistry, biology, chemistry, computer science, mechanical engineering, chemical engineering, veterinary science, and medicine. Many lack experience in standard aspects of microbiological techniques and biological, chemical, or even basic laboratory safety.

TABLE 38-2. Biohazard potential of typical biotechnology processes

Process	Hazard
Raw material handling (weighing, mixing, dissolving, fermentation)	Allergenic dusts or aerosols, skin contact, spillage, effluent contamination, off gases, dust
Biomass separation (centrifugation, filtration)	Aerosol, spillage, leakage, skin contact
Product purification (homogenization, centrifugation, concentration, dialysis, chromatography, blending, filtration, filling, freeze/spray drying)	Aerosols, spillage, leakage, skin contact, dust
Waste management	
Handling untreated effluent	Aerosols
Handling treated effluent	Skin contact

Adapted from Hambleton P, Bennett AM, Leaver G, Benbough JE. Biosafety monitoring devices for biotechnology processes. *Trends in Biotechnology* 1992;10:192–199.

Although the potential threat of infection in this work environment has long been appreciated by microbiologists, the number of nonmicrobiologists engaged in biotechnology activities is increasing. A concern exists that these researchers may not be sufficiently trained or motivated to take the necessary precautions to protect themselves, their colleagues, and the environment from biological hazards.

Why Are They at Risk?

What becomes clear is that the main cause of laboratory exposures is the worker (1). The worker is the one who performs experiments, operates equipment, handles animals, and, when needed, cleans up spills. Review of laboratory-acquired infection indicates that many (if not most) laboratory-associated illnesses could have been prevented if proper procedures and practices were followed. Pharmaceutical production lines are similar. This is supported by studies evaluating the human factor in laboratory accidents. In one such study (22), two groups with 33 people each were selected according to the presence or absence of involvement in accidents. Each participant was asked to fill out questionnaires concerning habits and attitudes. There were several differences between groups. The accident-free group showed greater concern about infectious agents, were aware of the hazards associated with their work, and realized the importance of proper attitudes in safety endeavors. This group placed prime importance on understanding and following safety regulations. On the other hand, the accident-involved group was characterized as risk-takers. There is a presumption that they are more likely to violate known safety regulations. These may reflect fundamental lifestyle choices. There were more nonsmokers and nondrinkers in the accident-free group.

These findings underscore the role behavioral factors can play in accidents and imply some associated limitations of risk assessment. One way to minimize risk is to modify unsafe behavior patterns.

Behavioral patterns of interest included the finding that men were involved in seven times more accidents than women (normalized to working hours). There was a difference in accident involvement between age groups as well. The rate in the 17- to 24-year-old group was approximately twice that of the 45- to 64-year-old group. Unfortunately, the biotechnology work force is young and innovative and falls into the higher accident group. If previous studies provide guidance, then the behavior patterns in laboratories and production facilities are worth close observation (22). We must also develop a better understanding as to types of work activities that are taking place. In the introduction of this chapter, biotechnology was defined in terms of the types of disciplines or specialties involved. Clearly, the technologies that have been developed have opened doors to many secrets of nature. These are the technologies that have captured our interest. Unfortunately, most of our attention has been focused on genetic engineering (recombinant DNA), and the importance of cell biology, protein engineering, and other applications with equal or greater likelihood for mischief to human health has been minimized.

WHAT ARE THE HAZARDS?

From a practical standpoint, there are three main groups of potential hazards associated with biotechnology: biological hazards, chemical hazards, and physical hazards.

Biological Hazards

Biohazards are associated with three properties of microorganisms:

- Potential for a few species to cause illness or disease
- Potential for undetected genotypic or phenotypic changes to alter a tested and approved process
- Ubiquity of organisms that can contaminate the system

Analysis of surveys (23–29) of laboratory-associated infections reveals that the actual causes for most laboratory-acquired illnesses are not known. Fewer than 20% of documented infections can be attributed to accidental contact, ingestion, or injection with infectious material. The remaining 80% have been attributed to unknown or unrecognized causes (24–30). These analyses suggest that personnel engaged in research are at a higher risk than personnel associated with diagnostic, educational, or industrial activities (Table 38-3). The risk to personnel who are in direct contact with the agent is higher than for personnel who are only remotely involved. Eighty percent of the 300 illnesses reviewed by Wedum et al. (29) at Fort Detrick involved trained laboratory personnel. Support personnel such as janitors, dishwashers, and maintenance and clerical workers were at lower risk. These results serve to confirm previous estimates reported by Sulkin and Pike (31).

Laboratory studies on the potential sources of infection have focused on the hazard potential of routine laboratory techniques (32–34). Because these studies suggest that most laboratory tech-

TABLE 38-3. Distribution of infection according to occupation

Personnel at risk	Percentage of infections: Study 1	Study 2
Principal scientists, technicians	82.3	78.1
Animal caretakers, janitors, dishwashers, maintenance personnel	13.7	10.3
Clerical personnel	3.7	6.6
Students	0	4.9

Adapted from Liberman DL, Harding AL. Biosafety overview. In: Liberman DL. *Biohazards management handbook,* 2nd ed. New York: Marcel Dekker Inc, 1995.

niques create aerosols, inhalation exposure to undetected infectious aerosols may contribute significantly to occupational illness among laboratory workers who handle infectious material (24,26,35–38).

Based on available data, preventive measures have been developed that provide safeguards for the protection of scientific and support personnel, the experiment, and the environment. These safeguards are collectively referred to as *containment practices* (12,35,37–39).

SIGNIFICANCE OF AEROSOLS

The health risks associated with biological aerosols depend on the nature of the hazard, the concentration, and on the size and related distribution of the aerosol particles in the lung. Most human-made aerosols and industrial dusts contain particles of a wide range of sizes. The size, shape, and density of the particle determine the site of deposition in the body. Any process, such as stirring or bubbling, results in the formation of a thread of film of liquid that can break down into small droplets and evaporate to form an aerosol. The size of the particles in an aerosol is critical in determining the length of time the particle will remain airborne, the site of deposition in the respiratory tract, the survival and infectivity of microorganisms, and the allergic response to dusts and proteinaceous material. In allergic responses, such as allergy to pollens and molds, larger size and greater concentration of aerosol particles are of significance. When the effect of the aerosol depends on a small number of droplets, such as in airborne infection, then the small particles are significant because of their greater number and the greater probability of being inhaled. For this reason, it is imperative that any monitoring and control measures are based on the understanding of the particle size of an aerosol or dust giving rise to the hazard (18).

Bioaerosols from biotechnology processes are likely to range in size from individual cells of process organisms to clumps of cells adhered together in a matrix of culture broth (19). All are able to be inhaled, but single cells and small clumps of cells are likely to be in the respirable range (with an aerodynamic-equivalent diameter of less than 4 micrometers) and capable of penetrating deep into the lung (19). Studies have suggested that the majority of aerosol particles emitted from fermentation are in the submicrometer range (40). Nonviable cells can present a toxic or allergenic risk. Factors affecting the viability of cells include environmental factors, such as temperature, humidity, sunlight, oxygen concentration; the presence of protecting cell culture; and the state of the organism itself (19).

Studies of potential sources of infection have demonstrated that nearly all routine bacteriologic and virologic procedures are capable of producing aerosols. Table 38-4 provides illustrative data on the number of viable particles recovered within 2 feet of a work area. These data are based on an extensive series of air-sampling determinations (33,34).

TABLE 38-4. Concentration and particle size of aerosols created during representative laboratory techniques

Operation	Number of viable colonies	Particle size (μm)
Mixing culture with:		
Pipette	6	3.5
Vortex mirror	0	0
Mixer overflow	9.4	4.8
Use of Waring blender:		
Top on during operation	119	1.9
Top removed after operation	1,500	1.7
Use of sonicator	6	4.8
Lyophilized cultures:		
Opened carefully	134	10
Dropped and broken	4,838	10

TABLE 38-5. Infectious dose for humans

Disease or agent	Dose[a]	Route of inoculation
Scrub typhus	3	Intradermal
Q fever	10	Inhalation
Tularemia	10	Inhalation
Malaria	10	Intravenous
Syphilis	57	Intradermal
Typhoid fever	10^5	Ingestion
Cholera	10^8	Ingestion
Escherichia coli	10^8	Ingestion
Shigellosis	10^9	Ingestion
Measles	0.2[b]	Inhalation
Venezuelan encephalitis	1[c]	Subcutaneous
Polio virus 1	2[d]	Ingestion
Coxsackie A21	18	Inhalation
Influenza A2	790	Inhalation

[a]Dose in number of organisms.
[b]Median infectious dose in children.
[c]Guinea pig infective dose.
[d]Median infectious dose.
Adapted from National Institutes of Health. *Laboratory safety monograph.* Bethesda, MD: National Institutes of Health, 1979.

The simple presence of organisms in the air is insufficient to cause disease. To initiate a respiratory infection, infectious aerosols must be deposited and retained within the respiratory tract. Studies have shown that particles in less than the 5-μm range deposit in both sections. The data in Table 38-4 indicate that particles of respirable size are generated by routine laboratory procedures.

Droplets smaller than 5 μm in size lose their liquid content rapidly and then become airborne. These dried particles are called droplet nuclei. They can remain suspended in air for long periods and can be carried by convective air currents (41) and building ventilation systems.

Table 38-4 indicates that standard laboratory procedures generate aerosols and therefore are potentially hazardous to the investigator and to other personnel in the vicinity.

The infectious dose of a number of etiologic agents is presented in Table 38-5. Given the concentrations of organisms per milliliter of culture fluid and the number of bacteria, viruses, and fungi that can be found in each milliliter of fluid, it is easy to understand the need to control aerosols when dealing with these agents.

POTENTIAL FOR UNDETECTED GENOTYPES OR PHENOTYPIC CHANGES TO ALTER A TESTED AND APPROVED PROCESS

Because of the relatively few generations of the organism involved, little opportunity exists for new genotypes to become established during the course of an experiment or a standard fermentation run (42). Although the potential for genetic change would seem enormous, any mutations that occurred would be selected against by the experimental or fermentation conditions, and unless some specific advantage was conferred, the mutant probably would not become established (43).

UBIQUITY OF CONTAMINANTS

Unlike mutations, if a contaminant entered that was able to maintain itself, it could disrupt the system in several ways. The contaminant could directly inhibit or interfere with the biocatalyst (enzyme, cell, or microorganism). It could destroy the catalyst or the product by using it as an energy source. In addition, the contaminant could introduce substances that are difficult to separate from the product, thereby rendering the product unusable. In practice, an industrial fermentation is unlikely to become contaminated with a highly pathogenic microorganism, because the environment inside the fermenter is so different from the human body that pathogenicity confers no selective advantage on the organism.

Biotechnologists may work with virtually any organism studied by conventional biologists. Remarkably few infectious diseases have been reported. The risk of work with engineered organisms may be of less risk than work with nonengineered organisms, because typical engineered organisms have been selected for properties unrelated to infectivity.

Historians of science may argue that biotechnology is not a new industry. Biotechnology began when humans first fermented honey and grapes for wine, or improved cultivated crops, or began breeding programs to select desirable traits in domesticated animals. This historical perspective is unassailable and unimportant. The public has a clear perception of biotechnology. It involves specialized research leading to products produced through molecular biology techniques. These use recombinant DNA and protein engineering processes that markedly increase the precision and shorten the time period required for genetic experimentation.

Health and safety professionals also recognize that this new industry is part of a long continuum of human endeavor. As with other high-tech industries that are now well established, biotechnology research and production may create risks for occupational illness. A significant challenge will be to anticipate the hazards of this work and prevent illnesses as new processes and products are introduced.

Because of health and safety concerns, research facilities for these activities are heavily engineered and rather expensive. Any operation that may generate a workplace aerosol or inadvertently release an organism to the environment is a candidate for containment. Containment is achieved through local barriers, building barriers, and personnel practices and procedures. Local barriers in biotechnology laboratories may include any or all of the items listed in Table 38-6 (7).

Biological safety cabinets may have an open front (class I and class II). Workers are protected by the air curtain formed when laminar air flow meets the air stream drawn into the front face opening. Gases and aerosols generated in the cabinet are carried into the air stream to the exhaust filter or the recirculation air filter. Class III cabinets, or glove boxes, have closed fronts and afford an additional level of protection. Work with dangerous agents is performed in class III cabinets, which have glove ports for access. All equipment necessary for work with dangerous organisms, including incubators, autoclaves, centrifuges, and even animal storage cages, may be contained within a series of contiguous class III cabinets (44). Routine maintenance and testing programs are critical for biological safety cabinets of all classes, as malfunctioning equipment may actually increase the risk of infection (45).

TABLE 38-6. Local barriers in biotechnology laboratories

Biological safety cabinets (classes I, II, and III)
Chemical fume hoods
Glove bags
Enclosed centrifuges
Enclosure for sonicators
Safety blenders
Enclosed fermentation equipment

TABLE 38-7. Laboratory support spaces with health and safety implications for biotechnology

Glass washing and autoclaving room
Bulk chemical and supply storage area
Laboratory washroom
Low-level-radiation waste-handling area
Radiation counting room and support area[a]
Equipment rooms
Waste-storage rooms
Biological waste incinerator[b]
Wastewater treatment systems
Animal facilities[c]
Interstitial spaces for ventilation
Dedicated access hallways for waste disposal and other maintenance tasks

[a]Smaller facilities often contract this activity to an outside vendor, who offers scintillation equipment and other radiation support facilities at a remote site.
[b]On-site incineration is economically desirable for large operations. A variety of clean air standards, which may change over time, have to be met.
[c]At large research institutions, animal housing facilities are often remote from research facilities. There is usually some need for temporary housing and handling on site as well.

Laboratory hoods work by the same general ventilation principle as the class I biosafety cabinets. A hood should be able to maintain a constant inward velocity at the sash face to move noxious chemicals away from biologists during operations. In addition, the movable sash should be positioned to provide barrier protection against chemical explosions, fires, and splashes. As with biological safety cabinets, laboratory hoods require balancing, routine testing, and maintenance.

Laboratory facilities are frequently laid out to meet the particular needs of a specific investigator or research and development enterprise. Concerns include conforming usage (zoning), transportation access, and compatibility of abutters and neighbors, as well as availability and constraints on utilities (46) (notably waste disposal). The presence of local regulations, especially those constraining the use or application of certain technologies, will be an important consideration for biotechnologists. These regulations are usually unrelated to the health and safety considerations described above. Laboratories are an obvious part of the facility, but insufficient attention may be paid to health and safety support spaces listed in Table 38-7.

Chemicals Common to the Biotechnology Industry

Common operations of biotechnology include gel electrophoresis, high-performance liquid chromatography (HPLC), and protein and nucleic acid engineering. Table 38-8 lists the chemicals frequently used by biotechnologists for HPLC. Although health-related incidents have not been the norm, those that have occurred commonly involved exposure to acetonitrile. Acetonitrile is a common solvent and extractant. It is toxic by any route of exposure, and massive exposures have been reported to cause death by cyanide asphyxiation after inhalation in workplaces. Intoxication and death after inhalation (47) or accidental ingestion (48,49) are delayed, sometimes for hours. Cyanide is only one of the toxicants liberated by acetonitrile metabolism, but it is probably the most important one. Thiocyanate production may also contribute to reported fatal outcomes. Survivors of acute exposures have suffered from a variety of reversible symptoms and findings affecting the central nervous system, blood, and possibly the kidneys (47).

Such dramatic outcomes have not been reported for exposed biotechnologists. Yet biologists and support staff, including cus-

TABLE 38-8. Chemicals used by biotechnologists for high-performance liquid chromatography (ranked by approximate usage)

Chemical	Primary toxicity
Methanol	Metabolic acidosis, optic neuropathy, CNS depression
Ammonium hydroxide	Strong irritant
Acetonitrile[a]	Cyanidelike
Methylene chloride	CNS, animal carcinogen
n-Hexane	Central and peripheral neurotoxicity
Dimethyl formamide	Liver
N-Methylpyrrolidone	Animal teratogen; heat decomposition to NO_x
Ethyl acetate	Relatively low toxicity, dermatitis
Trifluoroacetic acid	Strong irritant
Tetrahydrofuran	Irritant
Triethylamine	Irritant and sensitizer, CNS
Ethanol amine	Irritant and sensitizer, CNS
Acetic anhydride	Strong irritant
Dimethylaminopyridine	Irritant, heat decomposition to toxic fumes

CNS, central nervous system.
[a]Most common chemical causing health-related incidents to date in biotechnology research.

todial personnel, do not always have the training to recognize the dangers of their chemicals. The absence of life-threatening exposures to acetonitrile is likely due to relatively small quantities used so far by biotechnologists rather than to universally adequate training or workplace hygiene. There have been a number of less dramatic exposures to laboratory personnel, characterized by malaise, nausea, and headache, followed in at least two cases by subjective dyspnea. Blood gases were normal, save for evidence of hyperventilation, in two cases in which they were obtained. To our knowledge, neither cyanide nor thiocyanate levels have been obtained for exposures in a biotechnology setting. Blood cyanide and thiocyanate measurements are not considered to be well correlated with dose at lower levels of exposure in any case (50). One exposure was to a custodian who was inappropriately involved in the cleanup of a broken storage bottle. The short-term exposure limit of 60 ppm was likely exceeded. This worker experienced delayed, prolonged, and temporarily incapacitating anxiety once the toxic potential of acetonitrile was recognized. Episodes such as this illustrate the importance of training personnel in spill control protocols and restricting cleanup to trained personnel.

Other chemicals used in HPLC have toxic properties not always recognized by laboratory personnel. Methylene chloride (dichloromethane) is a multipurpose solvent used to remove paint or grease that is recognized as an animal (51) and possible human carcinogen (52,53). An often-mentioned additional hazard is metabolic conversion to carbon monoxide (54,55); this is probably an important hazard at higher doses more characteristic of exposures to paint strippers than to research laboratory workers. Skin absorption is an important route of exposure (56).

Of the common HPLC chemicals listed in Table 38-8, the following toxins are absorbed through skin: methanol (which is said to have caused deaths by skin absorption) (57), acetonitrile, methylene chloride, dimethylformamide, pyridines, and fluoroacetic acid. Trifluoroacetic acids are less toxic than the highly hazardous monofluoracetates (58,59), but are still capable of being absorbed through skin. Bipolar compounds such as dimethylformamide are particularly interesting in this regard, as they may enhance the entry of other toxic agents through their universal solvent activity, as well as by altering the natural barrier mechanisms of the skin. Skin permeability is particularly important to biotechnologists, who may appropriately use chemical hoods or other ventilation mechanisms of protection, but still expose their hands to a variety of chemicals. Table 38-9 lists some of the chemicals that might be encountered in laboratory reagent preparations. Amyl alcohol is frequently responsible for *odor calls,* when neighboring laboratory and office inhabitants become concerned by the presence of a fruity but distinctly chemical smell. Unstable compounds such as dimethyl sulfate (60) and hydrazine (61) are capable of causing spectacularly destructive incidents. Biotechnologists generally use small quantities of these chemicals. Chronic diseases related to exposure have not been seen in this population so far. Skin splashes, with accompanying burns or local irritation, have occurred.

TABLE 38-9. Reagents used in biotechnology laboratories, ranked by approximate usage

Chemical	Primary toxicity
Glacial acetic acid	Irritant
Hydrochloric acid	Severe irritant
Trichloroacetic acid	Irritant
Isoamyl alcohol	Low toxicity, irritant
Phosphoric acid	Irritant
Formaldehyde	Irritant, sensitizer, animal carcinogen
Glutaraldehyde	Irritant, sensitizer
Dimethyl sulfate	Severe irritant, animal carcinogen
Dimethyl sulfoxide	Central nervous depressant, gastrointestinal
Sulfuric acid	Severe irritant
Hydrazine	Severe irritant; toxic to liver, blood, nervous system, kidney
Cyanogen bromide	Metabolic asphyxiant, pulmonary toxicity
Hydrofluoric acid	Severe irritant

An ongoing challenge in research laboratory environments is to inculcate good personal hygiene and work practices, so that buffers are mixed in hoods with the sash down to prevent eye splashes, and personnel are not found working without lab coats, gloves, and safety glasses when they should be wearing them. As biotechnology moves from lab bench to production, the quantities of chemicals, including acetonitrile, will increase from volumes of less than a liter to 20 or more liters at a time. Spill control and potential exposure will become important planning challenges as scale increases.

Gel electrophoresis is used to examine DNA fragments. Chemicals used in the preparation and staining of polyacrylamide gel electrophoresis include:

- Acrylamide
- *N,N'*-Methylene-bisacrylamide
- Ammonium persulfate
- Ethidium bromide
- *N',N',N',N'*-Tetramethylethylenediamine
- Tris-acetate-ethylenediaminetetraacetate

Three of these deserve special comment:

Tetramethylethylenediamine is a severe eye irritant as well as a potential sensitizer. Ethidium bromide is used, in a combination with ultraviolet light, to visualize DNA bands by fluorescent staining. Biotechnologists have been sufficiently concerned by the mutagenic properties (62) of ethidium bromide that it is one of the first toxins to undergo partial characterization of DNA damage pattern (63). Another potential source of exposure comes during large-scale preparation of closed circular plasmid DNA, when ethidium bromide is added to cesium chloride gradients.

Acrylamide is a white, crystalline powder used to make polyacrylamide gel. Researchers have commonly made up their own gels from acrylamide powder, with potential for dust exposure during weighing, transferring, and mixing operations. During visits to molecular biology laboratories, it is common to see waste acrylamide powder around balances. Acrylamide may be the second most common potential source of toxic exposure for biotechnology researchers, including skin contact with powder and with gel preparations. It has been made available in gel form, which should reduce the hazard.

At high doses, acrylamide is an important human neurotoxin, the likely entry portal of which is through the skin. A characteristic contact dermatitis of the palms often precedes the neurologic syndrome. Nonspecific central nervous system signs such as fatigue and malaise also precede the classical progressive, symmetric, distal peripheral neuropathy (64,65). Neither the dermatitis nor the neurologic syndrome have so far been reported from molecular biology workplaces. The cumulative nature of acrylamide neuropathy (65,66) nevertheless dictates that skin exposure not be permitted. Furthermore, acrylamide has other, less appreciated toxic properties. It crosses the placenta and causes experimental reproductive loss and neurotoxic effects in neonates at doses insufficient to cause overt maternal toxicity (67). Acrylamide also causes direct testicular degeneration in exposed rodents (68) and is recognized as a genotoxin with primary mechanisms of heritable translocations and spermatic chromosomal clastogenesis (69). It is unequivocally an animal carcinogen at several sites (67), although there are inadequate data for deciding if this applies also to humans (70).

Given these toxic properties, it is distressing that biologists endure routine, voluntary dermal exposures. The most likely explanation for this behavior is inadequate education. Suggested standard policies for reducing acrylamide exposure are listed in Table 38-10.

An important procedure in cell research uses gene markers in selection techniques. Methotrexate is a folic acid antagonist that kills cells unable to express the gene product dihydrofolate reductase. Researchers can link a second gene of interest, such as insulin or growth hormone, to the gene for dihydrofolate reductase. Then cells surviving antimetabolite treatment inherit both the selected gene and the additional gene linked to it. This process is called *selection for the linked gene*.

Although any number of antimetabolites could have been used for linked gene selection, the initial work was carried out with methotrexate. Biologists have taken a generally benign view of methotrexate toxicity, perhaps because the product solutions contain only micromolar quantities. Methotrexate has been used in pharmacologic treatment of leukemia, several other neoplasms, nonmetastatic trophoblastic diseases, and psoriasis. The toxicity of folic acid antagonists, such as methotrexate, is correspondingly impressive. At therapeutic doses, it is a proven teratogen, affects male and female reproductive capability, and

TABLE 38-10. Policies for reducing acrylamide exposure

Policy	Advantage
Source reduction: purchase in smallest container in amount required.	Economic: saves on waste disposal
	Mixing without weighing
Weigh out in tared closeable containers in fume hood.	Reduces exposure during weighing
Purchase in solution.	Reduces exposure during weighing
	Reduces skin exposure
Use ventilated glove box or hood with a dedicated balance.	Bottle of powder open only under local exhaust
Require gloves to prevent skin exposure.	Reduces potential skin exposure

causes bone marrow aplasia, severe stomatitis, and other gastrointestinal symptoms that may be fatal. In addition, methotrexate is responsible for hepatotoxicity, nephrotoxicity, and immunosuppression (71). Work-related exposures should obviously be controlled vigorously for a known human reproductive hazard. Skin exposure is unacceptable under industrial conditions. Waste liquor from cell-growth media may be regarded as hazardous for regulatory purposes if it contains methotrexate.

Although occupational professionals would clearly prefer that some other, less human-cytotoxic chemical be used for selective resistance, it is most unlikely that important research, development, or production activities will use any other selective approach. The U.S. Food and Drug Administration regards methotrexate selection as a standard technique. Neither pharmaceutical companies nor independent researchers have incentives to find replacement methodologies. Potential exposure activities, such as weighing, mixing, and waste handling, must be carried out with sufficient planning and attention to occupational and environmental safety to prevent exposure.

Chilled water is used to meet the precise temperature and humidity conditions required for cell line production. Chemical hazards of chilled-water unit maintenance include exposure to a variety of corrosive or sensitizing chemicals, including strong alkaline and acid chemicals, amines, and hepatotoxic solvents, such as dimethylformamide. This problem is not unique to the biotechnology industry. Workers in power plants, industries, and office buildings also work with chilled-water units. Personnel have to control the chemical and biological hazards associated with servicing chilled-water systems. It is of obvious importance to install personal protective gear and a training program for chilled-water maintenance workers; manufacturers of chilled-water treatment chemicals are sometimes willing to collaborate in this process. Recirculating chilled-water units also pose a potential nuisance odor hazard. Such units often contain antifreeze additives such as ethylene glycol. Foul-smelling bacteria, such as *Clostridia glycoliticum*, may metabolize the antifreeze within standing chilled-water during intervals between operation. Any break in the chilled-water pipes releases the odorous metabolites. It is difficult and possibly unrealistic to persuade building inhabitants that the odor is not hazardous to health. Odors may finally be controlled when walls are scrubbed, furniture cleaned or repainted, and rugs replaced.

Recirculating chilled water is also a source of *Legionella pneumophila*, the organism responsible for Legionnaire's disease (72). Prevention of this work-related illness requires frequent biocidal treatments and routine microbiological sampling of treated water.

A frequently ignored chemical hazard common to research and production microbiology is cleanup. Scientists, technologists, and support staff such as glass washers are exposed to a variety of soaps and detergents. Some of these are phenolic based, some quaternary amines, and most can be sensitizing after long-term use.

A variety of potentially harmful chemicals is routinely used in other biotechnology laboratories. Biochemical laboratories use diazomethane, a potent alkylating agent, to convert fatty acids to their methyl esters to identify them in gas-liquid chromatography. Dimethyl sulfate is used as a reagent for the detection of guanines in DNA sequencing. Ethidium bromide is used to detect DNA in electrophoretic gels. Ethidium bromide intercalates into the DNA sequence and provides a fluorescent tag to mark the location of DNA. Ethyl methane sulfonate is used to induce mutation in strain improvement studies. Methotrexate, a chemotherapeutic agent, is used for selective resistance of cultures.

Tables 38-11 and 38-12 list chemical agents used by biotechnologists.

TABLE 38-11. Toxic chemicals found in biotechnology laboratories

Carbon tetrachloride
Chloroform
1,2-Dibromo-3-chloropropane
1,1-Dimethyl-ethylenimine
p-Dioxane
Ethylene dibromide
Propylenimine
Bromo-thyol methanesulfonate
Chloromethyl methyl ether
Diepoxybutane 1,1-dimethylhydrazine
1,2-Dimethylhydrazine
Ethyleneamine
Ethyl methanesulfonate
Hydrazines
Methylhydrazine
Methyl methanesulfonate
N-Nitrosodiethylamine
N-Nitrosodimethylamine
N-Nitrosodi-*n*-butylamine
N-Nitrosodi-*n*-propylamine
N-Nitroso-*N*-ethylurethane
N-Nitroso-*N*-methylurethane
N'-Nitrosopiperidine
Polychlorinated biphenyls
B-Propiolactone

TABLE 38-12. Chemical carcinogens (solids) frequently found in biotechnology laboratories

Ethionine
3 Methyl-4-amino-azobenzene
Urethane
N'-Acetoxy-2-acetylaminofluorene
N-Acetylaminofluorene
Aflatoxins complex
o-Aminoazotoluene
2-Aminofluorene
Benzo[a]pyrene
Chlorambucil
Cycasin
Diazomethane
Benzanthracene
7,12-Dimethyl-benzanthracene
4-Dimethyl-aminazabenzene
3,3-Dimethyl-benzidine
1,4-Dinitrosopiperazine
N-Hydroxy-2-acetylaminofluorene
Methotrexate
3-Ethylcholanthrene
4,4-Methylene-bis(2)-chloroaniline
Methyl-3-nitro-1-nitrosoguanidine
l–Naphthylamine
Formic acid (2-C4-methyl-2-thiazolyl) hydrazide
N-Nitroso-*N*'-ethylurea
N-Nitroso-*N*-methylurea
4-Nitroquinolone-*N*-oxide
Procarbazine
1,3-Propane sulfone
m-Toluenediamine
4-Aminobiphenyl
Benzidine
3,3-Dichlorobenzidine
3,3-Dimethexybenzidine
2-Naphthylamine
4-Nitrobiphenyl

Physical Hazards of Production Scale-Up

Biotechnology is a dynamic industry. There is no standard set of procedures or products. New products create new market niches. Competition is frequently based on new patents rather than cost control or marketing. Under these circumstances, manufacturers rush new discoveries from the laboratory to consumers without exploring other technologies that might facilitate production engineering. Most often, biotechnology production is a scaled-up version of laboratory methods.

Biologists may not appreciate that there are important physical hazards associated with scale-up activities (listed in Table 38-13). Laboratory scientists may fail to recognize that laboratory-grade materials do not support production technology. The lesson is learned when laboratory-grade tubing ruptures and an employee is burned. Steam burns are a fairly common problem. It is to be hoped that maturation of the industry will encourage more innovative use of production and industrial hygiene engineering, with reassessment of production technology. Other physical hazards include cuts, lacerations, and spills that often result from large glass bottles, which are heavy to lift and dangerous when dropped. A variety of heavy materials invites improved ergonomic approaches.

Shift work is required in biotechnology because microbial production and harvest do not follow human timetables. As a result, support workers work 12-hour days in some cyclic pattern such as 2 days on, 3 off, 3 on, and 2 off. The problems of shift work are well known and include an effect on virtually every organ system (73). Shift work is commonly thought to play a contributing role in industrial accidents. Although a typical biotechnology schedule appears more humane than shift work schedules commonly cited for other industries (74), the obligate round-the-clock nature of the work schedule may provide safety concerns in typically small, sparsely staffed enterprises.

Table 38-14 lists a cross section of organisms used in industrial applications. Of these, the vaccinia virus may be of considerable concern to immunosuppressed researchers, to their families and friends who may be immunosuppressed, and to exposed individuals with skin disorders.

In addition, there is a tendency toward host work with specific genes from dangerous organisms. As biotechnologists attempt to develop vaccines and other treatment strategies for serious diseases, researchers must grow these organisms before they can isolate specific genes. The National Institutes of Health (NIH) *Guidelines for Research Recombinant DNA Molecules* is an important resource for information about control of biohazards (75).

Another problem for biotechnologists is how to dispose of research organisms that have been radiolabeled. Strong public interest in biological waste and evolving infectious waste reg-

TABLE 38-13. Physical hazards of production activities

Type	Source
Burn	Pressurized steam, liquid nitrogen/acetone/dry ice
Hypothermia	Cold room (up to 12 hours continuously)
Electrical	Heavy equipment, electrophoresis units
Cuts	Glass bottles, glass bioreactors
Anoxic	CO_2 and N_2 lines
Ergonomic	Drums, large bottles, media preparation, and other scaled-up equipment
Repetitive trauma	Computer modeling
Shift work	24-hour microbial support (monitoring) of large-scale production; product isolation and purification

TABLE 38-14. Common host and vector organisms

Host	Vector
Escherichia cold k12	Plasmids, phage, shuttle vectors
Bacillus sp. (asporogenic strains)	Plasmids
Saccharomyces cerevisiae	Plasmids, shuttle vectors
Corynebacteria glutamicum	With and without plasmids
Streptomyces sp.	With and without plasmids
Mammalian tissue culture cells	Vaccinia virus, herpes virus, murine retrovirus, papillomavirus
Insect tissue culture cells	Baculovirus

ulations (76,77) requires that some acceptable form of biological decontamination be found. Chemical decontamination or usual modes of heat sterilization, such as incineration, are undesirable in this circumstance, because they only further disperse any radioactivity used to label research materials. A possible solution is the judicious use of filters within autoclave bag systems (78), so that steam sterilization can be accomplished without release of radioactivity. Waste disposal is but one of the safety and regulatory considerations for recombinant biologists who use radiolabeled materials. This broad topic is treated elsewhere in regard to human immunodeficiency virus (HIV) laboratories (79) and for microbiological laboratories in general (80).

EPIDEMIOLOGY OF BIOTECHNOLOGY EXPOSURE

No peer review data concerning population outcomes in biotechnology exist. The science is too new, the populations' individual sites too small, the movement of trained personnel from employer to employer too rapid, and the enthusiasm of scientist-entrepreneurs for nonproduct research too small to have encouraged any systematic looks at health outcomes among biotechnologists.

Epidemiologic studies are definitely needed. Cancer miniepidemics have been reported among scientists using recombinant technology (81–84). Cancer prevalence miniepidemics may indicate an underlying occupational health problem, or they may be simply the result of chance. Designed population studies are needed to decide whether there is an increased incidence of cancer or any other chronic disease outcome among biotechnologists. Studies showing the absence of excess disease would also be extremely important to the industry. Chemical and biological exposures of recombinant DNA work may vary greatly depending on the type of research or production activity. This is an impediment to epidemiologic research, because it may prove difficult to identify sizable populations with similar exposure for study, even if the research question is excess cancer.

Infectious diseases have not yet proved an especially important epidemiologic problem for recombinant biologists. The introduction of more dangerous research organisms is likely to change this pattern, however. Recombinant vaccine research with retroviruses or mycobacteria provides examples of evident infectious hazards. Even research with noninfectious genomes may incur the risk of misleading seroconversion. False seroconversions are already a concern of HIV researchers who work with noninfectious pieces of genome material.

To date, chemical and physical hazard exposures have resulted in acute rather than chronic or permanent problems. Informal reports indicate that transient malaise from acetonitrile overexposure, acid burns, and steam burns from ruptured lines are the most common problems. Support personnel may also have problems from shift work.

MEDICAL SURVEILLANCE FOR BIOTECHNOLOGY

Medical surveillance of workers involves the collection and use of medical information, biological monitoring, medical screening, or other health data for developing strategies for the prevention of disease. Biological monitoring is the use of tests of body fluids or skin to indicate exposure, and medical screening is the early detection of a health effect to prevent overt disease or to increase chances of recovery.

The potential occupational hazards associated with biotechnology laboratories will vary according to the microbial species, products, reagents, processes, and setting. Potential exposures in the biotechnology laboratory include biological agents, fermentation products, chemicals and solvents, carcinogens, radioactive materials, nonionizing radiation, animal handling, and musculoskeletal stresses (85). The most useful medical evaluations target the potential risks and workplace hazards (86).

Reviewing the specifics of the job descriptions and potential exposures is the first step. Program content and participation are then determined. The medical surveillance program must comply with federal, state, and local governmental regulations. Workers should be completely informed of the results of their medical evaluations. Records remain confidential and are released only with the employee's authorization. Authorization for release of information pertinent to the ability to perform job duties is usually obtained at the time of the preplacement examination. The human resource department and supervisor need to be notified only about medical conditions, restrictions, or accommodations as they relate to the individual's fitness to work (86).

The program usually includes a preplacement or baseline examination to determine whether the employee is at increased risk to self or others as the result of job activities or job-related exposures. The evaluation includes review of the prospective employee's job requirements and exposures; relevant medical and occupational history; and for those who require a more complete evaluation, a physical examination, laboratory testing, and serum storage. Individuals who should be included in the medical surveillance program are laboratory technicians who work with potentially hazardous agents, particularly at the biosafety level (BL) 3 or BL4; individuals handling teratogenic, carcinogenic, and mutagenic chemicals; individuals working with oncogenic and teratogenic microbial agents; animal caretakers; maintenance, custodial, and housekeeping staff; others who work in areas in which potential exposure to hazardous materials can occur; and individuals who by questionnaire reveal a medical condition that would increase their risk in handling certain agents (86).

The purposes of periodic monitoring of biotechnology workers include detecting evidence of exposure to biological or chemical hazards, detecting early clinical signs or symptoms of disease, assessing control measures, detecting changes in employee health status, and identifying patterns of disease indicating a workplace exposure. The periodic evaluations should focus on changes from the baseline exam as a result of potential exposures—such as the development of allergy—or signs and symptoms of adverse effects of infectious agents or biologically active agents. Exit evaluations are similar to baseline examinations, and usually a final serum sample is taken for banking at that time (86).

In the biotechnology industry, primary prevention is by hazard control, safe work practices, and immunizations. When working with biological agents, two key components of a medical surveillance program are determining the immune status of the employee and eliciting the employee's vaccination history.

Because many of the biological agents are opportunistic pathogens, an individual whose immune status is compromised should be advised to refrain from working with them. Employees should be offered vaccinations if available for the agents in use. All employees exposed to blood, body fluids, or tissue cultures should be offered hepatitis B vaccination (84).

Of particular concern is identifying underlying medical conditions, such as those that might alter host defenses, allergies, the inability to receive vaccinations, and reproductive risks of exposed workers. Risk factors need to be evaluated case by case, and recommendations must be based on the employee's personal health history and the job description. The employee should be fully informed about potential risks. Employment decisions should take into account input from the employee, the occupational medicine service, management, and possibly the employee's physician. The job description, the level of increased risk, and the opportunities for limiting exposure by restrictions and accommodations need to be considered. Responses may include a change in work processes, reassignment of specific tasks, job transfer, or additional protective measures. Recommendations for job restriction or accommodations should be appropriate for the current situation and avoid exclusion based on inaccurate presumptions of risk or future disabilities (86,87).

The Centers for Disease Control and Prevention (CDC)–NIH *Biosafety in Microbiological and Biomedical Laboratories* monograph (88,89) is based on the assumption of a population of immunocompetent individuals and recommends that the laboratory director not allow persons at increased risk of acquiring infections or for whom infections might be usually hazardous to enter the BL2 or higher laboratory or animal room.

Common conditions that could interfere with immune function include steroid treatment for medical conditions such as asthma or inflammatory bowel disease, acute viral infections, poorly controlled diabetes mellitus, severe alcoholism, pregnancy, or immunosuppressive therapy for cancer or connective tissue diseases. Medical interventions, such as offering Pneumovax to an asplenic worker, can target specific risks. Workers with chronic dermatitis, eczema, or psoriasis have an increased susceptibility to infection because of altered cutaneous defenses and therefore must wear gloves or avoid exposure to potentially infectious agents (86).

Reproductive hazards in the laboratory can include biological, chemical, and physical hazards that cause concerns about infertility, exposure during pregnancy, and adverse pregnancy outcomes. Risks may include exposure to anesthetic gases, radiation, ethylene oxide, cytotoxic drugs, and certain solvents. Chemical agents suspected of causing adverse outcome in animal experiment include chloroform, glycol ethers, and xylene (90).

Risks of animal handling include zoonoses, physical harm from bites or scratches, and cutaneous or inhalant allergic responses. Laboratory animal allergy is much more common than zoonotic infections. Table 38-15 lists illness associated with biotechnology processes. Reduction of exposure to animal allergens by engineering controls—such as proper ventilation, cages, protective clothing, gloves, and masks—and appropriate work practices is recommended for all personnel working with animals in order to avoid sensitization (86). In addition to allergies to animal dander or urine (aerosolized animal proteins), biotechnology workers can develop allergies to biological products derived from raw material, fermentation, cell culture products, or enzymes and chemicals (18). Table 38-16 lists fungi associated with biotechnology industries that can cause asthma, and Table 38-17 lists fungi associated with allergic alveolitis.

Medical surveillance for work with hazardous chemicals depends on the adverse effect of the specific chemicals involved. The Occupational Safety and Health Administration's (OSHA's) *Occupational Exposure to Hazardous Chemicals in Laboratories* requires employers to provide medical examinations for employees whenever an employee develops signs or symptoms consistent with a potential chemical exposure in the laboratory; or if exposure levels for an OSHA-regulated substance are above the actions level or permissible exposure limit and require medical surveillance; or whenever a spill, leak, or explosion occurs, increasing the likelihood of exposure.

TABLE 38-15. Noninfectious illness associated with biotechnology processes

Product/process	Illness
Antibiotics	Hemorrhagic rhinitis, cardiovascular disorders, opportunistic colonization (candidiasis)
Brewing	Dermatitis, malt fever
Citric acid production	Asthma, bronchitis, allergic contact dermatitis
Enzymes	Asthma, conjunctivitis, allergic contact dermatitis, and urticaria
Endotoxin	Flulike symptoms on inhalation, stomach pains and renal pains, immune system complement, and the coagulation system
Fungal fermentations	Asthma, bronchitis
Single-cell protein	Allergic responses, asthma, dermatitis
Steroids	Feminization (of men), hypertension, body-weight increase

Adapted from Hambleton P, Bennett AM, Leaver G, Benbough JE. Biosafety monitoring devices for biotechnology processes. *Trends in Biotechnology* 1992;10:192–199.

TABLE 38-16. Fungi and actinomycete spores implicated in occupational asthma and used in biotechnology

Source of allergen	Fungus implicated
Enzyme production (surface culture)	*Aspergillus flavus*
	Aspergillus awamori
Food protein culture	*Candida tropicalis*
Flour	*Alternaria* spp.
	Aspergillus spp.
Soup manufacturer	*Agaricus hisporus*
	Eboletus edulis
Cheese dairy	*Penicillium camembertii*

Adapted from refs. 99,100.

TABLE 38-17. Fungi implicated in allergic alveolitis used in biotechnology

Source of allergen	Fungus implicated
Malting barley	*Aspergillus fumigatus*
	Aspergillus clavatu
Citric acid fermentation	*Penicillium* spp.
	Aspergillus fumigatus
	Aspergillus niger
Cheese	*Penicillium casei*
Mushroom culture	*Pleurotus ostreaus*
	Pholiota nameko
Humidifiers	*Penicillium* spp.
	Acremonium spp.
	Aspergillus fumigatus

Adapted from ref. 100.

Monitoring for exposure to radioactive materials is typically performed by the use of film badges. Only individuals who exceed the acceptable limits for occupational exposures need to be in a medical surveillance program that monitors acute and chronic effects of radiation exposure (89). The Nuclear Regulatory Commission has specific requirements relate to the use of radioisotopes (91,92).

Routine monitoring tests that physicians perform are more likely to detect abnormalities that are preexisting and that are not work related. Evaluations typically include routine blood tests, complete blood count, liver function tests, and blood chemistry test and urine analysis, as well as a questionnaire to determine exposures, symptoms, and change of health status. These routine blood tests are not sensitive enough to identify early adverse effects of many exposures with long latency in the development of adverse effects. They are also not specific enough to be the initial pickup of either acute or chronic work exposure.

The effectiveness of a medical surveillance program may be limited by a number of factors, including the small size of the group understudy, variability of individual exposures, long latency from exposure to onset of adverse health effects, uncertainty of adverse health effects, uncertainty of the connection between an exposure and an effect, and lack of sensitivity or specificity of common medical screening tests to detect early changes of disease (86).

Biological monitoring tests for carcinogens include tests to determine exposure (e.g., urine testing for carcinogens, their metabolites, or mutagenicity); biological effects (e.g., DNA adducts); and preclinical response (e.g., chromosomal alterations or sister chromatid exchange and monoclonal antibodies to detect altered oncogene proteins capable of causing the malignant transformation of cells). Biological monitoring of workers exposed to carcinogens has been used mostly in the research setting but has not been very useful for individual evaluations or medical surveillance programs (86).

PRODUCT HAZARDS

Biotechnology workers in fermentation or cell culture production areas with purification processes encounter risks similar to the traditional pharmaceutical and chemical industries in that exposure to physiologically active products can cause medically significant side effects (86). Drug manufacture has been associated with adrenocortical suppression in workers exposed to their manufacture (93); gynecomastia in male workers and menstrual bleeding in female workers have been associated with the manufacture of oral contraceptives (94).

ENVIRONMENTAL CONTROLS AND PREVENTION OF EXPOSURE

Tables 38-6 and 38-7 review some of the facility requirements of the biotechnology industry. Although the information presented in these tables relates to worker health and safety, it turns out that a considerable portion of the biotechnology facility investment relates to protecting the larger community rather than workers. The public has reacted strongly to the intentional manipulation of genetic material at the molecular level, as opposed to the chance changes of natural selection in the environment or the intentional but less precise changes of traditional breeding programs. In the contrast to public fear, it may seem to health care professionals that workers bear the brunt of real risks but receive few of the resources intended for environmental health. BL3 designations are designed to protect the environment and the public from laboratory releases, rather than to protect workers within laboratories.

The role of health and safety professionals in improving this ironic situation involves education and engineering. Workers, from custodial personnel to Nobel scientists, require information about hazards and how to mitigate them. The present cavalier attitude toward acetonitrile and acrylamide can best be reversed with strong educational programs. Even highly goal-oriented scientists can be convinced to protect their hands from a potent skin-absorbable toxin. Availability of protection plays a role in this process. Gloves adequate to prevent penetration, lab coats, and safety goggles are as important for biologists as they are for chemists. Preengineered laboratory hoods, adequately vented biological cabinets, specially designed centrifuges, and frequent preventive maintenance of ventilation facilities are essential to the protection process. Industrial hygiene and biohazard monitoring should be continuous to discover unexpected breaks in containment.

Uncontained aerosols and skin exposures are of major concern in chemical and biological safety. Each process and procedure can be designed to prevent them, providing personnel have adequate education. Interestingly, this prudent safety measure is also critical to preventing contamination at production facilities, so that commercial needs dictate some critical safety measures at large-scale facilities.

CONTROL MEASURES

Preventive measures have been developed that provide some protection to at-risk workers. Containment represents the integration of personnel procedures and practices with laboratory design and engineering features to minimize the exposure of workers to hazardous or potentially hazardous agents or substances (88). By using increasingly stringent procedures and better-designed facilities, work can be conducted with a higher degree of safety on agents with greater potential risk (95–97). The objective of incorporating containment measures into the design of a research program is to minimize the potential for exposure of investigative and support personnel, as well as minimizing the escape from the laboratory of experimental materials that may pose a health hazard to the surrounding community or cause some ecologic perturbation.

CONTAINMENT PRACTICES AND PROCEDURES

To describe in detail all the specific practices and procedures that are used to prevent laboratory-acquired illness and control product contamination is difficult. These procedures vary and depend to a great extent on factors including the agent, type of experiment, equipment, facilities, and proficiency of personnel. Fortunately, there are a number of excellent reviews on this subject (95–97). Each laboratory that is involved with or contemplates the use of hazardous or potentially hazardous agents should develop protocols that address the specific safety concerns of that hazard. However, several basic practices and facility considerations are worth reviewing here.

Personnel Practices

The laboratory director should determine whether the use of a particular agent requires special entry provisions. When entry restrictions are necessary, a hazard warning sign incorporating the universal biohazard symbol should be posted on all access doors to the restricted area. This sign should identify the infectious agent(s) currently used, list name and telephone number of the responsible supervisor, and define specific requirements for entering the area.

As inadvertent ingestion is a potential route of exposure to microorganisms, supervisors should prohibit eating, smoking, and drinking. This prohibition should also be extended to chewing gum, using throat lozenges, and applying cosmetics in the laboratory. Nail biting is strongly discouraged, as this is another means of exposure to hand contamination. Hand washing provides another means of preventing ingestion of organisms and their spread to other surfaces. Hands should be washed after working with infectious microorganisms or cleaning up a spill. Clearly, mouth pipetting is not to be permitted. Mechanical pipetting devices are required. These devices are more accurate than standard pipettes and eliminate aspiration and ingestion as a source of laboratory-acquired illness. One must keep in mind that 13% of confirmed accidental infections were caused by aspiration as a result of mouth pipetting.

Protective Clothing and Equipment

A second group of protective practices includes the use of appropriate gloves, face protectors, and laboratory clothing. Gloves function to prevent the worker's hands, fingers, and nails from being contaminated. This helps to reduce the hazards associated with ingestion (hand-to-mouth transfer) or the penetration of material through broken or unbroken skin. Although relatively few organisms can penetrate unbroken skin, many experiments also involve chemicals and radionuclides; therefore, using gloves should be regarded as a minimum requirement.

The description of an accidental human vaccination (98) with vaccinia virus demonstrates the importance of proper procedures and practices. While studying the immunogenicity of vaccinia viral recombinants, which expressed two proteins of a second virus (vesicular stomatitis virus), one of the workers accidentally was exposed to the recombinant virus and seroconverted to the proteins under study.

Analysis of this incident indicated that the exposure occurred when some of the viral culture contaminated a cut on the worker's ring finger. The worker promptly washed the affected area. Unfortunately, hand washing was insufficient to prevent subsequent infection. The worker experienced a mild infection and developed antibodies to one of the vesicular stomatitis virus proteins, as well as to the vaccinia virus. This laboratory-acquired infection would have been prevented if the worker had worn gloves. This illness was not reported in the scientific literature because of its laboratory origins; instead, it was reported because it represented the first human efficacy data for a vaccinia vaccine delivery system. But for those interested in science and safety, this exposure reinforces the need to understand and appreciate the importance of personnel protection requirements.

Laboratory clothing is designed to keep street clothing, forearms, hair, or other exposed surfaces free of contamination. Wearing these items, especially lab coats, to the cafeteria, libraries, meetings, or to other buildings provides a mechanism for spreading contamination to others as well as to oneself. The use of laboratory clothing must be restricted to the laboratory and not worn outside the laboratory area.

Housekeeping

Well-defined housekeeping procedures and schedules are important in reducing the risks of working with biohazardous material and in protecting the integrity of the work activity. Housekeeping should be done in a manner that reduces or prevents the generation of aerosols. Although vacuuming with a system that exhausts through a HEPA filter or using of a two-bucket wet-mopping method is frequently recommended (12), they are excessive for level 1 or level 2 laboratories. In these areas, the use of a wet- or dry-mop procedure with floor-care products that contain appropriate disinfectants should be sufficient.

Clearly, for areas in which agents of higher hazard level are handled, cleaning techniques such as the two-bucket mopping method and HEPA-filtered vacuums can be and should be considered (12).

Work Surfaces

Work surfaces must be decontaminated daily and immediately after spills. This reduces the spread of contamination to one's person and at the same time reduces the potential for contaminating one's own or someone else's experiment or process.

Waste Management

All biological waste and contaminated equipment should be decontaminated or inactivated before disposal or reuse. This is especially true if known pathogens are involved. Contaminated materials such as fermenters, culture flasks, glassware, and laboratory equipment should be decontaminated before washing, reuse, or disposal. This again helps to protect personnel not directly associated with the laboratory activity (e.g., glassware workers, janitors, repair personnel, animal care technical support). Such personnel should never be exposed to contaminated materials without first being informed and thoroughly trained.

Care should be exercised whenever hypodermic needles and syringes are used. Twenty-five percent of laboratory illnesses that have defined causes were attributed to syringe mishaps (89). Hypodermic needles and syringes should only be used for the parenteral injection or aspiration of fluids. Only needle-locking syringes or units in which the needle is an integral part of the syringe should be used. Syringes and needles are discarded directly into a puncture-resistant container immediately after use and are neither clipped nor resheathed. The contents of the puncture-resistant container should be chemically inactivated or autoclaved, or both, before disposal. Contaminated broken glass also presents a hazard and must be decontaminated and disposed of properly. Decontaminated needles or other sharps still present a physical hazard that needs to be addressed.

Containment Equipment

The purpose of safety equipment is to provide physical containment to protect workers from exposure to aerosols or infectious agents. Properly maintained and used equipment provides a significant level of protection to the worker, but such equipment must always be tested to assure that it is functioning correctly. Safety devices that prevent the escape of aerosols into the laboratory environment are available. These include biological safety cabinets and a variety of air-tight enclosures designed to house various pieces of laboratory equipment, such as sonicators and centrifuges. The biological safety cabinet is the principal device used to provide physical containment of infectious aerosols.

There are three types of biological safety cabinets. The personnel protection provided by class I and class II cabinets is dependent on the maintenance of an adequate inward airflow. These cabinets provide only partial containment and are not adequate for containment of high-risk infectious agents (sometimes designated class IV organisms). This is because of the chance for inadvertent escape of aerosols across the open cabinet front. This type of escape is prevented when a class III cabinet (glove box) is used. Class III cabinets are designed to completely isolate the worker from the hazard, thus this cabinet provides the highest level of personnel and product protection available. When such a degree of containment is needed, most (if not all) procedures involving infectious agents can be contained within them. Class III cabinet systems have been designed as an interconnected network of individual cabinets that contain various pieces of equipment such as incubators, refrigerators, and centrifuges. Double-door autoclaves and pass-through chemical dunk tanks also have been included in cabinet networks to allow safe introduction and removal of supplies and equipment during the course of the work.

The class II cabinet is the most commonly used piece of containment equipment in the biomedical research laboratory. This unit is used in preference to class I cabinets because the latter does not provide protection to the research located in the work area. The class I cabinet, like the chemical fume hood, draws unfiltered room air into the work area. Protection of research materials from contamination is attained in a class II cabinet by the down-flow of HEPA-filtered air over the entire work space.

FACILITY DESIGN/PROGRAM REQUIREMENTS

NIH and CDC provide guidance for the selection of appropriate biosafety precautions (12,89) and specific information on laboratory hazards associated with a variety of agents and recommendations on practical safeguards and facility considerations that can significantly reduce the risk of laboratory-associated diseases.

In the event that the agent is not described in these documents, the reader should consult a second publication from CDC, titled *The Classification of Etiological Agents on the Basis of Hazard* (96). This is a useful document that provides a more extensive listing of organisms and their hazard classification than NIH/CDC publications.

For reference purposes, four biosafety levels are described in the NIH/CDC publication. Each corresponds to the containment requirements for the four classes of microorganisms (I, II, III, IV) in the CDC publication. The agents of minimal hazard are in class I or BL1, and dangerous and exotic microorganisms are in class IV or BL4. Each biosafety level specifies work practices, containment equipment, and facility design appropriate for the different hazard classes of microorganisms. The facility design requirements for each level and the type of work suitable are outlined below. Features such as ease of cleaning, impervious bench surfaces, sturdy furnishings, hand-washing sinks, and window screens (if windows can be opened) are incorporated into even the lowest level of containment.

Biosafety Level 1 Containment

At BL1 containment, the laboratory provides an environment for work with low-hazard agents that can be controlled by standard laboratory practice. Viable microorganisms not known to cause disease in healthy human beings are handled at this level. Work activity is routinely conducted on an open bench. No special design features are required, although laboratory space should be separated from general offices, food service, and patient areas.

This laboratory is suitable for experiments involving the following:

- Microorganisms of minimal or no biohazard potential under ordinary handling conditions [such agents are designated class I (95) by CDC, or BL1]
- Cell or tissue culture studies that do not involve infectious plant, animal virus, or recombinant DNA handled at the BL1 containment level
- Recombinant DNA research requiring BL1 containment (microorganisms in this latter class include *Escherichia coli* K12, *Saccharomyces cerevisiae*, *Bacillus subtilis*, and nonprimate cells)

Biosafety Level 2 Containment

A BL2 laboratory is identical in construction to the BL1 facility. Although work that does not produce significant aerosols can be conducted on an open bench, biological safety cabinets are frequently present, and if contamination control is important (e.g., to keep cultures clean), they should be used.

This laboratory is suitable for experiments involving the following:

- Microorganisms of low biohazard potential, such as those in class II or BL2
- Primate cells or tissue culture systems, or both
- Recombinant DNA research requiring BL2 physical containment
- Oncogenic viral systems research classified under low or moderate risk
- Certain suspected carcinogens and other toxic chemicals

The microorganisms handled in a BL2 laboratory include many of the indigenous infectious agents that produce disease in humans (e.g., *Staphylococcus*, *Streptococcus*, measles, polio, enteric and bloodborne pathogens). Most academic, diagnostic, or industrial laboratories operate at BL1 and BL2.

Biosafety Level 3 Containment

At BL3, one encounters a facility that includes special engineering design features and containment equipment. These facilities are usually separated from the general traffic flow by controlled access corridors, air locks, locker rooms, or other double-door entries. Biosafety cabinets are used for all technical manipulations that involve unsealed cultures. The surfaces of walls, floors, and ceilings are constructed to be sealed. This means that all penetrations are chalked, collared, or sealed to prevent leaks.

The ventilation system in this facility is designed to exhaust more air than is supplied, resulting in a directional airflow from outer clean corridors into the laboratory, in which the higher potential for contamination exists. The air is usually discharged to the outdoors and not recirculated to other parts of the building without appropriate treatment.

This laboratory is suitable for experiments involving the following:

- Microorganisms of moderate biohazards potential, such as those in class 3 or BL3
- Cell tissue culture experiments that involve large volumes or high concentrations of virus-infected cells (in which the virus is infectious for humans or requires BL3 containment)
- Recombinant DNA research requiring physical containment at BL3
- Nonrestricted carcinogens and other toxic chemicals

BL3 organisms differ from those at BL2 because there is a real potential for infection that is due to aerosol exposure. Organisms such as *Mycobacterium tuberculosis*, St. Louis encephalitis virus, and *Coxiella burnetii* belong in this category.

Biosafety Level 4 Facility

BL4s are extremely sophisticated facilities in terms of design. They provide a very high level of containment for research involving biological agents that present a life-threatening potential to the worker or may initiate a serious epidemic disease. The distinguishing characteristics are the use of barriers to prevent the escape of hazardous material to the environment and additional barriers to protect laboratory personnel.

Barriers that serve to isolate the laboratory area from the immediate area include

- Monolithic walls, floors, and ceilings, in which all penetrations such as air ducts, electrical conduits, and utility pipes are sealed to ensure the physical isolation of the laboratory area
- Air locks, through which supplies and materials can be brought safely into the facility
- Contiguous clothing change rooms and showers, through which personnel enter and exit the facility
- Double-door autoclaves to sterilize wastes and other materials before removal from the facility
- Biowaste treatment systems to sterilize liquid wastes
- Separate ventilation systems that control air pressures and airflow directions within the facility
- Treatment systems to decontaminate exhaust air before discharge into the atmosphere

A description of specific operational procedures and laboratory practices recommended for use in maximum containment facilities can be found in the monograph entitled *Safety and Operational Manual: High Containment Research Facility* (94). These facilities are usually operated by very well-trained workers who work under rigorous supervision.

This laboratory is suitable for experiments involving the following:

- Microorganisms of high biohazard potential, such as those classified as class IV or BL4 (or higher)
- Recombinant DNA molecules requiring physical containment at the BL4 level
- Human carcinogens

PRACTICAL CONSIDERATIONS

As indicated, these are extremely sophisticated facilities that can provide the highest level of containment for working with agents that have life-threatening potential. Any more detailed descriptions of these facilities and associated research activities are beyond the scope of this section.

Although four distinct biosafety levels are described, there are instances in which a combination of procedures from two different levels provide a safer work environment. An absence of information and experience regarding new microorganisms often stimulates laboratory personnel to select work practices that offer increased protection. Laboratory manipulations of HIV have prompted biosafety committees and safety personnel to take a hard look at containment practices. Based on observations that this virus does not have a documented aerosol route of exposure, the need to require containment of a BL3 facility does not seem critical at this time, and a BL2 facility is currently routinely used. BL3 work practices—in conjunction with factors including the appropriate safety equipment, safety centrifuge cups, and biosafety cabinets—do afford a greater margin of safety for personnel. The resultant hybrid containment of BL2+ provides a greater measure of safety for work with agents such as HIV. Hybrid containment levels should be considered when new or novel agents are first handled and limited laboratory-scale safety information is available.

EDUCATION AND TRAINING

All personnel who work with hazardous organisms or substances must receive sufficient information and training to enable them to work as safely as possible. This instruction should include a thorough review of the following areas: operations and procedures, with emphasis on material transfer and other possible sources or exposure; adverse health effects of specific work practices, detailing which are acceptable and unacceptable; engineering controls (hazard control ventilation and acceptable parameters); containment equipment (e.g., contained centrifuges, safety cabinets) in use or being considered for use; proper disposal of contaminated waste; decontamination of surfaces; and specific emergency procedures to be followed in the event of an accident or spill. Each member of the work team must be familiar with the biology of the system or process. Personnel must understand that human factors are associated with accidents, such as tiredness, haste, and inattentiveness.

The risks associated with work involving infectious agents are minimized when appropriate attention is given to all biological safety practices. Each person involved in such work must accept full responsibility for biological safety to protect him- or herself, colleagues, and the general public.

Although primary emphasis is placed on preventing laboratory-acquired infections in humans, there are a number of infectious agents that affect animals or plants. Release of such agents to animal colonies and the environment must be prevented with equal vigor. Foot and mouth disease of cattle is an example of an animal disease that is so contagious and so costly economically that research on it is confined to a single laboratory located on an island several miles from the mainland. Ectromelia (mousepox) and lymphocytic choriomeningitis are less dramatic but more important examples of agents that require careful procedures to prevent spread of infection to animal colonies. Ectromelia can destroy an animal research program, and lymphocytic choriomeningitis is extremely hazardous to animal handlers.

SUMMARY

The potential threat of infection in the laboratory has long been recognized by the medical microbiological community as an ever-present occupational hazard. Published reports of the occurrence of laboratory-acquired infections have served as reminders that the potential can easily become an actuality. They have pointed out the need for unremitting adherence to appropriate precautionary measures.

It is crucial that management provide laboratory facilities that are commensurate with the requirement for the work to be conducted in a safe manner. Considerable information has been accumulated that clearly indicates that nearly all routine laboratory procedures are capable of producing aerosols. Therefore, any operation that generates a significant aerosol or involves a human, animal, or plant pathogen—or some other agent that could disrupt the environment if inadvertently released—should be contained within safety equipment or facilities. These containment systems must be subjected to periodic inspection and certification to assure proper function.

In the laboratory, the procedures used should be appropriate for the highest level of risk to which personnel, the experiment, and the environment will be subjected. Such an approach avoids multiple practices and the constant retraining of personnel.

Physical containment is dependent on the safety awareness and the techniques of the investigative staff, the availability and proper use of safety equipment, and the design of the laboratory or facility. It should be recognized that physical controls alone cannot create a facility that is safe. Containment is achieved through the combination of equipment, engineering features, and the scrupulous adherence to good laboratory or facility practices. Poor work practices can override the protection provided by equipment and facility design and place all personnel in jeopardy. Poor practices relate to more than simply poor technique or bad technique (e.g., sonication on an open bench). Poor practice also includes rushing through activities without thinking, being easily distracted or constantly distracting one's colleagues, working alone at night, or—even worse—working alone at night and feeling ill or tired. The effect of these practices should not be underestimated; too many of the exposures to infectious materials occur under these conditions.

REFERENCES

1. Liberman DF. Identification and control of human health hazards associated with current and emerging technology. In: Draggen SS, Cohrssen JJ, Morrison RE, eds. *Environmental impacts on human health: the agenda for long-term research and development*. New York: Praeger, 1987:193–219.
2. Cooney CL. Bioreactors: design and operation. *Science* 1983;219:728–733.
3. US Congress, Office of Technology Assessment. Impacts of applied genetics: microorganisms, plants and animals. Washington: US Government Printing Office, 1984.
4. Demain AL. Industrial microbiology. *Science* 1981;214:987–995.
5. Lee SB, Ryan LJ Jr. Occupational health and safety in the biotechnology industry—a survey of practicing professionals. *Am Ind Hygiene Assoc J* 1996;57:381–386.
6. Litchfield JH. Single-cell proteins. *Science* 1983;219:740–746.
7. Jackson DA. DNA: template for an economic revolution. *Ann N Y Acad Sci* 1995;758:356–365.
8. Gherna RL. Preservation. In: Gerhardt P, ed. *Manual of methods for general bacteriology*. Washington: American Society for Microbiology, 1981:208–217.
9. Kennett RH. Freezing of hybridoma cells. In: Kennett RH, McKearn TJ, Bechtol KB, eds. *Monoclonal antibodies*. New York: Plenum Publishing, 1980.
10. Sargeant K, Evans CCT. Hazards involved in the industrial use of microorganisms. Brussels, Belgium: Commission of the European Communities, 1979.
11. Klibanov AL. Immobilized enzymes and cells as practical catalysts. *Science* 1983;219:722–727.
12. National Institutes of Health. Laboratory safety monograph. Bethesda, MD: National Institutes of Health, 1979.
13. Blakebrough M. Design of laboratory fermenters. In: Norris JR, Robbins DW, eds. *Methods in microbiology*, vol 1. New York: Academic Press, 1969:473–504.
14. Calam CT. Culture of microorganisms in liquid medium. In: Norris JR, Robbins DW, eds. *Methods in microbiology*, vol l. New York: Academic Press, 1969:255–326.
15. Cooney CL. Bioreactors: design and operation. *Science* 1983;219:728–733.
16. National Institutes of Health. Guidelines for research involving recombinant DNA activity. *Federal Register* 1983;48:24555–24581.
17. National Cancer Institute. Design of biomedical research facilities. Bethesda, MD: National Institutes of Health, 1979.
18. Hambleton P, Bennett AM, Leaver G, Benbough JE. Biosafety monitoring devices for biotechnology processes. *Trends Biotechnol* 1992;10:192–199.
19. Crook B. Methods of monitoring for process microorganisms in biotechnology [Review]. *Ann Occup Hyg* 1996;40:245–260.
20. Demain A. An overview of biotechnology. *Occup Med: State of the Art Reviews* 1991;6:157–168.
21. Ducatman A, Coumbis J. Chemical hazards in the biotechnology industry. *Occup Med: State of the Art Reviews* 1991;6:193–208.
22. Martin JC. Behavioral factors in laboratory safety: personnel characteristics and modification of unsafe acts. In: Fuscaldo AA, et al., eds. *Laboratory safety: theory and practice*. New York: Academic Press, 1980:321–342.
23. Grist NR. Hepatitis in clinical laboratories. *J Clin Pathol* 1980;33:471–473.
24. Grist NR. Epidemiology and control of virus infections in the laboratory. *Yale J Biol Med* 1982;55:213–218.
25. Harrington JM, Shannon HS. Survey of safety and health care in British medical laboratories. *Br Med J* 1977;1:626–628.
26. Phillips GB. Control of microbiological hazards in the laboratory. *Am Ind Hyg Assoc J* 1969;30:170–176.
27. Pike RM. Laboratory-associated infections: summary and analysis of 3,921 cases. *Health Lab Sci* 1976;13:105–114.
28. Pike RM. Past and present hazards of working with infectious agents. *Arch Pathol Lab Med* 1978;102:333–336.
29. Wedum AC, Barkley WE, Hellman A. Handling of infectious agents. *JAMA* 1972;161:1557–1567.
30. Pike RM, Sulkin SE, Chulze ML. Continuing importance of laboratory infections. *Am J Public Health* 1965;55:190–199.
31. Sulkin SE, Pike RM. Survey of laboratory acquired infections. *Am J Public Health* 1951;41:769.
32. Liberman DL, Harding AL. Biosafety overview. In: Liberman DL, ed. *Biohazards management handbook*, 2nd ed. New York: Marcel Dekker Inc, 1995.
33. Anderson RE, Stein L, Moss ML, Gross NH. Potential infectious hazards of common bacteriological techniques. *J Bacteriol* 1952;64:473–481.
34. Kenny MT, Sabel FL. Particle size distribution of *Serratia marcescens* aerosols created during common laboratory procedures and simulated laboratory accidents. *Appl Microbiol* 1968;16:146-150.
35. Reitman M, Wedum AC. Microbiological safety. *Public Health Rep* 1956;71: 659–665.
36. Barkley WE. Containment and disinfection. In: Gerhardt P, ed. *Manual of methods for general bacteriology*. Washington: American Society for Microbiology, 1981:487–503.
37. Hellman AM, Oxman N, Pollack R, eds. *Biohazards in biologic research*. Cold Spring Harbor, NY: Cold Spring Harbor Laboratory, 1973.
38. Strain BA, Groschel DHM. Laboratory safety and infectious waste management. In: Murray D, Baron J, Faller MA, Tenover FC, Yolken RH, eds. *Manual of clinical microbiology*, 6th ed. Washington: American Society for Microbiology, 1995:75-85.
39. US Department of Health and Human Services. Biosafety in microbiological and biomedical laboratories. Washington: US Government Printing Office, 1984. [HHS (CDC) publication no 84-8395].
40. Liberman DF. Facility description and personnel practices for research activity of comparable hazard. *Public Health Lab* 1980;37:118–129.
41. Hatch TF. Distribution and deposition of inhaled particles in respiratory tract. *Bacteriol Rev* 1961;25:230–240.
42. Juozaitis A, Huang YL, Willeke K, et al. Dispersion of respirable aerosols in a fermenter and their removal in an exhaust system. *Appl Occup Environ Hyg* 1994;9:552–559.
43. National Academy of Science. Introduction of recombinant DNA-engineered organisms into the environment: key issues. Washington: National Academy Press, 1987.
44. Leopold M. The commercialization of biotechnology. *Ann N Y Acad Sci* 1993;700:214–231.
45. National Institutes of Health. Laboratory safety monograph. Bethesda, MD: National Institutes of Health, 1979.
46. Clark RP, et al. Microbiological safety cabinets and laboratory acquired infection [Letter]. *Lancet* 1988;2:844–845.
47. Wolfe MI. Facility considerations. In: Liberman DF, Gordon J eds. *Biohazards management handbook*. New York: Marcel Dekker Inc, 1989:1–45.
48. Amdur ML. Accidental group exposure to acetonitrile. *J Occup Med* 1959;1:627–633.
49. Caravati EM, Litovitz TL. Pediatric cyanide intoxication and death from an acetonitrile-containing cosmetic. *JAMA* 1988;260:3470–3473.
50. Tanii H, Hashimato K. Studies on the mechanisms of acute toxicity of nitriles in mice. *Arch Toxicol* 1984;55:47–54.
51. Pozzani VC, Carpeter PC, Palm PK. An investigation of the toxicity of acetonitrile. *J Occup Med* 1959;1:634–642.
52. National Institutes of Health, National Toxicology Program. NTP technical report on the toxicology and carcinogenesis studies of dichloromethane in F344/N rats and B6C3Ft mice (inhalation studies). Bethesda, MD: National Institutes of Health, 1986. [NIH no 86-2562/NTP-TR 306].
53. Heame FT, Grose F, Pifer JW, et al. Methylene chloride mortality study: dose response characterization and animal model comparison. *J Occup Med* 1987;29:217–228.
54. Mirer FE, Silverstein M, Park R. Methylene chloride and cancer of the pancreas [Letter]. *J Occup Med* 1988;30:475–478.
55. Stewart RD, Fisher TN, Hosko MJ, et al. Experimental human exposure to methylene chloride. *Arch Environ Health* 1972;25:342–348.
56. Stewart RD, Hake CL. Paint-remover hazard. *JAMA* 1976;235:398–401.
57. Proctor NH, Hughes JP, Fischman ML, eds. *Chemical hazards of the workplace*. Philadelphia: JB Lippincott Co, 1988.
58. Henson EV. The toxicology of some aliphatic alcohols—part II. *J Occup Med* 1960,2:497–502.
59. Parmagianni L, ed. *Encyclopedia of occupational health and safety*. Geneva: International Labor Office, 1983.
60. Peters RA, Spencer H, Bidstrup PL. Subacute fluoroacetate poisoning. *J Occup Med* 1981;23:112–113.
61. Ip M, Wong KL, Wong KF, So SY. Lung injury in dimethylsulfate poisoning. *J Occup Med* 1989;31:141–143.
62. Sotaniemi E, Hirvonen J, Isomaki H, et al. Hydrazine toxicity in the human: report of a fatal case. *Ann Clin Res* 1971;3:30–33.
63. McCann J, Choi E, Yamusaki E, Ames BN. Detection of carcinogens as mutagens in the *Salmonella* microsome test. *Proc Natl Acad Sci U S A* 1975;72:5135–5139.
64. Cariello NF, Keohavong P, Sanderson BJS, Thilly WG. DNA damage produced by ethidium bromide staining and exposure to ultraviolet light. *Nucleic Acids Res* 1988;16:4157.
65. Garland TO, Patterson M. Six cases of acrylamide poisoning. *Br Med J* 1967;4:134–138.

66. Spencer PS, Schaumberg HH. A review of acrylamide neurotoxicity: properties, uses, and human exposure. *Can J Neurol Sci* 1974;1:143–150.
67. Takahashi M, Ohara T, Hashimoto K. Electrophysiological study of nerve injuries in workers handling acrylamide. *Int Arch Arbeitsmed* 1971;28:1–11.
68. Dearfield KL, Abernathy CO, Ottley MS, et al. Acrylamide: its metabolism, developmental and reproductive effects, genotoxicity, and carcinogenicity. *Mutat Res* 1988;195:44–77.
69. Hashimoto K, Sakamoto J, Tanii H. Neurotoxicity of acrylamide and related compounds and their effects on male gonads in mice. *Arch Toxicol* 1981;41:179–189.
70. Shiraishi Y. Chromosome aberrations induced by monomeric acrylamide in bone marrow and germ cells of mice. *Mutat Res* 1978;57:313–324.
71. Sobel W, Bond TW, Parsons TW, Brenner FE. Acrylamide cohort mortality study. *Br J Ind Med* 1986;43:785–788.
72. Klassen CD, Amdur MD, Doull J, eds. *Casarett and Doull's toxicology: the basic science of poisons*, 3rd ed. New York: Macmillan, 1986.
73. Muraca PW, Stout IE, Yu VL, Yee YC. Legionnaire's disease in the work environment: implications for environmental health. *Am Ind Hyg Assoc* 1988;49:584–590.
74. Rutenfranz J, Knouth P. Shift work. In: Zenz C, ed. *Occupational medicine: principle and practical applications*. Chicago: Year Book, 1988:1087–1095.
75. Krieger GR. Shift work studies provide clues to industrial accidents. *Occup Health Saf* 1987;(Jan):21–34.
76. National Institutes of Health. Guidelines for research regarding recombinant DNA molecules. *Federal Register* 1995:60:20726–20748.
77. Environmental Protection Agency. EPA guide for infectious waste management. Washington: US Department of Commerce, 1986. [NTIS PB86-199130, EPA/530 SW-86-014].
78. Environmental Protection Agency. Standards for the tracking and management of medical waste: interim final rule and request for comments. 40 *CFR* parts 22 and 259. *Federal Register* 1989 March 24;54:12326–12395.
79. Stinson MC, Galanek MS, Ducatman AM, Masse FX. Inactivation and disposal of human immunodeficiency virus and radioactive waste in a P3 facility. *Appl Environ Microbiol* 1990;56:264–268.
80. Stinson MC, Kuritzkes DR, Masse FX. Guidelines for an effective radiation safety program in a human immunodeficiency virus laboratory. *Health Phys* 1990;58:503–505.
81. Staiger JW. Techniques for safe handling of radioactive material. In: Miller B, ed. *Laboratory safety: principles and practices*. Washington: American Society for Microbiology, 1986:242–260.
82. Stark A. Cancer hazards in the recombinant laboratory. *Occup Med: State of the Art Reviews* 1991;6:311–321.
83. Swirsky G, et al. Ranking the potential carcinogenic hazards to workers from exposure to chemicals that are tumorigenic in rodents. *Environ Health Perspect* 1987;76:211–219.
84. Pasteur Institute invites worldwide help to track r-DNA-lab cancer risk In: *McGraw-Hill's Biotechnology Newswatch*, 1986:1–2.
85. Halperin WE, Frazier TM. Surveillance for the effects of workplace exposure. *Ann Rev Public Health* 1985;6:419–432.
86. Landrigan PL, Harrington JM, Elliot LJ. The biotechnology industry. In: Harrington JM, ed. *Recent advances in occupational health*. New York: Churchill Livingstone, 1984:3–13.
87. Goldman RH. Medical surveillance in the biotechnology industry. *Occup Med* 1991;6:209–225.
88. US Department of Health and Human Services, Centers for Disease Control and Prevention, National Institutes of Health. Biosafety in microbiological and biomedical laboratories. Washington: US Government Printing Office, 1988. [HHS (CDC) pub no 93-8395].
89. Barkley E, Richardson J, eds. Biosafety in microbiological and biomedical laboratories. Bethesda, MD: National Institutes of Health, Centers for Disease Control and Prevention, 1993. [HHS (CDC) 93-8395].
90. Welch LS. Decision making about reproductive hazards. *Semin Occup Med* 1986;1:97–106.
91. US Nuclear Regulatory Commission. Personal monitoring requirements. Washington: US Nuclear Regulatory Commission. [10 *CFR* 20.202].
92. US Nuclear Regulatory Commission. Nuclear regulatory commission rules and regulations. Washington: US Nuclear Regulatory Commission. [10 CFR].
93. Newton RW, Browning MCK, Ingal J, et al. Adrenal cortical suppression in workers manufacturing synthetic glucocorticoids. *BMJ* 1978;1:73–75.
94. Harrington JM, Stein GF, Rivers RV, DeMorales AV. The occupational hazards of formulating oral contraceptives: a survey of plant employees. *Arch Environ Health* 1978;33:12–14.
95. US Department of Health, Education and Welfare, Public Health Service. *Safety and operations manual: high containment research facility*. Bethesda, MD, National Cancer Institute, 1977.
96. *Classification of etiologic agents on the basis of hazard*. Atlanta: US Department of Health, Education and Welfare, Public Health Service, Centers for Disease Control, 1976.
97. Liberman DF. Facility description and personnel practices for research activity of comparable hazard. *Public Health Lab* 1980;37:118–129.
98. Jones L, Ristow S, Yilma T, Moss B. Accidental human immunization with vaccinia virus expressing nucleoprotein gene. *Nature* 1986;319:543.
99. Tarvainen K, Kanerva L, Tupasela O, et al. Allergy from cellulase and xylanase enzymes. *Clin Exp Allergy* 1991;21:609–615.
100. Lacey J, Crook B. Fungal and actinomycete spores and pollutants of the workplace and occupational allergens. *Ann Occup Hyg* 1988;32:515–533.

CHAPTER 39
Dental Health Care Hazards

Jacqueline Messite, Harriet S. Goldman, and Ana A. Taras

Dentists and dental health professionals comprise a sizable group at risk for multiple occupational exposures. Approximately 400,000 dental professionals are employed in dental offices, laboratories, nursing homes, hospitals, and outpatient care facilities. Of these, 105,248 are dentists in full-time private practice, with an additional 29,998 in part-time private practice (1). Approximately 92% of dentists employ at least one auxiliary person, including hygienists, chairside assistants, laboratory technicians, and secretarial and clerical personnel (2).

Although dental professionals are exposed to chemical, physical, and biological agents, the degree of exposure is commonly within limits set by the Occupational Safety and Health Administration (OSHA) (3). However, unacceptable hazards and exposures—including excessive amounts of mercury and waste anesthetic gases in the environment—have been found in a number of dental offices and clinics. In addition, several offices and clinics have been cited by OSHA for not following proper infection-control guidelines and for exposing office personnel to dangerous pathogens (4).

Dental practice is generally not considered to be a high-risk occupation, and the degree of exposure to chemical agents is not life-threatening. Depending on the type of toxic agent and the degree of exposure, however, the potential for increased morbidity does exist. This chapter reviews the major occupational exposures in the dental workplace and discusses recommended preventive measures.

CHEMICAL AGENTS

During the routine practice of dentistry, dentists and dental personnel are at risk for multiple exposures to chemical agents. Although considered benign at the levels of exposure experienced by most dental patients, prolonged or repeated exposure to many of these chemicals can result in adverse health effects to the dental staff. Acute exposures resulting from chemical releases in the workplace are also cause for concern. Well documented are the effects of exposure to mercury, a key ingredient in dental amalgam. Dental personnel can inadvertently inhale waste anesthetic gases, the long-term exposure to which has been associated with a variety of deleterious health effects. Operations involving dental alloys containing metals, such as nickel and beryllium, may also expose dental staff to potential health risks. Finally, a number of adverse health consequences may result after exposure to certain disinfectants, sterilants, and photographic materials.

Mitigation of the inherent risks associated with the practice of dentistry can be accomplished by simply creating a healthy workplace environment and encouraging safe work habits. By keeping abreast of up-to-date chemical and health hazard information, the dental team can take steps to minimize their exposure during various procedures. To this end, a variety of resources exists. Among the most important sources of information are the material safety data sheets (MSDSs) that present summarized information about the health hazards of the chemical substances in the workplace. Provided by the manufacturer, the MSDS contains information about the product's hazardous ingredients and physical and chemical characteristics. Fire and explosion hazard data, reactivity data, health hazard data, precautions for safe handling and use, and control measures are also included. Another important resource for dental staff is the product label. These references provide information on safe work practices, protective equipment, and procedures to follow in case of an emergency. State and local health departments and the National Institute for Occupational Safety and Health (NIOSH) also provide fact sheets about hazardous substances and the effects of exposures. The dental team should note that the 1988 OSHA hazard communication regulation requires employers to implement a written hazard communication program. This program mandates the labeling of hazardous materials and the updating of MSDSs.

In maintaining safe chemical exposure levels, dentists and dental personnel are bound by federal standards set by OSHA. Certain states, including New York and New Jersey, may set additional legal standards. NIOSH and the American Conference of Governmental Industrial Hygienists also develop recommended standards. All legal and recommended standards, however, should be considered as guides. To avoid any possible health effects, dental personnel must always attempt to keep their exposure to potentially hazardous chemicals as low as possible. Appendix 39-1 is a quick reference chart of some of the most common and potentially dangerous chemical hazards in the dental workplace.

Waste Anesthetic Gases

Administration of inhalation anesthesia in dental operatories has resulted in considerable exposure of dental personnel to waste anesthetic agents. Although anesthetic gases have long been used in medicine and dentistry, deleterious effects on those occupationally exposed were not reported until the 1960s. Subsequently, effects of exposure to these gases have received much attention from scientific and medical communities. Reported effects in humans include decrements in motor, perceptual, and cognitive skills; liver disease; cancer; spontaneous abortion; and birth defects in offspring.

NIOSH estimates that more than 100,000 dentists and dental assistants in the United States are directly exposed to trace concentrations of inhalation anesthetics every year. These gases include nitrous oxide, halothane, enflurane, and others. Studies (5) in dental operatories in the late 1970s indicated a mean concentration of 900 parts per million (ppm) of nitrous oxide in the breathing zone of the dentist, far in excess of the 50 ppm indicated by NIOSH as achievable during analgesic anesthesia. In 1986, Middendorf et al. found ambient concentrations of nitrous oxide ranging from 132 to 880 ppm in the breathing zone of surveyed dentists (6). Scavenging equipment was used in only 17 of the 27 dental operatories, and the major sources of exposure were identified as leaks around the mask and exhaled air from the patient's mouth. Nitrous oxide levels ranging from 3 to 239 ppm were found in 18 scavenged offices surveyed by Kugel et al. (7). The authors underscored the importance of using an adequate scavenging system that should be checked periodically.

Perceptual, cognitive, and motor skills were studied in 40 male medical and dental students exposed on two occasions of 4 hours each by inhalation to either air or 500 ppm nitrous oxide with 5 ppm halothane (8). Compared with responses after breathing air, responses after exposure to nitrous oxide and halothane showed statistically significant decrements in the performance of tasks in which attention was divided between auditory and visual signals, a visual tachistoscopic test, and a memory test involving digit span and recall of word pairs. After nitrous oxide alone, significant decrement in responses occurred on digit test span only. Measurable decrements in performance of volunteers during testing at concentrations as low as 50 ppm nitrous oxide with 1 ppm halothane were noted in subsequent studies. Similar effects were not seen with 25 ppm nitrous oxide and 0.5 ppm halothane (9).

Maternal and paternal exposures to waste anesthetic gases have resulted in statistically significant increases in spontaneous abortion. A large-scale epidemiologic survey (30,650 dentists and 30,547 chairside assistants) grouped subjects according to occupational exposure to inhalation anesthetics (10). The results showed a statistically significant 1.5-fold increase in the rate of spontaneous abortion among the wives of the exposed dentists. Exposed female assistants experienced a 1.7- to 2.3-fold increase in the rate of spontaneous abortions compared with the unexposed female dental assistants (10). A study of 7,000 female dental assistants in California found that high levels of exposure to nitrous oxide significantly affected fertility (11).

Exposure to waste anesthetic gases occurs primarily from leakage of gases from the anesthetic system, poor fit of the masks on patients, and improper work practices. In addition, cleansing (i.e., blowing out) the system after use can release considerable residual gas from the tubing into the environment, which contributes to staff exposure. To provide a safer workplace for those at risk for exposure to waste anesthetic gases, the following preventive measures should be implemented:

1. Use effective scavenging equipment and monitoring devices.
2. Regularly inspect anesthetic administration equipment for leaks.
3. Direct waste gas away from windows, ventilators, air-conditioning inlets, or other areas that might allow gases back into the office.
4. Maintain adequate ventilation.
5. Minimize conversation with patients.
6. Check for snug fit of face mask.
7. Maintain and service equipment regularly.

Mineral Dusts (Airborne Particulates)

Clinical dental procedures, such as high-speed grinding of silica-containing composite restoratives, the contouring of fused porcelain, and the polishing of metals and plastics with silica- or metallic oxide–containing materials, are routine in the dental work environment. Although the effects of these agents are not well characterized, the compositional and physical properties of some of the commonly used dust-producing minerals closely resemble the features of minerals, such as asbestos and silica, that have been identified as causative agents in dust diseases of the lungs (e.g., pneumoconioses).

Asbestos has been used chiefly as a binder in periodontal dressings and as a lining material for casting rings and crucibles. Airborne asbestos is known to cause pulmonary fibrosis (i.e., asbestosis), lung cancer, and mesothelioma of the pleura and peritoneum. Studies of airborne fibers of asbestos during preparation of gingivectomy packs have shown asbestos fibers in the atmosphere at inhalation levels of 3 ft (91 cm) above the height of the table (12). Concern for the potential danger to dental personnel from asbestos exposure has led the Council on Dental Therapeutics of the American Dental Association to eliminate this material from its program of Accepted Dental Therapeutics. Dentists should be aware of the occupational hazards surrounding asbestos and use packs that do not contain this material. Additionally, dentists should avoid sanding or drilling on countertops that may contain asbestos.

METALS

Beryllium

Exposure to beryllium, a highly toxic metal, can occur during the melting, grinding, buffing, and general lathing operations of beryllium-containing alloys in the preparation of prosthetic devices. Acute exposure to high concentrations of beryllium compounds can cause marked irritation of the eyes and respiratory tract, including the lung. Rom reported three cases of acute chemical pneumonitis in dental laboratory technicians analogous to acute berylliosis as described by Denardi in the 1940s (13). The technicians were overexposed from the grinding and melting of a nonprecious alloy containing 2% beryllium. All three technicians presented with dyspnea and reticulonodular infiltrates in their chest radiographs. Biopsies in these cases showed acute pneumonitis in one, interstitial fibrosis in another, and granulomas in the third. In addition, Rom reported finding two of seven personal samples for beryllium analysis taken on dental laboratory workers in Utah as being in excess of the OSHA permissible exposure limit.

Chronic exposure to beryllium can produce delayed-onset pulmonary granulomatosis and damage the liver, kidney, and circulatory system. Skin exposure can cause dermatitis, and beryllium metal or compounds implanted in lacerations may result in skin ulcers or granulomas.

Proper protective gloves, eye protection, and NIOSH-approved masks should be worn when casting, polishing, or grinding beryllium-containing alloys. Power suction methods rather than air hoses are recommended for cleaning machinery and removing dust from clothing. Wastes and contaminated clothing should be disposed of properly.

Mercury

The dental profession uses more than 100 tons of mercury each year (approximately 2 to 3 lb of mercury per dentist office) in dental restorations (14). Dental personnel are exposed to this metal through the contact or handling of mercury and mercury-containing compounds, and inhalation of mercuric vapors and respirable dusts. The greatest single source of mercury vapor contamination in the dental operatory is accidental spillage.

The literature on mercury contamination in the dental office is vast, and observations regarding safety range from reports of low risk to those of alarming danger. Several cases of mercury toxicity in dentists has been documented in the literature (15–17). Reported symptoms of chronic mercurialism include loss of appetite, nausea, diarrhea, speech disorders, ulceration of oral mucosa, gingivitis, central nervous system disturbances, nephritis, possible thrombocytopenia, and aplastic anemia.

At least 10% of all dental offices in the United States may have ambient mercury vapor levels above the NIOSH recommended threshold-limit value (TLV) of 0.05 mg per m^3 (18). Dentists, with average mercury blood levels from 5 to 10 ng per mL, have higher blood mercury levels than those of the general population (19,20). One comprehensive assessment of the magnitude of mercury exposure among dentists in the United States that measured urinary mercury concentrations in 4,272 dentists found a mean urinary mercury concentration of 14.2 μg per L (range 0 to 556 μg per L) (14). More than 90% of the dentists surveyed had urinary concentrations between 0 and 35 μg per L, and almost 5% had levels greater than 100 μg per L. At the American Dental Association's health screening after 1985, urinary mercury levels dropped more than 50% (21). Mean mercury concentrations in urine increased as the number of hours each week in practice increased, and those dentists who prepared their own silver amalgam mixture had a statistically significant higher exposure risk related to increased urinary mercury levels.

In a study by Ship and Shapiro (22), body mercury concentrations of a group of 300 practicing dentists were measured for long-term and short-term accumulation. Those dentists with high mercury accumulation, evidenced by x-ray fluorescence of the head and wrist (more than 40 μg per g), had neurologic and neuropsychological problems as well as deterioration in their visual graphic performance (23). The authors concluded that "the results of the study indicate that the current standards of mercury hygiene in dentistry are not consistent with safety in the dental office."

To investigate whether infants of mothers occupationally exposed to low levels of elemental mercury had increased mercury level, Wannay and Skjaerasen studied a group of 19 female dentists, dental assistants, and dental technicians, and compared them with a group of 26 nonexposed women (20). No measure of their workplace exposure was made, but it was inferred from other studies that the exposure was approximately the recommended TLV of 0.05 mg per m^3 or lower. Tissue analysis indicated that the mercury content of the placenta in the exposed group (24.5 ng per g) was twice that of the unexposed, and that the chorion and the amnion membrane showed corresponding differences between the exposed and the nonexposed group (21 and 11.5 ng per g for the chorion and 14.6 and 5.3 ng per g for the amnion membrane, respectively) (20). The placentas for both groups and the chorion in the exposed group contained more mercury than the corresponding erythrocytes and plasma; the amount of mercury in the blood of the mothers and infants in both groups at the time of delivery was similar (20). Another survey of approximately 40,000 dentists' spouses and assistants during a 10-year period reports no correlation between spontaneous abortion rates, congenital defects, and mercury exposure (24). A smaller study, however, suggests an association between mercury levels in hair and menstrual cycle or reproductive difficulties (25).

The key to prevention of mercury contamination is in reducing the risk of mercury escaping into the environment. Precautions to take in working with mercury should include the following:

1. Adequate ventilation.
2. Office monitoring for mercury vapor at least once a year, or more if contamination is suspected.
3. Personal monitoring.
4. Biological evaluation of all dental personnel at least once a year.
5. Use water spray and suction when grinding amalgam.
6. Proper amalgam handling using a no-touch technique—sealed amalgam capsules.
7. Proper mercury storage away from heat sources in unbreakable, tightly sealed, well-labeled containers.
8. Cleaning up spills immediately. Do not use a vacuum cleaner. A wash bottle top or a syringe can recover all visible droplets. Adhesive tape to clean up small spills can be used. Area should be decontaminated with sulfur-containing compounds (commercial suppressants).
9. Avoidance of skin contamination.

Nickel

The wider application of nickel-containing base metal alloys has sparked concern over the safety of this material in the dental environment. Nickel is used in the production of prosthetic devices, in which nickel content of the base alloy can range up to 81%. Exposure to nickel has been associated with lung and nasal cancer in certain nondental industrial settings, and NIOSH has designated the metal as a potential carcinogen. Nickel is also a powerful allergen, because approximately 10% of women and almost 1% of men are sensitive to this agent (26).

Sources of exposure to dental personnel include the inhalation or ingestion of the dust produced during the grinding of this material or the vapor produced by overheating during the casting procedure. Acute exposure to the dust and fumes can result in irritation to the eyes, mucous membranes, and respiratory system. Proper protective gloves, protective eyewear, and NIOSH-approved masks should be worn when fabricating or grinding nickel-containing alloys. The use of high-velocity evacuation systems is recommended. Although exposure to nickel can be minimized by adequate controls, the risk of allergic response may remain (27).

DISINFECTANTS AND STERILANTS

Dental personnel use a variety of agents to sterilize and disinfect instruments and equipment in the workplace. If not used properly, these chemicals can produce toxic reactions. The following disinfectants and sterilants may be found in the dental workplace.

Chlorine Solutions

Diluted chlorine solutions, such as sodium hypochlorite, are used in the dental work environment to disinfect surface areas, such as countertops, trays, and mirrors. Chlorine can be a severe irritant to the eyes, nose, throat, mucous membranes, and skin. Contact with eyes or skin may also cause severe burns. Chronic exposure to this chemical can lead to lung irritation, bronchitis, and dental erosion. Chlorine should only be used in well-ventilated areas, and proper protective gear should be worn.

Ethylene Oxide

Ethylene oxide (EtO), an alkylating agent, is used as a sterilant in dental offices. Exposure of dental personnel to EtO can occur when excessive quantities are released during routine use of sterilizers. NIOSH recommends that EtO in the workplace be regarded as a potential occupational carcinogen. This recommendation is based on results of animal studies demonstrating EtO to be associated with increased rates of leukemia, stomach cancer, and brain cancer. Evidence of mutagenicity in at least 13 biological species and epidemiologic investigations at worksites suggested an excess risk of cancer mortality among the EtO-exposed workers; however, updated metaanalysis of study cohorts has not demonstrated strong statistical risks (28–28c). In addition, EtO can cause skin, respiratory, and eye irritation; skin-sensitization; cutaneous burns; nausea; vomiting; diarrhea; and nervous system effects. Ethylene oxide also is a potential hazard to male and female reproduction (28). Dental staff performing sterilization operations with EtO should be informed of its potential toxicity, and exposure to this agent should be minimized. The following controls should be implemented when working with EtO (29):

1. Direct exhaust from sterilizers to a safe outdoor location.
2. Purge sterilizers with a sufficient amount of air before opening.
3. Ensure use of interlocks to prevent opening of sterilizers while they are being operated.
4. Check equipment for leakage or malfunctioning parts.
5. Use protective gloves and forceps to remove items from sterilizers.
6. Store in adequately ventilated areas in which sources of ignition are strictly controlled.

It is important to emphasize that when control is not assured, alternate means for sterilization should be considered.

Glutaraldehyde Solutions

Glutaraldehyde is used in solutions for sterilization of non–heat-resistant instruments and for disinfection of handpieces. This chemical can cause severe irritation to the eyes, nose, and throat at low concentrations in the air. Contact with glutaraldehyde solutions can severely burn the eyes and may cause permanent damage. According to the *Right to Know Handbook for Dental Clinical Staff*, produced by the City of New York Mayor's Office of Operations, Citywide Office of Occupational Safety and Health, and District Council 37 Education Fund, a 5% glutaraldehyde solution, at first use, can cause dermatitis at much lower concentrations on repeated exposures. Glutaraldehyde should be used in well-ventilated areas, and heavy-duty rubber gloves should be worn. Chemical residues of glutaraldehyde on instruments should be wiped clean with alcohol. OSHA has published a ceiling concentration of glutaraldehyde of 0.2 ppm (29 *CFR* 1910, January 9, 1989). Cold sterilization procedures use solutions of glutaraldehyde, ranging from 0.13% up to 2%. A 2% glutaraldehyde solution left uncovered can generate airborne breathing zone concentrations in excess of the 0.2-ppm ceiling limit set by OSHA. Proper ventilation and use of butyl rubber gloves instead of latex gloves are necessary to protect workers.

Phenols and Phenolic Compounds

Phenols and phenolic compounds are toxic substances that should be used with care for emergencies in the dental work environment. Skin irritation can occur on contact with 0.5% phenol solution. Skin contact with stronger solutions of phenol or phenol compounds is not immediately painful, but deep damage and even local gangrene can result. Extensive skin absorption can affect the central nervous system and the circulatory system, subsequently causing difficulty in breathing, ringing in the ears, tremors, and convulsions. Vapors can cause irritation of the nose and throat, nausea, and vomiting. Repeated exposure may damage the liver and kidney. Strict precautions must be instituted if work with this substance is necessary. Adequate ventilation must be present and protection given to the skin, eyes, and face.

ORGANIC CHEMICALS

Methyl Methacrylate

Methyl methacrylate is used in the production of prosthetic devices. The monomer component of methyl methacrylate is an irritant to the eyes, mucous membranes, skin, and respiratory system. The material can be absorbed through the skin and produce neurologic effects, such as finger and palmar paresthesia, pain, and whitening of fingers in cold (30). Contact with methyl methacrylate may cause dermatitis and eye irritation, and inhalation of the vapor causes salivation and respiratory irritation. Exposure to high concentrations can cause unconsciousness and death, but the agent's powerful odor should alert most dental workers to its presence.

Pregnant rats exposed to methacrylate esters demonstrated embryo and fetal toxicity and teratogenic effects (31). Exposure of a human to methacrylate vapors has resulted in a prompt decrease in gastric motor activity that lasts for 20 to 30 minutes after cessation of exposure (32).

When using this material, dental personnel should wear safety glasses and gloves, and work in a well-ventilated area or use a supplied air respirator to avoid breathing the vapor. Any spills should be cleaned up promptly, and any areas of skin contact washed thoroughly.

Alcohols

Most alcohols are of relatively low toxicity but can be hazardous without proper precautions. Solutions of isopropyl alcohol can cause skin irritation and dryness with direct contact. Vapors from this agent can also cause eye, nose, and throat irritation. At very high levels, isopropyl alcohol is considered a narcotic. Alcohols should be used only to remove chemical residues, and not used to disinfect or sterilize equipment and surfaces.

PHOTOGRAPHIC DEVELOPERS AND FIXERS

Dental personnel who come in contact with photographic developers and fixers can be exposed to a variety of chemicals. Staff who work with these agents should be aware of their potential hazards.

1. Hydroquinone, used in developers, can severely irritate the skin and burn the eye. Repeated exposure can stain and discolor the mucous membranes covering the eyes, possibly leading to permanent damage. Limited evidence shows that chronic exposure to hydroquinone may lead to adverse reproductive effects (33).
2. Sulfur dioxide can build up in tanks containing photographic fixers. At low levels, vapors can cause eye, nose, and throat irritation. Exposure to high levels may result in dyspnea, coughing, and choking. Repeated exposure can lead to nosebleeds and irritation of the throat and lungs.

Control measures in working with photographic chemicals should include use of protective eyewear and heavy-duty rubber gloves. Contact lenses should be avoided, as they may absorb vapors. Adequate ventilation is imperative, and spilled chemicals should be cleaned up immediately. Exposure to dry powder during solution preparation should be minimized, and skin that comes in contact with these chemicals should be washed off immediately with a pH-balanced soap.

ACIDS

Acids are used in dentistry in pickling solutions, and in acid etch solutions and gels. Skin contact with these corrosive chemicals can cause serious injury. Eye contact may lead to permanent eye damage and blindness. Inhalation of vapors can cause nose, throat, and lung irritation. Exposure to high concentrations of these substances may result in unconsciousness and even death. Phosphoric acid and sulfuric acids are commonly used in acid etch solutions. Hydrochloric acid, nitric acid, picric acid, and sulfuric acids are used in pickling solutions. Acetic acid is found in photographic solutions.

Dental personnel who work with acids should take the following precautions:

1. Use proper protective gloves and eyewear.
2. Allow adequate ventilation.
3. Wash any skin or eye contact immediately with running water for 5 to 10 minutes. Seek medical assistance.
4. In the event of a spill, keep neutralizing agents, such as a soda lime, or commercial acid spill cleanup kit available.
5. Handle solutions carefully. Avoid splashes. Always add water to acid when mixing.
6. Properly label and store all acid-containing solutions.
7. Use forceps to handle any object being treated in acids.

SOAPS AND DETERGENTS

On average, dental personnel wash their hands more than 15 times a day (34). Such frequent contact with soaps and detergents is the most common cause of contact dermatitis among dental workers. The most likely reason for these dermatoses is destruction of the protective layers of the epidermis. Consequently, hand cleaners that do not contain abrasives, defat the skin, cause allergic sensitization, and break down with storage should be used.

LATEX

Hypersensitivity to latex is a serious medical problem that is affecting an increasing number of health care workers as well as their patients. One study revealed a 12% prevalence of immediate-type latex allergy among professionals in a hospital-based dental practice. This is similar to that in other health care workers who use latex gloves frequently (35). The use of vinyl, neoprene, or other latex substitute gloves should solve the problem.

PHYSICAL AGENTS

Ionizing Radiation

A considerable benefit exists from the judicious use of radiographic examinations in dental practice to evaluate such clinical situations as caries, periodontal disease, cysts, and tumors of the jaws. However, dental personnel should be familiar with the effects of such exposure and the measures needed to reduce the potential hazards for themselves as well as for their patients. With the development of more sensitive fast-speed films, and better techniques, equipment, and monitoring devices, the exposure of dental personnel and patients has been reduced considerably. Such effects as leukemia and shortened lifespan noted in the early dental literature no longer represent a significant risk for dental personnel. Nevertheless, there can be no apathy in the concern for unnecessary radiation exposure. Constant vigilance is required to assure that all measures are being taken to reduce the exposure to as low as possible. The Center for Devices and Radiologic Health of the U.S. Public Health Service has published guidelines on when, what types of radiographs, and at what intervals dental radiographs should be taken (36).

Nonionizing Radiation

Blue light has replaced ultraviolet light in most offices and laboratories as a means of curing resins and sealants. It can cause thermal or photochemical injury to the retina.

Lasers are also a potential hazard in the dental office. The energy they generate can burn or alter the target tissue and should never be directed toward nontarget tissues, the eyes, or onto reflective surfaces. For blue light and lasers, sources for such exposure should be properly maintained, located, and shielded so that eye exposure and skin contact are minimized. Protective glasses are available.

INFECTIOUS AGENTS

The dental office is a site for transmission of infectious diseases. These infectious diseases are transmitted by the following (37):

1. Direct contact (contact at source, the patient's mouth).
2. Indirect contact (contact with items contaminated with patient's microbes, such as surfaces, hands, sharps).

3. Droplet infection (contact with sprays, splashes, aerosols, or spatter).

Microbial routes of entry include the following (38):

1. Inhalation (aerosols generated by high-speed drilling and prophylaxis procedures).
2. Ingestion (swallowing spattered droplets of blood and saliva).
3. Mucous membranes (spattering into eyes, nose, and mouth).
4. Breaks in skin.

Airborne illnesses consist of upper respiratory infections, including tuberculosis and pneumonia. Blood-borne diseases include hepatitis B, herpes, and acquired immune deficiency syndrome (AIDS). Table 39-1 is a chart on the transmission of the most common infectious diseases in the dental office.

Herpes Simplex

Herpes simplex infections are of great practical importance to dentists because lesions of the eyes and fingers produce temporary inability to practice (38). Repeated recurrences of ocular herpes can lead to blindness and permanent inability to practice (39). The disease, which is caused by two viruses—type 1 and type 2—is spread predominantly by direct contact. The virus is found in gingival saliva and throat swabs. Clinically, the disease appears initially as vesicles that then break down to form ulcers. They heal without scarring in 14 to 21 days. The disease orally affects all mucous membranes and the lips (i.e., cold sore or fever blister) and recurs throughout a person's lifetime.

It is estimated that anywhere from 30% to 80% of adults in the general population have been exposed to the virus, depending on socioeconomic status (40). In the dental population, the prevalence of herpes virus increases with age, and, therefore, the young dentist, because he or she has probably had less exposure to the virus, is most susceptible to infection. Although eye and lip lesions occur more often in the general population, finger infection occurs twice as frequently in practicing dentists (31).

Hepatitis B

Hepatitis B can be devastating to the dental professional. Transmission of the virus in dental personnel is primarily by direct contact with contaminated blood or saliva through a break in the skin of the hands, or possibly through the mucous membranes of the eyes, mouth, or nose. The organism can survive for days on countertops, switches, and other environmental surfaces. The incubation period is long, usually between 6 weeks and 6 months. Early symptoms include extreme fatigue, headaches, malaise, joint pain, fever, and finally jaundice. Work may be impossible for as long as 6 months (40). OSHA estimates that each year in the health care environment, without vaccinations against it, there are 6,000 to 7,000 new hepatitis B infections. Between 1,500 and 1,900 persons develop acute symptoms, 300 to 400 persons are hospitalized, and between 130 and 165 persons die each year if the disease is contracted (41).

The dental profession's risk of acquiring hepatitis B is four times that of the general population (40). The prevalence among dentists in 1988 was 28%, with an illness rate of 6% (42,43). It is

TABLE 39-1. Serious infectious diseases found in dentistry

Disease	Agent	Route of transmission	Incubation period	Potential complications
Acquired immunodeficiency syndrome	Virus	Contact from blood, other body fluids	6 mo to 15 yr	Death
Chicken pox	Virus	Saliva, blood, droplets	10–21 d	Conjunctivitis, shingles, encephalitis
Common cold	Virus	Saliva, blood, droplets	48–72 h	Temporary disability
Cytomegalovirus	Virus	Oral	2–8 wk	Birth defects, death
Gonorrhea	Bacteria	Mucous membrane contact	1–7 d	Arthritis, female sterility, infant blindness
Hepatitis A	Virus	Oral, fecal	2–7 wk	Disability
Hepatitis B	Virus	Saliva, blood, droplets	6 wk–6 mo	Chronic disability, carrier mode death
Hepatitis (non-A, non-B)	Virus	Saliva, blood, droplets	6 wk–5 mo	Chronic disability, death
Hepatitis delta	"Piggyback" virus	Blood, other routes under investigation	Not known	Death, chronic carrier
Hepatic conjunctivitis	Virus	Saliva, blood, droplets	6–10 wk	Blindness
Herpes simplex II	Virus	Mucous membrane contact, possible saliva, blood	Up to 2 wk, also latent	Painful lesions, disability, death in children
Herpetic whitlow	Virus	Saliva, blood, droplets	2–12 d, also latent	Extreme pain, disability
Infectious mononucleosis	Virus	Saliva, blood, droplets	4–7 wk	Temporary disability
Influenza	Virus	Saliva, droplets	1–3 d	Death
Legionellosis	Bacteria	Respiratory	2–10 d	Death
Measles (German)	Virus	Saliva, nasal, droplets	9–11 d	Congenital defects, infant death
Measles (rubeola)	Virus	Saliva, nasal, droplets	9–11 d	Temporary disability, encephalitis
Mumps (men)	Virus	Respiratory	14–25 d	Temporary disability, sterility
Pneumonia	Bacteria	Respiratory, blood	Varies with organism	Death
	Virus	Blood		
Staphylococcus infections	Bacteria	Saliva, droplets, nosocomial	4–10 d	Skin lesions, osteomyelitis, death
Streptococcus infections	Bacteria	Saliva, blood, droplets	1–3 d	Rheumatic heart, kidney problems, death
Syphilis	Bacteria	Mucous membrane contact, congenital	2–12 wk	Central nervous damage, death
Tetanus	Bacteria	Open wound	7–10 d	Disability, death
Tuberculosis	Bacteria	Saliva, droplets	Up to 6 mo, also latent	Disability, death

From Runnells RR. *Infection control in the former wet finger environment.* Salt Lake, UT: I.C. Publishers Press, 1984.

estimated that there were approximately 3,000 asymptomatic carriers among dentists. This is not surprising, because an office seeing 20 patients per day treats one active hepatitis-carrier patient in 7 working days (36,37). As of 1992, more than 85% of dentists reported hepatitis B vaccination, and serologic evidence of infection decreased to 9% (44).

Hepatitis C

Hepatitis C is also devastating to the dental professional and is becoming more of an emerging problem. Hollow-bore needles are often the vehicle for transmission. Although hepatitis B is more transmittable, hepatitis C is more likely to produce a carrier state. It is transmitted percutaneously (45).

Acquired Immunodeficiency Syndrome

AIDS, a disease with a near 100% mortality rate, is transmitted by a virus through direct contact with body fluids, specifically blood and semen. Saliva does not seem to be a transmitter. A devastating disease marked by a decrease in the immune response, AIDS leaves an individual susceptible to life-threatening opportunistic infections as well as to various cancers (46).

Since 1987, studies of more than 17,000 dental workers, many of whom cared for AIDS or high-risk patients, have shown only three dentists who had antibodies to human immunodeficiency virus (HIV). Two of them had no other risk factors (47–47b).

Of further interest is a report from the Centers for Disease Control and Prevention (CDC) that states at least three patients have been infected in the course of treatment by an HIV-infected dentist (48,48a). CDC investigation of the dental practice in which this occurred found serious deficiencies in infection-control practices. No written policy or training course on infection-control practices was provided for the staff by the dentist, and no office protocol existed for reporting injuries, such as needlesticks. Barrier precautions were used, but the dental practice did not have written protocol or a consistent pattern for operatory cleanup and instrument reprocessing.

Tuberculosis

Tuberculosis is a leading cause of death related to infectious diseases worldwide (49,50). Predominantly an airborne disease, the contaminated droplets are discharged into the air by a person with active disease. These droplets can remain suspended in the air for a period, ready to be inhaled by a susceptible individual, even after the infected person leaves the immediate area. It is caused by the *Mycobacterium tuberculosis* bacillus. If the initial lung lesions do not heal, active disease occurs. Symptoms include fatigue, cough, weight loss, fever, chills, night sweats, malaise, and loss of appetite (40). Approximately 15 million persons have been infected, 90% of whom are asymptomatic and do not develop active tuberculosis (39). For many years, tuberculosis has been declining, but the disease is again on the increase among specific groups: immigrants from areas in the world in which a high incidence of this disease exists and in which many have received no or inadequate therapy, HIV-positive individuals, migrant farm workers, Native Americans, and those living in inner city slum areas. Another cause for alarm is the rapid emergence of multidrug-resistant tuberculosis. CDC guidelines should be followed.

Some General Practice Guidelines

CHEMICAL AGENTS:

For each of the chemical processes or products used, the following should be considered:

- Do you know the generic name and potential toxic effects of each ingredient?
- Have you obtained material safety data sheets from the manufacturer?
- Are all employees aware of proper handling practices, precautions, and cleanup instructions for spills?
- Are all hazardous substances properly labeled and stored?
- Is proper protective equipment available and used as indicated?
- Are in-service training sessions carried out at least annually?
- Are you and your employees aware of signs and symptoms of accidental exposures?
- Are records kept of the dates, quantities, and names of all chemicals used?
- Is the office adequately ventilated?
- Are eating, drinking, and smoking prohibited in the work area?
- Do you and your employees always try to use the least toxic substance for any operation or procedure?
- Is an eye wash fountain present in case of emergencies?
- Is hazardous waste disposed of properly?

PHYSICAL AGENTS

Ionizing radiation

- Are you and your staff aware of the latest techniques and requirements for the safe use of radiation?
- Does your equipment meet the state and federal requirements in regard to the x-ray beam diameter and filtration, and do you minimize the time and amperage needed to obtain satisfactory results?
- Is your examination room set up to permit adequate distance (at least 6 feet or 2 meters) for the x-ray operator to stand when the equipment is functioning?
- Do you have an adequately screened and shielded area for your workload?
- Do you use x-ray holders or other devices to hold film in place?
- Do you provide patients with a lead apron?
- Do you only use high-speed film?
- Do you have a quality control program for developing and fixing solutions to assure consistent film quality?
- Do you have your office inspected periodically by qualified persons to ensure that all equipment and shielding are properly maintained?
- Have you considered personnel dosimeter measurements for you and your staff to assure control?

Nonionizing radiation

- Are the sources of this radiation properly maintained and serviced?
- Are the operators properly shielded from the exposure?

INFECTIOUS DISEASES

Prevention of transmission includes the following:

- Are all employees as well as the dentist properly vaccinated?
- Do you take a thorough medical history on all patients?
- Are handwashing guidelines being followed?
- Are proper barrier techniques being utilized? These include gloves, masks, glasses, gowns, and protection of environmental surfaces.
- Are sharps being disposed of properly?
- Are proper sterilization and disinfection modalities being utilized, including flushing of waterlines, air/water syringes, and handpieces?
- Are prosthetic appliances, casts, impressions, wax rims disinfected?
- Is contamination by droplets and spatter limited by the use of high-volume evacuation, proper patient positioning, and rubber dams?

Figure 39-1. Dental workplace checklist.

Transmission

With all these infectious diseases, the possibility for transmission in the dental profession is significant. However, the actual number of cases is difficult to determine because specific morbidity is lacking (51). It should be stressed, however, that all dental personnel should be familiar with infection-control procedures specified by CDC and the American Dental Association, and that these procedures should be rigorously enforced (52,53).

DENTAL WORKPLACE CHECKLIST

The keys to maintaining safety in the workplace are knowledge and prevention. If potential for exposure to harmful agents is minimized, then dental personnel reduce their risk for adverse health effects. Appropriate infection control mechanisms must be in place to assure prevention of infectious diseases. Figure 39-1 consists of a checklist that can serve as general practice guidelines in surveying a dental workplace.

REFERENCES

1. American Dental Association, Bureau of Economic Research and Statistics. *1991 distribution of dentists*. Chicago: American Dental Association, 1992.
2. American Dental Association, Bureau of Economic Research and Statistics. *1995 survey of dental practice*. Chicago: American Dental Association, 1996.
3. Messite J. Occupational safety and health in the dental workplace. In: Goldman HS, Messite J, eds. *Occupational hazards in dentistry*. Chicago: Year Book Medical Publishers, 1984.
4. Jakush J. OSHA pays dentists visit: dentists pay sometime later. *Am Dental Assoc News* 1989.
5. Whitcher CE, Zimmerman DC, Piziali RL. *Control of occupational exposure to N_2O in the dental operatory*. Cincinnati: US Department of Health, Education and Welfare, National Institute on Occupational Safety and Health, 1977. [Publication 77-171].
6. Middendorf PJ, Jacobs DE, Smith KA, Mastro DM. Occupational exposures to nitrous oxide in dental operatories. *Anesth Prog* 1986;33:91–97.
7. Kugel G, Norris L, Zive M. Nitrous oxide and occupational exposure: It's time to stop laughing. *Anesth Prog* 1989;36:252–257.
8. Bruce DL, Bach MJ, Arbit J. Trace anesthetic effects on perceptual, cognitive, and motor skills. *Anesthesiology* 1974;40:453–458.
9. Bruce DL, Bach MJ. *Trace effects of anesthetics gases on behavioral performance of operating personnel*. Cincinnati: US Department of Health and Human Services, Public Health Service, National Institute of Occupational Safety and Health, 1976. [Publication 76–169].
10. Cohen EN, et al. Occupational disease in dentistry and chronic exposure to trace anesthetic gases. *J Am Dental Assoc* 1980;101:21–31.
11. Rowland AS, Baird DD, Weinberg CR, Shore VL, Shy CM, Wilcox AJ. Reduced fertility among women employed as dental assistants exposed to high levels of nitrous oxide. *N Engl J Med* 1992;327:993–997.
12. Dyer MR. The possible adverse effects of asbestos in gingivectomy packs. *Br Dent J* 1967;122:507.
13. Rom WN, Lockey JE, Lee JS, et al. Pneumoconiosis and exposure of dental laboratory technicians. *Am J Public Health* 1984;74:1252–1257.
14. Naleway C, Sakaguchi R, Mitchell E, Muller T, Ayer WA, Hefferren JJ. Urinary mercury levels in US dentists, 1975–1983: review of health assessment program. *J Am Dental Assoc* 1985;111:37–42.
15. Merfield DP, Taylor A, Gemmell DM, Parrish JA. Mercury intoxication in a dental surgery following unreported spillage. *Br Dent J* 1976;141:179–186.
16. Symmington IS, Cross JD, Dale IM. Mercury poisoning in dentists. *J Soc Occup Med* 1980;30:37–39.
17. Shapiro IM, Cornblath DR, Sumner AJ, et al. Neurophysiological and neuropsychological function in mercury exposed dentists. *Lancet* 1982;2:1147–1150.
18. Mantyla DG, Wright OD. Mercury toxicity in the dental office: a neglected problem. *J Am Dental Assoc* 1976;92:1189.
19. Battistone GC, Hefferren JJ, Miller RA, Cutright DE. Mercury: its relation to the dentist's health and dental practice characteristics. *J Am Dental Assoc* 1976;92:1182–1188.
20. Goldman HS. Mercury: problems and control. In: Goldman HS, Hartman KS, Messite J, eds. *Occupational hazards in dentistry*. Chicago: Year Book Medical Publishers, 1984.
21. Naleway CA, Roxe D, Chouc HN, Muller T, Dabney J, Siddoque F. On site screening for urinary Hg concentrations and correlation with glomerular and renal tubular function. *J Public Health Dent* 1991;51:12–17.
22. Shipp II, Shapiro IM. Mercury poisoning in dental practice. *Compendium Continuing Education General Dentistry* 1983;4:107–110.
23. Wannay A, Skjaersen J. Mercury accumulation in placenta and fetal membranes: a study of dental workers and their babies. *Environ Phys Biochem* 1975;5:348–352.
24. Brodsky JB, Cohen EN, Whitches C, Brown BW Jr, Wu MV. Occupational exposure to mercury in dentistry and pregnancy outcome. *J Am Dental Assoc* 1985;111:779–790.
25. Sikorski R, Juskiewicz T, Paszkowski T, Szpregier-Juskiewicz T. Women in dental surgeries: reproductive hazards in occupational exposure to metallic mercury. *Int Arch Occup Environ Health* 1987;59:551–557.
26. National Institute of Dental Research. Workshop: biocompatibility of metals in dentistry. *J Am Dental Assoc* 1984;109:469–471.
27. Newman SM. The relationship of metals to the general health of the patient, the dentist and office staff. *Int Dent J* 1986;36:35–40.
28. Their R, Bolt HM. Carcinogenicity and genotoxicity of the ethylene oxide: new aspects and recent advances. *Crit Rev Toxicol* 2000;30:595–608.

28a. Walker VE, Wu KY, Upton PB, et al. Biomarkers of exposure and effect as indicators of potential carcinogenic risk arising from in vivo metabolism of ethylene to ethylene oxide. *Carcinogenesis* 2000;21:1661–1669.

28b. Teta MJ, Sielken RL Jr, Valdez-Flores C. Ethylene oxide cancer risk assessment based on epidemiological data: application of revised regulatory guidelines. *Risk Anal* 1999;19:1135–1155.

28c. Shore RE, Garnder MJ, Pannett B. Ethylene oxide: an assessment of the epidemiological evidence on carcinogenicity. *Br J Ind Med* 1993;50:971–997.

29. Cooley RL. Physical, chemical and thermal injuries. In: Goldman HS, Hartman KS, Messite J, eds. *Occupational hazards in dentistry*. Chicago: Year Book Medical Publishers, 1984.
30. Rajaniemi R, Tola S. Subjective symptoms among dental technicians exposed to the monomer methyl methacrylate. *Scand J Work Environ Health* 1985;11:281–286.
31. Singh AR, Lawrence WH, Autian J. Embryonic-fetal toxicity and teratogenic effects of a group of methacrylate esters in rats. *Appl Pharmacol* 1972;22:314–315.
32. Tansy MF, Benhoyem S, Probst S. The effects of methyl methacrylate vapor on gastric motor function. *J Am Dental Assoc* 1974;89:372–376.
33. New Jersey State Department of Health. *Hazardous substance fact sheet—hydroquinone*. Trenton, NJ: New Jersey State Department of Health, 1985.
34. Caruso RJ. Dermatitis: a dentist's occupational hazard. *N Y State Dental J* 1981;47:543–545.
35. Safadi G, Safadi T, Terezhalmy G, Taylor J, Battisto J, Milton A. Latex hypersensitivity: its prevalence among dental professionals. *J Am Dental Assoc* 1996;127:83–88.
36. US Department of Health and Human Services, Public Health Service, FDA. The selection of patients for x-ray examinations, dental radiographs examinations. Rockville, MD: 1987.
37. Miller CH, Palenik CJ. *Infection control and management of hazardous materials for the dental team*. St. Louis: Mosby, 1994.
38. Rowe NH, Neine CS, Kowalski CJ. Herpetic whitlow: an occupational disease of practicing dentists. *J Am Dental Assoc* 1982;105:471–473.
39. Hartman KS. Infectious and communicable diseases. In: Goldman HS, Hartman KS, Messite J, eds. *Occupational hazards in dentistry*, 9th ed. Chicago: Year Book Medical Publishers, 1994.
40. Burket LW. *Oral medicine, diagnosis and treatment*. Philadelphia: JB Lippincott Co, 1984.
41. Proceedings of the National Symposium on Hepatitis B and the Dental Profession. *J Am Dental Assoc* 1985;110:613–650.
42. Siew C, et al. Screening dentists for HIV and hepatitis B. *N Engl J Med* 1988;318:1400–1401.
43. Siew C, et al. Survey of hepatitis B exposure and vaccination in volunteer dentists. *J Am Dental Assoc* 1987;114:457–459.
44. Cleveland, Jennifer L. Hepatitis B vaccinations and infection among US dentists, 1983–1992. *J Am Dental Assoc* 1996;127:1385–1390.
45. Cottone JA, Terezhalmy, GT, Molinari JA. *Practical infection control in dentistry*, 2nd ed. Philadelphia: Williams & Wilkins, 1996.
46. Robertson P, Greenspan D. *Perspectives on oral manifestations of AIDS*. Littleton, MA: PSG Publishing, 1988.
47. Chenoweth CE, Gobetti JP. Postexposure chemoprophylaxis for occupational exposure to HIV in the dental office. *J Am Dent Assoc* 1997;128:1135–1139.

47a. Root-Bernstein RS. Dental and research transmission of acquired immune deficiency syndrome? Or, is there any evidence that human immunodeficiency virus is sufficient to cause acquired immune deficiency syndrome? *Med Hypotheses* 1996;47:117–122.

47b. Henderson DK. Postexposure chemoprophylaxis for occupational exposures to the human immunodeficiency virus. *JAMA* 1999;281:931–936.

48. Centers for Disease Control and Prevention. Update: transmission of HIV infection during an invasive dental procedure—Florida. *MMWR Morb Mortal Wkly Rep* 1991;40:21–27.

48a. Hardie J. AIDS and dentistry: a retrospective analysis of the Florida case. *J Can Dent Assoc* 1993;59:987–991,1000.

49. Centers for Disease Control. Tuberculosis—United States, 1984. *MMWR Morb Mortal Wkly Rep* 1985;34:229.
50. Woodruff G. Tuberculosis and the dentist. *Aust Dent J* 1957;2:7–12.
51. Zwemer J, Williams J. Dentists, health status and risks. *J Am Coll Dent* 1987;54:7–12.
52. Centers for Disease Control and Prevention. Recommended infection control practices for dentistry. *MMWR Morb Mortal Wkly Rep* 1986;35:237–242.
53. American Dental Association. Infection control recommendations for the dental office and the dental laboratory. *J Am Dental Assoc* 1996;127:672–679.

APPENDIX 39-1

Most Common and Potentially Dangerous Chemical Hazards in the Dental Workplace

Name	Sources of exposure	Health effects	Standards: OSHA (PEL)[a] TWA	OSHA (PEL)[a] STEL	NIOSH (REL)[a]	ACGIH (TLV)[b] TWA	ACGIH (TLV)[b] STEL	Preventive measures
Acetic acid	Photographic solutions	Eye, nose, throat, and skin irritation; bronchitis; skin and eye burns	10 ppm 25 mg/m^3	— —	10 ppm 25 mg/m^3	10 ppm 25 mg/m^3	15 ppm 37 mg/m^3	1. Use proper protective gloves and eyewear. 2. Allow adequate ventilation. 3. Wash any skin or eye contact immediately with running water for 5 to 10 min. Seek medical assistance. 4. In the event of a spill, keep neutralizing agents such as soda lime or commercial acid spill cleanup kit available. 5. Handle solutions carefully. Avoid splashing. Always add water to acid when mixing. 6. Properly label and store all acid-containing solutions. 7. Use forceps to handle any object being treated in acids.
Acetone	Solvents	Eye, nose, throat, mucous membrane and skin irritation; dermatitis; CNS depressant	1,000 ppm 2,400 mg/m^3	—	250 ppm 590 mg/m^3	750 ppm 1,780 mg/m^3	1,000 ppm 2,380 mg/m^3	Wear proper protective eyewear and gloves.
Asbestos	Lining materials for casting binders in periodontal dressings	Pulmonary fibrosis; lung cancer; mesothelioma Identified by NIOSH as a potential human carcinogen and by ACGIH as a confirmed human carcinogen	Action level of 100,000 fibers/m^3 TWA[c]	—	100,000 fibers/m^3[,c] TWA in a 400-L sample	Amosite Chrysotile Crocidolite Other forms	0.5 fibers/cc[c] 2 fibers/cc[c] 0.2 fibers/cc[c] 2 fibers/cc[c]	Wear proper protective eyewear, gloves, and NIOSH-approved mask.
Beryllium	Casting alloys	Dermatitis, eye irritation; pulmonary edema; pneumonitis; pulmonary granulomatosis (delayed onset) Identified by NIOSH as a potential human carcinogen and by ACGIH as a confirmed human carcinogen	0.002 ppm	0.005 ppm (30 min) 0.025 ppm (C)	Do not exceed 0.5 µg Be/m^3	0.002 mg/m^3	—	Wear proper protective eyewear, gloves, and NIOSH-approved mask. Use power suction methods to remove dust.
Calcium carbonate	Polishing agents	Eye, nose, throat, and respiratory irritation	15 mg/m^3 (total dust) 5 mg/m^3 (respirable fraction)	—	10 mg/m^3 (total dust) 5 mg/m^3 (respirable fraction)	10 mg/m^3	—	Wear proper protective eyewear, gloves, and NIOSH-approved mask.
Chlorine	Disinfectants	Eye, nose, throat, mucous membrane, and skin irritation; bronchitis; dermatitis; dental erosion	0.1 ppm 0.3 mg/m^3	—	0.5 ppm (C) 1.45 mg/m^3 (C)	0.5 ppm 1.5 mg/m^3	1 ppm 2.9 mg/m^3	Wear proper protective eyewear and gloves.
Chromium (metal)	Casting alloys	Dermatitis; histologic fibrosis of the lung	1 mg/m^3	—	0.5 mg/m^3	0.5 mg/m^3	—	Wear proper protective eyewear, gloves, and NIOSH-approved mask.
Cobalt (metal)	Casting alloys	Eye, nose, throat, and skin irritation; dermatitis; respiratory hypersensitivity	0.05 mg/m^3	—	—	0.02 mg/m^3	—	Wear proper protective eyewear, gloves, and NIOSH-approved mask.

(continued)

Name	Sources of exposure	Health effects	OSHA (PEL)[a]		NIOSH (REL)[a]	ACGIH (TLV)[b]		Preventive measures
			TWA	STEL		TWA	STEL	
Ethylene oxide	Sterilizing agents	Skin, respiratory, and eye irritation; skin sensitization; peritoneal cancer; leukemia; adverse reproductive effects	1 ppm	—	5 ppm (10 min/d C)	1 ppm	—	1. Direct exhaust from sterilizers to a safe outdoor location. 2. Purge sterilizers with a sufficient amount of air before opening. 3. Ensure use of interlocks to prevent opening of sterilizers while they are being operated. 4. Check equipment for leakage or malfunctioning parts. 5. Use protective gloves and forceps to remove items from sterilizers. 6. Store in adequately ventilated areas where sources of ignition are strictly controlled.
		Identified by NIOSH as a potential human carcinogen; by ACGIH as a suspected human carcinogen	1.8 mg/m³ (5 ppm excursion limit)		9 mg/m³ (10 min/d C) <0.1 ppm (0.18 mg/m³) TWA	1.8 mg/m³	—	
Glutaraldehyde	Sterilizing agents	Eye, nose, and throat irritation; dermatitis; contact with eye may cause severe burns	— —	— —	2 ppm (C) 5 mg/m³ (15 min)	— —	0.2 ppm (C) 0.82 mg/m³ (C)	Wear proper protective gloves.
Hydrogen fluoride	Etching agents for porcelain	Nose, throat, and respiratory irritation; bronchitis; burns	3 ppm	—	3 ppm 10-h TWA 2.5 mg/m³ 10-h TWA 6 ppm (C)	— —	3 ppm (C) 2.3 mg/m³ (C)	Wear proper protective eyewear and gloves.
Hydroquinone	Methacrylate and denture base resins; photographic solutions	Eye and skin irritation, conjunctivitis, and keratitis	2 mg/m³	—	2 mg/m³ (C)	2 mg/m³	—	Wear proper protective eyewear and gloves.
Isopropyl alcohol	Solvents, wiping agents	Eye, nose, throat, and skin irritation; dermatitis	400 ppm 980 mg/m³	500 ppm 1,225 mg/m³	400 ppm 980 mg/m³ ST 500 ppm 1,225 mg/m³	400 ppm 983 mg/m³	500 ppm 1,230 mg/m³	Wear proper protective gloves.
Mercury	Amalgam	Loss of appetite, nausea, diarrhea, speech disorders, ulceration of mucosa, gingivitis, central nervous system disorders, nephritis, thrombocytopenia, aplastic anemia	—	0.1 mg/m³	0.05 mg/m³ TWA	0.025 mg/m³	—	1. Adequate ventilation. 2. Office monitoring for mercury vapor at least once a year, more if contamination is suspected. 3. Personal monitoring. 4. Biological evaluation of all dental personnel at least once a year. 5. Work area with continuous, seamless sheet flooring that extends up the walls for 1 ft. Tiled or carpeted floors should be avoided. 6. Nonporous cabinet tops with protective edging or a border to confine spills to the area. 7. Proper amalgam handling, using a no-touch technique.

(continued)

Name	Sources of exposure	Health effects	Standards					Preventive measures
			OSHA (PEL)[a]		NIOSH (REL)[a]	ACGIH (TLV)[b]		
			TWA	STEL		TWA	STEL	
								8. Proper mercury storage away from heat sources in unbreakable, tightly sealed well-labeled containers. 9. Cleaning up spills immediately. *Do not use a vacuum cleaner.* A wash bottle trap or a syringe can recover all visible droplets. Adhesive tape to clean up small spills can be used. Area should be decontaminated with sulfur-containing compounds. 10. Avoidance of skin contamination. 11. Use face mask to avoid breathing amalgam dust.
Methyl alcohol	Denatured alcohol	Dermatitis, erythema, scaling, optic neuropathy, metabolic acidosis	200 ppm 260 mg/m^3 SKIN	250 ppm 310 mg/m^3	200 ppm 10-h TWA 260 mg/m^3 10-h TWA	200 ppm 262 ppm SKIN	250 mg/m^3 328 mg/m^3	Wear proper protective eyewear and gloves.
Methyl methacrylate	Denture base resins	Eye, mucous membrane, respiratory, and skin irritation; dermatitis	100 ppm 410 mg/m^3	— —	100 ppm 410 mg/m^3	100 ppm 410 mg/m^3	— —	Wear proper protective eyewear and gloves.
Nickel (metal)	Casting alloys	Eye, mucous membrane, and respiratory irritation; allergic responses; dermatitis Identified by NIOSH as a potential human carcinogen	1 mg/m^3	—	0.015 mg/m^3	1 mg/m^3	—	Wear proper protective eyewear, gloves, and NIOSH-approved mask.
Nitric acid	Pickling solutions	Nasal and lung irritation, skin and eye burns from splashes; dental erosion	2 ppm 5 mg/m^3	4 ppm 10 mg/m^3	2 ppm 10-h TWA 5 mg/m^3 10-h TWA	2 ppm 5.2 mg/m^3	4 ppm 10 mg/m^3	1. Use proper protective gloves and eyewear. 2. Allow adequate ventilation. 3. Wash any skin or eye contact immediately with running water for 5 to 10 min. Seek medical assistance. 4. In the event of a spill, keep neutralizing agents such as soda lime or commercial acid spill cleanup kit available. 5. Handle solutions carefully. Avoid splashing. Always add water to acid when mixing. 6. Properly label and store all acid-containing solutions. 7. Use forceps to handle any object being treated in acids.
Nitrous oxide	Nitrous oxide	Decrements in motor, perceptual, and cognitive skills; liver disease; cancer; spontaneous abortion, and birth defects in offspring	—	—	25 ppm TWA 46 mg/m^3	50 ppm 90 mg/m^3	— —	1. Use effective scavenging equipment and monitoring devices. 2. Regularly inspect anesthetic administration equipment for leaks.

(continued)

Name	Sources of exposure	Health effects	Standards: OSHA (PEL)[a] TWA	OSHA (PEL)[a] STEL	NIOSH (REL)[a]	ACGIH (TLV)[b] TWA	ACGIH (TLV)[b] STEL	Preventive measures
								3. Direct waste gas away from windows, ventilators, air conditioning inlets, or other areas that might allow gases back into the office. 4. Maintain adequate ventilation. 5. Minimize conversation with patients. 6. Check for snug fit of face mask. 7. Maintain and service equipment regularly.
Phenol	Disinfectants	Mouth, nose, throat, and skin irritation; liver and kidney damage; severe skin burns from contact	5 ppm 19 mg/m^3 SKIN	— —	5 ppm 10-h TWA 19 mg/m^3 10-h TWA 15.6 ppm (C) 60 mg/m^3 (C) SKIN	5 ppm 19 mg/m^3 SKIN	— —	Wear proper protective gloves. If potential for high exposures present, wear NIOSH-approved mask.
Phosphoric acid	Etching agents, phosphate cements	Nose, throat, and lung irritation; bronchitis, dermatitis; skin and eye burns from splashing	1 mg/m^3	3 mg/m^3	1 mg/m^3 3 mg/m^3 (STEL)	1 mg/m^3	3 mg/m^3	1. Use proper protective gloves and eyewear. 2. Allow adequate ventilation. 3. Wash any skin or eye contact immediately with running water for 5 to 10 minutes. Seek medical assistance. 4. In the event of a spill, keep neutralizing agents such as soda lime or commercial acid spill cleanup kit available. 5. Handle solutions carefully. Avoid splashing. Always add water to acid when mixing. 6. Properly label and store all acid-containing solutions. 7. Use forceps to handle any object being treated in acids.
Picric agents	Pickling agents	Eye, nose, and throat irritation; dermatitis; yellow-stained hair and skin	0.1 mg/m^3 SKIN	—	0.1 mg/m^3 0.3 mg/m^3 (STEL) SKIN	0.1 mg/m^3 SKIN	—	1. Use proper protective gloves and eyewear. 2. Allow adequate ventilation.

(continued)

Name	Sources of exposure	Health effects	Standards: OSHA (PEL)[a] TWA	OSHA (PEL)[a] STEL	NIOSH (REL)[a]	ACGIH (TLV)[b] TWA	ACGIH (TLV)[b] STEL	Preventive measures
								3. Wash any skin or eye contact immediately with running water for 5 to 10 min. Seek medical assistance. 4. In the event of a spill, keep neutralizing agents such as soda lime or commercial acid spill cleanup kit available. 5. Handle solutions carefully. Avoid splashing. Always add water to acid when mixing. 6. Properly label and store all acid-containing solutions. 7. Use forceps to handle any object being treated in acids.
Silver (metal)	Amalgam and casting alloys	Eye, nose, throat, and skin irritation; dermatitis	0.01 mg/m^3	—	0.01 mg/m^3	0.1 mg/m^3	—	Wear proper protective eyewear, gloves, and NIOSH-approved mask.
Sulfur dioxide	Tanks containing photographic mixers	Eye, nose, mucous membrane, and throat irritation; eye and skin burns	5 ppm 13 mg/m^3	— —	2 ppm 10-h TWA 5 mg/m^3 10-h TWA 5 ppm 13 mg/m^3 (STEL)	2 ppm 5.2 mg/m^3	5 ppm 13 mg/m^3	Wear proper protective eyewear and gloves.

Action Level, exposure concentration at which employers must initiate certain provisions of the recommended standard; ACGIH, American Conference of Governmental Industrial Hygienists; C, ceiling limit; NIOSH, National Institute for Occupational Safety and Health; OSHA, Occupational Safety and Health Administration; PEL, permissible exposure limit; REL, recommended exposure limit; SKIN, denotes skin designation; STEL, short-term exposure limit, calculated for a 15-minute period unless otherwise noted; TLV, threshold limit value; TWA, time-weighted average, calculated for an 8-hour workday unless otherwise noted.

[a]From NIOSH Guide to Chemical Hazards, June 1994.

[b]From *Threshold Limit Values and Biological Exposure Indices for 1995–1996* American Conference of Governmental Hygienists.

[c]Fibers >5μm long. Note: The American Dental Association's Council on Therapeutics eliminated asbestos from its program of accepted therapeutics in 1979.

CHAPTER 40

Toxic Hazards of Mining and Smelting

Jefferey L. Burgess, Paul J. A. Lever, and Raymond J. Schumacher

MINING

Mining is the process of removing mineral resources from the earth. Smelting involves the separation of metallic components of ores and production of metals. Mining is one of the most dangerous occupations. The National Safety Council reported that in the United States in 1995, there were 30 deaths per 100,000 mining workers (a category that includes quarrying as well as oil and gas extraction) as compared with 24 deaths per 100,000 workers for agriculture and 16 for construction workers (1). Most mining deaths are associated with trauma, such as crush injuries, fires, or explosions (2).

The majority of mining injuries are musculoskeletal in origin. For example, in 1994, mining work injuries involving days away from work resulted from trauma in more than 60% of cases (contact with objects and equipment 40.1%, falls 18.9%, transportation accidents 2.9%, slips/trips 1%, fire explosions 0.5%), overexertion in 26.1%, exposure to harmful substances 4.8%, repetitive motion 0.5%, and all others 5.3% of cases. The National Safety Council also reported 1994 annual incidence rates for mining occupational injuries (per 10,000 full-time workers) of 11.8 for disorders associated with repeated trauma, 6.6 for dust diseases of the lungs, 3.0 for skin diseases and disorders, 1.8 for disorders due to physical agents, 1.2 for respiratory conditions due to toxic agents, and 1.4 for all other occupational diseases (1). Mining hazards include exposure to mine gases and dusts, noise, vibration, extremes of temperature and humidity, and less-than-ideal ergometric conditions (3).

In the United States, mining activities are commonly subdivided into the following standard mine classifications:

- Surface metal/nonmetal (metal examples: placer gold mines, porphyry copper mines, iron mines, etc.; nonmetal examples: gypsum mines, asbestos mines, olivine mines)
- Underground metal/nonmetal (metal examples: copper mines, lead/zinc mines, gold mines, etc.; nonmetal examples: marble mines, chromite mines, salt mines)
- Surface coal (strip mining or open pit)
- Underground coal (long wall or conventional)
- Quarries, sand and gravel (e.g., stones quarries, gravel pits)

Most mines are unique in layout and operation, because the geologic environments in which they occur often differ in mineralogy, geologic structure, and physical properties. Therefore, the associated health hazards can differ considerably, even among mines extracting the same mineral.

In principle, the objective of any mine is to extract a geologic resource from the earth in the most economic manner. Surface metal/nonmetal mines are called *open pits* and are designed based on the principle that the value of each block of ore (economically viable part of the resource) extracted from the pit must pay for its mining and processing costs (plus profit margin required), including the cost of removing the waste above it. In coal, surface mines are generally strip mines. Here, if the coal seam is close enough to the surface, then long thin pits are constructed by removing the overburden above the coal, extracting the coal, and then filling the strip pit with overburden from the next pit (Fig. 40-1). In both types of mines, drilling and blasting techniques, extremely large extraction machines (shovels, draglines), as well as transportation equipment (trucks, conveyor belts), are often used. Quarries are often similar in operation to open pit-type mines and use the same types of equipment.

If the resource is too far below the surface to be mined economically as a surface mine, then underground mining methods are the alternative. In underground mining, the layout of the mine is strongly coupled to the geology and structure of the deposit; thus, many underground mines have unique designs. In general, access to the underground is through vertical shafts, inclined ramps, or adits (horizontal tunnel into the side of a hill). In metal and nonmetal mines, development tunnels are driven to the ore body, then large areas called *stopes* are constructed to extract the ore (Fig. 40-2). Many techniques are based on drill, blast, and load mining cycles, whereas others use mechanical

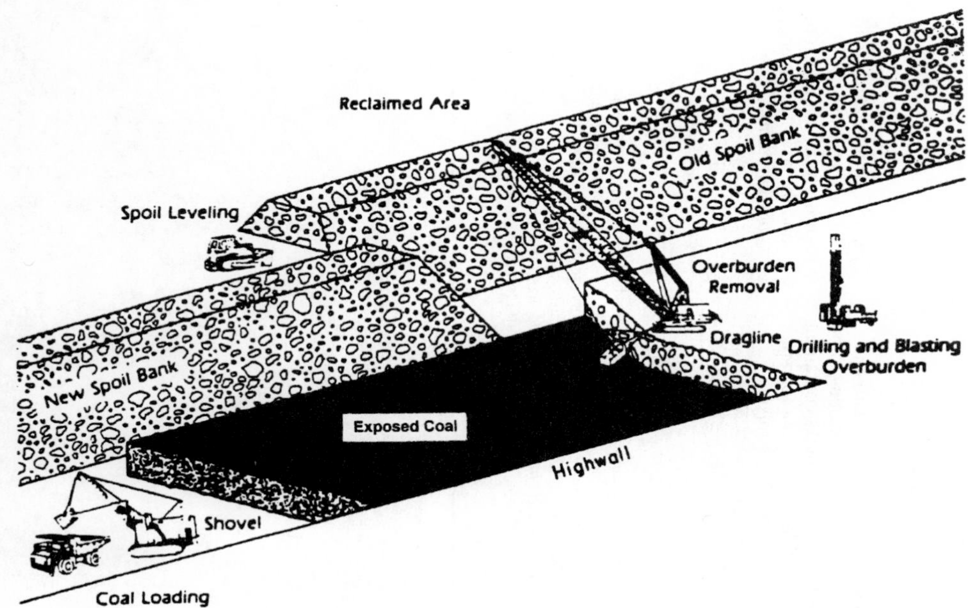

Figure 40-1. Surface mining, opencast method. (Reproduced with permission from Hartman HL. *SME mining engineering handbook,* vol. 1, 2nd ed. Littleton, CO: Society for Mining Metallurgy and Exploration, Inc., 1992.)

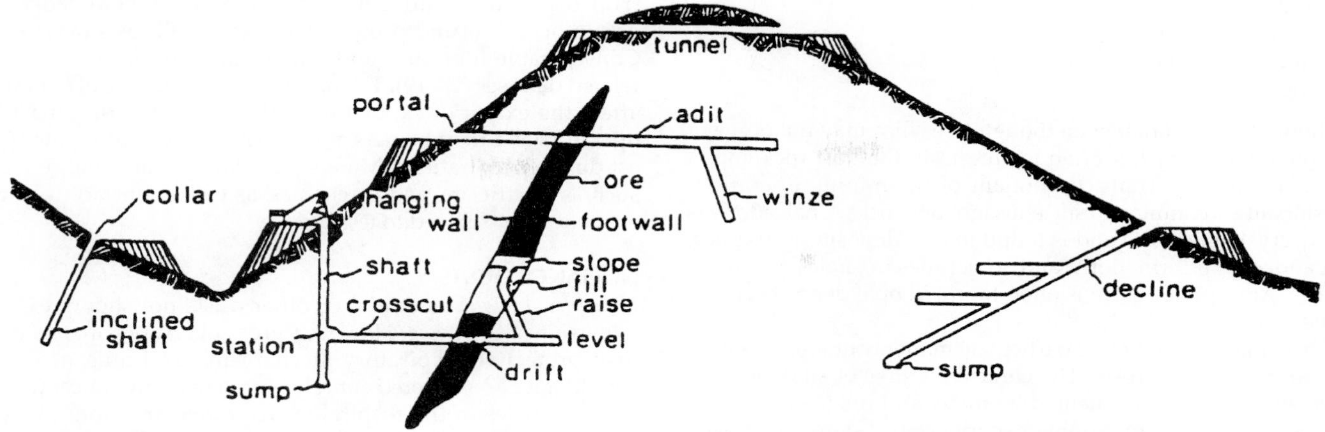

Figure 40-2. Underground mining, stoping method. (Reproduced with permission from Hartman HL. *SME mining engineering handbook,* vol. 1, 2nd ed. Littleton, CO: Society for Mining Metallurgy and Exploration, Inc., 1992.)

excavation machines, such as tunnel-boring machines. In coal, the tabular layout of coal seams and the softness of coal allows miners to use large electrically operated equipment to dig through the coal and transport it using conveyor belts to the surface. These machines can generate a large amount of dust and liberate gases from the coal and host rock. Thus, both underground metal and nonmetal and coal mines use large surface and underground fans to ventilate the workings.

General Mine Hazards

The pick and hammer were the major tools used in early mining methods. However, by the early 1900s, improved open pit and underground mining methods were already under development. New techniques often stressed the introduction of mechanization to improve productivity, which resulted in a decrease in manpower. These increases in mechanization often reduced the number of workers at risk, but also generated new problems such as increased dust levels, vibration, noise, and toxic gases. For example, the introduction of diesel motors produced new gases and particulates into the environment, and individuals were exposed to different explosive fumes through changes in explosive technology.

The mining community has attacked the toxic hazards problem in the mine environment using two approaches. The first is to improve the mine environment directly, and the second provides workers with protective equipment. Improvement in mine ventilation has been the most popular method for improving the underground environment, but continually increasing air velocity has practical limitations. The introduction of regulations—such as controlling the use of diesel engines and the storage and use of explosives—in addition to new techniques to suppress dust and control gases has helped to improve the mining environment.

The enforcement of all regulations for U.S. underground and surface mining operations is conducted by the Mining Safety and Health Administration (MSHA), and similar regulations have been established in other countries. The Federal Mine Safety and Health Amendments Act of 1977 is the basis for these regulations, which can be found in the *Code of Federal Regulations* (*CFR*) section 30. *CFR* 30 regulations allow employees to work for limited periods in concentrations of airborne contaminants that exceed permissible levels if they are protected with appropriate respiratory protective equipment. Respirators approved by National Institute for Occupational Safety and Health under *CFR* 42, part 84 are regulated. Thus, the use of materials such as respirators and protective clothing has also improved individual protection for workers. In general, surface mines have much lower overall exposures to toxic substances than experienced in underground mines, except possibly for exposure to dusts.

Mine Dusts

Dust hazards were severe in mining history and contributed to extensive deaths from dust-related diseases. Several important factors influence the probability of a miner's developing a dust-related illness, including the nature of the dust (e.g., mineralogy, particle size, toxicity), quantity of dust, length of exposure, period since first exposure, and individual susceptibility. In modern mines, dusts are still important because of safety issues related to reduced visibility, dust-induced chronic lung diseases, irritation effects, and other toxic effects.

Pneumoconioses are a set of lung diseases that include silicosis, asbestosis, coal-workers' pneumoconiosis, and other fibrotic lung diseases resulting from inhalation of dusts. This section contains an overview of mineral types, geologic factors, mine environments, and health issues related to the extensive topic of pneumoconiosis-producing dusts.

SILICA AND SILICOSIS

Exposure to dusts containing free silica (SiO_2) are associated with pulmonary injury. Free silica mineral species encountered in mining operations are quartz and tridymite, which are crystalline; cristobalite and chalcedony, which are microcrystalline; and diatomite and opal, which are amorphous. Exposure to silica dusts is possible whenever free silica is encountered in mining operations, and in particular during mining activities that include drilling, blasting, transportation, maintenance work, assaying, crushing, and milling.

Quartz is the most common mineral in the earth's crust and is often the major component of rocks encountered in mining and quarrying of the following materials:

- Base and precious metal ores in quartz-carbonate veins and some sedimentary and volcanic rocks
- Quartzite and sandstone
- Uranium ore in conglomerate and sandstone
- Placer deposits
- Mica
- Feldspar and mineral deposits in pegmatitic and granite rocks

- Coal
- Banded ironstone
- Sands and gravels
- Granites

It should be noted that even though free silica may not occur in the ore being mined, it often is present in the host rock and is therefore an important component of the mining operation. Cristobalite is common in siliceous igneous rocks. Chalcedony is finely crystalline silica and is found in coal deposits as nodules, in banded iron formations, and sometimes in shales and limestones. Amorphous silica is often found in opal deposits and in flints and cherts.

Prolonged inhalation of particulate matter containing free silica can result in silicosis. The clinical features of silicosis have been studied and documented by many authors (4–6) and will not be discussed here. Mining experience has shown that even though an individual can contract silicosis on the first dust exposure, the average time before detection is after 20 years of exposure (7,8). Silica dust remaining in the lungs may also cause silicosis many years after removal from the mining environment (9). Silica exposure has been associated with the development of chronic obstructive pulmonary disease, although this is a controversial finding (10). Exposure to crystalline silica may increase the incidence of lung cancer (11).

ASBESTOS AND ASBESTOS-RELATED DISEASES

Asbestos minerals are fibrous in nature and are subdivided into serpentine and amphibole classifications. The six main varieties of asbestos are chrysotile, which is serpentine, and tremolite, anthophyllite, actinolite, amosite, and crocidolite, which are amphibole. Chrysotile, amosite, crocidolite, and anthophyllite are the four that are of commercial value, and 95% of world production comes from chrysotile. The majority of asbestos is mined underground, where adequate ventilation and use of personal protective equipment are important in limiting exposure. It should be noted that during mining, the asbestos fibers are often bound together geologically, which limits the generation of the short fibers associated with asbestos-related diseases. However, the milling process breaks up the fibers and results in a considerably more dangerous environment.

Health effects from asbestos exposure have been well documented, and numerous review articles provide a detailed description of asbestos-related diseases (12–15). Asbestosis is the main threat to miners who have a prolonged exposure to elevated dust concentrations of all varieties of asbestos dust. Asbestos exposure increases the risk of primary lung cancer among miners (15). Primary malignant mesothelioma has been reported among crocidolite miners (16) but has been seen rarely when mining other asbestos varieties.

COAL AND COAL-RELATED PNEUMOCONIOSIS

Coal is generally ranked geologically according to criteria such as carbon content. The highest rank is anthracite, followed in decreasing order by bituminous coal, subbituminous coal, and lignite. The hardest coals have the highest ranks, contain the lowest amount of volatile matter, and generate the greatest amount of heat when burned. The coal rank and seam thickness often influence the type of dust exposure for the miner. Miners working in thin seams often have more contact during the mining process with rock strata adjacent to the coal seam. Many coal deposits can contain free silica in the shale and sandstone beds that neighbor the seam. Thus, the degree of hazard cannot be ascertained solely by knowledge of quartz with the coal itself.

Inhalation of coal mine dust can lead to coal workers' pneumoconiosis and silicosis, in addition to increased rates of industrial bronchitis and emphysema. Simple coal workers' pneumoconiosis and progressive massive fibrosis may occur. Considerable literature and data exist relating to these coal-related diseases (17–19). The place of work and type of operation affect the extent of exposure for the miner. Cutting machine operators and their helpers at the coal face experience the highest dust concentrations. Miners performing maintenance work, such as electricians and mechanics, as well as surface workers, are generally exposed to less dust.

NUISANCE DUSTS

Nuisance dusts are mineral or other dusts not shown to have adverse health effects. However, gross overexposure can overload protective respiratory mechanisms, and nuisance dusts should not be considered entirely harmless at any concentration. Dust particles in the respirable size range are more likely to result in adverse health effects. Examples of nuisance dusts found in mining include Portland cement, gypsum, kaolin, limestone, calcium carbonate, fibrous glass, and marble. These dusts are considered to be nuisance dusts if they do not contain any toxic impurities—for example, less than 1% quartz. Studies of exposure to dusts generated from mining or quarrying calcium carbonate rocks indicate little or no disease of the lungs (20). Free silica or silicates, which may be found with limestones and dolomites, can harm the lungs.

Radiation Exposures

Excess lung cancer has been well described in uranium miners (21). However, uranium mines are not the only mining environments in which radioactive contaminants are found. Measurements in gold, copper, lead and zinc, coal, limestone, phosphate, and more than 20 other types of mines have indicated significant radon daughter concentrations (22,23).

The radioactive decay chains of uranium and thorium are of concern in mining. Uranium is common in the earth's crust, and its decay chain includes radium (^{226}Ra), which is the parent of radon (^{222}Rn). The thorium decay chain contains an isotope of radon (^{220}Rn) called *thoron*, which can be a problem in any mine in which thorium minerals exist. Thoron behaves in the same manner as radon, and thorium daughters present the same cancer risk as radon daughters. A complete description of radon and radon daughter buildup and decay is available elsewhere (24).

In the underground mine atmosphere, radon and thoron concentrations vary considerably in space and time. In the steady-state geologic form, diffusion of thoron and radon is low. However, mining activities, such as blasting and material handling, can strongly influence concentrations (25). Even after mining is terminated, changes in barometric pressure can generate high radon concentrations. The control of airborne radiation can be attained by preventing or retarding their flow into the mine ventilation system by confinement techniques such as seals or bulkheads. Alternatively, ventilation can be used for diluting and removing the contaminated air.

Radiation monitoring is essential in mines to ensure an effective radiation control program. U.S. regulations (*CFR* 30, 57.5038) provide for an annual exposure limit of 4 working level months (WLM) for radon daughters (one working level month equals 170 hours of exposure to one working level). This relates to an average radon daughter concentration of 0.33 working level (WL), which equals 1.3×10^5 mev potential alpha energy from radon daughters per liter of air. In radon daughter environments exceeding 1.0 WL, respirators must be worn as a temporary measure (*CFR* 30, 57.5044), and respirators that remove radon and its daughters or provide fresh air must be worn in radon daughter

TABLE 40-1. Common mine gases

Gas	TLV-TWA[a]	Density[b]	Odor	Toxicity	Comments
Carbon dioxide	5,000 ppm	1.53	None	Asphyxiant	Toxic at higher concentrations
Carbon monoxide (whitedamp)	25 ppm	0.97	None	Chemical asphyxiant	Primarily from incomplete combustion
Hydrogen sulfide (stinkdamp)	10 ppm	1.19	Rotten eggs[c]	Irritant, chemical asphyxiant	Flammable range, 4–44%
Hydrogen	—	0.07	None	Flammable	Flammable range, 4–74%
Methane (firedamp)	—	0.55	None	Simple asphyxiant	Flammable range, 5–15%
Oxides of nitrogen	NO 25 ppm; NO_2 3 ppm	1.04; 1.58	Difficult to detect	Respiratory irritant	Poor warning properties, delayed pulmonary injury may occur
Radon	—	—	None	Carcinogenic	Not limited to uranium mines
Sulfur dioxide	2 ppm	2.26	Metallic	Irritant	Good warning properties

[a]American Conference of Governmental Industrial Hygienists Threshold Limit Value–Time Weighted Average.[31]
[b]Density of air = 1.
[c]Causes olfactory fatigue at concentrations exceeding 50 ppm.

concentrations higher than 10 WL (*CFR* 30, 57.5046). At least one radon daughter sample must be acquired in the exhaust airway of all U.S. mines and additional samples collected if a concentration greater than 0.1 WL is collected. Studies of MSHA data for 1985 through 1987 demonstrated 139 mines in the United States at a working level of 0.1 WL or more for radon daughter concentrations (23). Exposure of mine and mill workers to beta and gamma radiation has not been considered important for 0.1% to 1.0% grade U_3O_8 ores (26). However, there has been some concern of exceeding the 5 rem annual exposure level for external whole-body radiation when working with 1% to 5% U_3O_8 ores (27).

Mine Gases

The hazardous gases encountered in mines vary depending on the characteristics of the individual mine. Determinants include the mineral content of the ore, gases naturally present in the strata being mined, presence of organic debris, and mining equipment and procedures. Oxygen deficiency and excesses of carbon dioxide, carbon monoxide, methane, oxides of nitrogen, sulfur dioxide, hydrogen sulfide, diesel exhaust, and hydrogen are potential causes of miner morbidity and mortality. Common mine gases are listed in Table 40-1.

Oxygen deficiency, also known as *blackdamp*, can occur in poorly ventilated underground mines with decomposing organic material or reducing ores (3). Oxygen deficiency is defined by the Occupational Safety and Health Administration as less than 19.5% by volume (28). In individuals without significant underlying illness, respiratory symptoms occur at concentrations of less than 16% and unconsciousness at concentrations of less than 10% (29). Symptoms vary at a given oxygen concentration depending on the extent of worker exertion.

Carbon dioxide is a colorless gas with a slightly acid taste at high concentrations. Sources include mine personnel, flame safety lamps, fires, diesel engines, blasting operations, and occasionally coal and adjacent strata. Adverse health effects increase with higher concentrations. According to the U.S. Department of Labor's Mine Safety and Health Administration, 0.5% (5,000 ppm) increases ventilation, 3% doubles ventilation, and 10% is only tolerated for a few minutes at rest (29).

Carbon monoxide is a colorless, tasteless gas. Sources include diesel engines, fires, explosives, and offgassing from certain coals. Carbon monoxide acts as a chemical asphyxiant, interfering with oxygen transport by hemoglobin and through inhibition of the cytochrome oxidase system. Five hundred ppm (0.05%) can be fatal in 3 hours (29). The rate of interaction with blood increases with exertion.

Methane is the most common flammable gas found in mines and is produced primarily by coal and adjacent strata. Accumulation of methane has resulted in numerous explosions in underground and surface mines, and there have been more than 10,000 deaths in the last 60 years from methane-related explosions (29). Methane also acts as a simple asphyxiant by displacing oxygen from the air. Other hydrocarbons found in mines include ethane, propane, and acetylene, usually present in trace amounts. These also are potentially flammable and act as simple asphyxiants.

Oxides of nitrogen include nitrogen dioxide (NO_2), nitric oxide (NO), and nitrogen tetroxide (N_2O_4). They are formed at high temperatures by diesel and gasoline engines, fires, explosives, electrical discharge, and blasting. Because of their relatively low water solubility, they have poor warning properties. On inhalation they can reach the lower respiratory tract, causing delayed pulmonary damage.

Sulfur dioxide is a colorless irritating gas with a pungent sulfurous smell. Sources include fires that involve iron pyrites and blasting for certain sulfide ores. Sulfur dioxide is very water soluble and has good warning properties. It causes primarily upper respiratory tract and mucous membrane irritation, but at higher concentrations can also cause lower respiratory tract injury.

Hydrogen sulfide is a colorless, flammable, irritating gas, is heavier than air, and has an odor of rotten eggs at low concentrations. It is formed through blasting for sulfide ores and also occurs naturally in gas, oil, and coal fields. Hydrogen sulfide can act as an irritant as well as a chemical asphyxiant. Prolonged exposure increases the odor threshold through olfactory fatigue, which generally occurs above 50 ppm.

Diesel exhaust contains aldehydes, oxides of nitrogen, carbon monoxide, and particulates. Diesel exhaust is quite irritating and has been associated in some studies with an increased risk of lung cancer (30). Underground, scrubbers are used on diesel equipment to clean the exhaust. Hydrogen is colorless and tasteless and is not normally present in significant concentrations in mine air, except in the vicinity of battery-charging stations or after fires and explosions. Radon and radiation hazards are further described in the section Radiation Exposures.

General Safety Devices and Protective Equipment

The most appropriate solution for limiting exposure to toxic hazards is to use engineering control techniques. However, the dynamic nature of mines means that the layout is continually changing and the environmental engineering control techniques may not always work as planned. Monitoring programs are needed to determine the state of the environment, and personal protective equipment must often be used to protect miners, especially during times of transition.

Many mines use sophisticated sampling and measurement devices to determine gas and dust concentrations in the mine environment. To determine concentrations of harmful noxious or poisonous gases, *CFR* 30 requires detectors or laboratory analysis of mine air samples. Threshold limit values as specified by the American Conference of Government Industrial Hygienists are used to define acceptable limits (31). Handheld methane detectors, portable oxygen monitors, and flame safety lamps are used on a daily basis by miners. In underground coal mines, *CFR* 30 requires that regular testing for oxygen deficiency be made with an MSHA-approved and appropriately maintained permissible detector capable of detecting 19.5% oxygen with an accuracy of ± 0.5%. Handheld devices are commonly used for measuring concentrations of explosive gases, such as carbon monoxide (limit 2.5%), methane (limit 1.0%), hydrogen (limit 0.8%), hydrogen sulfide (limit 0.8%), acetylene (limit 0.4%), and propane (limit 0.4%). Detector tubes for measuring concentrations of toxic and noxious gases can be used in mines but are often only accurate within 25% of the actual reading. MSHA-approved portable self-contained detection instruments for gases such as nitric oxide and nitrogen dioxide can also be used. To determine dust exposures, a large array of MSHA-approved personal dust samplers are commonly used in U.S. mines.

Environmental monitoring systems are commonly found in underground coal mines and less frequently in underground metal and nonmetal mines, and have been used to continuously measure environmental parameters such as carbon monoxide, carbon dioxide, methane, hydrogen, oxides of nitrogen, hydrogen sulfide, and oxygen. If concentration limits for any of these parameters are approached or exceeded, then the monitoring system registers an alarm to alert the miners. In addition, if ventilation parameters such as airway pressures, airway velocities, and fan operations are also measured by the monitoring system, then the system can react to changes in the mine to maintain a healthy underground environment. It should be noted that atmospheric monitoring systems are not commonly found in surface mines, except possibly in enclosed surface structures, such as conveyor belt runs, mineral processing facilities, and workshops.

When engineering control techniques are not capable of maintaining a healthy mine environment, personal-protection devices can be used. For dust exposure, filter-type face masks are frequently used in the mining industry (32). Popular varieties of powered respirators include face masks, helmets, helmet air curtains, and canopy air curtains. The powered respirators are more often used at the mining face, where excessive dust generation can often be a problem. Abnormal gas conditions in underground mines can occur from outbursts of strata gases (carbon dioxide, methane, nitrogen), interruption of mine ventilation, fires, explosions, and excessive mining rates. In the event of an abnormal gas event, then respiratory protection using devices such as the gas mask, carbon monoxide self-rescuer, and self-contained self-rescuer must be provided. These are mostly temporary devices that allow the miner to escape from the affected working area. Self-contained breathing apparatuses are used primarily for rescue operations.

Mining Wastes

In 1990, mining and ore beneficiation processes generated an estimated 2 billion metric tons of solid waste in the United States, nearly one-half of which was unprocessed overburden removed to access ore. *Beneficiation* is crushing and grinding of ore to facilitate concentration of the raw material of interest by flotation. The waste product is slurried to impoundments that are an average of 500 acres in size. *Tailings* are the solid particulate result of evaporation at these sites. Only a small number of Comprehensive Environmental Response, Compensation, and Liability Act Superfund listings are minerals industry waste sites, said to be mostly a result of past rather than current industry practices (33).

The main focus of popular attention to mining wastes has been unsightly mounds of tailings and resulting airborne dust, although there is considerable potential for direct human toxicity by contamination of both ground- and surface water, which may be absorbed by crops or ingested by domestic animals or humans. Concentration of heavy metals in mine and tailings runoff water is enhanced by acidity in rain and inherent acidity of ores and tailings (34). Copper tailings may contain from a few ppm to several thousand ppm of arsenic, cadmium, chromium, copper, lead, zinc, beryllium, and silica. Gold, lead, and molybdenum tailings may additionally include other trace elements, such as silver, selenium, mercury, molybdenum, manganese, and iron (35). Airborne wastes, if uncontrolled, may also cause community toxicity. High indoor air radon concentrations have been documented in homes built on uranium tailings (36). In one of the most notorious examples of environmental exposure from mining wastes, an increase in cadmium concentration in rice was documented in the Jinsu River basin in Japan, downstream from a cadmium-zinc-lead mine. Ingestion of the rice was associated with epidemic Itai-Itai disease, consisting of severe bony deformities and chronic renal disease in villages with the highest rice-cadmium concentrations (37). An example of mineralogic composition of copper tailings is listed in Table 40-2.

TABLE 40-2. Mineralogical composition of copper cliff tailings

Feldspar	+50.0	M A1(Al,Si) O8, M = K, Na, Ca, Ba, NH4
Chlorite	20	M6(Al,Si)O10(OH)8, M = Mg, Fe2+, Fe3+, Mn
Quartz	10	SiO2
Pyroxenes	7	ABSi2O6, A = Na, Ca, Mg, Fe2+, B = Mg, Fe2+, Al
Biotite	7	K(Mg,Fe)3(Al,Fe)Si3O10(OH,F)2 (a mica)
Pyrrhotite	5.6	Fe1-xS
Magnetite	0.6	Fe3O4
Pentlandite	0.5	(Fe,Ni)9S8
Chalcopyrite	0.3	CuFeS2

Note: Zinc is also recovered from the ore, and although it isn't listed in the analysis, it is a significant soil contaminant around the plant.

SMELTING

The production of metals involves mining, concentration, and reduction to a metallic form. *Smelting* is defined as the melting or fusing of ores to separate the metallic components. Additional steps in the reduction of metals include roasting, calcining, sintering, converting, and refining, which are considered part of the overall smelting process.

There are two major smelting techniques: pyrometallurgy and hydrometallurgy. These techniques may be combined in smelter operations. A common preparatory step for pyro- and hydrometallurgy is concentrating the ore by crushing and using separation techniques. Pyrometallurgy involves heating of the ore to temperatures sufficient to reduce metal oxides to their

TABLE 40-3. Potential toxic exposures in smelters

Aluminum smelters
Carbon monoxide
Cryolite (Na_3AlF_6) dust
Fluoride (gaseous and particulate)
Polycyclic aromatic hydrocarbons
Sulfur dioxide
Copper smelters
Arsenic
Cadmium
Lead
Sulfur dioxide
Lead smelters
Arsenic
Cadmium
Chlorine gas
Copper
Lead
Sulfur dioxide
Zinc
Nickel smelters
Ammonia (hydrometallurgic process)
Carbon monoxide
Hydrogen sulfide
Nickel
Nickel carbonyl
Sulfur dioxide
Zinc smelters
Antimony
Arsenic
Cadmium
Carbon monoxide
Copper
Lead
Manganese
Zinc

metallic form. There are a variable number of steps in this process, depending on the specific ore and smelter. In hydrometallurgy, metal ores are processed through chemical treatments. The initial step is usually leaching, which may require the addition of electricity or heating. The ore may also be roasted before leaching. The leaching solution is then treated by electrolysis or further chemical treatment to reduce and remove the metals from solution.

The potential toxic exposures from smelters are numerous and vary among smelters. A partial list of potentially hazardous exposures is found in Table 40-3. The initial concentrating step and loading/unloading and transfer of the metal ores lead to particulate generation and the potential for worker exposure. Roasting, melting, and converting the metal ore can produce a variety of hazardous exposures, including sulfur dioxide and contaminants present in the ore (such as arsenic). The high temperatures and high noise level in the smelters also contribute to safety hazards. This chapter focuses on smelting of aluminum, copper, lead, nickel, and zinc.

Aluminum

Aluminum is produced primarily from bauxites, which contain a variable amount of alumina, kaolinite, and clay minerals. The bauxite is crushed, washed, and dried before refining. The bauxite is then heated and pressurized with caustic soda to form sodium aluminate, which is separated out and recovered.

Aluminum smelting involves reduction of alumina by an electrolytic process. The cathode is composed of coal and coal tar pitch. The anode is composed of coke and coal tar pitch and is used up as the electrolytic process continues. There are two major processes: Soderberg and prebake. The Soderberg process involves addition of coke and coal tar pitch to the anode in the smelter. It generally results in more worker exposure, with the horizontal-stud Soderberg cells emitting approximately six times more polycyclic aromatic hydrocarbons (PAHs) than vertical-stud cells (3). Prebakes are large carbon blocks that are manufactured outside the smelter and heated to remove the pitch and other contaminants in controlled conditions before transport. New smelters are almost entirely using the prebaked anodes, which produce less pollution and are more energy efficient.

In the smelter, alumina is dissolved in molten cryolite (Na_3AlF_6) baths called *pots*. Fluorspar (CaF_2) and aluminum fluoride (AlF_2) are added to reduce the melting temperature and to increase process efficiency (3). Alumina is added to the pots by opening a mechanically operated door after the surface crust is broken so the additional material can mix. A direct current is driven through the bath, maintaining a 960° to 980°C temperature, and the alumina is reduced to molten aluminum, which falls to the bottom of the bath. The aluminum metal is tapped every 24 to 48 hours by sucking it into a crucible. This process produces 99.8% pure aluminum.

Potential toxic hazards in the aluminum smelting industry include fluoride exposure from both gaseous and particulate sources, including cryolite dust, carbon monoxide, sulfur dioxide, and coal tar pitch volatiles (CTPVs), which include PAHs, heat stress, and electromagnetic radiation from the high direct current (DC) fields (3). The CTPVs and PAHs are produced from the consumption of the carbon and pitch anode. Sulfur dioxide, carbon monoxide, and carbon dioxide may also be produced from consumption of the anode. Typically, tapping, crust breaking, and anode changing are associated with increased exposure to emissions from the pots. Anode tenders have relatively greater exposures to sulfur dioxide and hydrogen fluoride than other smelter workers. Crane operators have the potential for significant toxic exposures and therefore often work in a contained cab with a separate ventilation system. Electrocution can occur if a worker touches the cathode leads and either another row of pots or the outside wall. Explosions can occur if a liquid container (e.g., a soda can or larger) is dropped into the pot, generates superheated steam, and explodes. Exposure to chlorine gas may occur in the casting plants, in which it is used to clean out casting furnaces (38). Noise exposure is the greatest in rod mills, although crust breakers may be as noisy as 95 dB.

Respiratory and carcinogenic effects have been described in aluminum smelter workers. Accelerated loss in lung function has been noted, although this problem may be prevented by improvements in working conditions (39). Although very controversial, both *de novo* asthma and exacerbation of underlying asthma have been reported. Hydrogen fluoride and other fluoride-containing chemicals have been implicated, along with respirable dust, sulfur dioxide, and CTPVs (38), and symptoms are seen in association with working close to fumes and dust when pot hoods are removed or during removal of hot anode blocks (40). Chronic obstructive pulmonary disease has also been associated with long-term exposure in aluminum smelters (38). The incidence of Shaver's disease, characterized by pulmonary fibrosis and emphysema, has been practically eliminated by improvements in workplace conditions through decreases in abrasive alumina and silica particulates. Elevated rates of bladder cancer and lung cancer have been reported (41).

Copper

Copper oxide or sulfide ore is usually ground in a ball mill to form a slurry, and additives are used to assist in the flotation of the copper-containing component. The separated component is then dried and transported for smelting as a 16% to 32% concentrate (3). Hydrometallurgic and pyrometallurgic smelting techniques are used. At most smelters, ore concentrate is roasted with air at approximately 1,000°F to remove impurities such as sulfur—and to a lesser degree, arsenic—by conversion to oxides. The resulting product is called *calcine*. Roaster emissions are run through electrostatic precipitators to separate out dust and aggregated fumes. The calcine is then heated with silica flux to high temperatures (greater than 2,000°F), usually in a reverberatory or electrical furnace, to convert copper oxide to copper sulfide and to further remove impurities. Other furnaces used include flash furnaces and Noranda reactors. In the furnaces, iron oxide is produced and rises up as slag, which is separated off. The copper matte is tapped and transported in large ladles to be poured into converters. In the converters, a silica flux is added, and air is blown through the mixture to convert the remaining iron sulfide to iron oxide (which is removed as slag) and to convert the copper sulfide to copper. Converter sulfur dioxide emissions are often collected for production of sulfuric acid, and copper-containing offgases are recovered and recycled. The more highly purified blister copper—named for the small bubbles of sulfur dioxide remaining in the copper—is then transferred to an anode furnace for additional refinement using air and natural gas. Electrolysis in a copper sulfate–sulfuric acid bath may be used to further purify the metal.

Potential exposures at copper smelters include arsenic, sulfur dioxide, lead, silica, heat, and noise, and to a lesser extent aromatic hydrocarbons, carbon monoxide, antimony, and cadmium. Most arsenic is transformed into arsenic trioxide during smelting. Copper smelter workers have been shown to have high urine arsenic concentrations (42). The greatest concentration of arsenic is found in flue dust, and thus those individuals collecting the dust and cleaning the flues are at high risk of exposure. Sulfur dioxide is produced during the oxidation of the copper ore, which contains an appreciable amount of sulfates. Inorganic sulfate-metal ion complexes have also been measured and may have different toxicologic properties than sulfur dioxide alone (43). Carbon monoxide is also formed from combustion. Dusts and fumes may contain silica, lead, cadmium, and molybdenum. Aromatic hydrocarbons may be produced during the use of electric furnaces and anode refining (44). Crane operators are at significant risk for exposure unless adequate respiratory protection is provided. Maintenance of ventilation and pollution control equipment can result in significant exposures to most of the hazardous materials previously described, often in a concentrated form. Areas requiring maintenance include flues, cyclones, wet-collectors, baghouses, electrostatic precipitators, and the acid plants. Maintenance is also required for general smelter operations and may potentially result in high exposures to contaminants.

Injuries reported in copper smelters have historically included acid skin burns, septum perforations from arsenic exposure, and inhalation injury from sulfur dioxide. An increase in lung cancer has been well documented (45–49), and work at the roasters and gas purifiers appears to carry a higher risk for developing lung cancer (50,51). Elevated lung cancer rates are felt to be related to cumulative arsenic exposure and not to sulfur dioxide exposure (52,53). Smelter arsenic exposure has also been correlated with respiratory cancer mortality (54), as well as increases in large intestine and bone cancer (55). Excesses in cardiovascular disease have also been reported (56). Raynaud's phenomenon and vasospastic reactivity have been described in association with smelter arsenic exposure (57).

Lead

Lead-bearing ore, primarily galena, is crushed and ground to a uniform size. Additives such as sodium carbonate, lime, copper sulfate, pine oil, cresylic acid, xanthate, and sodium cyanide may be used to prepare the lead concentrate (3). The concentrate is sintered to convert sulfur to sulfur dioxide and lead sulfide to lead oxide. The sinter is combined with coke and fed into a blast furnace, in which the lead is melted and reduced to its metallic form. The lead bullion is cooled, and most of the copper separates out. Any remaining copper is removed from the lead by the addition of sulfur before refining. Refining can be pyrometallurgic or hydrometallurgic, with the former predominating. The lead bullion is heated and oxidized to remove arsenic, antimony, and tin. Zinc is added to remove gold and silver, and then the zinc is removed by distilling at 600°C. The lead undergoes additional processing to remove impurities. Hydrometallurgic refining involves the use of fluorosilicates or molten sodium hydroxide and sodium nitrate (3).

The major toxic exposure in lead processing is lead dust. Additional potential hazards include exposure to arsenic, sulfur dioxide, cadmium, copper, indium, and zinc. Chlorine gas added to dezinc the lead may also pose an exposure hazard. Lead smelter workers have been reported to have increased renal disease, cerebrovascular disease, and adverse effects on spermatogenesis (58,59). Smelter lead exposure may result in a very slight increase of risk for some malignant neoplasms (60,61).

Nickel

Nickel-containing ores include sulfides, oxides, and silicates. The sulfide ores are concentrated through crushing, grinding, and flotation. Further processing varies but generally involves flotation, roasting, addition of flux and smelting, and either electrolysis or further chemical or pressure/heat treatment, depending on the associated metals found in the zinc-bearing ore. Roasting oxidizes iron sulfides to iron oxide and produces sulfur dioxide. Smelting typically occurs in reverberatory furnaces, and the matte is further processed in converters. The resulting mixture contains a number of different metals and is allowed to cool and crystallize. This is crushed and ground, and the nickel and copper sulfide components are removed and separated by flotation. The nickel sulfide is oxidized and may be treated with chlorination followed by hydrogen to remove copper and then reduce the nickel. Further purification can be achieved through electrolysis or combination with carbon monoxide to form nickel carbonyl, which is decomposed at higher temperatures to produce metallic nickel. Alternatively, hydrometallurgic processes may be used. Nickel oxide and nickel silicate ores are reduced using gypsum or sulfur-containing petroleum products during roasting and smelting and are further refined in converters. Hydrometallurgic procedures may also be used for these ores, involving the use of ammonia to leach the nickel, followed by further processing.

Potentially hazardous exposures can occur from the sulfur dioxide produced by the oxidation of sulfur or sulfates. In certain metallurgic processes, carbon monoxide and nickel carbonyl are used. Both are colorless and have poor warning properties, making these chemicals extremely hazardous. In hydrometallurgic smelting, ammonia is added under pressure to furnace matte to leach soluble metals, and hydrogen sulfide may be added to precipitate sulfide slurries. Exposure to nickel in smelters can result in allergic reactions, including dermatitis and rhinitis (62). Nickel refinery workers previously had a greatly elevated risk of mortality from lung cancer and carcinomas of the nasal sinus, but with improvements in working conditions, this increased mortality had resolved in at least one study (63).

Zinc

Zinc-bearing ore is usually in the sulfide form. It is concentrated through the use of crushing and grinding, followed by flotation using a small amount of pine oil and air agitation to float the mineral sulfides so they can be skimmed off. Additional flotation steps may be used to further concentrate the zinc. The zinc sulfide is converted to zinc oxide and sulfur dioxide through roasting, commonly in a fluidized-bed roaster. Sintering may follow in certain operations to remove contaminants and produce particles of a desired size. Contaminants produced in sintering may include cadmium and lead. Alternative processes are used for zinc oxide ores and secondary zinc-bearing metals, often using coal to reduce the zinc to a metallic form. Further processing involves the reduction of the zinc oxide through the combustion of coke and natural gas at temperatures of at least 1,000°C, producing volatilized metallic zinc and carbon monoxide. Hydrometallurgic processes are being used more frequently and involve leaching the zinc concentrate with sulfuric acid and further purification before electrolysis.

Exposure to zinc fume can result in metal fume fever. Lead, arsenic, and cadmium are common contaminants in zinc-bearing ores, and overexposure to these metals may occur. Often zinc and lead smelting are run in parallel. Most cadmium is produced from smelting and refining zinc ores, and zinc ore concentrates commonly contain 0.2% to 0.3% cadmium. Cadmium has been classified by International Agency for Research on Cancer as a confirmed human carcinogen (64). Copper, antimony, indium, germanium, and gallium may also be present and may be released during the smelting process. Lead, cadmium, and indium specifically may be volatilized during sintering. Zinc ores are also commonly found in the sulfide form, and sulfur dioxide is produced by oxidation during roasting. Carbon monoxide can be formed during zinc reduction.

Environmental Contamination

The effects of smelter emissions on nearby populations are well documented. Sulfur dioxide is a common waste gas from the smelting process. Many metals are present in complex with sulfates, and the oxidation during heating with oxygen produces sulfur dioxide. Other sulfur species are also produced during smelting and may be important respiratory irritants. The sulfur may complex with metal-containing aerosols, forming stable transition metal complexes, with the rate of formation dependent on the acidity of the mixture. Iron and copper complexed with sulfur dioxide have been measured in smelter plumes from copper and lead smelters (43), and these complexes may be more toxic than sulfur dioxide alone (65).

Soil and produce concentrations of cadmium, copper, and lead were found to increase with proximity to a smelter in Manitoba (66). Urinary arsenic levels were higher in residents living near a copper smelter than those living farther away, and this relationship was more marked in residents younger than 7 years old (67). Children aged 0 to 6 living within one-half mile of a copper smelter in Washington State had elevated urinary arsenic levels (68). In Port Pirie, Australia, blood lead concentrations of children were related to both soil lead concentration from a nearby smelter and father's employment at the smelter (69). Blood lead levels higher than 40 μg per dL were found in 53% of children aged 1 to 9 years living within 1.6 km of a lead smelter in El Paso, Texas (70). Blood lead levels in pregnant women were related to living distance from a large lead smelter (71). However, there was no relation of maternal blood lead with infant birthweight, length of gestation, or preterm delivery (72). Effects on animals are also found. The soil concentrations of copper, lead, and zinc were found to increase with proximity to a zinc smelter in Peru, and increased hepatic concentrations of arsenic, cadmium, lead, and manganese were found in sheep grazing near the smelter (73).

Reducing Toxic Exposures

Reducing worker exposure can be considered most easily during the design of a new smelter. Handling of crushed materials can be automated and contained to prevent spread of dusts. The use of hazardous materials can also be automated to minimize human exposure. Easy access for maintenance can be planned. Less toxic processes, such as using hydrometallurgy rather than pyrometallurgy, can decrease overall exposures. For established smelters, continued safety training and use of protective devices such as respirators can improve worker safety. Industrial hygiene surveys can identify exposure sources and suggest methods of minimizing exposures. Medical monitoring of employees can alert management to any occult problems and prevent the development of debilitating chronic diseases. This may include monitoring for heavy metals and periodic pulmonary function tests. Monitoring devices located near hazardous materials sources can be set to alarm if concentrations exceed set standards. More effective pollution control devices can decrease nearby population exposures. Additional improvements will most likely result from continued changes in smelter design and equipment, as well as from continued strengthening of occupational and environmental standards in association with adequate enforcement.

REFERENCES

1. National Safety Council. *Accident facts*, 1996 ed. Itasca, IL: National Safety Council, 1996.
2. US Department of Labor, Mine Safety and Health Administration. Injury experience in nonmetallic mineral mining, injury experience in metallic mineral mining. Information reports IR1233 and IR1234. Arlington, VA, 1996.
3. Burgess WA. *Recognition of health hazards in industry: a review of materials and processes*, 2nd ed. New York: John Wiley and Sons, 1995.
4. Ziskind M, Jones RN, Weill H. Silicosis. *Am Rev Respir Dis* 1976;113:643–665.
5. Van Ordstrand HS. Sarcoidosis and other masqueraders. *Ind Med Surg* 1964;33:209–212.
6. Schepers GWH. Theories and causes of silicosis. *Ind Med Surg* 1960;29:326–333, 359–369, 434–439.
7. Dix WB. McIntyre Research Foundation brief to the Royal Commission on the Health and Safety of Workers in Mines in Ontario; Feb 5, 1975.
8. Paterson JF. Silicosis in hardrock miners in Ontario. Toronto, Ontario: Ontario Ministry of Natural Resources, 1973. [Bull no 173].
9. Cowle JE. Health hazards of dust inhalation. *Canadian Mining J* 1970;91:61–67.
10. Oxman AD, Muir DC, Shannon HS, et al. Occupational dust exposure and chronic obstructive pulmonary disease: a systematic overview of the evidence. *Am Rev Respir Dis* 1993;148:38–48.
11. Anonymous. Occupational exposure to silica and cancer risk. *IARC Sci Publ* 1990;97:1–119.
12. Wright GW. Asbestos and health in 1969. *Am Rev Respir Dis* 1969;100:467–479.
13. National Institute for Occupational Safety and Health. Criteria for a recommended standard: occupational exposure to asbestos. Washington: US Government Printing Office, 1972.
14. Becklake MR. Asbestos-related diseases of the lung and other organs: their epidemiology and implications for clinical practice. *Am Rev Respir Dis* 1976;114:187–227.
15. Selikoff IJ, Bader RA, Bader ME, et al. Asbestos and neoplasia. *Am J Med* 1967;42:487–496.
16. Wagner JC, Sleggs CA, Marchand P. Diffuse pleural mesothelioma and asbestos exposure in the North Western Cape Province. *Br J Ind Med* 1960;17:260–271.
17. Jacobson G, Felson B, Pendergrass EP. Radiologic classification of the pneumoconioses. *Med Radiogr Photogr* 1968;44:18–24.

18. Doyle HN. The industrial hygiene of coal mining: recent directions. *Ann N Y Acad Sci* 1972;200:791–796.
19. Liddell FDK, May JD. Assessing the radiological progression of simple pneumoconiosis. London: National Coal Board Medical Service, 1976.
20. Parkinson NF. Silicosis in Canada. *AMA Arch Ind Health* 1955;12:56–63.
21. Samet J. Radon and lung cancer. *J Natl Cancer Inst* 1989;81:745–757.
22. US Mining Enforcement and Safety Administration. Evaluation of radioactive aerosols in United States underground coal mines. Information report IR1025. Arlington, VA: 1975.
23. National Institute for Occupational Safety and Health. *Criteria for a recommended standard: occupational exposure to radon progeny in underground mines*. Cincinnati: US Department of Health and Human Services, 1987. [Pub. no. 88-101].
24. Evans RD. Engineers guide to the elementary behavior of radon daughters. In: *Heath physics*, vol 17. New York: Pergamon, 1969:229–252.
25. Franklin JC, Droullard RF. Instrumentation developed by the Bureau of Mines for continuously monitoring radon and radon daughters. Transactions, Instrument Society of America. 1983;22:25–32.
26. Federal Radiation Council, Superintendent of Documents. Guidance for the control of radiation hazards in uranium mining. Federal Radiation Council Staff Report no 8 (rev). Washington: US Government Printing Office, 1967.
27. Mernagh JR, Chambers DB. Beat radiation protection consideration in the mining and milling of high grade uranium ore. Proceedings of the Occupational Radiation Safety in Mining, Canada Nuclear Association. Toronto: 1984:451–455.
28. US Code of Federal Regulations, Title 29, Part 1910.146(b).
29. US Department of Labor, Mine Safety and Health Administration. *Mine gases* [Safety manual no 2]. Arlington, VA: 1991.
30. Schenker MB, Smith T, Munoz A, et al. Diesel exposure and mortality among railroad workers: results of a pilot study. *Br J Ind Med* 1984;41:320–327.
31. American Conference of Governmental Industrial Hygienists. 1995–1996 *Threshold limit values for chemical substances and physical agents and biological exposure indices*. Cincinnati: American Conference of Governmental Industrial Hygienists, 1995.
32. Hustrulid WA, ed. *Underground mining method handbook*. Denver: Society of Mining Engineers of American Institute of Mining, Metallurgical, and Petroleum Engineers (AIME), 1982:1687–1710.
33. Ary TS. The importance of waste management regulations to the minerals industry. In: Yegulalp TM, Kim K, eds. *Proceedings of the First International Conference on Environmental Issues and Waste Management in Energy and Minerals Production*. Columbus, OH: Battelle Press, 1990:5–14.
34. Hwang S. An assessment of health and environmental impact of contaminant releases from a mine tailings pile. In: Yegulalp TM, Kim K, eds. *Proceedings of the First International Conference on Environmental Issues and Waste Management in Energy and Minerals Production*. Columbus, OH: Battelle Press, 1990:174–184.
35. Ferguson KD, Erickson PM. Pre-mine prediction of acid mine drainage. In: Salomons W, Förstner U, eds. *Environmental management of solid waste*. New York: Springer-Verlag, 1988:24–25.
36. Radon exposure assessment—Connecticut. *MMWR Morb Mortal Wkly Rep* 1989;38:713–715.
37. Asami T. Soil pollution by metals from mining and smelting activities. In: Salomons W, Förstner U, eds. *Chemistry and biology of solid waste: dredged material and mine tailings*. New York: Springer-Verlag, 1988:143–169.
38. Abramson MJ, Wlodarczyk JH, Saunders NA, Hensley MJ. Does aluminum smelting cause lung disease? *Am Rev Respir Dis* 1989;139:1042–1057.
39. Chan-Yeung M, Enarson DA, MacLean L. Longitudinal study of workers in an aluminum smelter. *Arch Environ Health* 1989;44:134–139.
40. O'Donnell TV, Welford D, Coleman ED. Potroom asthma: New Zealand experience and follow-up. *Am J Ind Med* 1989;15:43–49.
41. Ronneberg A, Andersen A. Mortality and cancer morbidity in workers from an aluminum smelter with prebake carbon anodes. Part II: cancer morbidity. *Occup Environ Med* 1995;52:250–254.
42. Yamauchi H, Takahashi K, Mashiko M, Yamamura Y. Biological monitoring of arsenic exposure of gallium arsenide and inorganic arsenic exposed workers by determination of inorganic arsenic and its metabolites in urine and hair. *Am Ind Hyg Assoc J* 1989;50:606–612.
43. Eatough DJ, Hansen LD. S(IV) chemistry in smelter produced particulate matter. *Am J Ind Med* 1980;1:435–448.
44. Stella F, ed. *Industry performance*. New York: Inform, 1979. Gomez M, Duffy R, Trivelli V, eds. *At work in copper: occupational health and safety in copper smelting*; vol 1.
45. Enterline PE, Marsh GM. Mortality studies of smelter workers. *Am J Ind Med* 1980;1:251–259.
46. Enterline PE, Marsh GM. Cancer among workers exposed to arsenic and other substances in a copper smelter. *Am J Epidemiol* 1982;116:895–911.
47. Enterline PE, Marsh GM, Esmen NA, et al. Some effects of cigarette smoking, arsenic, and SO_2 on mortality among US copper smelter workers. *J Occup Med* 1987;29:831–838.
48. Lee-Feldstein A. Arsenic and respiratory cancer in humans: follow-up of copper smelter employees in Montana. *J Natl Cancer Inst* 1983;70:601–609.
49. Lee-Feldstein A. Cumulative exposure to arsenic and its relationship to respiratory cancer among copper smelter employees. *J Occup Med* 1986;28:286–302.
50. Sandström A, Wall SGI, Taube A. Cancer incidence and mortality among Swedish smelter workers. *Br J Ind Med* 1989;46:82–89.
51. Sandström A, Wall SGI. Continued surveillance of cancer incidence among Swedish smelter workers. *Acta Oncologica* 1992;31:11–17.
52. Järup L, Pershagen G. Arsenic exposure, smoking, and lung cancer in smelter workers—a case-control study. *Am J Epidemiol* 1991;134:545–551.
53. Järup L, Pershagen G, Wall S. Cumulative arsenic exposure and lung cancer in smelter workers: a dose response study. *Am J Ind Med* 1989;15:31–34.
54. Lee-Feldstein A. A comparison of several measures of exposure to arsenic. *Am J Epidemiol* 1989;129:112–124.
55. Enterline PE, Day R, Marsh GM. Cancers related to exposure to arsenic at a copper smelter. *Occup Environ Med* 1995;52:28–32.
56. Axelson O, Dahlgren E, Jansson CD, et al. Arsenic exposure and mortality: a case-referent study from a Swedish copper smelter. *Br J Ind Med* 1978;35:8–15.
57. Lagerkvist G, Linderhom H, Nordberg GF. Vasospastic tendency and Raynaud's phenomenon in smelter workers exposed to arsenic. *Environ Res* 1986;39:465–474.
58. Alexander BH, Checkoway H, van Netten C, et al. Semen quality of men employed at a lead smelter. *Occup Environ Med* 1996;53:411–416.
59. Steenland K, Selevan S, Landrigan P. The mortality of lead smelter workers: an update. *Am J Public Health* 1992;82:1641–1644.
60. Steenland K, Boffetta P. Lead and cancer in humans: Where are we now? *Am J Ind Med* 2000;38:295–299.
60a. Lundstrom NG, Nordberg G, Englyst V, et al. Cumulative lead exposure I relation to mortality and lung cancer morbidity in a cohort of primary smelter workers. *Scan J Work Environ Health* 1997;23:24–30.
61. Anttila A, Heikkila P, Pukkala E, et al. Excess lung cancer among workers exposed to lead. *Scand J Work Environ Health* 1995;21:460–469.
62. US Department of Health, Education and Welfare. National Institute for Occupational Safety and Health. Criteria for a recommended standard: occupational exposure to inorganic nickel. Washington: US Government Printing Office, 1977. [Pub. no. 77-164].
63. Doll R, Matthews JD, Morgan LG. Cancers of the lung and nasal sinuses in nickel workers: a reassessment of the period of risk. *Br J Ind Med* 1977; 34:102–105.
64. International Agency for Research on Cancer. Cadmium and cadmium compounds. *IARC Monogr Eval Carcinog Risks Hum* 1993;58:119–237.
65. Amdur MO. Respiratory response of guinea pigs to sulfuric acid and sulfate salts. Presented at: US Environmental Protection Agency Symposium on Sulfur Pollution and Research Approaches, May 27–28, 1975.
66. Pip E. Cadmium, copper and lead in soils and garden produce near a smelter at Flin Flon, Manitoba. *Bull Environ Contam Toxicol* 1991;46:790–796.
67. Kalman DA, Hughes J, van Belle G, et al. The effect of variable environmental arsenic contamination on urinary concentration of arsenic species. *Environ Health Perspect* 1990;89:145–151.
68. Polissar L, Lowry-Coble K, Kalman DA, et al. Pathways of human exposure to arsenic in a community surrounding a copper smelter. *Environ Res* 1990;53:29–47.
69. Baghurst PA, Tong S, McMichael AJ, et al. Determinants of blood lead concentrations to age 5 years in a birth cohort study of children living in the lead smelting city of Port Pirie and surrounding areas. *Arch Environ Health* 1992;47:203–210.
70. Landrigan PJ, Gehlbach SH, Rosenblum BF, et al. Epidemic lead absorption near an ore smelter: the role of particulate lead. *N Engl J Med* 1975;292:123–129.
71. Graziano JH, Popovac D, Factor-Litvak P, et al. Determinants of elevated blood lead during pregnancy in a population surrounding a lead smelter in Kosovo, Yugoslavia. *Environ Health Perspect* 1990;89:95–100.
72. Factor-Litvak P, Graziano JH, Kline JK, et al. A prospective study of birthweight and length of gestation in a population surrounding a lead smelter in Kosovo, Yugoslavia. *Int J Epidemiol* 1991;20:722–728.
73. Reif JS, Ameghino E, Aaronson MJ. Chronic exposure of sheep to a zinc smelter in Peru. *Environ Res* 1989;49:40–49.

CHAPTER 41
Pneumoconioses

Feroza M. Daroowalla

The term *pneumoconiosis* is defined by the International Labour Office (ILO) as the accumulation of dust in the lungs and the tissue reactions to its presence. It refers to nonmalignant fibrosis and scarring of the lungs in reaction to environmental or occupational exposure to inorganic dusts, such as silica, asbestos, tin, and coal dusts (1). Dusts that result in fibrogenic pneumoconiosis are as follows:

Silica
- Cristobalite
- Quartz
- Tridymite

Mica
Graphite
Beryllium
Coal dust
Asbestos
Talc

Dusts that result in benign pneumoconioses are as follows:

Iron oxide (siderosis)
Tin ore (stannosis)
Barium compounds (baritosis)

Pneumoconiosis is classified as either simple or complicated [i.e., progressive massive fibrosis (PMF)]. In simple pneumoconiosis, the lesions are small and nodular, and are not usually associated with significant functional loss. Complicated pneumoconiosis is seen in a small percentage of individuals and involves large areas of lung in fibrosis, with associated functional compromise.

This chapter discusses lung disease related to exposures to coal, silica, silicates (mica, talc, kaolin), and cobalt.

COAL WORKERS' PNEUMOCONIOSIS

Introduction

Coal workers develop several different lung diseases that are referred to as *black lung*. These include simple coal workers' pneumoconiosis (CWP), PMF, silicosis, chronic airways obstruction, chronic industrial bronchitis, and emphysema.

Scope of Problem

The major producers of coal in 1990 were China, the United States, the former Union of Soviet Socialist Republics, and East Germany. CWP prevalence rates vary with time spent working and exposure, with rates between 2% to 32% in U.S. miners (2). These are underestimates, given the incomplete reporting of occupational illness in general and especially in these nations. Prevalence rates of PMF in the United States have decreased in the 1980s and 1990s. However, as of 1990, more than 1,500 death certificates in the United States mentioned the presence of CWP, and coal dust–related morbidity continues to be a problem in those who worked in the coal mines during the 1960s and 1970s (3).

Composition of Coal and Risk of Disease

The term *coal* refers to a group of rock material formed from fossilized plants occurring in a spectrum of forms, ranging from hard anthracite to friable lignite. Coal is classified by rank according to carbon content and combustibility. High-rank coal, such as anthracite with a 98% carbon content, presents a higher risk for the development of simple pneumoconiosis than lower-ranked materials, such as bituminous coal that is 90% to 95% carbon. In addition to the rank of coal, the cumulative dose of coal mine–dust exposure is an important risk factor for the development of simple pneumoconiosis. Tobacco use does not significantly affect the development of CWP. The risk of complicated pneumoconiosis is related to preexisting simple pneumoconiosis, cumulative dust exposure, and dust composition. Dust with greater than 15% quartz content is associated with silicosis (4,5).

Occupations at Risk

Coal is used as a fuel and in the production of coke, coal gas, coal tar compounds, and in the manufacture of fertilizers, food dyes, synthetic rubber, insecticides, and disinfectants.

Coal miners and workers involved in coal trimming, mining, and milling of graphite, making of carbon electrodes, and the manufacture and use of carbon black are susceptible to coal dust–related lung diseases. Coal miners, especially face workers, are exposed to the highest concentration of respirable airborne dusts, including carbon and silica. In addition to coal dust, coal miners are exposed to a variety of mineral dusts produced during the cutting of rock and dirt in the process of coal extraction. In underground mines, 30% to 40% of dust may be noncoal in origin, including approximately 5% silica. Those who are directly involved in rock cutting, surface drilling, or roof bolting may be exposed to dust with even higher contents of silica (6,7).

Clinical Features and Lung Function

Simple CWP is usually not associated with symptoms and is diagnosed on chest radiograph. Early in the course, however, a normal radiograph may obscure clinically and histologically significant disease. More advanced disease may be associated with dyspnea, productive cough, or melanoptysis. In some cases, emphysema or small airways disease may accompany the pneumoconiosis and produce changes on pulmonary function tests (PFTs), as well as symptoms of productive cough and dyspnea (5).

PMF, or complicated CWP, results in symptoms and functional impairment. Symptoms include dyspnea on exertion, cough production of black sputum, and wheezing. Progression of disease can result in pulmonary hypertension and cor pulmonale. Chest pain, digit clubbing, and hemoptysis are not seen (8).

Chronic airways obstruction is associated with coal mine work independent of radiographic CWP. It may be symptomatic and result in obstructive impairment on PFTs without significant radiographic changes (9,10). Generalized emphysema is observed in smoking and nonsmoking coal miners, and severity is related to the dose of mine dust. Bronchitis with chronic productive cough results from mucous gland enlargement and goblet cell proliferation caused by coal mine dust deposition (5,11).

Inadequate epidemiologic evidence exists to support a lung cancer risk with coal dust.

Radiographic Changes

Simple CWP is characterized by discrete rounded nodular densities, usually smaller than 3 mm in diameter, predominantly in the upper- and middle-lung zones. These densities are usually denoted as *p*- or *q*-type opacities, according to the ILO classification of chest radiographs for pneumoconiosis. Increased irregular densities can also be related to CWP and should be taken into consideration when evaluating a chest radiograph for the disease. Complicated CWP, or PMF, is characterized by larger opacities (larger than 10 mm), frequently bilateral and occurring in the upper- and middle-lung zones. They may form a sharp, lateral margin when surrounded by a zone of emphysematous lung.

The chest radiograph is not sensitive for early changes in pneumoconiosis that may be detected by more sensitive techniques, such as computed tomographs. To date, however, the computed tomograph scan is not used routinely for the diagnosis, rating, and management of CWP (12,13).

Pathology

The pathognomonic lesion on histology in simple CWP is a several-millimeter-wide (1 to 5 mm), rounded, pigmented lesion called the *coal dust macule*. Macules are initially distributed near the respiratory bronchioles in the upper lobes but can involve the lower lobes in time. Microscopic examination reveals collections of dust-filled macrophages with whorls of reticulin but minimal amounts of collagen. Adjacent alveolar walls are destroyed, leading to focal emphysematous change (14,15).

In complicated CWP or PMF, the lesions are 1 to 2 cm in diameter with extensive dust collection, and collagen and reticulin deposition. They occur in the upper lobes; may be bilateral, rounded, or irregular; and may contain cavities of black liquid. Accompanying changes of bronchitis and emphysema may be seen on pathologic examination (11).

Pathogenesis

The process begins when inhaled particles of dust with suitable diameter and aerodynamic characteristics deposit in the acinar units of the lung. These particles are engulfed by alveolar macrophages and removed to the hilar nodes. The macrophage and inflammatory cell response sets in motion a series of events that results in the release of free radicals and oxidative damage. The quality of the particles, particularly the quantity of quartz within, influences the intensity of the inflammatory response. The emphysema that frequently surrounds areas of coal macule or nodule formation is thought to be a result of the release of proteolytic enzymes (10).

Regulations

The Mine Safety and Health Administration of the U.S. Department of Labor established regulations in 1969 to limit mixed dust exposure in mines. These regulations were designed to prevent advanced CWP and, therefore, may not be protective for other respiratory conditions. The regulations differ based on the proportion of silica in the dust. The 8-hour time-weighted average (TWA) for dust with less than 5% silica is 2 mg per m^3. The 8-hour TWA is adjusted according to a formula (10 mg per m^3 per % silica) for dusts with greater than 5% respirable silica dust.

In nonmine settings, the Occupational Safety and Health Administration (OSHA) regulations apply. The 8-hour TWA limit is 2.4 mg per m^3 per (% SiO_2 + 2) if the respirable fraction is less than 5% SiO_2. The formula 10 per (% SiO_2 + 2) is used when the respirable fraction is greater than 5% SiO_2. The federal limit on dust was derived from studies that indicated that progression to category 2 (ILO classification) of chest radiograph would be prevented at dust exposure levels less than 2 mg per m^3. However, this does not take into account the possibility of disease and disease progression that may occur at lower dust levels without changes in chest radiograph (5,7).

Medical screening with periodic chest radiographs is mandated by U.S. federal regulations for all underground coal miners. In addition, miners with pneumoconiosis are entitled to increased frequency of personal environmental monitoring and the option to be transferred to an environment with less than or equal to 1 mg per m^3 of coal dust. Surveillance of workers for radiographic findings of disease allows early removal from exposure and is useful in simple pneumoconiosis, which is unlikely to progress in the absence of further exposure. Individuals with PMF should also be removed promptly from further exposure, although the disease may progress despite removal from dusty work. Chest radiograph surveillance, however, is not effective in predicting the development or the progression of disease in workers without radiographic changes, and ignores obstructive disease that may be invisible on chest radiograph. Therefore, it is important that a dust control program be implemented along with radiograph surveillance. Periodic screening with spirometry may also be undertaken to identify workers with accelerated loss of lung function and those who should limit their exposure to dust and to tobacco smoke (5,7).

Prevention and Management

Prevention of coal lung disease requires the reduction of dust levels and the duration of dust exposure. Dust control is achieved with ventilation, the use of water sprays, and mechanizing processes. Effective control goes hand in hand with dust monitoring. In the event that dust levels cannot be controlled, respirators or administrative restrictions on the number of hours worked must be used.

The principles of management include treating symptoms and complications, and facilitating compensation for disability. For those that have developed pneumoconiosis, medicines that relieve any airflow obstruction and treatment for hypoxemia or cor pulmonale are indicated. Periodic monitoring of spirometry and chest radiograph as well as evaluation of gas exchange is appropriate. Skin testing for tuberculosis should also be undertaken. Minimizing exposure to dust and tobacco once disease is diagnosed is necessary to prevent progression (5).

SILICOSIS

Introduction

Silicon dioxide or silica is a ubiquitous material in the earth's crust and exists in crystalline and amorphous forms. Crystalline silica, also referred to as *silica sand* or *free-silica*, occurs in three forms: quartz, cristobalite, and tridymite. Quartz is the most common and is a constituent of granite (30% silica), slate (40% silica), and sandstone (70% silica). Cristobalite and tridymite are formed when quartz or amorphous silica is heated to very high temperatures. Amorphous silica is noncrystalline and probably not toxic to the lungs. Examples of amorphous silica are diatomaceous earth, siliceous glass, opal, flint, and vitreous silica. Calcining of diatomaceous earth with heat in excess of 1,000°C results in the formation of cristobalite, which does have respiratory toxicity. This material is used as a filtering medium and in the food and beverage industry (16).

Diseases attributable or associated with the inhalation of free crystalline silica include silicosis, industrial bronchitis with airflow limitation, pulmonary and extrapulmonary tuberculosis, and lung cancer.

Scope of Problem

Silica-induced disease has been described since the times of Hippocrates and continues to be a prevalent disabling occupational lung disease today. In recognition of the hazards of silica, the joint ILO/World Health Organization Committee on Occupational Health undertook a program for global elimination of silicosis at its 1995 session. In developing nations, such as Colombia and India, prevalence estimates of silicosis range from 37% to 55%, with more than 1.5 million workers exposed in each country. In the United States, 4,313 deaths with silicosis listed on the death certificate were reported from 1979 to 1990. In a survey of four states, 447 confirmed cases were reported between 1988 and 1992. It is known that more than 250 workers die each year with silicosis in the United States. Estimates suggest that 100,000 of the 1 million workers in this country who are exposed to silica dust are at risk for developing silicosis. Although rates of silicosis are declining in developed nations as dust suppression and medical surveillance programs achieve their goals, the incidence rates in developing nations such as India, Thailand, China, and Bolivia may be on the rise (2,16). Clearly, worker morbidity and mortality related to silica are a contemporary and urgent issue in occupational health.

Exposure to Silica

The important elements in occupational and avocational exposures to silica are the free silica content of the dust aerosol, the concentration of particles in the inhaled air, the respirable proportion of the dust, and the duration of exposure. In general, exposure occurs when rock is drilled or removed from the earth, when silica-bearing stone is used to create other products, when silica-containing abrasives are used, when abrasives are directed at a stone surface, and when powdered silica is used as an additive or raw material in manufacturing. Occupations with exposure to silica are listed (17):

Hard rock mining
Tool grinding
Tunnel drilling
Knife sharpening
Stone quarrying (flint, slate)
Silica flour production
Stone crushing
Diatomaceous earth production
Granite monument carving
Glass manufacture
Stone sculpting
Plastics manufacture
Stone masonry
Paint manufacture
Foundry casting
Pottery, ceramics, clay
Ship building and repair
Soap and detergent manufacture
Foundry
Earth tunneling
Asphalt paving
Ceramic manufacture
Abrasive blasting

Radiographic and Clinical Findings

Silicosis is a fibrotic disease of the lungs caused by exposure to free crystalline silica. Four clinical and pathologic varieties of silicosis can be identified: chronic simple silicosis, PMF, accelerated silicosis, and acute silicosis (or silico-proteinosis).

CHRONIC SIMPLE (NODULAR) SILICOSIS

Chronic simple silicosis is a diffuse fibronodular disease that occurs after 20 to 40 years of exposure to dust with less than 30% quartz content. Pulmonary function is usually not impaired and neither is survival in the early stages of this disease. It is most commonly recognized as a radiographic abnormality of diffuse, rounded opacities 1 to 3 mm in diameter with an upper lobe predominance. Eggshell (i.e., thin and dense) calcification of hilar nodes is rare but characteristic. In general, the radiographic appearance is not a good indicator of clinical status in simple silicosis. As the disease progresses, symptoms of dyspnea and productive cough develop. PFTs may become representative of restrictive impairment with decreased diffusing capacity and hypoxemia with exercise. Chronic bronchitis symptoms are frequently seen in dust-exposed populations, and may accompany the symptoms and signs of fibrosis (18,19) (Figs. 41-1, 41-2).

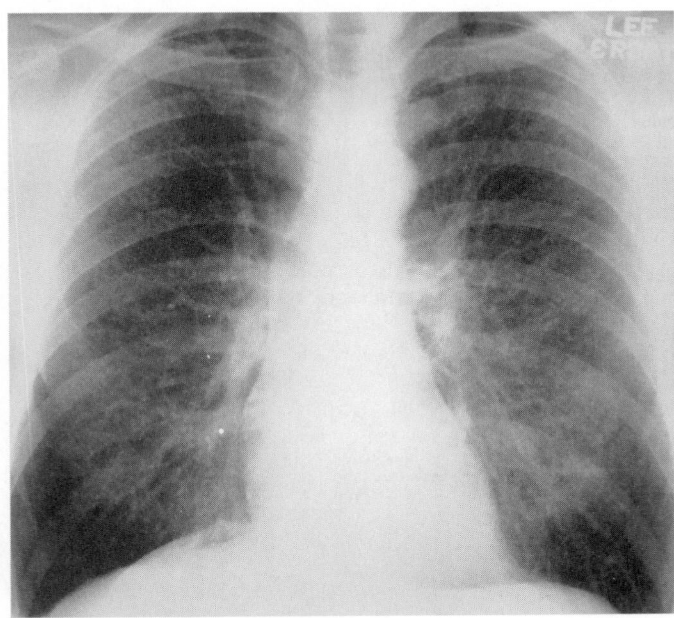

Figure 41-1. Chronic simple silicosis.

PROGRESSIVE MASSIVE FIBROSIS

PMF is a progression of simple silicosis in which the radiograph reveals large, irregular masses and volume loss in the upper lobes, basilar emphysema, and hilar retraction (Figs. 41-3, 41-4). PFTs reveal severe restriction or mixed obstruction and restriction, decreased pulmonary compliance, and hypoxemia. Symptoms include dyspnea on exertion of gradual onset and slow progression, often with associated bronchitis. This

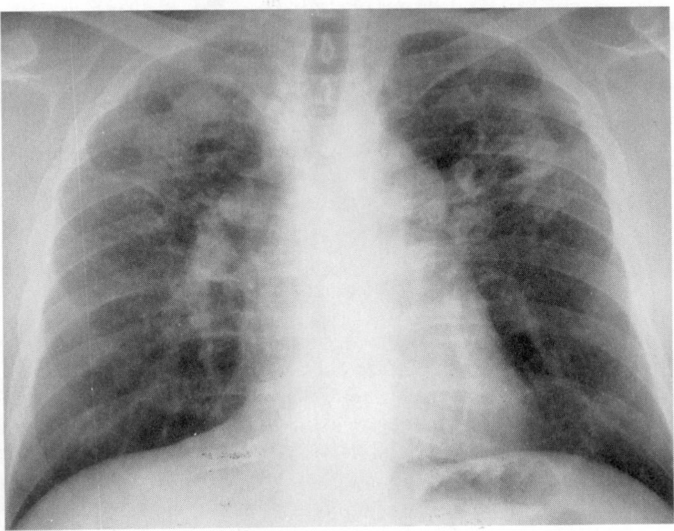

Figure 41-2. Chronic simple silicosis.

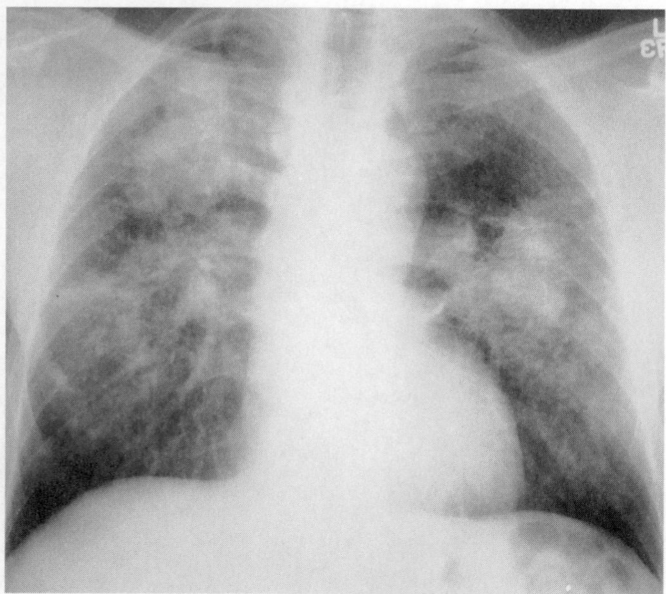

Figure 41-3. Progressive massive fibrosis.

presentation follows many years of exposure as reflected in the relatively advanced age of patients at presentation (older than 40 years of age) and may occur after exposure has ceased. The illness follows an insidious and progressive course despite discontinuation of exposure. Risk factors for developing PMF are high dust exposure level, history of tuberculosis, and an increased background level of small opacities on radiograph (18–20).

ACCELERATED SILICOSIS

Accelerated silicosis is an uncommon form of disease occurring after 2 to 5 years of intense free silica exposure with dusts of 40% to 80% quartz content. It presents clinically as dyspnea and radiographically as diffuse, small, irregular opacities or reticulonodular opacities in the middle-lung zones. It is almost uniformly fatal after several years (21,22).

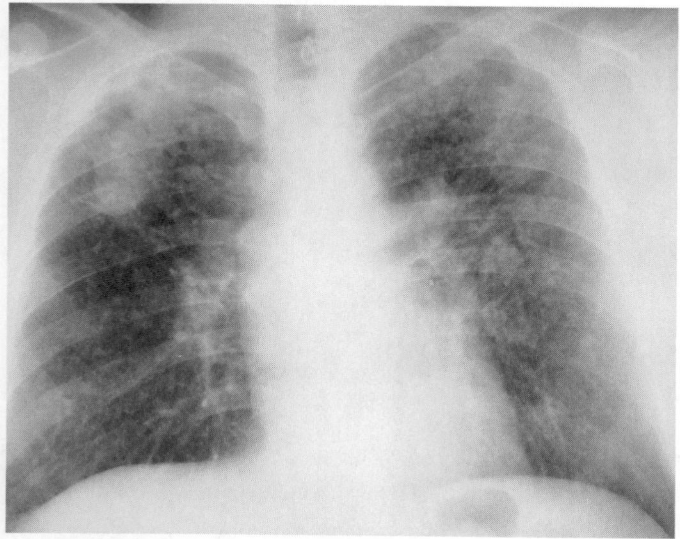

Figure 41-4. Progressive massive fibrosis.

ACUTE SILICOSIS (SILICOPROTEINOSIS)

This is a rare manifestation of disease that follows exposure to high concentrations of free silica or finely divided silica powder, such as that seen with sandblasters. The clinical presentation is that of rapidly progressive dyspnea and the onset of respiratory insufficiency within 1 to 3 years. The radiograph shows diffuse perihilar alveolar filling with ground-glass opacities. The pathologic finding is of progressive fibrosis accompanying alveolar filling with lipoproteinaceous exudate and cellular debris resembling pulmonary alveolar proteinosis. This entity usually results in death (16,17,23).

Differential Diagnosis

Diagnosis should be straightforward in an individual with a history of silica exposure, a chest radiograph showing nodular infiltrates, and PFTs with mild restrictive impairment in the case of simple silicosis. Sarcoidosis, idiopathic pulmonary fibrosis, rheumatoid lung, carcinomatous lymphangitis, and pulmonary hemosiderosis may be mistakenly diagnosed if the history of silica exposure is not adequately elicited. Acute and accelerated silicosis may resemble tuberculosis, chronic sarcoidosis, allergic alveolitis, or ankylosing spondylitis lung (17,19).

Pathology

On gross examination, the lungs have more pigmentation than usual, fibrous adhesions, and silicotic plaques over the pleural surfaces. The hilar nodes are enlarged with fibrotic nodules and are sometimes calcified. The characteristic fibrotic nodules are also found in the parenchyma of the lung, predominantly in apical and posterior regions of the lobes. In areas in which nodules have coalesced, cavitation may appear. Bullae representing emphysematous changes may surround areas of massive fibrosis (confluent nodules).

Microscopic examination of the silicotic nodule reveals a concentric arrangement of hyalinized collagen fibers, dust-laden macrophages, and peripheral reticulin fibers in the region of the respiratory bronchiole. The bronchioles and pulmonary vessels are involved and destroyed by the fibrosis. Silica particles are seen in the nodules as birefringent particles in polarized light (18).

The accelerated form of silicosis cannot be differentiated from chronic silicosis except for the additional appearance of thickened alveolar walls with proliferation of type II alveolar cells (17).

In acute silicosis, the alveolar spaces are filled with proteinaceous material consisting of phospholipids and surfactant, which stain with periodic acid–Schiff's reagent. The alveoli are lined by hypertrophic type II pneumocytes. In addition, the alveolar spaces contain desquamated pneumocytes, macrophages, and silica particles (17,18).

Pathogenesis

The process of fibrosis begins with the deposition of appropriately sized particles of crystalline silica in the alveolar spaces. The particle most likely to reach and be retained in the pulmonary acinus ranges from 0.5 to 3.0 μm in diameter. After deposition, the silica particles are phagocytosed by alveolar macrophages, which is a key event for the process that follows. The macrophages that have ingested the dust produce cytokines that recruit and activate T cells. The T cells then recruit and activate further populations of macrophages that stimulate fibroblasts to multiply and produce collagen. This process is amplified and perpetuated by the recruitment of other inflammatory cells, such as neutrophils, with enhanced production of fibrogenic factors. Death of the macrophage with release of silica particles, and reingestion by other macrophages, also plays a role in the perpetuation of the process (24).

Prevention

Primary prevention is the goal in silicosis, and begins with an increased awareness of silica-related disease and its use in industries. Engineering controls include the enclosure and isolation of processes, suppression of dust with water sprays, and ventilation. When high levels of dust are produced, as in sandblasting, workers should be protected with respirators or positive-pressure air supply equipment. A respirator program does not prevent all exposure and only achieves reduction in individual exposures. For a respirator program to be successful, it must be accompanied by an air monitoring program to make appropriate selection of respiratory protective equipment. Other administrative controls include finding silica substitutes for high dust jobs (16,25).

Management

No treatment exists for silicosis, and management of cases involves removal from further exposure to silica dust to minimize the chances of progression to massive fibrosis. In advanced disease, symptomatic treatment, such as oxygen supplements, bronchodilators, antibiotics, and treatment for cor pulmonale, should be provided. Treatment with inhaled aluminum powder, D-penicillamine, and polyvinyl pyridine-*N*-oxide has been used with varying amounts of success. The risk of side effects and the consideration of carcinogenic effects have limited the use of the latter two drugs. Lung transplantation and bronchopulmonary lavage have been used with limited success in patients with acute silicosis. Corticosteroids have not been found to be useful in simple silicosis or PMF. If steroids are used, however, prophylactic antituberculous drugs should also be administered. Tuberculosis in patients with silicosis is treated with the same drug regimen used in the remaining population. Infection and disease caused by *Mycobacterium avium-intracellulare* may require treatment with five or more drugs for lengthy periods (16,19).

Associated Illnesses

MYCOBACTERIAL AND OPPORTUNIST INFECTIONS

Tuberculosis and other nontuberculous mycobacterial infections occur more frequently among silicotics and those exposed to silica (without silicosis) than other individuals. This is especially true in workers with acute or accelerated silicosis, and in patients older than age 50 years. Mycobacterial infection occurs with increasing frequency as the extent of silicotic disease advances. In addition, those with disease caused by pure silica are more likely to have tuberculosis than those with disease caused by mixed dust. This predilection for mycobacterial infection is most likely related to the disabling and destructive effects on the alveolar macrophages by the silica dust in individuals with prior latent infection or with a risk of new exposure to tuberculosis (16,26–28).

Nontuberculous mycobacterial (NTM) disease is also becoming increasingly common in silicotics. One study found that in 22 of 83 silicotics with mycobacterial disease, 55% of cases were caused by NTM. The most commonly encountered NTM are *Mycobacterium kansasii*, *Mycobacterium intracellulare*, and *Mycobacterium scrofulaceum* (16,29).

Individuals with silicosis and more than two decades of crystalline silica exposure (without silicosis) should receive annual purified protein derivative (tuberculin) skin testing. The conversion of a skin test to positive (greater than 9-mm induration) without evidence of active disease is an indication for 1 year of prophylaxis with 300 mg daily of isoniazid. Mycobacterial disease should be suspected in any silicotic with rapid chest radiograph changes, or in individuals with new infiltrates or cavitation of preexisting nodules. Diagnosis may be difficult to make, as acid-fast staining of sputum smears can be falsely negative. In addition, constitutional symptoms may be mistaken for worsening silicosis rather than mycobacterial disease. Treatment with the four antituberculous drugs ethambutol, pyrazinamide, streptomycin, and rifampicin has been shown to be successful. Prevention of tuberculosis hinges on limitation of silica exposure and prompt chemoprophylaxis (16,30).

CONNECTIVE TISSUE DISEASES

Silicotics and individuals with high silica exposures have an increased prevalence of scleroderma and systemic sclerosis. The relationship with rheumatoid arthritis is not as strong. Silicotics may have positive serum levels of antinuclear antibodies and rheumatoid factor that may not be related to the occurrence of an arthritis. Mixed connective tissue disease and systemic lupus erythematosus have also been reported at higher rates in silicotics (31,32).

RENAL DISEASE

Silicon nephropathy has been described in association with silicosis and includes glomerulonephritis, nephrotic syndrome, and end-stage renal disease. Evidence exists of immune-mediated mechanisms in the silica-associated nephropathies. It is unclear whether a silica dose-dependent effect also plays a role in pathogenesis (16,33).

LUNG CANCER

The link between silicosis and pulmonary malignancy remains controversial. The difficulty in determining the association is in part because of confounding exposures in industry, such as radon, asbestos, and cigarette smoking.

Despite these difficulties, in 1996, the International Agency for Research on Cancer proposed that crystalline silica in the form of quartz and cristobalite from occupational sources be classified as a human carcinogen. The International Agency for Research on Cancer working group made these conclusions based on current epidemiologic literature. Although not all of the epidemiologic evidence demonstrated excess cancer risk, taken as a whole, the working group concluded that the studies support a finding of increased cancer risks from inhaled quartz and cristobalite (34,35).

The question of whether silica exposure results in an elevated risk of lung cancer in the absence of silicosis is still unanswered. It has been suggested that dust-related carcinogenicity may occur independent of fibrosis but this has yet to be proven conclusively. It might be that fibrogenesis predisposes to carcinogenesis or that the occurrence of the two diseases reflects a level of exposure to the causal agent (34,36,37).

REGULATIONS

The OSHA permissible exposure limit (PEL) for quartz is an 8-hour TWA of 10 mg per m^3 per (% SiO_2 + 2) for the respirable fraction and 30 per (% SiO_2 + 2) for the total quartz measurement. In addition, OSHA recommends that individuals chronically exposed to silica receive a baseline medical examination, chest radiograph, and PFTs (forced expiratory volume in 1 second, forced vital capacity, and diffusing capacity of the lungs for carbon monoxide). These should be repeated every 5 years in individuals with less than 20 years of exposure and repeated every 2 years for those with greater than 20 years of exposure. A chest radiograph should also be obtained on termination of employment. OSHA recommendations for medical management of a worker with an abnormal chest radiograph (classified as ILO class 1/0 or worse) are for placement in a mandatory respiratory protection program or a reevaluation of the current respiratory protection program. An examination by a lung physician should be procured and a decision made about monitoring requirements. Medical records are to be kept for at least 30 years after employees' termination of employment (17,38).

The American Conference of Governmental Industrial Hygienists suggested a threshold limit value in 1996 for the respirable fraction of crystalline silica of 0.05 mg per m^3 for cristobalite, 0.1 mg per m^3 for quartz, 0.05 mg per m^3 for tridymite, and 0.1 mg per m^3 of tripoli (for respirable quartz) (39).

PNEUMOCONIOSES ASSOCIATED WITH SILICATES

Talc

Talc is a magnesium silicate that exists in sheetlike crystalline forms or as fibers. Talc used in industrial settings can contain mixtures of silica, amphibole asbestos, tremolite, actinolite, and anthophyllite. Inhalation talc exposure can result in talco-asbestosis, talco-silicosis, and pure talcosis. Pure talcosis is found in occupational and nonoccupational settings associated with cosmetic use of talcum powder. Radiologic abnormalities include round or irregular opacities. On tissue examination, fibrosis, foreign body granulomas, and multinucleated giant cells are seen. Physiologic testing reveals normal, restrictive, or mixed restrictive and obstructive abnormalities in pulmonary function. Intravenous injection of materials contaminated with talc results in foreign body granulomatous reaction. The OSHA PEL for an 8-hour TWA is 20 million particles per cubic foot of air for talc without asbestos and less than 1% quartz (39–41).

Kaolin

Kaolin, also referred to as *china clay,* is an aluminum silicate. It is used in the manufacture of refractory ceramic bricks and fibers, and as filler in paints, plastics, and pharmaceuticals. Kaolin ore may contain silica and micas. In addition to the consequences of silica and mica exposure in kaolin workers, kaolin is thought to have fibrogenic activity on its own. Simple and complicated pneumoconioses can occur in kaolin workers. Irregular small opacities in all lung fields characterize the radiographic abnormalities seen with kaolin disease. PFTs in workers with simple pneumoconiosis can be normal or show mild restrictive abnormalities. Complicated disease can be accompanied by mixed or restrictive patterns. Pulmonary tissue examination reveals interstitial and nodular fibrosis and varies with the kaolin dust and quartz content of the lungs (39–41).

Mica

Mica consists of nine different species of silicates with less than 1% quartz that are colorless, odorless, and are in a nonfibrous plate form. The micas are used in the manufacture of plastics, in drilling, and in special paints. The major species used commercially are muscovite and phlogopite. Muscovite is a hydrated aluminum potassium compound sometimes called *white mica.* It is used in applications of its properties of transparency and heat and electricity resistance.

Pneumoconioses in mica mining and milling workers are generally thought to be caused by exposure to free silica and not directly to pure mica exposure. However, muscovite can result in a restrictive fibrotic disease in the pure form. The disease can appear in simple or complicated forms; the latter has larger lesions and more massive fibrosis. The radiographic pattern is that of fine nodularity linear densities and, possibly, pleural thickening. The OSHA PEL for mica with less than 1% crystalline silica is an 8-hour TWA of 20 million particles per cubic foot (39–41).

Vermiculite

Vermiculite has an aluminum iron magnesium silicate composition. It is used in insulation, fire-resistant materials, and as a carrier for fertilizer and other chemicals. In one study, vermiculite from a Montana mine was found to be contaminated with actinolite and tremolite asbestos. Workers in this mine experienced elevated risk of lung cancer, mesothelioma, and pleural and parenchymal abnormalities. Studies of populations at other mines seem to support findings that health effects of vermiculite are a result of contamination with tremolite and actinolite. Monitoring for amphibole contamination and for airborne dust characteristics and content are the chief ingredients of a surveillance program in industries using vermiculite (40–41).

HARD METAL DISEASE

The term *hard metal* refers to a group of metal alloys with characteristics of extreme hardness, resistance to wear, and tolerance of high temperatures. The group consists most commonly of tungsten carbide in a binder base. This binder is frequently cobalt. The cobalt is responsible for the health effects of hard metals (42–46).

Exposures

Exposure to hard metal occurs as it is formed from the powdered metal ingredients, as the hard metal is fashioned into tools, as hard metal tools are reconditioned or finished, and from aerosol inhalation of cobalt solubilized in metal working fluids, such as coolants. Cobalt exposure also occurs in the diamond polishing industry in which cobalt discs are used.

Health Effects

The respiratory health effects of cobalt include reversible airway obstruction or asthma, hypersensitivity pneumonitis, and pulmonary fibrosis. Only pulmonary fibrosis is discussed.

Pathology

Histologic examination reveals patchy involvement with fibrosis and areas of alveolitis. Microscopic examination reveals infiltration of the lung parenchyma with histiocytes and plasma cells with thickened alveolar septae. Usually, no granulomas exist in histology. In cases with alveolitis, the air spaces contain desquamated mononuclear cells and type II alveolar pneumocytes. A characteristic finding on tissue biopsy and bronchoalveolar lavage is of multinucleated giant cells.

Clinical Findings

Patients present with progressive cough and shortness of breath. Physical examination reveals tachypnea, finger clubbing, and basilar crackles. PFTs reveal reduced lung volumes, hypoxemia at rest and with exercise, and low diffusion capacity. Disease may progress to pulmonary hypertension and cor pulmonale. The chest radiograph may not show abnormalities in the early stages of symptoms. When abnormal, the radiograph presents with a reticulonodular pattern in the middle and lower zones, and sometimes with honeycombing.

Regulations

The PEL for cobalt is 50 μm per m^3 for a full-shift TWA.

Management

Once fibrosis has developed, treatment is limited to relief of symptoms. In the setting of a predominant alveolitis, however, corticosteroids may be successful in decreasing inflammation and symptoms. Because hypersensitivity pneumonitis plays a role in the pathogenesis of illness and because alveolitis is potentially reversible for some individuals, removal from further exposure is important (42).

REFERENCES

1. Anonymous. Pneumoconiosis redefined [Editorial]. *BMJ* 1972;2:552.
2. Attfield M, Wagner G. Coal. In: Harber P, Schenker MB, Balmes JR, eds. *Occupational and environmental respiratory disease*. St. Louis: Mosby, 1996; 23:362–372.
3. Althouse RB, Castellan RM, Wagner GR. Pneumoconiosis in the United States: highlights of surveillance data from NIOSH and other federal sources. *Occup Med* 1992;7:197–208.
4. Attfield MD, Morring K. An investigation into the relationship between coal workers' pneumoconiosis and dust exposure in US coal miners. *Am Ind Hyg Assoc J* 1992;53:486–492.
5. Petsonk EL, Attfield MD. Coal workers' pneumoconiosis and other coal-related lung disease. In: Rosenstock L, Cullen MR, eds. *Textbook of clinical occupational and environmental medicine*. Philadelphia: WB Saunders, 1994.
6. Amandus HE, Piacitelli G. Dust exposures at U.S. surface coal mines in 1982–1983. *Arch Environ Health* 1987;42:374–381.
7. Attfield M, Wagner GR. Coal. In: Harber P, Schenker MB, Balmes JR, eds. *Occupational and environmental respiratory disease*. St. Louis: Mosby–Year Book, 1996.
8. Soutar CA, Maclaren WM, Annis R, Melville AWT. Quantitative relations between exposure to respirable coal mine dust and coal workers' simple pneumoconiosis in men who have worked as miners but have left the coal industry. *Br J Ind Med* 1986;43:29–36.
9. Seixas NS, Robins TG, Attfield MD, Moulton LH. Exposure-response relationships for coal mine dust and obstructive lung disease following enactment of the Federal Coal Mine Health and Safety Act of 1969. *Am J Ind Med* 1991;21:715–734.
10. Seixas NS, Robins TG, Attfield MD, Moulton LH. Longitudinal and cross sectional analyses of exposure to coal mine dust and pulmonary function in new miners. *Br J Ind Med* 1993;50:929–937.
11. Douglas AN, Lamb D, Ruckley VA. Bronchial gland dimensions in coal miners: influence of smoking and dust exposure. *Thorax* 1982;37:760–764.
12. Collins HPR, Dick JA, Bennett JG, et al. Irregularly shaped small shadows on chest radiographs, dust exposure, and lung function in coal workers' pneumoconiosis. *Br J Ind Med* 1988;45:4–55.
13. International Labour Office. *Guidelines for the use of the international classification of radiographs of pneumoconiosis, rev ed*. Occupational safety and health series, no. 22 (rev 80). Geneva: International Labour Office, 1980.
14. Seaton A. Coal workers' pneumoconiosis. In: Morgan WKC, Seaton A, eds. *Occupational lung diseases*, 3rd ed. Philadelphia: WB Saunders, 1995.
15. Pneumoconiosis Committee of the College of American Pathology. Pathology standards for coal workers' pneumoconiosis: report of the Pneumoconiosis Committee of the College of American Pathology. *Arch Pathol Med* 1979;103:375–432.
16. Ad Hoc Committee of Scientific Assembly on Environmental and Occupational Health, American Thoracic Society. Adverse effects of crystalline silica exposure. American Thoracic Society statement. *Am J Respir Crit Care Med* 1997;155:761–765.
17. Davis GS. Silica. In: Harber P, Schenker MB, Balmes JR, eds. *Occupational and environmental respiratory disease*. St. Louis: Mosby–Year Book, 1996.
18. Silicosis and Silicate Disease Committee. Diseases associated with exposure to silica and nonfibrous silicate materials. *Arch Pathol Lab Med* 1988; 1112:673–720.
19. Seaton A. Silicosis. In Morgan WKC, Seaton A, eds. *Occupational lung diseases*, 3rd ed. Philadelphia: WB Saunders, 1995.
20. Ng TP, Cahan SL. Factors associated with massive fibrosis in silicosis. *Thorax* 1991;46:229–232.
21. Seaton A, Legge JS, Henderson J, Kerr KM. Accelerated silicosis in Scottish stonemasons. *Lancet* 1991;337:341–344.
22. Ziskind M, Weill H, Bailey WC, et al. Accelerated silicosis in sandblasters. *Chest* 1973;64:411.
23. Suratt PM, Winn WC, Brody AR, et al. Acute silicosis in tombstone sandblasters. *Am Rev Resp Dis* 1977;115:521–529.
24. Davis GS. Pathogenesis of silicosis: current concepts and hypothesis. *Lung* 1986;164:139–154.
25. Bates DV, Gotsch AR, Brooks S, Landrigan PJ, Handkinson JL, Merchant JA. Prevention of occupational lung disease. *Chest* 1992;102S:257S–276S.
26. Weber SL, Banks DE. Silicosis. In: Rosenstock L, Cullen MR, eds. *Textbook of clinical occupational and environmental medicine*. Philadelphia: WB Saunders, 1994.
27. Jones JG, Owen TE, Corrado HA. Respiratory tuberculosis and pneumoconiosis in slate workers. *Br J Dis Chest* 1967;61:138–143.
28. Snider DE. The relationship between tuberculosis and silicosis. *Am Rev Respir Dis* 1978;118:455–460.
29. Bailey WC, Brown M, Buechner HA, Weill H, Ichinose H, Ziskind M. Silico-mycobacterial disease in sandblasters. *Am Rev Respir Dis* 1974;110:115–125.
30. American Thoracic Society. Treatment of tuberculosis and tuberculosis infection in adults and children. *Am J Respir Crit Care Med* 1994;149:1359–1374.
31. Rustin MHA, Bull HA, Ziegler V. Silica associated systemic sclerosis is clinically, serologically and immunologically indistinguishable from idiopathic systemic sclerosis. *Br J Dermatol* 1990;123:725–734.
32. Sluis-Cremer GK, Hessel PA, Hnizdo E, Churchill AR. Relationship between silicosis and rheumatoid arthritis. *Thorax* 1986;41:596–601.
33. Steenland NK, Thun MJ, Ferguson CW, Port FK. Occupational and other exposures associated with male end-stage renal disease: a case control study. *Am J Public Health* 1990;80:153–159.
34. International Agency for Research on Cancer. Silica and some silicates. *IARC Monograph Carcinog Risk Hum* 1987;42:39–143.
35. International Agency for Research on Cancer. Silica, some silicates, coal dust and para-aramid fibrils. 1997;68:41–242.
36. Weill H, McDonald JC. Exposure to crystalline silica and risk of lung cancer: the epidemiologic evidence. *Thorax* 1996;51:97–102.
37. Amandus H, Costello J. Silicosis and lung cancer in U.S. metal miners. *Arch Environ Health* 1991;46:82–89.
38. Regulations for maximum permissible exposure levels of silica (quartz, cristobalite, tridymite, and tripoli). *Federal Register* 1989;54:2521–2523.
39. American Conference of Governmental Industrial Hygienists. Documentation of the threshold limit values and biological exposure indices. Cincinnati: American Conference of Governmental Industrial Hygienists, 1991.
40. Wakeman MA, Lockey JE. Other pneumoconioses. In: Rosenstock L, Cullen MR, eds. *Textbook of clinical, occupational and environmental medicine*. Philadelphia: WB Saunders, 1994.
41. Morgan WKC. Silicates and lung disease. In: Morgan WKC, Seaton A, eds. *Occupational lung diseases*, 3rd ed. Philadelphia: WB Saunders, 1995;13:238–307.
42. Morgan WKC. Other pneumoconioses. In: Morgan WKC, Seaton A, eds. *Occupational lung diseases*, 3rd ed. Philadelphia: WB Saunders, 1995.
43. Kelleher P, Pacheco K, Newman LS. Inorganic dust pneumonias: the metal-related parenchymal disorders. *Environ Health Perspect* 2000;108(Suppl 4):685–696.
44. Lison D. Human toxicity of cobalt-containing dust and experimental studies on the mechanism of interstitial lung disease (hard metal disease). *Crit Rev Toxicol* 1996;26:585–616.
45. Ding M, Shi X, Castranova V, Vallyathan V. Predisposing factors in occupational lung cancer: inorganic minerals and chromium. *J Environ Pathol Toxicol Oncol* 2000;19:129–138.
46. Wild P, Perdrix A, Romazini S, Moulin JJ, Pellet F. Lung cancer mortality in a site producing hard metals. *Occup Environ Med* 2000;57:568–573.

CHAPTER 42

Emerging Infectious Diseases

Rodney D. Adam

By the end of the 1960s, there was a great deal of optimism regarding the prospects for control and elimination of many of the common infections. Smallpox was on the verge of elimination. Highly effective vaccines were available for many of the common viral and bacterial infections, such as poliomyelitis, measles, rubella, mumps, tetanus, and diphtheria. Even for many of the important

TABLE 42-1. Newly identified agents of infectious diseases: 1977 to 1996

Date	Etiologic agent	Clinical illness
1977	Ebola virus	Ebola hemorrhagic fever
1977	*Legionella pneumophila*	Legionnaires' disease
1977	Hantaan virus	Hemorrhagic fever with renal syndrome
1977	*Campylobacter jejuni*	Colitis
1977	Hepatitis delta virus	Hepatitis, coinfection with hepatitis B
1978	*Clostridium difficile*	Antibiotic-associated colitis
1978	Astrovirus	Diarrhea
1980	Human T-cell lymphotropic virus-1	T-cell lymphoma—leukemia
1981	*Staphylococcus aureus*	Toxic shock syndrome
1982	Prions	Transmissible neurodegenerative disease
1982	*Escherichia coli* O157:H7	Hemorrhagic colitis; hemolytic uremic syndrome
1982	Human T-cell lymphotropic virus-2	Hairy cell leukemia
1982	*Borrelia burgdorferi*	Lyme disease
1983	Human immunodeficiency virus-1	Acquired immunodeficiency syndrome
1983	*Helicobacter pylori*	Gastritis and gastric and duodenal ulcers
1984	*Haemophilus influenzae aegyptius*	Brazilian purpuric fever
1985	*Enterocytozoon bieneusi*	Diarrhea in acquired immunodeficiency syndrome
1986	*Chlamydia pneumoniae*	Pneumonia, bronchitis, pharyngitis
1986	Human immunodeficiency virus-2	Acquired immunodeficiency syndrome (milder than human immunodeficiency virus-1)
1988	Human herpesvirus 6	Exanthem subitum
1989	*Ehrlichia chaffeensis*	Human monocytic ehrlichiosis
1989	Hepatitis C	Parenterally transmitted non-A, non-B hepatitis
1990	Hepatitis E	Enterically transmitted non-A, non-B hepatitis
1991	*Encephalitozoon hellum*	Keratoconjunctivitis in acquired immunodeficiency syndrome
1991	Guanarito virus	Venezuelan hemorrhagic fever
1992	*Rickettsia felis*	Murine typhuslike illness
1992	*Rickettsia japonica*	Rickettsial spotted fever
1992	*Tropheryma whippleii*	Whipple's disease
1992	*Vibrio cholerae* O139	New strain of epidemic cholera
1992	*Bartonella* (formerly *Rochalimaea*) *henselae*	Cat-scratch disease; bacillary angiomatosis
1993	*Septata intestinalis*	Diarrhea in acquired immunodeficiency syndrome
1993	Sin nombre virus	Hantavirus pulmonary syndrome
1993	*Cyclospora cayetanensis*	Diarrhea
1993	*Babesia* species	Febrile illness
1994	Sabia virus	Brazilian hemorrhagic fever
1994	Human herpesvirus-8	Kaposi's sarcoma
1994	*Ehrlichia equi*	Human granulocytic ehrlichiosis
1994	*Rickettsia japonica*	Spotted fever
1994	Human herpesvirus-7	Exanthem subitum, central nervous system disease
1994	Hepatitis F	Hepatitis
1995	Hepatitis G (also GB)	Hepatitis
1996	*Borrelia* species	Relapsing fever
1996	*Metorchis conjunctus*	Abdominal pain and eosinophilia

infections without available vaccines, such as malaria and tuberculosis, the incidence was dropping sharply, and there was considerable optimism regarding the potential for their total elimination. The surgeon general of the United States announced in 1967 that it was time to close the book on infectious diseases (1). A 1976 review that summarized the progress of the first two centuries of the United States in eradicating many of the common infectious diseases was slightly more restrained in its optimism (2). However, the subsequent two decades have yielded a large number of newly identified pathogens (Table 42-1) (3). These include diseases that appear to be truly new [e.g., human immunodeficiency virus (HIV)], diseases thought initially to be new but subsequently recognized to have been in existence for years [e.g., hantavirus pulmonary syndrome (HPS)], and previously known infections for which etiologic agents have been identified. In addition to the newly identified infectious disease agents, a number of other diseases that have reemerged are discussed, along with the reasons for their reemergence (Fig. 42-1). Not only has the variety of infectious agents expanded, but the infectious disease mortality in the United States rose by 58% from 1980 to 1992, and in 1992, infections trailed only cardiovascular disease and malignancies as causes of death (4).

The identification of new pathogenic agents has been accompanied by the discovery that infectious agents are associated with a number of diseases that have not classically been considered infectious. Many malignancies result from chronic infections, including lymphoma and nasopharyngeal carcinoma (Epstein-Barr virus), human T-cell leukemia/lymphoma virus-1 (HTLV-1), liver cancer (hepatitis B and C), cervical carcinoma (human papillomavirus), stomach cancer (*Helicobacter pylori*), and Kaposi's sarcoma [human herpesvirus-8 (HHV-8)]. Coronary atherosclerosis has been associated with *Chlamydia pneumoniae* and cytomegalovirus infections, renal failure (hemolytic-uremic syndrome) with *Escherichia coli* O157:H7, and peptic ulcer disease with *H. pylori* infection. The variety of conditions that have been found to have infectious etiologies is so great that an article was entitled "Are All Diseases Infectious?" (5).

Many of the newly emergent infections (Table 42-2) are seen because of their occurrence in association with the immunocompromised state caused by HIV infection. Infections such as *Pneumocystis carinii* pneumonia and cytomegalovirus retinitis were quite uncommon before the HIV epidemic, but are now commonplace. The opportunistic infections that have emerged primarily because of HIV infection and other forms of immunocompromised status form an extensive topic by themselves. Therefore, only a selected few of the HIV-associated infections are discussed in this chapter.

For the diseases that have been extant for many years and are now making a resurgence, the categorization as *reemergent* is somewhat arbitrary and may depend on the bias of the author. In this chapter, the general principles and reasons for changes in disease prevalence are discussed, and a few of the more dramatic examples of reemergent infections are examined in greater detail.

CATEGORIES OF EMERGING DISEASES

New Infections

Despite all the infections for which etiologic agents have been identified since 1976, it is likely that the only truly new pathogen is HIV. Although the exact timing and location of origin remain controversial, it appears likely that HIV originated in central Africa in the last half of the twentieth century and shares ancestry with simian immunodeficiency virus. Thus, the best guess at this time is that HIV originated from a monkey or ape virus that developed mutations, allowing its adaptation to the human host. The observation of a truly new infection of the magnitude of HIV has revealed new insights into epidemiologic patterns, and has demonstrated the complex interplay of human behavioral and social factors in the spread of the infection. The epidemic in equatorial

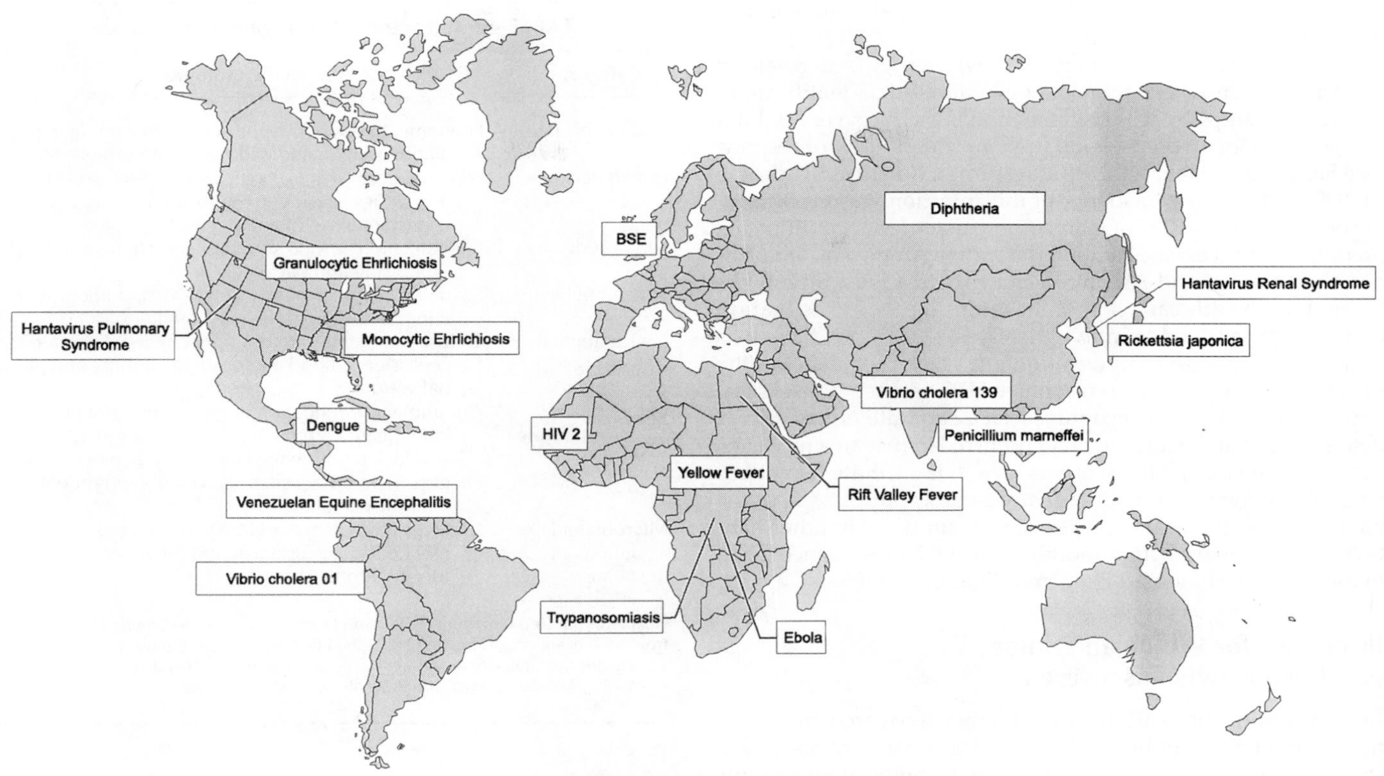

Figure 42-1. Geographic locations of selected emerging infections. BSE, bovine spongiform encephalopathy; HIV, human immunodeficiency virus.

Africa has spread predominantly as a result of heterosexual transmission of the infection within local population groups. In contrast, the epidemic in the United States and western Europe began predominantly as an infection of male homosexuals and was followed rapidly by its spread among parenteral drug users, with relatively limited spread into the remainder of the population. The spread of the epidemic in other areas has been facilitated by female prostitution. For example, in India, the proliferation of the HIV epidemic has followed the major truck routes, with truck drivers acquiring the infection via their contact with prostitutes, followed by transmission to prostitutes in other communities as well as transmission within the communities in which they live (6).

Newly Recognized Infections

A number of reasons exist to explain why some diseases that have been in existence for decades or longer may have evaded recognition until something happened to allow their detection. The most common reason is that clinical overlap with a more common disease prevents the identification of a disease as a distinct entity. Detection of the disease in question may then result when improved diagnostic testing allows better discrimination among disease entities. For example, the identification of hepatitis B surface antigen in 1973 quickly resulted in the discovery that some cases of transfusion-related hepatitis must have resulted from another agent, and eventually led to the discovery of hepatitis C in 1989. Similarly, the identification of hepatitis A allowed the discovery of hepatitis E as another cause of enterically transmitted (infectious) hepatitis. Sequence analysis of the small subunit (16S) ribosomal RNA of pathogenic agents has sometimes resulted in the discovery of distinct species of genera that were already known to cause human infection (7). These new agents include a new species of *Borrelia*, which causes relapsing fever in Spain (8), and spe-

TABLE 42-2. Selected reemergent infections

	Breakdown in public health	Change in organism (drug resistance, virulent clone)	Change in human host	Change in ecology of insect or animal vectors
Streptococcus pyogenes	—	×	—	—
Tuberculosis	×	×	×	—
Malaria	×	×	—	—
Yellow fever	×	—	—	—
Hantavirus pulmonary syndrome	—	—	—	×
African trypanosomiasis	×	—	—	—
Bovine spongiform encephalopathy	—	—	×	—
Lyme disease	—	—	×	×
Human immunodeficiency virus	—	—	×	—

cies of *Babesia*, newly identified as human pathogens in the western United States (9–11).

Alternatively, a disease may be newly recognized when its incidence increases to a frequency that allows its identification. A notable example of this phenomenon is the discovery of HPS in 1993. This infection presents with a sudden onset of respiratory failure associated with adult respiratory distress syndrome (ARDS). Thus, a low incidence of this infection was masked by the occurrence of ARDS of many other etiologies. In addition, its predominant occurrence among the Native Americans of northern New Mexico and Arizona was in an area with little high-technology health care, sometimes limiting the investigation that could be applied to individual cases. Only when there was a change in the ecosystem resulting in a greater incidence of the infection was it possible to recognize HPS as a separate clinical entity. After HPS was recognized as a separate entity, it was determined that the infection had occurred in that area for years, as well as outside the four corners area. It is a tribute to modern technology that the etiologic agent was promptly classified as a hantavirus on the basis of its serologic similarity to other hantaviruses, followed within months by sufficient sequence information to allow epidemiologic investigation of HPS.

Infections for Which an Etiology Has Been Newly Discovered

In addition to the truly new or newly discovered infection, numerous clinical entities that have characteristics suggestive of infectious diseases exist, but for which the etiologic agents remain unknown. For example, the epidemic occurrence of cases of Kawasaki syndrome suggests an infectious etiology, but no etiologic agent has yet been identified. Certain cases of chronic fatigue syndrome have occurred in epidemic fashion, suggesting an infectious etiology, but no infectious agent has been convincingly associated with this syndrome. The 1990s have been marked by the association of infectious agents with some diseases that have long been assumed to be infectious in nature as well as some diseases that were assumed to be noninfectious. For example, cat-scratch disease (CSD) has been assumed to be an infectious disease for decades, but it was not until 1992 that the etiologic agent was first cultured. It was initially called *Rochalimaea*, but later classified as a *Bartonella* on the basis of the sequence of the small subunit ribosomal RNA. Similarly, the agent of Whipple's disease has never been cultured *in vitro*, but the use of the polymerase chain reaction allowed its identification in 1991 (12) and its classification in 1992 as *Tropheryma whippleii*, an actinomycete (13).

REEMERGING DISEASES

Many infectious diseases are characterized by epidemic occurrence with substantial variation in incidence over months, years, or decades. Seasonality occurs when the variation is annual and is found in infections caused by influenza, enteroviral infections, malaria, tick-borne infections, and numerous others. Other infections cycle at longer, less-predictable intervals, such as cholera and measles. In general, the reasons for the periodicity of these infections is not well understood, but may be partially because of the degree of immunity within populations.

With the dramatic reduction in certain infectious diseases during the last half of the twentieth century because of improved living conditions, public health measures, immunization, and the use of antibiotics, it is sometimes difficult to determine whether a decreased incidence of any particular infection is because of these human-induced changes or is simply because of periodicity for a given infection. The reemergence of a number of infections has yielded insight into the answers for some of these questions.

TABLE 42-3. Factors in emergence of diseases

Categories	Specific examples
Societal events	Economic impoverishment, war or civil conflict, population growth and migration, and urban decay
Health care	New medical devices, organ or tissue transplantation, drugs causing immunosuppression, and widespread use of antibiotics
Food production	Globalization of food supplies, and changes in food processing and packaging
Human behavior	Sexual behavior, drug use, travel, diet, outdoor recreation, and use of child care facilities
Environmental changes	Deforestation and reforestation, changes in water ecosystems, flood and drought, famine, and global warming
Public health infrastructure	Curtailment or reduction in prevention programs, inadequate communicable disease surveillance, and lack of trained personnel (i.e., epidemiologists, laboratory scientists, vector- and rodent-control specialists)
Microbial adaptation and change	Changes in virulence and toxin production, development of drug resistance, and microbes as cofactors in chronic diseases

Adapted from Department of Health and Human Services, Centers for Disease Control and Prevention. Addressing emerging infectious disease threats: a prevention strategy for the United States. Atlanta: Department of Health and Human Services, Centers for Disease Control and Prevention, 1994.

Reasons for Emergence or Reemergence of Infections

ECOLOGICAL FACTORS

A number of diverse ecological factors may be important in the emergence or reemergence of a particular disease (Table 42-3). One of the more frequent examples involves changes that result in closer proximity between humans and vectors or animal hosts of zoonotic infections. It is likely that the recognition of Lyme disease in the United States in 1975 occurred because the increased urbanization of the deer population allowed a greater potential for tick-borne transmission to humans. Presumably, this same phenomenon led to the geographic spread of Lyme disease throughout the 1980s.

Climate changes potentially have a variety of effects on infectious disease transmission. Heavy rainfall in the southwestern United States in 1993 after 6 years of drought resulted in a proliferation of the deer mouse, bringing them into closer contact with humans, and led to the outbreak of HPS that was recognized in 1993 (14–16). In sub-Saharan Africa, epidemic transmission of meningococcal meningitis occurs during the dry season (17), whereas in tropical Africa, malaria transmission is the most intense during the rainy season because of the proliferation of the anopheline mosquitoes. The range of the *Aedes aegypti* mosquito, the vector of yellow fever, dengue, and other viral infections, is limited by climate because it does not tolerate freezing temperatures. Other vectors, such as the anopheline mosquitoes that transmit malaria, are found in greater numbers in warm, humid climates. In addition, the *Plasmodium* parasites are limited to temperatures of greater than 16°C, and the incubation period in the mosquito is substantially shortened as the temperature rises to 27°C. During the twentieth century, the earth's mean temperature has risen by 0.5°C. Whether this increase is human-induced remains highly controversial, but regardless of the etiology, continued warming could potentially allow extension of some of these so-called tropical diseases further into the regions that currently have more temperate climates. In the nineteenth and early twentieth centuries, diseases such as dengue and malaria were endemic in the United States, but disappeared, probably because of improvement in living standards. Cases of dengue have appeared in Texas in the setting of epidemic transmission south of the border in Mexico (18), but, in general, cases of dengue remain rare in the United States. The most important determinant for the respect of national borders shown by these infections is the socioeconomic status, with the climate playing a secondary role. Therefore, it is likely that an extension of the range of these diseases has the greatest impact on countries bordering the current endemic areas that have large numbers of people living in lower socioeconomic conditions (19).

Even earthquakes can have an important effect on infectious disease transmission, as demonstrated by a large outbreak of coccidioidomycosis in Ventura County, California, after an earthquake that occurred in 1994 (20). *Coccidioides immitis* is a fungus found in the soil in certain semiarid climates. Normally, the highest incidence is in the lower Sonoran desert of southern Arizona, northern Mexico, and the San Joaquin Valley of California. The earthquake allowed the fungus to be carried by dust clouds into an area that normally has very little coccidioidomycosis.

In some cases, the epidemiology of an infectious disease may change because of the introduction of a vector into a new area. In the 1980s, the *Aedes albopictus* mosquito was introduced into the United States from Japan via water in old tires. This mosquito is capable of transmitting dengue and eastern equine encephalitis (21,22), raising the concern that the epidemiology of these infections in the United States is changing.

MICROBIAL ADAPTATION

Soon after the introduction of penicillin, the first isolates of penicillinase-producing *S. aureus* were identified, and now approximately 95% of *S. aureus* isolates are resistant to penicillin. Isolates of *S. aureus* resistant to the antistaphylococcal penicillins (e.g., methicillin) have spread throughout the world and are frequent in some regions. Other organisms for which drug resistance has become an important problem include *Plasmodium falciparum*, *Plasmodium vivax*, *Mycobacterium tuberculosis*, *Streptococcus pneumoniae*, and *Enterococcus faecium*. In fact, isolates of *E. faecium* that are resistant to all available antimicrobial agents are now common. Drug resistance occurs by a number of mechanisms (23). This includes new enzymes able to degrade antibiotics, typically acquired by plasmids from other organisms, or may occur by stepwise increases in ability to pump the antibiotic out of the bacterial cell. The development of drug resistance may be a frequent event, sometimes occurring during the therapy of a single patient (e.g., *Mycobacterium tuberculosis*), or may be a rare event that occurred only once or very few times worldwide (e.g., *S. aureus* resistance to methicillin, *Plasmodium falciparum* resistance to chloroquine).

Organisms may also acquire new virulence factors by acquisition of the gene from other organisms or by mutation of existing genes. Probable examples of this include toxic shock production by *S. aureus* or *Streptococcus pyogenes*. HIV most likely adapted to humans from another primate host and is even able to adapt to different cell types within an individual human host because of its rapid mutation rate.

HUMAN BEHAVIOR

Throughout the centuries, human behavior has had a major impact on the occurrence of infectious diseases. As Semmelweis pointed out in the 1840s, the failure of physicians to wash their hands after doing autopsies and before their next delivery led to the uncontrolled transmission of the agent of puerperal fever in the obstetrics ward. The plague epidemic of the Middle Ages resulted in part from the crowded substandard living conditions that brought people into close proximity with rats and with each other. In the last half of the twentieth century, the sexual revolution in the United States and elsewhere, with its concomitant increase in numbers of sexual partners, led to increased frequencies of a number of sexually transmitted infections, including *Chlamydia trachomatis*, human papillomavirus, herpes simplex virus, and HIV. Even human diets can play an important role in the transmission of infectious diseases. Enteric and systemic pathogens that are commonly transmitted by food include *E. coli*, *Campylobacter jejuni*, *Shigella* sp., *Salmonella* sp., *Trichinella spiralis*, *Toxoplasma gondii*, *Listeria monocytogenes*, *Brucella* sp., and numerous others. The epidemic of transmissible neurodegenerative disease in the United Kingdom most likely resulted because cows fed on the remains of other cows who had died from bovine spongiform encephalopathy (BSE), resulting in a high prevalence of BSE in cattle; then, people were rarely infected after ingestion of meat from these cattle. Needless to say, the effect on the British cattle industry has been substantial.

BREAKDOWN IN PUBLIC HEALTH

The decreased mortality from infectious diseases in developed nations during the twentieth century has resulted far more from improved hygiene and public health measures than from the use of antimicrobial agents. However, sometimes dramatic reduction in disease frequency leads to disregard and even contempt for infectious agents that have the potential to cause substantial morbidity and mortality. Examples include the substantial increases in frequency and morbidity from pertussis that occurred in Europe and North America when the fear of vaccine side effects resulted in low immunization rates in entire populations. Revolution and war in a number of countries have led to high numbers of refugees living in conditions of poor hygiene, resulting in very high incidences of cholera and other enterically transmitted infections. In Russia, more lax immunization standards have led to a substantial decrease in the immunization rate, allowing a large outbreak of diphtheria in the 1990s. West African trypanosomiasis had been largely controlled by approximately 1960, but political instability, economic hardship, and warfare have substantially impaired the control efforts and led to a marked increase in the number of cases in rural Zaire, and most likely in other surrounding areas. The dismantling of tuberculosis control programs throughout the United States has played an important role in the current resurgence of tuberculosis.

SPECIFIC AGENTS OF DISEASE

Prions

The occurrence of a transmissible neurodegenerative disease called *kuru* was described in 1957 in Papua New Guinea (24). Epidemiologic evidence suggested that it was transmitted by cannibalism. A number of other similar neurodegenerative diseases have been described in humans (e.g., Creutzfeldt-Jakob disease, Gerstmann-Sträussler disease) and animals (e.g., scrapie, mink transmissible encephalopathy). These illnesses were initially considered to be slow virus diseases, but repeated attempts to isolate viral nucleic acid in association with these illnesses have failed, leading to the hypothesis in

1982 of a transmissible protein disease, called *prion* (25). The different forms of the disease now appear to be caused by abnormal structures of the PrP gene that replicates itself by inducing similar structural changes in the normal form of the protein, although the hypothesis remains highly controversial and some still believe that an unidentified virus is responsible for the disease (26).

Creutzfeldt-Jakob disease is the most commonly documented disease of this category in humans. A small portion is familial in nature, whereas most cases are sporadic. The typical age of onset for the sporadic cases is 60 years, but a few have resulted from corneal transplantation or growth hormone administration. In 1996, a new form of transmissible neurodegenerative disease was described in the United Kingdom in which people were affected at much younger ages (mean age, 29 years) than Creutzfeldt-Jakob disease, and the clinical presentation was significantly different (27). The epidemiologic evidence has suggested a link to ingestion of meat from cattle with BSE or mad cow disease, resulting in a major controversy in the United Kingdom as well as the remainder of Europe (28).

VIRUSES

Human Retroviruses

A 1980 review of RNA tumor viruses (retroviruses) concluded, "Retroviruses endemic to human populations have not been identified. (29)" However, the extensive basic retroviral research that had been done in the 1980s laid the foundation for the subsequent identification of the first human retrovirus to be identified. Ironically, it was the very same year that the first report of a human retroviral cause of cancer was published (HTLV-1) (30). The following year, the first clinical reports of acquired immunodeficiency syndrome (AIDS) were published (31,32), followed by an unprecedented international effort that resulted in the description of the etiologic agent 2 years later (33–35). In 1986, a form of HIV distinct enough to be considered a separate virus (HIV-2) was described (36).

Hemorrhagic Fever

Viral hemorrhagic fever may be caused by a variety of agents, including yellow fever, Ebola virus, Marburg virus, Lassa fever virus, and numerous others. A variety of agents of hemorrhagic fever have been identified [e.g., Guanarito virus (Venezuelan hemorrhagic fever) (37), Sabia virus (Brazilian hemorrhagic fever) (38)] or have been recognized in increased numbers or new locations (yellow fever, dengue, Ebola virus) during the 1990s. Although dengue typically causes an influenzalike illness, it may also cause hemorrhagic fever.

Hemorrhagic fever is characterized by an abrupt onset of fever, headache, and myalgias followed by bleeding manifestations, including petechiae hemorrhage and ecchymoses. Other systemic complications, including jaundice and central nervous system involvement, may also be seen. When death occurs, it is typically the result of multiorgan failure, including disseminated intravascular coagulation and jaundice. Other manifestations are more characteristic of some, but not all, viruses. For example, abdominal pain, diarrhea, and rash are very common with Ebola virus, but are not typical of the other causes of viral hemorrhagic fever.

The transmission of yellow fever by mosquitoes was documented by Walter Reed in 1900, and a highly effective vaccine was used for large-scale immunization beginning in 1937 (2). Two forms of transmission have been documented: (a) the urban form in which *Aedes aegypti* is the vector and humans provide the major reservoir of infection and (b) the jungle cycle in which a variety of *Aedes* mosquitoes are vectors, nonhuman primates provide the major reservoir, and humans are incidental hosts. Mosquito control programs along with vaccine use have allowed the elimination of yellow fever from North America and a substantial reduction in the number of cases in South America and Africa. The number of cases in Africa has substantially increased, however, with 18,735 cases reported from 1987 to 1991; this number is thought to represent less than 1% of the actual cases (39). Inadequate financial resources for vaccine purchase are probably a major contributor to this outbreak.

Dengue fever is a viral illness transmitted by the *Aedes aegypti* mosquito, and it is characterized by fever, chills, headache, and myalgias. The epidemiology and the frequent rash help to distinguish it from influenza. Less commonly, people develop a hemorrhagic syndrome in association with their infection. Four distinct serotypes of dengue exist, and dengue hemorrhagic fever typically occurs in someone with prior dengue caused by a different serotype, leading to the hypothesis that the immune response plays a key in the pathogenesis of dengue hemorrhagic fever. Although rare in the United States, dengue is common in Central America and the Caribbean islands, and cases have been documented in the border state of Texas (18). Dengue accounted for 7% of all hospitalizations (including 29% of admissions for febrile illnesses) for U.S. military troops during the first 6 weeks of a mission in Haiti in 1994 (40).

Ebola virus was first identified as a cause of epidemic hemorrhagic fever in Zaire and Sudan in 1976 (41,42), with a mortality of 90% for the strain found in Zaire. Then, with the exception of a few cases of a different strain, it was imported into the United States from the Philippines in 1989, and few cases were documented until 1995, when another large epidemic surfaced in Kikwit, Zaire. Although monkeys are susceptible to infection with Ebola virus, the severity of the illness they acquire casts doubt on the likelihood that they are the natural reservoirs for the virus; therefore, the epidemiology of the infection is poorly understood. It is known that person-to-person transmission can occur under conditions of close personal contact, and that medical personnel taking care of infected patients are at risk for acquisition of Ebola infection (43).

Viral hemorrhagic fever should be considered in any patient with a compatible clinical presentation, especially if a history of travel to an endemic area exists. When hemorrhagic fever is suspected, strict respiratory and contact isolation should be instituted, and the Centers for Disease Control and Prevention (or comparable organization for other countries) should be notified immediately.

Hantavirus Pulmonary Syndrome

In 1993, an outbreak of cases of severe respiratory failure in the four corners area of Arizona, New Mexico, Colorado, and Utah was thought initially to be pneumonic plague. It was soon shown that the illness was not plague, and screening of patient sera for reactivity with antigens from a large variety of pathogenic agents led to the discovery of cross-reactivity with the hantaviruses. Previously, other hantaviruses had been identified in the eastern United States but had not been associated with human disease, whereas the hantavirus agent of hemorrhagic fever with renal syndrome (HFRS) had been identified as an important cause of disease in Korea in 1978. Subsequently, it was determined that HPS was caused by a distinct member of the hantavirus family, and the deer mouse was identified as the vector for human infection. Molecular epidemiologic studies showed conclusively that the virus was not new, but had been endemic in the mouse population for years (16). Heavy rainfall in the spring had led to a tenfold increase in the number of deer mice and a consequently greater proximity to humans. Human infection frequently occurred after working in a building that had been contaminated by mouse droppings. After the outbreak in 1993, the incidence of the illness has substantially decreased, but scattered cases of HPS have been identified in the four corners area and in other parts of the United States (14).

Patients with HPS develop a sudden-onset fever and myalgias, followed by cough and dyspnea in several days, with evidence of pulmonary capillary leakage (ARDS) and hypotension (15). The complete blood cell count typically shows an elevated hematocrit, leukocytosis, and thrombocytopenia, and the absence of thrombocytopenia casts doubt on a potential diagnosis of HPS (14). The diagnosis of someone with suspected HPS can be established accurately by the detection of antibodies by enzyme-linked immunosorbent assay or Western blot. The treatment is supportive, and despite intensive care treatment, the mortality is 52% (44). The efficacy of intravenous ribavirin has been demonstrated for Lassa fever and possibly for HFRS. Patients with HPS have been treated with ribavirin, but its efficacy has not yet been demonstrated.

Since the identification of HPS, a number of other hantaviruses from throughout the world have been associated with HPS or HFRS (45) as well as encephalitis (46).

Human Herpesviruses

In 1986, a new virus was isolated from a patient with a lymphoproliferative disorder and was called *human B-lymphotrophic virus* (47), but has subsequently been named human herpesvirus-6 (HHV-6). Exanthem subitum has long been recognized as one of the common childhood viral exanthems, but it was not until 1988 that HHV-6 was identified as the etiologic agent of this infection (48). Patients with exanthem subitum typically present with 3 to 5 days of high fever and no localizing signs or symptoms, followed by the development of a maculopapular rash on the neck and trunk shortly after defervescence. Subsequently, HHV-6 has been found to be a common cause of acute febrile illness without rash in young children, including the frequent occurrence of febrile seizures. It also has been associated more rarely with meningitis and encephalitis, and has been proposed as an agent of disease in bone marrow transplant and other immunocompromised patients (49–51). Like the other herpesviruses, HHV-6 establishes a latent infection, and its role in this latter setting is less clear because of the difficulty in distinguishing between incidental and symptomatic reactivation of the virus.

HHV-7 is a virus that infects most people during early childhood. Its association with human disease is less conclusive, but it has been proposed as a cause of exanthem subitum (52) and of central nervous system disease (53).

The endemic occurrence of Kaposi's sarcoma in several regions of the world and its occurrence in the United States in HIV-infected homosexual men, but not in other HIV-infected patients raised the suspicion that Kaposi's sarcoma was caused in part by an infectious agent. This suspicion was substantiated when DNA from a new human herpesvirus was found in Kaposi's sarcoma lesions (54). This virus was characterized more completely and named HHV-8. Subsequent serologic surveys have yielded epidemiologic confirmation of the association between HHV-8 and Kaposi's sarcoma.

Hepatitis Viruses

Epidemiologically, the agents of viral hepatitis can be divided into two broad categories: (a) those with enteric transmission that are transmitted primarily by the fecal-oral route and (b) those that are transmitted parenterally and sexually. After the identification of the Australia antigen (now called *hepatitis B surface antigen*) of hepatitis B in 1965 and the subsequent identification of hepatitis B as an important cause of transfusion-related hepatitis, it became clear that there were other causes of transfusion-associated hepatitis. After screening of blood for hepatitis B markers (especially hepatitis B surface antigen), transfusion-associated hepatitis B was nearly eliminated. However, the incidence of transfusion-related hepatitis not caused by hepatitis B was as high as 18% in cardiovascular surgery patients (55). This so-called new form of hepatitis was termed *non-A, non-B hepatitis*. The virus could not be grown in culture, but was cloned by producing a large quantity of infectious virus in chimpanzees, followed by construction of a complementary DNA library and screening of this library with serum obtained from a patient with non-A, non-B hepatitis (56).

The identification of hepatitis C was followed rapidly by the development of serologic screening for hepatitis C (57), and application of these tests for diagnostic purposes and for screening of blood intended for transfusion. The currently available serologic tests detect antibodies to hepatitis C in at least 90% of potentially infectious blood donors, leading to a significant decrease in transfusion-associated hepatitis (58). Hepatitis C is also frequently transmitted through the use of contaminated needles by injecting drug users. Unlike hepatitis B, hepatitis C is rarely transmitted sexually in the absence of HIV coinfection. Spread within households also appears to be quite rare. However, a substantial number of cases exists for which a source cannot be identified.

In contrast to hepatitis B, in which approximately 10% of people infected as adults develop chronic infection, the frequency of chronic infection after infection with hepatitis C virus is at least 50% and possibly greater than 80%. Hepatitis C rarely causes fulminant hepatitis, but causes chronic indolent liver damage in many to most of those infected, with progression to chronic liver disease typically occurring in 20 or more years. Data indicate a strong correlation between chronic hepatitis C infection and the subsequent development of hepatocellular carcinoma; in at least some regions, the association of hepatitis C with hepatocellular carcinoma is greater than the association with hepatitis B.

In people with asymptomatic infection, no clear role for treatment exists, but some treatment with interferon-alpha is beneficial for some people with progressive hepatitis C infection. Liver transplantation remains an option for people with endstage hepatitis C liver disease; in fact, hepatitis C is one of the most frequent indications for liver transplantation.

A putative hepatitis F virus has been isolated, but little additional work has yet been published to confirm its association with human disease (59,60). Hepatitis GB was originally associated with acute hepatitis in a Chicago surgeon (61). Serum from the surgeon was used to transmit hepatitis to tamarin monkeys (62), and, in 1995, a viral agent that reacted with that serum was identified (63). Subsequently, a viral isolate called hepatitis G (64) was found to be so similar to one of the three genotypes of hepatitis GB (genotype C) that it is considered to be the same virus. A number of studies have found hepatitis G to be common in the United States and elsewhere, and commonly associated with blood transfusion, but its role as a cause of hepatitis has not yet been confirmed (65,66).

In a story parallel to that of transfusion-associated hepatitis, the identification of hepatitis A in 1973 as the major cause of enterically transmitted (infectious) hepatitis rapidly led to the conclusion that there must be other causes of enterically transmitted hepatitis. In 1983, viral particles were detected by immunoelectron microscopy in fecal samples of patients with enterically transmitted non-A hepatitis, and, subsequently, the virus was cloned in 1990 (67).

Endogenous transmission of hepatitis E has not yet been documented in the United States and is quite uncommon in developed countries. However, the infection has been documented in southern Asia, Africa, and Mexico. Infection frequently occurs through contaminated water, and symptoms typically develop 1 to 2 months after infection, with loss of appetite, nausea, vomiting, and general malaise. Fever and right upper quadrant pain may be present. The frequency of severe disease, including fulminant hepatitis and fatality, is similar or possibly somewhat greater than that of hepatitis A for most individuals. Hepatitis E is particularly severe when acquired in the third trimester of pregnancy, however, leading to a mortality rate of 20% in this setting.

Other Viruses

Other viral infections have shown a major resurgence. Rift Valley fever is caused by a mosquito-borne virus and is found in sub-Saharan Africa. It typically presents as an acute febrile illness and, in some people, causes retinitis, encephalitis, or hemorrhagic fever. After an absence of 12 years from Egypt, a marked increase in cases was seen in 1993, with an estimated 600 to 1,500 cases (68). In 1995, a large outbreak of Venezuelan equine encephalitis began in northwestern Venezuela, resulting in an estimated 13,000 human cases (69,70).

BACTERIA

Escherichia coli OH157:H7

E. coli, which produce a Shiga toxin (STEC), have been associated with hemorrhagic colitis in infected humans. The initial reports of *E. coli*–induced hemorrhagic colitis in 1983 and 1984 were associated with serotype OH157:H7 (71–73), and most subsequent cases and epidemics have been caused by the OH157:H7 serotype. *E. coli* OH157:H7 is a common cause of acute hemorrhagic colitis and is the most common cause of hemolytic uremic syndrome in the United States (74,75). Other serotypes of STEC have been associated with a similar syndrome (76). Most patients with STEC infection have acute abdominal pain with bloody diarrhea (77). Fecal leukocytes are typically absent, but may be found.

After infection, an incubation of 1 to 7 days (typically 3 to 4 days) is followed by the abrupt onset of cramping abdominal pain and diarrhea that becomes bloody within approximately 2 days. Fever is usually low grade or absent. Approximately 10% of patients develop hemolytic uremic syndrome or, less frequently, thrombotic thrombocytopenic purpura approximately 1 week (2 to 14 days) after the onset of the diarrhea (77). Younger children and the elderly are at particularly high risk for the development of hemolytic uremic syndrome. Most of the 3% to 5% of fatalities occur in people with this complication who are at the extremes of age. Of the survivors, approximately 5% have severe permanent sequelae, such as end-stage renal failure.

The diagnosis is established by isolation of the etiologic agent from cultures of fecal specimens. Identification of *E. coli* O157:H7 (or other serotypes) is not a standard part of the routine stool culture in most laboratories, but should be specifically requested in patients with bloody diarrhea or with hemolytic uremic syndrome. The yield is best in the first few days and falls off substantially for fecal specimens submitted after more than 1 week of illness.

No proven benefit exists from antimicrobial therapy; in fact, antimicrobial therapy may actually increase the risk of hemolytic uremic syndrome. The use of antimotility agents has been associated with a greater risk of adverse outcome and should be avoided (78).

Ehrlichiosis

In 1986, the first report of human monocytic ehrlichiosis was published (79). *Ehrlichia canis* was thought to be the etiologic agent initially, based on the morphologic features and immunologic cross-reactivity, but, subsequently, the etiologic agent was determined to be distinct from *E. canis* on the basis of sequence analysis of the 16S ribosomal sequence and was named *Ehrlichia chaffeensis* (80). The initial case of human infection by *E. chaffeensis* was identified when a man with a disease similar to Rocky Mountain spotted fever (RMSF), but without a rash, had inclusions in the leukocytes that looked like microorganisms (79). The primary site of infection for *E. chaffeensis* is the monocyte and tissue macrophage. The infection is most likely transmitted by the *Amblyomma americanum* tick and demonstrates the increased incidence in the summer months seen for other tick-borne infections. The cases of human monocytic ehrlichiosis have most commonly been documented in the southeastern and south central states of the United States, resulting in considerable overlap with the endemic region for RMSF. In fact, the incidence of ehrlichiosis in the southeastern United States is similar to that of RMSF.

People with ehrlichiosis usually have fever, headache, malaise, and myalgias. A minority of patients have gastrointestinal symptoms or rash. Laboratory evaluation typically shows leukopenia, thrombocytopenia, and elevated transferase levels. Monocytic inclusions are nearly diagnostic when found, but are only seen in a small number of cases. The leukopenia and lack of rash may also help to distinguish the illness from RMSF. The illness typically lasts 2 to 3 weeks, and may last longer. Severe illness and fatalities are not unusual. The diagnosis may be suspected on the basis of the clinical illness, especially when a history of tick exposure exists and may be confirmed by serologic testing. The polymerase chain reaction is also very promising (81), but is not yet available commercially. The evidence demonstrates that patients treated with a tetracycline or chloramphenicol have a better outcome (82), despite the observation that chloramphenicol has limited activity in an *in vitro* assay system. When ehrlichiosis is suspected on clinical grounds, treatment should not be delayed for serologic confirmation.

A similar illness has been documented in the upper midwestern states of Minnesota and Wisconsin (83) and in New York (84), but it is one in which morulae may be found in the neutrophils and no inclusions are found in the mononuclear leukocytes. Thus, the illness is called *human granulocytic ehrlichiosis*. As in human monocytic ehrlichiosis, patients have fever, headache, malaise, and myalgias, and typically do not have a rash. Anemia, thrombocytopenia, leukopenia, and elevated transaminase levels are found in most patients. Sequence analysis of the 16S ribosomal RNA of the etiologic agent has indicated that the organism is closely related to *Ehrlichia equi*, and perhaps is part of the same species group. Infected patients develop antibodies to *E. equi*, but not to *E. chaffeensis*. Treatment with doxycycline (and presumably other tetracyclines) appears to be effective.

The *Ehrlichia* sp. not only cause infection as single pathogens, but may also cause coinfection with other tick-borne organisms, such as the agents of Lyme disease or ehrlichiosis (85), potentially confusing the diagnosis of any one of these diseases.

Rickettsia

The first human infection with *Rickettsia felis* was described in 1992 in a patient with an illness similar to murine typhus (86). Although antigenically similar to *Rickettsia typhi*, it is genetically distinct. In Japan, a new rickettsial organism pathogenic to humans, *Rickettsia japonica*, has been identified as a cause of spotted fever (87). In addition, a number of cases of rickettsialpox, caused by *Rickettsia akari*, have been reported from New York City (88). Whether this represents an increase in the number of *R. akari* infections or simply improved recognition is not known.

Chlamydia pneumoniae

In 1986, a report of a new *Chlamydia psittaci* strain, TWAR, described the frequent association of this organism with acute pharyngitis, bronchitis, and "atypical pneumonia" in college students (89). Subsequently, this organism was found to be distinct enough from *C. psittaci* to be classified as a separate species, *C. pneumoniae*. A number of studies from the United States and Canada have identified *C. pneumoniae* as the cause of approximately 6% to 12% of cases of acute pneumonia, in inpatient and outpatient settings. In addition to this frequent occurrence of endemic disease, *C. pneumoniae* has also been associated with epidemic outbreaks of pneumonia. *C. pneumoniae* infection occurs infrequently in children younger than age 5 years, becomes common in older children and young adults, then falls in frequency for older adults. Transmission is human to human; in contrast to *C. psittaci*, zoonotic transmission has not been documented.

The most common clinical illnesses caused by *C. pneumoniae* are bronchitis and pneumonia (90). Low-grade fever and wheezing are common. Frequently, rales and rhonchi are heard on physical examination. The leukocyte count is usually normal, and the chest radiograph typically shows a single subsegmental infiltrate. Severe illness can occur, but most patients have relatively mild illnesses. The illness is relatively prolonged in comparison to other forms of pneumonia, frequently lasting 2 to 3 weeks. Pharyngitis is common in the initial stages of the illness, but is uncommon as the sole manifestation. Sinusitis has also been associated with acute infection, but it is not clear whether this is a primary *C. pneumoniae* sinusitis or a secondary bacterial process.

In addition to its role as a cause of acute respiratory disease, *C. pneumoniae* has also been proposed as a cause of coronary atherosclerosis and has actually been isolated from the coronary artery of a patient with severe atherosclerosis.

Infections with *C. pneumoniae* can be diagnosed by cell culture techniques, by polymerase chain reaction, or by serologic testing. These tests are now available commercially. No controlled trials of treatment have been reported, but erythromycin and the newer macrolides as well as the tetracyclines appear to be effective.

Helicobacter pylori

For years, excessive gastric acid production had been considered the hallmark of duodenal ulcer disease. Then, a 1984 report described the presence of curved bacilli in gastric biopsies of most patients who had chronic gastritis or duodenal or gastric ulcer (91). This bacterium was initially called *Campylobacter pyloridis* because of its morphologic resemblance to *C. jejuni*, but has since been named *Helicobacter pylori* (92,93).

Acute *H. pylori* infection results in approximately 1 week of nausea and upper abdominal pain, followed by the development of chronic inflammatory disease of the stomach or duodenum. More than 90% of cases of duodenal ulceration and 50% to 90% of gastric ulcers, including almost all those not associated with nonsteroidal antiinflammatory drug use or Zollinger-Ellison syndrome, are associated with *H. pylori* infection (92). Gastric malignancies are also associated with *H. pylori* infection, including gastric carcinoma as well as the relatively rare B-cell gastric lymphomas (mucosal-associated lymphoid tumors). Most mucosal-associated lymphoid tumors are associated with *H. pylori* infection, and some have regressed after successful treatment of *H. pylori* infection.

A number of methods are available to establish the diagnosis of infection caused by *H. pylori*. After acute infection, most patients develop immunoglobulin G (IgG) and IgM antibodies to the organism. The IgM response is transient, but IgG antibodies persist during active infection and decline after successful therapy, making antibody testing useful in the diagnosis of *H. pylori* infection as well as for response to therapy. *H. pylori* produces large quantities of urease; therefore, detection of urease production by the organism is useful for diagnostic purposes. After ingestion of radiocarbon-labeled urease, the breath of a patient can be monitored for the radiolabeled carbon. In addition, the organism can be detected in endoscopic specimens by detection of urease, by histologic detection of the organism in biopsy specimens, or by growth of the organism in cultures.

Effective antimicrobial therapy is remarkably effective in resolving the symptoms associated with *H. pylori* infection. Regimens consisting of a single agent are ineffective, however, requiring the use of combination therapy, usually with three agents. The agents used include bismuth subsalicylate, tetracycline, metronidazole, and amoxicillin. In addition, an agent that inhibits gastric acid secretion (H_2 blocker, omeprazole) speeds resolution of the symptoms and may improve the efficacy of antimicrobial therapy.

Bartonellosis

Several human infections are now attributed to agents in the genus *Bartonella*. The initial reports of fever and lymphadenopathy associated with the scratch of a cat were published in the early 1950s, and the clinical entity had been recognized even before then. The etiologic agent remained elusive until 1983, however, when the Warthin-Starry stain was used to demonstrate the presence of bacilli in histologic specimens of lymph nodes obtained from patients with CSD (94). In 1988, *Afipia felis* was proposed as the etiologic agent of CSD, but subsequent research showed that this initial association was incorrect and that the true etiologic agent was *Bartonella henselae* (formerly *Rochalimaea henselae*) (94). The reclassification from *Rochalimaea* to *Bartonella* was done when sequence analysis of the small subunit (16S) ribosomal RNA indicated marked similarity to *Bartonella bacilliformis*, the cause of bartonellosis (i.e., verruga peruana or Carrión's disease), a sandfly-borne disease found in the western Andes, primarily in Peru. In addition to the isolation of *B. henselae* from the lymph nodes of people with CSD, the organism has been isolated from asymptomatic cats and from a cat flea.

CSD is found throughout the world, but appears to be somewhat more prevalent in warm, humid climates. The prevalence of *B. henselae* bacteremia is high in cats of all ages, but is higher in frequency as well as density in kittens. Fleas are efficient vectors for transmission of *B. henselae* from one cat to another, but a role in transmission of the infection from cats to humans has not been clearly documented.

Human infection presents approximately 3 to 10 days after a feline scratch, typically from a newly acquired kitten, with a round, nontender red-brown papule at the sight of the scratch. The papule may last for days to a few weeks and is followed by tender lymph nodes within the lymph drainage pattern of the initial site of infection, which may later become fluctuant.

Other manifestations of *B. henselae* infection in the immunocompetent patient include Parinaud's oculoglandular syndrome, consisting of unilateral conjunctivitis and adenopathy after inoculation of the organism onto the conjunctiva. Encephalopathy and culture-negative endocarditis are other complications.

Disseminated disease may occur in immunocompetent and immunocompromised patients, and is seen most commonly in advanced HIV infection. *B. henselae* infection in patients with AIDS causes bacillary angiomatosis, which consists of numerous skin and subcutaneous vascular nodules. Infection may also involve the visceral organs, especially the liver; this manifestation is called *peliosis hepatis*.

The diagnosis of *B. henselae* infection may be documented by detection of the organism in histologic specimens from infected patients or by detection of antibodies to the infecting agent. Antimicrobial treatment is clearly effective in AIDS patients with bacillary angiomatosis or peliosis hepatis. The most effective agents are erythromycin and the newer macrolides, as well as the tetracyclines. In contrast, no convincing data exist suggesting that antimicrobial therapy has any impact on the natural course of CSD in the immunocompetent patient, although rifampin, ciprofloxacin, gentamicin, and trimethoprim/sulfamethoxazole may be somewhat effective.

Bartonella quintana (formerly *Rochalimaea quintana*) has been documented as the etiology of trench fever, a febrile illness that was notably common in the soldiers involved in trench warfare during World War I (95,96). With the development of new serologic and culture techniques, it has been possible to establish this organism as the etiology of febrile illness in homeless men, culture-negative endocarditis, as well as infection in AIDS patients similar to that caused by *B. henselae*. This organism appears to be transmitted by the body louse. The diagnosis can be established by isolation of the organism from the blood using alterations of available blood culture systems. A wide variety of antimicrobial agents are effective for treatment, including penicillin, tetracyclines, and the macrolides.

Tropheryma whippleii

Whipple's disease is a systemic infection in which the gastrointestinal manifestations tend to predominate. Patients with Whipple's disease, typically middle-aged men, present with diarrhea and weight loss, abdominal pain, and arthralgias. Less commonly, the central nervous system, heart, and other organ systems may be involved. In the early 1980s, bacilli were found in intestinal biopsy specimens, and patients were found to respond to treatment with trimethoprim/sulfamethoxazole and other antibiotics, so the disease was assumed to have an infectious etiology. Then, in 1991 (12) and 1992 (13), the sequence of the small subunit ribosomal RNA was obtained, allowing the classification of the causative agent as an actinomycete, *T. whippleii*.

Streptococcus pyogenes

Streptococcus pyogenes has long been a major cause of human morbidity and mortality. In the 1840s, Oliver Wendell Holmes and, a few years later, Ignaz Semmelweis described the contagious nature of puerperal fever. In the portion of the Viennese hospital in which Semmelweis worked, the maternal mortality was greater than 10% before the introduction of handwashing. The description of the clinical course and epidemiology of puerperal sepsis suggests that *S. pyogenes* was the major cause of puerperal sepsis and, consequently, the major cause of maternal mortality. The introduction of infection control procedures into obstetrics has resulted in a dramatic decline in the occurrence of puerperal sepsis and of *S. pyogenes* as an etiology. Subsequently, however, *S. pyogenes* has been recognized as the cause of rheumatic fever (97), poststreptococcal glomerulonephritis, cellulitis, and other skin and soft-tissue infections.

By the early 1980s, the incidence of rheumatic fever in the United States and other developed countries had declined to a level that prompted a reconsideration of the current treatment of pharyngitis (98–100). In addition, serious invasive disease caused by *S. pyogenes* was rarely seen. In the late 1980s, however, a resurgence of rheumatic fever in Utah (101) and Ohio (102,103) served as a warning that excessive complacency regarding this complication of *S. pyogenes* infection was not warranted. Shortly thereafter, reports of invasive infections caused by *S. pyogenes* in developed countries throughout the world began to appear (104). At least in the United States and Canada, some evidence exists that these invasive streptococcal infections are caused by a single clonal lineage of bacteria that has been widely dispersed over the last few years (105).

Patients with invasive *S. pyogenes* infections most commonly present with necrotizing infections involving the facial and muscular layers of the extremities (necrotizing fasciitis) (101). Bacteremia is common and may be seen in the absence of a soft-tissue focus of infection. A number of clinical features have suggested that toxin production is a key component of the infection, and, indeed, pyrogenic exotoxin A has been isolated from the majority of the bacterial isolates associated with invasive disease (104). Patients have profound systemic illness, including acute renal failure, coagulopathy, liver involvement, and ARDS. Frequently, a desquamative rash of the distal extremities occurs 1 to 2 weeks after the onset of illness, as seen in other toxin-mediated illnesses, such as staphylococcal toxic shock syndrome. The mortality rate is 30%, despite the occurrence of this infection in younger, otherwise healthy patients.

In patients presenting with soft-tissue infections, necrotizing fasciitis is suspected when the patient has a profound systemic illness, especially if renal failure, coagulopathy, or ARDS is present. The degree of edema is more impressive than that seen in routine cellulitis, whereas the degree of local erythema is frequently less, perhaps because the focus of infection is deeper in the necrotizing infection. Hospitalization and prompt medical and surgical therapy are essential. Because of the limited efficacy of penicillin and presumably other cell-wall-active antibiotics in animal models of necrotizing *S. pyogenes* infections, clindamycin in addition to penicillin is frequently recommended for therapy (104). Early surgical debridement is important in attaining a favorable outcome. When uncertainty exists about the nature of the infection, magnetic resonance imaging scanning may be useful in pointing to facial inflammation.

Vibrio cholerae

Cholera is a disease that has been known at least from the early nineteenth century and likely for millennia (106). In the 1840s, it was identified as a waterborne contagious disease, and in 1854, its association with curved bacteria was noted. Over the nineteenth and twentieth centuries, cholera has been characterized by a series of pandemics that began in Asia and subsequently spread throughout the world, each lasting for years to decades. The first began in 1817, whereas the seventh pandemic began in 1961 and is still continuing. *Vibrio cholerae* has been divided into

139 serotypes. The fifth and sixth pandemics were caused by the classic O1 serotype, whereas the seventh has been caused by a different biotype of the O1 serotype, called the *El Tor* biotype. This pandemic reached Peru in 1991 and has subsequently caused a large outbreak in many of the South American countries. Meanwhile, in 1992, a new epidemic of cholera began in eastern India and Bangladesh (107). This outbreak is caused by the newly identified serotype O139, and has been proposed as the eighth pandemic. The United States has been relatively spared from the cholera epidemics, but the number of cases reported from 1992 to 1994 was substantially increased from the previous 27 years (108). Most were acquired in Latin America and most were caused by the O1 serotype. The available parenteral vaccine is limited by an efficacy of approximately 50% and numerous side effects; in addition, it is effective only for the O1 serotype. Therefore, considerable effort has gone into the development of orally administered vaccines for the O1 and the O139 *V. cholerae* serotypes. Vaccines with greater than 80% efficacy have been developed for both serotypes, although they are not yet available for general use.

Cholera is characterized by the sudden onset of profuse watery diarrhea, accompanied by substantial fluid loss and, sometimes, hypovolemic shock. The mainstay of therapy consists of fluid replacement by the oral route when possible or by the parenteral route when necessary. In addition, the course of illness is shortened by appropriate antimicrobial therapy. The most commonly used antibiotic has been tetracycline, but the levels of resistance of *V. cholerae* to tetracycline in some parts of the world are high enough to preclude their routine use. The fluoroquinolones are highly effective, but are too expensive for many of the areas with a high incidence of cholera.

Mycobacterium tuberculosis

Mycobacterium tuberculosis has afflicted the human population for at least a millennium (109) and likely much longer. It is one of the most common causes of infectious morbidity and mortality in the world. It has also been an important disease in the United States, but the annual incidence had dropped from 84,304 in 1953 to 22,201 in 1985, and a seemingly realistic goal of tuberculosis eradication was being entertained (110). From 1985 to 1992, however, the annual number of cases actually increased to 26,673. This increase in tuberculosis cases is almost equally because of increased numbers of cases of tuberculosis in foreign-born and in HIV-infected individuals, whereas most of the increased mortality is caused by coinfection with *M. tuberculosis* and HIV. An increased prevalence of multidrug-resistant tuberculosis has also played an important role in the resurgence of tuberculosis in the United States, especially in HIV-infected patients for whom the efficacy of the second-line drugs is rather poor.

Resistance of *M. tuberculosis* to isoniazid and rifampin [multidrug resistance (MDR)] has been recognized as an important problem in certain regions, and has also played an important role in the resurgence of tuberculosis. The second-line drugs are clearly less effective, requiring a longer duration of therapy, and, even so, a much higher relapse and mortality rate exist in HIV-infected patients (111,112). The HIV epidemic as well as the breakdown in public health measures directed at tuberculosis control had allowed this problem to surface in New York City, and in 1991, the incidence of MDR reached a level of 19% (113). The recognition of MDR was followed by a greatly increased effort at case finding and especially directly observed therapy, an approach that has resulted in a significant decline in the rate of MDR from 19% down to 13% (114), providing a useful example for other cities and communities.

The seriousness of tuberculosis in the United States pales in comparison to the problem in developing countries. Tuberculosis is the most common single infectious cause of mortality in the world, with the bulk of those deaths occurring in developing areas (115), and is the seventh most common cause of death of all causes worldwide (116). Tuberculosis is the most common opportunistic infection in HIV-infected people in many parts of the world; in this setting, it is more difficult to recognize and to treat, and has increased potential for transmission to other individuals. Thus, tuberculosis is currently one of the most important public health problems worldwide.

Enterococcus species

The enterococci are relatively uncommon pathogens in otherwise healthy individuals, but in the hospital, they are a frequent cause of nosocomial infections, such as urinary tract infections, intraabdominal infections, and line-related bacteremias. The enterococci are inherently antibiotic resistant with minimal inhibitory concentrations (MIC) to penicillin that are approximately 100-fold higher than those of most streptococci. The treatment of choice for infections caused by these organisms is penicillin or ampicillin, and because these agents only have bacteriostatic activity for infections by the enterococci, gentamicin (or streptomycin) is also given when bactericidal activity is needed, such as for treatment of endocarditis. Throughout the 1980s, beta-lactam resistance, then aminoglycoside resistance, and, finally, vancomycin resistance developed in the United States, primarily in *E. faecium*. *Enterococcus faecalis* is the most common species to cause human infection, whereas *E. faecium* is the second most common but is more likely to be antibiotic resistant. The vancomycin-resistant enterococci are especially worrisome because no effective therapy exists for these organisms, and also because of concern that this antibiotic resistance may be transmitted to the streptococci or staphylococci. An investigational drug, quinupristin-dalfopristin (Synercid) demonstrates in vitro activity for vancomycin-resistant enterococci, but the rapid development of resistance in vitro (117) and during therapy (118,119) casts doubt on the ultimate role of this drug.

Streptococcus pneumoniae

S. pneumoniae has long been the most common bacterial cause of pneumonia, and is also one of the most common causes of otitis media, sinusitis, and meningitis. Until approximately 1980, *S. pneumoniae* remained exquisitely sensitive to penicillin throughout the world. Then, penicillin resistance of *S. pneumoniae* in Europe in the 1980s was followed in the 1990s by the rapid spread of penicillin-resistant pneumococci in the United States. Most of these isolates demonstrate intermediate resistance to penicillin (MIC 0.1 to 1.0) and can still be treated by high doses of penicillin; but, even these moderately resistant isolates may respond more slowly to therapy. For meningitis caused by these moderately resistant isolates, cefotaxime and ceftriaxone are frequently recommended because they more consistently penetrate the blood-brain barrier than penicillin. The frequency of colonization with *S. pneumoniae*, with at least intermediate resistance to penicillin, is greater than 20% to 30% in children in some regions of the United States (120). The availability of oral agents effective for treatment of otitis media caused by these isolates is quite limited, although clindamycin or high doses of amoxicillin may be effective. A smaller number of isolates are highly resistant to penicillin (MIC is greater than 2.0); vancomycin is the only agent that is consistently effective for these isolates. The proliferation of antibiotic-resistant *S.*

pneumoniae appears, in large part, to be because of the frequent use of oral antibiotics in children (treatment of otitis) and adults (treatment of upper respiratory infections). It is likely that this phenomenon can be resolved only by a marked reduction in the outpatient use of antibiotics.

FUNGI

Of the many fungal species that are known, few are truly pathogenic for immunocompetent human hosts, but many are occasionally pathogenic for the immunocompromised host. Even the fungi that are pathogenic for immunocompetent patients (e.g., *Coccidioides immitis* and *Histoplasma capsulatum*) are more likely to cause severe disease in the immunocompromised host. *C. immitis* and *H. capsulatum* commonly infect immunocompetent hosts in the geographic regions where they are found and are relatively uncommon causes of progressive disease. But, when people with advanced HIV infection acquire these infections, the likelihood of progressive disease is much higher (121).

One fungal organism that was rarely documented as a pathogen before the HIV epidemic is *Penicillium marneffei*. In Thailand and other parts of Southeast Asia, *P. marneffei* is one of the most common opportunistic infections documented in patients with advanced HIV infection (122,123). In a series from northern Thailand, *P. marneffei* infection was documented in 21% of AIDS patients (122). Patients present with fever and weight loss, and the majority have papular skin lesions that resemble molluscum contagiosum. The chest radiograph may show diffuse reticulonodular patterns. The organism may be demonstrated histologically from skin lesions or the bone marrow, and may be cultured from these sites as well as from the blood or sputum. Treatment with amphotericin B or itraconazole is usually effective.

PROTOZOA

A number of protozoan parasites are common etiologies of human intestinal infection and diarrhea (124), including agents such as *Entamoeba histolytica* and *Giardia lamblia*, which have been recognized for many years as intestinal pathogens, as well as organisms recognized as pathogens.

Cryptosporidium parvum was first described as a human pathogen in 1976 (125), but few cases were described until the high incidence of cryptosporidiosis in patients with advanced HIV infection was noted (126,127). *C. parvum* was first described as a pathogen for immunocompetent people in an outbreak of cryptosporidiosis in veterinary students (126). Subsequently, it was described as a common cause of diarrhea in children in day care centers and waterborne outbreaks of disease. National awareness of the importance of cryptosporidial infections was raised when a waterborne outbreak of cryptosporidiosis in Milwaukee affected an estimated 400,000 people (128).

The diarrhea in immunocompetent people usually lasts less than 1 week, but in patients with advanced HIV infection, the diarrhea may be profuse, lasting for months. The organism is not eradicated by antimicrobial therapy, although paromomycin, a nonabsorbed aminoglycoside, may offer transient benefit.

When *Cyclospora* infection was first documented in humans in 1979 in Papua New Guinea, it was thought to represent a new species of *Isospora* because each of the two sporocysts observed in each oocyst was thought to contain four sporozoites (129). Since 1985, organisms 8 to 10 μm in size, which are red with modified acid-fast stains and autofluoresce under UV light, have been reported with increasing frequency from humans worldwide (91,130). They have frequently been described as coccidian-like bodies, cyanobacteriumlike bodies, or blue-green algae. Data obtained from expatriates and tourists visiting Nepal confirmed that these organisms were responsible for diarrheal illness (130,131). In 1993, at the University of Arizona, the organisms were determined to belong to the genus *Cyclospora* when the oocysts were induced to excyst and found to have two sporocysts, each containing two sporozoites (132,133). *Cyclospora* is transmitted via the fecal-oral route and has been implicated as the etiology of a number of water- and foodborne outbreaks of diarrhea (124). Extraintestinal infection has not been documented, and the diarrhea is self-limited although it may last for weeks. Trimethoprim/sulfamethoxazole is effective in the treatment of *Cyclospora* infections (134).

The microsporidia comprise an entire phylum of obligate intracellular protozoan organisms (135,136). At least five genera (*Enterocytozoon*, *Encephalitozoon*, *Septata*, *Pleistophora*, and *Nosema*) as well as other unclassified microsporidia have been associated with human disease (136). They may cause intestinal infection and diarrhea (e.g., *Enterocytozoon*), corneal infection (e.g., *Nosema*), or encephalitis (e.g., *Encephalitozoon*). Some of the microsporidia may cause infection in immunocompetent patients, but most microsporidial infections (other than *Nosema*) occur in patients with advanced HIV infection.

Malaria has been recognized as a disease from biblical times, and has been described by Hippocrates and by Homer. Human malaria is caused by four species (*Plasmodium falciparum*, *Plasmodium vivax*, *Plasmodium ovale*, and *Plasmodium malariae*) and is transmitted by anopheline mosquitoes. Most human fatalities result from *P. falciparum* infection. In the United States, endogenous transmission was not interrupted until the 1940s. Subsequently, a malaria control campaign using mosquito control and malaria treatment strategies resulted in the near eradication of malaria from the Indian subcontinent by the early 1960s. However, initial optimism regarding the control of malaria was followed by insecticide resistance among mosquitoes and drug resistance of *P. falciparum*. Chloroquine resistance has been the most effective antimalarial drug in history and has been used since its development during World War II for the treatment of malaria. By the middle 1980s, however, *P. falciparum* throughout most of the world was resistant to chloroquine. The major exception is *P. falciparum* in Central America and the Caribbean islands (137,138), where it remains susceptible to chloroquine. In 1989, the first report suggesting the possibility of chloroquine resistance in *P. vivax* in the island of Irian Jaya/Papua New Guinea was published (139). Later studies have confirmed the chloroquine resistance, and have indicated that chloroquine resistance in *P. vivax* is such a problem that chloroquine is no longer effective in that area (140). Although mefloquine is still effective for chloroquine-resistant *P. vivax* infection, *P. falciparum* in northeastern Thailand has already become resistant to mefloquine, and the possibility of increasing levels of drug resistance in *P. falciparum* and *P. vivax* is an important concern.

African trypanosomiasis, or African sleeping sickness, is an infection found throughout equatorial Africa. Different subspecies of *Trypanosoma brucei* infect humans and a variety of animals and are transmitted from one host to another by the tsetse fly. The disease has had major implications for human health as well as a major economic impact, because domestic cattle cannot be raised throughout the entire tsetse fly belt. The human forms of the disease are West African and East African trypanosomiasis. East African trypanosomiasis, caused by *Trypanosoma brucei rhodesiense*, is primarily a zoonotic infection and humans are incidental hosts, whereas West African trypanosomiasis, caused by *Trypanosoma brucei gambiense*, is a human infection and nonhuman hosts have not been identified. In the early part of the twentieth century, African trypanosomiasis was the most important public health problem in equatorial Africa and accounted for a reduction in the population of Uganda from 6.5 to 2.5 million people (141). An active control program resulted in a dramatic reduction in the number of cases, however, so that by 1960, the lack of nonhuman reservoirs prompted optimism for the potential of the eradication of West African trypanosomiasis. However, the success of the 1950s was followed by revolutions and warfare in the 1960s and thereafter. This warfare and political instability resulted in a breakdown in the existing public health and disease control programs and a lack of money for the necessary drugs to treat infected people. The prevalence of the infection in portions of Zaire has reached 6% to 10%, and as high as 40% to 70% in some villages. The continued political instability in that region precludes great optimism for control of the infection in the foreseeable future.

Most of the helminths associated with human disease have been recognized for many years because they are easier to locate and identify than the microbial pathogens. Nevertheless, helminths previously not associated with human disease have been identified, such as a syndrome of abdominal pain, low-grade fever, and eosinophilia associated with the North American liver fluke, *Metorchis conjunctus*, after eating raw fish (142).

REFERENCES

1. Butler JC, Kilmarx PH, Jernigan DB, Ostroff SM. Perspectives in fatal epidemics [Review]. *Infect Dis Clin North Am* 1996;10:917–937.
2. Wishnow RM. The conquest of the major infectious diseases in the United States: a bicentennial retrospect [Review]. *Annu Rev Microbiol* 1976;30:427–450.
3. Satcher D. Emerging infections: getting ahead of the curve. *Emerg Infect Dis* 1995;1:1–6.
4. Pinner RW, Teutsch SM, Simonsen L, et al. Trends in infectious diseases mortality in the United States [See comments]. *JAMA* 1996;275:189–193.
5. Lorber B. Are all diseases infectious? [Review]. *Ann Intern Med* 1996;125: 844–851.
6. Bollinger RC, Tripathy SP, Quinn TC. The human immunodeficiency virus epidemic in India: current magnitude and future projections [Review]. *Medicine (Baltimore)* 1995;74:97–106.
7. Fredericks DN, Relman DA. Sequence-based identification of microbial pathogens: a reconsideration of Koch's postulates [Review]. *Clin Microbiol Rev* 1996;9:18–33.
8. Anda P, Sanchez-Yebra W, del Mar Vitutia M, et al. A new *Borrelia* species isolated from patients with relapsing fever in Spain [See comments]. *Lancet* 1996;348:162–165.
9. Persing DH, Herwaldt BL, Glaser C, et al. Infection with a *Babesia*-like organism in northern California. *N Engl J Med* 1995;332:298–303.
10. Thomford JW, Conrad PA, Telford SR III, et al. Cultivation and phylogenetic characterization of a newly recognized human pathogenic protozoan. *J Infect Dis* 1994;169:1050–1056.
11. Quick RE, Herwaldt BL, Thomford JW, et al. Babesiosis in Washington state: a new species of *Babesia*? *Ann Intern Med* 1993;119:284–290.
12. Wilson KH, Blitchington R, Frothingham R, Wilson JA. Phylogeny of the Whipple's-disease-associated bacterium. *Lancet* 1991;338:474–475.
13. Relman DA, Schmidt TM, MacDermott RP, Falkow S. Identification of the uncultured bacillus of Whipple's disease [See comments]. *N Engl J Med* 1992;327:293–301.
14. Simonsen L, Dalton MJ, Breiman RF, et al. Evaluation of the magnitude of the 1993 hantavirus outbreak in the southwestern United States. *J Infect Dis* 1995;172:729–733.
15. Duchin JS, Koster FT, Peters CJ, et al. Hantavirus pulmonary syndrome: a clinical description of 17 patients with a newly recognized disease. The Hantavirus Study Group [See comments]. *N Engl J Med* 1994;330:949–955.
16. Nichol ST, Spiropoulou CF, Morzunov S, et al. Genetic identification of a hantavirus associated with an outbreak of acute respiratory illness [See comments]. *Science* 1993;262:914–917.
17. Patz JA, Epstein PR, Burke TA, Balbus JM. Global climate change and emerging infectious diseases [See comments]. *JAMA* 1996;275:217–223.
18. Anonymous. Dengue fever at the US-Mexico border, 1995–1996. *MMWR Morb Mortal Wkly Rep* 1996;45:841–844.
19. Reiter P. Global warming and mosquito-borne disease in USA [Letter]. *Lancet* 1996;348:622.
20. Schneider E, Hajjeh RA, Spiegel RA, et al. A coccidioidomycosis outbreak following the Northridge, CA, earthquake. *JAMA* 1997;277:904–908.
21. Mitchell CJ, Niebylski ML, Smith GC, et al. Isolation of eastern equine encephalitis virus from *Aedes albopictus* in Florida. *Science* 1992;257:526–527.
22. Francy DB, Moore CG, Eliason DA. Past, present and future of *Aedes albopictus* in the United States [Review]. *J Am Mosq Control Assoc* 1990;6:127–132.
23. Gold HS, Moellering RC Jr. Antimicrobial-drug resistance [Review]. *N Engl J Med* 1996;335:1445–1453.
24. Gajdusek DC, Zigas V. Degenerative disease of the central nervous system in New Guinea: the endemic occurrence of "Kuru" in the native population. *N Engl J Med* 1957;257:974–978.
25. Prusiner SB. Novel proteinaceous infectious particles cause scrapie. *Science* 1982;216:136–144.
26. Mestel R. Putting prions to the test. *Science* 1996;273:184–189.
27. Will RG, Ironside JW, Zeidler M, et al. A new variant of Creutzfeldt-Jakob disease in the UK [See comments]. *Lancet* 1996;347:921–925.
28. Anderson RM, Donnelly CA, Ferguson NM, et al. Transmission dynamics and epidemiology of BSE in British cattle [See comments]. *Nature* 1996;382:779–788.
29. Bishop JM. The molecular biology of RNA tumor viruses: a physician's guide. *N Engl J Med* 1980;303:675–682.
30. Poiesz BJ, Ruscetti FW, Gazdar AF, Bunn PA, Minna JD, Gallo RC. Detection and isolation of type C retrovirus particles from fresh and cultured lymphocytes of a patient with cutaneous T-cell lymphoma. *Proc Natl Acad Sci U S A* 1980;77:7415–7419.
31. Anonymous. *Pneumocystis pneumonia*—Los Angeles. *MMWR Morb Mortal Wkly Rep* 1981;30:250–252.
32. Anonymous. Kaposi's sarcoma and *Pneumocystis pneumonia* among homosexual men—New York City and California. *MMWR Morb Mortal Wkly Rep* 1981;30:305–308.
33. Gelmann EP, Popovic M, Blayney D, et al. Proviral DNA of a retrovirus, human T-cell leukemia virus, in two patients with AIDS. *Science* 1983; 220:862–865.
34. Gallo RC, Sarin PS, Gelmann EP, et al. Isolation of human T-cell leukemia virus in acquired immune deficiency syndrome (AIDS). *Science* 1983; 220:865–867.
35. Barre-Sinoussi F, Chermann JC, Rey F, et al. Isolation of a T-lymphotropic retrovirus from a patient at risk for acquired immune deficiency syndrome (AIDS). *Science* 1983;220:868–871.
36. Kanki PJ, Barin F, M'Boup S, et al. New human T-lymphotropic retrovirus related to simian T-lymphotropic virus type III (STLV-IIIAGM). *Science* 1986;232:238–243.
37. Salas R, de Manzione N, Tesh RB, et al. Venezuelan haemorrhagic fever. *Lancet* 1991;338:1033–1036.
38. Lisieux T, Coimbra M, Nassar ES, et al. New arenavirus isolated in Brazil. *Lancet* 1994;343:391–392.
39. Robertson SE, Hull BP, Tomori O, Bele O, LeDuc JW, Esteves K. Yellow fever: a decade of reemergence [Review]. *JAMA* 1996;276:1157–1162.
40. Anonymous. Dengue fever among US military personnel—Haiti, September-November, 1994. *MMWR Morb Mortal Wkly Rep* 1994;43:845–848.
41. Anonymous. Ebola haemorrhagic fever in Zaire, 1976. *Bull World Health Organ* 1978;56:271–293.
42. Bres P. The epidemic of Ebola haemorrhagic fever in Sudan and Zaire, 1976. Introductory note. *Bull World Health Organ* 1978;56:245.
43. Baron RC, McCormick JB, Zubeir OA. Ebola virus disease in southern Sudan: hospital dissemination and intrafamilial spread. *Bull World Health Organ* 1983;61:997–1003.
44. Khan AS, Khabbaz RF, Armstrong LR, et al. Hantavirus pulmonary syndrome: the first 100 US cases. *J Infect Dis* 1996;173:1297–1303.
45. Schmalijohn C, Hjelle B. Hantaviruses: a global disease problem. *Emerg Infect Dis* 1997;3:95–104.
46. Sexton DJ, Rollin PE, Breitschwerdt EB, et al. Life-threatening Cache Valley virus infection. *N Engl J Med* 1997;336:547–549.
47. Josephs SF, Salahuddin SZ, Ablashi DV, Schachter F, Wong-Staal F, Gallo RC. Genomic analysis of the human B-lymphotropic virus (HBLV). *Science* 1986;234:601–603.
48. Yamanishi K, Okuno T, Shiraki K, et al. Identification of human herpesvirus-6 as a causal agent for exanthem subitum [See comments]. *Lancet* 1988; 1:1065–1067.
49. Singh N, Carrigan DR. Human herpesvirus-6 in transplantation: an emerging pathogen [Review]. *Ann Intern Med* 1996;124:1065–1071.
50. LaRocco MT, Burgert SJ. Infection in the bone marrow transplant recipient and role of the microbiology laboratory in clinical transplantation. *Clin Microbiol Rev* 1997;10:277–297.
51. Levy JA. Three new human herpesviruses (HHV6, 7, and 8). *Lancet* 1997; 349:558–563.
52. Tanaka K, Kondo T, Torigoe S, Okada S, Mukai T, Yamanishi K. Human herpesvirus 7: another causal agent for roseola (exanthem subitum). *J Pediatr* 1994;125:1–5.
53. Torigoe S, Koide W, Yamada M, Miyashiro E, Tanaka-Taya K, Yamanishi K. Human herpesvirus 7 infection associated with central nervous system manifestations. *J Pediatr* 1996;129:301–305.
54. Chang Y, Cesarman E, Pessin MS, et al. Identification of herpesvirus-like DNA sequences in AIDS-associated Kaposi's sarcoma [See comments]. *Science* 1994;266:1865–1869.

55. Prince AM, Brotman B, Grady GF, et al. Long-incubation post-transfusion hepatitis without serological evidence of exposure to hepatitis-B virus. *Lancet* 1974;2:241–246.
56. Choo QL, Kuo G, Weiner AJ, Overby LR, Bradley DW, Houghton M. Isolation of a cDNA clone derived from a blood-borne non-A, non-B viral hepatitis genome. *Science* 1989;244:359–362.
57. Kuo G, Choo QL, Alter HJ, et al. An assay for circulating antibodies to a major etiologic virus of human non-A, non-B hepatitis. *Science* 1989;244:362–364.
58. Cuthbert JA. Hepatitis C: progress and problems [Review]. *Clin Microbiol Rev* 1994;7:505–532.
59. Deka N, Sharma MD, Mukerjee R. Isolation of the novel agent from human stool samples that is associated with sporadic non-A, non-B hepatitis. *J Virol* 1994;68:7810–7815.
60. Bowden DS, Moaven LD, Locarnini SA. New hepatitis viruses: are there enough letters in the alphabet? [Review]. *Med J Aust* 1996;164:87–89.
61. Schlauder GG, Pilot-Matias TJ, Gabriel GS, et al. Origin of GB-hepatitis viruses [Letter]. *Lancet* 1995;346:447–448.
62. Deinhardt F, Holmes AW, Capps RB, Popper H. Studies on the transmission of human viral hepatitis to marmoset monkeys. I. Transmission of disease, serial passages, and description of liver lesions. *J Exp Med* 1967;125:673–688.
63. Simons JN, Pilot-Matias TJ, Leary TP, et al. Identification of two flavivirus-like genomes in the GB hepatitis agent. *Proc Natl Acad Sci U S A* 1995;92:3401–3405.
64. Linnen J, Wages J Jr, Zhang-Keck ZY, et al. Molecular cloning and disease association of hepatitis G virus: a transfusion-transmissible agent. *Science* 1996;271:505–508.
65. Alter MJ, Gallagher M, Morris TT, et al. Acute non-A-E hepatitis in the United States and the role of hepatitis G virus infection. Sentinel Counties Viral Hepatitis Study Team [See comments]. *N Engl J Med* 1997;336:741–746.
66. Alter HJ, Nakatsuji Y, Melpolder J, et al. The incidence of transfusion-associated hepatitis G virus infection and its relation to liver disease [See comments]. *N Engl J Med* 1997;336:747–754.
67. Reyes GR, Purdy MA, Kim JP, et al. Isolation of a cDNA from the virus responsible for enterically transmitted non-A, non-B hepatitis. *Science* 1990;247:1335–1339.
68. Arthur RR, el-Sharkawy MS, Cope SE, et al. Recurrence of Rift Valley fever in Egypt. *Lancet* 1993;342:1149–1150.
69. Anonymous. Venezuelan equine encephalitis—Colombia, 1995. *MMWR Morb Mortal Wkly Rep* 1995;44:721–724.
70. Rico-Hesse R, Weaver SC, de Siger J, Medina G, Salas RA. Emergence of a new epidemic/epizootic Venezuelan equine encephalitis virus in South America. *Proc Natl Acad Sci U S A* 1995;92:5278–5281.
71. Remis RS, MacDonald KL, Riley LW, et al. Sporadic cases of hemorrhagic colitis associated with *Escherichia coli* O157:H7. *Ann Intern Med* 1984; 101:624–626.
72. Pai CH, Gordon R, Sims HV, Bryan LE. Sporadic cases of hemorrhagic colitis associated with *Escherichia coli* O157:H7. Clinical, epidemiologic, and bacteriologic features. *Ann Intern Med* 1984;101:738–742.
73. Riley LW, Remis RS, Helgerson SD, et al. Hemorrhagic colitis associated with a rare *Escherichia coli* serotype. *N Engl J Med* 1983;308:681–685.
74. Tarr PI, Neill MA, Allen J, Siccardi CJ, Watkins SL, Hickman RO. The increasing incidence of the hemolytic-uremic syndrome in King County, Washington: lack of evidence for ascertainment bias. *Am J Epidemiol* 1989;129:582–586.
75. Martin DL, MacDonald KL, White KE, Soler JT, Osterholm MT. The epidemiology and clinical aspects of the hemolytic uremic syndrome in Minnesota [See comments]. *N Engl J Med* 1990;323:1161–1167.
76. Acheson DWK, Keusch GT. Editorial response: Shiga toxin-producing *Escherichia coli* serotype OX3:H21 as a cause of hemolytic-uremic syndrome. *Clin Infect Dis* 1997;24:1280–1282.
77. Boyce TG, Swerdlow DL, Griffin PM. *Escherichia coli* O157:H7 and the hemolytic-uremic syndrome [See comments]. [Review]. *N Engl J Med* 1995;333:364–368.
78. Cimolai N, Carter JE, Morrison BJ, Anderson JD. Risk factors for the progression of *Escherichia coli* O157:H7 enteritis to hemolytic-uremic syndrome [See comments]. *J Pediatr* 1990;116:589–592. [Published erratum appears in *J Pediatr* 1990 Jun;116(6):1008].
79. Maeda K, Markowitz N, Hawley RC, Ristic M, Cox D, McDade JE. Human infection with *Ehrlichia canis*, a leukocytic rickettsia. *N Engl J Med* 1987;316:853–856.
80. Anderson BE, Dawson JE, Jones DC, Wilson KH. *Ehrlichia chaffeensis*, a new species associated with human ehrlichiosis. *J Clin Microbiol* 1991;29:2838–2842.
81. Everett ED, Evans KA, Henry RB, McDonald G. Human ehrlichiosis in adults after tick exposure: diagnosis using polymerase chain reaction. *Ann Intern Med* 1994;120:730–735.
82. Dawson JE, Warner CK, Standaert S, Olson JG. The interface between research and the diagnosis of an emerging tick-borne disease, human ehrlichiosis due to *Ehrlichia chaffeensis* [See comments]. [Review]. *Arch Intern Med* 1996;156:137–142.
83. Bakken JS, Dumler JS, Chen SM, Eckman MR, Van Etta LL, Walker DH. Human granulocytic ehrlichiosis in the upper Midwest United States: a new species emerging? [See comments]. *JAMA* 1994;272:212–218.
84. Aguero-Rosenfeld ME, Horowitz HW, Wormser GP, et al. Human granulocytic ehrlichiosis: a case series from a medical center in New York state. *Ann Intern Med* 1996;125:904–908.
85. Mitchell PD, Reed KD, Hofkes JM. Immunoserologic evidence of coinfection with *Borrelia burgdorferi*, *Babesia microti*, and human granulocytic *Ehrlichia* species in residents of Wisconsin and Minnesota. *J Clin Microbiol* 1996;34:724–727.
86. Walker DH, Barbour AG, Oliver JH, et al. Emerging bacterial zoonotic and vector-borne diseases. Ecological and epidemiological factors [Review]. *JAMA* 1996;275:463–469.
87. Uchida T, Uchiyama T, Kumano K, Walker DH. *Rickettsia japonica* sp. nov., the etiological agent of spotted fever group rickettsiosis in Japan. *Int J Syst Bacteriol* 1992;42:303–305.
88. Kass EM, Szaniawski WK, Levy H, Leach J, Srinivasan K, Rives C. Rickettsialpox in a New York City hospital, 1980 to 1989 [See comments]. *N Engl J Med* 1994;331:1612–1617.
89. Grayston JT, Kuo CC, Wang SP, Altman J. A new *Chlamydia psittaci* strain, TWAR, isolated in acute respiratory tract infections. *N Engl J Med* 1986;315:161–168.
90. Kuo CC, Jackson LA, Campbell LA, Grayston JT. *Chlamydia pneumoniae* (TWAR) [Review]. *Clin Microbiol Rev* 1995;8:451–461.
91. Marshall BJ, Warren JR. Unidentified curved bacilli in the stomach of patients with gastritis and peptic ulceration. *Lancet* 1984;1:1311–1315.
92. Blaser MJ. *Helicobacter pylori* and the pathogenesis of gastroduodenal inflammation [Review]. *J Infect Dis* 1990;161:626–633.
93. Goodwin CS, Mendall MM, Northfield TC. *Helicobacter pylori* infection. [Review]. *Lancet* 1997;349:265–269.
94. Bass JW, Vincent JM, Person DA. The expanding spectrum of *Bartonella* infections. II. Cat-scratch disease [Review]. *Pediatr Infect Dis J* 1997;16:163–179.
95. Bass JW, Vincent JM, Person DA. The expanding spectrum of *Bartonella* infections: I. Bartonellosis and trench fever [Review]. *Pediatr Infect Dis J* 1997;16:2–10.
96. Maurin M, Raoult D. *Bartonella (Rochalimaea) quintana* infections [Review]. *Clin Microbiol Rev* 1996;9:273–292.
97. Stollerman GH. Rheumatic fever. *Lancet* 1997;349:935–942.
98. Gerber MA, Markowitz M. Management of *Streptococcal pharyngitis* reconsidered [Review]. *Pediatr Infect Dis* 1985;4:518–526.
99. Anonymous. Decline in rheumatic fever [Editorial]. *Lancet* 1985;2:647–648.
100. Shulman ST. The decline of rheumatic fever: what impact on our management of pharyngitis? [Editorial]. *Am J Dis Child* 1984;138:426–427.
101. Veasy LG, Wiedmeier SE, Orsmond GS, et al. Resurgence of acute rheumatic fever in the intermountain area of the United States. *N Engl J Med* 1987;316:421–427.
102. Hosier DM, Craenen JM, Teske DW, Wheller JJ. Resurgence of acute rheumatic fever. *Am J Dis Child* 1987;141:730–733.
103. Congeni B, Rizzo C, Congeni J, Sreenivasan VV. Outbreak of acute rheumatic fever in northeast Ohio. *J Pediatr* 1987;111:176–179.
104. Stevens DL, Tanner MH, Winship J, et al. Severe group A streptococcal infections associated with a toxic shock-like syndrome and scarlet fever toxin A [See comments]. *N Engl J Med* 1989;321:1–7.
105. Cleary PP, Kaplan EL, Handley JP, et al. Clonal basis for resurgence of serious *Streptococcus pyogenes* disease in the 1980s. *Lancet* 1992;339:518–521.
106. Kaper JB, Morris JG, Jr., Levine MM. Cholera [Review]. *Clin Microbiol Rev* 1995;8:48-86. [Published erratum appears in *Clin Microbiol Rev* 1995 Apr;8(2):316].
107. Anonymous. Large epidemic of cholera-like disease in Bangladesh caused by *Vibrio cholerae* O139 synonym Bengal. Cholera Working Group, International Centre for Diarrhoeal Diseases Research, Bangladesh [See comments]. *Lancet* 1993;342:387–390.
108. Mahon BE, Mintz ED, Greene KD, Wells JG, Tauxe RV. Reported cholera in the United States, 1992–1994: a reflection of global changes in cholera epidemiology. *JAMA* 1996;276:307–312.
109. Salo WL, Aufderheide AC, Buikstra J, Holcomb TA. Identification of *Mycobacterium tuberculosis* DNA in a pre-Columbian Peruvian mummy. *Proc Natl Acad Sci U S A* 1994;91:2091–2094.
110. Cantwell MF, Snider DE Jr, Cauthen GM, Onorato IM. Epidemiology of tuberculosis in the United States, 1985 through 1992 [See comments]. *JAMA* 1994;272:535–539.
111. Iseman MD. Treatment of multidrug-resistant tuberculosis [Review]. *N Engl J Med* 1993;329:784-791. [Published erratum appears in *N Engl J Med* 1993 Nov 4;329(19):1435].
112. Sepkowitz KA, Raffalli J, Riley L, Kiehn TE, Armstrong D. Tuberculosis in the AIDS era [Review]. *Clin Microbiol Rev* 1995;8:180–199.
113. Frieden TR, Sterling T, Pablos-Mendez A, Kilburn JO, Cauthen GM, Dooley SW. The emergence of drug-resistant tuberculosis in New York City [See comments]. *N Engl J Med* 1993;328:521–526. [Published erratum appears in *N Engl J Med* 1993 Jul 8;329(2):148].
114. Fujiwara PI, Cook SV, Rutherford CM, et al. A continuing survey of drug-resistant tuberculosis: New York City, April 1994. *Arch Intern Med* 1997;157:531–536.
115. Raviglione MC, Snider DE Jr., Kochi A. Global epidemiology of tuberculosis: morbidity and mortality of a worldwide epidemic [See comments]. *JAMA* 1995;273:220–226.
116. Murray CJL, Lopez AD. Mortality by cause for eight regions of the world: global burden of disease study. *Lancet* 1997;349:1269–1276.
117. Millichap J, Ristow TA, Noskin GA, Peterson LR. Selection of *Enterococcus faecium* strains with stable and unstable resistance to the streptogramin RP 59500 using stepwise in vitro exposure. *Diagn Microbiol Infect Dis* 1996;25:15–20.

118. Chow JW, Donahedian SM, Zervos MJ. Emergence of increased resistance to quinupristin/dalfopristin during therapy for *Enterococcus faecium* bacteremia. *Clin Infect Dis* 1997;24:90–91.
119. Chow JW, Davidson A, Sanford E III, Zervos MJ. Superinfection with *Enterococcus faecalis* during quinupristin/dalfopristin therapy. *Clin Infect Dis* 1997;24:91–92.
120. Anonymous. Drug-resistant *Streptococcus pneumoniae*—Kentucky and Tennessee, 1993. *MMWR Morb Mortal Wkly Rep* 1994;43:23–26.
121. Wheat J. Endemic mycoses in AIDS: a clinical review [Review]. *Clin Microbiol Rev* 1995;8:146–159.
122. Chariyalertsak S, Sirisanthana T, Supparatpinyo K, Nelson KE. Seasonal variation of disseminated *Penicillium marneffei* infections in northern Thailand: a clue to the reservoir? *J Infect Dis* 1996;173:1490–1493.
123. Duong TA. Infection due to *Penicillium marneffei*, an emerging pathogen: review of 155 reported cases [Review]. *Clin Infect Dis* 1996;23:125–130.
124. Marshall MM, Naumovitz D, Ortega Y, Sterling CR. Waterborne protozoan pathogens [Review]. *Clin Microbiol Rev* 1997;10:67–85.
125. Nime FA, Burek JD, Page DL, Holscher MA, Yardley JH. Acute enterocolitis in a human being infected with the protozoan *Cryptosporidium*. *Gastroenterology* 1976;70:592–598.
126. Current WL, Reese NC, Ernst JV, Bailey WS, Heyman MB, Weinstein WM. Human cryptosporidiosis in immunocompetent and immunodeficient persons. Studies of an outbreak and experimental transmission. *N Engl J Med* 1983;308:1252–1257.
127. Pitlik SD, Fainstein V, Garza D, et al. Human cryptosporidiosis: spectrum of disease. Report of six cases and review of the literature. *Arch Intern Med* 1983;143:2269–2275.
128. Mac Kenzie WR, Hoxie NJ, Proctor ME, et al. A massive outbreak in Milwaukee of *Cryptosporidium* infection transmitted through the public water supply [See comments]. *N Engl J Med* 1994;331:161–167. [Published erratum appears in *N Engl J Med* 1994 Oct 13;331(15):1035].
129. Ashford RW. Occurrence of an undescribed coccidian in man in Papua New Guinea. *Ann Trop Med Parasitol* 1979;73:497–500.
130. Hoge CW, Shlim DR, Rajah R, et al. Epidemiology of diarrhoeal illness associated with coccidian-like organism among travelers and foreign residents in Nepal. *Lancet* 1993;341:1175–1179.
131. Shlim DR, Cohen MT, Eaton M, Rajah R, Long EG, Ungar BL. An alga-like organism associated with an outbreak of prolonged diarrhea among foreigners in Nepal. *Am J Trop Med Hyg* 1991;45:383–389.
132. Ortega YR, Sterling CR, Gilman RH, Cama VA, Diaz F. *Cyclospora* species—a new protozoan pathogen of humans [See comments]. *N Engl J Med* 1993;328:1308–1312.
133. Ortega YR, Gilman RH, Sterling CR. A new coccidian parasite (*Apicomplexa: Eimeriidae*) from humans. *J Parasitol* 1994;80:625–629.
134. Hoge CW, Shlim DR, Ghimire M, et al. Placebo-controlled trial of co-trimoxazole for *Cyclospora* infections among travelers and foreign residents in Nepal [See comments]. *Lancet* 1995;345:691–693. [Published erratum appears in *Lancet* 1995 Apr 22; 345(8956):1060].
135. Weber R, Bryan RT. Microsporidial infections in immunodeficient and immunocompetent patients. *Clin Infect Dis* 1994;19:517–521.
136. Weber R, Bryan RT, Schwartz DA, Owen RL. Human microsporidial infections [Review]. *Clin Microbiol Rev* 1994;7:426–461.
137. Wyler DJ. Malaria chemoprophylaxis for the traveler [Review]. *N Engl J Med* 1993;329:31–37.
138. Wyler DJ. Malaria: overview and update [Review]. *Clin Infect Dis* 1993; 16:449–456.
139. Rieckmann KH, Davis DR, Hutton DC. *Plasmodium vivax* resistance to chloroquine? *Lancet* 1989;2:1183–1184.
140. Murphy GS, Basri H, Andersen EM, et al. *Vivax malaria* resistant to treatment and prophylaxis with chloroquine. *Lancet* 1993;341:96–100.
141. Ekwanzala M, Pepin J, Khonde N, Molisho S, Bruneel H, De Wals P. In the heart of darkness: sleeping sickness in Zaire. *Lancet* 1996;348:1427–1430.
142. MacLean JD, Arthur JR, Ward BJ, Gyorkos TW, Curtis MA, Kokoskin E. Common-source outbreak of acute infection due to the North American liver fluke *Metorchis conjunctus*. *Lancet* 1996;347:154–158.

CHAPTER 43

Diseases of International Travel and Remote Sites

Rodney D. Adam

Travelers to other countries and sometimes to different regions of their own countries have the potential for exposure to new infectious agents of disease. In general, these risks are magnified when the travel is to the developing or semideveloped countries. Some of these risks can be diminished by appropriate precautions before and during travel, whereas others can be dealt with more promptly if the risk is known.

Although this chapter deals primarily with infectious problems of travelers, it is important to remember that many noninfectious problems exist as well. In fact, the most common causes of death related to travel are not infectious. Rather, the most important causes of death related to travel are preexisting conditions, such as coronary heart disease or asthma, and trauma, including motor vehicle trauma and weapon-related trauma. Other noninfectious risks are less severe but still have the potential to interfere significantly with travel. These include jet lag and other sleep disorders, motion sickness, and altitude sickness.

A number of excellent resources are available for addressing the infectious problems of travel, including books primarily devoted to travel-related problems (1,2), reviews of specific travel-related entities, such as traveler's diarrhea (3) and malaria (4) prevention and treatment, and books (5) and reviews dealing specifically with immunization (6–8). The most helpful single source for travel-related questions is "Health Information for International Travelers" (1) that is published by the Centers for Disease Control and Prevention and updated every 1 or 2 years. The "Red Book" report of the Committee on Infectious Diseases is also very useful, but is only updated every 3 years (5). The Centers for Disease Control and Prevention also maintains an information telephone number, (404) 332–4559, and a Web site, http://www.cdc.gov, that provide up-to-date information on travel-related risks.

SYNDROMES AND SPECIFIC INFECTIONS

Traveler's Diarrhea

Traveler's diarrhea is the most common infectious complication of travel and occurs in approximately 20% to 50% of travelers to the developing countries (3), and somewhat less frequently in travelers to the semideveloped countries. Traveler's diarrhea is most commonly bacterial in etiology and is acquired by ingestion of contaminated food or water. Commonly implicated bacteria include *Escherichia coli*, *Shigella* species, *Campylobacter jejuni*, and *Salmonella* species. Viruses, especially Rotavirus, are also common. Less frequently, protozoan infections, including amebiasis, giardiasis, cryptosporidiosis, isosporiasis, or cyclosporiasis, are seen. In patients who present with acute onset of abdominal pain, fever, and bloody diarrhea, invasive bacteria or *Entamoeba histolytica* are the most likely etiologies. In contrast, the other protozoan etiologies of diarrhea are more indolent in their onset and may produce diarrhea and malabsorption with or without fluid loss.

In view of the resurgence of cholera in many parts of the world, including the Indian subcontinent, Africa, and South America, cholera should be considered in patients who present with watery diarrhea and fluid loss. Cholera is the only diarrheal illness for which a vaccine is currently available. Vaccination with a series of two injections results in an efficacy of 50% for a period of 3 to 6 months. This vaccine is only effective for the O1 strains of *Vibrio cholerae* and, thus, is ineffective for much of the cholera on the Indian subcontinent where the O139 serogroup is endemic. Although serious side effects are rare, fever, malaise, and pain at the injection site are very common and troubling side effects. No countries require the cholera vaccine for entry. For these reasons, the vaccine is seldom, if ever, indicated for travelers. Orally administered vaccines that are effective for the O1 and O139 serotypes have been shown to be safe and reasonably effective in field trials, but these vaccines are not yet available in the United States.

Despite appropriate food and water precautions, many people get traveler's diarrhea. Preventive therapy with antibiotics [e.g., doxycycline, trimethoprim/sulfamethoxazole (TMP/SMX)] or bismuth subsalicylate (Pepto-Bismol) is somewhat effective, but the benefit is limited enough that preventive therapy is usually not recommended because of the expense, inconvenience, toxicity, and potential for microbial resistance. A more prudent course includes traveler-initiated antibiotic therapy at the onset of diarrhea. Three components exist to the treatment of traveler's diarrhea:

1. Maintain adequate hydration by ingestion of fluids or intravenous therapy if necessary. Hydration is especially important in the case of cholera or other forms of diarrhea characterized by severe fluid loss. Packets for preparing oral rehydration solution are generally available. A packet intended for 1 L of oral rehydration solution contains sodium chloride (3.5 g), potassium chloride (1.5 g), glucose (20 g), and trisodium citrate (2.9 g).
2. Initiation of antibiotic therapy at the onset of diarrhea. Studies indicate that the fluoroquinolones (e.g., ciprofloxacin, ofloxacin, norfloxacin) are superior to other antibiotics, such as TMP/SMX (3,9). The fluoroquinolones are active against all the major bacterial etiologies of traveler's diarrhea, including *Escherichia coli*, *Shigella*, *Salmonella*, *Vibrio cholerae*, and *Campylobacter*, although the emergence of resistance has already been noted, especially for *Campylobacter*. A single 500-mg dose of ciprofloxacin (10), and probably a single dose of the other fluoroquinolones, is highly effective, lessening expense, antibiotic toxicity, and potential for development of bacterial resistance. The fluoroquinolones have not yet been approved for use in children younger than 18 years because of the development of arthropathy in juvenile test animals. Although this complication has never been documented in humans, caution would suggest that TMP/SMX be used rather than fluoroquinolones for children (past the neonatal period) or in breast-feeding women. Sulfonamides should be avoided in late pregnancy; thus, few good oral antimicrobial options exist for treatment of traveler's diarrhea in pregnancy.
3. Even in patients treated with antibiotics, evidence exists that symptoms resolve more quickly when an antimotility agent is used additionally (11,12). Studies have used loperamide (Imodium), which is available in the United States without a prescription. Antimotility agents should probably not be used in patients with dysentery and fever or bloody stools.

Further medical attention should be sought by patients who are severely ill or when the diarrhea persists. Persistent diarrhea suggests the possibility of resistant bacteria, protozoa (e.g., *Giardia lamblia*, *E. histolytica*, *Cryptosporidium*, *Cyclospora*, and *Isospora*), or other etiologies (e.g., tropical sprue). Because *G. lamblia* is a relatively common cause of persistent diarrhea, empiric treatment with metronidazole is sometimes initiated in travelers with persistent diarrhea. Metronidazole (although in a higher dose) is also effective for *E. histolytica* infection, whereas TMP/SMX is effective for *Cyclospora* or *Isospora* infection; no treatment is effective for *Cryptosporidium*.

Fever

Fever during international travel or after return from travel may merely indicate an illness not specifically related to travel. However, a number of febrile illnesses are associated with travel to different parts of the world and should be considered in the differential diagnosis of fever. Malaria is one of the most important considerations because of the life-threatening potential of *Plasmodium falciparum* infections and because malaria is readily treatable. Fever may also be the presenting manifestation of any one of a number of hemorrhagic fevers that are endemic in Africa and South America (e.g., Lassa, Ebola, Marburg). These viruses, however, are generally much less common than dengue or yellow fever. Other considerations include rickettsial infection, typhoid, African trypanosomiasis, relapsing fever, tuberculosis, or acute human immunodeficiency virus (HIV) infection. Localizing signs or symptoms may point to specific diagnosis and should be sought.

Dengue Fever

Dengue is common in parts of Central and South America as well as in much of southern Asia and was the cause of 30% of hospitalizations for febrile illness among military personnel in Haiti (13). Dengue is transmitted by the bite of an *Aedes aegypti* mosquito. After a 2- to 7-day incubation period, patients develop an abrupt onset of fever and chills, headache, myalgias, and arthralgias, followed by defervescence and a maculopapular skin rash in 3 to 6 days. Four different serotypes exist, and natural infection results in protection from only the homologous serotype. When a second infection with a heterologous serotype occurs, patients may develop dengue hemorrhagic fever that has a high mortality rate and is clinically similar to the other hemorrhagic fevers. No vaccine is yet available, but appropriate mosquito precautions decrease the likelihood of infection.

Yellow Fever

Yellow fever ranges in severity from asymptomatic or subclinical to life-threatening in nature. After a 3- to 6-day incubation, a sudden onset of fever, chills, headache, myalgias, and arthralgias is followed by complete resolution or progression to more severe disease that may include coagulopathy, jaundice, renal failure, or cardiac failure. Yellow fever occurs in the tropical and subtropical regions of South America, up to the Panama Canal zone, and in Africa (Fig. 43-1), where a major resurgence was documented through the 1980s to 1990s (14). Therefore, yellow fever immunization is generally indicated for travelers to these areas. Some of these countries require yellow fever vaccination for travelers entering from other countries that have yellow fever, even if the traveler has not been to an area of that country known to be endemic for yellow fever. Therefore, close attention should be given to the requirements of the individual countries. Because it is a live virus vaccine, a theoretical risk exists in immunocompromised patients; however, cases of severe vaccine-related illness have yet to be documented in these patients. The yellow fever vaccine is able to infect a developing fetus, but adverse effects on the fetus have not been documented. Therefore, pregnant women traveling to areas of low risk for yellow fever should be given a medical waiver, whereas pregnant women traveling to areas in which the risk of yellow fever is high should be given the vaccine. Severe encephalitis caused by yellow fever vaccine has been documented in infants younger than 4 months. Therefore, the vaccine is absolutely contraindicated for children younger than 4 months, and in general, the immunization should be delayed until after 9 months of age. Other adverse reactions are generally mild, but 2% to 5% of vaccinees develop mild systemic flu-like symptoms approximately 5 to 10 days after immunization. The immune response lasts for at least 10 years

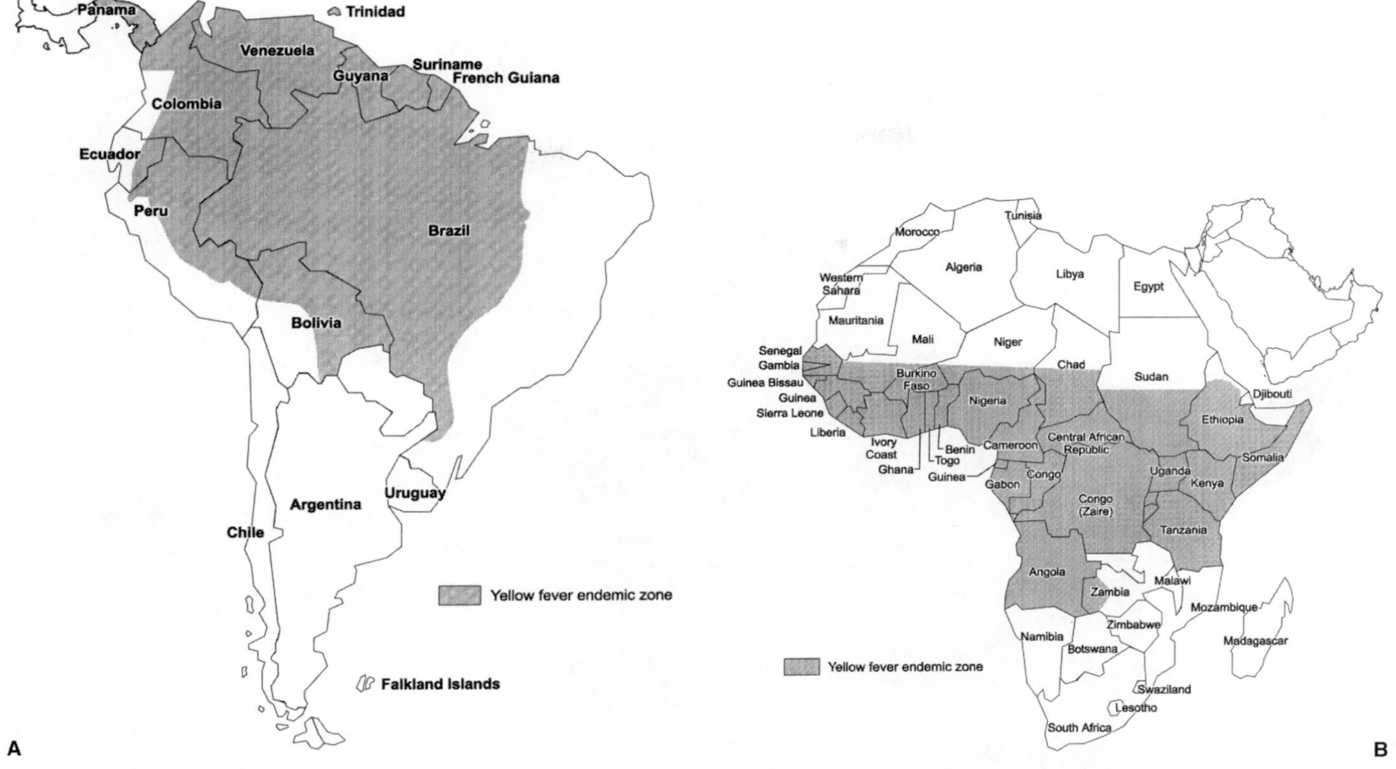

Figure 43-1. The areas of South America and Africa with yellow fever transmission are shown. **A:** Yellow fever in the Americas. The areas of South America and Panama with yellow fever transmission. **B:** Yellow fever in Africa. The areas of Africa Panama with yellow fever transmission. (Adapted from ref. 5, with permission.)

(and possibly a lifetime); reimmunization is recommended at 10-year intervals for travelers to endemic areas.

Typhoid Fever

Salmonella typhi, the cause of typhoid fever, is transmitted from human to human by direct contact or indirectly through contaminated food or water. Typhoid fever is common in much of the developing world and is characterized by high fever, prostration, and is frequently accompanied by septic shock. Diarrhea is present in a minority of cases. The organism can be cultured from fecal specimens in 50% of cases, but is cultured more reliably from blood or bone marrow samples. Serologic tests are commonly used, but have very poor sensitivity and specificity. Chloramphenicol and TMP/SMX have been the most commonly used therapeutic agents, but resistance of *S. typhi* to these drugs is an increasing problem. The fluoroquinolones and the third-generation cephalosporins (e.g., ceftriaxone) are more reliably effective when available.

Three vaccines are now available for prevention of typhoid, all of which have comparable efficacy, estimated at 50% to 80%. Phenol inactivated vaccine has been used for many years and consists of a series of two injections given 30 days apart. Local and systemic side effects are very common with this vaccine. Therefore, it has mostly been replaced in the United States by the two newer vaccines because of their markedly improved side-effect profiles. The oral vaccine consists of a live attenuated strain of *S. typhi* in a capsule form. One capsule is taken every other day on an empty stomach, for a total of four capsules. The vaccine must be refrigerated until used and is recommended only for patients older than 6 years of age. Duration of immunity is 5 years.

The new parenteral vaccine (Typhim Vi) results in only 2 years of protective immunity, but it remains a viable alternative to the oral vaccine because it can be given to children as young as 2 years of age, and because of the potential for improved compliance because of the single injection.

Malaria

Malaria may be caused by any one of four species of *Plasmodium* (*P. falciparum*, *P. vivax*, *P. ovale*, and *P. malariae*). *P. falciparum* and *P. vivax* are the most common and widespread species, and can be found in most regions in which malaria transmission occurs (Fig. 43-2). The major exception is West Africa, where *P. vivax* transmission is rare or nonexistent. West Africa has the highest malaria transmission rate in the world, with approximately 90% of cases caused by *P. falciparum* and most of the remainder by *P. ovale*. After the bite of an infected female anopheline mosquito, the sporozoites are rapidly transmitted to the liver. After an incubation period, which depends on the species (approximately 10 to 14 days), merozoites are released into the bloodstream, beginning the symptomatic portion of the infection. In the case of *P. vivax* and *P. ovale*, some of the organisms remain in the liver in a latent form, providing the opportunity for relapse months to years later. Malaria is characterized by high fever, chills, and headache. The fevers are classically seen every 2 (*P. falciparum*, *P. vivax*, and *P. ovale*) or 3 (*P. malariae*) days, but this pattern is frequently not seen. *P. falciparum* infection is of special concern, because it is frequently fatal in children and in nonimmune adults when treatment is not promptly administered.

Malaria may be prevented by avoidance of mosquitoes and by chemoprophylaxis (Table 43-1). Because *P. falciparum* is wide-

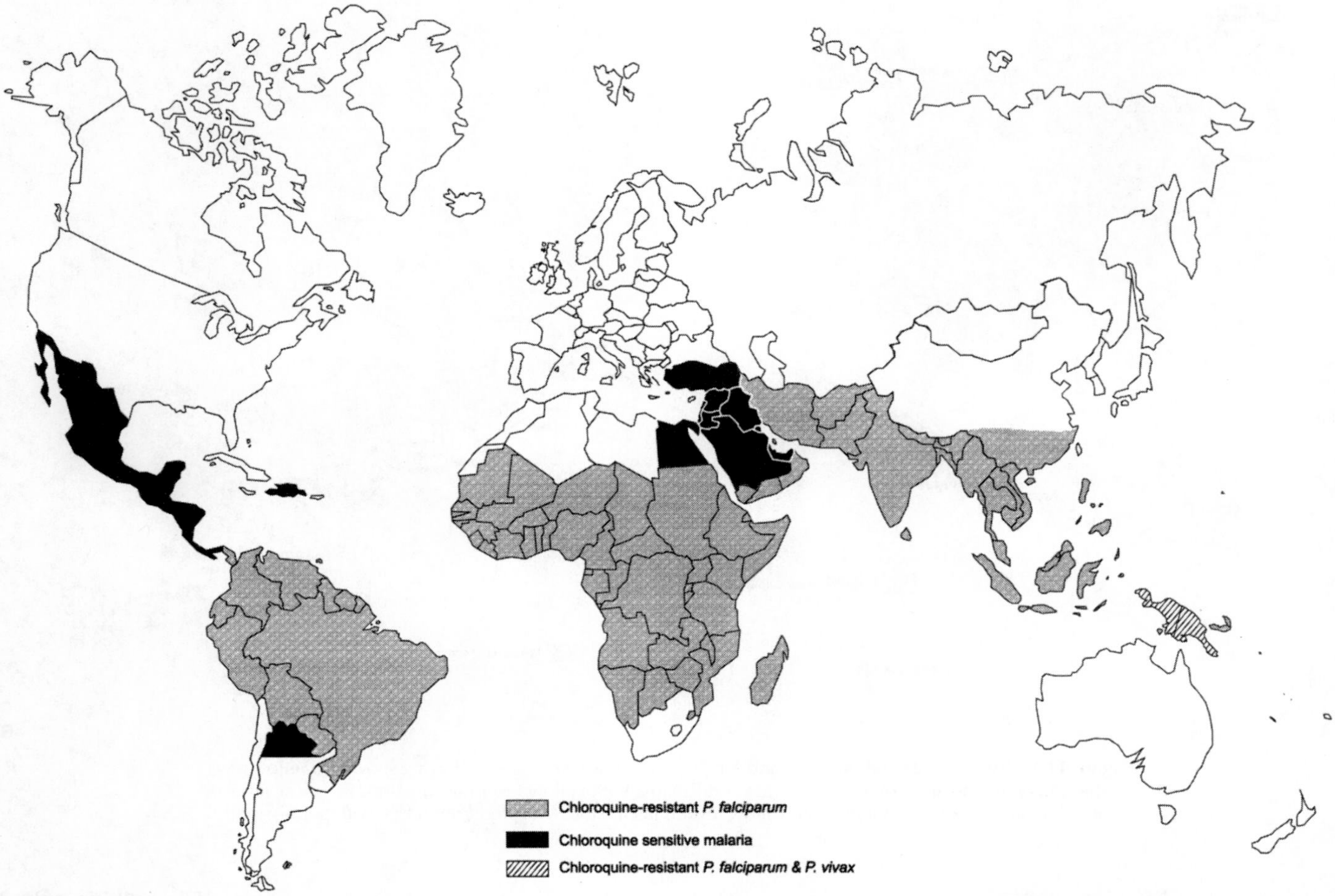

Chloroquine-resistant *P. falciparum*
Chloroquine sensitive malaria
Chloroquine-resistant *P. falciparum* & *P. vivax*

Figure 43-2. The countries of the world with malaria transmission. With the exception of China and Argentina, no attempt has been made to distinguish which regions within individual countries have malaria. (Adapted from ref. 5, with permission.)

spread and has the greatest potential for drug resistance and mortality, the preventive strategies are directed especially at prevention of *P. falciparum*. These strategies are also effective for the other species. As of 1997, *P. falciparum* in Central America (to the Panama Canal zone) and the Caribbean, as well as the Middle East, was still susceptible to chloroquine, making it the preventive drug of choice in these areas. Mefloquine is used in most of the remainder of the world, with the exception of northern Thailand, where doxycycline is used because of widespread mefloquine resistance. The other species of malaria remain susceptible to chloroquine (and the other drugs), with the exception that *P. vivax* on the island of New Guinea is now highly resistant to chloroquine. The available regimens are more than 95% effective (15), but malaria should still be considered as a potential source of fever, even in someone taking effective preventive therapy. Mefloquine occasionally causes sleep disturbance and other minor psychiatric side effects, but because this problem is more common when warning is given, it should not be overemphasized. Doxycycline is an equally effective alternate (15), but it must be taken every day; it has the potential for toxicity related to sun exposure, especially in light-skinned people; and it should generally not be used in children younger than 8 years because of the potential for tooth staining. Atovaquone/proguanil (Malarone) is the newest antimalarial drug and offers significant benefits compared to older antimalarial medications, particularly with regard to side effects.

The diagnosis of malaria can readily be established by examination of thick (for sensitivity) and thin (for morphology) blood smears, although the infection can be missed when the parasitemia is low or when the smear is taken between febrile episodes. Frequently, the etiologic agent can be determined on the basis of the morphology and epidemiology. When any doubt exists, *P. falciparum* should be assumed to be the etiologic agent, and all children or nonimmune adults should be hospitalized for treatment (see Table 43-1). For returning travelers who have had moderate to intense exposure to a relapsing malaria (*P. vivax* or *P. ovale*), a course of primaquine is up to 80% effective in preventing relapse (see Table 43-1).

Hepatitis

Hepatitis has a number of distinct viral etiologies and can be mimicked by a number of other viral or bacterial agents that incidentally involve the liver, as well as those infections that result in space-occupying lesions of the liver, such as amebiasis or echinococcosis. Hepatitis viruses are broadly divided into those that are transmitted by the fecal-oral route and those that are transmitted primarily by parenteral and sexual exposure. Hepatitis A is by far the most common form of enterically transmitted hepatitis throughout the world, and after traveler's diarrhea, may be the most common infection documented in travelers (16). Hepatitis E is also transmitted enterically and is similar to hepatitis A in its

TABLE 43-1. Malaria prevention and treatment

Type of malaria	Prevention[a–d]	Treatment[b–d]
Plasmodium falciparum resistant to chloroquine	Mefloquine, 250 mg (228 mg base) weekly (approximately 5 mg/kg for children) or Doxycycline, 100 mg daily (2 mg/kg for children) or Atovaquone/proguanil, 1 tablet (250 mg atovaquone/100 mg proguanil) daily, starting 1–2 d prior to entering a malaria-endemic area; 1 tablet daily while in area; and 1 tablet daily for 7 d after return.	Quinine, 650 mg (8.3 mg/kg) q 8 h for 3–7 d or Quinidine, 10 mg/kg (max 600 mg) loading dose over 1–2 h, then 0.02 mg/kg/h until oral Rx tolerated In addition to quinine or quinidine, give Fansidar, 3 tablets single dose; tetracycline, 250 qid for 7 d; doxycycline, 100 mg bid; mefloquine, 1,250 mg single dose; or clindamycin 900 mg tid for 3 d (dose should be adjusted appropriately for children) Single daily dose of 4 tablets for 3 d (dose should be adjusted for children and depends on body weight)
Plasmodium vivax resistant to chloroquine (island of New Guinea)	Mefloquine, 250 mg weekly (approximately 5 mg/kg for children) or Doxycycline, 100 mg daily (2 mg/kg for children)	Mefloquine, 1,250 mg single dose (25 mg/kg for children)
P. falciparum resistant to mefloquine (northern Thailand)	Doxycycline, 100 mg daily (2 mg/kg for children; no satisfactory prevention exists for children <8 yr)	Quinine, 650 mg (8.3 mg/kg) q 8 h for 7 d Quinidine, 10 mg/kg (max, 600 mg) loading dose over 1–2 h, then 0.02 mg/kg/h until oral Rx tolerated In addition to quinine or quinidine, give doxycycline, 100 mg bid, or clindamycin, 900 mg tid for 3 d [doses adjusted for children]
Chloroquine-sensitive malaria (e.g., Central America and Caribbean)	Chloroquine, 500 mg (300-mg base) weekly (8.3 mg; 5 mg base/kg/wk for children)	Chloroquine 1,000 mg (16.6 mg/kg for children) followed by one-half the initial dose in 6 h and in 1 and 2 d
Prevention of relapse after malaria exposure stops (*P. vivax* or *Plasmodium ovale*)	Primaquine, 26.3 mg (15 mg base) (0.5 mg; 0.3 mg base for children) daily for 2 wk	

Bid, twice a day; q, every; qid, four times a day; Rx, medication; tid, three times a day.
[a]Preventive therapy begins 1 to 2 weeks before entering malarious area and continues until 4 weeks after exposure stops.
[b]Doses given as the salt unless otherwise noted.
[c]The maximum pediatric dose should not exceed the adult dose.
[d]Doxycycline is not recommended for children younger than 8.

clinical presentation, except that pregnant women developing hepatitis E have a mortality rate as high as 20% in comparison with a much lower rate for hepatitis A. At this time, hepatitis E has only been documented in the developing countries, including Mexico and India.

Hepatitis A is usually asymptomatic when acquired at a young age (e.g., younger than 2 years). Therefore, in countries in which hepatitis A is highly endemic, most people acquire the infection early in life and clinical hepatitis is relatively uncommon in people growing up there, but is very common in tourists from countries with a low prevalence of hepatitis A.

Immune globulin (gamma globulin) given by the intramuscular route has been used for many years for the prevention of hepatitis A and is approximately 90% effective. The immune globulin must be repeated every 2 to 5 months, depending on the dose of immune globulin used initially.

Hepatitis A vaccine has an efficacy of 95%. After a single dose, most vaccinees have protective antibody levels within 2 weeks. The immune response to the initial dose lasts approximately 6 to 12 months, and lasts at least 10 years when the second dose is given 6 to 12 months after the first. The two available brands are inactivated vaccines, with the same adjuvant and preservative as well as similar dosing schedules, and can be used interchangeably (Table 43-2).

It is recommended that the immunization be given at least 1 month before travel and that immune globulin be given in addition to the vaccine when less time is available. However, most people develop adequate antibody levels within 2 weeks, and primate studies have confirmed protection from vaccine given up to 3 days after exposure to hepatitis A (17). The lack of human cases of hepatitis A more than 16 days after vaccination (18) also suggests the possibility of postexposure efficacy, because the incubation period of hepatitis A is usually longer than 1 month. Further studies should clarify whether immune globulin is needed in this setting or whether vaccination alone is sufficient.

The vaccine has not been approved for use in children younger than 2 years of age, and immune globulin is recommended for prevention of hepatitis in these younger children. However, most cases of hepatitis A infection in children younger than 2 years of age are asymptomatic. Therefore, it is not clear how much benefit can be obtained from using immune globulin in these younger children.

Hepatitis B and hepatitis C are the most commonly identified agents of parenteral and sexually transmitted hepatitis. Acute hepatitis B infection may remain asymptomatic or may result in fulminant life-threatening liver failure. In comparison to hepatitis A, the incubation period is somewhat longer, and the onset of symptoms tends to be somewhat more indolent in nature. Delta hepatitis (hepatitis D) is caused by a defective virus that can replicate only in the presence of hepatitis B surface antigen. Delta hepatitis should be considered in people with fulminant hepatitis B, as well as in patients known to be hepatitis B surface antigen carriers who present with an exacerbation of their preexisting hepatitis.

Universal immunization with hepatitis B is now being encouraged in the United States, but relatively few people have completed hepatitis B immunization. Because hepatitis B is transmitted primarily by sexual and parenteral routes, the vaccine is not routinely necessary for travelers. However, many

TABLE 43-2. Immunizations used for international travel

Vaccine	Efficacy	Vaccine type	Route and dose	Schedule for primary immunization	Timing of booster	Use in children	Use in pregnancy	Contraindications and major toxicities	Location and types of travel
Hepatitis A	95%	Inactivated	IM 1 mL (1,440 EL.U. for Havrix; 50U for Vaqta)	0 and 6–12 mo; protection for 6–12 mo after single dose	Unknown, >10 yr.	Not indicated for age younger than 2 yr. One-half dose for ages 2–18 yr.	Compare theoretical risk of vaccination with risk of disease.	—	Developing and semideveloped countries
Immune globulin (for hepatitis A prevention)	90%	Immunoglobulin	IM 0.2 mL/kg up to mL for exposure up to 3 mo	Single dose	N/A; give hepatitis A vaccine for more prolonged exposure.	Dosed by weight	Give when indicated, regardless of pregnancy.	—	Developing and semideveloped countries
Hepatitis B	90%	Subunit (HB_sAg)	IM 1 mL	0, 1, and 6 mo	Not recommended.	One-half dose for ages 0–19 yr; adult dose if mother is HB_sAg+; 95% efficacy for children.	Give when indicated, regardless of pregnancy.	—	Countries with high prevalence of HB_sAg; medical workers; likelihood of sexual or parenteral exposure
Typhoid vaccine	50%–80%	—	—	—	—	—	—	—	Developing countries; significant exposure to contaminated food or water
Oral		Live attenuated	Oral capsule	q.o.d. for 4 doses	5 yr	Not indicated for age younger than 6 yr.	Compare theoretical risk of vaccination with risk of disease.	—	—
Injectable (Typhim Vi)		Subunit (polysaccharide)	IM 0.5 mL	Single dose	2 yr	Not indicated for age younger than 2 yr.	Compare theoretical risk of vaccination with risk of disease.	—	—
Injectable (phenol inactivated)		Inactivated	SQ 0.5 mL	0 and 1 mo	3 yr	One-half dose for ages 6 mo–10 yr; not indicated for younger than 6 mo.	Use a less toxic vaccine.	Severe systemic and local complications are common.	—

Cholera	50%	Inactivated	SQ or IM 0.5 mL	0 and 1 mo	6 mo	—	—	Severe systemic and local complications are common.	Rarely, if ever, indicated
Neisseria meningitidis	Nearly 90% for serotypes in vaccine	Subunit (polysaccharide)	SQ 0.5 mL	Single dose	3 yr	Not indicated for age younger than 2 yr.	Compare theoretical risk of vaccination with risk of disease; risk is generally low in travelers.	—	Meningococcal belt of sub-Saharan Africa; Nepal and Mongolia
Japanese encephalitis	90%	Inactivated	SQ 1 mL	0, 7, and 28 d	3 yr	Not indicated for age younger than 1 yr; one-half dose for younger than 3 yr. Same as adult.	Compare theoretical risk of vaccination with risk of disease.	Anaphylaxis that can occur up to 7–10 d after immunization.	Southern Asia; rural areas with likelihood of substantial exposure
Rabies Preexposure	—	Inactivated	IM 1 mL or ID 0.1 mL	0, 7, and 21 or 28 d	2 yr or by serologic testing; postexposure prophylaxis with IM doses at d 0 and 3 are still necessary.	—	Compare theoretical risk of vaccination with risk of disease.	—	Developing countries; likelihood of exposure to animal bites
Postexposure	Nearly 100%		IM RIG 20 IU/kg + vaccine IM 1 mL	RIG: d 0; vaccine: d 0, 3, 7, 14, and 28	N/A		Give when indicated, regardless of pregnancy.		Potential exposure to rabies
Yellow fever	>95%	Live attenuated	SQ 0.5 mL	Single dose	10 yr recommended, but immunity may be lifetime.	Contraindicated when younger than age 9 mo.	Asymptomatic fetal infection occurs; should be avoided when the risk of infection is low, but given when the exposure is high.	Encephalitis in children younger than 4 mo; caution in immunocompromised patients.	Equatorial South America and Africa

EL.U., ELISA units; HB_sAg, hepatitis B surface antigen; ID, intradermal; IM, intramuscular; IU, international unit; N/A, not applicable; qod, every other day; RIG, rabies immune globulin; SQ, subcutaneous.

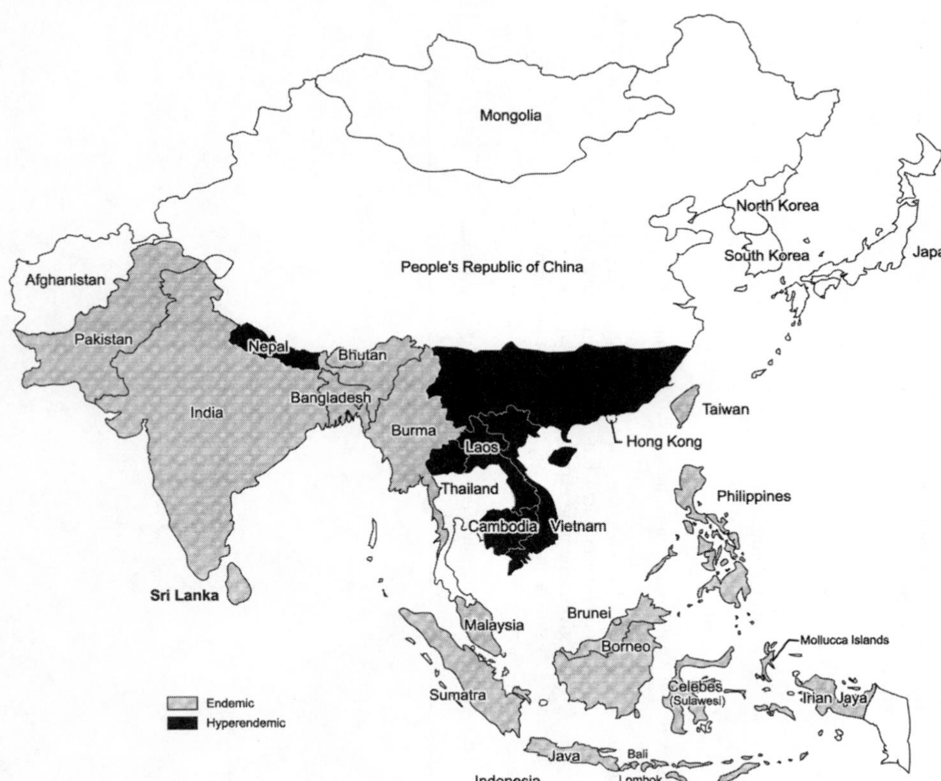

Figure 43-3. The countries with Japanese encephalitis transmission are shown. For the endemic regions (*gray*), no attempt has been made to distinguish which regions within individual countries have Japanese encephalitis. The areas of highest risk (hyperendemic regions) are shown in black. Countries with few cases, such as Korea, Russia, and Japan, were not included. (Adapted from ref. 5, with permission.)

parts of the world have substantially increased carrier rates for hepatitis B surface antigen, and travelers with sexual encounters in these areas, those using parenteral drugs, and medical workers are at increased risk for acquisition of hepatitis B and should be immunized. Because hepatitis D infection depends on the presence of hepatitis B surface antigen, hepatitis B vaccination also prevents hepatitis D.

No available vaccine exists for the prevention of hepatitis C, and development of a vaccine may be especially difficult because of the genetic diversity of hepatitis C. One study demonstrated efficacy of immune globulin with high titers of hepatitis C antibody for prevention of hepatitis C infection (19). However, serum that is seropositive for hepatitis C is excluded from the immune globulin available in the United States; therefore, efficacy would not be expected.

Japanese Encephalitis

Japanese encephalitis (JE) is transmitted by the bite of a number of species of *Culex* mosquitoes. The vector species in much of the endemic region feed predominantly at dusk and through the evening; thus, the risk during the daytime is less. JE is endemic to much of South Asia, extending from Pakistan through China in addition to Indonesia, the Philippines, and other Pacific islands (Fig. 43-3). Subclinical infection is common, but when encephalitis occurs, mortality is 30% and neurologic sequelae occur in 50% of the survivors.

The available vaccine is approximately 90% effective (20). The primary vaccination consists of a series of three injections on days 0, 7, and 28. The third dose can be given 2 weeks after the first dose, when time does not permit the longer interval. Local and systemic reactions occur in approximately 20% of vaccine recipients, and severe hypersensitivity reactions, such as erythema, angioedema, and anaphylaxis, occur in approximately 0.3% of vaccinees (21). These reactions most commonly occur within minutes after administering the vaccine but have sometimes occurred as long as 7 to 10 days after a dose. Therefore, it is recommended that patients be observed for one-half hour after administration of the vaccine and that travel be delayed for 10 days after completion of the series. Most travelers to endemic regions are at very low risk for acquisition of JE, and because of the toxicity, the vaccine should only be used for travelers at substantial risk of exposure to JE. The risk varies widely according to location of travel, time of year, and duration of time in the endemic area, and must be assessed on an individual basis. A detailed list of country and region-specific risk can be found in "Health Information for International Travel" (1).

Meningococcal Meningitis

Epidemics of infection caused by *Neisseria meningitidis* are especially common in the sub-Saharan region of Africa as well as the African countries of Kenya, Tanzania, and Burundi (Fig. 43-4). Epidemic meningococcal disease has also been noted in Nepal and Mongolia. In the United States, the most common meningococcal serotype is B, which is not represented in the available vaccine (the vaccine includes serogroups A, C, Y, and W-135). In contrast, the epidemic strains found in Africa are primarily A and C, which can be prevented by the vaccine. Although routine travelers are at relatively low risk for acquiring meningococcal meningitis, the vaccine is recommended for travelers to endemic regions.

Rabies

Domestic animals, especially dogs, in many of the developing countries have a high incidence of rabies. Although rabies vaccination is not routinely recommended for travelers, vaccination should be considered for long-term travelers and for those most likely to have contact with dogs. When dog bites do occur in these countries, they should be assumed to result in rabies expo-

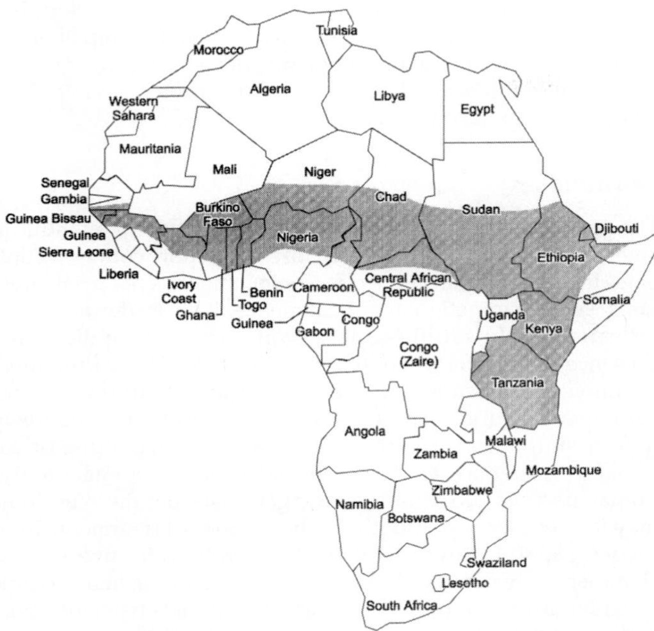

Figure 43-4. The meningococcal meningitis belt of Africa. (Adapted from ref. 5, with permission.)

sure. Preexposure immunization for rabies consists of a series of three intradermal or intramuscular injections at 0, 7, and 28 days. The intradermal route of administration uses one-tenth of the dose used for intramuscular administration, making it more economical. Although the intradermal route is effective for preexposure immunization, it is somewhat less effective for postexposure immunization. Postexposure rabies immunization in people who have completed a preexposure immunization schedule consists of two doses of intramuscular rabies vaccine on days 0 and 3. Rabies immune globulin is not used in this case. For postexposure rabies immunization in people without prior immunization, rabies immune globulin is used in addition to a series of five intramuscular doses of the vaccine on days 0, 3, 7, 14, and 28. One-half of the rabies immune globulin is generally injected into the bite wound area and the other one-half given by the intramuscular route, typically into the gluteus. Intramuscular vaccination is used for postexposure prophylaxis, because failures have been reported for intradermal vaccine. The response to rabies immunization is impaired in patients receiving chloroquine, and theoretical concern exists for the response in people receiving mefloquine because it is chemically similar; however, cases of impaired response have not been reported.

Sexually Transmitted Diseases

The incidence and prevalence of many of the sexually transmitted diseases (STDs) are much higher in many of the developing countries than in the developed countries. Certain types of travel have included sexual contact with prostitutes in the country of travel, leading to a high risk of STDs among these travelers. For example, gonorrhea goes untreated in many of the developing countries and is a major cause of female infertility and ectopic pregnancy, in addition to male urethral stricture. Chancroid is caused by *Haemophilus ducreyi* and is manifested primarily by genital ulceration and inguinal adenopathy. Hepatitis B is transmitted most commonly by sexual intercourse or vertically, and the carrier rate is high throughout Africa and southern Asia. In addition, the infections that are still highly prevalent in the developed countries, such as chlamydia, papillomavirus, herpes simplex virus, and syphilis, are common in developing countries as well. In the United States and western Europe, HIV infection continues to be transmitted primarily through male homosexual contact and parenteral drug use, but the transmission of HIV throughout most of the remainder of the world is predominantly by the heterosexual route. Data from Thailand suggest that the rate of female-to-male transmission of HIV is approximately 5% per sexual contact, in contrast to 0.1% per contact in the United States. The reasons for this great difference are not totally clear, but proposed explanations include differences in transmission potential for the different endemic viral isolates, lower rates of male circumcision, and higher rates of untreated STDs in the areas with high levels of heterosexual transmission. HIV2 is common in West Africa, but the transmission potential and virulence are much lower than for HIV1 (22,23). Condoms appear to be approximately 90% effective in decreasing HIV transmission when used consistently and correctly (24–26). In Thailand, the incidence of new HIV infections has actually been decreased by an aggressive campaign of STD treatment of prostitutes and condom use by their clients (27).

Tuberculosis

Tuberculosis is most commonly acquired by the aerosol route from patients with untreated cavitary pulmonary disease. It is found throughout the world but is more common in the developing countries. A resurgence throughout the world in the 1980s can be attributed to the HIV epidemic. HIV-infected patients are at increased risk for acquiring tuberculosis, more likely to relapse after treatment, and may be contagious in the absence of the usual signs of tuberculosis.

Travelers with the potential for increased exposure to tuberculosis (including medical workers) should have a tuberculin skin test before departure and approximately 2 to 3 months after return. If the skin test converts from negative to positive, appropriate workup and isoniazid therapy are initiated. A positive skin test is now considered to be 5, 10, or 15 mm of induration, depending on the *a priori* likelihood of tuberculosis and degree of immunocompromise (e.g., 5 mm is considered positive in an HIV-infected patient) (5).

Helminth Infections

Helminth infections, rare in the developed countries, are common throughout much of the remainder of the world. The intestinal helminths, such as *Ascaris* (roundworm), hookworm, whipworm, pinworm, and *Strongyloides* are especially common in children. *Ascaris*, whipworm, and pinworm are generally acquired by ingesting eggs via fecal contamination, whereas hookworm and *Strongyloides* infections result when larvae from the soil directly penetrate the human skin. These infections are relatively uncommon in adult travelers and typically cause little morbidity other than mild abdominal pain. Mebendazole and other anthelmintics are effective against these parasites.

Schistosoma species are trematodes that are transmitted to humans when the cercariae are released into the water from their intermediate hosts, which are species of freshwater snails. The cercariae then burrow directly through the skin and mature in the human intestine. Thus, infections are typically acquired by wading or swimming in freshwater in endemic areas [e.g., parts of South America (*S. mansoni*), Africa (*S. mansoni* and *S. hematobium*), and southern Asia (*S. japonicum* and *S. mekongi*)]. An acute infection syndrome 1 to 2 months after exposure (Katayama fever) has been reported in travelers with massive *S. japonicum* or *S. mansoni* infections, which consist of fever, chills, headache, cough, and occasional death (28). However, most of the morbidity is caused by chronic infection of the portal system with venous obstruction (*S. mansoni, S. japonicum*, and *S. mekongi*) or bladder scarring (*S. hematobium*) as a result of the schistosome eggs and the surrounding granulomatous inflammation. The morbidity is proportional to the worm and egg burden. Thus, microscopic examination of fecal or urine (*S. hematobium*) specimens is useful in establishing the diagnosis. Praziquantel and other anthelmintics are effective therapeutic agents.

The tissue nematodes are transmitted by the bites of infected insects. Onchocerciasis (*Onchocerca volvulus*) infection is transmitted by the black fly and is most common in West Africa. Generalized dermatitis and, less commonly, blindness (river blindness) may result; the manifestations are generally more severe in the case of prolonged or heavy infection. *Loa loa* (loiasis) is transmitted by the tabanid fly and is found primarily in parts of West Africa. Patients develop subcutaneous lesions (Calabar swellings), and sometimes the worm migrates across the ocular conjunctiva (eye worm). Treatment is with diethylcarbamazine. Lymphatic filariasis, most commonly caused by *Wuchereria bancrofti* or *Brugia malayi*, is found in parts of South Asia and equatorial Africa and is transmitted by mosquitoes. Acute infection may result in a tropical pulmonary eosinophilia syndrome, but most of the morbidity is because of the lymphatic obstruction that results from chronic infection. Treatment is with diethylcarbamazine or ivermectin, but treatment is of limited benefit after the development of lymphatic complications.

Cysticercosis is caused by the pork tapeworm (*Taenia solium*) for which humans are the definitive hosts and pigs are the intermediate hosts. Cysticercosis results when humans ingest the eggs from human fecal contamination and become accidental intermediate hosts. Months or years after the initial infection, focal cystic lesions form and eventually calcify. When these lesions form in the brain, cerebral cysticercosis results and is the most common cause of seizures in endemic areas. Treatment with praziquantel or albendazole (usually accompanied by corticosteroids) is somewhat effective.

Echinococcosis is most commonly caused by *Echinococcus granulosus*, a canine tapeworm whose natural intermediate hosts are sheep, other livestock, and wild animals. It is found in livestock areas throughout the world, including southern Europe, Latin America, Africa, and in northern Arizona and southern Utah in the United States. Human disease results when humans become accidental intermediate hosts as a result of ingesting eggs from material contaminated by feces of the definitive host. Cystic lesions develop in the liver, lungs, or sometimes other parts of the body over a period of months to years after infection. Albendazole is sometimes effective, but surgical excision is frequently required.

None of the invasive helminth infections is common in routine travelers, but may be found after longer stays in the endemic areas (e.g., in Peace Corps workers).

Eosinophilia

Moderate blood eosinophilia in a short-term traveler is often simply an incidental finding and may indicate atopic disease, such as asthma or an eosinophilic reaction to medication. However, when eosinophilia is high grade (more than 10% to 20%) or occurs in people with prolonged exposure to invasive helminth infections, there should be strong suspicion of helminth infection. Eosinophilia is especially common with infections caused by the tissue nematodes as well as schistosomiasis or strongyloidiasis, but is absent or low grade in cysticercosis or in echinococcosis. A number of diagnostic tests are available for evaluation of suspected helminth infections in patients with eosinophilia. The actual tests depend on which infections are most strongly suspected, but include stool examination for ova and parasite, skin snip or blood samples for detection of nematode microfilaria, or serologic tests for certain of the helminths. In general, the protozoan infections do not give significant eosinophilia.

Dermatoses

The presence of a skin rash or lesion in a traveler may indicate any one of a wide variety of diagnoses. The more common etiologies include routine cutaneous or subcutaneous bacterial infections, such as impetigo or subcutaneous abscess, dermatitis, or urticaria (29). In addition, many skin rashes may indicate the presence of specific travel-related infections. One of the most common is cutaneous larva migrans, especially in people sunbathing on the tropical beaches where dogs and cats roam freely (29). A migratory serpiginous rash occurs when a dog or cat hookworm penetrates the skin and becomes an accidental human parasite. No significant danger exists, but the symptoms may last for weeks or months in the absence of treatment. Topical or systemic treatment with thiabendazole is effective. Diffuse skin rashes are commonly seen in dengue and the hemorrhagic fever syndromes, the spotted fever forms of rickettsial infection, and measles. Focal lesions may be seen in cutaneous leishmaniasis and American or African trypanosomiasis. Calabar swellings may be seen in loiasis. Genital ulceration may indicate chancroid, herpes simplex, or syphilis.

Systemic Protozoan Infections

Leishmaniasis is a protozoan infection caused by a number of different species of *Leishmania*. These organisms are found in scattered locations throughout Central and South America, Africa, and Asia, as well as southern Europe. Infection occurs via the bite of an infected sand fly, which is generally a painful bite. In the cutaneous forms of leishmaniasis, a chronic ulcer develops at the site of the bite and may persist for years in the absence of specific therapy. Visceral or systemic leishmaniasis is less common but is found in certain regions of Brazil and Africa. Patients present with fever, wasting, and hepatosplenomegaly, sometimes mimicking disseminated tuberculosis or HIV infection. The mortality is very high in the absence of specific treatment. Occasionally, the cutaneous form of the disease responds to local heat treatment, but systemic therapy is generally required, and it is always required for visceral leishmaniasis. Pentavalent antimony is most commonly used for treatment, but amphotericin B is probably more effective and can be used to treat antimony failures. The antifungal azole drugs, such as ketoconazole and itraconazole, have also been used successfully.

Two forms of African trypanosomiasis exist: East and West African trypanosomiasis. East African trypanosomiasis is predominately a zoonotic infection, because its natural hosts consist of wild animals of East Africa. Infections in travelers are rare but may be seen in game hunters. People are infected through the bite of an infected tsetse fly. The bite is typically painful, and an ulcerative lesion develops at the site of the bite. In the absence of treatment, a febrile illness with parasitemia is followed by meningoencephalitis after a period of weeks to months; hence the term *African sleeping sickness*. The encephalitis is invariably fatal if left untreated. In contrast to East African trypanosomiasis, West African trypanosomiasis is predominately a human infection and is somewhat more indolent in nature. By the 1960s, it was almost eradicated from Africa but has made a major resurgence in the 1990s. Therefore, it is possible that travelers to the Congo (Zaire) and other parts of equatorial West Africa are at increased risk for exposure to West African trypanosomiasis. The diagnosis of African trypanosomiasis can be established by microscopic identification of the parasite in the initial ulcer, or in blood, cerebrospinal fluid, or bone marrow samples. Suramin and pentamidine are effective for treatment before the development of central nervous system (CNS) disease, but are ineffective for CNS disease. CNS infection is generally treated with arsenical compounds (e.g., melarsoprol), but these are accompanied by a high incidence of reactive encephalopathy. Difluoromethylornithine (DFMO) (eflornithine) is effective for West African trypanosomiasis with CNS involvement and is much safer, but is expensive and frequently not available in the endemic region.

American trypanosomiasis is a zoonotic protozoan infection found throughout the tropical regions of South and Central America and typically occurs in rural areas with primitive housing. Human infection results indirectly from the bite of a reduviid (kissing) bug. At the time of the bite, the bug defecates, and, because the wound is pruritic, parasites from the feces are frequently introduced into the skin by scratching. The parasites may also be directly introduced through the mucous membranes, such as the ocular conjunctiva. Most infections are initially asymptomatic, but an acute febrile illness with edema, malaise, lymphadenopathy, and occasionally myocarditis or meningoencephalitis may be seen, primarily in children. An asymptomatic chronic infection may result (with or without acute symptoms), with the eventual development of cardiomegaly with congestive heart failure and arrhythmias, as well as megaesophagus and megacolon. The parasites may be identified on blood smears during acute infection, but the diagnosis of chronic infection is usually established by serologic testing. Benznidazole is useful in the treatment of the acute infection, but no proven therapy exists for chronic infection.

REGIONS OF THE WORLD

Developed Countries

Western Europe, Canada, Australia, and New Zealand are developed countries that generally have health risks similar to those in the United States. Therefore, no specific travel-related precautions are necessary for protection from infectious diseases.

Developing and Semideveloped Regions

Other than Western Europe, United States, Canada, Australia, and New Zealand, the risk for acquiring certain infectious diseases is increased anywhere from a little to a great deal, depending on the specific country and setting within that country. Traveler's diarrhea may affect 20% to 50% of travelers to many of these regions. The risk for acquiring hepatitis A is also increased for most of the countries within this category, and preventive measures should be taken. Typhoid fever is found in many of these regions, but most tourists are at relatively low risk. The typhoid fever vaccine is especially recommended for those spending a prolonged period of time at their destination, or those for whom safe food and water are going to be more difficult to find. Travelers should also remember that rabies in dogs in most developing countries is substantially more common than in the developed countries. Preexposure rabies vaccination should be considered for people planning a prolonged stay. STDs are especially common in many of the developing countries; the risk of STDs is especially high in travelers who engage in sexual contact with prostitutes. Tuberculosis is especially common in many of the developing countries, and the frequency has been increasing because of the HIV epidemic and the common occurrence of coinfection with HIV and *Mycobacterium tuberculosis*. In many of the developing countries, testing of blood (for HIV or hepatitis) intended for transfusion is limited or unavailable, and needles are frequently reused. Therefore, considerable caution is warranted for these or other medical procedures.

South America

Malaria is found throughout South America (with the exception of most of Uruguay, Argentina, and Chile), and *P. falciparum* is chloroquine resistant except in northern Argentina. Yellow fever is found in most of the regions in which malaria is found. Chagas disease and cutaneous and visceral leishmaniasis are found in much of the northern one-half of South America, especially in the rural areas, but these infections are rare in routine travelers. A major outbreak of cholera has been centered in Peru. Localized outbreaks of viral encephalitis and hemorrhagic fever have been documented, including a widespread outbreak of Venezuelan equine encephalitis in Venezuela. Transmission levels of dengue are high in the northern portions of South America.

Central America, Mexico, and the Caribbean

Malaria is found in much of Central America and the Caribbean. *P. falciparum* remains susceptible to chloroquine, except east (South American side) of the Panama Canal. Dengue is common throughout much of this region. For purposes of yellow fever and malaria prevention, Panama east of the Canal Zone should be considered with South America.

Africa

Malaria is a substantial risk throughout most of Africa (with the exception of parts of South Africa and northern Africa); in fact, the level of malaria transmission in West Africa is the highest of anywhere in the world. Yellow fever is found throughout equatorial Africa. The meningococcal belt is located in the sub-Saharan region, and vaccination is generally recommended for travelers to this region (see Fig. 43-1). Travelers have been at low risk for acquisition of African trypanosomiasis (sleeping sickness), but a major resurgence at least in the Congo (Zaire) in the 1990s could lead to increased risk to travelers. Schistosomiasis (*S. mansoni* and *S. hematobium*) is endemic to parts of Africa; travelers to these regions should avoid freshwater swimming. Several of the tissue nematodes, including lymphatic filariasis, onchocerciasis, and loiasis (eye worm), are endemic in portions of Africa. These infections are uncommon in routine travelers, but have been documented as problems in longer-term travelers to the highly endemic areas, such as Peace Corps workers.

Middle East

Israel poses little increased risk of infectious diseases compared to the United States, but a risk of hepatitis A and traveler's diarrhea exists in most of the other Middle East countries, as well as malaria in limited areas. This is one of the few areas in which *P. falciparum* is still susceptible to chloroquine; however, cases of chloroquine-resistant *P. falciparum* acquired in Saudi Arabia were documented in 1997, raising the possibility that chloroquine may not continue to be of use in this area. Leishmaniasis (mostly cutaneous) is found in many parts of the Middle East.

South Asia

Malaria is found throughout most of South Asia, except that the risk is minimal in China, Taiwan, Hong Kong, and Singapore.

The cities of most other South Asia countries are malaria-free. In Thailand, the major area of risk is in the north (e.g., Chiang Mai), where the *P. falciparum* is resistant to the usual antimalarial drug, mefloquine. Meningococcal meningitis is found in Nepal. JE is found in much of South Asia; however, short-term travelers are at low risk for acquisition of JE.

North Asia and Eastern Europe

The tropical diseases, such as yellow fever and malaria, are not present in North Asia and Eastern Europe, but hepatitis A, traveler's diarrhea, and typhoid are common in some of these areas. Echinococcosis and cysticercosis are endemic in some regions, such as southeastern Europe; these tend to afflict long-term residents in the farming communities. In addition, immunization practices are inadequate in many portions of southeastern Europe and the countries of the former Soviet Union, leading to outbreaks of diphtheria, polio, and other vaccine-preventable diseases.

SPECIAL TRAVEL SITUATIONS

Pregnant and Breast-Feeding Women

A number of factors specific to pregnant or breast-feeding women who are traveling should be taken into account, including increased susceptibility to certain infections, known or theoretical complications of vaccines, and potential complications of medications. As a general rule, the inactivated vaccines are considered safe during pregnancy, but are frequently avoided unless the potential benefit clearly outweighs the risk of immunization. Of the vaccines especially used for travelers, the one vaccine in which any significant impact on pregnancy has been noted is the yellow fever vaccine. Fetal infection with yellow fever vaccine has been documented during pregnancy, but no adverse outcome on pregnancy has been observed. Therefore, it is recommended that pregnant women who are traveling to areas of high risk be vaccinated for yellow fever but that vaccination be deferred for low-risk exposures.

Known or theoretical contraindications to a variety of medications are used for prevention or treatment of travel-related infections. Chloroquine is the only medication used for malaria prophylaxis for which substantial safety data exist for all three trimesters of pregnancy. Enough safety data have accumulated so that mefloquine is recommended during the second and third trimesters of pregnancy. Although no specific complications of mefloquine have been noted during the first trimester, theoretical concern still exists regarding administration of mefloquine during this time. It is preferable that travel to areas of high risk for malaria transmission be delayed until after the first trimester, but if this is not possible, mefloquine probably represents the most satisfactory alternative (30). Doxycycline, an alternate drug for malaria prevention, causes bone and tooth deposits in the fetus when administered during late pregnancy and during the first few years of childhood. Therefore, doxycycline should be used during pregnancy only if the benefits clearly outweigh the known toxicity. Sulfonamides are known to displace bilirubin from albumin-binding sites and, therefore, have been associated with the development of kernicterus in some premature infants and may cause hemolysis in newborns with G6PD deficiency. Therefore, sulfonamide drugs, such as TMP/SMX, are generally avoided during late pregnancy and during the neonatal period. The fluoroquinolones, which are commonly used for treatment of traveler's diarrhea, have not yet been approved for use for children younger than 18 years because of the occurrence of arthropathy in animal studies. So far, this toxicity has not been observed in humans, but until these concerns are more completely resolved, the fluoroquinolones should be used during pregnancy, breast-feeding, or in children only when the benefits clearly outweigh the theoretical toxicity.

Pregnant women are at increased risk for acquisition of and morbidity from certain infections. Malaria during pregnancy may result in maternal or fetal anemia, spontaneous abortion, stillbirth, or low birth weight. Hepatitis E has a low mortality in the general population, but the mortality during pregnancy may be as high as 20%.

Children

Special considerations for children include different doses or toxicities for certain drugs, differences in indications or dosing for immunizations, and different susceptibilities to certain infections. The drugs that are of specific concern for use in children include doxycycline and mefloquine, which are used for malaria prophylaxis and the fluoroquinolones. Doxycycline is generally avoided in children younger than 8 years because of the potential for staining of teeth. Until the late 1990s, mefloquine was not recommended for use in children weighing less than 15 kg. However, this recommendation was not because of theoretical toxicity in children, but because of the difficulty in accurate dosing for children. No liquid formulation of the drug is available; therefore, the adult dose of 250 mg must be divided accurately enough to assure an adequate, yet nontoxic, dose for children.

Many of the immunization needs and regimens for children are different from those of adults and include different vaccine doses and minimum ages for vaccination. Most often, these minimum ages merely reflect the lack of data for younger ages. Yellow fever vaccine, however, has been documented as a cause of encephalitis in children younger than 4 months of age; the vaccine should never be used at ages younger than 4 months and only with very high-risk exposures for children 4 through 9 months.

Medical Workers

Medical workers are at an increased risk for exposure to certain infections because of their contact with patients. This includes those pathogens that can be transmitted by needle-stick injuries, especially hepatitis B; therefore, medical workers should be immunized for hepatitis B. Transmission of HIV occurs in approximately 0.3% of needle sticks from HIV-positive patients. The risk of HIV infection after a needle-stick injury from a patient known or suspected to be HIV infected can be decreased by 79% by initiating a course of zidovudine (AZT), 200 mg three times a day, immediately after the injury and continuing for 4 weeks (31). For higher-risk injuries, such as those involving larger quantities of blood, two [zidovudine and lamivudine (3TC)] or three (zidovudine, lamivudine, and the protease inhibitor indinavir) drugs are now recommended (32,33). Other infections characterized by bloodstream infections, such as malaria, trypanosomiasis, and viral hemorrhagic fevers, can also be transmitted parenterally. Medical workers are also at increased risk for acquiring infections that are transmitted by the respiratory route, most notably tuberculosis. Baseline tuberculin skin tests should be done before travel and repeated 2 to 3 months after returning, with administration of isoniazid if the skin test converts from negative to positive.

Immunocompromised Travelers

Immunocompromised travelers are of concern because of their potential for more severe illness caused by some pathogens, as well as actual or theoretical risk from some of the live vaccines. HIV-infected people are at a markedly increased risk for acquisition of severe tuberculosis. The severity of African and South American trypanosomiasis, leishmaniasis, and a number of bacterial infections may also be increased. Some of the same considerations apply to other immunocompromised patients, although most are less severely immunocompromised than HIV-infected patients.

The live vaccines that are commonly used for routine immunizations include measles, mumps, rubella, oral polio, and varicella vaccines. Immunocompromised people are at increased risk for paralytic poliomyelitis from the oral polio vaccine; therefore, inactivated polio vaccine should be used for these patients. The measles vaccine poses an increased risk for patients with advanced HIV infection and is frequently avoided during this time. However, natural measles infection is devastating during HIV infection, so the risk of vaccine toxicity must be weighed against the likely exposure to the natural infection. Varicella vaccine is associated with an increased risk of vaccine-associated varicella in immunocompromised patients. However, this complication generally is not life threatening, and again, the known risk of the vaccine must be weighed against the potential for severe disease caused by the natural infection.

Among the vaccines used especially in travelers, oral typhoid and yellow fever vaccines are live vaccines, and although no adverse reactions to oral typhoid or yellow fever vaccines have been noted in immunocompromised patients, these vaccines generally should be avoided unless the benefits clearly outweigh the risks. In the case of typhoid vaccine, the injectable vaccine provides a suitable alternative. BCG is seldom used in the United States, but is commonly used in many other countries. It has been documented as a cause of severe infection in immunocompromised patients and should be avoided.

Pneumococcal vaccine should be considered for immunocompromised travelers, although the response of immunocompromised patients is likely to be less satisfactory than for immunocompetent patients.

Long-Term Travelers

People traveling to remote areas for long periods of time are frequently at risk for infections that are very uncommon in travelers, especially when the travel is to remote areas with poor hygiene or significant exposure to insect vectors. The actual diseases vary greatly, not only with the country but also with the specific region of the country of travel; therefore, approaches to long-term travelers must be individualized.

PREVENTIVE MEASURES

Routine Immunizations

Many of the diseases that are prevented by routine immunizations in developed countries are still common in the underdeveloped countries; therefore, it is important that routine immunizations be updated in travelers. Diphtheria/pertussis/tetanus or tetanus/diphtheria immunization should be updated as appropriate for travelers. Diphtheria/pertussis/tetanus immunization is generally used up to age 6 and tetanus/diphtheria immunization after that age, with booster immunization every 10 years (sooner in the case of major trauma). Measles is especially common in many of the developing countries, and adequate protection of travelers born during or after 1957 should be assured. Those people born before 1957 are generally assumed to have already had measles and should be at low risk for acquisition of measles during travel. The efficacy of a single dose of measles vaccine is 95% to 98%, and this immunity probably lasts for life. Of those who do not respond to the initial vaccination, approximately one-half respond to a subsequent vaccination, a phenomenon that has engendered the use of two immunization doses for measles. It is reasonable, therefore, to offer a second measles vaccine to patients born after 1957 who have only received one measles vaccine.

Polio has been eradicated from the Western Hemisphere and from western and northern Europe. Therefore, polio vaccination is not indicated for travel to these areas. However, polio transmission continues in Asia, Africa, and southeastern Europe. For adults who have completed primary vaccination for polio, a single (once in a lifetime) dose of the oral or injectable vaccine is recommended when traveling to areas that still have polio. The incidence of paralytic polio from the oral vaccine is approximately 1 per 1 million, and occurs primarily after the first dose or in immunocompromised patients or immunocompromised household contacts of vaccinees. Therefore, the injectable polio vaccine is preferred for adults who have not completed the primary series or who have immunocompromised household members. For travelers with no prior polio immunization, the complete series of three doses should be administered when possible.

Younger children are at potential risk for invasive *Haemophilus influenza* B infections when traveling and should have *H. influenzae* vaccination. The indications for pneumococcal and influenza vaccines are similar for travelers as for people who remain in the United States or other developed countries. It should be remembered that influenza occurs almost exclusively in the winter, and that travel from the northern to the southern hemisphere may result in a different pattern of exposure that might otherwise be expected. In equatorial regions, relatively little seasonality of influenza transmission exists.

Immunizations Used Primarily for Travelers

A number of immunizations should be considered for travelers, depending on the location, duration, and other features of their travel (see Table 43-2). Hepatitis A is the most common vaccine-preventable disease in travelers and should be offered to all travelers older than 2 years of age who are traveling to developing or semideveloped countries. The risk of typhoid is significantly lower but should also be considered for travelers to these same areas, especially those with prolonged travel or potential for more intense exposure. Yellow fever vaccine should be administered to travelers to most of the tropical and subtropical areas of South America and Africa. Rabies, JE, meningococcal, and hepatitis B vaccines are used for selected travelers or locations of travel, and cholera vaccine should rarely, if ever, be used.

Chemoprophylaxis and Chemotherapy

Chemoprophylaxis and chemotherapy are used primarily for prevention of malaria and treatment of traveler's diarrhea. Obviously, other specific infections should be treated as appropriate. Preventive therapy with isoniazid should be administered to travelers with documented skin test conversion.

Insect Control

A number of important diseases, including malaria, yellow fever, dengue, and many forms of encephalitis (e.g., JE), are spread by mosquitoes and flies (e.g., leishmaniasis, African trypanosomiasis, onchocerciasis). Many of these insects bite at dusk, so the risk is highest at that time. In general, the risk of mosquito-borne infections is greater in rural than in urban areas. Exposure can be reduced in the following ways:

1. Remaining in enclosed or screened areas at dusk.
2. Protective clothing (hats, long-sleeved shirts, long pants) should be worn at all times and can be treated with permethrin-containing insect repellent for added protection.
3. Outside sleeping areas should be completely covered with mosquito netting. Ideally, the mosquito netting should be treated with permethrin.
4. Applying insect repellent containing 25% diethyltoluamide to exposed skin surfaces. (Higher concentrations are toxic and lower concentrations are less effective.)

Water and Food Precautions

Because the agents of traveler's diarrhea in addition to *S. typhi*, hepatitis A and E, brucellosis, and some of the intestinal helminths, are transmitted by the fecal-oral route, many of these infections can be prevented by avoidance of contaminated food and water.

Bottled carbonated beverages are usually safe and readily available, and provide the best approach for most short-term tourists. Bottled, noncarbonated water is probably safer than tap water in many places, but its safety cannot be assured. Use of ice, brushing of teeth with tap water, or drinking shower or swimming water should be avoided.

Boiling water for 1 minute, even at high altitudes, is very effective. In fact, 15 minutes at 65°C (150°F) kills most of the enterically transmitted pathogens. Coffee and tea are usually made with boiling or nearly boiling water and are generally safe to drink.

Halogenation with iodine or chlorine (iodine is preferable) is also quite effective for the viral and bacterial pathogens, but is less consistently effective for *G. lamblia*. This can be accomplished by adding five drops of 2% tincture of iodine (ten drops for cloudy or cold water) and allowing it to stand for at least 30 minutes (several hours for the cloudy water). Alternatively, tetraglycine hydroperiodide tablets (e.g., Globaline, Potable-Agua, Coghlan's) can be used according to the manufacturer's directions.

Bacteria and parasites can be removed by filtering through a pore size of 1 μm or less. Viruses are not removed by this method, but some filters have a charcoal adsorption system that removes at least some of the viruses. When using a filter, contamination of the outflow tract of the filter must be avoided. Fewer data exist concerning the efficacy of filtration; therefore, the other methods are generally preferred.

The risk for acquisition of infection from food varies widely with the type of food. Therefore, foods can be divided into risky or relatively safe categories. Boiled, baked, or fried foods have generally been heated long enough to destroy the enterically transmitted pathogens and can be considered relatively safe. However, the risk of food poisoning still exists from heat-stable toxins (e.g., *Staphylococcus aureus*). These foods can also be contaminated when stored improperly after being heated or when contaminated utensils are used. Fruits with a thick removable peel (e.g., citrus) are generally safe.

Foods that are not adequately heated to destroy the pathogens or in which contamination is allowed to occur after heating should be avoided. Unpasteurized dairy products (including soft cheeses) may transmit salmonellosis, brucellosis, or listeriosis. Undercooked meats are a potential source for trichinosis (especially pork), *Campylobacter* (especially poultry), salmonellosis (especially poultry), and other bacterial and parasitic infections. Raw fruits or vegetables are commonly contaminated with a variety of enterically transmitted viral, bacterial, protozoan, and helminthic agents as a result of handling or from the use of animal or human excrement as fertilizer.

Food from street vendors or buffets is frequently kept for long periods of time at the ideal incubation temperature for the enterically transmitted bacteria and should generally be avoided.

Some fish and shellfish found in the tropical areas of the West Indies, Pacific Ocean, and Indian Ocean contain heat-stable toxins (especially ciguatera toxins) with a variety of clinical manifestations. Barracuda and, to a lesser extent, red snappers, groupers, and other fish may contain the toxins.

Freshwater Swimming

Some of the bodies of freshwater in the tropical or subtropical regions have the snails that transmit schistosomiasis. Swimming or wading in these areas should be avoided.

Needles and Blood Transfusions

Needles are frequently reused in the developing countries, and often the techniques used are inadequate to assure complete sterilization. Blood and blood products in many of the developing countries are not adequately tested for HIV, hepatitis B and C, or other pathogens.

REFERENCES

1. Anonymous. *Health information for international travel 1996–97*. Atlanta: Centers for Disease Control and Prevention, 1997.
2. Thompson RE. *Travel and routine immunizations*. Milwaukee: Shoreland, 1997.
3. DuPont HL, Ericsson CD. Prevention and treatment of traveler's diarrhea [See comments] [Review]. *N Engl J Med* 1993;328:1821–1827.
4. Wyler DJ. Malaria chemoprophylaxis for the traveler [Review]. *N Engl J Med* 1993;329:31–37.
5. Committee on Infectious Diseases. *1997 red book: report of the committee on infectious diseases*. Elk Grove Village, IL: American Academy of Pediatrics, 1997.
6. Gardner P, Eickhoff T, Poland GA, et al. Adult immunizations, part 1. *Ann Intern Med* 1996;124:35–40.
7. Barnett ED, Chen R. Children and international travel: immunizations [See comments] [Review]. *Pediatr Infect Dis J* 1995;14:982–992.
8. Gardner P, Schaffner W. Immunization of adults [See comments] [Review]. *N Engl J Med* 1993;328:1252–1258.
9. Ericsson CD, Johnson PC, DuPont HL, Morgan DR, Bitsura JA, de la Cabada FJ. Ciprofloxacin or trimethoprim-sulfamethoxazole as initial therapy for travelers' diarrhea: a placebo-controlled, randomized trial. *Ann Intern Med* 1987;106:216–220.
10. Salam I, Katelaris P, Leigh-Smith S, Farthing MJ. Randomised trial of single-dose ciprofloxacin for travelers' diarrhoea [See comments]. *Lancet* 1994; 344:1537–1539.
11. Murphy GS, Bodhidatta L, Echeverria P, et al. Ciprofloxacin and loperamide in the treatment of bacillary dysentery. *Ann Intern Med* 1993;118:582–586.
12. Petruccelli BP, Murphy GS, Sanchez JL, et al. Treatment of traveler's diarrhea with ciprofloxacin and loperamide. *J Infect Dis* 1992;165:557–560.
13. Trofa AF, DeFraites RF, Smoak BL, et al. Dengue fever in U.S. military personnel in Haiti. *JAMA* 1997;277:1546–1548.
14. Robertson SE, Hull BP, Tomori O, Bele O, LeDuc JW, Esteves K. Yellow fever: a decade of reemergence [Review]. *JAMA* 1996;276:1157–1162.
15. Ohrt C, Richie TL, Widjaja H, et al. Mefloquine compared with doxycycline for the prophylaxis of malaria in Indonesian soldiers: a randomized, double-blind, placebo-controlled trial. *Ann Intern Med* 1997;126:963–972.
16. Steffen R, Rickenbach M, Wilhelm U, Helminger A, Schar M. Health problems after travel to developing countries. *J Infect Dis* 1987;156:84–91.
17. D'Hondt E, Purcell RH, Emerson SU, Wong DC, Shapiro M, Govindarajan S. Efficacy of an inactivated hepatitis A vaccine in pre- and postexposure conditions in marmosets. *J Infect Dis* 1995;171[Suppl 1]:S40–S43.
18. Werzberger A, Mensch B, Kuter B, et al. A controlled trial of a formalin-inactivated hepatitis A vaccine in healthy children [See comments]. *N Engl J Med* 1992;327:453–457.
19. Piazza M, Sagliocca L, Tosone G, et al. Sexual transmission of the hepatitis C virus and efficacy of prophylaxis with intramuscular immune serum globulin: a randomized controlled trial. *Arch Intern Med* 1997;157:1537–1544.
20. Hoke CH, Nisalak A, Sangawhipa N, et al. Protection against Japanese encephalitis by inactivated vaccines. *N Engl J Med* 1988;319:608–614.
21. Berg SW, Mitchell BS, Hanson RK, et al. Systemic reactions in U.S. Marine Corps personnel who received Japanese encephalitis vaccine. *Clin Infect Dis* 1997;24:265–266.
22. Markovitz DM. Infection with the human immunodeficiency virus type 2. [Review]. *Ann Intern Med* 1993;118:211–218.
23. Poulsen AG, Aaby P, Larsen O, et al. 9-year HIV-2-associated mortality in an urban community in Bissau, West Africa. *Lancet* 1997;349:911–914.
24. Deschamps MM, Pape JW, Hafner A, Johnson WD Jr. Heterosexual transmission of HIV in Haiti. *Ann Intern Med* 1996;125:324–330.

25. Saracco A, Musicco M, Nicolosi A, et al. Man-to-woman sexual transmission of HIV: longitudinal study of 343 steady partners of infected men. *J Acquir Immune Defic Syndr Hum Retrovirol* 1993;6:497–502.
26. de Vincenzi I. A longitudinal study of human immunodeficiency virus transmission by heterosexual partners. European Study Group on Heterosexual Transmission of HIV [see comments]. *N Engl J Med* 1994;331:341–346.
27. Nelson KE, Celentano DD, Eiumtrakol S, et al. Changes in sexual behavior and a decline in HIV infection among young men in Thailand [see comments]. *N Engl J Med* 1996;335:297–303.
28. Visser LG, Polderman AM, Stuiver PC. Outbreak of schistosomiasis among travelers returning from Mali, West Africa. *Clin Infect Dis* 1995;20:280–285.
29. Caumes E, Carriere J, Guermonprez G, Bricaire F, Danis M, Gentilini M. Dermatoses associated with travel to tropical countries: a prospective study of the diagnosis and management of 269 patients presenting to a tropical disease unit. *Clin Infect Dis* 1995;20:542–548.
30. Phillips-Howard PA, Wood D. The safety of antimalarial drugs in pregnancy [Review]. *Drug Saf* 1996;14:131–145.
31. Anonymous. Case-control study of HIV seroconversion in health-care workers after percutaneous exposure to HIV-infected blood: France, United Kingdom, and United States, January 1988–August 1994. *MMWR Morb Mortal Wkly Rep* 1995;44:929–933.
32. Anonymous. Update: provisional Public Health Service recommendations for chemoprophylaxis after occupational exposure to HIV. *MMWR Morb Mortal Wkly Rep* 1996;45:468–480.
33. Centers for Disease Control and Prevention. Public Health Service guidelines for the management of health-care worker exposures to HIV and recommendations for postexposure prophylaxis. *MMWR Morb Mortal Wkly Rep* 1998;47:1–33.

CHAPTER 44

Pulp and Paper Industry Hazards

Melanie A. Marty and Dennis J. Shusterman

The pulp industry in the United States annually produces approximately 54 million metric tons of cellulose material for the subsequent manufacture of paper, cardboard, and fiberboard, or almost one-quarter ton per capita (1). The process of transforming a corresponding volume of wood chips into pulp requires large-scale industrial facilities with major economic, environmental, and aesthetic impacts on adjoining communities. A long-standing public awareness of the nuisance quality of odorous air emissions from pulp mills has been joined by concerns regarding compounds of potential toxicologic significance in the mills' air and water effluent. In addition, intensive use of a variety of hazardous materials raises inevitable questions regarding worker health and safety.

PROCESS DESCRIPTION

Pulp mills function to extract and process cellulose fibers from wood, simultaneously removing unwanted constituents, such as lignin (wood's intercellular glue). The majority of pulp mills operating in the United States use the sulfate or *kraft* method. This method relies heavily on chemical digestion. Perhaps 20% of domestic pulp production involves nonkraft processes, including the groundwood, semichemical, and sulfite techniques (1). Because of the small fraction of production represented by each of these methods, our detailed consideration of production processes will be limited to kraft mills.

Figure 44-1 is a simplified process diagram for a kraft mill. Included in this representation are input (raw materials), output (product and by-products), and closed-loop (recycled) processes. The principal raw materials for the kraft process are

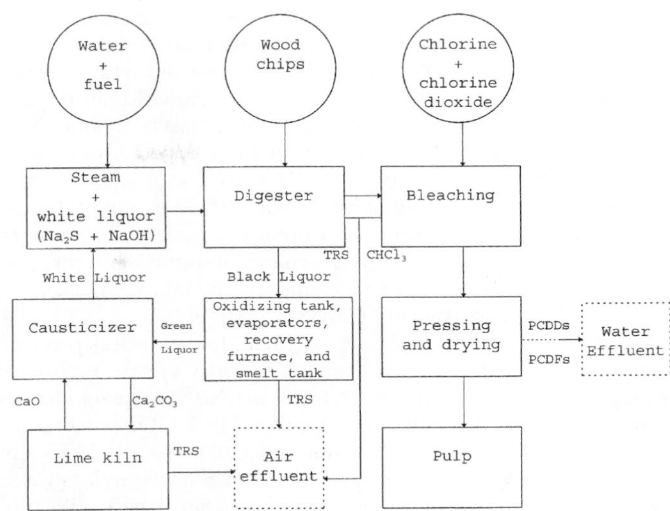

Figure 44-1. Process diagram for a kraft mill. PCDDs, polychlorinated dibenzo-*p*-dioxins; PCDFs, polychlorinated dibenzofurans; TRS, total reduced sulfur.

wood chips, water, fuel, and bleaching agents (most commonly chlorine and chlorine dioxide). Sodium sulfide (used in the digestion of the pulp) is recycled through operation of the recovery furnace, evaporators, and lime kiln; however, the escape of even a small fraction of the recirculating sulfur (as hydrogen sulfide, organic sulfides, and various mercaptans) gives pulp mill air emissions their characteristic odor.

The operation of a kraft pulp mill can be summarized this way: Wood chips are broken down by a combination of sodium sulfide (in basic solution) and heat. The resulting pulp is washed and bleached with a combination of molecular chlorine and chlorine dioxide or hypochlorite. The washed pulp is rolled and dried, and the dried pulp cut and baled for shipment. Wastewater from the bleaching process is typically discharged directly or with minimal treatment (e.g., an aerated stabilization basin) into a nearby body of water. Spent digester fluid is concentrated in evaporators and fed into the recovery furnace, which recycles solid sodium sulfide and combusts the dissolved lignin as a source of energy. A lime kiln recovers calcium oxide for regeneration of the caustic component of the digester fluid (2–4).

AIRBORNE EMISSIONS FROM KRAFT PULP MILLS

Irritant and Odorant Chemicals

Reduced sulfur compounds are remarkable for their odorant potency; the odor threshold of ethyl mercaptan, for example, has been measured as low as 0.01 parts per billion (ppb) (5). The U.S. Environmental Protection Agency (EPA), which has regulated pulp mill emissions since 1978, has formulated an aggregate measure of reduced sulfur gas emissions from pulp mills known as *total reduced sulfur (TRS)*. Principal sources of TRS emissions in pulp mills include the lime kiln and main recovery furnace (as stack gases) and various rooftop sources (e.g., offgasing from the digester). Operational upsets (e.g., breached seals on the digester) can produce significant transients in TRS emissions.

The single most prominent fraction of pulp mill TRS is hydrogen sulfide (H_2S). Published odor thresholds for H_2S range from 0.5 to 20 ppb, with a geometric mean of 8.1 ppb (5,6). Upper-respiratory irritation does not occur below approximately 10 parts per million (ppm). Objective signs of H_2S upper-respiratory irritation occur between 50 and 100 ppm. Concentrations in the range of

100 to 200 ppm produce olfactory fatigue, whereas 250 to 500 ppm exposures have been associated with pulmonary edema. Exposures in the 500- to 1,000-ppm range are associated with systemic toxicity, including confusion, dysequilibrium, convulsions, respiratory paralysis, and death (7). Systemic toxicity has been thought to occur via inhibition of the cytochrome oxidase system (in a manner analogous to cyanide), although a 1992 study documents hyperpolarization of neurons with normal Na^+/K^+ adenosine triphosphatase activity (8). Experimental human exposures to H_2S (2 ppm × 30 min) resulted in no significant change in pulmonary function among 26 male pulp mill workers and in only minor changes in a subset of asthmatics (two out of ten studied) (9).

Controversy exists regarding whether H_2S exposures produce subacute or chronic effects. The vast majority of case reports of severe H_2S intoxication (those involving loss of consciousness with or without convulsions) report either a fatal outcome or recovery without permanent sequelae (10,11). The World Health Organization defines chronic, low-level H_2S exposures as those occurring between 50 and 100 ppm and associates these with "lingering, largely subjective manifestations of illness" (12). In experimental systems, mice exposed to 100 ppm H_2S by inhalation for 2 hours a day over 4 days showed progressive inhibition of cerebral cytochrome oxidase activity (13), whereas guinea pigs exposed to 20 ppm of H_2S for 1 hour per day over 11 days showed significant lowering of phospholipid concentrations in the cerebral hemispheres and brainstem, but not in the cerebellum (14). The human health significance of these animal observations is unclear.

The other reduced sulfur gases of concern in pulp mill air emissions—methyl mercaptan, dimethyl sulfide, and dimethyl disulfide—have been less extensively studied than hydrogen sulfide but appear to exhibit the same general toxicologic properties (15,16). Reported odor thresholds for methyl mercaptan range from 0.02 to 42.00 ppb, with a geometric mean of 1.6 ppb; for dimethyl sulfide, the range is 1 to 20 ppb, with a mean value of 11 ppb; and for dimethyl disulfide, the corresponding values are 0.3, 90, and 41 ppb (5,6). The relative odorant potencies of these compounds exceed their irritant and systemic toxicity by an even greater factor than is the case for hydrogen sulfide, making it difficult for irritant or toxic exposures to occur, except in situations of impaired escape.

Approximately 600,000 tons of sulfur dioxide (SO_2) are emitted from pulp and paper manufacturing in the United States (17). The major sources are boilers used to generate steam and electricity. Kraft pulp mill recovery furnaces, lime kilns, and reduced sulfur gas oxidation units are also significant sources. In contrast to the reduced sulfur gases, sulfur dioxide—an odorant at greater than approximately 0.5 ppm and a respiratory irritant at greater than 2 ppm (5)—has relatively poor warning properties. Asthmatics may be sensitive to SO_2 concentrations as low as 0.25 to 0.3 ppm, particularly when exercising (18,19). Community monitoring for SO_2 is required under the federal Clean Air Act, but given the dilution factor from stack to community, it is more likely to pose a hazard to pulp mill workers than to the general public (20). For example, acute SO_2 overexposures among pulp mill workers have resulted in immediate fatalities and in the development of chronic, irreversible airflow obstruction, with or without bronchiolitis obliterans (21–23). Similarly, pulp mill workers who report having been exposed to leaks of chlorine or chlorine dioxide—two other irritant gases—appear to be at risk for developing subsequent obstructive pulmonary symptoms and spirometric abnormalities, as reviewed in the section Occupational Epidemiology for Kraft Pulp Mill Workers.

Combustion processes at pulp and paper mills result in the emissions of approximately 300,000 tons of nitrogen oxides per year in the United States (17). The major sources are boilers; minor sources include kraft mill recovery furnaces and lime kilns. Nitrogen oxides are irritant gases and major contributors to the formation of photochemical smog.

Table 44-1 summarizes the toxicology and occupational exposure standards for irritant and odorant chemicals used in (or emitted from) kraft pulp mills, including digester chemicals, bleaching agents, reduced sulfur gases, and sulfur dioxide. The occupational standard for hydrogen sulfide exposure, for example, has been set by the Occupational Safety and Health Administration at 20 ppm (ceiling value), based on the compound's irritancy (24). California treats H_2S as an ambient criteria pollutant with a 1-hour ambient standard of 30 ppb; this level was set at a multiple of the odor threshold calculated to produce an annoyance reaction in the public (25). Sulfur dioxide is regulated

TABLE 44-1. Irritant and odorant chemicals in the kraft pulp process

Source	Chemical	Toxicity	ACGIH TLV-TWA	OSHA PEL-TWA
Processing				
Digestion	Sodium sulfide	Caustic; skin, eye, and upper respiratory irritant	10 ppm	20 ppm[b] (H_2S)
			15 ppm[a] (H_2S)	—
	Sodium hydroxide	Caustic: skin, eye, and upper respiratory irritant	2 mg/m[a]	2 mg/m
	Anthraquinone	Phototoxic dermatitis	—	—
Bleaching	Chlorine gas	Upper and lower respiratory irritant	0.5 ppm	1.0 ppm[b]
			1.0 ppm[a]	—
	Chlorine dioxide	Upper and lower respiratory irritant	0.1 ppm	0.1 ppm
			0.3 ppm[a]	—
Effluent				
Air	Hydrogen sulfide	Odorant: upper and lower respiratory irritant; cellular poison	10 ppm	20 ppm[b]
	Methyl mercaptan	Odorant: upper and lower respiratory irritant; cellular poison	0.5 ppm	10 ppm[b]
	Dimethyl sulfide	Odorant: upper and lower respiratory irritant; cellular poison	—	—
	Dimethyl disulfide	Odorant: upper and lower respiratory irritant; cellular poison	—	—
	Sulfur dioxide	Upper and lower respiratory irritant; bronchoconstrictor	2 ppm	5 ppm
			5 ppm[a]	—

ACGIH, American Conference of Governmental Industrial Hygienists; OSHA, Occupational Safety and Health Administration; PEL-TWA, permissible exposure limit–(8-hour) time-weighted average (enforceable standard of OSHA); TLV-TWA, threshold limit value–(8 hour) time-weighted average (recommended standard of ACGIH).
[a]Short-term exposure limit—15-minute time-weighted average not to be exceeded during workday.
[b]Ceiling standard—Not to be exceeded at any time.
Adapted from American Conference of Governmental Industrial Hygienists. *Threshold limit values and biological exposure indices for 1996–1997.* Cincinnati: ACGIH, 1996; and U.S. Department of Labor Occupational Safety and Health Administration. Air contaminants: final rule. 29 *CFR* Part 1910. *Fed Regist* 1993;58(124):35338–35351.

at the federal level as a criteria pollutant, with an annual average limit of 0.03 ppm and a 24-hour standard of 0.14 ppm. California has a lower (0.05 ppm) 24-hour SO_2 standard, as well as a 0.25 ppm 1-hour limit. By contrast, the occupational exposure limit for SO_2 is 5 ppm averaged over 8 hours.

Industrial hygiene surveys of kraft pulp mills have documented peak H_2S levels within work areas to 20 ppm (with mean levels between 0.05 and 2.0 ppm) and peak methyl mercaptan levels to 15 ppm (mean levels between 0.07 and 3.7 ppm). Specific locations with high-exposure potential include the chip chute and evaporation vacuum pumps. Sulfur dioxide tends to be more of a problem in sulfite mills, with peak levels to 23 ppm (mean levels ranging from 0.05 to 5.7 ppm) (20). Because of the oxidizing environment of the recovery furnace and lime kiln, most H_2S entering these combustion devices is converted to sulfur dioxide. Given the further dilution of stack and fugitive emissions as they disperse off site, community exposures to reduced sulfur gases are generally in the low ppb range, greater than the odor threshold but less than levels known to produce objective irritant effects.

CHLORINATED COMPOUNDS

The major chlorinated hydrocarbon emitted into ambient air from bleached kraft pulp mills is chloroform. The EPA estimates that approximately 3,340 mg of chloroform per year is emitted from the pulp and paper industry, accounting for 40% of all chloroform air emissions in the United States (26). Chloroform is produced during the pulp bleaching process by the reaction of chlorine or chlorine compounds and lignins in the pulp suspension, followed by degradation of chlorinated lignins in the alkaline extraction stage. The chloroform subsequently evaporates into the air from the wastewater stream. Use of hypochlorite for bleaching pulp results in the greatest production of chloroform. Substitution of chlorine dioxide for hypochlorite salts has been suggested as a control measure for chloroform that would result in a 92% reduction in chloroform emissions from pulp mills (26).

Chloroform is acutely toxic at high concentrations (e.g., anesthetic concentrations of 5,000 ppm), producing adverse effects in the liver and kidney, the cardiovascular system, and the central nervous system. At concentrations in ambient air, one would not expect acute or chronic noncancer health effects to occur (27). The major concern in terms of public health is a potential increased risk of cancer from inhalation of chloroform in ambient air. Chloroform carcinogenic potency and classification are summarized in Table 44-2.

Other halogenated volatile organic compounds that may become airborne as a result of evaporation from wastewater include methylene chloride, trichloroethylene, tetrachloroethylene, carbon tetrachloride, bromodichloromethane, and chlorodibromomethane. All of these compounds are mutagenic, and the first four have tested positive in animal carcinogenicity bioassays. As is the case for chloroform, the major public health concern would be a potential increase in the risk of cancer from inhalation of these compounds in ambient air.

No studies have adequately documented concentrations of volatile halogenated organic compounds in ambient air near pulp mills. However, measurements of chloroform in many locations in California (not near pulp mills) indicate that chloroform is a ubiquitous contaminant of ambient air, with concentrations ranging from 0.13 to 1.8 μg chloroform per m^3 of air. The excess cancer risk could range to approximately 5 in 1 million from inhalation of chloroform in ambient air (27). The risk in a community surrounding a major source of chloroform, such as a pulp mill, could conceivably be higher.

The concentrations of 2,3,7,8-tetrachlorodibenzo-*p*-dioxin (TCDD) toxic equivalents in the stack gases of three kraft mill recovery furnaces were less than 0.01, 0.01, and 0.12 ng per dry standard cubic meter (dscm) at 3% O_2 (28). These data indicate that recovery furnaces are not as important a source of environmental polychlorinated dibenzo-*p*-dioxins (PCDDs) and dibenzofurans (PCDFs) as other combustion sources.

TABLE 44-2. Some carcinogens present in bleached kraft mill effluent

Compound	Class[a]	Cancer potency[b]
Benzene	A	2.9×10^{-2}
Carbon tetrachloride	B2	1.3×10^{-1}
Chloroform	B2	8.1×10^{-2}
1,2-Dichloroethane	B2	9.1×10^{-2}
Hexachlorobenzene	B2	1.7
Hexachlorodibenzodioxin	B2	$6.2 \times 10^{+3}$
Methylene chloride	B2	1.4×10^{-2}
2,3,7,8-Tetrachlorodibenzo-*p*-dioxin (and related congeners)	B2	$1.6 \times 10^{+5}$
Tetrachloroethylene	B2	5.1×10^{-2}
Trichloroethylene	B2	1.1×10^{-2}
2,4,6-Trichlorophenol	B2	2.0×10^{-2}

[a]Classification of carcinogen under the U.S. Environmental Protection Agency. A, sufficient evidence of carcinogenicity in humans and animals; B2, inadequate evidence of carcinogenicity in humans and sufficient evidence of carcinogenicity in animals.
[b]These cancer potency values, expressed in units of inverse dose $(mg/kg\text{-}day)^{-1}$, were derived by the U.S. Environmental Protection Agency. When multiplied by lifetime dose, the product is the theoretical lifetime risk of contracting cancer when exposed to the chemical at the given dose level.

Measurements of 2,3,7,8-TCDD toxic equivalents in workplace air at a bleaching plant and the paper and paperboard production lines of a paper mill ranged between 0.002 and 0.2 pg per m^3 (29). The only dioxin congeners quantifiable at the subpicogram per m^3 level were 1,2,3,6,7,8-hexachloro- and 1,2,3,4,6,7,8-heptachlorodibenzo-*p*-dioxin. No 2,3,7,8-TCDD was detected in any sample, and no PCDDs were detected at the bleaching plant. However, PCDFs were found at the bleaching plant with 2,3,7,8-tetrachlorodibenzofuran (TCDF) representing the majority (0.49 to 0.64 pg per m^3). Chlorinated furans were the major components in all samples from the paper and paperboard production lines. The highest concentration of a furan encountered on the paperboard production line was 1.9 pg per m^3 for 1,2,3,4,6,7,8-heptachlorodibenzofuran. The congener profile of the paper dust was mirrored in the air samples. This study indicates the potential for workplace inhalation exposure to PCDD/PCDF in the pulp and paper industry.

PARTICULATE EMISSIONS

Particulate emission sources at a pulp mill include the kraft recovery furnaces, lime kilns, smelt dissolving tanks, and power boilers, which are frequently wood fired (30). The typical kraft recovery furnace equipped with an electrostatic precipitator emits approximately 0.2 g particulate per m^3, mainly as sodium salts and black ash, with mass mean diameters on the order of 1.5 μm. Average emissions from existing lime kilns controlled with Venturi scrubbers are approximately 0.15 to 0.3 g particulate per m^3. Particulates from the lime kilns consist of relatively large (greater than 10 μm) particles of lime dust and small (mass mean diameter less than 1 μm) particles of sodium sulfate and sodium carbonate. Smelt dissolving tanks emit primarily sodium sulfate and sodium carbonate particles less than 1 μm in mass mean particle diameter at rates of approximately 0.1 g particulate per m^3.

EPA estimates the production of particulate from the recovery furnace at 0.5 to 12 kg per thousand kilograms (kkg) of product. Estimates for other units include 0.01 to 0.5 kg per kkg from smelt dissolving tanks, 0.15 to 2.5 kg per kkg from lime kilns, and 0.012 to 0.4 kg per kkg from power boilers (31).

The major health impacts of particulate emissions depends on the particle size distribution, air dispersion, and dilution, and possibly on the chemical composition of the particles. Few data exist that quantify particulate matter in the ambient air surrounding pulp mills. However, the potential exists for adverse respiratory health effects under appropriate meteorologic conditions, particularly from small particles (e.g., respirable particles 1 to 10 μm in diameter) of lime and sulfates that escape from the lime kilns and smelt tanks. A 1993 epidemiologic study demonstrates a link between particulate matter in ambient air and respiratory and cardiovascular morbidity and mortality, irrespective of the composition of the particles (32).

Waterborne Emissions from Kraft Pulp Mills

The kraft pulping process results in production of a large amount of contaminated water that is discharged—usually with little treatment—into a receiving body of water. The processes of wood digestion and subsequent bleaching produce an enormous number of chemicals, many of them chlorinated. Hundreds of these chemicals have been identified (33–36) and associated with a particular process or bleaching stage within the kraft mill (36–42). The compounds formed vary with the type of wood being processed as well as with the process itself. Among the compounds identified in bleached kraft pulp mill effluents are resin acids; organic acids and their chlorinated derivatives; small-chain volatile chlorinated organic compounds; chlorinated phenols, guaiacols, catechols, vanillins, benzenes, cymenes, aldehydes, ketones, thiophenes, and terpenes; and large polycyclic compounds, including PCDDs and PCDFs. Resin acids and fatty acids degrade readily; however, some chlorinated compounds persist in the aquatic environment (43). Abietan-18-oic acid and dehydroabietic acid are dominant resin acids identified in one study (35). It has been estimated that a kraft mill with production of 1,000 tons of pulp per day using conventional chlorine bleaching produces 50 to 65 tons of chlorinated organic substances per day and discharges 30 to 40 million gallons effluent per day (44–45). Estimation of the concentrations of some of these compounds in treated and raw effluent is found in Table 44-3.

Chlorophenolics, PCDD, and PCDF have been measured in suspended sediments downstream of pulp mills (46). Concentrations dropped between 200- and 1,000-fold after substitution of chlorine bleaching with chlorine dioxide bleaching. Several studies identified a number of compounds in river bottom sediment downstream from bleached kraft mill effluent (BKME) discharge. Fatty acids, resin acids, fichtelite, and dehydroabietin were detected in the ppm range (35). In addition, PCDD and PCDF have been identified in river bottom sediment. Switching from chlorine bleaching to chlorine dioxide and further to ozonation decreases the sediment load of chlorinated compounds. Chlorinated phenolics would drop much more rapidly than PCDD and PCDF because of the latter's resistance to degradation.

Concern has been building about the production of PCDDs and PCDFs in the pulp mill bleaching processes and the resulting environmental contamination with these highly toxic compounds. The EPA analyzed samples of fish from many bodies of water in the United States and noticed a correlation between levels of 2,3,7,8-tetrachlorodibenzo-*p*-dioxin in fish tissue and the frequency of pulp and paper manufacturing plants in the watershed of contaminated fish (47). The EPA and the paper industry conducted a joint study to document the extent of dioxins discharged by the industry. The study sampled effluent, sludges, and pulp at each of 104 pulp mills in the United States that bleach with chlorine for 2,3,7,8-TCDD and 2,3,7,8-TCDF (48). Median concentrations of 2,3,7,8-TCDD and 2,3,7,8-TCDF in bleached pulps were 6.4 and 18 ppt, respectively. Wastewater effluent median concentrations were 42 ppq 2,3,7,8-TCDD and 120 ppq 2,3,7,8-TCDF. Sludge contained 63 ppt 2,3,7,8-TCDD and 233 ppt 2,3,7,8-TCDF. Taking into account the volume of the product/waste streams, approximately one-third of the total TCDD and TCDF produced appears in each stream.

Keuhl and colleagues found that samples of sludge from seven pulp and paper mill plants contained 2,3,7,8-TCDD ranging from undetectable at 1 pg per g to 414 pg per g (49). The variability is probably the result of different process parameters at the different mills. Sludge from one mill was characterized further; this sample contained 1,860 pg octaCDD (chlorinated dibenzo-para-dioxin) per g, 800 pg 2,3,7,8-TCDF per g, 640 pg other TCDF per g, and 150 pg 2,3,7,8-TCDD per g. The presence of PCDDs and PCDFs in pulp mill sludge has raised concern about the practice of using pulp mill sludge to amend soil with concomitant contamination of the environment, particularly with respect to contamination of the agricultural food chain (50).

The pulp, filtrate, and fines from an 850 T per day bleached softwood kraft pulp mill contained approximately 90 to 100 pg 2,3,7,8-TCDF per g and approximately 10 pg 2,3,7,8-TCDD per g after the first chlorination stage (41). Gas chromatography and mass spectrometry chromatograms revealed that the predominant isomers were 1,2,7,8- and 2,3,7,8-TCDF and 2,3,7,8-TCDD. A 1988 study documented the presence of ppt levels of PCDDs and PCDFs in finished paper products, including newsprint, coffee filters, cosmetic tissue, and recycled scrap paper (51).

Several studies have shown that the pulp bleaching processes substantially influence the formation of chlorinated compounds (36,41,46,48,49,52–54). Substitution of chlorine dioxide for chlorine, a reduction in the ratio of chlorine to lignin, elimination of hypochlorite, and use of oxygen delignification result in significant drops in the production of PCDDs, PCDFs, chlorinated phenols, cymenes, and cymenenes.

The toxicity of kraft pulp mill effluents to fish has been extensively studied and is summarized in the following sections about effluents. There is a limited amount of published toxicologic data for a handful of the compounds present in pulp mill effluent. Mutagenicity and carcinogenicity of some important constituents of pulp mill effluent are reviewed in the sections below. A review describes other toxicologic endpoints of some constituents of BKME (28).

AQUATIC TOXICITY

The constituents of BKME considered to be most toxic to fish are resin acids, chlorinated phenolics, and low-molecular-weight chlorinated neutral compounds (55,56). In addition, decreased dissolved oxygen levels downstream affect the survival of aquatic organisms (35). 2,6-Dichlorohydroquinone and some polychlorodihydroxybenzenes have also been implicated as acute toxicants present in first chlorination stage effluents (39,57). The higher chlorinated phenolics are more toxic to a number of aquatic species than are the lower chlorinated phenolics (42).

Neutralized BKME (without further treatment) commonly has 96-hour median lethal concentration (LC_{50}) values ranging from 15% to 50% (vol/vol) (57). Exposures to various concentrations of BKME resulted in a number of adverse physiologic and biochemical changes in a variety of fish species (57–65). Adverse effects in fish have been noted in the laboratory and in the field in fish caught near effluent outflows. Such changes included decreased swimming speed and stamina, changes in respiration and arterial tension, changes in blood cell count, aberrant carbohydrate metabolism, elevated hepatic cytochrome P-450–dependent monooxygenase activities, impaired ion homeostasis, and pathologic changes in the gills and liver. Decreased resistance to skin parasites has been observed (64). Reproductive toxicity observed after exposure to BKME includes decreased egg hatch-

TABLE 44-3. Common contaminants of bleached kraft pulp mill effluents before and after biological treatment

Chemical	Pulp mill[a]	Untreated average concentration (μg/L)	Treated average concentration (μg/L)	%R[b]
Benzene	M	1	2	0
1,1,1-Trichloroethane	F	24	0	100
2,4,6-Trichlorophenol	M	11	5	55
	B	8	1	88
Chloroform	D	647	67	90
	M	1,405	12	99
	B	1,550	16	99
2,4-Dichlorophenol	M	4	4	0
	B	2	1	50
Dichlorobromomethane	D	1	0	100
	F	15	0	100
Pentachlorophenol	B	19	19	0
	F	8	1	88
Tetrachloroethylene	B	3	0	100
	F	1	0	100
Trichloroethylene	B	2	0	100
Abietic acid	D	11,800	1,467	88
	M	178	767	0
	B	1,043	119	89
	F	470	3	99
Dehydroabietic acid	D	3,500	520	99
	M	232	43	86
	B	861	123	86
	F	273	5	98
Isopimaric acid	D	887	380	57
	M	115	407	0
	B	107	21	80
	F	74	98	0
Pimaric acid	D	1,357	710	48
	M	157	430	0
	B	115	22	81
	F	63	0	100
Epoxystearic acid	D	817	0	100
Chlorodehydroabietic acid	D	1,433	473	67
	M	50	42	16
	B	78	11	86
	F	44	0	100
Dichlorodehydroabietic acid	M	57	39	32
	B	3	1	67
	F	6	0	100
Trichloroguaiacol	M	18	0	100
	B	1	0	100
	F	4	1	75
Tetrachloroguaiacol	M	11	0	100
	B	8	1	88
	F	7	3	57

[a]The data were obtained for various subcategories of bleached kraft pulp mills. B, bleached kraft pulp mills producing pulp for coarse paper uses, such as paperboard, tissue; D, bleached kraft pulp mills producing dissolving pulp, a highly refined pulp containing virtually no lignin used in the manufacture of rayon, cellophane, and cellulose acetate and nitrate; F, bleached kraft pulp mill producing fine pulp for use in printing and writing paper; M, bleached kraft pulp mill producing market pulp from wood not destined for a particular use and sold on the open market.
[b]%R—Approximate percent reduction in concentration by biological treatment. These are only approximations as they are taken from averages of a number of mills with variations in treatment. However, one can see that certain chemicals are biodegraded or volatilized more readily than others. Note the large variability in amount of chemical produced with the type of pulp produced.
Adapted from U.S. Environmental Protection Agency, 1984.

ability, decreased egg survival, developmental abnormalities, retarded growth and development, increased mortality, reduced sperm motility, and inhibited fertilization (66–72). Ecological tests of BKME demonstrated adverse effects in the marine bacterium *Photobacterium phosphoreum*, microalgae, and the water flea *Daphnia magna* (44,64,73). The highest toxicity was associated with the chlorine bleaching stage filtrates.

MUTAGENICITY OF CHEMICALS IN BLEACHED KRAFT PULP MILL EFFLUENT

Several investigators have reported that chlorination-stage effluent from bleaching of kraft pulp produced positive dose-related mutagenic responses in the Ames/*Salmonella* assay (55,74–77). The response was reduced on addition of rat liver S9 mix or after passage of the effluent through XAD-2 resin. Virtually all of the mutagenic activity was recovered in the neutral fraction, which contained compounds of moderate polarity.

Other investigators found that pulp mill effluent produces positive results in the SOS chromotest, microscreen phage induction assay, and the differential DNA repair test (43,77,78). Ozonation as a bleaching method results in lower mutagenicity in all test systems relative to chlorine dioxide bleaching. Activated sludge treatment of the ozone-bleached effluent further reduced mutagenicity (77). Polar water-soluble material from BKME produced at

TABLE 44-4. Some mutagenic constituents of bleached kraft mill effluent

Compound	Test[a]	Strain/cell[b]	Concentration[c]	Reference number
Neoabietic acid	Ames/*Salm*	TA1535, TA100, TA1538, TA98	250–1,000 μg/plate	81
	Reversion, Trp+	*S. cerevisiae* XV185-14C	100–1,000 μg/mL	88
1,1,2,3-Tetrachloro-2-propene	Ames/*Salm*	A1535, TA100, TA98	10 μg/plate	81
	Fluctuation	TA1535	0.2 μM	88
	Fluctuation	*E. coli* WP2	0.1 mM	82
	Reversion	*S. cerevisiae*	0.1–0.4 μL/mL	88
	Sister chromatid exchange	CHO	0.1 mM	82
	Chromosomal aberration	CHO	1.0, 5.0 mM	82
1,1,2,3,3-Pentachloropropene	Ames/*Salm*	TA1535, TA100	10 μg/plate	81
	Reversion, Trp+, Hom+	*S. cerevisiae*	0.1–0.2 μL/mL	88
1,2-dichloroethane	Ames/*Salm*, desiccator	TA1535, TA100	3–9 mg/plate	81
	Conversion, Trp+	*S. cerevisiae*, D7	0.001–0.1 μL/mL	88
1,3-dichloroacetone	Ames/*Salm*	TA1535	4.5 μg/plate[d]	76
	Conversion, Trp+	*S. cerevisiae*, D7	0.0001–0.01 μg/mL	88
2-chloropropenal	Ames/*Salm*	TA1535	0.1 μg/plate[e]	76
Trichloroethylene	Ames/*Salm*	TA1535	0.1 mg/plate	76
Monochloroacetaldehyde	Ames/*Salm*	TA1535	45 μg/plate	76
Trichloroacetaldehyde	Reversion Trp+	*S. cerevisiae* XV185-14C	50–1,000 μg/mL	88
3-chloro-4-(dichloromethyl)-5-hydroxy-2(5H)-furanone	Ames/*Salm*	TA100	4.5 μg/plate	83
	Chromosomal aberration	CHO	4.0 μg/mL	84
	Mitotic index	CHO	8.5 μg/mL	84
Acetovanillone	Reversion, Trp+, Hom+	*S. cerevisiae* XV185-14C	200–800 μg/mL	88
3-Chloro-*cis*-muconic acid	Reversion, Trp+, Hom+	*S. cerevisiae* XV185-14C	10–250 μg/mL	88
4,5-Dichlorocatechol	Reversion, Trp+, Hom+	*S. cerevisiae* XV185-14C	25–100 μg/mL	88
4,5-Dichloroguaiacol	Reversion, Trp+, Hom+	*S. cerevisiae* XV185-14C	25–75 μg/mL	88
Dichloromethane	Ames/*Salm*, desiccator	TA1535, TA100	0.5 mL/desiccator	81
Dibromochloromethane	Conversion, Trp+	*S. cerevisiae* D7	0.001–0.5 μL/ml	88
1,1,1, Trichloroethane	Ames/*Salm*, desiccator	TA1535, TA100	0.1–1.0 mL/desiccator	81
1,1,3-Trichloroacetone	Ames/*Salm*	TA100	0.01–0.05 μL/plate	74
	Conversion, Trp+	*S. cerevisiae* D7	0.001–0.1 μL/mL	88
1,1,1-Trichloroacetone	Conversion, Trp+	*S. cerevisiae* D7	0.001–0.1 μL/mL	88
1,1,1,3-Tetrachloroacetone	Reversion, His+	*S. cerevisiae* XV185-14C	0.0005–0.005 μL/mL	88
1,1,3,3-Tetrachloroacetone	Ames/*Salm*	TA100	0.01–0.05 μL/plate	74
	Conversion, Trp+	*S. cerevisiae* D7	0.0001–0.001 μL/mL	88
Pentachloroacetone	Ames/*Salm*	TA100	0.01–0.2 μL/plate	74
	Conversion, Trp+	*S. cerevisiae* D7	0.001–0.01 μL/mL	88
Hexachloroacetone	Ames/*Salm*	TA100	0.1–0.5 μL/plate	74
	Ames/*Salm*	TA1535	1.0 mg/plate	76
7-Oxodehydroabietic acid	Reversion, Trp+	*S. cerevisiae* XV185-14C	100–10,000 μg/mL	88
2,3,7,8-Tetrachloro-dibenzo-*p*-dioxin	Conversion	*S. cerevisiae*	?	91
	Cell transformation assay	BHK	0.025–0.250 μg/mL	94
	Mouse lymph mutation frequency	L5178Y	0.05–0.50 μg/mL	93

[a]Genotoxicity assay: Ames/*Salm*, the Ames assay using *Salmonella typhimurium* in a plate incorporation system; reversion, gene reversion assay using the yeast *Saccharomyces cerevisiae;* Conversion, gene conversion assay using *S. cerevisiae.* Loci that the reversion and conversion test systems examine are indicated in this column.
[b]The strains of *S. typhimurium* and *S. cerevisiae* are indicated in this column. Mammalian cell types used in sister chromatid exchange and cell transformation assays are CHO, Chinese hamster ovary cells; BHK, baby hamster kidney cells.
[c]Unless otherwise noted, the lowest concentration tested that produced at least a doubling in the mutation frequency, or concentration range over which a positive dose response was observed. Assays for volatile compounds were conducted by placing the compound in a desiccator containing plates of bacterial tester strains.
[d]This concentration of 1,3-dichloroacetone induced a 13-fold increase in mutation frequency relative to controls.
[e]This concentration of 2-chloropropenal induced a 20-fold increase in mutation frequency relative to controls.

a kraft mill absorbed by XAD-4 and XAD-8 resins was equally mutagenic as the whole effluent in the Ames assay without metabolic activation (79). The majority of the mutagenic activity was associated with NaOH eluents, which likely contain organic acids. Methanol eluents in the study were weakly mutagenic. Acidic and alkaline extracts of kraft mill effluent proved highly genotoxic in the SOS chromotest (78,79). The addition of S9 liver fraction containing monooxygenases reduced genotoxicity of alkaline extracts but increased the genotoxicity of suspended particulate matter extracts. The addition of liver S9 fraction also revealed the presence of nonpolar promutagenic compounds in BKME. Resin acids and chlorinated catechols and guaiacols may account for most of the genotoxicity of acidic extracts. Alkaline extracts contain chlorinated ketones and aliphatics.

Several chloroacetones and aldehydes were found to induce dose-related increases in mutation frequency in *Salmonella* (Table 44-4) (74,76). Douglas and colleagues (74) state that chloroacetones appear to be major contributors to mutagenic activity of chlorination stage effluents and that mutagenicity of a mixture of chloroacetones was greater than additive. However, levels of chloroacetones in chlorination stage effluents vary considerably. In addition, chloroacetones are labile in alkaline solution, and the contribution to mutagenicity of total pulp mill effluent may be pH dependent. A potent mutagen has been identified in BKME as 3-chloro-4-(dichloromethyl)-5-hydroxy-2(5H)-furanone (68). This compound is unstable at high pH and is therefore underrepresented in the typical alkaline extractions of BKME.

Other compounds present in BKME identified as mutagenic in the Ames/*Salmonella* assay are presented in Table 44-4 and include resin acids and chlorinated propenes, methanes, ethanes, and a furanone (76,80–84). 2,3,7,8-TCDD has been tested in the Ames/*Salmonella* test system and is generally regarded as non-mutagenic in bacteria (85–87).

Chlorination stage effluent concentrate was found to induce gene conversion, mitotic recombination, and aberrant colony formation in *Saccharomyces cerevisiae* strain D7 (75). Several constituents of pulp mill effluent—including chlorinated catechols, guaiacols, acetones, aldehydes, and propenes—are mutagenic in strains of *S. cerevisiae* (see Table 44-4), inducing reversions in strain XV185-14C in the absence of exogenous metabolic activating system (88,89). Several chlorinated acetones and ethanes, 2,3,7,8-TCDD, dibromochloromethane, and dichlorobromomethane produced gene conversion in *S. cerevisiae* strain D7 (89–91). Addition of S9 as an exogenous metabolic-activating system increased the activity of 1,1,3-trichloroacetone and trichloroacetaldehyde but not the other test compounds.

Priha and Talka found that certain fractions of BKME induced threefold increases in sister chromatid exchange in Chinese hamster ovary cells without metabolic activation (55). Several constituents of BKME induced increases in sister chromatid exchange, chromosomal aberrations, micronuclei formation, cell transformation, and mutation frequency, as well as changes in mitotic index in mammalian cell lines and vertebrates *in vivo* (see Table 44-4) (82,84,92–94).

CARCINOGENICITY OF CONSTITUENTS OF BLEACHED KRAFT MILL EFFLUENT

Several compounds identified in BKME are considered to be carcinogens by the EPA and the International Agency for Research on Cancer, including the volatile organic compounds chloroform, trichloroethylene, methylene chloride, ethylene dichloride, tetrachloroethylene, and benzene (95). These chemicals are volatilized into the air during effluent treatment and discharge. As such, some of the volatile organic compounds may be more important in terms of air contaminants than as water pollutants; however, the concentrations of chloroform, for example, are quite high in the effluent before dilution in receiving waters.

Other less volatile chlorinated carcinogens present in BKME include 2,4,6-trichlorophenol, pentachlorophenol, hexachlorobenzene, 2,3,7,8-tetrachlorodibenzodioxin, and hexachlorodibenzodioxins. The known carcinogens and their classification and approximate potencies are listed in Table 44-2. Of these carcinogens, the most potent are the PCDDs. Other toxic effects of a number of BKME constituents are reviewed by EPA (31).

HUMAN EXPOSURE: BIOCONCENTRATION AND BIOACCUMULATION IN FISH

Some of the compounds in BKME may reach the human food chain through bioaccumulation in fish. Rainbow trout bioconcentrated 2,4,6-trichlorophenol, trichloroguaiacol, and tetrachloroguaiacol in liver and muscle tissue (96). 2,4,6-trichlorophenol, 2,3,4,6-tetrachlorophenol, 4,5,6-trichloroguaiacol, 3,4,5,6-tetrachloroguaiacol, and pentachlorophenol were found at concentrations greater than 1 mg per mL in the bile of fish living 1 km from a pulp mill outflow (58,97). Resin acids (pimaric, isopimaric, abietic, and dehydroabietic acids) were also found in the bile at concentrations of approximately 1 mg per L. Resin acids and chlorophenolics were measurable in the bile of perch, roach, mountain whitefish, and long-nose sucker as far as 230 km downstream from the effluent outflow (46,97). 2,4-Dichlorophenol, 3,4-dichloroguaiacol, 2,4,6-trichlorophenol, pentachlorophenol, tetrachloroveratrole, and tetrachloroguaiacol were detected in mountain whitefish immediately downstream of a kraft mill (46). These compounds were not detected in fish upstream of the effluent outflow.

Concentrations of 2,4,6-trichlorophenol, 2,3,4,6-tetrachlorophenol, and pentachlorophenol in the plasma of lake trout exposed to simulated BKME were 50, 150, and 275 times higher than in the water (58). Bile concentrations of these compounds ranged to as much as 32,000 times (pentachlorophenol) higher than in the water. Measurements of chlorophenolics in the bile of mountain whitefish and long-nose sucker indicated bioconcentration factors of 10,000 to greater than 100,000 over water column concentrations (46). However, filet concentrations were much lower than bile, and chlorophenolics are readily excreted by the fish, so depuration is rapid.

Bioconcentration factors (BCFs) for a number of compounds—including chlorinated guaiacols, chlorinated aliphatics, and chlorinated benzenes—are tabulated in Suntio and colleagues (33). BCFs for several carcinogenic constituents of BKME are listed in this review, including those for benzene, chloroform, carbon tetrachloride, dichloromethane, and hexachlorobenzene. Pentachlorobenzene and hexachlorobenzene have the highest BCF (log of the BCF in rainbow trout ranges to 5.37). Other toxic compounds with notable BCFs listed in Suntio (33) include monochlorobenzene and dichloro-, trichloro-, and tetrachlorobenzenes. Lindstrom and Osterberg (37) state that approximately 10% to 15% of total organically bound chlorine in the bleach plant effluent is lipophilic and may pose hazard through bioaccumulation.

PCDDs and PCDFs are lipophilic compounds and are readily bioconcentrated in aquatic organisms. BCFs have been measured for 2,3,7,8-TCDD by a number of investigators and range from approximately 1,000 to upward of 86,000 (98–101). Variability in measured BCFs can be attributed to fat content, species, presence of humic material and sediment, and a host of other factors. Preliminary results of the EPA National Bioaccumulation Study revealed that PCDD and PCDF concentrations in fish sampled near pulp mill outflows were in the 10 to 200 ppt range (48). In addition to cancer risk from PCDDs and PCDFs, bioaccumulation of these compounds may present a risk of other toxic effects, including immunotoxicity, reproductive toxicity, and endocrine abnormalities (102–110). Cancer risks to humans from consumption of carcinogen-contaminated fish may be significant and would depend on a number of factors, including extent of recreational or commercial fishing of contaminated fish, an individual's fish consumption rate, extent of contamination, and validity of extrapolation of results from animal cancer bioassays to humans. The food chain may increase levels of PCDD and PCDF, as well as chlorinated phenolics for some species. Thus, bioaccumulation may be more important than bioconcentration from the water column as a source of human exposure to contaminated fish (46).

HUMAN EXPOSURE: DRINKING WATER

Swedish investigators observed long-range transport of chlorinated organic compounds originating from a 200,000 ton per year kraft pulp mill through a river basin with ultimate contamination of a public drinking water supply (111). In the finished drinking water, pulp mill effluent constituents accounted for more than 50% of the chlorinated organic compounds, and chlorination of the finished drinking water accounted for the rest. However, the chlorinated drinking water was more mutagenic in the Ames assay than diluted biotreated pulp mill effluent. Gas chromatography-mass spectrometry indicated that as many as 15% to 20% of the peaks in the drinking water intake seemed to originate from the pulp mill. Retention times of some peaks corresponded to sesquiterpenes and trichlorobenzene previously identified in kraft pulp mill effluent. Further study to characterize potential health impacts of BKME contamination of drinking water supplies is needed.

COMMUNITY EPIDEMIOLOGY NEAR KRAFT PULP MILLS

Numerous studies in the United States and Scandinavia have examined the health status of communities near kraft pulp mills. Health endpoints examined have included acute and chronic respiratory diseases and a variety of annoyance symptoms (including headaches, nausea, and eye and throat irritation). These studies implicate odorous pulp mill air emissions in the genesis of community annoyance reactions but are somewhat ambiguous on the question of respiratory tract irritation.

Jonsson and colleagues (112) conducted a community odor annoyance study in Eureka, California, downwind from two pulp mills. Odor annoyance was found to be positively related to odor exposure zone, as validated by olfactometry. A follow-up community symptom survey found that self-reported headache, sputum production (women only), and odor annoyance were related to residential proximity to pulp mills, but this relationship did not hold for a variety of other respiratory, gastrointestinal, or neurologic symptoms. Some respiratory and ocular symptoms actually showed an inverse relationship to odor exposure (i.e., they were more prevalent at greater distance from the mills) (113).

Deprez and colleagues (114) examined respiratory disease hospital admission rates in 66 Maine towns located between 0 and 15 miles from kraft pulp mills. Age- and sex-adjusted respiratory admission rates were positively related to unemployment rates and to the proportion of the town's work force employed at the local pulp mill, but distance between the mill and the geographic center of the town (regardless of the wind direction) did not explain variations in admission rates. Mikaelsson et al. (115) conducted an interview and clinical screening study in a sulfite (nonkraft) pulp mill community in northern Sweden; the principal air pollutants identified in the community were sulfur dioxide and chlorine. They found no community-wide excess prevalence of either asthma or chronic bronchitis compared with other regions in the country. On a case-by-case basis, however, both smoking and employment in the pulp mill were strong risk factors for chronic bronchitis. Stjernberg et al. (116,117) extended this study to include not only additional subjects, but also measures of community air quality. They again found no community-wide increase in asthma or bronchitis prevalence, with mean annual ambient levels of SO_2 averaging between 0.008 and 0.013 ppm (levels below the U.S. annual average standard of 0.03 ppm or the 24-hour standard of 0.14 ppm).

In the early 1990s, Jaakkola et al. (118), Marttilla et al. (119), and Haahtela et al. (120) studied communities surrounding (predominantly sulfate) pulp mills in Finland. In the first two (cross-sectional) studies, researchers documented self-reported respiratory symptoms among adults (118) and children (119) in three communities: one highly exposed, one moderately exposed, and one unexposed to pulp mill emissions. After correcting for various potential confounders, retrospective period prevalence rates (both 1- and 12-month) were found to be positively related to exposure for the following symptoms: eye irritation, nasal congestion, headache, breathlessness, and wheezing (118,119). In the last study, a moderately to highly exposed community was surveyed on two occasions: once during and once again 4 months after a documented pollution episode. Point prevalence rates (2-day reporting periods) were determined for various symptoms. Among the 45 individuals responding on both occasions, reports of eye or throat irritation, cough, and nausea were significantly higher during the polluted than nonpolluted period (120). Limitations of this study included a lack of control for seasonality and presence of an additional pollutant (mesityl oxide) during the pollution episode. Overall, the authors concluded that hydrogen sulfide, mercaptans, and organic sulfides appear to be capable of producing respiratory tract and mucous membrane irritation at lower exposure levels than previously documented, although none of the studies included objective measures of respiratory function.

OCCUPATIONAL EPIDEMIOLOGY FOR KRAFT PULP MILL WORKERS

The occupational health status of pulp mill workers has been studied for a variety of endpoints, including cancer, pulmonary function, skin diseases, and hearing impairment. For some health endpoints, findings have varied sufficiently across studies that there remains significant controversy regarding their interpretation. This is particularly true for cancer.

The effects of pulp mill work on pulmonary function have been receiving increasing attention and have been reviewed in detail (121). Community studies of chronic respiratory disease (in particular, bronchitis) near pulp mills have typically shown excesses in relationship to smoking and mill employment, but not to residence proximity to mills per se (114–117). On the other hand, the significance of pulp mill employment has been variable in those cross-sectional and longitudinal respiratory health studies that have been carried out among mill workers themselves. Combined survey and clinical studies conducted in New Hampshire (122) and British Columbia (123) failed to show a higher prevalence of chronic pulmonary disease in pulp mill workers than in the community at large. However, another Canadian study highlighted two specific kraft mill work activities—bleaching and maintenance—as possible risk factors for obstructive lung disease (124). The importance of episodic overexposures to chlorine gas in the genesis of asthmalike symptoms (reactive airways dysfunction syndrome or irritant-induced asthma) and in accelerated pulmonary function decline has since been highlighted by several investigators (125–131). Selected studies have also demonstrated the importance of smoking as a risk factor for respiratory disease within the pulp mill work force (132,133).

Chip pile workers at pulp mills have been shown to be exposed to high concentrations of airborne mold spores. Although few cases of hypersensitivity pneumonitis could be found in the Finnish occupational disease registries, a limited study there found a tendency toward subclinical pulmonary impairment among such workers who were precipitin positive for *Aspergillus fumigatus* (134). Attention to biological agents in the process water of paper mills has also led to studies of microbial aerosolization and respiratory tract colonization. One such study confirmed increased rates of nasal colonization by *Klebsiella pneumoniae* among workers so exposed but no concomitant increase in respiratory symptoms or illnesses (135).

Cancer mortality patterns among pulp mill workers have been examined in a number of cohort studies—yielding proportional mortality ratios and standardized mortality ratios—and in case-control studies and tumor registry–based standardized incidence ratio studies. A variety of methodologic limitations—including potential ascertainment bias, the healthy worker effect, and spurious correlations that are due to multiple statistical comparisons—exist. Accordingly, caution is indicated in the interpretation of individual study results.

Table 44-5 summarizes the results of four proportional mortality ratio, two standardized mortality ratio, three standardized incidence ratio, and five case-control studies of pulp or paper mill workers (136–149). In no case was the same malignancy

TABLE 44-5. Studies of cancer incidence and mortality in pulp mill workers

Reference number	136	137[a]	138	139	140[b]	141[c]	142	143	144	145[d]	146	147	148	149[e]
Study type	PMR	PMR	PMR	PMR	SMR	SMR	SIR	SIR	SIR		CC	CC	CC	CC
Malignancy														
Lymphopoietic		*												
Leukemias			**									(–)		
Lymphomas (especially Hodgkin's)	*													*
Lymphosarcoma	*			**	*									
Reticulosarcoma					*									
Genitourinary														
Bladder	*													
Gastrointestinal														
Pharyngeal			**											
Gastric	*		**		*									*
Pancreatic	*						*						(–)	*
Colorectal		*	**											
Respiratory														
Sinonasal										**	(–)			
Laryngeal			**											
Lung		**							**					
Mesothelioma								*						

*, nonsignificant excesses; **, significant excesses; (–), no association (case-control studies); CC, case control; PMR, proportional mortality ratio; SIR, standardized incidence ratio; SMR, standardized mortality ratio.
[a]Examined "pulp, paper, and paperboard mill workers."
[b]Found an excess of gastric cancers in sulfite mill workers.
[c]Examined "paper workers."
[d]Examined "paper and wood industries."
[e]Grouped all lymphoma types in one category.

found to be significantly elevated in more than one study. However, for two sites—gastric cancer and lymphosarcoma—there were one study each with significant excesses and at least two studies each with nonsignificant excesses. (One of the studies showing nonsignificant excess of gastric cancer was among workers in sulfite—but not sulfate—pulp mills.) Two reviews of this topic emphasize (a) the heterogeneity of findings across studies and (b) a general inadequacy of exposure assessment in most investigations (150,151).

Finally, a variety of cutaneous hazards also exists in pulp mills, including wet work and botanical allergens (152), phototoxic chemicals (e.g., anthraquinone) used in delignification (153), and cutaneous irritants used in slimicides (e.g., methylene-bis-thiocyanate, bis-1,4-bromoacetoxy-2-butene, and 2,3-dichloro-4-bromotetrahydrothiophene-1,1-dioxide) (154–155).

REFERENCES

1. American Paper Institute. US wood pulp data. New York: American Paper Institute, 1988.
2. Britt KW, ed. *Handbook of pulp and paper technology.* New York: Reinhold, 1964.
3. Minor J. Pulp. In: Grayson M, ed. *Kirk-Othmer encyclopedia of chemical technology,* vol 19. New York: John Wiley and Sons, 1983:379–419.
4. Teschke K, Demers P. Paper and pulp industry. In: *Encyclopedia of occupational health and safety,* 4th ed. Geneva: International Labor Office, 1997: Chapter 72.
5. Ruth JH. Odor thresholds and irritation levels of several chemical substances: a review. *Am Ind Hyg Assoc J* 1986;47:A142–A151.
6. Amoore JE, Hautala E. Odor as an aid to chemical safety: odor thresholds compared with threshold limit values and volatilities for 214 industrial chemicals in air and water dilution. *J Appl Toxicol* 1983;3:272–290.
7. Beauchamp RO, Bus JS, Popp JA, Craig JB, Andjelkovich DA. A critical review of the literature on hydrogen sulfide. *CRC Crit Rev Toxicol* 1984;13:25–97.
8. Reiffenstein RJ, Hulbert WC, Roth S. Toxicology of hydrogen sulfide. *Annu Rev Pharmacol Toxicol* 1992;32:109–134.
9. Jappinen P, Vilkka V, Marttila O, Haahtela T. Exposure to hydrogen sulfide and respiratory function. *Br J Ind Med* 1990;47:824–828.
10. Burnett WW, King EG, Grace M, Hall WF. Hydrogen sulfide poisoning: review of five years' experience. *Can Med Assoc J* 1977;117:1277–1280.
11. Deng J-F, Chang S-C. Hydrogen sulfide poisonings in hot-spring reservoir cleaning: two case reports. *Am J Ind Med* 1987;11:447–451.
12. World Health Organization. *Environmental health criteria,* vol 19. Geneva: World Health Organization, 1981.
13. Savolainen H, Tenhunen R, Elovaara E, Tossavainen A. Cumulative biochemical effects of repeated subclinical hydrogen sulfide intoxication in mouse brain. *Int Arch Occup Environ Health* 1980;46:87–92.
14. Haider SS, Hasan M, Islan F. Effect of air pollutant hydrogen sulfide on the levels of total lipids, phospholipids and cholesterol in different regions of the guinea pig brain. *Indian J Exp Biol* 1980;18:418–420.
15. Sandmeyer EE. Organic sulfur compounds. In: Clayton GD, Clayton FE, eds. *Patty's industrial hygiene and toxicology,* 3rd ed. New York: John Wiley and Sons, 1981:2061–2111.
16. Rose VE. Thiols. In: *International Labor Association. Encyclopedia of occupational health and safety,* vol 2. Geneva: International Labor Organization Press, 1983:2172–2173.
17. Pinkerton JE. Emissions of SO-2 and NO-x from pulp and paper mills. *Air and Waste* 1993;43:1404–1407.
18. Bethel RA, Erle DJ, Epstein J, Sheppard D, Nadel JA, Boushey HA. Effect of exercise rate and route of inhalation on sulfur dioxide-induced bronchoconstriction in asthmatic subjects. *Am Rev Respir Dis* 1983;128:592–596.
19. Horstman D, Roger LJ, Kehrl H, Hazucha M. Airway sensitivity of asthmatics to sulfur dioxide. *Toxicol Ind Health* 1986;2:289–298.
20. Kangas J, Jappinen P, Savolainen H. Exposure to hydrogen sulfide, mercaptans and sulfur dioxide in pulp industry. *Am Ind Hyg Assoc J* 1984;45:787–790.
21. Charan N, Myers C, Lakshminarayan S, Spencer T. Pulmonary injuries associated with acute sulfur dioxide inhalation. *Am Rev Respir Dis* 1979;119:555–560.
22. Woodford D, Coutu R, Gaensler E. Obstructive lung disease from acute sulfur dioxide exposure. *Respiration* 1979;38:238–245.
23. Galea M. Fatal sulfur dioxide inhalation. *Can Med Assoc J* 1964;91:345–347.
24. US Department of Labor, Occupational Safety and Health Administration. *Air contaminants—permissible exposure limits.* Washington: US Government Printing Office, 1989.
25. Amoore JE. *The perception of hydrogen sulfide odor in relation to setting an ambient standard.* Sacramento, CA: California Air Resources Board, 1985. [Contract A4-046-33].
26. US Environmental Protection Agency. *Survey of chloroform emission sources.* Research Triangle Park, NC: Office of Air Quality Planning and Standards, 1985. [EPA-450/3-85-026].
27. US Environmental Protection Agency. Health effect assessment for chloroform. Cincinnati, 1988.
28. US Environmental Protection Agency. *National dioxin study: tier 4—combustion sources.* Research Triangle Park, NC: Office of Air Quality Planning and Standards, 1987. [EPA-450/4-84-014h].

29. Rosenberg C, Kontsas H, Jappinen P, Tornaeus J, Hesso A, Vainio H. Airborne chlorinated dioxins and furans in a pulp and paper mill. *Chemosphere* 1994;29:1971–1978.
30. Pinkerton JE, Blosser RO. Characterization of kraft pulp mill particulate emissions: a summary of existing measurements and observations. *Atmos Environ* 1981;15:2071–2078.
31. US Environmental Protection Agency. *Paper production and processing—occupational exposure and environmental release study.* Cincinnati: US Environmental Protection Agency, Office of Research and Development, Industrial Environmental Research Laboratory, 1984. [EPA-600/2-84-120].
32. Ostro B. The association of air pollution and mortality: examining the case for inference. *Arch Environ Health* 1993;48:336–342.
33. Suntio LR, Shiu WY, Mackay D. A review of the nature and properties of chemicals present in pulp mill effluents. *Chemosphere* 1988;17:1249–1290.
34. Kringstad KP, Lindstrom K. Spent liquors from pulp bleaching. *Environ Sci Technol* 1984;15:236A–248A.
35. Wilkins AL, Singh-Thansi M, Langdon AG. Pulp mill sourced organic compounds and sodium levels in water and sediments from the Tarawera River, New Zealand. *Bull Environ Contam Toxicol* 1996;57:434–441.
36. Rantio T. Chlorohydrocarbons in pulp mill effluent and the environment II: Chlorcymenes and chlorocymenenes. *Chemosphere* 1996;32:239–252.
37. Lindstrom K, Osterberg F. Chlorinated carboxylic acids in softwood kraft pulp spent bleach liquors. *Environ Sci Technol* 1986;20:133–145.
38. Knuutinen J. Analysis of chlorinated guaiacols in spent bleach liquor from a pulp mill. *J Chromatogr* 1982;248:289–295.
39. McKague AB. Some toxic constituents of chlorination-stage effluents from bleached kraft pulp mills. *Can J Fish Aquat Sci* 1981a;38:739–743.
40. McKague AB. Phenolic constituents in pulp mill process streams. *J Chromatogr* 1981b;208:287–293.
41. Swanson SE, Rappe C, Malmstrom J, Kringstad KP. Emissions of PCDDs and PCDFs from the pulp industry. *Chemosphere* 1988;17:681–691.
42. Kovacs TG, Martel PH, Voss RH, Wrist PE, Willes RF. Aquatic toxicity equivalents factors for chlorinated phenolic compounds present in pulp mill effluents. *Environ Toxicol Chem* 1993;12:281–288.
43. Wong PTS, Chau YK, Ali N, Whittle DM. Biochemical and genotoxic effects in the vicinity of a pulp mill discharge. *Environ Toxicol Water Quality* 1994;9:59–70.
44. Bonsor N, McCubbin N, Sprague JB. Kraft mill effluents in Ontario: municipal-industrial strategy for abatement. Report for Technical Advisory Committee, Toronto, 1989.
45. Graves WC, Burton DT, Richardson LB. Effect of 20- to 30-day continuous exposure of treated bleach kraft mill effluent on selected freshwater species. *Bull Environ Contam Toxicol* 1980;25:651–657.
46. Owens JW, Swanson SM, Birkholz DA. Environmental monitoring of bleached kraft pulp mill chlorophenolic compounds in a northern Canadian river system. *Chemosphere* 1994;29:89–109.
47. US Environmental Protection Agency. *National dioxin study: tier 3, 5, 6, 7.* Washington: Office of Water Regulations and Standards, 1986.
48. US Environmental Protection Agency. *"The 104 Mill Study" summary report.* Washington: Office of Water Regulations and Standards, 1990.
49. Kuehl DW, Butterworth BC, De Vita WM, Sauer CP. Environmental contamination by polychlorinated dibenzo-*p*-dioxins and dibenzofurans associated with pulp and paper mill discharge. *Biomed Environ Mass Spectrom* 1987;14:443–447.
50. Olson LJ, Anderson HA, Jones VB. Landspreading dioxin-contaminated papermill sludges: a complex problem. *Arch Environ Health* 1988;43:186–189.
51. Beck H, Eckart K, Mathar W, Wittkowski R. Occurrence of PCDD and PCDF in different kinds of paper. *Chemosphere* 1988;17:51–57.
52. Axegard P, Renberg L. The influence of bleaching chemicals and lignin content on the formation of polychlorinated dioxins and dibenzofurans. *Chemosphere* 1989;19(1–6):661–668.
53. de Sousa F, Kolar M-C, Kringstad KP. Influence of chlorine ratio and oxygen bleaching on the formation of PCDFs and PCDDs in pulp bleaching, part 1: a laboratory study. *Tech Assoc Pulp Paper Ind J* 1989;72:147–153.
54. Heimburger SA, Blevins DS, Bostwick JH, Donnini GP. Kraft mill bleach plant effluents: recent developments aimed at decreasing their environmental impacts, part 1. *Tech Assoc Pulp Paper Ind J* 1988;71:51–60.
55. Priha MH, Talka ET. Biological activity of bleached kraft mill effluent (BKME) fractions and process streams. *Pulp Paper Can* 1986;87:143–147.
56. Leach JM, Thakore AN. Isolation and identification of constituents toxic to juvenile rainbow trout (*Salmo gairdneri*) in caustic extraction effluents from kraft pulp mill bleach plants. *J Fish Res Board Can* 1975;32:1249–1257.
57. Walden CC, Howard TE. Toxicity of pulp and paper mill effluents—a review. *Pulp Paper Can* 1981;82:115–124.
58. Oikari A, Lindstrom-Seppa P, Kukkonen J. Subchronic metabolic effects and toxicity of a simulated pulp mill effluent on juvenile lake trout, *Salmo trutta m. lacustris*. *Ecotoxicol Environ Saf* 1988;16:202–218.
59. Andersson T, Bengtsson B-E, Forlin L, Hardig J, Larsson A. Long-term effects of bleached kraft mill effluents on carbohydrate metabolism and hepatic xenobiotic biotransformation enzymes in fish. *Ecotoxicol Environ Saf* 1987;13:53–60.
60. Hardig J, Andersson T, Bengtsson B-E, Forlin L, Larsson A. Long-term effects of bleached kraft mill effluents on red and white blood cell status, ion balance, and vertebral structure in fish. *Ecotoxicol Environ Saf* 1988;15:96–106.
61. Woelke CE. Measurement of water quality with the Pacific oyster embryo bioassay. In: *Water quality criteria.* Philadelphia: American Society for Testing Materials, 1967.
62. Thakore AN, Howard TE. *Site of action of chemicals from pulp mill effluent that are toxic to fish.* Ottawa, Ontario: Canadian Forestry Service, 1976. [CPAR project no 488].
63. Couillard CM, Berman RA, Panisset JC. Histopathology of rainbow trout exposed to a bleached kraft pulp mill effluent. *Arch Environ Contam Toxicol* 1988;17:319–323.
64. Axelsson B, Norrgren L. Parasite frequency and liver anomalies in three-spined stickleback (*Gasterosteus aculeatus* L.) after long-term exposure to pulp mill effluents in marine mesocosms. *Arch Environ Contam Toxicol* 1991;21:505–513.
65. Lindstrom-Seppa P, Huuskonen S, Pesonen M, Muona P, Hanninen O. Unbleached pulp mill effluents affect cytochrome P450 monooxygenase enzyme activities. *Marine Environ Res* 1992;34:157–161.
66. Kovacs T. Effects of bleached kraft mill effluent on freshwater fish: a Canadian perspective. *Water Poll Res J Can* 1986;21:91–118.
67. Graves WC, Burton DT, Richardson LB, Margrey SL. The interaction of treated bleached kraft mill effluent and dissolved oxygen concentration on the survival of the developmental stages of the Sheepshead minnow (*Cyprinodon variegatus*). *Water Res* 1981;15:100–1011.
68. Vuorinen M, Vourinen PJ. Effects of bleached kraft mill effluent on early life stages of brown trout (*Salmo trutta* L.). *Ecotoxicol Environ Saf* 1987;14:117–128.
69. National Council on Air and Stream Improvement. Effects of biologically stabilized bleached kraft mill effluent on cold water stream productivity as determined in experimental streams—first progress report [Tech bull no 368]. New York: National Council of the Paper Industry for Air and Stream Improvement, 1982.
70. Tana J, Nikunen E. Impact of pulp and paper mill effluent on egg hatchability of pike (*Esox lucius* L.). *Bull Environ Contam Toxicol* 1986;36:738–743.
71. Burton DT, Hall WL, Klauda RJ, Margrey SL. Effects of treated bleached kraft mill effluent on eggs and prolarvae of striped bass (*Morone saxatalis*). *Water Res Bull* 1983;19:869–879.
72. Cherr GN, Shenker JM, Lundmark C, Turner KO. Toxic effects of selected bleached kraft mill effluent constituents on the sea urchin sperm cell. *Environ Toxicol Chem* 1987;6:561–569.
73. Nguyen TKO, Bengtsson B-E. Toxicity to microtox, micro-algae and duckweed of effluents from the Bai Bang Paper Company (BAPACP), a Vietnamese bleached kraft pulp and paper mill. *Environ Poll* 1995;90:391–399.
74. Douglas GR, Nestmann ER, McKague AB, et al. Mutagenicity of pulp and paper mill effluent: a comprehensive study of complex mixtures. *Environ Sci Res* 1983;27:431–459.
75. Kamra OP, Nestmann ER, Douglas GR, Kowbel DJ, Harrington TR. Genotoxic activity of pulp mill effluent in *Salmonella* and *Saccharomyces cerevisiae* assays. *Mutat Res* 1983;118:269–276.
76. Kringstad KP, Ljungquist PO, de Sousa F, Stromberg LM. Identification and mutagenic properties of some chlorinated aliphatic compounds in the spent liquor from kraft pulp chlorination. *Environ Sci Technol* 1981;15:562–566.
77. Helma C, Mersch-Sundermann V, Houk VS, et al. Comparative evaluation of four bacterial assays for the detection of genotoxic effects in the dissolved water phases of aqueous matrices. *Environ Sci Technol* 1996;30:897–907.
78. White PA, Rasmussen JB, Blaise C. Comparing the presence, potency, and potential hazard of genotoxins extracted from a broad range of industrial effluents. *Environ Mol Mutagen* 1996;27:116–139.
79. Rao S, Burnison BK, Rokosh DA, Taylor CM. Mutagenicity and toxicity assessment of pulp mill effluent. *Chemosphere* 1994;28:1859–1870.
80. Nestmann ER, Lee EG-H, Mueller JC, Douglas GR. Mutagenicity of resin acids identified in pulp and paper mill effluents using the *Salmonella*/mammalian microsome assay. *Environ Mutagen* 1979;1:361–369.
81. Nestmann ER, Lee EG-H, Matula TI, Douglas GR, Mueller JC. Mutagenicity of constituents identified in pulp and paper mill effluents using the *Salmonella*/mammalian-microsome assay. *Mutat Res* 1980;79:203–212.
82. Ellenton JA, Douglas GR, Nestmann ER. Mutagenic evaluation of 1,1,2,3-tetrachloro-2-propene, a contaminant in pulp mill effluents, using a battery of *in vitro* mammalian and microbial tests. *Can J Genet Cytol* 1981;23:17–25.
83. Holmbom BR. Isolation and identification of an Ames-mutagenic compound present in kraft chlorination effluents. *Tech Assoc Pulp Paper Ind J* 1981;64:172–174.
84. US Environmental Protection Agency. *Biological and chemical studies on 3-chloro-4-(dichloromethyl)-5-hydroxy-2(5H)-furanone: a potent mutagen in kraft pulp chlorination effluent and chlorinated drinking water.* Research Triangle Park, NC: Health Effects Research Laboratory, 1988.
85. Geiger LE, Neal RA. Mutagenicity testing of 2,3,7,8-tetrachlorodibenzo-*p*-dioxin in histidine auxotrophs of *Salmonella typhimurium*. *Toxicol Appl Pharmacol* 1981;59:125–129.
86. Gilbert P, Saint-Ruf G, Poncelet, F et al. Genetic effects of chlorinated anilines and azobenzenes on *Salmonella typhimurium*. *Arch Environ Contam Toxicol* 1980;9:533–541.
87. Mortelmans K, Haworth S, Speck W, et al. Mutagenicity testing of agent orange components and related chemicals. *Toxicol Appl Pharmacol* 1984;75:137–146.
88. Nestmann ER, Lee EG-H. Mutagenicity of constituents of pulp and paper mill effluent in growing cells of *Saccharomyces cerevisiae*. *Mutat Res* 1983;119:273–280.
89. Callen DF, Wolf CR, Philpot RM. Cytochrome P-450 mediated genetic activity and cytotoxicity of seven halogenated aliphatic hydrocarbons in *Saccharomyces cerevisiae*. *Mutat Res* 1980;77:55–63.
90. Nestmann ER, Lee EG-H. Genetic activity in *Saccharomyces cerevisiae* of compounds found in effluents of pulp and paper mills. *Mutat Res* 1985;155:53–60.

91. Bronzetti G, Zeiger E, Lee I, et al. Genetic effects of 2,3,7,8-tetrachlorodibenzo-*p*-dioxin (TCDD) in yeast *in vitro* and *in vivo*. In: Hutzinger O, Frei RW, Aerian E, Pocchiari F, eds. *Chlorinated dioxins and related compounds: impact on the environment.* Proceedings of a workshop held at the Instituto Superiore di Sanita, Rome, Italy, 22–24 October, 1980. New York: Pergamon Press, 1982:429–436.
92. Das RK, Nanda NK. Induction of micronuclei in peripheral erythrocytes of fish *Heteropneustes fossilis* by mitomycin C and paper mill effluent. *Mutat Res* 1986;175:67–71.
93. Rogers AM, Anderson ME, Back KC. Mutagenicity of 2,3,7,8-tetrachloro-dibenzo-*p*-dioxin and perfluoro-*n*-decanoic acid in L517BY mouse lymphoma cells. *Mutat Res* 1982;105:445–449.
94. Hay A, Ashby J, Styles JA, et al. The mutagenic properties of 2,3,7,8-tetra-chlorodibenzo-*p*-dioxin. *Am Chem Soc J Div Environ Chem* 1983;3:14–22.
95. International Agency for Research on Cancer. Overall evaluations of carcinogenicity: an updating of IARC monographs, volumes 1 to 42. *IARC Monogr Eval Carcinog Risk Hum Suppl* 1987;7.
96. Landner L, Lindstrom K, Karlsson M, Nordin J, Sorenson L. Bioaccumulation in fish of chlorinated phenols from kraft pulp mill bleachery effluents. *Bull Environ Contam Toxicol* 1977;18:663–673.
97. Oikari AOJ. Metabolites of xenobiotics in the bile of fish in waterways polluted by pulp mill effluents. *Bull Environ Contam Toxicol* 1986;36:429–436.
98. Corbet RL, Muir DCG, Webster GRB. Fate of 1,3,6,8-TCDD in an outdoor aquatic environment. *Chemosphere* 1983;12:523–527.
99. Isensee AR, Jones GE. Absorption and translocation of root and foliage applied 2,4-dichlorophenol, 2,7-dichlorodibenzo-*p*-dioxin, and 2,3,7,8-tetra-chlorodibenzo-*p*-dioxin. *J Agric Food Chem* 1971;19:1210–1214.
100. Yockim RS, Isensee AR, Jones GE. Distribution and toxicity of TCDD and 2,4,5-T in an aquatic model ecosystem. *Chemosphere* 1978;3:215–220.
101. Petty JD, Smith LM, Peterman PH, Mehrle PM, Buckler DR, Stalling DL. Bioconcentration of TCDD and TCDF by rainbow trout in a flow-through exposure. Presented at: Society of Environmental Toxicology and Chemistry Seventh Annual Meeting; November 2–5, 1986; Alexandria, VA.
102. Courtney KD, Moore JA. Teratology studies with 2,4,5-T and 2,3,7,8-TCDD. *Toxicol Appl Pharmacol* 1971;20:396–403.
103. Neubert D, Dillman I. Embryotoxic effects in mice treated with 2,4,5-trichlorophenoxyacetic acid and 2,3,7,8-tetrachlorodibenzo-*p*-dioxin. *Arch Pharmacol* 1972;272:243–264.
104. Sparschu GL, Dunn FL, Rowe VK. Study of the teratogenicity of 2,3,7,8-tetrachlorodibenzo-*p*-dioxin in the rat. *Food Cosmet Toxicol* 1971;9:405–412.
105. Murray FJ, Smith FA, Nitschke KD, Humiston CG, Kociba RJ, Schwetz BA. Three-generation reproduction study of rats given 2,3,7,8-tetrachloro-dibenzo-*p*-dioxin (TCDD) in the diet. *Toxicol Appl Pharmacol* 1979;50:241–252.
106. Schantz SL, Barsotti DA, Allen JR. Toxicological effects produced in nonhuman primates chronically exposed to fifty parts per trillion 2,3,7,8-tetrachlorodibenzo-*p*-dioxin (TCDD). *Toxicol Appl Pharmacol* 1979;48:A180.
107. Kociba RJ, Keyes DG, Beyer JE, et al. Results of a two-year chronic toxicity and oncogenicity study of 2,3,7,8-tetrachlorodibenzo-*p*-dioxin in rats. *Toxicol Appl Pharmacol* 1978;46:279–303.
108. Gorski JR, Muzi G, Weber LWD, et al. Some endocrine and morphological aspects of the acute toxicity of 2,3,7,8-tetrachlorodibenzo-*p*-dioxin (TCDD). *Toxicol Pathol* 1988;16:313–320.
109. Jones MK, Weisenburger WP, Sipes IG, Russell DH. Circadian alterations in prolactin, corticosterone, and thyroid hormone levels and down-regulation of prolactin receptor activity by 2,3,7,8-tetrachlorodibenzo-*p*-dioxin. *Toxicol Appl Pharmacol* 1987;87:337–350.
110. Kociba RJ, Cabey O. Comparative toxicity and biologic activity of chlorinated dibenzo-*p*-dioxins and furans relative to 2,3,7,8-tetrachlorodibenzo-*p*-dioxin (TCDD). *Chemosphere* 1985;14:649–660.
111. Wigilius B, Boren H, Grimvall A, Carlberg GE, Hagen I, Brogger A. Impact of bleached kraft mill effluents on drinking water quality. *Sci Total Environ* 1988;74:75–96.
112. Jonsson E, Deane M, Sanders G. Community reactions to odors from pulp mills: a pilot study in Eureka, California. *Environ Res* 1975;10:249–270.
113. Deane M, Sanders G. Health effects of exposure to community odors from pulp mills, Eureka, 1971. *Environ Res* 1977;14:164–181.
114. Deprez RD, Oliver C, Halteman W. Variations in respiratory disease morbidity among pulp and paper mill town residents. *J Occup Med* 1986;28:486–491.
115. Mikaelsson B, Stjernberg N, Wiman L-G. The prevalence of bronchial asthma and chronic bronchitis in an industrialized community in northern Sweden. *Scand J Soc Med* 1982;10:11–16.
116. Stjernberg N, Eklund A, Nystrom L, Rosenhall L, Emmelin A, Stromqvist L-H. Prevalence of bronchial asthma and chronic bronchitis in a community in northern Sweden: relation to environmental and occupational exposure to sulfur dioxide. *Eur J Respir Dis* 1985;67:41–49.
117. Stjernberg N, Rosenhall L, Eklund A, Nystrom L. Chronic bronchitis in a community in northern Sweden: relation to environmental and occupational exposure to sulfur dioxide. *Eur J Respir Dis* 1986;69:153–159.
118. Jaakkola JJ, Vilkka V, Marttila O, Jappinen P, Haahtela T. The South Karelia air pollution study: the effects of malodorous sulfur compounds from pulp mills on respiratory and other symptoms. *Am Rev Respir Dis* 1990;142:1344–1350.
119. Marttila O, Jaakkola JJ, Vilkka V, Jappinen P, Haahtela T. The South Karelia air pollution study: the effects of malodorous sulfur compounds from pulp mills on respiratory and other symptoms in children. *Environ Res* 1994;66:152–159.
120. Haahtela T, Marttila O, Vilkka V, Jappinen P, Jaakkola JJ. The South Karelia air pollution study: acute health effects of malodorous sulfur air pollutants released by a pulp mill [See comments]. *Am J Public Health* 1992;82:603–605.
121. Toren K, Hagberg S, Westberg H. Health effects of working in pulp and paper mills: exposure, obstructive airways diseases, hypersensitivity reactions, and cardiovascular diseases. *Am J Ind Med* 1996;29:111–122.
122. Ferris BG Jr, Burgess WA, Worcester J. Prevalence of chronic respiratory disease in a pulp mill and a paper mill in the United States. *Br J Ind Med* 1967;24:26–37.
123. Chan-Yeung M, Wong R, MacLean L, Tan F, Dorken E, Schulzer M, et al. Respiratory survey of workers in a pulp and paper mill in Powell River, British Columbia. *Am Rev Respir Dis* 1980;122:249–257.
124. Enarson DA, Johnson A, Block G, Maclean L, Dybuncio A, Schragg K, et al. Respiratory health at a pulpmill in British Columbia. *Arch Environ Health* 1984;39:325–330.
125. Charan NB, Lakshminarayan S, Myers GC, Smith DD. Effects of accidental chlorine inhalation on pulmonary function. *West J Med* 1985;143:333–336.
126. Kennedy SM, Enarson DA, Janssen RG, Chan-Yeung M. Lung health consequences of reported accidental chlorine gas exposures among pulpmill workers. *Am Rev Respir Dis* 1991;143:74–79.
127. Schwartz DA, Smith DD, Lakshminarayan S. The pulmonary sequelae associated with accidental inhalation of chlorine gas. *Chest* 1990;97:820–825.
128. Salisbury DA, Enarson DA, Chan-Yeung M, Kennedy SM. First-aid reports of acute chlorine gassing among pulpmill workers as predictors of lung health consequences. *Am J Ind Med* 1991;20:71–81.
129. Henneberger PK, Ferris BG Jr, Sheehe PR. Accidental gassing incidents and the pulmonary function of pulp mill workers. *Am Rev Respir Dis* 1993;148:63–67.
130. Bherer L, Cushman R, Courteau JP, et al. Survey of construction workers repeatedly exposed to chlorine over a three to six month period in a pulpmill: II. Follow up of affected workers. *Occup Environ Med* 1994;51:225–228.
131. Malo JL, Cartier A, Boulet LP, et al. Bronchial hyperresponsiveness can improve while spirometry plateaus two to three years after repeated exposure to chlorine causing respiratory symptoms. *Am J Respir Crit Care Med* 1994;150:1142–1145.
132. Poukkula A, Huhti E, Makarainen M. Chronic respiratory disease among workers in a pulp mill: a ten-year follow-up study. *Chest* 1982;81:285–259.
133. Huhti E, Ryhanen P, Vuopala U, Takkunen J. Chronic respiratory disease among pulp mill workers in an arctic area in Northern Finland. *Acta Med Scand* 1970;187:433–444.
134. Jappinen P, Haahtela T, Liira J. Chip pile workers and mould exposure: a preliminary clinical and hygienic survey. *Allergy* 1987;42:545–548.
135. Niemela SI, Vaatanen P, Mentu J, Jokinen A, Jappinen P, Sillanpaa P. Microbial incidence in upper respiratory tracts of workers in the paper industry. *Appl Environ Microbiol* 1985;50:163–168.
136. Milham S Jr, Demers RY. Mortality among pulp and paper workers. *J Occup Med* 1984;26:844–846.
137. Solet D, Zoloth SR, Sullivan C, Jewett J, Michaels DM. Patterns of mortality in pulp and paper workers. *J Occup Med* 1989;31:627–630.
138. Schwartz E. A proportionate mortality ratio analysis of pulp and paper mill workers in New Hampshire. *Br J Ind Med* 1988;45:234–238.
139. Svirchev LM, Gallagher RP, Band PR, Threlfall WJ, Spinelli JJ. Gastric cancer and lymphosarcoma among wood and pulp workers. *J Occup Med* 1986;28:264–265.
140. Robinson CF, Waxweiler RJ, Fowler DP. Mortality among production workers in pulp and paper mills. *Scand J Work Environ Health* 1986;12:552–560.
141. Ferris BG, Puleo S, Chen HY. Mortality and morbidity in a pulp and a paper mill in the United States: a ten-year follow-up. *Br J Ind Med* 1979;36:127–134.
142. Malker HS, McLaughlin JK, Malker BK, Stone BJ, Weiner JA, Ericsson JL, et al. Biliary tract cancer and occupation in Sweden. *Br J Ind Med* 1986;43:257–262.
143. Malker HSR, McLaughlin JK, Malker BK, Stone BJ, Weiner JA, Erickson JLE, et al. Occupational risks for pleural mesothelioma in Sweden, 1961–79. *J Natl Cancer Inst* 1985;74:61–66.
144. Jappinen P, Hakulinen T, Pukkala E, Tola S, Kurppa K. Cancer incidence of workers in the Finnish pulp and paper industry. *Scand J Work Environ Health* 1987;13:197–202.
145. Hayes RB, Gerin M, Raatgever JW, De Bruyn A. Wood-related occupations, wood dust exposure and sinonasal cancer. *Am J Epidemiol* 1986;124:569–577.
146. Fukuda K, Motomura M, Yamakawa M. Relationship of occupation with cancer of the maxillary sinuses in Hokkaido, Japan. *J Natl Cancer Inst Monogr* 1985;69:169–173.
147. Morton W, Marjanovic D. Leukemia incidence by occupation in the Portland-Vancouver metropolitan area. *Am J Ind Med* 1984;6:185–205.
148. Norell S, Ahlbom A, Olin R, Erwald R, Jacobson G, Lindberg-Navier I, et al. Occupational factors and pancreatic cancer. *Br J Ind Med* 1986;43:775–778.
149. Wingren G, Persson B, Thoren K, Axelson O. Mortality pattern among pulp and paper mill workers in Sweden: a case-referent study. *Am J Ind Med* 1991;20:769–774.
150. Hogstedt C. Cancer epidemiology in the paper and pulp industry. *IARC Sci Publ* 1990;104:382–389.
151. Toren K, Persson B, Wingren G. Health effects of working in pulp and paper mills: malignant diseases. *Am J Ind Med* 1996;29:123–130.
152. Storrs FJ. Dermatitis in the forest products industry. In: Maibach HI, Gellin GA, eds. *Occupational and industrial dermatology.* Chicago: Year Book, 1982:323–328.
153. Menezes Brandao F, Valente A. Photodermatitis from anthraquinone. *Contact Dermatitis* 1988;18:171–172.
154. Jappinen P, Eskelinen A. Patch tests with methylene-bis-thiocyanate in paper mill workers. *Contact Dermatitis* 1987;16:233.
155. Rycroft RJ, Calnan CD. Dermatitis from slimicides in a paper mill. *Contact Dermatitis* 1980;6:435–439.

CHAPTER 45

Hazardous-Waste Disposal and Waste Treatment

John A. Lowe

Past mismanagement of hazardous substances left the United States with a legacy of contaminated soil, groundwater, sediment, and surface water. In the early 1980s, several well-publicized cases of reported symptoms and adverse health effects in locations such as Love Canal, New York, and Times Beach, Missouri, caused people to cast suspicions over all sites where chemical wastes are treated, stored, and disposed. Congress responded with the passage or reauthorization of laws, such as the Comprehensive Environmental Response, Compensation and Liability Act (CERCLA), also known as *Superfund*, and the Resource Conservation and Recovery Act (RCRA). States also enacted waste site cleanup programs on the models of CERCLA and RCRA. By the late 1980s, a fairly standard set of approaches was developed for waste site investigation and cleanup (1,2). Estimates of the resources needed for cleanup of privately owned sites and sites on federal facilities ranged from $480 billion to $1 trillion, to be expended over 30 years (3). A thriving industry developed in hazardous-waste consulting, engineering, and construction services. Health risks associated with exposure to waste site contaminants also furthered the study of environmental epidemiology (4) and exposure analysis (5). These studies have advanced the understanding of waste site exposures and adverse effects in humans, but have been less successful in verifying that regulatory and engineering responses to hazardous-waste sites have produced changes in human exposures or shown measurable benefits to human health.

The process of managing and cleaning up hazardous-waste sites has undergone a transition since the 1980s. Congress delayed reauthorization of the Superfund law, which expired in 1994, reflecting some of the confusion about the nature of risks from hazardous-waste sites and what is needed to address them. Some of the cleanup costs are better understood, such as the Cold War mortgage (estimated to be $227 billion for cleanup of facilities managed by the U.S. Department of Energy that used to manufacture nuclear weapons). The time and expense associated with waste site cleanup have engendered controversy about the public health benefits associated with hazardous-waste site cleanup in relation to the costs involved. Problems have been encountered with understanding the relationship between exposure, health risks, site contaminants, and decision making regarding cleanup. These problems have helped spur advances in exposure assessment and environmental epidemiology, however, and have helped transform the debate about how to use risk assessment for decision making. Remediation of hazardous-waste sites has changed over time from cleanup (e.g., excavation of contaminated soils or pumping and treating contaminated groundwater) to management, using techniques such as bioremediation. Over time, hazardous-waste sites have transformed from a public health problem, to a regulatory and engineering problem, to a social problem concerning issues such as brownfields and environmental equity.

HAZARDOUS-WASTE SITES: NATURE OF THE PROBLEM

Identification of hazardous-waste sites is an initial step toward identifying the nature of their human health threats to surrounding communities and making decisions about remediation. Under CERCLA, the U.S. Environmental Protection Agency (EPA) developed the Comprehensive Environmental Response, Compensation and Liability Information System as a mechanism for identifying potential hazardous-waste sites. These sites would later undergo preliminary assessment and hazard ranking to evaluate the magnitude of their human health or ecological threat (4). More than 40,000 sites are listed in the Comprehensive Environmental Response, Compensation and Liability Information System inventory of sites potentially requiring cleanup. Most of these sites have undergone preliminary assessment, and 1,300 have been placed on the National Priority List (NPL) based on the potential presence of significant human health or ecological risks. Sites on the NPL have undergone further evaluation during the Remedial Investigation/Feasibility Study process to select an appropriate remedial alternative (i.e., cleanup strategy). Selected remedial alternatives then have been committed to action in a Record of Decision, with the actual cleanup being implemented during an engineering and construction phase referred to as *Remedial Design/Remedial Action* (1).

During reauthorization of CERCLA in 1986, Congress gave new authority to the Agency for Toxic Substances and Disease Registry (ATSDR), a part of the Centers for Disease Control and Prevention, to perform public health assessments at NPL sites. Public health assessments are ATSDR's principal device for identifying communities that need public health follow-up. Public health assessments are conducted using environmental contamination data provided primarily by EPA, health outcome data (e.g., birth defects) supplied by state health departments, and community-reported health concerns. Since 1986, the ATSDR has completed more than 1,700 public health assessments of communities around Superfund sites. Using public health assessments, ATSDR has completed an analysis of the demographic characteristics of persons residing around 93% of the current 1,300 NPL sites, and concluded that 11 million people live within 1 mile of an NPL site. An assessment in 1993 to 1994 concluded that approximately 60% of 136 sites have complete exposure pathways to nearby residents (6). Substances most commonly reported at Superfund sites were lead, trichloroethylene (TCE), toluene, benzene, polychlorinated biphenyls, chloroform, phenol, arsenic, cadmium, and chromium (7). Most were sites listed on the NPL based on potential threats to groundwater or drinking water supplies, followed by potential impacts to surface water or soil (4).

Studies performed to identify the potential magnitude of hazardous-waste site risks have evaluated potential health effects using surrogate measures of exposure such as proximity to sites (8). However, proximity to hazardous-waste sites or even the presence of exposure pathways does not necessarily translate to adverse effects on human health. Evaluation of the potential relationship between hazardous-waste sites and health effects is the objective of environmental epidemiology. Environmental epidemiology is the study of the effect on human health of physical, biological, or chemical factors in the external environment. By examining specific populations or communities exposed to different ambient environments, it seeks to clarify the relationship between these factors and human health (4).

SURVEY OF ENVIRONMENTAL EPIDEMIOLOGY STUDIES

Numerous epidemiologic studies have evaluated potential associations between adverse health effects in communities and hazardous-waste disposal (4,9–11). A summary of selected studies is presented in Table 45-1. Some studies attempted to use direct

TABLE 45-1. Summary of selected environmental epidemiological investigations of hazardous-waste sites

Study location	Author	Study design and period of observation	Numbers and types of subjects	Exposure measure	Major health endpoints	Reported outcomes
Hardeman County, Tennessee	Clark et al. 1982 (42)	Cross-sectional, 1978	49 residents at high exposure, 33 residents at intermediate exposure; reference group: 57 unexposed local residents	Carbon tetrachloride in well water; high exposure group had >150 μg/L; intermediate exposure group had <45 μg/L	Liver function	Transient abnormalities of liver function in exposed groups
Lowell, Massachusetts	Ozonoff et al. 1987 (43)	Cross-sectional, 1983	1,049 potentially exposed, reference group of 948 presumably exposed	Surrogate: based on residential distance from the site	Self-reported health problems	Increased prevalence of minor symptoms, irregular heartbeat, fatigue, bowel problems
Woburn, Massachusetts	Lagakos et al. 1986 (44)	Case-control, 1964–1983	20 childhood leukemia cases; reference group of 164 children in Woburn	Surrogate: residence in households served by contaminated wells	Childhood leukemia	Significant association with estimated exposure
Woburn, Massachusetts	Lagakos et al. 1986 (44)	Retrospective follow-up, 1960–1982	4,936 pregnancies among Woburn residents; internal reference	Surrogate: residence in households served by contaminated wells	Adverse pregnancy outcomes; childhood disorders	Association with perinatal deaths; eye/ear anomalies; CNS anomalies; association with kidney/urinary tract infection
Woburn, Massachusetts	Feldman et al. 1988 (45)	Clinical case-control, 1987	28 members of eight families with suspected neurotoxicity because of chronic exposure to TCE in contaminated water; reference group: 27 subjects exhibiting no signs of neurotoxicity or exposure to neurotoxicants	Surrogate: residence in households served by contaminated wells	Blink reflex measurement as indicator of neurotoxicity of TCE	Significant difference in mean blink reflex function when compared to reference group
Santa Clara County, California	California Department of Health Services, 1985 (46)	Retrospective follow-up, 1980–1982	1980–1981: pregnancies in one census tract served by contaminated water; reference group: pregnancies in one census tract not served by contaminated water 1981–1982: live births in a seven-census-tract study area served by contaminated water; reference group: live births in the rest of the county	Surrogate: residence in households served by contaminated water	1980–1981: pregnancy outcomes 1981–1982: congenital cardiac defects	1980–1981: significant excess of spontaneous abortions and congenital malformations 1981–1982: excess incidences of cardiac defects within and outside of the study area. No support for an association with solvent leaks
Santa Clara County, California	Swan et al. 1989 (47)	Retrospective follow-up, 1981–1983	106 babies with diagnosis of cardiac anomaly; born in the county during period of exposure to contaminated water; reference group: babies born in unexposed areas and during unexposed times	Surrogate: residence in households served by contaminated water	Cardiac anomalies	Increased prevalence of cardiac anomalies but temporal distribution suggests solvent leak not responsible
Clinton County, Pennsylvania	Budnick et al. 1984 (48)	Mortality, 1950–1979	Clinton County and three adjacent counties in Pennsylvania; reference groups: 1) Pennsylvania; 2) U.S. population	Surrogate: residence in the area	Bladder cancer mortality	Increased bladder cancer mortality in male resident population after 1970
Clinton County, Pennsylvania	Logue and Fox 1986 (49)	Cross-sectional, 1983	179 long-term residents in the area near the waste site	Surrogate: residence in the area	Self-reported health problems	Increased prevalence of skin problems and sleepiness
Hamilton, Ontario, Canada	Hertzman et al. 1987 (50)	Retrospective follow-up Workers: 1965–1980	Workers: 197 at the site; reference group: 235 nonlandfill outdoor workers from Hamilton Wentworth region	Workers: outdoor employment on or adjacent to the site		Workers: clusters of respiratory, skin, narcotic, and mood disorders
		Residents: 1976–1980	Residents: 614 households within 750 miles of edge of the landfill; reference group: 636 households in same air pollution region as the landfill	Residents: long/short-term residence in area during 1976–1980		Residents: confirmed association between landfill site exposure and mood, narcotic, skin, and respiratory conditions
Montreal, Quebec, Canada	Goldberg et al. 1995 (13)	Case-control, 1979–1989	Live births among residents of three postal zones within 2–4 km of the landfill site; represented exposure zones selected based on prevailing wind direction; reference group: comparable groups drawn from nonexposed areas on the Island of Montreal	Surrogate: proximity to the landfill and location relative to prevailing wind direction	Low birth weight, preterm birth, small for gestational age	Significant elevation in low birth weight and small for gestational age in high exposure zone

CNS, central nervous system; TCE, trichloroethylene.

measures of body burden (typically for lipophilic substances such as polychlorinated biphenyls or DDT) as a measure of exposure, though these exposure data often have limited availability. More commonly used are surrogate measures of exposure, such as proximity to the site, use of a drinking water supply near the site, or measurement of chemical concentrations in air, water, or food. Health-effects indicators often included self-reported symptoms obtained by questionnaires supplemented by physical or clinic examinations. Sometimes, occurrence rates are available from disease registries, particularly for cancer and reproductive outcomes. Cross-sectional and retrospective follow-up surveys are typical study designs.

For example, age-adjusted cancer mortality rates were evaluated in 339 U.S. counties containing hazardous-waste sites where there was evidence of contaminated groundwater providing a sole source of drinking water. Significant associations were observed for increased mortality rates from cancers in several sites of the body (principally gastrointestinal cancers) in counties with hazardous-waste sites compared with counties without hazardous-waste sites. The authors were unable to identify consistent spatial patterns that suggest a broad distribution of gastrointestinal cancers associated with hazardous-waste sites throughout the United States. However there appeared to be excess mortality from gastrointestinal cancers in the states forming EPA Region III (Delaware, Maryland, Pennsylvania, Virginia, and West Virginia). Other factors possibly contributing to the observed mortality included diet and occupational exposures (individuals potentially exposed to waste site contaminants also may have received workplace exposures at the same facilities) (8).

Although epidemiologic findings are still unfolding, when health data from many Superfund sites are evaluated in aggregate, proximity to hazardous-waste sites seems to be associated with a small-to-moderate increased risk of some types of birth defects and cancers (12). The National Research Council indicated in 1991 that "a decade after implementation of Superfund and despite congressional efforts to redirect the program, substantial public health concerns remain, and critical information of exposures and health effects with hazardous-wastes is still lacking" (4). Since then, several initiatives have transformed this picture. Significant research efforts have been initiated in the areas of exposure assessment and biomarkers to benefit the practice of environmental epidemiology and to improve decision making for hazardous-waste site cleanup. Hazardous-waste sites are being ranked in terms of health, ecological, and societal risks alongside disparate problems, such as air quality, surface water quality, drinking water protection, habitat restoration, ecosystem disruption, and global climate effects, to determine how limited resources should be allocated among them. Hazardous-waste sites also are viewed as a social problem with the emergence of environmental equity and brownfield development issues.

However, the presence of these broader issues has not diminished the importance of environmental epidemiology in addressing the risks associated with hazardous-waste sites. The Superfund Basic Research Program, funded through the National Institute for Environmental Health Sciences has sponsored a range of research advancing the field of environmental epidemiology. For example, a study at Boston University is incorporating case-control data from a study area into a Geographic Information System to evaluate the cancer risk associated with single and multiple geographically located exposures. A digitized representation of pertinent spatial (residence, exposure zones) and demographic (years of residence, age, sex) data then can be used to evaluate new analytic techniques to detect and verify spatial aggregation (hot spots or clusters) of adverse effects. At the University of California, Berkeley, the role of genetic differences in glutathione transferase enzymes is being investigated as it potentially relates to susceptibility to childhood leukemia, bladder cancer, and DNA damage by environmental pollutants. A case-control study also is being performed to investigate the relationship between environmental exposures and the risk of childhood leukemia, using molecular biology techniques to characterize the presence of genetic changes and possible effects of modifiers (e.g., tobacco smoke, diet) and to estimate the critical time of exposure. Clusters of childhood leukemia have been reported around hazardous facilities, including Superfund sites. Currently, little is known about the causes of childhood leukemia and what environmental exposures may cause the disease. Genetic damage may be inherited or occur *in utero* or after birth. Exposure to environmental carcinogens during any of these intervals is suspected to cause detrimental genetic change.

The investigation of cancer risks near a municipal solid waste landfill in Montreal, Quebec, Canada (13), illustrates the limitations of epidemiologic studies in evaluating the relationship between disposal sites and health risks with respect to the assessment of exposure. The principal exposure concern with the Miron Quarry municipal solid waste landfill was air emissions of volatile organic chemicals in landfill gas. Evidence of exposure to landfill gas emissions consisted of odor complaints from residents up to 1.5 km from the landfill, and measurement of methane concentrations in air near the landfill, ranging from 0 to 25 parts per million. The collection system detected numerous aromatic and chlorinated volatile hydrocarbons in landfill gas, at concentrations ranging from 1 to 218 mg per m^3 (note that these are not concentrations in ambient air potentially representing human exposure). Several of these chemicals were known or suspected human carcinogens, including benzene, vinyl chloride, TCE, tetrachloroethylene and methylene chloride. For purposes of evaluating cancer incidences, low-, medium-, or high-exposure zones were defined around the site based on proximity to the landfill and prevailing wind directions. Cancer cases were assigned to the exposure zones using data compiled in a nationwide cancer registry. The relative risks for cancers of the stomach, upper respiratory tract (trachea, bronchus, and lung) and liver were elevated slightly in the high-exposure zone closest to the landfill. The ratios were relatively significant from reference areas though the relative risks were small, ranging from 1.1 to 1.5. The strengths of this study are that the cancer incidences were estimated from a cancer registry that would reduce underreporting bias. The principal limitations are errors in exposure classification, inadequate control of potential confounding factors, and a relatively short period from first exposure (the landfill opened in 1968) to cancer onset (evaluated between 1981 and 1988).

The absence of exposure data creates significant difficulties in evaluating the relationship between the observed risk ratios and volatile organic compounds (VOCs) detected in landfill gas. In the late 1960s and mid-1970s, a growing body of evidence also indicated that pollutant exposure concentrations (those that humans actually come in contact with) could differ significantly from ambient measurements (14). The Total Exposure Assessment Methodology Study performed in the late 1980s showed that personal exposures to VOCs measured by personal sampling generally were greater than outdoor concentrations. This was due largely to elevated levels in indoor air at home or work. Specific sources included smoking or passive smoking (aromatic hydrocarbons), visiting dry cleaners (tetrachloroethane), visiting service stations (aromatic hydrocarbons), and occupation. In most cases, these specific sources far outweighed the impact of traditional major point sources (chemical plants, petroleum refineries, petrochemical plants) and area sources (dry cleaners and service stations) on personal exposure (15–17). Given the multiplicity of emissions sources of VOCs, exposure data in this case are a critical element in judging the relationship between emissions from a landfill and observed health effects.

ROLE OF EXPOSURE ASSESSMENTS IN MANAGING HAZARDOUS-WASTE SITES

Environmental epidemiology studies provide the most defensible data regarding the relationship between hazardous-waste site contaminants and human health effects. As discussed previously, epidemiology studies of hazardous-waste sites too often are insufficiently conclusive to allow decision makers to address problems with specific sites. With regard to hazardous-waste sites:

> Perhaps the single most perplexing problem in developing human health data related to toxic wastes sites is in the assessment of exposure experienced by the study population because it is seldom possible to have direct evidence of exposure in terms of body burden residues found in human tissues or fluids. Exposure often must be estimated from questionnaire data, employment records, and from air, water, and soil monitoring of the environment surrounding the dump site area. To further complicate matters, the toxicity of chemicals may vary over time or through transport. Researchers must contend with complex mixtures of chemicals and there have been few attempts to estimate health effects related to such exposure. Furthermore, chemicals are often nonspecific as they relate to a particular disease and outcome measurements may require long latency periods before disease assessment is possible. Finally, the size of populations living around hazardous waste sites is usually small, a situation that may result in studies with low statistical power and inconsistent results. (8)

A complete pathway of exposure must be present for adverse health effects to be associated with contaminants at a hazardous-waste site. A complete exposure pathway contains these five elements:

- Source (e.g., landfill, spill)
- Transport media (e.g., groundwater, air)
- Exposure point (e.g., drinking water well, food source, shower)
- Route of exposure (i.e., ingestion, inhalation, dermal absorption)
- Receptor population (e.g., families, schoolchildren) (2,18)

If any of these elements is missing, no complete pathway exists, and there is no human exposure to hazardous-waste site contaminants. The pathways of exposure to the surrounding populations are influenced by factors such as proximity of human populations, access to the site that influences the potential for on-site contact, the nature of human activities (drinking water supplies, food sources) that influence routes of exposure, and physical and chemical properties that influence the potential for contaminants to migrate from the site into offsite groundwater, surface water, or air. Assessment of human exposure is highly site-specific, accounting for the nature of the site (such as the local topography, soil conditions, geology, and hydrology), the physical and chemical characteristics of the wastes disposed there, and the characteristics of the surrounding populations and resources.

Exposure assessments are indispensable for the conduct of effective risk assessments, for the success of epidemiologic research, for the surveillance of environmental and health stresses in populations and ecosystems, and for development and evaluation of the efficacy of risk management activities. Risk management is synonymous with management of exposures (19). Exposure requires the simultaneous occurrence of two events: (a) the presence of an environmental toxicant at a particular point in space and time and (b) the presence of a person or persons at that same location and time. Peoples' activity patterns, eating and drinking habits, and lifestyle characteristics must be superimposed over concentration in environmental media before it is possible to derive realistic estimates of actual human exposure. Too often in the past, pollutant concentrations in a particular medium have been assumed to represent exposure, only for it to be found later that they did not provide an accurate picture because of modifying factors such as the time people spend indoors versus outdoors, food preparation and cooking, and use of bottled water instead of tap water. Experience has shown that exclusive reliance on central monitoring sites (e.g., urban air pollution monitoring sites or samples from drinking water reservoirs) and bulk sampling procedures (e.g., spot checks for pesticides in food for determining human exposures) is not adequate or sufficient in most cases, especially for potentially at-risk groups, such as migrant farm workers, subsistence fishermen, and farmers, and those who are more susceptible, including pregnant women and their fetuses and the infirm or elderly (5).

Because of the sense of urgency typically pervading many regulatory decisions, strong incentives exist for risk and exposure assessments to collect information that meets pressing regulatory needs. However, the amount of data generated with this narrow, short-term focus often outstrips the ability to interpret the data. This short-term focus also has not been matched by an effort to improve the quality of exposure and risk assessment (5). For example, EPA has used the reasonable maximum exposure (RME) scenario in risk assessments for making remedial action decisions at Superfund sites (2). RME is defined as the highest exposure that is reasonably expected to occur at a site. The intent of the RME is to develop a conservative estimate of exposure (i.e., well above the average case) that is still within the range of possible exposure (2). Examples of specific factors in the RME exposure scenario are exposure concentrations in soil, water, or air that are based on the upper 95% confidence limit on the mean concentration at a site. However, whether an estimated exposure rate is truly the "reasonable maximum" is open to question depending on the spatial distribution of contamination (hot spots) as it relates to frequency of contact and locations of potentially exposed individuals at the site.

This approach results in an exposure estimate with no consistent interpretation. For example, the calculated RME may be less-than-average exposure at one site, well above average at another, and a near-maximum exposure at a third, all depending on contaminant distribution and sampling locations (20,21). These problems lessen the credibility of exposure and risk assessments as decision-making tools for managing hazardous-waste sites.

For risk assessment to be perceived as a credible and reliable tool for decision making, EPA has identified the need for full characterization of health risks (22). Full characterization of health risks means that numeric estimates of human exposure and health risks must be accompanied by narrative that describes the nature of the data, assumptions, and parameters used in exposure estimation; characterizes the variability and uncertainty in exposure estimates; and provides a statement of the level of confidence in the exposure estimates. In this light, it is more important to develop a distribution of exposures in a population so that risk descriptors, such as high-end and central-tendency risk estimates, can be presented to risk managers. The high-end exposure estimate should be presented (22). High-end risk is a plausible estimate of the individual risk for those individuals at the upper end of the risk distribution. The intent of this descriptor is to convey an estimate of risk in the upper range of the distribution but to avoid estimates that are beyond the true distribution. High-end risk means risks above the ninetieth percentile of the population distribution, but not higher than the individual in the population who has the highest risk.

Current exposure assessment capabilities, however, are hampered by technical limitations in the currently available exposure measurement techniques, severe limitations of the currently available databases containing exposure and exposure-relevant data, reliance on numerous assumptions that have been proven incorrect or are not supported by common experience or direct observations, and by the current fragmentation and lack of coherence of available models for different media, pathways, or chemicals (19). Examples of exposure-related questions that may prove to be difficult to answer include (23)

- Measurements in an urban neighborhood show low levels of several chemicals. Are these abnormal levels because of a nearby source or are they typical for an urban environment?
- An exposure assessment, which combines estimates of concentrations in air, water, or soil with a scenario describing human activities, provides an estimate of chemical exposure associated with a particular situation. Is this estimate consistent with levels actually experienced by the population in question?
- Exposure estimates are developed in different ways. Some are estimates derived from an exposure scenario, some from short-term measurements, and some from body-burden measurements. Are these estimates correct?
- Members of a particular community experience exposures to a variety of chemicals during their daily routine. Are the individuals who are most highly exposed to one chemical also at the higher end of the exposure distribution for other chemicals, or are the exposures distributed more randomly across the population?

These questions have relevance for regulatory decisions, such as how to manage potential exposure to hazardous-waste site contaminants. They go to the heart of such matters as how to identify particular sources of exposure (particularly important in determining when to clean up a hazardous-waste site), whether regulatory action is based on exposure assessments that are overly conservative or reasonably representative of human populations, the reliability of exposure models used in regulatory decision making, and whether certain subpopulations experience disproportionately higher exposures and health risks—an important concern for the environmental justice movement (23).

TRANSITIONAL ISSUES IN HAZARDOUS-WASTE SITE MANAGEMENT

The dimensions of hazardous-waste site problems have changed since the passage of Superfund and RCRA in the late 1970s and early 1980s. Originally viewed as a public health problem (4), or a regulatory and engineering problem (1), hazardous-waste sites have acquired attributes of social problems (e.g., brownfields or the Cold War mortgage). Ongoing debate about how to address hazardous-waste sites has delayed congressional reauthorization of the Superfund law, which expired in 1994. Part of this debate involves the level of state or local involvement there should be in making cleanup decisions about hazardous-waste sites.

Concerns have arisen that the threats posed by some regulated substances (such as hazardous-waste site contaminants) might have been overstated and, conversely, that some unregulated substances might pose greater threats than originally believed. Questions also have been raised about the economic costs of controlling or remediating chemical contaminants that might pose extremely small risks. Debates about reducing risks and controlling costs have been fed by the lack of universal agreement among scientists about which methods are best for assessing risk to humans. However, considerable advances have been made in the sciences underpinning risk assessment (i.e., toxicology, geology, meteorology). Better data and increased understanding of biological mechanisms and of the behavior of chemicals in the environment should enable risk assessments that are less dependent on conservative default assumptions and more accurate as predictions of human risk (24). Further discussions have focused on developing a process for using risk assessment to make good risk management decisions and for actively engaging stakeholders in that process. A six-stage process has been proposed for risk management that can be scaled to the importance of a public health or environmental problem (25).

NATIONAL HUMAN EXPOSURE ASSESSMENT SURVEY

The perception is growing that exposure surveillance of the U.S. population benefits efforts to identify, assess, manage, and communicate health risks associated with environmental agents (5). The National Human Exposure Assessment Survey (NHEXAS) is a federal interagency activity intended to provide credible, reliable, and timely exposure-related information to decision makers. The goals of NHEXAS are to document the occurrence and distribution of chemical exposure, including geographical and temporal trends, understand the underlying causes of exposure for potentially at-risk subpopulations, and provide data and methods for linking information on exposures, doses, and health outcomes.

One principal objective of the NHEXAS is to test the validity of modeled exposure assessments. The methods of NHEXAS involve measurements using questionnaires, diaries, interviews, personal monitoring, and human tissue monitoring. The measured parameters include sociodemographic and residential characteristics, time-activity patterns, exposure factors (such as food or water consumption patterns), media concentrations (in air, water, food, soil, and dust), exposure concentrations (breathing zone air), and dose (body burden in blood, urine, and hair). These measurements are made with a population-based probability sampling design. The nature and intensity of these studies probably preclude their routine use. However, they should be useful for drawing inferences regarding potential sources of exposures for the general U.S. population and sensitive subpopulations, building reliable models of exposure, identifying biomarkers that can be used to monitor exposure of sensitive subpopulations, and providing a better exposure database for supporting environmental epidemiologic investigations.

BROWNFIELDS

As presently conceived, Superfund entails investigating the degree of contamination at each site, estimating the potential exposures and risks, establishing cleanup goals for soil and groundwater, comparing and choosing treatment technologies, litigating the allocation of liability among potentially responsible parties, and adhering to the maze of applicable local, state, and federal laws. The process is cumbersome, staggeringly expensive, and painfully slow. Selecting appropriate cleanup goals and developing plans for sites also engender much contention and resentment (26). One of the problems that may have inadvertently been created by the Superfund process is brownfields. Brownfields consist of land or buildings that are abandoned or underused where expansion or redevelopment is complicated in part because of the threat of known or potential contamination. Federal and state laws governing the treatment of these sites may require remediation (cleanup) of the property before redevelopment and can contribute to uncertain liability for property owners or users. As a result of these and other factors, redevelopment and reuse of these sites can be hindered. Redevelopment of brownfield sites is a particular problem in many central cities and inner suburbs of U.S. metropolitan areas that need to create jobs and attract commercial and industrial development. Because of this, a number of states and cities have developed programs to facilitate assessment, cleanup, and redevelopment of brownfields.

The exact number and environmental condition of brownfields in the country is unknown. Estimates range from tens of thousands to 450,000 sites. Information on the level of contamination of brownfields is limited. Some sites have anywhere from zero to low or moderate contamination to extremely hazardous conditions. Other sites have not been evaluated. Although the exact nature and extent of the problem is difficult to assess, most sites considered brownfields are not associated with extreme levels of contamination. They will never be considered for addition to the NPL or similar state priority lists. Because these sites do not pose a serious threat or warrant immediate federal attention, they become the responsibility of the states or municipalities where they are located. For this reason, states have taken an active role in identifying and confronting the barriers to promoting brownfield cleanup and redevelopment.

Because brownfields are known as potential hazardous-waste sites, a number of challenges to their cleanup and reuse exist. Uncertain liability associated with federal and state environmental laws is perhaps the most critical. The complicated and often overlapping nature of these laws creates an unclear picture of the real risk of liability and provides a barrier for redevelopment of a site. The costs of site characterization and cleanup, when added to the costs of development, also may be a barrier to investing in a brownfield site. Other uncertainties that may frustrate action on brownfields include specification of cleanup requirements and definition of the role for public involvement at brownfield sites. Finally, demand for these sites varies depending on the location, with some sites having limited redevelopment potential even after cleanup (27).

NATURAL ATTENUATION CONCEPTS AND MANAGEMENT OF CONTAMINATION

Superfund and RCRA corrective action programs share the common purposes of protecting human health and the environment from contaminated groundwaters and restoring those waters to a quality consistent with their current or reasonable expected future uses. Experience has shown that restoration to drinking water quality levels (or more stringent levels where required) may not always be achievable because of the limitations of available remediation technologies. Using microorganisms to degrade contaminants in groundwater (*in situ* bioremediation) has emerged as a new technology for groundwater remediation. Research has contributed greatly to understanding the biotic, chemical, and hydrologic parameters characteristic of the ideal candidate site for successful implementation of *in situ* bioremediation. These characteristics include (a) a homogeneous and permeable aquifer; (b) a contaminant originating from a single source; (c) a low groundwater gradient; (d) no free product; (e) no soil contamination; and (f) an easily degraded, extracted, or immobilized contaminant. Obviously, few sites meet these characteristics. However, development of information concerning site-specific geological and microbiological characteristics of the aquifer combined with knowledge about potential chemical, physical, and biochemical fates of the wastes present can be used to develop a bioremediation strategy for a less-than-ideal site (28).

Biological *in situ* treatment of aquifers is usually accomplished by stimulation of indigenous microorganisms to degrade organic waste constituents present at a site (29). The microorganisms are stimulated by injecting inorganic nutrients and, if required, an appropriate electron acceptor, into aquifer materials. However, effectiveness of inoculation into uncontrolled and poorly accessible environments, such as the subsurface, is much more difficult to achieve, demonstrate, and assess.

Bioremediation of an aquifer contaminated with organic compounds can be achieved by biodegradation of the compounds. In the case of aerobic metabolism, bioremediation can achieve complete mineralization of constituents to carbon dioxide, water, inorganic salts, and cell mass. With anaerobic metabolism, methane, carbon dioxide, and cell mass result. In the natural environment, however, a constituent may not be completely degraded. It may be transformed to an intermediate product or products that may be equally or more hazardous than the parent compound. For example, TCE is degraded through reductive dehalogenation to vinyl chloride (30), potentially increasing the risks associated with biodegradation of TCE in groundwater.

RISK ASSESSMENT IN TRANSITION

The transition in risk assessment has taken two forms. In one case, risk assessment for hazardous-waste sites has become highly standardized with well-developed guidelines. At the same time, the scope and role of risk assessment as a decision-making tool have expanded.

Current Practices: Risk Assessment Guidance for Superfund

Risk assessments for hazardous-waste sites, in their current form, are based on *Risk Assessment Guidance for Superfund (RAGS)*, a series of guidance documents developed by the EPA Office of Solid Waste and Emergency Response (2,31,32). These guidance documents promoted the use of the RME scenario for exposure assessment, the linearized-multistage model for assessing risks from carcinogen exposure (a no-threshold cancer risk assessment model), and the reference dose for other systemic effects, as the basis for risk management at Superfund sites. Added guidance, principally addressing exposure assessment techniques, has been developed by the EPA Office of Research and Development. These have included the EPA *Exposure Factors Handbook* and *Guidelines for Exposure Assessment* (33,34). Guidelines for using risk assessments based on the RAGS methodology have been developed by the Office of Solid Waste and Emergency Response. These risk management guidelines specify that remedial actions should achieve excess lifetime cancer risks ranging from 1 in 10,000 to 1 in 1,000,000 using risk assessments based on the RME scenario (35).

Some of the debate during congressional reauthorization of the Superfund law has revolved around how to achieve consistency in selection of remedial actions and in cleanup standards. The latter issue also involves achieving consistency in risk assessment methods. This has led to the development of Soil Screening Levels (SSLs), which are based on the guidelines published in RAGS. SSLs are risk-based soil contaminant concentrations (presented in units of mg of contaminant per kg of soil) that are derived based on future residential land use assumptions and associated exposure scenarios. It supports the identification of those portions of a site containing soils that are contaminated at levels that warrant a full evaluation of potential risk to support selection of a remedial option, and those portions containing soils that do not present risks warranting further analysis (i.e., those that can be screened out). These chemical-specific SSLs then are compared against concentrations of each contaminant of concern in site soils. Discrete areas of soils with contaminants at concentrations that fall below their respective SSL value can be eliminated from further investigation at the site. Although those site areas with any contaminants exceeding their SSL do not necessarily require remediation, they do require further evaluation to determine if removal or remedial action is necessary. Although SSLs are not cleanup standards, they can be used to delineate areas in soil with contaminants considered to pose health risks that warrant further evaluation (36).

SSLs do much to provide consistency in risk assessments and cleanup levels for hazardous-waste sites (20). However, the risk assessment approach underlying SSLs has several conceptual difficulties. Also, because SSLs are based on RME assumptions, they do not reflect the distribution of potential exposures and risks considered necessary to achieve full characterization of health risks. EPA guidelines state that risk assessments should strive for full characterization of health risks (22). SSLs represent the traditional approach, addressing uncertainty in risk assessment using conservative assumptions that err on the side of safety and tend to overstate the risks associated with environmental contaminants. Although a conservative risk assessment has the advantages of simplicity and high agency acceptability, these are often outweighed by its disadvantages: exaggeration of health risks, inadequate risk communication, and loss of scientific credibility. These problems can lead to misspent resources in controlling or remediating environmental hazards that are more perceived than real. Some of the alternatives that have been proposed to address this concern include use of tiered approaches to risk assessment and the use of probabilistic risk assessments.

RISK-BASED CORRECTIVE ACTION

The tiered approach to risk assessment is a feature of risk-based corrective action (RBCA) for petroleum release sites (37). RBCA is a consistent decision-making process developed for the assessment and response to petroleum releases based on protection of human health and the environment. RBCA offers a three-tiered approach for incorporating risk assessment in the corrective action process. Although developed originally to address petroleum releases, RBCA provides a framework that can be applied to assess and manage risks associated with different chemicals under a variety of site conditions. With RBCA, the extent of cleanup to be performed is risk-based, with assessment and corrective action activities tailored to site-specific conditions and nature of site risks. RBCA integrates risk assessment practice with site characterization activities and selection of remediation options to ensure that the chosen action is protective of health and the environment. Use of a tiered, risk-based approach, such as RBCA, can result in protective, yet cost-effective corrective actions.

The tier 1 evaluation is a risk assessment to develop concentrations in soil or water for various property use categories (e.g., residential, commercial, or industrial) and exposure pathways using conservative default exposure factors and assumptions. Tier 1 evaluations are tabulated for easy use and are compared directly with chemical concentrations measured in source areas. In a tier 2 evaluation, additional site characterization data and predictive modeling are used to estimate the extent of attenuation that may occur between the source area and a distant point of exposure such as a property boundary or a nearby residential well. The predictive modeling used is relatively simplistic, with model inputs limited to readily attainable data such as total porosity or soil bulk density. The models do not account for all relevant physical and chemical phenomena, resulting in predicted concentrations greater than are likely to occur (e.g., assuming steady-state or constant concentrations in the source area). The tier 3 evaluation relies on more sophisticated statistical techniques to evaluate site characterization data, refined analytical methods, such as hydrocarbon fingerprinting, more complex predictive modeling and site-specific exposure factors. A tier 3 evaluation may involve collection of significant additional site information and more extensive data assessment and modeling than are required for either a tier 1 or 2 evaluation. Examples of tier 3 activities include nonparametric statistical analyses, numeric groundwater modeling, laboratory studies to estimate leachability and biodegradation, surveys of activities of nearby populations, and probabilistic analyses to estimate the statistical distribution of exposure and risks associated with chemical concentrations at a given site.

Use of a tiered approach provides a user with an option to determine target levels for remediation based progressively on more realistic conditions, which may reduce the extent and cost of remedial action at the expense of added site characterization and assessment of data.

PROBABILISTIC RISK ASSESSMENT

The realization is growing that highly conservative risk assessments yield unrealistic estimates of the risks associated with hazardous-wastes, which exaggerate public concerns and cleanup actions beyond what is required to protect public health and the environment. One approach for improving risk assessments that is gaining acceptance is the use of probabilistic techniques. Probabilistic risk assessment holds the promise of making environmental decision-making risk-based, providing a better basis for communicating the nature of risks associated with hazardous-wastes, and improving the scientific credibility of risk assessment.

Some crucial limitations to the current RME approach exist. First, the combination of several upper-bound or worst-case assumptions means that the risk assessment is considering an exposure scenario with an extremely small likelihood of occurring. Second, with the mixture of average, upper-bound, and worst-case assumptions, risk managers have no way of knowing the degree of conservatism in a risk assessment (20). Current EPA guidelines for hazardous-waste site risk assessments reflect a deterministic analysis, which uses a point estimate for each assumption, resulting in a single estimate of risk. It is difficult to know the bounds of uncertainty surrounding that estimate, or the magnitude of conservatism in it. Probabilistic analysis provides a distribution of risk estimates, based on ranges or distribution of possible values for each assumption. The contrasts between deterministic and probabilistic (or stochastic) analyses are presented in Figures 45-1 and 45-2. One technique used to translate the uncertainty in assumptions into a distribution of risk estimates is Monte Carlo simulation. In this technique, the assumptions to the risk assessment model are transformed into input distributions. A large number of independent samples are collected from each distribution from which corresponding outputs (i.e., risk estimates) are calculated. With a large sampling, a distribution of risks is obtained. Summary statistics (such as mean, median, and confidence limits) and percentiles may then be estimated from the distribution. The distribution of risks from a Monte Carlo simulation then can reflect average or median risks, representing exposure scenarios with a reasonable likelihood of occurring, along with high-end risks, representing exposure scenarios that are less likely to occur (38–40).

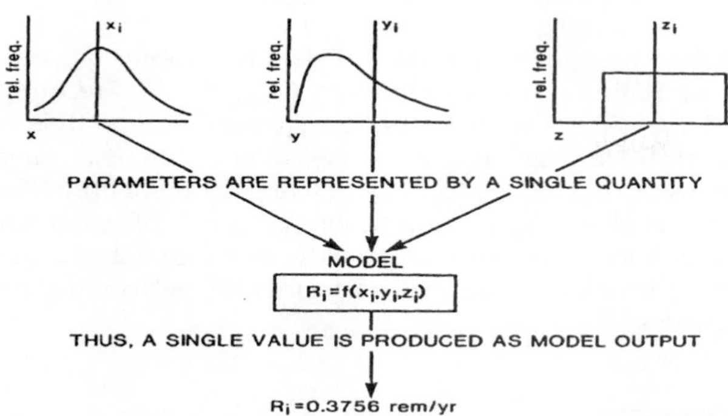
ALTHOUGH A RANGE OF VALUES ARE POSSIBLE FOR EACH INPUT PARAMETER IN A MODEL,
rel. freq.
PARAMETERS ARE REPRESENTED BY A SINGLE QUANTITY
MODEL
$R_i = f(x_i, y_i, z_i)$
THUS, A SINGLE VALUE IS PRODUCED AS MODEL OUTPUT
$R_i = 0.3756$ rem/yr

Figure 45-1. Exposure assessment based on deterministic methods. (From Hoffman FO, Miller CW. Uncertainties in environmental radiological assessment models and their implications in environmental radioactivity. Proceedings of the 19th Annual Meeting of the NCRP, April 6–7, 1983. Bethesda, MD: National Council on Radiation Protection and Measurements, 1983:110–138, with permission.)

FRAMEWORK FOR RISK ASSESSMENT AND RISK MANAGEMENT

The Commission on Risk Assessment and Risk Management was mandated by Congress in the Clean Air Act Amendments of 1990 "to make a full investigation of the policy implications and appropriate uses of risk assessment and risk management in regulatory programs under various Federal laws to prevent cancer and other chronic human health effects which may result from exposure to hazardous substances" (25,41). The work of the commission grew out of the recognition that as risk assessment has been growing more complex and sophisticated, the output of risk assessment for the regulatory process often seems too focused on refining assumption-laden, mathematic estimates of small risks associated with exposure to individual chemicals rather than on the overall goal—risk reduction and improved health status. The commission proposed a systematic, comprehensive framework that addresses various contaminants, media, and sources of exposure, and public values, perceptions, and ethics, as it keeps the focus on the risk management goal:

- Formulate the problem in broad context.
- Analyze the risks.
- Define the options.
- Make sound decisions.
- Take actions to implement the decisions.
- Perform an evaluation of the effectiveness of the actions taken.

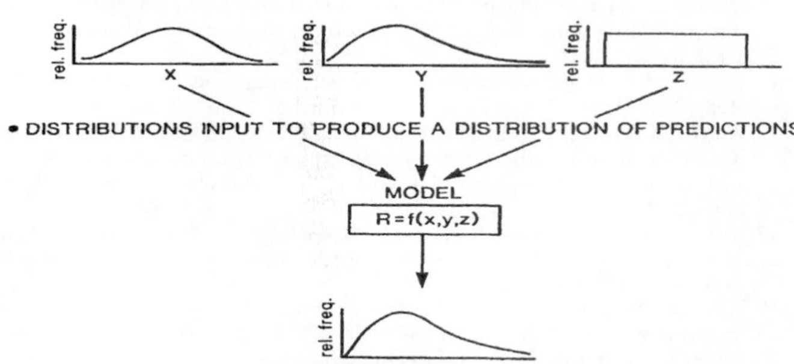
• UNCERTAIN PARAMETERS DESCRIBED AS RANDOM VARIABLES
rel. freq.
X
Y
Z
• DISTRIBUTIONS INPUT TO PRODUCE A DISTRIBUTION OF PREDICTIONS
MODEL
R = f(x,y,z)
PREDICTED VALUES (R)

Figure 45-2. Exposure assessment based on probabilistic (stochastic) method. (From FO Hoffman, Miller CW. Uncertainties in environmental radiological assessment models and their implications in environmental radioactivity. Proceedings of the 19th Annual Meeting of the NCRP, April 6–7, 1983. Bethesda, MD: National Council on Radiation Protection and Measurements, 1983:110–138, with permission.)

The framework explicitly embraces collaborative and early involvement of stakeholders. The process can be refined and its conclusions changed as important new information is acquired. The framework requires that a potential or current problem be put into a broader context of public health or environmental health. The interdependence of related multimedia problems also must be identified. The framework focuses on cumulative risks to human and environmental health. It also addresses the benefits, costs, and social, cultural, ethical, political, and legal dimensions of risk reduction options.

The framework documents examined the relationships between risk management and regulatory decision making, including the roles and processes of risk communications, methods for risk comparisons, uses of risk bright lines, such as a 1×10^{-6} excess lifetime cancer risk level, and the nature of administrative and judicial processes. Discussions of the limitations of risk assessment and economic analysis in risk management and the scope and role for peer review in risk assessment culminated in several recommendations for risk assessment practices for different regulatory agencies.

One of the problems with remedy selection under the Superfund law has been the inconsistent use of future land uses and of realistic exposure scenarios in risk assessments. A principal recommendation is that risk assessments and remedy selection should be based on reasonably anticipated current and future uses of a site. Initial inclusion of affected communities as partners in the investigation and remedy selection processes can improve the likelihood that the choice of a remedy reflects reasonably anticipated uses of the site and the wishes of the community. EPA should continue to use its 10^{-6} to 10^{-4} excess lifetime cancer risk range as a guide for site-specific, risk-based cleanup goals, related to future land use. It was recommended that risk assessments be based on realistic high-end exposure scenarios for screening assessments and descriptive or probabilistic distributions or ranges of exposure for refined risk assessment (41).

Three basic decision-making structural and functional problems have been identified with EPA risk assessments:

- Unjustified conservatism, often manifested as an unwillingness to accept new data or abandon default options
- Undue reliance on point estimates generated by risk assessment
- Lack of appropriate conservatism because of a failure to accommodate such issues as synergism, human variability, or unusual exposure conditions

Although EPA's risk assessment practices rely heavily on default assumptions, EPA never has articulated the scientific or policy basis of those options. Because of limitations on time, resources, scientific knowledge, and available data, the report concluded that EPA should retain its conservative, default-based approach to risk assessment for screening analysis in standard setting. Several recommendations have been offered to make this approach more effective:

- Use an iterative approach to risk assessment.
- Provide justification for defaults and establish a procedure that permits departure from defaults.
- When communicating information about risks to decision-makers and the public, identify the sources and magnitude of the uncertainty associated with risk estimates (24).

CONCLUSIONS

When Congress enacted the original Superfund law in 1980, there was little awareness of the extent of the problem created by years of inappropriate or inadequate hazardous-waste disposal practices. Originally, it was thought that Superfund would need to clean up just a few hundred sites. It was expected that the initial authorization of $1.6 billion plus reasonable expenditures by private companies would be sufficient. As of 1999, more than 1,300 sites with significant contamination have been identified. The universe of contaminated sites may range into several hundred thousand, a legacy of an earlier industrial era. Most of those sites are not so highly contaminated or complex as to require the attention and active management of the federal Superfund program. EPA, states, and others are working together on a range of approaches to address this array of contaminated sites. Many states administer voluntary cleanup programs that can return contaminated lands (brownfields) to productive reuse (41).

Of the 1,300 Superfund sites assessed by ATSDR from 1987 through December 1994, completed exposure pathways were identified at approximately 40% of sites. Although epidemiologic findings are still unfolding, when evaluated in aggregate (i.e., by combining health data from many Superfund sites), proximity to hazardous-waste sites seems to be associated with a small-to-moderate increased risk of some kinds of birth defects and, less well documented, some specific cancers. Gaps still exist in scientific knowledge about the toxicity, bioavailability, exposure, and human health effects of individual hazardous substances and mixtures of substances released from Superfund sites and during emergency releases. A particular need exists for data on levels of exposure to hazardous substances in community populations (6). These problems have promoted initiatives, such as the Superfund Basic Research Program, through the National Institute for Environmental Health Sciences, and NHEXAS, through several federal agencies, in an attempt to improve the ability to make decisions about hazardous-waste site cleanup.

Although environmental epidemiology provides the best scientific evidence regarding potential health effects associated with hazardous-waste sites, the limitations of epidemiologic research make it difficult to draw definitive conclusions about individual sites. Decision making regarding hazardous-waste site cleanup is likely to be based on risk assessment for the foreseeable future. However, risk assessment is but one element of environmental decision making. Other factors include applicable statutes, precedents established within the responsible government agencies, and good public policy. The limited resources available for environmental protection should be spent to generate information that helps risk managers to choose the best possible course of action among available options. The results of a risk assessment are not scientific estimates of actual risk. They are conditional estimates of the risk that could exist under specified sets of assumptions (24). Combined with other information—clinical, political, engineering, social, and economic—risk assessment can be useful for guiding decisions about hazardous-waste site cleanup. An iterative approach has been recommended as the best way to use limited time and resources for risk assessments.

Concern exists about the possible public reaction to iterative determinations of risk. Suppose that a first-tier, screening risk assessment of a contaminated site concludes that an upper-bound incremental lifetime cancer risk greater than 10^{-6} is possible. Later refined risk assessments of the same site conclude that the risk is likely to be less than 10^{-6}. The residents of the surrounding community have been told first that the site poses a risk to their health and now that it does not. It is unlikely that such apparently conflicting conclusions establish any credibility for a regulatory agency. Citizens remain suspicious and probably believe that the site constitutes a health hazard, despite messages to the contrary.

An iterative approach could still yield the risk-management decisions required under regulatory mandates in a resource-limited manner. At the same time, it could provide incentives for further research where it is warranted. A vast difference might exist between having the truth and having enough information to enable a risk manager to choose the best course of action from several options. This is probably a more useful course of action, given the time and resource constraints for performing risk assessments (41).

REFERENCES

1. US Environmental Protection Agency. *Guidance for conducting remedial investigation/feasibility studies under CERCLA*. Washington: Office of Emergency and Remedial Response, 1988.
2. US Environmental Protection Agency. *Risk assessment guidance for Superfund*, vol I: *Human health evaluation manual (Part A)*. Washington: Office of Emergency and Remedial Response, 1989. [EPA/540/1-89/002].
3. Russell M, Colglazier EW, English MR. *Hazardous waste remediation: the task ahead*. Knoxville: University of Tennessee, Waste Management Research and Education Institute, 1991.
4. National Research Council. *Environmental epidemiology*, vol 1. *Public health and hazardous waste*. Committee on Environmental Epidemiology. Washington: National Academy Press, 1991.
5. Sexton K, Callahan MA, Bryan EF, Saint CG, Wood WP. Informed decisions about protecting and promoting public health: rationale for a national human assessment survey. *J Expo Anal Environ Epidemiol* 1995; 5(3):229–232.
6. Johnson BL. Testimony of Barry L. Johnson, Assistant Administrator of the Agency for Toxic Substances and Disease Registry before the Water Resources and Environment Subcommittee Committee on Transportation and Infrastructure, US House of Representatives, Washington, DC, June 27, 1995. Available at: http://atsdr1.atsdr.cdc.gov:8080/test627.html.
7. Grisham JE. *Health aspects of the disposal of chemical wastes*. New York: Pergamon Press, 1986.
8. Griffith J, Riggan WB, Pellom AC. Cancer mortality in U.S. counties with hazardous waste sites and groundwater pollution. *Arch Environ Health* 1989;44(2):69–74.
9. Levine, R, Chitwood DD. Public health investigations of hazardous organic chemical disposal in the United States. *Environ Health Perspect* 1985;62:415–422.
10. Buffler PA, Crane M, Key MM. Possibilities of detecting health effects by studies of populations exposed to chemicals from waste disposal sites. *Environ Health Perspect* 1985;62:423–456.
11. Upton AC, Kneip T, Toniolo P. Public health aspects of toxic chemical disposal sites. *Annu Rev Public Health* 1989;10:1–25.
12. Agency for Toxic Substances and Disease Registry. *ATSDR report to Congress for fiscal years 1993–1995*. Atlanta: Office of Policy and External Affairs, 1996.
13. Goldberg MS, Al-Homsi N, Gouset L, Riberdy H. Incidence of cancer among persons living near a municipal solid waste landfill in Montreal, Quebec. *Arch Environ Health* 1995;50(6):416–424.
14. Ott WR. Total human exposure: basic concepts, EPA field studies and future research needs. *J Air Waste Manage Assoc* 1990;40:966–975.
15. Wallace LA, Pellizzari ED, Hartwell TD, Sparcino CM, Sheldon LS, Zelon H. Personal exposures, indoor-outdoor relationships, and breath levels of toxic air pollutants measured for 355 persons in New Jersey. *Atmos Environ* 1985;10:1651–1661.
16. Wallace LA. Major sources of benzene exposure. *Environ Health Perspect* 1989;82:165–169.
17. Hartwell TD, Pellizzari ED, Perrit RL, Whitmore RW, Zelon HS, Wallace LA. Comparison of volatile organic levels between sites and seasons for the Total Exposure Assessment Methodology (TEAM) Study. *Atmos Environ* 1987;21:2413–2424.
18. Agency for Toxic Substances and Disease Registry. Environmental data needed for public health assessments. Springfield, VA: National Technical Information Service, 1994.
19. US Environmental Protection Agency. *A Science Advisory Board report: human exposure assessment. A guide to risk ranking, risk reduction, and research planning*. Washington: Science Advisory Board, Indoor Air Quality/Total Human Exposure Committee, 1995. [EPA-SAB-IAQC-95-005].
20. US Environmental Protection Agency. *Review of the office of solid waste and emergency response draft risk assessment guidance for Superfund, human health evaluation manual*. Science Advisory Board, Environmental Health Committee, 1993. [EPA-SAB-EHC-93-007].
21. US Environmental Protection Agency. *Guidance for evaluating the technical impracticability of ground water restoration*. Washington: Office of Solid Waste and Emergency Response, 1993.

22. US Environmental Protection Agency. Guidance on risk characterization for risk managers and risk assessors. OSWER memorandum from F. Henry Habitch II, Deputy Administrator, February 26, 1992. (Also published as Appendix B in National Research Council, Committee on Risk Assessment of Hazardous Air Pollutants. *Science and Judgment in Risk Assessment*. Washington: National Academy Press, 1994.)
23. Callahan MA, Clickher RP, Whitmore RW, Kalton G, Sexton K. Overview of important design issues for a National Human Exposure Assessment Survey. *J Expo Anal Environ Epidemiol* 1995;5(3):257–282.
24. National Research Council. *Science and judgment in risk assessment*. Committee on Risk Assessment of Hazardous Air Pollutants. Washington: National Academy Press, 1994.
25. Commission on Risk Assessment and Risk Management. Framework for environmental health risk management, final report, vol 1. The Presidential/Congressional Commission on Risk Assessment and Risk Management. Available at: http://www.riskworld.com. Accessed 1997.
26. Graham JD, Sadowitz M. Superfund reform: reducing risk through community choice. *Issues Sci Technol* 1994;10(4):35–42.
27. Office of Technology Assessment. *The state of the states on brownfields: programs for cleanup and reuse of contaminated sites*. Washington: Technical Information Service, 1995.
28. Sims JL, Suflita JM, Russell HH. *In situ bioremediation of contaminated ground water: EPA groundwater issue*. Washington: Office of Solid Waste and Emergency Response, 1991. [EPA/540/S-92/003].
29. Thomas JM, Ward CH. In situ biorestoration of organic contaminants in the subsurface. *Environ Sci Technol* 1989;23:760–766.
30. Sims JL, Suflita JM, Russell HH. *Reductive dehalogenation of organic contaminants in soils and ground water: EPA groundwater issue*. Washington: Office of Solid Waste and Emergency Response, 1991. [EPA/540/4-90/054].
31. US Environmental Protection Agency. *Risk assessment guidance for Superfund*, vol I: *human health evaluation manual*. Supplemental guidance: standard exposure factors. Final draft. Washington: March 25, 1991.
32. US Environmental Protection Agency. *Risk assessment guidance for Superfund*, vol. I: *development of risk-based preliminary remediation goals*. [Interim publication 9285.7-01B]. Washington: Office of Emergency and Remedial Response, 1991.
33. US Environmental Protection Agency. *Exposure factors handbook*. Office of Research and Development, National Center for Environmental Assessment, U.S.E.P.A.; 1999 CD-ROM.
34. US Environmental Protection Agency. Final guidelines for exposure assessment. *Federal Register* 1992;57(104):22888–22938.
35. US Environmental Protection Agency. Role of the baseline risk assessment in Superfund remedy selection decisions. Memorandum from Don R. Clay, April 22, 1991. Washington: Office of Solid Waste and Emergency Response, 1991.
36. US Environmental Protection Agency. *Technical background document for soil screening guidance*. Washington: Office of Solid Waste and Emergency Response, 1996.
37. American Society for Testing and Materials. *Standard guide for risk-based corrective action applied at petroleum release sites*. West Conshohocken, PA: American Society for Testing Materials, 1995.
38. Burmaster DE, von Stackelberg K. Using Monte Carlo simulations in public health risk assessments: estimating and presenting full distributions of risk. *J Expo Anal Environ Epidemiol* 1991;1(4):491–512.
39. Thompson KM, Burmaster DE, Crouch EAC. Monte Carlo techniques for quantitative uncertainty analysis in public health risk assessments. *Risk Anal* 1992;12(1):53–63.
40. Smith RL. Use of Monte Carlo simulation for human exposure assessment at a Superfund site. *Risk Anal* 1994;14(4):433–439.
41. Commission on Risk Assessment and Risk Management. Risk assessment and risk management in regulatory decision-making, final report, vol. 2. The Presidential/Congressional Commission on Risk Assessment and Risk Management. Available at: http://www.riskworld.com. Accessed 1997.
42. Clark CS, Meyer CR, Gartside PS, et al. An environmental health survey of drinking water contamination by leachate from a pesticide waste dump in Hardeman County, Tennessee. *Arch Environ Health* 1982;37:9–18.
43. Ozonoff D, Colten ME, Cupples A, et al. Health problems reported by residents of a neighborhood contaminated by a hazardous waste facility. *Am J Ind Med* 1987;11:581–597.
44. Lagakos SW, Wessen BJ, Zelen M. An analysis of contaminated well water and health effects in Woburn, Massachusetts. *J Am Statist Assoc* 1986;81:583–596.
45. Feldman RG, Chirico-Post J, Proctor SP. Blink reflex latency after exposure to trichloroethylene in well water. *Arch Environ Health* 1988;43:143–148.
46. California Department of Health Services. *Pregnancy outcomes in Santa Clara County, 1980–1982: reports of two epidemiological studies*. Berkeley, CA: California Department of Health Services, 1985.
47. Swan SH, Shaw G, Harris JA, Neutra RR. Congenital cardiac anomalies in relation to water contamination, Santa Clara County, California, 1981–1983. *Am J Epidemiol* 1989;129:885–893.
48. Budnick LD, Sokal DC, Falk H, Logue JN, Fox JM. Cancer and birth defects near the Drake Superfund site, Pennsylvania. *Arch Environ Health* 1984;39:409–413.
49. Logue JN, Fox JM. Residential health study of families living near the Drake Chemical Superfund site in Lock Haven, Pennsylvania. *Arch Environ Health* 1986;41(4):222–228.
50. Hertzman C, Hayes M, Singer J, Highland J. Upper Ottawa street landfill site health study. *Environ Health Perspect* 1987;75:173–195.

CHAPTER 46

Hazards of Shipbuilding and Ship Repairing

Katherine L. Hunting and Laura S. Welch

Shipyard work involves construction and repair of merchant vessels; U.S. Navy and U.S. Coast Guard ships and submarines; non–self-propelled vessels, such as barges; offshore drilling rigs; and platforms. According to the national data from 1988, the U.S. shipbuilding and ship repair industry employs approximately 128,000 production workers, equally divided between Naval and private shipyards. This employment figure does not include supervisory, administrative, and professional workers, such as engineers (1).

The construction of a ship is a complex task, involving many trades and skills and the use of many hazardous substances. Much of the ship is constructed in a berth or a building dock; preliminary work is also done in offices and ancillary shops that are an integral part of the shipyard. In the shops, conditions are similar to those in engineering or manufacturing facilities, whereas work aboard ship is similar to construction conditions.

The basic construction of a ship's hull is accomplished by measuring, cutting, assembling, and welding steel plates. In the shop, the plate is cut to size, usually with flame cutting; formed to shape by cutting or rolling; and fabricated into subassemblies by welding. Subassemblies are then transferred to the building dock by cranes or vehicles; assembled by welding; finished with pneumatic chisels, gouging, or grinding; and sandblasted and painted. The ship is finished with the installation of plumbing, ventilation, machinery, flooring, berths, decking, and electronic equipment. Each of these tasks is performed by a different trade or set of trades, each with a unique set of hazards. Table 46-1 lists the primary shipyard trades and the proportion of shipyard workers represented in each occupational group.

TABLE 46-1. Major occupational groups, shipbuilding and ship repairing (production workers only)

Occupational group	Percent*
Welders	10.6
Machinists and machine tool operators	6.8
Pipefitters and insulators	6.8
Shipfitters	6.6
Electricians	5.9
Painters	5.1
Material movement and service workers	3.7
Sheet metal workers	3.5
Shipwrights, carpenters, and loftworkers	3.3
Marine trade helpers	3.0
Riggers	2.1
Electronic technicians and mechanics	1.6
Other tradeworkers	41.0
Total	100.0

*These data are from a 1986 survey of private U.S. shipyards that estimated 65,309 production workers in the private sector of the industry. Naval shipyards were not included in the survey; however, the distribution of trades is expected to be similar to private yards.
From the U.S. Department of Labor, Bureau of Labor Statistics.

DESCRIPTION OF SHIPYARD TRADES AND EXPOSURES

Because many readers may not be familiar with shipyard work, this section describes the work done by the most important shipyard trades. Exposures typically experienced by each trade also are discussed. It should be noted that the following descriptions are generalized; even among workers in the same trade, tasks and exposures vary considerably. The most important distinction, for most trades, is whether individuals work in the shop, aboard the ship (exterior or interior), or, as in some cases, in shipyard facilities ("maintenance" trade workers).

Welders

Welders join metals by heating them to high temperatures. These processes result in emissions of toxic fumes, dusts, gases, and vapors. The principal components of welding fumes from carbon steel are oxides of nitrogen and vaporized iron, which condenses to a fine dust (2). In addition, fumes from welding or cutting may contain ozone, carbon monoxide, zinc, fluorides, silica, lead, chromium IV, nickel, aluminum, beryllium, cobalt, copper, manganese, magnesium, vanadium, arsenic, or other metals (3). The composition of welding fumes varies, depending on the type of metal being welded, the presence of a coating on the metal, the welding technique, and the type of electrode and filler wire used. Ship hulls are typically constructed of carbon steel; alloys may, however, be used to construct the ship's superstructure (4) and for numerous specialty applications. Many different welding or cutting techniques, including gas metal arc, low hydrogen, submerged arc, gas tungsten, plasma arc, gas welding, gas/flame cutting, and arc air gouging, are used in shipyard work (5). Hand welding and machine welding, in which joints are welded without manual manipulation of the welding electrode or torch, are used in shipyard work (1).

Nonfume chemical exposures experienced by welders include decomposition products (most notably, phosgene) of organic solvents used to degrease metals before welding. Fuel gases, such as propane, acetylene, and hydrogen, may also be released. Physical hazards of welding work include electricity, heat, noise, vibration, ionizing radiation, and ultraviolet, visible, and infrared radiation (3).

Before the mid-1970s, shipyard welders were frequently exposed to asbestos. The highest exposures occurred when welders worked around delagging operations (removal of asbestos insulation) or in areas in which asbestos was being sprayed. Welders occasionally removed asbestos insulation themselves to weld fixtures into place. Also, welders typically used asbestos blankets for protection from sparks and hot metal slag (6).

Machinists

A machinist fabricates metal parts, mechanisms, or machines and may install ship machinery as well (1). Turners, planer operators, drillers, grinders, milling machine operators, press machine operators, and toolmakers are classified as machinists (7). Exposures include use of antioxidants, synthetic cutting fluids, cutting oils, chromates, greases, lubricants, rust inhibitors, and solvents.

Cutting oils vary in their content of polycyclic aromatic hydrocarbons, some of which are thought to be carcinogenic in humans (8). Machinists have a high risk of occupational dermatitis, on an irritant and an allergic basis, and may develop acne from cutting oils. Allergy may develop to additives and antimicrobial agents in the oils or synthetic fluids (9). Because of working in close proximity to other crafts during ship construction, shipyard machinists also have significant exposure to products used by other trades, including asbestos.

Pipefitters and Insulators

The marine pipefitter lays out, installs, and maintains a ship's piping systems, which include steam heat, power, hot water, hydraulic, air pressure, and oil supply pipes. This job includes laying out pipe sections, cutting and boring holes, operating shop machines for cutting and threading pipe fittings, and bolting or welding pipes together. A pipefitter's work involves installation and insulation of pipes. An insulator covers boilers, pipes, tanks, and refrigeration units with insulating materials. These materials include asbestos, man-made mineral fibers (MMMFs), cork, plastic, and magnesium; their purpose is to reduce loss or absorption of heat, prevent moisture condensation, and deaden sound (1). The most significant hazard for insulators and pipefitters in shipyards has been asbestos; 70% of pipefitters surveyed in 1975 had x-ray changes secondary to asbestos (10). Asbestos may now present during ship repair, but not during new construction. As MMMFs have replaced asbestos for shipyard applications, these exposures are of increasing concern to pipefitters and insulators, as well as to those who work near them in dusty environments.

Shipfitters

A shipfitter lays out and fabricates plates, bulkheads, frames, and other metal structural parts and braces them in position within the hull of the ship for riveting or welding (1). The most significant exposure to a shipfitter is the fumes from welding and cutting. These exposures may occur in the shop during fabrication; during hull construction, as structural parts are tack welded before permanent welding; or indirectly, from work near welders. Platers, a subgroup of shipfitters who mark and position steel plates ready for welding, often work in close proximity to welders (11). Like most other shipyard trades, shipfitters may have indirect asbestos exposure.

Electricians

A marine electrician installs and repairs wiring, fixtures, and equipment for shipboard electrical systems. The counterpart to this position is the maintenance electrician, who installs, maintains, and repairs equipment for the generation, distribution, or use of electric energy in the shipyard (1). Exposures of concern are solvents (formerly including benzene), metal fumes, fluxes, chlorinated biphenyls, epoxy resins, chlorinated naphthalenes, and electrical current (12). Electricians often must remove or replace insulation material and may also work in the vicinity of insulators (11). Electricians, particularly those who work aboard ship or in shipyard power plants, have had considerable exposure to asbestos. Many studies of shipyard workers, which have included electricians, have found an increased lung cancer risk. Electricians have also been found to have an increased risk of chest x-ray changes (6,13) and mesothelioma (14,15). Shipyard electricians have also been found to have increased rates of leukemia (12).

Painters

A painter applies paint, varnish, lacquer, or other finishes to the surfaces of the ship, primarily using brushes or spray guns. Maintenance painters perform similar work in the shipyard facilities (1). Before application of coatings, painters also prepare ship surfaces, removing scale, rust, and old paint. Surface preparation is done by abrasive blasting or by wiping surfaces with solvents (16,17). Shipyard painters are exposed to a wide variety of organic solvents, including aliphatic hydrocarbons, alcohols, ketones, glycol ethers, chlorinated hydrocarbons, and aromatic hydrocarbons. Benzene is present now only as a very low-level contaminant, but significant exposures were present before 1977. Painters are also potentially exposed to numerous metals and metal oxides, including lead, chromium, cadmium, nickel, and organic tins, that are used in coatings as antifouling agents (16). Metal exposures may occur as a result of paint removal operations; painters must be protected from exposure to lead dust when preparing red lead-painted surfaces (17,18). Painters may be exposed to silica if they sandblast or work in the vicinity of sandblasting operations. Work in confined spaces adds another hazardous element to painting work.

Painters working aboard ships, like workers in most other shipyard trades, are potentially exposed to asbestos and have been shown to be at risk of mesothelioma (14) and other asbestos-related diseases. Organic solvents impair nervous system function; solvent-exposed shipyard painters have been found to have increased acute neurologic symptoms (19,20), neurobehavioral performance decrements (20), and increased vibratory perception thresholds indicative of peripheral polyneuropathy (21). Other organ system effects have also been found in association with shipyard painting exposures. For example, epoxy resin systems contain irritating, and often sensitizing, compounds. Studies show increased hematologic and sperm abnormalities among shipyard painters exposed to ethylene glycol ethers (22,23).

Material Movement and Service Workers

This category of workers includes several different occupational groups whose exposures may vary depending on their work location. Crane operators run various types of cranes to hoist, move, and place materials, machines, and products within a shipyard. Guards, janitors, truck drivers, and forklift operators are also classified with material movement and service workers (1).

Sheet Metal Workers

A sheet metal worker fabricates, assembles, installs, and repairs sheet metal products and equipment (1). Welding exposures, which are particularly likely to occur among shop workers, are of concern. Sheet metal workers are also exposed to asbestos and MMMFs during shipboard installation or repair of ducts or other products. Because many ducts are fabricated with MMMF liners, exposure to MMMF dust often occurs during in-shop fabrication or during on-ship installation.

Shipwrights, Maintenance Carpenters, and Loftworkers

Shipwrights, maintenance carpenters, and loftworkers work with wood carpentry. The shipyard carpenter constructs and maintains woodwork and equipment, such as docks, structures to support ships in dry dock, bins, cribs, counters, partitions, framing, doors, floors, stairs, casings, and trim. Carpentry work is done in the shop and aboard the ships by shipwrights, and in the shipyard facilities by the maintenance carpenter (1). Shipyard carpenters have had significant exposures to asbestos, and are also exposed to wood dust, glues, and solvents. At the Portsmouth Naval Shipyard, for example, the solvents with which carpenters worked included xylene, toluene, acetone, methylene chloride, tetrachloroethane, methyl ethyl ketone, and (formerly) benzene (12). Loftworkers lay out full-scale models of the ship and construct templates and molds to be used as patterns and guides for layout and fabrication of various structural parts of ships (1). Loftworkers work in a separate shop area, the *mold loft*. As such, these workers are exposed to wood dust, glues, and solvents, but not generally to asbestos.

Riggers

A rigger's job involves movement of machinery, equipment, structural parts, and other heavy loads aboard ships. The job includes installation and repair of rigging and weight-handling gear on ships, and attaching necessary hoists and pulling gear to rigging to lift, move, and position heavy loads (1). As with other material movement workers, riggers' chemical exposures vary, depending on work occurring in their vicinity.

Electronics Technicians and Mechanics

Electronics workers install, maintain, repair, overhaul, construct, and test electronic equipment and related devices (1). This work is carried out in the shop and aboard the ship (where asbestos exposure may occur). Hazardous exposures include solvents used in cleaning components, electrical current, and electromagnetic radiation.

HEALTH EFFECTS OF SHIPYARD EXPOSURES

The major classes of shipyard hazards are summarized in Table 46-2. The many trades involved in building and repairing ships have differing exposures. Exposures to asbestos, radiation, and heat are widespread in the shipyard and common to many trades. This complex exposure picture makes it difficult to assess the health hazards to shipyard workers. Table 46-3 lists some of the most important occupational diseases that occur in shipyards. Although some of what we know about shipyard-related occupational diseases comes from shipyard worker health studies, much of what is known comes from health studies carried out among relevant trades in other industries.

A number of mortality studies have been carried out among shipyard worker populations. A limitation of these studies is that exposures have been evaluated by using the job title as a general indicator of exposure. For instance, cancer studies of welders may presume that increased risks are attributable to welding fume exposure without doing an assessment of the degree of asbestos or radiation exposure. Results of such stud-

TABLE 46-2. Major classes of shipyard hazards

- Physical hazards
  - Extremes of temperature
  - Oxygen deficiency in closed spaces
  - Ergonomic stress of work in confined spaces
  - Noise
  - Vibration
  - Ionizing radiation
  - Electricity
  - Airborne particles
- Chemical hazards
  - Diesel exhaust and other combustion products
  - Fumes and gases from welding and burning
  - Dusts from asbestos and other insulation, sandblasting
  - Vapors from paints, thinners, resins
  - Lead
  - Organic tins
  - Oils
  - Epoxy resin systems

TABLE 46-3. Occupational diseases of particular interest in shipyards

Conjunctivitis or keratitis from welding arcs
Deafness caused by pneumatic hammers, chippers, arc air gouging
Vibration white finger
Acute lung irritation from zinc, oxides of nitrogen, and ozone from welding and burning
Siderosis from welding
Silicosis from sandblasting
Solvent narcosis
Occupational asthma from epoxies and isocyanates
Asbestosis and asbestos-related cancers
Cataracts from lasers and ionizing radiation
Irritant contact dermatitis

Modified from Bridges VG, Campbell J, Howe W. Shipbuilding. In: Parmeggiani L, ed. *Encyclopedia of occupational health and safety*, 3rd ed. Geneva: International Labour Organization, 1983:2027–2032.

ies, therefore, should be interpreted with caution regarding causal exposures.

Welding

Welding work takes place in shops, during hull assembly, during interior construction, and in finishing phases. Trades involved with welding include welders, caulker/burners, boilermakers, platers, shipfitters, and sheet metal workers (11). Welders and boilermakers have the highest exposure to welding fumes. Caulker/burners and platers are also exposed, generally to a lesser degree. Workers in other trades are also exposed to welding fumes, as they often work in the vicinity of welding. In addition to fume proximity, factors such as work location (e.g., shop, open air, or confined space), provision of exhaust ventilation, and use of personal protective equipment modify exposure.

Health effects of welding exposures are specifically covered in a variety of sources (3,24,25).

Exposure to welding fumes while working in confined or other poorly ventilated areas can cause metal fume fever. This acute condition often resembles an upper respiratory infection, acute bronchitis, pneumonia, or upper gastrointestinal infection (3), and is relatively common. It has been estimated that nearly 40% of welders older than age 30 years have experienced metal fume fever (24). Pneumonitis has been less commonly reported in association with welding work; it may result from acute high-concentration exposures to nitrogen dioxide, ozone, and a number of metal fumes (3).

Chronic respiratory disease also occurs among welders. Siderosis, or *welder's lung*, is a benign condition resulting from the accumulation of iron oxides in the lung. Fibrosis may also develop in response to many other welding exposures (2,3,24).

Numerous studies have reported an increased risk of chronic bronchitis among smoking and nonsmoking welders compared with nonwelders (24), and a study of pulmonary function found an excess of small airways disease in shipyard arc welders (26). The risk is more pronounced among smokers (2,3). Shipyard welders appear to be at risk of developing obstructive chronic bronchitis; in other industries, welding has not been associated with obstructive changes. Sjögren (24) suggests that inhalation of air contaminants is higher for shipyard welders than for other welders because of their work in semiconfined or confined spaces.

Welding fumes may contain a variety of metals, such as chromium (VI) or nickel, that are either known or suspected carcinogens. Epidemiologic studies carried out in many occupational settings have found welding to be associated with a moderately increased risk of lung cancer (3,24). Several studies have specifically addressed the risk attributable to shipyard welding exposures and have found an excess risk of lung cancer among welders or other workers with welding exposures (7,11,27–31). Several of these papers controlled for smoking (7,29,31). Many shipyard welders have had substantial asbestos exposures, and it is not known how much of their observed excess risk of lung cancer is attributable to this versus welding exposures or to other possible carcinogens, such as ionizing radiation (29,31), although a definite risk exists for the welding exposure based on these studies. Shipyard welders (6,32) as well as other welders (24) have an increased risk of mesothelioma.

Epidemiologic evidence is equivocal for the relationship between welding and cancers at sites other than the lung (3,24). Cancers of concern include laryngeal, nasal, sinonasal, kidney, and other urinary tract organs. Stern et al. (12) noted an increased risk of leukemia among shipyard welders. Limited epidemiologic evidence (3) indicates that welders may have increased cardiovascular disease death rates, as well as increased risk of reproductive disorders (33).

Asbestos

Asbestos materials are now infrequently used in new ship construction, but were extensively used in vessels constructed before 1975. In Finland alone, it is estimated that 24,000 people have exposure to asbestos in shipyards (34). As a consequence, asbestos-related disease may appear in current workers from past exposures, and the potential exists for exposure in the repair of vessels constructed before 1975. Present-day exposure to asbestos is carefully regulated, and exposures are expected to be quite low when the work is carried out according to regulations.

Crocidolite, amosite, and chrysotile have been used extensively in shipyards since the beginning of the twentieth century. In shipyards in the United States, amosite was added to chrysotile just before and during World War II (10). Asbestos was used as insulation for pipes, boilers, and steam lines and in welders' blankets. Carpenters used asbestos board in constructing fireproof doors. Because of the confined spaces in ships and the overlapping of jobs and processes between trades, one must assume that all production workers who worked on the ship have had some exposure to asbestos. In addition, many shop workers have had asbestos exposure.

Dust concentrations were not measured to any degree in the 1940s and 1950s, but the mobile nature of the work resulted in dust concentrations that varied from day to day and from one part of a ship to another. In general, the process of removing insulation generates higher fiber counts than the application, and the highest fiber levels were present in the confined spaces of boiler and engine rooms. Samples taken during the removal of lagging had mean values of 171 fibers per mL in boiler rooms and 88 fibers per mL in engine rooms in one shipyard in England (32). Nicholson (35) conducted an integrated analysis of monitoring data in shipyards in the 1960s and estimated an overall time-weighted average for shipyard work at between 4 and 12 fibers per mL for fibers longer than 5 mm.

The well-recognized health hazards of asbestos exposure in shipyards and elsewhere include asbestosis, pleural fibrosis, lung cancer, and mesothelioma; increased rates of colon cancer, laryngeal cancer, and other cancers have been reported as well.

A survey of chest x-ray abnormalities in a large shipyard during the 1970s found that 46% of 1,000 shipyard production workers (most with more than 20 years of employment) had pleural or parenchymal changes compatible with asbestos disease (10). The prevalence of abnormalities ranged from 36% in carpenters and 40% in painters to 74% in pipefitters. The rates of abnormalities were even higher in workers engaged exclusively in ship repair in the same period; 86% of repair workers with 20 years or more of experience had pleural or parenchymal abnormalities (36). A cross-sectional survey of sheet metal workers found the risk of asbestosis was increased by shipyard employment compared to construction work outside of shipyards (37); these data suggest that the risk for nonmalignant asbestos lung disease is higher for all construction workers with a history of shipyard work.

Sandén et al. (38) found an increased odds ratio (OR) for lung cancer (OR, 2.3) and gastric cancer (OR, 1.4) among Swedish shipyard workers. Fletcher (39) found an incidence of lung cancer 2.5 times that expected in British shipyard workers. Edge (40) found a twofold-increased risk of lung cancer among men with pleural plaques in a British shipyard. Putoni and coworkers (41) found a standardized mortality ratio (SMR) for lung cancer of 2.2 in shipyard workers in Genoa. In a population-based case-control study of lung cancer, Blot et al. (42) found an odds ratio of 1.4 for shipyard work (10,15,43–46). Most of these studies attributed the increased risk to heavy asbestos exposure in shipyards; none included a detailed exposure assessment.

Shipyard workers experience an excess mortality rate because of mesothelioma (10,15,43–46). Selikoff et al. (10) found that 10% of deaths among 440 shipyard workers were from pleural or peritoneal mesothelioma. Kolonel et al. (15) reported eight cases of mesothelioma among 7,000 men followed prospectively after work in the Pearl Harbor Naval Shipyard. As discussed in the section Welding, studies of shipyard welders have found excess mortality from mesothelioma (6). Shipbuilding was also found to convey an increased risk of mesothelioma in a study using the Swedish Cancer Registry (32). Cases of mesothelioma were reported in nine different shipyard trades: laggers, painters, boilermakers, shipwrights, welders, electricians, fitters, plumbers, and joiners. Many of these trades do not work directly with asbestos, but work in proximity to workers using asbestos products. Because most cases of mesothelioma are attributable to asbestos exposure (47), one can conclude that all these trades—and, by analogy, other trades without daily use of asbestos products—have had significant asbestos exposure in shipyards.

Man-Made Mineral Fibers

MMMFs are used in ship construction as an insulating material and have been the primary substitute for asbestos in that application. Valić and coworkers (48) measured fiber counts during insulation work in shipbuilding and found that respirable fiber counts ranged from 2.6–35.0 fibers per mL in the engine room and 27.7 to 23.9 fibers per mL in the auxiliary engine rooms.

MMMFs have long been recognized as acute irritants to the skin and the respiratory tree. Several studies have investigated the chronic health effects of exposure to MMMFs. Cohort studies of disease incidence and mortality have been conducted in populations exposed to MMMFs. Bayliss et al. (49) studied the causes of death for a cohort of 14,000 men working in fibrous glass production and found an excess of deaths caused by nonmalignant respiratory disease. A case-control study within this cohort found an association between nonmalignant respiratory disease and exposure to small-diameter glass fibers. Enterline et al. (50) also found an excess of nonmalignant respiratory deaths in a cohort of 15,000 fibrous glass production workers. A nested case-control study of the Enterline cohort suggested the excess was attributable to smoking. Robinson et al. (51) also found an excess of deaths from nonmalignant respiratory disease. None of these cohort analyses found a dose-response relationship, and other mortality studies have not found such an excess of nonmalignant respiratory disease (52,53).

Two studies have found an increased prevalence of small opacities on chest x-rays in men exposed to MMMFs in fibrous glass production (54,55); Weill et al. demonstrated a dose-response relationship. Others have not observed this effect (56).

Several cross-sectional studies have investigated the prevalence of respiratory symptoms or pulmonary function abnormalities in workers exposed to MMMF. Sixt (57) found an increase in elastic recoil in sheet metal workers exposed to fibrous glass. Hill et al. (58) found an increase in spirometric abnormalities in a group exposed to fibrous glass, but without a dose-response relationship. A large study by Engholm and associates (59) found an increased rate of chronic bronchitis in 135,000 Swedish construction workers exposed to fibrous glass. Hunting et al. found an increased rate of chronic bronchitis in sheet metal workers who had the highest estimated exposure to MMMF (60). Several other cross-sectional studies, many in smaller populations, found no effect of MMMF exposure on either respiratory symptoms or pulmonary function.

MMMFs are classified as a IIB carcinogen by the International Agency for Research on Cancer (61). Animal studies have demonstrated that MMMFs introduced into the pleural or peritoneal space can cause cancer if their size and shape characteristics are similar to asbestos fibers. Stanton and coworkers (62) have described the characteristics of fibers that carry the most carcinogenic potential; most MMMF products have some proportion of fibers with these size characteristics. Two large epidemiologic studies, one in the United States (63) and one in Europe (64,65), have not shown a definite increase in lung or other cancers overall. In the European study, however, the subpopulation working with rock/slag wool did have an excess of lung cancer, whereas the U.S. study found an excess of lung cancer at one MMMF plant and not at others.

These studies as a whole suggest that MMMFs, and fibrous glass in particular, affect the respiratory tract, but no consistent pattern is present in the existing data. It is worth noting that the cohort studies were conducted in MMMF manufacturing facilities in which fiber counts are significantly lower than in secondary uses, such as insulation applications or sheet metal fabrication shops (66).

A few studies have specifically examined the health effects of MMMF in shipyards. Valić et al. (48) found that insulators without prior exposure to asbestos who worked with MMMFs had an increased frequency of nonspecific respiratory complaints and decreased values for midexpiratory flow (i.e., MEF50 and MEF75) compared with normal values. Smoking was not specifically controlled for in either analysis. Sandén and Järvholm (67) compared the frequency of respiratory symptoms and ventilatory function in 1,682 shipyard workers, with and without exposure to MMMFs. They found an increased frequency of chronic cough and phlegm among the men with MMMF exposure, but no difference in lung function. The men with MMMF exposure had a higher prevalence of pleural plaques; whether this was caused by MMMFs or to prior asbestos exposure could not be determined.

Physical Hazards

VIBRATION

Shipbuilding entails a great deal of metal working. One of the tools used for cutting metal is a chipping gun. This tool has caused many cases of vibration white finger disease (VWF) in shipyard chipper-grinders. VWF is occupationally induced Raynaud's phenomenon and usually results from the long-term use of hand-held vibrating tools. The disease worsens with continued exposure to vibration but does not remit with cessation of exposure; this makes prevention and early diagnosis very important. Since the early 1980s, more than 50 cross-sectional studies of hand-arm vibration have been published, but much still needs to be learned about the pathophysiology and quantitative assessment.

Shipyard workers exposed to hand-arm vibration include metal working trades, such as boilermakers, shipfitters, and sheet metal workers. Tools used include sanders, burring tools, drills, grinders, cutters, and various air-powered guns (68). Since approximately 1970, much of the cutting of metal has been performed with lasers, so the risk of VWF has decreased, but vibrating tools are still used for grinding and removing burrs. A good deal of ship construction is outside work and may entail exposure to cold environments; working in the cold may contribute to the development of VWF and certainly contributes to the degree of symptoms a worker experiences. In one study, 20% of shipyard workers using pneumatic chipping and grinding tools had VWF (69). In another, among workers with exposure to vibrating tools more than 32 hours per week, 71% of grinders had vascular symptoms and 84% had neurologic symptoms; there was a crude OR of 38 for vascular symptoms among the full-time pneumatic tool users (68).

Several investigators have suggested methods for early detection; changes in tool design have also been recommended to reduce the extent of VWF in many industries. Appropriate changes in a shipyard include the introduction of dampers, addition of vibration-absorbing handles to tools, and tool redesign (17). It is important to note that if the guidelines of the American Conference of Government Industrial Hygienists for vibration exposure (70) were applied to tools studied in one shipyard, chipping hammers, large burring machines, and other tools would be banned outright (68), pointing to an urgent need for better tool design.

NOISE

Pneumatic hammers, gouging tools, and chipping machines are sources of significant noise exposure in shipyards. Noise-induced hearing loss from such exposures has been well described (71).

TEMPERATURE

Because much ship construction is outside work, shipbuilding and repair entail exposure to extremes of hot and cold. In addition, work in confined spaces, such as ballast tanks, is common; these spaces can become extremely hot in summer.

Excessive heat exposure decreases workplace productivity and can also cause serious adverse health effects and even death. These adverse effects include the following (72,73):

1. ***Heat cramps***: When prolonged exposure to heat causes sweating that is not adequately replaced by fluid intake, muscle cramps may occur, even among trained athletes. The appropriate treatment is rest with fluid replacement.
2. ***Heat exhaustion***: Weakness, headache, nausea, and fainting may occur. Rest, removal to a cool area, and replacement of fluids with frequent small sips of liquids treat the condition or intravenous rehydration.
3. ***Heat stroke***: Dizziness, headache, irritability, nausea, and confusion are accompanied by hot, dry skin. Collapse, coma, renal failure, and death may occur. First aid must be immediate with rapid cooling of the affected person.

Other adverse effects include prickly heat, diminished work capacity, and perhaps decreased sperm quality (74). Sustained body temperature elevation is also known to adversely affect sperm production and pregnancy outcome.

Heat may contribute to safety hazards as well, because of decreased alertness. In addition, increased sweating may create slippery surfaces, fog safety eyewear, and otherwise make personal protective equipment difficult to wear.

Contributing factors to heat stress include ambient temperature, humidity, and the use of protective clothing. Protective gear, required for a number of jobs, including asbestos removal, welding, and work in confined spaces, may substantially increase the heat hazard by decreasing convective, evaporative, and radiant heat loss and by increasing workload. Working generates metabolic heat, ranging from 252 to 504 kJ per hour with light work (e.g., typing, desk work), 1,008 to 1,260 kJ per hour with heavy levels of work (e.g., painting), or 1,512 kJ per hour with extremely heavy work (e.g., climbing ladders, lifting 20 kg cases 10 times per minute) (73).

The adverse health effects of heat can be decreased by monitoring the response to heat stress and adapting workloads by increasing the number of workers performing a given task, increasing rest breaks, and providing cool areas and liquids. Accurate assessment of workloads and heat exposure should include industrial hygiene monitoring of wet bulb globe temperature and assessment of work site and of work practices (75).

CONFINED AND ENCLOSED SPACES

Confined spaces are areas into and out of which movement is difficult. Toxic or explosive gases can build up in confined spaces; they are not designed for continuous worker presence. Such spaces include ballast tanks, bilge tanks, missile tubes, tunnels, pipelines, and open-top spaces more than 4 ft (1.2 m) in depth. Enclosed areas are easier to get in or out of and include spaces such as pump stations. Three main dangers exist in confined spaces and enclosed areas: (a) toxic and corrosive vapors and fumes, (b) explosive gases and flammable substances, and (c) lack of oxygen.

A prime hazard of confined spaces is oxygen deficiency. The normal percentage of oxygen in air is 21%, but the chemical decomposition process plus heat and humidity often decrease oxygen in a confined space. Other gases, such as nitrogen and carbon dioxide, displace oxygen in the air. Workers should not enter any confined space in which the oxygen percentage is below 19.5%, unless they are equipped with a supplied air respirator.

The effects of oxygen deficiency are often difficult to identify, because one of the first signs is a feeling of well-being. As the level falls to 14% to 16%, a person begins to feel tired, weak, and light-headed. When levels drop to 6% to 10%, a worker rapidly loses consciousness and can die in minutes.

One toxic substance that accumulates in poorly ventilated areas is carbon monoxide (CO), a colorless, odorless gas. At lower levels, it causes headaches and dizziness; loss of consciousness occurs at higher levels. The OSHA permissible exposure limit for CO is 50 ppm.

Certain procedures and controls must be followed before workers enter any confined space or unventilated area. Strict written procedures must be established for entering confined spaces or enclosed areas in which gases can accumulate, and poorly ventilated areas must be routinely monitored for dangerous gas levels.

IONIZING RADIATION

Shipyard workers engaged in the construction and repair of nuclear-powered vessels may be exposed to ionizing radiation, in addition to other shipyard hazards. The primary source of ionizing radiation is exposure to corrosion products in the primary coolant system of the nuclear reactor; these corrosion products are neutron-activated by the reactor. Water in the reactor circulates through a closed piping system to transfer heat away from the reactor core to a heat exchange system; steam generated in the process of cooling the core is used as a power source for propulsion. Trace amounts of corrosion and wear products from the interior surface of the primary coolant system become radiation-contaminated; anyone handling the coolant water or the piping may be exposed. The coolant water contains several short-lived and longer-lived radionuclides. The most significant radiation source is cobalt-60, which has a half-life of 5.3 years (76).

Radiation exposure of shipyard workers occurs after reactor shutdown for repair and in shops in which contaminated components of the ship's materials are repaired. The shipyard workers are not directly exposed to uranium, and internal ingestion of radionuclides is not thought to be a significant factor. The first exposure to these radiation sources began in 1957 in the Groton shipyard, with the overhaul of a nuclear-powered submarine (76), and subsequently in other yards. At eight Naval and private shipyards studied by Matanoski (76), there were 35,000 nuclear shipyard workers with more than 0.5 rem of cumulative radiation exposure out of more than 106,000 total nuclear workers.

Ionizing radiation is known to cause acute radiation sickness, cataracts, and cancer at a variety of sites. The question with shipyards work in general is whether the radiation exposure has been sufficient to cause disease at the generally low-level exposures encountered in routine work. Specific shipyard studies have concentrated primarily on cancer.

Najarian and Colton (77) reported that shipyard workers in the Portsmouth Naval Shipyard in Kittery, Maine, had a fivefold increase in deaths from leukemia and a twofold increase in deaths from all cancers, using a PMR (proportionate mortality rate) analysis. This report prompted further and more extensive studies. Rinsky (27,78) and Stern (12) and their associates have reported the results of several studies of cancer in the same shipyard. A cohort study (78) did not find excess mortality for any cause in shipyard workers exposed to radiation; the authors attributed the difference in results between the PMR and SMR analyses to exposure misclassification. The SMR for leukemia was raised to 1.6 in the group with a lifetime exposure of at least 1 rem at least 15 years before death, but the confidence interval was 0.51 to 3.86. The SMR for lung cancer in the same group was 1.98. To further investigate these two findings, two case-control studies were conducted. One, investigating leukemia deaths (12), did not find an association with exposure either to solvents or radiation, but did find that electricians and welders had an excess risk. The other study investigated lung cancer deaths (27) and found that radiation workers were more heavily exposed to asbestos and welding fumes; controlling for these exposures to the extent possible reduced the risk from radiation. It was not possible to completely separate the effects from asbestos and radiation in this study.

Matanoski (76) studied the mortality of nuclear workers in eight shipyards and compared three groups: nonnuclear workers, nuclear workers with a cumulative dose of greater than 0.5 rem, and nuclear workers with a cumulative dose of less than 0.5 rem. No significant mortality differences were found between the groups for all causes, leukemia, lymphoma, or lung cancer.

These epidemiologic studies, taken together, do not provide clear information to determine whether exposure to ionizing radiation in shipyards elevates cancer risk to workers.

CONCLUSIONS

This chapter summarizes the toxic exposures encountered by workers building and repairing ships and the disease risks faced by these workers. Because of the variety of shipyard trades, exposures, and health risks, a work history is of the utmost importance to anyone providing clinical services to shipyard workers. Similarly, researchers in this field also need to obtain detailed information on the jobs performed by the individuals studied.

Clearly, the shipyard industry is hazardous, with numerous exposures to physical agents and chemical substances. The most important hazard in a historical sense has been asbestos; the most significant hazards in a prospective sense can be determined by existing and new construction technologies, and by the degree of attention to control of exposures.

REFERENCES

1. US Department of Labor, Bureau of Labor Statistics. *Industry wage survey: shipbuilding and repairing*, October 1986 (Bulletin 2295). Washington: US Government Printing Office, 1988.
2. Cotes JE. Occupational health today and tomorrow: a view from two shipyards. *J R Coll Physicians Lond* 1988;22:232–236.
3. National Institute for Occupational Safety and Health. *Criteria for a recommended standard: welding, brazing, and thermal cutting* (Publication no 88-110). Washington: US Department of Health and Human Services (NIOSH), 1988.
4. Bridges VG, Campbell J, Howe W. Shipbuilding. In: Parmeggiani L, ed. *Encyclopedia of occupational health and safety.* Geneva: International Labour Organization, 1983:2027–2032.
5. Burgess WA. Potential exposures in industry: their recognition and control. In: Clayton GD, Clayton FE, eds. *Patty's industrial hygiene and toxicology,* vol 1. New York: John Wiley and Sons, 1978:1149–1221.
6. McMillan GHG. The health of welders in naval dockyards: the risk of asbestos-related diseases occurring in welders. *J Occup Med* 1983;25:727–730.
7. Tola S, Källiomaki PL, Pukkala E, Asp S, Korkala ML. Incidence of cancer among welders, platers, machinists, and pipe fitters in shipyards and machine shops. *Br J Ind Med* 1988;45:209–218.
8. International Agency for Research on Cancer. Polynuclear aromatic hydrocarbons, part II: carbon blacks, mineral oils (lubricant base oils and derived products) and some nitroarenes. *IARC Mongr Eval Carcinog Risk Chem Hum* 1984;33:87–168.
9. Rycroft RJG. Cutting fluids, oils, and lubricants. In: Maibach HI, Gellin GA, eds. *Occupational and industrial dermatology.* Chicago: Year Book Medical Publishers, 1982:233–236.
10. Selikoff IJ, Lilis R, Nicholson WJ. Asbestos disease in United States shipyards. *Ann N Y Acad Sci* 1979;330:295–312.
11. Newhouse ML, Oakes D, Woolley AJ. Mortality of welders and other craftsmen at a shipyard in NE England. *Br J Ind Med* 1985;42:406–410.
12. Stern FB, Waxweiler RA, Beaumont JJ, et al. A case-control study of leukemia at a naval nuclear shipyard. *Am J Epidemiol* 1986;123:980–982.
13. Anton-Culver H, Culver BD, Kurosaki T. An epidemiologic study of asbestos-related chest x-ray changes to identify work areas of high risk in a shipyard population. *Appl Ind Hyg* 1989;4:110–118.
14. Malker HSR, McLaughlin JK, Malker BK, et al. Occupational risks for pleural mesothelioma in Sweden. *J Natl Cancer Inst* 1985;74:61–66.
15. Kolonel LN, Yoshizawa CN, Hirohata T, Myers BC. Cancer occurrence in shipyard workers exposed to asbestos in Hawaii. *Cancer Res* 1985;45:3924–3928.
16. Sparer J, Welch LS, McManus K, Cullen MR. Effects of exposure to ethylene glycol ethers on shipyard painters. I. Evaluation of exposure. *Am J Ind Med* 1988;14:497–507.
17. Kovshilo VE. Environmental hygiene in shipbuilding and ship repairing. In: International Symposium on Safety and Health in Shipbuilding and Ship Repairing. Safety and health in shipbuilding and ship repairing: proceedings of a symposium organized by the Government of Finland (and others), held in Helsinki, 30 August–2 September 1971. Geneva: International Labour Office, 1972:63–75.
18. Georgiev L. Exposure to dust and harmful chemicals in shipbuilding and ship repairing. In: International Symposium on Safety and Health in Shipbuilding and Ship Repairing. Safety and health in shipbuilding and ship repairing: proceedings of a symposium organized by the Government of Finland (and others), held in Helsinki, 30 August–2 September 1971. Geneva: International Labour Office, 1972:103–105.
19. Cherry N, Hutchins H, Pace T, Waldron HA. Neurobehavioural effects of repeated occupational exposure to toluene and paint solvents. *Br J Ind Med* 1985;42:291–300.
20. Valciukas JA, Lilis R, Singer RM, Glickman L, Nicholson WJ. Neurobehavioral changes among shipyard painters exposed to solvents. *Arch Environ Health* 1985;40:47–52.
21. Halonen P, Halonen JP, Lang HA, Karskela V. Vibratory perception thresholds in shipyard workers exposed to solvents. *Acta Neurol Scand* 1986;73:561–565.
22. Welch LS, Cullen MR. Effect of exposure to ethylene glycol ethers on shipyard painters. III. Hematologic effects. *Am J Ind Med* 1988;14:527–536.
23. Welch LS, Schrader SM, Turner TW, Cullen MR. Effects of exposure to ethylene glycol ethers on shipyard painters. II. Male reproduction. *Am J Ind Med* 1988;14:509–526.
24. Sjögren B. Effects of gases and particles in welding and soldering. In: Zenz C, ed. *Occupational medicine: principles and practical applications,* 3rd ed. St. Louis: Mosby–Year Book, 1994:917–925.

25. Zenz C, ed. *Occupational medicine: principles and practical applications*, 3rd ed. St. Louis: Mosby–Year Book, 1994.
26. Hjortsberg U, Orbaek P, Arborelius M. Small airways dysfunction among non-smoking shipyard arc welders. *Br J Ind Med* 1992;49:441–444.
27. Rinsky RA, Melius JM, Hornung RW, et al. Case-control study of lung cancer in civilian employees at the Portsmouth Naval Shipyard, Kittery, Maine. *Am J Epidemiol* 1988;127:55–64.
28. Schoenberg JB, Stemhagen A, Mason TJ, Patterson J, Bill J, Altman R. Occupation and lung cancer risk among New Jersey white males. *J Natl Cancer Inst* 1987;79:13–21.
29. Moulin JJ, Wild P, Haguenoer JM, et al. A mortality study among mild steel and stainless steel welders. *Br J Ind Med* 1993;50:234–243.
30. Simonato L, Fletcher AC, Andersen A, et al. A historical prospective study of European stainless steel, mild steel, and shipyard welders. *Br J Ind Med* 1991;48:145–154.
31. Danielsen TE, Langard S, Andersen A, Knudson O. Incidence of cancer among welders of mild steel and other shipyard workers. *Br J Ind Med* 1993;50:1079–1103.
32. Sheers G, Coles RM. Mesothelioma risks in a naval dockyard. *Arch Environ Health* 1980;35:276–282.
33. Bonde JP. Semen quality in welders exposed to radiation heat. *Br J Ind Med* 1992;49:5–10.
34. Huuskonen MS, Koskinen K, Tossavainen A, et al. Finnish Institute of Occupational Health asbestos program, 1987–1992. *Am J Ind Med* 1995;28:123–142.
35. Nicholson WJ. Case study: asbestos—the TLV approach. *Ann N Y Acad Sci* 1976;271:152–169.
36. Selikoff IJ, Nicholson WJ, Lilis R. Radiological evidence of asbestos disease among ship repair workers. *Am J Ind Med* 1980;1:9–22.
37. Welch LS, Michaels D, Zoloth SR. The National Sheet Metal Examination Group. The National Sheet Metal Worker Asbestos Disease Screening Program: radiologic findings. *Am J Ind Med* 1994;25:635–648.
38. Sandén A, Näslund PE, Järvholm B. Mortality in lung and gastrointestinal cancer among shipyard workers. *Int Arch Occup Environ Health* 1985;55:277–283.
39. Fletcher DE. A mortality study of shipyard workers with pleural plaques. *Br J Ind Med* 1972;29:142–145.
40. Edge JR. Incidence of bronchial carcinoma in shipyard workers with pleural plaques. *Ann N Y Acad Sci* 1979;330:289–294.
41. Putoni R, Vercelli M, Franco M, Valerio F, Santi L. Mortality among shipyard workers in Genoa, Italy. *Ann N Y Acad Sci* 1979;330:353–377.
42. Blot WJ, Morris LE, Stroube R, Tagnon I, Fraumeni JF Jr. Lung and laryngeal cancers in relation to shipyard employment in coastal Virginia. *J Natl Cancer Inst* 1980;65:571–575.
43. Enterline PE, Henderson VL. Geographic patterns for pleural mesothelioma deaths in the United States 1968–81. *J Natl Cancer Inst* 1987;79:31–37.
44. Lumley KPS. A proportional study of cancer registrations of dockyard workers. *Br J Ind Med* 1976;33:108–114.
45. McDonald AD, McDonald JC. Malignant mesothelioma in North America. *Cancer* 1980;46:1650–1656.
46. Vianna NJ, Maslowsky J, Roberts S, Spellman G, Patton RB. Malignant mesothelioma epidemiologic patterns in New York State. *J Occup Med* 1981;4:735–738.
47. Mossman BT, Gee JBL. Asbestos-related diseases. *N Engl J Med* 1989;320: 1721–1730.
48. Vali F, Beriti-Stahuljak D, Skuri Z, Cigula M. Exposure to man-made mineral fibers and respiratory effects in users industry: shipbuilding. *Acta Med Iugoslavica* 1986;40:21–29.
49. Bayliss DL, Dement JM, Wagoner JK, Blejer HP. Mortality patterns among fibrous glass production workers. *Ann N Y Acad Sci* 1976;271:324–335.
50. Enterline PE, Marsh GM. The health of workers in the MMMF industry. In: World Health Organization. Biological effects of man-made mineral fibers, vol 1. Proceedings of a WHO/International Agency for Research on Cancer conference, Copenhagen, Denmark, 20–22 April 1982. Copenhagen: World Health Organization Regional Office for Europe, 1982:311–339.
51. Robinson CF, Dement JM, Ness GO, Waxweiler RJ. Mortality patterns of rock and slag mineral wool production workers: an epidemiological and environmental study. *Br J Ind Med* 1982;39:45–53.
52. Shannon HS, Hayes M, Julian JA, Muir DCF. Mortality experience of glass fibre workers. *Br J Ind Med* 1984;41:35–38.
53. Saracci R, Simonato L. Man-made vitreous fibers and workers' health. *Scand J Work Environ Health* 1982;8:234–242.
54. Weill H, Hughes JM, Hammad YY, Glindmeyer HW, Sharon G, Jones RN. Respiratory health in workers exposed to man-made vitreous fibers. *Am Rev Respir Dis* 1983;128:104-112.
55. Nasr ANM, Ditchek T, Scholtens PA. The prevalence of radiographic abnormalities in the chests of fiber glass workers. *J Occup Med* 1971;13:371–376.
56. Wright GW. Airborne fibrous glass particles: chest roentgenograms of persons with prolonged exposure. *Arch Environ Health* 1968;16:175–181.
57. Sixt R, Bake B, Abrahamsson G, Thiringer G. Lung function of sheet metal workers exposed to fiber glass. *Scand J Work Environ Health* 1983;9:9–14.
58. Hill JW, Rossiter CE, Foden DW. A pilot respiratory morbidity study of workers in a MMMF plant in the United Kingdom. In: World Health Organization. Biological effects of man-made mineral fibres, vol 1. Proceedings of a WHO/International Agency for Research on Cancer conference, Copenhagen, Denmark, 20–22 April 1982. Copenhagen: World Health Organization, 1984:413–426.
59. Engholm G, Von Schmalensee G. Bronchitis and exposure to man-made mineral fibres in non-smoking construction workers. *Eur J Respir Dis* 1982;63[Suppl 118]:73–78.
60. Hunting KL, Welch LS. Occupational exposure to dust and lung disease among sheet metal workers. *Br J Ind Med* 1993;50:432–442.
61. Anonymous. Man-made mineral fibres. *IARC Monogr Eval Carcinog Risks Hum* 1988;43:39–171.
62. Stanton MF, Layard M, Tegeris A, et al. Relation of particle dimension to carcinogenicity in amphibole asbestoses and other fibrous minerals. *J Natl Cancer Inst* 1981;67:965–975.
63. Enterline PE, Marsh GM, Henderson V, Callahan C. Mortality update of a cohort of US man-made mineral fibre workers. *Ann Occup Hyg* 1987;31:625–656.
64. Saracci R, Simonato L, Acheson ED, et al. Mortality and incidence of cancer of workers in the man made vitreous fibres producing industry: an international investigation at 13 European plants. *Br J Ind Med* 1984;41:425–436.
65. Simonato L, Fletcher AC, Cherrie J, et al. The International Agency for Research on Cancer historical cohort study of MMMF production workers in seven European countries: extension of the follow-up. *Ann Occup Hyg* 1987;31:603–623.
66. Esmen NA, Sheehan MJ, Corn M, Engel M, Kotsko N. Exposure of employees to man-made vitreous fibers: installation of insulation materials. *Environ Res* 1982;28:386–398.
67. Sandén A, Järvholm B. Pleural plaques, respiratory symptoms and respiratory function in shipyard workers exposed to man-made mineral fibres. *J Soc Occup Med* 1986;36:86–89.
68. Letz R, Cherniack MG, Gerr F, Hershman D, Pace P. A cross sectional epidemiological survey of shipyard workers exposed to hand-arm vibration. *Brit J Ind Med* 1992;49:53–62.
69. National Institute for Occupational Safety and Health. *Vibration white finger disease in U.S. workers using pneumatic chipping and grinding hand tools. I: Epidemiology.* (Publication no 82-118). Cincinnati: US Department of Health and Human Services (NIOSH), 1982.
70. American Conference of Governmental Industrial Hygienists. *1990-1991 Threshold limit values for chemical substances and physical agents and biological exposure indices: hand-arm segmental vibration*. Cincinnati: American Conference of Governmental Industrial Hygienists, 1990:82–86.
71. Olishifski JB. Occupational hearing loss, noise, and hearing conservation. In: Zenz C, ed. *Occupational medicine: principles and practical applications*, 3rd ed. Chicago: Year Book Medical Publishers, 1988:274–323.
72. Keilblock AJ, Schutte PC. Physical work and heat stress. In: Zenz C, ed. *Occupational medicine: principles and practical applications*, 3rd ed. Chicago: Year Book Medical Publishers, 1988:334–356.
73. Eastman Kodak Company, Human Factors Section, Health Safety and Human Factors Laboratory. *Ergonomic design for people at work*, vol 1. New York: Van Nostrand–Reinhold, 1983.
74. Levine RJ, Bordson BL, Mathew RM, Brown MH, Stanley JM, Starr TB. Deterioration of semen quality during summer in New Orleans. *Fertil Steril* 1988;49:900–906.
75. National Institute for Occupational Safety and Health. Proceedings of a NIOSH workshop on recommended heat stress standards. (Publication no 81-108). Cincinnati: US Department of Health and Human Services (NIOSH), 1980.
76. Matanoski GM. *Health effects of low-level radiation in shipyard workers, final report*. Baltimore: The Johns Hopkins University Press, 1989. [Department of Energy contract no. DE-AC02-79EV10095].
77. Najarian T, Colton T. Mortality from leukemia and cancer in shipyard nuclear workers. *Lancet* 1978;i:1018–1020.
78. Rinsky RA, Zumwalde RD, Waxweiler RJ, et al. Cancer mortality at a naval nuclear shipyard. *Lancet* 1981;i:231–235.

CHAPTER 47

Health Care Facility Hazards

Steven Black and Monica Lambert Hultquist

Employees of health care facilities face a variety of occupational hazards. Although some of these stressors are common in many workplaces, others are more frequently or exclusively experienced by those working in health care settings. These hazards include acute or chronic exposure to chemicals, exposure to biological agents, physical exposure hazards, and psychosocial hazards.

PRESERVATIVES, STERILANTS, AND DISINFECTANTS

Formaldehyde

Formaldehyde has long been used in medical facilities as a preservative, a tissue fixative, and a disinfectant. Chemically, it is the lowest-molecular-weight aldehyde, containing a single carbon atom. It is a gas at room temperature, but is readily soluble in water. For nearly all medical applications, an aqueous preparation of formaldehyde, commonly known as *formalin*, is used. Commercial formalin preparations generally consist of 37% to 50% formaldehyde in water, with 8% to 15% methanol to prevent polymerization (1). Less concentrated solutions can be purchased or prepared as necessary for the specific application. Formaldehyde is also sold in a solid (i.e., polymerized) form called *paraformaldehyde* (2), which is sometimes used for laboratory purposes.

The fixative action of formaldehyde is a result of its ability to bind with and crosslink protein molecules and single-strand deoxyribonucleic acid chains. Its sterilizing and preservative effects are a result of similar reactions with bacterial cell walls and endotoxins (1).

Hospital employees with the greatest potential exposure to formaldehyde are pathologists, morticians, and laboratory personnel. Significant health effects can be caused from skin exposure to formalin solutions or inhalation of formaldehyde gas. Concentrated formalin solutions are strong skin irritants and are sensitizers even in weak solutions (3). The high sensitization power of formaldehyde can result in disseminated skin symptoms from only local skin contact or inhalation in very sensitive persons (3). Skin sensitivity has been linked to the direct irritating effects and true immunologic skin reactions (4).

Acute health effects of airborne formaldehyde are related to exposure concentration. Levels of less than 1 part per million (ppm) can cause eye, nose, and upper airway irritation and headaches (4). These irritating effects are severe at concentrations of approximately 12 ppm (1), and because of this, occupational exposures to greater concentrations do not occur under normal conditions. However, accidents and large spills can result in immediately dangerous airborne formaldehyde exposures. Concentrations up to 30 ppm lead to increased upper airway irritation, increased nasal resistance, lower airway obstruction, and chronic pulmonary obstruction. Exposures from 50 to 100 ppm cause pulmonary edema, inflammation, and pneumonia, and death occurs at levels of more than 100 ppm (4). Because of these dangers, areas must be evacuated in the event of large spills and cleaned up only by qualified persons with appropriate respiratory protection.

Chronic exposure to formaldehyde has been found to cause nasal cancer in rats (4), but only at concentrations that produce other cytotoxic effects in the nasal cavity. The American Conference of Governmental Industrial Hygienists (ACGIH) concluded in a review of epidemiologic studies that "the oncogenic potential of formaldehyde is a threshold phenomenon and that prevention of upper respiratory tract irritation and the associated regenerative hyperplasia should eliminate, for all practical purposes, any excess cancer risk posed by occupational formaldehyde exposure alone" (4). ACGIH lists formaldehyde as a suspected human carcinogen.

Other organizations also recognize the carcinogenic potential of formaldehyde. Based on reviews of animal studies, the National Institute for Occupational Safety and Health (NIOSH) recommended in 1981 that formaldehyde be handled in the workplace as a potential occupational carcinogen (2). The International Agency for Research on Cancer (IARC) labeled formaldehyde as a Group 2A agent, probably carcinogenic to humans (5).

Responding to the research, in 1992, the Occupational Safety and Health Administration (OSHA) lowered the 8-hour permissible exposure limit (PEL) to 0.75 ppm after a lengthy regulatory process (6). The new limit was designed to reduce the risk to workers for cancer, irritation of the eye, nose, and throat, and employee sensitization. The standard includes a short-term exposure limit of 2 ppm for 15-minute periods, and an action level of 0.5 ppm. The standard also includes detailed instructions concerning exposure monitoring, regulated areas, methods of compliance, personal protective equipment, hygiene protection, housekeeping, emergencies, and medical surveillance.

Control of formaldehyde exposures is a significant challenge for hospital health and safety personnel. Formerly routine tasks performed in the morgue or pathology laboratories can readily generate airborne concentrations exceeding the current short-term exposure limit (2 ppm). One example is the pathologic dissection of specimens preserved in formalin. Formaldehyde gas is readily released from formalin solution on the specimen, cutting board, and in the storage container. The exposure risk increases with increasing surface areas wetted with formalin solution. Techniques used to prevent overexposure to the pathologist include the following:

- Rinsing or soaking preserved specimen in water before dissection
- Keeping the lid on the storage container at all times except for removal and replacement of specimen
- Frequent or continuous rinsing of cutting board
- Local exhaust ventilation
- Good general room ventilation
- Respiratory protection (as a last resort)

Efforts to limit employee exposure to formalin have been greatly influenced by the 1992 OSHA standard. Primary control methods used by hospitals include local exhaust ventilation, installing automated tissue-processing equipment, and substitution of other chemicals. Work methods and procedures have also been modified to limit exposure times and concentrations. In procedures in which exposures still exceed legal limits, personal protective equipment, including gloves and respirators, is used to prevent overexposure.

Glutaraldehyde

Glutaraldehyde is a five-carbon dialdehyde that is readily soluble in water. Its primary function in medical facilities is as an antimicrobial agent that is effective at room temperature and pressure. Glutaraldehyde does not damage plastic or rubber parts and is often used to disinfect sensitive equipment, such as endoscopes. Glutaraldehyde is classified as a high-level disinfectant, meaning that it has a lethal action against all types of microorganisms except for high concentrations of bacterial spores (7). Other medical uses include developing of radiographic film, fixing tissue samples, and as a topical treatment for common warts and other skin conditions (8).

As a disinfectant, glutaraldehyde is sold as a 2% to 3% aqueous solution with a slightly acidic pH. Before use, the solution is activated by raising the pH to approximately 8.0 by adding a sodium bicarbonate solution. Activation greatly increases microbiocidal activity (3,7), but limits stability of the solution. The primary method of biocidal action appears to be interaction with cell surface amino groups, in combination with other effects (7).

Occupational exposure to hospital personnel occurs primarily during the disinfection of medical equipment with glutaraldehyde solutions, especially when the work is done by hand. Instruments are first washed to remove organic contamination. Next, the instruments are soaked in the glutaraldehyde solution for a prescribed length of time. Larger instruments, such as endoscopes, require larger soaking tanks, which increases the liquid surface area and evaporation rates. For endoscopes, glutaraldehyde solution must be forced through the narrow scope lumen using a syringe to ensure complete contact. This procedure increases the time an employee must spend near uncovered glutaraldehyde solution. Skin exposure can occur during the cleaning process, removal of items from the glutaraldehyde solution and transfer to a rinse sink, and during rinsing.

Inhalation of low concentrations (less than 1.0 ppm) of glutaraldehyde may cause irritation of the skin and mucous membranes (8). Glutaraldehyde is a contact irritant and sensitizer and can cause allergic contact dermatitis and eczema (3,9). Airborne concentrations of glutaraldehyde from 1.6 to 37.6 ppm have been shown to cause respiratory irritation in guinea pigs, but not respiratory sensitization (10). Airborne glutaraldehyde concentrations have also been shown to cause occupational asthma (11). In a nonoccupational exposure, glutaraldehyde causes bloody diarrhea and colitis in patients undergoing sigmoidoscopy with endoscopes that have not been properly rinsed after cleaning (1).

The NIOSH recommended exposure limit (REL) and the ACGIH threshold-limit value (TLV) are 0.05 ppm (0.2 mg per m^3). OSHA does not currently have a PEL. The ACGIH TLV is based on the irritation threshold of glutaraldehyde in humans (4).

Glutaraldehyde is much less volatile than formaldehyde. The vapor pressure of a 2% glutaraldehyde solution is 0.0012 mm Hg (4), giving a saturation vapor concentration of 5.2 ppm. However, the RELs are also low, and growing evidence exists in the literature that these levels might not protect against skin effects (including sensitization), respiratory irritation, and occupational asthma (9,11–14). One study, an epidemiologic investigation including 39 hospital employees exposed to glutaraldehyde and 68 unexposed employees, showed significant increases in skin and respiratory symptoms and headaches in the exposed group (12). Glutaraldehyde exposures of the exposed group were intermittent and at concentrations well below the Swedish short-term occupational exposure limit of 0.8 mg per m^3 (0.2 ppm).

Quantitating levels of skin exposure is much more difficult than measuring airborne concentrations. Because of glutaraldehyde's ability to produce allergic contact dermatitis, manufacturers recommend that gloves be worn during use. However, common latex examination gloves may be permeable to glutaraldehyde. In a study conducted by Johnson and Johnson of a 2% glutaraldehyde solution, breakthrough of glutaraldehyde through latex gloves (based on glove thickness) was observed between 1 and 4 hours (*unpublished letter*, 1997).

Because of uncertainties concerning safe exposure levels, work practices involving glutaraldehyde should be carefully controlled. Cleaning rooms should have good general air ventilation, and laboratory hoods or other local exhaust ventilation systems should be supplied if feasible. Local exhaust systems should be ducted out of the building or passed through a chemical filter capable of removing glutaraldehyde vapors. Glutaraldehyde containers should be kept covered at all times except for the insertion and removal of instruments. Employees should wear aprons, face splashguards, and gloves. Latex gloves should be avoided, and if used, they should be doubled and changed frequently. Automatic glutaraldehyde washers, which can considerably lower exposure times, airborne concentrations, and the possibility of skin contact, are commercially available for items such as endoscopes.

Ethylene Oxide

Ethylene oxide (EtO) is a colorless, flammable gas at room temperature and normal atmospheric pressure. In medical facilities, EtO is used in specially designed units as a sterilant for instruments and materials that are sensitive to steam sterilization. Traditionally, EtO was prepared with a chlorofluorocarbon (CFC) stabilization agent in a 12% EtO, 88% CFC mix (i.e., *88/12*) to reduce flammability and explosive hazards. Since the production ban of CFCs under the U.S. Environmental Protection Agency Clean Air Act, EtO has been used in mixtures with carbon dioxide, hydrochlorofluorocarbons, or as 100% EtO.

Only 0.02% of the 6 billion lb of EtO produced annually in the United States is used for sterilization purposes (4). However, because of the labor-intensive nature of the sterilization process, hospitals make up a major portion of workers exposed to ethylene oxide (4).

Acute exposures to high levels of EtO (greater than 100 ppm) cause nausea, headache, weakness, vomiting, drowsiness, incoordination, and general irritation (4). As a gas used at high process concentrations, such exposures can easily occur during accidents or improper use of equipment. In early studies on experimental dogs and rats, no effects were noted at long-term daily exposure levels of approximately 50 ppm, and only slight effects were noted at 100 ppm (15). The effects of low-level EtO exposures have been studied in greater detail in animals and humans. Concern was sparked by two long-term inhalation studies conducted on Fischer 344 rats that showed increases in brain tumors, mononuclear cell leukemia, and peritoneal mesothelioma, resulting from exposure levels as low as 10 ppm (16,17). Subsequent studies have shown EtO to be mutagenic in monkeys and carcinogenic in mice (4).

An association between EtO and cancer in humans was first suggested from two studies published in 1979 concerning EtO-exposed workers in Sweden (18,19). In the first study, excess cases of leukemia were noted among employees working with and around EtO sterilizers, and the second study recorded excess cancers, including leukemia, among workers in an EtO production plant. Since that time, the relationship between EtO and cancer has been widely studied. In a 1993 review and metaanalysis of ten epidemiologic studies concerning EtO and cancer, Shore concluded that the current data did not provide consistent and convincing evidence that EtO causes leukemia or non-Hodgkin's lymphoma, but that the issues were not resolved and required further studies of exposed populations (20). One case study also linked low-level EtO exposure to occupational asthma (21).

The IARC monograph for EtO published in 1994 classified EtO as a Group 1 agent, carcinogenic to humans (22). The evaluation was based on limited evidence of carcinogenicity in humans and sufficient evidence in experimental animals. IARC also listed EtO as a potential reproductive hazard. ACGIH classified EtO as a suspected human carcinogen in 1984 (4).

In response to the evidence of carcinogenicity, in 1984 OSHA promulgated a standard dedicated to controlling EtO exposure (23). The PEL was lowered from 50 to 1 ppm for an 8-hour time-weighted average exposure. An action level was defined as one-half the PEL (0.5 ppm). Also included was an excursion limit of 5 ppm for 15-minute average exposures. The remainder of the standard lists specific methods for measuring and limiting employee exposure, including sections on exposure monitoring, regulated areas, methods of compliance, respiratory protection and personal protective equipment, emergency situations, medical surveillance, communication of hazards to employees, record keeping, and observation of monitoring results.

The combined effects of a lower workplace exposure limit, more stringent environmental controls, and increased explosion hazards from the use of 100% EtO have necessitated better sterilizer designs. New EtO sterilizers are usually installed in specially designed rooms used only for the sterilizers and aeration equipment. The room is ventilated with dedicated systems separate from the rest of the building ventilation. Sterilizer exhaust is ducted directly to the outside and, increasingly, through abatement equipment (required in some states) before release to the atmosphere. EtO concentrations in the rooms are also continuously monitored by EtO gas detectors. However, proper work practices are still important to limit EtO exposure to within the current legal limits.

Sterilizers are designed to run between 2 and 5 hours (24), which includes gas contact and aeration times. However, 8 to 12 hours of additional mechanical aeration are required to allow residual EtO to diffuse out of the cloth and paper instrument packaging. This is often done in separate aerators to free up the sterilizer for new loads. Sterilization-area employees who transfer the medical instruments from the sterilizer to the aerators are potentially exposed to residual EtO. Actual exposure depends on the type of sterilizer, the type and amount of material sterilized, and the procedure and time taken to move items between the sterilizer and aerator. Carts should be used whenever possible to transport items from the sterilizers to aerators; carrying trays of items by hand positions items directly in the breathing zone of the employee and can dramatically increase exposure to EtO. Sterilizers should never be opened to retrieve a critical instrument or free up the sterilizer for a new load, a practice that sometimes occurs, before the minimum recommended aeration time.

Maintenance employees are also at risk of EtO exposure, primarily from changing out EtO cylinders used on 88/12 sterilizers. Exposure risk is greatest when opening sterilant supply lines while switching canisters. Lines must be purged before opening, and the equipment area should have good general air ventilation.

Disinfectants and Cleaning Agents

Several other chemicals are used in hospital environments as disinfectants, including alcohols, chlorine compounds, hydrogen peroxide, iodophors, peracetic acid, phenolics, and quaternary ammonium compounds (25). Many of these compounds are skin or respiratory irritants.

Chemically, quaternary ammonium compounds are organically substituted ammonium compounds in which the nitrogen atom has a valence of 5 (25). Several different compounds that fall under this category are in use, one of the most common being benzalkonium chloride. This compound has been linked to possible irritation or sensitivity reactions when used as a preservative in nasal sprays (26,27), but other studies have shown the effects are not conclusive (28). Lauryl dimethyl benzyl ammonium chloride (a specific quaternary ammonium compound) was also shown to be a cause of asthma in a pharmacist chronically exposed to residual vapors from a floor cleaner containing the compound (29).

HAZARDOUS MEDICATIONS

Antineoplastic Drugs

Antineoplastic drugs are increasingly used for the treatment of patients with a variety of malignant diseases. Adverse health effects, including mutagenicity, carcinogenicity, and teratogenicity, have been documented in patients therapeutically treated with antineoplastic drugs (30). Consequently, health effects of people who handle and administer them have also been studied. Occupational exposure has been documented from studies measuring urinary excretion of drugs by the employees who mixed or administered the drugs (31). Effects have also been found in pharmacists and nurses involved in mixing, administering, or otherwise handling the drugs. These effects include mutagenicity of urine (32), increases in chromosomal aberrations, and elevation of sister chromatid exchanges (33). Epidemiologic studies have shown increases in leukemia, and case studies of cancer have been reported in people preparing and handling the drugs (34,35).

In 1986, OSHA issued an instruction publication for employees occupationally exposed to antineoplastic drugs (36). Detailed guidelines are included for many issues involving work with cytoplastic drugs, including drug preparation, drug administration, patient care, waste disposal, spills, medical surveillance, and training and information dissemination. Primary recommendations include the use of protective gloves and disposable gowns for situations in which skin exposure is a possibility, and use of a Class II vertical flow containment hood, also called a *biological safety cabinet*, for preparing drugs.

OSHA considers the use of vertical flow containment hoods critical for preventing occupational exposure. In a vertical flow hood, filtered air comes in from the bottom of the hood, passes up through the work surface, and is captured and exhausted by the hood making up the top part of the cabinet. Using this system, the drugs are protected from microbiological contamination, and the preparer is protected from exposure. For the horizontal airflow work benches that are not favored by OSHA, filtered air is blown in from the back, across the work area, and then out the front of the bench past the person preparing the medications.

Although publication of the OSHA guidelines has increased use of protective measures to limit exposure, compliance with the guidelines in the United States is far from complete or universal (37,38). In addition, some latex gloves have been found to be permeable to anticancer drugs—in one case, within 15 minutes (39). In another study, multiple surface wipes of work area surfaces collected measurable quantities of an antineoplastic agent in a facility that followed the OSHA guidelines (30). The authors of this study called for further recognition of dermal exposures and ingestion as routes of exposure.

However, some studies indicate that the use of recommended control measures might limit the effects of occupational exposure. A British study showed no increase in mutagenicity between a group of pharmacists and nurses handling cytotoxic agents under recommended work procedures and a control group of nonexposed office workers (40). Also, a study of 1,282 Danish oncology department nurses occupationally exposed to antineoplastic drugs in well-controlled environments found no increase in miscarriages, malformations, low birth weight, or preterm birth (41). The authors suggested that the lack of reproductive effects might be attributable to good exposure-control measures.

Other Hazardous Drugs

Some drugs other than neoplastic agents also have been recognized as possible hazards to the occupationally exposed. In 1990, the American Society of Hospital Pharmacists defined a class of agents as hazardous drugs (42). The American Society of Hospital Pharmacists defined four characteristics that could be considered hazardous, including the following:

- Genotoxicity
- Carcinogenicity
- Teratogenicity or fertility impairment
- Serious organ or other toxic manifestations at low doses in experimental animal or treated patients

OSHA recognized this effort and expanded the guideline for cytotoxic drugs to include other hazardous drugs (43). OSHA lists some common drugs that are considered hazardous and recommends that professional judgment be used for new or experimental drugs in which chemical structure or activity indicates potential toxicity.

NITROUS OXIDE AND OTHER GENERAL ANESTHETICS

General anesthetic agents used in medical and dental operating rooms include nitrous oxide gas and several volatile liquids, including halothane, trichloroethylene, and isoflurane, among others. These agents are administered to patients as inhaled gases or vapors. Occupational exposure occurs from sources including exhaled air from the patient, openings around the face mask seal, leaks in the delivery or scavenging equipment, or spills of volatile liquid anesthetics. Concentrations of these waste gases in operating suites vary widely, depending on general ventilation (number of nonrecycled air changes per hour) and the use of waste gas scavenging devices that capture and remove air exhaled from the patient. Anesthesiologists and anesthetists are exposed to greater concentrations than other operating room personnel because of their proximity to the anesthesia machine and the patient (44).

The presence of waste anesthetic gases and possible health effects was given little attention until the late 1960s; nitrous oxide was listed as a simple asphyxiant by the ACGIH until 1977. Since that time, a number of epidemiologic studies of operating room personnel have shown increases in some health effects in subjects with chronic exposures (4). In a study sponsored by the American Society of Anesthesiologists and published in 1974, reproductive effects, including spontaneous abortion and congenital abnormalities, along with cancer, hepatic, and renal disease, were noted in operating room nursing staffs (45). Anesthetic gas scavenging systems were not in common use at the time of the study. Neurologic complaints, including numbness, tingling, and muscle weakness, have been seen in dentists with high exposure levels to nitrous oxide (46).

The ACGIH's TLV for nitrous oxide and halothane is 50 ppm (4). The TLV for nitrous oxide is the calculated safe level based on animal studies, and the halothane TLV is based on a comparison of toxicologic and use concentration data with trichloroethylene and chloroform. NIOSH has an REL of 25 ppm for nitrous oxide based on one report of decreased audiovisual performance of humans after exposure to 50 ppm nitrous oxide (47). For halothane, the NIOSH REL of 2 ppm is based on potential reproductive effects and the ability to maintain such levels in operating rooms (48).

Studies have shown significantly lower concentrations of waste anesthetic gases in operating rooms equipped with gas scavenging equipment compared to those without such devices. In a study of ten Canadian hospitals, all the mean daily concentrations of nitrous oxide measured in rooms without scavenging equipment were more than 25 ppm, whereas only 29% of rooms with some form of scavenging equipment were above this level (49). Another study showed that concentrations of halothane could be controlled to 0.02 ppm with a gas-tight anesthetic system (50). In a third study, nitrous oxide concentrations were measured in 30 operating rooms before and after the start of hygienic measures, including an inspection and repair of the nitrous oxide equipment, increasing general air ventilation, and use of a double mask scavenging system (51). Levels in surgery on adults fell from 61 to 90 ppm to 2 to 15 ppm; for children, they fell from 134 to 764 ppm to 8 to 42 ppm.

OTHER CHEMICAL HAZARDS

Methyl Methacrylate

Methyl methacrylate is a widely used chemical in the production of industrial polymers. In medical settings, the methyl methacrylate monomer is mixed with a powdered polymethyl methacrylate to form an acrylic bone cement. Because of the short setting time, mixing is usually done in the surgical suite.

Methyl methacrylate is a very strong skin sensitizer, and persons who have become sensitized can sustain allergic contact dermatitis from skin contact with the liquid or from touching acrylics that are not completely cured (3). Because methyl methacrylate is also a strong solvent, it may also penetrate rubber gloves. All skin contact should be avoided by people who must regularly work with methyl methacrylate. Difficulty in following this advice has been noted for surgeons and orthodontists, and sometimes an assistant must be used for handling and placing uncured polymer (52).

The OSHA PEL for methyl methacrylate vapor is 100 ppm. Inhalation overexposure is not a concern in operating rooms because of the relatively small amount used, the short exposure time, and the good general air ventilation used in surgical suites.

Data concerning methyl methacrylate was reviewed by IARC in 1994, and methyl methacrylate was listed as a group 3 agent, not classifiable as to its carcinogenicity to humans (22).

Latex

Latex is a term used in industry for a material's coating properties. A good example of this is in the paint industry, in which the name *latex paint* is used for many types of oil- and water-based paints, despite the fact that no natural latex rubber is in latex paint.

Natural rubber was discovered by native people in South and Central America. Later, it was exploited by the Europeans and when the vulcanization process was discovered. Large plantations were developed in Southeast Asia and Africa.

The common term of natural rubber latex (NRL) has come to refer to the material derived from the rubber tree (*Hevea brasiliensis*) that is used in industry, at home, and in the medical fields. The trees require 8 to 10 years to reach maturity before they can be tapped for natural latex. Approximately 150 adult trees produce approximately 100 g of solid natural latex per week. This makes approximately ten pairs of surgical gloves, or 1,500 pairs per acre.

NRL is a delicate, complicated intercellular arrangement of a highly anastomosed system of cells that synthesize the *cis*-1,4-polyisoprene. The isoprene subunit appears to be the backbone of biomolecules comprising natural latex rubber. These cells are called *lactiferous* or *laticifer cells*.

NRL products are used in a wide range of medical applications because of the unique combination of strength, flexibility, elasticity, tear resistance, and barrier qualities of natural rubber.

Latex Allergies

Latex allergies are a relatively new problem. NRL is an allergen. Because of OSHA's enforcement of the Centers for Disease Control and Prevention's (CDC) Standard Precautions to protect against biohazards, people are wearing latex gloves at a higher rate, accounting for an increase in latex allergies. It has been suggested that inferior gloves on the market are subjecting the people to higher concentrations of proteins in the latex gloves. Also, the use of powdered gloves is very common, and the powder absorbs the allergen and increases exposure potential. Direct contact with NRL is not necessary for the initiation of sensitization, indicating that at least some antigens may be aerosolized from the NRL gloves. The possibility exists that antigen may be carried on syringe needles from the rubber stoppers of multiple-use vials.

Allergic reactions may be delayed or immediate, are normally local, or may become systemic and can be potentially fatal. Hypersensitivity reactions are categorized into five groups. Latex allergic reactions are classified as type I and type IV only. Type I hypersensitivity is a protein allergy. The antigen in the IgE-mediated response is a latex protein or polypeptide, perhaps more than one.

The reactions to latex proteins are systemic, type I hypersensitivity immune reactions, in which a massive histamine release occurs. This results in a clinical manifestation of urticaria or anaphylaxis.

Urticaria can manifest as hives that are raised red wheels with blanched centers, and local swelling with onset in just a few minutes. Reduction may take several hours to days.

Anaphylaxis can result in facial swelling, difficulty in breathing, abdominal cramping, vomiting, rapid heartbeat, low blood pressure, shock, and death. Onset may only be a very few minutes and may progress very rapidly, requiring emergency treatment.

Type IV hypersensitivity is a delayed hypersensitivity reaction of cutaneous contact dermatitis caused not by latex, but by the chemicals added during rubber manufacture. These include accelerators to speed curing, such as mercaptobenzothiazole, dithiocarbamates, and antioxidants, such as *p*-phenylenediamine.

Type IV hypersensitivity (allergic contact dermatitis) is a cell-mediated immunologic reaction initiated by contact-sensitizing chemicals. No symptoms exist during the initial sensitization period. The acute response that follows subsequent exposure results in vesicles that elicit pain if scratched.

Chronic dermatitis, the result of prolonged, repeated exposure without the opportunity to heal, results in skin that is dry, cracked, and thickened. These symptoms may extend beyond the boundary of the gloves.

A careful history should also be obtained from every patient before any procedure involving contact with latex. Previous medical history, especially unexplained allergic or anaphylactic reactions during a medical procedure, may indicate sensitization.

Contact dermatitis is the most frequent symptom; respiratory tract symptoms are second. One should be suspicious if a patient is symptomatic on the job and then, after a period of time, is asymptomatic at home.

People who have a history of only mild latex-glove eczema rarely have anaphylactic events; however, a history of severe or worsening latex glove–induced eczema, urticaria, or work-related conjunctivitis, rhinitis, or asthma may indicate allergic sensitization and increased risk for more severe reactions in the future.

Food allergies known to coexist with latex sensitivities may be useful for identifying the risks of latex exposure. People who have allergies to any of the listed fruits may be more sensitive to latex. Proteins, avocados, bananas, chestnuts, and papaya have the highest degree of association with the others being listed as moderate:

Avocados
Apples
Bananas
Carrots
Celery
Chestnuts
Figs
Kiwi
Melons
Papaya
Potatoes
Peaches
Tomatoes

The use of screening tests for predicting anaphylaxis has vastly improved and is still evolving. The radioallergosorbent test uses a blood sample from a suspected NRL-sensitized individual. It measures specific IgE antibodies against NRL allergens. This method has an 80% sensitivity and 100% specificity in nonatopic individuals.

Nitrile gloves are a little more costly but are a good substitute. Vinyl gloves may also be used; however, the vinyl glove failure rate is much higher than that of the latex glove. Also, vinyl gloves are not suitable for infection control.

It is better to buy a known brand that has the protein levels on the label, which may be a little more costly. Some of the less costly gloves from Indochina and the Far East Asia regions have allergin levels of several hundred times those of domestic gloves.

Powdered gloves normally have a much higher level of protein that can be absorbed by the powder and transferred to the skin. When gloves are removed, the powder is aerosolized. When the next set of gloves is put on without washing the hands, the powder remains; allergens from the old and the new powder exist, thus increasing exposure.

U.S. Food and Drug Administration Recommendations for Health Care Workers

U.S. Food and Drug Administration recommendations for health care workers include taking general histories of patients, including questions about latex sensitivity. For surgical and radiology patients, spina bifida patients, and health care workers, this recommendation is especially important. Questions about itching, rash, or wheezing after wearing latex gloves or inflating a toy balloon may be useful.

If latex sensitivity is suspected, consider using devices made with alternative materials, such as nitrile, vinyl, or plastic. For example, a health professional could wear a nonlatex glove over the latex glove if the patient is sensitive. If the health professional and the patient are sensitive, a latex middle glove could be used. (Latex gloves labeled *hypoallergenic* may not always prevent adverse reactions.)

Whenever latex-containing medical devices are used, especially when the latex comes in contact with mucous membranes, be alert to the possibility of an allergic reaction.

If an allergic reaction does occur and latex is suspected, advise the patient of a possible latex sensitivity and consider an immunologic evaluation.

Advise patients to tell health professionals and emergency personnel about any known latex sensitivity before undergoing medical procedures. Consider advising patients with severe latex sensitivity to wear a medical identification bracelet.

The U.S. Food and Drug Administration is also asking health professionals to report incidents of adverse reactions to latex or other materials used in medical devices.

Latex Avoidance Procedures for Health Care Workers

By touching any latex object, the health care worker can transmit the allergen by hand to the patient. Latex avoidance procedures should be followed by health care workers to keep the powder from the gloves away from the patient, because the powder acts as a carrier for the latex protein. Therefore, to reduce the possibility of the latex protein becoming airborne, care must be taken not to snap gloves on and off or, better yet, powderless or nonlatex gloves should be used.

A readily available master list of latex-free devices and products should be kept and updated as necessary.

It is recommended to develop programs to educate health care workers in the care of latex-sensitive patients. This should include the development of educational programs for patients and their families in the care and precautions that should be taken to prevent latex exposure. This should encompass a first-aid protocol in the event of a severe reaction.

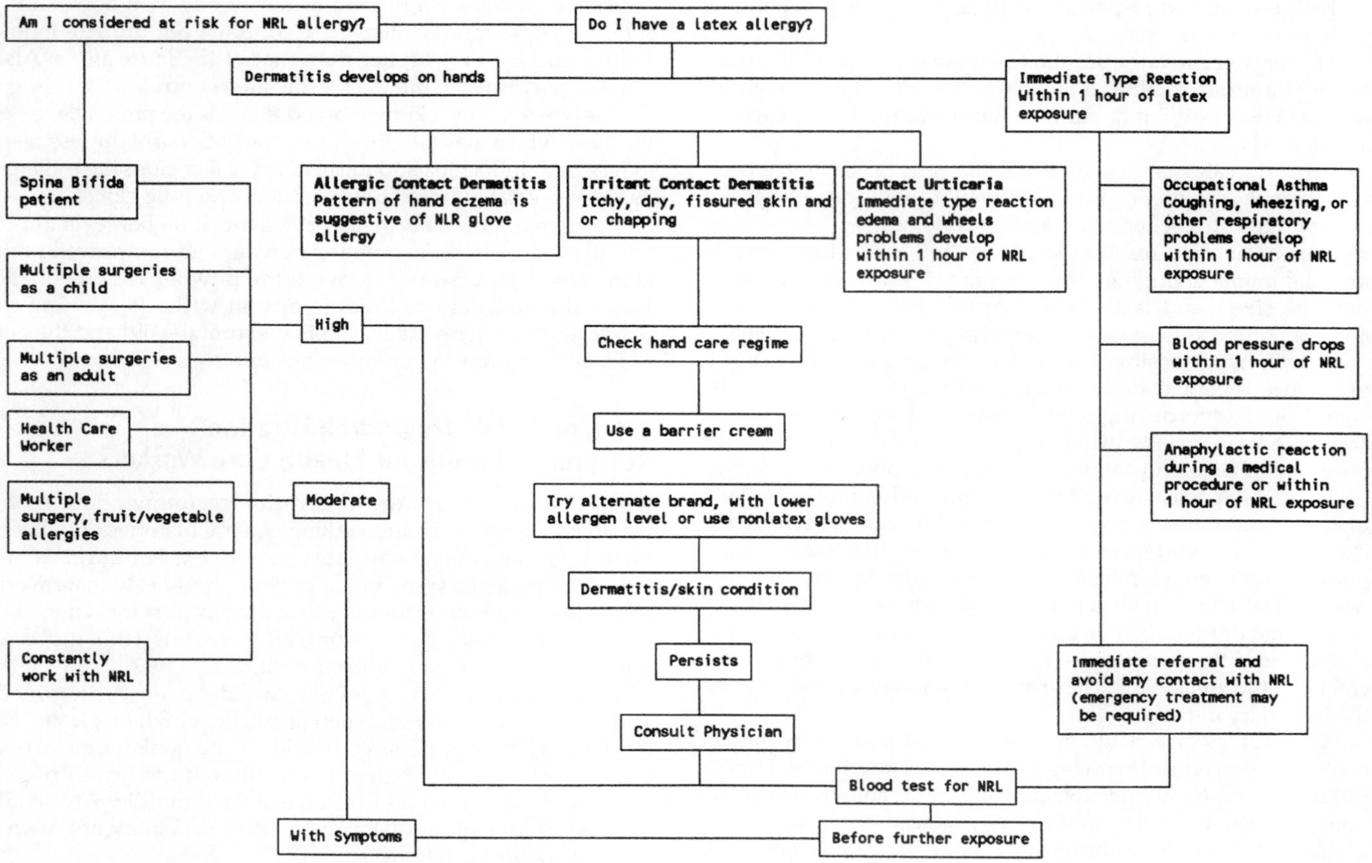

Am I considered at risk for NRL allergy?

Do I have a latex allergy?

Dermatitis develops on hands

Immediate Type Reaction Within 1 hour of latex exposure

Spina Bifida patient

Allergic Contact Dermatitis Pattern of hand eczema is suggestive of NLR glove allergy

Irritant Contact Dermatitis Itchy, dry, fissured skin and or chapping

Contact Urticaria Immediate type reaction edema and wheels problems develop within 1 hour of NRL exposure

Occupational Asthma Coughing, wheezing, or other respiratory problems develop within 1 hour of NRL exposure

Multiple surgeries as a child

High

Check hand care regime

Multiple surgeries as an adult

Blood pressure drops within 1 hour of NRL exposure

Health Care Worker

Use a barrier cream

Anaphylactic reaction during a medical procedure or within 1 hour of NRL exposure

Multiple surgery, fruit/vegetable allergies

Moderate

Try alternate brand, with lower allergen level or use nonlatex gloves

Dermatitis/skin condition

Constantly work with NRL

Persists

Immediate referral and avoid any contact with NRL (emergency treatment may be required)

Consult Physician

Blood test for NRL

With Symptoms

Before further exposure

Figure 47-1. Evaluation and management of latex allergy. Note: If any employee in the facility has a natural rubber latex allergy, type I or IV hypersensitivity, the entire facility should be using nonpowdered gloves.

Latex-sensitive patients should be protected from unintended exposures in the same manner as drug-sensitive patients. Some methods include "latex sensitive" wrist bands, door or bed signs, flagging of records, or latex alert tags on hospitalized patients' garments.

Patients with any latex allergy should be encouraged to wear medical alert bracelets, necklaces, or tags, regardless of the severity of their reactions, as the allergic reaction may convert from a local to a systemic one.

Private offices, clinics, and hospitals should be cognizant of possible risks to latex-sensitive patients and health care personnel. All products and medical procedures that come in intimate patient contact or are used by health care personnel must be reviewed for possible latex content. A readily available master list of items safe for sensitive patients may help avoid unintended exposures.

Patients with myelomeningocele (i.e., spina bifida) should be referred for elective surgical procedures to centers that have latex-free surgical suites available. Other patients with a history suggesting a high risk of anaphylaxis should be evaluated and appropriately tested before surgery, with recommendations to be made on a case-by-case basis.

Health care personnel who show signs of latex contact dermatitis or latex hypersensitivity should be encouraged to avoid continued exposure to natural latex products and to use either synthetic latex or nonlatex substitutes. Because the natural history of this condition is still unclear, however, some individuals have become anaphylactic-sensitive over time.

Patients and health care workers at risk should be cautioned about the risk of repeated reactions in situations of latex exposure, to include exposures in the hospital and outside the medical environment (Fig. 47-1).

Natural Latex Rubber

Natural latex rubber is produced from the processed sap of the rubber tree *H. brasiliensis*. Natural latex is widely used for medical products because of properties that include elasticity, durability, and resistance to viral penetration. However, latex products are increasingly found to cause skin irritation and other allergic reactions. These reactions have been linked to hypersensitivity to *H. brasiliensis* proteins that persist in the final latex product, in amounts as much as 2% by weight (53).

The American College of Physicians summarized the clinical symptoms of latex rubber allergy (54). They reported nonimmunologic, irritant dermatitis of the hand as the most common clinical presentation. Contact dermatitis type IV delayed-hypersensitivity reactions to rubber additives were reported as the most common immunologic manifestation of latex rubber allergy. Type I allergic responses, including contact urticaria, rhinoconjunctivitis, asthma, and anaphylaxis, were reported as less common manifestations. Increasing incidences of latex allergies have been reported since the mid-1980s. The American College of Allergy, Asthma, and Immunology reported that between 8% and 17% of exposed hospital employees internationally are at risk for latex reactions (55). Several theories for the increase have been postulated (56,57). These include the increased latex exposure because of the universal precautions; an increased number of new, inexperienced glove manufacturers; changes in manufacturing practices, including raw material washing techniques; and the use of cornstarch powder as a lubricant for gloves.

Exposure to the plant proteins in natural latex can occur from skin contact, contact with tissues during surgery, and inhalation of airborne allergens. Glove cornstarch powder absorbs latex allergens, and the particles can become airborne during glove removal (58). Exposure to airborne powder has been shown to cause increased airway resistance, acute rhinitis, conjunctivitis, and systemic reactions in persons sensitive to latex (53,58). Use of gloves with low allergen content or powder-free gloves is effective in reducing aeroallergen levels (54,59).

Several control measures are currently being implemented or discussed to protect persons already sensitive to latex and to prevent future sensitization. These measures include limiting the use of latex products, using latex gloves that have low protein concentrations, prohibiting powdered gloves, and substituting gloves and other devices with those made of other materials (55,57). Laws requiring the labeling of natural latex are recommended by some groups, and manufacturing methods that result in lower final concentrations of plant proteins are being examined.

BIOLOGICAL HAZARDS

Infectious Diseases

Infectious diseases are a common and often very serious threat to health care workers. All health care workers who come into contact with patients, their blood, or their body fluids are at risk for exposure to infectious agents (60–68). The spread of microorganisms in hospitals and health care facilities can occur by several routes of transmission. The most common routes are (a) airborne, (b) droplet, and (c) contact transmission (68).

Airborne transmission occurs by dissemination of small airborne droplet nuclei (5 mm or less) that contain microorganisms and remain suspended in air for an extended period of time. Disease may be transmitted when a susceptible host inhales the contaminated air. Microorganisms can also disseminate through air on dust particles and be carried through ventilation and air-conditioning systems (64,68).

Droplet transmission occurs when an infected source (i.e., patient) coughs, sneezes, or speaks, causing the generation of microorganism-containing droplets (5 mm or greater in size) that propel through the air and deposit on mucous membranes of a susceptible host (i.e., health care provider) (62,63).

Contact transmission, the most common route of nosocomial infection transmission in health care facilities, may be either *direct* or *indirect*. In direct-contact transmission, microorganisms are transferred when the infected source comes directly into bodily contact with the susceptible host. The indirect-contact mode of transmission involves the transfer of microorganisms from the source to the susceptible host via an intermediate object, such as contaminated gloves or instruments. Frequently, the spread of nosocomial infections from one patient to another is caused by the cross-contamination of a caregiver who has used poor handwashing techniques (68).

Infectious diseases may be viral, bacterial, or fungal in nature and may originate from a variety of different sources in health care facilities, including visitors, staff, equipment, and contaminated dusts and aerosols in ventilation systems, but most often from infected patients and their blood and body secretions (61,68).

EVOLUTION OF ISOLATION PRACTICES IN THE UNITED STATES

Recognition of the problem of disease spread in health care settings and attempts to control it occurred well before the beginning of the twentieth century. The earliest recommendations for isolation precautions date as far back as the 1870s in hospital handbooks that advised keeping infected patients physically separated from other patients (60). The evolution of practices to prevent disease transmission in health care institutions has been based on the growing knowledge of microorganisms, the findings of epidemiologic research studies, and the need for protection against the new multidrug-resistant microorganisms. Over the years, the CDC, OSHA, and other organizations have set forth recommendations and guidelines for prevention of infectious disease spread, including isolation practices in health care facilities.

In 1985, when acquired immunodeficiency syndrome began to reach epidemic proportions in the United States, dramatic changes in isolation practices were seen with the introduction of Universal Precautions. Universal Precautions (i.e., Blood and Body Fluid Precautions) were designed to reduce the risk of blood-borne pathogen transmission in health care facilities primarily through the use of barriers, such as gowns and gloves, when in contact with any patient's blood or body fluids (68). In 1987, Body Substance Isolation was introduced. This system recommended isolation of all potentially infectious moist body substances (e.g., blood, sputum, urine, feces, and wound drainage) of all patients, regardless of their known disease status, through the use of gloves and other barrier equipment (68,69).

In the early 1990s, the emergence of new multidrug-resistant microorganisms and the comeback of the tuberculosis (TB) epidemic brought new concerns to health care workers. A new, up-to-date system of isolation was needed and was set forth by the CDC and its Hospital Infection Control Practices Advisory Committee. This guideline is a two-tiered system intended to reduce transmission of blood-borne and other pathogens in health care facilities (68). The first part of the guideline, called *Standard Precautions*, synthesizes the major elements of Universal Precautions and Body Substance Isolation and applies them to all patients, regardless of their known infection status. They are to be used by all health care personnel when in contact with any patient's blood, body fluids, secretions, excretions, nonintact skin, and mucous membranes. Through the use of personal protective equipment (e.g., gloves, gowns, masks, and eyewear), stringent handwashing, and proper handling of soiled equipment, linens, specimens, and so forth, Standard Precautions are designed to prevent the spread of microorganisms from known and unknown sources of infection (68).

The second part of the guideline sets forth isolation practices to be used when coming in contact with patients with infections known to be transmitted via a specific route (e.g., airborne, droplet, or contact). These *Transmission-Based Precautions* outline specific isolation practices to be used in each situation in addition to Standard Precautions (68). Table 47-1 provides examples of specific conditions in which only Standard Precautions are to be used and when Transmission-Based Precautions should be used in addition to Standard Precautions.

OCCUPATIONAL SAFETY AND HEALTH ADMINISTRATION BLOOD-BORNE PATHOGENS STANDARD

In 1989, OSHA proposed a ruling on occupational exposure to blood-borne pathogens in health care facilities. In this ruling, OSHA recognized the significant risk that exposure to blood-borne pathogens presents to health care workers and set forth specific guidelines, based primarily on Universal Precautions, on dealing with this risk. In 1991, OSHA issued its final ruling on Occupational Exposure to Blood-Borne Pathogens (29 *CFR*,

TABLE 47-1. Conditions requiring transmission-based precautions and their corresponding specific isolation practices

Examples of illness/infections	Type of precaution	Specific isolation practices
Legionnaires' disease, bacterial or fungal meningitis, ringworm (dermatophytosis), coccidioidomycosis	Standard precautions only	Personal protective equipment when in contact with any blood or body fluid (except sweat); handwashing after glove removal, proper handling of used equipment and wastes, and employee adherence to occupational health and Occupational Safety and Health Administration's blood-borne pathogens standard
Tuberculosis, measles (rubeola), chickenpox (varicella), disseminated herpes zoster (varicella-zoster)	Airborne precautions and standard precautions	Patient placement in isolation room with negative pressure, 6 to 12 air changes per h, local exhaust ventilation equipped with high-efficiency particulate air filtration, and doors closed when occupied; employee respiratory protection (nonsurgical mask); limit patient transport and mask patient during transport; and all standard precaution practices
German measles (rubella), influenza, meningococcal meningitis, pertussis (whooping cough)	Droplet precautions and standard precautions	Patient placement in private room (no special ventilation required), doors may remain opened; employee respiratory protection when within 3 ft of patient (general surgical mask okay); employee personal protective equipment (e.g., gloves and gown); limit patient transport and mask patient when transporting; and all standard precaution practices
Ebola viral hemorrhagic fever, draining, infected wound abscess, pediculosis (lice), chickenpox (varicella)	Contact precautions and standard precautions	Patient placement in private room, no special ventilation; gown and gloves on entering room; strict handwashing after glove removal; limit patient transporting; proper handling of used equipment and wastes; and all standard precaution practices

Adapted from refs. 61–68.

Part 1910.1030). In short, the standard requires employers in any hospital or health care facility to do the following (61):

- Develop an exposure-control plan, identifying employees at risk of occupational exposure to blood-borne pathogens.
- Provide employee training on occupational risks, methods to reduce risks, and use of worker protection methods, including Universal Precautions and safe handling of contaminated linens, needles, and other wastes.
- Maintain records of employee training.
- Use warning labels and hazardous waste signs to identify hazards.
- Provide medical evaluation and treatment to employees after an exposure incident and maintain records of all exposures and treatments.
- Provide hepatitis B vaccine to employees at no cost.
- Provide suitable personal protective equipment to employees.

TUBERCULOSIS

After years of steadily declining as a major public health problem in America, the transmission of TB is once again on the rise and posing a greater-than-ever threat to the population and to health care providers (64,66,67).

Mycobacterium tuberculosis, the causal agent of TB, is a highly resistant, rod-shaped bacterium that is expelled and aerosolized in droplet form when an infected person coughs, sneezes, or talks (62,64). The droplets vary in size, but studies show that most of them are between 1 and 4 mm in diameter (65). These small droplets are capable of remaining suspended in air for long periods of time and have been shown to circulate through ventilation systems and spread into entire buildings (62,64). Various factors, including the nature of the bacteria, susceptibility of the host, and the conduciveness of the environment, affect the ability of the *Mycobacterium tuberculosis* organism to spread. The CDC identifies the following environmental factors as enhancing the transmission of TB (64):

- Contact between an infectious person and a susceptible host in small, enclosed spaces
- Inadequate ventilation, resulting in insufficient air dilution and removal of contaminants (specifically TB-infected droplet nuclei)
- Recirculation of air containing TB-infected droplet nuclei

In attempts to reduce risks of TB transmission in health care facilities, various state and federal agencies have set forth recommendations and guidelines. In 1993, OSHA issued its Draft Guidelines for Preventing the Transmission of Tuberculosis in Health Care Facilities that focuses on (a) risk assessment, (b) engineering controls, (c) administrative controls, (d) respiratory protection, (e) education and training, and (f) counseling, screening, and feasibility (66). These guidelines were finalized in 1995 (66a).

Some specific strategies recommended by OSHA, the CDC, and other agencies for the prevention of TB transmission in health care settings include the following (60–67a):

- Provide isolation of patients with known or suspected active TB infection in specially designed, designated isolation rooms.
- Equip isolation rooms with special ventilation systems (i.e., negative pressure relative to surrounding areas and separate local exhaust ventilation with HEPA filtration unit).
- Require all employees coming in contact with infectious patient to use Standard Precautions, accompanied by the appropriate transmission-based airborne precaution procedures.
- Use appropriate NIOSH- and Mine Safety and Health Organization (MSHA)–certified particulate filter respirators that prevent penetration of aerosolized particles in the 1- to 5-mm size range.
- Consider use of ultraviolet germicidal irradiation to destroy infectious droplets in isolation rooms.
- Provide adequate employee education, training, and record keeping.
- Offer appropriate screening (e.g., tuberculin skin tests), counseling, and treatment for occupation exposure cases.

Occupational Needlesticks

One of the largest biological threats to health care workers is infectious diseases contracted from occupational needlesticks. Approximately 1,000,000 accidental needlesticks occur in this country annually (70). All health care workers—nurses, physicians, and pharmacy, laboratory, and housekeeping personnel—are at risk for accidentally getting stuck by a needle that has been contaminated by a patient's blood or body fluids. Clinical and housekeeping activities that contribute to the risk of needlestick injuries include recapping needles, disposing of needles incorrectly, drawing blood or other body fluids, administering injectable medications, and handling trash and linens that contain sharps.

The resulting biological injury from an occupational needlestick can be extremely serious. Among the threats from percutaneous exposure to contaminated needles are transmission of various bacterial, viral, fungal, and parasitic infections. Two life-threatening pathogens commonly associated with needlesticks are the hepatitis B virus and the human immunodeficiency virus (HIV) (70–73). The CDC has estimated that needlestick injuries account for approximately 80% of reported occupational HIV exposures (71).

In addition to personal health risks, the financial cost of evaluation and treatment of workers who sustain needlestick injuries can be significant to the health care facility. Specific costs usually include the following:

- Personnel time (e.g., occupational health care nurses and physicians treating the worker, laboratory employees)
- Laboratory tests (e.g., HIV and hepatitis B antibody screening)
- Postexposure prophylactic treatments (e.g., hepatitis B vaccine and immune globulin, zidovudine therapy, counseling)

New CDC guidelines were published in 1998 and were further updated in January 2001 (73a,73b). These costs can vary, depending on the extent of the injury. One study estimated costs of a single needlestick injury to be approximately $400.00, not including additional costs for treatment should the injury result in transmission of HIV (73).

NEEDLESTICK PREVENTION

The most effective way to prevent health care workers' exposure to infectious diseases from needlesticks is to develop and implement a comprehensive needlestick prevention program. A 1988 study of blood-exposed health care workers found that 80% of the exposures were caused by needlesticks and concluded that 37% of these sticks could have been prevented if certain infection control precautions had been taken (72).

Many hospitals and major health care facilities now incorporate education on needlestick prevention into their infection control programs. An effective needlestick prevention program varies depending on the specific needs of the institution, but it might include the following:

1. Special equipment (e.g., sharps containers designed for safe needle and syringe disposal; safety designs on syringes and needle caps; needleless medication injectors)
2. Education and training (specialized in-service training for all health care workers that come in contact with contaminated needles)
3. Safe work practice protocols that are developed and monitored according to CDC and OSHA recommendations and guidelines for preventing infectious disease transmission in health care facilities (e.g., avoid needle recapping)

On November 6, 2000, the Needlestick Safety and Prevention Act was passed. This act mandated specific revisions of OSHA's bloodborne pathogens standard within six months (www.osha-slc.gov/needlesticks/index.html). The revised OSHA bloodborne pathogen standard specifically mandates consideration of safer needle devices as part of the reevaluation of appropriate engineering controls during the annual review of the employer's exposure control plan. It calls for employers to solicit frontline employee input in choosing safer devices. New provisions require employers to establish a log to track needlesticks rather than only recording those cuts or sticks that actually lead to illness and to maintain the privacy of employees who have suffered these injuries.

PHYSICAL HAZARDS

Radiation

Radiation refers to emission of energy in the form of rays, waves, or particles. It exists in many forms, including nonionizing radiation (e.g., radio waves, microwaves, and ultraviolet light) and ionizing radiation (e.g., beta particles, x-rays, and gamma rays). Nonionizing radiation has the ability to increase the temperature of a substance, whereas ionizing radiation has the ability to create ions in matter, thereby destroying or severely altering the material at the cellular level (74). Although both types of radiation may cause undesirable effects to the human body, ionizing radiation is of most concern because of its demonstrated capability to cause significant biological damage. For the sake of this discussion, the term *radiation* refers to ionizing radiation only.

The use of radiation for diagnostic, treatment, and research purposes in the health care industry is widespread. Radioactive solutions are administered to patients for various nuclear medicine studies, x-ray–emitting equipment is used for a host of radiological diagnostic procedures, and an array of radioactive elements are used to treat various forms of cancer. Although the use of radiation is of extreme importance to medical technology, it can present a considerable health threat to those who work around it. Health care workers who operate radiology equipment, handle radioactive materials, administer radiation therapy, or come into contact with patients who have received radionuclide therapy are at high risk for radiation exposure and contamination (74–76).

Biological effects to humans are caused by acute or chronic radiation exposures. Specific adverse effects are determined by the type, magnitude, and location (i.e., part or whole body) of exposure. Biological effects may range from mild local skin erythema and hair loss to blood cell abnormalities, severe genetic alterations, and death. In general, areas of the body that are most vulnerable to the effects of ionizing radiation are those with the highest cellular turnover, such as the hematopoietic, gastrointestinal, and reproductive systems (74,76).

Several terms have been used to express the effect of a dose of radiation. The radiation absorbed dose (rad) has been a common unit of dose since the 1950s and refers to the absorption of 100 ergs of energy per gram of tissue. The term *roentgen equivalent man* (rem) was developed in the early 1960s, when it was discovered that the biological effects of radiation depended on the type of radiation involved. The rem is used to express the effects of all types of ionizing radiation on a biologically equivalent basis and is equal to the dose in rad multiplied by the appropriate Radiation-Weighting Factor for the particular type of radiation (e.g., x-ray and gamma ray). In 1977, the term *sievert* (Sv) was introduced as an expression of radiation dose and is the most commonly used term today. One Sv is equal to 100 rem. One millisievert (mSv) is equal to 100 mrem (75).

As scientists learned more about the short- and long-term effects of radiation, systems of dose limits and recommendations were developed. The International Commission on Radiological Protection and the National Counsel on Radiation Protection and Measurements have been on the forefront of developing occupational and general public radiation exposure guidelines since 1928 (75). As more has been discovered about radiation's deleterious health effects, recommended limits have been reduced. Today, the National Counsel on Radiation Protection and Measurements recommends an effective occupational whole-body equivalent dose limit of 50 mSv (5 rem) per year, not to exceed 100 mSv in any 5-year period (77). This was the recommendation adopted by most regulatory agencies until 1991, when new data obtained from Hiroshima and Nagasaki radiation survivors suggested that the risk of ionizing radiation was 3 to 4 times greater than previously estimated (78). At this time, the International Commission on Radiological Protection reduced their occupational dose limit to 20 mSv per year, not to exceed 100 mSv in any 5-year period (76).

Health care institutions today are required by law to abide by restrictions and guidelines set forth by the International Commission on Radiological Protection and other government agencies regarding radiation protection. Compliance with these guidelines is generally well monitored by state radiation regulatory agencies as well as other organizations, such as the Joint Commission on Accreditation of Health Care Organizations (79,80).

In general, radiation protection programs in health care institutions are comprised of two basic elements: (a) environmental controls and (b) personal dosimetry (75,79). Environmental controls include all measurement and surveillance techniques to monitor and control the amount of radiation exposure that workers and the general public are receiving. Personal dosimetry is used to supplement environmental controls for workers who are subject to a significantly higher risk of external radiation exposure (e.g., radiology and nuclear medicine technicians). Here, a small radiation detector, such as a thermoluminescent film badge, is worn on the body of the worker. The dosimeter integrates the dose of radiation received over an extended period of time, thereby providing an estimation of exposure to the worker (74,79).

Back Injuries

Back injuries, particularly sprains and strains, have historically been a common complaint of health care workers (81–83). Studies have shown that health care workers most at risk for experiencing back injuries are those who lift and transport patients, such as nurses, nursing assistants, aides, and orderlies, in hospitals and nursing care facilities (82,84,85).

Studies comparing nursing occupations with other occupations in regard to incidence, prevalence, and causes of lower-back pain and injury have exposed the problem to be far greater among health care workers than for nearly any other group of workers (83,85). One study found that nurses, aides, and orderlies were 22.1 times more likely to file a back-injury claim than cashiers (85).

Worker's compensation records indicate that approximately 20% of all worker's compensation cases are related to back injuries (86). Furthermore, it has been estimated that this category makes up the second most expensive occupational affliction in terms of worker's compensation costs and treatment expenditures nationwide (87,88).

BACK INJURY PREVENTION AND CONTROL STRATEGIES

Approaches to prevention of back injuries in health care settings must include a combination of education, training, and the provision of adequate personnel and equipment. More specifically, an effective back safety program might include the following elements:

Education and instruction on good body mechanics:
- Proper lifting techniques
- Good posture

Training on use of available resources:
- Special lifting or sliding devices for transferring and lifting patients.
- Back support equipment (e.g., belts and support braces).
- Use of other personnel (e.g., encourage asking for assistance; not overestimating one's strength and ability to lift).
- Provide appropriate lifting devices and back support equipment and require use if necessary.
- Focus on ergonomic approaches that involve recognized hazardous aspects of the job and redesigning or altering them (via different equipment, task, environment, personnel) to make them safer (89,90).

Lasers

The term *laser* means "*l*ight *a*mplification by *s*timulated *e*mission of *r*adiation." Lasers are used for a variety of purposes in many different industries. In health care, lasers are used primarily for microscopic surgery and measuring blood elements. Laser beams, which are actually a form of radiation, are capable of focusing large amounts of energy on a very small surface area. This characteristic makes them useful in medicine as a tool to heat, cut, coagulate, and vaporize biological tissue.

The active medium used in lasing can be a liquid, solid, or gas. Laser output may be delivered as a continuous wave or in short bursts of energy or *pulses*. Most commonly used in the health care industry are the carbon dioxide, argon, and neodymium–yttrium-argon-garnet lasers (91–93).

The capability of lasers to alter biological tissue is precisely why lasers can pose a hazard to health care workers. By-products of lasers, or the laser plume, that consist of resulting particle debris, smoke, and vapors, present a hazard as well (91–93). Health hazards associated with lasers and laser plume include the following:

- Eye hazards (e.g., severe retinal damage, corneal scarring, and permanent loss of vision)
- Skin hazards (e.g., localized redness, mild to severe burns, incision of tissue)
- Respiratory hazards from laser plume (e.g., eye and mucous membrane irritation, respiratory ailments, fatigue, and nausea)
- Fire and electrical hazards

The American National Standards Institute, in recognizing the dangers associated with lasers, has developed a classification system to categorize lasers according to the severity of their potential hazard. The classes range from Class I (least severe hazard) to Class IV (most severe hazard), based on the wavelength and power of the laser beam (94). Every facility that uses Class III-B or Class IV lasers is required to have a trained laser safety officer on staff. It is the laser safety officer's responsibility to communicate, monitor, and enforce laser safety measures (92,94). These safety measures include the following:

- Engineering controls (to reduce or eliminate exposure at the source)
- Administrative controls (to prevent unsafe acts by employees)
- Personal protective equipment (to prevent injury if an exposure does occur)

PSYCHOSOCIAL HAZARDS

Stress Related to Shift Work, Decision Making, and High-Pressure Environment

Occupational stress does not exist exclusively in health care settings alone. Health care workers, however, are subject to a unique set of psychological stressors that are inherent in health care and may be exceptionally challenging. These stressors are often related to conflicts involving shift work, scheduling, life-and-death decision making, and dealing with critical legal and ethical dilemmas.

Shift work and prolonged odd-hour schedules are significant and very common sources of stress to health care workers. Shift work is more prevalent in the health care industry than in any other occupational sector (95). Approximately 10.3% of all health care workers work night shifts; more than one-half of whom are hospital workers—primarily nurses (95,96). All health care workers who work nights and rotating or prolonged shifts, including aides, technicians, security officers, and physicians, are at risk for experiencing the resulting ill effects. Shifts and schedules that disrupt normal sleep cycles and circadian rhythms have been shown to lead to an array of ailments, including sleep deprivation, fatigue, decreased mental acuity, gastrointestinal disorders, cardiovascular disease, and compromised job performance (97–100).

Sleep deprivation is one of the most common complaints among night and rotating-shift health care workers. Studies have shown that night nurses get less sleep than day- and evening-shift nurses and that their sleep patterns are broken up more than their average-shift–working coworkers (97,98). Physicians in postgraduate residency programs frequently work on-call and 24-hour shifts that allow them to get little or no sleep in 24-hour periods (97,101). Lack of sufficient rest can lead to many safety and job performance problems. Studies have shown that the frequency of accidents and mistakes occurring in health care facilities is greatest on night shifts (102). Sleep-deprived residents have demonstrated less ability to perform math (101). Furthermore, nurses who rotate shifts are perceived as less efficient and motivated by their supervisors than straight-shift workers (103).

Gastrointestinal ailments rank high on the shift worker complaint list as well. A NIOSH study of 1,750 nurses and nurse aides in nonsupervisory positions found that digestive disturbance was the most common reported health problem of night-shift and rotating-shift workers (100). Studies have suggested that the physiologic mechanism that associates shift work and gastrointestinal disorders involves alterations in adrenal secretions, digestive enzyme secretions, feeding patterns, and gastrointestinal motility (100,104,105). These are all factors that affect digestion and can be disrupted by shift work. The strain of working nights or rotating shifts has actually been shown to produce a stresslike response, creating preulcerative gastrointestinal conditions (104,105).

An association between cardiovascular disease and shift work has been demonstrated by several studies (106,107). Night- and rotating-shift workers have been found to have higher serum cholesterol and triglyceride levels than day-shift workers (106). In addition, they have been shown to have higher rates of cigarette smoking and less optimal dietary habits (106,107). Odd-shift workers also tend to have altered patterns of normal heart rate and blood pressure caused by disruptions in metabolism and circadian rhythms (107). These are all factors that contribute to the higher rate of heart disease among shift workers.

Another major source of stress to health care workers is the process of critical decision making. Frequently, critical life-or-death decisions must be made, often with little time and on the basis of inadequate information. For obvious reasons, this can put a great deal of pressure on the employees who are responsible for any detrimental repercussions resulting from their decision. Furthermore, as ethical and legal issues surrounding health care increase, the challenge of dealing with such situations becomes more and more stressful for those involved. In addition, particularly in acute care facilities, a sense of "anything can happen" often exists. This can cause feelings of lack of control and constant tension for workers. All of these factors help to contribute to a high-stress work environment that is very prevalent in health care settings.

INTERVENTION AND CONTROL STRATEGIES

Many factors may influence one's ability to deal with occupational stress, including one's personality, confidence level, degree of training and experience in the job, and overall emotional well-being and adaptability. Although removing stress-related conflicts from the job altogether is not possible, strategies exist that the health care institution can implement to control and ease the adverse effects imposed by stress and shift work. These strategies may include the following:

- Control frequency of shift work (shorter rotations or longer periods) and limit number of hours employees are allowed to work at night.
- Provide clockwise shift rotation (morning to afternoon, afternoon to nights).
- Control lighting in the environment for its positive effect on circadian rhythms of workers.
- Provide adequate facilities for nutritious meals during night shifts.
- Provide medical and physical fitness follow-ups for odd-shift workers.
- Offer emotional support and counseling to employees dealing with stress and shift-related problems.
- Create systems of shared leadership that provide workers with a channel for group problem solving with their peers as well as supervisors in a nonthreatening environment.
- Incorporate individual adaptability and preferences into scheduling when possible; take into account the wide variability in individuals' ability to cope and adapt to odd-hours shifts.
- Make adequate staffing a priority on all shifts, and supply back-up staff and on-call personnel in case of sick calls or other unforeseen staffing needs.
- Educate shift workers about the increased risk of health problems associated with shift work and how to reduce or cope with these risks.
- Provide shift workers with encouragement and opportunities to maintain physical fitness.
- Offer stress-reduction programs and free or low-cost mental health care plans for employees.
- Provide open-door policies and counseling for legal and ethical issues.

Violence

Workplace violence has been on the rise in many occupational settings. In health care environments, violent acts may be initiated by staff members, patients (particularly those who are confused, combative, or mentally ill), angry or irrational visitors, outside criminals, gang members, or drug addicts in search of narcotics. Health care settings at high risk for violent acts include psychiatric and mental health facilities, emergency departments, nursing homes and long-term care facilities, community health clinics, and hospitals (108–112).

Surveys of hospitals across the country report that the highest percentage of violent acts generally occurs in the emergency department (up to 43%), followed by psychiatric units (up to 41%) (110,111). They also found that general medical or surgical floors in hospitals have the fastest rising rate of violent incidences among all areas (110,112).

In emergency departments throughout the country, murders and hostage situations are reported on a regular basis (111). The high incidence of weapon carrying may be largely responsible for this. Studies report that approximately 8% to 15% of patients admitted to various emergency health care settings were carrying a lethal weapon (108,109).

In mental health care settings and general hospital medical or surgical units, violent acts are typically a result of psychiatric illness, substance abuse, disputes over hospital rules or pain management, and other social and family stress issues (109–111).

The underlying cause of violence in the health care setting is multifactorial. Social factors similar to those responsible for the general increase in societal crime contribute largely to the problem (110–112). More unique to the health care environment is that patients, families, and community members are usually experiencing a crisis situation, such as illness, injury, or death of a loved one. These situations foster feelings of desperation and loss of control, which lead to increased levels of stress and emotional instability. These factors may combine to provide an atmosphere that is more conducive to crime and violence.

PREVENTION AND CONTROL STRATEGIES

Aside from efforts to reduce overall crime in society, specific guidelines for crime and violence prevention in hospitals and other health care facilities must be followed if the problem is to be alleviated. Health care institutions must incorporate a comprehensive safety and security program that operates in cooperation with all employees and local law enforcement agencies. Elements of an effective program include administrative, engineering, and work practice controls as outlined:

Administrative controls:

- Provide ample well-trained security staff.
- Have a security program for visitors entering the facility (e.g., entrance with visitor passes only).
- Develop comprehensive, written emergency action plan for employees and provide mandatory in-service training.
- Provide special personal safety education training for community health employees going out into the field.
- Maintain relations with local police department for development and updating of emergency procedures and programs.

Engineering controls:

- Provide alarm systems and panic buttons easily accessible to employees in cases of emergency situations.
- Equip long hallways and concealed or high-risk areas with closed-circuit television monitors and curved mirrors for surveillance purposes.
- Install metal detection devices in emergency departments for identification of weapons on individuals entering the premises.
- Install bulletproof glass barriers in admitting, triage, and other high-risk public access areas.
- Provide separate, locked areas for employee restrooms and lounges, not accessible to the general public.
- Provide well-lighted, guarded staff and visitor parking areas.
- Limit public access to patient care areas—especially newborn maternity wards (e.g., no back elevator or stairway access to public).
- Offer handheld alarms and protection devices (e.g., pepper spray) to community health care workers out in the field.

Work practice controls:

- Wear nonprovocative, nondangerous clothing and jewelry.
- Carry narcotic and other keys well concealed but easily accessible.
- Notify other staff members of whereabouts at all times when leaving the work area.
- Do not enter parking lots and garages unattended, especially at night.
- Maintain constant awareness of surroundings and of emergency procedures for that area; keep up-to-date on all safety education and training; and instruct community health workers never to enter areas where they feel unsafe or threatened.

REFERENCES

1. Leslie GB. The toxicologic importance of formaldehyde and glutaraldehyde in the hospital environment. *Indoor Built Environ* 1996;5:132–137.
2. National Institute for Occupational Safety and Health. *Formaldehyde: evidence of carcinogenicity.* Current Intelligence Bulletin Number 34, 1981.
3. Camarasa JG. Health personnel. In: *Textbook of contact dermatitis*, 2nd ed. New York: Springer-Verlag, 1995:573–587.
4. American Conference of Governmental Industrial Hygienists. *Justification of the TLVs*. Cincinnati: American Conference of Governmental Industrial Hygienists, 1992.
5. International Agency for Research on Cancer. Wood dust and formaldehyde. *IARC Monogr Eval Carcinog Risks Hum* 1995;62.
6. Occupational Safety and Health Administration. Occupational exposure to formaldehyde. *Federal Register* 1992;57:22290.
7. Russell AD. Glutaraldehyde: current status and uses. *Infect Control Hosp Epidemiol* 1994;15:724–733.
8. Beauchanp RO, St. Clair MBG, Fennell TR, Clarke DO, Morgan KT. A critical review of the toxicology of glutaraldehyde. *Crit Rev Toxicol* 1992;22:143–174.
9. Bardazzi F, Melino M, Alagna G, Veronesi S. Glutaraldehyde dermatitis in nurses. *Contact Dermatitis* 1996;14:319–320.
10. Werley MS, Burleigh-Flayer HD, Ballantyne B. Respiratory peripheral sensory irritation and hypersensitivity studies with glutaraldehyde vapor. *Toxicol Ind Health* 1995;11:489–501.
11. Gannon PFG, Bright P, Campbell M, O'Hickey SP, Burge PS. Occupational asthma due to glutaraldehyde and formaldehyde in endoscopy and x ray departments. *Thorax* 1995;50:156–159.
12. Norback D. Skin and respiratory symptoms from exposure to alkaline glutaraldehyde in medical services. *Scand J Work Environ Health* 1988;14:366–371.
13. Calder IM, Wright LP, Grimstone D. Glutaraldehyde allergy in endoscopy units. *Lancet* 1992;339:433.
14. Leinster P, Baum JM, Baxter PJ. An assessment of exposure to glutaraldehyde in hospitals: typical exposure levels and recommended control measures. *Br J Ind Med* 1993;50:107–111.
15. Hine C, Rowe VK, White ER, Darmer KI, Youngblood GT. Epoxy compounds. In: *Patty's industrial hygiene and toxicology*, vol 2A, 3rd rev ed. New York: John Wiley and Sons, 1981:2141–2258.
16. Snellings WM, Weil CS, Maronpot RR. A two-year inhalation study of the carcinogenic potential of ethylene oxide in Fischer 344 rats. *Toxicol Appl Pharmacol* 1984;75:105–117.
17. Lynch DW, Lewis TR, Moorman WJ, et al. Carcinogenic and toxicologic effects of inhaled ethylene oxide and propylene oxide in F344 rats. *Toxicol Appl Pharmacol* 1984;76:69–84.
18. Hogstedt C, Malmqvist N, Wadman B. Leukemia in workers exposed to ethylene oxide. *JAMA* 1979;241:1132–1133.
19. Hogstedt C, Rohlen O, Berndtsson BS, Axelson O, Ehrenberg L. A cohort study of mortality and cancer incidence in ethylene oxide production workers. *Br J Ind Med* 1979;36:276–280.
20. Shore RE, Gardner MJ, Pannett B. Ethylene oxide: an assessment of the epidemiological evidence on carcinogenicity. *Br J Ind Med* 1993;50:971–997.
21. Verraes S, Michel O. Occupational asthma induced by ethylene oxide. *Lancet* 1995;346:1434–1435.
22. International Agency for Research on Cancer (IARC) working group on the evaluation of carcinogenic risks to humans: some industrial chemicals. Lyon, France: Feb. 15–22, 1994. *IARC Monogr Eval Carcinog Risks Hum* 1994;60:1–560.
23. Occupational Safety and Health Administration. OSHA ethylene oxide standard. *Federal Register* 1984;49:25734.
24. Rutala WA. Disinfection and sterilization of patient-care items. *Infect Control Hosp Epidemiol* 1996;17:377–384.
25. Rutala WA. Association for Professionals in Infection Control and Epidemiology (APIC) guideline for selection and use of disinfectants. *Am J Infect Control* 1996;24:313–342.
26. Ponder RD, Wray BB. A case report: sensitivity to benzalkonium chloride. *J Asthma* 1993;30:229–231.
27. Graf P, Hallen H. Effect on the nasal mucosa of long-term treatment with oxymetazoline, benzalkonium chloride and placebo nasal sprays. *Laryngoscope* 1996;106:605–609.
28. Bratt PM, Ainge G, Bowles JAK, et al. The lack of effect of benzalkonium chloride on the cilia of the nasal mucosa in patients with perennial allergic rhinitis: combined functional, light, scanning and transmission electron microscopy study. *Clin Exp Allergy* 1995;25:957–965.
29. Burge PS, Richardson MN. Occupational asthma due to indirect exposure to lauryl dimethyl benzyl ammonium chloride used in a floor cleaner. *Thorax* 1994;49:842–843.
30. McDevitt JJ, Lees PSJ, McDiarmid MA. Exposure of hospital pharmacists and nurses to antineoplastic agents. *J Occup Med* 1993;35:57–60.
31. Ensslin AS, Stoll Y, Pethran A, Pfaller A, Rommelt H, Fruhmann G. Biological monitoring of cyclophosphamide and ifosfamide in urine of hospital personnel occupationally exposed to cytostatic drugs. *Occup Environ Med* 1994;51:229–233.
32. Falck K, Grohn P, Sorsa M, Vainio H, Heinonen E, Holsti L. Mutagenicity in urine of nurses handling cytostatic drugs. *Lancet* 1979;1:1250–1251.
33. Oestreicher U, Stephan G, Glatzel M. Chromosome and SCE analysis in peripheral lymphocytes of persons occupationally exposed to cytostatic drugs handled with and without use of safety covers. *Mutat Res* 1990;242:271–277.
34. Levin L, Holly E, Seward J. Bladder cancer in a 39-year-old female pharmacist. *J Natl Cancer Inst* 1993;85:1089–1091.
35. Gavriele P, Airoldi M, Succo G, Brando V, Ruo Redda MG. Undifferentiated nasopharyngeal-type carcinoma in a nurse handling cytostatic agents. *Eur J Cancer B Oral Oncol* 1993;29B:153.
36. Occupational Safety and Health Administration, Office of Occupational Medicine. *Work practice guidelines for personnel dealing with cytotoxic (antineoplastic) drugs*. Washington: US Department of Labor, 1986. [OSHA instruction publication 8-1.1].
37. Valanis B, Vollmer WM, Labuhn K, Glass A, Corelle C. Antineoplastic drug handling protection after OSHA guidelines. *J Occup Med* 1992;34:149–155.

38. Valanis B, Driscoll K, McNeil V. Comparison of antineoplastic drug handling policies of hospitals with OSHA guidelines: a pilot study. *Am J Public Health* 1990;80:480–481.
39. Mader RM, Rizovski B, Steger GG Moser K, Rainer H, Dittrich C. Permeability of latex membranes to anti-cancer drugs. *Int J Pharm* 1991;68:151–156.
40. Cooke J, Williams J, Morgan R, Cooke P, Calvert R. Use of cytogenetic methods to determine mutagenic changes in the blood of pharmacy personnel and nurses who handle cytotoxic agents. *Am J Hosp Pharm* 1991;48:1199–1205.
41. Leinster P, Baum JM, Baxter PJ. An assessment of exposure to glutaraldehyde in hospitals: typical exposure levels and recommended control measures. *Br J Ind Med* 1993;50:107–111.
42. American Society of Hospital Pharmacists. ASHP technical assistance bulletin on handling cytotoxic and hazardous drugs. *Am J Hosp Pharm* 1990;47:1033–1049.
43. Anonymous. Controlling occupational exposure to hazardous drugs. In: *Occupational Safety and Health Administration (OSHA) technical manual*. Washington: US Department of Labor, 1995:V:1-1–V:3-24. [OSHA instruction TED 1.15].
44. Cohen EN. *Anesthesia exposure in the workplace*. Littleton, MA: PSG Publishing, 1980.
45. American Society of Anesthesiologists. Occupational disease among operating room personnel: a national study. Report of an ad hoc committee on the effects of operating room personnel. *Anesthesiology* 1974;41:321–340.
46. Brodsky JB, Cohen EN, Brown BW, Wu ML, Whitcher CE. Exposure to nitrous oxide and neurologic disease among dental professionals. *Anesth Analg* 1981;60:297–301.
47. Bruce DL, Bach MJ. Effects of trace anesthetic gases on behavioral performance of volunteers. *Br J Anesth* 1976;48:871–876.
48. National Institute for Occupational Safety and Health. *Criteria for a recommended standard—occupational exposure to waste anesthetic gases and vapors*. Springfield, VA: National Technical Information Service, 1977.
49. Sass-Kortsak AM, Wheeler IP, Purdham JT. Exposure of operating room personnel to anesthetic agents: an examination of the effectiveness of scavenging systems and the importance of maintenance programs. *Can Anaesth Soc J* 1981;28:22–28.
50. Berner O. Concentration and elimination of anesthetic gases in operating theaters: influence of anesthesia apparatus leakages. *Acta Anaesth Scand* 1978;22:46–54.
51. Schuyt HC, Verberk MM. Measurement and reduction of nitrous oxide in operating rooms. *J Occup Environ Med* 1996;38:1036–1040.
52. Rietschel RL, Fowler JF. Contact dermatitis in health personnel. In: *Fisher's contact dermatitis*, 4th ed. Baltimore: Williams & Wilkins, 1995:590–608.
53. Slater, JE, Mostello LA, Shaer C, Honsinger RW. Type I hypersensitivity to rubber. *Ann Allergy* 1990;65:411–414.
54. Sussman GL, Beezhold DH. Allergy to latex rubber. *Ann Int Med* 1995;122:43–46.
55. American College of Allergy, Asthma and Immunology. Position statement: latex allergy—an emerging healthcare problem. *Ann Allergy Asthma Immunol* 1995;75:19–21.
56. Charous BL. The puzzle of latex allergy: some answers, still more questions. *Ann Allergy* 1994;73:277–284.
57. Robbins J. Rubber gloves: peril for some. *The New York Times* 1997 Jan 29:B10.
58. Jaeger D, Kleinhans D, Czuppon AB, Baur X. Latex-specific proteins causing immediate-type cutaneous, nasal, bronchial, and systemic reactions. *J Allergy Clin Immunol* 1992;89:759–768.
59. Swanson MC, Bubak ME, Hunt LW, Yunginger JW, Warner MA, Reed CE. Quantification of occupational latex aeroallergens in a medical center. *J Allergy Clin Immunol* 1994;94:445–451.
60. Lynch T. *Communicable disease nursing*. St. Louis: Mosby, 1949.
61. Department of Labor, Occupational Safety and Health Administration. Occupational exposure to bloodborne pathogens, final rule. *Federal Register* 1991;56:64175–64182.
62. Wells WF. *Aerodynamics of droplet nuclei*. Cambridge, MA: Harvard University Press, 1955.
63. Louden RG, Roberts RM. Droplet expulsion from the respiratory tract. *Am Rev Respir Dis* 1967;95:435–442.
64. Centers for Disease Control and Prevention. Updated guidelines for preventing transmission of tuberculosis in health care settings with special emphasis on HIV-related issues. Draft no 5, 15 Jan 1993.
65. Riley RL, O'Grady F. *Airborne infection—transmission and control*. New York: Macmillan Press, 1961.
66. US Department of Labor, Occupational Safety and Health Administration. Draft guidelines for preventing the transmission of tuberculosis in health care facilities, 2nd ed: notice of comment period. *Federal Register* October 1993;58:52809–52854.
66a. Centers for Disease Control and Prevention. Essential components of a tuberculosis prevention and control program. Screening for tuberculosis and tuberculosis infection in high-risk populations. *MMWR Morb Mortal Wkly Rep* 1995;44:1–16.
67. Jarvis WR, Bolyard EA, Bozzi CJ. Respirators, recommendations, and regulations: the controversy surrounding protection of health care workers from tuberculosis. *Ann Intern Med* 1995;122:142–146.
67a. Centers for Disease Control and Prevention. Targeted tuberculin testing and treatment of latent tuberculosis infection. *MMWR Morb Mortal Wkly Rep* 2000;49:1–54.
68. Garner J. The Hospital Infection Control Practices Advisory Committee: guideline for isolation precautions in hospitals. *Infect Control Hosp Epidemiol* 1996;17(1):53–79.
69. Lynch P, Jackson MM, Cummings MJ, Stamm WE. Rethinking the role of isolation practices in the prevention of nosocomial infections. *Ann Intern Med* 1987;107:243–246.
70. Jagger, J. Introduction. In: Charney W, ed. *Essentials of modern hospital safety*, vol 3. Boca Raton, FL: CRC Press, 1994:vii–xi.
71. Centers for Disease Control and Prevention. Public Health Service statement of occupational exposure to human immunodeficiency virus, including considerations regarding zidovudine postexposure use. *MMWR Mortal Morb Wkly Rep* 1990;39:1–14.
72. Marcus R. CDC Cooperative Needlestick Surveillance Group: surveillance of health care workers exposed to blood from patients infected with the human immunodeficiency virus. *N Engl J Med* 1988;319:1118–1123.
73. Jagger J, Hunt E, Pearson RD. Estimated cost of needlestick injuries for six major needled devices. *Infect Control Hosp Epidemiol* 1990;11:584–588.
73a. Centers for Disease Control and Prevention. Public health service guidelines for the management of health-care worker exposures to HIV and recommendations for postexposure prophylaxis. *MMWR Morb Mortal Wkly Rep* 1998;47:1–28.
73b. Centers for Disease Control and Prevention. Serious adverse events attributed to nevirapine regimens for postexposure prophylaxis after HIV exposures—worldwide, 1997–2000. *MMWR Morb Mortal Wkly Rep* 2001;49:1153–1156.
74. Barnes EC. Ionizing radiation. In: *The industrial environment—its evaluation and control*. Washington: US Department of Health, Education, and Welfare, 1973.
75. Moeller DW. History and perspective on the development of radiation protection standards. In: Sinclair WK, ed. *Radiation protection today: the NCRP at sixty years*. Bethesda, MD: National Council on Radiation Protection and Measurements, 1990.
76. International Commission on Radiological Protection. *1990 recommendations of the ICRP (ICRP publication no. 60)*. Elmsford, NY: Pergamon Press, 1991.
77. *1987 NCRP recommendations on limits for exposure to ionizing radiation (report no. 91)*. Bethesda, MD: National Council on Radiation Protection, 1987.
78. Beir V. *Biological Effects of Ionizing Radiation Committee: health effects of exposures to low levels of ionizing radiation*. New York: National Academy Press, 1990.
79. Seeram E. *Radiation protection*. Philadelphia: Lippincott–Raven, 1997.
80. Joint Commission on Accreditation of Healthcare Organizations. *The Joint Commission 1995 accreditation manual for hospitals*, vol 1. Oakbrook Terrace, IL: Joint Commission on Accreditation of Healthcare Organizations, 1994.
81. Cust G, Pearson JCG, Mair A. The prevalence of low back pain in nurses. *Int Nursing Rev* 1972;19:169–179.
82. Harper P, Billet E, Gutowski M, SooHoo K, Lew M, Roman A. Occupational low-back pain in hospital nurses. *J Occup Med* 1984;27:518–524.
83. Owen BD, Damron C. Personal characteristics and back injury among hospital nursing personnel. *Res Nurs Health* 1984;7:305–313.
84. Jensen RC. Low back pain and back injury among health care workers. In: *American Conference of Governmental Industrial Hygienists. Occupational hazards to health care workers*. Cincinnati: American Conference of Governmental Industrial Hygienists; 1987:41–50.
85. Jensen RC. How to use workers' compensation data to identify high risk groups. In: Slote L, ed. *Handbook of occupational safety and health*. New York: John Wiley and Sons, 1987:364–403.
86. National Institute for Occupation Safety and Health. *Proposed national strategies for the prevention of leading work-related disease and injuries, part 1*. Washington: Association of Schools of Public Health, 1986.
87. Klein BP, Jensen RC, Sanderson LM. Assessment of workers compensation claims for back strains/sprains. *J Occup Med* 1984;26:443–448.
88. US Congress, Office of Technology Assessment. *Preventing illness and injury in the workplace*. Washington: Office of Technology Assessment, 1994. [OTA-H-256].
89. Pheasant S. *Ergonomics, work and health*. Gaithersburg, MD: Aspen Publishers, 1991.
90. Garg A, Owen BD. Reducing back stress to nursing personnel: an ergonomic intervention in a nursing home. *Ergonomics* 1992;35:1353–1375.
91. Anonymous. *Laser safety training manual*, 6th ed. Cincinnati: Rockwell Associates, 1984.
92. Anonymous. *Laser safety guide*. Toledo, OH: Laser Institute of America, 1992.
93. Rockwell RJ Jr. Controlling laser hazards. *Laser Applic* 1986;Sept:93–99.
94. American National Standards Institute. *Safe use of lasers in health care facilities*. New York: American National Standards Institute, 1996.
95. Mellor EF. Shiftwork and flextime: how prevalent are they? *Monthly Labor Rev* 1986;109:14–21.
96. Adams C. *Report of the hospital nursing personnel surveys*. Chicago: American Hospital Association, 1989.
97. US Congress, Office of Technology Assessment. *Biological rhythms: implications for the worker*. Washington: US Government Printing Office, 1991. [OTA-BA-463].
98. Torii S, Okudaira N, Fukuda H, et al. Effects of night shift on sleep patterns of nurses. *J Hum Ergol Suppl* 1982;11:233–244.
99. Fossey E. Shiftwork can seriously damage your health! *Prof Nurse* 1990; June:476–480.
100. Tasto DL, Colligan MJ, Skjei EW, Polly SJ. Health consequences of shiftwork. Cincinnati: National Institute of Occupational Safety and Health, 1978.
101. Leighton K, Livingston M. Fatigue in doctors. *Lancet* 1983;1:1280.
102. Monk TH. Shiftworker performance. *Occup Med* 1990;5:193–198.
103. Coffey LC, Skipper JK, Jung FD. Nurses and shiftwork: effects on job performance and job related stress. *J Adv Nurs* 1988;13:245–254.

104. Vener KJ, Szabo S, Moore JG. The effect of shiftwork on gastrointestinal function: a review. *Chronobiologia* 1989;16:421–449.
105. Segawa K, Nakazawa S, Tsukamato Y, et al. Peptic ulcer is prevalent among shiftworkers. *Dig Dis Sci* 1987;32:449–453.
106. Akerstsdt T, Knutsson A, Alfredsson L, Theorell T. Shiftwork and cardiovascular disease. *Scand J Work Environ Health* 1984;10:409–414.
107. Knutsson A, Akerstedt T, Jonsson BG, Osth-Gomer K. Increased risk of ischemic heart disease in shiftworkers. *Lancet* 1986;12:89–92.
108. Anderson AA, Ghali AY, Bansil RK. Weapon carrying among patients in a psychiatric emergency room. *Hosp Community Psychiatry* 1989;40:845–847.
109. Goetz RR, Bloom JD, Chenell SL, Moorehead JC. Weapons possession by patients in a university emergency department. *Ann Emerg Med* 1991;20:8–10.
110. Worthington K. Taking action against violence in the workplace. *Am Nurse* 1993;25:12–13.
111. Keep N, Gilbert, P. California Emergency Nurses Association's informal survey of violence in California emergency departments. *J Emerg Nurs* 1992;18:433–439.
112. U.S. Department of Labor, Bureau of Labor Statistics. *Occupational injuries and illnesses in the United States by industry (Bulletin 2379)*. Washington: US Department of Labor, 1991.

CHAPTER 48

Construction Industry Hazards

Laura S. Welch

Construction workers build, repair, renovate, modify, and demolish structures, including houses, office buildings, temples, factories, hospitals, roads, bridges, tunnels, stadiums, docks, airports, and more. In industrialized nations, construction is consistently ranked among the most dangerous occupations. Among industrial sectors in the United States, the death rate from work-related traumatic injuries in construction is exceeded only by such rates for mining or for agriculture, forestry, and fishing (1,2).

Occupational diseases are also an important cause of morbidity in construction workers (3,4). Table 48-1 summarizes the sentinel health events that may occur in construction workers, and what exposures can lead to these diseases. The sentinel health events list was developed to identify diseases that, if they occur, point to an opportunity for intervention and prevention of future cases. These diseases do not represent an exhaustive list of occupational disease in construction, but do illustrate the extent of the possible problem.

Estimates for the cost of injuries in construction in the United States range from $10 billion to $40 billion annually (5); at $20 billion, the cost per construction worker is $3,500 yearly. One cost indicator, worker's compensation premiums for three trades—carpenters, masons, and structural iron workers—averaged 28.6% of payroll nationally in mid-1994 (1). In addition to worker's compensation, liability insurance premiums and other indirect costs exist, including reduced work crew efficiency, clean-up (e.g., from a cave-in or collapse), or overtime necessitated by an injury; these indirect costs can exceed the worker's compensation claim for an injury by several multiples (6,7).

Construction often must be done in extreme heat or cold, in windy, rainy, snowy, or foggy weather, or at night. On-again, off-again work adds to the health risks, including the emotional toll of uncertainty about getting another job (8). In the United States, where no universal health insurance exists, intermittent employment and the high cost of health insurance mean that many con-

TABLE 48-1. Sentinel health events in construction

Condition	Industry/process/occupation	Agent
Asbestosis	Asbestos industries and utilizers	Asbestos
Bronchitis (acute), pneumonitis, and pulmonary edema caused by fumes and vapors	Arc welders, boilermakers	Nitrogen oxides, vanadium pentoxide
Chronic or acute renal failure	Plumbers	Inorganic lead
Contact and allergic dermatitis	Cement masons and finishers, carpenters, floor layers	Adhesives and sealants, irritants (e.g., cutting oils, phenol, solvents, acids, alkalis, detergents); allergens (e.g., nickel, chromates, formaldehyde, dyes, rubber products)
Extrinsic asthma	Woodworkers, furniture makers	Red cedar (plicatic acid) and other wood dusts
Histoplasmosis	Bridge maintenance workers	Histoplasma capsulatum
Inflammatory and toxic neuropathy	Furniture refinishers, degreasing operations	Hexane
Malignant neoplasm of scrotum	Chimney sweeps	Mineral oil, pitch, tar
Malignant neoplasm of nasal cavities	Woodworkers, cabinet and furniture makers, carpenters	Hardwood and softwood dusts, chlorophenols
Malignant neoplasm of trachea, bronchus, and lung	Asbestos industries and utilizers	Asbestos
Malignant neoplasm of nasopharynx	Carpenter, cabinetmaker	Chlorophenols
Malignant neoplasm of larynx	Asbestos industries and utilizers	Asbestos
Mesothelioma (malignancy of peritoneum and pleura)	Asbestos industries and utilizers	Asbestos
Noise effects on inner ear	Occupations with exposure to excessive noise	Excessive noise
Raynaud's phenomenon (secondary)	Jackhammer operator, riveter	Whole body or segmental vibration
Sequoiosis	Red cedar mill workers, woodworkers	Redwood sawdust
Silicosis	Sandblasters	Silica
Silicotuberculosis	Sandblasters	Silica and mycobacterium tuberculosis
Toxic encephalitis	Lead paint removal	Lead
Toxic hepatitis	Fumigators	Methyl bromide

Note: Lead exposure occurs in at least 23 construction-related industrial/occupational groups, including painting, contractors, bridge and highway construction, and demolition work. Extremely high levels of lead exposure have been documented for workers in these groups.
Reprinted from Sullivan P, Moon Bank K, Hearl F, Wagner G. Respiratory risk in the construction industry. In: Ringen K, Englund A, Welch LS, Weeks JL, Seegal J, eds. Health and safety in construction. *Occup Med* 1995;10(2):335–352, with permission.

struction workers and their families do not have health care coverage. Even when construction workers do work the 30 or 60 days needed to qualify for insurance coverage on a job—if coverage is available—they often cannot afford to maintain coverage from the time that job ends until they are eligible for coverage on another project. For workers who do have health care coverage, episodic employment, frequent changes of employer, and continuous changes in work site exposures and ambient conditions limit the clinician's or the researcher's ability to trace the individual's work history or exposures to hazards. Because of these factors, many of which are unique to construction, limited data exist on the extent or effect of toxic exposures in the construction industry. This chapter summarizes available data on toxic exposures, musculoskeletal disorders, and occupational lung disease in construction.

HAZARDOUS MATERIALS IN CONSTRUCTION

Construction workers use a wide range of materials, some of which are considered hazardous (4,9,10). Table 48-2 outlines the carcinogens that may be found on construction sites (11–13), and Table 48-3 shows the extent of sensitizing agents in the industry (14–16). Due to such hazards, medical surveillance of some workers may be necessary (17).

Lead exposure and lead toxicity are particularly important problems in the construction industry (17–31). The Occupational Safety and Health Administration (OSHA) estimates that nearly 1 million U.S. construction workers are exposed to lead on the job (32). Most (78%) of these workers are involved in commercial or residential remodeling and potentially are exposed to lead-based paint. In 1992, the National Institute for Occupational Safety and Health (NIOSH) reported on blood-lead levels in construction workers at eight bridge projects; their lead levels ranged from 51 to 160 mg per dL whole blood, and 26 (62%) workers with these blood-lead elevations worked in a containment structure (18). Increased lead testing of small children specified under the 1991 Centers for Disease Control and Prevention guidelines for the prevention of childhood lead poisoning has resulted in increased residential lead abatement activity and, thus, more potential risk of exposure to lead among workers and members of workers' households (33). The 1991 guidelines were updated in 1997 (33a) and can be found at www.cdc.gov/nceh/lead/guide/guide97.html.

In 1991, OSHA and NIOSH jointly issued recommendations intended to prevent lead exposure in construction (34). The document recommended using engineering controls, appropriate work practices, personal protective equipment (including respirators), and evaluation of the effectiveness of these measures by air and blood-lead monitoring. In 1992, NIOSH published an alert for preventing lead poisoning in construction workers (23). This publication identified high-risk activities associated with lead dust and fumes among bridge and structural steel workers: abrasive blasting, sanding, burning, cutting or welding on steel structures coated with lead paint, and the use of containment enclosures at these sites that could result in higher lead concentration.

Now, with the introduction of Title X with specifications for lead abatement, and the OSHA standard for lead in construction, the construction workforce and industry are undergoing major changes in the way work is performed and how employees are being protected from lead exposure. If lead is in the workplace, there must be strict adherence to the prevention, control, and monitoring principles of the OSHA standard. Continued surveillance for elevated blood-lead levels is crucial in assessing the overall condition and health of the construction workforce.

TABLE 48-2. Carcinogens relevant to construction

Substance	Uses or where encountered
C1: Established human carcinogens	
Beechwood dust	Joinery, circular saw on building sites
Benzene	Gasoline
Nickel compounds	Welding electrode
Oak wood dust	Joinery, circular saw on building sites
Tar, pitch	Road works
Zinc chromates	Old coatings
C2: Probable human carcinogens	
Benzo(a)pyrene	Road works, diesel engine emission, chimney sweeping
Cadmium compounds	Old coatings
Chromium (VI) compounds	Wood protection
Diesel engine emissions	Diesel engines
Hydrazine	Water treatment
C3: Suspected human carcinogens	
Dichloromethane	Stripper, solvent
Diphenylmethane-4,4'diisocyanate	Polyurethane
Formaldehyde	Conservation of dispersion products
Lead chromate	Old coatings
Wood dust (besides beechwood and oak wood dust)	Joinery, circular saw on building sites

Reprinted from Ruhl R, Kluger N. Hazardous materials in construction. In: Ringen K, Englund A, Welch LS, Weeks JL, Seegal J, eds. Health and safety in construction. *Occup Med* 1995;10(2):335–352, with permission.

TABLE 48-3. Areas of use of transdermal and sensitizing materials in construction

Substance	Transdermal (T) or sensitizing (S)	Areas of use
Benzene	T	Gasoline
Carbon tetrachloride	S	Solvent
Diphenylmethane-4,4'diisocyanate	S	Polyurethane
2-Ethoxyethanol	T	Solvent
Ethylbenzene	T	Solvent
Formaldehyde	S	Cleaning, disinfection
Hexamethylene diisocyanate	S	Polyurethane
Hydrazine	T,S	Water treatment
Isophorone diisocyanate	S	Polyurethane
Methanol	T	Solvent
2-Methoxyethanol	T	Solvent
Methyl methacrylate	S	Coating
Nickel	S	Welding electrode
Oil of turpentine	S	Solvent
Phenol	T	Solvent
Tin compounds	T	Wood protection
Toluene diisocyanate	S	Polyurethane
Wood dust	S	Joinery
Xylene	T	Solvent

Reprinted from Ruhl R, Kluger N. Hazardous materials in construction. In: Ringen K, Englund A, Welch LS, Weeks JL, Seegal J, eds. Health and safety in construction. *Occup Med* 1995;10(2):335–352, with permission.

WORK-RELATED MUSCULOSKELETAL DISORDERS

Construction workers have a high prevalence of musculoskeletal complaints described as pain, ache, and discomfort (35–61). In a Swedish study, early retirements resulting from these disorders were more common among construction workers than

TABLE 48-4. Key disorders and documented associated work postures, psychosocial factors, or trades

Disorder	Work posture, psychosocial factor, or trade
(Excess of) musculoskeletal problems	Carpenters, bricklayers, concrete workers, plumbers, machine and crane operators
Neck symptoms	Crane operators, electricians, insulators, painters, machine operators
Neck, shoulder symptoms	Machine operators, carpenters
Neck, shoulder pain	Using handheld machines, hands above shoulder level, reported high psychological stress
Shoulder symptoms	Using vibrating tools
Shoulder symptoms	Scaffolding erectors, insulators, painters, crane operators
Shoulder tendinitis	Rock blaster
Radiographic acromioclavicular joint osteoarthritis	Bricklayers, rock blasters
Acromioclavicular joint osteoarthritis	Heavy manual work, vibration exposure
Hand or wrist	Electricians, insulators, scaffolding erectors, sheet metal workers
Elbow and wrist osteoarthritis	Using pneumatic, percussive tools (chipping hammers, scalers)
Nerve entrapment of median nerve (carpal tunnel syndrome)	Repetitive, forceful work
Disk degeneration	Heavy manual work
Herniated disk	All construction
Herniated lumbar disk	Heavy manual work, motor vehicle drivers
Lower back pain	Using handheld machines
	Stooping
	Kneeling
	Reported high psychological stress
	High demand and low resources
Nonspecific lower back pain	Concrete workers (prefabricated)
	Roofers, carpet and floor layers, scaffolding erectors
Nonspecific lower back pain	Machine operators, carpenters
Sciatica	Concrete reinforcement workers
Hip (coxarthrosis)	Heavy manual work
Knee, hip osteoarthritis	All construction
Knee osteoarthritis	Heavy manual work
Radiologic knee osteoarthritis	Heavy shipyard industry (laborers)
Knee symptoms	Carpet and floor layers, plumbers, roofers
Thickening of prepatellar or superficial infrapatellar bursa	Carpet and floor layers
Bursitis (front of knee)	Carpet and floor layers

Reprinted from Holmstrom E, Moritz U, Engholm G. Musculoskeletal disorders in construction workers. In: Ringen K, Englund A, Welch LS, Weeks JL, Seegal J, eds. Health and safety in construction. *Occup Med* 1995;10(2):335–352, with permission.

other workers. During 1988 to 1989, 72% of all sick leaves in the construction industry in Sweden lasting more than 4 weeks were because of musculoskeletal disorders (35).

Epidemiologic studies on musculoskeletal disorders in construction workers are summarized in Table 48-4. Interview surveys conducted in Finland and Sweden studied the relationship between work and musculoskeletal disorders in construction workers. Carpenters, bricklayers, concrete workers, plumbers, and machine and crane operators had a significantly increased standardized morbidity ratio for musculoskeletal diseases. In Finland, neck and shoulder symptoms, lumbago, nonspecific lower back pain, and sciatica were more prevalent among machine operators and carpenters than sedentary workers (36,57), indicating that construction work is a risk factor.

Finnish investigations comparing machine operators and carpenters showed that machine operators have an increased age-adjusted relative risk for more persistent neck symptoms (43). Surveys found that shoulder symptoms occurred most frequently among scaffolding erectors, insulators, and painters (42,44,45). In another study, hand and wrist symptoms were experienced frequently by approximately one-half of a group of electricians (40).

Several studies summarized in Table 48-4 looked at the occurrence of specific medical disorders of the knee, back, and shoulders (41–53). A Finnish work analysis of carpet and floor laying and painting showed that carpet and floor layers kneeled, on average, 42% of the time in the observed work tasks. Among painters, kneeling was rare (57). One clinically verified knee disorder, bursitis in the front of the knee, was more frequent among carpet and floor layers than painters (58,59), suggesting kneeling and squatting as contributory factors. Ultrasonography showed thickening of the prepatellar or superficial infrapatellar bursa in 49% of the carpet and floor layers and in 7% of the painters (60). In addition, radiographic changes of the patella were more common among carpet and floor layers than among painters.

A study of bricklayers and rock blasters found that physical workload contributed to the development of radiographic osteoarthritis of the acromioclavicular joint, and exposure to vibration contributed to the development of shoulder tendinitis (39). Construction workers also have an increased relative risk for herniated disk, with an odds ratio of 2.4, compared to office workers (51). A clear association between severe lower back disorders, such as sciatica and herniated disk, and heavy work was proven in prospective studies in which heavy work was defined as construction work of some kind (46,51), whereas an association between nonspecific back pain and work load is less well established in construction workers (46,51,52).

OCCUPATIONAL LUNG DISEASES

Construction workers are exposed to a variety of hazardous agents that may pose risks to the respiratory system, including asbestos, silica, dust, synthetic vitreous fibers, cadmium, chromates, formaldehyde, resin adhesives, cobalt, metal fumes, creosote, gasoline, oils, diesel fumes, paint fumes and dusts, pitch, sealers, solvents, wood dusts and wood preser-

TABLE 48-5. Construction exposures identified by Occupational Safety and Health Administration as potentially resulting in respiratory effects

Lung cancer
Arsenic, inorganic (measured as arsenic)
Asbestos
Beryllium
Chromic acid and chromates
Coal tar pitch volatiles
Formaldehyde
Zinc chromates
Nonmalignant respiratory effects
Aluminum (pyrophoric powders)
Asphalt fumes
Bismuth telluride (selenium-doped)
Carbon black
Chlorine dioxide
Chromium (II) compounds (as chromium)
Chromium metal (as chromium)
Coal dust
Cotton dust
Dicyclohexyl methane-4,4-diisocyanate
Ethyl acrylate
Ferrovanadium dust
Fibrous glass
Grain dust (oat, wheat, barley)
Graphite, natural, respirable <1% quartz
Indium and compounds
Iron oxide (dust and fumes)
Mica, respirable dust containing <1% quartz
Mineral wool fiber
Nickel (soluble compounds)
Nitrogen oxide
Oxygen difluoride
Ozone
Paraquat, respirable dust
Silica
Soapstone
Sulfur dioxide
Sulfur tetrafluoride
Talc (containing no asbestos)
Tin oxide
Trimellitic anhydride
Wood dust
Yttrium

Reprinted from Sullivan P, Moon Bank K, Hearl F, Wagner G. Respiratory risk in the construction industry. In: Ringen K, Englund A, Welch LS, Weeks JL, Seegal J, eds. Health and safety in construction. *Occup Med* 1995;10(2):335–352, with permission.

vatives, and excessive cold. In 1992, as part of an update of exiting standards, OSHA identified agents for which exposure represented a risk for malignant or nonmalignant respiratory disease, as shown in Table 48-5. Table 48-6 lists the substances for which proposed limits are based on avoidance of respiratory effects.

Mortality

Since 1968, the National Center for Health Statistics has prepared data listing underlying and contributing causes of death (62). Industry and usual occupation codings on death certificates were reported by 25 states in 1985 to 1990. In this subset of all U.S. death certificates, there was a total of 286 deaths with asbestosis among decedents aged 15 and over with industry and occupation coding indicating construction work. Construction worker deaths from lung cancer, coal workers' pneumoconiosis, silicosis, malignant neoplasms of the pleura, and malignant neoplasms of the peritoneum are identified as being in excess (63).

Lung Cancer

Studies from several countries, using a variety of designs, have documented an increased risk of lung cancer among general construction workers (64–69), even after controlling for smoking (64,70–72). Painters and plasterers appear to be at increased risk of lung cancer (68,69,71–77). One factor may be cadmium, used as a pigment in paint. NIOSH has documented excess risk of lung cancer associated with cadmium exposure (78) and identified the construction industry as one area in which OSHA standards are needed to better protect workers. High potential for exposure may occur during unventilated renovation work. In addition, painters and plasterers may be exposed to acetone, acids, alkalis, benzene, chlorinated hydrocarbons, chromates, drying agents, paint strippers, oil base and resin paints, pigments, silica, solvents, thinners, and turpentine, as well as asbestos from spackling compounds and building restoration (68,74,76).

Selikoff and Seidman examined 4,951 deaths occurring from 1967 to 1986 among 17,800 male asbestos insulation workers in the United States and Canada and documented a statistically significant increase in lung cancer mortality (standardized mortality ratio of 375) (79). Finkelstein also documented increased risk of lung cancer among insulators (80). Sheet metal workers, who may be exposed to asbestos when working near insulators, are at increased risk of lung cancer (72,81). Structural metal workers also experience increased lung cancer risk (74,77).

Construction welders may be exposed to filler metals containing cadmium, fluxes containing fluorine compounds, and metal fumes including nickel and chromium. Several studies have found increased risk of lung cancer among welders in a variety of work settings (69,71,74,76,82).

Increased risk of lung cancer has been observed among stone masons, bricklayers, and tile setters (70,72,83). Masons, bricklayers, and cement finishers may be exposed to cobalt, epoxy resins, pitch, lime, and excessive cold. Masons may also be exposed to lung carcinogens, such as asbestos, silica, nickel, and hexavalent chromium (83). Other construction trades in which increased risk of lung cancer has been observed include electricians (68,74,76), carpenters and woodworkers (77), plumbers and pipe fitters, and roofers and mastic asphalt workers (69,72,76,84–86). Roofers are exposed to volatile materials vaporizing from heated asphalt, including polycyclic aromatic hydrocarbons from coal tar pitch and bitumen fumes (87).

Nasal Cancer

Woodworkers, cabinetmakers, and furniture makers experience excess risk of nasal cancer (88–90). Carpenters and joiners also appear to be at increased risk of developing nasal cancer (89,91). Carpenters and cabinetmakers may be exposed to wood dust, formaldehyde, solvents, toluene, wood preservative, shellac, stains, bleaches, resin and casein glues, oils, polishes, and insulation agents including asbestos. Given the rarity of nasal cancer, the evidence for a relationship between nasal cancer and occupational exposure to wood dust is compelling (90).

Several studies have also found an increased risk of nasal cancer among general construction workers (73,89,90,92–94).

Mesothelioma

Reports of mesothelioma among construction workers come from several countries (95–97). Mesothelioma has been observed among construction workers who worked as insulators (79,98), shipyard construction workers (65,97–99), carpenters, sheet metal workers, construction and maintenance workers, and electricians (65,81,98,100).

TABLE 48-6. Substances for which proposed limits are based on avoidance of respiratory effects

Chemical name	NIOSH recommended exposure limits[a]	OSHA permissible exposure limits[b]	1994–1995 ACGIH threshold limit values[c]	Species	Comments
Aluminum (pyrophoric powders)			5 mg/m^3 TWA		
Asphalt fumes	5 mg/m^3 ceiling (15-min) (total particulate)		5 mg/m^3 TWA		
Bismuth telluride (Se-doped)			5 mg/m^3 TWA	Dogs, rats, rabbits	Granulomatous lesions in lungs seen after 6 mo of exposure
Carbon black	3.5 mg/m^3 TWA; if PAHs are present, 0.1 mg/m^3 TWA	3.5 mg/m^3 TWA	3.5 mg/m^3 TWA		
Chlorine dioxide		0.1 ppm TWA	0.1 ppm TWA, 0.3 ppm STEL		
Chromium (II) compounds (as Cr)	0.5 mg/m^3 TWA	0.5 mg/m^3 TWA	0.5 mg/m^3 TWA		
Chromium (III) compounds (as Cr)	0.5 mg/m^3 TWA	0.5 mg/m^3 TWA	0.5 mg/m^3 TWA		
Chromium metal (as Cr)	0.5 mg/m^3 TWA	1 mg/m^3 TWA	0.5 mg/m^3 TWA		
Coal dust, <5% quartz		2.4 mg/m^3 TWA	2 mg/m^3 TWA	Humans	Calculated estimate of 10% probability of developing pneumoconiosis with fibrosis after 35 years of exposure to coal dust
Coal dust, >5% quartz		10 mg/m^3 % SiO_2+2	0.1 mg/m^3 TWA (as quartz)		
Cotton dust	200:g/m^3 TWA lint-free cotton dust	1 mg/m^3 TWA	0.2 mg/m^3 TWA		
Dicyclohexyl methane-4,4-diisocyanate			0.005 ppm TWA		
Ethyl acrylate		25 ppm TWA, Skin	5 ppm TWA, 15 ppm STEL		
Ferrovanadium dust	1 mg/m^3 TWA, 3 mg/m^3 STEL	1 mg/m^3 TWA, 3 mg/m^3 STEL	1 mg/m^3 TWA		
Fibrous glass	5 mg/m^3 TWA total fibrous glass		10 mg/m^3 TWA		
Grain dust (oat, wheat, barley)			4 mg/m^3 TWA	Humans	Chronic bronchitis, shortness of breath, reduced pulmonary function, increased incidence of respiratory symptoms
Graphite, natural, respirable <1% quartz		15 mppcf TWA	2 mg/m^3 TWA	Humans	Anthracosilicosis, similar to that seen in coal miners
Indium and compounds		0.1 mg/m^3 TWA	0.1 mg/m^3 TWA	Rats	Widespread alveolar edema after exposure to In_2O_2
Iron oxide (dust and fumes)		10 mg/m^3 TWA	5 mg/m^3 TWA		
Mica, respirable dust containing <1% quartz		20 mppcf TWA	3 mg/m^3 TWA	Humans	Signs and symptoms resembling silicosis and pneumoconiosis in 8 of 57 workers
Mineral wool fiber			10 mg/m^3 TWA		
Nickel (soluble compounds)	0.015 mg/m^3 TWA[d] (inorganic compounds)	1 mg/m^3 TWA	0.1 mg/m^3 TWA		
Nitrogen dioxide	1 ppm ceiling (15-min)	5 ppm ceiling	3 ppm TWA, 5 ppm STEL	Humans	Fatal pulmonary edema
Oxygen difluoride		0.05 ppm TWA	0.05 ppm ceiling	Laboratory animals	Lethal to a wide variety of laboratory species, causing pulmonary edema and hemorrhage after several hours of exposure
Ozone		0.1 ppm TWA	0.1 ppm ceiling	Humans, mice	Significant reduction in pulmonary vital capacity; damage to alveolar tissue

Paraquat		0.5 mg/m³ TWA, Skin	0.1 mg/m³ TWA (respirable) 0.5 mg/m³ TWA (total dust)	Humans	69 accidental deaths from pulmonary injury reported through 1972
Silica C amorphous, diatomaceous earth		20 mppcf	10 mg/m³ TWA		
Silica C amorphous, precipitate, and gel			10 mg/m³ TWA		
Silica C crystalline cristobalite	50:g/m³ TWA	250/% SiO_2+5 (as mppcf)	0.05 mg/m³ TWA	Dogs	Cellular infiltration of lung and fibrotic nodules in pulmonary lymph nodes
Silica C crystalline quartz, respirable	50:g/m³ TWA	250/% SiO_2+5 (as mppcf)	0.1 mg/m³ TWA	Humans	Accelerated loss of pulmonary function beyond effects of aging alone
Silica C crystalline tridymite (as respirable quartz dust)	50:g/m³ TWA	250/% SiO_2+5 (as mppcf)	0.05 mg/m³ TWA	Rats	Most active form of free silica when administered by intratracheal injection
Silica C crystalline tripoli (as respirable quartz dust)	50:g/m³ TWA	250/% SiO_2+5 (as mppcf)	0.1 mg/m³ TWA	Laboratory animals	Progressive nodular fibrosis
Silica, fused		250/% SiO_2+5 (as mppcf)	0.1 mg/m³ TWA (respirable dust)		
Soapstone C total dust		20 mppcf TWA	6 mg/m³ TWA		
Soapstone C respirable dust			3 mg/m³ TWA		
Sulfur dioxide	0.5 ppm TWA	5 ppm TWA	2 ppm TWA, 5 ppm STEL	Humans	Accelerated loss of pulmonary function
Sulfur tetrafluoride			0.1 ppm ceiling	Rats 4 h/d/ 10 d	Emphysema, marked clinical signs of respiratory impairment
Talc (containing no asbestos)		20 mppcf TWA	2 mg/m³ TWA (respirable dust)		
Tin oxide			2 mg/m³ TWA		
Trimellitic anhydride			0.04 mg/m³ ceiling	Rats	Intraalveolar hemorrhage (no exposure duration indicated)
Wood dust, hard			1 mg/m³ TWA		
Wood dust, soft			5 mg/m³ TWA 10 mg/m³ STEL		
Yttrium		1 mg/m³ TWA	1 mg/m³ TWA		

ACGIH, American Conference of Government Industrial Hygienists; mppcf, million particles per cubic foot; NIOSH, National Institute for Occupational Safety and Health; OSHA, Occupational Safety and Health Administration; PAH, polyaromatic hydrocarbon; ppm, parts per million; SiO_2, silicon dioxide; STEL, short-term exposure limit; TWA, time-weighted average.

[a]National Institute for Occupational Safety and Health time-weighted average limits are for 10 hour/day, 40 hour/week exposures unless otherwise specified, and its ceilings are peaks not to be exceeded for any period of time unless a duration is specified in parentheses.

[b]Occupational Safety and Health Administration's permissible exposure limits do not currently apply to agriculture; Occupational Safety and Health Administration's time-weighted average limits are for 8-hour exposures; its short-term exposure limits are for 15 minutes, unless otherwise specified, and its ceilings are peaks not to be exceeded for any period of time.

[c]American Conference of Government Industrial Hygienists sets threshold limit values. The threshold limit value–time-weighted average is for an 8-hour exposure; the "ceilings" are peaks not to be exceeded for any period of time during a working shift. These values are updated annually; readers should consult www.acgin.org for the most current values.

[d]National Institute for Occupational Safety and Health considers nickel a potential occupational carcinogen.

Reprinted from Sullivan P, Moon Bank K, Hearl F, Wagner G. Respiratory risk in the construction industry. In: Ringen K, Englund A, Welch LS, Weeks JL, Seegal J, eds. Health and safety in construction. *Occup Med* 1995;10(2):269–284, with permission.

TABLE 48-7. Prevalence rate and rate ratio of self-reported respiratory conditions among 1,785 white male construction workers ages 15 and older

Respiratory condition	Prevalence rate per 1,000 workers	Rate ratio
Lung cancer	1.7	1.31
Asbestosis	2.8	2.15
Asthma	19.6	0.82
Emphysema	25.8	1.34
Chronic bronchitis	24.1	1.30

Note: The rate ratio is the ratio of the rate in construction workers compared to the rate among other workers who participated in the survey.
Reprinted from Sullivan P, Moon Bank K, Hearl F, Wagner G. Respiratory risk in the construction industry. In: Ringen K, Englund A, Welch LS, Weeks JL, Seegal J, eds. Health and safety in construction. *Occup Med* 1995;10(2):269–284, with permission.

Morbidity

Surveillance data on respiratory disease incidence or prevalence among construction workers are limited. The Bureau of Labor Statistics, U.S. Department of Labor, collects occupational injury and illness data from the nation's private industry in accordance with a provision of the Occupational Safety and Health Act of 1970 (101). Respiratory conditions accounted for 14.3% of approximately 7,000 reported occupational illness cases among construction workers. NIOSH estimated the prevalence rate of reported respiratory conditions based on a national probability sample of construction workers from data collected through the National Health Interview Survey in 1988 (Table 48-7). Of the 42,487 respondents to this survey, 1,785 white male subjects indicated that they have work experience in the construction industry. Prevalence rates ranged from 1.7 to 25.8 per 1,000 white male construction workers for lung cancer and emphysema, respectively. Asthma was reported less frequently by construction workers than by the general population, but because sensitized individuals may voluntarily leave the construction workforce, the reported prevalence may be low because of a healthy worker effect.

Asbestosis

Asbestos has been recognized as a respiratory health risk for a number of construction trades (102,103). Occupational exposure to asbestos, and a diagnosis of asbestosis, occurs in many construction trades, particularly among those working as plumbers and pipe fitters (103), electricians, sheet metal workers, and insulators. Several studies have suggested that all construction workers may be at risk from asbestos-induced disease resulting from exposure associated with working adjacent to insulation workers (104,105). Although asbestos is no longer used in new residential or heavy construction, workers in the specialty trades (standard industrial classification of 17) may continue to be exposed to previously installed asbestos material during maintenance, renovation, addition, or demolition activities. Asbestos-containing fireproofing was sprayed on structural steel and other components of many U.S. high-rise buildings before it was banned in 1973 (81,105). Asbestos insulation was sprayed on ductwork. Asbestos cement, associated with fibrotic disease, has been used in roof tiles, roofing panels, wallboard, and domestic and industrial waste tanks. Use of spackle and taping compounds in drywall construction has been associated with asbestos exposure, with especially high exposure during sanding operations (106,107). Old vinyl flooring may also contain asbestos.

Silicosis

Occupational exposure to silica occurs in the construction industry among workers employed in concrete removal and demolition work, bridge and road construction, tunnel construction, and concrete or granite cutting, drilling, sanding, and grinding (108,109). Sandblasters and rock drillers are at increased risk from exposure to crystalline silica. Those working nearby in other trades on the same construction site may also be at risk from silica-related disease. In the United States, sand containing crystalline silica is still used in abrasive blasting operations for maintenance of structures, preparing surfaces for painting, or in forming decorative patterns during installation of building materials. The use of silica for abrasive blasting creates a high potential for silica exposure for the operator and for bystanders (110).

OSHA compliance monitoring data suggest that silica exposures within the construction industry continue to exceed recommended limits, and surveillance data based on the small number of silicosis cases recorded on death certificates in the United States suggest that some construction trades may be at increased risk for the disease. Evidence exists of silicosis risk among construction workers from international studies as well (98,111).

Bronchitis

Bronchitis has been reported among construction workers exposed to asbestos (112) and human-made mineral fibers (113,114), painters using spray application methods (115), and arc welders.

Chronic Obstructive Pulmonary Disease

Chronic obstructive pulmonary disease has been reported among tunnel construction workers, construction painters, sheet metal workers, and construction arc welders (115–117). Chronic nonspecific lung disease symptoms have been found among construction workers, woodworkers, and painters, even after adjusting for smoking and age (118–119). Specific exposures associated with excess risk of chronic nonspecific lung disease included heavy metals, mineral dust, and adhesives (120).

Occupational Asthma

Chan-Yeung reviewed agents and trades at risk for occupational asthma, including construction (121). Possible causal exposures include wood dust and welding flux. Welders are at increased risk of occupational asthma as a result of exposure to ammonium chloride fumes.

Inhalation Injury, Irritation, and Fevers

Painters may experience irritation of the respiratory system after exposure to acetone, amyl acetate, methyl ethyl ketone (2-butanone), and *n*-butyl lactate used as components or solvents in paints, varnishes, or lacquers (122). Cement workers may also be at risk of respiratory irritation from components of cement, including amyl acetate and methyl ethyl ketone (2-butanone). Welders are exposed to several respiratory irritants, including ammonium chloride and boron trifluoride in soldering flux. Metal fume fever has been reported with exposure to nickel, chromates, copper fumes, beryllium, cadmium, and other metal fumes that may be present during welding operations (123,124). Symptoms include upper respiratory tract irritation, metallic taste, nausea, and fever.

Respiratory Infection

Construction workers involved in excavation in tropical or subtropical areas may be at risk for nocardiosis, especially if they have another risk factor for the disease, such as lymphoma, deficient cell-mediated immunity, or immunosuppressive therapy. Road and bridge work and construction activities involving clearing of bird and bat roosts in river valleys in the eastern and central United States can result in histoplasmosis, a pneumonitis caused by respiratory infection occurring after inhalation of airborne fungal spores. The disease may be acute, inactive, or chronic, and can result in disability and death if untreated (125–128).

Elevated tuberculosis risk is found among silicotics (129). Legionnaires' disease has occasionally been reported in construction activities involving excavation or in the vicinity of cooling towers (130).

REFERENCES

1. Powers MB. Cost fever breaks. *Engineering News-Record* 1994;233(13):40–41.
2. Robinson C. Mortality patterns among construction workers in the United States. *Occup Med* 1995;10:269–284.
3. Markowitz S, Fisher E, Fahs M, et al. Occupational disease in New York State: a comprehensive reexamination. *Am J Ind Med* 1989;16:417–436.
4. Engholm G, Englund E. Morbidity and mortality patterns among construction workers in Sweden. *Occup Med* 1995;10:261–268.
5. Meridian Research. Worker protection programs in construction. Silver Spring, MD: Meridian Research, 1994. [OSHA contract J-9-F-1-0019].
6. Hinze J. *Indirect costs of construction accidents*. Austin, TX: Construction Industry Institute, 1991.
7. Levitt RE, Samelson NM. *Construction safety management*, 2nd ed. New York: John Wiley and Sons, 1993.
8. Ringen K, Englund A, Welch LS, Weeks JL, Seegal J. Why construction is different. *Occup Med* 1995;10:255–260.
9. Burkhart G, Schulte PA, Robinson C, et al. Job tasks, potential exposures, and health risks of laborers employed in the construction industry. *Am J Ind Med* 1993;24:413–425.
10. Ruhl R, Kluger N. Hazardous materials in construction. *Occup Med* 1995;10:335–352.
11. Carnevale F, Montesano R, Partensky C, Tomatis L. Comparison of regulations on occupational carcinogens in several industrialized countries. *Am J Ind Med* 1987;12:453–473.
12. Knecht U, Woitowitz H-J. Risk of cancer from the use of tar bitumen in road works. *Br J Ind Med* 1989;46:24–30.
13. Vainio H, Wilbourn J. Identification of carcinogens within the IARC monograph program. *Scand J Work Environ Health* 1992;18[Suppl 1]:64–73.
14. Jansen K, Ruhl R. Low-chromate cements—application and potential, II. International Colloquium on Industrial Medicine in the Building Trades. Baden-Baden, Germany, October 1992.
15. Jolanki R, Kanerva L, Estlander T, et al. Occupational dermatoses from epoxy resin compounds. *Contact Dermatitis* 1990;23(3):172–183.
16. Avnstorp C. Risk factors for cement eczema. *Contact Dermatitis* 1991;25:81–88.
17. Marino PE, Franzblau A, Lilis R, Landrigan PJ. Acute lead poisoning in construction workers: the failure of current protective standards. *Arch Environ Health* 1989;44:140–145.
18. Welch LS, Roto P. Medical surveillance for construction workers. *Occup Med* 1995;10:421–434.
19. National Institute for Occupational Safety and Health. Request for assistance in preventing lead poisoning in construction workers. Cincinnati: National Institute for Occupational Safety and Health, 1992. [NIOSH publication 91-116a].
20. Fischbein A, Leeds M, Solomon S. Lead exposure among iron workers in New York City: a continuing occupational hazard in the 1980s. *N Y State J Med* 1984;84:445–448.
21. Himmelstein J, Wolfson M, Pransky G, et al. Lead poisoning in bridge demolition workers—Massachusetts. *MMWR Mortal Morb Wkly Rep* 1989;38:687–694.
22. Landrigan PJ, Baker EL, Himmelstein JS, et al. Exposure to lead from the Mystic River Bridge: the dilemma of deleading. *N Engl J Med* 1982;306:673–676.
23. McCammon C, Daniels W, Hales T, Lee S. Lead exposure during lining of tanks with lead sheeting. *Appl Occup Environ Hyg* 1992;7:88–91.
24. Campbell BC, Baird AW. Lead poisoning in a group of demolition workers. *Br J Ind Med* 1977;34:298–304.
25. Pollock CA, Ibels LS. Lead intoxication in paint removal workers on the Sydney Harbour Bridge. *Med J Aust* 1986;145:635–639.
26. Rae CE, Bell CN, Ellion CE, Shannon M. Ten cases of acute lead intoxication among bridge workers in Louisiana. *Ann Pharmacother* 1991;25:932–937.
27. Risk I, Thurman D, Beaudoin D. Lead exposures among lead burners—Utah, 1991. *MMWR Mortal Morb Wkly Rep* 1992;41:307–310.
28. Stockbridge H, Daniell W. Lead poisoning among bricklayers—Washington state. *MMWR Mortal Morb Wkly Rep 1991*;40:169–171.
29. Sussell A, Tubbs R, Montopoli M. Occupational exposures during abrasive blasting removal of leadbased paint on a highway bridge. *Appl Occup Environ Hyg* 1992;7:497–503.
30. Waller K, Osorio AM, Maizlish N, Royce S. Lead exposure in the construction industry: results from the California Occupational Lead Registry, 1987 through 1989. *Am J Public Health* 1992;82:1669–1671.
31. Zimmer FE. Lead poisoning in scrap-metal workers. *JAMA* 1961;175:238–240.
32. Occupational Safety and Health Administration. Lead exposure in construction, interim final rule. *Federal Register* 1993;58:26590–26649.
33. Centers for Disease Control and Prevention. Preventing lead poisoning in young children: a statement by the Centers for Disease Control. Atlanta: Centers for Disease Control, 1991. [DHHS publication 99-2230].

33a. Centers for Disease Control and Prevention. Screening young children for lead poisoning: guidance for state and local public health officials. Atlanta: Department of Health and Human Services, Centers for Disease Control and Prevention, 1997.

34. Occupational Safety and Health Administration, National Institute for Occupational Safety and Health. Working with lead in the construction industry. Washington: Occupational Safety and Health Administration, National Institute for Occupational Safety and Health, 1991.
35. Holmstrom E, Moritz U, Engholm G. Musculoskeletal disorders in construction workers. *Occup Med* 1995;10:295–311.
36. Tola S, Riihimaki H, Videman T, et al. Neck and shoulder symptoms among men in machine operating, dynamic physical work and sedentary work. *Scand J Work Environ Health* 1988;14:299–305.
37. Holmstrom E, Lindell J, Moritz U. Low back and neck/shoulder pain in construction workers: physical and psychosocial risk factors. Part 2: relationship to neck/shoulder pain. *Spine* 1992;17:672–677.
38. Stenlund B, Goldie I, Hagberg M, Hogstedt C. Shoulder tendinitis and the relation to heavy manual work and exposure to vibration. *Scand J Work Environ Health* 1993;19:43–49.
39. Stenlund B, Goldie I, Hagberg M, et al. Radiographic osteoarthrosis in the acromioclavicular joint resulting from manual work or exposure to vibration. *Br J Ind Med* 1992;49:588–593.
40. Hunting KL, Welch LS, Cuccherini BA, Seiger LA. Musculoskeletal symptoms among electricians. *Am J Ind Med* 1994;25:149–163.
41. Gemne G, Saraste H. Bone and joint pathology in workers using hand-held vibrating tools. *Scand J Work Environ Health* 1987;13:290–300.
42. Stock S. Workplace ergonomic factors and the development of musculoskeletal disorders of the neck and upper limbs: a meta-analysis. *Am J Ind Med* 1991;19:87–107.
43. Andersson GBJ. Epidemiologic aspects on low-back pain in industry. *Spine* 1981;6:53–60.
44. Riihimaki H. Radiographically detectable degenerative changes of the lumbar spine among concrete reinforcement workers and house painters. *Spine* 1990;15:114–119.
45. Wickstrom G. Effects of work on degenerative back disease. *Scand J Work Environ Health* 1978;4[Suppl 1]:1–12.
46. Heliovaara M. Occupation and risk of herniated lumbar intervertebral disc or sciatica leading to hospitalization. *J Chronic Dis* 1987;40:259–264.
47. Kelsey JL. An epidemiological study of the relationship between occupations and acute herniated lumbar intervertebral discs. *Int J Epidemiol* 1975; 4:197–205.
48. Holmstrom E, Lindell J, Moritz U. Low back and neck/shoulder pain in construction workers: physical and psychosocial risk factors. Part 1: relationship to low back pain. *Spine* 1992;17:663–671.
49. Budorf A, Govaert G, Elders L. Postural load and back pain of workers in the manufacturing of prefabricated concrete elements. *Ergonomics* 1991;34:909–918.
50. Riihimaki H, Tola S, Videman T, Hanninen K. Low-back pain and occupation. A cross-sectional questionnaire study of men in machine operating, dynamic physical work and sedentary work. *Spine* 1989;14:204–209.
51. Riihimaki H, Wickstrom G, Hanninen K, Luopajarvi T. Predictors of sciatic pain among concrete reinforcement workers and house painters—a five-year follow-up. *Scand J Environ Health* 1989;15:415–423.
52. Bigos SJ, Spengler DM, Martin NA, et al. Back injuries in industry: a retrospective study. II. Injury factors. *Spine* 1986;11:246–251.
53. Lindberg H, Danielsson LG. The relation between labor and coxarthrosis. *Clin Orthop* 1984;191:159–161.
54. Vingard E, Alfredsson L, Goldie I, Hogstedt C. Occupation and osteoarthrosis of the hip and knee: a register based cohort study. *Int J Epidemiol* 1991; 20:1025–1031.
55. Kohatsu ND, Schurman DJ. Risk factors for the development of osteoarthrosis of the knee. *Clin Orthop* 1990;261:242–246.
56. Lindberg H, Montgomery F. Heavy labor and the occurrence of gonarthrosis. *Clin Orthop* 1987;214:235–236.
57. Kivimaki J, Riihimaki H, Hanninen K. Knee disorders in carpet and floor layers and painters. *Scand J Work Environ Health* 1992;18:310–316.
58. Kivimaki J. Occupationally related ultrasonic findings in carpet and floor layers' knees. *Scand J Work Environ Health* 1992;18:400–402.
59. Thun M, Tanka S, Smith SB. Morbidity from repeated knee trauma in carpet and floor layers. *Br J Ind Med* 1987;44:611–620.
60. Kivimaki J. Occupationally related ultrasonic findings in carpet and floor layers' knees. *Scand J Work Environ Health* 1992;18:310–316.
61. Rhiimaki H, Wickstrom G, Hanninen K, Luopajarvi T. Predictors of sciatic pain among concrete reinforcement workers and house painters—a five year follow-up. *Scand J Work Environ Health* 1989;15:415–423.

62. US Department of Health and Human Services, Public Health Service, National Center for Health Statistics. *Public use data documentation: multiple cause of death for ICD-9: 1987 data*. Hyattsville, MD: US Government Printing Office, 1989.
63. Robinson C, Halperin W, Alterman T, et al. Mortality patterns among construction workers in the United States. *Occup Med* 1995;10(2):269–283.
64. Blot WJ, Davies JE, Brown LM, et al. Occupation and the high risk of lung cancer in northeast Florida. *Cancer* 1982;50:364–371.
65. Coggon D, Pannett B, Osmond C, Acheson ED. A survey of cancer and occupation in young and middle aged men. I. Cancers of the respiratory tract. *Br J Ind Med* 1986;43:332–338.
66. Feldman JP, Gerber LM. Sentinel health events (occupational): analysis of death certificates among residents of Nassau County, NY between 1980–82 for occupationally related causes of death. *Am J Public Health* 1990;80: 158–161.
67. Harrington JM, Blot WJ, Hoover RN, et al. Lung cancer in coastal Georgia: a death certificate analysis of occupation—brief communication. *J Natl Cancer Inst* 1978;60:295–298.
68. Milne KL, Sandler DP, Everson RB, Brown SM. Lung cancer and occupation in Alameda County: a death certificate case-control study. *Am J Ind Med* 1983;4:565–575.
69. Ng TP. Occupational mortality in Hong Kong, 1979–1983. *Int J Epidemiol* 1988;17:105–110.
70. Buiatti E, Kriebel D, Geddes M, et al. A case control study of lung cancer in Florence, Italy. I. Occupational risk factors. *J Epidemiol Community Health* 1985;39:244–250.
71. Lerchen ML, Wiggins CL, Samet JM. Lung cancer and occupation in New Mexico. *J Natl Cancer Inst* 1987;79:639–645.
72. National Institute for Occupational Safety and Health. Occupational characteristics of white cancer victims in Massachusetts, 1971–1973. Cincinnati: National Institute for Occupational Safety and Health, 1984. [Publication No 84-109].
73. Neuberger M, Kundi M. Occupational dust exposure and cancer mortality C results of a prospective cohort study. *IARC Sci Publ* 1990;97:65–73.
74. Ronco G, Ciccone G, Mirabelli D, et al. Occupation and lung cancer in two industrialized areas of Northern Italy. *Int J Cancer* 1988;41:354–358.
75. Matanoski G. Mortality of workers in the painting trades. Proceedings of the Fourth National Cancer Institute/Environmental Protection Agency/National Institute for Occupational Safety and Health Collaborative Workshop: progress on joint environmental and occupational cancer studies, April 22–23, 1986. Rockville, MD: National Institutes of Health, 1988:137–143. [Publication no 88-2960].
76. Menck HR, Henderson BE. Occupational differences in rates of lung cancer. *J Occup Med* 1976;18(12):797–801.
77. Pukkala E, Teppo L, Hakulinen T, Rimpela M. Occupation and smoking as risk determinants of lung cancer. *Int J Epidemiol* 1983;12:290–296.
78. Stayner L, Smith R, Thun M, et al. A dose-response analysis and quantitative assessment of lung cancer risk and occupational cadmium exposure. *Ann Epidemiol* 1992;2:177–194.
79. Selikoff IJ, Seidman H. Asbestos-associated deaths among insulation workers in the United States and Canada, 1967–1987. *Ann N Y Acad Sci* 1991; 643:1–14.
80. Finkelstein MM. Analysis of mortality patterns and workers' compensation awards among asbestos insulation workers in Ontario. *Am J Ind Med* 1989;16(5):523–528.
81. Zoloth S, Michaels D. Asbestos disease in sheet metal workers: the results of a proportional mortality analysis. *Am J Ind Med* 1985;7:315–321.
82. Simonato L, Fletcher AC, Andersen A, et al. A historical prospective study of European stainless steel, mild steel, and shipyard welders. *Br J Ind Med* 1991;48:145–154.
83. Rafnsson V, Johannesdottir SG. Mortality among masons in Iceland. *Br J Ind Med* 1986;43:522–525.
84. Kaminski R, Geissert KS, Dacey E. Mortality analysis of plumbers and pipefitters. Cincinnati: National Institute of Occupational Safety and Health, 1979.
85. Lynge E, Thygesen L. Occupational cancer in Denmark: cancer incidence in the 1970 census population. *Scand J Work Environ Health* 1990;16[Suppl 2]:1–35.
86. Hansen ES. Mortality of mastic asphalt workers. *Scand J Work Environ Health* 1991;17:20–24.
87. Emmett EA. Cutaneous and ocular hazards of roofers. *Occup Med* 1986; 1:307–322.
88. Imbus HR, Dyson WL. A review of nasal cancer in furniture manufacturing and woodworking in North Carolina, the United States, and other countries. *J Occup Med* 1987;29:734–740.
89. Luce D, Leclerc A, Morcet JF, et al. Occupational risk factors for sinonasal cancer: a case-control study in France. *Am J Ind Med* 1992;21:163–175.
90. Mohtashamipur E, Norpoth K, Luhmann F. Cancer epidemiology of woodworking. *J Cancer Res Clin Oncol* 1989;115:503–515.
91. Vaughan TL. Occupation and squamous cell cancers of the pharynx and sinonasal cavity. *Am J Ind Med* 1989;16(5):493–510.
92. Comba P, Battista G, Belli S, et al. A case-control study of cancer of the nose and paranasal sinuses and occupational exposures. *Am J Ind Med* 1992;22:511–520.
93. Hall NEL, Rosenman KD. Cancer by industry: analysis of a population-based cancer registry with an emphasis on blue-collar workers. *Am J Ind Med* 1991;19(2):145–159.
94. Roush GC, Meigs JW, Kelly J, et al. Sinonasal cancer and occupation: a case-control study. *Am J Epidemiol* 1980;111:183–193.
95. Begin R, Gauthier JJ, Desmeules M, Ostiguy G. Work-related mesothelioma in Quebec, 1967–1990. *Am J Ind Med* 1992;22(4):531–542.
96. Chellini E, Fornaciai G, Merler E, et al. Pleural malignant mesothelioma in Tuscany, Italy (1970–1988). II. Identification of occupational exposure to asbestos. *Am J Ind Med* 1992;21:577–585.
97. Mowe G, Andersen A, Osvoll P. Trends in mesothelioma incidence in Norway. *Ann N Y Acad Sci* 1991;643:449–453.
98. Muscat JE, Wynder EL. Cigarette smoking, asbestos exposure, and malignant mesothelioma. *Cancer Res* 1991;51:2263–2267.
99. Tagnon I, Blot WJ, Stroube RB, et al. Mesothelioma associated with the shipbuilding industry in coastal Virginia. *Cancer Res* 1980;40:3875–3879.
100. Milham S. Mortality experience of the AFL-CIO United Brotherhood of Carpenters and Joiners of America, 1969–1970 and 1972–1973. Washington: US Government Printing Office, 1978. [NIOSH Publication no 78-152].
101. US Department of Labor, Bureau of Labor Statistics. Occupational injuries and illnesses in the United States by industry, 1991. Washington: US Government Printing Office, 1993.
102. Baker EL, Dagg T, Greene RE. Respiratory illness in the construction trades. I. The significance of asbestos-associated pleural disease among sheet metal workers. *J Occup Med* 1985;27(7):483–489.
103. Sprince NL, Oliver LC, McLoud TC. Asbestos-related disease in plumbers and pipefitters employed in building construction. *J Occup Med* 1985; 27:771–775.
104. Kilburn KH, Warshaw RH. Asbestos disease in construction, refinery, and shipyard workers. *Ann N Y Acad Sci* 1991;643:301–312.
105. Welch LS, Michaels D, Zoloth S. Asbestos-related disease among sheet-metal workers. Preliminary results of the National Sheet Metal Worker Asbestos Disease Screening Program. *Ann N Y Acad Sci* 1991;643:287–295.
106. Fischbein A, Rohl AN, Langer AM, Selikoff IJ. Drywall construction and asbestos exposure. *Am Ind Hyg Assoc J* 1979;40:402–407.
107. Verma DK, Middleton CG. Occupational exposure to asbestos in the drywall taping process. *Am Ind Hyg Assoc J* 1980;41:264–269.
108. Burns C, Ottoboni F, Mitchell HW. Health hazards and heavy construction. *Ind Hyg J* 1962;July–August:273–281.
109. National Institute for Occupational Safety and Health. ALERT—request for assistance in preventing silicosis and deaths in rock drillers. Cincinnati: Department of Health and Human Services, 1992. [Publication no 92-107].
110. National Institute for Occupational Safety and Health. ALERT—request for assistance in preventing silicosis and deaths from sandblasting. Cincinnati: Department of Health and Human Services, 1992. [Publication no 92-102].
111. Ng TP, Yeung KH, O'Kelly FJ. Silica hazard of caisson construction in Hong Kong. *J Soc Occup Med* 1987;37:62–65.
112. Hedenstierna G, Alexandersson R, Kolmodin-Hedman B, et al. Pleural plaques and lung function in construction workers exposed to asbestos. *Eur J Respir Dis* 1981;62:111–122.
113. Engholm G, von Schmalensee G. Bronchitis and exposure to man-made mineral fibres in non-smoking construction workers. *Eur J Respir Dis* 1982;63[Suppl 118]:73–78.
114. Hunting KL, Welch LS. Occupational exposure to dust and lung disease among sheet metal workers. *Br J Ind Med* 1993;50:432–442.
115. White MC, Baker EL. Measurements of respiratory illness among construction painters. *Br J Ind Med* 1988;45(8):523–531.
116. Schwartz DA, Baker EL. Respiratory illness in the construction industry-airflow obstruction among painters. *Chest* 1988;93(1):134-137.
117. Kilburn KH, Warshaw RH. Pulmonary functional impairment from years of arc welding. *Am J Ind Med* 1989;87(1):62–69.
118. Heederik D, Pouwels H, Kromhout H, Kromhout D. Chronic non-specific lung disease and occupational exposures estimated by means of a job exposure matrix: the Zutphen study. *Int J Epidemiol* 1989;18(2):382–389.
119. Heederik D, Kromhout H, Kromhout D, et al. Relations between occupation, smoking, lung function, and incidence and mortality of chronic non-specific lung disease: the Zutphen study. *Br J Ind Med* 1992;49:299–308.
120. Heederik D, Kromhout H, Burema J, et al. Occupational exposure and 25-year incidence rate of non-specific lung disease: the Zutphen study. *Int J Epidemiol* 1990;19(4):945–952.
121. Chan-Yeung M. Occupational asthma. *Chest* 1990;98(5):148S–161S.
122. Occupational Safety and Health Administration. Air contaminants: proposed rule. *Federal Register* 1992 June 12;57:26002–26601.
123. Moreton J. Fume hazards in welding, brazing and soldering. *Metal Construction Br Welding J* 1977;9:33–34.
124. Niemeier RW. Testimony on occupational exposure to cadmium, May 7, 1990. Cincinnati: National Institute for Occupational Safety and Health, 1990.
125. Bertolini R. *Histoplasmosis—a summary of the occupational health concern*. Hamilton, Ontario: Canadian Centre for Occupational Health and Safety, 1988. [Report no P88-8E].
126. George RB, Penn RL. Histoplasmosis. In: Sarosi GA, Davies SF, eds. *Fungal diseases of the lung*. Orlando, FL: Grune & Stratton, 1986:69–85.
127. Powell KE, Hammerman KJ, Dahl BA, Tosh FE. Acute reinfection pulmonary histoplasmosis. *Am Rev Respir Dis* 1973;107:374–378.
128. Sorley DL, Levin ML, Warren JW, et al. Bat-associated histoplasmosis in Maryland bridge workers. *Am J Med* 1979;67:623–626.
129. Weeks JL, Levy BS, Wagner GR, eds. *Preventing occupational disease and injury*. Washington: American Public Health Association, 1991:551.
130. Morton S, Bartlett CLR, Bibby LF, et al. Outbreak of legionnaires' disease from a cooling water system in a power station. *Br J Ind Med* 1986;43:630–635.

CHAPTER 49

Medical Waste and Blood-Borne Pathogen Exposures

John B. Sullivan, Jr., and Linda M. Micale

MEDICAL WASTE

Infectious waste is defined as that waste that is capable of producing infection or characterized by a pathogen that can produce human disease. Such wastes can include highly infectious pathogens, including hepatitis, human immunodeficiency viruses (HIV), pathogenic fungi, and other biological materials. Difficulties exist in characterizing biohazardous waste because of the large variety of material generated, the nature of the pathogens, the types of wastes and disposables, and the many different health care entities that generate such waste.

Most medical wastes are not infectious, but may be contaminated by biological fluids or blood that is infectious. Estimations are that only 15% of health care–generated waste is infectious, with the remaining 85% being a combination of disposable gloves, plastics, paper, needles, syringes, and other medical disposable items (1,2). The health care worker has the highest risk of infectivity and injury (3).

The familiar red bags and biohazard-labeled containers are common features of health care environments (Figs. 49-1 through 49-3). The contents of these waste containers vary considerably. In addition to the common sharps and needles, the addition of plastic disposables, latex products, and paper contribute greatly to the medical-waste load. Previous surveys indicate that large hospitals generate on the average 4.18 kg of waste per bed per day (6,063 tons per day based on 1.267 million hospital beds that existed in 1987 in the United States) (2). The U.S. Environmental Protection Agency (EPA) recognizes six broad categories of infectious waste:

1. Isolation wastes
2. Cultures, biologics, stocks of infectious agents
3. Human blood and blood products
4. Pathologic wastes

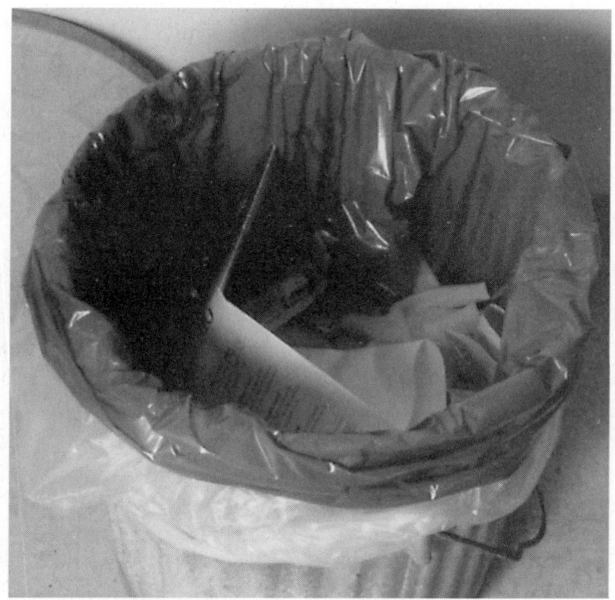

Figure 49-2. Red bag medical waste container.

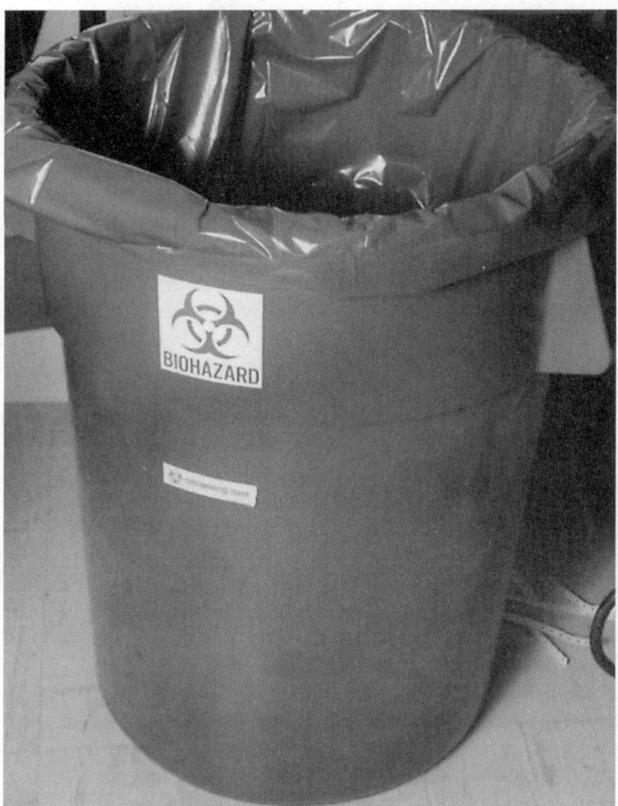

Figure 49-1. Typical biohazardous waste container showing the biohazard symbol.

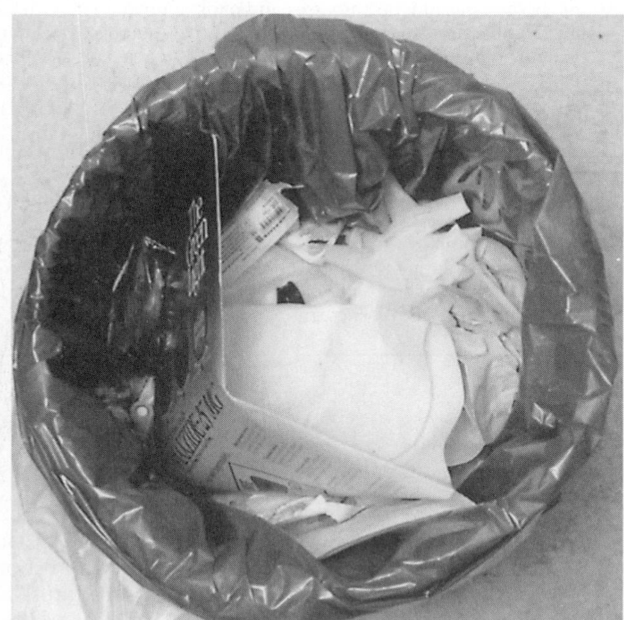

Figure 49-3. Red bag waste container showing variety of noninfectious items as content.

TABLE 49-1. Categorization of medical wastes

Isolation wastes

Isolation wastes involve materials that come into contact with blood, secretions, excretions, feces, and other biological fluids of patients with communicable diseases. This includes a variety of wastes, such as needles, disposable plastic items, gowns, masks, paper products, bandages, rubber drains, suture material, and tubing.

Cultures and stocks of infectious agents

Cultures and stocks of infectious agents have high concentrations of pathogens that are an important factor in risk management and are usually associated with pathology laboratories. Included are blood cultures, agar plates, and cultures of a variety of biological fluids that can serve as a medium of infectivity. Also included is a wide variety of pathogens. Culture media are usually sterilized before being discarded.

Blood and blood products

Blood should always be considered infectious. Common infectious problems include hepatitis, human immunodeficiency virus, malaria, rubella, measles, and others.

Autopsy and surgery wastes

Autopsy and surgery wastes are generated in hospital emergency departments, surgery, pathology departments, and autopsy areas. Included are body parts, tissues, biological fluids, organs, and secretions from infected or potentially infected patients. Such wastes may also contain plastic, metal, or cardboard. All surgical dressings from patients should be regarded as contaminated and sources of infection. In addition to gauze dressings and bandages of many varieties, these wastes include some biopsy and tissue specimens, cast materials, drapes, silastic tubing, needles, pads, biological fluids, metal instruments, and latex gloves.

Laboratory wastes

Laboratory wastes include all culture plates (glass and plastic), transfer devices, plastic tops, agar, paper, plastics used in automated chemical processes, autopsy wastes, blood and blood products, urine and blood containers, and glass tubes.

Sharps

Sharps include needles and other sharp objects, syringes, needles of all sizes, scalpel blades, pipettes, and broken glass. This category of waste materials has the highest risk of causing injury and transmission of disease.

Dialysis unit wastes

Dialysis unit wastes include sheets, towels, gloves, aprons, bandages, tubing, gloves, filters, and dialysis membranes. These wastes carry a high incidence of hepatitis.

Animal body parts

Animal body parts include carcasses and parts of dead animals, usually confined to research facilities or university settings. Parts may be infectious and contain experimental biological agents as well as experimental pharmaceuticals, including antineoplastic drugs, carcinogens, and potent immunosuppressants.

Discarded biologicals

Discarded biologicals include vaccines and drugs that are either outdated or used in animals and humans with infectious diseases. Also included could be antineoplastic drugs and discarded serum from multiple sources (human and animal).

Contaminated equipment

Contaminated equipment includes equipment and equipment parts that come into contact with infectious agents. Patient care equipment, filters, metals, plastics, rubber, cloth, and fabrics.

5. Contaminated sharps
6. Contaminated animal carcasses, body parts, and bedding

Waste by-products can be categorized as isolation wastes, cultures, blood and blood products, dialysis unit wastes, used hypodermic needles and syringes, pathology and autopsy wastes, discarded biologics, remains of surgical procedures, laboratory waste, contaminated disposables, and animal bedding and body parts (Table 49-1). Other components of medical wastes may include antineoplastic agents, radiopharmaceuticals, and the myriad plastics and papers that end up in the red containers.

The Centers for Disease Control and Prevention (CDC) differs slightly from the EPA and recognizes five categories of infectious medical waste (2):

1. Microbiological
2. Sharps
3. Blood
4. Pathologic
5. Contaminated animal carcasses

The CDC and the EPA also differ with respect to an optional waste category that the EPA identifies as surgical and autopsy wastes, contaminated wastes from laboratories and dialysis units, and contaminated equipment.

Many noninfectious materials are disposed of as biohazards because of the Occupational Safety and Health Administration (OSHA) regulations regarding blood-borne pathogens and universal precaution practices. Monetary savings can be realized by adopting the CDC guidelines and definitions as opposed to EPA guidelines (2).

Major sources of medical and infectious wastes are hospitals. However, given that more than 180,000 private physician offices, more than 98,000 dental offices, 16,400 nursing homes, 2,900 ambulatory health care centers, 650 ambulatory surgical centers, 860 dialysis units, and 225 blood banks exist, it is clear that the volume of wastes generated continues to increase (2). Also, as greater efficiencies in health care are necessary, the increase in ambulatory-generated waste may alter the overall nature of the waste streams (2).

Even the use of the terms *medical waste* and *infectious waste* have been debated regarding a determination of the correct label to apply to best categorize the hazard and nature of the waste streams.

The EPA and the CDC have published guidelines that differ on the designation and disposal of medical wastes. The CDC and the EPA agree on the definition of medical wastes as infectious waste in five categories but disagree on the one category of isolation wastes as being communicable. The EPA also has an optional medical waste that may be derived from sources such as surgical procedures, dialysis wastes, contaminated equipment, and autopsies. The EPA allows local responsible hospital or clinic authorities to decide whether these wastes should be managed as though they were infectious (2).

Disposal practices among large medical facilities, such as hospitals and large outpatient clinics, are fairly uniform. Policies for managing biohazards and medical waste, as well as disease prevention and infection control, are required by accrediting agencies and OSHA. Proper training of staff who handle infectious waste and compliance with OSHA standards on blood-borne pathogens and universal precautions is required.

Risk management issues regarding medical-waste generation and disposal involve needlesticks, mucous membrane exposures of workers, handling, storage, and transport. These items include initial disposal practices in clinical areas, storage in clinical areas, tracking of wastes, storage in depository areas, handling at the site of origin by employees of the facility as well as the transport company, transportation, and handling at the incineration facility.

OSHA has issued a standard relating to the regulation of occupational exposure to hepatitis B virus, HIV, and other blood- and biological fluid–transmitted pathogens. The standard applies to all occupational exposures to blood and other potentially infectious materials. The definition of *occupational exposure* is a reasonably anticipated skin, eye, mucous membrane, or parenteral contact with potentially infectious material that may result from the performance of an employee's duties. This standard requires employers to identify and document tasks in which an occupational exposure may occur. The employer is also required to have a written infection control plan. The OSHA standard establishes four compliance methods:

1. *General compliance*: OSHA has adopted the universal precautions recommended by the CDC.
2. *Engineering and work practice*: Serves to reduce exposures in the workplace by eliminating and controlling the hazard.
3. *Personal protective equipment*: Requires employers to provide and employees to use appropriate protective devices and garb, such as eye shields, gowns, gloves, head and foot coverings, and resuscitation devices to prevent exposure.
4. *Housekeeping*: Requires cleaning and disinfection of contaminated areas and items that contact potentially infectious media.

The OSHA standard requires employers to have an employee health program and offer hepatitis B vaccine to all employees who are exposed to potential sources one or more times per month. The health program must provide postexposure evaluation and medical follow-up of exposed employees. This evaluation includes potential HIV exposure evaluation. Postexposure evaluation must offer collection and testing of the source's blood (if permission is granted) and review of the source's medical records for risk factors. The employee's blood must also be tested and the employee offered counseling, appropriate treatment, and prophylaxis.

The OSHA standard requires appropriate labeling of containers of infectious waste and refrigerators containing blood and blood products, and containers used to transport and store potentially infectious materials. Training of employees who have occupational exposure is mandated. This training must include modes of transmission, safe practices to reduce exposures, personal protection, the use of personal protective devices, vaccines available, and explanation on how to handle an exposure and the medical evaluation. Medical record documentation of exposures is also necessary, and this must be kept confidential. Documentation of employee training is also included in the standard.

Infection Risks

Health care workers who come into contact with bodily fluids, secretions, blood, and blood products are at risk. Accidents are usually a result of injury from needles and syringes, splash exposures, or contamination of open wound sites or mucous membranes with biological fluids from a known, suspected, or unknown infectious source. A variety of infectious agents are recognized as etiologic sources for which health care workers are at risk (Table 49-2). Transmission of hepatitis B and HIV is the primary concern of health care personnel. Factors necessary to produce disease are as follows:

1. Presence of a pathogen
2. Presence of a host
3. Route of exposure for transmission
4. Exposure to the pathogen
5. Exposure to infective dose

Infective doses of some agents have been characterized. Prevention of disease is part of risk management, and practices of health care facilities to prevent disease from infectious hazardous materials must be part of risk management strategy. Overall, the risk of acquiring an infection from medical waste is very remote. Solid municipal waste is thought to be many-fold more microbially contaminated than medical waste (2).

TABLE 49-2. Human risks from medical waste

Bacteria
Bordetella pertussis
Mycobacterium tuberculosis
Treponema pallidum
Staphylococcus aureus
Streptococcus pyogenes
Neisseria meningococcus
Viruses
Human immunodeficiency virus (HIV)
Hepatitis B
Hepatitis A
Non-A, non-B hepatitis
Cytomegalovirus
Herpes simplex
Measles
Mumps
Rubella
Respiratory syncytial virus

STORAGE AND TRANSPORTATION OF WASTE

Other risk management issues involve the handling, storage, and transportation of medical waste. Medical waste is collected in either red bags or plastic sharps containers (Fig. 49-4). These smaller plastic collection containers are placed in large, 40-gallon plastic drums for transport and disposal, usually by incineration. These red 40-gallon drums are clearly marked with a biohazard symbol (Fig. 49-5). The transporting truck may not always be marked with any symbol or placard to indicate its contents. An accident involving such a transport truck could result in spills of medical wastes that may be a health hazard to responding fire and paramedical personnel. The transport vehicle is large enough to carry multiple drums stacked on top of each other.

MEDICAL-WASTE REGULATIONS

The EPA is charged with implementing the federal solid- and hazardous-waste management program under the Resource

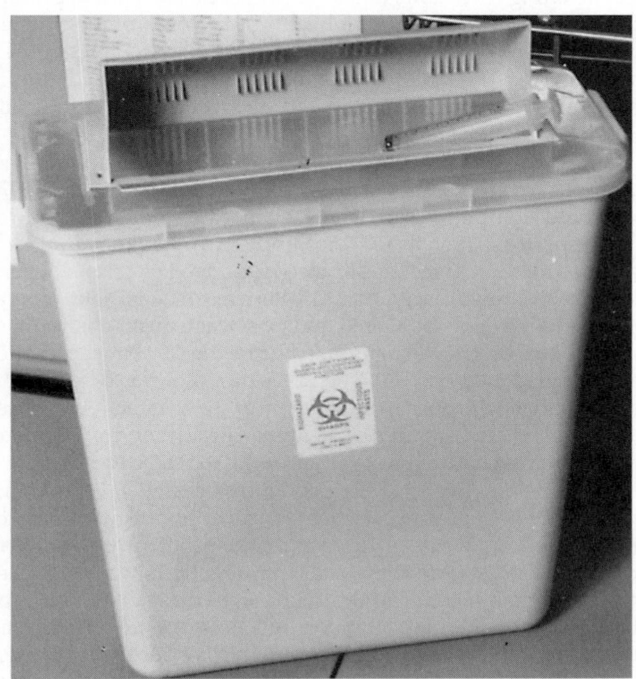

Figure 49-4. Sharps container.

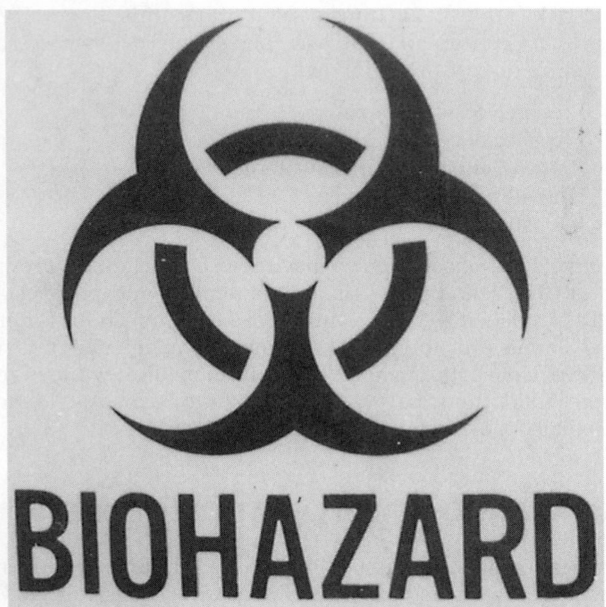

Figure 49-5. Biohazard symbol.

Conservation and Recovery Act (RCRA) of 1976 (4). RCRA amended the 1965 Solid Waste Disposal Act. Under RCRA, the EPA was mandated by the U.S. Congress to develop criteria for identifying and listing hazardous waste. EPA regulations encompass medical or infectious waste as a solid waste, although the agency did not regulate these wastes based on their potential health risks. Years after the passage of RCRA, the federal government has taken steps to reevaluate its position on medical waste.

In RCRA Section 1004, the Congress defined *hazardous wastes* as a "solid waste or combination of solid wastes which, because of its quantity, concentration, or physical, chemical, or infectious characteristics, may (a) cause or significantly contribute to an increase in mortality or an increase in serious irreversible, or incapacitating reversible, illness or (b) pose a substantial present or potential hazard to human health or the environment when improperly treated, stored, transported, or disposed of, or otherwise managed" (4). Solid wastes may be solid, semisolid, liquid, or contained gaseous material that is discarded or has fulfilled its intended use, with some exceptions noted in the law (5).

In response to their congressional mandate to identify and list hazardous wastes, the EPA proposed regulations in December 1978 that would have placed certain infectious wastes under the hazardous-waste provisions of RCRA, Subtitle C. The *Federal Register* described these as "infectious waste[s] generated by certain departments in health care facilities and veterinary hospitals, by laboratories handling etiologic agents, and by sewage treatment facilities, unless these wastes were sterilized or incinerated in accordance with specified methods" (6). The EPA's proposal was based on the rationale that improper management of these infectious wastes could result in a substantial risk to human health and environment. Such a risk was considered at variance with the objectives of RCRA.

Nevertheless, the EPA received approximately 60 comments on the 1978 proposal expressing concerns about the listing of these infectious wastes. Reportedly, insufficient information existed to establish that exposure to infectious wastes causes harm to human health (7). On the basis of these comments, the EPA postponed its rulemaking on infectious wastes and deleted the proposal in the final rules issued on May 19, 1980. The EPA decided instead to collect technical information and evaluate problems related to infectious waste management. In 1982 and 1986, the EPA published draft and final guidelines, respectively, concerning proper infectious waste handling and disposal rather than develop enforceable standards.

In 1997, the EPA published its final rule with standards of performance for hospital, medical, and infectious waste incinerators (see Standards for Incinerators section).

U.S. Environmental Protection Agency Guidelines for Infectious Waste Management

The 1986 EPA Guide for Infectious Waste Management provides recommendations aimed at reducing risks from managing infectious wastes. The guide addresses problems associated directly with their infectious characteristics and identifies the six broad categories of infectious wastes previously listed in the Medical Waste section. The guide cautioned that other characteristics that may render certain infectious wastes "hazardous" may also subject them to RCRA Subtitle C regulations.

The recommendations contained in this document generally follow accepted practices for safe waste management. The EPA suggested that generators develop a comprehensive system to handle wastes. To reduce health risks, these wastes should be segregated during handling and treatment, and packaged in containers appropriate for and compatible with the waste type. Additional packaging or rigid containment may be necessary to reduce risks during storage and transport, and care should be taken to prevent its impairment. Storage areas should be specially designated, and access should be restricted. Wastes should be treated before disposal to alleviate their infectious characteristics. Treatment may involve steam sterilization, chemical disinfection, and incineration. Compaction of the wastes should be avoided before treatment to ensure the integrity of the packaging; further, the agency noted that compaction may inhibit effective treatment. Although the EPA appeared to favor incineration, it did not preclude the use of other treatment alternatives. Disposal alternatives correspond to the treatment method selected by the generator and include discharge of treated liquids or ground-up solids to sewage systems, and land disposal of treated solids and incinerator ash.

The EPA did not intend for the guide to hinder states from passing laws and developing regulations to manage infectious wastes (6). Since the enactment of RCRA, many states passed hazardous-waste legislation that includes controls for infectious wastes. The EPA noted, however, that most requirements were general, involving facility licensing and treatment or disposal methods. Specific standards for risk management were not typically identified as of the 1986 document. The EPA invited states to use the guide as a reference source to assist in the development of their regulatory programs. The EPA's World Wide Web site (http://www.epa.gov) includes a list of state agencies that have medical-waste contacts.

The CDC has issued guidelines on medical-waste handling. The EPA and CDC definitions of infectious waste differ. The EPA guide identifies communicable disease isolation wastes as one of the six categories recommended for across-the-board controls. The CDC recommends that such waste be managed according to individual hospital policy. In addition, the CDC does not recognize the optional infectious wastes identified by the guide, including dialysis unit wastes and miscellaneous laboratory wastes. The difference reflects the persistent difficulty that the EPA and other entities have experienced when trying to quantify the potential for an infectious waste to transmit disease (8).

On November 12, 1987, the EPA met with health care experts to evaluate whether the agency should develop regulatory measures to handle infectious wastes (8). The panel agreed that contaminated needles, laboratory wastes, and bulk blood had the greatest potential for transmission of disease, although laboratory wastes and blood could be treated onsite to minimize risks;

the potential for exposures of all types increased in occupational settings; and public exposures were expected primarily from improper disposal practices. Given this belief, the panel suggested that employers should institute a suitable waste management program and properly train health care workers and infectious waste handlers, and that the EPA should consider working with OSHA to develop standards for these workers. The panel believed that small-quantity generators of infectious wastes should be evaluated in addition to traditional sources, such as hospitals. The panel's packaging and containment recommendations echoed those in the 1986 guide. The panel also suggested that a tracking program be implemented to monitor the path of infectious wastes from generation through transport, treatment, and disposal, although the risk-reduction value of such a program was seriously questioned. The principal role recommended for EPA at that time involved the development and dissemination of educational materials to improve risk management and public understanding of the infectious waste issue.

In June 1988, the EPA provided information on available literature, including the guide and a hospital combustion study (6). The *Federal Register* entry also contained a request for comment on the adequacy of the EPA's current definition of infectious wastes, potential risks from exposure, the role of the federal government in infectious waste management, and the appropriateness of exemptions for small-quantity generators. The infectious waste tracking system was noted as a means to reduce the potential of improper disposal of these wastes.

Medical-Waste Tracking

Improperly disposed wastes became an effective visual symbol of the nation's exacerbated solid-waste management problem. Further public concern focused on the risk of spreading the AIDS virus by indiscriminate disposal of contaminated syringes and other medical materials. The U.S. Congress reacted with the passage of the Medical Waste Tracking Act of 1988 (MWTA), PL 100-582 (9).

MWTA was a semivoluntary, 2-year pilot demonstration program (5) that amended the Solid Waste Disposal Act by adding Subtitle J. The act was originally written to apply to facilities that generate more than 50 lb of medical waste monthly in New York, New Jersey, Connecticut, and states along the Great Lakes. Unless they formally opt out of the program, these states had to provide written, uniform documentation in a chain-of-custody manner to track waste storage and disposal. Other states could be included in the program on petition by the governor of the state. The act provided compliance orders and substantial criminal and civil penalties to enforce its provisions for participating states.

MWTA Section 3 defined medical waste as "solid wastes generated in the diagnosis and treatment, or immunization of human beings or animals, in research pertaining thereto, or in the production or testing of biologicals" (10). Like previous EPA guidance, the act did not include hazardous wastes identified or listed under Subtitle C. The act also excluded household wastes, typically commercially available products, as defined under Subtitle C (11). Ten types of medical wastes were covered under the program (Table 49-3).

EPA regulations implementing MWTA were published in the *Federal Registers* of March 24, June 2, and August 24, 1989 (6,12,13). Whereas the March 24 entry described the demonstration program, the later entries noted changes in states covered by MWTA. Each of the Great Lakes states formally opted out of the program. The governor of Louisiana and the mayor of Washington, D.C., petitioned for inclusion but later requested deletion. The state of Louisiana had prepared its own regulations; the mayor of Washington, D.C., had reevaluated the ability of the city to implement the program before the second year of demonstration. Authorities in Rhode Island and Puerto Rico petitioned for and were granted inclusion in the program.

TABLE 49-3. Medical Waste Tracking Act application

1. Cultures and stocks of infectious agents, vaccines
2. Human tissues and organs
3. Blood and blood products
4. Needles, sharps, syringes, glass, blades
5. Wastes that contact blood of dialysis patients
6. Biological waste or discarded equipment that contacts blood or excretions, or secretions from humans or animals isolated secondary to communicable disease

The following items if they contact infectious agents:

7. Autopsy and surgical waste
8. Discarded equipment
9. Laboratory waste
10. Animal carcasses and bedding

At the conclusion of the demonstration program, Section 11008 of MWTA required the EPA to make a final report to the U.S. Congress on a range of topics, including types and sizes of generators, potential risks, costs associated with proper and improper waste management, changes in practices attributable to the program, effectiveness of treatment methods, existing controls and the potential for waste reduction, and the appropriateness of penalties for noncompliance. The demonstration program concluded in 1992.

The MWTA represented a first federal legislative effort to control infectious and medical wastes. Speakers at a hearing before the U.S. House of Representatives on July 25, 1989, testified of the need for a national, long-term solution to the problem of medical wastes. The usefulness of the demonstration program was questioned (8). Some speakers called for federal regulations, whereas others recommended a federal requirement for states to adopt permitting programs based on a federal model. It was reported that 22 states were already upgrading or enacting new programs to control medical wastes.

The U.S. General Accounting Office was preparing a report discussing findings of a medical-waste study conducted in a number of states (9). The U.S. General Accounting Office report was expected to confirm that states were taking a stronger role in medical and infectious waste management. Extensive problems were observed at federal facilities during the study. The study also found that hospital incinerators, often outdated and inefficient, may be unable to comply when EPA's regulations for these treatment and disposal units become effective. The U.S. General Accounting Office's effort did not report on the extent of the public health problem posed by infectious wastes.

In May 1990, the EPA released its first interim report to the U.S. Congress, *Medical Waste Management in the United States* (10–13). The report was generated as part of the requirements of MWTA. The EPA estimated that one-half million tons of "regulated medical wastes" were generated by 375,000 facilities. Most of these wastes (77%) are generated by hospitals. The EPA also characterized the wastes by types and described the range of management practices observed. The EPA could not readily define the impact of medical-waste handling and disposal on public health and the environment. Instead, the EPA proposed a detailed assessment coordinated with the Agency for Toxic Substances and Disease Registry. Such a study would be required, according to the EPA, before identifying the scope of a nationwide regulatory program to track medical-waste generation and disposal. Nevertheless, the scope of nationwide regulations is likely to include certain uniform labeling requirements, according to the report.

On June 25, 1995, the EPA removed portions of federal regulations that were no longer in effect, including 40 *CFR* Part 259 "Standards for the Tracking and Management of Medical Waste." Nonetheless, the EPA held seminars for facilities and operators as a follow-up to the information compiled through the MWTA. The seminars were available to facilities or operators that needed assistance in managing medical wastes, including air pollution control options, operator information, developing waste management plans, and selecting appropriate waste management options. Information from these seminars can be obtained through the EPA web site (http://www.epa.gov) or ordered as EPA document numbers (625/4-91/030).

Finally, entities seeking to control medical wastes eventually face the clouded line between RCRA-regulated hazardous wastes, MWTA medical wastes, and other environmental regulations. First, health care facilities have traditionally generated small quantities of hazardous wastes (between 100 and 1,000 kg per month) (4). Hazardous wastes generated include waste solvents, such as xylenes and acetones, and metal-containing wastes, such as mercury and silver solutions. Waste streams listed in RCRA regulations or that exhibit one of four hazardous-waste characteristics must be stored, treated, disposed of, or recycled in accordance with RCRA standards, regardless of their medical-waste status (5).

MEDICAL-WASTE INCINERATION

Incineration is the current method of disposal. However, incinerators with inadequate controls may produce emissions subject to air quality control laws. Generators may also be constrained in their treatment, storage, or disposal methods as a result of the EPA's plans to increase controls over disposal of treated medical wastes in sanitary landfills.

Medical-waste generators must know enough about their waste streams to segregate solid, medical, toxic, and hazardous components and handle them in accordance with all of the rules that may apply. Although rules controlling medical wastes may be fragmented and weak, public and legislative interest in the future of medical-waste management is likely to ensure that increased federal controls are instituted.

Special concerns regarding medical-waste incineration revolve around the nature of the plastics, the amount of paper products, moisture content, and metal content. Incineration reduces waste volume by approximately 90% and produces ash as a by-product. For 1,000 lb of medical waste incinerated, 200 lb of ash is produced (14).

Previous characterization of hospital medical waste has revealed the following approximate composition by weight (15):

Paper, 65%
Plastics, 30%
Moisture, 10%
Other, 5%

The plastic content of medical waste contributes to the load of chlorinated chemical emissions from incineration processes. Previous estimates of the plastic content of medical wastes have been approximately 30% (16,17). Plastics most commonly found in medical waste include:

Polyethylene
Polystyrene
Latex
Polyurethane
Polypropylene
Polyvinylchloride

Plastics containing varying amounts of nitrogen, sulfur, and chlorine, in addition to carbon, hydrogen, and oxygen:

	Polyethylene (Wt %)	Polyvinylchloride (Wt %)	Polyurethane (Wt %)
Nitrogen	0.06	0.08	5.98
Sulfur	0.03	0.14	0.02
Chlorine	Trace	45.32	2.42

Special concerns regarding medical wastes are radioactive wastes not segregated from bulk medical wastes, the presence of cytotoxic drugs, and metals.

By-Products of Incineration

Typical pollutants produced by hospital waste incineration can be characterized according to the size, efficiency, and temperature of the incinerator. Data available for large air-controlled incinerators in the United States and Canada reveal the following emission contaminants (Table 49-4):

Trace metals
Polycyclic organics
Low-molecular-weight organics
Acidic gases
Particulates
Carbon monoxide
Pathogenic organisms

By-products of incineration are related to the efficiency of the combustion process as well as the chemical nature of the medical wastes being incinerated. Time, temperature, turbulence, and dwell time are critical variables for proper incineration. The EPA currently recommends a 2-second dwell time for biomedical waste. Most available incinerator emission data come from larger hospital-controlled air incinerators. Most hospital incinerators have a 1-second dwell time and cannot meet the requirement. Incineration temperatures must be between 1,000° and 1,200°C (1,800° to 2,400°F) to destroy dioxins, furans, and antineoplastic agents.

ACID GASES

Acid gases consist mainly of hydrochloric acid, sulfur dioxide, and nitrogen dioxides. Chlorine is present in plastics found in syringes and other disposable products commonly used in med-

TABLE 49-4. The individual contaminants that can be expected to be present in medical waste incineration emissions

Trace metals	Low-molecular-weight organics
Arsenic	Ethane
Cadmium	Ethylene
Chromium	Propane
Iron	Trichlorotrifluoroethane
Manganese	Trichloroethylene
Lead	Tetrachloroethylene
Nickel	Propylene
Mercury	Acidic gases
Zinc	Sulfur dioxide
Vanadium	Hydrochloric acid
Selenium	Nitrogen oxides
Molybdenum	Hydrofluoric acid
Polycyclic organics	Others
Dioxins	Particulates
Furans	Carbon monoxide
	Pathogens
	Low-level radioactive

ical environments. Reacting with hydrogen during the combustion process, hydrochloric acid is formed. Hydrogen sources in medical waste include paper, plastics, and rubber and latex products, as well as any biological fluids and moisture. The high hydrogen content of medical wastes, along with the ready availability of chlorine from plastics, makes the generation of hydrochloric acid from incineration processes the predominant acid gas. Studies have reported that up to 65% of chlorine in medical waste is converted to HCl during combustion (17).

Sulfur present in medical waste is oxidized to SO_2 during incineration. The rate of production is proportional to the sulfur content. Because of the presence of high HCl content in emissions and the fact that HCl is a stronger acid, most alkaline compounds bind first with HCl, thus allowing for SO_2 to remain as an emission contaminant.

Nitrogen oxides formed during incineration of medical waste predominantly consist of NO. Oxidation of NO to NO_2 is limited in the combustion process. Most of the nitrogen oxides are formed in the combustion air via reaction of molecular nitrogen with oxygen.

TRACE METALS

Trace metal emission quantity is directly proportional to the amount of metal introduced into the incineration process. Sources include needles, surgical instruments, and other sharp objects. Plastics made of polyvinyl chloride contain cadmium. Inks on paper and wrappers contain lead, chromium, and cadmium. Metals may be deposited on particulates emitted from the incineration process. This is termed *fine particle enrichment*. Metals have been found predominantly in the respirable particulate fraction of incineration processes. Less particulate enrichment occurs at higher incineration temperatures. Other metals found in emissions are arsenic, manganese, nickel, mercury, antimony, selenium, tin, zinc, molybdenum, and vanadium. Controlling temperature and particulate size reduces metal enrichment of particulates that can be inhaled.

PARTICULATES

Particulates are produced by the incomplete combustion of wastes and entrapment of noncombustible items in emission gases. Sources of particulates include inorganic compounds, ash, and organometallics. Particulate emissions are largely inorganic compounds and are inorganic salts of metals and oxides. Up to 50% of these compounds are soluble in water. Water-soluble particulates are mainly sulfate salts of sodium, phosphorus, calcium, zinc, and ammonium. Insoluble particulates consist mainly of oxides, silica, and phosphate salts of aluminum, silica, calcium, lead, zinc, and iron. The fuel used in the incineration process itself can contribute to the particulate matter emitted. Large organic molecules can be formed in pyrolysis that contain an inorganic nucleus. As the residence time in the incineration process increases along with the temperature, particulate size decreases along with the volume of particulates emitted.

ORGANICS

Sources include the medical waste as well as the incinerator fuel used in the pyrolysis process. Waste emits water and organics as it is being heated during combustion. Volatile organic compounds escaping from the waste mass are pyrolyzed above the mass in the process. An efficient thermal process results in a high degree of CO_2 and water from the combustion of medical-waste organics.

DIOXINS AND FURANS

Data indicate that the formation of polychlorodibenzodioxins and polychlorodibenzofurans is related to the efficiency of the combustion process, as well as to the chlorine content of plastics being incinerated. Increased temperature and increased efficiency reduce the production of these compounds. The source of these polychlorinated organic compounds is largely the plastics found in medical wastes. Because the predominant content of medical waste appears to be plastics, these contaminants become a major by-product of incineration and must be specifically addressed in risk management. A low chlorine content in medical plastics helps to significantly reduce the dioxin and furan content of incinerator emissions. If the health facilities were to use plastics composed of polyethylene and polystyrene in place of polyvinyl chloride, the dioxin and furan pyrolysis by-products would be greatly reduced.

Dioxin and furan emissions can thus be controlled and reduced by creating optimal incineration conditions, controlling the oxidizing environment of incineration, and controlling the chlorine content of plastics incinerated.

OTHER ORGANICS

Intermediate organic compounds are products formed in the combustion of medical wastes, including chlorobenzenes and chlorophenols. These by-products are most likely intermediates in the production of polychlorinated biphenyls.

Low-molecular-weight organics are products of an incomplete combustion. Emissions of these compounds can be controlled by time, temperature, and turbulence factors in the incineration process.

CARBON MONOXIDE

A product of incomplete combustion, carbon monoxide emissions are regulated by state and federal standards.

RADIOACTIVES

Medical waste may contain some low-level radioactive contamination. Not all facilities in the survey segregate radioactive waste from other medical waste. This issue can best be addressed and risk minimized by requiring separation of radioactive waste from other waste at the site of origin.

Standards for Incinerators

In September 1997, the EPA promulgated standards for incinerators of hospital, medical, or infectious wastes under the Clean Air Act Amendments of 1990. They were effective March 1998 and apply to new and existing stationary units (40 *CFR* 60, subpart Ce, with amendments to subparts Cb–Cd). The rules used the definition of medical wastes found in the former MWTA to determine which incinerators should be included. The act's definition did not fully address all three terms, but it was deemed the most appropriate available for medical wastes. Hospital wastes are discards generated at a hospital. The definition of hospital wastes does not include human or animal corpses or parts that are intended for interment. Infectious agents are any organism, such as a virus or bacteria, that is capable of being communicated by invasion and multiplication in body tissues and capable of causing disease or adverse health impacts in humans (18).

Incinerators covered by this rule are required to reduce emissions of certain air pollutants to the maximum level that the EPA has determined to be achievable. Air pollutants covered by the rule include particulate matter, sulfur dioxide, hydrogen chloride, oxides of nitrogen, carbon monoxide, lead, cadmium, mercury, dioxins and dibenzofurans, and fugitive ash emissions. The EPA states that some of these pollutants are carcinogens and, at sufficient concentrations, can cause toxic effects after exposure (21). According to the EPA's web site, the rule is intended to reduce mercury emissions by 94% and dioxins by 95%. Other pollutants are expected to be reduced by 75% to 98%. When complying with these standards, facilities can consider the cost, energy requirements, and any non–air quality health and environmental impacts. The EPA requires states to develop plans to implement and enforce these emissions requirements for incinerators.

Facilities constructed after September 15, 1997, are required to prepare an analysis of the impacts of their facility on the surrounding area. The analysis must consider practicable air quality control alternatives that minimize potential risks to health and environment. The siting study involves a detailed list of data submittal requirements, identified in 40 *CFR* 60.58c. Controls for mercury and dioxins are specifically addressed at this time.

In addition to setting standards, the rule also includes a number of management requirements. Operators must have certain qualifications and complete a specified training program. Facilities are prohibited from operations unless the detailed criteria for training and qualifications are met. Waste management plans must be prepared to separate certain components of solid waste from the health care waste stream to reduce the amount of toxic emissions from incinerated waste (18). In 40 *CFR* 60.17, the EPA references and incorporates a publication by the American Hospital Association entitled *An Ounce of Prevention: Waste Reduction Strategies for Health Care Facilities*. The publication must be considered when preparing a waste management plan for covered incinerators. Finally, compliance and performance testing are required in 40 *CFR* 56c to determine whether the incinerator is functioning in accordance with EPA standards.

CONCLUSION

Health care facilities must comply with the EPA's RCRA regulations regarding medical waste. Also, hospitals must comply with the standards set by accrediting bodies regarding biohazards, infection control, and infectious waste management. Ambulatory health care facilities and smaller generators must also comply with RCRA regulations. Included in standards are protection of personnel, visitors, and patients; establishment of policy and procedures for waste management; personnel training; and review and evaluation of policy.

REFERENCES

1. Council on Scientific Affairs. Infectious medical wastes. *JAMA* 1989;262:1669–1671.
2. Rutala W. Management of infectious waste by U.S. hospitals. *JAMA* 1989;262:1635–1640.
3. Fleming D. Hazard control for infectious agents. *Occup Med* 1987;2:499–511.
4. Resource Conservation and Recovery Act, PL 94-580, 1976.
5. US Code of Federal Regulations, Title 40, Parts 261–265. Washington: US Government Printing Office, 1999.
6. US Environmental Protection Agency. Hazardous waste management system: identification and listing of hazardous waste; infectious waste management. *Federal Register* 1988:53(106).
7. US Environmental Protection Agency. Guide for infectious waste management (PB86-199130). Washington: National Technical Information Service, 1986.
8. Slavik N. Report on the proceedings of the EPA infectious management meeting. Washington: Environmental Protection Agency Headquarters, 1987.
9. US Congress. Medical Waste Tracking Act of 1988, PL 100-582, 1988.
10. Raupp J. *Health care institutions: the Resource Conservation and Recovery Act (RCRA)—the teenage years*. Scottsdale, AZ: Arizona Bar Association, 1989.
11. US Environmental Protection Agency. Standards for the tracking and management of medical waste. *Federal Register* 1989:54:12326.
12. US Environmental Protection Agency. Standards for the tracking and management of medical waste. *Federal Register* 1989:54:35189.
13. US Environmental Protection Agency, Office of Solid Waste. Medical waste management in the United States. First interim report to Congress, May 1990.
14. Brunner C, Brown C. Hospital waste disposal by incineration. *JAPCA* 1988;38:1297–1309.
15. Jenkins A. Evaluation test on a hospital refuse incinerator at St. Agnes Medical Center, Fresno, California. Fresno, CA: California Air Resource Board, Stationary Source Division, 1987.
16. Murnyak G, Gazenich D. Chlorine emissions from a medical waste incinerator. *J Environ Health* 1982;45:83–85.
17. Kaiser E, Carotti A. Municipal incineration of refuse with two percent and four percent additions of four plastics: polyethylene, polyurethane, polystyrene, and polyvinyl chloride. Proceedings of the 1972 National Incinerator Conference, June 1972.
18. US Environmental Protection Agency. Standards of performance for new stationary sources and emission guidelines for existing sources: hospital/medical/infectious waste incinerators. *Federal Register* 1997;62.

CHAPTER 50

Toxic Hazards of Firefighters and Combustion Toxicology

Linda H. Morse, Deborah J. Owen, Gary Fujimoto, and Robert J. Harrison

Fire fighting is hazardous work because it is performed in an uncontrollable environment. Fire, heat, and risk of explosion and structure collapse are dangers not amenable to an industrial safety specialist's careful quantification and control. Although dozens of studies exist of chemical exposures and their effects in stationary hazardous environments, such as oil refineries and auto body painting operations, there have been few actual studies of the environment that firefighters face during a working fire, the dose of toxins that enter the body from that environment, or the effects of the chemicals. Firefighter exposure to toxic chemicals occurs in four situations:

1. The traditional exposure to combustion and pyrolysis products in the course of fire fighting
2. Response to hazardous chemical spills and releases
3. Providing backup to law enforcement agencies during arrest of drug dealers and illegal drug laboratories
4. Exposure at the fire station to diesel exhaust, cigarette smoke, and cleaning supplies

Firefighters also have significant biological, physical, stress- and shift-work, and ergonomic hazards. Typical urban firefighters spend far more time in medical response and rescue work than actual fire fighting, exposing them to a variety of biological hazards. These include blood-borne pathogens, such as hepatitis B and C and human immunodeficiency virus; airborne microbes, including tuberculosis and meningococcus; Lyme disease from ticks; and potentially a wide variety of other agents. The "universal precaution" protection equipment (i.e., gloves, masks, and goggles) required by the Occupational Safety and Health Administration (OSHA) is frequently inadequate in roadside emergency accident situations.

A recognized problem is noise exposure documented to occur not only from sirens but also from engines and radios. Studies have documented significant noise-induced high-frequency hearing loss in professional firefighters from these exposures.

Psychophysiologic hazards of stress and shift work in firefighters is commonly assumed, although the effects are not well understood. Most urban professional firefighters work approximately ten 24-hour shifts per month. Many also work additional day jobs in between, placing them at risk for sleep deprivation and resultant accidents in an already dangerous occupation. Anxiety and depression from traumatic incidents are recognized as serious problems, with most departments now providing some type of postincident counseling for firefighters. The stress of constantly being awakened by alarms is one of the assumed causes of coronary artery disease in firefighters, although little scientific support exists.

TABLE 50-1. Incapacitating and irritant toxic by-products of fires

Toxins	Sources	Toxic effects
Hydrogen cyanide	From combustion of wool, silk, polyacrylonitrile, nylon, polyurethane, and paper	Binds to cytochrome oxidase and interferes with cellular respiration
Nitrogen dioxide and other oxides of nitrogen	Produced in small quantities from fabrics and in larger quantities cellulose nitrate and celluloid	Pulmonary irritant capable of causing immediate death as well as delayed injury to lungs
Hydrogen chloride	From combustion of polyvinyl chloride and some fire-retardant materials containing bromine	Respiratory irritants
Sulfur dioxide	From materials containing sulfur	An irritant, intolerable well below lethal concentrations
Isocyanates	From polyurethanes and polymers	Potent respiratory irritants and sensitizers are believed to be the major irritants in smoke produced by isocyanate-based urethanes
Acrolein	From pyrolysis of polyolefins, cellulose and wood-containing materials at temperatures approximately 400°C	Strong respiratory irritant

Finally, ergonomic problems are significant. The firefighters' workplace moves constantly, and work tools consist of turnout gear and self-contained breathing apparatuses (SCBA) weighing 50 lb, which are hot in addition to heavy. Hazardous materials team level A protection involves full-body encapsulation in chemical protective clothing that, at moderate work levels, can elevate core body temperatures within 15 minutes.

FIRE TOXICOLOGY

Firefighters are exposed to an array of chemical hazards in the fire environment. The chemical constituent of what is generally referred to as *smoke* is a complex mixture of compounds that are constantly evolving during a fire. These products of combustion vary depending on the material undergoing thermal degradation, the temperature of the fire, and the oxygen content.

The rapid proliferation of synthetic materials in homes and industries, such as plastics and high-technology materials, has changed the fire environment considerably since the 1970s. Hazardous materials incidents involving large quantities of toxic chemicals also often involve fires, leading to vaporization of toxic liquids and chemical mixtures.

Fires involving natural material, such as wood, paper, cotton, and other natural fibers, as well as fires involving plant materials, all produce massive quantities of carbon dioxide (CO_2) and carbon monoxide (CO). CO_2 acts as a simple asphyxiant by displacing oxygen and leads to hypoxemic states. CO acts as a chemical asphyxiant with an affinity for hemoglobin more than 200 times greater than for oxygen. The carboxyhemoglobin generated is incapable of transporting oxygen and inhibits the release of oxygen from oxyhemoglobin with a shift to the left in the oxygen dissociation curve. The half-life of carboxyhemoglobin at room air is 4 to 6 hours. This is shortened to 1 hour with 100% O_2 and 20 minutes at 3 atmospheres pressure (hyperbaric oxygen).

Burning wood and wood products produce various aldehydes, such as acetaldehyde, formaldehyde, and acrolein, which are irritants to the mucous membranes and lungs. Of these, acrolein is one of the most irritating and composes up to 8% of all aldehydes from vehicular and residential fires (1,2). Common household items, such as silk and wool, produce ammonia and cyanide (Table 50-1).

Other compounds produced during combustion and pyrolysis include various polycyclic aromatic hydrocarbons (PAHs) and volatile organic compounds. PAHs generated during combustion have irritant and carcinogenic potential. One of the best-known carcinogens is benzo(a)pyrene, although a variety of other carcinogenic PAHs are frequently present in the fire environment (3,4).

Although the combustion of synthetic products, such as plastics and rubber, is known to generate similar toxic products, certain products can be expected to liberate specific materials when burned. Polyvinyl chloride, a plastic compound used in household plumbing and various other products used in many pieces of furniture, is produced from isocyanates, which generate cyanide compounds along with hydrochloric acid. Neoprene on pyrolysis produces sulfur dioxide and hydrogen sulfide (5).

Teflon, which is a fluorinated synthetic, can cause polymer fume fever on overheating (generally a problem encountered during production) and can produce hydrofluoric acid as can other fluorinated compounds. Hydrofluoric acid is particularly important because of the toxic properties associated with the highly electronegative fluoride ion that attacks enzymes and cell membranes leading to necrotic ulcerated tissue. Although levels leading to systemic toxicity are not usually found in the fire environments, irritant effects from hydrofluoric acid vapor can be anticipated to affect the eyes and mucous membranes during fires.

Because of the unstable and unpredictable nature of the fire environment and the massive technical difficulties involved, very few studies have examined chemical exposures in the firefighters' environment, and those have been limited to a few common combustion products: CO_2, CO, HCN, HCl, NO_2 aldehydes, particulates, and halogenated solvents (2). The most exhaustive study used a portable vacuum cleaner to draw air through a variety of collection tubes inserted in the sides of the machine that hung from the waist of firefighters. Successful samples were obtained in 24 fires (6). All fires had one or more samples for the following classes of chemicals: acids, acid gases, gases, aromatic hydrocarbons, particulates, aldehydes, oxyhydrocarbons, furans, nitrohydrocarbons, metals, and halogenated hydrocarbons (Table 50-2). Of these, six known carcinogens were found: acrylonitrile, arsenic, benzene, benzopyrene, chromium, and vinyl chloride (Table 50-3).

TABLE 50-2. Samples and classes of chemicals obtained in 24 San Francisco fires

Samples	Classes of chemicals
Acids	Hydrogen chloride, hydrogen cyanide
Acid gases	Nitrogen dioxide
Gases	Carbon monoxide, carbon dioxide
Aromatic hydrocarbons	Benzene, toluene, xylene, aliphatics, ethane, propane
Particulates	Benzpyrene
Aldehydes	Acrolein benzaldehyde, formaldehyde
Oxyhydrocarbons	Phenol, alcohols, methylethyl ketone
Nitrohydrocarbons	Pyridine, acrylonitrile, benzonitrile
Metals	Lead, chromium, arsenic
Halogenated hydrocarbons	Chloroethane, bromomethane

TABLE 50-3. Carcinogens in samples from 24 San Francisco fires

Carcinogen (prevalence)	Target tissues
Acrylonitrile (3/24)	Stomach, colon, brain, lung
Arsenic (8/24)	Lung, skin
Benzene (12/24)	Hematopoietic system
Benzpyrene (24/24)	Skin, lung, brain
Chromium (10/24)	Lung
Vinyl chloride (8/24)	Lung, brain, liver

PULMONARY INJURY AND RESPIRATORY ABNORMALITIES

The inhalation of products of combustion can produce a range of injuries to the airway, including irritation of the upper airway, laryngospasm, bronchospasm, and alveolar injury with pulmonary edema. Smoke contains sensory irritants in the vapor phase and the particulate phase. Toxic gases, such as chlorine, hydrochloric acid, hydrofluoric acid, and acrolein, can be easily inhaled by victims in fires. In addition, pulmonary insufficiency can be produced by the inhalation of particulate matter and soot that have toxic chemicals adhering to their surfaces (7–9). Individuals who are in a closed environment are at high risk for inhalation of these products of combustion.

Symptoms and signs of smoke inhalation include tachypnea, cough, stridor, shortness of breath, bronchial spasm, rales, chest pain, and chest tightness, as well as central nervous system signs of headache, confusion, dizziness, and coma. Individuals who inhale smoke may also show signs of singed nasal hairs, carbonaceous soot sputum, or soot in the oropharynx. Burns of the face may also be present, as well as edema of the upper airway above the epiglottis.

Victims of fire and inhalational injury from by-products of combustion should be evaluated with arterial blood gases, methemoglobin concentrations, chest x-rays, electrocardiogram, spirometry, and, if necessary, bronchoscopy. Upper airway damage can result from thermal injury or edema from toxic gases and other by-products of combustion. Injury to the lower airways is not from heat but is secondary to toxic gases, free radicals, and small particles that can penetrate to lower airways and alveolar surfaces, carrying toxic by-products of combustion. Symptoms of lower respiratory tract injury include shortness of breath and bronchospasm, manifested by hypoxemia seen in arterial blood gases.

Early pulmonary responses can be demonstrated in victims of a fire environment because of decrements in the ratio of one-second forced expiratory volume (FEV_1) and the forced vital capacity (FVC) (7,8). Unconscious victims found in a fire environment have a greater chance of having a lower airway injury, because they have lost their protective mechanism of breath-holding and laryngospasm. The presence of facial burns or soot in the upper airway is not an indication of lower airway injury. Superheated air is rapidly cooled before reaching the lower respiratory tract because of the efficient heat-exchanging mechanism of the oropharynx and the nasopharynx (8). An exception to this is the inhalation of hot steam that contains 4,000 times the heat capacity of superheated air and can produce heat injury to the lower lungs. Smoke and heat can cause upper airway injury and tracheobronchitis, which can lead to upper airway obstruction.

Radiographic manifestations of smoke inhalation may not be apparent on the first chest x-ray. Radiologic findings are generally nonspecific, and most of the findings appear within the first 24 hours after the injury. The results of the admission chest x-ray may be normal, because pathology may require hours to develop. Pulmonary infiltrates may require several hours to be recognizable on a chest x-ray. The abnormalities seen on the chest x-ray may include alveolar edema and perivascular and peribronchial infiltrates, as well as interstitial edema (7). The acute effects of fire fighting on pulmonary function have been studied and have shown significant changes in spirometry after exposure to smoke (10). Routine fire fighting has been shown to cause acute decrements in FEV_1 and FVC and is being associated with an increase in airway responsiveness (11,12).

HAZARDOUS MATERIALS INCIDENTS

Toxic chemical spills and leaks are familiar to almost every professional fire department in the United States. Indeed, the 1990s have witnessed the development of a distinct new suboccupation, hazardous materials teams, with training materials routinely incorporated into new firefighter education.

More than 100,000 chemicals are used in U.S. industrial operations daily, with almost 2,000 new ones added each year. OSHA safety standards for work week exposure exist for approximately 500 substances. Standards for toxicity testing in new chemicals have only been in place since 1976. The vast majority of the chemicals used in industrial operations were put into use before passage of that law. Whereas a number of the larger chemical companies have gone back and tested particularly suspect chemicals, rigorous analysis is still applied to few chemicals used in industrial operations. Increasing use and transport have led to a rapid rise in the number of hazardous materials spills and leaks. The fire service has always been responsible for handling these incidents. Kales et al. describe 2 years' medical surveillance of the 40 members of the Boston-area hazardous materials team who responded to 56 incidents involving a wide range of chemical exposures, including plastics, rubbers and acrylics, metals, chlorine, acids, ammonia, and ethylene oxide (13).

The Agency for Toxic Substances and Disease Registry has characterized the general classes of chemicals and their frequency of involvement in hazardous materials releases with and without victims (Table 50-4) (14).

TABLE 50-4. Chemicals, grouped by categories, released in all events and in events with victims, January 1, 1990, through December 31, 1991

Chemical category	All events		Events with victims		
	Frequency	(%)[a]	Frequency	(%)[b]	(%)[c]
Acids	224	(12)	65	(19)	(29)
Ammonias	243	(13)	55	(16)	(23)
Bases	61	(3)	23	(7)	(38)
Chlorine	46	(3)	16	(5)	(35)
Cyanides	15	(1)	6	(2)	(40)
Herbicides	343	(19)	37	(11)	(11)
Insecticides	66	(4)	24	(7)	(36)
Metals	147	(8)	18	(5)	(12)
Polychlorinated biphenyls	65	(4)	1	(0.3)	(2)
Unclassified	312	(17)	39	(11)	(13)
Volatile organic compounds	307	(17)	39	(17)	(19)

[a]Percentage of all events.
[b]Percentage of events with victims.
[c]Percentage of events with victims within chemical category.
From ref. 14, with permission.

ILLEGAL DRUG LABORATORIES

A very hazardous task of the fire department is provision of backup to Drug Enforcement Agencies and local police agencies during the capture and arrest of criminals producing illegal drugs. The growth of the industrial chemical industry has been matched by a similar spurt, particularly in the 1980s, in so-called designer drug production. Illegal drugs such as heroin, marijuana, and cocaine are produced from natural plants, although the production operation (particularly cocaine) may require the use of chemicals. However, since the days of lysergic acid diethylamide (LSD) in the 1960s, production of illegal synthetic drugs has grown dramatically. Most frequently, production of illegal synthetic drugs requires a small amount of space (e.g., motel room or rented apartment), minimal equipment, and some chemical knowledge. Awareness of the danger of these drug laboratories in late 1989 led to law enforcement agencies' requesting that a fire department hazardous materials team be standing by during the dramatic (and often violent) forced entry and arrest action. In these situations, firefighters have been required to help handle chemical booby traps in addition to chemical identification containment and disposal. Firefighters are also exposed when inadequate knowledge or carelessness on the producer's part leads to a fire, explosion, or toxic chemical leak. Chemicals can be left behind after the production operation is over, and the fire department may be called to identify and remove them.

FIRE STATIONS

Traditionally, fire stations have received little health and safety attention. Understanding of the hazards of passive cigarette smoke has led to a ban on smoking in many fire stations. Many fire stations were built in the 1950s and 1960s, and indoor air quality issues are being raised by firefighters concerned about inadequate heating, ventilation, and air-conditioning system functioning. Research into the effects of diesel exhaust has resulted in attempts to capture the diesel exhaust from the fire fighting apparatus and vent it outdoors instead of into firefighters' living quarters. Washing machines for turnout gear are being demanded so that turnout gear can be decontaminated immediately after service. Increasing awareness of infectious diseases has led to numerous incidents of overzealous use of cleaning agents in fire stations. These agents (usually commercial products), if used inappropriately in undiluted or unventilated ways, can lead to pulmonary, skin, and eye irritation, and lead to reactive airways–related health problems.

PERSONAL PROTECTIVE GEAR

Standard personal protective equipment or *turnout gear* consists of 50 to 65 lb of boots, pants, jacket, helmet, gloves, and SCBA. Wearing this equipment increases body heat, respiratory rate and depth, and heart rate, which can significantly affect intake and transport of chemicals. Until approximately 1980, firefighters were not encouraged and, in fact, were frequently discouraged from wearing their SCBAs during any but the worst fires. Most departments did not even supply SCBAs to all members until the mid-1970s. Currently, SCBAs are frequently not worn during the takedown or overhaul period after the active fire has been extinguished. Wet bandanas are the standard respiratory protective equipment provided to wild-lands firefighters.

First responders to chemical incidents are most frequently the closest station, equipped with only standard gear, which may provide little protection to chemicals that can damage or penetrate the skin. Hazardous materials team members are now better equipped with complete occlusive suits and SCBA, but the suits add significant heat stress to the body. Universal precautions, latex gloves, goggles, and face masks may work well in controlled hospital conditions, but they often dislodge or tear in field circumstances. Concern has also been raised about latex allergy and anaphylaxis.

MEDICAL APPROACH TO ACUTE EXPOSURES

Acute exposures are primarily inhalational. Risk factors and signs suggestive of inhalation injury include enclosed space fires, burning synthetic materials, steam exposure, altered mental status, chest pain, age older than 40 years, and loss of consciousness. Firefighters should be asked whether an SCBA was used, for how long, and whether there were any episodes of equipment failure, such as running out of air. Was there a prolonged period of overhaul (the cleanup period after the knockdown phase of fire extinguishing) when protective equipment was not being used? Did the firefighter require supplemental oxygen at the scene because of minor symptoms of fatigue or smoke inhalation? If the firefighter is unconscious or unable to provide a coherent history, other firefighters should be asked about how and where the injured worker was found.

The medical evaluation of the firefighter after an inhalation injury requires multiple considerations and potentially several levels of consultation. Studies have shown that the incidence of inhalation injury increases with extent of the burn in fire victims. When burns involve more than 70% body surface area, studies have shown that roughly two-thirds of these individuals have inhalation injuries (15). However, firefighters using protective equipment and SCBA should also be evaluated based on symptoms suggesting inhalation injury rather than percentage of skin surface burned, because of their protective equipment.

Once basic life support systems have been stabilized and a full assessment has been made for thermal skin burns, evaluation for inhalation injury should ensue. The signs and symptoms that should suggest inhalation problems include individuals with hoarseness, cough, or respiratory stridor who have a history of any type of exposure to the fire environment in which the individual was not using SCBA or in which such systems failed because of malfunction or depletion of oxygen. Such injuries can be delayed up to 24 hours before laryngeal edema develops. Other data that should be considered in this assessment include any degree of hypoxemia on arterial blood gas analysis, the presence of carboxyhemoglobinemia (correcting for smokers and extrapolating back to determine the initial level of carboxyhemoglobin based on the half-life of 4 to 6 hours on room air), and the presence of singed hair or burns involving the nasopharynx. Any suggestion of an inhalation injury should prompt a visual evaluation of the upper airways with fiberoptic laryngobronchoscopy. A high level of suspicion should be maintained, because many firefighters minimize their symptoms. Hospitalization with close observation should be considered if laryngeal edema is suspected, because prompt endotracheal intubation is required for these individuals.

Inhalation injury carries serious prognostic implications. In a large cohort study, patients with inhalation injuries had mortality rates of 29% compared to rates of 2% in those without. Inhalation injury was associated with hospital stays three times longer when present among burn victims (16). Hyperbaric oxygen is indicated for significant CO toxicity. Carboxyhemoglobin determinations should be specifically requested and performed with cooximetry, because manual spectrophotometry has led to erroneously elevated CO hemoglobin levels in clinical situations (17).

Other considerations after inhalation exposures include cyanide determinations because of the presence of hydrogen cyanide in many fire environments. Assessment of these individuals must be made cautiously, because the induction of methemoglobin (with amyl and sodium nitrate used in the cyanide antidote kit) may be relatively contraindicated if severe hypoxemia is present.

In situations involving the combustion of fluorinated materials resulting in the generation of hydrofluoric acid vapor, treatment can be directed toward the irritant effects on the eyes, mucous membranes, and lungs. This can be treated with 1% calcium gluconate by irrigation for ocular injuries or 2.5% calcium gluconate by nebulization for inhalation injuries.

It is always important to evaluate each incident for specific substances or chemical exposures, because toxic effects of these materials may mandate directed treatment or monitoring of target organ systems. This certainly applies to hazardous materials incidents or industrial fires involving large quantities of specific compounds or products.

In the setting of acute toxic exposures, field decontamination and stabilization should be undertaken before emergency department transport. Information from coworkers regarding type and route of exposure is valuable. Because of delayed and unknown effects, any parameters outside the ordinary should lead to observation. The evaluating clinician must deliberate carefully before returning a firefighter to duty. Residual, mild CO poisoning effects, which might be well tolerated by an otherwise healthy individual returning home, could pose a serious danger to the firefighter and to others if the firefighter was called out to handle another incident. The best approach is to be conservative and cautious.

CHRONIC EXPOSURES

Because of the uncontrolled occupational environment and the varying nature of exposures, only a few studies that have examined firefighter morbidity or mortality exist. Moreover, many of the existing studies are flawed because of changes in the work environment during the study period or because of the comparison of firefighters to the general population (i.e., the superhealthy worker effect). Another flaw occurs when state or local worker's compensation statistics are used in areas in which presumptions exist. In California, for example, under the state worker's compensation statute, heart trouble is presumed to be work-related in law enforcement and fire fighting positions because of occupational stress. The same is true for cancer and pulmonary problems for firefighters. All studies using worker's compensation data show a high rate of cardiac and pulmonary disease and cancer in firefighters as a result (not necessarily scientifically founded).

The best-designed studies use police (another superhealthy worker group) as a control. In these studies, an elevated rate of chronic respiratory disease mortality has been identified. Several studies on the acute effects of fire fighting on the lungs show significant abnormalities of pulmonary function and methacholine challenge test results after exposure, persisting beyond the temporal period expected for an acute irritant airway reaction. These results are biologically plausible, given the highly irritating nature of many of the chemicals in a fire environment and hazardous material release incidence.

Harrison et al. found an elevated rate of airway reactivity in wild-lands firefighters in California (18). The study was an elegant design, monitoring pre- and postshift FEV_1 and pre- and postseason methacholine challenge tests in 41 firefighters. Brundt-Rauf found acute pulmonary effects in firefighters, and Shepard confirmed this monitoring with pre- and postshift spirometry at a busy downtown San Francisco fire station, again finding statistically significant decrements in pulmonary function after fires (11,19). Other studies have mixed results, although Kales's work again shows accelerated loss of pulmonary function (12). Interestingly, evaluation of firefighters at the Kuwait oil fires after the Gulf War revealed no change in pulmonary function, even though these U.S. oil fire specialist teams were in smoke 24 hours a day, just as wild-land firefighters (*personal communication*, D. Owens). Kales et al. also studied biochemical abnormalities in the blood, evaluating renal and liver function and so forth in their study of 40 firefighters; they found few biochemical abnormalities, and none of the markers was associated with specific toxic exposures (12).

Mortality Studies of Firefighters

A number of epidemiologic studies exist in the literature that address occupational mortality of firefighters (20,21). Guidotti reviewed the literature and compared the data to the associations for disease cited by the Industrial Disease Standards Panel of Ontario (20).

Guidotti studied the conclusions on lung cancer from some studies and concluded that the overall evidence does not support a presumption of increased risk. Golden and colleagues also noted that the majority of the studies showed no statistically significant excess risk of lung cancer (21). Firth et al. calculated standardized incidence ratios for male workers in New Zealand and found that firefighters had increased risk of lung cancer, although the results were not statistically significant (22). Because exposures to known lung carcinogens occur in firefighters, continued surveillance through clinical epidemiologic studies is warranted.

Guidotti studied the risk of genitourinary cancers and concluded that an association exists with kidney, ureter, and bladder cancer (20). Golden and colleagues also noted an increased risk of bladder cancer in the majority of studies they reviewed (21). Moreover, they found that a majority of the studies they reviewed showed an increased risk of prostate cancer. Vena and Fiedler found a significant excess of mortality from bladder cancer in a cohort study of the firefighters in Buffalo, New York (23). Specifically, they found that firefighters who worked more than 40 years had almost a sixfold risk. Guidotti also showed an increased risk in bladder cancer 40 to 49 years after entry (24). Sama et al. studied standardized morbidity odds ratios (SMORs) and found a statistically significant elevation for bladder cancer (SMOR, 159; 95% confidence interval, 102–250) (25). Because specific toxicants known to cause bladder cancer are associated with firefighter exposures, it is important that medical professionals working with firefighters encourage them to be vigilant in their use of SCBA and other protective equipment.

Golden and colleagues demonstrated that most of the published epidemiologic studies reported an increased risk estimate for leukemia (21). They also noted that an increased risk estimate exists for non-Hodgkin's lymphoma. Heyer et al. reported an excess mortality from leukemia in Seattle firefighters who had worked for 30 or more years (26). Feuer and Rosenman studied the proportionate mortality ratios (PMRs) in firefighters in New Jersey and found an elevated PMR for leukemia (PMR, 2.76) compared to police (27). In a death certificate study by Figgs et al., a significant association for firefighters and non-Hodgkin's lymphoma was demonstrated (28). Burnett and colleagues examined death certificates from 27 states through the National Occupational Mortality Surveillance system (29). They found elevated PMRs for leukemia (PMR, 171; 95% confidence interval, 118–240) and non-Hodgkin's lymphoma (PMR = 161; 95% confidence interval, 112–224) for firefighters younger than age 65 years. Benzene is known to be associated with an increased risk for acute myelogenous leukemia and has been documented in significant concentrations at fire sites.

Guidotti reported an association with cancer of the colon and rectum, as did Golden et al. (20,21). Although no published surveillance data exist regarding colon cancer in firefighters, the Phoenix Fire Department has been providing flexible sigmoidoscopies for firefighters and retirees older than age 45 years for the past 8 years. Preliminary review of 250 individuals revealed a nearly 20% incidence of polyps. No frank malignancies were detected, and the data are incomplete regarding the number of adenomatous polyps identified (*personal communication*, Richard Gerkin, MD, Phoenix Fire Department). Medical personnel working with firefighters should advise them of the recommendations of such organizations as the American Cancer Society and the United States National Cancer Institute that endorse screening with flexible sigmoidoscopy every 3 to 5 years in individuals older than age 50 years. Aronson and colleagues studied the mortality in Toronto firefighters and observed an increased risk of brain and other nervous system tumors (SMR, 201; 95% confidence interval, 110–337) (30). Tornling et al. studied the mortality in Stockholm firefighters and found an increased risk of brain tumors (SMR, 279; 95% confidence interval, 91–651) (31). Demers and colleagues studied Seattle and Tacoma firefighters and found an excess number of brain tumors (SMR, 2.09; 95% confidence interval, 1.23–3.28) (32). Grimes et al. conducted a proportionate mortality study of Honolulu firefighters and found a significant increased risk of death from brain cancer (33).

Golden and colleagues summarized the studies regarding skin cancer risk and firefighters and found that the majority showed an excess (21). Burnett et al. calculated a PMR of 163 (95% confidence interval, 115–223) for malignant neoplasms of the skin (29). Feuer and Rosenman found a significant excess of skin cancers compared to the U.S. population (PMR, 2.70) but not to the police population (PMR, 1.35) (27). Sama et al. also demonstrated a significant elevation of risk for melanoma (SMOR, 292; 95% confidence interval, 170–503) compared to the state population but not to the police population (SMOR, 138; 95% confidence interval, 60–319) (25).

Firth and colleagues demonstrated an increased risk for laryngeal cancer in New Zealand firefighters (22). Muscat and Wynder were unable to demonstrate an increased risk of laryngeal cancer in a case-control study (34).

Overall, firefighters appear to be at increased risk for several types of cancers. Some firefighters do not use their SCBA in certain situations, such as overhauling or when responding to outdoor fires. By using this information to educate firefighters about their risks, it may be possible to increase their compliance in the use of protective equipment.

Melius reviewed the data on cardiovascular disease in firefighters and found mixed results regarding mortality incidence (35). He felt that two important factors that must be considered as contributing to the risk of cardiovascular disease in firefighters were CO exposure and the extreme physical demands that are required to do the job. Guidotti also noted the unconvincing results in the mortality literature but suggested that clinical studies support a risk of myocardial infarction when extreme exertion is combined with CO exposure (20).

MEDICAL SURVEILLANCE

Because of the limited number of biological monitoring tests available and the huge number of possible occupational chemical exposures in fire fighting, medical surveillance should be oriented toward potential target organs as well as fitness-for-duty issues.

Examinations are now recommended by the National Fire Protection Association and mandated for hazardous materials team members by the OSHA 1910:120 hazardous waste regulation (36).

The baseline evaluation should include the following:

1. Complete medical history, including past and current problems; allergies; immunizations; review of systems.
2. Complete occupational history, including all jobs since high school, hobbies, and moonlighting or secondary jobs. (Firefighters quite frequently have secondary jobs with significant chemical exposures, such as house painting, construction work, and chimney cleaning.)
3. Documentation of personal exposure record and significant past exposures. (Actual copies of the personal exposure record or incident report should be photocopied for the chart.)
4. Complete physical examination, including careful musculoskeletal and neurologic evaluation.
5. Documentation of screening pulmonary function tests FEV_1, FVC, FEV_1/FVC, and a curve with a peak expiratory flow rate on a calibrated spirometer by a qualified technician from a pulmonary function facility or one holding National Institute of Occupational Safety and Health certification. These baseline records are critical to the individual and department for worker's compensation and epidemiologic purposes.
6. Documentation of hearing ability and risk factors (past or present) for hearing loss. Screening audiometry studies show a high rate of noise-induced hearing loss among firefighters.
7. Chest x-ray for baseline and comparison later if hospitalized or needing treatment.
8. Electrocardiogram for baseline, and comparison later if hospitalized or needing treatment.
9. Laboratory tests:
   - Urinalysis.
   - Stool occult blood: Occult blood tests should be part of routine evaluation.
   - Complete blood count with differential: Firefighters are frequently in low-oxygen situations in which anemia would pose a hazard. Also, fire fighting is associated with an elevated rate of hematopoietic cancers.
   - Chemistry panel: baseline for kidney and liver function (which may be damaged by toxic exposures) and lifestyle issues (liver function tests for alcohol, cholesterol, and triglycerides for fats and cholesterol intake).
   - Red blood cell cholinesterase: In any department responding to pesticide spills, a baseline is necessary. Two of the seven classes of pesticides inhibit cholinesterase. Because the range of normal is wide, a significant decline may be misread as still within normal limits, unless a baseline value exists for comparison.
   - Fitness testing: Some form of strength, agility, and endurance evaluation is usually required by the department before hire and, with increasing frequency, on a periodic basis. A fitness physiology laboratory is best equipped to provide the range of services. Alternatively, an exercise pulmonary test plus strength and flexibility testing through a hospital or physical therapy group can suffice. Cardiac treadmill tests are not indicated, because a high rate of false-positives exists in healthy asymptomatic adults.

Periodic Medical Surveillance Evaluations

National Fire Protection Association 1500 mandates periodic medical surveillance examinations; OSHA requires yearly evaluation for hazardous materials team members.

Periodic surveillance includes the following (every year for hazardous material if the firefighter is older than age 40 years, every 2 years if younger than age 40 years):

1. Update of medical history (review of systems, new problems, and new medications)
2. Update of occupational health history (past year)
3. Updated exposure records
4. Complete physical examination
5. Spirometry
6. Audiometry
7. Stool occult blood
8. Lipid panel alternating with general chemistry
9. Repeat strength endurance and agility testing

Records from these evaluations should be available 24 hours a day, in case the firefighter is injured and baseline data are needed. A copy of pertinent information and laboratory test results should also be given to the firefighter at the time of each examination.

Before retirement or leaving the department, a repeated or updated complete evaluation should be performed. Records of all prior evaluations and this exit evaluation must be saved for 30 years after the last visit, as all firefighters are exposed to carcinogens.

All contact with the firefighter must remain confidential, except for those incidents involving worker's compensation. Personal lifestyle and job hazards overlap so much in the profession that the clinician must win the trust of the firefighter to practice good medicine. (This is also in accordance with the American College of Occupational Medicine Code of Ethics and civil court rulings since the mid-1980s.)

HEALTH PROMOTION

Explanation of good personal lifestyle and occupational health habits should prove the most rewarding part of a clinician's interaction with firefighters. The same drive and competitive edge that led them into the fire service proves useful in health promotion. Initiation of cholesterol testing can lead to a competition among the firefighters as to whose level is lowest.

SUMMARY

Medical involvement with the fire fighting service includes not only provision of acute and chronic injury and disease care, but also involvement with other issues related to firefighter health and safety. Better studies are needed regarding the effects of multiple chemical exposures on morbidity and mortality, fitness, and cardiopulmonary response.

REFERENCES

1. Lowery WT, Juarez L, Petty CS, Roberts B. Studies of toxic gas production during actual structural fires in the Dallas area. *J Forensic Sci* 1985;30(1):59–72.
2. Decker WJ, Garcia-Cantu A. Toxicology of fires: an emerging clinical concern. *Vet Hum Toxicol* 1986;28(5):431–433.
3. Lowery WR, Peterson J, Petty CS, Badgett JL. Free radical production from controlled low-energy fires: toxicity considers. *J Forensic Sci* 1985;30(1):73–85.
4. Hartzell GE, Packham SC, Switzer WG. Toxic products from fires. *Am Ind Hyg Assoc J* 1983;44(4):248–255.
5. Alarie Y. The toxicity of smoke from polymeric materials during thermal decomposition. *Annu Rev Pharmacol Toxicol* 1985;25:325–347.
6. Morse L, et al. Firefighter health and safety. In: Rom WN. *Environmental and occupational medicine*. Boston: Little, Brown and Company, 1992:1197–1204.
7. Cohen MA, Guzzardi LJ. Inhalation of products of combustion. *Ann Emerg Med* 1983;12:628–632.
8. Cahalane M, Demling RH. Early respiratory abnormalities from smoke inhalation. *JAMA* 1984;251(6):771–773.
9. Ghilarducci DP, Tjeerdema RS. Fate and effects of acrolein. *Rev Environ Contam Toxicol* 1995;144:95–146.
10. Texidor HS, Rubin E, Novick GS, Alonso DR. Smoke inhalation: radiologic manifestations. *Radiology* 1983;149:383–387.
11. Sheppard D, Distenfano S, Morse L, Becker C. Acute effects of routine firefighting on lung function. *Am J Ind Med* 1986;9:333–340.
12. Large AA, Owens GR, Hoffman, LA. The short-term effects of smoke exposure on the pulmonary function of firefighters. *Chest* 1990;97:806–809.
13. Kales SN, Polyhronopoulous GN, Christiani DC. Medical surveillance of hazardous materials response firefighters: a two year prospective study. *J Occup Environ Med* 1997;39(3):238–247.
14. Hall HI, Dhara VR, Kaye WE, Price-Green P. Surveillance of hazardous substances releases and related health effects. *Arch Environ Health* 1994;49(1):45–48.
15. Monafo WW. Initial management of burns. *N Engl J Med* 1996;335:1581–1586.
16. Saffle JR, Davis B, Williams P. Recent outcomes in the treatment of burn injury in the United States: a report from the American Burn Association Patient Registry. *J Burn Care Rehabil* 1995;16:219–232.
17. Kales SN, Pentiuc F, Christiani DC. Pseudoelevation of carboxyhemoglobin levels in firefighters. *J Occup Med* 1994;36(7):752–756.
18. Materna BL, Jones JR, Sutton PM, et al. Occupational exposures in California wildlands firefighting. *Am Ind Hyg Assoc J* 1992;53(1):69–76.
19. Brant-Rauf PW, Fallon LF, Tarantini T, Idema C, Andrews L. Health hazards of firefighters: exposure assessment. *Br J Ind Med* 1988;45:606–612.
20. Guidotti TL. Occupational mortality among firefighters: assessing the association. *J Occup Environ Med* 1995;37:1348–1356.
21. Golden AL, Markowitz SB, Landrigan PJ. The risk of cancer in firefighters. *Occup Med* 1995;10:803–820.
22. Firth HM, Cooke KR, Herbison GP. Male cancer incidence by occupation: New Zealand, 1972–1984. *Int J Epidemiol* 1996;25:14–21.
23. Vena JE, Fiedler RC. Mortality of a municipal-worker cohort: IV, firefighters. *Am J Ind Med* 1987;11:671–684.
24. Guidotti TL. Mortality of urban firefighters in Alberta, 1927–1987. *Am J Ind Med* 1993;23:921–940.
25. Sama SR, Martin TR, Davis LK, Kriebel D. Cancer incidence among Massachusetts firefighters, 1982–1986. *Am J Ind Med* 1990;18:47–54.
26. Heyer N, Weiss NS, Demers P, Rosenstock L. Cohort mortality study of Seattle fire fighters: 1945–1983. *Am J Ind Med* 1990;17:493–504.
27. Feuer E, Rosenman K. Mortality in police and firefighters in New Jersey. *Am J Ind Med* 1986;9:517–527.
28. Figgs LW, Dosemeci M, Blair A. United States non-Hodgkin's lymphoma surveillance by occupation 1984–1989: a twenty-four-state death certificate study. *Am J Ind Med* 1995;27:817–835.
29. Burnett CA, Halperin W, Lalich NR, Sestito JP. Mortality among firefighters: a 27-state survey. *Am J Ind Med* 1994;26:831–833.
30. Aronson KJ, Tomlinson GA, Smith L. Mortality among firefighters in metropolitan Toronto. *Am J Ind Med* 1994;26:89–101.
31. Tornling G, Gustavsson P, Hogstedt C. Morality and cancer incidence in Stockholm firefighters. *Am J Ind Med* 1994;25:219–228.
32. Demers PA, Heyer NJ, Rosenstock L. Mortality among firefighters from three northwestern United States cities. *Br J Ind Med* 1992;49:664–670.
33. Grimes G, Hirsch D, Borgeson D. Risk of death among Honolulu firefighters. *Hawaii Med J* 1991;50:82–85.
34. Muscat JE, Wynder EL. Diesel exhaust, diesel fumes, and laryngeal cancer. *Otolaryngol Head Neck Surg* 1995;112:437–440.
35. Melius JM. Cardiovascular disease among firefighters. *Occup Med* 1995;10:821–827.
36. National Fire Protection Association. *1,582 medical requirements for firefighters, 1992*. Quincy, MA: National Fire Protection Association, 1992.

CHAPTER 51

Hazards of Wastewater Treatment Facilities, Sewage, and Sludge

Allen G. Kraut, Gary R. Krieger,
John B. Sullivan, Jr., and Melissa Gonzales

WASTEWATER, SEWAGE, AND SLUDGE

Wastewater is the water supply of a community after it has been used or fouled. Wastewater is composed of human sewage and water disposed of in domestic, industrial, and commercial use

TABLE 51-1. Typical composition of untreated domestic wastewater

Contaminants	Unit	Concentration		
		Weak	Medium	Strong
Solids, total	mg/L	350	720	1,200
Dissolved, total	mg/L	250	500	850
Fixed	mg/L	145	300	525
Volatile	mg/L	105	200	325
Suspended solids	mg/L	100	220	350
Fixed	mg/L	20	55	75
Volatile	mg/L	80	165	275
Settleable solids	mL/L	5	10	20
Biochemical oxygen demand, mg/L: 5-day 20%C (BOD_5, 20°C)	mg/L	110	220	400
Total organic carbon	mg/L	80	160	290
Chemical oxygen demand	mg/L	250	500	1,000
Nitrogen (total as N)	mg/L	20	40	85
Organic	mg/L	8	15	35
Free ammonia	mg/L	12	25	50
Nitrites	mg/L	0	0	0
Nitrates	mg/L	0	0	0
Phosphorus (total as P)	mg/L	4	8	15
Organic	mg/L	1	3	5
Inorganic	mg/L	3	5	10
Chlorides	mg/L	30	50	100
Sulfate	mg/L	20	30	50
Alkalinity (as $CaCO_3$)	mg/L	50	100	200
Grease	mg/L	50	100	150
Total coliform	No./100 mL	10^6–10^7	10^7–10^8	10^7–10^9
Volatile organic compounds	µg/L	<100	100–400	>400

Adapted from ref. 1, with permission.

for bathing, cooking, washing, and other activities that collect water streams in sewers or septic tanks (1).

The nature of wastewater depends on the collective streams. Wastewater contains suspended solids, inorganics, organic chemicals, biodegradable organic matter, pathogenic microorganisms, and metals (Table 51-1). Pathogenic microorganisms

TABLE 51-2. Types and numbers of microorganisms typically found in untreated domestic wastewater

Organism	Concentration number/mL
Total coliform	10^5–10^6
Fecal coliform	10^4–10^5
Fecal streptococci	10^3–10^4
Enterococci	10^2–10^3
Shigella	Present
Salmonella	10^0–10^2
Pseudomonas aeruginosa	10^1–10^2
Clostridium perfringens	10^1–10^3
Mycobacterium tuberculosis	Present
Protozoan cysts	10^1–10^3
Giardia cysts	10^1–10^2
Cryptosporidium cysts	10^0–10^2
Helminth ova	10^0–10^2
Enteric viruses	10^1–10^2

Adapted from ref. 1, with permission.

TABLE 51-3. Infectious agents potentially present in raw domestic wastewater

Bacteria
- *Escherichia coli* (enteropathogenic)
- *Legionella pneumophila*
- *Leptospira* (150 spp.)
- *Salmonella typhi*
- *Salmonella* (~1,700 spp.)
- *Shigella* (4 spp.)
- *Vibrio cholerae*
- *Yersinia enterocolitica*

Viruses
- Adenovirus (31 types)
- Enteroviruses (67 types—e.g., polio, echo, and coxsackieviruses)
- Hepatitis A
- Norwalk agent
- Reovirus
- Rotavirus

Protozoa
- *Balantidium coli*
- *Cryptosporidium*
- *Entamoeba histolytica*
- *Giardia lamblia*

Helminths
- *Ascaris lumbricoides*
- *Enterobius vermicularis*
- *Fasciola hepatica*
- *Hymenolepis nana*
- *Taenia saginata*
- *Taenia solium*
- *Trichuris trichiura*

Adapted from ref. 1, with permission.

and indicator pathogens are found in high concentrations per gram of raw sewage (Tables 51-2, 51-3). If allowed to accumulate and sit, untreated wastewater produces malodorous emissions as a result of decomposition of organic material.

The characteristics of wastewater have changed in the United States, with an increasing number of organic chemicals, such as pesticides, phenol, and chlorinated solvents, being added yearly. Concern over toxic volatile organic chemicals and release of odors has led to further regulation of treated wastewater.

The amount of biological and organic material present in wastewater determines the extent of treatment required at wastewater facilities and can be determined by three methods: (a) biochemical oxygen demand (BOD), (b) chemical oxygen demand, and (c) total organic carbon (1,2). The 5-day BOD (BOD_5) is a measurement of dissolved oxygen used by microorganisms in the oxidation of organic matter. BOD results are used to determine the quantity of oxygen required to biologically stabilize the organic material present, to determine the size of waste treatment facilities, to measure efficiency of treatment, and to determine compliance with wastewater discharge permits. Chemical oxygen demand measures the content of organic matter of wastewater. An oxidizing agent, such as potassium dichromate, is used to determine the oxygen equivalent of organic material present. Total organic carbon is applicable to small concentrations of organic material and can be rapidly performed.

Odors in domestic wastewater are caused by gases produced by decomposition of organic material or by chemicals added to wastewater. Hydrogen sulfide is the most characteristic chemical causing such odors and is produced by anaerobic microorganisms (Table 51-4).

Sludge is the biosolid produced during sewage treatment and contains between 0.25% and 12% solids, with the remainder

TABLE 51-4. Odorous compounds associated with untreated wastewater

Odorous compound	Chemical formula	Odor, quality	Odor threshold (ppm)	
			Detection	Recognition
Amines	$CH_{34}NH_2$, $(CH_3)_3H$	Fishy	None	—
Ammonia	NH_3	Ammoniacal	17	37
Chlorine	Cl_2	Pungent, irritant (mucous membranes)	0.080	0.314
Diamines	$NH_2(CH_2)_4NH_2$, $NH_2(CH_2)_5NH_2$	Decayed flesh	—	—
Dimethyl sulfide	$(CH_3)_2S$	Cabbagelike	0.001	0.001
Diphenyl sulfide	$(C_6H_5)_2SH$	Cabbagelike	0.0001	0.0021
Hydrogen sulfide	H_2S	Rotten eggs	<0.00021	0.00047
Indole	C_8H_7N	Fecal odor	0.0001	—
Mercaptans (e.g., methyl and ethyl)	CH_3SH, $CH_3(CH_2)SH$	Decayed cabbage	0.0003, 0.0005	0.001, 0.001
Mercaptans (e.g., *T* = butyl and crotyl)	$(CH_3)_3CSH$, $CH_3(CH_2)_3SH$	Skunk	—	—
Methyl amine	CH_3NH_2	Fishy or ammoniacal	4.7	—
Organic sulfides	$(CH_3)_2S$, $(C6H_5)_2S$	Rotten cabbage	—	—
Skatole	C_9H_9N	Fecal matter	0.001	0.019

Adapted from ref. 1, with permission.

being water (1). Sludge biosolids are by-products of the physical treatment, biological treatment, and precipitation of suspended solids in sewage and wastewater by chemicals in the wastewater treatment process. The typical composition and characteristics of sludge are shown in Table 51-5. Sludge contains health hazards consisting of pathogenic microorganisms, metals, organic chemicals, nitrates, and ammonia similar to sludge, but more concentrated depending on stage of treatment (Table 51-6). Sludge biosolids are divided into primary sludge and secondary sludge that differ in densities of pathogenic and indicator microorganisms (Tables 51-7, 51-8). Primary sludges are produced during the first phase of physical treatment of sewage and wastewater. Secondary sludge is the product of biological treatment of wastewater.

Sludge contains a higher content of pathogenic microorganisms than is present in raw sewage because of the concentrating of the treatment methods. Settling of larger microorganisms, such as helminths and adsorption of viruses onto biosolids, occurs during sludge formation, making sludge a potentially more hazardous waste because sewage microorganisms are more concentrated in sludge during treatment.

WASTEWATER TREATMENT PROCESS

Sewage is a mixture of liquids and solids of domestic and industrial origin that varies in composition from sewer to sewer and from hour to hour. Sewage collects through a system of sewer pipes—ranging from 20 cm to 3.5 m in diameter—that terminates in wastewater facilities (3).

Modern wastewater and sewage treatment facilities are designed to reduce the overall pollutants' organic content and pathogen content of wastewater streams before the treated water is discharged back into the environment. Untreated sewage and wastewater—with its high organic content—promotes microbial growth with consumption of its available oxygen content. Thus, sewage is relatively anaerobic, and when it contaminates water bodies it causes oxygen depletion, which produces

TABLE 51-5. Typical chemical composition and properties of untreated and digested sludge

Item	Untreated primary sludge		Digested primary sludge		Activated sludge, range
	Range	Typical	Range	Typical	
Total dry solids (TS), %	2–8	5	6–12	10	0.83–1.16
Volatile solids (% of TS)	60–80	65	30–60	40	59–88
Grease and fats (% of TS)					
Ether soluble	6–30	—	5–20	18	—
Ether extract	7–35	—	—	—	5–12
Protein (% of TS)	20–30	25	15–20	18	32–41
Nitrogen (N, % of TS)	1.5–4.0	2.5	1.6–6.0	3	2.4–5.0
Phosphorus (P_2O_5, % of TS)	0.8–2.8	1.6	1.5–4.0	2.5	2.8–11.0
Potash (K_2O, % of TS)	0–1	0.4	0–3	1	0.05–0.07
Cellulose (% of TS)	8–15	10	8–15	10	—
Iron (not as sulfide)	2–4	2.5	3–8	4	—
Silica ($SiOl_{122}$, % of TS) 15.0–20.0	—	10–20	—	—	—
pH	5–8	6	6.5–7.5	7	6.5–8.0
Alkalinity (mg/L as $CaCO_3$)	500–1,500	600	2,500–3,500	3,000	580–1,100
Organic acids (mg/L as HAc)	200–2,000	500	100–600	200	1,100–1,700
Energy content, BTU/lb	10,000–12,500	11,000	4,000–6,000	5,000	8,000–10,000

BTU, British thermal unit.
Adapted from ref. 1, with permission.

TABLE 51-6. Characteristics of biosolids and sludge produced during wastewater treatment

Biosolids or sludge	Description
Screenings	Screenings include all types of organic materials large enough to be removed on bar racks. The organic content varies, depending on the nature of the system and the season of the year.
Grit	Grit is usually made of the heavier inorganic solids that settle with relatively high velocities. Depending on the operating conditions, grit may also contain significant amounts of organic matter, especially fats and grease.
Scum/grease	Scum consists of the floatable materials skimmed from the surface of primary and secondary settling tanks. Scum may contain grease, vegetable and mineral oils, animal fats, waxes, soaps, food wastes, vegetable and fruit skins, hair, paper and cotton, cigarette tips, plastic materials, condoms, grit particles, and similar materials. The specific gravity of scum is less than 1.0 and usually around 0.95.
Primary sludge	Sludge from primary settling tanks is usually gray and slimy and, in most cases, has an extremely offensive odor. Primary sludge can be readily digested under suitable conditions of operation.
Sludge from chemical precipitation	Sludge from chemical precipitation with metal salts is usually dark in color, although its surface may be red if it contains much iron. Lime sludge is grayish brown. The odor of chemical sludge may be objectionable, but it is not as bad as primary sludge. Although chemical sludge is somewhat slimy, the hydrate of iron or aluminum in it makes it gelatinous. If the sludge is left in the tank, it undergoes decomposition similar to primary sludge, but at a slower rate. Substantial quantities of gas may be given off and the sludge density increased by long residence times in storage.
Activated sludge	Activated sludge generally has a brownish, flocculent appearance. If the color is dark, the sludge may be approaching a septic condition. If the color is lighter than usual, there may have been underaeration with a tendency for the solids to settle slowly. Sludge in good condition has an inoffensive earthy odor. The sludge tends to become septic rapidly and then has a disagreeable odor of putrefaction. Activated sludge digests readily alone or when mixed with primary sludge.
Trickling-filter sludge	Humus sludge from trickling filters is brownish, flocculent, and relatively inoffensive when fresh. It generally undergoes decomposition more slowly than other undigested sludges. When trickling-filter sludge contains many worms, it may become inoffensive quickly. Trickling-filter sludge digests readily.
Digested sludge (aerobic)	Aerobically digested sludge is brown to dark brown and has a flocculent appearance. The odor of aerobically digested sludge is not offensive; it is often characterized as musty. Well-digested aerobic sludge dewaters easily on drying beds.
Digested sludge (anaerobic)	Anaerobically digested sludge is dark brown to black and contains an exceptionally large quantity of gas. When thoroughly digested, it is not offensive, its odor being relatively faint and that of hot tar, burned rubber, or sealing wax. When drawn off onto porous beds in thin layers, the solids first are carried to the surface by the entrained gases, leaving a sheet of comparatively clear water. The water drains off rapidly and allows the solids to sink down slowly onto the bed. As the sludge dries, the gases escape, leaving a well-cracked surface with an odor resembling that of garden loam.
Composted sludge	Composted sludge is usually dark brown to black, but the color may vary if bulking agents—such as recycled compost or wood chips—have been used in the composting process. The odor of well-composted sludge is inoffensive and resembles that of commercial garden-type soil conditioners.
Septage	Sludge from septic tanks is black. Unless the sludge is well digested by long storage, it is offensive because of the hydrogen sulfide and other gases that it gives off. The sludge can be dried on porous beds if spread out in thin layers, but objectionable odors can be expected while it is draining unless it is well digested.

Adapted from ref. 1, with permission.

severe effects on aquatic life. To avoid such problems, sewage treatment facilities use three processes to treat wastewater (1,2):

- *Primary treatment*: A physical process involving separation of larger debris and solids followed by sedimentation
- *Secondary treatment*: A biological degradation using microorganisms to decompose suspended biosolids and reduce pathogen content
- *Tertiary treatment*: A physiochemical process that removes suspended solids and turbidity

TABLE 51-7. Densities of microbial pathogens and indicators in primary sludges

Type	Organism	Density (number per gram of dry weight)
Virus	Various enteric viruses	10^2–10^4
	Bacteriophages	10^5
Bacteria	Total coliforms	10^8–10^9
	Fecal coliforms	10^7–10^8
	Fecal streptococci	10^6–10^7
	Salmonella sp.	10^2–10^3
	Clostridium sp.	10^6
	Mycobacterium tuberculosis	10^6
Protozoa	*Giardia* sp.	10^2–10^3
Helminths	*Ascaris* sp.	10^2–10^3
	Trichuris vulpis	10^2
	Toxocara sp.	10^1–10^2

Adapted with permission from Gerba CP. Pathogens in the environment. In: Pepper I, Gerba C, Brusseau M, eds. *Pollution science*. San Diego: Academic Press, 1996.

TABLE 51-8. Densities of pathogenic and indicator microbial species in secondary sludge biosolids

Type	Organism	Density (number per gram of dry weight)
Virus	Various enteric viruses	3×10^2
Bacteria	Total coliforms	7×10^8
	Fecal coliforms	8×10^7
	Fecal streptococci	2×10^2
	Salmonella sp.	9×10^2
Protozoa	*Giardia* sp.	10^2–10^3
Helminths	*Ascaris* sp.	1×10^3
	Trichuris vulpis†	$<10^2$
	Toxocara sp.	3×10^2

Adapted with permission from Gerba CP. Pathogens in the environment. In: Pepper I, Gerba C, Brusseau M, eds. *Pollution science*. San Diego: Academic Press, 1996.

Primary Treatment

Primary (physical) treatment is the first step in wastewater treatment and involves passage of sewage through screens to remove large debris and physically separate large solids (1,2). A moving screen then separates smaller solids. Wastewater is then diverted to large grit tanks, in which heavier wastes, sand, and gravel settle to the bottom. From here, waste streams go into a sedimentation tank or clarifier. Materials lighter than water float to the top and are skimmed off. Partially purified sewage or primary sludge flows over the edge of the tank for further processing. In some cases, sewage is collected in septic tanks and transferred to treatment facilities for purification. Side streams from this primary treatment phase can contain high concentrations of total suspended solids, which can release odorous gases.

Colloidal particles, such as proteins and oily emulsions that do not naturally separate from sewage, may be coagulated by the addition of inorganic compounds, such as aluminum sulfate. Under appropriate pH conditions, the positive metal ions in the coagulant materials neutralize the negative charge of the colloid, promoting coagulation. Particles larger than 0.4 μm in diameter precipitate from solution (3).

Secondary Treatment

Secondary treatment refers to the biodegradation of sewage by aerobic or anaerobic bacteria. In this stage, remaining solids are decomposed, and the overall concentration of pathogenic microorganisms is reduced. To accomplish this, the stream is treated in either a sewage lagoon, filter bed, or aeration tank (1,2). Aerobic processes are divided into those that do and those that do not actively provide oxygen or air to the sludge.

A trickling filter bed is composed of stones or corrugated plastic sheets through which the wastewater drips (1,2). The wastewater effluent is pumped through a sweeping overhead sprayer or perforated pipes onto this bed. Microorganisms in this trickling bed degrade organic material in the water aerobically.

Aeration tank digestion, or activated sludge process, is the most common method used in the United States for secondary treatment (1,2). Aeration tanks are constructed of reinforced concrete and are open to the air. They are circular or rectangular and have inlet and outlet valves. Effluent from primary treatment processes is pumped into a tank with a slurry rich in bacteria. This slurry is called *activated sludge*. Air or oxygen is then pumped in to encourage bacterial growth, thus decomposing organic material present. After this, the sludge goes into a settling tank in which water is siphoned off the top and sludge is removed from the bottom (1,2). This secondary sludge is then removed.

Sewage lagoons are called *oxidation* or *stabilization ponds*. These serve as natural, shallow degradation ponds. Decomposition occurs over 1 to 4 weeks by natural means. The three categories of oxidation ponds are the following (1,2):

- *Aerobic pond*: A shallow lagoon or pond in which natural mixing occurs. The shallow levels allow light and oxygen to penetrate. Detention time is 3 to 5 days.
- *Aerated pond*: A pond 1 to 2 m deep that is mechanically mixed for aeration for less than 10 days.
- *Anaerobic pond*: A pond 1 to 10 m in depth that serves as pretreatment for wastes with high BOD, such as those containing heavy concentration of protein and suspended solids.

Activated aerobic processes accelerate sewage metabolism by providing additional oxygen to promote bacteria digestive activity. Under appropriate conditions, this process has a purification efficiency of greater than 95%. When oxygen is not actively added to the system, sewage remains in stabilization ponds, usually 3 to 4 m deep, for between 10 and 60 days. This process is used when sufficient space is available and the underlying soil can retain toxic effluents, preventing groundwater contamination.

Anaerobic sewage treatment takes place in closed steel digesters and is temperature dependent. Anaerobic treatment is less efficient than the aerobic processes but can provide methane as an energy source for the plant. This method is used to treat activated sludge or effluents from industries such as sugar processing, in which the amount of oxygen necessary to degrade sewage makes aerobic processes impractical (1–3).

In aerobic and anaerobic treatments, sewage must be examined by trained individuals to ensure that conditions are appropriate for waste degradation. Important considerations include the presence of adequate amounts of nitrogen, phosphorus, and trace elements; the absence of toxic metals; and optimal temperature and pH. The last step in secondary treatment is a disinfection process to remove residual bacteria. Protozoa and enteric viruses can survive many disinfectant chemicals. Ultraviolet light disinfection is being used more commonly than chlorine for this last step.

Settled sludge is then collected for concentration and disposal. Sludge materials can contain a variety of metal loads, which are regulated by the U.S. Environmental Protection Agency (EPA) before these materials can be applied to agricultural land (Table 51-9).

Tertiary Treatment

Tertiary sewage treatment is reserved for industrial sewage containing a higher percentage of nonbiodegradable contaminants. This treatment further reduces turbidity, suspended organics, nitrogen, phosphorus, metals, and pathogens. The process includes the steps of coagulation, filtration, activated carbon absorption of organic material, and further disinfection. A variety of chemical and physical reactions—most commonly precipitation, oxidation, and absorption—are used for additional purification. Ozone may be used in the process.

The precise mechanisms and compounds used are dependent on the pollutant in question. Lime is used in the precipitation of fluorides and phosphates in the fertilizer industry, cyanides are oxidized by adding sodium hypochlorite, and dyes may be adsorbed by using activated charcoal powder. Remain-

TABLE 51-9. Typical metal content in wastewater sludge

	Dry sludge, mg/kg	
Metal	Range	Median
Arsenic	1.1–230.0	10
Cadmium	1–3,410	10
Chromium	10–99,000	500
Cobalt	11.3–2,490.0	30
Copper	84–17,000	800
Iron	1,000–154,000	17,000
Lead	13–26,000	500
Manganese	32–9,870	260
Mercury	0.6–56.0	6
Molybdenum	0.1–214.0	4
Nickel	2–5,300	80
Selenium	1.7–17.2	5
Tin	2.6–329.0	14
Zinc	101–49,900	1,700

Adapted from ref. 1, with permission.

ing pathogens are killed by chlorination or oxygenation, allowing the purified water to be released or recycled (1–3). Tertiary treatment is necessary before discharge into bodies of water, for drinking water, or for irrigation purposes.

Sludge Processing

Accumulated sludge from sewage treatment is dewatered by sedimentation, centrifugal separation, or filtration to reduce bulk before deposition. This is called *thickening*. Sludge volume may also be reduced chemically, most commonly with ferric chloride or by bacterial digestion. Metal-containing sludge can be detoxified by treatment with sodium silicate, producing insoluble metal silicates. Treating organic content of sludge reduces odors and reduces pathogens. Sludge treatment involves the following general steps, from thickening to final disposal (1,2):

- *Thickening*: Water removal and volume reduction of sludge. Solids are allowed to settle by gravity or centrifugation.
- *Digestion*: A microbial process that stabilizes organic matter and reduces bacterial content because of high temperatures generated. Digestion can be aerobic or anaerobic. Anaerobic digestion occurs in covered tanks and produces methane gas. Aerobic digestion injects oxygen or air into open tanks. Aerobic digestion reduces odors but produces greater amounts of sludge for disposal.
- *Conditioning*: Involves further dewatering and thickening of sludge. Chemicals such as ferric chloride, alum, or lime are added to precipitate suspended particles.
- *Dewatering*: Involves pathogen destruction, odor control, gas production, and stabilizing organic matter. This is accomplished by air-drying, centrifugation, or vacuum filtration. Coagulation with alum, lime, or ferric chloride further removes pathogens and kills viruses.
- *Incineration and wet oxidation*: Volume and weight reduction, reduction of fuel requirements for incineration.
- *Final disposal*: Landfill, land application, incineration.

Sludge is disposed of in a number of ways, including incineration, ocean dumping, placement in a landfill, injection into deep wells, or use as fertilizer in agriculture (1,2). Odor-control problems associated with sludge-handling systems are significant. Several types of compounds produce sludge-related odor problems (see Table 51-4): (a) hydrogen sulfide (H_2S), which can be minimized if anaerobic conditions are controlled; (b) ammonia odors, which are generated at the pH levels typically encountered with lime stabilization of sludge; (c) ammonia releases, which happen during the alkaline, chemical-fixation process; (d) chlorine odors, which are residual from chlorine oxidation systems; and (e) organic acid odors.

HEALTH HAZARDS OF SEWAGE AND WASTEWATER TREATMENT

Sewage and wastewater treatment workers perform a number of tasks in a variety of conditions, ranging from monitoring electronic equipment in officelike settings to fixing pumps in confined spaces. Workers processing sewage and maintaining sewage systems are exposed to a variety of biological and toxicologic hazards. Although the standard focus of medical monitoring and surveillance may be on chemical and biological hazards, injury frequency rates for workers in wastewater facilities are typically higher than those for other industrial personnel; hence, typical safety issues should not be overlooked (4). Confined space entry, physical injury (including slips and falls), fires, electrical shock, and noise exposures are all safety and hygiene areas that can be sources of injuries.

Although no large-scale epidemiologic studies have been performed in sewage treatment workers, two small studies have revealed no increase in overall mortality (4,5). Both of these studies revealed some selected, but different, cancer sites with elevated standard mortality ratios. However, these increases were based on small numbers.

Many case reports and case series attest to the potential toxicologic hazards of sewage work (6–8). Several cases of death from toxic gases or asphyxiant gases in confined spaces are reported by the National Institute of Occupational Safety and Health and the Centers for Disease Control and Prevention (9).

Sewage workers have been shown to have more obstructive changes in lung function testing than controls (10). Although this has been postulated to be due to H_2S exposure (11), bacterial endotoxins may also have a role in this process (12).

The need for adequate biosafety procedures and protocols has been extensively evaluated by the American Industrial Hygiene Association in two monographs in 1995 and 1996 (13,14). A similar study that promoted guidelines for the assessment of bioaerosols was published by the American Conference of Government Industrial Hygienists in 1989 (14a). The Water Environment Federation has a three-volume manual, *Operation of Municipal Wastewater Treatment Plants*, which contains detailed occupational safety and health information and is probably the single best source of standard industry practice information (15).

Exposure health hazards occur through the following scenarios in wastewater treatment facilities:

- Exposure to chemicals necessary to process wastewater and sludge sewage
- Exposure to biologicals and pathogenic microorganisms
- Exposure to hazards produced by sewage and sludge decay
- Exposure to toxic wastes in the sewage or sludge
- Hazards of confined spaces

Hazards Related to Chemicals Used in the Treatment Process

Sewage treatment workers use more than 90 different chemical compounds in their work. Compounds routinely used include alkaline cleaners, organic solvents, disinfectants, chemicals for sewage treatment, alum, ferric chloride, ferric sulfate, ferrous sulfate, lime, laboratory reagents, paints, lubricants, hydraulic fluids, and pesticides (1).

Various organic solvent–based materials used in adhesives, cements, and cleaners can routinely cause skin and mucosal irritation and neurologic symptoms such as headache, lightheadedness, and fatigue. Some of these compounds also have specific organ toxicities.

A number of disinfectants—including alcohols, hydrogen peroxide, ammonia, liquid chlorine, ozone, and iodine—are used in wastewater facilities (Table 51-10). Workers must be warned that ammonia and chlorine should not be mixed, as pulmonary edema may result from inhalation of the resulting chloramines.

Aluminum sulfate alum and ferric chloride are chemicals commonly used in sewage treatment. Aluminum sulfate, a sewage coagulant, is irritating to the skin and mucous membranes and can produce sulfuric acid when mixed with water. Ferric chloride, a sludge dewatering agent, decomposes to hydrochloric acid in the presence of moisture or light. When either of these compounds is used, workers must wear protective equipment to avoid exposure to breakdown products.

A vast variety of laboratory chemicals including potassium iodide, potassium dichromate, and various acidic and basic

TABLE 51-10. Chemical applications in wastewater collection, treatment, and disposal

Application	Chemicals used[a]	Remarks
Collection		
Slime-growth control	Cl_2, H_2O_2	Control of fungi and slime-producing bacteria
Corrosion control (H_2S)	Cl_2, H_2O_2, O_3	Control brought about by destruction of H_2S in sewers
Corrosion control (H_2S)	$FeCl_3$	Control brought about by precipitation of H_2
Odor control	Cl_2, H_2O_2, O_3	Especially in pumping stations and long, flat sewers
Treatment		
Grease removal	Cl_2	Added before preaeration
BOD reduction	Cl_2, O_3	Oxidation of organic substances
pH control	KOH, $Ca(OH)_2$, NaOH	—
Ferrous sulfate oxidation	Cl_2[b]	Production of ferric sulfate and ferric chloride
Filter-ponding control	Cl_2	Residual at filter nozzles
Filter-fly control	Cl_2	Residual at filter nozzles, used during fly season
Sludge-bulking control	Cl_2, H_2O_2, O_3	Temporary control measure
Digester supernatant oxidation	Cl_2	—
Digester and Imhoff tank foaming control	Cl_2	—
Ammonia oxidation	Cl_2	Conversion of ammonia to nitrogen gas
Odor control	Cl_2, H_2O_2, O_3	—
Oxidation of refractory organic compounds	O_3	—
Disposal		
Bacterial reduction	Cl_2, H_2O_2, O_3	Plant effluent, overflows, and storm water
Odor control	Cl_2, H_2O_2, O_3	—

BOD, biochemical oxygen demand; H_2S, hydrogen sulfide.
[a] Cl_2, chlorine; H_2O_2, hydrogen peroxide; O_3, ozone; $FeCl_3$, ferric chloride; KOH, potassium hydroxide; $Ca(OH)_2$, calcium hydroxide; NaOH, sodium hydroxide.
[b] $6FeSO_4 \times 3Cl_2$ ø $2FeCl_3 + Fe_2(SO_4) + 42H_2O$.
Adapted with permission from Gerba CP. Pathogens in the environment. In: Pepper I, Gerba C, Brusseau M, eds. *Pollution science.* San Diego: Academic Press, 1996.

buffers are used to assess the efficiency of sewage processing. As the majority of persons performing laboratory testing have little or no formal training in chemistry, appropriate safety practices should be included in any testing instructions.

The largest classes of chemical compounds found in some sewage treatment plants are lubricants and hydraulic fluids. Used to service plant equipment, these compounds can cause dermatitis and folliculitis. Other potential hazardous exposures in treatment plants include pesticides used to control flies and rodents, mercury used in gauges and switches, and asbestos insulation materials.

Chlorine is used in wastewater treatment facilities for a wide variety of purposes, including disinfection, odor control, grease and scum removal, and chemical neutralization. Approximately 6% of U.S. chlorine production is used to chlorinate drinking water and sewage.

Workers potentially exposed to chlorine should be informed of its extreme toxicity and of the proper ways to handle this compound. Because of the risk of explosion, chlorine should not be added to sewage that contains ammonia, sulfur, or gasoline.

Full-face respirators are the minimal level of protection necessary for workers changing chlorine cylinders or tank car connections. Impermeable gloves and protective clothing must be worn when working with liquid chlorine. Emergency eyewash facilities should be located in areas in which chlorine is used or stored.

The odor threshold for chlorine is 0.02 ppm. Gaseous chlorine exposures cause nasal irritation at concentrations of 0.2 ppm and severe eye and nose irritation at concentrations between 1 and 3 ppm. Further symptoms include irritation of the throat, cough that may be productive of whitish or blood-tinged sputum, chest pain, and chest tightness. Systemic symptoms—including nausea, vomiting, dizziness, and stupor—may develop depending on the degree of exposure. Death due to pulmonary edema has occurred in overexposed individuals.

Acute restrictive and obstructive pulmonary function decrements have been reported in individuals surviving initial exposures. Most survivors, including those hospitalized, do not develop persistent pulmonary function abnormalities.

Workers overexposed to chlorine should be evaluated emergently. Those who remain symptomatic or show hypoxemia should be admitted to the hospital for observation and supportive treatment if necessary. Precautions should be taken against the possibility that workers may develop pulmonary toxicity a number of hours after the exposure has ended. Although steroids have been used and are thought by some to be helpful, clinical trials have been variable. Prophylactic antibiotics have not been proven to be efficacious in the management of chlorine toxicity.

Infectious Hazards

Pathogens in sewage and wastewater are numerous and include bacteria, viruses, protozoa (cryptosporidium, *Giardia*), and helminths (acanthamoeba) (see Tables 51-2; 51-3).

Disinfectants may not always kill protozoa present. Cryptosporidium is a one-celled protozoan parasite that is transmitted to humans by ingesting the oocysts excreted in the feces of infected mammals, primarily livestock. It has high resistance to disinfectants. In March and April 1993, an outbreak of cryptosporidium in the Milwaukee, Wisconsin, water supply system illustrated the vulnerability of conventionally treated public water supplies. In this episode, 400,000 people became ill with severe diarrhea after drinking cryptosporidium-contaminated water. In 1994, dozens of cases were reported in acquired immunodeficiency virus patients in Las Vegas, Nevada. However, some authors have pointed out that it is unclear whether there is an actual increase in the incidence of cryptosporidiosis and giardiasis or if the increased number of cases is the result of more sophisticated surveillance programs and improved detection methods (16). For example, polymerase chain reaction technology and the use of gene probes can now be used to detect a myriad of bacteria, viruses, and protozoa in various types of water sources (16).

Due to the increased public concern over parasitic contamination, an enhanced surface water treatment rule has been proposed in the United States, with similar efforts under way in Canada.

As opposed to the broader public health aspects of water treatment, there is an ongoing effort to evaluate wastewater treatment workers for possible overexposures to pathogens. An increased risk of self-limited diarrheal diseases has been seen in sewage treatment workers employed in various jurisdictions, especially in the first 5 years of employment.

AIRBORNE INFECTIOUS AGENTS AND BIOAEROSOLS

Sewage workers also have exposure to airborne infectious agents and endotoxin (16–18). These include bacteria, viruses, and fungi emitted from sewage and sludge sources in wastewater treatment plants that are pathogenic or can cause irritancy and allergic diseases. The study of bioaerosols spread around sewage treatment plants has shown high concentrations of various bacteria, mainly coliform, at different distances from emission sources. Microbiological analysis of colony-forming units per cubic meter (CFU/m^3) have demonstrated the presence of *Micrococcus, Streptococcus, Escherichia, Bacillus, Pseudomonas, Proteus, Staphylococcus*, and *Klebsiella*. Hemolytic pathogens found were *Streptococcus pyogenes, Streptococcus pneumoniae, Corynebacterium diphtheriae, Staphylococcus aureus, Streptococcus faecalis, Streptococcus agalactiae*, and *Corynebacterium pseudotuberculosis* (17,18). The numbers of CFUs found depended on the distance away from the emission source. For instance, the number of coliform bacteria varied approximately 2,000 CFU per m^3 near the emission source and approximately 300 CFU per m^3 at a distance of 25 m and 8 CFU per m^3 at 100 m (17,18). There was a rapid decrease in the number of coliform bacteria between 25 and 50 m from the source. It has been thought that coliform bacteria do not survive in the air long because of environmental factors such as ultraviolet radiation and temperatures. Studies have shown that coliform bacteria decrease rapidly as the distance from the source increases, whereas hemolytic bacteria are still found in the area at a distance of 100 m. Therefore, it is thought that hemolytic bacteria may be a reliable indicator of health hazards, more so than coliform bacteria.

Leptospirosis is a known occupational disease of sewer workers (19–21). Other parasitic infections, such as giardiasis, are also reported to be health hazards for sewage treatment workers (22). Although the general risk of hepatitis A infection in sewage treatment workers in North America is low, in certain locations and when community epidemics have occurred, occupational transmission has been noted (20,23). Exposure to human immunodeficiency virus (HIV) in wastewater treatment work has received careful evaluation. Casson et al. studied the survivability of HIV in raw wastewater and wastewater that had been subjected to a variety of treatments (24). Overall results demonstrated that infectious HIV was fairly stable in wastewater up to 12 hours but experienced a 2 to 3 log reduction in infectivity after 48 hours. To put this in perspective, under similar conditions, HIV survivability is considerably less than poliovirus by one to two orders of magnitude.

A variety of symptoms—particularly eye, ear, nose, and skin—have been reported in compost/sludge-exposed workers. The Water Environment Federation has extensively evaluated this problem for wastewater and sludge workers in a detailed 1991 publication (17).

The main strategies for worker protection are a combination of appropriate immunizations (e.g., hepatitis A and B for selected workers) and systems that promote good personal hygiene while at the workplace: (a) proper personal protective gear; (b) strict segregation of all eating/food service activities from plant operations; (c) work uniforms, daily changes, and adequate locker and shower facilities; and (d) close examination and follow-up of all cuts, abrasions, and skin rashes.

Bioaerosol exposures are not ubiquitous at a wastewater treatment facility but rather tend to be associated with sludge dewatering and indoor areas where aeration occurs. The Water Environment Federation recommends that periodic air monitoring should be performed; however, the difficulty in establishing this type of program should not be minimized, because the appropriate collection and interpretation of bioaerosol samples is not easy.

Toxic Hazards of Sewage and Sludge Decomposition

Sewer gases are a mixture of hydrogen sulfide, ammonia, methane, carbon dioxide, nitrogen, and other compounds (Table 51-11). Depending on their density, they may be located at the top or bottom of an enclosed space (Fig. 51-1) and create conditions immediately dangerous to life and health (9).

H_2S is a heavy gas that usually concentrates at the bottom of enclosed or confined spaces. Its characteristic rotten egg odor is easily detectable at levels of well less than 1 ppm. Olfactory paralysis or attenuation may occur at higher concentrations; hence, odor detection is not considered a reliable means of determining safe H_2S exposure levels.

H_2S is a potent irritant at higher concentrations and a toxic asphyxiant. Eye irritation may occur after several hours of exposure at the 10- to 20-ppm range. Higher levels of exposure produce keratoconjunctivitis or *gas eye*. Pulmonary edema may result from acute overexposures. H_2S reversibly inhibits the cytochrome oxidase system, blocking aerobic metabolism. At high concentrations, it directly produces toxic inhibition of the respiratory center, causing death from respiratory arrest. Treatment involves emergent response by cardiopulmonary resuscitation and induction of methemoglobinemia with intravenous nitrate. The induction of methemoglobinemia has been shown to be effective for cyanide poisoning, which has a similar mechanism of action as H_2S. However, only anecdotal cases are available. Hyperbaric oxygen treatment is proposed as an added treatment to induction of methemoglobinemia and has been anecdotally efficacious in some cases.

Low-level episodic H_2S exposures, which can be frequently detected by nearby residents of many wastewater treatment plants, represent more of a nuisance effect rather than an actual health impact. Low-level odors are usually assumed to be H_2S; however, EPA has identified 13 sulfur-bearing compounds, including H_2S, that have been identified at wastewater treatment facilities. The Water Environment Federation has extensively studied this issue and has an extensive chapter on this subject in volume II of their *Manual of Practice No. 11* for wastewater treatment plants (15).

Carbon monoxide may be introduced into sewer systems from fires or faulty equipment. Carbon monoxide's strong affinity for hemoglobin and its ability to shift the oxygen dissociation curve to the left make it a toxic asphyxiant gas. Carboxyhemoglobin concentrations of 10% can cause headache, and collapse and coma may occur at carboxyhemoglobin concentrations of 35% to 45%. Higher levels may lead to death.

Ammonia, a natural breakdown product of sewage, is irritating to the eyes and respiratory system. Because of its high solubility, ammonia first affects the upper airway. Respiratory distress follows exposures to levels greater than 100 ppm.

Methane—a highly flammable colorless, odorless gas—is produced by anaerobic digestion or the natural breakdown of sewage. Methane is lighter than air, and it collects at the top of

TABLE 51-11. Characteristics of common wastewater gases

Gas and chemical formula	Explosive limits (LEL/UEL)	OSHA[b] (ppm)	ACGIH (TLV)[a] TWA–STEL (ppm)		Common properties	Most common courses of exposure	Preferred method of testing
Chlorine Cl_2	Nonflammable	1 ceiling	0.5	1	Yellow-green color; pungent odor	Chlorine cylinders and feed line leaks	Chlorine detector
Hydrogen sulfide H_2S	4.3; 46	20 ceiling	10	15	Colorless, characteristic rotten egg odor at low levels	Sewer, sludge gas	H_2S detector, lead acetate paper and ampules
Ammonia NH_3	16; 25	50	25	35	Colorless, pungent	Sludge, sewer gas	Oxygen deficiency indicator, odor
Carbon monoxide CO	12.5; 74.2	50	25		Colorless, tasteless, odorless, nonirritating	Product of combustion	CO monitor
Carbon dioxide CO_2	Nonflammable	5,000	5,000	30,000	Colorless, odorless, acid taste at high levels	Sludge, sewer gas, combustion products	Oxygen deficiency indicator
Methane CH_4	5; 15	—	No limits providing sufficient oxygen available		Colorless, odorless, tasteless	Digestion of sludge	Combustible gas indicator, oxygen deficiency indicator
Nitrogen N_2	Nonflammable	—	—	—	Colorless, odorless, tasteless	Sewer and sludge gas	Oxygen deficiency indicator

ACGIH, American Conference of Government Industrial Hygienists; LEL/UEL, lower explosive limit/upper explosive limit; OSHA, Occupational Safety and Health Administration; ppm, parts per million; TLV, threshold limit value; TWA–STEL, time-weighted average, short-term exposure limit.
[a]ACGIH values, 1996. All values are 8-hour, time-weighted averages unless otherwise noted. Readers should consult the most current ACGIH values at www.acgih.org.
[b]Occupational Safety and Health Administration provisions, 29 *CFR* 1910.

enclosed spaces. A simple asphyxiant gas, it is only hazardous because of displacement of oxygen. Methane can spark or flame at air concentrations of 5%.

Carbon dioxide (CO_2) is colorless, odorless, and nonflammable. It concentrates at the bottom of enclosed spaces and at high concentrations may lead to oxygen deficiency. CO_2 narcosis may ensue after breathing air containing 7% to 10% CO_2 for a few minutes. Table 51-11 summarizes the characteristics of gases commonly encountered in the wastewater industry.

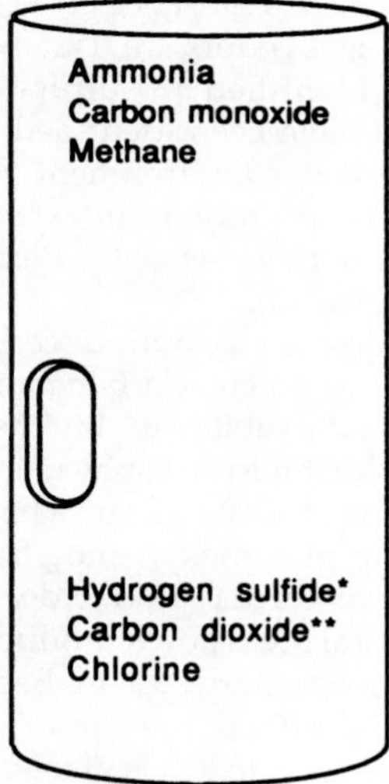

Figure 51-1. Location of highest concentrations of gases in a confined space, such as a container. *May rise in hot or humid conditions. **May rise if heated.

Workers may be exposed to mixtures of these gases when maintaining sludge digesters. Digester gas produced during anaerobic sludge digestion is composed primarily of methane (65%–70%) and CO_2 (25%–30%). Small amounts of nitrogen, hydrogen, oxygen, and hydrogen sulfide can also be present (15).

Hazards of Confined Spaces

Sewage systems and wastewater treatment facilities contain confined spaces that can be immediately dangerous to life and health because of lack of oxygen, explosive atmosphere, or toxic gases. Septic tanks are classic hazardous confined spaces. The three major hazards associated with working in confined spaces are oxygen deficiency, explosions, and the toxicities of gases present.

An oxygen concentration of 19.5% has been recommended as the lower limit, below which workers must use supplied air (9). The three prerequisites for explosion are (a) a combustible material, (b) air or another supporter of combustion, and (c) a source of ignition. Gases are combustible throughout a range of air mixtures, starting at the lower explosive limit, at which the minimal concentration of gas required to propagate a flame is available, and ending at the upper explosive limit, above which the concentration of oxygen no longer supports combustion. The lower and upper explosive limits are expressed in percent by volume in air at sea level.

Confined spaces have been classified into three classes based on their explosivity, oxygen level, and toxicity. Class A confined spaces are immediately dangerous to life; class B are dangerous but not immediately life threatening; and class C, although potentially hazardous, do not require modifications of work procedures (9). Classification is determined by the most hazardous existing condition.

Work procedures for confined spaces having A or B classifications require that before the initiation of work, trained individuals with fully charged self-contained breathing apparatus

TABLE 51-12. Types of confined spaces

Parameter	Class A	Class B	Class C
Characteristics	Immediately dangerous to life	Dangerous, but not immediately life-threatening	Potential hazard
Rescue procedures	At least two individuals fully equipped with life-support equipment. Maintenance of communication requires an additional person stationed within the confined space.	One individual fully equipped with life-support equipment, indirect visual or auditory communication with workers,	Standard procedures. Direct communication with workers outside the confined space.
Oxygen	≤10% or ≥25%	16.1%–19.4% 21.5%–24.9%	19.5%–21.4%
Explosivity toxicity	≥20% LEL Immediately dangerous to life and health	10%–19% LEL Greater than contamination level references in OSHA regulations	≤10% LEL Less than contamination level referenced in OSHA regulations

LEL, lower explosive limit; OSHA, Occupational Safety and Health Administration.
Adapted from ref. 9, with permission.

be present in case of emergency. Backup personnel should not enter confined spaces until adequate assistance has arrived. Failure to do so has led to a number of deaths (9) (Table 51-12).

The Centers for Disease Control and Prevention and the National Institute of Occupational Safety and Health review confined space injuries or death (9). Many are reported for sewers, wastewater facilities, and related confined spaces, such as pump stations, sewers, sludge tanks, septic tanks, digesters, manure pits, wells, filter tanks, water tanks, and recirculation pits (Table 51-13).

Hazards Related to Toxic Chemical Wastes in Sewage

Reports have identified toxic exposures to sewage workers after disposal of industrial wastes in sewage systems. Hexachlorocyclopentadiene was found to cause eye and throat irritation and headache in heavily exposed sewage treatment workers in Louisville, Kentucky (25). A mixture of waste compounds, consisting mostly of Stoddard's solvent and hydrochloric acid, caused a group of sewer repairmen to develop nausea, vomiting, dizziness, and eye and throat irritation (26).

Chronic effects of exposure to industrial compounds are less well documented in sewage treatment workers. Morgan et al. described increased risk of spontaneous abortion in the spouses of sewage treatment workers (27). Hexachlorocyclopentadiene was detected in urine of sewage treatment workers chronically exposed to sewage from a pesticide plant (28). Elevated levels of urinary mutagens have been reported in sewage treatment workers (29). Fertility, however, was not found to be affected in a study of workers chronically exposed to chemically contaminated sewer wastes (30).

TABLE 51-13. Selected confined space reported deaths

Location	IDLH condition	Work performed
Sewage digester: 2 deaths	Explosion from methane.	Sludge removal from bottom of 8-ft-deep tank.
Manure pit: 5 deaths	Methane and hydrogen sulfide (H_2S); asphyxiation.	Individuals entered to perform maintenance.
Sewer manhole: 1 death	Oxygen (O_2) deficiency 6% and methane 20%.	Worker entered to perform measurement.
Sewer manhole: 1 death	Oxygen-deficient atmosphere: O_2 5 ft down = 20.5% O_2 9 ft down = 14% O_2 13 ft down = 4%	Worker entered to install a plug.
Valve vault: 1 death	Oxygen deficiency; O_2 averaged 3.5%, nitrogen averaged 76.3%.	Entry of worker into underground vault 6 ft × 7 ft.
Digester: 2 deaths	Fire in enclosed space with 30-inch manhole entry.	6,400 cubic ft of enclosed space with 5-ft ceiling height.
Digester: 2 deaths	Drowning by raw sewage that flooded the enclosed space.	Workers repairing leaks and cleaning pump in 13 ft × 15 ft × 13 ft enclosed space.
Sewer line: 2 deaths	Carbon monoxide 2,000 ppm, O_2 level 19%.	Entry into newly constructed sewer line.
Clarifier tank: 1 death	Exposure to nitric acid, phosphoric acid, NCl, H_2SO_4, which was present in tank. Acids may have released toxic gases from sludge.	Workers entered tank to physically remove thick sludge. Tank had been previously descaled with chemicals.
Wastewater holding tank: 2 deaths	Workers poured 1.5 gallons H_2SO_4 plus action on organics to produce toxic gases.	Workers entered to unplug drain and replace elbow joint. Entry port was 18-in. diameter.
Sewage pump station: 4 deaths	Raw sewage and H_2S entered chamber from removed bolts of inspection valve.	Workers entered 50-ft-deep underground pumping station through metal shaft 3 ft in diameter. Underground space was 8 ft × 8 ft × 7 ft.
Sludge tank: 2 deaths	Sludge level 12 inches deep at bottom; H_2S 500 ppm.	Sampling of sludge in chamber 8 ft × 9 ft × 8 ft.

IDLH, immediately dangerous to life and health.
Adapted from ref. 9, with permission.

TABLE 51-14. Regulated pollutants in wastewater sludge

	Type of disposal or reuse				
Pollutant	Land application	Distribution and marketing	Monofilling	Surface disposal	Incineration
Aldrin	X	X			
Arsenic	X	X	X	X	X
Benzene			X	X	
Benzo(a)pyrene	X	X	X	X	
Beryllium					X
Bis(2-ethylhexylphthalate)			X	X	
Cadmium	X	X	X	X	X
Chlordane	X	X	X	X	
Chromium	X	X			X
Copper	X	X	X	X	
DDD/DDE/DDT		X	X	X	X
Dieldrin	X	X			
Dimethyl nitrosamine	X		X	X	
Heptachlor	X	X			
Hexachlorobenzene	X	X			
Hexachlorobutadiene	X	X			
Lead	X	X	X	X	X
Lindane	X	X	X	X	
Mercury	X	X	X	X	X
Molybdenum	X				
Nickel	X	X	X	X	X
PCB	X	X	X	X	
Selenium	X	X			
Toxaphene	X	X	X	X	
Trichloroethylene	X		X	X	
Total hydrocarbons					X
Zinc	X	X			

DDD, 1,1-dichloro-2,2-*bis*(p-chlorophenyl)ethane; PCB, polychlorinated biphenyls.
Adapted from ref. 1, with permission.

Multiple medical surveys of primary sewage treatment workers exposed to industrial sewage containing benzene, toluene, and other organic solvents revealed that significant numbers of workers reported acute central nervous system symptoms (lightheadedness, fatigue, increased sleep requirement, and headache) consistent with solvent or other chemical exposures (30a–30d).

TABLE 51-15. Typical waste compounds produced by commercial, industrial, and agricultural activities that have been classified as priority pollutants

Nonmetals	Ethylbenzene
Arsenic	Toluene
Selenium	Halogenated compounds
Metals	Chlorobenzene
Barium	Chloroethane
Cadmium	Dichloromethane
Chromium	Tetrachloroethene
Lead	Pesticides, herbicides, insecticides
Mercury	Endrin
Silver	Lindane
Organic compounds	Methoxychlor
Benzene	Toxaphene

Adapted from ref. 1, with permission.

Chemicals such as acids, which are added to wastes and may be used to descale tanks, can cause release of toxic gases from sludge. This can be lethal in confined spaces (31). Regulated pollutants contained in wastewater sludge are listed in Table 51-14, and priority pollutants are listed in Table 51-15.

PROTECTIVE MEASURES

Proper education and training are the most important aspects of any occupational safety and health program for sewage treatment workers to enable them to identify and limit potentially toxic exposures and conditions immediately dangerous to life and health (9,31).

Continuous air monitoring is used throughout wastewater facilities to warn of potential hazards. Stationary devices alarm at high levels of hydrogen sulfide and combustible gases and signal oxygen deficiency. Portable explosivity indicators used by workers before entering and during work in confined spaces measure relative combustibility compared with a suitable standard. Odor, particularly in sewage treatment plants, should not be relied on to detect toxic chemicals, as the smell of these materials may be masked by the presence of other compounds.

Individuals implementing occupational safety and health programs in sewage treatment plants should use the hierarchy of protection for other chemical exposures. Initial approaches to controlling exposures should include replacement of toxic compounds with less dangerous ones and engineering measures to lower exposures. Adequate sources of fresh air should be ensured wherever possible.

Because of the vast array of anticipated and unanticipated chemical exposures that can occur in treatment plants, workers must have access to and be trained in the use of respiratory protective equipment.

A large number of compounds used in sewage treatment plants are irritating to or absorbed through the skin. Protection from such exposure should be provided by chemical-resistant latex, neoprene, or rubber gloves. Shower and eyewash facilities should also be available in cases of emergency.

DISPOSAL OF TREATED SLUDGE AND WASTEWATER

The products of wastewater and sewage treatment are processed wastewater and processed sludge. The disposal of sludge materials has been the subject of intense scientific and EPA regulatory interest because of concerns related to residual pathogenic organisms and high metal loads (see Table 51-9). If these materials are applied to land near residential areas, high levels of public concern should be anticipated, and proactive educational information must be disseminated.

The majority of domestic sewage treatment or treated wastewater is released into natural bodies of water after secondary treatment. In some instances, when sewage has not been purified sufficiently, it is chlorinated or treated with ultraviolet light before release. Treated wastewater can be disposed of by discharge into bodies of water or by applying it to land-use purposes. Wastewater disposal practices include the following (1,2):

- *Low-rate irrigation*: A slow method of surface application to crops at a rate of 1.5 to 10.0 cm per week. This allows some wastewater to be taken up by crops while the remainder percolates through the soil. From 50% to 70% of water is taken up by crops. The remaining nitrogen and phosphorus present in this water must be appropriately managed to prevent groundwater pollution. Phosphorus is precipitated in the soil. Both are used by plants.
- *Overland flow*: Wastewater flows for a distance of 50 to 100 m along a 2% to 8% vegetated slope, usually grass covered. Water evaporates into the air and percolates through soil. Between 30% and 50% of phosphorus is retained in soil. Most of the nitrogen is released into the atmosphere by volatilization of ammonia and action of microbes. Remaining water is collected in a ditch at the base of the slope.
- *High-rate filtration or soil aquifer treatment*: Loading rates exceed 50 cm per week, and water percolates through soil for groundwater recharge. Soil must be finely textured for several meters in depth to remove viruses.
- *Wetland treatment*: Wetlands serve as an effective filtration for wastewater effluents. Artificially constructed wetlands can be used for this instead of natural wetlands. Wetlands are approximately a meter in depth or less and support aquatic life and vegetation. Vegetation helps filter water and provides a surface for bacteria attachment. The two types of constructed wetlands are (a) free-water system and (b) subsurface-flow system. The free-water system is like a natural wetland marsh. The subsurface-flow system is made up of channels with bottoms of sand or rock to support vegetation.

Sludge disposal methods include the following:

- *Land farming*: Land farming is the practice of sludge disposal onto agricultural land (1,2). The EPA issued regulations in 1993 requiring monitoring of pollutants from sludge used for land farming, such as lead and mercury, which can accumulate. The total metal load cannot be exceeded during the lifetime of farming (1,2). Land farming provides essential nutrients to agricultural land and reduces fertilizer need. Sludge contains nutrients of phosphorus, calcium, nitrogen, organic carbon, and magnesium, in addition to heavy metals that must be monitored as pollutants. Metals of concern are mercury, lead, arsenic, cadmium, nickel, chromium, and zinc. Sludge can contain organic chemicals such as pesticides, polyaromatic hydrocarbons, and solvents. Many of these are removed or degraded in the sludge treatment process. Sludge is high in nitrate content and ammonium. Nitrates can be leached from soil into groundwater, causing pollution. Water recharging an aquifer cannot exceed the EPA limit of nitrogen (NO_3^--N) of 10 mg per L.
- *Deep well injection*: This method disposes of sludge waste deep into the ground to minimize contact with humans. Waste with high concentrations of toxic compounds and wastes of large volume of liquid or slurry waste are chosen for this disposal method. Groundwater pollution can still occur from leakage and movement through soil to aquifers. Injection is usually into confining layers of rock to a depth of 200 to 4,500 meters.
- *Incineration*: Incineration of waste-containing toxic materials is closely regulated. Destruction of organic chemicals must exceed 99.99% (1,2). Incineration cannot be used for wastes with high water content, noncombustible solids, or those containing radioactive metals.
- *Immobilization*: Waste with high metal or radioactive content is immobilized or stabilized, such as with cement, before disposal. This prevents leaching and must meet the EPA's toxicity characteristics leaching procedure method (2). Wastes high in organic chemical content are not candidates for immobilization.
- *Discharge into bodies of water*: Liquid waste can be disposed of in large bodies of water if they meet certain criteria. A National Pollution Discharge Elimination System permit is required in the United States. The waste must meet water-quality standards of the EPA and be nonhazardous. Special permits are required for the discharge of wastes that exceed any limit.

LAND APPLICATION CONTROVERSIES

Despite considerable concern, the evidence for adverse health effects associated with wastewater or treated sludge applied for irrigation and fertilization purposes appears to be minimal (32–35). A 3-year prospective study involving application of treated sludge to farmland did not demonstrate any adverse health effects based on low rates and application. Similar results cannot be assumed with higher rates.

Another area of concern associated with sludge application is the problem of heavy metal loadings and accumulation of these metals in edible crops. Crops can take up metals that tend to accumulate in the roots and leaves (35). The fear is that direct ingestion of these crops would have an adverse effect on either humans or livestock. The uptake of sludge metals into crops is a complex scientific issue because soil properties—such as pH, redox, cation exchange capacity, and organic matter—can have a significant impact on metal uptake (35,36). Chaney has argued that it is possible to define a "no observed adverse effect level" quality sludge (36). This area continues to be actively researched and is the source of much controversy during public hearings and siting studies for land application of sludge-amended materials.

REFERENCES

1. Tchobanoglous G, Burton F. *Wastewater engineering: treatment, disposal, reuse*, 3rd ed. New York: McGraw-Hill, 1991.
2. Gerba C. Municipal waste and drinking water treatment. In: Pepper I, Gerba C, Brusseau M. *Pollution science*. New York: Academic Press, 1996.
3. Agamennome M. Waste water treatment and disposal. In: Parmeggiani L, ed. *Encyclopedia of occupational safety and health*. Geneva: International Labour Office, 1983.
4. Hadeed SJ. 1989 safety survey: injury rates drop to 15-year low. *Oper Forum* 1989;7,4,24.
5. Friis L, Edling C, Hagmar L. Mortality and incidence of cancer among sewage workers: a retrospective cohort study. *Br J Ind Med* 1993;50(7):653–657.
6. Lafleur J, Vena JE. Retrospective cohort mortality study of cancer among sewage plant workers. *Am J Ind Med* 1991;19(1):75–86.
7. Uragoda CG. A case of chlorine poisoning of occupational origin. *Ceylon Med J* 1970;15:223–224.
8. Adelson L, Sunshine I. Fatal hydrogen sulfide intoxication: report of three cases occurring in a sewer. *Arch Pathol* 1966;81:375–380.
9. Worker deaths in confined spaces: a summary of surveillance findings and investigative case reports. US Department of Health and Human Services, Centers for Disease Control and Prevention, National Institute of Occupational Safety and Health, 1994.
10. Kraut A, Lilis R, Marcus M, Valciukas J, Wolff M, Landrigan P. Neurotoxic effects of solvent exposure in sewage treatment workers. *Arch Environ Health* 1988;43:263–268.
11. Zuskin E, Mustajbegovic J, Schachter EN. Respiratory function in sewage workers. *Am J Ind Med* 1993;23(5):751–761.
12. Richardson DB. Respiratory effects of chronic hydrogen sulfide exposure. *Am J Ind Med* 1995;28(1):99–108.
13. Heinsohn PA, Jacobs RR, Concoby BA. American Industrial Hygiene Association biosafety reference manual, 2nd ed. Fairfax, VA: American Industrial Hygiene Association, 1995.
14. Dillon HK Heinsohn PA, Miller JD. *American Industrial Hygiene Association field guide for the determination of biological contaminants in environmental samples*, 2nd ed. Fairfax, VA: American Industrial Hygiene Association, 1996.

14a. American Conference of Governmental Industrial Hygienists. *Guidelines for the assessment of bioaerosols in the indoor environment*. Cincinnati: ACGIH, 1989.

15. Water Environment Federation. *Operation of municipal wastewater treatment plants, manual of practice*, no 11, 5th ed. Vol. I–III. Alexandria, VA: Water Environment Federation, 1996.
16. Emde KM, Mao H, Finch GR. Detection and occurrence of waterborne bacterial and viral pathogens. *Water Environ Res June* 1992;64(4):641–643.
17. Water Environment Federation. *Biological hazards at wastewater treatment facilities*. Special publication. Alexandria, VA: Water Environment Federation, 1991.
18. Kocwa-Haluch R. Comparison of the airborne spread of coliform bacteria around a sewage treatment plant. *Ann Agric Environ Med* 1996;3:13–17.
19. Laitinen S, Kangas J, Kotimaa M, et al. Workers' exposure to airborne bacteria and endotoxins at industrial wastewater treatment plants. *Am Ind Hyg Assoc J* 1994;55(11):1055–1060.
20. McCunney RJ. Health effects of work at waste water treatment plants: a review of the literature with guidelines for medical surveillance. *Am J Ind Med* 1986;9:271–279.
21. De Serres G, Levesque B, Higgins R, et al. Need for vaccination of sewer workers against leptospirosis and hepatitis A. *Occup Environ Med* 1995; 52:505–507.
22. Heap B, McCulloch M. Giardiasis and occupational risk in sewage workers. *Lancet* 1991;338:1152.
23. De Serres G, Laliberte D. Hepatitis A among workers from a waste water treatment plant during a small community outbreak. *Occup Environ Med* 1997;54:60–62.
24. Casson LW, Sorber CA, Palmer RH, Enrico A, Gupta P. HIV survivability in wastewater. *Water Environ Res* 1992;64(4):213–215.
25. Morse DL, Kominssky JR, Wisseman CL, Landrigan PJ. Occupational exposure to hexachlorocyclopentadiene: How safe is sewage? *JAMA* 1979;241:217–279.
26. Sewer collapse and toxic illness in sewer repairmen—Ohio. *MMWR Morb Mortal Wkly Rep* 1981;30:89–90.
27. Morgan RW, Kheifets L, Obrinsky DL, Whorton MD, Foliant DE. Fetal loss and work at a waste water treatment plant. *Am J Public Health* 1984;74:499–501.
28. Elia VJ, Clark CS, Majeti VA, et al. Hazardous chemical exposure at a municipal wastewater treatment plant. *Environ Res* 1983;32:360–371.
29. Scariett-Kranz JM, Babish JG, Stickland D, Goodrich RM, Lisk DJ. Urinary mutagens in municipal sewage workers and water treatment workers. *Am J Epidemiol* 1986;124:884–892.
30. Lemasters GK, Zenick H, Hertzberg V, et al. Fertility of workers chronically exposed to chemically contaminated sewer wastes. *Reprod Toxicol* 1991;5(1):31–37.

30a. Mulloy KB. Sewage workers: toxic hazards and health effects. *Occup Med* 2001;16:23–38.

30b. Rylander R. Health effects among workers in sewage treatment plants. *Occup Environ Med* 1999;56:354–357.

30c. Scarlett-Kranz JM, Babish JG, Strickland D, Lisk DJ. Health among municipal sewage and water treatment workers. *Toxicol Ind Health* 1987;3:311–319.

30d. Nethercott JR, Holness DL. Health status of a group of sewage treatment workers in Toronto, Canada. *Am Ind Hyg Assoc J* 1988;49:346–350.

31. National Safety Council. Atmospheres in sub-surface structures and sewers [Data sheet i-550-rev. 85]. Chicago: National Safety Council, 1985.
32. Brown RE. A demonstration of acceptable systems of land disposal of sewage sludge. [CS-805189]. Cincinnati: US Environmental Protection Agency, 1985.
33. Dorn CR. Municipal sewage sludge application on Ohio farms: health effects. *Environ Res* 1985;38(2):332–359.
34. Komsta-Szumska E. Environmental impact of sewage sludge on livestock: a review. *Vet Hum Toxicol* 1986;28(1):31–37.
35. Hattemer-Frey HA, Krieger GR, Lau V. An evaluation of the effect of some properties on root uptake of four metals: Superfund risk assessment. In: Hoddinott K, ed. *Soil contamination study*, 2nd vol. Fredericksburg, VA: American Society for Testing and Materials, 1996:149–158.
36. Chaney RL. Twenty years of land application research. Hazards of sewers, wastewater facilities and sludge materials. *Biocycle*. September 1990; 54–59.

CHAPTER 52

Agricultural Hazards

John B. Sullivan, Jr., Gary R. Krieger, Carlisle F. Runge, and Melissa Gonzales

AGRICULTURE MORBIDITY AND MORTALITY

Farming gives the impression of a healthy lifestyle. Farmers usually live far from congested and polluted urban areas and appear to be healthier than their urban counterparts. However, despite this idyllic existence, farming is associated with a high incidence of illness and mortality that makes it one of the most hazardous occupations.

The U.S. Department of Agriculture defines a farm as an area of land that could sell $1,000 worth or more of agricultural products per year. Agricultural labor is provided by 2.1 million farm

TABLE 52-1. Frequencies and fatality rates per 100,000 workers for the agricultural production and agricultural services sectors by cause of death, 1980–1989

	Agricultural production		Agricultural services	
Cause of death	Deaths	Rate (per 100,000 workers)	Deaths	Rate (per 100,000 workers)
Machinery	2,427	9.5	111	1.5
Motor vehicles	1,013	4.0	118	1.6
Electrocution	354	1.4	125	1.7
Environmental	318	1.2	41	0.6
Falling objects	316	1.2	206	2.9
Falls	258	1.0	101	1.4
Homicide	177	0.7	26	0.4
Suicide	136	0.5	21	0.3
Suffocation	131	0.5	3	<0.01
Air transport	121	0.5	42	0.6
Caught in or struck by flying objects	102	0.4	32	0.4
Drowning	83	0.3	25	0.3
Fires	74	0.3	3	<0.01
Poisoning	65	0.3	6	0.01
Explosions	53	0.2	8	0.01
Water transport	39	0.2	15	0.02
Other/unknown	156	0.6	21	0.03

Reprinted from ref. 3, with permission.

TABLE 52-2. Frequencies and fatality rates per 100,000 workers for the agricultural production and agricultural services sectors by gender and cause of death, and by age group and cause of death for men, 1980–1989

	Male								
	Age group (yr)								
Cause of death	16–24	25–34	35–44	45–54	55–64	65+	Total	Female total	Total
Machinery	4.3	5.6	6.3	9.8	13.8	31.9	9.7	0.2	7.8
Motor vehicles	3.3	3.7	3.3	4.4	4.9	8.1	4.2	0.4	3.5
Electrocution	0.9	1.5	1.9	2.8	2.4	4.1	2.0	0.1	1.6
Environmental	2.5	2.5	1.6	1.6	0.8	0.8	1.8	0.1	1.5
Falling objects	0.5	1.1	1.1	1.5	1.7	4.0	1.4	<0.1	1.1
Falls	0.6	0.7	1.0	1.2	2.0	4.0	1.3	0.2	1.1
Homicide	0.4	0.7	0.8	0.8	0.8	1.0	0.7	0.2	0.6
Suicide	0.2	0.8	1.1	1.0	0.5	0.1	0.6	<0.1	0.5
Suffocation	0.4	0.4	0.6	0.7	1.0	0.9	0.5	<0.1	0.5
Air transport	0.4	0.4	0.5	0.5	0.4	1.3	0.5	0.0	0.4
Caught in or struck by flying objects	0.4	0.5	0.5	0.4	0.7	0.6	0.4	<0.1	0.4
Drowning	0.5	0.4	0.4	.02	0.4	0.5	0.3	0.0	0.3
Fires	0.1	0.2	0.2	0.2	.04	1.1	0.3	<0.1	0.2
Poisoning	0.3	0.3	0.3	0.4	0.1	0.3	0.3	<0.1	0.2
Explosions	0.1	0.3	0.3	0.3	0.3	0.2	0.2	<0.1	0.2
Water transport	0.3	0.3	0.2	0.2	0.2	0.1	0.2	0.0	0.2
Other/unknown	0.2	0.5	0.5	0.7	1.3	1.5	0.7	<0.1	0.5

Reprinted from ref. 3, with permission.

owners, family members, and hired workers. As many as 25% of all farm workers are children younger than 16 years of age (1). The Office of Migrant Health of the Department of Health and Human Services estimates that between 2.7 and 5 million extra hired employees in agribusiness are seasonal and migrant workers, with approximately 30% being migrant (2).

Besides being involved in one of the most accident-prone occupations, farmers have higher incidences of certain types of cancers as well as higher incidences of morbidity and mortality from respiratory disease (3). Broader public health issues have also come to attention in the form of the spread of pesticides, chemicals, and other pollutants from farmland into groundwater, air, and soil.

In the United States, work-related fatalities in the agricultural sector are tracked by the National Safety Council, the Bureau of Labor Statistics, and the National Institute of Occupational Safety and Health (NIOSH). These three organizations estimate that the fatality rate in agricultural industry ranges from 17 to 42 deaths per 100,000 (3). Through their National Traumatic Occupational Fatalities surveillance system, NIOSH uses death certificates to monitor work-related fatalities. However, fatalities of juveniles in the agricultural industry younger than age 16 years are missed by this surveillance database.

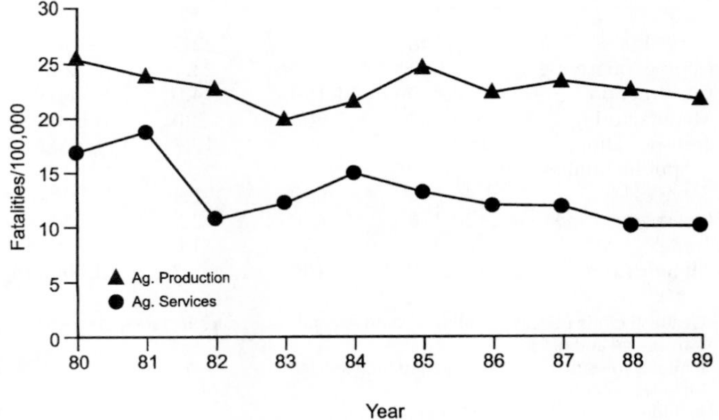

Figure 52-1. Mortality comparison of agricultural production and services sectors.

A survey of 6,727 deaths in agricultural production and services from 1980 to 1989 categorized cause of death (3) (Table 52-1). In this review, the male age-specific average annual death rate increased with increasing age (Table 52-2). Compared with the U.S. civilian working population—which had an average annual fatality rate of 7 deaths per 100,000, as reported by NIOSH from 1980 through 1989—the average annual fatality rate in the agricultural sectors was 22.9 deaths per 100,000 for production services and 12.6 per 100,000 for service sectors of agriculture (3) (Fig. 52-1). Machinery-related fatality tends to be higher for the agricultural production sector, whereas death from falling objects is higher in the service sector. The agricultural production sector shows a tenfold higher average annual death rate for machinery deaths during the period of 1980 to 1989 (3). Also, the agricultural services area had a six-fold higher fatality rate annually compared with civilian working populations as reported by NIOSH (3). Drowning, environmental causes, electrocutions, and other machinery-related deaths—such as caused by flying objects—had a twofold or higher difference in the average annual fatality rates for agricultural production and services sectors compared with the civilian working population (3).

Prevention of machinery-related deaths is a pressing need in the agricultural production and services industry, particularly among male farm workers. Also, black agricultural workers showed a higher risk for work-related fatalities in the agricultural production and services sectors than other ethnic groups.

Agriculture is a unique industry, because people of all ages are at risk. Farms are often worksites and homes, so even nonworkers can be exposed to hazards. Thus, it cannot be assumed that the majority of farm injuries and illnesses occurs with full-time farmers, because hired workers, spouses, young children, women, and retired and part-time farmers are also at risk.

The diversity of the workers differs from one area of the country to another, and within each area, agriculture workers differ from the workforce in other industries. For example, each year more than 300,000 agricultural laborers work in the state of California. These workers differ from the rest of the workforce in the state in the nature of their work, ethnic and cultural makeup, and socioeconomic and employment relationships. A significant portion are Mexican nationals who work transiently, moving to a new location as work becomes available. The great diversity of crops cultivated in California creates a multitude of job tasks, each of which may entail its own particular risk. Workers in southwestern states share these characteristics.

The workforces in the southeastern states differ in ethnic makeup and sociologic factors. Workers are often informally recruited by labor contractors and have no idea in whose field they are working. These factors combine to make it difficult to obtain valid data to ascertain the extent to which occupational health problems exist among migrant agricultural workers.

Agricultural workers in other regions have their own set of occupational exposures varying with crop selection and type of animal production. In the midwestern and north-central United States, where crops and harvesting practices differ, automated farm equipment is extensively used in the harvest of grains and cereals. Animal confinement systems, grain silos, and hay storage each have characteristic hazards and associated health effects.

Comparisons of respiratory disease rates for farmers and farm laborers show regional differences between Iowa and California; California showed an elevated rate relative to Iowa. Although the reason for this difference is not fully understood, the differences in the mobility and the socioeconomic and ethnic backgrounds of the worker populations and differences between crops and work practices are cited as potential explanations. For example, pesticide use is high in both areas; however, the crop mix is substantially different between the two states. Iowa has greater acreage of corn, whereas California has substantial commercial vegetable acreage. Thus, whereas California requires intensive applications of halocarbon fumigants for controlling nematodes, in Iowa this problem is typically controlled by granule-formulated organophosphates. Fumigant gases may be widely used in warehouses containing perishable crops; elemental sulfur dusts are used as miticides and fungicides, and large quantities of organophosphate and carbamates are applied to orchards, vineyards, and row crops.

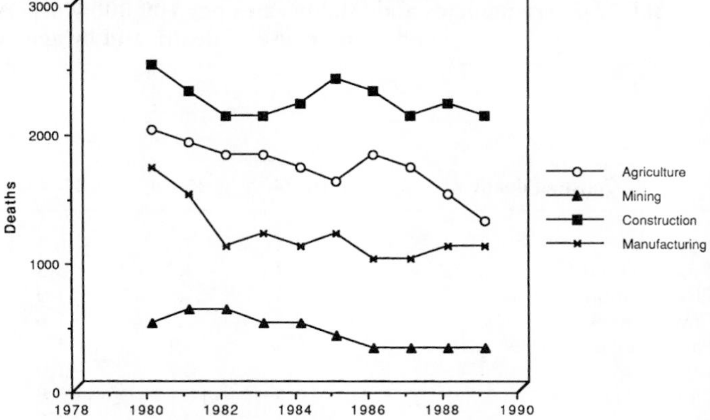

Figure 52-2. Work deaths by industry division, 1980–1989. (Reprinted with permission from National Safety Council. *Accident facts.* Chicago, IL: NSC, 1990.)

SPECIFIC HEALTH HAZARDS IN AGRIBUSINESS

Overall mortality for common diseases in farmers appears to be less than that for the general population; however, injuries and illness related to farming continue to rank with the mining, manufacturing, and construction industries (Fig. 52-2, Table 52-3). Morbidity and mortality figures may actually be underestimates, because agricultural facilities with fewer than 11 employees are exempt from the Occupational Safety and Health Administration's (OSHA) legal injury and illness reporting requirements, and more than 95% of farms have less than this number of employees (4).

The type of labor involved in farming gives rise to chronic musculoskeletal and joint injuries secondary to repetitive motion or vibration and hearing impairment from excess noise. Physical activity and manual labor are more characteristic of third world agribusiness, whereas developed countries use more mechanized approaches to labor. Exposures to toxic chemicals are also more common among agricultural laborers in developing countries.

Farm workers are exposed to a variety of chemicals, fertilizers, pesticides, and fumigants. Farmers have an increased incidence of lymphatic and hemopoietic, stomach, brain, prostate, lip, skin, and connective tissue cancers compared with other occupational groups. An excess mortality rate that is due to respiratory disorders is attributed to exposure to organic dust and bioaerosols. Skin disease in the form of mechanical trauma, overexposure to sunlight and chemicals, and dermatitis are other common occupational hazards of farming.

Unlike other industries that have access to specialized occupational health care and preventive services, the agriculture industry has traditionally lacked organized health and safety programs. This is especially true in third world countries or in the case of migrant farm workers.

Stressors of Agricultural Life

Farming is a highly stressful occupation. The National Safety Council indicates that of all workers, farmers and agricultural workers are more likely to die on the job than any other American worker (5). One out of 18 farm employees was injured in 1989 on farms, and one out of 19 employees was injured in 1990 on farms that had 10 or more employees (5).

Elevated levels of stress are a reason why farmers and agricultural workers may take shortcuts that compromise health

TABLE 52-3. Unintentional injuries at work by industry, United States—1990 [a]

	Workers (millions)	Deaths	Death rates (per 100,000 workers)	Disabling injuries
Agriculture[b]	3,348	770	22.5	150,000
Mining, quarrying[c]	562	130	23.1	20,000
Construction	8,479	1,190	14.0	400,000
Manufacturing	19,993	600	3.0	670,000
Transportation, public utilities	7,948	850	10.7	370,000
Services[d]	46,766	640	1.4	900,000
Government	20,118	470	2.3	580,000
Trade[e]	27,473	450	1.6	710,000
All industries	**134,688**	**5,100**	**3.8**	**3,800,000**

[a]Deaths include persons of all ages. Workers and death rates include persons 16 years of age and older.
[b]Includes forestry, fishing, and agricultural services.
[c]Includes oil and gas extraction.
[d]Includes finance, insurance, and real estate.
[e]Includes wholesale and retail trade.
Reprinted with permission from National Safety Council. Injury facts. Chicago, IL: NSC, 2000.

TABLE 52-4. Yearly summary of total injuries and fatalities by class code

Class code	1989	1990	1991	1992	1993	1994	1995
Nurseries—propagation and cultivation	4,918	4,521	4,484	3,959	3,259	2,639	23,780
Orchards—citrus and deciduous fruit	9,219	7,622	7,099	7,447	6,067	5,617	43,071
Poultry, eggs, hogs, sheep	1,373	1,321	1,309	1,133	850	777	6,763
Florists, cultivating, and gardening	1,818	1,839	1,751	1,673	1,371	1,140	9,592
Dairy farms	2,058	2,327	2,211	2,167	2,081	1,906	12,750
Stock farms and feed yards	1,422	1,395	1,147	995	896	776	6,631
Vineyards	5,994	5,928	5,928	5,574	5,642	4,921	33,987
Potato crops	689	636	618	542	518	489	3,492
Cotton farms	1,437	1,490	1,436	1,140	1,089	1,091	7,683
Orchards—nut crops	966	1,041	929	945	926	905	5,712
Farm machinery operation, contractors	1,075	1,011	989	865	883	752	5,575
Strawberry crops	986	1,301	1,255	1,089	1,024	825	6,480
Field crops	1,443	1,390	1,069	1,061	834	831	6,628
Truck farms	7,941	7,922	7,948	6,922	6,072	5,613	42,418
Cotton gins	381	336	330	275	316	269	1,907
Total	**41,720**	**40,080**	**38,503**	**35,787**	**31,828**	**28,551**	**216,469**

Reprinted with permission from Villarejo D. New approach to calculating risks: occupational injuries. *California Institute for Rural Studies* 1998;7(4):1–3.

and safety. Specific stressors in the agricultural environment include machinery problems, diseases, accidents, economic issues, and government regulations.

Fiscal and economic issues are prime stressors for farming families and the individuals working in the agricultural business (5). Other unique agricultural stressors are weather conditions, interpersonal relationships, and the perception of government interference in the farming business. The transition of the family farm to corporate farming has also tended to increase the stresses in the farming business. The economic contribution to farm-related stressors is demonstrated by the following 1995 data derived by the U.S. Department of Agriculture (6):

- Net farm income fell $13.6 billion from 1994 to 1995. Net value added was $12.5 billion less than in 1994, a 14.6% decline. Net value added represents the total value of the farm sector's output of goods and services and agriculture's addition to the national economic output.
- The value of agriculture's output of commodities and services before expenses fell by $4.8 billion.
- Total value of livestock production fell by $1.9 billion.
- Farm marketing receipts rose $5 billion.
- Net cash income declined.
- Production expenses rose for the third straight year.
- Feed expenditures followed grain prices and were $24.5 billion in 1995, up $1.9 billion from 1994.
- Agricultural chemical expenses rose $500 million to $7.7 billion despite drop in crop production.
- There were more hours worked along with increased wages paid.
- Total interest expenses jumped 8.1% to $12.8 billion.
- Cost of production increased, land values decreased, and commodity prices declined.

The family farm—along with the concept of a family business with a family growing up and living on a farm—slowly disappeared through the years, adding to the stress. Men and women who work in the agricultural and farming business have been showing increasing signs and symptoms of chronic stress (7,8). Studies on farmers in Washington State show that the high cost of machinery relative to production, government regulations in policy shifts, high debt load, poor return on investments, poor crops, and high interest rates were many of the self-reported stressors (6). Investigators divided these stressors into three areas: (a) economic, (b) environmental and machinery, and (c) operational.

In developing countries, more than 50% of the population is involved in agriculture and farming, whereas in industrialized nations, less than 5% of the population is involved in agricultural business. Because food must be provided to the world's population of 5 billion, agriculture remains an important contributor to the world economy. Despite this economic importance, farming as a business and way of life faces financial and political hardships.

Health Problems in Farming Production and Services

Agriculture is a diversified pursuit divided broadly into agricultural production and agricultural services. Injuries and fatalities also vary depending on the nature of the agribusiness (Table 52-4).

Machinery accidents, motor vehicle accidents, electrocution, and environmental exposures are some of the most common health risks farm workers face. Overall, risks can be categorized as follows:

- Trauma and injury
- Respiratory disease
- Toxic exposures to chemicals
- Cancer
- Skin disease
- Infections
- Hearing loss
- Neurologic disorders
- Repetitive muscle and joint disorders

Accidents and Trauma

Injuries and accidents in agriculture are related to farm equipment, falling objects, motor vehicles, electrocution, falls, drowning, and explosions (see Table 52-1). In the agricultural production area, machine-related accidents have the highest mortality rate, whereas falling objects cause the highest mortality rate in the agricultural services sector. Deaths from falling objects were caused by trees, limbs, or logs (3).

Power takeoff devices are particular problems causing injury to extremities and death. These devices transmit torque from a tractor to a device, such as an auger, a baler, or other machine having drive lines, drive shafts, and moving belts. Such power takeoff devices may not be adequately shielded, and clothing or extremities of workers can be snagged by the rapidly spinning shaft or belt. Entanglement of fingers, hands, legs, and arms can result in complete or partial traumatic amputation and crush injury. Avulsion of the scalp can result from hair entanglement. Blunt trauma and contusions can result to head, face, abdomen, or thorax.

Auger injuries are reported to cause as many as 50% of farm machinery–related deaths and 50% of amputations in children (9). An auger is a corkscrew device operating in an encasement that is used to transport corn, grain, or other products from the ground level to the top level of a silo or storage bin. Entanglement of clothes, hair, or extremities can result in serious injury or death. Augers have openings at the intake and output areas; children can reach in and become entrapped. Traumatic injuries secondary to augers are prone to infection as a result of deep tissue penetration of foreign material and microorganisms in the farm product. Fractures and amputation tend to be complicated by the nature of the mechanical trauma. Limb amputations in children tend to be more proximal, because children's limbs easily fit into the opening of the device.

Corn pickers consist of side-by-side rollers rotating in opposite directions. The rollers snap the ears of corn from the stalk and deposit them into a gathering chain or into an auger that transports the ears to the combine for removal of the husks. Corn-picker injuries are common and—in approximately 90% of the cases—leave a permanent disability, generally of the hand (10). Stalks that become jammed in the rollers have to be removed before the machine can continue to operate. Consequently, if the machine is not turned off, the rollers may snag the farm worker's hand or glove, causing crush and amputation injuries, degloving injuries, or partial and complete amputation of fingers and distal hand (11). Wounds are heavily contaminated with debris, dirt, and grease. In some situations, farm workers are forced to self-amputate a portion of their hand to disengage from the machine.

Corn-picker injuries are divided into type I, type II, and type III. Type I injuries are those in which all fingers and thumb are amputated. In type II injuries, the thumb is spared, but all the remaining fingers are lost. In type III injuries, the thumb and one finger remain vital. Also, farm workers may be at risk of a second hand trauma when trying to free an entrapped hand. Dislocations of the elbow and shoulder on the affected side, as well as ligament and tendon injuries, may also occur (12). Injuries from corn pickers result in infection in 50% of cases within the first 5 days of injury from *Klebsiella*, *Enterococcus*, *Pseudomonas*, *Escherichia coli*, and *Staphylococcus* (13). *Serratia* species have also been reported as causative of infections after corn-picker injuries (14).

The hay baler is another device that frequently causes trauma, injury, and death in farm workers. Hay balers have rollers and rotating belts, which tie hay that weighs as much as 2,000 pounds per bale. Hands and extremities can become entrapped in such devices, particularly when the rollers become jammed and the individual tries to relieve the jam. Traumatic amputations, fractures, degloving injuries, and evulsion injuries are common. Evulsion of the scalp can also occur if hair is caught in such a device. Farmers may also be hit by falling hay bales, causing crush injuries, vertebral fractures, sternal fractures, and particularly crushes of the twelfth thoracic vertebra. This fracture syndrome has been named *hay balers' fracture* (15).

Accidents related to tractors occur from rollover events and falls. Between 27% and 53% of fatal farm accidents involve tractors (16). The Centers for Disease Control and Prevention reports approximately 132 deaths as a result of tractor rollovers annually in the United States. Rollover protective devices provide tractors with protection in the event of a rollover. Rollover protective devices are effective in preventing tractor rollover–related fatalities and injuries, especially when used with harnesses or seat belts to keep the worker within a protected area. The Centers for Disease Control and Prevention reported in 1993 that 40% of workers involved in rollover accidents with no rollover protective devices died compared with 2% of those in cases in which protective devices were used.

Farm animals are another cause of accidents and injuries. Most of these are either bovine- or equine-related trauma. More than one-third of these injuries occurred on the first day the individual worked with the animal. Two-thirds of the accidents occurred when the animal was standing, walking, or running. Cattle account for 57% of injuries and horses for 27% of injuries (17). Other causes of injuries are falls from horses, kicks from aggressive animals, assaults from animals, or falls from animal-drawn vehicles. Kicks, bites, crush injuries, and falls are the common categories and mechanisms of injury. Preventive measures include restraining animals, avoiding close spaces with animals, moving slowly around animals, and taking care during milking.

Death by electrocution is another cause of death in farm workers and is almost evenly split between agricultural production and agricultural services (see Table 52-1). Electrocution deaths result from contact between irrigation equipment and power lines, or between other equipment and power lines.

Respiratory Disease

Farmers have a high incidence of respiratory disease compared with those in nonfarming occupations (18). Exposure to dust, vapors, and chemicals that cause pulmonary disease is common in farming. Declines in forced expiratory volume in one second (FEV_1) are associated with dusty environments, such as swine farming and hay and grain handling. Exposure to organic dust and bioaerosols is a major cause of respiratory disease in the agricultural business and farming.

ORGANIC DUSTS

Avoidance of antigen exposure and causative bioaerosols is crucial. Continued exposure to the inciting antigen can lead to clinical deterioration and permanent pulmonary fibrosis. Anecdotal reports indicate beneficial effects from systemic steroid therapy in acute hypersensitivity pneumonitis. Those who have been treated with steroids seem to show more rapid improvement in pulmonary function physiologic abnormalities, but there was no real difference between the treated and untreated groups 5 years later (19–22). In situations of progressive disease, a trial of steroid therapy is indicated. Inhaled steroids and β-agonists may be useful in individuals with chest symptoms.

Despite the different pathogenesis between organic dust toxic syndrome (ODTS) and hypersensitivity pneumonitis, it is difficult to separate these two syndromes by clinical symptoms and physical examination (Table 52-5). Both can present with cough, leukocytosis, fever, dyspnea, chills, malaise, myalgia, and pulmonary function decrements. ODTS is characterized by a history of high-level dust exposure with negative serology for precipitating serum antigens. The cause of ODTS is an acute inflammatory pulmonary response to inhaled dusts; there are usually no long-term sequelae. Hypersensitivity pneumonitis has a higher incidence in late winter and early spring. ODTS has a higher incidence in late summer and early fall. The prevalence rate for hypersensitivity pneumonitis in farming is thought to be 4.2 per 1,000 (23). The incidence of ODTS versus hypersensitivity pneumonitis is difficult to ascertain, given the common symptoms of both diseases. The incidence of ODTS is estimated to vary from 10 to 190 per 10,000 population at risk (24).

Chronic Bronchitis

Farmers have a high incidence of respiratory irritant exposure and chronic cough attributed to exposure to dusty environ-

TABLE 52-5. Comparison of toxic pneumonitis with hypersensitivity pneumonitis

Organic dust toxic syndrome	Hypersensitivity pneumonitis
History: Onset in 4–12 h after concentrated organic dust exposure over a short period of time (1 h or less)	**History:** Onset 4–8 h after exposure to antigens or antigen-contaminated environment
Signs/symptoms: Fever, chills, dyspnea, myalgias, headache, nonproductive cough, malaise, chest tightness	**Signs/symptoms:** Fever, chills, malaise, nonproductive cough, dyspnea, shortness of breath, chest tightness, myalgias, tachypnea, tachycardia; duration 12–36 h and disease may progress with permanent damage
Pulmonary examination: Normal or few scattered rales on pulmonary examination	**Pulmonary examination:** Rales
Complete blood cell count: Leukocytosis (>20,000/mm^3) with predominance of neutrophils	**Complete blood cell count:** Leukocytosis with lymphocytosis and eosinophils
Arterial blood gases: Mild hypoxemia with mild alveolar arterial gradient	**Arterial blood gases:** Mild to severe hypoxemia with an increased gradient
Serology: Negative serum precipitins	**Serology:** Positive serum precipitins to antigens
Bronchoalveolar lavage: Neutrophil predominance of neutrophils and macrophages, tumor necrosis factor present	**Bronchoalveolar lavage:** Lymphocytosis, ↑ fibronectin, ↑ albumin, ↑ angiotensin-converting enzyme, ↑ hyaluronic acid, ↑ CD8 T cells, ↑ CD4:CD8 ratio, ↑ natural killer cells
Chest x-ray: Normal or shows only mild interstitial infiltrate	**Chest x-ray:** Dense infiltrates, coarse opacities, Kerley-B lines, ground-glass appearance
Biopsy: Multifocal acute inflammation of terminal bronchioles, alveoli, and interstitial area with exudate of macrophages and neutrophils	**Biopsy:** Interstitial pneumonitis, fibrosis, granulomas
Pulmonary function tests: Mild restriction and mild diffusion defect	**Pulmonary function tests:** Severe restriction, obstruction, and decreased diffusion defect
	High-resolution computed tomography scan: May be normal early then show abnormal changes that include micronodules or diffuse parenchymal opacification; increased densities of parenchyma
Mechanism: Nonimmune-mediated inflammation	**Mechanism:** Immune-mediated type III and type IV hypersensitivity
Prognosis: Excellent; duration of 12–24 h, may last as long as 5–7 d; recovery generally in 24–48 h; no pulmonary fibrosis	**Prognosis:** Resolution of abnormal pulmonary function tests in 4–6 wk, untreated may require 6–12 mo to resolve after exposure removal; chronic disease results in restrictive/obstructive defects; fibrosis can occur with permanent injury

ments. The ambient air in and around various agricultural production, storage, and transportation facilities is laden with a variety of gases, dusts, suspended particles, and bioaerosols, which pose a respiratory risk. These include organic antigens such as pollen, fungal spores, animal danders, grain dust, and mites; synthetic chemicals such as fertilizers, insecticides, and herbicides; and toxic gases released from decomposing plant or animal material.

Chronic bronchitis is clinically recognized by chronic cough with sputum production and is reported in as many as 21% of farmers surveyed, with nonsmoking farmers apparently at a higher risk (25). Grain workers have a 49% prevalence of chronic bronchitis symptoms (25).

Grain workers also may have a dose-related decline in peak flow and FEV_1 after exposures of greater than 2 weeks. Risk of bronchitis increases with smoking and intensity of dust exposure. Farmers working with dairy cows, swine, and other animal confinement operations also experience higher rates of respiratory symptoms. Table 52-6 reviews the clinical differences between bronchitis and asthma.

Asthma and Bronchial Hyperreactivity

Barns, dairy houses, swine houses, grain handling, and animal confinement areas expose workers to high antigenic loads of organic dusts and chemicals. The indoor air of animal confinement areas can be heavily contaminated by organic dusts (26).

Agricultural workers may experience asthma that is immunoglobulin E (IgE) mediated or nonspecific bronchial hyperreactivity that is due to inflammation and irritancy. Acute respiratory symptoms and chronic symptoms with decrements in pulmonary function have been identified. Pulmonary function abnormalities include decreases in FEV_1, forced vital capacity (FVC), forced expiratory flow ($FEF_{25\%-75\%}$), and positive methacholine challenge (see Table 52-6).

Symptoms of asthma and airway hyperreactivity include cough, chest tightness, wheezing, and dyspnea. Those with allergic-induced asthma can develop wheezing within minutes after allergen exposure, or symptoms can be delayed for as long as 24 hours. Sensitization periods range from months to years. Those with allergic-mediated asthma do not require a high-level exposure to incite signs and symptoms. Pulmonary function tests in asthma show obstructive airflow patterns.

Asthma is an inflammatory disease with multiple causes. The pathophysiology basic to asthma is bronchospasm and airway obstruction caused by inflammation and airway edema. Asthma can be allergic mediated or nonallergic mediated. Nonallergic-

TABLE 52-6. Comparison of chronic bronchitis and asthma

Bronchitis	Asthma
Signs and symptoms: Cough with sputum production, chest tightness; symptoms occurring for 2 or more yr classified as chronic bronchitis	**Signs and symptoms:** Wheezing, cough, dyspnea within minutes of exposure or may be delayed as long as 24 h
Physical examination: May find diminished breath sounds, rhonchi, or rales	**Physical examination:** Bronchospasm—chest examination may be normal in between bouts; inspiratory/expiratory wheezes
Exposure history: Dusty environments, smoking; seen frequently in swine confinement workers; smoking worsens symptoms	**Exposure history:** Period of sensitization required for IgE-mediated asthma; once sensitized, extent of exposure to cause symptoms is minimal
Pulmonary function test: Decreased flow rates	**Pulmonary function test:** Decreased flow rates, FEV_1 and $FEF_{25\%-75\%}$; positive methacholine challenge

FEF, forced expiratory flow; FEV_1, forced expiratory volume in one second; IgE, immunoglobulin E.

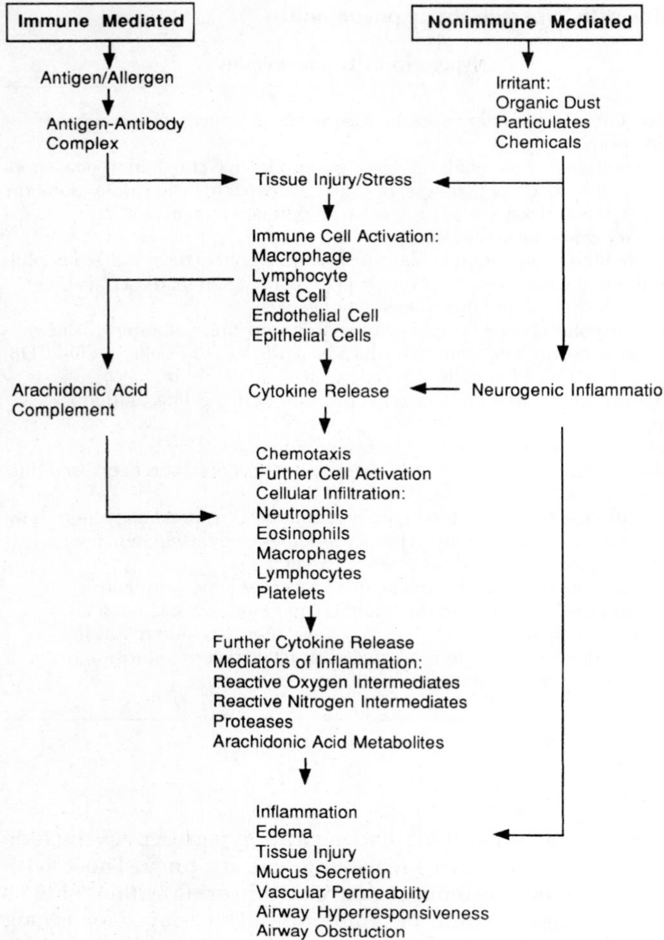

Figure 52-3. Inflammation pathways.

mediated asthma may range from mild nonspecific bronchial hyperactivity to more serious forms of reactive airways.

Asthma occurs in phases because of the multiple inflammatory-mediated reactions that occur after an inciting exposure (27) (Fig. 52-3). Acute asthma is clinically manifested by cough and wheezing after the initiation of an inflammatory cascade by either an IgE-mediated mechanism or a non–IgE-mediated mechanism. By either mechanism, proinflammatory vasoactive amines are released from IgE mast cells or macrophages which results in smooth muscle constriction and edema. Mucus is secreted into the airways, causing coughing and dyspnea. Longer term, the inflammation results in an infiltration of neutrophils, eosinophils, and basophils, which release additional mediators of inflammation (27). Within 12 hours, the number of lymphocytes and monocytes increases in lung tissue and may bring about more chronic forms of asthma via cytokine and arachidonic acid release. This late-phase response occurs from 2 to several days (27).

Inflammation causes disruption of the airway endothelial lining, which causes reflex coughing and bronchial hyperreactivity. The long-term response can leave airways sensitive to multiple, diverse environmental stimuli. Long-term inflammation is associated with changes in lung tissue architecture with fibrosis and hypertrophy of airway smooth muscle. This causes further airway thickening and obstruction.

Asthma has a circadian rhythm, with worsening of symptoms in the early morning hours between 3 a.m. and 5 a.m. BAL fluid shows increased inflammatory cells in nocturnal asthma (27). Asthmatic symptoms vary from mild to severe dyspnea, but wheezing and shortness of breath occurring in an episodic manner are characteristic. Because of this episodic occurrence of symptoms, peak flow measurements provide better information than pulmonary function tests.

Treatment of asthma is based on the disease severity and targeting the inflammation and bronchospastic activity. A systematic management program therapy for asthma is best after a step-care approach (Table 52-7). The goal is to control signs and symptoms and to avoid triggering exposures. Pharmacologic therapy without exposure avoidance does not benefit the patient. The prognosis of asthma caused by environmental exposures is directly related to the duration of exposure. Workers who are continually exposed can develop severe asthma lasting years (28). Also, engineering controls play an important role in controlling exposure.

Farmer's Lung Disease

Farmer's lung disease is a hypersensitivity pneumonitis caused by inhalation of material from moldy hay containing thermophilic actinomycetes bacteria (20–22). After handling moldy hay or crops, workers may experience acute onset of cough, dyspnea, and fever. In acute cases, symptoms are manifested 3 to 4 hours after exposure and may resemble viral infection clinically. Fatigue, fever, weight loss, malaise, and a nonproductive cough are major symptoms. However, the disease may develop gradually, producing permanent dyspnea and pulmonary impairment. A chest radiograph may show bilateral reticular interstitial patterns. Recurrence of symptoms when the worker is reexposed to moldy hay or grain indicates the diagnosis. Pulmonary function tests may show a loss of FVC and FEV_1, as well as ventilation-perfusion imbalance, which may produce hypoxemia.

Farmer's lung disease has been associated with thermophilic gram-positive actinomycetes, a filamentous bacteria that grows at temperatures between 30° and 65°C. The species identified as causative agents are:

- *Micropolyspora faeni* (*Faenia rectivirgula*)
- *Thermoactinomyces vulgaris* and *T. thalpophilus*
- *Saccharomonospora viridis*
- *Streptomyces griseus* and *S. albus*
- *Aspergillus fumigatus*

These bacteria thrive in hay that spontaneously heats from being moist. *T. thalpophilus* growing in hay produces an antibiotic that inhibits the growth of *T. vulgaris* (20). The presence of antibodies to *M. faeni* (*F. rectivirgula*) and *T. vulgaris* in affected patients may be identified. Antigens from these species are used to identify precipitin antibodies in the serum of ill workers. *A. fumigatus* precipitin antibodies are also occasionally found.

The heating of moist hay is essential for fungal and bacterial growth and spontaneously occurs in moist hay. With low water content, *Aspergillus glaucus* fungi are dominant and slowly increase the water content with their respiration. This allows for the proliferation of actinomycetes and other fungi. Spontaneous heating of hay substrate thus promotes growth of thermophilic species. To prevent molding of hay, the water content should be less than 20%. The spore count of moldy hay may exceed 100 million spores per g (20), whereas dry hay has less than 5 million spores per g (Table 52-8).

Cases of farmer's lung are geographic and seasonal where climatic conditions are conducive to the development of moldy hay. The prevalence of the disease is directly related to the rainfall in the area. Turning and stacking of hay in the field are

TABLE 52-7. Step-care therapy for asthma

	Signs/symptoms	Therapy	Response
Step 1	Mild intermittent asthma	β_2-bronchodilator: Available in short, intermediate, and long acting; albuterol, terbutaline, pirbuterol, metaproterenol, every 4–6 h	Reverses bronchoconstriction rapidly; does not prevent inflammation. Increasing use greater than every 4 h indicates loss of control and that inflammation requires more aggressive treatment.
		Anticholinergics: Inhaled ipratropium bromide	Slow onset of action; produces bronchodilation by reducing cholinergic tone of airway; has additive effect with β_2 agonists; is more effective in chronic obstructive pulmonary disease than for chronic asthma management.
Step 2	Mild persistent asthma	Inhaled β_2 agonist as needed not to exceed 3–4 times/d, plus one of the following:	Acute reversal of bronchospasm to relieve symptoms Pharmacologic agents to control inflammation:
		Inhaled corticosteroid (200–500 μg)	Glucocorticosteroids: Most potent antiinflammatory agent available; leads to ↑ mucous production, stabilizes vascular leakage, ↑ inflammatory cell release of mediators and cell activation, β_2 agonist response; used to control inflammation and gain remission of asthma (beclomethasone, triamcinolone, flunisolide)
		Inhaled cromolyn sodium	Cromolyn sodium: Inhibits inflammatory cell activation and mediator release; maximum clinical benefit may require weeks of therapy
		Inhaled nedocromil (tilade)	Nedocromil: Inhibits inflammatory cell activation and mediator release; maximum clinical benefit may require weeks of therapy
		Consider theophylline	Leukotriene antagonist: Zafirlukast (Accolate), an oral leukotriene inhibitor, blocks LTD_4 receptors; it attenuates the acute airway obstructive response to allergen
Step 3	Moderate persistent asthma	Inhaled corticosteroid (800–2,000 μg); long-acting β_2 bronchodilator; theophylline or oral β_2 agonist	Blocks inflammatory reactions; provides bronchodilation
Step 4	Severe persistent asthma	Inhaled corticosteroid 800–2,000 μg daily long-acting β_2 bronchodilator or sustained-release theophylline and/or long-acting oral β_2 agonist Oral corticosteroid long-term short-acting β_2 agonist as needed for relief of acute symptoms	Blocks inflammatory reactions; provides bronchodilation

much less of a hazard in terms of bioaerosol exposure. Exposure to bioaerosols is high in stored hay. Moldy hay is handled in opening bales for animal feeding or threshing and moving moldy grain. Most serious exposures occur in enclosed barns that have inadequate ventilation. Bioaerosol concentrations can reach 1×10^9–10^{10} spores per m^3. Exposure tends to be highest in winter and spring. Unloading moldy grain from silos creates similar hazards.

An increase in chronic cough, bronchitis, and decreased pulmonary functions has been seen in workers serologically positive to farmer's lung disease antigens. Chronic pulmonary symptoms have been positively correlated with the presence of positive antibody serology.

After termination of exposure, serum precipitin antibodies may persist for 3 to 5 years (20–22). Many past cases of farmer's lung disease were probably misdiagnosed and were actually ODTS.

TABLE 52-8. Characteristics of hay

Hay	H_2O content (%)	Maximum temperature (°C)	Spore content (millions/g)	
			Fungi	Actinomycetes
Very moldy	35–50	50–65	10–100	350–1,200
Moldy	20–30	35–45	2–60	3–250
Dry	15–20	22–26	0.1–7	0.5–8

Adapted with permission from ref. 20.

Animal Confinement Areas and Animal Wastes

Animal confinement areas represent multiple health hazards when large numbers of animals are raised in an enclosed structure with a limited amount of area provided per animal. Although it brings about a tremendous increase in productivity, the use of these confinement systems is associated with an increase in physical, chemical, and biological exposures to the agriculture worker. An estimated 700,000 workers are employed in livestock and poultry confinement operations (26). Confinement areas include poultry, swine, veal, beef, and dairy operations.

Exposures in confinement areas consist of organic dusts and toxic chemicals. Exposures can be high because of the relative crowding of animals, feeding, manure and animal waste disposal, and inadequacy of ventilation. The term *concentrated animal feeding operations* is applied to confinement areas (29). Animal wastes are part of the agricultural production cycle and therefore part of the cost of doing business. Animal agricultural waste is divided into range waste, pasture waste, and confined waste. Range and pasture waste are more dispersed into large areas. The confinement area concentrates wastes. Range and pasture animal waste can influence groundwater quality by increasing turbidity and fecal coliform content (29).

Agriculture pollution can be either point source or nonpoint source. Nonpoint contamination sources are those in which contaminants are not concentrated during production and do not pass through conduits for disposal such as pastures, feedlots, and more dispersed sources (29). Point sources concentrate contaminants and pass them through a pipeline, conduit, or canal for disposal. Point sources include indoor animal confinement areas, dairy operations, and lagoons or ponds containing animal waste. The Environmental Protection Agency (EPA) may designate some agricultural point sources of pollution as national pollution discharge elimination systems, requiring special permits depending on whether discharge occurs into navigable waters (29). *Navigable waters* is liberally defined as including all stream beds—even if they are dry—and irrigation canals that empty into water courses. Animal waste pollutants of concern include the following:

- Organic nitrates in the form of amino acids and proteins, which are converted to NH_4^+, then to nitrite (NO_2^-) and to nitrates (NO_3^- N)
- Animal urine containing urea, which breaks down to ammonia and carbon dioxide [ammonia (NH_3) may volatilize as a gas or be converted to NH_4^+]
- Phosphorus and phosphates, which are found in animal manure in organic and inorganic forms (organic phosphorus must be mineralized to inorganic phosphorus to be used by plants)
- Fecal coliform bacteria
- Pesticides
- High biochemical oxygen demand wastes (a measure of a substance's ability to contaminate the environment and utilize oxygen to oxidize organic material)
- Carbon dioxide, an asphyxiant in confined spaces
- Hydrogen sulfide, generated by anaerobic processes in manure
- Ammonia (NH_3) gas
- Methane (CH_4) gas

Preventing environmental contamination and avoiding soil and water contaminant spread by animal confinement facilities involves proper facility siting and waste management. Facility sites should be outside of flood plains, in areas in which the soil content is high in clay, and far enough from residences and public buildings to avoid complaints (29). Waste management also includes collection, conveyance, storage, and use of animal wastes. Solid wastes are physically removed, whereas liquid or semiliquid wastes are removed by conduits, canals, or pipes to a central collection point. Flush systems may be involved, which generate large volumes of wastewater. Animal waste is stored in evaporative ponds or storage ponds in which microbiological activity degrades organic waste material, allows for ammonia to volatilize, for NO_3^- to denitrify, and for water to evaporate (29). Storage ponds are designed to be either aerobic or anaerobic. Aerobic ponds allow for high O_2 levels to support aerobic bacteria, and anaerobic ponds support anaerobic bacteria.

Disposal of manure or manure sludge is usually by land application. However, before it can be applied, it is necessary to ascertain the concentration and types of toxic agents present, salt content, and nutrient content.

Animal confinement production workers have a high prevalence of respiratory symptoms: cough, excess sputum and phlegm production, wheezing, and irritation to the nose and throat. Feeds, organic dusts, animal waste, and proteins of animal origin are the greatest contributors to the total dust load, which reaches excessively high levels during feeding (26,30–33) (Table 52-9).

TABLE 52-9. Hazards of concentrated feeding operations

Organic dust	Proteases
Proteins: urine, dander, serum	Ammonia adsorbed to dust particulates
Fecal material	Infectious agents
Bacteria: gram negative	Insect parts
Fecal particles	Toxic chemicals
Fungi	Hydrogen sulfide
Pollen	Ammonia
Grain mites	Carbon dioxide
Endotoxin	Methane
1,3-β-glucan	Carbon monoxide

Human antibodies specific for feed dusts suggest an immunologic basis for the respiratory symptoms observed. Biological materials also contribute adversely to the effects on the respiratory tract. A single antigen has not been identified as the primary source of sensitization. To test for sensitization, it would be necessary to use a large antigen panel to assess the many types of dust present in barns and confinement systems.

A summary of the symptoms reported by swine confinement workers includes cough with sputum production, chest tightness, dyspnea, wheezing, malaise, fever, dizziness, myalgias and arthralgia, fatigue, and throat irritation (30). Pulmonary function studies have shown decrements in flow volumes as well as the parameters of FEV_1 and FEV_1/FVC. Using dust masks may help prevent work-related respiratory symptoms (34).

The incentive for energy production from methane released by anaerobic decomposition of wastes from animal confinement units has made liquid manure storage a frequent hazard of confinement systems. The uncontrolled activity of anaerobic and facultative microbes in stored manure produces metabolic byproducts, including as many as 150 different gases, many of which are known to be toxic (32). Air concentrations of methane, ammonia, carbon dioxide, carbon monoxide, and hydrogen sulfide can exceed chronic and short-term exposure limits if proper controls are not practiced and maintained. In addition to respiratory symptoms, workers are also subject to the central nervous system–depressant effects of carbon dioxide and the toxic effects of hydrogen sulfide and carbon monoxide. Displacement of atmospheric oxygen by the mixture of gases has led to asphyxiation, especially among workers entering confined spaces.

The development of hypersensitivity pneumonitis is a risk from exposure to airborne microorganisms and organic dusts. Significant amounts of suspended endotoxins from gram-negative bacteria are present in swine confinement units, poultry production and processing facilities, and airborne grain dusts (33). Endotoxins are thought to be responsible for pulmonary reactions in persons exposed to cotton dust and are also associated with headache, diarrhea, and other symptoms in compost workers.

An IgE-mediated asthmatic response can be precipitated by the exposure to a variety of organic agents. Pollen from cereal grains, dander from livestock, fungal antigens in grain dust and adhering to crops, or dust mites in organic dusts are among the most common causative agents for this type of response (35). Nonimmunologic asthmatic responses can also be elicited from exposure to various organic dust agents such as microorganisms, glucans, endotoxins, irritant dust, and chemical by-products of organisms.

Toxic gases can be generated in confined areas from urine and manure to levels that can cause illness or even death. Enclosed or confined structures, covered lagoons, and animal confinement areas with flow slats that accumulate wastes can be immediately dangerous to life and health (IDLH) as a result of toxic gas accumulation. Toxic gases are generated in manure pits and may be released when the manure is moved or stirred. Manure pits constitute confined spaces that can be IDLH. Gases can accumulate in the indoor air of animal confinement areas from wastes beneath the flooring of the houses. During manure agitation in pits, large amounts of hydrogen sulfide can be suddenly released and rise quickly to IDLH levels. Worker deaths have resulted when entering manure pits after emptying or when entering to repair equipment (36).

Respiratory illness from dusts and gases is related to the length of exposure. Those who work in confinement areas more than 2 hours daily and for 6 or more years are at greatest risk (26). More than 60% of veterinarians providing care to animals in confinement areas experience respiratory symptoms (26). Dust and toxic gases increase in winter months and during times of inadequate ventilation. Dust also increases dramatically when animals are fed, moved, or handled.

Swine confinement workers seem to have the worst health problems compared with others (26). Swine confinement dust concentrations average 3 to 6 mg per m^3 and may rise to 10 to 20 mg per m^3 in winter (26). Airborne concentrations of endotoxin, H_2S, CO_2, and CO may exceed recommended safe concentrations (26). As many as 70% of swine confinement workers experience respiratory symptoms. Symptoms tend to be worse in smokers and those with preexisting respiratory illness or allergies. Coughing, eye irritation, nasal irritation, and chest tightness commonly occur within 30 minutes of being in the swine confinement environment. Symptoms may abate in 24 to 48 hours after terminating exposure. In some cases, respiratory illness may become chronic. The majority of the cases of illness are thought not to be allergic, but more likely toxic inflammation.

Organic dust may cause ODTS. High H_2S concentrations of 100 to 400 ppm can produce eye irritation, cough, tracheobronchitis, dyspnea, and even pulmonary edema or death at higher concentrations.

As many as 25% of swine confinement workers experience chronic bronchitis with cough and chronic sputum production (26). Smokers have a greater prevalence and severity. Pulmonary function tests may show decrements throughout the day of exposure. BAL fluid shows a persistent leukocytosis.

Prevention of exposure and management of symptoms are crucial to prevent further illness. Engineering controls and ventilation changes are usually necessary to control dust and to prevent exposure to toxic gases. Dust masks and personal protective equipment are effective in preventing exposures. Education about manure pits and confined spaces is crucial.

Grain Dust

Grain dust consists of organic and inorganic material from cereals: wheat, barley, oats, rye, and maize. Twenty percent of grain dust is inorganic, of which the major component is quartz. Grain dust contains numerous contaminants, such as

- Grain kernel pieces
- Pieces of seeds
- Trichome particles
- Insect parts
- Endotoxins
- Mycotoxins
- Silica
- Plant enzymes
- Mite parts
- Bacteria (particularly gram negative)
- Mold and fungi (*Aspergillus, Absidia, Mucor, Taenia, Faenia, Penicillium, Ustilago*)
- Residues of pesticides, fungicides, herbicides, and fumigants

Grain dust can be broadly divided into two groups according to whether it is produced in harvesting or in storage. The microbial content of grain dust in harvesting contains large numbers of fungi hyphae, spores, and bacteria (20). *Cladosporium* species is the most abundant fungi. Other fungi include *Verticillium, Paecilomyces, Alternaria, Epioccumi, Ustilago,* and *Puccinia* (20). Farm workers may show positive skin tests to these fungi.

Stored grain changes in microbial content depending on moisture, aeration, and spontaneous heating during storage. As temperature and moisture content increase, the dominant microflora become thermophilic microorganisms. As moisture rises to between 30% to 50%, the temperature rises to approximately 65°C, and thermophilic fungi grow: *Absidia corymbifera, Mucor pusillus, Taenia vulgaris, Faenia rectivirgula,* and *Aspergillus fumigatus*. These fungi can cause respiratory illness, including hypersensitivity pneumonitis.

Grain dust is a product of grain handling. Grain dust levels tend to be in the range of 10 to 25 mg per m^3 with respirable dust ranging from 0.5 to 5 mg per m^3. Respirable dust tends to be higher with barley and wheat and lower with corn. Several processes in which workers are exposed range from working in grain elevators to transporting, milling, and baking (37). Grain elevators are sources of high particulate pollutants, both inside the elevator and outside. Dust levels vary between 5 and 50 mg per m^3, depending on ventilation effectiveness. Air particulates as high as 1,000 mg per m^3 have been recorded (37). Particles less than 10 μm are considered respirable, and as much as 10% of grain dust would fit this size (37). The components of grain dust vary with the grain and location. Grain dust possesses significant properties to induce inflammation and activation of the alternative complement pathway and activation of pulmonary macrophages (37).

Handling moldy grain can expose workers to high bioaerosol concentrations containing bacteria, fungi, mycotoxins, endotoxin, and 1,3-β-glucans. During storage, microorganisms colonize grains and plant material if water content is high (usually >14%) (23). As water content increases in stored grain, the temperature increases spontaneously because of metabolic activity. Temperatures of 65°C can be attained with water content greater than 35% (23). This creates a fire risk that is due to combustible compounds produced during microbiological growth.

Dominant microorganisms in stored grain are thermophilic fungi and actinomycetes, which produce easily aerosolized spores. The airborne concentration of fungi has been found to vary from 1×10^3 to 1×10^8 CFU per m^3, depending on the task or activity involving grain (Table 52-10) (23).

Clinical symptoms after exposure may vary depending on the composition and nature of the grain dusts inhaled. Skin irritation and pruritus are common symptoms after exposure to oat and barley dusts because of the trichome particles that penetrate the skin (37). A syndrome known as a *grain itch* is caused by a mite. Irritation of the eyes, nose, and upper airway are common symptoms after grain dust exposure (37).

TABLE 52-10. Airborne concentrations

Fungi	
Harvesting	10^5–10^7 CFU/m^3
Drying	10^3–10^5 CFU/m^3
Handling	10^4–10^6 CFU/m^3
Crushing	10^4–10^8 CFU/m^3
Bacteria/actinomycetes	
Harvesting	10^7–10^9 CFU/m^3
Handling	10^3–10^5 CFU/m^3
Crushing	10^7–10^9 CFU/m^3
Microorganisms	
Silo unloading	10^5–10^9 CFU/m^3
Microorganisms (cells/m^3)	
Harvesting	10^5–10^7 CFU/m^3
Drying	10^6 CFU/m^3
Unloading	10^7–10^9 CFU/m^3
Crushing	10^5–10^8 CFU/m^3

CFU, colony-forming unit.

Respiratory diseases after exposure to grain dusts vary from hypersensitivity pneumonitis to asthma and toxic pneumonitis. Chronic exposure results in airflow limitations evident on pulmonary function testing. Toxic pneumonitis, also known as *grain fever,* is an acute febrile illness occurring after exposure to dusts and is reported to occur in as many as 30% of farmers (37). Symptoms include malaise, cough, dyspnea, chills, and fever. Symptoms may last from hours to days.

Hypersensitivity pneumonitis (allergic alveolitis) is associated with the handling of moldy materials. This condition is not commonly associated with handling dry grain (37). Asthmatic reactions can be induced by both allergic and nonallergic causes. Overall, grain dust exposure can produce symptoms associated with chronic bronchitis, asthma, hypersensitivity pneumonitis, and chronic airflow limitations.

Cotton Dust: Byssinosis and Mill Fever

Pulmonary disease caused by chronic exposure to cotton dust is called *byssinosis*. Workers exposed to cotton dust slowly develop a chronic cough that is particularly worse on returning to work on Monday, with improvement over the weekend. Over time, the cough becomes worse and relenting with no weekend improvement (38). The term *byssinosis* characterizes symptoms related to chest discomfort and shortness of breath experienced by workers returning to work on Monday (38). Overall, respiratory symptoms experienced by cotton workers include low-grade fever, wheezing, chest tightness, and an initial dry cough followed by a productive cough with longer exposure and asthma (38).

Cotton lint is separated from the seed by cotton gins and formed into bales for transport to cotton mills. Dust can be generated during the stages of milling, while cotton is being cleaned and separated. Machines are used in this job and are isolated to prevent dust exposure to workers. But cleaning machinery can generate dust exposure and byssinosis. From the blowing machines, cotton moves to the carding room for final impurity removal while the cotton is combed. Worker exposure to cotton dust occurs during ginning and milling processes.

Cotton dust contains more than 1,000 different bacterial species plus various levels of endotoxin (39). Regional differences in bacterial flora and endotoxin levels exist. In California, the main bacterial species is *Bacillus*. In Mississippi and Texas, the bulk of bacteria is *Pseudomonas* species.

The pathophysiology of cotton dust exposure is an inflammatory response in the lungs that is caused by responses of pulmonary macrophages and the release of mediators of inflammation. The causative agents in cotton dust are thought to be products of the plant as well as endotoxin, molds, and numerous gram-negative or gram-positive bacteria. Plant products include histamine, phenols, epoxides, terpenoids, tannin, and lancinilene C7-methyl ether (38).

Affected workers have a decline in ventilatory capacity over the week's shift with increased prevalence of bronchitis. Mill fever characterizes the respiratory illness experienced by new workers in a cotton mill or those who experience illness on returning after a prolonged absence.

Byssinosis is generally referred to as the acute illness that develops on returning to work after being off work. New employees who develop illness acutely after beginning work generally leave and seek other employment. These acute symptoms can be duplicated by inhalational challenge with cotton dust (40). A shift of FEV_1 between 5% and 10% decrement is regarded as suggestive of byssinosis when accompanied by symptoms. An FEV_1 decline greater than 10% is considered diagnostic (40). Diffusion capacity remains normal.

Chronic effects and long-term exposure effects have been controversial. Dust exposure is thought to be associated with excess declines in FEV_1.

The current U.S. cotton dust standard of 0.2 mg per m^3 applies to picking, carting, and spinning (40). The level allowed in slashing and weaving is 0.750 mg per m^3 (40). Employees' preplacement exam should include FVC and FEV_1, which is repeated within 6 months of employment.

Pathophysiologically, cotton dusts cause release of histamine and other mediators of inflammation, which causes declines in FEV_1. Increased histamine metabolites are found in the urine of cotton dust–exposed subjects (40). Lancinilene C and lancinilene E-7 methyl ester are chemotactic agents isolated from water extracts of cotton. Tannin, a component of cotton dust, also induces an acute pulmonary inflammation with infiltration of neutrophils (40). Concentrations of endotoxin in cotton dust correlate better with byssinosis symptoms than do concentrations of respirable dust.

Silos and Silo Filler's Disease

Silos store animal feed (silage) but are also potential health hazards. Respiratory exposures to dusts, confined space, and trauma hazards exist. Silos can be relatively airtight and may be aboveground storage units, tower units, or below-ground units.

Silage is a fermented form of animal feed. The silo process squeezes air out from the stored grass or grain, creating a low O_2-content atmosphere. Remaining oxygen is consumed by plant cells. If moisture content is high, microbial growth can occur. The basic silo principle is that with an increasing anaerobic environment, lactate levels and organic acid levels increase and cause pH to decline, suppressing microbial growth and preventing spoilage. However, silage exposed to air becomes overgrown with a layer of bacteria and fungi, which can generate high aerosols of organic dust if disturbed.

Silos are classified according to location of the silage unloading area: top or bottom unloading. Bottom-unloading silos are closed when filled, and gases rapidly accumulate. Top-unloading silos are the most common and are unsealed. But silo gases still accumulate at the top and create a confined space hazard if entered. The silo process generates nitrogen dioxide (NO_2) starting within 24 hours after filling, which remains high for 96 hours or longer. Anyone who enters the silo during this time is exposed to this NO_2 hazard. NO_2 exposure can occur upon entry after 12 hours postfilling. Exposure can occur within the silo, in the chute up to the silo, or when crawling through the door onto the silage bed.

Silos are most hazardous at the time of recent filling and at unloading. During storage, silage in an anaerobic environment remains unspoiled. Silage at the top, though—in contact with oxygen—does spoil and develops a layer of fungal and bacterial contamination. Before unloading, the contaminated layer must be removed manually. This task exposes the worker to high organic dust and bioaerosol concentrations. Also, the head space above the silage is oxygen deficient and constitutes a confined space that can cause asphyxia if entered. The unloading mechanism at the base of a silo can also serve as a confined space.

Silo gases are much more concentrated in bottom-unloading units, creating situations that can be IDLH to workers who enter without proper respiratory protection.

The ambient atmosphere inside a silo is quickly depleted of O_2, whereas CO_2, NO_2, and dinitrogen tetroxide (N_2O_4) accumulate rapidly. NO_2 air concentrations range from 200 to 2,000 ppm. Because these gases are heavier than air, they remain just above the silage level for weeks, even after production of the toxic gases dwindles. NO_2 has a bleachlike odor with a slight yellow color that stains silage. The presence of dead birds in silos is a clue to deadly gases.

NO_2 production correlates with silage nitrate levels. Nitrate levels are highest in corn, Sudan grass, and sorghum. Nitrate levels in plants are also increased by moisture, heavy fertilization, cool and wet growing seasons, immaturity of plants at harvest, and cutting plants close to the ground (41). NO_2 levels exceeding 200 ppm have been measured within 1 week of silo filling.

Silo filler's disease was first described in a series of 17 cases seen at the Mayo Clinic over a period of 32 years. Silo filler's disease is a condition that results from NO_2 pulmonary exposure generated by silage, particularly corn. NO_2 is heavier than air and is released as a product of the oxidation of nitrate groups in silage and nitrogen-rich soils. As the silage decays in this manner, the silos in which it is stored begin to fill with the gas. NO_2 may reach IDLH concentrations sufficient to produce respiratory irritation and death. High NO_2 concentrations can cause acute pulmonary edema. NO_2 concentrations greater than 200 ppm can cause immediate loss of consciousness. Concentrations approximately 50 to 100 ppm cause eye and airway irritation. Prolonged exposure at these concentrations can damage respiratory epithelium and alveolar epithelium.

Gases released from decomposing fodder and other chemical agents used in agricultural practice pose a significant hazard to pulmonary function. Chlorine, sulfur dioxide, ozone, phosgene, herbicides such as paraquat, and fertilizers such as anhydrous ammonia can cause similar immediate irritation of the mucous membranes of the upper respiratory tract. If the exposure is great enough, delayed pulmonary edema may develop. Farmers who enter silos unprotected are at risk. Because NO_2 and CO_2 are heavier than air, they create confined space hazards.

Exposures to silo gases cause dizziness, loss of consciousness, dyspnea, chest tightness, wheezing, chest pain, cough, fever, myalgias, and pulmonary edema if high enough in concentration (42,43).

Potato Processing

Workers engaged in potato processing can be exposed to protein allergens, chlorogenic acid, fungi, bacteria, endotoxin, and other components of organic dust. Potato production includes unloading from trucks, washing, peeling, and blanching (steaming and sulfuration) of potato pulp before drying (44). In one study, 45.9% of workers reported respiratory symptoms: cough, dyspnea, chest pain, fever, nausea, headache; FEV_1 and FVC decreased over work shifts; and 67.2% of workers had positive precipitin antibodies to microbial antigens in the environment. Antibodies to *Agromyces ramosus*, *Alcaligenes faecalis*, and *Thermetobacter calcoaceticus* correlated with symptoms (44). Total dust air concentrations increased throughout production, finally exceeding 100 mg per m^3. Endotoxin air concentration, although initially low, rose dramatically through the final stages of production to levels ranging from 46 to 1,894 μg per m^3 (104–106 ng/m^3). Microorganism air concentrations ranged between 28 and 93 CFU × 10^3 of air. Dominant bacteria were *Corynebacterium xerosis*, *Arthrobacter*, *Microbacterium* spp., *Agromyces ramosus*, and *Brevibacterium linens*. Gram-negative bacteria were mainly *Pseudomonas* and *Acinetobacter*. *Aspergillus niger* was the predominant fungus (44).

Green Tobacco Sickness

Green tobacco sickness is an occupational illness occurring among workers who crop or harvest tobacco leaves that are damp from rain or dew. The incidence of the illness is regularly noted in the tobacco fields of North Carolina, where workers report headache, pallor, nausea, vomiting, and prostration after handling wet tobacco leaves. Symptoms resemble nicotine poisoning but may simulate organophosphate poisoning and heat exhaustion and thus may be treated inappropriately. The moisture on the tobacco leaves probably acts as a solvent for the nicotine, facilitating dermal absorption, especially as work clothing becomes wet (45). Sufficient urinary excretion of nicotine and its major metabolite, cotinine, has been observed in conjunction with the symptoms of green tobacco sickness. Workers who smoke rarely experience symptoms. This is probably due to the fact that smokers are more tolerant to the amount of nicotine they absorb while working on the harvest (46).

Barns

Barn environments differ on their degree of enclosure, ventilation, content, and levels of contamination. Barns may contain hay, grass, cows, and other farm animals, and thus present an organic dust hazard. The density of animals and type of activity in barns determines the degree of organic dust exposure. Barns contain feeds that can be contaminated with bacteria, fungi, endotoxins, and storage mites. Hay can be heavily contaminated with thermophilic actinomycetes and *Faenia rectivirgula*, causative agents of hypersensitivity pneumonitis.

Depending on the moisture content, the fungal spore counts and actinomycetes in hay vary greatly (see Table 52-8). Handling of hay is a major source of dust generation.

INFECTIOUS DISEASES IN AGRICULTURAL WORKERS

Infectious diseases represent a hazard to farm workers through zoonotic spread and as a secondary consequence of farm-related injury (Table 52-11). Skin trauma is a common injury that can result in secondary infections. Deep tissue injury from farming equipment can result in serious infections because of the presence of numerous microbial organisms in farm produce.

Bacterial diseases include the zoonotic infections of tularemia (*Francisella tularensis*), anthrax (*Bacillus anthracis*), brucellosis (*Brucella*), leptospirosis (*Leptospira interrogans*), plague (*Yersinia pestis*), and glanders (*Pseudomonas moller*). Soft tissue infections are usually caused by staphylococcus and streptococcus organisms.

Viral zoonosis includes rabies, viral encephalitis, cowpox virus, contagious ecthyma, and Hantavirus. Chlamydial infections include Rocky Mountain spotted fever (*Rickettsia rickettsii*), Q fever (*Coxiella burnetii*), and ornithosis (*Chlamydia psittaci*). Fungal infections include histoplasmosis, blastomycosis, coccidioidomycosis, and sporotrichosis.

CHEMICAL EXPOSURES

The use of chemicals—particularly fertilizers, rodenticides, pesticides, nematocides, acaricides, slimicides, fumigants, and herbicides—is pervasive in agriculture. Agriculture uses approximately 65% of the registered pesticides in the United States for the control of insect vectors and to reduce crop loss.

Pesticides have helped reduce disease in our environment through control of insects and improved living conditions. They have increased the amount of available food. Pesticides include organophosphates, carbamates, rodenticides, fumigants, herbicides, and fungicides. Additional agents include food preservatives and seed dressings.

TABLE 52-11. Infectious diseases associated with agriculture

Brucellosis (*Brucella* spp.)
Leptospirosis (*Leptospira interrogans*)
Toxoplasmosis (*Toxoplasma gondii*)
Rabies
Psittacosis
Tetanus (*Clostridium tetani*)
Anthrax (*Bacillus anthracis*)
Erysipelas (*Streptococci*)
Q-fever (*Coxiella burnetii*)
Ornithosis (*Chlamydia psittaci*)
Histoplasmosis (*Histoplasma*)
Blastomycosis
Coccidioidomycosis [Valley fever (*Coccidioides immitis*)]
Sporotrichosis
Tuberculosis
Salmonella dermatitis (*Salmonella dublin*)
Glanders (*Pseudomonas moller*)
Staphylococcus infections
Streptococcus infections
Staphylococcal and streptococcal infection
Echinococcosis
Salmonellosis (*Salmonella*)
Rocky Mountain spotted fever (*Rickettsia rickettsii*)
Tularemia (*Francisella tularensis*)
Ascariasis
Plague (*Yersinia pestis*)
Balantidiasis
Listeriosis (*Listeria monocytogenes*)
Viral encephalitis
Cowpox virus
Hantavirus
Giardiasis (*Giardia lamblia*)

Pesticide Exposure

Pesticide exposures have acute, chronic, and long-term health effects. Besides the classical organophosphate/carbamate cholinesterase inhibition–caused illness, other health concerns include dermatitis, pulmonary injury, carcinogenesis, renal disease, liver disease, reproductive toxicity, and neurologic and neurobehavioral toxicity.

A list of pesticides used in farming is presented in Table 52-12. The most commonly used agricultural pesticides are organophosphates, carbamates, and herbicides.

Two categories of workers are occupationally exposed to pesticides. The first group consists of those workers described as mixers, loaders, and applicators of pesticide formulations. A high rate of occupational injury in these workers is due to their acute exposure to high concentrations of pesticides at full strength. Illness is related to accidental spills and dermal or inhalation exposure. The second category consists of field workers who are exposed to pesticide residues on the foliage of crops and in soils of treated fields. The exposure of this group differs from that of the mixer-loader-applicator group in that it is a more chronic, low-dose exposure, primarily involving dermal absorption.

The pesticides most frequently implicated in acute field exposures have been the organophosphates and carbamates. These pesticides exert their primary and acute toxic effects by inhibiting acetylcholinesterase. A 60% depression in cholinesterase activity can produce relatively mild nonspecific symptoms, such as nausea, headaches, malaise, constriction of pupils, and an asthmalike tightness of the chest. Greater depressions of cholinesterase activity may produce pulmonary edema, unconsciousness, respiratory failure, and even death. Cholinesterase depressions resulting from carbamate exposures usually reverse more rapidly than those resulting from organophosphate exposure. Depression in plasma cholinesterase can also occur from pregnancy and birth control pills, which can make interpretation difficult if no symptoms are associated with exposure.

Symptoms of organophosphate or carbamate poisoning can range from mild to severe. The degree of symptoms is dependent on the nature of the pesticide and its toxicity, absorbed dose, and prior level of cholinesterase activity. Weakness, abdominal pain, nausea, diarrhea, vomiting, and visual changes are associated with mild toxicity. Workers who are chronically exposed to organophosphate and carbamate insecticides without proper protection can deplete their cholinesterase activity to seriously low levels and be at increased risk for developing poisoning, even after a mild exposure that would normally not be serious. These individuals are at an increased risk for other work-related accidents and injuries.

Workers can be poisoned from crop residues as well as from direct contact during application (47–50). The rationale behind the legal reentry intervals has been to prohibit entry into treated fields to allow sufficient decay of the pesticide, such that potential health risks should be mitigated.

A study of Nebraska farmers and pesticide applicators discovered that 30% of these individuals had significant reductions in serum cholinesterase activity, and 22% had pesticide poisoning symptoms (51). One example of poisoning occurred when a field crew began harvesting in a mevinphos (Phosdrin)-treated field 2 hours after the pesticide was applied. Members of the crew sought medical treatment for a variety of symptoms ranging from nausea and visual disturbances to chest pain and shortness of breath. Plasma cholinesterase levels were depressed 15%, and red blood cell cholinesterase was depressed almost 6%. Symptoms persisted for as long as 10 weeks after exposure, which was longer than the 14 days it took for cholinesterase levels to normalize (47).

In response to serious illnesses and deaths among agricultural pesticide applicators, the state of California introduced a medical surveillance requirement in 1974 (52). The primary goal of medical surveillance is to prevent the development of profound cholinesterase depression and pesticide toxicity. California employers are required to provide wash and change facilities, clean work clothing, and the use of closed mixing and loading systems for the most toxic pesticides. Medical surveillance is also required for all agricultural pesticide applicators whose exposure to cholinesterase-inhibiting pesticides in toxicity category I or II (Table 52-13) is expected to reach 30 hours in any 30-day period. Mixer and loaders exclusively using closed systems are exempt from this requirement. Workers are referred to a physician medical supervisor for baseline red blood cell and plasma cholinesterase determination not less than 30 days after the last exposure to a cholinesterase-inhibiting pesticide. Workers are retested during their exposure period to detect any probable pesticide overexposure. If red blood cell cholinesterase activity is depressed to 70% below baseline or plasma cholinesterase to 60% or below, the worker must be removed from exposure to organophosphate or carbamate pesticides. Removed workers may not resume handling cholinesterase-inhibiting pesticides until their cholinesterase activity levels have returned to at least 80% of baseline values. However, although the regulations also require enclosed mixing and loading systems or enclosed cabs and industrial hygiene measures in conjunction with medical supervision, surveys of workers demonstrated previously that cholinesterase depression exceeding the state's requirements for removal still existed (48).

The Federal Food, Drug, and Cosmetic Act originally established harvest intervals restricting the time between pesticide application and harvest, based on pesticide residue levels on

TABLE 52-12. Partial listing of pesticides

- Inorganic and organometallic pesticides
  - Barium carbonate
  - Sodium dichromate
  - Copper sulfate
  - Zinc chloride
  - Zinc phosphide
  - Cadmium chloride
  - Elemental mercury
  - Mercuric chloride
  - Thallium sulfate
  - Lead arsenate
  - Methylmercury
  - Ethyltin and related organotins
  - Bismuth subcarbonate
  - Bismuth subsalicylate
  - Antimony potassium tartrate
- Arsenical pesticides
  - Phosphorus
  - Elemental sulfur
  - Sodium selenate
  - Sodium fluoride
  - Sulfuryl fluoride
  - Zinc hexafluorosilicate
  - Sodium chlorate
  - Boric acid
- Pyrethrins, pyrethroids, and plant-derived pesticides
  - Pyrethrins
  - Phenothrin
  - Decamethrin
  - Cypermethrin
  - Cyfluthrin
  - Deltamethrin
  - Cyhalothrin
  - Fenvalerate
  - Cyfluthrinate
  - Fluvalinate
  - Tralomethrin
  - Tralocythrin
  - Permethrin
  - Resmethrin
  - Rotenone
  - Nicotine
  - Anabasine
  - Sabadilla and related compounds
  - Strychnine
  - Ricin
  - Blasticidin-*S*
- Propellants, solvents, and oil insecticides
  - Dichlorodifluoromethane
  - Kerosene
  - Tetralin
  - Xylene
- Fumigants and nematocides
  - Hydrogen cyanide and the cyanide salts
  - Acrylonitrile
  - Isobornyl thiocyanoacetate
  - Carbon disulfide
  - Aluminum phosphide and phosphine
  - Naphthalene
  - Epoxyethane
  - Methyl bromide
  - Dichloromethane
  - Chloropicrin
  - Boron trifluoride
  - Carbon tetrachloride
  - 1,2-Dibromoethane
  - 1,2-Dichloroethane
  - 1,1,1-Trichloroethane
  - Trichloroethylene
  - Tetrachloroethylene
  - 1,1-Dichloro-1-nitroethane
  - Dibromochloropropane
  - 1,3-Dichloropropene
  - 1,2-Dichloropropane
  - *p*-Dichlorobenzene
- Chlorinated hydrocarbon insecticides
  - DDT
  - Tetrachlorodiphenylethane (TDE)
  - Ethylan
  - Methoxychlor
  - γ-Hexachlorocyclohexane (lindane)
  - Chlordane
  - Heptachlor
  - Aldrin
  - Dieldrin
  - Endrin
  - Isobenzan
  - Endosulfan
  - Mirex
  - Chlordecone
  - Toxaphene
  - Kelthane
- Organophosphate pesticides
  - Mipafox
  - Dimefox
  - DFP
  - Malathion
  - Parathion-methyl
  - Demeton-methyl
  - Oxydemeton-methyl
  - Dichlorvos
  - Trichlorfon
  - Naled
  - Jodfenfos
  - Methidathion
  - Phenthoate
  - Phosphamidon
  - Pirimiphos-methyl
  - Temephos
  - Thiometon
  - Schradan
  - Merphos
  - Leptophos
  - Carejin
  - Edifenphos
  - Fonofos
  - Mevinphos
  - Azinphos-methyl
  - Bromophos
  - Dicapthon
  - Monocrotophos
  - Dicrotophos
  - Dimethoate
  - Endothion
  - Fenitrothion
  - Fenthion
  - Formothion
  - Parathion
  - Diazinon
  - Demeton
  - Phorate
  - Tetraethylpyrophosphate (TEPP)
  - Carbophenothion
  - Chlorfenvinphos
  - Chlorphoxim
  - Chlorpyrifos
  - Dialifos
  - Dichlofenthion
  - Dioxathion
  - Fensulfothion
  - Phosalone
  - Phoxim
- Carbamate pesticides
  - Carbaryl
  - Aldocarb
  - Propoxur
  - 3-Isopropylphenyl-*N*-methylcarbamate
  - 4-Benziothielyn-*N*-methylcarbamate
  - Bufencarb
  - Carbofuran
  - Dioxacarb
  - Isolan
  - Landrin
  - Methomyl
  - Mexacarbate
  - Oxamyl
  - Phencyclocarb
  - Promecarb
  - Bendiocarb
- Nitro compounds and related phenolic pesticides
  - 2,4-Dinitrophenol
  - Binapacryl
  - Dinocap
  - Dinoseb
  - Pentachlorophenol
  - TCDD
- Synthetic organic rodenticides
  - Sodium fluoroacetate
  - Fluoroacetamide
  - Fluoroethanol
  - Gliftor
  - MNFA
  - Pyraminyl
  - ANTU
  - Warfarin
  - Difenacoum
  - Brodifiacoum
  - Diphacinone
  - Chloralose
  - Norbormide
- Herbicides
  - 2,4-*D*-Dichlorophenoxyacetic acid
  - 2,3,5-Trichlorophenoxyacetic acid
  - MCPA
  - Silvex
  - Dicamba
  - TCA
  - Propanil
  - Phenmedipham
  - Cycloate
  - Molinate
  - Diuron
  - Dichlobenil
  - Ioxynil
  - Paraquat
  - Diquat
  - Atrazine
  - Prozapine
  - Simazine
  - Amitrole
  - Pyrazon
- Fungicides and biocides
  - Captan
  - Captafol
  - Tetrachlorophthalide
  - Dichloran
  - Quinotozene
  - 1-Chlorodinitrobenzene
  - Diphenyl
  - Thiram
  - Ziram
  - Maneb
  - Zineb
  - Benomyl
  - Thiabendazole
  - Thiophanate-methyl
  - Organotins (tributyltin)
- Miscellaneous pesticides
  - Chlorfenxon
  - Propargite
  - Azoxybenzene
  - Chlordimeform
  - Metaldehyde
  - Diethyltoluamide (DEET)
  - Busulfan
  - Chlorambucil
  - Thiotepa
  - Hexamethylmelamine
  - 5-Fluorouracil
  - Methotrexate
  - Porfiromycin

Adapted from Hayes W, Laws E. *Pesticides studied in man*, vol 1–3. San Diego: Academic Press, 1991.

TABLE 52-13. U.S. Environmental Protection Agency's toxicity categories for pesticides

Category	LD_{50}[a]
I	≤50 mg/kg
II	51–100 mg/kg
III	>500 mg/kg

[a]Animal, oral, and dermal median lethal dose.

foodstuffs, for the purpose of consumer protection. Today, it is the EPA that lists tolerance levels of residues on food under the Toxic Substances Control Act. The intervals themselves, however, are established by the individual states (53). Reentry intervals for the purpose of worker safety did not become a regulatory issue until the passage of the Occupational Safety and Health Act of 1970, which created OSHA, and the passage of the 1972 amendments to the Federal Insecticide, Fungicide and Rodenticide Act (FIFRA). OSHA became the first federal agency to propose pesticide reentry standards to protect the health of field workers. The first standards included 21 organophosphorous insecticides and five crops (citrus, peaches, grapes, tobacco, and apples). After protest from several agricultural groups, these standards were replaced within 6 weeks with less stringent standards, covering only nine organophosphates with intervals ranging from 1 to 3 days for wet areas and 14 days for dry areas (based on average rainfall greater or less than 25 inches) (54). In 1973, the federal court gave jurisdiction to set and administer reentry standards to the EPA. Final EPA reentry standards, published in the *Federal Register* in 1974, required 48-hour reentry intervals for 11 organophosphate pesticides, endrin, and endosulfan (55).

States were given the responsibility and authority to set additional restrictions to address local problems. California has been the only state to establish its own reentry standards, which require longer intervals of between 5 and 30 days (56). Even with these longer intervals, there have still been numerous cases of illnesses among field worker crews that were induced by contact with residues on leaf surfaces (57).

The extent to which field workers are adversely affected by contact exposure to pesticide residues is a controversial subject. Many factors or a combination of factors may be necessary to produce an actual episode of poisoning by residues. Also, the dose-response mechanisms are difficult to assess because of the great variation in the types of pesticides used, work rate, quantity of pesticide contacted, and individual metabolism. The use of biological markers, such as pesticide metabolites, has been attempted as a means of determining absorption. However, biological monitoring is costly and, as noted earlier, the agriculture workforce does not lend itself well to any long-term surveillance. In an effort to overcome this obstacle, exposure assessment models have been attempted for individual types of crops that involve similar maintenance and harvest so as to have similar exposure patterns. These models correlate the dislodgeable foliar residues available for contact with daily dermal dose rates of an average harvester. The result is an empiric transfer factor expressed in terms of quantity of residue per unit of body surface area (58). Thus far, transfer factors for tree fruits, such as citrus and peaches, are in the range of 4,000 to 30,000 cm^2 per hour. A substantial number of data need to be amassed under varying climatic conditions for the transfer factor to be an effective method of quantifying exposure without the use of biological monitoring.

The number of officially reported cases of residue-related illness is estimated to be only 1% to 2% of the actual number. Considerable indirect evidence suggests that farm workers are adversely affected by pesticide residues, but the true magnitude of the problem is uncertain because cases are largely undetected and grossly underreported. Important socioeconomic and cultural factors must be understood and carefully evaluated in any attempt to study this problem.

Monitoring Pesticide-Exposed Workers

Monitoring red blood cell acetylcholinesterase activity is the easiest and least expensive screening method for organophosphate and carbamate exposures. California requires acetylcholinesterase monitoring for category I and II chemicals (see Table 52-13). Assays are conducted in state-approved laboratories. However, there is still much variation among the different assays used. Also, results may be reported in different units. Without a baseline level of red blood cell acetylcholinesterase activity, interpretation can be difficult. California's approach to monitoring exposed employees is as follows (59):

- Workers handling type I or II organophosphate/carbamate in a closed system and who do not apply insecticides receive preexposure monitoring to establish a baseline.
- New employees handling insecticides are tested once every 30 days, with the first test performed within 3 days after working 7 or more days in any consecutive 30-day period. The next two tests are at 30-day intervals when regularly handling pesticides.
- Employees after the first three tests are tested every 60 days unless medical supervision requires otherwise in writing.

If the red blood cell cholinesterase level of activity falls below 70% of baseline or plasma cholinesterase falls below 60% of baseline, the worker must be removed from the work site and cannot return until both enzyme levels return to 80% of baseline. The dose-response curve of cholinesterase inhibition is steep; therefore, further exposure can result in much steeper declines in enzyme activity. For this reason, additional doses of a pesticide can cause precipitous dips in enzyme activity resulting in cholinesterase inhibition signs and symptoms (59).

Pesticide-Related Dermatitis

Pesticide-related dermatitis is a common occupational problem in agribusiness (60). Many pesticides are associated with contact dermatitis or allergic dermatitis (Table 52-14). Pesticides that are skin sensitizers include dithiocarbamates, pyrethrins, thioates, thiurams, parathion, and malathion. Contact dermatitis is also common after exposures to plants sprayed with pesticides. Contact dermatitis may also be related to the solvent used to dilute certain pesticides for application.

Allergic contact dermatitis is a type IV hypersensitivity reaction that can occur after repeated antigen exposure. Clinically, it is difficult to distinguish from an irritant contact dermatitis. Patch testing is useful in making a diagnosis of allergic contact dermatitis.

Herbicide Exposure

Herbicides are probably the most heavily used pesticides in agriculture. Exposure concern centers around chronic health effects and cancer. Herbicides are classified according to time of application:

- Preplanting—Applied before land is seeded
- Preemergency—Applied before unwanted weeds appear
- Postemergent—Applied after weeds appear

TABLE 52-14. Pesticides associated with contact dermatitis or allergic dermatitis

Contact dermatitis	Benomyl
Phenylmercuric nitrate	Captan
Dazomet	Captafol
Glyphosphate	Mancozeb
Atrazine	Folpet
Prozapine	Plandrel
Simazine	Chlorothalonil
Trichlorobenzyl	Dinobuton
2,4-Dichlorophenoxy acetic acid (2,4-D)	Ditalmifos
	Ethoxyquin
Choline chloride	Ethylene bisdithiocarbamates
Paraquat	Metam sodium
Diquat	Amitrole
Sulfur	Chloridazon
Triphenyl tin hydroxide	Phenmedipham
Tributyl tin oxide	Alachlor
Copper sulfate	Barban
Hexachlorobenzene	Dazomet
Chlorothalonil	Pyrethrum and pyrethroids
Chlorpyrifos	Arsenic compound
Carbaryl	Ethylene oxide
Methylbromide	Parathion
Allergic dermatitis	Methyl parathion
Fungicides	Malathion
Thiocarbamates	Naled
Ziram	Triphanatemethyl
Maneb	Propargite (miticide)
Zineb	Dinitrochlorobenzene
Thiram	

Adapted with permission from ref. 60.

Herbicide chemical classes used in agriculture are:

- Chlorophenoxy compounds (2,4-dichlorophenoxy acetic acid)
- Triazines (atrazine, simazine, prozapine)
- Bipiridyls (paraquat and diquat)
- Acetanilids (alachlor, metholalchlor)
- Organic acids (dicamba)
- Organic phosphorus compounds (glyphosate)

Although the overall acute toxicity of herbicides is low, some herbicides have serious health consequences after exposure. Overall, herbicides are skin irritants and can produce contact dermatitis or skin burns, or both.

The bipiridiyls (paraquat and diquat) can cause dermatitis, skin burns, and ocular burns on exposure. Paraquat is extremely toxic after ingestion. It can cause burns of the mouth and esophagus from nonspecific oxidant injury. Paraquat ingestion can also result in alveolitis and fatal pulmonary fibrosis. It can cause cardiac, hepatic, and renal damage. The lethal dose of paraquat appears to be 6 g, although many have died who have ingested less (60). Paraquat actively accumulates in alveolar cells of the lung, where it forms a free radical that reacts with oxygen. A reactive oxygen species—superoxide anion—is formed from this reaction, which is converted to hydrogen peroxide. The superoxide anion and peroxide then interact to produce lipid peroxidation injury of the alveolar cells that perpetuates itself. Paraquat skin exposure is associated with contact dermatitis, Bowen's disease, squamous cell carcinoma, fingernail discoloration, nail deformity, and nail loss (61).

Glyphosate in the formulated product can cause eye and skin irritation (59).

Cancer is a concern related to herbicide exposure. Reviews of epidemiologic studies focusing on lymphoma and soft-tissue sarcomas show relative risks of sarcoma after exposure to phenoxyacetic acid herbicides to range from 0.7 to 6.8 (61). The relative risk for non-Hodgkin's lymphoma ranged from 0.4 to 4.8. Studies related to multiple myeloma report an excess cancer risk associated with phenoxyacetic acid herbicides (61). Other associated cancers with exposure are leukemia, testicular cancer, and ovarian cancer (62). Farm workers mixing and applying herbicides had an eightfold increased risk for non-Hodgkin's lymphoma.

Other studies have not shown an increased cancer risk associated with herbicide exposure. One study reviewed animal, ecological, case-control, and historical cohort studies of the association between cancer and three chlorophenoxy herbicides and found no relationship between exposure and cancer (63). Another case-control study found no increased risk of multiple myeloma in those exposed to phenoxy herbicides (64).

Fumigant Exposure

Agricultural workers use fumigants to prevent spoilage of agricultural products in an enclosed area. Fumigants are gases or vapors and are also used in soil. Fumigants commonly used in agricultural environments include

- Ethylene dibromide
- Phosphine (zinc or aluminum phosphide)
- Carbon tetrachloride and carbon disulfide mixtures
- Malathion and methoxychlor mixtures
- Chloroform
- Methyl bromide
- Chloropicrin
- Ethylene dichloride
- Dichloropropene and dichloropropane mixtures
- Ethylene oxide
- Propylene oxide
- Dibromochloropropane
- Formaldehyde
- Hydrogen cyanide
- Acrylonitrile
- Sulfur dioxide
- Sulfuryl fluoride

Exposure to fumigants—such as chloropicrin,acrolein, formaldehyde, sulfuryl fluoride, and sulfur dioxide—can cause respiratory tract injury because they are strong irritants. Exposure can cause immediate upper airway irritation, bronchospasm, laryngospasm, and cough. Methyl bromide, phosphine, and ethyl oxide also cause irritant upper respiratory symptoms. Fumigants can also, depending on the exposure, produce multisystem damage with pulmonary edema, central nervous system depression, hepatotoxicity, and renal toxicity after high-level acute exposures. Skin exposure can result in dermatitis.

Methyl bromide, which is used to sterilize soil, is a potent neurotoxin. Methyl bromide also causes chemical burn injury in contact with the skin or eyes. Acrylonitrile exposure is associated with toxic epidermal necrolysis. Nail injury is also associated with exposure to 4,6-dinitro-*O*-cresol (60).

Phosphine is produced by the action of hydrogen with metallic phosphides such as zinc or aluminum phosphide. Phosphine is a toxic gas with fishlike odor (odor threshold 0.03 ppm). Toxic exposure causes nausea, diarrhea, vomiting, respiratory symptoms, cough, and dizziness. High exposure can cause pulmonary edema, liver damage, cardiovascular collapse, cardiac injury, cardiac necrosis, and dysrhythmias.

Sulfur dioxide is used as a fumigant in enclosed spaces and may be encountered in produce transported by truck. Levels of SO_2 may rise to concentrations IDLH in the enclosed back of a truck.

Fumigants are usually highly toxic but have little specificity for any particular organism. Generally, each fumigant has its own distinctive toxic properties.

Fungicide Exposure

Fungicides are used to control members of the ascomycetes, phycomycetes, basidiomycetes, and imperfect groups of organisms. Fungicides include sulfur, copper, mercury, tin, and zinc compounds, dithiocarbamates, carbamates, organophosphorous compounds, halogenated hydrocarbons, aromatic nitro compounds, quinones, anilines, phthalimides, pyrimidines, pyridines, triazines, thiodaoaxoles, and isoxazolones. Commonly used fungicide compounds include the following:

- Baycor
- Bayleton
- Captafol
- Copper sulfate
- Cycloheximide
- Dichlorophene
- Quintozene
- Benomyl
- Captan
- Chlorothalonil
- Pentachlorophenol
- Ziram
- Ferbam
- Maneb
- Zineb
- Mancozeb
- Fenarimol
- Folpet
- Hexachlorobenzene
- Tributyl tin oxide
- Triphenyl tin oxide
- Triphenyl tin fluoride
- Triphenyl tin hydroxide

Dithiocarbamates are carbamic acid derivatives lacking any anticholinesterase activity. Chemically, many of these compounds have a metal atom incorporated that helps name the fungicide:

- Maneb (Mn)
- Zineb (Zn)
- Ferbam (Fe)
- Ziram (Zn)

Maneb chronic exposure may cause parkinsonism because of its manganese content (65).

Captan is a known animal mutagen and carcinogen and is regulated as a probable human carcinogen. Captan has a chemical structure similar to thialidomine and may react with cells to produce thiophosgene, which is cytotoxic and binds to SH-, amino-, and OH-containing enzymes (66).

Rodenticide Exposure

Rodenticides—poisons used to control rodents—are highly toxic and nonspecific. These include strychnine, sodium fluoroacetate, zinc and aluminum phosphide, norbromide, fluoroacetamide, alphachloralose, brodifacoum, diphencoumarin, diphenacinone, and pindone. Long-acting anticoagulants brodifacoum, pindone, diphencoumarin, and diphenacinone are known as *super warfarins*, and human ingestion can result in an abnormal prothrombin time for months.

Fluoroacetic acid compounds (sodium fluoroacetate, fluoroacetamide, and *N*-methyl-*N*-(1-naphthyl-fluoroacetamide) combine with oxaloacetate to form fluorocitrate and to interfere with the Krebs cycle by preventing conversion of citrate to isocitrate (66).

Other Toxic Chemical Exposures

Farm workers can be exposed to other potential toxins besides pesticides and insecticides. Because of the nature of agribusiness, toxic chemicals can be generated by animal confinement practices, sludge, silage, manure, and microbiologicals (26,36,42,67). These chemicals include the following:

- Ammonia
- Carbon monoxide
- Hydrogen sulfide
- Nitrogen dioxide
- Methane

Confined space environments are high-risk factors for exposure to these chemicals.

CANCER, AGRICULTURE, AND PESTICIDE EXPOSURE

Agricultural workers tend to have an excess of several cancers (61,62,68):

- Lip
- Stomach
- Melanoma
- Prostate
- Brain
- Testicles
- Soft-tissue sarcoma
- Non-Hodgkin's lymphoma
- Hodgkin's disease
- Multiple myeloma
- Leukemia
- Cervix
- Uterus
- Thyroid

Despite these findings, farmers tend to have a low mortality for all other forms of cancer. In women on farms, there is an excess of cervical cancer and cancer of the uterus (68). Some cancers tend to be linked with geographic regions. Non-Hodgkin's lymphoma and lip and brain cancer excesses are localized to the central regions of the U.S. farming community (68). Also, excess bone and thyroid cancer were seen only in white men (68). There was excess stomach and cervical cancer among nonwhite women in the south.

Mortality studies in farming revealed an excess mortality for lymphoma and leukemia (69,70). Case-control studies from Iowa farming communities in the 1980s found an increased lymphocytic leukemia and multiple myeloma (71).

Investigations into the possible etiologies or associated risks have focused on pesticides. As an example, elevated risk for lymphosarcoma, reticulosarcoma, and other lymphomas in areas with heavy insecticide, herbicide, and fertilizer use has been noted (72).

Studies have examined the suspected link between cancers and pesticide exposure in farmers. Many pesticides have demonstrated carcinogenic and genotoxic properties in animals (Table 52-15). Of interest in implicating pesticide exposure as a potential

TABLE 52-15. Evidence for carcinogenicity of pesticides

Compound	Animal	Human	*In vitro*	IARC[a]	EPA[b]
Aldrin	Limited	Inadequate	Inadequate	3	C
Amitrole	Sufficient	Inadequate	Inadequate	2B	B2
a-Naphthylthiourea	Inadequate	Inadequate	—	3	C
Aramite	Sufficient	—	—	—	—
Arsenicals	Inadequate	Sufficient	Limited	1	A
Benzyl chloride	Limited	Inadequate	Limited	3	C
Benzotrichloride	Sufficient	Inadequate	Limited	2B	B2
Benzoyl chloride	Inadequate	Inadequate	Inadequate	3	C
Benzyl chloride	Limited	Inadequate	Sufficient	3	C
Captan	Limited	Insufficient	—	—	—
Carbon tetrachloride	Sufficient	Inadequate	Inadequate	2B	B2
Chlordane	Limited	Inadequate	Inadequate	3	C
Chlordimeform (metabolite)	No data	Insufficient	—	—	—
Chlorobenzilate	Limited	Insufficient	—	—	—
Chlorophenols	—	Limited	—	2B	B2
Chlorothalonil	Limited	Insufficient	—	—	—
Diallate	Limited	Insufficient			
1,2-Dibromochloropropane	Sufficient	—	—	—	—
p-Dichlorobenzene	Sufficient	No data	—	2B	B2
2,4-Dichlorophenoxyacetic acid esters	Inadequate	Inadequate	Inadequate	3	C
p,p'-Dichlorodiphenyltrichloroethane	Sufficient	Inadequate	Inadequate	2B	B2
Dicofol (Kelthane)	Limited	Insufficient	—	—	—
Dieldrin	Limited	Inadequate	Inadequate	3	C
Ethylene dibromide	Sufficient	Inadequate	Sufficient	2B	B2
Ethylene oxide	Limited	Inadequate	Sufficient	2B	B2
Ethylene thiourea	Sufficient	Inadequate	Limited	2B	B2
Fluomenturon	Inadequate	No evaluation	—	—	—
Formaldehyde	Sufficient	Inadequate	Sufficient	2B	B2
Heptachlor	Limited	Inadequate	Inadequate	3	C
Hexachlorobenzene	Sufficient	—	—	—	—
Kepone (chlordecone)	Sufficient	—	—	—	—
Lindane (γ-hexachlorocyclohexane)	Limited	Inadequate	Inadequate	3	C
Malathion	No evidence	No data	—	—	—
4-Chloro-2-methylphenoxy acetic acid	Inadequate	Inadequate	—	3	C
Methyl parathion	No evidence	No evidence	—	3	C
Mirex	Sufficient	—	—	—	—
Nitrofen	Sufficient	No data	—	—	—
Parathion	Inadequate	Insufficient	—	—	—
Pentachlorophenol	Inadequate	Inadequate	Inadequate	3	C
Phenoxy acids	—	Limited	—	2B	B2
ø-Phenylphenol	Limited	Insufficient	—	—	—
Piperonyl butoxide	No evidence	No evidence	—	—	—
Sulfallate	Sufficient	No data	—	—	—
2,3,4,8-Tetrachlorodibenzo-*p*-dioxin	Sufficient	Inadequate	Inadequate	2B	B2
Tetrachlorovinphos	Limited	Insufficient	—	—	—
Thiourea	Sufficient	—	—	—	—
Toxaphene	Sufficient	—	—	—	—
Trichlorfon	Inadequate	Insufficient	—	—	—
2,4,5-Trichlorophenol	Inadequate	Inadequate	No data	3	C
2,4,6-Trichlorophenol	Sufficient	Inadequate	No data	2B	B2
2,4,5-Trichlorophenoxyacetic acid	Inadequate	Inadequate	Inadequate	3	C
Vinyl chloride	Sufficient	Sufficient	Sufficient	1	A

[a]IARC, International Agency for Research on Cancer. Evidence is divided into the following categories: 1, evidence is sufficient to establish a causal relationship between the agent and human cancer; 2, agent or process is probably carcinogenic to humans; 2A, limited, almost sufficient evidence for carcinogenicity in humans; 2B, combination of sufficient evidence in animals and inadequate human data; and 3, cannot be classified according to carcinogenicity in humans.
[b]EPA, Environmental Protection Agency. Evidence is divided into the following groups: A, carcinogenic to humans (epidemiologic evidence supports a causal relationship); B, probably carcinogenic to humans (B1, epidemiologic evidence limited or the weight of evidence from animal studies is sufficient, or B2, evidence is sufficient from animal studies but epidemiologic studies provide inadequate evidence or no data); and C, possibly carcinogenic to humans (limited evidence from animal studies and no human data).
Reprinted with permission from ref. 70.

cause is the finding of cancer patterns among others exposed to pesticides in their occupations similar to those in farming. However, this pattern tends to break with lung cancer. Farmers tend to have a lower incidence of lung cancer compared with structural pesticide applicators, who have a higher-than-expected lung cancer mortality (73). In situations in which effects of tobacco use could be controlled, some studies have shown an increased lung cancer rate in farmers exposed to pesticides (74,75). The organochlorine pesticides chlordane, heptachlor, dieldrin, aldrin, lindane, and DDT have been scrutinized as potential causes of increased risk of cancer. However, reviews of most of the significant studies performed through the years show inconclusive evidence for carcinogenicity of these organochlorine pesticides (69,70).

Multiple epidemiologic studies examining the relationship of chemical exposures and cancers in agricultural workers have been performed. Difficulties are encountered in trying to assess the exposure to pesticides and determine any increases in relative cancer risks. Phenoxy herbicides, such as 2,4,5-trichlorophenoxyacetic acid (2,4,5-T) and 2,4-dichlorophenoxyacetic acid (2,4-D), have been extensively studied with respect to potential carcinogenesis (69,76–83). These herbicides had been contaminated with 2,3,7,8-tetrachlorodibenzo-*p*-dioxins, a known animal carcinogen. In June 2000, EPA proposed upgrading dioxin to a known human carcinogen after a multiyear reassessment that generated substantial scientific controversy. Multiple case-control and cohort studies of phenoxy herbicide-exposed agricultural workers published between 1979 and 1988 demonstrated widely ranging relative risks (76–83).

Swedish case-control studies published in 1981 indicated a six-fold increase in soft-tissue sarcoma and lymphoma in phenoxy acid– or chlorophenol-exposed workers (79). Studies in New Zealand and the United States published between 1986 and 1988—as well as Swedish studies in 1988 and 1989—demonstrated varying relative risks (81,82). Swedish studies in 1988 had shown only a 3.3-fold relative risk for sarcoma (69). A twofold relative risk for soft-tissue sarcoma was found in Italian rice field workers in a 1987 study (82). However, U.S. studies published in 1986 and 1987, along with New Zealand studies in 1984 and 1986, demonstrated a relative risk of only 1.0 (69,81–83). Swedish cohort studies differed from case-control studies and found a relative risk of only 0.9 for soft-tissue sarcoma, compared with the five- to sixfold relative risk in earlier Swedish studies involving herbicide exposure (69).

A 1986 study reported a twofold excess of non-Hodgkin's lymphoma among farmers who used phenoxyacetic acid herbicides (84). This study showed that risk increased with the days per year of use to above sevenfold excess for those reporting use for 21 days or more per year of 2,4-D. Similar associations for lymphoma and 2,4-D have been reported in other studies (85,86). Case-control studies in 1981 showed an increased relative risk of 6.0 for non-Hodgkin's lymphomas in phenoxy herbicide–exposed workers, but a 1989 Swedish study found a relative risk of only 1.6 (87,88). Other studies from New Zealand in 1987 and from Washington in 1987 failed to show an increased risk for lymphomas in persons exposed to phenoxy herbicides (81,83).

Brain cancer is significantly higher among vineyard workers exposed to pesticides than among the general population (89). Triazine is a heavily used herbicide, and exposure was associated with a two- to fourfold increased risk of ovarian cancer in Italian studies (90).

Many variables regarding exposure remain unknown: methods of herbicide application, dose absorbed, length of exposure, route of exposure, cofactors (such as presence of other chemicals or potential carcinogens), and genetic background. The increase in certain cancers in agricultural workers appears real; however, the exact etiology remains unknown. Pesticides associated epidemiologically with specific cancers are listed in Table 52-16.

TABLE 52-16. Pesticides and cancer associations reported in epidemiologic studies

Pesticide	Cancer
Phenoxyacetic acid herbicides	Non-Hodgkin's lymphoma, soft-tissue sarcoma, prostate, Hodgkin's disease, multiple myeloma, stomach, lung, nasal, and nasopharyngeal
2,4-dichlorophenoxy acetic acid	Non-Hodgkin's lymphoma, prostate
2,4,5-trichlorophenoxyacetic acid	Soft-tissue sarcoma
4-chloromethyl phenoxyacetic acid	Soft-tissue sarcoma
Triazine herbicides	Ovary
Atrazine	Ovary
Arsenical insecticides	Lung, skin, non-Hodgkin's lymphoma
Organochlorine insecticides	Leukemia, non-Hodgkin's lymphoma, soft-tissue sarcoma, pancreas, skin, lung, liver, breast, neuroblastoma, multiple myeloma
Chlordane	Lymphoma, lung, neuroblastoma
DDT	Leukemia, non-Hodgkin's lymphoma, Hodgkin's disease, pancreas, lung, liver, multiple myeloma, skin, soft-tissue sarcoma, breast
Lindane	Lymphoma, breast
Methoxychlor	Leukemia
Toxaphene	Lymphoma
Organophosphate insecticides	Non-Hodgkin's lymphoma, leukemia, lung
Crotoxyphos	Leukemia
Diazinon	Non-Hodgkin's lymphoma
Dichlorvos	Leukemia, non-Hodgkin's lymphoma
Famphur	Leukemia
Malathion	Non-Hodgkin's lymphoma

Reprinted with permission from ref. 73, p. 277.

PEDIATRIC CANCER AND PESTICIDE EXPOSURE

Studies have linked pesticide exposure of children to cancer. Childhood leukemia and neuroblastoma were linked with chlordane exposure (91,92). Occupational exposure of either parent to pesticides and use of pesticides in the home during childhood have been linked to acute myeloid leukemia (93). Non-Hodgkin's lymphomas were associated with household or garden pesticide use and indoor pesticide application (93,94).

Soft-tissue sarcomas in children have been associated with yard treatment with the pesticides 2,4-D, carbaryl, and diazinon (94). Wilms' tumor and brain cancers are reportedly linked with pesticide exposure and parental occupational exposure to pesticides (73).

REPRODUCTIVE TOXICITY, DEVELOPMENTAL TOXICITY, AND PESTICIDES

The genotoxic properties of some pesticides have triggered investigations into the potential for these chemicals to produce germ-cell–level defects that would be expressed as birth anomalies. In addition, the potential for endocrine disruption by those chemicals with androgenic or estrogenic properties could alter male to female sex ratio of birth anomalies.

Garry et al. (95) have studied the possibility that offspring of pesticide appliers might have increased risks of birth anomalies based on the observation that chromosome rearrangements occurred at the highest frequency in pesticide appliers who stored grain (95,96). This study reported several findings that, if confirmed, have important implications for pesticide/fungicide usage:

- Birth defect rates were increased in the offspring born to licensed private appliers, particularly those offspring conceived in the spring.

- Rates were higher in the general population residing in high-use chlorophenoxy herbicide/fungicide regions within Minnesota.
- Shifts in the male to female sex ratio of offspring with anomalies were observed.

Exposure to pesticides also is associated with a detrimental effect on male infertility. These findings will undoubtedly lead to additional research efforts in this emerging area of environmental health concern.

According to the EPA, *reproductive toxicity* is the occurrence of adverse effects on the reproductive system that may result from environmental exposures. *Developmental toxicity* is the occurrence of adverse effects on the developing organism that may result from exposure before conception, during prenatal development, or postnatally (73).

The nematocide dibromochloropropane was found to be a male reproductive toxin, and its production was terminated. Two male reproductive toxins are chlordecone (Kepone) and ethylene dibromide. Kepone production in the United States was terminated in 1977. Ethylene dibromide is still in use as a fumigant.

REGULATION OF PESTICIDES

The primary federal statute for the regulation of manufacturing, use, and distribution of pesticides is FIFRA, which was enacted in 1947. Since then, FIFRA was amended in 1972, 1975, and 1978. The EPA has had the responsibility to regulate pesticide use since 1970. Pesticide regulation first occurred under the Insecticide Act of 1910, which was a consumer protection measure against mislabeling and distribution of ineffective pesticides. FIFRA replaced this act. Pesticides are also regulated by the EPA under the following acts:

- Federal Environmental Pesticide Control Act
- Resource Conservation Recovery Act of 1972
- Comprehensive Environmental Response, Compensation and Liability Act (Superfund)
- Toxic Substances Control Act
- Clean Water Act
- Safe Drinking Water Act

A *pesticide* is defined under FIFRA as "any substance or mixture of substances intended for preventing, destroying, repelling, or mitigating any pest, and . . . any substance or mixture of substances intended for use as a plant regulator, defoliant, or desiccant." This definition includes insecticides, fungicides, herbicides, rodenticides, desiccants, disinfectants, defoliants, and nematocides. FIFRA requires all pesticides sold or distributed to be registered with the EPA. Once registered, FIFRA classifies the pesticide as general or restricted in use. The application and use of pesticides are tightly controlled by the EPA under FIFRA.

FIFRA prohibits the sale of unregistered pesticides, the production of pesticides by unregistered manufacturers, the use of adulterated pesticides, and the use of a pesticide in a manner inconsistent with its labeling. The EPA has the authority to enforce FIFRA by legal sanctions, including civil penalties, criminal fines, injunctions, product seizure, termination of product sales, or recalls. When evidence indicates that a particular pesticide may be a significant health hazard, the appropriate regulatory agency or agencies can take any of the following actions:

- Issue permissible exposure limits for the workplace
- Cancel registration and order withdrawal of the product from the market
- Place restrictions on use or application of the compound
- Set tolerance limits for pesticide residues on foodstuffs
- Cancel registration
- Establish maximum permissible contamination levels for the pesticides in drinking water

In addition to the regulation of pesticide use and application, FIFRA requires the pesticide manufacturer to be registered with the EPA. The EPA, under agreement with the Food and Drug Administration, establishes pesticide tolerance for raw foods and produce. Pesticides that might be considered food additives are controlled by the EPA under the Food, Drug, and Cosmetic Act. Once a pesticide is discarded, it becomes a hazardous waste and is then under regulation by the Resource Conservation Recovery Act and not FIFRA.

The 1978 amendment to FIFRA allows manufacturers of pesticides to have a waiver on submission of data demonstrating efficacy of their product, except when the product has a direct relation to or effect on public health. In addition, the 1978 amendment allows for public disclosure of the safety and health data regarding pesticide regulation. The 1978 amendment also transfers to states the responsibility to enforce pesticide use regulations if they can demonstrate that they possess the means to do so. The EPA reserves the right to revoke any state's responsibility for pesticide regulation if that state is unable or unwilling to enforce the regulations.

Regulation of a pesticide suspected to be a carcinogen is not uniformly applied by all federal agencies. However, these agencies have been consistent in regulating a substance when it is expected to cause an increase of more than four cases of cancer per 1,000 persons. If the expected increase in cancer is less than one in a million, then regulation is unlikely. Cost-effectiveness of regulation is also considered if the cost of regulation is anticipated to be less than $2 million per life saved.

REFERENCES

1. Cordes D, Rea D. Health hazards of farming. *Am Family Physician* 1988; 38(4):233–244.
2. Schenker MB, McCurdy SA. Occupational health among migrant and seasonal farm workers: the specific case of dermatitis. *Am J Ind Med* 1990;18:345–351.
3. Myers J, Hard D. Work related fatalities in the agricultural production and services sectors, 1980–89. *Am J Ind Med* 1995;27:51–63.
4. Purschwitz MA, Field WE. Scope and magnitude of injuries in the agricultural workplace. *Am J Ind Med* 1990;18:179–192.
5. Elkind T, Cody-Salter H. Farm stressors: the hazards of agrarian life. *Ann Agric Environ Med* 1994;1:23–27.
6. US Department of Agriculture. Farm business economic report, 1995. Economic Research Service, 1997.
7. Bultena G, Lasley P, Guler J. The farm crisis: patterns and impacts of financial distress among Iowa farm families. *Rural Sociology* 1986;51:436–448.
8. Walker J. Self-reported stress symptoms in farmers. *J Clin Psychol* 1988;1:10–16.
9. Letts R, Gammon W. Auger injuries in children. *Can Med J* 1978;118:519–522.
10. Campbell D, Brian R, Cooney W, Ilstrup D. Mechanical corn picker hand injuries. *J Trauma* 1979;19(9):678–681.
11. Gorsche T, Wood M. Mutilating corn picker injuries of the hand. *J Hand Surg* 1988;13a(3):423–427.
12. Proust A. Special injuries of the hand. *Emerg Med* 1993;11(3):767–779.
13. Melvin P. Corn picker injuries of the hand. *Arch Surg* 1972;104:26–29.
14. Cogbill TH, Steenlage ES, Landercasper J, Strutt PJ. Death and disability from agricultural injuries in Wisconsin: a 12-year experience with 739 patients. *J Trauma* 1991;31(12):1632–1637.
15. Mayba I. Hay baler's fracture. *J Trauma* 1984;24(3):271–273.
16. Purschwitz M, Field W. Scope and magnitude of injuries in the agricultural workplace. *Am J Ind Med* 1990;18:179–192.
17. Hoskin A, Miller T. Farm accident surveys: a 21 state summary with emphasis on animal related injuries. *J Safety Res* 1979;11(1):2–13.
18. Iverson M, Brink O, Dahl R. Lung function in a five year follow-up of farmers. *Ann Agric Environ Med* 1994;1:39–43.
19. Fogelmark B, Rylander R. (1-3)-β-D-Glucan in some indoor air fungi. *Indoor Build Environ* 1997;6:291–294.
20. Pickering C, Taylor A. Extrinsic allergic bronchioloalveolitis (hypersensitivity pneumonitis). In: Parkes R, ed. *Occupational lung disorders*, 3rd ed. Boston: Butterworth–Heinemann, 1994.
21. Balmes J. Hypersensitivity pneumonitis. In: Harber P, Schenker M, Balmes J, eds. *Occupational and environmental disease*. St. Louis: Mosby, 1996.

22. Murphy D, Morgan W, Seaton A. Hypersensitivity. In: Morgan D, Seaton A, eds. *Occupational lung diseases*, 3rd ed. Philadelphia: WB Saunders, 1995.
23. Eduard W. Exposure to non-infectious microorganisms and endotoxins in agriculture. *Ann Agric Environ Med* 1997;4:179–186.
24. Milanonski J, Sorenson W, Dutkiewicz J, Lewis D. Chemotaxis of alveolar macrophages and neutrophils in response to microbial products derived from organic dust. *Environ Res* 1995;64:59–66.
25. Zejda J, McDuffie H, Dosman J. Epidemiology of health and safety risks in agriculture and related industries—practical applications for rural physicians. *Western J Med* 1993;158(1):56–93.
26. Donham K. Respiratory disease hazards to workers in livestock and poultry confinement structures. *Semin Respir Med* 1993;14(1):49–59.
27. Bone R. Goals of asthma management. *Chest* 1996;109(4):1056–1065.
28. Bernstein D. Allergic reactions to workplace allergens. *JAMA* 1997;278(22): 1907–1913.
29. Freitas R, Burr M. Animal wastes. In: Pepper I, Gerba C, Brusseau M, eds. *Pollution science*. San Diego: Academic Press, 1996.
30. Katlia ML, Mantyjarvi RA, Ojanen TH. Sensitization against environmental antigens and respiratory symptoms in swine workers. *Br J Ind Med* 1981;38:344–348.
31. Donham KJ. Health effects from work in swine confinement buildings. *Am J Ind Med* 1990;17:17–25.
32. Donham KJ, Knapp LW, Monson R, Gustafson K. Acute toxic exposure to gases from liquid manure. *J Occup Med* 1982;24:142–145.
33. Clark S, Rylander R, Larson L. Airborne bacteria endotoxin and fungi in dust in poultry and swine confinement buildings. *Am J Ind Hyg Assoc J* 1983;44:537–541.
34. Zejda J, Hurst T, Barber E, et al. Respiratory health status in swine producers using respiratory protective devices. *Am J Ind Med* 1993;23:743–750.
35. Cockcroft DW, Dosman JA. Respiratory health risks in farmers. *Ann Intern Med* 1981;95:380–382.
36. US Department of Health and Human Services, Centers for Disease Control and Prevention, National Institute for Occupational Safety and Health. Worker deaths in confined spaces: a summary of surveillance findings and investigative case reports. 1994.
37. Hurst JS, Dosman JA. Characterization of health effects of grain dust exposures. *Am J Ind Med* 1990;17:27–32.
38. Rylander R. Health effects of cotton dust exposures. *Am J Ind Med* 1990; 17:39–45.
39. Chun D, Perkins H. Profile of bacterial genera associated with cotton from low endotoxin and high endotoxin growing regions. *Ann Agric Environ Med* 1997;4:233–242.
40. Morgan W. Byssinosis and related conditions. In: Morgan W, Seaton A, eds. *Occupational lung diseases*, Philadelphia: WB Saunders, 1995.
41. May J, Schenker M. Agriculture. In: Harber P, Schenker M, Balmes J, eds. *Occupational and environmental respiratory disease*. St. Louis: Mosby, 1996.
42. Lowry T, Schuman LM. Silo-filler's disease: a syndrome caused by nitrogen dioxide. *JAMA* 1956;162:153–160.
43. Moskowitz RL, Lyons HA, Cottle HR. Silo-filler's disease: clinical, physiological and pathological study of a patient. *Am J Med* 1964;36:457.
44. Dutkiewicz J. Bacteria, fungi and endotoxin as potential agents of occupational hazard in a potato processing plant. *Am J Ind Med* 1994;25:43–46.
45. Gehlbach SH, Williams WA, Perry LD, Woodall JS. Green tobacco sickness: an illness of tobacco harvesters. *JAMA* 1974;229:1880–1883.
46. Ghosh SK, Parikh JR, Govani VN, Roa MN, Kashyap SK, Chatterjee SK. Studies on occupational health problems in agricultural tobacco workers. *J Occup Med* 1980;29:113–117.
47. Coye MJ, Barnett PG, Midtline JE, Valesco AR, et al. Clinical confirmation of organophosphate poisoning of agricultural workers. *Am J Ind Med* 1986;10:399–409.
48. Brown SK, Ames RG, Mengle DC, et al. Cholinesterase activity depression among California agricultural pesticide applicators. *Am J Ind Med* 1989;15:143–150.
49. Spear RC, Poppendorf WJ, Spencer WF, Milby TH. Worker poisonings due to paraoxon residues. *J Occup Med* 1977;19:411–414.
50. Brown SK, Ames RG, Mengle CD. Occupational illnesses from cholinesterase-inhibiting pesticides among agricultural applicators in California 1982–1985. *Environ Health* 1989;44:34–39.
51. Weisenburger DD. Environmental epidemiology of non-Hodgkin's lymphoma in Eastern Nebraska. *Am J Ind Med* 1990;18:303–305.
52. State of California Department of Food and Agriculture. Medical supervision. Code of regulations, title 3, chapter 6, section 6728; 1989.
53. US Environmental Protection Agency. Harvest intervals. EPA code of federal regulations, title 40; 1989.
54. US Department of Labor, Occupational Safety and Health Administration. Emergency temporary standard for exposure to organophosphorous pesticides. *Federal Register* 1973;38:10715.
55. US Environmental Protection Agency. Farm workers dealing with pesticides. Proposed health-safety standards. *Federal Register* 1974;39:9457.
56. State of California Department of Food and Agriculture. Re-entry intervals. Code of regulations, title 3, chapter 6, section 6772; 1989.
57. Kahn E. Pesticide related illness in California farm workers. *J Occup Med* 1976;18:693–696.
58. Popendorf WJ, Leffingwell JT. Regulating OP residues for farm worker protection. *Residue Rev* 1982;82:125–201.
59. Wilson B, Sanborn J, O'Malley M. Monitoring the pesticide-exposed worker. *Occup Med* 1997;12(2):347–363.
60. O'Malley M. Skin reactions to pesticides. *Occup Med* 1997;12(2):327–345.
61. Blair A, Zahm S. Herbicides and cancer: a review and discussion of methodologic issues. *Recent Results Cancer Res* 1990;120:132–145.
62. Morrison H, Wilkins K, Semenciw R, et al. Herbicides and cancer. *J Natl Cancer Inst* 1992;84(24):1865–1874.
63. Bond G, Rossbacher R. A review of potential human carcinogenicity of the chlorophenoxy herbicides MCPA, MCPP and 2,4-DP. *Br J Ind Med* 1993;50:340–348.
64. Brown L, Burmeister LF, Evertt G, Blair A. Pesticide exposures and multiple myeloma in Iowa men. *Cancer Causes Control* 1993;4:153–156.
65. Ferraz H, Bertolucci P, Pereira J, et al. Chronic exposure to the fungicide maneb may produce symptoms and signs of CNS manganese intoxication. *Neurology* 1988;38:550–553.
66. Costa L. Basic toxicology of pesticides. *Occup Med* 1997;12(2):251–268.
67. Crook B, Cocker J, Gillanders E, Redmayne A, Jones K. Microbially derived toxic gases as a possible cause of an episode of ill health in forestry: case reports. *Ann Agric Environ Med* 1997;4:277–280.
68. Blair A, Dosemeci M, Heineman E. Cancer and other causes of death among male and female farmers from twenty-three states. *Am J Ind Med* 1993; 23:729–742.
69. Pearce N, Reif JS. Epidemiologic studies of cancer in agricultural workers. *Am J Ind Med* 1990;18:133–148.
70. Journal of the American Medical Association Council of Scientific Affairs. Cancer risks of pesticides in agricultural workers. *JAMA* 1988;260:959–966.
71. Burmeister LF. Cancer in Iowa farmers: recent results. *Am J Ind Med* 1990;18:295–301.
72. Staftlas AF, Blair A, Cantor KP, Hanrahan L, Anderson HA. Cancer and other causes of death among Wisconsin farmers. *Am J Ind Med* 1987;11:119–129.
73. Zahm S, Ward M, Blair A. Pesticides and cancer. *Occup Med* 1997;12(2):269–289.
74. Brownson R, Alavanja M, Chang J. Occupational risk factors for lung cancer among nonsmoking women—a case-control study in Missouri (United States). *Cancer Causes Control* 1993;4:449–454.
75. Swanson G, Lin CS, Burns P. Diversity in the association between occupation and lung cancer among black and white men. *Cancer Epidemiol Biomarkers Prev* 1993;2:313–330.
76. Blair A, Zahm SH. Methodologic issues in exposure assessment for case-control studies of cancer and herbicides. *Am J Ind Med* 1990;18:285–293.
77. Hardell L, Sandstrom A. Case-control study: soft-tissue sarcomas and exposure to phenoxyacetic acids or chlorophenols. *Br J Cancer* 1979;39:711–717.
78. Hardell L, Eriksson M, Lenner P, Lundgren E. Malignant lymphoma and exposure to chemicals, especially organic solvents, chlorophenols and phenoxy acids: a case-control study. *Br J Cancer* 1981;43:169–176.
79. Eriksson M, Hardell L, Berg NO, Moller T, Axelson O. Soft-tissue sarcomas and exposure to chemical substances: a case-referent study. *Br J Ind Med* 1981;38:27–33.
80. Hardell L. Relation of soft-tissue sarcoma, malignant lymphoma and colon cancer to phenoxy acids, chlorophenols and other agents. *Scand J Work Environ Health* 1981;7:119–130.
81. Smith AH, Pearce NE, Fisher DO, Giles HJ, Teague CA, Howard JK. Soft tissue sarcoma and exposure to phenoxyherbicides and chlorophenols in New Zealand. *J Natl Cancer Inst* 1981;73:1111–1117.
82. Vineis P, Terracini B, Ciccone G, et al. Phenoxy herbicides and soft-tissue sarcomas in female rice weeders. *Scand J Work Environ Health* 1986;13:9–17.
83. Woods JS, Polissar L, Severson RK, Heuser LS, Kulander BG. Soft-tissue sarcoma and non-Hodgkin's lymphoma in relation to phenoxyherbicide and chlorinated phenol exposure in western Washington. *J Natl Cancer Inst* 1987;78:899–910.
84. Hoar S, Blair A, Holmes F, et al. Agricultural herbicide use and risk of lymphoma and soft tissue sarcoma. *JAMA* 1986;256:1141–1147.
85. Zahm S, Weisenburger D, Babbit P, et al. A case-control study of non-Hodgkin's lymphoma and the herbicide 2,4-dichlorophenoxy acetic acid (2,4-D) in eastern Nebraska. *Epidemiology* 1990;1:349–356.
86. Wigle D, Semenciw R, Wilkens K, et al. Mortality study of Canadian male farm operators: non-Hodgkin's lymphoma mortality and agricultural practices in Saskatchewan. *J Natl Cancer Inst* 1990;82:575–582.
87. Wiklund K, Dich J, Holm LE. Risk of malignant lymphoma in Swedish pesticide appliers. *Br J Cancer* 1987;56:505–508.
88. Wiklund K, Lindefors BM, Holm LE. Risk of malignant lymphoma in Swedish agricultural and forestry workers. *Br J Ind Med* 1988;45:19–24.
89. Viel J, Challier B, Pitard A, Pobel, D. Brain cancer mortality among French farmers: the vineyard pesticide hypothesis. *Arch Environ Health* 1998;53(1):65–70.
90. Donna A, Crosignani P, Robutti F, et al. Triazine herbicides and ovarian epithelial neoplasms. *Scand J Work Environ Health* 1989;15:47–53.
91. Epstein S, Ozonoff D. Leukemias and blood dyscrasias following exposure to chlordane and heptachlor. *Teratog Carcinog Mutagen* 1987;7:527–540.
92. Infant P, Newton W. Prenatal chlordane exposure and neuroblastoma. *N Engl J Med* 1978;293:308.
93. Buckley J, Robison L, Swotinsky R, et al. Occupational exposures of parents of children with acute nonlymphocytic leukemia—a report from the children's cancer study group. *Cancer Res* 1989;49:4030–4037.
94. Leiss J, Savitz D. Home pesticide use and childhood cancer: a case-control study. *Am J Public Health* 1995;85:249–252.
95. Garry VF, Schreinemachers D, Harkins ME, Griffith J. Pesticide appliers, biocides and birth defects in rural Minnesota. *Environ Health Perspect* 1996;104:394–399.
96. Strohmer H, Boldizsar A, Plockinger B, et al. Agricultural work and male infertility. *Am J Ind Med* 1993;24:587–592.

CHAPTER 53
Indoor Environmental Quality and Health

John B. Sullivan, Jr., Mark D. Van Ert, Gary R. Krieger, and Bradford O. Brooks

Approximately 71 million employees work indoors in the United States and the U.S. Bureau of Labor Statistics estimates that more than 21 million of these are exposed to some degree of poor indoor environmental quality (1). The Occupational Safety and Health Administration (OSHA) estimates that 69,000 severe headaches and 105,000 respiratory problems may be caused by poor indoor environmental quality (1). Employees working in service industries, in wholesale and retail trades, and in government jobs make up the bulk of those at risk (Table 53-1) (1).

Changing energy use strategies in the 1970s resulted in construction of buildings with improved energy efficiencies and tighter sealing to prevent energy loss. As a consequence, health complaints relating to indoor environments began to increase, and the term *tight building* or *sick building syndrome* (SBS) was adopted to describe this problem. Complaints relating to the environment had previously been attributed to either poor working conditions or psychological factors. It soon became apparent, however, that health complaints could also be attributed to inadequate ventilation, mold overgrowth, lack of fresh air exchange, excess biological and chemical contaminants, dampness, or inadequate dilution of indoor contaminants (1–9). The phrase *poor indoor air quality* is used to describe environmental conditions indoors that can result in signs and symptoms attributable to the buildup of airborne contaminants. Such illness, however, is often multifactorial. Symptoms commonly expressed in cases of poor environmental air quality are as follows:

- Mucous membrane irritation
  - Eye irritation
  - Nasal symptoms
  - Throat irritation
  - Drying of mucous membranes
  - Drying of skin
  - Rashes
  - Sinus congestion
- Respiratory symptoms
  - Cough
  - Chest tightness
  - Sore throat
  - Voice changes and hoarseness
  - Asthma
  - Difficulty breathing
  - Bronchial hyperresponsiveness
- Constitutional
  - Nausea
  - Abdominal complaints
  - Myalgia
  - Arthralgia
- Neurologic and neurobehavioral
  - Headache
  - Fatigue
  - Dizziness
  - Lethargy
  - Difficulty concentrating
  - Memory problems

TABLE 53-1. Occupational Safety and Health Administration sites of poor indoor air quality

Occupational field	Employees working indoors	No. of buildings with air quality problems	No. of employees exposed to air quality problems
Agriculture, forestry, fishing	279,050	51,956	83,715
Mining	180,700	4,554	54,210
Construction	1,643,750	128,091	493,125
Manufacturing	5,748,000	77,573	1,724,400
Transportation	3,412,350	48,563	1,023,705
Wholesale and retail trade	15,744,000	384,466	4,723,200
Finance, insurance, real estate	7,248,150	104,863	2,174,445
Services	26,926,000	385,235	8,077,800
Government	9,473,561	173,100	2,842,068
Total	**70,655,561**	**1,358,400**	**21,196,668**

From ref. 1, with permission.

For example, increased incidences of allergic diseases, coughing, wheezing, shortness of breath, asthma, bronchitis, headaches, eye irritation, muscle aches, fever, chills, nausea, vomiting, and diarrhea are reported among children and adults exposed to indoor biological contaminants, but biologicals encompass a wide array of contaminants and biochemical by-products (1–9).

The World Health Organization (WHO) characterized SBS in 1983. Since then, health complaints associated with poor indoor air quality have been classified as either SBS or building-related illness. Although arbitrary and archaic, this classification serves to categorize illness as traceable or untraceable to a defined cause or source.

SBS defines a set of symptoms whose origin is uncertain or related to ill-defined factors in the environment. Affected individuals experience multiple and sometimes vague health complaints. In such cases, health complaints tend to cease when the individual leaves the site and recur when the individual reenters the site.

The term *building-related illness* applies to a definable medical condition able to be traced to a single source and documented by specific signs and symptoms consistent with a known disease. Examples include *Legionella pneumophila*, hypersensitivity pneumonitis caused by organic dusts and bioaerosols, carbon monoxide poisoning, and allergic-mediated asthma caused by identifiable allergens. The seriousness of building-related illness became apparent in the *Legionella pneumophila* infection of 182 American Legion members attending a convention in 1976 in Philadelphia, resulting in 29 fatalities. The dissemination of this bacterium from contaminated ventilation systems emphasizes the contribution of the multiple factors of humidity, biological growth, and ventilation to causing illness.

SOURCES AND CAUSES OF POOR ENVIRONMENTAL QUALITY

Studies indicate that vague complaints relating to mucous membrane irritation, respiratory symptoms, and headache occur more commonly in office environments (3,4,9,10). But sources and causes of such health complaints are multiple and can be difficult to identify. Investigations of these sites show that deterioration of the environmental quality indoors is most often caused by problems with airborne contaminants traceable to one or more of the following general sources:

- Chemical
- Biological
- Physical
- Psychosocial

A dynamic mixture of chemical, biological, and particulate pollutants arising from a variety of sources circulates in indoor air:

Chemical sources
  Chemicals volatilizing from building materials and furnishings
  Cleaning materials and disinfectants
  Chemicals emitted from office machines and materials
  Pesticides
  Tobacco smoke
  Combustion products from cooking and fireplaces
Physical sources
  Ventilation problems
  Dusts
  Particulates
  Fibers, such as asbestos or fiberglass
Biological sources
  Pollen
  Mold and fungus
  Biological by-products of microbes
  Bacteria
  Viruses
  Dander from pets
  Insects and insect parts
  Human skin particles
  Dust mites

These pollutants are influenced by air movement, ventilation, temperature, and humidity. Most of the chemical sources of indoor contaminants are comprised of volatile organic chemicals (VOCs). Analyses of indoor air samples demonstrate between 50 and 300 different VOCs present in low levels in nonindustrial environments, such as offices, homes, shopping centers, and malls (11–13) (Table 53-2).

Biological sources of indoor pollution include mold, fungus, pollen, spores, bacteria, viruses, and insects, such as dust mites and roaches. Water reservoirs and damp areas provide nutrient sources for microorganism growth. Relatively high humidity and moisture allow biological agents to amplify to levels that when disseminated indoors can trigger illness and allergies. Reports indicate that indoor dampness and mold growth are associated with increased respiratory illness in adults and children (5,7,8). High relative humidity also encourages growth in the dust mite population, which can cause allergies and asthma. More attention is being focused on biochemical products of microorganisms as potential causes of indoor-related respiratory illness, such as endotoxin, 1,3-β-glucan, mycotoxins, peptidoglycan, and VOCs emitted from fungi (9).

Physical factors, the third source of indoor-related illness, include dusts, fibers, particulates, and overall comfort factors, such as ventilation, lighting, temperature, humidity, noise, and vibration. Dust and particulate matter are ever present indoors. Each cubic meter of air contains small concentrations of millions of particulates, of which 99% are invisible to the eye (9).

Psychosocial factors, the fourth source of illness indoors, include elevated stress from perceived or real environmental threats and illness, lack of control over the environment, the nature of the work itself, and conflict arising from adversarial stances of management or coworkers. Psychosocial factors can be particularly complex. Frequently, however, some employees may be improperly labeled as *psychogenic* or their illness as *psychological* without a proper or thorough investigation of environmental causes (14–17).

TABLE 53-2. A partial list of volatile organic chemicals identified indoors

Xylenes	Chlorobenzene
Ethylbenzene	Pinene
Toluene	Carbon tetrachloride
1,1,1-Trichloroethane	Chloroform
1,1,2-Trichloroethane	1,2-Dichloroethane
Dichlorobenzenes	Methylene chloride
Styrene	1,2,4-Trimethylbenzene
Hexane	1,1-Dichloroethylene
2-Butanone	Naphthalene
1,1-Dichloroethane	1,3-Dichloropropane
Alkyl benzenes	1,3,5-Trimethylbenzene
Ethyltoluene	Hexanol
Methylcyclopentane	Heptadecane
2-Methylhexane	Ethyl acetate
Methylcyclohexane	Isopropylbenzene (cumene)
2,2,5-Trimethylhexane	*n*-Propylbenzene
Ethylene dibromide	1,2,3-Trimethylbenzene
Bromodichloromethane	Acetone
Methyl butyl ether	*n*-Heptane
Undecane	*n*-Butanol
Dodecane	Benzyl chloride
Decane	Dimethyl phthalate
Tridecane	1,1,2,2-Tetrachloroethane
Tetradecane	1,1,2,2-Tetrachlorethylene
m-Ethyltoluene	Dibutyl phthalate
Cyclohexane	Butyl acetate
3,4-Dimethylheptane	2-Ethoxyethelacetate
Pentadecane	1,4-Dimethylethylbenzene
Hexadecane	2-Propanol
1,2,4-Trichlorobenzene	2-Methylbutane
Nonanal	2,2,4-Trimethylpentane
Limonene	1,4-Dimethylcyclohexane
Nonane	Pyridine
Chloroethyl vinyl ether	Propane
4-Methyl-2-pentanone	2-Vinyl pyridine
Carbon disulfide	Diethyl phthalate
Benzene	Ethylene dichloride
Tetrachloroethylene (perchlorethylene)	Dichlorethylene
Trichloroethylene (trichloroethene)	Camphene
Octane	Isopropyl ether
	Trichlorofluoromethane (Freon)
	Methyl chloride

INDOOR ENVIRONMENTAL QUALITY AND COMFORT FACTORS

Overall comfort in the indoor environment of home or work directly affects perceptions of health. Research shows that human comfort levels in the work environment are second in importance only to satisfaction regarding the nature of the work itself (14). Human well-being indoors is a result of multiple interacting factors that collectively contribute to perceptions of comfort and indoor environmental quality. But these factors can also contribute to illness and discomfort indoors.

Energy Conservation

Energy conservation strategies dating from the 1970s have contributed to declining indoor air quality (4,8,10). Building design and operational changes focused on decreasing energy consumption to comply with goals of reducing American dependency on foreign energy sources. But energy-efficient buildings may sacrifice ventilation effectiveness to reduce overall energy costs (17–20). Such efforts may result in better-insulated buildings but reduce the performance capacity of ventilation systems. The overall result is often inadequate fresh air exchange for building occupants that allows airborne chemical contaminants and pollutants to concentrate.

Building Materials and Furnishings

Products used in construction contain chemicals that can outgas into the indoor environment. Building materials are constantly changing and new products are entering the market, so it is difficult to keep track of the large variety of volatile chemicals contained in these products. Building products, ranging from structural materials to coatings, contain chemicals that are emitted indoors (11–13,21). Emissions of VOCs from building materials depend on the nature of the material, the chemicals, and the location of the material in the structure. Emission rates can vary from an initial high release in minutes or hours to long-term degassing over weeks, months, and even years. Such products include wood, insulation, plastics, sealers, caulking, adhesives, paints, varnishes, waxes, finishes, lacquers, fabrics, and carpets.

Furnishings and fabrics can act as sinks to absorb airborne chemicals, releasing them slowly back into the indoor environment, depending on temperature, humidity, and ventilation. In general, warmer temperatures and higher humidity increase the rate of emission of VOCs.

HUMAN FACTORS

Human activity contributes to indoor contamination by introducing irritating cleaning agents, pesticides, solvents, tobacco smoke, particulates, dust, fibers, mold, and allergens. Humans also shed millions of skin particles and microbes indoors. Cooking and other combustion sources introduce carbon monoxide, nitrogen dioxide (NO_2), sulfur dioxide (SO_2), and particulates into indoor air (22,23). Computers, copiers, fax machines, laser printers, and other office machines emit volatile chemicals and ozone.

Smokers contribute to the indoor chemical and particulate pollutant load. Whereas environmental tobacco smoke (ETS) has previously been thought of as a nuisance to most nonsmokers, the U.S. Environmental Protection Agency (EPA) considers it to be a substantive risk factor for cancer and heart disease (24,25). The EPA classifies ETS as a group A carcinogen, meaning that it causes human cancer. Although the EPA's cancer conclusions are being questioned, ETS remains a prime contributor to cough, shortness of breath, and chest tightness in exposed asthmatics (26). ETS also contributes to significant formaldehyde exposure indoors (27,28).

VENTILATION SYSTEM

Up to 50% of poor indoor air quality cases can be traced to a ventilation problem (19,20). A properly functioning ventilation system provides adequate fresh air and dilutes and removes pollutants. It also balances indoor air quality with comfort. Ventilation is a dominant cost of building maintenance and energy use, and decreasing ventilation is sometimes used as a cost-saving measure. Such approaches, however, can lead to the buildup of pollutants indoors.

Breathing produces carbon dioxide (CO_2) as a by-product, and its concentration indoors is a useful measure of air freshness. Accumulation of CO_2 concentrations of more than 800 parts per million (ppm) of air indicates inadequate fresh air supply and can be associated with health complaints, such as fatigue, headache, lethargy, and general discomfort. The American Society for Heating, Refrigeration and Air-Conditioning Engineers (ASHRAE) recommends that indoor CO_2 concentrations do not exceed 1,000 ppm (19,20,29,30). Elevated CO_2 concentrations of more than 800 ppm, however, may signal the buildup of other indoor pollutants because of their inadequate removal or dilution. ASHRAE has issued a number of indoor air quality standards including 62-1999, Ventilation for Acceptable Indoor Air Quality (superseding 62-1989), and projects 62.1P and 62.2P.

Air ducts contaminated with dirt, dust, and moisture can provide sources for microbial growth that may cause illness. The 1976 discovery of legionnaires' disease in Philadelphia underscores the fact that serious illness and death can result from a contaminated ventilation system.

Humidity

Excessive moisture and dampness indoors increases the risk of childhood asthma and other respiratory symptoms (5,7,8). Relative humidity values indoors more than 60% are associated with overgrowth of fungus and bacteria that can contaminate ventilation systems, carpet, wall spaces, insulation, ceiling tiles, window seals, and other areas of the indoor environment. Humidity less than 20% can cause drying of skin and mucous membranes, leading to irritation. High relative humidity increases upper airway moisture, allowing dusts and water-soluble toxic chemicals to dissolve more easily, contributing to upper airway irritation, inflammation, and cough.

A humidity range of 45% to 50% is recommended by ASHRAE and the EPA (24). Properly functioning ventilation systems help to maintain relative humidity between 20% and 60% (20).

Noise and Vibration

Whereas *sound* applies to the form of energy that produces hearing, *vibration* is the term applied to nonaudible sensations of touch and feeling. Noise is an unpleasant sound.

Noise is generated by vibrations transmitted as mechanical energy through air, solid, or liquid. It includes a spectrum ranging from infrasound to audile sound to ultrasound. Sound is measured in frequency (cycles per second) called a *hertz* (Hz). As an example, a sound frequency of 100 Hz means the period of vibration is 1/100 of a second (0.01 seconds). The *wavelength* of sound is the distance it travels in one cycle. Wavelength is an important property of sound and ranges from high frequency to low frequency. The term *decibel* (dB) is used to express the level of loudness associated with sound. A decibel reference level of zero is assigned to the sound heard by a person with excellent hearing in a quiet location. A sound of 140 dB is considered a pain threshold (31,32). The human ear is more sensitive to high frequencies, and sounds audible to the human ear range from 35 to 20,000 Hz.

Excess or chronic noise can cause health effects (31,32). Low-frequency noise between 20 and 100 Hz can produce health complaints, ranging from general annoyance and distraction to physiologic and psychological effects (31,32). Noise less than 100 Hz can be felt as vibration. Vibrations that interact with body receptors of touch and pressure can interfere with human performance. Sounds in the 40- to 60-Hz range have effects on the respiratory system because of the resonance characteristics of the chest wall. Sound between 0.1 and 20 Hz can cause dizziness and nausea, but usually only in decibels less than 120 (31,32).

The level (loudness) and the nature (frequency) of noise are important in producing symptoms. Prolonged exposure to low-frequency noise can result in fatigue, headache, difficulty concentrating, nausea, disorientation, cough, dizziness, and digestive problems. Most of these health effects occur around 7 Hz. OSHA regulates occupational exposure to noise by the Noise Control Act of 1972 that established the Office of Noise Abatement and Control within the EPA. This act enforces noise control regulations for machines, railroads, interstate motor carriers, and aircraft. OSHA's threshold limit value (TLV) for noise is 85 dB for an 8-hour day or 80 dB for a 24-hour period. Hearing loss can occur in individuals exposed to 75 dB 8 hours per day over a lifetime (33).

Besides auditory effects, noise can cause physical and psychological health effects. Noise interferes with communication, can cause disturbances in sleep, induces stress, irritability, fatigue, and interferes with performance and productivity. The threshold for annoyance is approximately 30 to 40 dB. Excess noise can elevate blood pressure, cause irritability, decrease productivity, and be generally discomforting (32,33).

Lighting

Light is the portion of the electromagnetic spectrum visible to the human eye, and can affect physical and psychological health. Studies involving seasonal depression demonstrate a relationship between a person's mood and lighting. Visual stress can be caused by inappropriate lighting, inadequate contrast, or glare. In addition, suboptimal lighting can cause eye irritation, stress, fatigue, headaches, and affect moods and performance. Studies demonstrate that performance and satisfaction rise with an increase in luminescence. However, bright light can cause feelings of dissatisfaction (32,34).

Because a relationship exists between lighting design and energy use patterns, architects and engineers have sought to minimize energy consumption with increased use of natural light and more energy-efficient light sources. The health consequences of artificial lighting are a subject of much research, adding to the complexities of indoor comfort and health.

Odors and Irritancy

Odors may range from tolerable to objectionable, and odors that seem satisfactory to the human nose generally have not been a concern for the majority of people indoors. Frequently, odors are associated with respiratory symptoms and mucous membrane irritation. The common chemical senses (CCS) formed by trigeminal nerve endings in the nose and upper airways detect irritants, pungent chemicals, and irritating particulates. The olfactory nerves detect odors. Different chemicals give rise to different olfactory responses that may give rise to different human responses. Health complaints associated with odors are a complex issue, and some individuals may complain of odor intolerance or an increased sensitivity to certain odors from indoor sources.

Stress

Poor indoor air quality can be a chronic stressor. How an individual adapts or maladapts to such stresses determines if health problems develop. Stress also occurs when an individual cannot control the environmental source of their illness. If the environment is perceived to be a threat, fears can develop and stress levels may rise. Another common cause of stress is the conflict that often surrounds indoor air quality problems and the adversarial stances of supervisors toward an individual's complaints about air quality.

Other stressors include the nature of the job and negative employee relationships. Workplace stress continues to be a growing concern because of its high financial and health care. Stress from all causes is estimated to cost $150 billion a year in lost productivity and worker's compensation claims (16). Most stress claims are the result of cumulative events, not single events. Environmental stimuli, such as chemicals, odors, and irritants, and recurring illness from unknown sources can precipitate chronic stress in some susceptible individuals.

Activity and Clothing

The level of human activity indoors determines metabolic rate and, thus, is related to thermal comfort. ASHRAE publishes a table of metabolic rates associated with a variety of activities and levels of work. Most office workers are sedentary and ASHRAE's thermal comfort standards are based on this level of relative activity. Dissipation of heat caused by activity is necessary to maintain thermal comfort, and clothing is a prime factor related to heat loss or gain. ASHRAE has a table of clothing values for thermal comfort. These values are expressed as *clo* units of thermal resistance. One clo unit = 0.88°F × ft^2 × h/BTU (32). Various articles of clothing represent different clo values: trousers plus short-sleeve shirt = 0.5 clo units.

BIOLOGICAL MECHANISMS OF INDOOR ENVIRONMENT–RELATED ILLNESS

Pollutants, thermal comfort, humidity, adequacy of ventilation, and air movement combine to play interacting roles in perceptions of health in work and home environments. Studies estimate that between 20% and 35% of office workers perceive indoor air quality problems in their work environment (17–20). But health complaints, such as headache, sinus congestion, and fatigue, may be difficult to separate from general symptoms experienced by the overall population. Therefore, establishing a cause-effect relationship between the indoor environment and illness is often difficult because of the numerous variables involved (35). Also, the definition of what constitutes SBS varies. WHO recognized this difficulty and combined various definitions into a singular summary to describe the syndrome as follows (33):

1. A majority of occupants indoors report symptoms.
2. Symptoms appear more frequently in one building or part of a building than any other.
3. Six categories of symptoms cover the majority of health complaints:
   - Sensory irritation
   - Neurologic symptoms
   - General health symptoms
   - Skin irritation
   - Unspecific hypersensitivity reactions
   - Odor and taste problems
4. Mucous membrane, nose, eye, and throat irritations are the most frequently expressed symptoms.
5. Other symptoms tend to be less expressed.
6. No singular causality can be identified.

Still, patterns of illness can be correlated with environmental clues. Poor indoor environmental quality should at least be considered if typical symptomatology occurs in a site characterized by one or more of the following (Table 53-3):

- Presence of chemical odors
- Recent remodeling
- Newly constructed building
- Presence of moisture or water damage
- Heavy use of cleaning agents
- Indoor combustion sources
- Mold contamination and discoloration of walls and ceilings
- Musty or stale odors
- Excess dust or particulates on walls or other surfaces
- New carpet odors
- Office machines in unventilated areas or in direct sunlight

Affected persons express improvement of symptoms when they are away from work and over weekends, with recurrence of symp-

TABLE 53-3. Clues to potential indoor air quality problems

Odors
- Chemicals
- Musty
- Stale
- Tobacco smoke
- New carpet
- Pesticides
- Diesel or gasoline engine exhaust

Remodeled site or new building
- Paints
- Varnishes
- Glues
- Lacquers
- Thinners
- Adhesives
- Roofing materials
- New carpet
- Grouts
- Caulking
- Sealants
- Pressed woods
- Solvents

Office machines
- Placed in unventilated area
- In warm rooms
- Located in direct sunlight

Water and moisture damage
- In ventilation system
- In subbasements
- Involving floors, ceilings, or insulation
- Involving carpet or walls
- Involving wallboard or sheet rock

Combustion sources
- Tobacco smoke
- Fireplace flue not working properly or in need of cleaning
- Unvented gas heaters and gas appliances
- Internal combustion in a confined space
- Combustion sources near ventilation intake vent
- Space heaters unvented
- Charcoal grills indoors

Accumulation of dust and particulates
- On surfaces such as desks and walls
- In ventilation system
- On ventilation grills

Overuse of cleaning agents or disinfectants
- On large surface areas
- In poorly ventilated areas
- Containing irritating chemicals
- In small or confined spaces

Ventilation problems
- Poor air movement
- Stale air
- Microbial contamination
- Dirty vents
- Lack of air filtration
- Pollutant source near fresh air intake

Environmental factors
- Too humid
- Too warm
- Harsh or glaring light
- Excessive noise
- Vibrations

toms on returning to work. The time factor of exposure duration seems to be important in determining how quickly symptoms resolve in anecdotal cases. The longer the exposure, the slower the resolution of symptoms seems to occur. The search for biological models to explain the causes of these signs and symptoms has focused on the following mechanisms (11–14,22,23,35–40):

- Inflammation involving upper and lower airways
- Mucous membrane irritancy
- Neurobehavioral and neurologic effects of VOCs
- Allergic reactions and hypersensitivity to chemicals and biologicals
- Stress and psychological reactions
- Infections
- Effects of chemicals and biological toxins on the immune system

Inflammation and irritation of mucous membranes are primary mechanisms at the root of many indoor air quality–related health problems. Underscoring the complexity of the problem, environmental factors, such as temperature and humidity, can interact with airborne contaminants to trigger illness (35,36). Also, why some people are more susceptible than others may partially be explained by their atopic status and their heightened susceptibility to inflammation (36,37). Still, symptoms associated with poor indoor air quality are sometimes difficult to delineate from those caused by common allergies because allergens and nonallergens share similar pathways of inflammation and illness production.

Because humans breathe between 10,000 and 20,000 L of air daily, with most passing through the nose, upper airway, and respiratory tract, exposure to airborne contaminants is unavoidable (36). Thus, those with a predisposition to inflammation by either nonimmune stimuli or immune stimuli may be more prone to respiratory irritation and inflammation caused by airborne contaminants (37–39).

Irritancy and Pungency Caused by Airborne Contaminants

Airborne contaminants include particulates, bioaerosols, or chemicals, and respirable airborne particles of 10 μm in diameter or less can penetrate into the airways (see Fig. 52-3).

Detection of airborne chemicals and particulates by the nasal passages and upper airways involves the common chemical senses, a specialized network of nerves emanating from the trigeminal nerve with endings located in the face, eyes, and nasal passages (39,41,42) (Fig. 53-1). As the trigeminal nerve leaves the brain, it divides into three branches innervating both sides of the face and upper airways: the ophthalmic, the maxillary, and the mandibular. The ophthalmic branch innervates the interior part of the nose, the

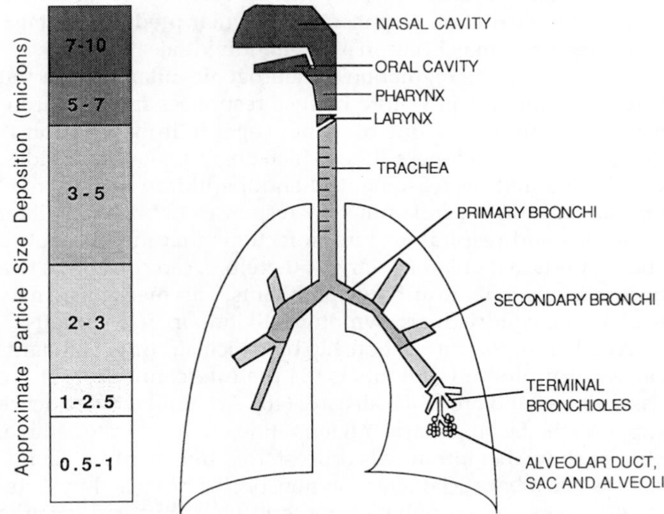

Figure 53-1. Schematic illustration of respiratory tract anatomy and approximate pattern of particle deposition.

conjunctiva, the cornea, and the iris of the eye. The maxillary branch innervates the posterior and inferior nasal passages. The mandibular branch innervates the tongue and the mouth. Activation of these chemical sensory pathways by airborne hazards serves to warn of danger by producing an irritancy reaction. If this CCS interaction with irritants is unregulated or a constant activation occurs, inflammation can result.

The CCS responds quantitatively and qualitatively to stimulation by chemical vapors and airborne particulates (39,43,44). Small changes in molecular structure among VOCs give rise to large differences in chemical potencies. The nerve receptors in the membranes of the nose and mouth are close to the surface, separated only by a thin film of moisture. Airborne chemicals can penetrate this moisture layer to react with nerve endings.

VOCs and low-molecular-weight chemicals can activate the CCS nerve receptors either by physical or by chemical reactions. Those that bind chemically produce a more potent reaction (39,41). Examples of such chemicals are formaldehyde, acrolein, chlorine, ozone, sulfur dioxide, and aldehydes.

The nerves of the CCS release neuropeptides in response to environmental irritants. This type of inflammatory response is termed *neurogenic inflammation* (39,41,43). Neuropeptides (also termed *neurokinins*) are found in nerve fibers of the nose, dental pulp, and the eyes and can be released by lung tissue. Therefore, volatile chemicals can produce irritant effects and release inflammatory neuropeptides at nerve sites around the body, throughout the nasal mucosa, lungs, and other sites that store such mediators (39,44,45). Neuropeptide release results in a cascade of events leading to more inflammation, swelling, pain, and the release of other inflammatory mediators from tissues, amplifying effects and producing symptoms:

Sneezing
Nasal stuffiness
Rhinorrhea
Facial pain
Eye irritation
Watery eyes
Headache
Sinus congestion
Cough
Fatigue
Throat irritation
Wheezing

Desensitization of these sensory nerves may also occur with a fading of the irritation response. No singular predictor dictates which response may occur in a given individual.

Disorders in the regulation of neurogenic inflammation can lead to prolonged and more intense responses from environmental stimulants. Control of neurogenic inflammation is through neutral endopeptidase, which degrades neuropeptides. Conditions that decrease neutral endopeptidase activity may increase neurogenic inflammatory responses (39,43,44). Irritant chemicals and respiratory viral infections that inhibit neutral endopeptidase regulatory activity, therefore, can contribute to a person's sensitivity to airborne pollutants. This mechanism may explain some individuals' symptoms to indoor air pollutants.

Another important relationship by which airborne pollutants cause respiratory symptoms is via the interconnection of the nasal airway and bronchial airways (46). Accumulating evidence supports the fact that nasal inflammation can aggravate asthma. Studies show that intranasal corticosteroid treatment for allergic rhinitis has a beneficial effect on nonspecific bronchial hyperresponsiveness and on asthma symptoms (46). Thus, induction of nasal inflammation by airborne contaminants is an important mechanism linked to lower airway respiratory symptoms.

CCS receptors respond to different types of stimuli besides chemical: thermal, mechanical, biologicals, particulates, dusts, and bioaerosols. At lower exposure levels, a summation effect occurs. That is, the more tissue and receptors that are exposed to irritants, the stronger the response. Time summation may also be an important event in symptom amplification from indoor pollutants.

Respiratory Irritation, Bronchial Hyperresponsiveness, and Asthma

The lungs also respond to airborne chemicals and hazards via inflammation. The surface epithelial cell layer of the lungs forms a physical barrier against inhaled toxins and hazards. These cells secrete a thin sterile moisture barrier over the surface of the lungs and bronchioles. Other specialized cells secrete a thick mucous layer on top of the water layer. Together, these layers form a gel phase that traps chemicals, particles, and dusts. The surface lining of the lower airway is made up of ciliated epithelial cells, forming a brush border that constantly pushes trapped substances toward the mouth where they can be expectorated or swallowed.

Besides epithelial cells that can release cytokines and other mediators of inflammation, nerve endings can be stimulated by irritants to cause bronchoconstriction. If the cell layer lining the airway is damaged by an inhaled hazard, nerve endings can react by constricting the airway. This may occur because of a high-level acute exposure or chronic low-level exposure. Also, pulmonary macrophages and epithelial cells release mediators in response to stimuli by irritants causing an inflammatory cascade resulting in an acute or chronic response (45,47,48).

Because the tissues of the airways form an interactive protective mechanism, irritants and toxins that affect one cell or tissue type affect others. Toxins and particulates that damage the protective mechanism and result in inflammation of the airway (referred to as toxic inflammation) can cause cough, shortness of breath, chest tightness, wheezing, and asthma. Once an inhaled hazard induces the inflammatory process, chemical mediators of inflammation are released by epithelial cells and macrophages [(interleukin (IL)-1, tumor necrosis factor-α (TFN-α), and IL-6]. Once released, these chemical mediators activate other cells, causing a cascade of inflammation (38,47,48).

Acute exposures produce inflammatory responses that differ from those of chronic exposures. Also, chronic exposures producing ongoing inflammation may result in pathologic alterations in airway tissues, including fibrosis and increased production of mucus (Fig. 53-2).

Exposure to airborne contaminants may also produce a hyperresponsiveness of the airways that can be either IgE mediated or non–IgE mediated. Some low-molecular-weight chemicals, such as acid anhydrides and isocyanates, may serve as haptens to generate type I immune-mediated asthma. Bioaerosols can act as antigens to cause type IV hypersensitivity reactions, such as hypersensitivity pneumonitis (see Chapters 25 and 97).

The term *reactive airways* or *nonspecific bronchial hyperresponsiveness* is used to describe nonimmune-mediated asthma caused by inhaled respiratory irritants. Once a person has developed reactive airways, exposure to chemically unrelated airborne irritants may trigger symptom onset via inflammation (49).

An entity termed *reactive airways dysfunction syndrome* has been described after a high-level exposure to irritant chemicals. Signs and symptoms of respiratory irritation occur quickly after such an exposure, with coughing, chest tightness, and throat burning. Reexposure to irritating vapors or fumes can precipitate symptoms of cough, wheezing, and shortness of breath. Pulmonary function tests may be abnormal but are usually reversible on treatment with a bronchodilator. Reactive airways dysfunction

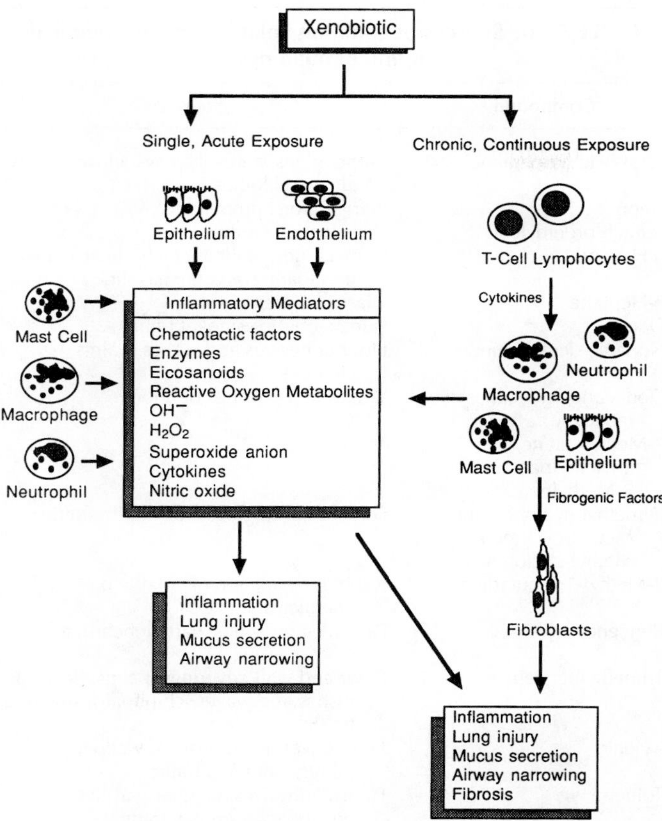

Figure 53-2. Pathways of xenobiotic-induced inflammatory events.

syndrome and other forms of hyperresponsive airways probably represent a spectrum of the same disease process and have as a common basis inflammation of the airway (38–40,47–49).

Another inflammatory syndrome of a nonallergic nature attributed to airborne pollutants is *reactive upper airways dysfunction*. It too has been described after an acute high-level exposure or after chronic low-level exposure to airborne contaminants (43). Reactive upper airways dysfunction is manifested by signs and symptoms of rhinitis (runny nose), nasal stuffiness, eye burning, sinus congestion, facial pain, and severe headache, almost of a migraine nature (see Table 53-3) (37,39,41,43).

Symptoms of bronchial hyperresponsiveness usually begin with cough, chest tightness, and may proceed to shortness of breath and wheezing. Such hyperreactive airways can last for weeks, months, or years, and is managed like asthma (49). Because of the lowered level of sensitivity of individuals with reactive airways or reactive upper airways dysfunction, common indoor air pollutants, such as perfumes, solvent vapors, tobacco smoke, physical irritants, bioaerosols, and irritating cleaning chemicals, can trigger respiratory reactions (49).

An important feature of upper and lower reactive airways is the potential loss of the protective cell surface barrier because of chronic inflammation. The loss of this protective lining increases the airway's susceptibility to chemical irritants and prolongs the disease process (43,49).

Irritant Vocal Cord Dysfunction

Irritant vocal cord dysfunction (IVCD) is a newly recognized medical disorder, often misdiagnosed as asthma (50). Cases of IVCD have occurred after acute high-level occupational or environmental exposures. Vocal cord dysfunction is a disorder of the larynx in which the vocal cords adduct inappropriately during an inspiration or expiration. Signs and symptoms and causes of IVCD are listed in Tables 53-4 and 53-5. The abnormality can occur in inspiration, expiration, or in both phases of the respiratory cycle. Patients with IVCD express a significant increase in chest complaints.

TABLE 53-4. Clinical criteria for vocal cord dysfunction

Irritant vocal cord dysfunction
- Documented absence of preceding vocal cord dysfunction or laryngeal disease
- Onset of symptoms after a single specific exposure or accident
- Exposure to an irritating gas, smoke, fume, vapor, mist, or dust
- Onset of symptoms within 24 h after exposure
- Symptoms of wheezing, stridor, dyspnea, cough, or throat tightness
- Abnormal direct laryngoscopy for vocal cord dysfunction either in the asymptomatic state, during symptoms, or with a provocative study
- Exclusion of other types of significant vocal cord disease

Non-irritant–induced vocal cord dysfunction
- Symptoms of wheezing, stridor, dyspnea, cough, or throat tightness
- Abnormal direct laryngoscopy for vocal cord dysfunction either in the asymptomatic state, during symptoms, or with a provocative study
- Exclusion of other types of significant vocal cord disease
- Absence of onset of symptoms after a single specific exposure or accident

Reprinted from ref. 50, with permission.

Vocal cord dysfunction often mimics asthma and, therefore, it is important to consider the diagnosis of IVCD in symptomatic patients after irritant exposures to distinguish it from hyperresponsive airways. The pathogenesis of IVCD is not known, but direct inflammation caused by irritants is suggested (50).

Vocal cord dysfunction may be associated with symptoms of panic, depression, and anxiety. Psychopathology can also occur. Chronic symptoms of sinusitis, rhinitis, and voice changes occur and can exacerbate vocal cord dysfunction (50).

The frequency of gastroesophageal reflux disease is higher in IVCD than other causes of vocal cord dysfunction (50). Gastroesophageal reflux disease must be managed appropriately to prevent acid reflux from causing further respiratory irritation and asthmatic episodes. The irritation caused by reflux of gastric acid onto the vocal cords may also have a role in the pathogene-

TABLE 53-5. Vocal cord dysfunction–associated symptoms

Symptom	Irritant vocal cord dysfunction	Vocal cord dysfunction	*P* Value
Wheeze	9/11 (82)	26/33 (79)	.83
Cough	11/11 (100)	31/33 (94)	.40
Shortness of breath	11/11 (100)	30/33 (91)	.30
Choking or throat tightness	9/10 (90)	22/26 (85)	.68
Chest pain or chest tightness	6/6 (100)	17/30 (57)	.04
Stridor	4/6 (67)	6/8 (75)	.73
Gastroesophageal reflux	7/10 (70)	19/32 (59)	.55
Voice changes	11/11 (100)	14/16 (88)	.22
Dysphagia	5/9 (56)	8/30 (27)	.44
Rhinosinusitis	8/11 (73)	30/33 (91)	.13

Note: Expressed as number of patients reporting symptom/number of patients for whom the symptom was adequately recorded, with percentage in parentheses.
Reprinted from ref. 50, with permission.

sis of IVCD. Gastric acid reflux produces distinct symptoms of hoarseness, persistent nonproductive cough, a sensation of pressure deep in the throat, and a continual need to clear the throat. Causes of IVCD are listed:

Ammonia
Flux fumes
Cleaning chemicals
Odors
Smoke
Organic solvents
Machine fluid
Ceiling tile dust
Sulfur dioxide

The differentiation and correct diagnosis of vocal cord dysfunction are important because therapy for vocal cord dysfunction is different from that for asthma, and patients may benefit from speech therapy to retrain muscles that cause laryngeal dysfunction or biofeedback. Vocal cord dysfunction does not seem to benefit from inhaled corticosteroids, bronchodilators, or leukotriene inhibitors.

VOLATILE ORGANIC CHEMICALS INDOORS AND HEALTH EFFECTS

VOCs are an important category of chemical compounds found in the air of most indoor environments. The term *VOC* defines a mixture of VOCs with highly variable chemical and physical properties. WHO defines classes of VOCs: semivolatile, volatile, and highly volatile. VOCs have melting points below room temperature and boiling points from 50° through 100°C to 240° through 260°C. Studies of volatile organic hydrocarbons found indoors indicate that they are low in concentration, usually in parts per billion or parts per million, but may become more concentrated than in a typical outdoor environment.

Characterization of the quantity and types of indoor air chemical contaminants has been undertaken using gas chromatography-mass spectrometry (GC-MS) in an effort to delineate the chemicals to which humans are exposed. From 50 to 300 VOCs can be detected by air samples in nonindustrial environments, including offices, homes, public buildings, shopping centers, and malls (Table 53-6). VOC sources include building materials, solvents, paints, furnishings, office machines, cleaning materials, human activity, pesticide spraying, and remodeling. In clean environments, the total volatile organic chemical (TVOC) load is much less than 1 mg per m^3, with individual VOCs less than 1% of any recognized exposure standard (11–13,51–54).

TABLE 53-6. Sources of common volatile organic chemicals found in buildings

Compound	Source
1,1,1-Trichloroethane	Carpet glues, aerosol sprays, cleaners, dry-cleaned clothes
Freon	Refrigerators, propellants
Tetrachloroethylene	Dry-cleaned clothes
n-Hexane	Carpet glues, wallpaper, chipboard, insulation foam, smoking, gasoline
n-Heptane	Glass cleanser, traffic
Octane	Paints, tobacco smoke, traffic
Nonane, decane, undecane	Floor adhesives and waxes, paints, cleaners
Dodecane, tridecane, tetradecane	Waxes and polishes of floor
2-Methylbutane, 2-Methylpentane, 3-Methylpentane	Traffic
Dimethyl-cyclopentane, Methyl-cyclopentane, Methyl-cyclohexane	Solvent-based glues and waxes, traffic
2-Methyl-1,3-butadiene	Rubbers, oxidation of volatile organic chemicals
Benzene	Paints, carpet glues, particleboard, tobacco smoke, traffic
Trimethylbenzenes	Floor and wall coverings, paints, floor varnishes and waxes, chipboard, smoking, traffic
Xylenes	Floor covering, adhesives, wallpaper, paints, smoking, traffic
Toluene	Paints, adhesives, lacquer parquet, cleaners, tobacco smoke, traffic
Naphthalene	Antimoth products
Ethanol	Cleaners, varnish, floor covering (linoleum, lacquer)
2-Butoxyethanol	Floor cleaners, paints, wax strippers, and varnish removers
Acetone	Glues, carpets, particleboard, drapes, bioeffluents
Cyclohexanone	Resins, waxes
Benzaldehyde, nonanal, decanal	Cleaners, chipboard, photochemical oxidation of volatile organic chemicals, Tenax
Butyl acetate, ethyl acetate	Floor covering (parquet, PVC flooring)
Acetic acid	Varnishes, silicon sealant
Benzoic acid	Floor detergent
Dodecanoic acid	Wood glue, varnishes
a-Pinene, terpenes	Cleaners, air fresheners, wood products
Limonene	Lemon-scented cleaners, air fresheners, polishes, waxes

PVC, polyvinyl chloride.
Reprinted from ref. 12, with permission.

Chemical Emissions from Office Products

Concern over the impact of manufacturing processes and product waste streams on the outdoor environment has resulted in a wide variety of innovations dedicated to the development of sustainable manufacturing and consumption. Manufacturers expend much time and resource implementing programs devoted to pollution prevention, design for disassembly, recycling and reuse of recycled materials, and waste stream minimization. This emphasis on manufacturing and waste stream environments, however, ignores an important environmental niche between manufacture and disposal. That unique environmental niche is the indoor environment surrounding product use. Concern for the outdoor environment has influenced many companies to spend more resources attempting to understand how a product affects a sanitary landfill than on how that same product affects the indoor environment and its human occupants. Although traditional product safety is a major concern for most manufacturers, the impact of a product on the indoor environment is complex.

Although U.S. efforts to minimize air and water pollution have met with measurable success, an increasing public concern exists over a new generation of pollution-related human illness in the office, home, and transportation environments. High-speed printers, copiers, visual display terminals, duplicators, microfiche, and blueprint machines are point sources of indoor contaminants that cannot be disregarded, especially when used in inadequately ventilated facilities. Most modern electronic products emit low levels of volatile organic compounds into the indoor environment. These fugitive emissions arise from plastics, solvents, coatings, adhesives, and encapsulans associated with manufacture, as well as consumable supplies, such as toners, inks, paper, transparency films, and labels.

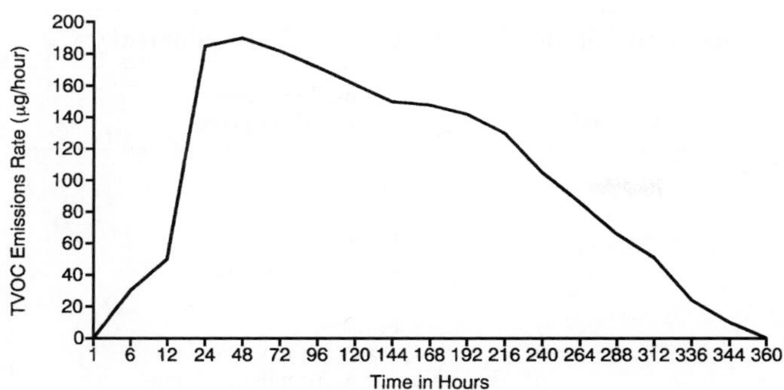

Figure 53-3. Bell-shaped chemical emissions profile from office electronic products. TVOC, total volatile organic chemical.

The newer an item of electronic equipment, the higher may be its potential rate of chemical emissions.

The chemical emission profile of an electronic product is largely dependent on the product itself. Those products that do not consume supplies (e.g., computers and monitors) typically produce a bell-shaped curve of emissions, resulting from a diffusion and evaporation of chemicals left over from manufacture that over time decrease to insignificance (Fig. 53-3). Those products that consume supplies (e.g., printers and photocopiers) typically produce higher levels of emissions, producing a sigmoidal curve that reaches a steady-state emission rate dependent on the supplies used and the duration and frequency of use (Fig. 53-4).

Whether a product's emissions impact significantly an indoor environment depends on two opposing factors: (a) the type and rate of chemical emitted, and (b) the rate and effectiveness of that environment's ventilation.

VOCs, ozone, and particulate emissions from electronic products can be measured in chambers or under field conditions. Clearly, chamber measurement in which variables, such as background VOC concentrations, temperature, humidity, air exchange rate, and mixing, can be controlled yields superior results. It is often impossible, however, to chamber-test certain products because of their size or mobility constraints. When field testing products for chemical emissions, it is essential to know product function and exhaust paths, ambient air VOC profiles, temperature, and humidity.

Whether samples are taken directly from products under field conditions, or are obtained from chamber studies, all sampling and analysis should be performed using validated and traceable techniques. Usually these techniques require GC-MS approaches to allow for the appropriate qualitative and quantitative resolution. Date requirements for product emission analyses include the chemical species involved, their concentration, and the rate at which they are emitted. These data can then be used to perform predictive modeling, formal quantitative risk assessments, and to determine the ventilation requirements associated with product use.

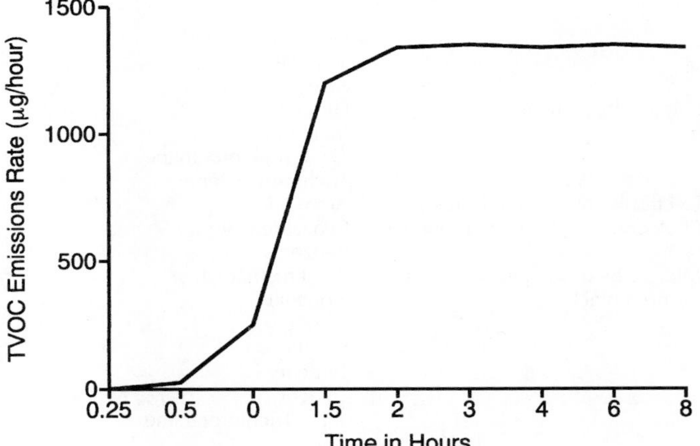

Figure 53-4. Sigmoidal chemical emissions profile from office products that consume supplies. TVOC, total volatile organic chemical.

Office and clerical work environments are common sites where poor indoor air quality frequently occurs (3,10–12,17). These offices are in modern or remodeled buildings and use computers, copiers, fax machines, laser printers, and paper products. They also depend on centrally controlled ventilation systems. Laser printers and copiers sitting in direct sunlight or in unventilated rooms release ozone and volatile irritant chemicals that can accumulate.

Carbonless copy paper is another source of chemical emissions in offices. The undersurface page of carbonless copy paper is coated with microcapsules of ink. The pH inside the capsule is acidic and the pH of the underlying sheets is alkaline. When the microcapsules are burst open by the pressure of writing or typing, the differences in the pHs cause color formation. Carbonless copy paper contains chemical allergens, solvents, and dyes that can produce eye irritation, rashes, and symptoms of respiratory irritation and allergy in office workers (55). Volatile organic chemicals and particulates from carbonless copy paper can accumulate in office environments because of the mass of paper used, handling of paper, filing, and shredding of documents. Adequate ventilation and control of paper dust and fibers can assist in preventing health complaints.

Chemical Emissions from Building Materials

Materials for building, remodeling, and construction vary from wet to dry. Most building products contain chemicals that can be emitted indoors (Table 53-7). Building products emit VOCs indoors at varying rates, and release is affected by volatility, temperature, humidity, air exchanges per hour, air circulation, reabsorbing sinks (reabsorbed by other materials in the environment to be slowly released over time), and air filtration (Table 53-8). Building products can be subdivided into short-term emitters versus long-term emitters.

Many covariables affect human response to low-level volatile chemicals, such as exposure duration, time of day, temperature, and humidity (35,53). Temperature and humidity act additively with the total volatile chemical load indoors to initiate symptoms (35).

Most outgassing of VOCs occurs when the building is new and slowly declines over time with a variety of half-lives, depending on the chemical, environmental factors, and the material. In addition, there may be odors associated with VOCs in a closed environment.

Building material, such as self-leveling-mortar containing casein, has been shown to release trace amounts of 2-ethyl-1-hexenol, ammonia, isoprophylamine, ethylamine, triethylamine, dimethylamine, trimethylamine, and dimethyl sulfide. Amines have been found in the 0.003- to .013-ppm range in indoor air after use of such mortar (56). In addition to the irritant effects from chemical emissions, an objectionable odor occurs because of the casein content of the mortar and possibly texturing materials for ceilings and outgassing of sulfhydryl compounds into the indoor environment (56).

The vapor emissions for building materials can vary from days to months and even up to years for formaldehyde emissions from particle board and pressed wood products (57). Sources of formaldehyde emissions are sealants, mortar, caulking compounds, paints, woods, plastics, vinyl products, foams,

TABLE 53-7. Volatile organic chemical emissions from building materials, interior furnishing, and office equipment

Material	Volatile organic chemicals emitted
Adhesives	Alcohols Amines Benzene Decane Dimethylbenzene Formaldehyde Terpenes Toluene Xylenes Nonane Undecane Dimethyloctane 2-Methylnonane *n*-Propylbenzene Limonene Pinene
Caulking compounds	Alcohols Alkanes Amines Benzene Diethylbenzene Formaldehyde Methylethylketone Xylenes Butyl propionate 2-Butoxyethanol Butanol Toluene Acetic acid Ethylbenzene nonane
Carpeting	Alcohols Formaldehyde 4-Methylethyl-benzene 4-Phenylcyclohexene Styrene
Ceiling tiles Chipboard Paneling Plywood Gypsum board Fiberboard	Alkanes Amines Benzene 3-Carene Formaldehyde Terpenes Toluene Acetone Hexanol Hexane Propanol Butanone Benzaldehyde Isopropanol 3-Methylpentane ethanol Methylethylketone Ethylbenzene *n*-Propylbenzene Limonene Pinene
Floor and wall coverings Wallpaper Linoleum floor covering Vinyl coatings	Acetates Alcohols Alkanes Amines Benzene Formaldehyde Undecane *n*-Propylbenzene Methyl styrene Xylenes 3-Methylpentane Toluene Heptane Ethylacetate Methylethlketone Ethylbenzene 4-Methyl-2-Pentanone Dodecane Nonane 1,2,3-Trimethylbenzene 1,2,4-Trimethylbenzene
Wood stains and varnishes Latex paints Polyurethane floor finish Floor lacquers	Acetates Acrylates Alcohols Alkanes Amines Benzenes Formaldehyde Limonene Polyurethane Toluene 2-Ethoxyethylacetates 2-Propanol Butanone Ethylbenzene Propylbenzene 1,1'-Oxybisbutane Butylpropionate Nonane Decane Undecane Methyloctane Dimethylnonane Trimethylbenzene *n*-Butanol Hexanol Xylene Nonane Dodecane
Appliances	Carbon monoxide Nitrogen dioxide Sulfur dioxide Polyaromatic hydrocarbons
Computers and video display terminals	*n*-Butanol 2-Butanol 2-Butoxyethanol Butyl-2-methylpropyl phthalate Caprolactam Cresol Diisooctyl phthalate Dodecamethyl cyclosiloxane 2-Thoxyethyl acetate Ethylbenzene Hexanedioic acid Toluene Xylene
Duplicating machines	Ethanol Methanol 1,1,1-Trichloroethane Trichloroethylene
Electrophotographic printers Photocopiers and related supplies Microfiche developers and blue-print machines	Ammonia Benzaldehyde Benzene Butyl methacrylate Nonanal Ozone Styrene Terpene Toluene 1,1,1-Trichloroethane

(continued)

TABLE 53-7. *(continued)*

Material	Volatile organic chemicals emitted
	Trichloroethylene
	Xylenes
	Zinc stearate combustion products
	Ammonium salts
	Polyolefin wax
	Carbon black
	Styrene-acrylate copolymer
Carbonless copy paper	Chlorobiphenyl
	Cyclohexane
	Dibutylphthalate
	Formaldehyde
	Kerosene
	Diethylethane
	Naphthalene
	Ammonia
Preprinted paper forms	Acetaldehyde
	Acetic acid
	Acetone
	Acrolein
	Benzaldehyde
	Butanol
	1,5-Dimethylcyclo-pentene
	2-Ethyl furan
	Heptane
	Hexamethyl cyclosiloxane
	Hexanal
	4-Hydroxy-4-methyl pentanone
	Isopropanol
	Paper dust
	Proprionaldehyde
	1,1,1-Trichloroethane
Typewriter correction fluids	Acetone
	1,1,1-Trichloroethane
Artificial essences fragrances	Nonane
	Decane
	Undecane
	Limonene
	Aromatic fragrances
	Ethylheptane
Room deodorants and fresheners	Acetaldehyde
	n-Butanol
	Ethylacetate
	Propylacetate
	Isobutylacetate
	Pinene
	Methylchloroform
	Isopropyl alcohol
	Isopropane/isobutane
	Triethylene glycol
	Propylene glycol
	Tertiary butyl alcohol
	Esters
	Terpenes
	Aldehydes
	Alcohols
	Brucine sulfate
	Propylene glycol
	Cyclomenaldehyde
	Benzyloacetate
	Hexanol
	Ether
	Lactones
	Acetols
	Resins
	Essential oils
	Hexylene glycol
	Nonylphenol
	Paradichlorobenzene
Sealants	Acetic acid
	Xylene
	Aliphatic hydrocarbons
	Toluene
	Petroleum hydrocarbons
	Hexane
	Methylethylketone
Cleaning agents and detergents	Pine oil
	Sodium hydroxide
	Ethylene glycol monobutyl ether
	Ethylenediamine tetraacetic acid
	Sodium carbonate
	Polyalkoxylated alcohol
	Sodium metasilicate
	Isopropanol
	Ethyl alcohol
	2-Butoxy ethanol
	Ammonium hydroxide
	Isobutane/propane
	Phosphoric acid
	Phosphates
	Dipropyleneglycol methyl ether
	Diethyleneglycol methyl ether
Glazing compound	Acetic acid
Dry cleaning	Trichloroethylene
	1,1,1-Trichloroethane
	Tetrachloroethylene
New clothing	Formaldehyde
Resins	Butylacrylate
Polymers	
Textile and leather finishes	
Carpet shampoo disinfectant	Pentachlorophenol
Wood preservative	Tetrachlorophenol
Fungicides	Pentachlorophenol
	Hexachlorobenzene
Insulation	Styrene
	Formaldehyde
	n-Propylbenzene pinene
Floor waxes	Trimethylcyclohexane
	α-Terpene
	Ethyltoluene
	o-Ethyltoluene
	m,p-Ethyltoluene
	m-Ethyltoluene
	1,2,3-Trimethylbenzene
	Decane
	Undecane
	Nonane
	Ethylmethylbenzene
	Dimethyloctane
Paint removers	Methylene chloride
Grease cleaner	Carbontetrachloride
Cleaning fluids	Trichloroethylene
	1,1,1-Trichloroethanol
	Ethylbenzene
	Xylene
	Undecane
Paint and lacquer solvents	Chlorobenzene
	Toluene
	Trichloroethylene
	Acetone
	Cyclohexane
	Xylene
	n-Butylbenzene
	Naphtha
Deodorizers	*o*-Dichlorobenzene
Moth balls	*m*-Dichlorobenzene
	p-Dichlorobenzene

(continued)

TABLE 53-7. *(continued)*

Material	Volatile organic chemicals emitted	Material	Volatile organic chemicals emitted
Moulding tape	Toluene	Carbon paper	Mineral oil
Edge sealing	Isobutanol		Stearic oil
	n-Butanol		Oleic oil
Jointing compound	Ethylbenzene		Carbon black
	Styrene		Nigrosine
	Xylene		Methyl violet
	n-Butanol		Crystal violet
	Isobutanol		Victoria blue
	Formaldehyde	Paints	Waxes
	Toluene		2-Ethyl-hexyl-acrylate
	Nonane		*N*-Methylol-acrylamide
	1,2,4-Trimetholbenzene		Pentaerythritol triacrylate
Heaters	Formaldehyde		Trimethylpropane triacrylate
Unvented gas heaters	Carbon monoxide		Tripropulene glycol triacrylate
Unvented gas ovens			Ethoxyethanol
Carpet—latex backed	Formaldehyde		Ethoxyethylacetate
	Xylene		Butylacrylate
	4-Phenylcyclohexene		Epoxy acrylate
Plastics	Propylacetate		Ethyl acrylate
	Dibutylphthalates		Titanium dioxide
			Latex

paper products, and insulation material. New homes release VOCs over a period of months, with a high concentration occurring immediately (Fig. 53-5) (Table 53-9) and then tapering off over a few months, with low levels persisting for years (57). Formaldehyde concentrations, however, tend to fluctuate, with higher indoor emissions occurring in warmer months (Fig. 53-6).

Human Studies of Volatile Organic Chemicals Indoors

Indoor air monitoring of homes and buildings free of health complaints show TVOC averaging much less than 1 mg per m^3 (11–13,51,53,54). These sites usually meet ASHRAE standards (62-1999) for ventilation, and health complaints are uncommon.

Human studies indicate that the average TVOC concentration in homes with indoor air quality problems ranges between 0.09 mg per m^3 and 13 mg per m^3 (11–13,51,53,54). Those with no problems average 0.36 mg per m^3, and range from 0.02 mg per m^3 to 1.7 mg per m^3. Human chamber studies show a TVOC threshold range for test subjects initiating symptoms between 0.2 mg per m^3 and 3 mg per m^3 (11–13,51,53,54). At a TVOC concentration more than 3 mg per m^3, discomfort and health complaints occur in test subjects (11–13,51–54). There were no health effects in test subjects at exposures less than 0.2 mg per m^3. At levels of 5 mg per m^3, objective and subjective health effects occurred. TVOC exposures of 8 mg per m^3 for 50 minutes caused irritation of mucosal membranes of the eyes and upper airways (11–13,51,53,54). Five human studies document sensory and neurobehavioral effects secondary to low levels of volatile chemicals indoors (51) (Table 53-10).

Headaches, neurobehavioral, and neurologic symptoms are noted in human test subjects at TVOC concentrations between 3 mg per m^3 and 25 mg per m^3 after an exposure of a few hours (51). Neurobehavioral performance tests confirm symptoms of drowsiness, fatigue, confusion, headache, and decreased attention occurring in subjects. Psychological performance tests indicate exposure-related impairment to learn new facts (51,53).

Neurologic symptoms associated with poor indoor air quality are puzzling and do not occur in every case of indoor air contamination. But in controlled human exposures, low-level mixtures of VOCs commonly found in indoor environments seem to be able to cause symptoms of irritancy and deficits in alertness, memory, and cognitive performance problems at concentrations below OSHA regulatory levels (51). A tendency to a stronger response in these studies was seen among prior SBS patients. Confusion, memory deficits, fatigue, drowsiness, and headache were associated with exposure to TVOC concentrations between 3 mg per m^3 and 25 mg per m^3 for only a few hours in test subjects (51), but seem to occur most often at the higher levels.

Overall, in most indoor environmental quality cases of the authors' experiences, neurologic symptoms usually tend to reverse quickly on leaving the contaminated environment. In some affected people, however, symptoms persist for no clear or plausible explanation. Theoretically, neurologic symptoms, such as fatigue and lethargy, might be explained by the action of inflammatory cytokines on the brain, but this remains to be proven (58,60).

Headache, fatigue, depression, anxiety, and chronic activation of the autonomic nervous system are adverse effects of chronic stressors of different varieties (61,62). Poor indoor air quality may also be acting as a chronic environmental stressor to cause such effects. Environmental exposures that escalate stress, to which people maladapt, may cause depression, irritability, mood alterations, difficulty concentrating, or difficulty sleeping (59,61,62). Identifying symptoms that are stress related and separating these from neurobehavioral toxicity require sophisticated neuropsychological testing.

Clinical cases report chronic fatigue and repeated respiratory infections associated with fungal contamination indoors (63). Airborne fungi and spores may incite inflammation via the 1,3-β-glucan component of their cell walls or release of VOCs (64). Thus, some environmental contaminants might serve as chronic stressors via activation of inflammation and activation of stress areas in the brain.

TABLE 53-8. Sources that emit volatile organic chemicals indoors at varying rates

Source	Volatile organic chemicals emitted	Rates µg/m$_2$
Building materials		
Plywood	Formaldehyde, terpenes, methylacetate, *n*-butanol, tetrachloroethylene, toluene, nonanol, *n*-undecane, tetradecane, naphthalene, *p*-dichlorobenzene, xylenes	40–2,400
Polystyrene foam	Styrene, ethylbenzene, aromatics	30–1,400
Rubber-backed nylon carpet	Toluene, benzene, *n*-decane, 4-phenycyclohexane	50–300
New vinyl flooring	Iso-alkanes, methylbenzenes, xylenes, ethylbenzene, toluene, 2-ethylhexanol, formaldehyde	120–43,000
Rubber floor covering	1,1,1-Trichloroethane, styrene, indene, 1,3/1,4-diisopropylbenzene, isodecane, acetophenone	410–1,400
Solvents and adhesives		
Solvent-based adhesives	Toluene, styrene, *n*-decane, *n*-undecane, cyclohexane, methylcyclopentane, alcohols	$5.1–16.5 \times 10^6$
Water-based adhesives	Nonane, decane, undecane, octane	$<10^4–2.1 \times 10^6$
Wall and flooring adhesive	Toluene, benzene, ethylacetate, styrene, ethylbenzene	2.5×10^6
Sealants	Methylethylketone, butylpropionate, 2-butoxyethanol, butanol, benzene, toluene	300–72,000
Wood stains	Nonane, decane, undecane, methyloctane, dimethylnonane, trimethylbenzene	17,000
Polyurethane varnish	Nonane, decane, undecane, methylethylketone, ethylbenzene, xylene	6,000
Solvent-based waxes and detergents	Alkanes, alkenes, terpenes	$<260 \times 10^6$
Water-based waxes and detergents	Alcohols, esters, alkoxyalcohols, terpenes, alcohols and acetates	1.2×10^5 to 1.2×10^6
Deodorizers	Nonane, decane, undecane, ethylheptane, limonene	$1.3–3.7 \times 10^6$
Liquid cleaner and disinfectant	Limonene, *p*-cymene, undecane, α-pinene, heptene, decane, nonane, heptane	1.1×10^6

Reprinted from Perry Rand Gee I. Vehicle emissions and effects on air quality: indoors and outdoors. *Indoor Environment* 1994;3:224–236, with permission.

Another study in nonsmoking adult volunteers with nonspecific bronchial reactivity who were exposed to VOC mixtures at zero, 2.5 mg per m^3, and 25 mg per m^3 showed a decline in forced expiratory volume in one second at 25 mg per m^3, a VOC concentration not uncommonly found indoors (65). Such findings support an inflammatory basis for the respiratory effects seen.

Other studies exposed subjects to VOC concentrations of 10 mg per m^3 of different compounds common to indoor air, controlling for humidity, air changes, skin temperature, air temperature, and exposure duration (51,53,54). These studies included measuring swelling of the nasal cavity, detection of odor, tear film stability, and examination for inflammatory cells in tear secretions of subjects. The results showed subjects experienced inflammation from exposures lasting more than 60 minutes, which was most pronounced at usual indoor temperatures (51). These subjects perceived air quality deterioration when the VOC concentration reached 8 mg per m^3, causing dryness, itching, burning of the eyes, and upper airway irritation. As the concentration increased, the adverse responses increased. Neurobehavioral and neurologic effects of confusion and fatigue occurred at TVOC concentrations of 25 mg per m^3 after an exposure lasting 3 and one-half hours. Thus, VOC exposure and air temperatures appear to be interdependent variables contributing to symptoms, and reduction of indoor temperatures can sometimes reduce VOC-related symptoms (51).

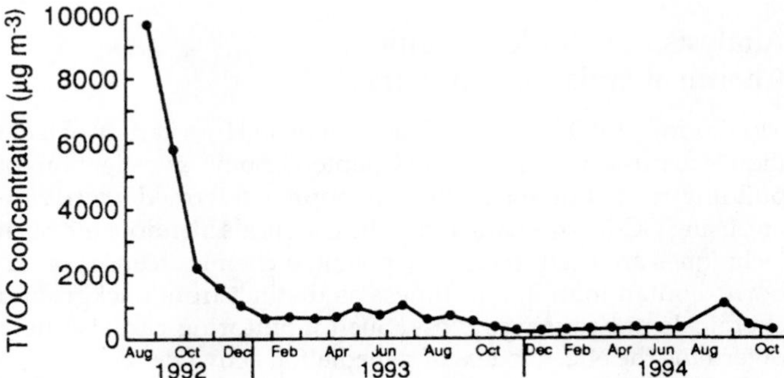

Figure 53-5. Total volatile organic chemical emissions profile from new home. TVOC, total volatile organic chemical. (From ref. 57, with permission.)

One double-blind study used 21 healthy subjects in comparison with a group of 14 subjects who had prior symptoms of SBS (53). The individuals who had prior symptoms had a tendency toward strong responses when exposed to low-level VOCs. Those with prior symptoms had exposure-related reductions in pulmonary functions, and both groups had an increased number of inflammatory cells in their tear fluids. Psychological performance tests indicated that the higher-exposure group had impaired ability to learn. The study concluded that low-level VOC exposure causes subjective complaints and objective effects in normal, healthy subjects, but more so in subjects who have had prior symptoms of SBS (53). Studies such as these demonstrate that the TVOC load in the environment probably plays an important role in initiating health complaints in a dose-related manner.

Gasoline refueling and driving expose people to VOCs in a confined environment (66). During refueling, the average TVOC in six studies ranged from 50 mg per m^3 to 150 mg per m^3. Gasoline emissions included *n*-pentane, *n*-butane, toluene, *m*- and *p*-xylene, and benzene. Main tailpipe emission of VOCs are methane, toluene, ethylene, *m*- and *p*-xylene, *n*-butane, and benzene (66). Inside automobiles, the VOC concentrations measured while driving were toluene (26 µg per m^3 to 56 µg per m^3), xylene (16 µg per m^3 to 23 µg per m^3), methylpentane (4 mg per m^3 to 18 mg per m^3), and benzene (9 µg per m^3 to 11 µg per m^3) (67,68).

In summary, symptoms of SBS appear to be able to be initiated in susceptible individuals when the total VOC concen-

TABLE 53-9. Whole house concentration (μg/m^{-3}) of total volatile organic chemicals during the first and second year

		Year 1 (August 3, 1992–August 3, 1993)			Year 2 (August 3, 1993–August 3, 1994)		Summer (March 16, 1993–September 28, 1993)	Winter (September 28, 1993–March 15, 1994)
House	Chemical	Mean	Max	Min	Mean	RSD (%)	Mean	Mean
1	TVOC	1,938	8,270	635	362	75	808	200
	Benzene	27	149	3	4	24	4	4
	Toluene	19	88	3	6	40	6	6
	Xylenes	81	289	59	25	59	42	16
	Undecane	75	261	32	18	61	34	10
	HCHO	59	122	29	42	33	63	37
2	TVOC	1,603	6,472	648	315	57	500	203
	Benzene	5	9	3	5	22	3	4
	Toluene	12	38	4	6	42	6	6
	Xylenes	64	227	32	21	48	36	15
	Undecane	70	276	32	17	54	33	11
	HCHO	51	91	28	37	48	52	28
3	TVOC	1,429	5,179	531	363	67	939	272
	Benzene	8	35	3	7	36	4	5
	Toluene	10	31	3	36	290	4	6
	Xylenes	30	94	14	20	136	19	8
	Undecane	57	176	26	16	59	39	10
	HCHO	41	106	17	40	43	53	30
4	TVOC	1,954	5,660	863	896	61	1,578	802
	Benzene	8	39	3	4	32	5	4
	Toluene	12	32	5	7	42	9	7
	Xylenes	33	85	16	45	183	25	26
	Undecane	82	202	41	37	61	70	31
	HCHO	43	111	15	45	45	59	35
Outside	TVOC	71	150	7	37	40	31	43
	Benzene	6	11	3	5	33	4	4
	Toluene	9	18	3	6	53	6	6
	Xylenes	7	11	4	4	40	4	5
	Undecane	4	24	6	1	20	2	1
	HCHO	3	5	2	2	63	3	2

HCHO, formaldehyde; RSD, relative standard deviation (i.e., standard deviation expressed as percentage of mean); TVOC, total volatile organic chemical.
Reprinted from ref. 57, with permission.

tration rises more than 3 mg per m^3 indoors (13,36,51,53,54). As the TVOC levels approach 25 mg per m^3, headache, psychological effects, fatigue, and adverse neurobehavioral effects are reported. Individuals with prior symptoms of SBS seem to have a tendency toward a stronger response in these studies. Thus, these studies provide guidelines for TVOC concentrations indoors that are associated with symptoms (Table 53-11). To relate TVOCs indoors to symptoms, however, it is important to convert TVOC measured in parts per million into mg/m^3 using the formula:

$$\text{mg/m}^3 = \frac{\text{ppm (molecular weight)}}{24.45}$$

Conversion of ppm to mg/m^3 allows the comparison of total VOC environmental contaminants using their average molecular weight to guidelines provided by human studies.

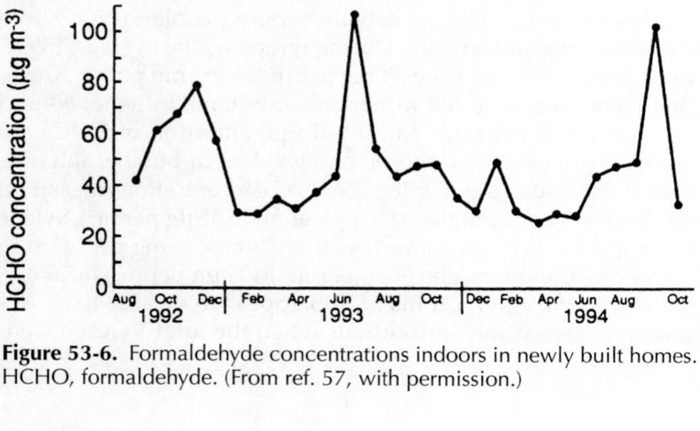

Figure 53-6. Formaldehyde concentrations indoors in newly built homes. HCHO, formaldehyde. (From ref. 57, with permission.)

Analysis of Volatile Organic Chemical Emissions Indoors

Monitoring of VOCs indoors is accomplished by a variety of techniques discussed extensively in Chapter 3. Some investigations of building-related illness include an approach termed *fingerprinting*, using GC-MS to characterize the chemicals in indoor air. Such techniques are used to identify potential chemical causes of airborne contamination and illness as distinct from background chemicals not causing illness. Such monitoring can also help determine the effectiveness of remediation activities.

Indoor VOC analysis in homes typically shows VOCs to be 10 times higher than those outdoors (57). Studies in homes show a variety of VOCs, from 85 detectable peaks up to 120 detectable peaks (57). VOC emissions and formaldehyde emission in homes studied are shown in Figures 53-5 and 53-6.

TABLE 53-10. Summary of five low-level indoor volatile organic chemical exposure experiments

Exposure		Population			
Type	mg/m^3	Type	Number of subjects	Measure of effects	Reference
Twenty-two volatile organic compounds	0, 5, 25	Randomly selected but sick building syndrome–sensitive	64	Subjective sensory responses, indications of neurologic effects, and changes in eye and nose liquids	1
Twenty-two volatile organic compounds	0, 1, 3, 8, 25	Randomly selected and healthy	25	Sensory symptoms, headache, and general well-being	2
n-Decane	0, 40, 140, 400	Random, healthy	63	Sensory symptoms, tear film stability, leukocytes in eye liquids	3
Twenty-two volatile organic compounds	0, 25	Healthy Sick building syndrome subjects	21 14	Sensory symptoms, lung function Leukocytes in eye liquids and nasal secretions, performance	4
Twenty-two volatile organic compounds	0, 25	Healthy males	76	Sensory symptoms, neurobehavioral tests	5

1. Molhave L, Bach B, Pedersen OF. Human reactions to low concentrations of volatile organic compounds. *Environment International* 1986;12:167–175.
2. Molhave L. The sick building syndrome (SBS) caused by exposures to volatile organic compounds (VOCs). In: Weekes DM, Gammage RB, eds. *The practitioner's approach to indoor air quality investigations.* Akron, Ohio: American Hygiene Association, 1990a.
3. Kjaergaard SK, Molhave L, Pedersen OF. Human reactions to indoor air pollutants: *n*-decane. *Environment International* 1989;15:473–482.
4. Kjaergaard SK, Molhave L, Pedersen OF. Human reactions to a mixture of indoor air volatile organic compounds. *Atmospheric Environment* 1991;25A:1417–1426.
5. Otto DA. Neurotoxic effects of controlled exposure to a complex mixture of volatile organic compounds. Research Triangle Park, NC: US Environmental Protection Agency, 1990. USA.EPA/600/1-90/001.

Adapted from ref. 51, with permission.

Basically, most materials tested in homes emitted VOCs. Major chemical classes of emissions found in chamber tests were C_9 to C_{14} aliphatic hydrocarbons, C_5 to C_{10} aldehydes, toluene, xylene, terpenes (α-pinene, limonene, carene), naphthalene, ethylacrylate, texanol (paints), 2,2,4-trimethyl-1,3-pentanediol (flooring materials), 4-methyl-2-pentanone, camphene, nonane, dichloromethane, pentane, 1,2,3,5-tetramethylbenzene, hexanal, pentanal, ethylbenzene, 4-ethyl-1-methylbenzene, undecane, limonene, terpinene, 1-methylnaphthalene, biphenyl, acenaphthene, and styrene (56).

Also, the composition of VOC mixture and emission rates change with time. Timber and woods are long-term sources of terpenes and aldehydes. Wood used for framing maintained a high VOC emission rate for 2 weeks (57). The TVOC emission profile is used to classify materials as short-term or long-term emitters and as high, moderate, or low VOC emitters (57) (Table 53-12):

- High emitters: TVOC 100 mg/m^2/hour
- Moderate emitters: TVOC 10 mg/m^2/hour
- Low emitters: TVOC 0.01 mg/m^2/hour

TABLE 53-11. Signs and symptoms of sick building syndrome correlated with volatile organic chemical concentration

Total volatile organic chemical concentration (mg/m^3)	Health effects
0–0.3	Clean environment
0.3–3	Odors, threshold for health complaints
3–10	Discomfort, irritation, inflammation, headache
10–25	Neurologic symptoms

It is important to be aware that the multiplicity of environmental factors, such as temperature, humidity, ventilation, air exchanges, the location and nature of the building material, and sinks, all influence VOC emissions and TVOC airborne concentrations in the indoor environment.

GC-MS fingerprinting can also be used to determine whether removal of a chemical source is associated with abatement of health effects. An example of this approach is shown by a case

TABLE 53-12. Classification of materials based on rate of volatile organic chemical emissions

Long-term volatile organic chemical emitters		
High	Moderate	Low
Water proof bituminous emulsion	Waterborne emulsion paints, putty, treated timber	Vinyl flooring, carpet, underlay, chipboard, bituminised fiberboard, asphalt, plywood, untreated timber
Short-term volatile organic chemical emitters		
High	**Moderate**	**Very low or not detectable**
Spray-on adhesive, acrylic adhesive, wood stain, gloss paints and undercoats, caulk	Foam sealant	Plasterboard, polyvinyl chloride skirting board

Adapted from ref. 57, with permission.

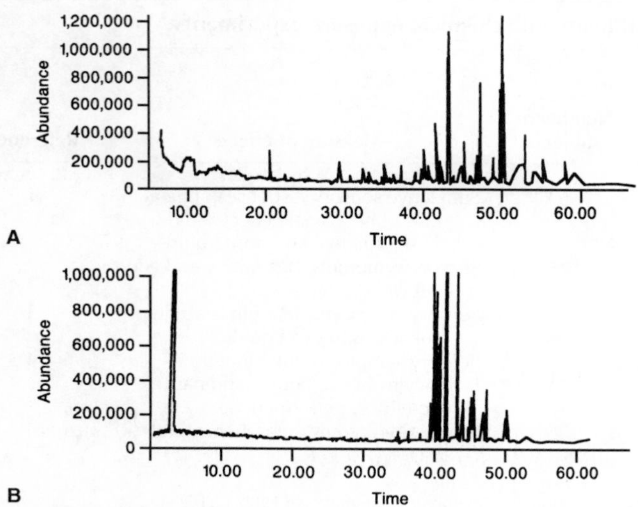

Figure 53-7. A: Identification of solvent in indoor air by gas chromatography–mass spectrometry. Air samples were collected in stainless steel canisters. A pesticide with a solvent-based carrier had been applied outside the home next to an exterior wall, and the occupants were experiencing irritant symptoms. **B:** Gas chromatography–mass spectrometry fingerprint of the solvent used with the pesticide confirms similar pattern to the samples collected indoors.

involving the presence of a solvent diluent of a pesticide that was injected along the perimeter of one area of a home. Indoor air samples collected in stainless steel canisters revealed a GC-MS fingerprint pattern similar to that of the solvent carrier. The presence of this petroleum solvent (Fig. 53-7A and B) was associated with irritant symptoms in the occupants. Attempts at remediation resulted in reduction of indoor air concentrations of the solvent after removal of exterior wall dirt where the pesticide was sprayed (Fig. 53-8A). Finally, cleaning the contaminated air return of the ventilation system resulted in almost total elimination of the airborne solvent as well as relief of health effects (Fig. 53-8B).

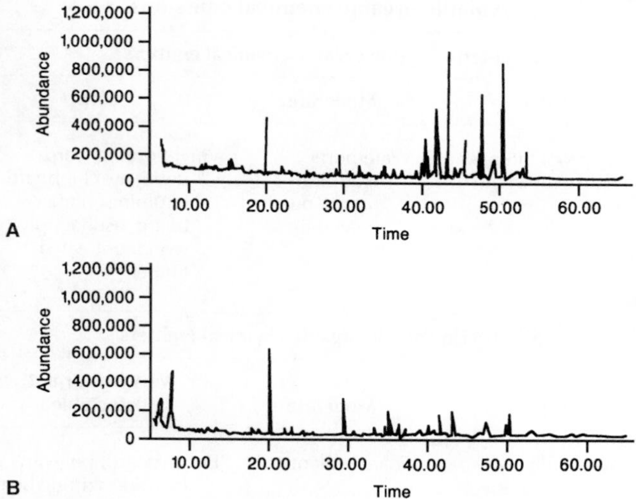

Figure 53-8. A: Repeat sampling results of the indoor air after removal of exterior wall soil contaminated with the pesticide and solvent. Results show failure to remediate contamination of the indoor air. **B:** Gas chromatography–mass spectrometry pattern demonstrates that cleaning of ventilation air duct returns in addition to removal of the exterior wall soil resulted in effective elimination of the air contaminant.

Volatile Organic Compounds in Human Blood

Human exposure to volatile chlorinated organic chemicals may result in low plasma concentrations of VOCs (69). Blood concentrations of volatile halogenated compounds may be higher in winter months, when residents spend most of their time indoors. Interpreting such plasma concentrations of organic chemicals is difficult in relationship to health complaints. The presence of such hydrocarbons in low concentrations is indicative of exposure from a wide variety of sources or environments, but does not necessarily constitute the existence of disease.

Sample collection can be a source of error in measuring VOCs in human blood. Studies show that VOC contaminants can be introduced into blood collection tubes (69). Studies have been performed to determine background VOC blood concentrations of nonoccupationally exposed individuals. Exposure to gasoline, tobacco smoke, and other sources of VOCs can account for levels in the parts per billion to parts per trillion range (69).

NEW CARPET

A variety of chemicals may volatilize from new carpets and the adhesives used to attach carpet to floors. The distinctive new carpet odor has been traced to the chemical 4-phenylcyclohexene (4-PC) (70,71). The source of 4-PC is styrene-butadiene rubber latex used to bind the backing of new carpet (Fig. 53-9). Production of styrene-butadiene rubber latex results in the formation of 4-PC as a chemical by-product via the Diels-Adler reaction. When isolated, 4-PC is a clear, oily liquid, possessing the distinctive new carpet odor (70,71).

Analysis of carpet pieces demonstrated that 4-PC was a common contaminant in several environments reported to cause health effects after new carpet had been installed (70,71). Acute and subacute exposure to low parts per billion of 4-PC may be responsible for symptoms of headaches, lethargy, and skin and mucous membrane irritation (72) (Table 53-13).

Air monitoring in office and home environments for 4-PC has revealed concentrations ranging from 0.3 to 40 parts per billion (ppb) (70,71). Data suggest that 4-PC air concentrations decay over several months from a high of 30 ppb to 1 or 2 ppb after carpet installation. Airborne concentrations of 5 ppb are odiferous. 4-PC concentrations less than 1 ppb have not been associated with illness after installation of new carpet in homes and work environments.

Studies of total VOC release from new carpet installation show a decline from the day of installation of approximately 11 mg per m^3 to approximately 1 mg per m^3 by 10 days (70,71). These TVOC levels exceed concentrations known to produce health complaints.

An investigation of an office space in which 21 of 34 workers complained of health effects showed 4-PC present as an air contaminant at 1.9 ppb as well as a variety of VOCs from the adhesive used to glue the carpet to the floor (72). Formalde-

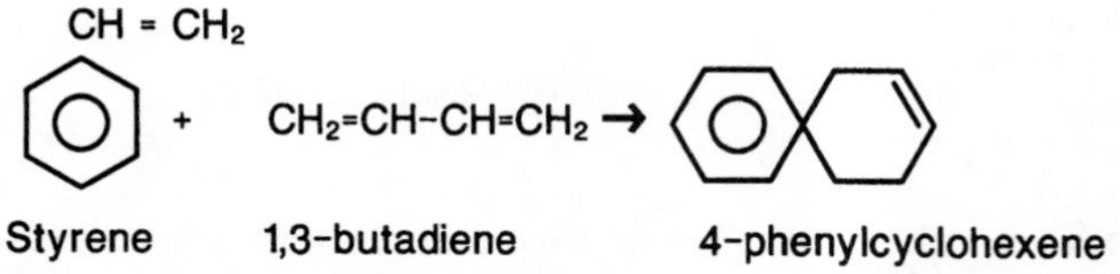

CH = CH_2 + CH_2=CH–CH=CH_2 →

Styrene 1,3-butadiene 4-phenylcyclohexene

Figure 53-9. Diels-Alder reaction of styrene with 1,3-butadiene to produce 4-phenylcyclohexene as a by-product of styrene-butadiene rubber production.

TABLE 53-13. Signs and symptoms in 21 of 34 workers with 1.9 parts per billion of 4-phenylcyclohexene plus other volatile organic chemicals in the environment

Signs and symptoms	Number of workers	Percentage
Headache	14	67
Throat soreness	11	52
Fatigue and lethargy	10	48
Upper airway irritation	7	48
Nausea	10	48
Ocular irritation	8	38
Dizziness	6	29
Chest tightness	6	29
Skin irritation	5	24
Visual disturbance	5	24
Unusual taste	4	19
Myalgias	4	19
Shortness of breath	3	14

Sullivan J, Van Ert M, Krieger G. Indoor air quality and human health. In: Sullivan J, Krieger G. *Hazardous materials toxicology: clinical principles of environmental health.* Baltimore: Williams & Wilkins, 1992.

hyde, detected at 0.03 ppm, was not considered to be a source of worker illness. New carpet had been installed in this work area 1 week before employees moved into the site. No other source of indoor air pollution was found. Chemical odors were noted by the majority of workers occupying the site almost immediately. Within a few weeks of occupancy, health complaints were registered by the majority of the employees. The first indication of a health problem occurred when one of the workers presented to an emergency department with severe headache, vomiting, and upper airway irritation. The patient reported that headaches and nausea began within 3 weeks of moving into the new building. The patient also complained of ocular and skin irritation. These symptoms lessened during off-work hours. Surveys revealed 21 of the 34 workers (62%) occupying the building site had adverse health effects (see Table 53-13).

Of the 21 patients with symptoms, 10 described some form of past allergic condition, such as hay fever or seasonal rhinitis. The other 11 had no previous allergic manifestations. Smoking was not allowed in the work site, and six of the 21 affected workers were smokers. The building was a one-story modular type with a large open area partitioned into smaller cubicles. The area housed clerical staff with video display terminals used in the previous work area. The entire work area was open except for two administrative offices.

The illness experienced by these employees is similar to that seen in other building-related illnesses with the exception of more pronounced headaches and lethargy. Headaches (67%) and lethargy (48%) may be the result of central nervous system effects of 4-PC at low air concentrations. Prominent mucous membrane irritant effects were also apparent; sore throat (52%), eye irritation (38%), chest tightness (29%), upper airway irritation (48%), cough (24%), and skin irritation (24%) accounted for a large number of complaints, indicating the irritant nature of the mixed chemical exposure.

It is evident that 4-PC may be a chemical that could pose significant health effects for office workers and homeowners exposed to new carpet emissions. The extent of these health effects is not entirely known, but appears to be similar to other indoor air pollutants except that clinical symptomatology occurs in the low parts per billion range. 4-PC decays over several weeks to months in the indoor environment and even after 3 to 6 months may be detected in the 1 to 2 ppb range. The level of this compound can be reduced in the indoor environment by steam cleaning carpet and simultaneously improving ventilation. Explanation to workers of the expected health effects along with assurance that this and other chemicals can be removed from the environment should be part of the management plan.

Such factors as where samples are taken may cause variability in measurements when assessing health complaints. Steam cleaning new carpet along with improving ventilation can reduce vapors to a tolerable level for most people.

CLEANING AGENTS AND DISINFECTANTS

Many cleaning agents and disinfectants can contribute to poor indoor air quality. Material data sheets for these agents should be available. Cleaning agents and disinfectants contain a variety of irritating and sensitizing chemicals that can cause eye irritation, respiratory irritation, exacerbate reactive airways symptoms, cause dermatitis, and may cause asthma. Irritant chemicals in disinfectants and cleaning agents are as follows:

- Benzalkonium chloride
- Benzoyl peroxide
- Isopropanol
- Formaldehyde
- Glutaraldehyde
- Phenol
- Alcohols
- Chlorine compounds
- Potassium permanganate
- Free iodine
- Povidone iodine
- Thimerosal
- Gentian violet
- Hexachlorophene
- Chlorhexidine
- Phenylphenol
- Ethyl alcohol
- Ethylenediamine tetraacetic acid
- Quaternary ammonium chlorides
- Cationic detergents
  - Octyldecyldimethyl ammonium chloride
  - Dioctyldimethyl ammonium chloride
  - Didecyldimethyl ammonium chloride
  - *n*-Alkyldimethylbenzyl ammonium chloride
- Nonionic surfactants
- Sodium metasilicate
- Fragrances
- Colorants

The use of these agents in poorly ventilated areas or on large surfaces in enclosed spaces may result in exposure of occupants to low levels of sensitizers, such as quaternary ammonium compounds, surfactants, and alkyl benzyl ammonium chloride. Contact and allergic dermatitis may occur after exposure to some chemicals in these products. Also, chronic exposure may cause bronchial hyperresponsiveness and airway inflammation.

Disinfectants and cleaning products can be responsible for chemical odors in addition to being a source of respiratory irritation. Chemicals in these products are amines, surfactants, cationic and anionic detergents, ammonia, acids, hypochlorites, phenols, alcohols, and caustics. Substituting these cleaning agents for less irritating agents can be helpful in eliminating indoor pollution sources.

INDOOR COMBUSTION SOURCES

Natural gas is used by approximately 50% of households, potentially exposing occupants to by-products of combustion. Besides gas appliances, other combustion sources are fireplaces, tobacco smoke, cooking, internal combustion machines, and charcoal fires. Pilot lights, cooking, and gas appliance use contribute to nitrogen dioxide indoors, a respiratory irritant. Common pollutant by-products of combustion are the following:

- Nitrogen dioxide
- Sulfur dioxide
- Formaldehyde
- Carbon dioxide
- Soot
- Particulates
- Volatile organic compounds

If wood stoves or coal stoves are not airtight, pollutants can escape indoors. Airflow patterns indoors may be altered, causing backdrafting of combustion by-products. Faulty design of fireplace flues can result in emission backdrafting.

CARBON MONOXIDE AND VEHICLE EXHAUST EMISSIONS

The most serious health threat from combustion is carbon monoxide. Thousands are seriously injured and killed yearly by this insidious poison. The following are carbon monoxide sources:

- Automobile exhaust
- Combustion processes
- Gas stoves
- Wood or coal stoves
- Fireplaces
- Tobacco smoke
- Charcoal cookers
- Space heaters
- Gas hot water heaters, unvented
- Unvented gas furnace
- Methylene chloride in paint remover

Intake vents located in loading docks, garages, or busy traffic areas can bring outside exhaust pollutants indoors. Buildings with many story levels may have a negative air pressure on the lower floors as compared to upper floors, which causes exhaust pollutants from outdoors to be drawn inside the lower levels.

Improperly ventilated natural gas appliances contribute to concentrations of carbon monoxide, nitrogen oxides, and formaldehyde indoors. Inefficient and improperly ventilated natural gas appliances have resulted in cases of carbon monoxide poisoning in the home. Charcoal grills release high levels of carbon monoxide indoors and can be particularly dangerous in small spaces.

Carbon monoxide is a deadly gas that is odorless, colorless, and heavier than air. It can quickly fill a small space, such as a mobile home or bedroom. Mild toxicity produces headache, nausea, dizziness, and drowsiness that tend to influence a person to fall asleep, not allowing escape from the deadly gas (Table 53-14).

Carbon monoxide poisoning may elude diagnosis because it mimics other illnesses, like gastroenteritis. Carbon monoxide exposure should be expected if more than one person in a household is sick with similar symptoms, especially if a gas heater or space heater has been recently turned on because of cold weather.

TABLE 53-14. Carbon monoxide poisoning: signs and symptoms with increasing levels in blood

Level of carbon monoxide in blood (%)	Signs and symptoms
10–20	Headache, shortness of breath
20–30	Severe headache, dizziness, nausea, vomiting, difficulty concentrating
30–40	Lethargy, fainting on exertion, visual and auditory disturbance, dizziness, chest pain, fainting
40–50	Rapid heart rate, fainting, heart attack, seizures
50–60	Coma, brain damage, cardiac arrest
70 or more	Death

FORMALDEHYDE

Formaldehyde is a common indoor contaminant and a known upper airway, eye, and skin irritant. Formaldehyde exposure has become such a concern that OSHA issued a new formaldehyde standard in 1993 for medical evaluation of exposed workers. OSHA set the permissible exposure limit (PEL) for formaldehyde at 0.75 ppm in 1993.

Formaldehyde has many sources: carpet, fabrics, pressed wood products, tobacco smoke, phenolic resins, plywood and binders in fiberglass insulation, cosmetics, food, and combustion by-products. In studies, formaldehyde airborne concentrations in homes ranged from 0.1 ppm to 0.5 ppm, with an average of 0.07 ppm (73–75).

Formaldehyde is a colorless gas at room temperature, but also can be found in a liquid or solid form. Low concentrations of formaldehyde are present in ambient air, primarily because of burning of petroleum fuels and automobile exhaust.

Formaldehyde emissions indoors from building materials is in the following order of decreasing emission rate: chipboard, carpet, plywood, plasterboard, bituminised fiberboard, 15-mm plywood, mineral wool insulation, and curtains (57).

Formaldehyde releasers are used as preservatives in many commercial products, including cleaning agents, shampoos, soaps, paints, lacquers, cutting oils, cosmetics, coloring agents, skin care products, toilet cleaners, automotive cleaning agents, disinfectants, dishwashing liquids, and descaling agents (Table 53-15).

It is impossible to escape formaldehyde exposure because it is contained in a normal diet. Smoked foods and foods prepared on grills can have high concentrations of formaldehyde, up to 1,000 ppm. Formaldehyde is common in fruit, such as apples and tomatoes, and is found in dairy products, vegetables, baked goods, and food preservatives.

The hazards of formaldehyde are mainly from inhalation and dermal contact. General exposure occurs through the use of formaldehyde-containing products, burning fuels, tobacco smoke, or formaldehyde releases as preservatives. Formaldehyde in the air at a home or work arises from burning of organic fuel, such as wood, coal, natural gas, oil, and gasoline or diesel fuel. Resins used as glues and adhesives in the manufacturing of wood products, such as furniture and paneling, are prime sources of formaldehyde. Formaldehyde is also used in the manufacture of carpets and permanent pressed clothing. Sidestream tobacco smoke is said to contain up to 40 ppm of formaldehyde (76).

Health effects from formaldehyde include upper airway irritation and eye irritation. Symptoms of throat irritation, fatigue, headache, eye irritation, and nausea have been reported in indoor air concentrations of formaldehyde between 0.1 and 1.0 ppm (74,75). The respiratory irritation threshold and ocular irritation threshold are 0.8 to 1.0 ppm (74,75). Because of formaldehyde's water solubility, it is absorbed in the upper airway and does not usually reach the lower airways. Some individuals, however, experience asthma exacerbations on exposure to formaldehyde. Patch testing can determine if a person has an allergic hypersensitivity skin reaction to formaldehyde.

TABLE 53-15. Examples of formaldehyde releasers in common products

- Benzylhemiformal
  - Cleaning agents
  - Polishes
- Bioban CS-1246
  - Cutting fluids
- Nitrobutyl morfoline
  - Cutting fluids
- Bromonitrodioxane
  - General cleaners
  - Dishwashing liquids
  - Automotive cleaners
- Bromonitropropanediol
  - Automotive cleaners
  - Dishwashing liquid
  - Disinfectants
  - General cleaners
- Chloroallylhexaminium chloride
  - Cleaning agents
  - Coloring agents
  - Paints and lacquers
  - Polishes
  - Shampoo
  - Hair care products
  - Soap and skin care products
- Diazolidinyl urea
  - Soap and skin care products
- Dimethylol urea
  - Cleaning agents
  - Cutting fluids
- Dimethylol dimethyl hydantoin
  - Shampoo, hair care products
  - Soap and skin care products
- Dimethoxymethane
  - Cleaning agents
- Formaldehyde
  - Cleaning agents
  - Coloring agents
  - Curing agents
  - Cutting fluids
  - Paints
  - Lacquers
  - Polishes
  - Shampoo
  - Hair products
  - Soap
  - Skin care products
  - Surface active agents
  - Toilet cleaners
- Hexamethylenetetramine
  - Cleaning agents
- Imidazolidinyl urea
  - Shampoo and hair care products
- *N*-Methylolchloroacetamide
  - Coloring agents
- *N*-Methylolethanolamine
  - Paints and lacquers
- Trihydroxyethylhexahydro *S*-triazine
  - Disinfectants
- Paraformaldehyde
  - Disinfectants
  - Descaling agents

ENVIRONMENTAL TOBACCO SMOKE

The burning of tobacco indoors introduces chemical pollutants and particulates. A report published in the *Journal of the American Medical Association* in 1992 reviewed evidence that exposure to ETS contributed to excess deaths from heart disease and cancer (24,25). If the epidemiologic evidence is valid, then ETS may be responsible for 35,000 to 40,000 excess deaths from heart disease annually (25). However, this estimate is based on 1980s data and is being questioned.

Tobacco smoke is made up of more than 4,000 toxic substances, including carcinogens (Table 53-16). The EPA has classified ETS as a group A carcinogen, meaning that sufficient evidence exists to prove that it causes cancer in humans (24). OSHA has also classified ETS as a potential occupational carcinogen.

Exposure to ETS exacerbates asthma, causing more than a 20% decline in forced expiratory volume in one second (26). ETS is an irritant of the eyes and upper airway also and is a significant source of formaldehyde exposure indoors (27).

NITROGEN OXIDES

Nitrogen oxide sources are burning of fossil fuels, industrial processes, and motor vehicles. NO_2, the most common of the oxides of nitrogen, is a reddish brown to yellow gas with an acrid irritating odor. Nitrogen oxides are involved in the photochemical generation of ozone.

Indoor exposure to nitrogen oxides occurs from gas-burning appliances, unvented furnaces, stoves, hot water heaters, tobacco smoke, kerosene space heaters, and influx of outdoor air contamination from vehicle exhaust.

Gas stoves are a principal source of nitrogen dioxide indoors and when a gas stove is used for cooking, the peak nitrogen dioxide concentration in a kitchen can be 1 ppm or higher.

Nitrogen oxides are insoluble in water and, therefore, can penetrate to the lower respiratory tract. Children are particularly susceptible to NO_2 because of their developing respiratory system. Studies have linked NO_2 exposure and increased respiratory illness in children (22,23). Low levels of NO_2 cause rhinorrhea, throat irritation, eye irritation, and cough. Asthmatics are sensitive to low NO_2 levels. Mild exposure causes shortness of breath, headache, cough, fatigue, nausea, and dizziness that can persist up to 2 weeks postexposure. Exposure to massive concentrations can produce severe lung damage, asphyxiation, laryngospasm, and death. The irritant effects of NO_2 do not occur until concentrates reach approximately 13 ppm (23).

After a severe exposure, individuals may develop permanent respiratory impairment. Exposure to NO_2 concentrations as low as 0.10 to 0.60 ppm can enhance airway responsiveness in asthmatics (77). At concentrations greater than or equal to 1.5 ppm, NO_2 increases airway reactivity in healthy subjects (78). Epidemiologic studies suggest an association between NO_2 exposure and the susceptibility to respiratory illness (79,80). Nitrogen dioxide exposure limits are as follows:

TLV [American Conference of Governmental Industrial Hygienists (ACGIH) 8-hour time-weighted average (TWA)], 3 ppm
PEL (OSHA 15-minute ceiling), 5 ppm
Immediately dangerous to life and health, 20 ppm
National Ambient Air Quality Standard (EPA annual average), 0.053 ppm

SULFUR OXIDES

The main source of SO_2 is burning of sulfur-containing fuels. SO_2 is a component of indoor and outdoor pollution arising from automobile exhaust. It is found in lower concentrations indoors than outdoors. The use of kerosene space heaters can generate significant concentrations of indoor SO_2.

SO_2 is soluble in water and tends to be absorbed in the upper respiratory tract. Nasal breathing filters out most inhaled SO_2, preventing its passage into more sensitive areas of the lungs. Mouth breathing tends to increase the amount of SO_2 that reaches the lungs.

SO_2 is highly irritating to the eyes and airways. Its odor is detectable at 0.5 ppm. Concentrations more than 6 ppm induce symptoms of irritation, including eye irritation, tearing, runny nose, coughing, shortness of breath, bronchospasm, chest tightness, and a choking sensation. Prolonged and chronic exposure to SO_2 can produce chronic bronchitis, airway inflammation, chronic cough, increased mucous excretion, and clearing of the throat. Massive exposure to SO_2 can result in severe permanent pulmonary damage. SO_2 concentrations in the indoor environment and outdoors in the air are associated with decreases in pulmonary functions. Exercise in polluted environments with low humidity increase health problems to those susceptible, such as asthmatics. SO_2 exposure limits are as follows:

TLV (ACGIH) (8-hour TWA), 2 ppm
PEL (OSHA 8-hour TWA), 5 ppm
Immediately dangerous to life or health, 100 ppm
National Ambient Air Quality Standard (EPA), 0.14 ppm

OZONE

Ozone (O_3) is a naturally occurring colorless or light blue gas with a pungent electrical-type odor. It is a potent chemical respiratory tract irritant and is the principal oxidant in photochemical smog. Exposures occur more commonly in urban and

TABLE 53-16. Examples of pollutants in the vapor phase of environmental tobacco smoke

Compound	Concentration/cigarette	Compound	Concentration/cigarette
Nitrogen	280–320 mg (56–64%)	Nicotine	1,000–3,000 μg
Oxygen	50–70 mg (11–14%)	Nornicotine	40–150 μg
Carbon dioxide	45–65 mg (9–13%)	Anatabine	5–15 μg
Carbon monoxide	14–23 mg (2.8–4.6%)	Anabasine	5–12 μg
Water	7–12 mg (1.4–2.4%)	Bipyridyls	10–30 μg
Argon	5 mg (1.0%)	*n*-Hentriacontane (*n*-$C_{31}H_{64}$)	100 μg
Hydrogen	0.5–1.0 mg	Total nonvolatile hydrocarbons	300–400 μg
Ammonia	10–130 μg	Naphthalenes	3–6 μg
Nitrogen oxides	100–600 μg	Phenanthrenes	0.2–0.4 μg
Hydrogen cyanide	400–500 μg	Anthracenes	0.05–0.1 μg
Hydrogen sulfide	20–90 μg	Fluorenes	0.6–1.0 μg
Methane	1.0–2.0 mg	Pyrenes	0.3–0.5 μg
Volatile alkanes	1.0–1.6 mg	Fluoranthenes	0.3–0.45 μg
Volatile alkenes	0.4–0.5 mg	Carcinogenic polynuclear aromatic hydrocarbons	0.1–0.25 μg
Isoprene	0.2–0.4 mg		
Butadiene	25–40 μg	Phenol	80–160 μg
Acetylene	20–35 μg	Other phenols	60–180 μg
Benzene	12–60 μg	Catechol	200–400 μg
Toluene	20–60 μg	Other catechols	100–200 μg
Styrene	10 μg	Other dihydroxybenzenes	200–400 μg
Volatile aromatic hydrocarbons	15–30 μg	Scopoletin	15–30 μg
Formic acid	200–600 μg	Cyclotenes	40–70 μg
Acetic acid	100–1,700 μg	Quinones	0.5 μg
Propionic acid	100–300 μg	Solanesol	600–1,000 μg
Methyl formate	20–30 μg	Neophytadienes	200–350 μg
Volatile acids	5–10 μg	Limonene	30–60 μg
Formaldehyde	20–100 μg	Other terpenes	200–250 μg
Acetaldehyde	400–1,400 μg	Palmitic acid	100–150 μg
Acrolein	60–140 μg	Stearic acid	50–75 μg
Volatile aldehydes	80–140 μg	Oleic acid	40–110 μg
Acetone	100–650 μg	Linoleic acid	60–150 μg
Volatile ketones	50–100 μg	Linolenic acid	150–250 μg
Methanol	80–180 μg	Lactic acid	60–80 μg
Volatile alcohols	10–30 μg	Indole	10–15 μg
Acetonitrile	100–150 μg	Skatole	12–16 μg
Volatile nitriles	50–80 μg	Quinolines	2–4 μg
Furan	20–40 μg	Benzofurans	200–300 μg
Volatile furans	45–125 μg	Stigmasterol	40–70 μg
Pyridine	20–200 μg	Sitosterol	30–40 μg
Picolines	15–80 μg	Campesterol	20–30 μg
3-Vinylpyridine	10–30 μg	Cholesterol	10–20 μg
Volatile pyridines	20–50 μg	Aniline	0.36 μg
Pyrrole	0.1–10 μg	Toluidines	0.23 μg
Pyrrolidine	10–18 μg	Other aromatic amines	0.25 μg
N-Methylpyrrolidine	2.0–3.0 μg	*N*-nitrosamines	0.34–2.7 μg
Volatile pyrazines	3.0–8.0 μg	Glycerol	120 μg
Methylamine	4–10 μg		
Aliphatic amines	3–10 μg		

Reprinted from US Department of Health and Human Services. Reducing the health consequences of smoking. Rockville, MD: Centers for Disease Control and Prevention, 1989, with permission.

suburban environments, particularly during air pollution alerts. O_3 is a common outdoor pollutant and is consumed in the transformation of nitrogen monoxide into nitrogen dioxide. Consequently, the levels of atmospheric ozone may be higher in rural areas as compared to urban areas.

O_3 concentrations are higher outdoors than indoors, but indoor levels can increase when windows or doors are open. Average concentrations indoors range from 0 to 0.02 ppm (0 to 40 mcg per m^3), with peak levels approaching 0.1 to 0.2 ppm (200 to 400 mcg per m^3). Photocopiers and laser printers can produce peak O_3 concentrations of 0.2 ppm indoors and breathing zone levels of approximately 0.10 ppm (81,82).

One-half of the U.S. population lives in areas that cannot meet or have not met federal ambient air quality standards for O_3. Therefore, millions of people are exposed to this respiratory irritant. O_3 is formed by the action of ultraviolet light on nitrogen oxides and hydrocarbons in the atmosphere. Because O_3 formation depends on ultraviolet radiation, its formation is greatest on warm and sunny days. In heavily populated areas, typically the pattern of O_3 formation occurs mainly in the late mornings, lasting until late afternoon or early evening. O_3 is also formed at higher altitudes by ultraviolet light action on oxygen. Environmental exposure limits and guidelines to ozone follow:

National Ambient Air Quality Standard, 0.12 ppm (1-hour average), 0.08 ppm (8-hour average)
TLV (ACGIH), 0.10 ppm (8-hour TWA)
PEL (OSHA), 0.10 ppm (8-hour TWA)
Immediately dangerous to life and health, 10 ppm

Ozone is used as a disinfectant and bleaching agent. Copiers, laser printers, and electrostatic air filters are sources of ozone indoors.

Ozone has a short half-life and, consequently, interaction with humans is limited to an air-fluid interface, such as the mucous membranes of the upper airway, the respiratory tract, or the eye. Because ozone has little water solubility, it can penetrate to deep areas of the respiratory tract. Fifty percent of ozone is taken up in the upper airway and nasal passages. O_3 that reaches the lower airways can actually be absorbed into the blood to a small degree. Because O_3 has a potent oxidizing agent, it can damage tissues.

Signs and symptoms of O_3 exposure are cough, headache, chest tightness, chest pain, chest tightness on deep inspiration, shortness of breath, a dry throat, wheezing, and difficulty breathing. O_3 has been documented to significantly impair the ability to perform sustained exercise, probably through the discomfort that it produces on inspiration during intensive periods of exercise. Other symptoms include extreme fatigue, somnolence, dizziness, insomnia, decreased ability to concentrate, acrid taste and smell, and eye irritation. If an individual increases his or her breathing rate or engages in exercise for long durations of exposure, symptoms can be provoked at O_3 concentrations lower than the federal ambient air quality standard.

Studies link ambient O_3 concentrations with exacerbation of asthma. In some people, acute respiratory responses to O_3 become attenuated with repeated daily exposures (see also Chapter 97).

Environmental Sampling for Biologicals

Sampling for biologicals in the indoor environment requires a strategy related to the health effects exhibited by the occupants and the characteristics of the environment as determined by inspection. Characterization of biological growth and bioaerosols may include analyses for some or all of the following:

- Microscopy (characterizing spores, pollen, or particulates)
- Species identification of microorganisms
- Airborne colony-forming units per cubic meter (CFU/m^3) of viable organisms
- Antigen content of dust
- 1,3-β-glucan in dust samples
- Peptidoglycan (gram-positive bacteria)
- Ergosterol analysis of spores
- Endotoxin
- Mycotoxin
- 3-hydroxy fatty acids/phospholipid ester-linked fatty acids

The physical and aerodynamic properties of bioaerosols affect their collection and assay. The aerodynamics of bioaerosols are determined by particle size, diameter, shape and density, hydrophobic or hydrophilic properties, electrical charges, and their chemical nature (83). For spherical particles, the aerodynamic properties are related mainly to their diameter. For elongated or spherical-shaped particles, the smallest diameter may better represent its aerodynamic properties.

Large particles fall faster than smaller ones. Therefore, collection assays may overestimate large particles compared to small particles. Also, small particles flow around a surface, whereas larger particles impact onto a surface. Hydrophilic particles may be more easily collected into a liquid impinger than hydrophobic particles, which would pass through the liquid. Also, more water-soluble particles dissolve in the liquid. The electrostatic charge also affects behavior of particles with respect to surface interaction. Charged particles may be more attracted to surfaces with opposite charges.

Sampling may be for viable fungi and bacteria, total fungi and bacteria, or fungal and bacterial chemical substances. When sampling for biological contaminants indoors, simultaneous sampling outside serves as a source of comparison and may also reveal an outdoor source of contamination.

Standard biological sampling for microorganisms is divided into the following:

1. *Representative sampling*: Refers to only a portion of a population of biologicals that are selected for a study, such as a single bacterial or fungal species.
2. *Observational sampling*: Involves onsite inspection and sensory perception of an expert to determine information about sources, dispersion, and exposure of individuals to biologicals. Observational sampling can result in immediate decisions regarding the health and safety of an environment and the relationship of signs and symptoms to environmental conditions.
3. *Bulk sampling*: Refers to collection of a physical sample on a surface or from a specifically identified biological source, such as in a ventilation system. Bulk sampling allows for determination of an amount of antigen per gram of dust. This, however, does not consider the total amount of dust in the environment or the amount that might be aerosolized. To have meaning, bulk samples must be collected from the primary source of the causative agent in the environment.
4. *Wipe or surface sampling*: With wipe or surface sampling, a defined area is swabbed and the swabbing material is treated in the same manner as the microporous filter. This, however, only gives a measure of concentration for a given area, not a volume of air. This technique may be useful for evaluating ventilation ducts.
5. *Dust sampling*: Similar to air sampling, except a coarser filter is used to collect dust. This indicates the concentration of viable fungi and bacteria adhering to dust, which may not be accounted for in other sampling techniques.
6. *Air sampling*: This is more representative of human exposure to bioaerosols. Variables of air sampling are the aerodynamics and the physical nature of the particles, electrical charge, and chemical nature. Collecting a sample representative of the bioaerosols in certain space over time to make determinations regarding health effects is critical to interpreting results and health implications. Particle size of biologicals can vary from less than 1 μm to more than 100 μm. Attempting to characterize the sample for such a range of particle sizes can be difficult with a single collecting device. Respirable bioaerosols of health concern, however, generally are from 0.1 μm to 10.0 μm in diameter. Focusing on these sizes provides a better human exposure representation.

AIR SAMPLING FOR BIOLOGICALS

Three ways in which viable fungi and bacteria may be collected from air follow:

1. *Filtration*: Involves drawing air through a microporous filter, resulting in microorganisms being intercepted by the filter. This filter is then placed in peptone water and shaken. This suspension is used to inoculate growth media or is serially diluted into the media and then spread onto culture plates. After incubation, the bacterial or fungal colonies are counted; each colony represents 1 CFU or viable organism. These data allow investigators to calculate the concentrations of airborne viable fungi and bacteria. Nonviable spores and microorganisms that can also cause health problems are not detected by this method.
2. *Impaction*: Involves drawing air through an impactor, an instrument that places a maximum limit on the size of par-

ticles collected. The air drawn through the impactor is impacted onto an agar plate, depositing fungi and bacteria. The agar plate is incubated and the resulting colonies are counted. This method underestimates the number of viable cells, because the force involved in sampling may destroy many of them.

3. *Liquid trapping*: Trapping of fungi and bacteria in a liquid is accomplished by bubbling air through water. Two instruments used are the impinger and cyclone scrubber. This causes airborne microorganisms to become entrained in the water that is then used to inoculate growth media. The media are then spread on culture plates and incubated, after which colonies are counted.

To determine the total fungal or bacterial count in air, not just viable count, microscopy may be used. Air is drawn through a microporous filter, and the filter is viewed under a microscope. This allows a visual count of viable and nonviable cells and spores.

Sampling time is another important feature. Continuous sampling over an exposure period of interest might be ideal; however, it may not be achievable. Many times sampling is done for a specified period, such as for 5 minutes.

SAMPLING FOR CHEMICALS

Because culturing techniques may significantly undercount viable organisms, assays for biochemicals derived from microorganisms are being investigated as a means to characterize biocontaminants. Research shows that fungal biomass may be determined by ergosterol analysis (84–86). Ergosterol is stable and is found in living and nonviable spores. Air is collected on a microspore titer and spores are extracted with methanol. Analysis is by gas-liquid chromatography–mass spectrometry or high-pressure liquid chromatography. One study showed 3.2 μg of ergosterol per milligram of spores. *Aspergillus* and *Penicillia* produce 1.4 μg per mg to 6.0 μg per mg.

A modified LAL analysis is used to assay for airborne (1,3)-β-glucan content (87–91), which research is showing can correlate with respiratory symptoms.

Volatile chemicals generated by fungi are being used to help determine fungal presence and the nature of fungal contamination indoors. Detection of 3-methylfuran indicates fungal growth and amplification (87,88). Detection of 1-octen-3-ol indicates dormant fungal mass. Geosmin presence indicates fungal mass presence and active growth (87,88). Volatile chemical by-products can be sampled with a portable air sampler (Anasorb 747 carbon tube). Samples should be obtained in areas of concern and near ventilation intakes outdoors with control samples. GC-MS with selected ion detector is used to analyze for volatile chemicals.

When sampling for airborne mycotoxins, a microporous filter should be the collection medium or, if sampling for mycotoxins in dust, a coarser filter may be used. After sampling, the mycotoxins are extracted from the filter and the extract is tested for cytotoxicity to certain cellular preparations (87,88). This reveals the presence or absence of mycotoxins but does not provide a quantitative measurement.

Endotoxin sampling is similar to mycotoxin sampling in the collection stage. Endotoxin is extracted from microporous filters or dust filters and may be analyzed in two ways: The extract may be analyzed for lipopolysaccharide content using GC-MS, or the extract may be analyzed using an LAL assay. Either approach may provide a quantitative measurement of endotoxin concentration (87,88).

Detection of dust mites may be accomplished by using two methods, microscopy and feces detection. A microscope with tenfold magnification should be used to identify mites, and samples for viewing should be collected from bedding and carpets. Detection of dust mite feces may also give an indication of the concentration of the population. This is performed by collecting dust and mixing with reagents that change color according to the amount of feces in the sample (87,88).

Spore traps can provide a continuous recording of spores that collect onto a greased tape that can run for days. This allows recording of four sizes and the analyses of spores, looking for fluctuations in concentrations and the nature of spores throughout a time course. Identification of fungal, bacterial, and spore species is critical to assessing health risks.

CULTURE MEDIA

Biological air sampling requires nutrient media, such as potato dextrose agars and blood protein agars. Potato dextrose agars are used to quantify airborne fungi, and blood protein agars are used to quantify airborne bacteria. The agars are used in conjunction with a high-flow air-sampling pump and a single-stage viable impactor. Air samples for each agar are collected over a 5-minute period.

The selection of culture medium is critical because different microbes may grow poorly or not at all in standard culture media and under certain conditions. Also, living organisms can be damaged by the collection technique and not grow. Air sampling for culture usually underestimates the true bioaerosol concentration (92). For comparison, air sampling should be conducted outdoors in close proximity to the fresh air intakes to service controls. Indoor air samples should be collected simultaneously near suspected sources of contamination before and after agitation of sources. Source agitation can produce a 1,000-fold increase in the indoor air bioaerosol concentrations.

Gravity or settling Petri dishes in culture media underestimate or may even fail to detect biological contaminants that can remain in the air for lengthy periods of time. Culture plate impactors used for bacterial sampling use general media, such as nutrient agar or casein soy peptone agar. Specialized media are sometimes used. Pathogenic bacteria grow best around 95°F (35°C). Thermophilic organisms grow best at 122°F (50°C) or higher, and most other common organisms grow between 25° and 30°C (77° and 86°F).

Legionella pneumophila may not be detected in air samples and, therefore, sampling from contaminated sources such as water is important to detect this organism.

Sampling of fungi is performed by plating air samples, bulk samples, or liquid samples onto appropriate culture media, such as potato dextrose, Sabouraud's dextrose, or malt extract agar. Malt extract agar has advantages because bacteria do not grow well on it, and it is also a medium that grows *Aspergillus* species. *Aspergillus fumigatus* generally grows at 45°C in incubation; otherwise, all other cultures for fungi are incubated at room temperature.

High-volume filtration sampling devices can be used to evaluate airborne antigens and mycotoxins. Volumetric sampling with sieve or slit impactors can be used over an interval of time in areas of suspected high fungal spore concentrations.

Air sampling is limited to detection of living microbial organisms, but nonliving particles can also produce illness and can be assayed. Nonliving biologicals, however, do not grow on culture media. Spore traps can be used to determine spore samples. Microscopy can assist in identifying particulates of biologicals. High-volume air samplers are required to collect enough airborne mycotoxins for detection by the analytical assay. Mycotoxin assay is by GC-MS.

Fungal spore counts are obtained by drawing air into a sampler and impacting them onto a moving sticky surface (Burkhard sport trap). The spores can be examined microscopically. Microporous filters are also used to sample spores. Spores are eluted from the filters and counted microscopically.

Guidelines for antigen environmental loads have only been established for dust mites. The detection of mycotoxins may only be achieved in a culture medium. In some instances, however, mycotoxin can be collected from dust. Antigen concentrations can be measured with radioimmunoassay or enzyme-linked immunoassays.

Interpreting Results of Microbiological Sampling

Microbiological sampling results can be difficult to interpret. Analytic methods are not consistent across laboratories, and an accreditation program for laboratories that perform bioaerosol analysis does not exist. The ACGIH and the American Industrial Hygiene Association have published reference manuals for biological sampling (87,88).

No TLVs exist for bacterial or fungal bioaerosol concentrations in interpreting indoor sampling results. However, guidelines do exist. Concentrations of total culturable bacteria outdoors are typically 100 to 1,000 CFU per m^3; however, these numbers can vary quite dramatically in different geographic regions (93). Data for viruses, as measured in plaque-forming units, are similarly variable. Proactive monitoring is discouraged because of the difficulty of data interpretation.

In general, assaying environments for biological contamination should combine air sampling, bulk sampling, and inspection to characterize the extent of contamination and make decisions regarding health hazards. Decisions to measure for chemical byproducts are individualized on a case-by-case basis.

Indoor concentrations of less than 100 CFU per m^3 are usually not a concern, whereas those more than 1,000 CFU per m^3 deserve further attention. Concentrations between 100 and 1,000 CFU per m^3 are subject to interpretation on a case-by-case basis. The presence of any single type of fungus in levels exceeding 500 CFU per m^3 indicates a potential contaminating source.

Some investigators recommend that indoor levels of nontoxic and nonpathogenic microorganisms should be less than or equal to 300 CFU per m^3. Also, no microorganism should contribute individually to more than 50 CFU per m^3 of the total, with the exception of *Cladosporium*. Levels of fungi greater than 300 CFU per m^3 require further investigation for potential inadequate air filtration, excess humidity, and potential contaminant sources. Fungi of levels 300 to 500 CFU per m^3 appear to be normal and do not represent a health effects threshold, but rather a threshold for further investigation (94). These investigators state that indoor to outdoor ratios involving fungal CFUs per m^3 are not acceptable for evaluating indoor bioaerosol concentrations. Rather, sampling should identify individual microorganism components and compare indoor to outdoor ratios. These conclusions are based on evaluation of more than 900 indoor samples that show fungal and bacterial bioaerosol concentrations ranging from 0 to 6,077 CFU per m^3, with an average of 157 CFU per m^3. Eighty-seven percent of the measurements were less than 300 CFU per m^3 and only 6% were greater than 500 CFU per m^3 (94). Thirty-seven genera of fungi were identified in these samples.

Frequently occurring fungi in this study were *Cladosporium*, yeast, hyphae, *Penicillium*, *Aspergillus*, *Alternaria*, and *Curvularia*. One hundred eighty-two outdoor samples had fungal and bacterial bioaerosols in concentrations ranging from 0 to 12,668 CFU per m^3, with an average of 860 CFU per m^3. One-third of these samples were less than 300 CFU per m^3 and 51% were more than 500 CFU per m^3. Thirty-three genera of fungi were identified in the outdoor samples (Tables 53-17 and 53-18). This study showed that the average fungal concentration of 157 CFU per m^3 indoors is more than five times less than the average outdoor concentration of 860 CFU per m^3.

The ACGIH recognizes an indoor to outdoor fungi ratio of 33%. This ratio has been questioned because outdoor bioaerosol concentrations vary considerably (94). Therefore, using the 33% indoor to outdoor ratio results in a recommended indoor concentration of bioaerosols that may be too liberal as an accepted concentration limit (94). Indoor and outdoor populations of bioaerosols should be similar, with indoor concentrations lower than outdoor concentrations for individual microorganisms. Thus, concentrations less than or equal to 200 CFU per m^3 may be considered typical for indoor bioaerosol concentrations.

Other studies have reported that airborne concentrations of indoor fungi exceeding 500 CFU per m^3 are abnormal and should be investigated (95). A problem exists, however, when trying to determine whether the indoor source is coming from the outdoors as opposed to an indoor contamination source. Indoor sources are most likely when a significant difference exists between indoor and outdoor bioaerosol concentrations.

Techniques used to control biologicals include isolation systems, high-efficiency particulate air (HEPA) filtration, ultraviolet lights, carbon adsorption, electrostatic precipitation, negative air ionization, and heating and dehydration. Future technologies

TABLE 53-17. Frequency of occurrence and average colony-forming units per cubic meter of indoor fungi

Observed	Frequency (%)	Average (colony-forming units per cubic meter)
Total	100	157
Cladosporium	77	92
Yeast	56	52
Sterile hyphae	56	29
Bacteria	52	28
Penicillium	50	48
Aspergillus	33	20
Alternaria	17	30
Curvularia	7	20
Acremonium	30	8
Epicoccum	3	8
Geotrichum	3	18
Phoma	2	7
Fusarium	2	16
Paecilomyces	2	9
Dendryphiella	2	5
Drechslera	2	13
Absidia	2	1
Chaetomium	2	6
Nigrospora	2	10
Actinomycetes	1	3
Monocillium	1	17
Cunninghamella	1	11
Monilia	1	5
Rhizopus	1	5
Trichoderma	1	10
Gilmaniella	1	3
Hansfordia	1	3
Hyalodendron	1	3
Mucor	1	8
Stemphylium	1	5
Botrytis	1	2
Pleospora	1	4
Humicola	1	23
Pithomyces	1	10
Unidentified	1	6
Stachybotrys	1	3
Ulocladium	1	4
Basipetospora	<1	2
Gliocladium	<1	5
Oidiodendron	<1	2
Aureobasidium	<1	8

Adapted from ref. 94, with permission.

TABLE 53-18. Frequency of occurrence and average colony-forming units per cubic meter of outdoor fungi

Observed	Frequency (%)	Average (colony-forming units per cubic meter)
Total	100	860
Cladosporium	85	570
Sterile hyphae	76	87
Yeast	58	126
Penicillium	52	120
Bacteria	46	58
Alternaria	38	58
Aspergillus	27	277
Geotrichum	20	91
Curvularia	12	71
Fusarium	12	74
Epicoccum	8	17
Drechslera	6	62
Acremonium	6	43
Phoma	5	31
Trichoderma	2	35
Cunninghamella	2	21
Paecilomyces	2	22
Pleospora	2	35
Basipetospora	2	15
Nigrospora	2	22
Monilia	1	89
Monocillium	1	56
Ulocladium	1	10
Botrytis	1	22
Phoma	1	24
Pithomyces	1	3
Rhizomucor	1	9
Rhizopus	1	7
Mucor	1	14
Humicola	1	14
Stachybotrys	1	7
Actinomycetes	1	106
Absidia	1	36
Aureobasidium	1	12
Chrysosporium	1	36
Gonatobotrys	1	24
Gliocladium	1	35

Adapted from ref. 94, with permission.

include passive solar exposure, photocatalytic oxidation, ultrasonic atomization, air ozonization, ultraviolet lasers, agglomerators, and virus detection systems.

VIRUSES

Assaying for the presence of viruses requires specialized culture media. Viral culture media are generally tissue cultures. If collection is delayed beyond an hour, the samples should be refrigerated.

VENTILATION AND INDOOR ENVIRONMENTAL QUALITY

The ventilation system or air-handling unit of an office or home is frequently referred to as the *HVAC* system. The HVAC consists of the mechanical and functional components of duct work, air filter, air conditioning, and heating unit. The primary functions of the HVAC are to maintain indoor air pollutants at a minimum, control odors, maintain oxygen and carbon dioxide levels at acceptable concentrations, provide humidifying, cooling and heating, and maintain overall comfort. Although ventilation systems for homes and offices share common features, an additional function for commercial sites is to maintain a balance of positive air pressure in work areas. This positive pressure forces air to circulate to prevent the build up of pollutants.

HVAC systems in commercial office buildings and some homes are installed to service zones. As the number and size of zones increase indoors, so does the cost of ventilation. A zone is typically defined by the presence of a thermostat. Zones also allow for individual control of the HVAC and, therefore, the comfort level of that zone.

The HVAC is frequently cited as a cause of indoor air quality problems. The National Institute for Occupational Safety and Health (NIOSH) categorized the following major causes of ventilation-related health problems in studies of more than 1,300 cases of poor indoor air quality (20):

- 50% of cases related to deficiencies in ventilation, lack of outside fresh air, poor air distribution, uncomfortable temperature, or uncomfortable humidity.
- 30% of cases related to indoor chemical or biological contaminants.
- 10% of cases were attributed to an outdoor pollutant introduced to the indoors.

NIOSH also discovered patterns in these cases:

- Forced ventilation was common in sites with health problems.
- Health complaints increased as people density indoors rose.
- Problem buildings were energy efficient, thus creating a tight envelope.
- Workers perceived little or no control over their environment.

Understanding HVAC functioning is critical to indoor air quality evaluations:

Outside air is supplied to the interior of the building via ventilation ducts.

Contaminated or used air is removed from the building interior through air return ducts, or a plenum, located in the ceiling or wall, to a central return duct.

A portion of stale air is then exhausted outside and an equal portion of fresh outdoor air is introduced through the air handler, mixing with and diluting any pollutants in the stale air.

The mixed air then passes through an air filter.

The air is then conditioned by heating or cooling through a cooling coil or heat exchanger.

The introduction of fresh air is balanced with the exit of stale air.

HVAC systems have an outside air intake on the top or side of a building that brings outdoor air inside. The outdoor air is then mixed with recirculated air from the occupied area. The mixed air usually passes through a filter to remove gross contaminants. This filtered air then passes through a fan that creates a positive pressure to force the air through coils that either cool or heat. A drain pan beneath the coils collects water that condenses on the cooling coil. Air leaving the coil may be humidified or dehumidified, depending on the circumstances. This conditioned air then moves through a ventilation duct at a speed of 10 to 20 mph to a distribution box. The supplied air then travels from the distribution box through small ducts to terminal ducts and diffusers and into the rooms. The supplied air migrates throughout the room and eventually enters an air return vent, also called a *plenum*, where it is recirculated or exhausted outdoors (20).

HVACs can be broadly divided into *constant air volume system* or *variable air volume system*. Constant air volume HVAC systems vary air temperature for comfort control, and, depending on the sophistication of the HVAC system, a single constant supply system can provide ventilation and comfort control in multiple zones. Thermostats allow for more individual control of comfort, but generally cause increased energy use.

Variable air volume HVACs control the amount of air delivered to the interior work space to maintain temperature. If temperatures are too high inside, the system delivers a higher volume of cooler air. Thus, airflow varies with the temperature. A variable volume HVAC is more energy efficient but may not always deliver enough outside fresh air. Sophisticated HVAC systems in modern office buildings may have combinations of multiple zones, variable air volumes, and complex duct work (20).

Ventilation processes can also be divided into *active* or *passive*. Homes frequently have active air exhaust features and passive air supply. Commercial building ventilation systems usually involve active exhaust and active air supply.

Inadequately functioning HVAC systems allow indoor contaminants to accumulate, contributing to stale and stagnant air, and may even introduce outdoor pollutants and allergens into the indoors, especially if the air is unfiltered. A frequently occurring problem is an imbalance in the flow of fresh air versus outflow of stale air. This can create *dead zones* of no air circulation indoors. These dead zones are essentially stale air that escapes being recirculated.

HVACs can be sources of moisture, allowing mold and other microorganisms to amplify and be circulated indoors. Over time, dust, dirt, and debris build up in the ventilation system. Proper maintenance can help prevent accumulated dirt and dust from being circulated indoors.

Indoor Air Quality Guidelines for Ventilation

ASHRAE has promulgated four standards dealing with the indoor environment:

- ASHRAE 62-1999: Ventilation for acceptable air quality with proposed 62.1P and 62.2P.
- ASHRAE 62-1989: Ventilation for acceptable air quality
- ASHRAE 52-1992: Thermal environmental conditions for human occupancy
- ASHRAE 52-1992: Air filtration

The ASHRAE standard (62-1999) on ventilation has as its objective to provide clean, fresh air in which contaminants do not exceed the limits set by the National Primary Ambient Air Quality Standard for outdoor air. This includes pollutants, such as sulfur dioxide, nitrogen dioxide, ozone, carbon dioxide, total particulates, lead, chlordane, and radon.

Whereas the ASHRAE standard is a practical guide oriented to providing comfort and air quality, it does not address air pollutant sources. If ASHRAE ventilation standards are met, however, and sources of pollutants controlled or eliminated, indoor contaminants are minimized to a level of comfort for the majority of people.

Ventilation systems have traditionally been designed to provide odor control and thermal comfort under the assumption that the air in a building is perfectly mixed. Increasing experience demonstrates that nonuniform mixing is common and that the task of predicting pollution transport produced by the ventilation systems is not simple. In the United States, building ventilation adequacy is measured and compared with ASHRAE guidelines.

To date, the home environment has escaped guidelines and regulations for indoor air quality, but is under consideration in 62.1P and 62.2P. Agencies in the United States and in other countries, however, are examining guidelines for residential indoor air quality.

ASHRAE standard 55-1992 provides the specific conditions in which 80% to 90% of indoor occupants should find the environment thermally comfortable. It does not address air quality or ventilation. The standard combines the variables of humidity, temperature, clothing, activity and movement, and radiant heat sources to achieve an 80% satisfaction rate among all indoor occupants and a 90% satisfaction rate for any one variable. ASHRAE standard 62-1989 actually addresses the relative humidity indoors, calling for a range of 30% to 60% (20).

ASHRAE standard 52-1992, Methods of Testing Air Cleaning Devices Used in General Ventilation for Removing Particulate Matter, establishes important factors in selecting air filters and filter rating procedures (20).

VENTILATION ADEQUACY

A major function of the ventilation system is maintaining fresh clean air to match the comfort needs of the number of people in a particular indoor environment. The concentration of CO_2 measured in parts per million in indoor air is used as a general measure of air freshness and adequacy of outdoor air delivery. It is a common measurement obtained by environmental consultants to test the adequacy of ventilation.

Outdoor CO_2 concentrations are always lower than those indoors. CO_2 build up in the interior of a home or office is dependent on the number of people in the site and the ability of the ventilation to replace stale air with fresh air. If the number of occupants in an indoor environment remains constant, then measuring CO_2 can assist in determining the quantity of outdoor air being delivered. Continuously monitoring CO_2 concentrations over days or weeks can generate confidence in the result because ventilation needs fluctuate with population demands. An electronic device is used to monitor CO_2 continuously in parts per million. Taking spot checks of the CO_2 may not be representative of the ventilation adequacy because CO_2 concentrations fluctuate and tend to be low in the morning hours and rise in the afternoon (Fig. 53-10). CO_2 can rise during the mid-morning if the space is operating with minimal airflow. As the interior of the building is cooled further, the CO_2 concentrations may fall by the afternoon. Reviewing CO_2 concentrations over a period of time can provide a better determination of the ventilation system performance. If the ventilation system is working adequately, then the CO_2 concentration inside in the early morning is close to the outdoor CO_2 value

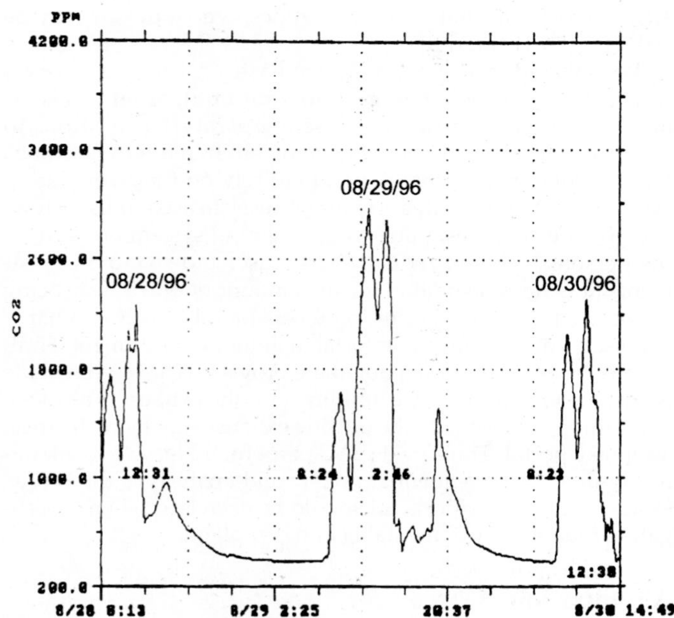

Figure 53-10. Carbon dioxide fluctuations indoors. Note the high levels, indicating inadequate ventilation.

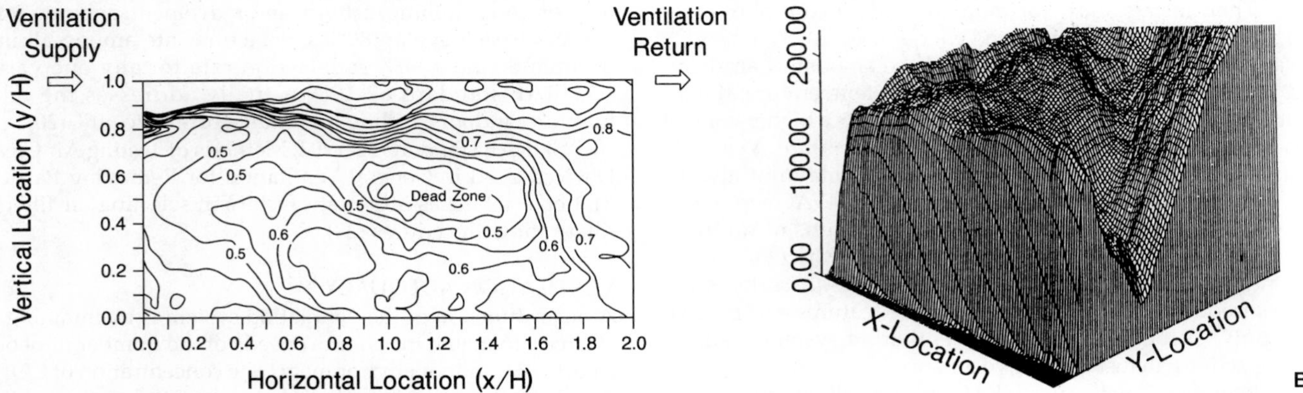

Figure 53-11. A: Two-dimensional mapping of the results of simulated airflow monitoring, identifying areas of no air movement. **B:** Three-dimensional model showing dead space areas representing little or no effective air movement as areas of depression. (Reprinted from Anderson R. Determination of ventilation efficiency based upon short-term tests. Golden, CO: US Department of Energy, National Renewable Energy Laboratory, 1988, with permission.)

at that time. If the CO_2 value is greater than the outdoor CO_2 value, then the ventilation may not be providing adequate fresh air.

CO_2 concentrations more than 800 ppm can be associated with health complaints. In many cases, people complain of headache, fatigue, and airway irritation when CO_2 levels exceed 800 ppm, signifying the buildup of pollutants. However, OSHA does not consider the CO_2 concentration indoors to be in violation of its regulatory control until levels rise more than 5,000 ppm. Such dichotomy between OSHA regulations and reality contribute to frequent conflict in some cases of poor indoor air quality.

One-half of NIOSH's indoor air quality health complaint investigations were related to inadequate ventilation. Although ventilation systems are designed primarily to provide control over thermal comfort, it has been assumed that airflow is evenly mixed by the ventilation system. This assumption, however, is not always true. Uniform distribution of fresh air via the ventilation systems for maximum dilution of indoor pollutants is not always a reality, and microenvironments of ventilation and distribution mismatches can occur. These mismatches can result in areas of poor air quality or dead zones, where the air may be stale (Fig. 53-11A and B).

With the advent of a strong emphasis on energy conservation, there has been a tendency to limit outdoor air intake as much as possible during adverse temperature conditions to avoid having to heat or cool incoming air. In modern buildings of tight construction that depend entirely on their ventilation system for outside air, this is relatively easy to accomplish. However, the persons designing the ventilating system are seldom the persons trying to reduce energy use, and so, after adjustments, it is not uncommon for the amount of outside air being introduced into the system to be considerably below what is necessary to maintain a comfortable indoor environment. Similar problems can occur if inadequate provisions have been made for exhausting air from the building or if the exhaust is blocked. In addition, occasionally the outside exhaust vent faces the fresh air intake portal. Thus, the HVAC perpetually recycles contaminated air. Careful sequential review and analysis of the HVAC system is always critical and should be exercised when investigating indoor environmental health complaints.

Air Filtration

Air filtration adds to the ability of the HVAC to prevent contaminants from entering indoor air. Depending on the type of air filter, the device may be more or less efficient in removing contaminants. The best filtration system is integrated with the ventilation system during building design. Retrofitting air filters to an older ventilation, however, can be easily achieved.

Most air filtration systems are designed to remove particulates, such as mold, pollens, spores, general allergens, dusts, and fibers. Some may remove chemicals and odors. Air filtration products range from single disposal filters to permanently installed air filtration systems. Filter efficiency is rated by its ability to retain particulates and dusts. The higher the efficiency rating, the more effective the filter is in retaining smaller and smaller particles that can penetrate deeply into the airways. Adequate air filtration helps to maintain a healthy environment by doing the following:

1. Preventing the entry of dust, particulates, and allergens into the indoors.
2. Preventing the accumulation of dirt and debris in the heating and cooling units, which would reduce performance and efficiency.
3. Preventing dust and dirt to accumulate in the ventilation ductwork, which can serve as a nutrient source for microbial growth.
4. Preventing entry of corrosion-producing pollutants, such as dust particles containing acid and alkaline chemicals.
5. Preventing entry of chemicals and odors from the outside.

Modern HVAC systems usually use two filters: a coarse filter that first removes large particles, followed by a finer filter to trap smaller dust.

Air filters come in a wide variety of designs and efficiencies with numerous suppliers. The type of filter should be based on a review of needs, filter efficiency, function, design and ease of installation, and maintenance. Filters vary from coarse to fine and inefficient to efficient. Coarse filters trap larger particles and are generally used as prefilters. Fine filters remove visible dust and irritant particulates. ASHRAE Standard 52 has two filter rating procedures:

1. *Dust spot efficiency test*: Used with filters that stop small particles.
2. *Arrestance test*: Used with filters that stop larger, coarse particles.

A filter with a high arrestance rating may be inefficient and ineffective in stopping small dust particles. The three performance characteristics applied to any filter are (a) filter efficiency in removing particles from the airflow, (b) airflow resistance caused by the filter, and (c) time interval between cleaning and filter replacement.

Dust and particulate filters: These are usually disposable fiberglass filters and are not efficient at trapping small particulate matter. They do not remove chemical vapors or odors unless combined with a carbon-impregnated medium. Particulate filters vary with respect to the size of the particulates trapped, ranging from coarse filtration to fine particulate filtration. The least effective consists of a coarse prefilter placed at the air intake of the air-conditioning unit. This type of filter stops only the largest of dusts and particulates. Fine particles and dust that are in the respirable range are not stopped by this type of filter. A fine particulate filter is recognized by its pleated construction, providing more surface area to entrap fine particles.

Media filters: These filters are made of paper or fabric stretched over a frame and arranged in a pleated fashion to enlarge the surface area of contact. Check for filter efficiency, because some of these filters can be porous and inefficient. Media filters may be carbon impregnated to absorb gases and vapors of chemicals. Some filter products contain antimicrobial treatment to prevent microbial growth on the filter itself. Activated charcoal has been used for many years to adsorb chemicals. Carbon filters basically contain a medium impregnated with activated charcoal, which provides a massive surface area to adsorb gases, odors, and chemical vapors. Carbon can adsorb many different chemicals, but adsorbs larger molecules best.

Electronic air filters: Three types exist:

1. *Self-charging filters*: These are made out of plastic fibers that create static electricity by airflow passing through the filter medium. The static electric charge attracts dusts and particulate matter, trapping them in the filter. Static electricity generated by air movement through such a filter medium does not generate ozone. These types of filters generally trap only coarser particles, and efficiency declines rapidly as airflow increases or humidity increases.
2. *Electrostatic precipitators*: These filters operate in two stages: (a) Dust and particulates pass through a prefilter and then a charged electrical field, which applies a negative or positive charge to the particle. (b) The second stage involves a precipitating or collection section of the filter, consisting of negatively charged or positively charged areas that attract and deposit the charged particles. The efficiency of these types of filters varies, and they produce ozone, an irritant. Some electrostatic filters are combined with other media, such as charcoal or a coarse particle filter, improving their function.
3. *Charged medial filters*: Made from a dielectric material, such as fiberglass or cellulose, stretched across a frame. A direct current voltage is applied to the dielectric, creating an electrostatic field. This type of filter is not efficient because the electric current is not strong enough to place a charge on most particles to entrap them.

HEPA: HEPA filtration was a technology developed by the Atomic Energy Commission to remove radioactive particles from the air in manufacturing plants. By definition, HEPA filtration must remove at least 99.7% of all airborne particles of 0.3 μm in diameter (one-three-hundredth the diameter of a human hair). Air filters of 85% efficiency filter out most irritants affecting health. Higher-efficiency filters require more energy use and higher costs, but the reduction of health problems compensates for this.

Negative ion generator: This type of system is not a true air filter. It generates negative ions in the indoor air that attach to particulates and dust suspended in air, causing them to take on a negative electrical charge. The charged particles then attach to surfaces in the indoor environment, such as walls and furniture, thus being eliminated from the air but not from the indoor environment. It should not be used as a substitute for proper air filtration because dusts and particulates are not removed from the indoors.

Air purifiers and negative ion generators are portable units designed to clean and purify air in a room of a home or office. Both can be helpful in reducing the pollutant load in a room. Air purifiers recycle air; they do not provide fresh air. Portable air purifiers that come in self-contained units for use in individual rooms of a home or office are available, and their specifications should be reviewed to insure the unit suits the individual's needs.

Ion generators have shown conflicting results on preventing symptoms of asthmatics and those with SBS. Neither air purifiers nor ion generators are substitutes for proper air filtration and adequate fresh air.

Heating, Ventilation, and Air-Conditioning Contamination by Microorganisms

Microorganisms, such as bacteria and fungi, are common in outdoor and indoor environments, and their presence in low levels in a ventilation system is considered normal. Problems occur, however, when they amplify to high levels that can then be transported indoors as a bioaerosol. Fungus and bacteria require nutrients to amplify, and dirt and moisture are such nutrient sources. Growth sites for biologicals include the following HVAC areas:

- Air filters
- Humidifiers
- Cooling coils
- Condensation pans
- Moisture and debris in ventilation ducts

The presence of active microbial organism growth in the ventilation system is a potential health problem. The presence of microorganism overgrowth should be suspected if one or more of the following is noted: (a) musty or foul odors are present, (b) a discoloration of surface areas—green, black, white, or pink, (c) a presence of moisture that is slimy or cloudy, or (d) moisture damage to carpet or walls associated with odors.

Elimination of microbial contamination growth involves (a) removal of dust and debris and moisture, (b) correcting the cause of contamination, (c) preventing the spread of microorganisms from the contaminated area, and (d) treating the contaminated area with an appropriate chemical biocide, if necessary.

Air sampling for microorganisms can verify an airborne contaminant problem that may affect health. Sampling and interpretation of results, however, should be performed by qualified experts.

The use of chemical biocides to kill contaminating microorganisms should be undertaken by qualified experts. Biocides are toxic and are controlled by the Federal Insecticide, Fungicide, and Rodenticide Act. Six classes of biocides exist, and four are allowed for use in HVAC systems:

1. Sterilants that kill 100% of all forms of microbes.
2. Disinfectants that eliminate 99.999% of infectious, pathogenic bacteria.
3. Sanitizers that reduce, but not necessarily eliminate, 99.9% of microbes.
4. Fungicides intended to inhibit growth of or kill fungus pathogenic to humans or animals.

The surface to be treated must be cleaned, then thoroughly washed with the biocidal agent. The surface should not be allowed to remain moist for more than 24 hours; otherwise, regrowth might occur. The EPA recommends that porous material, such as fiberglass insulation, that can serve as an amplifier source for microbe growth be first contained, then removed. Sanitizing such materials is virtually impossible.

Biocidal agents should only be applied by experts in a manner to minimize human exposure. These agents kill fungi and other microorganisms, and their proper use and efficacy require expert judgment. The manufacturer's instructions must be followed to avoid future problems.

Heating, Ventilation, and Air-Conditioning Codes and Professional Standards

Air concentrations of chemicals that result in SBS are usually two to three orders of magnitude less than PELs set by OSHA for a work site. OSHA PELs are based on air levels considered to be healthy for an industrial work environment and refer to airborne concentrations of substances to which employees can be exposed on a daily basis, without adverse health effects. OSHA does recognize that some workers may be more susceptible or hypersusceptible to much lower levels of chemicals than their standards. OSHA's PEL concept, however, is the only legally enforceable standard. Too many times an indoor environment has been judged to be clean based on such regulatory standards, yet the occupants continue to experience health problems.

In 1995, OSHA proposed the following regulations for indoor air quality for nonindustrial work sites, but these proposals have not yet been adapted (1). Specific guidelines that can help achieve high indoor air quality derived from OSHA's proposed standards are

- Keep CO_2 levels less than 800 ppm (25 to 30 cubic feet per minute of outside air).
- Keep relative humidity less than 60%.
- Obtain and maintain records on HVAC systems.
- Inspect, maintain, and operate HVAC systems in accordance with building codes in force at the time the building was constructed.
- Exhaust smoking areas to outdoors, and keep area under negative pressure.
- Provide local exhaust for specific pollutant emitters.

The growth of nonregulatory standards by professional organizations has helped to ensure better quality of air in home and work environments through HVAC design, construction, cleaning, maintenance, and quality of air delivered. Each of these organizations is dedicated to providing standards in its particular field to ensure a comfortable and healthy environment:

- *ASHRAE*: Ventilation standards for acceptable indoor air quality, ASHRAE standard 62-1999.
- *National Air Duct Cleaners Association*: Standard 1992-01 relates to standardized mechanical cleaning of nonporous air conveyance systems.
- *National Air Filtration Association*: Provides guides and technical assistance for proper air filtration.
- *North American Insulation Manufacturers Association*: Represents manufacturers of flexible duct liners and duckboard. The organization has produced guidelines for proper fabrication, installation, and maintenance of their members' products. The organization also provides fibrous glass duct construction standards.
- *Sheet Metal and Air Conditioning Contractor's National Association*: Has developed standards and guides governing the fabrication and installation of HVAC systems, HVAC Duct Construction Standard.
- *National Fire Protection Association*: Standard 90-A details construction materials, insulating materials, coatings, and other materials that may be used in construction and design of ventilation systems for fire safety.

Problems within the Heating, Ventilation, and Air-Conditioning System

HVAC systems are complex and have many mechanical parts with extensive branching duct work. Most HVAC problems can be categorized as mechanical, functional, or contamination.

- *Mechanical*: Examples are problems with fans, air handler units, air filters, or leaks around ventilation ducts.
- *Functional*: Examples are an imbalance of air, differences of air pressures within a building, insufficient fresh air, and exhaust air reentrainment, which causes odors.
- *Contamination*: Examples include dust, debris, mold, bacteria, or outside source brought indoors.

HVAC problems generally require the assistance of professionals, especially in large buildings. Ventilation specialists can use tracers or nontoxic smoke to evaluate airflow problems. A commonly used tracer is sulfur hexafluoride, which is chemically inert. Flow rates and air balances can be measured along with CO_2 concentrations to check for inadequate fresh air. Problems may arise in the following areas of the HVAC system, underscoring its complexity.

Outside air intake: A supply of outdoor air is drawn into an air intake vent and delivered to the air handler unit in the HVAC system either passively or actively to match the amount of stale air exhausted. The intake may be adjustable, so the amount of outside air admitted can be varied. The outdoor air supply delivered to the air handler unit of the HVAC system is presumed to be fresh and free of outdoor contaminants. This is not always the case. Outdoor air can be polluted by chemicals, pollens, automobile exhaust, and odors. Remember that the same chemicals outdoors can concentrate indoors.

The location of the intake vent is important to assuring fresh, clean air. Outdoor contaminants can be drawn indoors either by the air handler or through leakage in the ventilation system. The fresh air intake source should be away from any potential source of contaminants and pollutants, such as parked automobiles or trucks emitting vehicle exhaust near loading docks, exhaust from other combustible sources such as furnaces, or kitchens, or a congested urban area, street, or highway, or any other source of contamination and pollution.

Air supply ducts and distribution ducts: Ventilation ducts move outside air through the air handler and into the indoor space. Ventilation ducts can become contaminated by dust, moisture, microorganisms, and debris, which can be circulated into indoor air. Air leakage and imbalanced air pressure can occur. Normally occupied spaces in a building are under a slight positive pressure relative to return exhaust vents. This pressure differential allows air to move in the direction of the exhaust. Because the exhaust is under negative pressure relative to occupied spaces, any leaks around the return vents also draw air in from outside. If an occupied space does not maintain a positive air pressure relative to outdoors, then leaks can occur around doors and other potential leakage sites. Also, imbalance can result in areas of dead zones indoors, where stale air accumulates along with pollutants.

Air is distributed from the air-handling unit to the occupied indoor areas by multiple branching ventilation ducts. As the number of ducts increases, the rate of airflow in each decreases. The air enters through diffusers, which prevents the occupied areas from feeling drafty while mixing the air. The amount of air passing through a duct can be controlled by dampers, usually set to respond to a thermostat. Unless the system is set to deliver at least a minimum of air, some individual areas may get no air exchange during times when the thermostat does not call for temperature modification. Air blowing from the end of a duct can travel as a stream from an appreciable distance without mixing uniformly in a room, creating dead zones that allow contaminants to build up in the environment.

Fans: HVAC fans create air pressure that moves air through the ventilation system. The main fans are usually located just after the air filters. Other fans may be located near exhaust vents. Fans are selected to deliver a quantity of air to meet ventilation requirements. The amount of air in cubic feet per meter and air pressure is a function of fan speed. Mechanical or electrical problems with a fan can affect air pressure and airflow throughout the HVAC system and, therefore, through the indoor environment. Fans can also become contaminated with dust or biologicals. Fans can move large quantities of air but can only work against a small pressure gradient. Obstructions in the ventilating system can reduce airflow even if the fan is working properly.

Air handler: This should be inspected to insure that it is clean and free of dust, moisture, and debris. Moisture problems can be caused by water leaks into the air handler through gaps or spaces in sheet metal joints. Also, condensation of water vapor in the intake system can occur when it operates during cooler hours with relative humidity high. The cooling coil should also be inspected for water condensation and dirt and debris. Any water condensation can result in the growth of microorganisms. Inspection of the filters, the cooling coil, and the pan for moisture can help eliminate many problems with aeroallergens from mold growth and bacteria in this area.

The room housing the HVAC system's air handler is usually under negative pressure relative to the unit itself. Contaminants can be drawn into the system from this point. It is important to note if the air handler unit is located near any source of contamination or pollution. In commercial buildings, the intake areas and handlers may be near traffic or a loading dock area, which are sources of vehicle exhaust and odors.

Air filters: Air filters should be inspected and either replaced or maintained according to manufacturers' recommendations. Gaps around the filters allow contaminated air to bypass. Filters should be inspected to determine if they need replacement and whether the filter fits tightly within its housing. Dirt, debris, or moisture on a filter is a source of nutrients for amplification of microorganisms.

Cooling and dehumidifying coils: Air is passed over cooling coils. If the air temperature is cooled below the dew point, water condenses on the coils. If the water is not adequately drained and the coils are not kept clean, mold and other microorganisms can grow, becoming a source of contamination.

Heating devices: These depend on combustion, and the products of combustion should be vented to the outside. This may not be the case, and dangerous carbon monoxide can build up indoors. Other sources of heat might be electric heating coils, a furnace, a heat pump, or even the cooling coils of a dehumidifier. Heated surfaces remain dry and should only cause problems if they collect dust or if they leak. In some new buildings, heat is primarily supplied around the outer walls to balance heat loss. The remainder of the building receives heat from the occupants, office machines, and lights, which generate heat as a byproduct. In these situations, the main ventilation system is primarily called on for cooling.

Humidifier and evaporative cooler: In cold climates, heating outside air to comfortable temperatures reduces its relative humidity. Moisture is usually added to this dry air by spraying water into the airflow or passing the air over sources of moisture. Evaporative coolers pass warm, dry air through moist mats. As the water evaporates, it cools and humidifies the air. Moist surfaces support growth of biologicals and require maintenance and cleaning.

Air return: Rooms have a grillwork that allows air to move into return air ducts or plenums. These return vents may be located on the ceiling or near the floor. Even if a fan is present to aid this movement, measurable airflow in the room exists only close to the vent. It is quite common to use the space above a ceiling as the return air plenum. These grills should be inspected for dirt and dust, which could indicate buildup inside air vents.

Outside exhaust: In older buildings, sufficient air usually leaks out through cracks to make a general exhaust to the outside unnecessary. In newer buildings, exhausts are necessary. In addition to an exhaust on the main system, some local exhaust systems exist, which take air from a problem area (i.e., a restroom or a particular machine) and exhaust it to the outside. Most building codes require the restrooms and kitchens to have such exhaust ventilation.

Recirculation and air mixing: Because heating or cooling a building takes energy, and because draft-free temperature control requires that air entering offices be only a slightly different temperature than room air, it is the usual practice to circulate greater volumes of air than those needing to be drawn from the outside. Thus, ducts exist that allow much of the air returning from indoor areas to mix with outside air, pass through the filters, and return back into the indoors. A common ventilation in new buildings is the roof-mounted integrated unit that contains the intake, exhaust, and recirculating vents and controls. It is not uncommon that adequate makeup air has been neglected, particularly in manufacturing settings. Another common practice to save energy is to run the ventilating system only when the building is in use and for a limited period before and after hours. This may be automatically or manually controlled. This practice allows pollutants to build up, particularly over weekends.

Cooling towers: Cooling towers are used in commercial buildings to provide cool air. Warm water used in cooling towers favors the growth of biologicals, such as *Legionella pneumophila*, which is responsible for legionnaires' disease. Frequently, biocidal material is used to inhibit and control microbial growth. The proper cleaning and decontamination of cooling towers require the knowledge of professionals. Studies have shown that simple addition of biocides may be inefficient in controlling the growth of microorganisms. Dirt within the water and around the tower may make the biocide ineffective. If other organic materials are contaminating the system, then they can bind the biocide so it cannot reach concentrations to control microorganisms. The treatment of the cooling towers with chlorine-containing compounds has been more effective in controlling microorganisms.

Economizers: This is an energy-saving device that helps control the cooling of outside air coming indoors. Surveys should include a review of the economizer settings and testing of the operation of the economizer, including the damper movements. Economizers can result in lack of fresh air, allowing indoor air contaminants to build up.

EVALUATING INDOOR ENVIRONMENT-RELATED HEALTH PROBLEMS

Most businesses do not have a written and implemented indoor environmental quality plan that proactively addresses the indoor environment to prevent problems from arising. Affected employees usually have sought medical care for their symptoms long before the indoor environment is suspected. In other cases, employees may suspect that their work environment is causing their symptoms, but management ignores their claims. In these cases, workers may be blamed for being disgruntled or lazy. At this stage, adversarial relationships between company manage-

TABLE 53-19. Indoor air quality evaluation checklist

I. Building survey and environmental audit
  1. Building design and age
  2. Building location
  3. Building materials: exterior, mortar, flooring, ceilings, interior walls
  4. Interior furnishings: furniture, carpets, drapes, fabrics
  5. Interior finishing, paints, coatings, plastics
  6. Heating, ventilation, and air-conditioning: Location of intake and exhaust vents, coolers, last cleaning date, filters
  7. Recent renovations and changes to building
  8. Windows: Can they be opened and are they opened? Location of windows
  9. Movement of air mass when windows are opened

II. Interviews and health questionnaire
  1. Health survey and identification of ill workers
  2. Location of ill workers
  3. Location of workers relative to building alterations
  4. Identification of asthmatics and allergic individuals
  5. Description of syndrome
  6. Occurrence of syndrome relative to season
  7. Occurrence of syndrome relative to heating, ventilation, and air-conditioning

III. Pollution source identification
  1. Chemicals
  2. Volatiles, vapors, and semivolatile chemicals
  3. Cleaning agents
  4. Particulates, metals, dusts
  5. Biologics: mold, endotoxin, bacteria
  6. Inorganics
  7. Processes and reactions that produce pollutants
  8. Carbon monoxide and carbon dioxide
  9. Tobacco use
  10. Physical sources and thermal comfort factors (lighting, airflow, noise, humidity, temperature)
  11. Outside environmental sources (dust, odors, molds)
  12. Appropriate environmental monitoring

IV. Medical evaluation of employees
  1. Health evaluation
  2. Evaluation of signs and symptoms related to organ system
  3. Pulmonary functions if indicated
  4. Other studies as indicated

V. Remediation
  1. Heating, ventilation, and air-conditioning alterations and cleaning
  2. Engineering and technical controls
  3. Decontamination
  4. Removal of source
  5. Alteration of work habits
  6. Moving workers
  7. Control external sources
  8. Control psychogenesis

See EPA 1991 "Building Air Quality."

ment and the affected employees escalate, and employee trust regarding the company's ability or willingness to solve the problem wanes. Affected employees usually become angry and miss work. Some file worker's compensation claims at this point.

The evaluation of indoor environmental quality–related illness requires a systematic approach because of the complexity of potential causes. The objectives of the investigation are to gather information about the building, identify signs and symptoms of those with health complaints, locate and identify potential causes, determine work-relatedness of any illness, and remediate the cause by removing or isolating the source (Table 53-19).

Building Inspection

Regular building inspections can be preventive. Such an approach, however, is rare for a number of reasons. The building is usually leased, with the landlord off premise. Most business managers are not aware of what problems to look for in either preventing or reacting to a problem. In many cases, only a few workers are complaining of illness, and linking this with the indoor environment is usually not considered.

Building inspection involves collecting information about the site and its characteristics, and then performing a site survey. The inspection should be conducted by a qualified environmental specialist, such as an industrial hygienist, and includes the following basics:

1. Location of the building with respect to surrounding and outdoor sources of contamination.
2. Age of the building and construction materials.
3. Activities in the building.
4. HVAC system functioning, operation, filters, maintenance, and condition.
5. Adequacy of fresh air supply.
6. Number of occupants in affected areas.
7. Building maintenance, cleaning, and cleaning agents used.
8. Interior fabrics, building products, laser printers, copiers, drapes, carpets, and other sources of chemical emissions.
9. Presence of ETS.
10. Characterization and inspection of HVAC system, including humidification, location of ventilation ducts (exhaust and intake), movement of air, and air exchange.
11. Window locations and window openings.
12. Stagnant air and poor areas of air movement.
13. Physical factors, thermal comfort, lighting, noise, and humidity.
14. Dust and dirt on floors, desks, and in ventilation system.
15. Microbial contamination of ventilation system coolers and ducts.
16. Chemicals used in the environment.
17. Location of copying machines and other equipment in relationship to vents.
18. Renovations and building changes.
19. Changes to the immediate outdoor environment.
20. Location of outdoor air intake vents.
21. Odors.
22. Plumbing, water stains, and moisture damage areas.
23. Indoor pesticide application.

On concluding the building inspection, the investigators should provide a preliminary assessment of their findings, recommendations for changes, and recommendations for any further evaluations and monitoring. Easily identified causes of health complaints should be addressed immediately. At this phase, more in-depth investigation of particular problem areas may be conducted with appropriate monitoring.

Health Audit

A health questionnaire can be useful in determining the health status of employees and can help identify individuals who are manifesting symptoms associated with poor indoor environmental quality. The questionnaire should include location of the employee in the work site, dates the employee experienced illness, whether smoking is allowed, presence or absence of allergic conditions, and location where employees experience symptoms.

After employees complete the questionnaire, symptoms can be tabulated so the actual incidence and prevalence of illness can be determined and the location associated with symptoms identified. An example of a general health questionnaire is presented in the EPA's December 1991 publication, "Building Air Quality" (www.eps.gov/iaq/base).

TABLE 53-20. Checklist for ventilation problems

Yes	No	
❑	❑	Does the air in the room make people uncomfortable or sick?
❑	❑	Are odors present?
❑	❑	Is the space comfortable?
❑	❑	Too cold?
❑	❑	Too hot?
❑	❑	Too humid?
❑	❑	Too dry?
❑	❑	Can you feel the air moving or is the air stagnant?
❑	❑	Do office machines, copiers, printers, and such have adequate ventilation?
❑	❑	Is air distributed throughout the entire space?
❑	❑	Are dead zones of no air movement present?
❑	❑	Does the room have an air supply vent?
❑	❑	Does the room have an air return vent?
❑	❑	Is air moving out of the air supply vent? (Check with tissue paper.)
❑	❑	Is air moving into return vent? (Check with tissue paper.)
❑	❑	Are air vent diffusers open?
❑	❑	Is dust or dirt present on the air vent grill surfaces?
❑	❑	Does the heating, ventilation, and air-conditioning system operate when people are in the space?
❑	❑	Is the air intake of the ventilation system located near a contaminant source, such as a garage or vehicle parking area?
❑	❑	Has the heating, ventilation, and air-conditioning been inspected or cleaned recently?
❑	❑	Has the air filter been replaced or serviced?
❑	❑	Is there a lack of outside air?
❑	❑	Are there air pressure differences between rooms?
❑	❑	Is there excessive tobacco smoke?
❑	❑	Poorly vented heating equipment?
❑	❑	Poorly located intakes?
❑	❑	Is there visible mold, slime, or biological growth?
❑	❑	Is visible moisture or water present?
❑	❑	Is there water damage indoors?
❑	❑	Are cleaning chemicals stored in mechanical room or near air intake?
❑	❑	Is there deteriorated insulation around ventilation ducts?
❑	❑	Is there dirt debris in vents?
❑	❑	Is there improper exhaust ventilation?

See also EPA 1991 "Building Air Quality."

Identifying the prevalence rate of ill employees can help determine whether an excessive number of health complaints is related to a possible indoor air pollution cause. Because many individuals at a variety of times manifest a number of these vague complaints, however, it can be difficult to derive a true prevalence rate for indoor air pollution–related illness. Frequently, only one or a few individuals are voicing health complaints.

Strategies and Tactics

Symptoms can be generated by the buildup of low concentrations of multiple indoor contaminants, including off-gassing from building materials, emissions from office machinery, and solvents and other chemicals used in the office work and building maintenance. This synergy of low-level multiple pollutants is accentuated by a suboptimally performing HVAC system.

Because problems related to ventilation are responsible for 50% to 60% of indoor air quality problems, altering and adjustments in ventilation can result in improvement or resolution of symptoms (Table 53-20). The volume of fresh air should be increased if possible. Sometimes decreasing the occupancy numbers is helpful. Smoking should be eliminated totally. Local exhaust ventilation may also serve to reduce a pollutant source. Sometimes decreasing indoor temperature helps decrease volatile chemical emissions. Cleaning agents used indoors should be evaluated to determine if they contain irritants and sensitizers. If so, they should be replaced.

Inadequate outside air intake can be assessed by measuring the rise in CO_2 levels in the building over the day and subsequent fall in the evening with the building unoccupied but the ventilating system running at daytime levels. If the outside air intake is sufficient to adequately manage CO_2, it is assumed that other contaminants are managed also.

Temperature and humidity, and, if necessary, airflow at vents and return air grills, should also be checked. Although wet-and-dry bulb thermometers can be used, this level of accuracy is generally unnecessary. A desk thermometer and relative humidity meter should be adequate. Measurements for airflow assure that a vent is functioning and indicate if the airflow is directed in a suitable direction. In general, exact measurements of these parameters are less critical except in special circumstances.

These guidelines are based on whole building analysis rather than an analysis of the spatial distribution of the building's ventilation. Pollutant transport depends on building geometry, pollutant source characteristics, and thermo/fluid boundary conditions, such as flow rate, thermal stratification, duct location, and diffuser type. If the air in the room is well mixed, then the concentration can be predicted based on knowledge of the room ventilation rate, the pollutant source strength, and the concentration in the supply air. In situations in which the well-mixed assumption does not apply, knowledge of local concentration distributions is required to determine average ventilation system performance. Even if an acceptable average room concentration can be achieved at a given ventilation rate, the sensitivity of concentration to flow nonuniformities can produce localized areas (dead zones) with acceptably high concentration levels. As a result, a detailed knowledge of source strengths and local ventilation system performance is required to ensure that the ventilation system provides pollutant control at reasonable ventilation rates.

To properly evaluate indoor air problems, it is necessary to have some basic knowledge of ventilation. Because buildings are not constructed to contain air pressures significantly different from outside pressures, it is necessary to move air out of the building to move air into a building, and vice versa. If a system imbalance exists in a building, it may be noticeable when outside doors or windows are opened, resulting in a rush of air either into (excessive exhaust or insufficient intake) or out of (insufficient exhaust or excessive intake) the building. With the slight pressure difference between inside and outside, however, only as much air enters the building as is able to leave the building.

Inadequately functioning HVAC systems allow indoor contaminants to accumulate, contributing to stale and stagnant air, and may even introduce outdoor pollutants and allergens into the indoors, especially if the air is unfiltered. A frequently occurring problem is an imbalance in the flow of fresh air versus outflow of stale air. This can create dead zones of no air circulation indoors. These dead zones are essentially stale air that escapes being recirculated. HVACs can be sources of moisture, allowing mold and other microorganisms to amplify and be circulated indoors. Over time, dust, dirt, and debris build up in the ventilation system. Proper maintenance can help prevent accumulated dirt and dust from being circulated indoors.

Monitoring strategies for pollutants are based on the environmental assessment and health survey. Decisions regarding monitoring for VOCs and biologicals are driven by what is found on the inspection and the pattern of illness of the occupants. Monitored variables may include the following:

1. CO_2 (should be <800 ppm)
2. Relative humidity:

Winter 30% to 50%
Summer 40% to 60%
Plenum and ductwork <70%

3. Ambient air temperature (should meet ASHRAE standard 52-1992)
4. HVAC functioning and condition (should meet ASHRAE standard 62-1989)
5. TVOCs
6. Specific volatile chemicals
7. Combustion products, such as CO, NO_2, SO_2, and ozone
8. Biologicals, bioaerosols, and chemical by-products
9. Lighting level
10. Airflow: supply diffusers, return grills, and local exhaust systems
11. Airflow between spaces
12. Vertical air temperature
13. Air filtration
14. Noise and vibration

RADON INDOORS

Radon (radon-222), a naturally occurring nonreactive, colorless, odorless, and tasteless noble gas, is a product of the decay of trace amounts of uranium-238 found in soil and rock. Radon's eventual fate is to decay through a number of intermediates to lead-206, a stable end product. As a gas, radon can diffuse through soil and rock and enter home environments. In certain geographic areas, concentrations of radon can be higher in indoor environments compared to those outdoors.

Natural uranium found in the earth contains a predominance of the isotope ^{238}U. Uranium-238 decays through a series of isotopes, one of which is radium-226. Radium-226, an alpha emitter, and its daughter products are responsible for a large fraction of alpha emissions received by humans from the environment (96). Radium-226 present in soil and rock decays with a half-life ($t_{1/2}$) of 1,622 years to radon-222, which has $t_{1/2}$ of 3.8 days. Radon decay results in the generation of short-lived α- and β-emitting progeny. After six decay steps that produce isotopes with half-lives from 1.6×10^{-4} seconds to 26.8 minutes, the isotope of lead-210 is reached with a $t_{1/2}$ of 22 years (96). Lead-210 decays with a $t_{1/2}$ of 238 days to stable lead-206.

Because radon is a gas, it diffuses from its point of origin through soil and can enter a home or building via cracks or pipes. The porosity of the soil helps to determine its transfer. Thus, radon can move by diffusion and pressure differences into basements and indoor spaces. Radon-222 decays by alpha-particle emission to radon daughters: polonium-218 (radon A), lead-214 (radon B), bismuth-214 (radon C), polonium-214 (radon C^1) (97). Radon is not a health hazard by itself, instead health hazards are caused by the radon decay products (daughters) that emit alpha particles. Daughters are chemically active and can attach to particles, surfaces, and human tissue (98–100). Polonium-218 and polonium-214 are daughters that emit alpha particles.

A difference exists between radon activity indoors and exposure to harmful radon daughters. Radon activity is measured in either curies or becquerels, and typical air concentrations are expressed in terms of picocuries per liter or becquerels per cubic meter. Soil contains approximately 1 pCi of radium per g, which provides an emission of 0.5 pCi of radon per square meter per second (100). Outdoor radon concentrations average 0.20 pCi per m^3 (greater than Bq per m^3), and typical indoor air concentrations are 1.2 pCi per L (945 Bq per m^3) (97,100).

Radon exposure is expressed in terms of working levels (WL) or working levels per month (WLM), an accumulation measurement. One WL is any combination of radon daughters in 1 L of air that results in the release of 1.3×10^5 MeV of alpha energy (97). In general, 1 pCi of radon per L is equivalent to 0.005 WL (97,100). The WLM assumes 170 hours per month of exposure (not dose) (100).

Occupational exposure to radon in the United States was reduced from 12 WLM per year to 4 WLM per year in 1971 (98). The level for remediation activity in the home environment is considered to be 2 WLM per year (98). As of 1989, EPA monitoring has shown radon concentrations to be less than 4 pCi per L in 74% of homes across the United States (100).

The relationship of exposure to radon and actual dose of radon and its daughters remains complex. Therefore, most assays are designed to measure radon rather than the biologically active daughters. As mentioned previously in this section, radon is not hazardous by itself; instead, radon daughters that emit alpha particles create a health hazard when they attach to dusts and other aerosols because of their electrical charge and are inhaled, depositing in the tracheobronchial tree.

It is estimated that 9.25×10^{20} Bq per m^3 of radon is released from the earth on an annual basis (97). Variation in atmospheric radon concentration is dependent on meteorologic conditions and amount released from the soil. Outdoor radon concentrations are highest at midnight, with minimum concentrations occurring at noon because of air mixing.

The airborne radon concentration in a home is a factor of the earth surrounding the home containing radon gas, air changes per hour in the home, amount of radon in water and in natural gas, and construction of the home (100). Radon can diffuse through cracks in foundations and walls, openings for plumbing, and cinder block (100). Radon does not pass easily through solid concrete foundations. WHO has set limits of radon at 0.11 WL for existing buildings (100).

Ventilation reduces indoor radon concentrations if air exchanges average approximately four times per hour. Because this volume of air exchange is not easily achieved, radon concentration indoors exceeds that outdoors. Radon exposure also arises from contaminated water and natural gas and can be released from rock materials used to build houses. Action in the home is recommended if radon concentrations exceed 400 Bq per m^3 (11 pCi/L).

Health effects from excessive radon daughter exposure relate mainly to an increased risk of lung cancer from alpha particle exposure. Most studies of the relationship of lung cancer and radon exposure are from uranium miners. Studies indicate that all forms of lung cancer are increased by radon exposure (98). Also, the contribution of smoking to lung cancer is a confounding factor in determining the exact etiology. Radon exposure and smoking are thought to increase the risk of lung cancer tenfold over nonsmokers (98).

Over the lifetime of an individual, exposure to 1 WLM per year is thought to increase the number of deaths from lung cancer by a factor of 1.5 over the current rate in men and women (99). The National Council on Radiation Protection and Measurements has published guidelines on remediation and control of radon in indoor environments (National Council on Radiation Protection and Measurements report no. 77, 1984).

PSYCHOSOCIAL ASPECTS OF INDOOR AIR QUALITY

The presence of illness in the workplace can be unsettling to employees, stimulate anxieties about possible toxic exposures, and accentuate worker stress. An indoor environmental quality investigation can generate strong emotional responses, especially if results are negative but illness continues. The overall effect leaves building occupants discouraged, suspicious, and unconvinced that the problem has been discovered and a proper solution found. Stress- and anxiety-related symptoms can occur after suspected exposure or actual exposure of employees to unknown environmental health threats. Thus, psychosocial factors are important to consider when investigating indoor environmental quality problems. Some of these are as follows:

- The environment itself
- Boredom associated with the job
- Pressure to produce
- Everyday relationship between labor and management
- Lack of communication and social support within the work environment
- Adversarial relationship between employees and management because of environmental quality problems

Stress and Environmental Threats

In the 1950s, Dr. Hans Selye expressed the concept that stress was a general response of living organisms to external or internal stimuli, which he termed *stressors*. Dr. Selye observed that chronic stress could lead to exhaustion, organ system failure, and even death. He confirmed what has been known for centuries, that stressful thoughts and feelings affect our physical well-being.

The phenomenon of acute reactions or triggering of symptoms when rechallenged with a stressor has been observed in animals and is termed the *generalized adaptation syndrome* by Selye in his 1950 book, *Stress*. The term *generalized* was introduced because he was able to show that chemicals and other stressors also lead to a maladaptive response.

The physiologic basis of stress involves interconnections between the brain and other areas of the body via the hypothalamic-pituitary-adrenal (HPA) axis. When activated, epinephrine, norepinephrine, and corticosteroid secretions increase. Whereas the stress response, referred to as the *fight or flight* reaction, is essential for well-being and survival, chronic stress can result in illness.

Poor indoor environmental quality can be a chronic stressor. The concept of pollutants as activators of the stress mechanism has research support. Biomarkers in the brain have been found that indicate that brain cells are activated in response to stressors.

Exposures to chemicals may evoke expression of brain biomarkers indicative of neuronal excitation response to stress. Pyrethroid insecticides administered intraperitoneally in animal models evoke c-Fos and c-Jun protein biomarkers in brain neurons in the thalamus, hypothalamus, hippocampus, and cortex to varying degrees (101). C-Fos and c-Jun proteins are transcription factors encoded by rapidly inducible protooncogenes (102,103). Such markers indicate changes in neuron activity and programming. C-Fos expression in homogenates is demonstrated after the administration of lindane. This expression of c-Fos and c-Jun biomarkers reflects an intense and lasting neuronal excitation. Such markers appear in the cells of the brain, which are functionally activated by stressors of all varieties. With the use of c-Fos and c-Jun markers, scientists can study areas of the brain that are activated by adverse stimuli (104).

Animals studied using conditioned stressors (stressors that produce fear or anxiety without pain or without some kind of insult) at the time of exposure show activation of areas in the hypothalamus that contain corticotropin-releasing hormones. Other areas activated in the studies included the amygdala, the basal ganglia, and thalamic nuclei (101–104). The areas of the brain activated by stressors are associated with the HPA and the sympathetic nervous system. The HPA pathway, thus, may be activated by a variety of stressors (physical, chemical, and psychological).

Stress can have effects on the human immune system although the neuroendocrine responses of the central nervous system are activated by the HPA (105–109). Although stress responses can cause release of endogenous opioids, cortisol, and catecholamines, which may alter the humoral and cellular immune system, this immune response is not chemically induced immunotoxicity, but rather a physiologic response of the immune system to stressors.

Studies show that stress can elevate numbers of T cells and B cells, impair responsiveness of lymphocytes to mitogens, decrease CD4 to CD8 (T helper to T suppressor) ratios, increase natural killer (NK) cell populations, and decrease NK cell activity (110–113). Individuals treated with β-adrenergic antagonist drugs, such as propranolol, show inhibition of immune alterations after stressful episodes (114).

Mood and anxiety disorders and other psychiatric conditions are associated with immune alterations. It is reported that a linear relationship exists between severity of depression and immune compromise, including a marked reduction in the response to mitogens by lymphocytes, reduced NK cell activity, and alteration of immune cell numbers, primarily an increase in CD8 T cell lymphocytes (113).

Marital discord, bereavement, and other such stressors are associated with immunosuppression and higher antibody titers to Epstein-Barr virus, lower NK cell activity, and reduced lymphocyte response to mitogens (111,112,115,116). The chronic stress of providing care to family members with debilitating disease is associated with decreases in CD4 T cells, lower helper to suppressor cell ratios, and increased antibody titers to Epstein-Barr virus (115,116). Bereavement, depression, and anxiety activate neuroendocrine functions, which reduce NK cell activity and reduce T cell numbers with CD4 markers.

Individuals under stress show higher titers of Epstein-Barr viral capsid antigen IgG. Plus, negative moods depress mitogen stimulation of lymphocytes. Studies also show that stressors increase the number of CD8 marker T cells, CD16/56 cells (NK cells), decrease mitogen response, and increase numbers of B cells (CD19) within 5 minutes of the stressor (106–108,117). These immune changes can persist for hours.

Chronic stress acts opposite of acute stress in producing immune function changes. Chronic stress reduces NK cell numbers and activity, whereas acute stress elevates NK cell numbers and activity. Acute stress elevates lymphocyte subsets. In contrast, chronic stress decreases lymphocyte mitogen responsiveness. Research has shown that moderate exercise modulates the effects of chronic diseases and has positive effects on immune function (118). Relaxation methods also positively modulate the immune system through stress reduction (114).

Chronic stress and associated somatic, behavioral, and psychological responses outlast their initiating cause, with symptoms persisting for long periods of time. Also, chronic stress is associated with a loss of personal control over one's health (119). Efforts to increase a patient's sense of control over aspects of their health should have positive health effects.

Control or lack of control is another feature affecting perceptions of stress, health, and well-being. Loss of control over one's environment, especially when it is suspected as a cause of illness, increases stress levels. In contrast to the industrial or occupational environment, residential environments allow significant personal control of thermal comfort factors as well as ventilation.

Psychogenic Illness

Certain features exist that suggest a psychogenic origin of indoor environmental problems as opposed to contaminant-induced illness (120–122):

1. An incidence of the problem in areas that are not consistent with ventilation patterns in the workplace or the environment.
2. A temporal sequence of events that is not consistent with ventilation flow patterns and ventilation flow rates or chemical sources.
3. An absence of medical findings compatible with exposures.
4. Outbreak of illness consistent with person-to-person transmission rather than transmission from a source.
5. Severe symptoms of sudden onset among a number of people, particularly if the symptoms begin after leaving the source of exposure or do not resolve on leaving the work site.
6. Moderate to severe symptoms that are unrelated to the nature of a contaminant found.
7. A diversity of symptoms without collaborating objective findings.
8. The discovery of individuals who are affected, not because they are near the source of the exposure, but rather become affected after learning of the exposure or learning that someone else is exhibiting signs of illness.
9. Pattern of the illness after a classic epidemic curve in which conversation is the vector of spread.
10. Managerial or supervisory change or changes in work flow or production volume, including deadline requirements.

The term *psychogenesis* has emotional connotations, and its cavalier use can further adversarial relations between management and workers in the investigation of indoor environment illness.

In general, organizations whose employees are more prone to develop psychogenic illness are generally rigid and authoritarian, with poor communication between workers and management (121,122). Workers may not believe that management is serious about the problem, and the worker believes he or she has an inability to control environmental conditions. Multiple stresses can affect a worker's ability to relate to the environment. These stresses may be fear of loss of job, external forces, and the thought of environmental contamination (123).

Threat of exposure to toxins can add to anxiety. Workers may become alarmed if they believe that a chemical contamination in an environment may cause them long-term health consequences. Also, heightened concern occurs if the source of the potential problem, such as an odor, cannot be established or identified and remediated.

Odors in the environment can create anxieties and stress. The psychologic responses to indoor air quality problems may relate more to an odor of a chemical than to its toxic effects. Odors, such as sulfur odors, odors of rotten eggs, or odors of chemicals or hydrocarbons, can be distressing to workers.

The relationship of management and employee can be greatly tested during these times. Sending workers to an emergency department unnecessarily may further serve to intensify anxiety. The use of a knowledgeable, single-source professional can help to prevent distortion of facts and decrease rumors. Closing the workplace is not recommended unless a serious and significant threat to the health of the workers exists. Once a workplace has been closed, it is difficult to reopen again.

Communication should be open and should be timely. Because rumor is the most common source of information, rumors should be dispelled by having frequent meetings and open discussions with employees regarding the investigation. Communication with the media may be important in some situations in which a public health concern is present. The media, if not properly educated, can help foster sensationalism and rumor.

WORK-RELATEDNESS OF POOR INDOOR ENVIRONMENTAL PROBLEMS

Illness associated with poor indoor environmental quality may range from vague and subjective to objective and easily recognizable. Environmental monitoring and investigations, however, may not produce evidence of a source.

Despite these difficulties, a medical condition, disease, or illness can be said to be work-related if the following criteria are met (124):

1. An employee-employer relationship exists.
2. The event is causally related to the work activity or work environment.
3. Medical conditions exist that are compatible with health effects secondary to exposure to an environment, chemical, industrial site, or other agents in question.
4. There was previously or is presently a sufficient exposure to agents in the work environment to produce illness or disease.
5. A preexisting disease is exacerbated by a previous or present work site exposure.
6. Evidence supports an occupational etiology.

Impairment and Disability

Impairment is present if an exposure results in a reduction or loss of use of a body part or reduction of function of a body system. This functional limitation may or may not prevent the individual from meeting the demands of his or her life's activities or conditions of employment. Disability results from a permanent impairment that cannot be overcome through retraining, use of accommodative procedures, or rehabilitation. Medical conditions, such as asthma, may result in episodic expressions of impairment. The medical condition may also result in a permanent impairment expressed on an episodic basis.

Individuals with health problems secondary to poor indoor environmental quality may fall under protection of the Americans with Disabilities Act (ADA), especially if one or more of their major life activities is substantially limited. Poor indoor air quality may be a reason why an employee may not be productive or be able to continue working in a specific environment. Accommodations may be required to make the environment healthy and safe for affected individuals, or the affected person may need to be relocated to another area of the work site or building.

The ADA, signed into law in 1990, has the purpose of eliminating discrimination against disabled individuals with the enforcement of federal law. Title I of the ADA applies to employment issues of qualified, disabled individuals. Disability is defined as mental or physical impairment that substantially limits one or more major life activities. Major life activities are defined as those activities that an average individual can perform with few or no difficulties. Under the ADA, employers are responsible for making reasonable accommodations to qualified individuals capable of performing essential functions of the job.

REFERENCES

1. US Department of Labor, Occupational Safety and Health Administration. Indoor air quality. *Federal Register* April 5 1994;59(65):15968–16039.
2. Dales R, Burnett R, Zwanenburg H. Adverse health effects among adults exposed to home dampness and molds. *Am Rev Respir Dis* 1991:143:505–509.
3. Amalkin R, Martinez K, Marinkovich V, et al. The relationship between symptoms and IgG and IgE antibodies in an office environment. *Environ Res* 1998;76:85–93.
4. Norback D, Wieslander G, Bjornsson E, et al. Eye irritation, nasal congestion, and facial skin itching in relation to emissions from newly painted indoor surfaces. *Indoor Built Environ* 1996;5:270–279.

5. Dales R, Zqanenburg H, Burnch R, et al. Respiratory health effects of home dampness and molds among Canadian children. *Am J Epidemiol* 1991; 134:196–203.
6. Menzies D, Bourbeau J. Building related illness. *N Engl J Med* 1997;337(21): 1524–1531.
7. Verhoeff A, Van Strien R, Van Wijnen J, et al. Damp housing and childhood respiratory symptoms—the role of sensitization to dust mites and molds. *Am J Epidemiol* 1995;141:103–110.
8. Waegemaekers M, Van Wageningen N, Brunckreef B, et al. Respiratory symptoms in damp homes. *Allergy* 1989;44:1–7.
9. Seltzer J, ed. Effects of the indoor environment on health. *Occup Med: State of the Art Reviews* 1995;10(1):1–245.
10. Middaugh A, Pinney S, Linz D. Sick building syndrome: medical evaluation of two work forces. *J Occup Med* 1992;34(12):1197–1203.
11. Lagoudi A, Loizidou M, Asimakopoulos D. Volatile organic compounds in office building, 1. Presence of volatile organic compounds in the indoor air. *Indoor Built Environ* 1996;5:341–347.
12. Lagoudi A, Loizidou M, Asimakopoulos D. Volatile organic compounds in office building, 2. Identification of pollution sources in indoor air. *Indoor Built Environ* 1996;5:348–354.
13. Holcomb L, Seabrook B. Indoor concentrations of volatile organic compounds: implications for comfort, health and regulation. *Indoor Environ* 1995;4:7–26.
14. Bauer R, Greve K, Besch EL, et al. The role of psychological factors in the report of building-related symptoms in sick building syndrome. *J Consult Clin Psychol* 1992;60(2):213–219.
15. Cameron L, Leventhal E, Leventhal H. Seeking medical care in response to symptoms and life stress. *Psychosom Med* 1995;57:37–47.
16. Lehmer M, Bentley A. Treating work stress: an alternative to workers' compensation. *J Occup Environ Med* 1997;39(1):63–67.
17. Mendell M, Smith A. Consistent pattern of elevated symptoms in air conditioned office buildings: a reanalysis of epidemiologic studies. *Am J Public Health* 1990;80:1193–1199.
18. Diasty R, Olson P. Improving indoor air quality through healthy building envelope design and systems selection. *Indoor Environ* 1995;2:285–290.
19. Rolloos M. HVAC systems and indoor air quality. *Indoor Environ* 1993;2:204–212.
20. Burton J. General ventilation of nonindustrial occupancies. In: Plog B, Niland J, Quinlan P, eds. *Fundamentals of industrial hygiene*, 4th ed. Itasca, IL: National Safety Council, 1996; 595-618.
21. Girman JR. Volatile organic compounds and building bake-out. In: Cone JE, Hodgson MJ, eds. *Occup Med: State of the Art Reviews* 1989;4:695–712.
22. Linaker C, Chauhan A, Inskip H, et al. Distribution and determinants of personal exposure to nitrogen dioxide in school children. *Occup Environ Med* 1996;53:200–203.
23. Strom J, Alfredsson L, Malmfors T, Selroos O. Nitrogen dioxide: causation and aggravation of lung diseases. *Indoor Environ* 1994;3:58–68.
24. Steenland K. Passive smoking and the risk of heart disease. *JAMA* 1992;7(1):94–99.
25. Humble C, Croft J, Gerber A, Casper M, Hames C, Tyroler H. Passive smoking and 20-year cardiovascular disease mortality among non-smoking wives, Evans County, Georgia. *Am J Public Health* 1990;80:599–601.
26. Stankus R, Menon P, Rando RJ, et al. Cigarette smoke-sensitive asthma: challenge studies. *J Allergy Clin Immunol* 1988;82(3)(1):333–338.
27. Godish T. Formaldehyde exposure from tobacco smoke—a review. *Am J Public Health* 1989;79:1044–1045.
28. Hodgson MJ. Environmental tobacco smoke and the sick building syndrome. In: Cone JE, Hodgson MJ, eds. *Occup Med: State of the Art Reviews* 1989;4:735–740.
29. Stricker S. Physiological responses to elevated carbon dioxide levels in buildings. *Indoor Built Environ* 1997;6:301–308.
30. Turner W. Ventilation. *Occup Med: State of the Art Reviews* 1995;10(1):41–57.
31. Burt T. Sick building syndrome: acoustic aspects. *Indoor Built Environ* 1996;5:44–59.
32. Levin H. Physical factors in the indoor environment. *Occup Med: State of the Art Reviews* 1995;19(1): 59–94.
33. World Health Organization. Indoor air pollutants: exposure and health effects. Copenhagen, Denmark: World Health Organization, 1983.
34. Sandstrom M, Lyskov E, Berglund A, et al. Neurophysiological effects of flickering light in patients with perceived electrical hypersensitivity. *J Occup Environ Med* 1997;39(1):15–22.
35. Molhave L. Controlled experiments for studies of the sick building syndrome. *Ann N Y Acad Sci* 1992;641:46–55.
36. Molhave L, Liu Z. Sensory and physiological effects on humans of combined exposures to air temperatures and volatile organic compounds. *Indoor Air* 1993;3:155–169.
37. Bascom R, Kesavanathan J, Swift D. Human susceptibility to indoor contaminants. *Occup Med: State of the Art Reviews* 1995;10(1):119–132.
38. Frew J. The immunology of respiratory allergies. *Toxicol Lett* 1996;86:65–72.
39. Damgard G. Mechanisms of activation of the sensory irritant receptor by airborne chemicals. *Toxicology* 1991;21(3):183–208.
40. Schook L, Laskin D, eds. *Xenobiotics and inflammation*. San Diego: Academic Press, 1994.
41. Cometto-Muniz J, Cain W. Relative sensitivity of the ocular trigeminal, nasal trigeminal, and olfactory systems to airborne chemicals. *Chemical Senses* 1995;20(2):191–198.
42. Cometto-Muniz J, Cain W. Thresholds for odor and nasal pungency. *Physiol Behavior* 1990;48:719–725.
43. Meggs WJ. RADS and RUDS—the toxic induction of asthma and rhinitis. Clin Toxicol 1994;32(5):487–501.
44. Dusser D, Djokic T, Borson D, Nadel J. Cigarette smoke induces bronchoconstrictor hyperresponsiveness to substance P and inactivates airway neutral endopeptidase in the guinea pig. *J Clin Invest* 1989;84:900–906.
45. Farley J. Inhaled toxicants and airway hyperresponsiveness. *Annu Rev Pharmacol Toxicol* 1992;32:67–88.
46. Mygind N, Dahl R, Nielsen L. Effect of nasal inflammation and of intranasal anti-inflammatory treatment on bronchial asthma. *Respir Med* 1998;92:547–549.
47. Hirsch F, Kroemer G. The immune system and immune modulation. In: Kresina T, ed. *Immune modulating agents*. New York: Marcel Dekker Inc, 1998.
48. Kapsenberg M. Chemicals and proteins as allergens and adjuvants. *Toxicol Lett* 1996;86:79–83.
49. Lemanske R, Busse W. Asthma. *JAMA* 1997;278(22):1855–1873.
50. Perkner J, Fennelly KP, Balkissoon R, et al. Irritant-associated vocal cord dysfunction. *J Occup Environ Med* 1998;40(2):136–143.
51. Molhave L. Volatile organic compounds, indoor air quality and health. *Indoor Air* 1991;4:357–376.
52. Morrow L, Ryan C, Hodgson M, Robin N. Alterations in cognitive and psychological functioning after organic solvent exposure. *J Occup Med* 1990;32(5):444–450.
53. Kjaergaard S, Molhave L, Pedersen O. Human reactions to a mixture of indoor air volatile organic compounds. *Atmos Environ* 1991;25A(8):1417–1426.
54. Molhave L, Damgaard Nielsen G. Interpretation and limitations of the concept "total volatile organic compounds" (TVOC) as an indicator of human responses to exposures of volatile organic compounds (VOC) in indoor air. *Indoor Air* 1992;2:65–77.
55. La Marte F, Merchant J, Casale T. Acute systemic reactions to carbonless copy paper associated with histamine release. *JAMA* 1988;260:242–243.
56. Lundholm M, Larrell G, Mathiasson L. Self-leveling mortar as a possible cause of symptoms associated with "sick building syndrome." *Arch Environ Health* 1990;45:135–140.
57. Crump D, Squire R, Yu C. Sources and concentrations of formaldehyde and other volatile organic compounds in the indoor air of four newly built unoccupied test houses. *Indoor Built Environ* 1997;6:45–55.
58. Silberstein S. Advances in understanding the pathophysiology of headache. *Neurology* 1992;42(2):6–10.
59. Leher P, Isenberg S, Hochron S. Asthma and emotion: a review. *J Asthma* 1993;30:5–26.
60. Smith T, Hewson A. Neuroendocrine-induced immune modulation and autoimmunity. In: Kresina T. *Immune modulating agents*. New York: Marcel Dekker Inc, 1998.
61. Bachen E, Marsland A, Manuck S, Cohen S. Psychological stress and immune competence. In: Kresina T. *Immune modulating agents*. New York: Marcel Dekker Inc, 1998.
62. Williams R. Somatic consequences of stress. In: *Neurobiological and clinical consequences of stress—from normal adaption to post-traumatic stress disorder*. Philadelphia: Lippincott–Raven, 1995.
63. Auger P, Gourdeau P, Miller JD. Clinical experience with patients suffering from a chronic fatigue-like syndrome and repeated respiratory infections in relation to airborne molds. *Am Jr Ind Med* 1994;25:41–42.
64. Fogelmark B, Rylander R. (1→3)-β-Glucan in some indoor air fungi. *Indoor Built Environ* 1997;6:291–294.
65. Harving H, Dahl R, Molhave L. Lung function and bronchial reactivity in asthmatics during exposure to volatile organic compounds. *Am Rev Respir Dis* 1991;143:751–754.
66. Becher R, Hongslo JK, Jantunen MJ, Dybing E. Environmental chemicals relevant for respiratory hypersensitivity: the indoor environment. *Toxicol Lett* 1996;86:155–162.
67. Wixtrom R, Brown S. Individual population exposures to gasoline. *J Exp Anal Environ Epidemiol* 1992;2:23–78.
68. Weisel C, Lawryck N, Lioy P. Exposure to emissions from gasoline within automotive cabins. *J Exp Anal Environ Epidemiol* 1992;2:79–96.
69. Ashley D, Bonin M, Cardinali F, McCraw J, Wooten J. Measurement of volatile organic compounds in human blood. *Environ Health Perspect* 1996;104[Suppl 5]:871–877.
70. Van Ert MD, Clayton JW, Crabb CL, Walsh DW. Identification and characterization of 4-phenylcyclohexene—an emission product of new carpeting. Presented at: American Industrial Hygiene conference in San Francisco, May 1988.
71. Vogelman I, Clayton JW, Crutchfield CD, Van Ert MD. Evaluation of 4-phenylcyclohexene concentrations in home and chamber environments. Presented at the American Industrial Hygiene conference in San Francisco, May 1988.
72. Van Ert MD, Sullivan JB. Personal data. University of Arizona, Tucson.
73. Stock T, Mendez S. A survey of typical exposure to formaldehyde in Houston area residences. *Am Ind Hyg Assoc J* 1985;46:313–317.
74. Bender J, Mullin L, Graepel G, Wilson W. Eye irritation response of humans to formaldehyde. *Am Ind Hyg Assoc J* 1983;44:463–465.
75. Schacter N, Tosun T, Beck G. A study of respiratory effects from exposure to 2 ppm formaldehyde in healthy subjects. *Arch Environ Health* 1986;41: 229–239.
76. US Environmental Protection Agency, Office of Health and Environmental Assessment. Respiratory health effects of passive smoking: lung cancer and other disorders. Washington: US Environmental Protection Agency, 1992.
77. Mohsenin V. Airway responses to nitrogen dioxide in asthmatic subjects. *J Toxicol Environ Health* 1987;22:371–380.

78. Frampton M, Morrow P, Cox C, et al. Effect of nitrogen dioxide exposure on pulmonary function and airway reactivity in normal humans. *Am Rev Respir Dis* 1991;143:522–527.
79. Rossi O, Kinnula V, Tienari J. Association of severe asthmatic attacks with weather, pollen and air pollutants. *Thorax* 1995;48:244–248.
80. Goings S, Kulle T, Bascom R, et al. Effect of nitrogen dioxide on susceptibility to influenza—a virus infection in healthy adults. *Am Rev Respir Dis* 1989;139:1075–1081.
81. Allen R, Wadden R, Ross E. Characterization of potential indoor sources of ozone. *Am Ind Hyg Assoc J* 1978;39:466–471.
82. Hansen T, Andersen B. Ozone and other air pollutants from photocopying machines. *Am Ind Hyg Assoc J* 1986;47:659–665.
83. Burge H. Aerobiology of the indoor environment. *Occup Med: State of the Art Reviews* 1995;10(1):27–40.
84. Gessner M, Chauvet E. Ergosterol-to-biomass conversion factors for aquatic hypomycetes. *Appl Environ Microbiol* 1993;59:502–507.
85. Setiz L, Sauer R, Burroughs H, et al. Ergosterol as a measure of fungal growth. *Phytopathology* 1979;69:1202–1203.
86. Miller J, Young J. The use of ergosterol to measure exposure to fungal propagules in indoor air. *Am Ind Hyg Assoc J* 1997;58:39–43.
87. Dillon HE, Heinsohn PA, Miller JD, eds. *Field guide for the determination of biological contaminants in environmental samples*, 2nd ed. Fairfax, VA: American Industrial Hygiene Association, 1996.
88. American Conference of Governmental Industrial Hygienists. Guidelines for the assessment of bioaerosols in the indoor environment. Cincinnati: American Conference of Governmental Industrial Hygienists, 1989.
89. Rylander R. Airway responsiveness and chest symptoms after inhalation of endotoxin or (1→3)-β-D-glucan. *Indoor Built Environ* 1996;5:106–111.
90. Rylander R. Airborne (1→3)-β-D-glucan and airway disease in a day-care center before and after renovation. *Arch Environ Health* 1997;52(4):281–285.
91. Goto H, Yuasa F, Rylander R. (1→3)-β-D-glucan in indoor air—its measurement and in vitro activity. *Am J Ind Med* 1994;25:81–83.
92. Seltzer J. Biologic contaminants. *Occup Med* 1995;10(1):1–25.
93. Muilenburg ML. The outdoor environment. In: Burge HA, ed. *Bioaerosols*. Boca Raton, FL: CRC Press, 1995.
94. Robertson L. Monitoring viable fungal and bacterial bioaerosol concentrations to identify acceptable levels for common indoor environments. *Indoor Built Environ* 1997;6:295–300.
95. Reynolds S, Streifel A, McJilton C. Elevated airborne concentrations of fungi in residential and office environments. *Am Ind Hyg Assoc J* 1990;51:601–604.
96. Eisenbud M. In: *Environmental radioactivity*, 3rd ed. San Diego: Academic Press, 1987.
97. Mettler F, Upton A. *Medical effects of ionizing radiation*, 2nd ed. Philadelphia: WB Saunders, 1995.
98. Harley N, Samet JM, Cross FT, Hess T, Muller J, Thomas D. Contribution of radon and radon daughters to respiratory cancer. *Environ Health Perspect* 1986;70:17–21.
99. Fabrikault J. Shelter and indoor air in the twenty-first century—radon, smoking, and lung cancer risks. *Environ Health Perspect* 1990;89:275–280.
100. Council on Scientific Affairs. Radon in homes. *JAMA* 1987;258:668–672.
101. Hassouna I, Wickert H, El-Elaimy I, et al. Systemic application of pyrethroid insecticides evokes differential expression of c-Fos and c-Jun in rat brains. *Neurotoxicology* 1996;17(2):415–432.
102. Hoffman G, Smith M, Berbalis J. C-Fos and related immediate early gene products as markers of activity in neuroendocrine systems. *Frontiers Neuroendocrinol* 1993;14:173.
103. Rabin B, Pezzone M, Kusnecov A, Hoffman G. Identification of stressor activated areas in the central nervous system. *Methods Neurosci* 1995;24:185.
104. Pezzone M, Lee W, Hoffman G, et al. Activation of brain stem catecholaminergic neurons by condition and uncondition aversive stimuli as revealed by c-fos immunoreactivity. *Brain Res* 1993;608:310.
105. Blalock J, Smith E. Human leukocyte interferon (HuIFN-α) potent endorphin-like opioid activity. *Biochem Biophys Res Commun* 1981b;101:472–478.
106. Kiecolt-Glaser J, Glaser R. Psychoneuroimmunology and health consequences: data and shared mechanisms. *Psychosom Med* 1995;57:269–274.
107. Herbert T, Cohen S, Marsland A, Bachen E, et al. Cardiovascular reactivity and the course of immune response to an acute psychological stressor. *Psychosom Med* 1994;56:337–344.
108. O'Leary A. Stress, emotion, and human immune function. *Psychol Bull* 1990;108(3):363–382.
109. Zakowski S, McAllister C, Deal M, Baum A. Stress, reactivity, and immune function in healthy men. *Health Psychol* 1992;11(4):223–232.
110. Kusnecov A, Rabin B. Stressor induced alterations of immune function—mechanisms and issues. *Int Arch Allergy Immunol* 1994;105:107.
111. Esterling B, Antoni M, Kumar M. Emotional repression, stress disclosure responses and Epstein-Barr viral capsid antigen titers. *Psychosom Med* 1990;52:392–410.
112. Kiecolt-Glaser J, Speicher C, Holliday J, Glaser R. Stress and the transformation of lymphocytes by Epstein-Barr virus. *J Behav Med* 1984;7:1.
113. Khan M, Sansoni P, Silverman E, et al. Beta adrenergic receptors on human suppressor, helper, and cytolytic lymphocytes. *Biochem Pharmacol* 1986;35:1137.
114. Bachen E, Manuck S, Cohen S, et al. Adrenergic blockade ameliorates cellular immune responses to mental stress in humans. *Psychosom Med* 1995;57:366–372.
115. Kiecolt-Glazer J, Glaser R, Shuttleworth E, et al. Chronic stress and immunity in family care givers of Alzheimer's disease victims. *Psychosom Med* 1987;49:523–535.
116. McKinnon W, Weisse C, Reynolds C, et al. Chronic stress, leukocyte subpopulations and humoral response to latent viruses. *Health Psychol* 1989;8:389–402.
117. Heninger G. Neuroimmunology of stress. In: Friedman MJ, Charney DS, Deutch AY, eds. *Neurobiological and clinical consequences of stress: from normal adaptation to PTSD*. Philadelphia: Lippincott–Raven Publishers, 1995.
118. Irwin M, Mascovich A, Gillin C, et al. Partial sleep deprivation reduces natural killer cell activity in humans. *Psychosom Med;* 1994:56:493–498.
119. Peterson C, Stunkard A. Personal control and health promotion. *Soc Sci Med* 1989;28(8):819–828.
120. Guidotti T, Alexander R, Fedoruk M. Epidemiologic features that may distinguish between building-associated illness outbreaks due to chemical exposure or psychogenic origin. Brief Communication from building-associated outbreaks. *J Occup Med* 1987;29:148–150.
121. Boxer PA. Indoor air quality: a psychosocial perspective. *J Occup Med* 1990; 32:425–443.
122. Olkinuora M. Psychogenic epidemics and work. *Scand J Work Environ Health* 1984;10:501–504.
123. Colligan MJ. The psychological effects of indoor air pollution. *Bull N Y Acad Med* 1981;57:1014–1026.
124. Department of Health, Education, and Welfare. *A guide to work-relatedness of disease*. Cincinnati: National Institute for Occupational Safety and Health, 1979. [DHEW (NIOSH) Publication no 79-216].

SECTION

V

Specific Health Hazards and Toxins

CHAPTER 54

Hydrogen Cyanide and Inorganic Cyanide Salts

Steven C. Curry and Frank A. LoVecchio

SOURCES AND PRODUCTION

Hydrogen Cyanide

Hydrogen cyanide (HCN) has a boiling point of 27.7°C, allowing it to be found as a gas or liquid in the workplace (Table 54-1). As a gas, it is explosive, colorless, and has a faint odor that is variously described as bitter almonds, sweet, pungent, or metallic. Liquid HCN is a colorless or a bluish white solution that has a similar odor because of the release of HCN gas into surrounding air. Although most persons are able to smell HCN, the minority identify it as being similar to bitter almonds. Furthermore, wide individual variations in odor threshold and rapid olfactory fatigue make it possible for an entire group of persons to be exposed to toxic concentrations of HCN without anyone noticing any abnormal odor (1–3).

The main method used in manufacturing HCN in the United States involves reacting ammonia and methane in controlled conditions. HCN is also manufactured by reacting sodium carbonate with coke-oven gas, by reacting cyanide salts with mineral acids, by reacting ammonia with air and natural gas, and from the decomposition of formamide (4).

HCN is sold as a gas and is available as technical-grade liquids of various percentages. It is sold or transported in bottles, drums, cylinders, and tanks. Almost all grades of HCN contain a stabilizer, such as phosphoric acid, to prevent decomposition and explosion. Impure or unstable HCN can undergo spontaneous exothermic polymerization with explosive violence (4).

Inorganic Cyanide Salts

A number of inorganic cyanide salts are commercially available, and the more commonly used ones are summarized in Table 54-2. Sodium, potassium, and calcium cyanide [$Ca(CN)_2$] account for the majority of industrial consumption and are described in more detail.

Sodium and potassium cyanide are crystalline, white solids at room temperature. The three main methods of commercial production are reacting sodium or potassium carbonate with carbon and ammonia, reacting HCN with sodium or potassium hydroxide, or using a process involving coke-oven gas (4,5).

NaCN and KCN are sold as powders, flakes, granules, pillow-shaped 1-oz (28-g) blocks, or pellets or as aqueous solutions. On the commercial scale, solid NaCN and KCN are packed in steel or fiber drums before shipping. Aqueous solutions are shipped in tanks by truck or rail (4).

$Ca(CN)_2$ is manufactured by heating calcium cyanamide with a source of carbon in electric furnaces at temperatures greater than 1,000°C. $Ca(CN)_2$ is sold on the commercial scale as flakes or blocks (4,5).

Sites, Industries, and Businesses Associated with Exposures

HCN and inorganic cyanide salts are used in a wide variety of commercial processes. The National Institute of Occupational Safety and Health (NIOSH) estimates that 20,000 workers are exposed daily to NaCN alone (4). When one considers the plethora of cyanogenic compounds found in industry, tens of thousands of workers potentially come in contact with cyanide every working day.

Hydrogen Cyanide Formation from Cyanide Salts

The release of excessive amounts of HCN gas into the breathing zone of workers can result in collapse and death within seconds to minutes. Whereas workers frequently are aware of the potential danger when using liquid or gaseous HCN, they typically are unaware of the great potential for formation of lethal quantities of HCN from processes using cyanide salts.

When most inorganic cyanide salts come in contact with mineral acids, large quantities of HCN are formed and are released into the atmosphere. Using NaCN and hydrochloric acid as an example

$$NaCN + HCl \rightarrow HCN + NaCl$$

Two common scenarios for generation of HCN include the accidental mixing of acid and cyanide solutions in electroplating baths and the accidental pouring of cyanide waste solutions into acid waste containers or into other waste solutions with pHs less than 10.5 to 11.

Even less recognized by workers is the potential for generation of large quantities of HCN simply from mixing water-soluble cyanide salts with water. NaCN, for example, dissolves in water according to the following equilibrium:

$$NaCN \longleftrightarrow Na^+ + CN^-$$

Sodium cyanide is relatively soluble in water, and large quantities of free CN^- ions are formed. However, the pK_a of HCN is relatively high at 9.3. Therefore, CN^- splits water to form HCN according to the following reaction:

$$CN^- + H_2O \longleftrightarrow HCN + OH^-$$

TABLE 54-1. Chemical and physical properties of hydrogen cyanide

Molecular formula	HCN
Atomic weight	27.03
Physical form	Liquid or gas
Boiling point	27.7°C for a 96% solution
Freezing point	−16.8°C for a 96% solution
Color	Colorless to tint of blue
Odor	Variously described as bitter almond, metallic, sweet; not detectable by many persons with wide variation in odor threshold
Water solubility	Very miscible
Density	0.7 g/mL for a 96% solution
Vapor density	0.93 (air = 1)
Vapor pressure	807 mm Hg
Flashpoint	−17.8°C (closed cup)
Lower explosive limit	6% by volume in air
Upper explosive limit	41% by volume in air
pK_a	9.3 at 25°C
1 mg HCN/m^3	0.906 ppm
1 ppm HCN	1.104 mg/m^3

In the case of NaCN, the entire reaction becomes:

$$NaCN + H_2O \longleftrightarrow HCN + NaOH$$

The percentage of cyanide converted to HCN in aqueous solutions of cyanide salts is dependent on the pH of the solution, as illustrated in Figure 54-1. HCN's pK_a of 9.3 makes it necessary for pHs to be more than 10.5 to 11 to prevent formation and release of significant quantities of HCN.

An employee who does nothing but add a cyanide salt to pure water (pH 7) or to tap water can initially cause the generation of lethal quantities of HCN before enough hydroxide (e.g., NaOH) is formed to raise pH and limit HCN formation. Simply using a stream of water to clean up a spill of cyanide salts (e.g., rinsing them into a drain or mopping the floor) can result in serious poisonings and fatalities. Poisonings and deaths from the inhalation or dermal absorption of HCN have occurred when workers contaminated with powdered inorganic cyanide salts have decontaminated themselves in water showers, but continued to wear wet clothing rather than undress (6).

Metal Extraction and Recovery

Aqueous solutions of cyanide are able to complex with gold and silver to form compounds that remain soluble in alkaline solutions of cyanide salts. On the smallest scale, a person may reclaim gold and silver in his or her home by placing old jewelry in small jars of alkaline cyanide solutions. On the largest scale, copper mines maintain lakes and ponds containing hundreds of thousands of gallons of aqueous alkaline cyanide salts for extracting gold, silver, and other metals from impure ore. Operations of intermediate scale involve crushing waste products containing precious metals (e.g., circuit boards, transistors, used x-ray film) and then agitating them in rotary drums containing alkaline cyanide solutions.

Once the desired metal has moved into solution by complexing with cyanide, the metal is extracted back out of solution by various methodologies, including electroplating the metal out of solution onto a cathode.

The most commonly used cyanide salts in metal leeching operations are NaCN, KCN, and $Ca(CN)_2$ (4). Because cyanide is converted to HCN in aqueous solutions of these salts at pHs near and less than the pK_a of HCN, solutions are kept alkaline, with typical pHs ranging from 10.5 to 12. This often involves the addition of sodium or potassium hydroxide.

In metal reclaiming operations, several sources of exposure to cyanide salts exist. Skin contact with granular cyanide salts can occur during the preparation of leeching solutions. Improper techniques may allow for skin contact with alkaline cyanide solutions (7,8) during the leeching process from splashing of the solution out of the mixing container, from reaching into the solution to retrieve work pieces or to agitate the mixture, or from mists created above tanks of metal-cyanide solution during the electroplating phase. Contamination of air with significant amounts of granular cyanide salts (9) or with fine mists of cyanide solutions (10,11) may also result in inhalation and mucous membrane contact (mouth, throat, nose, large airways) with cyanide.

Electroplating

In electroplating operations, a metal-cyanide salt is dissolved in an electroplating bath containing pieces that are to be plated serving as cathodes. As current flows through the bath, the metal is reduced and deposited on the desired substrate. Many different metals can be plated in this manner, including gold, silver, copper, cadmium, zinc, tin, and indium.

Scenarios for employee contact with cyanide in electroplating operations are the same as those from metal reclaiming operations. Most electroplating baths contain NaCN or KCN in addition to the metal-cyanide, making it mandatory that plating solutions be kept at alkaline pHs. However, some gold electroplating operations can be performed at neutral or mildly acidic pHs if sodium or potassium cyanoaurite ($Na[Au(CN)_2]$ or $K[Au(CN)_2]$) is used as the source of gold in the bath. During normal electroplating operations, sodium and potassium cyanoaurite do not release large quantities of HCN when dissolved in water or weak acids, although adequate ventilation is required to prevent accumulation of HCN. It has been suggested that death after suicidal ingestion of $Na[Au(CN)_2]$ does not appear to be from cyanide poisoning (12). If significant quantities of sodium or potassium cyanoaurite mix with strong mineral acids, however, large amounts of HCN can be quickly formed.

Pesticides

Cyanide compounds are used in agricultural and horticultural pest control. Cyanide fumigation powders containing NaCN or $Ca(CN)_2$ are sprinkled on floors or down rodent burrows. In the presence of water, HCN is released and reaches lethal concentrations in air. In the case of $Ca(CN)_2$, moisture in the air is enough to allow for significant HCN formation by the following formulas:

$$Ca(CN)_2 + H_2O \rightarrow Ca(OH)CN + HCN$$

$$Ca(OH)CN + H_2O \rightarrow Ca(OH)_2 + HCN$$

Earlier in the twentieth century, death from HCN exposure during fumigation was not rare. For example, five sailors died after dropping cyanide eggs into vats of acid while fumigating a ship (13). In 1935, Cousineau and Legg reported that one human death occurred for every 2,000 cyanide fumigations in Detroit (14).

Metal Hardening

The penetration of a metal's surface by nascent carbon and nitrogen results in a hardened, weather-resistant exterior. One method to achieve this end is called *cyaniding*, and involves heating the metal in a liquid solution, such as NaCN, NaCl, and Na_2CO_3 in the presence of atmospheric oxygen (4,5).

At temperatures more than 50°C, NaCN decomposes to formate and ammonia:

TABLE 54-2. Chemical and physical properties of selected cyanide salts

Compound	Molecular formula	CAS number	Atomic weight	RTECS number	Synonyms	Comments
Ammonium cyanide	NH_4CN	12211-52-8	44.1	—	—	Very soluble in cold H_2O; decomposes at 36°C to form HCN and NH_3
Barium cyanide	$Ba(CN)_2$	542-62-1	189.4	CQ8785000	Barium dicyanide; UN 1565 (DOT)	Very soluble in H_2O
Cadmium cyanide	$Cd(CN)_2$	542-83-6	164.5	—	—	Solubility in H_2O 1.7 g/100 mL at 15°C
Calcium cyanide	$Ca(CN)_2$	592-01-8	92.1	EW0700000	Calccyanide; UN 1575 (DOT)	Releases HCN in H_2O or humid air
Copper (I) cyanide	CuCN	544-92-3	89.6	GL7150000	Cuprous cyanide	Almost insoluble in H_2O; decomposed by H_2NO_3
Copper (II) cyanide	$Cu(CN)_2$	14763-77-0	115.6	GL7175000	Cupric cyanide; copper cyanamide; UN 1587 (DOT)	Insoluble in H_2O
Gold (I) cyanide	AuCN	506-65-0	223	—	Aurous cyanide; gold monocyanide	Insoluble in H_2O or dilute acids; releases HCN when heated in HCl; dissolved by aqua regia; ignition causes formation of metallic gold and CN
Gold (II) cyanide	$Au(CN)_2$	535-37-5	275.05	—	Auric cyanide; gold tricyanide	Usually found as trihydrate $Au(CN)_2(H_2O)_3$ with a molecular weight of 329.1; very soluble in H_2O; decomposes at 50°C
Lead cyanide	$Pb(CN)_2$	592-05-2	259.2	OG0175000	C.I. pigment yellow 48; UN 1620 (DOT)	Slightly soluble in cold H_2O; soluble in hot H_2O
Mercury (II) cyanide	$Hg(CN)_2$	592-04-1	252.6	OW1515000	Mercuric cyanide; cyanuria; UN 1636 (DOT)	Solubility in cold H_2O of 9.3 g/100 mL
Potassium cyanide	KCN	151-50-8	65.1	TS8750000	Cyanide of potassium; UN 1680 (DOT)	Solubility in cold H_2O of 50 g/mL; yields HCN on contact with H_2O or acids
Potassium cyanoaurite	$K[Au(CN)_2]$	13967-50-5	288.1	—	Gold potassium cyanide; potassium aurocyanide; potassium dicyanoaurate (I); aurate (1–), bis(cyano-C-), potassium	Less HCN liberated from aqueous or weakly acidic solutions than with other water-soluble salts
Silver cyanide	AgCN	506-64-9	133.9	VW3850000	UN1684 (DOT)	Almost insoluble in H_2O and dilute acid, *but* dilute HCl causes formation of HCN and $AgCl_2$
Sodium cyanide	NaCN	143-33-9	49.0	VZ7525000	Cyanide of sodium	Solubility in cold H_2O of 48 g/100 mL; yields HCN on contact with water or dilute acids
Sodium cyanoaurite	$Na[Au(CN)_2]$	15280-09-8	272.0	—	Gold sodium cyanide; sodium dicyanoaurate (I); aurate (1–), bis(cyano-C)-, sodium	Less HCN liberated from aqueous and weakly acidic solutions than with other salts
Zinc cyanide	$Zn(CN)_2$	557-21-1	117.4	ZH1575000	Zinc dicyanide	Insoluble in H_2O; readily releases HCN on contact with mineral acids

CAS, Chemical Abstracts Service; HCN, hydrogen cyanide; RTECS, Registry of Toxic Effects of Chemical Substances; DOT, U.S. Department of Transportation.

$$NaCN + 2\ H_2O \rightarrow NH_3 + HCOONa$$

The presence of NaCl in the cyanide solution retards NaCN's decomposition to ammonia and formate. NaCl, however, enhances the hydrolysis of NaCN to HCN at temperatures less than 80°C.

Skin contact with hot solutions can result in burns, allowing for enhanced absorption of cyanide through injured skin. Splashes or mists of cyanide solution allow for mucous membrane, inhalational, and skin exposure to cyanide. Of course, if the pH of the solution falls, HCN can be released in large quantities, especially in the presence of heat and NaCl.

MISCELLANEOUS USES OF CYANIDE

Table 54-3 lists various commercial applications for cyanide. $Ca(CN)_2$ is used as a cement stabilizer. Cyanides are essential for the synthesis of various inorganic and organic chemicals, including plastics and rubbers.

Many metal polishes contain NaCN or KCN. Poisonings were reported in the early 1900s when workers rubbed tar-

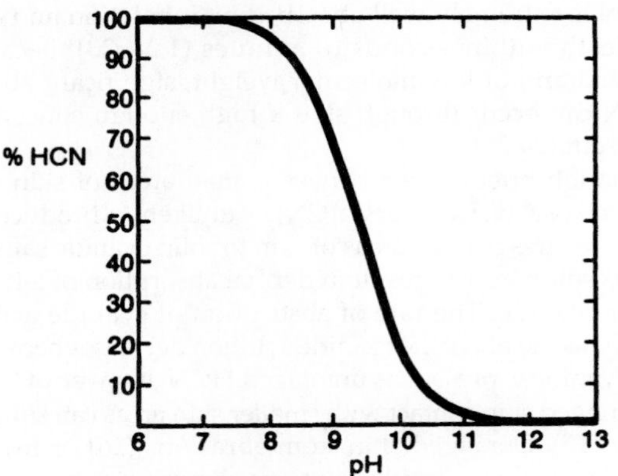

Figure 54-1. Percentage of cyanide present as hydrogen cyanide in an aqueous solution of a cyanide salt is dependent on the pH of the solution. The pK_a of hydrogen cyanide is 9.3. HCN, hydrogen cyanide.

TABLE 54-3. Occupations of manufacturing process associated with cyanide exposure

Dyeing	Metal hardening
Printing	Paper production
Soldering	Cement stabilizer
Metallurgy	Chemical synthesis
Fumigators	Rubber manufacturing
Firefighting	Leather manufacturing
Photography	Plastics manufacturing
Electroplating	Synthetic fiber production
Metal polishing	Precious metal extraction
Mirror making	Pesticide workers and manufacturing

nished silver with chunks of cyanide salts or removed silver stains from their hands by vigorously rubbing skin with pieces of KCN (15). Of course, the ingestion of a cyanide-containing metal polish can result in severe poisoning and death (16).

HCN is commonly found in smoke (17–19), including that from cigarettes. The burning of most organic compounds containing carbon and nitrogen can generate HCN under the correct conditions (20). Firefighters are commonly exposed to atmospheres containing significant quantities of HCN, and cyanide poisoning may be a major factor in death from smoke inhalation, especially in fires involving plastics.

CLINICAL TOXICOLOGY OF EXPOSURE

Route of Exposure

The main routes of exposure to cyanide in the industrial setting are from skin contact and inhalation (4). Exposure to air containing cyanide dust or mists of aqueous cyanide salts may also allow for significant mucous membrane contact. The placing of contaminated hands into the mouth or the inhalation of dusts or mists may also allow for swallowing and gastrointestinal absorption of cyanide compounds.

Because cyanide salts are rapidly absorbed from mucous membranes, symptoms after acute inhalation of or mucous membrane contact with toxic concentrations of cyanide salts may begin within seconds to a few minutes after exposure (7,9). A worker who accidentally receives a mouthful of aqueous or powdered cyanide may quickly collapse. However, the absorption of cyanide from the gastrointestinal tract is slower, allowing for delayed toxicity if cyanide compounds are swallowed, assuming survival after initial mucous membrane contact with the poison.

HCN is extremely well absorbed by inhalation and can produce death within seconds to minutes (1,21–23). Because it is unionized and of low molecular weight, significant absorption of HCN can occur through skin if high enough concentrations are present (24,25).

Although brief contact between small areas of skin and dry, powdered NaCN, KCN, or $Ca(CN)_2$ is unlikely to produce toxicity, short exposures of large areas of skin to solid cyanide salts or their aqueous solutions can result in dermal absorption of lethal quantities of cyanide. The rate of absorption of cyanide across skin increases as the pH of the cyanide solution decreases because more of the cyanide is present as unionized HCN at lower pHs (6).

Prolonged skin contact with smaller skin areas can still produce toxicity (15). Damaged skin from abrasions (26) or from burns caused by alkaline cyanide solutions allows for increased dermal absorption of cyanide. In contrast to the rapid onset of symptoms from the inhalation of HCN, the onset of symptoms after large, acute dermal exposures sometimes may be delayed for as long as 30 minutes if decontamination has not been effective, especially if the worker continues to wear wet, contaminated clothing (6).

In many instances, several routes of exposure to cyanide may exist. A 19-year-old male who collapsed after a bag of powdered KCN burst in his face probably experienced inhalational, dermal, and mucosal contact with the powder (9). One male died and two males were found comatose after working in a truck that threw $Ca(CN)_2$ powder 24 ft at a height of 6 ft onto grapevines (27). Probable exposures included inhalational, mucosal, and dermal contact with the powder as well as inhalation of HCN formed when $Ca(CN)_2$ reacted with water vapor.

Metabolism

Humans detoxify cyanide by transferring sulfane sulfur [$R\text{-}SO_{(x)}\text{-}S^-$] to cyanide, thus converting it to thiocyanate (SCN^-). Thiocyanate is excreted in the urine with an elimination half-life of approximately 2.5 days in those with normal renal function (28).

Two main enzymes are thought to be capable of converting cyanide to thiocyanate (29,30). The first is rhodanese (thiosulfate sulfurtransferase, EC 2.8.1.1), an enzyme restricted to mitochondria. Rhodanese is found in various tissues, especially liver, kidney, and skeletal muscle. The most commonly described reaction catalyzed by rhodanese involves the transfer of a sulfur atom from thiosulfate ($S_2O_3^{2-}$), a source of sulfane sulfur, to cyanide:

$$CN^- + S_2O_3^{2-} \rightarrow SCN^- + SO_3^{2-}$$

The second enzyme capable of forming thiocyanate transfers sulfur from mercaptopyruvate to cyanide and is named β-mercaptopyruvate-cyanide sulfurtransferase (EC 2.8.1.2).

$$HSCH_2COCOO^- + CN^- \rightarrow SCN^- + CH_3COCOO^-$$

In addition to being found in liver and kidneys, this latter enzyme is also found within erythrocytes (30).

Although rhodanese has traditionally been credited with cyanide's detoxication, current data indicate that this may not in fact be true. Thiosulfate, a substrate for rhodanese, is thought to be unable to penetrate the inner mitochondrial membrane where rhodanese is located (31,32). Ballantyne and others (30,31,33) suggest an overall scheme whereby numerous sulfur sources are acted on by various sulfurtransferases, including rhodanese and mercaptopyruvate sulfurtransferase, to form sulfur, which then complexes with albumin in blood. A nonenzymatic reaction of the sulfane-albumin complex with cyanide may actually account for thiocyanate formation. This hypothesis is in keeping with kinetic studies suggesting that cyanide detoxication takes place in a volume of distribution similar to blood volume (34).

However, other data clearly demonstrate that the albumin-sulfane complex appears to play a minor role in the *in vivo* detoxication of cyanide. In bloodless rats in which blood is replaced by a fluorocarbon emulsion, sodium thiosulfate still efficiently antagonizes cyanide (35). In the absence of blood or circulating albumin, cyanide's detoxication can only be attributed to sulfurtransferase reactions occurring in tissue sites other than blood.

Out of these disparate data, investigators agree that sulfane sulfur, such as thiosulfate, is required for and greatly accelerates detoxication of cyanide by converting cyanide to thiocyanate, regardless of mechanism.

Cyanide is rapidly taken up and sequestered by red blood cells (36,37). Such action does not appear to enhance the metabolism of cyanide, but might act to partially lessen toxicity by preventing the diffusion of cyanide out of blood into tissues.

Cyanide's affinity for the cobalt ion (Co^{2+}) causes it to combine with hydroxocobalamin to form cyanocobalamin, which is then excreted in the urine and bile. This route of detoxication normally plays a minor role in acute cyanide poisoning. The administration

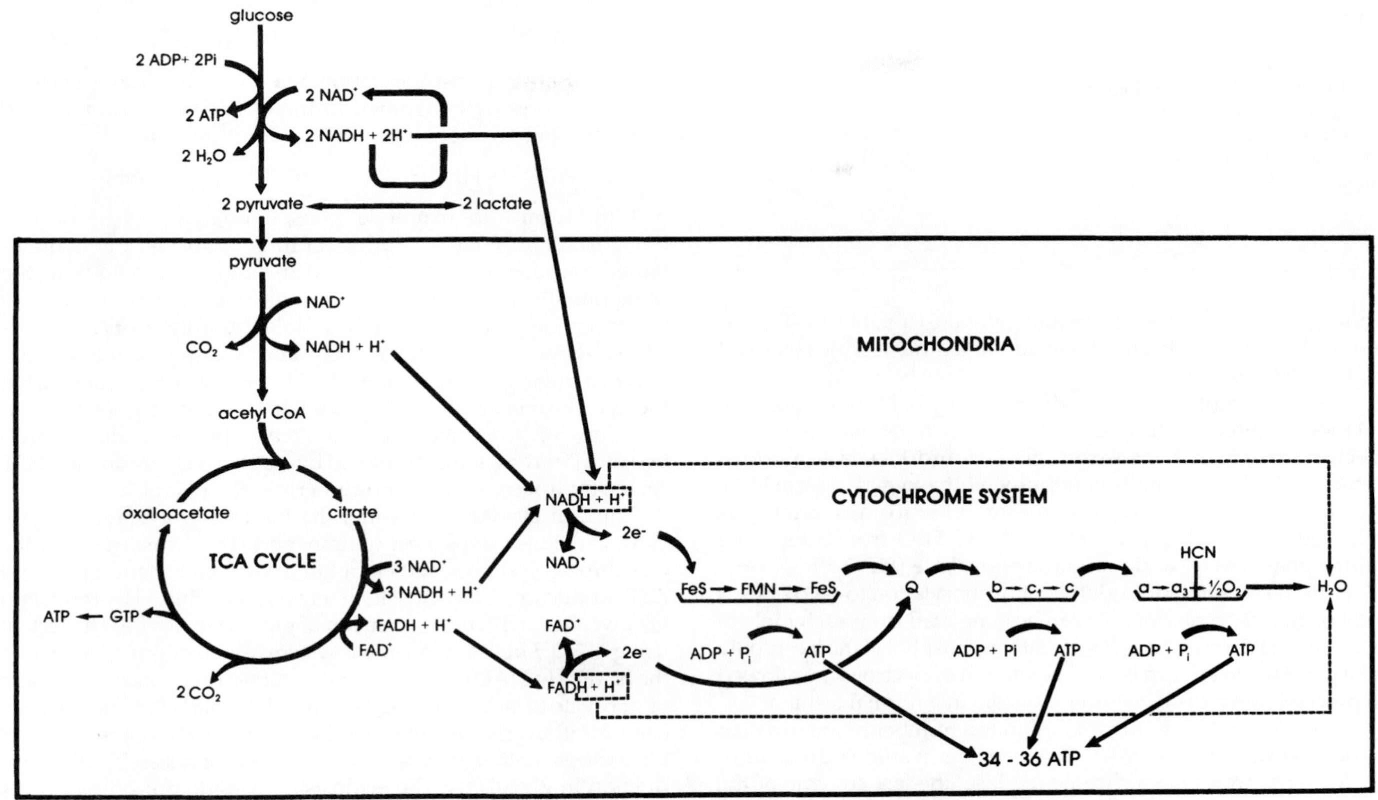

Figure 54-2. Simplified, schematic diagram of cellular adenosine triphosphate production. a, cytochrome a; a_3, cytochrome a_3; acetyl CoA, acetyl coenzyme A; ADP, adenosine diphosphate; ATP, adenosine triphosphate; b, cytochrome b; c, cytochrome c; c_1, cytochrome c_1; FAD^+, oxidized flavin adenine dinucleotide; FADH, reduced flavin adenine dinucleotide; FeS, iron-sulfur protein; FMN, flavin mononucleotide; GTP, guanosine triphosphate; NAD^+, oxidized nicotinamide adenine dinucleotide; NADH, reduced nicotinamide adenine dinucleotide; P_i, inorganic phosphate; Q, coenzyme Q; TCA cycle, tricarboxylic acid cycle (Krebs cycle).

The conversion of 1 mol glucose to 2 mol pyruvate via glycolysis produces a net 2 mol adenosine triphosphate. Normally, pyruvate enters the mitochondrion where it is metabolized in the tricarboxylic acid cycle (Krebs cycle) to produce reduced nicotinamide adenine dinucleotide and reduced flavin adenine dinucleotide. Electrons donated by reduced nicotinamide adenine dinucleotide and reduced flavin adenine dinucleotide are transported down the cytochrome system and eventually onto oxygen. Energy released during electron transport is harnessed to generate the great majority of the cell's adenosine triphosphate (oxidative phosphorylation). Depending on the mechanism by which reduced nicotinamide adenine dinucleotide from glycolysis is shuttled into the mitochondrion, a total of 36 to 38 mol adenosine triphosphate (including the indirect synthesis of adenosine triphosphate from guanosine triphosphate in the tricarboxylic acid cycle and adenosine triphosphate generated in glycolysis) can be generated from each mole of glucose.

Cytochrome oxidase comprises cytochrome a and cytochrome a_3. Hydrogen cyanide combines with cytochrome a_3 of cytochrome oxidase and interrupts electron transport, causing a decline in oxygen consumption and oxidative phosphorylation. Adenosine triphosphate production in glycolysis (glucose to lactate) becomes an increasingly important pathway for adenosine triphosphate synthesis as oxidative phosphorylation is impaired. Although lactate concentrations rise in cyanide poisoning, they are not responsible for metabolic acidosis (see text).

of large amounts of hydroxocobalamin, however, is used as antidotal therapy in some countries (38). Hydroxocobalamin is not available in suitable form for this purpose in the United States.

Pathophysiology

The major immediate energy source for living cells is adenosine triphosphate (ATP). ATP is mainly produced either in the cytoplasm via glycolysis or through oxidative phosphorylation in the mitochondrion (Fig. 54-2).

In glycolysis, two moles of ATP are generated from the metabolism of each mole of glucose to pyruvate. Glycolysis can proceed in the absence of oxygen as long as pyruvate is converted to lactate, regenerating nicotinamide adenine dinucleotide (NAD^+). Unfortunately, the minimal amount of ATP produced in glycolysis does not support life except in selected tissues (e.g., erythrocytes).

In the mitochondrion, pyruvate from glycolysis is decarboxylated before combining with oxaloacetate to form citrate, the first step in the tricarboxylic acid cycle (Krebs cycle). Citrate then

TABLE 54-4. Partial list of enzymes inhibited by cyanide

Xanthine oxidase
Carbonic anhydrase
Nitrite reductase
2-Keto-4-hydroglutarate aldolase
Acetoacetate decarboxylase
Cytochrome oxidase
Succinate dehydrogenase
Glutamic acid decarboxylase

Adapted from refs. 31 and 39, with permission.

undergoes a series of reactions that generate CO_2, H_2O, GTP, and reduced nicotinamide and flavin adenine dinucleotides (NADH and FADH, respectively).

The major route of ATP production is by oxidative phosphorylation in mitochondria. In the inner mitochondrial membrane, electrons are transferred from NADH and FADH to various cytochromes before finally combining with oxygen to form H_2O. As electrons are transferred among cytochromes, energy is released and used to generate ATP and H_2O from adenosine diphosphate (ADP) and inorganic phosphate (HPO_4^{2-}).

With the addition of oxidative phosphorylation to glycolysis, a total of 36 to 38 moles of ATP can be generated from each mole of glucose. ATP production via oxidative phosphorylation can only take place when oxygen is present and when electrons are allowed to proceed down the cytochrome system in a normal fashion.

Cyanide combines with and inhibits a number of mammalian enzymes (31,39) (Table 54-4). However, it is cyanide's great affinity for ferric iron in cytochrome oxidase, the last enzyme of the cytochrome system, that appears to account for the majority of its toxicity. At physiologic pH, most cyanide in the body is present as HCN. By combining with cytochrome oxidase, HCN prevents electron transport in the cytochrome system, bringing oxidative phosphorylation and the majority of the cell's ATP production to a halt (see Fig. 54-2) (34). Cyanide's ability to inhibit glutamate decarboxylase may result in a fall in brain γ-aminobutyric acid (GABA) concentrations and contribute toward convulsions (40).

A metabolic acidosis and fall in oxygen consumption always accompany serious cyanide poisoning. The metabolic acidosis deserves particular discussion because most authors have incorrectly attributed acidosis to elevated circulating lactate concentrations resulting from glycolytic conversion of glucose to lactate. Unquestionably, as ATP production via oxidative phosphorylation is impaired, the conversion of glucose to lactate via glycolysis is accelerated and becomes an important source of ATP, resulting in elevated lactate concentrations. However, ATP production via the conversion of glucose to lactate is not acidifying; it does not produce a net increase in the number of hydrogen ions (41–43). For example, Gevers (44) illustrated glycolysis at pH 8.2:

$$\text{glucose} + 2\,ADP^{3-} + 2\,HPO_4^{2-} + 10\,H^+ \rightarrow$$
$$2\,\text{lactate}^- + 2\,ATP^{4-} + 2\,H_2O + 10\,H^+$$

The amounts of ATP and lactate generated in glycolysis certainly vary according to cellular pH and concentrations of available substrates (42). However, the fact that glycolytic production of lactic acid and ATP is not acidifying holds true regardless of pH (42,45,46).

An understanding of the generation of ATP in oxidative phosphorylation and of ATP's hydrolysis in metabolic processes explains the metabolic acidosis accompanying cyanide poisoning. Viable cells use ATP as an energy source by hydrolyzing ATP to ADP and phosphate. The hydrolysis of ATP results in the net production of hydrogen ions (42). Again, pH and concentrations of available substrates influence dissociation of hydrogen ions from ATP, ADP, and phosphate. A net increase in hydrogen ion concentration always occurs from the hydrolysis of ATP.

$$ATP^{4-} + 4\,H^+ + H_2O \rightarrow ADP^{3-} + HPO_4^{2-} + 5\,H^+$$

In oxidative phosphorylation via the cytochrome system, hydrogen ions are consumed in the opposite reaction as ATP and water are generated from ADP and phosphate:

$$ADP^{3-} + HPO_4^{2-} + 5\,H^+ \rightarrow ATP^{4-} + H_2O + 4\,H^+$$

With regard to oxidative phosphorylation, when normal homeostatic mechanisms are operating, a normal pH is maintained because ATP is being used throughout the body at the same rate it is being produced in mitochondria. In other words, hydrogen ion production via the cellular hydrolysis of ATP is balanced by the ability of the cytochrome system to use hydrogen ions in aerobic generation of ATP (45). When electron transport in the cytochrome system is impaired and oxidative phosphorylation slows or stops, hydrogen ions created by the cellular hydrolysis of ATP are no longer buffered by aerobic ATP production (42). As the hydrogen ion concentration rises, the pH falls.

Thus, in cyanide poisoning, the binding of cyanide to cytochrome oxidase stops electron transport. This impairment of the cytochrome system results in a fall in oxygen consumption and ATP production. Cells must then rely on anaerobic ATP production via glycolysis with the conversion of glucose to lactate. The lack of using NADH in the cytochrome system also results in elevation of the NADH to NAD ratio, a factor that serves to enhance conversion of pyruvate to lactate (42). Although cellular and circulating lactate concentrations rise, the elevated lactate levels are not responsible for acidosis. Rather, they serve as a marker for anaerobic ATP production in glycolysis. The acidosis of cyanide poisoning occurs because cells hydrolyze ATP generated in glycolysis, producing H^+, while, at the same time, the ability to buffer hydrogen ions via oxidative phosphorylation is impaired. In fact, any metabolic or physiologic imbalance resulting in a greater hydrolysis of ATP than synthesis of ATP in oxidative phosphorylation can result in metabolic acidosis, whether it be from impaired oxidative phosphorylation or excessive ATP consumption by tissue (42,45).

Acute Cyanide Poisoning

Several reasons exist why cyanide poisoning is mainly characterized by dysfunction of the cardiovascular and central nervous system. In the face of acidosis and falling ATP concentrations from impaired oxidative phosphorylation, organs most sensitive to energy deprivation (brain, heart) are affected first. Cytochrome oxidase in the heart is also more sensitive to inhibition by cyanide (47). Finally, cyanide concentrations are higher in brain and myocardium than in other organs at the time of death (31).

Central nervous system abnormalities range from agitation and anxiety to confusion, lethargy, coma, convulsions, and cerebral death. Initial stimulation of carotid body receptors by relatively low concentrations of cyanide results in tachypnea. However, lethal concentrations of cyanide rapidly produce apnea.

Cardiovascular toxicity early in cyanide poisoning results in tachycardia and, at times, hypertension. In more serious or lethal poisonings, hypotension, bradyarrhythmias, heart blocks, ventricular arrhythmias, and asystole develop. Wexler and colleagues (48) recorded electrocardiographic changes in 16 males who received intravenous injections of up to 0.2 mg cyanide per kg body weight (one subject experienced a "momentary dim-out"). Respiratory stimulation was immediately preceded by sinus arrests lasting from 0.88 to 4.2 seconds, which were thought to be vagally mediated. Immediately after sinus arrests, irregularities in sinus rhythms with slowing of heart rates occurred for periods of a few seconds to as long as 2 minutes. This was then followed by gradual accelerations of heart rates to levels higher than control values. These investigators also reported on electrocardiographic changes in four males executed by inhalation of HCN. Among various arrhythmias reported, a progressive shortening of the ST segment was noted until, terminally, the T wave originated on the R wave. This T on R phenomenon has since been noted in other cases of severe cyanide poisoning (49).

Nonspecific findings accompanying many cases of cyanide poisoning include diaphoresis, weakness, nausea, and vomiting (23). Other abnormalities resulting from impaired ATP production include rhabdomyolysis, renal failure, hepatic necrosis, and adult respiratory distress syndrome (31,50,51).

Because of their alkaline nature, solid or aqueous solutions of cyanide salts can produce corrosive injury when coming in contact with moist mucosal surfaces, including the gastrointestinal tract. Severe skin burns can also occur after acute dermal contact with alkaline cyanide solutions (8).

Patients who survive severe poisoning may be left with permanent neurologic deficits, including lesions in the basal ganglia (52,53). Lesions in the basal ganglia are not specific for cyanide, but are seen after severe hypoxemia or after poisoning by many metabolic toxins, including carbon monoxide and methanol.

The minimal amount of HCN required to produce death in humans is not definitely known as most acute poisonings are secondary to massive overdoses. Fatal doses of HCN vary among different species, making exact extrapolation to humans difficult. In general, these animal data indicate that prolonged exposures to HCN concentrations more than 90 parts per million (ppm) are incompatible with life, and concentrations ranging from 10 to 45 ppm may produce a plethora of symptoms with thresholds in each species difficult to determine with certainty (4).

Commonly reported dose-response relationships in humans for inhalation of HCN usually have been referenced to a 1931 publication by Flury and Zernik (54), or to other authors who, in turn, reference Flury and Zernik. However, Flury and Zernik referred to data by Lehmann and Hess that cannot be located (4). McNamara (55) has since pointed out that Lehmann worked almost entirely with rabbits, a species more sensitive to HCN than humans.

From cases of human exposures in which air concentrations of HCN have been reported, several generalizations can be made. Headache, metallic taste, and other minor symptoms may develop after several minutes of exposure to 10 to 30 ppm HCN in breathing air (4). Death may occur within 1 hour when breathing 100 ppm HCN (4,31), and fatalities have been reported after exposure to more than 300 ppm for a few minutes. Survival has been reported after a 90-second exposure to HCN at an estimated concentration of 453 to 557 ppm, and after 3 minutes' exposure to 500 ppm HCN (21,22). Ballantyne has suggested an inhalational 5-minute median lethal concentration(LC_{50}) for HCN of 680 ppm, and a 30-minute LC_{50} of 200 ppm (31).

The lethal oral dose of HCN is estimated to be approximately 50 mg in an adult. Oral ingestion of 5 mL of 20% hydrocyanic acid has been fatal. Lethal oral doses of KCN or NaCN are estimated to be 200 to 300 mg. However, survival has been reported after much larger ingestions, with intensive supportive care (49,50,56).

Chronic Exposures

Skin contact with aqueous solutions of cyanide salts can be irritating because of the alkaline pH of such liquids (57,58). Prolonged contact with alkaline cyanide solutions may result in severe corrosive burns (8). Deep burns from cyanide-containing electroplating solutions may require several weeks to heal, possibly because of metals also present in the bath. Topical contact with HCN may produce a blotchy rash of the face (4). Dermatitis associated with gold cyanide electroplating has also been attributed to hydrazine present in plating solutions (59). Some authors believe that allergic reactions to metals in the solutions or to cyanide itself may contribute to dermatitis (60).

Cyanide salts are also irritating to the upper respiratory tract. Chronic nasal mucosal irritation and ulceration of the nasal septum have been noted in electroplaters (61,62). Caution must be taken before attributing such changes to cyanide, however, because many metals used in electroplating operations (e.g., chromium, nickel) can cause identical findings. Cohen reported no irritating effects in electroplaters breathing air cyanide concentrations of 0.006 mg per m^3 (63).

Several authors have discussed the possibility of chronic systemic cyanide poisoning resulting from industrial exposure to cyanide (64–67). Suggested disorders resulting from long-term, low-level cyanide exposure have included headache, weakness, dysgeusia, vomiting, abdominal pain, chest pain, and nervousness. After an extensive review of the world's literature, NIOSH concluded that convincing evidence for chronic cyanide poisoning from regular exposures to air cyanide concentrations less than 10 ppm is lacking (4). Almost all such symptoms are subjective (e.g., headache, nausea, nervousness) and can be produced by a multitude of stress factors in any working environment. In most reports describing chronic cyanide poisoning, cyanide levels in air were not reported or were reported as area measurements that may not have reflected cyanide concentrations in the breathing zone near plating baths or other cyanide solutions. In some reports describing electroplating operations, articles suggest such poor housekeeping that dermal contact with cyanide solutions seemed likely. Most important, reports using control groups of workers with whom to compare symptoms are the exception.

Some workers may experience recurrent signs and symptoms of mild cyanide poisoning (e.g., headache, lightheadedness, nausea, metallic or bitter almond taste) each time they work for significant amounts of time in air containing cyanide concentrations more than 10 to 20 ppm. Furthermore, repeated episodes of acute, severe cyanide poisoning may be accompanied by serious neurotoxicity and result in permanent neurologic deficits (23). Although no convincing data exist to suggest permanent effects from working in air containing 10 ppm cyanide, NIOSH recognized that some workers did develop a constellation of subjective symptoms when working in air with average cyanide concentrations between 7 and 10 ppm. Partly because transient exposures to air cyanide concentrations far more than 10 ppm can occur when 8-hour time-weighted average concentrations are 5 ppm, NIOSH recommended that the 8-hour time-weighted average permissible exposure limit for all cyanide be changed to a 10-minute ceiling limit of 5 mg per m^3 in 1976 (4).

Thiocyanate competes with iodine for thyroidal uptake, potentially producing hypothyroidism (68,69). Because of thiocyanate's long elimination half-life, concern has been raised that accumulation of thiocyanate in those chronically exposed to cyanide may result in goiters (70,71). El Ghawabi reported mild to moderate thyroid enlargement in 36 electroplaters exposed to cyanide for many years (71). Air concentrations of cyanide averaged between 6.4 and 10.4 ppm. Nevertheless, Hartung (72) notes that the occurrence of thyroid abnormalities after long-term cyanide exposures has been only rarely reported. In fact, rats sensitive to goitrogenic agents that were fed food containing up to 300 ppm HCN did not develop changes in the thyroid, even though tissue levels of thiocyanate were elevated (73). Finally, others have suggested that smoking (a source of cyanide) has more of an influence on urinary thiocyanate levels than occupational exposure to cyanide at concentrations less than 8 ppm (74). This implies that occupational exposures to cyanide less than 8 ppm are no more likely to produce thyroid disease than smoking.

No data could be located to suggest that occupational exposure to cyanide is carcinogenic or mutagenic.

The continuous subcutaneous infusion of NaCN into gravid Golden Syrian hamsters was embryofetotoxic during organogenesis, especially with regard to neural tube development (75). However, even at the lowest cyanide dose, some maternal toxicity was evident. No data could be located suggesting that maternal exposures to cyanide concentrations that do not produce maternal toxicity are embryofetotoxic. However, studies in this area are notably lacking.

Diagnosis

In blood, most cyanide is concentrated within red blood cells, making red cell cyanide concentrations many-fold higher than those in plasma (36,37). Plasma cyanide is in equilibrium with tissue cyanide and reliably correlates with tissue cyanide levels (37,76). The higher levels of cyanide found in red cells are more easily measured, and red cell cyanide concentrations correlate with those in plasma and tissue. This explains why red blood cell cyanide concentrations can be used to confirm the diagnosis of cyanide poisoning.

It is important to note that cyanide levels as commonly performed by laboratories do not provide accurate measurements of whole blood cyanide concentrations. During acidification of whole blood during analysis, oxyhemoglobin released from red cells combines with thiosulfate in plasma or serum to generate HCN (36). Reported whole blood cyanide levels, then, may be many-fold higher than actual values and may easily mislead the physician into thinking that cyanide toxicity is present when it is not. In fact, whole blood cyanide levels actually correlate better with serum or plasma SCN^- concentrations than with HCN concentrations. Whole blood cyanide concentrations, therefore, should not be ordered because of their inaccuracy as commonly performed.

Because, in part, whole blood cyanide concentrations usually fail to reflect whole blood cyanide levels, there have been tremendous variations in what have been reported to be lethal or near-lethal whole blood cyanide concentrations. Other factors contributing to this inconsistency include the time after the onset of poisoning that blood samples were obtained, whether any antidotes for cyanide were administered, and the instability of cyanide in stored blood or in postmortem tissue (1,77–79).

Early metabolic disturbances from cyanide toxicity (e.g., metabolic acidosis) begin to appear at red blood cell cyanide concentrations of approximately 1 mg per L (80). Obvious cyanide toxicity is apparent when red blood cell cyanide concentrations reach approximately 5 mg per L.

When confronted with a patient suspected to be experiencing cyanide poisoning, physicians must make decisions regarding therapy before results of cyanide levels are available. Other physical and laboratory data must be examined for clues to the diagnosis of cyanide poisoning.

An anion gap metabolic acidosis is invariably present in serious cyanide poisoning. Although the arterial lactate concentrations may be elevated, the lactate concentration frequently does not account for the entire anion gap or base deficit because lactate is not actually responsible for acidosis.

The fall in oxygen consumption accompanying cyanide poisoning can allow for increased oxygen content of peripheral and mixed venous blood (79,81,82). The presence of bright red venous blood or retinal veins, then, suggests the possibility of cyanide poisoning (83). However, many persons experiencing cyanide poisoning are cyanotic (53,84,85). Although arterial PO_2 can be normal in cyanide poisoning, low cardiac output and intrapulmonary shunting in any patient with severe shock can cause arterial hypoxemia, including those experiencing cyanide poisoning.

Cardiovascular and metabolic parameters obtained from invasive monitoring with systemic and pulmonary artery catheters may reveal changes compatible with either sepsis, hepatic failure, or cyanide poisoning. All three conditions can cause a metabolic acidosis, hypotension, a fall in oxygen consumption, a rise in mixed venous oxygen content, and a fall in the arterial-venous oxygen content difference.

The toxicologic differential diagnosis of cyanide poisoning includes methemoglobinemia (when cyanosis is present), asphyxia (e.g., inert gases, methane), and poisonings by sulfide, azide, arsine, phosphine, phenol, methyl halides, and carbon monoxide. Unfortunately, any intoxication characterized by the sudden onset of seizures may be accompanied by hypotension, hypoxemia, and a metabolic acidosis, making the differential diagnosis large (e.g., monomethylhydrazine, cicutoxin, isoniazid, strychnine). However, sudden unexpected collapse into unconsciousness or convulsions accompanied by metabolic acidosis and decreased oxygen consumption in spite of adequate oxygen delivery makes one lean toward the diagnosis of cyanide or sulfide poisoning.

MANAGEMENT OF ACUTE TOXICITY

Antidotal Strategy

In the United States, the two main antidotal strategies for treating cyanide poisoning are the induction of methemoglobinemia with amyl nitrite or sodium nitrite, and the enhancement of conversion of cyanide to thiocyanate by the administration of sodium thiosulfate.

Cyanide binds to cytochrome oxidase because of its attraction to its ferric iron (Fe^{3+}). Normal hemoglobin contains ferrous iron (Fe^{2+}), explaining why cyanide does not significantly bind to this pigment. When iron of reduced hemoglobin is oxidized to the ferric state, methemoglobin is formed. Because methemoglobin cannot carry oxygen and shifts the hemoglobin-oxygen dissociation curve to the left, the body has extensive mechanisms for maintaining methemoglobin levels within erythrocytes less than 1% to 2% (i.e., 1% to 2% of all heme pigments are in the met form). In the absence of anemia, methemoglobin fractions of 20% to 30% are tolerated without life-threatening symptoms in the healthy person (86).

Sodium nitrite and amyl nitrite overwhelm the erythrocyte with oxidant stress, raising methemoglobin concentrations. This source of circulating ferric iron then competes with cytochrome oxidase for binding by cyanide, causing cyanide to dissociate from cytochrome oxidase in tissue and to move into blood, where it combines with methemoglobin in erythrocytes to form cyanmethemoglobin (34) (Fig. 54-3).

The historically suggested dose of sodium nitrite for adults without anemia is 10 mL of a 3% solution (300 mg) over several minutes. This dose has remained unchanged from that originally suggested and reiterated by Chen (87). Although circulating methemoglobin fractions of 25% to 40% (assuming no anemia) have been advocated to be most effective (88–90), these recommended levels of methemoglobinemia are based mainly on simply producing the highest fraction of methemoglobinemia that can be achieved in the nonanemic patient without seriously compromising oxygen delivery. This degree of methemoglobinemia is rarely achieved with recommended doses of sodium nitrite (87,88). For example, Moser reported peak methemoglobin fractions in humans of only 10.1% after intravenous administration of 400 mg sodium nitrite and of 17.5% after 600 mg of sodium nitrite (91). Kiese and Weger reported that methemoglobin fractions rose to a mean of 7% in six volunteers receiving sodium nitrite 4 mg per kg (88). A single volunteer who received sodium nitrite 12 mg per kg developed a methemoglobin fraction of 30%.

Sodium nitrite is also a relatively slow methemoglobin-producing agent. Thirty minutes may be required to raise met-

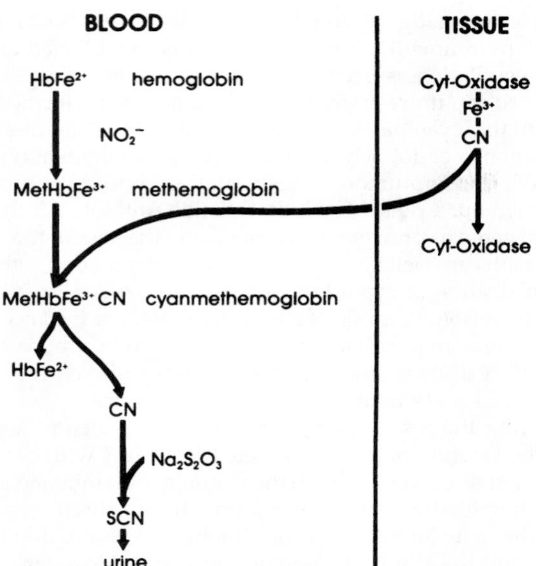

Figure 54-3. Antidotal strategy for cyanide poisoning. Cyanide binds to ferric iron on cytochrome oxidase in tissue, producing cyanide poisoning. Nitrite converts a fraction of circulating ferrous hemoglobin to ferric methemoglobin. Because cyanide's binding to cytochrome oxidase and methemoglobin is reversible, ferric iron of methemoglobin competes with cytochrome oxidase for binding by cyanide. Cyanide moves out of tissue and into erythrocytes as it binds with methemoglobin to form cyanmethemoglobin. Conversion of cyanide released from cyanmethemoglobin to thiocyanate is markedly enhanced by the administration of sodium thiosulfate. $HbFe^{2+}$, ferrous hemoglobin; NO_2^-, nitrite; $MetHbFe^{3+}$, methemoglobin; CN^-, cyanide; $Na_2S_2O_3$, sodium thiosulfate; SCN^-, thiocyanate; Fe^{3+}, ferric.

hemoglobin fractions to 7% after sodium nitrite 4 mg per kg, and 60 minutes may be required to reach 30% after sodium nitrite 12 mg per kg (88). Despite the slow onset of relatively low-grade methemoglobinemia after the administration of 300 mg sodium nitrite, the combination of sodium nitrite and sodium thiosulfate remains superior to more rapid methemoglobin-forming agents (32), possibly because of a more sustained methemoglobinemia produced by nitrite (32). Furthermore, the fact that dramatic improvements in symptoms have occurred well before methemoglobin levels have peaked (81,92) also suggests that mechanisms other than methemoglobin production may be important in nitrite's antidotal action (32,93).

Sodium thiosulfate is a source of sulfane sulfur that enhances the conversion of cyanide to thiocyanate. Thiosulfate generally is not given alone in the treatment of symptomatic cyanide poisoning because of what has been believed to be a slow action as compared with sodium nitrite (animal data concerning the speed with which thiocyanate reverses cyanide poisoning are conflicting) (94,95). Furthermore, although induction of nonlethal methemoglobinemia can rapidly reverse serious cyanide poisoning, cyanide eventually is released from cyanmethemoglobin, at least partly by reduction of cyanmethemoglobin to normal hemoglobin (96). Coadministration of sodium thiosulfate with sodium nitrite, therefore, ensures cyanide's rapid conversion to thiocyanate as it is released from cyanmethemoglobin (see Fig. 54-3). The combination of sodium nitrite and sodium thiosulfate increases the required lethal dose for cyanide up to 13 times in some animal models as compared to increases of three- to fourfold when each agent is given alone (97).

The main adverse effect from sodium or amyl nitrite is vasodilation and hypotension (89). Nitrite-induced hypotension, in part, has caused physicians in the military or in other countries to switch to or investigate other antidotes in the treatment of cyanide poisoning. These include other methemoglobin-producing agents, such as 4-dimethylaminophenol (98), or cyanide-chelating agents, such as cobalt edetate (99) and hydroxocobalamin (38).

Data exist suggesting that vasodilation actually may be beneficial in cyanide poisoning. Vasodilators that do not produce methemoglobinemia (e.g., phenoxybenzamine, chlorpromazine) are only slightly protective against cyanide when given alone. These vasodilators, however, significantly enhance the antidotal effect of thiosulfate in animal models (100,101). Other data indicate that vasodilation plays a relatively unimportant role as compared with methemoglobin induction in explaining the antidotal effect of nitrite. The injection of erythrocytes exposed to nitrite *in vitro* and then washed free of excess nitrite provides a degree of protection equivalent to that produced by nitrite directly injected into animals poisoned with cyanide (96).

The administration of 100% oxygen along with nitrite and thiosulfate to poisoned animals enhances survival over animals breathing room air. Animal studies reveal no advantage of hyperbaric oxygen therapy over the administration of 100% oxygen at one atmosphere (102).

Solutions A and B is an antidotal strategy mentioned only to be condemned. Solution A is 15.8% ferrous sulfate in 3% citric acid. Solution B is 6% sodium carbonate. Extensive research has been unsuccessful in determining the origin of this antidotal strategy (103). However, it has been recommended that two solutions be mixed together in equal parts and drunk immediately after the oral ingestion of cyanide. Ferrous iron liberated from the reaction of solution A with solution B is supposed to combine with cyanide in the gut to form relatively harmless ferrocyanide, preventing serious cyanide toxicity. Unfortunately, no animal or human data exist to justify its use. Unpublished data in small groups of rats indicate that the antidote is effective if given within 60 seconds of the instillation of cyanide into the stomach by a plastic tube. The administration of the antidote after 60 seconds has no effect (103). Furthermore, a human drinking cyanide absorbs significant, if not lethal, quantities in the mucous membranes of the mouth and throat. Callaghan and Halton (103) concluded, "The preparation and administration of the unproved A and B remedy would delay the institution of measures with proved antidotal value. Therefore, we discourage the use of solutions A and B because the origin, theoretical basis and efficacy of this remedy reside primarily in folklore myth, not in proved antidotal action."

α-Ketoglutarate, an intermediate in the Krebs cycle, binds cyanide and inhibits its availability at the tissue level (104). Pretreatment with intraperitoneal and subcutaneous α-ketoglutarate in mice results in mild decreases in plasma cyanide levels and lethality when compared to pretreatment with sodium nitrite and sodium thiosulfate (105). Hume et al. reported a dose-response improvement in survivability when α-ketoglutarate and sodium thiosulfate were combined before exposure to HCN. When α-ketoglutarate was administered 2 minutes after a median lethal dose of cyanide, however, it resulted in only a 1.6-fold improvement in survival (106). The clinical applicability of using α-ketoglutarate as antidotal therapy has not been established.

Dihydroxyacetone restores cyanide-inhibited mitochondrial respiration *in vitro* (107). The use of dihydroxyacetone as a pretreatment before poisoning with cyanide was effective; however, it was of minimal value when administered 2 minutes later (106).

Nitric oxide, a naturally occurring vasodilator, is formed *in vivo* from sodium nitrite and is responsible for nitrite-induced vasodilation (108). Nitric oxide also may cause formation of methemoglobin (109). However, nitric oxide is difficult to study because of its short half-life of 10 to 15 seconds (110). Diethylamine/nitric oxide, a long-acting nitric oxide–releasing complex, improved survivability when mice were pretreated before the administration of cyanide (111). Nitric oxide's role as antidotal therapy remains experimental.

TABLE 54-5. Initial pediatric dosage of sodium nitrite based on hemoglobin concentration

Hemoglobin concentration (g/100 mL)	3% Sodium nitrite solution (mL/kg)
7.0	0.19
8.0	0.22
9.0	0.25
10.0	0.27
11.0	0.30
12.0	0.33
13.0	0.36
14.0	0.39

Adapted from ref. 90, with permission.

Lilly Cyanide Antidote Kit

The Lilly Cyanide Antidote Kit (Eli Lilly and Company, Indianapolis, IN) contains breakable amyl nitrite pearls for induction of methemoglobinemia by inhalation as well as injectable solutions of sodium nitrite and sodium thiosulfate.

The inhalation of amyl nitrite is meant to be a temporizing measure until sodium nitrite can be given intravenously. A crushed pearl is held in front of the patient's nose and mouth, or in front of an intake valve of a ventilation bag for 30 seconds of every minute. Amyl nitrite pearls are rather ineffective at producing methemoglobinemia as compared with intravenous sodium nitrite (87), and it is far more important to adequately ventilate and oxygenate the patient than to administer amyl nitrite by inhalation.

Sodium nitrite should be given as soon as intravenous access is established. The adult dose is 10 mL of a 3% solution (300 mg). The administration of an entire ampule (10 mL) of 3% sodium nitrite to a small child can produce overwhelming, lethal methemoglobinemia (90). The same is true for an adult experiencing significant anemia. Children without anemia can receive 0.33 mL of 3% sodium nitrite per kilogram body weight, up to 10 mL. If a child's hemoglobin concentration is known, Table 54-5 can be consulted for more specific doses.

After the administration of intravenous sodium nitrite, 50 mL of 25% sodium thiosulfate should be administered intravenously to adults over several minutes. The pediatric dose is 1.65 mL of 25% sodium thiosulfate per kilogram body weight (90).

If signs of cyanide poisoning persist for 30 minutes or recur after an initial response to the antidote kit, sodium nitrite and sodium thiosulfate doses may be repeated. Although some authorities suggest that one-half the initial dose be used, this author's experience is that two doses of 300 mg sodium nitrite given as close as 10 minutes apart do no not produce methemoglobin fractions more than 20% in otherwise healthy, nonanemic adults. Nevertheless, it is highly recommended that total hemoglobin and methemoglobin concentrations be rapidly measured, when possible, before repeating a dose of sodium nitrite to be sure that dangerous methemoglobinemia does not occur, especially in children.

Medical Management

When it is suspected that a worker is unconscious from exposure to cyanide, the most important task for those not yet affected is to protect themselves and immediately leave the area. Rescue of an incapacitated victim should only be performed by personnel equipped with protective clothing or suits, respirators, and devices that can quickly measure cyanide concentrations in air (e.g., Draeger Tubes, National Draeger). Rescue personnel should not enter areas containing more than 200 ppm HCN unless they are wearing gas-tight suits (4). After the victim has been moved to a safe environment, an airway should be established and adequate ventilation assured, preferably with 100% oxygen. Direct mouth-to-mouth resuscitation should not be performed if it is thought that cyanide was orally ingested. Rather, bag-mask-valve ventilation or endotracheal intubation and bag ventilation should be used. Cardiopulmonary resuscitation should be initiated in those without a pulse. The Lilly Cyanide Antidote Kit should be administered as previously described and the patient transported to a health care facility after dermal decontamination. Other than administration of cyanide antidotes and oxygen, treatment of cyanide poisoning is one of supportive care. For instance, severe acidosis may require correction with sodium bicarbonate. Adult respiratory distress syndrome may require positive-pressure ventilation and continuous positive airway pressure.

During the rescue and resuscitation of a victim, personnel must be careful not to contaminate themselves with cyanide by coming in direct contact with the victim's contaminated clothing or with spilled cyanide compounds. In unconscious patients, after the institution of cardiopulmonary resuscitation (if indicated) and the administration of nitrite and thiosulfate, all contaminated clothing should be cut off the patient, and the victim should be thoroughly decontaminated with water.

The victim who experiences an acute dermal exposure to significant quantities of powdered or aqueous cyanide and remains alert should immediately undergo thorough water decontamination in a shower for several minutes and should immediately remove all clothing, including shoes and socks.

A person who only has inhaled HCN gas but has escaped to a safe environment without becoming seriously ill is not in danger of developing delayed onset of more serious symptoms (1).

BIOLOGICAL MONITORING

Red blood cell and plasma cyanide concentrations are generally used in the diagnosis of acute cyanide poisoning rather than in routine biological monitoring. Urinary and plasma thiocyanate concentrations have been reported to be higher in workers exposed to cyanide than in control subjects. However, smoking and diet also influence thiocyanate concentrations in plasma and urine, making interpretation difficult (74). No studies exist demonstrating that routine monitoring of red blood cell and plasma cyanide levels, plasma thiocyanate concentrations, or urinary thiocyanate excretions adds any information to that obtained from air cyanide concentrations and inspection of the work site to ensure good housekeeping and work practices. In their recommended standard for HCN and inorganic cyanide salts, NIOSH made no recommendations for biological monitoring (4).

Environmental Monitoring

Various manufacturers provide industry with real-time air cyanide monitors. Such monitors sound alarms when predetermined concentrations of cyanide in air are detected.

National Draeger provides Draeger Tubes that can be used for rapid, portable grab sampling. These tubes quantify air cyanide concentrations between 2 and 25 mg per m^3.

A NIOSH method (112) for measurement of air cyanide concentrations involves drawing air through a cellulose-ester membrane filter and then through a bubbler containing 10 mL 0.1 N potassium hydroxide. Cyanide eluted from the filter with 0.1 N KOH and cyanide in the bubbler are quantified using an ion-specific electrode. This method does not distinguish between gaseous HCN and particulate cyanide salts.

Exposure Limits

The American Conference of Governmental Industrial Hygienists has set a ceiling limit for sodium, potassium, and $Ca(CN)_2$ at 5 mg per m^3 measured as cyanide. For HCN, the organization has set a ceiling limit of 4.7 ppm.

OSHA has set a permissible exposure limit for cyanide salts at 5 mg per m^3, and for HCN at 10 ppm.

NIOSH has recommended a 10-minute ceiling value for NaCN, KCN, and $Ca(CN)_2$ of 5 mg per m^3 measured as cyanide, and a 10-minute ceiling value for HCN of 4.7 ppm.

REFERENCES

1. Peden NR, Taha A, McSorley PD, et al. Industrial exposure to hydrogen cyanide: implications for treatment. *BMJ* 1986;293:538.
2. Gonzales ER. Cyanide evades some noses, overpowers others. *JAMA* 1982; 248:2211.
3. Curry AS. Cyanide poisoning. *Acta Pharmacol Toxicol* 1963;20:291–294.
4. US Department of Health, Education, and Welfare, National Institute for Occupational Safety and Health. Criteria for a recommended standard for occupational exposure to hydrogen cyanide and cyanide salts. National Institute for Occupational Safety and Health, 1976. [NTIS PB-266-230].
5. Homan EF. Reactions, processes and materials with potential for cyanide exposure. In: Ballantyne B, Marrs TC, eds. *Clinical and experimental toxicology of cyanides*. Bristol: IOP Publishing, 1987:1–21.
6. Dugard PH. The absorption of cyanide through human skin in vitro from solutions of sodium cyanide and gaseous HCN. In: Ballantyne B, Marrs TC, eds. *Clinical and experimental toxicology of cyanides*. Bristol: IOP Publishing, 1987:127–137.
7. Muller-Hess B. Intoxication caused by absorption of hydrocyanic acid through the skin. *Muerch Med Wocheschr* 1942;89:492.
8. Tovo S. Poisoning due to KCN absorbed through skin. *Minerva Med* 1955;75: 158–161.
9. Thomas TA, Brooks JW. Accidental cyanide poisoning. *Anaesthesia* 1970;25: 110–114.
10. Smith AR. Cyanide poisoning. *N Y Dept Labor Ind Bull* 1932;11:169–170.
11. Young MA. Health hazards of electroplating. *J Occup Med* 1965;7:348–352.
12. Wright IH, Vesey CJ. Acute poisoning with gold cyanide. *Anaesthesia* 1986; 41:936–939.
13. Stock PG, Monier-Williams GW. Preliminary report on the use of hydrogen cyanide for fumigation purposes. Reports on Public Health and Medical Subjects, no 19. London: Ministry of Health, 1923.
14. Cousineau A, Legg FG. Hydrocyanic acid gas and other toxic gases in commercial fumigation. *Am J Public Health* 1935;25:277–294.
15. McKelway JI. Three cases of poisoning by potassium cyanide. *Am J Med Sci* 1905;129:684–688.
16. Kreig A. Cyanide poisoning from metal cleaning solutions. *Ann Emerg Med* 1987;16:582–584.
17. Levine MS, Radford EP. Occupational exposures to cyanide in Baltimore fire fighters. *J Occup Med* 1978;20:53–56.
18. Jones J, McMullen J, Dougherty J. Toxic smoke inhalation: cyanide poisoning in fire victims. *Am J Emerg Med* 1987;5:318–321.
19. Wetherell HR. The occurrence of cyanide in the blood of fire victims. *J Forensic Sci* 1966;11:167–173.
20. Ballantyne B. Hydrogen cyanide as a product of combustion and a factor in morbidity and mortality from fires. In: Ballantyne B, Marrs TC, eds. *Clinical and experimental toxicology of cyanides*. Bristol: IOP Publishing, 1987:248–291.
21. Barcroft J. The toxicity of atmospheres containing hydrocyanic acid gas. *J Hyg* 1931;31:1–34.
22. Bonsall JL. Survival without sequelae following exposure to 500 mg/m^3 of hydrogen cyanide. *Hum Toxicol* 1984;3:57–60.
23. Carmelo S. New contributions to the study of subacute-chronic hydrocyanic acid intoxication in man. *Rass Med Ind* 1955;24:254–271.
24. Drinker P. Hydrocyanic acid gas poisoning by absorption through the skin. *J Ind Hyg* 1932;14:1–2.
25. Walton DC, Witherspoon MG. Skin absorption of certain gases. *J Pharmacol Exp Ther* 1926;26:315–324.
26. Ballantyne B. Comparative acute toxicity of hydrogen cyanide and its salts. In: Lindstrom RE, ed. *Proceedings of the fourth annual chemical defense bioscience review.* Maryland: US Army Medical Research Institute of Chemical Defense, 1984.
27. Johnstone RT. *Occupational medicine and industrial hygiene*. St. Louis: Mosby, 1948:130–135.
28. Schulz V, Bonn R, Kindler J. Kinetics of elimination of thiocyanate in 7 healthy subjects and 8 subjects with renal failure. *Klin Wochenschr* 1979;57:243–247.
29. Sorbo B. Thiosulfate sulfurtransferase and mercaptopyruvate sulfur-transferase. In: Greenberg DM, ed. *Metabolic pathways, vol. VII. Metabolism of sulfur compounds*. New York: Academic Press, 1975:433–456.
30. Westley J, Adler A, Westley L, et al. The sulfur transferases. *Fundam Appl Toxicol* 1983;3:377–382.
31. Ballantyne B. Toxicology of cyanides. In: Ballantyne B, Marrs TC, eds. *Clinical and experimental toxicology of cyanides*. Bristol: IOP Publishing, 1987:41–126.
32. Way JL, Sylvester D, Morgan RL, et al. Recent perspectives on the toxicodynamic basis of cyanide antagonism. *Fundam Appl Toxicol* 1984;4:S231–S239.
33. Vennesland B, Castric PA, Conn EE, et al. Cyanide metabolism. *Fed Proc* 1982;41:2639–2648.
34. Way JL. Cyanide intoxication and its mechanism of antagonism. *Annu Rev Pharmacol* 1984;24:451–481.
35. Piantadosi CA, Sylvia AL. Cerebral cytochrome a, a_3 inhibition by cyanide in bloodless rats. *Toxicology* 1984;33:67–79.
36. Vesey CJ, Wilson J. Red cell cyanide. *J Pharm Pharmacol* 1978;30:20–26.
37. McMillan DE, Svoboda AC. The role of erythrocytes in cyanide detoxification. *J Pharmacol Exp Ther* 1982;221:37–42.
38. Jouglard J, Nava G, Botta A, et al. A propos d'une intoxication aigue par le cyanure traitee par l'hydroxocobalamine. *Marseille Med* 1974;12:617–624.
39. Solomonson LP. Cyanide as a metabolic inhibitor. In: Vennesland B, Conn EE, Knowles CJ, et al., eds. *Cyanide in biology*. London: Academic Press, 1981:11–28.
40. Tursky T, Sajter V. The influence of potassium cyanide poisoning on the aminobutyric acid level in rat brain. *J Neurochem* 1962;9:519–523.
41. Krebs HG, Woods HG, Alberti KGMM. Hyperlactataemia and lactic acidosis. *Essays Med Biochem* 1975;1:81–103.
42. Mizock BA. Lactic acidosis. *DM* 1989;35:233–300.
43. Zilva JF. The origin of acidosis in hyperlactataemia. *Ann Clin Biochem* 1978;15:40-43.
44. Gevers W. Generation of protons by metabolic processes in heart cells. *J Mol Cell Cardiol* 1977;9:867–874.
45. Mizock BA. Controversies in lactic acidosis. *JAMA* 1987;258:497–501.
46. Johnston DG, Alberti KGMM. Acid-base balance in metabolic acidoses. *Clin Endocrinol Metab* 1983;12:267–285.
47. Ballantyne B. An experimental assessment of the diagnostic potential of histochemical and biochemical methods for cytochrome oxidase in acute cyanide poisoning. *Cell Mol Biol* 1977;22:109–123.
48. Wexler J, Whittenberger JL, Dumke PR. The effect of cyanide on the electrocardiogram of man. *Am Heart J* 1947;34:163–173.
49. DeBush RF, Seidl LG. Attempted suicide by cyanide. *Calif Med* 1969; 110:394–396.
50. Graham DL, Laman D, Theodore J, et al. Acute cyanide poisoning complicated by lactic acidosis and pulmonary edema. *Arch Intern Med* 1977;137:1051–1055.
51. Brivet F, Delfraissy JF, Duche M, et al. Acute cyanide poisoning: recovery with non-specific supportive therapy. *Intensive Care Med* 1983;9:33–35.
52. Uitti RJ, Rajput AH, Ashenhurst EM, et al. Cyanide-induced Parkinsonism: a clinicopathologic report. *Neurology* 1985;35:921–925.
53. Peters CG, Mundy JVB, Rayner PR. Acute cyanide poisoning. *Anaesthesia* 1982;37:582–586.
54. Flury F, Zernik F. HCN (hydrocyanic acid, prussic acid). In: *Noxious gases—vapors, mist, smoke and dust particles*. Berlin: Verlag von Julius Springer, 1931:400–415.
55. McNamara BP. Estimates of the toxicity of hydrocyanide acid vapor in man. Edgewood Arsenal technical report EB-TR-76023. US Department of the Army; 1976.
56. Miller MH, Toops TC. Acute cyanide poisoning. Recovery with sodium thiosulfate therapy. *J Indiana State Med Assoc* 1951;44:1164.
57. Braddock WH, Tingle GR. So-called cyanide rash in gold mine mill workers. *J Ind Hyg* 1930;12:259–264.
58. Nolan JW. Potassium cyanide poisoning. *JAMA* 1908;50:365.
59. Wrangsjo K, Martensson A. Hydrazine contact dermatitis from gold plating. *Contact Dermatitis* 1986;15:244–245.
60. Mathias CGT. Contact dermatitis from cyanide plating solutions. *Arch Dermatol* 1982;118:420–422.
61. Elkins HB. *The chemistry of industrial toxicology*, 2nd ed. New York: John Wiley and Sons, 1959:94–95.
62. Barsky MH. Ulcerations of the nasal membranes and perforation of the septum in a copper plating factory—unusual and sudden incidence. *N Y State J Med* 1937;37:1031–1034.
63. Cohen SR, Davis DM, Kramkowski RS. Clinical manifestations of chromic acid toxicity—nasal lesions in electroplate workers. *Cutis* 1974;13:558–568.
64. Blanc P, Hogan M, Mallin K, et al. Cyanide intoxication among silver-reclaiming workers. *JAMA* 1985;253:367–371.
65. Saia B, DeRosa E, Galzigna L. Remarks on the chronic poisoning from cyanide. *Med Lav* 1970;61:580–586.
66. Radojicic B. Determining thiocyanate in urine of workers exposed to cyanides. *Arh Hig Rada Toksikol* 1973;24:227–232.
67. Chandra H, Gupta BN, Bhargava SK. Chronic cyanide exposure—a biochemical and industrial hygiene study. *J Anal Toxicol* 1980;4:161–165.
68. Wollman SH. Nature of the inhibition by thiocyanate of the iodide concentrating mechanism of the thyroid gland. *Am J Physiol* 1956;186:453–459.
69. Wood JL. Biochemistry. In: Newman AA, ed. *Chemistry and biochemistry of thiocyanic acid and its derivatives*. New York: Academic Press, 1975:156–221.
70. Wuthrich F. Chronic cyanide poisoning as industrial intoxicant. *Schweiz Med Wochenschr* 1954;84:105–107.
71. El Ghawabi SH, Gaafar MA, El-Saharti AA, et al. Chronic cyanide exposure: a clinical, radioisotope, and laboratory study. *Br J Ind Med* 1975;32:215–219.
72. Hartung R. Cyanides and nitriles. In: Clayton GD, Clayton FE, eds. *Patty's industrial hygiene and toxicology*, 3rd ed., vol. 2C. New York: John Wiley and Sons, 1982:4845–4900.
73. Howard JW, Hanzal RF. Chronic toxicity for rats of food treated with hydrogen cyanide. *J Agric Food Chem* 1955;3:325–329.

74. Maehly AC, Swensson A. Cyanide and thiocyanate levels in blood and urine of workers with low-grade exposure to cyanide. *Int Arch Arbeitsmed* 1970;27:195–209.
75. Doherty PA, Ferm V, Smith RP. Congenital malformations induced by infusions of sodium cyanide in the Golden hamster. *Toxicol Appl Pharmacol* 1982;64:456–464.
76. Ballantyne B. Artifacts in the definition of toxicity by cyanides and cyanogens. *Fundam Appl Toxicol* 1983;3:400–408.
77. Ballantyne B, Marrs TC. Post-mortem features and criteria for the diagnosis of acute lethal cyanide poisoning. In: Ballantyne B, Marrs TC, eds. *Clinical and experimental toxicology of cyanides*. Bristol: IOP Publishing, 1987:217–247.
78. Ballantyne B. In vitro production of cyanide in normal human blood and the influence of thiocyanate and storage temperature. *Clin Toxicol* 1977;11:173–193.
79. Hall AH, Rumack B. Clinical toxicology of cyanide. *Ann Emerg Med* 1986; 15:1067–1074.
80. Pasch T, Schulz V, Hoppelshauser G. Nitroprusside-induced formation of cyanide and its detoxication with thiosulfate during deliberate hypotension. *J Cardiovasc Pharmacol* 1983;5:77–85.
81. Shragg TA, Albertson TE, Fisher CJ. Cyanide poisoning after bitter almond ingestion. *West J Med* 1982;136:65–69.
82. Johnson RP, Mellors JW. Arterialization of venous blood gases: a clue to the diagnosis of cyanide poisoning. *J Emerg Med* 1988;6:401–404.
83. Buchanan IS, Dhamee MS, Griffiths FED, et al. Abnormal fundal appearances in a case of poisoning by a cyanide capsule. *Med Sci Law* 1976;16:29–32.
84. Wesson DE, Foley R, Sabatini S, Wharton J, Kapusnik J, Kurtzman NA. Treatment of acute cyanide intoxication with hemodialysis. *Am J Nephrol* 1985;5:121–126.
85. Lasch EE, El Shawa R. Multiple cases of cyanide poisoning by apricot kernels in children from Gaza. *Pediatrics* 1981;68:5–7.
86. Curry SC. Methemoglobinemia. *Ann Emerg Med* 1982;11:214–221.
87. Chen KK, Rose CL. Nitrite and thiosulfate therapy in cyanide poisoning. *JAMA* 1952;149:113–119.
88. Kiese M, Weger N. Formation of ferrihemoglobin with aminophenols in the human for the treatment of cyanide poisoning. *Eur J Pharmacol* 1969;7:97–105.
89. Vogel SN, Sultan TR, Ten Eyck RP. Cyanide poisoning. *Clin Toxicol* 1981;18: 367–383.
90. Berlin CM. The treatment of cyanide poisoning in children. *Pediatrics* 1970; 46:793–796.
91. Moser P. Zur wirkung von nitrit auf rote blutzellen des menschen. *Arch Exp Pathol Pharmakol* 1950;210:60–70.
92. Hall AH, Doutre WH, Ludden T, Kulig KW, Rumack BH. Nitrite/thiosulfate treated acute cyanide poisoning: estimated kinetics after antidote. *J Toxicol Clin Toxicol* 1987;25:121–133.
93. Way JL, Leung P, Sylvester DM, Burrows G, Way JL, Tamulinas C. Methemoglobin formation in the treatment of acute cyanide intoxication. In: Ballantyne B, Marrs TC, eds. *Clinical and experimental toxicology of cyanides*. Bristol: IOP Publishing, 1987:402–412.
94. Aw TC, Bishop CM. Letter. *J Soc Occup Med* 1981;31:173–175.
95. Friedberg KD, Shukla UR. The efficiency of aquocobalamine as an antidote in cyanide poisoning when given alone or combined with sodium thiosulfate. *Arch Toxicol* 1975;33:103–113.
96. Kruszyna R, Kruszyna H, Smith RP. Comparison of hydroxylamine, 4-dimethylaminophenol and nitrite protection against cyanide poisoning in mice. *Arch Toxicol* 1982;49:191–202.
97. Chen KK, Rose RL, Clowes GHA. Methylene blue (methylthionine chloride), nitrites and sodium thiosulphate against cyanide poisoning. *Proc Soc Exp Biol Med* 1933;31:250–251.
98. Weger NP. Treatment of cyanide poisoning with 4-dimethylamino-phenol (DMAP)—experimental and clinical overview. *Fundam Appl Toxicol* 1983;3:387–396.
99. Dodds C, McKnight C. Cyanide toxicity after immersion and the hazards of dicobalt edetate. *BMJ* 1985;291:785–786.
100. Gurrows GE, Way JL. Antagonism of cyanide toxicity by phenoxybenzamine [Abst]. *Fed Proc* 1975;36:534.
101. Way JL, Burrows GE. Cyanide intoxication: protection with chlorpromazine. *Toxicol Appl Pharmacol* 1976;36:1–5.
102. Way JL, End E, Sheehy MH, et al. Effect of oxygen on cyanide intoxication IV. Hyperbaric oxygen. *Toxicol Appl Pharmacol* 1972;22:415–421.
103. Callaghan JM, Halton DM. Solutions A and B: cyanide antidote or folklore myth? *J Soc Occup Med* 1988;38:65–68.
104. Moore SJ, Norris JC, Ho IK, et al. The efficacy of α-ketoglutaric acid in the antagonism of cyanide intoxication. *Toxicol Appl Pharmacol* 1986;82:40–44.
105. Bhattacharya R, Vijayayaraghavan R. Cyanide intoxication in mice through different routes and its prophylaxis by α-ketoglutarate. *Biol Environ Sci* 1991;4:452–459.
106. Niknahad H, O'Brien PJ. Antidotal effect of dihydroxyacetone against cyanide toxicity in vivo. *Toxicol Appl Pharmacol* 1996;138:186–191.
107. Niknahad H, Khan S, O'Brien PJ. Hepatocyte injury resulting from the inhibition of mitochondrial respiration at low oxygen concentrations involves reductive stress and oxygen activation. *Chem Bio Interact* 1995;98:1–18.
108. Robinson CP, Baskin SI, Franz DR. The mechanism of action of cyanide on the rabbit aorta. *J Appl Toxicol* 1985;5:372–377.
109. Blough NV, Zafiriou OC. Reaction of superoxide with nitric oxide to form peroxonitrile in alkaline aqueous solution. *Inorgan Chem* 1985;24:3502–3504.
110. Furchgott RF. Role of endothelium in response to vascular smooth muscle. *Circ Res* 1983;53:557–573.
111. Baskin SI, Nealley EW, Lempka JC. Cyanide toxicity in mice pretreated with diethylamine nitric oxide complex. *Hum Exp Toxicol* 1996;15:13–18.
112. Eller PM, ed. *National Institute for Occupational Safety and Health manual of analytical methods*, 3rd ed. [NIOSH publication no. 84-100, NTIS PB85-179018]. Cincinnati: National Institute for Occupational Safety and Health, 1984.

CHAPTER 55
Hydrogen Sulfide

Jou-Fang Deng

CHEMICAL AND PHYSICAL PROPERTIES

Hydrogen sulfide (H_2S) (Chemical Abstracts Service registry number 7783-06-4) occurs in a variety of natural and industrial settings. It exists as a gas under normal conditions. It may be liquefied, however, by reduced temperature or increased pressure. Synonyms for hydrogen sulfide include dihydrogen monosulfide, dihydrogen sulfide, hydrogen sulphide, hydrosulfuric acid, sewer gas, stink damp, sulfur hydride, and sulfuretted hydrogen (1).

H_2S is a colorless, irritant, and asphyxiant gas. It is generally stable when properly stored in cylinders at room temperature. However, in the air, it is flammable and explosive and may be ignited by static discharge. It does not polymerize. It may react with metals, oxidizing agents, and acids, such as nitric acid, bromine pentafluoride, chlorine trifluoride, nitrogen triiodide, nitrogen trichloride, oxygen difluoride, and phenyldiazonium chloride. When heated to decomposition, it emits highly toxic sulfur oxide fumes. The general chemical and physical properties of H_2S are listed in Table 55-1 (1–3).

SITES, INDUSTRIES, AND BUSINESSES ASSOCIATED WITH EXPOSURES

H_2S is one of the principal compounds involved in the natural cycle of sulfur in our environment. Natural sources constitute approximately 90% of the atmospheric burden of H_2S (4). It is found in the environment in volcanic gases, marshes, swamps, sulfur springs, and other geothermal sources, and as a product of bacterial action during the decay of plant and animal protein (2,5,6). H_2S generation can be expected whenever oxygen is depleted, and organic material containing sulfate is present (7). For example, in India and Sri Lanka, H_2S is produced as a by-product in the process by which

TABLE 55-1. Physical and chemical properties of hydrogen sulfide

Molecular formula	H_2S
Molecular weight	34.08
Boiling point	–60.33°C
Specific gravity, 0°C	1.54 g/L
Vapor pressure, 25°C	19.6 atm
Melting point	–85.49°C
Vapor density	1.19
Autoignition temperature	250°C
Explosive range in air	4.5–45.5%
Color	Colorless
Conversion factors	1 mg/m^3 = 0.717 ppm 1 ppm = 1.394 mg/m^3

Adapted from references 1–3.

coconut fibers are separated from the husk. This procedure involves the decomposition of husks in shallow ponds, and H_2S is produced as a result of microbiologic decay. It occurs in most petroleum and natural gas deposits and also in many mines. As a result, it is a potential health hazard to workers involved in drilling, mining, smelting, or processing operations (2).

H_2S is used in the manufacturing of chemicals; in metallurgy; as an analytical reagent; as an agricultural disinfectant; as an intermediate for sulfuric acid, elemental sulfur, sodium sulfide, and other inorganic sulfides; as an additive in extreme pressure lubricants and cutting oils; and as an intermediate for organic sulfur compounds (1). Large quantities of H_2S are used in the production of heavy water, which is used as a moderator in some nuclear power reactors.

In other industries, H_2S is produced as an undesirable byproduct. In manufacturing processes, it is formed whenever elemental sulfur or certain sulfur compounds are present with organic chemicals at high temperature (8). Examples include petroleum refineries, natural gas plants, petrochemical plants, coke oven plants, kraft paper mills, viscose rayon manufacture, sulfur production, iron smelters, food processing plants, and tanneries. In the tanning industry, H_2S is produced in the process by which hair or wool is removed from the hides.

TABLE 55-2. Occupations with potential exposure to hydrogen sulfide

Animal fat and oil processors	Lead removers
Animal manure removers	Lithographers
Artificial-flavor makers	Lithopone makers
Asphalt storage workers	Livestock farmers
Barium carbonate makers	Metallurgists
Barium salt makers	Miners
Blast furnace workers	Natural gas production and processing workers
Brewery workers	Painters using polysulfide caulking compounds
Bromide-brine workers	Papermakers
Cable splicers	Petroleum production and refinery workers
Caisson workers	Phosphate purifiers
Carbon disulfide makers	Photoengravers
Cellophane makers	Pipeline maintenance workers
Chemical laboratory workers, teachers, students	Pyrite burners
Cistern cleaners	Rayon makers
Citrus root fumigators	Refrigerant makers
Coal gasification workers	Rubber and plastics processors
Coke oven workers	Septic tank cleaners
Copper ore sulfidizers	Sewage treatment plant workers
Depilatory makers	Sewer workers
Dyemakers	Sheepdippers
Excavators	Silk makers
Felt makers	Slaughterhouse workers
Fermentation process workers	Smelting workers
Fertilizer makers	Soapmakers
Fishing and fish processing workers	Sugar beet and cane processors
Fur dressers	Sulfur spa workers
Geothermal power drilling and production workers	Sulfur products processors
Gluemakers	Synthetic fiber makers
Gold ore workers	Tank gagers
Heavy metal precipitators	Tannery workers
Heavy water manufacturers	Textiles printers
Hydrochloric acid purifiers	Thiophene makers
Hydrogen sulfide production and sales workers	Tunnel workers
Landfill workers	Utility hole and trench workers
Lead ore sulfidizers	Well diggers and cleaners
	Wool pullers

From ref. 2, with permission.

In many instances, H_2S has been found together with other substances, such as carbon disulfide, methane, and sulfur dioxide; however, it can exist by itself. Generally, H_2S is not found in high concentrations in the ambient air. Occasional catastrophic releases in processing and transport have exposed the general public to concentrations high enough to elicit toxic symptoms and death. Such accidents can be anticipated under the condition whenever sulfur-containing chemicals react with acid (e.g., sodium sulfhydrate reacts with acid sewage) (9,10).

The National Institute for Occupational Safety and Health (NIOSH) estimated in 1977 that approximately 125,000 employees in 73 industries were potentially exposed to hydrogen sulfide in the United States. The occupations of which employees may be exposed to H_2S are listed in Table 55-2 (2).

Because it is heavier than air, H_2S tends to accumulate in low-lying areas. This property is responsible for many of the poisonings occurring during oil drilling, manure sewage handling, and wastewater treatment processes. Most of the instances of H_2S poisonings are occupational. In the United States, H_2S is present in fatal concentrations in 4% to 14% of some natural gas at the well head; gas field leaks and resulting poisonings account for many of the fatalities related to H_2S exposures (2). In the high sulfur oil fields of Wyoming and western Texas, 26 persons died from exposure to H_2S between October 1, 1974, and April 28, 1976 (11). In addition to petroleum refining, other industries, such as heavy water manufacturing, hide tanning, rubber vulcanizing, rayon manufacturing, pelt processing, manure refuse and sewage, fishing, hospital, and wastewater treatment, have also reported H_2S poisonings (3). Acute H_2S poisoning is not solely an occupational hazard. Occasional community-wide accidents have also been reported. The most dramatic and serious event occurred in 1950 at Poza Rica, Mexico. The flare apparatus on a gas well malfunctioned and large quantities of H_2S were released into the atmosphere. Within 3 hours, 320 residents were hospitalized and 22 died (12).

CLINICAL TOXICOLOGY

Route of Exposure, Absorption, Metabolism, and Elimination

The kinetics of H_2S have been partially characterized in animal studies. In environmental and occupational exposures, the lung rather than the skin is the primary route of absorption (13,14). The dermal absorption of H_2S is minimal (15,16). Results from animal inhalation studies indicate that H_2S is distributed in the body to the brain, liver, kidneys, pancreas, and small intestine (17). With the body, H_2S is metabolized by oxidation, methylation, and reaction with metallo- or disulfide-containing proteins. Orally, intraperitoneally, and intravenously administered H_2S is primarily oxidized and directly excreted as either free sulfate or conjugated sulfate in the urine (18). The importance of methylation in the detoxification processes of H_2S, however, is unknown (19). The reaction of H_2S with vital metalloenzymes, such as cytochrome oxidase, is the likely toxic mechanism of H_2S (7,20). Reaction with nonessential proteins may also serve as a detoxification pathway (21,22). Systemic poisoning occurs when the amount of H_2S absorbed exceeds that which can be detoxified and eliminated (14,23). Because of its rapid oxidation in the blood, H_2S is not considered a cumulative poison (14,24,25). The fact that low concentrations of the gas [e.g., 20 parts per million (ppm)] can be tolerated for long periods without harm is also an indication that, at lower concentrations, potential cumulative action is unlikely (26).

No animal data are available regarding the exhalation of H_2S after inhalation exposure. In animals, the excretion of H_2S by the lungs is minimal after parenteral administration of H_2S (26–28).

TABLE 55-3. Physiologic effects of human exposure to H_2S

Physiologic effects	Concentration (parts per million)
Odor intensity	
Threshold	0.02
Minimally perceptible	0.13
Faint but readily perceptible	0.77
Easily noticeable, moderate	4.6
Safe for 7-hour exposure	20
Strong, unpleasant but not intolerable	27
Eye and respiratory tract irritation is noticeable	50
Olfactory fatigue level	100
Olfactory nerve paralysis	150
Prolonged exposure may cause pulmonary edema	250
Dizziness, breathing ceases in few minutes	500
Unconscious quickly, death results if not rescued promptly	700
Rapid collapse and respiratory paralysis	1,000
Imminent death	5,000

Adapted from ref. 3, with permission.

Because rescue personnel have developed H_2S poisoning shortly after starting mouth-to-mouth resuscitation on victims who had been poisoned, however, it is likely that significant H_2S is excreted from the lungs (9).

Acute Toxicity

PHYSIOLOGIC EFFECTS AND GENERAL TOXICOLOGY

H_2S is an irritant and an asphyxiant gas. The physiologic and toxic effects associated with various concentrations of H_2S exposure are listed in Table 55-3, and are summarized in the following paragraph.

H_2S is well known by its characteristic odor similar to rotten eggs. The perception threshold of this odor varies individually; however, 0.13 ppm has been generally accepted as the threshold. At a concentration of 50 ppm, H_2S acts as an irritant on the mucous membranes of the eyes and the respiratory tract. Its irritant action on the eye produces keratoconjunctivitis, known as *gas eye*. When inhaled, H_2S exerts an irritant action throughout the entire respiratory tract; the deeper structures experience the greatest damage. The irritant action and odor similar to rotten eggs often provide the first warning of H_2S exposure. At more than 150 ppm, the gas exerts a paralyzing effect on the olfactory apparatus. If an exposed person is not aware of this effect, it could jeopardize life. Prolonged exposure to moderate concentrations (250 ppm) may cause pulmonary edema. At concentrations more than 500 ppm, drowsiness, dizziness, excitement, headache, unstable gait, and other systemic symptoms occur within a few minutes. Sudden loss of consciousness without premonition, anxiety, or sense of struggle are characteristic of acute exposure at concentrations more than 700 ppm. At concentrations of 1,000 to 2,000 ppm, H_2S gas is rapidly absorbed through the lung into the blood. Initially hyperpnea occurs, followed by rapid collapse and respiratory inhibition. At higher concentrations, H_2S exerts an immediate paralyzing effect on the respiratory centers. When the concentration reaches 5,000 ppm, imminent death almost always results. Generally speaking, imminent death caused by asphyxia can happen at any time when the concentration reaches 1,000 ppm or more, unless spontaneous respiration is reestablished or artificial respiration is promptly provided (3).

TARGET ORGAN TOXICITY

The main target organs or systems for H_2S include the olfactory apparatus, eyes, respiratory system, and nervous system. However, other organs, such as the heart, digestive system, and endocrine system, may also be affected (29–33).

Effect on Olfactory Apparatus. The typical rotten eggs odor of H_2S is detectable by olfaction at low concentrations, between 0.02 and 0.13 ppm. The odor intensity may be perceived differently by individuals, however, when the ambient concentration is less than 30 ppm. Less than this concentration, no known human health consequence is related to the exposure. The characteristic odor of H_2S, as long as it is perceptible, provides a useful warning signal because the odor threshold is much lower than the toxic level. When the concentration reaches 100 ppm, however, olfactory fatigue occurs (2,33,34). Once the concentration reaches 150 ppm, H_2S exerts a paralyzing effect on the olfactory apparatus, and its natural signal of warning is lost (24,26,32). These effects may occur gradually on exposure to small amounts of this gas or quite rapidly where lethal concentrations of the gas are present (35,36). Odor of H_2S is, therefore, an unreliable warning signal at elevated concentrations because of rapid paralysis of the olfactory apparatus (14,23,24).

Effect on Eyes. The direct action of H_2S on mucous membranes is usually observed first by symptoms of eye irritation, resulting from local inflammation of the conjunctiva and cornea (3). Conjunctivitis or gas eye was first described by workers in the petroleum industry (3). Acute inflammation of conjunctiva accompanied by lacrimation and mucopurulent exudate is not uncommon. In severe cases, corneal erosion with blurred vision may also occur. Occasionally, corneal ulceration may occur, resulting in impaired vision (24). Because the cornea is affected, together with the conjunctiva in many instances, keratoconjunctivitis rather than conjunctivitis more accurately describes the ophthalmologic effects of H_2S exposure (37–39). In general, irritation of the eyes occurs at a concentration of H_2S of 50 ppm; however, conjunctivitis or sore eyes have been observed on exposures in the range of 5 to 100 ppm (40,41).

Effect on Respiratory System. At low concentrations, the irritant effects of H_2S are more prominent on the eyes and olfactory apparatus. However, prolonged exposure to concentrations as low as 50 ppm may cause inflammation and dryness of the respiratory tract (23,24,42). The irritant effect of H_2S extends rather uniformly throughout the entire respiratory tract, resulting in rhinitis, pharyngitis, laryngitis, bronchitis, and pneumonia (25). Cough, sore throat, hoarseness, runny nose, and chest tightness are the most common symptoms of exposure between 50 and 250 ppm. However, in acute massive exposure, symptoms of respiratory irritation may not appear, either because of the shortness of the exposure or because they are obscured by the more prominent, systemic effects. Apparently, irritating symptoms vary with the duration and intensity of the exposures.

Pneumonia resulting from H_2S exposure is thought to partially result from impaired ciliary activity and alveolar macrophage dysfunction (43,44). In an *in vitro* study, using sections of rabbit trachea exposed to H_2S in an environmentally controlled chamber, either 600 ppm for 5 minutes or 400 ppm for 10 minutes resulted in cessation of ciliary movement (43). In the rat, H_2S exposure to 45 ppm for 4 or 6 hours decreased the ability of the lungs to inactivate *Staphylococcus epidermidis* deposited by aerosol. The reduced *Staphylococcus* inactivation was considered to be because of an impaired alveolar macrophage function caused by the H_2S exposure (44). These findings may partially explain the mechanism of pneumonia occurring after H_2S poisoning. Because H_2S can penetrate the alveoli, pulmonary edema is not uncommon after prolonged exposure to H_2S in concentrations exceeding 250 ppm (23). In acute massive exposure, systemic poisoning by H_2S results in paralysis of the respiratory center of the brain. On acute exposures at concentrations more than 1,000 ppm, respiratory paralysis followed by imminent death may occur at any time (14,23,25). Autopsy findings from those individuals experiencing an instantaneous death after H_2S exposure reveal no characteristic signs, indicating that asphyxia rather than a direct mucous membrane irritant effect predominates in an acute massive exposure of H_2S.

Effect on Nervous System. The central nervous system effects of H_2S have been considered to be a result of enzyme poisoning at the cellular level. After rapid absorption from the alveoli, H_2S is transported quickly to the brain. Central nervous system depression symptoms, such as drowsiness, fatigue, and dizziness, may occur with environmental exposure at 200 ppm. As the concentration reaches 500 ppm, headache, weakness of extremities, spasms, nausea, agitation, dizziness, and staggering may become more prominent. This may be followed by rapid loss of consciousness and respiratory paralysis as the concentration rises more than 1,000 ppm (24,25). At higher concentrations of H_2S, rapid respiratory paralysis and death may occur at any moment without any warning symptoms. Delirium, coma, and convulsions along with other neurologic symptoms may also occur in certain conditions of acute exposures (9,14,24,25,31,33,45). Clinical observations show that many victims recover completely from an unresponsive status in the settings of acute massive H_2S poisoning. However, irreversible damage to the nervous system associated with prominent sequelae after H_2S poisoning is not uncommon (23,24,30,31).

Effect on Other Organs or Systems. Studies regarding the health effects of H_2S on the other organs or systems are limited. Electrocardiogram tracings indicative of cardiac arrhythmia, myocardial ischemia, and myocardial infarction have been observed in cases of H_2S intoxication (10,29,30,46,47). Acute poisoning of rabbits with H_2S caused changes in ventricular repolarization, whereas subacute poisoning led to cardiac arrhythmia. A decrease in the reactivity of adenosine triphosphate phosphohydrolase and the reduced nicotinamide adenine dinucleotide phosphate oxidoreductase in myocardial cells was also noted, indicating a direct toxic effect of H_2S on myocardial cells (48). These findings are predictable because H_2S exerts its poisoning effects at the cellular level in a manner similar to cyanide. In H_2S poisoning, the gastrointestinal and endocrine systems may also be affected, producing symptoms of nausea, vomiting, diarrhea, abdominal cramps, gastric burning, and irregular menstruation (31–33,49). Several studies have examined the effect of 5 ppm H_2S on exercising men and women. Five ppm was selected because it is the concentration at one-half the occupational exposure limit (50,51). None of the subjects reported any adverse health effects subsequent to the exposure; however, some mild biochemical changes occurred in parameters that were markers for anaerobic and aerobic metabolism.

CLINICAL SYNDROME

The mechanism of H_2S poisoning is similar to that of other sulfides and cyanides. Similar to cyanide, H_2S is a potent inhibitor of cytochrome oxidase, resulting in tissue hypoxia (52). In purified preparations of cytochrome oxidase, sulfide has proven more potent than cyanide (53).

Clinically, acute H_2S intoxication can be defined as the effects from a single exposure to massive concentrations of H_2S that rapidly produce signs of unconsciousness and respiratory distress. Concentrations exceeding 700 ppm produce such acute effects. *Subacute H_2S intoxication* is the term applied to the effects of continuous exposure to concentrations ranging from 100 to 700 ppm for up to several hours. In this range of exposure, eye irritation is the most commonly observed effect. However, pulmonary edema may be a more important and potentially fatal complication of subacute H_2S intoxication (54). The following two cases illustrate typical presentations of acute massive and subacute intoxication by H_2S (54).

Case 1: Acute Massive Intoxication. A 40-year-old healthy man collapsed immediately after having descended into a hot-spring reservoir for regular maintenance work to clean precipitant debris. Four men who remained outside the manhole went down one by one to rescue him and also collapsed suddenly after smelling a strong odor of rotten eggs down at the bottom. One died on the scene; the other four were resuscitated and sent to a hospital. They presented to the hospital emergency room with an odor of rotten eggs and were unconscious but agitated, vomiting, tachypneic, cyanotic, with clammy skin and gray-greenish sputum. During their hospitalization, aspiration pneumonia and keratoconjunctivitis were noted in three of them. They recovered completely without any significant sequelae (54).

Case 2: Subacute Intoxication. A 30-year-old man collapsed in a hot-spring reservoir after he and an 18-year-old man had been shoveling the precipitant debris at the bottom for 2 hours. At the emergency room, both presented with tachypnea. Diffuse rhonchi, rales, and wheezing were audible throughout their chests. Their chest films showed infiltrates characteristic of pulmonary edema, bilaterally. Both developed refractory respiratory failure and died within 12 hours after the exposure (54).

The severity and variety of clinical manifestation and outcomes related to acute massive exposure of H_2S have been described extensively. The following acute clinical manifestations and outcomes are illustrated: (a) death caused by acute respiratory arrest, (b) successful resuscitation from recurrent apnea and pulmonary edema, (c) initial unconsciousness followed by tachypnea and complete recovery, (d) recovery from simple pulmonary edema without systemic involvement, and (e) unconsciousness followed by mild symptoms after recovery. One striking observation in the study was the predominance in frequency and severity of the systemic neurologic manifestations over the local irritative effects. This finding is quite typical in the instances of acute massive H_2S intoxication (9). In 221 cases of exposure to H_2S associated with the oil, gas, and petrochemical industries in Canada, the overall mortality was 6%; three-fourths of all victims experienced a period of unconsciousness, and 12% were comatose. A high proportion of patients had other neurologic signs and symptoms, including altered behavior patterns, confusion, vertigo, agitation, or somnolence. Respiratory tract effects were second in frequency only to neurologic manifestations. Forty percent of all patients required some form of respiratory assistance, and 15% of all patients developed pulmonary edema. Less severely affected patients complained primarily of headache, sore eyes, or gastrointestinal upsets. Some clinical observations reported that victims of H_2S poisonings may survive with neurologic sequelae; however, Burnett et al. did not find any recognizable neurologic sequelae among survivors (31).

Chronic and Long-Term Effects

The health effects of long-term exposures to low concentrations of H_2S are still uncertain. A preliminary study done in Rotorua, New Zealand, a major recreational center, showed that no chronic health impairment could be identified after long-term exposure to H_2S to 0.005 to 1.9 ppm (55). Other reports suggest that prolonged exposure to H_2S with concentrations less than 50 ppm over long periods may produce a chronic form of poisoning (25,56). Such a chronic intoxication is a subjective state, characterized by certain neurasthenic symptoms, such as fatigue, headache, dizziness, and irritability (57). Some authors have suggested that chronic symptoms and signs actually reflect recurring acute or subacute toxic exposures (7).

CARCINOGENICITY, MUTAGENICITY, TERATOGENICITY, AND EFFECTS ON REPRODUCTION

No published reports exist of carcinogenesis, mutagenesis, or teratogenesis attributable to H_2S exposure.

Management of Toxicity

TREATMENT

General Supportive Care. In acute H_2S intoxication, cessation of respiration is an immediate threat to life. Accordingly, the provision of artificially assisted respiration on an emergency basis is absolutely critical. Hence, moving the victim to fresh air and starting respiratory and cardiovascular support should be done immediately. Because many instances occurred in which the rescuers were overcome by H_2S, rescuers should wear a self-contained breathing apparatus. Mouth-to-mouth resuscitation is not recommended (9). After being moved away from the site, the victim needs to be monitored for respiratory distress and neurologic, ophthalmologic, and possible cardiovascular complications. If the victim is not breathing, cardiopulmonary resuscitation should be started immediately. Because oxygen can enhance the metabolism of sulfide and may benefit the injured tissue, it should be supplied as quickly as possible.

Induction of Methemoglobinemia. Because the poisoning mechanism of H_2S is similar to that of cyanide, induction of methemoglobinemia by the nitrite antidote method, a common treatment for cyanide poisoning, has also been proposed in the treatment of H_2S poisoning (10,58–60). In laboratory animals, the therapeutic induction of methemoglobinemia has been shown to have protective and antidotal effects against sulfide as well as against cyanide (20). Clinically, several cases have been reported that were successfully treated by this method in conjunction with vigorous supportive care (10,59,60). Overall, however, the success rate of the nitrite antidote method for sulfide poisoning has not been as clearly established as for cyanide treatment, and the value of this method has been questioned. Beck et al. believe that the methemoglobinemia protocol is too slow to detoxify the sulfides when compared with oxyhemoglobin. They suggest that breathing oxygen-enriched air is the only effective antidote (61).

To induce methemoglobinemia, the literature suggests beginning with a 3% sodium nitrite intravenous injection. However, if the sodium nitrite is not ready for injection, amyl nitrite by inhalation 15 to 30 seconds of every minute is recommended. Once 10 mL of 3% sodium nitrite is available, it can be injected intravenously over a 2- to 4-minute period for an adult. If signs and symptoms of systemic poisoning continue or recur, the nitrite injection should be repeated with one-half the dose. Cyanide antidote kits have been available in industrial and hospital settings for the purpose of methemoglobinemia induction. The thiosulfate solution contained in these kits, however, has not been recommended in the treatment of H_2S poisoning.

Hyperbaric Oxygen Therapy. Hyperbaric oxygen therapy has been proposed for severe H_2S poisoning (62,63). Successful treatment by this regimen has been reported in two patients. The first patient was unconscious with pulmonary edema on presentation. After 300 mg sodium nitrite was injected, he could open and close his eyes on command but still showed decerebrate posturing of his right arm on painful stimuli. He was extubated immediately after hyperbaric oxygen therapy (2.5 atmospheres absolute oxygen) for 90 minutes. Three hours after leaving the emergency room, he was eating a soft diet. He was discharged 48 hours later after another two sessions of hyperbaric oxygen therapy (62). The second patient was also unconscious on presentation. He received a total of 750 mg sodium nitrite by intravenous injection, without clinical response. Hyperbaric oxygen therapy was started 10 hours after H_2S exposure. After the first hyperbaric oxygen therapy session, the patient was more alert and able to follow simple commands (63). It was proposed that hyperbaric oxygen therapy would increase oxyhemoglobin levels and tissue oxygen concentrations, thus allowing oxygen to better compete with sulfide for binding sites on the cytochrome oxidase system and also enhancing the catalytic oxidation of sulfide. Also, hyperbaric oxygen therapy could minimize the damage of injured tissue by optimum supportive care (63). Because hyperbaric oxygen therapy has been used only in the treatment of H_2S poisoning, more clinical evaluations are needed before drawing any conclusion. However, this method can be considered as an extension of the vigorous general supportive care that has been reemphasized by many investigators.

In 1985, 250 cases of exposure to H_2S in Alberta, Canada, were reviewed and compared with the study done in 1977 (64). It was found that (a) the fatality rate decreased from 6% to 2.8%, (b) the unconsciousness rate at hospital arrival decreased from 13% to 2%, (c) the hospital admission rate fell from 51% to 22%, and (d) a relative decrease existed in the accident worker's compensation claim rate (17.4%). These findings were consistent with an impact of increased awareness of the dangers of H_2S, improved first aid treatment at the site of exposure, and the vigorous supportive care in the clinic or hospital.

Although the Canadian study does not conclusively demonstrate the efficacy of vigorous general supportive care in the treatment of H_2S poisonings, its findings suggest that such an approach may be the most appropriate treatment.

DIAGNOSIS

The diagnostic criteria for environmental poisoning include a history of exposure, an appropriate clinical syndrome, and the presence of the suspected chemical and its metabolites in body fluids. The diagnosis of H_2S poisoning relies primarily on the history of exposure, the presence of the smell of rotten eggs, and the fairly specific clinical syndrome. The presence of darkening of copper and silver coins in the pockets or of discolored jewelry provides supporting evidence of exposure to H_2S (2). The clinical picture of acute massive H_2S poisoning is usually typical, as the case given in the Clinical Syndrome section demonstrates. Because the plasma concentrations of sulfhemoglobin do not reflect the degree of H_2S exposure, their values in the clinical setting have never been confirmed. So far, no laboratory test is considered valuable for diagnostic use in clinical practice. However, urinary thiosulfate and blood sulfide anion determination are useful in a forensic setting (65).

EXPOSURE LIMITS, ENVIRONMENTAL AND BIOLOGICAL MONITORING, AND MEDICAL SURVEILLANCE

Exposure Limits

No federal ambient air or emission standards for H_2S are presently in place in the United States. Several states, however, have standards, which are described in Table 55-4 (4).

The Occupational Safety and Health Administration permissible exposure limit for H_2S is a ceiling concentration of 20 ppm

TABLE 55-4. Ambient air quality standards for H_2S

State	Concentration (parts per million)	Averaging time
California	0.03	1 h
Connecticut	0.2	8 h
Kentucky	0.01	1 h
Massachusetts	0.014	24 h
Montana	0.03	30 min
Nevada	0.24	8 h
New York	0.10	1 h
Pennsylvania	0.10	1 h
Texas	0.08	30 min
Virginia	0.16	24 h

From ref. 4, with permission.

for 15 minutes or a maximum allowable peak of 50 ppm for 10 minutes. NIOSH has recommended a reduced standard of 10 ppm ceiling for 10 minutes, and that work areas in which the concentration of H_2S exceeds 50 ppm be evacuated. The American Conference of Governmental Industrial Hygienists recommends a threshold limit value of 10 ppm as an 8-hour time-weighted average and a short-term exposure limit of 15 ppm (1,4).

Environmental Monitoring

Most H_2S poisonings have occurred in the places where it is commonly used or produced. Because these exposures are predictable and can be prevented, an environmental monitoring system may warn exposed workers of their overexposure and is valuable for prevention.

H_2S has lower and upper explosive limits of 4.3% and 45.5%, respectively, and an autoignition temperature of 260°C. Appropriate procedures and precautions must be taken to avoid the occurrence of fire and explosion. The storage and disposal of H_2S must comply with all local, state, and federal regulations. Efforts should be made to avoid or minimize the formation and accumulation of H_2S, for example, by the use of refrigeration on fishing boats and maintenance of adequate airflow rates in sewers and storage areas.

Engineering controls should be used to keep airborne H_2S less than concentrations at which it is hazardous to the health of workers. To confirm that H_2S concentrations are less than the evacuation limit and to prevent worker exposure to H_2S at hazardous concentrations, a continuous real-time monitoring of workplace air usually is required in addition to periodic personal breathing zone air sampling. For breathing zone air samples, NIOSH recommends that a midget impinger be used and that the methylene blue method be used for H_2S analysis (2). At the work site, a fixed H_2S detector system must have a two-stage, spark-proof alarm, with a lower triggering level of 10 ppm to warn workers that H_2S is more than the ceiling limit, and a higher triggering level of 50 ppm to signal workers to evacuate the area and to obtain respiratory protection for rescue or repair efforts or for carrying out contingency plans. Fixed H_2S monitors should also automatically trigger supplementary ventilation of the workplace. Portable H_2S monitors and detector tubes may also be supplementally used as needed. Continuous monitoring can protect the workers, however, only when it is combined with an alerting and alarm system, adequate ventilation, respiratory protection, and other appropriate measures. Respiratory protection (self-contained breathing apparatus) is needed when the engineering controls are in the process of being installed or when they fail and need to be supplemented. Such respirators may also be used for operations that require entry into tanks or closed vessels and in emergency situations. These respirators should be immediately accessible to employees in emergency situations. The workers must be advised of the hazards of exposure to H_2S and trained in the use of respiratory protective devices and in the administration of artificial respiration (2).

Biological Monitoring

Biological monitoring is not of value in preventing harmful effects of H_2S exposure. Most of the effects that have been associated with H_2S exposure are not cumulative but arise from sudden, comparatively brief exposures at high concentrations or from repeated exposures to individually bearable concentrations (2).

Medical Surveillance

NIOSH recommends that preplacement examinations be given to employees who are potentially exposed to H_2S (2). These examinations must specifically assess the worker's ability to use respiratory protection (66). These examinations should be made available at 3-year intervals to all workers exposed to H_2S at concentrations more than the ceiling concentration limit. Individuals exposed to H_2S at concentrations more than 50 ppm should be examined promptly by a physician (2).

REFERENCES

1. Environmental Protection Agency. *Hydrogen sulfide: chemical profiles*. Washington: Environmental Protection Agency, 1985.
2. National Institute for Occupational Safety and Health. Criteria for a recommended standard: occupational exposure to hydrogen sulfide. [DHEW publication no (NIOSH) 77–158]. Washington: US Government Printing Office, 1977.
3. Beauchamp RO Jr, Bus JS, Popp JA, Boreiko CJ, Andjelkovich DA. A critical review of the literature on hydrogen sulfide toxicity. *CRC Crit Rev Toxicol* 1984;13:25–97.
4. Environmental Protection Agency. *Health assessment document for hydrogen sulfide, review draft*. Washington: Environmental Protection Agency, 1986 [PB 87–117420].
5. Cooper RC, Jenkins D, Young LY. *Aquatic microbiology laboratory manual*. Austin, TX: University of Texas, 1976.
6. Mercado SG. Geothermo-electric project of Cerro-Priete: contamination and basic protection. Proceedings of the second UN symposium on the development and use of geothermal resources. San Francisco: 1975:1386–1393.
7. National Research Council, US Subcommittee on Hydrogen Sulfide. *Hydrogen sulfide*. Baltimore: University Park Press, 1979.
8. Macaluso P. Hydrogen sulfide. In: *Kirk-Othmer encyclopedia of chemical technology*, 2nd ed. New York: John Wiley and Sons, 1969;19:375–389.
9. Kleinfeld M, Giel C, Rosso A. Acute hydrogen sulfide intoxication: an unusual source of exposure. *Ind Med Surg* 1964;33:656–660.
10. Peters JW. Hydrogen sulfide poisoning in a hospital setting. *JAMA* 1981;246: 1588–1589.
11. Pettigrew GL. *Preliminary report on hydrogen sulfide exposure in the oil and gas industry*. Dallas: US Department of Health, Education, and Welfare, Public Health Service, Dallas Regional Office, 1976.
12. McCabe LC, Clayton GD. Air pollution by hydrogen sulfide in Poza Rica, Mexico. An evaluation of the incident of Nov 24, 1950. *Arch Ind Hyg Occup Med* 1952;6:199–213.
13. Burgess WA. Potential exposures in industry: their recognition and control. In: Clayton GD, ed. *Patty's industrial hygiene and toxicology*. New York: John Wiley and Sons, 1978;1:1149–1222.
14. Yant WP. Hydrogen sulfide in industry: occurrence, effects and treatment. *Am J Public Health* 1930;20:598–608.
15. Laug EP, Draize JH. The percutaneous absorption of ammonium hydrogen sulfide and hydrogen sulfide. *J Pharmacol Exp Ther* 1942;76:179–188.
16. Walton DC, Witherspoon MG. Skin absorption of certain gases. *J Pharmacol Exp Ther* 1925;26:315–324.
17. Voigt GE, Muller P. The histochemical effect of hydrogen sulfide poisoning. *Acta Histochem* 1955;1:223–239.
18. Curtis CG, Bartholomew TC, Rose FA, Dodgson KS. Detoxication of sodium 35-S-sulfide in the rat. *Biochem Pharmacol* 1972;21:2313–2321.
19. Weisiger RA, Jakoby WB. S-Methylation: thiol S-methyltransferase. In: Jakoby WB, ed. *Enzymatic basis of detoxification*. New York: Academic Press, 1980;2:131.
20. Smith RP, Gosselin RE. Hydrogen sulfide poisoning. *J Occup Med* 1979; 21:93–97.
21. Smith RP, Kruszyna R, Kruszyna H. Management of acute sulfide poisoning: effects of oxygen, thiosulfate, and nitrite. *Arch Environ Health* 1976; 31:166–169.

22. Smith RP, Gosselin RE. The influence of methemoglobinemia on the lethality of some toxic anions. *Toxicol Appl Pharmacol* 1964;6:584–592.
23. Milby TH. Hydrogen sulfide intoxication: review of the literature and report of unusual accident resulting in two cases of nonfatal poisoning. *J Occup Med* 1962;4:431–437.
24. Ahlborg G. Hydrogen sulfide poisoning in shale oil industry. *Arch Ind Hyg Occup Med* 1951;3:247–266.
25. Haggard HW. The toxicology of hydrogen sulfide. *J Ind Hyg* 1925;7:113–121.
26. Evans CL. The toxicity of hydrogen sulfide and other sulfides. *J Exp Physiol* 1967;52:231–248.
27. Gunina AI. Transformation of sulfur-35-labeled hydrogen sulfide introduced into blood. *Dokl Akad Nauk SSSR* 1957b;112:902–904.
28. Susman JL, Hornig JF, Thomas SC, Smith RP. Pulmonary excretion of hydrogen sulfide, methanethiol, dimethyl sulfide, and dimethyl disulfide in mice. *Drug Chem Toxicol* 1978;1:327–333.
29. Kaipainen WJ. Hydrogen sulfide intoxication: rapidly transient changes in the electrocardiogram suggestive of myocardial infarction. *Ann Med Intern Fenn* 1954;43:97–101.
30. Kemper FD. A near-fatal case of hydrogen sulfide poisoning. *Can Med Assoc J* 1966;94:1130–1131.
31. Burnett WW, King EG, Grace M, Hall WF. Hydrogen sulfide poisoning: review of five years' experience. *Can Med Assoc J* 1977;117:1277–1280.
32. Gafafer WM, ed. Occupational disease: a guide to their recognition. [Publication no 1097]. Washington: US Department of Health, Education, and Welfare, 1964:163.
33. Poda GA. Hydrogen sulfide can be handled safely. *Arch Environ Health* 1966;12:795–800.
34. Jones JP. Hazards of hydrogen sulfide gas [Abst]. 23rd Annual Gas Measurement Institute 1975;16.
35. Adelson L, Sunshine I. Fatal hydrogen sulfide intoxication. *Arch Pathol* 1966;81:375–380.
36. Johnstone RT, Saunders WB, eds. *Occupational disease and industrial medicine*. Philadelphia: WB Saunders, 1960.
37. Carson MB. Hydrogen sulfide exposure in the gas industry. *Ind Med Surg* 1963;32:63–64.
38. Nesswetha W. Eye damage through sulfur interactions. *Arbeitsmed Sozialmed Arbeitshyg* 1969;4:288–290.
39. Masure R. Keratoconjunctivitis of viscose rayon fibers: a clinical and experimental study. *Rev Belge Pathol Med Exp* 1950;20:297–341.
40. American Conference of Governmental Industrial Hygienists. Hydrogen sulfide. In: *Documentation of the threshold limit values*, 6th ed. Cincinnati: American Conference of Governmental Industrial Hygienists, 1991.
41. Elkins HB. Hydrogen sulfide. In: *The chemistry of industrial toxicology*. New York: John Wiley and Sons, 1950.
42. Mitchell CW, Yant WP. Correlation of the data obtained from refinery accidents with a laboratory study of H_2S and its treatment. *US Bureau of Mines Bulletin* 1925;231:59–79.
43. Cralley LV. The effect of irritant gases upon the rate of ciliary activity. *J Ind Hyg Toxicol* 1942;24:193–198.
44. Rogers RE, Ferin J. Effects of hydrogen sulfide on bacterial inactivation in the rat lung. *Arch Environ Health* 1981;36:261–264.
45. Henkin RI. Effects of vapor phase pollutants on nervous system and sensory function. In: Finkel AJ, Duel WC, eds. *Clinical implications of air pollution research*. Acton, MA: Publishing Sciences Group, 1976.
46. Ravizza AG, Carugo D, Cerchiari EL. The treatment of hydrogen sulfide intoxication: oxygen versus nitrites. *Vet Hum Toxicol* 1982;24:241–242.
47. Vathenen AS, Emberton P, Wales JM. Hydrogen sulfide poisoning in factory workers [Letter]. *Lancet* 1988;1:305.
48. Kosmider S, Rogala E, Pacholek A. Electrocardiographic and histochemical studies of the heart muscle in acute experimental hydrogen sulfide poisoning. *Arch Immunol Ther Exp* 1967;15:731–740.
49. Vasileva IA. Effect of small concentrations of carbon disulfide and hydrogen sulfide on the menstrual function of women and the estrual cycle of experimental animals. *Gig Sanit* 1973;7:24–27.
50. Bhambhani Y, Burnham R, Snydmiller G, et al. Comparative physiological responses of exercising men and women to 5 ppm H_2S exposure. *Am Ind Hyg Assoc J* 1994;55:1030–1035.
51. Bhambhani Y, Burnham R, Snydmiller G, et al. Effects of 5 ppm H_2S inhalation on biochemical properties of skeletal muscle in exercising men and women. *Am Ind Hyg Assoc J* 1996;57:464–468.
52. Albaum HG, Tepperman J, Bodonsky O. Spectrophotometric study of competition of methemoglobin and cytochrome oxidase for sulfide in vitro. *J Biol Chem* 1946;163:641–647.
53. Nicholls P. The effect of sulfide on cytochrome aa3, isosteric and allosteric shifts of the reduced A-peak. *Biochim Biophys Acta* 1975;396:24–35.
54. Deng JF, Chang SC. Hydrogen sulfide poisonings in hot-spring reservoir cleaning: two case reports. *Am J Ind Med* 1987;11:447–451.
55. Siegel SM, Penny P, Siegel BZ, Penny D. Atmospheric hydrogen sulfide levels at the Sulfur Bay Wildlife area, Lake Rotorua, New Zealand. *Water Air Soil Pollut* 1986;28:385–391.
56. Mitchell CW, Davenport SJ. Hydrogen sulfide literature. *Public Health Rep* 1924;39:1–13.
57. Illinois Institute for Environmental Quality. Hydrogen sulfide health effects and recommended air quality standard. Chicago: Environmental Resource Center, 1974. [IIEQ doc no 74–24, NTIS no PB 233 843].
58. Chen KK, Rose CL. Nitrite and thiosulfate therapy in cyanide poisoning. *JAMA* 1952;149:113–119.
59. Vannatta JB. Hydrogen sulfide poisoning: report of four cases and brief review of the literature. *J Okla State Med Assoc* 1982;75:29–32.
60. Stine RJ, Slosberg B, Beacham BE. Hydrogen sulfide intoxication: a case report and discussion of treatment. *Ann Intern Med* 1976;85:756–758.
61. Beck JF, Bradbury CM, Connors AJ, Donini JC. Nitrite as an antidote for acute hydrogen sulfide intoxication. *Am Ind Hyg Assoc J* 1981;42:805–809.
62. Whitcraft DD, Bailey TD, Hart GB. Hydrogen sulfide poisoning treated with hyperbaric oxygen. *J Emerg Med* 1985;3:23–25.
63. Smilkstein MJ, Bronstein AC, Pickett HM, Rumack BH. Hyperbaric oxygen therapy for severe hydrogen sulfide poisoning. *J Emerg Med* 1985;3:27–30.
64. Arnold IM, Dufresne RM, Alleyne BC, Stuart PJ. Health implication of occupational exposures to hydrogen sulfide. *J Occup Med* 1985;27:373–376.
65. Kangas J, Savolainen H. Urinary thiosulfate as an indicator of exposure to hydrogen sulfide vapor. *Clin Chim Acta* 1987;164:7–10.
66. National Institute for Occupational Safety and Health. *Guide to industrial respiratory protection*. Washington: US Government Printing Office, 1987. [DHHS Publication no. (NIOSH) 87–116].

CHAPTER 56
Carbon Monoxide

Donna L. Seger and Larry W. Welch

SOURCE OF EXPOSURE

Carbon monoxide (CO) is a leading cause of poisoning morbidity and mortality in the United States. In 1995, the American Association of Poison Control Centers Annual Report recorded 19,253 CO exposures. Only 394 of these exposures were intentional, and 47 of the exposures were fatal (1). The majority of unintentional exposures is the result of a malfunctioning heating source, occupational exposure, or fire. The difficulty in diagnosing CO intoxication in less obvious situations causes the morbidity from CO to be grossly underestimated (2).

Steel industry workers, miners, auto mechanics, warehouse storage and loading facility workers, as well as firefighters, may be exposed to high concentrations of CO. Although malfunctioning equipment is frequently the cause of exposure to high levels of CO, inadequate ventilation of the area may be the critical factor in the development of toxicity. Occupational Safety and Health Administration guidelines limit exposure to no more than 50 parts per million (ppm) over an 8-hour time-weighted average. Fires in rooms with natural polymeric materials may cause CO concentrations of up to 50,000 ppm. The National Institute for Occupational Safety and Health considers CO concentrations of 1,500 ppm to be immediately dangerous to life or health (3).

Methylene chloride (CH_2Cl_2), a simple halogenated hydrocarbon, is found in industrial products, such as paint strippers, insecticides and other fumigants, aerosol propellants, and Christmas tree bubble lights. CH_2Cl_2 is absorbed dermally and by inhalation. It is highly lipid soluble, slowly released from adipose tissue and hepatically metabolized to carbon dioxide (70%) and CO (30%). Exposure to CH_2Cl_2 may result in carboxyhemoglobin (COHb) saturations of 10% to 50%, which can peak up to 8 hours after exposure. Mental status changes immediately after the exposure are likely to be attributable to the solvent, but later neurologic symptoms should be attributed to CO. Serum COHb should be obtained in this setting, and treatment administered should be that for CO poisoning. Uncontrolled exposures in individuals working with paint strippers may be fatal (4).

Atmospheric CO varies in urban areas and depends on weather conditions and individual activity. Concentrations may vary from 1 ppm in rural areas to 140 ppm in urban areas with heavy traffic.

The majority of atmospheric CO (approximately 60%) comes from vehicular fuel combustion (diesel fumes contain little CO). Ice-surfacing machines, propane-powered vehicles (trucks and forklifts), and industrial processes (coke ovens and solid waste incinerators) add to atmospheric CO. Smoke from house and forest fires can contain up to 10% CO. Atmospheric CO is removed through migration to the upper atmosphere, oxidation to carbon dioxide, and reduction to methane by microorganisms (5).

Home sources of CO, such as oil-powered furnaces and natural gas (space heaters, ovens, and fireplaces), add minimally to atmospheric CO but may cause CO poisoning in the event of malfunction or inadequate ventilation. The production of CO can be greatly increased by incorrect air-fuel mixture (i.e., faulty ventilation of combustion gases caused by leaks, cracks, or inadequate fresh air intake). Proper oxygenation is required to prevent incomplete combustion of natural gas. A danger of natural gas is that warning irritating vapors do not occur when combustion is incomplete and high levels of CO are present (6).

PHYSIOLOGY

CO uptake is determined by many variables, such as the concentration of CO in the inspired air and the duration of exposure, the ventilatory rate, pulmonary diffusing capacity, exposure, and the rate of endogenous CO production. CO is excreted by the lungs at a rate dependent on the patient's minute volume. CO elimination is complex, and elimination time also appears to depend on length of exposure, and whether the exposure was continuous or intermittent (5,6).

Physiologic CO is formed from endogenous degradation of hemoglobin and nonhemoglobin heme-yielding serum COHb saturations of 0.5% in healthy individuals. These saturations may be as high as 4% to 6% in patients with increased red cell breakdown (e.g., acute hemolytic anemia, polycythemia, and blood transfusions). Cigarette smoking may cause COHb saturations of 5% to 10% (6).

The half-life of COHb is approximately 4.5 hours in room air oxygen concentrations (21%) at 1 atm. Delivering 100% oxygen at atmospheric pressure reduces the half-life. A pressure of 3 atm reduces the CO elimination half-life to 23 minutes. These values vary between individuals.

PATHOPHYSIOLOGY AND MECHANISM OF TOXICITY

To date, no single mechanism has been accepted as explaining the clinical picture of CO toxicity, which includes the development of delayed neuropsychiatric sequelae. Proposed mechanisms include hypoxia-ischemia, cytochrome oxidase inhibition resulting in cellular toxicity, and CO-mediated brain lipid peroxidation.

Carbon monoxide is a tasteless, colorless, odorless gas that rapidly diffuses across alveolar-capillary membranes and binds to hemoglobin with an affinity 250 times greater than that of oxygen. Increasing blood COHb saturation decreases the number of hemoglobin sites available to bind oxygen. Normally, a decreased number of oxygen-hemoglobin binding sites (e.g., simple anemia) decreases the affinity of hemoglobin for oxygen, which shifts the oxyhemoglobin curve to the right. However, CO causes an allosteric change in the oxyhemoglobin complex, which increases the affinity of oxygen for hemoglobin and shifts the oxyhemoglobin dissociation curve to the left. Tissue hypoxia causes acidosis, which shifts the oxyhemoglobin dissociation curve back to the right (7). This mechanism of reduced oxygen carrying and delivery of oxygen by hemoglobin was the original theory of CO toxicity.

However, CO also binds to cytochrome oxidase, causing cellular hypoxia. Approximately 10% to 15% of total body CO is bound to extravascular proteins, such as myoglobin, cytochrome oxidase, cytochrome P-450, catalase, and peroxidases. The rate of dissociation from cytochrome oxidase is slow, raising the possibility that CO may cause a prolonged adverse effect despite transient hypoxia. Cellular compensations may include increasing electron flow through uninvolved cytochrome molecules (8).

The relationship between carboxyhemoglobin and the partial pressure of oxygen in the blood is expressed by the Haldane equation:

$$\frac{\text{COHb}}{\text{O}_2\text{Hb}} = (m)\frac{P\text{CO}}{P\text{O}_2}$$

Because of the high affinity of CO for hemoglobin (240 times that of O_2, the higher the partial pressure of O_2, the faster the decline in COHgb. The mass effect of a very high PaO_2 as can be attained by hyperbaric oxygen is

21% O_2 (room air) – PaO_2 100 mm Hg = 0.3 mL O_2/100 mL blood
100% O_2 = PaO_2 673 mm Hg = 2 mL O_2/100 mL blood
2 atm (hyperbaric) = 4.3 mL O_2/100 mL blood

Because CO also binds to other heme-containing proteins, such as cardiac myoglobin and cytochrome enzymes, it is probable that the Haldane effect would also occur at these sites to displace CO.

Some of the evidence for cellular toxicity may be found in a study performed in 1976 (9). Goldbaum transfused dogs with red blood cells highly saturated with CO to produce COHb of 60% to 70%. This extremely elevated saturation caused no signs of toxicity. However, direct inhalation of CO in control animals resulted in death at COHb saturations of 57% to 64%. Goldbaum concluded that dissolved CO freely enters tissues, binds to cytochrome oxidase, and causes toxicity. The CO complexed with red blood cells did not immediately equilibrate with plasma and tissue, which explains the lack of toxicity in the transfused animals. Vital signs and arterial blood gases were not monitored, however, and autopsies were not performed. Therefore, tissue hypoxia and hypotension may explain the results. Goldbaum's conclusions were questioned when a study in which animals whose blood was replaced by perfluorocarbon emulsions (capable of carrying large quantities of oxygen) survived indefinitely despite CO administration (10). Subsequently, Piantadosi's experiments revealed that CO may form a ligand with cerebral cytochrome oxidase, causing impaired mitochondrial function even at low concentrations of CO. He proposed the pathophysiologic difference between CO hypoxia and hypoxic or oligemic hypoxia was because of this impaired mitochondrial function (11).

Differing opinions contend that CO toxicity can be explained by hypoxia, hypotension induced by hypoxia, and CO binding to cardiac myoglobin (carboxymyoglobin), which depresses myocardial contractility. Supporting evidence for hypoxia as the primary cause of toxicity is (a) postanoxic encephalopathy explains the inability of blood COHb saturations at presentation to predict delayed neurologic sequelae and (b) cerebral pathologic changes that occur after CO exposure (parenchymal necrosis in areas of cerebral gray matter) are similar to the neuropathologic changes that occur after hypoxia (12,13). Bilateral necrosis of the globus pallidus is a hallmark of CO poisoning, but it should be noted that this lesion occurs in other hypoxic-ischemic settings as well. Other areas that may be affected are cerebral cortex, hippocampus, cerebellum, and substantia nigra (14).

Cerebral white matter lesions, also seen in CO poisoning, occur when ischemia is superimposed on hypoxia but do not occur as a result of hypoxia alone. Hypoxia-induced cerebral vasodilation (which maintains cerebral perfusion) is prevented if hypotension occurs concurrently. Ischemia is far more damaging to the central nervous system than simple hypoxia. Lesions in primates after CO exposure are anatomically indistinguishable from hypoxic-ischemic lesions (15).

Research reveals that brain lipid peroxidation (i.e., degradation of unsaturated fatty acids after peroxide generation) occurs after CO exposure (16). Coma from hypotension-induced cerebral hypoperfusion occurs in rats that subsequently demonstrate brain lipid peroxidation at autopsy. In animal models, hypotension is required to produce late neurologic effects and lipid peroxidation (17–19). The role of lipid peroxidation, the factors that initiate this cascade, and its relation to clinical features of toxicity are unknown. Additionally, evidence exists that CO may be a neural messenger and a direct activator of guanylate cyclase, a smooth muscle relaxer (20,21).

The roles and interactions of cytochrome oxidase inhibition, hypoxia-ischemia, and lipid peroxidation are intertwined and appear difficult to separate.

DELAYED NEUROPSYCHIATRIC AND BEHAVIORAL SEQUELAE

After CO exposure, an abrupt onset of neurologic and psychiatric deterioration may follow a recovery period of several weeks. The first case involving delayed sequelae was described in 1926. A 58-year-old woman had a seemingly normal recovery after CO-induced coma. One month later, she became disoriented, mute, developed a parkinsonian syndrome, and subsequently died. Autopsy revealed bilateral necrosis of the globus pallidus and widespread demyelination of the entire subcortical white matter. Subsequent case reports have documented delayed onset of gross neurologic impairments, such as akinesia, parkinsonism, psychosis, amnesia, apathy, apraxia, dementia, mutism, urinary and fecal incontinence, and gait disturbances, as well as subtler deficits, such as intellectual deterioration, memory impairment, and personality changes, in patients who were asymptomatic or had apparent resolution of symptoms at the time of exposure (22–24).

Retrospective reviews report that the incidence of delayed neurotoxicity ranges from 2% to 43%. Neither clinical nor laboratory parameters (including blood COHb saturation) predict which patients will develop delayed sequelae. An unanswered question is whether patients with cognitive function deficits at the time of the exposure are at risk for delayed sequelae, or whether these deficits are acute effects of exposure to CO. Volunteers exposed to CO (COHb less than 20%) may demonstrate temporary mental impairment (8,25–28).

Only standardized, quantifiable neuropsychological test batteries reveal deficits in attention and concentration, eye-hand coordination, manual dexterity, pure motor speed, reaction time, memory, and reasoning (29). Messier and Myers (30) have developed a CO neuropsychological screening battery that detects differences between the CO-exposed patient and the unexposed person. Bedside testing does not include this battery (30). Cognitive deficits may be present in patients who are asymptomatic and have normal physical examination results. Furthermore, outcome may vary greatly depending on other exposure parameters, such as age, severity of poisoning, and preexisting physical conditions.

Behavior and personality disturbances, often subtle or transient, occur after many neurotoxin exposures, including CO. Because these changes may occur in the absence of cognitive or sensorimotor changes, they may be misdiagnosed as being reactive or a preexisting condition. For example, depression after the exposure may be reactive depression or depression induced by the neurochemical or structural central nervous system changes caused by the poisoning. Diagnosis is difficult because behavioral and psychiatric disturbances may occur after a cogent period lasting from several days to weeks (16).

DIAGNOSIS AND EVALUATION OF POISONING

The diagnosis of CO poisoning may be suggested by the circumstances that caused the patient to seek medical attention. CO poisoning must be considered in patients with smoke inhalation or who were in a closed space during a fire, as well as patients who present with a flulike illness during the winter. History must include environmental and occupational exposures as well as the use of home-heating materials and recreational activities (e.g., indoor ice skating, recreational boats, and riding in the back of pick-up trucks) (31–33).

The acute and chronic effects of CO can mimic many neurologic or psychiatric illnesses. Symptoms resembling multiple sclerosis, parkinsonism, Korsakoff's amnestic syndrome, bipolar disorder, schizophrenia, and hysterical conversion reaction have been reported. Headache, fatigue, malaise, nausea, vomiting, or diarrhea, however, may be the only complaints on presentation. Respiratory distress is unusual, even in patients who complain of chest pain and exhibit tachycardia and tachypnea. Routine physical examination is frequently unremarkable. Skin color is more likely to be cyanotic or pale, not the cherry-red coloration that may be a postmortem finding. Signs of smoke inhalation (singed nasal hairs or eyebrows and soot in the oral cavity or sputum) should alert one to the potential development of airway obstruction from thermal and chemical injury, pulmonary edema, and chemical pneumonitis (34).

The nervous system and heart have the highest metabolic requirements for oxygen and are most susceptible to oxygen deprivation. Abnormalities of basal ganglia function are characteristic of CO neurotoxicity. Basal ganglia function is involved in planning, staging, and execution of movements. Insults to this area cause tremor, decreases in motor speed, slowed reaction time, poor manual dexterity, decreased eye-hand coordination, and poor sequencing of complex motor movements. Detailed psychometric testing is necessary to reveal deficits of this nature (30).

Typically, tachycardia occurs in an attempt to compensate for tissue hypoxia. In healthy individuals, dilatation of the coronary vessels caused by CO-induced tissue hypoxia meets the increased cardiac oxygen requirements. In patients with coronary artery disease, however, exacerbation of angina and arrhythmias can occur with a blood COHb of less than 10% (35).

Patients with coronary artery disease are at increased risk for myocardial infarction immediately after exposure or several days later. An electrocardiogram should be obtained in any potentially significant poisoning and in all patients with a history of coronary artery disease.

Although an elevated blood COHb provides an unequivocal marker of exposure, it is not a reliable indicator of the severity of the poisoning. Conversely, a normal blood COHb may be present in clinically severe poisoning by the time that a patient presents to the hospital. Carboxyhemoglobin saturations are misleading when taken in isolation because one needs to take into account the following variables: length of time of exposure, peak COHb saturation, delay between CO exposures and blood sampling, interim use of supplemental oxygen, age, metabolic rate, pulmonary function, and physical activity. Various tables have attempted to correlate symptoms and signs at presentation to blood COHb saturations (Table 56-1). Most tables suggest that patients with COHb saturations of 20% may develop headache and experience dyspnea on exertion, that

TABLE 56-1. Carbon monoxide poisoning: signs and symptoms with increasing levels in blood

Level of carbon monoxide in blood	Signs and symptoms
10–20%	Headache Shortness of breath
20–30%	Severe headache, dizziness Nausea Vomiting Difficulty concentrating
30–40%	Lethargy Fainting on exertion Visual Auditory disturbance Dizziness Chest pain Fainting
40–50%	Rapid heart rate, fainting Heart attack Seizures
50–60%	Coma Brain damage Cardiac arrest
70% or more	Death

saturations of 30% to 40% are associated with ataxia and dizziness, and that saturations greater than 50% result in syncope, seizures, and coma. However, clinical case reports have clearly demonstrated these tables are inconsistent, at best, and that blood COHb saturations correlate poorly with the severity of the acute poisoning and the likelihood of complications. Therefore, the severity of CO poisoning cannot be based solely on CO saturation (36,37).

Laboratory findings may be deceptively normal even in severe CO intoxications. Because arterial oxygen pressure (PaO_2) is a measure of oxygen dissolved in plasma, it is not affected by changes in hemoglobin saturation. As a result, the PaO_2 may be normal, whereas hemoglobin oxygen saturation is decreased. Lactic acid and glucose may be elevated as well as serum enzyme activities (creatine kinase, lactate dehydrogenase, alanine transferase, aspartate transferase).

The role of neuroimaging techniques in the evaluation of CO poisoning has yet to be determined. Bilateral or unilateral low-density lesions of the globus pallidus or of the white matter may be seen on computerized tomography (CT) of the brain. Clinical neurologic abnormalities may not correlate with the anatomic localization seen on CT. Topographic analysis of electroencephalogram mapping and technetium-99m-hexamethyl propylamine oxime brain single-photon emission computed tomography has demonstrated regional cerebral blood flow anomalies in the temporoparieto-occipital region in CO poisoning, which are the watershed areas of the major cerebral arteries (38). Scans with abnormal results cannot be correlated with clinical signs or symptoms. Anomalies similar to those found after CO exposure are also found in postanoxic syndrome, hypoglycemia, cerebral infarction, Alzheimer's, and Parkinson's. Xenon-enhanced CT studies of CO-exposed patients reveal a decrease in cerebral blood flow in frontal, temporal, and basal ganglia areas, even in patients with complete resolution of symptoms (39). Whether patients with regional cerebral blood flow anomalies have a higher incidence of delayed sequelae or require further treatment to prevent development of a delayed syndrome is unknown. After exposure, a lag period of 2 to 3 days may occur before either CT or magnetic resonance imaging reveals abnormalities (40).

MANAGEMENT

Initial treatment of CO poisoning involves removal of the patient from the source of exposure and institution of basic life support measures. One hundred percent oxygen should be administered to facilitate dissociation of CO from the hemoglobin molecules. Although rebreather masks are typically used to deliver 100% oxygen, these masks do not have a tight seal and deliver only 55% to 60% oxygen. Endotracheal intubation and mechanical ventilation with 100% oxygen should be initiated if the patient is unconscious. As acidosis shifts the oxyhemoglobin dissociation curve to the right to increase tissue oxygen delivery, bicarbonate administration should be withheld except in cases of life-threatening acidosis.

The role of hyperbaric oxygen (HBO) in treating symptoms and signs of CO toxicity at the time of exposure to prevent delayed sequelae is unknown. HBO causes a high oxygen tension that rapidly displaces CO from the blood and tissues and dissolves enough oxygen in the plasma to meet the body's metabolic needs, even in the absence of functioning hemoglobin. HBO prevents lipid peroxidation in CO-exposed animals. Technetium-99m-hexamethyl propylamine oxime brain single-photon emission computed tomography imaging pre- and post-HBO reveals that HBO improves perfusion of and metabolism in the CO-affected brain (38). It is not known how HBO compares to normobaric oxygen in shortening the duration of symptoms and signs of toxicity in acute poisoning and in helping it prevent delayed neurologic sequelae (provided structural brain damage has not occurred). No conclusive evidence exists that shortening the duration of clinical features of toxicity diminishes the severity of delayed sequelae because no controlled trials have been reported. Nor have there been any controlled studies that included appropriate psychometric testing on follow-up that compared the effectiveness of HBO and normobaric oxygen administration. One of the problems is the lack of clinical or laboratory prognostic indicators to determine which patients will develop late neuropsychiatric sequelae. Irrefutably, patient prognosis and indications for HBO are not wholly dependent on COHb saturation. The value of delayed HBO in the prevention and mitigation of delayed neuropsychiatric sequelae days to weeks after exposure is unproved.

Published recommendations that comatose patients or patients with blood COHb saturations greater than 40% should undergo HBO are empiric in origin and are not based on scientific evidence. Other historical empiric recommendations for HBO include any resulting neurologic deficit (other than headache), including disorientation and focal neurologic signs; history of loss of consciousness or syncope; cardiac ischemia; dysrhythmia; or electrocardiographic evidence of ischemia after CO exposure, seizures or history of seizure, metabolic acidosis, pulmonary edema, or pregnancy in women who are symptomatic (41). No evidence and many questions exist as to whether the following patients need HBO: patients with a headache or dizziness after CO exposure, children, or asymptomatic patients with COHb saturations greater than 10%.

Infants and children have an increased susceptibility to CO toxicity because of their higher metabolic rate and higher tissue oxygen demand. Clinically, children seem to have an increased incidence of lethargy and syncope at lower COHb concentrations than adults. Delayed neurologic sequelae have been reported (42). Neuropsychological (NP) testing is difficult in children younger than 7 years of age. Although no specific guidelines exist for children, use of HBO should be considered in children who have been exposed to CO (27).

The fetus is extremely susceptible to CO toxicity. The fetal oxyhemoglobin dissociation curve lies to the left of the adult curve and is shifted more to the left by CO. After maternal exposure to CO, fetal COHb saturations continue to rise for several

TABLE 56-2. Maryland Institute for Emergency Medical Services Systems indications for hyperbaric oxygen

Coma
Neurologic impairment as evidenced by neuropsychological testing or other means
Cardiovascular involvement
Serum carboxyhemoglobin levels of more than 40%
Pregnancy carboxyhemoglobin levels of more than 15%
Ischemic heart disease in association with serum carboxyhemoglobin levels of more than 20%
Recurrent symptoms up to 3 weeks after original treatment with surface oxygen
Symptoms that do not resolve after 6 hours of continuous 100% surface oxygen

hours and equilibrate at a COHb saturation 10% higher than maternal COHb. The half-life of fetal COHb is 15 hours. Analysis of case reports suggests a fetal mortality of 36% to 67% after maternal exposure. Autopsy evidence of basal ganglia and gray matter lesions, tone impairment, mental deterioration, and multiple anomalies in children after *in utero* exposure suggest that CO is a teratogen. Pregnancy does not create a risk that is greater than usual when undergoing HBO. HBO should be considered in all pregnant women exposed to CO (43,44).

Recommended diving schedules vary from 3 atm for 45 minutes repeated every 6 hours, depending on the clinical picture, to 2 atm for 90 minutes repeated every 6 hours, depending on the clinical picture. No proof exists that repeated sessions are better than single sessions or that 3 atm is preferable to 2 atm. In fact, pressures more than 2.5 atm may cause cerebral capillary leakage and perivascular edema (45–47).

Complications of HBO are usually minimal. Ear barotrauma and ear pain, sinus pain, and tooth pain are common complaints. Oxygen toxicity seizures occur infrequently. Patients with obstructive lung disease may lose their hypoxic drive. Patients may complain of claustrophobia, but this does not have life-threatening consequences. Emesis may occur (45).

The approach to the CO-poisoned patient is to perform NP testing at the time of presentation after the exposure. Patients with abnormal results are maintained on 100% oxygen or undergo HBO until deficits resolve. Many factors are considered in determining treatment options. A patient's willingness to be placed in a single chamber, hemodynamic stability, age, neurologic deficits, severity of symptoms, and NP abnormalities are the most important factors. This approach requires the ability to perform NP testing at the time of presentation after the exposure, which is not possible in many settings. Lack of valid studies makes a standard approach to the CO patient difficult, and management varies significantly among treating physicians (Table 56-2).

Most states now have a hyperbaric facility either within the state or nearby. The Divers Alert Network at Duke University [Durham, NC: (919) 684-8111] provides emergency consultation and maintains a list of all available chambers. Cost may be a consideration, and the decision to refer a patient to a chamber should be made by the individual clinician. A consultation with the toxicologist at the nearest Regional Poison Center and with the physician at the nearest chamber may be of benefit.

REFERENCES

1. Litovitz TL, Felberg L, White S, et al. AAPC annual report. *Am J Emerg Med* 1995;14(5):487.
2. Caplan Y, Thompson B, Levine B, et al. Accidental poisoning involving carbon monoxide, heating systems, and confined spaces. *J Forensic Sci* 1986;1:117.
3. Shusterman DJ. Clinical smoke inhalation injury: systemic effects. *Occup Med* 1993;8(3):469.
4. Horowitz BZ. Carboxyhemoglobinemia caused by inhalation of methylene chloride. *Am J Emerg Med* 1986;1:48.
5. Jackson DL, Menges H. Accidental carbon monoxide poisoning. *JAMA* 1980;243(8):772.
6. Winter PM, Miller JN. Carbon monoxide poisoning. *JAMA* 1976;236(13):1502.
7. Coburn RF, Forster RE, Kane PB. Considerations of the physiological variables that determine the blood carboxyhemoglobin concentration in man. *J Clin Invest* 1965;44:1899.
8. Ball E, Stritmatter C, Cooper O. The reaction of cytochrome oxidase with carbon monoxide. *J Biol Chem* 1951;193:635.
9. Goldbaum LR, Ramirez RG, Absalon KB. What is the mechanism of carbon monoxide toxicity? *Aviat Space Environ Med* 1975;46:1289.
10. Yokoyama K. Effect of perfluorochemical (PFC) emulsion on acute carbon monoxide poisoning in rats. *Jpn J Surg* 1978;4:342.
11. Piantadosi CA. Carbon monoxide, oxygen transport, and oxygen metabolism. *J Hyperbaric Med* 1987;2(1):27.
12. Olson KR. Carbon monoxide poisoning: mechanisms, presentation, and controversies in management. *J Emerg Med* 1984;1:233.
13. Ginsberg MD. Carbon monoxide intoxication: clinical features, neuropathology, and mechanisms of injury. *J Toxicol Clin Toxicol* 1985;23:281-288.
14. Ginsberg M. Carbon monoxide. In: Spencer P. Schaumberg, eds. *Experimental and clinical neurotoxicology.* Baltimore: Williams & Wilkins, 1980:374.
15. Ginsberg MD, Myers RE, McDonagh BF, et al. Experimental carbon monoxide encephalopathy in the primate. *Arch Neurol* 1974;30:209.
16. Thom SR. Carbon monoxide-mediated brain lipid peroxidation in the rat. *J Appl Physiol* 1990;68:997.
17. Okeda R, Funata N, Takano T, et al. The pathogenesis of carbon monoxide encephalopathy in the acute phase—physiological and morphological conditions. *Acta Neuropathol* 1981;54:1.
18. Okeda R, Funata N, Takano T, et al. Comparative study on pathogenesis of selective cerebral lesions in carbon monoxide poisoning and nitrogen hypoxia in cats. *Acta Neuropathol* 1982;56:265.
19. Shang J, Piantadosi CA. Mitochondrial oxidative stress after carbon monoxide hypoxia in the rat brain. *J Clin Invest* 1992;90:1193.
20. Verma A, Hirsch DJ, Glatt CE, et al. Carbon monoxide: a putative neural messenger. *Science* 1993;259:381.
21. Utz J, Ullrich V. Carbon monoxide relaxes ileal smooth muscle through activation of guanylate cyclase. *Biochem Pharmacol* 1991;41:1195.
22. Smith JS, Brandon S. Morbidity from acute carbon monoxide poisoning at three-year follow-up. *Br Med J* 1973;1:318.
23. Lugaresi A, Montagna P, Morreale A, et al. "Psychic akinesia" following carbon monoxide poisoning. *Eur Neurol* 1990;30:167.
24. Hart IK, Kennedy PGE, Adams JH, et al. Neurological manifestation of carbon monoxide poisoning. *Postgrad Med J* 1988;64:213.
25. Choi IS. Delayed neurologic sequelae in carbon monoxide intoxication. *Arch Neurol* 1983;40:433.
26. Norkol DM, Kirkpatrick JN. Treatment of acute carbon monoxide poisoning with hyperbaric oxygen: a review of 115 cases. *Ann Emerg Med* 1983;14:1168.
27. Laties V. Carbon monoxide and behavior. *Arch Neurol* 1980;167:68.
28. Stewart RD, Peterson JE, Baretta ED, et al. Experimental human exposure to carbon monoxide. *Arch Environ Health* 1970;21:154.
29. Hartman D. *Neuropsychological toxicology: identification and assessment of human neurotoxic syndrome.* New York: Pergamon Press, 1988:244.
30. Messier LD, Myers R. A neuropsychological screening battery for emergency assessment of carbon-monoxide-poisoned patients. *J Clin Psych* 1991;47:675.
31. Silvers SM, Hampson NB. Carbon monoxide among recreational boaters. *JAMA* 1995;274:1614.
32. Johnson CJ, Moran JC, Paine SC, et al. Abatement of toxic levels of carbon monoxide in Seattle ice skating rinks. *Am J Public Health* 1975;65:1087.
33. Hampson NB, Norkool DM. Carbon monoxide poisoning in children riding in the back of pickup trucks. *JAMA* 1992;267:538.
34. Lowe-Ponsfort FL, Henry JA. Clinical aspects of carbon monoxide poisoning. *Adverse Drug React* 1989;4:217.
35. Sheps DS, Herbst MC, Henderliter AL, et al. Production of arrhythmias by elevated carboxyhemoglobin in patients with coronary artery disease. *Ann Intern Med* 1990;113:343.
36. Smith SR, Steinberg S, Gaydos JC. Errors in derivations of the Coburn-Forster-Kane equation for prediction carboxyhemoglobin. *AIHAJ* 1996;57:621.
37. Vremon HJ, Mahoney JJ, Stevenson DK. Carbon monoxide and carboxyhemoglobin. *Adv Pediatr* 1995;42:303.
38. Denays R, Makhoul E, Dachy B, et al. Electroencephalographic clinical smoke inhalation mapping and 99m Tc HMPAO single-photon emission computed tomography in carbon monoxide poisoning. *Ann Emerg Med* 1994;24(5):947.
39. Sesay M, Bidabe AM, Guyot M, et al. Regional cerebral blood flow measurements with xenon-CT in the prediction of delayed encephalopathy after carbon monoxide intoxication. *Acta Neurol Scand* 1996;[Suppl]166:22.
40. Choi IS, Kim SK, Lee SS, et al. Evaluation of outcome of delayed neurologic sequelae after carbon monoxide poisoning by technetium-99m hexamethylpropylene amine oxime brain single photon emission computed tomography. *Eur Neurol* 1995;35:137.
41. Myers RAM, Snyder SK, Linberg S, et al. Value of hyperbaric oxygen in suspected carbon monoxide poisoning. *JAMA* 1981;246:2478.
42. Klees M, Heremans M, Dougan S. Psychological sequelae to carbon monoxide intoxication in the child. *Sci Total Environ* 1985;44:165.

43. Hill EP, Hill JR, Power GG, et al. Carbon monoxide exchanges between the human fetus and mother: a mathematical model. *Am J Physiol* 1977;232:311.
44. Elkharrat D, Raphael JC, Korach JM, et al. Acute carbon monoxide intoxication and hyperbaric oxygen in pregnancy. *Int Care Med* 1991;17:289.
45. Hyperbaric oxygen therapy: a committee report. Bethesda, MD: Undersea and Hyperbaric Medical Society, 1986.
46. Leach RM, Rees PJ, Wilmshurst P. Hyperbaric oxygen therapy. *BMJ* 1998; 317:1140–1143.
47. Grim PS, Gottlieb LJ, Boddie A, Batson E. Hyperbaric oxygen therapy. *JAMA* 1990;263:2216–2220.

CHAPTER 57
Methemoglobin-Forming Compounds

Donna L. Seger and Christina E. Hantsch

Methemoglobinemia is an important consideration in the differential diagnosis of the cyanotic patient, especially one unresponsive to oxygen therapy. Clinical symptoms of methemoglobinemia are secondary to tissue hypoxia, as methemoglobin cannot transport oxygen. An understanding of the physiology and pathophysiology is required to diagnose and manage patients with methemoglobinemia.

PHYSIOLOGY AND PATHOPHYSIOLOGY

Hemoglobin contains four heme molecules; each heme molecule contains iron in the reduced, ferrous (Fe^{2+}) state. Oxyhemoglobin and deoxyhemoglobin are the two normal conformations of hemoglobin. Oxyhemoglobin is the product of reversible binding of oxygen to hemoglobin. This binding involves an electron shift and oxidation of iron to the ferric (Fe^{3+}) state. When oxygen subsequently is released, deoxyhemoglobin (ferrous iron) is restored. Although the majority of oxyhemoglobin is reduced in this manner, 3% of oxyhemoglobin undergoes autoxidation (i.e., the oxygen is released from the heme pocket as a superoxide radical) (1). The iron of the involved heme group remains in a ferric (Fe^{3+}) state. The resultant hemoglobin molecule is methemoglobin. The ferric iron of the involved heme group typically binds to a water molecule ($HbFe^{3+}$-H_2O) or a hydroxyl ion ($HbFe^{3+}$-OH–) and, therefore, cannot transport oxygen. The conformational change associated with autoxidation also increases the affinity of the other heme groups for oxygen. Consequently, the oxyhemoglobin dissociation curve is shifted to the left and, for a given oxygen tension, tissue oxygenation is decreased (2–4).

Under normal physiologic conditions, 1% to 2% of erythrocyte protein is methemoglobin. Biochemical mechanisms within the erythrocyte continually convert methemoglobin to hemoglobin via reduction reactions. The Embden-Meyerhof glycolytic pathway and the hexose monophosphate shunt supply the necessary energy (2,3,5,6).

The Embden-Meyerhof glycolytic pathway generates the electron donor (reducing agent) nicotine adenine dinucleotide (NADH) (Fig. 57-1). Normally, 95% of methemoglobin reduction occurs via NADH. NADH-cytochrome b_5 reductase[1] facilitates electron transfer from NADH to cytochrome b_5 and then to methemoglobin (Fig. 57-2). During the neonatal period, NADH-cytochrome b_5 reductase activity is low (1,3). This, in combination with higher susceptibility of fetal hemoglobin to oxidant stress, increases the risk of methemoglobinemia in infants (1,3,4,7).

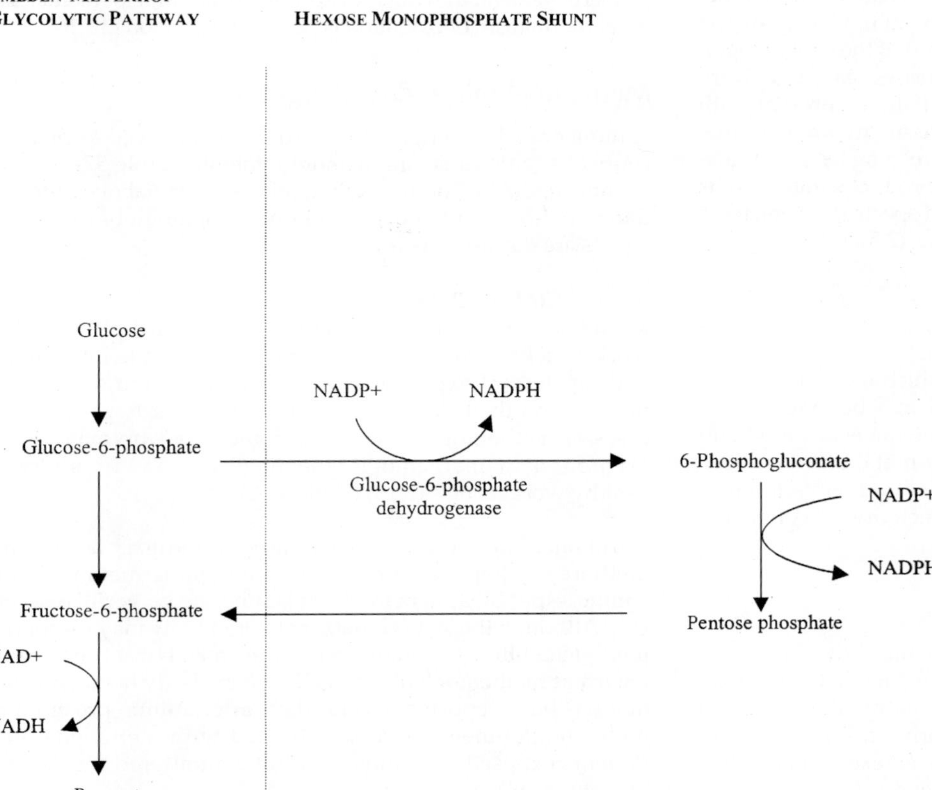

Figure 57-1. The Embden-Meyerhof glycolytic pathway and the hexose monophosphate shunt.

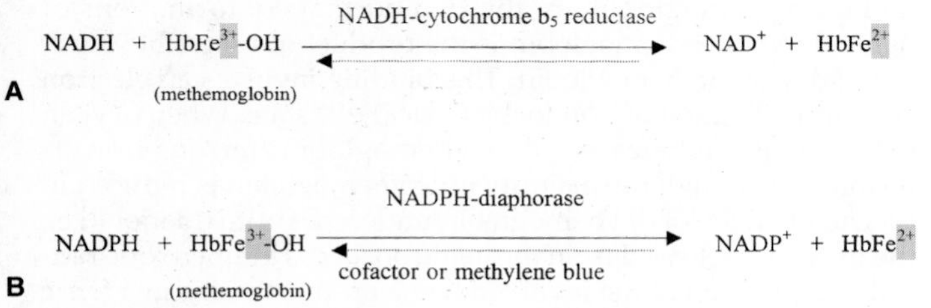

A

NADH-cytochrome b_5 reductase

$NADH + HbFe^{3+}\text{-}OH \rightleftarrows NAD^{+} + HbFe^{2+}$

(methemoglobin)

B

NADPH-diaphorase

$NADPH + HbFe^{3+}\text{-}OH \rightleftarrows NADP^{+} + HbFe^{2+}$

(methemoglobin) cofactor or methylene blue

Figure 57-2. A: NADH-dependent reduction pathway. **B:** NADPH-dependent reduction pathway.

In the hexose monophosphate shunt, glucose-6-phosphate dehydrogenase (G6PD) reduces nicotine adenine dinucleotide phosphate to NADPH (see Fig. 57-1). Up to 5% of methemoglobin reduction uses this electron donor. NADPH-diaphorase[1] transfers an electron from NADPH to an intermediate compound and finally to methemoglobin. Methylene blue, the antidote for methemoglobinemia, acts via this pathway (see Fig. 57-2) (1–3,5–7). Details on the mechanism of action of methylene blue are reviewed in the Management section of this chapter.

An inherited defect of the hexose monophosphate shunt is G6PD deficiency. This deficiency prevents the production of NADPH and renders methylene blue therapy ineffective. It does not increase the risk of methemoglobinemia development in affected individuals (2,3,8).

SULFHEMOGLOBINEMIA

In rare circumstances, agents that typically induce methemoglobinemia instead cause sulfhemoglobinemia. Sulfhemoglobin results from incorporation of sulfur into the heme pocket. As with methemoglobin, the altered heme group of sulfhemoglobin is unable to transport oxygen. The conformation change of sulfhemoglobin is irreversible. As opposed to the change with methemoglobin, however, it decreases the oxygen affinity of the unaffected heme groups and results in a shift of the oxyhemoglobin dissociation curve to the right and increases oxygen delivery to tissue for a given oxygen saturation. Patients present with cyanosis but no associated symptoms of tissue hypoxia. Sulfhemoglobinemia is rarely life-threatening. Screening tests (see Analytical Information section of this chapter) produce similar results to those of methemoglobinemia. Advanced spectrophotometry is necessary to differentiate the two conditions (2,5,7).

ETIOLOGY

Methemoglobinemia, a clinical state in which more than 1% to 2% of total hemoglobin is methemoglobin, may be congenital or acquired. The majority of methemoglobinemia is acquired and occurs when an exogenous agent or its metabolite oxidizes hemoglobin. Abnormal hemoglobin structure (hemoglobin M disease) and decreased reducing enzyme activity are congenital causes of methemoglobinemia (7).

Congenital Methemoglobinemia

Hemoglobin M is abnormal hemoglobin caused by amino acid substitution on the alpha or beta chain of the hemoglobin molecule. In all variants of this hemoglobinopathy, the abnormal hemoglobin maintains iron in the ferric form causing methemoglobinemia. Neither intrinsic mechanisms nor exogenous reducing agents (e.g., ascorbic acid, methylene blue) reduce the methemoglobin. This condition is transmitted as an autosomal dominant inheritance pattern. The homozygous state, which has 100% methemoglobin, is incompatible with life. Patients with heterozygous hemoglobin M are cyanotic but asymptomatic. They maintain 25% to 30% methemoglobin (1,2,5,9).

Inadequate synthesis or abnormal structure decreases enzyme activity. Congenital deficiency of NADH-cytochrome b_5 reductase is the most common enzyme deficiency causing methemoglobinemia. In this condition, only the NADPH-methemoglobin reductase pathway and nonenzymatic routes reduce methemoglobin to hemoglobin. Both the homozygous and heterozygous states are compatible with life.

Individuals with homozygous NADH-cytochrome b_5 reductase deficiency have 10% to 50% methemoglobin. Although cyanotic, these individuals are usually asymptomatic until 40% methemoglobin is approached. At higher values, exertional dyspnea, easy fatigue, and headache may occur. This is in contrast to patients with acquired methemoglobinemia who are more symptomatic with similar methemoglobin percentages. Daily oral doses of methylene blue or ascorbic acid effectively maintain total methemoglobin at less than 10%. Individuals with heterozygous NADH-cytochrome b_5 reductase deficiency maintain a physiologic amount of methemoglobin. Individuals with either heterozygous or homozygous enzyme deficiency are predisposed to acquired methemoglobinemia when exposed to oxidant substances (1,2,5,9).

Congenital deficiency of NADPH-reductase occurs infrequently. As this enzyme system is a minor methemoglobin reducing system, individuals with this condition do not suffer from methemoglobinemia (1,9).

Acquired Methemoglobinemia

Acquired methemoglobinemia occurs when an exogenous agent or its metabolite oxidizes hemoglobin at a rate that exceeds normal enzymatic capacity for hemoglobin reduction (1,3,10). Continued exposure, prolonged half-life, and/or metabolites with oxidative properties extend the course of acquired methemoglobinemia. The exact mechanism of oxidation is poorly understood (2,7,10).

Methemoglobin-Inducing Agents

A number of industrial and environmental as well as pharmaceutical agents cause methemoglobinemia (Table 57-1). Some agents are direct oxidants, while others are metabolized to oxidants. A few of the more common methemoglobin-inducing agents are discussed below.

INDUSTRIAL AGENTS

Methemoglobinemia is an occupational hazard primarily for workers within the chemical industry (11). Acute inhalational and/or dermal exposures to aromatic compounds (aniline, nitrites, and their derivatives) cause the majority of industrial cases of methemoglobinemia. Chronic exposure may induce asymptomatic methemoglobinemia (2% to 5%) in otherwise healthy workers (4,7,12,13) (Table 57-2).

Aniline. Aniline is commonly used in industry as an intermediate in chemical syntheses. The hepatic metabolites of aniline, especially phenylhydroxylamine, are powerful oxidants (14). Although the symptomatic patient initially may respond to methylene blue, prolonged zero-order metabolism may cause recurrent methemoglobinemia (15). Heinz body hemolytic anemia has been reported several days after aniline-precipitated methemoglobinemia that was treated with methylene blue. Patients exposed to aniline should be monitored for delayed hemolysis (16).

TABLE 57-1. Methemoglobin-inducing agents: industrial, environmental, and pharmaceutical (2,4,8)

Acetanilid	Nitroglycerin (glyceryl trinitrate)
Acetophenetidin	Nitrophenol
Alloxans	Nitrosobenzene
Alpha naphthylamine	Ozone
Aminophenols	Pamaquine®
Ammonium nitrate	Para-aminopropiophenone
Amyl nitrite	Para-bromoanaline
Aniline	Para-chloraniline
Aniline dyes	Para-dichloroamine
Anilinoethanol	Para-nitroaniline
Antipyrine	Para-toluidine
Arsine	Pentaerythritol tetranitrate
Benzene	Phenacetin
Benzocaine	Phenols
Butyl/isobutyl nitrite	Phenylazopyridine (Pyridium®)
Chloranilines	Phenylenediamine
Chlorates	Phenylhydrazine
Chlorobenzene	Phenylhydroxylamine
Chloromethylaniline	Phenytoin (Dilantin®)
Chloronitrobenzene	Piperazine
Cobalt preparations	Plasmoquine
Crayons, wax (red or orange)	Prilocaine
Dapsone	Primaquine
Diaminodiphenylsulfone	Prontosil
Diesel fuel additives	Propitocaine
Dimethylamine	Pyridine
Dimethylaniline	Pyrogallol
Dinitrobenzene	Quinones
Dinitrophenol	Resorcinol
Dinitrotoluene	Shoe dye/polish
Hydrogen peroxide	Silver nitrate
Hydroquinone	Sodium nitrite
Hydroxylacetanilid	Sodium nitroprusside
Hydroxylamine	Spinach
Inks	Sulfonamides
Kiszka	Sulfanilamide
Lidocaine	Sulfapyridine
Menthol	Sulfathiazole
Meta-chloraniline	Sulfonal
Methylacetanilid	Sulfones
Methylene blue	Tetranitromethane tetronal
Monochloroaniline	Tetralin
Naphthylamines	Toluenediamine
Naphthalene	Toluidine
Nitrates	Toluylhydroxylamine
Nitrites	Trichlorocarbanilide (TCC)
Nitrobenzene	Trinitrotoluene
Nitrofurans	Trional
Nitrogen oxide	Vegetables (carrots and spinach)

ENVIRONMENTAL AGENTS

Poorly constructed wells, shallow wells, and other polluted water supplies are a major environmental source of methemoglobin-inducing substances. Nitrates and nitrites are common well contaminants especially in agricultural areas where nitrogen-based fertilizers are used. Other sources of nitrates are organic animal waste and sewer systems. Microorganisms in the water or soil oxidize organic nitrogen to ammonia and then to nitrate (17) (see Table 57-2).

Nitrates and Nitrites. Nitrates, not direct oxidants themselves, are reduced to nitrites (direct oxidants) in the liver or bowel. In the liver, reduction occurs via glutathione–organic nitrate reductase. In the bowel, reduction occurs via nitrate reductase systems of intestinal microorganisms such as *Escherichia coli, Pseudomonas aeruginosa*, and *Acinetobacter* (18). The chief sources of nitrate body burden are vegetables (cauliflower, spinach, and broccoli). Other sources include cured meats, fruits, juices, milk products, and bread. Increased contamination of drinking water is increasing dietary intake of nitrates. By Environmental Protection Agency standards, the maximal permissible nitrate level in drinking water is 45 ppm NO_3^- or 10 ppm NO_3^-N (17–20).

Infant cyanosis from methemoglobinemia due to well-water nitrates was first described by Comly in 1945 (21). Infants are particularly susceptible to nitrate-induced methemoglobin formation for a number of reasons. First, infants have a decreased capacity to secrete gastric acid. The higher gastric pH is incapable of destroying bacteria that convert nontoxic nitrates to methemoglobin-producing nitrites (8). Infants also consume larger amounts of nitrate relative to total hemoglobin concentration. This is because they maintain a greater fluid intake per body weight and per gram of hemoglobin, which increases the relative amount of ingested well-water nitrates. Also, water is frequently boiled before it is used to dilute infant formula; boiling concentrates the nitrates. Finally, infants have lower NADH-cytochrome b_5 reductase activity and higher susceptibility to oxidant stress (1,3–5,7,20–23).

PHARMACEUTICAL AGENTS

Many pharmaceutical agents have been reported to increase methemoglobin production.

Nitroglycerin. Standard doses of nitrate preparations, whether oral, sublingual, transdermal, or intravenous, do not produce clinically significant percentages of methemoglobin (24–26). However, methemoglobinemia should be considered when intravenous nitroglycerin is infused at a high dose for a prolonged period or administered to a patient with anemia, hepatic dysfunction, or renal dysfunction. The severity of coronary artery disease that may mandate such administration also may make the patient intolerant of any increase in methemoglobin percent (27–30).

Amyl nitrite, butyl nitrite, and other volatile nitrites are popular inhalants among certain populations. Users of these products claim they delay and prolong orgasm. Known as "rush," "poppers," and "snappers," these preparations can cause potentially fatal methemoglobinemia when inhaled or ingested. Inhalation of volatile nitrites can also cause massive hemolysis in the presence of an intrinsic erythrocyte defect (i.e., G6PD deficiency) presumably due to nitrite ion–induced oxidative destruction of the erythrocyte (31–34).

Dapsone. Dapsone (4, 4-diaminodiphenylsulfone) is a synthetic sulfone structurally similar to the sulfonamides. For years dapsone was prescribed for the treatment of leprosy, dermatitis herpetiformis and malaria prophylaxis (in the combination drug Maloprim). Today, there are many additional indications. It is currently used for treatment of *Pneumocystis carinii* pneumonia (35). The role of dapsone in the treatment of brown recluse spider bites is being investigated (36,37).

Dapsone, itself not an oxidizing agent, is hydroxylated to a metabolite which is an oxidant and capable of causing methemoglobinemia. Dapsone's elimination half-life is 10 to 50 hours with therapeutic administration; after an overdose, the half-life may be as long as four days (38, 39). Consequently, methemoglobinemia following ingestion of dapsone may be prolonged and require repeated treatment with methylene blue. As an alternative to bolus doses, continuous infusion of methylene blue has been successfully used (38,39). Dapsone overdose may also cause sulfhemoglobinemia and hemolysis (36,37). Administration of multiple-dose activated charcoal shortens the half-life of dapsone following overdose (40).

TABLE 57-2. Selected industrial and environmental methemoglobin-inducing agents and their sources/uses

Agent	Sources/uses
Aminophenol	Photographic developers
	Hair dye
	Manufacture of pharmaceuticals
Ammonium nitrate	Chemical cold packs
Aniline	Dye production
	Manufacture of pharmaceuticals
	Photographic developers
	Shoe polish
	Resins
	Varnish
	Perfumes
	Organic chemical syntheses
Arsine	Organic chemical syntheses
	Solid state electronic components
	Metal smelting by-product
Butyl/isobutyl nitrite	Room deodorizer propellant
Chlorobenzene	Paint solvent
	Color printing
	Dry-cleaning industry
Cobalt	Electroplating
	High-speed steels
Dimethylamine	Manufacture of pharmaceuticals
	Stabilizer in gasoline
	Soap and surfactant production
	Insecticide and fungicide production
Dimethylaniline	Analytical reagent
	Dye precursor
Dinitrotoluene	Manufacture of explosives
	Manufacture of dyes
Hydrogen peroxide	Bleaching agent (textiles and paper)
	Rocket fuel
	Disinfectant
Hydroquinone	Photographic developers
	Pharmaceutical precursor
	Leaves of blueberry, red whortleberry, cranberry, bearberry
	Stabilizer in paints, varnishes, motor oils
	Rubber processing chemical intermediate
Hydroxylamine	Production of rubber synthetics
	Photographic developer solutions
Naphthalene	Moth repellent
	Chemical and dye manufacturing
Nitrates and nitrites (inorganic)	Contaminated well water
	Meat preservatives
	Vegetables
	Industrial salts
	Contaminants of nitrous oxide anesthesia canisters
Nitroglycerin	Manufacture of dynamite
Phenol	Plastic surgery face peels
	Management of spasticity
	Detergent disinfectants
Phenylene diamine	Dyeing of furs
	Hair dye
	Photographic developers
Pyridine	Agricultural chemical syntheses
	Solvent
Quinone	Tanning hides
	Dye manufacture
	Fungicide manufacture
Resorcinol	Tanning
	Manufacture of resorcinol-formaldehyde resins
	Manufacture of explosives, dyes, cosmetics, adhesives
Tetranitromethane	Oxidizer in rocket propellant

Adapted from refs. 2, 3, 5, 12, and 13.

ANESTHETIC AGENTS

Lidocaine is not a direct oxidant, and the mechanism by which it produces methemoglobinemia is unknown. Therapeutic doses of intravenous lidocaine increase methemoglobin percentage but not to a clinically significant range. However, methemoglobinemia should be considered when large doses of lidocaine are administered (41).

Benzocaine is another local anesthetic that is not a direct oxidant but has been reported to induce methemoglobinemia. The oxidant effect may be through an *N*-hydroxy derivative (3). Many commercially available products contain up to 20% benzocaine. These include dermatologic ointment, anesthetic lubricant for rectal suppository, endotracheal tube, or esophageal stethoscope, topical teething preparation, and pharyngeal spray (Cetacaine) (42). Many routes of exposure have caused methemoglobinemia in children (43–45). Topical pharyngeal anesthetic use of benzocaine has also been reported to cause methemoglobinemia in adults (46,47).

Phenazopyridine. Phenazopyridine (Pyridium), an azo dye, has been used as a genitourinary analgesic since the 1920s. Both methemoglobinemia and Heinz body hemolytic anemia have been reported following chronic phenazopyridine administration or acute toxic ingestion (8,48).

CLINICAL SIGNS AND SYMPTOMS OF ACQUIRED METHEMOGLOBINEMIA

The hallmarks of methemoglobinemia are cyanosis and chocolate-brown blood. The cyanosis may be present in the absence of symptoms of hypoxia. The fraction of methemoglobin and the rapidity of its development, as well as the preexisting condition of the individual, determine symptom severity. Patients (nonanemic and otherwise healthy) with less than 15% methemoglobin are usually asymptomatic. Major hypoxic symptoms occur with 55% or more. There is a high rate of mortality associated with methemoglobin over 70%. Fortunately, methemoglobinemia of that severity is seldom seen (2,5). Symptoms typically associated with specific values are listed in Table 57-3.

In assessing the cyanotic patient, central cyanosis must be differentiated from peripheral cyanosis. With peripheral cyanosis, discoloration is due to reduced perfusion of distal regions and is

TABLE 57-3. Signs and symptoms associated with acquired methemoglobin percentages (nonanemic, otherwise healthy individuals)

Methemoglobin percent	Signs/symptoms
0–15	None
15–20	Chocolate-brown blood
	Cyanosis
20–45	Anxiety
	Exertional dyspnea
	Weakness
	Fatigue
	Dizziness
	Lethargy
	Headache
	Syncope
	Tachycardia
45–55	Depressed level of consciousness
55–70	Stupor/coma
	Seizure
	Bradycardia
	Dysrhythmia
>70	Cardiovascular collapse
	Death

seen especially in the nailbeds and the nose. With central cyanosis, discoloration is due to an inadequate amount of oxyhemoglobin in arterial blood and is seen in the mucous membranes of the mouth, lips, and conjunctivae. Only 1.5 g per dL of methemoglobin produces cyanosis equivalent to that produced by 5.0 g per dL of deoxyhemoglobin, or 0.5 g per dL of sulfhemoglobin (48–50).

The most frequent cause of central cyanosis is cardiopulmonary disease. Therefore, physical evaluation of the cyanotic patient must focus on the chest and cardiac examinations. Diagnostic aids include the chest radiograph, electrocardiogram, and arterial blood gas measurements. If these studies are normal, other causes of central cyanosis must be considered. Administration of 100% oxygen is indicated when cyanosis is present. Cyanosis unresponsive to administration of 100% oxygen in a patient with normal or high arterial oxygen tension should make the clinician consider methemoglobinemia (or sulfhemoglobinemia) (1,5,50).

ANALYTICAL INFORMATION

In emergent situations or when formal blood analysis is not available, several tests can screen for methemoglobinemia. First, a drop of blood placed on filter paper will appear a chocolate-brown color if more than 15% methemoglobin is present. Second, the chocolate-brown color of methemoglobin is not altered when exposed to oxygen whereas normal venous blood turns bright red when exposed to oxygen. Third, if methemoglobin is present, blood will turn pink when diluted with deionized water (1:100) and mixed with a crystal of potassium cyanide (KCN) due to the formation of cyanomethemoglobin (2,44,50).

The results of arterial blood gas (ABG) analyses and oximeters must be interpreted carefully. In most hospitals, ABG results are reported with calculated oxygen saturation (SaO_2) based on the measured partial pressure of oxygen (PaO_2). The PaO_2 (the amount of oxygen dissolved in plasma) and the calculated saturation are unaffected by the presence of methemoglobin or other abnormal hemoglobin. Bedside pulse oximeters only detect the wavelengths of deoxyhemoglobin and oxyhemoglobin. They report an oxygen saturation that does not reflect the presence of methemoglobin, carboxyhemoglobin, or sulfhemoglobin. The oxygen saturation may be reported as normal even with significant methemoglobinemia. In contrast, CO-oximeters detect the wavelengths of deoxyhemoglobin and oxyhemoglobin as well as abnormal hemoglobins. The reported oxygen saturation is the ratio of oxyhemoglobin to total hemoglobin (oxyhemoglobin, deoxyhemoglobin, methemoglobin, sulfhemoglobin, and carboxyhemoglobin). The appropriate (low) oxygen saturation will be reported for patients with methemoglobinemia (3,51). Many CO-oximeters, however, do not distinguish between methemoglobin and sulfhemoglobin. The more advanced spectrophotometric analysis of newer CO-oximeters differentiates these two abnormal hemoglobins and determines true methemoglobin as a percentage of total hemoglobin (2,5). Unfortunately, such spectrophotometric equipment may not be readily available. Falsely low methemoglobin values may be reported if there is a delay between phlebotomy and laboratory analysis as the oxidation and reduction of methemoglobin continue at varying rates *in vitro* (8).

Knowledge of total hemoglobin concentration is important. Hypoxia will occur at lower methemoglobin percentages in anemic patients due to decreased total oxygen carrying capacity. A peripheral smear should be analyzed for the presence of hemolysis (2,5,44).

MANAGEMENT

As in all clinical situations, the priority in management of acquired methemoglobinemia is attention to the patient's airway, breathing, and circulation. For poisoned patients, the next priority is prevention of further exposure. This includes removal from the environment if the exposure route is inhalational, dermal decontamination if the exposure is cutaneous, and consideration of gastric decontamination if the exposure is oral. Enhancement of tissue oxygenation is the goal of treatment. Oxygen should be administered to all cyanotic patients. Fluids and buffer administration will increase tissue perfusion and correct acidosis that is common in patients with significant hypoxia. Blood methemoglobin percentage should be obtained. Other causes of cyanosis must be considered. Appropriate evaluation for coexisting toxicity of the etiologic agent needs to be undertaken (2,5).

Many patients with methemoglobinemia are asymptomatic or have minor symptoms that are relieved by supplemental oxygen alone. Methemoglobinemia resolves spontaneously with a half-life of 55 minutes unless there is ongoing accelerated production.

Antidote Therapy

METHYLENE BLUE

The antidote of choice for methemoglobinemia is methylene blue (methylthionine chloride). Administration of methylene blue is indicated in symptomatic patients. This typically happens with 30% methemoglobinemia or greater but can be seen at lower values especially if there is coexisting anemia or another condition worsened by hypoxia (e.g., coronary artery disease, emphysema) (10). Methylene blue provides an exogenous intermediate for NADPH-diaphorase reduction and increases its activity (6). NADPH-diaphorase transfers an electron to methylene blue to form leukomethylene blue. Leukomethylene blue accelerates the reduction of ferric iron to ferrous iron in the hemoglobin molecule. Methemoglobinemia usually resolves within 1 to 2 hours. This oxidation-reduction cycle between methylene blue and leukomethylene blue is reversible. When low concentrations of methylene blue are present, erythrocyte reduction of methemoglobin occurs; when high concentrations of methylene blue are present, formation of methemoglobin occurs. Methylene blue is ineffective if, as with G6PD deficiency, there is an inadequate supply of NADPH. Severe hemolysis may instead result due to the oxidant stress (7,10).

The recommended dose of methylene blue is 1 to 2 mg per kg (0.1 to 0.2 mL per kg of a 1% solution) administered intravenously in normal saline over a period of 5 to 10 minutes. If symptoms of hypoxia have not improved within an hour of administration of methylene blue, the dose should be repeated. With apparent refractory cases, however, a second methemoglobin measurement and hematocrit should be obtained. Potential causes of continued hypoxia and lack of response to methylene blue include G6PD deficiency, NADPH-diaphorase deficiency, and sulfhemoglobinemia. Since only 10% to 20% methemoglobinemia produces discoloration, cyanosis may persist despite resolution of symptoms. Additionally, methylene blue is a dye that imparts a bluish discoloration to the skin. Side effects of methylene blue administration include dizziness, headache, confusion, nausea, vomiting, abdominal and precordial pain, dysuria, tremor, tachycardia, and electrocardiogram changes. Infiltration of methylene blue can cause tissue necrosis (52). Although available, oral methylene blue has unpredictable, slow absorption and its use should be limited to congenital methemoglobinemia (2,53).

The cumulative dose of methylene blue should not exceed 5 to 7 mg per kg in the acute period. Higher doses of methylene blue increase methemoglobin production and cause hemolytic anemia with Heinz body formation. Repeated doses of methylene blue should not be withheld if the patient remains symptomatic or if ongoing exposure to the etiologic agent cannot be prevented. Continuous infusion of 1 mg per kg per hour methylene blue has been effective in the treatment of recurrent methemoglobinemia following dapsone ingestion (38,39).

The safety of methylene blue for administration in pregnancy has not been established. The only clinical information on fetal exposure is from previous obstetric use of methylene blue in amniocentesis and diagnosis of premature rupture of membranes. An association with intestinal atresia and fetal death following second trimester exposure has been reported (54–56). Neonatal methemoglobinemia, hemolytic anemia, hyperbilirubinemia, and jaundice have been attributed to late gestational exposure (52,57–59).

TOLUIDINE BLUE

Toluidine blue is another antidote for methemoglobinemia. The recommended dose is 2 to 4 mg per kg intravenously and it can be repeated after 30 minutes if clinically indicated. Toluidine blue increases the activity of the NADPH-reduction pathway. Although toluidine blue is reported to have superior efficacy to methylene blue, it is only available in Germany. Fetal exposure may cause mutagenesis. Like methylene blue, it is not effective for treatment of sulfhemoglobinemia or methemoglobinemia in G6PD-deficient patients (52).

ASCORBIC ACID

Ascorbic acid reacts directly with oxidant compounds and reduces them within the erythrocyte. It has no place in the treatment of acquired methemoglobinemia, because the rate at which it reduces methemoglobin is slower than the normal intrinsic mechanism. Ascorbic acid administration is indicated only when methemoglobinemia is caused by a hereditary enzyme deficiency (2,3,7,42,43).

GLUTATHIONE AND *N*-ACETYLCYSTEINE

Glutathione, an intracellular antioxidant and cofactor in many enzymatic pathways, reduces methemoglobin by a slow, nonenzymatic process. It does not acutely reduce methemoglobin in patients with acquired methemoglobinemia. It is not an effective antidote even for congenital methemoglobinemia because exogenous glutathione cannot enter cells (1,2,5,60).

N-acetylcysteine (NAC) has been considered as an alternative treatment for methemoglobinemia, especially in G6PD-deficient patients in whom methylene blue is relatively contraindicated. In addition to glutathione restoration, substitution for glutathione and independent antioxidant properties have been proposed as the mechanism(s) of action of NAC in methemoglobinemia. Currently, there is no clinical evidence to support the use of NAC in methemoglobinemia (60).

EXCHANGE TRANSFUSION AND HYPERBARIC OXYGEN

Exchange transfusion and hyperbaric oxygen have been proposed as alternative therapies in the management of methemoglobinemia. The suggested benefit of exchange transfusion is repletion of hemoglobin as well as reduction of the concentration of the etiologic agent. Hyperbaric oxygen maximizes the dissolved oxygen content of blood. Further study is needed to assess effectiveness. These modalities may have a greater role in the treatment of patients with poor response, or contraindication, to methylene blue (2,3,5,10).

SUMMARY

Methemoglobinemia is typically an acquired condition resulting from exposure to an oxidizing agent. Central cyanosis unresponsive to oxygen administration is the classic clinical presentation. Symptoms result from tissue hypoxia. Other toxic manifestations of the etiologic agent may be present and require treatment.

An understanding of the pathophysiology of methemoglobinemia is essential to prompt diagnosis and treatment of the patient with methemoglobinemia. Antidotal therapy with methylene blue may be life-saving and methemoglobinemia should therefore be considered in the appropriate clinical setting.

REFERENCES

1. Mansouri A, Lurie AA. Concise review: methemoglobinemia. *Am J Hematol* 1993;42:7–12.
2. Curry S. Methemoglobinemia. *Ann Emerg Med* 1982;11:214–221.
3. Coleman MD, Coleman NA. Drug-induced methaemoglobinaemia. *Drug Safety* 1996;14(6):394–405.
4. Griffin JP. Methaemoglobinaemia. *Adverse Drug React Toxicol Rev* 1997;16(1): 45–63.
5. Hall AH, Kulig KW, Rumack BH. Drug- and chemical-induced methaemoglobinaemia. *Toxicol Man Rev* 1986;1:253–260.
6. Beutler E. Energy metabolism and maintenance of erythrocytes. In: Beutler E, Lichtman MA, Coller BS, Kipps TJ, eds. *Williams' hematology*, 5th ed. New York: McGraw-Hill, 1995:394–403.
7. Beutler E. Methemoglobinemia and other causes of cyanosis. In: Beutler E, Lichtman MA, Coller BS, Kipps TJ, eds. *Williams' hematology*, 5th ed. New York: McGraw-Hill, 1995:654–663.
8. Green E, Zimmerman RC, Ghurabi WH, et al. Phenazopyridine hydrochloride toxicity: a cause of drug-induced methemoglobinemia. *J Am Coll Emerg Phys* 1979;8:426–431.
9. Lukens J. The legacy of well-water methemoglobinemia. *JAMA* 1987;20: 2793–2795.
10. Price D. Methemoglobinemia. In: Goldfrank LR, Flomenbaum NE, Lewin NA, Weisman RS, Howland MA, Hoffman RS, eds. *Goldfrank's toxicologic emergencies*, 4th ed. New York: Appleton & Lange, 1990:1169–1180.
11. Beer ST, Bradberry SM, Vale JA. The use of methylene blue in occupational methaemoglobinaemia. Presented at EAPCCT Scientific Meeting, Oslo, 1997.
12. Bradberry SM, Whittington RM, Parry DA, et al. Fatal methemoglobinemia due to inhalation of isobutyl nitrite. *J Toxicol Clin Toxicol* 1994;32(2):179–184.
13. Hathaway GJ, Proctor NH, Hughes JP, et al. The chemical hazards. In: Hathaway GJ, Proctor NH, Hughes JP, Fischman ML, eds. *Chemical hazards of the workplace*, 3rd ed. New York: Van Nostrand–Reinhold, 1991.
14. Harrison JH, Jollow DJ. Contribution of aniline metabolites to aniline-induced methemoglobinemia. *Mol Pharmacol* 1987;32:423–431.
15. Kearney TE, Manoguerra AS, Dunford JV. Chemically induced methemoglobinemia from aniline poisoning. *West J Med* 1984;140:282–286.
16. Harvey JW, Keitt AS. Studies of the efficacy and potential hazards of methylene blue therapy in aniline-induced methemoglobinemia. *Br J Hematol* 1983;54:29–41.
17. Kross BC, Ayebo A, Hall A, et al. Nitrate/nitrite toxicity. In: *Agency for Toxic Substance Disease Registry: Case studies in environmental medicine*, 1991.
18. Murad F. Drugs used for the treatment of angina: organic nitrates, calcium-channel blockers, and beta-adrenergic antagonists. In: Goodman, Gilman A, Rall T, Nies A, Taylor P, eds. *The pharmacological basis of therapeutics*, 8th ed. New York: Pergamon Press, 1990:764–774.

19. Dixon DS, Reisch RF, Santinga PH. Fatal methemoglobinemia resulting from ingestion of isobutyl nitrite, a "room odorizer" widely used for recreational purposes. *J Forensic Sci* 1981;3:587–593.
20. Johnson CJ, Bonrud PA, Dosch TL, et al. Fatal outcome of methemoglobinemia in an infant. *JAMA* 1987;40:2796–2797.
21. Comly HH. Cyanosis in infants caused by nitrates in well water. *JAMA* 1987;20:2788–2792.
22. Fan AM, Wilhite CC, Book SA. Evaluation of the nitrate drinking water standard with reference to infant methemoglobinemia and potential reproductive toxicity. *Regul Toxicol Pharmacol* 1987;7:135–148.
23. May RB. An infant with sepsis and methemoglobinemia. *J Emerg Med* 1985;3:261–264.
24. Arsura E, Lichstein E, Guadagnino V, et al. Methemoglobin levels produced by organic nitrates in patients with coronary artery disease. *J Clin Pharmacol* 1984;24:160–164.
25. Paris PM, Kaplana RM, Stewart RD, et al. Methemoglobin levels following sublingual nitroglycerin in human volunteers. *Ann Emerg Med* 1986;15:171–173.
26. Saxon SA, Silverman ME. Effects of continuous infusion of intravenous nitroglycerin on methemoglobin levels. *Am J Cardiol* 1985;56:461–464.
27. Bojar RM, Rastegar H, Payne DD, et al. Methemoglobinemia from intravenous nitroglycerin: a word of caution. *Ann Thorac Surg* 1987;43:332–334.
28. Zurick AM, Wagner RH, Starr NJ. Intravenous nitroglycerin, methemoglobinemia, and respiratory distress in a postoperative cardiac surgical patient. *Anesthesiology* 1984;61:464–466.
29. Kaplan KJ, Taber M, Teagarden JR, et al. Association of methemoglobinemia and intravenous nitroglycerin administration. *Am J Cardiol* 1985;55:181–183.
30. Robicsek F. Acute methemoglobinemia during cardiopulmonary bypass caused by intravenous nitroglycerin infusion. *J Thorac Cardiovasc Surg* 1985;90:931–934.
31. O'Toole JB, Robbins GB, Dixon DS. Ingestion of isobutyl nitrite, a recreational chemical of abuse, causing fatal methemoglobinemia. *J Forensic Sci* 1987;6:1811–1812.
32. Laaban JP, Bodenan P, Rochemaure J. Amyl nitrite poppers and methemoglobulinemia. *Ann Intern Med* 1985;103:804–805.
33. Bogart L, Bonsignore J, Carvalho A. Massive hemolysis following inhalation of volatile nitrites. *Am J Hematol* 1986;22:327–329.
34. Shesser R, Mitchell J, Edelstein S, et al. Methemoglobinemia from isobutyl nitrite preparations. *Ann Emerg Med* 1981;10:262–264.
35. Reiter WM, Cimoch PJ. Dapsone-induced methemoglobinemia in a patient with *P. carinii* pneumonia and AIDS. *N Engl J Med* 1987;317:1740–1741.
36. Linakis JG, Shannon M, Woolf A, et al. Recurrent methemoglobinemia after acute dapsone intoxication in a child. *J Emerg Med* 1989;7:477–480.
37. Iserson KV. Methemoglobinemia from dapsone therapy for a suspected brown spider bite. *J Emerg Med* 1985;3:285–288.
38. Berlin G, Brodin B, Hilden J. Acute dapsone intoxication: a case treated with continuous infusion of methylene blue, forced diuresis and plasma exchange. *J Toxicol Clin Toxicol* 1985;22:537–548.
39. Dawson AH, Whyte IM. Management of dapsone poisoning complicated by methaemoglobinaemia. *Med Toxicol Adverse Drug Exp* 1989;4:387–392.
40. Bradberry SM, Vale JA. Multiple-dose activated charcoal: a review of relevant clinical studies. *J Toxicol Clin Toxicol* 1995;33(5):407–416.
41. Weiss LD, Generalovich T, Heller M, et al. Methemoglobin levels following intravenous lidocaine administration. *Ann Emerg Med* 1987;16:323–325.
42. Rodriguez LF, Smolik LM, Zbehlik AJ. Benzocaine-induced methemoglobinemia: report of a severe reaction and review of the literature. *Ann Pharmacother* 1994;28:643–649.
43. Kellett PB, Copeland CS. Methemoglobinemia associated with benzocaine-containing lubricant. *Am Soc Anesthesiol* 1983;59:463–464.
44. Gentile DA. Severe methemoglobinemia induced by a topical teething preparation. *Pediatr Emerg Care* 1987;3:176–178.
45. Seibert RW, Seibert JJ. Infantile methemoglobinemia induced by a topical anesthetic, Cetacaine. *Laryngoscopy* 1984;94:816–817.
46. Spielman FJ, Anderson JA, Terry WC. Benzocaine-induced methemoglobinemia during general anesthesia. *J Oral Maxillofac Surg* 1984;42:740–743.
47. Buckley AB, Newman A. Methemoglobinemia occurring after the use of a 20% benzocaine topical anesthetic prior to gastroscopy. *Gastrointest Endosc* 1987;6:466–467.
48. Zimmerman RC, Green ED, Ghurabi WH, et al. Methemoglobinemia from overdose of phenazopyridine hydrochloride. *Ann Emerg Med* 1980;9:147–149.
49. Mayo W, Leighton K, Robertson B, Ruedy J. Intraoperative cyanosis: a case of dapsone-induced methaemoglobinaemia. *Can J Anaesth* 1987;34:79–82.
50. Jaffe ER. Methemoglobinemia in the differential diagnosis of cyanosis. *Hosp Pract* 1985;92–110.
51. Barker SJ, Tremper KK, Hyatt J. Effects of methemoglobinemia on pulse oximetry and mixed venous oximetry. *Anesthesiology* 1989;70:112–117.
52. Meredith TJ, Jacobsen D, Haines JA, et al. Methylene blue and toluidine blue. In: *IPCS/CEC evaluation of antidotes series*, vol 2: *antidotes for poisoning by cyanide*. Cambridge, England: Cambridge University Press, 1993.
53. Bradberry SM. The use of methylene blue in acquired methemoglobinemia. Presented at EAPCCT Scientific Meeting, Oslo, 1997.
54. Nicolini U, Monni G. Intestinal obstruction in babies exposed in utero to methylene blue. *Lancet* 1990;336:1258–1259.
55. Van Der Pol JG, Wolf H, Boer K et al. Jejunal atresia related to the use of methylene blue in genetic amniocentesis in twins. *Brit J Obstet Gynaecol* 1992;99:141–143.
56. Kidd SA, Lancaster PAL, Anderson JC et al. Fetal death after exposure to methylene blue dye during mid-trimester amniocentesis in twin pregnancy. *Prenat Diagn* 1996;16:39–47.
57. Vincer MJ, Allen AC, Evans JR, et al. Methylene-blue-induced hemolytic anemia in a neonate. *CMAJ* 1987;136:503–504.
58. McEnerney JK, McEnerney LN. Unfavorable neonatal outcome after intraamniotic injection of methylene blue. *Obstet Gynecol* 1983;61(3):35S–37S.
59. Crooks J. Haemolytic jaundice in a neonate after intra-amniotic injection of methylene blue. *Arch Dis Child* 1982;57:872–886.
60. Wright RO, Magnani M, Shannon MW, et al. *N*-acetylcysteine reduces methemoglobin in vitro. *Ann Emerg Med* 1996;28:499–503.

CHAPTER 58

Halogenated Solvents, Trichloroethylene, and Methylene Chloride

Donald G. Barceloux

This review covers the health effects of the following halogenated solvents: 1,2-dichloroethane (ethylene dichloride), 1,2-dichloroethylene (acetylene dichloride), dichloromethane (methylene chloride), 1,2-dichloropropane (propylene dichloride), tetrabromoethane (acetylene tetrabromide), tetrachloroethane (acetyl tetrachloride), tetrachloroethylene (perchloroethylene), tetrachloromethane (carbon tetrachloride), 1,1,1-trichloroethane, trichloroethylene, trichloromethane (chloroform), and 1,1,2-trichloro-1,2,2-trifluoroethane (chlorofluorocarbon-113).

Knowledge of these chemicals and their health effects is not complete enough to delineate all the effects of exposure to these chemicals. Knowledge regarding the health effects of these solvents is primarily based on the following: (a) case reports of both single, acute overdose and chronic overexposure, (b) epidemiologic studies of workers, and (c) animal experiments. The medicinal use of some of these solvents (e.g., trichloroethylene, tetrachloroethylene, tetrachloromethane, and trichloromethane) provides limited data on the human effects of these chemicals. The collection of data on solvents must be interpreted both cautiously and critically to determine the health effects of these solvents. Case reports demonstrate only a temporal relation between exposure and health effects. This type of information depends heavily on the ability of the author to document exposure to the toxin and to exclude other causes of the illness. Even though numerous similar case reports make causation more tenable, only a well-controlled epidemiologic study can confirm an association between a chemical and a health effect (1).

The validity of an epidemiologic study depends on the study design (i.e., type of study, adequate sample size, appropriate goals, and relevant individuals), assignment (i.e., response rate, dropout rate, selection bias), assessment (i.e., measures of outcome, information bias, confounding variables), interpretation (i.e., clinical importance, appropriate interpretation), and extrapolation (i.e., appropriate conclusion and range of data, direct applicability to new population). Many studies on halogenated solvents lack accurate data on actual concentrations and on the duration of exposure. Even assuming that epidemiologic studies demonstrate a clear association between a chemical and the health effect, the determination of true causation depends on satisfying certain principles of causation listed by Hill and known as the Hill Criteria (2).

All of the desired data are never available, and, therefore, the determination of causation depends on a careful analysis of existing medical data based on critiques of the validity of the human studies and the adequacy of animal data. A thorough evaluation of the accumulated animal and human data on these halogenated solvents allows a determination of many, but not all, of the health effects of these chemicals.

MEDICINAL HISTORY

Most of these halogenated solvents were discovered in the 1800s and were initially investigated as anesthetic agents. Flourens first used trichloromethane as an animal anesthetic in 1847, and later that year Simpson performed surgery on humans with trichloromethane anesthesia (3). Over the next 100 years, trichloromethane was the anesthetic of choice until other drugs with less cardiac and hepatic toxicity replaced trichloromethane after World War II. The nefarious use of trichloromethane as an anesthetic continues as a means of incapacitating victims (4). Halogenated solvents tested for use as anesthetics and discarded during the 1800s included the following (with adverse side effects in parentheses): 1,2-dichloroethane (excessive salivation, convulsive movements, postoperative blue-gray corneal opacities), tetrachloromethane (cardiac depression, prolonged recovery times), 1,1,1-trichloroethane (moderate hypotension, ventricular dysrhythmias during hypoxia and during hypercarbia), dichloromethane (excessive clonic movements, lack of muscle relaxation), and 1,2-dichloroethylene (excessive flammability). Of these chemicals, only trichloromethane and tetrachloromethane were associated with the development of hepatic and renal toxicity during their use as an anesthetic.

Damage to the trigeminal nerve complicated the use of trichloroethylene as a narcotic in the early 1900s, and this discovery led to the use of this agent for the treatment of *tic douloureux*. Treatment was suspended in the 1930s because of the lack of efficacy, but cranial neuropathies appeared again after the use of trichloroethylene as an anesthetic in the 1940s. Otherwise, the incidence of adverse effects generally was low after the use of trichloroethylene as an anesthetic (5). In 1977, the U.S. Food and Drug Administration (FDA) banned the use of trichloroethylene as a general anesthetic and as a surgical disinfectant.

Hall introduced tetrachloromethane as an anthelmintic for the treatment of hookworm in 1921. For the next 10 years, thousands of patients, particularly in the South Pacific, received small doses (3 to 10 mL in adults) of tetrachloromethane. Although this chemical was an effective agent, serious reactions occurred in a few patients, particularly alcoholics and poorly nourished children. These susceptible patients developed liver necrosis, renal damage, and gastrointestinal hemorrhage (6). Subsequently, tetrachloroethylene became a substitute for tetrachloromethane as a treatment for hookworm and pinworm. More than 50,000 cases of hookworm were treated with doses of up to 8 mL of tetrachloroethylene (maximum average adult dose), with surprisingly few side effects other than giddiness and lightheadedness (7).

Tetrachloroethylene was not considered an adequate substitute for trichloromethane anesthesia because of its mucous membrane–irritating properties, poor volatility, and inadequate muscle relaxation (8). 1,1,2,2-Tetrachloroethane was not considered for medicinal use because the hepatic toxicity of this compound was well known in the United States by 1922. Willcox reported the development of a toxic hepatitis in airplane factory workers in 1914 at the Hindon airplane factory that was similar to the experience in Germany, where tetrachloroethane was used as a solvent for the cellulose acetate sprayed over the linen that covered German airplanes (9).

CHEMISTRY

Table 58-1 lists the chemical data for each of the halogenated solvents. Evaluation of the toxicity of each of these halogenated solvents should include an analysis of the toxicity of the respective isomers, which may differ substantially in their ability to cause human illness. The isomer 1,1-dichloroethane (ethylidene chloride) is approximately five times less toxic than 1,2-dichloroethane in subchronic animal studies (10).

Dichloroethylene exists in the following three forms: (a) 1,1-dichloroethylene, (b) *cis*-1,2-dichloroethylene, and (c) *trans*-1,2-dichloroethylene. Based on animal studies, 1,1-dichloroethylene possesses greater hepatic toxicity than the other chlorinated ethylene compounds (11) and this isomer also produces a unique pattern of hepatocellular injury. The anesthetic action of the *trans* isomer appears twice as potent as the *cis* isomer of 1,2-dichloroethylene based on inhalation studies in rats (12).

The 1,1,2 isomer of trichloroethane produces more profound central nervous system (CNS) depression than 1,1,1-trichloroethane, and the former isomer probably causes more hepatic toxicity than 1,1,1-trichloroethane based on animal experiments that demonstrate 1,1,2-trichloroethane produces as much liver damage as tetrachloromethane (13).

PHYSICOCHEMICAL PROPERTIES

Generally these chemicals are clear, colorless liquids that are nonflammable and possess characteristically sweet, chloroformlike odors and slight mucous membrane–irritating properties. They are usually highly volatile, slightly soluble in water, but highly miscible in most of the organic solvents. The exceptions to the poor flammability rule of these halogenated solvents are 1,2-dichloroethane, 1,2-dichloroethylene, and the thermal decomposition product of trichloroethylene, dichloroacetylene. Table 58-2 lists the odor properties of these chemicals. The odors of these chemicals are generally not noticeable enough to allow workers to detect levels above recommended workplace standards, but levels that are immediately dangerous to the workers' health usually can be smelled.

EXPOSURE

Uses

All of these halogenated solvents have commercial applications in addition to those that result from their ability to dissolve lipophilic material. Changes in the volume of the particular chemicals produced depend not only on their physicochemical properties but also on their recognized toxicity. Tetrachloroethylene replaced trichloroethylene as a dry cleaning and degreasing agent because of concern about hepatotoxicity and environmental contamination by the latter. Commercial production of 1,1,1-trichloroethane has increased substantially. This chemical is an excellent degreasing agent and probably produces less toxicity than other chlorinated hydrocarbons because of the minor biotransformation of 1,1,1-trichloroethane in the human body. The FDA banned the use of trichloromethane as an active or inactive ingredient in human or drug products as of July 29, 1976. Similarly, domestic uses of tetrachloromethane were banned in the United States in 1970, and the use of this chemical as a grain fumigant was stopped in 1986. 1,2-Dichloroethane is no longer registered for agricultural use in the United States or in Canada. The use of dichloromethane is decreasing as well. In 1989, the FDA banned the use of dichloromethane in hairsprays, and, in 1996, Sweden banned the occupational use of

TABLE 58-1. Chemical data of halogenated solvents

Chemical Abstracts name	**1,2-Dichloroethane**
CAS registry number	107-06-2
NIOSH number	KI0525000
Structural formula	H H | | Cl — C — C — Cl | | H — H
Synonyms	α- or β-Dichloroethane, 1,2-bichloroethane, ethane dichloride, sym-dichloroethane dichloroethylene, ethylene chloride, ethylene dichloride, EDC, glycol dichloride
Trade names	Dutch liquid, Dutch oil, Freon 150, Brocide, ENT 1656, Borer-Sol, Destroxol, Gaze Olefiant, Dichloremulsion
Molecular formula	$C_2H_4Cl_2$
Molecular weight	98.9
Chemical Abstracts name	**1,2-Dichloroethene**
CAS registry number	540-59-0
NIOSH number	KV9360000
Structural formula	H H | | C = C | | Cl Cl
Synonyms	1,2-Dichloroethylene, acetylene dichloride, sym-dichloroethylene, dichloro-1,2-ethylene (French), 1,2-dichloraethan (German), 1,2-DCE
Trade names	Dioform
Molecular formula	$C_2H_2Cl_2$
Molecular weight	96.95
Chemical Abstracts name	**Dichloromethane**
CAS registry number	75-09-2
NIOSH number	PA8050000
Structural formula	H | Cl — C — Cl | H
Synonyms	DCM, methane dichloride, methylene bichloride, methylene dichloride, methylene chloride
Trade names	Aerothene MM, Solmethine, Freon 30, Narkotil, Solaesthin
Molecular formula	CH_2Cl_2
Molecular weight	84.93
Chemical Abstracts name	**1,2-Dichloropropane**
CAS registry number	78-87-5
NIOSH number	TX9625000
Structural formula	H Cl Cl | | | H — C — C — C — H | | | H H H
Synonyms	α- or β-Dichloropropane, propylene chloride, propylene dichloride, 1,2-dichloropropane, bichlorure de propylene (French)
Trade names (pure compound)	ENT 15406, NCI-C55141
Trade names (insecticide formulations)	D-D (Shell Oil Company), Dorlone, Dowfume, Telone, Vidden D (Dow Chemical Company), Terr-o-cide (Great Lakes Chemical Corp.), Vorlex (Nor-Am Agricultural Products)
Molecular formula	$C_3H_6Cl_3$
Molecular weight	112.99
Chemical Abstracts name	**1,1,2,2-Tetrabromoethane**
CAS registry number	79-27-6
NIOSH number	KI8225000
Structural formula	Br Br \ | HC — CH / | Br Br
Synonyms	Acetylene tetrabromide, sym-tetrabromoethane, 1,1,2,2-tetrabroomethaan (Dutch), 1,1,2,2-tetra-bromoetano (Italian), 1,1,2,2-tetrabromaethan (German)
Trade names	Muthmann's liquid, AI3-08850
Molecular weight	345.7
Chemical Abstracts name	**1,1,2,2-Tetrachloroethane**
CAS registry number	79-34-5
NIOSH number	KI8575000
Structural formula	Cl Cl | | H — C — C — H | | Cl Cl
Synonyms	1,1,2,2-Tetrachloroethane, sym-tetrachloroethane, S-tetrachloroethane, acetylene tetrachloride, dichloro-2,2-dichloroethane, 1,1-dichloro-2,2-dichloroethane, 1,1,2,2-tetracloroetano (Italian), 1,1,2,2-tetrachloroethane (French), 1,1,2,2-tetrachloroaethan (German), 1,1,2,2-tetrachloorethaan (Dutch)
Molecular formula	$C_2H_2Cl_4$
Molecular weight	167.84
Chemical Abstracts name	**Tetrachloroethene**
CAS registry number	127-18-4
NIOSH number	KX3850000
Structural formula	Cl Cl \ / C = C / \ Cl Cl
Synonyms	Carbon dichloride, ethylene tetrachloride, carbon bichloride, perchloroethylene, tetrachloroethane, tetrachloroethylene, 1,1,2,2-tetrachloroethane, per, perc, perchlor
Molecular formula	C_2Cl_4
Molecular weight	165.8
Chemical Abstracts name	**Tetrachloromethane**
CAS registry number	56-23-5
NIOSH number	FG4900000
Structural formula	Cl | Cl — C — Cl | Cl
Synonyms	Carbona, tetrachlorocarbon, carbon chloride, carbon tet, methane tetrachloride, perchloromethane, tetrachlormethan (German), tetrachloure de carbone (French), tetrachlorometano (Italian)
Trade names	Freon 10, benzioform, univerm, tetrasol, fluikoids, fasciolin Halon 104, vermostricid

(continued)

TABLE 58-1. *(continued)*

Chemical Abstracts name	**1,1,1-Tetrachloroethane**
CAS registry number	71-55-6
NIOSH number	KJ2975000
Structural formula	Cl H | | Cl — C — C — H | | Cl H
Synonyms	α-Trichloroethane, methyl chloroform, trielene, trichloroethane, methyl trichloromethane, 1,1,1,-trichloroetano (Italian), 1,1,1-trichloraethan (German), 1,1,1-trichloorethaan (Dutch), aerothene TT, chloroethene, chlorothene NU, chlorothene VG alpha-T, TCEA, TCA, NCI-CA4626
Isomer	Ethane, 1,1,1-trichloro-1,1,2-trichloroethane, beta-trichloroethane, beta-T, NCI-C04579, vinyl trichloride
Molecular formula	$C_2H_3Cl_3$
Molecular weight	133.41
Chemical Abstracts name	**Trichloromethane**
CAS registry number	67-66-3
NIOSH number	FS9100000
Structural formula	Cl | H — C — Cl | Cl
Synonyms	Chloroform, formyl trichloride, methane trichloride, methenyl chloride, methenyl trichloride, methyl trichloride, trichloroform, trichlorometano (Italian), chloroforme (French), chloroformio (Italian), trichloormethaan (Dutch)
Trade names	Freon 20, R20, R20 (refrigerant)
Molecular formula	$CHCl_3$
Molecular weight	119.38
Chemical Abstracts name	**Trichloroethene**
CAS registry number	79-01-6
NIOSH number	KX4550000
Structural formula	Cl Cl \\ / C = C / \\ H Cl
Synonyms	Acetylene trichloride, trichloroethylene, ethylene trichloride, ethenyl trichloride, TCE, Tri, 1,1,2-trichloroethylene, trichloroethylenum, trichloroethylen (German), trichloroethylene (French), trichloroetilene (Italian), trichlooretheen (Dutch)
Chemical formula	C_2HCl_3
Molecular weight	131.4
Chemical Abstracts name	**1,1,2-Trichloro-1,2,2-trifluoroethane**
CAS registry number	76-13-1
NIOSH number	KJ4000000
Structural formula	F Cl | | Cl — C — C — F | | Cl F
Synonyms	Trichlorotrifluoroethane, 1,1,2-trichloro-1,2,2-fluoroethane
Trade names	Freon 113, FC-113
Molecular formula	$C_2Cl_3F_3$
Molecular weight	187.37

CAS, Chemical Abstracts Service; NIOSH, National Institute for Occupational Safety and Health.

this chemical. The production of 1,2-dichloropropane decreased substantially since the 1980s because its agricultural use is no longer permitted in the United States. 1,1-Dichlorethylene (vinylidene dichloride) is produced in much larger quantities than 1,2-dichloroethylene because of its use in the production of monoacrylic fibers and copolymers; however, only the latter is used as a solvent. The London Amendment to the Montreal Protocol progressively limits the production of 1,1,2-trichloro-1,2,2-trifluoroethane as well as other fluorocarbons. Table 58-3 lists the commercial uses of these halogenated solvents.

Impurities

Most technical and commercial grades of halogenated solvents contain impurities (e.g., other chlorinated hydrocarbons) and stabilizers (e.g., antioxidants, acid receptors). The concentration of these impurities rarely exceeds 1% to 3% of the total liquid. Stabilizers present in 1,1,1-trichloroethane include nitromethane, butanols, 1,4-dioxane, butylene oxide, 1,3-dioxolane, and *n*-methylpyrrole. Stabilizers (e.g., amines, epoxides, esters) are added to tetrachloroethylene to prevent the formation of hydrochloric acid from moisture and light. Individual impurities rarely exceed 100 mg per kg of trichloroethylene, and total impurities usually do not exceed 1 g per kg trichloroethylene (14). Impurities include tetrachloromethane, trichloromethane, 1,2-dichloroethane, *cis*- and *trans*-1,2-dichloroethylene, pentachloroethane, 1,1,1,2-tetrachloroethane, 1,1,2,2-tetrachloroethane, 1,1,1-trichloroethane, 1,1,2-trichloroethane, 1,1-dichloroethylene, bromodichloroethylene, tetrachloroethylene, bromodichloromethane, and benzene.

Reactions

The formation of the toxic contaminant dichloroacetylene resulted from the use of trichloroethylene as an anesthetic agent in closed systems with alkali absorbers and as a cleaning solvent in submarines and space capsules. In the workplace, dichloroacetylene production resulted from the use of trichloroethylene on moist alkaline materials such as concrete (15). Significant decomposition of trichloroethylene into dichloroacetylene and phosgene occurs at temperatures higher than 60°C (16). When contaminated by traces of trichloroethylene, the vaporization of tetrachloroethylene over sodium hydroxide also may generate dichloroacetylene. In sunlight, trichloromethane oxidizes to phosgene in the presence of strong oxidizing agents (e.g., chromic acid produced phosgene and chlorine gas from trichloromethane). Pyrolysis of vapors of trichloromethane higher than 450°C produces hydrochloric acid and various chlorinated hydrocarbons, including tetrachloroethane and tetrachloroethy-

TABLE 58-2. Odor properties

Solvent chemical name	Common name	Levels (ppm)		Characteristics
		Threshold[a]	Obvious	
1,2-Dichloroethane	Ethylene dichloride	6–110	180	Chloroformlike
1,2-Dichloroethylene	Acetylene dichloride	17	—	Acrid, ethereal
Dichloromethane	Methylene chloride	150–500	800	Pleasant, chloroform
1,2-Dichloropropane	Propylene dichloride	>0.25	130–190	Unpleasant, chloroform
Tetrabromoethane	Acetylene tetrabromide	—	—	Pungent, camphor
Tetrachloroethane	Acetylene tetrachloride	1.5	—	Pungent, chloroform
Tetrachloroethylene	Perchloroethylene	5–50	>100	Ethereal, chloroform
Tetrachloromethane	Carbon tetrachloride	100–200	250	Chloroform
1,1,1-Trichloroethane	—	16–400	800	Chloroform
Trichloroethylene	TCE	20–80	>100	Chloroform
Trichloromethane	Chloroform	50–200	—	Chloroform
1,1,2-Trichloro-1,2,2-trifluoroethane	FC-113	350–1000	—	Sweet

ppm, parts per million.
[a]Odor thresholds reported in the medical literature vary considerably based on the following variables: (a) chemical purity, (b) definition of odor response, (c) size and number of trials, and (d) method of presentation of stimulus.

TABLE 58-3. Commercial uses of halogenated solvents

Halogenated solvent	Commercial use
1,2-Dichloroethane	Vinyl chloride production, chemical intermediate, lead scavenger, solvent
1,2-Dichloroethylene	Chemical intermediate, low temperature extractant (caffeine, perfumes), solvent (printed circuits, fats, phenol, camphor, natural rubber, lacquer, thermoplastics)
Dichloromethane	Degreasing agent, paint/varnish remover, blowing agent for urethane foams, solvent extractant (drugs, coffee), fumigant (grain, fruits)
1,2-Dichloropropane	Chemical intermediate (tetrachloroethylene, tetrachloromethane), solvent, soil fumigation (with dichloropropene), lead scavenger, metal degreaser
Tetrabromoethane	Solvent, gauge fluid, flotation agent, catalyst, refractive liquid
Tetrachloroethane	Solvent, mothproofing textiles, paint/varnish/rust remover, immersion liquid (crystallography), determination of theobromine in cacao
Tetrachloroethylene	Grain fumigation, chemical intermediate (chlorofluorocarbons), veterinary anthelmintic, heat exchange fluid
Tetrachloromethane	Chemical intermediate (Freon 11, Freon 12), fire extinguishing agent, grain fumigant, solvent, metal degreaser, flammability suppressant, paint manufacturing, gasoline additive, semiconductor production, refrigerant
1,1,1-Trichloroethane	Cleaning solvent, electrical machinery, plastics, textile spotting fluid, chemical intermediate, coolant, lubricant, inks, drain cleaners
Trichloroethylene	Vapor degreasing, typewriter correction fluid, low temperature heat transfer fluid, fire retardant, chemical intermediate, polyvinyl chloride manufacturing, extractant, lacquer/adhesive
Trichloromethane	Chemical intermediate (Freon 22), cleaning agent, insecticidal fumigant, solvent
1,1,2-Trichloro-1,2,2-trifluoroethane	Solvent (electrical, electronics), dry cleaning

lene. Thermal decomposition of 1,1,1-trichloroethane occurs at temperatures less than 260°C, whereas large amounts of hydrogen chloride and trace amounts of phosgene form at temperatures above that level (17). Vapor formation and thermal oxidative degradation at high temperatures may produce phosgene, carbon monoxide, and hydrochloric acid from tetrachloroethylene. The addition of weak acids to tetrachloroethane produces trichloroethylene, whereas the addition of strong alkalis causes the formation of the flammable toxin dichloroacetylene. Contact of dichloromethane with common metals at room temperature usually produces no significant decomposition, although prolonged heating with water at 79°C causes the formation of methyl chloride, methanol, hydrochloric acid, formic acid, and some carbon monoxide. Thermal decomposition of products containing dichloromethane as a result of open flames includes hydrogen chloride, and, to a lesser extent, phosgene (18). With light, air, or moisture, 1,2-dichloroethylene gradually decomposes to form hydrochloric acid in a similar manner as 1,2-dichloroethane. Unstabilized tetrachloroethylene decomposes slowly in water to yield trichloroacetic and hydrochloric acids.

Sources

None of the halogenated solvents is a natural constituent of the environment. Human exposure occurs primarily as a result of the volatilization of these chemicals to air during commercial use, and, to a lesser extent, secondary to the contamination of groundwater near industrial sites. The relatively low partition coefficients of these halogenated solvents suggest that these chemicals probably are not easily transferred from the environment into the food chain.

DICHLORO- SOLVENTS

The primary source of 1,2-dichloroethane is volatilization of this chemical from industrial processes, and, to a lesser extent, from leaded fuel. Levels of 1,2-dichloroethane in suburban and rural areas usually are below detection, whereas levels in urban areas generally are below 0.2 parts per billion (ppb) 1,2-dichloroethane. Typical levels in office buildings in the United States average approximately 1 ppb 1,2-dichloroethane (19). Levels near point sources (e.g., vinyl chloride plants) may be one to two times higher. 1,2-Dichloroethane is not a frequent contaminant of food or water.

Almost all of the dichloromethane released in the air results from the volatilization of dichloromethane during commercial or consumer uses. For the general population, air is the major source of exposure to dichloromethane with levels ranging from 0.07 to 0.29 μg dichloromethane per m^3 in remote areas to 15 μg dichloromethane per m^3 in urban areas. Higher levels (e.g., 43 μg dichloromethane per m^3) have occurred near hazardous-waste sites (20). Most table-ready food has levels below 1 part per million (ppm) dichloromethane.

Exposure of the general population to dichloroethylene occurs primarily through inhalation of urban air and the ingestion of contaminated drinking water. This chemical is a frequent low-level contaminant of urban air with concentrations ranging from 0.013 to 0.076 ppb 1,2-dichloroethylene (21). Contamination of groundwater may result from the leaching of contaminated-waste disposal sites or from the anaerobic biodegradation of more highly chlorinated ethenes and ethanes released into the groundwater.

TRICHLORO- SOLVENTS

Air and, to a lesser extent, contaminated water and food are the major sources of exposure to trichloroethane for the general population. Urban air may contain levels in the range of ppb, and drinking water may contain ng per L to μg per L 1,1,1-trichloroethane. Typical concentrations in air in rural areas are less than 0.2 ppb 1,1,1-trichloroethane, whereas mean levels in urban areas range from 0.1 to 1.0 ppb 1,1,1-trichloroethane (22). The concentration of 1,1,1-trichloroethane indoors usually exceeds the level of 1,1,1-trichloroethane outdoors. Although background levels of 1,1,1-trichloroethane in water are low (i.e., <1 ppb), high levels of contamination may occur in groundwater near industrial sources or near waste disposal sites.

The primary source of exposure to trichloroethylene for the general population is contact with water or food contaminated with trichloroethylene. This chemical is a contaminant of both natural and processed food with higher levels present in meats, margarine, and beverages. The mean level for positive samples from a survey of groundwater averaged approximately 1 to 2 ppb trichloroethylene (23). Although trichloromethane is a naturally occurring chemical, anthropogenic sources account for most of the trichloromethane present in the environment. Exposure of the general population to trichloromethane results primarily from inhalation and ingestion of food and drinking water. Background levels of trichloromethane in remote regions average approximately 0.02 ppb, whereas mean levels in the ambient air near U.S. cities range from 0.02 to 2.00 ppb trichloromethane (24). The level of trichloromethane in indoor air depends primarily on the amount of water used and on the ability of trichloromethane to evaporate from the water. Only a small amount of trichloromethane is released directly in water compared with the amount of trichloromethane produced by the chlorination of water. A yearlong study of drinking water in the United States demonstrated a median level of 14 μg trichloromethane per L (25). In a survey of 549 food samples, approximately 55% contained detectable levels of trichloromethane ranging from 2 to 830 μg trichloromethane per kg with a mean level of 71 μg trichloromethane per kg (26). Low levels of trichloromethane generally appear in fish, poultry, and meat.

TETRACHLORO- SOLVENTS

Ingestion of drinking water and inhalation of ambient air are the primary means of exposure to tetrachloromethane for the general population. The estimated daily intake of tetrachloromethane for the average person is much greater (i.e., 0.1 μg/kg) from ambient air compared with water (0.01 μg/kg). Most foods do not contain tetrachloromethane. Most tetrachloromethane released into the environment results from the volatilization of this chemical during production processes. Typical ambient outdoor levels in rural areas average approximately 0.13 ppb tetrachloromethane compared with mean and maximum urban levels of 0.19 ppb and 1.4 ppb tetrachloromethane, respectively (27). Indoor levels may exceed outdoor levels of tetrachloromethane. In a study of homes in several U.S. cities, the indoor levels averaged 0.16 ppb tetrachloromethane and reached up to 1.4 ppb tetrachloromethane (28).

Approximately 80% to 85% of the tetrachloroethylene produced in the United States is released in the environment, mostly as a result of evaporative losses from dry cleaning and from industrial plants. Average ambient air levels in the United States range from 0.16 ppb tetrachloroethylene in rural areas to 1.30 ppb tetrachloroethylene near sources of tetrachloroethylene emission (29). A survey of 13 dry-cleaning plants detected air levels that ranged from 1 to 138 ppm tetrachloroethylene with the highest levels occurring in shops that require the physical transfer of tetrachloroethylene-saturated clothing from washing machines to dryers (30). Tetrachloroethylene may migrate through soil to groundwater, but the release of tetrachloroethylene to groundwater is small (i.e., <1% of total release) compared with the release of tetrachloroethylene to the atmosphere. Approximately 25% of water supplies in the United States contains tetrachloroethylene with concentrations in positive samples ranging from 0.01 to 1,500 ppb tetrachloroethylene.

CHLOROFLUOROCARBON-113

Inhalation is the main means of exposure to 1,1,2-trichloro-1,2,2-trifluoroethane. In remote regions of the United States, the median concentration was 241 ng 1,1,2-trichloro-1,2,2-trifluoroethane per m^3 compared with a level of 2,376 ng 1,1,2-trichloro-1,2,2-trifluoroethane per m^3 recorded in Los Angeles (31).

ENVIRONMENTAL FATE

The atmosphere is the main environmental sink for these chemicals because of their high vapor pressure. These solvents are relatively resistant to direct photolysis in the atmosphere, and, therefore, degradation of these chemicals usually occurs by their reaction with hydroxyl radicals. The majority of these chemicals have short half-lives in the atmosphere that limit transfer of these solvents from the troposphere to the stratosphere. The exceptions are trichloroethane, tetrachloroethane, tetrachloromethane, and 1,1,2-trichloro-1,2,2-trifluoroethane with half-lives in the troposphere of 5 to 10 years, less than 2 years, 15 to 100 years, and 86 to 100 years, respectively. The contribution of these chemicals to the depletion of ozone in the stratosphere remains to be determined, although the contribution of the former two chemicals is small compared with the latter two. The high vapor pressure of these solvents also limits the contamination of surface water, although some of these chemicals migrate rapidly through soil to contaminate groundwater. Based on the current level of understanding, existing contamination of the environment by these halogenated solvents has not produced documented adverse health effects; however, some of these chemicals are common groundwater contaminants, and few data exist on the long-term health effects.

Dichloro- Solvents

Because of the moderate persistence (i.e., atmospheric half-life of 1.5 to 4.0 months) of dichloroethane in the atmosphere, long-range transport from point sources is possible. After evaporation, dichloroethane undergoes photooxidation. Although dichloroethane may produce chlorine radicals that interact with ozone in the stratosphere, this solvent probably does not contribute significantly to the depletion of the ozone layer, because the predicted rate of this reaction is three times less than a similar reaction with chlorofluorocarbon-11 (32). Dichloroethane evaporates quickly from running water because of its high volatility and low water solubility. Large spills of dichloroethane may contaminate groundwater because it leaches quickly through soil. Biodegradation of dichloroethane is slow (33), and, consequently, this solvent may persist in groundwater for months to years after contamination.

Most of the dichloromethane released into the environment partitions into the atmosphere, where photochemical degradation produces hydroxyl radicals that persist approximately 6 months (34). This chemical does not contribute significantly to photochemical smog or depletion of ozone in the stratosphere. Dichloromethane leaches easily from soil to groundwater; however, the rapid degradation of this chemical in soil limits the migration of dichloromethane from accidental spills.

Elimination of 1,2-dichloroethylene from the atmosphere is rapid (i.e., half-lives of 8.0 and 3.6 days for the *cis* and *trans* isomers, respectively) as a result of their reaction with hydroxyl radicals produced by photolysis (35). Experimental data suggest that the reaction of 1,2-dichloroethylene with ozone is too slow to produce significant depletion of ozone in the stratosphere (36). 1,2-Dichloroethylene undergoes slow reductive dechlorination under anaerobic conditions with a half-life up to 11 years for the *cis* isomer (37).

The major release sites of dichloropropane from industrial sources are to the atmosphere and soil. Partial volatilization of dichloropropane occurs in soil with the rest of this solvent leaching into subsurface soil and to groundwater. The principal methods of elimination are groundwater hydrolysis and anaerobic biotransformation, but these processes are slow, and, therefore, dichloropropane persists in groundwater for long periods.

Trichloro- Solvents

The atmospheric lifetime of trichloroethylene is relatively short (approximately 10 days) as a result of photoreduction by hydroxyl radicals, and, consequently, trichloroethylene is not a persistent chemical in the atmosphere unless continual release of trichloroethylene occurs. However, trichloroethylene is highly mobile in soil, and the chemical decomposition of trichloroethylene in sealed water may be long (i.e., 25 years) based on *in vitro* studies. Consequently, the trichloroethylene released into the soil migrates readily to groundwater, where this chemical may remain for months to years. Dichloromethane, vinyl chloride, 1,2-dichloroethylene, and chloroethane are potential degradation products of the anaerobic transformation of trichloroethylene in the soil (38).

1,1,1-Trichloroethane is one of the most stable and least reactive of all the chloroethanes. In the troposphere, the long half-life (i.e., 5 to 10 years) and lack of direct photochemical degradation allow migration of this chemical from the troposphere to the stratosphere (39). The potential of trichloroethane to deplete the ozone in the stratosphere is one order of magnitude less than comparable amounts of trichlorofluoromethane (chlorofluorocarbon-11) (40). The chemical degradation rate of trichloroethane is slow with 1,1-dichloroethane being the major product of anaerobic degradation. Depending on temperature, the observed half-life of trichloroethane in water ranges from 0.5 to 3.0 years.

The high vapor pressure of trichloromethane causes the rapid volatilization of this chemical from industrial sources and surface water. Because trichloromethane is relatively nonreactive, long transport of this chemical from industrial sources is possible. The calculated half-life of trichloromethane ranges from 80 to 180 days.

Tetrachloro- Solvents

Tetrachloroethane is relatively inert, with a half-life in the atmosphere exceeding 800 days (41). The adsorption of tetrachloroethane to soil is weak, and, therefore, tetrachloroethane leaches easily into groundwater; however, levels of this chemical in drinking water range from undetectable to less than 1 ppb.

Products of the photochemical reaction of tetrachloroethylene with hydroxyl radicals include phosgene and carbon tetrachloride. The estimated half-life of tetrachloroethylene in the troposphere is approximately 100 to 250 days; however, the reaction of tetrachloroethylene with ozone is slow, and, consequently, current levels of tetrachloroethylene probably do not contribute significantly to the depletion of ozone in the stratosphere (42). Experimental data indicate that tetrachloroethylene has little potential to accumulate in the food chain.

Tetrachloromethane degrades in the atmosphere by slow photolysis to chlorine, carbon dioxide, carbon monoxide, and hydrogen chloride with an estimated half-life ranging from 15 to 100 years. Few data are available regarding the biotransformation of tetrachloromethane. This solvent is relatively resistant to photodegradation and oxidation in water. Consequently, this chemical may persist in water for extended periods. Data on the fate of tetrabromomethane in the atmosphere are very limited.

Chlorofluorocarbon-113

1,1,2-Trichloro-1,2,2-trifluoroethane is very resistant to decomposition in the lower atmosphere (i.e., troposphere), and transport to the stratosphere occurs slowly, where the lifetime of this chemical reaches up to 100 years. Almost all releases of this chemical partition into the atmosphere because of its limited water solubility and high volatility. After slow transport to the stratosphere, intense UV radiation dechlorinates 1,2-trichloro-1,2,2-trifluoroethane, and the chlorine atoms act as a catalyst to convert ozone to oxygen.

DOSE EFFECT

Inhalation

All of the halogenated solvents are CNS depressants that produce dose-related changes in mental function and in the level of consciousness depending on the individual chemical and the duration of exposure. Table 58-4 lists the ambient air levels considered safe by the U.S. Occupational Safety and Health Administration and the American Conference of Governmental Industrial Hygienists (ACGIH). The threshold limit value time-weighted average (TLV-TWA) is the level at which an average worker may be repeatedly exposed (i.e., 40 hours a week) without experiencing adverse effects. The TLV short-term exposure limit (TLV-STEL) is the concentration at which workers can undergo short-term exposure without experiencing (a) sufficient narcosis to produce an increased incidence of accidental injury or reduced work efficiency, (b) chronic or irreversible tissue damage, or (c) eye or upper respiratory tract irritation. The TLV-STEL is a supplemental acute exposure limit to the TLV-TWA, which primarily addresses chronic injury. The low TLV-TWAs of 1,2-dichloroethane, tetrachloromethane, and trichloromethane result from their carcinogenic properties in animals, whereas the low levels for tetrabromoethane, tetrachloromethane, and tetrachloroethane evolve from their potent toxicity to the liver. A cross-sectional study of 135 workers exposed to concentrations as high as 11 ppm tetrachloromethane over 5 years demonstrated statistically significant ($p < .05$) increases in the serum level of alanine aminotransaminase and in γ-glutamyl transferase when compared with controls; however, no clinically significant, dose-dependent reduction of liver function was detected (43).

When the TLV-STEL is exceeded, neuropsychological testing indicates that changes in psychomotor performance (e.g., manual dexterity) precede decrements in cognitive performance (e.g.,

TABLE 58-4. Recommended exposure limits and irritant levels[a]

	U.S. Occupational Safety and Health Administration			American Conference of Governmental and Industrial Hygienists		
	PEL-TWA (ppm)	STEL (ppm)	Skin designation	TLV-TWA	Skin designation	Eye/upper respiratory tract irritation
1,2-Dichloroethane	1[b]	2	–	10	–	NA
1,2-Dichloroethylene	200	–	–	200	–	NA
Dichloromethane	25	125	–	50	–	2,300
1,2-Dichloropropane	75	110	–	75	–	NA
Tetrabromoethane	1[c]	–	–	–	–	1
Tetrachloroethane	1[c]	–	+	1	+	14–33
Tetrachloroethylene	25	–	–	50	–	100–600
Tetrachloromethane	2[b]	–	–	5	+	NA
Trichloroethane	350	450	–	350	–	1,000
Trichloroethylene	50	200	–	50	–	400–1,000
Trichloromethane	2[b]	–	–	10	–	4,000
1,1,2-Trichloro-1,2,2-trifluoroethane	1,000	1,250	–	1,000	–	NA

–, none; +, present; NA, not available; PEL, permissible exposure limit; ppm, parts per million; STEL, short-term exposure limit; TLV, threshold limit value; TWA, time-weighted average.
[a]Readers should check www.osha.gov and www.acgih.org for the most current values.
[b]Based on carcinogenic properties.
[c]Based on hepatorenal toxicity.

learning and memory). Manual dexterity was reduced after 3 hours of exposure to 300 and 500 ppm trichloroethylene (44). After a 3-hour exposure to 800 ppm dichloromethane, significant deficits in psychomotor tasks (e.g., simple and choice reaction times, reduced tapping speed, and impaired coordination and steadiness) developed in human volunteers (45). Measures of cognitive performance (e.g., reproduction of visual patterns, learning and retention of nonsense syllables) did not deteriorate after 2 hours of exposure to concentrations up to 1,000 ppm dichloromethane (46). In general, mild exposures cause varying degrees of inebriation, headache, lightheadedness, weakness, irritability, and nausea, whereas exposure to higher levels produces slurred speech, poor coordination, giddiness, confusion, lethargy, and ataxia, depending on the individual potency of the chemical and the duration of exposure. Levels of 10,000 to 25,000 ppm trichloroethane, trichloroethylene, trichloromethane, and dichloromethane produce coma in humans within a short period. Animal studies indicate that levels of approximately 100,000 to 200,000 ppm 1,1,2-trichloro-1,2,2-trifluoroethane are required to produce coma and convulsions, but these concentrations are so high that asphyxia may contribute to the CNS changes (47).

Dermal

Most of these chemicals do penetrate human skin but in insufficient quantities to substantially add to the body burden of the halogenated solvents. Exceptions to this generalization include tetrachloroethane and tetrachloromethane. The ACGIH adds a skin notation to these substances that refers to the potential contribution to the overall body burden from their transcutaneous absorption.

Oral

Limited data are available on the dose-related effects of the ingestion of halogenated solvents. Substantial variation may occur between individual subjects as a result of susceptibility (e.g., ethanol-induced liver disease, malnutrition): A 5 1/2-year-old girl died from hepatorenal failure after ingesting 1 mL of tetrachloromethane, whereas a 29-year-old man survived a 100-mL ingestion of tetrachloromethane with supportive care and hemodialysis (48). Case reports suggest that both 1,2-dichloroethane and 1,1,2,2-tetrachloroethane are highly toxic. A fatal hepatorenal syndrome developed in a 14-year-old boy who ingested approximately 50 mL of dichloroethane (49). The ingestion of 28 to 57 mL of tetrachloroethane by a 20-year-old man resulted in coma, respiratory depression, then death approximately 15 hours after ingestion (50). The estimated lethal oral dose in humans is approximately 3 to 5 mL (7 g) of trichloroethylene per kg body weight, and a report in the Russian literature attributes a death to the ingestion of 50 mL of trichloroethylene. Based on case reports, ingestion of 0.5 mL of trichloroethylene per kg body weight can produce significant CNS depression (51,52). The ingestion of an estimated 8 to 10 mL of tetrachloroethylene in a 6-year-old, 22-kg boy induced coma requiring 5 days of respiratory support (53).

TOXICOKINETICS

Absorption

The pulmonary route is the main source of excessive exposures to the halogenated solvents. These chemicals are generally well absorbed through both the lungs and gastrointestinal tract. The amount of absorption depends on the speed of transfer of the chemical through the pulmonary capillaries into the blood (i.e., blood/air partition coefficient) and the concentration of the chemical in the blood. This buildup depends primarily on the rate of metabolism, because distribution of the solvents to lipid-rich tissue is generally slow. The greatest percentage of trichloroethylene is absorbed during the first few minutes, although the absolute quantity absorbed increases with increasing ventilation. Rapid metabolism and a relatively high blood/air partition coefficient (approximately 15) explains the relatively complete absorption of trichloroethylene (54). Excellent absorption of tetrachloroethylene occurs across the capillary membranes of the pulmonary bed in part because of its extremely high blood/air partition coefficient (approximately 145). Peak blood levels are reached immediately after inhalation ceases (55). In humans, the lungs absorb approximately 25% of an inhaled dose of 300 ppm trichloroethane for 6 hours (56). After exposure to 100 to 200 ppm dichloromethane for 2 to 4 hours, initial absorption of this solvent is rapid, but absorption reaches steady-state conditions within 1 to 2 hours, probably because of the limited solubility of dichloromethane in the blood (57).

The low peak levels of chlorofluorocarbons in the arteries compared with the total dose administered via inhalation suggest that absorption by the lungs is slow, as determined by animal studies (58). Case reports of human exposure and animal data suggest that oral absorption of trichloroethylene, trichloromethane, tetrachloroethylene, dichloromethane, dichloroethane, tetrachloroethane, and tetrabromoethane is rapid and substantial. Gastrointestinal absorption is generally less complete than pulmonary absorption. Whereas 2 to 6 mL of oral tetrachloroethylene produces drowsiness, inhalation of approximately 5 mL of tetrachloroethylene vapors produces anesthesia. The gastrointestinal absorption of trichloroethane and dichloroethylene appears less complete than other halogenated solvents, and absorption of 1,1,2-trichloro-1,2,2-trifluoroethane is poor. The dermal absorption of most halogenated solvents is not sufficient to produce toxicity by itself, but the transcutaneous absorption of tetrachloroethane and tetrachloromethane may contribute to the total body burden of these chemicals. Transcutaneous absorption of dichloroethane in guinea pigs produced a steadily increasing blood level of trichloroethylene that suggested the possibility of accumulating toxicity after dermal exposure to dichloroethane (59).

Distribution

Once absorbed, halogenated solvents distribute rapidly to tissue based on their lipid content and individual tissue/blood partition coefficients. The highest concentrations generally appear in the fat, brain, and blood. With inhalation, peak blood levels occur soon after inhalation ceases, whereas with oral administration, peak levels occur 1 to 2 hours afterward. Animal and human studies indicate that accumulation of these chemicals in fat generally is not substantial after chronic exposure unless concentrations are high. An exception is tetrachloroethylene, which accumulates because of its markedly prolonged biological half-life. Some of these halogenated solvents (e.g., trichloroethylene, trichloromethane, dichloroethane) cross the placenta and may accumulate in the fetus.

Metabolism

The extent and type of metabolism vary among the halogenated solvents. Substantial biotransformation of these chemicals occurs in the human body after exposure to dichloroethane, dichloropropane, tetrachloroethane, and trichloroethylene. This transformation generally occurs in the liver via the cytochrome P-450 oxidative pathway. Glutathione conjugation is an alternate common pathway. Animal studies indicate that the body extensively metabolizes dichloroethane depending on the amount administered. Although the exact intermediate has not been identified, evidence in animal studies indicates that the episulfonium ion formed via the glutathione conjugation pathway is the major toxic intermediary *in vivo*. Subsequently, the biotransformation of this intermediary produces the suspected carcinogen (32). The toxic intermediary of tetrachloroethane metabolism has not been identified. Hydrolytic cleavage of the carbon chlorine bond via dichloroacetic acid to glyoxylic acid subsequently forms the end product, carbon dioxide. A minor pathway produces trichloroethylene and another one produces tetrachloroethylene. Figure 58-1 demonstrates the biotransformation of trichloroethylene. The cytochrome P-450 mixed function oxidase system converts tri-

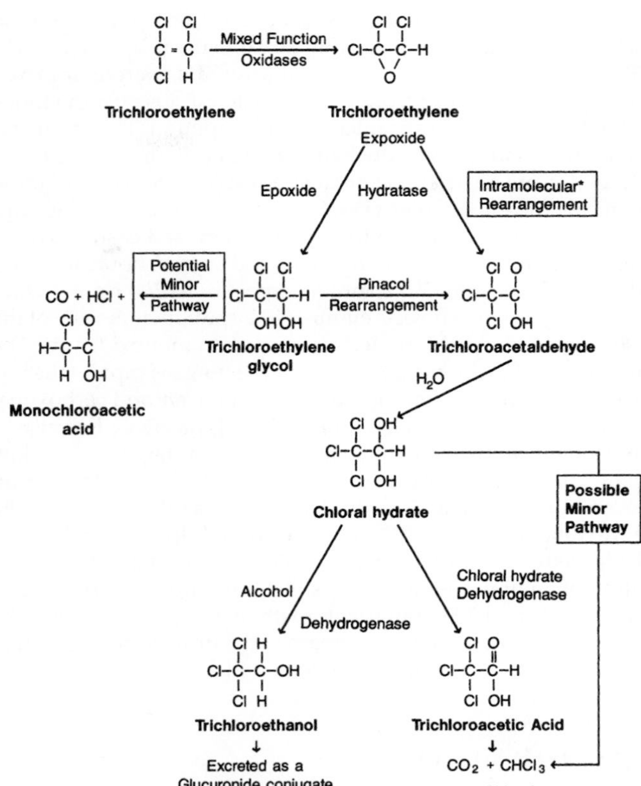

Figure 58-1. Metabolism of trichloroethylene. *, major pathway.

chloroethylene into an epoxide, which subsequently rearranges to trichloroacetylaldehyde and then chloral hydrate. Another pathway, which operates only at high doses, leads to the formation of dichloroacetyl chloride and dichloroacetic acid. Substantial species variation occurs in the ability to use these alternate pathways (60). Trichloroethane and tetrachloromethane undergo comparatively less transformation, but these solvents produce toxic intermediates that probably produce hepatotoxicity by the formation of free radicals. The major metabolic pathway of dichloromethane involves formation of carbon monoxide by the hepatic microsomal cytochrome P-450 mixed function oxidase system (61). This reaction requires both molecular oxygen and reduced nicotinamide adenine dinucleotide phosphate to form formyl chloride, which then decomposes to carbon monoxide. Animal studies suggest that this pathway is easily saturated, indicating that metabolism is dose-dependent. Metabolic enzymes of tetrachloroethylene become saturated after exposure to levels of approximately 400 ppm (500 to 600 mg body burden) (62). Substantial variation in the metabolic rate of some compounds (e.g., tetrachloroethylene) exists between species, with a much higher rate in mice and rats than in humans (63).

The body metabolizes only small amounts of trichloromethane and tetrachloroethylene. The major metabolite of the former is trichloroethanol, whereas the major metabolites of the latter are trichloroacetic acid and oxalic acid. Trichloroethanol is a metabolic product of chloral hydrate and of trichloroethylene as well as tetrachloroethylene and trichloroethane. Little if any metabolism of 1,1,2-trichloro-1,2,2-trifluoroethane occurs in the body.

Elimination

Pulmonary excretion and liver metabolism are the two major routes of elimination for halogenated solvents. Humans eliminate more than 90% of an absorbed dose of trichloroethane unchanged through the lungs after an exposure to approximately 200 ppm trichloroethane (64). Similarly, rats excrete approximately 70% to 90% of an orally administered dose via the lungs within the first 72 hours as unchanged compound. The estimated elimination half-lives of unchanged trichloroethane and tetrachloroethylene are triexponential as a result of excretion of these chemicals from the blood vessel–rich tissue, muscle tissue, and fat compartment. Excretion from poorly perfused tissue (i.e., fat) averaged 53 hours for trichloroethane and 55 to 65 hours for tetrachloroethylene. After 7.5 hours of exposure to 200 ppm dichloromethane, human subjects eliminated approximately 30% of the absorbed dose of dichloromethane as carbon monoxide (65). The elimination of dichloromethane from the lungs is rapid, whereas the elimination of carbon monoxide from the air and carboxyhemoglobin from the blood is more gradual, probably because of the delayed release of dichloromethane from fat stores. At low doses, the liver metabolizes approximately 70% to 90% of an absorbed dose of trichloroethylene, whereas the lungs excrete approximately 10% to 20% of the absorbed dose as unchanged trichloroethylene. Pulmonary excretion is less after the administration of an oral dose in animals. After workplace exposures of between 100 and 200 ppm trichloroethylene, approximately 30% to 50% of an absorbed dose appears in the urine as trichloroethanol and 10% to 30% as trichloroacetic acid.

PATHOPHYSIOLOGY

Central Nervous System

CNS depression develops after exposure to high doses of all of the halogenated solvents, and most deaths result from respiratory depression and subsequent hypoxia. The exact mechanism of CNS depression has not been delineated, but the most plausible explanation is a change in membrane fluidity that subsequently alters neural transmission. Pathologic examinations of animals exposed to lethal concentrations of halogenated solvents generally do not demonstrate significant histologic damage to the brain after acute overdose (66,67). Cranial neuropathies that follow exposure to trichloroethylene as a degreasing agent or as an anesthetic probably result from the decomposition product, dichloroacetylene (68). No pathologic studies have detected such neuropathies after exposure to pure trichloroethylene. Histologic studies of rabbits and mice exposed to concentrations of dichloroacetylene ranging from 19 to 300 ppm demonstrated extensive cranial nerve damage, particularly in the sensory nucleus of the trigeminal nerve (69). Compared with case reports of human exposures resulting in cranial neuropathies, this experimental evidence revealed less distinctive evidence of damage in the cranial nuclei and relatively more damage in other areas of the brain.

Whether any of the other halogenated solvents produce permanent neurologic damage after chronic exposure is unproven. These chemicals belong to the class of organic solvents that has been associated with the development of neurobehavioral changes (i.e., organic solvent syndrome) based on epidemiologic studies primarily from Scandinavia. Better exposure data and improved studies are needed before these chlorinated solvents can be linked to the development of permanent neurologic changes in humans. Biochemical changes in the brain have been detected in animals after chronic exposure to trichloroethane. Mongolian gerbils exposed continuously to 70 ppm trichloroethane developed reduced DNA concentrations in the posterior cerebellar hemisphere, anterior cerebellar vermis, and hippocampus. After a 3-month exposure to trichloroethane, Mongolian gerbils demonstrated an increased concentration of glial fibrillatory acetic protein in the sensory motor cerebral cortex at levels of 210 and 1,000 ppm trichloroethane, but not at levels of 70 ppm trichloroethane. The S-100 protein concentrations decreased in the frontal cerebral cortex after exposure to 210 ppm trichloroethane but not at 70 or 1,000 ppm trichloroethane (70). The S-100 protein is a marker of an increase in astroglial cells; the glial fibrillatory acetic protein is the main subunit of astroglial filaments, and, therefore, glial fibrillatory acetic protein is found mainly in fibrillatory astrocytes. This same group also found changes in the brains of Mongolian gerbils exposed to trichloroethylene, dichloromethane, and tetrachloroethylene. The clinical significance of these biochemical changes remains unclear because (a) no consistent dose effect was present, (b) changes were not detected in the same areas of the brain, and (c) behavior abnormalities did not correlate with the areas of the brain demonstrating biochemical changes. Hence, these studies do not fulfill the principles of causation necessary to prove neurotoxicity. Further animal studies and epidemiologic data are necessary to delineate what permanent effects, if any, exposure to halogenated solvents at current workplace standards cause in the brain.

Liver

Tetrachloroethane, tetrachloromethane, and trichloromethane are classic hepatotoxins. Animal studies indicate that tetrachloroethane is relatively more toxic to the liver than either trichloromethane or tetrachloromethane (71). These hepatotoxins produce acute fatty infiltration, centrilobular necrosis, and cirrhosis in animals after chronic exposure. Those animal studies demonstrate substantial variability both in the binding and in subsequent hepatotoxicity of trichloromethane depending on animal species, genetic strain, sex, and age compared with the more consistent pattern of hepatotoxicity caused by tetrachloroethane and tetrachloromethane. This difference in animal toxicity correlates with the clinical experience in which trichloromethane produced substantially fewer cases of hepatotoxicity compared with tetrachloroethane and tetrachloromethane.

Tetrachloromethane produces its toxicity as a result of the formation of trichloromethyl free radicals and lipid peroxidation (72). Although early animal experimentation suggested that trichloroethylene was moderately hepatotoxic, later work suggests that the hepatotoxic effects of exposure to trichloroethylene are minimal (73). Liver damage is an uncommon complication of animal experimentation after both acute and chronic exposure to trichloroethylene. Tetrachloroethylene, trichloroethane, and dichloromethane are weak hepatotoxins. Animal studies suggest that liver abnormalities occur after exposure to these halogenated solvents only at levels far above those required to produce CNS symptoms (i.e., mild intoxication). Similarly, high-dose, subacute, and chronic animal studies of dichloroethane and of dichloropropane demonstrate some mild histologic changes (e.g., cloudy swelling, fatty degeneration of the liver) but no significant hepatic dysfunction despite doses far exceeding recommended levels (71,74).

Pathologic examination of animals repeatedly exposed to saturated concentrations (approximately 50 ppm) of tetrabromoethane for 15 minutes per day up to 92 days revealed congestion, vacuolation, fatty degeneration, and some necrosis of the liver, along with reparative effects that suggested the possibility of mild to moderate cirrhosis (75). These animal studies indicate that tetrabromoethane should be considered in the same category of hepatotoxins as tetrachloroethane, tetrachloromethane, and trichloromethane.

Kidney

The halogenated solvents that produce hepatotoxicity also tend to produce less dramatic changes in the kidneys. The most common histologic abnormality after exposure to these chemicals is cloudy swelling of the tubular epithelium, particularly the convoluted tubule. Results of animal experimentation on the renal system are somewhat conflicting for trichloroethylene, in part because of the propensity for nephrotoxins to contaminate exposure to this chemical. Animal studies indicate that trichloroethylene is a weak nephrotoxin (76). 1,2-Dichloroethane is an exception to the general rule in that this chemical produces the most prominent histologic changes (slight degeneration to complete necrosis of the tubular epithelium, interstitial edema, and hemorrhage) in the kidney of rats after fatal exposures (77).

Cardiovascular System

The halogenated solvents are CNS depressants and are, therefore, capable of producing vasodilatation and hypotension. Animal studies of trichloroethane indicate a two-phased depression of blood pressure after exposure to 8,000 to 25,000 ppm trichloroethane. Initially, both systolic and diastolic blood pressure decrease sharply, with a corresponding increase in myocardial contractility and cardiac output. A marked decrease in heart rate, myocardial contractility, and stroke volume characterizes the terminal phase (78). Cardiac sensitization (multiple ventricular beats in excess of controls or ventricular fibrillation) developed in 3 of 18 dogs exposed to 5,000 ppm trichloroethane after the intravenous injection of 8 mg of epinephrine per kg body weight and in all dogs exposed to 10,000 ppm trichloroethane (79). Trichloroethylene and 1,1,2-trichloro-1,2,2-trifluoroethane, but not trichloromethane, demonstrate similar cardiac sensitization. The animal model of epinephrine-induced dysrhythmias has been used to explain sudden death in the workplace after exercise and exposure to halogenated solvents. This model does not, however, duplicate sympathomimetic stimulation after stressful situations. In the latter situation, the adrenal medulla releases epinephrine and adrenergic transmitters (i.e., norepinephrine appears in the adrenergic terminals of the sympathetic nerves). Furthermore, the volume of sympathomimetic amines released after endogenous stimulation (e.g., approximately 0.004 mg per kg per minute in humans) is approximately one order of magnitude less than the volume released after experimental administration (e.g., 0.05 mg per kg per minute) (80). The development of ventricular dysrhythmias after halogenated solvent exposure is not well documented in the workplace, but animal studies suggest that dysrhythmias occur after exposure to high doses (i.e., 5,000 ppm) of these chemicals. The body converts dichloromethane to carbon monoxide, and the resultant decrease in oxygen delivery may exacerbate preexisting cardiovascular disease (e.g., dysrhythmias, chest pain, myocardial ischemia) in workers. In animal studies, high doses of dichloroethane or dichloropropane may produce adrenocortical hemorrhage (81), and, therefore, acute adrenal insufficiency may contribute to death in these animals.

Lung

The halogenated solvents display varying degrees of upper respiratory tract irritation but seldom produce alveolar damage. Some animals (e.g., rabbits and rats) exposed to 1,000 ppm dichloromethane for periods up to 6 months develop gross pulmonary congestion, edema, and some focal necrosis of the lung (82). One study of rats gavaged with 0.25 mL of tetrachloromethane in mineral oil per kg body weight demonstrated intraalveolar fibrin, intramural clots, endothelial sloughing, and necrosis of granular pneumocytes in the exposed animals (83). These changes suggested a direct tetrachloromethane-induced toxicity to the authors, but their work has not been duplicated to exclude confounding factors such as mineral oil aspiration.

Eye

These halogenated solvents generally produce mild chemical conjunctivitis in the eyes of animals given injections of these chemicals, depending on the concentration. Exposure to high concentrations of these chemicals in the air generally does not produce persistent changes. Blue-gray corneal opacities developed in dogs after the systemic, but not intraocular, administration of dichloroethane. No similar cases of corneal opacities have been reported in humans.

Postmortem Findings

Postmortem examination of patients who died immediately after overexposure to halogenated solvents generally demonstrate only nonspecific findings. The most common finding on autopsy of patients who died from trichloroethane exposure is acute passive congestion of the viscera with petechial hemorrhages in the brain and lungs (84). Pathologic changes demonstrated on the autopsies of patients dying from hepatotoxicity after exposure to tetrachloromethane include fatty degeneration and centrilobular necrosis of the liver, degeneration of the proximal and distal convoluted tubules and loops of Henle (i.e., acute tubular necrosis without involvement of the glomeruli), acute myocarditis, adrenal hemorrhage, gastrointestinal bleeding, pulmonary hemorrhage, and edema (85). CNS changes usually reflect either underlying disease or the effects of hepatorenal failure (86). In contrast to animal studies, postmortem examination of suicidal poisonings from tetrachloroethane do not demonstrate significant hepatic or renal pathology. Death occurs approximately 10 to 20 hours after suicidal ingestion of a fatal amount of tetrachloroethane. Dissection and histologic examination of adrenals were not reported. These autopsy reports indicate that hepatorenal failure is not the etiology of death in acute tetrachloroethane-induced deaths, in contrast to those dying from chronic tetrachloroethane poisoning.

CLINICAL PRESENTATION

Acute Systemic Toxicity

All halogenated solvents are classic CNS depressants that may produce some initial excitation followed by depression of the CNS. The type and onset of symptoms depend on the duration of exposure, concentration, exposure history, minute ventilation, and individual susceptibility. After inhalation of high doses of these chemicals, the rapid onset of CNS depression may occur, manifested by dizziness, ataxia, headache, fatigue, lethargy, nausea, and abdominal pain and progressing to stupor, apnea, coma, and death. After exposure to high concentrations, symptoms may develop rapidly within minutes; and, similarly, after removal from exposure, recovery is rapid (i.e., 30 minutes unless hypoxic damage or trauma occurs). Exposure to tetrachloroethylene is an exception because of its prolonged elimination time. Neurologic signs and symptoms after ingestion of trichloroethylene or tetrachloroethylene may be delayed several hours and include mental confusion, disorientation, poor concentration, dysarthria, ataxia, incontinence, urinary retention, amnesia, dysphasia, and numbness. Prolonged coma may follow the ingestion of tetrachloroethylene, and delayed dysrhythmias (over 24 hours) may develop after the ingestion of large amounts of trichloroethylene in patients who display CNS depression (87). Dichloromethane possesses direct CNS effects independent of the production of carboxyhemoglobin. Furthermore, patients with cardiopulmonary disease may be particularly susceptible to the effects of dichloromethane-induced carboxyhemoglobinemia. A 66-

year-old man developed an anterior myocardial infarction after a 3-hour exposure to a paint remover containing 80% dichloromethane (88). Recovery is usually complete within 24 hours unless the exposure produced secondary damage (i.e., myocardial ischemia, hypoxia) or the neurotoxin dichloroacetylene was present in the environment.

The hepatotoxic halogenated solvents (i.e., tetrachloroethane, tetrachloromethane, trichloromethane, tetrabromoethane, dichloroethane, and dichloropropane) produce initial narcotic effects followed by the development of hepatorenal dysfunction. The exact presentation depends on the dose and individual susceptibility. Symptoms of the hepatorenal phase (i.e., vomiting, nausea, abdominal pain, edema, jaundice, fever, chills, diarrhea, anorexia, epistaxis, dyspnea) typically begin several days after exposure and progress depending on the severity of toxicity. Renal dysfunction typically occurs concurrently with hepatic damage, although the severity of renal damage rarely may exceed hepatic dysfunction. Surviving patients typically do not develop either hepatic or renal sequelae. The development of hepatic failure after exposure to other halogenated solvents is rare and poorly documented probably due in part to predisposing conditions that cause individual hypersensitivity. The ingestion of these chemicals—trichloroethylene in particular—may produce substantial gastrointestinal irritation.

Pulmonary damage usually does not result from exposure to halogenated solvents unless known pulmonary irritants (e.g., phosgene, hydrogen chloride) contaminate the environment (89).

Central Nervous System

The lack of good exposure data and well-designed epidemiologic studies complicates the interpretation of data available on the chronic neurologic sequelae of exposure to halogenated solvents. Although none of these pure chemicals is a recognized neurotoxin, early case reports and uncontrolled epidemiologic studies associated workplace exposure to trichloroethylene (90,91), tetrachloroethylene (92,93), and dichloromethane (94) with a high prevalence of nonspecific CNS symptoms (e.g., headache, irritability, emotionality, personality changes, fatigue, and anxiety). Chronic overexposure (i.e., 200 to 400 ppm tetrachloroethylene) was associated with an excessive number of the following symptoms: headache, fatigue, lightheadedness, vomiting, and upper respiratory tract irritation (95).

Early reports of neurologic sequelae (optic neuritis, cerebellar degeneration, cerebral hemorrhages) after chronic exposure to tetrachloromethane are not documented well enough to separate the direct toxic effects of tetrachloromethane from other causes. Individual case reports associate the development of peripheral neuropathies with workplace exposure to trichloroethane (96,97), 1,1,2-trichloro-1,2,2-trifluoroethane (98), and trichloroethylene (99). Additionally, a case report associated the development of an encephalopathy with exposure to trichloroethane (100). Small, epidemiologic studies of workers exposed to levels of tetrachloroethylene and to trichloroethane below current workplace standards have not detected deleterious effects on clinical symptoms (101), mortality (102,103), or neurobehavioral performance (104).

The present data on animal studies, case reports, and epidemiologic studies do not support a causal link between the development of chronic neurologic symptoms and exposure to halogenated solvents below established TLV-TWA concentrations. Determination of whether these neurologic symptoms result from exposure to organic solvents (i.e., organic solvent encephalopathy) depends on whether problems with study design flaws and inadequate neuropsychological testing can be overcome.

Gastrointestinal Tract

The replacement of hepatotoxic halogenated solvents with less toxic ones, along with improved industrial hygiene standards, led to a marked decrease in the number of reported cases of hepatotoxicity after exposure to the hepatotoxic halogenated solvents. Rare case reports have associated the development of hepatitis with exposure to trichloroethylene (105,106), trichloroethylene and trichloroethane (107), and tetrachloroethylene (108). Liver biopsies typically demonstrate centrilobular necrosis in these cases, although fatty degeneration and necrosis of the midzonal areas also were present. Considering the large number of workers exposed to these halogenated solvents, the number of case reports of liver damage is exceedingly small. Clinical reports and cases series on tetrachloroethylene generally associate biochemical changes in the liver only at levels exceeding 100 ppm tetrachloroethylene (109). Occupational exposure to trichloroethylene also has been associated with the development of pneumatosis cystoides intestinalis (multiple gas-filled cysts within the intestinal wall) (110).

Skin

The halogenated solvents are defatting agents that may produce chronic irritation as a result of their defatting properties. They are not known to produce sensitization in the skin. A syndrome called *degreaser's flush* has been described and results from ethanol-induced vasodilatation of superficial skin vessels. This skin response maximizes approximately 30 minutes after exposure to trichloroethylene and resolves by approximately 60 minutes (111).

Reproductive Abnormalities

None of the halogenated solvents is a recognized teratogen, but human data are inadequate to make final determinations. Evidence for teratogenesis independent of maternal toxicity after exposure to trichloromethane is limited in rats but absent in mice and rabbits (112). Although trichloroethylene crosses the placenta in animals, teratogenesis has not yet been demonstrated in either animals or humans. Similarly, trichloroethane passes the placental barrier and probably also distributes into the highly lipid breast milk, but no observable effects on implantation, litter size, fetal absorption, or incidence of skeletal or visceral malformations were evident after rodents were exposed to 75 ppm trichloroethane 7 hours per day on days 6 to 15 of gestation (113). Similarly, tetrachloroethylene is not teratogenic in animals; however, this chemical is fetotoxic in animals at doses that are toxic to the mother. This same study demonstrated no teratologic effects after exposure to 300 ppm tetrachloroethylene 7 hours daily during days 6 through 15 of gestation, but a significant increase in the incidence of resorptions among the fetal population appeared. An epidemiologic study associated the presence of halogenated hydrocarbons in contaminated well water with an increased incidence of major cardiac malformations in children born to mothers who lived near these wells (114). The lack of a direct dose-response relationship and the complexity of the exposure data, however, limit extrapolation to the specific teratogenic effects of halogenated hydrocarbons.

Carcinogenicity

The U.S. National Toxicology Ninth Report on Carcinogens (Revised January 2001) lists the following five halogenated solvents as suspected carcinogens: tetrachloromethane, 1,2-dichloroethane, dichloromethane, tetrachloroethylene, and trichloromethane (115). This category implies that these chemicals may be reasonably anticipated to be human carcinogens based on (a) evidence of carcinogenicity from studies in humans that cannot exclude chance, bias, or confounding, but appear credible; or (b) sufficient evidence of carcinogenicity from studies of animals which indicate an increased incidence of malignant tumors (i) in multiple species or strains, (ii) in multiple experiments, or (iii) to an unusual degree with regard to the incidence, site, or type of tumor. The basis for these chemicals primarily results from data in animals. Although human data are limited, epidemiologic studies to date have failed to detect consistent, dose-related elevations of cancer rates in workers exposed to these chemicals (116). Considerable variation exists between species in the development of neoplasms—especially liver tumors—after exposure to these five solvents. Differences in peroxisome induction and metabolism account for some of these differences, which complicate the extrapolation of animal studies to the actual risk in humans, who are exposed to much lower doses than experimental animals (117).

Similarly, the International Agency for Research on Cancer lists these five chemicals in their group B category—agents that are possibly carcinogenic in humans. This category applies to those chemicals for which sufficient evidence of carcinogenicity exists in experimental animals, but inadequate evidence of carcinogenicity exists in humans.

The other halogenated solvents are listed as chemicals that are not classifiable according to their carcinogenicity to humans and are not suspected carcinogens. Some controversy surrounds the classification of carcinogenicity to humans from exposure to trichloroethylene, partly because of differences in metabolism between different species (118). The high metabolic rate of B6C3F1 mice contributes to the unique susceptibility of these animals to the development of tumors (119). A U.S. National Toxicology Program study using uncontaminated trichloroethylene at a dose of 1 g trichloroethylene per kg body weight demonstrated a significant increase in the incidence of hepatocellular carcinomas in B6C3F1 mice of both sexes. However, the failure to detect significant excesses of cancer in human epidemiologic studies (120) may result from the fact that the metabolic pathways leading to the formation of proximate carcinogens are not activated at low doses when trichloroethylene follows first-order kinetics.

LABORATORY

Biochemical Abnormalities

The most serious abnormalities of serum chemistry result from hepatorenal failure after exposure to the hepatotoxic halogenated solvents and include elevated serum hepatic aminotransferase, bilirubin, alkaline phosphatase, ammonia, creatinine, and lactate levels. A prolonged prothrombin time may lead to hemorrhage and to a reduced hemoglobin level. Hypoglycemia may complicate liver failure. Maximum elevations of serum hepatic aminotransferase develop between 1 and 3 days after exposure in nonfatal cases and generally return to normal within 2 weeks. Renal dysfunction is indicated by rising serum creatinine, and reduced urinary flow may accompany hepatic failure. The most sensitive indicator of hepatic dysfunction after exposure to trichloroethane is an elevation of the urinary bilinogen (121). Abnormalities may appear several days after exposure and remain a week after exposure.

Dysrhythmias may develop up to 24 hours after a large ingestion of trichloroethylene. Premature ventricular contractions are the most common dysrhythmias; however, bradycardia, conduction disturbance, and serious ventricular dysrhythmias may occur during acute intoxication. Trichloroethylene and tetrachloromethane are radiopaque, and these chemicals may appear on abdominal x-rays after ingestion (122). Other blood abnormalities include hypercalcemia complicating the course of the ingestion of dichloroethane and progressive monocytosis associated with chronic poisoning by tetrachloroethane (123).

Biochemical abnormalities after exposure to dichloromethane are unusual except for those relating to the formation of carbon monoxide (i.e., carboxyhemoglobinemia, acidosis). Carboxyhemoglobin levels may not be a good indicator of toxicity, in part because the lungs excrete the carbon monoxide dissolved in venous plasma before it reaches the systemic (arterial) circulation (124). Furthermore, dichloromethane produces direct CNS depression independent of the carboxyhemoglobin level, and, therefore, CNS effects are not directly related to the carboxyhemoglobin level.

Neurologic Testing

Studies in volunteers indicate that acute exposure to approximately 1,000 ppm trichloroethylene causes changes in reaction time, manual dexterity, and attention scores. No specific neurologic or neuropsychological test (attention, mood, short-term memory, executive function) is consistently abnormal in workers chronically exposed to trichloroethylene or tetrachloroethylene. Without baseline testing, the specificity of neuropsychological testing is poor. A study of 65 dry cleaners revealed a statistically significant difference in scores on visual reproduction pattern recognition and in pattern memory of workers in the high-exposure group (>3 years) compared with the low-exposure group (125). The detected differences were subclinical, and no significant differences were detected in tests of mood, psychomotor speed, simple attention, and executive function. Another study demonstrated subclinical differences in memory, perceptual seed, attention, and intellectual impairment (digit symbol) after adjustment for age, gender, and intelligence (126). Nakatsuka and colleagues did not detect any significant impairment of color vision in a study of 64 dry cleaners chronically exposed to tetrachloroethylene (127); however, Cavalleri and coworkers demonstrated some subclinical color loss, primarily in the blue-yellow range, in a cohort of 35 dry cleaners with relatively low exposure (mean, approximately 6 ppm tetrachloroethylene) (128). Patients exposed to the contaminant dichloroacetylene may develop abnormalities of the visual fields and trigeminal evoked potentials (129).

Analytical Methods

The method recommended for the determination of halogenated solvents in the occupational setting is the National Institute for Occupational Safety and Health activated charcoal method for collection and concentration, and subsequent solvent (carbon disulfide) extraction of the charcoal with gas chromatographic analysis of the extractant. Gas chromatography with electron capture has now largely replaced the Fujiwara colorimetry test for the determination of halogenated solvents in biological samples. Either solvent extraction of samples or head space methods may be used. Use of the Fujiwara method may produce false-positive results because of the presence of other halogens (e.g., chlorine, iodine, fluorine, and bromine). Photodetection with a halide meter possesses the same drawbacks. The biotransformation of trichloroethylene, tetrachloroethylene, and trichloroethane results in varying levels of trichloroacetic acid in the urine, and false positives may result if other chemicals, including chloral hydrate, are not excluded as potential sources of trichloroacetic acid.

Human Levels

Because of the ubiquitous presence of halogenated solvents in our environment, blood samples may contain detectable levels of these solvents without occupational exposure (130). Human data are too limited to establish definite dose-effect levels for these halogenated solvents. Some data are available from experimental human exposures to levels of halogenated solvents in the workplace. Additionally, some data from postmortem analysis of patients dying of suicidal and accidental overexposure to these chemicals are available (131,132).

Health Surveillance

BIOLOGICAL MONITORING

Table 58-4 lists the current workplace standards for environmental levels of the halogenated solvents. Monitoring the level of chemicals in the air evaluates the potential contaminants to which a worker is exposed but does not measure the actual dose received by the worker. The latter depends on work practices, protective equipment, and actual location in relation to the source of exposure. Biological monitoring attempts to more accurately measure the dose the worker received, although, because of individual variation, biological monitoring should be applied to a group and not to an individual. The ACGIH developed biological exposure limits as an aid to supplement environmental monitoring.

The end-exhaled air concentration of tetrachloroethylene drops rapidly after cessation of exposure during the first 30 minutes, and then decreases slowly. Sixteen hours after exposure ceases, the end-exhaled air concentration of tetrachloroethylene reaches approximately 8% of the inhaled level, assuming repeated exposures (133). The concentration of tetrachloroethylene in exhaled air within the first hour, then, represents recent exposure, whereas concentrations the following morning or weekend more closely approximate the exposure as a TWA (134). After workplace exposure to tetrachloroethylene, the concentration of trichloroacetic acid rises in the blood for the first 24 hours and then declines with a half-life of approximately 80 hours (135). The ACGIH's biological exposure limit is 7 mg trichloroacetic acid per L urine at the end of the workweek or 10 ppm tetrachloroethylene in end-exhaled air collected before the shift after at least 2 consecutive work days.

The measurement of trichloroethane in exhaled air before the work shift (i.e., 16 hours after the cessation of exposure after at least 2 consecutive days) is the most specific biological measure of exposure to trichloroethane. The biological exposure limit recommended by the ACGIH is 40 ppm trichloroethane; however, substantial individual variation exists (e.g., body fat, physical activity). The sample should be collected as soon as possible and immediately refrigerated because of the rapid decline of trichloroethane. Measurement of urinary trichloroacetic acid is a less specific measure of the dose of trichloroethane in workers, but the urinary trichloroacetic acid is an accurate measure of the extent of trichloroethane exposure (136). The ACGIH recommended biological exposure limit for trichloroethane in urine is 10 mg of trichloroacetic acid per L voided at the end of the workweek. This measurement is only a screening test and is not a specific measure of exposure because other chlorinated hydrocarbons produce trichloroacetic acid.

Trichloroethanol levels in exhaled air, blood, and urine are also indicators of the TWA during the preceding several days because approximately 30% to 50% of an absorbed dose of trichloroethylene is metabolized to trichloroethanol. Measurements of trichloroacetic acid or trichloroethanol in the urine or blood are the recommended methods to monitor exposure to trichloroethylene. The ACGIH recommends a concentration of 4 g of free trichloroethanol per L of blood collected at the end of the workweek as a biological limit of trichloroethylene exposure. The biological exposure limit for trichloroacetic acid in the urine is 100 mg per g creatinine. Data must be interpreted cautiously because of confounding factors, such as ethanol consumption, racial differences, time of sampling, and coexposure to other solvents. Monitoring of trichloroethylene in end-exhaled air is primarily a test to confirm an excessive exposure to this chemical, when the origin of elevated levels of trichloroacetic acid and of trichloroethanol is unclear. After exposure ceases, the end-exhaled concentration of trichloroethylene declines in a multiexponential fashion; therefore, end-exhaled air samples collected soon after exposure ceases indicate recent exposure, whereas the level present in end-exhaled air of trichloroethylene several hours after exposure ceases represents an average of the preceding several days. Concentrations exceeding 0.4 ppm trichloroethylene in an end-exhaled air sample collected 16 hours after the last exposure suggest an excessive exposure.

Blood carboxyhemoglobin levels probably should not exceed 5% in workers exposed to dichloromethane. This carboxyhemoglobin level approximates the concentration obtained after a workday exposure to 100 ppm dichloromethane in resting nonsmokers (137). After absorption of dichloromethane, the pulmonary excretion of unchanged dichloromethane is small (i.e., <5%) and rapid. Sampling (i.e., nonsmokers only) should occur either within 2 hours of the exposure when steady-state levels appear, or 16 hours after the last shift (i.e., preshift level).

MEDICAL MONITORING

Preplacement physical examinations should focus on establishing a baseline for kidney and cardiac function as well as detecting preexisting conditions (e.g., arteriosclerotic heart disease, liver dysfunction, chronic skin conditions, alcoholism) that may predispose the worker to toxic effects of halogenated solvents. Periodic medical examinations should be designed to detect alterations in CNS function (e.g., impairment of perceptual speed, reaction time, and manual dexterity), hepatic dysfunction, gastrointestinal symptoms, and dermatitis. The extent of routine laboratory analyses (serum hepatic transaminases, urinalysis, serum creatinine) depends on the judgment of the physician regarding the severity of the exposure based on workplace practice, environmental monitoring, and biological exposure limits.

TREATMENT

First Aid

DERMAL

Damage to the skin usually results either from prolonged skin contact or from chronic defatting of the skin. Contaminated clothing should be removed and the affected area washed with soap and copious amounts of water.

EYE

Halogenated solvents are direct irritants to the epithelium of the eye, and installation of these compounds into the eye results in irritation of the conjunctiva and damage to the corneal epithelium. Spontaneous recovery usually occurs. Corneal abrasions and some turbidity may appear initially. After direct installation of these chemicals into the eye, the eye should be irrigated thoroughly for at least 15 minutes and medical attention sought if erythema or irritation persists.

ORAL

Existing data on oral exposures to halogenated solvents are too limited to confidently predict the exact level at which decontamination measures should be instituted. Table 58-5 lists the recommended quantities of halogenated solvents at which decontamination measures are appropriate. These guidelines

TABLE 58-5. Recommendations for decontamination

Solvent	Ingested amount[a]
1,2-Dichloroethane	One swallow
1,2-Dichloroethylene	Large, intentional ingestion
Dichloromethane	Large, intentional ingestion
1,2-Dichloropropane	>One swallow
Tetrabromoethane	>Several swallows
Tetrachloroethane	One swallow
Tetrachloroethylene	Several swallows
Tetrachloromethane	One swallow
Trichloroethane	Large, intentional ingestions
Trichloroethylene	>One swallow
Trichloromethane	One swallow
1,1,2-Trichloro-1,2,2-trifluoroethane	Usually not necessary

Note: These recommendations are estimates based on the limited data available and may change when better data become available.
[a]One swallow in a 2-year-old child and an adult is approximately 5 mL and 20 mL, respectively. Large, intentional ingestions usually exceed 120 to 150 mL in adults. These levels are based on pure substances. For products containing more than one substance, the decision to use decontamination measures should be based on the most toxic substance present in the blend at a concentration exceeding 10% to 20%.

apply only when the ingestion occurs less than 1 hour before the initiation of treatment and the patient does not display a lack of gag reflex, coma, or convulsive activity. After the administration of ipecac syrup, the patient should be observed in the upright position to minimize the hazard of aspiration. The indication of emesis after the ingestion of chlorinated hydrocarbons has not been associated with the development of aspiration pneumonitis. Dichloromethane is a mucous membrane irritant, and dilution with water or milk after ingestion should be initiated after the oral administration of small amounts of this chemical.

INHALATION

The immediate danger from large exposures to halogenated solvents is CNS and respiratory depression. The victim should be moved from the contaminated environment as soon as safely possible. The adequacy of respiration should be evaluated in the patient with altered mental status and oxygen and artificial ventilation begun as needed. For unconscious patients, the pulse should be checked, and cardiopulmonary resuscitation should be initiated if the pulse is absent. Medical attention should be sought for victims with any alteration of mental status or with respiratory difficulty.

Acute Management

STABILIZATION

The treatment of exposure to these chemicals is primarily supportive. Respiratory depression and dysrhythmias represent the greatest immediate danger to life after exposure. The adequacy of oxygenation should be assessed initially and arterial blood gases drawn if indicated. Patients with altered mental status or those reporting dyspnea should receive supplemental oxygen and be monitored with a pulse oximeter. Hypotension initially should be treated with volume expansion and then vasopressors as needed. Symptomatic patients should be monitored for the development of dysrhythmias. Although sympathomimetic drugs should be administered with caution, their use in the clinical setting should not be avoided if indicated. Sensitization of the myocardium occurs at levels higher than 5,000 ppm in animal studies, levels that are unlikely to occur in the clinical setting because of the rapid elimination of these solvents from the lungs. Lidocaine is the initial antiarrhythmic of choice, with beta blockers being a second-line drug for ventricular ectopy. Hypotension usually responds to removal of the patient from exposure and volume expansion. Persistent hypotension necessitates a search for other causes (myocardial infarction, trauma, excessive volume depletion). Animal studies indicate that adrenal hemorrhage may occur after exposure to high concentrations of some halogenated solvents (i.e., dichloroethane, dichloropropane). Accordingly, acute adrenocortical insufficiency should be considered in any patient in whom hypotension or vascular collapse supervenes or who does not respond to the usual supportive measures. The diagnosis of adrenal apoplexy should be confirmed by serum cortisol levels before treatment. Once a blood specimen has been collected, treatment should begin with intravenous hydrocortisone in a dose of 200 to 300 mg during the first 24 hours.

DECONTAMINATION

No clinical studies support the clinical use of any decontamination measure after exposure to halogenated solvents. Table 58-5 lists estimated quantities of ingested solvents that may benefit from decontamination. These levels are only estimates because of the lack of data; therefore, these recommendations may change as more data appear. Ipecac syrup is the emetic of choice at a dose of 15 mL for 1- to 3-year-old children and 30 mL for patients older than 10 years. The induction of emesis generally is not recommended beyond 1 hour because these compounds are rapidly absorbed, and the effectiveness of decontamination measures rapidly diminish after 1 hour. Contraindications to the use of ipecac syrup include the presence of marked lethargy, loss of the gag reflex, coma, and convulsions. Lavage with saline is an alternative method of decontamination; however, the poor water solubility of these chemicals may limit this method's effectiveness. The administration of activated charcoal is a reasonable alternative to ipecac syrup and lavage, but few data are available on the adsorptive capacity of activated charcoal for hydrocarbons. Although activated charcoal binds many drugs, some hydrocarbons do not adsorb well to activated charcoal (138).

ENHANCEMENT OF ELIMINATION

Because most of these chemicals are excreted through the lungs, good ventilation should be maintained. Hyperventilation (three times the normal minute volume) has been recommended for an ingestion of more than 1.2 mL of tetrachloroethylene per kg body weight, or blood levels greater than 10 μg tetrachloroethylene per mL. In a 6-year-old boy, hyperventilation reduced the initial elimination half-life of tetrachloroethylene from 160 to 30 minutes, but this therapy did not alter the slower, terminal elimination half-life. Hemodialysis may be necessary for the development of renal failure; however, hemodialysis removes only small amounts of tetrachloromethane from the blood (139). The elimination of other halogenated solvents by hemodialysis or hemoperfusion has not been studied. The high lipophilic characteristics of these solvents argue against the efficacy of hemodialysis.

Although the use of hyperbaric oxygen for 6 hours improved the survival of rats administered oral doses of tetrachloromethane (140), and case reports note a successful outcome after the use of hyperbaric oxygen (141,142), the use of hyperbaric oxygen in this setting remains experimental. A 32-year-old worker was found unconscious in a poorly ventilated area after exposure to a paint preparation containing approximately 25% dichloromethane (143). The initial carboxyhemoglobin level was 5.4% and rose to 13% despite 46 minutes of hyperbaric oxygen administered 1 hour after admission. Although the authors felt that hyperbaric oxygen was beneficial, the clinical course did not correlate well with the carboxyhemoglobin level, and the neurologic effects probably resulted from the direct CNS effects of dichloromethane rather than the effects of carbon monoxide.

ANTIDOTES

A single case report documented the survival of a 61-year-old man after the ingestion of a lethal dose of 250 mL of tetrachloromethane after the use of intravenous *n*-acetylcysteine (144). Theoretically, this antidote restores glutathione levels and prevents the formation of toxic intermediates; however, clinical data are not adequate to support the use of *n*-acetylcysteine in this situation, and, therefore, administration of *n*-acetylcysteine for a patient who overdoses on tetrachloromethane remains experimental. Although no antidotes have been studied for the treatment of trichloromethane intoxication, the depletion of glutathione stores after overdose with this chemical suggests that *n*-acetylcysteine would be as effective as the administration of *n*-acetylcysteine after tetrachloromethane administration.

SUPPORTIVE CARE

Potential complications of exposure to halogenated solvents include cardiac dysrhythmias, aspiration pneumonia, chemical hepatitis (delayed), and hypoxic encephalopathy. Symptomatic patients should be monitored for the development of dysrhythmias, and patients who ingest large amounts of these compounds should be monitored for 24 hours to detect the delayed development of dysrhythmias. Patients exposed to high concentrations of these chemicals should receive a chest x-ray, arterial blood gas, electrocardiogram, and measurement of serum creatinine and hepatic transaminases. Profuse diarrhea may exacerbate electrolyte imbalance and predispose the patient to dysrhythmias. Consequently, generous intravenous fluid replacement should be given and serum electrolytes monitored at least daily. Patients exposed to large concentrations of the hepatotoxic halogenated solvents (dichloroethane, tetrabromoethane, tetrachloroethane, trichloromethane, and tetrachloromethane) should be followed for at least 3 days to detect the development of hepatorenal failure. Serial hematocrits and stool guaiac tests are necessary only for those patients who develop abnormalities in coagulation and therefore are predisposed to the development of gastrointestinal bleeding. Supportive care includes the treatment of renal failure with dialysis and hepatic failure with fresh frozen plasma, vitamin K, low-protein diet, neomycin, lactulose, and careful fluid and electrolyte balance. These patients may benefit from total parenteral nutrition. Carboxyhemoglobin levels should be obtained from patients exposed to dichloromethane, but these levels do not necessarily accurately reflect the clinical status of the patient. The use of 100% oxygen or hyperbaric oxygen has not been well studied after dichloromethane exposure. Although treatment of high levels (e.g., >30%) of carboxyhemoglobin with hyperbaric oxygen is reasonable (145), no data indicate that morbidity or mortality is directly related to the carboxyhemoglobin level.

REFERENCES

1. Magos L. Thoughts on life with untested and adequately tested chemicals. *Br J Ind Med* 1988;45:721–726.
2. Hill AB. The environment and disease: association or causation? *Proc R Soc Med* 1965;58:295–300.
3. Gilman AG, Goodman LS, Rall TW, et al, eds. *The pharmacological basis of therapeutics*, 8th ed. New York: Macmillan, 1990:261.
4. Nashlelsky MB, Dix JD, Adelstein EH. Homicide facilitated by inhalation of chloroform. *J Forensic Sci* 1995;70:134–138.
5. Ostlere G. The role of trichloroethylene in general anesthesia. *BMJ* 1948;1:195–196.
6. Lamson PD, Minot AS, Robbins BH. The prevention and treatment of carbon tetrachloride intoxication. *JAMA* 1921;90:345–349.
7. Lambert SM. Hookworm disease in the South Pacific, ten years of tetrachlorides. *JAMA* 1933;100:247–248.
8. Foot EB, Bishop K, Apgar V. Tetrachloroethylene as an anesthetic agent. *Anaesthesiology* 1943;4:283–292.
9. Willcox WH. An outbreak of toxic jaundice due to tetrachloroethane poisoning. A new type amongst aeroplane workers. *Lancet* 1915;1:544–547.
10. Hoffman HT, Birnstiel H, Jobst P. On the inhalation toxicity of 1,1- and 1,2-dichloroethane. *Arch Toxicol* 1971;27:248–265.
11. Reynolds ES, Moslen MT. Damage to hepatic cellular membranes by chlorinated olefins with emphasis on synergism and antagonism. *Environ Health Perspect* 1977;21:137–147.
12. Smyth HF. Hygienic standards for daily inhalation. The Donald E. Cummings Memorial lecture. *Am Ind Hyg Q* 1956;17:129–185.
13. Royal Society of Chemistry. Organo-chlorine solvents. Health risks to workers. Brussels Commission of the European Communities publ. no. EUR 10531EN, 1986:131–146.
14. International Programme on Chemical Safety. Environmental health criteria 50. Trichloroethylene. Geneva: World Health Organization, 1985.
15. Greim H, Wolff T, Hofler M, et al. Formation of dichloroacetylene from trichloroethylene in the presence of alkaline material. Possible cause of intoxication after abundant use of chloroethylene-containing solvents. *Arch Toxicol* 1984;56:74–77.
16. Firth JB, Stuckey RE. Decomposition of trilene in closed circuit anaesthesia. *Lancet* 1945;1:814–816.
17. Crummett WB, Stenger VA. Thermal stability of methyl chloroform and carbon tetrachloride. *Ind Eng Chem Analyst (Edn)* 1956;48:434.
18. National Institute for Occupational Safety and Health (NIOSH). Recommended standard for occupational exposure to methylene chloride. Department of Health, Education, and Welfare (NIOSH) publ. no. 76–138. Cincinnati: Department of Health, Education, and Welfare, 1976.
19. International Programme on Chemical Safety. *Environmental health criteria 176. 1,2-Dichloroethane*, 2nd ed. Geneva: World Health Organization, 1995.
20. Harkov R, Giante SJ, Bozelli JW, LaRegina JE. Monitoring volatile organic compounds at hazardous and sanitary landfills in New Jersey. *J Environ Sci Health* 1985;20(Part A):491–502.
21. Agency for Toxic Substances and Disease Registry. *Toxicological profile for 1,2-dichloroethene*. Atlanta: US Department of Health and Human Services, Public Health Service, ATSDR, 1990.
22. Agency for Toxic Substances and Disease Registry. *Toxicological profile for 1,1,1-trichloroethane*. Atlanta: US Department of Health and Human Services, Public Health Service, ATSDR, 1990.
23. Westrick JJ, Mello JW, Thomas RF. The groundwater supply survey. *J Am Water Works Assoc* 1984;76:52–59.
24. Singh HB, Salas LJ, Stiles RE. Distribution of selected gaseous organic mutagens and suspected carcinogens in ambient air. *Environ Sci Technol* 1982;16:872–880.
25. Krasner SW, McGuire MJ, Jacangelo JG, Patania NL, Reagan KM, Aieta EM. The occurrence of disinfection by-products in U.S. drinking water. *J Am Water Works Assoc* 1989;81:41–53.
26. Daft JA. Determination of fumigants and related chemicals in fatty and non-fatty food. *J Agric Food Chem* 1989;37:560–564.
27. Simmonds PG, Cunnold DM, Alyea FN, et al. Carbon tetrachloride lifetimes and emissions determined from daily global measurements during 1978–1985. *J Atmospheric Chem* 1988;7:35–58.
28. Wallace LA. Personal exposures, indoor and outdoor air concentrations and exhaled breath concentrations of selected volatile organic compounds measured for 600 residents of New Jersey, North Dakota, North Carolina and California. *Toxicol Environ Chem* 1986;12:215–236.
29. Agency for Toxic Substances and Disease Registry. *Toxicological profile for tetrachloroethylene*. Atlanta: US Department of Health and Human Services, Public Health Service, ATSDR, 1993.
30. Solet D, Robis TG, Sampaio C. Perchloroethylene exposure assessment among dry cleaning workers. *Am Ind Hyg Assoc J* 1990;51:566–574.
31. International Programme on Chemical Safety. *Environmental health criteria 133. Fully halogenated chlorofluorocarbons*. Geneva: World Health Organization, 1990.
32. International Programme on Chemical Safety. *Environmental health criteria 62. 1,2-Dichloroethane*. Geneva: World Health Organization, 1987.
33. Corapcioglu MY, Hossain MA. Ground-water contamination by high-density immiscible hydrocarbon slugs in gravity-driven gravel aquifers. *Ground Water* 1990;28:403–412.
34. Rayez JC, Rayez MT, Halvick P, Duguay B, Lesclaux R. A theoretical study of the decomposition of halogenated alkoxy radicals. I. Hydrogen and chlorine extrusions. *J Chem Phys* 1987;34:619–629.
35. Hazardous Substances Data Bank. *1,2-Dichloroethylene*. Bethesda, MD: National Library of Medicine, National Institutes of Health, US Department of Health, 1997.
36. Atkinson R, Aschmann SM, Goodman MA. Kinetics of the gas-phase reaction of nitrate radicals with a series of alkynes, haloalkenes, and alpha, beta-unsaturated aldehydes. *Int J Chem Kinet* 1987;19:299–308.
37. Agency for Toxic Substances and Disease Registry. *Toxicological profile for 1,2-dichloroethene*. Atlanta: US Department of Health and Human Services, Public Health Service, ATSDR, 1990.
38. Parsons F, Wood PR, DeMarco J. Transformation of tetrachloroethane and trichloroethane in microcosms and groundwater. *J Am Water Works Assoc* 1984;76:56–59.
39. Midgley PM. The production and release to the atmosphere of 1,1,1-trichloroethane (methyl chloroform). *Atmos Environ* 1989;23:2663–2665.
40. International Programme on Chemical Safety. *Environmental health criteria 136. 1,1,1-Trichloroethane*. Geneva: World Health Organization, 1992.
41. Singh HB, Salas LJ, Smith AJ, Shigeishi H. Measurements of some potentially hazardous organic chemicals in urban environments. *Atmos Environ* 1981;15:601–612.

42. Atkinson R, Carter WPL. Kinetics and mechanisms of the gas-phase reactions of ozone with organic compounds under atmospheric conditions. *Chem Rev* 1984;84:437–470.
43. Tomenson JA, Baron CE, O'Sullivan JJ, Edwards JC, Stonard MD, Walker RJ, Fearnley DM. Hepatic function in workers occupationally exposed to carbon tetrachloride. *Occup Environ Med* 1995;52:508–514.
44. Stopps GJ, McLaughlin M. Psychophysiological testing of human subjects exposed to solvent vapors. *Am Ind Hyg Assoc J* 1967;28:43–50.
45. Winneke G. The neurotoxicity of dichloromethane. *Neurobehav Toxicol Teratol* 1981;3:391–395.
46. Gamberle F, Annwall G, Hultengren M. Exposure to methylene chloride. II. Psychological functions. *Scand J Work Environ Health* 1975;1:95–103.
47. Hygenic Guide Series. 1,1,2-Trichloro-1,2,2-trifluoroethane (trifluorotrichloroethane, fluorocarbon No. 113). *Am Ind Hyg Assoc J* 1968;29:521–525.
48. Fogel RD, Davidman M, Poleski MH, et al. Carbon tetrachloride poisoning treated with hemodialysis and total parenteral nutrition. *CMAJ* 1984;128:560–561.
49. Yodaiken RE, Babcock JR. 1,2-Dichloroethane poisoning. *Arch Environ Health* 1973;26:281–284.
50. Mant AK. Acute tetrachloroethane poisoning. A report on two fatal cases. *BMJ* 1953;1:655–656.
51. Stephens JA. Poisoning by accidental drinking of trichloroethylene. *BMJ* 1945;2:218–219.
52. Eichert H. Trichloroethylene intoxication. *JAMA* 1936;106:1952–1954.
53. Koppel C, Arendt U, Koeppe P. Acute tetrachloroethylene poisoning, blood elimination kinetics during hyperventilation therapy. *Clin Toxicol* 1985;23:103–115.
54. Monster AC. Differences in uptake, elimination and metabolism in exposure to trichloroethylene, 1,1,1-trichloroethane and tetrachloroethylene. *Int Arch Occup Environ Health* 1979;42:311–317.
55. Pegg DG, Zempel JA, Braun WH, et al. Distribution of tetrachloroethylene following oral and inhalation exposure in rats. *Toxicol Appl Pharmacol* 1979;51:465–474.
56. Nolan RJ, Freshour NL, Rick DL, et al. Kinetics and metabolism of inhaled methyl chloroform (1,1,1-trichloroethane) in male volunteers. *Fundam Appl Toxicol* 1984;4:654–662.
57. Divencenzo GD, Yanno FJ, Astill FJ. Human and canine exposures to methylene chloride vapor. *Am Ind Hyg Assoc J* 1972;33:125–135.
58. Shangel L, Koss R. Determination of fluorinated hydrocarbon propellants in blood of dogs after aerosol administration. *J Pharm Sci* 1972;61:1445–1449.
59. Jakobson I, Wahlberg JE, Holmberg B, et al. Uptake via the blood and elimination of 10 organic solvents following epicutaneous exposure of anesthetized guinea pigs. *Toxicol Appl Pharmacol* 1982;63:181–187.
60. Kimbrough RD, Mitchell FL, Houk VN. Trichloroethylene: an update. *J Toxicol Environ Health* 1985;15:369–383.
61. Kubic VL, Anders MW. Metabolism of dihalomethanes to carbon monoxide. III. Studies on the mechanism of reaction. *Biochem Pharmacol* 1978;27:2349–2355.
62. Monster AC, Boersman G, Steenweg H. Kinetics of tetrachloroethylene in volunteers: influence of exposure concentration and waste load. *Int Arch Occup Environ Health* 1979;72:303–309.
63. Reitz RH, Gargas ML, Mendrala AL, Schumann AM. *In vivo* and *in vitro* studies of perchloroethylene metabolism for physiologically based pharmacokinetic modeling in rats, mice, and humans. *Toxicol Appl Pharmacol* 1996;136:289–306.
64. Fernandez JG, Droz PO, Humbert BE, Caperos JR. Trichloroethylene exposure. Simulation of uptake, excretion, and metabolism using a mathematical model. *Br J Ind Med* 1977;34:43–55.
65. DiVincenzo GD, Kaplan CJ. Uptake, metabolism and elimination of methylene chloride vapor by humans. *Toxicol Appl Pharmacol* 1981;59:130–140.
66. Kranz JC Jr, Park CS, Ling JSL. Anesthesia LX. The anesthetic properties of 1,1,1-trichloroethane. *Anaesthesia* 1959;20:635–640.
67. Adams EM, Spencer HC, Rowe UK, et al. Vapor toxicity of trichloroethylene determined by experiments on laboratory animals. *AMA Arch Ind Hyg Occup Med* 1951;4:469–481.
68. Barret L, Torch S, Leray C, Sarlieve L, Saxod R. Morphometric and biochemical studies in trigeminal nerve of the rat after trichloroethylene and dichloroacetylene oral administration. *Neurotoxicology* 1992;13:601–614.
69. Reichert D, Lieboldt G, Hanschlar G. Neurotoxic effects of dichloroacetylene. *Arch Toxicol* 1976;37:23–38.
70. Karkson JE, Rosengren LE, Kjellstrand P, et al. Effects of low dose inhalation of three chlorinated aliphatic organic solvents on deoxyribonucleic acid in gerbil brains. *Scand J Work Environ Health* 1987;13:453–458.
71. Wright WH, Schaffer JM. Critical anthelmintic tests of chlorinated alkyl hydrocarbons and a correlation between the anthelmintic efficacy, chemical structure and physical properties. *Am J Hyg* 1932;16:325–428.
72. Kalf GF, Post GB, Synder R. Solvent toxicology. Recent advances in the toxicology of benzene, the glycol ethers, and carbon tetrachloride. *Annu Rev Pharmacol Toxicol* 1987;27:399–427.
73. Waters EM, Gerstner HB, Huff JE. Trichloroethylene 1. An overview. *J Toxicol Environ Health* 1977;2:671–707.
74. Heppel LA, Neal PA, Perrin TL, et al. The toxicity of 1,2-dichloroethane (ethylene dichloride). V. The effect of daily inhalations. *J Ind Hyg Toxicol* 1946;28: 113–120.
75. Tray MG. Effect of exposure to the vapors of tetrabromoethane (acetylene tetrabromide). *AMA Arch Ind Hyg Occup Med* 1950;2:407–419.
76. US National Toxicology Program (NTP). *Technical report on the carcinogenesis studies of trichloroethylene (without epichlorhydrin) in F 344/n rats and BCF mice*. Research Triangle Park, NC: National Institutes of Health, publ. no. 83–1979, NTP TR 243, 1983.
77. Spencer HC, Rowe VK, Adams EM, et al. Vapor toxicity of ethylene dichloride determined by experiments on laboratory animals. *Arch Ind Hyg Occup Med* 1951;4:482–493.
78. Herd PA, Lipsky M, Martin HF. Cardiovascular effects of 1,1,1-trichloroethane. *Arch Environ Health* 1974;28:227–233.
79. Reinhart CF, Mullins LS, Maxfield ME. Epinephrine-induced cardiac arrhythmia-potential of some common industrial solvents. *J Occup Med* 1973;15:953–955.
80. Back KC, Van Stee EW. Toxicology of halo alkane propellants and fire extinguishants. *Annu Rev Pharmacol Toxicol* 1977;17:83–95.
81. Heppel LA, Neal PA, Perrin TL, et al. The toxicity of 1,2-dichloroethane (ethylene) III. Its acute toxicology and the effect of protective agents. *J Pharmacol Exp Ther* 1945;84:53–63.
82. Heppel LA, Neal PA. Toxicology of dichloromethane (methylene chloride) III. Its effects on running activity in the male rat. *J Ind Hyg Toxicol* 1944;26:17–21.
83. Gould VE, Smuckler EA. Alveolar injury in acute carbon tetrachloride intoxication. *Arch Intern Med* 1971;128:109–117.
84. Hatfield TR, Mayleoski RT. A fatal methyl chloroform (trichloroethane) poisoning. *Arch Environ Health* 1970;20:279–281.
85. Moon HD. The pathology of fatal carbon tetrachloride poisoning with special reference to the histogenesis of the hepatic and renal lesions. *Am J Pathol* 1950;26:1041–1057.
86. Cohen MM. Central nervous system in carbon tetrachloride intoxication. *Neurology* 1957;7:238–244.
87. Thomas G, Baud FJ, Galliot M, et al. Clinical and kinetic study of 4 cases of acute trichloroethylene intoxication. *Vet Hum Toxicol* 1987;29[Suppl 2]:97–99.
88. Stewart RD, Hake CL. Paint remover hazard. *JAMA* 1976;235:398–401.
89. English JM. A case of probable phosgene poisoning. *BMJ* 1964;1:38.
90. Bardodej Z, Vyskocil J. The problem of trichloroethylene in occupational medicine. *AMA Arch Ind Health* 1956;13:581–592.
91. El Ghawabi SM, Mansoor MB, El Gamel AA, et al. Chronic trichloroethylene exposure. J *Egypt Med Assoc* 1973;56:715–724.
92. Coler HR, Rossmiller HR. Tetrachloroethylene exposure in a small industry. *AMA Arch Ind Hyg Occup Med* 1953;8:227–233.
93. Gold J. Chronic perchloroethylene poisoning. *Can Psychiatr Assoc J* 1969; 14:627–630.
94. Collier H. Methylene dichloride intoxication in industry. A report of two cases. *Lancet* 1936;1:594–595.
95. Cai S-X, Huang M-Y, Chen Z, Liu Y-T, Jin C, Watanabe T, et al. Subjective symptom increase among dry-cleaning workers exposed to tetrachloroethylene vapor. *Ind Health* 1991;29:111–121.
96. House RA, Liss GM, Wills MC. Peripheral sensory neuropathy associated with 1,1,1-trichloroethane. *Arch Environ Health* 1994;49:196–199.
97. Liss GM. Peripheral neuropathy in two workers exposed to 1,1,1-trichloroethane. *JAMA* 1988;260:2217.
98. Raffi GB, Violante FS. Is freon 113 neurotoxic? A case report. *Int Arch Occup Environ Health* 1981;49:125–127.
99. Mitchell ABS, Parsons-Smith BG. Trichloroethylene neuropathy. *BMJ* 1969;1:422–423.
100. Kelafant GA, Berg RA, Schleenbaker R. Toxic encephalopathy due to 1,1,1-trichloroethane exposure. *Am J Ind Med* 1994;25:439–446.
101. Kramer CG, Ott MG, Fulkerson JE, Hicks N. Health of workers exposed to 1,1,1-trichloroethane; a matched-pair study. *Arch Environ Health* 1978;33: 331–342.
102. Katz RM, Jowett D. Female laundry and dry cleaning workers in Wisconsin: a mortality analysis. *Am J Public Health* 1981;71:305–307.
103. Blair A, Decoufle P, Grauman D. Causes of death among laundry and dry cleaning workers. *Am J Pub Health* 1979;69:508–511.
104. Tuttle TC, Wood GD, Crether CB, et al. A behavioral and neurological evaluation of dry cleaners exposed to perchloroethylene. Cincinnati: Department of Health, Education, and Welfare, National Institute for Occupational Safety and Health, publ. no. 77–214, 1977.
105. Priest RJ, Horn RC. Trichloroethylene intoxication. A case of acute hepatic necrosis possibly due to this agent. *Arch Environ Health* 1965;11:361–365.
106. McCurrey RJ. Diverse manifestations of trichloroethylene. *Br J Ind Med* 1988;45:122–126.
107. Theile DL, Eigenbrodt EH, Ware AJ. Cirrhosis after repeated trichloroethylene and 1,1,1-trichloroethane exposure. *Gastroenterology* 1982;83:926–929.
108. Meckler LC, Phelps DK. Liver disease secondary to tetrachloroethylene exposure. A case report. *JAMA* 1966;197:144–145.
109. Gennari P, Naldi M, Motta R, et al. Gamma-glutamyl-transferase isoenzyme pattern in workers exposed to tetrachloroethylene. *Am J Ind Med* 1992;21:661–671.
110. Sato A, Yamaguchi K, Nakajima T. A new health problem due to trichloroethylene: pneumatosis cystoides intestinalis. *Environ Health* 1987;42:144–147.
111. Stewart RD, Hake CL, Peterson JE. "Degreaser's flush" dermal response to trichloroethylene and ethanol. *Arch Environ Health* 1974;29:1–5.
112. Barlow SM, Sullivan FM. *Reproductive hazards of industrial chemicals*. London: Academic Press, 1982.

113. Schewtz TA, Leong BKJ, Gehring PJ. The effect of maternally inhaled trichloroethylene, perchloroethylene, methyl chloroform, and methylene chloride on embryonal and fetal development in mice and rats. *Toxicol Appl Pharmacol* 1975;32:84–96.
114. Goldberg SJ, Lebowitz MD, Graver EJ. An association of human congenital cardiac malformations and drinking water contaminants. *J Am Coll Cardiol* 1990;16:155–164.
115. US National Toxicology Program. *Ninth annual report on carcinogens.* Research Triangle Park, NC: National Institute of Environmental Health Sciences, Public Health Service, US Department of Health and Human Services, January 2001.
116. Weiss NS. Cancer in relation to occupational exposure to perchloroethylene. *Cancer Causes Control* 1995;6:257–266.
117. Maronpot RR, Anna CH, Devereux TR, Lucier GW, Butterworth BE, Anderson MW. Considerations concerning the murine hepatocarcinogenicity of selected chlorinated hydrocarbons. *Prog Clin Biol Res* 1995;391:305–323.
118. Templin MV, Stevens KD, Stenner RD, Bonate PL, Tuman D, Bull RJ. Factors affecting species differences in the kinetics of metabolites of trichloroethylene. *J Toxicol Environ Health* 1995;44:435–447.
119. Bolt HM. Pharmacokinetic factors and their implication in the induction of mouse liver tumors by halogenated hydrocarbons. *Arch Toxicol* 1987;[Suppl 10]:190–203.
120. Axelson O, Selden A, Andersson K, Hogstedt C. Updated and expanded Swedish cohort study on trichloroethylene and cancer risk. *J Occup Med* 1994;36:556–562.
121. Stewart RD. Methyl chloroform intoxication. Diagnosis and treatment. *JAMA* 1971;215:1789–1792.
122. Bagnasco FM, Stringer B, Muslim AM. Carbon tetrachloride poisoning. *N Y State J Med* 1978;78:646–647.
123. Minot GR, Smith LW. The blood in tetrachloroethane poisoning. *Arch Intern Med* 1921;28:687–702.
124. Langehennig PL, Seeler RA, Berman E. Paint removers and carboxyhemoglobin. *N Engl J Med* 1976;295:1137.
125. Echeverria D, White RF, Sampaio C. A behavioral evaluation of PCE exposure in patients and dry cleaners: a possible relationship between clinical and preclinical effects. *J Occup Environ Med* 1995;37:667–680.
126. Seeber A. Neurobehavioral toxicity of long-term exposure to tetrachloroethylene. *Neurotoxicol Teratol* 1989;11:579–583.
127. Nakatsuka H, Watanabe T, Takeuchi Y, et al. Absence of blue-yellow color vision loss among workers exposed to toluene or tetrachloroethylene, mostly at levels below occupational exposure limits. *Int Arch Occup Environ Health* 1992;64:113–117.
128. Cavalleri A, Gobba F, Paltrinieri M, Fantuzzi G, Righi E, Aggazzotti G. Perchloroethylene exposure can induce color vision loss. *Neurosci Lett* 1994;179:162–166.
129. Leandri M, Schizzi R, Scielzo C, Favale E. Electrophysiological evidence of trigeminal root damage after trichloroethylene exposure. *Muscle Nerve* 1995;18:467–468.
130. Hamijimiragha H, Ewers V, Jansen-Rosseck R, et al. Human exposure to volatile halogenated hydrocarbons from the general environment. *Int Arch Occup Environ Health* 1986;58:141–150.
131. Baselt RC. *Disposition of toxic drugs and chemicals in man,* 2nd ed. Davis, CA: Biomedical Publications, 1982.
132. Ellenhorn ME, Barceloux DG. *Medical toxicology: diagnosis and treatment of human poisoning.* New York: Elsevier Science, 1988.
133. US Environmental Protection Agency (EPA). *Health assessment document for perchloroethylene.* Washington: EPA; 1985. EPA publ. no. 60/8-82-005F.
134. Monster AC. Biological monitoring of chlorinated hydrocarbon solvents. *J Occup Med* 1986;28:583–588.
135. Monster AC, Boersma G, Steenweg H. Kinetics of tetrachloroethylene in volunteers; influence of workload and exposure concentration. *Int Arch Occup Environ Health* 1979;42:303–309.
136. Imbriani M, Ghittori S, Pezzagno G, et al. 1,1,1-Trichloroethane (methyl chloroform) in urine as biological index of exposure. *Am J Ind Med* 1988;13:211–222.
137. Astrand I, Ovrum P, Carlsson A. Exposure to methylene chloride. I. Its concentration in alveolar air and blood during rest and exercise and its metabolism. *Scand J Work Environ Health* 1975;1:78–94.
138. Laass W. Therapy of acute oral poisonings by organic solvents. Treatment by activated charcoal in combination with laxatives. *Arch Toxicol* 1980;[Suppl 4]:406–409.
139. Nielson VK, Larsen J. Acute meal failure due to carbon tetrachloride poisoning. *Acta Med Scand* 1965;178:363–374.
140. Burk RF, Reiter R, Lane JM. Hyperbaric oxygen protection against carbon tetrachloride hepatotoxicity in the rat. Association with altered metabolism. *Gastroenterology* 1986;90:812–818.
141. Truss CD, Killanberg PG. Treatment of carbon tetrachloride poisoning with hyperbaric oxygen. *Gastroenterology* 1982;82:767–769.
142. Burkhart KK, Hall AH, Gerace R, Rumack BH. Hyperbaric oxygen treatment for carbon tetrachloride poisoning. *Drug Safety* 1991;6:332–338.
143. Rioux JP, Meyers RAM. Hyperbaric oxygen for methylene chloride poisoning: report on two cases. *Ann Emerg Med* 1989;18:691–695.
144. Mathieson PJ, Williams G, MacSweeney JE. Survival after massive ingestion of carbon tetrachloride treated by intravenous infusion of acetylcysteine. *Hum Toxicol* 1985;4:627–631.
145. Rudge FW. Treatment of methylene chloride induced carbon monoxide poisoning with hyperbaric oxygenation. *Mil Med* 1990;155:570–572.

CHAPTER 59
Benzene and Other Hematotoxins

Richard D. Irons

The cells of the blood fulfill a variety of critical functions for the individual including transport of oxygen, host resistance, and hemostasis. Toxic responses involving the blood often involve a reduction in the number of circulating cells, either as a result of direct destruction or decreased production and release. Among the most frequently encountered blood dyscrasias secondary to drug or chemical exposure are thrombocytopenias, which may result from direct destruction frequently as a result of drug-induced immune complex formation, or decreased production resulting from bone marrow suppression.

A characteristic of anemias or cytopenias associated with chemicals or drugs is that individual responses vary widely both with respect to the severity and the nature of abnormality encountered following toxic exposure. Most blood dyscrasias secondary to drug or chemical exposure are transient and resolve upon withdrawal of the toxin. However, persistent and even fatal blood dyscrasias (e.g., cytopenias, myelodysplasias, and aplastic anemia) are not uncommon in cases of chronic severe bone marrow depression and have a well-established tendency to progress to acute leukemia.

In recent years it has become increasingly appreciated that myelodysplastic syndrome (MDS) and acute myelogenous leukemia (AML) are stages in the progression of a common transformation process that is frequently observed following cancer chemotherapy with alkylating agents or following chronic exposure to high concentrations of benzene (1,2). Moreover, many historical references to aplastic anemia occurring as a consequence of chronic exposure to hematotoxic agents may with hindsight have been more appropriately diagnosed as MDS.

HEMATOPOIESIS

Hematopoiesis is a process of cell amplification and differentiation in which a very small number of stem cells give rise to progressively more differentiated progenitor cells that in turn give rise to mature blood cells (Fig. 59-1).

The earliest hematopoietic progenitor cell is the pluripotent stem cell (PSC), which can give rise to progenitor cells in all blood cell lineages but has very limited proliferative activity itself. PSCs also possess the unique capacity of self-regeneration, and after embryogenesis, maintain exclusive responsibility for the production of blood cells throughout life.

In the normal adult, hematopoiesis occurs in the bone marrow and is largely restricted to scattered clusters of hematopoietic cells in the proximal epiphyses of the long bones, skull, vertebrae, pelvis, ribs and sternum. Even under conditions of extreme hematopoietic stress, such as occurs following bone marrow transplantation, extramedullary hematopoiesis in spleen, liver, and lymph nodes occurs only rarely in humans.

The hematopoietic precursor cells of the bone marrow and the mature cells of the blood exist in a dynamic equilibrium in which the senescence and destruction of mature blood cells are balanced by the production and release of new cells. In the average adult, destruction and replacement amount to between 200 and 400 billion cells per day. The rate of cell division in morphologically identifiable precursor cells in the bone marrow approaches

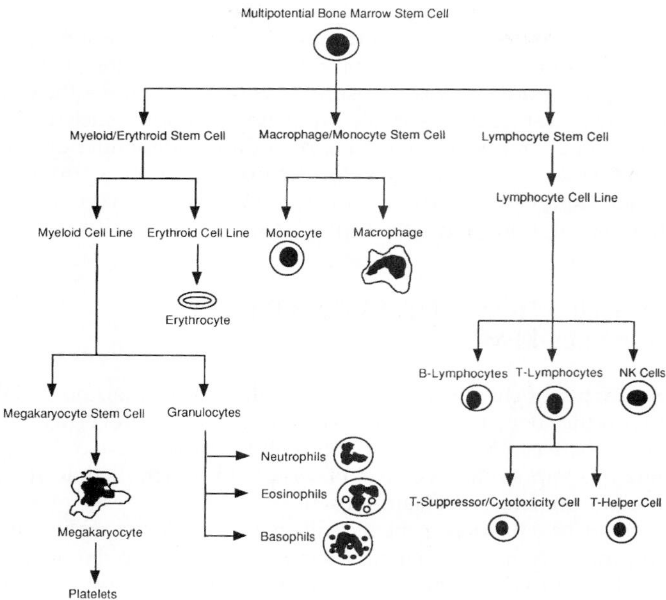

Figure 59-1. Blood cell differentiation. NK, natural killer.

the maximum for mammalian cells. Transient insults to the bone marrow may be readily accommodated by alterations in the proliferation of committed differentiating precursor cells. However, the physiologic response to prolonged insult to the bone marrow must eventually result in alterations in the differentiation of clonogenic progenitor cells, the activation of an increased proportion of normally resting stem cell populations, or both.

EPIDEMIOLOGY OF LEUKEMIAS

In the United States there are approximately 24,000 new cases of leukemia a year, which represent about 3% of all malignancies. AML and its variants account for 46% of all leukemias; chronic myelogenous leukemia (CML), 14%; acute lymphatic leukemia (ALL), 11%; and chronic lymphatic leukemia (CLL), 29%. These numbers are generally comparable among Western countries. In adults, AML constitutes almost 90% of all acute leukemias (3).

All known etiological agents together are responsible for a very small fraction of the overall incidence of leukemia, the vast majority of which arise *de novo* in the absence of any history of drug, radiation, or chemical exposure (4). Leukemia secondary to treatment of other malignant diseases, such as ovarian carcinoma, breast cancer, multiple myeloma, and chronic lymphocytic leukemia, is well documented because of the ability to obtain detailed follow-up and accurate exposure histories in patients receiving previous radiation or alkylation therapy (5–10).

Secondary AML, involving M1, M2, M4, or M6 subtypes, is a well-established phenomenon and is by far the most predominant hematopoietic malignancy arising as a consequence of cancer treatment (11,12). AML has also been observed following immunosuppressive therapy for nonneoplastic disorders, although it should be noted that immunosuppressive therapy resulting in AML has frequently included multiple alkylating agents and/or radiation therapy (13).

Isolated reports of other types of leukemias arising secondary to chemotherapy have appeared (14–16); however, in view of the very small numbers of cases and inconsistent pattern, it has been suggested that these represent coincidental occurrences (17).

CML has been observed following radiation and has been reported secondary to combined radiation-chemotherapeutic paradigms (18–20). However, it is noteworthy that in over 2,000 confirmed cases of leukemia secondary to radiation and/or chemotherapy reported in the world literature, CML has not been documented as occurring secondary to chemotherapy alone. In previous studies of Hodgkin's disease, treatment employing combined paradigms in which radiotherapy was followed by chemotherapy was particularly potent at inducing secondary AML, the cumulative risks of treatment approaching 10% (21–23). The frequency of occurrence of secondary AML varies depending on the treatment paradigms employed but generally ranges between 0.3% and 20% (17,21–24).

There are a number of serious difficulties that frustrate attempts to study hematopoietic malignancies secondary to chemical exposure in addition to their relative scarcity. For years there has been growing recognition among hematologists and hematopathologists of the clinical and biological importance of classifying hematopoietic and lymphoid neoplasms on the basis of individual cell types. At the same time there has remained a tendency on the part of epidemiologists to combine these relatively rare neoplasms into broad categories in order to have sufficient numbers to permit epidemiologic analysis.

This tendency to combine or "lump" different nosologic categories together in order to derive sufficient analytical power can be misleading if the etiology and pathogenesis of the diseases are different. This problem is compounded by the major classification scheme of the *International Classification of Diseases* (*ICD*), which refers to only three major categories of lymphoid neoplasms (i.e., lymphosarcoma and reticulosarcoma, 200; Hodgkin's disease, 201; and lymphatic leukemia, 204). This scheme encourages the combination of acute and chronic myeloid leukemias (205), and frustrates efforts to use the morphologically based French-American-British Cooperative Group (FAB) classification of leukemias (25). Although the most recent edition (*ICD-9*) provides for increased subtyping, in part to accommodate more relevant nosology, the major classification scheme that forms the basis for most of the available epidemiologic literature remains biologically archaic.

The advent of cell and molecular biology has led to increased classification and subtyping of hematopoietic and lymphoid neoplasms based on pheno- and genotypic analysis. In conducting retrospective studies, differences and ambiguities between the current and older literature will continue to serve as a source of frustration for several years to come. In the Western world, and for most of the developing world as well, variations in the differential diagnosis of AML subtypes do not represent a major source of confusion. However, as variations and improvements in diagnostic criteria have occurred, disparities with respect to disease classification have increased between the current and older literature and from one country or geographical region to another.

One salient example is a continuing ambiguity over the differential diagnosis of CML and MDS. While the evidence linking the development of MDS and AML with chemical or drug exposure is unequivocal, the same has not been convincingly demonstrated for CML. CML is a malignant myeloproliferative disorder of a hematopoietic stem cell that is characterized by the presence of the Philadelphia (Ph^1) chromosome. Transformed cells in CML can give rise to myeloid, erythroid, megakaryocyte or B lymphoid precursors (26–28). The Ph^1 chromosome represents a shortened chromosome 22 (22q-) arising from a reciprocal translocation t(9;22)(q34;q11) and is present in over 95% of patients with CML. The molecular lesion is associated with the transposition of the *c-abl* gene from chromosome 9 to a specific segment of chromosome 22, known as the break cluster region (*bcr*) (29). *Bcr-abl* fusion proteins form abnormal stable complexes with cytoplasmic signaling proteins that result in abnormal activation of $p21^{ras}$ (30–32). This results in abnormal activation of a cytokine regulatory signal in the target cell associated with the origin of CML. Even in the small number of patients with presumptive CML who are Ph^1-negative, a significant number possess the *bcr-abl* molecular rearrangements found in Ph^1-positive CML (33–35).

Because the morphological and cytological parameters of CML can be difficult or impossible to distinguish from myelodysplastic syndrome (MDS), cytogenetic or molecular analysis is important in the classification of patients with the disease. In one study of 25 cases originally classified as Ph^1-negative CML, cytogenetic examination resulted in 24 cases being reclassified as MDS or other myeloproliferative disorders distinct from CML (36). Comparisons of the incidence of CML and MDS and their respective reporting frequencies are problematic in the absence of detailed cytogenetic or molecular evaluation using banded chromosome analysis or techniques such as reverse transcriptase-polymerase chain reaction (RT-PCR) or fluorescence *in situ* hybridization (FISH).

Case reports are useful in drawing attention to a potential problem or suggesting a possible relationship between exposure and disease. A major strength of case reports is that the clinical diagnosis is usually well documented. On the other hand, a major weakness is that a reliable exposure history is exceedingly difficult to obtain. As a result, details of exposure are usually circumstantial or anecdotal and not quantifiable. Rarely, if ever, is chemical exposure documented even remotely as well as the diagnosis (37). By definition, case histories or collections of case histories are cumulative, and the case selection process is not random. Therefore, it is impossible to assign with any certainty "the denominator" in comparing the incidence of an exposure-disease relationship relative to the general population. Case reporting is subjective, and susceptible to such influences as the perception or suspicion of an association between a disease and exposure to a given agent, and even the potential legal consequences of such an association (37). Such biases are not always subtle. There are instances where the authors have forthrightly admitted that the motivation for publishing a collection of case histories was to influence medicolegal proceedings (38), and there are "collections" of case histories that have actually been abstracted from court records (39).

Case reports, either isolated or collected, are important for suggesting a possible relationship between exposure and disease and for providing a rationale for the conduct of more rigorous and detailed studies. Yet despite their importance in this regard, they cannot be used to establish a causal relationship. Lack of accurate exposure data is often the factor limiting the value of quantitative epidemiologic studies. The virtual absence of reliable exposure data in case reports places even more severe restraints on their utility. Often the alleged exposure is isolated, transient, separated by months or years from the onset of the disease, or not characterized at all. Casual accounts of past chemical exposures are not an adequate substitute for personnel monitoring or industrial hygiene measurements.

Quantitative retrospective or prospective epidemiology studies have the advantage of being able to establish a causal association between a given exposure and disease. Nevertheless, individual epidemiology studies often lack sufficient sample size to be definitive on their own. If the incidence of the disease is rare in the study population, several independent studies may be necessary in order to establish a clear pattern between exposure to a specific agent and a particular disease. Under these conditions, meaningful comparisons between studies can often be obscured by inconsistency in the nosologic classifications used, differences in the assignment of subjects to exposure groups, or confounding exposures to different combinations of agents.

Although quantitative epidemiology studies can establish the relationship between occupational exposure and increased incidence of a disease, inability to reliably quantitate the exposure is often still a major weakness, especially in retrospective studies. Attempts to use job classification schemes as a surrogate for exposure often assume that risk is cumulative and that the product of duration and exposure concentration defines the risk of disease rather than specific exposure conditions, such as the regimen or frequency of exposure and dose-dependency. For some compounds, such as 2,4-dichlorophenoxyacetic acid (2,4-D) and benzene, there is evidence to suggest that cumulative assumptions may be inappropriate.

OCCUPATIONS, HEMATOTOXICITY, AND LEUKEMIA

A number of chemicals have been evaluated for their potential to produce bone marrow toxicity or leukemia. However, associations between certain occupations and increased risk of leukemia or lymphoma have been observed for which the nature of the causative agent remains obscure.

Increased incidence of leukemia in workers in the rubber and tire industry has consistently been reported in epidemiology studies (40,41). In the absence of reliable exposure data, an assumed role for benzene served as a point of departure in a number of case reports and reviews, including one by this author (42). However, rubber and tire manufacture represents a complex setting in which simultaneous exposures to a variety of agents occur, and findings in subsequent studies have not proven to be consistent with the benzene hypothesis (43). Benzene exposure is associated with an increased risk of AML; whereas, in the rubber industry in particular, excesses are seen in lymphocytic as well as nonlymphocytic leukemias (44).

Checkoway and coworkers evaluated the specific association of leukemia and solvent exposure in the rubber industry and found that risk of lymphocytic leukemia was stronger for other solvents (e.g., carbon tetrachloride and carbon disulfide) than for benzene (45). An increased incidence of leukemia, primarily AML, has been observed among welders (46–48), and an increased incidence of lymphatic/hematopoietic neoplasms has been reported among plumbers (49). Although metal fumes, solvents, and flux have been hypothesized to be involved, the causative agent(s) remains a mystery.

A role for specific chemical exposure in the development of multiple myeloma has been frequently suggested, but no association between a specific chemical and multiple myeloma has been convincingly established. Even for high-dose γ-radiation, which traditionally has been thought to be a causal factor associated with the development of multiple myeloma in atom bomb survivors, follow-up analysis of atomic bomb survivors does not reveal an excess risk for multiple myeloma (50).

Other associations have been variously reported between environmental or occupational influences and the risk of developing multiple myeloma with differing degrees of confidence. These include asbestos—weakly positive to positive (51–53); auto/diesel exhaust—positive (54,55); and use of multivitamins, antacids, or laxatives—weakly positive to positive (52). A particularly consistent association has been observed between farming, exposure to meat products, use of fertilizers (51,54–58), and exposure to wood dust (54,57,58). These associations are significant in that they are consistent with the long-suggested role for chronic stimulation of the lymphoreticular system in the development of multiple myeloma (59).

A particularly intriguing and potentially serious problem in occupational medicine relates to the effects of extended space flight on hematologic and immunologic function. A consistent observation on U.S. and Soviet space flights has been a postflight reduction in circulating red blood cell mass and a decrease in cell-mediated immune function (60,61). Crew members returning from Spacelab 1 experienced an average 13% decrease in RBC and nearly a 9% reduction in hemoglobin concentration. These changes were preceded by a precipitous depression in peripheral reticulocytes, which was less than half of normal by day 7 of the mission and reached a nadir of −60.9% on landing day. This decrease in red cell mass, which is somewhat attenuated on longer missions, appears to involve both decreased erythrocyte lifespan and a suppression of erythropoiesis. Initial hypotheses to explain these effects included hyperoxia and a decrease in the production of erythropoietin by the kidney. Nevertheless, subsequent experiments have demonstrated that the clinical effects occur in the absence of elevated oxygen, and studies have failed to find a significant decrease in serum erythropoietin levels during space flight.

Additional studies have provided evidence that hypogravity adversely influences lymphocyte function, including a decrease in cell density–dependent T-lymphocyte response *in vitro* (62,63). Lymphocyte activation requires cell-cell contact, lymphokine production and release, and receptor-lymphokine interactions that lead to cell proliferation. Regulation of hematopoietic precursor cells is known to involve similar interaction between growth factors and receptors present on growth factor–dependent cells. Therefore, hematopoietic cells as well are likely to be susceptible to a variety of influences in the space environment, including hypogravity, radiation, environmental contaminants, and microbial flora. However, the long-term biological significance of these effects and the potential influence of the space flight environment on hematopoiesis and resistance to infectious disease remain unclear.

CYTOPENIAS AND BLOOD DYSCRASIAS

In recent years a great deal of attention has been focused on leukemias secondary to chemical exposure. In contrast, relatively little concern has been paid to other blood dyscrasias arising under similar circumstances. This is a disturbing trend when one considers the relatively dismal prognosis of secondary aplastic anemia or MDS quite independent of the tendency of survivors to go on to develop acute leukemia.

Until recently, reporting practices for hematologic dyscrasias have been much less uniform and reliable than for leukemias. If ascertaining the frequency of secondary leukemia is attended with serious difficulties, determining the incidence of other blood dyscrasias secondary to chemical exposure has been tantamount to impossible. Until very recently there have been no authoritative studies on the frequency of blood dyscrasias in the general population. However, Buffler and coworkers have recently completed a study of age-specific rates of myelodysplastic syndrome occurring in males over a 5-year period on the upper Texas Gulf Coast. Results of this study suggest that while the age-adjusted rate of myelodysplasias is relatively low (i.e., 2 to 2.8 per 100,000), there are marked differences in the age-specific incidence, ranging from 0.061 per 100,000 for whites and Hispanics 20 to 29 years of age to 19.59 per 100,000 for the 70 to 79 age group (PA Buffler, *personal communication*).

Another source of confusion concerns variations in the nosologic criteria used to differentiate individual cytopenias, aplastic anemia, pancytopenia, hypoplastic anemia, aleukemic leukemia, myelodysplastic syndrome, and refractory anemia. For example, the incidence of myelodysplastic syndrome may be seriously underestimated by classifications employing the use of such terms as *Ph^1-negative* CML (36). In one ongoing follow-up study of approximately 2,000 employees and retirees engaged in chemical manufacturing, the incidence of myelodysplastic syndrome cases appears to be about 36 per 100,000 (64). If one employs age-specific incidence data obtained in the Buffler study as a denominator for comparison with the general population, these results suggest an elevation in the incidence of myelodysplastic syndrome in an occupational setting. Moreover, recent studies of Chinese workers reveal an increased incidence of myelodysplastic syndrome in individuals occupationally exposed to benzene.

Benzene

Benzene is a colorless, highly flammable volatile liquid discovered in 1825 by Faraday. The source of most benzene is petroleum refining. However, benzene is also a by-product of combustion processes and is a common environmental pollutant found in automobile emissions and from evaporation of gasoline (65).

Benzene's primary use is as an intermediate in production of other chemicals such as ethylbenzene. It is also used for numerous industrial processes and in the formation of synthetic rubbers, lubricants, dyes, pharmaceutical agents, agricultural chemicals, glues, and paints. Benzene is a component of gasoline. Benzene concentrations in gasoline are generally less than 2% by volume in the United States, but in other countries the concentration may be as high as 5% (66).

BENZENE EXPOSURE SOURCES

Occupational exposures to benzene occur in the rubber industry, oil refining, chemical plants, shoe manufacturing, gasoline storage facilities and gasoline service stations. Benzene is ubiquitous in the environment and is found in ambient air, indoor air, water, and human blood samples (67) (see Chapter 28).

Blood concentration of benzene in occupational settings has been studied. The mean occupational benzene exposure for 167 workers studied was 186 ng per L (58 ppb). The range was from 5 to 1,535 ng per L. The mean blood benzene level in all of these workers was 420 ng per L at the end of the shift, and 287 ng per L the next morning following the shift (67). The mean blood level of 243 control subjects was 165 ng per L, indicating the ubiquitous environmental presence of benzene. Mean blood benzene concentrations were significantly higher in smokers than in nonsmokers, as compared to both the general population and in the exposed workers.

Nonsmoking workers occupationally exposed to benzene at environmental levels lower than 100 ng per L and the nonsmoking general population exposed to environmental benzene have similar blood benzene concentrations (67). The comparison between environmental and blood benzene concentrations in nonsmoking workers demonstrated that the benzene level was higher in blood (584 ng per L) than in the atmosphere of the workplace (186 ng per L) with the blood environment ratio being about 3 to 1 (584/186) (67). Also, the benzene level in venous blood was lower than in arterial blood.

Smoking substantially increases blood benzene concentrations. The daily intake of benzenes from a single cigarette varies from 5.9 to 73 μg (68). Nonsmokers who live with smokers have a 30% to 50% higher benzene level in the breath than do the nonsmokers who do not live with a smoker.

The environmental levels of the air benzene concentrations found in various locations are listed in Table 59-1. Benzene environmental contamination is detected in surface waters in the United States and has been found at a median concentration of 5 ppb. Benzene is also found in ocean water at 5 to 40 ppt (parts per trillion) and contaminated coastal water at 50 to 175 ppt (69,70).

Benzene exposure can also occur via ingestion of contaminated food products, but food intake is estimated at less than 1% of the average daily benzene intake of the general population (71).

In the air of urban areas, it is believed that close to 85% of the benzene emissions originate from automobiles. Individuals are exposed to benzene both inside of an automobile while driving and

TABLE 59-1. Benzene air concentrations

Indoor	1.8 ppb
Gas station	<1.0–3.2 ppb
Urban air	4–160 ppb
Rural air	0.16–3.50 ppb
Chemical plant	14 ppb
Refinery	9 ppb

Note: See Chapter 28 for additional data.
Adapted from Gist G, Burg J. Benzene—A review of the literature from a health effects perspective. *Toxicol Ind Health* 1997;13(6):661–713.

outside in the ambient air. Studies have shown that benzene concentrations inside of an automobile vary depending on the driving conditions and the density of traffic. Moving from a parking lot into normal traffic on an urban roadway increased the indoor benzene concentration from 17 to 62.3 μg per m^3 (72). Variables that affected the benzene concentration inside of an automobile included interior smoking and the presence of a catalytic converter. Benzene concentrations were much higher in automobiles without catalytic converters. With inside smoking, the benzene concentration rose from 28.2 to 91 μg per m^3. Also, toluene was present and its airborne concentration rose from 86.2 to 279.4 μg per m^3.

It is important to note that the indoor air of a vehicle contains both benzene and toluene concentrations derived from smoking and from the use of gasoline. In one automobile study, the indoor benzene and toluene concentrations were assayed in an urban parking lot with no traffic in an automobile with a catalytic converter, and then with an automobile without the catalytic converter. The indoor vehicle concentration levels of benzene in the first experiment increased from 15.2 to 174 μg per m^3, and from 97.7 to 560 μg per m^3 for toluene. In the second experiment, benzene increased from 19 to 386 μg per m^3 and toluene rose from 102 to 1,0148 μg per m^3.

Benzene regulatory limits are as follows:

- U.S. Occupational Safety and Health Administration permissible exposure limit = 1 ppm
  Short-term exposure limit (STEL) (15 min) = 5 ppm
- American Conference of Governmental Industrial Hygienists threshold limit value = 0.5 ppm
  STEL (15 min) = 2.5 ppm
- National Institute for Occupational Safety and Health recommended exposure limit = 0.1 ppm
  STEL = 1 ppm
- Immediately dangerous to life and health = 500 ppm

ABSORPTION, METABOLISM, AND EXCRETION OF BENZENE

Benzene is absorbed from respiratory, gastrointestinal, and dermal routes. Respiratory uptake varies from 47% to 80% (66), and dermal absorption has been estimated to range from 0.05% to 0.2% (73).

To exert its hemotoxic effects, benzene must be metabolized (74,75). The metabolism of benzene is shown in Figure 59-2.

Benzene is metabolized via a series of oxidation steps involving the benzene ring by the cytochrome P-450 monooxygenase enzyme system. Several metabolic steps are required to produce the toxic metabolites. The major benzene metabolite produced by the liver P-450 enzyme system is phenol. Phenol is then further oxidized by the P-450 enzyme system to hydroquinone. Both hydroquinone and phenol can be conjugated in the liver to nontoxic products, or can diffuse into bone marrow. Once in bone marrow, phenol and hydroquinone can be acted upon by the myeloperoxidase-dependent enzyme system, which metabolizes hydroquinone to a reactive benzoquinone, stimulated by the presence of phenol (Fig. 59-3). Benzoquinone has been shown to be both myelotoxic and clastogenic.

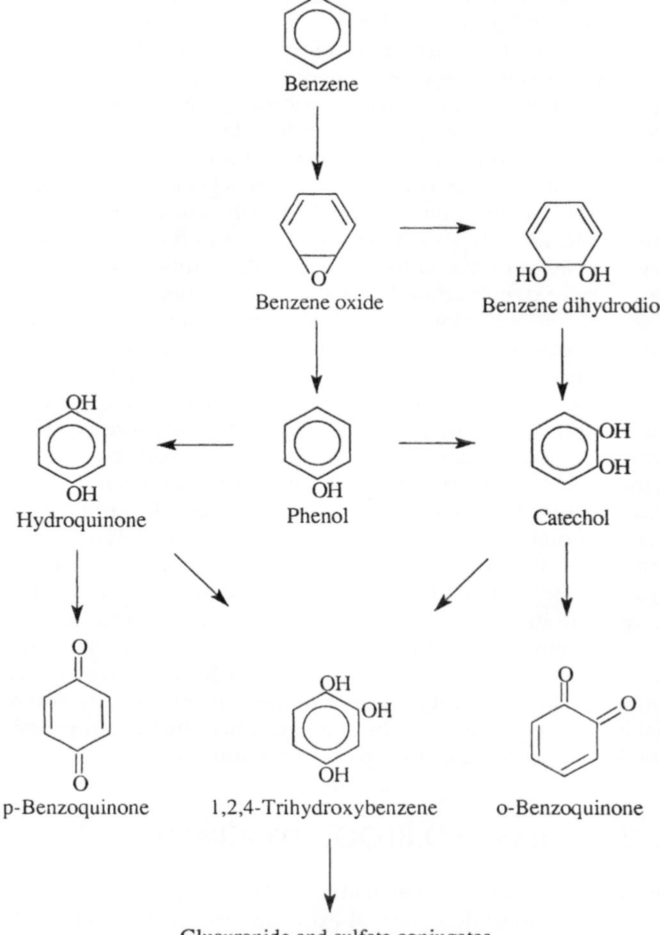

Figure 59-2. Benzene metabolism.

The major metabolites of benzene metabolism are phenol, hydroquinone, and catechol. These metabolites are interactive and can affect the rate of each other's metabolism because they are substrates for the P-450 enzyme system. The route of exposure has little effect on the subsequent metabolism of benzene to hemotoxic metabolites.

Both ethanol and toluene alter benzene metabolism (76–78). Workers exposed to a combination of benzene and toluene produce a significantly lower urinary phenol excretion than those exposed to either benzene or toluene alone (77). Toluene decreases the toxicity of benzene in animals and interferes with benzene metabolism in humans. Studies of benzene-exposed workers show that the formation of phenol and quinol, but not catechol, is suppressed when the individual is also expressed to toluene. Conversely, formation of hippuric acid and *o*-cresol from toluene is reduced by coexposure to benzene (77).

In animal models, the coexposure of benzene and toluene reduces the extent of DNA damage by 50%, compared to benzene alone (78). Thus, there appears to be a protective effect of toluene on the hematotoxicity and genotoxicity of benzene.

The multiple metabolic pathways for benzene provide opportunities for modulating its metabolism and myelotoxicity. Animal studies indicate that the metabolites of benzene are related to the dose, and that the profile of the urinary metabolites can serve as an indicator of the amount of benzene flowing through metabolic

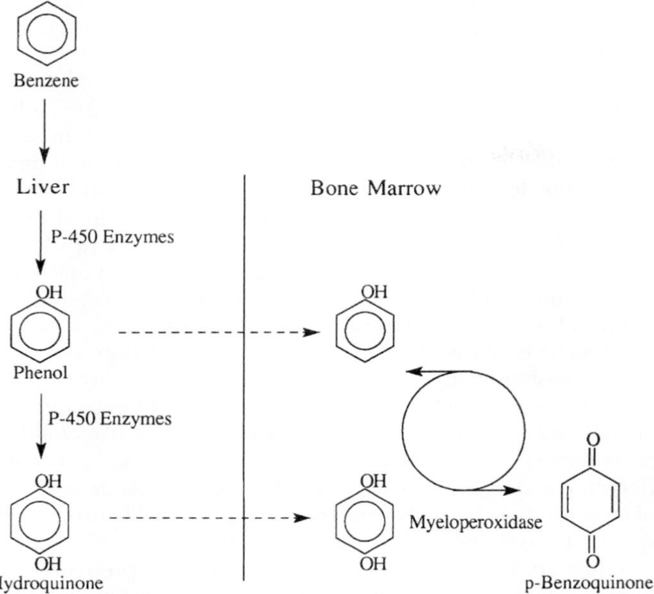

Figure 59-3. Benzene-induced myelotoxicity.

pathways. Due to the interactive effects of benzene with its metabolites at high exposure concentrations, the parent compound benzene may inhibit metabolism of phenol to hydroquinone (75).

Animal studies indicate that there is a competitive inhibition among benzene and its metabolites, with a decrease in total hydroquinone conjugates and an increase in phenol conjugates formed with exposure to increasing doses of benzene. The phenol metabolite seems to be a pivotal metabolite in the metabolism of benzene because it can undergo oxidation to hydroquinone and also be conjugated by glucuronyl transferases and sulfur transferases. If the phenol metabolite has a greater opportunity for conjugation compared with oxidation, benzene toxicity may be reduced. Thus, if the metabolic milieu has a greater abundance of conjugating enzymes compared to oxidative enzymes, the toxicity of benzene can be reduced.

Because no single benzene metabolite reproduces the myelotoxic and hematotoxic effects of exposure to benzene, the mechanisms of toxicity remain somewhat speculative. Studies have shown that myeloperoxidase in bone marrow cells metabolizes hydroquinone to 1,4-benzoquinone. Benzoquinone is a highly reactive compound with hemotoxic effects (Table 59-2). The conversion of hydroquinone to 1,3-benzoquinone involving a 2-electron oxidation process dependent upon the presence of myeloperoxidase and hydrogen peroxide. Also, this metabolism is stimulated by the presence of phenol (79). The concentration of phenol has to be higher than that of the hydroquinone for this stimulation to occur, but the myeloperoxidase-dependent hydroquinone metabolism occurs when the phenol to hydroquinone ratio was as low as 1.3 (75). When the ratio rose above 10, the metabolism was much more significant.

It has been speculated that the mechanism by which phenol stimulates the oxidation of hydroquinone involves the enzymatic oxidation of phenol to a phenoxy radical, which then oxidizes the hydroquinone to a semiquinone radical. The oxidation of hydroquinone to a semiquinone is a rate-limiting step in the oxidation of hydroquinone to benzoquinone.

BIOLOGICAL MONITORING OF BENZENE

The common biological marker for benzene exposure is based on the measurement of urinary phenol. However, studies have shown that urinary phenol as a biomarker may be unreliable for low-level benzene exposure less than 5 ppm (80). Other biological markers include urinary hydroquinone and unmetabolized benzene both in urine and blood. *S*-phenylmercapturic acid was shown to be a specific and sensitive biomarker, but gas chromatography-mass spectrometry is required (81). Other studies have shown that trans, trans-muconic acid was a useful biological marker for benzene exposure between 1 and 68 ppm (82). Another study demonstrated that trans, trans-muconic acid appeared to be the most reliable of the benzene metabolites to employ for low-level benzene exposure monitoring between 0.25 and 3.5 ppm (83).

TABLE 59-2. 1,4-Benzoquinone toxicity

Binds to DNA
Interferes with microtubule assembly
Inhibits RNA and DNA synthesis
Causes single-stranded DNA breaks
Causes SCE in human lymphocytes
Causes chromosomal fragmentation during all division
Inhibits cell division
Interferes with stromal cell growth in bone marrow
Interferes with lymphocyte blastogenesis

SCE, sister chromatid exchange.
Adapted from ref. 75.

BENZENE TOXICITY

Benzene has been recognized as a hematotoxin for more than 100 years. High benzene exposure has been known to cause aplastic anemia, bone marrow suppression and pancytopenia in animal models. Benzene is associated with immunological effects, causes damage to bone marrow stem cells, and DNA damage to human lymphocytes. Epidemiological studies have demonstrated an increased risk of leukemia, aplastic anemia, and other hematological abnormalities in populations occupationally exposed to benzene. The most common form of benzene hematotoxicity is depression of hematopoietic cells both in the peripheral blood and in the bone marrow. All cell linages erythroid, myeloid and lymphoid are susceptible to the toxic effects of benzene. The lymphoid line of cells is the most sensitive.

IMMUNOTOXIC EFFECTS OF BENZENE

Benzene- and benzene metabolite–induced alterations in cellular and humoral immunity have been demonstrated in animal studies. The effects of benzene inhalation on T- and B lymphocytes and immune responses in mice were studied with exposures to 50 ppm or 200 ppm benzene vapor for six hours a day for 7 or 14 consecutive dates. The ratio and absolute number of T- and B lymphocytes in the blood and spleen were decreased after a 7-day exposure at 50 ppm benzene. The B-lymphocyte depression was shown to be dose dependent and exceeded that of the T-lymphocyte depression. Also, the ability to form antibodies was suppressed at all benzene exposure concentrations. However, the cell-mediated immune response measured by contact sensitivity was actually enhanced (84).

Benzene and its five metabolites, muconic acid, hydroquinone, catechol, *p*-benzoquinone and benzenetriol, have been shown to produce DNA damage in human lymphocytes (85). Other studies in humans have examined the effects of benzene exposure on the generation of interleukin-1 (IL-1). In one study using controls, a population of mechanics was exposed to low level of benzenes from fuels. Their exposure was assessed by measurements of workplace ambient air benzene concentration and urinary benzene metabolites. The level of exposure of these mechanics to the benzene from the fuels was below 1 ppm. IL-1α

production was not decreased in mechanics exposed to benzene from fuels and no correlation between IL-1α concentrations and red blood cell counts were found (86). This study used the generation of IL-1α as a sensitive biomarker for benzene-induced aplastic anemia. It had been hypothesized that benzene inhibited the cleavage of the precursor to IL-1α and that the lack of mature IL-1α is responsible for benzene-induced bone marrow suppression. Bone marrow macrophages also play a potential role in the pathological process, and are an important source of IL-1. Macrophages are also sensitive to the toxic effects of benzene metabolites. Although in this study, vehicle mechanics had been exposed to benzene more often than the control subjects, their IL-1α production was the same as that of control subjects.

Because bone marrow macrophage dysfunction and deficient IL-1 production have been reported for patients with aplastic anemia, other studies examined whether or not benzene exposures involved interference in development of IL-1. Hydroquinone has been known to prevent the proteolytic conversion of pre–IL-1α to the mature cytokine by calpain (87). This study supported observations in the mouse model that benzene-induced bone marrow cell depression results from a lack of IL-1α caused by inhibition of calpain by benzoquinone, the protease required for converting pre–IL-1α to its active cytokine. Thus, hydroquinone, due to its oxidation in the macrophage to benzoquinone, can inhibit the proteases involved in converting pre–IL-1α and pre–IL-1α to mature biologically active cytokines in the mouse model (87).

Other studies have shown effects of benzene and quinone metabolites on RNA synthesis, in lymphocytes and on the production of IL-2 (88). The effect on lymphocytes exposed to benzene is a dose-dependent inhibition of RNA synthesis. Also, exposure of lymphocytes to benzene metabolites hydroquinone or *p*-benzoquinone results in a dose-dependent inhibition of RNA synthesis in lymphocytes.

Human studies of the effects of benzene on phytohemagglutinin (PHA) stimulation of lymphocytes have been performed. In this study, 66 male workers in a refinery were compared to 33 controlled workers in the same refinery not known to be exposed to benzene. Lymphocyte responsiveness to phytohemagglutinin, a measure of lymphocyte blastogenesis, was studied and the results showed there was no difference between the exposed group and the control group (89).

Other studies, involving gasoline pump mechanics compared to 15 controls, were investigated with lymphocyte micronucleus assays in differential leukocyte counts of the peripheral blood smear. Stimulation of lymphocytes in the study was by phytohemagglutinin and pokeweed mitogen. The exposed pump mechanics had increased frequencies in sizes of micronuclei in the pokeweed mitogen–stimulated lymphocyte cultures but not in those stimulated with phytohemagglutinin. Also, the studies showed that the leukocyte count was significantly higher in the gasoline-exposed group. Exposure was a time-weighted average of 1 mg per m^3 of benzene with peak levels of 20 mg per m^3 (90).

Other studies have examined the effects of benzene and its metabolites on macrophage function and the ability of macrophage to be activated for host defense (91). In one study, benzene had no effect on macrophage function or activation. However, the metabolites of benzene, catechol, hydroquinone, benzoquinone, and benzenetriol had effects on macrophage function and activation. Benzoquinone inhibited a broad range of macrophage functions including release of hydrogen peroxide, FC-receptor–mediated phagocytosis, interferon-α (IFN-α) priming for tumor cytolysis, and bacterial lipopolysaccharide (LPS) triggering of cytolysis (91). Hydroquinone inhibited hydrogen peroxide release in priming for cytolysis and benzenetriol inhibited phagocytosis and cytolytic priming. Catechol inhibited the release of hydrogen peroxide from macrophages. The results suggest that benzene metabolites alter macrophage function through various mechanisms.

Studies have shown that benzene increases susceptibility of mice to *Listeria monocytogenes* and tumor graphs (92,93). Studies have also sought to determine the concentrations of inhaled benzene that interfere with immune responses in animal models. Results demonstrated that short-term inhalation of benzene (6 days' exposure to 10 ppm and 6 days' exposure to 31 ppm) produced immune depressant effects (94). Exposure to 10 ppm of benzene resulted in a significant depression of lipopolysaccharide-induced B-cell stimulation. Also, phytohemagglutinin-induced blastogenesis was depressed at 31 ppm.

Benzene is an established leukemogen and has been shown to induce chromosomal damage in human lymphocytes. *In vitro* studies with benzene metabolites, hydroquinone, 1,4-benzoquinone, phenol, and catechol resulted in significant increases in micronuclei formation. Hydroquinone resulted in a larger increase in micronuclei compared to phenol, catechol, and 1,4-benzoquinone treatment of *in vitro* human lymphocytes. Thus, it appears that hydroquinone may be a major contributor to clastogenicity (95).

Other studies have shown inhibition of IFN-γ production by benzene and benzene metabolites (96). Exposure to benzene or its metabolites can alter lymphocyte subpopulations, inhibit IL-2 synthesis, depress mitogen-stimulated blastogenesis of B lymphocytes and T lymphocytes, and affect maturation of lymphopoietic cells. IFN-γ enhances B-cell maturation, augments histocompatibility antigen expression, activates natural killer cells, and induces differentiation of cell types. Studies show that dihydroxy and diketo metabolites of benzene inhibited IFN-γ production. However, benzene and phenol had no inhibitory effect on IFN-γ production at the concentrations tested. A dose-dependent inhibition of IFN-γ production was seen following exposure of spleen cells to hydroquinone and *p*-benzoquinone. Other studies have shown that hydroquinone inhibits bone marrow pre–B-cell maturation (97). Other results have shown that short-term exposure to hydroquinone blocks maturation stages of B-cell differentiation in the bone marrow.

The effect of hydroquinone on IL-1 secretion by human monocytes *in vitro* has also been studied (98). This exposure of human monocytes to micromolar concentrations of hydroquinone for 2 hours resulted in a dose-dependent reduction of IL-1 secretion. Hydroquinone also inhibited RNA and protein synthesis in a dose-dependent manner. The study concluded that hydroquinone contributes to myelotoxicity of benzene in humans by inhibiting the production of cytokines involved in the regulation of hematopoiesis by mononuclear phagocytes.

Other studies have shown that hydroquinone prevents conversion of pre–IL-1α to the cytokine in bone marrow stromal macrophages. In animal studies, stromal macrophages exposed to benzene for 2 days were incapable of processing the pre–IL-1α to the mature cytokine when stimulated in culture with lipopolysaccharide (99). Other studies have examined decreases in calpain content in bone marrow–derived macrophages as a mechanism underlying hydroquinone-induced decreases in pre–IL-1α conversion. Hydroquinone, at concentrations not cytotoxic, decreased the total calpain activity of macrophages between 14% and 30%. Calpain-2 levels were decreased by 50% after treatment with hydroquinone. Thus, decreased calpain-2 may represent a potential mechanism of hydroquinone-induced inhibition of pre–IL-1α processing (100).

BENZENE AND LEUKEMIAS

On the basis of scientific evidence, benzene remains the only major industrial chemical for which a clear causal relationship with leukemia, specifically AML, has been established. Nevertheless, a number of agents have been reported to produce anemia, cytopenias, leukemia, or lymphoma for which the quality and quantity of supporting evidence vary widely. Among these are lead, arsenic, radium, ethylene oxide, pesticides (e.g., chlordane, heptachlor, and the phenoxy herbicides), ethylene glycol, trinitrotoluene (TNT), and 1,3-butadiene. For most of these chemicals the results of different studies are contradictory, and many suffer from weak methodology and inadequate statistical power. In this context, it appears that generalizations about the hematotoxicity of classes of compounds may be imprudent in the absence of more reliable information.

An important consideration in study design is that the actual number of affected individuals is quite small. The gloomy predictions of previous risk assessments notwithstanding, the actual demonstrated incidence of leukemia and blood dyscrasias does not represent a large proportion of the individuals exposed even in populations chronically exposed to a known human leukemogen, benzene. Wong recently analyzed the risks of developing AML in workers exposed to benzene (101). He reported relative risks on the order of 100 for individuals exposed to extremely high concentrations (400 ppm per year) but no significant excess risks were observed below 200 ppm per year. These results are actually consistent with those previously reported by Rinsky et al., who reported a statistically significant excess in leukemia above 200 ppm per year (102). For virtually all other occupational or environmental agents, the evidence for leukemogenesis remains questionable.

The hypothesis that benzene exposure is associated with the development of multiple myeloma (MM) has been a frequent theme in the occupational literature (103). Nevertheless, aside from the frequency with which benzene has been hypothesized to cause multiple myeloma, the associations are weak, studies inconsistent, and a causal relationship has not been convincingly demonstrated. Both positive (52,104,105) and negative associations (51,55,58,106,107) have been reported between exposure to benzene and/or employment in the petroleum industry and an increased risk of multiple myeloma, although the majority of studies have observed either very weak (56,109–111) or no association (54,57,101,111–115). Rinsky et al. reported four cases of multiple myeloma versus 1.4 expected in a benzene-exposed pliofilm cohort (102). However, more recent follow-up studies of the same cohort have reported no significance between benzene exposure and an increased risk of developing multiple myeloma in the face of an increasing risk for AML (101,115).

OTHER HEMATOTOXINS

Lead

The changing patterns of lead (Pb) use in society have modulated the prevailing forms of Pb toxicity encountered in modern times. Lead poisoning was one of the most predominant hazards of past centuries; it has even been suggested to have contributed to the fall of the Roman Empire (116). Cases of moderate to severe Pb poisoning in which anemia is present have declined dramatically in recent years. However, chronic Pb poisoning as an occupational hazard is far from extinct. Painters exposed to Pb-contaminated dust pose a particular problem. The most significant effects of chronic Pb poisoning are those involving the central nervous system (CNS). For example, organic lead compounds, such as tetraethyl- and tetramethyl lead, which have been widely employed as gasoline additives, are potent neurotoxins. Anemia, which can be clinically significant as well, is usually a late manifestation of chronic Pb intoxication and is moderate unless there is a severe hemolytic component. In both experimental and clinical experience, hematological abnormalities associated with Pb toxicity are confined to the erythrocytes. Lead-induced anemia is brought about by two major mechanisms: interference with erythropoiesis by the inhibition of heme synthetase and δ-amino-levulinic acid (ALD) dehydrase, and direct binding of Pb to the erythrocyte membrane resulting in increased fragility. In many cases, the latter can be documented only with great difficulty. Pb is distinguished by its ability to produce selective suppression of erythropoiesis while generally sparing other cell lineages. In the bone marrow, there is a marked maturation arrest in erythropoiesis, accompanied by an increase in the number of erythroblasts. Polychromatophilic erythroblasts often exhibit basophilic stippling, which usually can be demonstrated in bone marrow cells even when not present in circulating erythrocytes. From a clinical point of view, it should be appreciated that basophilic stippling can be a prominent feature but is not as specific or sensitive for Pb poisoning as once thought, and, in fact, is uncommon in workers exposed to the current permissible exposure limit (PEL) (50 μg per m^3). The anemia associated with Pb poisoning can be moderately severe but is usually mild in industrial poisoning cases. Erythrocytes may be hypochromic, and there is usually a moderate reticulocytosis. A decrease in Fe utilization can usually be demonstrated. Elevations in bone marrow or erythrocyte porphyrin levels may occur early as a result of Pb toxicity to mitochondria, although their rise in urine usually is not an early indicator of Pb intoxication. Historically, urinary ALD output has been employed as a diagnostic indicator in cases of suspected Pb poisoning (117); however, today blood Pb measurements are used almost exclusively. The marginal evidence suggesting that Pb might be a human carcinogen has been the subject of debate (118–120). However, there is no indication that exposure to Pb is associated with hematopoietic or lymphoid malignancies.

Arsenic

Acute arsenic (As) poisoning is rarely occupational in origin and usually occurs via food or drink (121). Megaloblastic disturbances in hematopoiesis have been reported in acute arsenic poisoning, which may be accompanied by a marked reduction in leukocyte count (122). However, it would appear that hematopoietic toxicity is a relatively minor aspect of the multiple toxic effects of this metal. In cases of acute poisoning, elevations of As can be found in urine, which is the main route of excretion. It should be kept in mind that urinary excretion of As is rapid and the half-life of the metal in blood extremely short (~1 to 3 days). Arsenic determination in hair can be a useful quantitative parameter when exposure is thought to have occurred. Urine concentrations correlate better with chronic exposure.

Increased mortality in workers occupationally exposed to arsenicals has been reported due to leukemia (unclassified) in one study (123) and to lymphoma and Hodgkin's disease—but *not* leukemia—in another (124). Taken together, these observations are by no means conclusive because the study results are inconsistent, the number of cases in each study is exceptionally small, and the likelihood of confounding exposures is great in both.

Radium

Occupational exposure to radium (Ra) no longer poses a significant health hazard, but Ra poisoning in the dial-painting industry during the first quarter of this century represents a classic but tragic episode in the history of occupational medicine. A landmark retrospective study of 634 women employed in this industry between 1915 and 1929 was reported by Polednak et al. (125). The affected population comprised virtually all women who were employed in the Ra dial industry prior to 1930. The major source of exposure was ingestion of Ra paint by workers who would lick the brushes used to paint luminous watch dials in order to maintain a fine point on the brush. Some inhalation of radon daughters and Ra dust is thought to have occurred as well. Depending on the age at first exposure, mortality ratios associated with "bone cancer" ranged between 81 and 250, reflecting the bone-seeking nature of ^{226}Ra. Excess deaths due to leukemia and "diseases of the blood and blood-forming organs" were also noted, with mortality ratios of 2.13 and 3.91 observed for each, respectively. Although the number of leukemias is small (i.e., 3), the pattern of ^{226}Ra deposition and the marked increase in bone-related cancers, together with reports of aplastic anemia, anemia, and leukopenia in earlier studies of Ra workers (126–129), suggest that a causal relationship may exist.

Ethylene Oxide

Ethylene oxide is a direct-acting epoxide and alkylating agent employed as an intermediate in chemical manufacture and used extensively as a gaseous sterilization agent. Exposures to ethylene oxide are most likely to occur in a hospital setting during the loading and unloading of sterilization chambers and the offgassing of recently sterilized items. Ethylene oxide is clearly a biologically reactive agent, with chronic exposure associated with mutagenic and cytogenetic effects in humans and experimental animals (130). Even so, evidence in support of ethylene oxide as a human leukemogen is extremely limited.

In 1979 Hogstedt and coworkers reported two cases of leukemia and one lymphoma among a small group of Swedish workers exposed to ethylene oxide and potentially exposed to a variety of other agents as well (131,132). Similarly, Theiss et al. reported a nonsignificant excess of deaths due to leukemia (i.e., 2 observed versus 1.1 expected) in potentially exposed workers (133). These results are contrasted by those of Morgan et al., who found no leukemia deaths among 767 workers with potential exposure to ethylene oxide (134). As noted by Austin and Sielkin, limitations inherent in all of these studies include inconsistent results, small cohort sizes, small numbers of observed and expected events, and inadequate quantitative exposure data (130).

Glycol Ethers

The glycol ethers are a class of compounds that are used extensively in industry as solvents in the manufacture of varnishes, latex paints, dyes, inks, and antifreeze compounds. They are generally regarded as being of low toxicity. Previous case reports have suggested that glycol ethers may be hematotoxic to humans. In a cross-sectional survey of employees involved in glycol ether manufacture, no differences in hematological parameters were observed between an exposed versus a control population (135). More recently, Welch and Cullen studied the effect of exposure to glycol ethers on shipyard painters (136). No significant differences in the means of hematologic variables were noted between exposed and nonexposed groups, and no correlation with cumulative exposure was established. However, a small proportion of the exposed group presented as anemic and granulocytopenic according to the criteria used in the study. In another study, motivated by the referral of a printer with aplastic anemia, Cullen et al. examined bone marrow injury in a small group of lithographers exposed to glycol ethers (137). Peripheral blood counts, including differential and platelet counts, were normal; yet bone marrow biopsies revealed various abnormalities including myeloid hypoplasia, stromal cell injury, and sideroblastosis in three of seven exposed workers. The lack of consistency between the results of these studies, together with the small number of exposed workers examined, provides an inadequate base upon which to draw any sweeping conclusions. While there is insufficient evidence to conclude that exposure to glycol ethers results in blood or bone marrow toxicity, common sense dictates that exposure to these agents should be minimized.

Trinitrotoluene

Occupational exposure to trinitrotoluene (TNT) was historically associated with the munitions industry, and hematotoxicity resulting from wartime exposure to TNT has previously been reviewed by Scott et al. (138). The major route of exposure was via the skin and occurred during the hand loading of artillery shells. Although aplastic anemia has been reported as a consequence of TNT exposure, dermatitis, gastritis, toxic hepatitis, hemolytic anemia, and methemoglobinemia are all more common in cases of TNT poisoning.

Aromatic Solvents

An occasional misstatement in the secondary literature notwithstanding, benzene is the only primary aromatic solvent with hematotoxic properties. Neither the clinical nor the experimental literature will support an association between the alkylbenzenes, toluene, or xylenes and blood dyscrasias or leukemia. The explanation for such marked differences in the hematotoxicity of benzene and substituted benzenes is almost certainly related to major differences in the metabolism and bioactivation of these compounds. It is well established in experimental models that toluene, when present in relatively high concentrations, will actually protect against benzene-induced bone marrow toxicity by competing for primary metabolism.

1,3-Butadiene

1,3-Butadiene (BD) is a colorless gas that is used in the production of styrene-butadiene or polybutadiene rubber. Styrene-butadiene rubber was introduced as a substitute for natural rubber during WWII and has subsequently become a mainstay of the rubber industry. Early studies in experimental animals and in humans indicated very little acute or cumulative toxicity associated with exposure to BD. Subsequently, several epidemiology studies have examined the potential relationship between occupational exposure to BD and cancer, but to date the results have proved to be inconsistent and contradictory. These studies show no consistent pattern with respect to either the duration of exposure or disease and in the aggregate fail to demonstrate an increase in hemopoietic neoplasms in butadiene-exposed workers. The first such study of synthetic rubber workers suggested that the incidence of leukemia was marginally increased in one of two plants, but only in workers with short-term exposure, not long-term exposure (139). Another study of butadiene monomer workers revealed an increase in NHL but *not* leukemia, again only in short-term workers (140). One possible explanation is that this study is confounded by the previous employment histories of the study population. Still, a third study of SBR workers found a deficit in lymphopoietic cancers compared with that expected in the total cohort and no increase in leukemia, but an increase in leukemia in a case-control study within the same cohort (141–143). At present, the contradiction between these two studies remains unexplained, although methodologic considerations are likely to play an important role. In the case-control study, the exposure status of cases was characterized as either "never exposed" or "ever exposed" to butadiene. Subsequent analysis has suggested that the statistical significance of the findings would disappear upon reassignment of exposure status for only one case (143).

The most recent study of SBR workers, representing the largest evaluation of BD-exposed workers to date is that of Delzell et al. (144). Relative risks of developing leukemia of unspecified type ranged between 2 and 3, while no other increases in cancer were observed related to employment in the SBR industry. Excess mortality was primarily associated with laboratory and SBR maintenance workers. Several characteristics of this study raise the possibility that confounding exposures in SBR production may play a role in the observed results. These include the relatively low risk, the absence of any leukemia cases encountered in workers exposed to BD monomer alone, and the lack of any apparent dose-response relationship.

Studies of BD toxicity and carcinogenicity in experimental animals suggest that there are marked species differences in susceptibility to BD (145–148). Many strains of laboratory mouse are uniquely susceptible to the development of T-cell lymphoma/leukemia (TL), either spontaneously or as a result of chemical or radiation exposure. In contrast, T-cell leukemias or lymphomas are relatively uncommon in humans or rats, are not easily induced by radiation, and are not generally associated with chemotherapy of chemical exposure. Rats are relatively resistant to BD toxicity. The compound has proven to be carcinogenic in that species only at high exposure concentrations, and there is no evidence of hematotoxicity in rats exposed to the chemical. On the other hand, subacute exposure to BD in mice results in a megaloblastic anemia, and chronic exposure results in an increased incidence of a variety of neoplasms, most spectacularly a 60% incidence of lymphatic leukemia.

The sensitivity of the mouse to the development of TL appears to correlate with the susceptibility of an early hematopoietic progenitor cell is not found in human bone marrow, and that appears to be more important in explaining differences in susceptibility to TL than more modest species differences in the tissue-specific metabolism of xenobiotics (149,150). This cell is uniquely susceptible to functional suppression by murine leukemogens, such as radiation, 1,3-butadiene, and the AIDS drug, ddC. As a result, murine TL does not appear to be an appropriate biological model for hazard identification in humans.

Chlordane and Heptachlor

In recent years, the pesticide field has been plagued with an abundant but confusing literature that is confounded by exposure to multiple agents and replete with contradiction. Many of the apparent contradictions between studies may be explained by differences in the identification of chemicals involved, measures of exposure employed, and the size of the cohorts examined.

Chlordane and heptachlor have received a great deal of attention because of their wide use as insecticides. Nevertheless, human studies are contradictory and fail to support a consistent association between these two agents and toxicity to the blood and bone marrow. The evidence suggesting that chlordane and heptachlor produce blood dyscrasias and leukemia is largely derived from a small number of case reports of aplastic and hypoplastic anemia for which the association of disease with exposure to these agents appears tenuous, together with a collection of cases assembled from the "nonscientific literature" (e.g., litigation records) (39,151). These cases are taken from anecdotal sources (152). These are contrasted by quantitative epidemiology studies, both prospective and retrospective, as well as a case-control study of 60 cases of aplastic anemia (153) that have not found an increased incidence of leukemias or aplastic anemia in workers engaged in the production or application of these two chemicals (154–156). At the present time, it appears reasonable to conclude that, both on the basis of the experimental and human literature, an association between chlordane or heptachlor and hematotoxicity amounts to not much more than a hypothesis.

Phenoxy Herbicides

The chlorophenoxy herbicides are an important class of compounds, the principal examples of which are 2,4-dichlorophenoxyacetic acid (2,4-D), 2,4,5-trichlorophenoxyacetic acid (2,4,5-T), and 4-chloro-2-methylphenoxyacetic acid (MCPA). These compounds are among the most widely used herbicides in agriculture and first received wide notoriety in the 1960s as a result of the use of Agent Orange (a mixture of chlorophenoxy compounds) as a defoliant in the Vietnam War. An emotional controversy has surrounded the contamination of Agent Orange, as well as commercial preparations of some of these herbicides, with chlorinated dibenzodioxins, most significantly 2,3,7,8-tetrachlorodibenzo-*p*-dioxin (TCDD). A number of reviews have attempted to summarize the evidence concerning the potential leukemogenicity of the phenoxy herbicides. However, these have served only to highlight the difficulties in evaluating a group or class of compounds for which individual representatives and/or their potential contaminants may have differing toxic profiles (157).

Following the first report by Hardell and Sandstrom in 1979, a number of case-control and retrospective cohort studies have attempted to examine the potential relationship between exposure to phenoxy herbicides and non-Hodgkin's lymphoma (NHL) (158). The majority of studies have evaluated exposure to the phenoxyacetic acid herbicides as a group with largely inconsistent and contradictory results. Hardell et al. reported an increased risk of both Hodgkin's and non-Hodgkin's lymphoma for the phenoxy herbicides, although no difference in risk was observed between those individuals exposed to products likely to contain TCDD as a contaminant and those not likely to contain TCDD (159). Woods et al. found a small increase in the risk of NHL among farmers but not in other occupations potentially exposed to 2,4-D (160). These studies were contrasted by the results of Pearce who found no increase in NHL among New Zealand workers exposed to 2,4,5-T (161). A relatively large number of retrospective cohort studies of workers exposed to phenoxy herbicides have been reported over the last decade, which, when taken together, suggest no increase in NHL (157). However, two recent case-control studies of farmers in Kansas (162) and Nebraska (163) reveal a pattern that suggests that the use of 2,4-D in an agricultural setting increases the risk of NHL among persons frequently handling the chemical. These studies included histopathological review of all cases. The Nebraska study further suggests that the risk of NHL increases with the degree of exposure to 2,4-D, as indicated by the application method and time spent in contaminated clothing, but not with the number of years of use. The small numbers of subjects in these studies is a limiting factor in evaluating the independent risks of 2,4-D, organophosphate insecticides, and fungicides, all of which are in common use in the farming industry.

REFERENCES

1. Vogelstein B, Fearon ER, Hamilton SR, et al. Genetic alterations during colorectal-tumor development. *N Engl J Med* 1988;319:525–532.
2. Varmus H, Weinberg RA. *Genes and the biology of cancer.* New York: Scientific American Library, 1993.
3. Jandl JH. *Blood: textbook of hematology.* Boston: Little, Brown and Company, 1987:1–1214.
4. Alderson M. The epidemiology of leukemia. *Adv Cancer Res* 1980;31:1–76.
5. Karchmer RK, Amare M, Larsen WE. Alkylating agents as leukemogens in multiple myeloma. *Cancer* 1974;33:1103–1107.
6. Canellos GP, Arseneau JC, DeVita VT. Second malignancies complicating Hodgkin's disease in remission. *Lancet* 1975;1:947–949.
7. Catovsky D, Galton DA. Myelomonocytic leukemia supervening on chronic lymphocytic leukemia. *Lancet* 1971;1:478–479.
8. Pedersen-Bjergaard J, Nissen NI, Sorensen HM, et al. Acute non-lymphocytic leukemia in patients with ovarian carcinoma following long-term treatment with treosulfan (=dihydroxybusulfan). *Cancer* 1980;45:19–29.

9. Greene MH, Harris EL, Gershenson DM, et al. Melphalan may be a more potent leukemogen than cyclophosphamide. *Ann Intern Med* 1986;105:360–367.
10. Rosner F, Grunwald HW. Hodgkin's disease and acute leukemia: report of eight cases and review of the literature. *Am J Med* 1975;58:339–353.
11. Bennett JM, Catovsky D, Daniel MT, et al. Proposed revised criteria for the classification of acute myeloid leukemia. *Ann Intern Med* 1985;103:626–629.
12. Levine EG, Bloomfield CD. Leukemias and myelodysplastic syndromes secondary to drug, radiation, and environmental exposure. *Semin Oncol* 1992;19:47–84.
13. Grunwald HW, Rosner F. Acute leukemia and immunosuppressive drug use: a review of patients undergoing immunosuppressive therapy for non-neoplastic diseases. *Arch Intern Med* 1979;139:461–466.
14. Falkson HC, Portugal MA, Falkson G. Leukaemia in Hodgkin's disease. *S Afr Med J* 1976;50:1429–1431.
15. Ali NO, Janes WO. Malignant myelosclerosis (acute myelofibrosis). Report of two cases following cytotoxic chemotherapy. *Cancer* 1979;43:1211–1215.
16. Cuny G, Penin F, Guerci O, et al. Maladie di Hodgkin associee a une leucose aigue. *Ann Med Nancy* 1973;12:1103–1110.
17. Rosner F, Grunwald HW. Chemicals and leukemia. In: Henderson ES, Lister TA, eds. *Leukemia*. Philadelphia: WB Saunders, 1990:271–287.
18. Tucker MA, D'Angio GJ, Boice JD Jr, et al. Bone sarcomas linked to radiotherapy and chemotherapy in children. *N Engl J Med* 1987;317:589–593.
19. Tucker MA, Coleman CN, Cox RS, Varghese A, Rosenberg SA. Risk of second cancers after treatment for Hodgkin's disease. *N Engl J Med* 1988;318:76–81.
20. Wierda D, Irons RD, Greenlee WF. Immunotoxicity in C57BL/6 mice exposed to benzene and Aroclor 1254. *Toxicol Appl Pharmacol* 1981;60:410–417.
21. Coleman CN, Williams CJ, Flint A, et al. Hematologic neoplasia in patients treated for Hodgkin's disease. *N Engl J Med* 1977;297:1249–1252.
22. Reimer RR, Hoover R, Fraumeni JF Jr, Young RC. Acute leukemia after alkylating-agent therapy of ovarian cancer. *N Engl J Med* 1977;297:177–181.
23. Pedersen-Bjergaard J, Larsen SO. Incidence of acute nonlymphocytic leukemia, preleukemia, and acute myeloproliferative syndrome up to 10 years after treatment of Hodgkin's disease. *N Engl J Med* 1982;307:965–971.
24. Bergsagel DE, Phil D, Bailey AJ, et al. The chemotherapy of plasma-cell myeloma and the incidence of acute leukemia. *N Engl J Med* 1979;301:743–748.
25. World Health Organization. ICD-9, *International Classification of Diseases for Oncology*, 2nd ed. Geneva: WHO, 1990.
26. Fialkow PJ, Jacobson RJ, Papayannopoulou T. Chronic myelocytic leukemia: clonal origin in a stem cell common to the granulocyte, erythrocyte, platelet and monocyte/macrophage. *Am J Med* 1977;63:125–130.
27. Fialkow PJ, Denman AM, Singer JW, Jacobson RJ, Lowenthal MN. Human myeloproliferative disorders: clonal origin in pluripotent stem cells. In: Clarkson B, Marks PA, Till JE, eds. *Differentiation of normal and neoplastic hematopoietic cells*. Cold Spring Harbor, NY: Cold Spring Harbor Laboratory, 1978:131–144.
28. Fialkow PJ, Denman AM, Jacobson RJ, Lowenthal MN. Chronic myelocytic leukemia: origin of some lymphocytes from leukemic stem cells. *J Clin Invest* 1978;62:815–823.
29. Groffen J, Stephenson JR, Heisterkamp N, de Klein A, Bartram CR, Grosveld G. Philadelphia chromosomal breakpoints are clustered within a limited region, *bcr*, on chromosome 22. *Cell* 1984;36:93–99.
30. Puil L, Liu J, Gish G, et al. Bcr-Abl oncoproteins bind directly to activators of the Ras signalling pathway. *EMBO J* 1994;13:764–773.
31. Tauchi T, Boswell HS, Leibowitz D, Broxmeyer HE. Coupling between p210bcr-abl and Shc and Grb2 adaptor proteins in hematopoietic cells permits growth factor receptor-independent link to ^{ras} activation pathway. *J Exp Med* 1994;179:167–175.
32. Duronio V, Welham MJ, Abraham S, Dryden P, Schrader JW. p21^{ras} activation via hemopoietin receptors and c-kit requires tyrosine kinase activity but not tyrosine phosphorylation of p21^{ras} GTPase-activating protein. *Proc Natl Acad Sci U S A* 1992;89:1587–1591.
33. Kurzrock R, Blick MB, Talpaz M, et al. Rearrangement in the breakpoint cluster region and the clinical course in Philadelphia-negative chronic myelogenous leukemia. *Ann Intern Med* 1986;105:673–679.
34. Bartram CR, Kleihauer E, de Klein A, et al. C-abl and bcr are rearranged in a Ph1-negative CML patient. *EMBO J* 1985;4:683–686.
35. Kurzrock R, Gutterman JU, Talpaz M. The molecular genetics of Philadelphia chromosome-positive leukemias. *N Engl J Med* 1988;319:990–998.
36. Pugh WC, Pearson MN, Vardiman JW, Rowley JD. Philadelphia chromosome-negative chronic myelogenous leukaemia: a morphological reassessment. *Br J Haematol* 1985;60:457–467.
37. Young NS. Drugs and chemicals as agents of bone marrow failure. In: Testa NG, Gale RP, eds. *Hematopoiesis: long term effects of chemotherapy and radiation*. New York: Marcel Dekker Inc, 1988:131–157.
38. Girard R, Mallein ML, Fourel R, Tolot F. Lymphose et intoxication benzolique professionnelle chronique. *Arch Mal Prof* 1966;27:781–786.
39. Epstein SS, Ozonoff D. Leukemias and blood dyscrasias following exposure to chlordane and heptachlor. *Teratogenesis Carcinog Mutagen* 1987;7:527–540.
40. Andjelkovic D, Taulbee J. Mortality experience of a cohort of rubber workers, 1964–1973. *J Occup Med* 1976;18:387–394.
41. Delzell E, Monson RR. Mortality among rubber workers: V. processing workers. *J Occup Med* 1982;24:539–545.
42. Irons RD. Benzene toxicology update. *J Appl Toxicol* 1982;2:57–58.
43. Monson RR, Fine LJ. Cancer mortality and morbidity among rubber workers. *J Natl Cancer Inst* 1978;61:1047–1053.
44. McMichael AJ, Spirtas R, Kupper LL, Gamble JF. Solvent exposure and leukemia among rubber workers: an epidemiologic study. *J Occup Med* 1975;17:234–239.
45. Checkoway H, Wilcosky TC, Wolf PH, Tyroler HA. An evaluation of the associations of leukemia and rubber industry solvent exposures. *Am J Ind Med* 1984;5:239–249.
46. Silverstein MN, Maizlish N, Park R, Mirer F. Mortality among workers exposed to coal tar pitch volatiles and welding emissions: an exercise in epidemiologic triage. *Am J Public Health* 1985;75:1283–1287.
47. Stern FB, Waxweiler RA, Beaumont JJ, et al. A case-control study of leukemia at a naval nuclear shipyard. *Am J Epidemiol* 1986;123:980–992.
48. Stern RM. Cancer incidence among welders: possible effects of exposure to extremely low frequency electromagnetic radiation (ELF) and to welding fumes. *Environ Health Perspect* 1987;76:221–229.
49. Kaminski R, Geissert KS, Dacey E. Mortality analysis of plumbers and pipefitters. *J Occup Med* 1980;22:183–189.
50. Preston DL, Kusumi S, Tomonaga M, et al. Cancer incidence in atomic bomb survivors. Part III: Leukemia, lymphoma and multiple myeloma, 1950–1987. *Radiat Res* 1994;137:S68–S97.
51. Morris PD, Koepsell TD, Daling JR, et al. Toxic substance exposure and multiple myeloma: a case-control study. *J Natl Cancer Inst* 1986;76:987–995.
52. Linet MS, Harlow SD, McLaughlin JK. A case-control of multiple myeloma in whites: chronic antigenic stimulation, occupation, and drug use. *Cancer Res* 1987;47:2978–2981.
53. Kagan E, Jacobson RJ. Lymphoid and plasma cell malignancies: asbestos-related disorders of long latency. *Am J Clin Pathol* 1983;80:14–20.
54. Flodin U, Fradriksson M, Persson B. Multiple myeloma and engine exhausts, fresh wood, and creosote: a case-referent study. *Am J Ind Med* 1987;12:519–529.
55. Eriksson M, Karlsson M. Occupational and other environmental factors and multiple myeloma: a population based on case-control study. *Br J Ind Med* 1992;49:95–103.
56. Cuzick J, Stavola BD. Multiple myeloma—a case-control study. *Br J Cancer* 1988;57:516–520.
57. McLaughlin JK, Linet MS, Stone BJ, Blot WJ, Fraumeni JF Jr., Malker HSR, Weiner JA, Ericsson JLE. Multiple myeloma and occupation in Sweden. *Arch Environ Health* 1988;43:7–10.
58. Boffetta P, Stellman SD, Garfinkel L. A case-control study of multiple myeloma nested in the American Cancer Society prospective study. *Int J Cancer* 1989;43:554–559.
59. Farhangi M, Osserman EF. Biology, clinical patterns, and treatment of multiple myeloma and related plasma-cell dyscrasias. In: Twomey JJ, Good RA, eds. *The immunopathology of lymphoreticular neoplasms*. New York: Plenum Publishing, 1978:641–718.
60. Kimzey S. The effects of extended space flight on hematologic and immunologic systems. *J Am Med Wom Assoc* 1975;30:218–232.
61. Leach CS, Johnson PC. Influence of space flight on erythrokinetics in man. *Science* 1984;225:216–219.
62. Cogli A, Bechler B, Muller O, Hunzinger H. Effect of microgravity on lymphocyte activation. ESA SP-1091, European Space Agency: 1988.
63. Steele KJ. Zero gravity and the immune system: a challenge to man's survival in space. *Analog Science Fiction/Science Fact* 1989;191:36–50.
64. Coles S, Bennett J, Ross C. Medical surveillance for leukemia at a petrochemical manufacturing complex: four-year summary, 1991. (Unpublished).
65. Runion H, Scott L. Benzene exposure in the United States, 1978–1983: an overview. *Am J Ind Med* 1985;7:385–393.
66. Gist G, Burg J. Benzene—a review of the literature from a health effects perspective. *Toxicol Ind Health* 1997;13:661–713.
67. Brugnone F, Perbellini L, Romeo L, et al. Benzene in environmental air and human blood. *Int Arch Occup Environ Health* 1998;71:554–559.
68. Brunnenan K, Kagan M, Cox J. Analysis of 1,3-butadiene in other selected gas phase components in cigarette mainstream and sidestream smoke by gas chromatography—mass selective detection. *Carcinogenesis* 1990;11:1863–1868.
69. Staples C, Werner A, Hoogheen T. Assessment of priority pollutant concentrations in the United States using the STORET database. *Environ Toxicol Chem* 1985;4:131–142.
70. Sauer T. Volatile organic compounds in open ocean and coastal waters. *Org Geochem* 1981;3:91–101.
71. Hattemer-Frey H, Travis C, Land M. Benzene: environmental partitioning and human exposure. *Environ Res* 1990;53:221–232.
72. Davoli E, Cappellini L, Moggi M. Online monitoring of benzene air concentrations while driving in traffic by means of isotopic dilution gas chromatography/mass spectrometry. *Int Arch Occup Environ Health* 1996;68:262–267.
73. Franz T. Percutaneous absorption of benzene, Advances in modern toxicology VI, applied toxicology of petroleum hydrocarbons. Princeton, NJ: Princeton Scientific Publishers:61–70.
74. Irons R. Quinones as toxic metabolites of benzene. *J Toxicol Environ Health* 1985;16:673–378.
75. Medinsky M, Kenyon E, Schlosser P. Benzene: a case study in parent chemical and metabolite interactions. *Toxicology* 1995;105:225–233.
76. Medinsky M, Schlosser P, Bond J. Critical issues in benzene toxicity and metabolism: the effect of interactions with other organic chemicals on risk assessment. *Environ Health Perspect* 1994;102[Suppl 9]:119–124.
77. Inoue O, Seiji K, Watanabe T, et al. Mutual metabolic suppression between benzene and toluene in man. *Int Arch Environ Health* 1988;60:15–20.
78. Plappert U, Barthel E, Seidel H. Reduction of benzene toxicity by toluene. *Environ Mol Mutagen* 1994;24:283–292.

79. Eastmond D, Smith M, Irons R. An interaction of benzene metabolites reproduces the myotoxicity observed with benzene exposure. *Toxicol Appl Pharmacol* 1987;91:85–95.
80. Ong C, Lee B. Determination of benzene and its metabolites: application in biological monitoring of environmental and occupational exposure to benzene. *J Chromatogr A* 1994;660:1–22.
81. van Stittert N, Boogaart P, Beulink G. Application of the urinary *S*-phenylmercapturic acid test as a biomarker for low levels of exposure to benzene in industry. *Br J Ind Med* 1993;50:460–469.
82. Ong C, Kok P, Lee B, et al. Evaluation of biomarkers for occupational exposure to benzene. *Occup Environ Med* 1995;52:528–533.
83. Ong C, Kok P, Ong C, et al. Biomarkers of exposure to low concentrations of benzene: a field assessment. *Occup Environ Med* 1996;53:328–333.
84. Aoyama K. Effects of benzene inhalation on lymphocyte subpopulations and immune response in mice. *Toxicol Appl Pharmacol* 1986;85:92–101.
85. Anderson D, Yu T, Schmezer P. An investigation of the DNA damaging ability of benzene and its metabolites in human lymphocytes using the comet assay. *Environ Mol Mutagen* 1995;26:305–314.
86. Hotz P, Carbonnelle P, Scheiff J. Interleukin-1 alpha hematological examination in mechanics exposed to low benzene concentrations. *Int Arch Occup Environ Health* 1998;71:19–28.
87. Niculescu R, Bradford H, Colman R, et al. Inhibition of the conversion of pre-interleukin-1 alpha and -1 beta to mature cytokines by *p*-benzoquinone, a metabolite of benzene. *Chem Biol Interact* 1995;98:211–222.
88. Post G, Snyder R, Kalf G. Inhibition of RNA synthesis in interleukin-2 production in lymphocytes in vitro by benzene and its metabolites, hydroquinone and *p*-benzoquinone. *Toxicol Lett* 1995;29:161–167.
89. Yardley-Jones A, Anderson D, Jenkinson P. Effect of occupational exposure to benzene on phytohemagglutinin (PHA) stimulated lymphocytes in man. *Br J Ind Med* 1988;45:516–522.
90. Hogstedt B, Holmen A, Karlsson A, et al. Gasoline pump mechanics had increased frequencies and sizes of micronuclei in lymphocytes stimulated by pokeweed mitogen. *Mut Res* 1991;263:51–55.
91. Lewis J, Odom B, Adams D. Toxic effects of benzene and benzene metabolites on mononuclear phagocytes. *Toxicol Appl Pharmacol* 1988;92:246–254.
92. Rosenthal G, Snyder C. Modulation of the immune response to *Listeria monocytogenes* by benzene inhalation. *Toxicol Appl Pharmacol* 1985;80:502–510.
93. Rosenthal G, Snyder C. Inhaled benzene reduces aspects of cell mediated tumor surveillance in mice. *Toxicol Appl Pharmacol* 1987;88:5–43.
94. Rosen M, Snyder C, Albert R. Depressions in B- and T-lymphocyte mitogen induced blastogenesis in mice exposed to low concentrations of benzene. *Toxicol Lett* 1984;20:343–349.
95. Yager J, Eastmond D, Robertson M. Characterization of micronuclei induced in human lymphocytes by benzene metabolites. *Cancer Res* 1990;50:393–399.
96. Cheung S, Nerland D, Sonnenfeld G. Inhibition of interferon gamma production by benzene and benzene metabolites. *J Natl Cancer Inst* 1988;80:1069–1072.
97. King A, Landreth K, Wierda D. Hydroquinone inhibits bone marrow pre-B cell maturation in vitro. *Mol Pharmacol* 1987;32:807–812.
98. Carbonnelle P, Lison D, Leroy J, Lauwerys R. Effect of benzene metabolite, hydroquinone on interleukin-1 secretion by human monocytes in vitro. *Toxicol Appl Pharmacol* 1995;132:220–226.
99. Renz J, Kalf G. Role for interleukin-1 (IL-1) and benzene induced hematotoxicity: inhibition of conversion of pre-IL-1α to mature cytokine in murine macrophages by hydroquinone and prevention of benzene induced hematotoxicity in mice by IL-1 α. *Blood* 1991;78:938–944.
100. Miller A, Schattenberg D, Malkinson A. Decreased content of the IL-1 alpha processing enzyme calpain in murine bone marrow-derived macrophages after treatment with the benzene metabolite hydroquinone. *Toxciol Lett* 1994;74:177–184.
101. Wong O. Risk of acute myeloid leukaemia and multiple myeloma in workers exposed to benzene. *Occup Environ Med* 1995;52:380–384.
102. Rinsky RA, Smith AB, Hornung RW, et al. Benzene and leukemia: an epidemiologic risk assessment. *N Engl J Med* 1987;316:1044–1050.
103. Goldstein BD. Is exposure to benzene a cause of human multiple myeloma? *Ann N Y Acad Sci* 1990;609:225–234.
104. Thomas TL, Waxweiler RJ, Moure-Eraso R, Itaya S, Fraumentti F. Mortality patterns among workers in three Texas oil refineries. *J Occup Med* 1982;24:135–141.
105. Aksoy M, Erdem S, Dinçol G, Kutlar A, Bakioglu I, Hepyüksel T. Clinical observations showing the role of some factors in the etiology of multiple myeloma. *Acta Haematol* 1984;71:116–120.
106. Theriault G, Goulet L. A mortality study of oil refinery workers. *J Occup Med* 1979;21:367–370.
107. Paci E, Buiatti E, Costantini AS, et al. Aplastic anemia, leukemia and other cancer mortality in a cohort of shoe workers exposed to benzene. *Scand J Work Environ Health* 1989;15:313–318.
108. Reference deleted by author.
109. Blot WJ, Brinton LA, Fraumeni JF Jr, Stone BJ. Cancer mortality in U.S. counties with petroleum industries. *Science* 1977;198:51–53.
110. Decoufle P, Blattner WA, Blair A. Mortality among chemical workers exposed to benzene and other agents. *Environ Res* 1983;30:16–25(abst).
111. Ott MG, Townsend JC, Fishback WA, Langner RA. Mortality among individuals occupationally exposed to benzene. *Arch Environ Health* 1978;Jan/Feb:3–10.
112. Rushton L, Alderson MR. An epidemiological survey of eight oil refineries in Britain. *Br J Ind Med* 1981;38:225–234.
113. Wen CP, Tsai SP, McClellan WA, Gibson RL. Long-term mortality study of oil refinery workers. *Am J Epidemiol* 1983;118:526–542.
114. Bond GG, McLaren EA, Baldwin CL, Cook RR. An update of mortality among chemical workers exposed to benzene. *Br J Ind Med* 1986;43:685–691.
115. Paxton MB, Chinchilli VM, Brett SM, Rodricks JV. Leukemia risk associated with benzene exposure in the Pliofilm cohort: I. Mortality update and exposure distribution. *Risk Anal* 1994;14:147–154.
116. Gilfillen SC. Lead poisoning and the fall of Rome. *J Occup Med* 1965;7:53–60.
117. Albahary C. Lead and hemopoiesis: the mechanism and consequences of the erythropathy of occupational lead poisoning. *Am J Med* 1972;52:367–377.
118. Cooper WC, Gaffet WR. Mortality of lead workers. *J Occup Med* 1975;17:100–107.
119. Kang HK, Infante PF, Carra JS. Occupational lead exposure and cancer. *Science* 1980;207:935–936.
120. Cooper WC. Occupational lead exposure: what are the risks? *Science* 1980;208:129–131.
121. Landrigan PJ. Arsenic—state of the art. *Am J Ind Med* 1981;2:5–14.
122. Nordberg GF, Pershagen G, Lauwerys R. *Inorganic arsenic—toxicological and environmental aspects.* Odense, Denmark: Department of Community Health and Environmental Medicine, Odense University, 1979.
123. Axelson O, Dahlgren E, Jansson C-D, Rehnlund SO. Arsenic exposure and mortality: a case-referent study from a Swedish copper smelter. *Br J Ind Med* 1978;35:8–15.
124. Ott MG, Holder BB, Gordon HL. Respiratory cancer and occupational exposure to arsenicals. *Arch Environ Health* 1974;29:250–255.
125. Polednak AP, Stehney AF, Rowland RE. Mortality among women first employed before 1930 in the U.S. radium dial-painting industry. *Am J Epidemiol* 1978;107:179–195.
126. Martland HS, Conlon P, Knef JD. Some unrecognized dangers in the use and the handling of radioactive substances. *JAMA* 1925;85:1769–1776.
127. Martland HS. Microscopic changes of certain anemias due to radioactivity. *Arch Pathol* 1926;2:465–472.
128. Martland HS. Occupational poisoning in manufacture of luminous watch dials. *JAMA* 1929;92:466–473.
129. Martland HS. The occurrence of malignancy in radioactive persons. A general review of data gathered in the study of the radium dial painters, with special reference to the occurrence of osteogenic sarcoma and the inter-relationship of certain blood diseases. *Am J Cancer* 1931;15:2435–2516.
130. Austin SG, Sielken RL. Issues in assessing the carcinogenic hazards of ethylene oxide. *J Occup Med* 1988;30:236–245.
131. Hogstedt C, Malmqvist N, Wadman B. Leukemia in workers exposed to ethylene oxide. *JAMA* 1979;241:1132–1133.
132. Hogstedt C, Rohlén O, Berndtsson BS, Axelson O, Ehrenberg L. A cohort study of mortality and cancer incidence in ethylene oxide production workers. *Br J Ind Med* 1979;36:276–280.
133. Theis AM, Frentzel-Beyme R, Link R, et al. Mortality study on employees exposed to alkylene oxides (ethylene oxide/propylene oxide) and their derivatives. In: Proceedings of the Symposium on Prevention of Occupational Cancer, Helsinki, 1981.
134. Morgan RW, Claxton KW, Divine BJ, Kaplan SD, Harris VB. Mortality among ethylene oxide workers. *J Occup Med* 1981;23:767–770.
135. Cook RR, Bodner KM, Kolesar RC, et al. A cross-sectional study of ethylene glycol monomethyl ether process employees. *Arch Environ Health* 1982;37:346–351.
136. Welch LS, Cullen MR. Effect of exposure to ethylene glycol ethers on shipyard painters: III. Hematologic effects. *Am J Ind Med* 1988;14:527–536.
137. Cullen MR, Rado TA, Waldron JA, Sparer J, Welch LS. Bone marrow injury in lithographers exposed to glycol ethers and organic solvents used in multicolor offset and ultraviolet curing printing processes. *Arch Environ Health* 1983;38:347–354.
138. Scott JL, Cartwright GE, Wintrobe MM. Acquired aplastic anemia: an analysis of thirty-nine cases and review of the pertinent literature. *Medicine* 1959;38:119–172.
139. Meinhardt TJ, Young RJ, Hartle RW. Epidemiologic investigations of styrene-butadiene rubber production and reinforced plastics production. *Scand J Work Environ Health* 1978;4[Suppl 2]:240–246.
140. Divine BJ. An update on mortality among workers at a butadiene facility—preliminary results. *Environ Health Perspect* 1990;86:119–128.
141. Matanoski GM, Schwartz L. Mortality of workers in styrene-butadiene polymer production. *J Occup Med* 1987;29:675–680.
142. Santos-Burgoa C, Matanoski GM, Zeger S, Schwartz L. Lymphohematopoietic cancer in styrene-butadiene polymerization workers. *Am J Epidemiol* 1992;136:843–854.
143. Matanoski GM, Santos-Burqua C, Schwartz L. Mortality of a cohort of workers in the styrene-butadiene polymer manufacturing industry (1943–1982). *Environ Health Perspect* 1990;86:107–117.
144. Delzell E, Sathiakumar N, Hovinga M, et al. A follow-up study of synthetic rubber workers. *Toxicology* 1996;113:182–189.
145. Irons RD, Stillman WS, Cloyd MW. Selective activation of endogenous ecotropic retovirus in hematopoietic tissues of B6C3F1 mice during the preleukemic phase of 1,3-butadiene exposure. *Virology* 1987;161:457–462.
146. Irons RD, Smith CN, Stillman WS, Shah RS, Steinhagen WH, Leiderman LJ. Macrocytic-megaloblastic anemia in male NIH Swiss mice following repeated exposure to 1,3-butadiene. *Toxicol Appl Pharmacol* 1986;85:450–455.
147. Irons RD, Smith CN, Stillman WS, Shah RS, Steinhagen WH, Leiderman LJ. Macrocytic-megaloblastic anemia in male B6C3F1 mice following chronic exposure to 1,3-butadiene. *Toxicol Appl Pharmacol* 1986;83:95–100.

148. Irons RD, Cathro HP, Stillman WS, Steinhagen WH, Shah RS. Susceptibility to 1,3-butadiene-induced leukemogenesis correlates with endogenous ecotropic retroviral background in the mouse. *Toxicol Appl Pharmacol* 1989;101:170–176.
149. Melnick RL, Kohn MC. Mechanistic data indicate that 1,3-butadiene is a human carcinogen. *Carcinogenesis* 1995;16:157–163.
150. Bond JA, Recio L, Andjelkovich D. Epidemiological and mechanistic data suggest that 1,3-butadiene will not be carcinogenic to humans at exposures likely to be encountered in the environment or workplace. *Carcinogenesis* 1995;16:165–171.
151. Infante PF, Epstein SS, Newton F. Blood dyscrasias and childhood tumors and exposure to chlordane and heptachlor. *Scand J Work Environ Health* 1978;4:137–150.
152. Furie B, Trubowitz S. Insecticides and blood dyscrasias: chlordane exposure and self-limited refractory megaloblastic anemia. *JAMA* 1976;235:1720–1722.
153. Wang HH, Grufferman S. Aplastic anemia and occupational pesticide exposure: a case-control study. *J Occup Med* 1981;23:364–366.
154. Shindell S, Ulrich S. Mortality of workers employed in the manufacture of chlordane: an update. *J Occup Med* 1986;28:497–501.
155. Shindell S. The author replies. *J Occup Med* 1987;29:909–911.
156. MacMahon B, Monson RR, Wang HH, Zheng T. A second follow-up of mortality in a cohort of pesticide applicators. *J Occup Med* 1988;30:429–432.
157. Bond GG, Bodner KM, Cook RR. Phenoxy herbicides and cancer: insufficient epidemiologic evidence for a causal relationship. *Fundam Appl Toxicol* 1989;12:172–188.
158. Hardell L, Sandstrom A. A case control study: soft tissue sarcomas and exposure to phenoxyacetic acids or chlorophenols. *Br J Cancer* 1979;39:711–717.
159. Hardell L, Eriksson M, Lenner P, Lundgren E. Malignant lymphoma and exposure to chemicals, especially organic solvents, chlorophenols and phenoxy acids: a case-control study. *Br J Cancer* 1981;43:169–176.
160. Woods JS, Polissar L, Severson RK, Heuser LS, Kulander BG. Soft tissue sarcoma and non-Hodgkin's lymphoma in relation to phenoxyherbicide and chlorinated phenol exposure in western Washington State. *J Natl Cancer Inst* 1987;78:899–910.
161. Pearce N. Phenoxy herbicides and non-Hodgkin's lymphoma in New Zealand: frequency and duration of herbicide use. *Br J Ind Med* 1989;46:143–144.
162. Hoar SK, Blair A, Holmes FF, et al. Agricultural herbicide use and risk of lymphoma and soft-tissue sarcoma. *JAMA* 1986;256:1141–1147.
163. Zahm SH, Weisenburger DD, Babbitt PA, et al. A case-control study of non-Hodgkin's lymphoma and the herbicide 2,4-dichlorophenoxyacetic acid (2,4-D) in eastern Nebraska. *Epidemiology* 1990;1:349–356.

CHAPTER 60

Polychlorinated Biphenyls and Other Polyhalogenated Aromatic Hydrocarbons

Peter G. Shields, John Whysner, and Kenneth H. Chase

POLYCHLORINATED BIPHENYLS

Polychlorinated biphenyls (PCBs) comprise a closely related group of synthetic chlorinated compounds manufactured in the United States under the trade name Aroclor (1,2) and in other countries under other trade names (Table 60-1). PCBs were widely used in the electrical utility industry but had other applications as well. Aroclor formulations vary by degree of chlorination and congener content. Figure 60-1 shows the structure of PCBs with the numbering system for chlorine substitution. Two hundred nine theoretical congeners exist, but commercial mixtures do not contain significant quantities of most of these. The congeners are identified by the position of the chlorine on the ring and a standardized notation was adopted by the International Union of Pure and Applied Chemists. Toxicologic properties vary according to the number and position of the chlorines. Positions 2, 6, 2', and 6', which are adjacent to the bond between the two biphenyl rings, are "ortho"; whereas positions 3, 5, 3', and 5' are "meta"; and positions 4 and 4' are "para." Some PCB congeners are coplanar because the chlorinated configuration allows both phenyl rings to have a parallel spatial orientation.

TABLE 60-1. Commercial polychlorinated biphenyl mixtures

Manufacturer	Trade name	Identifier	Percent chlorine by weight
Monsanto Co. (USA)	Aroclor	1242	42
		1248	48
		1254	54
		1260	60
		1016	41
Farbenfabricken Bayer (Germany)	Clophen	A30	42
		A50	54
		A60	60
Kanegatuchi Co. (Japan)	Kanechlor	300	42
		400	48
		500	53
		600	60
Prodelec Co. (France)	Pyralene	3010	42
		1476	54
Caffarro Co. (Italy)	Apirolio	None	42

Aroclors are classified by a four-number system beginning with 12 (i.e., referring to 12 carbon atoms) and ending with the percentage, by weight, of chlorine (e.g., Aroclor 1260 has 60% chlorine by weight) (see Table 60-1). The exception is Aroclor 1016, which is the most recently produced and contains approximately 41% chlorine by weight. For all these mixtures, an overlap of congeners is present, so that, for example, pentachlorobiphenyls are present in Aroclor 1242, 1248, 1254, and 1260, but in very different percentages. Environmentally detectable PCBs may not be the same as the parent commercially produced Aroclors, because individual congeners have different partitioning, uptake, and retention properties in environmental matrices, and differences in environmental degradation pathways exist (3). In past occupational exposures and certain environmental situations, however, the preponderance of a particular Aroclor may be inferred by the congener pattern.

During the 1970s, concern regarding the continued unrestricted use of PCBs surfaced because of their environmental persistence and toxicity in laboratory animals (4–6). Monsanto voluntarily halted production, and Congress banned further manufacture in 1979, limiting the distribution of PCBs under the Toxic Substances Control Act (40 *CFR* 761.20). Since then, environmental levels and food contamination have substantially decreased (7).

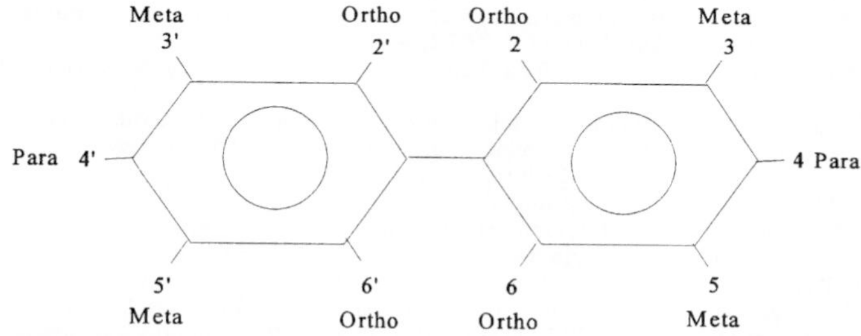

Figure 60-1. Structure of a polychlorinated biphenyl molecule. Chlorine substitution can occur at any numbered position. The meta, para, and ortho positions are shown.

Absorption, Metabolism, and Excretion

A detailed description of PCB pharmacokinetics in animals should take into consideration the complexity of various Aroclor compositions and also genetically determined differences across species; however, certain general properties of PCBs can be described. PCBs can be absorbed through the skin, lungs, and gastrointestinal tract (8). Dermal absorption is the major route in occupational groups (9), whereas ingestion is the major route in reported environmental exposures (10–13). PCBs are transported by the bloodstream to the liver and muscle, where they are redistributed to adipose tissue. An equilibrium is established under which partitioning among tissues remains relatively constant for a given species. Elimination of PCBs is slow, and even low levels of absorption can lead to bioaccumulation.

PCBs are metabolized in the liver to form hydroxylated phenolic compounds (14–16). They can be excreted as such, or as methylsulfinyl or glucuronide metabolites formed via other metabolic pathways (17). Proposed arene-oxide intermediates also may be hydrolyzed to form dihydrodiols or glutathione conjugates (3), which can then be metabolized to catechols or methyl sulfonyl metabolites, respectively. The rate of formation of metabolic products varies depending on the congener and animal species. Dogs and rodents metabolize PCBs relatively quickly compared with primates (15). Excretion is via the biliary tract to feces or via the urine.

PCBs induce cytochrome P-450 enzymes in various organs of laboratory animals, including liver, lung, and small intestine (3,18). This induction may alter the metabolism of other chemicals but may have only minor effects on the metabolism of PCBs. Different P-450 enzymes are induced depending on the number and position of chlorine atoms within the PCB congener (e.g., meta and para versus ortho substitution) (3). Induction varies widely across species (3,14,17,19,20). The coplanar congeners cause the greatest induction of aryl hydrocarbon hydroxylase, compared with mono-ortho–substituted compounds, and then other congeners (3,21). Other PCBs, however, primarily induce other P-450s. In an *in vitro* model, rat cells were more sensitive compared with human cells, and the pattern of cytochrome P-450 induction can be different (22). When comparing different Aroclor mixtures and congeners, the effects of the Aroclors on aryl hydrocarbon hydroxylase activity have been primarily attributed only to a few congeners (23).

The half-life of PCBs varies by congener but is shorter in experimental animals than humans and is generally less for lower-chlorinated congeners. In a small group of occupationally exposed persons, the serum half-life was reported to be 6 to 7 months for Aroclor 1242 and 33 to 34 months for Aroclor 1260 (24). In another study (25), the half-life in workers for lower-chlorinated congeners was 2.6 years, while for higher chlorinated congeners it was 4.6 years. Children have been reported to metabolize PCBs faster than their mothers, as the half-life for Kanechlor 500 (similar to Aroclor 1254) in blood was 2.8 years in children compared with 7.1 years in mothers (26). The mean half-life in blood for 2,3',4',4,5-pentachlorobiphenyl was 9.8 months, whereas the half-life for 2,3,3',4,4'-pentachlorobiphenyl was 6.7 months (27). The elimination rate of PCBs in the body also might be related to the body burden, where higher levels are cleared faster (28). An overview of studies (29) concluded that substantial variation exists in reported half-lives among all studies published, but that estimates of less than 1 year and more than 10 years are probably not accurate.

Body burdens in humans depend on many factors including route and length of exposure, place of residence, gender, age, and possibly extent of alcohol consumption (11,30–35). Worldwide levels in various tissues have been summarized (36). The average PCB level for nonoccupationally exposed persons is estimated to be approximately 7 parts per billion (ppb) with a range up to 30 (32). In contrast, occupationally exposed persons can have PCB blood levels up to 3,300 ppb (37). Adipose levels are generally less than 3 parts per million (ppm) in the general population, but levels up to 33 ppm have been reported in the occupational setting (34,37,38). The National Human Adipose Tissue Survey found that levels above 3 ppm in the general population have been decreasing over a 10-year period ending in 1983; however, the prevalence of any detectable level has been increasing (33). PCBs can be detected in many organs of the body, and levels vary depending on fat content; on a lipid basis, levels in different organs are similar (13). The partitioning coefficient between adipose tissue and blood varies from 100 to 1 to 190 to 1, depending on PCB body burdens (34,38–40). Partitioning coefficients were also reported for brain to liver to fat of 1 to 3.5 to 81 in necropsy samples from Denmark (8). PCBs also are present in placental cord blood (41) and breast milk (42,43). Levels in breast milk are positively associated with increased age, omnivorous diet, and fish consumption, and negatively associated with Quetelet index [weight/(length)^2] and the amount of lactation (44).

Effects in Laboratory Animals

PCBs produce relatively little acute toxicity. The dose required to produce death in 50% of treated animals ranges from 0.5 g per kg to 11.3 g per kg, depending on the Aroclor and animal species (8). Carcinogenic and noncarcinogenic toxic responses vary widely among species (8,45). Monkeys, guinea pigs, and minks are relatively sensitive compared with rodents (46).

Subacute and chronic exposures in laboratory animals lead to a variety of effects, occurring as a syndrome (i.e., a constellation of signs and symptoms that do not appear separately). For example, progressive weight loss, chloracne, alopecia, skin edema, swelling around the eyes, lymphoid and thymic involution, hepatomegaly, bone marrow depression, and reproductive dysfunction commonly occur together (8,47,48). Rats and mice, unlike primates, do not develop facial edema, alopecia, or chloracne. Some of these effects are associated with the coplanar congeners, which are considered to be agonists for the aryl hydrocarbon-receptor signal transduction pathway, and segregate in genetically inbred mice with and without receptor responsiveness (3,16). Mono-ortho–substituted coplanar congeners cause a similar toxic syndrome, although to a lesser extent than coplanar congeners (21). It is likely that the parent PCB congeners are responsible for the toxic effects in laboratory animals, rather than reactive metabolites.

Neurologic and behavioral effects have been reported in laboratory mice and monkeys following prenatal, neonatal, or early postnatal exposures to PCBs. Exposures in adult laboratory animals generally do not produce measurable toxicity except for a few effects that are reversible (49,50). After prenatal exposure, monkeys can become hyperactive in early life and show other signs or toxicity (51,52).

The target organ for PCB tumorigenicity in animals is the liver. Monkeys, guinea pigs, and minks are relatively sensitive compared with rodents (46). Three studies report that Aroclor 1260 or Clophen A60 induce hepatocellular carcinomas in laboratory mice and rats exposed to large doses over a lifetime (53–55). Aroclor 1254 and Kanechlor 500 at high doses also led to a small incidence of hepatocellular carcinoma (56,57). A reevaluation of published studies (58) using uniform pathologic criteria indicates that the potency of the PCB mixtures depends on the chlorination, and not all exposures should be considered equivalent. One study in laboratory rodents showed that Aroclors 1242 and 1016, in addition to 1260 and 1254, can induce a dose-related increase in liver tumors

(59). It should be noted that, in spite of the morphologic appearance, these lesions do not otherwise display malignant behavior; for example, it has not been demonstrated that animals with these tumors live longer than controls and metastases (54,55).

Laboratory animal studies show that PCBs act as modifying agents after exposure to known carcinogens. In carcinogenesis models, they can act as tumor promoters or inhibitors; that is, they can increase or decrease, respectively, tumor incidence resulting from prior exposures to DNA-reactive carcinogens (8,14,60–67). In laboratory animals, PCBs have been shown to promote hepatocellular tumors and preneoplastic lesions following ingestion of *N*-nitrosamines (60,62,63,68,69) and azo dyes (70), and also lung tumors after exposure to *N*-nitrosamines (71). They also inhibit these tumors if the animals are treated with PCBs before carcinogen exposure (61,64,72,73). PCBs also can inhibit the transplantability and growth of tumorigenic cells (74,74a).

Effects in Humans

Many studies of persons exposed to PCBs exist, including persons with high occupational exposures (75). Several publications report various effects in humans related to PCB exposure, although dermal irritation and chloracne are the only consistent findings of clinical significance (75), and these are limited to workplace exposures. A critical review (76) of studies investigating environmental exposures did not suggest any adverse health effects, whereas the results are equivocal in the occupational setting. Caution must be used when reviewing studies, especially those that involve early occupational exposures before 1950 or heated PCBs, because the exposures might have involved chlorinated compounds other than PCBs, such as chloronaphthylenes and polychlorinated dibenzofurans (PCDFs).

Chloracne is a follicular skin eruption characterized by pinhead- to pea-sized, straw-colored cysts (77). Comedo formation is often present. The lesions have a unique distribution pattern, which involves the face, shoulders, abdomen, scrotum, penis, and ears. In contrast to typical acne, the nose is spared in chloracne. Skin biopsies may not be helpful for diagnosis, especially in chronic cases (77). Individual lesions also tend to last longer than typical acne and can recur. Chloracne does not occur due to skin exposure but occurs as a result of systemic absorption. It is thought that chloracne typically occurs in persons with PCB blood levels greater than 200 ppb (78,79), except in those cohorts in which exposures to other chlorinated compounds such as chloronaphthylenes or dibenzofurans also have occurred (80). Fischbein and colleagues reported that a group of workers suffered hyperpigmentation, hyperkeratosis, and chloracne, but the relationship to PCB exposure was uncertain because PCB body burdens did not correlate with dermatologic findings (81). Chloracne has not been associated with environmental exposures (11,12). Separate from chloracne, PCBs can cause a transient dermatitis with contact, although this may be due to stabilizers or epoxides contained in the PCB mixtures (75).

Alterations in blood liver–associated enzyme levels among workers have been reported in several studies, but liver function measured through bilirubin, albumin, or prothrombin times is not affected (34,38,74,82). Although differences were reported for the mean levels of serum alanine aminotransferase, aspartate aminotransferase, and γ-glutamyl transpeptidase between exposed and unexposed workers, the group means and most individual levels were well within laboratory reference ranges (34,37,74,82). The clinical significance of these findings remains uncertain because workers do not develop clinical manifestations of hepatitis or other liver disease, although one study of Italian workers exposed to Pyralene (similar to Aroclor 1242) reported an unexpected incidence of hepatomegaly (79).

Several studies have correlated serum lipid levels with blood PCB levels. Chase and colleagues found a statistically significant age-adjusted positive association of plasma PCB levels with triglycerides but not cholesterol (34). Smith et al. investigated 228 workers and found a significant correlation for PCBs with high-density lipoprotein cholesterol (37). Kreiss et al. (83) and Baker (84) investigated groups of people who were environmentally exposed to both PCBs and dichlorodiphenyl-trichloroethane and reported positive correlations of serum PCB values with serum cholesterol and triglycerides. Although it was initially postulated that PCBs might have caused an abnormal lipid metabolism, other reports suggest that any correlation reflects PCB affinity for serum lipids (47,74,82,85,86). Furthermore, cardiovascular disease, the major health effect that would be predicted from abnormal lipid levels, has not been shown to increase in the PCB-exposed cohorts (87–89).

Other PCB-related health effects have been suggested in certain studies but have not been confirmed in the scientific literature. An association between PCB exposure and symptoms such as headache, fatigue, and nervousness has been reported in two studies that were not formally controlled (10,90). These findings were not reported in six others (34,37,38,79,91,92). One study noted a positive association between serum PCB levels and blood pressure (93), but this finding was later characterized as uncertain by the same author (32). Additionally, this finding was not identified in ten other studies (three specifically reported the results of blood pressure measurements, whereas numerous others reported normal physical examinations) (34,37,38,79,84,91,92,94–96). Alterations in pulmonary function testing of workers exposed to PCBs have been reported in one study (97) but not duplicated in another that investigated the same group of workers (98), and these alterations were not associated with symptoms or chest radiographic findings. Another study on a different group of workers did not find pulmonary function abnormalities in relation to PCB levels (74). Neurologic findings were reported in one study (37) but not in others (34,37,94,95). One study of psychosocial effects in persons living near a PCB contamination and remediation area was consistent with psychosocial effects due to concerns of health effects, but the psychosocial effects were not related to actual environmental exposure (99).

Reported reproductive effects in women occupationally or environmentally exposed to PCBs have included lower infant birth weight, smaller head circumference, shortened gestational age, and early impairment of psychomotor development (100–102). Possible confounding variables were tobacco use and other environmental contaminants. In all of these studies, the mean differences between exposed and nonexposed groups were small; therefore, the clinical significance of these reports is uncertain. Maternal serum and cord blood PCB levels were not associated with premature rupture of fetal membranes (103), and spontaneous fetal death was not associated with exposure through consumption of fish (104). In one study (105) of children whose PCB maternal levels and intellectual function were measured at age 11 years in relation to birth levels, it was reported that IQ decreased 6.2 points in those with the highest PCB levels. Reading mastery was reportedly decreased as well. Several methodologic problems limit the validity of the conclusions in this study, including low participation rates that might select for children whose parents are aware of reading problems and know that their children were exposed to PCB, the use of a composite score for PCB exposure from different biological matrices rather than from a consistent source, and levels of lead and mercury were shown to affect intellect in this same study group. Although the Jacobson publication (105) reported that the effects were due to prenatal exposure, another study excluded this cause (106).

In 1968 and again in 1978, persons in Japan and Taiwan, respectively, ingested relatively large amounts of PCBs, PCDFs, quarterphenyls, and terphenyls via accidental contamination of rice oil. These contamination cases are known as the *Yusho* and *Yu Cheng* episodes, respectively. In each case, the oil was used for cooking and was consumed over several months. It has been determined that exposure to the PCDFs, rather than to PCBs, was more likely to be responsible for the toxic effects of the oil (107–111). Various health effects were described, including dermatologic, neurologic, hepatic, and ocular manifestations (112–116). Children are reported to have cognitive and developmental impairment (117–120). Yu Cheng mortality studies have shown that, although the overall and cancer-related mortalities were reported to be decreased compared with the general population, death from cirrhosis increased (121,122). Hepatitis infections and alcohol use were not considered in the analyses, however, and other methodologic issues make any conclusions tenuous. Owing to the primary involvement of PCDFs in the etiology of the Yusho and Yu Cheng episodes, these studies should not be used to assess potential PCB-related health effects.

Epidemiologic studies have investigated the causes of death in workers with long-term continuous exposure to high levels of PCBs (87–89,123). These reports fail to demonstrate consistently increased death rates for all causes of death, cancer deaths, or any individual cause of death when compared with the expected number for the general population. One study reported an increased rate of hematologic neoplasms, but most of those individuals described had been exposed for a relatively short period before the diagnosis, and no dose-response relationship could be identified (88). This finding was not duplicated in two other studies (87,89). An increased rate of liver, biliary, and gallbladder cancer also has been reported (87), but a dose-response relationship could not be identified, and other evidence suggests that these tumor types should not be analyzed as a group. An excess of malignant melanoma was found in another study (123) of capacitor workers. Although a proportional hazards model was developed based on exposure, no relation to exposure and melanoma could be found. It should be noted that investigators from the same institution (124) wrote that the available exposure data did not lend itself to establishing an exposure-response relationship, and that the results were not corroborated by other studies. In summary, no consistent findings exist among several different occupational studies, which leads to the conclusion that positive associations in any individual study were due to chance—statistical analysis notwithstanding—or confounding factors.

Several studies have focused on associations between PCB body burdens and breast cancer. Three small case series studies were reported in the literature; one study found an association between breast cancer and total PCB adipose tissue levels (125), whereas two others did not (126,127). Wolff and coworkers (128) published the report of a nested case-control study of women enrolled in the New York University Women's Health Cohort Study. They found that in 68 cases (compared with 171 matched controls), serum PCBs were borderline elevated in cases (mean difference, 1.0 ng per mL), but the paired difference was not statistically significantly different. Several methodologic factors limit this study, and another larger cohort study (129) did not replicate these findings. Also, breast cancer has been studied in several occupational cohorts, in which women are exposed to much greater amounts of PCBs than are in the environment, with no reported increased breast cancer risk (130).

Genotoxicity

The effects of PCBs at the genetic level have been widely investigated. Overwhelming evidence demonstrates that the PCBs are not mutagenic (8,14). DNA binding has been reported in crude studies, although a specific nucleotide adduct has not been identified (131–134).

Regulatory Information

PCBs were banned for use in open systems in 1976 and in closed systems beyond 1979 (40 *CFR* 761.210). Transformers that con-

TABLE 60-2. Regulatory and recommended limit values

Media	Agency	Polychlorinated biphenyls	Limit	Comment	Reference
Food	Food and Drug Administration	Any Aroclor	2.0 ppm	Fish	*Federal Register* 1984;49(100):21214–21520
Water	Environmental Protection Agency (EPA)	Any Aroclor	0.0005 mg/L		EPA, 1994
	National Academy of Sciences (NAS)	Any	0.05 and 0.35 mg/L	7-d and 24-h SNARL	NAS, 1980
Air	National Institute of Occupational Safety and Health (NIOSH)	Aroclor 1242 and 1254	1 μg/m^3	Occupational exposure	NIOSH Criteria Document, 1977
		Aroclor 1242	10 mg/m^3	Immediately dangerous to life and health	NIOSH, 1990
		Aroclor 1254	5 mg/m^3	Immediately dangerous to life and health	NIOSH, 1990
	American Conference of Governmental Industrial Hygienists (ACGIH)	Aroclor 1242	1 mg/m^3	Skin, occupational exposure	ACGIH, 1990
		Aroclor 1254	0.5 mg/m^3	Skin, occupational exposure	ACGIH, 1990
	Occupational Safety and Health Administration	Aroclor 1242	1 mg/m^3	Occupational exposure	29 *CFR* 1910.100
		Aroclor 1254	0.5 mg/m^3	Occupational exposure	29 *CFR* 1910.100
Soil	Toxic Substances Control Act	Any Aroclor	50 ppm		40 *CFR* 761.210
	EPA	Any Aroclor	10–25 ppm		*Federal Register* (4/87)

ppm, parts per million; SNARL, suggested no adverse response level.

tain more than 500 ppm are considered PCB transformers. Levels between 25 and 500 ppm are considered "contaminated." Environmental and occupational exposures are regulated by several state and federal agencies. Exposure limit values are presented in Table 60-2. The International Agency for Research on Cancer considers that human studies for PCBs provide limited to inadequate evidence of carcinogenicity, whereas animal studies have been considered to provide sufficient evidence.

POLYBROMINATED BIPHENYLS

Polybrominated biphenyls (PBBs) have been used primarily as flame retardants. Their structure is similar to PCBs, but bromine, rather than chlorine, is substituted for hydrogen. With one exception, PBBs are not widespread environmental contaminants. This exception occurred in 1974 when PBBs (commercially produced as Firemaster) were accidentally mixed into livestock feed because of confusion with magnesium oxide (marketed as Nutrimaster) (4). Contamination was limited to persons living in Michigan. No human clinical illness has been causally linked to this PBB exposure (4). Although medical complaints and altered neurobehavioral studies were reported in presumably exposed Michigan residents versus Wisconsin controls, the symptoms and biological studies were not correlated with body burdens (4,135). Blood testing did not reveal clinical abnormalities (4,31). One occupational study reported chemical, but not clinical, evidence of hypothyroidism (136). Immune system parameters have been measured in Michigan residents, and, although several alterations have been reported in humoral and cell-mediated immunity, they were not correlated with PBB body burden (137). Other studies have assessed lymphocyte function in relation to PBB levels, and no correlations were found (138). PBBs are thought to have a stronger potential to cause chloracne compared with PCBs (77).

The effects of PBB exposure in laboratory animals are similar to the effects seen with PCBs (4,139). PBBs without meta-para-bromine substitutions are metabolized more than other PBBs (140). Rats are more sensitive to PBB-cytochrome P-450 induction compared with humans (141). PBBs may cause hepatocellular carcinoma in rodents (142). It also has been reported that the major contaminant in the Firemaster mixture described above is relatively nontoxic (143). PBBs, similar to PCBs, promote preneoplastic and neoplastic lesions in the rodent liver (143–145). The International Agency for Research on Cancer determined that studies have provided sufficient evidence to document cancer in laboratory animals, but insufficient evidence still exists for cancer in humans.

CHLORINATED BENZENES

Chlorinated benzenes are a group of compounds used as solvents, pesticides, herbicides, fungicides, and in a number of organic chemical syntheses. They are cyclic aromatic compounds with one to six substituted chlorine atoms. Exposure to these compounds occurs mainly in the occupational setting, but levels have been detected in a variety of environmental media, including air, soil, food, and water. Higher degrees of chlorination result in lower water solubility, flammability, and volatility (146). Thus, the ability to become airborne or leach from soil is variable. Chlorinated benzenes are lipophilic, so bioaccumulation in animal and human tissues occurs (although to a much lesser extent than other chlorinated aromatic hydrocarbons).

Limited information is available on the pharmacokinetics and toxicity of chlorinated benzenes in animals or humans. Animal studies indicated that, once absorbed into the body, P-450 metabolic enzymes in the liver convert these compounds into chlorinated phenols via an arene oxide intermediate (147,148). The chlorophenols are excreted in the urine and feces as sulfur intermediates (149) or combine with cellular proteins after further detoxification (148,150). Binding to cellular proteins allows for additional metabolism and dechlorination (147,150).

Chlorinated benzenes and metabolites have been detected in blood, adipose tissue, urine, and exhaled air of persons without known occupational exposures (33). The National Human Adipose Tissue Survey reported detectable levels of chlorobenzene, 1,2-dichlorobenzene, and 1,4-dichlorobenzene in 96%, 63%, and 100%, respectively, of samples tested. These levels were correlated with age (35). For hexachlorobenzene, 100% of samples tested had detectable levels, with a median of 0.31 ppm in 1983 (33). Levels in humans have reportedly been decreasing over a 10-year period during the 1970s and 1980s. Retention time in humans is predicted to be 15 years (151).

The major known health effect of chlorinated benzenes is the development of porphyria cutanea tarda, which was reported in the 1950s when persons in Turkey ingested grain contaminated with up to 0.2 g of hexachlorobenzene (152). Some resulting health effects reportedly persisted up to 20 years. Occupational cohorts exposed to chlorinated benzenes have not been reported to suffer porphyria cutanea tarda (146).

Isolated case reports and small studies exist for other health effects of chlorinated benzenes (146). A study on persons accidentally exposed to 1,2-dichlorobenzene used as a pesticide reported dizziness, headache, fatigue, nausea, and eye and mucous membrane irritation. The workers had a statistically significantly elevated number of clastogenic chromosomal alterations in the peripheral leukocytes (8.9% vs. 2% in controls) (153). Other studies have found clastogenic effects in persons exposed to 1,2,4,5-tetrachlorobenzene (154). Anecdotal cases exist linking chlorinated benzenes to aplastic anemia, chronic lymphocytic leukemia, acute myelogenous leukemia, hemolytic anemia, and methemoglobinemia (153).

An epidemiologic association between chlorinated benzenes and human cancer has not been established. Studies in animals noted an association of liver and kidney carcinoma, as well as adrenal and parathyroid adenomas with hexachlorobenzene and dichlorobenzene, but not with other chlorobenzenes. *In vitro* genotoxicity studies of chlorinated benzenes generally have been negative (155).

REFERENCES

1. Lloyd JW, Moore RM, Woolf BS, Stein HP. Polychlorinated biphenyls. *J Occup Med* 1975;18:109.
2. Durfee RL. Production and usage of PCBs in the United States. In: Proceedings of the National Conference on Polychlorinated Biphenyls, Chicago, 1975:103–107. Washington: US Environmental Protection Agency.
3. Safe SH. Polychlorinated biphenyls (PCBs): environmental impact, biochemical and toxic responses, and implications for risk assessment. *Crit Rev Toxicol* 1994;24:87–149.
4. Kimbrough, RD. Human health effects of polychlorinated biphenyls (PCBs) and polybrominated biphenyls (PBBs). *Ann Rev Pharmacol Toxicol* 1987;27:87–111.
5. Kutz FW, Strassman SC. Residues of polychlorinated biphenyls in the general population of the United States meeting. Proceedings of the National Conference on PCBs. 1975;(abst).
6. Price HA, Welch RL. Occurrence of polychlorinated biphenyls in humans. *Environ Health Perspect* 1972;1:73–78.
7. Fensterheim RJ. Documenting temporal trends of polychlorinated biphenyls in the environment. *Regul Toxicol Pharmacol* 1993;18:181–201.
8. Agency for Toxic Substances and Disease Registry. *Selected PCBs (Aroclor-1260, -1254, -1248, -1242, -1232, -1221, and -1016).* Washington: Agency for Toxic Substances and Disease Registry, US Public Health Service, 1987:1–136.
9. Lees PSJ, Corn M, Breysse PN. Evidence for dermal absorption as the major route of body entry during exposure of transformer maintenance and repairmen to PCBs. *Am Ind Hyg Assoc J* 1987;48:257–264.
10. Humphrey HEB. Population studies of PCBs in Michigan residents. *PCBs: Human and Environmental Hazards* 1983;21:299–311.

11. Mussalo-Rauhama H, Moilanen R. Influence of diet and other factors on the levels of organochlorine compounds in human adipose tissue in Finland. *J Toxicol Environ Health* 1984;13:689–704.
12. Fiore BJ, Anderson HA, Hanrahan LP, Olson LJ, Sonzogni WC. Sport fish consumption and body burden levels of chlorinated hydrocarbons: a study of Wisconsin anglers. *Arch Environ Health* 1989;44:82–88.
13. Kimbrough RD. Polychlorinated biphenyls (PCBs) and human health: an update. *Crit Rev Toxicol* 1995;25:133–163.
14. Safe S. Polychlorinated biphenyls (PCBs): mutagenicity and carcinogenicity. *Mutat Res* 1989;220:31–47.
15. Sipes IG, Slocumb ML, Perry DF, Carter DE. 4,4'-Dichlorobiphenyl: distribution, metabolism, and excretion in the dog and monkey. *Toxicol Appl Pharmacol* 1980;55:554–563.
16. Safe S. Toxicology, structure-function relationship, and human and environmental health impacts of polychlorinated biphenyls: progress and problems. *Environ Health Perspect* 1992;100:259–268.
17. Sipes IG, Schnellmann RG. Biotransformation of PCBs: metabolic pathways and mechanisms. *Environmental Toxin Series* 1987;1:97–110.
18. Ueng T, Alvares AP. Selective induction and inhibition of liver and lung cytochrome P-450–dependent monooxygenases by the PCBs mixture, Aroclor 1016. *Toxicology* 1985;35:83–94.
19. Abdel-Hamid FM, Moore JA, Matthews HB. Comparative study of 3,4,3',4'-tetrachlorobiphenyls in male and female rats, and female monkeys. *J Toxicol Environ Health* 1981;7:181–191.
20. McConnell EE. Comparative toxicity of PCBs and related compounds in various species of animals. *Environ Health Perspect* 1985;60:29–33.
21. Chu I, Villeneuve DC, Yagminas A, et al. Toxicity of PCB 77 (3,3',4,4'-tetrachlorobiphenyl) and PCB 118 (2,3',4,4',5-pentachlorobiphenyl) in the rat following subchronic dietary exposure. *Fundamen Appl Toxicol* 1995;26:282–292.
22. Dubois M, DeWaziers I, Thome JP, Kremers P. P450 induction by Aroclor 1254 and 3,3',4,4'-tetrachlorobiphenyl in cultured hepatocytes from rat, quail and man: interspecies comparison. *Comp Biochem Physiol C Pharmacol Toxicol Endocrinol* 1996;113C:51–59.
23. Hong C, Bush B, Xiao J, Qiao H. Toxic potential of non-ortho and mono-ortho coplanar polychlorinated biphenyls in Aroclors, seals, and humans. *Arch Environ Contam Toxicol* 1993;25:118–123.
24. Steele G, Stehr-Green P, Welty E. Estimates of the biological half-life of polychlorinated biphenyls in human serum. *N Engl J Med* 1986;314:926–927.
25. Phillips DL, Smith AB, Burse VW, Steele GK, Needham LL, Hannon WH. Half-life of polychlorinated biphenyls in occupationally exposed workers. *Arch Environ Health* 1989;44:351–354.
26. Yakushiji T, Watanabe I, Kuwabara K, et al. Rate of decrease and half-life of polychlorinated biphenyls (PCBs) in the blood of mothers and their children occupationally exposed to PCBs. *Arch Environ Contam Toxicol* 1984;13:341–345.
27. Chen PH, Luo ML. Comparative rates of elimination of some individual polychlorinated biphenyls from the blood of PCB-poisoned patients in Taiwan. *Food Chem Toxicol* 1982;20:417–425.
28. Ryan JJ, Levesque D, Panopio LG, Sun WF, Masuda Y, Kuroki H. Elimination of polychlorinated dibenzofurans (PCDFs) and polychlorinated biphenyls (PCBs) from human blood in the Yusho and Yu-Cheng rice oil poisonings. *Arch Environ Contam Toxicol* 1993;24:504–512.
29. Shirai JH, Kissel JC. Uncertainty in estimated half-lives of PCBs in humans: impact on exposure assessment. *Sci Total Environ* 1996;187:199–210.
30. Wolff MS, Fischbein A, Thornton J, Rice C, Lilis R, Selikoff IJ. Body burden of polychlorinated biphenyls among persons employed in capacitor manufacturing. *Int Arch Occup Environ Health* 1982;49:199–208.
31. Kreiss K, Roberts C. Serial PBB levels, PCB levels, and clinical chemistries in Michigan's PBB cohort. *Arch Environ Health* 1982;37:141–147.
32. Kreiss K. Studies on populations exposed to polychlorinated biphenyls. *Environ Health Perspect* 1985;60:193–199.
33. Mack GA, Mohadjer L. Baseline estimates and time trends for beta-benzene hexachloride, hexachlorobenzene, and polychlorinated biphenyls in human adipose tissue 1970-1983. Washington: US Environmental Protection Agency, Office of Toxic Substances, Exposure Evaluation Division, 1985:i-A–30.
34. Chase KC, Wong O, Thomas D, Berney BW, Simon RK. Clinical and metabolic abnormalities associated with occupational exposure to polychlorinated biphenyls (PCBs). *J Occup Med* 1982;24:109–114.
35. Lordo RA, Dinh KT, Schwemberger JG. Semivolatile organic compounds in adipose tissue: estimated averages for the U.S. population and selected subpopulations. *Am J Public Health* 1996;86:1253–1259.
36. Mes J. PCBs in human populations. In: Waid JS, ed. *PCBs and the environment.* Boca Raton, FL: CRC Press, 1987:39–61.
37. Smith AB, Schloemer J, Lowry LK, et al. Metabolic and health consequences of occupational exposure to polychlorinated biphenyls. *Br J Ind Med* 1982;39:361–369.
38. Emmett EA, Maroni M, Schmith JM, Levin BK, Jefferys J. Studies of transformer repair workers exposed to PCBs. I. study design, PCB concentrations, questionnaire, and clinical examination results. *Am J Ind Med* 1988;13:415–427.
39. Wolff MS, Thornton J, Fischbein A, Lilis R, Selikoff IJ. Disposition of polychlorinated biphenyl congeners in occupationally exposed persons. *Toxicol Appl Pharmacol* 1982;62:294–306.
40. Brown JF Jr, Lawton RW. Polychlorinated biphenyl (PCB) partitioning between adipose tissue and serum. *Bull Environ Contam Toxicol* 1984;33:277–280.
41. Yakushiji T, Watanabe I, Kuwabara K, et al. Long-term studies of the excretion of polychlorinated biphenyls (PCBs) through the mother's milk of an occupationally exposed worker. *Arch Environ Contam Toxicol* 1978;7:493–504.
42. Frank R, Rasper J, Smout MS, Braun HE. Organochlorine residues in adipose tissues, blood and milk from Ontario residents, 1976–1985. *Can J Public Health* 1988;79:150–158.
43. Mussalo-Rauhamaa H, Pyysalo H, Antervo K. Relation between the content of organochlorine compounds in Finnish human milk and characteristics of the mothers. *J Toxicol Environ Health* 1988;25:1–19.
44. Albers JMC, Kreis IA, Liem AKD, van Zoonen P. Factors that influence the level of contamination of human milk with poly-chlorinated organic compounds. *Arch Environ Contam Toxicol* 1996;30:285–291.
45. Tryphonas L, Charbonneau S, Tryphonas H, et al. Comparative aspects of Aroclor 1254 toxicity in adult cynomolgus and rhesus monkeys: a pilot study. *Arch Environ Contam Toxicol* 1986;15:159–169.
46. Gillette DM, Corey RD, Helferich WG, et al. Comparative toxicology of tetrachlorobiphenyls in mink and rats. *Fundamen Appl Toxicol* 1987;8:5–14.
47. Allen JR, Carstens LA, Barsotti DA. Residual effects of short-term, low-level exposure of nonhuman primates to polychlorinated biphenyls. *Toxicol Appl Pharmacol* 1974;30:440–451.
48. Allen JR, Abrahamson LJ, Norback DH. Biological effects of polychlorinated biphenyls and triphenyls on the subhuman primate. *Environ Res* 1973;6:344–354.
49. Seegal RF, Bush B, Brosch KO. Polychlorinated biphenyls induce regional changes in brain norepinephrine concentrations in adult rats. *Neurotoxicology* 1985;6:13–24.
50. Rosin DL, Martin BR. Neurochemical and behavioral effects of polychlorinated biphenyls in mice. *Neurotoxicology* 1981;2:749–764.
51. Silkworth JB, Grabstein EM. Polychlorinated biphenyl immunotoxicity: dependence on isomer planarity and the Ah gene complex. *Toxicol Appl Pharmacol* 1982;65:109–115.
52. Silkworth JB, Antrim L, Kaminsky LS. Correlations between polychlorinated biphenyl immunotoxicity, the aromatic hydrocarbon locus, and liver microsomal enzyme induction in C57BL/6 and DBA/2 mice. *Toxicol Appl Pharmacol* 1984;75:156–165.
53. Kimbrough RD, Squire RA, Linder RE, Strandberg JD, Montali RJ, Burse VW. Induction of liver tumors in Sherman strain female rats by polychlorinated biphenyl Aroclor 1260. *J Natl Cancer Inst* 1975;55:1453–1459.
54. Norback DH, Weltman RH. Polychlorinated biphenyl induction of hepatocellular carcinoma in the Sprague-Dawley rat. *Environ Health Perspect* 1985;60:97–105.
55. Schaeffer E, Greim H, Goessner W. Pathology of chronic polychlorinated biphenyl (PCB) feeding in rats. *Toxicol Appl Pharmacol* 1984;75:278–288.
56. Liddell FDK, Gibbs GW, McDonald JC. Radiological changes and fibre exposure in chrysotile workers aged 60–69 years at Thetford mines. *Ann Occup Hyg* 1982;26:889–898.
57. Ito N, Nagasaki H, Makiura S, Arai M. Histopathological studies on liver tumorigenesis in rats treated with polychlorinated biphenyls. *Gann* 1974; 65:545–549.
58. Moore JA, Hardisty JF, Banas DA, Smith MA. A comparison of liver tumor diagnoses from seven PCB studies in rats. *Regul Toxicol Pharmacol* 1994;20:362–370.
59. US Environmental Protection Agency (EPA). *PCBs: cancer dose-response assessment and application to environmental mixtures.* Washington: EPA, 1996:i–77.
60. Oesterle D, Deml E. Promoting effect of polychlorinated biphenyls on development of enzyme-altered islands in livers of weaning and adult rats. *J Can Res Clin Oncol* 1983;105:141–147.
61. Makiura S, Aoe H, Sugihara S, Hirao K, Arai M, Ito N. Inhibitory effect of polychlorinated biphenyls on liver tumorigenesis in rats treated with 3'-methyl-4-dimethylaminoazobenzene, *N*-2-fluoroenylacetamide, and diethylnitrosamine. *J Natl Cancer Inst* 1974;53:1233.
62. Nishizumi M. Effect of phenobarbital, dichlorodiphenyltrichloroethane, and polychlorinated biphenyls on diethylnitrosamine-induced hepatocarcinogenesis. *Gann* 1979;70:835–837.
63. Nishizumi M. Radioautographic evidence for absorption of polychlorinated biphenyls through the skin. *Ind Health* 1976;14:41–44.
64. Nishizumi M. Reduction of diethylnitrosamine-induced hepatoma in rats exposed to polychlorinated biphenyls through their dams. *Gann* 1980; 71:910–912.
65. Deml E, Oesterle D, Wiebel FJ. Benzo[a]pyrene initiates enzyme-altered islands in the liver of adult rats following single pretreatment and promotion with polychlorinated biphenyls. *Cancer Lett* 1983;19:301–304.
66. Yoshimura H, Yoshihara S, Koga N, et al. Inductive effect on hepatic enzymes and toxicity of congeners of PCBs and PCDFs. *Environ Health Perspect* 1985;59:113–119.
67. Edelman DA. Exposure to asbestos and the risk of gastrointestinal cancer: a reassessment. *Br J Ind Med* 1988;45:75–82.
68. Preston BD, Van Miller JP, Moore RW, Allen JR. promoting effects of polychlorinated biphenyls (Aroclor 1254) and polychlorinated dibenzofuran-free Aroclor 1254 on diethylnitrosamine-induced tumorgenesis in a rat. *J Natl Cancer Inst* 1981;66:509–515.
69. Pereira MA, Herren SL, Britt AL, Khoury MM. Promotion by polychlorinated biphenyls of enzyme altered foci rat liver. *Cancer Lett* 1982;15:185–190.
70. Kimura NT, Kanematsu T, Baba T. Polychlorinated biphenyl(s) as a promotor in experimental hepatocarcinogenesis in rats. *Z Krebsforsch Klin Onkol Cancer Res Clin Oncol* 1976;87:257–266.
71. Anderson LM, Logsdon D, Ruskie S, et al. Promotion by polychlorinated biphenyls of lung and liver tumors in mice. *Carcinogenesis* 1994;15:2245–2248.
72. Hayes MA, Roberts E, Safe SH, Farber E, Cameron RG. Influences of different polychlorinated biphenyls on cytocidal, mitoinhibitory, and nodule-selecting activities of *N*-2-fluorenylacetamide in rat liver. *J Natl Cancer Inst* 1986;76:683–691.

73. Hori M, Fujita K, Yamashiro K, et al. Influences of polychlorinated biphenyls (PCB) and PCB-like chemicals on 20-methylcholanthrene-induced mouse skin carcinogenesis. *Fukuoka Igaku Zasshi* 1985;76:92–98.
74. Emmett EA, Maroni M, Jefferys J, Schmith J, Levin BK, Alvares A. Studies of transformer repair workers exposed to PCBs: II. Results of clinical laboratory investigations. *Am J Ind Med* 1988;14:47–62.
74a. US Environmental Protection Agency. *PCBs: Cancer dose-response assessment and application to environmental mixtures*. Washington: US Environmental Protection Agency, National Center for Environmental Assessment, Office of Research and Development, September 1996:1–83.
75. James RC, Busch H, Tamburro CH, Roberts SM, Schell JD, Harbison RD. Polychlorinated biphenyl exposure and human disease. *J Occup Med* 1993;35:136–148.
76. Swanson GM, Ratcliffe HE, Fischer L. Human exposure to polychlorinated biphenyls (PCBs): a critical assessment of the evidence for adverse health effects. *Regul Toxicol Pharmacol* 1995;21:136–150.
77. Coenraads P, Brouwer A, Kees O, Tang N. Chloracne: some recent issues. *Dermatol Clin* 1994;12:569–576.
78. Ouw HE, Simpson GR, Siyali DS. Use and health effects of Aroclor 1242, a polychlorinated biphenyl, in an electrical industry. *Arch Environ Health* 1976;31:189–194.
79. Maroni M, Colombi A, Arbosti G, Cantoni S, Foa V. Occupational exposure to polychlorinated biphenyls in electrical workers. II: health effects. *Br J Ind Med* 1981;38:55–60.
80. Good CK. A cutaneous eruption in marine electricians due to certain chlorinated naphthalenes and diphenyls. *Arch Dermatol Syph* 1943;48:251–257.
81. Fischbein A, Rizzo JN, Solomon SJ, Wolff MS. Oculodermatological findings in workers with occupational exposure to polychlorinated biphenyls (PCBs). *Br J Ind Med* 1985;42:426–430.
82. Lawton RW, Ross MR, Feingold J, Brown JF Jr. Effects of PCB exposure on biochemical and hematological findings in capacitor workers. *Environ Health Perspect* 1985;60:165–184.
83. Kreiss K, Zack MM, Kimbrough RD, Needham LL, Smrek AL, Jones BT. Cross-sectional study of a community with exceptional exposure to DDT. *JAMA* 1981;245:1926–1930.
84. Baker EL, Landrigan PJ, Glueck CJ, et al. Metabolic consequences of exposure to polychlorinated biphenyls (PCB) in sewage sludge. *Am J Epidemiol* 1980;112:553–563.
85. Emmett EA. Polychlorinated biphenyl exposure and effects in transformer repair workers. *Environ Health Perspect* 1985;60:185–192.
86. Guo YL, Emmett EA, Pellizzari ED, Rohde CA. Influence of serum cholesterol and albumin on partitioning of PCB congeners between human serum and adipose tissue. *Toxicol Appl Pharmacol* 1987;87:48–56.
87. Brown DP. Mortality of workers exposed to polychlorinated biphenyls: an update. *Arch Environ Health* 1987;42:333–339.
88. Bertazzi PA, Riboldi L, Pesatori A, Radice L, Zocchetti C. Cancer mortality of capacitor manufacturing workers. *Am J Ind Med* 1987;11:165–176.
89. Gustavsson P, Hogstedt C, Rappe C. Short-term mortality and cancer incidence in capacitor manufacturing workers exposed to polychlorinated biphenyls (PCBs). *Am J Ind Med* 1986;10:341–344.
90. Fischbein A, Wolff MS, Lilis R, Thornton J, Selikoff IJ. Clinical findings among PCB-exposed capacitor manufacturing workers. *Ann N Y Acad Sci* 1979;320:703–715.
91. Takamatsu M, Oki M, Maeda K, Inoue Y, Hirayama H, Yoshizuka K. PCBs in blood of workers exposed to PCBs and their health status. *Am J Ind Med* 1984;5:59–68.
92. Stehr-Green PA, Welty E, Steele G, Steinberg K. Evaluation of potential health effects associated with serum polychlorinated biphenyl levels. *Environ Health Perspect* 1986;70:255–259.
93. Kreiss K, Zack MM, Kimbrough RD, Needham LL, Smrek AL, Jones BT. Association of blood pressure and polychlorinated biphenyl levels. *JAMA* 1981;245:2505–2509.
94. Stehr-Green PA, Ross D, Liddle J. A pilot study of serum polychlorinated biphenyl levels in persons at high risk of exposure in residential and occupational environments. *Arch Environ Health* 1986;41:240–244.
95. Acquavella JF, Hanis NM, Nicolich MJ, Phillips SC. Assessment of clinical, metabolic, dietary, and occupational correlations with serum polychlorinated biphenyl levels among employees at an electrical capacitor manufacturing plant. *J Occup Med* 1986;28:1177–1180.
96. Akagi K, Okumura M. Association of blood pressure and PCB level in yusho patients. *Environ Health Perspect* 1985;59:37–39.
97. Warshaw R, Fischbein A, Thornton J, Miller A, Selikoff IJ. Decrease in vital capacity in PCB-exposed workers in a capacitor manufacturing facility. *Ann N Y Acad Sci* 1979;320:277–283.
98. Lawton RW, Ross MR, Feingold J. Spirometric findings in capacitor workers occupationally exposed to polychlorinated biphenyls (PCBs). *J Occup Med* 1986;28:453–456.
99. Dunn JT, Taylor SM, Elliott SJ, Walter SD. Psychosocial effects of PCB contamination and remediation: the case of Smithville, Ontario. *Soc Sci Med* 1994;39:1093–1104.
100. Fein GG, Jacobson JL, Jacobson SW, Schwartz PM, Dowler JK. Prenatal exposure to polychlorinated biphenyls: effects on birth size and gestational age. *J Pediatr* 1984;105:315–320.
101. Gladen B, Rogan WJ, Hardy P, Thullen J, Tingelstad J, Tully M. Development after exposure to polychlorinated biphenyls and dichlorodiphenyl dichloroethene transplacentally and through human milk. *J Pediatr* 1988;113:991–995.
102. Taylor PR, Stelma JM, Lawrence CE. The relation of polychlorinated biphenyls to birth weight and gestational age in the offspring of occupationally exposed mothers. *Am J Epidemiol* 1989;129:395–406.
103. Ron M, Cucos B, Rosenn B, Hochner-Celnikier D, Hadani-Ever P, Pines A. Maternal and fetal serum levels of organochlorine compounds in cases of premature rupture of membranes. *Acta Obstet Gynecol Scand* 1988;67:695–697.
104. Mendola P, Buck GM, Vena JE, Zielezny M, Sever LE. Consumption of PCB-contaminated sport fish and risk of spontaneous fetal death. *Environ Health Perspect* 1995;103:498–502.
105. Jacobson JL, Jacobson SW. Intellectual impairment in children exposed to polychlorinated biphenyls in utero. *N Engl J Med* 1996;335:783–789.
106. Huisman M, Koopman-Esseboom C, Fidler V, et al. Perinatal exposure to polychlorinated biphenyls and dioxins and its effect on neonatal neurological development. *Early Hum Dev* 1995;41:111–127.
107. Kunita N, Kashimoto T, Miyata H, Fukushima S, Hori S, Obana H. Causal agents of yusho. *Am J Ind Med* 1984;5:45–58.
108. Kashimoto T, Miyata H, Kunita S, et al. Role of polychlorinated dibenzofuran in yusho (PCB poisoning). *Arch Environ Health* 1981;36:321–326.
109. Masuda Y, Yoshimura H. Polychlorinated biphenyls and dibenzofurans in patients with yusho and their toxicological significance: a review. *Am J Ind Med* 1984;5:31–44.
110. Nagayama J, Masuda Y, Kuratsune M. Determination of polychlorinated dibenzofurans in tissues of patients with yusho. *Food Cosmet Toxicol* 1977;15:195–198.
111. Kashimoto T, Miyata H, Kunita N. The presence of polychlorinated quaterphenyls in the tissues of yusho victims. *Food Cosmet Toxicol* 1981;19:335–340.
112. Wong C, Chen C, Cheng P, Chen P. Mucocutaneous manifestations of polychlorinated biphenyls (PCB) poisoning: a study of 122 cases in Taiwan. *Br J Dermatol* 1982;107:317–323.
113. Lu Y, Wong P. Dermatological, medical, and laboratory findings of patients in Taiwan and their treatments. *Am J Ind Med* 1984;5:81–115.
114. Chia L, Chu F. Neurological studies on polychlorinated biphenyl (PCB)-poisoned patients. *Am J Ind Med* 1984;5:117–126.
115. Hirota Y, Hirota T. Blood polychlorinated biphenyls and manifestation of symptoms in chronic "Yusho" patients. *Fukuoka Igaku Zasshi* 1995;86:247–255.
116. Hsu MM, Mak C, Hsu C. Follow-up of skin manifestations in Yu-Cheng children. *Br J Dermatol* 1995;132:427–432.
117. Lai T, Guo Y, Yu M, Ko H, Hsu C. Cognitive development in Yucheng children. *Chemosphere* 1994;29:2405–2411.
118. Guo YL, Chen Y, Yu M, Hsu C-C. Early development of Yu-Cheng children born seven to twelve years after the Taiwan PCB outbreak. *Chemosphere* 1994;29:2395–2402.
119. Chen YJ, Guo Y, Hsu C, Rogan WJ. Cognitive development of Yu-Cheng ("oil disease") children prenatally exposed to heat-degraded PCBs. *JAMA* 1992;268:3213–3218.
120. Yu MM, Hsu C, Guo YL, Chen S, Luo J. Disordered behavior in the early-born Taiwan Yu-Cheng children. *Chemosphere* 1994;29:2413–2422.
121. Yu M, Guo YL, Hsu C-C, Rogan WJ. Increased mortality from chronic liver disease and cirrhosis 13 years after the Taiwan "Yu-Cheng" ("oil disease") incident. *Am J Ind Med* 1997;31:172–175.
122. Hsieh S, Yen Y, Lan S, Hsieh C, Lee C. A cohort study on mortality and exposure to polychlorinated biphenyls. *Arch Environ Health* 1996;51:417–424.
123. Sinks T, Steele G, Smith AB, Watkins K, Shults RA. Mortality among workers exposed to polychlorinated biphenyls. *Am J Epidemiol* 1992;136:389–398.
124. Mazzuckelli LF, Schulte PA. Notification of workers about an excess of malignant melanoma. *Am J Ind Med* 1993;23:85–91.
125. Falck F, Ricci F, Wolff MS, Godbold J, Deckers P. Pesticides and polychlorinated biphenyl residues in human breast lipids and their relation to breast cancer. *Arch Environ Health* 1992;47:143–146.
126. Unger M, Kiaer H, Blichert-Toft M, Olsen J, Clausen J. Organochlorine compounds in human breast fat from deceased with and without breast cancer and in a biopsy material from newly diagnosed patients undergoing breast surgery. *Environ Res* 1984;34:24–28.
127. Dewailly E, Dodin S, Verreault R, et al. High organochlorine body burden in women with estrogen receptor-positive breast cancer. *J Natl Cancer Inst* 1994;86:232–234.
128. Wolff MS, Toniolo PG, Lee EW, Rivera M, Dubin N. *Blood levels of organochlorine residues and risk of breast cancer.* J Natl Cancer Inst 1993;85:648–652.
129. Krieger N, Wolff MS, Hiatt RA, Rivera M, Vogelman J, Orentreich O. Breast cancer and serum organochlorines: a prospective study among white, black, and Asian women. *J Natl Cancer Inst* 1994;86:589–599.
130. Adami H, Lipworth L, Titus-Ernstoff L, et al. Organochlorine compounds and estrogen-related cancers in women. *Cancer Causes Control* 1995;6:551–566.
131. Wong A, Basrur P, Safe S. The metabolically mediated DNA damage and subsequent DNA repair by 4-chlorobiphenyl in Chinese hamster ovary cells. *Res Commun Chem Pathol Pharmacol* 1979;24:543.
132. Morales NM, Matthews HB. In vivo binding of 2,3,6,2',3',6'-hexachlorobiphenyls and 2,4,5,2',4',5'-hexachlorobiphenyls to mouse liver macromolecules. *Chem Biol Interact* 1979;27:99–110.
133. Oakley GG, Robertson LW, Gupta RC. Analysis of polychlorinated biphenyl-DNA adducts by 32P-postlabeling. *Carcinogenesis* 1996;17:109–114.
134. McLean MR, Robertson LW, Gupta RC. Detection of PCB adducts by the 32P-postlabeling technique. *Chem Res Toxicol* 1996;9:165–171.
135. Anderson HA, Lilis R, Selikoff IJ, Rosenman KD, Freedman S, Valciukas JA. Unanticipated prevalence of symptoms among dairy farmers in Michigan and Wisconsin. *Environ Health Perspect* 1978;23:217–226.

136. Bahn AK, Mills JL, Snyder PJ, et al. Hypothyroidism in workers exposed to polybrominated biphenyls. *N Engl J Med* 1980;302:31–33.
137. Bekesi JG, Roboz JP, Fischbein A, Mason P. Immunotoxicology: environmental contamination by polybrominated biphenyls and immune dysfunction among residents of the state of Michigan. *Cancer Detect Prev Suppl* 1987;1:29–37.
138. Silva J, Kauffman CA, Simon DG, et al. Lymphocyte function in human exposed to polybrominated biphenyls. *J Reticuloendothel Soc* 1979;26:341–347.
139. Henck JW, Mattsson JL, Rezabek DH, Carlson CL, Rech RH. Developmental neurotoxicity of polybrominated biphenyls. *Neurotoxicol Teratol* 1994;16:391–399.
140. Borlakoglu JT, Wilkins JPG. Correlations between the molecular structures of polyhalogenated biphenyls and their metabolism by hepatic microsomal monooxygenases. *Comp Biochem Physiol Pharmacol Toxicol Endocrinol* 1993;105C:113–117.
141. Merrill JC, Beck DJ, Kaminski DA, Li AP. Polybrominated biphenyl induction of cytochrome P450 mixed function oxidase activity in primary rat and human hepatocytes. *Toxicology* 1995;99:147–152.
142. Kimbrough RD, Groce DF, Korver MP, Burse VW. Induction of liver tumors in female Sherman strain rats by polybrominated biphenyls. *J Natl Cancer Inst* 1981;66:535–542.
143. Sleight S. Effects of PCBs and related compounds on hepatocarcinogenesis in rats and mice. *Environ Health Perspect* 1985;60:35–39.
144. Rangga-Tabbu CR, Sleight SD. Development of preneoplastic lesions in the liver and nasal epithelium of rats initiated with *N*-nitrosodimethylamine or *N*-nitrosopyrrolidine and promoted with polybrominated biphenyls. *Food Chem Toxicol* 1992;30:921–926.
145. Rezabek MS, Sleight SD, Jensen RK. Short-term oral administration of polybrominated biphenyls enhances the development of hepatic enzymes: altered foci in initiated rats. *J Toxic Environ Health* 1987;20:347–356.
146. Agency for Toxic Substances and Disease Registry. *Toxicological profile for polychlorinated biphenyls*. Atlanta: US Department of Health and Human Services, Public Health Service, ATSDR, September 1997.
147. Stewart FP, Smith AG. Metabolism of the "mixed" cytochrome P-450 inducer hexachlorobenzene by rat liver microsomes. *Biochem Pharmacol* 1986;35:2163–2170.
148. Stewart FP, Smith AG. Metabolism and covalent binding of hexachlorobenzene by isolated male and female rat hepatocytes. *Biochem Pharmacol* 1987;36:2232–2234.
149. Tanaka A, Sato M, Tsuchiya T, Adachi T, Niimura T, Yamaha T. Excretion, distribution, and metabolism of 1,2,4-trichlorobenzene in rats. *Arch Toxicol* 1986;59:82–88.
150. Ommen BV, Adang AEP, Brader L, Posthumus MA, Muller F, Van Bladeren PJ. The microsomal metabolism of hexachlorobenzene. *Biochem Pharmacol* 1986;35:3233–3238.
151. Burton MAS, Bennett BG. Exposure of man to environmental hexachlorobenzene (HCB): an exposure commitment assessment. *Sci Total Environ* 1987;66:137–146.
152. Peters H, Cripps D, Gocmen A, Bryan G, Erturk E, Morris C. Turkish epidemic hexachlorobenzene porphyria. *Ann N Y Acad Sci* 1986;514:183–190.
153. Zapata-Gayon C, Zapata-Gayon N, Gonzalez-Angulo A. Clastogenic chromosomal aberrations in 26 individuals accidentally exposed to ortho dichlorobenzene vapors in the National Medical Center in Mexico City. *Arch Environ Health* 1982;37:231–235.
154. Kiraly J, Szentesi I, Ruzicska M, Czeize A. Chromosome studies in workers producing organophosphate insecticides. *Arch Environ Contam Toxicol* 1979;8:309–319.
155. Brusick DJ. Genotoxicity of hexachlorobenzene and other chlorinated benzenes. *Sci Publications* 1985;77:393–397(abst).

CHAPTER 61

Polychlorodibenzodioxins and Polychlorodibenzofurans

John S. Andrews, Jr., Larry L. Needham, and Donald G. Patterson, Jr.

SOURCES AND PRODUCTION

Polychlorinated dibenzo-para-dioxins (polychlorinated dibenzo-*p*-dioxins, or PCDDs) and polychlorinated dibenzofurans (PCDFs) each have two or more chlorine atoms attached to a triple-ring structure as a nucleus. In PCDDs, two benzene rings are connected through a pair of oxygen atoms. In PCDFs, two benzene rings are connected through an oxygen atom and a carbon-to-carbon bond.

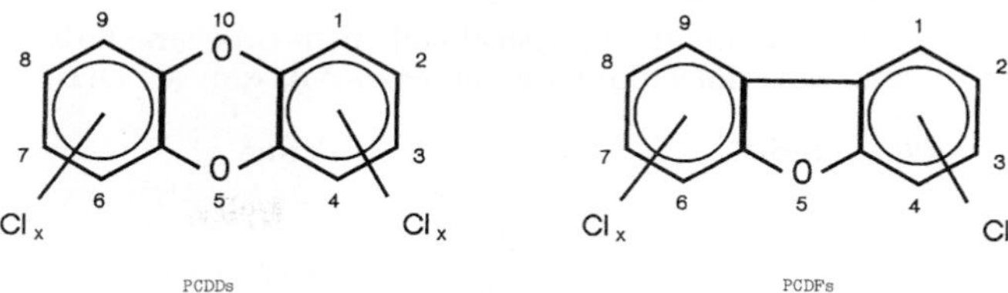

Figure 61-1. General structures of polychlorinated dibenzo-*p*-dioxins (PCDDs) and polychlorinated dibenzofurans (PCDFs). The carbon atoms are numbered using standard nomenclature. Chlorine atoms (Cl_X) may be substituted for hydrogen atoms at any of the numbered carbon atoms.

A chlorine atom may be substituted for hydrogen on any carbon atom in the two benzene rings. Theoretically, 74 different PCDDs and 134 different PCDFs are possible. The general structures of these compounds and the numbering of their atoms are shown in Figure 61-1.

The chemical names of these compounds depend on the number and location of the chlorine atom substitutions for hydrogen atoms. The common name for the PCDDs is *dioxins* and the common name for PCDFs is *furans*.

PCDDs and PCDFs exist as contaminants of other products and as contaminants adhering to particulates. None of these compounds is known to be made by living organisms. Because of their high lipid solubility, these compounds are easily incorporated into the lipid-containing tissues of fish, animals, and humans.

Physical and chemical characteristics of each PCDD and PCDF are slightly different. For many of the congeners, no data are available. The physical and chemical characteristics of the biologically significant PCDDs and PCDFs (those with four or more chlorine atoms) are summarized in Table 61-1. The known physical and chemical characteristics of the individual PCDDs and PCDFs are given in the Agency for Toxic Substances and Disease Registry's *Toxicological profile for chlorinated dibenzo*-p-*dioxins* (1).

EXPOSURE SOURCES: OCCUPATIONAL AND ENVIRONMENTAL

PCDDs and PCDFs are not produced for commercial purposes but occur as trace contaminants in several chemical processes, primarily during the synthesis of chlorinated phenols; for example, 2,3,7,8-tetrachlorodibenzo-*p*-dioxin (2,3,7,8-TCDD) is a byproduct in the synthesis of 2,4,5-trichlorophenol, an intermediate compound formed during the production of 2,4,5-trichlorophenoxyacetic acid and hexachlorophene. Trace levels of PCDDs and PCDFs are also formed during the bleaching of wood pulp to make white paper and white paper products, the incineration of chlorine-containing waste materials, and the combustion of leaded gasoline. PCDDs and PCDFs have also been found in soil, food (e.g., meat, fish, dairy products), human milk (2), and cigarette smoke (3). From specimens collected in fiscal year 1987 (October 1, 1986, through September 30, 1987), Orban and coworkers (4) estimated that the U.S. population had an average adipose tissue concentration of 5.38 pg 2,3,7,8-TCDD per g of lipid [1 pg = 1×10^{-12} g, expressed in parts per trillion (ppt)].

CLINICAL TOXICOLOGY

Route of Exposure

Ingestion, inhalation, and dermal absorption are all thought to be routes of exposure to PCDDs and PCDFs. Exposure for most individuals is small, comes from a variety of sources, and is via a vari-

TABLE 61-1. Summary of physical and chemical characteristics of tetra-octa polychlorinated dibenzo-*p*-dioxins (PCDDs)

Characteristic	Value
Molecular weight	322.0–459.8
Color	Colorless, white, or no data
Physical state	Solid, crystalline solid, or no data
Melting point	175°–332°C
Boiling point	446.5°–510°C. No data for penta or hexa PCDDs.
Density	
at 20°C	No data
at 25°C	1.827 g/mL for 2,3,7,8-TCDD; others unknown
Odor	No data
Odor threshold	
Water	No data
Air	No data
Water solubility	
at 20°C	0.4×10^{-6} to 1.9×10^{-3} mg/L
at 25°C	2.27×10^{-9} to 6.3×10^{-4} mg/L or no data
Organic solvents	For 2,3,7,8-TCDD: Agent Orange, *o*-dichlorobenzene, chlorobenzene, benzene, chloroform, acetone For octa CDD: acetic acid, anisole, chloroform, dioxane, *o*-dichlorobenzene, diphenyl oxide, pyridine, xylene For others: unknown
Partition coefficients	
Log K_{ow}	6.6–13.37 or no data
Log K_{oc}	No data
Vapor pressure at 25°C	8.25×10^{-13} to 4.0×10^{-3} mm Hg
Henry's law constant	1.31×10^{-6} to 1.0×10^{-4} atm•m³/mole
Autoignition temperature	No data
Flashpoint	No data
Flammability limits	No data
Conversion factors in air; at 25°C, 760 mm Hg	Tetra: 1 mg/m³ = 0.0759 ppm; 1 ppm = 13.17 mg/m³ Penta: 1 mg/m³ = 0.0686 ppm; 1 ppm = 14.58 mg/m³ Hexa: 1 mg/m³ = 0.0625 ppm; 1 ppm = 15.99 mg/m³ Hepta: 1 mg/m³ = 0.0575 ppm; 1 ppm = 17.39 mg/m³ Octa: 1 mg/m³ = 0.0532 ppm; 1 ppm = 18.81 mg/m³
Explosive limits	No data

atm•m³, cubic meters atmosphere; CDD, chlorinated dibenzo-*p*-dioxin; ppm, parts per million; TCDD, tetrachlorodibenzo-*p*-dioxin.
Adapted from ref. 1, with permission.

ety of exposure routes. It is generally accepted that approximately 98% of human exposure comes from food (5). Exposure has also occurred from the use of hexachlorophene, from herbicide use, from exposure to PCDD- and PCDF-containing industrial wastes, from incinerators, and from industrial and transportation incidents. In occupational settings, exposure has occurred in chemical manufacturing processes and from handling the wastes from these processes. The predicted average daily intake of 2,3,7,8-TCDD has been estimated at 0.047 ng per day (1 ng = 1×10^{-9} g) (Table 61-2).

Data are incomplete on the absorption of PCDDs and PCDFs in humans from various routes of exposure. A study of PCDD and PCDF absorption in four breast-fed human infants showed that, for most congeners, the absorption is found to be over 95% (6). One animal study showed that bioavailability is strongly influenced by the matrix in which the compound occurs (7).

TABLE 61-2. Predicted average daily intake of 2,3,7,8-tetrachlorodibenzo-*p*-dioxin in the United States

Source	Daily intake (ng/day)	Percentage of total daily intake
Air	0.001	2
Water	6.5×10^{-6}	<0.01
Food	0.046	98
Produce	(0.005)	(11)
Milk	(0.013)	(27)
Meat	(0.023)	(50)
Fish	(0.005)	(10)
Total intake	0.047	100

Adapted from refs. 1 and 15, with permission.

Although the absorption of 2,3,7,8-TCDD from oily soil at Times Beach, Missouri, was shown to be greater than 50%, absorption from nonoily New Jersey soil was less than 1% (8). Nonetheless, many risk assessments assume 100% absorption, which introduces a safety factor.

The toxicity of PCDDs and PCDFs differs greatly depending on the location and number of chlorine atom substitutions in the compound. 2,3,7,8-TCDD, which is the most toxic of the known congeners in animals, is an unusual molecule because it is symmetric across both the horizontal and vertical axes. It is a very stable, lipophilic compound that lacks reactive functional groups. Using 2,3,7,8-TCDD as a reference, the toxicity of the chlorinated dibenzo-*p*-dioxins and dibenzofurans decreases with both a decreasing and an increasing number of chlorine atoms. Compounds with chlorine substitutions at the 2, 3, 7, and 8 positions in each isomer group are the most toxic.

The relative potency of these compounds in various cell and animal models has been assessed, and Toxicity Equivalency Factors (TEFs) have been derived. The TEF approach has been successful in predicting the effects in animal studies (9). Whereas 2,3,7,8-TCDD has a TEF of 1, other PCDDs and PCDFs have TEFs that are some fraction of 1. For example, pentachlorodibenzo-*p*-dioxins with chlorine substituted at 2, 3, 7, 8, and one additional position have TEFs of 0.5 (Table 61-3). The total toxic equivalency of a mixture of PCDDs and PCDFs is the sum of the products of the concentration and TEF for each congener in the mixture. Estimated average daily total toxic equivalencies from PCDDs and PCDFs from a typical state-of-the-art municipal waste incinerator have been estimated at 0.0003 ng per day (Table 61-4).

Distribution

In the steady state, PCDDs and PCDFs are thought to equilibrate in the body based on the tissues' lipid content. Serum 2,3,7,8-TCDD levels on a lipid-adjusted basis have been found to be highly correlated with lipid 2,3,7,8-TCDD levels (11). Levels of various PCDDs and PCDFs in the general U.S. population are shown in Table 61-5. Tissues with less lipid, such as the liver, have been found to have one-tenth the 2,3,7,8-TCDD concentration as adipose tissue on a total weight basis (12). The liver fraction of the total PCDD and PCDF body burden decreases as the overall body concentration of PCDD and PCDF decreases (13). For a given body burden, the adipose tissue concentrations vary in a manner inversely proportional to the mass of the adipose tissues.

TABLE 61-3. Toxicity equivalency factors (TEFs) of polychlorinated dibenzo-*p*-dioxins (PCDDs) and polychlorinated dibenzofurans (PCDFs)

PCDDs	TEFs[a]
DiCDDs	0.001
TriCDDs	0.01
2,3,7,8-TCDD	1
Other tetra TCDDs	0.01
2,3,4,7,8-Penta CDD[b]	0.1
2,3,7,8-Hexa CDD[b]	0.1
2,3,7,8-Hepta CDD[b]	0.01
Octa CDD	0.0001
PCDFs	**TEFs[a]**
DiCDFs	Nontoxic
TriCDFs	0.01
2,3,7,8-Tetra CDF	0.05
1,2,3,7,8-Penta CDF	0.05
2,3,4,7,8-Penta CDF	0.5
2,3,7,8-Hepta CDF[b]	0.01
Octa CDF	0.0001

CDD, chlorinated dibenzo-*p*-dioxin; CDF, chlorinated dibenzofuran; TCDD, tetrachlorodibenzo-*p*-dioxin.
[a] U.S. Environmental Protection Agency recommended values, derived from ref. 10.
[b] Any isomer that contains chlorine in the 2,3,7,8 positions.

Metabolism

Little is known about the metabolism of these compounds in humans. A generalized scheme has been put forth for the biotransformation of PCDDs based on *in vivo* studies in other mammals (14).

The half-life of some of these compounds in humans can be measured not in hours, days, weeks, or months, but in years. Some animal studies of 2,3,7,8-TCDD have shown that a large proportion of the administered compound persists in an unmetabolized form in the liver, suggesting that toxicity is due to the compound itself and not to a metabolite (15). Metabolic studies in various species have shown that 2,3,7,8-TCDD gives rise to monohydroxy, dihydroxy, and monomethoxy metabolites. Administration of these metabolites from dogs to guinea pigs showed that the metabolites were at least 100 times less acutely toxic than 2,3,7,8-TCDD itself (16).

TABLE 61-4. Estimated average daily intake of toxic equivalencies (TEQs) of polychlorinated dibenzo-*p*-dioxins and polychlorinated dibenzofurans due to a typical state-of-the art municipal incinerator

Exposure pathway	Daily intake of TEQs (ng/day)	Percentage of daily intake
Inhalation	1.3×10^{-4}	43
Ingestion	1.1×10^{-4}	37
Mother's milk	5.7×10^{-5}	19
Dermal absorption	2.2×10^{-6}	1
Total intake	3×10^{-4}	100

Adapted from refs. 1 and 15, with permission.

TABLE 61-5. Polychlorinated dibenzo-*p*-dioxin and polychlorinated dibenzofuran concentrations in adipose tissue from composite samples on a lipid basis

Compound	Minimum (pg/g)	Median (pg/g)	Maximum (pg/g)
2,3,7,8-TCDD	<0.98	6.54	15.1
2,3,7,8-TCDF	0.893	1.89	3.88
1,2,3,7,8-PeCDD	<2.44	10.2	24.4
1,2,3,7,8-PeCDF	<0.066	0.249	1.42
2,3,4,7,8-PeCDF	<0.264	9.21	29.2
1,2,3,7,8,9-HxCDD	<3.86	11.5	22
1,2,3,7,8,9-HxCDF	<0.29	0.341	1.98
1,2,3,6,7,8-HxCDD	13.3	76.1	174
1,2,3,4,7,8-HxCDF	<3.11	7.3	17
1,2,3,6,7,8-HxCDF	<0.556	5.03	14.3
2,3,4,6,7,8-HxCDF	<0.337	0.479	2.49
1,2,3,4,6,7,8-HpCDD	20.9	11	230
1,2,3,4,6,7,8-HpCDF	<1.15	17.7	32.5
1,2,3,4,7,8,9-HpCDF	<0.731	0.715	1.74
OCDD	152	838	1630
OCDF	<0.68	1.19	13.2

HpCDD, heptachlorodibenzo-*p*-dioxin; HpCDF, heptachlorodibenzofuran; HxCDD, hexachlorodibenzo-*p*-dioxin; HxCDF, hexachlorodibenzofuran; OCDD, octochlorodibenzo-*p*-dioxin; OCDF, octochlorodibenzofuran; PeCDD, pentachlorodibenzo-*p*-dioxin; PeCDF, pentachlorodibenzofuran; TCDD, tetrachlorodibenzo-*p*-dioxin; TCDF, tetrachlorodibenzofuran.
Note: Not detected (ND) concentrations are replaced by half of the detection limit.
Adapted from refs. 1 and 4, with permission.

Elimination

Elimination of these compounds is generally assumed to occur slowly by loss of the lipid-containing materials to which the PCDDs and PCDFs are attached. Michalek and colleagues estimated the half-life of 2,3,7,8-TCDD in 213 enlisted military personnel who handled Agent Orange as 8.7 years with a 95% confidence interval (CI) of 8.0 to 9.5 years (17). Four other studies showed the half-life of 2,3,7,8-TCDD in humans to be 7 years or more (18–21); the primary route of elimination was the feces (19). The half-life of PCDDs and PCDFs in humans may vary from 3.0 years for 1,2,3,4,6,7,8-heptachlorodibenzofuran to 19.6 years for 2,3,4,7,8-pentachlorodibenzo-*p*-dioxin (20).

SIGNS, SYMPTOMS, AND SYNDROMES

Acute

The most prominent acute manifestation of toxicity that has been shown in humans is chloracne, an acnelike condition that takes months or years to disappear (22–25). Clinically, this skin lesion is characterized by hyperplasia and hyperkeratosis of the interfollicular epidermis, hyperkeratosis of the sebaceous follicles, and squamous metaplasia of the sebaceous glands that form cysts and keratinaceous comedones in a typical distribution (26). Data are not yet available to determine the amount, route, or duration of exposure that is necessary to cause chloracne. Serum samples from exposed persons in Seveso, Italy, have shown that all children who had serum 2,3,7,8-TCDD levels greater than 11,000 ppt based on lipid content developed chloracne. A 16-year-old girl with serum levels of 800 ppt developed chloracne, whereas a 15-year-old boy with levels of 10,400 ppt did not. Chloracne was not seen in adults who had serum levels in the range of 1,770 to 9,140

TABLE 61-6. Health effects associated with exposure to 2,3,7,8-tetrachlorodibenzo-*p*-dioxin and body burdens in humans

Duration of exposure (yr)	System	Effect	Reference
<1	Dermal	Chloracne in children	28
<1	Reproductive	No increased risk of spontaneous abortion	29
15	Gastrointestinal	No increased risk of clinical gastrointestinal disease	30
15	Hepatic	No increased risk of clinical hepatic disease	30
NS	Dermal	Chloracne in 5 out of 7 individuals	31
11	Dermal	Chloracne	32
6.5	Immunologic	Immunosuppression	33
15	Neurologic	No increased risk for peripheral neuropathy	34
<1	Reproductive	Change in sex ratio of children	35
15	Reproductive	Increased prevalence of high luteinizing hormone and low testosterone levels	36
NS	Genotoxicity	No chromosome aberrations or sister chromatid exchanges	37
1	Cancer	Increased cancer mortality risk	38
NS	Cancer	Increased cancer mortality rate	39
20	Cancer	Increased cancer mortality rate	40

NS, not stated.
Reprinted from ref. 1, with permission.

ppt (27). Health effects from a variety of studies are shown in Table 61-6.

Other less consistently reported effects from dioxin exposure in humans include asthenia, headaches, pain in the extremities (25), peripheral neuropathy (40), ulcers (41), altered liver function (42), enzyme induction (43), altered lipid metabolism (44–46), developmental problems (47), and abnormal urinary porphyrin patterns (48). Immune system dysfunction (49) and altered T-cell subsets (50,51) have been reported by some investigators but not others (52,53). Epidemiologic studies show an increase in several liver enzymes associated with 2,3,7,8-TCDD exposure, but these increases did not exceed what are considered normal values for these enzymes, and they disappeared over several years (54). A study of workers with high serum 2,3,7,8-TCDD did not find an elevated risk for porphyria cutanea tarda or porphyrinuria (55). A case-control study of Vietnam veterans with testicular cancer was not consistent with the hypothesis that Agent Orange was a risk factor for the testicular cancer (56).

Studies with human cell lines have shown various enzyme inductions (57,58). Lymphocyte proliferative responses studied in workers with increased body burdens of 2,3,7,8-TCDD and other PCDDs and PCDFs showed that these body burdens did not induce any medically significant changes in the capacity for proliferation of lymphocytes, measured as 3H-thymidine incorporation (59).

Human breast cell culture lines have been used to study the effects of 2,3,7,8-TCDD *in vitro* (58). Treatment of cultures of spontaneously immortalized human epidermal cells with 2,3,7,8-TCDD sensitized them to carcinogen toxicity, and TCDD strongly stimulated the expression in cells of P-450 1A1 and 1B1, enzymes that are important for xenobiotic metabolism (60).

Studies in Wistar rats and mice engrafted with human fetal thymus and liver tissue fragments show that the human thymus serves as a target for TCDD and that both the human and Wistar rat thymus display comparable sensitivities to the toxic action of TCDD (61). A review article concludes that the first intrathymic target cell for the action of 2,3,7,8-TCDD is the thymus cortical epithelial cell (62).

2,3,7,8-TCDD has been shown to be extremely toxic in some animal species. For example, the range of the oral lethal concentration that kills 50% of test animals (LC_{50}) in guinea pigs is 0.6 to 2.0 µg per kg (63); in the hamster, the LC_{50} ranges from 1,000 to 5,000 µg per kg. Other findings in animals include enzyme induction (64–66), altered liver function (67,68), altered lipid metabolism (69,70), porphyria (71,72), decreased host resistance to infectious diseases and suppressed humoral and cell-mediated immune responses (73), and decreased thymus weight (74). The immunologic effects have been shown to be on an aryl hydrocarbon receptor–dependent process (73).

The most common finding after lethal exposure for animals is a loss of body weight and a "wasting away syndrome" (67). In Missouri, horses unintentionally exposed to 2,3,7,8-TCDD–contaminated waste oil exhibited a progressive deterioration in health, including anorexia, listlessness, loss of body weight, dermatitis, emaciation, weakness, unsteady gait, and chronic cough (75). Similar findings were seen in dogs and cats (75).

Chronic and Long-Term Effects

The weight of evidence from human and animal studies suggests that adverse human health effects may be caused by chronic or long-term exposure to PCDDs and PCDFs. The only teratogenic effect suggested in humans is an increased prevalence of neural tube defects (76). 2,3,7,8-TCDD has been shown to be teratogenic in rats and mice, however (71,77). Doses as low as 0.25 µg per kg for 10 days in rats have been shown to be fetotoxic (78). In animals, 2,3,7,8-TCDD also has been shown to be immunotoxic and an inducer of microsomal enzymes (79).

In a study of birth defects carried out on 15,291 births in Seveso, Italy, from January 1, 1977, to December 31, 1982 (80), 26 births were observed in the most highly contaminated area. None of the offspring showed any major structural defects, although two had mild defects (a female with a flat hemangioma—7 by 6 mm—and a female with a small periurethral cyst). The data collected failed to demonstrate any increased risk of birth defects associated with 2,3,7,8-TCDD exposure, but the number of exposed pregnancies was small (2,900 from exposed areas, of which only 461 were from the most highly contaminated areas). Mocarelli and colleagues showed that a greater-than-expected number of female infants was born to parents who had been exposed to 2,3,7,8-TCDD at Seveso (81). The mechanism for this increase is not known.

A cytogenic study performed by Tenchini and colleagues on 25 induced abortions from women exposed to 2,3,7,8-TCDD showed no evidence of chromosomal aberrations (82).

A retrospective cohort study of workers in a chemical plant in Hamburg, Germany, investigated the relationship between mortality (all causes, cancer, cardiovascular diseases, ischemic heart diseases) and exposure to PCDDs and PCDFs (83). The total mortality was elevated in all dose groups. The highest relative risk (RR) was observed for the highest 2,3,7,8-TCDD decile (RR = 2.43, 95% CI = 1.80 to 3.29). Mortality due to cancer and ischemic heart diseases showed dose-dependent relations with TCDD and all PCDDs and PCDFs combined. The highest RRs for cancer (RR = 3.3, 95% CI = 2.05 to 5.31) and ischemic heart disease (RR = 2.48, 95% CI = 1.32 to 4.66) were observed in the highest PCDD- and PCDF-exposed group. This study suggests a strong dose-dependent relationship between exposure to PCDDs and PCDFs and mortality due to cancer and ischemic heart disease mortality.

Whether data show that 2,3,7,8-TCDD is carcinogenic in humans is strongly debated. Two studies considered by some researchers to be important show a 5- to 7-times elevation in soft tissue sarcoma in persons with occupational exposure to phenoxy herbicides or chlorophenols (84,85). These compounds were assumed to contain 2,3,7,8-TCDD. Mortality studies of American Vietnam veterans, however, have not shown any increase in carcinogenesis (86). A summary of existing human studies suggests that only the studies by the Centers for Disease Control and Prevention's (CDC) National Institute for Occupational Safety and Health may have the power to identify an association between cancer and TCDD (87).

Although 2,3,7,8-TCDD has been shown to be carcinogenic in rats (0.1 μg per kg per day) and mice (0.5 to 2.0 μg per kg per week) (71,88), these results do not resolve whether this compound acts as an initiator or a promoter. The majority of all carcinogenicity studies suggest that this compound is not genotoxic and that it is not likely, therefore, to be an initiator. No definite proof exists (89).

MANAGEMENT OF TOXICITY OR EXPOSURE

Persons with recent exposure to PCDDs or PCDFs should have the chemicals removed from their skin as quickly as possible to prevent additional absorption of the compounds. Exposed persons should be asked for an exposure history, including onset of exposure, duration of exposure, and type of exposure. Physical examinations, including a thorough examination of the skin, should be given. Routine laboratory blood and liver tests should be carried out. In most situations, however, evidence of exposure and disease relatable to the exposure is lacking. Because chloracne is the only human effect documented thus far, no other specific abnormality can be considered pathognomonic for exposure.

No specific treatments have been recommended for routine exposure. No routine clinical test is available to measure PCDDs and PCDFs in sera or other human tissues. Serum levels of 2,3,7,8-TCDD and other PCDDs and PCDFs can be measured using gas chromatography-mass spectrometry (90,91). Although, in highly exposed persons, 2,3,7,8-TCDD has been found in serum specimens as small as 1 mL, research laboratories usually need 50 mL of serum to give an accurate serum PCDD or PCDF level.

MEDICAL AND/OR BIOLOGICAL MONITORING INCLUDING INSTRUMENTATION AND/OR METHODS

Serum tests for PCDDs and PCDFs are currently expensive ($1,000 or more) because much work must be done to rid specimens of interfering substances, and considerable effort must be expended to ensure good quality control of the testing. The equipment necessary to test for these compounds in the parts per quadrillion range is also expensive, approaching $700,000. A listing of the analytical methods is given in the *Toxicological profile for chlorinated dibenzo-p-dioxins* published by the Agency for Toxic Substances and Disease Registry (1). Although various methods are listed in the document, most investigators in the field use methods based on those of Patterson and colleagues at CDC's National Center for Environmental Health (90,92).

OCCUPATIONAL AND ENVIRONMENTAL REGULATIONS

Table 61-7 gives selected regulations and guidelines applicable to PCDDs and PCDFs. The U.S. Environmental Protection Agency (EPA) has said that a 10^4 to 10^7 excess cancer risk exists (one excess cancer case per 10,000 to 10,000,000 persons) when 2.2×10^{-8} to 2.2×10^{-11} mg per L of 2,3,7,8-TCDD is present in the water (103). The U.S. Food and Drug Administration considers that no serious health concerns exist if 2,3,7,8-TCDD levels in fish are below 25 ppt (1,104). The National Institute for Occupational Safety and Health considers 2,3,7,8-TCDD a potential occupational carcinogen that should be controlled to the fullest extent possible (1,105). EPA, CDC, and the U.S. Food and Drug Administration have carried out risk assessments for 2,3,7,8-TCDD. Human intake values estimated by each agency as corresponding to an estimated cancer risk of 1×10^6 (one excess cancer case per 1,000,000 persons) are 6.4 fg per kg per day (EPA), 27.6 fg per kg per day (CDC), and 57.2 fg per kg per day (Food and Drug Administration) (1 fg = 1×10^{-15} g) (1). EPA is currently reevaluating its risk assessment for 2,3,7,8-TCDD and the other PCDDs and PCDFs.

TABLE 61-7. Regulations and guidelines for polychlorinated dibenzo-*p*-dioxins

International
- The International Agency for Research on Cancer classified 2,3,7,8-TCDD as a probable human carcinogen (93).
- The World Health Organization listed a tolerable daily intake for 2,3,7,8-TCDD of 10 pg/kg/d (94).
- The Health Council of the Netherlands gave a health-based exposure limit (2,3,7,8-TCDD or total toxic equivalency factor) of 1 pg/kg/d (95).

United States
- The U.S. Environmental Protection Agency listed 2,3,7,8-TCDD as a Hazardous Air Pollutant (96).
- A permit is required for the underground injection of 2,3,7,8-TCDD–containing wastes designated as hazardous under the Resource Conservation and Recovery Act (97).
- The Department of Transportation listed dioxins as hazardous material subject to requirements for packaging, labeling, and transportation (98).
- Ocean dumping of 2,3,7,8-TCDD is prohibited except when in trace amounts (99).
- The Toxic Substances Control Act regulates the use, disposal, and distribution in commerce of process wastewater treatment sludges intended for land application from pulp and paper mills using chlorine- or chlorine derivative–based bleaching processes (100).
- The National Institutes for Occupational Safety and Health of the Centers for Disease Control and Prevention listed 2,3,7,8-TCDD as a potential human carcinogen (101).
- The National Academy of Sciences listed an acceptable daily intake of 2,3,7,8-TCDD from water of 10^{-4} μg/kg/d (102).
- The U.S. Food and Drug Administration said that fish with 2,3,7,8-TCDD levels greater than 50 parts per trillion should not be consumed (103).

TCDD, tetrachlorodibenzo-*p*-dioxin.

EXPOSURE CONTROLS

EPA has listed dioxin-containing wastes as acute hazardous wastes, defined as "wastes that are so hazardous that they may, either through acute or chronic exposure, cause or significantly contribute to an increase in serious-irreversible or incapacitating-reversible illness regardless of how they are managed" (1,106). Effective November 8, 1986, EPA prohibited further land disposal of certain dioxin-containing hazardous wastes (1,107).

ENVIRONMENTAL FATE AND TRANSPORT

PCDDs and PCDFs have entered the environment by a variety of means, including the use of herbicides, bleaching, incineration, and combustion. Once there, they are remarkably stable, and many of these compounds, especially those substituted with chlorine at the 2,3,7,8 carbon positions, bioaccumulate in the human food chain. Sources of dioxin include food, milk (including human milk), air, the pesticide 2,4,5-trichlorophenoxyacetic acid, and dust contaminated with PCDDs or PCDFs from waste disposal or incineration. PCDDs and PCDFs are not very water-soluble but tend to attach to particles. Thus, they are not often found in significant amounts in groundwater, surface water, or drinking water. However, because of the variety and ubiquitous sources of small amounts of PCDDs and PCDFs, these compounds can be found at ppt levels in the lipid-containing tissues of humans, especially of persons living in industrialized countries (5–8).

ENVIRONMENTAL AND OCCUPATIONAL MONITORING

Persons need not be monitored for levels of PCDDs and PCDFs in their blood, serum, or adipose tissue unless they are thought to have been excessively exposed. Analytical methods are referenced and described in references 1, 90, and 92 as discussed in the section Medical and/or Biological Monitoring Including Instrumentation and/or Methods.

Routine environmental monitoring of soil, air, and water for PCDDs and PCDFs is not indicated. Analytical methods for any needed environmental measurements of PCDDs or PCDFs have been described (1). Environmental media that can be analyzed include air, air from contaminated buildings, birds, car exhaust, cigarettes, cigarette smoke and ash, drinking water, fly ash, fog (water and particles), foods (including fish and crab), fuel oils, gaseous waste effluents, groundwater, incinerator stack emissions, landfill leachate, pottery clay, pyrolized transformer oil, reactor residues, sediment, sludge, soil, and still bottoms. Samples are collected in containers, often quartz fiber filter/polyurethane foam. Various procedures are used to eliminate contaminants. Specimens are then analyzed for PCDDs and PCDFs by high-resolution gas chromatography followed by high- or low-resolution mass spectrometry.

ACKNOWLEDGMENTS

Special thanks to Dr. Hanna Pohl who supplied information from a draft of the updated *Toxicological profile for chlorinated dibenzo-*p*-dioxins* being prepared by the Agency for Toxic Substances and Disease Registry and to Dr. Charles Xintaras and Jeanne Bucsela who reviewed and edited drafts of this chapter. Preparation of this chapter was supported in part by funds from the Comprehensive Environmental Response, Compensation, and Liability Act trust fund.

REFERENCES

1. Agency for Toxic Substances and Disease Registry. Toxicological profile for chlorinated dibenzo-*p*-dioxins (update). PB/99/121998. Atlanta: US Department of Health and Human Services, Public Health Service, ATSDR, September 1999.
2. Schecter A, Ryan JJ, Constable JD. Polychlorinated dibenzo-*p*-dioxin and polychlorinated dibenzofuran levels in human breast milk from Vietnam compared with cow's milk and human breast milk from the North American Continent. *Chemosphere* 1987;16:2003–2016.
3. Muto H, Takizawa Y. Dioxins in cigarette smoke. *Arch Environ Health* 1989; 44:171–174.
4. Orban JE, Stanley JS, Schwemberger JG, et al. Dioxins and dibenzofurans in adipose tissue of the general U.S. population and selected subpopulations. *Am J Public Health* 1994;84:439–445.
5. Beck H, Eckart K, Mathar W, Wittkowski R. PCDD and PCDF body burden from food intake in the Federal Republic of Germany. *Chemosphere* 1989;18: 417–424.
6. Dahl P, Lindstrom G, Wiberg K, Rappe C. Absorption of polychlorinated biphenyls, dibenzo-*p*-dioxins and dibenzofurans by breast-fed infants. *Chemosphere* 1995;30:2297–2306.
7. Poiger H, Schlatter C. Influence of solvents and adsorbents on dermal and intestinal absorption of 2,3,7,8-tetrachlorodibenzo-*p*-dioxin. *Food Cosmet Toxicol* 1980;18:477–482.
8. McConnell EE, Lucier GW, Rumbaugh RC, et al. Dioxin in soil: bioavailability after ingestion by rats and guinea pigs. *Science* 1984;223:1077–1079.
9. Birnbaum LS. Use of toxic equivalency factors for risk assessment for dioxins and related compounds. *Toxicology* 1995;105:391–401.
10. US Environmental Protection Agency. Exposure and human health reassessment of 2,3,7,8-tetrachlorodibenzo-*p*-dioxin (TCDD) and related compounds. Parts I and II. Washington: US Environmental Protection Agency, National Center for Environmental Assessment, Office of Research and Development, September 2000.
11. Patterson DG Jr, Needham LL, Pirkle JL, et al. Correlation between serum and adipose tissue levels of 2,3,7,8-tetrachlorodibenzo-*p*-dioxin in 50 persons from Missouri. *Arch Environ Contam Toxicol* 1988;17:139–143.
12. Leung H-W, Wendling JM, Orth R, et al. Relative distribution of 2,3,7,8-tetrachlorodibenzo-*p*-dioxin in human hepatic and adipose tissues. *Toxicol Lett* 1990;50:275–282.
13. Carrier G, Brunet RC, Brodeur J. Modeling of the toxicokinetics of polychlorinated dibenzo-*p*-dioxins and dibenzofurans in mammalians, including humans. II. Kinetics of absorption and disposition of PCDDs/PCDFs. *Toxicol Appl Pharmacol* 1995;131:267–276.
14. Van den Berg M, DeJongh J, Poiger H, et al. The toxicokinetics and metabolism of polychlorinated dibenzo-*p*-dioxins (PCDDs) and dibenzofurans (PCDFs) and their relevance for toxicity. *Crit Rev Toxicol* 1993;24:1–74.
15. Hattemer-Frey HA, Travis CC. Comparison of human exposure to dioxin from municipal waste incineration and background environmental contamination. *Chemosphere* 1989;18:643–649.
16. Poiger H, Weber H, Schlatter C. Special aspects of metabolism and kinetics of TCDD in dogs and rats. Assessment of toxicity of TCDD-metabolite(s) in guinea pigs. In: Hutzinger O, Frei RW, Merian E, Pocchiari F, eds. *Chlorinated dioxins and related compounds. Impact on the environment.* New York: Pergamon Press, 1982:317–325.
17. Michalek JE, Pirkle JL, Caudill SP, et al. Pharmacokinetics of TCDD in veterans of Operation Ranch Hand: 10-year follow-up. *J Toxicol Environ Health* 1996;47:209–220.
18. Pirkle JL, Wolfe WH, Patterson DG Jr, et al. Estimates of the half-life of 2,3,7,8-tetrachlorodibenzo-*p*-dioxin in Vietnam veterans of Operation Ranch Hand. *J Toxicol Environ Health* 1989;27:165–171.
19. Poiger H, Schlatter C. Pharmacokinetics of 2,3,7,8-TCDD in man. *Chemosphere* 1986;15:1489–1494.
20. Flesch-Janys D, Becher H, Gurn P, et al. Elimination of polychlorinated dibenzo-*p*-dioxins and dibenzofurans in occupationally exposed persons. *J Toxicol Environ Health* 1996;47:363–378.
21. Needham LL, Gerthoux PM, Patterson DG Jr, et al. Half-life of 2,3,7,8-tetrachlorodibenzo-*p*-dioxin in serum of Seveso adults: interim report. *Organohalogen Compounds* 1994;21:81–85.
22. Dunagin WG. Cutaneous signs of systemic toxicity due to dioxins and related chemicals. *J Am Acad Dermatol* 1984;10:688–700.
23. Crow KD. Chloracne and its potential clinical implications. *Clin Exp Dermatol* 1981;6:243–257.
24. Tindall JP. Chloracne and chloracnegens. *J Am Acad Dermatol* 1985;13:539–558.
25. Suskind RR. Chloracne and associated health problems in the manufacture of 2,4,5-T. In: Report to the Joint Conference of the National Institute of Environmental Health Sciences and International Agency for Research on Cancer. Lyon, France: World Health Organization, 1978.
26. Taylor JS. Environmental chloracne: update and overview. *Ann N Y Acad Sci* 1979;320:295–307.
27. Centers for Disease Control and Prevention. Preliminary report: 2,3,7,8-tetrachlorodibenzo-*p*-dioxin exposure to humans, Seveso, Italy. *MMWR Morb Mortal Wkly Rep* 1988;37:733–736.
28. Mocarelli P, Needham LL, Marocchi A, et al. Serum concentrations of 2,3,7,8-tetrachlorodibenzo-*p*-dioxin and test results from selected residents of Seveso, Italy. *J Toxicol Environ Health* 1991;32:357–366.

29. Wolfe WH, Michalek JE, Miner JC, et al. Paternal serum dioxin and reproductive outcomes among veterans of Operation Ranch Hand. *Epidemiology* 1995;6:17–22.
30. Calvert GM, Hornung RW, Sweeney MH, et al. Hepatic and gastrointestinal effects in an occupational cohort exposed to 2,3,7,8-tetrachlorodibenzo-*p*-dioxin. *JAMA* 1992;267:2209–2214.
31. Schecter A, Ryan JJ, Papke O, et al. Elevated dioxin levels in the blood of male and female Russian workers with and without chloracne 25 years after phenoxyherbicide exposure: the UFA "Khimprom" incident. *Chemosphere* 1993;27:253–258.
32. Jansing P-J, Korff R. Blood levels of 2,3,7,8-tetrachlorodibenzo-*p*-dioxin and gamma-globulins in a follow-up investigation of employees with chloracne. *J Dermatol Sci* 1994;8:91–95.
33. Tonn T, Esser C, Schneider EM, et al. Persistence of decreased T-helper cell function in industrial workers 20 years after exposure to 2,3,7,8-tetrachlorodibenzo-*p*-dioxin. *Environ Health Perspect* 1996;104:422–426.
34. Sweeney MH, Fingerhut MA, Arezzo J, et al. Peripheral neuropathy after occupational exposure to 2,3,7,8-tetrachlorodibenzo-*p*-dioxin (TCDD). *Am J Ind Med* 1993;23:845–858.
35. Egeland GM, Sweeney MG, Fingerhut MA, et al. Total serum testosterone and gonadotropins in workers exposed to dioxins. *Am J Epidemiol* 1994;139:272–281.
36. Zober A, Ott M, Fleig I, et al. Cytogenic studies in lymphocytes of workers exposed to 2,3,7,8-TCDD. *Int Arch Occup Environ Health* 1993;65:157–161.
37. Fingerhut MA, Halperin WE, Marlow DA, et al. Cancer mortality in workers exposed to 2,3,7,8-tetrachlorodibenzo-*p*-dioxin. *N Engl J Med* 1991;324:212–218.
38. Ott MG, Zober A. Cause specific mortality and cancer incidence among employees exposed to 2,3,7,8-TCDD after a 1953 reactor accident. *Occup Environ Med* 1996;53:606–612.
39. Manz A, Berger J, Dwyer JH, et al. Cancer mortality among workers in chemical plant contaminated with dioxin. *Lancet* 1991;338:959–964.
40. Filippini G, Bordo B, Crenna P, Massetto N, Musicco M, Boeri R. Relationship between clinical and electrophysiological findings and indicators of heavy exposure to 2,3,7,8-tetrachlorodibenzo dioxin. *Scand J Work Environ Health* 1981;7:257–262.
41. Suskind RR, Hertzberg VS. Human health effects of 2,4,5-T and its toxic contaminants. *JAMA* 1984;251:2372–2380.
42. Poland AP, Smith D, Metter G, Possick P. A health survey of workers in a 2,4-D and 2,4,5-T plant with special attention to chloracne, porphyria cutanea tarda, and psychologic parameters. *Arch Environ Health* 1971;22:316–327.
43. Jaiswal AK, Nebert DW, Eisen HW. Comparison of aryl hydrocarbon hydroxylase and acetanilide 4-hydroxylase induction by polycyclic aromatic compounds in humans and mouse cell lines. *Biochem Pharmacol* 1985;34:2721–2731.
44. Oliver RM. Toxic effects of 2,3,7,8-tetrachlorodibenzo-1,4-dioxin in laboratory workers. *Br J Ind Med* 1975;32:49–53.
45. Axelson O. The health effects of phenoxy acid herbicides. In: Herrington JM, ed. *Recent advances in occupational health*. Edinburgh: Churchill Livingstone, 1984:253–266.
46. Calvert GM, Wilie KK, Sweeney MH, Fingerhut MA, Halperin WE. Evaluation of serum lipid concentrations among U.S. workers exposed to 2,3,7,8-tetrachlorodibenzo-*p*-dioxin. *Arch Environ Health* 1996;51:100–107.
47. Birnbaum LS. Developmental effects of dioxins and related endocrine disrupting chemicals. *Toxicol Lett* 1995;82–83:743–750.
48. Doss M, Sauer H, von Tieperman R, Colombi AM. Development of chronic hepatic porphyria (porphyria cutanea tarda) with inherited uroporphyrin decarboxylase deficiency under exposure to dioxin. *Int J Biochem* 1984;16: 369–373.
49. Hoffman RE, Stehr-Green PA, Webb KB, et al. Health effects of long-term exposure to 2,3,7,8-tetrachlorodibenzo-*p*-dioxin. *JAMA* 1986;255:2031–2038.
50. Knutsen AP. Immunologic effects of TCDD exposure in humans. *Bull Environ Contam Toxicol* 1984;33:673–681.
51. Knutsen AP, Roodman ST, Evans RG, et al. Immune studies in dioxin-exposed Missouri residents: Quail Run. *Bull Environ Contam Toxicol* 1987;39:481–489.
52. Evans RG, Webb AP, Roodman ST, et al. A medical follow-up of the health effects of long-term exposure to 2,3,7,8-tetrachlorodibenzo-*p*-dioxin. *Arch Environ Health* 1988;43:273–278.
53. Webb KB, Evans RG, Knutsen AP, et al. Medical evaluation of subjects with known body levels of 2,3,7,8-tetrachlorodibenzo-*p*-dioxin. *J Toxicol Environ Health* 1989;28:183–193.
54. Mocarelli P, Marocchi A, Brambilla P, Gerthoux P, Young DS, Mantel N. Clinical laboratory manifestations of exposure to dioxin in children: a six-year study of the effects of an environmental disaster near Seveso, Italy. *JAMA* 1986;256:2687–2695.
55. Calvert GM, Sweeney MH, Fingerhut MA, et al. Evaluation of porphyria cutanea tarda in U.S. workers exposed to 2,3,7,8-tetrachlorodibenzo-*p*-dioxin. *Am J Ind Med* 1994;25:559–571.
56. Bullman TA, Watanabe KK, Kang HK. Risk of testicular cancer associated with surrogate measures of Agent Orange exposure among Vietnam veterans on the Agent Orange Registry. *Ann Epidemiol* 1994;4:11–16.
57. Kiyohara C, Hirohata T, Masuda Y. Effects of polychlorinated dibenzo-*p*-dioxin and dibenzofuran congeners in human lymphoblastic cells on aryl hydrocarbon hydroxylase activity. *Chemosphere* 1995;31:3673–3680.
58. Dohr O, Vogel C, Abel J. Different response of 2,3,7,8-tetrachloro-dibenzo-*p*-dioxin (TCDD)-sensitive genes in human breast cancer MCF-7 and MDA-MB 231 cells. *Arch Biochem Biophys* 1995;321:405–412.
59. Neubert T, Maskow L, Delgado I, Helge H, Neubert D. Chlorinated dibenzo-*p*-dioxins and dibenzofurans and the human immune system. 2. In vitro proliferation of lymphocytes from workers with quantified moderately-increased body burdens. *Life Sci* 1995;56:421–436.
60. Walsh AA, deGraffenried LA, Rice RH. 2,3,7,8-Tetrachlorodibenzo-*p*-dioxin sensitization of cultured human epidermal cells to carcinogenic heterocyclic amine toxicity. *Carcinogenesis* 1995;16:2187–2191.
61. De Heer C, Schuurman HJ, Liem AK, et al. Toxicity of 2,3,7,8-tetra-chlorodibenzo-*p*-dioxin (TCDD) to the human thymus after implantation in SCID mice. *Toxicol Appl Pharmacol* 1995;134:296–304.
62. De Heer C, De Waal EJ, Schuurman HJ, et al. The intrathymic target cell for the thymotoxic action of 2,3,7,8-tetrachlorodibenzo-*p*-dioxin. *Exp Clin Immunogenet* 1994;11:86–93.
63. Esposito MP, Tiernan TO, Dryden FE. Dioxins. Washington: Environmental Protection Agency, 1980. [EPA-600-2-80-197.]
64. Poland A, Glover E. 2,3,7,8-Tetrachlorodibenzo-*p*-dioxin: a potent inducer of delta-aminolevulinic acid synthetase. *Science* 1973;179:476–477.
65. DeVito MJ, Birnbaum LS, Farland WH, Gasiewicz TA. Comparisons of estimated human body burdens of dioxin-like chemicals and TCDD body burdens in experimentally exposed animals. *Environ Health Perspect* 1995;103:820–831.
66. Safe SH. Modulation of gene expression and endocrine response pathways by 2,3,7,8-tetrachlorodibenzo-*p*-dioxin and related compounds. *Pharmacol Ther* 1995;67:247–281.
67. Courtney KD, Putnam JP, Andrews JE. Metabolic studies with TCDD (dioxin) treated rats. *Arch Environ Contam Toxicol* 1978;7:385–396.
68. Kociba R, Keyes DG, Beyer JE, Carreon RM, Gehring PJ. Long-term toxicologic studies of 2,3,7,8-tetrachlorodibenzo-*p*-dioxin (TCDD) in laboratory animals. *Ann N Y Acad Sci* 1979;320:397–404.
69. Gasiewicz TA, Neal RA. 2,3,7,8-Tetrachlorodibenzo-*p*-dioxin tissue distribution, excretion, and effects on clinical parameters in guinea pigs. *Toxicol Appl Pharmacol* 1979;51:329–339.
70. Cunningham HM, Williams DT. Effect of tetrachlorodibenzo-*p*-dioxin on growth rate and the synthesis of lipids and proteins in rats. *Bull Environ Contam Toxicol* 1972;7:45–51.
71. Kociba RJ, Keyes DG, Beyer JE, et al. Results of a two-year chronic toxicity and oncogenicity study of 2,3,7,8-tetrachlorodibenzo-*p*-dioxin in rats. *Toxicol Appl Pharmacol* 1978;46:279–303.
72. Kociba RJ, Keeler PA, Park CN, Gehring PJ. 2,3,7,8-Tetrachloro-dibenzo-*p*-dioxin (TCDD): results of a 13-week oral toxicity study in rats. *Toxicol Appl Pharmacol* 1976;35:553–574.
73. Kerkvliet NI. Immunological effects of chlorinated dibenzo-*p*-dioxins. *Environ Health Perspect* 1995;103[Suppl 9]:47–53.
74. Vos JG, Moore JA. Suppression of cellular immunity in rats and mice by maternal treatment with 2,3,7,8-tetrachlorodibenzo-*p*-dioxin. *Int Arch Allergy Appl Immunol* 1974;47:777–794.
75. Case AA, Coffman JR. Waste oil: toxic for horses. *Vet Clin North Am* 1973;3: 273–277.
76. Field B, Kerr C. Herbicide use and incidence of neural-tube defects. *Lancet* 1979;1:1341–1342.
77. Courtney KD, Moore JA. Teratology studies with 2,4,5-trichloro-phenoxyacetic acid and 2,3,7,8-tetrachlorodibenzo-*p*-dioxin. *Toxicol Appl Pharmacol* 1971;20:396–403.
78. Khera KS, Ruddick JA. Polychlorodibenzo-*p*-dioxins: perinatal effects and the dominant lethal test in Wistar rats. *Adv Chem Ser* 1973;120:70–84.
79. Vos JG, Moore JA, Zinkl JG. Effect of 2,3,7,8-tetrachloro-dibenzo-*p*-dioxin on the immune system of laboratory animals. *Environ Health Perspect* 1973;5:149–162.
80. Mastroiacovo P, Spagnolo A, Marni E, Meazza L, Bertollini R, Segni G. Birth defects in the Seveso area after TCDD contamination. *JAMA* 1988;259:1668–1672.
81. Mocarelli P, Brambilla P, Mario Gerthoux P, et al. Change in sex ratio with exposure to dioxin [Letter]. *Lancet* 1996;348:348–409.
82. Tenchini ML, Crimaudo C, Pacchetti G, Mottura A, Agosti S, De Carli L. A comparative cytogenetic study on cases of induced abortions in 2,3,7,8-tetrachlorodibenzo-*p*-dioxin exposed and nonexposed women. *Environ Mutagen* 1983;5:73–86.
83. Flesch-Janys D, Berger J, Gurn P, et al. Exposure to polychlorinated dioxins and furans (PCDD/F) and mortality in a cohort of workers from a herbicide-producing plant in Hamburg, Federal Republic of Germany. *Am J Epidemiol* 1995;142:1165–1175.
84. Hardell L, Sandstrom A. Case-control study: soft tissue sarcomas and exposure to phenoxyacetic acids or chlorophenols. *Br J Cancer* 1979;39:711–717.
85. Ericksson M, Hardell L, Berg NO, Moller T, Axelson O. Soft-tissue sarcomas and exposure to chemical substances: a case-referent study. *Br J Ind Med* 1981;38:27–33.
86. Centers for Disease Control and Prevention. Vietnam Experience Study. Postservice mortality among Vietnam veterans. *JAMA* 1987;257:790–795.
87. Scheuplein RJ, Bowers JC. Dioxin: an analysis of the major human studies. Comparison with animal-based cancer risks. *Risk Anal* 1995;15:319–333.
88. National Toxicology Program. Carcinogenesis bioassay of 2,3,7,8-tetrachlorodibenzo-*p*-dioxin in Osborne-Mendel rats and $B6C3F_1$ mice (gavage study). Research Triangle Park, NC: National Toxicology Program, 1982. Technical Report Series no. 209 (NTP-80-31).
89. Shu HP, Paustenbach DJ, Murray FJ. A critical evaluation of the use of mutagenesis, carcinogenesis, and tumor promotion data in a cancer risk assessment of 2,3,7,8-tetrachlorodibenzo-*p*-dioxin. *Regul Toxicol Pharmacol* 1987;7:57–88.
90. Patterson DG Jr, Hampton L, Lapeza CR Jr, et al. High-resolution gas chromatographic/high-resolution mass spectrometric analysis of human serum

on a whole-weight and lipid basis for 2,3,7,8-tetrachloro-dibenzo-*p*-dioxin. *Anal Chem* 1987;59:2000–2005.
91. Nygren M, Hansson M, Sjostrom M, et al. Development and validation of a method for determination of PCDDs and PCDFs in human blood plasma. A multivariate comparison of blood and adipose tissue levels between Vietnam veterans and matched controls. *Chemosphere* 1988;17:1663–1692.
92. Patterson DG Jr, Furst P, Alexander LR, et al. Analysis of human serum for PCDDs/PCDFs: a comparison of three extraction procedures. *Chemosphere* 1989;19:89–96.
93. International Agency for Research on Cancer (IARC) monographs on the evaluation of carcinogenic risks to humans. Overall evaluations of carcinogenicity: an updating of IARC monographs volumes 1 to 42. Lyon, France: World Health Organization, International Agency for Research on Cancer, 1987. IARC monograph supplement F.
94. Consultation on tolerable daily intake from food of PCDDs and PCDFs. Summary report. Bilthoven, the Netherlands: World Health Organization, 1991.
95. Health Council of the Netherlands. Dioxins: polychlorinated dibenzo-*p*-dioxins, dibenzofurans and dioxin-like polychlorinated biphenyls. Health Council of the Netherlands, Council on Risk Evaluation and Substances/Dioxins, 1996.
96. Public Law 549. 101st Congress, 2nd Session. (November 15, 1990). Amendments to the Clean Air Act. Section 112 (U.S. Code 42USC7412), Hazardous Air Pollutants. Washington: US Government Printing Office, 1990.
97. US Environmental Protection Agency. Underground injection control program. Code of Federal Regulations. 40 *CFR* 144.1.
98. US Department of Transportation. List of hazardous substances and reportable quantities. Code of Federal Regulations. 49 *CFR* 172.101.
99. US Environmental Protection Agency. Ocean dumping: constituents prohibited as other than trace contaminants. Code of Federal Regulations. 40 *CFR* 227.6.
100. Regulation of land application of sludge from pulp and paper mills using chlorine and chlorine derivative bleaching processes. Code of Federal Regulations. 40 *CFR* 744.
101. National Institute for Occupational Safety and Health recommendations for occupational safety. Cincinnati: US Department of Health and Human Services, Public Health Service, Centers for Disease Control and Prevention, National Institute for Occupational Safety and Health, Division of Standards Development and Technology Transfer, 1992.
102. Drinking water and health: part II. Washington: National Academy of Sciences, Safe Drinking Water Committee, National Academy Press, 1977:508–513.
103. US Environmental Protection Agency. 2,3,7,8-Tetrachlorodibenzo-*p*-dioxins. Health advisory. Washington: Office of Drinking Water; March 31, 1987.
104. US Environmental Protection Agency. Health assessment document for polychlorinated dibenzo-*p*-dioxins. Washington: Office of Health and Environmental Assessment, 1985. [EPA report no. 600/8-84-014.]
105. National Institute for Occupational Safety and Health. 2,3,7,8-Tetrachlorodibenzo-*p*-dioxin. Atlanta: US Department of Health and Human Services, Public Health Service, Centers for Disease Control, National Institute for Occupational Safety and Health, 1984. Current intelligence bulletin 40.
106. US Environmental Protection Agency. Hazardous waste management system: dioxin-containing wastes. *Federal Register* 1985;50:1978–2006.
107. US Environmental Protection Agency. Hazardous waste management system: land disposal restrictions. *Federal Register* 1986;51:40572–40677.

CHAPTER 62

Inorganic Acids and Bases

Christopher H. Linden

SOURCES AND PRODUCTION

Definitions, Concepts, and Nomenclature

Acids and bases (or alkali) are classes of chemicals belonging to the more general category of substances known as corrosives or caustics. Inorganic or mineral acids and bases, in contrast to their organic counterparts (see Chapter 63), do not contain carbon atoms. The term *acid* is derived from the Latin word for sour (*acidis*), which describes the taste of acidic compounds such as vinegar. *Alkali* is derived from the Arabic word for the ashes of a plant (*al kali*). A base was initially defined as a substance capable of reacting with an acid to form a neutral compound or salt.

The term *corrosive* originally referred only to substances (primarily acids) that had the ability to attack (corrode) metals. It now denotes all compounds (acids, bases, and other classes of chemicals) that cause tissue injury as a result of nonspecific chemical reactions. *Caustic*, a term once used exclusively in reference to biologically toxic bases, is now considered synonymous with *corrosive*.

According to the electrolytic dissociation theory developed by Ostwald and Arrhenius in the 1880s, acids and bases are compounds that dissociate on solution in water to produce positively charged hydrogen ions (H^+ or protons) and negatively charged hydroxide ions (OH^-), respectively. A more comprehensive definition, proposed separately but almost simultaneously by Bronsted and Lowry in 1923, defines an acid as a compound that has a tendency to donate (lose) a proton and a base as one that has a tendency to accept (gain) a proton.

Acids and bases can be classified as monobasic, dibasic, tribasic, etc., according to the number (n) of dissociated H^+ or OH^- ions per molecule of the parent compound. A molar (M) solution contains 1 gram molecular weight of an acid or base per L of water (or other solvent). Its normality (N), the number of gram equivalent weights of H^+ or OH^- in a liter, is n × the molarity.

Acids and bases also can be classified according to their charge or lack of it. Molecular acids and bases are neutral (e.g., hydrochloric acid, sodium hydroxide), cationic ones are positively charged (e.g., HSO_4^+), and anionic ones are negatively charged (e.g., HSO_4^-).

Acidity or alkalinity of a solution is commonly measured by one of two methods: determination of the *pH* or neutralization by titration. The pH, defined as the negative logarithm (base 10) of the H^+ ion concentration ($pH = -\log_{10} [H^+]$), can be calculated from the H^+ ion concentration (measured electrometrically by a hydrogen or glass electrode) or determined directly by an indicator dye that changes color at a known pH (e.g., litmus paper).

The pH of pure water at 25°C is 7 and is defined as neutral. Solutions with a pH less than 7 are said to be acidic and those with a pH greater than 7 are considered basic. Solutions with extremes of pH (less than 2 or more than 12) are said to be strongly acidic or strongly basic. Some common solutions and their pH values are shown in Table 62-1. It should be remembered that, because of the logarithmic transformation, solutions that differ by 1 pH unit have a 10-fold difference in H^+ ion concentration.

The second way to measure the acidity (or alkalinity) of an aqueous solution is to add incremental amounts of a known concentration (normality) of a strong acid or strong base (defined below) until a neutral or physiologic pH is reached. The number of equivalents of OH^- (or H^+) required for neutralization is known as the buffering capacity, titratable (or free) acidity or alkalinity, and the titratable acid/alkaline reserve (TAR). It represents the amount of acid or base (in charged or dissociated form) that is available for reacting with tissue.

Reactions involving acids and bases can be expressed as equilibria with constants that define the position of the equilibrium. For the dissociation of an acid or base in water, the concentration of water is orders of magnitude higher than that of other reactants. By convention, it is incorporated into the respective dissociation constants (K_a and K_b). In addition, because the extent of dissociation varies greatly between different acids and bases (*K* values range from less than 10–20 to more than 10^8), it is customary to express equilibrium constants in terms of their negative logarithm (base 10), the pK_a or pK_b. Logarithmic transformation of equilibrium equations (i.e., the Henderson-Hasselbach equation) shows that the pK_a of an acid (or the pK_b of a base) is the pH (or pOH) at which equal concentrations of an acid (or base) and its conjugate or base (or

TABLE 62-1. pH of some common solutions

Solution	pH
Concentrated (37%) HCl	−1.1
1.0 M HCl	0
0.1 M HCl	1.0
0.01 M HCl	2.0
Gastric juice	1.2–3.0
Citrus juices	1.8–4.0
Vinegar	2.4–3.4
Carbonated beverages	2.5–3.5
Wines	2.8–3.8
Beer	4.0–5.0
Black coffee	5.0
Normal saline	5.0–5.5
Lactated Ringer's	6.5
Intracellular fluid	6.1–6.9
Milk	6.3–6.6
Distilled water	7.0
Tap water	6.5–8.0
Blood	7.4
Interstitial fluid	7.4
Seawater	7.5
Tears	7.3–7.7
Bile	8.0
Liquid antacids	8.0–10.0
Limewater	10.5
Household ammonia	11.0–12.0
Household bleach	11.0–12.0
0.01 M NaOH	12.0
0.1 M NaOH	13.0
1 M NaOH	14.0
Saturated NaOH	15.0

acid) are present. The pK_a of a base is the pH at which equal concentrations of base and its conjugate acid are present, and it equals 14 minus the pK_b.

From a chemical perspective, strong acids and strong bases are those that are essentially completely dissociated in water. They have high dissociation constants (>1) and either low (<0) or high (>14) pK_a values, respectively. Weak acids and bases are incompletely dissociated in water. They have lower dissociation constants, and pK_a values between 0 and 14. Examples of each, in order of decreasing acid strength (increasing base strength) are shown in Table 62-2. Some common names for acids and bases are listed in Table 62-3.

Chemical Forms

Acids and bases exist as salts and anhydrides as well as in pure form. A salt is a compound formed by replacing some, but not all, H^+ or OH^- ions of an acid or base by another ion or radical (e.g., sodium bisulfate, $NaHSO_4$ is a salt of sulfuric acid, H_2SO_4). An acid or basic anhydride is an oxide of a metalloid or a metal, respectively, that can combine with water to form an acid or base [e.g., magnesium oxide, MgO, is the anhydride of magnesium hydroxide, $Mg(OH)_2$]. In general, acid and basic salts and anhydrides have the same properties as the corresponding acid and base.

Chemical Reactions

Acids and bases, particularly the strong ones, are highly reactive compounds. With the exception of open reactions involving bicarbonate (HCO_3), in which the evolution of gaseous

TABLE 62-2. Inorganic acids and bases

Name	Chemical formula	pK_a[a]
Strong acids (pK_a<0)		
Perchloric	$HClO_4$	
Permanganic	$HMnO_4$	
Bromic	$HBrO_3$	
Chloric	$HClO_3$	
Nitric	HNO_3	
Iodic	HIO_3	
Hydrobromic	HBr	
Hydrochloric	HCl	
Hydriodic (hydrotic)	HI	
Sulfuric	H_2SO_4	
Pyrophosphoric	$H_4P_2O_7$	
Pyrosulfuric	$H_2S_2O_7$	
Chromic	CrO_3	
Weak acids		
Hypophosphoric	H_3PO_2	1.1
Periodic	HIO_4	1.6
Sulfurous	H_2SO_3	1.8
Sulfuric	HSO_4	1.9
Selenic	H_2SeO_4	1.9
Phosphoric	H_3PO_4	2.1
Arsenic	H_3AsO_4	2.3
Tellurous	H_2TeO_3	2.4
Selenious	H_2SeO_3	2.5
Phosphorous	H_3PO_3	2.7
Nitrous	HNO_2	3.3
Hydrofluoric	HF	3.4
Carbonic	H_2CO_3	6.5
Sulfurous	HSO_3	6.9
Hydrogen sulfide	H_2S	7.0
Hypochlorous	HClO	7.5
Telluric	$Te(OH)_6$	7.7
Ammonium ion	NH_4^+	9.2
Boric	H_3BO_3	9.2
Hydrocyanic	HCN	9.3
Silver ion	Ag^+	10.0
Hydrogen peroxide	H_2O_2	11.6
Water	H_2O	15.8
Weak bases		
Calcium carbonate	$CaCO_3$	5.7
Hydrazine	N_2H_4	8.0
Ammonia	NH_3	9.3
Ammonium hydroxide	NH_4OH	9.3
Magnesium hydroxide	$Mg(OH)_2$	10.0
Silver hydroxide	$Ag(OH)_2$	10.0
Arsenic trioxide	As_2O_3	10.0
Lead hydroxide	$Pb(OH)_2$	11.0
Zinc hydroxide	$Zn(OH)_2$	11.0
Calcium hydroxide	$Ca(OH)_2$	11.6
Barium hydroxide	$Ba(OH)_2$	11.7
Strong bases (pK_a>14)		
Cesium hydroxide	CsOH	
Lithium hydroxide	LiOH	
Potassium hydroxide	KOH	
Rubidium hydroxide	RbOH	
Sodium hydroxide	NaOH	
Calcium carbide	C_2Ca	
Calcium oxide	CaO	
Sodium carbonate	Na_2CO_3	
Potassium carbonate	K_2CO_3	
Sodium hypochlorite	NaClO	
Sodium hypophosphate	$Na_4P_2O_6$	
Sodium metasilicate	Na_2SiO_3	
Sodium silicate	$Na_2Si_3O_7$	
Trisodium phosphate	Na_3PO_4	

[a]Approximate values at 25°C. For bases, the pK_a is that of the conjugate acid and pK_b = 14 − pK_a.

TABLE 62-3. Common names of some acids and bases

Common name	Chemical name
Aquafortis	Nitric acid
Aqua regia (nitromuriatic acid)	Mixture of hydrochloric and nitric acids
Baking soda	Sodium bicarbonate
Bleach	Sodium hypochlorite
Caustic potash	Sodium hydroxide
Caustic soda	Potassium hydroxide
Chalk (Paris white)	Calcium carbonate
Lime	Calcium oxide
Limestone	Calcium carbonate
Lye	Sodium or potassium hydroxide
Magnesia	Magnesium oxide
Muriatic acid	Hydrochloric acid
Oil of vitriol	Sulfuric acid
Slaked lime	Calcium hydroxide
Soda ash (washing soda)	Sodium carbonate
Soda lime	Mixture of sodium hydroxide and lime
Soluble glass (water glass)	Sodium silicate
Spirit of Hartshorn (ammonia water)	Ammonium hydroxide
Spirits of salts	Hydrochloric acid

CO_2 results in cooling, reactions involving acids and bases generally produce heat. Reactions between strong acids and bases often produce large amounts of heat (that of neutralization) and can sometimes be explosive. Similarly, the hydration of anhydrides tends to have a large heat of solution and be highly exothermic. The amount of heat (that of dilution and solution) generated when acids, bases, or their salts are added to water tends to be small. But it can be much greater when water is added to an acid, base, or salt, particularly when concentrated forms of strong acids or bases are involved. When used as oxidizing or reducing agents, acids and bases may react violently with compounds or materials being treated.

Chemical reactions involving acids are notorious for producing hazardous gases. Reactions with metals may liberate hydrogen gas, potentially resulting in a fire or explosion upon exposure to an ignition source (e.g., flame or spark). Hydrazine itself is highly flammable. Reactions involving aqueous solutions of the halogen acids may be accompanied by the evolution of a halogen gas (e.g., bromine, chlorine) as well as an acid gas. The actions of acids on sulfur-containing compounds (e.g., drain cleaning) may result in the liberation of hydrogen sulfide and sulfur oxide gases. Reactions of acids with arsenic, phosphorous, and antimony compounds may liberate arsine (AsH_3), phosphine (PH_3), and stibine (SbH_3) gas, respectively. Mixing an acid with a cyanide salt can produce cyanide gas. Combining bleach (sodium hypochlorite) with an acid may produce chlorine gas (1,2); combining it with ammonia may result in the evolution of chloramine gases (NH_2Cl and $NHCL_2$) (3,4). Saturated or concentrated solutions of strong acids also spontaneously may release acid fumes, particularly when heated.

Physical Forms

Most acids and bases are crystalline solids in pure form at room temperature. A few are gases (e.g., the halogen acids, hydrogen cyanide, hydrogen sulfide, and ammonia) or liquids (e.g., hydrazine). All are readily soluble in water and exist as aqueous

TABLE 62-4. Industries, occupations, and processes involving potential exposure to acids and bases

Acids
- Acrylonitrile polymerization
- Astringent manufacturing
- Candle manufacturing
- Chemical synthesis (arsenites, chlorides, nitrates, phosphates)
- Dental cement production and use
- Disinfection/disinfectant manufacturing
- Electronics manufacturing
- Explosives manufacturing
- Felt hat production
- Fertilizer manufacturing
- Glass making/working
- Glue manufacturing
- Jewelry manufacturing
- Mirror manufacturing
- Paper manufacturing
- Plumbing
- Nitroglycerin manufacturing
- Scale removal (boilers, gas and oil wells)
- Sugar refining
- Watch manufacturing
- Woodworking

Bases
- Baking powder manufacturing
- Case hardening
- Cement/mortar/plaster manufacturing
- Compositors
- Degreasing
- Laundry working
- Masonry
- Optics manufacturing
- Printing
- Railroad shop work
- Refrigeration
- Soap manufacturing

Acids and bases
- Aircraft manufacturing/maintenance
- Automobile maintenance/body work
- Bleach manufacturing
- Bronzing
- Cellulose manufacturing
- Chemical manufacturing
- Cloth preparation/sizing
- Dye manufacturing
- Electroplating
- Enameling
- Engraving
- Etching
- Food presentation
- Foundry work
- Fur processing
- Furniture polishing
- Galvanizing
- Laboratory work
- Metal production/working (cleaning, pickling, pitting, polishing, tempering)
- Mercerizing
- Mordanting
- Oil drilling
- Ore drilling
- Painting
- Petroleum refining
- Pharmacist
- Photograph developing
- Rocket fuel production
- Rubber manufacturing
- Synthetic fiber manufacturing
- Tanning of leather
- Wire-making

solutions. They generally can be stored in glass or plastic containers but not in metal or rubber ones. Acid and basic salts and anhydrides are primarily solids. Most are hygroscopic and absorb moisture from air if left uncovered. Commercial products may contain combinations of acids or bases (or their derivatives) and other chemicals.

EXPOSURE SOURCES AND DEMOGRAPHICS

Because of their chemical reactivity, acids and bases are used ubiquitously in manufacturing, arts and crafts, and in the home. Industrial activities involving potential exposure to acids and bases are listed in Table 62-4. Common household products containing these compounds are listed in Table 62-5.

Nearly 100,000 exposures to acids and bases were reported to poison centers in the United States in 1995 (5). The actual number of exposures is probably several times greater. Industrial and avocational exposures are usually accidental and involve skin, eye, and inhalational exposure. Ingestion is most commonly accidental (e.g., environmental exploration by tasting in toddlers; misidentification of drinkable liquids by adults) but may sometimes be intentional (i.e., suicidal). Although more in vogue in past centuries (6), the use of acid for murder (e.g., poisoned beverages) or malicious disfigurement (e.g., vitriol throwing) continues to be reported (7). Acids and bases have also been used in recent incidents of product tampering (e.g., intentional adulteration of food and personal hygiene products).

TABLE 62-5. Some household products containing acids and bases

Product	Active ingredient(s)
Automatic dishwasher detergents	Sodium carbonate, metasilicate, and phosphates
Batteries	
Automotive	Sulfuric acid
Alkaline	Hydroxides of alkali metals
Bleach	Chlorine/sodium hypochlorite
	Hydrogen peroxide
Clinitest®	Sodium hydroxide
Denture cleaners	Hydrogen peroxide (generated from perborate and persulfate)
Drain cleaners	Sodium hydroxide
	Acids (nitric, sulfuric)
Dyes (hair)	Ammonia
Dyes/stains (wood, metal)	Acids (especially nitric)
Glass/metal cleaners	Acids (especially nitric)
	Ammonia
Laundry detergents	Sodium silicate, perborate, percarbonate, sulfate, and phosphates
Mildew removers	Sodium hydroxide and hypochlorite
Oven cleaners	Sodium hydroxide
Paint removers	Sodium hydroxide
Pool/spa disinfectants	Hydrobromic, hydrobromous, hydrochloric, and hypochlorous acids
Portland cement	Calcium, silicon, ferric, aluminum, and magnesium oxides
Roach insecticides	Boric acid
Rust removers	Acids, especially hydrofluoric
Toilet bowl cleaners	Ammonia
	Acids (hydrochloric, phosphoric, sodium bisulfate)
	Bases (sodium carbonate, silicates)

CLINICAL TOXICOLOGY

Local Effects

From a biological perspective, acids and bases are capable of causing damage to any cells with which they come in contact, and hence, are classified as primary irritants. The injuries they cause are often referred to as chemical burns. Their ability to react with tissue is high and nonselective so effects are generally limited to the sites of exposure: external or internal body surfaces such as the skin, eyes, and respiratory and gastrointestinal (GI) tracts. Pulmonary injury may result from the aspiration of ingested liquids and the inhalation of gases, dusts, and vapors.

Primary irritants can be characterized as weak, strong, or corrosive according to their biological potency. Federal legislation (8) mandates that commercial products containing such agents that have been deemed hazardous by the U.S. Consumer Product Safety Commission (9) bear a label containing a signal word which reflects their relative toxicity (Table 62-6). Labels also must identify ingredients, the nature of their toxicity, first-aid measures, and a "keep out of reach of children" statement.

Pathologically, the gross appearance of tissue damaged by acids and bases is different. Acids typically produce coagulation necrosis with eschar formation, whereas bases cause liquefaction necrosis with tissue softening (10–21). With acids and bases, epithelial sloughing with ulceration may ensue. Tissue injury begins within seconds of contact, progresses rapidly over the first few minutes, and then slowly for a period of several hours to several days (22). In general, bases tend to cause more cellular damage than acids (23–25). Injured tissue first heals by way of granulation tissue formation (at several days to several weeks postexposure) and later by scar and stricture formation (beginning approximately 3 weeks postexposure).

Effects at the cellular level include protein precipitation (albuminate formation) by acids and protein dissolution, lipid (membrane) emulsification, and fat saponification by bases. Oxidation-reduction reactions appear to be the underlying mechanism. The generation of free radicals (e.g., amines, oxygen, thiols) also may play a role. These reactions are accompanied by the production of heat. Production of heat tends to be greater with acids than with bases and when solid formulations are involved. Although heat theoretically may cause additional injury, its effects are thought to be minor compared with those caused by chemical reactions.

Histologically, cell necrosis, microvascular thrombosis, and leukocyte and bacterial invasion are seen early in the course of injury by acids and bases. Later, granulation tissue formation occurs, followed by fibroblast proliferation, neovascularization, and connective tissue formation.

The extent of tissue destruction depends on the dose, formulation, contact time of the acid or base, and the nature and premorbid condition of the tissue involved (10,22). The greater the dose and the longer the exposure, the more severe the resultant injury. The dose, which depends on the pK_a concentration and

TABLE 62-6. Labeling requirements for corrosive commercial products

Classification	Signal word	Definition
Weak irritant	"Caution"	Irritating to mucosa
Strong irritant	"Warning"	Irritating to mucosa and skin
Corrosive	"Danger"	May cause severe burns, permanent damage, or death—vapor harmful

volume of the acid or base, is reflected by the pH and TAR. For a given molar concentration and volume, the greater the strength of an acid or base (i.e., the more extreme its pK_a, the greater its potency). And for a given agent, as either its volume or concentration (e.g., pH or pOH) increases, so do its TAR and tissue toxicity. Debate continues, however, as to whether pH or TAR best predicts the relative potency of different acids and bases (26,27). Solids and highly viscous liquids tend to cause more severe but also more localized injury than liquids and gases. Mucosal surfaces are more susceptible to damage than skin. Diseased, immature, or aged tissues are thought to be more susceptible than healthy adult ones.

From a clinical perspective, acids and bases can be considered strong (i.e., potent) if they have a pK_a of less than 2 or more than 12 (see Table 62-2) (18,28). In practical terms, small volumes of solutions of strong acids and bases (even dilute ones) or of those with extremes of pH (less than 2 or more than 12), and large volumes of solutions of weak acids or bases or of those of intermediate pH, all have the potential for causing significant tissue damage. In contrast to their more concentrated industrial counterparts, household ammonia (5% to 10%), bleach (3% to 6% sodium hypochlorite), and hydrogen peroxide (3%) are relatively nontoxic. Occasionally, however, they may cause severe injuries. Similarly, liquid dishwashing and laundry detergents are relatively innocuous whereas automatic dishwashing detergents are not (29).

Systemic Effects

As a rule, acids and bases are not absorbed into the systemic circulation, and their effects remain localized to sites of initial contact. Exceptions (i.e., absorbable agents) include the anions of some acids (e.g., arsenic and other heavy metals, cyanide, fluoride), ammonia, hydrazine, and perhaps large doses of ingested acids. The disposition and systemic toxicity of anions are discussed in Chapters 4 and 22. The systemic effects observed in patients with large ingestions of strong acids may be because of the direct action of absorbed acid or complications of local injury such as hypoxia, shock, and intestinal ischemia or necrosis (30,31). Although rare, similar toxicity also has been described after the ingestion of alkali (32) and central nervous system (CNS) effects have been reported after exposure to acid fumes (33).

Ammonia may be absorbed from the lungs and the intestines (34–36). Blood ammonia levels may be transiently elevated after the inhalation or ingestion of large doses. They usually remain normal (less than 30 mg per dL), however, because absorbed ammonia is rapidly taken up by all metabolically active tissues where it is used in amino acid transamination reactions. In the liver, excess ammonia is converted to urea. Small amounts are excreted in expired air and urine, but hepatic metabolism is the primary route of elimination. Hyperammonemia associated with liver failure and inborn errors of metabolism is primarily the result of the inability to metabolize ammonia that is normally produced in the GI tract by way of bacterial action on nitrogenous wastes. The CNS is the principal target organ.

Hydrazine can be absorbed through the skin and through the respiratory and gastrointestinal tracts (37–41). It is widely distributed to tissues but its metabolic fate is not clear. Target organs include the lungs, liver, kidneys, CNS, and possibly red blood cells, coagulation-fibrinolytic pathways, and the immune system. Numerous enzymes, such as those involved in glucose, amino acid, ammonia, and lipid metabolism, also are affected. The antidotal activity of vitamin B_6 (pyridoxine) against CNS toxicity suggests that hydrazine inhibits enzymes requiring this agent as a cofactor (e.g., those involved in γ-aminobutyric acid synthesis). Hydrazine is eliminated from the blood with a half-life of approximately 2 hours. It is slowly excreted in the urine.

SIGNS AND SYMPTOMS

Acute Toxicity

Primary target organs for acids and bases are the eyes, skin, and respiratory and GI tracts. Involvement of more than one target organ is not uncommon. Signs and symptoms depend on the site of exposure. Systemic toxicity may sometimes accompany surface injuries.

EYE EXPOSURE

Eye injury may occur after contact with liquid, solid, mist, fume, or gaseous forms of an acid or base (42–46). Acid exposures result in pain, photophobia, blepharospasm, tearing, and conjunctival injection. Local or diffuse clouding of the cornea and conjunctiva may occur. Central corneal injuries (those along the visual axis) can result in decreased visual acuity. In severe cases, the lens epithelium and the entire thickness of the cornea may be involved. Epithelial sloughing with corneal ulceration and perforation also can occur. Uveitis, manifested by pain that is unrelieved with topical anesthetics and increases over time, decreased visual acuity, abnormal pupil size, shape, or reactivity, and a "cell and flare reaction" of the anterior chamber (leukocyte infiltration and smoky-appearing aqueous humor), may develop several days after exposure.

Ophthalmic injuries caused by bases tend to be more severe and progressive than those caused by acids. They also have a greater tendency to result in late complications. Ammonium hydroxide is especially potent in its ability to penetrate corneal tissues. Mild exposures present with signs and symptoms of conjunctivitis similar to those described for acids. Diffuse or localized vascular thrombosis and edema of the conjunctiva and sclera may give them a porcelain white appearance. Edema (clouding), softening (keratomalacia), sloughing, and ulceration of the cornea may be seen. Ulcerations may continue to progress for many days. As with acid injuries, those involving the central cornea or anterior chamber can result in decreased acuity of vision. In severe cases, corneal perforation, uveitis, increased intraocular pressure, and lens destruction can occur.

SKIN EXPOSURE

Corrosive burns of the skin may develop after exposure to solutions of acids or bases, liquid hydrazine, or high concentrations of acid or ammonia gas (7,34,35,39–41,46–53). They also may occur after prolonged exposure to dry cement powder (e.g., when it spills into the cuffs of work boots) (7,54) or during attempts to remove particulate matter from the skin by washing or flushing with water. Although the skin, because of its keratinization, is more resistant to corrosive injury than mucosal surfaces, all degrees of injury may be seen.

Mild to moderate (partial thickness) burns from acids and bases resemble thermal burns and cause pain, tenderness, edema, and erythema. Blistering is uncommon, but sloughing may occur. Blanching may sometimes be noted with acid injuries.

Severe (full thickness) acid burns are characterized by a firmly adherent, stiff (leathery) eschar that is insensate. Associated discoloration of the skin may occur: typically white or gray with sulfuric acid, yellow-brown with nitric acid, and green with hydrochloric acid. Wounds may appear black if significant intradermal bleeding occurs (because of red cell lysis and heme iron pigmentation). Spontaneous eschar separation usually occurs approximately 4 weeks after exposure. With severe alkali burns, the skin feels soapy and appears white to dark brown, and the eschar is initially pliant and soft. It may ulcerate or later become dry and friable.

Burns resulting from dermal exposure rarely extend beyond the subcutaneous fat layer. Because of evaporative cooling, those caused by anhydrous or liquid ammonia may be accompanied by frostbite (49). The reaction of hydrogen peroxide with tissue results in the liberation of oxygen. The use of this agent for wound irrigation can cause subcutaneous emphysema and systemic oxygen (gas bubble) embolism (55,56).

INHALATIONAL EXPOSURE

Respiratory tract injury to the nose, mouth, pharynx, larynx, tracheobronchial tree, and pulmonary parenchyma may follow exposure to acid gases or fumes, ammonia gas, hydrazine fumes, and dusts of acids or bases (33–35,39–41,48–50,57–65). Symptoms after mild exposures include burning pain involving the nose, mouth, throat, and chest. Erythema and injection of mucosal surfaces may be seen. In severe cases, dysphagia, hoarseness, coughing, dyspnea, weakness, dizziness, and syncope may be noted. Edema, stridor, and drooling are indicative of severe upper airway injury. A lateral soft-tissue neck x-ray may reveal laryngeal or periglottic edema.

With mild exposures, lung sounds are usually normal. Wheezing, rales, rhonchi, and frothy or bloody sputum indicate moderate to severe pulmonary injury. Associated findings may include tachypnea, tachycardia, fever, hypoxia, and cyanosis. A chest x-ray may show diffuse or patchy infiltrates, atelectasis, or pulmonary edema with a normal size heart. Pneumomediastinum, pneumothorax, and pneumatoceles also may be seen. Pulmonary function testing may reveal evidence of small airway obstruction. Radioisotope (e.g., 133-xenon) lung ventilation scanning may show delayed washout of gas in areas of small airway destruction.

ASPIRATION

Aspiration may occur during the act of swallowing an acid or base or upon the subsequent regurgitation or vomiting of the ingested material (28,52,65–81). It also has been reported after an assault to the face (82). The pulmonary injury is similar to that seen after aspiration of gastric contents but it is often more severe. All areas of the respiratory tract may be involved. Perhaps because bases generally have higher viscosity and lower volatility than acids, damage caused by their aspiration tends to be limited to the upper airway. Signs, symptoms, and ancillary test findings are similar to those after inhalation exposure.

INGESTION

Ingestion of corrosives may cause injury to any area of the GI tract from the mouth to the proximal small bowel (10–25,29,66–131). One or more sites may be affected. Distal injuries may occur without coexistent oral lesions (98,105,113,123,124). Solids, ingested alone or with a liquid, tend to stick to mucosal surfaces and cause severe injury to localized areas of the mouth, esophagus, and, less often, the stomach. Liquids generally cause more diffuse damage of variable severity.

Statistically, ingested bases tend to injure the esophagus more often and more severely than the stomach. With acids, the converse is true. So many exceptions exist that these generalizations do not reliably predict toxicity in a particular individual. The limited amount of hydrochloric acid normally present in the stomach is insufficient to neutralize even small volumes of a strong or concentrated base. Conversely, the squamous epithelium of the esophagus, although slightly alkaline, offers little protection against the effects of strong or concentrated acids. And finally, although relatively resistant to injury, the acid-producing areas of the body of the stomach are not always spared from damage when strong or concentrated agents are ingested.

TABLE 62-7. Endoscopic grading of esophageal and gastric injury because of corrosives

Grade	Depth	Appearance
I	Superficial	Mucosal hyperemia and edema
II	Transmucosal	Blistering, sloughing, or ulcerative lesions of mucosa with or without involvement of superficial muscle layers
III	Transmural	Ulcerative lesions extending into deep muscle layers, serosa, or beyond

Areas of the GI tract most prone to injury are those at (or immediately proximal to) points of anatomical narrowing: the cricopharyngeal, aortic/left mainstem bronchus (retrocardiac), and diaphragmatic/lower sphincter areas of the esophagus, and the antral/pyloric regions of the stomach.

Oropharyngeal burns cause pain, drooling, muffled or slurred speech, and dysphagia. Examination may reveal erythema, edema, ulcerations, or gray to white discoloration, particularly of the posterior mouth and pharynx. Symptoms of esophageal involvement may include chest pain, drooling, dysphagia, and vomiting. Those of stomach and small bowel injury include abdominal pain and tenderness (epigastric or generalized). Vomiting or regurgitation may also occur with GI injuries.

Statistically, oropharyngeal lesions, vomiting, drooling, and stridor are associated with the presence of significant injuries to the upper GI tract (105,113,123,124,130,131). Vomiting is highly predictive of severe esophageal burns. Other findings are less specific. As the number of these findings increases, so does the likelihood of a significant injury. Conversely, their collective absence virtually excludes such injuries. It should be noted, however, that these associations apply only to children with unintentional exposures. Adults, particularly those with suicidal ingestions, may have severe injuries in the absence of these findings.

Severity of esophageal and gastric burns is best assessed by endoscopy (Table 62-7) (132). The extent (i.e., surface area) of injury may be small or large, patchy or diffuse, and may involve multiple anatomical sites. Accurate assessment of the depth of ulcerative lesions may be difficult because of adherent exudates. Necrotic tissue may appear black, apparently because of iron pigmentation resulting from hemorrhage, erythrocyte hemolysis, and hemoglobin destruction.

Because of the greater risk of iatrogenic esophageal perforation associated with the use of rigid endoscopes, flexible fiberoptic endoscopy is the procedure of choice. The use of a flexible endoscope also may obviate the need for general anesthesia and allows for more complete evaluation of organs distal to the esophagus. The admonition that the endoscope not be passed beyond the most proximal site of transmucosal (or deeper) esophageal injury because of the risk of causing an iatrogenic perforation arose in the era when rigid endoscopy was the only technique available for the nonoperative evaluation of GI injuries. It is no longer relevant. With carefully performed flexible endoscopy, the full extent of gastric and duodenal damage can be safely assessed despite the presence of concomitant esophageal injuries.

Accurate assessment of the severity and extent of esophageal and gastric burns is important for prognostic purposes. Patients with superficial (grade 1) burns are not at risk for stricture formation, whereas this complication has been noted in 40% to 100% of patients with transmural (grade 3) lesions. Patients with transmucosal (grade 2) burns also may develop strictures but the risk appears to be low. Esophageal or gastric perforation occurs exclusively in patients with transmural burns (unless diagnostic or therapeutic interventions are causative or contributory).

Optimal timing of initial endoscopy is a matter of continued debate. If endoscopy is performed shortly after ingestion, the extent and severity of injuries may be underestimated. Conversely, if it is performed long after ingestion, the opportunity for tailoring initial therapy to the extent of injury is lost. The performance of endoscopy between 6 and 24 hours after ingestion is most often recommended and appears to be a reasonable compromise. In patients with severe symptoms, it is prudent to perform endotracheal intubation before endoscopy to avoid potential airway problems (e.g., aspiration, obstruction). Repeat endoscopy may be useful in assessing the progression of injury and the response to treatment.

Although contrast esophagography (cinefluoroscopy) also may identify esophageal injuries, it is less sensitive than endoscopy for accurate diagnostic assessment (103). Hence, immediately after exposure, it should be used only as an adjunct to endoscopy. However serial radiographic studies may be useful for assessing the subsequent course of injury and healing. Contrast esophagography and upper GI radiographs also may be used to confirm suspected perforation or stricture formation. Because of potential extravasation, the lower tissue toxicity of water-soluble (ionic or nonionic) contrast agents makes them preferable to barium for the evaluation of suspected perforations (despite their relative disadvantage in terms of x-ray clarity).

Findings on esophagography in patients with acute corrosive injury can be divided into those indicative of mucosal disruption and those indicative of motility disorders (133,134). Radiographic manifestations of mucosal injury include blurring or irregularities (e.g., scalloping or straightening) of esophagogastric margins because of superficial ulceration, sloughing, and pseudomembrane formation; linear or plaquelike retention of contrast caused by deep ulceration; and extravasation of contrast in cases of perforation. Mucosal bullae may occasionally be visualized (135). Radiographic patterns indicating altered motility include atonic dilation, atonic rigidity with narrowing, and uncoordinated or otherwise abnormal peristaltic contractions. Only patients with the latter two patterns appear to be at risk for stricture formation.

Esophageal and gastric perforation may result in mediastinitis or peritonitis. The former is suggested by fever, severe chest pain, respiratory distress, pleural rub, Hammond's crunch, and mediastinal widening with a pleural effusion (usually left-sided) on chest x-ray. Esophageal perforation also may result in pneumomediastinum or pneumothorax. Peritonitis is suggested by fever, abdominal tenderness, guarding, rebound, rigidity, and absent bowel sounds. Free air below the diaphragms on chest or abdominal x-ray may be noted in patients with stomach or bowel perforations. GI gangrene with intramural and intravascular gas (e.g., in portal veins and mesenteric arteries) has also been reported (136). Rupture of the stomach (because of gastric distention caused by the evolution of carbon dioxide gas) may develop after the ingestion of sodium bicarbonate (137). Systemic oxygen embolization can occur in the absence of gangrene or perforation after the ingestion of concentrated hydrogen peroxide (138,139).

Severe gastric and small bowel injuries often result in marked third spacing of peritoneal fluid as manifest by abdominal distention and signs of hypovolemia or shock. A rapid and thready pulse, hypotension, increased or decreased respirations, pallor, diaphoresis, and depressed sensorium may be noted. Shock may occur in the absence of GI bleeding. Acute hemorrhage is, in fact, uncommon.

SYSTEMIC TOXICITY

Severe injuries caused by the ingestion of acids may be accompanied by metabolic acidosis, hemolysis, coagulopathy, hyponatremia, and renal toxicity (30,101,115). Metabolic acidosis also may occur in patients with severe GI damage caused by bases (32). Hyperphosphatemia and hypocalcemia have been reported after the ingestion of phosphoric acid (140). The chronic ingestion of sodium bicarbonate may result in metabolic alkalosis, hypernatremia, hypokalemia, hypochloremia, hyporeninemia, hypovolemia, and hypertension (141). The intravenous injection of large amounts of bleach may cause acute hemolysis, hyperkalemia, hypoxia, and cardiopulmonary arrest (142,143).

Coma, bradycardia, hypotension, pulmonary edema, acidosis, liver dysfunction and coagulopathy may be seen after the ingestion of large amounts of ammonia (36,144). The serum ammonia, blood urea nitrogen, and amylase levels may be elevated. The inhalation of ammonia from ampules (smelling salts) initially causes decreased respirations, increased blood pressure, and sometimes bradycardia (145). Prolonged ammonia inhalation causes the blood pressure to decrease. Ammonia inhalation also may cause anaphylactoid reactions (146).

Hypotension, weakness, excited behavior, tremor, lethargy, ataxia, nystagmus, coma, fever, hyperglycemia, hypoglycemia, hepatitis (fatty degeneration), peripheral neuropathy, nephritis, and renal tubular necrosis may result from acute or chronic hydrazine exposure (37–41,147–150). Seizures, hemolysis, and methemoglobinemia have been noted in animals but not in humans. The onset of systemic hydrazine toxicity may be delayed 14 hours or longer after skin exposure.

Chronic and Long-Term Effects

TARGET ORGAN EFFECTS

Sequelae of severe acid burns of the eye include corneal vascularization, corneal scarring (cicatrix), and the formation of adhesions between the eyeball and eyelid (symblepharon) (43–45). Severe eye injury caused by bases may result in vascularization, scarring, thickening (pannus), and persistent edema of the cornea, anterior chamber synechiae (adhesions between the iris and cornea or lens), cataracts, glaucoma, and symblepharon (42–45). Blindness may occur in both instances.

Full-thickness skin burns may result in indolent ulcers and permanent scarring. They usually remain sterile until approximately 2 to 3 weeks after injury (52).

Severe inhalational injuries may cause persistent hoarseness, pulmonary fibrosis, bronchiectasis, and chronic obstructive airway disease (33,57,60,63). Chronic neurobehavioral dysfunction also has been reported (33).

Severe oral burns may result in chronic pain, ageusia or dysgeusia, and slurred speech. Severe GI burns (i.e., those that are deep, circumferential, or extensive) may lead to esophageal strictures and pyloric stenosis. Esophageal strictures can be graded according to severity and extent (91).

Chronic skin exposure to low doses of corrosives, particularly bases, may result in a contact or eczematous dermatitis with erythema, drying, fissuring, and scaling. Electroplaters chronically exposed to acid fumes, particularly those of chromic acid, may develop ulcerations or perforations (chrome holes) of the nasal septum (151). Chromium compounds also can cause allergic or hypersensitivity dermatitis, asthma, and pneumonitis. Hydrazine has been reported to cause hypersensitivity dermatitis and a lupus erythematosus–like syndrome (38–40,152).

TERATOGENESIS

No adverse effects of acids and bases on the human fetus have been reported. Hydrazine is mutagenic in a variety of *in vitro* test systems.

CARCINOGENESIS

Lung cancer has been associated with chronic exposure to chromium compounds (153). Epidermoid carcinoma of the nasal septum after direct contact with an ammonia-oil mixture has been reported (154). An increased incidence of pulmonary adenocarcinoma has been found in rodents, but not humans, exposed to hydrazine (155). No evidence exists to support an association between the chronic inhalation of acid mists and respiratory tract cancer (156,157). Squamous cell carcinoma of the esophagus and stomach may occur 20 to 40 years after damage caused by ingested bases and acids, respectively (158–160).

Management of Exposures

To prevent secondary casualties, corrosive or acid-resistant protective clothing (e.g., head gear, goggles, gloves, jumpsuits, boots) should be worn by rescuers of those involved in industrial or traffic accidents, particularly where explosion, fire, or significant chemical spills or leaks have occurred. The same is true for those involved with environmental clean-ups. Respiratory protection using self-contained breathing apparatus also may be necessary. A positive pressure oxygen source (e.g., Scott Air Pack, Scott Health and Safety, Monroe, NC) generally is preferable to one using a demand valve (e.g., minimum safety apparatus). Dilution or neutralization of spilled material never should be performed without first investigating and excluding the possibility that such actions may precipitate a dangerous chemical reaction (e.g., explosion, toxic gas evolution).

CLINICAL EVALUATION

Because the severity of injury caused by acids and bases relates directly to the duration of exposure, decontamination should initially take precedence over performing a detailed physical examination. Only resuscitative measures are of higher priority. Although most exposures result in immediate symptoms, a history of exposure may itself be sufficient reason to initiate decontamination measures. Victims of industrial or transportation accidents may require additional evaluation for injuries because of physical trauma. When the history fails to reveal the identity of the offending agent and symptoms suggest exposure to a corrosive, determining the pH of the chemical involved may be helpful in identifying it as an acid or base.

Eye Exposure. The presence or absence of tearing and the appearance of the eyelids, their sulci, surrounding skin, conjunctivae, sclerae, corneas, and fundi should be noted when eyes have been exposed to acids or bases. The location of any abnormalities should be clearly documented [i.e., by drawing a picture of the eye(s) or referring to the position on the corneal surface as if it were the face of a clock]. Pupil size, shape, and reactivity, tear pH [e.g., by applying pHydrion® (MicroEssential Laboratory, Brooklyn, NY) paper to the lower conjunctival sulcus], and visual acuity also should be noted. Examination of the eye surfaces under ultraviolet light after the instillation of fluorescein should be performed in all cases. Slit lamp examination of the anterior chamber should be performed in patients with corneal, pupillary, or visual abnormalities.

Skin Exposure. Location, size, color, texture, and sensibility of any visible lesions or areas of discomfort should be noted if skin has been exposed to acids or bases. Assessment of patients with burns involving more than 10% of the body surface area should include complete vital signs, general physical examination, cardiac monitoring, and routine laboratory tests (e.g., blood count, coagulation profile, serum chemistries, urinalysis). The distal neurovascular status of extremities with circumferential or extensive burns should be documented.

Inhalation Exposure. Evaluation should focus on the assessment of airway potency and respiratory function. Vital signs (especially the respiratory rate), skin color (e.g., the presence or absence of peripheral or generalized cyanosis), the ability to speak and swallow offered liquid as well as oral secretions, the appearance of the oropharyngeal mucosa, the quality of the voice, and the presence of abnormal upper or lower airway sounds should be noted. The adequacy of oxygenation should be assessed by oximetry or arterial blood gas analysis. Laryngoscopy and soft-tissue neck radiographs should be performed in patients with evidence of upper airway injury who do not require immediate intubation (see treatment section below). Patients with respiratory symptoms or abnormal breathing sounds should have a chest x-ray and bedside pulmonary function testing [e.g., peak flow by a Wright spirometer (Clement-Clarke International, Harlow, Essex, UK) or forced expiratory volume in 1 second by a computerized spirometer]. Patients with abnormal vital signs, chest pain, respiratory distress, or hypoxia also should be evaluated by a 12-lead electrocardiogram (ECG) and routine laboratory studies.

Ingestion. Patients who have ingested acids or bases first should be assessed for the possibility of concomitant respiratory tract injury. The presence or absence of oropharyngeal burns, vomiting, drooling, and stridor and the location of any pain, either continuous or on swallowing, should be documented. The neck should be examined for tenderness and crepitus. Abdominal findings, including bowel sounds and abdominal girth (distention), should be noted.

Endoscopy should be used liberally. It is recommended in all patients with signs or symptoms of upper GI tract injury. It also should be strongly considered in asymptomatic patients with intentional ingestions of acids or bases that are considered strong or have extremes of pH (i.e., less than 2 or greater than 12). Patients with indications for endoscopy, particularly those with abnormal vital signs, chest or abdominal pain, respiratory symptoms, and peritoneal signs, should have cardiac monitoring, an ECG, x-rays (e.g., neck, chest, abdomen), arterial blood gas analysis, and routine laboratory studies (including coagulation studies, blood count, type and cross-match, routine chemistries, liver and renal function tests, and urinalysis). Patients with intentional ingestions generally should have a toxicology screen (qualitative analysis of urine and serum) to rule out other exposures.

Systemic Toxicity. In addition to the focused examinations noted above, all patients, especially those with systemic complaints or exposures to corrosives that are known to cause systemic toxicity, should have a complete physical examination. Particular emphasis should be placed on the assessment of neurologic function and the exclusion of potential but possibly occult organ dysfunction (e.g., by ECG, laboratory testing, x-rays).

TREATMENT

Advanced life support measures should be instituted as necessary. As always, ensuring patency of the airway, adequate oxygenation and ventilation, and normal circulatory function are the highest priorities. Decontamination is next. Therapies designed to limit local toxicity are specific to the route of exposure. In some instances (e.g., exposure to hydrocyanic acid or acid anions containing heavy metals), the early institution of antidotal or enhanced elimination (i.e., chelation) therapy also may be necessary.

Eye Exposure. The involved eye(s) should immediately be irrigated with copious amounts of fluid (161). Patients at non-medical facilities should be instructed to flush their eye(s) with tap water for 10 to 20 minutes. They should either pour water into the eye from a drinking glass or rinse the eye with slow running water from a faucet or shower head. If water is not available, milk or any clear, drinkable fluid may be used.

Patients who are at a medical facility should initially have their eye(s) irrigated with normal saline or lactated Ringer's solution (at least 2 L per eye or for 20 minutes for those with visible corneal, conjunctival, or scleral lesions). Intravenous tubing with or without a scleral attachment is useful for this purpose. The irrigating solution should be allowed to flow by gravity. Alternatively, irrigation may be accomplished using commercially available ophthalmic solutions applied as a low-pressure stream from a squeeze bottle. Because normal saline and lactated Ringer's solutions are slightly acidic, they can themselves cause mild eye irritation. Lactated Ringer's solution tends to be better tolerated, perhaps because of its more physiologic pH (see Table 62-1). Lactated Ringer's solution also is theoretically preferable to normal saline because it is buffered (i.e., resists changes in pH).

If possible, the tear pH should be determined before irrigation. Searching for pH paper should not, however, cause decontamination to be delayed. The instillation of a topical ophthalmic anesthetic, such as proparacaine or tetracaine, also is recommended before irrigation because it is difficult for patients to keep their eyes open and cooperate with irrigation unless anesthesia is provided. Finally, any visible particulate material adherent to the surfaces of the eye should be removed manually (e.g., via cotton-tipped swab, eye spud, or forceps) before irrigation. After irrigation, the tear pH should be checked or rechecked. If it falls outside the 5 to 8 pH range, additional irrigation is indicated.

Any patient with corneal, conjunctival, scleral, or lid lesions should be referred to an ophthalmologist for further evaluation and treatment. Specific treatment for corneal injuries may include the use of hydrophilic (gelatinous) contact lenses, eye patching, topical antibiotics, cycloplegics, mydriatics, drugs for the control of intraocular pressure, and topical or systemic therapy with agents that modulate collagen synthesis. For example, ascorbic acid, citric acid, corticosteroids, calcium disodium ethylenediaminetetraacetic acid (EDTA), sodium EDTA, *N*-acetylcysteine, and D-penicillamine may be used for alkali injuries (44,45). Because many of these therapies are controversial or experimental, they should only be used by, or on the direction of, an ophthalmologist.

Skin Exposure. Exposed skin should immediately be irrigated with saline, tap water, milk, or another clear drinkable liquid for a minimum of 10 to 20 minutes for acids and 30 to 60 minutes for bases. Although dilute acetic acid (e.g., vinegar) has been reported to be more effective than water for alkali injuries (162), the use of neutralization therapy remains controversial (see Ingestion section below). Any particulate material should be removed manually before wetting. Wound care (e.g., topical antibiotics, debridement, grafting) and intravenous fluid therapy are the same as those for thermal injuries.

Inhalation Exposure. After removal of the victim from the source of exposure, cool, humidified, high-flow oxygen should be provided. The oxygen dosage subsequently can be adjusted according to the results of pulse oximetry or arterial blood gas analysis. Patients with mild signs and symptoms usually can be treated with oxygen by face mask, whereas those with evidence of moderate-to-severe injury may require oxygen therapy by endotracheal tube (57,60,63). Indications for intubation include CNS depression (confusion or coma); respiratory distress with stridor, drooling, or cyanosis; hypoxia (PO_2 <60) that is not rapidly correctable by oxygen (with or without continuous positive airway pressure); and respiratory insufficiency (PCO_2 >50). In patients with oropharyngeal or laryngeal edema, blind nasal intubation or the use of a fiberoptic laryngoscope may be successful when the glottis cannot be directly visualized. Cricothyroidotomy may be necessary if the trachea cannot otherwise be intubated.

Patients with mild to moderate laryngeal edema may improve after the administration of racemic epinephrine (by aerosol inhalation). An early but brief course of systemic corticosteroids (e.g., 2 mg per kg per day of methylprednisolone i.v. in divided doses for 24 to 48 hours) also may be helpful. Patients with wheezing should be treated with standard asthma medications (e.g., beta-adrenergic agonists). Although steroids may be useful for refractory reactive airway disease, they are not indicated solely for the treatment of pneumonitis or pulmonary edema. Pulmonary edema may respond to positive end expiratory pressure ventilation but diuretics should be avoided. Aggressive tracheal suctioning may be necessary to remove secretions. Antibiotics should be used to treat documented pulmonary infection rather than prophylactically. Pending the results of sputum Gram's stain and culture, empiric therapy should include coverage for *Staphylococcus aureus* and gram-negative organisms and oral flora. Cefazolin, cefoxitin, or cefuroxime are reasonable choices for the empiric treatment of patients with leukocytosis, fever, purulent sputum, or infiltrates on chest x-ray.

Ingestion. Dilution of the ingested agent should be accomplished as soon as possible (15–21). Dilution is intended to decrease the concentration of corrosive and to minimize effects because of potential exothermic reactions. It is contraindicated in patients with signs of esophageal or gastric perforation. Traditionally, milk and tap water have been the preferred agents (163,164). The volume administered should be limited to a maximum of 5 mL per kg because greater amounts may increase the risk of inducing vomiting and reexposing the esophagus, which has a wall that is much thinner than that of the stomach, to gastric contents. In addition, the increased intraluminal pressure generated by vomiting theoretically could increase the risk of perforation.

Use of weak acids (e.g., carbonated beverages, citrus juices, vinegar) as diluents for ingested alkali remains controversial (163–169). Although these agents are more effective than milk or water in neutralizing the pH, neutralization is accompanied by the production of heat that could lead to superimposed thermal injury. In addition, carbon dioxide released after the ingestion of carbonated beverages theoretically could lead to gastric distention and increase the risk of vomiting and perforation.

Experimental data indicate that the heat generated by neutralization is small (less than 3°C) when liquid alkali are involved (168) but may be greater when solid formulations are neutralized (163,166,167). Although it is unknown what effect, if any, the role of heat plays in the pathogenesis of tissue injury, it is quite clear that the efficacy of dilutional (170,171) and neutralization (168) therapy is maximal if performed within 5 minutes of exposure and rapidly declines thereafter. Hence, the awake, alert patient immediately should be given any clear, drinkable beverage if milk and water are not available. Until further information becomes available, lemon juice and vinegar, however, should be avoided (166,167).

Orogastric nasogastric intubation for the purpose of gastric aspiration, lavage, or the administration of diluents to patients who cannot or will not drink them is also controversial (15–21,164). A theoretical risk exists of this procedure producing an iatrogenic esophageal or gastric perforation at the site of deep (transmural or transmucosal) lesions. However, the vast majority of iatrogenic perforations occur during attempts at therapeutic dilation of stenoses. In more than 5,000 patients with corrosive ingestion (all the cases reported in the references cited in this chapter), only three perforations occurred sooner than 24 hours after ingestion. All were spontaneous. All were present at time of initial presentation and none was caused by the insertion of a gastric tube for decontamination. In addition, the author has noted extremes of gastric fluid pH as long as 12 hours after large ingestions (at the time of endoscopy). For these reasons, immediate gastric intubation followed by aspiration, dilution, and lavage is recommended for patients who have ingested more than one swallow of a strong acid or base in liquid form and present within 1 to 2 hours of ingestion.

This approach long has been advocated for acid ingestions, but only recently for those involving bases (18,164). Because solids may stick to mucosal surfaces and cause relatively greater local injury, the risk of perforation theoretically is higher. Hence, gastric intubation is not recommended for the decontamination of patients who have ingested solid acids or bases.

If gastric intubation is performed, a small-bore tube (e.g., 10F catheter in children and 18F catheter in adults) should be gently inserted to minimize mechanical trauma. One to 2 L of milk or tap water usually is sufficient for gastric lavage. Because of the risk of water intoxication, normal saline is recommended for lavage in children under 2 years of age. The volume of lavage fluid aliquots should be kept small (approximately 5 mL per kg) to avoid regurgitation into the esophagus. Lavage should continue until the effluent has a pH of 5 to 7. Commercially available gastric tubes with a pH sensor [e.g., GrapHprobe, (Zinetics Medical, Salt Lake City, UT)] are ideal for this purpose. Alternatively, the pH of the lavage effluent can be determined by pH paper.

Activated charcoal does not effectively adsorb acids or bases and obscures endoscopic visualization and assessment of injury. Unless an ingested agent is likely to cause systemic toxicity (e.g., hydrocyanic acid, hydrazine, acids, or salts with heavy metal anions), charcoal administration is not recommended.

Subsequent management includes continued supportive care, symptomatic treatments, and measures intended to prevent complications (i.e., strictures and perforations). The efficacy of corticosteroids in preventing esophageal strictures remains controversial. Experimental studies suggest that steroids are effective in inhibiting collagen synthesis and preventing alkali-induced strictures if they are given prophylactically (172,173). However, their efficacy when administered after the insult has not been clearly demonstrated. Although analyses of all data favor the use of steroids (21,174), only one controlled clinical trial has shown steroids to be beneficial (114), whereas two others have found them to be ineffective (77,99).

Strictures that develop in patients treated with steroids may be easier to subsequently dilate than those that develop in patients not treated with steroids (121). On the other hand, steroids may increase the incidence of perforation, infectious complications, and death (if antibiotics are not given concurrently). They may inhibit wound healing and mask signs of mediastinitis and peritonitis (80,121,172). For optimal efficacy and minimal risk, steroids should be given as soon after ingestion as possible. They should not be used without concurrent antibiotic therapy or if a suspicion of esophageal or GI perforation exists. The efficacy of steroids in preventing esophageal and gastric outlet strictures resulting from acid burns has not been studied.

Until further data become available, the following approach is suggested. Patients with suspected esophageal burns should be given an intravenous dose of a broad spectrum of antibiotic (e.g., ampicillin or a first- or second-generation cephalosporin) and a corticosteroid (e.g., methylprednisolone, 2 mg per kg) on presentation. These medications can be continued or discontinued depending on the degree and extent of esophageal injury noted on endoscopy and the preference of the specialist (e.g., gastroenterologist or general, pediatric, ear-nose-throat, or thoracic surgeon) who performs it. Even when a gastroenterologist does the endoscopy, surgical consultation is advised. This prevents delays in treatment should operative management become necessary.

Patients without visible injury on endoscopy, and those having only superficial (grade 1) mucosal lesions or limited transmucosal (grade 2) lesions are not at risk for stricture formation or perforation. Hence, antibiotics and steroids are neither of potential benefit nor of potential harm and should be discontinued. These patients can be discharged (with outpatient follow-up) or referred for psychiatric evaluation provided they are able to take oral fluids. Antacids, H2-blockers, analgesics, and sucralfate may be given for symptomatic relief.

Patients with extensive or circumferential transmucosal (grade 2) lesions or shallow transmural (grade 3) injury are at significant risk for stricture formation but negligible risk for perforation. Hence, steroids may be of benefit without being potentially harmful and should be continued. Such patients should be given nothing by mouth and provided with parenteral fluids or hyperalimentation until they are able to swallow their own secretions. Symptomatic therapy as mentioned above should be provided. Antibiotics should be continued for 3 to 5 days post-ingestion or until the patient is free of pain and able to swallow. Although the optimal dose is unknown, 2 mg per kg per day of intravenous methylprednisolone or oral prednisone, given in divided doses every 4 to 6 hours for 1 week and then tapered over the next 2 weeks, is generally recommended.

Patients with deep or extensive transmural (grade 3) lesions are at high risk for perforation and stricture formation. In addition, steroids have not been shown to be effective in preventing strictures in such patients (23,77,80). Because the risk of steroids is substantial and their benefit unlikely, they also should be discontinued in patients with these findings. Such patients should be given intravenous antibiotics, analgesics, and H2 blockers, such as cimetidine, but nothing by mouth. Patients with actual or suspected perforations and those with shock, acidosis, or peritoneal findings suggesting extensive tissue necrosis should be treated in a similar manner. In patients with mediastinitis or peritonitis, antibiotic coverage should be extended to cover oral anaerobes and bowel flora (e.g., with clindamycin, metronidazole, or an aminopenicillin). Operative management (i.e., drainage, debridement, diversion procedures, resection) and nutritional support via enteral (i.e., feeding jejunostomy) or parenteral hyperalimentation also may be necessary (175–177).

Other agents inhibit that collagen synthesis (e.g., β-aminopropionitrile, D-penicillamine, *N*-acetylcysteine) are effective in preventing strictures in experimental animals but the clinical use of these agents has not yet been reported (178–180). Similarly, mucosal protective agents, such as sodium polyacrylate and sucralfate, appear to limit tissue injury and prevent subsequent strictures in animal models but their value in reducing injuries in human poisonings remains unknown (180–182).

Mechanical measures also have been used to prevent or treat strictures. Indwelling esophageal stents (Silastic tubes) may be placed at the time of endoscopy and left in place for approximately 2 weeks in an attempt to prevent stricture formation. Alternatively, nasogastric tubes or string may be placed in the esophagus to maintain a patent lumen and facilitate bouginage in the event that strictures subsequently develop (183–185). Because the use of these procedures may lead to reflux esophagitis and increase the risk of esophageal perforation, their efficacy is controversial (13).

Patients who develop strictures can be treated by either bouginage or surgery (e.g., esophageal resection or replacement by colonic interposition) (175,177,186). Dilation therapy should be delayed until at least 4 weeks after ingestion. If it is performed earlier, it is associated with an increased risk of iatrogenic perforation.

TABLE 62-8. Threshold limit values for some acids and bases

Substance	ACGIH TWAs (ppm)	ACGIH TWAs (mg/m³)	ACGIH STELs (ppm)	ACGIH STELs (mg/m³)	NIOSH RELs (ppm)	NIOSH RELs (mg/m³)	OSHA PELs (ppm)	OSHA PELs (mg/m³)
Ammonia	25	17	35	24	50	34.8 (C, 5 min)	50	35 (TWA, 8 h)
Calcium carbonate	—	10	—	—	—	—	—	—
Calcium hydroxide	—	5	—	—	—	5 (TWA, 8 h)	—	—
Calcium oxide	—	2	—	—	—	—	—	5 (TWA, 8 h)
Chromic acid	—	—	—	—	—	0.025 (TWA, 10 h) 0.05 (C, 5 min)	—	0.1 (C, 0 min)
Hydrazine	0.1	0.13	—	—	0.03 (C, 2 h)	0.04	1	1.3 (TWA, 8 h)
Hydrogen bromide	3 (C)	9.9 (C)	—	—	3 (C)	—	3 (TWA, 8 h)	—
Hydrogen chloride	5 (C)	7.5 (C)	—	—	5 (C)	—	5 (C)	—
Hydrogen peroxide	1	1.4	—	—	—	—	—	—
Nitric acid	2	5.2	4	10	2	5 (TWA, 10 h)	2	5 (TWA, 8 h)
Phosphoric acid	—	1	—	3	—	—		1 (TWA, 8 h)
Portland cement (dust)	—	10	—	—	—	—	—	—
Potassium hydroxide	—	2 (C)	—	—	—	—	—	—
Sodium bisulfite	—	5	—	—	—	—	—	—
Sodium hydroxide	—	2 (C)	—	—	—	2 (C, 15 min)	—	2 (TWA, 8 h)
Sulfuric acid	—	1	—	3	—	1 (TWA, 10 h)	—	1 (TWA, 10 h)

ACGIH, American Conference of Governmental Industrial Hygienists; C, ceiling limit; NIOSH, National Institute for Occupational Safety and Health; OSHA, Occupational Safety and Health Administration; PEL, permissible exposure limit; ppm, parts per million; REL, recommended exposure limit; STEL, short-term exposure limit; TWA, time-weighted average. Note: ACGIH TWAs are concentrations that produce no adverse effect on repeated exposure during an 8-hour workday and 40-hour work week; STEL concentrations are the 15-minute TWAs that should not be exceeded; Cs denote the concentration that should not be exceeded at any time. NIOSH and OSHA time limits for TWA and Cs are noted in parentheses.

Systemic Toxicity. Treatment of systemic effects is primarily supportive: maintenance of physiologic, hematologic, and biochemical homeostasis by standard measures. In certain cases, agent-specific therapy also may be necessary. Treatments of cyanide, hydrogen sulfide, and heavy metal poisoning are discussed in other chapters [Chapters 54 (cyanide), 55 (hydrogen sulfide), and 71–74 (metals)].

Elimination of ammonia can be enhanced by hemodialysis but this therapy is unlikely to be necessary in patients with normal liver and kidney function. Since hydrazine appears to cause a functional pyridoxine deficiency, patients with systemic hydrazine poisoning, particularly those with neurologic dysfunction, should be given supplemental pyridoxine (vitamin B_6) (147,148,187). Although the optimal dose is unknown, 25 mg per kg i.v. is usually recommended. This dose can be repeated in several hours if there is an incomplete, transient, or no response.

BIOLOGICAL AND ENVIRONMENTAL FATE AND MONITORING

Biological exposure indices and soil and water monitoring parameters are not applicable to acids and bases because these agents readily decompose (i.e., undergo neutralization reactions) on exposure to tissues and environmental compounds.

OCCUPATIONAL AND ENVIRONMENTAL REGULATIONS

Workplace standards for atmospheric exposure limits to acids and bases have been established only for a small number of agents (Table 62-8) (188–190). Direct eye, skin, or GI tract exposure to industrial or household products containing concentrated or strong acids or bases (excluding small amounts present in foods, cosmetics, or toiletries) should be completely avoided.

REFERENCES

1. Gapany-Gapanavicius M, Yellin A, Almog S, Tirosh M. Pneumomediastinum: a complication of chlorine exposure from mixing household cleaning agents. *JAMA* 1982;248:349–350.
2. Reisz GR, Gammon RS. Toxic pneumonitis from mixing household cleaners. *Chest* 1986;89:49–52.
3. Pinkus JL. Monochloramine hazard from a mixture of household clean solutions. *N Engl J Med* 1965;272:1133.
4. Dooms-Goossens A, Gevers D, Mertens A, Vanderheyden D. Allergic contact urticaria due to chloramine. *Contact Dermatitis* 1983;9:319–320.
5. Litovitz TL, Felberg L, White S, et al. 1995 Annual Report of the American Association of Poison Control Centers Toxic Exposure Surveillance System. *Am J Emerg Med* 1996;14:487–537.
6. Polson CJ, Green MA, Lee RM, eds. *Clinical toxicology.* 3rd ed. Philadelphia: JB Lippincott Co, 1984:243–259.
7. Leonard LG, Scheulen JJ, Munster AM. Chemical burns: effect of prompt first aid. *J Trauma* 1982;22:420–423.
8. Federal Hazardous Substances Act (1976, with amendments in 1981). 15 *USC* 1261 et seq.
9. US Consumer Protection Safety Committee. Report of the Toxicology Advisory Board. Washington: TAB, USCPSC, 1982.
10. Dafoe CS, Ross CA. Acute corrosive esophagitis. *Thorax* 1969;24:291–294.
11. Allen R, Thoshinsky M, Stallone R, Hunt TK. Corrosive injuries of the stomach. *Arch Surg* 1970;100:409–413.
12. Tewfik TL, Schloss MD. Ingestion of lye and other corrosive agents—a study of 86 infants and child cases. *J Otolaryngol* 1980;9:72–77.
13. Kirsh MM, Ritter F. Caustic ingestion and subsequent damage to oropharyngeal and digestive passages. *Ann Thora Surg* 1926;21:74–82.

14. Kirsh MM, Peterson A, Brown JW, Orringer MB, Ritter F, Sloan H. Treatment of caustic injuries of the esophagus: a ten year experience. *Ann Surg* 1978;188:675–678.
15. Bikhazi HB, Thompson ER, Shumrick DA. Caustic ingestion: current status. *Arch Otolaryngol* 1969;89:112–115.
16. Knopp R. Caustic ingestions. *J Am Coll Emerg Phys* 1979:329–336.
17. Tucker JA, Yarington CT. The treatment of caustic ingestion. *Otolaryngol Clin North AM* 1979;12:343–350.
18. Penner GE. Acid ingestion: toxicology and treatment. *Ann Emerg Med* 1980;9:374–379.
19. Friedman EM, Lovejoy FH. The emergency management of caustic ingestions. *Emerg Med Clin North Am* 1984;2:77–86.
20. Howel JM. Alkaline ingestions. *Ann Emerg Med* 1986;15:820–825.
21. Wason S. Coping swiftly and effectively with caustic ingestions. *Emerg Med Rep* 1989;10:25–32.
22. Leape LL, Ashcraft RW, Scarpelli DG, Holder DG. Hazard to health: liquid lye. *N Engl J Med* 1971;284:578–581.
23. Hawkins DB, Demeter MJ, Barnett TE. Caustic ingestion: controversies in management: a review of 214 cases. *Laryngoscope* 1980;90:98–109.
24. Jakobsson SW, Rajs J, Jonsson JA, et al. Poisoning with sodium hypochlorite solution. Report of a fatal case, supplemented with an experimental and clinico-epidemiological study. *Am J Forensic Med Pathol* 1991;12:320–327.
25. Zargar Sa, Kochhar R, Nagi B, et al. Ingestion of strong corrosive alkalis. Spectrum of injuries to upper GI tract and natural history. *Am J Gastroenterol* 1992;87:337–341.
26. Hoffman RS, Howland MA, Kamerow HN, et al. Comparison of titratable acid/alkaline reserve and pH in potentially caustic household products. *Clin Toxicol* 1989;27:241–261.
27. Boldt GB, Carroll RG. Titratable acid/alkaline reserve is not predictive of esophageal perforation risk after caustic exposure. *Am J Emerg Med* 1996; 14:106–108.
28. Vancura EM, Clinton JE, Ruiz E, Krenzelok EP. Toxicity of alkaline solutions. *Ann Emerg Med* 1980;9:118–122.
29. Muhlendahl KEV, Oberdisse U, Krienke EG. Local injuries caused by accidental ingestion of corrosive substances by children. *Arch Toxicol* 1978;39:299–314.
30. Linden CH, Berner JM, Kulig K, Rumach BH. Acid ingestion: toxicity following systemic absorption. *Vet Hum Toxicol* 1983;25[Suppl 1]:66(abst).
31. Grief F, Kaplan O. Acid ingestion: another cause of disseminated intravascular coagulopathy. *Crit Care Med* 1986;14:990–991.
32. Okonek S, Bierbach H, Atzpodien W. Unexpected metabolic acidosis in severe lye poisoning. *Clin Toxicol* 1981;18:225–230.
33. Kilburn KH. Effects of a hydrochloric acid spill on neurobehavioral and pulmonary function. *J Occup Envir Med* 1996;38:1018–1025.
34. National Institute for Occupational Safety and Health (criteria document for a recommended standard): Occupational exposure to ammonia. DHEW 74-136. Washington: Government Printing Office, 1974:1–88.
35. International Programme on Chemical Safety: Ammonia. Environmental Health Criteria 54. Geneva: World Health Organization, 1986:1–210.
36. Linden CH, Rumack BH, Galle SJ. Systemic toxicity following household ammonia ingestion. *Vet Hum Toxicol* 1984;26[Suppl 2]:59(abst).
37. Comstock CC, Lawson LH, Green EA, Oberst FW. Inhalation toxicity of hydrazine vapor. *Arch Ind Hyg Occup Med* 1954;10:476–490.
38. Clark DA, Bairrington JD, Bitter HL, et al. Pharmacology and toxicology of propellant hydrazines. Aeromedical review 11–68. Brooks Air Force Base, TX: USAF School of Aerospace Medicine, Aerospace Medical Division, 1968:1–126.
39. National Institute for Occupational Safety and Health (Criteria document for a recommended standard). Occupational exposure to hydrazines. DHEW 78–172. Washington: Government Printing Office, 1978:1–269.
40. Reinhardt CF, Brittelli MR. Heterocyclic and miscellaneous nitrogen compounds. In: Clayton GD, eds. *Patty's industrial hygiene and toxicology.* New York: John Wiley and Sons, 1981:2791–2800.
41. International Programme on Chemical Safety. *Hydrazine. Environmental Health Criteria 68.* Geneva: World Health Organization, 1987:1–89.
42. Pfister KR, Koski J. Alkali burns of the eye: pathophysiology and treatment. *South Med J* 1982;75:417–422.
43. Tripathi RC, Tripathi BJ. The eye: chemical injuries, toxins, and poisons. In: Riddell RH, ed. *Pathology of drug-induced and toxic diseases.* New York: Churchill Livingstone, 1982:432–456.
44. McCulley JP, Moore TE. Chemical injuries of the eye. In: Leibowitz HM, ed. *Corneal disorders: clinical diagnosis and management.* Philadelphia: WB Saunders, 1984:471–478.
45. Parrish CM, Chandler JW. Corneal trauma: chemical injuries. In: Kaufman HE, McDonald MB, Barron BA, Waltman SR, eds. *The cornea.* New York: Churchill Livingstone, 1988:608–644.
46. Vilogi J, Whitehead B, Marcus SM. Oven-cleaner pads: new risk for corrosive injury. *Ann J Emerg Med* 1985;3:412–414.
47. Girard LJ, Alford WE, Felman GL, Williams B. Severe alkali burn. *Trans Am Acad Ophthalmol Otolaryngol* 1970;74:788–803.
48. Helmers S, Top FH, Knapp LW. Ammonia injuries in agriculture. *J Iowa Med Soc* 1971;61:271–280.
49. Birken GA, Fabri PJ, Carey LC. Acute ammonia intoxication complicating multiple trauma. *J Trauma* 1981;21:820–822.
50. Arwood R, Hammond J, Ward GG. Ammonia inhalation. *J Trauma* 1985;25:444–447.
51. Early SH, Simpson RL. Caustic burns from contact with wet cement. *JAMA* 1985;254:528–529.
52. Sawhney CP, Kaushish R. Acid and alkali burns: considerations in management. *Burns* 1989;15:132–134.
53. Wang XW, Davies JWL, Sirvent RLZ, Robinson WA. Chromic acid burns and acute chromium poisonings. *Burns* 1985;11:181–184.
54. Skiendzielewski JJ. Cement burns. *Ann Emerg Med* 1980;9:316–318.
55. Bassan MM, Dudai M, Shalev O. Near-fatal systemic oxygen embolism due to wound irrigation with hydrogen peroxide. *Postgrad Med J* 1982;58:448–450.
56. Sleigh JW, Linter SPK. Hazards of hydrogen peroxide. *BMJ* 1985;291:1706.
57. Close LG, Catlin FI, Cohn AM. Acute and chronic burns of the respiratory tract. *Arch Otolaryngol* 1980;106:151–158.
58. Hajel R, Janigan DT, Landrigan PL, et al. Fatal pulmonary edema due to nitric acid fume inhalation in three pulp-mill workers. *Chest* 1990;97:487–489.
59. Walton M. Industrial ammonia gassing. *Br J Ind Med* 1973;30:78–86.
60. Montague TJ, Macneil AR. Mass ammonia inhalation. *Chest* 1980;77:496–498.
61. Flury KE, Dines DE, Rodarte JR, Rodgers R. Airway obstruction due to the inhalation of ammonia. *Mayo Clin Proc* 1983;58:389–393.
62. Sobonya R. Fatal anhydrous ammonia inhalation. *Hum Pathol* 1977;8:293–299.
63. O'Kane GJ. Inhalation of ammonia vapour: a report of the management of eight patients during the acute stages. *Anaesthesia* 1983;38:1208–1213.
64. Oberst FW, Comstock CC, Hackley EB. Inhalational toxicity of ninety percent hydrogen peroxide vapor-acute, subacute, and chronic exposures of laboratory animals. *Arch Ind Hyg Occup Med* 1954;10:319–327.
65. Kaelin RM, Kapaaci Y, Tschopp JM. Diffuse interstitial lung disease associated with hydrogen peroxide inhalation in a dairy worker. *Am Rev Respir Dis* 1988;137:1233–1235.
66. Moulin D, Bertrand JM, Buts JP, Nyakabasa M, Otte JB. Upper airway lesions in children after accidental ingestion of caustic substances. *J Pediatr* 1985;106:408–410.
67. Giusti GV. Fatal poisoning with hydrogen peroxide. *Forensic Sci* 1973;2:99–100.
68. Yarington CT. Ingestion of caustic: a pediatric problem. *J Pediatr* 1965;67: 674–677.
69. Moore WR. Caustic ingestions: pathophysiology, diagnosis, and treatment. *Clin Pediatr* 1986;25:192–196.
70. Wasserman RL, Ginsburg CM. Caustic substance injuries. *J Pediatr* 1985;107: 169–174.
71. Schild JA. Caustic ingestion in adult patients. *Laryngoscope* 1985;95:1199–1201.
72. Adam JS, Birck HG. Pediatric caustic ingestion. *Ann Otol Rhinol Laryngol* 1982;91:656–658.
73. Cardona JC, Daly JF. Management of corrosive esophagitis: analysis of treatment, methods, and results. *N Y State J Med* 1964;64:2307–2313.
74. Feldman M, Iben AB, Hurley EJ. Corrosive injury to the oropharynx and esophagus: eighty-five consecutive cases. *Calif Md* 1973;118:6–9.
75. Borja AR, Ransdell HT, Thomas TV, Johnson W. Lye injuries of the esophagus: analysis of ninety cases of lye ingestion. *J Thorac Cardiovasc Surg* 1969; 57:533–538.
76. Ferguson MK, Migliore M, Staszak VM, Little AG. Early evaluation and therapy of caustic esophageal injury. *Am J Surg* 1989;157:116–120.
77. Anderson KD, Rouse TM, Randolph JG. A controlled trial of corticosteroids in children with corrosive injury of the esophagus. *N Engl J Med* 1990;323:637–640.
78. Moazam F, Talbert JL, Miller D, Mollitt DL. Caustic ingestion and its sequelae in children. *South Med J* 1987;80:187–190.
79. Wason S. Coping swiftly and effectively with caustic ingestions. *J Emerg Med* 1985;2:175–182.
80. Oakes DD, Sherck JP, Mark JB. Lye ingestion clinical patterns and therapeutic implications. *J Thorac Cardiovasc Surg* 1982;83:194–204.
81. Middelkamp JN, Ferguson TB, Roper CL, Hoffman FD. The management and problems of caustic burns in children. *J Thorac Cardiovasc Surg* 1969; 57:341–346.
82. Hallagan LF, Smith M. Profound atelectasis following alkaline corrosive airway injury. *J Emerg Med* 1994;12:23–25.
83. Lopez GP, Dean BS, Krenzelok EP. Oral exposure to ammonia inhalants: a report of 8 cases. *Vet Hum Toxicol* 1988;30:350(abst).
84. Ernest RW, Leventhal M, Luna R, Martinez H. Total esophagogastric replacement after ingestion of household ammonia. *N Engl J Med* 1963;268:815–818.
85. Norton RA. Esophageal and antral strictures due to ingestion of household ammonia: report of two cases. *N Engl J Med* 1960;262:10–12.
86. Chassin JL, Slattery LR. Jejunal stricture due to ingestion of ammonia. *JAMA* 1953;152:134–136.
87. Gonzalez LL, Zinninger MM, Altemeier WA. Cicatricial gastric stenosis caused by ingestion of corrosive substances. *Ann Surg* 1962;156:84–89.
88. Meyer CT, Brand M, DeLuca VA, Spiro HM. Hydrogen peroxide colitis: a report of three patients. *J Clin Gastroenterol* 1981;3:31–35.
89. Landau GD, Saunders WH. The effect of chlorine bleach on the esophagus. *Arch Otolaryngol* 1968;80:174–176.
90. French RJ, Tabb HG, Rutledge LJ. Esophageal stenosis produced by ingestion of bleach. *South Med J* 1970;63:1140–1144.
91. Pike DG, Peabody JW, Davis EW, Lyons WS. A re-evaluation of the dangers of Chlorox ingestion. *J Pediatr* 1963;63:303–305.
92. Yarington CT, Bales GA, Frazer JP. A study of the management of caustic esophageal trauma. *Ann Otol Rhinol Laryngol* 1964;73:1130–1135.
93. Okonek S, Reinecke HJ, Krienke EG, et al. Poisoning by hypochlorite-containing disinfectants: a retrospective analysis of 594 cases of poisoning. *Dtsch Med Wochenschr* 1984;109:1874–1877(abst).
94. Fatti L, Marchand P, Crawshaw GR. The treatment of caustic strictures of the esophagus. *Surg Gynecol Obstet* 1956;102:195–206.
95. Davis LL, Raffensperger J, Novak GM. Necrosis of the stomach secondary to ingestion of corrosive agents: report of three cases requiring total gastrectomy. *Chest* 1972;62:48–51.

96. Adams JT, Skucas J. Corrosive jejunitis due to ingestion of nitric acid. *Am J Surg* 1980;139:282–285.
97. Abramson AL. Corrosive injury to the esophagus: result of ingesting some denture cleanser tablets and powder. *Arch Otolaryngol* 1978;104:514–516.
98. Krenzelok EP, Clinton JE. Caustic esophageal and gastric erosion without evidence of oral burns following detergent ingestion. *J Am Coll Emerg Phys* 1979;8:5–7.
99. Cello JP, Fogel RP, Boland CR. Liquid caustic ingestion: spectrum of injury. *Arch Intern Med* 1980;140:501–504.
100. Subbarao KSVK, Kakar AK, Chandrasekhar V, Anathakrishnan N, Banerjee A. Cicatrical gastric stenosis caused by corrosive ingestion. *Aust NZ J Surg* 1988;58:143–146.
101. Soni N, O'Rourke I, Pearson I. Ingestion of hydrochloric acid. *Med J Aust* 1985;142:471–472.
102. Stannard MW. Corrosive esophagitis in children: assessment by esophagogram. *Am J Dis Child* 1978;132:596–599.
103. Mansson I. Diagnosis of acute corrosive lesions of the aesophagus. *J Laryngol Otol* 1978;92:499–504.
104. Cullen ML, Klein MD. Spontaneous resolution of acid gastric injury. *J Pediatr Surg* 1987;2:550–551.
105. Gaudreault P, Parent M, Mcguigan MA, Chicoine, Lovejoy FH. Predictability of esophageal injury from signs and symptoms: a study of caustic ingestion in 378 children. *Pediatrics* 1983;71:767–770.
106. Sugawa C, Mullins RJ, Lucas CE, Leibold WC. The value of early endoscopy following caustic ingestion. *Surg Gynecol Obstet* 1981;153:553–556.
107. Welsh JJ, Welsh LW. Endoscopic examination of corrosive injuries of the upper gastrointestinal tract. *Laryngoscope* 1978;88:1300–1309.
108. Postlethwait RW. Chemical burns of the esophagus. *Surg Clin North Am* 1983;63:915–924.
109. Buntain WL, Cain WC. Caustic injuries to the esophagus: a pediatric overview. *South Med J* 1981;74:590–593.
110. Steigmann F, Dolehide R. Corrosive gastritis. *N Engl J Med* 1956;245:981–986.
111. Symbas PN, Viasis SE, Hatcher CR. Esophagitis secondary to ingestion of caustic material. *Ann Thorac Surg* 1983;36:73–77.
112. Aaron E, Taylor W, Mills LJ, Platt MR. Corrosive burns of the esophagus and stomach: a recommendation for an aggressive surgical approach. *Ann Thorac Surg* 1986;41:276–283.
113. Crain EF, Gershel JC, Mezey AP. Caustic ingestions: symptoms as predictors of esophageal injury. *Am J Dis Child* 1984;138:863–865.
114. Jordan FT. Diagnosis and treatment of acid gastric burns. *New Phys* 1976; 25:70–74.
115. Warren JB, Griffin DJ, Olson RC. Urine sugar reagent tablet ingestion causing gastric and duodenal ulceration. *Arch Intern Med* 1984;144:161–162.
116. Fisher RA, Echhauser ML, Radivoyevitch M. Acid ingestion in an experimental model. *Surg Gynecol Obstet* 1985;161:91–99.
117. Webb WR, Koutras P, Ecker RR, Sugg WL. An evaluation of steroids and antibiotic in caustic burns of the esophagus. *Ann Thorac Surg* 1970;9:95–102.
118. Meredith JW, Kon ND, Thompson JN. Management of injuries from liquid lye ingestion. *J Trauma* 1988;28:1173–1180.
119. Cleveland WW, Chandler JR, Lawson RB. Treatment of caustic burns of the esophagus: early esophagoscopy and adrenocortical steroids. *JAMA* 1963;186:262–264.
120. Viscomi GJ, Beekhuis GJ, Whitten CF. An evaluation of early esophagoscopy and corticosteroid therapy in the management of corrosive injury of the esophagus. *J Pediatr* 1961;59:356–360.
121. Haller JA, Andrews HG, White JJ, Tamer A, Cleveland WW. Pathophysiology and management of acute corrosive burns of the esophagus: results of treatment in 285 children. *J Pediatr Surg* 1971;6:578–584.
122. Klein J, Olson KRR, McKinney HE. Caustic injury from household ammonia. *A J Emerg Med* 1985;3:320.
123. Previtera C, Giusti F, Guglielmo M. Predictive value of visible lesions (cheeks, lips, oropharynx) in suspected caustic ingestion: may endoscopy reasonably be omitted in completely negative pediatric patients? *Pediatr Emerg Care* 1990;6:176–178.
124. Christesen HBT. Prediction of complications following unintentional caustic ingestion in children. Is endoscopy always necessary? *Acta Paediatr* 1995;84:1177–1180.
125. Kynaston JA, Patrick MK, Shephard RW, et al. The hazards of automatic-dishwasher detergent. *Med J Austral* 1989;151:5–7.
126. Madarikan BA, Lari J. Ingestion of dishwasher detergent by children. *Brit J Clin Pract* 1990;44:35–36.
127. Dickson KF, Caravati EM. Hydrogen peroxide exposure—325 exposures reported to a regional poison center. *Clin Toxicol* 1994;32:705–714.
128. deFerron P, Gossot D, Azoulay D, et al. Esophagogastric injuries by liquid chlorine bleach in adults. *Dig Surg* 1988;5:148–150.
129. Zargar SA, Kochhar, Nagi B, et al. Ingestion of corrosive acids. Spectrum of injury to upper gastrointestinal tract and natural history. *Gastroenterol* 1989;97:702–706.
130. Vergauwen P, Moulin D, Buts JP, et al. Caustic burns of the upper digestive and respiratory tracts. *Europ J Pediatr* 1991;150:700–705.
131. Gorman RL, Khin-Maung-Gyi MT, Klein-Schwartz W, et al. Initial symptoms as predictors of esophageal injury in alkaline corrosive ingestions. *Am J Emerg Med* 1992;10:189–192.
132. Zargar SA, Kochhar R, Mehta S, et al. The role of fiberoptic endoscopy in the management of corrosive ingestion and modified endoscopic classification of burns. *Gastrointest Endosc* 1991;37:165–169.
133. Muhletaler CA, Gerlock AJ, de Soto L, Halter SA. Acid corrosive esophagitis: radiographic findings. *Am J Radiol* 1980;134:1137–1141.
134. Kuhn JR, Tunell WP. The role of initial cineesophagography in caustic esophageal injury. *Am J Surg* 1983;146:804–806.
135. Levitt R, Stanley R, Wise L. Gastric bullae—an early roentgen finding in corrosive gastritis following alkali ingestion. *Radiology* 1975;115:597–598.
136. Fink DW, Boyden FM. Gas in the portal veins: a report of two cases due to ingestion of corrosive substances. *Radiology* 1966;87:741–743.
137. Mastrangelo MR, Moore EW. Spontaneous rupture of the stomach in a healthy adult man after sodium bicarbonate ingestion. *Ann Intern Med* 1984;101:650–651.
138. Luu TA, Kelley MT, Strauch JA, et al. Portal vein gas embolism from hydrogen peroxide. *Ann Emerg Med* 1992;21:1391–1393.
139. Christensen DW, Faught WE, Black RE, et al. Fatal oxygen embolism after hydrogen peroxide ingestion. *Crit Care Med* 1992;20:543–544.
140. Caravati EM. Metabolic abnormalities associated with phosphoric acid ingestion. *Ann Emerg Med* 1987;16:904–906.
141. Thomas SH, Stone CK. Acute toxicity from baking soda ingestion. *Am J Emerg Med* 1994;12:57–59.
142. Froner GA, Rutherford GW, Rokeach M. Injection of sodium hypochlorite by intravenous drug users (letter). *JAMA* 1987;258:325.
143. Hoy RH. Accidental systemic exposure to sodium hypochlorite (Chlorox) during hemodialysis. *Am J Hosp Pharm* 1981;38:1512–1514.
144. Schmidt FC, Vallencourt DC. Changes in the blood following exposure to gaseous ammonia. *Science* 1948;108:555–556.
145. Zitnik RS, Burchell HB, Shepherd JT. Hemodynamic effects of inhalation of ammonia in man. *Am J Cardiol* 1969;24:187–190.
146. Herrick RT, Herrick S. Allergic reaction to aromatic ammonia inhalant ampule. *Am J Sports Med* 1983;11:28.
147. Keirklin JK, Watson M, Bondoc CC, Burke JF. Treatment of hydrazine-induced coma with pyridoxine. *N Engl J Med* 1976;249:938–939.
148. Harati Y, Naikan E. Hydrazine toxicity, pyridoxine therapy, and peripheral neuropathy. *Ann Intern Med* 1986;104:727–729.
149. Sotaniemi E, Hirvonen J, Isomaki H, Takkunen J, Kaila J. Hydrazine toxicity in the human: report of a fatal case. *Ann Clin Res* 1971;3:30–33.
150. Reid FJ. Hydrazine poisoning. *BMJ* 1965;2:1246.
151. Lindberg E, Hedensterna G. Chrome plating: symptoms, findings the upper airways, and effects on lung function. *Arch Environ Health* 1983;38:367–374.
152. Reidenberg MM, Durant PJ, Harris RA, DeBoccardo G, Lahita R, Steuzel KH. Lupus erythematosus-like disease due to hydrazine. *Am J Med* 1983;75:365–370.
153. Langard S, Vigander T. Occurrence of lung cancer in workers producing chromium pigments. *Br J Ind Med* 1983;40:71–74.
154. Shimkin MB, de Lorimier AA, Mitchell JR, Burroughs TP. Appearance of carcinoma following single exposure to a refrigeration ammonia-oil mixture. *Arch Ind Hyg Occ Med* 1954;9:186–193.
155. Wald N, Boreham J, Doll R. Bonsall J. Occupational exposure to hydrazine and subsequent risk of cancer. *Br J Ind Med* 1984;41:31–34.
156. Sathiakumar N, Delzell E, Amoateng-Adjepong Y, et al. Epidemiologic evidence on the relationship between mists containing sulfuric acid and respiratory tract cancer. *Crit Rev Toxicol* 1997;27:233–251.
157. Swenberg JA, Beauchamp RO. A review of the chronic toxicity, carcinogenicity, and possible mechanisms of inorganic acid mists in animals. *Crit Rev Toxicol* 1997;27:253–259.
158. O'Donnell CH, Abbott WE, Hirshfield JW. Surgical treatment of corrosive gastritis. *Am J Surg* 1949;78:251–255.
159. Appelqvist P, Salmo M. Lye corrosion carcinoma of the esophagus: a review of 63 cases. *Cancer* 45:2655–2658.
160. Parkinson AT, Haidak GL, McInerney RP. Verrucous squamous cell carcinoma of the esophagus following lye stricture. *Chest* 1970;57:489–492.
161. Rost KM, Jaeger RW, deCastro FJ. Eye contamination: a poison center protocol for management. *Clin Toxicol* 1979;14:295–300.
162. Woodward D. Irrigation with acetic acid. *Ann Emerg Med* 1989;18:911.
163. Rumack BH, Burrington JD. Caustic ingestions: a rational look at diluents. *Clin Toxicol* 1977;11:27–34.
164. Okada Y, Iway A, Kobayashi H. Gastric lavage solution for ingestion of corrosive agents. *Jpn J Acute Med* 1987;11:75–80.
165. Leape L. New liquid lye drain cleaners. *Clin Toxicol* 1974;7:109–114.
166. Maull KI, Osmand AP, Maull CD. Liquid caustic ingestions: an *in vitro* study of the effects of buffer neutralization and dilution. *Ann Emerg Med* 1985;14: 1160–1162.
167. Lacouture PG, Gaudreault P, Lovejoy FH. Clinitest table ingestion: an *in vitro* investigation concerned with initial emergency management. *An Emerg Med* 1986;15:143–146.
168. Homan CS, Maitra SR, Lane BP, et al. Effective treatment for acute alkali injury to the esophagus using weak-acid neutralization therapy: an *ex-vivo* study. *Acad Emerg Med* 1995;2:952–958.
169. Smilkstein MJ. Should we add an acid to an alkali injury? For now, let's remain neutral! *Acad Emerg Med* 1995;2:945–946.
170. Homan CS, Maitra SR, Lane BP, et al. Effective treatment of acute alkali injury of the rat esophagus with early saline dilution therapy. *Ann Emerg Med* 1993;22:178–182.
171. Homan CS, Maitra SR, Lane BP, et al. Histopathologic evaluation of the therapeutic efficacy of water and milk dilution for esophageal acid injury. *Acad Emerg Med* 1995;2:587–591.
172. Hallet JA, Bachman K. The comparative effect of current therapy on experimental caustic burns of the esophagus. *Pediatrics* 1964;34:236–245.

173. Knox WG, Scott JR, Zintel H, Guthrie R, McCabe RE. Bouginage and steroids used singly or in combination in experimental corrosive esophagitis. *Ann Surg* 1967;166:930–941.
174. Howell JM, Dalsey WC, Hartsell FW, et al. Steroids for the treatment of corrosive esophageal injury: a statistical analysis of past studies. *Am J Emerg Med* 1992;10:421–424.
175. Meredith JW, Kon ND. Management of injuries from liquid lye ingestion. *J Trauma* 1988;28:1173–1180.
176. Horvath OP, Tibor O, Gabriella Z. Emergency esophagogastrectomy for treatment of hydrochloric acid injury. *Ann Thorac Surg* 1991;52:98–101.
177. Wu M, Lai W. Surgical management of extensive corrosive injury of the alimentary tract. *Surg Gynecol Obstet* 1993;177:12–16.
178. Thompson JN. Corrosive esophageal injuries: II. An investigation of treatment methods and histochemical analysis of esophageal strictures in a new animal model. *Laryngoscope* 1987;97:1191–1202.
179. Lui A, Richardson M, Robertson WO. Effects of *N*-acetylcysteine on caustic burns. *Vet Hum Toxicol* 1985;28:316(abst).
180. DiCostanzo J, Noirelerc M, Jouglard J, et al. New therapeutic approach to corrosive burns of the upper gastrointestinal tract. *Gut* 1980;21:370–375.
181. Ehrenpreis ED, Leiken JB, Ehrenpreis S, Goldstein JL. Use of sodium polyacrylate in rat gastrointestinal alkali burns. *Vet Hum Toxicol* 1988;30:135–138.
182. Reddy AN, Budhraja M. Sucralfate therapy for lye-induced esophagitis. *Am J Gastroenterol* 1988;83:71–73.
183. Mills LJ, Estrera AS, Platt MR. Avoidance of esophageal stricture following severe caustic burns by the use of an intraluminal stent. *Ann Thorac Surg* 1979;28:60–65.
184. Reyes HM, Lin CY, Schlunk FF, Replogle RL. Experimental treatment of corrosive esophageal burns. *J Pediatr Surg* 1974;9:317–327.
185. Wijburg FA, Heymans HS, Urbanns NA. Caustic esophageal lesions in childhood: prevention of stricture formation. *J Pediatr Surg* 1989;24:171–173.
186. Butler C, Madden JW, Davis WM, et al. Morphologic aspects of experimental esophageal lye strictures II. Effects of steroid hormones, bougienage, and induced lathyrism on acute lye burns. *Surgery* 1977;81:431–435.
187. Cornish HH. The role of vitamin B in the toxicity of hydrazine. *Ann N Y Acad Sci* 1969;166:136–145.
188. Centers for Disease Control and Prevention. *MMWR* 1986;35:1–33S.
189. NIOSH Recommendations for occupational safety and health. Compendium of policy documents and statements. Cincinnati, Department of Health and Human Services, National Institute for Occupational Safety and Health, Pub. No. 92-100, 1992.
190. American Conference of Governmental Industrial Hygienists. Threshold limit values and biological exposure indices for 1996–1997. Cincinnati: ACGIH, 1996.

CHAPTER 63

Organic Acids and Bases

Hon-Wing Leung and Dennis J. Paustenbach

ORGANIC ACIDS: SOURCES AND PRODUCTION

Organic acids constitute a very wide range of chemicals and have numerous industrial applications. Many occur naturally in the body and are biochemical intermediates in metabolic processes. The most common organic acids contain a dissociable hydrogen ion from a carboxyl functional group bound to an aliphatic (e.g., acetic acid), olefinic (e.g., acrylic acid), or aromatic hydrocarbon moiety (e.g., benzoic acid). Organic acids with the carboxyl group are referred to as *carboxylic acids.* Longer-chain aliphatic carboxylic acids are also known as *fatty acids.* Compounds containing a dissociable hydrogen ion from a hydroxyl group may be classified as organic acid as well; however, their acid strength is generally less than that of the carboxylic acids. Examples of organic acids containing the hydroxyl group include the phenols (carbolic acid), glycols, naphthols, glycerols, and catechols (1).

Industrial Uses

Fatty acids are constituents of oil and waxes. Organic acids are used in the production of fibers, resins, plastics, and dyestuffs. They are important intermediates in the manufacture of pharmaceuticals, cosmetics, and food additives (2). Many carboxylic acids are generally recognized as safe by the U.S. Food and Drug Administration and are used as food additives. Carboxylic acids are commonly prepared from the oxidation of the corresponding aldehydes.

Routes of Exposure and Exposure Sources

The physical form of organic acids may range from a liquid to a waxy solid. The shorter-chain organic acids are liquid at room temperature, whereas the longer-chain acids (i.e., more than 10 carbons) tend to be solids. Table 63-1 lists the physicochemical properties of selected organic acids. Exposure via inhalation is largely determined by the vapor pressure of the organic acids. Short-chain organic acids, such as formic, acetic, and propionic acids, are more volatile and, therefore, present a greater potential for inhalation exposure. Direct contact of organic acids with exposed body surfaces may produce primary irritation. The eyes, skin, and the mucous membrane of the respiratory tract are particularly susceptible.

CLINICAL TOXICOLOGY

Metabolism

Aliphatic monocarboxylic acids are metabolized by beta oxidation to acetate or butyrate, which is further converted to CO_2 and water via the citric acid cycle. Metabolism of certain medium-chain acids may proceed by omega oxidation, which produces dicarboxylic acid. Omega oxidation does not normally occur with acids having more than 12 carbons unless the capacity for beta oxidation is saturated or blocked because of substituents in the alpha or beta positions. Organic acids with alpha substituents are not readily metabolized and are eliminated in the urine after conjugation with glucuronide (3,4).

Acute Toxicity

The primary health effect after single exposure to organic acids is irritation of the eyes, skin, and other mucous membranes. The ability of an organic acid to irritate tissues is a function of both its molecular weight and water solubility. As long as the compound is soluble in water, its potential to irritate increases with increasing molecular weight, except for the first member of the aliphatic series, formic acid. High-molecular-weight organic acids are not water soluble and are not irritants. The degree of irritation is predominantly governed by the strength of the acid, its water solubility, and its ability to penetrate the skin. The shorter-chain acids are relatively strong acids and can produce corrosion. Generally, substances with a pH less than 2 are strong corrosives; however, pH is not the sole determinant of potency. Other factors include concentration, molarity, and complexing ability of the anion (5). The relative strength of an organic acid is measured by its equilibrium dissociation constant, K_a; or, more conveniently, this is expressed as the negative decadic logarithm, denoted pK_a. For organic acids, the lower the pK_a, the stronger the acid and vice versa. The presence of substituent groups on an organic acid may markedly affect its acidity. Electron-withdrawing substituents, such as halogens (F, Cl, Br, I) and nitro (NO_2) groups, disperse the negative charge and stabilize the anion, thus increasing acidity. In contrast, electron-releasing substituents, such as alkyl and hydroxyl groups, intensify the negative charge, destabilize the anion, and thus decrease acidity (1). For this reason, chloroacetic acid and trichloroacetic acid are stronger acids than acetic acid, while propionic and acetic acids

TABLE 63-1. Physicochemical properties of organic acids

	CAS no.	Molecular weight	Melting point (°C)	Boiling point (°C)	Solubility in water (g/mL)	pK_a1	pK_a2	Vapor (mm Hg)	Pressure (°C)
Saturated acids									
Formic	64-18-6	46	8	101	Miscible	3.75	—	35	20
Acetic[a]	64-19-7	60	17	118	Miscible	4.76	—	11.4	20
Propionic[a]	79-09-4	74	−21	141	Miscible	4.87	—	3.3	28
Butyric[a]	107-92-6	88	−8	164	Miscible	4.82	—	0.8	20
Isobutyric	79-31-2	88	−47	155	0.2	4.86	—	1	15
Valeric	109-52-4	102	−34	186	0.033	4.84	—	1	42
Isovaleric	503-74-2	102	−29	176	0.042	4.78	—	1	34
Caproic	142-62-1	116	−5	205	0.011	4.87	—	1	72
Isocaproic	646-07-1	116	−33	201	Slightly	4.84	—	—	—
2-Methylvaleric	97-61-0	116	—	194	0.006	4.78	—	0.02	20
2-Ethylbutyric	88-09-5	116	−32	194	Slightly	4.73	—	0.08	20
Heptanoic	111-14-8	130	−8	223	0.002	4.88	—	1	78
Caprylic	124-07-2	144	17	240	0.011	4.9	—	1	78
2-Ethylhexanoic	149-57-5	144	—	228	Slightly	—	—	0.03	20
Nonanoic	112-05-0	158	13	254	Insoluble	4.95	—	1	108
Capric	334-48-5	172	32	268	Insoluble	—	—	1	128
Undecylenic	122-37-8	186	30	284	Insoluble	—	—	1	101
Lauric	143-07-7	200	44	225	Insoluble	—	—	1	121
Myristic	544-63-8	228	54	250	Insoluble	—	—	1	142
Palmitic	57-10-3	256	64	267	Insoluble	—	—	1	154
Stearic	57-11-4	284	69	291	0.0003	—	—	1	174
Oxalic	144-62-7	90	189	157	0.083	1.46	4.4	0.54	105
Malonic	141-82-2	104	136	—	1.54	2.8	5.85	—	—
Succinic[a]	110-15-6	118	189	235	0.08	4.17	5.64	0.03	47
Malic[a]	6915-15-7	134	131	—	0.56	3.4	5.05	—	—
Thiomalic	70-49-5	150	154	—	0.5	—	—	—	—
Tartaric[a]	87-69-4	150	171	—	1.33	2.93	4.23	—	—
Adipic[a]	124-04-9	146	153	338	0.014	4.43	5.52	1	160
Citric[a]	77-92-9	192	153	—	0.59	3.08	4.75	—	—
Pimelic	111-16-0	160	106	272	0.05	4.47	5.42	—	—
Suberic	505-48-6	174	144	300	0.0016	—	—	—	—
Azelaic	123-99-9	188	106	287	0.0024	4.53	5.33	1	178
Sebacic	111-20-6	202	135	295	0.001	4.59	5.59	—	—
Unsaturated acids									
Propiolic	471-25-0	70	18	144	Miscible	1.89	—	11	55
Acrylic	79-10-7	72	13	141	Miscible	4.25	—	3	20
Crotonic	107-93-7	86	72	185	0.055	4.69	—	0.2	20
Methacrylic	79-41-4	86	16	162	Slightly	4.66	—	0.7	20
Pentanoic	591-80-0	100	23	188	Slightly	4.6	—	20	93
Hexanoic	1191-04-4	114	94	—	—	4.73	—	14	183
Sorbic[a]	110-44-1	112	134	228	0.0025	4.77	—	<0.01	20
Undecylenic	112-38-9	184	24	275	Insoluble	—	—	10	160
Linolenic	1955-33-5	278	−11	157	Insoluble	—	—	0.05	125
Linoleic	2197-37-7	280	−5	202	Insoluble	—	—	16	229
Elaidic	112-79-8	282	45	288	Insoluble	—	—	100	288
Oleic	112-80-1	282	13	234	Insoluble	—	—	10	225
Ricinoleic	141-22-0	298	5	245	Insoluble	—	—	10	226
Arachidonic	506-32-1	304	−49	163	Insoluble	—	—	—	—
Maleic	110-16-7	116	139	—	Freely	1.83	6.09	—	—
Fumaric	110-17-8	116	287	—	0.0063	3.03	4.44	1.7	165
Mesaconic	498-24-8	130	204	250	0.027	3.09	4.75	—	—
Citraconic	498-23-7	130	93	—	Freely	2.29	6.15	—	—
Itaconic	97-65-4	130	172	—	0.083	3.85	5.45	—	—
Aconitic	499-12-7	174	130	198	0.5	2.8	4.46	—	—

CAS, Chemical Abstracts Service.
[a]Substances generally recognized as safe by the U.S. Food and Drug Administration.

are weaker acids than formic acid. A correlation between the strength of organic acids and their potential to cause irritation has been established (6). A similar relationship of pK_a and acute skin irritation in humans for a homologous series of benzoic acid derivatives also has been reported (7).

The oral median lethal doses of some common organic acids in the rat are shown in Table 63-2. The most common toxic response resulting from acute exposure to organic acids is irritation. Irritation is a localized inflammatory reaction of the mucous membranes or epithelium. It is characterized by the presence of erythema and edema. Exposure to strong organic acids can produce a burning sensation in the eyes and respiratory tract. Contact with skin can cause dermatitis. Dermal ulceration with eschar formation may ensue in prolonged exposure with potent organic acids (8). The escharotic response results from the desiccating action that causes a coagulation of the pro-

TABLE 63-2. Oral median lethal doses of organic acids in the rat

Saturated acids	g/kg	Unsaturated acids	g/kg
Formic	1.83	Propiolic	0.15
Acetic	3.42	Acrylic	1.77
Propionic	3.43	Crotonic	0.7
Butyric	4.58	Methacrylic	5.83
Isobutyric	0.28	Pentanoic	0.47
Valeric	1.45	Sorbic	5.28
Isovaleric	2.6	Linolenic	>3.2
Caproic	5.97	Linoleic	>3.2
Isocaproic	3	Maleic	0.71
2-Methylvaleric	2.4	Fumaric	10.7
2-Ethylbutyric	2.03	Undecylenic	>2.5
Heptanoic	7	Citraconic	1.32
Caprylic	5.68		
2-Ethylhexanoic	2.3		
Capric	3.32		
Lauric	12		
Palmitic	>2		
Stearic	>5		
Oxalic	0.43		
Malonic	1.31		
Succinic	2.26		
Malic	>3.2		
Thiomalic	1.2		
Citric	11.7		
Pimelic	7		

teins in the superficial tissue. The coagulative necrosis of acid burns restricts further penetration into deep tissues.

Death may occur from inhalation exposure to organic acids when escape is impossible, such as in emergencies within confined spaces. Generally, the irritative properties of acids provide ample warning to limit the exposure such that temporary discomfort or annoyance is elicited. However, certain individuals may develop a tolerance to repeated high concentrations of organic acids. This phenomenon has been referred to in the medical literature as *adaptation*, *desensitization*, *olfactory fatigue*, or *accommodation*. Such unusual diseases as acid-etched teeth and perforated skin lesions are examples of this phenomenon (9). Although these diseases are only of historic interest in the United States, they may still exist in less-developed nations.

Sensitization

Unsubstituted aliphatic acids are not sensitizers in humans (10). Certain substituted organic acids, such as iodoacetic acid, have been reported to be sensitizers. The aromatic organic acid, benzoic acid, is a mild irritant and an occasional skin sensitizer. Because it is a solid at room temperature and has a low vapor pressure, however, it poses a lesser human health hazard compared with other more volatile sensitizers.

Chronic Toxicity

Organic acids rarely induce chronic toxic effects. Unlike other highly reactive molecular structures, such as nitroso or epoxide groups, the carboxylic acid group does not readily interact with DNA or other tissue macromolecules. Organic acids are expected to have low carcinogenic potential, and, accordingly, only a few have been tested in cancer bioassays.

Methanoic Acid

Methanoic acid is commonly known as *formic acid*. It is also called *formylic* and *hydrogen carboxylic acid*. The major hazard of methanoic acid exposure is severe burns to the skin, eyes, or mucosal surfaces. Lacrimation, nasal discharge, cough, laryngeal discomfort, erythema, and blistering may occur depending on exposure concentrations. Exposure to 0.3 to 42.0 parts per million (ppm) methanoic acid vapor for 1 hour was reported to be more irritating than the same concentration of formaldehyde (11). Methanoic acid was not clastogenic in the Chinese hamster ovary cells (12). No pathologic changes were noted in the skin of mice painted with 8% methanoic acid for 50 days (13). Male and female rats dosed with 0.2% to 0.4% of the calcium salt of methanoic acid in the drinking water for three successive generations developed no adverse effects in growth, fertility, and organ functions (14). A worker accidentally splashed with methanoic acid developed severe dyspnea and dysphagia and died within 6 hours (15). Because methanoic acid can inhibit cellular respiration, workers with cardiovascular diseases are especially predisposed to the effects of methanoic acid (16). The threshold limit value established by the American Conference of Governmental Industrial Hygienists (ACGIH) for methanoic acid is 5 ppm as an 8-hour time-weighted average.

Ethanoic Acid

Ethanoic acid is commonly known as *acetic acid*. It is also called *ethylic* and *methanecarboxylic acid*. Ethanoic acid was not clastogenic in the Chinese hamster ovary cells (12). Rats given 390 mg per kg per day ethanoic acid in the drinking water for 4 months had body weight loss but not at a dose of 195 mg per kg per day (17). Gastric lesions were seen in rats fed 4.5 g per kg per day of ethanoic acid in the diet for 30 days (18). In a study of five workers exposed to 80 to 200 ppm ethanoic acid vapor for 7 to 12 years, the principal findings were blackening and hyperkeratosis of the skin of the hands, conjunctivitis, pharyngitis, and erosion of the exposed teeth (19). The threshold limit value established by the ACGIH for ethanoic acid is 10 ppm as an 8-hour time-weighted average.

Propanoic Acid

Commonly known as *propionic acid*, this organic acid is also called *methylacetic* and *ethanecarboxylic acid*. Propanoic acid was not active in a battery of *in vitro* genotoxicity tests (20). No remarkable changes were seen in rats fed 5% propanoic acid for 110 days (21). A no-observed-effect level of 1 mg per kg per day was established from a study in rats fed propanoic acid for 6 months (22). Rats fed a diet containing 4% propanoic acid developed forestomach tumors believed to have resulted from increased cellular proliferation (23). The threshold limit value established by the ACGIH for propanoic acid is 10 ppm as an 8-hour time-weighted average.

Butanoic Acid

Butanoic acid is commonly known as *butyric acid*. It is also called *ethylacetic* and *1-propanecarboxylic acid*. Butanoic acid is less irritating than propanoic acid (24). No mortality was observed in rats exposed for 8 hours to air saturated with butanoic acid vapor (25). Butanoic acid was not active in a battery of *in vitro* genotoxicity tests (26). Rats, mice, and hamsters fed a diet containing 4% butanoic acid for 7 days developed forestomach lesions (27). No gastric lesions were found in rats fed 1% to 10% butanoic acid for up to 500 days (21). No developmental toxicity was observed in rats treated with 133 mg per kg per day butanoic acid during days 6 to 15 of gestation (28). Continuous inhalation of up to 200 mg per m^3 of butanoic acid in rats for 7 months produced a slight pulmonary reaction but no other histologic changes. The suggested maximum exposure concentration for butanoic acid in Russia is 100 mg per m^3 (24).

Pentanoic Acid

Pentanoic acid is commonly known as *valeric acid*. It is also called *propylacetic* and *1-butanecarboxylic acid*. No mortality occurred in rats exposed for 8 hours to air saturated with pentanoic acid vapor (25). No significant changes were seen in rats and rabbits exposed to 200 to 300 mg per m^3 of pentanoic acid for 6 months (29). No remarkable change was observed in the glandular stomach of rats fed 5% pentanoic acid (21). Rats exposed continuously to pentanoic acid vapor for 97 days had no adverse changes (30). No developmental toxicity was observed in rats treated with 100 mg per kg per day pentanoic acid during days 6 to 15 of gestation (28). The maximum allowable concentration for pentanoic acid in Russia is 5 mg per m^3 (31).

Hexanoic Acid

Hexanoic acid is commonly known as *caproic acid*. It is also called n-*hexoic* and *2-butylacetic acid*. Rats exposed to air saturated with hexanoic acid for 8 hours experienced no fatalities (25). No adverse changes were observed in rats fed 2% to 8% hexanoic acid in the diet for 3 weeks (32). The maximum allowable concentration in Russia for hexanoic acid is 5 mg per m^3 (31).

Heptanoic Acid

Heptanoic acid is commonly known as *heptylic acid*. It is also called *enanthic* and *1-hexanecarboxylic acid*. Mice receiving 125 mg per kg per day of heptanoic acid by intraperitoneal injection died within 2 to 4 days after dosing (33).

Octanoic Acid

Octanoic acid is commonly known as *caprylic acid*. It is also called n-*octylic acid* and *1-heptanecarboxylic acid*. Octanoic acid is not mutagenic in the bacterial or yeast assays with or without metabolic activation (34). Rats fed 6% octanoic acid in the diet for 9 weeks experienced 45% mortality (35); however, only slight effects were observed in rats fed a diet containing 10% octanoic acid for 10 days (36). No developmental toxicity was observed in rats treated with 1,500 mg per kg per day octanoic acid during days 6 to 15 of gestation (28). No skin irritation or sensitization was reported in human volunteers given 1% octanoic acid in an occluded patch test (37).

Nonanoic Acid

Nonanoic acid is commonly known as *pelargonic acid*. It is also called *pelargic* and *1-octanecarboxylic acid*. Rats fed a diet of 4.17% nonanoic acid for 4 weeks had no discernible effects (38). A 12% solution of nonanoic acid in petrolatum produced no irritation or sensitization in humans (39).

Decanoic Acid

Decanoic acid is commonly known as *capric acid*. It is also called *decylic* and *1-nonanecarboxylic acid*. No mortality was observed in rats exposed for 8 hours to saturated decanoic acid vapor (40). Decanoic acid (1% in petrolatum) did not produce irritation or sensitization when applied to human skin (41,42). No gastric lesions were seen in rats fed 10% decanoic acid in the diet for 150 days (21).

Dodecanoic Acid

Dodecanoic acid is commonly known as *lauric acid*. It is also called *duodecylic* and *1-undecanecarboxylic acid*. Dodecanoic acid produced neither irritation nor sensitization when applied to human skin (43). No adverse effects were seen in rats fed 10% dodecanoic acid in the diet for 18 weeks (44). Rats fed 10% dodecanoic acid in the diet for 150 days developed no stomach lesions (21). Mice injected subcutaneously with up to 5 mg of dodecanoic acid three times per week for 4 weeks and observed for 24 months had no increased incidence of tumors compared with controls (45).

Tetradecanoic Acid

The common name of tetradecanoic acid is *myristic acid*. It is also known as *crodacid* and *1-tridecanecarboxylic acid*. Tetradecanoic acid was a moderate irritant when applied to human skin (45). Treatment of rats with 10% tetradecanoic acid in the diet for 33 days did not significantly alter body weight; however, evidence of increased erythrocyte fragility was present (46).

Hexadecanoic Acid

The common name of hexadecanoic acid is *palmitic acid*. It is also known as *cetylic* and *1-pentadecanecarboxylic acid*. Hexadecanoic acid was a mild irritant when applied to human skin (47). Rats fed 10% hexadecanoic acid for 150 days developed no stomach lesions (21). Atherosclerotic lesions were noted in rats fed 6% hexadecanoic acid for 16 weeks (35). No tumors were reported for mice injected subcutaneously three times per week with up to 5 mg of hexadecanoic acid (45).

Octadecanoic Acid

Octadecanoic acid is commonly called *stearic acid*. It is also known as *cetylacetic* and *1-heptadecanecarboxylic acid*. Octadecanoic acid was not active in a battery of *in vitro* genotoxicity tests (48). Rats fed a diet containing 3,000 ppm octadecanoic acid for 30 weeks had an erratic weight gain, but no pathologic lesions in all of the organs examined (49). No sarcomas at the injection site were noted in mice injected subcutaneously with 0.5 mg octadecanoic acid once weekly for 6 months and observed for 21 months (50).

The toxicology of other aliphatic carboxylic acids is similar to those described for the saturated monocarboxylic acids. Generally, the health effects are characterized by low acute toxicity. The potential for irritation is much higher with the shorter-chain members in the series; for example, oxalic and malonic acids are relatively strong irritants, whereas pimelic and sebacic acids are not irritants. The presence of a second carboxyl group, as in oxalic acid, increases its acidity compared with formic acid. The dicarboxylic acids are less extensively metabolized than the monocarboxylic acids. In fact, oxalic and malonic acids are mainly excreted unchanged. Some reports suggest that acrylic, crotonic, and methacrylic acids may have sensitization potential.

ORGANIC BASES: SOURCES, PRODUCTION, AND INDUSTRIAL USES

Chemical compounds that are classified as organic bases are generally amines. They contain one or more amino (NH_2) functional groups that serve as proton acceptors, thus the basicity. They may be aliphatic amines (e.g., methylamine), aliphatic alcohol amines (e.g., ethanolamine), aromatic amines (e.g., aniline), or alicyclic amines (e.g., cyclohexylamine). The aliphatic amines can be further classified as primary, secondary, and tertiary amines depending on the number of alkyl side chains attached to the nitrogen of the amino moiety. Similar to the fatty acids, the longer-chain aliphatic amines are called fatty amines. A variety of alkylamines are naturally occurring in certain vegetables, fishes, cheeses, and bread (3,4), and some alkanolamines, such as monoethanolamine (MEA), *N*-methylethanolamine, and *N,N*-dimethylethanolamine, are metabolic intermediates in the biosynthesis of membranes and the neurotransmitter acetylcholine.

Aliphatic and aromatic amines are fundamental to industries producing explosives, pharmaceuticals, rubber chemicals, and dyes. They are also important intermediates in the manufacture of pesticides, plastics, and paints (2). The alkanolamines have found uses in such diverse areas as gas treating, metal working, industrial cleansers, and lubricants. The lower aliphatic amines are made by reacting ammonia with alcohols, aldehydes, or ketones. Alternatively, hydrogen cyanide is reacted with an alkene to yield an amide, which is then hydrolyzed to form the amine.

CLINICAL TOXICOLOGY

Routes of Exposure

The lower alkylamines, such as methylamine, are gases or volatile liquids and have high water solubility. They have a distinctive ammoniacal odor resembling that of decaying fish. The higher-molecular-weight alkylamines are less volatile, odorless, and sparingly soluble in water. The physicochemical properties of selected organic bases are shown in Table 63-3.

Like the organic acids, the shorter-chain organic bases possess the greatest potential for inhalation exposure because of their higher volatility. Many organic bases can be absorbed through the skin and produce systemic effects. Aqueous solutions of organic bases are highly irritating, and prolonged contact can cause injury to the eyes, skin, and respiratory tract. Certain organic bases, such as ethyleneamine, have been shown to be skin as well as respiratory sensitizers (51,52).

Metabolism

The organic amines are metabolized by the amine oxidases to ammonia and the corresponding aldehyde. The ammonia is converted to urea and excreted in the urine. The aldehyde is acted on by aldehyde dehydrogenase to the respective carboxylic acid, which is further metabolized as discussed earlier. The rate of deamination is faster with primary amines than secondary amines, and tertiary amines are more slowly oxidized than straight-chain amines. The rate of oxidation depends on the alkyl chain length, ranging from nil with methylamine to a maximum with hexylamine, and decreases with further increase in chain length (3,4). Certain alkanolamines may mimic their natural substrate, MEA, in the biosynthesis of membrane lipids, resulting in the production of aberrant phospholipids (53).

Acute Toxicity

The acute oral toxicity of the organic bases ranges from slightly to moderately toxic. The oral median lethal doses of selected organic bases in rats are shown in Table 63-4. Similar to the organic acids, the most significant acute effect of the organic bases is irritation. Exposure to concentrated vapor produces severe inflammation of the respiratory tract and pulmonary edema in laboratory animals. Exposure of the eyes to the vapors of certain organic bases [e.g., dimethylamine (54) and dimethylethanolamine (55)] has been associated with the condition clinically known as *glaucopsia*, a blue-gray vision in which vision is temporarily fogged due to a transient increase in corneal thickness. Prolonged skin contact to the organic bases can cause severe burns. Unlike the coagulative necrosis of acid burns, organic bases cause a liquefaction of the proteins in the superficial tissues, which allows penetration of the bases deep into the underlying dermal structure. Severe corneal damage resulting in blindness can occur to the eyes in prolonged contact with liquid organic bases. The irritative effects of organic bases are attributed to their alkalinity. Generally, the primary amines are more irritating than the secondary amines, which in turn are more irritating than the tertiary amines. The irritating potential decreases as the alkyl chain length increases. The alkanolamines generally are less irritating than the corresponding alkylamines.

Certain alkylamines mimic the action of bioactive amines, such as histamine and catecholamines, and may cause hemodynamic changes. The arylamines, such as aniline, produce methemoglobinemia. Secondary amines can react with nitrite to form nitrosamines, which are potent animal carcinogens. Some polyamines, especially ethylenediamine (EDA), diethylenetriamine (DETA), and triethylenetetramine (TETA), are strong skin sensitizers and may also cross-react with one another to elicit allergic dermatoses (56). Some alkyleneamines (e.g., EDA, TETA), alicyclic amine (piperazine), and alkanolamines (*N,N*-dimethylethanolamine, *N,N*-diethylethanolamine, aminoethylethanolamine) may be respiratory sensitizers (57–61). Hepatic, renal, and cardiac system injuries have been observed in laboratory animals given high doses of organic bases (62,63). In typical industrial exposures, however, acute local effect (i.e., irritation) predominates.

Alkylamines

The most salient toxicity associated with the exposure to this class of organic bases is skin, eye, and respiratory tract irritation. One distinctive effect associated with the exposure to the vapors of many alkylamines—ethylamine, dimethylamine, and triethylamine in particular—is that of glaucopsia. This visual disturbance results from a transient thickening of the corneal epithelium. Affected individuals experience haziness of vision followed by marked difficulty in visual discrimination accompanied by a partial loss of color discrimination in which objects take on a blue or gray coloration. These symptoms may be followed by the development of a halo effect around bright objects. A few subjects may develop photophobia. These effects usually resolve without treatment within 24 hours. However, after intense exposures, the corneal epithelial swelling may take several days to clear. Although glaucopsia is an entirely reversible process that does not do any permanent physical or functional injury to the eyes, the symptoms may impair the performance of skilled tasks. Exposures to alkylamine vapors in the workplace, therefore, should be carefully controlled. Table 63-5 gives the current occupational exposure limits for the alkylamines adopted by the ACGIH. Because of the paucity of long-term toxicity data on the alkylamines, the rationale of the exposure limits for these compounds is based largely on their irritative or other acute toxic effects in animals and by analogy to one another.

Alicyclic Amines

Two important members of this class of organic bases are cyclohexylamine and piperazine.

CYCLOHEXYLAMINE

Humans acutely exposed to cyclohexylamine in an industrial environment have reported symptoms of drowsiness, anxiety, and nausea (64). Cyclohexylamine is known to have sympathomimetic

TABLE 63-3. Physicochemical properties of organic bases

	CAS no.	Molecular weight	Melting point (°C)	Boiling point (°C)	Solubility in water (g/mL)	pK_a1	pK_a2	Vapor (mm Hg)	Pressure (°C)
Alkylamines									
Methylamine	74-89-5	31	–94	–6	Very	10.7	—	1,500	25
Dimethylamine	124-40-3	45	–93	7	Very	10.7	—	1,500	10
Trimethylamine	75-70-3	59	–117	3	Very	9.8	—	760	3
Ethylamine	75-04-7	45	–81	17	Miscible	10.7	—	400	3
Diethylamine	119-89-7	73	–48	56	Miscible	11	—	195	20
Triethylamine	121-44-8	101	–115	89	Freely	10.8	—	54	20
Propylamine	107-10-8	59	–83	49	Soluble	10.6	—	400	31
Di-*n*-propylamine	142-84-7	101	–63	111	Soluble	11	—	30	25
Isopropylamine	75-31-0	59	–101	34	Miscible	10.6	—	460	20
Diisopropylamine	108-18-9	101	–61	84	Slightly	11	—	70	20
n-Butylamine	109-73-9	73	–50	78	Miscible	10.7	—	72	20
Di-*n*-butylamine	11-92-2	129	–60	160	Soluble	10.6	—	2	20
Tri-*n*-butylamine	102-89-9	185	–70	214	Insoluble	—	—	20	100
Isobutylamine	78-81-9	73	–85	68	Miscible	10.8	—	100	19
n-Amylamine	110-58-7	87	–55	104	Soluble	—	—	—	—
Isoamylamine	107-85-7	87	—	95	Soluble	—	—	—	—
n-Hexylamine	111-26-2	101	–19	133	0.012	10.6	—	7	20
n-Heptylamine	111-68-2	115	–18	157	Slightly	—	—	—	—
2-Ethylhexylamine	104-75-6	130	—	142	0.0025	—	—	—	—
Octadecylamine	124-30-1	270	—	232	Insoluble	—	—	—	—
Allyamine	107-11-9	57	—	58	Miscible	9.7	—	—	—
Diallylamine	24-02-7	97	–88	111	0.086	9.3	—	—	—
Triallylamine	1102-75-9	137	–70	155	0.0025	8.3	—	—	—
Polyamines									
Ethylenediamine	107-15-3	60	9	116	Freely	10.7	7.6	10	22
N,N-Diethylethylenediamine	100-36-7	116	—	145	Very	7.7	10.5	4	20
1,3-Propanediamine	109-76-2	74	–24	135	Soluble	—	—	—	—
1,2-Propanediamine	78-90-0	74	–37	120	Miscible	6.6	9.7	8	20
1,4-Butanediamine	110-60-1	88	27	158	Very	9.2	10.8	—	—
1,3-Butanediamine	590-88-5	88	—	142	—	—	—	—	—
1,5-Pentanediamine	462-94-2	102	9	178	Soluble	10.3	9.1	—	—
1,6-Hexanediamine	124-09-4	116	41	204	Freely	11.8	10.8	—	—
Triethylenediamine	280-57-9	112	158	174	0.45	3	8.7	—	—
Diethylenetriamine	111-40-0	103	–3	207	Miscible	4.4	9.2	0.2	20
Triethylenetetramine	112-24-3	146	–35	277	Miscible	3.3	6.7	<0.01	20
Tetraethylenepentamine	112-57-2	189	–46	319	Miscible	3	4.7	<0.01	20
Pentaethylenehexamine	4067-16-7	232	–29	300	Miscible	—	—	<0.01	20
Alicyclic amines									
Cyclohexylamine	108-91-8	99	–18	134	Miscible	10.7	—	—	—
Dicyclohexylamine	101-83-7	181	–0.1	256	Slightly	10.4	—	—	—
N,N-Dimethylcyclohexylamine	98-94-2	127	–77	159	0.011	—	—	3	25
Piperazine	110-85-0	86	42	113	Miscible	5.3	9.8	6.65	20
Aminoethylpiperazine	140-31-8	129	–59	221	Miscible	—	—	0.009	20
Hydroxyethylpiperazine	103-76-4	130	–10	246	Miscible	—	—	0.004	20
Alkanolamines									
Ethanolamine	141-43-5	61	11	171	Miscible	9.5	—	520	20
Diethanolamine	111-42-2	105	28	269	0.96	8.9	—	0.37	20
Triethanolamine	102-71-6	149	21	335	Miscible	7.8	—		20
								0.0047	
Propanolamine	156-87-6	75	—	187	Miscible	—	—	—	—
Isopropanolamine	78-96-6	75	—	160	Miscible	—	—	—	—
N,N-Dimethylisopropanolamine	108-16-7	103	—	98	Miscible	—	—	14.7	20
Triisopropanolamine	122-20-3	191	—	305	Very	—	—	—	—
N-Methylethanolamine	109-83-1	75	–5	160	Miscible	—	—	0.48	20
N,N-Dimethylethanolamine	108-01-0	89	–59	135	Miscible	—	—	4.4	20
N-Ethylethanolamine	110-73-6	89	—	169	Miscible	—	—	—	—
N,N-Diethylethanolamine	100-37-8	117	–78	163	Miscible	—	—	1.3	20
Diisopropylethanolamine	96-80-0	145	–63	192	0.0548	—	—	0.26	20
N,N-Dibutylethanolamine	102-81-8	173	—	229	0.004	—	—	—	—
Methyldiethanolamine	105-59-9	119	–21	247	Miscible	—	—	<0.01	20
Ethyldiethanolamine	139-87-7	133	—	246	Miscible	—	—	—	—
t-Butylethanolamine	4620-70-6	117	43	118	Miscible	—	—	0.17	20
t-Butyldiethanolamine	2160-93-2	161	45	270	Miscible	—	—	0.0002	20

CAS, Chemical Abstracts Service.

TABLE 63-4. Oral median lethal doses of organic bases in the rat

Organic base	g/kg
Alkylamines	
Methylamine	0.15
Dimethylamine	0.7
Ethylamine	0.4
Diethylamine	0.54
Triethylamine	0.46
Propylamine	0.57
Dipropylamine	0.93
Diisopropylamine	0.77
Butylamine	0.5
Dibutylamine	0.55
Tributylamine	0.54
Diisobutylamine	0.26
Amylamine	0.47
Dipentylamine	0.27
2,2'-Diethyldihexylamine	1.64
Allylamine	0.11
Diallylamine	0.58
Triallylamine	1.31
2-Ethylbutylamine	0.39
2-Ethylbutylamine	0.39
Alkanolamines	
Ethanolamine	1.9
Diethanolamine	1.75
Triethanolamine	8.4
Isopropanolamine	4.26
N,N-Dimethylisopropanolamine	1.89
Triisopropanolamine	6.5
N-Methylethanolamine	1.65
N,N-Dimethylethanolamine	2.08
N-Ethylethanolamine	1.48
N,N-Diethylethanolamine	1.3
N,N-Dibutylethanolamine	1.07
Propanolamine	2.83
Methyldiethanolamine	1.87
t-Butyldiethanolamine	2.83
Polyamines	
Ethylenediamine	1.46
1,3-Propanediamine	0.35
1,2-Propanediamine	2.23
1,3-Butanediamine	1.35
Diethylenetriamine	1.71
Triethylenetetramine	4.34
Tetraethylenepentamine	3.25
Pentaethylenehexamine	>5
Alicyclic amines	
Cyclohexylamine	0.71
Dicyclohexylamine	0.37
Piperazine	2.83
Aminoethylpiperazine	2.14
Hydroxyethylpiperazine	5.66

effects akin to those of the catecholamines (65). In a reproduction study, mice fed a diet of 0.5% cyclohexylamine experienced growth retardation. Pregnancy rate, number of live fetuses, and fetal body weight were all reduced (66). In a multigeneration reproductive toxicity study, significant incidence of testicular atrophy and reduction of litter size were seen in rats given 150 mg per kg per day of cyclohexylamine (67). Cyclohexylamine has been widely tested for mutagenicity, teratogenicity, and carcinogenicity, because it is a metabolite of the artificial sweetener sodium cyclamate. The data have been critically reviewed and no evidence of these effects has been demonstrated (68).

PIPERAZINE

Rats fed piperazine in the diet at an average dosage of 2.06 g per kg per day for 7 days had decreased body weight and slightly increased kidney weight (69). Some biochemical changes were observed in rats given a piperazine dosage of 150 mg per kg per day by gavage for 30 days (70). Degenerative changes in the liver and kidney were seen in rats fed 0.3% to 1.0% piperazine in their diets for 90 days (71). No adverse effect was observed in beagle dogs fed a diet containing 1,500 ppm piperazine dihydrochloride from week 1 to 5 and 3,700 ppm from week 6 to 13 (72). No teratogenic effects were reported in mice given a gavage dosage of 1,000 mg per kg per day piperazine dihydrochloride during gestation days 6 to 15 (73). Piperazine, therefore, has low systemic toxicity. The predominant hazards from occupational exposure are dermatitis (74) and respiratory sensitization (59).

TABLE 63-5. Occupational exposure limits for organic bases adopted by the American Conference of Governmental Industrial Hygienists in 2000

Amine	Threshold limit value (mg/m³) 8-hour TWA	15-minute STEL	Ceiling
Methylamine	6.4	19	—
Dimethylamine	9.2	27.6	—
Trimethylamine	12	36	—
Ethylamine	9.2	27.6	—
Diethylamine	15	45	—
Triethylamine	4.1	12	—
Isopropylamine	12	24	—
Diisopropylamine	21	—	—
Butylamine	—	—	15
Cyclohexylamine	41	—	—
Ethylenediamine	25	—	—
Diethylenetriamine	4.2	—	—
Ethanolamine	7.5	15	—
Diethanolamine	2	—	—
Triethanolamine	5	—	—
N,N-Diethylethanolamine	9.6	—	—

STEL, short-term exposure limit; TWA, time-weighted average.

Polyamines

In addition to being severe skin and eye irritants, the polyamines—typified by EDA, DETA, and TETA—are reported to be skin sensitizers as well.

ETHYLENEDIAMINE

Reports suggest that exposure to EDA may be associated with the induction of occupational asthma (51,57). In a two-generation study, no reproductive toxicity was found in rats fed a diet including an EPA dosage of 0.5 g per kg per day (75), nor was teratogenicity evident in rats given 1 g per kg per day EDA in the diet or in rabbits given 80 mg per kg per day by gavage during organogenesis (76,77). EDA was not genotoxic in a variety of *in vitro* and *in vivo* test systems (78). A lifetime skin painting study in mice and a dietary feeding study in rats established that EDA was not oncogenic (79,80).

DIETHYLENETRIAMINE

The subchronic toxicity of DETA was evaluated in a 90-day dietary study in the rat. Concentrations of 7,500 and 15,000 ppm DETA resulted in dose-related pathologic effects in the liver and kidney. A no-observable-effect level was established as 1,000 ppm (81). DETA was inactive in a series of *in vitro* and *in vivo* genotoxicity tests (78). DETA was tested in lifetime dermal painting studies in mice and was not found to be carcinogenic (82).

TRIETHYLENETETRAMINE

Mice, rats, and rabbits given oral dosages of TETA at 0.8 or 4.0 mg per kg per day for 10 months developed central nervous system effects (83). Mice and rats were fed a diet containing up to 3,000 ppm TETA for 92 days. Increased frequencies of lung inflammation and hepatic fatty infiltration were seen in the mouse. In rats, the only effect noted was a reduced liver copper level (84). TETA was positive in the Ames test, the forward gene mutation test, the sister chromatid exchange, and the unscheduled DNA synthesis test with the Chinese hamster ovary cells, but was negative in the *in vivo* mouse micronucleus test and the *Drosophila* sex-linked recessive lethal test (78). TETA administered orally produced embryofetal toxicity and teratogenicity in mice and rats (85,86). These effects, however, were secondary to severe copper deficiency resulting from the chelating action of TETA (86,87). When TETA was administered percutaneously to the rabbit, it did not produce any developmental effects, even in the presence of severe maternal toxicity (88). TETA was not carcinogenic in a lifetime skin painting study in mice (82).

Alkanolamines

The most commonly used alkanolamines in industry are MEA, diethanolamine (DEA), and triethanolamine (TEA). The toxicologic properties of the alkanolamines generally resemble those of the alkylamines. The main biological effects are local irritation of the skin, eyes, and respiratory tract. The irritation potential decreases with increasing chain length. Whereas MEA is corrosive to the skin and eye, DEA causes only minor irritation, and TEA is not irritating. The toxicology of the alkanolamines was reviewed (89,90). Available data indicate that DEA is the most toxic alkanolamine from the standpoint of systemic toxicity. This may be because MEA is a normal biochemical intermediate in membrane phospholipid metabolism, and DEA is structurally similar enough to MEA to interfere with this function, whereas TEA may be sufficiently dissimilar to MEA to act as a substrate.

MONOETHANOLAMINE

Continuous exposure of rats, guinea pigs, and dogs to 66 to 102 ppm MEA for 3.5 to 13 weeks produced lung inflammation and damage to the liver and kidney (91). Liver and kidney effects were also seen in rats given 0.64 g per kg per day MEA in the diet for 90 days. The no-observed-effect level was 0.32 g per kg per day (25). The percutaneous application of 4 mg per kg per day MEA to rats resulted in nonspecific histologic changes in the heart and lung. Hepatotoxic manifestations included fatty degeneration of the liver parenchyma and subsequent focal necrosis (92). Hepatotoxic effect was also reported in a case of human poisoning to MEA (92). MEA was negative in a battery of *in vitro* tests for genotoxicity (89). One report suggested that MEA at 50 to 350 mg per kg per day given to pregnant rats by gavage during the period of organogenesis might produce embryopathic and teratogenic (hydroureter and hydronephrosis) effects (93). A subsequent study, however, showed no evidence of embryotoxic or teratogenic effects in rats similarly treated with up to 450 mg per kg per day MEA (94). In addition, no developmental toxicity was observed in studies with the rat and rabbit dosed percutaneously with 225 and 75 mg per kg per day MEA, respectively (95).

DIETHANOLAMINE

Rats exposed to 6 ppm DEA by inhalation for 13 weeks experienced growth rate depression, increased lung and kidney weights, and some deaths (96). Rats and mice treated with DEA in drinking water and by dermal application for 90 days developed anemia and adverse effects in the liver, kidney, brain, and heart (97,98). Rats exposed to aerosols of DEA for 90 days developed upper respiratory tract irritation; anemia; and effects in the liver, kidney, and testes. The level at which no effects were observed was 15 mg per m^3 (99). The developmental toxicity potential of DEA has been evaluated in both rats and rabbits. No teratogenic effects were seen in rats treated with 1,500 mg per kg per day by cutaneous contact or with 200 mg per m^3 6 hours per day during day 6 to 15 of gestation by aerosol inhalation exposure (100,101). Furthermore, no developmental toxicity was observed in rabbits similarly dosed with 350 mg per kg per day (102). DEA was inactive in a variety of *in vitro* and *in vivo* genotoxicity tests (89). The National Toxicology Program is testing DEA for carcinogenicity. Preliminary pathologic findings indicate that no evidence of neoplasm exists in the rat, but increased incidences of liver and kidney tumors were seen in the mouse. DEA was negative when tested in transgenic mice.

TRIETHANOLAMINE

In a 90-day percutaneous toxicity study, mice treated with TEA up to 2.3 g per kg per day produced only slight epidermal hyperplasia at the site of application but no other systemic effects (103). In other subchronic toxicity studies (25,104), the most commonly reported effects were in the liver and kidney. No embryofetal toxicity was observed in pregnant rats given 1,125 mg per kg per day TEA orally during organogenesis (105). In mating trial studies, percutaneous treatment with 500 mg per kg per day and 2,000 mg per kg per day TEA in rats and mice, respectively, for 10 weeks before mating, during breeding, and through gestation and lactation for females had no effects on reproductive functions (106). TEA was negative in a battery of *in vitro* and *in vivo* genotoxicity tests (89). A cancer bioassay in rats given drinking water containing up to 2% TEA for 2 years demonstrated that TEA was toxic to the kidneys but was not carcinogenic (107). Similarly, no evidence of carcinogenicity was observed in mice given drinking water containing 2% TEA for 82 weeks or treated percutaneously with TEA for 14 to 18 months (108,109). An increased incidence of lymphoid tissue tumors was reported in mice fed a diet containing 0.03% to 0.3% TEA (110). This finding is questionable because of flaws in the study, including an unusually low incidence of lymphoid tumors in the controls and the fact that the diet may have been contaminated with a nitrosamine. The National Toxicology Program is testing TEA for carcinogenicity. Preliminary pathologic findings have produced no evidence of neoplasm in rats, but an increased incidence of liver tumors was seen in female mice. The validity of this finding is questionable because the mice in this bioassay were infected with the bacterium *Helicobacter hepaticus*, which is a known cause of liver tumors in the mouse.

MANAGEMENT OF TOXICITY

The principal clinical manifestation of overexposure to organic acids and bases is irritation and corrosion. Ingestion causes severe, burning pain to the mouth, pharynx, and stomach, followed by vomiting and diarrhea of dark precipitated blood. Asphyxia may occur from edema of the glottis. After initial recovery, onset of fever may suggest mediastinitis or peritonitis from perforation of the stomach. Symptoms of skin contact are severe pain with dermal staining. The burn may penetrate the full thickness of the skin. The damage by organic bases is generally more severe than by organic acids because organic bases can solubilize the superficial proteins, which then allow the penetration of the organic bases into deep tissues. To control exposure while handling organic acids and bases, proper gloves should be worn and all exposed skin surfaces should be covered with protective clothing. Inhalation exposure to organic acids or bases causes irritation of the respiratory tract, which may be followed by pulmonary edema with tightness in the chest, dyspnea, and cyanosis. Prolonged exposure may cause erosion of the teeth. Inhalation exposure to certain organic bases has been linked to the induction of respiratory system allergies including occupational asthma.

Exposure of the eyes can produce erythema, conjunctivitis, iritis, and damage to the cornea. The symptoms are tearing, pain, and photophobia (111). Exposure of the eyes to vapors of some organic bases can lead to glaucopsia. Although this condition does not produce any permanent effects on vision, the symptoms may impair the ability to undertake coordinated activities and may render the affected individual more susceptible to physical accidents. The incidence of glaucopsia could be higher in those individuals wearing contact lenses owing to accumulation of the organic base under the lens. The use of contact lenses while handling volatile organic bases should therefore be discouraged. The most effective measures to avoid the development of respiratory sensitization and glaucopsia from exposure to airborne organic bases are adequate ventilation and engineering controls to reduce vapor concentrations. The use of eye protection, such as goggles and full-face respiratory protective equipment, is also highly recommended.

No specific antidotes exist for organic acid and base poisoning. Treatment involves the customary regimen of stabilization, decontamination, and supportive care. Oxygen may be recommended if airway complications arise from pulmonary edema and excessive swelling. If an organic acid or base is ingested, immediate dilution with milk or water within 30 minutes of exposure is indicated; however, neutralization with weak acids or bases should not be attempted because the exothermic reaction may aggravate the existing injury. Emesis is contraindicated because of reexposure of the esophagus. Activated charcoal is ineffective because it does not adsorb organic acids or bases. In the case of skin contact, removal of all contaminated clothes and copious irrigation of the exposed skin with saline are the treatments of choice. Exposed eyes should be irrigated for at least 30 minutes. For glaucopsia, prolonged washing of the eyes should be discouraged because excessive hydration may exacerbate the corneal epithelial swelling. The visual disturbance usually clears in 24 hours without treatment; however, those with established glaucopsia should be advised not to undertake potentially physically incapacitating tasks, including driving a motorized vehicle.

REFERENCES

1. Neckers DC, Doyle MP. *Organic chemistry.* New York: John Wiley and Sons, 1977.
2. Gosselin RE, Smith RP, Hodge HC, Braddock JE. *Clinical toxicology of commercial products*, 5th ed. Baltimore: Williams & Wilkins, 1984.
3. Lehninger A. *Principles of biochemistry.* New York: Worth Publishers, 1982.
4. Stryer L. *Biochemistry.* San Francisco: Freeman, 1981.
5. Marzulli FN, Maibach HI. *Dermatotoxicology*, 3rd ed. New York: Hemisphere, 1989.
6. Leung HW, Paustenbach DJ. Setting occupational exposure limits for irritant organic acids and bases based on their equilibrium dissociation constants. *Appl Ind Hyg* 1988;4:115–118.
7. Berner B, Wilson DR, Guy RH, Mazzenga GC, Clarke FH, Maibach HI. The relationship of pK_a and acute skin irritation in man. *Pharm Res* 1988;5:660–663.
8. Adams RM. *Occupational contact dermatitis.* Philadelphia: JB Lippincott Co, 1984.
9. Hunter D. *The diseases of occupations*, 6th ed. Boston: Little, Brown and Company, 1978.
10. Peterson JE. *Industrial health.* Englewood Cliffs, NJ: Prentice-Hall, 1977.
11. Amdur MO. The response of guinea pigs to inhalation of formaldehyde and formic acid alone and with a sodium chloride aerosol. *Int J Air Pollut* 1960;3:201–220.
12. Morita T, Takeda K, Okumura K. Evaluation of clastogenicity of formic acid, acetic acid and lactic acid on cultured mammalian cells. *Mutat Res* 1990; 240:195–202.
13. Frei JV, Stephens P. The correlation of promotion of tumour growth and of induction of hyperplasia in epidermal two-stage carcinogenesis. *Br J Cancer* 1968;22:83–92.
14. Malorny G. Acute and chronic toxicity of formic acid and formates. *Z Ernahrungswiss* 1969;9:332–339.
15. von Oettingen WF. The aliphatic acids and their esters—toxicity and potential dangers. *Arch Ind Health* 1959;20:517–522.
16. Liesivuori J, Kettunen A. Farmer's exposure to formic acid vapor in silage making. *Ann Occup Hyg* 1983;27:327–329.
17. Sollman T. Studies of chronic intoxications on albino rats. III. Acetic and formic acids. *J Pharmacol Exp Ther* 1921;16:463–474.
18. Mori K. Production of gastric lesions in rats by acetic acid feeding. *Gann* 1952;43:433–466.
19. Parneggiani L. *Encyclopedia of occupational health and safety.* Geneva: International Labor Office, 1983.
20. Basler A, von der Hude W, Scheutwinkel M. Screening of the food additive propionic acid for genotoxic properties. *Food Chem Toxicol* 1987;25:287–290.
21. Mori K. Production of gastric lesions in the rat by the diet containing fatty acid. *Jpn J Cancer Res* 1953;44:421–427.
22. Shchepetova GA. Hygienic standards for propionic acid and sodium propionate in water bodies. *Gig Sanit* 1970;35:96–98.
23. Clayson DB, Iverson F, Nera EA, Lok E. Early indicators of potential neoplasia produced in the rat forestomach by non-genotoxic agents: the importance of induced cellular proliferation. *Mutat Res* 1991;248:321–331.
24. Stasenkova KP, Kochetkova TA. Toxicologic characteristics of butyric acid. *Toksikol Movykh Prom Khim Veshchestv* 1962;4:19–28.
25. Smyth HF, Carpenter CP, Weil CS. Range-finding toxicity data: list IV. *Arch Ind Hyg Occup Med* 1951;4:119–122.
26. Ishidate M, Sofuni T, Yoshikawa K, et al. Primary mutagenicity screening of food additives currently used in Japan. *Food Chem Toxicol* 1984;22:623–636.
27. Harrison PT, Grasso P, Badescu V. Early changes in the forestomach of rats, mice and hamsters exposed to dietary propionic and butyric acid. *Food Chem Toxicol* 1991;29:367–371.
28. Narostsky MG, Francis EZ, Kavlock RJ. Continued evaluation of structure-activity relationships in the developmental effects of aliphatic acids in rats. *Teratology* 1991;43:433.
29. Egorov YL, Kasparov AA, Zakharov VM. Toxicology of synthetic fatty acids. *Uchen Zap Mosk Nauchn-Issled Inst Gig* 1961;9:40–46.
30. Dubrovskaya FI, Lukina IP. Effect of small concentrations of valeric acid vapors on experimental animals (white rats). *Gig Sanit* 1966;31:7–10.
31. Cook WA. *Occupational exposure limits worldwide.* Akron, OH: American Industrial Hygiene Association, 1987.
32. Moody DE, Reddy JK. Hepatic peroxisome (microbody) proliferation in rats fed plasticizers and related compounds. *Toxicol Appl Pharmacol* 1978;45:497–504.
33. Fassett DW, Irish DD. *Industrial hygiene and toxicology*, vol II, 2nd ed. New York: Wiley-Interscience, 1963.
34. *Mutagenic evaluation of caprylic acid.* Kensington, MD: Litton Bionetics, Inc., National Technical Information Service, 1976. [Project report PB257-872].
35. Renaud S. Thrombogenicity and atherogenicity of dietary fatty acids in rat. *J Atheroscler Res* 1968;8:625–636.
36. Narayana Rao M. The effect of steam volatile fatty acids on calcium metabolism in normal growing rats. *Indian J Med Res* 1954;42:37–42.
37. Opdike DLJ. Monographs on fragrance raw materials: caprylic acid. *Food Cosmet Toxicol* 1981;19:237–254.
38. Dryden LP, Hartman AM. Effect of vitamin B12 on the metabolism in the rat of volatile fatty acids. *J Nutr* 1971;101:589–592.
39. Opdyke DU. Monographs on fragrance raw materials: pelargonic acid. *Food Cosmet Toxicol* 1978;16:839–841.
40. Smyth HF, Carpenter CP, Weil CS, Pozzani UC, Striegel JA. Range-finding toxicity data: list VI. *Am Ind Hyg Assoc J* 1962;23:61–68.
41. Opdyke DU. Monographs on fragrance raw materials: capric acid. *Food Cosmet Toxicol* 1979;17:735–742.
42. Stillman MA, Maibach HI, Shalita AR. Relative irritancy of free fatty acids of different chain length. *Contact Dermatitis* 1975;1:65–69.
43. Cosmetic, Toiletry and Fragrance Association. Final report on the safety assessment of oleic acid, lauric acid, palmitic acid, myristic acid and stearic acid. Cosmetic Ingredients Review. *J Am Coll Toxicol* 1987;6:321–401.
44. Fitzhugh OG, Schouboe PJ, Nelson AA. Oral toxicities of lauric acid and certain lauric acid derivatives. *Toxicol Appl Pharmacol* 1960;2:59–67.
45. Swern D, Wieder R, McDonough M, Meranze DR, Shimkin MB. Investigation of fatty acids and derivatives for carcinogenic activity. *Cancer Res* 1970;30:1037–1046.
46. Elson CE, Voichick SJ. Dietary-induced alterations in the fatty acids of rat bone marrow. *Lipids* 1970;5:698–701.
47. Drill VA, Lazar P. *Cutaneous toxicity.* New York: Academic Press, 1977.
48. Leifer Z, Kada T, Mandel M, Zeiger E, Stafford R, Rosenkranz HS. An evaluation of tests using DNA repair-deficient bacteria for predicting genotoxicity and carcinogenicity. *Mutat Res* 1981;87:211–297.
49. Deichmann WB, Radomski JL, MacDonald WE, Kascht RL, Erdmann RL. The chronic toxicity of octadecylamine. *Arch Ind Health* 1958;18:483–487.
50. van Duuren BL, Katz C, Shimkin MB, Swern D, Weider R. Replication of low-level carcinogenic activity bioassays. *Cancer Res* 1972;32:880–881.
51. Lam S, Chan-Yeung M. Ethylenediamine-induced asthma. *Am Rev Respir Dis* 1980;121:151–155.
52. Baer R, Ramsey DL, Biondi E. The most common contact allergens. *Arch Dermatol* 1973;108:74–78.

53. Mathews JM, Garner CE, Matthews HB. Metabolism, bioaccumulation, and incorporation of diethanolamine into phospholipids. *Chem Res Toxicol* 1995;8:625–633.
54. Akesson B, Bengtsson M, Floren I. Visual disturbances after industrial triethylamine exposure. *Int Arch Occup Environ Health* 1986;57:297–302.
55. Leung HW, Tyl RW, Ballantyne B, Klonne DR. Developmental toxicity study in Fischer 344 rats by whole-body exposure to *N,N*-dimethylethanolamine vapor. *J Appl Toxicol* 1996;16:533–538.
56. Paustenbach DJ, Leung HW. Techniques for assessing the health risks of dermal contact with chemicals in the environment. In: Wang RGM, Knaak JB, Maibach HI, eds. Boca Raton, FL: CRC Press, 1993:343–385.
57. Aldrich FD, Stange AW, Geesaman RE. Smoking and ethylenediamine sensitization in an industrial population. *J Occup Med* 1987;29:311–314.
58. Fawcett IW, Newman Taylor AJ, Pepys J. Asthma due to inhaled chemical agents—epoxy resin systems containing phthalic acid anhydride, trimellitic acid anhydride and triethylenetetramine. *Clin Allergy* 1977;7:1–14.
59. Hagmar L, Bellander T, Bergoo B, Simonsson BG. Piperazine-induced occupational asthma. *J Occup Med* 1982;24:193–197.
60. Gadon ME, Melius JM, McDonald GJ, Orgel D. New-onset asthma after exposure to the steam system additive 2-diethylaminoethanol. *J Occup Med* 1994;36:623–626.
61. Vallieres M, Cockcroft DW, Taylor DM, Dolovich J, Hargreave FE. Dimethylethanolamine-induced asthma. *Am Rev Respir Dis* 1977;115:867–871.
62. Brieger H, Hodes WA. Toxic effects of exposure to vapors of aliphatic amines. *Arch Ind Hyg Occup Med* 1951;3:287–291.
63. Pozzani UC, Carpenter CP. Response of rats to repeated inhalation of ethylenediamine vapors. *Arch Ind Hyg Occup Med* 1954;9:223–226.
64. Watrous RM, Schulz HN. Cyclohexylamine, *p*-chloronitrobenzene, 2-aminopyridine: toxic effects in industrial use. *Ind Med Surg* 1950;19:317–320.
65. Elchelbaum M, Hengstmann JH, Rost HD, Brecht T, Dengler HJ. Pharmacokinetics, cardiovascular and metabolic actions of cyclohexylamine in man. *Arch Toxicol* 1974;31:243–263.
66. Kroes R, Peters PWJ, Berkvens JM, Verschuuren HG, De Vries T, Van Esch GJ. Long-term toxicity and reproduction study (including a teratogenicity study) with cyclamate, saccharin and cyclohexylamine. *Toxicology* 1977;8:285–300.
67. Oser BL, Carson S, Cox GE, Vogin EE, Sternberg SS. Long-term and multigeneration toxicity studies with cyclohexylamine hydrochloride. *Toxicology* 1976;6:47–65.
68. International Agency for Research on Cancer. Some non-nutritive sweetening agents—cyclamate: Lyon, France. *Monogr Eval Carcinog Risk Chem Hum* 1980;22:55–109.
69. *Range-finding toxicity and 7-day dietary inclusion studies*. Export, PA: Union Carbide Corporation Bushy Run Research Center, 1976. [Project report 39-102].
70. Raj RK. Effects of 30-day feeding of piperazine on rats. *Indian J Physiol Pharmacol* 1973;17:387–389.
71. *Results of dietary feeding of anhydrous piperazine and piperazine dihydrochloride in rats*. Midland, MI: Dow Chemical Company, 1957. [Project report T35.22-9-4].
72. *Thirteen-week dietary toxicity study in dogs*. Vienna, VA: Hazleton Laboratories, 1975. [Project report 819-102, 1975].
73. *Teratogenic study with piperazine dihydrochloride in CD-1 Swiss mice*. Northbrook, IL: Industrial Biotest Laboratories, 1976. [Project 8533-08519].
74. Calman CD. Occupational piperazine dermatitis. *Contact Dermatitis* 1975; 1:126.
75. Yang RS, Garman RH, Weaver EV, Woodside MD. Two-generation reproduction study of ethylenediamine in Fischer 344 rats. *Fundam Appl Toxicol* 1984;4:539–546.
76. DePass LR, Yang RH, Woodside MD. Evaluation of the teratogenicity of ethylenediamine dihydrochloride in Fischer 344 rats by conventional and pair-feeding studies. *Fundam Appl Toxicol* 1987;9:687–697.
77. Price CJ, George JD, Marr MC, Myers CB, Heindel JJ, Schwetz BA. Developmental toxicity evaluation of ethylenediamine (EDA) in New Zealand White (NZW) rabbits. *Teratology* 1993;47:432–433.
78. Leung HW. Evaluation of the genotoxic potential of alkyleneamines. *Mutat Res* 1994;320:31–43.
79. DePass LR, Fowler EH, Yang RSH. Dermal oncogenicity studies on ethylenediamine in male C3H mice. *Fundam Appl Toxicol* 1984;4:641–645.
80. Hermansky SJ, Yang RSH, Garman RH, Leung HW. Chronic toxicity and carcinogenicity studies of ethylenediamine dihydrochloride by dietary incorporation in Fischer 344 rats. *Food Chem Toxicol* 1999;37:765–776.
81. Leung HW, van Miller JP. Effects of diethylenetriamine dihydrochloride following 13 weeks of dietary dosing in Fischer 344 rats. *Food Chem Toxicol* 1997;35:481–487.
82. DePass LR, Fowler EH, Weil CS. Dermal oncogenicity studies on various ethyleneamines in male C3H mice. *Fundam Appl Toxicol* 1987;9:807–811.
83. Stavreva M. Toxicity and mechanism of action of triethylenetetramine (TETA) used as a siccative and anticorrosive epoxide protective coating. *Khigiena i Zdraveopazvane* 1979;22:179–182.
84. Greenman DL, Morrissey RL, Blakemore W, et al. Subchronic toxicity of triethylenetetramine dihydrochloride in B6C3F1 mice and F344 rats. *Fundam Appl Toxicol* 1996;29:185–193.
85. Tanaka H, Inomata K, Arima M. Teratogenic effects of triethylenetetramine dihydrochloride on the mouse brain. *J Nutr Sci Vitaminol* 1993;39:177–188.
86. Keen CL, Cohen NL, Lonnerdal B, Hurley LS. Teratogenesis and low copper status resulting from triethylenetetramine in rats. *Proc Soc Exp Biol Med* 1983;173:598–605.
87. Tanaka H, Yamanouchi M, Imai S, Hayashi Y. Low copper and brain abnormalities in fetus from triethylenetetramine dihydrochloride-treated pregnant mouse. *J Nutr Sci Vitaminol* 1992;38:545–554.
88. Tyl RW, Fisher LC, Troup CM, et al. Developmental toxicity evaluation of triethylenetetramine by occluded cutaneous application in New Zealand White rabbits. *J Toxicol Cut Ocular Toxicol* (in press).
89. Knaak JB, Leung HW, Stott WT, Busch J, Bilsky J. Toxicology of mono-, di-, and triethanolamine. *Rev Environ Contam Toxicol* 1996;149:1–85.
90. Ballantyne B, Leung HW. Acute toxicity and primary irritancy of alkylalkanolamines. *Vet Human Toxicol* 1996;38:422–426.
91. Weeks MH, Downing TO, Musselman NP, Carson TR, Groff WA. The effects of continuous exposure of animals to ethanolamine vapor. *Am Ind Hyg Assoc J* 1960;21:374–381.
92. Jindrichova J, Urban R. Acute monoethanolamine poisoning. *Pracov Lek* 1971;9:314–317.
93. Mankes RF. Studies on the embryopathic effects of ethanolamine in Long Evans rats: preferential embryopathy in pups contiguous with male siblings in utero. *Teratog Carcinog Mutag* 1986;6:403–417.
94. Liberacki AB, Hellwig J. Evaluation of the pre-, peri-, postnatal toxicity of monoethanolamine in rats following repeated oral administration during organogenesis. *Fundam Appl Toxicol* 1997;40:158–162.
95. Liberacki AB, Neeper-Bradley TL, Breslin WJ, Zielke GJ. Evaluation of the developmental toxicity of dermally applied monoethanolamine in rats and rabbits. *Fundam Appl Toxicol* 1996;31:117–123.
96. Hartung R, Rigas LK, Cornish HH. Acute and chronic toxicity of diethanolamine. *Toxicol Appl Pharmacol* 1970;17:308.
97. Melnick RL, Mahler J, Bucher JR, et al. Toxicity of diethanolamine. 1. Drinking water and topical application exposures in F344 rats. *J Appl Toxicol* 1994;14:1–9.
98. Melnick RL, Mahler J, Bucher JR, Hejtmancik M, Singer A, Persing RL. Toxicity of diethanolamine. 2. Drinking water and topical application exposures in B6C3F1 mice. *J Appl Toxicol* 1994;14:11–19.
99. Gamer AO, Mellert W, Gans G, Deckardt K, Kaufmann W, Hildebrand B. *Diethanolamine: 90-day liquid aerosol inhalation study in Wistar rats*. Ludwigshafen, Germany: BASF Aktiengesellschaft, 1996. [Project report 50I0075/93011].
100. Neeper-Bradley TL. *Definitive developmental toxicity evaluation of diethanolamine administered cutaneously to CD (Sprague-Dawley) rats*. Export, PA: Union Carbide Corporation Bushy Run Research Center, 1992. [Project report 54-563].
101. *Study of the prenatal toxicity of diethanolamine in rats after inhalation*. Ludwigshafen, Germany: BASF Aktiengesellschaft, 1993. [Project report 31R0233/90010].
102. Neeper-Bradley TL, Kubena MF. *Diethanolamine: developmental toxicity study of cutaneous administration to New Zealand White rabbits*. Export, PA: Union Carbide Corporation Bushy Run Research Center, 1993. [Project report 91N0136].
103. DePass LR, Fowler EH, Leung HW. Subchronic dermal toxicity study of triethanolamine in C3H/HeJ mice. *Food Chem Toxicol* 1995;33:675–680.
104. Hejtmancik M, Mezza L, Peters AC, Athey PM. *The repeated dose study of triethanolamine*. Columbus, OH: Battelle Columbus Laboratories, 1985.
105. Pereira M, Barnwell P, Bailes W. *Screening of priority chemicals for reproductive hazards: monoethanolamine, diethanolamine and triethanolamine*. Cincinnati: Environmental Health Research and Testing, Inc, 1987. [Project report ETOX-85-1002].
106. *Mating trial dermal study of triethanolamine*. Columbus, OH: Battelle Columbus Laboratories, 1988.
107. Maekawa A, Onodera H, Tanigawa H, et al. Lack of carcinogenicity of triethanolamine in F344 rats. *J Toxicol Environ Health* 1986;19:345–357.
108. Konishi Y, Denda A, Kazuhiko U, et al. Chronic toxicity carcinogenicity studies of triethanolamine in B6C3F1 mice. *Fundam Appl Toxicol* 1992;18:25–29.
109. Kostrodymova GM, Veronin VM, Kostrodymov NN. The toxicity during the combined action and the possibility of carcinogenic and cocarcinogenic properties of triethanolamine. *Gig Sanit* 1976;3:20–25.
110. Hoshino H, Tanooka H. Carcinogenicity of triethanolamine in mice and its mutagenicity after reaction with sodium nitrite in bacteria. *Cancer Res* 1978;38:3918–3921.
111. Ellenhorn MJ, Barceloux DG. *Medical toxicology: diagnosis and treatment of human poisoning*. New York: Elsevier Science, 1988.

CHAPTER 64
Hydrofluoric Acid Exposures

Edward P. Krenzelok

Hydrofluoric acid (HF) is a corrosive agent with unique chemical properties that has the potential to produce significant toxicity even after dermal exposure to seemingly small amounts and low concentrations. In contrast to most toxic exposures, nearly 90% of HF exposures result in the development of some toxic sequelae, and

TABLE 64-1. Composite national hydrofluoric acid exposure data 1992–1995

All reported poisoning exposures	7,565,191
All reported hydrofluoric acid exposures	9,831
Adults	63.4%
Accidental	98.1%
Treated in health care facility	74.9%
Outcome (severity)	
No effect	11.7%
Minor effect	52.9%
Moderate effect	33.6%
Major effect	1.8%
Fatalities (3)	0.03%

From refs. 1–4.

approximately 75% of patients require treatment in a health care facility (Table 64-1) (1–4). Although HF has a variety of industrial applications, exposures are not confined to the workplace, and a considerable percentage of incidents occur in the home (5). Regardless of the location of the incident, most HF exposures result from the failure to adhere to safety and treatment recommendations and from a lack of knowledge about the chemical itself.

SOURCES AND PRODUCTION

HF, known by a variety of synonyms (Table 64-2), is an inorganic acid produced when calcium fluoride reacts with sulfuric acid at high temperatures. HF is available as both a liquid and gas, and the liquid form is colorless and found in both the anhydrous and aqueous forms (Table 64-3). Ammonium fluoride and ammonium bifluoride are also common sources of HF (6). Anhydrous HF is highly reactive with water and boils at 19.4°C, whereas aqueous HF is not as reactive but spontaneously fumes at concentrations in excess of 48% (7). In all forms, HF is 1,000 times more undissociated than hydrochloric acid (8). The anhydrous and highly concentrated aqueous forms are considered to be strong acids, and the low-concentration aqueous solutions are weak acids.

TABLE 64-2. Hydrofluoric acid synonyms

- HF
- HFA
- Hydrogen fluoride solution
- Hydrofluoric acid solution
- Hydrofluoric acid
- Aqueous hydrofluoric acid
- Fluoric acid solution
- Anhydrous hydrogen fluoride
- Anhydrous hydrofluoric acid
- Hydrogen fluoride
- Hydrofluoride
- Hydrofluoric acid gas
- Fluohydric acid
- Fluoric acid
- Fluohydric acid gas
- Fluohydric acid
- NIOSH/RTECS MW 7875000
- CAS Registry Number 7664-39-3
- STCC Number
  - 49 300 22 Hydrofluoric acid solution
  - 49 300 24 Hydrofluoric acid, anhydrous
  - 49 300 20 Hydrofluoric acid and sulfuric acid mixtures
- EPA Hazardous Waste Number U134
- EPA Pesticide Chemical Code 045601
- UN Numbers/DOT
  - UN 1790 Hydrofluoric acid solution not >60%
  - UN 1052 Hydrogen fluoride, anhydrous
  - UN 1786 Hydrofluoric/sulfuric acid mixtures
- Caswell Number 484
- OHM/TADS Number 7216750

CAS, Chemical Abstracts Service; DOT, U.S. Department of Transportation; EPA, U.S. Environmental Protection Agency; NIOSH/RTECS MW, National Institute for Occupational Safety and Health/Registry of Toxic Effects of Chemical Substances; OHM/TADS, Oil and Hazardous Materials Technical Assistance Data System; STCC, Standard Transportation Commodity Code; UN, United Nations.

TABLE 64-3. Liquid forms and common concentrations of hydrofluoric acid

Form	Concentration (%)
Anhydrous	100
Aqueous	70
Reagent grade	5–52
Commercial products	0.5–70.0
Household	8

OCCUPATIONAL USES

HF was first used artistically to etch glass in 1670, and, since then, the use of HF has expanded to include a multitude of industrial applications (Table 64-4). The spectrum of industries using HF in industrial and commercial processes places a large number of workers at a substantial risk of being exposed to this highly toxic substance. HF is used in massive quantities in the petrochemical industry and thousands of kilograms of HF are capable of being released into the environment as a consequence of industrial accidents (9–11). HF exposure limits and workplace standards are listed in Table 64-5.

TABLE 64-4. Industrial applications of hydrofluoric acid

Industry	Application
Aerosol	Propellants
	Solvents
Agriculture	Insecticide/fertilizer production
Aluminum	Manufacture of aluminum chloride
	Reduction of aluminum oxide
Atomic energy	Production of uranium tetrafluoride
	Purification of isotopes
Brewery	Control fermentation
	Cleaning
Ceramic	Etching and glazes
Dental	Control dentinal sensitivity
	Dental prosthetics
Foundries	Removal of sand/scale from castings
Glassware	Etching/frosting/polishing
Laundry/textile	Stain removal
	Trace metal removal
Leather	Tanning process
Masonry	Cleaning sandstone, marble, brick, etc.
Metal	Cleaning/polishing
	Stainless steel pickling
	Welding with fluoride flux
Ophthalmology	Corneal repair
Petrochemical	Production of high-octane fuels
Pharmaceutical	Drug/dye production
Semiconductor industry	Wet etching of silicon wafers for microelectronic circuits and computer chips

TABLE 64-5. Hydrofluoric acid exposure limits and workplace standards

Standards	Exposure limit
Personal standards	
Threshold limit value ceiling	3 ppm (2.3 mg/m^3)
Short-term exposure limit (15 min)	6 ppm
Permissible exposure limit (8-h time-weighted average)	3 ppm
Odor threshold	0.04–0.13 ppm
Immediately dangerous to life and health	30 ppm
Biological Exposure Index (BEI)	
Before shift:	3 mg/g creatinine/sampling time
End of shift:	10 mg/g creatinine/ sampling time
Environmental standards	
Superfund Amendments and Reauthorization Act Title III standards	
Reportable quantity	100 lb
Threshold planning quantity	100 lb
Safe Drinking Water Act	Maximum contaminant level 4 mg/L

ppm, parts per million.

MECHANISMS, PROCESSES, AND REACTIONS LEADING TO EXPOSURE

HF is designated as a hazardous chemical in the Federal Hazardous Substances Act. The extensive toxicity profile, which is not universally appreciated, creates a high-risk environment when HF is used in occupational applications. Human carelessness (including the failure to read hazard text before use) and the failure to comprehend and recognize the basic physicochemical properties of HF are the primary epidemiologic factors that lead to HF exposures.

Human Factors

Noncompliance with usage recommendations and precautionary information accounted for 62% of all HF exposures in one series that involved predominately the home or nonoccupational use of HF (5). Workers commonly handle HF without taking safety precautions and wearing the appropriate safety equipment. This is best exemplified by the frequency of hand exposures, which occur when thin surgical-type latex gloves are used during HF application instead of heavier natural rubber, neoprene, nitrile, or polyvinyl chloride handwear, which are less likely to puncture and are more impervious to HF penetration. The failure to read and comply with product labels, the development of complacency that may occur during long accident-free periods, and the lack of continuing safety education by employers all may lead to HF exposure. Additional factors predisposing to exposures include inadequate ventilation at the site of use, placing HF solutions in improperly marked or unmarked containers, unauthorized use of industrial-strength HF at home, and cottage industry applications such as ceramics where the craftsman may have little knowledge of HF's toxicity.

Physicochemical Factors

The majority of individuals who use HF are not chemists who are familiar with its chemical and toxic properties but rather workers who use it for a specific purpose. Their knowledge of HF's physicochemical properties is limited to a single application. Leakage may occur when HF is improperly stored in stoneware or steel containers, because HF dissolves silica found in stoneware and is corrosive to steel (12). Explosions, due to the accumulation of gaseous materials, may occur when HF is stored in improper containers. Hydrogen gas evolves when HF is in contact with steel, and a gaseous form of silicon tetrafluoride may be produced when HF is stored in glass containers (12). Splash exposures may result when HF is transferred from the original to alternative containers. Explosive potential can also be achieved when concentrated HF is admixed with alkali or aqueous substances.

Anhydrous HF must be stored under pressure or at low temperatures because it boils at 19.4°C (13,14). HF fumes at concentrations in excess of 48% (13,14). Therefore, highly concentrated forms of HF easily produce vapors that can contaminate the workplace if the HF is not used under hoods or in appropriately ventilated areas. The ability to fume at moderate concentrations and relatively low temperatures creates ideal conditions after a spill for the development of extensive environmental hazards owing to vapor cloud formation.

Industrial applications include the use of HF in concentrations ranging from less than 1% to 100%. Although workers realize that concentrated HF is highly toxic, many workers may not be aware of HF's ability to produce serious injury in concentrations of less than 10%. When low concentrations are used, therefore, safety precautions may not be exercised. The severity of injury from HF exposure is partially concentration-dependent, because concentrated HF generally produces more severe and immediate toxicity. HF handlers should understand the potential for toxicity at all concentrations and realize that no common percentage can be regarded as safe.

CLINICAL TOXICOLOGY OF EXPOSURE

The severity of the toxic sequelae associated with HF exposures is dependent on the extent, duration, and route of exposure; concentrations of HF; temporal relationship of the exposure to decontamination and local and/or systemic treatment; and numerous other factors. Regardless of the influence of these factors, the clinical toxicology at the cellular level is the same.

Dermal Exposure

The majority of HF exposures is dermal, and more than 70% of all HF exposures involve the hands and specifically the digits (5). HF is 1,000 times less dissociated than hydrochloric acid. Being largely un-ionized, HF is capable of penetrating the skin and proceeding through lipid barriers to deeper subcutaneous tissue, even bone. This is in contrast to other chemical burns, as well as thermal burns, which are limited to the duration of the exposure (15). Tissue destruction secondary to HF is prolonged, because concentrated HF has sufficient free hydrogen ions that produce immediate corrosive effects and penetrate to subcutaneous tissue (8,16). Dilute solutions (10% to 20%) rarely produce immediate external corrosive effects and manifest their toxicity in delayed fashion (up to 24 hours) after sufficient HF has penetrated to the subcutaneous tissue (8,16). With high concentrations, the process may be less insidious, and death has occurred in only 1 to 2 hours after dermal exposure (17). The delayed presentation of clinical symptoms may produce complacency regarding the toxic potential of the exposure and result in an underestimation of the seriousness of the exposure (6). This is especially true after exposures to HF congeners, such as ammonium fluoride–containing products, which are converted to HF as a slower dissociation process (6). Once absorbed, HF distributes systemically, and the fluoride ion dissociates from the hydrogen (18,19). Free fluoride ion complexes with calcium and other cations, such as magnesium, rendering them ineffective in their physiologic functions and producing severe metabolic derangement (20–23). Bone demineralization and necrosis occur, and, as calcium becomes physiologically compromised, potassium is released from nervous tissue, resulting in the development of severe pain (21,24). Exposures to significant amounts of HF may produce profound hypocalcemia and effect cyclic adenosine monophosphate production sufficiently so as to produce serious arrhythmias and resultant hemodynamic compromise (6,24–26). Hypocalcemia may develop in precipitous fashion (25). Profound hypomagnesemia has been associated with exposure to HF precursors ammonium fluoride and ammonium bifluoride (6). The combination of marked hypocalcemia and hypomagnesemia may produce life-threatening cardiac arrhythmias such as ventricular fibrillation (6). Hyperkalemia may occur as a consequence of Na-K adenosine triphosphatase impairment and the extracellular release of potassium from erythrocytes (26,27). These effects can occur from small surface area exposures to high HF concentrations or from larger surface areas with low concentrations, depending on the total amount of HF absorbed. Dermal exposure, therefore, can produce local effects as well as serious systemic toxicity, even fatalities.

Inhalation Exposure

The clinical toxicology of inhalation exposure parallels that of dermal exposures with two exceptions: The toxic effects may have a more rapid onset, and pulmonary compromise may develop. Inhalation exposures to HF are rare and are generally the result of an explosion or substantial spill. The likelihood of HF being an inhalation hazard (other than in an explosion) decreases in proportion to reductions in concentration below 50%, because the partial pressure decreases accordingly (12). HF is water soluble, and small amounts are effectively scrubbed out by the upper respiratory tract, thereby preventing the extension of pathology beyond that region as demonstrated in studies involving nasal-breathing rats (28). These exposures are not likely to produce bronchospasm or pulmonary edema; however, because HF is so irritating, the inhalation of volatile fractions of concentrated HF can rapidly produce bronchospasm, chemical pneumonitis, and pulmonary edema and can progress to death (12,29,30). Furthermore, systemic absorption of HF can produce complexation of calcium and magnesium and can result in cardiovascular compromise (6,24).

Ocular Exposure

Explosions and splash incidents commonly result in dermal as well as ocular exposures. The eye is exquisitely sensitive to acids, and HF has corrosive properties that are similar to other acids. HF can denude corneal and conjunctival epithelium producing corneal edema and conjunctival ischemia (31). Inorganic acids, with the exception of HF, rarely penetrate beyond the corneal stroma because they produce coagulation necrosis, which limits the extent of penetration in all cases except for exposure to the most concentrated acids (32,33). HF, being highly un-ionized, is able to penetrate ocular tissue, precipitate cations, and produce rapid opacification and severe damage to the anterior anatomy of the eye (31,34). Systemic toxicity is unlikely after exposure limited solely to the eye.

Ingestion

Occupational exposures to HF principally involve the dermal, ocular, and inhalational routes. Ingestions in this setting are rare, and the majority of reported cases are suicide attempts. Fatal outcomes are common, but survival has been reported (26). The systemic clinical toxicology of ingested HF is the same as with the other routes of exposure. In addition to the established cellular toxicity, the corrosive nature of HF may produce superficial erosion, transmural erosion, or both, of the oropharyngeal and gastric mucosa (20,35). Aspiration may occur during the ingestion process and produce irritant effects in the pulmonary tree.

TOXICOKINETICS

Absorption

As a highly un-ionized moiety, HF is able to penetrate through physiologic barriers and is absorbed systemically via any route of exposure. HF has a low pK_a (3.8), which helps to maintain HF in the un-ionized state, which further facilitates rapid gastric absorption (35,36).

Metabolism

After HF is absorbed via any route, it eventually dissociates to free hydrogen and fluoride ions. The fluoride ion is not metabolized by any of the body's metabolic processes (36).

Elimination

The elimination toxicokinetics of HF have not been established; however, it appears to be a first-order process (37–39). Data on therapeutic doses of fluoride in healthy and osteoporotic patients indicate that approximately 50% of a daily dose of fluoride is eliminated via the urine, the feces account for 6% to 10%, and perspiration may account for the elimination of 13% to 23% of a daily dose (36). Tests conducted in occupationally exposed individuals suggest that urinary fluoride elimination occurs for at least 12 hours (38). The evaluation of workers who produced aluminum fluoride revealed that the fluoride ion had a mean half-life of 9 hours (range, 6.5 to 13.5 hours, n = 8) (40). The half-life appears to be linked to the delayed dissociation of aluminum and fluoride. Fluoride elimination, therefore, may be shorter after exposure to HF. Renal compromise can occur within 30 minutes of exposure to highly concentrated HF, further reducing the elimination of HF (20,29,30). One patient with dermal exposure to anhydrous HF eliminated approximately 75% of the total renal excretion during the first 24 hours after exposure (41).

SIGNS, SYMPTOMS, AND SYNDROMES FROM TOXIC EXPOSURE

Acute Toxicity

A variety of factors influence the acute local and systemic toxicity of HF exposures. The most significant factor influencing acute systemic toxicity is the total amount of fluoride ion absorbed. In dermal exposures, this is a function of the duration of the exposure, the total surface area affected, and the concentration of the HF. Fatalities have resulted after facial exposure (2.5% of the total body surface area) to anhydrous HF (42). Similarly, lower concentrations to larger surface areas or over prolonged periods may produce serious toxicity and even death (8,43). The implementation of treatment may also influence patient outcome. Rapid decontamination of externally exposed patients may reduce the absorption of HF and reduce local and systemic toxicity.

Dermal Toxicity

In 1943, the National Institutes of Health classified HF burns into three categories based solely on the concentration of HF (16). These guidelines do not take factors such as total affected surface area or the duration of the exposure into consideration. HF solutions not exceeding 20% may have a delay of up to 24 hours before producing erythema and pain. Burns from solutions with concentrations in the range of 20% to 50% are apparent within 1 to 8 hours after the exposure. Solutions of more than 50% HF produce immediate pain and tissue destruction. Although these guidelines are old, a general correlation exists between the concentration of HF and the onset of symptoms, especially with the highly concentrated solutions. However, symptoms from exposure to dilute solutions may occur more rapidly than these guidelines suggest.

Exposures to dilute solutions that go untreated have the potential to produce serious tissue damage. Dilute solutions usually produce delayed severe pain with or without initial erythema. The pain may intensify and be characterized as a burning or throbbing sensation, and the affected area may suffer tissue destruction, which may include the presence of whitish to black desiccated and hardened skin (eschar) secondary to coagulation necrosis (8,14,21,22). Single or coalescent bullae may develop, but this is the exception after the exposure to dilute solutions (8,44). Concentrated solutions produce a more rapid onset of symptoms manifest by intense pain and rapid tissue destruction. Blister formation is common, and tissue destruction may result in the development of deep subcutaneous necrosis, destruction of fingernail beds, severe scar formation, and the necessity of amputation of an affected digit (8,14,21,22). In significant hand exposures, HF penetration may produce tendonitis and carpal tunnel syndrome. Serious systemic toxicity and death can result from dermal exposures.

Inhalation Toxicity

HF is a respiratory irritant, and the inhalation of even low concentrations can produce minor irritation to the mucous membranes of the upper respiratory tract. The severity of irritation and the potential for severe toxic insults to the respiratory tract increases as the concentration of the inhaled HF increases. Concentrations in excess of 48% are known to fume, increasing the volatile fraction of HF, which is capable of being inhaled. High concentrations may produce severe chemical pneumonitis, bronchospasm, bronchial swelling (which may obstruct the airway), hemorrhagic pneumonitis, and pulmonary edema (12,22,29,30). Fatalities have been reported secondary to the inhalation of concentrated HF (29,30). As with dermal exposures, HF inhalation may produce serious systemic toxicity.

Ocular Toxicity

Consistent with the dermal and inhalation routes of exposure, the severity of ocular toxicity is dependent on the concentration of HF and the length of the exposure. Mild conjunctival irritation occurs in rabbits after exposure to 0.5% HF (32). Dilute solutions have produced delayed toxicity as long as 4 days after the exposure and have the potential to produce severe ocular toxicity (33). Characteristically, ocular exposures to HF produce the immediate onset of severe pain, corneal erosion, and a conjunctival and corneal inflammatory response resulting in vascularization and scarring of the cornea (32,33,45,46). The globe may perforate, and surrounding tissue including tear ducts and the eyelids may be adversely affected (46,47). Systemic toxicity is an unlikely outcome.

Ingestion Toxicity

HF has the potential to produce corrosive effects consistent with other acids. The corrosiveness increases as the concentration of the HF solution increases. Ingestion of HF produces pain and erosion of the mucous membrane of the mouth, esophagus, and stomach (48). The ingestion of an HF-containing rust remover available to consumers resulted in the development of spontaneous emesis, severe metabolic acidosis, hypotension, and death 90 minutes after the ingestion (35). The postmortem analysis revealed the presence of hemorrhagic pulmonary edema and diffuse hemorrhagic gastritis without the presence of ulceration. Systemic toxicity may occur in addition to the toxic local manifestations associated with HF ingestion.

Rectal Toxicity

Although not an expected route of exposure in the occupational setting, extensive tissue damage occurs after the inadvertent rectal administration of HF. Severe rectosigmoidal mucosal ulceration and the development of modest hypocalcemia have been described (49,50).

Systemic Toxicity

Only the ocular route has not been associated with the development of systemic toxicity from HF exposures. Electrolyte and acid-base abnormalities such as hypocalcemia, hypomagnesemia, hyponatremia, hyperkalemia, hyperphosphatemia, and metabolic acidosis may result from the absorption of HF (6,14,20,24,25,35,41–43,48,51,52). The risk of developing hypocalcemia and the attendant electrolyte abnormalities is dependent on the degree of exposure to HF. The risk increases as the affected body surface area, the HF concentration, or both increase. The following conditions are thought to predispose the patient to the development of hypocalcemia: 1% surface area with 50% HF, 5% surface area with any concentration HF, and inhalation of 60% HF (52). The resultant effects of systemic fluorosis are cardiovascular insults such as hypotension, ventricular arrhythmias, and asystole (24,36,52). Renal toxicity has been reported (29,30).

CHRONIC AND LONG-TERM EFFECTS

Chronic exposure to subacute amounts has a low index of toxicity (53,54). Three men exposed on a daily basis to 80% HF to remove glass from the surface of platinum in a ventilated hood had increased urinary levels of fluoride but no evidence of systemic fluorosis (53). The repeated exposure and absorption of 10 to 80 mg of fluoride per day may produce systemic fluorosis initially evident on radiographs as increased bone density due to fluoride deposition in bone, eventually leading to osteosclerosis due to the replacement of calcium by fluoride in the bone (36,55). Ligaments and joints may calcify, restricting mobility and producing severe pain. This condition can be crippling. Other manifestations of chronic fluorosis include anorexia, nausea, vomiting, diarrhea or constipation, shortness of breath, stiffness and diffuse rheumatic pain, malaise, and headache (36,55).

No evidence exists to suggest that HF is either teratogenic or carcinogenic.

MANAGEMENT OF TOXICITY

Paramount to the successful management of any HF exposure is cessation of the exposure, by removing the patient from the toxic environment, and decontamination. HF is rapidly absorbed, and any delay in decontaminating the patient increases the severity of the exposure. Only in cases in which life support is essential should decontamination be delayed temporarily. Life-threatening hypocalcemia may develop in precipitous fashion in patients with extensive surface area exposure or exposure to even small amounts of HF. Serum electrolytes should be determined expeditiously in these patients and vigorous calcium replacement may be necessary.

Clinical Examination

Before the examination, the treating physician and all assisting individuals should protect themselves from exposure to HF. Multiple layers of latex gloves, gowns, footwear covers, and other protective materials should be used. All contaminated clothing should be placed in heavy plastic bags or containers and marked accordingly. Care should be taken to supervise these containers to prevent housekeeping personnel from being contaminated. Supportive care and decontamination should be instituted before performing the routine examination. The diagnosis of HF poisoning is usually easy because exposure is known and the toxidrome of delayed onset of pain and erythema is characteristic. Intentional or occupational exposures associated with high morbidity may not be as readily apparent. The presence of hypocalcemia and hypomagnesemia may help to confirm a suspected diagnosis. The presence of an elevated serum fluoride concentration may also be helpful.

Affected areas should be examined for the presence of erythema, bullae, and burns. All contiguous anatomic regions should be examined, including skinfolds and areas covered by hair for evidence of toxicity. Dilute solutions may produce external evidence of toxicity in a delayed fashion. The absence of burns, therefore, does not rule out a toxic exposure unless the substance contained high concentrations of HF. After sufficient time has passed, affected areas are intensely painful, and palpation of those areas is not necessary to elicit a response regarding the presence of pain. The affected area is generally well-demarcated, and that information should be descriptively and artistically documented.

Patients suffering from ocular exposures should have a slit lamp examination after their eyes have been thoroughly irrigated. An ophthalmologist should be consulted.

Patients with significant inhalation exposures present with signs of respiratory compromise. The airway should be secured via endotracheal intubation if necessary. A thorough evaluation of respiratory function is essential. Pulmonary edema can be delayed, but it is unlikely to occur without the presence of severe upper respiratory tract irritation.

Those who ingest HF should have an extensive examination of the oropharyngeal cavity, and, unless the solution is very dilute, the patient's examination should include endoscopic evaluation of the esophagus and the stomach. These steps should be undertaken after sufficient immediate dilution of the stomach contents with water, milk, or 10% calcium gluconate solution. The induction of emesis is contraindicated. The rapid absorption of HF may produce early systemic toxicity, which may necessitate emergent life support and delay the examination.

Treatment

The focus of treatment is life support, decontamination, inactivation of the fluoride ion, and treatment of specific problems. As with all poisonings, if necessary, an airway must be secured, breathing supported, and the cardiovascular system maintained. Intravenous access should be established as soon as possible in patients with the potential to develop systemic toxicity. The patient should be thoroughly decontaminated. After successful completion of these initial steps, a regional poison information center should be consulted regarding the current therapy of HF exposures. The cornerstone of therapy involves the use of complexing agents, such as the divalent cations calcium and magnesium, as well as other agents that inactivate the fluoride ion. The most contentious issue is the means of delivering the complexing agent; topical, intraarterial, regional intravenous perfusion, and digital injection are among the techniques and routes of administration that are used to treat the HF-exposed patient. The first rule of therapy is "to do no harm." Dermal decontamination and the topical use of the appropriate fluoride complexing agent should be attempted as indicated. The use of invasive techniques such as digital injection and intraarterial administration of calcium should not be undertaken unless necessary. Serious iatrogenic injury can occur, especially when those utilizing the therapy are unfamiliar with the technique or if the improper solution or concentration is used (56,57).

DERMAL EXPOSURE

Table 64-6 details the basic management of dermal HF exposures. All contaminated clothing must be removed, and the affected areas should be irrigated immediately and continuously with large volumes of lukewarm tap water for at least 15 minutes. Survival after total body immersion has been reported, most likely owing to expeditious decontamination (58). Rapid decontamination is critical to successful patient outcomes (59). After irrigation has been completed, efforts should be made to prevent the absorption of any HF that remains on the skin. A variety of topical agents that purportedly complex with the fluoride ion and prevent its absorption have been used. They include the use of the cationic agent benzalkonium chloride, magnesium salts (magnesium sulfate, gluconate, hydroxide), and calcium salts (gluconate and acetate).

The data are generally conflicting as they relate to nearly all of the complexing agents except calcium gluconate. Many of the data are derived from animal studies that use pig, rabbit, and rat skin. No case-controlled studies that compare all of these modalities exist for humans. Studies have not conclusively proven benzalkonium chloride and magnesium salts to be more effective than thorough irrigation with water (45,60). One study, however, demonstrates the efficacy of quaternary amine com-

TABLE 64-6. Basic management of dermal hydrofluoric acid exposures

1. Terminate hydrofluoric acid exposure
2. Life support—IV access if necessary
3. External decontamination of the patient
   - Caregivers should protect themselves from exposure
   - Remove contaminated clothing and store safely
   - Irrigation of affected region(s)
     - Water or normal saline
   - Prevent absorption of HF
     - Calcium gluconate gel
   - Obtain electrolytes—emphasis on serum calcium
   - Analgesics as appropriate
4. If no pain relief consider parenteral calcium therapy
   - Options include:
     - Subcutaneous injections
     - Intraarterial calcium administration
     - Regional perfusion therapy
5. Debridement of affected region(s) as indicated

pounds (61). Calcium acetate wraps have been found to be effective in an animal model (57). The efficacy of magnesium hydroxide antacid was not statistically different from that of calcium gluconate in a study using lagomorphs (62). The majority of data, however, suggests that the liberal application of calcium gluconate gel to the affected area(s) immediately after irrigation is completed may be the most efficacious topical therapy (8, 22,43,57,62–64). Calcium gluconate gel, prepared as a 2.5% concentration in a water-miscible jelly base is the most common form in which to administer this type of topical therapy. Hand exposures are most easily treated by placing the calcium gluconate gel into a latex surgical glove and then placing the hand into the glove.

Despite the apparent effectiveness of topical calcium gluconate gel, topical therapies have limited usefulness because they do not penetrate the skin and are unable to reverse the toxic subcutaneous effects of the fluoride ion. One possible exception is the use of dimethyl sulfoxide in combination with 10% calcium gluconate. The dimethyl sulfoxide serves as a vehicle to carry calcium gluconate and allow penetration through dermal lipid barriers into the subcutaneous tissue as demonstrated in animal studies, but these data have not been applied to the use of dimethyl sulfoxide/calcium gluconate in human HF exposures (61,65). Patients presenting to emergency departments who experience delayed onset of pain after the use of less concentrated solutions of HF may respond to the topical application of calcium gluconate gel. Patients who show no response, as indicated by the relief or significant reduction of pain within 45 minutes, may need to be treated with parenteral administration of calcium gluconate.

Three types of parenteral treatments exist: local infiltration therapy, intraarterial infusion, and regional intravenous perfusion. Local infiltration therapy is based on the principle of injecting small amounts of calcium gluconate into the affected subcutaneous tissue, usually a digit. Conceptually, the calcium precipitates the fluoride ion in the form of insoluble calcium fluoride. This inactivates the fluoride ion and stops both the tissue destruction and the associated pain. Calcium gluconate is injected into the subcutaneous tissue using a 25- to 30-gauge needle, not exceeding a total injected volume of 0.5 mL per cm^2 (8,14,22,48). The procedure is painful and often difficult to perform in a patient who is already experiencing a great deal of discomfort. The successful endpoint of treatment is the elimination of pain. To facilitate the injection process, local block anesthesia is often instituted. This technique is controversial because it eliminates the resolution of pain as an endpoint of therapy, but it may be more humane because patients are in severe pain. Subungual exposure is a common problem because 72% of all exposures involve the fingers (5). Infiltration therapy may not be effective, and nail removal may be necessary; however, patients who are exposed to less than 10% HF may not need nail removal (66). The pain may persist for several days, but evidence suggests that no serious long-term sequelae develop. Performed properly, this procedure has gained widespread acceptance owing to its success in resolving pain and the relatively simple nature of the technique compared with the use of the intraarterial calcium infusion.

Improperly performed, local infiltration therapy has many attendant dangers. The procedure is extremely painful and may result in patients refusing care and subsequently developing more toxicity. Care must be exercised to refrain from administering large amounts of calcium gluconate. Excessive administration may produce a compartment syndrome that can result in vascular compromise, ultimately worsening the tissue destruction caused by the HF. Historically, 10% calcium gluconate has been used to inject the subcutaneous tissue. Five percent calcium gluconate, however, may be a better choice and may reduce the possibility of any tissue irritation from the higher concentration of calcium gluconate (42,57,67,68). Calcium chloride is very irritating and even corrosive to tissues and should never be used for local infiltration purposes (14).

Intraarterial calcium administration has been successful in the management of extremity exposures to HF (69–72). Compared with infiltration therapy, its disadvantages are that it requires hospital admission, is not universally available, and is invasive (intraarterial therapy should not be used by individuals who are inexperienced in its use). It requires that either calcium gluconate or calcium chloride be infused via the artery that provides the vascular supply to the affected area. After an arteriogram has confirmed which artery to use, the calcium salt is infused over 4 hours using a parenteral infusion pump. A common treatment regimen recommends the administration of 10 mL of a 10% solution of either calcium gluconate or calcium chloride mixed in 50 mL of 5% dextrose solution (71). Pain generally resolves by the conclusion of the infusion. If the pain returns, the infusion should be repeated. If pain resolution does not occur, another arteriogram should be performed to assess whether the cannulated artery is perfusing the affected tissue. The potential complications associated with intraarterial therapy should be considered before using this technique. Extravasation of calcium salts may cause local or regional tissue damage. Multiple attempts to cannulate an artery may produce local trauma. Only physicians competent in this technique should perform it.

Preliminary data indicate that the regional intravenous perfusion of an affected region with calcium gluconate may be effective (73,74). Patients experiencing HF exposure symptoms had the affected limb exsanguinated, and then a pneumatic tourniquet was inflated to 50 mm above the patients' systolic blood pressure. Ten percent calcium gluconate was administered intravenously in 30 to 40 mL of normal saline, and the ischemia was maintained for 20 to 25 minutes. Success (as indicated by pain reduction) occurred in most patients and thereby did not necessitate the use of intraarterial injection in those with a successful outcome. Further study is necessary to determine whether this technique is a suitable alternative to intraarterial injection in most cases.

Another alternative approach used in the animal model is the administration of intravenous magnesium sulfate (75,76). Studies have shown this technique to be more effective than conventional intradermal calcium gluconate therapy. Additional research must be done to determine whether a role for this modality exists.

OCULAR EXPOSURE

In the event of ocular exposure, contact lenses should be removed if present. The affected eye(s) should be irrigated with large volumes of lukewarm tap water or normal saline for a minimum of 15 minutes. A variety of antidotal irrigation solutions have been evaluated, and none has been found to be more efficacious than water or normal saline (32). Ointments and solutions containing benzalkonium chloride and calcium and magnesium salts have not been effective and have actually produced more severe ocular injury (32). Given the high affinity of calcium for fluoride, lactated Ringer's solution may have an application in ocular irrigation. Ocular irrigation with 1% calcium gluconate solution and frequent instillation of 1% calcium gluconate eyedrops have been recommended and were successful in some case reports but have not been studied (31,34,58). Subconjunctival injection of calcium gluconate or calcium chloride has been both toxic and unsuccessful. Immediate aggressive irrigation (even exposures to dilute solutions of HF) is the most effective ocular treatment modality.

INHALATION EXPOSURE

Therapy for inhalation exposure should be directed at supportive care. Humidified oxygen should be administered. Because HF is corrosive, primary consideration should be directed at maintaining an airway. Nebulized calcium gluconate has been suggested, but only limited evidence suggests that it is an effective therapy (22,43,77). With the routine use of HF in the petrochemical industry, nebulized calcium gluconate is available at some refineries as emergent therapy for HF inhalation incidents (77).

INGESTION EXPOSURE

Immediate dilution with water or milk (may precipitate the fluoride) is essential for ingestion exposure. If the ingestion is within the previous 90 minutes and emesis has not occurred, gastric lavage with a small-bore nasogastric tube may be efficacious (48). This procedure may prevent the absorption of inordinate amounts of HF and reduce systemic toxicity. Although lavage is generally not recommended when corrosives have been ingested, the nature of HF's systemic toxicity and its rapid absorption and often fatal outcome eliminate the contraindication of lavage. The use of calcium-containing lavage solutions may provide added benefit (78). Syrup of ipecac–induced emesis is contraindicated, and no evidence exists to support the use of activated charcoal, which may actually obscure endoscopic evaluation of the patient.

LABORATORY DIAGNOSIS

Although fluoride levels may be obtained, the diagnosis of HF toxicity is largely historical and clinical, because the dermal exposure syndrome is classic and in concert with a history of using HF. It is an easy diagnosis to make. Patients who are nonresponsive and have suffered dermal exposure to concentrated forms of HF may have obvious burns and the presence of hypocalcemia (reports of calcium levels as low as 2.2 mg per dL), hypomagnesemia, and hyperkalemia (42). Urine and blood fluoride levels are of little value in acute HF toxicity but may serve to provide confirmation of exposure in diagnostically challenging cases. They may identify individuals who have been chronically exposed with excessive fluoride exposure, subacute fluorosis, or overt fluorosis. Urinary fluoride monitoring should be conducted intermittently in individuals with chronic occupational exposure to HF, because it is an effective indicator of occupational exposure to HF (37–40).

REFERENCES

1. Litovitz TL, Holm KC, Clancy C, Schmitz BF, Clark LR, Oderda GM. 1992 annual report of the American Association of Poison Control Centers Toxic Exposure Surveillance System. *Am J Emerg Med* 1993;11:494–555.
2. Litovitz TL, Clark LR, Soloway RA. 1993 annual report of the American Association of Poison Control Centers Toxic Exposure Surveillance System. *Am J Emerg Med* 1994;12:546–584.
3. Litovitz TL, Felberg L, Soloway RA, Ford M, Geller R. 1994 annual report of the American Association of Poison Control Centers Toxic Exposure Surveillance System. *Am J Emerg Med* 1995;13:551–597.
4. Litovitz TL, Felberg L, White S, Klein-Schwartz W. 1995 annual report of the American Association of Poison Control Centers Toxic Exposure Surveillance System. *Am J Emerg Med* 1996;14:487–537.
5. El Saadi MS, Hall AH, Hall PK, Riggs BS, Augenstein WL, Rumack BH. Hydrofluoric acid dermal exposure. *Vet Hum Toxicol* 1989;31:243–247.
6. Klasner AE, Scalzo AJ, Blume C, Johnson P, Thompson MW. Marked hypocalcemia and ventricular fibrillation in two pediatric patients exposed to a fluoride-containing wheel cleaner. *Ann Emerg Med* 1996;28:713–718.
7. Mansdorf SZ. Anhydrous hydrofluoric acid. *Am Ind Hyg Assoc J* 1987;48:A452.
8. Edelman P. Hydrofluoric acid burns. State of the art reviews. *Occup Med* 1986;1:89–103.
9. Himes JE. Occupational medicine in Oklahoma: hydrofluoric acid dangers. *J Okla State Med Assoc* 1989;82:567–569.
10. Wing JS, Sanderson LM, Brender JD, Perrotta DM, Beauchamp RA. Acute health effects in a community after a release of hydrofluoric acid. *Arch Environ Health* 1991;46:155–160.
11. Dayal HH, Baranowski T, Li Y, Morris R. Hazardous chemicals: psychological dimensions of the health sequelae of a community exposure in Texas. *J Epidemiol Community Health* 1994;48:560–568.
12. Mayer L, Guelich J. Hydrogen fluoride (HF) inhalation and burns. *Arch Environ Health* 1963;7:445–447.
13. Shaw JB. Hydrofluoric acid. *Dent Tech* 1987;40:4–5.
14. Caravati EM. Acute hydrofluoric acid exposure. *Am J Emerg Med* 1988;6:143–150.
15. Herbert K, Lawrence JC. Chemical burns. *Burns* 1989;15:381–384.
16. Division of Industrial Hygiene, National Institutes of Health. Hydrofluoric acid burns. *Ind Med* 1943;12:634.
17. Chan KM, Svancarek WP, Creer M. Fatality due to acute hydrofluoric acid exposure. *Clin Toxicol* 1987;25:333–339.
18. Gutknecht J, Walter A. Hydrofluoric acid and nitric acid transport through lipid bilayer membranes. *Biochim Biophys Acta* 1981;644:153–156.
19. Craig RD. Hydrofluoric acid burns of the hands. *Br J Plast Surg* 1964;17:5359.
20. Menchel SM, Dunn WA. Hydrofluoric acid poisoning. *Am J Forensic Med Pathol* 1984;5:245–248.
21. Anderson WJ, Anderson JF. Hydrofluoric acid burns of the hand: mechanism of injury and treatment. *J Hand Surg* 1988;13A:52–57.
22. MacKinnon MA. Hydrofluoric acid burns. *Dermatol Clin* 1988;6:67–74.
23. Stremski ES, Grande GA, Ling LJ. Survival following hydrofluoric acid ingestion. *Ann Emerg Med* 1992;21:1396–1399.
24. Mullett T, Zoeller T, Bingham H, et al. Fatal hydrofluoric acid cutaneous exposure with refractory ventricular fibrillation. *J Burn Care Rehabil* 1987;8:216–219.
25. Greco RJ, Hartford CE, Haith LR, Patton ML. Hydrofluoric acid-induced hypocalcemia. *J Trauma* 1988;28:1593–1596.
26. Sheridan RL, Ryan CM, Quinby WC, Blair J, Tompkins RG, Burke JF. Emergency management of major hydrofluoric acid exposures. *Burns* 1995;21:62–64.
27. McIvor M, Cummings C, Mower M, et al. Sudden cardiac death from acute fluoride intoxication: the role of potassium. *Ann Emerg Med* 1987;16:777–781.
28. Stavert DM, Archuleta DC, Behr MJ, Lehnert BE. Relative acute toxicities of hydrogen fluoride, hydrogen chloride, and hydrogen bromide in nose- and pseudo-mouth-breathing rats. *Fundam Appl Toxicol* 1991;16:636–655.
29. Braun J, Stob H, Zober A. Intoxication following the inhalation of hydrogen fluoride. *Arch Toxicol* 1984;56:50–54.
30. Watson AA, Oliver JS, Thorpe JW. Accidental death due to inhalation of hydrofluoric acid. *Med Sci Law* 1973;13:277–279.
31. Rubinfeld RS, Silbert DI, Arentsen JJ, Laibson PR. Ocular hydrofluoric acid burns. *Am J Ophthalmol* 1992;114:420–423.
32. McCulley JP, Whiting DW, Petitt MG, Lauber SE. Hydrofluoric acid burns of the eye. *J Occup Med* 1983;25:447–450.
33. Hatai JK, Weber JN, Doizaki K. Hydrofluoric acid burns of the eye: report of possible delayed toxicity. *J Toxicol-Cut Ocular Toxicol* 1986;5:179–184.
34. Bentur Y, Tannenbaum S, Yaffe Y, Halpert M. The role of calcium gluconate in the treatment of hydrofluoric acid eye burn. *Ann Emerg Med* 1993;22:1488–1490.
35. Manoguerra AS, Neuman TS. Fatal poisoning from acute hydrofluoric acid ingestion. *Am J Emerg Med* 1986;4:362–363.
36. Houts M, Baselt RC, Cravey RH. Fluoride. In: *Courtroom toxicology.* New York: Matthew Bender, 1985.
37. Kono K, Yoshida Y, Yamagata H, Watanabe M, Shibuya Y, Doi K. Urinary fluoride monitoring of industrial hydrofluoric acid exposure. *Environ Res* 1987;42:415–420.
38. Kono K, Yoshida Y, Watanabe M, Orita Y, Dote T, Bessho Y. Urine, serum and hair monitoring of hydrofluoric acid workers. *Int Arch Occup Environ Health* 1993;65:S95–S98.
39. Kono K, Yoshida Y, Watanabe M, et al. Serum fluoride as an indicator of occupational hydrofluoric acid exposure. *Int Arch Occup Environ Health* 1992;64:343–346.
40. Pierre F, Baruthio, Diebold F, Biette P. Effect of different exposure compounds on urinary kinetics of aluminum and fluoride in industrially exposed workers. *Occup Environ Med* 1995;52:396–403.
41. Burke WJ, Hoegg UR, Phillips RE. Systemic fluoride poisoning resulting from a fluoride skin burn. *J Occup Med* 1973;15:39–41.
42. Tepperman PB. Fatality due to acute systemic fluoride poisoning following a hydrofluoric acid skin burn. *J Occup Med* 1980;22:691–692.
43. Trevino MA, Herrmann GH, Sprout WL. Treatment of severe hydrofluoric acid exposures. *J Occup Med* 1983;25:861–863.
44. Shewmake SW, Anderson BG. Hydrofluoric acid burns: a report of a case and review of the literature. *Arch Dermatol* 1979;115:593–596.
45. Carney SA, Hall M, Lawrence JC, Ricketts CR. Rationale of the treatment of hydrofluoric acid burns. *Br J Ind Med* 1974;31:317–321.
46. Grant WM. *Toxicology of the eye,* 2nd ed. Springfield, IL: Charles C Thomas Publisher, 1974:557–559.
47. Vaughan D, Asbury T. *General ophthalmology,* 11th ed. Los Altos, CA: Lange, 1986:340.
48. Poisindex Editorial Staff. Hydrofluoric acid. In: Rumack BH, ed. *Poisindex,* Vol 90. Denver, CO: Micromedex, 1996.
49. Foster DE, Barone JA. Rectal hydrofluoric acid exposure. *Clin Pharm* 1989;8:516–518.
50. Cappel MS, Simmon T. Fulminant acute colitis following a self-administered hydrofluoric acid enema. *Am J Gastroenterol* 1993;88:122–126.

51. Mayer TG, Gross PL. Fatal systemic fluorosis due to hydrofluoric acid burns. *Ann Emerg Med* 1985;14:149–153.
52. Greco RJ, Hartford CE, Haith LR, Patton ML. Hydrofluoric acid-induced hypocalcemia. *J Trauma* 1988;28:1593–1596.
53. White DA. Hydrofluoric acid—a chronic poisoning effect. *J Soc Occup Med* 1980;30:12–14.
54. Brown MG. Fluoride exposure form hydrofluoric acid in a motor gasoline alkylation unit. *Am Ind Hyg Assoc J* 1985;46:662–669.
55. Waldbott GL. Toxicity from repeated low-grade exposure to hydrogen fluoride—case report. *Clin Toxicol* 1978;13:391–402.
56. Dowbak G, Rose K, Rohrich RJ. A biochemical and histologic rationale for the treatment of hydrofluoric acid burns with calcium gluconate. *J Burn Care Rehabil* 1994;15:323–327.
57. Dunn BJ, MacKinnon MA, Knowlden NF, et al. Hydrofluoric acid dermal burns: an assessment of treatment efficacy using an experimental pig model. *J Occup Med* 1992;34:902–909.
58. Sadove R, Hainsworth D, Van Meter W. Total body immersion in hydrofluoric acid. *S Med J* 1990;83:698–700.
59. Conway EE, Sockolow R. Hydrofluoric acid burn in a child. *Pediatr Emerg Care* 1991;7:345–347.
60. Bracken WM, Cuppage F, McLaury RL, Kirwin C, Klaassen CD. Comparative effectiveness of topical treatments for hydrofluoric acid burns. *J Occup Med* 1985;27:733–739.
61. Seyb ST, Noordhoek L, Botens S, Mani MM. A study to determine the efficacy of treatments for hydrofluoric acid burns. *J Burn Care Rehabil* 1995;16:253–257.
62. Kurkhart KK, Brent J, Kirk MA, Baker DC, Kulig KW. Comparison of topical magnesium and calcium treatment for dermal hydrofluoric acid burns. *Ann Emerg Med* 1994;24:9–13.
63. Chick LR, Borah G. Calcium gluconate gel therapy for hydrofluoric acid burns of the hand. *Plast Reconstr Surg* 1990;86:935–940.
64. Kono K, Yoshida Y, Watanabe M, et al. An experimental study on the treatment of hydrofluoric acid burns. *Arch Environ Contam Toxicol* 1992;22:414–418.
65. Zachary LS, Reus W, Gottlieb J, Heggers JP, Robson MC. Treatment of experimental hydrofluoric acid burns. *J Burn Care Rehab* 1986;7:35–39.
66. Roberts JR, Merigian KS. Acute hydrofluoric acid exposure [Letter]. *Am J Emerg Med* 1989;7:125–126.
67. Kirkpatrick JJR, Enion DS, Burd DAR. Hydrofluoric acid burns: a review. *Burns* 1995;21:483–493.
68. Upfal M, Doyle C. Medical management of hydrofluoric acid exposure. *J Occup Med* 1990;32:726–731.
69. Velvart J. Arterial perfusion for hydrofluoric acid burns. *Hum Toxicol* 1983;2:233–238.
70. Pegg SP, Siu S, Gillett G. Intra-arterial infusions in the treatment of hydrofluoric acid burns. *Burns* 1985;11:440–443.
71. Vance MV, Curry SC, Kunkel DB, Ryan PJ, Ruggeri SB. Digital hydrofluoric acid burns: treatment with intraarterial calcium infusion. *Ann Emerg Med* 1986;15:890–896.
72. Siegel DC, Heard JM. Intra-arterial calcium infusion for hydrofluoric acid burns. *Aviat Space Environ Med* 1992;63:206–211.
73. Graudins A, Burns MJ, Aaron CK. Regional intravenous perfusion of calcium gluconate for upper-extremity hydrofluoric acid burns. *Ann Emerg Med* 1996;28:566(abst).
74. Henry JA, Hla KK. Intravenous regional calcium gluconate perfusion for hydrofluoric acid burns. *Clin Toxicol* 1992;30:203–207.
75. Williams JM, Hammad A, Cottington EC, Harchelroad FC. Intravenous magnesium in the treatment of hydrofluoric acid burns in rats. *Ann Emerg Med* 1994;23:464–469.
76. Cox RD, Osgood KA. Evaluation of intravenous magnesium sulfate for the treatment of hydrofluoric acid burns. *Clin Toxicol* 1994;32:123–136.
77. Lee DC, Wiley JF, Snyder JW. Treatment of inhalational exposure to hydrofluoric acid with nebulized calcium gluconate. *J Occup Med* 1993;35:470.
78. Larsen MJ, Jensen SJ. Inactivation of hydrofluoric acid by solutions intended for gastric lavage. *Pharmacol Toxicol* 1991;68:447–448.

CHAPTER 65
Ozone

Michael J. Lipsett

SOURCES AND PRODUCTION

Ozone (triatomic oxygen or O_3) is a naturally occurring, colorless to bluish gas with a characteristic odor associated with electrical discharges (1,2). A reactive oxidant, ozone is a potent respiratory tract irritant. Some of ozone's physical properties are listed below.

Molecular weight	48
Boiling point	–112°C
Melting point	–193°C
Density	1.66 (air = 1)
Solubility in water	0.49 mL per 100 mL at 0°C

Ozone was identified as the principal oxidant in photochemical air pollution in the early 1950s and has received considerable media attention because of the enormous difficulty and economic costs associated with controlling its formation in the troposphere and because of the destructive effects of human activities on stratospheric ozone, which protects earth from high-energy UV radiation. Thousands of published reports refer to the formation, toxicology, and epidemiology of ozone exposure: This chapter can only touch on some of the more salient aspects of the extensive research on this substance. For the interested reader, the topics discussed below have been reviewed recently in exhaustive detail by the U.S. Environmental Protection Agency (EPA) preliminary to the 1997 revision of the federal ambient air quality standard for ozone (3).

EXPOSURE SOURCES: ENVIRONMENTAL AND OCCUPATIONAL

Because ozone is formed through natural atmospheric processes, low-level exposure is ubiquitous. At higher concentrations, ozone occurs in the environmental and occupational settings listed in Table 65-1.

Ozone is formed naturally in the stratosphere by the action of solar radiation on molecular oxygen (O_2). The maximum concentration is found at an altitude of approximately 75,000 feet, but ozone can be detected at altitudes up to approximately 300,000 feet. Stratospheric ozone prevents high-energy UV radiation from penetrating the atmosphere. Many terrestrial life forms would be unable to survive without this ozone "shield." Reports that chlorofluorocarbons, other human-made haloge-

TABLE 65-1. Environmental and occupational sources of exposure to ozone

Environmental
Stratosphere (up to 10 ppm)
Troposphere (photochemical reactions, lightning)
Occupational
Electric arc welding
Disinfectant (drinking water, food in cold storage rooms, sewage treatment)
Industrial waste treatment
Oxidizing agent in chemical manufacturing
Peroxide manufacturing
Deodorizing agent (air, sewer gas, feathers)
Bleaching agent (paper pulp, oils, textiles, waxes, flour, starch, sugar)
Aging of liquor and wood
Mercury vapor lamps
High-voltage electrical equipment
Linear accelerators
X-ray generators
Indoor ultraviolet sources
Photocopy machines
Electrostatic air cleaners
Contamination of high-altitude aircraft cabins
Residential
Ozone-generating air purifiers
Electrostatic air cleaners

ppm, parts per million.
From refs. 1,3–7, with permission.

nated organic chemicals, and oxides of nitrogen intermittently deplete large sections of stratospheric ozone (particularly over Antarctica) precipitated unprecedented international cooperation in phasing out the use of the most destructive chlorofluorocarbons. In the troposphere, human activities are major sources of ozone precursors, although these precursors are also generated by natural processes. Background levels (nonanthropogenic) of ozone in the troposphere averaging up to 50 parts per billion (ppb) are due to intrusion of stratospheric ozone into the lower atmosphere, to the action of lightning on molecular oxygen, and to chemical reactions involving naturally occurring oxides of nitrogen and organic compounds, such as biogenic methane and other volatile organic compounds (3).

Ozone in photochemical smog is formed by the action of solar UV radiation on nitrogen oxides and reactive hydrocarbons, both of which are emitted by motor vehicles and many industrial sources. The basic reaction sequence involves the photolysis of nitrogen dioxide (NO_2) into nitric oxide (NO) and oxygen atoms (O). The latter react with O_2 to form ozone. NO, however, rapidly scavenges ozone, regenerating NO_2 and O_2, as summarized in the following reactions, in which M represents any nearby molecule that can absorb the energy of the reaction:

$$NO_2 + h\nu\ (295 \le \lambda < 430\ \text{nm}) \rightarrow NO + O$$

$$O + O_2 + M \rightarrow O_3 + M$$

$$NO + O_3 \rightarrow NO_2 + O_2$$

Little accumulation of ozone occurs in a steady state; however, many reactive organic compounds (primarily of human origin) facilitate the oxidation of NO to NO_2 by alternative mechanisms. These reactions reduce the scavenging effect of NO, allowing ozone levels to increase (3).

Driven by photochemical reactions, ozone formation tends to be greatest on warm, sunny days. The diurnal pattern of tropospheric ozone formation in populated areas is generally characterized by a broad peak lasting from the late morning until the late afternoon or early evening, although large-scale transport of ozone and its precursors may result in elevated ozone concentrations extending over thousands of square miles, including rural areas far removed from the precursor sources. Numerous meteorologic and other factors (e.g., thermal inversion height, wind speed and direction, and addition of other ozone precursors along an air-mass trajectory) affect the temporal ozone patterns downwind, so that peak concentrations may occur anytime from noon until late in the evening (4). Because ozone is the principal oxidant found in photochemical smog, exposure occurs most commonly by breathing air in urban and suburban environments. In 1996, the EPA estimated that more than 130,000,000 people lived in areas that violated the revised federal ambient air quality standard for ozone (5).

Indoor ozone levels tend to equal outdoor concentrations, but at lower levels because of the compound's ready destruction on indoor surfaces. Nevertheless, indoor-outdoor ratios as high as 0.8 have been reported (6). Because people spend most of their time indoors, overall exposure to ozone may in some circumstances be dominated by the indoor component (7). Structures with low ventilation rates (e.g., weatherized homes or office buildings) or those with activated carbon air filtration generally have substantially lower indoor/outdoor ratios (<0.1 to approximately 0.25) (6). Nonindustrial indoor sources include devices using high-voltage or UV light, such as photocopy machines, electrostatic air cleaners, and laser printers (8). In one industrial hygiene study of ozone emissions from indoor sources, residential electrostatic air cleaners produced little ozone, whereas photocopiers created indoor peak concentrations of up to 0.20 parts per million (ppm) (8). In another survey of the breathing zones of photocopier operators, peak ozone concentrations exceeded 0.10 ppm, but most machines generated concentrations less than 0.05 ppm (9). Ozone-generating devices have been marketed as indoor air "purifiers" to large numbers of consumers for residential use. Such devices have been found, under experimental conditions of limited ventilation, to produce indoor ozone concentrations that far exceed occupational and environmental air quality standards (10).

Commercially used ozone is typically manufactured by electronic irradiation of air. Because of the high cost of shipping ozone, it is usually manufactured on-site (1). Common occupational exposures to ozone have been reported to occur in electric arc welding, sewage and water treatment, in industries that use ozone as an oxidizing agent, and in aircraft cabins (11–14). During the 1980s, however, aircraft exposures decreased drastically as airlines installed ozone converters in ventilation systems and began listing tropopause heights in flight plans and alerting pilots to modify flight paths, if needed, to avoid cabin ozone contamination (Dr. William Wells, United Airlines, *personal communication*). Persons in outdoor occupations, particularly those requiring physical exertion and elevated ventilation rates (e.g., farming and construction), may experience exposures sufficient to produce respiratory symptoms or lung function decrements (15). Although ozone exposure may occur in a variety of worksites (see Table 65-1), published reports of acute occupational intoxication are uncommon.

CLINICAL TOXICOLOGY

Route of Exposure

Owing to its high chemical reactivity, the half-life of ozone gas in liquid or solid media is negligible (16). Thus, ozone uptake is generally limited to anatomic sites of air-liquid interface (e.g., the mucous membranes of the respiratory tract and eye).

Absorption

Ozone is a strong oxidant and reacts with tissues or extracellular substances throughout the respiratory tract. Its relatively low solubility facilitates delivery to the lower respiratory tract, the target site of greatest clinical significance, although systemic absorption is limited by ozone's reactivity.

Ozone absorption in the respiratory tract has been studied using a variety of approaches, which generally have produced results that are reasonably consistent (3). Approximately 40% to 50% of inspired ozone is taken up in the nasopharynx of resting humans, whereas approximately 90% to 95% or more of the ozone reaching the lower respiratory tract is removed, principally in the conducting airways, for a total respiratory tract uptake of approximately 90% (range of estimates, 76% to 97%) (3,17–20). Gerrity et al. reported that oral or oronasal (compared with exclusively nasal) breathing resulted in small, but statistically significant, increases in extrathoracic uptake of ozone in tidal-breathing human subjects (17). In contrast, Kabel et al., using a technique of bolus inhalation of ozone, reported greater uptake efficiency of nasal versus oral breathing (21). Two studies reported no differences in ozone-induced changes in pulmonary function or respiratory symptoms among volunteers breathing orally, oronasally, or nasally, when ozone was administered via a face mask (22,23). These reports suggest that ozone is scrubbed more or less equally by the nose and mouth. Increases in ozone removal efficiency are associated directly with concentration and inversely with breathing rate (17). Continuous ozone inhalation decreases the absorption efficiency of the central airways, facilitating increased delivery of ozone to the deep lung (20). This presumably occurs because of depletion of reactive mucus substrates in the airway. Reduction of tidal volume, a common functional response to ozone exposure, results in a significant decline in lower respiratory tract uptake of ozone (17). Increasing ventilation rates decrease absorption by the upper and lower airways, enhancing ozone penetration to the deep lung (18).

The magnitudes of symptomatic and functional responses to acute ozone exposure are roughly proportional to the effective dose delivered to the lung (i.e., concentration × duration of exposure × minute ventilation) (24–26). Enhanced responses to ozone associated with increasing concentration and ventilation have been extensively documented (3,9,27). The importance of duration of exposure has been recognized only since the 1990s. In chamber studies using ozone concentrations ranging from 0.08 to 0.12 ppm, exposures of up to 6.6 hours with moderate exercise resulted in a progressive increase in respiratory symptoms and a concomitant decline in several indices of pulmonary function (28–30). The incremental effects of multihour ozone exposures combined with the likelihood of such exposures occurring among children playing and adults working outdoors formed one of the principal foundations for the EPA's revision of the federal ambient air quality standard from a 1-hour average of 0.12 ppm to an 8-hour average of 0.08 ppm (31). Of the effective dose variables, ozone concentration appears to be most influential, followed by ventilation and duration (32,33).

Metabolism

Ozone uptake represents reactive absorption, which is related to the quantity of oxidizable material along the luminal surfaces of the respiratory tract. One study indicates that ozone's reactivity prevents it from penetrating very far; little can pass through a lipid bilayer, and none can pass through a cell (34). Thus, its pulmonary and extrapulmonary effects (see, for example, references 35 and 36) must be effected by reaction products. Ozone is capable of reacting with all hydrocarbons but reacts most rapidly with unsaturated compounds such as mono- and polyunsaturated fatty acids and major components of the pulmonary epithelial lining fluid (ELF) and cell membranes. Although ozone itself is not a radical, its toxicity is considered to be mediated via free radicals, directly through oxidative reactions that produce radicals, such as OH·, or through radical-dependent generation of cytotoxic molecules, including aldehydes, hydrogen peroxide, and ozonides (37). Although ozone can oxidize thiol, amine, alcohol, and aldehyde functional groups on cell proteins (reacting most rapidly with cysteine, methionine, tyrosine, tryptophan, and histidine), lipid peroxidation is one of its principal toxic effects, initiated through such free radical reactions (37,38). Support for a free radical mechanism comes from several studies showing that vitamin E retards or prevents ozone's effects on polyunsaturated fatty acids *in vitro*, and that vitamin E–deficient experimental animals are more susceptible to ozone toxicity. It is not known, however, whether supplemental vitamin E in the diet can protect humans against ozone's effects (39).

The ELF, consisting of approximately 90% lipid and 10% protein, provides the first line of defense against noxious substances such as ozone (37). Where the ELF is attenuated or absent, ozone may react directly with epithelial cells. Within the ELF, high concentrations of water-soluble antioxidants, including urate, ascorbic acid, and reduced glutathione, scavenge ozone and protect against oxidation of macromolecules. When the oxidative burden overwhelms the initial line of defense, vitamin E acts as part of a backup system, interrupting the propagation of free radical reactions (37). Pryor and colleagues proposed that lipid oxidation products, particularly ozonides, are the likely initial mediators of ozone toxicity, because these are known to be formed in ELF, are somewhat stable and diffuse more easily into the cytoplasm than protein oxidation products, and have been shown to elicit some of the initial events in the inflammatory cascade, such as activation of epithelial membrane phospholipases (40). Epithelial membrane phospholipases are responsible for release of arachidonic acid, which can be metabolized to a variety of proinflammatory prostaglandins (PGs) and leukotrienes. The production of inflammatory mediators results in the margination into the airway of activated neutrophils, which release proteolytic enzymes and additional reactive oxygen species, amplifying the local oxidative stress.

Free radical reactions in the cell membrane result in denaturation of unsaturated fatty acid side chains and the creation of additional organic free radicals. Peroxidation of membrane structural lipids results in predictable effects: increased membrane permeability; leakage of essential electrolytes and enzymes; inhibition of intracellular metabolism; and swelling and disintegration of mitochondria, lysosomes, and other organelles (41). Consistent with these observations, increased airway permeability due to ozone exposure has been reported in experimental animals and in human volunteers (42,43). Severe damage results in cell lysis and necrosis.

SIGNS, SYMPTOMS, AND SYNDROMES

Acute Symptoms and Physiologic Effects

Acute human responses to ozone have been characterized in scores of controlled exposure studies, most of which involve comparison of exercising human volunteers' responses to ozone versus clean air exposures (3). Respiratory symptoms caused by exposure to ozone concentrations comparable to ambient levels include cough, substernal pain on deep inspiration, shortness of breath, chest tightness, throat irritation, wheeze, and dyspnea (Table 65-2). Nonrespiratory symptoms reported in controlled exposure studies have also included headache, nausea, and malaise (44). Earlier occupational case reports and a controlled study representative of occupational but not ambient exposures suggest a more severe spectrum of effects, including (in addition to the above) somnolence and extreme fatigue, dizziness, insomnia, decreased ability to concentrate, cyanosis, pulmonary edema, acrid taste and smell, and eye irritation (2,45–48). Higher concentrations of ozone (3.2 to 12 ppm) cause fatal pulmonary edema

TABLE 65-2. Symptoms and signs reported in humans exposed to ambient concentrations of ozone in controlled settings

Respiratory symptoms (cough, substernal pain on inspiration, dyspnea, chest tightness, throat irritation, wheeze)
Impaired exercise performance
Decreased pulmonary function (FVC, FEV_1, FEF_{25-75}, peak flow, tidal volume)
Increased specific airway resistance
Increased ventilation rate
Upper and lower respiratory tract inflammation
Increased airway reactivity
Increased epithelial permeability
Altered tracheobronchial clearance

FEF_{25-75}, forced midexpiratory flow rate (25% to 75%); FEV_1, forced expiratory volume in 1 second; FVC, forced vital capacity.

and hemorrhage in experimental animals (45,49). The dearth of published reports of severe respiratory outcomes in humans, however, suggests that occupational exposures sufficient to induce such effects must be quite rare. In contrast, epidemiologic studies examining a variety of mild to severe outcomes indicate that members of the general population are likely to be susceptible to the acute toxicity of ozone.

Many studies document ozone's ability to significantly impair sustained exercise (50–54). Inspiratory discomfort is thought to be a principal reason for the diminution of exercise performance (53,54).

Acute exposure to ozone produces marked effects on pulmonary mechanics and airway reactivity. Established consequences of ozone exposure in chamber studies include decreases in inspiratory capacity, forced vital capacity (FVC), forced expiratory volume in 1 second (FEV_1), peak flow, and tidal volume and increased specific airway resistance (SR_{aw}) and frequency of respiration (3,27). Some of these responses can be blocked by pretreatment with atropine and are thought to be mediated by the parasympathetic nervous system (55). The effects on FVC and FEV_1 are due to individuals' inability to inspire fully, which is probably primarily attributable to stimulation of bronchial C fibers with an additional contribution from rapidly adapting receptors, resulting in reflex inhibition of inspiratory muscle contraction (56,57). Although animal toxicology studies indicate that the principal site of ozone-related damage is the junction of the conducting airways and the gas-exchange zone, few studies have carefully investigated ozone's effects on flow in the small airways. Weinmann and coworkers, however, reported that ozone exposure also significantly decreases forced midexpiratory flow rate (25% to 75%) (corrected for ozone-induced changes in FVC) on a more prolonged time course than its effects on lung volume (FVC), consistent with the timing of an inflammatory response in the small airways (58–60). This finding has yet to be replicated by other investigators.

Increased airway reactivity after ozone exposure is associated with significant increases in neutrophils and molecular markers of inflammation in the airways, indicating the potential importance of inflammation as both a consequence and an amplifier of ozone toxicity in humans and experimental animals (61–63). The temporal coincidence of inflammation and airway hyperresponsiveness does not necessarily imply a simple causal relationship, because some animal studies have shown increased ozone-induced airway responsiveness without a neutrophil influx (3). Dose-related increases in a variety of cellular and biochemical indicators of inflammation in the terminal bronchioles and alveoli, sampled by bronchoalveolar lavage (BAL), have been consistently reported in adult volunteers at exposure levels as low as 80 ppb (61,64,65). Markers of cell injury and inflammation that have been reported to be significantly increased in BAL and proximal airway lavage of ozone-exposed humans include neutrophils (up to approximately eightfold more than control levels), lactate dehydrogenase, PGE_2, $PGF_2\alpha$, thromboxane B_2, interleukin-6 (IL-6), IL-8, fibronectin, albumin, fibrinogen and other coagulation factors, complement fragments, plasminogen activator, granulocyte-macrophage colony-stimulating factor, α_1-antitrypsin, and others (60,64–66). Both airway epithelial cells and resident macrophages are capable of releasing many of these proinflammatory mediators after ozone exposure (27). Pretreatment of human volunteers with indomethacin, a cyclooxygenase inhibitor, reduces ozone's effects on FEV_1 and FVC but not on airway responsiveness, indicating that products of arachidonic acid metabolized by cyclooxygenase are important in the induction of the former but not the latter effects (67,68).

Ozone-related inflammatory responses occurring in the central airways and upper respiratory tract of humans have been reported as well (66,69). Nasal lavage has been used to examine such effects epidemiologically, and, although the effects of ozone exposure per se cannot be isolated from those of other unmeasured pollutants in these studies, it is a likely contributor to the inflammatory changes detected. Multiple nasal lavages of school children in Germany during the ozone season (May to October) indicated significant associations between increased ozone concentrations and the concentrations of neutrophils in lavage fluid as well as myeloperoxidase and eosinophilic cationic protein, markers for activation of neutrophils and eosinophils, respectively (70). Massive epithelial cell shedding and significantly increased neutrophil counts in serial nasal lavages, accompanied by persistently abnormal nasal mucosal findings by rhinoscopic examination, were found in young security guards from a non-polluted area who were temporarily assigned to outdoor duties in Mexico City, where the principal pollutant was ozone (71).

Considerable interindividual variability in functional and symptomatic responsiveness to ozone exists, with up to 25% to 30% of study populations demonstrating markedly greater effects than other subjects. For example, for a given dose of ozone, intersubject differences in FEV_1 decrements may be tenfold or greater. That the functional changes are highly reproducible over periods from 3 weeks to 14 months suggests the existence of an intrinsic responsiveness to ozone (72–74). The degree of ozone responsiveness, as measured by decrements in FEV_1 or FVC, does not correspond to the extent of ozone-related inflammation, as measured by BAL or airway lavage (66,75). If the principal mechanism underlying decrements in FVC and FEV_1 is neurally mediated, then the extent of ozone-related spirometric decrements may be related more to a given subject's intrinsic nociceptive responsiveness than to the degree of injury. Some investigators found an inverse relationship between airway inflammation and functional responses, suggesting perhaps that greater ozone sensitivity measured spirometrically is protective against further injury (66,75,76). In contrast, Balmes and colleagues found in 1996 that the extent of ozone-related inflammation was positively correlated ($r = 0.67$) with small increases in SR_{aw}, a measure of large-airway caliber, which they suggested could be due to mucosal edema, among other factors (75).

The determinants of individual ozone susceptibility are not well understood. Ozone responsiveness, as measured by various lung function measures, decreases with increasing age (77,78). Observations that women may be more responsive to a given dose of ozone than men have been inconsistent (59,79–81), as have reports that women may be more susceptible to ozone's effects during the follicular phase of their menstrual cycle, corresponding to a trough in the levels of circulating progesterone, which has antiinflammatory effects (59,82). Blacks have smaller lungs than whites of the same height, and it has been hypothesized that blacks could therefore receive a greater ozone dose per unit of lung tissue than whites for a given inhaled volume. In the only large study examining ozone susceptibility in black and white young men and women, Seal and coworkers found no significant overall differences among the four race and gender groups exposed to five concentrations of ozone (from 0.12 to 0.40 ppm), although black men experienced significant FEV_1 decrements at 0.12 ppm, whereas this did not occur in the other groups below 0.18 ppm (79). Although this finding suggests a possible racial difference in ozone susceptibility, no significant differences were found among the four groups in FEV_1 at ozone exposure concentrations greater than 0.18 ppm, and none were found at any concentration for SR_{aw} or cough (the other measured outcome variables). In a few controlled exposure studies, children appear to experience decreases in pulmonary function comparable in magnitude to those observed in adults but do not report symptoms to the same extent (83–85). Although this apparent difference in symptom reporting may represent real differences in somatic perception, it may also be the result of the relatively low mean ozone concentrations to which the children were exposed.

Cigarette smokers demonstrate less functional and symptomatic responsiveness to ozone than nonsmokers, possibly due in part to the increased intraluminal quantities of mucus available to react with inhaled ozone (74). Self-selection is also likely to play a role, however: Individuals who can tolerate cigarette smoking in the first place are likely to be resistant to a variety of irritant stimuli. Cessation of smoking for at least 6 months appears to increase somewhat certain functional responses to ozone (86).

One report suggests that a history of allergies or asthma, greater baseline airway reaction to pharmacologic bronchoconstrictors, and self-reported sensitivity to air pollution appear to be associated with susceptibility to acute exposure to ozone (87). Subjects with a history of allergic rhinitis, however, did not differ from nonallergic subjects in ozone-related symptoms or lung function indices, except for a slightly, but significantly, greater increase in SR_{aw} (88).

Because asthma is characterized by chronic inflammation and hyperresponsiveness of the airways, it has been hypothesized that the additional burden of inflammation due to ozone exposure could cause a worsening of this condition. Numerous epidemiologic studies have linked ambient ozone concentrations with exacerbations of asthma, measured as increases in symptom reporting, medication use, emergency room visits, and hospital admissions (89–97). In contrast, controlled exposure studies of 1 to 4 hours suggest that, at low levels (up to 0.2 ppm), mild asthmatics do not appear to experience either ozone-related lung function decrements or respiratory symptoms to a markedly greater extent than nonasthmatic subjects (98–100). At a higher exposure concentration (0.40 ppm) and effective dose, however, asthmatics had reduced lung function suggestive of bronchoconstriction compared with healthy controls, although the immediate symptomatic responses were similar in intensity (101). The discrepancy between the epidemiologic and the controlled exposure studies may be related to several factors experienced by the asthmatics in the epidemiologic studies: (a) greater effective doses, mainly related to duration of exposure; (b) comorbidities, such as intercurrent respiratory infections, which serve as exclusion criteria in the controlled exposure studies; (c) a broader spectrum of baseline illness severity: Participants in the controlled exposure studies generally tend to be mild asthmatics who are relatively (if not completely) asymptomatic at the initiation of the experiment, producing a kind of selection bias; and (d) exposure to allergens or other pollutants.

Some controlled exposure studies indicate that asthmatics exhibit responses suggesting increased susceptibility to ozone in relation to nonasthmatic subjects. In 1996, Horstman and colleagues reported that, after prolonged exposure to 160 ppb ozone for 7.6 hours under conditions meant to simulate outdoor work or play, atopic asthmatics experienced progressively greater bronchoconstriction than nonasthmatics as measured by FEV_1 and FEV_1/FVC, corrected for effects of exercise (102). As with nonasthmatics, considerable intersubject variability existed, with the functional and symptomatic response to asthma corresponding to baseline asthma severity. Asthmatics with more severe disease and those who may be experiencing a flare of their condition are routinely excluded from controlled exposure studies; this study suggests that such individuals could be at even greater risk from ozone exposure. Scannell et al. found that, for a given exposure to ozone, mild asthmatics had significantly greater inflammation than nonasthmatics, measured as percent neutrophils and total protein in BAL fluids, even though no significant differences were present in either symptomatic or functional responses between the groups (100). Similarly, McBride et al. reported ozone-related increases in markers of inflammation in nasal lavage fluid of asthmatic, but not healthy, adults after 90 minutes of exposure to 240 ppb ozone, at which concentration neither study group showed significant changes in pulmonary function (103). This is consistent with other findings that ozone-related injury and inflammation may occur in the absence of effect on standard spirometric measures of lung function (75).

The effects of ozone on individuals with other chronic respiratory conditions have not been extensively investigated. A few controlled exposure studies suggest that chronic obstructive pulmonary disease (COPD) does not appear to enhance respiratory sensitivity to ozone (3,104–106). Whether this is due to the general decline in ozone-responsiveness seen in older individuals; to poor exercise tolerance, which results in low ventilation rates and a low effective ozone dose delivered to the lungs; to the increased quantities of airway mucus available to react with inhaled ozone; or to other factors is not known. In 1997, Gong and colleagues reported the results of a small study of subjects with mainly emphysematous COPD, who would (at least theoretically) have less airway mucus than COPD patients whose illness is characterized more by the presence of chronic bronchitis (107). In 4-hour exposures to 240 ppb ozone involving light intermittent exercise, the researchers found a significantly decreased FEV_1 in nine COPD subjects in comparison with ten healthy elderly controls, but little effect on FVC, SR_{aw}, respiratory symptoms, or arterial oxygen saturation. The total FEV_1 decrements after 4 hours of ozone exposure (representing a combination of the effects of ozone and of exercise) averaged 19% in men with COPD versus 2% in healthy elderly subjects. Although the exposure conditions were more extreme than in prior studies, the results of this investigation suggest that some individuals with COPD may also be considered at increased risk from exposure to ambient levels of ozone, particularly because such individuals have little functional reserve.

In many individuals, acute pulmonary responses to ozone become attenuated with repeated daily exposures. In controlled chamber studies, maximal responses are generally observed on the second day of exposure, but on subsequent days, very few or no ozone-related effects may be present (108–112). In a laboratory setting, such "tolerance" or "adaptation" to ozone toxicity typically persists for several days to a week after cessation of exposure but may last up to approximately 3 weeks (109–111). One report suggests that attenuation of responses can also occur in adults with mild asthma, albeit at a slower rate than in subjects without asthma (113). Ozone-related increases in airway reactivity do not appear to attenuate with repeated daily exposures to the same extent as functional and symptomatic responses (114). In adult residents of Los Angeles, a seasonal variability in response to ozone is present that suggests longer-term adaptation (115). Such adaptation to repeated exposure may favor the development of chronic effects. Rats exposed to ozone at 0.35, 0.50, and 1.0 ppm for several days demonstrated "adaptation" to ozone's effects on several measures of lung function but also showed evidence of progressive inflammation and damage to tissue in the deep lung (116). In one report of 16 healthy young adult male volunteers exposed to 0.4 ppm for 2 hours per day for 5 consecutive days and then once again after 10 or 20 days, evidence of partial attenuation of the inflammatory response was found. For example, ozone-induced increases in several conventional inflammatory markers in BAL fluid (percent polymorphonuclear leukocytes, IL-6, PGE_2, and neutrophil elastase) were attenuated after 5 consecutive days of exposure. In contrast, indicators of cellular damage (lactate dehydrogenase, total BAL fluid protein, and percent epithelial cells), as well as the neutrophil chemotactic cytokine IL-8, showed no attenuation after repeated ozone exposure, indicative of ongoing cellular damage (3,117).

Controlled exposure studies, although useful for understanding some aspects of pollutant toxicity, cannot capture the complexity of real-world exposures or the diversity of potential human responses. Nevertheless, several studies have investigated interactions between exposures to ozone and other pollutants or bioaerosols. Brief exposure to low levels of ozone (120 ppb for 1 hour or less) appears to make the asthmatic lung more susceptible to the effects of subsequent challenge with other irritants (SO_2) or aeroallergens (pollens) (118–120). Bascom and coworkers found that subjects with histories of allergic rhinitis who were exposed to either ozone (0.5 ppm for 4 hours) or clean air before nasal challenge with antigen showed a dramatic ozone-induced mixed inflammatory cell influx (sevenfold increase in neutrophils, tenfold increase in mononuclear cells, and 20-fold increase in eosinophils) but no significant differences in antigen-induced respiratory symptoms, inflammatory cells, or mediators in nasal lavage fluid (121). In contrast, Jörres et al. found that ozone preexposure resulted in small, but statistically significant, increases in airway responsiveness to subsequent challenge with aeroallergen in subjects with allergic rhinitis (120). Ozone exposure not only elicits an inflammatory response in the nasal airways but also apparently has a priming effect on allergen-related responses of asthmatics, in that lesser quantities of intranasally applied allergen extract (in this case, house dust mite) were required to elicit nasal symptoms after ozone versus clean air preexposure (122). In this same report, ozone preexposure was also linked with increased quantities of eosinophilic cationic protein (an indicator of eosinophil activation), neutrophils, and IL-8 in nasal lavage fluid after subsequent challenge with allergen.

Most studies investigating responses to joint exposures of ozone and other pollutants have not found much of an effect on lung function or spirometry beyond that attributable to ozone itself, either in asthmatics or healthy volunteers (3,27). Copollutants studied in such experiments have included sulfur dioxide, NO_2, sulfuric acid, nitric acid, and carbon monoxide. Some studies involving multihour exposures to low levels of ozone (80 to 180 ppb) in combination with or after exposure to sulfuric acid particles (100 μg per m^3) suggest that combined exposure results in enhanced decrements in lung function in some asthmatics relative to nonasthmatics but without concomitant changes in respiratory symptoms (123,124). In one occupational case report, several months of low-level exposure to ozone (approximately 0.04 ppm) and to small quantities of copper oxide particles produced by high voltage electrical discharges in a television tube manufacturing factory reportedly caused severe asthma in a worker with a childhood history of this disease (125).

Numerous epidemiologic studies have linked ambient ozone levels with a variety of adverse respiratory outcomes acutely, including decrements in lung function, increased risks of emergency room visits and hospital admissions for respiratory diagnoses, and increased daily mortality. Such investigations primarily have been time-series analyses, which examine associations between fluctuations in air pollution in relation to the occurrence of adverse health outcomes while controlling for other time-varying factors (primarily daily temperature and other meteorologic factors, measured copollutants, seasonality, and day-of-week effects). Investigations of both children and adults indicate that exposure to low-level, ambient ozone concentrations is associated with small, transient lung function decrements (15,126–134). In one report by Brauer and colleagues, analysis of twice-daily spirometry of adult agricultural workers indicated a significant relationship between FEV_1 and FVC in an area in which the mean and maximum ozone concentrations were 40 and 84 ppb, respectively (15). These effects on lung function appear to persist past the day on which the insult occurred (15,129,134). In one study of an air pollution episode lasting several days, during which maximum daily ozone concentrations fluctuated between 0.12 and 0.185 ppm, peak flow decrements in some children lasted up to a week after the episode ended (134).

Although effects on lung function may occur in the absence of an ozone-related effect on respiratory symptoms, other studies have linked daily ozone levels not only with symptoms, but also with emergency room visits and hospital admissions for respiratory causes (135–141). Others have not detected significant associations between ozone and various respiratory outcomes (142,143). These discrepant results may be related to differences in concentrations of ozone and copollutants, the extent of covariation among the predictor variables, statistical power considerations, exposure and outcome measurement error, and differences in statistical modeling. In epidemiologic studies such as these, covariation between multiple pollutants and (more important) temperature make it difficult to determine unique effects of ozone. In general, asthma exacerbations have been more consistently linked than other health outcomes with ambient ozone concentrations (89–97).

Several time-series studies have demonstrated a relationship between ambient ozone levels and daily mortality (144–146). Reported ozone-associated increases in daily mortality have been on the order of a few percent. Anderson and colleagues, for example, reported an increase of 3.6% for cardiovascular mortality corresponding to a 29-ppb increase in the 8-hour measured average concentration of ozone during a study period when the maximum 8-hour average concentration of ozone was 94 ppb (144). The ozone-mortality relationship has been observed more clearly in relatively low-ozone cities such as London and Philadelphia, whereas no independent effect of ozone on daily mortality could be demonstrated in such high-ozone metropolitan areas as Mexico City or São Paolo, Brazil (147,148). Although ambient ozone was reported to be linked with daily mortality in Los Angeles, this association was found to diminish to nonsignificance in a later study when a measure of particulate air pollution (PM10) was also included in the regression model (149,150). A recent metaanalysis of daily mortality in several European cities (London, Athens, Barcelona, Paris, Amsterdam, Basel, Geneva, and Zurich) suggests a small, but consistent, increase in the pooled relative risk (RR) of daily mortality associated with modest increases in ambient ozone levels (RR = 1.029 for a 50-μg per m^3 increase in ozone, 95% confidence interval = 1.01 to 1.049). Inclusion of a particulate matter term in the regression model had only a slight impact on the ozone RR (150a). Considerations regarding the variability of results among ozone morbidity studies apply to the mortality studies as well. In addition, mortality studies are likely to be affected more by the age distributions and the prevalence of serious preexisting diseases in the populations under study. If these associations represent a causal relationship, the underlying mechanisms are by no means clear. Although low-level ozone exposure can initiate respiratory tract inflammation in exercising individuals at concentrations as low as 80 ppb, it is unlikely that this represents a threshold of effect (65). Rats exposed to ozone exposure (0.25 ppm for 5 days) have been reported to have evidence of peroxidation reactions in the heart and brain, which could contribute to human mortality if this were to occur in people with preexisting cardiovascular conditions (36).

Eye irritation occurring during smog episodes is mainly due to other photochemical oxidants, such as peroxyacetylnitrate, not to ozone (151,152). In industrial settings, however, eye and nasal irritation may occur (153). Concentrations greater than 2 ppm have been reported to be irritating to normal human eyes within minutes (154).

In animal studies, many effects on both local and systemic immunity have been documented, although most of these have occurred when ozone exposure concentrations far exceeded those to which humans are routinely exposed (155). Studies of mice exposed even briefly (2 to 3 hours) to ozone concentrations at or below the federal ambient air quality standard of 0.12 ppm have shown significantly decreased resistance to bacterial, but not viral, respiratory infections (156–161). A limited number of epidemiologic and clinical studies have generally failed to detect an effect of ozone or oxidant air pollution on respiratory infections in humans, although this issue has not been adequately investigated (162–165).

Pathology

Ozone damages tissues throughout the respiratory tract, depending on the pattern of breathing, exposure concentration, and duration. At high concentrations, ozone may cause desquamation of the airways and pulmonary edema (166). At sublethal concentrations (up to 1.0 ppm), airway epithelial cells are also damaged, but the principal site of injury is the central portion of the pulmonary acinus. Type I alveolar and ciliated bronchiolar cells appear to be particularly susceptible to ozone toxicity, with damage evident as early as 4 hours of exposure (167). Inflammatory responses at the junction of the conducting airways and the gas exchange zone have been reported consistently in studies of rodents, dogs, and nonhuman primates. Continued exposure over several days results in replacement of type I by type II cells as well as hypertrophy and hyperplasia of nonciliated cuboidal cells in the bronchiolar epithelium (168,169). When animals are allowed to recover in clean air from acute and subacute exposures, all of these lesions appear to be reversible (168,169).

As noted earlier, several investigators have measured markers of inflammation in the upper and lower respiratory tracts of ozone-exposed volunteers. BAL fluid from these subjects showed large increases in polymorphonuclear cells, other inflammatory mediators, and protein concentrations consistent with a transudation of serum (61,64,65). The latter finding suggests increased pulmonary vascular permeability, one of the hallmarks of inflammation, and tends to corroborate earlier work demonstrating increased permeability of the respiratory epithelium, as measured by technetium-99m–labeled diethylenetriamine pentaacetic acid clearance (170). Aris et al. took bronchial biopsies from the right upper lobe carina of volunteers 18 hours after acute exposure to either clean air or ozone (0.20 ppm for 4 hours) and found a significant neutrophil influx into the bronchial mucosa and epithelium after ozone exposure (66). This report is the first to provide histopathologic documentation of inflammation in human airways after ozone exposure and is consistent with similar findings in ozone-exposed monkeys, dogs, and guinea pigs (66).

Chronic Toxicity

Because ozone exposure produces injury and inflammation acutely, one of the principal uncertainties about ozone toxicity is the relationship between repeated exposures and chronic respiratory disease. As noted earlier, with short-term repetition of exposure (up to a week), an attenuation of functional, symptomatic, and inflammatory responses exists, in the presence of continuing biochemical evidence of cellular damage (116). The extent to which this attenuation plays a role in long-term studies is unknown. In a 3-month study of nonhuman primates, however, the degree of inflammation after 90 days was less than that observed after 7 days (171). This may be a consequence of the greater resistance of the altered epithelial cell population to environmental insults. Exposure of guinea pigs and rats to a relatively high ozone concentration (approximately 1.0 ppm) for 268 days caused a chronic bronchiolitis, with bronchiolar fibrosis, pneumonitis, "mild to moderate" emphysema, and occasional epithelial lesions in the trachea and major bronchi (172). Exposure of rats to substantially lower concentrations (between 0.12 and 0.25 ppm) resulted in less severe but still significant changes in the terminal bronchioles and alveolar septa, as well as a distribution of inflammation similar to that observed in acute exposures (173,174). Chronic exposures of monkeys showed changes in nasal epithelial secretory product, respiratory bronchiolitis (with inflammatory thickening of the bronchiolar wall and hypertrophy and hyperplasia of nonciliated cuboidal cells in the bronchiolar epithelium), and other changes, including the development of hyperplastic nodules that persisted after the cessation of exposure (171,175,176).

These animal experiments demonstrate that chronic exposure to ozone concentrations found in typical urban air results in centriacinar inflammation and small airway structural changes. Supporting human evidence is provided in an autopsy study in which postmortem lung specimens of 107 youths dying suddenly in the Los Angeles area showed a variety of airway and centriacinar lesions characteristic of oxidant damage (177). Because the investigators were not able to obtain data on smoking, occupational histories, or other potentially relevant exposures, this study can be viewed as suggestive only. Other lines of evidence support the notion that repeated ozone exposure may result in chronic lung disease, including the observations that ozone inactivates human α_1-antiproteinase inhibitor, increases the susceptibility of elastin to proteolysis by neutrophil elastase *in vitro*, and appears to cause the synthesis and deposition of abnormal collagen in rat lung (178–180). In one study in which adult male rats were exposed to an ozone regimen meant to mimic Los Angeles (continuous background of 0.06 ppm for 22 hours per day, with a 9-hour ramped spike up to a peak of 0.25 ppm for 5 days per week, for up to 78 weeks), the animals manifested small (<10%) but significant lung function decrements consistent with a restrictive pattern without evidence of abnormal or excess collagen deposition (181). Although the principal lesions produced by chronic ozone exposure are in the distal lung, diffuse emphysematous or fibrotic changes generally have not been observed in experimental animals.

Ozone exposure may result in indirect chronic respiratory effects. In an experiment reported by Pinkerton et al., rats were continuously exposed to a typical diurnal ozone pattern (0.06 ppm, with a gradual increase to and decrease from 0.25 ppm), 5 days a week for 6 weeks, then were exposed to aerosolized asbestos. One month later, the ozone-exposed rats had significantly more asbestos in their lungs than controls, suggesting that realistic ozone exposure concentrations may retard clearance of asbestos or other carcinogens (182).

Few epidemiologic studies have attempted to examine chronic effects of ozone exposure on lung function or symptoms (3). Several studies suggest the existence of significant associations of photochemical oxidant or ozone exposure with an accelerated decline in lung function and with symptoms of chronic respiratory disease in nonsmokers (183–188). A longitudinal study of nonsmoking Seventh Day Adventist adults in California also suggests a relationship between ambient ozone concentrations and incidence of asthma in men, but not women, and an association between chronic ozone exposure and asthma symptom severity (187–188b). The interpretability of these studies is limited, however, by problems in long-term exposure assessment, the high covariation between ozone and other pollutants (notably particles), issues of selection bias due to loss to follow-up (184,185), and systematic error involving lung function measurements (184). The Seventh Day Adventist studies used innovative refinements of exposure assessment, but the collinearity between ozone and particles in the areas under study still obscures the magnitude of the specific contribution of ozone (3). One cross-sectional survey of approximately 3,300 schoolchildren in 12 communities in southern and central California suggests effects of chronic ozone exposure on several lung function measures but not on the prevalence of asthma, bronchitis, cough, or wheeze (188). Peak ozone concentrations were most strongly associated with decreased FEV_1 and FVC in girls with asthma and in boys who spent more time outdoors.

Genetic Toxicity and Carcinogenicity

Ozone has been reported to be genotoxic in a variety of assay systems, but experimental results are inconsistent (3). Careful control of experimental conditions, however, is critical: Ozone's reactivity, toxicity, and physical state (as a gas) make it difficult to detect ozone-related genotoxicity in the absence of significant toxicity, particularly in *in vitro* assays (189). Many investigations have used relatively high ozone concentrations, raising concerns about experimental artifacts. Still, effects reported include mutations in *Escherichia coli* and *Salmonella typhimurium*, dominant lethal mutations in *Drosophila melanogaster*, plasmid DNA strand breakage, sister chromatid exchange, and chromatid and chromosome breaks in cultured human lymphocytes (189). For example, alveolar macrophages from rats exposed for 6 hours to 0.27 and 0.80 ppm ozone showed evidence of chromatid (but not chromosomal) breakage (190). In human subjects exposed to 0.5 ppm ozone for 6 to 10 hours, a threefold increase in chromatid-type aberrations persisted for up to 6 weeks (191). In contrast, no significant changes in chromosome or chromatid breaks were observed in lymphocytes of subjects exposed to 0.4 ppm ozone for 4 hours (192). Also, cultured human epidermal cells exposed to 5 ppm ozone for 10 minutes showed no evidence of DNA strand breakage (193).

In one experiment, arylamines found in tobacco smoke (e.g., naphthylamine and toluidine isomers) were transformed by 1-hour exposures to low levels of ozone (0.1 to 0.4 ppm) into unidentified stable products capable of causing single-strand DNA breaks in cultured human lung cells (194). Only 15 minutes of exposure to 0.10 ppm ozone was needed to change 1-naphthylamine (15 micromolar) into products capable of causing an equivalent of 100 rads of DNA damage. This work implies an increased risk of genetic toxicity not only to cigarette smokers, but also to those exposed to arylamines (and possibly other substances) in environmental tobacco smoke and in various industries in which ozone may also be present.

Brief (5-minute) exposure to 5 ppm ozone induces neoplastic transformation in cell culture, an effect enhanced by ionizing and nonionizing radiation (195,196). Repeated ozone exposure (0.7 ppm for 40 minutes) of cultured rat tracheal cells biweekly for 4.5 weeks caused preneoplastic changes that were not observed in rats exposed to ozone (0.14, 0.6, or 1.2 ppm) 6 hours per day for up to 4 weeks (197). Although some studies suggest that chronic ozone exposure may facilitate the development of benign pulmonary adenomas in mice and other hyperplastic nodules in nonhuman primates, few tests of carcinogenicity have been performed (175,189,198). The U.S. National Toxicology Program conducted a 2-year bioassay of groups of 50 male and 50 female rats and mice exposed to 0, 0.12, 0.50, or 1.00 ppm ozone, for 6 hours per day, five days a week, and a similar lifetime bioassay without the 0.12-ppm exposure concentration (189). The National Toxicology Program found no evidence of carcinogenicity in rats in either the 2-year or the lifetime assays, but found increased numbers of combined alveolar/bronchiolar adenomas and carcinomas in the exposed versus the control mice, which were interpreted qualitatively as "equivocal" and as "some evidence" for carcinogenic activity in the males and females, respectively. No concentration-response relationship was observed.

One report from the Seventh Day Adventist cohort study reported a strong association of ambient ozone exposure with lung cancer in males but not females. During the follow-up period (1977 to 1992), exposure to ambient ozone for 551 hours per year when the concentration exceeded 100 ppb was associated with an RR of lung cancer of 4.19 (95% confidence interval = 1.81 to 9.69). In this report, other air pollutants (PM10 and sulfur dioxide) were also associated with increased risks of lung cancer. Although this was a carefully executed study, these results were based on small numbers of lung cancer deaths (n = 18 for men and 12 for women) in this nonsmoking population (198a). Ozone exposure may enhance or retard lung tumorigenesis by other agents in rodents, depending on the exposure protocol (197,199). In a companion study to the National Toxicology Program bioassay (described earlier), ozone exposure of male rats (0.5 ppm for 6 hours per day, 5 days per week for 105 weeks) did not affect the incidence of lung tumors induced by subcutaneous injection of a known carcinogen, 4-(*N*-methyl-*N*-nitrosamino)-1-(3-pyridyl)-1-butanone, when compared with rats exposed to clean air.

Although ozone's ability to cause free radical formation and inflammation suggests that it may be genotoxic (either directly or indirectly) and potentially carcinogenic or cocarcinogenic in animals and humans, limited evidence supports this notion. Ozone may also affect the integrity of immune system defenses against tumor development and progression (200,201).

MANAGEMENT OF TOXICITY OR EXPOSURE

Diagnosis of ozone-related toxicity is based on a probable history of exposure and recognition of symptoms compatible with exposure. Because ozone symptomatology may mimic several cardiorespiratory illnesses, the differential diagnosis includes influenza, the common cold, sinusitis, asthma, bronchopneumonia, pulmonary embolism, and myocardial infarction (47). Asthmatic episodes triggered by ozone should be treated according to standard protocols. Although ozone is theoretically capable of causing pulmonary edema in humans, the scarcity of published reports indicates that it is very uncommon. Severe industrial overexposure should be managed like other acute inhalational injury, with supportive treatment. Except in these unusual instances, ozone-related symptoms are self-limited after termination of exposure, with recovery in milder cases generally occurring within hours. Symptomatic treatment includes analgesics for headache and chest pain and cough suppressants if indicated. Some reports of industrial ozone toxicity indicate a more prolonged convalescence, with resolution of symptoms occurring over 1 to 2 weeks (47).

MEDICAL OR BIOLOGICAL MONITORING

Ozone's high chemical reactivity combined with the rarity of severe intoxication does not make it a practical candidate for biological monitoring.

OCCUPATIONAL AND ENVIRONMENTAL REGULATIONS

Environmental and occupational standards governing exposure to ozone are displayed in Table 65-3.

TABLE 65-3. Environmental and occupational ozone exposure standards

Organization	Standard	Parts per million	mg/m^3
EPA NAAQS	1 h	0.12	0.23
	8 h[a]	0.08	0.15
OSHA-PEL	TWA	0.10	0.20
NIOSH-REL	IDLH	10	20
ACGIH TLV	Ceiling	0.10	0.20

ACGIH TLV, American Conference of Governmental and Industrial Hygienists, threshold limit value; EPA NAAQS, U.S. Environmental Protection Agency, national ambient air quality standard; IDLH, immediately dangerous to life and health; NIOSH-REL, National Institute for Occupational Safety and Health, recommended exposure limit; OSHA-PEL, U.S. Occupational Safety and Health Administration, permissible exposure limit; TWA, 8-hour time-weighted average.

[a]Promulgated July 18, 1997.

Notes: IDLH defined by NIOSH as "the maximum concentration from which, in the event of respirator failure, one could escape within 30 minutes without a respirator and without experiencing any escape-impairing or irreversible health effects" (202). As of this writing, ACGIH has also proposed to add three 8-hour TWA recommendations: 0.05 ppm for heavy work, 0.08 ppm for moderate work, and 0.10 ppm for light work.

EXPOSURE CONTROLS

Avoidance of exposure is the best management strategy. In the occupational setting, this means providing adequate engineering controls (e.g., entirely enclosed processes or local exhaust ventilation), thorough worker education about recognition of ozone-related symptoms and about appropriate work practices (use of personal protective equipment, such as an ozone-decomposing respirator, when adequate ventilation is impractical), and strict adherence to health and safety rules. In the context of environmental exposures, individuals should be advised to avoid aerobic exercise during peak ozone hours, pay attention to the air quality information provided by the print and broadcast media, and heed health advisories accompanying the declaration of a smog alert. As noted earlier, however, signs and symptoms of ozone toxicity have been demonstrated to occur in exercising adults at ozone concentrations as low as the revised federal ambient air quality standard (0.08 ppm) (31).

ENVIRONMENTAL FATE AND TRANSPORT

Ozone is continuously generated and degraded in the stratosphere and the troposphere. It has been estimated that background concentrations of ozone in the U.S. during daylight hours (7-hour average) probably fall between 25 and 45 ppb, including ozone of natural origin and that associated with human activities. Long-range transport of O_3 and its precursors is common, as its lifetime in the troposphere may be as long as 1 to 2 months. As noted earlier, ozone can be degraded by reaction with many surfaces. In addition, numerous atmospheric chemical reactions involve ozone transformation. Ozone reacts with NO to form O_2 and NO_2 (see Exposure Sources: Environmental and Occupational). UV radiation (λ<320 nm) photolyzes O_3 to molecular oxygen and an excited state oxygen atom, which can then react with water vapor to form the hydroxyl radical (OH·), the principal species responsible for degrading most volatile organic compounds in the troposphere. The hydroxyl radical can also react with NO_2 to form nitric acid. Ozone can react with NO_2 to form molecular oxygen and the nitrate radical (NO_3), which readily photolyzes and participates in a variety of other reactions. The atmospheric chemistry of ozone has been extensively investigated and has been the subject of a thorough review by the EPA, from which the preceding paragraph is excerpted (3).

ENVIRONMENTAL AND OCCUPATIONAL MONITORING

Ozone is routinely measured by chemiluminescence or ultraviolet photometry. The EPA has designated gas-phase chemiluminescence as the reference method for ozone monitoring. Ambient air is mixed in a chamber with ethylene, which reacts with ozone to produce an electronically excited species that emits visible light. A photomultiplier detects the light and produces a current directly proportional to the ozone concentration over the range of 1 ppb to at least 1 ppm. This signal is then amplified and displayed or read directly on a recorder. Although no interference from common atmospheric pollutants occurs, water vapor exerts positive interference of approximately 3% per percent water by volume at 25°C (3).

Equivalent methods designated by the EPA include UV photometry and gas-solid chemiluminescence (3). UV photometry measures light absorbed (at $\lambda = 254$ nm) by the sample in a chamber of known optical path length. To create a zero air sample, an airstream is diverted through an internal ozone scrubber before directing it through the absorption cell. After a specified interval, another sample (in which the ozone is to be measured) passes directly into the absorption cell. The ozone concentration is calculated from the difference in the transmittances measured. The ozone detection limit using UV photometry has been reported to be 5 ppb. Although ambient water vapor does not appear to affect measured ozone concentrations, aromatic compounds that also absorb UV light at 254 nm (e.g., styrene, nitrotoluene, and other organics) may exert small positive interferences in routine air monitoring (3). Given that many of these potential interferents are photochemically reactive, however, the extent to which they actually interfere with ambient ozone measurement is likely to be small, although this issue has not been examined in detail.

Gas-solid chemiluminescence has a similarly high degree of specificity and low detection limit, but is rarely used for ambient ozone monitoring. Chemiluminescence is produced by the reaction of ozone with rhodamine B adsorbed on activated silica. The intensity of the chemiluminescence is proportional to the concentration of ozone (3).

Several passive sampling devices to measure personal exposures to ozone have been developed during the past decade (3,203–205). Such devices have been used primarily for research purposes but may find wider applicability in the future.

REFERENCES

1. Sax NI, Lewis RJ. *Hawley's condensed chemical dictionary*, 11th ed. New York: Van Nostrand–Reinhold, 1987.
2. Jaffe LS. The biological effects of ozone on man and animals. *Am Ind Hyg Assoc J* 1967;28:267–277.
3. US Environmental Protection Agency. *Air quality criteria for ozone and related photochemical oxidants* (3 vols). Research Triangle Park, NC: US Environmental Protection Agency, 1996. EPA-600/P-93/004cF.
4. Lioy PJ, Dyba RV. Tropospheric ozone: the dynamics of human exposure. *Toxicol Ind Health* 1989;5:493–504.
5. Office of Air Quality Standards and Planning. Review of national ambient air quality standards for ozone. Assessment of scientific and technical information. OAQPS Staff Paper. Research Triangle Park, NC: US Environmental Protection Agency, 1996. EPA-452/R-96-007.
6. Wechsler CJ, Shields HC, Nalk DV. Indoor ozone exposures. *JAPCA* 1989;39: 1562–1568.
7. Liu L-JS, Koutrakis P, Suh HH, Mulik JD, Burton RM. Use of personal measurements for ozone exposure assessment: a pilot study. *Environ Health Perspect* 1993;101:318–324.

8. Allen RJ, Wadden RA, Ross ED. Characterization of potential indoor sources of ozone. *Am Ind Hyg Assoc* J 1978;39:466–471.
9. Hansen TB, Andersen B. Ozone and other air pollutants from photocopying machines. *Am Ind Hyg Assoc J* 1986;47:659–665.
10. Kissel JC. Potential impact of deliberately introduced ozone on indoor air quality. *J Exposure Anal Environ Epidemiol* 1993;3:155–164.
11. US Department of Transportation, Federal Aviation Administration, Perkins PJ, Holdeman JD, Nastrom GD. *Simultaneous cabin and ambient ozone measurements on two Boeing 747 airplanes*, vol I. Washington: US Government Printing Office, 1979. FAA-EE-79-05.
12. US Department of Health, Education, and Welfare, National Institute for Occupational Safety and Health, Key MM, Henschel AF, Butler J, Ligo RN, Tabershaw IR. *Occupational diseases. A guide to their recognition*. Washington: US Printing Office, 1977:428-430.
13. Morgan WKC, Seaton A. *Occupational lung diseases*, 3rd ed. Philadelphia: WB Saunders, 1995:570–584.
14. Reed D, Glasser S, Kaldor J. Ozone toxicity symptoms among flight attendants. *Am J Ind Med* 1980;1:43–54.
15. Brauer M, Blair J, Vedal S. Effect of ambient ozone exposure on lung function in farm workers. *Am J Respir Crit Care Med* 1996;154:981–987.
16. World Health Organization. Ozone and other photochemical oxidants. In: *Air quality guidelines for Europe*. Copenhagen, Denmark: World Health Organization Regional Office for Europe, 1987:315–326.
17. Gerrity TR, Weaver RA, Berntsen J, House DE, O'Neil JJ. Extrathoracic and intrathoracic removal of ozone in tidal breathing humans. *J Appl Physiol* 1988;65:393–400.
18. Hu S-C, Ben-Jebria A, Ultman JS. Longitudinal distribution of ozone absorption in the lung: quiet respiration in healthy subjects. *J Appl Physiol* 1992;75:1655–1661.
19. Gerrity TR, Biscardi F, Strong A, Garlington AR, Brown JS, Bromberg PA. Bronchoscopic determination of ozone uptake in humans. *J Appl Physiol* 1995;79:852–860.
20. Asplund, PT, Ben-Jebria A, Rigas M, Ultman JS. Longitudinal distribution of ozone absorption in the lung: effect of continuous inhalation exposure. *Arch Environ Health* 1996;51:431–438.
21. Kabel JR, Ben-Jebria A, Ultman JS. Longitudinal distribution of ozone absorption in the lung: comparison of nasal and oral quiet breathing. *J Appl Physiol* 1994;77:2584–2592.
22. Adams WC, Schelegle ES, Shaffrath JD. Oral and oronasal breathing during continuous exercise produces similar responses to ozone inhalation. *Arch Environ Health* 1989;44:311–316.
23. Hynes B, Silverman F, Cole P, Corey P. Effects of ozone exposure: a comparison between oral and nasal breathing. *Arch Environ Health* 1988;43:357–360.
24. Hu S-C, Ben-Jebria A, Ultman JS. Longitudinal distribution of ozone absorption in the lung; effects of respiratory flow. *J Appl Physiol* 1994;77:574–583.
25. Silverman F, Folinsbee LJ, Barnard J, Shephard RJ. Pulmonary function changes in ozone-interaction of concentration and ventilation. *J Appl Physiol* 1976;41:859–864.
26. Adams WC, Savin WM, Christo AE. Detection of ozone toxicity during continuous exercise via the effective dose concept. *J Appl Physiol* 1981;51:415–422.
27. Committee of the Environmental and Occupational Health Assembly of the American Thoracic Society. Health effects of outdoor air pollution. *Am J Respir Crit Care Med* 1996;153:3–50.
28. Folinsbee LJ, McDonnell WF, Horstman DH. Pulmonary function and symptom responses after 6.6 hour exposure to 0.12 ppm ozone with moderate exercise. *J Air Pollut Control Assoc* 1988;38:28–35.
29. Horstman DH, Folinsbee LJ, Ives PJ, Abdul-Salaam S, McDonnell WF. Ozone concentration and pulmonary response relationships for 6.6-hour exposures with five hours of moderate exercise to 0.08, 0.10 and 0.12 ppm. *Am Rev Respir Dis* 1990;142:1158–1163.
30. McDonnell WF, Kehrl HR, Abdul-Salaam S, et al. Respiratory responses of humans exposed to low levels of ozone for 6.6 hours. *Arch Environ Health* 1991;46:145–150.
31. US Environmental Protection Agency. National ambient air quality standards for ozone: final rule. *Federal Register* 1997 July 18 1997:62:38855–38896.
32. Hazucha M. Relationship between ozone exposure and pulmonary function changes. *J Appl Physiol* 1987;62:1671–1680.
33. Dreschler-Parks DM, Horvath SM, Bedi JF. The "effective dose" concept in older adults exposed to ozone. *Exp Gerontol* 1990;25:107–115.
34. Pryor WA. How far does ozone penetrate into the pulmonary air/tissue boundary before it reacts? *Free Rad Biol Med* 1992;12:83–88.
35. Buckley RD, Hackney JD, Clark K, et al. Ozone and human blood. *Arch Environ Health* 1975;30:40–43.
36. Ruhman I-U, Massaro GD, Massaro D. Exposure of rats to ozone: evidence of damage to heart and brain. *Free Rad Biol Med* 1992;12:323–326.
37. Kelly FJ, Mudway I, Krishna MT, Holgate ST. The free radical basis of air pollution: focus on ozone. *Respir Med* 1995;89:647–656.
38. Mustafa MG. Biochemical basis of ozone toxicity. *Free Rad Biol Med* 1990;9:245–265.
39. Pryor WA. Can vitamin E protect humans against the pathological effects of ozone in smog? *Am J Clin Nutr* 1991;53:702–722.
40. Pryor WA, Squadrito GL, Friedman M. A new mechanism for the toxicity of ozone. *Toxicol Lett* 1995;82/83:287–293.
41. Man SFP, Hulbert WC. Airway repair and adaptation to inhalation injury. In Loke J, ed. *Pathophysiology and treatment of inhalation injuries*. New York: Marcel Dekker Inc, 1988:1–47.
42. Kehrl HR, Vincent LM, Kowalsky RJ, et al. Ozone exposure increases respiratory epithelial permeability in humans. *Am Rev Respir Dis* 1987;135:1124–1128.
43. Miller PD, Gordon T, Warnick M, Amdur MO. Effect of ozone and histamine on airway permeability to horseradish peroxidase in guinea pigs. *J Toxicol Environ Health* 1986;18:121–132.
44. Lippmann M. Health effects of ozone: a critical review. *J Air Pollut Control Assoc* 1989;39:672–695.
45. Stokinger HE. Ozone toxicology: a review of research and industrial experience: 1954–1964. *Arch Environ Health* 1965;10:719–731.
46. Griswold SS, Chambers LA, Motley HL. Report of a case of exposure to high ozone concentrations for two hours. *Arch Ind Health* 1957;15:108–110.
47. Nasr AN. Ozone poisoning in man: clinical manifestations and differential diagnosis. A review. *Clin Toxicol* 1971;4:461–466.
48. Kleinfeld M, Giel CP. Clinical manifestations of ozone poisoning: report of a new source of exposure. *Am J Med Sci* 1956;231:638–643.
49. Stokinger HE. Evaluation of the hazards of ozone and oxides of nitrogen. *Arch Ind Health* 1957;15:181–197.
50. Schelegle ES, Adams WC. Reduced exercise time in competitive simulations consequent to low level ozone exposure. *Med Sci Sports Exerc* 1986;18:408–414.
51. Wayne WS, Wehrle PF, Carroll RE. Oxidant air pollution and athletic performance. *JAMA* 1967;199:151–154.
52. Gong H Jr, Bradley PW, Simmons MS, Tashkin DP. Impaired exercise performance and pulmonary function in elite cyclists during low-level ozone exposure in a hot environment. *Am Rev Respir Dis* 1986;134:726–733.
53. Adams WC. Effects of ozone exposure at ambient air pollution episode levels on exercise performance. *Sports Med* 1987;4:395–424.
54. Folinsbee LJ, Silverman F, Shephard RJ. Decrease of maximum work performance following ozone exposure. *J Appl Physiol* 1977;42:531–536.
55. Beckett WS, McDonnell WF, Horstman DH, House DE. Role of the parasympathetic nervous system in acute lung response to ozone. *J Appl Physiol* 1985;59:1879–1885.
56. Hazucha MJ, Bates DV, Bromberg PA. Mechanism of action of ozone on the human lung. *J Appl Physiol* 1989;67:1535–1541.
57. Coleridge JCG, Coleridge HM, Schelegle ES, Green JF. Acute inhalation of ozone stimulates bronchial C-fibers and rapidly adapting fiber receptors in dogs. *J Appl Physiol* 1993;74:2345–2352.
58. Weinmann GG, Bowes SM, Gerbase MW, Kimball AW, Frank R. Response to acute ozone exposure in healthy men. Results of a screening procedure. *Am J Respir Crit Care Med* 1995a;151:33–40.
59. Weinmann GC, Weidenbach-Gerbase M, Foster WM, Zacur H, Frank R. Evidence for ozone-induced small-airway dysfunction: lack of menstrual-cycle and gender effects. *Am J Respir Crit Care Med* 1995b;152:988–996.
60. Weinmann GC, Liu MC, Proud D, Weidenbach-Gerbase M, Hubbard W, Frank R. Ozone exposure in humans: inflammatory, small and peripheral airway responses. *Am J Respir Crit Care Med* 1995c;152:1175–1182.
61. Seltzer J, Bigby BG, Stulbarg M, et al. O_3-induced change in bronchial reactivity to methacholine and airway inflammation in humans. *J Appl Physiol* 1986;60:1321–1326.
62. Hulbert WM, McLean T, Hogg JC. The effect of acute airway inflammation on bronchial reactivity in guinea pigs. *Am Rev Respir Dis* 1985;132:7–11.
63. Holtzman MJ, Fabbri LM, O'Byrne PM, et al. Importance of airway inflammation for hyperresponsiveness induced by ozone. *Am Rev Respir Dis* 1983;127:686–690.
64. Koren HS, Devlin RB, Graham DE, et al. Ozone-induced inflammation in the lower airways of human subjects. *Am Rev Respir Dis* 1989;139:407–415.
65. Devlin RB, McDonnell WF, Mann R, et al. Exposure of humans to ambient levels of ozone for 6.6 hours causes cellular and biochemical changes in the lung. *Am J Respir Cell Mol Biol* 1991;4:72–81.
66. Aris RM, Christian D, Hearne PQ, Kerr K, Finkbeiner WE, Balmes JR. Ozone-induced airway inflammation in human subjects as determined by airway lavage and biopsy. *Am Rev Respir Dis* 1993;148:1363–1372.
67. Ying RL, Gross KB, Terzo TS, Eschenbacher WL. Indomethacin does not inhibit the ozone-induced increase in bronchial responsiveness in human subjects. *Am Rev Respir Dis* 1990;142:817–821.
68. Schelegle ES, Adams WS, Siefkin AD. Indomethacin pretreatment reduces ozone-induced pulmonary function decrements in human subjects. *Am Rev Respir Dis* 1987;138:1350–1354.
69. Graham D, Henderson F, House D. Neutrophil influx measured in nasal lavages of humans exposed to ozone. *Arch Environ Health* 1988;43:228–233.
70. Frischer TM, Kuehr J, Pullwitt A, et al. Ambient ozone causes upper airways inflammation in children. *Am Rev Respir Dis* 1993;148:961–964.
71. Calderon-Garciduenas L, Rodriguez-Alcaraz A, Garcia R, et al. Human nasal mucosal changes after exposure to urban pollution. *Environ Health Perspect* 1994;102:1074–1080.
72. McDonnell WF, Horstman DH, Abdul-Salaam S, House DE. Reproducibility of individual responses to ozone exposure. *Am Rev Respir Dis* 1985;131:36–40.
73. Gliner JA, Horvath SM, Folinsbee LJ. Pre-exposure to low ozone concentrations does not diminish the pulmonary function response on exposure to higher ozone concentrations. *Am Rev Respir Dis* 1983;127:51–55.
74. Frampton MW, Morrow PE, Torres A, Cox C, Voter KZ, Utell MJ. Ozone responsiveness in smokers and nonsmokers. *Am J Respir Crit Care Med* 1997;155:116–121.
75. Balmes JR, Chen LL, Scannel C, et al. Ozone-induced decrements in FEV1 and FVC do not correlate with measures of inflammation. *Am J Respir Crit Care Med* 1996;153:904–909.

76. Schlegele ES, Siefkin AD, McDonald RJ. Time course of ozone-induced neutrophilia in normal humans. *Am Rev Respir Dis* 1991;143:1353–1358.
77. McDonnell WF, Muller KE, Bromberg PA, Shy CM. Predictors of individual differences in acute response to ozone exposure. *Am Rev Respir Dis* 1993;147:818–825.
78. Dreschler-Parks DM, Bedi JF, Horvath SM. Pulmonary function responses of young and older adults to mixtures of O_3, NO_2, and PAN. *Toxicol Ind Health* 1989;5:505–517.
79. Seal E Jr, McDonnell WF, House DE, et al. The pulmonary response of white and black adults to six concentrations of ozone. *Am Rev Respir Dis* 1993;147:804–810.
80. Messineo TD, Adams WC. Ozone inhalation effects in females varying widely in lung size: comparison with males. *J Appl Physiol* 1990;69:96–103.
81. Hazucha MJ, Folinsbee LJ, Seal E, Bromberg PA. Lung function response of healthy women after sequential exposures to NO_2 and O_3. *Am J Respir Crit Care Med* 1994;150:642–647.
82. Fox SD, Adams WF, Brookes KA, Lesley BL. Enhanced response to ozone exposure during the follicular phase of the menstrual cycle. *Environ Health Perspect* 1993;101:242–244.
83. Avol EL, Linn WS, Shamoo DA, et al. Respiratory effects of photochemical oxidant air pollution in exercising adolescents. *Am Rev Respir Dis* 1985;132:619–622.
84. Avol EL, Linn WS, Shamoo DA, et al. Short-term respiratory effects of photochemical oxidant exposure in exercising children. *J Air Pollut Control Assoc* 1987;37:158–162.
85. McDonnell WF, Chapman RS, Leigh MW, Strope GL. Respiratory responses of vigorously exercising children to 0.12 ppm ozone exposure. *Am Rev Respir Dis* 1985;132:875–879.
86. Emmons K, Foster WM. Smoking cessation and acute airway response to ozone. *Arch Environ Health* 1991;46:288–295.
87. Hackney JD, Linn WS, Shamoo DA, Avol EL. Responses of selected reactive and nonreactive volunteers to ozone in high and low pollution seasons. In: Schneider T, Lee SD, Wolters GJR, Grant LD, eds. *Atmospheric ozone research and its policy implications*. Proceedings of the third US-Dutch International Symposium, Nijmegen, the Netherlands, May 9–13, 1988. Amsterdam: Elsevier Science, 1989:311–318.
88. McDonnell WF, Horstman DH, Abdul-Salaam S, Raggio LJ, Green JA. The respiratory responses of subjects with allergic rhinitis to ozone exposure and their relationship to nonspecific airway reactivity. *Toxicol Ind Health* 1987;3:507–517.
89. Whittemore AW, Korn EL. Asthma and air pollution in the Los Angeles area. *Am J Public Health* 1980;70:687–696.
90. Schoettlin CE, Landau E. Air pollution and asthmatic attacks in the Los Angeles area. *Pub Health Rep* 1961;76:545–548.
91. Ostro BS, Lipsett MJ, Mann JK, Braxton-Owens HB, White MC. Air pollution and asthma exacerbations among African-American children in Los Angeles. *Inhal Toxicol* 1995;7:711–722.
92. Cody RP, Weisel CP, Birnbaum G, Lioy PJ. The effect of ozone associated with summertime photochemical smog on the frequency of asthma visits to hospital emergency departments. *Environ Res* 1992;58:184–194.
93. Weisel CP, Cody RP, Lioy PJ. Relationship between summertime ambient ozone levels and emergency department visits for asthma in central New Jersey. *Environ Health Perspect* 1995;103[Suppl 2]:97–102.
94. Romieu I, Meneses F, Ruiz S, Sienra JJ, Huerta J. Effects of air pollution on the respiratory health of asthmatic children living in Mexico City. *Am J Respir Crit Care Med* 1996;154:300–307.
95. White MC, Etzel RA, Wilcox WD, Lloyd C. Exacerbation of childhood asthma and ozone pollution in Atlanta. *Environ Res* 1994;65:56–68.
96. Thurston GD, Ito D, Hayes CG, Bates DV, Lippmann M. Respiratory hospital admissions and summertime haze air pollution in Toronto, Ontario: consideration of the role of acid aerosols. *Environ Res* 1994;65:271–290.
97. Delfino RJ, Coate BD, Zeiger RS, Seltzer JM, Street DH, Koutrakis P. Daily asthma severity in relation to personal ozone exposure and outdoor fungal spores. *Am J Respir Crit Care Med* 1996;154:633–641.
98. Koenig JQ, Covert DS, Morgan MS, et al. Acute effects of 0.12 ppm ozone or 0.12 ppm nitrogen dioxide on pulmonary function in healthy and asthmatic adolescents. *Am Rev Respir Dis* 1985;132:648–651.
99. Linn WS, Buckley RD, Spier CE, et al. Health effects of ozone exposure in asthmatics. *Am Rev Respir Dis* 1978;117:835–843.
100. Scannell C, Chen L, Aris RM, et al. Greater ozone-induced inflammatory responses in subjects with asthma. *Am J Respir Crit Care Med* 1996;154:24–29.
101. Kreit JW, Gross KB, Moore TB, Lorenzen TJ, D'Arcy J, Eschenbacher WL. Ozone-induced changes in pulmonary function and bronchial responsiveness in asthmatics. *J Appl Physiol* 1989;66:217–222.
102. Horstman DH, Ball BA, Brown J, Gerrity T, Folinsbee LJ. Comparison of pulmonary responses of asthmatic and nonasthmatic subjects performing light exercise while exposed to a low level of ozone. *Toxicol Ind Health* 1995;11:369–385.
103. McBride DE, Koenig JQ, Luchtel DL, Williams PV, Henderson WR Jr. Inflammatory effects of ozone in the upper airways of subjects with asthma. *Am J Respir Crit Care Med* 1994;149:1192–1197.
104. Kehrl HR, Hazucha MJ, Solic JJ, Bromberg PA. Responses of subjects with chronic obstructive pulmonary disease after exposures to 0.3 ppm ozone. *Am Rev Respir Dis* 1985;131:719–724.
105. Solic JJ, Hazucha MJ, Bromberg PA. The acute effects of 0.2 ppm ozone in patients with chronic obstructive pulmonary disease. *Am Rev Respir Dis* 1982;125:664–669.
106. Linn WS, Shamoo DA, Venet TG, et al. Response to ozone in volunteers with chronic obstructive lung disease. *Arch Environ Health* 1983;38:278–283.
107. Gong H Jr, Shamoo DA, Anderson KR, Linn WS. Responses of older men with and without chronic obstructive pulmonary disease to prolonged ozone exposure. *Arch Environ Health* 1997;52:18–25.
108. Farrell BP, Kerr HD, Kulle TJ, Sauder LS, Young JL. Adaptation in human subjects to the effects of inhaled ozone after repeated exposure. *Am Rev Respir Dis* 1979;119:725–730.
109. Linn WS, Medway DA, Anzar UT, et al. Persistence of adaptation to ozone in volunteers exposed repeatedly for six weeks. *Am Rev Respir Dis* 1982;125:491–495.
110. Horvath SM, Gliner JA, Folinsbee LJ. Adaptation to ozone: duration of effect. *Am Rev Respir Dis* 1981;123:496–499.
111. Kulle TJ, Sauder LS, Kerr HD, Farrell BP, Bermal MS, Smith DM. Duration of pulmonary function adaptation to ozone in humans. *Am Ind Hyg Assoc J* 1982;43:832–837.
112. Folinsbee LJ, Bedi JF, Horvath SM. Respiratory responses in humans repeatedly exposed to low concentrations of ozone. *Am Rev Respir Dis* 1980;121:431–439.
113. Gong H Jr, McManus MS, Linn WS. Attenuated response to repeated daily ozone exposures in asthmatic subjects. *Arch Environ Health* 1997;52:34–41.
114. Folinsbee LJ, Horstman DH, Kehrl HR, Harder S, Abdul-Salaam S, Ives PJ. Respiratory responses to repeated prolonged exposure to 0.12 ppm ozone. *Am J Respir Crit Care Med* 1994;149:98–105.
115. Linn WS, Avol EL, Shamoo DA, et al. Repeated laboratory ozone exposures of volunteer Los Angeles residents: an apparent seasonal variation in response. *Toxicol Ind Health* 1988;4:505–520.
116. Tepper JS, Costa DL, Lehman JR, Weber MF, Hatch GE. Unattenuated structural and biochemical alterations in the rat lung during functional adaptation to ozone. *Am Rev Respir Dis* 1989;140:493–501.
117. Devlin RB, Folinsbee LJ, Biscardi F, et al. Inflammation and cell damage induced by repeated exposure of humans to ozone. *Inhal Toxicol* 1997;9:211–235.
118. Koenig JQ, Covert DS, Hanley QS, van Belle G, Pierson WE. Prior exposure to ozone potentiates subsequent response to sulfur dioxide in adolescent asthmatic subjects. *Am Rev Respir Dis* 1990;141:377–380.
119. Molfino NA, Wright SC, Katz I, et al. Effect of low concentrations of ozone on inhaled allergen responses in asthmatic subjects. *Lancet* 1991;338:199–203.
120. Jorres R, Nowak D, Magnussen H. The effect of ozone exposure on allergen responsiveness in subjects with asthma or rhinitis. *Am J Respir Crit Care Med* 1996;153:56–64.
121. Bascom R, Naclerio RM, Fitzgerald TK, Kagey-Sobotka A, Proud D. Effect of ozone inhalation on the response to nasal challenge with antigen of allergic subjects. *Am Rev Respir Dis* 1990;142:594–601.
122. Peden DB, Setzer RW, Devlin RB. Ozone exposure has both a priming effect on allergen-induced responses and an intrinsic inflammatory action in the nasal airways of perennially allergic asthmatics. *Am J Respir Crit Care Med* 1995;151:1336–1345.
123. Linn WS, Shamoo DA, Anderson KR, Peng R-C, Avol EL, Hackney JD. Effects of prolonged, repeated exposure to ozone, sulfuric acid, and their combination in healthy and asthmatic volunteers. *Am J Respir Crit Care Med* 1994;150:431–440.
124. Frampton MW, Morrow PE, Cox C, et al. Sulfuric acid aerosol followed by ozone exposure in healthy and asthmatic subjects. *Environ Res* 1995;69:1–14.
125. Lee HS, Wang YT, Tom KT. Occupational asthma due to ozone. *Singapore Med J* 1989;30:485–487.
126. Kinney PL, Ware JH, Spengler JD, Dockery DW, Speizer FE, Ferris BG. Short-term pulmonary function change in association with ozone levels. *Am Rev Respir Dis* 1989;139:56–61.
127. Spektor DM, Lippmann M, Lioy PJ, et al. Effects of ambient ozone on respiratory function in active normal children. *Am Rev Respir Dis* 1988;137:313–320.
128. Higgins ITT, D'Arcy JB, Gibbons DI, Avol EL, Gross KB. Effect of exposures to ambient ozone on ventilatory lung function in children. *Am Rev Respir Dis* 1990;141:1136–1146.
129. Spektor DM, Thurston GD, Mao J, He D, Hayes C, Lippmann M. Effects of single- and multi-day ozone exposure on respiratory function in active normal children. *Environ Res* 1991;55:107–122.
130. Castillejos M, Gold DR, Dockery D, Tosteson T, Baum T, Speizer FE. Effects of ambient ozone on respiratory function and symptoms in Mexico City schoolchildren. *Am Rev Respir Dis* 1992;145:276–282.
131. Spektor DM, Lippmann M, Thurston GD, et al. Effects of ambient ozone on respiratory function in healthy adults exercising outdoors. *Am Rev Respir Dis* 1988;138:821–828.
132. Hoek G, Fischer P, Brunekreef B, Lebret E, Hofschreuder P, Mennen MG. Acute effects of ambient ozone on pulmonary function of children in the Netherlands. *Am Rev Respir Dis* 1993;147:111–117.
133. Neas LM, Dockery DW, Koutrakis P, Tollerud DJ, Speizer FE. The association of ambient air pollution with twice daily peak expiratory flow rate measurements in children. *Am J Epidemiol* 1995;141:111–122.
134. Lioy PJ, Vollmuth TA, Lippmann M. Persistence of peak flow decrement in children following ozone exposures exceeding the national ambient air quality standard. *J Air Pollut Control Assoc* 1985;35:1068–1071.
135. Berry M, Lioy PJ, Gelperin K, Buckler G, Klotz J. Accumulated exposure to ozone and measurement of health effects in children and counselors at two summer camps. *Environ Res* 1991;54:135–150.
136. Ostro BD, Lipsett MJ, Mann JK, Krupnick A, Harrington W. Air pollution and respiratory morbidity among adults in Southern California. *Am J Epidemiol* 1993;137:691–700.

137. Ostro BD, Lipsett MJ, Mann JK, Braxton-Owens HB, White MC. Air pollution and asthma exacerbations among African-American children in Los Angeles. *Inhal Toxicol* 1995;7:711–722.
138. Delfino RJ, Murphy-Moulton AM, Burnett R, Brook JR, Becklake MR. Effects of air pollution on emergency room visits for respiratory illnesses in Montreal, Quebec. *Am J Respir Crit Care Med* 1997;155:568–576.
139. Thurston GD, Ito K, Hayes CG, Bates DV, Lippmann M. Respiratory hospital admissions and summertime haze air pollution in Toronto, Ontario: consideration of the role of acid aerosols. *Environ Res* 1994;65:271–290.
140. Burnett RT, Dales RE, Raizenn ME, et al. Effects of low ambient levels of ozone and sulfates on the frequency of respiratory admissions to Ontario hospitals. *Environ Res* 1994;65:172–194.
141. Schwartz J. Air pollution and hospital admissions for respiratory disease. *Epidemiology* 1996;7:20–28.
142. Braun-Fahrlander C, Ackermann-Liebrich U, Schwartz J, Gruehm HP, Rutishauser M, Wanner HU. Air pollution and respiratory symptoms in preschool children. *Am Rev Respir Dis* 1992;145:42–47.
143. Schwartz J. Air pollution and hospital admissions for the elderly in Birmingham, Alabama. *Am J Epidemiol* 1994;139:589–598.
144. Anderson HR, Ponce de Leon A, Bland JM, Bowen S, Strachan DP. Air pollution and daily mortality in London:1987–1992. *BMJ* 1996;312:665–669.
145. Sartor F, Demuth C, Snacken R, Walckiers D. Mortality in the elderly and ambient ozone concentration during the hot summer, 1994, in Belgium. *Environ Res* 1996;72:109–117.
146. Moolgavkar SH, Luebeck EG, Hall TA, Anderson EL. Air pollution and daily mortality in Philadelphia. *Epidemiology* 1995;6:476–484.
147. Borja-Aburto VH, Loomis DP, Bangdiwala SI, Shy CM, Rascon-Pacheco RA. Ozone, suspended particulates, and daily mortality in Mexico City. *Am J Epidemiol* 1997;145:258–268.
148. Saldiva PHN, Pope CA III, Schwartz J, et al. Air pollution and mortality in elderly people: a time-series study in Sao Paulo, Brazil. *Arch Environ Health* 1995;50:159–163.
149. Kinney PL, Ozkaynak H. Associations of daily mortality and air pollution in Los Angeles County. *Environ Res* 1991;54:99–121.
150. Kinney PL, Ito K, Thurston GD. A sensitivity analysis of mortality/PM-10 associations in Los Angeles. *Inhal Toxicol* 1995;7:59–69.
150a. Touloumi G, Katsouyanni K, Zmirou D, et al. Short-term effects of ambient oxidant exposure on mortality: a combined analysis within the APHEA [Air Pollution and Health: a European Approach] project. *Am J Epidemiol* 1997; 146:177–185.
151. Wilson KW. Survey of eye irritation and lacrimation in relation to air pollution. La Jolla, CA: Copley International Corporation (Prepared for the Coordinating Research Council, New York), 1974.
152. Hammer DL, Hasselblad V, Portnoy B, Wherle PF. Los Angeles student nurse study: daily symptom reporting and photochemical oxidants. *Arch Environ Health* 1974;28:255–260.
153. Challen PJR, Hickish DE, Bedford J. An investigation of some health hazards in an inert-gas tungsten-arc welding shop. *Br J Ind Med* 1957;15:276–282.
154. Grant WM. *Toxicology of the eye*, 3rd ed. Springfield, IL: Charles C Thomas Publisher, 1986:693–694.
155. Jakab GJ, Spannhake EW, Canning BJ, Kleeberger SR, Gilmour MI. The effects of ozone on immune function. *Environ Health Perspect* 1995;103[Suppl 2]:77–89.
156. Selgrade MJK, Illing JW, Starnes DM, Stead AG, Menache MG, Stevens MA. Evaluation of effects of ozone exposure on influenza infection in mice using several indicators of susceptibility. *Fund Appl Toxicol* 1988;11:169–180.
157. Wolcott JA, Zee YC, Osebold JW. Exposure to ozone reduces influenza disease severity and alters distribution of influenza viral antigens in murine lungs. *Appl Environ Microbiol* 1982;44:723–731.
158. Coffin DL, Blommer EJ. Alteration of the pathogenic role of streptococci group C in mice conferred by previous exposure to ozone. In: Silver IH, ed. *Aerobiology. Proceedings of the Third International Symposium held at the University of Sussex, England*. London: Academic Press, 1970:54–61.
159. Ehrlich R, Findlay JC, Gardner DE. Effects of repeated exposures to peak concentrations of nitrogen dioxide and ozone on resistance to streptococcal pneumonia. *J Toxicol Environ Health* 1979;5:631–642.
160. Gardner DE. Oxidant-induced enhanced sensitivity to infection in animal models and their extrapolations to man. *J Toxicol Environ Health* 1984;13:423–439.
161. Miller FJ, Illing JW, Gardner DE. Effect of urban ozone levels on laboratory-induced respiratory infections. *Toxicol Lett* 1978;2:163–169.
162. Pearlman ME, Finklea JF, Shy CM, Van Bruggen J, Newill VA. Chronic oxidant exposure and epidemic influenza. *Environ Res* 1971;4:129–140.
163. Wayne WS, Wehrle PF. Oxidant air pollution and school absenteeism. *Arch Environ Health* 1969;19:315–322.
164. Durham WH. Air pollution and student health. *Arch Environ Health* 1974;28:241–254.
165. Henderson FW, Elliott DM, Orlando GS. The immune response to rhinovirus infection in human volunteers exposed to ozone. In: Lee SD, Mustafa MG, Mehlman MA, eds. *International symposium on the biomedical effects of ozone and related photochemical oxidants*. Princeton, NJ: Princeton Scientific Publishers, 1983:253–254.
166. Coffin DL, Stokinger HE. Biological effects of air pollutants. In: Stern AC, ed. *Air pollution*, 3rd ed. vol II. London: Academic Press, 1977:231–360.
167. Evans JM, Oxidant gases. *Environ Health Perspect* 1984;55:85–95.
168. Plopper CG, Chow CK, Dungworth DL, Brummer M, Nemeth TJ. Effects of low levels of ozone on rat lungs. II. Morphological responses during recovery and reexposure. *Exp Mol Pathol* 1978;29:400–411.
169. Chow CK, Hussain MZ, Cross CE, Dungworth DL, Mustafa MG. Effect of low levels of ozone on rat lungs. I. Biochemical responses during recovery and reexposure. *Exp Mol Pathol* 1976;25:182–188.
170. Kehrl HR, Vincent LM, Kowalsky RJ, et al. Ozone exposure increases respiratory epithelial permeability in humans. *Am Rev Respir Dis* 1987;135:1124–1128.
171. Eustis SL, Schwartz LW, Kosch PC, Dungworth DL. Chronic bronchiolitis in nonhuman primates after prolonged ozone exposure. *Am J Pathol* 1981; 105:121–137.
172. Stokinger HE, Wagner WD, Dobrogorski OJ. Ozone toxicity studies. III. Chronic injury to lungs of animals following exposure at a low level. *Arch Ind Health* 1957;16:514–522.
173. Barry BE, Miller FJ, Crapo JD. Effects of inhalation of 0.12 and 0.25 parts per million ozone on the proximal alveolar region of juvenile and adult rats. *Lab Invest* 1985;53:692–704.
174. Crapo JD, Barry BE, Chang LY, Mercer RR. Alterations in lung structure caused by inhalation of oxidants. *J Toxicol Environ Health* 1984;13:301–321.
175. Fujinaka LE, Hyde DM, Plopper CG, Tyler WS, Dungworth DL, Lollini LO. Respiratory bronchiolitis following long-term ozone exposure in bonnet monkeys: a morphometric study. *Exp Lung Res* 1985;8:167–190.
176. Harkema JR, Plopper CG, Hyde DM, St. George JA, Dungworth DL. Effects of an ambient level of ozone on primate nasal epithelial muco-substances. *Am J Pathol* 1987;127:90–96.
177. Sherwin RP, Richters V. Centriacinar region (CAR) disease in the lungs of young adults, a preliminary report. In: Berglund RL, Lawson DR, McKee DJ, eds. *Tropospheric ozone and the environment*. Pittsburgh, PA: Air & Waste Management Association, 1991:178–196.
178. Johnson DA. Ozone inactivation of human alpha 1-antiproteinase inhibitor. *Am Rev Respir Dis* 1980;121:1031–1038.
179. Rieser KM, Tyler WS, Hennessy SM, Dominiguez JJ, Last JA. Long-term consequences of exposure to ozone. II. Structural alterations in lung collagen of monkeys. *Toxicol Appl Pharmacol* 1987;89:314–322.
180. Winters RS, Burnette-Vick BA, Johnson DA. Ozone, but not nitrogen dioxide, fragments elastin and increases its susceptibility to proteolysis. *Am Rev Respir Crit Care Med* 1994;150:1026–1031.
181. Costa DL, Tepper JS, Stevens MA, et al. Restrictive lung disease in rats exposed chronically to an urban profile of ozone. *Am J Respir Crit Care Med* 1995;151:1512–1518.
182. Pinkerton KE, Brody AR, Miller FJ, Crapo JD. Exposure to low levels of ozone results in enhanced pulmonary retention of inhaled asbestos fibers. *Am Rev Respir Dis* 1989;140:1075–1081.
183. Detels R, Tashkin DP, Sayre JW, et al. The UCLA population studies of chronic obstructive lung disease. IX. Lung function changes associated with chronic exposure to photochemical oxidants; a cohort study among never-smokers. *Chest* 1987;92:594–603.
184. Detels R, Tashkin DP, Sayre JW, et al. The UCLA population studies of CORD: X. A cohort study of changes in respiratory function associated with chronic exposure to SOx, NOx, and hydrocarbons. *Am J Public Health* 1991;81:350–359.
185. Tashkin DP, Detels R, Simmons M, et al. The UCLA population studies of chronic obstructive respiratory disease. XI. Impact of air pollution and smoking on annual change in forced expiratory volume in one second. *Am J Respir Crit care Med* 1994;149:1209–1217.
186. Euler GL, Abbey DE, Hodgkin JE, et al. Chronic obstructive pulmonary disease symptom effects of long-term cumulative exposure to ambient levels of total oxidants and nitrogen dioxide in California Seventh-Day Adventist residents. *Arch Environ Health* 1988;43:279–285.
187. Abbey DE, Petersen F, Mills PK, Beeson WL. Long-term ambient concentrations of total suspended particulates, ozone and sulfur dioxide and respiratory symptoms in a nonsmoking population. *Arch Environ Health* 1993;48:33–46.
188. Greer JR, Abbey DE, Burchette RJ. Asthma related to occupational and ambient air pollutants in nonsmokers. *J Occup Med* 1993;35:909–915.
188a. Peters JM, Avol E, Navidi W, et al. A study of twelve southern California communities with differing levels and types of air pollution. I. Prevalence of respiratory morbidity. *Am J Respir Crit Care Med* 1999;159:760–767.
188b. Peters JM, Avol E, Gauderman WJ, et al. A study of twelve southern California communities with differing levels and types of air pollution. II. Effects on pulmonary function. *Am J Respir Crit Care Med* 1999;159:768–775.
189. National Toxicology Program. *Toxicology and carcinogenesis studies of ozone and ozone/NNK in F344/N rats and B6C3F1 mice (inhalation studies)*. Technical Report Series No. 440. US Department of Health and Human Services, Public Health Service. Research Triangle Park, NC: National Institutes of Health, 1994.
190. Rithidech K, Hotchkiss JA, Griffith WC, Henderson RF, Brooks AL. Chromosome damage in rat pulmonary alveolar macrophages following ozone inhalation. *Mutat Res* 1990;241:67–73.
191. Merz T, Bender MA, Kerr HD, Kulle TJ. Observations of aberrations in chromosomes of lymphocytes from human subjects exposed to ozone at a concentration of 0.5 ppm for 6 and 10 hours. *Mutat Res* 1975;31:299–302.
192. McKenzie WH, Knelson JH, Rummo NJ, House DE. Cytogenetic effects of inhaled ozone in man. *Mutat Res* 1977;48:95–102.
193. Borek C, Ong A, Cleaver JE. DNA damage from ozone and radiation in human epithelial cells. *Toxicol Ind Health* 1988;4:547–553.
194. Kozumbo WJ, Agarwal S. Induction of DNA damage in cultured human lung cells by tobacco smoke arylamines exposed to ambient levels of ozone. *Am J Respir Cell Mol Biol* 1990;3:611–618.

195. Borek C, Zaider M, Ong A, Mason H, Witz G. Ozone acts alone and synergistically with ionizing radiation to induce in vitro neoplastic transformation. *Carcinogenesis* 1986;7:1611–1613.
196. Borek C, Ong A, Mason H. Ozone and ultraviolet light act as additive cocarcinogens to induce in vitro neoplastic transformation. *Teratog Carcinog Mutagen* 1989;9:71–74.
197. Thomassen DG, Harkema JR, Stephens ND, Griffith WC. Preneoplastic transformation of rat tracheal epithelial cells by ozone. *Toxicol Appl Pharmacol* 1991;109:137–148.
198. Hassett C, Mustafa MG, Coulson WF, Elashoff RM. Murine lung carcinogenesis following exposure to ambient ozone concentrations. *J Natl Cancer Inst* 1985;75:771–777.
198a. Abbey DE, Nishino N, McDonnell WF, et al. Long-term inhalable particles and other air pollutants related to mortality in nonsmokers. *Am J Respir Crit Care Med* 1999;159:373–382.
199. Witschi H. Effects of oxygen and ozone on mouse lung tumorigenesis. *Exp Lung Res* 1991;17:473–483.
200. Zelikoff JT, Kraemer G-L, Vogel C, Schlesinger RB. Immunomodulating effects of ozone on macrophage functions important for tumor surveillance and host defense. *J Toxicol Environ Health* 1991;34:449–467.
201. Li AF-Y, Richters A. Ambient level ozone effects on subpopulations of thymocytes and spleen T lymphocytes. *Arch Environ Health* 1991;46:57–63.
202. Reference deleted by author.
203. Monn C, Hangartner M. Passive sampling for ozone. *J Air Waste Manage Assoc* 1990;40:357–361.
204. Grosjean D, Hisham MWM. A passive sampler for atmospheric ozone. *J Air Waste Manage Assoc* 1992;42:169–173.
205. Koutrakis P, Wolfson JM, Bunyaviroch A, Froelich SE, Hirano K, Mulik JD. Measurement of ambient ozone using a nitrite-coated filter. *Anal Chem* 1993;65:209–214.

CHAPTER 66

Oxides of Nitrogen and Sulfur

Michael J. Lipsett

NITROGEN OXIDES

Sources and Production

Nitrogen oxides are reactive substances that encompass nitric oxide, nitrogen dioxide, and nitrogen tetroxide. These compounds occur together in dynamic equilibrium and collectively are termed *NO_x* or *nitrous fume*. Other members of the larger family of nitrogen oxides are nitrous oxide, peroxyacetyl nitrates, nitrites, nitroso compounds, nitrogen-containing acids, nitrogen peroxide, dinitrogen trioxide, and dinitrogen pentoxide.

Below 21°C, NO_2 exists as a liquid, principally as its dimer, N_2O_4. Increasing temperature favors the formation of NO_2 over N_2O_4 at equilibrium, although at ambient temperatures and concentrations, small quantities of NO_2 are likely to be present as N_2O_4 (1). NO is oxidized in ambient air to form NO_2, which therefore is always present when NO is detected. Both NO_2 and NO are reactive free radicals; their physical characteristics are presented in Table 66-1 (1–3).

Exposure Sources

Both NO and NO_2 are formed naturally as a result of bacterial metabolism of nitrogenous compounds and, to a lesser extent, from fires, volcanoes, and fixation by lightning. The main human-generated source of NO_x pollution of ambient air is fossil fuel combustion in motor vehicles and industry, particularly in the generation of electricity. High-temperature combustion results in oxidation of atmospheric N_2, first to NO and then to NO_2. Nitrogen in such fossil fuels as coal can be oxidized to NO_2 under oxygen-rich combustion conditions, whereas molecular nitrogen (N_2) tends to be formed preferentially with a fuel-rich mixture. The efficiency of thermal NO_x formation depends on combustion temperature, the air to fuel ratio, residence time in the combustion chamber, and other factors (4).

TABLE 66-1. Synonyms and physical properties of nitric oxide and nitrogen dioxide

	Nitric oxide	Nitrogen dioxide
Synonyms	Nitrogen monoxide Mononitrogen monoxide	Nitrogen peroxide Nitrogen tetroxide
Molecular weight (g/mol)	30.01	46.01
Melting point (°C)	−163.6	−11.2
Boiling point (°C)	−151.8	21.2
Physical state	Colorless gas	Reddish-brown gas, yellowish-brown liquid (N_2O_4)
Density (air = 1)	1.04	1.58
Solubility (g/100 g H_2O)	0.006	Reacts with water to form nitric and nitrous acids

From refs. 1–3, with permission.

The generation of tropospheric ozone and other photochemical oxidants is initiated with photolysis of NO_2, whereas NO acts as an ozone scavenger. Motor vehicle emissions near busy streets can result in high local NO_x concentrations. The typical diurnal NO_x pattern consists of a low background concentration, with morning and late afternoon spikes resulting from rush-hour traffic (5). Annual average concentrations of NO_2 in urban areas typically range between 10 and 50 parts per billion (ppb), whereas half-hour and 24-hour averages as high as 450 and 210 ppb, respectively, have been reported (5).

Commercial production of NO_2 involves oxidation of NO. Occupational settings commonly associated with exposures to nitrogen oxides involve production, transportation, and use of nitric acid (Table 66-2) (6–10). Contact of HNO_3 with organic material (e.g., in nitration of cotton) or certain metals (e.g., in acid dipping, pickling, and etching) produces NO_2. This production also may occur accidentally from spillage of HNO_3, which liberates NO_2 fumes after contact with paper, wood, or other organic material (11). NO_2 is also a by-product generated in the manufacture of many chemicals, including dyes, lacquers, explosives, and celluloid. Combustion of fossil fuels in enclosed or inadequately ventilated spaces, such as underground mines or skating rinks, also can result in NO_2 accumulation. Acetylene or electric arc welding causes the formation of nitrogen oxides through the oxidation of atmospheric nitrogen, which can result in toxic NO_2 concentrations in enclosed working environments.

Exposure to NO_2 is a hazard also in agriculture. Silo filler's disease is due to inhalation of NO_2 evolving from crops (e.g., alfalfa or corn) stored in a silo or pit for later use as feed for livestock (12). Nitrates in plants ferment and form nitrites, which form nitrous acid (HNO_2) on reaction with organic acids. HNO_2 decomposes and yields NO, which then is oxidized to NO_2. The latter can attain high concentrations near the surface of silage in silos [up to several thousand parts per million (ppm)] (13,14). Burning of propane or kerosene to add heat and carbon dioxide to the air in greenhouses produces NO_x concentrations of up to 3.5 ppm (5).

Commercial production of NO involves passage of air through an electric arc or oxidation of ammonia over platinum

TABLE 66-2. Occupational and nonoccupational occurrence and exposure to nitrogen oxides

Occupational
- Combustion of fossil fuels (e.g., automobile garages, ice-resurfacing machines in skating rinks, other internal combustion engines, boilers)
- Nitric acid production, transportation, and use (e.g., acid dipping of brass and copper, cleaning of copper or aluminum vats)
- Arc welding and other electric arc fixation of nitrogen
- Agriculture and horticulture (silo filling, fuel combustion in greenhouses)
- Decomposition of aqueous nitrous acid
- High-temperature oxidation of ammonia
- Chemical manufacturing uses (production of dyes and lacquers, agent of nitration and oxidation, catalyst, inhibitor of acrylate polymerization)
- Manufacture or use of explosives
- Missile fuel oxidizer
- Mining (diesel exhaust, shot-firing at coal seams)
- Firefighting (including exposure to smoke from burning plastics, shoe polish, nitrocellulose film, or fossil fuels)
- Medical administration of nitric oxide

Nonoccupational
- Gas- and oil-fired heaters and other household appliances
- Kerosene heaters
- Ice-skating rinks
- Ambient air pollution (motor vehicle exhaust, industrial boilers)
- Cigarette smoke

From refs. 6–10, with permission.

gauze. NO is used in a variety of industrial processes, including HNO_3 production, as a bleaching agent for rayon, as an oxidant in organic chemical reactions, and as a stabilizer (against free radical decomposition) for methyl ether and other materials (2).

Although NO has been viewed traditionally as an industrial toxin and air pollutant, it was demonstrated in the late 1980s to be identical with endothelium-derived relaxing factor and since then has been shown to have multiple essential roles in normal physiology. NO has been administered commonly as a selective vasodilator in patients with pulmonary hypertension, acute lung injury, and other disorders; health care workers in intensive care units are likely to be exposed to low levels of both NO and NO_2 (15). An intensive care simulation of NO administration produced measured levels of 30 to 45 ppb NO_2 and 210 to 240 ppb NO, both well below occupational exposure standards (16). However, in the same investigation, patients receiving high-dose NO [70 ppm; inspired oxygen concentration = 1] would have inhaled NO_2 concentrations of 6 ppm, exceeding both occupational and environmental standards (16).

Although regulatory attention has focused on outdoor or occupational exposure to NO_x, significant human exposure occurs in nonoccupational indoor settings (17–19). Concentrations of NO_2 indoors generally are lower than outdoor levels, although the opposite can occur in the presence of indoor sources. Gas-burning appliances, such as unvented furnaces and stoves, are the chief sources of nitrogen oxides indoors, although tobacco smoke and kerosene space heaters can also be contributing factors (8,18,20–22). For nonsmokers, exposure to residential tobacco smoke is likely to be of minor importance in personal NO_2 exposure in comparison with other sources (23). When a gas stove is used for cooking, peak 1-hour NO_2 kitchen concentrations can approach or even exceed 1 ppm (5). In urban areas with substantial vehicular pollution, infiltration of ambient NO_2 also may play a significant role in indoor exposures (18). Numerous reports have documented toxic concentrations of NO_2 (up to several parts per million) in ice-skating rinks (23–31).

Absorption, Metabolism, and Excretion

Inhalation is the predominant route of exposure to nitrogen oxides, although occasional accidental spills of N_2O_4 (e.g., used as missile fuel) may cause contact between the skin and mucous membranes and the liquid (7). Overt dermal and mucous membrane toxicity from such contact results in chemical burns.

As with ozone, NO_2 uptake in the respiratory tract is a function of reactive absorption occurring near the gas-liquid interface of the pulmonary epithelium. Its low water solubility allows penetration to the lower respiratory tract, the principal site of toxicity, but kinetics of absorption appear to be determined more by chemical reactivity than by solubility. Healthy volunteers exposed briefly to 0.29 to 7.20 ppm NO_2 absorbed between 81% and 92%, a finding based on comparison of NO_2 concentrations in inhaled and exhaled air (32). Asthmatics exposed at rest to 0.3 ppm NO_2 through a mouthpiece absorbed 72%, the amount increasing to 87% with exercise (33). After a short (7- to 9-minute) exposure of rhesus monkeys to radiolabeled NO_2, ^{13}N activity (measured at the thorax) remained virtually unchanged during the immediate postexposure period, although during the same interval, the activity of ^{125}Xe (a nonreactive gas used as a control) dropped to near-baseline levels, indicating that NO_2 or its reaction products had been bound within the respiratory tract (34). Uptake of NO_2 from the pulmonary airspace appears to be saturable and highly temperature-sensitive, suggesting that reactions with lung surface constituents represent an important, if not the sole, mechanism of NO_2 absorption (35,36). At concentrations of less than 10 ppm, NO_2 uptake appears to follow first-order kinetics (36).

Postlethwaite and Bidani (36) and Postlethwaite et al. (37) postulated that NO_2 uptake is governed mainly by reaction with constituents of the pulmonary surface-lining layer (SLL), which covers both the conducting airways and the alveolar surfaces. Little, if any, NO_2 is likely to diffuse through the extracellular SLL unreacted. Thus, NO_2-related toxicity, like ozone, probably is initiated via a cascade mechanism triggered by its primary reaction products.

Theoretically, reactions of NO_2 within the SLL could involve (i) reaction with intrapulmonary water to form HNO_3 and HNO_2, respectively, (ii) addition to double bonds, or (iii) hydrogen abstraction to produce HNO_2 and an organic radical (34,36). At physiologic pH, hydrogen abstraction is thought to predominate. In perfused rat lung, most absorbed NO_2 was converted to nitrite ion, presumably via formation and subsequent dissociation of HNO_2, with little formation of HNO_3 or nitrate (38). In addition, the driving force of NO_2 absorption *in vitro* appears to be the presence of oxidizable substrates (37). These observations and other evidence suggest that simple physical solubility or diffusion is unlikely to be as important in NO_2 uptake as chemical reactivity (36). Most absorbed NO_2 enters blood as nitrite ion, which then is oxidized to nitrate and is excreted in the urine (39,40). However, some absorbed NO_2 may participate in other reactions, possibly including nitrosation of amines to form nitrosamines (40).

NO is minimally soluble in water, but it is well absorbed via inhalation (i.e., between 85% and 93%) and has been proposed as a test gas for alveolar-capillary diffusion (32,41,42). NO's affinity for hemoglobin is more than 1,000 times greater than that of carbon monoxide. On absorption in blood, NO rapidly forms nitrosylhemoglobin, which is converted into methemoglobin. In the presence of methemoglobin reductase and oxygen in red blood cells, hemoglobin can be regenerated, resulting in nitrate and nitrite formation. Most inhaled NO is excreted as nitrate in the urine within 48 hours. Other metabolites include molecular nitrogen, urea, and ammonia (41,43). Some inhaled NO reacts with oxygen to form NO_2, which is metabolized to nitrite and nitrate, as described (43).

Physiologic Role of Nitric Oxide

NO plays an essential role in normal physiology. Synthesized endogenously from L-arginine by macrophages, neutrophils, endothelial cells, neurons, and other cell types, NO acts as a local transcellular messenger, activating guanylate cyclase, which catalyzes cyclic guanosine monophosphate synthesis. Air exhaled by healthy humans contains approximately 3 ppb NO and has been reported to reach peak concentrations of up to 300 ppb after breath holding for 1 minute (44). NO modulates a variety of physiologic functions via the NO–cyclic guanosine monophosphate signal transduction mechanism, including smooth-muscle reactivity (particularly vasorelaxation), inhibition of platelet adhesion and aggregation, intestinal ion transport, renal sodium transport, neurotransmission, and other processes (45). On diffusion into the intravascular space, NO binds avidly to hemoglobin (as noted), limiting the extent of its biological activity.

Clinical Toxicology

The relatively low solubility of NO_2 allows penetration to the lower respiratory tract, the principal site of toxicity. Described as "sweetish, acrid" (46) or "bleach" (47), the odor of NO_2 has been reported to be detectable at levels ranging from 0.04 to 5.00 ppm, whereas mucous membrane irritation becomes perceptible at somewhat higher concentrations (1 to 13 ppm) (9,46–49). Individuals unfamiliar with the visual or olfactory characteristics of NO_2 or in whom olfactory fatigue develops unwittingly may inhale large volumes of this gas, putting them at risk for delayed-onset lower respiratory toxicity (50). The severity of injury depends on the volume of gas inhaled; NO_2 concentration appears to be more important in this regard than is ventilation rate or duration of exposure. However, significant respiratory toxicity has occurred among vigorously exercising hockey players when NO_2 concentrations were likely to have been lower than the current occupational exposure limits. Mild intoxication may induce transient nonspecific symptoms, including dyspnea, cough, headache, fatigue, nausea, vertigo, and somnolence, which ordinarily dissipate over the ensuing hours to days but may persist for up to 2 weeks without clinically detectable pulmonary findings. Exposure to massive concentrations of nitrogen oxides may cause sudden death from laryngospasm or bronchospasm (51).

Between these extremes is a multiphasic course of disease that can be fatal if untreated. Affected individuals may experience a variety of acute symptoms, including dyspnea, cough, wheeze, chest pain, palpitations, weakness, diaphoresis, nausea, vomiting, headache, and eye irritation during or shortly after exposure. Exposed individuals have described a "choking" or "smothering" sensation (52). Removal to fresh air often alleviates symptoms, a relief that may induce some individuals to forego seeking medical care. However, after an interval of a few hours (usually 4 to 12), such persons may present with chemical pneumonitis or frank pulmonary edema, with dyspnea, tachypnea, cyanosis, cough, bronchospasm, hemoptysis, substernal pain, rales, and tachycardia (9,50,53–58). A chest radiograph taken soon after nitrogen oxide exposure may be normal and does not rule out the subsequent development of pulmonary edema. Laboratory findings may include decreased arterial oxygen saturation, leukocytosis, and elevated C-reactive protein (27).

Arterial hypoxemia observed at this stage may be due not only to an impaired diffusion capacity secondary to alveolar edema but to ventilation-perfusion defects and, in some cases, to methemoglobinemia resulting from the reaction of nitrite ions with hemoglobin (51). Although the normal limit for methemoglobinemia is less than 1%, concentrations of 2% to 3% have been reported among arc welders and up to 44% in postmortem blood samples from persons exposed to silo gas (59). Metabolic acidosis may be present. Although systemic hypotension can result from nitrate- or nitrite-induced vasodilatation, this finding is not common. The early appearance of findings characteristic of pulmonary edema is indicative of severe exposure and a worse prognosis. Except in cases of massive exposures, most individuals receiving appropriate, timely therapy will survive NO_2-induced pulmonary edema. Still, in the past, the case-fatality rate—nearly 30%—has been substantial (51).

After apparent recovery from the acute illness, some patients may develop bronchiolitis obliterans approximately 10 to 30 days after the exposure. This delayed manifestation of severe respiratory symptoms may occur also in the absence of a prior episode of pulmonary edema (53,58,60). Typically, this relapse is heralded by fever and chills, with rapid deterioration of the patient's condition. Other presenting symptoms may include fatigue, progressive shortness of breath and dyspnea, tachypnea, cough, hemoptysis, chest tightness, and cyanosis (9,51,55,58). Auscultation reveals bilateral inspiratory rales and expiratory wheezes, although occasionally affected persons may exhibit minimal or no unusual findings (9,60). Laboratory findings may include arterial hypoxemia, neutrophilic leukocytosis, and an elevated sedimentation rate (60). Chest radiographs may show a patchy distribution of pneumonitis or, more commonly, diffuse nodular infiltrates similar to those seen in miliary tuberculosis, with confluence of nodules in severe cases (11,50,60). Pathologic examination of open-lung biopsy and of autopsy specimens demonstrates an inflammatory exudate with fibrinous organization, a condition that may occlude the lumen of small bronchi and bronchioles (58,60,61). Pulmonary function tests during the initial acute stage demonstrate reduced lung volumes and diffusing capacity: These findings tend to be more severe during the delayed stage, during which a marked alveolar-arterial oxygen gradient is characteristic (11).

Nonoccupational exposures to NO_2 may result also in clinically significant respiratory toxicity. Several outbreaks of acute respiratory illness among ice hockey players, cheerleaders, and spectators have followed exposure to emissions from ice-resurfacing machines (known as *Zambonis*, after their inventor) (24–28,62). NO_2-related effects reported among hockey players and referees have ranged from symptoms of mild respiratory irritation to noncardiogenic pulmonary edema. In one incident in Minnesota, at least 116 individuals experienced respiratory symptoms (including cough, chest pain, hemoptysis, shortness of breath) during or shortly after a hockey game (24). The cheerleaders and hockey players had symptoms more severe than those of the spectators in the bleachers, presumably because of their increased activity levels and ventilation rates relative to the spectators and because NO_2 is denser than air, favoring the accumulation of higher concentrations near the ice. Many affected individuals also reported headaches, which were likely due to intoxication by CO rather than to NO_2. A similar incident in Wisconsin resulted in 63 cases of respiratory illness among high school students (25). In these and other episodes reported, NO_2 was not measured concurrently with exposure, but testing indicated that concentrations would have been in the range of 1 to 4 ppm, below the occupational exposure standard. As even controlled exposure studies of NO_2 in this concentration range generally have failed to detect effects of this gas in healthy individuals (other than small increases in airway reactivity), the incidence of NO_2-related intoxication in ice arenas illustrates the importance of ventilation rate and duration of exposure in determining toxicity. In the hockey player reports, most patients had delayed onset of serious symptoms, having experienced only minimal or mild respiratory symptoms during the games (24–28).

Effects of acute exposures to low levels of NO_2 have been examined extensively in human volunteers in controlled chamber studies. Healthy subjects may experience changes in lung function in response to short exposures at concentrations exceeding 1.5 to 2.0 ppm but typically not below 1 ppm. However, clear interindividual and interstudy differences are seen in regard to sensitivity (63–66). Exposure to 5 ppm NO_2 for 2 hours also has been reported to result in a modestly increased alveolar-arterial oxygen gradient (64). Exposure of healthy volunteers to 1 or 2 ppm NO_2 for up to 3 hours caused modest but statistically significant decreases in hemoglobin, hematocrit, and red blood cell cholinesterase, with a significant increase in peroxidized red blood cell lipids observed at the higher exposure concentration (67). The clinical implications for humans repeatedly exposed to low levels of NO_2 are unclear.

In two studies of older subjects with chronic obstructive pulmonary disease, exposure to 0.3 ppm NO_2 for 2 or 4 hours resulted in small decreases in the forced expiratory volume over 1 second (FEV_1) or forced vital capacity (FVC) or both, without accompanying symptoms (68,69). Another study involving a 4-hour exposure at 0.30 ppm, as well as others involving higher concentrations for shorter periods, found no such effects (70–72).

Exposure to as little as 0.1 to 0.6 ppm NO_2 has enhanced airway reactivity transiently in some asthmatics in controlled exposure studies, but the numerous studies examining this outcome also have been somewhat inconsistent (73–80). The interstudy discrepancies are likely to be related to differences in baseline disease severity of the study subjects and to differences in study protocols (exposure durations and concentrations, intensity of exercise, methods of assessing airway reactivity). Although few of these studies have found any immediate symptoms or changes in lung function after low-level NO_2 exposures, one implication of the increased airway reactivity is that asthmatics may be rendered more susceptible to aeroallergens or other respiratory irritants. A metaanalysis of results of controlled exposure studies found that resting exposures to low levels of NO_2 seemed to favor the development of increased airway reactivity, whereas protocols involving exercise were less likely to do so (81). Possibly exercise itself may render the lung somewhat refractory to bronchoconstrictive challenge, or NO_2 may, via formation of nitrite, induce smooth-muscle relaxation at the higher inhaled volumes accompanying exercise (81).

At higher concentrations (91.5 ppm), NO_2 increases airway reactivity in healthy subjects (82,83). The mechanism underlying increased reactivity attributable to NO_2 exposure is not well understood but appears to be blocked by oral pretreatment with ascorbic acid (84). Increased airway reactivity often is associated with inflammation. In controlled studies of humans, bronchoalveolar lavage (BAL) fluid obtained after subjects' exposure to 2.25 to 5.00 ppm NO_2 for 20 minutes showed increased numbers of mast cells and lymphocytes relative to baseline levels, whereas no significant inflammatory response occurred at lower exposure concentrations (85–88). Studies also found slightly increased numbers of neutrophils and lymphocytes but no increase in mast cells in BAL fluid from nonsmoking subjects exposed to 3.5 ppm NO_2 for 20 minutes (89). In a study of 8 healthy adults exposed to 2 ppm NO_2 or filtered air for 4 hours, exposure to NO_2 resulted in an inflammatory response consisting of increased neutrophils, interleukin-6, interleukin-8, α_1-antitrypsin, and tissue plasminogen activator in bronchial washings (representative of the airways) but not in BAL fluid (more representative of the alveoli than the bronchi) (90). These investigators also reported a subtle effect on small airway caliber consistent with their findings of inflammation but no effect on conventional measures of central airway function (e.g., FEV_1). In contrast, Vagaggini et al. (68) found that a 2-hour exposure at 0.3 ppm to NO_2 failed to induce an inflammatory response in healthy subjects, asthmatics, or patients with chronic obstructive pulmonary disease as measured by examination of postexposure nasal lavage and induced sputum, which tends to be representative of more proximal airways than BAL.

From these experiments, NO_2 exposure appears to be able to elicit increased airway reactivity and a modest inflammatory response at concentrations lower than occupational exposure limits; however, inflammation is less likely to occur at levels commonly encountered in nonoccupational settings. Inflammation observed after single exposures may attenuate with repetition. In one experiment involving 20-minute exposures of 10 healthy volunteers to 4 ppm NO_2 every other day (six times total), the inflammatory responses reported after single exposures using similar concentrations were not observed when BAL was performed after the final exposure (91). However, these investigators did observe small, but statistically significant, changes in T-lymphocyte subsets in the subjects' BAL fluid and reductions in the numbers of B cells and natural killer cells. More recently, 4-hour exposures of 12 healthy nonsmoking adults to 2 ppm NO_2 on four consecutive days resulted in attenuation of acute pulmonary function decrements (FEV_1 and FVC) and of acute changes in antioxidants (ascorbic acid, uric acid, and glutathione) in BAL fluid; however, neutrophils and myeloperoxidase were increased in bronchial washings after the NO_2 as compared with control (air) exposures (92). This experiment suggests that repeated exposures to NO_2 at concentrations observed in occupational settings may result in persistent neutrophilic inflammation.

Other studies suggested that exposure to low concentrations of NO_2 may increase the response of allergic individuals to inhalant antigens. For example, Tunnicliffe et al. (93) found that eight allergic asthmatics exposed randomly to clean air, 100 or 400 ppb NO_2 for 1 hour, then to a fixed dose of house dust mite antigen experienced small but significant decreases in FEV_1 after exposure to 400 (but not 100) ppb NO_2 in comparison with clean air. Other investigators have reported that 6-hour exposures of mild atopic asthmatics to a combination of 200 ppb sulfur dioxide and 400 ppb NO_2 resulted in decreases ranging from 37% to 63% in the dose of dust mite antigen challenge required to produce a 20% fall in FEV_1 as compared to antigen challenge after clean air exposure (94,95). This effect was maximal at 24 hours and persisted at least 24 to 48 hours after the exposure (95). These studies suggested that exposures to concentrations of NO_2 that can be encountered in everyday life (near gas stoves or in heavy traffic) may potentiate the effects of exposure to allergens in atopic asthmatics.

In immunotoxicologic studies of animal models, acute exposure to NO_2 has been reported to affect many host defenses against infection. Alveolar macrophages taken from experimental animals exposed to NO_2 concentrations ranging from 0.3 ppm to more than 10 ppm demonstrate changes in morphology and functional abilities. Other reported effects include decreased intrapulmonary killing of microorganisms and changes in systemic immune responses to specific antigens. Both structural and functional dimensions of ciliary clearance are impaired by NO_2 exposure in experimental animals, including decreased ciliary motility and beat frequency, changes in ciliary morphology, and decreased numbers of cilia (96–106).

Studies of individual components of human respiratory defenses are fewer in number. Brief exposures of human volunteers to low levels of NO_2 (1.5 or 3.5 ppm) produced marked ciliostasis (observed *in vivo* with fiberoptic bronchoscopy 45 minutes after exposure) that returned to normal levels after 24 hours (107). Similarly, dose-related decreases in ciliary beat frequency were reported in a human epithelial cell line exposed to concentrations ranging from 100 to 2,000 ppb NO_2 (108). Studies of the effects of NO_2 on human alveolar macrophages (AM) have been less consistent. Pinkston et al. (109) exposed AM extracted from BAL fluid obtained from 15 healthy adult volunteers to 5, 10, and 15 ppm NO_2 for 3 hours and found no effect on cell viability or on several immunoregulatory functions. In contrast, Helleday et al. (89) reported a trend ($p = .052$) toward decreased AM phagocytosis of yeast particles by AM extracted by BAL from nonsmoking subjects exposed to 3.5 ppm × 20 minutes. Frampton et al. (110) found that AM retrieved by BAL from four of nine subjects exposed for 3 hours to 0.6 ppm NO_2 showed decreased ability to inactivate influenza virus *in vitro* ($p < .07$), although no such effects were observed with an exposure protocol involving three 15-minute spikes of 2 ppm NO_2 superimposed on a continuous (3-hour) exposure to 0.05 ppm. In an experiment involving six exposures (one every other day) of 10 healthy volunteers to 4 ppm NO_2 before BAL, Sandström et al. (91) found no significant effect of NO_2 on the proportion of AM capable of phagocytosis of yeast, although the total number of AM recovered was reduced. The limited experimental data suggest that effects of NO_2 exposure on human defenses against infection still are poorly understood.

Acute and subacute NO_2 exposures (typically at concentrations ≥1 ppm) increase susceptibility to infection in experimental animals after aerosol challenge with a variety of respiratory pathogens, including bacteria, viruses, and mycoplasma (96–98,111). Subchronic exposure to a lower concentration of NO_2 (0.5 ppm) reportedly increased mortality from bacterial infection in rodents, although more recent investigations could not replicate these results (98,112). Superimposing short (1-hour) NO_2 spikes on a lower continuous background exposure, in concentrations similar to those occurring in urban environments, enhanced NO_2-related effects on infectivity in mice (113).

Few researchers have examined whether NO_2 exposure affects the integrated operation of human respiratory defenses against infection. Goings et al. (114) administered attenuated, live influenza virus intranasally to 152 volunteers exposed to clean air or 1, 2, or 3 ppm NO_2 for 2 hours on 3 consecutive days, with viral challenge occurring on the second day. Although infection rates were higher in two of the NO_2-exposed volunteers than in members of the control groups, the differences were not statistically significant; however, the investigators calculated that their study design probably had only approximately 21% power to detect a significant difference in infection rates.

Several epidemiologic investigations suggested associations between both ambient and indoor NO_2 concentrations and respiratory illnesses. Recent studies indicated associations between daily measurements of ambient NO_2 and small (but significant) decrements in lung function in asthmatics and increased risks of asthma emergency room visits, although the evidence is not entirely consistent (115–118). Some epidemiologic studies suggest an association between gas stove usage (which produces NO_2 and other combustion products) and an increased incidence of respiratory illness and decreased lung function in children, although results of studies examining this issue also are not consistent (119–125). Recent studies in which 1- or 2-week NO_2 residential concentrations were measured found no relationship between NO_2 and the incidence of respiratory infections in infants and preschool children (121,122). Another found an odds ratio of 2.2 [95% confidence interval (CI), 1.0 to 4.8] for respiratory symptoms in schoolchildren associated with having a gas stove in the home, even after adjustment for 4-day NO_2 concentrations, suggesting that other combustion emissions or peak NO_2 concentrations (not captured adequately in multiday averages) may be important (125). This study also found a dose-response relationship of marginal statistical significance ($p = .09$) between respiratory symptoms and NO_2 levels. However, epidemiologic investigation of the relationship between putative NO_2 exposure and respiratory illness is difficult: A variety of study design constraints (mainly concerning assessment and classification of exposure) tend to bias against finding an effect. Nevertheless, a metaanalysis of 11 epidemiologic studies suggested that exposure to NO_2 from residential gas stove usage (resulting in an estimated long-term increase of 30 µg per cubic meter or 16 ppb NO_2) increases the odds of respiratory illness and symptoms in children by approximately 20% (126).

The extent to which gas stove usage may contribute to induction or exacerbation of asthma or asthmalike symptoms has not been examined as extensively. In one recent study, use of a gas stove on a given day was found to increase the risk of exacerbation of respiratory symptoms in adults with moderate to severe asthma (127). In a large cross-sectional study of young adults in Great Britain, use of a gas stove for cooking was associated with significantly increased risks for a variety of asthma-related symptoms during the preceding year, including wheeze, wheeze with breathlessness, waking with chest tightness and shortness of breath, and asthma attacks in women but not men (128). Women who used a gas stove for cooking were observed also to have reduced lung function (measured as FEV_1 or as FEV_1/FVC) relative to those who did not (128). Although other studies have not detected such clear-cut relationships, these studies suggested that indoor exposure to NO_2 and possibly other gas stove emissions may adversely affect some individuals with preexisting asthma, either directly or through interaction with other environmental exposures.

Possibly, NO_2 exposure also may increase the risk of developing asthma: In a large case-control study of asthma in 3- and 4-year-old children, personal 24-hour NO_2 monitoring of a subsample of the participants suggested an approximately tenfold increase in risk of asthma in children whose personal exposure was greater than 15 ppb per day versus those whose exposure was lower, when controlling for numerous other recognized risk factors (129). The presence of animals in the house dramatically elevated such odds ratios, suggesting that, consistent with some of the controlled-exposure studies described earlier, NO_2 exposure may affect susceptible individuals' responses to aeroallergens (130).

In comparison with the voluminous documentation of NO_2 toxicity, relatively little information exists regarding adverse effects associated with inhalation of NO. Smokers are exposed routinely to several hundred parts per million NO in cigarette smoke, which does not appear to precipitate significant acute toxicity (131). Probably the most important effect of acute NO exposure is its ability to form methemoglobin, which is the basis for current occupational exposure limits (132). Because NO is synthesized endogenously and plays vital roles in normal physiology, a variety of deactivation mechanisms exist. As noted, NO has been used therapeutically (at concentrations of up to 100 ppm) as a selective pulmonary vasodilator in acute lung injury and other conditions (133).

Given its role in normal physiology, NO inhalation appeared to be markedly less noxious than NO_2 in experimental animals: One rodent toxicology study suggested that NO is at least 30 times less toxic (134). Brief exposures of rats to up to 1,500 ppm (for 15 minutes) or 1,000 ppm (for 30 minutes) produced no detectable histopathologic effects in the lungs, whereas exposure to 25 ppm NO_2 (for 30 minutes) caused mild to moderate inflammation (134). However, animals exposed to 1,000 ppm for 30 minutes became cyanotic and died shortly thereafter, presumably because of methemoglobin formation. In 14-day exposures of rabbits to 5 ppm NO, the principal pathologic findings in the lungs were edema of the alveolar-capillary membrane and of the walls of small arteries without evidence of inflammation, suggesting that the reported effects took place only after absorption and initial metabolism of NO (135).

Controlled-exposure studies of humans suggested moderate bronchoconstriction with concentrations of NO at 20 ppm and higher, with lesser effects of questionable biological significance observed at a concentration of 1 ppm (136,137). As noted, NO inhalation also produces selective pulmonary vasodilatation, which has proved useful therapeutically.

CHRONIC TOXICITY

Severe, symptomatic NO_2 intoxication after acute exposure has, on occasion, been linked with persistent respiratory impairment, with symptoms of chronic bronchitis, and with spirometric evidence of an obstructive or a restrictive defect (51,52,138,139). Lingering nonrespiratory symptoms from acute overexposure to NO_x are infrequent; however, several survivors of a massive rocket fuel spill reported headache and other subjective neuropsychiatric complaints for up to 1 year after the accident (7). Prolonged exposure to concentrations of NO_2 in excess of exposure limits results in focal emphysema in experimental animals. The evidence regarding whether such an effect may occur also in occupationally exposed humans is mixed (140,141). Acute exposure of healthy nonsmokers to 3 or 4 ppm NO_2 for several hours resulted in a 45% reduction of α_1-protease inhibitor activity in BAL fluid, although this finding could not be replicated at lower concentrations (1.5 ppm continuously for 3 hours or 0.05 ppm with three 2-ppm spikes) (142,143).

In a prospective California study of approximately 6,000 nonsmoking Seventh Day Adventists, Abbey et al. (144) found that average ambient NO_2 concentrations were not related to development of new cases of symptoms of chronic obstructive airway disease, cancer, myocardial infarction, or all-cause mortality. In the Adventist study, NO_2 concentrations were interpolated from fixed-site monitoring stations and, in some analyses, included a correction for indoor NO_2 concentrations. Another report on the mortality experience of the same cohort between 1977 and 1992 found no relationship between mean ambient NO_2 concentrations and all-cause mortality, cardiopulmonary mortality, and nonmalignant respiratory disease but did note an increased relative risk of lung cancer in women (relative risk, 2.81 for an interquartile range of 19.78 ppb NO_2; 95% CI, 1.15 to 6.89) but not in men. The latter may represent a chance finding, as it was based on only 12 lung cancer deaths in women (145).

A cross-sectional study of approximately 9,700 Swiss adults indicated that chronic exposure to NO_2, respirable particulate matter (PM), and SO_2 were associated with decreased lung function, although the high covariation among the pollutants limited the investigators' ability to segregate the effects of the individual pollutants (146). The results of this study are consistent with a longitudinal study of lung function among long-term residents of several areas in southern California, in which the greatest declines in FEV_1 over a 5- to 6-year period were observed among adults living in an area characterized by high levels of nitrogen oxides and sulfates, moderate levels of SO_2, and low levels of photochemical oxidants (147). A recent cross-sectional survey of approximately 3,300 schoolchildren in 12 communities in southern and central California suggested that chronic exposure to particles (measured as PM 10 and PM 2.5), and NO_2 adversely affected several lung function measures in girls but not in boys, who appeared to be affected more strongly by ambient ozone concentrations (148,149). In contrast, NO_2 exposure was not related to the prevalence of respiratory symptoms in girls (asthma, bronchitis, cough, or wheeze) but was associated with the prevalence of wheeze in boys (odds ratio, 1.47 for an interquartile range of 25 ppb; 95% CI, 1.04 to 2.09).

Although, in general, epidemiologic studies have not identified an independent effect of long-term exposures to ambient NO_2 (measured at fixed monitoring sites), this failure may be due to the greater spatial inhomogeneities associated with NO_2 than with several other pollutants (e.g., ozone) and to the frequent occurrence of indoor sources of NO_2, both of which tend to produce relatively greater measurement error and a bias against detecting an effect.

Repeated exposures to NO_2 may carry systemic consequences. NO_2 has been demonstrated to cause a variety of effects on the immune system (150,151). In an interesting series of reports, low-level exposure to NO_2 was shown to facilitate the development of melanoma metastases in the lungs of mice, probably through capillary endothelial cell injury, formation of microthrombi, and effects on the immune response (152–154). Furthermore, NO_2 is a free radical and has been shown to be genotoxic in a variety of *in vitro* assays, as has its metabolite nitrite (but not nitrate) (155). NO_2 inhalation may, therefore, be carcinogenic or cocarcinogenic; however, little evidence supports this proposition, although NO_2 exposure was linked with induction of pulmonary adenomas in a susceptible strain of mice (155). Another possibility is that a variety of products formed by reactions with NO_2 *in vivo* (nitrosamines) or in the atmosphere (nitroarenes) may pose genotoxic or carcinogenic risks, although the evidence for this hypothesis is even slimmer (155).

MECHANISMS OF RESPIRATORY TOXICITY AND PATHOLOGY

The toxicity of NO_2 is thought to be due to initiation of lipid peroxidation and to oxidation of cellular proteins and reducing substances (156). NO_2 can oxidize a variety of biological molecules, generating free radicals that can undermine the structural and functional integrity of cell membranes, enzymes and other proteins (particularly those containing thiol groups), nucleic acids, and other biomolecules. Vitamin E, a membrane-associated free radical scavenger, can diminish NO_2-induced lipid peroxidation (157). As is seen also in ozone toxicity, peroxidation of the cell membrane causes effects that have been well characterized: increased membrane permeability, leakage of essential electrolytes and enzymes, inhibition of cellular metabolism, and swelling and disintegration of intracellular organelles, including mitochondria, lysosomes, and endoplasmic reticulum (158).

Cells sustaining the greatest damage from sublethal concentrations of NO_2 (2 to 17 ppm) are type I alveolar and ciliated cells in the bronchiolar epithelium, principally at the junction of the terminal airways and the gas exchange tissue (159). In the continued presence of NO_2, repair processes result in hyperplasia of cuboidal epithelial cells derived from type II cells, clearance of cellular and amorphous debris, interstitial thickening, and an inflammatory response. The new cells have a substantially lower surface-to-volume ratio and are more resistant to the effects of NO_2. These histologic changes are reversible if animals are allowed to recover in clean air (159).

Animal experiments involving low-level exposures (2 ppm or less) for durations of weeks to several years demonstrated a constellation of findings that are relatively consistent among several species, representing various degrees of tissue damage and repair. As is true of acute sublethal lung injury, the site of greatest injury is the junction of the airways and the alveoli. Typical changes include evidence of lipid peroxidation, type I cell damage with type II cell proliferation, increased alveolar permeability, and increased production of antioxidant enzymes (160,161). Continuous exposure for several weeks to higher concentrations (30 ppm) produces a transient acute bronchiolitis and alveolitis, which subsequently evolve into a patchy centriacinar emphysema, with remodeling of alveoli and small airways and mild interstitial fibrosis (162,163). The development of focal emphysema may be attributable to the accumulation of a significant elastase burden in the lung secondary to neutrophil recruitment and degranulatijon (162).

MANAGEMENT OF TOXICITY OR EXPOSURE

As delayed onset of severe respiratory toxicity is well documented, in all instances in which significant exposure is likely to have occurred, affected patients should be observed for at least 48 hours, even if asymptomatic and exhibiting a normal chest radiograph. Management of NO_2 inhalation is complicated by the occurrence of similar symptoms of respiratory distress (dyspnea, tachypnea, cough, and hypoxemia). These symptoms represent three stages of disease due to three separate pathophysiologic phenomena (acute bronchospasm, pulmonary edema, and bronchiolitis obliterans), which may be observed in sequence or alone (56). In the initial acute phase, the diagnosis may not be obvious and will depend on eliciting a history suggestive of nitrogen oxide exposure. CO toxicity may complicate the management if affected individuals were exposed in a setting involving combustion. In an agricultural context, acute farmer's lung (due to hypersensitivity to thermophilic actinomycetes and often presenting as an influenza-like illness) usually can be distinguished from NO_2 intoxication by a history indicating that the silo air was dusty and that the crop had not been ensiled recently (12). Other elements of the differential diagnosis would include asthma, bronchitis, pneumonia, pulmonary embolus, inhalation of another toxicant, myocardial infarction, and left ventricular failure. Once an appropriate diagnosis has been made, the management of the acute phase consists mainly of supportive care (as for any toxic inhalation): oxygen, bronchodilators, hemodynamic monitoring, ventilatory support (as needed), and close observation to detect any deterioration in an affected patient's respiratory status. Use of the minimum oxygen concentration has been recommended to maintain arterial oxygenation, as hyperoxia may exacerbate the oxidant injury induced by NO_2 (164). If methemoglobinemia is present, it may exacerbate hypoxemia and should be treated with methylene blue, 1 to 2 mg per kg intravenously (165).

The mainstays of therapy of the phases of pulmonary edema and a later relapse (bronchiolitis obliterans) involve treatment with oxygen (as dictated by the patient's blood gas profile), α-agonists as needed, and corticosteroids. Pulmonary edema is of the increased permeability type and generally should be treated as are other acute lung injuries (166). Although no controlled clinical trials have tested the efficacy of systemic steroid administration, numerous case reports indicate that such treatment results in dramatic improvement; otherwise, death from progressive respiratory failure may occur (11,13,53,58,138). Some authors recommend continuation of oral corticosteroids for 6 to 8 weeks after a severe initial episode to retard or abort the proliferative cellular phase of bronchiolitis (9,51). According to one recent report, the use of corticosteroids reduced the incidence of this complication of NO_2 exposure to such an extent that "bronchiolitis obliterans has become a rare disease" (164).

Medical or Biological Monitoring

The American Council of Governmental Industrial Hygienists recommends that for such methemoglobin inducers as NO, workers' blood should be sampled during or at the end of the shift and the biological exposure index for methemoglobin in blood should not exceed 1.5% of an individual's hemoglobin (132).

Occupational and Environmental Regulations

Relevant occupational and environmental exposure standards are listed in Table 66-3. Given the potential severity of overexposure to nitrogen oxides, the best management strategy is prevention, principally through engineering controls and work practices but also through worker education. In particular, workers should be trained to seek medical attention even if an exposure did not seem excessive, because delayed onset of severe lower respiratory injury may occur in the absence of symptoms concurrent with or shortly after exposure. Welders should be provided with adequate ventilation or protective respiratory equipment. Entry into a silo within 1 to 2 weeks after filling should be avoided; if this is not possible, the silo should be vented before entry. Farm workers should be educated about the hazards of entering a recently filled silo, including not only appropriate safety practices but visual and olfactory cues to the recognition of NO_2 and of symptoms due to exposure to silo gas. Warning notices should be posted prominently, and children never should be permitted to play near a silo (12).

Recommendations to prevent NO_2 (and CO) intoxication in ice arenas include (i) regular maintenance and inspection of ice-resurfacing machines and heating systems, (ii) provision of adequate ventilation throughout the entire arena, particularly near the ice surface, (iii) appropriate air monitoring while the arena is in use, and (iv) education of arena owners and operators about the potential hazards of the Zamboni machine. Alternatively, use of an electric or battery-operated ice-resurfacing machine could be considered (25). A recent report indicates that installation of a lambda sensor–controlled fuel supply and metallic catalyst in propane- or gasoline-fueled ice resurfacers has the potential to reduce NO_x and other emissions by more than 90% at a fraction of the cost of a new electric resurfacer (167).

The National Institute for Occupational Safety and Health (NIOSH) has recommended that, except for respiratory protec-

TABLE 66-3. Occupational and environmental exposure limits for nitrogen dioxide and nitric oxide

	Organization	Standard	Parts per million	Milligrams per cubic meter
Nitrogen dioxide	OSHA-PEL	Ceiling[a]	5	9
	NIOSH-REL	IDLH	20	37
	ACGIH TLV	TWA	3	5.6
	STEL	STEL	5	9.4
	EPA NAAQS	Annual	0.053	0.1
Nitric oxide	OSHA-PEL	TWA	25	31
	NIOSH-REL	IDLH	100	123
	ACGIH TLV	TWA	25	31

ACGIH TLV, American Conference of Governmental Industrial Hygienists, threshold limit value; EPA NAAQS, U.S. Environmental Protection Agency, national ambient air quality standard; IDLH, immediately dangerous to life and health; NIOSH-REL, National Institute for Occupational Safety and Health, recommended exposure limit; OSHA-PEL, U.S. Occupational Safety and Health Administration, permissible exposure limit; STEL, short-term exposure limit; TWA, 8-hour time-weighted average.

[a]Ceiling values should not be exceeded at any time.

Notes: *IDLH* defined by NIOSH to refer to a condition "that poses a threat of exposure to airborne contaminants when that exposure is likely to cause death or immediate or delayed permanent adverse health effects or prevent escape from such an environment" (168).

STEL defined by ACGIH as "a 15-minute TWA which should not be exceeded at any time during a workday even if the 8-hour TWA is within the TLV-TWA." It is recommended that exposures up to the STEL should last no longer than 15 minutes and occur no more than four times daily.

tion at concentrations equal to or greater than 100 ppm, protective clothing is not necessary for predictable exposures to NO. In contrast, protective clothing and goggles are required in the presence of any possibility of skin or eye contact with NO_2 (or more importantly, N_2O_4). Any nonimpervious clothing contaminated with NO_2 (or N_2O_4) should be removed immediately. Eyewash and quick-drench equipment should be available for immediate use, if necessary. NIOSH recommends several classes of respirators for protection against inhalation toxicity, depending on the predicted exposure scenario (168).

Environmental Fate and Transport

Both NO and NO_2 are generated continuously by natural processes and human activities. The main atmospheric sink for NO involves conversion to NO_2 by photochemical processes and direct oxidation (169). NO_2 can be reconverted to NO by photolysis and can be converted to a variety of other nitrogen oxides. One of the principal sinks for NO_2 is conversion to HNO_3 by reaction with the hydroxyl radical:

$$NO_2 + OH^- + M \rightarrow HNO_3 + M$$

where M represents any energy-absorbing molecule, such as nitrogen or oxygen. Another series of nocturnal reactions converts NO_2 to HNO_3 as follows:

$$NO_2 + O_3 \rightarrow NO_3 + O_2$$

$$NO_2 + NO_3 \rightarrow N_2O_5$$

$$N_2O_5 + H_2O \rightarrow 2HNO_3$$

where NO_3 is the nitrate radical. Some HNO_3 reacts with alkaline compounds, such as ammonia, to form ammonium nitrate and other salts. Nitrate particles are removed from the atmosphere by both wet and dry deposition (169).

Environmental and Occupational Monitoring

PASSIVE SAMPLING

The Palmes tube is a diffusion-controlled passive sampler used widely in the workplace and in indoor air quality studies (170). Palmes tubes are made of acrylic with three grids impregnated with triethanolamine (TEA) and secured at one end with a plastic cap. The other end is sealed with a similar cap except during the sampling period. The stability of the TEA-NO_2 complex allows the lapse of long periods between sampling and analysis. Analysis involves adding an aqueous reagent mixture (sulfanilamide and *N*-1-naphthylamide-diamine-dihydrochloride) to the tube, then measuring the absorption of the resulting reddish-orange solution at 540 nm using a spectrophotometer (170). Modifications of this technique are using ion chromatography rather than spectrophotometry or using stainless steel rather than acrylic tubes (171,172).

NO can be measured also by using two Palmes tubes simultaneously, one to measure NO_2 directly, the other (containing an additional chromic acid–impregnated disc to convert NO to NO_2) to measure the NO_x concentration (NO_2 + NO). The NO concentration is obtained by subtraction, correcting for the differential diffusion capacities of these gases (173).

Yanagisawa and Nishimura (174) developed a badge-type personal sampler containing several layers of hydrophobic filters through which NO_2 diffuses before binding to a TEA-coated cellulose filter. The filter then is analyzed colorimetrically at 540 nm after extraction with *N*-1-naphthylamide-diamine-dihydrochloride and sulfanilic and phosphoric acids. This sampler can be used also to measure NO by replacing some of the hydrophobic filters with glass fiber filters containing a strong oxidant, such as chromium trioxide (174).

ACTIVE SAMPLING

One method commonly used for measuring NO_2 in the workplace involves drawing a known volume of air through a tube containing a TEA-impregnated molecular sieve. Aqueous TEA then is used to desorb the sample, followed by ion chromatographic analysis of the resultant nitrite (175). Measurement of NO is based on a similar principle but requires a three-tube sampling train to trap any NO_2 in the sample, followed by oxidation of NO to NO_2, which then is adsorbed by the TEA-impregnated molecular sieve in the third tube. The material in the third tube is analyzed as nitrite (as described) (176).

Active ambient measurements of NO_x can be conducted using a variety of techniques, including chemical luminescence (CL), absorption spectroscopy, laser-induced fluorescence, and several methods of wet chemical analysis. Gas-phase CL is the method used most commonly for ambient air monitoring, as it has been designated the standard reference method by the U.S. Environmental Protection Agency. It is the only method discussed here (177).

CL measures NO directly; therefore, NO_2 must be converted to NO before analysis. Although several methods exist for converting NO_2 to NO, techniques other than photolysis may generate significant interferences from other nitrogen-containing compounds in the air (178). Within the CL monitor, excess ozone is generated and added to the sample airstream to oxidize NO (including both NO in ambient air and the reduced NO_2) to an electronically excited $NO_2\cdot$. The latter emits photons of characteristic wavelengths (greater than 600 nm), which are counted by a photomultiplier tube. The NO concentration is proportional to the intensity of the light detected; however, because NO exists in ambient air in equilibrium with NO_2, the measured concentration represents NO_x. To obtain the ambient NO_2 concentration, another sample is measured without passing through the NO_2-NO converter. The instrument then subtracts this value from the NO_x measurement to yield the NO_2 concentration.

SULFUR OXIDES

Sources and Production

SO_2 is the only one of the four recognized monomeric sulfur oxides detectable at appreciable concentrations in the atmosphere. It is a highly irritating, colorless, soluble gas with a pungent odor and taste. In contact with water, it forms sulfurous acid, which accounts for its significant irritancy to eyes, mucous membranes, and skin. Physicochemical characteristics of SO_2 are listed in Table 66-4 (3,179).

As an outdoor air pollutant, SO_2 originates principally in combustion of sulfur-containing fuels, particularly in power plants, and in roasting of metal sulfide ores. In ambient air, SO_2 is oxidized at a rate of 0.5% to 10.0% per hour to sulfur trioxide, which, because of its strong affinity for water, is hydrated rapidly to form sulfuric acid (H_2SO_4) (5). Although elevated levels of SO_2 have been associated with widespread illness in air pollution catastrophes, much of the morbidity and mortality may have been due to particles with which SO_2 was associated. Concern about SO_2 as an air pollutant has focused recently on its capacity to induce bronchoconstriction in asthmatics and other sensitive individuals and on its role as a precursor in the formation of acid aerosols.

In the absence of human activities, background concentrations of ambient SO_2 are fairly low, in the range of 1 ppb. Maxi-

TABLE 66-4. Synonyms and physical properties of sulfur dioxide

Synonyms	Sulfurous acid, anhydride sulfurous anhydride, sulfurous oxide, sulfur superoxide
Molecular weight (g/mol)	64.07
Melting point	–72.7°C
Boiling point	–10°C
Physical state	Colorless gas with pungent or suffocating odor
Density (air = 1)	2.3
Solubility (g/100 g H_2O)	22.8 at 0°C, 8.5 at 25°C

From refs. 3 and 179, with permission.

mum hourly averages in U.S. urban settings typically are less than 100 ppb, although in the past, hourly averages exceeding 1.5 to 2.0 ppm have been reported in the vicinity of large nonferrous metal smelters (169). In nonoccupational settings, SO_2 generally is found at concentrations substantially lower indoors than outside; however, the use of kerosene space heaters can generate significant indoor concentrations (8).

Exposure Sources

Sources of exposure to SO_2 are listed in Table 66-5 (6,180–182). SO_2 contact with the air-liquid interface of the eyes and through inhalation are the principal clinically significant modes of exposure, although contact with liquid SO_2 occasionally may occur and can cause frostbite (180).

Absorption, Metabolism, and Excretion

SO_2 is highly soluble in water and, therefore, is absorbed efficiently in the upper respiratory tract. Two factors affecting the efficiency of absorption are the mode of breathing (oral versus oronasal) and the ventilation rate. The nose filters out most inhaled SO_2, preventing its passage to sensitive irritant receptors at and below the larynx (183,184). At rest, most people (approximately 85%) breathe through the nose, providing protection against the pulmonary toxicity of SO_2 (185). Mouth breathing, particularly at higher airflow rates, substantially increases the fraction of SO_2 reaching the lung (183). Thus, voluntary hyperventilation or exercise at a level of exertion requiring oronasal breathing lowers the threshold for SO_2-induced respiratory symptoms and bronchomotor responsiveness (185–187). Deep lung penetration and toxicity are enhanced by oxidation and adsorption to submicrometer acidic particles (188).

TABLE 66-5. Occupational and nonoccupational occurrence and exposure to sulfur dioxide

Combustion of sulfur-containing fossil fuels (notably in power plants and oil refineries)
Ore smelting
Roasting pyrites
Chemical manufacturing (primarily sulfuric acid but also chlorine dioxide, sodium sulfate, thionyl chloride, sulfites, and other uses)
Reducing agent and antioxidant
Bleaching agent in paper, pulp, wool, and textile manufacturing
Metal and ore refining
Portland cement manufacturing
Disinfectant in wineries, breweries, and food processing
Fumigant for grain
Food preservative (to increase shelf life, prevent discoloration, and preserve flavor of produce and shrimp)
Refrigerant
Solvent extraction of lubricating oils
Glass manufacturing
Roadside flares

From refs. 6 and 180–182, with permission.

Water rapidly dissolves SO_2 and forms ions of hydrogen, bisulfite, and sulfite, which exist in equilibrium as follows:

$$SO_2 + H_2O \rightarrow HSO_3^- + H^+ \quad pK_a = 1.86$$

$$HSO_3^- \rightarrow SO_3^= + H^+ \quad pK_a = 7.2 \text{ (189)}$$

Because of the high relative humidity and the ubiquity of water in the airway surfaces, the direct effects of SO_2 on the respiratory tract cannot be studied easily in the absence of water. Although hydrolysis occurs rapidly, the toxicity of SO_2 may be due to the gas itself and to bisulfite, sulfite, and hydrogen ions (189). At the airway surface, the ratio of bisulfite to sulfite ions is likely to be approximately 5 to 1, and some research suggests that bisulfite is a more potent bronchoconstrictor (in asthmatics) than is sulfite ion (189,190). Bisulfite ion reacts with many biological molecules via nucleophilic substitution, and sulfur-containing free radicals also may produce cellular damage (191). The quantities of hydrogen ion produced during inhalation of SO_2 are less than the acid concentrations required to produce bronchoconstriction in mild asthmatics (190). At higher concentrations that would be more characteristic of occupational than of environmental exposures, however, hydrogen ion may play a more prominent role in causing toxicity.

Radiolabeled SO_2 absorbed into the blood from the respiratory tract of experimental animals was distributed throughout the body, concentrating in the liver, spleen, kidneys, and esophagus (192,193). It is metabolized to a variety of sulfur-containing compounds and is excreted principally via the urine as sulfate (192). Significant quantities of SO_2 have been retained for a week or more in the lungs and trachea of experimental animals (193).

Clinical Toxicology

ACUTE TOXICITY

Because of its high solubility, SO_2 is extremely irritating to the eyes and upper respiratory tract, warning the exposed individual to escape before serious damage occurs. The odor is detectable at 0.5 ppm, although concentrations above 6 ppm have been reported to produce instantaneous mucous membrane irritation (10). Symptoms include ocular irritation and lacrimation, rhinorrhea, cough, shortness of breath, chest tightness or discomfort, and a choking sensation. Lower respiratory symptoms often are associated with SO_2-induced bronchoconstriction.

Numerous controlled-exposure investigations have demonstrated that SO_2 increases specific airway resistance. Responsiveness to this substance varies widely: Some asthmatics and atopics appear to be much more susceptible than do other populations tested (194–197). Studies in animals and humans indicated that SO_2 induces vagal reflex bronchoconstriction; however, in asthmatics and others sensitive to the effects of SO_2, additional mechanisms appear to be operative (189,194,195,198–200). Exercise (or voluntary oral hyperventilation) and low humidity augment the responses observed in asthmatics (187,201–204). With moderate exercise or hyperventilation, lower respiratory symptoms or bronchomotor effects (or both) have been observed consistently in asthmatics after short exposures (several minutes) to SO_2 concentrations of 0.5 ppm and higher, in some cases in the range of 0.2 to 0.3 ppm, all substantially below the current threshold limit value (196,197,203,205). Even among asthmatics, susceptibility to SO_2 varies widely; one investigation of adult asthmatics suggested a sevenfold range in susceptibility (197).

Little research has been conducted into the determinants of SO_2 susceptibility. One pilot study found no differences in results of lung function testing or nasal lavage in black versus white adult asthmatics exposed to SO_2 in a controlled setting (206). In another study of mild versus moderate to severe asthmatics, the latter group manifested SO_2-induced bronchoconstriction modestly greater than that in the milder asthmatics; however, because the more severe asthmatics started with less functional reserve, such exposures in real life could produce effects that are more severe clinically (196). In experimental settings, SO_2-induced bronchospasm in asthmatics often appears to be reversible within a half-hour, even without treatment; however, a number of study subjects have required rescue bronchodilator administration. In a case report involving exposure to SO_2 (as well as other toxicants) in the smoke of a roadside flare, a paramedic with mild asthma developed status asthmaticus necessitating hospitalization and intubation (182).

Preexposure to a low concentration of ozone (0.12 ppm) for 45 minutes potentiates the bronchoconstrictive effect of an otherwise subthreshold dose of SO_2 in adolescent asthmatics, suggesting the potential for interaction with other pollutants commonly found in urban environments (207). The bronchoconstrictive effects of SO_2 in asthmatics can be mitigated to varying degrees by prior administration of several asthma medications, including albuterol, salmeterol, nedocromil, cromolyn sodium, and theophylline (208–212).

Occasional reports have cited industrial accidents in which severe pulmonary injury occurred from relatively brief exposure to high concentrations of SO_2. Charan et al. (213) reported that an accident in a paper mill resulted in death within minutes for two workers whose lungs were found to have extensive sloughing of bronchial and bronchiolar mucosa and hemorrhagic alveolar edema. Galea (214) reported a case of an employee who died 17 days after a 15- to 20-minute exposure to SO_2 at a pulp and paper mill. Initially, this worker's symptoms consisted of ocular irritation and pain on inspiration, both of which subsided within a few days. However, 1.5 weeks later, he presented with a productive cough, dyspnea, wheeze, and bilateral rales, which progressed despite aggressive therapy. Autopsy findings included extensive tracheobronchitis, mucous hypersecretion, bronchiolitis obliterans, and diffuse alveolar damage.

Woodford et al. (215) described a clinical course reminiscent of severe intoxication by NO_2 in an individual exposed to SO_2 in an enclosed space for approximately 15 to 20 minutes. Within 2 days, this individual developed pulmonary edema, which improved with treatment. Two weeks after the accident, he experienced respiratory symptoms consistent with bronchiolitis obliterans; no confirmatory biopsy was obtained.

Sodium metabisulfite, which is used to prevent discoloration of shrimp in commercial trawlers, releases SO_2 in the presence of wet ice in a ship's hold. Atkinson et al. (181) reported the deaths of two shrimper crewmen who were likely to have been exposed to SO_2 released during the application of sodium metabisulfite. On autopsy, gross examination showed foamy edema throughout the tracheobronchial tree and alveoli.

Increased ambient SO_2 concentrations have been linked epidemiologically with both acute morbidity and mortality. In December 1952, approximately 4,000 excess deaths and substantial morbidity were attributed to an air pollution episode in which SO_2 averaged 0.95 ppm and PM (measured as British Smoke) was measured at concentrations up to approximately 4 mg per cubic meter (24-hour average) (216). In this and several other episodes, the excess illness and deaths clearly were associated with the air pollution mixture, although the relative etiologic roles of SO_2, PM, aerosol acidity, or other unmeasured pollutants have not been delineated clearly.

Numerous other time-series analyses of potential effects of lower levels of pollution indicate associations of a variety of adverse outcomes with SO_2, particles, and aerosol acidity and with other pollutants, although the associations with SO_2 are not always consistent or statistically significant. In addition to increases in daily mortality, outcomes linked with SO_2 include modest decrements in lung function, increased risks of respiratory symptoms, and hospital admissions for respiratory illness (including asthma and chronic obstructive pulmonary disease) (217–225). Some of these associations have been reported even at 24-hour SO_2 averages less than 0.1 ppm. In the absence of a convincing mechanistic explanation for direct SO_2 toxicity at low ambient concentrations, likely this substance is serving as an indicator for a complex mixture of pollutants, including perhaps acid sulfates, other particles, or unmeasured pollutants. In some analyses using particles or ozone as well as SO_2 in the regression models, the SO_2 effect diminishes substantially (221,225). This finding would suggest that the apparent SO_2 effect may in some cases be due to covariation with particles or other pollutants. Other analyses, however, suggest effects related to SO_2 but not particles, indicating that the explanation is not so simple (218,220).

CHRONIC TOXICITY

Prolonged exposure of dogs to high concentrations of SO_2 (200 ppm) causes a syndrome similar to human chronic bronchitis and involving chronic airway obstruction, airway inflammation, and symptoms of cough and mucous hypersecretion. However, unlike humans with the disease, this animal model exhibits decreased airway responsiveness to inhaled bronchoconstrictor agents (226,227). When exposed to 15 ppm using the same experimental protocol, the animals demonstrated none of these effects (227). With few exceptions, chronic exposure of animals to SO_2 does not produce observable adverse effects at concentrations lower than 20 ppm (189,228).

In humans, some survivors of massive SO_2 exposure have shown a chronic, obstructive defect and bronchial hyperreactivity in serial pulmonary function studies (213,215,229–231). Some of these workers also showed symptoms consistent with a diagnosis of chronic bronchitis, although for most of these individuals, cigarette smoking is likely to have played a contributory role (230). The extent to which recurrent occupational or environmental exposures to SO_2 produce adverse effects in humans is not clear, however, partly because both contexts usually contain confounding exposures to particulates or other irritants. Although some investigations suggested that occupational SO_2 exposure (even at levels below the current threshold limit value) is associated with increased upper and lower respiratory symptoms and decrements in various spirometric indices, other studies have not (228,232–234).

The International Agency for Research on Cancer concluded that evidence of SO_2 carcinogenicity to humans was inadequate and that evidence in experimental animals was limited (235). These conclusions were based on a review of more than a dozen epidemiologic studies of workers exposed to SO_2 in a variety of industries, none of which clearly indicated an increased risk of cancer attributable to SO_2 exposure, and several experimental studies in which significant increases of lung tumors were found in female mice exposed to SO_2 alone and in rats exposed to SO_2 in conjunction with the recognized carcinogen benzo[a]pyrene. Overall, the International Agency for Research on Cancer concluded that SO_2 was not classifiable as a human carcinogen (235).

MANAGEMENT OF TOXICITY OR EXPOSURE

Severe injury by SO_2 is rare, owing perhaps to its strong intrinsic warning properties. Treatment is symptomatic: Topical administration of sodium bicarbonate solution aerosol may alleviate eye or respiratory mucous membrane irritation (11). Respiratory support may be indicated in cases in which the exposed individual was trapped or was otherwise unable to escape the exposure. Systemic corticosteroids can be beneficial in acute SO_2-induced lung injury, although less published evidence supports their use than in the case of NO_2 (J. Balmes, *personal communication*). Asthmatic episodes triggered by SO_2 exposure should be treated with bronchodilator administration, if necessary.

Occupational and Environmental Regulations

Relevant occupational and environmental exposure standards are listed in Table 66-6. Given the potential severity of overexposure to SO_2, the best management strategy is prevention, principally through engineering controls and work practices but also through worker education. If exposure to liquid SO_2 is foreseeable, the NIOSH recommends frostbite precautions, including appropriate eye protection and personal protective clothing, and quick-drench facilities and eyewash fountains (168). In situations likely to produce exposure to gaseous SO_2 at concentrations exceeding current occupational standards, the NIOSH recommends several alternative means of respiratory protection, including chemical cartridge, powered air purifying, and supplied-air respirators (168). However, as discussed, some asthmatics and others with reactive airways may experience respiratory symptoms even when SO_2 concentrations are in compliance with existing workplace standards.

Environmental Fate and Transport

SO_2 is removed from the atmosphere primarily by wet or dry deposition in the gas phase or via oxidation to H_2SO_4, with formation of sulfate aerosols. In the gas phase, SO_2 is removed by dry deposition, primarily on vegetation, and by dissolution in water vapor in clouds, rain, fog, and dew to form dilute sulfurous acid. One of the principal atmospheric sinks for SO_2 is oxidation to H_2SO_4 by direct reaction with oxygen, by catalytic oxidation (e.g., with manganese or carbon catalysts), or by photochemical processes involving OH^- and peroxy radicals. Direct oxidation is slow in relation to the latter processes and plays a minor role in the conversion of SO_2 to sulfates. H_2SO_4 reacts with atmospheric ammonia to form ammonium sulfate, ammonium bisulfate, letovicite, and a variety of salts with ammonium nitrate. H_2SO_4 and its salts are the main constituents of acidic deposition (popularly known as *acid rain*) in the eastern United States and Canada (169).

TABLE 66-6. Occupational and environmental exposure limits for sulfur dioxide

Organization	Standard	Parts per million	Milligrams per cubic meter
OSHA-PEL	TWA	5	13
NIOSH-REL	IDLH	100	266
ACGIH TLV	TWA	2	5.2
STEL	STEL	5	13
EPA NAAQS	24 h	0.14	0.37

ACGIH TLV, American Conference of Governmental Industrial Hygienists, threshold limit value; EPA NAAQS, U.S. Environmental Protection Agency, national ambient air quality standard; IDLH, immediately dangerous to life and health; NIOSH-REL, National Institute for Occupational Safety and Health, recommended exposure limit; OSHA-PEL, U.S. Occupational Safety and Health Administration, permissible exposure limit; STEL, short-term exposure limit; TWA, 8-hour time-weighted average.

Notes: *IDLH* defined by NIOSH to refer to a condition "that poses a threat of exposure to airborne contaminants when that exposure is likely to cause death or immediate or delayed permanent adverse health effects or prevent escape from such an environment" (168).

STEL defined by ACGIH as "a 15-minute TWA which should not be exceeded at any time during a workday even if the 8-hour TWA is within the TLV-TWA." It is recommended that exposures up to the STEL should last no longer than 15 minutes and occur no more than four times daily.

Environmental and Occupational Monitoring

Different monitoring techniques are used to measure SO_2 in ambient air versus occupational settings. The pararosaniline method is the U.S. Environmental Protection Agency's reference method for determining compliance with primary and secondary national ambient air quality standards (236). This process involves passing a measured volume of air through a solution of potassium tetrachloromercurate, which reacts with SO_2 in the airstream to form a stable complex. Subsequently, the latter is reacted with pararosaniline dye and formaldehyde to form pararosaniline methyl sulfonic acid, the optical density of which is measured spectrophotometrically and is related directly to the initial concentration of SO_2 in the air sample. Several methods are available for determining levels of SO_2 in the workplace, most of which rely on ion chromatography for analysis (237).

REFERENCES

1. National Research Council. *Nitrogen oxides.* Washington: National Academy Press, 1977:4–19.
2. Budavari S, ed. *The Merck index,* 11th ed. Rahway, NJ: Merck & Co, 1989.
3. Weast RC. *Handbook of chemistry and physics,* 69th ed. Cleveland: CRC Press, 1988.
4. Seinfeld JH. *Atmospheric chemistry and physics of air pollution.* New York: John Wiley and Sons, 1986:79–86.
5. World Health Organization. *Air quality guidelines for Europe.* European Series No. 23. Copenhagen: World Health Organization Regional Publications, 1987.
6. Sax NI, Lewis RJ. *Hawley's condensed chemical dictionary,* 11th ed. New York: Van Nostrand–Reinhold, 1987.
7. Yockey CC, Eden BM, Byrd RB. The McConnell missile accident: clinical spectrum of nitrogen dioxide exposure. *JAMA* 1980;244:1221–1223.
8. Leaderer BP. Air pollutant emissions from kerosene space heaters. *Science* 1982;218:1113–1115.
9. Tse RL, Bockman AA. Nitrogen dioxide toxicity. Report of four cases in firemen. *JAMA* 1970;212:1341–1344.
10. Schwartz DA. Acute inhalational injury. In: Rosenstock L, ed. *Occupational pulmonary disease.* Philadelphia: Hanley & Belfus, 1987:297–318.
11. Ross JAS, Seaton A, Morgan WKC. Toxic gases and fumes. In: Morgan WKC, Seaton A, eds. *Occupational lung diseases,* 3rd ed. Philadelphia: WB Saunders, 1995:568–596.
12. Douglas WW, Hepper NGG, Colby TV. Silo-filler's disease. *Mayo Clin Proc* 1989;64:291–304.
13. Lowry T, Schuman LM. "Silo-filler's disease"—a syndrome caused by nitrogen dioxide. *JAMA* 1956;162:153–160.
14. Cummins BT, Raveney FJ, Jesson MW. Toxic gases in tower silos. *Ann Occup Hyg* 1971;14:275–283.
15. Goldman AP, Cook PD, Macrae DJ. Exposure of intensive-care staff to nitric oxide and nitrogen dioxide. *Lancet* 1995;345:923–924.
16. Williams TJ, Salamonsen RF, Snell G, Kaye D, Esmore DS. Preliminary experience with inhaled nitric oxide for acute pulmonary hypertension after heart transplantation. *J Heart Lung Transplant* 1995;14:419–423.
17. Spengler JD, Duffy CP, Letz R, Tibbetts TW, Ferris BG. Nitrogen dioxide inside and outside 137 homes and implications for ambient air quality standards and health effects research. *Environ Sci Tech* 1983;17:164–168.
18. Spengler J, Schwab M, Ryan PB, et al. Personal exposure to nitrogen dioxide in the Los Angeles basin. *J Air Waste Manag Assoc* 1994;44:39–47.
19. Marbury MC, Harlos DP, Samet JM, Spengler JD. Indoor residential NO_2 concentrations in Albuquerque, New Mexico. *J Air Pollut Control Assoc* 1988;38:392–398.
20. Borland C, Higenbottam T. Nitric oxide yields of contemporary UK, US, and French cigarettes. *Int J Epidemiol* 1987;16:31–34.
21. Linaker CH, Chauhan AJ, Inskip H, et al. Distribution and determinants of personal exposure to nitrogen dioxide in school children. *Occup Environ Med* 1996;53:200–203.

22. Lindvall T. Health effects of nitrogen dioxide and oxidants. *Scand J Work Environ Health* 1985;11(Suppl 3):10–28.
23. Berglund M, Bråbäck L, Bylin G, Jonson J-O, Vahter M. Personal NO_2 exposure monitoring shows high exposure among ice-skating schoolchildren. *Arch Environ Health* 1994;49:17–24.
24. Hedberg K, Hedberg CW, Iber C, et al. An outbreak of nitrogen dioxide–induced respiratory illness among ice-hockey players. *JAMA* 1989;262:3014–3017.
25. Smith W, Anderson T, Anderson HA, Remington PL. Nitrogen dioxide and carbon monoxide intoxication in an indoor ice arena—Wisconsin, 1992. *MMWR Morb Mortal Wkly Rep* 1992;41:383–385.
26. Morgan WKC. Zamboni disease. Pulmonary edema in an ice hockey player. *Arch Intern Med* 1995;155:2479–2480.
27. Karlson-Stiber C, Höjer J, Sjöholm Ö, Bluhm G, Salmonson H. Nitrogen dioxide pneumonitis in ice hockey players. *J Intern Med* 1996;239:451–456.
28. Soparkar G, Mayers I, Edouard L, Hoeppner VH. Toxic effects from nitrogen dioxide in ice-skating arenas. *CMAJ* 1993;148:1181–1182.
29. Brauer M, Spengler JD. Nitrogen dioxide exposures inside ice skating rinks. *Am J Public Health* 1994;84:429–433.
30. Lee K, Yanagisawa Y, Spengler JD, Nakai S. Carbon monoxide and nitrogen dioxide exposures in indoor ice skating rinks. *J Sports Sci* 1994;12:279–283.
31. Paulozzi LJ, Spengler RF, Vogt RL, Carney JK. A survey of carbon monoxide and nitrogen dioxide in indoor ice arenas in Vermont. *J Environ Health* 1993;56:23–25.
32. Wagner H-M. Absorption of NO and NO_2 in MIK and MAK concentrations during inhalation. *Staub-Reinhalt Luft* 1970;30:25–26.
33. Bauer MA, Utell MJ, Morrow PE, Speers DM, Gibb FR. Inhalation of 0.30 ppm nitrogen dioxide potentiates exercise-induced bronchospasm in asthmatics. *Am Rev Respir Dis* 1986;134:1203–1208.
34. Goldstein E, Goldstein F, Peek NF, Parks NJ. Absorption and transport of nitrogen oxides. In: Lee SD, ed. *Nitrogen oxides and their effects on health.* Ann Arbor, MI: Ann Arbor Science Publishers, 1983:143–160.
35. Postlethwaite EM, Bidani A. Reactive uptake governs the pulmonary air space removal of inhaled nitrogen dioxide. *J Appl Physiol* 1990;68:594–603.
36. Postlethwaite EM, Bidani A. Mechanisms of pulmonary NO_2 absorption. *Toxicology* 1994;89:217–237.
37. Postlethwaite EM, Langford SD, Jacobson LM, Bidani A. NO_2 reactive absorption substrates in rat pulmonary surface lining fluids. *Free Radic Biol Med* 1995;5:553–563.
38. Postlethwaite EM, Bidani A. Pulmonary disposition of inhaled NO_2–nitrogen-isolated rat lungs. *Toxicol Appl Pharmacol* 1989;98:303–312.
39. Postlethwaite EM, Mustafa MG. Fate of inhaled nitrogen dioxide in isolated perfused rat lung. *J Toxicol Environ Health* 1981;7:861–872.
40. Ewetz L. Absorption and metabolic fate of nitrogen oxides. *Scand J Work Environ Health* 1993;19(Suppl 2):21–27.
41. Yoshida K, Kasama K. Biotransformation of nitric oxide. *Environ Health Perspect* 1987;73:201–206.
42. Meyer M, Piiper J. Nitric oxide (NO), a new test gas for study of alveolar-capillary diffusion. *Eur Respir J* 1989;2:494–496.
43. Kosaka H, Uozumi M, Tyuma I. The interaction between nitrogen oxides and hemoglobin and endothelium-derived relaxing factor. *Free Radic Biol Med* 1989;7:653–658.
44. Persson MG, Wiklund NP, Gustafsson LE. Endogenous nitric oxide in single exhalations and the change during exercise. *Am Rev Respir Dis* 1993;148: 1210–1214.
45. Hobbs AJ, Ignarro LJ. The nitric oxide–cyclic GMP signal transduction system. In: Zapol WM, Bloch KD, eds. *Nitric oxide and the lung.* New York: Marcel Dekker Inc, 1997:1–57.
46. Ruth JH. Odor thresholds and irritation levels of several chemical substances: a review. *Am Ind Hyg Assoc J* 1986;47:A142–151.
47. American Industrial Hygiene Association. *Odor thresholds for chemicals with established occupational health standards.* Akron, OH: American Industrial Hygiene Association, 1989.
48. Bylin G, Lindvall T, Rehn T, Sundin B. Effects of short-term exposure to ambient nitrogen dioxide concentrations on human bronchial reactivity and lung function. *Eur J Respir Dis* 1985;66:205–217.
49. Amoore JE, Hautala E. Odor as an aid to chemical safety: odor thresholds compared with threshold limit values and volatilities for 214 industrial chemicals in air and water dilution. *J Appl Toxicol* 1983;3:272–290.
50. Lindquist T. Nitrous gas poisoning among welders using acetylene flame. *Acta Med Scand* 1944;119:210–243.
51. Horvath EP, doPico GA, Barbee RA, Dickie HA. Nitrogen dioxide–induced pulmonary disease: five new cases and a review of the literature. *J Occup Med* 1978;20:103–110.
52. Leib GMP, Davis WN, Brown T, McQuiggan M. Chronic pulmonary insufficiency secondary to silo-filler's disease. *Am J Med* 1958;24:471–474.
53. Jones GR, Proudfoot AT, Hall JI. Pulmonary effects of acute exposure to nitrous fumes. *Thorax* 1973;28:61–65.
54. Hirotani T, Maenaka Y, Yamamoto S, Kobayashi K. Adult respiratory distress syndrome caused by inhalation of oxides of nitrogen. *Keio J Med* 1987;36:315–320.
55. Milne JEH. Nitrogen dioxide inhalation and bronchiolitis obliterans. *J Occup Med* 1969;538–547.
56. Guidotti TL. The higher oxides of nitrogen: inhalation toxicology. *Environ Res* 1987;15:443–472.
57. Fleming GM, Chester EH, Montenegro HD. Dysfunction of small airways following pulmonary injury due to nitrogen dioxide. *Chest* 1979;75:720–721.
58. Moskowitz RL, Lyons HA, Cottle HR. Silo filler's disease. *Am J Med* 1964; 36:457–462.
59. Fleetham JA, Tunnicliffe BW, Munt PW. Methemoglobinemia and the oxides of nitrogen [Letter]. *N Engl J Med* 1978;298:1150.
60. Lowry T, Schuman LM. "Silo-filler's disease"—a syndrome caused by nitrogen dioxide. *JAMA* 1956;162:153–160.
61. McAdams AJ. Bronchiolitis obliterans. *Am J Med* 1955;19:314–322.
62. Anonymous. Ice hockey lung: NO_2 poisoning. *Lancet* 1990;335:1191.
63. von Nieding G, Wagner HM, Casper H, Beuthan A, Smidt U. Effect of experimental and occupational exposure to NO_2 in sensitive and normal subjects. In: Lee SD, ed. *Nitrogen oxides and their effects on health.* Ann Arbor, MI: Ann Arbor Science Publishers, 1980:315–331.
64. von Nieding G, Wagner HM. Experimental studies on the short-term effect of air pollutants on pulmonary function in man: two-hour exposure to NO_2, O_3, and SO_2 alone and in combination. In: Kasuga S, Suzuki N, Yamada T, et al., eds. *Proceedings of the Fourth International Clean Air Congress.* Tokyo: 1977:5–8.
65. Linn WS, Solomon JC, Trim SC, et al. Effects of exposure to 4 ppm nitrogen dioxide in healthy and asthmatic volunteers. *Arch Environ Health* 1985; 40:234–239.
66. Bylin G. Health risk evaluation of nitrogen oxide. Controlled studies on humans. *Scand J Work Environ Health* 1993;19(Suppl 2):37–43.
67. Posin C, Clark K, Jones MP, et al. Nitrogen dioxide inhalation and human blood biochemistry. *Arch Environ Health* 1978;33:318–324.
68. Vagaggini B, Paggiaro PL, Giannini D, et al. Effect of short-term NO_2 exposure on induced sputum in normal, asthmatic, and COPD subjects. *Eur Respir J* 1996;9:1852–1857.
69. Morrow PE, Utell MJ, Bauer MA, et al. Pulmonary performance of elderly normal subjects and subjects with chronic obstructive pulmonary disease exposed to 0.3 ppm nitrogen dioxide. *Am Rev Respir Dis* 1992;145:291–300.
70. Hackney JD, Linn WS, Avol EL, et al. Exposures of older adults with chronic respiratory illness to nitrogen dioxide. A combined laboratory and field study. *Am Rev Respir Dis* 1992;146:1480–1486.
71. Linn WS, Shamoo DA, Spier CE, et al. Controlled exposure of volunteers with chronic obstructive pulmonary disease to nitrogen dioxide. *Arch Environ Health* 1985;40:313–317.
72. Kerr HD, Kulle TJ, McIlheny ML, et al. Effects of nitrogen dioxide on pulmonary function in human subjects: an environmental chamber study. *Environ Res* 1979;19:392–404.
73. Orehek J, Massari JP, Gayrard P, Grimaud C, Charpin J. Effect of short-term, low-level nitrogen dioxide exposure on bronchial sensitivity of asthmatic patients. *J Clin Invest* 1976;57:301–307.
74. Roger LJ, Horstman DH, McDonnell W, et al. Pulmonary function, airway responsiveness, and respiratory symptoms in asthmatics following exercise in NO_2. *Toxicol Ind Health* 1990;6:155–171.
75. Kleinman MT, Bailey RM, Linn WS, et al. Effects of 0.2 ppm nitrogen dioxide on pulmonary function and response to bronchoprovocation in asthmatics. *J Toxicol Environ Health* 1983;12:815–826.
76. Mohsenin V. Airway responses to nitrogen dioxide in asthmatic subjects. *J Toxicol Environ Health* 1987;22:371–380.
77. Avol EL, Linn WS, Peng RC, Valencia G, Little D, Hackney JD. Laboratory study of asthmatic volunteers exposed to nitrogen dioxide and to ambient air pollution. *Am Ind Hyg Assoc J* 1988;49:143–149.
78. Rubinstein I, Bigby BG, Reiss TF, Boushey HA Jr. Short-term exposure to 0.3 ppm nitrogen dioxide does not potentiate airway responsiveness to sulfur dioxide in asthmatic subjects. *Am Rev Respir Dis* 1990;141:381–385.
79. Hazucha MJ, Ginsberg JF, McDonnell WF, et al. Effects of 0.1 ppm nitrogen dioxide on airways of normal and asthmatic subjects. *J Appl Physiol* 1983; 54:730–739.
80. Salome CM, Brown NJ, Marks GB, et al. Effect of nitrogen dioxide and other combustion products on asthmatic subjects in a home-like environment. *Eur Respir J* 1996;9:910–918.
81. Folinsbee LJ. Does nitrogen dioxide exposure increase airways responsiveness? *Toxicol Ind Health* 1992;8:273–283.
82. Frampton MW, Morrow PE, Cox C, Gibb FR, Speers DM, Utell MJ. Effect of nitrogen dioxide exposure on pulmonary function and airway reactivity in normal humans. *Am Rev Respir Dis* 1991;143:522–527.
83. Mohsenin V. Airway responses to 2.0 ppm nitrogen dioxide in normal subjects. *Arch Environ Health* 1988;43:242–246.
84. Mohsenin V. Effect of vitamin C on NO_2-induced airway hyperresponsiveness in normal subjects. *Am Rev Respir Dis* 1987;136:1408–1411.
85. Sandström T, Anderson MC, Kolmodin-Hedman B, Stjernberg N, Angstrom T. Bronchoalveolar mastocytosis and lymphocytosis after nitrogen dioxide exposure in men: a time-kinetic study. *Eur Respir J* 1990;3:138–143.
86. Sandström T, Stjernberg N, Eklund A, et al. Inflammatory cell response in bronchoalveolar lavage fluid after nitrogen dioxide exposure of healthy subjects: a dose-response study. *Eur Respir J* 1991;3:332–339.
87. Frampton MW, Finkelstein JN, Roberts NJ Jr, Smeglin AM, Morrow PE, Utell MJ. Effects of nitrogen dioxide exposure on bronchoalveolar lavage proteins in humans. *Am J Respir Cell Mol Biol* 1989;1:499–505.
88. Rubinstein I, Reiss TF, Bigby BG, Stites DP, Boushey HA Jr. Effects of 0.60 ppm nitrogen dioxide on circulating and bronchoalveolar lavage lymphocyte phenotypes in healthy subjects. *Environ Res* 1991;55:18–30.

89. Helleday R, Sandström T, Stjernberg N. Differences in bronchoalveolar cell response to nitrogen dioxide exposure between smokers and nonsmokers. *Eur Respir J* 1994;7:1213–1220.
90. Devlin RB, Horstman DP, Gerrity TR, et al. Inflammatory response in humans exposed to 2.0 ppm nitrogen dioxide. *Inhal Toxicol* 1999;11:89–109.
91. Sandström T, Helleday R, Bjermer L, Stjernberg N. Effects of repeated exposure to 4 ppm nitrogen dioxide on bronchoalveolar lymphocyte subsets and macrophages in healthy men. *Eur Respir J* 1992;5:1092–1096.
92. Blomberg A, Krishna MT, Helleday R, et al. Persistent airway inflammation but accommodated antioxidant and lung function responses after repeated daily exposure to nitrogen dioxide. *Am J Respir Crit Care Med* 1999;159:536–543.
93. Tunnicliffe WS, Burge PS, Ayres JG. Effect of domestic concentrations of nitrogen dioxide on airway responses to inhaled allergen in asthmatic patients. *Lancet* 1994;344:1733–1736.
94. Devalia JL, Rusznak C, Herdman MJ, Trigg CJ, Tarraf H, Davies RJ. Effect of nitrogen dioxide and sulphur dioxide on airway response of mild asthmatic patients to allergen inhalation. *Lancet* 1994;344:1668–1671.
95. Rusznak C, Devalia JL, Davies RJ. Airway response of asthmatic subjects to inhaled allergen after exposure to pollutants. *Thorax* 1996;51:1105–1108.
96. Rose RM, Fuglestad JM, Skornik WA, et al. The pathophysiology of enhanced susceptibility to murine cytomegalovirus respiratory infection during short-term exposure to 5 ppm nitrogen dioxide. *Am Rev Respir Dis* 1988;137:912–917.
97. Parker RF, Davis JK, Cassell GH, et al. Short-term exposure to nitrogen dioxide enhances susceptibility to murine respiratory mycoplasmosis and decreases intrapulmonary killing of *Mycoplasma pulmonis*. *Am Rev Respir Dis* 1989;140:502–512.
98. Pennington JE. Effects of automotive emissions on susceptibility to respiratory infections. In: Watson SY, Bates RR, Kennedy D, eds. *Air pollution, the automobile, and public health.* Washington: National Academy Press, 1988:499–518.
99. Schlesinger RB. Comparative toxicity of ambient air pollutants: some aspects related to lung defense. *Environ Health Perspect* 1989;81:123–128.
100. Suzuki T, Ikeda S, Kanoh T, Mizoguchi I. Decreased phagocytosis and superoxide anion production in alveolar macrophages of rats exposed to nitrogen dioxide. *Arch Environ Contam Toxicol* 1986;15:733–739.
101. Moldéus P. Toxicity induced by nitrogen dioxide in experimental animals and isolated cell systems. *Scand J Work Environ Health* 1993;19(Suppl 2):28–36.
102. Jakab GJ. Modulation of pulmonary defense mechanisms by acute exposures to nitrogen dioxide. *Environ Res* 1987;42:215–228.
103. Dawson SV, Schenker MB. Health effects of inhalation of ambient concentrations of nitrogen dioxide. *Am Rev Respir Dis* 1979;120:281–292.
104. Heller RF, Gordon RE. Chronic effects of nitrogen dioxide on cilia in hamster bronchioles. *Exp Lung Res* 1986;10:137–152.
105. Amoruso MA, Witz G, Goldstein BD. Decreased superoxide anion radical production by rat alveolar macrophages following inhalation of ozone or nitrogen dioxide. *Life Sci* 1981;28:2215–2221.
106. Aranyi C, Fenters J, Ehrlich R, Gardner D. Scanning electron microscopy of alveolar macrophages after exposure to oxygen, nitrogen dioxide, and ozone. *Environ Health Perspect* 1976;16:180.
107. Helleday R, Huberman D, Blomberg A, Stjernberg N, Sandström T. Nitrogen dioxide exposure impairs the frequency of the mucociliary activity in healthy subjects. *Eur Respir J* 1995;8:1664–1668.
108. Devalia JL, Sapsford RJ, Cundell DR, Rusznak C, Campbell AM, Davies RJ. Human bronchial epithelial cell dysfunction following *in vitro* exposure to nitrogen dioxide. *Eur Respir J* 1993;6:1308–1316.
109. Pinkston P, Smeglin A, Roberts NJ, Gibb FR, Morrow PE, Utell MJ. Effects of *in vitro* exposure to nitrogen dioxide on human alveolar macrophage release of neutrophil chemotactic factor and interleukin-1. *Environ Res* 1989;47:48–58.
110. Frampton MW, Smeglin AM, Roberts NJ, Finkelstein JN, Morrow PE, Utell MJ. Nitrogen dioxide exposure *in vivo* and human alveolar macrophage inactivation of influenza virus *in vitro*. *Environ Res* 1989;48:179–192.
111. Ehrlich R, Findlay JC, Gardner DE. Health effects of short-term inhalation of nitrogen dioxide and ozone mixtures. *Environ Res* 1977;14:223–231.
112. Ehrlich R, Henry MC. Chronic toxicity of nitrogen dioxide: I. Effect on resistance to bacterial pneumonia. *Arch Environ Health* 1968;17:860–865.
113. Graham JA, Gardner DE, Blommer EJ, House DE, Menache MG, Miller FE. Influence of exposure patterns of nitrogen dioxide and modifications by ozone on susceptibility to bacterial infectious disease in mice. *J Toxicol Environ Health* 1987;21:113–125.
114. Goings SAJ, Kulle TJ, Bascom R, et al. Effect of nitrogen dioxide on susceptibility to influenza A virus infection in healthy adults. *Am Rev Respir Dis* 1989;139:1075–1081.
115. Moseholm L, Taudorf E, Frosig A. Pulmonary function changes in asthmatics associated with low-level SO_2 and NO_2 air pollution, weather, and medicine intake. *Allergy* 1993;48:334–344.
116. Rossi OVJ, Kinnula VL, Tienari J, Huhti E. Association of severe asthma attacks with weather, pollen, and air pollutants. *Thorax* 1993;48:244–248.
117. Castellsague J, Sunyer J, Saez M, Anto JM. Short-term association between air pollution and emergency room visits for asthma in Barcelona. *Thorax* 1995;50:1051–1056.
118. Ostro BD, Lipsett MJ, Mann JK, Braxton-Owens H, White MC. Air pollution and asthma exacerbations among African-American children in Los Angeles. *Inhal Toxicol* 1995;7:711–722.
119. Speizer FE, Ferris B, Bishop YM, Spengler JD. Respiratory disease rates and pulmonary function in children associated with NO_2 exposure. *Am Rev Respir Dis* 1980;121:3–10.
120. Koo LC, Ho JHC, Ho CY, et al. Personal exposure to nitrogen dioxide and its association with respiratory illness in Hong Kong. *Am Rev Respir Dis* 1990;141:1119–1126.
121. Samet JM, Lambert WE, Skipper BJ, et al. Nitrogen dioxide and respiratory illnesses in infants. *Am J Respir Crit Care Med* 1993;148:1258–1265.
122. Braun-Fahrländer C, Ackermann-Liebrich U, Schwartz J, Gnehm HP, Rutishauser M, Wanner HU. Air pollution and respiratory symptoms in preschool children. *Am Rev Respir Dis* 1992;145:42–47.
123. Samet JM, Marbury MC, Spengler JD. Health effects and sources of indoor air pollution: I. *Am Rev Respir Dis* 1987;136:1486–1508.
124. Keller MD, Lanese RR, Mitchell RI, Cote RW. Respiratory illness in households using gas and electricity for cooking. *Environ Res* 1979;19:504–515.
125. Respiratory symptoms in children and indoor exposure to nitrogen dioxide and gas stoves. *Am J Respir Crit Care Med* 1998;158:891–895.
126. Hasselblad V, Eddy DM, Kotchmar DJ. Synthesis of environmental evidence: nitrogen dioxide epidemiology studies. *J Air Waste Manag Assoc* 1992;42:662–671.
127. Ostro BD, Lipsett MJ, Mann JK, Wiener MB, Selner J. Indoor air pollution and asthma. *Am J Respir Crit Care Med* 1994;149:1400–1406.
128. Jarvis D, Chinn S, Luczynska C, Burney P. Association of respiratory symptoms and lung function in young adults with use of domestic gas appliances. *Lancet* 1996;347:426–431.
129. Infante-Rivard C. Childhood asthma and indoor environmental factors. *Am J Epidemiol* 1993;137:839–344.
130. Infante-Rivard C. Nitrogen dioxide and allergic asthma [Letter]. *Lancet* 1995;345:931.
131. Dupuy PM, Frostell CG. Bronchial effects of nitric oxide. In: Zapol WM, Bloch KD, eds. *Nitric oxide and the lung.* New York: Marcel Dekker Inc, 1997:285–311.
132. American Conference of Governmental Industrial Hygienists. *1996 TLVs and BEIs. Threshold limit values for chemical substances and physical agents. Biological exposure indices.* Cincinnati: American Conference of Governmental Industrial Hygienists, 1996.
133. Zapol WM, Bloch KD, eds. *Nitric oxide and the lung.* New York: Marcel Dekker Inc, 1997.
134. Stavert DM, Lehnert BE. Nitric oxide and nitrogen dioxide as inducers of acute pulmonary injury when inhaled at relatively high concentrations for brief periods. *Inhal Toxicol* 1990;2:53–67.
135. Hugod C. Ultrastructural changes of the rabbit lung after a 5 ppm nitric oxide exposure. *Arch Environ Health* 1979;34:12–17.
136. Gustafsson LE. Experimental studies on nitric oxide. *Scand J Work Environ Health* 1993;19(Suppl 2):44–49.
137. Kagawa J. Respiratory effects of 2-hr exposures to 1.0 ppm nitric oxide in normal subjects. *Environ Res* 1982;27:485–490.
138. Becklake MR, Goldman HI, Bosman AR, Freed CC. The long-term effects of exposure to nitrous fumes. *Am Rev Tuberc* 1957;76:398–409.
139. Muller B. Nitrogen dioxide intoxication after a mining accident. *Respiration* 1969;26:249–261.
140. Kennedy MCS. Nitrous fumes and coal-miners with emphysema. *Ann Occup Hyg* 1972;15:285–300.
141. Robertson A, Dodgson J, Collings P, Seaton A. Exposure to oxides of nitrogen: respiratory symptoms and lung function in British coalminers. *Br J Ind Med* 1984;41:214–219.
142. Mohsenin V, Gee JBL. Acute effect of nitrogen dioxide exposure on the functional activity of $alpha_1$-proteinase inhibitor in bronchoalveolar lavage fluid of normal subjects. *Am Rev Respir Dis* 1987;136:646–650.
143. Johnson DA, Frampton MW, Winters RS, Morrow PE, Utell MJ. Inhalation of nitrogen dioxide fails to reduce the activity of human lung $alpha_1$-proteinase inhibitor. *Am Rev Respir Dis* 1990;142:758–762.
144. Abbey DE, Colome SD, Mills PK, Burchette R, Beeson WL, Tian Y. Chronic disease associated with long-term concentrations of nitrogen dioxide. *J Expo Anal Environ Epidemiol* 1993;3:181–202.
145. Abbey DE, Nishino N, McDonnell WF, et al. Long-term inhalable particles and other air pollutants related to mortality in nonsmokers. *Am J Respir Crit Care Med* 1999;159:373–382.
146. Ackermann-Liebrich U, Leuenberger P, Schwartz J, et al. Lung function and long term exposure to air pollutants in Switzerland. *Am J Respir Crit Care Med* 1997;155:122–129.
147. Tashkin DP, Detels R, Simmons M, et al. The UCLA population studies of chronic obstructive respiratory disease: XI. Impact of air pollution and smoking on annual change in forced expiratory volume in one second. *Am J Respir Crit Care Med* 1994;149:1209–1217.
148. Peters JM, Avol E, Navidi W, et al. A study of twelve southern California communities with differing levels and types of air pollution: I. Prevalence of respiratory morbidity. *Am J Respir Crit Care Med* 1999;159:760–767.
149. Peters JM, Avol E, Gauderman WJ, et al. A study of twelve southern California communities with differing levels and types of air pollution: II. Effects on pulmonary function. *Am J Respir Crit Care Med* 1999;159:768–775.
150. Azoulay-Dupuis E, Bouley G, Moreau J, Muffat-Joly M, Pocidalo J. Evidence for humoral immunodepression in NO_2-exposed mice: influence of food restriction and stress. *Environ Res* 1987;42:446–454.
151. Kuraitis KV, Richters A. Spleen cellularity shifts from the inhalation of 0.25–0.35 ppm nitrogen dioxide. *J Environ Pathol Toxicol Oncol* 1989;9:1–11.
152. Richters A. Effects of nitrogen dioxide and ozone on blood-borne cancer cell colonization of the lungs. *J Toxicol Environ Health* 1988;25:383–390.

153. Richters A, Richters V. Nitrogen dioxide (NO_2) inhalation. Formation of microthrombi in lungs and cancer metastasis. *J Environ Pathol Toxicol Oncol* 1989;9:45–51.
154. Richters A, Richters V, Alley WP. The mortality rate from lung metastases in animals inhaling nitrogen dioxide (NO_2). *J Surg Oncol* 1985;28:63–66.
155. Victorin K. Genotoxicity in health risk evaluation of nitrogen oxides. *Scand J Work Environ Health* 1993;19(Suppl 2):50–56.
156. Sagai M, Ichinose T. Lipid peroxidation and antioxidative protection mechanism in rat lungs upon acute and chronic exposure to nitrogen dioxide. *Environ Health Perspect* 1987;73:179–189.
157. Calabrese EJ, Horton HM. The effects of vitamin E on ozone and nitrogen dioxide toxicity. *World Rev Nutr Diet* 1985;46:124–147.
158. Man SFP, Hulbert WC. Airway repair and adaptation to injury. In: Loke J, ed. *Pathophysiology and treatment of inhalation injuries.* New York: Marcel Dekker Inc, 1988:1–47.
159. Evans MJ. Oxidant gases. *Environ Health Perspect* 1984;55:85–95.
160. Crapo JD, Barry BE, Chang LY, Mercer RR. Alterations in lung structure caused by inhalation of oxidants. In: Miller FJ, Menzel DB, eds. *Fundamentals of extrapolation modeling of inhaled toxicants: ozone and nitrogen dioxide.* Washington: Hemisphere Publishing, 1984:301–321.
161. Morrow PE. Toxicological data on NO_2: an overview. In: Miller FJ, Menzel DB, eds. *Fundamentals of extrapolation modeling of inhaled toxicants: ozone and nitrogen dioxide.* Washington: Hemisphere Publishing, 1984:205–227.
162. Glasgow JE, Pietra GG, Abrams WR, Blank J, Oppenheim DM, Weinbaum G. Neutrophil recruitment and degranulation during induction of emphysema in the rat by nitrogen dioxide. *Am Rev Respir Dis* 1987;135:1129–1136.
163. Freeman G, Crane SC, Stephens RJ, Furiosi NJ. Pathogenesis of the nitrogen dioxide–induced lesion in the rat lung: a review and presentation of new observations. *Am Rev Respir Dis* 1968;98:429–443.
164. Douglas WW, Colby TV. Fume-related bronchiolitis obliterans. In: Epler GR, ed. *Diseases of the bronchioles.* New York: Raven Press, 1994:187–213.
165. Rom WN, Barkman H. Respiratory irritants. In: Rom WN, ed. *Environmental and occupational medicine.* Boston: Little, Brown and Company, 1983:273–283.
166. Flick MR. Pulmonary edema and acute lung injury. In: Murray JF, Nadel JA, eds. *Textbook of respiratory medicine.* Philadelphia: WB Saunders, 1988:1359–1409.
167. Pennanen AS, Salonen RO, Eklund T, Nylund N, Lee K, Spengler JD. Improvement of air quality in a small indoor ice arena by effective emission control in ice resurfacers. *J Air Waste Manag Assoc* 1997;47:1087–1094.
168. National Institute for Occupational Safety and Health. *NIOSH pocket guide to chemical hazards.* Washington: US Government Printing Office, 1994.
169. Godish T. *Air quality,* 2nd ed. Chelsea, MI: Lewis Publishers, 1991:23–62.
170. Palmes ED, Gunnison AF, DiMattio J, Tomczyk C. Personal sampler for nitrogen dioxide. *Am Ind Hyg Assoc J* 1976;37:570–577.
171. Miller DP. Ion chromatographic analysis of Palmes tubes for nitrite. *Atmos Environ* 1984;18:891–892.
172. Miller DP. Low-level determination of nitrogen dioxide in ambient air using the Palmes tube. *Atmos Environ* 1988;22:945–947.
173. Palmes ED, Tomczyk C. Personal sampler for NO_x. *Am Ind Hyg Assoc J* 1979; 40:588–591.
174. Yanagisawa Y, Nishimura H. A badge-type personal sampler for measurement of personal exposure to NO_2 and NO in ambient air. *Environ Int* 1982;8:235–242.
175. Occupational Safety and Health Administration. *Nitrogen dioxide in workplace atmospheres (ion chromatography) (Method ID-182).* Salt Lake City: Occupational Safety and Health Administration Salt Lake City Analytical Laboratory, 1991.
176. Occupational Safety and Health Administration. *Nitric oxide in workplace atmospheres (ion chromatography) (Method ID-190).* Salt Lake City: Occupational Safety and Health Administration Salt Lake City Analytical Laboratory, 1991.
177. *Code of Federal Regulations, part 50.* Washington: US Government Printing Office, 1996.
178. Fehsenfeld FC, Drummond JW, Roychowdhury UK, et al. Intercomparison of NO_2 measurement techniques. *J Geophys Res* 1990;95:3579–3597.
179. Beliles RP, Beliles EM. Phosphorus, selenium, tellurium, and sulfur. In: Clayton GD, Clayton FE, eds. *Patty's industrial hygiene and toxicology,* vol II, part A. New York: John Wiley and Sons, 1993:783–829.
180. Von Burg R. Toxicology update: sulfur dioxide. *J Appl Toxicol* 1995;16:365–371.
181. Atkinson DA, Sim TC, Grant JA. Sodium metabisulfite and SO_2 release: an under-recognized hazard among shrimp fishermen. *Ann Allergy* 1993; 71:563–566.
182. Federman JH, Sachter JJ. Status asthmaticus in a paramedic following exposure to a roadside flare: a case report. *J Emerg Med* 1997;15:87–89.
183. Frank NR, Yoder RE, Brain JD, Yokoyama E. SO_2 absorption by the mouth and nose under conditions of varying concentration and flow. *Arch Environ Health* 1969;18:315–322.
184. Speizer FE, Frank NR. The uptake and release of SO_2 by the human nose. *Arch Environ Health* 1966;12:725–728.
185. Kleinman MT. Sulfur dioxide and exercise: relationships between response and absorption in upper airways. *J Air Pollut Control Assoc* 1984;34:32–37.
186. Bethel RA, Erle DJ, Epstein J, Sheppard D, Nadel JA, Boushey HA. Effect of exercise rate and route of inhalation on sulfur dioxide–induced bronchoconstriction in asthmatic subjects. *Am Rev Respir Dis* 1983;128:592–596.
187. Sheppard D, Saisho A, Nadel JA, Boushey HA. Exercise increases sulfur dioxide–induced bronchoconstriction in asthmatic subjects. *Am Rev Respir Dis* 1981;123:486–491.
188. Amdur MO. Aerosols formed by oxidation of sulfur dioxide. Review of their toxicology. *Arch Environ Health* 1971;23:459–468.
189. Sheppard D. Mechanisms of airway responses to inhaled sulfur dioxide. In Loke J, ed. *Pathophysiology and treatment of inhalation injuries.* New York: Marcel Dekker Inc, 1988:49–66.
190. Fine JM, Gordon T, Sheppard D. The roles of pH and ionic species in sulfur dioxide- and sulfite-induced bronchoconstriction. *Am Rev Respir Dis* 1987;136:1122–1126.
191. Neta P, Huie RE. Free-radical chemistry of sulfite. *Environ Health Perspect* 1985;64:209–217.
192. Yokoyama E, Yoder RE, Frank NR. Distribution of ^{35}S in the blood and its excretion in urine of dogs exposed to $^{35}SO_2$. *Arch Environ Health* 1971;22:389–395.
193. Balchum OJ, Dybicki J, Meneely GR. The dynamics of sulfur dioxide inhalation, absorption, distribution, and retention. *Arch Ind Health* 1960;21:564–569.
194. Sheppard D, Wong WS, Uehara CF, Nadel JA, Boushey HA. Lower threshold and greater bronchomotor responsiveness of asthmatic subjects to sulfur dioxide. *Am Rev Respir Dis* 1980;122:873–878.
195. Snashall PD, Baldwin C. Mechanisms of sulphur dioxide induced bronchoconstriction in normal and asthmatic man. *Thorax* 1982;37:118–123.
196. Linn WS, Avol EL, Peng RC, Shamoo DA, Hackney JD. Replicated dose-response study of sulfur dioxide effects in normal, atopic, and asthmatic volunteers. *Am Rev Respir Dis* 1987;136:1127–1134.
197. Horstman D, Roger LJ, Kehrl H. Hazucha M. Airway sensitivity of asthmatics to sulfur dioxide. *Toxicol Ind Health* 1986;2:289–298.
198. Nadel JA, Salem H, Tamplin B, Tokiwa Y. Mechanism of bronchoconstriction during inhalation of sulfur dioxide. *J Appl Physiol* 1965;20:164–167.
199. Nadel JA, Salem H, Tamplin B, Tokiwa Y. Mechanism of bronchoconstriction during inhalation of sulfur dioxide: reflex involving vagus nerves. *Arch Environ Health* 1965;10:175–178.
200. Field PI, Simmul R, Bell SC, Allen DH, Berend N. Evidence for opioid modulation and generation of prostaglandins in sulphur dioxide (SO_2)-induced bronchoconstriction. *Thorax* 1996;51:159–163.
201. Sheppard D, Eschenbacher WL, Boushey HA, Bethel RA. Magnitude of the interaction between the bronchomotor effects of sulfur dioxide and those of dry (cold) air. *Am Rev Respir Dis* 1984;130:52–55.
202. Linn WS, Shamoo DA, Anderson KR, Whynot JD, Avol EL, Hackney JD. Effects of heat and humidity on the responses of exercising asthmatics to sulfur dioxide exposure. *Am Rev Respir Dis* 1985;131:221–225.
203. Linn WS, Venet TG, Shamoo DA, et al. Respiratory effects of sulfur dioxide in heavily exercising asthmatics. *Am Rev Respir Dis* 1983;127:278–283.
204. Bethel RA, Sheppard D, Epstein J, Tam E, Nadel JA, Boushey HA. Interaction of sulfur dioxide and cold dry air in causing bronchoconstriction in asthmatic subjects. *J Appl Physiol* 1984;57:419–423.
205. Balmes JR, Fine JM, Sheppard D. Symptomatic bronchoconstriction after short-term inhalation of sulfur dioxide. *Am Rev Respir Dis* 1987;136:1117–1121.
206. Heath SK, Koenig JQ, Morgan MS, Checkoway H, Hanley QS, Rebolledo V. Effects of sulfur dioxide exposure on African-American and Caucasian asthmatics. *Environ Res* 1994;66:1–11.
207. Koenig JQ, Covert DS, Hanley QS, Van Belle G, Pierson WE. Prior exposure to ozone potentiates subsequent response to sulfur dioxide in adolescent asthmatic subjects. *Am Rev Respir Dis* 1990;141:377–380.
208. Koenig JQ, Marshall SG, Horike M, et al. The effects of albuterol on SO_2-induced bronchoconstriction in allergic adolescents. *J Allergy Clin Immunol* 1987;79:54–58.
209. Gong H, Linn WS, Shamoo DA, et al. Effect of inhaled salmeterol on sulfur dioxide–induced bronchoconstriction in asthmatic subjects. *Chest* 1996; 110:1229–1235.
210. Bigby B, Boushey H. Effects of nedocromil sodium on the bronchomotor response to sulfur dioxide in asthmatic patients. *J Allergy Clin Immunol* 1993;92:195–197.
211. Myers DJ, Bigby B, Boushey H. The inhibition of sulfur dioxide–induced bronchoconstriction in asthmatic subjects by cromolyn sodium is dose dependent. *Am Rev Respir Dis* 1986;133:1150–1153.
212. Koenig JQ, Dumler K, Rebolledo V, Williams PV, Pierson WE. Theophylline mitigates the bronchoconstrictor effects of sulfur dioxide in subjects with asthma. *J Allergy Clin Immunol* 1992;89:789–794.
213. Charan NB, Myers CG, Lakshminarayan S, Spencer TM. Pulmonary injuries associated with acute sulfur dioxide inhalation. *Am Rev Respir Dis* 1979;119:555–560.
214. Galea M. Fatal sulfur dioxide inhalation. *Can Med Assoc J* 1964;91:345–347.
215. Woodford DM, Coutu RE, Gaensler EA. Obstructive lung disease from acute sulfur dioxide exposure. *Respiration* 1979;38:238–245.
216. American Thoracic Society. Health effects of outdoor air pollution. *Am J Respir Crit Care Med* 1996;153:3–50.
217. Dockery DW, Ware JH, Ferris BG, Speizer FE, Cook NR, Herman SM. Change in pulmonary function in children associated with air pollution episodes. *J Air Pollut Control Assoc* 1982;32:937–942.
218. Charpin D, Kleisbauer JP, Fondarai J, Graland B, Viala A, Gouezo F. Respiratory symptoms and air pollution changes in children: the Gardanne coal-basin study. *Arch Environ Health* 1988;43:22–27.
219. Derrienic F, Richardson S, Mollie A, Lalloch J. Short-term effects of sulphur dioxide pollution on mortality in two French cities. *Int J Epidemiol* 1989; 18:186–197.
220. Hatzakis A, Katsouyanni K, Kalandidi A, Day N, Trichopoulos D. Short-term effects of air pollution on mortality in Athens. *Int J Epidemiol* 1986;15:73–81.
221. Spix C, Heinrich J, Dockery D, et al. Air pollution and daily mortality in Erfurt, East Germany. *Environ Health Perspect* 1993;101:518–526.

222. Dab W, Medina S, Quenel P, et al. Short-term respiratory health effects of ambient air pollution: results of the APHEA project in Paris. *J Epidemiol Community Health* 1996;50(Suppl 1):S42–S46.
223. Peters A, Goldstein IF, Beyer U, et al. Acute health effects of exposure to high levels of air pollution in Eastern Europe. *Am J Epidemiol* 1996;144:570–581.
224. Touloumi G, Samoli E, Katsouyanni K. Daily mortality and "winter type" air pollution in Athens, Greece—a time series analysis within the APHEA project. *J Epidemiol Community Health* 1996;50(Suppl 1):S47–S51.
225. Schwartz J. Short-term fluctuations in air pollution and hospital admissions of the elderly for respiratory disease. *Thorax* 1995;50:531–538.
226. Shore SA, Kariya ST, Anderson K, et al. Sulfur dioxide–induced bronchitis in dogs. Effects on airway responsiveness to inhaled and intravenously administered methacholine. *Am Rev Respir Dis* 1987;135:840–847.
227. Scanlon PD, Seltzer J, Ingram RH, Reid L, Drazen JM. Chronic exposure to sulfur dioxide. Physiologic and histologic evaluation of dogs exposed to 50 or 15 ppm. *Am Rev Respir Dis* 1987;135:831–839.
228. National Institute for Occupational Safety and Health. *Criteria for a recommended standard: occupational exposure to sulfur dioxide.* Washington: US Government Printing Office, 1974:16, 20–26.
229. Härkönen H, Nordnam H, Korhonen O, Winblad I. Long-term effects of exposure to sulfur dioxide. *Am Rev Respir Dis* 1983;128:890–893.
230. Piirilä PL, Nordman H, Korhonen OS, Winblad I. A thirteen-year follow-up of respiratory effects of acute exposure to sulfur dioxide. *Scand J Work Environ Health* 1996;22:191–196.
231. Rabinovitch S, Greyson ND, Weiser W, Hoffstein V. Clinical and laboratory features of acute sulfur dioxide inhalation poisoning: two-year follow-up. *Am Rev Respir Dis* 1989;139:556–558.
232. Archer VE, Gillam JD. Chronic sulfur dioxide exposure in a smelter: II. Indices of chest disease. *J Occup Med* 1978;20:88–95.
233. Osterman JW, Greaves IA, Smith TJ, Hammond SK, Robins JM, Theriault G. Respiratory symptoms associated with low level sulphur dioxide exposure in silicon carbide production workers. *Br J Ind Med* 1989;46:629–635.
234. Rom WN, Wood SD, White GL, Bang KM, Reading JC. Longitudinal evaluation of pulmonary function in copper smelter workers exposed to sulfur dioxide. *Am Rev Respir Dis* 1986;133:830–833.
235. International Agency for Research on Cancer. Sulfur dioxide and some sulfites, bisulfites, and metabisulfites. *IARC Monogr Eval Carcinog Risks Hum* 1992;54:131–188.
236. Reference method for the determination of sulfur dioxide in the atmosphere (pararosaniline method). *Code of Federal Regulations, Part 50, Appendix A.* Rev. 1996 Jul 1.
237. National Institute for Occupational Safety and Health. *NIOSH manual of analytical methods*, 4th ed. Washington: US Government Printing Office, 1994.

CHAPTER 67

Gasoline and Oxygenated Additives

Neill K. Weaver

Gasoline (mogas, motor spirit, petrol) is the generic name for the complex flammable mixture of paraffins, olefins, naphthenes, and aromatic hydrocarbons that serves as the principal fuel for the spark-activated internal combustion engine. In 1992, the world's apparent consumption of gasoline was 267 billion gallons. The United States accounts for nearly one-half of the world's motor vehicle registration and motor fuel consumption. In 1994, U.S. gasoline consumption was approximately 118 billion gallons, with 266 million motor vehicles (138 million passenger cars) driven nearly 2.4 trillion miles (1–3).

CHEMICAL CHARACTERISTICS AND COMPOSITION

Hydrocarbons

Gasoline is a complex mixture of hydrocarbons. The hydrocarbons are predominantly in the range of C5 to C10 (overall, C4 to C14) and include alkanes (paraffins), alkenes (olefins), naphthenes (cycloparaffins), and aromatics (Fig. 67-1) (4). The wide ranges of hydrocarbon types normally present in the liquid phase of commercial gasoline are shown in Table 67-1, along with their approximate levels in the vapor phase. With respect to molecular composition, gasoline theoretically contains more than 1,500 specific compounds, including isomers (5). Analysis by gas chromatography and mass spectrometry generally results in the identification of 150 to 180 individual compounds (6,7). The most prominent compounds (2% by weight or greater) found in a typical U.S. commercial gasoline are shown in Table 67-2. From the toxicologic viewpoint, the low concentrations of benzene (1% to 2% in most U.S. gasolines but somewhat higher—4% to 5%—in certain reformulated and European gasolines) and *n*-hexane (1% to 6%) are noteworthy (8,9). Only a few compounds (e.g., toluene) approach or exceed 10% concentra-

Type	Name	Formula	Structure
Alkanes (Paraffins)	n-Octane	n-C_8H_{18}	
(Isoparaffins)	Iso-octane 2,2,4-Trimethylpentane	i-C_8H_{18}	
Alkenes (Olefins)	Hexene	C_6H_{12}	
Naphthenes (Cycloparaffins)	Cyclohexane	C_6H_{12}	
Aromatics	Toluene	C_7H_8	

Figure 67-1. Types and examples of gasoline hydrocarbons.

TABLE 67-1. Composition of gasoline[a]

	Liquid phase (range)	Vapor phase (approximate concentration)
Hydrocarbon class		
Alkanes/naphthalenes	30–90%	90%
Aromatics	10–50%	2%
Alkenes	6–9%	9%
Additives		
1975 Organolead	± 39/gallon	<0.004%[b]
Ethylene dichloride (EDC)	150–300 ppm	0.15 ppm
Ethylene dibromide (EDB)	80–150 ppm	0.08 ppm
1989 Organolead (EDC and EDB not used)	<0.05 g/gallon	0.004%
Methyl tertiary butyl ether	10%	6%

[a]By volume (except organolead).
[b]Undetectable.

TABLE 67-2. Hydrocarbon compounds detected in U.S.-finished gasoline at ≥2 weight %

Chemical	Weight %	
	Estimated range	Weighted average
Toluene	5–22	10
2-Methylpentane (+ isomers)	4–14	9
n-Butane	3–12	7
Iso-Pentane	5–10	7
n-Pentane	1–9	5
Xylene (3 isomers)	1–10	3
2,2,4-Trimethlypentane	<1–8	3
n-Hexane	<1–6	2
n-Heptane	<1–5	2
2,3,3-Trimethylpentane	<1–5	2
2,3,4-Trimethylpentane	<1–5	2
3-Methylpentane	<1–5	2
Benzene	<1–4	2
2,2,3-Trimethylpentane	<1–4	2
Methylcyclopentane	<1–3	2
2-Methyl-2-butene	<1–2	2

tion; most of the 100 or more specific chemicals occur at dilute levels of 1%.

Although small quantities of natural gasoline sometimes are separated during production of crude oil, commercial gasolines are manufactured in petroleum refineries by blending four to eight component streams from processing units (Table 67-3) (4–6). Because gasoline is formulated to meet performance specifications (Table 67-4), its chemical composition and physical properties vary considerably, depending on the nature of the crude oil, refinery processing methods, and product qualities desired (10–12). A number of contaminants, including water, metals, particulate matter, and heterocyclics (nitrogen, sulfur, and oxygen compounds) are removed from the hydrocarbon streams to improve performance.

Additives

Gasoline also contains a number of additives; those commonly used and the purpose they serve are shown in Table 67-5 (6). Oxygenates, including such compounds as methyl tertiary butyl ether (MTBE), ethanol, methanol, and tertiary butyl alcohol, are added to gasoline as octane enhancers and antiknock agents (13). The amounts of oxygenates added are known to vary widely. MTBE has been used since 1979. In 1994, 2.2 billion gallons were blended into approximately 20% of U.S. gasoline.

TABLE 67-3. Streams used to blend a prototype gasoline (API P5-6)

Stream	CAS number	Volume %
Light catalytic cracked naphtha	64741-55-5	7.6
Heavy catalytic cracked naphtha	64741-55-4	44.5
Light catalytic reformed naphtha	64741-63-5	21.3
Light alkylate naphtha	64741-66-8	22

CAS, Chemical Abstracts Service.

TABLE 67-4. Gasoline performance specifications

Compositional feature	Function
Octane rating	Antiknock
Antiicing	Minimize stalls of cold engine
Seasonal front-end volatility	Quick-starting
Full boiling range volatility	Warm-up acceleration
Back-end volatility	Complete combustion (limit engine deposits)
Oxidation stability	Storage life (minimize gum formation)

MTBE at 10% concentration in liquid gasoline has been shown to result in a concentration of approximately 6% in vapor phase.

Prior to 1985, gasoline contained lead alkyls (tetraethyl tetramethyl at levels of 1.5 to 3.0 g per gallon (0.4 to 0.8 g per L) to increase octane number and suppress preignition. In 1985, the level was reduced to 0.5 g per gallon (0.13 g per L) and, in 1986, regulatory controls brought about a further reduction to 0.1 g per gallon (0.03 g per L). Now U.S. unleaded gasolines contain 0.05 g or less of lead per gallon (0.02 g per L).

The scavenging agents ethylene dichloride (EDC) and ethylene dibromide (EDB) prevent the accumulation of lead deposits in the engine. Former levels of EDC and EDB, which were 150 to 300 and 80 to 150 parts per million (ppm), respectively, have been reduced, consequent to lower lead levels. Calculated airborne concentrations of lead and the scavengers EDC and EDB, based on the higher levels in use more than a decade ago, are shown in Table 67-1. Such levels no longer occur because organolead has been phased out.

Other additives are present in very dilute amounts (5 pounds per 1,000 barrels). In the processing of finished gasoline, additives are blended in enclosed systems, so that worker exposures are unlikely to occur.

The Clean Air Act amendments of 1990 required the phasing-in of more stringent national vehicle tailpipe emission standards and the use of reformulated gasolines in the nine cities that most seriously exceeded air quality standards, beginning in 1995. An oxygenated fuel is defined to have 2.7 weight per dL oxygen; (e.g., 11 vol per dL MTBE). In general, the reformulated gasolines contain oxygenates (MTBE, 12% to 14% liquid volume) and have compositional changes that include significant reductions in aromatics (including benzene), olefins, and sulfur and a reduction in Reid vapor pressure. These modifications have resulted in consistent and significant reductions amounting to 25% to 40% in tailpipe emissions of total hydrocarbons, nonmethane organic gases, carbon monoxide, oxides of nitrogen, total toxins, and evaporative losses (13).

TABLE 67-5. Additives typically used in motor gasoline

Purpose	Agent
Antiknock	Tetraethyl/tetramethyl lead
Lead scavengers	Ethylene dichloride/dibromide
Detergents	Amines
Antirust agents	Sulfonates
Antioxidants	Aminophenols
Antiicing	Alcohols, glycols
Upper cylinder lubricants	Light mineral oils
Oxygenates	Methyl tertiary butyl ether Ethanol, methanol

PHYSICAL PROPERTIES

Volatility, Water Solubility, and Other Physical Features

Selected physical properties of motor gasoline are shown in Table 67-6 (10–12). The volatility of the hydrocarbon constituents is controlled by the nominal boiling-point ranges. The octane number, which is adjusted in accordance with engine requirements and marketing strategies, actually is determined by a trial run of the gasoline sample in a specially constructed test engine. Approximate motor octane numbers are listed for typical regular- and premium-grade gasolines. The Reid vapor pressure is controlled to meet seasonal (temperature) and geographic (altitude) needs; the "high end" may be subject to regulatory limits [11 pounds per square inch (0.8 kg per square centimeter) or less] to reduce vapor losses to the atmosphere.

With respect to solubility in water, the paraffinic hydrocarbons are highly insoluble, whereas certain aromatic compounds (e.g., benzene) are somewhat soluble. Oxygenates (MTBE, alcohols) present in certain blends are miscible and will be extracted into a water column. Factors relevant to the explosion hazard of gasoline include its ready volatility at ambient temperatures: One gallon (3.7 L) of liquid gasoline forms more than 20 cubic feet (0.56 cubic meters) of vapor at 15.5°C and 1 atmosphere. An additional hazard factor is gasoline's explosive range of vapor (1 to 6 vol per dL) and the low flash point of the vapor. Other physical items listed in Table 67-6 have the following exposure implications: (i) liquid gasoline, being less dense than water, floats on an aquatic surface; (ii) gasoline vapor, with more than twice the density of air, displaces oxygen in a confined space; and (iii) gasoline's low viscosity enhances evaporation by rapid spreading on (and running off of) a surface. The odor threshold of gasoline is 0.06 to 0.08 ppm, with an odor recognition threshold of 0.15 to 0.20 ppm.

Gasoline Vapor Phase and Liquid Phase

Important differences exist in the hydrocarbon composition of gasoline vapor as compared with liquid gasoline. The molecular components of gasoline distribute into the volatile phase in relation to their individual boiling points and vapor pressures. During the process of evaporation from liquid to vapor phase, the low carbon-containing compounds (the "light" hydrocarbons with low boiling points, C3 to greater than C5) evaporate quickly and reach relatively high concentration in the vapor mixture, whereas the higher carbon compounds (with higher boiling points) evaporate slowly, resulting in low concentration levels. Overall, the vapor phase is composed principally of alkanes and naphthenes (approximately 90% by volume), whereas the aromatics, which potentially are more toxic, are reduced to approximately 2% (see Table 67-1; Figs. 67-2, 67-3) (14,15). After the addition of MTBE to gasoline, vapor phases will contain lower concentrations of MTBE.

Analysis of gasoline vapor during loading of tanker trucks at a U.S. bulk station revealed that C3 to C5 compounds constituted more than 75% by volume of the total hydrocarbon vapor; similar studies at European worksites showed an average of 90% of C3 to C5 compounds. These findings are particularly significant in evaluating the potentially toxic effects of gasoline vapor because of the low toxicity exhibited by the C3 to C5 compounds. Benzene, a compound for which there is cause for concern, has levels in gasoline vapor that usually are less than 1 mg per cubic meter in U.S. samples and that may be somewhat

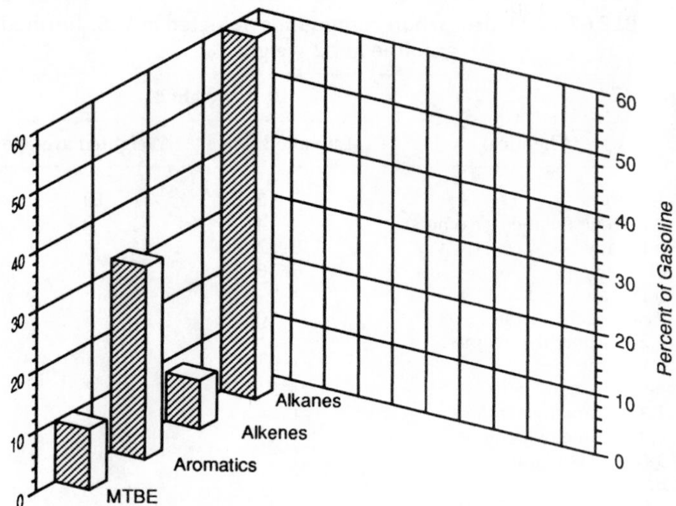

Figure 67-2. Liquid phase of gasoline. MTBE, methyl tertiary butyl ether.

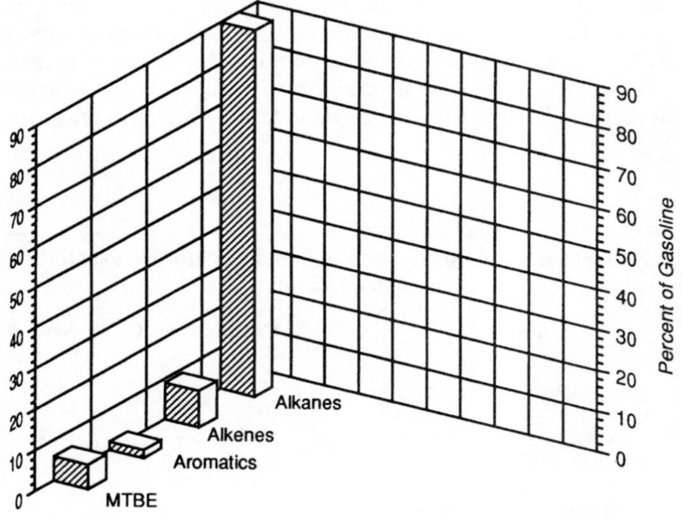

Figure 67-3. Vapor phase of gasoline. MTBE, methyl tertiary butyl ether.

TABLE 67-6. Physical properties of commercial motor gasoline

Boiling point range	
United States	50–200°C
Europe	25–220°C
Aviation gasoline (Avgas)	25–170°C
Density	0.7–0.8 g/cm³
Kinematic viscosity (at 20°C)	1 centistokes
Reid vapor pressure	8–15 psi (0.4–0.9 atm)
Vapor density (air = 1)	2–5
Octane number regular grade	91–93
ASTM premium grade	96–99
Flash point	–46°C
Explosive/ignition range (vapor concentration in air)	1.3–6.0% by volume
Solubility in water	
Paraffinic hydrocarbons	Highly soluble
Aromatic hydrocarbons	Somewhat soluble
Oxygenates	Soluble

ASTM, American Society for Testing and Materials; atm, atmosphere.

higher in European samples (8,9). Concentrations of organolead additives, along with the scavengers EDC and EDB, were too low to be detected in breathing-zone air samples for tank truck loaders working with leaded gasoline (14). Analyses of other compounds with recognized toxic effects—*n*-hexane, toluene, and xylenes—revealed exposure levels well below their established exposure limits.

SITES, INDUSTRIES, AND BUSINESSES ASSOCIATED WITH EXPOSURE

Although the operations of a modern petroleum refinery are highly complex, the processing methods involved in the manufacture of gasoline are well characterized (4–6,10,11). Operational procedures usually are highly successful in maintaining refinery streams in a closed system of pipes and vessels. Nevertheless, the refinery air contains low levels of hydrocarbon vapor, the result of fugitive emissions and multiple small releases, leaks, and spills. The same hydrocarbon compounds in gasoline are present in the refinery atmosphere, but their relative proportions are different and variable to some degree throughout the refinery. Refinery workers are exposed to the mixture of hydrocarbons generally present in refinery air, and employee exposures to gasoline vapor potentially occur at any point downstream, from the final blending site for the finished gasoline to the retail outlet (usually a gasoline pump in a service station).

Approximately 300 petroleum refineries and 140,000 service stations and gasoline retail outlets are found in the United States (16). Gasoline distribution systems use a wide variety of transport facilities and devices, including pipelines, ocean-going tankers, barges, railway tank cars, tanker wagon trucks, drums, and canisters (including those carried by hand). Runion (17) identified the operating conditions during which access to hydrocarbon streams and vapors are prone to occur, with resultant employee exposures:

- Operational start-ups, shutdowns, and mishaps
- Turnarounds and other maintenance activities
- Gauging, sampling, and analysis
- Worker entry into tanks, vessels, and unit structures
- Product, catalyst, or process chemical transfer; loading and unloading
- Waste treatment for handling activities (not closed processes)

Extensive monitoring programs for workers potentially exposed to gasoline vapor have been reported (6,15,17–20; R. Diakun, *personal communication,* 1983). Exposures, expressed as total hydrocarbon for 8-hour time-weighted average (TWA) periods, are shown in Table 67-7 for selected petroleum worker assignments and worksites. Overall, the highest exposures were measured during marine loading operations; intermediate levels were experienced by driver salespeople loading road tankers; and service station employees and refinery workers had low-level exposures.

Studies of exposure to benzene (a toxic component and a possible surrogate marker for gasoline) and to MTBE (at sites using reformulated gasoline) among service station attendants and operators revealed average levels of less than 0.1 ppm benzene and less than 1 ppm MTBE (20).

With respect to community exposures, the levels of benzene determined near service stations, bulk terminals, and refineries were in the low parts-per-billion range (generally, less than 10 ppb), leading to the conclusion that refineries and chemical plants do not contribute to total exposures in any discernible way (21). During self-serve automobile refueling, average benzene levels were 164 to 1,100 ppb. As these exposures are infrequent and of short duration (usually 2 minutes), the possibility of health implications remains questionable.

TABLE 67-7. Exposure of airborne gasoline constituents in selected U.S. operations and occupations

Operation/occupation	Total mean hydrocarbon concentration (TWA, mg/m^3)
Refinery workers	15
Driver salespeople	39
Service station attendants	4–23
Marine loading	246
Loading of tanker trucks	
Top, no vapor recovery	46
Bottom, with vapor recovery	40
Gasoline truck drivers	46

TWA, 8-hour time-weighted average.

GROUNDWATER CONTAMINATION BY GASOLINE

Environmental releases of gasoline are associated with its production, transportation, and storage. These occurrences may be characterized as originating83 either at point sources (e.g., from storage tanks) or at non–point sources (e.g., storm water runoff). Storage tanks are the principal cause of point source releases. Natural processes operative in reducing gasoline contaminants in groundwater include evaporation at the air interface, adherence to soil particles, dilution as the contaminated water column moves away from the pollution source, and bacterial biodegradation. Remediation treatment practices include "pump and treat," air sparging, soil vapor extraction, and carbon adsorption.

The presence of gasoline components in household water results in potential exposure by ingestion and by inhalation and skin absorption while bathing and showering. In homes that have had a contaminated water source, benzene levels have been measured, and the levels generally are less than 1 ppb. However, contaminated homes may have levels in excess of 20 ppb, with peak concentrations in the bathroom while showering in excess of 160 ppb (21).

Because of their solubility, oxygenates may be present in relatively high concentration in water equilibrated with an oxygenated fuel. For a gasoline with 10% MTBE, laboratory water equilibrium concentrations were observed to be higher than 3,600 ppm MTBE, whereas total benzene, toluene, ethylbenzene, and xylene was 114 ppm. Because it is less biodegradable and less likely to be sorbed to aquifer soils, dissolved MTBE is considered to be more mobile in groundwater than are benzene, toluene, ethylbenzene, and xylene compounds. Because MTBE travels with the water column, it may be the first compound detected (by taste, odor, or chemical analysis) downgradient from a gasoline release. Taste and odor thresholds for MTBE in water are low (40 to 140 µg per L) and are within the range of the U.S. Environmental Protection Agency draft health advisory for drinking water. This facilitates early detection of impaction of water supplies with MTBE.

The application of industrial hygiene measures and engineering controls has resulted in significant reductions in worker exposures through the years. Incentives for even more use of controls include not only further reductions in worker exposures but the prevention of vapor releases to the atmosphere (where certain hydrocarbon compounds contribute to the formation of photochemical smog) and provision of economic benefits by limiting product losses.

CLINICAL TOXICOLOGY

Gasoline is the aggregate of myriad individual chemical substances, and consideration of its absorption, biotransformation, and excretion is exceedingly complicated. Consequently, observations pertinent to the clinical toxicology of gasoline focus on the whole gasoline, on selected components (naphtha), or on one or more specific compounds because of inherent toxicity (benzene) or as a "marker" (2,2,4-trimethylpentane) that serves as a surrogate for the entire complex mixture.

Routes of Exposure

Gasoline exposures occur by skin contact (with potential percutaneous absorption), ingestion (often associated with aspiration), and inhalation of the vapor (19). Of these various mechanisms, the inhalation route is by far the most important. Hydrocarbons in the C3 to C10 range are transferred across the alveolar lining of the lungs fairly readily, across the mucosa of the gastrointestinal tract to a lesser degree, and across the skin barrier least of all.

Gasoline's disagreeable taste and odor generally serve to prevent the swallowing of this liquid or severely limit the quantity ingested. However, the gagging and choking associated with the swallowing attempt often cause aspiration of the liquid gasoline into the respiratory tract, which is far more serious.

Exposure situations that result in skin contact with gasoline, usually from a spill or splash, invariably involve inhalation of vapor as well; the latter exposure is much more important with respect to systemic absorption. Experimental studies of the percutaneous absorption of benzene and isooctane demonstrate very limited transport across the skin (22,23). Franz (23) found absorption of benzene through the skin of palm and forearm of human volunteers after a brief (10- to 20-second) exposure to pure benzene to be 0.003 and 0.002 μL per square centimeter, respectively. Topical application of isooctane in the monkey resulted in the absorption of 0.003 μL per square centimeter; similar application to human skin *in vitro* resulted in absorption of 0.006 μL per square centimeter.

Distribution, Biotransformation, and Excretion

Because of high lipid solubility, hydrocarbons tend to accumulate in tissues in proportion to their fat content (principally brain, adrenal glands, bone marrow, and liver). Because hydrocarbons are relatively inert biochemically, most are excreted unchanged through the lungs; a small fraction may be excreted in urine, but this route is restricted by the low solubility of the hydrocarbons in water. However, oxidative metabolism allows some aromatic hydrocarbons to be eliminated as water-soluble urinary biotransformation products conjugated with sulfuric acid, glycine, or glucuronic acid (24–26). The oxidative pathway for *n*-hexane to a neurotoxic intermediate is well documented. However, this mechanism is notably unique: Other hydrocarbons do not exhibit this form of neurotoxicity.

Signs, Symptoms, and Syndromes from Toxic Exposure

Knowledge of the toxicity of gasoline may be derived from the individual hydrocarbon compounds present in gasoline, from hydrocarbon mixtures that are components of gasoline (refinery streams, naphthas, solvents), or from the whole gasoline itself. Although the importance of information derived from specific compounds and components is acknowledged, the following discussion relates to experimental studies of and clinical observations about whole commercial gasoline and its vapor. Other fuels (liquefied natural gas and propane, alcohols, gasohols, and reformulated gasoline) with end uses similar to those of gasoline are excluded from consideration. Except for the toxic effects resulting from organolead compounds after rather extraordinary exposure patterns to leaded gasoline, no distinctions of toxicologic significance are made regarding gasolines, which differ with respect to additive packages, blends, grades, or commercial brands.

Experimental Studies in Animals

Although toxicity studies in animals (e.g., rodents) have limited applicability to humans, the usefulness of such studies in addressing clinical toxicity is recognized widely. Gasoline has been investigated extensively by standardized experimental procedures in laboratory animals. Key findings of the bioassay program conducted largely with technical and financial support of the American Petroleum Institute are summarized in Table 67-8 (27,28).

Overall, a low order of toxicity for gasoline is demonstrated by various test procedures, which show that a high (18-mg-per-kg) oral dose is required to induce mortality (median lethal dose); mortality is absent on acute and subacute dermal exposures; skin and eye irritation is minimal; dermal sensitization is absent; and survival and clinical and pathologic observations are normal in subchronic and chronic inhalation studies. The slight increase in number of hepatocellular tumors in female mice in the chronic inhalation experiment is of questionable significance, as this lesion is a rather common finding in bioassay studies with this species and gender. However, the induction of tubular nephropathy and renal cancers in male rats after chronic exposure to wholly vaporized gasoline by inhalation has been a subject of intense investigation and warrants additional comment.

A metabolic pathway that has been demonstrated for hydrocarbons is unique for the male rat (29,30). Branched-chain alkanes (isoparaffins) with six or more carbon atoms are bound to a male rat–specific protein, α_2-microglobulin. The protein-hydrocarbon complex is deposited in cells in the proximal tubule of the kidney, leading to cellular degeneration and regeneration. The lesion is reversible but, if protracted, as in chronic inhalation exposure, continuing cell turnover ultimately results in nongenetic tumor promotion. This metabolic process is not operative in animals lacking the α_2-microglobulin (mice, dogs, guinea pigs, primates of either gender, and female rats). On this basis, the male rat model of renal carcinogenesis is deemed inappropriate for humans.

A large number of publications have reported experimental studies of hydrocarbons, and a critical review of findings reveals some disparities and even contradictions in results. Such discrepancies are not surprising in view of the variability of test substances (often ill-defined, sometimes inappropriate or nonrepresentative), test procedures, and protocols, and levels of quality assurance used in conducting the research. Nevertheless, the bioassay studies provide an information base of considerable utility in evaluating the potential toxicity of gasoline in humans.

Acute Toxicity

In a 1941 review of gasoline intoxication, Machle (31) noted that despite a paucity of reports, clinical cases of poisoning had occurred after the commercial use of petroleum distillates; he predicted that intoxications would become more frequent as a

TABLE 67-8. Bioassay findings—reference gasoline

Test	Species	Results
Acute oral toxicity	Rat	LD_{50} = 18.85 mL/kg
Acute dermal toxicity	Rabbit	0% mortality at 5 mL/kg
Subchronic dermal toxicity	Rabbit	0% mortality at 8 mL/kg
Primary eye irritation	Rabbit	Nonirritating
Primary dermal irritation	Rabbit	Slightly irritating
Dermal sensitization	Guinea pig	Nonsensitizing
Mutagenesis assays		
Ames *Salmonella*	—	Negative
In vitro lymphoma	Mouse	Negative
In vivo bone marrow cytogenetics	Rat	Negative
Reproductive assays (inhalation 400 and 1,600 ppm)		
Dominant lethal teratogenesis	Mouse Rat	Negative Negative
Chronic dermal carcinogenicity (50 μL twice/wk/lifetime)	Mouse	No tumor induction No systemic effects
Subchronic inhalation (0, 400, and 1,500 ppm, 6 h/d, 5 d/wk, 90 d)	Rat Monkey	Survival, clinical, and pathology examinations normal, except tubular nephropathy in male rat
Chronic inhalation (0, 67, 292, and 2,056 ppm 6 h/d, 5 d/wk, lifetime)	Rat, mouse	Survival, clinical, and pathology examinations normal, except tubular nephropathy in male rat
Immunoassays		
30-d inhalation (1,500 and 3,000 ppm)	Rat, rabbit	No treatment-related antigene and antibodies in sera, urine
Lung and kidney tissues from chronic and subchronic inhalation studies	Rat, monkey	No antibasement membrane antibodies

LD_{50}, median lethal dose.

consequence of increasing opportunities for harmful exposure along with expanding distribution and use of gasoline. The following year, in evaluating the toxicity of gasoline vapor, Drinker et al. (32) described gasoline as a "very innocuous substance." Consideration of its harmful effects necessitates distinguishing the fires and explosion hazard and intoxications resulting from accidental spills and releases, inappropriate use, intentional misuse, and inhalation abuse from those occurring during manufacture, distribution, and intended use as a fuel for the internal combustion engine.

The principal hazard of gasoline clearly is its flammability, unassociated with toxicity (11). Despite a formidable safety effort, flashes, fires, and explosions still occur. Burns experienced by adolescents may occur in association with gasoline abuse ("sniffing") (33).

INHALATION TOXICITY OF GASOLINE VAPORS

The inappropriate use of gasoline as a solvent for degreasing and cleaning purposes poses a frequent risk for short-term vapor exposure. Although the principal concerns for gasoline vapor relate to its irritant effects and its actions as a depressant for the central nervous system (CNS) by way of its narcotizing (anesthetic) properties, the fact that high concentrations in a confined space may act as a simple asphyxiant by displacement of oxygen should not be overlooked.

The toxic effects of gasoline vapor are related to the inherent toxicity of its individual components, possible interactions (synergism, addition, or inhibition), their concentration in the vapor phase, and the duration of exposure. Human experience for exposures for various levels and periods are summarized in Table 67-9 (8,34,35). In general, exposures in the range of 250 to 1,000 ppm cause irritation to eyes, nose, and throat and produce headache, dizziness, flushed face, dysphagia, slurred speech, nausea, anorexia, dullness, and mental confusion.

Exposure to 1,000 to 5,000 ppm for 15 to 60 minutes may cause CNS depression and feelings of anesthesia. More severe intoxication is associated with vomiting, miosis, delirium, cyanosis, coma, clonic convulsions, and respiratory depression. Inhalation exposure to more than 5,000 ppm may cause rapid loss of consciousness and death. More than 10,000 ppm may cause microhemorrhages and blood vessel damage in body organs.

Tetraethyl lead absorption during exposure to leaded gasoline is not significant in acute exposures, and lead intoxication is not likely.

Methyl Tertiary Butyl Ether. MTBE has been studied alone and in combination with gasoline in rodents via intravenous, intraperitoneal, cutaneous, and inhalation routes and was found to be only slightly toxic (35). The toxicity of gasoline does not appear to be altered by the addition of 10% to 15% MTBE. Clinical symptoms in rats and mice exposed to MTBE at 29,000 mg per cubic meter in air for 6 hours over 13 consecutive days included CNS depression (anesthetic effects) and mild irritation; the observed symptoms were reversible, and no mortality occurred. Negative studies were reported after bioassays for reproductive effects (36).

TABLE 67-9. Human experience: exposure to gasoline vapors

Concentration (ppm)	Exposure time	Effect
5,000–16,000	5 min	Lethal
10,000	4 min	Dizziness
10,000	10 min	Intoxication
3,000	15 min	Dizziness
1,000	1 h	Dizziness, headache, nausea
1,000	30 min	Eye irritation only
500	1 h	Eye irritation only
160–270	8 h	Eye irritation only

Interestingly, MTBE has been used in humans as an experimental therapeutic agent by infusion into the gallbladder or bile duct to dissolve gallstones. The gallbladder concentrated MTBE in a manner to dissolve cholesterol gallstones effectively with minimal systemic absorption. No serious side effects were observed in treated patients. On the basis of currently available exposure and toxicity information, MTBE as an additive in gasoline appears unlikely to pose a human health hazard.

Ethylene Dichloride. Repeated exposures to EDC in an occupational environment have been associated with anorexia, nausea, vomiting, epigastric pain, irritation of mucous membranes, and liver and kidney dysfunction (37,38). Hepatotoxicity can occur after inhalation exposure in humans. Marked fatty degeneration in monkeys was demonstrated at exposure of 400 ppm for 8 to 12 days. No effect in monkeys was demonstrated after exposure to 100 ppm for up to 14 days. Guinea pigs exposed to 400 ppm for 14 days showed slight parenchymatous degradation of the liver. Acute poisonings may occur with exposure concentrations of 75 to 125 ppm. Increases in hepatic enzymes have been observed in human exposure cases. Centrilobular hepatic necrosis has been observed on autopsy of a 51-year-old man who died after an inhalation exposure in a confined space (33). This case was remarkable for the elevation of serum ammonia, serum transaminases (serum glutamic-oxaloacetic and serum glutamic-pyruvic transaminase), lactate dehydrogenase, and creatine phosphokinase isoenzymes. In addition, elevation of mitochondrial ornithine carbonyl transferase and mitochondrial glutamic-oxaloacetic transaminase was observed, which indicates that EDC can cause mitochondrial damage.

Ethylene Dibromide. Exposure to EDB at concentrations of 10 to 40 ppm for 6 hours per day in rats and mice, 5 days per week for 105 days, demonstrated increased tumors in the nasal cavity, respiratory tract, mammary glands, and spleen. Also, a decrease in fertility occurred, owing to abnormal development of sperm (39).

Notably, the role of MTBE and other oxidants (methanol, ethanol) in reformulated gasoline continues to evolve, and the use of scavenging agents (EDC and EDB) has been discontinued, owing to the phase-out of leaded gasoline in the United States (see Additives under Chemical Characteristics and Composition).

Fatalities after Gasoline Inhalation and Inhalational Abuse. During the 3-year period 1993 to 1995, the American Association of Poison Control Centers, serving an average population in excess of 200 million, reported 5,700,000 human exposure incidents, 2,116 with fatal outcomes. Gasoline exposure accounted for 61,449 incidents, 6 resulting in fatalities (Table 67-10) (40–42). Information was available for four of the gasoline-related deaths: Two occurred in infants (ages 15 and 18 months) with exposure by aspiration-ingestion; the other two were youths (ages 14 and 20 years) with exposure by inhalation abuse.

The likely mechanism of sudden death is cardiac arrhythmia (ventricular fibrillation leading to asystole). Experimental studies suggested that myocardial irritability is induced as a direct toxic effect of volatile hydrocarbons, by release of catecholamines, and by interaction of the two processes. Such fatal events have been noted more frequently as a consequence of sniffing solvents containing high concentrations of aromatic and halogenated hydrocarbons rather than of sniffing gasoline (43).

Effects of extraordinary exposure levels and patterns experienced as a consequence of inhalation abuse warrant separate consideration. Inhalation abuse occurs commonly in teenagers and delinquent juveniles. Although more than 50 publications relating to the subject have appeared during the last decade, no comprehensive investigation of the disorder has appeared, doubtless owing to the elusive nature of the abusers. Exposure patterns in abuse cases vary widely; four to six inhalations of concentrated vapor (probably at levels of tens of thousands of parts per million) are reported to induce a "high" lasting for a few to several hours; serious abusers may engage in the practice several times daily for protracted periods (44,45). Sniffing and other forms of repeated overexposure can lead to CNS depression, hallucinations, encephalopathy, ataxia, Gilles de la Tourette's disease, convulsions, retrobulbar neuritis, encephalitis, and conditions similar to those of multiple sclerosis. Neurologic manifestations reported in association with gasoline toxicity include vertigo, nystagmus, dementia, and peripheral neuropathy.

Well-documented cases of lead encephalopathy have been reported, the result of intense and persistent sniffing of leaded gasoline (46,47). The clinical picture includes a variety of behavioral changes and central and peripheral neuropathies; abnormalities of neurologic evaluation and blood chemistries (parameters related to lead intoxication) are present. The syndrome likely is due to an admixture of severe and cumulative hydrocarbon and organic and inorganic lead toxicities and predictably will disappear when leaded gasoline no longer is available.

Both acute and chronic effects of gasoline toxicity in abusers are likely to be confounded by other factors leading to impaired health: malnutrition, chronic infection, emotional and psychiatric disorders, medical neglect, and stressful lifestyle. In view of the evidence indicating widespread practice of abuse, the apparent infrequency of occurrence of serious health effects suggests a remarkable tolerance for gasoline vapor on the part of the abusers.

INGESTION AND ASPIRATION OF GASOLINE

Because of gasoline's unpalatability, adults rarely drink large amounts, even in suicide attempts. Dysfunction of the swallowing reflex from vapor-liquid gasoline results in choking and gagging, so that aspiration is prone to occur. Hence, aspiration properly is considered an almost inevitable accompaniment of ingestion.

The most common cause of gasoline ingestion in adults is oral suction to initiate siphoning (48,49). In children, ingestion accidents occur as a result of improper storage of gasoline in beverage bottles (50).

TABLE 67-10. American Association of Poison Control Centers Toxic Exposure Surveillance System

Year	No. participating centers	Population served (million)	No. human exposures	Total fatalities	No. gasoline exposures	Gasoline fatalities
1993	84	181.3	1,751,000	626	19,200	2
1994	65	215.9	1,926,000	766	20,965	3
1995	67	218.5	2,023,000	724	21,284	1
Total	—	—	5,700,000	2,116	61,449	6

Gasoline exhibits a low level of toxicity on the gastrointestinal tract. In contrast, entry of even a small amount (1 mL) into the respiratory tract causes severe pneumonitis; the low kinematic viscosity and surface tension facilitate spreading on mucosal and alveolar surfaces, which may be accentuated by gasping and coughing. The resulting chemical pneumonitis is severe and may be fatal, especially in infants and children.

Gasoline is absorbed relatively poorly from the intestinal tract; binding of hydrocarbons with food and intestinal contents and acceleration in transit time due to irritant effects may reduce absorption further. Machle (31) noted the disparity in reports of a single oral dose fatal to humans (apparently approximately 7.5 g per kg), as deaths had been reported to occur from as little as 10 g, but recovery had followed ingestion of 250 g (32). The disparity may have been due to the unrecognized presence and extent of aspiration pneumonitis. A few cases of intravascular hemolysis have been reported as an uncommon systemic manifestation after ingestion of gasoline (51).

DERMAL EFFECTS

Ordinarily, skin contact with gasoline results from a splash or spill, which quickly spreads into a thin layer of liquid and promptly evaporates; this process produces no ill effects. In contrast, immersion incidents, during which the skin is in prolonged contact with gasoline (e.g., an unconscious subject lying in a pool of liquid), may result in a severe chemical burn. Such lesions involve partial or even full thickness of the skin, the effects being altogether similar to those of a thermal burn (52,53). An occluded patch test with gasoline never should be carried out, as severe ulceration results from persistent skin contact with the liquid hydrocarbon under the patch.

Repeated skin contact with gasoline may cause a chronic dermatitis due to defatting of the skin. Such repeated contacts ordinarily should not occur but are seen occasionally as a result of careless handling or inappropriate use of gasoline as a solvent (cleaning or degreasing agent). Although skin sensitization to gasoline components theoretically is possible, contact dermatitis rarely occurs.

OCULAR EFFECTS

Exposure of the eyes to a splash of liquid gasoline or high vapor concentrations causes conjunctival irritation, but the effects are temporary.

Chronic and Long-Term Effects

The conventional view or assumption that long-term health effects due to gasoline were absent or negligible was based on many decades of experience, which included extensive health evaluation programs (including periodic examinations and surveillance of morbidity and mortality in petroleum workers) without evidence of occupationally related disease. However, what was recognized is that conditions related to contact with gasoline might exist but be obscured within the general ill-health patterns afflicting populations at large. Such concerns focused particularly on the possibility that gasoline vapor exposures have a causal role in chronic renal disease and in cancer. The former issue has been addressed by health monitoring and the latter by epidemiologic studies in petroleum workers.

POSSIBLE RENAL EFFECTS

Gasoline vapor exposures in the occupational setting have been considered a possible cause of impaired renal function (54,55). However, the studies linking renal disease (other than transitory urinary findings) to chronic gasoline vapor inhalation involve subjects with likely exposures to other known nephrotoxic agents (halogenated hydrocarbon solvents, metals, etc.). Such confounding is noted also in anecdotal reports attributing Goodpasture's syndrome to gasoline; an etiologic role for gasoline in Goodpasture's syndrome appears unlikely when serial cases are examined. Extensive periodic examination programs for gasoline workers have not disclosed evidence of impaired renal function, nor have uremia and end-stage renal disease been reported as significant causes of death in the epidemiologic studies.

After the 1984 report by MacFarland et al. (27) about the induction of kidney tumors in male rats and increased liver tumors in female mice from wholly vaporized gasoline, concern was expressed that gasoline might be carcinogenic in humans. Further research indicated that the hyperplastic and neoplastic kidney lesions in male rats are due to accumulation of hyaline deposits in the proximal tubule of the kidney. This accumulation is secondary to α_2-microglobulin, a low-molecular-weight protein that is synthesized in large amounts in the liver. This protein, which is unique to the male rat, binds to branched alkanes and is excreted by the glomerulus and reabsorbed, but the renal lysosomal complex is unable to metabolize this compound, and hyaline droplets accumulate (see Experimental Studies in Animals). Therefore, this form of renal neoplasia most likely is not relevant in regard to human risk (29). The significance of the occurrence of liver tumors in the B6C3F1 female mouse also is questionable, as this mouse has a high frequency of spontaneous liver tumors.

EPIDEMIOLOGIC STUDIES

More than 20 publications covering cohort mortality studies (including follow-up) of petroleum workers have appeared. Four articles (56–59) have reviewed and evaluated these studies; the article by Wong and Raabe (59) presented a metaanalysis of cancers by tumor site. Only one of the cohort studies focused on workers whose predominant exposure was gasoline (three distribution centers in the United Kingdom). The others involved general refinery workers, whose exposures were to volatile hydrocarbons present in the ambient air of refineries (which might serve as a surrogate for gasoline vapor). As actual exposure levels were unknown, worker classification by job assignment provided a crude index of exposure.

In general, the findings in multiple epidemiologic investigations demonstrated a "healthy-worker effect" in refinery employees, with overall mortality rates considerably lower than those of comparison populations. Among petroleum workers, mortality from circulatory, respiratory, digestive, and genitourinary diseases were consistently lower than that in the general population.

Although overall cancer death rates were low, some inconsistency was noted with respect to cancer incidence at certain specific sites; increased occurrence of tumors involving skin, brain, pancreas, prostate, kidney, and the hemopoietic system (leukemia) was reported in some cohorts (but not in a majority). In assessing cancer occurrence in relation to gasoline exposure, the International Agency for Research on Cancer concluded, "There is inadequate evidence for the carcinogenicity in humans of gasoline" and "[g]asoline is possibly carcinogenic for humans" (6).

The general conclusions derived from clinical observations, health monitoring, and epidemiologic investigations are reassuring in that no definite evidence of occupationally related chronic health effects has been demonstrated in petroleum workers (and, by inference, in workers exposed to gasoline). The ultimate question of whether chronic low-level exposure to gasoline vapor can cause disease (particularly cancer of specific sites) remains unresolved. Perhaps efforts to accumulate a sizable "downstream" gasoline-worker population and more extensive case-control investigations will provide a more definitive answer. However, recent cohort and nested case-control studies of marketing and marine distribution workers, considered to represent the occupational segments with highest gasoline exposure in the petroleum industry, have concluded that exposure to gasoline at levels experienced by the cohort is not a significant risk factor for leukemia (all cell types), acute myeloid leukemia, kidney cancer, or multiple myeloma (60,61).

MANAGEMENT OF GASOLINE INTOXICATION

Procedures selected for diagnostic examination and treatment of gasoline intoxication depend on the nature of exposure and must be individualized for particular cases. Because no antidote or specific therapy exists for hydrocarbon intoxication, treatment is symptomatic and supportive. The following general measures warrant consideration and may be found useful as initial or early treatment in appropriate clinical situations.

Inhalation

Most patients who are overcome (anesthetized) by breathing high levels of gasoline vapor recover promptly on removal from the contaminated site. Patients with more severe CNS depression may require resuscitation, oxygen, and breathing assistance. All patients should be observed for relapse and followed up for possible complications. In severe, chronic abuse cases with encephalopathy, the possibility of lead intoxication from inhalation of leaded gasoline vapor must be considered, because specific chelation therapy may be extremely important to expedite recovery.

Ingestion

Emesis should not be induced. Evacuation of stomach contents by gastric tube is not indicated because of the danger of aspiration unless the airway is protected by a cuffed endotracheal tube. If vomiting occurs, measures to minimize aspiration (Trendelenburg or left lateral decubitus position) should be used. The administration of activated charcoal slurry and a cathartic may be considered. Gasoline also will act as a cathartic. A chest radiograph and pulse oximetry can be useful in determining whether pulmonary aspiration has occurred. The chest radiograph may not show signs of infiltrates for several hours after aspiration. Aspiration pneumonitis is managed by standard accepted procedures and therapy.

Skin

After contact with liquid gasoline (splash or spill), thorough cleansing with soap and water is all that is necessary. Chemical burns due to protracted immersion are treated as a thermal burn.

Eyes

Ocular irritation after exposure to liquid gasoline or its concentrated vapor is relieved by irrigation.

ENVIRONMENTAL MONITORING

In environmental monitoring for gasoline vapor exposure, sampling and analytic procedures are available to determine the concentration of total hydrocarbons and selected compounds collected at the sample site (62). Worksite or breathing-zone air samples are drawn through a high-volume collection tube in which activated charcoal or polymer entraps the hydrocarbons present. The analytic procedure involves desorption followed by capillary gas chromatography with a flame ionization detector.

Exposure Limits

The adopted values established by the American Conference of Governmental Hygienists (63) are the 8-hour TWA, 300 ppm (890 mg per cubic meter), and the short-term exposure limit, 500 ppm (1,480 mg per cubic meter). Similar values established by the U.S. Occupational Safety and Health Administration (64) are the 8-hour TWA, 300 ppm (900 mg per cubic meter) and the short-term exposure limit, 500 ppm (1,500 mg per cubic meter).

Biological Monitoring

The procedures used for environmental monitoring may be adapted for breath analysis. A qualitative pattern of hydrocarbon compounds can serve as a "fingerprint" for identification of gasoline exposure, and the quantitative determination of selected "marker" compounds can serve for derivation of an estimate of exposure severity. Similarly, the hydrocarbon content of blood and serum can be established, but with greater difficulty. These techniques have been used rather extensively in research, but their application to clinical and occupational settings has been limited.

PREVENTION OF HEALTH EFFECTS

During its normal course of manufacture, distribution, and use as a fuel, gasoline is contained largely within enclosed systems. Although opportunities exist for release of liquid and vapor at a number of transfer points, exposures are controlled so that the likelihood of toxic reactions is negligible or nonexistent. Potentially hazardous exposures usually occur as a result of accidental spills and releases, improper containment, careless handling, inappropriate use, or intentional abuse. Obviously, education—perhaps assisted by additional regulation and enforcement—will have a major role in the further reduction of harmful exposures to gasoline.

REFERENCES

1. American Petroleum Institute. *Basic petroleum data book. Petroleum industry statistics.* Washington: American Petroleum Institute, 1996:16.
2. Energy Information Administration, Office of Energy Markets and End Use. *International energy annual 1993.* Washington: US Department of Energy, 1995.
3. Motor Vehicle Manufacturer's Association. *Motor vehicle facts and figures.* Detroit: Motor Vehicle Manufacturer's Association, 1994.
4. Domask WG. Introduction to petroleum hydrocarbons. Chemistry and composition in relation to petroleum-derived fuels and solvents. In: Mehlman MA, Hemstreet GP, Thrope JJ, Weaver NK, eds. *Renal effects of hydrocarbon toxicology,* vol. 7. Princeton, NJ: Princeton Scientific Publishers, 1984:1–27.
5. King RW. Petroleum: its composition, analysis and processing. In: Weaver NK, ed. *State of the art reviews: occupational medicine in the petroleum industry.* Philadelphia: Hanley & Belfus, 1988:409–431.
6. International Agency for Research on Cancer. Gasoline. Occupational exposures in petroleum refining: crude oil and major petroleum fuels. *IARC Monogr Eval Carcinog Risks Hum* 1989;45:159–201.
7. Maynard JB, Sanders WN. Determination of the detailed hydrocarbon composition and potential atmospheric reactivity of full range motor gasolines. *J Air Pollut Control Assoc* 1969;19:505–527.
8. Runion HE. Benzene in gasoline. *Am Ind Hyg Assoc J* 1975;36:338–350.
9. CONCAWE (developed by the Task Force on Exposure to Benzene). Exposure to atmospheric benzene vapor associated with motor gasoline. Report No. 2/81. Den Haag: The Oil Companies' International Study Group for Conservation of Clean Air and Water—Europe, 1981.
10. Bell HS. *American petroleum refining,* 3rd ed. New York: Van Nostrand, 1945.
11. Eckardt RE. Petroleum and petroleum products. In: Parmeggiani L, ed. *Encyclopaedia of occupational health and safety,* 3rd ed. Geneva: International Labour Office, 1983.

12. American Society for Testing and Materials. *Specifications for automotive gasoline. Annual book of ASTM standards*, vol. 05.01 (D439). Philadelphia: American Society for Testing and Materials, 1988.
13. Sawyer RF. Trends in auto emissions and gasoline composition: international symposium on the health effects of gasoline. *Environ Health Perspect* 1993:101(Suppl 6):5–12.
14. McDermott JH, Killiany SE. Quest for a gasoline TLV. *Am Ind Hyg Assoc J* 1978;39:110–117.
15. CONCAWE [developed by Special Task Force CH (STF-14)]. A survey of exposure to gasoline vapor. Report No. 4/87. Den Haag: The Oil Companies' International Study Group for Conservation of Clean Air and Water—Europe, 1981.
16. Anderson RO. *Fundamentals of the petroleum industry.* Norman, OK: University of Oklahoma Press, 1984.
17. Runion HE. Occupational exposures to potentially hazardous agents in the petroleum industry. In: Weaver NK, ed. *State of the art reviews: occupational medicine in the petroleum industry.* Philadelphia: Hanley & Belfus, 1988:409–431.
18. Rappaport SM, Selvin S, Waters MA. Exposures to hydrocarbon components of gasoline in the petroleum industry. *Appl Ind Hyg* 1987;2:148–154.
19. Weaver NK. Gasoline toxicology—implications for human health. In: Maltconi C, Selikoff IJ, eds. *Living in a chemical world. Occupational and environmental significance of industrial carcinogens,* vol 534. New York: New York Academy of Sciences, 1988.
20. Hartle R. Exposure to methyl tert-butyl ether and benzene among service station attendants and operators: international symposium on the health effects of gasoline. *Environ Health Perspect* 1993:101(Suppl 6):23–26.
21. Akland GG. Exposure of the general population to gasoline: international symposium on the health effects of gasoline. *Environ Health Perspect* 1993:101(Suppl 6):27–32.
22. Blank IH, McAuliffe DJ. Penetration of benzene through human skin. *J Invest Dermatol* 1985;85:522–526.
23. Franz TJ. *Absorption of petroleum products across the skin of monkey and man.* API MBSD res. publ. 32-32749. Washington: American Petroleum Institute, 1984.
24. Gerarde HW, Ahlstrom DB. Toxicologic studies on hydrocarbons. XI. Influence of dose on the metabolism of mono-*n*-alkyl derivatives of benzene. *Toxicol Appl Pharmacol* 1966;9:185–190.
25. Gerarde HW. *Toxicology and biochemistry of aromatic hydrocarbons.* Amsterdam: Elsevier Science, 1960.
26. International Program on Chemical Safety. *Environmental health criteria 20. Selected petroleum products.* Geneva: World Health Organization, 1982.
27. MacFarland HN, Ulrich CE, Holdsworth CE, et al. A chronic inhalation study with unleaded gasoline vapor. *J Am Coll Toxicol* 1984;3:231–248.
28. Scala RA. Motor gasoline toxicity. *Fundam Appl Toxicol* 1988;10:553–562.
29. Short BG, Swenberg JA. *Pathologic investigations of the mechanism of unleaded gasoline–induced renal tumors in rats,* vol 8. Research Triangle Park, NC: Chemical Industry Institute of Toxicology, 1988:1–6.
30. Garg BD, Olson MJ, Li LC, Roy AK. Phagolysosomal alterations induced by unleaded gasoline in epithelial cells of the proximal convoluted tubules of male rats: effect of dose and treatment duration. *J Toxicol Environ Health* 1989;26:101–118.
31. Machle W. Gasoline intoxication. *JAMA* 1941;117:1965–1971.
32. Drinker P, Yaglow CP, Warren MF. The threshold toxicity of gasoline vapor. *J Ind Hyg Toxicol* 1943;25:225–232.
33. Cole M, Herndon DN, Desai MH, Abston S. Gasoline explosions, gasoline sniffing: an epidemic in young adolescents. *J Burn Care Rehabil* 1986;7:532–534.
34. Davis A, Schafer LJ, Bell ZG. The effects on human volunteers of exposure to air containing gasoline vapor. *Arch Environ Health* 1960;1:548–554.
35. Reese E, Kimbrough RD. Acute toxicity of gasoline and some additives. *Environ Health Perspect* 1993:101(Suppl 6):115–132.
36. American Petroleum Institute. *Reproduction, teratogenesis (rat and mouse).* Report nos. 32-30329, 32-30326, 32-30237. Washington: American Petroleum Institute, 1984.
37. Agency for Toxic Substances and Disease Registry. *Toxicological profile for 1,2-dichloroethane.* Atlanta: US Department of Health and Human Services, Public Health Service, ATSDR, 1989.
38. Nouchi T, Miura H, Kanayama M, Mizuguchi O, Takano T. Fatal intoxication by 1,2-dichlorethane—a case report. *Int Arch Occup Environ Health* 1984;54:111–113.
39. Toxicology update. *Appl Toxicol* 1989;9:203–210.
40. Litovitz TL, Holm KC, Clancy C, Schmitz BF, Clark LR, Oderda GM. 1992 annual report of the American Association of Poison Control Centers National Data Collection System. *Am J Emerg Med* 1993;11:494–555.
41. Litovitz TL, Clark LR, Soloway RA. 1993 annual report of the American Association of Poison Control Centers National Data Collection System. *Am J Emerg Med* 1994;12:546–84.
42. Litovitz TL, Felberg L, Soloway RA, Ford M, Geller R. 1994 annual report of the American Association of Poison Control Centers National Data Collection System. *Am J Emerg Med* 1995;13:551–97.
43. Litovitz TL. Myocardial sensitization following inhalation abuse of hydrocarbons. In: Weaver NK, ed. *State of the art reviews: occupational medicine in the petroleum industry.* Philadelphia: Hanley & Belfus, 1988:567–568.
44. Watson JM. Solvent abuse by children and young adults: a review. *Br J Addict* 1980;75:27–36.
45. Fortenberry JD. Gasoline sniffing [Review]. *Am J Med* 1985;79:740–744.
46. Edminster SC, Bayer MJ. Recreational gasoline sniffing: acute gasoline intoxication and latent organic lead poisoning. *J Emerg Med* 1985;3:365–370.
47. Coulehan JL, Hirsch W, Brillman J, et al. Gasoline sniffing and lead toxicity in Navajo adolescents. *Pediatrics* 1983;71:113–117.
48. Schwartz WK. Gasoline ingestion [Letter]. *JAMA* 1979;242:1968–1969.
49. Lacouture P, McGuigan M, Lovejoy FH. Gasoline ingestion after the great blizzard [Letter]. *N Engl J Med* 1978;298:1037.
50. Banner W, Walson PD. Systemic toxicity following gasoline aspirations. *Am J Emerg Med* 1983;3:292–294.
51. Stockman JA. More on hydrocarbon-induced hemolysis [Letter]. *J Pediatr* 1977;90:848.
52. Simpson LA, Cruse CW. Gasoline immersion injury. *Plast Reconstr Surg* 1981;67:54–57.
53. Hansbrough JF, Zapata-Sirvent R, Dominic W, et al. Hydrocarbon contact injuries. *J Trauma* 1985;25:250–252.
54. Viau C, Bernard A, Lauwerys R, et al. A cross-sectional survey of kidney function in refinery employees. *Am J Ind Med* 1987;11:177–187.
55. Phillips SC, Petrone RL, Hemstreet GP. A review of the non-neoplastic kidney effects of hydrocarbon exposures in humans. In: Weaver NK, ed. *State of the art reviews: occupational medicine in the petroleum industry.* Philadelphia: Hanley & Belfus, 1988:495–510.
56. Savitz DA, Moure R. Cancer risk among oil refinery workers: a review of epidemiologic studies. *J Occup Med* 1984;26:662–670.
57. Harrington JM. Health experience of workers in the petroleum manufacturing and distribution industry: a review of the literature. *Am J Ind Med* 1987;12:475–497.
58. Delzell E, Austin H, Cole P. Epidemiologic studies in the petroleum industry. In: Weaver HK, ed. *State of the art reviews: occupational medicine in the petroleum industry.* Philadelphia: Hanley & Belfus, 1988:455–474.
59. Wong O, Raabe GK. Critical review of cancer epidemiology in petroleum industry employees with a quantitative meta-analysis by cancer site. *Am J Ind Med* 1989;15:283–310.
60. American Petroleum Institute. *A mortality study of marketing and marine distribution workers with potential exposure to gasoline in the petroleum industry.* Publ. no. 4555. Washington: American Petroleum Institute, 1992.
61. Wong O, Trent L. *A nested case-control study of kidney cancer, leukemia, and multiple myeloma in a cohort of land-based terminal workers exposed to gasoline in the petroleum industry.* Publ. no. 45551. Washington: American Petroleum Institute, 1994.
62. CONCAWE [developed by Analytical Working Group of the Special Task Force on Gasoline Vapor Exposure (H/STF-14)]. Method for monitoring exposure to gasoline vapor in air. Report no. 8/86. Den Haag: The Oil Companies' International Study Group for Conservation of Clean Air and Water—Europe, 1986.
63. American Conference of Governmental Industrial Hygienists. *Threshold limit values and biological exposure indices for 1990–91.* Cincinnati: American Conference of Governmental Industrial Hygienists, 1990:25.
64. US Department of Labor, Occupational Safety and Health Administration. Air contaminants: final rule. *Federal Register* 1989 Jan 15;54:2332–2983.

CHAPTER 68
Crude Oil

Charles E. Lambert, Donald M. Molenaar, Charles R. Clark, and Jill Ryer-Powder

Crude oil, a naturally occurring mixture, is one of the world's most important raw materials owing to its position as a major source of the world's energy and the main feed stock for the petrochemical industry (1,2). Worldwide production of crude oil has been estimated at approximately 60 million barrels per day (3–5). Most of this production is transported to oil refineries, where it is used as feed stock.

CHEMICAL CHARACTERISTICS AND COMPOSITION

Crude oil is basically the remains of prehistoric plants and animals deposited in the sediments of ancient swamps, lakes, and oceans. Over the millennia, these organic-rich sediments have been buried and subjected to high temperatures and pressures. These processes serve to transform the biogenic components of the sediments into a complex mixture of hydrocarbons referred

TABLE 68-1. Crude oil classification

Crude type	Description
Sour crude	Likely to have high sulfur content
Sweet crude	Likely to have low sulfur content
Paraffinic base	Large number of straight chain hydrocarbons
Cycloparaffinic base (naphthenic)	Large concentration of saturated rings with side chains predominating
Aromatic base	Large concentration of aromatic compounds
Mixed base	No major type predominating

to as *crude oil* (6). Crude oil composition can vary widely from one deposit to another. Depending on the source, varying amounts of sulfur, nitrogen, oxygen, and trace amounts of metals such as vanadium and nickel can also be incorporated into these compounds.

At a molecular level, crude oil is composed primarily of varying amounts of straight and branched-chain paraffins, cycloparaffins, and monocyclic and polycyclic aromatic hydrocarbons. *Paraffins* are defined as having saturated carbon-hydrogen bonds and can be present as linear nonbranched compounds, linear branched compounds, and cyclic branched compounds. The cycloparaffins are also known as *naphthenic compounds*. Aromatic compounds are those containing at least one benzene ring. Whereas some of these compounds contain a single benzene ring (e.g., alkylbenzenes), others contain two benzene rings (naphthalene derivatives) or polycyclic or polynuclear aromatic hydrocarbons, which contain multiple fused benzene rings (e.g., chrysene, benzopyrene). The aromatic compounds can contain varying amounts of nitrogen (e.g., indoles and quinolines), oxygen (e.g., benzofuran), and sulfur (e.g., benzothiophene, dibenzothiophene), which can greatly influence the reactivity and toxicity of the compound.

As might be expected from such a complex mixture, the distribution of carbon compounds in crude oil is very broad. The carbon number (i.e., number of carbon atoms in the compound) of hydrocarbons found in crude oil ranges from 1 to more than 50 (7). Gary (8) proposes a general elemental composition of crude oil of 84% to 87% carbon, 11% to 14% hydrogen, 0% to 3% sulfur, and 0.2% nitrogen. Focusing on the aromatic compounds, the International Agency for Research on Cancer (IARC) states that the benzene composition of various crude oils ranges from 0.01% to 1.00% and of polycyclic aromatic hydrocarbons from 0.2% to 7.0%. As noted earlier, metals such as nickel, vanadium, iron, lead, and copper may also be present in crude oil but at much lower concentrations than that of benzene [generally only a few parts per million (ppm)] (9). Physicochemical parameters of crude oil also vary depending on the specific source of the crude oil. For example, crude oil boils in the temperature range of 0° to more than 1,000°C and has flash points in the range of –7° to –31°C.

TABLE 68-2. Typical levels of various compounds in crude oils

Type of crude oil	Typical composition of 250–300°F fraction				
	% Paraffins	% Naphthenes	% Aromatics	% Wax	% Asphalt
Paraffinic	45–60	20–30	15–25	1–10	0–5
Naphthenic	15–25	65–75	10	Trace	0–5
Aromatic	5	60–75	20–25	0–0.5	0–20

TABLE 68-3. Physical characteristics of crude oil

Characteristic	Description
Color	Red, brown, or black
Viscosity	From fluid as water to tarlike
Odor	From nil to rotten egg
Pour point	0° to 100°F (–17° to 38°C)
Gravity	<10 to >50 API gravity; 0.8 to 1.0 specific gravity

API, American Petroleum Institute.

Crude oils can be classified according to their hydrocarbon and sulfur content. Table 68-1 presents a description of each of the crude oil classifications. The typical levels of various compounds in crude oils is presented in Table 68-2.

Crude oils vary widely in appearance and consistency depending on their source, owing to the various numbers and proportions of molecular types, the arrangement of molecules, and the size of hydrocarbons. Crude oils range from yellowish brown, mobile liquids to black, viscous semisolids (10). The hydrocarbons in crude oil may be gaseous, liquid, or solid, under normal conditions of temperature and pressure (10). Generally, at ambient temperatures, compounds with molecules containing up to 4 carbon atoms are gaseous, those with 5 to 20 carbon atoms are liquid, and those with more than 20 carbon atoms are solid (10). The gaseous and solid compounds are dissolved in the liquid fraction of crude oil (10). The nature of the crude oil governs the nature of the products that can be manufactured from it and their suitability for special applications (10). For example, a naphthenic crude oil will be more suitable for the production of tar for roadways, whereas a paraffinic crude oil will be better suited for wax. A naphthenic crude oil can yield lubricating oils with viscosities that are sensitive to temperature (10). Table 68-3 presents the physical characteristics of crude oil.

EVALUATION OF PHYSICAL AND CHEMICAL CHARACTERISTICS

Evaluation of crude oils as feed stock for particular refineries is accomplished using relatively simple analytic tests. Each crude oil is compared with other available feed stocks on the basis of the following characteristics (8):

- *Gravity, American Petroleum Institute (API)*: The density of petroleum oils is expressed in terms of API gravity rather than specific gravity. It is related to specific gravity in such a fashion that an increase in API gravity corresponds to a decrease in specific gravity. Crude oil gravity may range from less than 10 API to more than 50 API. API gravity always refers to the liquid sample at 60°F (15.6°C) (8).
- *Sulfur content*: The value of crude oil is influenced to the greatest extent by API gravity and sulfur content. Sulfur content varies from less than 0.1% to greater than 5.0%. The term *sour crude* refers to a crude with high sulfur content, whereas *sweet crude* refers to a crude with low (0.5%) sulfur content (8).
- *Pour point*: The pour point, expressed in degrees Fahrenheit, indicates the point at which the crude oil stops flowing. This point indicates the relative paraffinicity and aromaticity of the crude. The lower the pour point, the lower is the paraffin content and the greater is the content of aromatics (8).
- *Carbon residue*: The carbon residue value indicates the asphalt content of the crude and the quantity of the lubricating oil fraction that can be recovered. It is determined by distillation

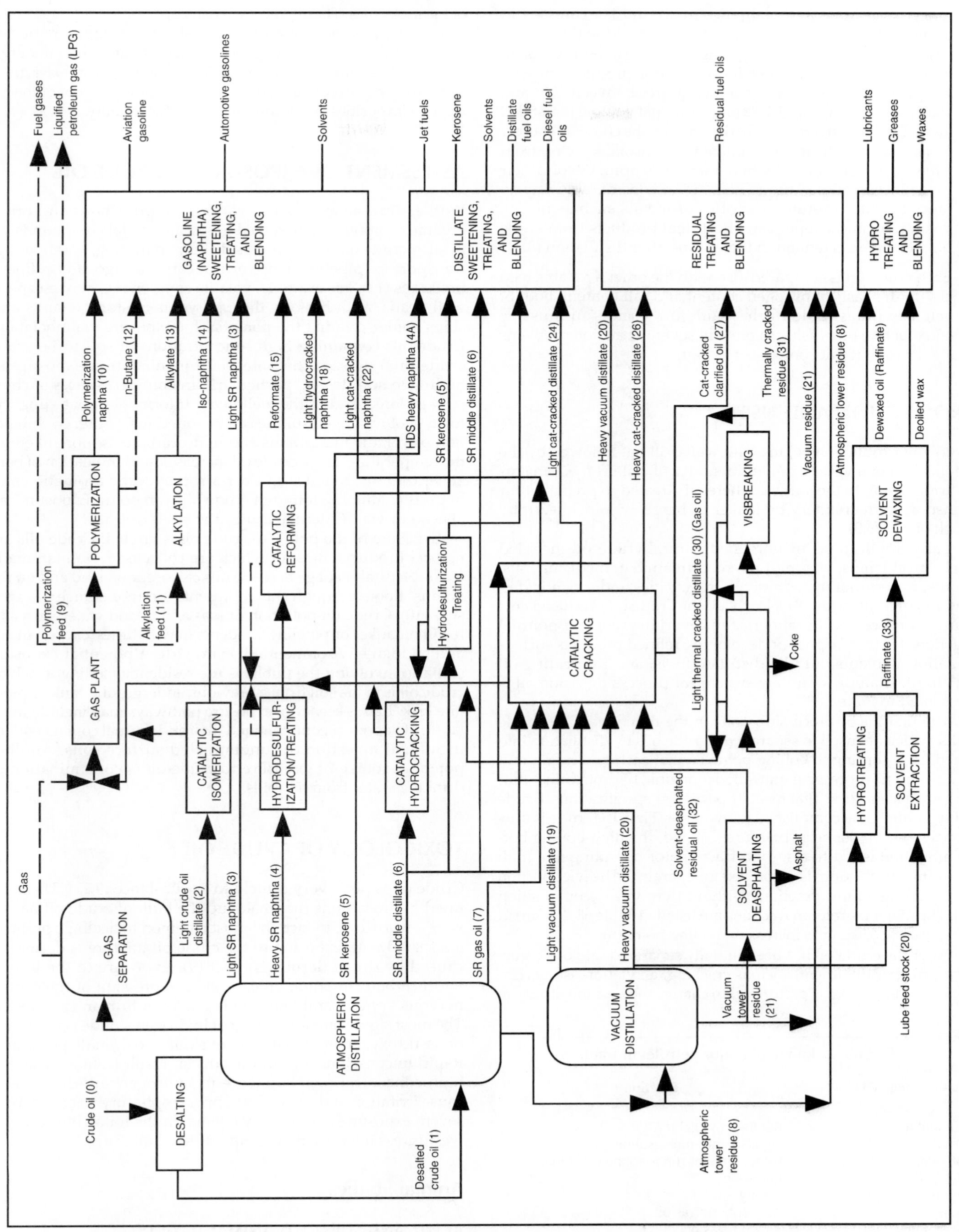

Figure 68-1. Flow system for processing crude oil. The numbers in parentheses represent the sequential steps in crude oil processing. Lt, light; HDS, hydrodesulfurization; Hvy, heavy; SR, straight run. (Reproduced from US Department of Labor, Occupational Health and Safety Administration, OSHA instruction TED 1.15 CH-1. May 24, 1996. Washington: Office of Science and Technology Assessment, 1996.)

to a coke residue in the absence of air and is expressed in terms of the weight percentage of carbon residue (11).

- *Distillation range*: The boiling range of the crude provides an indication of the quantities of the various products present. When crude oil is heated to temperatures between 200° and 450°F, between 20% and 40% of the original volume is distilled away. Distillation fraction size depends on the crude oil source.
- *Metals content*: The metals content of crude oils can vary from a few parts per million to more than 1,000 ppm. Despite their low concentrations, the metals are of considerable importance because minute quantities of metals such as nickel, vanadium, and copper can affect final products from crude oil. Most metals remain in the residue after distillation (8).

Each crude oil is compared also with the other available feed stocks on the basis of nitrogen content and salt content, both of which are undesirable in the crude oil. Crude oil must be desalted before processing to prevent severe corrosion problems that will result if salt content is too high.

PRODUCTION AND USE

Crude oil production begins with well drilling, followed by the application of a variety of natural and artificial lift mechanisms to bring the oil to the surface. There it is treated to prepare it for transport to the refinery by tanker or barge, by pipeline, or by truck or rail (6,9).

Early applications of unrefined natural crude oil included fuel for oil lamps, heating fuel, road treatment, medicinal oils, paints, waterproofing, adhesives, insecticides and rodenticides, and tool manufacture (9). Nearly all the crude oil produced currently is processed in refineries into various fuel and nonfuel fractions for the purpose of developing refined products such as gasoline, solvents, middle distillate fuels, and lubricating oil (9,10). An example of a flow system for processing crude oil is presented in Figure 68-1.

The first major processing units in the refinery are the crude stills, which are used to separate the crude oils by distillation into fractions according to boiling point, so that each processing unit (e.g., catalytic processing unit, alkylation unit, hydrotreating unit) will have feed stocks that meet its particular specifications. Crude oil separation is accomplished in two steps. First, the crude is fractionated at atmospheric pressure. Second, the high-boiling bottom fraction is fed to a second fractionator operating at a high vacuum. The vacuum is employed to separate the heavier portion of the crude oil into fractions without pyrolytic decomposition (8). The major petroleum fractions are listed in Table 68-4 in broad categories according to increasing boiling point (8).

After the crude oil has been initially separated into basic fractions, further treatment, such as cracking, alkylation, isomerization, and reforming, is performed to change the size and structure of the molecules. These process usually are carried out to produce solvent streams and to improve the yield and octane of hydrocarbons useful in gasoline. These converted streams then undergo additional treatment and separation processes, such as extraction, hydrotreating, sweetening, dewaxing, and physical separation, to remove impurities and improve the product quality.

TABLE 68-4. Range of major petroleum fractions

Boiling range (°F)	Fraction
Ambient temp	Butanes and lighter
90–220	Light straight-run gasoline
180–400	Heavy straight-run gasoline (naphtha)
330–540	Kerosene
420–640	Light gas oil
550–830	Atmospheric gas oil
750–1,050	Vacuum gas oil
>1,000	Vacuum-reduced crude

ASSESSMENT OF EXPOSURE TO CRUDE OIL

Workers can be exposed to various hydrocarbons and other organic compounds, dissolved gases, and metal compounds (9) in such crude oil operations as drilling, pumping, and treating; transport by pipeline, ship, or rail cars; storage; and refinery processes (12). For example, volatile components may escape at well heads, at pumps, or through vents in storage tanks and ships' tanks, creating the potential for exposure via inhalation. Crude oils containing high concentrations of sulfur (i.e., sour crude oils) present the potential for inhalation exposure to hydrogen sulfide gas, particularly in confined spaces such as storage tanks and at the well head. Information regarding the toxicity of hydrogen sulfide can be found in Chapter 55. Inhalation of volatile mercaptans and hydrocarbons is more likely as the temperature of the crude oil increases, and inhalation of benzene, toluene, xylene, and certain polycyclic aromatic compounds commonly found in crude oils can occur. Exposure can also occur via the dermal route after spills or leaks.

Exposure of the public to crude oil is limited. Crude oils are natural products, most of which are collected from man-made wells. Natural seepage of crude oils can occur on land and on the oceans' floor, although this represents a minor source of exposure (10). Crude oil pollution of seas and inland waterways as a result of tanker or pipeline accidents may, at times, cause a major and sudden environmental hazard (10). A potential exposure scenario involving the public is the residential setting in which crude oil is in the soil from a previous underground tank or pipeline leak. In this scenario, exposure pathways may include inhalation of vapors or contaminated dust and dermal contact with or incidental ingestion of contaminated surface soils. Another potential source of exposure to crude oil is contamination of drinking water from oil spills.

TOXICOLOGY OF CRUDE OIL

Crude oil is not a very acutely toxic substance (9,13). The saturated hydrocarbons that make up the bulk of crude oil have a very low toxicity. In fact, the most common toxicologic problem associated with exposure to the crude oil mixture is dermatitis caused by direct dermal contact (9). Exposure to the lighter hydrocarbons in crude oil can cause depression of the central nervous system, and benzene is a known human carcinogen. The most significant toxic effect of hydrogen sulfide is inhibition of tissue oxygenation in a manner similar to cyanide poisoning. Rapid unconsciousness and death can result from exposure to high concentrations. Exposure to hydrogen sulfide can also cause irritation of the eyes and upper respiratory tract and, with severe exposures, pulmonary edema. In the following sections, we address the toxicity data for crude oil mixtures.

Animal Studies

ACUTE AND SUBACUTE ANIMAL TOXICITY

The toxicity of crude oil has been examined in laboratory animals in a number of acute oral and dermal studies. Acute expo-

TABLE 68-5. Summary of crude oil carcinogenicity studies in laboratory animals

Animal	Dose regimen	Effects	Reference
Mice	Two crude oils (differing in hydrocarbon character, nonhydrocarbon type, and use for end products), 50 mg applied to back 2 times weekly for 80 wk	Skin tumor development in 20–38% of mice	(25)
Mice	Crude oil, 25 mg applied to back 3 times weekly for 21 wk	Squamous cell carcinoma in 84% of mice; fibrosarcoma in 54% of mice	(20)
Mice	Paraffinic-asphaltic base, naphthenic, or another (unspecified) crude, 0.2 mL applied to skin for 52 wk	Skin tumor yield between 0% and 5%	(22, as cited in 9)
Mice	Crude oil applied to skin 3 times weekly for 6 mo, then 2 times weekly for life	Papilloma development in 10% of mice	(5, as cited in 9)
Mice	In 3 groups of 30 mice, skin application 2 times weekly for 10 mo	No squamous cell tumors observed; skin angiosarcoma development in 2 mice	(27, as cited in 9)
Mice	Crude oil, 3, 6, 12, or 25 mg applied to shaved skin 2 times weekly for 30 wk	No skin tumors	(23, as cited in 9)
Mice	Composite petroleum sample, 25 mg applied to shaved skin 3 times weekly for 22 wk	No skin tumors	(23, as cited in 9)
Mice	Composite petroleum sample, 0, 0.08, 0.3, 0.4, or 2.0 mg applied to shaved skin 3 times weekly for 24 mo	Skin carcinoma development in 4 of the mice treated with highest dose	(23, as cited in 9)
Mice	Two types of crude oil, 50 µL applied to clipped dorsal skin 2–3 times weekly (duration not specified)	No skin tumors	(19, as cited in 9)
Mice	Crude oil, 0.08, 0.3, 0.4, or 2.0 mg applied to shaved skin 3 times weekly for 24 mo	No skin tumors	(24, as cited in 9)
Mice	Two types of crude oil, 50 mg applied to skin 2 times weekly for 80 wk	Squamous cell tumor development in 38% of animals treated with paraffinic oil; skin tumor development in 20% of animals treated with naphthenic crude	(21, as cited in 9)
Mice	Crude oil, 50 mg applied to skin 2 times weekly for 80 wk	Tumor incidence 20%	(21, as cited in 9)
Mice	Crude oil, 5 mg applied to skin 3 times weekly for 78 wk	Skin tumor development in 92% of animals	(21, as cited in 9)
Mice	Crude oil, 2.5- and 5.0-mg applications to skin 3 times weekly for life	Tumor development	(28)
Mice	Crude oil, 0.17, 1.7, and 16.8 mg applied to back 3 times weekly for life	Skin tumor development in 0%, 20%, and 78% of animals, respectively	(26)
Rabbits	Three types of crude oil, 0.3 mL applied to skin 2 times weekly for 52 wk	Skin tumor development in 2 of 30 rabbits	(22, as cited in 9)
Rabbits	Crude oil, applied 3 times weekly to surface of one ear for 6 mo followed by 2 times weekly for life	Papilloma development in 6 of 8 rabbits and tumor development in 1 rabbit	(5, as cited in 9)
Rabbits	Crude oil, applied to skin 3 times weekly for 10–17 mo	Papilloma development	(27, as cited in 9)

sure to high concentrations of crude oil via the oral route can cause gastrointestinal, liver, and kidney effects and irritation (11,14,15). Dermal and oral lethal dose tests have demonstrated a low order of toxicity to mice, rats, and rabbits (median lethal dose greater than 5 g per kg) (16).

REPRODUCTIVE SYSTEM AND DEVELOPMENTAL STUDIES

Reproductive system and developmental studies have been conducted in rats. In a study by Kahn et al. (17), administration of (i) 5 mL per kg of crude oil on gestation day 3, 6, 11, 15, or 17, or (ii) 1 or 2 mL per kg daily on gestation days 6 through 16, or (iii) 2 to 10 mL per kg on gestation day 6 resulted in an increased number of resorptions and decreased fetal weight and length as well as decreased maternal body weight. A dose of 5 mL per kg to pregnant rats on gestation day 11, 15, or 17 resulted in induction of placental and fetal hepatic enzyme systems (18). These effects are seen only at doses that are maternally toxic. No developmental abnormalities have been reported from exposure to crude oil.

CHRONIC TOXICITY TO ANIMALS

Crude oil has not been evaluated in chronic studies in animals by routes other than dermal. Dermal carcinogenesis studies in mice, cited by the IARC, did not provide adequate details for a complete carcinogenicity evaluation and are classified as "limited" (9). The IARC has rated the human evidence as "inadequate," leading to an overall evaluation that crude oil is "not classifiable as to its carcinogenicity to humans" (9).

Table 68-5 provides a summary of the crude oil carcinogenicity studies performed in laboratory animals (5,9,19–28). It is evident from the table that the incidence and prevalence of tumors differ between studies. Most likely, this is the result of the use of different sources of crude oil and the concentration and duration of exposure.

Human Studies

ACUTE AND SUBACUTE HUMAN TOXICITY

The major acute effect of crude oil on humans is depression of the central nervous system from inhalation of the lighter, more volatile hydrocarbons contained in crude oil. This effect is reversible after cessation of exposure, even at high concentrations. Dermal contact may result in skin irritation (9).

CHRONIC HUMAN HEALTH EFFECTS

Information on chronic human health effects from exposure to crude oil is available only from epidemiologic studies of occupationally exposed individuals. These studies have focused mainly on refinery workers; very few studies have focused specifically on humans' exposure to crude oil. Studies of refinery workers may not be appropriate to assess risk from exposure to crude oil because refinery workers may be exposed to many products and chemicals used in the refinery process. Prolonged exposure of workers in oil fields resulted in obvious adverse effects on the skin, such as dermatitis and hyperpigmentation,

TABLE 68-6. Summary of epidemiology studies involving exposure to crude oil

Protocol	Results	Reference
Case-control study for men employed in oil industry	An elevated risk for lung cancer was found for black men more than 53 years old who had been employed in petroleum exploration and production. The ratio associated with crude oil exploration and drilling was threefold among persons older than 62 years (no information on cigarette smoking).	(30, as cited in 9)
Case-control study for men employed in oil industry (reanalysis of risk of lung cancer in relation to work in petroleum mining and refining industry)	OR for lung cancer associated with employment in petroleum industry was 1.2. OR for welders, operators, boiler makers, painters, and oil-field workers was 2.3 (no information on cigarette smoking).	(31, as cited in 9)
Case-control study of 347 hospital patients with germ cell tumor of the testis—petroleum and natural gas extraction workers	OR for testicular cancer and petroleum and gas workers was 2.3 (i.e., excess risk for testicular cancer was observed).	(32)
Case-control study of 81 cases of testicular cancer and petroleum and natural gas extraction workers	No excess risk for testicular cancer was found (OR, 0.5).	(33)
Population-based case-control study for male cancer patients with known occupational exposure to petroleum hydrocarbons	A moderate to strong statistical association with rectal (OR, 3.7) and squamous cell lung cancers (OR, 3.5) was found.	(34)
Case-control study of oil-field workers	Increased risk of myelogenous leukemia was found among oil and gas production workers.	(35)

OR, odds ratio.

perhaps confounded by overexposure to sunlight (29, as cited in ref. 10). Those epidemiologic studies that have examined the relationship between crude oil exposure and cancer present conflicting results (Table 68-6) (30–35). For example, the finding of testicular cancer in one study (32) was not confirmed in another study (33). In a study citing lung cancer as an effect related to exposure to crude oil (30, as cited in ref. 9), the researchers failed to control for subjects' smoking practices.

The IARC has evaluated the human epidemiologic data for cancer and, as previously discussed, determined that there is "inadequate evidence" for carcinogenicity of crude oil in humans. Given this evaluation of the human evidence, in conjunction with the IARC's limited evaluation of animal evidence, overall crude oil cannot be classified as to its carcinogenicity to humans (group 3). A summary of the epidemiologic studies cited by the IARC (9) and available in the literature is presented in Table 68-6.

ABSORPTION, DISTRIBUTION, METABOLISM, AND EXCRETION

Consideration of the chemical and physical properties of crude oil permits some understanding of its absorption. The volatile compounds will enter the body primarily by inhalation. Lung absorption will be governed mainly by the air-blood partition coefficients of these materials. Absorption of the low-volatility to nonvolatile components will occur mainly after ingestion in the digestive system, with very high-molecular-weight species passing through unchanged.

The metabolism of some of the components of crude oil has been studied extensively. These materials are oxidized via oxidative transformation. The majority of these reactions are catalyzed by monooxygenase enzymes of the P-450 family and increase water solubility by hydroxylation for excretion through the kidneys. Some of the metabolic products can enter the body's energy cycles after further metabolism (36).

Compounds may be excreted in urine after metabolism or, if volatile, in exhaled air as the parent compound after cessation of exposure. Very high-molecular-weight compounds are eliminated in the feces after passing through the digestive system.

ENVIRONMENTAL TOXICOLOGY

It is beyond the scope of this chapter to provide a detailed assessment of all the environmental issues associated with crude oil. When crude oil is released to water, the more volatile hydrocarbons can evaporate quickly. The heavier components of crude oils can sink and move below the surface or along the bottom of the water body. The movement of water can create an emulsion of the water and oil. Oil remaining on the surface of the water eventually forms tar balls or patches of surface oil that drift ashore or break up into small pieces and sink to the bottom (1).

On exposure to air, water, or sunlight, crude oil can change composition. Approximately 10% of crude oil evaporates. Less than 5% of crude oil dissolves in water. Hydrocarbons exposed to sunlight can be converted to polar oxidized compounds (1). Crude oil is also degraded by microbial metabolism.

Crude oil can affect plants and animals by physical contact with the plant or animal, by toxic effects, and through habitat destruction. The toxicity of crude oil to animals is believed to be due both to the lighter and more soluble hydrocarbons and the polycyclic aromatic hydrocarbons.

GUIDELINES, STANDARDS, AND OCCUPATIONAL SAFETY

Currently, no federal or state regulatory occupational or public health standards exist for crude oil. However, as crude oil is processed and refined, many of the resulting products are controlled by existing federal or state standards and criteria. At least 30 states have set specific soil cleanup levels or guidelines based on the total petroleum hydrocarbon (TPH) measurement (37). These levels or guidelines are set independently of or in combination with standards for benzene, toluene, ethylbenzene, and xylenes or polynuclear aromatic hydrocarbons. The levels range from background to 10,000 ppm TPH in soil (38). Many states have adopted a level of 100 ppm TPH in soil (38). Neither the American Conference of Government Industrial Hygienists nor the Occupational Safety and Health Administration has developed an occupational exposure limit for crude oil.

Adherence to health and safety precautions is important for anyone working with petroleum hydrocarbons. The potential for fire exists where flammable vapors from spills or releases can reach a source of ignition. Gloves and protective eyewear should be worn for dermal and eye protection (7). When there is the potential for exposure to hydrogen sulfide gas or to high concentrations of vapor or mist (e.g., in the head space of storage vessels), respirators should be worn. Hard hats should always be worn in the refinery area. In operations involving exposure to crude oil, industrial hygienists typically monitor for benzene, toluene, xylene, hydrogen sulfide, and total hydrocarbons.

REFERENCES

1. Albers PH. The effects of petroleum on different stages of incubation in bird eggs. *Bull Environ Contam Toxicol* 1978;19:624–630.
2. American Petroleum Institute. *Facts about oil*. Washington: American Petroleum Institute, 1984:8–9.
3. American Petroleum Institute. *Basic petroleum data book: petroleum industry statistics*, vol 7, no. 3. Washington: American Petroleum Institute, 1987.
4. Anderson RO. *Fundamentals of the petroleum industry*. Norman, OK: University of Oklahoma Press, 1984.
5. Antonov AM, Lints AM. The blastomogenic action of natural Saratov oil. *Probl Oncol* 1960;6:1629–1634.
6. Baker AM, Baker R, Cyrus C, et al. Production. In: Gerding M, ed. *Fundamentals of petroleum*, 3rd ed. Austin, TX: Petroleum Extension Service, 1986:176–245.
7. Clayton GD, Clayton FE. *Patty's industrial hygiene and toxicology*, vol 2B, 4th ed. New York: John Wiley and Sons, 1994.
8. Gary JH, Handwerk G. *Petroleum refining technology and economics*, 2nd ed. New York: Marcel Dekker Inc, 1984:16.
9. International Agency for Research on Cancer. Occupational exposures in petroleum refining: crude oil and major petroleum fuels. *IARC Monogr Eval Carcinog Risks Hum* 1989;45:159–201.
10. World Health Organization. *Environmental health criteria 20: selected petroleum products*. Geneva: World Health Organization, 1982.
11. Khan S, Irfan M, Rahimtula AD. The hepatotoxic potential of a Prudhoe Bay crude oil: effect on mouse liver weight and composition. *Toxicology* 1987: 46:95–105.
12. Suess MJ, Grefen K, Reinisch DW, eds. *Ambient air pollutants from industrial sources*. Amsterdam: Elsevier Science, 1985:279–282.
13. Beck LS, Hepler DI, Hansen KL. The acute toxicology of selected petroleum hydrocarbons. In: MacFarland HN, Holdsworth CE, MacGregor JA, Call RW, Lane ML, eds. *Advances in modern environmental toxicology: Vol 6. Applied toxicology of petroleum hydrocarbons*. Princeton, NJ: Princeton Scientific Publishers, 1984:1–16.
14. Khan S, Rahman SM, Payne JF, Rahimtula AD. Mechanisms of petroleum hydrocarbon toxicity: studies of the response of rat liver mitochondria to Prudhoe Bay crude oil and its aliphatic, aromatic, and heterocyclic fractions. *Toxicology* 1986:42:131–142.
15. Khan S, Payne JF, Rahimtula AD. Mechanisms of petroleum hydrocarbon toxicity: destruction of liver microsomal and mitochondrial calcium pump activities by Prudhoe Bay crude oil. *J Biochem Toxicol* 1986:1:31–43.
16. Stubblefield WA, McKee RH, Kapp RW Jr, Hinz JP. An evaluation of the acute toxic properties of liquids derived from oil sands. *J Appl Toxicol* 1989;9:59–65.
17. Khan S, Martin M, Rahimtula AD, Payne JF. Effect of a Prudhoe Bay crude oil on hepatic and placental drug metabolism in rats. *Can J Physiol Pharmacol* 1987;65:2400–2408.
18. Khan S, Martin M, Payne JF, Rahimtula AD. Embryotoxic evaluation of a Prudhoe Bay crude oil in rats. *Toxicol Lett* 1987;38:109–114.
19. Bingham E, Barkley W. Bioassay of complex mixtures derived from fossil fuels. *Environ Health Perspect* 1979;30:157–163.
20. Clark CR, Walter MK, Ferguson PW, Katchen M. Comparative dermal carcinogenesis of shale and petroleum-derived distillates. *Toxicol Ind Health* 1988;4:11–22.
21. Coomes RM, Hazer KA. Statistical analyses of crude oil and shale oil carcinogenic test data. In: MacFarland HN, Holdsworth CE, MacGregor JA, Call RW, Lane ML, eds. *Advances in modern environmental toxicology: vol 6. Applied toxicology of petroleum hydrocarbons*. Princeton, NJ: Princeton Scientific Publishers, 1984:167–186.
22. Hieger I, Woodhouse DL. The value of the rabbit for carcinogenicity tests on petroleum fractions. *Br J Cancer* 1952;6:293–299.
23. Holland JM, Rahn RO, Smith LH, Clark BR, Chang SS, Stephens TJ. Skin carcinogenicity of synthetic and natural petroleums. *J Occup Med* 1979;21:614–618.
24. Holland JM, Wolf DA, Clark BR. Relative potency estimation for synthetic petroleum skin carcinogens. *Environ Health Perspect* 1981;38:149–155.
25. Lewis SC, King RW, Cragg ST, Hillman DW. Skin carcinogenic potential of petroleum hydrocarbons: crude oil, distillate fractions, and chemical class subfractions. In: MacFarland HN, Holdsworth CE, MacGregor JA, Call RW, Lane ML, eds. *Advances in modern environmental toxicology: Vol 6. Applied toxicology of petroleum hydrocarbons*. Princeton, NJ: Princeton Scientific Publishers, 1984:139–150.
26. Renne RA, Smith LG, Tolley HD. *Health effects of synthetic fuels. Pacific Northwest Laboratory annual report for 1981 to the DOE Office of Energy Research*. Richland, WA: Pacific Northwest Laboratory, 1982.
27. Shapiro DD, Getmanets IY. Blasomeogenic properties of petroleum of different sources [in Russian]. *Gig Sanit* 1962;27:38–42.
28. Wilson JS, Holland LM. Periodic response difference in mouse epidermis chronically exposed to crude oils or BaP: males vs. females. *Toxicology* 1988;50:83–94.
29. Schwartz L, Julipan L, Peck S. Dermatoses caused by petroleum. In: *Occupational diseases of the skin*, 2nd ed. London: Kimpton, 1947:232–258.
30. Gottlieb MS, Pickle LW, Blot WJ, Fraumeni JF Jr. Lung cancer in Louisiana: death certificate analysis. *J Natl Cancer Inst* 1979;63:1131–1137.
31. Gottlieb MS. Lung cancer and the petroleum industry in Louisiana. *J Occup Med* 1980;22:384–388.
32. Mills PK, Newell GR, Johnson DE. Testicular cancer associated with employment agriculture and oil and natural gas extraction. *Lancet* 1984;1:207–210.
33. Sewell CM, Castle SP, Hull HJ, Wiggins C. Testicular cancer and employment in agriculture and oil and natural gas extraction. *Lancet* 1986;1:553.
34. Siemiatycki J, Dewar R, Nadon L, Gerin M, Richardson L, Wacholder S. Associations between several sites of cancer and twelve petroleum-derived liquids: results from a case-referent study in Montreal. *Scand J Work Environ Health* 1987;13:493–504.
35. Sathiakumar N, Delzell E, Cole P, Brill I, Frisch J, Spivey G. A case control study of leukemia among petroleum workers. *J Occup Environ Med* 1995;37:1269–1277.
36. Timbrell JA. *Principles of biochemical toxicology*. London: Taylor and Francis, 1982.
37. Oliver T, Kostecki P. State by state summary of cleanup standards. *Soils* 1992:14–24.
38. Michelsen T, Boyce CP. Cleanup standards for petroleum hydrocarbons: Part 1. Review of methods and recent developments. *J Soil Contamination* 1993;2:109–124.

CHAPTER 69
Middle Distillates and Residual Fuels

Charles R. Clark, Jill Ryer-Powder, Charles E. Lambert, and Donald M. Molenaar

Middle distillates are petroleum products used to fuel many types of engines, lamps, heaters, furnaces, and stoves, and used as solvents (1). These distillates represent the fraction of crude oil that boils in the middle range. They are distinguished from one another primarily by their boiling-point ranges, chemical additives, and uses. Examples of middle distillates include kerosene, home heating oil, most diesel fuels, and jet fuel. Residual fuels generally are the heavier fraction in the distillation process that produces the middle distillates; therefore, they boil at a higher temperature than do middle distillates. Some examples of residual fuels include marine diesel fuel (MDF) and bunker fuel. Because of the differences in their composition, middle distillates and residual fuels are discussed separately in this chapter.

MIDDLE DISTILLATE FUEL PRODUCTS: CHARACTERIZATION AND USE

Middle distillate fuels are complex hydrocarbon mixtures derived from crude oil. They typically have boiling points ranging between 175° and 375°C. The composition of middle distillates varies with the original crude source and the refinery streams from which they are blended (2). Aliphatic and aromatic hydrocarbons are the major constituents of middle distillates. Some orefinic hydrocarbons also may be present. The complexity of the mixture increases rapidly with increasing boiling point

TABLE 69-1. Physical and chemical characteristics of middle distillates

	Aviation turbine fuels: jet A, jet A-1, jet B (ASTM D 1655)[a]	Kerosene: no. 1-K, no. 2-K (ASTM D 3699)[b]	Diesel fuel oil: grade low-sulfur no. 1-D; grade low-sulfur no. 2-D; grade no. 1-D; grade no. 2-D (ASTM D 975)[a]	Gas turbine fuel oils: no. 0-GT, no. 1-GT, no. 2-GT (ASTM D 2880)[b]	Marine fuels: DMX, DMA, DMB, DMC (ASTM D 2069)[a]	Fuel oils: no. 1, no. 2, grade no. 4 light (ASTM D 396)[a]
Synonyms	Jet fuel, JP-1, JP-5, JP-7, JP-8, kerosene, jet kerosene	N/A	Kerosene, diesel oil, diesel fuel, diesel fuel oil no. 1 or 2, diesel oil no. 1 or 2, no. 1 or 2 diesel, diesel fuel no. 1 or 2	N/A	N/A	Kerosene, coal oil, range oil, distillate fuel oil, furnace oil, gas oil, home heating oil no. 1 or 2, burner oil no. 1 or 2, fuel oil no. 1 or 2
Boiling range (°C)	175–300	175–375	175–375	175–375	175–375	175–375
Flashpoint (°C minimum)[c]	38	38	38 for no. 1; 52 for no. 2	38	43 for DMX, 60 for DMA, DMB, DMC	38
Vapor pressure at 21°C (mm Hg)	2.12–26.40	2.12–26.40	2.12–26.40	2.12–26.40	2.12–26.40	2.12–26.40
Solubility in water at 20°C (mg/L); organic solvents	5; miscible	5; miscible	5; miscible	5; miscible	5; miscible	5; miscible

ASTM, American Society of Testing Materials; JP, jet propulsion; N/A, not available.
[a]*Annual Book of American Society of Testing Materials Standards*, vol 05.01.
[b]*Annual Book of American Society of Testing Materials Standards*, vol 05.02.
[c]Minimum specifications in American Society of Testing Materials Standards.

as a result of the increasing number of atoms in a molecule and the number of structural isomers.

Middle distillates typically contain minor amounts of sulfur, nitrogen, and oxygen-containing molecules (1). They also may contain very low concentrations of additives [typically fewer than 1,000 parts per million (ppm)] added to enhance a specific fuel performance feature.

Table 69-1 presents the six classes of middle distillates with their official American Society of Testing Materials (ASTM) designation, other names that have been used to refer to the same products, and physical and chemical characteristics of toxicologic importance. The ASTM Committee D-2 on Petroleum Products and Lubricants has developed a mass spectrometry method for middle distillates (3). This method provides information sufficient to distinguish relatively minor differences in composition.

Exposure to Middle Distillates

The major sources of public exposure to middle distillates include use of kerosene heaters, refueling of diesel vehicles, and accidental spills. Inhalation of vapors and dermal contact are the major routes of exposure, although inhalation of vapors is limited by the low volatility of middle distillates. In the workplace, inhalation and dermal contact also are the primary routes of exposure to middle distillate fuels. Dermal exposure probably occurs to a greater extent. The determination of vapor concentrations in the workplace has been confined largely to the estimation of total hydrocarbons.

In the petroleum industry, exposures to the middle distillate fuel products are limited, owing to a combination of closed processing systems, outdoor operations, and low middle distillate volatility. Some dermal and inhalation exposure may occur during maintenance operations. Middle distillate materials sometimes are used in drilling muds in crude oil and natural gas–drilling operations. The route of exposure during these operations typically is skin contact. Middle distillates are used also as "cutters" or thinning solvents for the transportation of highly viscous petroleum products, such as asphalt. In these instances, the material may be distilled off and recycled or allowed to evaporate on use. No exposure limits have been set specifically for middle distillates.

Absorption, Distribution, Metabolism, and Excretion

Limited data are available to evaluate the absorption, distribution, metabolism, or excretion of middle distillates after exposure in humans. Because hydrocarbons generally are lipophilic, the lower-molecular-weight components (i.e., short-chain hydrocarbons) are likely to be absorbed. On the basis of animal data (4–8) and human case studies (9,10), absorption of diesel fuel can be assumed to occur by the dermal, inhalational, and oral routes of exposure. In acute animal toxicity studies, many of the symptoms of overexposure were reversible. This finding suggests that the retention of components in body tissues is limited. The hydrocarbon components of middle distillates are metabolized readily by the liver and are not expected to have long biological half-lives. The metabolism of middle distillates is likely to be oxidative in nature, resulting in compounds with increased water solubility. These metabolic products of middle distillates likely are eliminated in part by the kidney.

Animal Toxicity

Animal median lethal concentration tests of middle distillate fuels demonstrate a low order of acute oral and dermal toxicity. In rats, oral median lethal concentration values of more than 60 mL per kg for jet fuel JP-5, more than 5 g per kg for jet fuel JP-4, and 7.5 g per kg for diesel fuel have been reported (11–14). An acute dermal toxicity test in the rabbit showed no mortality at 5 mL per kg for middle distillate fuels (12). A primary eye irritation test in rabbits showed minimal irritation; however, prolonged skin contact can cause severe irritation (12). Single oral doses of JP-5 as low as 1 mL per kg produced behavioral effects in rats (15).

American Petroleum Institute–sponsored sensitization tests of middle distillate materials, in which 0.5 mL was applied to the skin of guinea pigs, did not produce any evidence of sensitization except for a weak response by a hydrodesulfurized middle distillate (12). No developmental effects were found in the fetuses of female rats that were exposed by inhalation during gestation to vapors of either no. 2 home heating oil or diesel fuel (16,17). Mice exposed dermally to JP-5 for 13 weeks (18) and rats exposed via inhalation to diesel fuel aerosol (19) did not demonstrate any histologic changes in their reproductive systems.

Several subchronic dermal toxicity studies of 2 to 3 weeks' duration have examined a variety of middle distillate materials using rabbits (1). The only effect seen was severe skin irritation.

Inhalational exposures of rats, mice, and dogs to jet fuel concentrations ranging from 150 to 1,000 mg per cubic meter for between 90 days and 60 weeks produced effects on the kidney, liver, blood, and nasal mucosa (6,20–24). The most obvious changes were seen in the kidneys of exposed male rats, which developed hyaline droplet nephropathy. This effect occurs only in male rats and has been found to be related to the presence in these animals of a low-molecular-weight protein called *α_2-globulin*. Available evidence indicates that humans do not possess this protein and are not likely to experience these effects (25). Exposed female mice experienced liver changes. Mild liver effects were reported also in rats and dogs. Other effects of exposure included mild changes in the blood, mild nasal inflammatory changes in the rats, and moderately decreased body weight gain in rats.

An inhalational study of intermittent 8-month exposures to 2,500 or 5,000 mg per cubic meter of JP-4 reported only organ weight changes in male rats exposed to the high-dose level and a transient increase in red blood cell fragility in female dogs (24). Decreased body weight was reported for male rats exposed to 500 or 1,000 mg per cubic meter intermittently for 1 year (26,27).

Skin-painting carcinogenesis bioassays constitute the majority of chronic toxicity studies on middle distillate fuel streams. The data show that middle distillate fuels, as a class, are weak to moderate skin carcinogens in mice, producing tumor incidences in the 5% to 30% range. Mean tumor latencies are greater than 70 weeks (typically 90 to 100 weeks) (13,18,28–37). Middle distillates, with the exception of cracked stocks (38), do not appear to be mutagenic and have been shown to be tumor-promoting substances, as opposed to initiators (29,31,33–35,39–41). Chronic skin irritation is suspected strongly of being a necessary prerequisite for tumor promotion by many substances (3,33,40,42–44). Suppression of chronic irritation in mouse skin has been demonstrated to suppress the tumor response as well (40,45–47).

Human Toxicity

The human toxicity data regarding middle distillate fuel streams indicate that middle distillate materials are moderate to severe skin irritants after prolonged and repeated contact. The mechanism is thought to operate through defatting of lipid components of the skin. The middle distillates have a low viscosity and surface tension, rendering aspiration after ingestion a potential hazard. Aspiration may result in substantial damage to the pulmonary tissue.

Human and animal studies suggest that transient depression in central nervous system function (dizziness, drowsiness, headache, and fatigue) may result from exposure to high concentrations of vapors. No evidence substantiates long-term nervous system damage. Chronic inhalation and oral or dermal exposures to high concentrations of jet fuel by workers has been reported to cause fatigue, depressed mood, lack of initiative, dizziness, sleep disturbances, and impairment of attention and sensorimotor speed (48). Although the psychiatric and psychological examination of these workers with long-term exposure to jet fuel indicated some differences from controls on subjective measures, clinical neurologic examinations (including electroencephalographic and nerve conduction) showed negligible differences. Furthermore, population selection issues, small sample size, and lack of control for exposure to other chemicals do not allow generalization about the observed effects.

Epidemiologic studies of occupationally exposed refinery workers often are not appropriate to assess the risk from exposure to middle distillates, because refinery workers may be exposed to many other products and chemicals used in the refinery process. The few epidemiologic studies that focus on middle distillate exposures did not provide conclusive evidence for carcinogenicity (49). Although the International Agency for Research on Cancer (IARC) (26) determined that occupational exposures to fuel oils during petroleum refining probably are carcinogenic in humans, the problem has not been studied sufficiently to make definitive statements about specific middle distillate fuels. The IARC concluded that jet fuel, distillate diesel fuels, and distillate fuel oils are not classifiable as to their carcinogenicity in humans (group 3): Either insufficient data exist or existing data are conflicting. The IARC made these evaluations on the basis of their judgment of inadequate human and limited or inadequate animal evidence. In formulating these overall evaluations, the IARC noted the limited evidence for carcinogenicity in experimental animals of straight-run kerosene and one sample of a hydrotreated kerosene (26).

Guidelines, Standards, and Occupational Safety

The U.S. Occupational Safety and Health Administration developed a permissible exposure limit for petroleum distillates (naphtha) of 400 ppm (29 *CFR* 1910.1000). The National Institute for Occupational Safety and Health has a time-weighted average (TWA) for petroleum distillates (naphtha) of 350 mg per cubic meter, a ceiling reference exposure level of 1,800 mg per cubic meter, and a level of immediate danger to life and health of 10,000 ppm (50,51). These limits were developed for the naphtha fractions of petroleum distillates, which are more volatile than are middle distillates. The moderate vapor pressure of middle distillates renders attaining a vapor concentration of 10,000 ppm difficult. The Occupational Safety and Health Administration's permissible exposure limit of 5 mg per cubic meter (8-hour TWA) for oil mists has been used also when exposure to middle distillate aerosols is anticipated. The American Conference of Governmental Industrial Hygienists has proposed an 8-hour TWA of 100 mg per cubic meter for diesel fuel and kerosene.

Under the U.S. Department of Transportation's Hazardous Material Transportation Act, fuel oils are designated as hazardous materials that are subject to requirements for packaging, shipping, and transporting (49 *CFR* 172.101, appendix A). Under the Marine Protection Research and Sanctuaries Act of the U.S. Environmental Protection Agency (EPA), ocean dumping of oils of any kind known or suspected to be carcinogens, mutagens, or teratogens is prohibited except when they are present as trace contaminants (40 *CFR* 227.6). Under the EPA's Clean Water Act, oil and grease are designated as conventional pollutants (1).

No reference dose or cancer slope factor is published in the EPA's Integrated Risk Information System (52) or Health Effects Assessment Summary Tables (53) for middle distillates. A reference dose of 0.02 mg per kg per day for no. 2 diesel fuel has been published by Ryer-Powder et al. (54,55).

RESIDUAL FUEL OILS: CHARACTERIZATION AND USE

Residual or heavy fuel oils are composed of residues from various refining processes, including atmospheric and vacuum distillation, vacuum thermal cracking, catalytic cracking, and hydrocracking. Residues often are blended with such middle distillate diluents as kerosene to reduce viscosity. Residual fuel oils are used as fuels in industrial and commercial power plant boilers and furnaces, marine boilers, marine and railroad diesel engines, and blast furnaces (48). Table 69-2 presents the four ASTM classes of residual fuels with their official ASTM designations, synonyms, and physical and chemical characteristics of toxicologic importance (56).

The residual fuel oils are complex mixtures of relatively high-molecular-weight hydrocarbons. They are blended from fractions that boil at temperatures between 350° and 650°C. The molecular weights of the constituents can range from approximately 300 to more than 1,000. Residual fuel oils contain asphaltenes, polar aromatics, aromatics, saturated hydrocarbons, and heteromolecules containing sulfur, oxygen, nitrogen, and metals (26). If blended with catalytic cracked residues, they may contain appreciable polynuclear aromatic hydrocarbons (26).

Acute and Subacute Toxicity

Symptoms from acute exposure to residual fuel oils include mild irritation of the eyes and skin. If the oils are ingested, aspiration is a potential hazard. Residual fuel oils, however, generally have a low order of acute and subacute oral and dermal toxicity. Studies of four different lots of no. 6 fuel oil (varying in sulfur content and specific gravity) demonstrated in rats acute oral median lethal doses (LD_{50}s) of more than 25 mL per kg. Acute dermal toxicity tests demonstrated no mortality at 5 mL per kg. The different lots of no. 6 fuel oil ranged from nonreactive to mildly positive in guinea pig dermal sensitization tests. Primary dermal irritation and primary eye irritation tests showed this oil to be slightly to minimally irritating in rabbits (45). In subacute dermal LD_{50} studies, three different lots of this oil were applied to the skin of eight rabbits at 8 mL per kg for 24 hours per day, 5 days per week for 2 weeks (45). Mortality ranged from 0% to 38%. Application of a fourth lot caused 62.5% mortality at a dose of 1.0 mL per kg. Animals in all groups exhibited dermal irritation, weight loss, and severe liver pathology.

Male and female mice were dosed dermally with 2,000 to 40,000 mg per kg of MDF for 14 consecutive days (33). Dosages greater than 20,000 mg per kg resulted in 100% mortality. Inflammation and skin lesions were reported. No treatment-related mortality was observed in mice administered MDF 250 to 4,000 mg per kg by dermal application 5 days per week for 13 weeks. Those in the group given a dose of 4,000 mg per kg exhibited a chronic dermatitis at the site of application.

Continuous 90-day inhalational exposure to 50 or 300 mg per cubic meter of MDF produced results similar to those with other middle distillates (20,23), including hyaline droplet nephropathy and reduced body weight gain in male rats at both doses. Increased lung and liver inflammation also was observed in female mice. The only changes (all mild) noted in dogs were increased osmotic fragility of red blood cells, increased frequency of cytoplasmic vacuolization of hepatocytes (due to accumulation of excess glycogen), and elevated blood urea nitrogen.

Chronic Toxicity

Chronic toxicity studies have been conducted with MDF. MDF produced kidney lesions in mice treated dermally three times per week for 60 weeks (6). Kidney lesions were not observed in a second dermal study in which mice were treated with up to 500 mg per kg MDF diluted in acetone five times per week for 103 weeks (18).

Skin carcinogenicity studies have been conducted with residual fuel oils. MDF applied dermally to mice has resulted in skin tumors (6,18). Blended fuel oils (obtained by adding differing amounts of catalytically cracked clarified oil) applied to mouse skin produced skin tumors, and some of these oils have been shown to be tumor initiators (34). Tumor frequency increased and latency decreased as concentration of cracked residue in the

TABLE 69-2. American Society of Testing Materials' names of residual fuels and physical and chemical characteristics of toxicologic importance

	Diesel fuel oil grade no. 4-D (ASTM D 975)[a]	Gas turbine fuel oils: no. 3-GT, no. 4-GT (ASTM D 2880)[b]	Marine residual fuels: FMA-0, RMB-10, RMC-10, RMD-15, RMB-25, RMF-25, RMG-35, RMH-35, RMK-35, RML-35, RMH-45, RMK-45, RML-45, RMH-55, RML-55 (ASTM D 2069)[a]	Fuel oils: no. 4, no. 5 (light), no. 5 (heavy), no. 6 (ASTM D 396)[a]
Synonyms	Diesel oil, diesel fuel oil no. 1 or 2, diesel oil no. 1 or 2	N/A	Marine boiler fuels, bunker fuel oil, bunker C fuel oil	Residual fuel oil, industrial fuel oil, marine boiler fuels, power station fuel oil, bunker fuel oil, bunker C fuel oil
Boiling range (°C)	350–650+	350–650+	150–650+	350–650+
Flash point (°C minimum)[c]	55	55 for no. 3-GT; 66 for no. 4-GT	60	55 for no. 4 and no. 5; 60 no. 6
Vapor pressure at 21°C (mm Hg)	<0.01	<0.01	<0.01	<0.01

ASTM, American Society of Testing Materials; N/A, not available.
[a]*Annual Book of American Society of Testing Materials Standards*, vol 05.01.
[b]*Annual Book of American Society of Testing Materials Standards*, vol 05.02.
[c]Minimum specifications in American Society of Testing Materials Standards.

fuel increased (57). The IARC has classified residual fuel oils and MDF as possibly carcinogenic to humans (group 2B) on the basis of limited evidence of cancer in animals (26).

Guidelines, Standards, and Occupational Safety

No exposure guidelines or standards are specific to residual fuels. Those cited in the chapter for the middle distillates are applicable also to residual fuels.

REFERENCES

1. Agency for Toxic Substances and Disease Registry. *Toxicological profile for fuel oils.* Atlanta: US Department of Health and Human Services, Public Health Service, ATSDR, 1993.
2. US Air Force. *The installation restoration program toxicology guide,* vol 4. Contract no. 1981-A076-A1. DOE interagency agreement no. 1891-A076-A1. Wright Patterson Air Force Base, OH: Harry G. Armstrong Aerospace Medical Research Laboratory, Aerospace Medical Division, Air Force Systems Command, 1989.
3. Argyris TS, Slaga TJ. Promotion of carcinomas by repeated abrasion in initiated skin of mice. *Cancer Res* 1981;41:5193–5195.
4. Chu I, Rinehart W, Hoffman G, et al. Subacute inhalation toxicity of a medium-boiling coal liquefaction product (154–378°C) in the rat (part III). *J Toxicol Environ Health* 1989;28:195–204.
5. Dalbey WS, Lock S, Garfinkel S, Jenkins R, Holmberg R, Guerin M. Inhalation exposures of rats to aerosolized diesel fuel. In: MacFarland HN, Holdsworth CE, MacGregor JA, et al., eds. *The toxicology of petroleum hydrocarbons.* Washington: American Petroleum Institute, 1982:13–25.
6. Easley JR, Holland JM, Gipson LC, Whitaker MJ. Renal toxicity of middle distillates of shale oil and petroleum in mice. *Toxicol Appl Pharmacol* 1982;65:84–91.
7. Kainz RJ, White LE. Depressant effects associated with the inhalation of uncombusted diesel vapor. In: MacFarland HN, Holdworth CE, MacGregor JA, Call RW, Lane ML, eds. *Advances in modern environmental toxicology: Vol 6. Applied toxicology of petroleum hydrocarbons.* Princeton, NJ: Princeton Scientific Publishers, 1984.
8. Parker GA, Bogo V, Young RW. Acute toxicity of petroleum- and shale-derived distillate fuel, marine: light microscopic, hematologic, and serum chemistry studies. *Fundam Appl Toxicol* 1986;7:101–105.
9. Crisp AJ, Bhalla AK, Hoffbrand BJ. Acute tubular necrosis after exposure to diesel fuel. *BMJ* 1979;2:177.
10. Rodriguez PE, Latour Perez J, Aller Alvarezz JL, Alix J, Alix Y. Diesel fuel pneumonia. Presentation of a case. *Rev Clin Exp* 1976;143:397–400.
11. Beck LS, Jepler DI, Hasen KL. The acute toxicology of selected petroleum hydrocarbons. In: MacFarland HN, Holdworth CE, MacGregor JA, Call RW, Lane ML, eds. *Advances in modern environmental toxicology: vol 6. Applied toxicology of petroleum hydrocarbons.* Princeton, NJ: Princeton Scientific Publishers, 1984:1–16.
12. American Petroleum Institute. *Results of toxicological studies.* API publ. no. 45591. Washington: American Petroleum Institute, 1994.
13. Clark CR, Walter MK, Ferguson PW, Katchen M. Comparative dermal carcinogenesis of shale and petroleum-derived distillates. *Toxicol Ind Health* 1988;4:11–22.
14. Parker GA, Bogo V, Young RW. Acute toxicity of conventional versus shale-derived JP5 jet fuel: light microscopic, hematologic, and serum chemistry studies. *Toxicol Appl Pharmacol* 1981;57:302–317.
15. Bogo V, Young RW, Hill TA, Cartledge RM, Nold J, Parker GA. Neurobehavioral toxicology of petroleum- and shale-derived jet propulsion fuel no. 5 (JP-5). In: MacFarland HN, Holdworth CE, MacGregor JA, Call RW, Lane ML, eds. *Advances in modern environmental toxicology: vol 6. Applied toxicology of petroleum hydrocarbons.* Princeton, NJ: Princeton Scientific Publishers, 1984:17–32.
16. American Petroleum Institute. *Teratology study in rats: diesel fuel.* Doc. no. FYI-AX-0183-0230. Washington: American Petroleum Institute, 1979.
17. Beliles RP, Mecler FJ. Inhalation teratology of jet fuel A, fuel oil, and petroleum naphtha in rats. In: MacFarland HN, ed. *Proceedings of the symposium on the toxicology of petroleum hydrocarbons, Washington, DC, May 1982.* Washington: American Petroleum Institute, 1983:233–238.
18. National Toxicology Program, National Institutes of Health. *Toxicology and carcinogenesis studies of marine diesel fuel and JP-5 Navy fuel (CAS no. 8008-20-6) in B6C3F1 mice (dermal studies).* Technical report series no. 310. NIH publ. no. 86-2566. Research Triangle Park, NC: US Department of Health and Human Services, 1986.
19. Lock S, Dalbey W, Schmoyer R, et al. *Chemical characterization and toxicologic evaluation of airborne mixtures—inhalation toxicology of diesel fuel obscurant aerosol in Sprague-Dawley rats: Final report, phase 3. Subchronic exposures.* Oak Ridge, TN: Oak Ridge National Laboratory, 1984.
20. Bruner RH. Pathologic findings in laboratory animals exposed to hydrocarbon fuels of military interest. In: Mehlman MA, Hemstreet P III, Thorpe JJ, Weaver NK, eds. *Advances in modern environmental toxicology: vol 7. Renal effects of petroleum hydrocarbons.* Princeton, NJ: Princeton Scientific Publishers, 1984:133–140.
21. Gaworski CL, MacEwen EH, Vernot RH, Burner RH, Cowan MJ Jr. Comparison of the subchronic inhalation toxicity of petroleum and oil-shale JP-5 fuels. In: MacFarland HN, Holdworth CE, MacGregor JA, Call RW, Lane ML, eds. *Advances in modern environmental toxicology: vol 6. Applied toxicology of petroleum hydrocarbons.* Princeton, NJ: Princeton Scientific Publishers, 1984:33–47.
22. MacEwen JD, Vernot EH. *Toxic Hazards Research Unit annual technical report AD-A147-8577.* Springfield, VA: National Technical Information Service, 1984.
23. MacEwen JD, Vernot EH. *Toxic Hazards Research Unit annual technical report AD-A161-5582.* Springfield, VA: National Technical Information Service, 1985.
24. MacNaughton MG, Uddin DE. Toxicology of mixed distillate and high-energy synthetic fuels. In: Mehlman MA, Hemstreet P III, Thorpe JJ, Weaver NK, eds. *Advances in modern environmental toxicology: vol 7. Renal effects of petroleum hydrocarbons.* Princeton, NJ: Princeton Scientific Publishers, 1984:121–132.
25. US Environmental Protection Agency. Alpha 2u-globulin: association with chemically induced renal toxicity and neoplasia in the male rat. (Prepared for the Risk Assessment Forum, EPA/625/3-91/019F.) Washington: US Environmental Protection Agency, 1991.
26. International Agency for Research on Cancer Working Group on the Evaluation of Carcinogenic Risks to Humans. Occupational exposures in petroleum refining; crude oil and major petroleum fuels. *IARC Monogr Eval Carcinog Risks Hum* 1989;45:1–322.
27. MacEwen JD, Vernot EH. *Toxic Hazards Research Unit annual technical report AD-A110-5873.* Springfield, VA: National Technical Information Service, 1981.
28. American Petroleum Institute. *Lifetime dermal carcinogenesis bioassay of refinery streams in C3H/HeJ mice (API 135r).* API Health and Environmental Sciences Department report 36-31364. Washington: American Petroleum Institute, 1988.
29. American Petroleum Institute. *Short-term dermal tumorigenesis study of selected petroleum hydrocarbons in male CD-1 mice, initiation and promotion phases.* API Health and Environmental Sciences Department report 36-32643. Washington: American Petroleum Institute, 1988.
30. Blackburn GR, Deitch RA, Schreiner CA, Mackerer CR. Predicting carcinogenicity of petroleum distillation fractions using a modified *Salmonella* mutagenicity assay. *Cell Biol Toxicol* 1986;2:63–84.
31. Gehart JM, Hatoum NS, Halder CA, Warne TM, Schmitt SL. Tumor initiation and promotion effects of petroleum streams in mouse skin. *Fundam Appl Toxicol* 1988;11:76–90.
32. Lewis SC, King RW, Cragg ST, Hilman DW. Skin carcinogenic potential of petroleum hydrocarbons: crude oils, distillate fractions and chemical class subfractions. In: Mehlman MA, ed. *Applied toxicology of petroleum hydrocarbons.* Princeton, NJ: Princeton Scientific Publishers, 1984:139–150.
33. McKee RH, Plutnick RT, Przygoda RT. The carcinogenic initiating and promoting properties of a lightly refined paraffinic oil. *Fundam Appl Toxicol* 1989;12:748–756.
34. Skisak C. The role of chronic acanthosis and subacute inflammation in tumor production in CD-1 mice by petroleum middle distillates. *Toxicol Appl Pharmacol* 1991;109:399–411.
35. US Environmental Protection Agency, Office of Toxic Substances. *Preliminary evaluations of initial TSCA section 8(e) substantial risk notices, January 1987–December 1988: Report 8EHQ-1288-0773.* Washington: US Environmental Protection Agency, 1988:470–472.
36. US Environmental Protection Agency, Office of Toxic Substances. *Preliminary evaluations of initial TSCA section 8(e) substantial risk notices, January 1987–December 1988: Report 8EHQ-1288-0775.* Washington: US Environmental Protection Agency, 1988:476–479.
37. US Environmental Protection Agency, Office of Toxic Substances. *Preliminary evaluations of initial TSCA section 8(e) substantial risk notices, February 1, 1983–December 31, 1984: Report 8EHQ-0683-0480.* Washington: US Environmental Protection Agency, 1983:49–51.
38. Conaway CC, Schreiner CA, Cragg ST. Mutagenicity evaluation of petroleum hydrocarbons. In: MacFarland HN, Holdworth CE, MacGregor JA, Call RW, Lane ML, eds. *Advances in modern environmental toxicology: vol 6. Applied toxicology of petroleum hydrocarbons.* Princeton, NJ: Princeton Scientific Publishers, 1984:89–106.
39. Marino DJ, Finkbone HN, Strother DE, Mast RW, Furedi EM. Tumor initiation and promotion activity of straight run and fractionated kerosenes [abstract 776]. Presented at the 1990 Society of Toxicology meetings, Miami, FL, 1990.
40. Skisak CM, Furedi-Machacek EM, Schmitt SS, Swanson MS, Vernot EH. Chronic and irritation/promotion skin bioassays of petroleum refinery streams. *Environ Health Perspect* 1994;102:82–87.
41. Slaga TJ, Triplett LL, Fry RJM. *Chemical characterization and toxicologic evaluation of airborne mixtures. Tumorigenicity studies of diesel fuel-2, red smoke dye, and violet smoke dyes in the SENCAR mouse skin tumorigenesis.* Report no. AD-A159 728/5:29. Springfield, VA: National Technical Information Service, 1986.
42. Argyris TS. Tumor promotion by abrasion induced epidermal hyperplasia in the skin of mice. *J Invest Dermatol* 1980;75:360–362.
43. Frei JV, Stephens P. The correlation of promotion of tumor growth and induction of hyperplasia in epidermal two-stage carcinogenesis. *Br J Cancer* 1968;22:83–92.
44. Hergenhahn M, Murstenberger G, Opferkuch HJ, Adolf W, Mack H, Hecker E. Biological assays for irritant tumor-initiating and promoting activities. *J Cancer Res* 1982;104:31–39.
45. Belman S, Troll W. The inhibition of croton oil–promoted mouse skin tumorigenesis by steroid hormones. *Cancer Res* 1972;32:450–454.

46. Ghadially FN, Green HN. The effect of cortisone on chemical carcinogenesis in the mouse skin. *Br J Cancer* 1954;8:291–295.
47. Slaga TJ, Scribner JD. Inhibition of tumor initiation and promotion by anti-inflammatory agents. *J Natl Cancer Inst* 1973;51:1723–1725.
48. Knave B, Olson BA, Elofsson S, et al. Long-term exposure to jet fuel: II. A cross-sectional epidemiologic investigation on occupationally exposed industrial workers with special reference to the nervous system. *Scand J Work Environ Health* 1978;4:19–45.
49. US Environmental Protection Agency. *Oral reference doses and oral slope factors for JP-4, JP-5, diesel fuel, and gasoline.* (Memorandum from Joan S. Dollarhide to Carol Sweeney.) Washington: US Environmental Protection Agency, 1992.
50. National Institute for Occupational Safety and Health. *NIOSH pocket guide to chemical hazards.* Publ. no. 84-100, method 1550. Cincinnati: National Institute for Occupational Safety and Health, 1990.
51. National Institute for Occupational Safety and Health. *NIOSH recommendations for occupational safety and health: compendium of policy documents and statements.* DHHS (NIOSH) publ. no. 92–100. Cincinnati: National Institute for Occupational Safety and Health, 1992.
52. US Environmental Protection Agency. *Integrated risk information system (IRIS).* Washington: US Environmental Protection Agency, 1996.
53. US Environmental Protection Agency. *Health effects assessment summary tables (HEAST).* Washington: Office of Solid Waste and Emergency Response, US Environmental Protection Agency, May 1995.
54. Ryer-Powder JE, Custance SR, Sullivan MJ. Determination of reference doses of mineral spirits, crude oil, diesel fuel number 2, and lubricating oil. Presented at the Society of Petroleum Engineers Sixty-Eighth Annual Technical Conference and Exhibition, Houston, TX, October 3–6, 1993.
55. Ryer-Powder JE, Sullivan MJ. Update on the derivation of an oral reference dose for diesel fuel no. 2. In: Kostecki PT, Calabrese EJ, Barkan CPL, eds. *Principles and practices for diesel contaminated soils*, vol 3. Amherst, MA: Amherst Science Publishers, 1994.
56. American Society for Testing and Materials. Standard specifications for fuel oils (ASTM D 396-86). In: *Annual book of ASTM standards*, vol 05.10. Philadelphia: American Society for Testing and Materials, 1986:210–215.
57. Bingham E, Trosset RP, Warshawsky D. Carcinogenic potential of petroleum hydrocarbons. A critical review of the literature. *J Environ Pathol Toxicol* 1980;3:483–563.

CHAPTER 70

Petroleum Lubricants, Asphalt, and Coke

Donald M. Molenaar, Charles R. Clark, Charles E. Lambert, and Jill Ryer-Powder

LUBRICATING OILS

Lubricating oils, also called *mineral oils*, are petroleum hydrocarbon derivatives formulated to reduce friction between surfaces in relative motion. They may also serve other secondary purposes, including heat transfer, metal processing, corrosion protection, and medicinal and food uses. Lubricating oils are composed of a complex mixture of hydrocarbons and are produced from the vacuum distillation of the residues from the crude oil distillation process. Lubricating oils include lubricating oil base stocks, technical white oils, white oils, and medicinal oils. The major difference between these oils is the severity of treatment applied to each after initial vacuum distillation. Most lubricating and specialty oils sold today are produced by blending a small number of lubricating oil base stocks and additives (1).

Chemical Characteristics and Composition

Lubricating oil production begins with the residual material left from the atmospheric distillation process, which yields the lighter gasoline and middle distillate fractions. Vacuum distillation of this residuum produces gas oils and the lubricating oil fractions, which undergo further processing (hydrotreating, solvent extraction, dewaxing, etc.) to remove impurities and improve certain physical properties. Lubricating oil base stocks contain between 17 and 40 carbons and are composed of paraffins, cycloparaffins (naphthenes), alkyl benzenes, naphthenobenzenes, multiring aromatics, thiophenes, and polar compounds. Lubricating oils boil at a temperature ranging between 570° and 1,000°F (2) and range in appearance from thin, easily flowing spindle oils to thick cylinder oils (2). Additives are typically used to meet the desired qualifications for the final product. Examples of lubricating oil additives are presented in Table 70-1 (J. Ryer-Powder, *personal communication*, 1996). As is evident from the table, additives are present in small amounts and do not make a large contribution to the toxicity of lubricating oils.

Depending on the source, lubricating oils may be described as paraffinic or naphthenic. Paraffinic crude oils are characterized mainly by high wax content, high natural viscosity index (low rate of change in viscosity with temperature), and relatively low aromatic hydrocarbon content. Naphthenic crude oils are normally low in wax and relatively high in cycloparaffins and aromatic hydrocarbons. Most crude oils contain some polynuclear aromatic hydrocarbons (PAHs); however, treatment in the refinery is sufficiently thorough to remove the PAHs, resulting in low PAH content in the finished product. The actual composition and appearance of lubricating oils depend on the source of the crude oil and the manufacturing and treatment processes used.

Evaluation of Chemical Characteristics

The chemical and physical characteristics of lubricating oils are important factors in determining the best use for these oils. Viscosity, viscosity index, and distillation temperature are critical characteristics of these base oils. The higher the viscosity index, the less change in viscosity occurs with temperature. Other properties considered important are pour point, oxidation resistance, flash point, boiling temperature, and acidity.

A system for defining lubricating oils and other refinery streams, based on the petroleum crude oil refinery process, was adopted in 1978 under the U.S. Toxic Substances Control Act and in 1981 under the Commission of the European Communities' Sixth Amendment to the Dangerous Substances Directive—European Inventory of Existing Commercial Chemical Substances. Each stream is defined on the basis of petroleum crude oil type, viscosity, and process and is identified by a Chemical Abstracts Service registry number, which identifies its last refining process (3).

Production and Use

The first step in the processing of lubricating oils is separation on the crude oil distillation units of the individual fractions according to viscosity and boiling range (1). The raw lubricating oil fractions from most crude oils contain components that have undesirable characteristics for finished lubricating oils (1). These raw lubricating oil fractions must be refined further and treated to obtain base oils with the qualities and specifications needed for the various applications. Treatment processes include acid treatment, solvent extraction, hydrofinishing, and a solvent dewaxing process (2). Each process, treatment, and resulting characteristic is explained in Table 70-2. The severity of the processes applied to lubricating oils has a major impact on their toxicity.

TABLE 70-1. Functions and examples of typical lubricating oil additives

Additive	Typical percentage in oil	Function	Example
Dispersants	3–6	Diesel detergency Sludge and varnish control	Polyisobutenyl succinimides of highly polar polyamines
Metal detergents	1–3	Diesel detergency Rust control	Overbased calcium and magnesium sulfonates
Antioxidants	0.8–1.5	Oxidation control	ZDDP
Antiwear agents	0.8–1.5	Valve-train wear control Cylinder or ring wear control Bearing wear control	ZDDP
Friction modifiers	0.5–1.0	Fuel economy	Hydroxylated octadecylamine
Viscosity modifiers	5–11	High-temperature viscosity Dispersiveness	Polymethacrylates
Biocides	0.05–0.50	Control of bacterial and fungal growth	Boron compounds, phenol and chlorophenol derivatives, triazenes

ZDDP, zinc dialkyldithiophosphate.

Assessment of Exposure to Lubricating Oil

The World Health Organization (WHO) (2) has identified the most common lubricating oil product categories and market applications (Table 70-3). Human exposure to lubricating oils varies according to intended use. The major routes of exposure in the industrial setting include inhalation of mists and dermal contact. Vapor inhalation does not represent a significant exposure route, as condensation to mist occurs during vaporization into room-temperature air. Exposure to mists can occur during such operations as metal-working, for which the lubrication oil is used during cutting and grinding. Dermal exposure to waste oil can occur when engine oils are changed during routine maintenance. There is limited potential for exposure to hydraulic fluids, turbine oils, engine oils, and other oils that are used in closed systems. White oils, which are highly refined to remove aromatics and other impurities, are considered to be nontoxic. They are used in food and textile machinery and as direct food additives. Lubricating oils may change in physical and chemical characteristics over the course of time, depending on their use, and such changes may alter their toxicity. For example, used motor oil may contain soot, PAHs, and metals that were not present in the unused motor oil.

Animal Toxicity

ACUTE AND SUBACUTE TOXICITY

The acute toxicity of lubricating oil has been examined in laboratory animals in a number of studies. Naphthenic and paraffinic base stocks were found to be of low toxicity when administered to animals by oral and dermal routes of exposure (4). Oral median lethal doses (LD_{50}s) of more than 5 g oil per kg of body weight in rats and a dermal LD_{50} of more than 5 g per kg in rabbits have been reported. Dermal tests in guinea pigs showed no evidence of sensitization. Eye and skin tests on rabbits revealed slight to no irritation as a result of exposure to lubricating oils. In subacute dermal tests, rabbits treated with 5 g per kg three times weekly for a period of 3 weeks developed skin irritation and inflammation.

The results of unpublished animal studies suggest that lubricating oils do not present a reproductive or developmental toxicity hazard. White oils and a lubricant base stock have been evaluated in separate developmental toxicity studies in pregnant rats treated by the dermal route from gestational days 0 through 19. No adverse effects on maternal reproductive parameters or offspring viability or development were observed. Slight dermal irritation from daily oil treatment did not affect reproductive outcome. Analysis of maternal blood and placenta and fetal tissue for radiolabeled residue of the base stock indicated that very small quantities of the oil crossed the placenta but did not appear to be toxic or to bioaccumulate (Mobil Business Resources Corp, *unpublished data*, 1996).

A dermal reproductive toxicity study, using the same white oil in male and female rats treated from 10 weeks before mating through mating, gestation, and lactation, did not produce any adverse effects on reproductive performance of either gender, maternal body weight or food consumption, gestation, delivery, or litter size. It also did not cause toxicity to the fetus *in utero* or retard survival or development of the offspring during lactation (Mobil Business Resources Corp, *unpublished data*, 1996).

An oral reproductive toxicity study in rats was conducted with a neutral lubricant base oil. All animals were dosed via gav-

TABLE 70-2. Processes for refining and treating distillate fractions

Process	Treatment	Resulting characteristic
Acid treatment	Mixing of oil with sulfuric acid and centrifugation of acid sludge, followed by mixing of oil with absorbent clay and filtration	Reduced carbons and sludge-forming tendencies; improved color, odor, and stability
Solvent extraction	Extraction of aromatics from oil fractions, producing a low-aromatic or aromatic-free refined and a high-aromatic extract	Improved viscosity index
Hydrofinishing	Introduction of hydrogen to remove sulfur and olefins, diolefins, and aromatic compounds	Improved viscosity index; improved color and oxygen stability and lowered organic acidity
Solvent dewaxing	Separation of slack wax from base oil fractions obtained from paraffinic crude oil residues	Lowered pour point

TABLE 70-3. Categories of lubricating oil products

Lubricating oil product	Types of lubricating oils used in formulation
Industrial lubricating oils	Highly refined paraffinic base oils
Lubricants for internal combustion engines of various types	Highly refined paraffinic base oils
Crankcase, compressor, gear, and turbine oils	Highly refined paraffinic base oils
Greases for bearings and other purposes	Naphthenic or paraffinic base oils
Hydraulic, transformer, insulating, heat-transmission oils	Naphthenic base oils
Metal-working oils: cutting, grinding, rolling, drilling, drawing oil	Light-viscosity, solvent-refined, paraffinic, or naphthenic base oils
Textile oils	Light- to medium-viscosity oils derived from base oils that either have been highly refined or have undergone limited refining
Waxes of various grades and purity	Paraffinic base oil
Medicinal white oil used for medicinal and food-grade applications	Severely refined naphthenic or paraffinic distillates

Adapted from ref. 2, with permission.

age daily for a minimum of 14 days prior to mating, throughout mating, and until the day prior to necropsy. Female rats were dosed through gestation and lactation until necropsy on lactation day 4. Male rats underwent necropsy after the breeding period and after 30 days of dosing. No evidence of reproductive, developmental (by viability, external appearance, and necropsy), or neonatal toxicity was attributed to treatment with this base oil (Chevron, *unpublished report* no. WIL-187007, 1995).

CHRONIC TOXICITY

In a 90-day rat study with dietary exposure to six mineral oils, rats exhibited increased liver weights, increases in liver enzyme activity, tissue accumulation of mineral hydrocarbon, and the development of granulomatous tissue in the liver. Rats also had lymph node effects consisting of increased weight, accumulation of mineral hydrocarbon, and histiocytosis. These effects were noted only at the highest dose used in the study (1,500 mg per kg) (5). Another set of studies conducted by Exxon Biomedical Sciences, Inc. (6), demonstrated a no-observable-adverse-effect level when 4,350 mg per kg per day of medicinal white oil was administered to rats via oral gavage, indicating that white oils are practically nontoxic even in large doses.

Unrefined lubricating oils are known to produce skin tumors in laboratory animals (7–12). Studies have shown that skin cancer is associated with the presence of PAHs (13), some of which are known to be carcinogenic. Solvent-extracted and severely hydrotreated lubricant base oils from which the PAHs are removed do not normally induce skin cancer in mice (7,13–16). Studies by Blackburn et al. (17) and Roy et al. (18) have demonstrated a correlation among mutagenicity, skin cancer, and PAH content. These studies demonstrated that solvent residue eliminated both mutagenicity and skin cancer with a database of more than 120 compounds (17,18).

The International Agency for Research on Cancer (IARC) (3) categorizes mineral oils into eight classes on the basis of the refining history and has evaluated carcinogenicity on the basis of the animal and human evidence. This agency has found sufficient evidence for carcinogenicity in experimental animals for untreated vacuum distillates, acid-treated oils, and aromatic oils, including extracts from solvent treatment of distillates and the high-boiling fraction of catalytically cracked oils, mildly solvent-refined oils, mildly hydrotreated oils, and some gasoline engine oils. In contrast, it found inadequate evidence of carcinogenicity in experimental animals for severely hydrotreated oils and used and unused formulated products. The IARC also found limited evidence of carcinogenicity in experimental animals for cutting oils, whereas no evidence of carcinogenicity was found in experimental animals for severely solvent-refined oils and white oils. Finally, the agency found sufficient evidence of carcinogenicity in studies with mineral oils containing various additives and impurities that have been used in historical occupations such as mule spinning, metal machining, and jute processing (3). The relevance of these findings to modern industrial practices and uses of mineral oils is not clear. The reader is referred to the IARC monograph titled "Polynuclear Aromatic Compounds: Part 2, Carbon Blacks, Mineral Oils, and Some Nitroarenes" (3) for a complete description of toxicity studies involving several different lubricating oils.

Human Toxicity

ACUTE AND SUBACUTE TOXICITY

It is generally agreed that mineral base oils, lubricating oils, and greases have a low order of toxicity when ingested by humans (19). Exposure of the eyes, skin, and respiratory tract to such substances may cause slight irritation. Clinical studies on the effects of mineral oils after ingestion by humans indicate that the principal concern is aspiration (20). Gastrointestinal symptoms on ingestion may include abdominal cramps and diarrhea.

CHRONIC TOXICITY

Chronic occupational exposure to lubricating oils is not common owing to their use in closed systems. However, in some instances, such as cutting and grinding operations, workers can be exposed to oil mists via inhalation and dermal exposure (21). Prolonged or repeated skin contact may produce skin irritation and dermatitis. Severely refined lubricating oils have not been shown to cause eye or skin irritation, except with prolonged, repeated exposure (22). Inhaled mineral oil is taken up rapidly by alveolar macrophages and is transferred to the regional lymph nodes. Mineral oils are metabolized via hydroxylation and carboxylation and enter the fatty acid cycle in the body. However, when this metabolic capability is overwhelmed, mineral oil can be deposited in the interstitial tissue and the lymph nodes, where it induces a cellular reaction. According to the WHO (2), if the exposure is sufficiently high and of long duration, fibrosis may occur.

Ingestion of mineral oils has been evaluated in epidemiologic studies and case studies. Boyd and Doll (23) conducted a case-control study of cancers of the stomach and large bowel associated with mineral oil or other laxative use. The use of mineral oil had the highest association with gastrointestinal cancer, although it was considered unlikely that this material could be an important cause of such cancer (13). A case-control study conducted by Higginson (24) did not confirm the positive correlation between mineral oil use and large-intestinal cancer reported by Boyd and Doll (23). In a clinical case study, prolonged ingestion of mineral oil over a number of years resulted in oil deposition in the small intestine, abdominal lymph nodes, liver, spleen, and lungs (24a).

Although European studies have reported an association between cutting oil exposure and skin and scrotal cancer (25,26), studies in the United States suggest that the occurrence of these cancers after exposure to cutting oil is very low. It has been suggested that the differences in cancer occurrence may be due to improvements in additives and the fact that the term *mineral oil* in Great Britain has been used interchangeably with *heavy* or *aromatic oil* (22). More recently, a mortality study sponsored by the United Auto Workers and General Motors suggested a link between cutting oils or machining fluids and various forms of cancer (e.g., esophageal, laryngeal, and rectal). The study evaluated workplace exposures from 1940 to 1984. Because the composition of these materials has changed substantially since 1940, and because the most notable effects were seen among those with work histories dating back to that time, the relevance of these findings to present-day exposures is uncertain (27).

Guidelines, Standards, and Occupational Safety

The American Conference of Governmental Industrial Hygienists (ACGIH) has developed a threshold limit value (TLV) for oil mist of 5 mg per cubic meter as an 8-hour time-weighted average (TWA) and a short-term exposure limit of 10 mg per cubic meter. In April 1996, the ACGIH proposed to establish a mineral oil mist TLV-TWA of 5 mg per cubic meter for total mist and a TLV-TWA of 5 mg per cubic meter for oil containing the sum total of 15 polycyclic aromatic hydrocarbons listed as carcinogens by the National Toxicology Program. The U.S. Occupational Safety and Health Administration (OSHA) has developed a permissible exposure limit of 5 mg per cubic meter as an 8-hour TWA.

The carcinogenicity classification of mineral oils is addressed in interpretive guidance to the OSHA Hazard Communication Standard (28,29). OSHA bases its classification of mineral oils on the results of the IARC review of carcinogenicity (3). According to OSHA, hydrotreated base oils are classified on the basis of their processing history, and solvent-refined base stocks are classified on the basis of their viscosity index after processing. Mildly hydrotreated base stocks (defined as having been processed at a pressure of 800 pounds per square inch or less at temperatures up to 800°F) are considered as possibly carcinogenic. Severely hydrotreated base stocks are considered to be noncarcinogenic. OSHA considers solvent-refined base stocks to be carcinogenic if they have a viscosity index of less than 85 after processing.

Currently, no federal or state regulatory standard or criterion applies to remediation of lubricating oil from soil. At least 30 states have set specific soil cleanup levels or guidelines based on the total petroleum hydrocarbon (TPH) measurement (30). These levels or guidelines are set alone or in combination with standards for benzene, toluene, ethylbenzene, and xylenes or PAHs. These levels range from background to 10,000 parts per million (ppm) TPH in soil (31). Many states have adopted a soil cleanup level of 100 ppm TPH in soil (31).

PETROLEUM COKE

Petroleum coke is the carbonaceous deposit that remains after redistillation and further processing of various residues left from the refining process. (Note that the term *coke* can refer also to a product derived from coal. This product is not the same as that derived from crude oil.) The process of coking involves a severe method of thermal cracking used to upgrade heavy residuals into lighter products or distillates. The feed stocks for the coking process include residual oil, clarified oil, tars and, occasionally, wastewater and sludges. Coking produces straight-run gasoline (coker naphtha), various middle distillate fractions used as catalytic cracking feed stocks, and coke (32).

Coke usually contains water and some liquid hydrocarbon. Before it is used, the coke must be dried. The process of crushing and heating coke to remove the liquid material is called *calcining*. Most petroleum coke is produced as hard, porous, irregular-shaped lumps ranging in size from 20 inches down to fine dust (1). This type of coke is called *sponge coke* (or *green coke*). The main uses for sponge coke are in the manufacture of electrodes and anodes, as a carbon source for carbides, and in the manufacture of graphite. A second form of coke, *needle coke*, has an elongated crystalline structure. Needle coke requires special coker feeds and more severe operating conditions, but its low electrical resistance makes it preferable to sponge coke in the manufacture of electrodes.

Chemical Characteristics

The composition of petroleum coke depends on the feed stock. Typically, it contains 85% to 97% fixed carbon, 0.2% to 2.5% sulfur, and 6% to 15% volatile matter (1,33). Metals such as arsenic, vanadium, nickel, selenium, iron, and boron may also be present (1,33). A typical analysis of petroleum coke includes tests for benzene extractables, which is an indication of the amount of PAHs. In tests conducted by the American Petroleum Institute, such benzene extractables as benzo(a)pyrene, benzo(e)pyrene, benzo(g,h,i)perylene, benzo(a)anthracene, and dibenzo(a,h)anthracene ranged from approximately 0.15% to 2.10%.

Exposure Assessment

Humans can be exposed to hazardous gases associated with coking operations (i.e., hydrogen sulfide, carbon monoxide, and trace PAHs). When coke is moved as a slurry, oxygen depletion may occur within confined spaces (such as storage silos) because the wet carbon can adsorb oxygen. Wastewater from the coking process may contain oil, sulfides, ammonia, or phenol and may be highly alkaline. Exposure to dust may occur during or after the coke-drying process. The use of personal protective equipment and adherence to safe work practices are necessary to avoid exposures to chemicals and other hazards such as heat and noise that are associated with the coking process.

Acute Toxicity

Given coke's high inert-carbon content, the acute toxicity of coke is low. On the basis of its physical and chemical characteristics, contact with the eyes and skin may cause irritation. Inhalation also may cause irritation of the respiratory tract, but toxicity via the oral and dermal routes is expected to be low.

Chronic Toxicity

A chronic inhalation study using petroleum coke was conducted on rats and monkeys. In this study, three groups of animals were exposed to clean air or 10.2 mg per cubic meter or 30.7 mg per cubic meter of petroleum coke dust for 2 years. No gross toxic effects were noted in the monkeys. In rats, a dose-dependent inflammatory response was seen in the lungs (34).

A dermal carcinogenicity study was conducted in mice in which two types of petroleum coke (delayed-process coke and fluid-process coke) diluted to 25% in mineral oil and applied three times weekly for the lifetime of the mice did not produce skin tumors. The only observed effect was an increased incidence of epidermal acanthosis (thickening of the skin) (35).

In a study conducted by Lipscomb and Lee (36), the effects of coke dust on respiratory function were evaluated in workers involved in petroleum coke production. A medical history, pulmonary function tests, and chest radiographs were obtained. Abnormal pulmonary function tests were significantly related to the amount of exposure to coke dust in 10% of the workers. However, the study did not stipulate the type of dust monitored (green or calcined coke). No evidence of pneumoconiosis, chronic bronchitis, or emphysema was noted.

Guidelines, Standards, and Occupational Safety

Currently, no federal or state regulatory, occupational, or public health standards are extant for petroleum coke. Generally, the occupational guidelines for particulates are used. The ACGIH has set a TLV-TWA of 10 mg per cubic meter for inhalable total particulates and a TLV-TWA of 3 mg per cubic meter for respirable particulates.

ASPHALT (BITUMEN)

Asphalt, also known as *bitumen*, is an extremely complex mixture of high-molecular-weight hydrocarbons having greater than 25 carbons and high carbon-to-hydrogen ratios. It also contains small amounts of various metals, such as nickel, iron, or vanadium. It is produced from the residue of distillation of crude oil or by separation as the raffinate from a residual oil in a deasphalting or carbonization process (13). The distillation residuum may be further processed by air blowing, solvent precipitation, or blending of other refining streams to achieve the desired physical properties (37). The major uses of asphalt include road paving and roofing. It is used also as a coating for electrical and sound insulation and corrosion protection and in municipal drinking water reservoirs (13).

Note that petroleum-derived asphalts are chemically and toxicologically distinct from coal tar pitches, which have similar uses. Coal tar pitches are manufactured by the high-temperature carbonization of bituminous coals and differ from asphalt substantially in composition and physical characteristics. Coal tar pitches contain higher levels of carcinogenic PAHs and are typically more toxic than petroleum-derived asphalts.

Chemical Characterization

Asphalt consists of compounds that typically boil at temperatures exceeding 1,000°F. The chemical composition of asphalt depends on the source of crude oil, which varies in sulfur and aromatic content. Asphalt is composed of high-molecular-weight combinations of alkanes, cycloalkanes, aromatics, and heteromolecules containing sulfur, oxygen, nitrogen, and heavy metals (e.g., vanadium, nickel, iron) (38). PAHs in asphalt are determined by the levels of PAH in the feed stock. Asphalt often is diluted with vacuum gas oils, distillate aromatic extracts, or clarified slurry oil (39). Additives used in asphalt include organic antistrip agents, silicone oil, elastomers, polymers, antioxidants, kerosene, and diesel fuel.

Exposure Assessment

Aside from walking or riding on asphalt pavement and roads, the general population does not normally come into contact with asphalt. However, the general population can experience negligible exposure to fumes from heated asphalts for short periods during road-building or roof-covering operations or from weathered run-off from roads (2). Occupational exposure may occur from repeated dermal contact with asphalt, accidental splashing with hot asphalt, or inhalation of asphalt fumes.

Research has been conducted to determine the levels of exposure to asphalt fumes that may be encountered in asphalt's manufacture and use and to establish the character and potential hazard of such fumes. Data are available from the Asphalt Institute regarding the content of PAHs from emissions of petroleum asphalt (40). This study demonstrated that emissions contained very low levels (maximum of 340 mg per cubic meter) of PAHs. The major PAH was pyrene, and the concentrations of benzo(a)pyrene ranged from 3 to 22 mg per cubic meter. In a study of the exposure of asphalt paving workers, particulate emission levels (principally mineral dusts) ranged from 0.15 to 3.46 mg per cubic meter (41). Emissions from roofing kettles have also been studied (42). A high-volatility asphalt in the kettle emitted particulates in concentrations between 0.25 and 12.60 mg per cubic meter. The benzene-soluble portion of the collected particulates consisted predominantly of innocuous hydrocarbons: paraffins, cycloparaffins, and one- to three-ring aromatics. PAHs were less than 0.05% of the total benzene solubles (38).

Animal Toxicity

No available literature addresses the acute toxicity of asphalt. However, WHO indicates that it is considered to be low (2). Several studies have been conducted regarding the potential for skin and lung carcinogenicity. Little success was achieved in early experiments that attempted to produce either skin tumors in mice and rabbits exposed to petroleum road asphalts or lung tumors in rats and guinea pigs exposed to fumes of petroleum roofing asphalt (13,43). Studies conducted by Kireeva (44) in which six different grades of asphalt were tested in mouse skin-painting assays demonstrated very few tumors. This is in contrast to the strong carcinogenicity of coal tar pitch in similar tests (13). In studies by Simmers et al. (45–48), tumors were observed in mice exposed via dermal contact to diluted asphalt or steam-refined asphalt, whereas no tumors appeared after dermal exposure to air-refined asphalt. Bingham and Feasley (49) observed only one benign tumor after skin application of straight-run asphalt, but they observed malignant and benign tumors after skin application of a thermal asphalt.

Thayer et al. (50) studied the dermal carcinogenicity of laboratory-generated emissions from asphalt and coal tar in mice. The emissions were generated by heating the asphalt and coal tar samples at 450° or 605°F, temperatures reported to be substantially higher than those used in asphalt paving operations, and were condensed to provide the material used in the bioassay. These condensates, when diluted and applied repetitively to the skin of mice, produced squamous cell carcinomas and papillomas. The relevance of this study to human exposure scenarios is not clear. In chronic inhalation studies in mice and guinea pigs, asphalt fumes did not induce tumors (51,52).

Human Toxicity

Acute dermal or inhalation exposure may cause irritation to the skin or respiratory tract. Prolonged and repeated exposure to asphalt has caused redness, peeling, neck discoloration, and throat and eye irritation (13). Although several epidemiologic studies have been conducted in an attempt to correlate exposure to asphalt with cancer, these studies are of limited value because workers usually are grouped by their exposure to any asphalt-like material, including coal tar.

Henry (53) performed an analysis of 3,753 cases of skin cancer reported in the United Kingdom between 1920 and 1945. He identified only one case in which asphalt might have been involved—a road worker for 23 years who had also been exposed to coal tar.

Hoogendam (54) reviewed the health status and causes of death of individuals who had worked in an asphalt production facility in a refinery. Exposure ranged from days to 40 years. No significant differences between the health pattern of this population and the control group were apparent, and no cases of skin tumors were encountered.

Baylor and Weaver (55) studied the health of 462 asphalt workers in 25 refineries and compared the data with those for 379 controls. Each subject had been engaged in asphalt work for at least 5 years, the average being 15.1 years. No significant health differences were noted between the two groups.

In an epidemiologic study involving roofers, no statistical increase in lung cancer mortality was found with up to 19 years of exposure to asphalt (8,56). Exposure for 20 years or longer was associated with elevated death rates from lung cancers and cancers at other sites.

Two studies performed by Hansen (1989 and 1991, as cited in ref. 37) have drawn considerable interest because of their findings of increased risks of lung and digestive tract cancers among study populations of workers in Denmark's mastic asphalt industry. The term *mastic asphalt* refers to a low-volume specialty asphalt product that is applied at high temperatures by workers positioned on their hands and knees. Neither the composition of mastic asphalt nor the work practices used in its application bear any resemblance to U.S. asphalt materials or operations.

The IARC currently is conducting a retrospective cohort and nested case-control study of cancer mortality and incidence in an international study population of asphalt workers from seven European countries (37). This study is being conducted because the IARC believes that the current available epidemiologic data are inconclusive. This study should be completed by 1998.

Guidelines, Standards, and Occupational Safety

The ACGIH has set a TLV of 5 mg per cubic meter as a TWA for exposure to asphalt fumes (57). The National Institute for Occupational Safety and Health has set a recommended exposure limit of 5 mg per cubic meter (total particulates) for asphalt fumes as a 15-minute ceiling limit. The institute has also published a draft consensus document that calls for paving equipment ventilation systems to reduce asphalt fume exposures by 80% (58).

REFERENCES

1. Gary JH, Handwerk GE. *Petroleum refining—technology and economics*, 2nd ed. New York: Marcel Dekker Inc, 1984.
2. World Health Organization. *Selected petroleum products*. Environmental health criteria 20. Geneva: World Health Organization, 1982.
3. International Agency for Research of Cancer. Polynuclear aromatic compounds: 2. Carbon blacks, mineral oils and some nitroarenes. *IARC Monogr Eval Carcinog Risks Hum* 1984;33:35–85.
4. American Petroleum Institute. *Results of toxicological studies*. API publ. no. 45591. Washington: American Petroleum Institute, Jan 1994.
5. Worrell NR. *A 90-day feeding study in the rat with six different white mineral oils, three different mineral waxes and coconut oil*. API publ. no. 4560. Washington: American Petroleum Institute, 1992.
6. Exxon Biomedical Sciences, Inc. Subchronic oral gavage study in rats, project 301970. Laboratory reports 84MRL131 and 84MRL118. Florham Park, NJ: Exxon Biomedical Sciences, Inc., 1984.
7. Gradiski D, Blachere A, Vinot J , Zissu D, Limasset JC, Lafontaine M. The carcinogenic effect of a series of petroleum-derived oils on the skin of mice. *Environ Res* 1983;32:258–268.
8. Hammond EC, Selikoff IJ, Lawther PL, Seidman H. Inhalation of benzpyrene and cancer in man. *Ann N Y Acad Sci* 1976;271:116–124.
9. Jepsen JR, Stoyanov S, Unger M, Clausen J, Christensen HE. Cutting fluids and their effects on the skin of mice. An experimental study with special reference to carcinogenicity. *Acta Pathol Microbiol Scand [A]* 1977;85:731–738.
10. McKee RH. The dermal carcinogenic potential of unrefined and hydrotreated lubricating oils. *J Appl Toxicol* 1989;9:265–270.
11. Roe FJC, Carter RL, Taylor W. Cancer hazard from mineral oil used in the processing of jute. *Br J Cancer* 1967;21:695–702.
12. Twort CC, Ing HR. Investigations on carcinogenic agents [in German]. *Z Krebsforsch* 1928;27:308–351.
13. Bingham E, Trosset R, Warshawsky D. Carcinogenic potential of petroleum hydrocarbons. A critical review of the literature. *J Environ Pathol Toxicol* 1980;3:483–563.
14. Doak SM, Brown VK, Brown PF, Smith JD, Roe FJ. The carcinogenic potential of twelve refined mineral oils following long term topical application. *Br Med J* 1983;48:429–436.
15. Halder CA, Warne TM, Little RQ, Gavin PJ. Carcinogenicity of petroleum lubricating oil distillates: 1. Effects of solvent-refining, hydroprocessing, and blending. *Am J Ind Med* 1984;5:265–274.
16. McKee RH, Przygoda R. The genotoxic and carcinogenic potential of engine oils and highly refined lubricating oils. *Environ Mutagen* 1987;9(Suppl 8):72(abst).
17. Blackburn GR, Deitch RA, Schreiner CA, Mackerer CR. Predicting carcinogenicity of petroleum distillation fractions using a modified *Salmonella* mutagenicity assay. *Cell Biol Toxicol* 1986;2:63.
18. Roy TA, Johnson SW, Blackburn GR, Mackerer CR. Correlation of mutagenic and dermal carcinogenic activities of mineral oils with polycyclic aromatic compound content. *Fund Appl Toxicol* 1988;10:466–476.
19. Gerarde HW. *Toxicology and biochemistry of aromatic hydrocarbons in commercial solvents*. Amsterdam: Elsevier Science, 1960.
20. Jampolis RW, McDonald JR, Clagett OT. Mineral oil granuloma of the lungs: an evaluation of methods for identification of mineral oil tissue. *Int Abstr Surg* 1953;97:105–119.
21. Gellin GA. Cutting fluids and skin disorders. *IMS Ind Med Surg* 1970;39:65–70.
22. Clayton GD, Clayton FE. *Patty's industrial hygiene and toxicology*, vol 2B. New York: John Wiley and Sons, 1991.
23. Boyd JT, Doll R. Gastro-intestinal cancer and the use of liquid paraffin. *Br J Cancer* 1954;8:231–237.
24. Higginson J. Etiological factors in gastrointestinal cancer in man. *J Natl Cancer Inst* 1966;37:527–545.

24a. Nochomovitz LE, Uys CJ, Epstein S. Massive deposition of mineral oil after prolonged ingestion. *S Afr Med J* 1975;13:2187–2190.

25. Catchpole WM, Macmillan E, Powell H. Specifications for cutting oils with special reference to carcinogenicity. *Ann Occup Hyg* 1971;14:171–179.
26. Waterhouse JH. Cutting oils and cancer. *Ann Occup Hyg* 1971;14:161–170.
27. Eisen EA, Tolbert PE, Monson RR, Smith TJ. Mortality studies of machining fluid exposure in the automobile industry: I. A standardized mortality ratio analysis. *Am J Ind Med* 1992;22:809–824.
28. US Department of Labor, Occupational Safety and Health Administration. Rules and regulations, 29 *CFR* part 1910. Hazard communication: interpretation regarding lubricating oils. *Federal Register* 1985 Dec 20:50: 51852–51854.
29. US Department of Labor, Occupational Safety and Health Administration. Rules and regulations, 29 *CFR* 1910.1200. Hazard communication: final rule. 59 *Federal Register* 6126; 1994 Feb 6.
30. Oliver T, Kostecki P. State by state summary of cleanup standards. *Soils* 1992;(Dec):14–24.
31. Michelson T, Boyce CP. Cleanup standards for petroleum hydrocarbons: 1. Review of methods and recent developments. *J Soil Contam* 1993;2:109–124.
32. US Department of Labor, Occupational Health and Safety Administration. Petroleum refining processes. OSHA instruction TED 1.15 CH-1, section III: chapter 2. Washington: Office of Science and Technology Assessment, 1996, May 24.
33. CONCAWE 1993. Petroleum coke. Report no. 93/105. Den Haag: The Oil Companies' International Study Group for Conservation of Clean Air and Water, 1993.
34. Klonne DR, Burns JM, Halder CA, Holdsworth CE, Ulrich CE. Two-year inhalation study of petroleum coke in rats and monkeys. *Am J Indust Med* 1987;11:375–389.
35. American Petroleum Institute. *Carcinogenic potential of petroleum coke and process products*. Washington: American Petroleum Institute, 1982.
36. Lipscomb J, Lee S. Health hazard evaluation report no. HETA 81-421-1251. Port Arthur, TX: Great Lakes Carbon Corporation, 1981. [As cited in CONCAWE, 1990].
37. Asphalt Industry Environmental Oversight Committee (AIEOC). Presentation on asphalt fumes to the TLV Committee, American Conference of Governmental Industrial Hygienists, October 5, 1996.
38. King RW, Puzinauskas VP, Holdsworth CE. *Asphalt composition and health effects: a critical review*. API technical publication. Washington: American Petroleum Institute, 1984.
39. Puzinauskas VP, Corbett LW. Differences between petroleum asphalt, coal-tar pitch and coal tar. Research report no. 75-1. College Park, MD: Asphalt Institute, 1978.
40. Puzinauskas VP, Corbett LW. Report on emissions from asphalt hot mixes. Research report no. 75-1A. College Park, MD: Asphalt Institute, 1975.

41. Puzinauskas VP. Exposures of paving workers to asphalt emissions. Research report no. 80-1. College Park, MD: Asphalt Institute, 1980.
42. Puzinauskas VP. Emissions from asphalt roofing kettles. Research report no. 79-2. College Park, MD: Asphalt Institute, 1979.
43. Wallcave L, Garcia H, Feldman R, Lijinsky W, Shubik P. Skin tumorigenesis in mice by petroleum asphalts and coal tar pitches of known polynuclear aromatic hydrocarbon content. *Toxicol Appl Pharmacol* 1971;18:41–52.
44. Kireeva IS. Carcinogenic properties of coal-tar pitch and petroleum asphalts used as binders for coal briquettes. *Hyg Sanit* 1968;33:35–40.
45. Simmers MH, Podolak E, Kinosite R. Carcinogenic effects of petroleum asphalt. *Proc Soc Exp Biol Med* 1959;101:266–268.
46. Simmers MH. Cancers from air-refined and steam-refined asphalt. *Ind Med Surg* 1965;34:255–261.
47. Simmers MH. Cancers in mice from asphalt fractions. *Ind Med Surg* 1965;34:573–577.
48. Simmers MH. Tumors from asphalt fractions injected into mice. *Ind Med Surg* 1966;35:889–894.
49. Bingham E, Feasley CF. Carcinogenic properties of experimental electrode binders. Unpublished thesis, University of Cincinnati, 1972.
50. Thayer PS, Menzies DT, Von Thuna PC, Miller A. *Roofing asphalts, pitch and UVL carcinogenesis.* Cincinatti: National Institute for Occupational Safety and Health, 1981.
51. Hueper WC, Payne WW. Carcinogenic studies on petroleum asphalt, cooling oil and coal tar. *Arch Pathol* 1960;70:372–384.
52. Simmers MH. Petroleum asphalt inhalation by mice. *Arch Environ Health* 1964;9:727–734.
53. Henry SA. Occupational cutaneous cancer attributable to certain chemicals in industry. *Br Med Bull* 1947;4:389–401.
54. Hoogendam I. *Health checks on asphalt workers.* Inten. Rep. Med. Div. The Hague: Shell International Petroleum Co, 1962.
55. Baylor CH, Weaver NK. A health survey of petroleum asphalt workers. *Arch Environ Health* 1968;17:210–214.
56. Selikoff IJ. Roofers study. In: Industrial Health Foundation. *Proceedings of the symposium on particulate polycyclic organic matter (coal tar pitch volatiles), April 29–30, 1975.* Pittsburgh: Carnegie-Mellon Institute of Research, 1976:78–85.
57. Argyris TS, Slaga TJ. Promotion of carcinomas by repeated abrasion in initiated skin of mice. *Cancer Res* 1981;41:5193–5195.
58. National Institute of Occupational Safety and Health. Engineering control guidelines for hot mix asphalt pavers, no. 61 *CFR*, 51708. Atlanta: National Institute of Occupational Safety and Health, 1996.

CHAPTER 71
Arsenic

Luke Yip and Richard C. Dart

SOURCE, PRODUCTION, COMMON NAMES, AND USES

Arsenic is ubiquitous in the environment. Exposure to arsenic may come from natural sources (groundwater, arsenic-containing mineral ores), industrial processes (semiconductor manufacturing, burning of fossil fuels or wood treated with arsenic preservatives, metallurgy, glass clarification, smelting and refining of metals and ores), commercial products (wood preservatives, pesticides, herbicides, fungicides, fire salts), food (seafood, kelp, wine, tobacco), or intentionally administered sources with either a benevolent intent (antiparasitic drugs, folk remedies, and such naturopathic remedies as "Asiatic pill," *kushtay*, yellow root) or a malevolent intent (suicidal or homicidal attempts) (1). Today, acute arsenic poisoning most commonly is the result of an accidental ingestion or the result of suicidal or homicidal intent. Ingestion of contaminated well water, opium inhalation, smelting of metals, and combustion of fossil fuels can result in chronic toxicity. Large-scale hazardous material incidents involving arsenic have not occurred in the United States. However, the potential for small- or large-scale exposures exists, and the health effects could be severe, as evidenced by the poisoning of 12,131 Japanese children who consumed arsenic-tainted dry milk. The incident caused 130 deaths (2).

In the United States, arsenic has been used primarily in insecticides, with the concentrated liquid forms having extreme potential toxicity to humans. The highest worker exposures in the insecticide industry have been reported to occur in the mixing, screening, drying, bagging, and drum-filling operations (3). Regulatory restrictions, especially for home products, have reduced this problem dramatically (4). Smelting of metals, especially copper, has produced high arsenic exposures at workplaces (4,5). Increased arsenic levels also have been demonstrated in populations located near smelting plants (6). Similarly, arsenic-containing products are used as herbicides, desiccants in the cotton industry, wood preservatives, and animal feed additives. Arsenic has been used also in chemical warfare agents (5). More recent industrial release of arsenic has occurred in the semiconductor industry (7). Arsenic in the form of gallium arsenide (GaAs) is used as a dopant, speeding transmission in microcomputer chips used in communications equipment, scientific instruments, and the computer industry (8). It may be released from chips for hours after their manufacture (9). GaAs particulates are toxic in animal models, and arsine is used in GaAs production. The risks posed by this source currently are unknown. An extensive review of arsenic sources has been published (10).

CHEMICAL AND PHYSICAL FORMS

Arsenic has a molecular weight of 74.9 and is classified as a transition element or metalloid because it commonly complexes with metals but also reacts with carbon, hydrogen, and oxygen. Arsenic compounds can be classified into three major groups: inorganic, organic, and arsine gas. The latter is discussed separately in this chapter (see Arsine Gas). The three most common valence states are the metalloid [elemental (0) oxidation state], the arsenite [trivalent (+3) state], and the arsenate [pentavalent (+5) state]. Both arsenite and arsenate forms are highly soluble in water.

The toxicity of arsenic compounds varies considerably. In general, the arsenicals can be arranged in their order of decreasing toxicity: inorganic trivalent compounds, organic trivalent compounds, inorganic pentavalent compounds, organic pentavalent compounds, and elemental arsenic (11). Trivalent arsenic generally is two- to tenfold more toxic than is pentavalent arsenic. In rodents, the oral median lethal dose of arsenic trioxide (trivalent) in solution ranges from 10 to 60 mg per kg. Humans appear to be an order of magnitude more sensitive, and the minimum oral lethal human dose probably is between 10 and 300 mg.

Some marine organisms and algae contain large amounts of organic arsenic, sometimes known as *fish arsenic*. It is seen in the form of arsenobetaine, a trimethylated arsenic compound, and of arsenocholine. Arsenobetaine and arsenocholine are excreted unchanged in the urine, with total clearance in approximately 2 days, and exert no known toxic effects in humans. Most commercially available compounds containing arsenic are produced from arsenic trioxide (5). Organic arsenic–containing compounds include arsanilic acid, methylarsonic acid, dimethylarsinic acid (cacodylic acid, DMA), and arsenobetaine (4).

SITES, INDUSTRIES, AND BUSINESSES ASSOCIATED WITH EXPOSURES

The microelectronics industry represents an increasing source of arsenic exposure (Table 71-1). Both inorganic arsenic and arsine are used in the manufacture of computer chips for communications

TABLE 71-1. Sites, industries, and businesses associated with exposures

Business or industry	Mechanism	Example
Acute exposure		
Pesticide spraying	Food and water contamination	Inorganic arsenicals
Microelectronic manufacture	Air contamination by gas or particulates	Arsine, arsenic oxides, gallium arsenide
Arsenical products	Food and water contamination	Beer, soy water, milk
War gases	Air contamination	Lewisite, others
Chronic exposure		
Microelectronic manufacture	Air contamination by gas or particulates	Arsine, arsenic oxides, gallium arsenide
Smelting of nonferrous ores	Air, water contamination	Gold, copper
Fossil fuel combustion	Air, water contamination	Coal, oil shale
Phosphate detergents	Water, food contamination	Milk, others
Leaching of mine tailings and smelter	Water contamination	Residue piles
Copper leach liquors	Water contamination	Hazardous waste
Pesticide application	Air, water, food contamination	Agriculture
Arsenical manufacturing	Air, water contamination	Sheep dip factory, insecticides, herbicides, fungicides, algicides, wood preservatives
Cotton harvesting	Air, water contamination	Cotton gin operation
Food additives	—	Poultry

equipment, scientific equipment, and computers. Several steps in manufacture could expose workers to arsenic, especially if equipment malfunctions occur. In such cases, either air contamination or physical contamination can occur. In addition, preliminary studies have suggested that in industrial GaAs chip manufacture, air contamination by arsenic exceeds recommended limits and should be considered a source for arsenic toxicity (8).

The potential for hazardous material incidents exists in many of the aforementioned industries. Accidents involving the source materials (i.e., arsine canisters or containers of arsenic oxide powders) may expose workers and the surrounding population. Although mass exposures have not yet occurred, isolated deaths from industrial exposures have been reported (12).

ORGANIC AND INORGANIC ARSENIC

Routes of Absorption and Toxic Exposure

INHALATION

The major routes of arsenic entry into the human body are ingestion and inhalation. The amount of arsenic absorbed by inhalation is thought to be in the 60% to 90% range. Airborne arsenic particles usually occur in the As_2O_3 form (5) and may be inhaled, deposited in the upper airways, and swallowed after mucociliary clearance, thereby resulting in gastrointestinal (GI) absorption rather than in pulmonary inhalation (4,13). Documented biological effects after respiratory exposure to arsenic concentrations previously believed to be benign raise serious questions about the safety of even minor inhalation exposure (4). Further evaluation of this aspect of arsenic exposure is needed (4).

Inhalation of elemental arsenic, arsenic compounds, or arsine can occur during several stages of semiconductor manufacture. Wafer manufacture requires handling of elemental arsenic. Arsenic oxides are produced during the heating process. Arsine gas is used as a dopant to introduce arsenic into the wafer. A worker can be exposed during accidents or by handling materials contaminated during the manufacturing process. High-risk areas include ampule loading and breakout, ingot slicing and sandblasting, and epitaxial reactor loading and cleaning (8).

INGESTION

Soluble forms of ingested arsenic are well absorbed (60% to 90%) from the GI tract (5). Organic arsenic compounds in food and medication also are well absorbed (14,15). Most reported cases of acute arsenic toxicity result from ingestion (4). In addition, particulate arsenic may be cleared by the pulmonary mucociliary apparatus and swallowed, thus becoming a source of GI exposure.

SKIN ABSORPTION

Little information is available concerning the chemical form, conditions for absorption, kinetics, or other information needed to evaluate the significance of skin absorption in specific populations (4). However, toxic systemic effects have been reported from rare occupational accidents in which arsenic trichloride or arsenic acid was splashed on workers' skin (16).

Pharmacokinetics of Exposure

After absorption, arsenic is bound to proteins in the blood and is redistributed to the liver, spleen, kidneys, lungs, and GI tract within 24 hours. Clearance from these tissues is dose-dependent. Two to four weeks after exposure ceases, most of the arsenic remaining in the body is found in keratin-rich tissues, such as skin, hair, and nails.

In vivo, interconversion of arsenite and arsenate takes place. Both forms of arsenic undergo biomethylation in the liver to monomethylarsonic acid (MMA) and DMA. The methylation process may represent detoxification because the metabolites exert less acute toxicity in experimental lethality studies. The liver's efficiency in methylation decreases with increasing arsenic dose. When the methylating capacity of the liver is exceeded, exposure to excess levels of inorganic arsenic results in increased retention of arsenic in soft tissues.

Arsenic is eliminated from the body primarily by renal excretion. Urinary arsenic excretion begins promptly after absorption and, depending on the amount of arsenic ingested, urinary excretion may remain elevated for 1 to 2 months. After low-level exposure to inorganic arsenic, most of the urinary arsenic is present in the form of methylated metabolites. Mahieu et al. (17) demonstrated in humans that after acute intoxication by inorganic arsenic, arsenic is excreted in the urine as inorganic arsenic, MMA, and DMA, but the proportion of these metabolites varies over time. During the first 2 to 4 days after intoxication, arsenic is excreted mainly in the inorganic form. This is followed by a progressive increase of the proportion excreted as MMA and DMA. The time at which arsenic is excreted primarily as its methylated metabolites would depend on the severity and duration of the intoxication. Pentavalent arsenic is cleared more rapidly than is trivalent arsenic. Because arsenic is cleared quickly from the blood, blood levels may attain "normal" status, although urine levels may remain markedly elevated. Renal dysfunction may be a major impediment to normal elimination of arsenic compounds.

Inorganic arsenic can cross the human placenta: High levels of arsenic were found at postmortem examination in a neonate born after acute maternal arsenic intoxication (18).

Pathophysiology of Exposure

Arsenicals appear to produce multiorgan injury by two major mechanisms. Arsenic's overt toxicity is believed to be related to its reversible binding to sulfhydryl groups, leading to the inhibition of critical sulfhydryl-containing enzyme systems. Trivalent arsenite is particularly potent in this regard. The pyruvate and succinate oxidation pathways are particularly sensitive to arsenic inhibition. Dihydrolipoate, a sulfhydryl cofactor, appears to be a principal target. Normally, dihydrolipoate is oxidized to lipoate via a converting enzyme, dihydrolipoate dehydrogenase. Arsenic reacts with both dihydrolipoate and dihydrolipoate dehydrogenase, preventing the formation of lipoate. Lipoate is involved in the formation of key intermediates in the Krebs cycle. As a result of lipoate depletion, the Krebs cycle and oxidative phosphorylation are inhibited. Without oxidative phosphorylation, cellular energy stores in the form of adenosine triphosphate (ATP) are depleted, resulting in metabolic failure and cell death.

The other mechanism by which arsenic is believed to produce cellular injury is termed *arsenolysis*. Pentavalent arsenate can substitute competitively for phosphate in biochemical reactions. During oxidative phosphorylation, energy is produced and stored in the form of ATP. The stable phosphate ester bond in ATP can be replaced by an arsenate ester bond. However, the high energy stored in the arsenate ester bond is wasted, as it is and is hydrolyzed rapidly. Cellular respiration will be stimulated in a futile attempt to restore this lost energy. In effect, trivalent arsenicals inhibit critical enzymes in the Krebs cycle, also leading to inhibition of oxidative phosphorylation, and pentavalent arsenicals uncouple oxidative phosphorylation by arsenolysis. This results in the disruption of cellular oxidative processes and leads to endothelial cellular damage. The fundamental lesion seen clinically is loss of capillary integrity, resulting in increased permeability of blood vessels and tissue hypoxia, which leads to generalized vasodilation, transudation of plasma, hypovolemia, and shock.

Clinical Toxicology: Signs, Symptoms, and Syndromes

ACUTE TOXICITY

Clinical effects of acute arsenic poisoning usually involve multiorgan systems, in particular the GI tract and the cardiovascular, respiratory, hematologic, neurologic, renal, and dermatologic systems (Table 71-2). The bone marrow, skin, and peripheral nervous system may develop chronic toxicity after acute or chronic exposure. Thus, an acute poisoning may cause both acute and chronic syndromes.

Gastrointestinal Tract. Symptoms usually begin within 30 minutes after a serious arsenic ingestion, but onset may be delayed by ingestion with food. The most prominent clinical finding associated with acute arsenic poisoning probably is related to the GI tract. Some forms of arsenic are corrosive. Acute ingestion may lead to oral irritation, a burning sensation in the mouth and throat, and dysphagia. A metallic taste or a garlicky odor on the breath (or both) have been described but often are absent. Nausea, vomiting, diarrhea, and abdominal pain are common. The toxic effects of arsenic on the GI mucosal vasculature are vasodilation, transudation of fluid into the bowel lumen, mucosal vesicle formation, and sloughing of tissue fragments. Rupture of vesicles may cause bleeding, profuse watery stools ("rice-water stools"), and a protein-losing enteropathy. In serious cases, hemorrhagic gastroenteritis may ensue within minutes to hours after acute ingestion. Nausea, vomiting, and severe hemorrhagic gastroenteritis can lead to profound intravascular volume loss, resulting in hypovolemic shock, the major cause of mortality and morbidity. Aggressive resuscitation with crystalloids, colloids, and blood products with intensive hemodynamic monitoring may be required.

TABLE 71-2. Manifestations of acute arsenic poisoning

Bodily system affected	Symptom or sign	Time of onset
Systemic	Thirst	Minutes
	Hypovolemia, hypotension	Minutes to hours
Gastrointestinal system	Garlic or metallic taste	Immediate
	Burning mucosae	Immediate
	Nausea and vomiting	Minutes
	Diarrhea	Minutes to hours
	Abdominal pain	Minutes to hours
	Hematemesis	Minutes to hours
	Hematochezia, melena	Hours
	Rice-water stools	Hours
Hematopoietic system	Red cell hemolysis	Minutes to hours
	Hematuria	Minutes to hours
	Isolated blood element decrease (i.e., lymphopenia)	Several weeks
	Pancytopenia	Several weeks
Pulmonary system (primarily in inhalational exposures)	Cough	Immediate
	Dyspnea	Minutes to hours
	Chest pain	Minutes to hours
	Pulmonary edema	Minutes to hours
Liver	Jaundice	Days
	Fatty degeneration	Days
	Central necrosis	Days
Kidneys	Proteinuria	Hours to days
	Hematuria	Hours to days
	Acute renal failure	Hours to days
Central nervous system	Confusion, delirium	Hours
	Encephalopathy	Minutes to hours
	Seizures	Minutes to hours
Peripheral nervous system	Sensory and motor neuropathy	Several weeks

Cardiovascular System. Electrocardiographic (ECG) changes after arsenic ingestion include nonspecific ST- and T-wave changes, sometimes mimicking ischemia or hyperkalemia and QTc prolongation (19–22). These ECG abnormalities are reported to occur in approximately one-half the patients who experience arsenic poisoning. These ECG changes may be evident from 4 to 30 hours after ingestion and may persist up to 8 weeks (20–22).

Five cases of arsenic-induced torsades de pointes have been reported (23–26). In all these cases, QTc prolongation was evident on the admission electrocardiogram, peripheral neuropathy was a prominent finding on physical examination at the time of hospital admission, and the polymorphic ventricular tachydysrhythmias ultimately were self-limited. Although documentation specified when during the hospital course the torsades de points was observed, the time between arsenic exposure and the onset of cardiac dysrhythmias remains speculative.

Anyone with arsenic intoxication necessitating hospitalization should be admitted to an intensive care unit (ICU). Extended cardiac monitoring for ventricular dysrhythmias is indicated for all patients whose electrocardiogram reveals QTc prolongation. When a prolonged QTc interval is evident, type IA antidysrhythmic cardiac medications should be avoided, as these drugs may themselves cause further QTc prolongation and worsen the atypical ventricular tachycardia (24). Lidocaine, magnesium, and isoproterenol have been used with limited success in the management of arsenic-induced torsades de pointes (23,24,26). A transvenous pacemaker for overdrive pacing may be necessary (23,24).

Respiratory System. Cough, dyspnea, and chest pain may develop after arsenic exposure by the pulmonary route (5). Pulmonary edema may occur, especially in cases of inhalation. Noncardiogenic pulmonary edema may occur from increased capillary permeability, and cardiogenic pulmonary edema may occur from myocardial depression.

Hematopoietic System. Either acute or chronic arsenic poisoning may affect the hematopoietic system. Reversible bone marrow depression with pancytopenia, particularly leukopenia, may occur. This has been observed to reach a nadir at 1 to 2 weeks, with recovery beginning 2 to 3 weeks later. However, it is chronic arsenic intoxication that usually is associated with severe hematopoietic derangements. A wide variety of hematologic abnormalities have been described (27–32):

- Anemia
- Absolute neutropenia
- Thrombocytopenia
- Relative eosinophilia: more common than absolute eosinophilia
- Basophilic stippling, increased bone marrow vascularity, and rouleau formation

Moderate anemia may be normochromic and normocytic or hypochromic and microcytic and, in the studies cited, was due in part to an increase in hemolysis and disturbed erythropoiesis-myelopoiesis (27–32). Reticulocytosis with predominant normoblastic erythropoiesis was evident. Accelerated pyknosis of the normoblast nucleus, *karyorrhexis*, is characteristic of arsenic poisoning, and the typical cloverleaf nuclei may be evident (33).

Hematologic findings may appear within 4 days after arsenic ingestion (33) and, in the absence of any specific therapy, erythrocytes, leukocytes, and thrombocytes can return to normal values within 2 to 3 weeks after arsenic exposure is discontinued (27). Symptomatic treatment with blood product transfusions and antibiotics were necessary only for severe anemia, bleeding, or infections (27–32).

Neurologic System. Usually, neuropathy is not the initial complaint associated with acute arsenic poisoning. Polyneuropathy associated with arsenic toxicity has been described as an axonal-loss sensorimotor polyneuropathy (sensory and motor conduction responses of low amplitude or that cannot be elicited, often with preserved motor conduction velocities).

The onset of neuropathy has been reported to occur 1 to 3 weeks after the presumed arsenic exposure (34,35). Clinical presentation may range from mild paresthesia with preserved ambulation to distal weakness, quadriplegia, and respiratory muscle insufficiency. Arsenical neuropathy is a diffuse, symmetric, painful sensorimotor neuropathy, with the sensory component being more prominent in a stocking-and-glove distribution (35,36). This polyneuropathy begins in the peripheral extremities and may progress in an ascending fashion to involve proximal arms and legs. Dysesthesias begin in the lower extremities, with a severe painful burning sensation occurring in the soles of the feet. Accompanying loss of vibration and positional sense causes a gait disturbance, followed by the loss of pinprick, light touch, and temperature sensation. Motor dysfunction is characterized by the loss of deep tendon reflexes, muscle weakness, and wasting. In severe poisoning, ascending weakness and paralysis may involve the respiratory muscles, resulting in neuromuscular respiratory failure (37,38). In the upper extremities, the ulnar and median nerves are affected most commonly. Researchers have reported that many of the patients with arsenical neuropathy initially were thought to have Landry-Guillain-Barré disease (34,38). The differentiation between the two conditions is based on clinical and laboratory findings in that arsenical neuropathy rarely involves the cranial nerves, sensory manifestations are more prominent, weakness in the distal portions of the extremities is more severe, and the cerebrospinal fluid protein levels usually are less than 100 mg per dL (34,35). Patients with polyneuropathy associated with severe arsenic poisoning should be observed closely for respiratory dysfunction, as aggressive ventilatory support may be needed. Neuromuscular respiratory failure may be delayed 1 to 2 months after the initial presentation.

Altered neurologic functions include confusion, delirium, encephalopathy, seizures, coma, and death (34,35). Cases of toxic encephalopathy associated with elevated arsenic levels slowly resolving over months to years have been described (39,40). However, encephalopathy may be permanent.

Renal System. The fundamental lesion in arsenic toxicity is the loss of capillary integrity, and increased glomerular capillary permeability may result in proteinuria. However, the kidneys are relatively spared from the direct toxic effects of arsenic. Hypovolemic shock associated with prominent GI symptoms may lead to hypoperfusion of the kidneys and result in oliguria, acute tubular necrosis, and renal insufficiency or failure.

The kidneys are the main route of excretion for arsenic compounds. Normal, functioning kidneys can excrete more than 100 mg of arsenic in the first 24 hours (41). Owing to shock and decreased glomerular filtration rate and depending on the body's arsenic burden, peak urinary arsenic excretion often may be delayed by 2 to 3 days. Hemodialysis (initiated 24 to 96 hours after ingestion) has been reported to remove approximately 4 mg of arsenic over a 4-hour period in patients with established renal failure (42,43). Only small amounts of arsenic should be expected to be removed by dialysis, because minimal amounts of arsenic are left in the central compartment once tissue distribution and equilibration are complete. This would limit the usefulness of hemodialysis when normal renal function is present. However, hemodialysis may be considered in acute arsenic poisoning in which renal failure coexists (42,43).

Skin. Few acute skin changes except flushing are found with arsenic poisoning, although chronic skin changes from acute exposure may develop. Eczematoid lesions of variable severity may develop (5). Dermal changes occurring most frequently in arsenic-exposed humans are hyperpigmentation, melanosis, hyperkeratosis, warts, and skin cancer (4,5,44). The lesions usually appear 1 to 6 weeks after the onset of illness. In most cases, a diffuse, brawny desquamation develops over the trunk and extremities that is dry, scaling, and nonpruritic. Patchy hyperpigmentation—dark brown patches with scattered pale spots sometimes described as raindrops on a dusty road—occurs particularly on the eyelids, temples, axillae, neck, nipples, and groin.

Arsenical hyperkeratosis usually appears as cornlike elevations, less than 1 cm in diameter, occurring most frequently on the palms of the hands and soles of the feet. Most cases of arsenical keratoses remain morphologically benign for decades; in other cases, marked atypia (precancerous) develops and appears indistinguishable from Bowen's disease, an *in situ* squamous cell carcinoma. Skin lesions will take several years to manifest the characteristic pigmented changes and hyperkeratoses, whereas skin cancer will not become evident for up to 40 years.

Brittle nails, the surface of which is marked by transverse white bands (leukonychia striata arsenicalis transversus), have been associated with arsenic poisoning; the characteristic bands are known as *Reynolds-Aldrich-Mees lines* (45–47). This finding reflects transient disruption of nail plate growth during acute poisoning. Leukonychia striata arsenicalis transversus takes approximately 5 to 6 weeks to appear over the lunulae after acute poisoning (34). Thinning of the hair and patchy or diffuse alopecia also are associated with arsenic poisoning (46,48).

Besides being a chemical irritant, arsenic may function as a contact allergen. Low, noncaustic skin exposures may result in vesiculation in sensitized people (4). Mucous membrane irritation and ulceration involving the face, cornea, nasal septum, and respiratory tract also may occur (49).

CHRONIC AND LONG-TERM TOXICITY

The bone marrow, skin, and peripheral nervous system may become involved after acute or chronic exposure (Table 71-3). Aplastic anemia has been documented. Acute myelogenous leukemia has been reported after chronic exposure (28). Chronic ingestion of inorganic arsenic has been strongly associated with an increased risk of skin cancer in humans (50,51). Arsenic-induced skin cancer occurs mostly in unexposed areas, such as the trunk, palms, and soles. More than one type of skin cancer may occur in affected individuals. In order of decreasing frequency, the types of skin cancers reported most commonly are Bowen's disease, squamous cell carcinomas, basal cell carcinomas, and combined forms (50,51). Hyperkeratosis and hyperpigmentation usually are present in patients with dermal malignancies. An excess of respiratory cancer in arsenic-exposed workers has been reported (52,53), although recent additional monitoring of these patients raised questions of whether a significant excess of lung cancer existed (54). The U.S. Occupational Safety and Health Administration has linked arsenic to cancer of skin, lungs, lymph glands, and bone marrow (55). Arsenic has been associated also with bladder, kidney, prostate, and liver cancer (56).

Peripheral vascular disease and associated gangrene (so-called Blackfoot disease) have been reported to result from arsenic poisoning (57). Elevation of hepatic transaminases also has been noted in several reports (52,58).

Inorganic arsenic is teratogenic after administration of large doses in rodents. However, whether toxic effects will be observed at permissible exposure limits is uncertain, owing to a current lack of evidence (59).

TABLE 71-3. Manifestations of chronic arsenic poisoning

Bodily system affected	Symptom or sign
Systemic	Thirst
	Hypovolemia, hypotension
Skin, mucous membranes	Eczema
	Hyperkeratosis, palms and soles
	Warts
	Melanosis or vitiligo (or both)
	Mucous membrane irritation, ulceration
	Alopecia
	Squamous cell cancers
Gastrointestinal system	Stomatitis
	Diarrhea
Hematopoietic system	Leukopenia
	Anemia
	Pancytopenia
	Acute myelogenous leukemia
Kidneys	Acute renal failure
Central nervous system	Confusion, delirium
	Encephalopathy
	Seizures
Peripheral nervous system	Sensory and motor neuropathy

Clinical Features. A temporal appearance of organ system injury seems to be associated with arsenic poisoning. In certain cases, after a delay of minutes to hours, severe hemorrhagic gastroenteritis becomes evident and may be accompanied by cardiovascular collapse or death. Bone marrow depression with leukopenia may appear within 4 days of arsenic ingestion and usually reaches a nadir at 1 to 2 weeks. Encephalopathy, congestive cardiomyopathy, noncardiogenic pulmonary edema, and cardiac conduction abnormalities may occur several days after improvement of the initial GI manifestation. Sensorimotor peripheral neuropathy may become apparent several weeks after resolution of the initial signs of intoxication.

Laboratory Features. Arsenic is a general cellular poison that affects most organ systems of the body to some degree. Thus, laboratory tests should include a complete blood count with peripheral smear; analysis of levels of electrolytes, liver enzymes, creatine phosphokinase, arterial blood gas, and blood and urine arsenic; a renal profile with urine analysis; electrocardiography; and chest and abdominal radiography. Nerve conduction velocity studies may be indicated if peripheral neurologic symptoms are present. Some arsenic compounds, particularly those of low solubility, are radiopaque and, if ingested, may be visible on abdominal radiography. (See also Biological Monitoring, in the section Arsine Gas.)

Probably the most important diagnostic test is urinary arsenic measurement. Urine arsenic levels may be measured as a spot sample (i.e., the concentration in a single voided urine specimen, reported in micrograms per liter). Urine arsenic levels may be measured also as a timed urine collection (i.e., the concentration in urine collected over a 12- to 24-hour period, reported in micrograms per 12 or 24 hours). The quantitative 24-hour urine collection is considered the most reliable. In an emergency situation, the spot urine sample may be of value. Normal total urinary arsenic values are less than 50 μg per L or less than 25 μg per 24 hours. In the first 2 to 3 days after acute symptomatic intoxication, total 24-hour urinary arsenic excretion typically exceeds several thousand micrograms and spot urine concentrations are greater than 1,000 μg per L; depending on the severity, these values may not return to baseline levels for weeks. Recent ingestion of seafood may elevate urinary arsenic values markedly for the next 48 hours. Therefore, an important approach is to record carefully the patient's dietary history over the last 48 hours, when only total urinary arsenic is measured. Speciation of the urinary arsenic can be performed in some laboratories; otherwise, the urinary arsenic test should be repeated in 2 to 3 days. Whole-blood arsenic, normally less than 1 μg per dL, may be elevated early on in acute intoxication. However, blood levels decline rapidly to normal values despite elevated urinary arsenic excretion and continuing symptoms.

Elevated arsenic content in hair and nail segments, normally less than 1 part per million (ppm), may persist for months after urinary arsenic values have returned to baseline. However, caution must be exercised in interpreting the arsenic content obtained from hair and nails, because the arsenic content of these specimens may be increased by external contamination. (See also Environmental Monitoring, in the section Arsine Gas.)

Toxicologic Management

The current management of acute arsenic poisoning relies on supportive care and chelation therapy. As in all life-threatening emergencies, the general management of arsenic poisoning begins with elimination of further exposure to the toxic agent and provision of basic and advanced life support, focusing on maintenance of a patent airway, adequate ventilation, and cardiovascular support. Anyone requiring hospitalization because of arsenic intoxication should be admitted to the ICU. Consultation with a regional poison center and a clinical toxicologist is recommended to assist with the management of the patient.

DECONTAMINATION

Gastric lavage should be performed after an acute arsenic ingestion and should be considered if the ingestion has been within the last 24 hours, as some arsenicals of low solubility may be retained in the stomach for a prolonged period. Frequently, seriously poisoned patients will already have vomited. Activated charcoal and cathartics may be used, but their efficacy is unclear. Data from *in vitro* and *in vivo* animal studies suggested that inorganic arsenicals are not bound well to activated charcoal (60). On evidence of a heavy metal burden on an abdominal radiograph, whole-bowel irrigation with a polyethylene glycol electrolyte solution may rapidly help to clear the GI tract of the metallic load. However, the absence of radiopacities on an abdominal radiograph is nondiagnostic, and whole-bowel irrigation still should be considered in the presence of a definite history that a poorly soluble arsenical has been ingested.

After dermal exposure, clothing should be removed, and the skin should be cleaned for all arsenic exposures. After decontamination of the skin, standard symptomatic skin care is used to treat dermatitis, ulcers, and other skin lesions (5).

SUPPORTIVE MEASURES

Aggressive monitoring of intravascular volume status should be performed in an ICU. Volume should be replaced as clinically indicated, first by isotonic crystalloid administration and then by colloids and specific blood products. Vasopressors are recommended for refractory hypotension.

No data indicate specific measures to prevent dysrhythmias. Dysrhythmias should be treated according to the accepted guidelines of the advanced cardiac life support. Type IA antidysrhythmic agents should be avoided in the presence of a prolonged QTc interval on the electrocardiogram.

The management of arsenical polyneuropathy should include both symptomatic treatment for pain and physical therapy and rehabilitation. In cases of progressive sensorimotor dysfunction, particularly ascending weakness, respiratory muscle function should be monitored carefully. On evidence of impending neuromuscular respiratory failure, aggressive supportive measures should be initiated in a timely fashion.

Potential renal failure, in part due to hemolysis and hemoglobinuria, should be managed by maintaining good renal perfusion evident by a urine output of 1 to 2 mL per kg per hour. Although urine alkalinization has been suggested to prevent deposition of red blood cell (RBC) breakdown products, no credible evidence supports this recommendation.

CHELATION

In addition to supportive therapy, a chelating agent often is used for treating arsenic poisoning. Dimercaprol [2,3-dimercapto-1-propanol (British anti-Lewisite, or BAL)] is the traditional chelating agent that has been used clinically in arsenic poisoning. In humans and animal models, the antidotal efficacy of BAL has been shown to be most effective when it was administered promptly (i.e., minutes to hours) after acute arsenic exposure (61,62). In cases of suspected acute symptomatic intoxication, treatment should not be delayed while specific laboratory confirmation is awaited. BAL is administered parenterally as a deep intramuscular injection. The initial dose is 3 to 5 mg per kg every 4 hours, gradually tapering to every 12 hours over the next several days. As the patient improves, an oral agent may be substituted, such as succimer, a water-soluble analog of BAL (63–65). In the United States, succimer is available only in an oral formulation. This restriction precludes its use in acute severe arsenic intoxication when shock, vomiting, gastroenteritis, and splanchnic edema limit GI absorption. For patients with stable GI and cardiovascular status, a dosing regimen of 10 mg per kg every 8 hours for 5 days, reduced to every 12 hours for another 2 weeks, may be employed. D-Penicillamine also has been reported to be a successful treatment in cases of acute pediatric arsenic toxicity (66–68). Oral D-penicillamine, 25 mg per kg every 6 hours (to a maximum of 1 g per day), should be used if BAL or succimer is unavailable or if the patient is unable to tolerate either of these medications.

Reservations concerning the use of BAL and D-penicillamine recently have been raised. In rabbits, treatment with BAL 1 hour after administration of arsenite was found to increase brain arsenic levels (69). Penicillamine's ability to chelate arsenic effectively has been described as ineffective or inferior to the water-soluble BAL analogs (70).

The therapeutic endpoints of chelation are poorly defined. Usually, 24-hour urinary arsenic excretion is followed before, during, and after chelation with continued chelation therapy until the urinary arsenic excretion is less than 25 μg per 24 hours. Alternatively, when more than 90% of the total arsenic excreted in the urine can be demonstrated to be in the form of MMA and DMA, endogenous biomethylation and detoxification may obviate the need for continued chelation (17). This is likely to occur during the recovery period, when urinary inorganic arsenic concentration has declined to less than 100 μg per 24 hours or the total blood arsenic level is less than 200 μg per L (17,71).

Chelation treatment seems to show variable results on neurotoxicity, and some debate concerns the efficacy of chelation therapy in the treatment of arsenic-induced neuropathy (34–36,72). Early chelation therapy may prevent incipient peripheral neuropathy in some patients. However, the value of chelation in the treatment of an established arsenic neuropathy has not been demonstrated. In cases of chronic symptomatic arsenic intoxication with high urinary arsenic excretion, an empiric course of chelation may be warranted.

HEMODIALYSIS

If oliguria or renal failure develops, hemodialysis should be considered; otherwise, it contributes minimally to arsenic clearance as compared with the normally functioning kidneys. Arsenic and arsenic chelates are excreted in the urine (43).

ARSINE GAS

Arsine gas (hydrogen arsenide) is a colorless, nonirritating, inflammable gas with a garlicky odor; it is considered to be the most toxic of the arsenicals. The characteristic garliclike odor is an unreliable warning for arsine gas exposure, and hazardous effects may occur below the odor threshold (73). Arsine gas exposure usually occurs in the industrial-occupational setting, which includes smelting and refining of metals and ores, galvanizing, soldering, etching, lead plating, metallurgy, burning of fossil fuels, and microelectronic semiconductor production (in which computer chips made of GaAs are etched with strong acids) (8,74).

Pathophysiology

Arsine gas poisoning is related to its affinity to bind with RBCs, which causes a rapid and severe Coombs' test–negative hemolytic anemia. The exact mechanism by which arsine gas is lytic to the RBC has not been elucidated definitively. However, *in vitro* and animal studies indicate that hemolysis requires the presence of oxygen (75); that a reduction in the RBCs' glutathione concentration is time- and concentration-dependent on arsine gas exposure (76–78); and that an inverse correlation exists between the level of reduced glutathione and the extent of hemolysis (76,77). These findings are consistent with a mechanism of oxidative stress–induced damages to the RBCs, resulting in hemolysis.

Toxic concentrations of arsine gas appear to have deleterious effects on the kidneys. Postulated mechanisms of arsine gas–induced renal failure include direct toxic effect of arsine on renal tubular cell respiration; hypoxia due to the hemolytic anemia; and massive release of the arsenic-hemoglobin-hepatoglobin complex, which precipitates in the tubular lumen and exerts a toxic effect on the nephron (79). Depending on its severity, renal failure may be evident by 72 hours from the time of exposure (74).

Clinical Presentation

Arsine gas poisoning presents a clinical picture much different from the other arsenicals. The severity and the time to manifestation of arsine gas poisoning depend on the concentration and duration of the exposure. After an acute massive exposure, death may occur without the classic signs and symptoms of arsine poisoning. After low-concentration exposures, arsine gas is believed to be cleared rapidly and efficiently from plasma into the RBCs. However, after high-concentration exposures, the arsine gas load may exceed the binding capacity of the erythrocytes, and the gas may damage vital organs directly. This could explain how death would occur after arsine gas poisoning before the classic signs and symptoms are evident. In cases in which signs and symptoms of arsine gas poisoning develop over time, the associated morbidity and mortality are, in part, related to the consequences of its hematologic and renal effects. In general, after a significant exposure to arsine gas, usually a delay of 2 to 24 hours ensues before symptoms of arsine gas poisoning become apparent (74). Initial complaints include dizziness, malaise, weakness, dyspnea, nausea, vomiting, diarrhea, headache, and abdominal pain (74,80). Dark-red discoloration of the urine, hemoglobinuria, or hematuria frequently appears 4 to 12 hours after inhalation of arsine gas (74,80). Depending on the severity of the exposure, reddish staining of the conjunctiva and duskily bronzed skin may become apparent within 12 to 48 hours (80). However, the sensitivity of this sign is unclear. The conjunctival and skin discoloration are due to the presence of hemoglobin. This condition should be distinguished from jaundice, which is due to the presence of bilirubin (80). The triad of symptoms—abdominal pain, hematuria, and bronze-tinted skin—are recognized as characteristic clinical features (74). Low-level arsine exposure also may cause chronic arsenicalism (74).

In a report by Josephson et al. (73), ECG changes associated with arsine poisoning were characterized by high peaked T waves, particularly in the precordial leads. The most pronounced T-wave change occurred between the second and the twelfth day after exposure, and this was not influenced by the severity of the exposure. The severity of illness did not correlate with the height of the T wave. No delay was evident in atrioventricular or intraventricular conduction times. T-wave amplitude normalized on the weekly follow-up electrocardiogram. The exact etiology of the ECG change remains speculative.

Management

Management of arsine gas poisoning begins with removing an affected patient from the source of exposure while ensuring that rescue personnel are not exposed. Treatment is focused on restoring the intravascular RBC concentration, monitoring serum potassium, preventing further renal insult, and providing aggressive supportive care. Patients requiring hospitalization for arsine poisoning should be admitted to the ICU. In cases of acute and severe arsine poisoning, exchange transfusion has been advocated (81,82) as the most efficient and effective means of management and is considered the treatment of choice (74). Maintaining good urine output (1 to 2 mL per kg per hour) is important at all times. Urine alkalinization has been recommended to prevent deposition of RBC breakdown products in the kidneys. In situations in which there is evidence of renal insufficiency or failure, both exchange transfusion and hemodialysis may be required; exchange transfusion would restore the intravascular RBC concentration and simultaneously remove erythrocyte debris and arsenic-hemoglobin complexes (81). Hemolysis due to arsine gas poisoning can be a dynamic process, with continued hemolysis for days in untreated patients (82). Some researchers have suggested that with early diagnosis of arsine gas poisoning and prompt institution of exchange transfusion, the incidence of renal damage and long-term renal insufficiency may be reduced (82,83).

The results from using BAL in the treatment of acute arsine poisoning have been disappointing (80,84,85); BAL does not appear to afford protection against arsine-induced hemolysis. Whether BAL would be beneficial in subacute or chronic arsine poisoning remains speculative (74). Arsine gas may cause chronic effects similar to those caused by the other arsenicals, and resultant peripheral neuropathy has been reported, as have liver and renal injury (5).

BIOLOGICAL MONITORING

Biological monitoring offers the advantage of more accurately determining or revealing an affected individual's exposure. However, the underlying concept is that performed accurately, the test depicts the degree of toxicity being experienced. For some metals, this correlation is good; for others, it is poor. Blood arsenic levels have been shown to correlate poorly with arsenic exposure; whereas urinary arsenic excretion correlates better with arsenic exposure. Correlation of urinary arsenic to airborne arsenic was demonstrated (86). Urinary arsenic excretion ranges from 0.01 to 1.00 mg per L. However, normal values in most laboratories range from 0.01 to 0.15 mg per L (87). This outcome is affected by dietary intake of arsenic-rich foods. It can take 48 hours for urinary levels to return to normal after ingestion of arsenic-rich foods (87).

Instead of total arsenic determinations, which are influenced highly by such recent arsenic ingestions as seafood, levels of

TABLE 71-4. Standards and regulations for inorganic arsenic

Agency	Focus	Level	Comment
ACGIH	Air in workplace	200 μg/m^3	Advisory; 8-h TWA
EPA	Air in environment	N/A	Under review
	Water	50 ppb	Regulation; maximum contaminant in drinking water
FDA	Food	0.5–2.0 ppm	Regulation; applies to animals treated with veterinary drugs
NIOSH	Air in workplace	2 μg/m^3	Advisory; 15-min ceiling limit
OSHA	Air in workplace	10 μg/m^3	Regulation; PEL over 8-h workday

ACGIH, American Conference of Governmental Industrial Hygienists; EPA, U.S. Environmental Protection Agency; FDA, U.S. Food and Drug Administration; N/A, nonapplicable; NIOSH, National Institute for Occupational Safety and Health; OSHA, U.S. Occupational Safety and Health Administration; PEL, permissible exposure limit; TWA, 8-hour time-weighted average.

methylated derivatives of arsenic can be determined in the urine. Airborne inorganic arsenic is converted to methylated derivatives before urinary excretion (13). MMA and DMA account for much of arsenic excretion (88). These levels are not influenced by the presence of organic arsenic from marine origin (8). Exposures below the National Institute for Occupational Safety and Health–recommended level of 2 μg per cubic meter will not increase urinary levels above the baseline level (8).

Analysis of hair or nail arsenic content exemplifies many of the problems involved in biological monitoring of arsenic. Arsenic may accumulate during periods of exposure. As a result, such analysis has been concluded to be useful for monitoring arsenic toxicity. However, arsenic appears to prefer the sulfhydryl-rich environment of the hair and nails; thus, accumulation may represent exposure, not toxicity. In addition, environmental contamination of the exterior of these structures can lead to a falsely high estimation of exposure. Finally, the particular laboratory performing the analysis affects the reliability of results (89,90). If specimens are collected and analyzed properly and the results are interpreted appropriately, hair or nail arsenic levels may aid in the diagnosis of arsenic toxicity.

Arsenic hair levels are similar between men and women and among various hair colors. However, the hair of black women appears to have a significantly increased arsenic content as compared to that of other groups (90).

ENVIRONMENTAL MONITORING

Environmental monitoring of arsenicals is performed to identify workplace exposure without requiring direct sampling from individuals involved. Several concepts must be borne in mind in interpreting environmental monitoring. First, the results can be only as accurate as the sampling and analytic procedures used. Arsenic often is present in minute quantities that require processing and concentration procedures. Second, exposure and toxicity are not the same. An exposed individual may not develop toxicity, whereas another individual may develop toxicity to minimal exposures.

Choice of sample may be a major concern. Vegetation and other materials may be coated in arsenic-containing dust. A decision must be made concerning inclusion or exclusion of the dust in the sample analyzed. Arsenic-containing solutions may contain suspended material that may or may not have to be removed before analysis (4). Water, urine, and other aqueous samples should be analyzed within hours or should be frozen and stored.

Levels in natural waters decrease with time (91). Because trace concentrations usually are involved, preconcentration of the specimen may be necessary. Conversion of arsenic to arsine, coprecipitation with iron (III) hydroxide, distillation as arsenic (III) chloride, and extraction have been used (91). Oxidation to convert organic compounds to inorganic compounds may be necessary. In air samples, arsenic usually is associated with small particulates. However, variable amounts of the arsenic in air samples may be volatile and might not be collected on sample air filters (91). In general, all aspects of the analysis of arsenic in the environment should be considered carefully before sampling is performed.

Exposure Limits

The reported minimum lethal exposure to arsenic has been 1 mg per kg of ingested arsenic in a child (92). Acute ingestion of 200 mg of arsenic trioxide may be fatal in an adult (Table 71-4). For arsine gas, the threshold limit value and 8-hour time-weighted average equal 0.05 ppm. Immediate death has occurred at exposure to 150 ppm (93).

SUMMARY

Always a serious threat to health, arsenic is becoming more threatening as its technologic applications increase. Experience in other countries shows that contamination of food and water can lead to severe, widespread consequences. As with many diseases, the diagnosis of arsenic toxicity often requires a suspicious mind on the part of physicians. This is particularly true of the neurologic manifestations that only partially may resolve with treatment. Once a diagnosis is made, effective therapy exists in the new dimercapto chelating agents.

REFERENCES

1. Kosnett M. Arsenic toxicity. In: Kreiss K, ed. *Case studies in environmental medicine*, no. 5. Atlanta: Agency for Toxic Substances and Disease Registry, June 1990.
2. Yamashita N, Doi M, Nishio M. Recent observations of Kyoto children poisoned by arsenic tainted dry milk. *Jpn J Hyg* 1972;27:364.
3. Patty FA. *Industrial hygiene and toxicology*, 2nd ed. New York: John Wiley and Sons, 1962.
4. National Academy of Sciences. *Medical and biologic effects of environmental pollutants, arsenic.* Washington: National Research Council, National Academy of Sciences, 1977.
5. Ishinishi N, Tsuchiya K, Vahter M, Fowler BA. Arsenic. In: Friberg L, Nordberg GF, Vouk V, eds. *Handbook on the toxicology of metals.* Amsterdam: Elsevier Science, 1986.
6. Baker EL Jr, Hayes CG, Landrigan PJ, et al. A nationwide survey of heavy metal absorption in children living near primary copper, lead, and zinc smelters. *Am J Epidemiol* 1977;106:261–273.
7. Webb DR, Sipes IG, Carter DE. In vitro solubility and in vivo toxicity of gallium arsenide. *Toxicol Appl Pharmacol* 1984;76:96–104.
8. Harrison RJ. Gallium arsenide. State of the art reviews. *Occup Med* 1986;1:49–58.
9. Ungers LJ, Jones JH, McIntyre AJ, McHenry CR. Release of arsenic from semiconductor wafers. *Am Ind Hyg Assoc J* 1985;46:416–420.
10. Buchanan WD. *Toxicity of arsenic compounds.* Amsterdam: Elsevier Science, 1962.
11. Gorby MS. Arsenic poisoning. *West J Med* 1988;149:308–315.

12. Wald PH, Becker CE. Toxic gases used in the microelectronics industry. State of the art reviews. *Occup Med* 1986;1:105–117.
13. Smith TJ, Crecelius EA, Reading JC. Airborne arsenic exposure and excretion of methylated arsenic compounds. *Environ Health Perspect* 1977;19:89–93.
14. Crecelius EA. Changes in the chemical speciation of arsenic following ingestion by man. *Environ Health Perspect* 1977;19:147–150.
15. Bettley FR, O'Shea JA. The absorption of arsenic and its relation to carcinoma. *Br J Dermatol* 1975;92:563–568.
16. Garb LG, Hine CH. Arsenical neuropathy: residual effects following acute industrial exposure. *J Occup Med* 1977;19:567–568.
17. Mahieu P, Buchet JP, Roels HA, et al. The metabolism of arsenic in humans acutely intoxicated by As_2O_3. Its significance for the duration of BAL therapy. *Clin Toxicol* 1981;18:1067–1075.
18. Lugo G, Cassady G, Palmisano P. Acute maternal arsenic intoxication with neonatal death. *Am J Dis Child* 1969;117:328–330.
19. Gousios AG, Adelson L. Electrocardiographic and radiographic findings in acute arsenic poisoning. *Am J Med* 1959;27:659–663.
20. Weinberg SL. The electrocardiogram in acute arsenic poisoning. *Am Heart J* 1960;60:971–975.
21. Barry KG, Herndon EG Jr. Electrocardiographic changes associated with acute arsenic poisoning. *Med Ann DC* 1962;31:25–27.
22. Glazener FS, Ellis JG, Johnson PK. Electrocardiographic findings with arsenic poisoning. *Calif Med* 1968;109:158–162.
23. St Petery J, Gross C, Victorica BE. Ventricular fibrillation caused by arsenic poisoning. *Am J Dis Child* 1970;120:367–371.
24. Goldsmith S, From AH. Arsenic-induced atypical ventricular tachycardia. *N Engl J Med* 1980;303:1906–1908.
25. Little RE, Kay GN, Cavender JB, et al. Torsade de points and T-U wave alternans associated with arsenic poisoning. *PACE* 1990;13:164–170.
26. Beckman KJ, Bauman JL, Pimental PA, et al. Arsenic-induced torsade de pointes. *Crit Care Med* 1991;19:290–292.
27. Kyle RA, Pease GL. Hematologic aspects of arsenic intoxication. *N Engl J Med* 1965;273:18–23.
28. Kjeldsberg CR, Ward HP. Leukemia in arsenic poisoning. *Ann Intern Med* 1972;77:935–937.
29. Westnoff DD, Smaaha RJ, Barnes A Jr. Arsenic intoxication as a cause of megaloblastic anemia. *Blood* 1975;45:214–246.
30. Selzer PM, Ancel MA. Chronic arsenic poisoning masquerading as pernicious anemia. *West J Med* 1983;139:219–220.
31. Chan KM, Mathews WS. Acute arsenic overdose. *Lab Med* 1990;21:649–652.
32. Rezuke WN, Anderson C, Pastuszak WT, et al. Arsenic intoxication presenting as a myelodysplastic syndrome: a case report. *Am J Hematol* 1991;36:291–293.
33. Limarzi LR. The effects of arsenic (Fowler's solution) on erythropoiesis. *Am J Med Sci* 1943;206:334–347.
34. Heyman A, Pfeiffer JB, Willett RW, et al. Peripheral neuropathy caused by arsenical intoxication. *N Engl J Med* 1956;254:401–409.
35. Jenkins RB. Inorganic arsenic and the nervous system. *Brain* 1966;89:479–498.
36. Chhuttani PN, Chawla LS, Sharma TD. Arsenic neuropathy. *Neurology* 1967;17:269–274.
37. Greenberg C, Davies S, McGowan T, et al. Acute respiratory failure following severe arsenic poisoning. *Chest* 1979;76:596–598.
38. Donofrio PD, Wilbourn AJ, Albers JW, et al. Acute arsenic intoxication presenting as Guillain-Barré-like syndrome. *Muscle Nerve* 1987;10:114–120.
39. Fincher RM, Koerker RM. Long-term survival after acute arsenic encephalopathy. *Am J Med* 1987;82:549–552.
40. Bolla-Wilson K, Bleecker ML. Neuropsychological impairment following inorganic arsenic exposure. *J Occup Med* 1987;29:500–503.
41. Fesmire FM, Schauben JL, Roberge RJ. Survival following massive arsenic ingestion. *Am J Emerg Med* 1988;6:602–606.
42. Gilbertson A, Vaziri ND, Mirahamadi K, et al. Hemodialysis of acute arsenic intoxication with transient renal failure. *Arch Intern Med* 1976;136:1303–1304.
43. Vaziri ND, Upham T, Barton CH. Hemodialysis clearance of arsenic. *Clin Toxicol* 1980;17:451–456.
44. Shannon RL, Strayer DS. Arsenic-induced skin toxicity. *Hum Toxicol* 1989;8:99–104.
45. Reynolds ES. An account of the epidemic outbreak of arsenical poisoning occurring in beer-drinkers in the North of England and the Midland Counties in 1900. *Lancet* 1901;1:166–170.
46. Aldrich CJ. Leuconychia striata arsenicalis transversus. *Am J Med Sci* 1904;127:702–709.
47. Mees RA. The nails with arsenical polyneuritis. *JAMA* 1919;72:1337.
48. Ayres S Jr, Anderson NP. Cutaneous manifestations of arsenic poisoning. *Arch Dermatol* 1934;30:33–43.
49. Uhde GI. Arsenic eye burns. *Am J Ophthalmol* 1946;29:1090–1093.
50. Jackson R, Grainge JW. Arsenic and cancer. *Can Med Assoc J* 1975;113:396–401.
51. Renwick JH, Harrington JM, Waldron HA, et al. Long-term effects of acute arsenical poisoning. *J Soc Occup Med* 1981;31:144–147.
52. Lee AM, Fraumeni JF. Arsenic and respiratory cancer in man: an occupational study. *J Natl Cancer Inst* 1969;42:1045–1052.
53. Ott MG, Holder BB, Gordon HL. Respiratory cancer and occupational exposure to arsenicals. *Arch Environ Health* 1974;29:250–255.
54. Sobel W, Bond GG, Baldwin CL, Ducommun DJ. An update of respiratory cancer and occupational exposure to arsenicals. *Am J Ind Med* 1988;13:263–270.
55. Anonymous. *Health hazards of inorganic arsenic.* Washington: US Occupational Safety and Health Administration, 1979.
56. Chen CL, Kuo TL, Wu MM. Arsenic and cancers. *Lancet* 1988;1:414–415.
57. Tseng W-P. Effects and dose-response relationships of skin and Blackfoot disease with arsenic. *Environ Health Perspect* 1977;19:109–119.
58. Axelson O, Dahlgren E, Jansson C-D, Rehnlund SO. Arsenic exposure and mortality: a case-referent study from a Swedish copper smelter. *Br J Ind Med* 1978;35:8–15.
59. Council on Scientific Affairs. Effects of toxic chemicals on the reproductive system. *JAMA* 1985;253:3431–3437.
60. Al-Mahasneh QM, Rodgers GC, Benz FW, et al. Activated charcoal as an adsorbent for inorganic arsenic. *Vet Hum Toxicol* 1990;32:351.
61. Eagle M, Magnuson HJ. The systemic treatment of 227 cases of arsenic poisoning (encephalitis, dermatitis, blood dyscrasias, jaundice, fever) with 2,3 dimercaptopropanol (BAL). *J Clin Invest* 1946;25:420–441.
62. Eagle M, Magnuson HJ, Fleischman R. The systemic treatment of experimental arsenic poisoning (Mapharsen, Lewisite, phenyl arsenoxide) with BAL. *J Clin Invest* 1946;25:451–466.
63. Aposhian HV, Carter DE, Hoover TD, Hsu C, Maiorino RM, Stone E. DMSA, DMPS and DMPA—as arsenic antidotes. *Fundam Appl Toxicol* 1984; 4:858–870.
64. Graziano JH. Role of 2,3-dimercaptosuccinic acid in the treatment of heavy metal poisoning. *Med Toxicol* 1986;1:155–162.
65. Fournier L, Thomas G, Garnier R, et al. 2,3-Dimercaptosuccinic acid treatment of heavy metal poisoning in humans. *Med Toxicol* 1988;3:499–504.
66. Kuruvilla A, Bergeson PS, Done AK. Arsenic poisoning in childhood an unusual case report with special notes on therapy with penicillamine. *Clin Toxicol* 1975;8:535–540.
67. Peterson RG, Rumack BH. D-penicillamine therapy of acute arsenic poisoning. *J Pediatr* 1977;91:661–666.
68. Watson WA, Veltri JC, Metcalf TJ. Acute arsenic exposure treated with oral D-penicillamine. *Vet Hum Toxicol* 1981;23:164–166.
69. Hoover TD, Aposhian HV. BAL increases the arsenic-74 content of rabbit brain. *Toxicol Appl Pharmacol* 1983;70:160–162.
70. Kreppel H, Reichl FX, Forth W, Fichtl B. Lack of effectiveness of D-penicillamine in experimental arsenic poisoning. *Vet Hum Toxicol* 1989;31:1–5.
71. Mahieu P, Buchet JP, Lauwerys R. Evolution clinique et biologique d'une intoxication orale aigue par l'anhydride arsenieux et considerations sur l'attitude therapeutique. *J Toxicol Clin Exp* 1987;7:273–278.
72. Le Quesne PM, McLeod JG. Peripheral neuropathy following a single exposure to arsenic. *J Neurol Sci* 1977;32:437–451.
73. Josephson CJ, Pinto SS, Petronella SJ. Arsine: electrocardiographic changes produced in acute human poisoning. *Arch Ind Hyg* 1951;4:43–52.
74. Fowler BA, Weissberg JB. Arsine poisoning. *N Engl J Med* 1974;291:1171–1174.
75. Graham AF, Crawford TBB, Marrian GF. The action of arsine on blood: observations on the nature of the fixed arsenic. *Biochem J* 1946;40:256–260.
76. Pernis B, Magistretti M. A study of the mechanism of acute hemolytic anemia from arsine. *Med Lavoro* 1960;51:37–41.
77. Peterson DP, Bhattacharyya MH. Hematological response to arsine exposure: quantitation of exposure response in mice. *Fundam Appl Toxicol* 1985;5:499–505.
78. Blair PC, Thompson MB, Bechtold M, et al. Evidence for oxidative damage to red blood cells in mice induced by arsine gas. *Toxicology* 1990;63:25–34.
79. Muehrcke RC, Pirani CL. Arsine-induced anuria: a correlative clinicopathological study with electron microscopic observations. *Ann Intern Med* 1968;68:853–866.
80. Macaulay DB, Stanley DA. Arsine poisoning. *Br J Ind Med* 1956;13:217–221.
81. McKinstry WJ, Hickes JM. Emergency-arsine poisoning. *Arch Ind Health* 1957;16:32–41.
82. Teitelbaum DT, Kier LC. Arsine poisoning: report of five cases in the petroleum industry and a discussion of the indications for exchange transfusion and hemodialysis. *Arch Environ Health* 1969;19:133–141.
83. Uldall PR, Khan HA, Ennis JE, et al. Renal damage from industrial arsine poisoning. *Br J Ind Med* 1970;27:372–377.
84. Kensler CJ, Abels JC, Rhoads CP. Arsine poisoning, mode of action and treatment. *J Pharmacol Exp Ther* 1946;88:99–108.
85. Pino SS, Petronella SJ, Johns DR, et al. Arsine poisoning: a study of thirteen cases. *Arch Ind Hyg* 1950;1:437–451.
86. Nelson MK. Arsenic trioxide production. In: Carnow BW, ed. *Health effects of occupational lead and arsenic exposure.* Washington: US Government Printing Office, 1976.
87. Dickerson OB. Arsenic. In: Waldron HA, ed. *Metals in the environment.* New York: Academic Press, 1980.
88. Buchet JP, Lauwerys R, Roels H. Comparison of the urinary excretion of arsenic metabolites after a single oral dose of sodium arsenite, monomethylarsonate, or dimethylarsinate in man. *Int Arch Occup Environ Health* 1981;48:71–79.
89. Sky-Peck HH, Joseph BJ. The use and misuse of human hair in trace metal analysis. In: Brown SS, Savory J, eds. *Chemical toxicology and clinical chemistry of metals.* New York: Academic Press, 1983.
90. Savoie JY, Weber JP. Evaluating laboratory performance via an interlaboratory comparison program for toxic substances in blood and urine. In: Brown SS, Savory J, eds. *Chemical toxicology and clinical chemistry of metals.* New York: Academic Press, 1983.
91. *Arsenic.* Geneva: World Health Organization, 1981:27–30.
92. Woody NC, Kometani JT. BAL in the treatment of arsenic ingestion of children. *Pediatrics* 1948;1:372–378.
93. Ellenhorn MJ, Barceloux DG. *Medical toxicology.* New York: Elsevier Science, 1988:1013.

CHAPTER 72
Mercury

Luke Yip, Richard C. Dart, and
John B. Sullivan, Jr.

Mercury (atomic weight, 200.6) is a member of the class II family of metals. The chemical symbol, Hg, is derived from the Greek word *hydrargyros*, meaning "water silver." This is perhaps its best description, as it is the only metal that maintains a liquid state at room temperature.

Mercury is a naturally occurring metal that is mined chiefly as mercuric sulfate (HgS) in cinnabar ore. It is converted into three primary forms, each with a distinct toxicology: elemental [metallic (O) oxidation state] mercury; inorganic [mercurous (Hg^{1+}), mercuric (Hg^{2+})] mercury salts; and organic (alkyl, phenyl) mercury. Elemental mercury is also called *quicksilver* or *hydrargyrum*. Included among the elemental mercury compounds are any ionic compounds that can decompose into mercury vapor in the occupational setting. Mercurous mercury usually is combined to form salts that dissociate slowly in water or body fluids to form Hg^{2+} and Hg^0. Organic mercury consists of two subcategories: long-chain alkyl and aryl mercurial compounds and short-chain alkyl compounds, which include methyl and ethyl mercury. The dialkyl derivatives of the short-chain group become toxic after the loss of one alkyl group. The pattern and severity of mercury toxicity are highly dependent on the form of mercury and route of exposure, mostly because of different pharmacokinetic profiles. Chronic exposure to any form of mercury may result in toxicity. Table 72-1 lists inorganic and organic mercurial compounds and their uses.

SITES, INDUSTRIES, AND BUSINESSES ASSOCIATED WITH EXPOSURE

Approximately 70,000 U.S. workers are exposed to mercury annually (1). The general population is exposed to mercury mainly via food such as fish (1). Anthropogenic release of mercury into the environment from human-related activities is estimated to be 2,000 metric tons per year, mainly from mining and ore smelting (1).

Elemental mercury occurs as a part of the earth's natural geochemistry, comprising 0.05 µg per g of the earth's crust. Mercury is also released into the environment through mining and industrial discharge and the combustion of fossil fuels. In the atmosphere, mercury concentrations range from 3.9 ng per cubic meter over remote nonmineralized areas up to 50 ng per cubic meter over mineralized areas. Surface soils may contain 20 to 625 ng per g. Ocean water ranges from 3 ng per L in open sea to 5 to 6 ng per L in coastal waters. The bulk of mercury in the oceans is apparently from natural sources such as volcanic eruptions and volatilization or solubilization of rocks, soils, and sediments (1).

Surface water contains less than 50 ng of mercury per L. Industrial and mining activities have increased the environmental flux of mercury from a concentration of 25,000 tons to 40,000 tons per year, with one-third of this flux returning to land and two-thirds to the oceans. Methylation of mercury by microorganisms such as *Methanobacterium* greatly increases the transport of mercury in the environment, which also can lead to the bioaccumulation of mercury in fish and thus, eventually, to deposition in humans.

TABLE 72-1. Inorganic and organic mercurial compounds and their uses

Inorganic	Ammoniated mercury ($HgNH_2Cl$)—antiseptic
	Mercuric acetate [$Hg(OOC_2H_3)_2$]—catalyst in organic synthesis, pharmaceuticals
	Mercuric arsenate ($HgNH_3O_4$)—waterproofing and antifouling paints
	Mercuric benzoate [$Hg(C_7H_5O_2)_2$]—antisyphilitic
	Mercuric bromide ($HgBr_2$)—medicinal use
	Merbromin (Mercurochrome; 25% mercury + 20% bromine)—antiseptic cream
	Mercurous chloride (calomel, mercury monochloride, Hg_2Cl_2)—a laxative
	Mercuric chloride (corrosive sublimate, mercury bichloride)—antiseptic solution
	Mercury cyanate [fulminate of mercury, $Hg(CNO)_2$]—explosive
	Mercuric cyanide [$Hg(CN)_2$]—antiseptic, photography
	Mercuric oxide, red (red or yellow precipitate Hg^0)—pigment, dry batteries
	Mercuric potassium cyanide—silvering glass, in mirrors
	Mercuric sulfide (cinnabar, red vermilion, Chinese red)—used in tattoos, combined with cadmium sulfide
	Mercuric salicylate (salicylate mercury)—topical antiseptic
	Mercuric acetate [$Hg(OOC_2H_3)_2$]
	Sublimate ($HgCl_2$)
Organic	Thimerosal (Merthiolate; 49% mercury)
	Alkyl mercury fungicides: dialkyl mercury, ethyl mercury
	Phenyl mercury fungicides ($PhHg^+$): phenyl mercury
	Alkoxyalkyl mercury fungicides: methoxyethyl mercury
	Mercurial diuretics (Mersalyl, Chlormerodrin)

TABLE 72-2. Products and industries associated with potential mercury exposure

Elemental mercurials
- Dental medicine
- Batteries
- Barometers
- Boiler makers
- Calibration instruments
- Caustic soda production
- Carbon brush production
- Ceramics
- Chloralkali production
- Ultrasonic amplifiers
- Direct current meters
- Infrared detectors
- Electrical apparatus
- Electroplating
- Fingerprint detectors
- Silver and gold extraction
- Jewelry
- Fluorescent, neon, and mercury arc lamps
- Manometers
- Paints
- Paper pulp manufacturing
- Photography
- Pressure gauges
- Thermometers
- Semiconductor solar cells

Inorganic mercurials
- Disinfectants
- Paints and dyes
- Explosives
- Fireworks manufacturing
- Fur processing
- Ink manufacturing
- Chemical laboratory workers
- Percussion caps and detonators
- Spermicidal jellies
- Tannery workers
- Wood preservatives
- Tattooing materials
- Taxidermists
- Vinyl chloride production
- Mercury vapor lamps
- Antisyphilitic agents
- Thermoscopy
- Silvering in mirrors
- Photography
- Perfumery and cosmetics
- Acetaldehyde production

Organic mercurials
- Bactericides
- Embalming preparations
- Paper manufacturing
- Farmers
- Laundry and diaper services
- External antiseptics
- Fungicides
- Insecticide manufacture
- Seed handling
- Wood preservatives
- Germicides

TABLE 72-3. Mercury regulations and guidelines

Agency	Description	Concentration
International: WHO		
Guidelines	Drinking-water guideline values (applies to all forms of mercury)	0.001 mg/L
Regulations	Permissible tolerable weekly intake	5 μg/kg total 3.3 g/kg CH_3Hg
United States		
Regulations: Air		
OSHA	Alkyl compounds—PEL, TWA	0.01 mg/m^3
	Inorganic mercury (skin)	0.05 mg/m^3—TWA
	Alkyl compounds	0.03 mg/m^3 (skin)—STEL
Guidelines		
Air		
ACGIH	Ceiling-alkyl compounds—STEL	0.03 mg/m^3
	Alkyl compound—TWA	0.01 mg/m^3
	Aryl compounds	0.1 mg/m^3
	Metallic mercury and inorganic compounds	0.025 mg/m^3
NIOSH	Aryl or inorganic mercury as mercury—REL for occupational exposure (8-h TWA)	0.1 mg/m^3 ceiling (skin)
	Mercury (organo) alkyl compounds	0.01 mg/m^3—TWA
	Mercury vapor as mercury	0.03 mg/m^3 (skin)—STEL 0.05 mg/m^3 (skin)—TWA
Water		
EPA	Inorganic mercury—Lifetime Health Advisory (adult)	0.002 mg/L
	Inorganic mercury—Longer-Term Health Advisory (adult)	0.002 mg/L
	Drinking water equivalent level	0.002 mg/L
	Mercury and phenylmercuric acetate—Ambient Water Quality Criteria for Human Health	
	Water and fish	0.05 μg/L
	Fish only	0.051 μg/L
	Mercury and phenylmercuric acetate as mercury—Ambient Water Quality Criteria for Aquatic Organisms	
	Acute (1-h average)	Marine: 1.8 μg/L; freshwater: 1.4 μg/L
	Chronic (4-d average)	Marine: 0.94 μg/L; freshwater: 1.77 μg/L
	National Primary Drinking Water Regulations	
	MCLGs for inorganic compounds	0.002 mg/L
	MCL for inorganic compounds	0.002 mg/L
Food		
FDA	Action level for poisonous or deleterious substances in human food and animal feed—fish, shellfish, crustaceans, other aquatic animals (fresh, frozen, or processed)	1 ppm
	Bottled water	0.002 mg/L

ACGIH, American Conference of Governmental Industrial Hygienists; EPA, U.S. Environmental Protection Agency; FDA, U.S. Food and Drug Administration; IRIS, integrated risk information system; MCL, maximum contamination level; MCLG, maximum contamination level goal; NIOSH, National Institute for Occupational Safety and Health; OSHA, U.S. Occupational Safety and Health Administration; PEL, permissible exposure limit; ppm, parts per million; REL, recommended exposure limit; STEL, short-term exposure limit; TWA, time-weighted average; WHO, World Health Organization.
From ref. 2, with permission.

World production of mercury is approximately 8,000 tons per year. Two predominant extraction techniques are used in commercial production. Mercury can be extracted from cinnabar (mercury sulfide) by firing the ore in retorts with either lime or iron and collecting the liberated mercury vapor by condensation. Alternatively, in direct furnaces, sulfur dioxide formation releases mercury. Italy, Mexico, Spain, and the Soviet Union are the major mercury-producing countries. There are also ore deposits in Yugoslavia, Canada, Algeria, Japan, China, New Zealand, California, Oregon, Washington, and Nevada.

Mercury is predominantly used in the manufacture of electric meters, industrial control instruments, and dry batteries, in the production of chloralkali, in antimildew paints, as catalysts and fungicides, and to a lesser degree, in pharmaceuticals and for general laboratory use. The largest number of exposed workers are employed in health services, dental medicine, the chemical products industry, electrical equipment manufacturing, chloralkali production, and mining (1).

In the past, mercury was used in the felt hat industry and in fingerprinting. However, these applications are no longer practiced. Using mercury to extract gold and silver has also become less common. Agricultural use of mercury as a fungicide and for seed dressings increases the potential for environmental contamination and for possible accidental ingestion. Organic mercurial compounds have been used for medicinal purposes such as diuretics, external antiseptics, and laxatives. Table 72-2 lists potential occupational exposures to the various forms of mercury.

Mercury vapor is released from volcanoes and the earth's crust, from industrial uses, incineration and burning of fossil fuels, and mining operations, and from degradation of mercury-containing products. Atmospheric mercury finds its way back to earth in precipitation. Ultimately, mercury reaches the oceans

TABLE 72-4. Events and regulatory decisions associated with methyl mercury

1953	In Minamata, Japan, 111 people die or suffer nervous system damage from consuming fish from waters severely polluted by mercury from industrial discharges.
1965	In Niigata, Japan, 120 people are poisoned by consuming fish polluted by methyl mercury.
1969	The EPA sets a 0.5-ppm limit for total mercury in fish.
1969	Swedish researchers discover that methyl mercury accumulates in fish.
1969	The FDA sets a 0.5-ppm action level as the maximum safe limit for total mercury in fish. Action levels are the limit at or above which the FDA will act to remove a product from the market.
1971–1972	A methyl mercury poisoning outbreak occurs in Iraq when seed grain treated with a methyl mercury fungicide is ingested. Children born to mothers who were pregnant at the time they ate the grain were found to experience neurologic effects, delayed development, and delayed motor skills.
1979	The FDA raises the mercury action level to 1 ppm based, in part, on a National Marine Fisheries Service study that showed this level would adequately protect consumers.
1980	The WHO publishes a study on methyl mercury toxicity that states that "the general population does not face a significant health risk from methyl mercury."
1984	The FDA changes the basis for enforcement of the mercury action level from total mercury to methyl mercury.
1984	The NIEHS and Rochester University begin a study in the Seychelles Islands, where fish is a major source of protein, to track prenatal exposure to methyl mercury and effects on the fetus.
1991	Under mandate of the Clean Air Act amendments, the EPA begins an assessment of an acceptable level of methyl mercury in fish to be completed by 15 December 1993.
1992	The NIEHS and Odense University begin a study of methyl mercury effects on a fish-eating population in the Faroe Islands.
1993	The Sierra Club and the Natural Resources Defense Council sue the EPA to complete and release its methyl mercury report. The EPA is granted a 1-yr extension.
1994	The EPA delays release of its report. The environmental groups sue again. The EPA is ordered to submit its report by 15 April 1995.
1995	The EPA misses the deadline for release of its report. EPA officials say the delay is due to waiting for additional data from the Seychelles studies.
1995–1996	Initial results of the Seychelles studies show no major health problems. Initial results of the Faroe Islands study, released in 1994, however, indicate neuropsychological dysfunction in children with increased methyl mercury exposure levels.
1996	The EPA has yet to release its final report, although the agency has called for a stricter standard for methyl mercury in fish of 0.1 μg/kg body wt/d.

EPA, U.S. Environmental Protection Agency; FDA, U.S. Food and Drug Administration; NIEHS, National Institute of Environmental Health Science; WHO, World Health Organization.
Adapted from Wheeler M. Focus: measuring mercury. *Environ Health Perspect* 1996;104:826–831.

and other bodies of water, where microorganisms convert it to methyl mercury by bacteria that produce methane. Once methylated, mercury is released from the microorganisms and bioaccumulates up the food chain.

Mercury and mercury-containing compounds are on the list of toxic chemicals in Section 313 of the Emergency Planning and Community Right-to-Know Act of 1986. Table 72-3 summarizes the regulatory data with regard to all mercury compounds in the occupational and nonoccupational environment. Table 72-4 summarizes the events and regulatory decisions associated with methyl mercury (2).

CLINICAL TOXICOLOGY

The general mode of toxicologic action involves the covalent binding of mercury to sulfhydryl groups, inactivating enzymes of cellular function and metabolism of carbohydrates at the pyruvic acid level (3). Binding also occurs to carboxyl, amide, amine, and phosphoryl groups. The high affinity of mercury for sulfhydryl groups as well as other biochemical moieties explains its toxic manifestations and basic toxic mechanism.

Mercury toxicology is divided according to mercury's form: elemental, inorganic, or organic. Elemental mercury is liquid at room temperature and readily vaporizes. Of the inorganic mercury compounds, the divalent mercuric salts are the most commonly encountered poison. The organic mercury compounds can be divided into those that are stable in living organisms and those that are broken down, such as phenyl mercury and methoxyalkyl mercury compounds (3).

Elemental Mercury

Various instruments contain elemental mercury, including thermometers, manometers, barometers, switches, pumps, and special surgical tubes (Miller-Abbott, Canter, Kaslow). Dental amalgam is prepared with elemental mercury and contains approximately 50% elemental mercury by weight. Personnel in the occupational setting who are potentially exposed include chloralkali mercury cell operators; electroplaters; explosives manufacturers; laboratory personnel; pesticide and fungicide production and application workers; manufacturers of batteries and mercury vapor lamps; miners; processors of cinnabar, gold, silver, copper, and zinc; and metallurgists. Exposures to mercury vapor from elemental mercury spill, work hazard, home gold ore purification, accidental heating of metallic mercury, and vacuum cleanup of a mercury spill have also been reported (4–7).

ABSORPTION, METABOLISM, AND EXCRETION

When ingested, elemental mercury is poorly absorbed (less than 0.01%) from the intact and normally functioning gastrointestinal (GI) tract. Elemental mercury is the only metal that exists in liquid form at standard temperature and pressure. Owing to a very low vapor pressure of 0.0012 mm Hg, metallic mercury can evaporate slowly at room temperature or rapidly when heated, saturating the air at 13 to 18 mg per cubic meter at 24°C (77°F). A small spill in an enclosed space (e.g., bedroom) can also produce high levels of mercury in the air because of its low vapor pressure. Mercury vapor is insoluble in water. Elemental mercury is readily oxidized in the presence of oxygen.

Exposure to elemental mercury predominantly occurs through inhalation of the vaporized metal. A small fraction of the inhaled dose is expired, but most of the mercury vapor crosses the alveolar membrane and is absorbed quickly into the circulation. Approximately 75% of the inhaled dose is retained (8,9). The absorbed elemental mercury vapor rapidly diffuses into the red blood cells (RBCs) and tissues, where it undergoes oxidation to the mercuric ion and binds to ligands in the RBCs (10). However, a certain amount of the dissolved vapor persists in the plasma to reach the blood–brain barrier, which it crosses readily (11,12). Once in the brain tissue, the dissolved mercury vapor is oxidized to mercuric ion, which is trapped within the central nervous system (CNS), where it is available for binding tissue ligands (10). Elemental mercury vapor also is easily transported across the placenta (13,14).

Elemental mercury vapor is eliminated from the body mainly as mercuric ion by the urine and fecal routes. Exhalation of mercury vapor and secretion of mercuric ions in saliva and sweat do occur and contribute to the elimination process. The rate of excretion is dose-dependent. Elemental mercury follows a biphasic elimination rate, initially rapid, then slow, with a biological half-life in humans of approximately 60 days.

The pulmonary system and CNS are the primary target organs of elemental mercury vapor poisoning. Damage to the respiratory system results from acute inhalation exposure to high concentrations of elemental mercury vapor, which acts as a direct airway irritant and a cellular poison (4–6,14–21). Pulmonary toxicity is characterized by exudative alveolar and interstitial edema, erosive bronchitis and bronchiolitis with interstitial pneumonitis, and desquamation of the bronchial epithelium. The ensuing obstruction results in alveolar dilatation, interstitial emphysema, pneumatocele formation, pneumothorax, and mediastinal emphysema.

In the CNS, a cumulative toxic effect occurs as the inhaled elemental mercury vapor is oxidized to mercuric ion, leading to progressive CNS dysfunction. Mercuric ion has an affinity to bind and react to sulfhydryl moieties of proteins, leading to nonspecific inhibition of enzyme systems and pathologic alteration of cellular membranes.

Ingestion. Although elemental mercury is poorly absorbed from the GI tract (22), systemic absorption of mercury is possible in the presence of any bowel abnormality affecting mucosal integrity, impeding normal motility and transit. In addition, inflammatory bowel disease or enteric fistula has been reported to allow for prolonged elemental mercury exposure and the conversion of metallic mercury to an inorganic absorbable ion (23). Another potential problem involving the GI tract with elemental mercury is that it can be retained in the appendix, resulting in local inflammation, perforation, and the consequent possibility of systemic mercury intoxication; as such, appendectomy has been recommended (24–26).

Subcutaneous injection of elemental mercury may cause a local fibrous reaction, local abscess, granuloma formation, systemic embolization, and systemic absorption with toxic manifestations (27–31).

Intravenously injected elemental mercury has been reported to cause pulmonary and systemic mercury embolization, associated with an elevated blood mercury level, which often was without sequelae (27,32–36). However, mercury embolism in the lung is the greatest cause of fatality in suicide attempts from injection of metallic mercury. Renal damage also is possible, with white blood cells appearing in the urine. This condition either can resolve itself spontaneously or may lead to renal failure. Extravasation of mercury at the injection site can produce a severe local inflammatory reaction (35). Granuloma formation with fibrosis and inflammation as a result of systemic mercury absorption has also been reported (37).

Inhalation. Acute intense inhalation exposure to elemental mercury in a confined or poorly ventilated space may result in death. Typically, toxic effects develop within several hours after acute toxic inhalation exposure. The initial effects include fever, chills, headache, dyspnea, gingivostomatitis, nausea, vomiting, metallic taste in the mouth, paroxysmal cough, tachypnea, chest tightness, diarrhea, and abdominal cramps (6,14,16,19). These may subside within 2 to 7 days or, in severe cases, may progress to interstitial pneumonitis, bilateral infiltrates, atelectasis, noncardiogenic pulmonary edema, interstitial pulmonary fibrosis, and death (4,5,18,19,38,39). In addition, such complications as subcutaneous emphysema, pneumomediastinum, and pneumothorax may occur.

Children younger than 30 months seem to be particularly susceptible to such exposures (21). This difference in age-related outcome results from the direct effect of mercury vapor on the lung. Contact with the distal portion of the lung, where absorption is almost complete, can lead to exudative alveolar and interstitial edema. Obstruction from bronchial epithelium desquamation may develop and possibly result in severe ventilation-perfusion defects and hypoxemia. The obstruction is proportionately greater in infants than in older children and adults and results in alveolar dilation, interstitial emphysema, pneumatocele formation, pneumothorax, and mediastinal emphysema (21). In one case, 22-year follow-up of a patient after aspiration of elemental mercury showed progressive fibrosis with pleural effusions, pulmonary granulomas, and bronchiectasis, probably resulting from the effects of local irritation. The fibrosis, however, may have minimized systemic absorption of sequestered mercury, as the patient demonstrated no evidence of acute or chronic systemic toxic reaction (40).

CHRONIC ELEMENTAL MERCURY EXPOSURE

Chronic intoxication from inhalation of mercury vapor produces a classic triad of gingivostomatitis, tremor, and neuropsychiatric disturbances. Mercurial tremor has been described as both static and intentional. Static or resting tremor occurs when the muscle is at rest and is a fine, trembling motion, most evident in the upper extremities. Intentional or ataxic tremor occurs when there is purposeful movement of an extremity or as an aggravation of an established static tremor. Traditionally, five degrees of tremor have been described:

1. Static tremor that is most pronounced with arms stretched and the fingers spread
2. Static tremor associated with intentional aggravation that minimally affects delicate motor activities
3. Static and intentional tremor that interferes with fine-motor activities (e.g., writing)
4. Tremors interfering with gross-motor function
5. Concussion mercurialis, a generalized and intense tremor that prevents daily activities and that occasionally occurs as sudden bursts of episodic duration, tetanus mercurialis, or shakes

Neuropsychiatric manifestations, termed *erythism,* include fatigue, insomnia, anorexia, and memory dysfunction. There may be an insidious change in mood that include shyness, withdrawal, depression, loss of confidence, nervousness, irritability, timidity, and a tendency to resent being observed, combined with a burst of quick temper of unusual degree for the individual affected and frequent blushing.

Evidence of visual disturbances includes a brown light reflex from the anterior capsule of the lens, opacities of the lens, and vascular changes at the corneoscleral junction (41).

The clinical course that has been reported to follow aspiration of elemental mercury ranges from no acute respiratory symptoms (42) to cough and mild dyspnea (40,43,44), acute pneumonitis (45), and progressive cough with copious amounts of frankly bloody sputum production, which led to respiratory compromise and death (46). In each case (except for the patient that died), the patient recovered without any significant respiratory sequelae attributable to the aspiration misadventure and remains asymptomatic. However, in two patients, systemic absorption of the aspirated elemental mercury was suggested by elevations in the patients' 24-hour urinary mercury concentration (42,43). Neither one of the patients was symptomatic otherwise. Elemental mercury was consistently evident on chest radiographs taken on follow-up examination, which occurred anywhere from 1 month to 20 years after the initial event (40,44). In one case, 22 years after mercury aspiration postmortem findings in the lungs included globules of elemental mercury surrounded by extensive fibrosis and granuloma formation (40).

Acrodynia (from the Greek words for "extremity" or "extreme" and "pain") refers to a now rare idiosyncratic reaction caused by chronic mercury exposure. Acrodynia primarily occurs in infants and children and is characterized by pain in the extremities often accompanied by pinkish or red discoloration, swelling, and desquamation ("pink disease"), anorexia, insomnia, irritability or apathy, lethargy, profuse sweating (which often leads to malaria-type rashes), photophobia, hypertension, hypotonia, abnormal sensations, and a generalized erythematous rash.

Subclinical changes in peripheral nerve function and renal function have been reported. However, frank neuropathy and nephropathy are rare. Parkinsonian states, dysarthria, and a syndrome resembling amyotrophic lateral sclerosis have also been noted (41).

A correlation exists between mercury exposure and the urinary excretion of mercury. Occupational exposures of mercury that produce neurologic effects such as tremors are associated with urinary concentrations of mercury of 200 µg per L of urine (47). These symptoms usually are reversible after exposure is terminated. Electromyography and nerve conduction studies may demonstrate impairment of peripheral nerves in workers chronically exposed to mercury vapor. Urine mercury concentrations greater than 200 µg per L have been associated with tremors and poor hand-eye coordination (48). Tremors have also been seen with a blood mercury concentration of 1 to 2 µg per dL (47).

DIAGNOSIS

Diagnosis depends on integrating characteristic findings with a history of known or potential exposure and the presence of elevated whole blood mercury concentration and urinary mercury excretion. Abdominal radiographs may be used to document the extent of the GI contamination after elemental mercury ingestion.

Radiographs of the injection site may help to define the extent of the infiltrated mercury. Chest radiography and computed axial tomography may be useful in determining the location of systemic embolization.

Whole blood and urinary mercury concentrations are useful in confirming exposure. In most people without occupational exposure, the whole blood mercury concentration is less than 2 µg per dL, and urinary mercury concentration is less than 10 µg per L. A quantitative 24-hour urinary mercury excretion, usually less than 50 µg per 24 hours, probably is the most useful tool in diagnosing acute exposure. A urinary mercury concentration between 30 and 50 µg per L may be associated with subclinical neuropsychiatric effects; between 50 and 100 µg per L, with early subclinical tremor; in excess of 100 µg per L, with overt neuropsychiatric disturbances; and greater than 200 µg per L, with true tremors.

MANAGEMENT

The chief priority in managing mercury poisoning is to identify and eradicate the source of elemental mercury exposure and to institute control measures to prevent repeated intoxication.

Treatment of Elemental Mercury Ingestion. In cases in which elemental mercury ingestion has been documented, whole-bowel irrigation with polyethylene glycol electrolyte solution or surgical removal of the affected areas of the colon may be considered, depending on radiographic evidence of mercury retention, elevated blood or urine mercury concentrations, and the patient's clinical status. Repeat abdominal radiographs may be used to document the effectiveness of whole-bowel irrigation or to follow the progress of the ingested metallic mercury.

Treatment of Elemental Mercury Injection. Local wound management of the injection sites should include prompt excision of all readily accessible subcutaneous areas in which metallic mercury is demonstrated, copious saline irrigation to remove metallic mercury droplets, and suction removal of the mercury (49). Surgical excision of mercury granulomas has also been recommended (37). Injection of dimercaprol [2,3-dimercapto-1-propanol (British anti-Lewisite, or BAL)] into the wound is not recommended as it appears to delay wound healing (50).

Treatment of Elemental Mercury Inhalation. Patients acutely exposed to elemental mercury vapor have the potential to develop respiratory failure due to severe pulmonary toxicity, and so these patients should be monitored closely. Chest radiographs, arterial blood gases, and pulmonary function should be monitored in patients with pulmonary symptoms. Supplemental oxygen and bronchodilators should be administered as needed. Progressive deterioration of respiratory function may require aggressive airway management with tracheal intubation, mechanical ventilation, and positive end-expiratory pressure. Early treatment with corticosteroids has been used in an attempt to reduce the complication of pulmonary fibrosis (21). However, neither corticosteroids nor prophylactic antibiotics have proved benefits in the management of elemental mercury vapor–induced pulmonary complications.

Patients who have aspirated elemental mercury should be managed in a similar fashion. Vigorous suctioning, postural drainage, and good pulmonary toilet may assist expectoration of aspirated mercury (40,43). In addition, bronchoscopy may be indicated.

Chelation. In addition to supportive therapy, mercury poisoning often is treated with a chelating agent. The metal-chelator complex is water-soluble and can be excreted in the urine, bile, or both and, to some extent, can be removed by hemodialysis.

Chelating agents that are commercially available in the United States for use in mercury poisoning are BAL, succimer [2,3-dimercaptosuccinic acid (DMSA)], and D-penicillamine. The choice of chelator depends on the form of mercury involved and the presenting signs and symptoms of the patient.

It is believed that BAL, with its two sulfhydryl groups, forms a stable ring-structure chelate with mercury and successfully competes with the sulfhydryl groups in the body. BAL can be administered only by intramuscular injection. The BAL-mercury complex is excreted in both the urine and feces. Measuring the urinary mercury concentration helps to assess the effects of chelation therapy. It has been stated that BAL and its metal chelate dissociate in an acid medium and that maintenance of an alkaline urine may protect the kidneys during chelation therapy (51).

Some researchers suggest that in patients with glucose-6-phosphate dehydrogenase deficiency, BAL should be administered with caution because it may cause hemolysis (52,53). The side effects of BAL appear to be dose-dependent, with an incidence of greater than 50% at a dose of 5 mg per kg of body weight (52). The reported adverse side effects include pain at the injection site; systolic and diastolic hypertension with tachycardia; nausea; vomiting; headache; burning or constricting sensation in the mouth, throat, and eyes; lacrimation; salivation;

rhinorrhea; muscle aches; tingling of the extremities; pain in the teeth; sense of constriction in the chest; abdominal pain; sterile or pyogenic abscesses at the site of injection; and feeling of anxiety or unrest. In addition to these side effects, a febrile reaction may occur in children. These signs and symptoms were most severe within 30 minutes after administration of BAL and usually dissipate within 1.0 to 1.5 hours. The undesirable side effects may be lessened by the use of epinephrine or by pretreatment with antihistamine or ephedrine (53).

DMSA is a chelating agent used in the treatment of intoxication with several heavy metals. A water-soluble analog of BAL, DMSA enhances the urinary excretion of mercury, lead, and arsenic and has an insignificant effect on elimination of the endogenous minerals calcium, iron, and magnesium. Minor increases in zinc and copper excretion may occur. Oral DMSA is rapidly but variably absorbed, with peak blood levels occurring between 1 and 2 hours after ingestion. The drug is predominantly cleared by the kidneys, with peak urinary elimination of the parent drug and its metabolites occurring at between 2 and 4 hours. Reported adverse effects of DMSA include GI disturbances (anorexia, nausea, vomiting, diarrhea), a mercaptanlike odor to the urine, rashes, mild to moderate neutropenia, and mild reversible increases in hepatic transaminase levels. Currently in the United States, DMSA is available only in an oral formulation.

D-Penicillamine is also an orally active chelating agent. It is excreted primarily in the urine. Acute allergic reactions that sometimes are encountered early in the course of therapy include fever, rashes, leukopenia, eosinophilia, thrombocytopenia, and occasionally, renal tubular damage, proteinuria, and nephrotic syndrome. Because this chelator expresses cross-sensitivity with penicillin, patients allergic to penicillin should not be given D-penicillamine. Pyridoxine antagonism has been demonstrated, but such clinical effects after chelation therapy are rare (54). D-Penicillamine may facilitate the absorption of mercury from the GI tract and so should not be given when there is evidence that mercury remains in the GI tract.

BAL and D-penicillamine have both been used in the treatment of acute and chronic poisoning from mercury vapor. The use of BAL in elemental mercury poisoning has been discouraged after animal studies showed that BAL may redistribute mercury to the brain from other tissue sites (55–57). Because the brain is a target organ in elemental mercury poisoning, it would seem prudent not to use BAL. DMSA appears to incite fewer side effects and induce more efficient mercury excretion as compared with D-penicillamine. Available data also suggest a role for DMSA in enhancing urinary mercury excretion and reducing nephrotoxicity after GI absorption of elemental mercury (58). In cases of mercury vapor poisoning for which chelation therapy is considered, DMSA appears to be the logical choice. The initial recommended dose of DMSA is 10 mg per kg of body weight every 8 hours, tapering to every 12 hours over the next several days. DMSA can be administered via nasogastric tube in severe poisoning cases in which endotracheal intubation is required.

The therapeutic endpoints of chelation are poorly defined. Probably the only objective measurable effect of chelation therapy is enhanced urinary excretion of mercury. A potential endpoint for chelation may be when the patient's urinary mercury concentration approaches baseline.

Although the use of chelators is recommended to increase mercury excretion and relieve target organs of metal burden, the use of BAL has not been proved to affect the course of elemental mercury–induced respiratory failure, and the effect of DMSA on clinical outcome has not yet been fully studied. No role has been defined for multiple-dose activated charcoal, hemoperfusion, or hemodialysis in removing elemental mercury.

Inorganic Mercury

Acute inorganic mercury poisoning is usually the result of intentional or accidental ingestion. Most of the literature on inorganic mercury poisoning deals with mercuric chloride (mercuric bichloride, $HgCl_2$). In animals, the median lethal dose of mercuric chloride is approximately 1 mg per kg of body weight intravenously or intraperitoneally. In adults, the lethal dose of mercuric chloride has been estimated to be between 1 and 4 g.

Mercurials have been used and are available for a variety of purposes, including medicinal agents (antiparasitics, anthelminthics, antiseptics, antipruritics, disinfectants), paint, stool fixatives, permanent-wave hair solutions, teething powder, button batteries, fungicides and biocides, folk remedies [e.g., among Mexican-Americans for *empacho*, a chronic stomach ailment, and among Asians (in Chinese herbal patent medications)], and in occult practices (among Latin-American and Caribbean natives). Fortunately, the medicinal uses for mercurials have been replaced by less toxic drugs. However, topical antiseptics containing mercury are still being used.

ABSORPTION, METABOLISM, AND EXCRETION

Absorption of inorganic mercury salt from the GI tract is dose-dependent. Seven to fifteen percent of an oral dose is absorbed, whereas large amounts remain bound to the GI mucosa. Insoluble compounds may be oxidized to more soluble compounds, resulting in enhanced absorption. After absorption, the salt dissociates into the ionic form and is initially distributed between RBCs and plasma. Distribution of mercury within the body and within the organs varies widely. It has been demonstrated by an animal autoradiographic study that mercuric ion accumulates predominantly in the renal cortex (59). Mercuric ion does not appear to cross the blood–brain barrier or the placental barrier significantly. However, the autoradiographic study revealed that the brain does take up mercury slowly and retains it for a longer period than in the kidney (59). Mercuric ion is eliminated from the body mainly by the urinary and fecal routes, with small amounts appearing in the saliva and sweat. The rate of excretion is dose-dependent. Inorganic mercury follows a biphasic elimination rate, being initially rapid and then slowing, with a biological half-life in humans of approximately 60 days.

The target organs of inorganic mercury poisoning are the GI tract and the kidneys. The caustic property of the inorganic mercurials could cause damage throughout the GI tract, including corrosive stomatitis, necrotizing esophagitis, gastritis, and ulcerative colitis. Postmortem examination of patients who died within 48 hours of ingestion of inorganic mercurials showed severe hemorrhagic necrosis of the upper GI wall (60). Nephrotoxicity after inorganic mercury poisoning resulted from acute tubular necrosis of the distal portions of the proximal convoluted tubules and incited a brief diuresis followed by acute oliguric renal failure and uremia (60,61). Oliguria or anuria has been noted to develop within 24 hours in 50% of acute overdoses (62–65). The CNS usually is spared because only small amounts of mercuric ion can cross the blood–brain barrier. However, cases of CNS toxicity have been described with chronic mercury ingestion.

CLINICAL TOXICOLOGY

The clinical effects of acute inorganic mercury poisoning can be divided into the initial local corrosive effect on the GI tract followed by the injury that occurs at the site of excretion, the kidneys. Depending on the amount ingested, the GI symptoms that follow may vary from mild gastritis to severe necrotizing ulceration of the intestinal mucosa, which can be fatal within a few hours (66). Ingestion of 100 mg of inorganic mercury has been reported to be associated with a bitter metallic taste in the mouth, a sense of constriction about the throat, substernal burning, gastritis, abdominal pains, nausea, and vomiting (61). A serious acute inorganic mercury ingestion may cause the abrupt onset of hematemesis, hemorrhagic gastroenteritis, and abdominal pain. The patient may die within hours from shock and peripheral vascular collapse due to fluid and electrolyte losses (62). Intestinal necrosis may ensue. In addition, massive bleeding from the colon has been reported to occur as late as 8 to 9 days after ingestion (60). Most of the bleeding in the latter case came from the rectum, which was the most severely involved section of the colon. Such injuries to the GI tract can lead to massive fluid, electrolyte, and blood loss that result in shock and death.

Acute inorganic mercury ingestion may lead to acute oliguric renal failure due to acute tubular necrosis. Invariably, those patients who develop renal involvement initially have severe GI symptoms (66). Typically, oliguric renal failure occurs within 72 hours of ingestion and, as such, the initial GI symptoms may be resolving although renal toxicity may not yet be apparent (60,66). Spontaneous resolution of acute toxic anuria with renal tubular regeneration may be expected to occur between 8 and 12 days after inorganic mercury ingestion (67), with clinical recovery (if it occurs) occurring between 9 to 14 days after ingestion (60,66).

The chronic effects of inorganic mercury exposure are similar to those of elemental mercury exposure. Evidence exists of long-term behavioral impairment after low-level chronic exposure to inorganic mercury (68). Workers exposed to inorganic mercury exhibit subclinical psychomotor and neuromuscular changes that make difficult ascertainment of the full effects of chronic inorganic mercury intoxication (69,70).

DIAGNOSIS

As with elemental mercury exposure, diagnosis depends on integrating characteristic findings with a history of known or potential exposure and the presence of elevated whole blood mercury concentration and urinary mercury excretion. Inorganic mercury may be visualized on an abdominal radiograph as radiopaque foreign bodies in the GI tract. A positive radiograph would confirm a diagnosis, but the absence of radiopaque substances is not diagnostic. See Elemental Mercury, Diagnosis for information on whole blood and urinary mercury concentrations.

Relationships between urinary mercury concentration and clinical findings have generally been based on chronic exposure. Severity of symptoms varies widely even among individuals, and the correlation between urinary mercury concentration and symptoms often is poor.

Whole blood mercury concentrations in excess of 50 µg per dL in acute inorganic mercury poisoning often are associated with gastroenteritis and acute renal tubular necrosis.

MANAGEMENT

Treatment of Inorganic Mercury Ingestion. In acute inorganic mercury ingestions, GI decontamination should be performed to minimize absorption and to decrease the corrosive effect of the ingested inorganic salt. As with the ingestion of any corrosive substance, inducing emesis is discouraged. Elective tracheal intubation may be prudent before attempting GI decontamination. Gastric lavage should be performed with caution, as the GI tract may have already been severely damaged. Endoscopy is recommended if corrosive injury (drooling, dysphagia, abdominal pain) is suspected. A theoretically reasonable but not rigorously studied approach calls for the use of a protein gastric lavage solution (1 pint skim milk with 50 g glucose, 20 g sodium bicarbonate, and 3 eggs beaten into a mixture) to bind the mercury, along with rinsing the stomach with egg white or concentrated human albumin after the lavage (55). Activated charcoal, 1 g per kg of body weight, as a slurry may also be used, as 1 g of charcoal is capable of binding 850 mg of mercuric chloride (55).

In cases that exhibit radiographic evidence of radiopaque foreign bodies in the GI tract and in which no evidence of gastroenteritis exists, bowel irrigation with polyethylene glycol electrolyte solution should be considered. Repeat abdominal radiographs may be used to document the effectiveness of bowel irrigation.

In a serious inorganic mercury ingestion, the initial GI injury may result in severe fluid, electrolyte, and blood loss. Aggressive monitoring of the patient's volume status should be undertaken. Intravascular and GI losses should be replaced by the appropriate administration of crystalloid, colloid, and blood products. An indwelling Foley catheter should be placed to monitor the urine output carefully; urine output should be maintained at 1 to 2 mL per kg per hour. Distinguishing between oliguria due to inadequate volume resuscitation or replacement and oliguria due to toxic nephropathy and resulting renal failure is important. Invasive hemodynamic monitoring may be necessary.

Aggressive surgical intervention may be required in patients experiencing severe gastric necrosis or in whom hemorrhagic ulcerative colitis becomes life threatening (60,71). It has been suggested that the rectum be resected at the time of colectomy, when indicated for controlling hemorrhage from the colon (60).

Chelation. The effectiveness of BAL depends on the promptness of administration and adequate dosing (66,72–74). The most effective interval within which to administer BAL has been reported to be fewer than 4 hours after mercury ingestion (73). Because prompt intervention is paramount in reducing renal injury, expedient chelation therapy would be prudent in suspected cases of acute inorganic mercury poisoning. Chelation should not be withheld while laboratory confirmation of mercury poisoning is awaited. DMSA is also effective, but the capacity of the GI tract to absorb orally administered DMSA may be impaired by hemorrhagic gastroenteritis, hemodynamic instability, and splanchnic edema. Once the GI and cardiovascular status have been stabilized, chelation with DMSA may be substituted for BAL. The empiric recommended dosing of BAL is 3 to 5 mg per kg every 4 hours for 2 days, followed by 2.5 to 3.0 mg per kg every 6 hours for the next 2 days and then every 12 hours for 7 more days.

Once renal damage has occurred from inorganic mercury poisoning, therapy should be directed at the acute renal failure that may ensue. Hemodialysis should be used to support the patient through the oliguric or anuric renal failure period. A potential problem arises with continued BAL therapy in patients who develop renal insufficiency, because the kidneys are one of the main routes by which BAL-Hg is eliminated. In such circumstances, BAL therapy may be judiciously continued as there is some evidence from animal studies that a significant fraction of BAL-Hg is excreted also in the bile. Some studies indicate that hemodialysis may contribute to the elimination of BAL-Hg in patients with renal failure (63,74,75). In a patient who is in renal failure but is otherwise stable and has a functional GI tract, DMSA may be an alternative to BAL.

Organic Mercury

The organomercurials are compounds in which the mercury atom is joined to a carbon atom via a covalent bond. It is the relative stability of this covalent bond that determines the toxicology of the organic mercury compounds. The organomercurials can be classified as short-chain alkyl (methyl, ethyl, and propyl mercury), long-chain alkyl, and aryl (phenyl) mercury compounds. In aryl compounds, mercury is joined by a carbon link to an aromatic ring, such as benzene or toluene. The aryl and long-chain mercury compounds behave toxicologically similarly to inorganic mercury (47). In general, the short-chain alkyl group, particularly methyl mercury, is considered the most toxic of the organomercurials.

Although inorganic mercury toxicity has been known and described for centuries, organic mercury toxicity was described only relatively recently. The first organic mercurials were used in chemical research. Diethyl mercury injections were used for the treatment of syphilis beginning in 1887 but soon were abandoned because of severe CNS effects. Around 1913, organic mercury compounds were noted to induce a diuresis, which led to the development of mercurial diuretics. These agents were used for more than 30 years before they were replaced by less toxic drugs. The antifungal and antibacterial properties of organomercurials prompted their use as seed dressings and ointments.

Organic mercurials are used chiefly as preservatives and antiseptics. Methyl, ethyl, and phenyl compounds are used as seed dressings to inhibit fungal growth and delay germination. Misuse of treated seed has been the most common cause of poisoning from organic mercury. Examples of such compounds are monomethyl mercury chloride, ethyl mercuric chloride, methyl mercuric iodide, and chloromethyl mercury. Merbromin (Mercurochrome), the first organic mercurial antiseptic, still is used routinely. Phenylmercuric acetate (PMA), phenylmercuric nitrate, phenylmercuric borate, thimerosal, and Mercurochrome are all mercurial antiseptics found predominantly in ophthalmic products such as eyedrops and contact lens solutions. They are also found in vaccines, immunoglobulins, nasal sprays, and lyophilized powders.

PMA normally is used in the powder form as a seed dressing and in paper manufacturing. Another seed dressing, methyl mercuric dicyanamide, takes a liquid form. Aerosolization can occur with either the dust or liquid forms.

Microorganisms in soil and water can methylate inorganic mercury to form organic mercury. A nonenzymatic methylation of Hg^{+2} ions by methylcobalamin, a by-product of bacterial synthesis, is the postulated mechanism.

Potential sources of exposure to organic mercury include herbicides, fungicides, germicides, and timber preservatives. However, organic mercury exposure is primarily dietary. In the general population, the major source of exposure to methyl mercury is through the consumption of predatory fish (e.g., pike, tuna, and swordfish). Major incidents of human poisoning with methyl mercury have occurred (Minamata and Iraq epidemics), with devastating outcomes. Acute ingestion of 10 to 60 μg per kg of body weight of methyl mercury may be lethal, and chronic daily ingestion of 10 μg per kg of body weight may be associated with adverse neurologic and reproductive effects.

Ingestion of cereals treated with organic mercurial fungicides for planting and of fish from mercury-polluted streams and rivers are major sources of dietary organic mercury exposure. Consumption of game birds or their eggs from areas in which methyl mercury fungicides are used can result in exposure.

Disinfectant makers, fungicide makers, seed handlers, farmers, lumberjacks, pharmaceutical industry workers, and wood preservers may be exposed to organic mercury compounds in their occupations. In the paper industry, organic mercury compounds are used to control slime.

Another source of organic mercury compound exposure is pharmaceutical product use. Vaginal contraceptive jellies and suppositories may contain PMA, phenylmercuric nitrate, or other organic mercurials that are easily absorbed. Thimerosal in ophthalmic products may cause blepharoconjunctivitis and punctate keratitis in contact lens users, but no systemic toxicity has been reported.

Latex paints may contain phenylmercuric acetate as a preservative. Beginning August 20, 1990, the U.S. Environmental Protection Agency announced that no mercury-containing compounds could lawfully be added to interior latex paint. However, paint produced before that time may still be sold.

ABSORPTION, METABOLISM, AND EXCRETION

Organic mercury compounds can be subdivided into two classes on the basis of their mechanism of metabolism: short-chain alkyl mercury compounds, and aryl and long-chain mercury compounds. Cleavage of the carbon-mercury bond occurs at differing rates after absorption. The aryl and long-chain mercury bonds are readily broken *in vivo* to yield inorganic mercury. Thus, aryl and long-chain mercury toxicity is similar to the toxicity of inorganic mercury. In contrast, short-chain mercurials have a strong, stable carbon-mercury bond that is cleaved slowly, and the inorganic mercury does not play a role in the toxicity of alkyl mercury. All tissues except muscle and blood biotransform organic mercury to an inorganic form. Inorganic mercury is oxidized to the divalent cation in the lungs, RBCs, and liver. This cation, in turn, can be reduced to the elemental form to be exhaled as metallic mercury vapor.

GI absorption of organic mercurials is more complete than that of the inorganic compounds because of their increased lipid solubility. Organic mercury antiseptics undergo limited skin penetration; however, in rare cases, such as topical application to an infected omphalocele, intoxication has resulted. The short-chain alkyl mercury compounds are lipid-soluble and volatile. Consequently, highly efficient absorption can occur through inhalation, ingestion, or dermal exposure, as in the case of methyl mercury. Approximately 80% of inhaled short-chain mercury salt vapors are absorbed. Absorption of aerosols depends on particle size.

More than 90% of methyl mercury is absorbed from the GI tract, as compared with only 15% of inorganic mercury (48). Methyl mercury also crosses the placenta, accumulates in the fetus, and is excreted in toxic amounts in breast milk (76). It is readily lipid-soluble and distributes widely throughout the body (77). Blood levels equilibrate with tissue levels, making blood a clinical indicator of exposure. In the blood, more than 90% of methyl mercury is found in the red cells, with whole blood–to–plasma ratios of 200 to 300 to 1 (78). Methyl mercury is distributed slowly from the blood to the body. Although uniformly distributed, it concentrates in the liver, kidney, blood, brain, hair, and epidermis. Newly formed hair avidly incorporates methyl mercury in direct proportion to the blood concentration and so is sometimes used as monitoring medium. The amount of methyl mercury in brain tissue, although less than in liver and kidney, is greater than the amount of mercury found in brain tissue in cases of inorganic mercury poisoning.

In humans, nearly 10% of the body's methyl mercury burden is in the brain, and the biological half-life of methyl mercury is approximately 70 days (79). Methyl mercury readily crosses the blood–brain barrier as well as the placental barrier (80). In animal studies, the dissociation between the carbon and mercury bond of methyl mercury is very slow (78), whereas phenyl mercury undergoes rapid breakdown to inorganic mercury within 24 hours (77,81). In humans, the major route of excretion of methyl mercury is in the feces, with less than 10% appearing in the urine (82). Methyl mercury is also secreted in the bile. A portion undergoes enterohepatic circulation, whereas the remainder is converted to the inorganic form by the intestinal flora. Extensive enterohepatic recirculation may account for the long biological half-life of this compound (83). This long half-life equates to an excretion rate of 1% per day of the total body burden.

Tissue distribution of aryl and long-chain mercurials resembles that of methyl mercury initially. After 1 week, however, the tissue distribution is more akin to inorganic mercurials (10).

Phenyl mercury is an aryl mercury compound that is metabolized *in vivo* to inorganic mercury and is eliminated primarily fecally for the first few days, with some excretion of the parent compounds in the urine. Later, this shifts to predominantly urinary excretion of inorganic mercury.

CLINICAL TOXICOLOGY

Mercury has an affinity to bind to, or reacts with, sulfhydryl moieties of proteins, leading to nonspecific inhibition of enzyme systems and pathologic alteration of cellular membranes. Likewise, mercury can bind to primary and secondary amine, amide, carboxyl, and phosphoryl groups. Methyl mercury inhibits the sulfhydryl-containing enzyme choline acetyl-transferase, which catalyzes the final step in acetylcholine's synthesis (47).

The CNS is particularly vulnerable to the toxic effects of methyl mercury. This is attributed to the high lipid solubility of methyl mercury, which results in rapid access across the blood–brain barrier. However, lipid-soluble complexes have not been detected. Methyl mercury is secreted in bile conjugated to glutathione. It may then be transported across the blood–brain barrier as a complex with cysteine by a specific membrane carrier, which may be attributable to its resemblance to an endogenous substrate. The resultant neuronal damage is predominantly located within the cerebellar granular layer, the calcarine fissure of the occipital area, an d the precentral gyrus. Methyl mercury has been shown to alter brain ornithine decarboxylase (ODC) levels. ODC is an enzyme associated with cellular maturity, and neurotransmitter uptake at the presynaptic and postsynaptic adrenergic receptor sites (84). Methyl mercury is also a potent teratogen and reproductive toxin.

Important aspects of methyl mercury toxicity include its predisposition for the CNS, its insidious onset, and its poor prognosis. The classic triad of methyl mercury poisoning is dysarthria, ataxia and constricted visual fields (85). Other signs and symptoms include paresthesias, hearing impairment, and progressive incoordination, loss of voluntary movement, and mental retardation. Perinatal exposure to methyl mercury has caused mental retardation and a cerebral palsy–type syndrome in offspring.

Most of the detailed information regarding organic mercury toxicity has been derived from methyl mercury poisoning cases. Methyl mercury is a cumulative poison, and no distinct differences appear to exist between acute and chronic methyl mercury poisoning. After acute methyl mercury intoxication, symptoms usually are delayed for several weeks or months. Typically, symptoms worsen for 3 to 10 years, during which time cases may be misdiagnosed as other diseases. Because the cases identified by Harada were atypical of the Hunter-Russell syndrome, Harada named them *chronic Minamata disease* (23). The delayed appearance of symptoms may be related to consumption of low levels of methyl mercury for a prolonged period.

Respiratory Effects. Organic mercurials are mucous membrane irritants. They may cause blistering of the oropharynx and nasopharynx. Significant absorption can occur via inhalation.

Gastrointestinal Effects. Methyl mercury does not usually produce GI effects. Ethyl mercury poisoning can produce nausea, vomiting, diarrhea, and abdominal cramps. Phenyl mercury may produce stomatitis and gum discoloration.

Renal Effects. Clinical nephrotoxicity has not been observed in human methyl mercury poisoning. Mercurial diuretics, methoxyethyl mercury, ethyl mercury, and phenyl mercury compounds have caused renal toxicity, including nephrotic syndrome, albuminuria, and renal failure. An autoimmune response to a mercury-protein complex has been hypothesized.

Dermal Effects. Dermatitis consisting of erythroderma and pruritus, initially affecting the hands, arms, and face but followed by involvement of the trunk and legs, has been described in patients exposed to mercury during all three Iraqi epidemics. It was believed to occur from direct cutaneous contact. Blistering similar to second-degree burns can occur from contact with aryl mercury compounds. Cutaneous application of Mercurochrome to burns has been associated with toxicity and death in children.

Hematologic Effects. Mercurial diuretics have been associated with thrombocytopenia and agranulocytosis, and phenyl mercury has caused neutropenia. Phenyl mercury is much less toxic than methyl mercury because it is less volatile, crosses the placenta and blood–brain barrier more slowly, and is more rapidly excreted. Its pattern of toxicity is intermediate between alkyl and inorganic mercury.

Teratogenicity. All forms of mercury cross the placenta into the fetal circulation. Elemental mercury passes more readily than inorganic mercury compounds, but organic alkyl mercury compounds pass with the greatest ease owing to their relatively higher lipid solubility. Maternal exposure usually occurs from the consumption of foodstuffs treated with methyl mercury. However, inhalation and skin absorption are also possible routes of exposure to other forms of mercury. The phytotoxic effects of mercury were first noted in women who were undergoing treatment for syphilis with mercury and were observed to have a high frequency of spontaneous abortion. Congenital damage has been reported in infants whose mothers were unaware of their exposure to methyl mercury during pregnancy because they experienced no ill effects. In contrast, some mothers have shown signs and symptoms of mercury intoxication whereas their infants did not, although abnormal neurologic signs in affected infants became more obvious over time.

The alkyl mercury concentrations in fetal RBCs are 30% higher than in maternal RBCs, and fetal tissue levels are twice the maternal tissue levels (47). Blood mercury levels of infants will be maintained by transmission of methyl mercury via maternal milk, which has 5% of the mercury concentration of maternal blood.

Methyl mercury is a teratogen in rats, mice, cats, hamsters, and humans. Organic mercury rapidly crosses the placental barrier, accumulating in the fetus (86). Twenty-five infants born during the Minamata epidemic had a cerebral palsy–like syndrome with severe mental retardation, cerebellar symptoms (ataxia, intention tremor, nystagmus, dysmetria), hypersalivation, hyperkinesia (chorea, athetosis), limb deformities, strabismus, and seizure disorders. Their mothers, although heavy fish eaters, experienced mild or no symptoms. Fetal hemoglobin, although increasing fetal susceptibility, may protect the mother by its stronger affinity for methyl mercury than the mother's hemoglobin. Moreover, *congenital Minamata disease*, as it sometimes is known, occurs at lower exposure levels of methyl mercury than those associated with adult toxicity. Autopsy data demonstrated cortical and cerebellar atrophy and hypoplasia, corpus callosum hypoplasia, and demyelination of the pyramidal tract (86,87). This diffuse brain involvement differs from those changes seen in the adult. Microtubule-dependent neuronal migration and cell division may be inhibited. Methyl mercury appears to bind alpha- and beta-tubulin proteins avidly, inhibiting the polymerization of microtubules. The observed arrest in late mitosis is consistent with microtubule inhibition. This inhibition is specific to small amounts of organic mercury (86).

EPIDEMICS OF ORGANIC MERCURY EXPOSURES

The largest number of cases of human poisoning from organic mercurials has resulted from ingestion of contaminated foods. Epidemics have occurred in Minamata Bay and Niigata, Japan, Iraq, Pakistan, Guatemala, Ghana, New Mexico, and the Soviet Union (87).

Minamata Bay in 1956 and the Agano River, Niigata, Japan, in 1964 were polluted by the mercury effluent from factories using inorganic mercuric chloride catalysts in acetaldehyde and vinyl chloride processing (87). Inorganic mercury was methylated by the microflora of the bay and concentrated as it moved up the food chain. Methyl mercury was discovered in samples of the effluent, proving that the factory process itself methylated the inorganic mercury. Fish absorbed methyl mercury both by eating contaminated food and directly through their gills. Fish have an excretion half-life of several hundred days, which allows the organic mercury to accumulate to concentrations 1,000 times greater than that in the surrounding water. This fact resulted in mercury levels as high as 50 parts per million (ppm) in fish and 85 ppm in shellfish. Affected individuals probably ingested up to 4 mg of mercury per day, which is 40 times the estimated safe daily intake, as fish was a dietary staple.

In northern Iraq in 1956 and central Iraq in 1960, people ate wheat grain treated with the fungicide Granosan-M (7.7% ethyl mercury-*p*-toluene sulfonanilide), intended for seed use (87). The largest epidemic occurred in Iraq in 1971 through 1972, from ingestion of homemade breads made from wheat seed treated with phenylmercuric acetate, methyl mercury dicyanamide, methyl mercury acetate, and ethyl mercury (87). The epidemic included 6,500 poisoning cases and 450 deaths. Three New Mexico children in 1969 developed organic mercury toxicity after consumption of meat from a hog feed seed grain treated with cyanomethyl mercury guanidine (Panogen).

The Minamata Bay and Iraqi epidemics have better defined the clinical presentation of methyl mercury poisoning (47):

- Psychological: difficulty concentrating, short- and long-term memory loss, emotional volatility, depression, decreased intellectual abilities, and ultimately, coma
- Cerebellar: generalized ataxia with stumbling gait, dysdiadochokinesia, and lack of coordination
- Sensory: numbness and stocking-glove paresthesias of distal extremities and mouth, deafness, tunnel vision, visual field constriction, scanning speech with slurring, and dysphagia
- Motoric: spasticity; tremors of hands, face, or legs; and weakness proceeding to paralysis

The initial symptoms are fatigue and perioral or extremity paresthesias, followed by difficulty with hand movements. Sensation and visual disturbances occur next. Electrocardiographic abnormalities (ST-segment changes) were noted in approximately one-third of cases from the last Iraqi poisoning (87).

Ingestion of ethyl mercury–treated seed resulted in the 1956 and 1960 Iraqi poisonings (87). Characterization of the clinical syndrome of the affected patients revealed distinct differences from methyl mercury toxicity. Involvement of the kidneys, GI tract, and skin were more representative of inorganic mercury toxicity. Patients exposed to the ethyl mercury–treated seed experienced from polydipsia, polyuria, proteinuria, abdominal pain with nausea and vomiting, and pruritus, especially involving the palms, soles, and genitals, often progressing to an exfoliative dermatitis. Although patients exhibited slurred speech and ataxia, mentation was not affected. Deep musculoskeletal pains and frequent electrocardiographic changes (ST depression, T-wave inversion, prolonged QT and PR intervals, and ectopy) also were reported.

DIAGNOSIS

Diagnosis of organic mercury toxicity depends on integration of characteristic findings with a history of known or potential exposure and the presence of an elevated whole blood mercury concentration, which may reflect recent exposure. Although an occupational and exposure history is necessary, a complete physical examination, including a thorough neurologic examination, should also be performed. Patients should be evaluated for the presence of a tremor, pathologic reflexes, hyperreflexia, abnormal cerebellar function (especially ataxic gait, Romberg's sign, and finger-to-nose test), constriction of visual fields, nystagmus, dysarthric speech, short- and long-term memory, and impaired hearing. Neuropsychiatric and nerve conduction studies as well as electromyography should be considered.

Whole blood is the best sample for organic mercury testing as it is concentrated in RBCs. Methyl mercury undergoes biliary excretion and enterohepatic recirculation, with 90% eventually being excreted in the feces. Therefore, urinary mercury measurements are not useful. Blood levels for mercury are normally less than 2 µg per dL and should not exceed 5 µg per dL. Whole blood mercury concentrations in excess of 20 µg per dL have been associated with symptoms (e.g., paresthesias).

Hair levels of mercury were used extensively in investigating the Minamata epidemic. Normally, hair mercury levels average 2 to 15 ppm, but those afflicted with the disease had levels between 100 and 700 ppm. Hair levels have been used to document temporally remote exposures. However, because of concern about external contamination, hair analysis is not used routinely.

Electromyography and nerve conduction velocities may be useful in determining neurologic effects on peripheral nerves.

β-Acetyl glucosaminidase (a lysosomal enzyme) and retinol-binding protein (a low-molecular-weight protein) in renal tubular cells are being studied as sensitivity indicators of subclinical renal dysfunction from inorganic mercury exposure. β-Acetyl glucosaminidase and retinol-binding protein are research tools, and whether they are clinically useful as an indicator of renal damage has not yet been determined.

MANAGEMENT

Supportive Therapy for Organic Mercury Intoxication. Treatment of organic mercurial intoxication is primarily supportive. After organic mercurials have been ingested acutely, gastric lavage should be performed. Administration of activated charcoal may be beneficial. A successful way to decrease the rate of methyl mercury absorption is to introduce a nonabsorbable mercury-binding substance (polythiol resin) into the GI tract so as to interrupt the enterohepatic recirculation of methyl mercury (88,89). Repeated oral administration of a polythiol resin in methyl mercury intoxication may be beneficial. Limited data suggest that oral neostigmine may improve motor strength in patients with moderate to severe chronic methyl mercury intoxication (89).

Chelation. Chelation with BAL has been ineffective in treating neurologic symptoms due to methyl mercury poisoning

(90), and the use of BAL in organic mercury poisoning has been discouraged since animal studies (55–57) showed that BAL may redistribute mercury to the brain from other tissue sites. Because the brain is a target organ in organic mercury poisoning, it would seem prudent not to use BAL. Animal studies involving other chelators suggest that DMSA is effective in reducing the brain concentration of methyl mercury (91), and DMSA treatment prevented the development of cerebellar damage in methyl mercury–poisoned animals (92). However, in humans, DMSA's effect on clinical outcome has not yet been studied fully.

Hemodialysis, peritoneal dialysis, hemoperfusion, and forced diuresis are of little value, as methyl mercury is distributed widely and in large volume and a considerable amount of methyl mercury resides within the RBCs.

BIOLOGICAL MONITORING

Individuals who are occupationally exposed to mercury should undergo periodic physical examinations and 24-hour urinary mercury determinations at 6-month to 1-year intervals. If air monitoring reveals mercury levels within the upper half of the threshold limit value (TLV), employees should undergo physical examination and a repeat urinary mercury level determination. Any worker in whom the TLV is exceeded should be examined immediately and submit to a urinary mercury determination. Hair analysis cannot be recommended at this time because of the concern with external contamination.

Blood level monitoring is the best measure of recent exposure to inorganic and elemental mercury. It is not a measure of the total body burden, however. Organic mercurials, which are more lipid-soluble than inorganic forms, tend to concentrate in RBCs. A plasma-RBC mercury ratio of 1 to 1 is believed to be indicative of inorganic mercury; a plasma-RBC mercury ratio of 1 to 10 suggests organic mercury toxicity. A history and physical examination help to make the diagnosis of organic mercury intoxication. Symptoms may be seen with a methyl mercury blood concentration of 3 to 5 µg per dL.

Urine mercury concentrations may be significantly altered by disinfectants and other products. Assessing the total body burden of mercury can be accomplished by a chelation challenge using D-penicillamine. A fourfold increase in a 24-hour mercury concentration over baseline may suggest a body burden. Because abundant sulfhydryl groups are found in hair, mercury levels in hair may be 250 to 300 times the RBC concentration.

ENVIRONMENTAL MONITORING

Prevention is the best management of toxicity in the occupational setting. Appropriate ventilation of work areas in which dust, vapor, or aerosol exposure is possible should prevent toxic accumulation. Personal and area air sampling of the environment should be routinely performed. Industrial hygiene surveys can be conducted to monitor levels of mercury. In enclosed areas and occupational settings, mercury vapor concentrations can be detected with electronic devices such as a mercury vapor analyzer. Ambient air concentrations as low as 0.001 mg per cubic meter can be detected. The National Institute for Occupational Safety and Health (NIOSH) recommends an air-sampling method using a solid sorbent media, low flow rate, and flameless atomic absorption for detection of elemental mercury concentrations. The complete procedure for this analysis is outlined in Method 6000 of the *NIOSH Manual of Analytic Methods*.

The mercury decontamination procedure for buildings includes removal of carpets and several cleanings of floors, walls, and solid surfaces with a product containing a metallic mercury sulfide–converting powder, a chelating compound, and a dispersing agent. A polyurethane coating then is applied to all floor surfaces.

The recommended threshold limit value for an 8-hour time-weighted average (TLV-TWA) for mercury vapor and for inorganic and nonalkyl organic mercurials is 0.05 mg per cubic meter in the United States and the European Community. The ceiling value (TLV-C) for mercury vapor is 0.1 mg Hg per cubic meter in the United States, and for methyl- and ethyl mercury, the TLV-TWA is 0.01 mg per cubic meter. In Russia, the TLV-C values are 0.01 mg per cubic meter for mercury vapor and 0.005 mg per cubic meter for alkyl mercury (2). It has been noted that an air concentration of mercury of 0.05 mg per cubic meter corresponds to a urinary concentration of approximately 50 µg per L and blood concentrations of approximately 30 to 35 µg per L (3).

The U.S. Environmental Protection Agency's suggested ambient air level for population exposure is less than 10 to 20 ng per cubic meter. Atmospheric discharges from industrial facilities are not to exceed 2.3 kg per day from chloralkali plants or smelters and 3.2 kg per day from sludge incineration and drying. Mercury discharge into waterways from chloralkali plants is regulated to the limit of 140 mg for every 1,000 kg of product. The maximum allowable mercury concentration in fish is 0.3 mg per kg in the United States, Finland, and Sweden (2).

The maximum (ceiling) methyl mercury level, which cannot be exceeded at any time during the work period, is 0.04 mg per cubic meter. A separate area for eating and smoking should be provided. Respirators and protective clothing should be used during cleaning and maintenance operations and spills. Preemployment and periodic physical examinations should be conducted, with emphasis on vision (especially visual fields), CNS, renal function, and skin.

The American Conference of Governmental Industrial Hygienists makes yearly recommendations of airborne concentrations of substances to which workers can be exposed day after day without adverse effects. These TLVs can refer to a TWA, a short-term exposure limit (STEL), or a ceiling. The TLV-TWA is an average concentration for a normal 8-hour day and 40-hour week to which workers can be exposed without adverse effect. The TWA-STEL is the maximum exposure concentration allowable during a 15-minute period in an 8-hour day. Exposure to the TWA-STEL should occur no more than four times daily, with an hour-long interval between exposures. A TWA-C is the maximum allowable airborne concentration at any time during the 8-hour work period that must not be exceeded.

The U.S. Occupational Safety and Health Administration (OSHA) is entrusted with setting and enforcing workplace standards. OSHA receives guidance from NIOSH and the American Conference of Governmental Industrial Hygienists in formulating these levels. Permissible exposure limits (PELs) are the legally mandated guidelines established by OSHA. Usually, TWAs and PELs are the same. However, differences may exist, as TWAs are updated yearly, whereas PELs are updated infrequently.

REFERENCES

1. Agency for Toxic Substances and Disease Registry. Potential for human exposure. In: *Toxicological profile for mercury*. Atlanta: US Department of Health and Human Services, Public Health Service, ATSDR, April 1993.
2. Agency for Toxic Substances and Disease Registry. Regulations and advisories. In: *Toxicological profile for mercury*. Atlanta: US Department of Health and Human Services, Public Health Service, ATSDR, April 1993.

3. Berlin M. Mercury. In: Friberg L, Nordberg G, Vouk V, eds. *Handbook on the toxicology of metals*, vol 2. New York: Elsevier Science, 1986.
4. Tennant R, Hohnston HJ, Wells JB. Acute bilateral pneumonitis associated with the inhalation of mercury vapor. *Conn Med* 1961;25:106–109.
5. Jaeger A, Tempe JD, Haegy JM, Leroy M, Porte A, Mantz JM. Accidental acute mercury vapor poisoning. *Vet Hum Toxicol* 1979;215:62–63.
6. Snodgrass W, Sullivan JB, Rumack BH. Mercury poisoning from home gold ore processing. *JAMA* 1981;246:1929–1931.
7. Schwartz JG, Snider TE, Montiel MM. Toxicity of a family from vacuumed mercury. *Am J Emerg Med* 1992;10:258–261.
8. Hursh JB, Clarkson TW, Cherian MG, Vostal JJ, Mallie RV. Clearance of mercury (Hg-197, Hg-203) vapor inhaled by human subjects. *Arch Environ Health* 1976;31:302–309.
9. Cherian MG, Hursh JB, Clarkson TW, Allen J. Radioactive mercury distribution in biological fluids and excretion in human subjects after inhalation of mercury vapor. *Arch Environ Health* 1978;33:109–114.
10. Clarkson TW. The pharmacology of mercury compounds. *Annu Rev Pharmacol* 1972;12:375–406.
11. Magos L. Mercury-blood interaction and mercury uptake by the brain after vapor exposure. *Environ Res* 1967;1:323–337.
12. Magos L. Uptake of mercury by the brain. *Br J Ind Med* 1968;25:315–318.
13. Clarkson TW, Magos L, Greenwood MR. The transport of elemental mercury into fetal tissues. *Biol Neonate* 1972;21:239–244.
14. Lien DC, Todoruk DN, Rajani HR, Cook DA, Herbert FA. Accidental inhalation of mercury vapor: respiratory and toxicologic consequences. *Can Med Assoc J* 1983;129:591–595.
15. Campbell JS. Acute mercurial poisoning by inhalation of metallic vapor in an infant. *Can Med Assoc J* 1948;58:72–75.
16. Matthes FT, Kirschner R, Yow MD, Brennan JC. Acute poisoning associated with inhalation of mercury vapor: report of four cases. *Pediatrics* 1958; 22:675–688.
17. Teng CT, Breenan JC. Acute mercury vapor poisoning: a report of four cases with radiographic and pathologic correlation. *Radiology* 1959;73:354–361.
18. Hallee TJ. Diffuse lung disease caused by inhalation of mercury vapor. *Am Rev Respir Dis* 1969;99:430–436.
19. Jung RC, Aaronson J. Death following inhalation of mercury vapor at home. *West J Med* 1980;132:539–543.
20. Moutinho ME, Tompkins AL, Rowland TW, Banson BB, Jackson AH. Acute mercury vapor poisoning: fatality in an infant. *Am J Dis Child* 1981;135:42–44.
21. Jaffe KM, Shurtleff DB, Robertson WO. Survival after acute mercury vapor poisoning. *Am J Dis Child* 1983;137:749–751.
22. Wright N, Yeoman WB, Carter GF. Massive oral ingestion of elemental mercury without poisoning. *Lancet* 1980;1(8161):206.
23. Bredfeldt J, Moeller D. Systemic mercury intoxication following rupture of a Miller-Abbott tube. *Am J Gastroenterol* 1978;69:478–480.
24. Birnbaum W. Inflammation of the vermiform appendix by metallic mercury. *Am J Surg* 1947;74:494–496.
25. Crikelair GF, Hiratzka T. Intraperitoneal mercury granuloma. *Ann Surg* 1953;137:272–275.
26. Ernst E. Metallic mercury in the gastrointestinal tract. *Acta Chir Scand* 1985;151:651–652.
27. Conrad ME, Sanford JP, Preston JA. Metallic mercury embolization—clinical and experimental. *Arch Intern Med* 1957;100:59–65.
28. Hill DM. Self-administration of mercury by subcutaneous injection. *BMJ* 1976;1:342–343.
29. Rachman R. Soft tissue injury by mercury from a broken thermometer. *Am J Clin Pathol* 1974;61:296–300.
30. Krohn IT, Solof A, Mobini J, Wagner DK. Subcutaneous injection of metallic mercury. *JAMA* 1980;243:548–549.
31. Zillmer EA, Lucci KA, Barth JT, Peake TH, Spyker DA. Neurobehavioral sequelae of subcutaneous injection with metallic mercury. *J Toxicol Clin Toxicol* 1986;24:91–110.
32. Celli B, Kahn MA. Mercury embolism of the lung. *N Engl J Med* 1976;295: 883–885.
33. Ambre JJ, Welsh MJ, Svare CW. Intravenous elemental mercury injection: blood levels and excretion of mercury. *Ann Intern Med* 1977;7:451–453.
34. Chitkara R, Seriff NS, Kinas HY. Intravenous self-administration of metallic mercury in attempted suicide; report of a case with serial roentgenographic and physiologic studies over an 18-month period. *Chest* 1978;73:234–236.
35. Oliver RM, Thomas MR, Cornaby AJ, Neville E. Mercury pulmonary emboli following intravenous self-injection. *Br J Dis Chest* 1987;81:76–79.
36. Torres-Alanis O, Garza-Ocanas L, Pineyro-Lopez A. Intravenous self-administration of metallic mercury: report of a case with 5-year follow-up. *Clin Toxicol* 1997;35:83–87.
37. Netscher DT, Friedland JA, Guzewicz RM. Mercury poisoning from intravenous injection: treatment by granuloma excision. *Ann Plast Surg* 1991;26: 592–596.
38. Lilis R, Miller A, Lerman Y. Acute mercury poisoning with severe chronic pulmonary manifestations. *Chest* 1985;88:306–309.
39. Levin M, Jacobs J, Polos PG. Acute mercury poisoning and mercurial pneumonitis from gold ore purification. *Chest* 1988;94:554–556.
40. Dzau VJ, Szabos S, Chang YC. Aspiration of metallic mercury: a 22-year follow-up. *JAMA* 1977;238:1531–1532.
41. Adams CR, Ziegler DK, Lin JT. Mercury intoxication simulating amyotrophic lateral sclerosis. *JAMA* 1983;250:642–643.
42. Tsuji HK, Tyler GC, Redington JV, Kay JH. Intrabronchial metallic mercury. *Chest* 1970;57:322–328.
43. Wallach L. Aspiration of elemental mercury: evidence of absorption without toxicity. *N Engl J Med* 1972;287:178–179.
44. Janus C, Klein B. Aspiration of metallic mercury: clinical significance. *Br J Radiol* 1982;55:675–676.
45. Schulz E. Roentgenolgische studien nach aspiration von mettalischen quecksilber. *Fortschr Gev Rontgenstr Nuklearmed* 1958;89:24–30.
46. Zimmerman JE. Fatality following metallic mercury aspiration during removal of a long intestinal tube. *JAMA* 1969;208:2158–2160.
47. Agency for Toxic Substances and Disease Registry. Health effects. In: *Toxicological profile for mercury.* Atlanta: US Department of Health and Human Services, Public Health Service, ATSDR, April 1993.
48. Shapiro IM, Cornblath DR, Sumner AJ, et al. Neurophysiologic and neuropsychologic functions of mercury exposed dentists. *Lancet* 1982;1:1147–1150.
49. Bleach N, McLean LM. The accidental self-injection of mercury: a hazard for glass-blowers. *Arch Emerg Med* 1987;4:53–54.
50. Baruch AD, Hass A. Injury to the hand with metallic mercury. *J Hand Surg* 1984;9A:446–448.
51. Klaassen CD. Heavy metals and heavy metal antagonists. In: Gilman AG, Goodman LS, Rall TW, Murad F, eds. *The pharmacological basis of therapeutics*, 7th ed. New York: Macmillan, 1985:1605–1627.
52. Eagle M, Magnuson HJ. The systemic treatment of 227 cases of arsenic poisoning (encephalitis, dermatitis, blood dyscrasias, jaundice, fever) with 2,3-dimercaptopropanol (BAL). *J Clin Invest* 1946;25:420–441.
53. Tye M, Siegel JM. Prevention of reaction to BAL. *JAMA* 1947;134:1477.
54. Jaffe IA. The antivitamin B_6 effect of penicillamine: clinical and immunological implications. *Adv Biochem Psychopharmacol* 1972;4:217–226.
55. Berlin M, Ullrebg S. Increased uptake of mercury in mouse brain caused by 2,3-dimercaptopropanol. *Nature* 1963;197:84–85.
56. Berlin M, Lewander T. Increased brain uptake of mercury caused by 2,3-dimercaptopropanol (BAL) in mice given mercuric chloride. *Acta Pharmacol* 1965;22:1–7.
57. Canty AJ, Kishimoto R. British anti-Lewisite and organo mercury poisoning. *Nature* 1972;253:123–125.
58. Kosnett M, Dutra C, Osterloh J, et al. Nephrotoxicity from elemental mercury: protective effects of dimercaptosuccinic acid. *Vet Hum Toxicol* 1989;31:351.
59. Berlin M, Ullrebg S. Accumulation and retention of mercury in the mouse. *Arch Environ Health* 1963;6:589–601.
60. Sanchez-Sicilia L, Seto DS, Nakamoto S, Kolff WJ. Acute mercurial intoxication treated by hemodialysis. *Ann Intern Med* 1963;59:692–706.
61. Schreiner GE, Maher JF. Toxic nephropathy. *Am J Med* 1965;38:409–449.
62. Winek CL, Fochtman FW, Bricker JD, Wecht CH. Fatal mercuric chloride ingestion. *Clin Toxicol* 1981;18:261–266.
63. Leumann EP, Brandenberger H. Hemodialysis in a patient with acute mercuric intoxication: concentrations of mercury in blood, dialysate, urine, vomitus and feces. *Clin Toxicol* 1977;11:301–308.
64. Tubbs R. Membranous glomerulonephritis associated with mercuric chloride solutions: case report and review of the literature. *BMJ* 1982;77:409–413.
65. Datyner ME, Cox PA. Inorganic mercury poisoning. *Anesth Intensive Care* 1981;6:459–463.
66. Troen P, Kaufman SA, Katz KH. Mercuric bichloride poisoning. *N Engl J Med* 1951;244:459–463.
67. Fishman AP, Kroop IG, Leiter HE, et al. A management of anuria in acute mercurial intoxication. *N Y State J Med* 1948;48:2363–2396.
68. Williamson AM, Teo RK, Sanderson J. Occupational mercury exposure and its consequences for behaviour. *Int Arch Occup Environ Health* 1982;50:273–286.
69. Miller JM, Chaffin DB, Smith RG. Subclinical psychomotor and neuromuscular changes in workers exposed to inorganic mercury. *Am Ind Hyg Assoc J* 1975;36:725–733.
70. Rosenman KD, Valciukas JA, Glickman L, Meyers BR, Cinotti A. Sensitive indicators of inorganic mercury toxicity. *Arch Environ Health* 1986;41:208–215.
71. Sauder PH, Livardjani F, Jaeger A, et al. Acute mercury chloride intoxication. Effects of hemodialysis and plasma exchange on mercury kinetics. *J Toxicol Clin Toxicol* 1988;26:189–197.
72. Gilman A, Allen RP, Philips FS, et al. The treatment of acute systemic mercury poisoning in experimental animals with BAL, thosorbitol and BAL glucoside. *J Clin Invest* 1946;26:549–556.
73. Longcope WT, Luetscher JA Jr, Calkins E, et al. Clinical uses of 2,3-dimercaptopropanol (BAL). *J Clin Invest* 1946;25:557–567.
74. Doolan PD, Hess WC, Kyle LH. Acute renal insufficiency due to bichloride of mercury. *N Engl J Med* 1953;249:273–276.
75. Maher JF, Schreiner GE. The dialysis of mercury and mercury-BAL complex. *Clin Res* 1959;7:298–299.
76. Amin-Zaki L, Elhassani S, Majeed MA, Clarkson TW, Doherty RA, Greenwood M. Intra-uterine methylmercury poisoning in Iraq. *Pediatrics* 1974;54:587–595.
77. Gage JC. Distribution and excretion of methyl and phenyl mercury salts. *Br J Ind Med* 1964;21:197–202.
78. Aberg B, Ekman L, Falk R, Greitz U, Persson G, Snihs JO. Metabolism of methylmercury (^{203}Hg) compounds in man. *Arch Environ Health* 1969;19:478–484.
79. Suzuki T, Matsumoto N, Miyama T, et al. Placental transfer of mercuric chloride, phenylmercuric acetate and methylmercury acetate in mice. *Ind Health* 1967;5:149–155.
80. Norseth T, Clarkson TW. Studies on the biotransformation of ^{203}Hg-labeled methylmercury chloride in rats. *Arch Environ Health* 1970;21:717–727.

81. Miller VL, Klavano PA, Csonka E. Absorption, distribution and excretion of phenyl mercuric acetate. *Toxicol Appl Pharmacol* 1960;2:344–352.
82. Ekman L, Greitz V, Magi A, et al. Metabolism and retention of methyl-203-mercury nitrate in man. *Nord Med* 1968;79:450–456.
83. Norseth T, Clarkson TW. Intestinal transport of ^{203}Hg-labeled methylmercury chloride. *Arch Environ Health* 1971;22:568–577.
84. Slotkin TA, Bartolome J. Biochemical mechanisms of developmental neurotoxicity of methylmercury. *Neurotoxicology* 1987;8:65–84.
85. Hunter D, Bonford RR, Russell DS. Poisoning by methylmercury compounds. *Q J Med* 1940;9:193–213.
86. Harda H. Congenital Minamata disease: intrauterine methylmercury poisoning. *Teratology* 1978;18:285–288.
87. Gerstner BH, Huff JE. Selected case histories and epidemiology examples of human poisonings. *Clin Toxicol* 1977;11:131–150.
88. Clarkson TW, Small H, Norseth T. The effect of a thiol containing resin on the gastrointestinal absorption and fecal excretion of methylmercury compounds in experimental animals. *Fed Proc* 1971;30:543.
89. Bakir F, Damluji SF, Amin-Zaki L, et al. Methylmercury poisoning in Iraq: an interuniversity report. *Science* 1973;181:230–241.
90. Hay WJ, Rickards AG, McMenemey WH, Cumings JN. Organic mercurial encephalopathy. *J Neurol Neurosurg Psychiatry* 1963;26:199–202.
91. Aaseth J. Recent advance in the therapy of metal poisoning with chelating agents. *Hum Toxicol* 1983;2:257–272.
92. Magos L, Peristianis GC, Snowden RT. Postexposure preventive treatment of methylmercury intoxication in rats with dimercaptosuccinic acid. *Toxicol Appl Pharmacol* 1978;45:463–475.

CHAPTER 73
Lead

James P. Keogh and Leslie V. Boyer

CHEMICAL AND PHYSICAL PROPERTIES

Lead (atomic number, 82; atomic weight, 207.21) is a gray, soft, heavy metal widely distributed in the earth's crust. It exists in nature as a mixture of three isotopes—^{206}Pb, ^{207}Pb, and ^{208}Pb—and forms compounds with a valence state of +2 and +4 (Table 73-1). Lead melts at a temperature of 327°C and boils at 1,740°C. Because of its low melting point, it was one of the first metals smelted and used by ancient humans.

TABLE 73-1. Lead compounds

Lead compound	Chemical symbol	Molecular weight
Lead, metal	Pb	207.19
Lead acetate	$Pb(C_2H_3O_2)_2$	325.28
Lead arsenate	$Pb_3(AsO_4)_2$	899.4
Lead azide	$Pb(N_3)_2$	291.23
Lead carbonate (basic white lead)	$2PbCO_3Pb(OH)_2$	775.6
Lead chloride	$PbCl_2$	278.1
Lead chromate (chrome yellow)	$PbCrO_4$	323.18
Lead molybdate	$PbMoO_4$	367.13
Lead nitrate	$Pb(NO_3)_2$	331.2
Lead monoxide	PbO	223.19
Lead oxide (red)	Pb_3O_4	685.57
Lead sesquioxide	Pb_2O_3	462.38
Lead suboxide	Pb_2O	430.38
Lead peroxide	PbO_2	239.19
Lead oxychloride	$PbCl_2 \cdot 2PbO$ (mineral yellow)	519.29
Lead silicate	$PbSiO_3$	283.27
Lead sulfate	$PbSO_4PbO$	526.44
Lead sulfide	PbS	239.25
Lead stearate	$Pb(C_{18}H_{35}O_2)_2$	774.15
Tetraethyl lead	$Pb(C_2H_5)_4$	323.44
Tetramethyl lead	$Pb(CH_3)_4$	267.33

Lead is exploited commercially from a variety of ores, the most abundant of which is galena. When used as a metal, most commonly it is alloyed with tin, antimony, or arsenic. It forms a variety of inorganic compounds, many of which are brightly colored. Tetraethyl lead and tetramethyl lead are the only two organic compounds in common use (1).

SITES, INDUSTRIES, AND BUSINESSES ASSOCIATED WITH EXPOSURE

World production of lead totals approximately 9 million metric tons annually. In the United States, approximately 11 million metric tons of lead are consumed, approximately 5 million metric tons of which are produced from mining and approximately 6 million metric tons of which are recovered from scrap (principally from recycled batteries) (1). Sites, processes, and industries associated with lead exposures are presented in Table 73-2.

Lead is extracted from the ore first by a mechanical separation process involving flotation. The enriched ore then is smelted. After primary smelting, the lead bullion still contains significant amounts of other metals and undergoes a further step of refining.

Secondary lead smelters reclaim scrap lead. Storage batteries and lead-sheltered cable are the products recycled most commonly. Because the average lead storage battery has a useful life of only approximately 2 years and 80% of the lead in batteries is recycled, this process of secondary smelting provides one-third of the lead for new products each year. Approximately one-half of all lead produced is used to produce lead storage batteries, such that lead forms the metal grids, and lead oxide is used as a paste within the battery. Sheet lead is used to line chemical reaction vessels, for waterproofing and soundproofing, and for radiation shielding. Lead alloys are used as solders and to sheathe power and telephone cables from moisture.

Compounds of lead are used extensively for paints and coatings. The use of lead additives in residential paint was banned in the United States in 1977 because of the danger of childhood lead poisoning. Lead-containing pigments still are used for outdoor paint products because of their bright colors and weather-resistant properties. "Red lead" (Pb_3O_4) is used extensively as a

TABLE 73-2. Sites and industries associated with lead exposure

Lead smelting
Battery manufacturing
Welding and cutting operations
Construction and demolition
Rubber manufacturing
Plastics manufacturing
Printing
Firing ranges
Radiator repair
Soldering of lead products
Production of gasoline additives
Zinc smelting
Solid waste combustion
Organic lead production
Copper smelting
Ore crushing and grinding
Frit manufacturing
Paint and pigment manufacturing

TABLE 73-3. Reported cases of adult lead poisoning by industry

Industry (SIC code)	No. of cases (%)	No. of cases with blood Pb >70 µg/dL (%)
Electric and electronic equipment (36)	462 (35)	15 (21)
Primary metal industries (33)	433 (33)	15 (21)
Chemical products (28)	87 (7)	0 (0)
Stone clay and glass (32)	83 (6)	2 (2)
Auto repairs (75)	47 (4)	4 (5)
Special trade contractors (17)	39 (3)	11 (15)
Heavy construction (16)	23 (2)	13 (18)
All others	153 (10)	11 (18)
Total	1,327	71

SIC, Standard Industrial Code.
Note: Data were available from only those four states (New York, New Jersey, California, Texas) that required reporting of elevated lead levels by laboratories in 1987. Adapted from *MMWR Morb Mortal Wkly Rep* 1989;38:644.

rustproofer and primer for structural steel. Lead azide is used in primers and explosives (2). Tetraethyl lead and, to some extent, tetramethyl lead are used as antiknock additives in gasoline. The popularity of leaded gasoline has greatly declined in the United States, but it still is being used in other countries.

The great diversity of lead-containing processes and products results in many ways in which workers can be exposed (Table 73-3). Processes of burning, blasting, grinding, or sanding applied to lead-painted or -coated surfaces are the most common causes of uncontrolled exposures.

ENVIRONMENTAL AND OCCUPATIONAL LEAD EXPOSURE

Exposure of the general population to lead occurs from lead in air, water, food, and soil. Air lead concentrations range from 7.6×10^{-5} µg per cubic meter in very remote areas to more than 10 µg per cubic meter near direct emission sources, such as a smelter (3). Urban air sampling has revealed an average maximum concentration of 0.36 µg per cubic meter from 147 sites in 1984 (3). With the introduction and use of non-lead-containing gasoline, the atmospheric content of lead in the United States has declined since 1983 (3).

The lead content of surface water in the United States varies between 5 and 30 µg per L (3), with the higher concentrations in urban areas. Sources of lead at the tap include the lead solder in pipe joints or lead pipes within homes, the contributions of which may be increased by the effects of low-pH water on the joints or pipe involved (3). The U.S. Environmental Protection Agency (EPA) proposed a limit in drinking water of 5 µg lead per L. It is estimated that 20% of the American population consumes drinking water with lead concentrations exceeding 20 µg per L (4). Lead occurs in such foods as dairy products, meat, fish, poultry, grains, and cereals (3). The baseline intake of lead on a daily basis via consumption of food and water varies between 5 and 15 µg per day across all age groups (3). There is significantly higher soil and dust intake in children. The concentration of lead in soil results from both the natural occurrence of lead in crystal layers and human activities that produce lead. In urban areas, lead levels may be as high as 2,000 to 10,000 µg per g (ppm) of soil near roads (3). Naturally occurring concentrations of lead in soil range from fewer than 10 µg to up to 30 µg per g (3). Near smelters, the lead level in soil may be as high as 60,000 µg per g (3).

Household Sources and Consumer Products Associated with Exposure

Household sources of lead include paint, soil, dust, food, water, cosmetics, art materials, toys, and hobbies (5). Despite the cessation of use of leaded paint by 1977, household paint and dust remain the most significant sources of childhood lead exposure in the United States because of the large number of homes that were built during the lead-paint era and remain in use. Many years of peeling and chipping household paint may result in accumulations of lead in house dust and soil, causing an ongoing hazard even after overpainting or abatement have reduced the availability of wall paint itself. In the United States, approximately 83% of private housing units and 86% of public housing units built before 1980 contain at least some lead paint (6). A home environmental score based on visual rating of surfaces (from intact to peeling) and x-ray fluorescence for lead content may be related quantitatively to blood lead levels in children living in lead-contaminated homes (7).

Precipitated lead from air pollution also contributes to lead in dust and soil. Increased soil lead levels in communities in which lead mining and smelting occur have been associated with elevated blood lead levels, particularly in small children (8). Reduction in the use of leaded gasoline by 99.8% in the United States between 1976 and 1990 has reduced the largest source of general community exposure both in ambient air and in dust in and around homes (9).

Parental occupation also may contribute to childhood lead dust exposure (e.g., lead miners, who bring lead dust home on skin and clothes) (8). An increased prevalence of lead poisoning has been associated with poverty and with black and Hispanic demographics (10,11). This greater prevalence may be due to greater dust and soil lead burden as well as lead paint residues in older or dilapidated housing.

Contamination of community and domestic water systems by the use of lead piping or lead solder in pipes remains a problem in some areas. The number of food and soft-drink cans sealed with lead solder declined from 47.0% in 1980 to 0.9% in 1990 (9). With the reduction of lead in air and the elimination of lead solder from food and beverage cans, lead contamination of food greatly decreased during the 1980s in the United States (12).

Steady declines in lead emissions, combined with the discontinuation of use of lead in household paint, have resulted in declining average lead levels among American children over the past several decades. Phase 1 of the Third National Health and Nutrition Examination Survey indicated that among U.S. children from ages 1 through 5, the prevalence of lead levels exceeding 25 µg per dL dropped from 9.3% in the 1970s to 0.5% in the 1980s. The prevalence of blood lead levels higher than 10 µg per dL during the same years dropped from 88.2% to 8.9% (9), with a further drop in the 1990s to 4.4% (10).

Absorption, Metabolism, and Excretion

As a fume or fine particulate, lead is absorbed readily through the lungs. It is not absorbed as well from the gastrointestinal (GI) tract in adults (20% to 30%), but children absorb as much as 50% of dietary lead. Inorganic lead is not absorbed through intact skin, but organic lead compounds (tetraethyl lead, tetramethyl lead) can be. Absorption from the lungs depends on the size of the particulate. Particles in the 0.5- to 5.0-µm range are most likely to be deposited in the alveoli, where they can be absorbed. Larger particles that are entrapped in the larger airways are likely to be swallowed and may lead to GI absorption.

Absorption of ingested lead is influenced by its form, particle size, and iron and calcium absorption (13). After absorption into the blood stream, almost all lead is carried bound to the red cell. Lead is distributed extensively throughout tissues, with highest concentrations in bone, teeth, liver, lung, kidney, brain, and spleen (2). With prolonged exposure over time, most absorbed lead ends up in bone. Lead appears to be substituted for calcium in the bone matrix and is not known to cause any deleterious effect on bone itself. Bone storage may act as a "sink," protecting other organs, but bone is also a long-term storage depot, allowing the chronic accumulation of lead in the body and can provide a source for remobilization of lead and continued toxicity after exposure has ceased.

Lead crosses the blood–brain barrier and concentrates in the gray matter of the brain. Lead also readily crosses the placenta. Because pregnancy is a period during which maternal calcium stores are mobilized, a significant amount of lead may be transferred simultaneously to the developing fetus (14).

In adults, lead is excreted by the kidney at a rate of approximately 30 μg per day (15). With increasing body stores, this amount may rise considerably but rarely is more than 200 μg per day (16,17). Excretion may be due both to glomerular filtration and (in part) to shedding of tubular epithelial cells, in which the lead tends to concentrate (18).

The extent of fecal excretion in humans is uncertain. Early lead balance studies by Kehoe (15) indicated that fecal lead nearly matched daily oral intake of lead. The extent to which this fecal lead content represents merely unabsorbed lead rather than true excretion is not clear. In rats, bile has been shown to be a major route of excretion after intravenous administration of lead. The importance of this route in humans is unclear (19).

The kinetics of the uptake, distribution, and equilibration of lead in blood, bone, and soft tissue are complex (20). Models invoking three compartments that correspond more or less anatomically to blood, soft tissue, and bone storage are useful but not always satisfactory in predicting changes in tissue levels under all conditions. With initial exposure to a high dose, the blood lead level may rise and fall relatively quickly, but some of the decline in blood lead may be due to redistribution rather than excretion. Once a significant burden has been stored in bone, absorbed lead has a remarkably long half-life, as long as 10 years in some studies (21). In such a situation, blood lead levels (and, presumably, tissue lead levels as well) may remain elevated for decades after an exposure has ceased. Although chelating agents increase urinary excretion, they also may alter the exchange between body compartments (e.g., across the blood–brain barrier) (22). The clinical signs and symptoms of lead toxicity are summarized in Tables 73-4 and 73-5.

TABLE 73-4. General signs and symptoms of lead toxicity

Mild and moderate signs and symptoms
- Fatigue
- Irritability
- Lethargy
- Paresthesias
- Myalgias
- Abdominal pain
- Tremor
- Headache
- Vomiting
- Weight loss
- Constipation
- Loss of libido

Severe signs and symptoms
- Motor neuropathy
- Encephalopathy
- Seizures
- Coma
- Severe abdominal cramping
- Epiphyseal lead lines in children
- Renal failure

TABLE 73-5. Spontaneous and elicited symptoms of lead poisoning in adults

Symptom	No. of patients with this complaint: No. spontaneously described (%)	No. examiner-elicited (%)	Total (%)
Headache	25 (53)	2 (4)	27 (57)
Irritability	15 (32)	13 (28)	28 (60)
Memory loss	4 (9)	14 (29)	18 (60)
Decreased memory span	2 (4)	9 (19)	11 (23)
Lassitude	22 (47)	2 (4)	24 (51)
Insomnia	8 (17)	5 (11)	13 (28)
Decreased libido	6 (13)	12 (25)	18 (38)
Anorexia	7 (15)	5 (11)	12 (26)
Nausea	8 (17)	3 (6)	11 (23)
Abdominal pain	9 (19)	3 (7)	12 (26)
Constipation	2 (4)	7 (15)	9 (19)
Arthralgias	14 (30)	8 (17)	22 (47)
Myalgias	10 (21)	4 (9)	14 (30)
Paresthesias	9 (19)	4 (9)	13 (28)
Motor weakness	5 (11)	2 (4)	7 (15)

Note: Symptoms from a series of 47 men presenting with elevated lead levels to the University of Maryland Occupational Health Project.
Adapted from ref. 12.

CLINICAL TOXICOLOGY

Acute Toxicity

Under conditions of extremely high respiratory exposure to lead, an acute encephalopathy can develop, accompanied by renal failure and severe GI symptoms (23). In most cases, however, lead is absorbed more slowly over weeks to months, and the clinical course is subacute or chronic.

Chronic and Long-Term Toxicity

Absorbed lead is toxic to a variety of enzyme systems. Lead has affinity for sulfhydryl groups and is toxic to zinc-dependent enzyme systems. Two enzymes in heme synthesis are affected (i.e., inhibited) by lead: δ-aminolevulinic acid dehydrase (ALA-D), a cytoplasmic enzyme, and ferrochelatase, a mitochondrial enzyme (4). Interference with ALA-D is dose-related and occurs at blood lead concentrations between 10 and 20 μg per dL. Interference with ALA-D is complete at blood lead concentrations of 70 and 90 μg per dL (4). Ferrochelatase catalyzes the transfer of iron from ferritin into protoporphyrin and forms heme (4). Ferrochelatase inhibition by lead results in an increase in coproporphyrin excretion in urine and an increase of protoporphyrin in red blood cells (4). Erythrocyte protoporphyrin concentrations in adults will be elevated at blood lead concentrations of 25 to 30 μg per dL (4). Heme synthesis is essential not only to hemoglobin but to synthesis of cytochromes needed for all oxidative metabolism throughout the organism.

Lead also interferes with enzymes important in maintaining the integrity of membranes and affecting steroid metabolism (24). Concentrations of neurotransmitters have been shown to be affected in a number of studies (25). Vitamin D synthesis in renal tubular cells is affected by lead, owing to an interference with a heme-containing

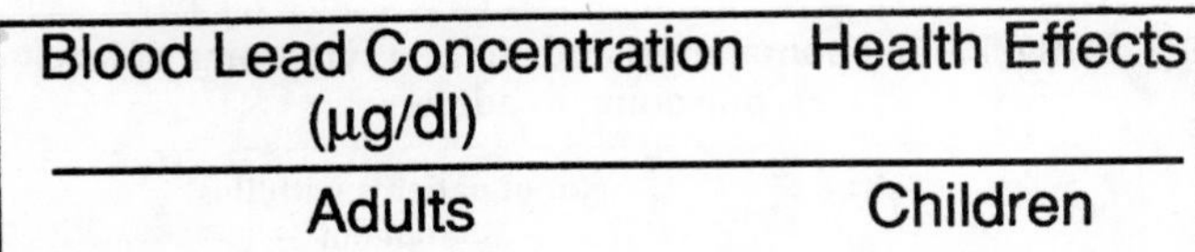

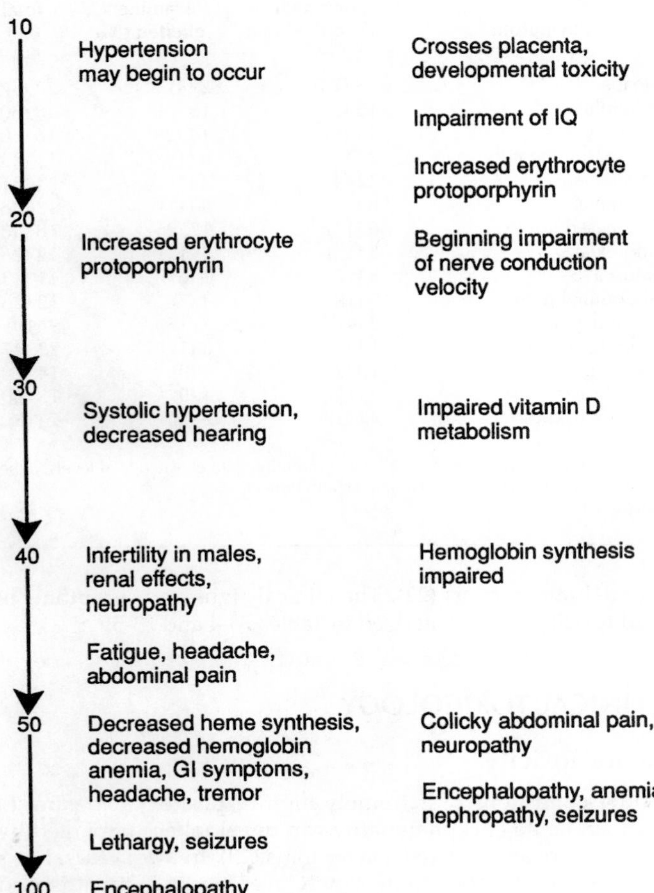

Figure 73-1. Range of lead-induced health effects in adults and children.

hydroxylase enzyme that converts 25-hydroxyvitamin D to 1,25-hydroxyvitamin D (26). The health effects of lead can range from subclinical to overt disease (Fig. 73-1; Tables 73-6, 73-7).

CENTRAL NERVOUS SYSTEM

Effects in Adults. Central nervous system (CNS) effects can develop after a brief intense exposure or more gradually with lower levels of exposure. Acute encephalopathy, characterized by diffuse pathologic changes and cerebral edema, usually is associated with high blood lead levels (more than 150 µg per dL). A subacute or chronic encephalopathy affecting both cognitive function and mood is seen more commonly than the acute form. Headaches and lassitude are common early symptoms of lead intoxication. Sleep disturbance, often with early morning awakening, irritability, and loss of libido, also are elicited frequently by recording of a thorough history. Because of the nonspecific nature of these early CNS symptoms, patients frequently do not seek medical attention and, when they do, often are not given correct diagnoses. Cessation of exposure and chelation therapy often have a favorable effect on these symptoms; however, in severe cases, some level of symptoms may persist.

CNS effects are not confined to those patients who become symptomatic. Studies of lead-exposed workers have shown abnormalities on psychometric testing results, including cognitive difficulty and visuomotor problems (27–32). Baker et al. (33,34) demonstrated that exposed brass foundry workers whose blood lead levels were in the range of 40 to 60 µg per dL had impaired neurobehavioral function. The prevalence of abnormalities was correlated to an index of lead exposure integrated over time. A striking reduction in lead exposure and blood lead levels in the workforce was accompanied by a corresponding improvement in function among those in the exposed group but not the controls (33,34). In Sweden, Mantere et al. (32) showed that psychometric and nerve condition abnormalities developed in workers newly exposed to lead as blood lead levels rose above 30 µg per dL.

Early after the introduction of tetraethyl lead as a gasoline additive, numerous cases of severe encephalopathy developed among workers at tetraethyl lead production facilities. Both the rapidity and severity of these intoxications probably were related to dose absorbed, as organic lead can be absorbed readily through the skin and can pass easily across the blood–brain barrier (26,35).

Effects in Children. Over the past several decades, epidemiologic studies have demonstrated that chronic, low-level lead poisoning may lead to CNS injury among children younger than 5 years. Needleman et al. (36) evaluated a range of psychological tests in a cohort of children, comparing the lead content of deciduous teeth with school performance. Children with higher levels of lead absorption showed a marked deficit in school performance as compared to that in controls. An 11-year follow-up study showed deficits in CNS functioning and a pattern of social failure that persisted into young adulthood in the children with higher lead exposures (37). Relatively low chronic blood lead levels have been associated also with poor gross and fine motor development (38). In 1997, 890,000 U.S. children were estimated to have blood lead levels at or exceeding 10 µg per dL (39), the level above which subtle CNS effects are suspected to occur. Data from the Centers for Disease Control and Prevention's (CDC's) Childhood Blood Level Surveillance program showed that the proportion of children tested with blood lead levels greater than 10 µg per dL decreased from 10.5% in 1996 to 7.6% in 1998. The proportions of children with blood lead levels greater than 15 µg per dL and 20 µg per dL also decreased (41a).

Few studies have examined the long-term effects of childhood lead poisoning. A study by White et al. (41) among 34 Boston subjects and 20 matched controls 50 years after diagnosis of symptomatic lead poisoning suggested that a permanent pattern of cognitive dysfunction may result from lead poisoning in the first several years of life. The study authors suggested that cognitive deficits among previously lead-poisoned adults may explain lower occupational achievement in this group. Ongoing release of skeletal stores of lead may contribute also to CNS injury later in life, when mobilization of these stores occurs during pregnancy, lactation, or osteoporosis. Acute lead poisoning may produce encephalopathy both in children and in adults. Ataxia, altered state of consciousness, and seizures have been reported in children with blood lead levels higher than 100 µg per dL, although predicting which children with such levels will develop these side effects is impossible (42).

PERIPHERAL NERVOUS SYSTEM

Lead causes a peripheral neuropathy that affects primarily the motor nerves and appears to be mainly axonal (25). Clinically, the neuropathy is more severe in the upper rather than the lower extremity and may cause more severe effects on the dominant side. Although the classic wristdrop of so-called painter's palsy has become rare, subclinical neuropathy has been demonstrated

TABLE 73-6. Summary of lowest observed effect levels for key lead-induced health effects in adults

Lowest observed effect level [blood lead (μg/dL)]	Heme synthesis and hematologic effects	Neurologic effects	Renal effects	Reproductive effects	Cardiovascular effects
100–120	—	Encephalopathic signs and symptoms	—	—	—
80	Anemia	Encephalopathy symptoms	Chronic nephropathy	—	—
60	—	—	—	Reproductive effects in women	—
50	Reduced hemoglobin production	Overt subencephalopathic neurologic symptoms	—	—	—
40	Increased urinary ALA and elevated coproporphyrins	Peripheral nerve dysfunction (slowed nerve conduction)	—	—	—
30	—	—	—	Altered testicular function	Elevated blood pressure (white men, aged 40–59)
25–30	Erythrocyte protoporphyrin elevation in men	—	—	—	—
15–20	Erythrocyte protoporphyrin in women	—	—	—	—
<10	ALA-D inhibition	—	—	—	—

ALA, aminolevulinic acid; ALA-D, aminolevulinic acid dehydrase.
From ref. 3, with permisison.

in a number of populations of exposed workers, with effects beginning at levels of blood lead well within what had been regarded in the past as acceptable for industrial workers (32). Lead targets motor axons and produces axonal degeneration and segmental demyelination (14). Studies have demonstrated slowed conduction in small motor fibers of the ulnar nerve to be a sensitive marker of subclinical lead neurotoxicity (26,43,44). Decreases in ulnar nerve motor conduction velocity are seen at blood lead concentrations of 30 to 40 μg per dL. In addition to this form of polyneuropathy, lead absorption predisposes individuals to nerve entrapment, such as carpal tunnel and tarsal tunnel syndromes (30,31).

HEMATOPOIETIC SYSTEM

Anemia in lead poisoning results both from impairment of hemoglobin production and from changes in red cell membranes. Hemoglobin levels may remain in a normal range despite moderately severe intoxication, because enzyme induction may compensate for the effects of lead. The effect of the intoxication may become apparent only when stress is placed on the erythrocyte (e.g., after blood donation) (45). A noticeable rise in hemoglobin concentration is common when lead intoxication resolves. With more severe intoxication, a normochromic, normocytic anemia develops, characterized by the presence of basophilic stippling of erythrocytes on a blood smear. Severe

TABLE 73-7. Summary of lowest observed effect levels for key lead-induced health effects in children

Lowest observed effect level [blood lead (μg/dL)]	Heme synthesis and hematologic effects	Neurologic effects	Renal effects	Gastrointestinal effects
80–100	—	Encephalopathic signs and symptoms	Chronic nephropathy (aminoaciduria, etc.)	Colic and other overt symptoms
70	Anemia	—	—	—
60	—	Peripheral neuropathies	—	—
50	—	—	—	—
40	Reduced hemoglobin synthesis	Peripheral nerve dysfunction (slowed NCVs)	—	—
	Elevated coproporphyrin	CNS cognitive effects	—	—
	Increased urinary ALA	—	—	—
30	Erythrocyte protoporphyrin elevation	Altered CNS electrophysiologic responses, effect on IQ	Vitamin D metabolism interference	—
15	ALA-D inhibition	MDI deficits, reduced gestational age and birth weight (prenatal exposure)	—	—
	Py-5-N activity inhibition	—	—	—
10	—	—	—	—

ALA, aminolevulinic acid; ALA-D, aminolevulinic acid dehydrase; CNS, central nervous system; IQ, intelligence quotient; MDI, mental development index; NCVs, nerve conduction velocities; Py-5-N, pyrimidine-5'-nucleotidase.
From ref. 3, with permission.

anemia often is a result of the superimposition of a hemolytic process caused, presumably, by membrane changes (24).

GASTROINTESTINAL TRACT

Although GI symptoms are fairly prominent in the clinical presentation of lead toxicity, little is known about the mechanism by which pain and colic are produced. They are presumed to be related to effects on the autonomic ganglia of the GI tract. Transaminase elevations are reported occasionally in lead intoxication but, despite the relatively high concentration of lead in the liver, seemingly little evidence of impaired function exists (24).

RENAL SYSTEM

For centuries, lead exposure has been associated with the development of hypertension, renal failure, and gout (46). Studies of "moonshine" drinkers in Alabama have shown that gout, hypertension, and renal failure are common outcomes of lead intoxication by this route (47). Renal effects of lead have been studied extensively in humans and in experimental animals. Lead accumulates in the proximal tubular cells, a process that explains the marked effect on urate excretion. In addition, Fanconi's syndrome (proteinuria, aminoaciduria, and phosphaturia) has been described as the result of lead accumulation. Inclusion bodies have been demonstrated in renal tubular cells on biopsy. These inclusions are thought by some to represent binding of lead by a renal binding protein that may mitigate the effects of lead on the cell's function (48). As toxicity progresses, a chronic interstitial nephritis may develop, in some cases progressing to end-stage renal failure.

A study by Wedeen (44) has shown increased body burdens of lead in a population of veterans with hypertension and renal failure. This finding has raised the possibility that some cases of unexplained renal failure may be caused by previously unrecognized lead poisoning. However, this finding was not duplicated in a study of members of a health maintenance organization in California (49,50). Lead interferes with the renin-aldosterone system (24), and this interference may play a role in the development of hypertension that is seen as a sequela of lead poisoning.

Few studies have examined the renal effects of lead in children. A study among Romanian children who were aged 3 to 6 years and had average blood lead levels of 34 µg per dL showed a statistically significant relationship between blood lead concentration and *N*-acetyl-β-D-glucosaminidase (NAG) activity in urine (57).

CARDIOVASCULAR SYSTEM

Large-scale mortality studies of individuals in the lead-smelting and battery industries have strongly supported the link between lead and hypertension. In an American population who worked between 1946 and 1970, most workers had mean blood levels in the range of 40 to 70 µg per dL. An increase occurred in deaths from renal disease and from hypertensive cardiovascular disease (52). Mortality studies in the United Kingdom and Australia show a similar pattern (53,54). Not all studies of occupational groups have shown an association between blood pressure and lead absorption (55). Little is known about the natural history of the development of hypertension in lead poisoning, its pathophysiology and relation to renal effects, and the effects of intervention.

PULMONARY SYSTEM

Although a recent report has identified pneumoconiosis in lead miners, no reports have cited pulmonary dysfunction among other intoxicated populations. The changes seen in miners may be due to exposure to silica in the ore (56).

ENDOCRINE SYSTEM

Lead has been shown to cause decreased serum thyroxine levels, effects on adrenal hormones, and changes in vitamin D levels. However, the mechanisms and clinical significance of such effects have not been elucidated (24).

REPRODUCTIVE SYSTEM

Women. Occupational exposure to lead, both maternal and paternal, has been associated with decreased fertility, spontaneous abortion, stillbirth, and increased infant mortality (57). Only a few modern epidemiologic studies have addressed lead's effects on reproductive outcome in women. These studies suggest that the increase in spontaneous abortions seen among populations who work in lead-related industries may not be seen at the lower doses of lead encountered in community exposure (58).

Lead readily crosses the placenta and accumulates in the fetus (15). Bellinger et al. (59) correlated the results of developmental assessments in 249 two-year-old children with cord blood lead levels taken at birth. These levels had an inverse relationship with developmental scores, and this effect was seen at levels as low as the 10- to 20-µg-per-dL range.

Men. Studying lead exposure effects on the male reproductive system has been somewhat easier than studying similar effects in women. Lancranjan et al. (60) demonstrated decreased sperm counts and increased numbers of abnormal sperm in battery-plant workers. Some evidence of an effect was seen even among the plant's office workers, who had blood lead levels that averaged 23 µg per dL. Workers also reported a marked increase in sexual dysfunction. A study among Italian battery-plant workers showed similar findings and supported a direct toxic effect on spermatogenesis rather than an effect mediated by endocrine changes (61).

Management of Toxicity in Children

SCREENING

Although lead-poisoned children may present for evaluation of failure to thrive, frequent vomiting, anemia, or encephalopathy, physicians in practice today far more commonly will encounter infants and toddlers who appear completely asymptomatic despite blood lead levels in the 1- to 25-µg-per-dL range. For this reason, the CDC in 1997 recommended screening of all children at risk for lead poisoning, using the whole-blood lead level as the diagnostic standard (62). Blood lead levels, rather than erythrocyte protoporphyrin, now are accepted as the primary screening test, because the latter is not sufficiently sensitive to detect blood lead levels lower than 25 µg per dL, the previously accepted standard (63).

With the national decline in average blood lead level, the goal of universal blood lead screening among young children is likely to be replaced by targeted screening. High-risk groups that may be targeted include black, low-income, urban, and Hispanic children (64); those with pervasive developmental disorders (65); and those living in geographic regions associated with older housing (66).

The use of standardized screening questionnaires for identification of children at risk for lead poisoning has been proposed but is hindered by the low sensitivity and negative predictive value of most screening questions. Community-specific questionnaires may be of some value, but these must be tested locally before they are used in place of universal blood lead screening (67).

TABLE 73-8. Classification of childhood lead poisoning and suggested treatment

Class	Blood lead (µg/dL)	Suggested interpretation and action
I	≤9	Normal; rescreen as indicated
IIA	10–14	Educate parents, rescreen in 3 mo, report to health department for community statistics
IIB	15–19	Educate parents, test for and correct iron deficiency, rescreen in 3 mo; if level persists, proceed as for class III
III	20–44	Retest within 1 mo, complete medical evaluation, consider chelation therapy
IV	45–69	Retest within 48 h, complete medical evaluation, begin environmental assessment and medical treatment, including chelation, within 48 h
V	≥70	Medical emergency: retest immediately; hospitalize and begin treatment immediately, identify and remove source of lead

From ref. 63, with permission.

MEDICAL EVALUATION

Young children presenting with possible lead poisoning should be assessed for recognizable sequelae and correlates of exposure. These include a history of such behavioral factors as pica (which increases hand-mouth exposure) and home environmental factors that suggest the availability of lead. Sequelae of poisoning may include lethargy, vomiting, irritability, developmental delay, and failure to thrive, but what must be borne in mind is that most children with low-level poisoning will have no overtly apparent signs or symptoms.

The whole-blood lead level test now is considered the standard for diagnosis of childhood lead poisoning. A classification system based on blood level has been established by the CDC (Table 73-8) (62). Once an elevated blood lead level has been recognized, the extent of the workup depends on an affected child's particular environmental and medical conditions. In most cases, a complete blood count and serum iron determination are indicated. Abdominal radiography may reveal recently ingested paint chips as radiodensities. Long-bone films may show growth arrest lines in children with chronic exposure.

TREATMENT

Treatment of lead poisoning may involve source abatement, behavior modification programs, dietary manipulations, and chelation. CDC treatment guidelines, based on lead poisoning classification (62), are outlined in Table 73-8.

Abatement. Separation of poisoned children from the source of ongoing exposure is the first priority in treatment. Although in many cases simple cleanup measures are effective, in severe cases abatement may involve prolonged hospitalization and the evaluation and removal of siblings to alternative living arrangements. In some cities, health authorities have developed "safe houses" in which families can live until hazards are abated. Because removing lead-containing paint in a poorly controlled fashion often can leave an affected home more contaminated with lead dust than prior to the removal, strict supervision of lead abatement is critical. Guidelines have been developed by the federal department of Housing and Urban Development (68) and should be applied if lead in residential paint exceeds 1.0 µg per square centimeter [5,000 parts per million (ppm)] when found on friction-impact surfaces, on protruding surfaces within 3 feet of floor or ground, or in deteriorated condition on any surface (69). Abatement and interim control methods should be instituted also where soil levels exceed 400 ppm and where indoor dust levels exceed 100 µg per square foot (on floors), 500 µg per square foot (on interior window sills), 800 µg per square foot (in window troughs), and 800 µg per square foot (exterior surface) (69).

A retrospective study of St. Louis children with blood lead levels greater than 25 µg per dL showed a greater decline in mean blood lead levels among children whose homes underwent abatement procedures than among those whose homes did not. This effect was more pronounced among children with higher blood lead levels (greater than 35 µg per dL) than lower (25 to 34 µg per dL) (70). A modest decline in blood lead level occurs after abatement of outdoor soil by greater than 1,000 ppm (71), but children who live in homes with elevated floor-dust lead levels do not appear to benefit from soil abatement alone (72). Children living in homes that underwent abatement prior to the 1991 change in CDC blood lead guidelines remain at risk of low-level lead poisoning under the new definition, suggesting that improvement in home lead abatement technology may be necessary (73).

Effective September 6, 1997, federal law mandates the disclosure of lead-related information on sale of all pre-1978 housing in the United States. Under Title X, Section 1018, a home purchaser must receive a lead information pamphlet, the seller must disclose all known lead hazards, purchasers are allowed a 10-day period for lead inspection, and all sales contracts must contain a lead warning statement (74).

Dietary Interventions. For children with blood lead levels in the 10- to 25-µg-per-dL range, specific environmental sources may not be identified readily. To reduce the bioavailability of trace ingested lead in such cases, several dietary manipulations have been suggested. These include consumption of regular meals, correction of iron deficiency, and increased consumption of calcium and phosphorus. Frequent food consumption over the course of the day (regular meals plus snacks) may inhibit the absorption of lead because of lead chelators and precipitators naturally present in food; in addition, increased caloric intake may help children with failure to thrive. Lead poisoning and iron deficiency frequently coexist, and animal studies suggest that iron may be a competitive inhibitor of GI lead absorption (75). Higher dietary iron intake has been associated with lower blood lead levels among urban preschool children (76). Dietary calcium appears to inhibit the GI absorption of luminal lead by binding to and displacing it from common mucosal carriers, and phosphorus binds lead in the small intestine to form an insoluble complex (75).

Chelation. Since the release of the CDC's 1991 guidelines for the management of lead poisoning in young children (62), the use of oral and parenteral agents for the chelation of lead has been reconsidered. In 1995, the Committee on Drugs of the American Academy of Pediatrics reviewed the evidence for the use of chelators and recommended that they not be prescribed for children with blood lead levels of less than 25 µg per dL. Those children with levels between 25 and 45 µg per dL should not receive chelation therapy routinely but may benefit from use of oral chelators in cases in which elevated lead levels persist despite environmental intervention. Children with lead levels between 45 and 70 µg per dL should undergo chelation, usually with oral succimer, and those with encephalopathy or with levels in excess of 70 µg per dL should be admitted to the hospital for parenteral therapy with $CaNa_2$–ethylenediaminetetraacetic acid ($CaNa_2$-EDTA) and dimercaprol [2,3-dimercapto-1-propanol (British anti-Lewisite, or BAL)] (77).

Succimer (Chemet), or 2,3-dimercaptosuccinic acid (DMSA), appears to be effective in the short-term reduction of moderately elevated blood lead levels (78,79). It was approved by the U.S. Food and Drug Administration as an orally effective chelating agent for lead poisoning in children for blood lead concentrations in excess of 45 μg per dL. It was not approved for use in children with blood lead levels of less than 45 μg per dL, but this decision was made principally to prevent the misuse of chelation in children for whom environmental investigation and remediation have not occurred (80).

Succimer is available in 100-mg doses. The recommended dose for children is 10 mg per kg orally, three times daily (30 mg per kg per day) for 5 days, then twice daily (20 mg per kg per day) for the next 14 days. After this 19-day course, a 2-week rest is recommended before resumption of treatment, unless blood lead concentrations remain unacceptably high.

Reports of succimer toxicity have been rare and include a decrease in plasma zinc concentrations and a transient elevation in serum glutamic-pyruvic transaminase. The major adverse effect is gastrointestinal and includes nausea and vomiting. Rashes have been reported in 4% of patients. The strong sulfur odor of any of the thiol chelators renders the medication unpalatable to many patients. The course may be repeated if needed, with an appropriate drug-free interval of 2 weeks.

For severely ill children requiring hospitalization, the management of pediatric lead poisoning has been described in detail by Chisolm (81) and Chisolm and Barltrop (82) and by Piomelli et al. (83). With blood lead levels higher than 70 μg per dL or signs of encephalopathy, therapy involves a combination of agents, beginning with BAL, 45 mg per kg intramuscularly every 4 hours. Adequate urinary output should be established by hydration, after which $CaNa_2$-EDTA, 1,500 mg per square meter per 24 hours, should be added to the treatment by continuous infusion in normal saline or dextrose and water. $CaNa_2$-EDTA may be administered intramuscularly also in divided doses every 4 hours. This combined therapy is continued for 5 days. Liver and renal functions should be monitored during this combined therapy. A second course of therapy may be required if the blood lead concentration rebounds. Rebound can best be assessed 2 days after combined therapy. In up to 50% of patients treated, BAL produces toxic or adverse side effects, such as rash, fever, and hypertension. Other adverse effects include nausea, vomiting, and headache. $CaNa_2$-EDTA does not appear to reduce overall body lead burden for children with moderate lead poisoning when the pretreatment levels are considered (84).

Management of Toxicity in Adults

DIFFICULTIES IN DIAGNOSIS

Recognition of lead poisoning in the adult depends on a high incidence of suspicion and careful recording of a patient history. The infrequency of diagnostic signs and the nonspecific nature of the symptoms frequently lead to misdiagnosis. Although lead poisoning usually has an insidious onset, symptoms may present suddenly and dramatically after a brief but intense exposure. Intense respiratory exposure can be produced by cutting or abrasive blasting of lead-coated steel or by use of powered sanding equipment on lead-painted surfaces. Severe acute disease has been seen also with ingestion of contaminated food (85) or other lead-containing products and recently was described from intravenous injection of contaminated methamphetamine (23). In this setting, patients may develop an acute encephalopathy that can mimic other neurologic or psychiatric illnesses. Acute colic may be mistaken for appendicitis or other intraabdominal catastrophe.

More commonly, symptoms develop insidiously over weeks to months as the dose accumulates. An affected patient's history may suggest any of a number of GI, rheumatologic, or psychiatric illnesses. Diagnosis depends on careful history recording to reveal a possible source of exposure. In most cases, workers in a primary lead-producing or lead-using industry will be aware of the exposure and well may be under medical surveillance. Workers in smaller industries and in construction in which exposures often are uncontrolled are at great risk and may be totally unaware of their exposure. In this situation, the care with which the physician records an occupational and environmental history is critical.

Processes that most commonly cause lead poisoning in adults are those involving disruption of painted or rustproofed surfaces. These can include burning or sanding of lead-containing paint, cutting or blasting of structural steel, and welding or burning of rustproofed steel. Secondary smelting, including the reclaiming of batteries and telephone cables, frequently is conducted by small businesses with little awareness of hazards to workers. Indoor firing ranges may expose occupants to high levels of lead when ventilation in the building is imperfect. Hobbies, including stained-glass work and ceramics, also can pose a risk. The use of lead-glazed pottery for food or beverages can pose a threat of which affected individuals may be unaware.

Physical findings usually are of little help in diagnosis. Motor weakness may be detectable, and signs of peripheral nerve entrapment may be present. Gingival lead lines, the development of which depends on the presence of some degree of pyorrhea, rarely are seen. Routine laboratory work may reveal decreased hemoglobin and hematocrit, but severe anemia is not seen commonly. The classic sign of basophilic stippling rarely is seen. After closure of the epiphyses, lead lines in bone no longer develop.

Measurement of blood lead level and free erythrocyte porphyrin (FEP) or zinc protoporphyrin (ZPP) is the key to diagnosis. Because the test is technically difficult, use of a laboratory that routinely and regularly measures blood lead is important. Local health officials or the poison center may be of help in identifying the appropriate laboratory. The U.S. Occupational Safety and Health Administration (OSHA) maintains a list of laboratories certified to perform measurements for medical surveillance.

TREATMENT

The first step in treatment must be to identify patients' exposure, to identify any other individuals (family members or coworkers) who also may have been exposed, and to intervene to stop the exposure. Involvement of local health officials may be essential to confirm the route of exposure and to identify and assess all those at risk. Under no circumstances should affected individuals return to the work or home activity that caused the poisoning until all risk of further exposure has been eliminated.

Chelation therapy is indicated for the treatment of severe symptoms, such as intractable headache, irritability, and other personality changes; myalgias or arthralgias; and abdominal colic. End-organ damage, as evidenced by neuropathy or nephropathy, also is an indication for intervention. Even in the absence of symptoms, markedly elevated blood lead levels may be an indication for therapy. In some severe situations, instituting therapy before test results return may be appropriate as long as other treatable etiologies in the differential diagnosis have been considered. With less acutely ill patients, a number of factors should be considered in deciding on the need for chelation. In cases with minimum symptoms, only cessation of exposure may be necessary. When an affected patient has persisting symptoms, history and laboratory values may provide information about prognosis. The blood lead level, which is sensitive to recent exposure and to current mobilization of lead from bone stores, should be interpreted in the context of the history of exposure. Many cases permit rendering some judgment about how long exposure is likely to have been going on and to offer some clue as to the time required to excrete the toxic burden without chelation. Because FEP and ZPP will rise after a moderate postexposure period and then will decline slowly, they can be a clue in this process. If the entire period of exposure to lead was relatively short, the current blood lead is relatively low, and the symptoms are relatively mild, stopping the exposure and treating the symptoms may be all that is needed. At any given blood lead level, the more slowly the dose has been accumulated and the greater the FEP or ZPP level, the longer the symptoms are likely to persist. Chelation therapy may shorten the symptomatic period in such a situation, but repeated courses of treatment may be necessary. Because bone stores may be remobilized by therapy, blood lead levels often rebound after each course of treatment. As body burden is reduced, blood levels rebound more slowly and to lower levels.

Although chelation therapy has demonstrated its value for treating severe symptomatic intoxication, as yet no controlled studies have examined its effects. Controversy remains about its value in the setting of asymptomatic or mildly symptomatic intoxication. Although removing lead as rapidly and thoroughly as possible is theoretically attractive, chelating agents may cause unintended harm by redistributing lead into organs or organelles. Resolution of this issue may have to await controlled trials. Chelation therapy never should be given prophylactically nor given to a patient in whom lead absorption may be continuing. Once a decision to undertake therapy has been made, therapy should be continued until symptoms have improved and lead levels remain at an acceptable level.

$CaNa_2$-EDTA has been the mainstay of therapy in the past. Although succimer (DMSA) is not yet specifically approved for use in adults, it has proved to be an efficacious therapeutic agent in treating lead poisoning, and it is the drug of first choice for most patients. Dimercaprol and penicillamine are used much less frequently since succimer became available.

In the presence of severe encephalopathy or when blood lead levels exceed 100 μg per dL, treatment should begin with a combination of succimer and $CaNa_2$-EDTA. If affected patients cannot take succimer orally or it otherwise is contraindicated, dimercaprol can be used intramuscularly with the EDTA. For less emergent situations or as a continuation of initial therapy, either EDTA or succimer alone may be used.

$CaNa_2$-EDTA has low toxicity and a low rate of side effects when used in appropriate dosage. Although varied regimens are in use, exceed 2 g of $CaNa_2$-EDTA daily is unwise in adults. $CaNa_2$-EDTA should be given intravenously no more rapidly than 1 g over 1 hour, and slower infusions generally are preferred to minimize the risk of hypercalcemia. Excretion is mainly urinary.

Toxic effects of $CaNa_2$-EDTA include renal tubular necrosis, which is reversible on discontinuation of therapy; rash; febrile reactions; fatigue; thirst; myalgia; chills; and (rarely) cardiac dysrhythmias. Electrocardiographic monitoring rarely is indicated in adults. Doses of $CaNa_2$-EDTA should be reduced in the presence of renal failure. Although intramuscular injection of $CaNa_2$-EDTA is efficacious, it is exceedingly painful in adult doses. Oral $CaNa_2$-EDTA is not effective and may increase lead absorption.

Because repeated daily doses of $CaNa_2$-EDTA typically produce gradually decreasing amounts of urinary lead excretion, therapy typically is continued for 5 days and then is interrupted to assess effect and to watch for rebound. Blood levels should be assessed after each round of therapy and weekly thereafter to determine whether rebound is occurring and whether further therapy is warranted.

DMSA, an oral analog of dimercaprol, is given orally. The recommended adult course, 10 mg per kg three times daily for 5 days followed by 10 mg per kg twice daily for 14 days, usually produces impressive reductions in blood lead levels. As with EDTA, rebound can occur, and repeated courses may be necessary. This dose results in an appreciable rate of side effects—in particular nausea and vomiting—that require cessation of the drug. Rashes and elevation of transaminases also have been reported, and preexisting liver abnormalities are a relative contraindication. For patients with normal liver function, DMSA probably is the drug of first choice. Patients trade the increased risk of reversible side effects and the unpleasantness of the regimen (which, for adults, involves swallowing as many as seven pungent capsules three times daily) for the advantages of outpatient treatment that is more rapidly efficacious.

Dimercaprol is thick and oily and must be administered by deep intramuscular injection. The usual dose is 45 mg per kg given intravascularly every 4 hours. Up to 50% of patients will have some adverse reaction after receiving a dose of 45 mg per kg. Side effects include hypertension and tachycardia, which is dose-related. Rash is common along with nausea, vomiting, headache, and paresthesias. BAL is 50% excreted in bile and can be used if renal compromise is present.

D-Penicillamine is an oral chelator that effectively increases urinary lead excretion. It is administered in either 125- or 250-mg dosage forms. The usual dose is 25 to 35 mg per kg per day in four divided doses. The typical adult dose is 250 mg four times daily by mouth for 10 days. Adverse effects of D-penicillamine include hypersensitivity reactions and renal toxicity. Blood dyscrasias, such as leukopenia, thrombocytopenia, and eosinophilia, also have occurred (80). Liver and renal functions should be monitored during therapy.

EXPOSURE LIMITS AND ENVIRONMENTAL MONITORING

Air

The EPA has established national primary and secondary air quality standards of 1.5 μg of lead per cubic meter of air as an arithmetic mean averaged over a calendar quarter (40 *CFR* 50.12).

Water

The federal Clean Water Act established a water quality criterion for lead at 50 μg of lead per L for domestic water supplies. The same limit is the National Primary Drinking Water Maximum Contaminant Level. The Safe Drinking Water Act requires suppliers of lead-contaminated water to notify customers of any lead content in their water and to describe the potential hazards of lead, what the water system is doing about it, and whether to seek an alternative supply of water (52 *CFR* 41534). In most U.S. settings, the principal source of lead contamination of drinking water is not the source waters or the transmission system but the use of lead-containing solder in domestic plumbing. Especially with acidic water, substantial leaching can occur as water sits in household pipes. Some states and municipalities have banned lead-containing solder for use in water supply pipes. The EPA has recommended that the level of 50 μg per L be lowered to 5 μg per L.

Gasoline

The use of organic lead additives in gasoline has been declining since the 1970s and has nearly been eliminated in the United States. Leaded gasoline still is permitted for farm equipment and for some marine use. As leaded gasoline was the single largest source of lead absorption to which the general population was exposed, the removal of lead from gasoline resulted in dramatic decreases in the average blood lead levels of the population.

Waste Disposal

Lead is treated as a hazardous waste under the Resource Conservation and Recovery Act (40 *CFR* 260).

Consumer Product Safety

Lead-containing paint and certain consumer products bearing lead-containing paint have been banned by the U.S. Consumer Products Safety Commission. "Lead-containing" is defined by the presence of more than 0.06% lead by weight of the paint or the dried surface (42 *CFR* 44199; 43 *CFR* 8515). Lead paint continues to be used in some exterior applications, and interior surfaces painted prior to 1975 are suspect. Lead content can be checked from paint chips, from dust in window wells, or by the use of an x-ray fluorescence detector that can read dirpectly from surfaces. Lead paint removal is regulated by Housing and Urban Development guidelines and by state and local regulations (60,61).

U.S. Occupational Safety and Health Administration Regulations

The OSHA lead standard sets a permissible exposure level for lead of 50 µg per cubic meter of air for an 8-hour time-weighted average (Table 73-9). An action level of 30 µg per cubic meter also is provided, above which an employer is obligated to provide training, protective clothing, washing facilities, and medical surveillance. The standard also requires that an employer remove from exposure any workers whose lead levels are markedly elevated or who are believed by a physician to need such removal. Workers whose blood lead levels are 50 µg per dL must be removed immediately from the exposure. Workers whose blood lead levels exceed 40 µg per dL must undergo medical evaluation (63). (These blood lead removal levels were set in 1978, and accumulating evidence of the dangers of lead at lower doses has rendered them increasingly obsolete. Therefore, OSHA is discussing bringing its rules up to date.)

Where it has been enforced, the lead standard has resulted in dramatic decreases in cases of intoxication and in average levels of blood lead among workers. After it became apparent that some of the worst poisonings were taking place in construction and demolition, the OSHA standard was extended to cover these industries in 1996. Organic lead compounds were excluded from these regulations and, at present, are covered only by the older standard of 200 µg per cubic meter of air.

TABLE 73-9. Regulatory limits for lead exposure

Agency	Sample or medium	Concentration	Regulation
OSHA	Air	50 µg Pb/m^3	Permissible exposure limit for an 8-h workday
ACGIH	Air	150 µg Pb/m^3	Time-weighted average for 40-h work week
EPA	Air	1.5 µg Pb/m^3	3-mo average
EPA	Water	50 µg Pb/L	Consideration being given to lowering this to 5 µg/L
OSHA	Blood	60 µg/dL	Removal from exposure
OSHA	Blood	40 µg/dL	Medical evaluation required
CDC (EPA)	Blood	10–15 µg/dL	Level of concern in children

ACGIH, American Conference of Governmental Industrial Hygienists; CDC, Centers for Disease Control and Prevention; EPA, U.S. Environmental Protection Agency; OSHA, U.S. Occupational Safety and Health Administration.
[a]Anticipated reduction for 1991.
Adapted from Agency for Toxic Substances and Disease Registry, U.S. Department of Health and Human Services, Public Health Service, 1999.

Other Public Health Regulations

A number of states require the reporting of cases of lead poisoning in children or adults to health authorities. Encouraged by the National Institute of Occupational Safety and Health and the Centers for Disease Control, most states now require laboratories to report all elevated blood lead levels to begin surveillance for excessive lead exposure and frank poisonings. Some local governments conduct screening programs to detect elevated lead levels among children.

REFERENCES

1. Woodbury WD. Lead. In: *Minerals yearbook 1987.* Washington: Bureau of Mines, US Department of Commerce, 1987:541–567.
2. Stokinger HE. The metals. In: Clayton GD, Clayton FE, eds. *Patty's industrial hygiene and toxicology.* New York: Wiley Interscience, 1981:1687–1728.
3. Agency for Toxic Substances and Disease Registry. *Toxicological profile for lead.* US Department of Health and Human Services, Public Health Service, ATSDR, July 1999.
4. Landigan P. Current issues in the epidemiology and toxicology of occupational exposure to lead. *Environ Health Perspect* 1990;89:61–66.
5. National Research Council. *Measuring lead exposure in infants, children, and other sensitive populations.* Washington: National Academy Press, 1993.
6. Office of Pollution Prevention and Toxics. Report on the National Survey of Lead-Based Paint in Housing: base report. Report no. EPA/747-R95-003. Washington: US Environmental Protection Agency, Office of Pollution Prevention and Toxics, 1995.
7. Markowitz ME, Bijur PE, Ruff HA, Balbi K, Rosen JF. Moderate lead poisoning: trends in blood lead levels in unchelated children. *Environ Health Perspect* 1996;104:968–972.
8. Cook M, Chappell WR, Hoffman RE, Mangione EJ. Assessment of blood lead levels in children living in a historic mining and smelting community. *Am J Epidemiol* 1993;137:447–455.
9. Blood lead levels—United States, 1988–1991. *MMWR Morb Mortal Wkly Rep* 1994;43:545–548.
10. Update: blood lead levels—United States, 1991–1994. *MMWR Morb Mortal Wkly Rep* 1997;46:141–146.
11. Sargent ID, Brown MJ, Freeman JL, Bailey A, Goodman D, Freeman DH. Childhood lead poisoning in Massachusetts communities: its association with sociodemographic and housing characteristics. *Am J Public Health* 1995;85:528–534.
12. Maryland Department of Health and Mental Hygiene. *Lead poisoning: strategies for prevention.* Baltimore: Maryland Department of Health and Mental Hygiene, 1984.
13. Watson WS, Hume R, Moore MR. Oral absorption of lead and iron. *Lancet* 1989;8:236–237.
14. Baltrop D. Transfer of lead to the human foetus. In: Baltrop D, Burland WL, eds. *Mineral metabolism in paediatrics.* Philadelphia: FA Davis Co, 1968:135–150.
15. Kehoe RA. Toxicological appraisal of lead in relation to the tolerable concentration in the ambient air. *J Air Pollut Contain Assoc* 1969;19:690–700.
16. Forni A, Cambiaghi G, Secchi GC. Initial occupational exposure to lead. *Arch Environ Health* 1976;31:73–78.
17. Chisolm JJ, Barrett MB, Harrison HV. Indicators of internal dose of lead in relation to derangement in heme synthesis. *Johns Hopkins Med J* 1975;137:612.
18. Bennett WM. Lead nephropathy. *Kidney Int* 1985;28:12–20.
19. Arai F, Yamamura Y, Yamauchi H, Yoshida M. Biliary excretion of dimethyl lead after administration of tetraethyl lead in rabbits. *Sangyo Igaku* 1983;25:175–180.
20. Rabinowitz MB, Wetherill GW, Kopple JD. Kinetic analysis of lead metabolism in healthy humans. *J Clin Invest* 1976;58:260–270.
21. Christoffersson JO, Ahlgren L, Schute A, Skerfving S, Mattson S. Decrease of skeletal lead levels in man after end of occupational exposure. *Arch Environ Health* 1986;41:312–318.
22. Cory-Slechta DA, Weiss B, Cox C. Mobilization and redistribution of lead over the course of calcium disodium ethylene diamine tetraacetate chelation therapy. *J Pharmacol Exp Ther* 1987;243:804–813.

23. Chandler DB, Norton RL, Kauffman KW, et al. Lead poisoning associated with methamphetamine use, Oregon 1988. *MMWR Morb Mortal Wkly Rep* 1989;38:830–831.
24. Cullen MR, Robins JM, Eskenazi B. Adult inorganic lead intoxication: presentation of 31 new cases and a review of recent advances in the literature. *Medicine* 1983;62:221–247.
25. Krigman MR, Bouldin TW, Mushak P. Lead. In: Spencer PS, Schaumberg HH, eds. *Experimental and clinical neurotoxicology.* Baltimore: Williams & Wilkins, 1980.
26. Goyer R. Lead toxicity: from overt to subclinical to subtle health effects. *Health Perspect* 1990;86:177–181.
27. Stollery BT, Banks HA, Broadbent DE, Lee WR. Cognitive function in lead workers. *Br J Ind Med* 1989;46:698–707.
28. Hogstedt C, Hane M, Agrell, Bodin L. Neuropsychological test results and symptoms among workers with well defined long term exposure to lead. *Br J Ind Med* 1983;40:99–105.
29. Valciukas JA, Lilis R, Singer R, Fischbein A, Anderson HA, Glickman L. Lead exposure and behavioral changes: comparison of four occupational groups with different levels of lead absorption. *Am J Ind Med* 1980;1:421–426.
30. Bleecker ML, Lindgren KN, Ford DP. Differential contribution of current and cumulative indices of lead dose to neuropsychological performance by age. *Neurology* 1997;48:639–645.
31. Kajiyama K, Doi R, Sawada J, et al. Significance of subclinical entrapment of nerves in lead neuropathy. *Environ Res* 1993;60:248–253.
32. Mantere P, Hanninen H, Hernberg S, Luukkonen R. A prospective follow-up study on psychological effects in workers exposed to low levels of lead. *Scand J Work Environ Health* 1984;10:43–50.
33. Baker EL, Feldman RG, White RA, et al. Occupational lead neurotoxicity: a behavioral and electrophysiological evaluation. *Br J Ind Med* 1984;41:352–361.
34. Baker EL, Feldman RG, White RA, et al. Occupational lead in neurotoxicity: improvement in behavioral effects after reduction of exposure. *Br J Ind Med* 1985;42:507–516.
35. Walsh TJ, Tilson HA. Neurobehavioral toxicology of the organoleads. *Neurotoxicology* 1984;5:67–86.
36. Needleman HL, Gunnoe C, Leviton A, et al. Deficits in psychological and classroom performance of children with elevated dentine lead levels. *N Engl J Med* 1979;300:689–695.
37. Needleman HL, Schell A, Bellinger D, Leviton A, Allred EN. The long term effects of exposure to low doses of lead in childhood. *N Engl J Med* 1990;322:83–88.
38. Dietrich KN, Berger OG, Succop PA. Lead exposure and the motor developmental status of urban six-year-old children in the Cincinnati Prospective Study. *Pediatrics* 1993;91:301–307.
39. Centers for Disease Control and Prevention. Erratum. *MMWR Morb Mortal Wkly Rep* 1997;46:60.
40. Centers for Disease Control and Prevention. Blood lead levels in young children—United States and selected states, 1996—1999. *MMWR Morb Mortal Wkly Rep* 2000;49:1133–1137.
41. White RF, Diamond R, Proctor S, Morey C, Hu H. Residual cognitive defects 50 years after lead poisoning during childhood. *BMJ* 1993;50:613–622.
42. Davoli CT, Serwint JR, Chisolm JJ. Asymptomatic children with venous lead levels >100 mg/dl. *Pediatrics* 1996;98:965–968.
43. Seppalainen A, Hernsberg S, Rock B. Relationship between blood lead levels and nerve conduction velocities. *Neurotoxicology* 1979;1:313–332.
44. Wedeen RD. In vivo tibial XRF measurement of bone lead. *Arch Environ Health* 1990;45:69–71.
45. Grandjean P, Jensen BM, Sand SH, Jorgensen PI, Antonsen S. Delayed blood regeneration in lead exposure: an effect on reverse capacity. *Am J Public Health* 1989;79:1385–1388.
46. Wedeen RP. *Poison in the pot.* Carbondale, IL: Southern Illinois University Press, 1984.
47. Morgan JM, Ball GV, Oh SJ, et al. Lead poisoning. *South Med J* 1972;65:278–288.
48. Goering PL, Fowler BA. Mechanisms of renal lead-binding protein protection against lead inhibition of delta-aminolevulinic acid dehydratase. *J Pharmacol Exp Ther* 1985;234:365–371.
49. Batumen V, Landy E, Maesaka JK, Wedeen RP. Contribution of lead to hypertension with renal impairment. *N Engl J Med* 1983;309:17–21.
50. Osterloth JD, Selby JV, Bernard BP, et al. Body burdens of lead in hypertensive nephropathy. *Arch Environ Health* 1989;44:304–310.
51. Verberk MM, Willems TEP, Verplanke AJW, De Wolff FA. Environmental lead and renal effects in children. *Arch Environ Health* 1996;51:83–87.
52. Cooper WC, Wong O, Kheifets L. Mortality among employees of lead battery plants and lead-producing plants, 1947–1980. *Scand J Work Environ Health* 1985;11:331–345.
53. Fanning D. A mortality study of lead workers, 1926–1985. *Arch Environ Health* 1988,43:247–251.
54. McMichael AJ, Johnson HM. Long-term mortality profile of heavily exposed lead smelter workers. *J Occup Med* 1982;24:375–378.
55. Parkinson DK, Hodgson MJ, Bromet EJ, Dew MA, Connell MM. Occupational lead exposure and blood pressure. *Br J Ind Med* 1987;44:744–748.
56. Masjedi MR, Estineh N, Bahadori M, Alavi M, Sprince NL. Pulmonary complications in lead miners. *Chest* 1989;96:18–21.
57. Harbison RD. *Hamilton & Hardy's Industrial Toxicology,* 5th ed. St. Louis, MO: Mosby, 1998.
58. Murphy MJ, Graziano JH, Popovac D, et al. Past pregnancy outcome among women living in the vicinity of a lead smelter in Kosovo, Yugoslavia. *Am J Public Health* 1990;80:33–35.
59. Bellinger D, Leviton A, Waternaux C, Needleman H, Rabinowitz M. Longitudinal analyses of prenatal and postnatal lead exposure and early cognitive development. *N Engl J Med* 1987;316:1037–1043.
60. Lancranjan I, Popescu HI, Gavanescu O, Klepsch I, Serbanescu M. Reproductive ability of workmen occupationally exposed to lead. *Arch Environ Health* 1975;30:396–401.
61. Assennato G, Baser ME, Molinini R, et al. Sperm count suppression without endocrine dysfunction in lead exposed men. *Arch Environ Health* 1986; 41:387–390.
62. Centers for Disease Control and Prevention. Screening young children for lead poisoning: guidance for state and local public health officials. Centers for Disease Control and Prevention, November 1997.
63. Turk DS, Schonfeld OJ, Cullen M, Rainey P. Sensitivity of erythrocyte protoporphyrin as a screening test for lead poisoning. *N Engl J Med* 1992;326:137–138.
64. Diermayer M, Hedberg K, Fleming D. Backing off universal childhood lead screening in the USA: opportunity or pitfall? *Lancet* 1994;344:1587–1588.
65. Shannon M, Graef JW. Lead intoxication in children with pervasive developmental disorders. *Clin Toxicol* 1996;34:177–181.
66. Targeted screening for childhood lead exposure in a low prevalence area—Salt Lake County, Utah, 1995–1996. *JAMA* 1997;277:1508–1509.
67. Rooney BL, Hayes EB, Allen BK, Strutt PJ. Development of a screening tool for prediction of children at risk for lead exposure in a Midwestern clinical setting. *Pediatrics* 1994;93:183–187.
68. US Housing and Urban Development. Lead-based paint: interior guidelines for hazard identification and abatement. *Federal Register* 1990;55:14556–14789.
69. Guidance on identification of lead-based paint hazards. *Federal Register* 1995;60(175).
70. Staes C, Matte T, Copley CG, Flanders D, Binder S. Retrospective study of the impact of lead-based paint hazard remediation of children's blood lead levels in St. Louis, Missouri. *Am J Epidemiol*1994;39:1016–1026.
71. Weitzman M, Aschengrau A, Bellinger D, Jones R, Hamlin JS, Beiser A. Lead-contaminated soil abatement and urban children's blood lead levels. *JAMA* 1993;269:1647–1654.
72. Aschengrau A, Beiser A, Bellinger D, Copenhafer D, Weitzman M. The impact of soil lead abatement on urban children's blood lead levels: phase II results from the Boston Lead-in-Soil Demonstration Project. *Environ Res* 1994;67:125–148.
73. Swindell SL, Charney E, Brown MJ, Delaney J. Home abatement and blood lead changes in children with class III lead poisoning. *Clin Pediatr* 1994;33:536–541.
74. Title X, Section 1018 (disclosure rule). *Federal Register* 1996;61(45).
75. Sargent ID. Role of nutrition in the prevention of lead poisoning in children. *Pediatr Ann* 1994;23:636–642.
76. Hammad TA, Sexton M, Langenberg P. Relationship between blood lead and dietary iron intake in preschool children: a cross-sectional study. *Ann Epidemiol* 1996;6:30–33.
77. Committee on Drugs, American Academy of Pediatrics. Treatment guidelines for lead exposure in children. *Pediatrics* 1995;96:155–160.
78. Besunder JB, Anderson RL, Super DM. Short-term efficacy of oral dimercaptosuccinic acid in children with low to moderate lead intoxication. *Pediatrics* 1995;96:683–687.
79. Liebelt EL, Shannon M, Graef JW. Efficacy of oral meso-2,3-dimercaptosuccinic acid therapy for low-level childhood plumbism. *J Pediatr* 1994;124:313–317.
80. Liebelt EL, Shannon MW. Oral chelators for childhood lead poisoning. *Pediatr Ann* 1994;23:616–619.
81. Chisolm JJ. Treatment of lead poisoning. *Mod Treat* 1971;8:593–612.
82. Chisolm JJ, Barltrop D. Recognition and management of children with increased lead absorption. *Arch Dis Child* 1979;54:249–262.
83. Piomelli S, Rosen JF, Chisolm JJ, Graef JW. Management of childhood lead poisoning. *J Pediatr* 1984;105:523–532.
84. Markowitz ME, Bijur PE, Ruff H, Rosen JF. Effects of calcium disodium versenate ($CaNa_2$-EDTA) chelation in moderate childhood lead poisoning. *Pediatrics* 1993;92:265–271.
85. Hershko C, Abrahamov A, Moreb J, et al. Lead poisoning in a West Bank Arab village. *Arch Intern Med* 1984;144:1969–1973.

CHAPTER 74
Cadmium

Michael P. Waalkes, Zakaria Z. Wahba, and Richard E. Rodriguez

Cadmium is a highly toxic transition (heavy) metal; human exposure to cadmium has been and continues to be a major concern. Cadmium is a highly cumulative toxic agent, and it is estimated to have a biological half-life in humans in excess of

20 years. Cadmium exposure has been shown to have adverse effects on a variety of tissues and is linked with various chronic diseases, including carcinogenesis and osteomalacia. Cadmium usage has increased dramatically during the past 40 to 50 years and continues, gradually, to increase. Only a small portion of the yearly production of cadmium ever is recycled. Thus, the known and suspected effects of cadmium and its continued industrial usage reinforce the view that cadmium poses a significant threat to the human population and the environment (1–7).

PHYSICAL PROPERTIES AND PRODUCTION

Properties and Chemical Forms

Cadmium is a silvery, crystalline metal resembling zinc. It is tarnished only slightly by air or water. Metallic cadmium exists in a hexagonal, closely packed arrangement in which each atom has 12 nearest neighbors, 6 surrounding it in its own closely packed layer and 3 above and 3 below this layer. In this structure, each layer is a plane of symmetry, and the set of nearest neighbors of each atom has D_{3h} symmetry (8). Cadmium has oxidation states of 0, +1, and +2, with the latter being the most common. Highly unstable but strongly reducing dimers of Cd^{1+} can be obtained by irradiation of aqueous solutions. The physical properties of cadmium are listed in Table 74-1 (9,10).

The stereochemistry of cadmium is a direct result of the *d* shell configuration. No ligand field stabilization exists, as the outer *d* shell of cadmium is complete. Thus, the stereochemistry of cadmium compounds is determined solely by size, electrostatic forces, and covalent bonding forces. Cadmium's coordination numbers include four (tetrahedral), five (trigonal by pyramidal), and six (octahedral), although the coordination number of most cadmium-organo compounds usually is two.

Cadmium is a member of division A of analytic group II, which consists of the common metals, the ions of which form chlorides. The chlorides are insoluble in dilute acid, but their sulfides are precipitated by hydrogen sulfide in 0.3 *M* hydrochloric acid. This property permits the separation and identification of cadmium from other heavy metals of analytic group II. Cadmium forms numerous divalent compounds, including oxides, hydroxides, sulfides, selenides, tellurides, and halides. Complex anions can be formed with halides in aqueous solution. Complex cations with ammonia and amine ligands are well defined and are obtained as crystalline salts.

TABLE 74-1. Physical properties of cadmium

Property	Value
Atomic number	48
Atomic weight	112.41
Electronic structure	2.18.81.2
Outer configuration	4d10 5s2
Oxidation states	0, +1, +2
Reduction potential	Cd^{2+}/Cd
Volts	–0.40
Density (g/cm^3) at 20°C	8.65
Melting point	320.9
Boiling point	767
Radii of divalent ion (A)	0.93

Reprinted from refs. 9 and 10, with permission.

Production, Natural Occurrence, and Common and Chemical Names

Cadmium is found in the rare mineral element greenockite and in CdS and Otavite. Both forms are found in zinc and zinc and lead–rich ores. Cadmium usually is recovered as a by-product of zinc refining. Other materials that contain cadmium are hawleyite (cadmium sulfite), xanthrocroite, cadmoselite (cadmium selenide), and monteporrite (cadmium oxide). Most of the cadmium produced comes from zinc smelters and from sludge obtained from the electrolytic refining of zinc. In 1973, world production of cadmium was 17 million kg, whereas U.S. production was 3.36 million kg (11). More recent figures indicate that world production has risen, although the U.S. remains a major supplier and consumer of cadmium (5).

Pure cadmium is produced from several sources, including the sintering of flue dusts and the roasting of zinc ores and as a by-product of slag zinc. In the smelting of cadmium-containing zinc ores, the two metals are reduced together. Owing to the fact that cadmium is more volatile than is zinc, the two compounds can be separated by fractional distillation. Because cadmium is less active than is zinc, electrolytic separation also can be accomplished (12,13).

BATTERIES

Cadmium is used as the negative electrode in long-lasting nickel-cadmium batteries. This use of cadmium has grown considerably in recent years (5). These batteries are rechargeable and are very important in biomedical applications (12).

ELECTROPLATING

A significant part of the cadmium produced is used in electroplating such metals as iron and steel, although this application has diminished in recent years (5). As cadmium is not corroded easily, it is an excellent protective agent and much better than zinc for this purpose. Metals coated with cadmium are dipped in an electrolytic bath containing tetracyanocadmate ions $[Cd(CN)4]^2$. A two-electron reduction occurs, yielding metallic cadmium, a cyanide anion:

$$[Cd(CN)4]^2 + 2e^- \rightarrow Cd + 4CN$$

The baths provide 20% of the cadmium that is electroplated, and the cadmium anode consumes the other 80%. The most important applications of cadmium electroplating are in the automotive and aircraft industries. Other applications include electronic parts, marine equipment, and industrial machinery (12,14).

PLASTICIZERS

Another large consumer of cadmium is the plastics industry. Cadmium salts of long-chain fatty acids admixed with barium salts serve as stabilizers for plastics. Substituted cadmium phosphonium chloride has been used by the rubber industry as an additive. When added to plastics, cadmium provides stability against heat and light (5).

PIGMENTS

Cadmium is used as a component of pigments used in manufacturing plastics, ceramics, and glass (5). The paint industry uses CdS, CdSe, and CdO in a mixture for use as pigments. Pure CdO is used in phosphors (15).

ALLOYS

Cadmium is used in making a number of alloys, such as Woods metal (12.5% Cd; melting point, 65.5°C) and Lipowitz alloy (10% Cd; melting point, 70°C). Alloys containing cadmium (99% cadmium in combination with nickel-silver or copper) are used for bearings, because high speeds and temperatures would be excessive for tin and lead alloys. Other alloys are used for soldering aluminum. The cadmium content of these alloys varies from 10% to 95%. Alloys with a low melting point are used in fire protection, fusible links, fusible cores for foundry molds, bending pipes and then sections, soldering, and sealing.

NUCLEAR INDUSTRY

Cadmium is very important in the nuclear industry, although this industry constitutes a minor aspect of cadmium consumption. Cadmium absorbs neutrons very well and thus is used in making neutron shields and rods for use in controlling the chain reaction of nuclear reactors.

Synthesis of Industrially Used Cadmium Compounds

The Chemical Abstracts Service lists 152 cadmium compounds in their chemist database (formerly known as *Toxlist*). These compounds contain cadmium as a major element in the compound infrastructure or as a trace element. Next we provide a partial list of cadmium compounds, with their synthesis and principal uses.

CADMIUM ACETATE

Cadmium acetate is a result of the reaction of cadmium nitrate with acetic anhydride. It is used for producing iridescent effects on porcelains and pottery. It also serves as a reagent for the determination of sulfur, selenium, and tellurium in cadmium electroplating. Textile manufacturers use cadmium acetate for dying and printing, and the petroleum industry uses it for the purification of mercaptans from crude oils and gasolines.

CADMIUM CARBONATE

Cadmium carbonate originates from the reaction of cadmium hydroxide and carbon dioxide. Its uses include its application as a lawn and turf fungicide, as a wettable powder in combination with organic fungicides. It also is used in the preparation of high-purity, specialized chemicals, such as phosphors for use in monitors.

CADMIUM CHLORIDE

Cadmium chloride originates in the reaction of cadmium metal, cadmium oxide, or carbonate in hydrochloric acid and evaporating to dryness. It is used in pesticides and nonpasture fungicides and is found in photographic material, in phosphors, in electronic coatings for vacuum tubes, and in the manufacture of special mirrors and production of lubricants. Cadmium chloride has applications in dyeing and in calico printing of textiles.

CADMIUM FLUROBORATE

Cadmium fluroborate is the product of the reaction of aqueous fluroboric acid and cadmium metal, carbonate, or oxide. A principal use is its function in electroplating.

CADMIUM FLUORIDE

Cadmium fluoride is produced by the reaction of cadmium carbonate and hydrofluoric acid. Uses for cadmium fluoride include its addition as an ingredient in glass and in nuclear reactor rods.

CADMIUM NITRATE

Cadmium nitrate arises as a result of the reaction of cadmium oxide with nitric acid. It is used in the manufacture of nickel-cadmium batteries and as a turf fungicide.

CADMIUM OXIDE

Cadmium oxide is prepared by the distillation of cadmium metal from graphite retort and subsequent reaction of vapor with air. The functions in which it is used include electroplating, the production of cadmium electrodes for alkaline batteries, and the synthesis of other cadmium compounds.

CADMIUM SULFATE

Cadmium sulfate results from the reaction of cadmium metal, oxide, carbonate, or sulfide in sulfuric acid. It is found in the production of plastic stabilizers (polyvinyl chlorides) and of pigments.

CADMIUM SULFIDE

One of the most versatile of the cadmium compounds, cadmium sulfide is used in the production of pigments (yellow to deep maroon) and to increase heat stability in plastics, colored vulcanized rubber, and epoxy resins. It also is found in imprinting inks for alkali resistance, in paints that are resistant to hydrogen sulfide blacking, and in phosphors for cathode-ray tube screens. Additional uses for cadmium sulfide include phosphorescent tapes and markers, watch and instrument dials, interior decorations, theatrical decorations, x-ray fluorescent screens, and body temperature gradient detectors. A medical use for cadmium sulfide is as an active ingredient in shampoos designed to treat seborrheic dermatitis of the scalp.

INDUSTRIES AND OCCUPATIONS ASSOCIATED WITH EXPOSURES

The major businesses associated with potential cadmium exposure are shown in Table 74-2. These include the primary production industries, such as cadmium smelting (3,5). Lead and zinc smelting also can be a source of cadmium exposure. The electroplating industry is another major (although diminishing) source of exposure, because cadmium fumes can be generated during the electroplating process (3,5). The processing involved in manufacture of cadmium-nickel batteries also can lead to worker exposure, owing to proximity to cadmium dust (3). Cadmium fumes generated by welding of cadmium-plated materials are extremely dangerous and are the primary cause of acute fatal poisonings (3). In alloy production using cadmium, such as copper-cadmium and silver-cadmium alloy manufacture, significant exposures can occur (3). The production of plastic stabilizers and

TABLE 74-2. Occupations with potential cadmium exposure

Alloy production	Pigment production and use
Battery production	Plastics production
Brazing	Plating
Coating	Printing
Diamond cutting	Semiconductor and superconductor production
Dry color formulation	Sensor production
Electroplating	Smelting and refining
Electrical contact production	Solar cell production
Enameling	Soldering
Engraving	Stabilizer production
Glasswork	Textile printing
Laser cutting	Thin film production
Metallizing	Transistors production
Paint production and use	Welding
Pesticide production and use	
Phosphorus production	

Reprinted from ref. 5, with permission.

cadmium pigments also can lead to exposure (3). The production of jewelry using silver-based solder containing cadmium is another documented source of industrial exposure, owing to the generation of cadmium oxide fumes in the process (5,16,17).

Major anthropogenic environmental exposure sources include the use of sewage sludge as fertilizer, manufacture and use of phosphate-based fertilizers, incineration of waste and wood, coal combustion, and oil and gasoline combustion (2,5). Natural sources of environmental exposure include volcanic particles, wind-blown dust, and forest fires (2,5).

CLINICAL TOXICOLOGY OF CADMIUM EXPOSURE

Routes of Exposure

Exposure to cadmium in human populations occurs both through the natural environment and in the workplace. Although occupational exposure was the most prominent form in the past, significant exposures have occurred also through the environment. Hence, both types of exposures must be considered relevant in a discussion of clinical toxicology.

ENVIRONMENT

Generally, cadmium occurs naturally in the environment as a sulfide deposit. Increased industrial use, starting at the beginning of the twentieth century, gave rise to increases in production of cadmium from a few tons per year to nearly 18,000 tons in 1975 (2,4,5). Cadmium is dispersed widely, and contamination of soil, water, and air frequently has occurred through mining, refining, and smelting operations. Other significant sources of environmental cadmium include the combustion of fossil fuels, municipal waste incineration, and agricultural practices (e.g., the use of phosphate fertilizers and sludge amendment for soils) (2,3). Use of cadmium in batteries, alloys, paints, and plastics also contributes to environmental levels and thus to human exposure (2,3).

Oral exposure to cadmium is the major route in nonindustrially exposed individuals; food consumption constitutes the primary environmental source of cadmium for the nonsmoking general population (2). The cadmium content of different foodstuffs ranges from 0.001 to 1.3 parts per million (ppm), and the average intake from food and water is estimated at from 10 to 30 μg daily (2). In highly polluted areas, this level can rise to as high as 400 μg daily of cadmium intake (2,4,5). Meat by-products, especially liver and kidney, can be high in cadmium. In certain areas, shellfish and seafood also can contain elevated levels of cadmium. Vegetable products generally contain levels of cadmium greater than those in meat-based foodstuffs (15). Exposure to cadmium by way of contaminated water that was used for irrigation of rice has been associated with Itai-Itai (or "ouch-ouch") disease, a multisystem disorder with characteristic severe osteomalacia. This phenomenon occurred in Japan and affected primarily postmenopausal, multiparous women (2).

Inhalation of cadmium is a major source of cadmium intake for the general population. Average concentrations of cadmium in air are estimated as follows: rural areas, less than 1 to 6 ng per cubic meter; urban areas, 5 to 50 ng per cubic meter; and industrial areas, 20 to 700 ng per cubic meter (18). Cadmium intake by inhalation in the general population averages 0.02 μg per day and can be as high as 2.0 μg per day in highly polluted areas. Thus, even with highly polluted atmospheric conditions, food still is the main cadmium source in the general population.

An additional source of respiratory cadmium intake is cigarette smoking, as the tobacco plant readily absorbs cadmium from soil. Estimates maintain that a one-pack-a-day smoker can potentially absorb 2 μg of cadmium daily, owing to smoking (2,15). Seemingly, second-hand smoke likely may contribute to cadmium burden in nonsmokers.

OCCUPATION

Estimates indicate that more than 0.5 million workers are exposed to cadmium in U.S. workplaces (5). This figure includes workers in primary cadmium industries, such as ore smelting, and those in secondary industries, where exposure potential is lower. Welding is a primary example of the latter.

Inhalation is the predominant route of exposure to cadmium in occupational settings. Secondary oral exposure may occur under conditions of poor industrial hygiene, such as storage of food or eating in contaminated areas, but exposure from such sources is minor in comparison to that by direct inhalation. Dermal exposures to cadmium under most conditions probably are not a significant risk factor, particularly where appropriate industrial hygiene is observed. Cigarette smoking must be considered a significant augmentation to industrial cadmium exposure. External contamination of cigarettes with cadmium in the workplace has been shown to increase worker exposure significantly (2).

Inhalation exposure to various chemical and physical forms of cadmium can occur. Typically, during ore smelting, cadmium oxide fumes are inhaled, whereas inhalation of mist and dust of cadmium cyanate or cadmium chloride can occur during electroplating operations (4,5).

Historically, workplace air concentrations of cadmium were very high, with values detected in the range of mg per cubic meter (4,5). Over the past several decades, increased awareness of the toxic potential and resultant improvements in industrial hygiene have decreased these concentrations of cadmium considerably, typically below suggested or mandated occupational limits. Because of this change, overt intoxications resulting from inhalation under occupational conditions now are rare (16,17).

Absorption, Metabolism, and Excretion

ABSORPTION

Absorption of cadmium depends primarily on the route of exposure and secondarily on the compound in question. Most salts of cadmium are absorbed poorly from the gastrointestinal (GI) tract. Estimates maintain that only approximately 5% of ingested cadmium is absorbed, although various conditions, including dietary status and iron deficiency anemia, can elevate this percentage (2,19). The absorption of cadmium from the GI tract does not appear to differ between the genders (19). Cadmium has a relatively long transit time in the GI tract, possibly owing to uptake of cadmium by the mucosal cells (19).

Absorption from the respiratory system, however, is fairly different. Whereas the GI tract absorbs only approximately 5% of the cadmium presented to it, depending on the *in vivo* solubility of the inhaled compound, more than 90% of the cadmium deposited deep in the lung can be absorbed (5,18). The ability of the lung to absorb cadmium must be considered in assessing actual exposure levels. Cadmium absorbed from the pulmonary system clearly will reach and can affect other distant organ systems. For instance, chronic nephrotoxicity is a well-documented result secondary to chronic inhalation of cadmium (2–5).

METABOLISM

Once absorbed, cadmium is bound to red blood cells and serum albumin. Serum cadmium is taken up very rapidly by soft tissues, primarily liver and kidney, and has a very high volume of distribution indicative of the rapid tissue concentration (1,3,20).

Typically, more than 50% of the body burden of cadmium will be found in the liver and kidney. The half-life of cadmium is thought to be very long, and accumulation occurs within these tissues (1). A critical concentration of cadmium is postulated to exist within the kidney; once this is exceeded, cadmium-induced nephropathy will occur (1,2). Human newborns have very low tissue levels of cadmium, as the placenta appears to be an effective barrier to cadmium; however, fetal exposure will occur with increasing maternal exposure (1,21).

Cadmium is not biotransformed in the classic sense of the term. Furthermore, once absorbed, cadmium is excreted only very slowly. However, biological defense mechanisms to reduce the toxic potential of cadmium do exist. A key aspect of the metabolism of cadmium is the low-molecular-weight, metal-binding protein metallothionein, which is synthesized in response to cadmium exposure (2,4). After synthesis, metallothionein will bind cadmium with a very high affinity and apparently render it toxicologically inert (1,2,4), at least when the complex remains intracellular. Hence, cadmium is detoxified by long-term storage rather than by biotransformation or enhanced elimination. Liver and kidney tissues have a high capacity for metallothionein synthesis (22), and, soon after absorption, most of the cadmium will be found predominantly in the liver and kidney (1,2). Hence, the metabolism of cadmium is involved intimately with metallothionein. Zinc treatment prior to normally toxic or lethal doses of cadmium in animals will prevent toxic effects of cadmium (4,23,24), probably owing to zinc's ability to induce metallothionein.

Indeed, cadmium appears frequently to follow the biological pathways of zinc metabolism and, to a lesser extent, calcium. For instance, cadmium frequently will be taken up by cells through mechanisms normally devoted to zinc uptake (25–27). On the molecular level, many of the toxic effects of cadmium are thought to be due to its replacement of zinc in biological systems. Zinc deficiency states modify cadmium distribution and potentially enhance cadmium toxicity (28).

Cadmium is stored in association with metallothionein for long periods. However, cadmium in association with metallothionein is thought to be the actual species toxic to the kidneys. Cadmium-metallothionein is highly nephrotoxic and will induce an acute proximal tubular necrosis characteristic of long-term exposure to ionic forms of cadmium (29,30). Circulating cadmium-metallothionein appears to be taken up specifically by the proximal tubule when it is degraded, and the cadmium is released in locally high concentrations. Rodents treated chronically with cadmium salts do not exhibit nephropathy until after serum levels of cadmium-metallothionein have become significantly elevated. The source of cadmium-metallothionein is thought to be the liver, from which (with continued cadmium exposure) it eventually is lost. Monitoring serum cadmium-metallothionein thus may be a possible predictor of nephrotoxicity onset; however, this hypothesis has not been tested directly.

EXCRETION

Once absorbed, cadmium is excreted very poorly. This observation is consistent with cadmium's very long biological half-life, estimated at between 25 and 30 years in humans (2). After absorption, the prominent route of cadmium elimination occurs via the urine; therefore, urinary cadmium is thought to be a reflection of body burden (1,2). The onset of cadmium-induced nephropathy is followed by a marked increase of urinary cadmium in the form of cadmium-metallothionein complex (2,30). Otherwise, cadmium is eliminated unchanged.

Approximately 95% of ingested cadmium will be eliminated in the feces owing to the poor level of cadmium absorption from the GI tract. Thus, fecal cadmium consists almost exclusively of unabsorbed cadmium. Although some cadmium that had been absorbed into the mucosa may be added to fecal cadmium through mucosal turnover, it would represent a very small portion of the total fecal content (19). In sufficient quantities, oral cadmium is a very powerful emetic, and this too could be considered as a form of elimination of unabsorbed cadmium.

Signs, Symptoms, and Syndromes

ACUTE TOXICITY

Routes of Exposure and Target Organs. Acute intoxication with cadmium can occur from either ingestion or inhalation. Such intoxication does, however, require relatively high concentrations. Acute cadmium exposure typically is most toxic to the tissue with which it has initial contact (i.e., the lung from inhalation and the GI tract from ingestion). With sufficient dose, however, renal and hepatic involvement can occur from either route of cadmium exposure.

Ingestion. Typical symptoms of oral intoxication with cadmium include nausea, vomiting, abdominal cramping and pain, diarrhea, increased salivation, tenesmus, and choking. Cadmium also is a very powerful emetic. Depending on the level of consumption, recovery from a single oral exposure can be rapid and apparently without long-term effects. This finding has been reported from cases in which intoxication occurred from consumption of contaminated drinks containing up to 16 mg of cadmium per L (31). However, death has occurred with higher oral doses of cadmium (32). In addition to the foregoing symptoms, hemorrhagic gastroenteritis, hepatic and renal (particularly cortical) necrosis, cardiomyopathy, and metabolic acidosis have been associated with high oral cadmium exposure (2,32).

Inhalation. Exposure to high levels of cadmium fumes by inhalation also can lead to intoxication (33–35). Signs and symptoms of acute cadmium poisoning after inhalation include (in order of frequency) nasopharyngeal irritation, chest pain, headache, dizziness, cough, dyspnea, vomiting, nausea, chills, weakness, and diarrhea (33). Sustained hyperpyrexia can occur in severe exposure cases and typically is associated with a poor prognosis (33). These symptoms are essentially those suggestive of metal fume fever. An antemortem diagnosis of cadmium intoxication rests on obtaining a knowledge of the conditions and, if possible, agent of exposure (34). An unpleasant metallic taste in the mouth, which is enhanced by cigarette smoking, occasionally occurs in exposed workers during or immediately after exposure (33). Cadmium fume pneumonitis frequently is accompanied by a pulmonary edema (occasionally hemorrhagic) of noncardiac origin (33). Fully 20% of all cases of cadmium-induced chemical pneumonitis are estimated to be fatal owing to fulminant interstitial pulmonary edema (33,34). Hepatic necrosis and bilateral renal cortical necrosis also occur in severe exposure cases (2,29). Later, pulmonary fibrosis can develop and result in a persistent restrictive ventilatory defect (33).

CHRONIC TOXICITY

Target Organs and Systems. The chronic toxic (noncarcinogenic) effects associated most clearly with cadmium exposure occur in the pulmonary system and in the kidney. Pulmonary system effects are associated exclusively with inhalation exposure, whereas renal effects appear after oral or inhalation exposures. Secondarily, chronic cadmium exposure has been associated with skeletal system toxicity, hypertension, and cardiovascular disease and carcinogenesis in the lung.

Pulmonary System. The chronic pulmonary effect of cadmium in humans typically is manifested as an obstructive lung disease (1,2). A significant increase in deaths caused by respiratory disease in cadmium-exposed workers has been seen repeatedly in epidemiologic studies (1,2,5). The disease state results from a chronic bronchitis, progressive fibrosis of the lower airways, and alveolar damage resulting in emphysema (2,5,6). Pulmonary physiologic assessment indicates a reduced vital capacity and an increased residual volume. Dyspnea also is a common complaint in exposed individuals. The level of obstructive disease appears to be related to the duration and level of cadmium exposure (1,2).

Less frequently, lung cancer has been associated with chronic cadmium inhalation (5), although not all epidemiologic studies have reported such an association (5,6). Such studies frequently are complicated by concurrent exposure to metals other than cadmium and cigarette smoking. Recent studies have, however, allowed elimination of such mitigating factors in human cadmium carcinogenesis studies (5). The recent production of malignant pulmonary tumors (adenocarcinomas) in rodents chronically exposed to cadmium via inhalation supports these human data (5,36), and cadmium now has been accepted as a human carcinogen (5). Pulmonary tumors produced by cadmium are primarily adenocarcinomas.

Renal System. The chronic renal effects of cadmium are characterized by proximal tubular necrosis and dysfunction and can occur after chronic oral or inhalation exposure (1,2). The manifestations of cadmium-induced nephropathy include low-molecular-weight proteinuria, aminoaciduria, and glucosuria and frequently are accompanied by increased cadmium in the urine (1,2). The lesions are most pronounced in the renal cortex. Cadmium complexed with metallothionein may be the actual etiologic agent (see Metabolism).

Nephropathy is thought to occur when the renal cortical cadmium concentration exceeds a "critical" level of 200 μg per g (2). The average level of cadmium in the renal cortex in nonoccupationally exposed individuals is approximately 15 to 30 μg at age 50; however, renal cortical levels in nonpolluted areas of Japan range from 50 to 125 μg per g of tissue (15). Cigarette smoking can double renal cortical cadmium concentration (15). Thus, even in the general population of nonoccupationally exposed individuals, a very small margin of safety exists for cadmium exposure and nephropathy.

The proteinuria induced by chronic cadmium exposure is characterized by low-molecular-weight proteins that normally would be reabsorbed in the proximal tubular elements (1,2). The most prominent protein found is β_2-microglobulin. Several other low-molecular-weight proteins are present, including retinol-binding protein and lysozyme (1,2). Higher-molecular-weight proteins, such as albumin, indicative of glomerular effects in cadmium-exposed workers, also are present occasionally (37). The renal effects of cadmium are not seen exclusively in workers who have been exposed occupationally, and a low-molecular-weight proteinuria in the general population has been seen with environmental exposure to cadmium (38).

A single study has associated occupational cadmium exposure with renal cancer (39). This finding, however, has not been confirmed by other studies in human populations or in rodent testing. Exposure to multiple agents, of which cadmium was only one, may have been an important factor in the development of renal carcinogenesis (39).

Skeletal System. Cadmium intoxication can have dramatic effects on calcium homeostasis and metabolism and can increase calcium excretion. Osteomalacia and osteoporosis accompanied by bone pain are part of the syndrome Itai-Itai disease, which appears to have resulted from cadmium intoxication in a group of Japanese women in the 1940s (1,2). Typically, the victims were postmenopausal and multiparous and presented with severe bone deformities and chronic nephropathy (1,2). Beyond cadmium exposure, nutritional deficiencies (particularly vitamin D deficiency) are thought also to have been possible contributors to this syndrome (1,2).

Cardiovascular System. Hypertension after chronic cadmium exposure has been shown in rodent models (1,2). The mechanism of this effect is unknown and could be linked to renal, cardiac, or direct vasoconstrictive effects of cadmium. In humans, an increased rate of mortality from cerebrovascular disease has been detected in populations living in cadmium-polluted areas and having cadmium-induced nephropathy (40).

Carcinogenesis and Teratogenesis. In several epidemiologic studies, cadmium exposure in the workplace has been linked to carcinogenesis in various tissues, including the lungs, the prostate, the kidneys, and the stomach (5,6). A few studies have indicated an association between cadmium levels in food or drinking water and prostatic cancer (41). Several epidemiologic studies, however, produced negative results in associating cadmium with human carcinogenesis (5,6). Evidence in animal studies indicated that cadmium can be a very potent carcinogen and suggested that tumors of the lung (36), prostate, testes, and injection site (42,43) are induced in rats or mice by cadmium injections or ingestion. On the basis of accumulating evidence in the lungs in humans (5) and strong supportive evidence of pulmonary carcinogenicity in rodents, cadmium now is considered a human carcinogen (5). The mechanism by which cadmium is carcinogenic is essentially unknown.

Teratogenic effects of cadmium have not been observed in humans. However, cadmium has been shown to be a potent teratogen in animal models. Its teratogenic effects mimic those produced by zinc deficiency.

Management of Toxicity

CLINICAL EXAMINATION

Signs and symptoms of cadmium intoxication depend on the route of exposure. Local irritation is one of the major signs of acute cadmium toxicity, whether it be irritation of the GI tract after oral exposure or irritation of the respiratory system after inhalation.

Acute cadmium inhalation may cause irritation to the upper respiratory system and trigger chest pains, nausea, and dizziness. In cases of excessive inhalation of cadmium fumes (usually cadmium oxide) and dust, severe signs may develop, such as loss of ventilatory capacity with a corresponding increase in residual lung volume; fatal pulmonary edema; or residual emphysema with peribronchial and perivascular fibrosis (44). Dyspnea is the most frequent complaint of patients with cadmium-induced lung disease.

In the case of acute intoxication after oral exposure, symptoms usually include some signs of irritation of the GI tract, including nausea, vomiting, excessive salivation, diarrhea, and abdominal cramping. Death can result from hemorrhagic gastroenteritis (32). Acute high-dose oral ingestion also may be accompanied by signs of liver and kidney damage, hypoproteinemia with hypoalbuminemia, and metabolic acidosis (26). Renal tubular dysfunction can occur after either chronic pulmonary or GI exposure to the metal (1,2). In fact, renal dysfunction can occur long after withdrawal of cadmium exposure, indicating that the progressive nature of this disorder is based on release of biological stores of previously accumulated cadmium. A low-molecular-weight proteinuria indicative of proximal tubular damage is the hallmark of cadmium-induced renal dysfunction.

In advanced cases of cadmium intoxication, secondary manifestations, including severe osteoporosis and osteomalacia, have occurred. This form of cadmium intoxication has been seen industrially after inhalation of cadmium and after long-term ingestion of contaminated food. Cadmium-induced bone diseases occur mainly at the later stages of cadmium poisoning. Affected patients are likely to have had kidney disease before the bone damage occurs. The diagnosis of osteoporosis or osteomalacia (or both) is based on blood analysis of calcium, phosphate, and alkaline phosphate and on radiography of the skeleton, particularly the long bones, pelvis, and ribs (3). Severe bone pain also is common in such cases. Cadmium-induced bone loss is seen more frequently in postmenopausal women who have had multiple pregnancies.

LABORATORY DIAGNOSIS

Among the critical target organs in cadmium exposure, the most sensitive are the kidneys (45). Renal dysfunction is a common sign of cadmium toxicity, resulting from accumulation of cadmium in the renal cortex (1–3). The concentration of cadmium in blood and urine may reflect the cadmium level in the entire body and could predict the level of renal dysfunction. Interpretation of blood and urine levels may be complicated by recent exposures or smoking (or both). Renal function can be evaluated by determining levels of urinary albumin, creatinine, β_2-microglobulin, and total protein.

The main biochemical finding in cadmium toxicity is proteinuria subsequent to renal damage. The proteinuria has been postulated to result from cadmium transported to proximal tubules bound to metallothionein (29,30). The best indicator of cadmium-induced nephropathy appears to be β_2-microglobulin (1,2). Recent attention has been given to studies of urinary levels of retinol-binding proteins as an indicator of cadmium exposure. The determination of retinol-binding proteins has certain advantages over that of β_2-microglobulin, as it avoids interference from the pH of the urine (45,46).

In suspected cases of Itai-Itai disease, radiographic examinations of bones, particularly radius, ulna, femur, and humerus, are indicated, especially if an affected patient suffers from generalized pain and deformities of the lower extremities (50).

TREATMENT

The treatment of acute and chronic cadmium intoxication remains primarily palliative; no specific treatment alternatives are available. Additionally, no clear data support use of chelation therapy in humans as an effective means of therapeutic intervention in acute cadmium intoxication. However, treatment with calcium disodium–ethylenediaminetetraacetic acid ($CaNa_2$-EDTA) has been suggested as possibly effective when administered immediately after exposure to cadmium (47), as such treatment increases the urinary excretion of cadmium in rodents. The suggested dosage of $CaNa_2$-EDTA is 75 mg per kg of body weight per day in three to six divided doses for 5 days, and the total dose of $CaNa_2$-EDTA per 5-day course should not exceed 500 mg per kg of body weight per day (48). A second 5-day course may be given after at least 2 days without treatment after the first regimen (48). Standard precautions in the use of chelation therapy should be observed, and urinary cadmium content should be monitored.

In chronic exposure, the effectiveness of chelation therapy for cadmium poisoning is questionable. This limitation is due to the long half-life of cadmium in humans resulting from the ability of cadmium to induce and bind to metallothionein with very high affinity (49). Once metallothionein is synthesized in large amounts (24 to 48 hours after initial exposure), chelation is thought to be ineffective. Experimental studies of animals have shown that the interval after cadmium exposure plays an important role in the effectiveness of chelation therapy, as follows. As an alternative, to alleviate the problem of sites inaccessible to most chelators, a combination chelation therapy employing a water-soluble and lipid-soluble combination of 2,3-dimercapto-1-propanol [British anti-Lewisite (BAL)] and diethylenetriamine pentaacetic acid was used in rodents (50). In general, chelation therapy may be effective if the chelator is given very shortly after initial cadmium exposure, because a rapid decrease in the effectiveness of such therapy ensues with increasing time after the exposure. This effect probably is due to distribution of the metal to sites that are not reached by the chelators (51) and to increased synthesis of the high-affinity cadmium-binding protein metallothionein. Therefore, chelation therapy must take place as soon as possible after exposure.

In cases of Itai-Itai disease and some other cases of cadmium exposure associated with osteoporosis, vitamin D has been given to patients in large doses for long periods (months). The purpose of this primarily palliative therapy was the alleviation of some of the painful symptoms due to bone loss (2,46). An example of the dosage that was used is 100,000 IU of vitamin D_2 orally every day for 10 days (46). After discontinuation for 10 days, similar doses of vitamin D_2 were given again for 10 days. In addition, 300,000 IU of vitamin D_2 or vitamin D_3 was given 8 times annually by intramuscular injection. Anabolic steroid also was given orally and intramuscularly. Total doses of vitamin D given for approximately 1 year were 14,000,000 IU of vitamin D_2 and 2,100,000 IU of vitamin D_3 parenterally (46). Treatment with large doses of vitamin D and anabolic steroids by oral and parenteral administration resulted in gradual clinical improvement. Thus, in cases of bone disease, treatment with calcium and vitamin D or its metabolite (Calcitriol) can be somewhat helpful in restoring bone function.

OCCUPATIONAL AND ENVIRONMENTAL EXPOSURE MONITORING

The Occupational Safety and Health Administration issued two final cadmium standards in 1992, establishing a new permissible exposure limit for occupational exposure to cadmium at 5 µg per cubic meter as an 8-hour time-weighted average. This new standard covers general industry, the maritime industry, agriculture, and the construction industries (29 *CFR* 1910, 1915, 1926, and 1928). These new regulations also set standards for medical surveillance using three biological monitoring parameters—urinary cadmium, urinary β_2-microglobulin, and blood cadmium—thereby establishing criteria for worker removal from exposure (Table 74-3).

Urinary cadmium and β_2-microglobulin are standardized to creatinine levels in the urine. Urinary cadmium concentrations reflect long-term exposure and provide an estimate of the total cadmium body burden; urinary β_2-microglobulin is an indicator of renal tubular dysfunction; and blood cadmium is a measure of recent cadmium exposure, usually within the previous few months. The combination of these three biological monitoring parameters is used to classify employees of one of three categories requiring ongoing medical surveillance. The three categories—A, B, and C—correspond to a minimum, intermediate, or enhanced level of medical surveillance required (52). The action limit of airborne cadmium is 2.5 µg per cubic meter.

Cadmium appears to be eliminated by a two-compartment model with a rapid blood decline of 2 to 12 months and a half-

TABLE 74-3. U.S. Occupational Safety and Health Administration cadmium standard of biological monitoring and results categories

Biological marker	Monitoring result categories: Normal (category A)	Discretionary removal (category B)	Mandatory removal (category C)[a]
Cadmium in urine (μg/g creatinine)	≤3	>3 and ≤15	>15
β_2-Microglobulin (μg/g creatinine)	≤300	>300 and ≤1,500[b]	>1,500
Cadmium in blood (μg/L whole blood)	≤5	>5 and ≤15	>15

[a]Mandatory removal levels in category C for 1999.
[b]If an employee's β_2-microglobulin levels exceed 1,500 μg/g creatinine, for mandatory medical removal to be required (see Appendix A, Table B of the standard), either the employee's urinary cadmium level also must be greater than 3 μg/g creatinine or the blood cadmium level also must be greater than 5 μg/L whole blood.
Adapted from ref. 52.

life of approximately 100 days on the average (52). A second, slower elimination rate has an estimated half-life of 7.4 to 16.0 years and evinces a wide variation among individuals. This same two-compartment model has been observed also in a population of individuals with cadmium urinary excretions exhibiting an initial rapid decline followed by a slower decline, where the second slower elimination rate is 2 to 5 months (52).

Urinary cadmium concentration is influenced by the concentration of cadmium in the kidney and by the tubular dysfunction caused by cadmium nephrotoxicity. The contribution of smoking to cadmium concentrations in the blood or urine does not result in values outside of monitoring category A.

The current cadmium standard provides up to 18 months of medical removal protection. This period allows for making decisions as to affected workers' capacity for returning to a cadmium-exposure job. The decision to lift a restriction on a worker's ability to return to work is based on the return of abnormal biological monitoring results to normal levels. However, other indicators that physicians might use to make this determination include not only biological monitoring results but indications of end-organ damage and other health factors of affected workers that could have an impact on their health if the workers were allowed to return to the exposure.

Cadmium is a cumulative toxin and concentrates in the renal cortex. The first manifestation of cadmium-induced nephrotoxicity is renal tubular dysfunction associated with increased urinary excretion of low-molecular-weight protein, such as β_2-microglobulin and retinol-binding proteins. Also possible, but not seen as often, is an effect on the glomerulus leading to increased urinary excretion of higher-molecular-weight proteins, such as albumin, immunoglobulin G, and transferrin. To prevent nephrotoxic effects and other toxic manifestations of cadmium, an upper limit of 300 μg per g of creatinine for the urinary concentration both of β_2-microglobulins and of retinol-binding protein in the urine has been proposed (53).

The risk of abnormal tubular reabsorption of microproteins increases when the amount of cadmium in the body accumulates to the point that cadmium urinary concentrations exceed 10 μg of cadmium per g of creatinine (53). Irreversible cadmium-induced tubular proteinuria has been demonstrated in workers exposed to cadmium even after cessation of exposure (53). Also, cadmium-induced microproteinuria has been found to be predictive of an exacerbation of age-related decline of the glomerular filtration rate. Some indications suggest that the renal tubular toxic effects of cadmium are reversible provided that, at the time the exposure was reduced or terminated, the microproteinuria was mild (a β_2-microglobulin in the urine of less than 1,500 μg per g of creatinine) and the urinary cadmium values had never exceeded 20 μg of cadmium per g of creatinine (53). With severe microproteinuria (β_2-microglobulins in the urine greater than 1,500 μg per g of creatinine) in combination with urinary cadmium values exceeding 20 μg per g of creatinine, cadmium-induced renal tubular dysfunction was progressive despite cessation of cadmium exposure (53).

Proteinuria and glycosuria appear to be the most common signs of cadmium exposure, with renal disease due to industrial exposure. In addition, measurement of hypercalciuria, aminoaciduria, increased uric acid excretion with hypouricemia, and hypertension have been used (1–3). Neutron-capture x-ray analysis involving transportable measurement systems has been used to evaluate the amount of the metal that has accumulated in the liver and kidneys of workers employed in cadmium smelter plants (54,55). However, this method is limited by its level of detection (56). The critical level of cadmium in renal cortex has been suggested possibly to range from 215 to 390 μg per L (49,56). Measurement of levels of metallothionein in urine has been proposed as a specific finding indicative of cadmium nephropathy and may prove of value in diagnosis of exposure to cadmium (57).

Monitoring of cadmium exposure in humans generally has involved the assessment of cadmium levels in the blood or urine. Urinary cadmium is thought at least to provide a good index of excessive cadmium exposure (1,2). Blood concentrations of cadmium in nonexposed individuals typically are less than 10 μg per L. The largest portion of cadmium in blood (70%) is localized within the red blood cell (57). *In vivo* neutron activation analysis has been used also to determine tissue burdens of cadmium, particularly in the liver and kidneys, although this would not be sensitive enough to determine levels in the general population (1,57). In the assessment of cadmium-induced nephropathy, urinary levels of β_2-microglobulin frequently are used, although this method is nonspecific for cadmium and rather a general indicator of renal dysfunction (57). Urinary levels of β_2-microglobulin are increased only after the onset of renal pathology and hence are not predictive. Blood cadmium concentrations in symptomatic workers with pulmonary and renal toxicity vary widely (between 18 and 73 μg per L) (57). Recently, researchers have proposed that urinary metallothionein levels should be monitored to assess cadmium exposure, as these levels correlate with cadmium tissue levels (as determined better by neutron activation than by urinary levels of β_2-microglobulin (58). The predictive value of metallothionein determination is as yet unknown; however, it clearly is a more specific test.

Environmental Monitoring

Environmental surveying with stationary samplers has helped to establish exposure levels of various metals, including cadmium, in workplace air and in ambient air (3). However, more accurate assessment of individual exposures is obtained by the use of personal samplers (3). Caution should be exercised with respect to personal sampler data with cadmium, because personal habits can lead to an inaccurate assessment of environmental exposure. Such habits include cigarette smoking, which can result in oral contacts with contaminated hands or cigarettes and can cause substantially increased exposure in a manner that would not be detected by personal monitors (3).

Exposure Limits

Most countries have not set legal limits for the maximum daily intake of cadmium from food consumption. The World Health Organization (WHO) has proposed a provisional tolerable weekly intake of cadmium of 7 mg per kg (5). Japan has set the maximum concentration of cadmium in rice at 0.4 mg per kg. WHO guidelines place maximum levels in drinking water at 3 µg per L, whereas in the United States, the maximal level allowed is 10 µg per L (5). Cadmium and cadmium compounds are not allowed in cosmetic products in the countries of the European Economic Community (5).

The WHO recommends that cadmium exposure from respirable dust should be well below 20 µg per cubic meter in occupational settings. A complete listing of occupational regulations and guidelines concerning exposure in occupational settings is available in a previously published work (5).

REFERENCES

1. Goyer RA. Toxic effects of metals. In: Doull J, Klaassen CD, Amdur MO, eds. *Casarett and Doull's toxicology: the basic science of poisons.* New York: Macmillan, 1991:634–638.
2. Friberg L, Elinder CG, Kjellstrom T, Nordberg GF, eds. *Cadmium and health.* Cleveland: CRC Press, 1986.
3. Friberg L, Nordberg GF, Vouk VB, eds. *Handbook on the toxicology of metals.* Amsterdam: Elsevier Science, 1986.
4. Goering PL, Waalkes MP, Klaassen CD. Toxicology of cadmium. In: Goyer RA, Cherian MG, eds. *Handbook of experimental pharmacology: toxicology of metals,* vol 115. New York: Springer-Verlag, 1994:189–214.
5. Beryllium, cadmium, mercury, and exposures in the glass manufacturing industry. *IARC Monogr Eval Carcinog Risks Hum* 1993;58:1–415.
6. International Agency for Cancer Research. Some metals and metallic compounds. *IARC Monogr Eval Carcinog Risks Hum* 1980;23:1–415.
7. Waalkes MP. Metal carcinogenesis. In: Goyer RA, Klaasen CD, Waalkes MP, eds. *Metal toxicology.* San Diego: Academic Press, 1995:47–69.
8. Cotton FA, Wilkinson G. *Advanced inorganic chemistry: a comprehensive text,* 4th ed. New York: John Wiley and Sons, 1980.
9. Dean JA, ed. *Lange's handbook of chemistry,* 11th ed. New York: McGraw-Hill, 1973.
10. Weast RC, ed. *CRC handbook of chemistry and physics,* 60th ed. Boca Raton, FL: CRC Press, 1979.
11. Fairbridge RW, ed. *The encyclopedia of geochemistry and environmental sciences,* vol 4A. New York: Van Nostrand–Reinhold,1974:99–100.
12. Hebergall WH, Schmidt FC, Holtzclaw HF Jr. *College chemistry with analytical analysis,* 5th ed. Lexington, MA: DC Heath Company, 1976.
13. International Agency for Cancer Research. Some inorganic and organometallic compounds. *IARC Monogr Eval Carcinog Risk Chem Hum* 1976;2:274–299.
14. Walker R. Use and production of cadmium electrodeposits. *Met Finish* 1973;72:59–64.
15. International Agency for Cancer Research. Cadmium, nickel, some epoxides, miscellaneous industrial chemicals and general considerations on volatile anesthetics. *IARC Monogr Eval Carcinog Risk Chem Hum* 1980;11:39–70.
16. Baker EL, Coleman C, Peterson WA, Landrigan PL, Holtz JL. Subacute cadmium intoxication in jewelry workers: an evaluation of diagnostic procedures. *Arch Environ Health* 1979;34:173–177.
17. Garry VF, Pohlman BL, Wick MR, Garvey JS, Zeisler R. Chronic cadmium intoxication: tissue response in an occupationally exposed patient. *Am J Ind Med* 1986;10:153–161.
18. Waalkes MP, Oberdorster G. Cadmium carcinogenesis. In: Foulkes EC, ed. *Metal carcinogenesis.* Boca Raton, FL: CRC Press, 1990.
19. Shaikh ZA, Smith JC. Metabolism of ingested cadmium in humans. In: Holmstedt B, Lauwerys R, Mecier M, Roberfroid M, eds. *Mechanisms of toxicity and hazard evaluation.* Amsterdam: Elsevier Science, 1980:569–574.
20. Klaassen CD. Pharmacokinetics in metal toxicity. *Fundam Appl Toxicol* 1981;1:353–357.
21. Kuhnert PM, Kuhnert BR, Bottoms SF, Erhard P. Cadmium levels in maternal blood, fetal cord blood, and placental tissues of pregnant women who smoke. *Am J Obstet Gynecol* 1982;142:1021–1025.
22. Waalkes MP, Klaassen CD. Concentration of metallothionein in major organs of rats after administration of various metals. *Fundam Appl Toxicol* 1985;128:591–595.
23. Gunn SA, Gould TC, Anderson WAD. Effect of zinc on cancerogenesis by cadmium. *Proc Soc Exp Biol Med* 1964;115:653–657.
24. Gunn SA, Gould TC, Anderson WAD. Specificity in protection against lethality and testicular toxicity from cadmium. *Proc Soc Exp Biol Med* 1968;128:591–595.
25. Waalkes MP, Poirier LA. Interactions of cadmium with interstitial tissue of the rat tests: uptake of cadmium by isolated interstitial cells. *Biochem Pharmacol* 1985;34:2513–2518.
26. Stacey NH, Klaassen CD. Cadmium uptake by isolated rat hepatocytes. *Toxicol Appl Pharmacol* 1980;55:448–455.
27. Failla ML, Cousins RJ, Mascenik MJ. Cadmium accumulation and metabolism by rat liver parenchymal cells in primary monolayer culture. *Biochim Biophys Acta* 1979;538:63–72.
28. Waalkes MP. Effects of dietary zinc deficiency on the accumulation of cadmium and metallothionein in selected tissues of the rat. *J Toxicol Environ Health* 1986;18:301–313.
29. Cherian MG, Goyer RA, Delaquerriere-Richardson L. Cadmium-metallothionein-induced nephropathy. *Toxicol Appl Pharmacol* 1976;38:399–404.
30. Dudley RE, Gammal LM, Klaassen CD. Cadmium-induced hepatic and renal injury in chronically exposed rats: likely role of hepatic cadmium-metallothionein in nephrotoxicity. *Toxicol Appl Pharmacol* 1985;77:414–426.
31. Nordberg GF. Cadmium metabolism and toxicity. *Environ Physiol Biochem* 1972;2:7–36.
32. Wiśiewska-Knypl JM, Jablońska J, Myślak Z. Binding of cadmium on metallothionein in man: an analysis of a fetal poisoning by cadmium iodide. *Arch Toxicol* 1971;28:46–55.
33. Dumphy B. Acute occupational cadmium poisoning: a critical review of the literature. *J Occup Med* 1967;9:22–26.
34. Barnhart S, Rosenstock L. Cadmium chemical pneumonitis. *Chest* 1984;86: 789–791.
35. Patwardhan JR, Finckh ES. Fatal cadmium-fume pneumonitis. *Med J Aust* 1976;1:962–966.
36. Takenaka S, Oldiges HK, Hochrainer D, Obserdorster G. Carcinogenicity of cadmium aerosols in Wistar rats. *J Natl Cancer Inst* 1983;70:367–373.
37. Bernard A, Roels H, Hubermont G, Buchet JP, Masson PL, Lauwerys RR. Characterization of the proteinuria in cadmium-exposed workers. *Int Arch Occup Environ Health* 1976;38:19–30.
38. Shigamatsu I. Epidemiological studies on cadmium pollution in Japan. Proceedings of the First International Cadmium Conference. *S F Metal Bull* 1978.
39. Kolonel LN. Association of cadmium with renal cancer. *Cancer* 1976;37: 1782–1787.
40. Nogawa K, Kobayashi E, Honda R. A study of the relationship between cadmium concentrations in urine and renal effects of cadmium. *Environ Health Perspect* 1979;28:161–168.
41. Bako G, Smith ESO, Hanson J, Dewar R. The geographical distribution of high cadmium concentrations in the environment and prostate cancer in Alberta. *Can J Public Health* 1982;73:92–94.
42. Waalkes MP, Rehm S, Riggs CW, et al. Cadmium carcinogenesis in the male Wistar [Crl:(WI)BR] rats: dose-response analysis of tumor induction in the prostate and testes and at the injection site. *Cancer Res* 1988;48:4656–4663.
43. Waalkes MP, Rehm S, Riggs CW, et al. Cadmium carcinogenesis in the male Wistar [Crl:(WI)BR] rats: dose-response analysis of effects of zinc on tumor induction in the prostate and in the testes and at the injection site. *Cancer Res* 1989;49:4282–4288.
44. Zavon MR, Meadow CD. Vascular sequelae to cadmium fume exposure. *Am Ind Hyg Assoc J* 1970;31:180–182.
45. Roels H, Lauwerys R, Buchet JP, et al. In vivo measurement of liver and kidney cadmium in blood and urine. *Environ Res* 1981;26:217–240.
46. Nogawa K, Ishizaki A, Fukushima M. Studies on the women with acquired Fanconi syndrome observed in the Ichi River Basin polluted by cadmium. *Environ Res* 1975;10:280–307.
47. Cantilena LR, Klaassen CD. Decreased effectiveness of chelation therapy for Cd poisoning with time. *Toxicol Appl Pharmacol* 1982;63:173–180.
48. Klaassen CD. Heavy metals and heavy-metal antagonists. In: Gilman AG, Goodman LS, Rall TW, Murad F, eds. *Goodman and Gilman's the pharmacological basis of therapeutics,* 7th ed. New York: Macmillan, 1986:1605–1627.
49. Vallee BL. Historical review and perspectives. In: Kagi JHR, Nordberg M, eds. Metallothionein. *Experientia Suppl* 1979;34:19–40.
50. Cherian MG, Rodgers K. Chelation of cadmium from metallothionein in vivo and its excretion in rats repeatedly injected with cadmium chloride. *J Pharmacol Exp Ther* 1982;222:699–704.
51. Waalkes MP, Watkins JB, Klaassen CD. Minimal role of metallothionein in decreased chelator efficacy for cadmium. *Toxicol Appl Pharmacol* 1983;68:392–398.
52. McDiarmid M, Freeman C, Grossman E, Martonic J. Follow-up of biologic monitoring results in cadmium workers removed from exposure. *Am J Ind Med* 1997;32:261–267.
53. Roels H, Assche F, Oversteyns M, et al. Reversibility of microproteinuria in cadmium workers with incipient tubular dysfunction after reduction of exposure. *Am J Ind Med* 1997;31:645–652.
54. Al-Haddad IK, Chettle DR, Fletcher JG, Fremlin JG. A transportable system for measurement of kidney cadmium in vivo. *Int J Appl Radiat Isotope* 1981;32:109–112.
55. Thomas BJ, Harvey TC, Chettle DR, McLellan JS, Fremlin JH. A transportable system for the measurement of liver cadmium in vivo. *Phys Med Biol* 1979;24:432–437.
56. Roels H, Lauwerys R, Cardenne AN. The critical level of cadmium in human renal cortex: a reevaluation. *Toxicol Lett* 1983;15:357–360.
57. Carson B, Ellis H, McCann J. *Toxicology and biological monitoring of metals in humans.* Chelsea, MI: Lewis Publishers, 1987.
58. Tohyama C, Shaikh ZA, Nogawa K, Kobayashi E, Honda R. Elevated urinary excretion of metallothionein due to environmental cadmium exposure. *Toxicology* 1981;20:289–297.

CHAPTER 75
Copper

Donald C. Fisher

SOURCES AND PRODUCTION

Chemical Forms

Copper is a group IB metal that forms two series of compounds: copper (I) (cuprous) and copper (II) (cupric) compounds. Metallic copper is fairly resistant to corrosion and is not attacked by dry air, water, or nonoxidizing acid. Table 75-1 lists basic properties of copper. Copper I oxide (Cu_2O) occurs naturally as the reddish mineral cuprite. Copper II oxide is black and is obtained by heating copper metal in air. In moist air, copper becomes coated with green basic carbonate (1). Sulfide ores of copper, principally chalcopyrite ($CuFeS_2$) and chalcocite (Cu_2S), are the predominant forms mined and processed in the United States. The copper content of these ores usually is less than 1%. Table 75-2 lists the most common copper compounds, their common names, and predominant uses (1–3).

Sites, Industries, and Businesses Associated with Exposures

Copper was the first metal used by humans and appears to have been discovered on the island of Cyprus around 2500 BC (4). Copper salts have been used therapeutically for more than 2,000 years, and copper sulfate was a popular murder weapon and abortifacient in France in the mid-nineteenth century (5). As of 1994, 1.8 million metric tons were produced in the United States, primarily in Arizona, Utah, New Mexico, Montana, and Michigan. The United States produces 19% of the world's copper output, which exceeds 9.4 million metric tons annually. Chile, the United States, Canada, and Russia are the principal producers (6). Mined ores of copper are concentrated by a flotation process and then are refined. Smelting consists of applying sufficient heat (1,100° to 1,600°C) to concentrate the metal and fuse the remaining gangue (waste ore) into slag (7). Some of the workers who encounter significant amounts of copper and copper compounds are asphalt makers, fungicide and insecticide workers, and welders (8,9). Environmental exposure occurs primarily from ingestion of drinking water with high copper concentrations and accidental or intentional ingestion of copper sulfate (10,11).

CLINICAL TOXICOLOGY

Routes of Exposure

Copper is an essential element in mammalian systems. Illness occurs when diet is deficient or intake is excessive. The principal route of exposure is through ingestion, but inhalation of copper dust and fumes occurs in industrial settings. Toxicity has resulted from treatment of burns using topical copper compounds (12). Copper has been reported to be absorbed internally from prostheses, intrauterine devices, hemodialysis units using copper-containing equipment (12), and copper azide impregnation of the skin after an explosion (13).

TABLE 75-1. Properties of copper

Atomic weight	63.5
Specific gravity	8.92
Melting point	1,083°C
Boiling point	2,567°C

TABLE 75-2. Common copper compounds and uses

Compound (common name)	Uses
Cupric oxide (black copper oxide)	Catalyst, batteries, electrodes, desulfurizing oils, paints, insecticides, ceramic colorant, artificial gems, welding flux
Cuprous oxide (red copper oxide)	Fungicide, antifouling paint, photoelectric cells, catalyst, pigment for glass and glazes, in brazing paste
Cupric acetate, basic (verdigris)	Manufacture of pigments, fungicide, fabric dye, artificial flowers, catalyst
Cupric acetoarsenate (Paris, French, emerald, Schweinfurt, parrot, or Vienna green)	Insecticide, marine pigment, wood preservative
Cupric arsenite (Swedish or Scheele's green)	Pigment, wood preservative, fungicide, insecticide, rodenticide
Cupric borate	Pigment, fireproofing, wood preservative, fungicide, insecticide
Cupric carbonate, basic (Bremen blue or green)	Seed treatment, fungicide, pyrotechnics, pigment, feed additive, in Burgundy mixture
Cupric chloride	Catalyst, mordant, petroleum desulfurizing and deodorizing agent, inks, electroplating, photography, pyrotechnics, pigments, wood preserving, disinfectant, feed additive
Cupric chromate (VI)	Fungicide, seed protectant, wood preserving, mordant, textile preservative
Cupric hydroxide (copper hydrate)	Manufacture of rayon, battery electrodes, other Cu salts (mordant, pigment, fungicide, insecticide, feed additive, catalyst, paper treatment)
Cupric nitrate	Photocopying, colorant, mordant, finishing agent for copper, zinc, and aluminum metal, wood preservative, herbicide, fungicide, pyrotechnics; catalyst for solid rocket fuel and organic reactions
Cupric sulfate, pentahydride (bluestone, blue vitriol, Roman vitriol)	Fungicide, algicide, bactericide, herbicide, feed additive, in Bordeaux solution, mordant, dye preparation, tanning, wood preservative, electroplating, inks, pigments, photography, pyrotechnics
Cuprous cyanide	Electroplating, insecticide, fungicide, antifouling paints, polymerization catalyst
Cupric tungstate (VI); cuprous selenide	Semiconductors

Absorption, Metabolism, and Elimination

ABSORPTION

Adults ingest 1.2 to 5 mg of copper per day, approximately one-half of which is absorbed (14). After ingestion, maximum absorption of copper occurs in the stomach and jejunum. Absorption through the intestinal wall is facilitated by active transport, although the exact mechanism is unknown. Copper is bound initially in the serum to albumin and transcuprein, then later is bound more firmly to ceruloplasmin, which binds more than 75% of circulating copper (15). In acute poisoning, copper is bound also to metallothionein in the liver and kidney (16). Absorption is increased in copper deficiency and is impaired in small-bowel disease. Zinc and molybdenum inhibit the intestinal absorption of copper. Copper is distributed throughout the body but is stored primarily in liver, muscle, and bone. Normal serum levels are approximately 1 mg per mL. Serum levels increase with age, but no increase occurs in tissue stores (14). In all mammals, copper is an essential trace element involved in fundamental cellular respiration, free radical defense, connective tissue synthesis, iron metabolism, and neurotransmission. Copper-dependent enzymes include cytochrome oxidase, superoxide dismutase, lysyl oxidase, and dopamine β-hydroxylase (17,18).

METABOLISM

Absorbed copper initially is bound to albumin and is transported from the gastrointestinal tract to the liver. There it is transferred to ceruloplasmin, which is the primary transport vehicle for incorporating copper into the copper-dependent enzymes. Urinary excretion is enhanced by increased molybdenum intake, cirrhosis, and biliary obstruction (19).

ELIMINATION

Copper is eliminated principally through the feces after excretion into the bile, which is copper's primary excretory route. Biliary copper is absorbed poorly. The plasma half-life for radiocopper (^{87}Cu) is 17 to 18 hours, whereas the half-life for whole-body ceruloplasmin copper is 145 hours (20). Zinc stimulates the production of metallothionein, which in turn increases the elimination of copper (18). Urinary excretion of copper is low in humans. Healthy adults have urinary concentrations of less than 100 μg per 24 hours. A daily intake of 2 mg of copper results in a urinary concentration of between 11 and 48 μg per 24 hours (21).

Signs, Symptoms, and Syndromes

ACUTE TOXICITY

Because copper is an essential element, toxicity is uncommon, as with all essential elements. Acute copper toxicity is rare and usually is not serious. Most reports of acute toxicity are from suicidal ingestion of copper sulfate. However, death is rare, owing to copper sulfate's emetic properties. Mild forms of poisoning produce only nausea, vomiting, diarrhea, and malaise and have been described in patients poisoned by eating or drinking from copper-containing vessels (22,23) or from a soft-drink dispenser (24). Symptoms associated with severe poisoning usually follow the order of metallic taste, nausea, vomiting (sometimes of blue-green vomitus), hematemesis, diarrhea, melena, hypotension, coma, oliguria, jaundice, and death (25–29).

Skin. Contact dermatitis due to copper is rare (30). However, its occurrence can be substantiated by careful patch testing (31). Eczematous dermatitis (32) and urticaria (33) have been associated with use of copper intrauterine devices. Greenish discoloration of the hair has been seen in blond or lightly pigmented individuals exposed to copper dust or copper-tainted water used for shampooing or swimming (34,35). Copper-8-quinolinolate and copper resinate (from rosin) are potential allergic sensitizers (30).

Eye. Impregnation of the eye with elemental copper or copper alloys is called *chalcosis corneae*. This brownish or greenish-brown discoloration of the cornea, lens, or iris may occur after penetrating injuries with copper fragments. Copper sulfate, copper acetoarsenite, and verdigris (oxidized copper) cause irritation and inflammation but no permanent damage. Copper chloride and copper cyanide plating bath can cause severe reactions and permanent opacifications (36).

Respiratory System. Chronic exposure to copper dust and fumes in the industrial setting can lead to upper respiratory complaints and physical findings in workers. These findings include metal fume fever and ulceration and perforation of the nasal septum (9). No permanent lung changes have been reported from copper-related metal fume fever, and the illness does not return after cessation of exposure. Long-term exposure to dust in copper refining was not associated with chronic obstructive pulmonary disease or small airway disease in a case-control study (37). Chronic exposure to sprayed copper sulfate solution (Bordeaux solution) has been reported to cause pulmonary interstitial disease and adenocarcinoma of the lung in vineyard sprayers (vineyard sprayer's lung; see Syndromes for greater detail of metal fume fever and vineyard sprayer's lung).

Gastrointestinal Tract. The predominant findings of acute copper sulfate poisoning are gastrointestinal. These findings include nausea, vomiting, diarrhea, hematemesis, melena, and jaundice. Patients who developed intense jaundice from centrolobular necrosis after massive acute copper sulfate poisoning had a more fulminant course than did patients with milder jaundice from intravascular hemolysis (25). Indian childhood cirrhosis and idiopathic copper toxicosis appear to originate from the same, as yet unidentified genetic defect that leads to toxic accumulations of copper in the liver of children (38,39). This disease process may be enhanced by excessive copper ingestion (40). Workers who developed vineyard sprayer's lung also developed extensive liver pathology, including angiosarcoma. (These pathologic findings are described in greater detail in Syndromes.)

Renal System. Renal abnormalities have been observed after copper sulfate ingestion. Hematuria, rising blood urea nitrogen, and oliguria frequently were observed in a large series of poisonings (25). A picture of acute tubular necrosis was observed on urinalysis and renal biopsy. Intravascular hemolysis, but not hypotension, preceded development of acute tubular necrosis. Oliguria occurred in all 14 patients with hematuria, and 3 died.

Neurologic System. Although Wilson's disease brings about insult to the basal ganglia (see Chronic Toxicity and Long-Term Effects), no evidence substantiates neurologic injury from acquired copper toxicity. Coma observed in acute copper sulfate poisoning probably results from uremia (9).

Hematologic System. Hemolytic anemia accompanies severe acute copper sulfate poisoning (25) and additionally, follows burn treatment with copper sulfate and hemodialysis using copper-containing dialyzing equipment (41). Hemolytic anemia also occurs sporadically in Wilson's disease. The hemolysis is precipitous in these situations. For some individuals, hemolysis alone probably leads to mild jaundice, as compared with those who develop centrolobular necrosis of the liver. A similar abrupt hemolytic crisis has been seen also in several animal species with acute and chronic copper poisoning (5).

CHRONIC TOXICITY AND LONG-TERM EFFECTS

Acquired chronic copper toxicity, with the exception of that in vineyard sprayer's lung, has not been established firmly. Chronic disease from excessive copper storage is epitomized by Wilson's disease, an inherited, autosomal recessive error in copper metabolism. The disease is characterized by excess copper deposition in most organs, especially the liver, kidneys, brain, and eyes. Wilson's disease also is termed *hepatolenticular degeneration*, owing to the prominent effects on the liver (cirrhosis) and eye (Kayser-Fleischer rings). Excellent therapeutic results are obtained after treatment with D-penicillamine to chelate excess copper (5). The preferred maintenance treatment is 150 mg of zinc orally per day (42).

SYNDROMES

Metal Fume Fever. Chronic recurrent inhalation of copper fumes and dust can lead to nasal septal perforation and a systemic illness known as *metal fume fever.* This illness is characterized by nasal congestion, fever up to 39°C, chills, malaise, and shortness of breath. The symptoms generally develop after repeated exposure during the work week, tending to diminish toward the end of the week, only to return more prominently on reexposure after the weekend. This phenomenon has led to the term *Monday morning fever* (2,43). The illness is postulated to result from immune mechanisms (44), but no reports of chronic toxicity exist. All symptoms resolve after removal from exposure. A similar illness has been described in a patient undergoing hemodialysis. The symptoms resolved after a copper-containing part was removed from the dialysis unit (45).

Vineyard Sprayer's Lung. Vineyard sprayer's lung disease occurred when Bordeaux solution (1% to 2% solution of copper sulfate neutralized with lime) was chronically sprayed by Portuguese vineyard workers. These workers developed interstitial pulmonary disease, including histiocytic granulomas with associated nodular fibrohyaline scars containing abundant copper. The progression toward pulmonary fibrosis was highly variable among individuals, and a high incidence of adenocarcinoma, particularly alveolar cell carcinoma, was observed. Extensive liver damage also was noted. Biopsies revealed fibrosis, micronodular cirrhosis, angiosarcoma, and portal hypertension (46,47).

TERATOGENESIS

Copper ions cause irreversible immobilization of sperm *in vitro*, and intrauterine devices increase endometrial copper concentrations (48). High levels of copper given to mice during pregnancy caused increased fetal mortality and produced central nervous system malformations (49). No teratogenic effects attributed to copper have been observed in humans.

CARCINOGENESIS

With the exception of adenocarcinoma of the lung and angiosarcoma of the liver seen in patients with vineyard sprayer's lung, no evidence corroborates carcinogenesis from copper exposure (49). Excess lung cancer found in copper smelter workers has been shown to be caused by arsenic exposure (50), although increased lung cancer deaths have been observed in association with low arsenic concentrations in copper ore (51).

Management of Toxicity

CLINICAL EXAMINATION

Recording of a careful medical history is essential in leading practitioners to a suspicion of copper poisoning in acutely ill patients. The history should contain questions relevant to intentional poisoning with copper salts and to ingestion of food and drink, especially acidic beverages or alcohol prepared in copper-containing vessels. Persons acutely poisoned by copper (especially copper sulfate) should be evaluated initially for nausea, vomiting, and diarrhea. Blue-green vomitus is diagnostic. Investigation for abnormal liver and renal function and for hemolytic anemia should be conducted. Vital signs and urine output should be monitored frequently for hypotension and oliguria. The medical history is also the cornerstone of investigating dermatitis suspected to arise from copper. Inquiry as to exposure to copper salts at work, use of copper-containing jewelry, or use of a copper intrauterine device should be conducted. Patch testing may be necessary to confirm the diagnosis. A history of delayed onset of fever, chills, shortness of breath, and malaise after exposure to copper fumes should lead to the suspicion of metal fume fever. Fever, rigorous chills, diaphoresis, and wheezing may be noted on physical examination.

LABORATORY DIAGNOSIS

Laboratory findings in severe acute copper sulfate poisoning include abnormal hepatocellular function, hyperbilirubinemia (both direct and indirect), elevated blood urea nitrogen and creatinine, hematuria and cellular casts on urinalysis, anemia, positive stool guaiac, elevated serum copper (greater than 500 µg per dL), and ceruloplasmin.

Findings during episodes of metal fume fever include leukocytosis, abnormal pulmonary function study results (small airway obstruction, reduced lung volumes and carbon dioxide diffusing capacity), peribronchiolar cuffing, hazy infiltrates on chest radiography, and elevated urine copper levels (52).

TREATMENT

Removal from exposure generally is sufficient to resolve most illnesses associated with copper toxicity. This is especially true for metal fume fever and dermatitis, although the latter also may require application of topical corticosteroid preparations (7). Green hair from exogenous copper can be treated effectively with shampoos containing D-penicillamine (34).

In severe acute poisoning, emesis should not be induced and rarely is necessary, owing to spontaneous vomiting. Dilution with 4 to 8 ounces of milk or water is indicated after ingestion or prior to gastric lavage. After any seizure activity is controlled, gastric lavage may be indicated. If necessary to prevent further absorption, activated charcoal may be administered and followed by a cathartic (53). In symptomatic patients, either intravenous calcium disodium–ethylenediaminetetraacetic acid or intramuscular dimercaprol should be given as soon as feasible. D-Penicillamine may be given after initial chelation treatment with dimercaprol (27). Hemodialysis alone is not effective (49). Treatment of eye injuries includes vigorous irrigation with normal saline. Ophthalmologic referral is indicated for severe elemental copper, copper chloride, or copper cyanide plating bath injuries to the eye (36).

BIOLOGICAL MONITORING: BLOOD, SERUM, AND URINE CONCENTRATIONS

Normal blood concentrations of copper are reported to approach 1 mg per mL (21). The mean value in women is slightly higher than that in men. Copper concentration in serum or plasma varies with individuals, and diurnal variations can occur. One study reported plasma copper concentrations ranging from 0.89 to 1.37 mg per mL in healthy men and 0.87 to 1.53 mg per mL in healthy women. Ninety-five percent of the copper in plasma is in ceruloplasmin. Erythrocytes also contain a significant portion of copper found in blood in the form of an enzyme, superoxide dismutase (21).

Ceruloplasmin is one of the acute-phase reactant proteins and increases in acute and chronic inflammatory conditions. It is elevated also in patients taking estrogens and birth control pills and in those who are pregnant or have cirrhosis, cancer, or thyrotoxicosis. Increased serum concentrations of copper are found in individuals with such liver diseases as primary biliary cirrhosis and other cholestatic diseases (54).

Under conditions of extremely high copper dust levels (464 mg per cubic meter), urinary copper is elevated to approximately twice normal levels. However, at air concentrations near current exposure limits (1 mg per cubic meter) (55), biological monitoring is not warranted (43). Biological limit values cannot be established, owing to lack of reliable exposure, dose, and effect relationships (56).

OCCUPATIONAL AND ENVIRONMENTAL REGULATIONS

The Occupational Safety and Health Administration permissible exposure limit, the National Institute for Occupational Safety and Health–recommended exposure limit, and the American Congress of Government Industrial Hygienists' threshold limit value are 1 mg per cubic meter for copper dust and mist. The permissible exposure limit and threshold limit value for copper fumes are 0.1 mg per cubic meter and 0.2 mg per cubic meter, respectively. The U.S. Environmental Protection Agency has determined that lake and stream water should contain no more than 1 part per million (ppm) and drinking water no more than 1.3 ppm of copper. The National Academy of Sciences recommends 2 to 3 mg of copper per day as a safe and adequate daily intake for adults.

ENVIRONMENTAL FATE AND TRANSPORT

Copper is found in the earth's crust at approximately 70 ppm and in sea water at 0.001 to 0.02 ppm. Mining and smelting are the primary anthropogenic sources. Acidic soil conditions contribute to solubility and increased transport, although appreciable mobilization occurs only at pH less than 3 in organic soils. Low pH and the passage of soft water through copper pipes can produce high levels in drinking water; however, only 1% of U.S. drinking water samples exceed the U.S. Environmental Protection Agency standard (52).

ENVIRONMENTAL AND OCCUPATIONAL MONITORING

Copper fume and dust levels should be measured to ensure compliance with Occupational Safety and Health Administration standards. Remonitoring should be performed for any changes in work practices or plant processes that could cause a rise in air concentrations. For patients suspected of having nonoccupational overexposure to copper, an environmental evaluation should consist of measuring copper in drinking water, nonprescription remedies and supplements, and investigation of dietary practices, such as drinking acidic beverages from copper-containing vessels.

REFERENCES

1. Budavari S, ed. *The Merck index,* 12th ed. Rahway, NJ: Merck & Co, 1996.
2. Beliles RP. The metals. In: Patty FA, ed. *Industrial hygiene and toxicology,* 4th ed. New York: Wiley-Interscience Publishers, 1994.
3. Scheinberg HI. Copper, alloys and compounds. In: *Encyclopedia of occupational health and safety,* 2nd ed. Geneva: ILO Press, 1984.
4. Joralemon IB. *Copper: the encompassing story of mankind's first metal.* Berkeley, CA: Howell-North Books, 1973.
5. Owens CA. *Copper deficiency and toxicity: acquired and inherited, in plants, animals, and man.* Park Ridge, NJ: Noyse Publications, 1981.
6. Bureau of the Census. *Statistical abstracts of the U.S., 1989,* 109th ed. Washington: US Department of Commerce, 1989.
7. Wagner WL. *Environmental conditions in U.S. copper smelters.* Washington: National Institute of Occupational Safety and Health, 1975.
8. National Institute of Occupational Safety and Health. *Occupational diseases: a guide to their recognition.* Washington: US Department of Health, Education, and Welfare, 1977.
9. Cohen SR. Environmental and occupational exposure to copper. In: Nriagu JO, ed. *Copper in the environment: Part II. Health effects.* New York: John Wiley and Sons, 1979.
10. Gulliver JM. A fatal copper sulfate poisoning. *J Anal Toxicol* 1991;15:341–342.
11. Sontz E, Schwieger J. The "green water" syndrome: copper-induced hemolysis and subsequent acute renal failure as consequences of a religious ritual. *Am J Med* 1995;98:311–315.
12. Goyer RA. Toxic effects of metals. In: Klassen CD, Amdur MO, Doull J, eds. *Toxicology: the basic science of poisons,* 5th ed. New York: McGraw-Hill, 1996.
13. Bentur Y, Koren G, McGuigan M, Spielberg SP. An unusual skin exposure to copper; clinical and pharmacokinetic evaluation. *Clin Toxicol* 1988;26:371–380.
14. Owens CA. *Physiological aspects of copper: copper in organs and systems.* Park Ridge, NJ: Noyse Publications, 1982.
15. Luza SC, Speisky HC. Liver copper storage and transport during development: implications for cytotoxicity. *Am J Clin Nutr* 1996;63:812S–820S.
16. Kurisaki E, Kuroda Y, Sato M. Copper-binding protein in acute copper poisoning. *Forensic Sci Int* 1988;38:3–11.
17. Harris ZL, Gitlin JD. Genetic and molecular basis for copper toxicity. *Am J Clin Nutr* 1996;63:836S–841S.
18. Vulpe CD, Packman S. Cellular copper transport. *Annu Rev Nutr* 1995; 15:293–322.
19. Abdel-Mageed AB, Oehme FW. A review of the biochemical roles, toxicity and interactions of zinc, copper and iron: II. Copper. *Vet Hum Toxicol* 1990;32:230–234.
20. Marceau N. The use of radiocopper to trace copper metabolic transfer and utilization. In: Nriagu JO, ed. *Copper in the environment: Part II. Health effects.* New York: John Wiley and Sons, 1979.
21. Aaseth J, Norseth T. Copper. In: Friberg L, Nordberg G, Vouk V, eds. *Handbook on the toxicology of metals,* 2nd ed. New York: Elsevier Science, 1986:233–254.
22. Ross AI. Vomiting and diarrhea due to copper in stewed apples. *Lancet* 1955;2:87–88.
23. Wyllie J. Copper poisoning at a cocktail party. *Am J Public Health* 1957;47:617.
24. Witherell LE, Watson WN, Giguere GC. Outbreak of acute copper poisoning due to soft drink dispenser. *Am J Public Health* 1980;70:1115.
25. Chuttani HK, Gupta PS, Gulati S, Gupta DN. Acute copper sulfate poisoning. *Am J Med* 1965;39:849–854.
26. Chugh KS, Sharma BK, Singhal PC, Das KC, Datta BN. Acute renal failure following copper sulfate intoxication. *Postgrad Med J* 1977;53:18–23.
27. Jantsch W, Kulig K, Rumack BH. Massive copper sulfate ingestion resulting in hepatotoxicity. *Clin Toxicol* 1984;22:585–588.
28. Akintonwa A, Mabadeje AFB, Odutola TA. Fatal poisonings by copper sulfate ingested from "spiritual water." *Vet Hum Toxicol* 1989;31:453–454.
29. Lamont DL, Duflou JAL. Copper sulfate: not a harmless chemical. *Am J Forensic Med Pathol* 1988;9:226–227.
30. Adams RM. *Occupational skin disease,* 2nd ed. San Diego: Grune & Stratton, 1990.
31. van Joost T, Habets JMW, Stolz E, Naafs B. The meaning of positive patch tests to copper sulfate in nickel allergy. *Contact Dermatitis* 1988;18:101–102.
32. Barranco VP. Eczematous dermatitis caused by internal exposure to copper. *Arch Dermatol* 1972;106:386–387.
33. Barkoff JR. Urticaria secondary to a copper intrauterine device. *Int J Dermatol* 1976;15:594–595.
34. Mascaró JM Jr, Ferrando J, Fontarnau R, Torras H, Dominguez A, Mascaró JM Sr. Green hair. *Cutis* 1995;56:37–40.
35. Sticherling M, Christophers E. Why hair turns green. *Acta Derm Venereol* 1993;73:321–322.
36. Grant WM. *Toxicology of the eye,* 3rd ed. Springfield, IL: Charles C Thomas Publisher, 1986.
37. Ostiguy G, Vaillancourt C, Bégin R. Respiratory health of workers exposed to metal dusts and foundry fumes in a copper refinery. *Occup Environ Med* 1995;52:204–210.
38. Scheinberg IH, Sernlieb I. Wilson disease and idiopathic copper toxicosis. *Am J Clin Nutr* 1996;63:842S–846S.
39. Adelson JQ. Indian childhood cirrhosis is a result of copper hepatotoxicity—in all likelihood. *J Pediatr Gastroenterol Nutr* 1987;6:491–492.
40. Müller T, Feichtinger H, Berger H, Müller W. Endemic Tyrolean infantile cirrhosis: an ecogenetic disorder. *Lancet* 1996;347:877–880.
41. Manzler AD, Schreiner AW. Copper-induced acute hemolytic anemia: a new complication of hemodialysis. *Ann Intern Med* 1970;73:409–412.
42. Sandstead HH. Requirements and toxicity of essential trace elements, illustrated by zinc and copper. *Am J Clin Nutr* 1995;61(Suppl):621S–624S.
43. Zenz CL. *Occupational medicine, principles and practice,* 3rd ed. New York: Elsevier Science, 1994.
44. Andrews AC, Lyons TD. Binding of histamine and antihistamine to bovine serum albumin by mediation with Cu (II). *Science* 1957;126:561.
45. Lyle WH, Payton JC, Hui M. Hemodialysis and copper fever. *Lancet* 1973;1:1324–1325.
46. Pimentel JC, Marques F. "Vineyard sprayer's lung": a new occupational disease. *Thorax* 1969;24:678–688.
47. Pimental JC, Menezes AP. Liver granulomas containing copper in vineyard sprayer's lung: a new etiology of hepatic granulomatosis. *Am Rev Respir Dis* 1975;111:189–195.
48. Holland MK, White IG. Heavy metals and human spermatozoa: III. The toxicity of copper ions for spermatozoa. *Contraception* 1988;38:685–695.
49. Agarqal K, Sharma A, Talukder G. Effects of copper on mammalian cell components. *Chem Biol Interact* 1989;69:1–16.
50. Lee AM, Fraumeni JF. Arsenic and respiratory cancer in man: an occupational study. *J Natl Cancer Inst* 1969;42:1045–1049.
51. Chen R, Wei L, Huang H. Mortality from lung cancer among copper miners. *Br J Ind Med* 1993;50:505–509.

52. Armstrong C, Moore L, Hackler R, et al. An outbreak of metal fume fever, diagnostic use of urinary copper and zinc determinations. *J Occup Med* 1983;25:886–888.
53. Hazardous Substances Data Bank. *Copper.* National Library of Medicine. http://toxnet.nlm.nih.gov
54. Wallach J. *Interpretation of diagnostic tests,* 6th ed. New York: Little, Brown and Company, 1996.
55. American Congress of Government Industrial Hygienists. *Threshold limit values and biological exposure indices for 1995–1996.* Cincinnati: American Congress of Government Industrial Hygienists, 1995.
56. Lauwerys RR, Hoet P. *Industrial chemical exposure, guidelines for biological monitoring,* 2nd ed. Ann Arbor, MI: Lewis Publishers, 1993.

CHAPTER 76
Zinc

Donald C. Fisher

SOURCES AND PRODUCTION

Zinc is a bluish-white soft metal placed in group IIB of the periodic table. It is always divalent. Table 76-1 lists its basic properties. In dry air, it is highly resistant to attack except at temperatures exceeding 225°C. In moist air, attack proceeds at room temperature. A light-gray film of hydrated basic carbonate forms on the surface in the presence of CO_2 and protects the metal from further corrosion. When heated to temperatures higher than 500°C, zinc volatilizes into small zinc oxide particles that rapidly flocculate as they cool, forming fumes. The principal mineral of zinc is sphalerite. Zinc constitutes approximately 0.02% of the earth's crust and is distributed widely. It is a relatively poor conductor of electricity and heat (1–3).

SITES, INDUSTRIES, AND BUSINESSES ASSOCIATED WITH EXPOSURE

Zinc has been used as an alloy with copper and tin since ancient times but probably was not recognized as a separate entity until the fifteenth century. Early Egyptian and other Mediterranean peoples may have used zinc as a topical ointment. Commercial production of zinc began in the eighteenth century (3). As of 1994, 6.8 million metric tons were produced worldwide, of which the United States contributed 5%. Chile, Canada, Australia, and Russia are the principal producers. After 1991, zinc was no longer considered a strategic metal, and the sale of the national defense stockpiles was authorized (4).

Zinc ore is processed by crushing and then concentrating to 50% to 60% metal by flotation. This concentrate is roasted to remove sulfur and then is processed further by either smelting or electrolytic refining. Smelted zinc contains impurities of other metals (lead, copper, and cadmium) and is suitable for galvanizing, spraying, annealing, and painting. Electrolytic refining produces high-grade zinc (in excess of 99.99% pure) suitable for alloys and die casting (1–4).

TABLE 76-1. Properties of zinc

Atomic weight	65.38
Specific gravity	7.14
Melting point	419.4°C
Boiling point	907°C

TABLE 76-2. Common zinc compounds and their uses

Compound (common name)	Uses
Zinc acetate	Wood preserving, mordant, glazes, reagent
Zinc carbonate	Pigment, feed additive, manufacture of porcelains, pottery, rubber
Zinc chloride	Deodorant, disinfectant, wood preservative, fireproofing, soldering flux, cement, mordant, petroleum refining, textile treatment, vulcanizing rubber, solvent for cellulose; manufacture of activated carbon, paper, glues, and dye
Zinc chromate (VI), hydroxide (zinc yellow, buttercup yellow)	Pigment in paint, oil, varnish, linoleum, rubber
Zinc cyanide	Electroplating, removing NH_2 from gas
Zinc fluoride	Fluoridation of organic compounds, glazes, enamels, wood preserving, electroplating; manufacture of phosphors for fluorescent lights
Zinc oxide (flowers of zinc, philosopher's wool, zinc white)	Pigments, cements, glass, tires, glue, matches, white ink, reagent, photocopy paper, flame retardant, semiconductor, fungicide, cosmetics, dental cements
Zinc phosphide	Rodenticide
Zinc silicate	Television screens, neon lights
Zinc stearate	Tablet and rubber manufacture; cosmetic and pharmaceutical powders; ointments, waterproofing, releasing agent in manufacture of plastics
Zinc sulfate (white vitriol, zinc vitriol)	Mordant, wood preserving, paper bleaching, reagent, manufacture of Zn salts, electrodeposition of Zn
Zinc sulfide (zinc blende)	Pigment (manufacture of luminous dials, x-ray and television screens)

Metallic zinc is used principally in galvanizing iron and steel to prevent corrosion and oxidation. Zinc metal also is die-cast for automotive components, electrical equipment, tools, hardware, toys, and fancy goods. Alloys of zinc include combinations with lead, cadmium, iron, tin, copper, aluminum, magnesium, and titanium. Alloys generally enhance zinc's galvanizing and die-casting characteristics (1–4). Table 76-2 lists important zinc compounds and their main uses (1–6). Of these compounds, zinc oxide is used most widely. Some of the occupations involving exposure to zinc and zinc compounds are alloy makers, embalmers, petroleum refinery workers, and welders and solderers.

CLINICAL TOXICOLOGY

Routes of Exposure

The most common route of exposure to zinc is that of diet. Inhalation of zinc fumes and dust occurs in some of the aforementioned industrial settings. Absorption occurs across broken epithelium when zinc oxide is applied to treat burns or wounds (3).

Absorption, Metabolism, and Elimination

ABSORPTION

Absorption of zinc occurs throughout the intestine but mainly in the jejunum (7). The mechanism of passage through the gastrointestinal mucosa is not understood completely but involves metallothionein binding or other zinc-protein complexes in luminal cells. Absorption ranges from 25% to 90% after ^{65}Zn oral administration in humans and is influenced by dietary factors. Zinc absorption is decreased when consumed with some vegetable proteins, calcium, and phosphorus but is increased when consumed with animal proteins (3). Prasad (8) noted that, after oral administration of ^{65}Zn, measurable zinc levels were found in the blood within 15 to 20 minutes, with peak levels in 2 to 4 hours. Plasma and serum levels were higher than in whole blood (8).

METABOLISM

Significant concentrations occur in the pancreas, prostate, kidney, liver, muscles, and retina. As many as 300 enzymes require zinc for optimal function. Zinc also interacts with proteins to regulate DNA and RNA synthesis and to modulate neurotransmission. It is required for growth hormone, helps to maintain cell membrane structural integrity, and retains antioxidant properties by inducing metallothionein production (7).

ELIMINATION

Zinc's biological half-life exceeds 300 days. A total of 70% to 80% of ingested zinc is excreted in the feces via bile and pancreatic secretions, which are enhanced by dietary protein of plant origin. Urinary and sweat excretion together account for roughly 15% but, in hot climates, 25% can be excreted by sweating alone. Breast milk also contains significant concentrations of zinc (2,3,7,8).

Signs, Symptoms, and Syndromes

ACUTE TOXICITY

Acute symptoms of oral zinc poisoning are primarily gastrointestinal. Symptoms include nausea, vomiting, abdominal pain, diarrhea, and hematemesis. Fever also is reported. With supportive care, zinc toxicity usually is self-limited, and resolution of symptoms occurs in a matter of hours or days.

Skin. Owing to its caustic action, zinc chloride can cause ulcerations and dermatitis of the exposed skin (9). Zinc pyrithione, a common constituent of shampoos, and zinc diethyldithiocarbamate contained in rubber prosthetic sleeves also are reported to cause dermatitis, as confirmed by patch testing (10,11). Zinc oxide dust may give rise to papular, pustular eczema by blocking sebaceous glands (2).

Eye. Both zinc chloride and zinc sulfate can cause significant eye injuries. Redness and persistent discomfort occur after exposure to concentrated solutions of either salt. Within 6 days, a discrete stromal opacity of the cornea develops, along with irregularity of the overlying epithelium. Lens opacities, iritis, and glaucoma may occur after splashing of concentrated (50%) zinc chloride solution (12).

Respiratory System. Most zinc salts irritate mucous membranes of the upper respiratory tract after inhalation. Cough and dyspnea followed by the gradual onset of adult respiratory distress syndrome and death, resulting from delayed pulmonary vascular fibrosis, have been reported with inhalation of zinc chloride smoke from smoke bombs (13,14). Inhalation of zinc oxide dust and fumes can produce metal fume fever; however, no changes in lung function occur between pre–work shift and post–work shift values or between early and late work-week values (15).

Gastrointestinal System. Gastrointestinal effects occur after ingestion of zinc chloride and zinc phosphide or from drinking acidic beverages from galvanized containers (2). These effects include abdominal pain, nausea, vomiting, diarrhea, and hematemesis. Zinc chloride has been found to cause esophagitis (16,17) and mucosal burns of the stomach (18). The toxicity of zinc phosphide probably is due to release of phosphine, which occurs on contact with water and is accelerated by an acidic environment (19,20). Nausea, vomiting, and jaundice occur after intravenous zinc poisoning (21).

Renal System. Microhematuria has been reported after zinc chloride ingestion (16). Acute tubular necrosis, probably due to hypoxia, was found in soldiers after fatal adult respiratory distress syndrome caused by zinc chloride smoke inhalation (22). Oliguria and renal failure occurred after iatrogenic intravenous overadministration of zinc sulfate (21).

Neurologic System. Lethargy follows ingestion of zinc chloride (16–18,23) and elemental zinc (23). Symptoms are reversible with treatment. Fatigue is associated with zinc metal fume fever (24).

Hematologic System. Chronic ingestion of high doses of supplemental zinc (more than 100 mg per day) gives rise to sideroblastic anemia and leukopenia from induced copper deficiency. The anemia and leukopenia reverse, with or without copper replacement, after cessation of zinc supplements (25,26). Leukocytosis can occur in zinc metal fume fever (see Syndromes).

CHRONIC AND LONG-TERM EFFECTS

Other than producing corneal and lens opacities after ocular zinc salt injury and anemia from zinc-induced copper deficiency, zinc toxicity does not result in any known chronic effects.

SYNDROMES: METAL FUME FEVER

Exposure to freshly generated zinc oxide fumes, usually from welding of galvanized iron, commonly leads to metal fume fever. The syndrome consists of a sweet metallic taste, dry cough, shortness of breath, fatigue, myalgias, fever, and chills beginning 4 to 12 hours after exposure. Other terms for the syndrome include *brass ague*, *brass chills*, *spelter shakes*, *zinc chills*, and *Monday morning fever*. Fever may reach 40°C and is followed by profuse diaphoresis and rigorous shakes. The white cell count may reach 20,000 during the illness. Symptoms generally persist for 1 to 3 hours but, even in severe cases, total recovery occurs within 24 to 48 hours. No long-term sequelae are observed. Tolerance is gained rapidly after repeat exposures but also is lost quickly, such that a more pronounced manifestation of the illness occurs after short duration of nonexposure followed by reexposure (hence the term *Monday morning fever*) (2,5,24). Cytokine production in bronchoalveolar lavage fluid corresponds to temporal and dose-dependent clinical findings after zinc oxide inhalation (27).

TERATOGENICITY AND CARCINOGENICITY

Zinc toxicity appears not to be teratogenic, although zinc deficiency is (28).

Testicular teratomas and seminomas as well as lung reticulosarcomas have occurred in birds and rodents when insoluble zinc salts in high concentrations are injected into these tissues. Zinc chromate is a suspected human carcinogen owing to hexavalent chromium (29,30). However, no evidence substantiates zinc carcinogenicity in humans (28).

Management of Toxicity

CLINICAL EXAMINATION

Evaluating patients with acute onset of nausea, vomiting, and abdominal pain after ingestion of solder flux, moss killer, or disinfectants should lead clinicians to suspect zinc chloride poisoning. Drinking acidic beverages from galvanized containers is a potential source of elemental zinc toxicity. Examination of the upper gastrointestinal tract should be conducted for mucosal burns and bleeding if hematemesis or guaiac-positive stools are encountered or if symptoms include abdominal or chest pain. Urine output must be monitored. When inhalation of zinc chloride or zinc phosphide is suspected, careful examination of the lungs and upper respiratory tract is warranted. Special consideration should be given to delayed-onset pulmonary edema, which may not develop until several days after acute inhalation of zinc chloride smoke. In patients with anemia and normal iron stores, chronic abuse of zinc-containing multivitamins or zinc supplements should be considered.

LABORATORY DIAGNOSIS

After acute zinc chloride ingestion, abnormal laboratory values have included elevations in serum zinc, glucose, amylase, lipase, and alkaline phosphatase. Serum zinc levels may be elevated slightly during bouts of metal fume fever (179 µg per dL; normal, 55 to 150 µg per dL) (24). Metal fume fever also causes leukocytosis (up to 20,000 white blood cells per cubic centimeter), with a left shift, and may elevate the lactate dehydrogenase level. Pulmonary function may be diminished, and patchy infiltrates on radiography may be seen during the episode. All findings return to normal during recovery (2,5).

In zinc-induced copper deficiency anemia, serum copper, ceruloplasmin, hemoglobin, hematocrit, red cell indices, and reticulocyte count are depressed. Serum zinc may be either normal or elevated. Serum iron level and total iron-binding capacity are normal. Ringed sideroblasts are seen on peripheral blood smears (26).

TREATMENT

Treatment for acute zinc toxicity is supportive. After oral ingestion of zinc or zinc salts, treatment should be directed toward control of nausea, vomiting, and diarrhea. Induced emesis, gastric lavage, or activated charcoal usually are unnecessary but may be useful in cases of substantial ingestion of zinc tablets or capsules. In the case of zinc phosphide, water should not be given with ipecac or gastric lavage, and activated charcoal should be mixed with sorbitol instead of water to minimize liberation of phosphine (19). Fluid and electrolyte imbalances must be corrected. Upper gastrointestinal mucosal burns should be treated with H_2 receptor antagonists, sucralfate, or antacids. Calcium disodium–ethylenediaminetetraacetic acid (16,17) and dimercaprol (21) have been successful in lowering serum zinc levels.

Supportive care also is indicated for acute zinc chloride inhalation. This may require ventilatory support with positive end-expiratory pressure, antibiotics, steroids, and maintenance of cardiac output. Inhalation of zinc oxide fumes and development of metal fume fever require nonspecific treatment after the patient has been removed from exposure, adequate engineering controls have been ensured, or an appropriate personal protective device has been provided. Treatment of zinc-induced copper deficiency requires discontinuation of supplemental zinc and therapy with oral or intravenous copper if necessary.

BIOLOGICAL MONITORING: BLOOD, PLASMA, AND URINE

For workers repeatedly exposed to zinc or zinc salts, preplacement and periodic examinations should include recording of a baseline history, a physical examination, a complete blood count, and spirometry. Zinc concentrations in humans are highest in the prostate and retina (500 mg per kg). High levels are found also in bone, kidney, liver, muscle, and pancreas (7). Concentrations of zinc in serum and plasma are near 1 µg per mL (100 µg per dL). The zinc concentration in blood is fivefold higher than that in plasma, owing to zinc concentration in erythrocytes (31).

TABLE 76-3. U.S. Occupational Safety and Health Administration permissible exposure limits for zinc compounds

Compound	TWA (mg/m^3)	STEL (mg/m^3)
Zinc chloride fumes	1	2
Zinc chromate (as CrO_3)	0.01	—
Zinc oxide fumes	5	10
Zinc oxide dust		
Total dust	10	—
Respirable fraction	5	—
Zinc stearate		
Total dust	10	—
Respirable fraction	5	—

STEL, short-term exposure limit; TWA, 8-hour time-weighted average.

Urinary excretion of zinc in humans not occupationally exposed is approximately 0.5 mg per 24-hour urine collection (29). Occupational exposure to zinc can produce a plasma concentration of 1.4 µm per mL and urinary concentrations of 800 µg per gram of creatinine (29). Biological limit values cannot be established, owing to lack of reliable exposure and dose-and-effect relationships (32).

OCCUPATIONAL AND ENVIRONMENTAL REGULATIONS

The recommended daily allowance for zinc is 15 mg per day for men, 12 mg per day for women, 10 mg per day for children, and 5 mg per day for infants. The U.S. Environmental Protection Agency recommends no more than 5 ppm in drinking water. Table 76-3 lists the U.S. Occupational Safety and Health Administration's permissible exposure limits, which include the 8-hour time-weighted average and the short-term exposure limit, for zinc chloride, zinc chromate, zinc dust and fumes, and zinc stearate dust and fumes.

EXPOSURE CONTROLS

Workplace zinc fumes should be maintained at less than 5 mg per cubic meter by engineering controls, such as appropriate exhaust ventilation. Use of personal protective devices (respirators) should be limited to short exposures that occur during performance of unusual jobs (5). Monitoring should be carried out any time for changes in work process or procedure that may cause an increase in zinc fumes or dusts.

ENVIRONMENTAL FATE AND TRANSPORT

Zinc is found in the earth's crust at approximately 40 mg per kg. The principal anthropogenic sources are mining and refining, primarily from blasting, crushing, and wet flotation. Significant soil contamination is found only near point sources.

REFERENCES

1. Cumpston AG. Zinc, alloys and compounds. In: *Encyclopedia of occupational safety and health,* 2nd ed. Geneva: International Labor Office Press, 1984.
2. Beliles RP. The metals. In: Patty FA, ed. *Industrial hygiene and toxicology,* 4th ed. New York: Wiley-Interscience Publishers, 1994.
3. National Research Council, Committee on medical and biologic effects of environmental pollutants. *Zinc.* Baltimore: University Park Press, 1979.
4. US Bureau of Mines. Salient zinc statistics. Washington: 1994.

5. Zenz CL. *Occupational medicine, principles and practice,* 3rd ed. New York: Elsevier Science, 1994.
6. National Institute of Occupational Safety and Health. *Occupational diseases: a guide to their recognition.* Washington: US Department of Health, Education, and Welfare, 1977.
7. Walsh CT, Sandstead HH, Prasad AS, Hewberne PM, Fraker PJ. Zinc. Health effects and research priorities for the 1990s. *Environ Health Perspect* 1994;102(Suppl 2):5–46.
8. Prasad AS. *Zinc metabolism.* Springfield, IL: Charles C Thomas Publisher, 1966.
9. Adams RM. *Occupational skin diseases,* 2nd ed. San Diego: Grune & Stratton, 1990.
10. Nigam PK, Tyagi S, Saxena AK, Misra, RS. Dermatitis from zinc pyrithione. *Contact Dermatitis* 1988;19:219.
11. Baptista A, Barros MA, Azenha A. Allergic contact dermatitis on an amputation stump. *Contact Dermatitis* 1992;26:140–141.
12. Grant WM. *Toxicology of the eye,* 3rd ed. Springfield, IL: Charles C Thomas Publisher, 1986.
13. Marrs TC, Colgrave HF, Edginton JAG, Brown RFR, Cross NL. The repeated dose toxicity of a zinc oxide/hexa-chloroethane smoke. *Arch Toxicol* 1988;62:123–132.
14. Homma S, Jones R, Qvist J, Zapol WM, Reid L. Pulmonary vascular lesions in the adult respiratory distress syndrome caused by inhalation of zinc chloride smoke: a morphometric study. *Hum Pathol* 1992;23:45–50.
15. Marquart H, Staid T, Heederik D, Visschers M. Lung function of welders of zinc-coated mild steel: cross-sectional analysis and changes over five consecutive work shifts. *Am J Ind Med* 1989;16:289–296.
16. Chobanian SJ. Accidental ingestion of liquid zinc chloride: local and systemic effects. *Ann Emerg Med* 1981;10:91–93.
17. Potter JL. Acute zinc chloride ingestion in a young child. *Ann Emerg Med* 1981;10:267–269.
18. Hedtke J, Daya MR, Nease G, Burton BT. Local and systemic toxicity following zinc chloride ingestion [abst]. Presented at the American Academy of Clinical Toxicology annual meeting, Atlanta, October 11–14, 1989.
19. Mack RB. A hard day's knight: zinc phosphide poisoning. *N C Med J* 1989; 50:17–18.
20. Casteel SW, Bailey EM. A review of zinc phosphide poisoning. *Vet Hum Toxicol* 1986;28:151–154.
21. Brocks A, Reid H, Glazer G. Acute intravenous zinc poisoning. *BMJ* 1977;1: 1390–1391.
22. Hjortso E, Qvist J, Thomsen JL, et al. ARDS after accidental inhalation of zinc chloride smoke. *Intensive Care Med* 1988;14:17–24.
23. Murphy JV. Intoxication following ingestion of elemental zinc. *JAMA* 1970;212:2119–2120.
24. Noel NE, Ruthman JC. Elevated serum zinc levels in metal fume fever. *Am J Emerg Med* 1988;6:609–610.
25. Prasad AS. Essentiality and toxicity of zinc. *Scand J Work Environ Health* 1993;19(Suppl 1):134–136.
26. Fiske DN, McCoy HE, Kitchens CS. Zinc-induced sideroblastic anemia: report of a case, review of the literature, and description of the hematologic syndrome. *Am J Hematol* 1994;46:147–150.
27. Blanc PD, Boushey HA, Wong H, Wintermeyer SF, Bernstein MS. Cytokines in metal fume fever. *Am Rev Respir Dis* 1993;147:134–138.
28. Leonard A, Ferber GB, Leonard F. Mutagenicity, carcinogenicity and teratogenicity of zinc. *Mutat Res* 1986;168:343–353.
29. American Congress of Governmental Industrial Hygienists. *Threshold limit values and biological exposure indices for 1995–1996.* Cincinnati: American Congress of Governmental Industrial Hygienists, 1995.
30. Dalager NA, Mason TJ, Fraumeni JF, Hoover R, Payne WW. Cancer mortality among workers exposed to zinc chromate paints. *J Occup Med* 1989;22:25–29.
31. Elinder C. Zinc. In: *Handbook on the toxicology of metals,* 2nd ed. New York: Elsevier Science, 1986:664–679.
32. Lauwerys RR, Hoet P. *Industrial chemical exposure: guidelines for biological monitoring,* 2nd ed. Ann Arbor: Lewis Publishers, 1993.

CHAPTER 77
Nickel

F. William Sunderman, Jr.

CHEMICAL AND PHYSICAL FORMS

Nickel (atomic number, 28; atomic weight, 58.7; boiling point, 2,732°C; specific gravity, 8.9 at 25°C) was discovered and named by Cronstedt in 1751. It is the twenty-fourth element in order of natural abundance in the earth's crust. Nickel from natural sources is a mixture of five stable isotopes; nine unstable nickel isotopes have also been identified. Nickel comprises 5% to 50% of the weight of meteorites, and an abundance of nickel helps to distinguish meteorites from other minerals. Major deposits of nickel ores are located in Australia, Canada, Cuba, Indonesia, New Caledonia, and Russia. Ores of commercial importance are either oxidic (e.g., laterite ores, which contain mixed Ni-Fe oxides) or sulfidic [e.g., pentlandite, $(NiFe)_9S_8$]. Annual worldwide production of nickel is approximately 70 million kg.

Nickel exists in five major forms: (i) elemental nickel and its alloys, (ii) inorganic, water-soluble nickel compounds, (iii) inorganic, water-insoluble nickel compounds, (iv) organic, water-insoluble nickel compounds, and (v) nickel carbonyl. The oxidation states of nickel include 0, +1, +2, +3, and +4, but the prevalent valences are 0 [e.g., in nickel metal, nickel alloys, and $Ni(CO)_4$] and +2 [e.g., in $NiCl_2$, $NiSO_4$, $Ni(OH)_2$, and NiO]. Because the nickel atom has unpaired electrons in two outer 3d orbitals, nickel can undergo redox reactions that involve one-electron transfers. As a consequence, nickel compounds participate in free-radical reactions that contribute to their toxicity and carcinogenicity.

Nickel is a silver-white, lustrous, hard, malleable, ductile, ferromagnetic metal that is relatively resistant to corrosion and is a fair conductor of heat and electricity. In crystalline compounds, nickel commonly is found either in the α-form (with a hexagonal lattice), or in the β-form (with a cubic lattice). In aqueous solutions, nickel exists principally as hexaquonickel ion $[Ni(H_2O)^{2+}]$, which is emerald green in color. Nickel monoxide occurs in two major forms, each of which exhibits different properties: black NiO, which is chemically reactive and readily yields nickel salts on contact with mineral acids, and green NiO, which is relatively inert and refractory to solubilization in dilute acids. Nickel carbide is a heat-resistant compound used to coat the turbine vanes of high-compression jet engines. Nickel carbonyl is a colorless liquid that boils at 43°C and decomposes at 60°C, producing carbon monoxide and finely powdered metallic nickel. $Ni(CO)_4$ decays spontaneously in air, with a half-life of approximately 30 minutes. The volatility and lipid solubility of $Ni(CO)_4$ enable it to cross cell membranes, and the redox reactivity of $Ni(CO)_4$ contributes to its high toxicity.

EXPOSURE SOURCES

Industrial operations that entail particular exposures of workers to nickel include the following: mining, roasting, smelting, and electrowinning nickel ores and concentrates; casting, grinding, and polishing nickel alloys (e.g., stainless steel, Monel metal, Nichrome); producing and processing nickel salts; electroplating; arc welding, plasma spraying, and flame cutting; fabricating Ni-Cd batteries; producing molds for the hollow-glass industry; making coins, jewelry, cutlery, and medical or dental implants; applying nickel glazes to ceramics; painting with nickel pigments (e.g., yellow nickel titanate); manufacturing electrical resistors, magnetic tapes, and computer components; producing and using nickel catalysts (e.g., Raney nickel) for hydrogenation of soaps, fats, and oils; using $Ni(CO)_4$ as a gaseous intermediate in the Mond reaction for nickel refining, as a catalyst for organic syntheses, or as a vehicle for vapor-deposition of nickel; producing cement; incinerating or reprocessing nickel-containing wastes; and combusting fossil fuels (1).

ENVIRONMENTAL EXPOSURES

Water Sources

Nickel enters groundwater and surface waters from dissolution of rocks and soils, biological cycles, atmospheric fallout, industrial processes, and waste disposal (1). Nickel leached from dump sites can contribute to nickel contamination of the aquifer, with potential ecotoxicity. Most inorganic nickel compounds are relatively soluble at pH values of less than 6.5, whereas nickel exists predominantly as insoluble hydroxides at pH values in excess of 6.7. Therefore, acid rain has a tendency to mobilize nickel from soil and increase the nickel concentration in groundwater, leading eventually to increased uptake and possible toxicity in microorganisms, plants, and animals. Sea water contains 0.1 to 0.5 μg of nickel per L. Surface waters average 15 to 20 μg of nickel per L and drinking water usually contains less than 20 μg of nickel per L. Drinking water occasionally has much higher nickel concentrations, owing to pollution of the water supply or leaching from nickel-containing pipes and nickel-plated faucets. For example, the nickel concentrations in municipal water samples collected in 1989 at five locations in Sudbury, Ontario, Canada, averaged 109 μg per L (range, 65 to 179 μg per L), attributable to local deposits of nickel ore and pollution from nickel mines and smelters (2).

Air Sources

Nickel enters the atmosphere from natural sources (e.g., volcanic emissions and windblown dusts produced by weathering of rocks and soils), combustion of fossil fuels, emissions of mining and refining operations, metal consumption in industrial processes, and incineration of wastes (1). Atmospheric concentrations of nickel in urban areas often are related to the consumption of fossil fuels as, for example, the nickel content of coal ranges from 4 to 24 mg per kg. Substantial atmospheric emissions of nickel are derived from fly-ash released from coal-fired power plants; nickel derived from petroleum is released into the environment in automotive exhaust fumes. As a result of such factors, atmospheric nickel concentrations in the United States are substantially lower in rural areas (average, 6 ng per cubic meter) than in towns and cities (average, 17 ng per cubic meter in summer, 25 ng per cubic meter in winter). Cigarette smoking can increase the amount of inhaled nickel by as much as 4 μg per pack of cigarettes (1).

Other Sources

The dietary intake of nickel by adult persons averages approximately 165 μg per day but may reach 900 μg per day in diets rich in oatmeal, cocoa, chocolate, nuts, and soya products (1,3,4). Wearing or handling of jewelry, coins, and utensils that are fabricated from nickel alloys or that have nickel-plated coatings can induce allergic dermatitis (5). Nickel salts of fatty acids (e.g., nickel laurate), used in paper coatings for pressure-sensitive forms, are another source of contact dermatitis. Implantation of nickel-containing prostheses or iatrogenic administration of nickel-contaminated medications or media (e.g., albumin, radiocontrast agents, hemodialysis fluids) leads to parenteral exposures, which can cause acute toxicity and immunologic disturbances (1,2,6–8).

ABSORPTION, METABOLISM, AND ELIMINATION

In fasting human volunteers who ingested an oral dose of $NiSO_4$ (12 to 50 μg per kg of body weight, added to drinking water), the alimentary absorption of nickel averaged 27% [standard deviation (SD), ± 17] of the dose. However, when the $NiSO_4$ was mixed with food, the volunteers absorbed only 0.7% (SD, ± 0.4) of the oral dose. Thus, the alimentary absorption of nickel is greatly influenced by dietary constituents (4).

In nickel refinery workers, inhaled nickel dust is retained in the nasal sinuses and lungs for many years after the cessation of exposure; some of the nickel is slowly absorbed, as evidenced by sustained hypernickelemia in retired refinery workers (9). Studies of acutely poisoned workers and animal experiments show that inhaled $Ni(CO)_4$ vapor is absorbed rapidly via the lung and enters erythrocytes, where the compound undergoes conversion to Ni^{2+} and carbon monoxide (10). During extracorporeal hemodialysis, traces of Ni^{2+} in hemodialysis fluid are absorbed into the plasma, owing to the chelating action of plasma albumin (2,11).

The metabolism and distribution of Ni^{2+} in humans have been fitted by a two-compartment toxicokinetic model (4,12). In human plasma, Ni^{2+} is bound to ultrafilterable constituents (e.g., histidine), albumin, and nickeloplasmin (an α_2-macroglobulin) (13). On the basis of analyses of tissues obtained at autopsy from human subjects without known occupational exposures to nickel, the mean nickel concentrations of tissues are ranked here in order of highest to lowest concentration: lung, thyroid, adrenal gland, kidney, heart, liver, brain, spleen, and pancreas (14,15). In adult humans, the body burden of nickel is estimated to average approximately 0.5 mg per 70 kg (i.e., approximately 7.3 μg per kg of body weight) (16). In tissue cytosol, nickel is bound to several proteins and peptides (17,18). Rodent studies indicate that Ni^{2+} induces metallothionein synthesis in kidney and liver, but Ni^{2+} evidently does not bind to metallothioneins in these tissues (19).

Urine is the major route for elimination of absorbed nickel. In 50 healthy persons without occupational exposures, urinary nickel excretion averaged 2.6 (SD, ± 1.4) μg per day (3). In volunteers who ingested $NiSO_4$, the renal nickel elimination half-time averaged 28 (SD, ± 9) hours; the renal clearance of nickel absorbed from drinking water averaged 8.3 (SD, ± 2.0) mL per minute per 1.73 square meters of body surface area (4). Most nickel in food remains unabsorbed in the alimentary tract and passes through into the feces, averaging 158 (SD, ± 75) μg per day (4). Nickel concentrations in postmortem samples of human bile range from 1 to 3 μg per L, suggesting that biliary excretion of nickel may be quantitatively significant (14). Sweat, saliva, gastric and intestinal secretions, hair, dermal detritus, fingernails, mother's milk, menses, and the placenta are minor routes or vehicles for nickel elimination in humans (3,20,21).

CLINICAL TOXICOLOGY

Respiratory exposure is of paramount importance in nickel carcinogenesis. The respiratory, oral, and parenteral exposure routes are important for acute nickel toxicity (e.g., inhalation of $Ni(CO)_4$; ingestion of nickel-contaminated beverages and foods; implantation of nickel-containing devices; administration of nickel-contaminated medications). Dermal exposure is primarily responsible for nickel dermatitis, although oral or parenteral exposures to nickel can potentiate hand eczema in nickel-sensitive persons (22).

Acute Nickel Carbonyl Poisoning

Accidental inhalation of $Ni(CO)_4$ generally causes acute toxic effects in two stages, immediate and delayed (23–26). The immediate symptoms (e.g., headache, vertigo, nausea, vomiting, insomnia, irritability) usually last a few hours, followed by an asymptomatic interval of 12 hours to 5 days, before the onset of delayed pulmonary, cardiac, and neurologic symptoms (e.g., tightness of the chest, nonproductive cough, dyspnea, cyanosis, tachycardia, palpitations, sweating, visual disturbances, vertigo, weakness, lassitude). The delayed symptoms often mimic viral pneumonia. In cases of severe $Ni(CO)_4$ poisoning, deaths have occurred 4 to 13 days after exposure. Autopsies have revealed pulmonary hemorrhage, proteinaceous alveolar exudate, interstitial pneumonitis, damage to alveolar lining cells, and denudation of bronchial epithelium. Pathologic lesions (e.g., parenchymal degeneration, edema, punctate hemorrhages) have also been noted in the brain, liver, kidney, adrenal glands, and spleen. In survivors, the recovery period tends to be protracted, with lassitude and dyspnea persisting up to 6 months (23–26).

Acute Nickel Pneumonitis

Accidental inhalation of metallic nickel particles can cause acute pneumonitis. For example, a welder died from acute respiratory distress syndrome after inhalation of a finely particulate nickel fume that was produced by a metal arc-welding process (27). The authors of the report on this event stressed that workers should wear respiratory protective equipment while welding with nickel wire electrodes.

Acute Toxicity from Divalent Nickel

Acute Ni^{2+} toxicity occurred when 32 electroplating workers accidentally drank water contaminated with $NiSO_4$ and $NiCl_2$ (1.6 g of nickel per L) (28). Twenty of the workers promptly developed symptoms (e.g., nausea, vomiting, abdominal discomfort, diarrhea, giddiness, lassitude, headache, cough, shortness of breath) that generally ceased within a few hours, but symptoms persisted for 1 to 2 days in seven cases. In workers with symptoms, the estimated nickel doses ranged from approximately 0.5 to 2.5 g. All the subjects recovered rapidly, without evident sequelae, and returned to work by the eighth day after exposure. Acute Ni^{2+} toxicity also occurred when 23 hemodialysis patients were exposed to nickel-contaminated dialysis fluid, owing to leaching of a nickel-plated heating tank (6). Symptoms (nausea, vomiting, weakness, headache, palpitations) developed during the dialysis treatment and generally lasted a few hours, but symptoms persisted for 2 days in some subjects; no adverse sequelae were noted.

Chronic Toxicity

ALLERGIC AND IMMUNOLOGIC EFFECTS

Allergy to nickel alloys and nickel compounds is one of the most common causes of contact dermatitis throughout the world; positive dermal patch tests to nickel occur in 7% to 10% of women and 1% to 3% of men in the general population (5,22). Dermal sensitization frequently occurs from exposures to nickel-containing coins, jewelry, watch cases, and clothing fasteners. Nickel dermatitis typically begins as a papulovesicular erythema of the hands, forearms, earlobes, or other areas of skin that contact nickel alloys, and spreads secondarily to areas (usually symmetric) that are distant from the contact sites. The erythematous lesions become eczematous and eventually undergo lichenification. Pompholyx (i.e., dyshidrotic eczema) is the predominant type of nickel-induced dermatitis, characteristically affecting the sides of the fingers, the palms, and sometimes the soles. Nickel hypersensitivity can cause pulmonary asthma, eosinophilic pneumonitis, conjunctivitis, inflammatory reactions around nickel-containing implants (e.g., orthopedic prostheses, dental inlays or bridges, cardiac valve prostheses, pacemaker wires), and anaphylactoid reactions after parenteral injection of nickel-contaminated medications (1,3).

RESPIRATORY EFFECTS

Chronic respiratory insufficiency may develop as a consequence of acute $Ni(CO)_4$ poisoning (26). In workers in nickel refineries, plating shops, or welding shops, inhalation of irritant nickel-containing dusts and aerosols may contribute to chronic respiratory diseases, including asthma, bronchitis, and pneumoconiosis (29). The workers may develop hypertrophic rhinitis, sinusitis, nasal polyposis, nasal septal perforations, and anosmia. Incidences of such nonneoplastic respiratory diseases in nickel-exposed workers have not been thoroughly studied, and the etiologic role of nickel is often unclear, as the affected workers generally are exposed to sundry dusts and vapors in addition to nickel compounds (29).

RENAL EFFECTS

Workers who are heavily exposed to soluble nickel compounds may develop mild renal tubular dysfunction, as evidenced by increased urinary excretion of β_2-microglobulin and *N*-acetylglucosaminidase (30,31).

REPRODUCTIVE EFFECTS

Increased incidences of congenital defects and spontaneous or threatened abortion were observed in a study of 758 Russian women who were employed in a nickel hydrometallurgy refining plant (32). Congenital malformations were present in 17% of live-born infants of the nickel-exposed mothers, as compared to 6% of live-born infants of a reference population of female construction workers. A sixfold increase in the relative risk of cardiovascular defects was noted in the infants of nickel-exposed women. Spontaneous and threatened abortions were noted in 16% and 17%, respectively, of all pregnancies in the nickel-exposed workers, as compared with 9% and 8%, respectively, in the reference group. In light of these findings and the teratogenic effects of nickel compounds for rodents and other animals (33), further investigations are needed of the adverse reproductive effects in nickel-exposed women.

CARCINOGENESIS

Epidemiologic studies have demonstrated increased mortality from carcinomas of the lung and nasal cavities in nickel refinery workers who were chronically exposed to inhalation of nickel-containing dusts and fumes from roasting, smelting, and electrolysis processes (34). Increased risks of other malignant tumors, including carcinomas of the larynx, kidney, prostate, and stomach and soft-tissue sarcomas, have occasionally been noted, but the statistical significance of these findings is doubtful. The respiratory tract cancers in nickel refinery workers have been associated with inhalation exposures to nickel compounds with low aqueous solubility (e.g., αNi_3S_2, NiO), as well as soluble nickel compounds (e.g., $NiSO_4$). Based on an evaluation of these epidemiologic studies, the International Agency for Research on Cancer Working Group on the Evaluation of the Carcinogenic Risks to Humans concluded: "There is sufficient evidence in humans for the carcinogenicity of nickel sulfate and of the combinations of nickel sulfides and oxides encountered in the nickel refining industry. There is inadequate evidence in humans for the carcinogenicity of nickel and nickel alloys." Based on an overall evaluation of human and animal data, the International Agency for Research on Cancer Working Group classified nickel compounds as carcinogenic to humans (group 1) and metallic nickel as possibly carcinogenic to humans (group 2B) (35).

A study of workers at a Norwegian nickel refinery points to a multiplicative effect of the risk of lung cancer from smoking and exposure to nickel compounds (36). An investigation of respiratory tract cancers in former workers at a Canadian nickel sinter plant demonstrated that the excess risk of death from cancers of the lung or nasal cavities continued for as long as 30 to 40 years after leaving the sinter plant (34). Remarkably, a person's age at first exposure to nickel had no effect on the risk of death from either lung or nasal cancers. The sustained risks of death from respiratory tract cancer in nickel refinery workers, even after nickel exposure has ceased, may reflect long-term persistence of carcinogenic nickel compounds in the respiratory tract mucosa (9,37,38).

Clinical Management

ACUTE NICKEL CARBONYL POISONING

After accidental exposure to $Ni(CO)_4$, the victim should be quickly transported to a hospital, after removal of contaminated clothing, institution of life support measures, and administration of oxygen (23,24). The immediate therapy is similar to that for acute carbon monoxide poisoning. Hyperglycemia and glycosuria typically develop after exposure to $Ni(CO)_4$. An acute exposure to $Ni(CO)_4$ is classified as *mild* if the initial 8-hour urine collection reveals a nickel concentration of less than 100 μg per L; *moderate* if the nickel concentration in the initial 8-hour urine collection is greater than 100 but less than 500 μg per L; and *severe* if the nickel concentration is greater than 500 μg per L. Patients in the moderate and severe categories of acute $Ni(CO)_4$ poisoning should be treated immediately with a chelating drug, sodium diethyldithiocarbamate (DDC) (23,24). The beneficial effect of DDC in acute $Ni(CO)_4$ poisoning has been attributed to diminution of the pulmonary nickel burden (39).

ACUTE POISONING FROM DIVALENT NICKEL

Presumptive diagnosis of acute Ni^{2+} poisoning is based on the clinical history and analysis of nickel in the exposure medium (28). The immediate supportive treatment is to maintain body temperature, because Ni^{2+} impairs thermoregulation, and to induce diuresis by administration of intravenous fluids, because Ni^{2+} is eliminated primarily via the urine. Confirmation of the diagnosis rests on quantitative determinations of nickel in body fluids, usually serum and urine.

In 20 electroplating workers (mentioned earlier) who developed acute symptoms after ingesting Ni^{2+}-contaminated water, the serum nickel concentrations averaged 286 μg per L (range, 13 to 1,340 μg per L), and urine nickel concentrations averaged 5.8 mg per L (range, 0.23 to 37.0 mg per L) on the day after exposure (28). For comparison, the reference intervals for nickel concentrations in healthy, nonexposed persons ranged from less than 0.05 to 1.10 μg per L in serum and 0.5 to 6.1 μg per L in urine. Ten severely exposed workers were treated by intravenous infusion of isotonic sodium chloride solution at 150 mL per hour for 3 days. The half-time for urinary elimination of nickel in these subjects averaged 27 hours (SD, ± 7), which was significantly shorter than the mean half-time of 60 ± 11 hours in subjects with less severe symptoms who did not receive intravenous fluids. Transient hyperbilirubinemia, proteinuria, and reticulocytosis occurred in some patients, but all recovered uneventfully (28).

Hemodialysis would be the therapy of choice for patients with acute Ni^{2+} poisoning, if renal function fails, or if cardiotoxicity and neurotoxicity become life-threatening. In contrast to $Ni(CO)_4$ poisoning, chelation with DDC would not be advised in severe Ni^{2+} toxicity, as DDC enhances the cerebral uptake of Ni^{2+} in rodents (40,41).

BIOLOGICAL AND MEDICAL MONITORING

Biological Monitoring

Urine is the most practical specimen for biological monitoring of occupational, environmental, or iatrogenic exposures to nickel compounds. In industrial workers, urine collections generally are performed at the end of the work shift, after the subject has washed and changed clothes. The urine is voided directly into an acid-washed plastic cup, with care to avoid nickel contamination. The advantages of urine are as follows: (i) A metal-free container is the only collection equipment that is needed; (ii) the collection procedure is painless and noninvasive; and (iii) nickel concentrations in urine specimens from healthy, nonexposed persons exceed the detection limits of electrothermal atomic absorption spectrometry with Zeeman background correction. Nickel concentrations are approximately eight-fold higher in urine than in serum. The disadvantages of urine as a specimen for biological monitoring of nickel exposures include (i) high matrix variability, (ii) fluctuating specific gravity, (iii) inaccurate timing of urine collections, and (iv) possible contamination from nickel-containing dust on the clothing (3,42). Urine specimens are acidified before freezing to minimize loss of nickel by adsorption on the container or on urine sediment. Ancillary tests include measurements of urine specific gravity or creatinine, so that urinary nickel concentrations can be normalized to a specific gravity of 1.024, or expressed per gram of creatinine (3,42).

The advantages of serum for biological monitoring of nickel exposures include controlled sample collection, low matrix variation, and little diurnal fluctuation, but a disadvantage is that nickel concentrations in serum specimens from healthy, nonexposed persons often are below the analytic detection limit. In patients with renal insufficiency who are treated by extracorporeal hemodialysis, urine seldom is available, so serum is the specimen of choice. To obtain serum specimens for nickel analysis, blood may be collected through a plastic intravenous cannula into an acid-washed plastic syringe. Alternatively, a steel needle can be employed, provided the first few milliliters of blood are discarded, having served to flush the needle. Plasma can be used in lieu of serum, but anticoagulants may pose problems; tests are needed to verify that heparin is free of nickel contamination or that ethylenediaminetetraacetic acid does not cause analytic interference. Analysis of nickel concentration in whole blood has little practical advantage for biological monitoring and is subject to matrix interference from iron in hemoglobin (3,42).

Feces are the best specimen for monitoring oral nickel intake. However, disadvantages of fecal nickel analyses include the problems of collecting feces for 3 to 5 days, pooling and homogenizing the specimens, digesting the samples with concentrated acids, and extracting nickel as a chelate into a solvent prior to analysis by electrothermal atomic absorption spectrometry. Nickel concentrations in saliva, hair, fingernails, sweat, milk, and blood lymphocytes sometimes are assayed in clinical investigations, but such tests seldom are practical for routine biological monitoring. Analysis of expired breath may be useful to detect $Ni(CO)_4$ after its inhalation (3,42).

Biological monitoring of nickel exposures is relatively free of problems from individual variability or lifestyle factors. Population surveys have not shown any significant differences between men and women or any age dependence of adults in regard to nickel concentrations in urine or serum. In one large study, smoking was associated with a slight elevation of urinary nickel concentration (43) but, in another study, no difference was noted between the serum nickel concentrations of smokers versus nonsmokers (44). In one study, alcohol consumption had no effect on urinary nickel concentrations (43) whereas, in another study, alcohol consumption was attended by slight elevation of serum nickel concentrations (44). Consumption of nickel-rich foods (especially chocolate) can cause mild elevation of urinary nickel concentrations, but this effect is insufficient to bias biological monitoring of nickel exposures (45).

Reviews on nickel analysis provide recommendations about specimen collection, transport, and storage, instrumental tech-

TABLE 77-1. Reference values for nickel concentrations in serum and urine of persons without occupational exposures to nickel compounds

Authors (reference)	Fluid	No. of subjects	Nickel concentration (mean ± SD) nmol/L	μg/L
Nixon et al. (47)	S	38	2.4 ± 1.5	0.14 ± 0.09
Gammelgaard and Veien (50)	S	20	2.4 ± 2.5	0.14 ± 0.15
Grandjean et al. (44)	S	162	4.1 ± 2.8	0.24 ± 0.16
Minoia et al. (51)	U	878	15 (2–66)[a]	0.9 (0.1–3.9)[a]
Angerer and Lehnert (52)	U	123	16 ± 24	0.9 ± 1.4
Ulrich et al. (53)	U	31	29 ± 17	1.7 ± 1.0

S, serum; SD, standard deviation; U, urine.
[a]Range of values.

niques, and quality assurance procedures (3,46–49). As the sensitivity of analytic methods has improved and nickel contamination has been reduced, the reference values for nickel concentrations in body fluids of healthy, nonexposed persons have gradually diminished. The reference values in Table 77-1 are illustrative of recent reports (44,47,50–53). Based on a critical evaluation of published data for nickel determinations in body fluids, the upper limit for serum nickel concentration is approximately 1 μg per L and the upper limit for urinary nickel concentration is approximately 6 μg per L in persons without occupational exposure (54).

Biological monitoring of nickel exposures is influenced by the elimination kinetics of nickel, which depend on the exposure routes and the chemical properties of the nickel compounds, especially in respect to aqueous solubility. Studies in nickel refineries have shown that biological monitoring programs can identify both individual workers who fail to adhere to recommended work practices and groups of workers with elevated nickel exposures (55,56). Nickel concentrations in urine or serum specimens from workers with inhalation exposures to soluble nickel salts (e.g., $NiCl_2$, $NiSO_4$) are generally proportional to the exposure levels and reflect the amount of nickel absorbed during the 1 or 2 preceding days. Absence of increased values usually indicates nonsignificant exposure, and presence of increased values should be a signal to reduce the exposure. In contrast, in workers with inhalation exposures to nickel powders, nickel alloys, and poorly soluble nickel compounds (e.g., αNi_3S_2, NiO), nickel concentrations in urine and serum specimens reflect the combined influences of recent exposures and long-term accumulation, as well as the bioavailability of the nickel species. In such workers, increased concentrations of nickel in body fluids generally are indicative of significant nickel absorption and should be a signal to reduce the exposures to the lowest levels attainable by current technology; absence of increased values does not necessarily indicate freedom from the health risk (e.g., cancers of the nasal cavities and lungs) that have been associated with chronic exposures to such compounds (3,42).

Medical Monitoring

Certain diagnostic tests may assist in detecting the pathologic sequelae of nickel exposures (3,42). These tests include (i) a dermal patch test and lymphocyte transformation assay to detect nickel allergy; (ii) urine β_2-microglobulin and *N*-acetylglucosaminidase assays to detect nephrotoxicity; (iii) pulmonary function tests; (iv) radiographic imaging of the lungs, mediastinum, and nasal cavities to detect pneumonitis, sinusitis, and tumors; and (v) biopsy and exfoliative cytology to detect respiratory tract dysplasia and neoplasia. Preneoplastic and neoplastic histologic abnormalities of the nasal mucosa have been observed in brush biopsy samples from nickel refinery workers, and malignancy-associated changes, including premalignant dysplasia, have been detected by imaging cytometry of nasal smears stained by the Papanicolaou technique (57). Preliminary reports have been published of enhanced tumor-associated antigens, oncogene expression, cytogenetic anomalies, and DNA-protein cross-links in blood specimens from nickel-exposed workers, but such findings require further clinical evaluation.

OCCUPATIONAL EXPOSURE REGULATIONS

Atmospheric limits for occupational exposures to nickel metal and sparingly soluble nickel compounds in various nations are as follows:

- 1 mg per cubic meter: Australia, Canada, Japan, Netherlands, United States
- 0.5 mg per cubic meter: Denmark, Germany, Russia, Sweden, United Kingdom
- 0.1 mg per cubic meter: Norway

The atmospheric limits for occupational exposures to soluble nickel compounds are as follows:

- 1 mg per cubic meter: Denmark, Japan, United States (Occupational Safety and Health Administration)
- 0.1 mg per cubic meter: Australia, Canada, Netherlands, Norway, Sweden, United Kingdom, United States (American Conference of Governmental Industrial Hygienists)
- 0.05 mg per cubic meter: Germany
- 0.005 mg per cubic meter: Russia

The atmospheric exposure limits for occupational exposure to $Ni(CO)_4$ are as follows:

- 7 μg nickel per cubic meter: Japan, United States
- 0.12 mg nickel per cubic meter: Australia
- 0.24 mg nickel per cubic meter: Germany
- 0.35 mg nickel per cubic meter: Canada, United Kingdom

In Germany, nickel metal, nickel sulfides and sulfidic ores, nickel oxides, and nickel carbonate, as they occur during production and use, are considered to be carcinogens, so that no Maximale Arbeitsplatz Konzentrationen limit has been established; only a technical guideline has been provided (58–61).

REFERENCES

1. Sunderman FW Jr, ed. Nickel in the human environment. *IARC Monogr Eval Carcinog Risks Hum* 1984;53:1–530.
2. Hopfer SM, Fay WP, Sunderman FW Jr. Serum nickel concentrations in hemodialysis patients with environmental exposure. *Ann Clin Lab Sci* 1989;19:161–167.
3. Sunderman FW Jr, Aitio A, Morgan LG, Norseth T. Biological monitoring of nickel. *Toxicol Ind Health* 1986;2:17–78.
4. Sunderman FW Jr, Hopfer SM, Sweeney KR, Marcus AH, Most BM, Creason J. Nickel absorption and kinetics in human volunteers. *Proc Soc Exp Biol Med* 1989;191:5–11.
5. Lidén C, Menné T, Burrows D. Nickel-containing alloys and platings and their ability to cause dermatitis. *Br J Dermatol* 1996;134:193–198.
6. Webster JD, Parker TF, Alfery AC, et al. Acute nickel poisoning by dialysis. *Ann Intern Med* 1980;92:631–633.
7. Leach CA Jr, Sunderman FW Jr. Hypernickelemia following coronary arteriography, caused by nickel in the radiographic contrast medium. *Ann Clin Lab Sci* 1987;17:137–144.
8. Sunderman FW Jr. Biological monitoring of metal exposures from joint implants. In: Buchhorn GH, Willert HG, eds. *Technical principles, design, and safety of joint implants.* Seattle: Hogrefe & Huber Publishers, 1994:184–187.

9. Torjussen W, Andersen I. Nickel concentrations in nasal mucosa, plasma, and urine in active and retired nickel workers. *Ann Clin Lab Sci* 1979;9:289–298.
10. Mikehyev MI. Distribution and excretion of nickel carbonyl. *Gig Trud Prof Zab* 1971;15:35–38.
11. Hopfer SM, Linden JV, Crisostomo MC, Catalanatto FA, Galen M, Sunderman FW Jr. Hypernickelemia in hemodialysis patients. *Trace Element Med* 1985;2:68–72.
12. Sunderman FW Jr. Toxicokinetics of nickel in humans. In: Nieboer E, Aitio A, eds. *Nickel and human health: current perspectives*. New York: John Wiley and Sons, 1992:69–76.
13. Nomoto S, Sunderman FW Jr. Presence of nickel in alpha-2 macroglobulin isolated from human serum by high performance liquid chromatography. *Ann Clin Lab Sci* 1988;18:78–84.
14. Rezuke WN, Knight JA, Sunderman FW Jr. Reference values for nickel concentrations in human tissues and bile. *Am J Ind Med* 1987;11:419–426.
15. Seemann J, Wittig P, Kollmeier H, Rothe G. Analytische Bestimmung von Cd, Pb, Zn, Cr und Ni in Humangewebe. *Lab Med* 1985;9:294–299.
16. Bennett BG. Environmental nickel pathways to man. *IARC Monogr Eval Carcinog Risks Hum* 1984;53:487–495.
17. Sarkar B. Nickel metabolism. *IARC Monogr Eval Carcinog Risks Hum* 1984;53:367–384.
18. Templeton DM, Sarkar B. Nickel binding to the C-terminal fragment of a peptide from human kidney. *Biochim Biophys Acta* 1986;884:382–386.
19. Sunderman FW Jr, Fraser CB. Effects of $NiCl_2$ and diethyldithiocarbamate on metallothionein in rat liver and kidney. *Ann Clin Lab Sci* 1983;13:489–495.
20. Centeno JA, Pestaner JP, Nieves S, Ramos M, Mullick FG, Kaler SG. The assessment of trace element and toxic metal levels in human placental tissues. In: Collery P, et al., eds. *Metal ions in biology and medicine*, vol 4. Paris: John Libby Eurotext, 1996:522–524.
21. Gammelgaard B, Peters K, Menné T. Reference values for nickel concentrations in human finger nails. *J Trace Elem Electrolytes Health Dis* 1991;5:121–123.
22. Maibach HI, Menné T, eds. *Nickel and the skin: immunology and toxicology.* Boca Raton, FL: CRC Press, 1989.
23. Sunderman FW, Sunderman FW Jr. Nickel poisoning VIII. Dithiocarb: a new therapeutic agent for persons exposed to nickel carbonyl. *Am J Med Sci* 1958;236:26–31.
24. Sunderman FW. The treatment of acute nickel carbonyl poisoning by sodium diethyldithiocarbamate. *Ann Clin Res* 1971;3:182–185.
25. Vuopala U, Huhti E, Takkunen J, Huikko M. Nickel carbonyl poisoning. Report of 25 cases. *Ann Clin Res* 1970;2:214–222.
26. Shi Z. Acute nickel carbonyl poisoning: a report of 179 cases. *Br J Ind Med* 1986;43:422–424.
27. Rendall REG, Phillips JI, Renton KA. Death following exposure to fine particulate nickel from a metal arc process. *Ann Occup Hyg* 1994;6:921–930.
28. Sunderman FW Jr, Dingle B, Hopfer SM, Swift T. Acute nickel toxicity in electroplating workers who accidentally ingested a solution of nickel sulfate and nickel chloride. *Am J Ind Med* 1988;14:257–266.
29. US Environmental Protection Agency. Health assessment document for nickel and nickel compounds. EPA report no. 600/8-83/012FF. Washington: US Environmental Protection Agency, 1986.
30. Sunderman FW Jr, Horak E. Biochemical indices of nephrotoxicity, exemplified by studies of nickel nephropathy. In: Brown SS, Davies DS, eds. *Organ-directed toxicity: chemical indices and mechanisms.* London: Pergamon Press, 1981:52–64.
31. Vyskocil A, Senft V, Viau C, Cizkova M, Kohout J. Biochemical renal changes in workers exposed to soluble nickel compounds. *Hum Exp Toxicol* 1994;13:257–261.
32. Chashschin VP, Artunina GP, Norseth T. Congenital defects, abortion, and other health effects in nickel refinery workers. *Sci Total Environ* 1994;148: 287–291.
33. Sunderman FW Jr, Reid MC, Shen SK, Kevorkian CB. Embryotoxicity and teratogenicity of nickel compounds. In: Clarkson TW, Nordberg GF, Sager PR, eds. *Reproductive and developmental toxicity of metals.* New York: Plenum Publishing, 1983:399–416.
34. Doll R, et al. Report of the international committee on nickel carcinogenesis in man. *Scand J Work Environ Hlth* 1990;16[Suppl]:9–84.
35. Nickel and nickel compounds. *IARC Monogr Eval Carcinog Risks Hum* 1990;49:257–445.
36. Andersen A, Berge SR, Engeland A, Norseth T. Exposure to nickel compounds and smoking in relation to incidence of lung and nasal cancer among nickel refinery workers. *Occup Environ Med* 1996;53:708–713.
37. Muir ECF, Jadon N, Julian JA, Roberts RS. Cancer of the respiratory tract in nickel sinter plant workers: effect of removal from sinter plant exposure. *Occup Environ Med* 1994;51:19–22.
38. Kaldor J, Peto J, Easton D, Doll R, Hermon C, Morgan L. Models for respiratory cancer in nickel refinery workers. *J Natl Cancer Inst* 1986;77:841–848.
39. Tjalve H, Jasim S, Oskarsson A. Nickel mobilization by sodium diethyldithiocarbamate in nickel-carbonyl-treated mice. *IARC Monogr Eval Carcinog Risks Hum* 1984;53:311–320.
40. Oskarsson A, Tjalve H. Effects of diethyldithiocarbamate and penicillamine on the tissue distribution of ^{63}Ni in mice. *Arch Toxicol* 1980;45:45–52.
41. Belliveau JF, O'Leary GP, Cadwell L, Sunderman FW Jr. Effect of diethyldithiocarbamate on nickel concentrations in tissues of $NiCl_2$-treated rats. *Ann Clin Lab Sci* 1985;15:349–350.
42. Sunderman FW Jr. Nickel. In: Clarkson TW, Friberg L, Nordberg GF, Sager PR, eds. *Biological monitoring of toxic metals.* New York: Plenum Publishing, 1988:265–282.
43. Alessio L, Apostoli P, Crippa M. Influence of individual factors and personal habits on the levels of biological indicators of exposure. *Toxicol Lett* 1995;77:93–103.
44. Grandjean P, Nielsen GD, Jorgensen J, Horder M. Reference intervals for trace elements in blood: significance of risk factors. *Scand J Clin Lab Invest* 1992;52:321–337.
45. Sunderman FW Jr, Hopfer SM, Crisostoma MC, Stoeppler M. Rapid analysis of nickel in urine by electrothermal atomic absorption spectrophotometry. *Ann Clin Lab Sci* 1986;16:219–230.
46. Sunderman FW Jr, Hopfer SM, Crisostomo MC. Nickel analysis by atomic absorption spectrometry. *Methods Enzymol* 1988;158:382–391.
47. Nixon DE, Moyer TP, Squillace DP, McCarthy JT. Determination of serum nickel by graphite furnace atomic absorption spectrometry with Zeeman-effect background correction: values in a normal population and a population undergoing dialysis. *Analyst* 1989;114:1671–1674.
48. Templeton DM. Measurement of total nickel in body fluids. Electrothermal atomic absorption methods and sources of preanalytical variation. *Pure Appl Chem* 1994;66:357–372.
49. Cornelis R, Heinzow B, Herber RFM, et al. Sample collection guidelines for trace elements in blood and urine. *J Trace Elements Med Biol* 1996;10:103–127.
50. Gammelgaard B, Veien NK. Nickel in nails, hair and plasma from nickel-hypersensitive women. *Acta Dermatol Venereol* 1990;70:417–420.
51. Minoia C, Sabbioni E, Apostoli P, et al. Trace element reference values in tissues from inhabitants of the European community: I. A study of 46 elements in urine, blood and serum of Italian subjects. *Sci Total Environ* 1990;95:89–105.
52. Angerer J, Lehnert G. Occupational chronic exposure to metals: II. Nickel exposure of stainless steel welders: biological monitoring. *Int Arch Occup Environ Health* 1990;62:7–10.
53. Ulrich L, Sulcova M, Spacek L, Neumanova E, Vladar M. Investigation of professional nickel exposure in nickel refinery workers. *Sci Total Environ* 1991;101:91–96.
54. Templeton DM, Sunderman FW Jr, Herber RFM. Tentative reference values for nickel concentrations in human serum, plasma, blood, and urine: evaluation according to the TRACY protocol. *Sci Total Environ* 1994;148:243–251.
55. Hogetveit AC, Barton RT, Andersen I. Variations of nickel in plasma and urine during the work period. *J Occup Med* 1980;22:597–600.
56. Morgan LG, Rouge PJC. Biological monitoring in nickel refinery workers. *IARC Monogr Eval Carcinog Risks Hum* 1984;53:507–520.
57. Reith AK, Reichborn-Kjennerud S, Aubele M, Jutting U, Gais P, Burger G. Biological monitoring of chemical exposure in nickel workers by imaging cytometry of nasal smears. *Analyt Cell Pathol* 1994;6:9–21.
58. Sunderman FW Jr. Mechanisms of nickel carcinogenesis. *Scand J Work Environ Health* 1989;15:1–12.
59. Hertel RF, Maass T, Müller VR. *Nickel: environmental health criteria.* Geneva: World Health Organization, 1991;108:1–383.
60. Nieboer E, Nriagu JO. *Nickel and human health: current perspectives.* New York: John Wiley and Sons, 1992:1–680.
61. *Safe use of nickel in the workplace.* Toronto: Nickel Development Institute, 1994:1–65.

CHAPTER 78

*Platinum and Related Metals: Palladium, Iridium, Osmium, Rhodium, and Ruthenium**

Peter L. Goering

Platinum and the Pt-group metals—palladium, rhodium, ruthenium, iridium, and osmium—are grouped into two triads within group VIII of the periodic table of elements. The first triad, consisting of the lighter elements (Ru, Rh, and Pd), is directly above the triad consisting of the heavier elements (Os, Ir, and Pt). These elements, collectively termed the *platinoids*, are of high commercial value because of their great resistance to most corrosive agents. The platinoids and their alloys appear in

*The views stated in this chapter are not to be construed as official policy of the U.S. Food and Drug Administration.

the chemical, petroleum, electrical, nuclear power, and automotive industries and in jewelry. Pt salts are used as catalysts in automotive and chemical industries. The metals in this group generally are nontoxic in the metallic state, but the soluble halide salts (particularly of Pt) and osmium tetroxide are highly reactive. Exposure to these elements results in hypersensitivity allergic reactions in susceptible individuals.

Pt, like gold, is a biologically nonessential metal being used clinically: Pt complexes for cancer chemotherapy and gold complexes for rheumatoid arthritis. The Pt chemotherapeutic compounds (e.g., cisplatin and carboplatin) are used to treat testicular, ovarian, bladder, prostate, thyroid, head, and neck tumors that are unresponsive to standard chemotherapy. The use of these compounds is limited because renal, gastrointestinal, hematologic, and otologic toxicities may occur. The platinoids are not essential elements in mammals.

SOURCES AND PRODUCTION

Chemical Forms

Many complex salts of the Pt metals exist, but the most common are platinum chloride (platinum tetrachloride, platinic chloride, $PtCl_4$); platinum dichloride (platinous chloride, $PtCl_2$); platinum dioxide (platinic oxide, PtO_2); and platinum sulfate [platinic sulfate, $Pt(SO_4)_2$]. Water-soluble Pt salts possessing reactive halogenated ligands eliciting strong hypersensitivity allergic reactions include ammonium and sodium chloroplatinates; sodium, potassium, and ammonium tetrachloroplatinates; and sodium, potassium, and ammonium hexachloroplatinates (Table 78-1) (1).

The platinoids form an important group of commercial metal alloys. Many of these alloys, such as Pt-Ir, are used for applications in which high corrosion resistance is needed. Uses of other alloys include Pt black (catalyst), Pt-Co (permanent magnets), and Pt-Rh (catalyst) (2). In clinical medicine, the two chemotherapeutic Pt complexes used most widely are *cis*-diaminedichloroplatinum(II) (cisplatin) and *cis*-diamine(1,1-cyclobutane dicarboxylato)platinum(II) (carboplatin).

The oxidation states of Pt most biologically relevant in chemical complexes are 2+ (II) and 4+ (IV). The coordination chemistry of Pt(II) complexes is square-planar, whereas that of Pt(IV) complexes is octahedral. These complexes are very stable, forming covalent attachments to various ligands that are relatively inert to ligand substitution (3). Others report that the square-planar (but not the octahedral) configuration is highly labile (4).

Other platinoids possess valence states ranging from 2+ to 8+. In biological media, Rh, Ru, and Ir (but not Pd and Os) form stable compounds with a coordination number of 6 and an octahedral configuration. Simple salts, such as chlorides, bromides, and sulfates, and complex hexamine and tetramine salts of the platinoids are water-soluble (4).

Ru can exhibit valence states from +2 to +8, but +3 is the most common. $Ru(OH)_2$, $RuCl_4$, and RuO_2 are stable and water-soluble, but generally the trivalent salts are not soluble. Rh forms salts with valence states +2, +3, and +4. The chloride, nitrate, and sulfate salts and the soluble hexachloro complexes are trivalent (4).

Pd salts are water-soluble and form divalent and tetravalent salts. Pd compounds include palladium chloride, palladium iodide, palladium oxide, palladium nitrite, and palladium nitrate. Pd coordination complexes have not been demonstrated to be present in biological systems. Ir forms divalent, trivalent, and tetravalent compounds. Divalent halide and sulfate salts are water-soluble, as are the anionic hexachloroiridates and hexaoxaloiridates (4).

Stable forms of Os exhibit valences of +3, +4, and +8. The tri- and tetrahalides and tetroxides are water-soluble, and OsO_4^{2-} is slightly soluble (4).

TABLE 78-1. Common platinum compounds

Compound	Formula
Hexachloroplatinic acid	$H_2[PtCl_6]$
Sodium tetrachloroplatinic acid	Na_2PtCl_4
Ammonium hexachloroplatinic acid	$(NH_4)_2PtCl_6$
Sodium hexachloroplatinic acid	Na_2PtCl_6
Platinic chloride (Pt tetrachloride)	$PtCl_4$
Platinous chloride (Pt dichloride)	$PtCl_2$
Platinic oxide	PtO_2
Platinic sulfate	$Pt(SO_4)_2$

Physical Forms

Metallic Pt is available in several forms: powder (Pt black); single crystalline solids; wire (0.05 to 0.005 diameter); and other compositions used for electronics, metallizing, and decorating ceramics and metals (5). Powdered Pt black is finely divided metallic Pt and is flammable when exposed to air. Soluble salts exist and are the most toxic forms. The other platinoids exist as fumes and dusts in metallic form, and the soluble salts exist as crystalline solids (5).

EXPOSURE SOURCES: ENVIRONMENTAL, OCCUPATIONAL, AND CLINICAL

World production of new platinoid metals (not recycled) was reported in 1988 to be approximately 200 tons. Pt and Pd constitute 45% each of that amount, Rh and Ru approximately 4% each, and Os and Ir less than 1% each (6,7). These elements are dispersed widely worldwide, but the most economically significant deposits occur at parts per million (ppm) levels in ores that contain significant deposits of copper and nickel. The main geographic sites for obtaining ore containing platinoid metals are in Sudbury, Ontario, Canada; the Bushveld Igneous Complex, South Africa; near Norils'k, Siberia, and in the Kola Peninsula, Russia (3). Russia and South Africa produce 90% of all mined Pt. Other deposits are found in the Ural Mountains (Russia), in Colombia, and in some of the western United States (8). Compound mineral species include sperrylite ($PtAs_2$); cooperite (PtS); and braggite (Pt, Pd, Ni)S (3,8).

Table 78-2 lists the industries and businesses in which Pt and Pt metals are used, with the percentage of total based on 1985

TABLE 78-2. Industries, businesses, and processes associated with platinoid exposure

Industry, business, or process
Primary production (mining and refining)
Recycling platinoid-containing products for extraction
Automotive
Electrical
Petroleum refining
Chemical
Ceramics, glass
Jewelry, arts
Dentistry
Pharmaceutical

estimates (9). The platinoids are of such value that end products are recycled to extract these metals. Most of the commercial applications exploit the catalytic activities, nobility (resistance to oxidation), and strength (at high temperatures) of these elements. The chemical industry uses Pt-Rh catalysts for production of nitric acid and spinnerets for rayon, glass fiber, and Plexiglas manufacture. The electrical industry uses Pd contacts and Pt-Ir spark plugs. Pt is used for jewelry and surgical implants. The pharmaceutical industry produces some drugs and vitamins with Pt catalysts, mostly in hydrogenation or dehydrogenation reactions. Pt, Pd, and Rh are used as catalysts in the automotive industry, which dominates use of this metal (approximately 50%) as a result of serving as a component of catalytic converters for air pollution abatement (3,5,10). These metals catalyze the oxidation of combustion by-products, which reduces the amount of hydrocarbons, carbon monoxide, and nitrogen oxides emitted into the environment (7).

Alloys of Pt-Ir are the most important commercial alloys because they are harder and more resistant to chemical attack than is Pt alone. Such alloys are used for jewelry, electrical contacts, fuse wire, and hypodermic needles. Pt-Co alloys have been developed into powerful magnets and are used in hearing aids, self-winding watches, and dental alloys (9). Uses for other Pt alloys include dentistry, electroplating, and surgical wire (2). Pd also is used in dental alloys (11,12).

Research laboratories are the major consumers of Os in the form of osmium tetroxide which, when reduced, serves as a black tissue stain for electron microscopy. Osmium-carbohydrate polymers exhibit potent antiinflammatory properties in experimental studies (13). Soluble salts of Rh are used in electroplating, and metallic Rh is used in the manufacture of high-reflectivity mirrors.

Most unintentional exposure to platinoid metals is due to poor industrial and occupational hygiene. Platinoid metals are mined, refined, and used as components in a number of commercial chemical processes; thus, workers can be exposed at any number of steps during production. In these production and manufacturing steps, workers can be exposed through inhalational, dermal, and oral routes.

Ore mined for platinoid metal extraction is concentrated initially by crushing and flotation and then is smelted to produce a copper-nickel sulfide matte containing the platinoid metals. After further concentration processes, the metal-rich substance is refined in hydrochloric acid and chlorine. After distillation, Pt solutions are treated with ammonium chloride to precipitate ammonium hexachloroplatinate, which is redissolved and refined (14). Hexachloroplatinic(IV) acid is the starting material for most Pt compounds and preparations.

Industrial processing of platinoids may lead to inadvertent exposures. The petroleum industry uses Pt as a catalyst in a proprietary process known as *platforming*, in which Pt catalyzes the isomerization of hydrocarbons in gasoline to increase its octane content. "Platfining" and "platreating" are proprietary processes for the treatment of hydrocarbon mixtures to remove deleterious material, such as sulfur and nitrogen, to aid in the synthesis of hydrocarbons for petrochemical production (5).

Os poisoning occurs via inhalation of OsO_4, which readily vaporizes from aqueous solutions at room temperature. The alloy Os-Ir readily releases OsO_4 vapor at the high temperatures used for annealing processes (4).

Exposure to Pt complexes may occur in the clinical situation. Cisplatin is a very effective chemotherapeutic agent for treating a variety of solid tumors. Since its introduction into clinical practice in 1972, cisplatin administered alone or in combination with other chemotherapeutic agents has assumed a major role in the treatment of malignant testicular tumors and ovarian cancers (15,16). Cisplatin also may be useful alone or in combination in treating other solid tumors, such as carcinomas of the bladder, lung, head and neck, endometrium, esophagus, and stomach. The compound has demonstrated some activity in treating lymphomas and osteogenic sarcomas (15,16). The cisplatin analog carboplatin has been approved for use in the treatment of small-cell lung cancer and recurrent ovarian cancer (17). Carboplatin exhibits fewer toxic side effects than does cisplatin but possesses comparable antitumor efficacy. Radioisotopic forms of the Pt-group metals, such as ^{103}Pd, ^{192}Ir, and ^{109}Ru, are used clinically for brachytherapy, the technique of implanting irradiation sources directly into tumors (18).

CLINICAL TOXICOLOGY

Route of Exposure

With the exception of those investigating Pt compounds, very few experimental reports describe the biochemistry, metabolism, and toxicology of the platinoids and their salts in mammalian systems. Several available clinical studies evaluated inadvertent human exposures to Pt salts via the inhalational and dermal routes. The antitumor compounds cisplatin and carboplatin are administered intravenously and have been well studied. Studies of the metabolism of platinoids deal mostly in radioactive salts obtained from nuclear fission products. From the viewpoint of clinical toxicology, the most important human routes of exposure to the platinoids are inhalation and dermal contact, with oral exposure being much less significant. These exposures occur primarily in occupations that use platinoid metals (e.g., Pt separation plants and catalyst manufacture). No evidence corroborates excessive exposure of the general population to the platinoids as a result of environmental mobilization and excessive emissions from mining and refining practices. This results, at least in part, from the commercial value and high prices of these metals, which drive industrial practices toward retrieving and recycling to minimize the loss of these metals. Despite these practices, elevated soil concentrations of Pt group metals (Pt, Pd, and Rh) have been reported near highways, most likely attributable to the exhaust of these metals from automobile catalytic converters (19). The highest soil levels of the Pt group metals are reported near urban roads with high traffic densities, and lower levels occur next to rural and suburban roads with lower traffic densities (20).

Absorption, Distribution, and Elimination

ABSORPTION

Absorption of the platinoids from inhalational and dermal routes is high (4). Oral absorption of the platinoids is very low. Studies using experimental animals have shown that absorption of the platinoids via parenteral routes (subcutaneous, intramuscular, intraperitoneal) other than intravenous is negligible, with significant retention of metal salts at the injection sites (4).

DISTRIBUTION

After inhalation, a majority of the dose of platinoid metals and salts is retained in the lungs and respiratory tract. After intravenous injection, most platinoids distribute to soft tissues, mainly kidney, liver, muscle, and spleen (4). Very little evidence substantiates long-term accumulation of the platinoids in these tissues, except for Ru, which is retained in bone.

As cisplatin is not effective when administered orally, some studies have used intravenous bolus injections. These studies have demonstrated that the drug has an initial plasma half-life of 25 to 50 minutes, followed by a slower phase with a half-life of 58 to 73 hours. Approximately 90% of the Pt in blood is protein-bound 2 to 4 hours after administration (21). Concentrations of the non-protein-bound and, thus, biologically active form of cisplatin decline much more rapidly in plasma, with the initial alpha-phase half-life of 8 to 30 minutes and the slower phase from 40 to 48 minutes. By 4 to 5 hours, non-protein-bound drug accounts for less than 2% to 3% of total circulating Pt (22). Cisplatin distributes primarily to kidney, liver, intestines, and testes, and a small percentage is capable of penetrating the central nervous system. Elevated levels of Pt persist in liver and kidney for 2 to 4 weeks (21,22).

In vivo, cisplatin can react with water in a nonenzymatic manner to form monoaquo and diaquo species after dissociation of the chloride groups (15). These metabolites extensively bind to protein (more than 90%) and thus have minimal cytotoxicities, but the non-protein-bound, ultrafilterable reactive species are cytotoxic.

The pharmacokinetic behavior of Pt administered as the cisplatin analog carboplatin differs strikingly from Pt administered as cisplatin. Carboplatin is well tolerated and does not induce nephrotoxicity. Thrombocytopenia is the major dose-limiting side effect. The pharmacokinetic differences between the two drugs most likely are related to the difference between the bidentate leaving group present in carboplatin as opposed to the two chlorine groups in cisplatin, the latter being more susceptible to hydrolysis (Fig. 78-1). In addition, carboplatin binds to plasma proteins much more slowly and much less avidly than does cisplatin. Ultrafilterable (non-protein-bound) Pt in carboplatin has a much longer half-life (170 versus 30 minutes) than does cisplatin (23).

EXCRETION

Excretion of the platinoid salts after intravenous injection occurs mainly via urine. Approximately 20% to 45% of a dose of Pt, Rh, and Ru is excreted within 24 hours, and 80% of the dose is excreted in urine in 1 week. Orally administered platinoids are excreted primarily in feces (4).

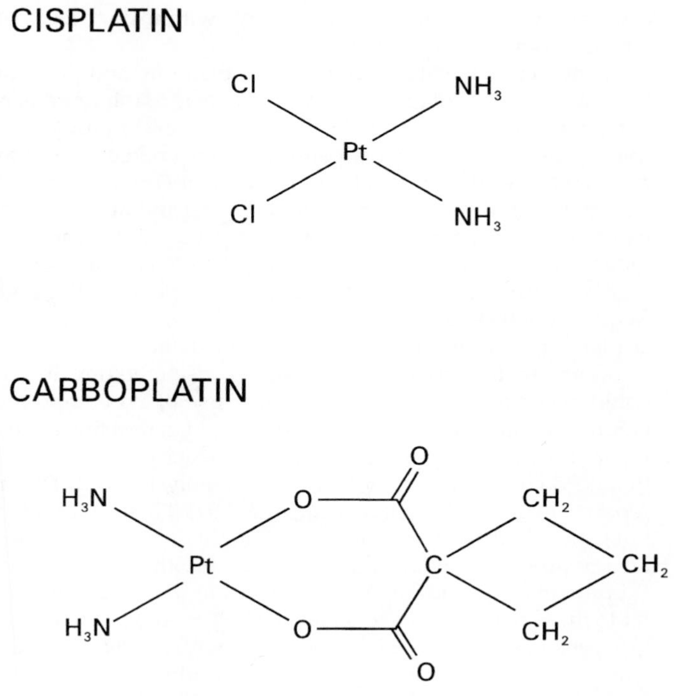

CISPLATIN

CARBOPLATIN

Figure 78-1. Basic structures of the chemotherapeutic platinum compounds cisplatin and carboplatin.

Excretion of cisplatin is biphasic and occurs primarily via the urinary route. Approximately 20% of an intravenous bolus injection of cisplatin is excreted in urine during the initial 6 hours, with 40% to 50% of the dose recovered in urine within 5 days. Elimination kinetics change when cisplatin is administered by infusion; the plasma half-life is reduced, and more drug is excreted (21,24). A higher percentage of a dose of carboplatin than cisplatin is excreted in the urine (25), and most of the dose is excreted during the initial 24 hours after injection (26).

Signs, Symptoms, and Syndromes from Exposure

ACUTE TOXICITY

After inhalation and dermal exposures, Pt oxides, and soluble Pt salts can act as irritants or sensitizers (allergens). Pt refinery workers with work-related respiratory symptoms have a high probability of having Pt salt allergy. Aerosols of ammonium tetrachloroplatinite(II) and ammonium hexachloroplatinate(IV) and airborne dust particles that contain the salts of these acids are the main occupational sensitizing agents. Metallic elemental Pt seems to be inert, with an exception possibly being the very fine powdered form. The latency period of sensitization may last for weeks or several months but could take years of working with Pt compounds prior to its occurrence (6).

After sensitization has taken place, signs and symptoms of exposure by the inhalational and dermal routes are asthma, conjunctivitis, urticaria, dermatitis, and eczema (Table 78-3). Exposure to Pt salts in the workplace has been associated with the onset of occupational asthma; a high proportion of workers who develop sensitivity to Pt previously were insensitive to other environmental allergens (27,28). A syndrome formerly termed *platinosis* can manifest the following symptomatology: lacrimation, sneezing, rhinorrhea, cough, dyspnea, bronchial asthma (from chloroplatinates), and cyanosis (29). The term *platinosis* is misleading in that it suggests the presence of pneumoconiosis and fibrosis, neither of which has been described as part of the Pt allergy syndrome. A more correct description for this syndrome is "allergy to Pt compounds containing reactive halogen ligands" (10,14,30). These aforementioned symptoms may be mediated via an immediate (type 1) hypersensitivity or via a delayed (type IV) hypersensitivity reaction (the latter occurring within 24 hours). The common skin lesions appear mainly between the fingers and in the antecubital fossae. The dermatitis reported in Pt refinery workers has been classified in the past as a type IV reaction (contact dermatitis); however, the dermatitis seen is of a primary irritant type, such as would follow exposure to strong acids and

TABLE 78-3. Clinical signs and symptoms of platinum allergy after inhalational, dermal, and ocular exposure

Upper respiratory	Lacrimation
Rhinorrhea	Redness
Sneezing	Itching
Itching of nose, throat, palate	Photophobia
Nasal congestion	Dermal
Lower respiratory	Urticaria
Cough	Angioedema
Dyspnea	Eczema
Asthmatic wheezing	Contact dermatitis
Cyanosis	Pruritus
Ocular	Systemic
Conjunctivitis	Lymphocytosis
Edema	Eosinophilia

Adapted with permission from ref. 9.

alkalis (30). As is the case with occupational asthma caused by exposure to various allergens, workers have reported continuing symptoms despite removal from the source of exposure (28,31).

The allergic reaction described is classified as a type I immediate hypersensitivity because it has been shown to be mediated by immunoglobulin E (IgE), including release of histamine from mast cells. The Pt complexes are too small to be allergens and must combine with a large-molecular-weight carrier, such as human serum albumin, to form a hapten capable of eliciting specific antibodies. Although IgE antibodies mediate the immediate reaction after reexposure, IgG antibodies are responsible for the delayed effects (6).

Cisplatin is a widely used chemotherapeutic agent with an antitumor activity mainly attributed to covalent binding to DNA (intrastrand cross-links between adjacent purines) and inhibition of DNA replication (32). Early clinical trials with cisplatin revealed that nephrotoxicity was the major dose-limiting effect that occurred in approximately two-thirds of patients. The incidence of this effect has been reduced markedly by the use of pretherapy hydration and diuretics, by altering the dosing regimen, or by both modalities (33). In humans, acute tubular necrosis is evident in the third segment (*pars recta*) of the proximal tubule (the distal convoluted tubule) and the collecting duct. In animal and human studies, cisplatin nephrotoxicity is manifested clinically by elevations in blood urea nitrogen and serum creatinine; proteinuria; enzymuria (as site-specific enzymes serve as biomarkers for specific damaged tubule cell populations); hyperuricemia; decreased creatinine clearance, glomerular filtration, and renal plasma flow; and increased urinary excretion of β_2-microglobulin (15,34).

The exact mechanism by which cisplatin-induced renal injury is produced is not clear. The main cell type damaged by cisplatin is the proximal convoluted tubule, although many other sites along the nephron may be injured. The role that the Pt atom itself plays in the nephrotoxic response is unclear. Administration of cisplatin and transplatin results in comparable renal concentrations of Pt; however, only the *cis* isomer is nephrotoxic (and has antitumor activity), indicating that the geometry of these complexes is important in the development of renal injury. Furthermore, the functional groups of the Pt complexes can modify the nephrotoxic effect significantly. These findings have supported the conclusion that cisplatin nephrotoxicity is related to the formation of an electrophilic metabolite, such as an aquated or hydroxylated form of cisplatin (34). Evidence for several mechanisms exists, including covalent binding of reactive metabolites to tissue macromolecules, such as proteins, lipids, or nucleic acids (34). Cisplatin has been shown to bind to sulfhydryl-containing cellular constituents, and toxicity may be related to decreases in cellular glutathione, formation of cytotoxic platinum-methionine complexes, or both (35). Cisplatin toxicity may be related to production of free radicals, such as superoxide anion, and lipid peroxidation (36–38). The mitochondrion is the primary organelle damaged by cisplatin in renal cells, and the associated cellular events include depletion of glutathione, increased lipid peroxidation, and disruption of calcium homeostasis (39,40).

Other effects associated with cisplatin use are gastrointestinal disturbances, myelosuppression, allergic reactions, and electrolyte disturbances. Cisplatin most likely will induce gastrointestinal disturbances manifested as nausea and vomiting, but diarrhea is uncommon (21,33). Mild to moderate myelosuppression occurs in most patients with transient leukopenia and thrombocytopenia. Hypersensitivity reactions to cisplatin and carboplatin are rare, but several case reports have described effects that range from skin rashes and facial edema to bronchoconstriction, tachycardia, hypotension, and anaphylaxis (41–43). The primary electrolyte alteration has been hypomagnesemia, which may be related to toxic action on kidney tubule ion transport processes (15,21).

Despite possessing comparable antitumor efficacy, the cisplatin analog carboplatin has been shown to be less toxic except for myelosuppression (44,45). Concomitant high-dose antiemetic treatment and extensive hydration are not necessary with carboplatin.

Generally, very few studies have reported cases of adverse human health effects associated with occupational or environmental exposure to Ru, Rh, Ir, and Pd (6); however, Ru tetroxide fumes are highly injurious to both lungs and eyes. The compound can be classified as a respiratory irritant because nasal ulcerations and discoloration of respiratory mucous membranes can occur (4,6). Industrial poisoning from Ir and Rh is rare. A recent case report describes an Ir chloride worker who developed respiratory tract symptoms and contact urticaria (46). Results from an Ir-Cl skin-prick test were positive, and Pt allergy was excluded via a negative result from a Pt skin-prick test. In general, exposure to Rh compounds does not result in Pt-type allergic reactions (4,6).

Metallic Os is considered biologically inert; however, exposure to OsO_4 vapors in industrial and laboratory settings can result in extreme ocular and respiratory inflammation and irritation and in acute conjunctivitis. Other signs and symptoms include headache, bronchoconstriction, difficulty in breathing, respiratory tract irritation, tracheal epithelium necrosis, bronchitis, and interstitial pneumonia (1,4,6,16). Ocular irritation occurs at low vapor concentrations. Continuous or higher exposures may cause lacrimation and visual disturbances (appearance of "rings" around lights).

CHRONIC TOXICITY

Target Organ Effects. Chronic occupational exposure to Pt compounds may exacerbate Pt hypersensitivity reactions, especially in atopic individuals. Reproductive toxicity is associated with long-term cisplatin use. Cisplatin used for chemotherapy alone and in combination with other chemotherapeutic agents has been shown to cause azoospermia in humans within 2 months after initiation of treatment (15). Recovery of sperm counts occurred in a majority of patients within 1.5 to 2.0 years after cessation of treatment.

Many heavy metals (lead, mercury, thallium, and gold) are neurotoxic, and cisplatin is known to be toxic to the central and peripheral nervous systems (15,21). Peripheral neuropathies (paresthesias) are the most common neurotoxicities and are reversible after discontinuation of treatment (15). Hematologic effects, which occur from 6 to 26 days after initiation of treatment, include hypomagnesemia, leukopenia, and thrombocytopenia (33). Ototoxicity caused by cisplatin often is irreversible and is manifested by tinnitus and hearing loss in the high-frequency (4,000- to 8,000-Hz) range (15,21,33). Long-term use of cisplatin may result in irreversible kidney damage.

Although industrial Pd poisoning is considered rare, toxicity could occur by prolonged therapeutic use of Pd compounds (4,6,16). A colloidal form of Pd has been used in the clinical treatment of tuberculosis, gout, and obesity. Toxicity from these colloidal Pd compounds may be due to hemolysis (4,6,16). Some reports have described skin sensitization to Pd in the workplace, but generally these compounds are thought not to pose a serious allergy problem similar to that associated with Pt salts (4,6,16). Pd-protein conjugates do not have antigenic determinants similar to those of Pt-protein conjugates (6). Some reports have cited skin sensitization (a type IV hypersensitivity) to Pd due to exposure in a research laboratory and to dental alloys (12,47).

OsO_4 has been used in Europe for 30 to 40 years for the treatment of rheumatoid arthritis, but its use is controversial.

Chronic toxicity from Os may occur after intraarticular injection, which results in Os accumulation in liver, spleen, heart, and kidneys. Damage to the kidney can occur (6,13).

Carcinogenesis and Mutagenesis. No reports have cited increased cancer risk from occupational exposure to Pt compounds. Although cisplatin is an effective antitumor agent in humans and experimental animals, it has been reported to increase the frequency of lung adenomas and to induce skin papillomas and carcinomas in mice (16). In a lifetime exposure study, a minimally significant increase in malignant tumors, primarily of the lymphoma-leukemia type, was found in mice given access to 5 ppm of either Rh or Pd (chloride salts) in drinking water (48).

Cisplatin and other Pt compounds are strong mutagens in bacterial systems, including the *Salmonella typhimurium* revertant tests (49,50). The compound induces chromosomal aberrations and increases in sister chromatid exchanges in cultured cells (16). After hydrolysis of the cisplatin chloride groups to form activated species, the Pt complex can react with DNA, forming both intrastrand and interstrand cross-links. The N(7) group of guanine is highly reactive, and the lesion demonstrated most readily to result in cytotoxicity involves intrastrand cross-links between adjacent guanines (15,21). Certain Pt(II), Pd(II), Rh(I), and Rh(III) complexes have been shown to be mutagenic in bacterial systems (51,52).

Management of Toxicity

CLINICAL EXAMINATION

Clinical signs and symptoms (see Table 78-3) of Pt exposure and toxicity via inhalational and dermal routes are those of classic allergic reactions and include irritation of the eyes and nose; cough, dyspnea, wheezing, and cyanosis; skin sensitization; and lymphocytosis (1,9).

Careful clinical diagnosis is needed to differentiate an asthmalike attack due to Pt salts from other causes of asthma and from upper airway obstruction by tumor, laryngeal edema, endobronchial disease, acute left ventricular failure, and eosinophilic pneumonias. Sensitization dermatitis due to Pt salts must be differentiated from primary irritant dermatitis, nummular eczema, atopic dermatitis, pustular eruptions of the palms and soles, psoriasis, herpes simplex and zoster, drug eruptions, and erythema multiforme (1).

Signs and symptoms of OsO_4 exposure include lacrimation, visual disturbances, conjunctivitis, headache, cough, dyspnea, and dermatitis. The visual disturbances that result from Os vapor exposure are perceived by the patient as a ring around lights. Diagnoses should be differentiated from other causes of conjunctivitis and mucous membrane irritation, such as viral infection of the upper respiratory tract and allergies. If involvement of the tracheobronchial tree is detected, the symptoms should be differentiated from cardiogenic pulmonary edema and viral or bacterial pneumonia (1).

LABORATORY DIAGNOSIS

In cases of asthma suspected to be induced by the platinoids, the following laboratory tests are recommended: electrocardiogram, sputum Gram's stain and culture, total serum IgE levels, and differential white blood cell count (1). Lymphocytosis and eosinophilia have been reported (1,10,14). Arterial oxygen saturation and arterial blood gases should be monitored. Lung function using spirometry also should be assessed (14,30).

The major dose-limiting effect from the use of cisplatin is nephrotoxicity; however, this can be controlled by varying dosing regimens and providing hydration (21). Renal diagnostic and function tests, such as blood urea nitrogen, serum creatinine, proteinuria, enzymuria, creatinine clearance, and glomerular filtration rate, will aid in evaluating the extent of nephrotoxicity. The primary toxic effect associated with the newer cisplatin analog carboplatin is myelosuppression (44,45). Thus, white blood cell counts should be monitored for potential toxicity related to cisplatin or carboplatin.

SPECIAL DIAGNOSTIC TESTS

In general, Pt allergy exists until proved otherwise when a worker exposed to Pt salts or chloroplatinic acid presents classic allergic symptoms (10). The diagnosis is based on a history of work-related symptoms, positive results from a skin-prick test with Pt salts, or a positive outcome on bronchial challenge test with Pt salts (10,14,27,30). (These tests are described briefly in the following sections.) More details of these tests can be found in several reports (27,28,53,54). Interested readers should consult with occupational health experts who are familiar or have experience with these tests and understand the relative advantages and disadvantages of each. In workers who develop Pt-induced allergy and asthma, positive results on skin-prick tests, bronchial hyperreactivity, and asthma symptoms may decrease with time after removal from exposure, but some level of allergy can persist for long periods (28,54). A brief algorithm that illustrates the use of special tests to confirm the diagnosis of Pt salt hypersensitivity is presented in Figure 78-2.

Skin-Prick Test. The skin-prick test uses any of three Pt salts: ammonium hexachloroplatinate [$(NH_4)_2PtCl_6$]; sodium tetrachloroplatinate (Na_2PtCl_4); or sodium hexachloroplatinate (Na_2PtCl_6). These Pt salts can be tested, using a titration method if necessary, by incorporating concentrations ranging from 10^{-9} to 10^{-3} g per mL. The test is performed easily and is rapid and reproducible. Small aliquots of the test solutions are placed on the volar surface of the forearm, then a 26-gauge hypodermic needle is inserted through the test solution into the epidermis, which is pricked gen-

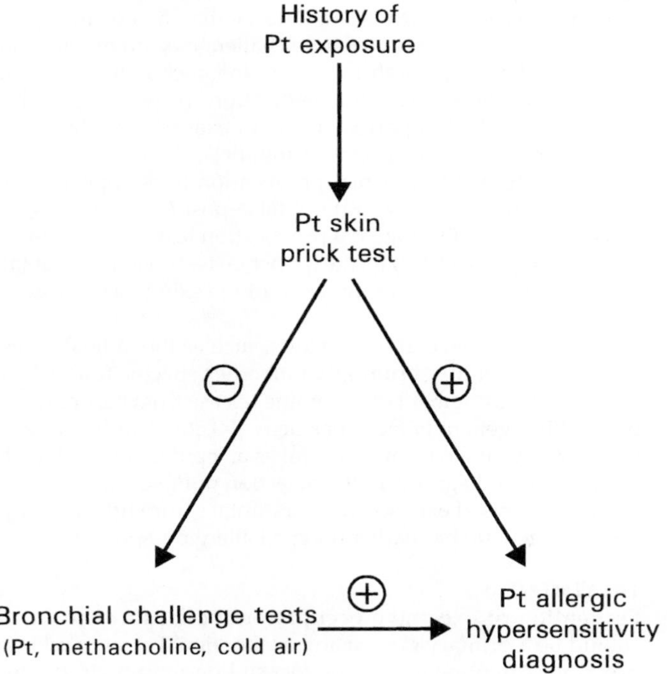

Figure 78-2. Algorithm for confirmation of a platinum salt–induced allergic hypersensitivity diagnosis.

tly in an upward direction. Control tests are performed using 0.9% NaCl as a negative control and histamine (0.1%) as a positive control. A definite wheal-and-flare reaction is diagnostic. A positive skin-prick test result is defined as one with a wheal diameter equal to or greater than the histamine control response (27,54).

The sensitization of workers due to repeated skin-prick testing is rare at the concentrations used for the test (10,14,27,30); however, no study has been designed to evaluate this. In one study, skin-prick tests with Pt salts caused mild systemic reactions not requiring treatment (27). Nonetheless, patients should be monitored carefully for any systemic reactions during these tests.

A skin-prick test using Pt salts exhibits a higher degree of specificity than sensitivity (27). Thus, the test is more effective at correctly excluding those who do not have Pt allergy (low false-positive response rate) but may not identify all those with Pt allergy, a limitation that results in a higher false-negative response rate. Negative skin-prick test results with Pt do not exclude allergy diagnosis.

Bronchial Challenge Tests. A bronchial challenge (or provocation) test may be used for workers who have negative results on skin-prick tests with Pt salts but present with clinical symptomatology suggestive of Pt exposure (27). Extreme caution and careful clinical decision making should be exercised for subjects who may have experienced a systemic side reaction during the skin-prick tests. The bronchial provocation tests should be conducted in a clinical setting in which emergencies can be addressed properly. The Pt salt solutions used for skin-prick testing may be used for the bronchoprovocation test; however, Na_2PtCl_2 should be used, owing to the limited solubility of $(NH_4)_2PtCl_6$ in physiologic solutions. Plethysmography is used to monitor lung function, including forced expiratory volume, specific airway resistance, and specific airway conductance. Lung respiratory parameters must be monitored carefully to ensure that these functions are not compromised seriously. Aerosolized solutions of Pt salts are inhaled using positive pressure (e.g., a jet nebulizer) (27). A positive change in bronchoreactivity is defined as a significant decrease in airway conductance (27) or increased airway resistance (55).

Other bronchial provocation tests that assess nonspecific bronchial hyperreactivity include challenges with methacholine (27) or cold air (54). Both methacholine, a cholinergic agonist, and cold air cause bronchoconstriction. In workers with Pt-induced bronchial hyperreactivity, an exacerbated decrease in airway conductance can occur using these challenge tests.

In one study, Pt bronchial provocation tests appeared to be highly specific (i.e., a low rate of false-positive responses) (27). Sensitivity of the Pt bronchial provocation tests was higher than that of skin-prick tests (i.e., the bronchial tests had a rate of false-negative responses lower than that of the skin-prick test).

Other Tests. Several *in vitro* tests, such as the radioallergosorbent test to identify serum IgE antibodies specific to Pt-Cl complexes, or measurement of histamine release from basophils, may be used but generally lack specificity (53,56). A radioallergosorbent test appears to be more useful as an epidemiologic tool than for individual diagnosis in the detection of Pt-specific antibodies in large cohorts of exposed workers. Total serum IgE also may be used as a general biomarker of type I allergic responses.

TREATMENT

Prevention of excessive occupational exposures to Pt salts should be a primary goal of any occupational safety and health program. Attention should be focused on minimizing occupational exposures with proper clothing and ventilation so that invasive procedures are not necessary. Should workers become sensitized to Pt or Pt-group metals, prompt removal from the workplace exposure source is important. For treatment of excessive inhalational and dermal exposures to the platinoids, appropriate procedures should be initiated, such as removal from the source of exposure, irrigation of eyes, and water washing of contaminated areas of skin. Treatments for contact dermatitis and bronchospasm may be initiated (1,10,30,33).

Preventive measures that should be undertaken to limit inhalational and dermal exposures include adequate workplace ventilation; use of mechanical filter respirators, rubber gloves, and protective clothing; and better personal hygiene. Those individuals with allergies or sensitization should be removed from the source (29). Studies have demonstrated that, in general, atopic individuals (i.e., those sensitive to common environmental allergens) are sensitized to the platinoids more quickly than are nonatopic individuals (6). Workers in these facilities should be monitored on a regular basis through use of several test procedures (see Biological Monitoring) as part of an industrial hygiene surveillance program. High standards of workplace isolation in Pt processing must be met so that workers do not come into direct contact with a liquid, fume, dust, or solid containing Pt salts.

Use of antihistamines for Pt allergy is controversial but can provide temporary relief of some of the upper respiratory symptoms (10,14). Bronchodilators can alleviate acute bronchospasm but are of no long-term benefit. As Pt salt sensitivity is an allergy and symptoms develop only after exposure, the best treatment requires cessation of exposure (14).

To treat excessive exposure to OsO_4 vapors, affected patients should be removed from the exposure source, eyes should be flushed with water if they were exposed, and the skin washed thoroughly. If OsO_4 is ingested and an affected patient is conscious, vomiting can be induced. For dermatitis, treatment modalities for contact dermatitis may be instituted. After severe exposure, hospitalization may be necessary for approximately 3 to 4 days to allow examination for onset of delayed pulmonary edema. Treatment modalities for common respiratory irritants may be used (1).

During cisplatin therapy, all test values of renal and hematopoietic function, in addition to auditory acuity, should be monitored. Slow infusion of cisplatin can reduce toxicity while maintaining efficacy. When used alone, the intravenous dose of 100 mg per square meter once every 4 weeks has been used (21). The dosage must be reduced when given in combination with other chemotherapeutic agents. To prevent nephrotoxicity, several interventions may be indicated and are reviewed by Anand and Bashey (57). Avoidance of other nephrotoxic drugs and hydration of affected patients is recommended: infusion of 1 to 2 L of fluid for 8 to 12 hours prior to treatment has been described as appropriate. Hydration is continued to ensure that glomerular filtration and urinary output are adequate. Concurrent administration of a diuretic, such as furosemide or mannitol, has been advocated to maintain renal output and to reduce nephrotoxicity (21,57,58).

Reduction of nephrotoxicity has been achieved via other intervention regimens. The coadministration of chloride salts to induce chloruresis may improve the therapeutic index of cisplatin via decreased renal activation of cisplatin chloride groups to cytotoxic hydroxyl or aquated species (59). Inducing chloruresis and maintaining hydration may allow for a doubling of the cisplatin dose, thus increasing antitumor efficacy and reducing dose-limiting nephrotoxicity; however, other systemic toxicities (myelosuppression, nausea, ototoxicity, and peripheral neuropathy) still may occur (60).

Other experimental protective approaches to reduce cisplatin nephrotoxicity, evaluated in laboratory animal studies or in humans in early clinical trials, involve free radical scavengers, antioxidants, compounds with high affinities for heavy metals (e.g., the sulfhydryl-containing chelator), diethyldithiocarbamate (21,61), and sulfhydryl-group reducing agents, such as tiopronin [*N*-(2-mercaptoproprionyl)-glycine] and dithiothreitol (62,63). These various interventions show promise in reducing cisplatin nephrotoxicity while maintaining its antitumor efficacy. Sodium thiosulfate binds covalently with cisplatin *in vitro* and inhibits cisplatin nephrotoxicity when administered concomitantly to experimental animals (64), and it may be effective clinically (65,66). The neutralization by sodium thiosulfate occurs primarily in the kidneys, not the plasma; thus, a larger proportion of drug can be delivered to the tumor (57). Dithiocarbamate analogs given prior to cisplatin can reduce the nephrotoxicity of cisplatin while not affecting antitumor efficacy, by a mechanism involving the shift of Pt excretion from the kidney to the biliary route (61). Amifostine (WR-2721), an aminothiol compound, administered prior to cisplatin infusion protects against nephrotoxicity and the myelosuppressive and neurotoxic effects associated with high cisplatin dosages (67). Other interventions involving sulfhydryl reactions that result in neutralization of cisplatin nephrotoxicity include treatment with glutathione and induction by bismuth of renal metallothionein, a rapidly synthesized, metal-binding protein (57,68). Treatment with glutathione has been shown to protect against cisplatin nephrotoxicity and neurotoxicity in experimental animals (69).

BIOLOGICAL MONITORING

Determination of plasma concentrations of Pt may be useful for monitoring a therapeutic regimen and in preventing toxicity after cisplatin administration. The flameless graphite furnace atomic absorption spectrophotometry (GFAAS) methods are advantageous for determining Pt levels in biological fluids (e.g., cisplatin monitoring) because of their high sensitivity, rapidity, and expediency (Table 78-4). A technique for Pt analysis using electrothermal atomic absorption spectrophotometry can be performed by injection of plasma samples (70,71) directly into the graphite furnace. The limit of detection for the method is 0.07 µg per mL. Pt is not detected in the plasma of normal subjects at the sensitivity level of this technique. Residue from the destruction of organic matter in the plasma may interfere with the analysis at lower Pt concentrations, but use of a deuterium background corrector reduces this effect. The matrix effect can be reduced further by dilution of plasma specimens with a detergent, such as 1% Triton X-100. This detergent reportedly aids in a more uniform drying of the sample while minimizing Pt loss during atomization. This technique was reported to involve an assay in which diluted plasma can be injected directly into the furnace with a total analysis time of less than 2 minutes. The assay is moderately sensitive (detection limit, 0.05 µg per mL), precise (coefficient of variance, less than 4.3%), and linear (r >0.9922) in the ranges of 0.05 to 4.0 µg per mL for Pt in cisplatin (72).

A GFAAS method (see Table 78-4) is available for determining Pt in urine after dilution with dilute nitric acid (73). A report by Shearan and Smyth (73) describes the determination of Pt in urine by differential pulse polarography (DPP) after dilution with boric acid–ethylene diamine buffer and adjustment to alkaline pH. The limits of detection for both methods are equal, but the recoveries are low: 31% and 44% using DPP and GFAAS, respectively. The low recovery most likely is due to the strong association of inorganic Pt with urinary constituents that are not broken down either through complexing (in DPP) or by acid digestion (in GFAAS).

In GFAAS, the proper conditions for drying, ashing, and atomization steps must be optimized. A gradual multistep drying program is necessary to ensure complete drying for reproducible absorbance. The ashing step must be regulated carefully so as to remove the effects of the matrix with minimal loss of Pt (72,73).

Using precolumn derivatization with diethyldithiocarbamate (74), researchers developed a high-performance liquid chromatography (HPLC) assay (see Table 78-4) with high sensitivity (detection limit, 2.5 µg per mL) to study the pharmacokinetics of ultrafilterable Pt (the cytotoxic and biologically active forms) in plasma of patients receiving a continuous infusion of cisplatin. The sample preparation requires minimal sample manipulation, and a 20-fold increase in sensitivity over GFAAS methods can be achieved. A clinically useful HPLC method has been developed also for measuring Pt as the parent drug or its metabolites in urine of patients administered Pt chemotherapeutic agents (75). It can circumvent many of the matrix interferences associated with other analytic techniques. The HPLC methods are advantageous because they are rapid and inexpensive, require minimal sample preparation, and are suited for analyzing large numbers of samples.

An extremely sensitive method employing adsorptive voltammetry detection has been reported for determination of Pt in urine, blood, and plasma (76,77); the detection limits reported in these studies are in the range of 0.02 to 0.2 ng per L, which represents an increase in sensitivity of several orders of magnitude above previously described methods. Levels of Pt were detected in body fluids of nonoccupationally exposed individuals; thus, this method would be useful for monitoring Pt workers.

TABLE 78-4. Methods used for monitoring of platinum in biological specimens

Technique	Matrix	Detection limit (µg/mL)	Precision (CV %)	Range of linearity (µg/mL)	Recovery (%)	Reference
GFAAS	Plasma	0.07	8	0.2–2.0	NR	(70)
GFAAS	Plasma	0.05	2.8	0.05–4.0	81	(72)
GFAAS	Urine	0.4	NR	0.2–1.0	44	(73)
DPP	Urine	0.4	NR	0.2–1.0	31	(73)
HPLC	Plasma	0.0025	7.3	0.0025–1.0	100	(74)
HPLC	Urine	0.025	2.5	0.025–0.5	97	(75)
AV	Plasma, blood, urine	0.2 ng/L	NR	NR	NR	(77)
AV	Blood	0.02 ng/L	NR	NR	94	(76)
NAA	Tissue	0.3 g/mL	6	NR	NR	(78)
ICP-MS	Tissue	0.05	NR	NR	98	(79)

AV, adsorptive voltammetry; DPP, differential pulse polarography; GFAAS, graphite furnace atomic absorption spectrophotometry; HPLC, high-performance liquid chromatography; ICP-MS, inductively coupled plasma–mass spectrometry; NAA, neutron activation analysis; NR, not reported.

Determination of tissue Pt that has been described (see Table 78-4) uses radiochemical neutron activation analysis (NAA) (78) and inductively coupled plasma–mass spectrometry (79). The methods are an order of magnitude less sensitive than are the GFAAS methods described and are very time-consuming and tedious. Although impractical for therapeutic monitoring, the NAA method allows for the determination of approximately 20 additional trace elements; thus, the study of multielement interactions during Pt exposure is possible. Treatment with cisplatin has been shown to alter levels of some essential elements in plasma (e.g., the magnesium level is lowered) (15,21).

OCCUPATIONAL MONITORING

To monitor the occupational environment for Pt, air is drawn through a cellulose ester filter 25 mm in diameter for approximately 2 hours. Subsequently, the filter is treated with hydrochloric acid to dissolve soluble Pt salts. The solution is analyzed for Pt by GFAAS or by inductively coupled plasma–atomic emission spectroscopy. Insoluble Pt salts and metal then are determined after dissolution in 50% aquaregia and evaporation to dryness several times with hydrochloride followed by either of the analytic atomic methods described. The same procedure is followed to monitor the occupational environment for Rh. NAA, inductively coupled plasma atomic emission spectroscopy, and GFAAS may be used to analyze the other platinoids (6).

Soil concentrations of Pt group metals (Pt, Pd, and Rh) have been analyzed using inductively coupled plasma–mass spectrometry or NAA (19,80).

OCCUPATIONAL EXPOSURE LIMITS

Exposure limits are necessary for Pt and the platinoids because of their potent sensitizing properties, not so much because of their systemic toxicities (7). Current American Conference of Governmental Industrial Hygienists (ACGIH) threshold limit values (TLV) and time-weighted averages (TWA)—8 hours per day, 40 hours per week—for metallic Pt dusts and soluble Pt salts are 1.0 and 0.002 mg per cubic meter, respectively (2,81). The TLV for Pt salts was set at a level to prevent respiratory effects and is believed to provide protection against sensitization; however, it does not offer protection to a previously sensitized individual. The U.S. Occupational Safety and Health Administration (OSHA) permissible exposure limit (PEL) and the National Institute for Occupational Safety and Health (NIOSH) recommended exposure limit (REL) for soluble Pt salts also are 0.002 mg per cubic meter.

The current recommended ACGIH TLV/TWA for Rh metal and insoluble Rh compounds (as Rh) is 1.0 mg per cubic meter (81), and the TLV/TWA for soluble Rh salts is 0.01 mg per cubic meter (81). These TLVs were set at levels to prevent possible allergic effects. The OSHA PEL and the NIOSH REL for Rh metal and insoluble Rh compounds are set at 0.1 mg per cubic meter, and the OSHA PEL and NIOSH REL for soluble Rh salts are set at 0.001 mg per cubic meter (81).

The current ACGIH TLV/TWA for exposure to osmium tetroxide is 0.0016 mg per cubic meter, or 0.0002 ppm, as Os (8,81). This TLV/TWA was set at a level to prevent irritation of the eyes or respiratory tract. The TLV–short-term exposure limit is 0.0047 mg per cubic meter, or 0.0006 ppm, as Os (81). The OSHA PEL and NIOSH REL for Os are set at 0.002 mg per cubic meter. No occupational exposure limits (TLVs) have been recommended for Pd, Ir, Ru, and their compounds.

REFERENCES

1. Proctor NH, Hughes JP, Fischman M. *Chemical hazards of the workplace.* Philadelphia: JB Lippincott Co, 1988:393–436.
2. Sax NI, Lewis RJ. *Hawley's condensed chemical dictionary,* 11th ed. New York: Van Nostrand–Reinhold, 1987:926–928.
3. McBryde WAE. Platinum and its compounds. In: Hampel CA, Hawley GG, eds. *The encyclopedia of chemistry,* 3rd ed. New York: Van Nostrand–Reinhold, 1973:865–867.
4. Venugopal B, Luckey TD. Toxicity of group VIII metals. In: Venugopal B, Luckey TD, eds. *Metal toxicity in mammals,* vol 2. New York: Plenum Publishing, 1978:273–305.
5. Hawley GG. *The condensed chemical dictionary,* 9th ed. New York: Van Nostrand–Reinhold, 1977:691–692.
6. Seiler HG, Sigel H. *Handbook on toxicity of inorganic compounds.* New York: Marcel Dekker Inc, 1988:341–344, 501–574.
7. Renner H, Schmuckler G. Platinum-group metals. In: Merian E, ed. *Metals and their compounds in the environment.* New York: VCH-Verlag, 1991:1135–1151.
8. Hammond CR. The elements. In: Weast RC, Astle MJ, Beyer WH, eds. *CRC handbook of chemistry and physics.* Boca Raton, FL: CRC Press, 1986:B5–B43.
9. Kawata Y, Shiota M, Tsutsui H, Yoshida Y, Sasaki H, Kinouchi Y. Cytotoxicity of Pd-Co dental casting ferromagnetic alloys. *J Dent Res* 1981;60:1403–1409.
10. Boggs PB. Platinum allergy. *Cutis* 1985;35:318–320.
11. Hermesch CB, Voss JE, Bales DJ, Mayhew RB. A clinical evaluation of a high-copper alloy containing palladium. *J Indiana Dent Assoc* 1982;61:1315.
12. Van Ketel WG, Niebber C. Allergy to palladium in dental alloys. *Contact Dermatitis* 1981;7:331–357.
13. Maugh TH. New ways to use metals for arthritis. *Science* 1981;212:430–431.
14. Jacobs L. Platinum salt sensitivity. *Nurs RSA* 1987;2:34–37.
15. Loehrer PJ, Einhorn LH. Cisplatin. *Ann Intern Med* 1984;100:704–713.
16. Goyer RA. Toxic effects of metals. In: Klaassen CD, ed. *Casarett and Doull's toxicology: the basic science of poisons,* 5th ed. New York: McGraw-Hill, 1996:725–726.
17. Paraplatin approved for recurrent ovarian cancer. *J Pharm Technol* 1989;5:83.
18. Brady LW, Micaily B, Miyamoto CT, Heilmann HP, Montemaggi P. Innovations in brachytherapy in gynecologic oncology. *Cancer* 1995;76(Suppl 10):2143–2151.
19. Heinrich E, Schmidt G, Kratz K-L. Determination of platinum-group elements (PGE) from catalytic converters in soil by means of docimasy and INAA. *Fresenius J Anal Chem* 1996;354:883–885.
20. Farago ME, Kavanagh P, Blanks R, et al. Platinum metal concentrations in urban road dust and soil in the United Kingdom. *Fresenius J Anal Chem* 1996;354:660–663.
21. Calabresi P, Chabner BA. Chemotherapy of neoplastic diseases. In: Gilman AG, Rall TW, Nies AS, Taylor P, eds. *Goodman and Gilman's the pharmacological basis of therapeutics,* 8th ed. New York: Pergamon Press, 1990:1249–1251.
22. Balis FM, Holcenberg JS, Bleyer WA. Clinical pharmacokinetics of commonly used anticancer drugs. *Clin Pharmacokinet* 1983;8:202–232.
23. Curt GA, Grygiel JJ, Curden BJ, et al. A phase I and pharmacokinetic study of diamminecyclobutane-dicarboxylatoplatinum (NSC 241240). *Cancer Res* 1983;43:4470–4473.
24. Madias NE, Harrington JT. Platinum nephrotoxicity. *Am J Med* 1978;65:307–314.
25. Van Echo DA, Egotin MJ, Whitacre MY, Olman EA, Aisner J. Phase I clinical and pharmacologic trial of carboplatin daily for 5 days. *Cancer Treat Rev* 1984;68:1103–1114.
26. Egorin MJ, Van Echo DA, Tipping SJ, et al. Pharmacokinetics and dosage reduction of *cis*-diamine(1,1-cyclobutane dicarboxylate)platinum in patients with impaired renal function. *Cancer Res* 1984;44:5432–5438.
27. Merget R, Schultze-Werninghaus G, Bode F, Bergmann E, Zachgo W, Meier-Sydow J. Quantitative skin prick and bronchial provocation tests with platinum salt. *Br J Ind Med* 1991;48:830–837.
28. Merget R, Reineke M, Rueckmann A, Bergmann E, Schultze-Werninghaus G. Nonspecific and specific bronchial responsiveness in occupational asthma caused by platinum salts after allergen avoidance. *Am J Respir Crit Care Med* 1994;150:1146–1149.
29. Plunkett ER. *Handbook of industrial toxicology.* New York: Chemical Publishing Co, 1976:341–342.
30. Hughes EG. Medical surveillance of platinum refinery workers. *J Soc Occup Med* 1980;30:27–30.
31. Baker DB, Gann PH, Brooks SM, Gallagher J, Bernstein IL. Cross-sectional study of platinum salts sensitization among precious metal refinery workers. *Am J Ind Med* 1990;18:653–664.
32. Chu G. Cellular responses to cisplatin: the roles of DNA-binding proteins and DNA repair. *J Biol Chem* 1994;269:787–790.
33. Ellenhorn MJ, Barceloux DG. *Medical toxicology—diagnosis and treatment of human poisoning.* New York: Elsevier Science, 1988:1055–1056.
34. Goldstein RS, Mayor GH. Minireview—the nephrotoxicity of cisplatin. *Life Sci* 1983;32:685–690.
35. Tosetti F, Rocco M, Fulco RA, et al. Serial determination of platinum, protein content, and free sulfhydryl levels in plasma of patients treated with cisplatin or carboplatin. *Anticancer Res* 1988;8:381–386.
36. Sodhi A, Gupta P. Increased release of hydrogen peroxide and superoxide anion by murine macrophages in vitro after cisplatin treatment. *Int J Immunopharmacol* 1986;8:709–714.
37. Sugihara K, Gemba M. Modification of cisplatin toxicity by antioxidants. *Jpn J Pharmacol* 1986;40:353–355.

38. Dobyan DC, Bull JM, Strebel FR, Sunderland BA, Bulger RE. Protective effects of *O*-(beta-hydroxyethyl)-rutoside on cisplatinum-induced acute renal failure in the rat. *Lab Invest* 1986;55:557–563.
39. Zhang J-G, Lindup WE. Role of mitochondria in cisplatin-induced oxidative damage exhibited by rat renal cortical slices. *Biochem Pharmacol* 1993;45: 2215–2222.
40. Zhang J-G, Lindup WE. Role of calcium in cisplatin-induced cell toxicity in rat renal cortical slices. *Toxicol In Vitro* 1996;10:205–209.
41. Lee TC, Hook CC, Long HJ. Severe exfoliative dermatitis associated with hand ischemia during cisplatin therapy. *Mayo Clin Proc* 1994;69:80–82.
42. Weidmann B, Mulleneisen N, Bojko P, Niederle N. Hypersensitivity reactions to carboplatin. *Cancer* 1994;73:2218–2222.
43. Sood AK, Gelder MS, Huang SW, Morgan LS. Anaphylaxis to carboplatin following multiple previous uncomplicated courses. *Gynecol Oncol* 1995;57: 131–132.
44. Calvert AH, Harland SJ, Newell DR, et al. Early clinical studies with *cis*-diamine-1,1-cyclobutane dicarboxylate platinum(II). *Cancer Chemother Pharmacol* 1982;9:140–147.
45. Koeller JM, Trump DL, Tutsch KD, Earhart RH, Davis TE, Tormey DC. Phase I clinical trial and pharmacokinetics of carboplatin (NSC 241240) by single monthly 30-minute infusion. *Cancer* 1986;57:222–225.
46. Bergman A, Svedberg U, Nilsson E. Contact urticaria with anaphylactic reactions caused by occupational exposure to iridium salt. *Contact Dermatitis* 1995;32:14–17.
47. Munro-Ashman D, Munro D, Hughes TH. Contact dermatitis from palladium. *Trans St. Johns Hosp Dermatol Soc* 1969;55:196–197.
48. Schroeder HA, Mitchener M. Scandium, chromium(VI), gallium, yttrium, rhodium, palladium, indium in mice. Effects on growth and life span. *J Nutr* 1971;101:1431–1438.
49. Coluccia M, Correale M, Fanizzi FP, et al. Mutagenic activity of some platinum complexes: chemical properties and biological activity. In: Merian E, Frei RW, Hardi W, Schlatter C, eds. *Carcinogenic and mutagenic metal compounds.* New York: Gordon and Breach, 1985:467–474.
50. Uno Y, Morita M. Mutagenic activity of some platinum and palladium complexes. *Mutat Res* 1993;298:269–275.
51. Warren G, Abbott E, Schultz P, Bennett K, Rogers S. Mutagenicity of a series of hexacoordinate rhodium(III) compounds. *Mutat Res* 1981;88:165–173.
52. Aresta M, Treglia S, Collucia M, Correale M, Giordano D, Moscelli S. Mutagenic activity of transition-metal complexes: relation structure-mutagenic and antibacterial activity for some Pd(II), Pt(II) and Rh(I) complexes. In: Merian E, Frei RW, Hardi W, Schlatter C, eds. *Carcinogenic and mutagenic metal compounds.* New York: Gordon and Breach, 1985:453–466.
53. Biagini RE, Bernstein IL, Gallagher JS, Moorman WJ, Brooks S, Gann PH. The diversity of reaginic immune responses to platinum and palladium metallic salts. *J Allergy Clin Immunol* 1985;76:794–802.
54. Brooks SM, Baker DB, Gann PH, et al. Cold air challenge and platinum skin reactivity in platinum refinery workers: bronchial reactivity precedes skin prick response. *Chest* 1990;97:1401–1407.
55. Biagini RE, Moorman WJ, Lewis TR, Bernstein IL. Ozone enhancement of platinum asthma in a primate model. *Am Rev Respir Dis* 1986;134:719–725.
56. Murdoch RD, Pepys J, Hughes EG. IgE antibody responses to platinum group metals: a large scale refinery survey. *Br J Ind Med* 1986;43:37–43.
57. Anand AJ, Bashey B. Newer insights into cisplatin nephrotoxicity. *Ann Pharmacother* 1993;27:1519–1525.
58. Pinzani V, Bressolle F, Haug IJ, Galtier M, Blayac JP, Balmes P. Cisplatin-induced renal toxicity and toxicity-modulating strategies: a review. *Cancer Chemother Pharmacol* 1994;35:1–9.
59. Earhart RH, Martin PA, Tutsch KD, Erturk E, Wheeler RH, Bull FE. Improvement in the therapeutic index of cisplatin (NSC 119875) by pharmacologically induced chloruresis in the rat. *Cancer Res* 1983;43:1187–1194.
60. Corden BJ, Fine RL, Ozols RF, Collins JM. Clinical pharmacology of high-dose cisplatin. *Cancer Chemother Pharmacol* 1985;14:38–41.
61. Basinger MA, Jones MM, Gilbreath SG, Walker EM Jr, Fody EP, Mayhue MA. Dithiocarbamate-induced biliary platinum excretion and the control of *cis*-platinum nephrotoxicity. *Toxicol Appl Pharmacol* 1989;97:279–288.
62. Zhang J-G, Zhong LF, Zhang M, Ma XL, Xia YX, Lindup WE. Amelioration of cisplatin toxicity in rat renal cortical slices by dithiothreitol in vitro. *Hum Exp Toxicol* 1994;13:89–93.
63. Zhang J-G, Lindup WE. Tiopronin protects against the nephrotoxicity of cisplatin in rat renal cortical slices in vitro. *Toxicol Appl Pharmacol* 1996;141:425–433.
64. Uozumi J, Litterst CL. The effect of sodium thiosulfate on subcellular localization of platinum in rat kidney after treatment with cisplatin. *Cancer Lett* 1986;32:279–283.
65. Markman M, Cleary S, Howell S. Nephrotoxicity of high-dose intra-cavitary cisplatin with intravenous thiosulfate protection. *Eur J Cancer Clin Oncol* 1985;21:1015–1018.
66. DeBroe ME, Wedeen RP. Prevention of cisplatin nephrotoxicity. *Eur J Cancer Clin Oncol* 1986;22:1029–1031.
67. Treskes M, Van der Vijgh WJF. WR2721 as a modulator of cisplatin and carboplatin-induced side effects in comparison with other chemoprotective agents: a molecular approach. *Cancer Chemother Pharmacol* 1993;33:93–106.
68. Kondo Y, Satoh M, Imura N, Akimoto M. Tissue-specific induction of metallothionein by bismuth as a promising protocol for chemotherapy with repeated administration of *cis*-diaminedichloroplatinum(II) against bladder cancer. *Anticancer Res* 1992;12:2303–2308.
69. Cavaletti G, Minoia C, Schieppati M, Tredici G. Protective effects of glutathione on cisplatin neurotoxicity in rats. *Int J Radiat Oncol Biol Phys* 1994; 29:771–776.
70. Baselt RC. Platinum. In: Baselt RC, ed. *Analytical procedures for therapeutic drug monitoring and emergency toxicology,* 2nd ed. Littleton, MA: PSG Publishing Co, 1987:238–239.
71. LeRoy AF, Wehling HL, Sponseller HL, et al. Analysis of platinum in biological materials by flameless atomic absorption spectrophotometry. *Biochem Med* 1977;18:184–191.
72. El-Yazigi A, Al-Saleh I. Rapid determination of platinum by flameless atomic absorption spectrophotometry following the administration of cisplatin to cancer patients. *Ther Drug Monit* 1986;8:318–320.
73. Shearan P, Smyth MR. Comparison of voltammetric and graphite furnace atomic absorption spectrometric methods for the direct determination of inorganic platinum in urine. *Analyst* 1988;113:609–612.
74. Reece PA. Sensitive high-performance liquid chromatographic assay for platinum in plasma ultrafiltrate. *J Chromatogr* 1984;306:417–423.
75. Bannister SJ, Sternson LA, Repta AJ. Urine analysis of platinum species derived from *cis*-dichlorodiammineplatinum(II) by high-performance liquid chromatography following derivatization with sodium diethyldithiocarbamate. *J Chromatogr* 1979;173:333–342.
76. Nygren O, Vaughan GT, Florence TM, Morrison G, Warner IM, Dale LS. Determination of platinum in blood by adsorptive voltammetry. *Anal Chem* 1990;62:1637–1640.
77. Messerschmidt J, Alt F, Toelg G, Angerer J, Schaller KH. Adsorptive voltammetric procedure for the determination of platinum baseline levels in human body fluids. *Frensenius J Anal Chem* 1992;343:391–394.
78. Tjioe PS, Volkers KJ, Kroon JJ, DeGoeij JJM, The SK. Determination of gold and platinum traces in biological materials as a part of a multielement radiochemical activation analysis system. In: Merian E, Frei RW, Hardi W, Schlatter C, eds. *Carcinogenic and mutagenic metal compounds.* New York: Gordon and Breach, 1985:171–182.
79. Minami T, Ichii M, Okazaki Y. Comparison of three different methods for measurement of tissue platinum levels. *Biol Trace Elem Res* 1995;48:37–44.
80. Parent M, Vanhoe H, Moens L, Dams R. Determination of low amounts of platinum in environmental and biological materials using thermospray nebulization inductively coupled plasma–mass spectrometry. *Fresenius J Anal Chem* 1996;354:664–667.
81. American Conference of Governmental Industrial Hygienists. *Threshold limit values for chemical substances in the work environment.* Cincinnati: American Conference of Governmental Industrial Hygienists, 1996.

CHAPTER 79
Beryllium

Lee S. Newman and Lisa A. Maier

Although beryllium is an excellent metal for use in high-technology applications, it produces a number of adverse health effects primarily targeting the lung, lymphatics, and skin. As the fourth lightest element, with an atomic weight of 9.02, beryllium has a low density (1.85 g per cubic centimeter), a high melting point, a high stiffness-to-weight ratio, high tensile strength, and a low coefficient of thermal expansion. These properties render it extremely attractive for applications in aerospace, nuclear weapons, electronics, automobiles, and other industries (Table 79-1). Exposure to beryllium also occurs during the extraction of the mineral from its ores—beryl and bertrandite—and during the processing of beryllium into metal alloys and ceramic prod-

TABLE 79-1. Industrial settings with potential beryllium exposure

Aerospace	Nuclear weapons manufacture
Automotive parts	Precision machining
Ceramics	Refractories
Computer parts	Smelters
Dental alloy preparation	Tool and die manufacture
Electronics	Welding
Mining of beryl ore	

ucts. Even the machining of metal alloys that contain less than 2% beryllium can cause significant lung disease.

Although beryllium is found in soils and coal, air concentrations generally are extremely low even in major urban centers. Occupational inhalational exposures represent the major source of exposure resulting in illness.

ABSORPTION, METABOLISM, AND EXCRETION

When beryllium enters the lungs or penetrates the skin, it injures these and other organs by at least two major toxicologic pathways: through its stimulation of cellular immunity and by direct chemical effects that induce inflammation. Skin disease due to beryllium exposure can result from cutaneous inoculation with beryllium splinters, contamination of open wounds, or cutaneous contact with beryllium salts leading to dermatitis. Although skin contact can be a significant cause of morbidity, the principal route of toxicity for beryllium is by inhalation. Inhalational injury can result from exposure to fumes (beryllium oxides) or to respirable dust of beryllium oxides, metal, salts, or alloy. Even beryllium-copper, beryllium-aluminum alloys, and newer materials that are combinations of beryllium metal plus beryllium oxide generate airborne levels of beryllium sufficient to cause disease. Although a definitive study of exposure results has not been published, exposure to beryl or bertrandite has not been shown to cause disease; however, beryllium ore workers can become sensitized to beryllium.

Beryllium particles obey the basic principles of particle deposition in the lung. Most likely, beryllium's chemical properties influence the toxic effect produced. Particle size, solubility, and form (high temperature–fired oxide versus low temperature–fired oxide) influence the development of the pulmonary immune response and disease. Most inhaled beryllium can be cleared by the lung's mucociliary escalator and alveolar macrophages. Of the remaining beryllium, some is translocated to regional lymph nodes. However, a significant amount of beryllium remains lodged in the pulmonary interstitium even decades after exposure has ceased. Beryllium is distributed principally to liver, bone, and kidney. The bulk of excretion occurs through the urine. Beryllium is absorbed poorly through the gastrointestinal tract, rendering this a less likely route of exposure.

EXPOSURE LIMITS AND MONITORING

The number of workers with potential beryllium exposure in the United States remains unknown, with some estimates indicating that up to 800,000 individuals have been exposed. This number is supported by the fact that many individuals who have seemingly trivial exposures—bystanders, security guards, plant office workers, and spouses and children of beryllium workers—are at risk for developing beryllium sensitization and chronic beryllium disease (CBD). Thus, the definition of *beryllium exposure* and of *beryllium worker* should be kept broad.

Disease rates for CBD have been estimated at 2% to 16% of exposed workers, depending on the group studied. In most studies, the average is 2% to 6%, with the higher rates being associated with particular work tasks. For example, machinists in both the ceramics and nuclear weapons manufacturing industries have been found to have increased risks for developing beryllium sensitization and disease. The exact exposure-response relationship for CBD, although still under investigation, does not appear to be strictly linear. Both dose and duration of beryllium exposure have been associated with increased risk of sensitization and disease in some studies. This is most apparent with the acute pneumonialike illness (acute pneumonitis) that occurs at high exposures (more than 25 μg per cubic meter). In contrast, CBD develops in workers with seemingly low levels of exposure, after exposure periods as short as 2 months, and at levels at or below the current permissible exposure limit (PEL). Thus, beryllium's effects appear to be dose- and work task–dependent.

Nonetheless, other factors seem to modify the impact of beryllium. For example, tobacco smoking may reduce the risk of beryllium sensitization, raising the question of a possible protective effect from smoking. Genetic susceptibility to beryllium also contributes to disease risk, as discussed later (see Beryllium Sensitization).

The establishment of PELs for beryllium is linked to the birth of the nuclear age. The current beryllium exposure standard was introduced by the Atomic Energy Commission in 1949 because of beryllium's use in the manufacture of nuclear weapons. That standard remains in place, although the U.S. Department of Energy is considering a revised policy to reduce exposure and to mandate medical surveillance. The U.S. Occupational Safety and Health Administration has adopted the Atomic Energy Commission occupational exposure limit of 2 μg per cubic meter for an 8-hour time-weighted average, with a peak permissible level of 25 μg per cubic meter. In the air surrounding factories (environmental standard), beryllium levels are not to exceed 0.01 μg per cubic meter per 24-hour period. This is the famous "taxicab standard" (so named because it was drafted in the back seat of a taxicab), which was extrapolated from information about the toxicity of beryllium as compared to other metals. This standard has eliminated most cases of acute beryllium pneumonitis, although a report described a case that occurred in a dental technician working with beryllium dental alloys in 1984. The standard's effectiveness in eliminating CBD is less impressive. Recent studies show that CBD continues to occur in modern beryllium industries at a rate of approximately 6%, even in plants that are able to document that they have maintained exposures near or below 2 μg per cubic meter. Thus, adherence to the existing standard does not afford full protection from CBD.

The beryllium standard continues to be examined by federal agencies, including the U.S. Department of Energy. Until such time as a new standard is promulgated, beryllium-using industries would be well advised to keep beryllium exposures to levels that are as low as reasonably achievable (well below 2 μg per cubic meter).

TOXICOLOGIC STUDIES IN ANIMALS

Although the human was the first unwitting "animal model" of beryllium disease, toxic, immunologic, carcinogenic, and genotoxic effects have been observed in a wide number of animal species and cell types. When administered intravenously, soluble beryllium salts complex with plasma proteins. Beryllium is absorbed poorly through the gastrointestinal tract of most animal species, rendering ingestion an unlikely route of toxic exposure. Beryllium has been shown to alter the structure and function of the liver, interfering with various liver enzyme induction pathways. Toxic effects on immune effector cells, including macrophages and lymphocytes, also have been observed and may contribute to the immunotoxicity that occurs (as described in the next section).

Neoplasms have been observed in many animal models after many forms of beryllium exposure, including osteosarcomas in rabbits and lung neoplasms in rats, nonhuman primates, and other species. Mechanistically, beryllium has been shown to block the entry of cells into the cell cycle, to alter the fidelity of DNA replication, to alter hormone-regulated gene expression, and to bind directly to nuclear proteins that regulate gene expression.

Immunotoxicity

Over the last 50 years, numerous animal models have been developed to examine the inflammatory and immunologic effects of beryllium. Inhalational or tracheal instillation of beryllium in a number of forms has been shown repeatedly to produce lung injury that ranges from an acute pneumonitis to mononuclear cell infiltration and formation of granulomas with varying degrees of fibrosis in rodents, dogs, and nonhuman primates. In a set of interesting and carefully designed studies, Haley et al. challenged beagle dogs with beryllium oxides and evaluated pathologic and immunologic responses longitudinally. Over the course of 1 year, the dogs developed granulomas, fibrosis, and lymphocytic interstitial infiltrates in the lungs. Helper T lymphocytes accumulated in the lungs and were shown to mount a lymphocytic proliferative response to beryllium when stimulated with beryllium salts *in vitro*, a response analogous to that of human lymphocytes seen in CBD. Unlike human disease, the pathologic and immunologic reactions in the dog appear to resolve spontaneously, as occurs in other animal models. Mouse and guinea pig strains that differ only in their major histocompatibility complex loci differ in their immune responses to beryllium, suggesting that the response to beryllium is, in part, under genetic control.

Carcinogenicity

Multiple studies in multiple species using multiple forms of beryllium and a variety of routes of administration have shown that beryllium is carcinogenic, producing osteosarcomas and lung cancer.

CLINICAL TOXICOLOGY

Beryllium's effects on humans take several forms, as summarized in Table 79-2. The principal forms are skin disease, acute lung disease, chronic lung disease, and cancer. As the respiratory diseases are the most common, they constitute the majority of the discussion in this section.

TABLE 79-2. Principal human health effects of beryllium

Organ system	Consequence
Skin	Contact dermatitis
	Subcutaneous granulomatous nodules
Eyes	Conjunctivitis
	Corneal ulceration
Oral cavity	Gingivitis
Respiratory system	Rhinitis
	Nasal perforation
	Bronchitis, bronchiolitis
	Acute pneumonitis
	Chronic beryllium disease
	Lung cancer
Lymphatic-hematologic system	Hilar and mediastinal adenopathy
	Beryllium sensitization
	Lymphopenia
Heart	Cardiomyopathy
Gastrointestinal system	Granulomatous hepatitis
Kidney	Nephrolithiasis
	Hypercalcemia, hypercalciuria
Rheumatologic system	Hyperuricemia

Pulmonary Effects

Beryllium-related respiratory effects range from acute inhalational injury with tracheitis, bronchitis, and pneumonitis to beryllium sensitization and CBD. A number of patients with acute beryllium disease survived the acute pneumonitis only to develop the chronic form of disease later.

Exposure to high concentrations of beryllium can cause inflammation of the upper and lower respiratory tract, airways, and bronchioles. Upper airway symptoms include epistaxis, facial pain, swelling of the nasopharyngeal region and, in some cases, nasal perforation. Acute tracheobronchitis can accompany the pneumonitis. This disorder may have either an abrupt or a subacute onset and likely is related to dose of exposure, beryllium solubility, and other properties of the inhaled beryllium material. Symptoms include chest pain, dry cough, and shortness of breath. Rhonchi may be heard on chest auscultation. Chest radiography may simply show an increase in peribronchial markings. Recovery is said to occur over the span of a month, although the disorder can become chronic.

The manifestations of acute beryllium pneumonitis are nonspecific and mimic other inhalational injuries. Affected individuals may develop blood-tinged sputum, chest pain, burning sensation in the chest, dyspnea on exertion, or dyspnea at rest. They also experience myalgias, anorexia, and fever. Clinical presentation may be either acute or subacute, with cyanosis, tachycardia, tachypnea, and rales on lung examination. Hypoxemia is found commonly, with evidence of low lung volumes (restriction). Chest radiography may be normal, show bilateral alveolar infiltrates, or display more fulminant pulmonary edema. Radiographic changes typically occur within a few weeks of the onset of symptoms. History of a recent high beryllium exposure, usually under upset conditions, favor this diagnosis.

Histopathologically, a nongranulomatous pneumonitis is seen, with nonspecific inflammatory infiltrates composed of neutrophils and more chronic inflammatory cells (mononuclear cells and lymphocytes) in the airways and interstitium associated with interalveolar edema and bronchiolitis. In approximately 17% of cases, acute pneumonitis progresses into a granulomatous pneumonitis consistent with CBD.

The principal therapeutic approach is to remove affected individuals from exposure. Corticosteroids may be used empirically, but no documentation exists to substantiate their efficacy. Oxygen, rest, and in some cases, ventilatory support may be required. The signs and symptoms of the acute pneumonitis may resolve within several weeks to months. In its most severe form, acute beryllium pneumonitis is fatal.

Beryllium Sensitization

Beryllium sensitization holds the mechanistic key to both skin effects and chronic lung effects of beryllium. A number of lines of evidence indicate that beryllium acts as an antigen that induces a hypersensitivity cellular immune response. In 1951, Curtis demonstrated that patients with CBD developed a cutaneous delayed-type hypersensitivity reaction when their skin was patch-tested with beryllium salts. Some individuals develop granulomas in the dermis at the skin-patch test sites. The *in vitro* corollaries of this delayed-type hypersensitivity response have been documented in numerous studies.

When peripheral blood or bronchoalveolar lavage (BAL) cells have been cultured in the presence of beryllium salts, lymphocytes that possess the ability to recognize beryllium as an antigen will proliferate. This observation forms the basis of the beryllium lymphocyte proliferation test (BeLPT) now used widely to detect CBD and to define beryllium sensitization. Beryllium sensitization itself can be defined as a beryllium-specific immune response measured by the blood BeLPT, BAL BeLPT, or beryllium skin-patch testing. The BeLPT discriminates CBD from other granulomatous diseases. Its role in diagnosis and disease detection in industry is discussed in Diagnostic Evaluation.

The immunopathogenesis of beryllium sensitization and disease revolves around beryllium's ability to trigger beryllium-specific T cells. Saltini et al. have shown that the cellular immune response to beryllium is class II major histocompatibility complex–dependent. Antigen-presenting cells present the beryllium to T lymphocytes that then, in turn, enter the cell cycle and divide. Beryllium-reactive T-cell clones probably recognize the antigen via their T-cell antigen receptor. Likely, beryllium acts as a hapten (i.e., beryllium combined with peptide), although the exact form of the antigen moiety remains unknown. After antigen presentation and T-cell recognition, a variety of the immune effector cells become activated. These lymphocytes, macrophages, and mast cells (among others) will differentiate, proliferate, accumulate at the site of beryllium deposition, and promote an inflammatory-immunologic response. They do so in part by releasing key cytokines and growth factors, including tumor necrosis factor–α, interleukin-6, interleukin-2, and interferon-γ. These cytokines serve to enhance the inflammatory and immune response. Beryllium appears to have both nonspecific adjuvant activity and antigen-specific properties.

The tendency to develop beryllium sensitization may be linked not only to exposure but to genetics. For example, Richeldi et al. and Rossman et al. demonstrated that patients who are beryllium-sensitized and who have CBD differ from exposed nondiseased individuals, on the basis of presence of particular amino acid substitutions in key positions on human leukocyte antigen (HLA) molecules. Such allelic differences have been found both in HLA-DP and HLA-DR loci. Because HLA class II molecules are involved in antigen presentation to T cells via the T-cell antigen receptor, genetic differences in HLA have been hypothesized to define an individual's susceptibility to beryllium sensitization and disease. Regardless of an individual's genetics, beryllium sensitization does not occur unless the individual has been exposed to beryllium. Beryllium sensitization precedes the formation of granulomas and clinical illness. What is not known at this time is how often sensitization progresses into disease. However, even with removal from exposure, individuals who are beryllium-sensitized can progress into clinical illness over time.

The use of the blood BeLPT as a medical screening tool in industry has defined a population of exposed workers who mount the cell-mediated, antigen-driven immune response to beryllium but in whom no pathologic or clinical features of CBD are found. These individuals are defined as *beryllium-sensitized.* They are asymptomatic, have normal lung function, normal exercise tolerance, normal chest radiograph results, and lung biopsies that do not show granulomas. The rate of beryllium sensitization without disease in a small number of published studies ranges from 1% to 3%. Sensitized individuals must remain under close medical scrutiny and should be reexamined at regular intervals for signs of clinical progression. Some individuals may have equivocal blood BeLPT results. In these individuals, sensitization may be confirmed using beryllium sulfate patch testing.

CHRONIC BERYLLIUM DISEASE

Clinical Signs and Symptoms

CBD, also known as *chronic berylliosis*, is a systemic granulomatous condition that typically affects the lungs and thoracic lymph nodes. Unlike the acute form of lung disease, CBD usually develops many years after first exposure and follows a typically indolent course with insidious symptom onset. On average, CBD develops 6 to 10 years after exposure has ceased, but the disorder has been seen to occur with a latency greater than 30 years and with as little as 2 months of exposure.

Unless the disease is detected early while patients are asymptomatic, most individuals with CBD develop fatigue, nonproductive cough, gradual onset of shortness of breath, and varying degrees of chest pain. Weight loss, anorexia, fevers, night sweats, and arthralgias are seen commonly. Clinical signs include bibasilar dry rales on chest auscultation, cyanosis, digital clubbing, lymphadenopathy, signs of right ventricular failure and cor pulmonale, and skin lesions. In early, more subtle stages of this condition, the only clinical findings may be a few fine bibasilar crackles heard on lung auscultation. Other organs that can be affected include the liver, myocardium, lymph nodes, and skin.

With the increasing use of the blood BeLPT as a screening tool in industry, subclinical cases of CBD are being recognized. Affected individuals with CBD often are asymptomatic and have normal chest radiograph results and normal lung function but, if examined carefully, will be found to have abnormal gas exchange during exercise capacity testing. Additionally, they sometimes have subtle nodular lesions on thin-section computed tomography (CT) and demonstrate granulomatous inflammation in their lungs. Subclinical disease progresses over time into more obvious clinical disease. Biochemical abnormalities include hyperuricemia, nonspecific elevations of serum immunoglobulins reflecting a polyclonal gammopathy, lymphopenia, and an elevated serum angiotensin-converting enzyme activity.

Pulmonary Physiology

In CBD, pulmonary function abnormalities may take several forms including (i) a predominantly obstructive pattern found in one-third of affected individuals; (ii) a restrictive pattern with decreased lung volumes usually seen in more advanced disease in one-fourth of such individuals; (iii) reduced diffusing capacity for carbon monoxide (DL_{CO}), often with normal lung volumes and normal airflow in approximately one-third of cases; and (iv) a mixed pattern of obstruction and restriction, with varying degrees of gas exchange derangement. More recent studies have found that the DL_{CO} is insensitive. Exercise tolerance testing is a more sensitive indicator, especially if arterial blood gas levels are assessed during the test. Patients with CBD demonstrate reduced exercise tolerance, decreased oxygen consumption, an abnormal fall in oxygen levels, and an abnormal widening of the alveolar-arterial oxygen gradient. Their exercise usually is limited by their ventilatory capacity. As the disease progresses, such individuals become increasingly inactive and may develop secondary cardiovascular deconditioning, which further limits their exercise capacity. Some patients with CBD exhibit normal exercise physiology. Nonetheless, exercise tolerance testing is the most sensitive tool for evaluating and studying the disease, especially at its early stages.

Radiographic and Imaging Abnormalities

Chest radiographic results in early CBD are normal. As the disease progresses, the radiograph shows diffuse bilateral infil-

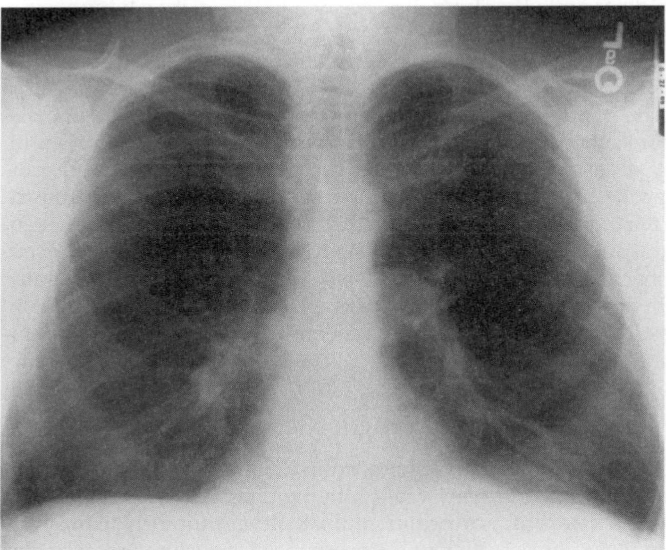

Figure 79-1. Chest radiograph from a patient with chronic beryllium disease illustrating typical findings of nodular parenchymal densities and hilar lymphadenopathy. Radiography results usually are normal when patients are detected through workplace screening with the beryllium lymphocyte proliferation test.

trates with hilar lymphadenopathy. Middle and upper lung field small opacities are most common and may appear irregular or rounded (Fig. 79-1). The nodules usually are categorized in the International Labour Organization scheme as small *p* or *q* opacities. With advancing disease, the chest radiograph shows increasingly widespread fibrosis and honeycombing. In a minority of patients, pleural abnormalities, which probably represent subpleural fibrosis and granuloma formation, are seen adjacent to areas of dense parenchymal involvement. Chest radiographs are an insensitive screening tool for CBD. Disease usually is physiologically and symptomatically obvious by the time that a chest radiograph result becomes abnormal.

Thin-section CT is more sensitive than is the plain chest radiograph. One recent study found abnormalities on CT in 10 of 13 CBD patients with normal chest radiographic results. The most common CT abnormalities are small nodules that typically track along bronchovascular sheaths, ground-glass opacification, thickened septal lines suggesting fibrosis, hilar lymph adenopathy, and bronchial wall thickening. Interestingly, bronchial wall thickening can be seen in CBD nonsmokers. The CT and chest radiographic abnormalities are somewhat nonspecific but, when taken together with tests such as the blood BeLPT, can be used to confirm the diagnosis without using invasive testing.

Bronchoalveolar Lavage

Suspected cases of CBD are confirmed best by bronchoscopy with BAL. Washing of cells from a segment of the lung usually reveals an increase in the total number of white blood cells with large numbers of lymphocytes. BAL cells can be tested for their ability to proliferate when exposed to beryllium salts *in vitro* (BAL BeLPT). Although this test often is considered the gold-standard immunologic test for CBD, some individuals who have CBD will have negative BAL BeLPT, usually because of the inhibitory effect of tobacco smoke on antigen presentation in the lung. Nonetheless, in cases generating a doubtful diagnosis, BAL is the procedure of choice.

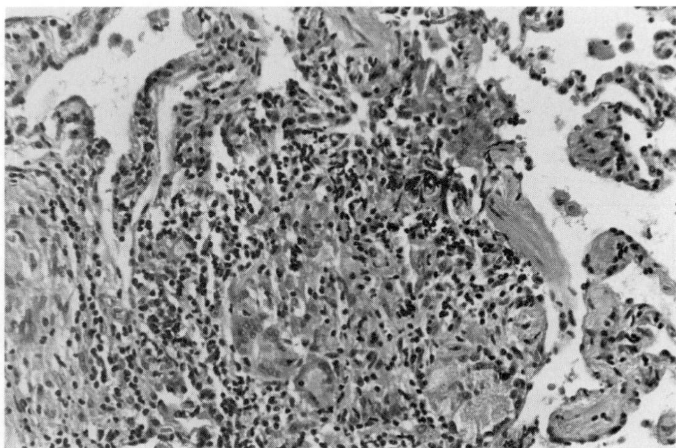

Figure 79-2. Lung histopathologic specimen in chronic beryllium disease showing typical noncaseating granulomas encapsulated by varying degrees of fibrosis. Other areas of lung parenchyma may show mononuclear cell infiltration. (Hematoxylin and eosin, 20× magnification)

Pathologic Features

The histopathologic alterations in the lungs or other organs in CBD range from diffuse mononuclear cell infiltration of the lung interstitium to the typical well-defined, noncaseating granulomas that exhibit varying degrees of pulmonary fibrosis (Fig. 79-2). In the lungs, the granulomas accumulate primarily in the interstitium and in bronchial submucosa. Biopsies should be cultured and stained for the presence of acid-fast bacilli and fungi. Granulomas can be found also in regional lymph nodes and, rarely, in the liver and in abdominal and cervical lymph nodes. Bronchoscopy with transbronchial lung biopsy usually is the best method of obtaining tissue.

Diagnostic Evaluation

Figure 79-3 illustrates the recommended diagnostic approach to CBD. Historically, the diagnostic criteria for CBD hinged on the presence of four of six criteria, including one of the first two: (i) beryllium exposure history, (ii) elevated beryllium levels in tissue or urine, (iii) chest radiographic result abnormalities, (iv) restrictive or obstructive physiology or abnormal DL_{CO}, (v) histopathologic findings consistent with CBD, and (vi) clinical course consistent with chronic respiratory illness. These were relatively nonspecific criteria. Measurement of beryllium in biological specimens usually does not establish the diagnosis and has technical limitations, especially in attempts to measure urine levels. Analysis of beryllium levels within lung tissue no longer is considered necessary for the diagnosis since the advent of superior immunologic assays that are both specific and sensitive.

With the introduction of transbronchial lung biopsy, BAL, and improvements in the blood and BAL BeLPT, the diagnostic criteria for CBD have changed. The diagnosis now is based on the demonstration of (i) a beryllium-specific immune response using blood or BAL BeLPT or beryllium salt patch testing and (ii) histopathologic changes consistent with CBD. Although a history of beryllium exposure is helpful, documentation of that exposure no longer is essential in establishing the diagnosis, as the BeLPT is highly specific and confirms exposure. The BeLPT can be performed using either blood or BAL cells, by exposing those cells to beryllium salts in culture (Fig. 79-4). In principle, if T lymphocytes that possess "memory" for beryllium antigen are present, they will start to proliferate *in vitro* when beryllium sulfate is added to the cell culture medium. Alternatively, if an

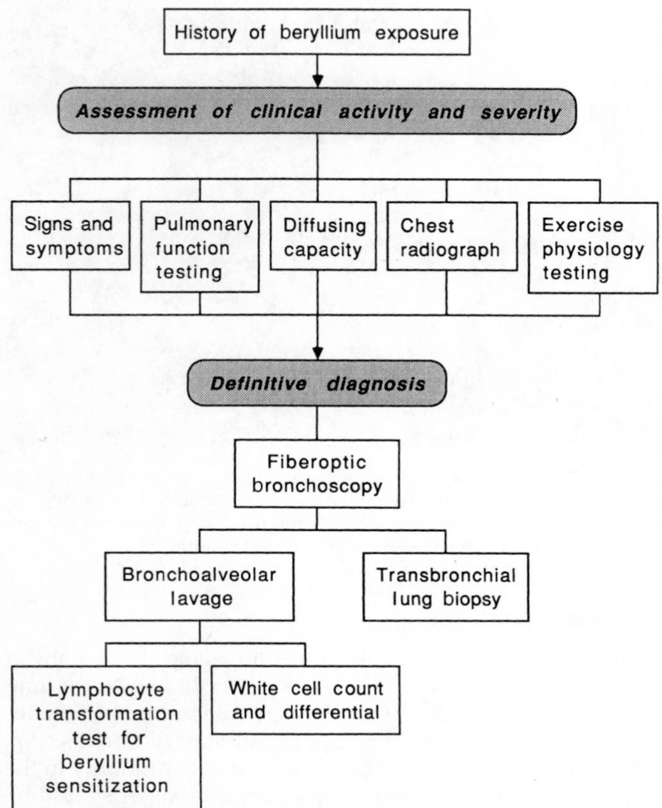

Figure 79-3. Recommended diagnostic approach to chronic beryllium disease. Goals of the evaluation in suspected cases of beryllium disease are twofold: to evaluate the level of impairment (usually due to lung involvement) and to make a definitive diagnosis (with the aid of the beryllium lymphocyte proliferation test and transbronchial lung biopsies).

affected individual's cells do not recognize beryllium as an antigen, they will not proliferate. Proliferation is assessed by placing the cells in 96-well microtiter plates, adding a range of beryllium sulfate concentrations to these cultured cells, and in the last 24 hours of culture, adding a radiolabeled DNA precursor. Cells are harvested, and the amount of radioactivity in the cells is measured. The degree of radioactivity of the cells correlates with the degree of proliferation that has occurred. Patients with sarcoidosis and other lung diseases will have negative lymphocyte responses to beryllium.

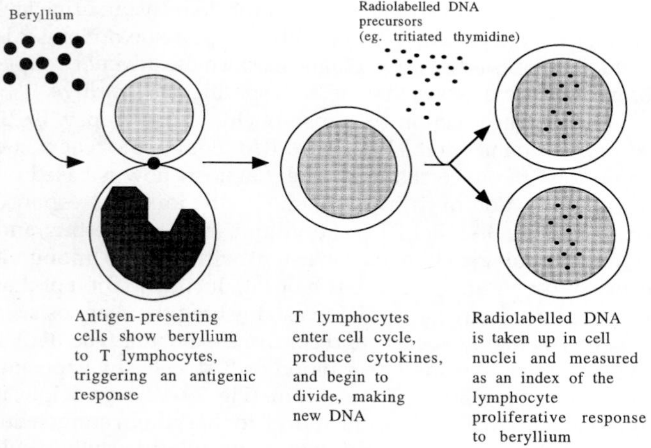

Figure 79-4. Beryllium lymphocyte proliferation test (see text for details).

Individuals now can receive diagnoses at early stages of CBD, prior to the appearance of clinical signs, symptoms, or exercise abnormalities. The immunologic tests distinguish CBD from other interstitial lung disorders, such as sarcoidosis and hypersensitivity pneumonitis. The BeLPT corrects misdiagnoses and helps to direct therapeutic interventions, such as removal from exposure. Nonetheless, the blood BeLPT misses between 10% and 20% of CBD cases. The BAL BeLPT can be affected by tobacco smoking. If equivocal or borderline blood BeLPT results are not clearly normal or abnormal on repeat, beryllium patch testing can be performed as a means of confirming that sensitization has occurred.

Natural History and Prognosis

CBD follows a variable clinical course. Some affected individuals remain stable for many years, although most experience gradual progression of symptoms and of physiologic dysfunction. Smaller subsets suffer much more rapid deterioration over the course of a few years, ultimately leading to respiratory insufficiency. Mortality rates range from 5% to 38%. The disease generally worsens if not treated. A small number of patients may improve spontaneously after exposure ceases, although many patients develop disease even decades after their last exposure. Both removal from exposure and medical treatment are recommended, although the long-term effectiveness of these interventions is not known. Early detection of the subclinical form of CBD may improve the management and change the natural history of this condition and is a subject of an ongoing longitudinal study.

Treatment

There is no cure for CBD. The goal is to prevent the disease by preventing exposure. For those individuals who have contracted CBD, the goals are to reduce morbidity and mortality. Corticosteroids slow disease progression. No randomized controlled trials have been conducted, but large clinical case series have shown the efficacy of corticosteroids as a means of reducing symptoms and improving lung function. Baseline evaluation, prior to the initiation of corticosteroids, should include chest radiography; thin-section CT; complete pulmonary function tests with assessment of lung volumes, spirometry, and DL_{CO}; and exercise physiology testing, preferably with arterial blood gas measurements. Patients who have subclinical disease may not require treatment initially but should receive careful follow-up for evidence of progression. Indications for treatment include the presence of severe symptoms, abnormal gas exchange, decreased exercise tolerance, and abnormal lung physiology. Patients who show a progressive decline in any of these tests should be considered for treatment, as should any individual who demonstrates pulmonary hypertension or cor pulmonale secondary to CBD.

Typical starting doses of corticosteroids are similar to those used to treat sarcoidosis (e.g., prednisone, 0.5 to 0.6 mg per kg of ideal body weight on a daily or alternate-day basis). After 3 to 6 months of this regimen, response to therapy should be reassessed, and the prednisone dose should be tapered to the minimum effective dose. Treatment usually is required for the rest of an affected individual's life. Disease relapses when steroids are withdrawn completely. Patients should be cautioned about the long-term side effects of corticosteroids and should be monitored and treated for those consequences.

Other adjunctive therapy includes the appropriate use of supplemental oxygen, diuretics to treat right ventricular failure, and in some cases, the use of inhaled steroids for those individuals who have severe cough and symptomatic obstructive physiology. Patients should be immunized to prevent influenza and pneumococcal infection. Antibiotics may be needed to treat bronchitis or pneumonia. If patients fail to respond to corticosteroids, other immunosuppressive agents may be helpful, although no formal studies have analyzed "salvage" therapy. As in sarcoidosis, anecdotal evidence suggests that methotrexate (5 to 15 mg orally per week) has a steroid-sparing effect.

SKIN DISEASE

When they come in contact with the skin, beryllium salts can cause acute or chronic contact dermatitis. This condition is another form of cell-mediated hypersensitivity. The dermatitis usually resolves with cessation of exposure. The acute dermatologic findings may be associated also with conjunctivitis and upper respiratory tract symptoms.

Chronic skin ulceration can develop if beryllium is inoculated accidentally into the skin, either as a metal splinter or as embedded particles in contaminated wounds. Some affected individuals develop wartlike granulomatous papules that contain beryllium. Resolution of such lesions is achieved by aggressive, recurrent debridement or by excision. The degree of active inflammation in these skin lesions can wax and wane. Affected individuals typically report that their papules rise and fall and become more or less painful and erythematous over time but that they never disappear completely until they are excised.

Recently, beryllium-containing dental prostheses have been shown to cause oral contact dermatitis. Beryllium patch tests in affected individuals confirmed beryllium sensitization. Patients who react to beryllium alloys in their dental crowns or bridges may develop chronic gingivitis and bleeding gums. Interestingly, beryllium preferentially deposits near the surface of nickel-chromium-beryllium dental alloys, and the beryllium has been shown to leach out of the dental prostheses into surrounding tissues.

CARCINOGENESIS

In animal studies, beryllium causes cancer in many different species, including lung cancer in rats and osteogenic carcinoma in rabbits. Histologic tumor types vary from adenocarcinoma to predominantly bronchoalveolar carcinoma. Large epidemiologic studies demonstrated an increased risk of lung cancer among workers exposed heavily to beryllium, such as those who have had acute beryllium disease. The standardized mortality ratios (SMR) for lung cancer are 1.37 to 1.97 for production workers and 3.14 for individuals with acute beryllium disease. Although some of the older studies have been criticized on methodologic grounds, more recent studies of historical data sets have confirmed an association between beryllium and lung cancer in humans, prompting the International Agency for Research on Cancer to reclassify beryllium as a class 1 human carcinogen. In one study of U.S. Beryllium Case Registry cases, the lung cancer risk in individuals with acute and chronic beryllium disease showed an SMR of 2.00. Those with more acute disease (presumably higher exposure) had a higher risk (SMR, 2.32) as compared to those with CBD (SMR, 1.57). In a separate study of beryllium-exposed workers, after adjusting for smoking, an increased risk of lung cancer was observed (SMR, 1.26).

DISEASE PREVENTION

Acute beryllium pneumonitis has been eliminated largely by attempts to adhere to the beryllium exposure standard. However, CBD continues to plague workers in industries that require specialized beryllium-based parts. More traditional modes of medical surveillance have been replaced by immune biomarkers. The blood BeLPT renders beryllium disease screening and surveillance more specific and more sensitive. It has a high positive predictive value, and both its positive and negative predictive values are superior to clinical evaluation, spirometry, and chest radiography. Chest radiographs identify a small number of additional cases of CBD that may be missed by blood BeLPT. The blood test identifies approximately 80% to 90% of cases.

Beryllium-exposed workers should undergo periodic testing, approximately every 2 years. High-risk areas can be identified by analyzing the frequency of disease or sensitization according to job task, job title, building, and the like. In several studies, machinists have been found to have rates of disease (10% to 16%) higher than those of other employees. New cases of disease and sensitization are detected with repeat periodic screening using the blood BeLPT, especially when it focuses on high-risk processes and manufacturing areas. Beryllium disease occurs even in segments of industry that work exclusively with beryllium-copper or other beryllium-containing alloys. Thus, these companies should be held to the same standards of exposure protection and medical surveillance.

Early studies in neighborhoods near beryllium manufacturing plants showed that disease occurred in areas surrounding such plants, where the ambient air levels were as low as 0.01 μg per cubic meter. Case series in the Japanese beryllium industry have found cases of CBD occurring below the PEL of 2 μg per cubic meter. More recent studies in the ceramics and metal reclamation industries—including a modern beryllium ceramics plant—showed that sensitization and CBD occur in plants where the measured median air concentrations are below the PEL of 2 μg per cubic meter. Apparent adherence to this standard is not sufficiently protective. The best opportunities for prevention of disease are (i) to substitute safer materials wherever possible; (ii) to use engineering and industrial hygiene standards that aim for the lowest possible, reasonably achieved beryllium levels, preferably at least one-tenth of the PEL; (iii) to use administrative controls that reduce the number of beryllium-exposed workers; (iv) to conduct a medical screening program to detect sensitization and disease early; (v) to educate and enlist the help of beryllium workers in developing safer work practices; and (vi) to restrict the egress of beryllium outside the workplace by enforcing good hygienic practices (e.g., clothing and shoe exchanges).

SUGGESTED READING

1. Bobka CA, Stewart LA, Engelken GJ, et al. Comparison of *in vivo* and *in vitro* measures of beryllium sensitization. *J Occup Environ Med* 1997;39:540–547.
2. Cullen MR, Kominsky JR, Rossman MD, et al. Chronic beryllium disease in a precious metal refinery. Clinical, epidemiologic, and immunologic evidence for continuing risk from exposure to low level beryllium fume. *Am Rev Respir Dis* 1987;135:201–208.
3. Epstein PE, Dauber JH, Rossman MD, Daniele RP. Bronchoalveolar lavage in a patient with chronic berylliosis: evidence for hypersensitivity pneumonitis. *Ann Intern Med* 1982;97:213–216.
4. Freiman DG, Hardy HL. Beryllium disease: the relation of pulmonary pathology to clinical course and prognosis based on a study of 130 cases from the US Beryllium Case Registry. *Hum Pathol* 1970;1:25–44.
5. Kreiss K, Miller F, Newman LS, Ojo-Amaize EA, Rossman MD, Saltini C. Chronic beryllium disease: from the workplace to cellular immunology, molecular immunogenetics, and back. *Clin Immunol Immunopathol* 1994;71:123–129.
6. Kreiss K, Mroz MM, Newman LS, Martyny J, Zhen B. Machining risk of beryllium disease and sensitization with median exposures below 2 μg/m^3. *Am J Ind Med* 1996;30:16–25.
7. Kreiss K, Mroz MM, Zhen B, Martyny JW, Newman LS. Epidemiology of beryllium sensitization and disease in nuclear workers. *Am Rev Respir Dis* 1993;148:985–991.
8. Kreiss K, Newman LS, Mroz MM, Campbell PA. Screening blood test identifies subclinical beryllium disease. *J Occup Med* 1989;31:603–608.
9. Kreiss K, Wasserman S, Mroz MM, Newman LS. Beryllium disease screening in the ceramics industry: blood test performance and exposure-disease relations. *J Occup Med* 1993;35:267–274.

10. Kriebel D, Brain JD, Sprince NL, Kazemi H. The pulmonary toxicity of beryllium. *Am Rev Respir Dis* 1988;137:464–473.
11. Mroz MM, Kreiss K, Lezotte DC, Campbell PA, Newman LS. Re-examination of the blood lymphocyte transformation test in the diagnosis of chronic beryllium disease. *J Allergy Clin Immunol* 1991;88:54–60.
12. Newman LS. To Be^{2+} or not to Be^{2+}: relating immunogenetics to occupational exposure. *Science* 1993;262:197–198.
13. Newman LS. Beryllium lung disease: the role of cell-mediated immunity in pathogenesis. In: Dean JH, Luster MI, Munson AE, Kimber I, eds. *Immunotoxicology and immunopharmacology*, 2nd ed. New York: Raven Press, 1994:377–393.
14. Newman LS. Significance of the blood beryllium lymphocyte proliferation test (BeLPT). *Environ Health Perspect* 1996;104:953–956.
15. Newman LS, Buschman DL, Newell JD Jr, Lynch DA. Beryllium disease: assessment with CT. *Radiology* 1994;190:835–840.
16. Newman LS, Kreiss K, King TE Jr, Seay S, Campbell PA. Pathologic and immunologic alterations in early stages of beryllium disease: re-examination of disease definition and natural history. *Am Rev Respir Dis* 1989;139:1479–1486.
17. Newman LS, Lloyd J, Daniloff E. The natural history of beryllium sensitization and chronic beryllium disease. *Environ Health Perspect* 1996;104:937–943.
18. Richeldi L, Sorrentino R, Saltini C. HLA-DPb1 glutamate 69: a genetic marker of beryllium disease. *Science* 1993;262:242–244.
19. Tinkle SS, Schwitters PW, Newman LS. Cytokine production by bronchoalveolar lavage cells in chronic beryllium disease. *Environ Health Perspect* 1996;104:969–971.

CHAPTER 80
Chromium

Robert J. Geller

SOURCES, PRODUCTION, AND USES

As mined, chromium is found most commonly as chromite ore, chromium oxide complexed with iron in the form $FeO{\cdot}Cr_2O_3$. Chromite ore typically also contains aluminum and magnesium oxides and may, in addition, contain titanium or vanadium oxides (or both) in varying quantities (1). Chromium is present in its trivalent state in chromite ore.

Chromium compounds are used widely in industry: in pigments (33%), metal surface plating (25%), leather tanning (25%), and textile production (10%). Photographic processes and catalyst production are other prominent uses.

CHEMICAL AND PHYSICAL FORMS

Chromium has a molecular weight of 52. Generally, it is present as a solid, although one notable exception is chromyl chloride, a hexavalent chromium compound that is a fuming liquid.

The chemical and toxicologic properties of chromium differ markedly, depending on the valence state of the metal. Chromium occurs in its metallic state (valence 0) and in valence states +2 through +6, but only the trivalent (+3) and hexavalent (+6) states are commonly found forms. Chromium in its +2 state frequently oxidizes rapidly to the +3 form, and the +4 and +5 states are found only as intermediates in the conversion between the +3 and +6 states. Some of the chromium compounds of industrial significance are included in Table 80-1.

SITES AND INDUSTRIES ASSOCIATED WITH EXPOSURE

A compilation of data provided by the U.S. National Institute for Occupational Safety and Health (NIOSH) (2) and the articles cited in this chapter indicate that a variety of industries involve chromium use. Table 80-2 is a partial list of such industries and occupational sites in which exposure to chromium is possible.

TABLE 80-1. Some common chromium compounds

Divalent (Cr^{2+})	
Chromous chloride	$CrCl_2$
Chromous sulfate	$CrSO_4$
Trivalent (Cr^{3+})	
Chromic oxide	Cr_2O_3
Chromic sulfate	$Cr_2[SO_4]_3$
Chromite ore	$FeO{\cdot}Cr_2O_3$
Hexavalent (Cr^{6+})	
Chromium trioxide	CrO_3
Chromic acid	H_2CrO_4
Chromic acid anhydrides	
Sodium chromate	Na_2CrO_4
Potassium chromate	K_2CrO_4
Dichromates	
Sodium dichromate	$Na_2Cr_2O_7$
Potassium dichromate	$K_2Cr_2O_7$
Ammonium dichromate	$(NH_4)_2Cr_2O_7$

Chromium toxicity has been studied frequently in the chrome-plating and chromium chemical manufacture industries. These studies, because of their cohort design, inherently involved occupational settings in which exposure levels were higher than presently are allowable (2,2a–d). Also, these studies did not always distinguish between similar—although not identical—jobs. Hard chrome plating (intended for protection of the surface) involves the application of a chrome finish denser than that of bright chrome plating (intended for application of a bright decorative surface), yet the two were not always studied separately.

CLINICAL TOXICOLOGY

Routes of Absorption and Exposure

INHALATION

Metallic chromium and chromous or chromic salts (valences 0, +2, +3) are absorbed minimally after inhalation. Local pulmonary deposition of these salts has been reported after exposure but without evidence of adverse systemic effects (2,3).

Inhalation of highly water-soluble hexavalent chromium salts, such as chromic acid, sodium dichromate, and potassium dichromate, may result in substantial systemic absorption. Less

TABLE 80-2. Industries likely to use chromium compounds

Anodizing
Color television picture tube manufacture
Copper etching
Glass working
Lithography
Metal plating
Metal working
Oil purification
Photoengraving
Photography
Portland cement use
Stainless steel grinding
Textile production
Welding

water-soluble salts are unlikely to produce systemic effects but may produce pulmonary effects (1).

INGESTION

Trivalent chromium salts are absorbed after ingestion, but only 1% to 25% of the dose ingested is absorbed (4). The extent of absorption varies with the particular salt ingested and the circumstances of ingestion. Hexavalent salts are converted by gastric juices to the trivalent form prior to absorption (5).

DERMAL ABSORPTION

Trivalent salts generally are absorbed poorly through intact skin (1). Once the dermal barrier is broken, however, absorption may occur. Hexavalent salts generally are absorbed well topically through intact skin.

Toxicokinetics

On the basis of rat models using ^{51}Cr compounds, chromium has been found to have complex multicompartment kinetics. Rats that received single doses of chromium chloride, a trivalent compound, displayed triphasic elimination, with half-lives of 0.5 days, 5.9 days, and 83.4 days (6). A different group of investigators found chromium chloride(III) to have an average half-life of 91.8 days, as compared to an average half-life of 22.2 days for sodium chromate(VI) (7).

Rats administered intratracheal ^{51}Cr-labeled lead chromate (an insoluble hexavalent salt) were compared to rats given intratracheal sodium chromate (a soluble hexavalent salt), in terms of their clearance of ^{51}Cr from the blood. Both groups were noted to display biphasic elimination. The shorter half-life was noted to be 2.4 days for the insoluble lead chromate and 4.6 days for the soluble sodium chromate (8).

These data suggest that hexavalent and trivalent chromium compounds are handled differently *in vivo*. The principal carrier protein for chromium compounds is transferrin; albumin transports chromium to a lesser extent. Chromium compounds pass through many tissue compartments, including the red blood cell, kidney, liver, spleen, and bone. It is likely that passage through some of these compartments is measured in days to weeks, but passage may be only a matter of hours through other compartments (9,9a).

Signs and Symptoms

ACUTE TOXICITY

Hexavalent Chromium Compounds. After oral or dermal exposure, hexavalent chromium compounds, including chromic acid and the chromates and dichromates, are potentially the most toxic of the chromium compounds commonly encountered. Ingestion of dichromates has proved fatal in 6 of 13 cases collected in one review (10); the oral lethal dose is estimated to be 0.5 to 5.0 g (11).

Skin. Hexavalent chromium compounds may be absorbed percutaneously, even through intact skin. On contact with skin, hexavalent chromium compounds act as both irritants and sensitizers. After local exposure to either airborne particles or contaminated surfaces, chromate dust or chromic acid mist has caused nasal lesions that progress, in some cases, to ulceration ("chrome ulcers") and even perforation of the nasal septum (12,13). These initial lesions have been described as "discrete areas of nasal irritation which burned intensely when the affected nostril was manually collapsed" (12). More severe lesions present an erythematous weeping and crusted appearance. In one study of chromic acid workers, the incidence and severity of nasal injury was related both to length of exposure and to the laxity of industrial hygiene practiced by individual workers (12).

After cutaneous exposure to chromic acid, erosions of the skin may occur. These "chrome holes" initially appear as papular lesions, either singly or grouped, with central ulceration. With progression, adjacent soft tissues become eroded as well (12).

Allergic contact dermatitis from chromates has been observed widely. Dermatitis may develop after exposure of sensitive individuals to even low levels of chromates (14). Furthermore, chromate sensitivity has proved fairly persistent once developed (15,16). In one study, 92% of the study patients with dichromate sensitivity induced by exposure to Portland cement continued to display contact dermatitis 10 years after they initially developed symptoms (15).

Once induced, chromate sensitivity may produce difficulty in multiple settings. Contact with textiles colored with chromate-based pigments can be sufficient to exacerbate the dermatitis. The wearing of leather shoes tanned with chromates can produce dermatitis of the feet if the feet are allowed to remain sweaty. "Housewives' eczema" may be largely a chromate sensitivity phenomenon, as detergents and bleaches in some areas contain more than trace amounts of chromate salts (14).

Gastrointestinal System. Gastric secretions convert hexavalent chromium to trivalent chromium after ingestion; the trivalent form is absorbed more readily from the gastrointestinal tract (5). In this process, however, the gastric and intestinal mucosa are in grave danger of severe erosive injury. Even small ingestions of dichromates have resulted in hemorrhagic gastroenteritis and death (17,18).

Renal System. Acute renal failure is common after large oral ingestions of hexavalent chromium compounds and after dermal exposure (19). Acute renal failure can occur after a dermal burn of 10% body surface area or less. While at work, a 28-year-old man experienced a burn to the left calf with a concentrated chromic acid solution. The area was irrigated immediately with water; however, full-thickness burns covering 1% of body surface area developed over the next few days. He developed nausea and vomiting within 1 hour of exposure and complete anuria within 24 hours. Laboratory evaluations 4 days after exposure were remarkable for a blood urea nitrogen level of 82.0 mg per dL and a serum creatinine level of 14.7 mg per dL. The patient's sodium level was 132.0 mEq per L; potassium, 4.9 mEq per L; calcium, 9.1 mg per dL; phosphorus, 5.0 mg per dL; and uric acid, 7.6 mg per dL. The patient's white blood count was 12.4 per cubic millimeter; platelets numbered 240,000; hemoglobin measured 15.5 g per dL; hematocrit measured 46%; and lactate dehydrogenase was 1,274 units per L. Renal ultrasonography showed no evidence of obstruction. A diagnosis of acute tubular necrosis secondary to acute chromium intoxication was made. Two weeks after exposure, the patient required hemodialysis three times weekly.

This case illustrates the potential for serious chromium intoxication and acute renal failure after chromic acid burns. Whereas the smallest burn previously reported in the literature to result in acute renal failure covered 10% of the body surface area, this patient's burn covered only 1% of the body surface area (ten times smaller than that previously reported to result in acute chromium intoxication) (20).

Pulmonary System. Inhalation of hexavalent chromium salts may result in pulmonary sensitization (2). Inhaled concentrated chromic acid mist has been reported to result in pulmonary edema, which may be delayed up to 72 hours after exposure (21).

Asthma has been reported in workers after repeated exposure to chromium compounds (over 3 months to 9 years) (22). However, the exact nature of the chromium compounds inhaled by these workers was not characterized. Occupational asthma from chromium has been reproduced on bronchial challenge testing with chromic sulfate, a trivalent chromium compound, in four patients, all of whom were ex-smokers (22).

Chronic inhalation of hexavalent chromium compounds presents an increased risk of lung cancers (see Carcinogenesis and Long-Term Health Effects). Adult respiratory distress syndrome has been reported after substantial ingestion (18).

Hepatic System. Hepatic dysfunction has been observed only rarely after exposure to chromic acid (2).

Trivalent Chromium. Trivalent chromium is absorbed poorly by inhalation and through intact skin, resulting in a low order of systemic toxicity. However, should trivalent chromium gain access to the systemic circulation, toxic effects may develop. For example, a 70% total body thermal burn from hot chromic sulfate mixed with sulfuric acid produced chromium poisoning with acute renal failure (23).

Inhalation of trivalent chromium salts can cause occupational asthma. In one case, immunoglobulin E antibodies to chromic sulfate were demonstrated (24). Pneumoconiosis has been observed also after exposure to chromite ore dust (4,25).

CARCINOGENESIS AND LONG-TERM HEALTH EFFECTS

Chronic inhalation of hexavalent chromium presents an increased risk of lung cancers, with the degree of risk depending on the particular salts and their solubility under biological conditions, on the circumstances of exposure, and on such concomitant risk factors as cigarette smoking. Chromate compounds that are insoluble or poorly soluble in water appear to be more potent pulmonary carcinogens as compared to chromates with high water solubility. Zinc chromate is the most potent carcinogen among the chromates commonly found in industrial settings; calcium chromate and lead chromate pose a lesser risk (1,9,26–34). Nonetheless, the NIOSH considers all hexavalent chromium compounds to be potential human carcinogens (21).

At this point, although agreement is not unanimous, trivalent chromium compounds and metallic chromium generally are considered to be either very weak carcinogens or noncarcinogenic.

GENOTOXICITY

A review of some 650 genotoxicity tests using a variety of methodologies was published by de Flora et al. (26). These authors found positive results in 88% of the 450 tests of hexavalent chromium compounds, as compared with 23% positive results with trivalent chromium compounds (9,26,27,29,33).

Management of Toxicity

CLINICAL MANAGEMENT

No matter what the route of exposure, the initial approach to an affected individual includes a brief assessment of clinical status followed by support of basic cardiopulmonary functions. Once the airway has been stabilized and cardiopulmonary support has been instituted as indicated, further measures can be considered.

TABLE 80-3. Ascorbic acid dosage for treatment of hexavalent chromium ingestion

Salt	Dose of ascorbic acid per gram of ingested chromium salt
Chromic acid, chromic trioxide	3.85
Sodium dichromate	2.9
Potassium dichromate	2.62
Ammonium dichromate	3

Ingestion

Decontamination. Emesis generally should *not* be induced in the patient exposed to chromium via ingestion, owing to the potential corrosive effects of the chromium compound and the potential for rapid deterioration of the patient. Usually, ascorbic acid should be administered orally or nasogastrically, if the patient is seen while the chromium compound is still in the stomach. Ascorbic acid has been shown to ameliorate the effects of topical human exposure to chromates (35) and to reduce toxicity after ingestion in rats if given within 2 hours of exposure (35). Ascorbic acid functions chemically to reduce Cr^{6+} to Cr^{3+}, the form less toxic to the gastric and intestinal mucosa. The dosage of ascorbic acid recommended for several hexavalent salts is shown in Table 80-3 (19).

Dilution of the ingested agent may be appropriate if dilution can be accomplished within minutes after ingestion, particularly if the ingested material's pH is fairly low (e.g., chromic acid) or fairly high (e.g., ammonium dichromate). Dilution may be accomplished with water or with fluids that also serve as demulcents, such as milk. The use of demulcent compounds (e.g., antacids, corn starch, or milk) in addition to those used for dilution has been recommended (19) and seems reasonable but has not been studied formally.

Gastric lavage to reduce the ingested dose may be desirable if chromium is likely to be present in the stomach. The potential benefit of lavage (removal of some of the ingested caustic toxin) must be weighed against the associated risk (perforation of the esophagus or stomach by the tube), particularly because some degree of injury already may have occurred. If the decision to proceed with lavage is made, a soft tube is preferable. Lavage using such antacids as magnesium hydroxide has been suggested, but no studies have demonstrated the efficacy of antacids relative to the use of water. Activated charcoal has not been studied experimentally in the treatment of chromate poisoning and would not be anticipated to be beneficial.

Elimination Enhancement. Exchange transfusion was effective in reducing blood chromium levels 67% in one case of chromium poisoning, using 10.9 L of blood (23). Existing evidence does not allow the conclusion that exchange transfusion generally should be employed, however.

Hemodialysis and charcoal hemoperfusion do not substantially enhance chromium removal from the body if renal function remains normal (18,36). However, if renal failure ensues, hemodialysis may be necessary for management of the renal failure itself.

Treatment. Fluid balance must be maintained. Affected patients should be monitored carefully for evidence of gastrointestinal bleeding, methemoglobinemia, hemolysis, coagulopathy, seizures, or pulmonary dysfunction. Appropriate supportive measures should be employed as indicated.

If hemolysis develops, alkaline diuresis may be indicated to reduce the possibility of further renal injury. Methemoglobinemia should be treated with methylene blue if the methemoglobin level exceeds 30% or if signs or symptoms of methemoglobinemia are present.

Chelation with ethylenediaminetetraacetic acid and British anti-Lewisite does not seem to be of clinical benefit (17,37). *N*-acetylcysteine increased chromium clearance and reversed oliguria in rats poisoned with potassium dichromate, but no published accounts have cited human experience using *N*-acetylcysteine (37).

Inhalation. After inhalation of hexavalent or trivalent chromium compounds, patients should be removed from further exposure and assessed carefully. If respiratory distress or cyanosis is noted, oxygen should be administered. Bronchospasm should be treated with bronchodilators; selective β_2-agonists, such as albuterol, are the agents of initial choice.

If the inhaled agent was concentrated chromic acid, continued observation and assessment should be considered, to note any development of pulmonary edema up to 72 hours after exposure. Similar precautions after the inhalation of other concentrated hexavalent, highly soluble chromium compounds are prudent.

Dermal Absorption. In cases of dermal absorption, the skin should be irrigated copiously with water. The affected area should be evaluated for the presence of chemical or thermal burns, and treatment should be provided as indicated.

The topical application of a freshly made 10% ascorbic acid solution (35,38) or of a barrier cream containing 2% glycine and 1% tartaric acid (39) has proved beneficial in some industrial settings in reducing the consequences of topical exposure to hexavalent chromium compounds.

LABORATORY STUDIES

Specific measurement of chromium or chromate levels after exposure has not been shown to have prognostic or therapeutic value. However, it may allow further documentation of exposure and assessment of the efficacy of measures used to enhance elimination (1).

BIOLOGICAL MONITORING

Methods for monitoring biological exposure have been recommended by the American Conference of Governmental Industrial Hygienists (40). That agency has published two biological exposure index (BEI) measures for hexavalent chromium compounds as a water-soluble fume. One BEI monitors the increase in total chromium in urine during a work shift, with an upper limit of 10 µg per g of creatinine. The other BEI samples the total urinary chromium at the end of the shift at the end of the work week, with an upper limit of 30 µg per g of creatinine (40).

Confounding factors must be addressed prior to institution of any biological monitoring. These factors include the difficulty of accurate and precise laboratory measurement and the possibility of sample contamination during collection and storage.

Studies show that the predominant form of chromium recovered in blood and tissues, even after exposure to hexavalent chromium, is trivalent chromium, because the hexavalent (Cr^{6+}) form is reduced to the trivalent form in tissues in biological media. Reduction of Cr^{6+} to Cr^{3+} decreases the entry of chromium into cells and lessens intracellular and DNA damage. Ascorbic acid and glutathione, both intracellularly and extracellularly, act as reductants for hexavalent chromium. Trivalent chromium is excreted mostly in the urine. In the opinion of some, using trivalent chromium levels in the urine is not the most reasonable biological monitoring approach (41).

Some researchers maintain that chromium determination in erythrocytes is a more useful estimation of the body burden of hexavalent chromium after exposure. This belief is based on the assumption that only Cr^{6+} is able to enter the red blood cell membrane because it exceeds plasma reduction capacity or because it has entered the red blood cells before reduction to Cr^{3+} has taken place. Assessing chromium levels in urine and in whole blood and monitoring workers with possible exposure to hexavalent chromium has been conducted. Some believe that chromium concentration in the red blood cell is the best measure of hexavalent chromium burden (41). When low chromium levels are found in the erythrocytes along with high urine chromium concentrations, extracellular reduction of hexavalent chromium is assumed to be sufficient for detoxification. In unexposed individuals, chromium concentrations in red blood cells up to 1 µg per L were detected. Values above this level suggest hexavalent chromium exposure. Thus, chromium level measurement in red blood cells appears to be a better measure of the hexavalent chromium burden of the body.

Once hexavalent chromium has penetrated into erythrocytes, it is reduced to Cr^{3+} and cannot escape the cell. Thus, hexavalent chromium compounds essentially are stored in red blood cells for their life span, allowing the identification of strong and weak reducers in response to hexavalent chromium exposure. Miksche and Lewalter (41) suggested erythrocyte monitoring of chromium in parallel with urine monitoring of chromium.

EXPOSURE LIMITS

The U.S. Occupational Safety and Health Administration recommends limits in its final rule—permissible exposure limits—on a time-weighted average basis (42). The American Conference of Governmental Industrial Hygienists recommends its threshold limit values (40) on a time-weighted average basis. Recommendations from both agencies are found in Table 80-4. NIOSH has declared that certain air concentrations are immediately dangerous to life and health (Table 80-5) (43).

SUMMARY

Chromium toxicity varies with particular chromium compounds. Metallic chromium and divalent and trivalent chromium compounds generally are less toxic than are hexavalent chromium compounds, although all may cause dermal sensiti-

TABLE 80-4. OSHA and ACGIH recommended exposure limits for chromium compounds

Chromium compound	OSHA PEL	ACGIH TLV
Metallic chromium	1.0 mg Cr/m^3	0.5 mg Cr/m^3
Divalent chromium compounds	0.5 mg Cr/m^3	0.5 mg Cr/m^3
Trivalent chromium compounds	0.5 mg Cr/m^3	0.5 mg Cr/m^3
Hexavalent chromium compounds		
Water-soluble	0.1 mg CrO_3/m^3	0.05 mg CrO_3/m^3
Water-insoluble	0.1 mg CrO_3/m^3	0.01 mg CrO_3/m^3
Chromic acid (ceiling)	0.1 mg CrO_3/m^3	0.05 mg CrO_3/m^3
Chromite ore	—	0.05 mg Cr/m^3

ACGIH, American Conference of Governmental Industrial Hygienists; OSHA, U.S. Occupational Safety and Health Administration; PEL, permissible exposure limit; TLV, threshold limit value.
Note: Please check most current recommendations.

TABLE 80-5. Air concentrations considered immediately dangerous to life and health by National Institute for Occupational Safety and Health standards

Chromium compound	Concentration
Metallic chromium	250 mg Cr/m^3
Insoluble chromium salts	500 mg Cr/m^3
Soluble divalent salts	250 mg Cr/m^3
Soluble trivalent salts	25 mg Cr/m^3
Hexavalent chromium compounds and chromic acid	15 mg CrO_3/m^3

zation. Hexavalent chromium compounds are dangerous after acute substantial exposure and may be hazardous also after chronic exposure to lower concentrations. Certain hexavalent chromium compounds have been demonstrated to be carcinogenic; all hexavalent compounds are potential carcinogens.

The optimal treatment for chromium toxicity lies in its prevention, with the use of good industrial hygiene practices and use of proper workplace industrial controls. Once toxicity develops, however, the ideal therapy has not yet been found.

REFERENCES

1. Sawyer HJ. Chromium and its compounds. In: Zenz C, ed. *Occupational medicine*, 3rd ed. St. Louis: Mosby, 1994:487–495.
2. Tabershaw IR, Utidjian HMD, Kawahara BL. Chromium and its compounds. In: Kay MM, ed. *Occupational diseases: a guide to their recognition.* Washington: National Institute for Occupational Safety and Health, 1977:352–354.

2a. Agency for Toxic Substances and Disease Registry. *Toxicologic profile for chromium compounds.* Atlanta: US Depatement of Health and Human Services, Public Health Service, ATSDR, 2000.

2b. Becker N. Cancer mortality among arc welders exposed to fumes containing chromium and nickel. Results of a third follow-up: 1989–1995. *J Occup Environ Med* 1999;41:294–303.

2c. Gibbs HJ, Lees PS, Pinsky PF, Rooney BC. Lung cancer among workers in chromium chemical production. *Am J Ind Med* 2000;38:606.

2d. Gibbs HJ, Lees PS, Pinsky PF, Rooney BC. Clinical findings of irritation among chromium chemical production workers. *Am J Ind Med* 2000;38:127–131.

3. Proctor NH, Hughes JP, Fischman ML, et al. Chromium. In: Proctor NH, Hughes JP, Fischman ML, et al., eds. *Chemical hazards of the workplace*, 2nd ed. Philadelphia: JB Lippincott Co, 1988:155–158.
4. Baselt RC, Cravey RH. *Disposition of toxic drugs and chemicals in man*, 4th ed. Foster City, CA: Chemical Toxicology Institute, 1995:168–170.
5. DeFlora S, Badolati GS, Serra D, et al. Circadian reduction of chromium in the gastric environment. *Mutat Res* 1987;192:169–174.
6. Mertz W, Roginski EE, Reba RC. Biological activity and fate of trace quantities of intravenous chromium(III) in the rat. *Am J Physiol* 1965;209:614–618.
7. Sayato Y, Nakamuro K, Matoni S, Ando M. Metabolic fate of chromium compounds: comparative behavior of chromium in the rat administered with $Na_2{}^{51}CrO_4$ and $^{51}CrCl_3$. *J Pharm Dynam* 1980;3:17–23.
8. Bragt PC, van Dura EA. Toxicokinetics of hexavalent chromium in the rat after intratracheal administration of chromates of different solubilities. *Ann Occup Hyg* 1983;27:315–322.
9. Katz SA, Salem H. The toxicology of chromium with respect to its speciation: a review. *J Appl Toxicol* 1993;13:277–224.

9a. US Environmental Protection Agency. *Toxiocological review of hexavalent chromium.* Washington: Environmental Protection Agency, 1998.

10. Bader TF. Acute renal failure after chromic acid injection. *West J Med* 1986;144:608–609.
11. Kaufman DB, DiNicola W, McIntosh R. Acute potassium dichromate poisoning. *Am J Dis Child* 1970;119:374–376.
12. Cohen SR, Davis DM, Kramkowski RS. Clinical manifestations of chromic acid toxicity. *Cutis* 1974;13:558–568.
13. Lee HS, Goh CL. Occupational dermatosis among chrome platers. *Contact Dermatitis* 1988;18:89–93.
14. Fisher AA. Blackjack disease and other chromate puzzles. *Cutis* 1976;18:21–22, 35.
15. Burrows D. Prognosis in industrial dermatitis. *Br J Dermatol* 1972;87:145–148.
16. Breit R, Turk RBM. The medical and social fate of the dichromate allergic patient. *Br J Dermatol* 1976;94:349–351.
17. Ellis EN, Brouhard BH, Lynch RE, et al. Effects of hemodialysis and dimercaprol in acute dichromate poisoning. *J Toxicol Clin Toxicol* 1982;19:249–258.
18. Iserson KV, Banner W, Froede RC, et al. Failure of dialysis therapy in potassium dichromate poisoning. *J Emerg Med* 1983;1:143–149.
19. Sharma BK, Singhal PC, Chugh KS. Intravascular hemolysis and acute renal failure following potassium dichromate poisoning. *Postgrad Med J* 1978;54:414–415.
20. Stoner RS, Tong TG, Dart RC, Sullivan JB. Acute chromium intoxication with renal failure after 1% body surface area burns from chromic acid [Abstract]. Presented at the American Academy of Clinical Toxicology (AACT) Annual Scientific Meeting, Baltimore, MD, October 1–4, 1988.
21. Riggs BS. Chromium. In: *Poisindex,* vol 91. (CD-ROM version.) Englewood, CO: Micromedex, 1996.
22. Park HS, Yu HJ, Jung KS. Occupational asthma caused by chromium. *Clin Exp Allergy* 1994;24:676–681.
23. Kelly WF, Ackrill R, Day JP, et al. Cutaneous absorption of trivalent chromium: tissue levels and treatment by exchange transfusion. *Br J Ind Med* 1982;39:397–400.
24. Novey HS, Habib M, Wells ID. Asthma and IgE antibodies induced by chromium and nickel salts. *J Allergy Clin Immunol* 1983;72:407–412.
25. Mancuso TF, Hueper WC. Occupational cancer and other health hazards in a chromate plant. *Ind Med Surg* 1951;20:358–363.
26. de Flora S, Bagnasco M, Serra D, et al. Genotoxicity of chromium compounds: a review. *Mutat Res* 1990;238:99–172.
27. Langård S. Role of chemical species and exposure characteristics in cancer among persons occupationally exposed to chromium compounds. *Scand J Work Environ Health* 1993;19(Suppl 1):81–89.
28. Abe S, Ohsaki Y, Kimura K, et al. Chromate lung cancer with special reference to its cell type and relation to the manufacturing process. *Cancer* 1982; 49:783–787.
29. Braver ER, Infante P, Chu K. An analysis of lung cancer risk from exposure to hexavalent chromium. *Terat Carcinog Mutagen* 1985;5:365–378.
30. Farkas I. WHO-coordinated international study on the health effects of occupational exposure of welders to chromium and nickel. *Nutr Res* 1985; (Suppl 1):683–689.
31. Hayes RB, Sheffet A, Spirtas R. Cancer mortality among a cohort of chromium pigment workers. *Am J Ind Med* 1989;16:127–133.
32. Langård S. One hundred years of chromium and cancer: a review of epidemiological evidence and selected case reports. *Am J Ind Med* 1990;17:189–215.
33. Norseth T. The carcinogenicity of chromium and its salts [Editorial]. *Br J Ind Med* 1986;43:649–651.
34. Svensson BG, Englander V, Akesson B, et al. Deaths and tumors among workers grinding stainless steel. *Am J Ind Med* 1989;15:51–59.
35. Samitz MH. Prevention of occupational skin diseases from exposure to chromic acid and chromates: use of ascorbic acid. *Cutis* 1974;13:569–574.
36. Behari JR, Tandon SK. Chelation in metal intoxication: VIII. *Clin Toxicol* 1980;16:33–40.
37. Banner W, Koch M, Capin DM, et al. Experimental chelation therapy in chromium, lead, and boron intoxication with *n*-acetylcysteine and other compounds. *Toxicol Appl Pharmacol* 1986;83:142–147.
38. Milner JE. Ascorbic acid in the prevention of chromium dermatitis. *J Occup Med* 1980;22:51–52.
39. Romaguera C, Grimalt F, Vilaplana J, et al. Formulation of a barrier cream against chromate. *Contact Dermatitis* 1985;13:49–52.
40. American Conference of Governmental Industrial Hygienists. *1995–96 Threshold limit values for chemical substances and physical agents and biological exposure indices (BEIs).* Cincinnati: American Conference of Governmental Industrial Hygienists, 1995.
41. Miksche L, Lewalter R. Biological monitoring of exposure to hexavalent chromium in isolated erythrocytes. In: Mendelsohn M, Peters J, Normandy M, eds. *Biomarkers and occupational health.* Washington: Joseph Henry Press, 1995.
42. US Occupational Safety and Health Administration, Department of Labor. Air contaminants, final rule: no. 29 *CFR* 1910. *Federal Register* 1989;54(12): 2332–2983.
43. National Institute for Occupational Safety and Health, US Department of Health and Human Services. *Pocket guide to chemical hazards.* (CD-ROM version.) Englewood, CO: Micromedex, 1996.

CHAPTER 81
Manganese

Raquel L. Gibly and John B. Sullivan, Jr.

SOURCES AND PRODUCTION

Chemical and Physical Forms

Manganese (molecular weight, 54.9) is a reddish gray or silvery soft metal, a member of group VII of the periodic table. It is the tenth most abundant metal in the earth's crust, at an average concentration of 1,000 parts per million (ppm). Mn is the nineteenth most abundant seawater metal at 1 part per billion (ppb) and is the fourth most widely used metal in the world (1,2). It is contained in various ores, including the oxides pyrolusite, braunite, manganite,

TABLE 81-1. Common names and chemical formulas for some manganese compounds and products

Common name	Formula	CAS number	Physical properties	Trade names	Common uses
Manganese	Mn	7439-96-5	Reddish gray, silvery	Mangacat, Mangan	
Manganese acetate	$C_4H_6O_4 \cdot Mn$	638-38-0	Pale red crystals	Diacetyl manganese	Food packaging
Manganese acetyl acetonate	$C_{10}H_{14}O_4Mn$	14024-58-9			Experimental tumorigenic compound
Manganese(II) chloride (1:2)	ClMn	7773-01-5	Cubic, pink crystals		Experimental mutagen
Mn dimethyl dithiocarbamate	$C_3H_7NS_2 \cdot {}^1\!/_2Mn$	15339-36-3			Pesticide
Manganese dioxide	MnO_2	1313-13-9	Tetragonal crystals	Mn black, cement black	Powerful oxidizer
Manganese EDTA complex	$C_{10}H_{12}MnN_2O_8 \cdot 2H$	55448-20-9			
Mn(II) ethylene-*bis*-dithiocarbamate	$C_4H_7N_2S_4 \cdot Mn$	12427-38-2	Yellow powder or crystals	Manam, Maneb, Manzate, Aamangan, Vancide	Fungicide
Manganese trifluoride	F_3Mn	7783-53-1	Red mass, monolithic crystals		Fluorinating agent
Manganese(II) oxide	MnO	1344-43-0	Grass-green powder	Cassel green	
Manganese(III) oxide	Mn_2O_3	1317-34-6	Black powder	Cassel brown, walnut stain	
Manganese(II) sulfate (1:1)	$O_4S \cdot Mn$	7785-87-7	Reddish crystals	Man-Gro, Sorba-Spray Mn	
Mn tricarbonyl methylcyclopentadienyl	$C_9H_7MnO_3$	12108-13-3		Antiknock-33, MMT, MCT	
Potassium permanganate	$MnO_4 \cdot K$	7722-64-7	Dark purple crystals	Condy's crystals, Cairox	Topical antibacterial chemical reagent

CAS, Chemical Abstract Services; EDTA, ethylenediaminetetraacetic acid.
Adapted with permission from refs. 1 and 4.

hausmannite, and psilomelane; hauserite, a sulfide; manganesespat, a carbonate; and tephroite, a silicate (1). The most commercially important of these is pyrolusite, which is made up primarily of manganese dioxide (Table 81-1) (1,3,4). Mn can be found as manganous and manganic salts, manganese sulfate, and manganese oxide (ore). Solid ore, powder, dust, and fumes are found as sulfides and oxides. Mn is soluble in water and dilute acid.

Suppliers and Uses

Australia, Brazil, Gabon, and South Africa supply 90% of the world market for Mn, other sources being Canada, Chile, China, Cuba, India, Ghana, Morocco, and Russia. Low-grade deposits are found in the United States.

Predominant uses for Mn are in the production of steel and iron alloys such as ferromanganese, silicomanganese, manganin, and spielgeleisen (15% to 30% manganese). Silicomanganese (between 65% and 68% Mn) is an alloy consisting of silicon and Mn (5). Because Mn is moderately reactive and brittle, it is found in Heusler alloys (18% to 25% manganese) with copper and aluminum or zinc. Many iron and steel manufacturing processes require the addition of Mn to molten iron to reduce the iron oxide content by the formation of manganese oxide. Manganese oxide dissolves readily in molten slag and is easily separated from the iron. Mn also is used to reduce the oxygen and sulfur content of molten steel, thereby increasing ductility.

Iron and steel alloys made with Mn demonstrate increased durability and corrosion resistance as compared to those that do not contain manganese. Steel Mn alloys are more malleable than others when forged. Mn may be produced from ferrous scrap that is used in the production of electric and open-hearth steel (5).

Mn and its compounds are used in paints, varnishes, inks, dyes, matches, pyrotechnics, bleaching agents, laboratory reagents, motor oils, fertilizers, disinfectants, and welding rods. Manganous acetate is used in fertilizers, leather tanning, and dyeing, as a drying agent for linseed oil, and as a decolorizer and coloring agent in the manufacture of glass and ceramics (1). Manganese carbonate has medicinal uses and is found also in the pigment manganese white. Manganese dioxide is used as a depolarizer in the manufacture of dry-cell batteries. Manganese sulfate is found in red pottery glaze and is used as a fertilizer for vines and tobacco. It also is used in veterinary medicine to prevent perosis in poultry. Manganese ethylene-*bis*-dithiocarbamate (Maneb) is a widely used commercial fungicide. Methylcyclopentadienyl manganese tricarbonyl (MMT) is an organic antiknock agent used in unleaded gasoline in Canada and is one of several organomanganese compounds that have been proposed for this use (1,6). In the United States, MMT has been used as an octane enhancer in leaded gasoline (Table 81-2) (1,7,8). It also serves as an additive in machine, diesel, and fuel oils. Potassium permanganate is highly bactericidal and fungicidal and is used in water purification (2).

Physiologic Sources and Uses

Mn is resident in both plants and animals. It is found most abundantly in whole grains and cereal products and in lesser amounts in tea, fruits, vegetables, dairy products, meats, poul-

TABLE 81-2. Common sources of exposure to manganese and its compounds

Substance	Use or source
Manganese metal	Alloy in feromanganese, silicomanganese, and manganin; Heusler alloys
Manganous acetate	Dyeing, leather tanning, fertilizers
Manganese dioxides	Mining, smelting, refining of manganese ore; dry-cell batteries, matches, pyrotechnics, fertilizers, drugs, glass and ceramics
Manganese salts	Paints, varnishes, inks, dyes
Manganese sulfate	Pottery glaze, fertilizer
Permanganate compounds	Decolorizer and pigment in glass and ceramic; oxidizing agent in chemical industry
Methylcyclopentadienyl manganese tricarbonyl (MMT or MCT)	Antiknock agent in lead-free gasoline

Adapted with permission from refs. 1 and 8.

TABLE 81-3. Recommended daily allowances (RDA) for manganese

Age (yr)	RDA
Adults (>18)	2.0–5.0 mg/day[a]
Adolescents (11–18)	2.0–3.0 mg/day
Children (1–10)	1.0–2.0 mg/day
Infants (0.5–1.0)	0.6–1.0 mg/day
Infants (0.0–0.5)	0.3–0.6 mg/day

[a]No changes for pregnancy or lactation.
From ref. 9, with permission.

try, and fish (9). It is supplemented in infant formulas and parenteral nutrition preparations. The average adult ingests between 4 and 10 mg per day (2,10).

Mn is an essential trace element necessary for the functioning of many enzyme systems, including pyruvate carboxylase (a metalloenzyme), arginase, phosphatase, and lipid and mucopolysaccharide synthetases (1). The skeletal system contains approximately 43% of the body's Mn, with the remainder found in such soft tissues as liver, pancreas, kidneys, brain, and central nervous system (CNS) (1). Mn is transferred across the placenta (10) and can be transferred in breast milk, with a mean concentration in breast milk of 7 to 120 μg per L (11).

The National Research Council (9) has set provisional daily intake recommendations for dietary Mn (Table 81-3). Mn deficiency has not been demonstrated in humans (1).

OCCUPATIONAL AND ENVIRONMENTAL SOURCES OF EXPOSURE

The most common victims of Mn toxicity are workers exposed to large amounts of Mn dust: miners, welders, and workers in dry-cell battery plants, steel alloy plants, and ceramic plants (12). Artists are also exposed to Mn through paint pigments (especially blues, purples, and greens) and metalwork (13). Toxic exposures have been reported from ingestion of drinking water contaminated by mining operations and improperly discarded lead-acid batteries. Combustion of MMT causes an increase in airborne Mn concentrations (7).

CLINICAL TOXICOLOGY

Routes of Exposure

Because Mn and its compounds are found readily as dusts, fumes, and solutes in groundwater, the primary routes of Mn exposure are inhalation and oral ingestion. Significant dermal absorption is not apparent, although contact dermatitis has been reported (1).

The rate of Mn absorption depends on intestinal Mn concentration and the body's total Mn load (1). Iron deficiency states and low-protein dietary states have been associated with increased absorption of oral Mn (10,14–16). Increased dietary calcium or phosphorus decreases Mn absorption (10).

Alveolar absorption occurs at a continuous slow rate and depends on Mn body reserves (1). After inhalational exposure, passive diffusion of inhaled Mn into the pulmonary capillary vascular system occurs. Studies have shown that a portion of inhaled Mn is transferred to the gastrointestinal tract and absorbed there, demonstrating significant gastrointestinal absorption even with inhalational exposures (17).

Distribution, Metabolism, and Elimination

DISTRIBUTION

Ingested Mn^{2+} is oxidized to Mn^{3+} in the alkaline medium of the duodenum (18). Only the Mn^{3+} cationic form of Mn seems to be well absorbed. Some absorbed Mn^{3+} is conjugated with bile in the liver and reexcreted into the intestine to undergo enterohepatic circulation (10). The exact mechanism of Mn absorption from the gastrointestinal tract remains unknown, and studies have not demonstrated whether active or passive transport systems are involved (18). On reaching the serum, Mn complexes with the β_1-globulin transmanganin, which is involved in its serum transport (1,18,19).

Mn concentrates in mitochondrial-rich tissues, where it alters calcium homeostasis and increases oxidation (20). The highest concentrations of Mn are found (in descending order) in bone marrow, brain, kidney, pancreas, and liver (10). Nearly 40% of the body's Mn pool is concentrated in the bone marrow. Mn is known to affect the color of one's hair and conjunctivae and can be found in these tissues as well. This element also is found bound to the porphyrin complex in erythrocytes.

Mn acts on the basal ganglia, the major pathologic change in human manganism being degeneration of the medial segment of the globus pallidus, with subsequent neuronal loss and gliosis (21). To a lesser extent the caudate nucleus and the putamen are involved. The substantia nigra rarely is involved, which allows the pseudoparkinsonism of manganism to be differentiated from true Parkinson's disease (22). Also, the Lewy bodies commonly seen in true Parkinson's disease rarely are evident in manganism (2).

The substantia nigra seems to be more commonly involved with manganism in animals than in humans, but this may be due to the higher levels of Mn used in the animal experiments (20). Decreased levels of catecholamines and serotonin in the corpus striatum and depletion of dopamine by Mn-mediated autoxidation seem to be the basic pathophysiologic defects (20,23). Mild CNS effects may also result from functional disturbances in postsynaptic striatal or pallidal neurons without profound dopamine depletion (24). Other CNS actions of manganese include promotion of free radical formation, decreased cortical glucose consumption, decreased γ-aminobutyric acid and substance P, and impairment of oxidative metabolism (21).

METABOLISM

Manganese does not appear to pass through the cytochrome P-450 or glucuronidation pathways, and elimination does not require active metabolism.

ELIMINATION

Mn excretion is not affected by the presence or absence of other metal ions. Absorbed Mn (Mn^{3+}) rapidly appears in bile fluid and undergoes enterohepatic circulation followed by excretion. Small amounts of Mn can be found in pancreatic fluid, with only extremely small amounts detectable in urine (less than 6% of absorbed dose). The major route of Mn excretion (up to 99%) is via the feces (17,18). Mn is also found in hair, which serves as a minor excretory pathway (25).

The half-life ($t_{1/2}$) of Mn has been studied in humans and depends on a person's health and previous exposure to Mn. Plasma Mn levels after intravenous injection showed a $t_{1/2}$ of 1.34 minutes in normal individuals, 2.03 minutes in healthy Mn miners, and 1.44 minutes in patients with chronic Mn poisoning (25). Whole blood $t_{1/2}$ for the same population was 1.28, 2.19, and 1.33 minutes, respectively (25). The whole body $t_{1/2}$ was 15.0 to 37.5 days, and was again dependent on the health and exposure status of the individual, with normal individuals having the slowest clearance rates and heavily exposed individuals having faster rates of clearance (25). Mn homeostasis is strictly regulated in the human body, such that rates of excretion always exceed absorption. Therefore, long-term accumulation of Mn is minimal in aging humans (1).

Signs, Symptoms, and Syndromes

GENERAL CLINICAL TOXICOLOGY

Mn is the least toxic of the essential metals (1). Toxicity of this element is related to its oxidation state and its parent compound. In general, the higher the oxidation state of Mn, the more toxic the compound. The exception is Mn^{2+}, which is two and a half to three times more toxic than Mn^{3+}. The anion in a Mn salt also acts as a predictor of toxicity, with manganese citrate being more toxic than (in descending order) manganese chloride, sulfate, or acetate (1).

Acute exposure syndromes can occur immediately, whereas chronic toxic signs and symptoms may be delayed 6 months or as late as 24 years after exposure has begun (12). Reports in the literature date back as far as 1837 when Dr. John Couper described changes in workers who inhaled manganese oxides (12). Mn has also been used historically as a purgative and a cutaneous cure for scabies and similar skin afflictions (12).

ACUTE TOXICITY

Acute exposure to Mn may produce multiple pulmonary syndromes ranging from a collection of flulike symptoms, termed *metal fume fever* (MFF), to manganese pneumonitis or pneumonia (1,26,27). MFF is caused by the inhalation of minute particles of metal dust (0.05 to 0.1 μm) that penetrate deeply into the respiratory tract and reside in the alveoli (27). MFF has been seen with the inhalation of Mn, magnesium, and other metal dusts. Once in the respiratory tract, the metal particles activate macrophages, which, in turn, cause the release of pyogenes, which cause local inflammatory and vasoactive reactions. Mn metal dust does not cause direct structural damage, and the signs and symptoms of MFF are reversible and without permanent sequelae.

Symptoms of MFF often begin with increased thirst and a metallic taste in the mouth. They then progress to include fever, chills, sweating, nausea, throat irritation, cough, headache, myalgias, and arthralgias. These symptoms usually manifest at the beginning of the work week, several hours after the exposure begins, and often remit by the weekend as tolerance is exhibited. Episodes usually are self-limiting and resolve within 36 hours of cessation of exposure (13). Tolerance may be acquired after continuous exposure, suggesting some form of immunologic response (27). Treatment is supportive care only.

Mn pneumonitis or pneumonia has been described in workers exposed to Mn ore, dry-cell battery production, and potassium permanganate manufacturing processes (28,29). Either of these conditions is more severe than MFF and may require antibiotic and bronchodilator therapy (29). Each condition is characterized by the onset of dyspnea, and fever. Expectoration is minimal. Acute radiographic changes consistent with pneumonia or lung hemorrhage are seen. The pneumonitis appears to be due to direct damage to respiratory epithelium as well as an immunodepressant action (29). Manganese dioxide has been shown to depress humoral immunity, alveolar macrophage function, and phagocytic activity (30,31). Manganic pneumonia is associated with a high mortality rate (1). Episodes of Mn pneumonitis place workers at risk for developing hyperreactive airway disease with long-term sequelae and chronic pulmonary disease (32).

TABLE 81-4. Chronic manganese poisoning: signs and symptoms

Stage I (prodromal)	Stage II (intermediate)
Anorexia	Abnormal gait
Asthenia	Clumsiness
Ataxia	Compulsive laughing or crying
Hallucinations	Confusion
Insomnia	Expressionless facies
Irritability	Increased sleepiness
Memory deficits	Worsening speech disorder
Nervousness	**Stage III (manganism)**
Poor coordination	Dementia
Sleepiness	Emotional lability
Speech impairment	Frontal-lobe dysfunction
Manganese mania	Parkinsonian-like syndrome
Aggressive behavior	Asthenia
Incoherent talk	Hypotonia
Mental excitement	Muscular hypertonia or rigidity
	Shuffling gait
	Fine tremor (worse with intention)
	Severe retropulsion
	Sexual impotence

Adapted from refs. 1, 2, 12, and 22.

Acute exposure to Mn appears to be the least toxic to the CNS as compared to all other metals, and acute CNS toxicity has not been reported. Rather, long-term, continuing exposure is necessary for the development of CNS toxicity from Mn.

CHRONIC TOXICITY

In chronic Mn poisoning, CNS effects predominate. The major effects are associated with both psychiatric and neurologic dysfunction. Psychiatric changes usually precede the motor changes, but motor deficits can occur without any other components (2).

Chronic Mn poisoning may be divided into three stages: prodromal, intermediate, and established (or manganism; Table 81-4) (12). Most often, cognitive dysfunction and emotional disturbance occur prior to severe motor and neurologic dysfunction and are the hallmarks of the prodromal phase. Symptoms of this phase include asthenia, anorexia, nonspecific muscular pain, nervousness, irritability, uncontrolled violent outbursts, insomnia, decreased libido, impotence, and labile affect (2,21). The psychological and neuromotor manifestations, known as *manganese mania* or *locura manganica*, vary widely in both intensity and duration (2,33). The intermediate phase is marked by the beginning of compulsive inappropriate laughter or crying, clumsy movement, exaggerated lower-limb reflexes, speech disorders, masque manganese (expressionless facies), visual hallucinations, sialorrhea, and confusion. Reports of visions, chasing cars, and unexplained physical violence are common. In all cases, the patients understood that they were behaving irrationally or experiencing hallucinations but were unable to correct their own dysfunctional states (10,12,28).

During the established phase, subjective and objective symptoms intensify. The patient exhibits a Parkinson's disease–like picture and is said to be experiencing manganism (2,12,22). One of the most common physical complaints is generalized muscular weakness followed by difficulty in walking, stiffness, and impaired speech (up to and including muteness). The difficulty in walking includes impairment of propulsion and retropulsion, often noted when the patient is walking downhill. The patient may characteristically continue to accelerate until he or she is stopped by running into an obstacle. Malingering may be ruled out by the striking degree of retropulsion such that, if a patient is pushed from the front, he or she will collapse completely without attempting to protect himself or herself from a backward fall (25,28). The most common neurologic signs are a masklike, expressionless face, decreased postural reflexes, increased muscle tone, and a slow and shuffling forward gait without associated arm movement, accompanied by an anteriorly flexed trunk. Samples of handwriting demonstrate marked micrographia. Tremors may be noted and are usually fine, small-amplitude resting tremors seen with hyperextension of the arms and hands. These tremors become exaggerated on movement (17,28).

Whether certain factors predispose an individual to the development of CNS toxicity remains controversial. Some factors that have been suggested to influence such toxicity are genetic and metabolic predispositions, nutritional status, age, anemia, and alcohol use (12).

Other symptoms of manganism include nephritis, cirrhosis of the liver, muscular fatigue, anorexia, and sexual impotence (1).

REPRODUCTIVE TOXICITY

Mn interferes with reproductive function by inhibiting energy synthesis in the seminiferous tubules of the testis and causing progressive damage with terminal calcification to the seminiferous tubules (34,35). It does not affect steroidogenesis. Interestingly, Mn has a positive effect on sperm motility, probably through the activation of adenylyl cyclase activity or via direct effects on ion channels (36).

Malformations including stillbirth, talipes equinovarus, cleft lip, imperforate anus, cardiac defects, pulmonary defects, syndactyly, and deafness, as well as motor disorders, have been noted in the Gryoote islanders of New South Wales who are chronically exposed to high levels of environmental Mn (14,37). In a study of mice, maternal toxicity of manganese(II) chloride registered a no observable adverse effect level of 4 mg per kg per day, whereas the no observable adverse effect level of embryo or fetal toxicity was 2 mg per kg per day (38).

CARCINOGENESIS

One case of carcinogenesis (carcinoma of the lung) has been reported after Mn exposure, but evidence of widespread induction of carcinogenesis among large group populations is lacking (39).

Management of Toxicity

CLINICAL EXAMINATION AND TREATMENT

Acutely exposed patients should be removed from the source of Mn exposure and decontaminated as the exposure and condition warrants (40). Rescue personnel should wear appropriate gloves, boots, and goggles. Special attention should be directed to an exposed individual's respiratory system, with monitoring of airway, breathing, and circulatory status. Supplemental oxygen and intravenous fluids should be administered as necessary. Specific detoxification methods or agents are not available. Chelating agents have not been found to affect tissue levels significantly or to change the symptoms of Mn intoxication (7).

Acute treatment for MFF and pneumonitis is based on the clinical status of the patient. MFF patients usually require only removal from the exposure and supportive treatment. Mn pneumonitis or pneumonia may necessitate antibiotic therapy, with bronchodilator treatment as appropriate. A patient's condition should be monitored with chest radiography and pulmonary function testing. Long-term monitoring for the development of reactive airways disease should be initiated.

Chronically exposed patients require a complete toxicologic history and physical examination with special attention to the neurologic system. A comprehensive occupational history should be obtained. No effective treatment exists for chronic Mn poisoning of the CNS, although various therapeutic agents have been suggested.

Levodopa (L-DOPA), a dopamine precursor, and 5-hydroxytryptophan, a serotonin precursor, have been proposed (41). Therapeutic benefits of improving rigidity, hypokinesia, postural reflexes, balance, and dystonia have been shown with various L-DOPA regimens (range, 4.8 to 8.0 g per day) up to a maximal dose of 8.0 g per day in six divided doses (41). One patient given 3 g of L-DOPA exhibited increased hypotonia, weakness, and tremor but markedly improved with administration of a 3-g dose of 5-hydroxytryptophan (41). These studies have been challenged with newer studies showing no effect of L-DOPA and suggesting no more than a placebo effect of this medication in manganism (22). That L-DOPA is ineffective in manganism is logical as the nigrostriatal pathway is unaffected in human Mn intoxication (22). Trihexyphenidyl and paraaminosalicylic acid have both been used, but more data are needed before recommendations can be made (2,13). Low-protein diets have also been suggested to improve symptoms of chronic Mn poisoning (42).

LABORATORY DIAGNOSIS

Patients acutely exposed to Mn should undergo a full biochemical analysis including complete blood count, blood urea nitrogen, creatinine, and calcium level determinations, liver profile, and urinalysis (spot sample or 24-hour collection). Serum Mn concentration should be obtained, although toxicity does not seem to correlate with serum concentration (Table 81-5).

The reference range for whole blood adult Mn concentration is 8.0 to 18.7 µg per L (43), with most bound in the erythrocyte porphyrin complex. The reference range for serum Mn concentration is 0.3 to 1.3 µg per L (43).

Urinary Mn levels may be indicative of recent exposures (days to weeks), with the normal level being less than 10 mg per L (reference range, 0.5 to 9.8 mg per L) (43). Biological exposure limits allow up to 50 mg per L for occupational exposure (44).

Tissue burden and serum concentrations of Mn do not correlate with symptomatology, and symptoms can occur and progress even after excess metal is cleared from the tissues (2,17). Therefore, serum, whole blood, and urine levels of Mn may be normal in acute or chronic intoxication and cannot be used to predict severity of disease or future progression (2,25,28). This is in contrast to Wilson's disease or lead encepha-

TABLE 81-5. Laboratory and diagnostic testing in manganese toxicity

Laboratory or diagnostic test	Abnormal findings
Urinary levels	>10 mg/L (up to 50 mg/L for occupational exposure)
Whole blood levels	>19 mg/L (normal reference range, 8.0–18.7 mg/L)
Serum levels	>1.3 mg/L (normal reference range, 0.3–1.3 mg/L)
Electroencephalographic parameters	Low-amplitude, weakened rhythms
Neuropsychiatric testing	Decreased memory, decreased reaction time, decreased motor coordination
Computed tomography scan, magnetic resonance imaging	Radiodense accumulations of manganese in affected areas; abnormalities in globus pallidus, caudate nucleus, putamen
Positron emission tomography	Normal fluorodopa scan

Data compiled from refs. 2, 12, 24, 43, and 44.

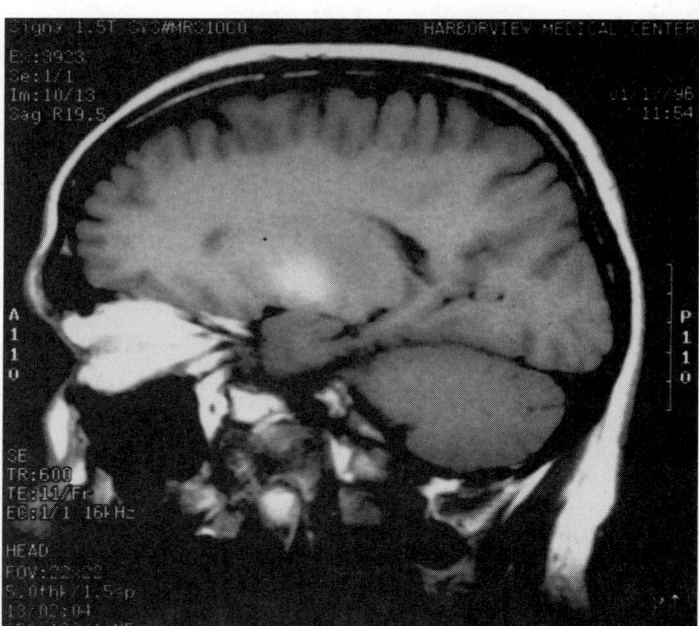

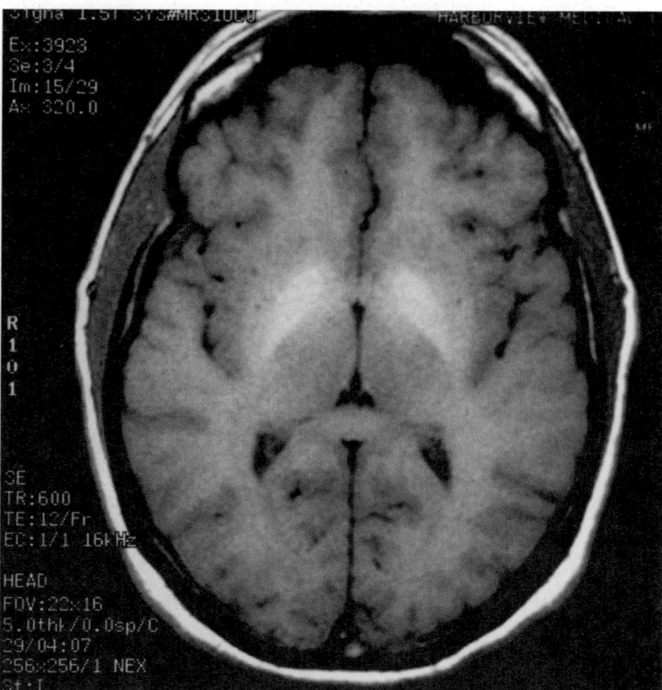

Figure 81-1. Magnetic resonance imaging scans reveal accumulations of the radiodense manganese in affected areas of the brain.

lopathy, in which serum levels do serve as markers for the degree of illness or as confirmatory evidence for diagnosis.

Increased exposure to Mn can lead to significant calcium loss via stool and result in lowered serum calcium levels. Metabolic activation of chondroitin sulfate synthetase, polysaccharide polymerase, and galactotransferase has been described in Mn excess (45).

Liver dysfunction (increased Golgi bodies, dilated biliary canaliculi) has been reported in isolated cases of Mn toxicity, but no confirmatory evidence for chronic liver toxicity or significant hepatic disorders is extant (13,33). No documented cases of nephrotoxicity are associated with Mn toxicity (10,28). Interference with hematopoiesis has been reported, and leukopenia, anemia, and monocytosis have all been seen, although none of these conditions has been clinically significant (1,33).

Chronically exposed patients must undergo a thyroid profile and vitamin B_{12} and folate level determinations to assist in the differential diagnosis of other neurologic diseases. Hair sample analysis may provide a better picture of chronic exposure over months to years. Because hair grows, on average, 1 cm per month, concentration patterns along hair segments could be used to determine long-term exposure patterns. Mn testing in hair has been known to be affected by hair color, nutritional status, and artificial hair treatments such as dying and waving (44).

SPECIAL DIAGNOSTIC TESTS

Computed tomography or magnetic resonance imaging of the brain may be necessary to rule out other possible CNS disease states that could mimic chronic Mn poisoning symptom complexes. Both computed tomography and magnetic resonance imaging should show accumulations of the radiodense Mn in the affected areas of the brain (Fig. 81-1). Positron emission tomography is also helpful in differentiating manganism from parkinsonism, with a fluorodopa positron emission tomography scan being normal in the Mn-poisoned patient and abnormal in the patient with Parkinson's disease (2,24).

Electroencephalography should also be performed. Electroencephalographic parameters consistent with Mn toxicity are nonspecific and include decreased amplitude and weakened rhythms (12).

Most patients suspected of chronic Mn poisoning should have a complete neuropsychological evaluation administered by a neuropsychologist with experience in toxicologic syndromes. The testing battery should be constructed from existing neuropsychological tests and should include tests of motor functions, response speeds, and memory. Rating scales for mood and subjective symptoms should also be included (12,46). Frequent testing of exposed individuals should occur, and group comparisons may be necessary to determine effects (46). Tests from the Swedish Performance Evaluation System seem to work well and can be used for comparability, as this system has been used in many studies on the neurotoxic effects of Mn (46,47).

MEDICAL MONITORING

The purposes of a medical monitoring program for Mn toxicity are early intervention into a pathophysiologic process to prevent further injury and screening for exposures to prevent disease. Medical monitoring for Mn toxicity must be targeted at establishing exposure through biological monitoring to prevent prodromal disease changes. In addition to biological monitoring, because Mn neurotoxicity resembles Parkinson's disease, some of the tools and techniques used to monitor Parkinson's disease may be applicable for Mn toxicity (Fig. 81-2). Twenty-four hour urine Mn assays are more useful for assessing acute (rather than chronic) exposures. Combined hair and urine analyses would be useful for determining internal Mn exposure.

Neuropsychological testing is sensitive in detecting early neurotoxicity changes from many different toxins. Because Mn toxicity symptoms do not correlate well with exposure levels or tissue levels, early intervention with sensitive testing methods is

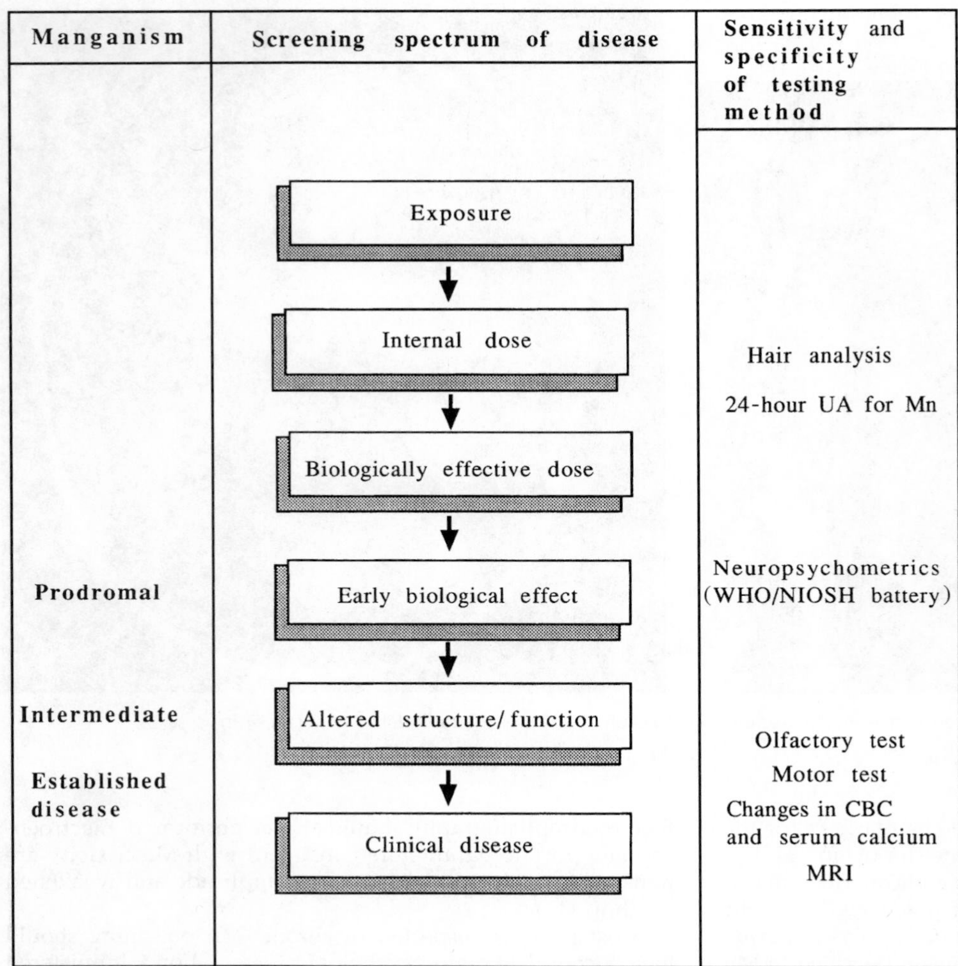

Manganism
Screening spectrum of disease
Sensitivity and specificity of testing method
Exposure
Internal dose
Hair analysis
24-hour UA for Mn
Biologically effective dose
Prodromal
Early biological effect
Neuropsychometrics (WHO/NIOSH battery)
Intermediate
Altered structure/function
Established disease
Clinical disease
Olfactory test
Motor test
Changes in CBC and serum calcium
MRI

Figure 81-2. Medical screening for manganese exposure and toxicity. Biological monitoring is the cornerstone, to prevent prodromal disease changes. In addition to biological monitoring, because manganese neurotoxicity resembles Parkinson's disease, some of the tools and techniques used to monitor Parkinson's disease may be applicable for manganese toxicity. CBC, complete blood cell count; MRI, magnetic resonance imaging; NIOSH, National Institute for Occupational Safety and Health; UA, urinary analysis; WHO, World Health Organization.

crucial. The World Health Organization and National Institute for Occupational Safety and Health (NIOSH) advocate a core battery of tests selected for their sensitivity to neurotoxic effects. Included in this neuropsychological battery are the following tests (12,46): aiming, simple reaction time, dexterity test, digit symbol test, Benton visual retention test, digit span, and profile of mood states. Testing is divided into sensory, motor, cognitive, and affect or personality areas. Neurotoxic syndromes can be complex, and confounding factors (preexisting disease, psychological problems, drug abuse) can alter findings. Neuropsychological testing complements other diagnostic measures.

One combination testing battery using olfactory detection (smell test), the Beck Depression Index, and motor testing demonstrated a 94% specificity and sensitivity in diagnosing Parkinson's disease (12,46). Such a battery might be able to detect intermediate or late changes in Mn toxicity.

OCCUPATIONAL AND ENVIRONMENTAL REGULATIONS AND EXPOSURE LIMITS

The U.S. Occupational Safety and Health Administration established a permissible exposure limit for inhalational exposure to Mn compounds (measured as Mn) at 1 mg per cubic meter (12). The ceiling air concentration limit is 5 mg per cubic meter, which should never be exceeded during any part of the workday. If instantaneous air monitoring is not available, then the ceiling value must be assessed as a 15-minute time-weighted average (TWA). Neurologic effects have been noted with levels as low as 2.5 mg per cubic meter (12).

The NIOSH-recommended exposure limit for Mn compounds (measured as Mn) is 1 mg per cubic meter, and the short-term exposure limit (STEL) is 3 mg per cubic meter (48). A concentration considered to be immediately dangerous to life or health has been established as 500 mg per cubic meter (48).

The American Conference of Governmental Industrial Hygienists (ACGIH) threshold limit value time-weighted average (TLV-TWA) for Mn fumes is 5 mg per cubic meter, which represents the TLV-TWA for welding fumes in general (49). No ACGIH STEL value exists for fumes. The ACGIH TLV-TWA for Mn is 0.2 mg per cubic meter, with a STEL of 3 mg per cubic meter (49).

The NIOSH has established a TWA exposure limit for MMT of 0.1 mg per cubic meter for dermal exposure. The ACGIH TLV-TWA for MMT (as Mn skin exposure) is 0.1 mg per cubic meter (49), whereas the OSHA ceiling limit for MMT is 5 mg per cubic meter.

High levels of Mn salts in water impart a bitter taste and give the water a brackish look (50). The public drinking water standard for Mn is 0.05 mg per L, which is based on aesthetic changes in water purity and not on established levels of toxicity (50). Levels of 0.3 to 2.16 mg per L have been shown not to cause symptoms (51), and levels up to 1,320 g per L have been found in drinking water (50). In the United States, no clearly defined level of toxic exposure in drinking water has yet been determined.

ENVIRONMENTAL MONITORING

Air samples for Mn air concentration determinations should be analyzed by the inductively coupled plasma method as described in the NIOSH Manual of Analytical Methods (48,52).

REFERENCES

1. Venugopal B, Luckey TD. Toxicity of group VII metals. In: *Metal toxicity in mammals,* vol 2. New York: Plenum Publishing, 1978:261–271.
2. Calne DB, Chu NS, Huang CC, Lu CS, Olanow W. Manganism and idiopathic parkinsonism: similarities and differences. *Neurology* 1994;44:1583–1586.
3. Sittig M. *Handbook of toxic and hazardous chemicals and carcinogens*, 2nd ed. Park Ridge, NJ: Noyes Publications, 1985:559–560.
4. Gosselin RE, Smith RP, Hodge HC. *Clinical toxicology of commercial products*, 5th ed. Baltimore: Williams & Wilkins, 1984.
5. Saric M, Markicevic A, Hrustic O. Occupational exposure to manganese. *Br J Ind Med* 1977;34:114–118.
6. Lynam DR. Environmental assessment of MMT fuel additives. *Sci Total Environ* 1990;40:49–50.
7. Sanchez DJ, Gomez M, Domingo JL, Llobet JM, Corbella J. Relative efficacy of chelating agents on excretion and tissue distribution of manganese in mice. *J Appl Toxicol* 1995;15:285–288.
8. Wilkenfeld M. Metal compounds and rare earths. In: Rom WN, ed. *Environmental and occupational medicine*, 2nd ed. Boston: Little, Brown and Company, 1992:815–830.
9. Food and Nutrition Board, National Research Council. *Recommended dietary allowances*, 10th ed. Washington: National Academy of Sciences, 1989:195–246.
10. Cotzias GC. Manganese in health and disease. *Physiol Rev* 1958;38:503–532.
11. Vuori E. A longitudinal study of manganese in human milk. *Acta Paediatr Scand* 1979;68:571–573.
12. Hartman DE. *Neuropsychological toxicology*, 2nd ed. New York: Plenum Publishing, 1995.
13. Lesser SH, Weiss SJ. Art hazards. *Am J Emerg Med* 1995;13:451–458.
14. Kilburn CJ. Manganese malformations and motor disorders: findings in a manganese-exposed population. *Neurotoxicology* 1987;8:421–430.
15. Pollack S, George JN, Reba RC, Kauman RM, Crosby WH. The absorption of nonferrous metals in iron deficiency. *J Clin Invest* 1965;44:1470–1473.
16. Gruden N. Iron-59 and manganese-54 retention in weanling rats fed iron-fortified milk. *Nutr Rep Int* 1982;25:849–858.
17. Mena I, Horiuchi K, Burke K, Cotzias GC. Chronic manganese poisoning. Individual susceptibility and absorption of iron. *Neurology* 1969;19:1000–1006.
18. Cotzias GC. Manganese versus magnesium: why are they so similar *in vitro* and so different *in vivo*? *Fed Proc* 1961;20:98–103.
19. Sandstead HH. Some trace elements which are essential for human nutrition: zinc, copper, manganese and chromium. *Prog Food Nutr Sci* 1975;1:371–391.
20. Meco G, Bonifati V, Vanacore N, Fabrizio E. Parkinsonism after chronic exposure to the fungicide Maneb (manganese ethylene-*bis*-dithiocarbamate). *Scand J Work Environ Health* 1994;20:301–305.
21. Mergler D, Huel G, Bowler R, et al. Nervous system dysfunction among workers with long-term exposure to manganese. *Environ Res* 1994;64:151–180.
22. Lu CS, Huang CC, Chu NS, Calne DB. Levodopa failure in chronic manganism. *Neurology* 1994;44:1600–1602.
23. Florence TM, Stauber JL. Neurotoxicology of manganese. *Lancet* 1988;1:363.
24. Wolters AC, Huang CC, Clark C, et al. Positron emission tomography in manganese intoxication. *Ann Neurol* 1989;26:647–651.
25. Cotsias GC, Horiuchi K, Fuenzalida S, Mena I. Chronic manganese poisoning: clearance of tissue manganese concentrations with persistence of the neurological picture. *Neurology* 1968;18:376–382.
26. Piscator M. Health hazards from inhalation of metal fumes. *Environ Res* 1976;11:268–270.
27. Week JL, Levy BS, Wagner GR. *Preventing occupational disease and injury.* Washington: American Public Health Association, 1991:422–425.
28. Rodier J. Manganese poisoning in Moroccan mines. *Br J Ind Med* 1955;12:21–35.
29. Davis TAL. Manganese pneumonitis. *Br J Ind Med* 1946;3:111–135.
30. Bergstrom R. Acute pulmonary toxicity of manganese dioxide. *Scand J Work Environ Health* 1977;3(Suppl 1):1–41.
31. Adkins BN, Luginbuhl GH, Miller FJ, Gardner DE. Increased pulmonary susceptibility to streptococcal infection following inhalation of manganese oxide. *Environ Res* 1980;23:110–120.
32. Brooks SM, Weiss MA, Bernstein IL. Reactive airways dysfunction syndrome (RADS). Persistent asthma syndrome after high level irritant exposures. *Chest* 1985;88:376–384.
33. Mena I, Marin O, Fuenzolida S, Cotzias GC. Chronic manganese poisoning: clinical picture and manganese turnover. *Neurology* 1967;17:128–136.
34. Iman Z, Chandra SV. Histochemical alterations in rabbit testis produced by manganese chloride. *Toxicol Appl Pharmacol* 1975;32:534–544.
35. Laskey JW, Rehnberg GL, Hein JF, Carter SD. Effects of chronic manganese (Mn_3O_4) exposure on selected reproductive parameters in rats. *J Toxicol Environ Health* 1982;9:677–687.
36. Magnus O, Brekke I, Abyholm T, Purvis K. Effects of manganese and other divalent cations on progressive motility of human sperm. *Arch Androl* 1990;24:159–166.
37. Cawte J. Emic accounts of a mystery illness: the Gryoote Eylandt syndrome. *Aust N Z J Psychiatry* 1984;18:179–187.
38. Sanchez DJ, Domingo JL, Llobet JM, Keen CL. Maternal and developmental toxicity of manganese in the mouse. *Toxicol Lett* 1993;69:45–52.
39. Rab S. Squamous cell lung cancer in dry battery worker. *JPMA J Pak Med Assoc* 1990;40:49–50.
40. Bronstein AC, Currance PL. *Emergency care for hazardous material exposures.* St. Louis: Mosby, 1988:191–192.
41. Mena I, Court J, Fuenzalida S, Papavasiliou PS, Cotzias GC. Modification of chronic manganese poisoning: treatment with L-dopa or 5-OH tryptophan. *N Engl J Med* 1970;282:5–10.
42. Mena I, Cotzias GC. Protein intake and treatment of Parkinson's disease with levodopa. *N Engl J Med* 1975;292:181–184.
43. Peitz NW, ed. *Clinical guide to laboratory tests*, 2nd ed. Philadelphia: WB Saunders, 1990:8–680.
44. Foo SC, Khoo NY, Heng A, et al. Metals in hair as biological indices for exposure. *Arch Occup Environ Health* 1993;65:S83–S86.
45. Burch RE, Hahn HKJ, Sullivan JF. Aspects of the roles of zinc, manganese, copper in human nutrition. *Clin Chem* 1975;21:501–520.
46. Iregren A. Using psychological tests for the early detection of neurotoxic effects of low level manganese exposure. *Neurotoxicology* 1994;15:671–678.
47. Lucchini R, Selis L, Folli D, et al. Neurobehavioral effects of manganese in workers from a ferroalloy plant after temporary cessation of exposure. *Scand J Work Environ Health* 1995;21:143–149.
48. US Department of Health and Human Services. *NIOSH pocket guide to chemical hazards.* DHHS publication no. 94-116. Cincinnati: NIOSH Publications, 1994:190–193.
49. American Conference of Governmental and Industrial Hygienists. *Threshold limit values for chemical substances and physical agents and biological exposure indices.* Cincinnati: American Conference of Governmental and Industrial Hygienists, 1996.
50. Kondakis XG, Makris N, Leotsinidis M, Prinou M, Papapetropoulos T. Possible health effects of high manganese concentration in drinking water. *Arch Environ Health* 1989;44:175–178.
51. Vieregge P, Heinzow B, Korf G, Teichert HM, Schleifenbaum P, Mosinger HU. Long term exposure to manganese in well water has no neurological effects. *Can J Neurol Sci* 1995;22:286–289.
52. Eller PM, Cassinelli ME, eds. *NIOSH manual of analytical methods for monitoring occupational exposures to toxic substances in air and biological samples.* Cincinnati: NIOSH Publications, 1994.

CHAPTER 82

Vanadium, Titanium, and Molybdenum

John G. Benitez and Ernesto Cortes-Belen

Vanadium, titanium, and molybdenum frequently are used together in the steel and alloy industries and frequently are used in different chemical compounds for different industries. This chapter discusses each metal separately, although very often all three are found together or with other metals and alloys.

VANADIUM TOXICITY

Sources and Production

Vanadium is one of the most common trace elements in nature, found as relatively insoluble salts and usually in the trivalent state (1). It is extracted from mineral deposits of carnotite, phosphate rock, titaniferous magnetite, and vanadiferous clays. Vanadium exists in fossil fuels in varying small amounts (2,3). At a global level, environmental levels of vanadium have increased owing to human activity (4). Vanadium is an essential trace element for normal human growth and nutrition. Deficiency of vanadium results in increased hematocrit levels, increased blood and bone marrow iron, and decreased blood lipid levels (5,6).

Production of vanadium requires first that it be extracted from the ores, slags, and boiler residues that contain vanadium in a low state of oxidation. Conversion to water-soluble vanadate ($NaVO_3$) requires that the ores, slags, and residues be roasted with salt, soda ash, or sodium sulfate. The resultant product then is leached with water or soda ash solution, and sometimes this process is followed by a further leaching with dilute acid. Ores that exist with oxidized vanadium, such as carnotite, may be leached with acid directly without roasting. The resulting precipitate is sodium polyvanadate and can be treated by solvent extraction or ion exchange to separate any impurities. With titaniferous magnetite, the roasting and leaching process may be used, but a common procedure used in the Soviet Union and South Africa is to smelt the magnetite and produce a pig iron containing vanadium. After the pig iron is blown with oxygen, the vanadium is recovered in the slag as vanadium pentoxide. The slag then can be roasted and leached as described or can be used directly to produce ferrovanadium. Purification of vanadium is achieved by various other procedures in which vanadium pentoxide, vanadium trichloride, or vanadium trioxide is reduced with other elements, such as calcium, magnesium, sodium, carbon, or aluminum. To produce pure metal (99.95%), impure grades of vanadium are refined by an electrolytic process (2).

Vanadium forms compounds in a bi-, tri-, tetra-, or pentavalent state. Its chemistry is similar to that of phosphorus (5). Pentavalent vanadium commonly is seen as the oxide V_2O_5, and it reacts with halides to form such pentavalent halides as $VOCl_3$, VOF_3, and $VOBr_3$. Reaction of the metal with fluorine yields the trivalent halide VF_3. Reduction of vanadium pentoxide with ammonia forms the tetravalent oxide VO_2. Dissolution of VO_2 in acids produces salts, such as $VOSO_4$ and $VOCl_2$. Vanadium tetrachloride (VCl_4) is produced by chlorination of vanadium at 300°C. When vanadium pentoxide is reduced with ammonia or hydrogen at 650°C, the trivalent oxide V_2O_3 is formed. The chloride is the result of reduction of VCl_4. Bivalent vanadium oxide is prepared by the reduction of vanadium pentoxide with hydrogen at 1,700°C (2).

Occupational and Environmental Exposure Sources

Vanadium is found in several industries. See Table 82-1 for further details. Exposure to vanadium pentoxide is the most common form of vanadium exposure studied. Other exposures occur much less frequently and, as a result, data are limited in regard to other chemical forms of vanadium. The usual route of entry is by inhalation of dust, although dust entry through the gastrointestinal tract also can occur. Direct ingestion or parenteral exposure is uncommon but has occurred in experimental situations. Workers who use vanadium pentoxide are at risk when inhaling fine dust, because fine particulate matter may penetrate deeper into the tracheobronchial tree (2,7). Exposures in industries occur with liberation of dust during the mining and processing of ores, the cleaning and maintenance of furnaces and boilers, use in the chemical industries, and use during the manufacture of steels and alloys (8).

TABLE 82-1. Industries using vanadium

Industry	Compound used
Steel and alloy manufacture	Ferrovanadium, aluminum, vanadium alloy
Iron and steel industries	Vanadium carbides
Flame cutting, brazing, welding	Steel, titanium, and vanadium alloys
Chemical production (catalyst)	Vanadium pentoxide
Dye manufacture	Vanadium salts, ammonium metavanadate
Polymers, synthetic rubbers, ceramics, electronics	Vanadium oxychloride, tetrachloride, and triacetylacetonate
Boiler repair and cleaning	Vanadium pentoxide
Pacemaker batteries	Vanadium pentoxide

Clinical Toxicology

ROUTES OF EXPOSURE

Foods from both plant and animal sources incorporate varying amounts of vanadium. Seafood tends to incorporate vanadium to a greater extent than do other foods. Foods contain vanadium in the range of a few parts per billion and probably play no part in acute toxicity (2). Industrial exposure to vanadium occurs through the respiratory system (3,9). Some vanadium is ingested orally through the trapping of dusts in the oropharynx and nasopharynx. Salts are absorbed poorly in the intestine, where only approximately 1% is absorbed (2).

DISTRIBUTION AND ELIMINATION

Of the vanadium that is absorbed, only a small amount enters bone and is mobilized more slowly than in other tissues. Vanadium is detected in a number of tissues: liver, lung, kidney, bone, spleen, thyroid, brain, fat, hair, bile, blood, urine, lower small and large intestines, and omentum (2,5). No vanadium has been detected in the human aorta, brain, muscle, ovary, or testis. The normal human serum concentration is 0.67 ng per mL (range, 0.26 to 1.3) (2).

Vanadium is excreted rapidly through the urine (91%), with 60% of an absorbed amount excreted within 24 hours. The remainder is excreted in the feces (9%) (2,5).

SIGNS, SYMPTOMS, AND SYNDROMES

Acute Toxicity. Acute exposure to vanadium oxide dusts is associated with acute upper and lower airway irritation (10). Conjunctivitis, rhinitis, and pharyngitis commonly occur within 0.5 hours of exposure and up to 12 hours after the exposure. Cough, wheezing, dyspnea, and substernal soreness occur with more severe exposures (3,5,7,9). A green-black discoloration of the tongue sometimes occurs. The discoloration results from simple exposure of the tongue mucosa to vanadium powder (9).

Reversible airway disease is a consequence of exposure to vanadium dust. Airway narrowing, with decreases in the forced vital capacity and the forced expiratory volume, can be detected within 24 hours of exposure. Complete reversal of these compromises to pulmonary function occurs in 8 to 10 days, and no long-term changes in pulmonary function test results have been observed (3,9,11).

Although vanadium interferes with the Na-K pump, causing renal dysfunction in animals, no studies or case reports support this effect in humans (1,12,13).

Chronic Toxicity. No chronic pulmonary effects of exposure have been demonstrated to date (2). Animal studies suggest a possible role of vanadium in renal toxicity and arterial hypertension, but that role has not been confirmed (14,15). Vanadium is both mutagenic and clastogenic in animal studies, although no human effect has been shown (3,16). Reduced live births in animals are reported to result from exposure (17).

Excessive amounts of vanadium have been suggested but not confirmed as a factor in manic-depressive illness. Elevated concentrations are found in plasma and hair of affected individuals (18).

Vanadium increases the glucose transport mechanism and inhibits gluconeogenesis in animals fed with vanadium supplements over several weeks. This hypoglycemic effect has not been demonstrated in humans (19–23).

Persistent upper abdominal pain, anorexia, nausea, and weight loss have been reported with oral intake of 22.5 mg vanadium per day for a period of 5 months (24,25).

MANAGEMENT OF TOXICITY OR EXPOSURE

Differentiating vanadium pulmonary toxicity from infection or allergy of the respiratory tract is difficult in that presenting signs and symptoms are similar. A specific vanadium exposure history must be elicited from affected individuals. Examination may reveal a patient with clear watery discharge from the eyes and nose. Mucosal surfaces may be erythematous. Auscultation of lung fields will reveal rhonchi or wheezing.

Treatment is supportive, and patient counseling may be necessary to ensure that no permanent damage will develop (2). Experimental animal data show that some chelators may help to remove the body burden of vanadium, although dialysis has not been clinically necessary after vanadium exposure (26).

Medical and Biological Monitoring. The laboratory is not helpful in determining or verifying exposure. Complete blood cell counts and chest radiographs usually are normal (10). Measuring urinary vanadium concentration may be helpful, especially if exposure was recent (less than 2 weeks). Monitoring of these levels over 5 to 7 days should be sufficient to detect a decrease if a patient was removed from the source or the source was controlled (3,8,9,27). Vanadium can be measured by spectrometry, atomic absorption spectrometry, inductively coupled plasma atomic emission spectrometry, inductively coupled plasma mass spectrometry, neutron activation analysis, and voltammetric methods, although flame atomic absorption and graphite furnace flame atomic absorption spectrometry are the most common measurement modalities (28).

Occupational and Environmental Regulations. Permissible exposure limits are listed in Table 82-2. Reversible airway disease and acute upper airway irritation may be minimized by keeping dust and fume exposure low.

Exposure Controls. Environmental protection should include measures to decrease dust formation, to minimize skin and eye contact, and to prevent dust accumulation. Warning labels on all containers used for vanadium products should include cautions indicating skin, eye, and respiratory irritation hazards. Ventilation protection should be required (8,10,27).

Environmental Fate and Transport

Vanadium is released from fossil fuels (2,3). With vanadium's increasing use in the steel and alloy industries and the use of fossil fuels, environmental levels of vanadium have increased (4). One estimate of particulate-bound emissions (anthropogenic) is 0.9×10^{11} g per year, which compares to the natural emissions from earth (0.8×10^{11} g per year). Soluble vanadium is estimated to increase ocean concentrations by approximately 4.4×10^{11} g per L per year, which is two orders of magnitude less than vanadium concentration in our present oceans (4). Vanadium is absorbed by many aquatic species (bivalves, crustaceans, echinoderms, polychaetes, and ascidians), although no specific effects were noted in species that seem to concentrate this element in the greatest degree (29,30).

TABLE 82-2. Vanadium permissible exposure limits

Agency	Limits
ACGIH TLV	0.05 mg/m^3 respirable dusts or fumes
OSHA TWA	0.5 mg/m^3 dust ceiling; 0.1 mg/m^3 fumes
NIOSH	0.05 mg/m^3 15-min ceiling

ACGIH, American Conference of Governmental Industrial Hygienists; NIOSH, National Institute for Occupational Safety and Health; OSHA, U.S. Occupational Safety and Health Administration; TLV, threshold limit value; TWA, 8-hour time-weighted average.

Environmental and Occupational Monitoring

Monitoring of particle size and concentration should be undertaken in the work environment. Personal monitor sampling also should be performed when possible (2).

TITANIUM TOXICITY

Sources and Production

Titanium is one of the most common components of the earth's crust, being ninth in abundance. It occurs naturally as ilmenite (iron titanate) and rutile (titanium dioxide) (31,32).

Titanium forms four distinct oxides: titanium monoxide (TiO), dititanium trioxide (Ti_2O_3), titanium dioxide (TiO_2), and titanium trioxide (TiO_3). In construction, titanium alloys are used with aluminum, iron, manganese, chromium, molybdenum, or vanadium (31).

Titanium slag is produced by smelting ilmenite in an electric furnace. Titanium dioxide content typically is 70% to 85%. Titanium dioxide is made by chlorinating ore at temperatures of 850° to 1,000°C. Impurities are removed chemically and through fractional distillation. The resulting titanium tetrachloride is converted to titanium dioxide by burning titanium tetrachloride in air or oxygen at temperatures of 1,200° to 1,370°C. Aluminum chloride is added to ensure near-total conversion to rutile (32).

Occupational and Environmental Exposure Sources

Titanium commonly is used in titanium alloys for military and commercial airplane parts. In addition, titanium frequently is used as a white pigment for a wide range of paints, paper, inks, plastics, and the like (Table 82-3).

Exposure results from breathing titanium dioxide dust. Possible exposure to intermediate products in titanium dioxide production (e.g., titanium tetrachloride) also may occur (33). Because of lack of data regarding human experience with other forms of titanium, discussion is limited to titanium dioxide. Exposure may occur at any stage: in the mining of ores, in the preparation of titanium oxide, and in any of the listed industries in which the powder is stored and used.

TABLE 82-3. Industries using titanium

Industry	Compound used
Military aircraft, missiles	Ferrotitanium
Flame cutting, brazing, welding	Steel, titanium, and vanadium alloys
Pulp-paper production (protective surface)	Titanium metal
Paint industries (white pigment)	Titanium dioxide
Commercial airplane parts	Titanium alloy
Flame retardant for wood	Titanium dioxide

Clinical Toxicology

ROUTES OF EXPOSURE

Titanium dioxide inhalation is the most common route of exposure. Ingestion is certainly possible when some dust accumulates on mucosal surfaces of the oropharynx and nasopharynx.

DISTRIBUTION, METABOLISM, AND ELIMINATION

No data are available regarding oral absorption of titanium. Pulmonary retention of titanium dioxide particles is well documented in several studies. Titanium dioxide is found in the lymphatics and regional nodes that drain the lungs, indicating a slow removal by this process (32). Titanium and other metals dissolve into surrounding tissues from metal alloy implants (34). Titanium is excreted renally (35).

SIGNS, SYMPTOMS, AND SYNDROMES

Acute Toxicity. Titanium dioxide is an irritant to the upper airway, as are other nuisance dusts (36). No evidence indicates that it induces an acute inflammatory reaction at commonly seen exposure concentrations (37). Inhalation of titanium tetrachloride may lead to inhalational injury, resulting in chemical pneumonitis and airway irritation. However, injury most likely results from the halide ion (7). In workers with preexisting chronic obstructive airway disease, titanium dioxide inhalation may exacerbate symptoms. Affected individuals may complain of irritated eyes and pharynx, and examination will reveal inflamed mucosal surfaces. Coughing is a frequent finding, although rhonchi and rales usually are absent unless underlying pulmonary or cardiac disease is present (36).

Chronic Toxicity. Titanium dioxide dust is retained in the lungs. Particles of this dust are found also in the regional nodes draining the lungs, suggesting that these particles are cleared slowly by the lymphatics (32). Little evidence indicates that titanium dioxide promotes a chronic inflammatory reaction in the lungs (37). However, in a case report, hypersensitivity to titanium was demonstrated. The affected patient had granulomatous disease of the lungs, and particulate matter that was found consisted of aluminum, titanium, zinc, nickel, and silicates. Causal relation between the titanium and the granulomatous disease was not proved (38). Inconclusive evidence demonstrates an increased incidence of chronic bronchitis and loss of ventilatory function (7,32). Titanium dioxide dust currently is considered to be merely a nuisance dust that results only in upper airway irritation (37). Titanium dissolved from alloy implants has been associated with increased release of inflammatory mediators and increased bone resorption with evidence of fibrosis. Mild chronic inflammatory changes in the adjacent tissues occur, but no clinical significance has been demonstrated (39,40).

No data are available regarding human genetic effects, and very limited epidemiologic data about carcinogenicity are available. That findings of carcinogenicity are as yet inconclusive most likely is attributable to the fact that workers are exposed to other chemicals (asbestos, silica) either prior to or during their current jobs. Pulmonary fibrosis seen in some affected workers may be due to the presence of silicon compounds (32). Recent animal data support the conclusion that titanium dioxide is a nuisance dust and does not produce any increased incidence of cancer rates (41).

MANAGEMENT OF TOXICITY OR EXPOSURE

Titanium dioxide is an irritant dust; therefore, management of exposure is supportive. Exposed workers should be removed from the environment, and supportive pulmonary care should be provided.

TABLE 82-4. Titanium permissible exposure limits

Agency	Limits
ACGIH TLV (8-h shift)	10 mg/m^3 total dust
OSHA TWA	15 mg/m^3

ACGIH, American Conference of Governmental Industrial Hygienists; OSHA, U.S. Occupational Safety and Health Administration; TLV, threshold limit value; TWA, 8-hour time-weighted average.

Medical and Biological Monitoring. Most laboratory tests (e.g., complete blood counts, analysis of serum electrolyte levels, and radiographs) are not helpful. Assessment of serum and urinary titanium levels help to identify recent exposure (36). Atomic absorption spectrometry and hydrogen peroxide methods now are used commonly to measure titanium in air and in biological specimens (35). Histochemical methods, electron microscopy or electron probe analysis, x-ray microanalysis, x-ray fluorescence, and optic emission spectrography are other procedures used for titanium determination.

Occupational and Environmental Regulations. Permissible exposure limits for exposure are listed in Table 82-4. Acute upper airway irritation may be reduced by keeping exposure to titanium dust at low limits.

Exposure Controls. Good industrial hygiene and monitoring of the environment should limit employee exposure to titanium dust. If employees must work in an environment with high titanium dioxide dust levels and poor ventilation, respirators should be used (36).

Environmental Fate and Transport

The average titanium concentration in the earth's crust is approximately 4.4 g per kg (31). Industrial effluents eventually may enter surface waters. Titanium halide effluents inhibit algal growth, whereas titanium oxalate–containing effluents minimally decrease algal growth, even at high concentrations (42).

Environmental and Occupational Monitoring

As is accomplished for testing exposure to other metals, monitoring of particle size and concentration should be performed when the working environment is evaluated. Biological monitoring of exposed personnel should be undertaken.

MOLYBDENUM TOXICITY

Sources and Production

Molybdenum is obtained from such ores as molybdenite (MoS_2), wulfenite ($PbMoO_4$), and powellite [$-Ca(MoW)O_4$]. Molybdenite is the most common and is obtained directly by mining and also as a by-product in some copper-mining operations. Molybdenite is roasted to molybdic oxide (MoO_3). Molybdic oxide then is converted to ammonium molybdate ($[NH_2]Mo_2O_7$). Several molybdenum products can be produced, because molybdenum forms compounds with various valence states: 0, +2, +3, +4, +5, and +6. Examples of these products are molybdenum

TABLE 82-5. Industries using molybdenum

Industry	Compound used
Steel	Molybdic oxide
Dry lubricant	Purified molybdenite or molybdenum sulfide
Color printing and pigment	Zinc molybdate
Electroplating	$Mo(OH_3)$
Aircraft industry (superalloys)	Molybdenum alloys
Powder metallurgy or vacuum-arc-cast metal	Molybdic acid or ammonium molybdate
Catalysts	Molybdenum powder or molybdenum acetylacetylacetonate
Feed stock	Molybdenum powder

dioxide and trioxide; molybdenum pentachloride ($MoCl_5$); and nitrogen, sulfur, and oxygen chelates (31).

Differences in toxicity occur if some compounds are more soluble than others. Insoluble molybdenum compounds include metallic molybdenum, molybdenum disulfide (MoS_2), and lead molybdate ($PbMoO_4$). Soluble compounds include molybdenum trioxide (MoO_3), ammonium molybdate, ammonium paramolybdate [$(NH_4)_6Mo_7O_{24}$–$4H_2O$], calcium molybdate ($CaMoO_4$), and sodium molybdate dihydrate (Na_2MoO_4–$2H_2O$) (43,44).

Occupational and Environmental Exposure Sources

Common uses of molybdenum include metallurgy, such as its use in alloys, and as a catalyst for the chemical industry. Exposure commonly occurs in the mining and processing of ores (Table 82-5).

Molybdenum and its compounds may be inhaled by breathing dust, and they may be absorbed also by skin contact. The more soluble the compound, the more toxic its manifestations are. Exposure may occur during the liberation of dust from mining and the processing of ore, from the grinding of metals or alloys, from oxyacetylene cutting, and from dust from its various compounds (31,43,44).

Clinical Toxicology

ROUTES OF EXPOSURE

Exposure to molybdenum and related compounds usually occurs via the inhalation of dust. If these compounds are water-soluble, absorption is increased, and toxicity may be greater than that from non-water-soluble compounds. Because of this property, skin absorption may occur. Gastrointestinal absorption is approximately 50% of an ingested amount and depends on the water solubility of the compound involved (31).

DISTRIBUTION, METABOLISM, AND ELIMINATION

Molybdenum is present in humans, with an average adult content of 9 mg (45). Molybdenum is contained principally in liver, kidney, small intestine, adrenal glands, fat, and blood. The major portion contained in the liver is contained in a nonprotein cofactor bound to the mitochondrial membrane. It may be moved to an apoenzyme, transforming it into an active enzyme (46). Human whole blood levels average approximately 5 ng per mL (45).

More than 50% of molybdenum is excreted primarily through the kidneys. Approximately 6% is excreted through the bile when excess molybdenum is present (31,46,47).

SIGNS, SYMPTOMS, AND SYNDROMES

Acute Toxicity. Molybdenum products may cause acute toxicity in humans, but adequate studies reporting such effects are lacking. Workers involved in producing molybdenum oxide have demonstrated a higher rate of headaches, backaches, aching joints, and nonspecific skin and hair changes (31,48). Increases in serum uric acid and ceruloplasmin also are noted (31,48). Fumes from arcing molybdenum metal cause respiratory irritation in animals. Molybdenum trioxide may cause irritation to mucous membranes (eyes, nose, throat). It also has caused weight loss and digestive disturbances in animals, which are secondary to decreased copper in serum (an effect from a high molybdenum concentration in blood). However, few data have addressed this effect in humans (43,44,49,50).

Chronic Toxicity. Data are extremely limited in regard to chronic toxicity from molybdenum and its compounds. Some workers had changes on radiographs, suggesting pneumoconiosis, but no long-term effects have been found attributable directly to molybdenum (31,34). Vitallium, an alloy of chromium, cobalt, and molybdenum, is implicated in producing pneumoconiosis in dental technicians. Such individuals are exposed by working with this alloy in the molding, cutting, and polishing of prosthetic parts. However, attributing pulmonary fibrotic changes to a specific metal or combination of metals is difficult in these cases (51). Kidney disease and liver dysfunction are reported after exposure in animals but not in humans (43,44). No changes in tissue growth rates are noted with alloys containing molybdenum (52). One rat model suggested decreased growth plate proliferation (53). Systemic lupus erythematosus (antinuclear antibody–negative) has been associated with a delayed-type hypersensitivity to molybdenum, but no causal link was established (54). In summary, molybdenum may cause a pneumoconiosis in susceptible individuals, but definitive data are lacking.

MANAGEMENT OF TOXICITY OR EXPOSURE

Persons exposed to hazardous concentrations of molybdenum should be removed from further exposure. Treatment is symptomatic, and no specific therapy is available for removal of molybdenum from tissues. Treatment of joint complaints is supportive.

Medical and Biological Monitoring. Laboratory measurement of serum and urinary molybdenum levels may be performed, but levels do not correlate with signs or symptoms. Serum uric acid and ceruloplasmin levels may be elevated (48). In the evaluation of airborne, soluble compounds of molybdenum, the National Institute for Occupational Safety and Health recommends atomic absorption spectrometry using nitrous oxide–acetylene flame (55). Other methods for measuring molybdenum levels are electron paramagnetic resonance spectroscopy, the dithiol method, and neutron activation.

Occupational and Environmental Regulations. Permissible exposure limits are listed in Table 82-6. As inhalation appears to be the primary route of exposure, control of dust and fumes is required.

Exposure Controls. Prevention of exposure is the mainstay in preventing toxicity, including good process enclosures with general dilution ventilation and local exhaust ventilation. The National Institute for Occupational Safety and Health and U.S. Occupational Safety and Health Administration recommend that workers exposed to insoluble molybdenum compounds wear personal protective equipment designed to limit dust, mist, or fume inhalation (43). Workers exposed to soluble com-

TABLE 82-6. Molybdenum permissible exposure limits

Agency	Limits
ACGIH TLV	5 mg/m^3 (soluble); 10 mg/m^3 (insoluble)
OSHA TWA	5 mg/m^3 (soluble); 15 mg/m^3 (insoluble)

ACGIH, American Conference of Governmental Industrial Hygienists; OSHA, U.S. Occupational Safety and Health Administration; TLV, threshold limit value; TWA, 8-hour time-weighted average.

pounds need impervious clothing, gloves, face shields, and other appropriate clothing as necessary to prevent skin contact (44). However, no data are available regarding skin effects or clinical effects from this route of absorption (55).

Environmental Fate and Transport

Molybdenum content in soil usually registers between 0.1 and 10.0 mg per kg. Leafy vegetables have a high content of the metal. Ash contains 10 to 40 μg per g of molybdenum. Air concentrations of molybdenum were up to 4 mg per cubic meter during Mo-steel production at a Russian steel mill. Water concentration varies from 0.5 μg per L (rivers) to up to 20.0 μg per L (ocean) (56).

Environmental and Occupational Monitoring

Monitoring of particle size and concentration should be undertaken in air and personal air sampling, especially during mining and processing of ore (56).

REFERENCES

1. Phillips TD, Nechay BR, Heidelbaugh ND. Vanadium: chemistry and the kidney. *Fed Proc* 1983;42:2969–2973.
2. Zenz C. Vanadium and its compounds. In: Zenz C, ed. *Occupational medicine,* 3rd ed. St Louis: Mosby–Year Book, 1994:584–594.
3. Kiviluoto M. Observations on the lungs of vanadium workers. *Br J Ind Med* 1980;37:363–366.
4. Hope BK. A global biogeochemical budget for vanadium. *Sci Total Environ* 1994;141:1–3.
5. Hosokawa S, Yoshida O. Vanadium in chronic hemodialysis patients. *Int J Artif Organs* 1990;13:197–199.
6. Hopkins LL, Mohr HE. Vanadium as an essential nutrient. *Fed Proc* 1974;33:1773–1775.
7. Nemery B. Metal toxicity and the respiratory tract. *Eur Respir J* 1990;3:202–219.
8. National Institute for Occupational Safety and Health and US Occupational Safety and Health Administration. Occupational health guideline for vanadium pentoxide dust. In: *Occupational health guidelines for chemical hazards.* Cincinnati: National Institute for Occupational Safety and Health and US Occupational Safety and Health Administration, 1978.
9. Lees REM. Changes in lung function after exposure to vanadium compounds in fuel oil ash. *Br J Ind Med* 1980;37:253–256.
10. Levy BS, Hoffman L, Gottsegen S. Boilermakers' bronchitis. Respiratory tract irritation associated with vanadium pentoxide exposure during oil-to-coal conversion of a power plant. *J Occup Med* 1984;26:567–570.
11. Musk AW, Tees JG. Asthma caused by occupational exposure to vanadium compounds. *Med J Aust* 1982;1:183–184.
12. Dafnis E, Sabatini S. Biochemistry and pathophysiology of vanadium. *Nephron* 1994;67:133–143.
13. Janiszewska G, Gachowicz L, Jaskoski D, Gromadzinska E. Vanadium inhibition of human parietal lobe ATPases. *Int J Biochem* 1994;26:551–553.
14. Boscolo P, Carmignani M, Volpe AR, et al. Renal toxicity and arterial hypertension in rats chronically exposed to vanadate. *Occup Environ Med* 1994;51:500–503.
15. Granadillo VA, Tahan JE, Salgado O, et al. The influence of blood levels of lead, aluminum and vanadium upon arterial hypertension. *Clin Chim Acta* 1995;233:47–59.
16. Owusu-Yaw J, Cohen MD, Fernando SY, Wei CI. An assessment of the genotoxicity of vanadium. *Toxicol Lett* 1990;50:327–336.
17. Ganguli S, Reuland DJ, Franklin LR, et al. Effects of maternal vanadate treatment on fetal development. *Life Sci* 1994;55:1267–1276.
18. Naylor GJ. In: *Metals ions in neurology and psychiatry.* New York: Alan R. Liss, 1985:99.
19. Brichard SM, Henquin JC. The role of vanadium in the management of diabetes. *Trends Pharmacol Sci* 1995;16:265–270.
20. Sprietmma JE. Diabetes can be prevented by reducing insulin production. *Med Hypotheses* 1994;42:15–23.
21. Harland BF, Harden-Williams BA. Is vanadium of human nutritional importance yet? *J Am Diet Assoc* 1994;94:891–894.
22. Hamel FG, Solomon S, Jespersen AS, et al. Alteration of tissue vanadium content in diabetes. *Metab Clin Exp* 1993;42:1503–1505.
23. McNeill JH, Battell M, Cam M, et al. Oral vanadium and lowering of blood glucose. *Diabetes* 1994;43:1268–1270.
24. Nielsen FH. Vanadium in mammalian physiology and nutrition. *Met Ions Biol Syst* 1995;31:543–573.
25. Kucera J, Byrne AR, Mravcova A, Lener L. Vanadium levels in hair and blood of normal exposed persons. *Sci Total Environ* 1992;115:191–205.
26. Domingo JL, Gomez M, Llobet JM, Corbella J. Chelating agents in the treatment of acute vanadyl sulphate intoxication in mice. *Toxicology* 1990;62:203–211.
27. National Institute for Occupational Safety and Health and US Occupational Safety and Health Administration. Occupational health guideline for vanadium pentoxide fume. In: *Occupational health guidelines for chemical hazards.* Cincinnati: National Institute for Occupational Safety and Health and US Occupational Safety and Health Administration, 1978.
28. Seiler HG. Analytical procedures for the determination of vanadium in biological materials. *Met Ions Biol Syst* 1995;31:671–688.
29. Kustin K, Robinson WE. Vanadium transport in animal systems. *Met Ions Biol Syst* 1995;31:511–542.
30. Zorba MA, Jacob PG, Al-Bloushi, Al-Nafisi R. Clams as pollution bioindicators in Kuwait's marine environment: metal accumulation and depuration. *Sci Total Environ* 1992;120:185–204.
31. Elinder CG, Zenz C. Other metals and their compounds. Titanium and its compounds. In: Zenz C, ed. *Occupational medicine,* 3rd ed. St Louis: Mosby–Year Book, 1988:613.
32. International Agency for Research of Cancer. Titanium dioxide. *IARC Monogr Eval Carcinog Risks Hum* 1989;47:307–326.
33. Fayerweather WE, Karns ME, Gilby P, Chen J. Epidemiological study of lung cancer mortality in workers exposed to titanium tetrachloride. *J Occup Med* 1992;34:164–169.
34. Sunderman FW. Carcinogenicity of metal alloys in orthopedic prostheses: clinical and experimental studies. *Fundam Appl Toxicol* 1989;13:205–216.
35. Stonkinger HE. Titanium. In: Clayton GD, Clayton FE, eds. *Patty's industrial hygiene and toxicology,* vol 2, 3rd ed. New York: John Wiley and Sons, 1982: 1968–1981.
36. National Institute for Occupational Safety and Health and US Occupational Safety and Health Administration. Occupational health guideline for titanium dioxide. In: *Occupational health guidelines for chemical hazards.* Cincinnati: National Institute for Occupational Safety and Health and US Occupational Safety and Health Administration, 1978.
37. Driscoll KE, Lindenschmidt RC, Maurer JK, et al. Pulmonary response to silica or titanium dioxide: inflammatory cells, alveolar macrophage-derived cytokines, and histopathology. *Am J Respir Cell Mol Biol* 1990;2:381–390.
38. Redline S, Barna BP, Tomashefski JF, Abraham JL. Granulomatous disease associated with pulmonary deposition of titanium. *Br J Ind Med* 1986;43:652–656.
39. Haynes DR, Rogers SD. The differences in toxicity and release of bone mediators induced by titanium and cobalt-chromium-alloy wear particles. *J Bone Joint Surg Am* 1993;75:825–834.
40. Torgersen S, Gjerdet NR, Erichsen ES, Bang G. Metal particles and tissue changes adjacent to miniplates. A retrieval study. *Acta Odontol Scand* 1995; 53:65–71.
41. Bernard BK, Osheroff MR, Hofmann A, Mennear JH. Toxicology and carcinogenesis studies of dietary titanium dioxide–coated mica in male and female Fischer 344 rats. *J Toxicol Environ Health* 1990;29:417–429.
42. Wong SL, Nakamoto L. Detection and toxicity from pulp and paper effluents. *Bull Environ Contam Toxicol* 1995;55:878–885.
43. National Institute for Occupational Safety and Health and US Occupational Safety and Health Administration. Occupational health guideline for molybdenum and insoluble molybdenum. In: *Occupational health guidelines for chemical hazards.* Cincinnati: National Institute for Occupational Safety and Health and US Occupational Safety and Health Administration, 1978.
44. National Institute for Occupational Safety and Health and US Occupational Safety and Health Administration. Occupational health guideline for soluble molybdenum compounds (as molybdenum). In: *Occupational health guidelines for chemical hazards.* Cincinnati: National Institute for Occupational Safety and Health and US Occupational Safety and Health Administration, 1978.
45. Sardesai VM. Molybdenum: an essential trace element. *Nutr Clin Pract* 1993;8:277–281.
46. Goyer RA. Toxic effects of chemicals. In: Klassen CD, Amdur MO, Doull J, eds. *Casarett and Doull's toxicology,* 3rd ed. New York: Macmillan, 1986:582–635.
47. Hosokawa S, Yoshida O. Role of molybdenum in chronic hemodialysis patients. *Int J Artif Organs* 1994;17:567–569.
48. Walravens PA, Moure-Eraso R, Solomons CC, et al. Biochemical abnormalities in workers exposed to molybdenum dust. *Arch Environ Health* 1979;34:302–308.
49. Ladefoged O, Storap M. Copper deficiency in cattle, sheep, and horses by excess molybdenum from fly ash. *Vet Human Toxicol* 1995;37:63–65.
50. Gengelbach GP, Ward JD, Spears JW. Effects of dietary copper, iron and molybdenum on growth and copper status of beef cows and calves. *J Anim Sci* 1994;72:2722–2727.

51. De Vuyst P, Vande Weyer R, De Coster A, et al. Dental technician's pneumoconiosis, a report of two cases. *Am Rev Respir Dis* 1986;133:316–320.
52. Goldring SR, Flannery MS, Petrison KK, et al. Evaluation of connective tissue cell responses to orthopedic implant materials. *Connect Tissue Res* 1990;29:77–81.
53. Parry NM, Phillipo M, Reid MD, et al. Molybdenum induced changes in the epiphyseal plate. *Calcif Tissue Int* 1993;53:180–186.
54. Federman M, Morell B, Graetz G, et al. Hypersensitivity to molybdenum as a possible trigger of ANA-negative systemic lupus erythematosus. *Ann Rheum Dis* 1994;53:403–405.
55. Stonkinger HE. Molybdenum. In: Clayton GD, Clayton FE, eds. *Patty's industrial hygiene and toxicology,* vol 2, 3rd ed. New York: John Wiley and Sons, 1982:1806–1819.
56. Elinder CG, Zenz C. Other metals and their compounds. Molybdenum and its compounds. In: Zenz C, ed. *Occupational medicine,* 3rd ed. St Louis: Mosby–Year Book, 1988:606–607.

CHAPTER 83
*Selenium**

David J. Thomas and Miroslav Styblo

OVERVIEW

Since the time that selenium was demonstrated to be biologically essential in mammals (1), researchers have identified several critical functions for this metalloid. Selenium is present as selenocysteine at the active sites of enzymes, including glutathione peroxidase, type I iodothyronine deiodinase, and a novel thioredoxin reductase (2–4). Endemic selenium deficiency in humans has occurred in some areas of China (5), as seen in Keshan disease and Kaschin-Beck disease, and during courses of total parenteral nutrition and in low-birth-weight infants (6). Recent work shows that the cardiomyopathy seen in Keshan disease may be due to increased virulence of cardiomyopathic coxsackievirus in a selenium-deficient host (7). The increased virulence of coxsackievirus in selenium-deficient mice has been attributed to an increased rate of mutation in the viral genome (8). Selenium is also a modifier of the metabolism and toxicity of organic compounds and of metals (9,10). Finally, selenium dietary intake affects the development and progression of many types of cancers. A recent intervention study suggested that selenium supplementation may affect cancer incidence and mortality in humans (11). If selenium supplementation is an effective mode of chemoprevention, possibly the incidence of acute and chronic intoxication will increase, owing to misuse of the metalloid as a dietary supplement.

SOURCES AND PRODUCTION

Selenium (atomic number, 34; Chemical Abstracts Service chemical luminescence number, 7782-49-2) is a metalloid that has an atomic mass of 78.96 and exists in at least four oxidation states in nature. Selenate (6+), selenite (4+), elemental selenium (0), and selenide (2–) are found in soils and vary in availability for translocation and incorporation into plants. Commercially, selenium is extracted from anode slime produced in electrolytic copper refining and from flue dust of pyrite burners (12,13).

*This manuscript has been reviewed in accordance with the policy of the National Health and Environmental Effects Research Laboratory, U.S. Environmental Protection Agency, and has been approved for publication. Approval does not signify that the contents necessarily reflect the views and policies of the Agency, nor does mention of trade names or commercial products constitute endorsement or recommendation for use.

EXPOSURE SOURCES

Concentrations of selenium in soils vary from 0.03 parts per million (ppm) to more than 30 ppm in regions with seleniferous soils (14,15). Regions with such soils include the upper Great Plains of the United States and Enshi County, Hubei Province, People's Republic of China. Plants of the genera *Astragalus, Haplopappus, Machaeranthera,* and *Stanleya* are primary selenium bioaccumulators, and their presence may identify regions of increased soil selenium concentrations (14). The concentration of selenium in surface water and groundwater usually is fairly low (less than 10 µg per L); however, regions with seleniferous soils may have elevated selenium levels in water. Irrigation drainage water can contain extremely high concentrations of selenium (16). Air concentrations of selenium generally are low (less than 10 ng per cubic meter) and derive at least in part from burning of selenium-containing fossil fuels (15). Overall, the contribution of respired selenium to the body burden of selenium is small. However, inhalation of gaseous selenium, selenium-laden aerosols, or particulate selenium can produce acute or chronic toxicity in humans (17–23).

Table 83-1 (5,14,17,24–27) lists occupational uses and environmental conditions in which excessive selenium exposure might occur. Although selenium exposure usually is well controlled in industrial settings, the potential for selenium intoxication exists. Exposure to excessive amounts of selenium by ingestion of selenium-contaminated food or by inhalation of selenium-containing aerosol also can occur. Excessive exposure to selenium by ingestion of selenium supplements (26) or by use of a selenium-containing shampoo (24) are unusual but documented events.

Chronic selenium poisoning has been described in North American and Chinese populations. During the 1930s, the health status of individuals residing in regions with seleniferous soils in Nebraska, South Dakota, and Wyoming was examined (28). Icteroid discoloration of skin, changes in fingernails, gastrointestinal disorders, and discoloration and decay of teeth were common signs and symptoms in individuals with the highest levels of selenium in urine (more than 200 µg per L). Notably, chronic selenium

TABLE 83-1. Possible occupational and environmental sources of selenium exposure

Source or site	Use
Industrial	
Glass manufacturing	Decolorizer and pigment
Pigment and glaze production	Colorant in dyes and glazes
Printing and etching	Inks
Steel production and fabrication	Steel alloys and copper alloys
Electrical devices and insulation	Photoelectric cells and rectifiers, gaseous electrical insulator (SeF_6)
Rubber production	Antioxidant and accelerator
Copper refining	H_2Se production in copper refining
Plastic production	Colorant
Environmental	
Ingestion of Se-containing plant and animal material	
Inhalation of Se-containing aerosol or gas	
Iatrogenic	
Self-medication with Se-containing supplements	
Use of Se-containing antidandruff shampoo	

Adapted from refs. 5, 14, 17, and 24–27.

intoxication of horses, pigs, and cows also occurred in this area. Historically, selenium intoxication in domestic animals has been termed both *alkali disease* and *blind staggers*. As noted by Raisback et al. (29), alkali disease is induced by excessive intake of selenium; the consumption of water with a high concentration of sulfate is the probable cause of blind staggers.

CLINICAL TOXICOLOGY

Routes of Exposure, Distribution, Metabolism, and Elimination

Organic selenium compounds [e.g., selenomethionine (SeMet)] are absorbed almost fully in the human intestine (30); the gastrointestinal absorption of selenite in humans is lower (44% to 70%) (31). Large differences in dietary selenium intakes have little effect on the extent of gastrointestinal absorption of this element (32). At extremes, daily intakes of selenium in diet range from 10 to 20 μg per day (in areas in which selenium deficiency has been recognized) up to approximately 5,000 μg per day (in seleniferous regions). A "safe and adequate" dietary intake of selenium probably ranges from approximately 50 to 200 μg per day (33), and this intake probably is achieved by most individuals in the United States. Notably, a daily intake of up to 724 μg of selenium by residents of the seleniferous region of the Great Plains of the United States has not been associated with evidence of chronic selenium toxicity (34).

Absorption of selenium from the respiratory tract has been examined. For a selenium aerosol with a 0.5-μm median mass aerodynamic diameter, the rate of clearance is 0.48 m^3 of air per hour (35). The solubility of respired selenium compounds apparently affects the rate of lung absorption. Long-term occupational exposure to elemental selenium dust can lead to very high concentrations of selenium in the lung (20). The toxicity of H_2Se is limited by its rapid decomposition in air to elemental selenium and water; hence, the risk from environmental exposure to this gas is relatively small (36). Chronic selenium poisoning has occurred after prolonged inhalation of selenium released by coal burning (37).

Skin absorption of selenium has not been studied extensively. In rats, a skin absorption rate for a sodium selenite solution of 10% per hour has been reported (38). Some selenium compounds (e.g., selenium oxychloride) are potent vesicants, producing severe burns at the site of application (39), and dermal application of selenium oxychloride can be lethal in dogs (40). Increased urinary excretion of selenium by human volunteers after dermal application of a selenium sulfide–containing lotion has been reported (41). A case report of signs and symptoms consistent with selenium poisoning in a woman using a selenium sulfide–containing shampoo suggested that significant dermal absorption can occur (24). Eye irritation can occur with chronic exposure to H_2Se (25).

Besides similarities between the metabolism of selenium and sulfur (42), the most striking aspects of selenium metabolism are the biological reduction of selenate (6+) and selenite (4+) to selenide (2–) and the subsequent excretion of selenide-containing compounds. At least two reactions in this reductive pathway are catalyzed by glutathione reductase and require glutathione and nicotinamide adenine dinucleotide phosphate (43). The end product of this phase of metabolism is the production of H_2Se. Selenide is a reactive species that forms complexes with metals (10). Further, H_2Se can be metabolized to dimethylselenide, a volatile compound that is lost in expired air. Dimethylselenide has a distinctive garliclike odor, and exhalation of this agent accounts for the garliclike odor of the breath characteristic of selenium intoxication. Dimethylselenide is metabolized to trimethylselenonium ion, which is excreted in urine.

The systemic kinetics of selenium in humans have been described (44,45). Urinary loss is the major route for excretion of selenium. The whole-body retention of selenium in human volunteers is longer after ingestion of selenium methionine than after ingestion of selenite (46), suggesting that its fate is influenced by chemical form. A depletion-repletion study in young men indicated that intake of approximately 70 μg of selenium per day is needed to maintain body selenium stores (47).

Signs, Symptoms, and Syndromes

Table 83-2 (17–23,26,48–61) summarizes data regarding the acute and chronic toxicity of selenium in certain affected humans. (It contains a description of the exposure scenario and provides data regarding the clinical course and modes of treatment.) The embryotoxic or teratogenic potency of selenium in mammals is not established clearly. A recent study in long-tailed macaques that received up to 300 μg of SeMet per day by nasogastric intubation throughout pregnancy provided evidence of maternal toxicity and associated fetal growth retardation; however, no teratogenic or gross morphologic changes in progeny have been attributed to SeMet exposure *in utero* (62). In contrast, selenium-containing compounds are teratogenic in birds. Exposure of mallards to high dietary concentrations of selenite (10 ppm) or of SeMet (25 ppm) reduced egg yield and inhibited embryonic growth. SeMet is more teratogenic than is selenite (63). In aquatic birds exposed to high environmental selenium levels at Kesterson Reservoir in northern California, similar patterns of congenital malformations have been noted (64). Shamburger (65) reviewed the extensive literature on the mutagenicity of a variety of selenium-containing compounds in eukaryotes. Recent studies found that inorganic and organic selenium compounds induce chromosomal abnormalities in cultured human peripheral blood lymphocytes (66,67).

The role of selenium in carcinogenesis is a topic of great interest. For humans, the International Agency for Research on Cancer classified selenium and selenium compounds as class 2B carcinogens and selenium sulfide as a group 3 carcinogen (68). Selenium can increase tumor yield in some exposure scenarios (69). Conversely, selenium also can inhibit development of chemically and virally induced tumors (10,70,71). In human populations, the relation between selenium intake and cancer risk remains a topic of great interest. Ecologic studies of selenium contents of foodstuffs and prevalence of certain tumors suggested an inverse relation between these variables (72). The hypothesis that an inadequate intake of selenium increases the risk of cancer has been examined in many studies (73–75). Intervention trials in which the diets are supplemented with selenium alone or in combination with other nutrients have been used to test the effect of selenium nutrition on the incidence of cancer.

A recent study tested whether supplementation of the diet with selenium affected the incidence of cancer (11). In that study, subjects received orally either 200 μg of selenium (as yeast selenium) per day or placebo and were studies for an average of 6.4 years. Although this study initially examined the effect of selenium supplementation on incidences of basal cell and squamous cell carcinomas of the skin, additional analyses showed that selenium supplementation significantly reduced total cancer mortality, total cancer incidence, and the incidences of colorectal, lung, and prostate cancers. Given current interest in the reduction of cancer risk by dietary modification, further studies of the effects of selenium supplementation on cancer incidence can be expected.

TABLE 83-2. Selenium intoxication in affected humans

Exposure	Signs and symptoms	Treatment and clinical course	Study
Acute intoxication			
Se fume exposure (workers exposed in the smelting of Se-coated rectifier plates)	Intense irritation of eyes, nose, and throat; garliclike breath odor	Symptomatic treatment of respiratory distress; no noted long-term effects	18
Se oxide fume inhalation (fire in factory producing Se-containing rectifiers; workers exposed for less than 20 min)	Immediate irritation of upper respiratory tract and bitter taste in mouth; secondary symptoms after 2–12 h (chills, nausea, vomiting, headaches); pneumonitis in 5 of 28 exposed workers	Symptomatic and supportive treatment; no reported long-term effects of exposure	19
Selenious acid ingestion (ingestion of gun-bluing solution by 3-year-old boy)	Coma, hypotension, excessive salivation, and strong garliclike breath odor	Gastric intubation and aspiration of stomach contents, and mechanical ventilation; death about 2 hours after ingestion of gun-bluing solution	48
Sodium selenate ingestion (ingestion of sheep drench by 15-year-old girl)	Strong garliclike breath odor, diffuse T-wave ECG flattening, and increased SGOT and serum alkaline phosphatase activities	Vomiting induced with gastric lavage and forced diuresis; treatment with vitamin C, BAL, and diazepam; complete recovery with discharge on hospital day 17	49
Hydrogen selenide inhalation (24-year-old man exposed during transfer of hydrogen selenide)	Severe dyspnea with pneumomediastinum, restrictive and obstructive airway disease	Symptomatic treatment with oxygen, theophylline, hydrocortisone; impaired postexposure function at 3 yr	21
Selenious acid ingestion (ingestion of gun-bluing solution by 52-year-old woman with suicidal intent)	Vomiting, garliclike breath odor, hypotension and pulmonary edema, adult respiratory distress syndrome, increased serum aspartate aminotransferase activity	Supportive and symptomatic therapy, administration of BAL on day 2 after exposure to treat possible copper intoxication; death 8 days after exposure; autopsy findings of acute small-bowel infarction, consolidation in lungs, centrilobular necrosis in liver, and papillary necrosis in kidney	50
Selenious acid ingestion (ingestion of gun-bluing solution by 2-year-old boy)	Second-degree burns of esophagus and stomach; coma; cardiomyopathy and intestinal distention; metabolic acidosis, hemoconcentration, hyperglycemia, leukocytosis	Vomiting induction, mechanical ventilation; improving condition until day 4 after exposure, at which time acute respiratory distress developed; infection with *Legionella dumoffii* not responsive to treatment; death on day 17 after ingestion	51
Eruptive explosion of selenious acid-caustic soda mixture (second-degree burns on face, frontal thorax, and upper legs of 44-year-old worker)	Pulmonary edema, unstable blood pressure, garliclike breath odor	Death within 90 min of exposure; autopsy findings of hyperemia of trachea and bronchi and hemorrhagic alveolar edema in lungs	52
Selenious acid ingestion (ingestion of gun-bluing solution by 40-year-old woman with suicidal intent)	Vomiting, diarrhea, delusional stupor, tachycardia, hypotension, anuria	Cardiac arrest at 8 h after exposure; autopsy findings of pulmonary edema and pleural effusion, interstitial edema in the kidney, necrosis of proximal tubules, and glomerular dilatation	53
Selenious acid ingestion (ingestion of gun-bluing solution by 2-year-old girl)	Vomiting, diarrhea, muscle spasm and restlessness, excessive salivation, hypertension, tachycardia	Parenteral fluids; complete recovery	54
Chronic intoxication (occupational and environmental sources)			
Hydrogen selenide inhalation (workers exposed for approximately 1 mo in a metal-etching and printing operation)	Nausea and vomiting, metallic taste and garliclike breath odor, fatigue and dizziness	Se-containing ink replaced in printing operation; resolved signs and symptoms	17
Se exposure from ingestion of raw or boiled fruit of *Lecythis ollaria*, the monkey's coconut (coco de mono)	Nausea and vomiting, generalized hair loss within 2 wk, gray transverse lines in nails	Resolution of signs and symptoms after cessation of exposure	55
Se fume and dust exposure (71-year-old man exposed for 50 years in Se refinery)	Reddish orange hair, reddish fingernails	Autopsy findings of high concentrations of Se in lungs, hair, and nails	20
Endemic Se intoxication (ingestion of plant food grown on seleniferous soil in Enshi County, Hubei Province, People's Republic of China)	Nail and hair loss; skin lesions with reddish pigmentation; increased dental caries; peripheral anesthesia, acroparesthesia, hemiplegia	Change in food supply to reduce Se consumption	56
Hydrogen selenide inhalation (21-year-old woman exposed chronically and intermittently for 1 yr in research laboratory)	Chronic diarrhea with lower-quadrant abdominal pain; bitter metallic taste and garliclike breath odor; granular conjunctivitis, dental caries	Resolution of signs and symptoms after cessation of exposure	22
Se dust exposure (40 workers processing Se cake in a copper refinery)	Garliclike breath odor, respiratory tract irritation, muscle and joint pain; approximately one-third of workers anemic	Resolution of signs and symptoms after cessation of exposure; increased hemoglobin after cessation of exposure	57
Selenious acid ingestion (intermittent ingestion of gun-bluing solution by 46-year-old man with homicidal intent)	Diarrhea, garliclike breath odor, hair loss, purple-red discoloration at the base of nails	Resolution of signs and symptoms after cessation of exposure	58

(continued)

TABLE 83-2. *(continued)*

Exposure	Signs and symptoms	Treatment and clinical course	Study
Se dust exposure (exposure of 31-year-old man in manufacture of photocopying machines)	Generalized hair loss, fragility of nails	Resolution of signs and symptoms after cessation of exposure	23
Chronic intoxication (iatrogenic or self-medication)			
Dietary Se supplementation ingestion (ingestion by 17-year-old boy and 11-month-old girl with cystic fibrosis of over-the-counter Se yeast complex supplement)	Vomiting, decreased appetite and weight loss, electrolyte abnormalities in 17-year-old; respiratory distress, dehydration, electrolyte abnormalities in 11-month-old	Recovery of 17-year-old after supportive therapy to correct electrolyte imbalance; development of hypocalcemia, tetany, hypotension in 11-month-old, with death on day 7 of hospitalization; autopsy findings of severe fatty liver, microscopically normal kidneys with some calcium deposits	59
Dietary Se supplementation ingestion (self-medication with an over-the-counter preparation; 23 cases in the United States)	Nausea and vomiting, changes in nails and hair, watery diarrhea, abdominal pain, garliclike breath odor	Improperly compounded Se-containing preparation (182 times the amount of Se stated by manufacturer)	60
Se supplementation in clinically hypothyroid children (hypothyroid children from region of endemic cretinism receive orally 50 µg of Se as selenomethionine daily for 2 mo)	Decreased serum T_3, T_4, and free T_4 after 2 mo of supplementation: evidence of adverse effect use of Se supplementation and iodine in hypothyroid subjects	Partial reversal of effects of Se on serum T_3, T_4, and free T_4 after treatment with iodine-containing supplement	61
Dietary Se supplementation ingestion (self-medicated 36-year-old man taking over-the-counter preparation)	Generalized hair loss, paresthesia, diarrhea, fatigue, yellowish white and red transverse lines in nails	Cessation of self-medication, hair regrowth, reversal of paresthesia, improperly compounded Se-containing preparation (500–1,000 times the amount of Se stated by manufacturer)	26

BAL, British anti-Lewisite; ECG, electrocardiograph; SGOT, serum glutamic-oxaloacetic transaminase.

Management of Toxicity or Exposure

Although most signs and symptoms are nonspecific, the presence of a garliclike odor of the breath may be an important clue to excessive selenium exposure, particularly in cases of chronic selenium intoxication (76). However, other possible causes of the garliclike odor that must be considered in differential diagnosis are excessive exposure to phosphorous, tellurium, arsenic, lewisite, pyridine, dimethyl sulfoxide, or garlic (22). As summarized in Table 83-2, treatment of selenium intoxication is largely symptomatic. Sources of exposure must be identified, and steps must be taken to control exposure. In cases of acute intoxication, such as those occurring after the accidental or suicidal ingestion of selenium-containing gun-bluing solution, emesis is contraindicated, and the potential benefit of gastric lavage to remove selenium must be carefully evaluated (77). Although dimercaptopropanol has been used to treat acute selenate poisoning (49), use of chelating agents generally is not supported. Indeed, dimercaptopropanol treatment may increase the toxicity of selenium (48). The high incidence of mortality in children who ingest gun-bluing solution strongly argues that better therapeutic approaches are needed.

MEDICAL AND BIOLOGICAL MONITORING

The need for a selective and sensitive indicator of selenium intoxication recently was noted by an expert panel (78). Laboratory diagnosis of selenium intoxication currently involves determination of the concentration of selenium in blood, erythrocytes, plasma or serum, urine, and hair or nails. Methods used for the determination of selenium contents of biological samples include fluorometric analysis (79), atomic absorption spectrophotometry (80), neutron activation analysis (81), and isotope dilution gas chromatography–mass spectrometry (82). A variety of studies have examined the relation among selenium intake, the concentration of selenium in blood, and the excretion of selenium in urine (83). An early study in selenium refinery workers suggested 100 µg of selenium per L as a maximum allowable concentration in urine (84). However, on the basis of more recent results obtained in seleniferous areas of China and the United States, urinary output of selenium between 600 and 1,000 µg per day may indicate overexposure (83). Urinary output of selenium increases with increasing daily intake of selenium, suggesting that monitoring of urinary selenium concentration would provide data on exposure (85,86).

A blood selenium concentration greater than 0.6 µg per mL has been suggested to be evidence of excessive exposure. In a case of fatal acute selenious acid poisoning in a 2-year-old boy (51), a plasma selenium concentration of 2.85 µg per mL was detected. Studies in a population residing in a seleniferous region of China have provided data regarding tissue selenium concentrations during chronic exposure to selenium (87). In those studies, an estimated daily intake of 910 µg of selenium was associated with the development of signs of selenosis (as exemplified by pathologic changes in fingernails). This level of selenium intake was associated with a blood selenium concentration of 1.05 µg per mL. Therefore, a reliable report of high plasma or blood selenium concentration should trigger immediate concern and intervention.

Hair is a biological medium that might be of use in monitoring chronic selenium exposure. A high correlation between blood and hair selenium concentrations has been reported (56), but the correlation between hair selenium concentration and tissue concentrations of selenium is not well understood (88). Potential confounding of the value of hair selenium concentration by the use of selenium-containing shampoos or by surface contamination with atmospheric selenium has been noted (89). "Normal" selenium concentration in serum is lower in young children than in adults, and it reaches adult levels at approximately 10 years of age (90). This observation may be important in assessing the significance of a particular blood or serum selenium concentration in an affected child.

TABLE 83-3. Occupational and environmental regulations and guidelines for selenium

Agency	Guideline	Reference
Occupational		
NIOSH	TWA for Se and Se compounds, 0.2 mg/m^3	92
ACGIH	TLV for Se and Se compounds (as Se), 0.2 mg/m^3	93
	TLV for Se hexafluoride (as Se), 0.05 ppm	
OSHA	PEL, TWA for Se compounds (as Se), 0.2 mg/m^3	93
	PEL, TWA for Se hexafluoride (as Se), 0.05 ppm	
Environmental		
WHO	Guideline for drinking-water Se, 0.01 mg/L	78
NRC	RDA for Se	96
	Men, 0.07 mg/day	
	Women, 0.055 mg/day	
	General, 8.7 × 10^{-4} mg/kg/day	
EPA	Reference dose for Se, 0.005 mg/kg/day	97

ACGIH, American Conference of Governmental Industrial Hygienists; EPA, U.S. Environmental Protection Agency; NIOSH, National Institute for Occupational Safety and Health; NRC, National Research Council; OSHA, U.S. Occupational Safety and Health Administration; PEL, permissible exposure limit; RDA, recommended dietary allowance; TLV, threshold limit value; TWA, time-weighted average; WHO, World Health Organization.

Measurement of erythrocyte or plasma glutathione peroxidase activity probably is not useful as an indicator of excessive selenium exposure. The activity of this enzyme is near maximum at normal levels of selenium intake (91). Reduced whole blood glutathione peroxidase activity has been associated with high dietary intake of selenium (85); in acute selenious acid poisoning, only a small increase in plasma glutathione peroxidase activity accompanied a very high plasma selenium concentration (54).

Occupational and Environmental Regulations

Table 83-3 (78,92–97) summarizes a variety of regulations and guidelines that have been developed for safe and acceptable levels of exposure to selenium and selenium compounds. Primary emphasis in setting the threshold limit value for industrial settings is to prevent irritation of eyes and mucous membranes (93). A recent addition to this list is the reference dose (RfD) for selenium developed by the U.S. Environmental Protection Agency (98). An RfD is an estimate of a daily exposure of a human population that is likely to be without an appreciable risk of adverse health effects during a lifetime of exposure. Often, an RfD is used in risk management to assess the hazard posed by chronic exposure to a specific chemical.

Exposure Controls

Suggestions for the control of exposure to selenium in the workplace have been summarized by Plunkett (99). Adequate ventilation, protective clothing and goggles, and respiratory protection are recommended. Selenium-contaminated eyes or skin can be treated acutely by washing with water or with a 10% aqueous solution of sodium thiosulfate.

ENVIRONMENTAL FATE AND TRANSPORT

The cycling of selenium through the environment has been described (13,100). The methylation of inorganic selenium by environmental microorganisms is an unusual aspect of the cycling of this metalloid (101). However, the quantitative significance of methylated selenium compounds in the cycling of selenium in the environment is unclear. Selenium is incorporated into selenoanalogs of sulfur-containing amino acids in both plants and animals (102,103).

ENVIRONMENTAL AND OCCUPATIONAL MONITORING

Beliles and Beliles (104) have summarized procedures for sampling for selenium in the atmosphere. Gases and vapors containing selenium can be scrubbed through hydrobromic acid (40% to 48%) that contains 5% to 10% free bromine. H_2Se can be collected in soda lime (sodium hydroxide and lime), and selenium dioxide can be collected in water in a midget impinger. Analysis of selenium by atomic absorption spectrophotometry with an argon-hydrogen flame and an electrodeless discharge lamp is recommended (80). Methods for the analysis of selenium in biological matrices have been described (79–82).

REFERENCES

1. Schwarz K, Foltz CM. Selenium as an integral part of factor 3 against dietary necrotic liver degeneration. *J Am Chem Soc* 1957;79:3292–3293.
2. Rotruck JT, Pope AL, Ganther HE, et al. Selenium: biochemical role as a component of glutathione peroxidase. *Science* 1973;179:585–590.
3. Burk RF, Hill KE. Regulation of selenoproteins. *Ann Rev Nutr* 1993;13:65–81.
4. Tamura T, Stadtman TC. A new selenoprotein from human lung adenocarcinoma cells: purification, properties, and thioredoxin reductase activity. *Proc Natl Acad Sci U S A* 1996;93:1006–1011.
5. Guang-Qi Y. Research on selenium-related problems in human health in China. In: Combs GF, Levander OA, Spallholz JE, Oldfield JE, eds. *Selenium in biology and medicine.* New York: Van Nostrand–Reinhold, 1987:9–32.
6. Van Vleet JF, Ferrans JJ. Etiologic factors and pathologic alterations in selenium–vitamin E deficiency and excess in animals and humans. *Biol Trace Elem Res* 1992;33:1–21.
7. Beck MA, Kolbeck PC, Rohr LH, Shi Q, Morris VC, Levander OA. Increased virulence of a human enterovirus (coxsackievirus B3) in selenium-deficient mice. *J Infect Dis* 1994;170:351–357.
8. Beck MA, Shi Q, Morris VC, Levander OA. Rapid genomic evolution of a non-virulent coxsackievirus B3 in selenium-deficient mice results in selection of identical virulent isolates. *Nat Med* 1995;1:433–436.
9. Wendel A, Reiter R. Modulation of xenobiotic metabolism in mouse liver by dietary selenium. In: Combs GF, Spallholz JE, Levander OA, Oldfield JE, eds. *Selenium in biology and medicine.* New York: Van Nostrand–Reinhold, 1987:283–290.
10. Whanger PD. Selenium in the treatment of heavy metal poisoning and chemical carcinogenesis. *J Trace Elem Electrolytes Health Dis* 1992;6:209–221.
11. Clark LC, Combs GF Jr, Turnbull BW, et al. Effects of selenium supplementation for cancer prevention in patients with carcinoma of the skin. A randomized controlled trial. *JAMA* 1996;276:1957–1963.
12. MacKenzie FT, Lantzy RJ, Patterson V. Global trace metal cycles and predictions. *Math Geol* 1979;11:99–142.
13. GESAMP (IMO/FAO/UNESCO/WMO/WHO/IAEA/UN/UNEP). Joint group of experts on the scientific aspects of marine pollution). Review of potentially harmful substances: arsenic, selenium, and mercury. *Rep Stud GESAMP* 1986;28:134–169.
14. Committee on Medical and Biologic Effects of Environmental Pollutants, Division of Medical Sciences Assembly of Life Sciences National Research Council. *Selenium.* Washington: National Academy of Sciences, 1976:1–40.
15. Bennett BG, Peterson PJ. Assessment of human exposure to environmental selenium. In: Combs GF, Levander OA, Spallholz JE, Oldfield JE, eds. *Selenium in biology and medicine.* New York: Van Nostrand–Reinhold, 1987:608–618.
16. Fan AM, Book SA, Neutra RR, Epstein DM. Selenium and human health implications in California's San Joaquin Valley. *J Toxicol Environ Health* 1988;23:539–559.
17. Buchan RF. Industrial selenosis. *Occup Med* 1947;3:439–456.
18. Clinton M Jr. Selenium fume exposure. *J Ind Hyg Toxicol* 1947;29:225–226.
19. Wilson H. Selenium oxide poisoning. *N C Med J* 1962;23:73–75.
20. Diskin CJ, Alper JC, Fliegel SE. Long-term selenium exposure. *Arch Intern Med* 1979;139:824–826.
21. Schecter A, Shanske W, Stenzler A, Quintilian H, Steinberg H. Acute hydrogen selenide inhalation. *Chest* 1980;77:554–555.
22. Alderman LC, Bergin JJ. Hydrogen selenide poisoning: an illustrative case with review of the literature. *Arch Environ Health* 1986;41:354–358.

23. Srivastava AK, Gupta BN, Bihari V, Guar JS. Generalized hair loss and selenium exposure. *Vet Hum Toxicol* 1995;37:468–469.
24. Ransome JW, Scott NM, Knoblock EC. Selenium sulfide intoxication. *N Engl J Med* 1961;264:384–385.
25. Robin JP. Safety and health aspects of selenium and tellurium in a copper refinery. In: *Proceedings of the International Symposium on Industrial Uses of Selenium and Tellurium*, 3rd ed. Darien, CT: Selenium-Tellurium Development Association, 1984:28–56.
26. Clark RF, Strukle E, Williams SR, Manoguerra AS. Selenium poisoning from a nutritional supplement. *JAMA* 1996;275:1087–1088.
27. Lewis DR. Dopant materials used in the microelectronics industry. *Occup Med* 1986;1:35–47.
28. Smith MI, Franke KW, Westfall BB. The selenium problem in relation to public health. *Public Health Rep* 1936;51:1496–1505.
29. Raisbeck MR, Dahl ER, Sanchez DA, Beldin EL, O'Toole D. Naturally occurring selenosis in Wyoming. *J Vet Diagn Invest* 1993;5:84–87.
30. Griffiths NM, Stewart RDH, Robinson MF. The metabolism of (^{75}Se) selenomethionine in four women. *Br J Nutr* 1976;35:372–382.
31. Thomson CD, Stewart RDH. The metabolism of (^{75}Se) selenite in young women. *Br J Nutr* 1974;32:47–57.
32. Schrauzer GN, White DA. Selenium in human nutrition: dietary intakes and effects of supplementation. *Bioinorg Chem* 1978;8:303–318.
33. Levander OA. The global selenium agenda. In: Hurley LS, Keen CL, Lonnerdal B, Rucker RB, eds. *Trace elements in man and animals*, vol 6. New York: Plenum Publishing, 1988:1–6.
34. Longnecker MP, Taylor PR, Levander OA, et al. Selenium in diet, blood, and toenails in relation to human health in a seleniferous area. *Am J Clin Nutr* 1991;53:1288–1294.
35. Medinsky MA, Cuddihy RG, Griffith WC, Weissman SH, McClellan RO. Projected uptake and toxicity of selenium compounds from the environment. *Environ Res* 1985;365:181–192.
36. Glover JR. Selenium and its industrial toxicology. *Ind Med Surg* 1970;39:50–54.
37. Whanger PD. China, a country with both selenium deficiency and toxicity: some thoughts and impressions. *J Nutr* 1989;119:1236–1239.
38. Dutkiewicz T, Dutkiewicz B, Balcerska I. Dynamics of organ and tissue distribution of selenium after intragastric and dermal administration of sodium selenite. *Bromatol Chem Toksykol* 1972;4:475–481.
39. Cerwenka EA, Cooper C. Toxicology of selenium and tellurium and their compounds. *Arch Environ Health* 1961;3:161–200.
40. Moxon AL. Selenium poisoning. *Physiol Rev* 1943;23:305–337.
41. Farley J, Skelly EM, Weber CB. Percutaneous absorption of selenium sulfide. *J Environ Sci Health* 1986;A21:571–582.
42. Levander OA. Selected aspects of the comparative metabolism and biochemistry of selenium and sulfur. In: Prasad AS, Oberleas D, eds. *Trace elements in human health and disease*, vol 2. New York: Academic Press, 1976:135–163.
43. Ganther HE. Metabolism of hydrogen selenide and methylated selenides. In: Draper HH, ed. *Advances in nutritional research.* New York: Plenum Publishing, 1979:107–129.
44. Janghorbani M, Christensen MJ, Nahapetian A, Young VR. Selenium metabolism in healthy adults: 2. Quantitative aspects using the stable isotope $^{74}SeO_3^{2-}$. *Am J Clin Nutr* 1982;35:647–654.
45. Patterson BH, Zech LA. Development of a model for selenite metabolism in humans. *J Nutr* 1992;22:709–714.
46. Cavalieri RR, Scott KG, Sairenji E. Selenite [^{75}Se] as a tumor-localizing agent in man. *J Nucl Med* 1966;7:197–208.
47. Levander OA, Sutherland B, Morris VC, King JC. Selenium balance in young men during selenium depletion and repletion. *Am J Clin Nutr* 1981;34:2662–2669.
48. Carter RF. Acute selenium poisoning. *Med J Aust* 1966;1:525–528.
49. Civil IDS, McDonald MJA. Acute selenium poisoning: case report. *N Z Med J* 1978;87:354–356.
50. Pentel P, Fletcher D, Jentzen J. Fatal acute selenium toxicity. *J Forensic Sci* 1985;30:556–562.
51. Nantel AJ, Brown M, Dery P, Lefebvre M. Acute poisoning by selenious acid. *Vet Hum Toxicol* 1985;27:531–533.
52. Schnellman B, Raithel HJ, Schaller KH. Acute fatal selenium poisoning: toxicological and occupational medical aspects. *Arch Toxicol* 1986;59:61–63.
53. Matoba R, Kimura H, Uchima E, et al. An autopsy case of acute selenium (selenious acid) poisoning and selenium levels in human tissues. *Forensic Sci Int* 1986;31:87–92.
54. Lombeck I, Menzel H, Frosch D. Acute selenium poisoning of a 2-year-old child. *Eur J Pediatr* 1987;146:308–312.
55. Kerdel-Vegas F. The depilatory and cytotoxic actions of "coco de mono" (*Lecythis ollaria*) and its relationship to chronic selenosis. *Econ Botany* 1966;20:187–195.
56. Yang G, Wang S, Zhou R, Sun S. Endemic selenium intoxication of humans in China. *Am J Clin Nutr* 1983;37:872–881.
57. Holness DL, Taraschuk IG, Nethercott JR. Health status of copper refinery workers with special reference to selenium exposure. *Arch Environ Health* 1989;44:291–297.
58. Ruta DA, Haider S. Attempted murder by selenium poisoning. *BMJ* 1989;299:316–317.
59. Snodgrass W, Rumack BH, Sullivan JB, et al. Selenium: childhood poisoning and cystic fibrosis. *Clin Toxicol* 1981;18:211–220.
60. Anonymous. Toxicity of superpotent selenium. *FDA Drug Bull* 1984;14:19.
61. Contempre B, Je D, Bebe N, Thilly CH, Diplock AT, Vanderpas J. Effects of selenium supplementation in hypothyroid subjects of a iodine and selenium-deficient area: the probable danger of indiscriminate supplementation of iodine-deficient subjects with selenium. *J Clin Endocrinol Metab* 1991;73:213–215.
62. Tarantal AF, Willhite CC, Lasley BL, et al. Developmental toxicity of L-selenomethionine in *Macaca fascicularis*. *Fundam Appl Toxicol* 1991;16:147–160.
63. Hoffman DJ, Heinz GH. Embryotoxic and teratogenic effects of selenium in the diet of mallards. *J Toxicol Environ Health* 1988;24:477–490.
64. Ohlendorf HM, Kilness AW, Simmons JL, et al. Selenium toxicosis in wild aquatic birds. *J Toxicol Environ Health* 1988;24:67–92.
65. Shamberger RJ. The genotoxicity of selenium. *Mutat Res* 1985;154:29–48.
66. Khalil AM. The induction of chromosome aberrations in human purified peripheral blood lymphocytes following in vitro exposure to selenium. *Mutat Res* 1989;224:500–506.
67. Khalil AM, Maslat AO. Chromosome aberrations, sister chromatid exchanges, and cell-cycle kinetics in human peripheral blood lymphocytes exposed to organoselenium in vitro. *Mutat Res* 1990;232:227–232.
68. International Agency for Research on Cancer. Some aziridine, *N*-, *S*-, and *O*-mustards and selenium. *IARC Monogr Eval Carcinog Risk Chem Hum* 1975; 9:1–268.
69. Possible enhancement of carcinogenesis in an animal model. *Nutr Rev* 1989; 47:173–175.
70. Milner JA. Effect of selenium on virally induced and transplantable tumor models. *Fed Proc* 1985;44:2568–2572.
71. Dorgan JF, Schatzkin A. Antioxidant micronutrients in cancer prevention. *Hematol Oncol Clin North Am* 1991;5:43–68.
72. Clark LC, Kantor KP, Allaway WH. Selenium in forage crops and cancer mortality in U.S. counties. *Arch Environ Health* 1991;46:37–42.
73. Stampfer MJ, Coldnitz GA, Willett WC. The epidemiology of selenium and cancer. *Cancer Surv* 1987;6:623–633.
74. Nomura A, Heilbrun LK, Morris JS, Stemmerman GN. Serum selenium and the risk of cancer, by specific site. *J Natl Cancer Inst* 1987;79:103–108.
75. Knekt P, Aromaa A, Maatela J. Serum vitamin E, serum selenium and the risk of gastrointestinal cancer. *Int J Cancer* 1990;42:846–850.
76. Hogberg J, Alexander J. Selenium. In: Friberg L, Nordberg GF, Vouk VB, eds. *Handbook on the toxicology of metals*, 2nd ed. Amsterdam: Elsevier Science, 1986:482–520.
77. Mack RB. The fat lady enters stage left: acute selenium poisoning. *N C Med J* 1990;51:636–638.
78. World Health Organization. *Selenium, in trace elements in human nutrition and health.* Geneva: World Health Organization, 1996:105–122.
79. Koh TS, Benson TH. Critical reappraisal of fluorometric method for determination of selenium in biological materials. *J Assoc Off Anal Chem* 1983; 66:918–926.
80. National Institute of Occupational Safety and Health. *Manual of analytical methods*, 3rd ed. Cincinnati: National Institute of Occupational Safety and Health, 1984.
81. Koirtyohann SR, Morris JS. General review of analytical methods. Some metals: As, Be, Cd, Cr, Ni, Pb, Se, Zn. *IARC Monogr Eval Carcinog Risks Hum* 1986;71:159–170.
82. Lewis SA. Determination of selenium in biological matrices. *Methods Enzymol* 1988;158:391–402.
83. Magos L, Berg GG. Selenium. In: Clarkson TW, Friberg L, Nordberg GF, Sager PR, eds. *Biological monitoring of toxic metals.* New York: Plenum Publishing, 1988:383–405.
84. Glover JR. Selenium in human urine: a tentative maximum allowable concentration for industrial and rural populations. *Ann Occup Hyg* 1967;10:3–14.
85. Valentine JL, Faraji B, Kang HK. Human glutathione peroxidase activity in cases of high selenium exposures. *Environ Res* 1988;45:16–27.
86. Elinder CG, Gerhardsson L, Oberdoerster G. Biological monitoring of toxic metals—overview. In: Clarkson TW, Friberg L, Nordberg GF, Sager PR, eds. *Biological monitoring of toxic metals.* New York: Plenum Publishing, 1988:63–65.
87. Yang G, Yin S, Zhou R, Gu L, Yan B, Liu Y. Studies of the safe maximal daily dietary Se intake in a seleniferous area in China: II. Relation between Se intake and the manifestation of clinical signs and certain biochemical alterations in blood and urine. *J Trace Elem Electrolytes Health Dis* 1989;3:123–130.
88. Cheng YD, Zhuang GS, Tan MG, et al. Preliminary study of correlation of Se content in human hair and tissues. *J Trace Elem Exp Med* 1988;1:19–21.
89. Fan AM, Chang LW. Human exposure and biological monitoring of methylmercury and selenium. In: Dillon HK, Ho MH, eds. *Biological monitoring of exposure to chemicals: metals.* New York: John Wiley and Sons, 1991:223–241.
90. Lockitch G. Selenium: clinical significance and analytical concepts. *Crit Rev Clin Lab Sci* 1989;27:483–541.
91. Lloyd B, Robson E, Smith I, Clayton BE. Blood selenium concentrations and glutathione peroxidase activity. *Arch Dis Child* 1989;64:352–356.
92. National Institute of Occupational Safety and Health. *Recommendations for occupational safety and health.* Washington: Department of Health and Human Services, 1992.
93. American Conference of Governmental Industrial Hygienists. *Documentation of the threshold limit values and biological exposure indices.* Cincinnati: American Conference of Governmental Industrial Hygienists, 1993.
94. Occupational Safety and Health Administration. Code of federal regulations: 29 *CFR*, 1910. Washington: US Occupational Safety and Health Administration, 1992.
95. Environmental Protection Agency. Code of federal regulations: 40 *CFR*, 141. Washington: Environmental Protection Agency, 1991.

96. National Research Council. *Recommended daily allowances*, 10th ed. Washington: National Academy of Sciences Press, 1989.
97. Environmental Protection Agency. *Selenium reference dose.* Integrated Risk Information System (IRIS) Online Database. Washington: Environmental Protection Agency, 1997.
98. Velazquez SF, Poirier KA. Problematic risk assessments for drinking water contaminants: selenium, aldicarb, and nickel. In: *Water contaminants and health: integration of exposure assessment, toxicology, and risk assessment.* New York: Marcel Dekker Inc, 1994:467–495.
99. Plunkett ER. *Handbook of industrial toxicology*, 3rd ed. New York: Chemical Publishing, 1987.
100. Wade MJ, Davis BK, Carlisle JS, Klein AK, Valoppi LM. Environmental transformation of toxic metals. *Occup Med* 1993;8:575–601.
101. Chau YK, Wong PTS, Silverberg BA, Luxon PL, Bengert GA. Methylation of selenium in the aquatic environment. *Science* 1976;192:1130–1131.
102. Yasumoto K, Suzuki T, Yoshida M. Identification of selenomethionine in soybean protein. *J Agric Food Chem* 1988;36:463–467.
103. Behne D, Weiss-Novak C, Kalcklösch M, Westphal C, Gessner H, Kyriakopoulos A. Studies on the distribution and characteristics of new mammalian selenium-containing proteins. *Analyst* 1995;120:823–825.
104. Beliles RP, Beliles EM. Phosphorus, selenium, tellurium, and sulfur. In: Clayton GD, Clayton FE, eds. *Patty's industrial hygiene and toxicology*, 4th ed, vol 2A. New York: John Wiley and Sons, 1993:783–829.

CHAPTER 84
Aluminum

J. Fergus Kerr and Joanne Mary Dalgleish

Aluminum is the third most common element, making up approximately 8% of the earth's crust. It is the most abundant metal and, owing to its affinity with oxygen, it exists naturally only in the oxidized form, particularly alumina (Al_2O_3). It is found also in many other minerals, especially in silicates, and is present in rocks and soils in the form of gems, such as ruby, sapphire, and turquoise. The naturally occurring, industrially important forms are alum (hydrated aluminum sulfate), bauxite, cryolite, corundum, and kaolin (1).

Aluminum is present in the air as aluminosilicates, usually in combination with dust particles. It occurs also in water, where amounts will vary depending on local geographic conditions.

SOURCES, USES, AND PRODUCTION

The production of aluminum metal requires three major steps. The first is the refining of bauxite by the Bayer process, resulting in alumina (aluminum oxide). The second step is electrolytic reduction of alumina by the Hall-Heroult process to produce aluminum; the final step is the casting of aluminum into ingots (2). During the Bayer process, bauxite ($Al_2O_3 \cdot H_2O$) is digested at high temperature and pressure in a caustic soda solution. The hydrate that is produced then is crystallized and calcined in a kiln to produce alumina. In the second step (the Hall-Heroult process), an electrolytic process involving carbon electrodes and cryolite flux reduces alumina to aluminum metal. The oxygen from the alumina passes to the carbon anode, reacting to form carbon dioxide and carbon monoxide. Two electrolytic cells may be used: a prebake cell or a Soderberg cell. In the final casting step, molten aluminum is poured into molds to form aluminum ingots. Pure aluminum is covered by a protective oxide coating (3,4). During the production of electrodes, some waste is produced. For smelters using the prebake process, polycyclic aromatic hydrocarbons are the result; for smelters using the Soderberg cell, coal tar pitch, petroleum coke, and some polycyclic aromatic hydrocarbons remain (2).

EXPOSURE SOURCES

The general population is exposed to aluminum through food, water, the inhalation of contaminated dust particles, and the use of some consumer products, such as deodorants and antiperspirants, antacids, and the like.

Environment

Dust from ores, rocks, and soils serves as the largest source of particle-borne aluminum (5). This dust results from such natural processes as weathering and volcanoes and from such human activities as mining. Approximately 13% of atmospheric aluminum results from human-based emissions associated with coal combustion, aluminum smelting, and other industrial activities through which ores and fuels are processed (6). Levels in the air vary, depending on sampling location, the level of human activities, and atmospheric conditions. Background levels range from 0.005 to 0.18 mg per cubic meter (5).

Aluminum is also naturally present in water. Surface runoff, tributary inflow, groundwater seepage, and human-based effluent may increase levels (7). The use of aluminum compounds in water purification processes also may increase water aluminum content (8). The aluminum concentration in natural waters is pH-dependent. High aluminum content in surface water is not seen unless the pH is less than 5. In general, surface water with a pH greater than 5.5 will have an aluminum concentration of less than 0.10 mg per L (5).

Aluminum has been detected at a mean soil concentration of 5,840 mg per kg from National Priority List and non–National Priority List hazardous-waste sites (9). Mining wastes, coal combustion, and aluminum smelting are the major contributors to nonnatural aluminum soil content (10). Other investigators have shown a wide range of soil concentrations, depending on the sampling location, varying from 700 mg per kg to more than 100,000 mg per kg (5).

Industry

Aluminum as a structural material is found in the construction, aircraft, and automotive industries. Many metal alloys also contain aluminum. Overhead power lines and electrical conductors contain aluminum. Some other uses include cooking utensils, decorations, highway signs, foil, dentures, and fencing.

Alum has been used for many thousands of years as a mordant for dyes and in the tanning of animal skins. Natural aluminum minerals, such as bentonite and clays, are used in water purification and in the brewing and paper industries (Table 84-1).

Food

As a contaminant, aluminum is found in naturally occurring and processed foods. Concentrations vary according to geographic area and on the specific food and processing method (5). Foods with the highest concentrations of aluminum tend to be those that contain aluminum as an additive (e.g., processed cheese) and grain-based products (11). The tea plant demonstrates the broad variation of aluminum concentrations in food plants. The usual concentration range is 0.378 to 2.445 mg per L but, because the tea plant is able to tolerate acidic soil in which aluminum is more readily available, levels in the leaves may accumulate up to 10,000 mg per kg (12). Cooking with aluminum utensils or the storage of foods in aluminum foil can increase the food's content of aluminum, particularly if foods are moist, salty, or acidic. One study found that the use of conditioned aluminum pans to prepare food resulted in food concentrations of between 0.24 and 125.0 mg per kg (13).

TABLE 84-1. Uses of aluminum

Aluminum form	Use
Aluminum metal	Automotive industry Aerospace industry Construction Metal alloys Electrical industry Cooking utensils Decorations Foil Fencing
Bentonite-zeolite	Water purification Sugar refining Brewing industry Paper manufacture
Aluminum sulfate	Water purification Dyes Tanning
Aluminum borate	Glass and ceramic production
Aluminum chloride	Rubber manufacturing Lubricants Wood preservatives Cosmetics
Aluminum chlorohydrate	Antiperspirants, deodorants
Aluminum hydroxide	Antacids Pharmaceutical industry
Aluminum phosphate	Antacids
Aluminum carbonate	Antacids
Aluminum silicate	Antacids Dental cement
Aluminum isoproxide	Paint industry Soap manufacturing Textile waterproofing
Aluminum trioxide	Absorbent Abrasive

Medicine

In ancient times, alum was used in different preparations to aid the healing of ulcers and to relieve dysentery (1). Alum's predominant present-day use is in the hydroxide form, providing relief from the pain of peptic ulceration and acidic reflux. Aluminum hydroxide is used also to lower serum phosphate levels in patients with chronic renal failure. The hydroxide form commonly is mixed with adsorbed vaccines to increase their potency and to reduce side effects (14).

ABSORPTION, METABOLISM, AND EXCRETION

The normal dietary intake of aluminum varies between 3 and 5 mg per day, with only approximately 15 μg being absorbed into the splanchnic circulation (15). In humans, the total body burden is kept to approximately 30 mg, with the bulk of the regulation being done by the kidneys, which excrete most of the 15 μg (16). Total body aluminum does not appear to increase with age (17). The form in which aluminum is ingested is a major determining factor in the amount absorbed. Aluminum phosphate and aluminum hydroxide are both absorbed poorly (18). Aluminum citrate is absorbed more readily. The citrate forms a tight complex with aluminum, preventing the formation of hydroxides or phosphates in the gastrointestinal tract (19).

Inhaled aluminum either is exhaled immediately or is trapped in the lung without penetrating further. Workers exposed to aluminum fumes, however, show a marked increase in urinary aluminum excretion, suggesting significant absorption across the alveolar membrane (20). Significant systemic absorption of aluminum through the skin has not been reported.

Within the body, aluminum is bound primarily to transferrin (21). Normal human plasma levels are approximately 10 μg per L, with a range of 2.1 to 42.0 μg per L being reported (14). Within the body, aluminum tends to concentrate in bone, spleen, heart, and liver (17). Brain aluminum can be high in patients who have chronic renal failure and are undergoing oral or parenteral loading of aluminum, but this has not been seen in subjects having large parenteral exposures and normal kidney function (22,23). The uremic state does not appear to affect the compartmentalization of aluminum in other tissues. The altered aluminum distribution in uremic patients may be related in part to a coexisting hyperparathyroid state (24).

Animal studies have demonstrated that only 3.9% of the plasma aluminum is filtered at the glomeruli, owing to its extensive plasma protein binding (25). Healthy individuals appear able to excrete the small amount of aluminum usually absorbed. Patients with renal impairment are known to be able to accumulate aluminum in excessive amounts. What is unknown is whether healthy individuals exposed to high aluminum loads may accumulate aluminum owing to an overwhelming of the normal excretory mechanisms. Biliary excretion also is reported, although the fraction excreted by this route is small (26).

CLINICAL TOXICOLOGY

Pulmonary System

Although bauxite is the principal source of aluminum, it is not associated with any defining pulmonary disease process that is distinctive and confined to its exposure (27).

Smelter operations in general embody five major job categories: pot room workers, carbon plant workers, workers involved in cathode production, and those workers engaged in casting and in maintenance. The type and extent of exposures in each work environment are different. Fluoride particles, carbon monoxide, coke impurities, and alumina are common exposures for pot room workers. Carbon plant workers have minimal fluoride exposure but are exposed to coke and coal-tar pitch compounds. Cathode workers and those in casting or maintenance are exposed to only insignificant amounts of alumina.

In 1936, Frostad (28) first demonstrated the existence of asthma or an asthmalike condition in Norwegian aluminum plant workers. Since then, numerous reports and scientific papers have reaffirmed the existence of this phenomenon in a number of countries, particularly Norway, Holland, France, Australia, and Canada (9). In general, it is not a clearly characterized illness, but affected workers typically describe wheezing, tightness in the chest, shortness of breath, and cough. Often, forced expiratory volume in 1 second (FEV_1) is reduced. The prevalence of pot room asthma varies greatly, with reports ranging from 0% to 39% (29). The results of studies investigating FEV_1 also have been variable. In two studies that used non–pot room workers from the same refinery as that employing the controls, reductions in FEV_1 were the same for test subjects and controls (30,31). However, a comparison against external controls identified a significant difference (32,33).

Occupational asthma secondary to alumina exposure could play a role in pot room asthma; however, these airway responses could be the result also of nonspecific bronchoconstriction induced by irritant pot room fumes.

Aluminosis is the development of pulmonary fibrosis after exposure to respirable particles of aluminum metal. Given this metal's propensity for complexing with oxygen, the circumstances in which this occurs are rare. The harmful effects of metallic aluminum powder first were described by Goralewski (34) in 1947 in a group of German workers employed in the manufacture of aluminum powder. Their illnesses demonstrated cough, fever, shortness of breath, and lethargy. Chest radiographs revealed some shadows and, on occasion, pneumothorax. In those patients undergoing histologic examination, fibrotic changes were detected. Similar cases of fibrosis were reported by a number of authors (35–37). In general, aluminosis does not occur in the absence of exposure to high dust concentrations in conjunction with the use of mineral oil–based lubricants (which tended to be used in the early part of the last century). The aluminum industry no longer uses any lubricant other than stearin (a fatty acid–based lubricant), which binds tightly with aluminum, forming aluminum stearate, and avoids direct exposure of the reactive sites to water (38).

A number of studies have shown an increased standardized mortality rate for aluminum exposure and lung cancer (29), the highest standardized mortality rate being 180. Some of these studies, however, are not controlled for cigarette smoking. In one report, excess lung cancers were found in the exposed group and correlated with a tar-years index and with years of aluminum production (39). Simonato (40) found that those workers in plants using the Soderberg process had an increase in lung cancer risk, again correlating with the tar-years index.

Cardiovascular System

Alfrey (17) has shown that aluminum accumulates in cardiac muscle. Elliott et al. (41) reported that 4 of 12 patients with dialysis encephalopathy and no history of ischemic heart disease died after a sudden cardiac event characterized by pulmonary edema. The authors theorized that because aluminum inhibits enzyme systems involving adenosine triphosphate and magnesium, these patients may have suffered from a relative depletion in myocardial magnesium. Epidemiologic studies of aluminum industry workers have failed to show a significant increased risk of death from cardiovascular disease (42,43).

Neurologic System

In 1921, Spofforth (44) reported a patient who presented with memory loss, tremor, and impaired coordination and apparently was aluminum poisoned. However, it was not until Alfrey et al. (45) reported in 1972 on a neurologic syndrome in patients undergoing long-term dialysis that aluminum-related neurologic disease generated widespread interest.

In their group of patients, Alfrey et al. (45) described dementia, speech impairment, coordination difficulty, and facial grimacing with electroencephalographic changes. Some patients progressed to seizures and death in 1 to 15 years. After this report, a number of other centers involved in renal dialysis reported similar findings. Initial hypotheses included dopamine deficiency and slow infectious agents along with toxicologic causes (45–48). In 1976, Alfrey et al. (46) followed up their report by measuring aluminum levels in brains from encephalopathic dialysis patients. Control subjects had aluminum levels of 2.2 parts per million (ppm), whereas encephalopathic patients had 25 ppm. Uremic patients who died of other causes had levels of approximately 6.5 ppm. Other studies have shown elevated serum aluminum levels in patients under long-term dialysis (47).

Although aluminum now is accepted widely to play a role in the development of dialysis encephalopathy syndrome, what is not certain is whether the toxicity is a result of increased tissue aluminum levels alone or results from a combination with enzyme inhibition or even alterations in postsynaptic cholinergic neurotransmission (48). Aluminum has been shown by a number of authors to have various effects on brain biochemistry and molecular function. Some of these findings are tabulated in Table 84-2 (49–56).

TABLE 84-2. Biochemical and molecular actions of aluminum

Decreased synaptosomal uptake of glutamic acid, γ-aminobutyric acid, and glycine (49)
Interactions with brain calmodulin (an intracellular calcium-binding protein), possibly changing calcium-dependent processes (50)
Reported interactions between aluminum and glycolytic enzymes, with a reduction in cerebral glucose use (51)
Binding to (Leu)-enkephalin, an endogenous central nervous system peptide (52)
Possible interference with brain cytochrome oxidase activity (53)
Inhibition of dihydropteridine reductase, important in maintaining cerebral concentrations of tetrahydrobiopterin, which is required in the manufacture of some neurotransmitters (54)
Inhibition of cholinergic neurotransmission (55)
Alterations in the metabolism of cyclic adenosine monophosphate and 5'-cyclic guanosine monophosphate (56)

In 1907, Alzheimer described neurofibrillary tangles and senile plaques, now recognized as the classic histologic changes associated with Alzheimer's disease. The disease is marked clinically by a progressive deterioration in learning, memory, judgment, language, and motor function. Aluminum is one of many competing theories in the etiology of this crippling illness. The metal has been demonstrated in the neurofibrillary tangle and the amyloid cores of the senile plaques (57,58). Some families demonstrate an autosomal dominant trait–inherited Alzheimer's disease. In the affected persons of these families, point mutations in the beta-amyloid precursor protein gene have been identified. Further, those patients who have high blood levels of aluminum and are undergoing dialysis may develop increased staining for amyloid precursor protein in cortical neurones; hence, aluminum may induce beta-amyloid deposition in the brain (59). Other theories regarding the possible role of aluminum in Alzheimer's disease include a defect of transferrin binding, releasing free aluminum to accumulate in the brain (60); reduction in the activity of choline acetyltransferase (61); and (according to more recent evidence) aluminum interaction with nucleic acid polyphosphates (62). Finally, some inconclusive epidemiologic data report a higher prevalence of Alzheimer's disease in areas with higher aluminum levels in drinking water (63).

As well as Alzheimer's disease and dialysis encephalopathy syndrome, amyotrophic lateral sclerosis and Parkinsonism have been linked to aluminum exposure (64), although the evidence supporting this link is limited.

Hematologic System

Anemia is well known in association with chronic renal disease, with no single etiologic factor being the cause. Contributing factors are a reduction in the synthesis of erythropoietin, hemolysis, derangements in iron metabolism, uremia, and possibly, aluminum. In 1978, Elliott et al. (65) first demonstrated a relationship between aluminum exposure and anemia in humans. Building on this finding, Short et al. (66) described a severe microcytic hypochromic anemia not due to iron deficiency in patients undergoing dialysis. Aluminum affects hemoglobin synthesis (67); although the exact mechanism remains to be elucidated, it may involve iron saturation of transferrin-binding sites or inhibition of δ-aminolevulinic acid dehydratase (or both processes). The anemic changes described have been demonstrated in the special population of patients who have chronic renal failure and are undergoing treatment. No workplace studies have demonstrated a significant hematologic effect from aluminum exposure.

Skeletal System

Individuals who are suffering from chronic renal failure and undergo dialysis tend to retain phosphate, which may result in ectopic calcium deposition and osteitis fibrosa cystica. Aluminum hydroxide is administered to control this hyperphosphatemia; however, excessive use results in low phosphate states, interfering with bone mineralization, and culminates in osteomalacia (68). The link between the development of osteomalacia and aluminum was demonstrated by Ward et al. (69), who showed a significant difference in the incidence of osteomalacia in comparing a small sample of patients dialyzed using deionized water as opposed to tap water treated with water softener (69). The mechanisms by which aluminum interferes with the normal physiologic functioning of bone are complex. Factors identified at present include a reduction in osteoblast number and function (70) and an inhibition of parathyroid hormone secretion (71).

Developmental and Reproductive Effects

Human data about the developmental effects of aluminum are limited to the development of encephalopathy with aluminum accumulation in premature infants who were undergoing dialysis for renal failure and who received intravenous fluids contaminated with aluminum (72). Animal studies have not shown developmental abnormalities (73). No human or animal study has demonstrated any effect of aluminum on reproductive capabilities.

Management of Toxicity

PREVENTION

In an industrial setting, the cornerstone of treatment is prevention. The measures that execute this effectively are not specific for aluminum but are those used commonly to prevent exposure to respirable dust and fumes. Hence, prevention includes appropriate engineering controls and the wearing of personal protective equipment as necessary.

Prevention is critical also for those individuals at special risk, especially patients who have chronic renal failure and undergo dialysis or treatment for hyperphosphatemia. Initially, the source of exposure should be identified. Variations in the severity of aluminum toxicity in patients with chronic renal failure has been shown to correlate with the presence of high levels of aluminum in tap water. In some cases, these high levels are the result of water purification methods used in specific localities. The use of aluminum-free water for dialysis has been shown to result in significant clinical improvement (74,75). No safe level of aluminum in dialysate has been demonstrated. Purification of water can be undertaken by one of two methods—deionization or reverse osmosis—with the latter being preferred. The use of aluminum-containing phosphate-binding gels in this high-risk group of patients may lead also to aluminum toxicity. Calcium citrate has been recommended as an alternative phosphate binder in chronic renal failure patients; however, it may lead to increased absorption of aluminum from foodstuffs (19). Calcium carbonate with small quantities of aluminum is used commonly in clinical practice.

Aluminum's relatively large volume of distribution and high percentage of protein binding negate the effective use of extracorporeal elimination methods. Chelating agents, particularly deferoxamine, are used to aid the removal of aluminum once its level has become toxic. Deferoxamine has a high affinity for aluminum, and 100 mg can potentially bind 4.1 mg Al^{3+} (76). The aluminum-deferoxamine complex has a molecular weight of 587 Da and can be dialyzed. Deferoxamine is not absorbed well orally and must be administered parenterally. The use of a deferoxamine challenge test is recommended to estimate a body's aluminum load. In patients with chronic renal failure, the use of deferoxamine has resulted in clinical improvement in encephalopathy, osteodystrophy, and anemia (67,77,78).

In 1991, McLachlan et al. (79) reported a 2-year controlled trial involving 48 patients who had Alzheimer's disease and were given deferoxamine, 125 mg intramuscularly every 12 hours, 5 days weekly. The results, when compared to results in groups receiving lecithin, 500 mg twice daily, and in patients receiving no treatment, suggested that the progress of the Alzheimer's disease was slowed (79).

On the basis of current data, the use of deferoxamine can be recommended in the setting of aluminum toxicity in patients who have chronic renal failure and are undergoing dialysis. The use of deferoxamine in an occupational or industrial setting has not been reported; because of these insufficient data, its routine use cannot be recommended.

MEDICAL MONITORING

The abundance of aluminum in the environment and the measurement of potentially small concentrations mean that contamination of samples is an important issue. Recent improvements in analytic methods have allowed the clarification of normal aluminum values. Normal human serum (or plasma) aluminum is less than 10 μg per L (80). Serum is preferred, as this eliminates the need to obtain aluminum-free anticoagulant, which otherwise is a potential source of contamination. Urine, body tissues, dialysate, and tap water also may be analyzed for aluminum. Whichever specimen is collected, all items used during the collection, preparation, and final assay should be checked for their potential contribution of aluminum. Of the many analytic methods in existence, the most common and widely recommended is graphite furnace atomic absorption spectrometry. Other methods include flame atomic absorption spectrometry, neutron activation analysis, and inductively coupled plasma-atomic emission spectrometry. Graphite furnace atomic absorption spectrometry is particularly useful for measuring low levels of aluminum (micrograms per liter) in biological specimens (9,81).

OCCUPATIONAL AND ENVIRONMENTAL REGULATIONS

The U.S. Occupational Safety and Health Administration set a permissible exposure limit–time-weighted (8-hour) average for total aluminum metal dust of 15 mg per cubic meter, with the respirable fraction being 5 mg per cubic meter (Table 84-3). The U.S. Environmental Protection Agency also set a limit (0.01 ppm) on the tolerance for residues of the fumigant phosphine in or on all raw agricultural commodities resulting from preharvest treatment of pest burrows with aluminum phosphide. The concern here is for toxicity from phosphine. Water is regulated with a proposed maximum contaminant level of 0.05 mg of aluminum per L. The current European and World Health Organization directive specifies a maximum acceptable concentration of 0.2 mg per L. The Environmental Protection Agency has set guidelines to protect freshwater aquatic life, for water pH that ranges between 6.5 and 9.0, with a 4-day average concentration limit for aluminum of 87 μg per L.

TABLE 84-3. U.S. Occupational Safety and Health Administration permissible exposure limit–8-hour time-weighted average for aluminum

Aluminum form	OSHA PEL/TWA
Aluminum metal	
Total dust	15 mg/m^3
Respirable fraction	5 mg/m^3
Pyro powders	5 mg/m^3
Welding fumes	5 mg/m^3
Soluble salts	2 mg/m^3
Alkyls	2 mg/m^3
Aluminum oxide	
Total dust	10 mg/m^3
Respirable fraction	5 mg/m^3

OSHA, U.S. Occupational Safety and Health Administration; PEL, permissible exposure limit; TWA, 8-hour time-weighted average.

ENVIRONMENTAL FATE AND TRANSPORT

Aluminum is a relatively reactive element, complexing with water and compounds rich in electrons, such as fluoride, chloride, phosphate, sulfate, and nitrate. Its transport within the environment is determined by the chemical state and associations it has and by the characteristics of the medium in which it is found. At a pH of 5.5 or greater, naturally occurring aluminum is undissolved. As a general rule, decreasing the environmental pH will result in greater mobility. In this respect, the presence of acid rain or acid mine drainage has raised concerns. At a pH of between 5 and 6, aluminum complexes with phosphate and is removed from solution. Considerable variability is seen in the ability of plants to accumulate aluminum. The tea plant (*Symplocos spicata*) is a unique instance, being able to grow in very acidic soils where it may act as an aluminum sink, and its leaf levels of this element may rise to 10,000 mg per kg (12). The bioconcentration in fish also has been studied, with the accumulation being a function of water quality and pH (82).

The main toxicity of aluminum generally is confined to susceptible populations, particularly neonates and patients with chronic renal failure. It may manifest itself as osteodystrophy, microcytic anemia, or dialytic encephalopathy. Its role in Alzheimer's disease remains unclear. What is known is that aluminum accumulates in a number of body organs, including the brain's gray matter. The current belief is that regardless of the route of exposure, aluminum is not the cause of Alzheimer's disease but that once the process has begun, aluminum is deposited in neurons and senile plaques and may take part in cellular breakdown (83).

REFERENCES

1. Ulmer DD. Toxicity from aluminium antacids. *N Engl J Med* 1976;254:218–219.
2. Dinman BD. Aluminum, alloys, and compounds. *Encyclopedia of occupational health and safety,* vol 1. 1983:131–135.
3. King SW, Savory J, Wills MR. Clinical biochemistry of aluminum. *Crit Rev Clin Lab Sci* 1981;14:1–20.
4. International Agency for Research on Cancer. Polynuclear aromatic compounds: 3. Industrial exposures in aluminium production, coal gasification, coke production, and iron and steel founding. *IARC Monogr Eval Carcinog Risks Hum* 1984;34:37–64.
5. Sorenson JRJ, Campbell IR, Tepper LB, Lingg RD. Aluminum in the environment and human health. *Environ Health Perspect* 1974;8:3–95.
6. Lantzy RJ, MacKenzie FT. Atmospheric trace metals: global cycles and assessment of man's impact. *Geochim Cosmochim Acta* 1979;43:511–526.
7. Eisenreich SJ. Atmospheric input of trace metals to Lake Michigan (USA). *Water Air Soil Pollut* 1980;13:287–302.
8. Qureshi N, Malmberg RH. Reducing aluminum residuals in finished water. *J Am Water Works Assoc* 1985;77:101–108.
9. Agency for Toxic Substances and Disease Registry. *Toxicological profile for aluminum.* Washington: US Department of Health and Human Services, Public Health Service, ATSDR, 1992.
10. Gabler RC Jr, Stoll RL. *Removal of leachable metals and recovery of alumina from utility coal ash.* NTIS/PB83–191650. Washington: US Department of the Interior, Bureau of Mines, 1983.
11. Pennington JAT, Jones JM, Vanderveen JE. Aluminum in total diet study foods and diets. Proceedings of the seventy-first annual meeting of the Federation of American Societies for Experimental Biology, Washington, DC, March 29–April 2, 1987. *Fed Proc* 1987;46:1002.
12. Lewis TE, ed. Introduction. In*: Environmental chemistry and toxicology of aluminum.* Chelsea, MI: Lewis Publishers, 1989:1–2.
13. Greger JL, Goetz W, Sullivan D. Aluminum levels in food cooked and stored in aluminum pans, trays and foil. *J Food Prot* 1985;48:772–777.
14. Reynolds JEF, ed. Aluminium hydroxide. *The extra pharmacopoeia,* 29th ed. London: Pharmaceutical Press, 1989:1075–1077.
15. Monteagudo FSE, Cassidy MJD, Fold PI. Recent developments in aluminium toxicology. *Med Toxicol* 1989;4:1–16.
16. Alfrey AC. Aluminum intoxication. *N Engl J Med* 1984;310:1113–1115.
17. Alfrey AC. Aluminum metabolism in uremia. *Neurotoxicology* 1980;1:43.
18. Martin RB. The chemistry of aluminum as related to biology and medicine. *Clin Chem* 1986;32:1797.
19. Slanina P, Frech W, Ekstrom LG, Loof L, Slorach S, Cedergren A. Dietary citric acid enhances absorption of aluminum in antacids. *Clin Chem* 1986;32:539.
20. Mussi I, Calzaferri G, Buratti M, Alession L. Behavior of plasma aluminum levels in occupationally exposed subjects. *Int Arch Environ Health* 1984;54:155.
21. Rahman H, Channon SM, Skillen AW, Ward MK, Kerr DNS. Protein binding of aluminum in normal subjects and in patients with chronic renal failure. *Proc Eur Dialysis Transplant Assoc* 1984;21:360–365.
22. Sedman A, Klein G, Merritt R, et al. Evidence of aluminum loading in infants receiving intravenous therapy. *N Engl J Med* 1985;312:1337.
23. Klein GL, Alfrey AC, Miller N, et al. Aluminum loading during total parenteral nutrition (part A). *Am J Clin Nutr* 1982;35:1425.
24. Alfrey AC, Sedman A, Chan YL. The compartmentalization and metabolism of aluminum in uremic rats. *J Lab Clin Med* 1985;105:227.
25. Henry DA, Goodman WG, Nudleman RK, et al. Parenteral aluminum administration in the dog: I. Plasma kinetics, tissue levels, calcium metabolism, and parathyroid hormone. *Kidney Int* 1984;25:362–369.
26. Williams JW, Vera SR, Peters TG, et al. Biliary excretion of aluminum in aluminum osteodystrophy with liver disease. *Ann Intern Med* 1986;104:782–785.
27. Morgan WKC, Dinman BD. Pulmonary effects of aluminum. In: Gitelman HJ, ed. *Aluminum and health: a critical review.* New York: Marcel Dekker Inc, 1989:203–234.
28. Frostad EW. Fluoride intoxication in Norwegian aluminum plant workers. *Tidsskr Nor Laegeforen* 1936;56:179–182.
29. Abramson MJ, Wlodarczyk JH, Saunders NA, Hensley MJ. Does aluminum smelting cause lung disease? *Am Rev Respir Dis* 1989;139:1042–1057.
30. Chan-Yeung M, Wong R, MacLean L, et al. Epidemiologic health study of workers in an aluminum smelter in British Columbia. Effects on the respiratory system. *Am Rev Respir Dis* 1983;127:465–469.
31. Field GB, Milne J. Occupational asthma in aluminum smelters. *Aust N Z J Med* 1975;5:475.
32. Chan-Yeung M, Enarson DA, MacLean L, Irving D. Longitudinal study of workers in an aluminum smelter. *Arch Environ Health* 1989;44:134–139.
33. Kilburn KH. Re-examination of longitudinal studies of workers. *Arch Environ Health* 1989;44:132–133.
34. Goralewski G. Die Aluminiumlunge: eine neue Gewerbeerkrankung. *Z Gesamte Inn Med* 1947;2:665–673.
35. Mitchell J. Pulmonary fibrosis in an aluminium worker. *Br J Ind Med* 1959;16:123–125.
36. McLaughlin AIG, Kazantis G, King E, et al. Pulmonary fibrosis and encephalopathy associated with the inhalation of aluminium dust. *Br J Ind Med* 1962;19:253–263.
37. Jordan JW. Pulmonary fibrosis in a worker using an aluminium powder. *Br J Ind Med* 1961;18:21–23.
38. Dinman BD. Aluminum in the lungs: II. The pyro powder conundrum. *J Occup Med* 1987;29:869–876.
39. Gibbs GW, Horwitz I. Lung cancer mortality in aluminum reduction plant workers. *J Occup Med* 1979;21:347–353.
40. Simonato L. Carcinogenic risk in the aluminum production industry: an epidemiological overview. *Med Lav* 1981;72:266–276.
41. Elliott HL, MacDougall AI, Fell GS. Aluminium toxicity syndrome. *Lancet* 1978;1:1203.
42. Milham S Jr. Mortality in aluminum reduction plant workers. *J Occup Med* 1979;21:475–480.
43. Mur JM, Moulin JJ, Meyer-Bisch C, et al. Mortality of aluminum reduction plant workers in France. *Int J Epidemiol* 1987;16:257–264.
44. Spofforth J. Case of aluminium poisoning. *Lancet* 1921;1:1301.
45. Alfrey AC, Mishell JM, Burks J, et al. Syndrome of dyspraxia and multifocal seizures associated with chronic hemodialysis. *Trans Am Soc Artif Intern Organs* 1972;18:257–261.
46. Alfrey AC, Le Gendre GR, Kaehny WD. The dialysis encephalopathy syndrome. Possible aluminum intoxication. *N Engl J Med* 1976;294:184–188.
47. McKinney TD, Basinger M, Dawson E, Jones MM. Serum aluminum levels in dialysis dementia. *Nephron* 1982;32:53–56.

48. Hewitt CD, Savory J, Wills MR. Aspects of aluminum toxicity. *Clin Lab Med* 1990;10:403–422.
49. Wong PCL, Lai JCK, Lim L, Davison AN. Selective inhibition of L-glutamate and gamma-aminobutyrate transport in nerve ending particles by aluminum, manganese and cadmium chloride. *J Inorg Biochem* 1981;14:253–260.
50. Siegel N, Huang A. Aluminum interaction with calmodulin. Evidence for altered structure and function from optical and enzymatic studies. *Biochem Biophys Acta* 1983;744:36–45.
51. Lai JCK, Blass JP. Inhibition of brain glycolysis by aluminum. *J Neurochem* 1984;42:438–446.
52. Siegel N. Molecular aspects of aluminum toxicity. *Am J Kidney Dis* 1985;6:353–357.
53. Ondreika R, Ginter E, Kortus J. Chronic toxicity of aluminum in rats and mice and its effects on phosphorous metabolism. *Br J Ind Med* 1966;23:305–312.
54. Altmann R, Al-Salihi F, Butler K, et al. Serum aluminum levels and erythrocyte dihydropteridine reductase activity in patients on hemodialysis. *N Engl J Med* 1987;317:80–84.
55. Yates CM, Simpson J, Russell D, Gordon A. Cholinergic enzymes in neurofibrillary degeneration produced by aluminum. *Brain Res* 1980;197:269–274.
56. Johnson GVW, Jope RS. Aluminum alters cyclic AMP and cyclic GMP levels but not presynaptic cholinergic markers in rat brain in vivo. *Brain Res* 1987;403:1–6.
57. Perl DP, Brody AR. Alzheimer's disease: x-ray spectrometric evidence of aluminum accumulation in neurofibrillary tangle-bearing neurons. *Science* 1980;208:297–299.
58. Murray JC, Tanner CM, Sprague SM. Aluminum neurotoxicity: a re-evaluation. *Clin Neuropharmacol* 1991;14:179–185.
59. Higgins GA. The regulation of the amyloid gene in Alzheimer's disease: possible environmental influences. In: Walton L, ed. *Alzheimer's disease and the environment.* RSM Round Table Series No. 26. London: Royal Society of Medicine, 1991:17–23.
60. Farrar G, Hodgkins P, Altmann P, Blair JA. A biochemical mechanism for Alzheimer's disease. In: Walton L, ed. *Alzheimer's disease and the environment.* RSM Round Table Series No. 26. London: Royal Society of Medicine, 1991:53–59.
61. Coyle JT, Prince DL, DeLong MR. Alzheimer's disease: a disorder of cortical cholinergic innervation. *Science* 1983;219:1184–1190.
62. Lukiw WJ, Kruck TPA, Crapper McLachlan DR. Aluminum and the nucleus of nerve cells. *Lancet* 1989;1:781.
63. Martyn C. Aluminum in water and its possible relationship to Alzheimer's disease. In: Walton L, ed. *Alzheimer's disease and the environment.* RSM Round Table Series No. 26. London: Royal Society of Medicine, 1991:87–94.
64. Perl DP, Gajdusek DC, Garruto RM, Yanagihara RT, Gibbs CJ Jr. Intraneuronal aluminum accumulation in amyotrophic lateral sclerosis and Parkinsonism-dementia of Guam. *Science* 1982;217:1053–1055.
65. Elliott HL, Dryburgh F, Fell GS, Sabet S, MacDougall AI. Aluminum toxicity during regular hemodialysis. *BMJ* 1978;1:1101–1103.
66. Short AIK, Winney RJ, Robson JS. Reversible microcytic hypochromic anemia in dialysis patients due to aluminum intoxication. *Proc Eur Dialysis Transplant Assoc* 1980;17:226–233.
67. Altmann P, Plowman D, Marsh F, Cunningham J. Aluminum chelation therapy in dialysis patients: evidence for inhibition of hemoglobin synthesis by low levels of aluminum. *Lancet* 1988;I:1288–1291.
68. Clarkson EM, Luck VA, Hynson WV, et al. The effect of aluminum hydroxide on calcium, phosphorous, and aluminum balances, the serum parathyroid hormone concentration and the aluminum content of bone in patients with chronic renal failure. *Clin Sci* 1972;43:519–531.
69. Ward MK, Ellis HA, Feest TG, et al. Osteomalacic dialysis osteodystrophy: evidence for a water borne etiological agent, probably aluminum. *Lancet* 1978;1:841–845.
70. Dunstan CR, Evans RA, Hills E, Wong SYP, Alfrey AC. Effect of aluminum and parathyroid hormone on osteoblasts and bone mineralization in chronic renal failure. *Calcif Tissue Int* 1984;36:133–138.
71. Morrissey J, Rothstein M, Mayor G, Slatopolsky E. Suppression of parathyroid hormone secretion by aluminum. *Kidney Int* 1983;23:699–704.
72. Polinsky MS, Gruskin AB. Aluminum toxicity in children with chronic renal failure. *J Pediatr* 1984;105:758–761.
73. Cranmer JM, Wilkins JD, Cannon DJ, et al. Fetal-placental-maternal uptake of aluminum in mice following gestational exposure: effect of dose and route of administration. *Neurotoxicology* 1986;7:601–608.
74. Kerr DNS, Ward MK, Arze RS, et al. Aluminum-induced dialysis osteodystrophy: the demise of Newcastle bone disease? *Kidney Int* 1986;29:S58–S64.
75. Platts MM, Anastassiades E. Dialysis encephalopathy: precipitating factors and improvement in prognosis. *Clin Nephrol* 1981;15:223–228.
76. Swartz RD. Deferoxamine and aluminum removal. *Am J Kidney Dis* 1985;6:358–364.
77. Ackrill P, Ralston AJ, Day JP, Hodge KC. Successful removal of aluminum from a patient with dialysis encephalopathy. *Lancet* 1980;2:692–693.
78. Malluche HH, Smith AJ, Abreo K, Fangere MC. The use of deferoxamine in the management of aluminum accumulation in bone in patients with renal failure. *N Engl J Med* 1984;311:140–144.
79. McLachlan DRC, Dalton AJ, Kruck TPA, et al. Intramuscular deferoxamine and Alzheimer's disease. *Lancet* 1991;337:1304–1308.
80. Savory J, Wills M. Analytical techniques for the analysis of aluminum. In: Gitelman HJ, ed. *Aluminum and health: a critical review.* New York: Marcel Dekker Inc, 1989:1–26.
81. Gardiner PE, Stoeppler M. Optimization of the analytical conditions for the determining of aluminum in human blood plasma and serum by graphite furnace atomic absorption spectrometry: 2. Assessment of the analytical method. *J Anal At Spectrom* 1987;2:401–404.
82. Cleveland L, Little EE, Wiedmeyer RH, et al. Chronic no-observed-effect concentrations of aluminum for brook trout exposed in low-calcium, dilute acidic water. In: Lewis TE, ed. *Environmental chemistry and toxicology of aluminum.* Chelsea, MI: Lewis Publishers, 1989.
83. Winship KA. Toxicity of aluminum: a historical review (part 2). *Adverse Drug React Toxicol Rev* 1993;12:177–211.

CHAPTER 85
Thallium

John B. Sullivan, Jr.

Thallium, which belongs to the aluminum family of metals, was discovered in 1861 by William Crookes. Thallium toxicity was recognized in 1863 and is related to divalent lead (1). Thallium (atomic number, 81; atomic weight, 204.4) is a soft, malleable, blue-white metal. Its name derives from a green spectral line identified by the term *thallos*. Thallium is a reactive metal that, when exposed to air, superficially oxidizes and forms a coating of thallium oxide (Tl_2O). At higher temperatures, it reacts with a green flame to form thallium(III) oxide (Tl_2O_3).

Thallium has oxidation states of 1+ and 3+ and generally is used in the salt form. After exposure to air, the elemental metal forms a brown-black oxide (2). Thallium is a highly reactive metal and is soluble in acids. The metal forms monovalent and trivalent salts. Thallium salts are colorless, odorless, and tasteless when dissolved in water. The metal is found mainly in the sulfate salt form (Tl_2SO_4).

SOURCES, USES, AND PRODUCTION

Thallium is ubiquitous in nature and occurs in sulfide ores of a variety of heavy metals in low concentrations. It is naturally present in the environment and also occurs from artificial processes. Thallium is found in the United States and Brazil in the minerals of lorandite and crookesite, it is a by-product of cadmium production, and it is recovered from lead and zinc smelting flue dust (2). Thallium is found in nature as the sulfate salt form and is found in potash, lead and zinc ores, and fossil fuels. In contact with water the metal forms thallium hydroxide. Thallium is insoluble in alkali bases and dissolves slowly in hydrochloric acid, forms alloys with other metals, and reacts and forms amalgamates with mercury. Organothallium compounds are stable only in the trivalent form. Thallium is present in the earth's crust, and at least 18 thallium compounds are known (Table 85-1).

Thallium's production worldwide occurs in small quantities because of its limited consumption. However, it is used in varied manufacture: electronics; specialized optical glasses; low-temperature thermometers; special highly resistant glass containing thallium and selenium; crystals for infrared instruments; electronic devices for semiconductors (as the cation in a tetragonal crystalline form and as thallium oxide) (3) and scintillation counters; mercury lamps; corrosion-resistant alloys with lead, zinc, silver, and antimony; organic reaction catalysts; and radioisotopes for physics and industry. In the field of medicine, thallium is used in equipment for scintigraphy of heart, liver, thyroid, and testes and for the diagnosis of melanoma. Additional uses include imitation jewelry, pyrotechnics, pigments

TABLE 85-1. Thallium and thallium compounds

Chemical name	Chemical formula
Thallium	Tl
Thallium acetate	$TlC_2H_3O_2$
Thallium aluminum sulfate	$TlAl(SO_4)_2$ $12H_2O$
Thallium bromide	$TlBr$
Thallium carbonate	Tl_2CO_3
Thallium chloride	$TlCl$
Thallium trichloride	$TlCl_3$
Thallium ethylate	$TlOC_2H_5$
Thallium fluoride	TlF
Thallium trifluoride	TlF_3
Thallium hydroxide	$TlOH$
Thallium iodide	TlI
Thallium nitrate	$TlNO_3$
Thallium nitrate trihydrate	$Tl(NO_3)_3$ $3H_2O$
Thallium(I) oxide	Tl_2O
Thallium(III) oxide	Tl_2O_3
Thallium sulfate	Tl_2SO_4
Thallium sulfide	Tl_2S

and dyes, and wood preservatives. Recently, thallium has found utility in the superconductor industry.

EXPOSURE SOURCES

Thallium is released into the environment from industrial processes. Concentrations of approximately 700 µg per cubic meter occur in emissions from coal-powered plants (4). Cement plants exhaust up to 2,500 µg per cubic meter into the air. Thallium that volatilizes from cement production condenses on ash particles that can contain up to 50 mg of thallium per kg of ash (4). Mine tailings are another environmental source of contamination and can release thallium into rivers and surface waters. The soil around cement-producing factories and smelters and brick production facilities has been found to contain up to 27 mg per kg of thallium (4). Thallium concentrates in vegetables and fruits and in animals but not to a great extent. Point sources of environmental distribution include coal-powered plants, cement production plants, and smelting operations, the major sources of thallium being emissions in the ashes produced. The public is exposed to thallium via copper, zinc, cadmium, and lead smelters. Drinking water contamination with thallium may occur in the area of smelting operations (2). Atmospheric thallium is present as the elemental form, oxide, or sulfate.

Thallium salts first were introduced as pesticides in Germany in 1920 (1). These initial compounds contained approximately 2% thallium sulfate (5). The persistence of thallium in the environment, along with its cumulative effect as a poison, rendered it an ideal rodenticide. In the late nineteenth century, thallium was used widely as a therapeutic agent for syphilis, tuberculosis, and dysentery and as a depilatory agent (1,5,6).

Thallium salts as rodenticides were restricted in 1965 in the United States. However, developing countries continue to make available thallium-containing pesticides. Compounds containing 3.5% to 5.0% thallium sulfate were available in the 1950s in the southeastern United States for control of ants and roaches. In the 1960s, thallium-containing rodenticides in the United States typically contained between 1% and 3% thallium sulfate. In 1965, household use of thallium preparations was banned by the U.S. Department of Agriculture.

Inhalation of contaminated air and ingestion of contaminated fruit are sources of low-level human exposure. Thallium exposures can occur from accidental and suicidal ingestion of the salt forms. Exposure also occurs from inhalation in a work area or ingestion of contaminated foods. Exposure to flue dust from pyrite roasting and from lead, copper, zinc, and cadmium smelting (2) can result in dermal contamination, as can inhalation of dust containing thallium. Absorption of thallium occurs through inhalation, ingestion, and dermal contact. Because thallium is a cumulative poison, it can be absorbed through both the skin and the gastrointestinal (GI) tract.

CLINICAL TOXICITY

Absorption, Metabolism, Distribution, and Elimination

Thallium is absorbed through intact skin, by inhalation, and by the GI route. Absorption in animal models has been demonstrated to be very rapid after dermal, oral, or inhalation routes, with almost 100% bioavailability.

After absorption, thallium is distributed intracellularly, with the kidneys having the highest concentrations, mainly in the renal medulla (2). Concentrations are found also in cardiac tissue and liver. Thallium concentrates in hair. The metal's concentration in adipose tissue and brain tissue is low (7). It distributes equally between red blood cells and plasma (7) and crosses the placenta into the fetus but in amounts much smaller than those present in maternal tissues.

Thallium is eliminated mainly via the GI tract and kidneys after first-order kinetics. The excretion of thallium in urine is associated with the urinary excretion of potassium (7). Potassium and thallium replace each other in the sodium- and potassium-activated adenosine triphosphatase pump; thus, thallium accumulates intracellularly while displacing potassium. The elimination of thallium in urine is slow, lasting weeks, despite the concentration of thallium in the kidneys (7). Thallium plasma concentrations generally remain low despite high urine and fecal content. In human cases of poisoning, the excretion of thallium occurs very slowly over several weeks to months. The elimination of thallium in humans differs from animals, and the rate of excretion is lower in humans than in animals. Thallium is eliminated also through hair and sweat. The biological half-life of thallium in humans is estimated to be approximately 10 days, and values up to 30 days have been reported (4).

Acute Toxicity

Although thallium salts are tasteless, odorless, and colorless, they are highly toxic. Poisoning from thallium has occurred owing to suicidal ingestion of rodenticides and thallium compounds used in homicide attempts and from its use as an abortifacient. Lethal oral doses are estimated to be between 6 and 40 mg per kg (4). Thallium poisoning presents with a triad of gastroenteritis, polyneuropathy, and alopecia. Initial symptoms after oral ingestion include anorexia, nausea, vomiting, metallic taste, abdominal pain, and GI bleeding. Later symptoms include constipation, continued GI bleeding, psychoses, seizures, and neuropathy (Table 85-2). A characteristic of thallium poisoning is the extreme sensitivity that develops in the lower extremities, with painful polyneuritis and paresthesias. Hallucinations, lethargy, delirium, and psychoses are seen. Alopecia generally occurs within a few weeks of poisoning, and white stripes on the nails (Mee's lines) may be noted within this same period. Causes of death generally are related to the central nervous system and cardiac and renal system effects. In cases of toxicity, thallium can be monitored in urine, blood, and hair.

TABLE 85-2. Signs and symptoms of thallium toxicity

- Acute toxicity
  - Coma
  - Ataxia
  - Tremor
  - Paralysis
  - Psychosis
  - Seizures
  - Cardiac dysrhythmias
  - Electrocardiographic changes (similar to those in hypokalemia)
  - Nausea
  - Vomiting
  - Abdominal pain
  - Gastrointestinal bleeding
  - Renal tubular necrosis
  - Renal failure
  - Elevated liver enzymes
  - Hepatic necrosis
- Chronic toxicity
  - Distal neuropathy
  - Cranial nerve neuropathy
    - Ptosis, ophthalmoplegia, retrobulbar neuritis, facial neuritis, oculomotor nerve weakness
  - Psychosis, depression
  - Distal paresthesias
  - Distal motor weakness
  - Ascending neuropathy
  - Polyneuritis
  - Ataxia
  - Fatigue
  - Psychosis
  - Emotional changes
  - Dermatitis, skin erythema, scaly skin
  - Diffuse proliferative glomerulonephritis
  - Nail changes, Mee's lines
  - Fatty infiltration of liver
  - Constipation
  - Renal failure
  - Lens opacities
  - Autonomic nervous system dysfunction
    - Vagal nerve lesion
    - Carotid sinus lesion
    - Sympathetic ganglion lesion
  - Muscle atrophy
  - Abnormal electromyelographic and nerve conduction study results

Postmortem examinations have shown mucosal hemorrhages in the intestines, heart, and endocrine glands; degenerative changes in renal glomeruli and renal tubules; fatty degeneration of nerve ganglion cells; damage to nerve axons; and disintegration of nerve myelin sheaths (4).

After acute exposure (usually by the oral route), the initial manifestations are nausea and vomiting. GI symptoms may subside and can be followed in approximately 7 to 14 days by abdominal pain, constipation, bloating sensation, and GI bleeding (8). Coma, delirium, hallucinations, bleeding, and seizures may occur early if the exposure is severe. People have died from hypotension, GI hemorrhage, and cardiac effects within 8 to 10 hours after thallium ingestion.

NEUROTOXICITY

Neurologic symptoms usually begin from the second or subsequent weeks after exposure and consist of ataxia, tremors, paresthesias, cognitive defects, and polyneuritis, usually in the lower extremities (8). Peripheral neuropathy is mixed and symmetric, with distal nerves affected more than are proximal nerves. Thallium affects longer axons first.

Involvement of the autonomic nervous system can occur with vagal nerve damage, carotid sinus denervation, and sympathetic ganglia lesions, resulting in signs and symptoms of autonomic dysfunction (4). Retrobulbar neuritis with visual impairment can develop along with optic atrophy (4). Painful neuritis of the lower extremities may be severe.

Multiple sites of nerve involvement are apparent on electrophysiologic studies and microscopy. Muscle stretch reflexes usually are present until late in the clinical course. Cranial nerves may be involved, and affected patients may manifest ptosis, facial paralysis, and disconjugate gaze (9). Neurologic effects can be persistent and permanent. Psychological and emotional changes can occur, with intense depression and psychosis. Recovery is slow and requires months.

In fatal cases of thallium poisoning, neuropathologic workup reveals cerebral edema and petechial hemorrhages in the white matter, parietal areas, and subthalamic areas (4). Degeneration of ganglia occurs, with axon damage and disintegration of myelin sheaths. Direct damage to the autonomic nervous system can account for tachycardia, fever, blood pressure changes, orthostatic hypotension, urinary retention, constipation, and cardiac arrhythmias (4). A symmetric mixed peripheral neuropathy occurs, distal nerves being affected more than proximal nerves and with lesser degrees of effect on nerves with shorter axons, such as the cranial nerves (4). Demyelination of the dorsal columns of the spinal cord also have been found on postmortem examination (4). Vagal nerve damage may result in tachycardia, paralytic ileus, and hypertension (8). Electromyelographic and nerve conduction studies demonstrate varying results. Nerve conduction studies may give normal results early in the course. Conduction velocities of faster fibers have been found to be abnormally low in some cases. Abnormal results in electromyelographic and nerve conduction studies are found.

OCULAR TOXICITY

Retrobulbar neuritis can develop and persist for months. Optic atrophy also may occur, along with involvement of ocular motor muscles. Acuity should be tested, as lens opacities sometimes are found. Such opacities usually are peripheral and symmetric bilaterally.

GASTROINTESTINAL TRACT TOXICITY

After exposure, elevated liver enzymes can occur along with hepatic necrosis and fatty infiltration of the liver. Hyperemia, congestion of the mucosa, hemorrhages in the mucosa of the stomach and intestinal tract, and swelling of mucosal cells have been noted on autopsy (4).

DERMATOTOXICITY

Dermal changes include erythema, anhidrosis, and injury to sebaceous glands (8,9). Diaphoresis may occur late in the disease course. Scaly skin also is common in thallotoxicosis. Interference in nail growth for several weeks and Mee's lines may be seen (8).

Alopecia is a classic finding after thallium poisoning. Involvement of the skin includes crusted eczematous lesions, acne, scaling skin, loss of eyelashes, follicular plugging, and eosinophilic keratohyalin granules in the epidermis. Sebaceous glands sometimes become necrotic.

Pustular lesions can occur on the face, and folliculitis may be noted. Hyperkeratosis and hypergranulosis can be evident in some affected patients (4). Alopecia generally is not permanent, and the hair that regrows is stronger than that which is lost.

RENAL TOXICITY

Renal biopsies in thallium-poisoned patients have shown diffuse proliferative glomerulonephritis, with immunofluorescence for immunoglobulin G, immunoglobulin M, and C3 (4). On autopsy, the kidneys may be found to be hyperemic and dull red and to have tubular swelling and degeneration of glomeruli.

CARDIOTOXICITY

Hemorrhagic myocardial lesions have been found on autopsy after thallium poisoning. Hematologic changes include anemia, leukocytosis, eosinophilia, thrombocytopenia, and lymphopenia (4). Hypertension, dysrhythmias, tachycardia, and electrocardiographic changes occur. Involvement of the autonomic nervous system contributes to cardiac effects. Abnormal urinary concentrations of catecholamines may occur with autonomic nervous system damage (4).

Chronic and Long-Term Effects

Recovery from thallotoxicosis can take many months, and residual neuropathy may persist. Chronic exposure to thallium is rare, and reported cases usually involved weakness and pain in the legs, hair loss, and psychological disturbances. Alopecia may not resolve for months after poisoning (8).

TERATOGENICITY AND CARCINOGENICITY

Thallium crosses the placenta and distributes to the fetus, but in small amounts as compared with maternal concentrations. It can induce symptoms of thallium intoxication in newborn babies (4). In some instances of maternal poisoning, no effects were found in children of pregnant women who were thallium-toxic (8,9). Premature births have occurred, and neonates exhibited low birth weight, alopecia, and Mee's lines (4).

The teratogenic effect of thallium compounds has been demonstrated in animals. Achondroplastic malformations in chickens, reduced fetal body weight, hydronephrosis, and vertebral body absence in rats have been noted.

Thallium has not been classified as a carcinogen in animals or humans. Very little information is available about the immunotoxic effects induced by thallium.

Management of Toxicity

No effective chelating agent is available to combat thallium poisoning. None of the traditional chelating agents—2,3-dimercapto-1-propanol [British anti-Lewisite (BAL)], calcium disodium–ethylenediaminetetraacetic acid, D-penicillamine, and dimercaptosuccinic acid—has shown any efficacy in thallotoxicosis or increasing the elimination of thallium in poisoning cases. Diethyldithiocarbamate (dithiocarb) and diphenylthiocarbazone (dithizone) have been studied as potential thallium-chelating agents in animals (10–12). After these animal studies and, in some cases, human trials, these chelators were discarded as ineffective. In fact, some patients demonstrated clinical deterioration, with increasing coma and electroencephalographic changes after dithiocarb administration in thallotoxicosis (11,12). Dithiocarb apparently formed a lipophilic complex with the thallium ion, which allowed for increased central nervous system concentration of thallium.

Because animal and human studies have shown that administration of potassium resulted in an increase in urinary excretion of thallium and increases in plasma thallium concentrations, current therapy for thallotoxicosis involves a combination of the oral administration of potassium chloride plus activated charcoal (10). Potassium and thallium are interchangeable metals across the cell membrane. Thallium can replace potassium in the sodium- and potassium-activated adenosine triphosphatase pump. Thus, administration of potassium will help to push thallium from its intracellular site into the extracellular area and plasma, permitting urinary and fecal excretion (8,10). Use of potassium alone may result in a worsening of clinical symptoms despite a decrease in thallium half-life, owing to redistribution of thallium from plasma (8).

Potassium ferric-cyanoferrate II (Prussian blue) also has been found to be effective in thallotoxicosis (13–16). Prussian blue, an inorganic pigment, has been administered orally in doses of 250 mg per kg daily dissolved in 50 mL of 15% mannitol divided twice daily (10 g twice daily having been administered for cases of thallium poisoning) (2,14,15). Prussian blue is not absorbed by the GI tract. The potassium in Prussian blue substitutes for thallium, and the thallium then is adsorbed by the remaining Prussian blue lattice in the GI tract and is excreted fecally. Prussian blue thus acts as an ion exchange medium for thallium.

Because the administration of potassium and activated charcoal has been successful in increasing the total body elimination of thallium, and should Prussian blue not be available, the administration of a combination of oral potassium chloride and activated charcoal is recommended. This therapy has proved to be successful in severe thallium cases managed by the author. The dose of potassium chloride is 20 mEq four times daily with activated charcoal, 20 to 30 g four times daily. A cathartic usually is required, owing to the constipating effect of thallium. This therapy may proceed for several weeks to several months during monitoring of clinical improvement and decreasing urinary thallium concentrations.

Thallium's half-life in blood has been reported to be between 11 and 15 days in the absence of treatment. With Prussian blue treatment, the half-life is abbreviated to between 2.3 and 3.7 days.

DIAGNOSIS AND BIOLOGICAL MONITORING

Among unexposed individuals, thallium in the urine may vary by 0.3 to 0.4 μg per L, mean urinary thallium concentrations in early-morning urine samples ranging from 0.13 to 1.69 μg per L (4). In individuals living near a point source of thallium, urine concentration ranges up to 5.2 μg per L (4). For cement workers, urinary concentrations are in the range of 0.3 to 8.0 μg per L; for foundry workers, they are 0.3 to 10.5 μg per L (4). Generally, concentrations in the urine below 5 μg per L are not likely to be associated with adverse health effects (4). Urinary values in excess of 500 μg per L have been associated with clinical toxicity (4).

Diagnosis can be difficult without appropriate exposure history. Certain signs and symptoms are characteristic of thallium poisoning, such as alopecia and polyneuritis. Concentrations of thallium can be confirmed in blood and urine. Urinary thallium concentrations are higher than are blood concentrations. Because renal excretion is one of the main elimination routes for thallium, a 24-hour urine sample quantitating thallium is the most helpful in ascertaining exposure.

The administration of 40 mEq of potassium chloride orally to a patient prior to a 24-hour urine collection will increase the urinary excretion of thallium and help to confirm the diagnosis (9).

ENVIRONMENTAL FATE AND TRANSPORT

Atmospheric contamination by thallium occurs at such point sources as cement-making plants, smelters, and plants that use coal for power. The air of six large American cities was found to contain 0.04 to 0.19 ng per cubic meter of thallium. Thallium is volatile at high temperatures and is not retained by emission control facilities. The fly ash from most of the point sources is the major contaminant source for the environment. Increased concentrations of thallium in water generally occur from waste material effluents from tailing ponds of mining operations. Concentration of thallium in soils ranges from 0.1 to 1.7 mg per kg of soil. Soil contamination occurs through point sources of waste generation, such as smelters, power-generating plants, brick works, and cement-manufacturing plants.

Thallium can contaminate both plants and fish via pollutant sources. The metal can inhibit the nitrification of soil by soil bacteria and, in plants, concentrates in the chlorophyll-containing regions. Hence, thallium can interfere with the oxygen production of plants. Aquatic plants and invertebrates can be affected by environmental concentrations of the metal. Wildlife intoxication has occurred due to wide-scale use of thallium as a rodenticide.

The U.S. Environmental Protection Agency calculates the general population air exposure to thallium at approximately 0.48 ng per cubic meter. Generally, less than 1 μg of thallium is found in the United States.

Thallium is retained in soil with large amounts of clay, organic material, iron oxides, and manganese oxides (4). As soil pH increases, thallium uptake by vegetation increases (4). In acid soils, thallium can be leached to groundwater and surface water. Thallium in most water sources takes the monovalent form; however, the oxidized trivalent thallium form also may exist. Thallium can bioconcentrate but usually does not magnify up the food chain to a great degree. In the average human diet, food generally contains less than 1 mg per kg of thallium. Also, humans take in less than 5 μg per day of thallium (4). Air concentration of thallium in the workplace generally is less than 22 μg per cubic meter in smelting operations (4).

EXPOSURE LIMITS

The American Conference of Governmental Industrial Hygienists and the U.S. Occupational Safety and Health Administration have adopted a threshold limit value of 0.1 mg per cubic meter for thallium. The acceptable daily intake of thallium is calculated to be 15.4 mg per day, according to the U.S. Environmental Protection Agency.

REFERENCES

1. Bendl BJ. Thallium poisoning: report of a case successfully treated with dithizone. *Arch Dermatol* 1969;100:443–445.
2. Kazantzis G. Thallium. In: Friberg L, Nordberg GF, Vouk V, eds. *Handbook on the toxicology of metals,* 2nd ed. Amsterdam: Elsevier Science, 1986:549–567.
3. Sleight AW. Chemistry of high-temperature super-conductors. *Science* 1988;242:1519–1527.
4. *Thallium: environmental health criteria.* IPCS 182. Geneva: World Health Organization, 1996.
5. Chamberlain PH, Stavinoha WB, Davis H, Kniker WT, Panos TC. Thallium poisoning. *Pediatrics* 1958;22:1170–1182.
6. Papp JP, Gay PC, Dodson VN, Pollard MH. Potassium chloride treatment in thallotoxicosis. *Ann Intern Med* 1969;71:119–123.
7. Lund A. Distribution of thallium in the organism and its elimination. *Acta Pharmacol Toxicol* 1956;12:251–259.
8. Saddique A, Peterson CD. Thallium poisoning: a review. *Vet Hum Toxicol* 1983;25:16–22.
9. Smith DH, Doherty RA. Thallotoxicosis: report of three cases in Massachusetts. *Pediatrics* 1964;34:480–490.
10. Lund A. The effect of various substances on the excretion and the toxicity of thallium in the rat. *Acta Pharmacol Toxicol* 1956;12:260–268.
11. Boak RL, Schmidtke RP, Wallach JD, Davis LE, Niemeyer KH. Thallium intoxication: a specific antidote, supportive therapy and clinical evaluation. *Vet Med* 1965;12:1227–1231.
12. Kamerbeek HH, Rauws AG, ten Ham M, van Heijst ANP. Dangerous redistribution of thallium by treatment with sodium diethyldithiocarbamate. *Acta Med Scand* 1979;189:149–154.
13. Special communication: thallium poisoning. *Clin Toxicol* 1972;5:89–93.
14. Van Der Merwe CF. The treatment of thallium poisoning: a report of 2 cases. *S Afr Med J* 1972;2:960–961.
15. Kamerbeek HH, Rauws AG, ten Ham M, van Heijst ANP. Prussian blue in therapy of thallotoxicosis. *Acta Med Scand* 1971;189:321–324.
16. Heydlauf H. Ferric-cyanoferrate(II): an effective antidote in thallium poisoning. *Eur J Pharmacol* 1969;6:340–344.

CHAPTER 86

Intermetallic Semiconductors: Arsine, Phosphine, and Inorganic Hydrides

Dean E. Carter and John B. Sullivan, Jr.

The intermetallic semiconductors are composed of equimolar ratios of group III and group V elements. The intermetallic semiconductor used most commonly is gallium arsenide (GaAs), followed in decreasing frequency by gallium phosphide (GaP) and indium phosphide (InP). However, any combination of the group III elements—aluminum, gallium, and indium—with the group V elements—phosphorus, arsenic, and antimony—should be called *semiconductors* as long as they exist in a 1:1 molar ratio of group III:group V (e.g., AlGaAs with a composition of 0.5 mol Al, 0.5 mol Ga, and 1.0 mol As). Research in this area may yield a variety of semiconductors with special applications.

The group III–to–group V intermetallic semiconductors are crystalline solids of high density. They can be prepared by condensing vapors of the elemental forms of the metalloids; thus, GaAs can be characterized as Ga(0)As(0). It can be prepared also from gallium trichloride and arsenic trihydride (arsine) and thus can be characterized as Ga(+III)As(–III). The exact chemical forms of the elements in an intermetallic compound do not appear to be as important for its toxicity as the chemical forms of its dissolution products.

The inorganic hydrides also include some of the group III and group V elements because these elements are used as dopants for silicon-based semiconductors: arsine (AsH_3), phosphine (PH_3), stibine (SbH_3), diborane (B_2H_6), and silane (SiH_4). In addition to being known by their common names, they can be described as the hydride of the element (e.g., antimony hydride). All these materials are gases at room temperature. P, B_2H_6, and SiH can autoignite in air at elevated temperatures, and they may represent a hazard from explosion or combustion. All these compounds may react rapidly with oxidants, and the possibility of explosive reactions after accidental release must be considered. The hydrides of P, As, and presumably, Sb can be formed from hydrolysis of a metallic phosphide, arsenide, and stilbide, respectively. For example, AsH_3 can be generated from acid and zinc arsenide. Generally, AsH_3 is thought to be formed when arsenides, such as GaAs, react with acids, and this activity is thought to represent a potential route of human exposure. However, studies have shown that AsH_3 is formed only when GaAs reacts with concentrated hydrochloric acid (1). Such other common acids as sulfuric, nitric, or perchloric acids did not form AsH_3. Human exposures are more likely to occur from reduction of arsenic oxides in forming AsH_3; this occurs when the arsenic oxide comes in contact with acid and a metallike Al or zinc, as might be found in metal recovery operations.

PH_3 can be formed during the machining (e.g., cutting, grinding, and polishing) of such phosphides as GaP and InP when water-cooled processes are used (2). It can be produced also when GaP and InP are annealed in hydrogen atmospheres and alkaline media. SbH_3 gas may be formed during annealing of In-Sb-type semiconductors in a hydrogen atmosphere and during processing of In-Sb with nonoxidizing acids. Although not all the conditions that might form such toxic hydrides as phosphine, AsH_3, and SbH_3 have been investigated completely, formation of such hydrides always should be considered when etching processes are involved.

SITES, INDUSTRIES, AND BUSINESSES ASSOCIATED WITH EXPOSURES

The aforementioned materials are used primarily in the microelectronics industry. GaAs has been used most often for optoelectronic devices over the past two decades. GaAs-related devices include light-emitting diodes, optical communications transmitters, and solid-state semiconductor lasers. GaAs may find use as a photovoltaic solar cell material. Several favorable properties as compared with silicon-based devices suggest that GaAs may find applications in military, space, telecommunications, and supercomputing systems. Potential applications include high-frequency microwave and millimeter-wave telecommunications, satellite communications, ground- and space-based radar, electronic warfare, and intelligent weapons. Other applications could include cellular telephones, high-definition television, and automobile and aircraft instrument displays and controls (3).

GaAs components are manufactured in four major steps: ingot growth, wafer processing, epitaxial growth, and device fabrication. In one process, GaAs is formed by heating stoichiometric quantities of elemental Ga and As in a sealed quartz ampule. Crystal growth is achieved in a reactor by one of several techniques. Exposure to GaAs can occur during ampule breakout, in which the quartz tube is broken and particles are released; during cleaning and maintenance operations for quartz glassware; and during cleaning of the reactors. The ends of the large crystal (called an *ingot*) are cropped, and the ingot is lathed; then it is mounted onto a holder for wafer slicing. Once sliced, the wafers are lapped to a desirable thickness, are chemically cleaned, and are polished. Worker exposure to GaAs particles may be expected during these cropping, slicing, lapping, polishing, back-lapping, and wafer-saving steps.

During the manufacture of devices, epitaxial growth processes form thin layers of GaAs that contain the circuits. These processes involve the chemical reaction of Ga and As species to deposit GaAs on the surface of the wafer, and this is followed by chemical etching to define the path of the circuits. For example, vapor-phase epitaxy uses the reaction at high temperature between gallium halides and AsH_3 (or arsenic halides). Exposure to particles can occur during epitaxial reactor cleaning and maintenance. GaAs device fabrication includes nitride and silox deposition, photolithography, plasma or wet etching (or both), diffusion, metallization, back-lapping, and final test (3). Some of these processes may generate solutions containing soluble Ga and As products. Contact with such would result in exposure to Ga and As salts.

The inorganic hydride gases may be used in a large number of the manufacturing processes for electronic devices. These gases commonly are found in substantial quantities in microelectronic manufacturing facilities. The electronics industry has established elaborate controls for AsH_3 gas use, so the likelihood of exposure is small but, in several cases, AsH_3 was generated from As-containing waste or metal recovery operations (4). Many metal ores contain As as an impurity; thus, AsH_3 may be generated in metal industries, in nonferrous metal refineries, and in the manufacture of silicon steel, when the ores contact acid in the presence of certain metals. Accidental generation of AsH_3 has occurred in some unusual circumstances; transmission casings splashed with As pesticides generated AsH_3 during a cleaning operation that involved dipping the casings in an alkaline solution contained in a metal tank (5).

ANIMAL TOXICOLOGY

The toxic effects from the intermetallic semiconductors occur primarily after inhalational exposure, although oral exposure to high doses also may result in toxicity. Only GaAs has been studied in any detail, in studies of experimental animals. A GaAs dose of 30 mg per kg, introduced into the lung by intratracheal administration, produced in the body enzymatic changes characteristic of soluble As compounds; equivalent changes were observed only when 1,000 mg per kg was given by oral administration (6). The cumulative absorption of GaAs from the lung as measured by the amount of As found in blood and urine was approximately 10% to 20% of the administered dose, and this appeared over a period of several days (7). This absorption was fairly constant over the dose range of 10 to 100 mg per kg (6).

After oral administration, the amount of GaAs absorbed appeared to depend on dose in the range of 10 to 1,000 mg per kg; at 1,000 mg per kg, less than 1% was absorbed, but the percentage of the dose absorbed rose to almost 10% at a dose of 10 mg per kg. All these results are based on As data, because no Ga was detected in either blood or urine. Lung and fecal analyses found more Ga than As, suggesting that Ga was absorbed less well from the lung than was As and that greater amounts of Ga were cleared from the lung by mucociliary mechanisms and subsequently were swallowed.

Dermal absorption of GaAs does not appear to be a problem, but GaAs exposure to the conjunctival sac of the eye caused a reaction in the mucous membranes (8).

The absorption of GaAs appeared to be accompanied by the formation of arsenic oxide. The urinary metabolites of GaAs in the hamster were the same as those found after inorganic As exposure (arsenite, arsenate, monomethylarsonic acid, and dimethylarsinic acid), and the quantities found were intermediate to those found after arsenite and arsenate administration (7).

Excretion of As absorbed from GaAs is probably as rapid as that found after inorganic As administration; reports indicate that approximately 35% of the soluble sodium arsenite is excreted within 48 hours in humans (4). GaAs is absorbed slowly from the lung, so As excretion is expected to continue for several weeks after GaAs exposure. GaAs remaining in the lung is eliminated slowly; a single intratracheal dose of 100 mg per kg was excreted in approximately 3 months and had a half-life in the range of 2 weeks (7).

With the exception of InAs, which seems to have solubility properties similar to those of GaAs (9), little is known about the bioavailability, metabolism, or excretion of the other group III–to–group V intermetallic compounds. Their bioavailability should depend on their dissolution rates in water and on chemical properties that would govern their oxidation rates. Experiments with GaAs showed the presence of oxides of As on the surface of the GaAs crystal after exposure to aqueous solutions, suggesting that oxidation may be necessary for the dissolution of these compounds (10).

Exposure to the hydride gases (phosphine, AsH_3, SbH_3, SiH, and B_2H_6) occurs mainly via the inhalational route. Absorption of AsH_3 should be fairly efficient, owing to its substantial solubility in water (1,10). Apparently, AsH_3 is absorbed unchanged after inhalation, because it has unique effects on red blood cells, but eventually it breaks down to release inorganic As in the body (11). Little appears to be known about the bioavailability, metabolism, or excretion of these compounds. Controlled studies of these compounds have been complicated by the toxic nature of these substances and by the form they take (i.e., gases).

The group III–to–group V intermetallic compounds have a low order of acute lethality after oral or intratracheal administration in animals. The oral median lethal dose (LD_{50}) of GaAs in mice and rats was reported to be greater than 15 g per kg (12). The threshold for acute effects after intragastric administration was reported as 7.0 g per kg (8). A threshold for acute effects of inhalation of GaAs aerosol for 4 hours was 152.5 mg per cubic meter using a variety of toxic indicators (7). A dose of 200 mg per kg GaAs was given to rats by intratracheal instillation without having lethal effects (13). Roschina (14) reported an LD_{50} of 3.7 g per kg for indium antimonide powder given to white mice by intraperitoneal administration in peach oil (14). The oral LD_{50} for indium arsenide was stated to be greater than 15 g per kg, and the threshold for acute effects after a single 4-hour inhalational exposure was 139 mg per cubic meter (12,15). Tarasenko and Fadeev (16) reported an oral LD_{50} of 8 g per kg for GaP in mice (7).

Lung changes appear within a week after a single exposure to GaAs. A GaAs dose of 100 mg per kg given by intratracheal instillation to rats resulted in type II pneumocytic hyperplasia, alveolar proteinosis, and interstitial pneumonia as determined by histopathologic examination (17). An inflammatory response was indicated also by enzyme activity changes in bronchopulmonary lavage studies. Significant increases were found in total lung weight and lung lipid, protein, and DNA content. Similar, but less severe, effects were seen at 30 mg per kg, and at 2.5 mg per kg, the biochemical effects were essentially absent. Indium antimonide was reported to cause desquamative and interstitial pneumonia in the lungs after 25 mg was administered by intratracheal instillation to unspecified animals and for an unspecified duration (14).

Studies in hamsters and rats showed testicular toxicity at 7.7 mg GaAs per kg, administered intratracheally twice weekly for a total of 16 times (18,19). GaAs caused testicular spermatid retention and epididymal sperm reduction in both species. Exposure of mice for 24 hours to a single intratracheal administration of GaAs at 200 mg per kg was shown to suppress antibody production and other T cell–mediated immunologic functions (20). The significance of these effects to human toxicity is unknown.

HUMAN TOXICOLOGY

Gallium Arsenide and Arsine

AsH_3 gas is a very toxic, colorless, nonirritating gas with a garlic odor. The fatality rate from AsH_3 gas exposure is reported to be as high as 25% (21). The hemolysis associated with acute AsH_3 exposure is characterized by a latent period, the length of which is inversely proportional to the extent of exposure. Inhalation of 250 parts per million (ppm) of AsH_3 is quickly lethal, inhalation of up to 50 ppm for 30 minutes may produce death, and 10 ppm can be lethal after a longer exposure period. A massive release of AsH_3 into a work environment has the potential to produce numerous casualties.

Clinically, the signs and symptoms of acute poisoning are those consistent with acute and massive hemolysis and secondary multiple organ effects, such as acute renal failure and pulmonary edema (22). Initially, effects are painless hemoglobinuria, dizziness, weakness, nausea, vomiting, abdominal cramping, and tenderness. After a latent period, usually 2 to 24 hours, jaundice accompanied by anuria or oliguria from renal failure may occur. Evidence of bone marrow depression also has been reported. A triad of hemolysis, abdominal pain, and hematuria is classic for AsH_3 poisoning (21). Individuals with preexisting renal or cardiac disease or hypersensitivity to hemolytic agents resulting from a congenital deficiency of reduced erythrocyte glutathione are potentially more sensitive to the effects of AsH_3.

The mechanism of AsH_3 toxicity is unclear because of several changes that occur in the cell, not all of which may be necessary for toxicity to occur. AsH_3 toxicity is cell-specific; erythrocytes and hepatocytes are targets, but cells from the lung, kidney, and heart are not, despite the fact that signs of AsH_3 poisoning can involve all those organs. Red cell hemolysis requires hemoglobin and oxygen; the presence of methemoglobin and carbon monoxide reduces the extent of hemolysis.

Treatment of AsH_3 toxicity consists of immediate removal of affected individuals from the exposure. Clinical evaluation for hemolysis by examination of plasma for elevation of free hemoglobin, hematuria, and fragmentation of erythrocytes should be conducted. Alkalinization of the urine may help to prevent acute renal failure in the event of hemolysis. Exchange transfusion also may be helpful should hemolysis occur. The use of heavy metal chelators is not of value in treating the acute toxic effects of AsH_3. The AsH_3-hemoglobin complex is not dialyzable; thus, exchange transfusion represents the only truly definitive therapy (21). Exchange transfusion is recommended if hemolysis is occurring and an elevated free plasma hemoglobin is in excess of 1.5 mg per dL (21). Recovery depends on the supportive care rendered, extent of exposure, and secondary pathology due to the hemolysis.

Unpublished reports of human exposures to AsH_3 have found large quantities of the metabolites of arsenic oxides in the urine. *In vitro* experiments have found arsenic oxides after the addition of AsH_3 to human red blood cells. As organs other than the blood are more sensitive to arsenite toxicity (as compared to AsH_3), the use of heavy metal chelators for As may be considered to treat the chronic toxic effects due to the metabolites of AsH_3 [arsenite, As (III) oxide]. What must be understood clearly is that the use of chelating agents in AsH_3 poisoning never has been tested.

A threshold limit value and time-weighted average (TLV/TWA) for workplace exposure to AsH_3 is 0.05 ppm (0.16 mg per cubic meter). This is the concentration to which nearly all workers can be exposed repeatedly without adverse effect, on the basis of an 8-hour TWA, during a working lifetime. This TLV was adopted by the American Conference of Governmental Industrial Hygienists (ACGIH) in 1977. The federal Occupational Safety and Health Administration (OSHA) also uses 0.05 ppm as the permissible exposure level. Notably, the documentation for this value provides little human exposure–response information. Multiple reasons explain this lack of documentation, two of which are that AsH_3 is colorless, nonirritating, and odorless at less than 1 to 2 ppm and that intermediate doses are followed by a significant latency period between exposure and hemolytic response. Thus, exposure may be undetected, and airborne concentrations remain undetermined.

Chronic, low-level exposure to AsH_3 in workers may result in higher-than-usual excretion of urinary As of more than 50 µg per L of urine (21), even when dietary intake is considered. A correlation has been found between urinary As excretion and chronic exposure to AsH_3 gas well below accepted regulatory standards. Further investigation is required to determine the long-term health hazards of chronic, low-level AsH_3 gas exposure.

The animal database associated with the TLV provides little quantitative dose-response information on the hemolytic effects of AsH_3 exposure. Lethality in mice exposed to AsH_3 concentrations ranging from 8 to 800 ppm has been evaluated. Hematologic responses were evaluated in mice exposed to 5 to 26 ppm

AsH_3 for 1 hour. The results range from a no-effect level of 5 ppm to a lethal concentration of 26 ppm. This concentration range is extremely narrow and represents less than a tenfold difference for the 1-hour exposure studied. Systemic effects from the As formation absorbed from the lung into the general circulation should be expected. GaAs administered to the lung caused some changes indicating toxicity to the liver and kidney; blood aminolevulinic acid dehydratase was decreased within 3 days of administration; liver and kidney aminolevulinic acid dehydratase was inhibited; and urinary aminolevulinic acid was increased 3 to 6 days after exposure (13). Effects in kidneys, liver, and spleen also were noted after indium antimonide administration, but no details were described (14).

Phosphine

PH_3 is produced by the reaction of hydrogen with metallic phosphides, such as aluminum phosphide, zinc phosphide, or GaP. Aluminum and zinc phosphides are fumigants. PH_3 is a colorless gas with a fishlike odor at air concentrations greater than 2 ppm (21). It is acutely toxic, and detection of dangerous amounts is difficult even though its odor threshold is 0.03 ppm (23). The TLV recommended by OSHA is 0.3 ppm, with a short-term exposure limit of 1 ppm (21).

Symptoms of PH_3 exposure to average concentrations of less than 10 ppm include diarrhea, nausea and vomiting, cough and tightness of the chest, dyspnea, paresthesia, tremor, ataxia, headache, and dizziness. More severe poisoning results in pulmonary edema, cardiovascular collapse, jaundice with elevated liver enzymes, myocardial injury with an elevated MB-creatine phosphokinase fraction of cardiac enzymes, and cardiac dysrhythmias. Mortality from severe poisoning is high.

A death was reported from exposure to concentrations of 8 ppm PH_3 for 1 to 2 hours per day (24). Death attributed to PH_3 poisoning occurs after ingestion of aluminum phosphide in suicide attempts. Oral doses equivalent to 2 or more grams of PH_3 gas have caused deaths. In such cases, clinical signs consisted of gastritis, altered sensorium, and vascular failure, with cardiac arrhythmia in some cases (25). Postmortem examination showed pulmonary edema, gastrointestinal mucosal congestion, and petechial hemorrhages on the surface of liver and brain. Histopathologic changes included desquamation of the epithelium of the bronchioles, vacuolar degeneration of hepatocytes, dilation and engorgement of hepatic central veins, and sinusoids and areas showing nuclear fragmentation.

The mechanism of PH_3 toxicity is not understood. The toxin produces local irritating and systemic effects. Treatment is supportive, and no definitive therapeutic intervention exists.

Stibine

SbH_3 antimony hydride is produced by the action of hydrogen on metallic Sb. It is a colorless gas with an OSHA TLV of 0.1 ppm. SbH_3 exposure by inhalation produces red blood cell hemolysis. It is also a lung irritant and causes subsequent injury to kidneys and liver. Signs and symptoms of poisoning include hemolysis, hemoglobinuria, hematuria, nausea, vomiting, jaundice, shock, and renal failure. Treatment is supportive. The use of exchange transfusion would be recommended along the same guidelines as those applicable to AsH_3 toxicity if hemolysis is occurring.

Diborane and Higher Boron Hydrides

Boron hydrides have been used as high energy sources and are very reactive compounds. Decaborane ($B_{10}H_{14}$) has been used as a rocket propellant, and its toxicity involves mainly the central nervous system with excitation and depression (26). The boron hydrides generally are very reactive, strong reducing agents, and they react readily with organic amines, alcohols, ketones, halogenated hydrocarbons, and unsaturated hydrocarbons (27). B_2H_6 is the only boron hydride that is a gas at normal pressures and temperature (27). Boranes are soluble in hydrocarbons and are slightly soluble in water. B_2H_6 hydrolyzes rapidly in water to hydrogen and boric acid. Amine boranes are very stable. Pentaborane (B_5H_9) and $B_{10}H_{14}$ hydrolyze very slowly (27). Boranes are fuels sources, fuel additives, initiators of rubber vulcanization, fungicides and bactericides, and initiators of ethylene, styrene, vinyl, and acrylic polymerization (27).

B_2H_6 is produced by reacting lithium aluminum hydride with boron fluoride. B_2H_6 is a colorless gas with a nauseating odor detectable at 2 to 4 ppm (21). B_2H_6 is a fire and explosive hazard and may autoignite in air at temperatures exceeding 104° to 120°F (40° to 45°C) (21).

Inhalational exposure to B_2H_6 results in hydrolysis to boric acid and hydrogen. The upper airway would be expected to be a main target of B_2H_6. However, systemic toxicity, with pulmonary edema, also can occur. In addition, B_2H_6 contact with air produces higher hydrides that will have toxicity different from that of boric acid.

Acute toxicity with B_2H_6 produces respiratory irritation, pneumonitis, and if exposure is severe, pulmonary edema. Human health effects from subacute exposure to B_2H_6 have been reported in occupational settings and have included chest tightness, cough, headache, nausea, chills, dizziness, extreme fatigue, and obtundation after a relatively small exposure to the gas (27). These symptoms may occur soon after exposure or can be delayed for up to 24 hours. Exposure may result also in fever, tremors, and muscle fasciculations. Animals exposed to toxic concentrations die from respiratory complications (27). Hypotension, bradycardia, and cardiac dysrhythmias were noted in animal studies. On autopsy, the lungs of these animals showed pulmonary edema and hemorrhage (27). Male rats were exposed for 8 weeks to 0.11 or 0.96 ppm of B_2H_6 for 6 hours per day, 5 days per week by inhalation. The lung changes showed dose-dependent effects indicating that the hyperenergia of type II cells with proliferation or hypertrophy without histopathologic changes occurred even in rats exposed to 0.11 ppm (28). The authors commented that the TLV of 0.1 ppm may not be protective enough for human exposure.

B_2H_6 has a distinctive rotten-egg odor that alerts workers to the exposure. The odor threshold is reported to be approximately 3 ppm. The TLV for B_2H_6 is 0.1 ppm. Therefore, if the odor is detected, the TLV could be violated. Massive inhalational exposure of B_2H_6 can be expected to produce pulmonary damage, pneumonitis, pulmonary edema, and maybe other systemic organ effects on the heart, liver, and kidneys. Treatment is mainly supportive care.

The other boranes—B_5H_9 and $B_{10}H_{14}$—have toxicity that differs from that of B_2H_6. $B_{10}H_{14}$ is a white solid, and B_5H_9 is a liquid. B_5H_9 has a detectable garliclike odor at 0.8 ppm. $B_{10}H_{14}$ has an odor threshold described as "chocolatelike and unpleasant" at 0.7 ppm (27). Both B_5H_9 and $B_{10}H_{14}$ can produce toxicity via inhalation, ingestion, or dermal exposure. Both are soluble in hydrocarbons but not water. $B_{10}H_{14}$ does not hydrolyze readily to boric acid. A direct negative inotropic cardiac effect has been demonstrated in animals secondary to $B_{10}H_{14}$ exposure (27). Other animal studies have demonstrated hypotension after $B_{10}H_{14}$ exposure. Apparently, the reducing power of the borane hydrides parallels their toxicity. B_5H_9 produces acute animal toxicity consisting of tremors, convulsions, ataxia, corneal opacities, coma, and death (27). $B_{10}H_{14}$ also produces seizures in animal models.

Clinical human cases of higher borane hydride toxicity have involved stupor, seizures, dizziness, disorientation, hyperexcitability, leukocytosis, hyperglycemia, elevated blood urea nitrogen, and liver damage (27). Dizziness, headache, fatigue, muscle spasm, and drowsiness appear to be common symptoms appearing early in humans after exposure to these compounds. Interestingly, symptoms may occur early or can be delayed for as long as 24 hours (27). Symptoms may last 1 to 3 days. Muscle spasms may be prominent and involve large muscle groups. Renal and liver toxicities have been mild in reported cases (27).

Changes in neurotransmitter concentrations with inhibition of norepinephrine, dopamine, and serotonin metabolism have been attributed to $B_{10}H_{14}$ and B_5H_9 (28). Neurologic and neuropsychological symptoms occurring after B_5H_9 exposure include confusion, impaired concentration, and recent memory deficits and may persist for days after exposure (28). Mild cognitive defects on neuropsychometric examinations have been reported after B_5H_9 exposure (29).

Silane

SiH_4 is a carrier gas used in the microelectronics industry. The main hazards of SiH_4 gas are fire, explosions, and asphyxiant conditions in confined spaces.

CHRONIC AND LONG-TERM HEALTH EFFECTS

Not much is known about the long-term effects of exposure to group III–to–group V intermetallic compounds. Inhalation of GaAs aerosol by rats and guinea pigs at 12 mg per cubic meter for 4 months showed some fibrosis, epithelial degeneration in the kidney and convoluted tubules, and fatty degeneration of the liver (8,12). On the basis of results from single-dose studies, these changes are reasonable. Other long-term effects that might be expected would be those resulting from the dissociation of the intermetallic into its corresponding oxides. Thus, repeated exposure to GaAs would be expected to show long-term effects associated with low doses of gallium oxide and arsenic oxide. Gallium oxide does not appear to show systemic toxicity after repeated inhalation or oral exposure, but the long-term effects of arsenic oxides are well known (and described in Chapters 33 and 71).

The long-term effects of the hydrides have not been well studied either. PH_3 does not appear to have cumulative effects, but no well-controlled repeated-dose studies have examined such effects. Chronic AsH_3 exposure results in a progressive decline in the red blood cell number and in the hemoglobin. Mice and rats exposed to concentrations as low as 0.5 ppm for 90 days (6 hours per day, 5 days per week) produced a regenerative anemia secondary to the hemolysis. Increased concentrations of methemoglobin were found in mice exposed to 2.5 ppm AsH_3 for 90 days (30). Mice exposed to levels as low as 0.5 ppm for 14 days showed that AsH_3 inhalation had marked effects on the murine immune system, and these effects implicated the T cell as a sensitive target (31). The results of these animal studies must be considered when the effects of human exposure are evaluated.

BIOLOGICAL MONITORING

No well-characterized biological monitors are specific for any of these compounds. The biological monitors for absorbed Sb should prove useful for compounds containing Sb (e.g., indium antimonide, SbH_3); however, the absorbed Sb may not permit accurate relation to the lung burden of intermetallic compounds. Blood and urine analyses are used as biological monitors for Sb. Values for normal individuals have been reported for blood (3 µg per L), serum (0.3 µg per L), and 24-hour urinary excretion (0.5 to 2.6 µg per L). Levels exceeding these may indicate exposure to Sb, although quantitative data relating exposure to urinary levels are incomplete (32).

Urinary As levels generally are used as a biological monitor for As exposure if care is taken to eliminate the exposure to "seafood" forms of As. Large quantities of As in the form of arsenobetaine may be ingested with seafood, and although arsenobetaine contributes to the total As levels, it has a low toxicity and does not originate from the exposure to inorganic As. Affected workers usually are asked to refrain from eating seafood 3 to 4 days before being tested for As, and the levels determined reflect workplace exposure to inorganic As compounds. Inorganic forms of As and their metabolites can be analyzed separately from one another and arsenobetaine, but only a few laboratories can provide the analysis. Urinary levels from normal inorganic As exposure should be less than 50 µg per L (32). However, urinary inorganic As levels must be used for exposure to intermetallic arsenide or AsH_3 (or both), but they do not reflect the potential hazard because of dietary contributions to As levels. Neither the hazard to the lung from intermetallic arsenide inhalation nor the hemolytic potential from AsH_3 are well assessed by urinary As levels. Preliminary indications from *in vitro* experiments (personal data, Dean E. Carter) with AsH_3 and erythrocytes suggest that changes in red blood cell structure (burr cells and spheroechinocytes) precede hemolysis by almost 30 minutes and may be useful as an indicator of AsH_3 effects after acute exposures.

No definitive data exist with regard to the biological monitoring of Ga or In (33).

OCCUPATIONAL AND ENVIRONMENTAL REGULATIONS

No specific exposure limits have been formulated for any of the group III–to–group V intermetallic compounds. The National Institute of Occupational Safety and Health (NIOSH) issued an alert and recommended that the exposure to GaAs be controlled by observing the NIOSH-recommended exposure limit for inorganic As (2 µg per cubic meter of air as a 15-minute ceiling) (33,34). NIOSH also recommended that the concentration of GaAs in air be estimated by determination of As. For Sb and compounds, a TLV of 0.5 mg of Sb per cubic meter was recommended by the ACGIH in 1980 (ACGIH, TLV–biological exposure index, 1997) (24).

For PH_3, a TLV of 0.3 ppm (0.42 mg per cubic meter) and a short-term exposure limit of 1 ppm (approximately 1.4 mg per cubic meter) are recommended (ACGIH, 1997) (24). A TLV of 0.05 ppm (0.2 mg per cubic meter) as As is recommended by ACGIH for AsH_3 (24). The OSHA standard for exposure to AsH_3 is 0.05 ppm (0.2 mg per cubic meter of air) as a TWA in any 8-hour work shift of a 40-hour week. A TLV of 0.1 ppm (approximately 0.5 mg per cubic meter) and a short-term exposure limit of 0.3 ppm (approximately 15 mg per cubic meter) are recommended by ACGIH for SbH_3 (24).

EXPOSURE CONTROLS AND ENVIRONMENTAL AND OCCUPATIONAL MONITORING

During the production of GaAs, some facilities have exceeded airborne As limits, depending on the control procedures applied (34). Examples of control procedures are the use of isolated areas, special ventilation, personal respirators, and careful cleaning procedures.

Air and water levels of inorganic As should be monitored in a manner consistent with local, state, or federal regulations.

REFERENCES

1. Scott N, Carter DE, Fernando Q. Reaction of gallium arsenide with concentrated acids: formation of arsine. *Am Ind Hyg Assoc J* 1989;50:379–381.
2. Knizek M. Toxicology risks during manufacture and processing of AIII-BV type semiconductors. *Electrotchnike Cas* 1978;29:152–157.
3. McIntyr AJ, Sherin BJ. Gallium arsenide processing and hazard control. *Solid State Technol* 1989;7:101–104.
4. Ishinishe N, Tsuchiya K, Vahter M, Fowler BA. Arsenic. In: Friberg L, Nordberg GF, Vouk VB, eds. *Handbook on the toxicology of metals,* 2nd ed, vol 2. Amsterdam: Elsevier Science, 1986:43–830.
5. Risk M, Fuortes L. Chronic arsenicalism suspected from arsine exposure: a case report and literature review. *Vet Hum Toxicol* 1991;33:590–595.
6. Webb DR, Sipes IG, Carter DE. In vitro solubility and in vivo toxicity and gallium arsenide. *Toxicol Appl Pharmacol* 1984;76:96–104.
7. Rosner MH, Carter DE. Metabolism and excretion of gallium arsenide and arsenic oxides by hamsters following intratracheal instillation. *Fundam Appl Toxicol* 1987;9:730–737.
8. Fadeev AI. Materials on substantiation of the MAC for gallium arsenide in the air of workplaces. *Gig Tr Prof Zabol* 1980;3:45–47.
9. Yamauchi H, Takahashi K, Yamamura Y, Fowler BA. Metabolism of subcutaneous administered indium arsenide in the hamster. *Toxicol Appl Pharmacol* 1992;116:66–70.
10. Pierson B, Van Wagenen S, Nebesny K, Fernando Q, Scott N, Carter DE. Dissolution of crystalline gallium arsenide in aqueous solutions containing complexing agents. *Am Ind Hyg Assoc J* 1989;50:455–459.
11. National Institute for Occupational Safety and Health. *Arsine (arsenic hydride) poisoning in the workplace.* Current Intelligence Bulletin 32. DHEW (NIOSH) publication no. 79-142. Washington, DC: US Department of Health, Education and Welfare, National Institute for Occupational Safety and Health, 1979.
12. Fadeev AI. Toxicity of some compounds of arsenic with rare metals. *Aktual Probl Gig Tr* 1978;32–35.
13. Goering PL, Maronpot RR, Fowler BA. Effect of intratracheal gallium arsenide on delta-aminolevulinic acid dehydratase in rats: relationship to urinary excretion of aminolevulinic acid. *Toxicol App Pharmacol* 1988;92:179–193.
14. Roschina TA. Toxicological characteristics of indium antimonide and gallium arsenide: new semiconducting materials. *Gig Tr Prof Zabol* 1966;10(5):30–33.
15. Fadeev AI, Borobeva RS, Akinfieva TA. Toxicity of intermetallic compounds. *Met Gigien Aspekty Otseni Ozdorovleniya Okruzh Sredy M* 1983:246–251.
16. Tarasenko NY, Fadeev AI. Occupational health problems related to the industrial use of gallium and indium compounds. *Gig Sanit* 1980;45(10):13–16.
17. Webb DR, Wilson SE, Carter DE. Comparative pulmonary toxicity of gallium arsenide, gallium (III), oxide and arsenic (III) oxide intratracheally instilled into rats. *Toxicol Appl Pharmacol* 1986;82:405–416.
18. Omura M, Hirata M, Tanaka A, et al. Testicular toxicity evaluation of arsenic-containing binary compound semiconductors, gallium arsenide and indium arsenide, in hamsters. *Toxicol Lett* 1996;89:123–129.
19. Omura M, Tanaka A, Hirata M, et al. Testicular toxicity of gallium arsenide, indium arsenide and arsenic oxide in rats by repetitive intratracheal instillation. *Fundam Appl Toxicol* 1996;32:72–78.
20. Burns LA, Munson AE. Gallium arsenide selectively inhibits T cell proliferation and alters expression of CD25 (IL-2R/p55). *J Pharmacol Exp Ther* 1993;265:178–186.
21. Wald P, Becker C. Toxic gases used in the microelectronics industry. State of the art reviews. *Occup Med* 1986;1(1):105–117.
22. Landrigan P, Costello R, Stringer W. Occupational exposure to arsine. *Scand J Work Environ Health* 1982;8:169–177.
23. Fluck E. The odor threshold of phosphine. *J Air Pollut Control Assoc* 1976;26:795.
24. American Conference of Governmental Industrial Hygienists. *Documentation of the threshold limit values,* 4th ed. Cincinnati: American Conference of Governmental Industrial Hygienists, 1980; 1995 supplement.
25. Misra UK, Tripathi AK, Pandey R, Bhargwa B. Acute phosphine poisoning following ingestion of aluminum phosphides. *Hum Toxicol* 1988;7:343–345.
26. Naeger L, Leibman K. Mechanisms of decaborane toxicity. *Toxicol Appl Pharmacol* 1972;22:517–527.
27. Rousch G. The toxicology of the boranes. *J Occup Med* 1959;1:46–52.
28. Nomiyama T, Omae K, Ishizuka C, et al. Evaluation of the subacute pulmonary and testicular inhalation toxicity of diborane in rats. *Toxicol Appl Pharmacol* 1996;138:77–83.
29. Hart R, Silverman J, Garretson L, Schulz C, Hamer R. Neuropsychological function following mild exposure to pentaborane. *Am Ind Med* 1984;6:37–44.
30. Blair PC, Bechtold M, Thompson MB, Moorman CR, Moorman MP, Fowler BA. Evidence for oxidative damage to erythrocytes in rats and mice induced by arsine gas. *Toxicologist* 1988;8:19.
31. Rosenthal GJ, Fort MM, Germolec DR, et al. Effects of subchronic exposure to arsine on immune functions and host resistance. *Toxicologist* 1988;8:19.
32. Elinder CG, Gerhardsson L, Oberdoerster G. Biological monitoring of toxic metals—overview. In: Clarkson TW, Friberg L, Nordberg GF, Sager PR, eds. *Biological monitoring of toxic metals.* New York: Plenum Publishing, 1988:1–71.
33. National Institute for Occupational Safety and Health. *1988: Reducing the potential risk of developing cancer from exposure to gallium arsenide in the microelectronics industry.* DHHS publication no. 88–100. Publications dissemination, DSDTT. Cincinnati: National Institute for Occupational Safety and Health, 1987.
34. Sheehy JW, Jones JH. Assessment of arsenic exposures and controls in gallium arsenide production. *Am Ind Hyg Assoc J* 1993;54:61–69.

CHAPTER 87

Oxidizers, Reducing Agents, and Other Highly Reactive Chemicals

John B. Sullivan, Jr.

OXIDATION-REDUCTION REACTIONS

In an oxidation-reduction reaction, the electrons of one substance transfer to another substance. The reducing agent gives up electrons, and the oxidizing agent gains electrons. Oxidizers and reducing chemicals can be highly reactive, stimulate or enhance combustion of other materials, or be explosive (Table 87-1). Occurrence of an explosion depends on the rapidity of the oxidation-reduction reaction. Oxidizing-reducing materials require specific warning labels. The rapidity with which a chemical undergoes oxidation-reduction reactions determines its health hazard (1).

The chemical characteristics of oxidizers allow them to react with a large number of other substances. Oxidizing agents can be hazardous and react violently with organic materials by contributing oxygen for further combustion. When oxidizing agents react, they can release large amounts of heat and cause ignition of other materials, particularly organic materials. Oxidizing agents that contain oxygen are unstable when exposed to heat and can propagate fire. In addition, oxidizers and reducing agents may decompose explosively when heated; may explode on being heated or when involved in fire; may react violently with hydrocarbon fuels; may, in the form of runoff, create a fire or explosion hazard; and may result in burns or death when inhaled or ingested or brought into contact with skin. Oxidizers or reducing agents involved in fires have the potential to produce irritating, corrosive, or toxic gases, and toxic or flammable vapors may accumulate in confined spaces. In addition to creating a potential for explosion and burn injury, systemically absorbed oxidizing agents may cause methemoglobinemia, hemolysis, dermal injury, and pulmonary injury. Among the common oxidizers are ammonium nitrate, organic peroxides, hydrogen peroxide, halogen gases, perchlorates, chlorates, chlorites, hypochlorites, ammonium compounds, nitrates, nitrites, chromium oxidizers, permanganates, and hydrazine (Table 87-2).

Oxidation reduction differs from combustion. Combustion is the process by which two or more substances chemically unite accompanied by evolution of heat and light. Many substances other than oxygen are capable of supporting the combustion process. Fuel, heat, and oxygen are the three essential components necessary to sustain a fire. Many highly reactive compounds are combustible (see Table 87-1).

TABLE 87-1. Highly reactive chemicals

- Oxidizers
  - Amyl nitrate
  - Aluminum nitrate
  - Ammonium dichromate
  - Ammonium persulfate
  - Barium chlorate
  - Barium chlorate, wet
  - Barium nitrate
  - Barium perchlorate
  - Barium permanganate
  - Barium peroxide
  - Bromates, inorganic
  - Cesium nitrate
  - Calcium chlorate
  - Calcium chlorite
  - Calcium nitrate
  - Calcium perchlorate
  - Calcium permanganate
  - Calcium peroxide
  - Borate-chlorate mixture
  - Chlorate-borate mixture
  - Chlorate–magnesium chloride mixture
  - Magnesium chloride–chlorate mixture
  - Chlorate, wet
  - Chlorates, inorganic
  - Chromic acid, solid
  - Chromic acid mixture, dry
  - Chromium trioxide, anhydrous
  - Didymium nitrate
  - Ferric nitrate
  - Lead nitrate
  - Lead perchlorate
  - Lead perchlorate, solid
  - Lead perchlorate, solution
  - Lithium hypochlorite, dry
  - Lithium hypochlorite mixture
  - Lithium hypochlorite mixtures, dry
  - Magnesium bromate
  - Magnesium nitrate
  - Magnesium perchlorate
  - Magnesium peroxide
  - Ammonium sulfate nitrate
  - Nitrate
  - Nitrates, inorganic
  - Perchlorate
  - Perchlorates, inorganic
  - Permanganate
  - Permanganates, inorganic
  - Peroxides, inorganic
  - Potassium bromate
  - Potassium chlorate
  - Potassium nitrate
  - Potassium nitrate–sodium nitrite mixture
  - Sodium nitrite–potassium nitrate mixture
  - Sodium nitrite mixture
  - Potassium nitrite
  - Potassium perchlorate
  - Potassium permanganate
  - Potassium persulfate
  - Silver nitrate
  - Sodium bromate
  - Sodium chlorate
  - Sodium nitrate
  - Potassium nitrate–sodium nitrate mixture
  - Sodium nitrate–potassium nitrate mixture
  - Sodium nitrite
  - Sodium perchlorate
  - Sodium permanganate
  - Sodium persulfate
  - Strontium nitrate
  - Strontium perchlorate
  - Urea hydrogen peroxide
  - Urea peroxide
  - Zinc ammonium nitrite
  - Zinc chlorate
  - Zinc nitrate
  - Zinc permanganate
  - Calcium hypochlorite, dry
  - Calcium hypochlorite mixture, dry, with more than 39% available chlorine (8.8% available oxygen)
  - Perchloric acid, with not more than 50% acid
  - Lead dioxide
  - Lead peroxide
  - Ammonium nitrate, with not more than 0.2% combustible substances
  - Ammonium nitrate, with organic coating
  - Hydrogen peroxide, aqueous solution, with not less than 20% but not more than 60%
  - Hydrogen peroxide (stabilized as necessary)
  - Ammonium nitrate fertilizers
  - Ammonium nitrate fertilizers with calcium carbonate
  - Ammonium nitrate fertilizers, with ammonium sulfate
  - Ammonium nitrate mixed fertilizers
  - Ammonium nitrate fertilizer with not more than 0.4% combustible material
  - Ammonium nitrate fertilizer
  - Bleaching powder
  - Calcium hypochlorite mixture, dry, with more than 10% but not more than 39% available chlorine
  - Ammonium nitrate, liquid (hot concentrated solution)
  - Potassium chlorate, aqueous solution
  - Potassium chlorate, solution
  - Sodium chlorate, aqueous solution
  - Calcium chlorate, aqueous solution
  - Calcium chlorate, solution
  - Beryllium nitrate
  - Dichloroisocyanuric acid, dry
  - Dichloroisocyanuric acid salts
  - Potassium dichloro-*s*-triazinetrione, dry
  - Sodium dichloroisocyanurate
  - Sodium dichloro-*s*-triazinetrione
  - Sodium percarbonates
  - Trichloroisocyanuric acid, dry
  - Trichloro-*s*-triazinetrione, dry
  - (mono)-(Trichloro)-tetra-(monopotassium dichloro)-penta-*s*-triazinetrione, dry
  - Zinc bromate
  - Thallium chlorate
  - Chloric acid
  - Chloric acid, aqueous solution, with not more than 10% chloric acid
  - Nitrites, inorganic
  - Barium bromate
  - Chromium nitrate
  - Copper chlorate
  - Lithium nitrate
  - Magnesium chlorate
  - Manganese nitrate
  - Nickel nitrate
  - Nickel nitrite
  - Thallium nitrate
  - Zirconium nitrate
  - Barium hypochlorite, with more than 22% available chlorine
  - Calcium hypochlorite, hydrated, with not less than 5.5% but not more than 10% water
  - Hydrogen peroxide, aqueous solution, with not less than 8% but less than 20% hydrogen peroxide
  - Oxidizing liquid
  - Oxidizing substances, liquid
  - Hydrogen peroxide and peroxyacetic acid mixture, with acid(s), water, and not more than 5% peroxyacetic acid, stabilized
  - Chlorates, inorganic, aqueous solution
  - Perchlorates, inorganic, aqueous solution
  - Hypochlorites, inorganic
  - Bromates, inorganic, aqueous solution
  - Permanganates, inorganic, aqueous solution
  - Persulfates, inorganic
  - Persulfates, inorganic, aqueous solution
  - Percarbonates, inorganic
  - Nitrates, inorganic, aqueous solution
  - Nitrites, inorganic, aqueous solution
- Unstable oxidizers
  - Ammonium perchlorate
  - Chlorites, inorganic
  - Guanidine nitrate
  - Lithium peroxide
  - Sodium chlorite
  - Strontium chlorate
  - Strontium chlorate, solid
  - Strontium chlorate, solution
  - Strontium peroxide
  - Tetranitromethane
  - Zinc peroxide
  - Perchloric acid, with more than 50% but not more than 72% acid
  - Hydrogen peroxide, aqueous solution, stabilized, with more than 60% hydrogen peroxide
  - Hydrogen peroxide, stabilized
  - Ammonium nitrate fertilizers with phosphate or potash
  - Potassium superoxide
  - Sodium superoxide
  - Ammonium chromate
- Water-reactive oxidizers
  - Potassium peroxide
  - Sodium peroxide
- Organic peroxides
  - Acetyl acetone peroxide
  - Acetyl benzoyl peroxide
  - Acetyl cyclohexanesulfonyl peroxide
  - Acetyl peroxide
  - Benzoyl peroxide
  - *tert*-Butyl cumene peroxide
  - *tert*-Butyl cumyl peroxide
  - *tert*-Butyl isopropyl benzene hydroperoxide
  - *tert*-Butyl hydroperoxide, not more than 80% in di-*tert*-butyl peroxide and/or solvent
  - *tert*-Butyl hydroperoxide
  - *tert*-Butyl peroxyacetate
  - *tert*-Butyl peroxybenzoate
  - *tert*-Butyl monoperoxymaleate
  - Di-*tert*-butyl peroxide
  - *tert*-Butyl peroxyisopropyl carbonate
  - *tert*-Butyl peroxyisononanoate
  - *tert*-Butyl peroxy-3,5,5-trimethylhexanoate
  - Di-(*tert*-butylperoxy)phthalate
  - *tert*-Butyl peroxypivalate
  - 2,2-Di-(*tert*-butylperoxy)butane
  - 1,3-Di-(2-tert-butylperoxy-isopropyl)benzene and 1,4-Di-(2-tert-butylperoxy-isopropyl)benzene mixtures
  - 1,4-Di-)2-tert-butylperoxy-isopropyl)benzene and 1,3-Di-(2-tert-butylperoxy-isopropyl)benzene mixtures
  - *p*-Chlorobenzoyl peroxide
  - Cumene hydroperoxide
  - Cyclohexanone peroxide, not more than 72% in solution

(continued)

TABLE 87-1. *(continued)*

Cyclohexanone peroxide, not more than 90% and not less than 10% water
Decanoyl peroxide
Dicumyl peroxide
Di-(2-ethylhexyl)-peroxydicarbonate
p-Menthane hydroperoxide
Lauroyl peroxide
Methyl isobutyl ketone peroxide
Isononanoyl peroxide
Caprylyl peroxide
Caprylyl peroxide, solution
Octanoyl peroxide
Pelargonyl peroxide
Paracetic acid, solution
Peroxyacetic acid, solution
Propionyl peroxide
Isopropyl percarbonate, unstabilized
Isopropyl peroxydicarbonate
Succinic acid peroxide
Tetralin hydroperoxide
2,4-Dichlorobenzoyl peroxide
n-Butyl-4,4-di-(*tert*-butylperoxy)valerate
tert-Butyl peroxyisobutyrate
tert-Butyl peroxy-2-ethylhexanoate
tert-Butyl peroxydiethylacetate
1,1-Di-(*tert*-butylperoxy)-3,3,5-trimethyl cyclohexane
Di-(1-hydroxycyclohexyl)-peroxide
Dibenzyl peroxydicarbonate
Di-(sec-butyl)peroxydicarbonate
Dicyclohexyl peroxydicarbonate
Di-(4-*tert*-butylcyclohexyl)-peroxydicarbonate
2,5-Dimethyl-2,5-di-(*tert*-butylperoxy)hexane
2,5-Dimethyl-2,5-di-(2-ethyl-hexanolyperoxy)hexane
2,5-Dimethyl-2,5-di-(*tert*-butylperoxy)hexyne-3
2,5-Dimethyl-2,5-di-(*tert*-butylperoxy)hexyne-3, with not more than 52% peroxide inert solid
1,1,3,3-Tetramethylbutyl hydroperoxide
1,1,3,3-Tetramethylbutyl peroxy-2-ethylhexanoate
Pinane hydroperoxide
Diacetone alcohol peroxides
Dicetyl peroxydicarbonate
3,3,6,6,9,9-Hexamethyl-1,2,4,5-tetraoxacyclononane
2,2-Di-(4,4-di-*tert*-butyl-peroxycyclohexyl)propane
Butyl peroxydicarbonate
Diisopropylbenzene hydroperoxide
2,5-Dimethyl-2,5-di(benzoylperoxy)hexane
2,5-Dimethyl-2,5-dihydroperoxy hexane, with not more than 82% water
Dimethylhexane dihydroperoxide, with 18% or more water
Dimethyl peroxydicarbonate
Di-*n*-propyl peroxydicarbonate
tert-Butyl peroxyneodecanoate
2,2-Dihydroperoxypropane
1,1-Di-(*tert*-butylperoxy)-cyclohexane
Diisobutyryl peroxide
tert-Butyl peroxycrotonate
Ethyl-3,3-di(*tert*-butyl-peroxy)butrate
Ethyl-3,3-di(*tert*-butyl-peroxy)butrate, not more than 77% in solution
Methyl ethyl ketone peroxide
tert-Butyl peroxydiethylacetate, with *tert*-butyl peroxybenzoate
tert-Butyl peroxyisobutyrate
Distearyl peroxydicarbonate
Di-(2-methylbenzoyl)peroxide
tert-Butyl peroxyneodecanoate
Dimyristyl peroxydicarbonate
tert-Butyl peroxy-3-phenylphthalide
Di-(3,5,5-trimethyl-1,2-dioxolanyl-3)peroxide
Ethyl-3,3-di-(*tert*-butylperoxy) butyrate
3-Chloroperoxybenzoic acid
Organic peroxides, mixtures
2,2-Di-(*tert*-butylperoxy)-propane
1,1-Di-(*tert*-butylperoxy)-cyclohexane
tert-Butyl peroxy-2-ethylhexanoate, with 2,2-do-(*tert*-butylperoxy) butane
tert-Butyl peroxy-2-ethylhexanoate, not more than 50% with phlegmatizer
Diisotridecyl peroxydicarbonate
tert-Butyl peroxybenzoate
tert-Amyl peroxyneodecanoate
Dimyristyl peroxydicarbonate, not more than 42%, in water
Lauroyl peroxide, not more than 42%, stable dispersion, in water
Di-(4-*tert*-butylcyclohexyl)-peroxydicarbonate
Dicetyl peroxydicarbonate, not more than 42%, in water
Cyclohexanone peroxide, not more than 72% as a paste
1,1-Di-(*tert*-butylperoxy)-cyclohexane
tert-Amyl peroxy-2-ethylhexanoate
Organic peroxides (including trial quantities)

Self-reacting chemicals
3-Chloro-4-diethylamino-benzenediazonium zinc chloride
Diphenyloxide-4,4'-disulfohydrazide
Diphenyloxide-4,4'-disulphohydrazide
1,1'-Azodi-(hexahydrobenzonitrile)
5-*tert*-Butyl-2,4,6-trinitro-*m*-xylene
4-[Benzyl(ethyl)amino]-3-ethoxybenzenediazonium zinc chloride
Sodium 2-diazo-1-naphthol-4-sulfonate
Sodium 2-diazo-1-naphthol-5-sulfonate
2-Diazo-1-naphthol-4-sulfochloride
2-Diazo-1-naphthol-5-sulfochloride
Azodicarbonamide

PEROXIDES

Peroxides are chemical compounds that contain the –O–O– linkage and may be inorganic [e.g., hydrogen peroxide (H_2O_2)] or organic (Fig. 87-1). Organic peroxides are extremely hazardous compounds (Table 87-3). Ethers, which tend to react and form explosive peroxides, are made up of two groups of hydrocarbons linked by oxygen.

Hydrogen Peroxide

Pure H_2O_2 is a colorless liquid. It is used as a bleaching agent for paper and textiles, as a rocket fuel, and as a general disinfectant. Human toxicity occurs through inhalation, intravenous injection, dermal contact, and ingestion. Ingestion of H_2O_2, especially concentrates of 35% or greater, can cause rapid coma, vomiting, acute gas emboli with cerebral infarction, cardiac embolization, arterial embolism, rupture of stomach or esophagus (or of both), seizure, and death. Treatment by hyperbaric oxygen is proposed and should be attempted. However, data regarding hyperbaric oxygen's specific value are lacking (2).

H_2O_2 is completely miscible with water and is sold commercially as a solution in concentrations of 3%, 35%, 50%, 70%, and 90%. The Department of Transportation designates H_2O_2 as a detonator and oxidizer and as a corrosive material. Potential exposure to H_2O_2 occurs in industrial settings in the manufacturing of various chemicals, such as acetone, and in production of antiseptics, benzoyl peroxide, disinfectants, and pharmaceuticals. H_2O_2 is incompatible with some metals (i.e., iron, copper, brass, bronze, bromium, zinc, lead, manganese, and silver). The level immediately dangerous to life and health (IDLH) is 75 parts per million (ppm), and the short-term exposure limit (STEL) is 2 ppm (3 mg per cubic meter).

H_2O_2 is an irritant of the skin, eyes, and mucous membranes from direct contact of all solutions or as a concentrated vapor or aerosolized mist. Burning sensations and erythema of the skin can occur after contact with solutions of H_2O_2. Concentrations higher than 30% can result in dermal burns and blisters. Dermal contact will produce a bleaching effect, and, if the H_2O_2 is not diluted sufficiently, can result in dermal burns, vesicular eruption, and skin edema. Exposure to high mist concentrations of H_2O_2 can result in pulmonary edema, coma, convulsions, and seizures.

H_2O_2 can undergo explosion and violent decomposition if it is contaminated by incompatible metals. It accelerates combustion of other materials, owing to its oxidizing effect. H_2O_2 is also an explosive hazard when mixed with organic compounds. Solutions greater than 35% have the ability to decompose spontaneously and thus present an explosion hazard. H_2O_2 concentrations of less than 35% undergo spontaneous decomposition but not in a violent manner. Such stabilizers as sodium pyrophosphate are added to prevent decomposition.

Heating H_2O_2 to 144°C (291°F) can cause violent decomposition. As H_2O_2 is a source of oxygen, solutions of 35% and 50% or more can cause ignition of combustible materials without other ignition sources. This peroxide compound is one of the strongest

TABLE 87-2. Common oxidizers

Perchloryl fluoride	ClO_3F
Hexachlorodiphenyl oxide	$C_{12}H_4Cl_6O$
Sodium chlorate	$NaClO_3$
Sodium chlorite	$NaClO_2$
Sodium hypochlorite	$NaClO$
Perchloric acid	$HClO_4$
Chloric acid	$HClO_3$
Chlorous acid	$HClO_2$
Hypochlorous acid	$HClO$
Chlorine	Cl_2
Fluorine	F_2
Bromine	Br_2
Iodine	I_2
Bromine pentafluoride	BrF_5
Chlorine trifluoride	ClF_3
Chlorine dioxide	ClO_2
Oxygen difluoride	OF_2
Nitrogen trifluoride	NF_3
Hydrogen peroxide	H_2O_2
Benzoyl peroxide	$(C_6H_5CO)_2O_2$
Peracetic acid	$CH_3CO\text{–}O\text{–}O\text{–}COCH_3$
Methyl ethyl ketone peroxide	—
Oxygen	O_2
Concentrated sulfuric acid	H_2SO_4
Concentrated nitric acid	HNO_3
Osmium tetroxide	OSO_4
Quinone	$C_6H_4O_2$
Tetranitromethane	$C(NO_2)_4$
Permanganates	MnO_4^-
Dichromates	$Cr_2O_7^-$
Ozone	O_3
Stannic salts	—

oxidizing agents known. Most organic materials will combust on contact with H_2O_2 and can release toxic by-products.

Organic Peroxides

Organic peroxides (R–O:O–R) are the most hazardous of the oxidizing agents (1). These compounds are very sensitive to heat or friction, are highly unstable, and constitute a serious explosion and fire hazard (see Table 87-3). They are sensitive to thermal and physical trauma that can cause a combustion and violent composition to the point of detonation. The weakness of the organoperoxide bond is responsible for the instability of these agents. Their –O–O– bond is broken easily by heat, sunlight, or friction-forming reactive free peroxo radicals. Organic peroxides are used in the production and processing of reinforced plastics, plastic film, and synthetic rubber. They are used also in other processes requiring bleaching, such as those in the textile, printing, and pharmaceutical industries. Fires involving organic peroxides should be controlled by carbon dioxide or halon agents rather than by water. Common organic peroxides include benzoyl peroxide, peracetic acid, cumene hydroperoxide, and methyl ethyl ketone peroxide. Ingestion of organic peroxides can result in acute vomiting, abdominal pain, gastroesophageal injury, gastrointestinal tract bleeding, and hepatic damage.

BENZOYL PEROXIDE

Benzoyl peroxide is a crystalline solid that can explode when heated. The molecular formula of benzoyl peroxide is $C_6H_5CO\text{–}O\text{–}COC_6H_5$. It has a threshold limit value (TLV) of 5 mg per cubic meter. Benzoyl peroxide is an irritant of the mucous membrane and eyes and can cause skin sensitization and irritation of the respiratory tract. The major health hazards from benzoyl peroxide are respiratory, ocular, and dermal injury. Benzoyl peroxide produces dermatitis and intense irritation of eyes, skin, and mucous membranes. It will explode suddenly when heat is applied.

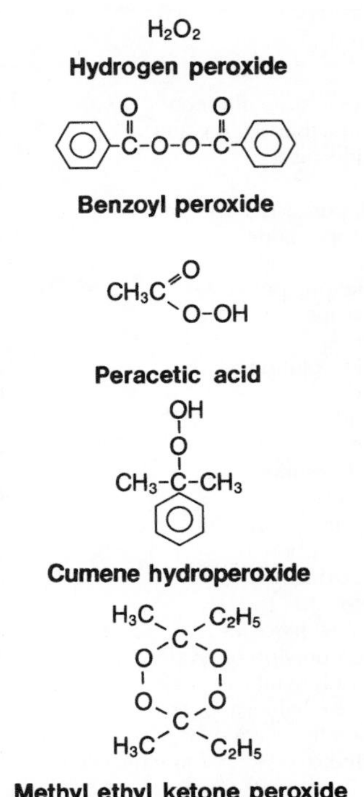

Figure 87-1. Chemical composition of peroxides.

PERACETIC ACID

Peracetic acid, also known as *acetyl hydroperoxide*, is used as a bactericide, fungicide, and sterilizing agent and is extremely explosive at temperatures of 100°C (230°F).

CUMENE HYDROPEROXIDE

Cumene hydroperoxide is used in the plastics industry and for the production of phenol. It decomposes to acetone and phenol in the presence of acids.

METHYL ETHYL KETONE PEROXIDE

Methyl ethyl ketone peroxide is a colorless liquid used in polymerization reactions and as a curing agent for polyester resins. It is a severe irritant of eyes, lungs, and mucous membranes. Animal data show that methyl ethyl ketone peroxide can produce gastrointestinal tract chemical burns and pulmonary hem-

TABLE 87-3. Hazards of organic peroxides

May explode from heat or contamination
May ignite combustibles
May be ignited by heat, sparks, or flames
May burn rapidly with flare-burning effect
Possible explosion from heated containers
Possible explosion from shock or friction in some
Possibly sensitive to temperature rises above a "control temperature" in some
Possible corrosive or toxic gases produced by fire
Possibly severe burns, injuries, and oxygen emboli from ingestion in organs (e.g., central nervous system)

orrhage on surface contact with the lungs. It also can cause hepatic injury on ingestion.

HALOGEN GASES AND HALOGENATED OXIDIZERS

Halogen Gases

Halogen gases (Cl_2, F_2, Br_2, and I_2) are strong oxidizing and corrosive agents. Chlorine and fluorine exist in a gaseous state. Bromine is a liquid, and iodine is a solid.

BROMINE

Bromine (Br_2; atomic number, 35; atomic weight, 79.9) is a reddish brown, dark, volatile liquid and is very corrosive and a strong oxidizing material. It is used in the manufacture of gasoline antiknock compounds, such as 1,2-dibromomethane, and in fire retardants, pharmaceuticals, and pesticides.

Bromine reacts with aqueous ammonium, aluminum, titanium, mercury, potassium, and other metals to produce combustible hazards. The TLV of bromine is 0.1 ppm, with a STEL of 0.3 ppm. The IDLH concentration is 10 ppm.

Human toxicity of bromine is due to its effects on the respiratory system, eyes, mucous membranes, and skin. Bromine gas in a 10-ppm concentration is severely irritating. High bromine concentrations produce dizziness, headache, nosebleeds, and severe irritation of the eyes and throat. Bromine is such a strong irritant that it can produce upper airway edema and pulmonary edema on inhalation of high concentrations. Skin burns can occur from liquid bromine spills. Bromine initially causes a cooling effect on the skin; after a delay, it will produce a burning sensation that can progress to deep chemical burns and brown discoloration of the skin.

Bromine is a liquid at standard conditions. At room temperature, bromine volatilizes and forms a red vapor that is a strong irritant. It is moderately soluble in water but very soluble in nonpolar solvents. Bromine tends to form singly charged negative ions (Br–). Hydrogen bromide (HBr) is a strong acid in aqueous solutions. Hypobromous acid (HOBr) results from the hydrolysis of bromine with H_2O and exists only in aqueous solutions. It is an oxidizing agent. Bromine monofluoride (BrF) is unstable and decomposes spontaneously at 50°C to form Br_2, BrF_3, and BrF_s (3). Methylbromide (CH_3Br) is a well-known organic bromide that has high neurotoxicity and is used as a soil fumigant.

CHLORINE

Chlorine (atomic number, 17; atomic weight, 35.4) is a green-yellow gas and is very irritating. It has a TLV of 1 ppm and a STEL of 3 ppm. Chlorine is a very powerful irritant of the eyes, skin, mucous membranes, and lungs. Chlorine inhalation can produce burning of the throat, chest, and eyes, difficulty in breathing, bronchospasm, and pulmonary edema. A concentration of 1,000 ppm can be rapidly fatal.

Chlorine gas is used in a variety of chemical processes and as a bleaching agent. It also is used commonly in swimming pools as a disinfectant. Chlorine is only slightly soluble in water and very soluble in alkaline solutions. It is a nonflammable gas but a strong oxidizer. As a bleaching agent, it often is used in the pulp and paper and the textile industries and in the formation of a variety of inorganic and organic chlorinated compounds. Chlorine is incompatible with other combustible substances and with fine particulates of metals. The National Institute for Occupational Safety and Health (NIOSH) has recommended a ceiling limit of 0.5 ppm for a 15-minute period of exposure.

TABLE 87-4. Oxychlorinated acids and oxychlorinated salt oxidizers

HClO or HOCl	Hypochlorous acid (weak acid)
$HClO_2$	Chlorous acid (weak acid)
$HClO_3$	Chloric acid (strong acid)
$HClO_4$	Perchloric acid (strong acid)
NaClO	Sodium hypochlorite
$NaClO_2$	Sodium chlorite
$NaClO_3$	Sodium chlorate
$NaClO_4$	Sodium perchlorate
$Ca(OCl_2)$	Calcium hypochlorite

Chlorine exhibits a readiness to form singly charged negative ions and, as such, behaves as an electron acceptor (an oxidizer). The electron affinity of chlorine is the greatest of all the halogen gases (3). Chlorine reacts with water to form hydrochloric acid, reacts with metal oxides to form oxychlorides, and reacts with salts of metals to form chlorides. Four oxides of chlorine exist: chlorine(I) oxide (photosensitive; Cl_2O); chlorine(II) oxide (ClO_2); chlorine hexoxide (Cl_2O_6); and chlorine heptoxide (Cl_2O_7). Oxychlorinated acids and oxychlorinated salt oxidizers are listed in Table 87-4.

Hypochlorous acid (HOCl or HClO) is formed by the action of chlorine (Cl_2) with water:

$$Cl_2 + H_2O \leftrightarrow HClO\ H_3O^+ + Cl^-$$

Once formed, hypochlorous acid undergoes a variety of reactions:

$$HClO + HCl \leftrightarrow Cl_2 + H_2O$$

$$HClO \rightarrow 2HCl + O_2$$

$$4HClO \leftrightarrow 2H_2O + 2Cl_2O \text{ (explosive chlorine monoxide)}$$

Chlorine monoxide is an explosive by-product of hypochlorous acid decomposition. Free chlorine can be released by the action of an oxidizing agent with hydrochloric acid (oxidizer + $HCl \rightarrow Cl_2 + H_2O$ + salt).

Calcium hypochlorite ($CaCl_2O_2$) is used for "shock treatment" to kill biologicals contaminating swimming pools and other water sources. Another chlorinating agent, trichloro-*s*-triazinetrione (TST) is also employed as a so-called shocking agent.

Cases of toxic gas production and explosive reactions after additions of these compounds to swimming pools have been reported (4). An explosive interaction between TST and calcium hypochlorite can occur. TST, which releases chlorine slowly, catalyzes a more rapid release of chlorine from calcium hypochlorite (4). TST forms cyanuric acid and hypochlorous acid, which react with the hypochlorite and chloride ions produced by calcium hypochlorite and rapidly form chlorine gas and heat in an explosive manner (4). Residues of TST in water are sufficient to catalyze this violent reaction when calcium hypochlorite is added. The addition of organic matter, such as algae in a water source, may enhance the explosive reaction.

TST undergoes a variety of chemical reactions, producing such toxic by-products as cyanuric acid, hypochlorous acid, and hydrochloric acid when exposed to water (4). The dry chemical may explode with the addition of water that contains organic material, producing aerosolized chemical particulates that may be inhaled. Depending on their size, particles may reach alveolar areas and produce pulmonary edema and severe pulmonary burns. Burns to the skin also can occur owing to water reaction of the compound during water decontamination. Further burns to the eyes and upper airways can result from contact with powder and particulate (4).

Different water-chlorinating chemicals should not be mixed, owing to the risks of rapidly producing large amounts of chlorine and of possible explosions. Water should not be added to chlorinator powder to render it more soluble, and chlorinator chemicals should be added with caution only to large quantities of water.

Common agents that cause release of chlorine include water-chlorinating chemicals, calcium hypochlorite ($CaCl_2O_2$) and TST ($Cl_3CNCO_3 + 3H_3O$); chlorine dioxide (ClO_2), a biocidal agent; and salts of dichloroisocyanuric acid.

Organic material, hydrocarbons, ammonia, and hydrogen will burn spontaneously on exposure to chlorine gas. A mixture of ammonia (NH_3) plus chlorine can produce nitrogen trichloride, an unstable explosive compound:

$$12NH_3 + 6Cl_2 \rightarrow 9NH_4Cl_3 + NCl_3 \text{ (explosive)} + N_2$$

TST plus ammonia, which may be present owing to biologicals or organic material in contaminated water, also can generate chlorine rapidly, an activity that triggers a reaction with NH_3 to produce the explosive gas nitrogen trichloride:

$$2(Cl_3CNCO)_3 + 3H_2O \rightarrow NCl_3 \text{ (explosive)} + 3(NCOH)$$

Hypochlorites. Chlorine reaction with alkalis produces hypochlorites. Sodium hypochlorite is bleach. Household bleach is approximately 5% sodium hypochlorite.

Hypochlorite salts are used as bleaching agents, disinfectants, and deodorants and occur in solid form or in aqueous solutions. Hypochlorites reacting with organic material spontaneously combust. Water accelerates this reaction (Table 87-5).

Calcium hypochlorite, as a swimming pool disinfectant, should not be mixed with small amounts of water prior to its addition to swimming pools, owing to the potential of an explosion and rapid release of chlorine gas. Calcium hypochlorite or TST mixed with algaecides or fungicides, ammonium, or organic material can burst into flames spontaneously. Hypochlorites also should not be mixed with muriatic acid in a concentrated form outside a large volume of water, owing to rapid and explosive formation of chlorine gas.

Hypochlorous Acid. Prepared by the reaction of chlorine monoxide (Cl_2O) with water (H_2O), hypochlorous acid (HClO or HOCl) is a yellow solution that decomposes in sunlight. It is a powerful oxidizing and bleaching agent.

Perchloric Acid. Perchloric acid ($HClO_4$) is a colorless, fuming, oily liquid that mixes readily with water. Cold, dilute perchloric acid reacts with such metals as zinc and iron and produces flammable hydrogen gas (4) plus a perchlorate. Concentrated, hot perchloric acid is a powerful oxidizing agent and explodes violently in contact with carbon-containing compounds, such as charcoal, paper, or alcohol.

TABLE 87-5. Hazards of chlorite mixtures

Chlorite + organic material = flammable
Chlorite + ammonia = explosive nitrogen chloride
$12NH_3 + 6Cl_2 \rightarrow 9NH_4CL_3 + N_2 + NCl_3$
Chlorite + sulfur → sodium sulfide (explosive), chlorine, sulfur dioxide
$2NaClO_2 + 3S \rightarrow Cl_2 + 2SO_2 + Na_2S$
Chlorite + metal particulates → explosion
$4Al + 3NaClO_2 \rightarrow 2Al_2O_3 + 3NaCl$
$2Mg + NaClO_2 \rightarrow 2MgO + NaCl$
Chlorite + hydrochloric acid → chlorine vapors
$Ca(OCl_2) + 4HCl \rightarrow CaCl_2 + 2H_2O + 2Cl_2$
Chlorite + TST → explosive nitrogen chloride + chlorine vapors

Chloric Acid. Chloric acid ($HClO_3$) reacts explosively with organic material. It is prepared by reacting chlorine with hot caustic substances (3).

FLUORINE

Fluorine (F_2; atomic number, 9; atomic weight, 18.99) is a pale yellowish gas and a very strong oxidizing agent. This gas is used in the production of fluorinated organic and inorganic compounds. It is a strong oxidizer used in rocket fuel. Fluorine is one of the strongest oxidizing agents known. It is incompatible with water, nitric acid, and other oxidizing materials. The TLV of fluorine is 0.1 ppm. It has an IDLH level of 5 ppm. The American Conference of Governmental Industrial Hygienists (ACGIH) recommends a TLV of 1 ppm and a STEL of 2 ppm.

Fluorine causes both chemical and thermal burns. It is a very severe irritant of the lungs, mucous membranes, skin, and eyes. The reaction of this gas with moisture produces hydrofluoric acid. Fluorine in high concentrations can produce laryngospasm and pulmonary edema. Exposure to lower concentrations (approximately 25 ppm) can result in sore throat, difficulty in breathing, chest pain, and cough. Dermal and eye burns can occur secondary to fluorine skin exposure.

Fluorine exhibits a readiness to form singly negative ions (F–). Electron affinity is less than that of bromine and chlorine. However, fluorine has the highest negative oxidation potential of an ion in relation to its elemental form. That is because of its greater reactivity in aqueous solution owing to lower energy of hydration and lower energy of dissociation (3).

Fluorine reacts violently with hydrogen as temperature increases. It reacts with all metals; in reaction with sulfur, silicon, carbon, and antimony, it will ignite (3). Rubidium, cesium, and potassium form trifluorides. Fluorine shipment requires a special permit, and it must be transported in a nonliquefied compressed gas state in seamless steel or nickel cylinders.

Unstable compounds of oxygen and fluorine are O_4F_2, O_3F_2, O_2F_2, and OF_2. Hydrogen fluoride is the most stable of hydrogen halides and is a very strong acid.

Organofluorine compound reactivity depends on the degree of fluorine substitution. The more highly substituted organofluorines tend to be more reactive, whereas the less substituted compounds usually are less reactive.

Halogenated Oxides

IODINE

Iodine (I_2; atomic number, 53; atomic weight, 126.9) is a purple solid with a sharp odor. Its vapor is violet. Iodine is used in the manufacture of organic materials and pharmaceuticals as well as in the photography industry. It has a TLV of 0.1 ppm.

Iodine is a strong irritant of the mucous membranes, respiratory tract, eyes, and skin. Ocular exposure can result in intense pain and blepharitis. Ingestion of 2 to 3 g of iodine is said to be possibly fatal and can result in a syndrome of tachycardia, parotitis, bronchitis, and difficulty in sleeping.

Iodine is incompatible with gaseous or aqueous ammonium, acetylene, powdered aluminum, and other active metals. In contact with the skin it can produce hypersensitivity and burns.

Iodine readily sublimes from its crystal solid state to a violet vapor (3). It is insoluble in water but soluble in alcohol, ether, carbon disulfide, and carbon tetrachloride (4). Iodine readily forms charged ions (I–) but has the lowest electron affinity of the four halogen gases. It also is the most electropositive of the halogens and functions in the I^+ form in some compounds, such as iodine perchlorate.

Iodine pentoxide (I_2O_5), a white compound, is the only binary combination with oxygen. Hydrogen iodide is the least stable of the four common halogen halides, rendering it a strong reducing agent (3).

Oxyacids of iodine are hypoiodous acid, idodic acid, and periodic acids. Hypoiodous acid is a strong oxidant. Hydroiodic acid is a colorless solution formed when hydrogen iodide gas is dissolved in water.

PERCHLORYL FLUORIDE

Perchloryl fluoride, with a TLV of 3 ppm and a chemical formula of ClO_3F, is a gas used in organic synthesis to produce fluorinated organic compounds. It is also a strong oxidizing agent and is used in rocket fuels and as an insulator (1). Perchloryl fluoride is a strong irritant of the eyes, mucous membranes, and lungs. In high concentrations, it can produce pulmonary edema and methemoglobinemia. Exposure to toxic concentrations can produce weakness, syncope, headache, and severe respiratory tract irritation and pulmonary edema. Skin contact from the liquid form can produce burns. Clinical symptomatology includes dizziness, headache, cyanosis, and syncope. Perchloryl fluoride is incompatible with compounds that are combustible, strong bases, amines, metal particulates, and other oxidizable materials. The IDLH level of perchloryl fluoride is 385 ppm (1).

CHLORATES

Potassium, sodium, and ammonium chlorates ($ClO–_3$) are strong oxidizing agents found in pyrotechnics, gunpowder, matches, flares, and fuses. The combination of organic material and chlorates forms a combustible mixture that can burst into flames. When chlorates are mixed with sulfur and charcoal, spontaneous combustion can occur. Chlorates also explode and ignite spontaneously when mixed with finely ground metals. Systemic effects include hemolysis, methemoglobinemia, and renal damage.

PERCHLORATES

Perchlorates ($ClO–_4$) are stabler than are hypochlorites, chlorites, and chlorates. They have slower chemical reactivity, and so transporting and storing them are less hazardous. Perchlorates react with organic matter and produce an ignition process. Perchloric acid ($HClO_4$) is both an oxidizer and a corrosive material. Perchlorates can cause methemoglobinemia after exposure. Perchloric acid is one of the strongest mineral acids and, as such, is both a corrosive and an oxidizer.

BROMINE PENTAFLUORIDE

Bromine pentafluoride (BrF_5) is a dense, colorless liquid with a boiling point of 40°C. It is a strong oxidizer and corrosive material. It is used as an oxidizer in liquid rocket propellants. Bromine pentafluoride is a strong irritant of the eyes, skin, and other mucous membranes. For this liquid, the ACGIH has recommended a TLV of 0.1 ppm and a STEL of 0.3 ppm.

CHLORINE TRIFLUORIDE

Chlorine trifluoride (ClF_3) is a green-yellow liquid that also can be a gas. It has a sweet irritating odor and a boiling point of 11°C. It is both a strong oxidizing agent and a corrosive agent. The TLV for chlorine trifluoride is 0.1 ppm, and its IDLH level is 20 ppm. It is used in rocket fuel, in nuclear reactor fuel processing, and as an incendiary agent. Human exposure occurs mainly from skin contact and inhalation. It is a very strong irritant of the eyes, respiratory system, and mucous membrane. The hydrolysis of chlorine trifluoride produces chlorine and hydrogen fluoride and chlorine dioxide. Human toxic effects also are related to these hydrolysis products.

CHLORINE DIOXIDE

Chlorine dioxide (ClO_2) is a yellow to slightly yellow gas with a very sharp, pungent odor. Used as a bleach in water purification and also as a disinfectant and fungicide, it is a strong oxidizing agent. It is incompatible with other combustible materials, organic matters, and solvents. The chlorine dioxide TLV is 0.1 ppm, and the ACGIH-recommended STEL is 0.3 ppm. Its IDLH level is 10 ppm. Chlorine dioxide is a severe ocular, mucous membrane, and respiratory irritant. Exposure to concentrations of up to 1 ppm has been fatal.

OXYGEN DIFLUORIDE

Oxygen difluoride (OF_2) is a rocket propellant and oxidizing agent. It is a colorless gas with a TLV of 0.05 ppm and is a potent irritant of mucous membranes and the respiratory tract.

AMMONIUM COMPOUNDS

The ammonium compounds are represented by ammonium nitrate and ammonium nitrite. Ammonium nitrate is a synthetic fertilizer and also has been used in formulations of dynamite since 1933. The two grades of ammonium nitrate are the fertilizer grade and an explosive grade. Both pose different hazards relative to their decomposition and explosivity. Ammonium agents that are oxidizers are ammonium nitrate, ammonium nitrite, ammonium chlorate, ammonium perchlorate, ammonium permanganate, ammonium dichromate, ammonium peroxydisulfate, ammonium picrate, sodium nitrate, ethylene glycol dinitrate, and *n*-propyl nitrate.

***Ammonium Nitrate*.** Ammonium nitrate is found in a variety of forms, such as fertilizer and explosives. The decomposition of ammonium salt oxidizing agents is explosive. When these compounds are exposed to heat, they can explode. The heating of ammonium nitrate produces decomposition into a variety of chemical products. At low temperatures, ammonium nitrate decomposes to nitrous oxide and water. When exposed to high temperatures, ammonium nitrate becomes explosive. It is incompatible also with powered metals, charcoal, and sulfur. When ammonium nitrate is heated in an enclosed area that retains the products of decomposition, a dangerous explosion can occur.

Ammonium Picrate. Ammonium picrate is a picric acid ammonium derivative used in explosives, pyrotechnics, and rocket propellants. Ammonium picrate is considered to be highly explosive and reacts with metal and sodium nitrite. The compound has a bitter taste and demonstrates the same properties as picric acid. It can be absorbed through the skin and can produce nausea, vomiting, diarrhea, staining of the skin, dermatitis, circular eruptions of the skin, coma, and seizures. On decomposition, it emits nitrogen oxide.

CHROMATES, CHROMIUM METALS, AND CHROMIUM SALTS

Chromium, with a 6+ (hexavalent) oxidation state, includes four compounds: metallic chromates, metallic dichromates, chromium trioxide, and chromyl chloride. The hexavalent chromium compounds are severe irritants of the lungs, eyes, mucous membranes, nose, and throat. These compounds are also the most toxic of the chromium compounds. Exposure to chromate dust can produce nasal ulcerations and perforations, epistaxis, respiratory irritation, bronchospasm, renal failure, dermatitis, skin sensitization, skin discoloration, and skin ulceration. Prolonged exposure also can result in dental erosions.

Chromic Acid

Chromic acid (H_2CrO_4) is a strong hexavalent oxidizing agent. Chromic acid and the chromates are incompatible with other combustible materials, organic materials, or readily oxidizable materials, such as paper, sulfur, and aluminum. Chromic acid and chromates have an IDLH level of 30 mg per cubic meter. NIOSH has recommended a TLV for chromic acid of 0.05 mg per cubic meter. The federal TLV for hexavalent chromium compound is 0.05 mg per cubic meter. Chromic acid is used as a metal and glass cleaner prior to electroplating. It is a highly toxic compound that can produce dermal burns resulting in systemic absorption with acute renal failure. Dermal burns of less than 3% can produce renal failure. Contact with the eyes can produce severe corneal injury. Dermatitis from chromic acid can vary from erythematous rash to eczematous lesions.

Chromyl Chloride

Chromyl chloride (CrO_2C1_2) is a red liquid produced by addition of concentrated hydrochloric acid and sulfuric acid to potassium dichromate.

Ammonium Dichromate

Ammonium dichromate [$(NH_4)_2Cr_2O_7$] can undergo thermal decomposition and produce a violent conflagration. It is a strong oxidizing agent and flammable solid.

Chromium Trioxide

Also known as chromium anhydride (CrO_3), chromium trioxide is a solid that may be produced also as a red liquid.

PERMANGANATES

Permanganate is the manganese atom in the 7+ oxidation state ($MnO-_4$). Ammonium permanganate (NH_4MnO_4) is a very strong oxidizing agent that can explode violently when exposed to heat. Permanganate salts are very strong oxidizing agents. Permanganate solutions are used as coating on magnesium alloys as protectants from corrosion.

POTASSIUM PERSULFATE

Potassium persulfate ($K_2S_2O_8$) is a crystalline white material that decomposes below 100°C. It is a very strong oxidizing agent and is used as a bleaching agent and as a polymerization catalyst. It is incompatible with combustible materials, organic materials, and other oxidizable materials, sulfur, metallic dust, aluminum dust, chlorates, and perchlorates. The ACGIH has recommended a TLV of 2 mg per cubic meter for this agent. Potassium persulfate reacts with moisture to produce ozone and sulfuric acid, which can incite an explosion in a closed container.

REDUCING CHEMICALS

Reducing agents are chemicals that lose electrons in oxidation-reduction reactions. The rapidity with which a chemical undergoes an oxidation-reduction reaction determines its hazard level. Several reducing agents are known to be hazardous owing to their extreme reactivity and to their clinical toxicity:

- Hydrazine
- Monomethylhydrazine
- Hydroxylamine
- Decaborane
- Pentaborane
- Boron trifluoride
- Boron tribromide
- Lithium hydride

Many of these agents are used as rocket propellants and fuels and in a variety of other industrial processes requiring strong reducing chemical properties.

Hydrazine

Hydrazine ($H_2N{\cdot}NH_2$) is a colorless fuming liquid and a reducing agent (3). This flammable liquid (producing a violet flame) is used as a rocket fuel. It is used also as a boiler water treatment for scavenging oxygen, in the preparation of anticorrosive materials, in manufacturing insecticides, plastics, rubber compounds, textile-treating agents, dyes, and pharmaceuticals, and as an antioxidant.

The IDLH level for hydrazine is 80 ppm. It is incompatible with oxidizing agents, H_2O_2, nitric acid, metal oxides, and strong acids and carries a hazard label warning of its corrosive properties. This agent is unstable, its decomposition being hastened by copper and iron. Hydrazine decomposes rapidly with heat:

$$2N_2H_4 \rightarrow 2NH_3 + N_2 + H_2$$

Mixed with air, hydrazine bursts into flame and explodes:

$$N_2H_4 + O_2 \rightarrow N_2 + 2H_2O$$

Hydrazine does not react with water; thus, fires can be controlled with water. Organic compounds of hydrazine include monomethylhydrazine and dimethylhydrazine, which are flammable. Dimethylhydrazine [$(CH_3)_2NNH_2$] is a rocket propellant with liquid oxygen.

Hydrazine should be stored to avoid any contact with oxidizing material, such as perchlorates, peroxides, permanganates, chlorates, nitrates, and strong acids, and with H_2O_2 and metal oxides, because a violent reaction can occur on contact with these materials. As hydrazine is a flammable liquid, it should be stored away from ignition sources. On decomposition, it gives off toxic nitrogen oxide combustion products. It is toxic by inhalational routes and can be absorbed also through the skin. Owing to its marked corrosive properties, it can cause chemical burns of the skin. Clinical toxicity includes methemoglobinemia, vomiting, tremors, seizures, liver necrosis, and hemolysis.

The vapor density of hydrazine is 1.1 (that of air being 1). It reacts exothermically and very violently with metal oxides and oxidizing agents, owing to its powerful reducing capabilities. Hydrazine vapors may cause irritation of the mucous membranes, eyes, nose, throat, and upper respiratory tract. Inhalation of vapors can produce coughing, shortness of breath, and pulmonary edema. Exposure to the eyes can produce temporary blindness. Acutely breathing the vapors will cause intense irritation of the mucous membrane and lungs and can cause nausea, vomiting, and dizziness. Higher vapor concentrations can produce tremors, seizures, and comas with hemolysis. Liquid splashes to the eyes can produce corneal injury and burns, whereas splashes to the skin can produce severe burns, dermatitis, and skin sensitization.

Hydrazine concentrations greater than 25% can produce severe burns and eye injury. Hydrazine can penetrate the skin and eye readily, and contact areas should be diluted immediately with water. Skin contact can result in itching and suppurative eczema after exposure.

Hydrazine is a probable human carcinogen and has been shown to produce lung and liver cancers and leukemia in animals. Workers who are to be in contact with hydrazine should undergo medical surveillance, including a complete blood count, liver and kidney function tests, pulmonary function tests, and neurologic evaluation, prior to placement.

The U.S. Occupational Safety and Health Administration (OSHA) permissible exposure limit (PEL) with a skin notation is 0.1 ppm. NIOSH recommends a ceiling limit of 0.04 mg per cubic meter over a 2-hour period. NIOSH also recommends an IDLH concentration of 80 ppm. Hydrazine has an odor that resembles ammonia gas. The odor threshold of hydrazine is 3.7 ppm and serves as a warning of exposure.

Hydroxylamine

Hydroxylamine (H_2NOH), a colorless, odorless crystalline solid, is a reducing agent used in organic synthesis (synthetic rubbers and graphic developing solutions) and in the production of acrylonitrile. It is explosive and flammable and produces toxic combustion by-products of nitrous oxides. Hydroxylamine may explode when exposed to heat or flames. Hydroxylamine is irritating to the skin, eyes, and mucous membrane and can cause dermatitis. It also produces methemoglobinemia. It is corrosive to the skin and mucous membranes on contact. Its TLV has not been established.

Monomethylhydrazine

Monomethylhydrazine (CH_3NHNH_2) is a fuming, colorless liquid that has an ammonia odor and boils at 88°C. It is flammable and is also known as *methylhydrazine*. Monomethylhydrazine has been used as a rocket propellant and as a solvent. It is incompatible with metal oxides and oxidizing materials, such as H_2O_2. The ceiling limit value of monomethylhydrazine is 0.2 ppm, and its IDLH level is 5 ppm. Monomethylhydrazine is a strong eye, mucous membrane, and upper respiratory irritant. It can produce symptoms of vomiting, respiratory irritation, and neurologic symptoms of tremors, ataxia, and seizures and methemoglobinemia on systemic absorption.

Boron Hydride

Boron hydride (B_2H_6) is known also as *diborane*. This strong reducing agent is used in rubber manufacturing and for high-energy fuels, including rocket fuel. The class of boron hydrides is very corrosive to synthetic rubbers and natural rubbers. Diborane has a TLV of 0.1 ppm and is a very strong pulmonary irritant. It has a sickening odor of rotten eggs; the odor detection threshold for diborane is 3.3 ppm. Because it is highly flammable as a gas (which is colorless), diborane should be protected against physical damage and stored in a refrigerated area that is well ventilated.

Diborane should not be allowed to come into contact with oxidizing agents, such as halogens, H_2O_2, or oxygen. It produces highly toxic combustion products. The IDLH inhalation limit is 40 ppm. The OSHA PEL is 0.1 mg per cubic meter (0.1 ppm as a time-weighted average). The ACGIH recommends a TLV of 0.1 ppm. The NIOSH IDLH value is 40 ppm.

Persons exposed to diborane present with chest tightness, cough, and difficulty in breathing. Its recognition odor at 3.3 ppm helps to avoid further injury. However, chronic exposure to diborane may produce olfactory fatigue. High concentrations can produce severe pulmonary irritation and pulmonary edema.

Decaborane

Decaborane ($B_{10}H_{14}$) is a colorless, crystalline, solid reducing agent with a pungent odor. It is flammable and is used in rocket propellants and as a vulcanizing agent in rubber manufacturing. It is incompatible with oxidizers, water, and halogenated hydrocarbons. The TLV for decaborane is 0.05 ppm with a dermal absorption warning. Its IDLH level is 20 ppm. Clinical toxicity is manifested by central nervous system stimulation, hyperexcitability, headaches, muscle tremors, and seizures. Decaborane can be absorbed via the skin. Early symptoms of exposure consist of dizziness, nausea, headaches, and muscle tremors; seizures occur with more severe intoxication. Symptoms usually subside in 24 to 48 hours, but fatigue may remain for up to 12 to 14 days. Neurobehavioral changes also may occur after exposures.

Pentaborane

Pentaborane (B_5H_9) is a colorless volatile liquid that ignites spontaneously in air. It hydrolyzes in water and decomposes at 150°C. Its TLV is 0.005 ppm, with an IDLH value of 3 ppm. Pentaborane is a strong reducing agent used in rocket fuel and as a gasoline additive. It is incompatible with oxidizers, halogenated hydrocarbons, and halogens. It can be absorbed by the inhalational and dermal routes. Pentaborane is the most toxic of the boron hydrides and can produce central nervous system excitation, muscle tremors, seizures, and hiccups. Early symptoms of toxicity consist of dizziness, headache, confusion, hiccups, ataxia, and tremors. Symptoms may be delayed 24 to 48 hours. Severe symptoms include coma, seizures, and neurobehavioral changes. Convulsions can occur rapidly after toxic exposure and present as opisthotonos and tonic contractions of facial muscles, neck muscles, abdomen, and extremities. Liver necrosis has occurred after exposure.

Lithium Hydride

Lithium hydride (LiH) is a reducing agent and a severe irritant of the skin, eyes, and mucous membranes. It takes the form of white crystals and has a TLV of 0.025 mg per cubic meter. Lithium hydride is a flammable solid and is dangerous when wet. It can be used as a desiccant. It is incompatible with other oxidizing agents, halogenated hydrocarbons, acids, and water. Its IDLH value is 15 mg per cubic meter. Lithium hydride can cause severe burns on skin and ocular contact. Systemic absorption can produce muscular tremors, nausea, and confusion. Ingestion also can produce burns of the esophagus and mouth. Powdered lithium hydride can ignite spontaneously in humid air or on contact with mucous membrane surfaces or moist skin surfaces and can result in thermal and alkaline burns.

Boron Tribromide

Boron tribromide (BBr_3) is a fuming liquid that boils at 90°C. It is a highly corrosive reducing agent used as a catalyst in organic chemical synthesis. The ACGIH recommends a TLV of 1 ppm. Hydrolysis produces hydrogen bromide, and the toxicity of boron tribromide is that of hydrogen bromide. Hydrogen bromide has a ceiling limit of 5 ppm. It is a gas and strong irritant of the eyes, lungs, and mucous membranes and may cause chemical burns by contact with vapors of the gas.

Boron Trifluoride

Boron trifluoride (BF_3) is a colorless, nonflammable gas used as a fumigant and a catalyst. It is a highly reactive gas with fire-retardant and antioxidant properties. When exposed to air, boron trifluoride forms a white fume. It is highly reactive with alkalis and moist air. Clinical toxicity consists of severe irritant effects of the eyes, lungs, and mucous membranes, and it can produce epistaxis. Boron trifluoride has an exposure ceiling limit of 1 ppm.

Epichlorohydrin

Epichlorohydrin (C_3H_5ClO) is highly reactive and flammable (Fig. 87-2). It is used in the manufacturing of epoxy resins, glycol, plasticizers, dye stuffs, lubricants, adhesives, pharmaceuticals, and oil emulsification products. Epichlorohydrin is a solvent for resins, gums, cellulose, esters, paints, and lacquers. It is used also as a stabilizer in chlorine-containing products, such as rubber, solvents, and pesticides.

Epichlorohydrin is a colorless liquid with a chloroformlike odor. Its vapor density equals 1.7 (that of air being 1.0). The compound is released into the environment through its use in various processes and industries. It is biodegradable, and bioaccumulation is negligible (5).

Epichlorohydrin is absorbed rapidly via skin contact, inhalation, or ingestion and is metabolized quickly. It is a strong irritant, and skin contact may cause burns and blisters that can be delayed. Epichlorohydrin is a skin sensitizer. Vapors and liquid are pulmonary irritants. Inhalation can cause pulmonary edema, vomiting, nausea, and inflammation. Animal studies demonstrate renal tubular and cortical necrosis. However, these renal effects have not been reported in studies of humans (5).

Eye and nasal irritation occurs at air concentrations of 76 mg per cubic meter (5). Skin spills can result in burns delayed from 10 minutes to several hours (5), even without initial appearance of erythema. Dermal lesions include burns, blisters, ulceration, erosions, and sensitization. Epichlorohydrin penetrates leather and rubber gloves. Asthma and bronchitis have been reported after vapor inhalation (5). Fatty degeneration of the liver has been reported after exposure (5).

Epichlorohydrin-air mixtures of 3.8% to 21.0% epichlorohydrin per volume of air are explosive in excess of 34°C and can be ignited by hot surface contact or flame at a distance because of the chemical's vapor density. Contact of epichlorohydrin with strong bases, acids, zinc, aluminum, metal chlorides, alcohols, trichloroethylene, isopropylamine, and oxidizing agents can cause fires or explosions. Burning epichlorohydrin produces a mist of hydrogen chloride, phosgene, and carbon monoxide. The chemical may polymerize rapidly if its container is exposed to a fire and explodes. It should be stored in a cool, dry room. The PEL for this chemical is 10 mg per cubic meter, the TLV-time-weighted average is 10 mg per cubic meter, and the OSHA STEL is 20 mg per cubic meter.

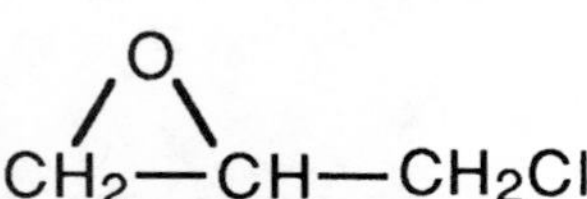

Figure 87-2. Chemical composition of epichlorohydrin.

WATER-REACTIVE AND SELF-REACTIVE CHEMICALS

Water-reactive and self-reactive chemicals include organometals, metal dusts, alkali metals (e.g., sodium, potassium, lithium), and numerous other compounds. Many reactive chemicals release toxic gases when they contact water (Table 87-6): chlorine, hydrogen chloride, phosphine, hydrogen fluoride, nitrogen dioxide, ammonia, hydrogen sulfide, hydrogen iodide, and hydrogen bro-

TABLE 87-6. Materials that create toxic vapors on contact with water

Material	Toxic vapor produced
Methyldichlorosilane	HCl
Methyltrichlorosilane	HCl
Trichlorosilane	HCl
Calcium phosphide	PH_3
Aluminum phosphide	PH_3
Lithium amide	NH_3
Magnesium aluminum phosphide	PH_3
Sodium phosphide	PH_3
Stannic phosphides	PH_3
Lithium hypochlorite, dry (oxidizer)	Cl_2 HCl
Lithium hypochlorite mixture (oxidizer)	Cl_2 HCl
Lithium hypochlorite mixtures, dry (oxidizer)	Cl_2 HCl
Potassium cyanide	HCN
Sodium cyanide	HCN
Zinc phosphide	PH_3
Acetyl bromide	HBr
Acetyl chloride	HCl
Aluminum bromide, anhydrous	HBr
Aluminum chloride, anhydrous	HCl
Antimony pentafluoride	HF
Calcium hypochlorite, dry (oxidizer)	Cl_2 HCl
Calcium hypochlorite mixture, dry (oxidizer), with more than 39% available chlorine (8.8% available oxygen)	Cl_2 HCl
Chromium oxychloride	HCl
Fluorosulfonic acid	HF
Phosphorus pentachloride	HCl
Silicon tetrachloride	HCl
Thionyl chloride	HCl SO_2
Acetyl iodide	HI
Magnesium diamide	NH_3
Magnesium phosphide	PH_3
Potassium phosphide	PH_3
Strontium phosphide	PH_3
Nitrosylsulfuric acid	NO_2
Iodine pentafluoride	HF
Ammonium hydrosulfide, solution	NH_3 H_2S
Ammonium sulfide, solution	NH_3 H_2S
Lithium nitride	NH_3
Uranium hexafluoride, fissile	HF
Aluminum phosphide pesticide	PH_3
Chlorine dioxide, hydrate, frozen	Cl_2

mide. Such toxic vapors can injure tissues directly and can produce toxic metabolic effects.

Self-reactive chemicals undergo self-decomposition or self-ignition that can be triggered by heat, friction, impact, or chemical reactions. These chemicals may burn violently or explode.

REFERENCES

1. Meyers E. *Chemistry of hazardous materials.* Englewood Cliffs, NJ: Prentice-Hall, 1977.
2. Sherman SJ, Boyer L, Sibley W. Cerebral infarction immediately after ingestion of hydrogen peroxide solution. *Stroke* 1994;25(5):1065–1067.
3. Considine D, Considine G. *Encyclopedia of chemistry.* New York: Van Nostrand–Reinhold, 1984.
4. Martinez T, Long C. Explosion risk from swimming pool chlorinators and review of chlorine toxicity, clinical toxicology. *J Toxicol Clin Toxicol* 1995;33(4):349–354.
5. World Health Organization. *Epichlorhydrin—environmental health criteria 33.* Geneva: World Health Organization, 1984.

CHAPTER 88

Metal Oxides

Francis J. Farrell

Metal oxides produce four types of lung disease: metal fume fever, chemical pneumonitis, hypersensitivity pneumonitis, and occupational asthma (1). Metal fume fever, a common acute industrial disease, is caused by the inhalation of oxides of metals, especially zinc. The first description was published by Potissier in 1822 (2). It was first described by Thackrah in 1831 among brass founders in England (3). Gardner, in 1848, gave the first report in the United States (4). The disease is also known as *brazier's disease, spelter shakes, brass chills, zinc chills, welder's ague, copper fever, Monday fever, foundry fever, the smothers,* and *galvo* (5–12). Various metal oxides can cause this syndrome, but the most common are oxides of zinc, copper, brass (copper and zinc alloy), and magnesium (13–21). Less common culprits are manganese, antimony, silver, tin, selenium, aluminum, nickel, vanadium, chromium, stainless steel, cadmium, lead, iron, cobalt, mercury, and arsenic.

INDUSTRIAL EXPOSURES

Metal fume fever occurs most commonly among welders. According to one report, of welders aged 20 to 59 years, 31% have had metal fume fever (18). However, it also may occur among zinc smelters, brass solderers, brass foundry workers, chrome electroplaters, chrome welders (from hexavalent chromic oxide fumes), iron galvanizers, molten metal fabricators, metal grinders, manufacturers of steel alloys, and those who work near electric furnaces that are used to melt metals.

Zinc oxide is extremely volatile at relatively low temperatures, and therefore a large amount of zinc oxide fume (powder) is produced during welding on galvanized metal and in the smelting process. The zinc oxide particles formed range in size from 0.2 to 1.0 µm. The small particle size allows the zinc oxide to pass into the smaller bronchial alveoli. Typically, the syndrome of metal fume fever begins 4 to 12 hours after sufficient exposure to freshly formed fumes of zinc oxide (22).

Welding is a process of joining metals in which adherence is produced by heating the metals to the appropriate temperature. Brazing is a form of welding. In these processes are a number of similar techniques such as oxygen cutting and arc gouging. The latter method is used for removing metal. Several types of welding exist and are reviewed next.

Arc Welding

"Arc welding occurs when the arc electrode is brought in contact with the work piece. A high temperature arc is thus initiated between them. The heat generated by the arc is controlled by current and the length of the arc. When these two are correct, the tip of the electrode and the base metal beneath it are melted. As the electrode tip melts, globules are pinched off, passing through the arc to be deposited in the molten puddle of the base metal. At the same time, the (flux) coating also melts to stabilize the arc and provide a gaseous shield against atmospheric contamination caused by oxygen and nitrogen. The cooling liquefied flux also provides a shield against contamination of the weld bead" (23).

MANUAL METAL ARC

Manual metal arc (MMA; also called *stick welding*) is a form of electric welding that uses a flux-coated, consumable stick electrode. The part to be welded and the consumable wire electrode represent two electrodes that are attached to an AC or DC power supply. When the electrodes are near one another, the electric arc is established. The metal bead is deposited, and joining occurs.

Vaporization of the electrode constituents produces a complex particulate fume by condensation. Also, the electrode itself and the flux both produce fume. Fumes are solid particles generated by condensation from the gaseous state, generally after volatilization from molten metals and often accompanied by a chemical reaction such as oxidation. Fumes flocculate and sometimes coalesce (24).

The flux-coated electrode has an antioxide effect, which allows the welds to have physical properties equal to or exceeding those of the parent metal (23). The flux or coating materials on the electrode provide an automatic cleansing and deoxidizing action on the molten weld. As the coating burns in the arc, it releases a gaseous inert atmosphere that protects the molten end of the electrode as well as the molten weld pool (23).

MMA fumes consist of chains and clusters of submicrometer particles and glassy, coated spheres up to 10 µm in diameter (25). Approximately 20% of MMA fume is deposited initially in the lungs of laboratory animals, and the balance is exhaled depending on particle size (25).

METAL INERT GAS

A second type of electric arc welding, metal inert gas welding, uses a gas-shielded consumable wire electrode. The welding torch has a center of consumable wire. Next to the electrode on the torch is a flow of inert gas such as helium, argon, carbon dioxide, or a blend of these gases (26), which results in high metal fume concentrations. The gas is used to prevent the formation of oxides and nitrides with the weld metal, which weakens the weld ductility and tensile strength.

In metal inert gas welding, there is no flux, and hence the fume is less complex than that produced by MMA. Chains are formed by condensation, which are submicron in diameter and may be as long as 100 µm (25). These chains are made up of oxide-encapsulated metals.

Gas Welding

In gas welding, the torch flame is generated by oxygen-gas fuel. Filler rods coated with flux release metal fumes. Electrodes may be made of stainless steel, copper, brass, bronze, aluminum, or lead. Bronze is an alloy of copper and tin to which other metallic substances, especially zinc, sometimes are added. Bronze is hard, sonorous, and sometimes brittle. It is used for statues, bells, and cannons, the proportion of the respective ingredients being varied to meet the particular requirements. Brass, on the other hand, is a yellowish metal that is essentially an alloy of copper and zinc. The type of electrode depends on the type of metal being welded.

CLINICAL TOXICOLOGY

Zinc Oxide Exposure

When zinc or its alloys are heated to temperatures exceeding 930°F, particles of zinc up to 1 μm in diameter are formed (27). Inhaled trace particles less than 1 μm in diameter cause the acute febrile illness known as *metal fume fever*, which is common in welders who work on various types of nonferrous metals or ferrous metals alloyed with or coated with other metals. Zinc fume from galvanized coatings is the most common cause. However, aluminum, antimony, nickel, selenium, silver, and tin metal fumes are produced in all high-temperature industrial operations such as welding. The submicrometer particles are deposited in different parts of the respiratory tract, but up to 50% of the inhaled particles are deposited in the lower regions (28). Individual variations occur depending on the breathing rate and tidal volume and whether inhalation is by nose or mouth. Metals are retained in the lung, cleared, or swallowed, or pass through the pulmonary tissues via the blood or lymph, and thus systemic absorption occurs (28).

Zinc is used to retard corrosion and impart a desirable surface texture. The zinc coating (galvanizing) is applied either by dipping the metal piece in a bath of molten zinc or by electroplating (23). Because the zinc oxide is highly volatile at relatively low temperatures, operations involving molten metals and galvanized metal can produce large amounts of zinc oxide fume, which is a dense white smoke. The U.S. Occupational Safety and Health Administration limit and threshold limit value (TLV) for 1980 for zinc oxide and zinc chloride are 5 and 1 mg per cubic meter, respectively (29).

Cadmium Oxide Exposure

Exposure to cadmium should always be considered in the differential diagnosis of metal fume fever, because of its potential seriousness. Cadmium is a lustrous white metal and has broad industrial uses ranging from electroplating to solder used in welding and brazing (30). It is a ubiquitous trace element, nonessential for human nutrition but present in the environment, especially in sea water, drinking water, meat, certain grains, and many dairy products (31). More than 10 million pounds of cadmium are used industrially in the United States each year. The metal is used in the manufacture of electrical conductors, bearings, ceramics, pigments, vapor lamps, dental prosthetics, and storage batteries; for rustproofing of tools and other steel articles; and as a component in various alloys. The photographic plating, rubber, motor, aircraft, and battery industries all use cadmium, and it is a by-product of zinc smelting (32). Cadmium is highly resistant to corrosion. Oxyacetylene burning and welding or soldering of cadmium-containing metal is especially hazardous where ventilation is inadequate. This has become a common health hazard: For example, coppersmiths and plumbers soldering copper tubing may be heavily exposed to cadmium. Serious problems may occur without recognition, because most workers are not aware of the potential toxicity of cadmium and therefore take no precautions against it (31). In addition, the initial symptoms of cadmium exposure usually are not sufficiently severe to cause individuals to seek medical attention.

The acute inhalation of cadmium fumes can cause both metal fume fever and chemical pneumonitis. Patterson (33) described three stages of lung damage in rats after inhalation of cadmium oxide: (i) acute pulmonary edema within 24 hours and lasting 3 days; (ii) proliferative interstitial pneumonitis 3 to 10 days after exposure, with epithelial and fibroblastic proliferation in lung parenchyma; and (iii) permanent lung damage consisting of perivascular and peribronchial fibrosis. Initially, acute exposure symptoms resemble metal fume fever but, after 24 hours, instead of improvement in the patient's condition, pulmonary edema and chemical pneumonitis occur. The condition may resolve over 7 days but, in 20% of cases, the dyspnea is progressive and may be accompanied by wheezing or hemoptysis; in these cases, death occurs 5 to 7 days after exposure (28,30,32). After cadmium oxide has been inhaled, months may pass before a patient's pulmonary function studies return to normal. Chronic poisoning may also produce disease, including emphysema (32). The vapor pressure at its melting point (320°C) is very significant, and hence a concentration of 50,000 times the safe limit can easily be produced when cadmium is melted.

The current Occupational Safety and Health Administration standard for cadmium dust is 200 μg per cubic meter as an 8-hour time-weighted average and 600 μg per cubic meter as a maximum ceiling. The American Conference of Governmental Industrial Hygienists recommended a ceiling limit for cadmium oxide fumes of 50 μg per cubic meter and an 8-hour time-weighted average standard for cadmium dust and salts (as cadmium) of 50 μg per cubic meter (29).

Metal Fume Fever

CLINICAL DIAGNOSIS

Metal fume fever has been described as resembling a flulike illness or acute malaria (34). The onset of this syndrome occurs 4 to 6 hours after sufficient exposure. Early signs and symptoms are shaking chills, weakness, muscle and joint aches, sweating, and high fever (35). The presenting symptoms are a metallic or sweet taste in the mouth, frequently accompanied by dryness and thirst. Throat irritation, dyspnea with occasional coughing, and wheezing occur (36), as may weakness, fatigue, and shortness of breath. Leukocytosis may occur during the acute period. In addition to low-grade fever, physical examination may reveal rales and wheezing (5,29,36), although bradycardia or tachycardia is rare. On occasion, persons exposed experience pleuritic chest pains and, rarely, paresthesias (6). A macular rash rarely is present (5). Hoarseness, vomiting, headaches, lethargy, sweating, and joint pain are noted sometimes. The episode runs its course in 24 to 48 hours, and a temporary period of tolerance (a day or two afterward) may ensue—hence the name *Monday fever*. Usually, no long-term complications are present, and the syndrome can recur frequently without major physiologic damage, although this point is somewhat controversial (37,38).

LABORATORY DIAGNOSIS

Arterial blood gas analyses frequently show hypoxemia, depending on the severity of exposure. The chest radiograph usually is normal but, in severe exposure, may show pneumonitis or pulmonary edema. Pulmonary function studies may be normal or may reveal a decrease in forced vital capacity but rarely show an obstructive pattern (39). Occasionally, the diffusing capacity of carbon monoxide is decreased (40). Bronchoalveolar lavage studies exhibit an increase in tumor necrosis factor and interleukin-6 and -8 in humans (41). Interleukin-1 (IL-1) also

TABLE 88-1. Laboratory findings in metal fume fever

- Leukocytosis
- Hypoxemia on arterial blood gas analysis
- Possible demonstration of pneumonitis or pulmonary edema on chest radiograph after severe exposure, although usually normal
- Lowered forced vital capacity (restrictive) on spirometry; rarely obstructive
- Decreased diffusing capacity of carbon monoxide
- Increased lactate dehydrogenase level
- Possibly elevated urinary or serum metal levels, although usually not helpful
- Pulmonary shunting
- Increased tumor necrosis factor, interleukin-6, and interleukin-8 in bronchoalveolar lavage fluid

may be involved (41). In some cases, the lactate dehydrogenase level is elevated (36). If zinc is involved, the serum zinc level may be increased. Determination of urinary zinc levels usually is not helpful. Urinary copper may be increased if copper exposure is the cause but, in general, serum or urinary metal determinations are of little help in the diagnosis. There may be evidence of pulmonary shunting (Table 88-1) (5).

Because no specific laboratory or physical findings exist to establish a diagnosis, the clinician must rely on a careful history. The symptoms may resemble a flulike illness, malaria, or septicemia. Hence, the diagnosis may escape early detection. Frequently, because of the incubation time, symptoms may occur after the workday has ended, and the patient may not seek medical attention. The best clues to an early diagnosis are a history of exposure, a metallic taste, and nasal irritation (36).

MANAGEMENT

The treatment of metal fume fever is supportive. Intravenous steroids may be given in severe cases, and intravenous theophylline and inhaled bronchodilators may be administered to alleviate wheezing. Oxygen is helpful, but antibiotics have proved to be of little value. Monitoring is generally recommended for a 24-hour period depending on the severity of the chemical syndrome (Table 88-2). Pulmonary function tests usually revert to normal within this time frame but, on occasion, may remain abnormal for long periods (6). One case report describes a "disabling pneumopathy" that occurred after recurrent metal fume fever (42). Myocardial and skeletal muscle injuries were reported in one case (43). Exposure to zinc fumes is not considered to be teratogenic or carcinogenic.

PATHOPHYSIOLOGIC FEATURES

The exact cause of metal fume fever is unknown, although some interesting immunologic associations have been made. Nonetheless, it generally is thought that this syndrome does not have an immunologic basis, because prior exposure is not required (Table 88-3) (2). One theory states that the presence of finely divided and dispersed metallic oxide in the lung destroys the microorganisms of the lower respiratory passages, thereby liberating endotoxins into the alveolar capillaries and causing an acute febrile response. Once this sterilization has occurred, it renders the lower respiratory tract "immune" to further fume exposure until sufficient time has elapsed to allow the reaccumulation of organisms (21). The accumulation of zinc particles in the alveoli and resident macrophages, resulting in metal fume fever and, eventually, pulmonary fibrosis, has been demonstrated in rats (44).

TABLE 88-2. Treatment guidelines for exposure to metal fumes

- Terminate exposure.
- Administer oxygen by mask.
- Provide supportive pulmonary care.
- Administer inhalation therapy with bronchodilators if indicated for bronchospasm.
- Administer theophylline loading and maintenance doses as necessary for adjunct management of bronchospasm.
- Observe symptomatic individuals for 24 hours.
- Consider use of corticosteroids in severe cases.
- Avoid use of antibiotics as these agents are of no value except in secondary infection.
- Check creatine phosphokinase and cardiac enzyme levels as indicated.

TABLE 88-3. Metal fume fever mechanism theories

- Modification of lung proteins by absorption, foreign protein reactions, endotoxins, or a nonspecific response to interleukin-1 (19–21,46)
- Immune complex disease (40,59)
- Accumulation in alveolar macrophages of metal particles that interfere with phagocytosis (44)
- Hypersensitivity pneumonitis (1,48)
- Delayed immunoglobulin E reaction (51)
- Increased tumor necrosis factor, interleukin-6, and interleukin-8 in bronchoalveolar lavage fluid; possibly, increased interleukin-1 also (41)

It is well known that the macrophage produces IL-1 in a response to a variety of nonspecific stimuli, including immune complexes, lipopolysaccharides, leukotrienes, and IL-2 (45). Synonyms for IL-1 include *endogenous pyrogen*, *hemopoietin-1*, and *catabolin*. IL-1 is an inflammatory cytokine produced primarily by macrophages. IL-1α is membrane-bound, whereas IL-1β is secreted. Therefore, IL-1 secretion's net effect is to contain invaders. Hence, it represents a primitive protective system, but too much secretion can result in disease. For example, massive infection can cause shaking chills and fever that resemble septicemia or metal fume fever. Hence, metal fume fever may be due to the nonspecific protective action of stimulated macrophages producing IL-1. Blanc et al. (41) have recently demonstrated also an increase of tumor necrosis factor, IL-6, and IL-8 in bronchoalveolar lavage fluid after zinc exposure (41). Although no one knows exactly how long it takes for the macrophage to recover after discharge, it is tempting to speculate that this time period would represent the refractory interval seen in metal fume fever.

A number of researchers suggested that metal fume fever was caused by a modification of lung protein attributable to the zinc fumes, which then was absorbed and produced a foreign protein reaction (20,44,46). Mueller and Seger (40) suggested the possibility that immune complexes were formed, resulting in the symptoms. Migally et al. (44) demonstrated that zinc particles accumulate in the alveoli and resident macrophages and suggested that these events result in metal fume fever and, eventually, pulmonary fibrosis.

In guinea pigs exposed to the current TLV of zinc at 5 mg per cubic meter, functional, morphologic, and biochemical changes indicative of an inflammatory reaction involving mainly the peripheral airways were noted (47). Infiltration of the proximal portion of the alveolar ducts in the adjacent alveoli was noted, characterized by interstitial thickening, increased pulmonary macrophages, and neutrophils. A mixed cellular infiltrate of macrophages, lymphocytes, and neutrophils was found. Pulmonary flow resistance increased and remained increased for 24 hours. Compliance decreased below that of controls for 48 hours, and resistance increased. The latter was believed to be attributable to abnormalities in the small airways. Edema and premature closing of the small airways was thought to contrib-

TABLE 88-4. Types of hypersensitivity pneumonitis

Antigen	Antigen source	Name of disorder
Thermophilic actinomycetes		
Micropolyspora faeni	Moldy hay	Farmer's lung
	Mushroom compost	Mushroom worker's lung
Thermoactinomyces vulgaria	Moldy sugarcane	Bagassosis
	Moldy hay	Farmer's lung
	Mushroom compost	Mushroom worker's lung
Thermoactinomyces sacchari	Moldy compost	Mushroom worker's disease
	Bagasse	Bagassosis
Thermoactinomyces candidus	Contaminated home humidifier and air-conditioning ducts	Humidifier lung
Thermoactinomyces virdis	Cattle	Fog fever
	Moldy cork	Suberosis
	Vineyards	Vineyard sprayer's lung
	Ventilation system	
True fungi		
Aspergillus clavatus	Moldy malt	Malt worker's lung
	Moldy barley	Farmer's lung
Aspergillus fumigatus	Moldy cheese	Cheese washer's lung
	Moldy hay	Farmer's lung
Cryptostroma corticale	Moldy maple logs	Maple bark disease
	Maple bark	Maple bark stripper's lung
Graphium sp.	Moldy wood dust (especially redwood)	Sequoiosis
Pullularia sp.	Moldy wood dust	Sequoiosis
	Water and steam	Sauna taker's lung
Alternaria sp.	Moldy wood pulp	Wood pulp worker's disease
Mucor stolonifer	Moldy paprika pods	Paprika slicer's lung
Penicillium caseii	Cheese mold	Cheese worker's lung
	Humidifier water	Humidifier lung
Cephalosporium sp.	Humidifier water	Humidifier lung
Penicillium frequentans	Moldy cork dust	Suberosis
Aspergillus versicolor		Dog house disease
Lycoperdon		Lycoperdonosis
Animal causes		
Furrier's lung		
Pigeon serum proteins	Pigeon droppings	Pigeon breeder's disease
Duck proteins	Feathers	Duck fever
Turkey proteins	Turkey products	Turkey handler's disease
Parrot serum proteins	Parrot droppings	Budgerigar fancier's disease
Chicken proteins	Chicken products	Feather plucker's disease
Bovine and porcine proteins	Pituitary snuff	Pituitary snuff taker's lung
Rat serum protein	Rat urine	
Bat serum protein	Bat droppings	Bat lung
Insect products		
Ascaris siro (mite)	Dust	
Sitophilus granarius (wheat weevil)	Contamination grain	Miller's lung
Amebae		
Naegleriaruberi	Contaminated water	
Acanthamoeba polyphaga	Humidifier water	Humidifier lung
Acanthamoeba castellani		
Vegetable products (unknown)	Sawdust (redwood, maple, red cedar)	Sequoiosis
	Cereal grain	Grain measurer's lung
	Dried grass and leaves	Thatched roof disease
	Tobacco plants	Tobacco grower's disease
	Tea plants	Tea grower's disease
	Cloth wrappings of mummies	Coptic disease
Chemicals, drugs, metals		
Toluene diisocyanate	Urethane foam	
Nitrofurantoin	Iatrogenic	
Sodium cromolyn	Iatrogenic	Sodium cromolyn lung
Hydrochlorothiazide	Iatrogenic	
Hard metals		Hard metal disease
Zinc		
Beryllium		
Pauli's reagent		Pauli's reagent lung
Thermotolerant bacteria		
Bacillus subtilis enzymes	Detergent	Detergent worker's lung
Bacillus cereus	Humidifier water	Humidifier lung

ute to decreased compliance. Lung volumes were decreased after exposure, probably owing to edema and cellular infiltration. These latter manifestations were considered to be responsible for the decrease in the diffusing capacity of carbon monoxide and for the resultant hypoxemia.

On the basis of previously cited studies, some authors have speculated that metal fume fever might be a form of hypersensitivity pneumonitis (1,48,49). Hypersensitivity pneumonitis, a flulike illness occurring 6 to 8 hours after exposure, usually to organic dust, has been reported to occur also after exposure to cobalt and beryllium (50) and to zinc (Table 88-4) (1,48,49). The symptoms in each case are very similar.

Hypersensitivity Pneumonitis

Hypersensitivity pneumonitis (extrinsic allergy alveolitis) actually represents a group of lung diseases affecting the small airways, the alveoli, and the interstitium. These diseases are caused by a variety of inhaled organic dusts but also by other agents (see Table 88-4). Sensitization to the particular antigen—which may be animal or plant proteins, microorganisms, fungi, organic dust, and occasionally, low-molecular-weight chemicals as well as metals—occurs.

The several forms of hypersensitivity pneumonitis are acute, subacute, and chronic. The condition usually is associated in the acute stage with precipitating antibodies to the particular antigen. The classic acute features are fever, myalgia, and lethargy 4 to 8 hours after exposure to the offending antigen. This presentation usually is accompanied by chest tightness or wheezing, a dry cough, and dyspnea. Generally, the symptoms improve within 24 hours in the absence of additional exposure. Physical examination reveals fever, tachycardia, and dyspnea. Occasionally, rales or wheezing is noted but, more often, auscultation of the chest is clear. Leukocytosis may occur. Pulmonary function studies reveal a restrictive defect. On repeated exposure, chronic interstitial lung disease may develop.

The chest radiograph is variable but may demonstrate a pattern resembling pulmonary edema. Activated T cells are increased in the bronchoalveolar lavage fluid. Pathologically, there may be numerous noncaseating, sarcoidlike granulomas, usually associated with giant cells (2). Infiltration with monocytes (e.g., lymphocytes, plasma cells, and histiocytes) also may be noted. Alveolar macrophages are increased. Some patients may exhibit hypersensitivity pneumonitis but have no precipitins, whereas other patients have precipitins but no disease. The exact pathogenesis is not known, although complement activation is believed to play a part and, in some cases, the immune mechanism may be immune complex formation. The alternate complement pathway may be activated. Hence, the common features between hypersensitivity pneumonitis and metal fume fever can be seen.

Farrell reported a case of angioedema and urticaria as acute and late-phase reactions to zinc fume exposure (51). The patient also had associated metal fume fever–like symptoms. Hives and angioedema developed immediately and in a delayed fashion in a 34-year-old man after he had welded zinc at his job; the exposure resulted in an associated metal fume fever–like reaction 6 to 8 hours later. The author found it conceivable that a delayed-type immunoglobulin E mechanism was involved. Mast cell degranulation in human skin causes both immediate and late-phase allergic reactions (52–54). The mediators released cause an influx of neutrophils and eosinophils at the site, which in turn initiates a more chronic inflammatory reaction of mononuclear cells (55). It has been postulated that basophils attracted to the site during the immediate allergic reaction, rather than mast cells, are stimulated to degranulate during the late-phase reaction (56). Also, mast cells might be restimulated to release additional mediators during the late-phase reaction. Human neutrophil–derived histamine-releasing activity (HRA-N), as described by White and Callender (1985), is released spontaneously by neutrophils (57). Only certain immunoglobulin E molecules interact with HRA-N to produce the late-phase reaction, and this heterogeneity explains why some patients have a late-phase reaction and others do not (57,58).

Kaplan and Zelichman (17) reported a case of a welder who developed dyspnea and hives within 15 minutes after acetylene welding with a rod containing iron, carbon, manganese, phosphorus, sulfur, silicon, chromium, and vanadium. This was proven by challenge testing. An interesting aspect of the case was that the patient had a history of metal fume fever previously but did not develop metal fume fever symptoms after the challenge. This too was suggestive of an immunologic reaction.

BIOLOGICAL AND ENVIRONMENTAL MONITORING

In conclusion, biological monitoring should be undertaken in workers, and workers should adhere strictly to established permissible exposure limits and TLVs. To prevent metal fume fever, adequate ventilation should be ensured in work areas where metals are heated to extreme temperatures that could incite the formation of oxide fumes. The diagnosis of cadmium chemical pneumonitis should always be considered because of its potential seriousness.

REFERENCES

1. Malo JL, Cartier JA. Occupational asthma due to fumes of galvanized metal. *Chest* 1987;92:375–377.
2. Morgan WKC, Seaton A. *Occupational lung disease*, 2nd ed. Philadelphia: WB Saunders, 1984:575.
3. McMillan G. Metal fume fever. *Occup Health* 1986;38:148–149.
4. Zenz C. Other metals. In: *Occupational medicine*, 2nd ed. Chicago: Year Book Medical Publishers, 1988:645–646.
5. Dula D. Metal fume fever. *J Am Coll Emerg Phys* 1978;7:448.
6. Anseline P. Zinc fume fever. *Med J Aust* 1972;2:316–318.
7. Asher F. *Hamilton & Hardy's industrial toxicology*, 4th ed. Littleton, CO: PSG Publishers, 1983:146–148.
8. Papp J. Metal fume fever. *Postgrad Med* 1968;43:160–163.
9. Stake J. Metal fume fever in ferro-chrome workers. *Cent Afr J Med* 1977; 23:25–28.
10. Smith C. Metal fume fever—a case review. *Occup Health Nurs J* 1980;28:23–25.
11. Fishburn CW, Zenz C. Metal fume fever—a report of a case. *J Occup Med* 1969;11:142–144.
12. Hopper W. Case report—metal fume fever. *Postgrad Med* 1978;5:123–124.
13. Drinker P. Certain aspects of the problem of zinc toxicity. *J Ind Hyg Toxicol* 1922;8:177–197.
14. Hammond JW. Metal fume fever in the crushed stone industry. *J Ind Hyg Toxicol* 1944;24:117–119.
15. Glass WI. Mercury fume fever. *N Z Med J* 1970;71:297–298.
16. Drinker K, Drinker P. Metal fume fever V—results of the inhalation by animals of zinc and magnesium oxide fumes. *J Ind Hyg Toxicol* 1928;10:56.
17. Kaplan I, Zelichman I. Urticaria and asthma from acetylene welding. *Arch Dermatol* 1963;88:188–194.
18. Ross R. Welders metal fume. *J Soc Occup Med* 1974;24:125–129.
19. Sayers RR. Metal fume fever and its prevention. *Public Health Rep* 1938;24:1080–1086.
20. Koelsch F. Metal fume fever. *J Ind Hyg Toxicol* 1923;8:87–97.
21. Kuh J, Collen M, Kuh C. Metal fume fever. *Permanente Found Med Bull* 1946;4:145–151.
22. Key MM, Henschel AF, Butler J, Ligo RN, Tabershaw IR. *Occupational diseases: a guide to their recognition*. Washington: US Department of Health, Education, and Welfare, Government Printing Office, 1977:408–410.
23. *Arc electrode manual*, 4th ed. Lake Zurich: Jefferson Publications (no. 13).

24. Levy BS, Wegman DH. *Occupational health.* Boston: Little, Brown and Company, 1983:471.
25. Hewitt PJ, Ray CN. Some difficulties in the assessment of electric arc welding fume. *Am Ind Hyg Assoc J* 1983;44:727–732.
26. Burgess WA. Potential exposures in industry—their recognition and control. In: Clayton G, Clayton F, eds. *Patty's industrial hygiene and toxicology.* New York: John Wiley and Sons, 1978:1172–1178.
27. Stokinger HE. *Industrial hygiene and toxicology,* 2nd ed. New York: John Wiley and Sons, 1967:1183,1186,1187.
28. Piscator M. Health hazards from inhalation of metal fumes. *Environ Res* 1976;11:268–270.
29. Rom W. *Environmental and occupational medicine.* Boston: Little, Brown and Company, 1983:503.
30. Barnart S, Rosenstock L. Cadmium chemical pneumonitis. *Chest* 1984;86: 789–791.
31. Johnson J, Kilburn K. Cadmium-induced metal fume fever—results of inhalation challenges. *Am J Ind Med* 1983;4:533–540.
32. Louria D, Joselow MM, Browder AA. The human toxicity of certain trace metals. *Ann Intern Med* 1972;76:307–319.
33. Patterson JC. Studies on toxicity of cadmium: pathology of cadmium poisoning in man and experimental animals. *J Ind Hyg Toxicol* 1947;29:294–301.
34. Doig AT, Challen PJR. Respiratory hazards in welding. *Ann Occup Hyg* 1964;7:223–231.
35. Sturgis CC, Drinker P, Thomson RM. Metal fume fever, part 1: clinical observations on the effect of the experimental inhalation of zinc oxide by two apparently normal persons. *J Ind Hyg* 1927;9:88–97.
36. Armstrong CW, Moore LW, Hackler RL, Miller B Jr, Strouble RB. An outbreak of metal fume fever—the diagnostic use of urinary copper and zinc determinations. *J Occup Med* 1983;12:886–888.
37. Drinker P, Thomson RM, Finn JL. Metal fume fever, part 4: threshold doses of zinc oxide, preventive measures, and the chronic effects of repeated exposures. *J Ind Hyg* 1927;9:331–345.
38. Roto P. Asthma, symptoms of chronic bronchitis and ventilatory capacity among cobalt and zinc production workers. *Scand J Work Environ Health* 1980;6[Suppl 1]:1–49.
39. Anthony JS, Zamel N, Aberman A. Abnormalities in pulmonary function after brief exposure to toxic metal fumes. *Can Med Assoc J* 1978;119:586–588.
40. Mueller EJ, Seger DL. Metal fume fever—a review. *J Emerg Med* 1985;2:271–274.
41. Blanc PD, Boushey HA, Wong H, Wintermeyer SF, Berstein MS. Cytokines in metal fume fever. *Am Rev Respir Dis* 1993;147:134–138.
42. Hartman AL, Hartman W, Buhlmann AA. Magnesium oxide as a cause of metal fume fever. *Schweiz Med Wochenschr* 1983;113:776–770.
43. Shusterman D, Neal E. Skeletal muscle and myocardial injury associated with metal fume fever. *J Fam Pract* 1986;23:159–160.
44. Migally N, Murphy RC, Doye A, Zambernad J. Changes in pulmonary alveolar macrophages in rats exposed to oxide of zinc and nickel. *J Submicrosc Cytol* 1982;14:621–626.
45. Strober W, James S. The interleukins. *Pediatr Res* 1988;24:111–119.
46. Amdur MO, McCarthy JF, Gill MW. Respiratory response of guinea pigs to zinc oxide fume. *Am Ind Hyg Assoc J* 1982;43:887–889.
47. Lam HF, Conner MW, Rogers AE, Fitzgerald S, Amdur MO. Functional and morphologic changes in the lungs of guinea pigs exposed to freshly generated ultrafine zinc oxide. *Toxicol Appl Pharmacol* 1978;78:29–38.
48. Trudeau C, Malo JL, Cartier A. Hypersensitivity pneumonitis after exposure to zinc. In: *Proceedings of the American Academy of Allergy and Immunology Annual Meeting,* 1989;173(abstr 6).
49. Ameille J, Brechot JM, Brochard P, Capron F, Dore MF. Occupational hypersensitivity pneumonitis in a smelter exposed to zinc fumes. *Chest* 1992; 101:862–863.
50. Mandel J, Baker B. Recognizing occupational lung disease. *Hosp Pract* 1989;24:21–30.
51. Farrell FJ. Angioedema and urticaria as acute and late-phase reaction to zinc fume exposure, with associated metal fume fever–like symptoms. *Am J Ind Med* 1987;12:331–337.
52. Lemanske RF Jr, Kaliner M. Mast cell–dependent late-phase reactions. *Clin Immunol Rev* 1981–82;1:547–548.
53. Lemanske RF Jr, Kalinger MA. Late-phase allergic reactions. *Int J Dermatol* 1983;22:401–409.
54. Lemanske RF Jr, Guthman DA, Oertel H, Barr L, Kaliner M. The biologic activity of mast cell granules, part 6: the effect of vinblastine-induced neutropenia on rat cutaneous late-phase reactions. *J Immunol* 1983;130:2837–2842.
55. Kaliner MA. Late-phase reactions. *N Engl Regional Allergy Proc* 1986;7:236–240.
56. Nacleno RM, Proud D, Togias AG, et al. Inflammatory mediators in late antigen-induced rhinitis. *N Engl J Med* 1985;313:65–70.
57. Warner JA, Pienkowski MM, Plaut M, Norman PS, Lichtenstein LM. Identification of histamine releasing factor(s) in the late phase of cutaneous IgE-mediated reactions. *J Immunol* 1986;136:2583–2587.
58. Orchard MA, Kagey-Sobotka A, Proud D, Lichtenstein LM. Basophil histamine release induced by a substance from stimulated human platelets. *J Immunol* 1986;136:2240–2244.

CHAPTER 89

Organometals

Claus-Peter Siegers and John B. Sullivan, Jr.

WATER-REACTIVE AND PYROPHORIC ORGANOMETALS

Organometals react violently with water, ignite spontaneously in air, and are flammable. As such, they present clear health hazards (1,2). Materials that spontaneously combust on exposure to air are termed *pyrophoric.*

Organometals are volatile liquids with unique toxicity and high chemical reactivity. These compounds contain a metal covalently bound to the carbon atom of an organic group in one of the following forms: (i) metals covalently bound to the carbon atom of an alkyl organic group, (ii) alkyl or aryl metallic compounds of electropositive metals forming an ionic compound, and (iii) compounds containing metals that are bound to aromatic rings, alkenes, or alkynes (1).

The organic group attached to a metal atom depends on the valence state of the metal. Carbonyl compounds contain the carbonyl group C = O, which imparts increased acidity and also provides a site for nucleophilic addition (3). The activity of a carbonyl group toward nucleophiles is due to the presence of the oxygen in the carbonyl group that imparts a tendency for a positive charge on the carbon (3).

Organometals are hazardous, owing to their toxicity and combustible properties. Those compounds that are relevant as environmental and occupational human health risks are listed in Table 89-1.

In general, organometallic toxicity is due to interaction with sulfhydryl groups. Most of these compounds are highly reactive with water in addition to being pyrophoric.

The clinical toxicity of organometals differs markedly from their inorganic counterparts. Owing to the organic nature of these compounds, they can penetrate into the central nervous system. The shorter-chain alkyl organometallic compounds are more toxic than are longer-chain compounds of the same type. Also, the body may metabolize each of these substances differently, attempting to cleave the metal-carbon bond. An example of this is the alkylmercury compound in which methylmercury is much stabler than ethylmercury. The conversion of methylmercury to inorganic mercury does not appear to be critical in determining the general toxicity of this compound. The aryl and alkoxyalkylmercury compounds, however, are less toxic than is the alkyl compound, and their conversion to inorganic mercury does appear to be critical in conferring their toxicity.

The toxicity of the metal in question can be altered by the ligand formation. As the organometal is absorbed systematically, it either must dissociate into the free cation or must exist in its complexed form.

HAZARDS OF ORGANOMETALS

Organometals are used in a variety of industrial chemical reactions, including syntheses and polymerization reactions. Approximately 50 organometallic compounds are used commercially. The U.S. Department of Transportation lists organometals as hazardous materials for transportation under the classification of pyrophoric liquids or solids (2). Most organometals are shipped as regulated hazardous materials. As an example, all

TABLE 89-1. Organometals

Organometal	Physiochemical properties and reactivity
Nickel carbonyl (C_4NiO_4)	Colorless, volatile liquid; oxidizes in air and is explosive
Tetraethyl lead (C_8H_2OPb)	Flammable colorless liquid; not pyrophoric; does not react with water
Methylmercury (C_2H_6Hg)	Colorless, volatile, flammable liquid; insoluble in water
Iron pentacarbonyl (C_5FeO_5)	Colorless to yellow, oily liquid; pyrophoric in air; insoluble in water
Trimethylaluminum [$Al(CH_3)_3$]	Liquid that undergoes spontaneous combustion in air; explosive; decomposes violently in water
Tri(isobutyl)aluminum [$Al(C_4H_9)_3$]	Colorless liquid; unstable above 165°F; pyrophoric; violently reacts with water
Triethylaluminum [$Al(C_2H_5)_3$]	Colorless liquid; ignites when exposed to air; reacts violently with water; used as incendiary munitions
Chlorodiethylaluminum [$(C_2H_5)_2AlCl$]	Colorless to light volatile liquid; ignites when exposed to air; reacts violently with water to form HCl gas and aluminum oxide
Ethyldichloroaluminum [$Al(C_2H_5)_2Cl_2$]	Colorless volatile liquid; ignites when exposed to air; reacts violently with water to form HCl gas, aluminum oxide
Dimethylcadmium [$(CH_3)_2Cd$]	Colorless liquid; explosive and decomposes at temperatures higher than 212°F; pyrophoric; decomposes in water
Tetramethyltin [$Sn(CH_3)_4$]	Colorless liquid; highly volatile; insoluble in water; thermally stable up to 750°F
Diethylzinc [$(C_2H_5)_2Zn$]	Highly flammable in air; extremely disagreeable odor; highly reactive with water
Ethylsodium (C_2H_5Na)	Highly reactive with water and forms flammable ethane
Dimethylarsine chloride [$(CH_3)_2ASCl$]	Highly flammable, colorless liquid; produces highly toxic vapor on exposure to air; offensive odor
Tributyltin [$Sn(C_4H_9)_3H$]	Highly irritating to skin, eyes, and mucous membranes; can produce chemical burns on prolonged contact
Dibutyltin [$Sn(C_4H_9)_2H_2$]	Thymic atrophy in animal studies; immunotoxin; reactive with water and can produce chemical burns
Trimethyltin [$Sn(CH_3)_3H$]	Reactive with water; colorless liquid; may produce chemical burns on contact
Triphenyltin [$Sn(C_6H_5)_3$]	Colorless liquid; reactive with water
Tetraphenyltin [$Sn(C_6H_5)_4$]	Colorless liquid; minimal fire hazard
Diethyltin [$Sn(C_2H_5)_2H_2$]	Colorless liquid; reactive with water; thymic atrophy in animal studies; immunotoxin
Ethyl lithium (C_2H_5Li)	Colorless liquid; violently reacts with water to generate heat and LiOH; spontaneously flammable in air
Phenyl lithium (C_6H_5Li)	Colorless liquid; reacts violently with water to form LiOH and heat; spontaneously flammable in air
Methyl lithium (CH_3Li)	Colorless liquid; spontaneously flammable in air; reacts violently with water to form heat plus LiOH
Trimethylphosphine [$(CH_3)_3P$]	Spontaneously flammable in air

organoaluminum compounds react violently with water. Tetraethyl lead (C_2H_5) is a flammable liquid but does not react with water. Because most organometallic compounds are pyrophoric liquids, they are shipped as solutions in organic solvents.

Diethyl zinc and ethyl sodium react with water to produce ethane, a dangerous flammable gas. Water-reactive organometallic compounds, such as ethyl sodium and the organoaluminum compounds, increase a fire's intensity when water is used as an extinguisher (2). Carbon dioxide usually is employed to extinguish fires involving organometallic compounds. Also, sand or graphite can be used to help to extinguish organometallic fires (2).

ORGANOLEAD COMPOUNDS

Sources, Production, and Exposure

Tetraethyl lead, also known as *tetraethylplumbane* or *lead tetraethyl*, has a formula of $C_8H_{20}Pb$ and a molecular weight of 323.45. Tetraethyl lead does not occur naturally; it is prepared by the reaction of PbC_{12} with ethyl zinc or Grignard reagent, via heating of C_2H_5Cl and sodium-lead alloy in an autoclave (4–7). Tetraethyl lead can be produced also from ethylene and hydrogen using triethylaluminum. Alternate syntheses use nonhalide compounds.

Tetraethyl lead is a colorless, flammable liquid that burns with an orange-colored flame with a green margin. It is insoluble in water, is soluble in benzene, ether, and gasoline, and is slightly soluble in alcohol. It does not react with water. The tetraalkyllead compounds tetraethyl lead and tetramethyl lead are used as gasoline additives to prevent "knocking" in engines.

Exposure to tetraethyl lead is greatest for workers in refineries and gas stations and for mechanics and other members of the automobile industry. Ubiquitous exposure results from gasoline exhaust, which is the largest source of lead exposure overall; however, most organic lead is converted to its inorganic form on combustion. National programs designed to limit sales of leaded gasoline have resulted in dramatic decreases in urban air lead concentrations (6).

Clinical Toxicology

The toxic effects and organ distribution of alkyllead compounds differ from those of inorganic lead. Tetraethyl lead and tetramethyl lead are dealkylated rapidly by the liver to the trialkyl metabolites, which are responsible for clinical toxicity. The trialkyl intermediates are biodegraded only slowly to inorganic lead (8–11).

In contrast to inorganic lead, the alkyl compounds are absorbed rapidly by inhalation or by the intact skin and are distributed to the central nervous system. Inhalational abuse of leaded fuel is a cause of alkyllead-induced encephalopathy (8–11).

Symptoms of Toxic Exposure

The toxic effects of alkyllead in the form of trimethyl or triethyl compounds present as neuropsychiatric or neurobehavioral manifestations as compared with those of inorganic lead. Acute intoxication is characterized by symptoms of hallucinations, delusions, excitement, or insomnia, which may progress to convulsions and delirium in fatal cases (8–11). Alopecia also may occur in some cases. Toxic effects of chronic exposure to alkyllead are similar to those of inorganic lead compounds (8–11). Employees at a tetraethyl lead manufacturing facility showed associations between higher chronic lead exposure and poorer scores in a number of neurobehavioral tests (particularly manual dexterity and learning) (12).

Management of Toxicity

Treatment of organolead intoxication includes the administration of metal-chelating agents that decrease blood lead and substantially increase urinary lead excretion. However, this procedure is controversial, as alkylleads are not chelatable and the therapy probably does not influence central nervous system symptoms (13). Hospitalized gasoline sniffers have a high degree of mortality, owing to sepsis after pulmonary aspiration. Respiratory care, therefore, is crucial for the survival of such patients.

Oral ingestion of fuel containing tetraethyl lead must be treated as an ingestion of organic solvents. Pulmonary aspiration may occur secondary to ingestion. Gastric lavage should be attempted only if the airway can be protected adequately with a cuffed endotracheal tube. Cathartics may aid in gastrointestinal elimination acutely.

Biological monitoring of environmental or occupational exposure to alkyllead compounds is the same as for inorganic lead, thus creating difficulty in differentiating the causes of lead burdening.

ORGANOMERCURY COMPOUNDS

Sources, Production, and Exposure

Methylmercury (dimethylmercury) has a chemical formula of C_2H_6Hg and a molecular weight of 230.66. Dimethylmercury is an environmental contaminant found, together with monomethyl mercury compounds, in fish and birds (14,15). It arises from bioconversion of naturally occurring inorganic mercury and subsequent enrichment in the food chain. Dimethylmercury is a colorless, volatile, flammable liquid. It is soluble in ether and alcohol and is insoluble in water. Methylmercury is the most toxicologically important organomercury compound. Other members of these compounds include ethylmercury, phenylmercury, and the alkoxyalkylmercury compounds.

Exposure to organic mercury results from handling alkylmercury-containing fungicides and algaecides in the agricultural industry and medical use of alkylmercury-containing ointments or diuretics that are obsolete. Nutritional exposure results from ingestion of fish-based diets, exacerbated in cases in which seafood is contaminated with anthropogenic organomercurials (14–16).

Clinical Toxicology

Inhalation of alkylmercury vapor is the main cause of acute intoxication. Chronic exposure results from ingestion of alkylmercury-contaminated food.

In contrast to elemental mercury, organic mercury compounds are absorbed rapidly and completely by the lungs, gastrointestinal tract, and the skin because of their high lipid solubility. The absorption of methylmercury, even mixed with food, is approximately 95% in adults.

A major difference among the organomercurials is that the stability of the carbon-mercury bond *in vivo* varies considerably. Thus, the alkylmercury compounds are much more resistant to biodegradation than are either phenylmercury or alkoxyalkylmercuric compounds.

The biodistribution of organic mercury compounds, in particular short-chain alkylmercuries, is unlike that of inorganic mercury. Although both forms of mercury distribute preferentially to the kidneys, the concentration in brain and blood is substantially higher for methylmercury. As a consequence, toxic manifestations of inorganic mercury are renal, whereas those for methylmercury are referable to the central nervous system. Phenylmercury and alkoxyalkylmercuric compounds do not produce central nervous system manifestations, owing to their biological instability.

Methylmercury is eliminated mainly in the feces as a result of biliary excretion and exfoliation of intestinal epithelial cells. Intestinal reabsorption occurs owing to hepatobiliary recirculation. The enterohepatic recirculation of methylmercury can be interrupted by the oral application of a polythiol resin, which increases fecal excretion.

Symptoms of Toxic Exposure

Two epidemic cases of poisoning, one in Japan's Minamata Bay (after ingestion of shellfish from methylmercury-contaminated waters) and the other in Iraq (after ingestion of fungicide-treated grain), shed significant light on the pathologic courses of chronic and acute methylmercury poisoning, respectively (17).

Regardless of the chemical form of exposure, the highest concentration of mercury occurs in the kidneys. However, the kidneys are the primary target organs for toxicity only in the case of inorganic mercury. The toxic effects of exposure to short-chain alkylmercury compounds center on the central nervous system. Central nervous system toxicity includes tremors, confusion, hallucinations, and delusional activity (18–21).

Tremor is seen also in inorganic mercury toxicity. Neuropsychiatric symptoms occur in methylmercury intoxication and in toxicity from inorganic mercury. Symptoms include paresthesias and visual field constriction, the most specific finding in Minamata disease (chronic methylmercury intoxication). At higher exposure levels, other sensory defects occur, such as hearing and vestibular function loss and defects in smell and taste. Other neurologic effects of toxic exposure to methylmercury are incoordination, paralysis, and abnormal reflexes (18–21). Moreover, behavioral abnormalities, including spontaneous fits of laughter and crying and intellectual deterioration, are specific for methylmercury poisoning (18–21).

Mercury readily crosses the placenta into fetal tissue regardless of the chemical form of exposure. Fetal intoxication by way of the mother has been documented in cases of methylmercury poisoning (22). Cerebral palsy is the most common presentation. An affected mother is much less sensitive than is the developing fetus, and newborns also show particular sensitivity (17). Methylmercury thus is an important developmental toxin, sometimes with effects becoming apparent only decades after the initial exposure.

Experimental studies showing a renal carcinogenic action of methylmercury have given rise to concerns about the genotoxic effects of these compounds. These effects have been shown only in male rodents, however, and no epidemiologic or clinical data exist to justify this concern (23).

Management of Toxicity

In acute events, lavage, cathartics, and charcoal can be administered to prevent absorption. Elimination can be promoted by polythiol resins that interrupt the enterohepatic circulation. Metal-chelating agents also can be used to eliminate mercury. Dimercaprol (British anti-Lewisite) is contraindicated in organic mercury intoxication, because it favors the uptake of mercury into the brain. D-Penicillamine, or better, its *N*-acetyl derivative, has been recommended as more effective and less toxic in the treatment of methylmercury poisoning. The more water-soluble and less toxic derivative of dimercaprol—2,3-dimercapto-1-propanesulfonate (DMPS)—has been shown to be more effective in methylmercury poisoning than several other chelators currently used. 2,3-Dimercaptosuccinic acid also is efficacious as a chelator in treating toxicity from mercury. DMPS was used to treat the 1971 victims of methylmercury poisoning in Iraq (24). The half-life of methylmercury was 10 days during DMPS therapy, as opposed to 26 days for those receiving D-penicillamine, and 17 days for those receiving *N*-acetyl-DL-penicillamine (24).

The primary aim of chelation therapy is to prevent the development of neuropsychiatric symptoms before they occur. In measurements of the half-life of methylmercury in blood, the fastest elimination rate was achieved by DMPS. Although chelators do not affect significantly the outcome of poisoning that results in a neuropsychiatric syndrome, therapy is recommended nonetheless.

ORGANOALUMINUM COMPOUNDS

Sources, Production, and Exposure

Organoaluminum compounds include trimethylaluminum, triethylaluminum, triisobutylaluminum, chlorodiethylaluminum, and dichloroethylaluminum. Trialkylaluminum compounds are colorless liquids at room temperature, sensitive to oxidation and hydrolysis in air. They are very reactive when exposed to water and are used as incendiary agents for military purposes.

Alkylaluminum halides of industrial importance are chlorodiethylaluminum and dichloroethylaluminum. The halides are colorless, volatile liquids or low-melting solids; they are less sensitive to oxidation on exposure to air. The halogen aluminum bonds are cleaved by water and alcohol. Alkylaluminum compounds are used as catalysts in polymerization processes and occur as intermediates in organic syntheses. Exposure to alkyl aluminum may occur in workers by inhalation or dermal contact. The trialkylaluminum compounds are pulmonary irritants after inhalation and are corrosive to the skin and mucosal membranes. However, as they are highly reactive in both air and water, they practically never gain systemic access to exert internal toxicity.

Symptoms of Toxic Exposure

Dermal or mucosal contact with trialkylaluminum can cause severe corrosive injury. After inhalation of vapor, irritation of the bronchoalveolar mucosa occurs. In severe cases, pulmonary edema may develop, often after a delay of several days. After eye contact, immediate rinsing with clear water is necessary to prevent ocular injury. Pulmonary toxicity is managed symptomatically.

ORGANOARSENIC COMPOUNDS

Sources, Production, and Exposure

Organoarsenic compounds include dimethylarsine (also known as *cacodyl*, from the Greek word *caco*, meaning "bad" or "ill"), cacodylic acid, arsenic trimethyl, arylarsenic and alkylarsenic halides, and arsenphenolamine. Dimethylarsine is a highly flammable, colorless liquid that, on exposure to air, produces a highly toxic vapor with an offensive odor.

Arsenphenolamine (arsaminol, arsphenamine, Salversan) was used historically as an antisyphilitic drug but no longer is acceptable treatment. It is a light-yellow, hygroscopic powder that oxidizes on exposure to air, becoming darker and more toxic.

Diphenylchloroarsine (Clark I), diphenylcyanarsine (Clark II), methyldichloroarsine, ethyldichloroarsine, bis(2-chlorovinyl)chloroarsine (Lewisite), and bis(2-chloroethyl)sulfide (Lost) were used in World War I as poison gases. Among the cacodyls, hydroxydimethylarsine oxide has been used as an herbicide.

Arsenical poison gases for military use are condemned by most nations of the world; nevertheless, exposure might be possible during the production of such gases, in handling, or in decontamination of hazardous worksites. Cacodylic acid and its salts used as herbicides may give rise to intoxications after inhalation or dermal contact. Fish and other seafoods represent an important dietary source for organic arsenicals, presumably because of food chain enrichment (24).

Clinical Toxicology

Acute intoxication is a result of inhalation of arsenic-containing poison gases. Chronic exposure to alkylarsenic compounds can result from ingestion of food contaminated with herbicides. Inhalation of arsenical gases produces immediate irritation of the bronchoalveolar mucosa and, in severe cases, the development of acute pulmonary edema. Dermal and ocular injury also occur, with blistering of the skin. Arsenical gases have a garliclike odor and are less toxic than are the arsenic halides. Chronic exposure to arsenical gases in herbicide-contaminated food intake may give rise to symptoms of chronic arsenic intoxication: gastrointestinal disorders, paresthesias, rashes, hyperpigmentation, peripheral neuropathy, and blood dyscrasias.

The pathology of poisoning by organic arsenicals appears qualitatively similar to poisoning by the inorganic forms. However, despite the fact that organic arsenicals have been used as poison gases, the toxicities of most other organic arsenicals are considerably lower than those of inorganic arsenicals of the same valence state. Indeed, methylation of inorganic arsenic is considered an important physiologic detoxification mechanism (25,26).

Management of Toxicity

Acute intoxication with arsenical gases or cacodyls is managed in a fashion similar to that involving other pulmonary irritants. Drug therapy of acute or chronic poisoning with organic arsenicals is the same as that involving inorganic arsenic compounds; however, because of their lower toxicity, the therapy sometimes can produce more symptoms than the poison (1). Dimercaprol, 2,3-dimercaptosuccinic acid, and DMPS are effective as therapeutic chelators.

NICKEL CARBONYL

Sources, Production, and Exposure

Nickel tetracarbonyl has a molecular weight of 170.73 and a chemical formula of $Ni(CO)_4$. It is a colorless, yellow to clear volatile liquid that oxidizes in the air and can ignite. It is soluble in alcohol, benzene, chloroform, acetone, and carbon tetrachloride. Nickel carbonyl is highly flammable and volatilizes at room temperature (2). This liquid is formed by nickel or its compounds in the presence of carbon monoxide, a reaction that considerably simplifies the process of industrial nickel refining. It is shipped in compressed gas cylinders and reacts with oxidizers, chlorine, nitric acid, oxygen, butane, and (explosively) with liquid bromine. Its vapor is heavier than air and can travel along floors to ignition sources (vapor density, 5.9).

Toxic exposures to nickel carbonyl outside an occupational setting are rare. Occupational exposure to nickel carbonyl occurs primarily during nickel refining, but it may occur also in the electroplating and electronics industries. The routes of exposure are mainly inhalation and absorption of the liquid after dermal contact. Nickel carbonyl and its vapor are decomposed by heat to carbon monoxide and nickel (the Mond process). Nickel carbonyl is highly explosive, and vapors in air can explode at 20°C (27). Vapors can explode in a closed space, and containers can explode if heated (27). Nickel carbonyl reacts slowly with air to produce nickel oxide.

Clinical Toxicology

After inhalation, nickel carbonyl is absorbed rapidly by the lungs and binds to erythrocytes and plasma albumin. It is distributed to various tissues, including muscle, fat, bone, connective tissue, intestine, liver, brain, and blood (27,28). After dietary exposure, excretion of nickel occurs mainly via the feces. Inhalation of nickel carbonyl results in the appearance of high amounts of urinary nickel; only minor amounts appear in the stools. Biodegradation of nickel carbonyl to nickel and carbon monoxide is important with respect to symptoms of toxicity after exposure. Nickel carbonyl has a musty odor, with an odor threshold of 1 part per million (ppm). The OSHA permissible exposure limit for this substance is 0.001 ppm. This is also the concentration that is immediately dangerous to life and health (28). Chronic effects of nickel carbonyl observed in nickel refinery workers include rhinitis, sinusitis, perforation of the nasal septum, and bronchial asthma.

Nickel carbonyl is the most toxic of the nickel compounds. An atmospheric exposure of 30 ppm for 30 minutes has been estimated to be lethal in humans (28,29). Initial symptoms of acute toxicity include giddiness, headache, vomiting, and shortness of breath. Delayed symptoms occurring in 12 to 24 hours are dyspnea, cyanosis, leukocytosis, hyperthermia, and acute chemical pneumonitis (28,29). Delirium and other central nervous symptoms also may appear. Death from a toxic exposure may occur between 2 and 13 days (21–23). Pathotoxicologic alterations found in the lungs include interstitial edema, fibroblast immigration, and capillary injury. Hepatic injury also can occur (28,29). Vapors are irritating to the eyes and mucous membranes. Dermal contact with the liquid can produce dermatitis and burns, resulting in absorption of the compound and systemic toxicity (28,29).

Nickel compounds as a group are human carcinogens. Because their carcinogenic activity appears to be related directly to their ability to enter cells, nickel carbonyl should be considered a particularly hazardous substance in this respect (30). Chronic exposure to nickel carbonyl has been implicated in cancer of the lungs and nose. These epidemiologic findings have been confirmed by inhalational exposure in experimental animals. Tobacco smoke also may contain significant amounts of nickel carbonyl.

An increased incidence of carcinomas of the lungs in nickel carbonyl–exposed workers has been detected only in England and was not confirmed by epidemiologic data from other countries (Germany, United States, Canada, France, Finland, Soviet Union). This has been explained by a coexposure of workers in England to arsenic-containing sulfuric acid. Often, because workers are exposed also to other nickel compounds, determining the compound that acts as the primary carcinogen is not possible. However, on the basis of experimental data, nickel carbonyl must be classified as carcinogenic for humans.

The increase of nickel in the urine has been used clinically to confirm an exposure. Urinary concentrations exceeding 0.5 mg per L are considered to be serious. Monitoring of carboxyhemoglobin in blood also may be relevant to explain signs of toxicity, because nickel carbonyl is metabolized to carbon monoxide.

Management of Toxicity

Acute intoxication with nickel carbonyl can be managed by such metal-complexing agents as dimercaprol or, better, diethyldithiocarbamate trihydrate (dithiocarb) (31–33). Daily oral doses of dithiocarb, 25 to 50 mg per kg, or dimercaprol, 3 mg per kg, every 4 hours are recommended in cases of severe intoxication (31–33). Otherwise, management is symptomatic.

Nickel carbonyl exposure can be monitored by measuring urinary levels of nickel (more than 0.5 mg per L). Environmental exposure is monitored by gas detector tubes.

IRON PENTACARBONYL

Sources, Production, and Exposure

Iron carbonyl (pentacarbonyliron; C_5FeO_5) has a molecular weight of 195.90 and is a colorless to yellow oily liquid. It is pyrophoric in air, burning to Fe_2O_3, and it decomposes by light to $Fe_2(CO)_9$ and carbon monoxide. It is practically insoluble in water, readily soluble in most organic solvents (ether, acetone, ethyl acetate), and slightly soluble in alcohol.

Iron carbonyl is prepared from iron, iron compounds, and carbon monoxide. It is used in the manufacture of powdered iron cores for high-frequency coils applied in the radio and television industry. It is used also as an antiknock agent in motor fuels and as a catalyst in organic reactions.

The risk of exposure to iron pentacarbonyl exists mainly for workers in the chemical industry. Routes of exposure are by inhalation or dermal contact. As a lipid-soluble compound, it is absorbed rapidly and may decompose to iron and carbon monoxide.

Clinical Toxicology

Acute toxicity of iron pentacarbonyl is similar to that of nickel carbonyl. Chronic exposure may result in iron overload, with the consequence of secondary hemochromatosis. Iron pentacarbonyl as a lipophilic compound is absorbed rapidly after dermal contact.

Iron pentacarbonyl is a pulmonary irritant and can produce pulmonary edema on inhalation. It also affects the central nervous system and may cause liver and kidney damage.

Management of Toxicity

For acute intoxication, the treatment of pulmonary edema and shock is of primary importance. Iron overload may be reduced by treatment with deferoxamine, an iron-chelating agent. The intravenous dose should not exceed 15 mg per kg per hour. Environmental or occupational exposure to iron pentacarbonyl is monitored by gas detector tubes. The exposure threshold limit value is 0.1 ppm, with a short-term exposure limit of 0.2 ppm.

ORGANOTIN COMPOUNDS

Organotin toxicity ranges from the very toxic trialkyltins to the less toxic dialkyltin and monoalkyltin compounds. Shorter-chain alkyltins appear overall to be more toxic than are longer-chain alkyltins. Tributyltin is a fungicide used in exterior paint (34,35). Tributyltin oxide is both a solid and a liquid, and human exposures can occur from inhalation and from skin absorption. The organotin compounds produce irritation of the eyes, mucous membranes, throat, and skin (35).

Exposure to tributyltin can produce irritation of the eyes, throat, and mucous membrane; conjunctivitis; nausea; headache; vomiting; and wheezing (35). Dermal contact of a solution or a solid can produce chemical burns and necrosis (35). Bis(tributyltin) oxide has fungicidal properties and has found use in interior and exterior paints. Case reports of toxicity from residential dwellers demonstrate tributyltin's continued use in paints (35). Pruritic and erythematous vesicular rashes have occurred after skin contact with paint containing tributyltin (35).

Tributyltin has been shown to cause immunosuppression, anemia, and weight loss in animals. Owing to its toxic effects, tributyltin is used as a biocide in exterior paints only, not in interior paints. The state of Washington has banned its use in interior house paint, owing to cases of toxicity.

The organotin compounds are biocides in many products and processes that require preservation, such as wood, leather, paper, paint, and textiles. Tributyltin, triphenyltin, and tetraorganotin are incompatible with strong oxidizers. All organotin compounds, especially tributyltins and dibutyltins, produce severe dermal injury and burns. Intense itching, inflammation, and erythema can occur on exposure. The lesions that develop generally are diffuse and erythematous and heal quickly after exposure is terminated. Exposure to the eyes can produce lacrimation, conjunctivitis, and conjunctival edema.

Trialkyltin and tetraalkyltin compounds are neurotoxic and can cause headache, dizziness, photophobia, vomiting, muscle weakness, and flaccid paralysis. Triphenyltin is a hepatotoxin. The typical organotins are triethyltin, dibutyltin, tributyltin, and triphenyltin. These compounds exist in the form of triethyltin iodide, dibutyltin chloride, tributyltin chloride, triphenyltin acetate, and bis(tributyltin) oxide. Trimethyltin and triethyltin are the most toxic of alkyltin compounds and produce specific neurotoxicity (34,35). The pattern of poisoning is very similar to that seen with tetraethyl lead (or triethyllead). Animals receiving injections of trialkyltin compounds develop aggressive behavior within 48 hours of dosing. Lesions are found in the hippocampus, pyriform cortex, amygdaloid nucleus, and cortex (31). In addition to behaving aggressively, animals developed irritability and tremor (36). Cerebral edema occurs in some animals after dosing with triethyltin (36).

Ingestion of triethyltin can produce neurologic symptoms of severe headache, vertigo, photophobia, visual disturbances, abdominal pain and vomiting, urinary retention, paralysis, and psychic disturbances (34–36). Persistent neurologic sequelae include diminished visual acuity, sensory loss, focal anesthesia, flaccid paralysis, incontinence, and cerebral edema.

Triphenyltin is a hepatotoxin that, in some occupational exposures, has produced hepatic damage with hepatomegaly and elevated liver enzymes (36). Triphenyltin is also a dermal irritant producing urticarial disruption, and toxic exposure can produce other effects, such as headache, nausea, vomiting, and blurred vision (34).

Trimethyltin has produced hyperexcitability and neurologic and behavioral changes in animals; seizures have been reported in some animal studies. In humans, trimethyltin toxicity has been manifested with memory loss, anorexia, confusion, decreased vigilance, disorientation, aggressiveness, and seizures (34–36).

The organotin compounds are known to have immunotoxic properties in animals (37). The major effect appears to occur in the cell-mediated immune responses (37). Although many organotins are extremely cytotoxic, the effects of dibutyl and dioctyltin appear to be highly specific (38). Both these compounds inhibit antibody responses to T-cell, but not B-cell, mitogens. They also produce thymus atrophy and decrease in thymocytes. Trimethyltin dichloride has shown histopathologic changes in the organ weight of the thymus and spleen of 50% to 60% (37). Also, animal studies demonstrated a decrease in T-cell–dependent antibody response and B-cell lymphocyte proliferation of 60% to 80% (37). In addition, trimethyltin affected cellular immunity and was shown to have an 80% decrease in T-lymphocyte proliferation from mitogen stimulation (37). Tributyltin has immunotoxic effects in animal species. Rats orally fed tributyltin oxide showed decreases in the lymphoid organ weight, such as the thymus (thymic atrophy) and spleen; a decrease in white blood cell count; and decreased lymphocyte counts. Animals fed triphenyltin also show immunotoxic effects, such as decreases in the weight of thymus, spleen, and lymph nodes, and a decrease in B-cell lymphocyte proliferation; delayed hypersensitivity reactions; a decrease in T-cell lymphocyte proliferation response to mitogen; and a decreased host resistance (37,38).

REFERENCES

1. Vouk V. General chemistry of metals. In: Friberg L, Nordberg G, Vouk V, eds. *Handbook of the toxicology of metals*, vol 1. New York: Elsevier Science, 1986:14–35.
2. Meyer E. *Chemistry of hazardous materials*. Englewood Cliffs, NJ: Prentice-Hall, 1977.
3. Morrison R, Boyd R. *Organic chemistry*, 2nd ed. Boston: Allyn & Bacon, 1966.
4. Beattie AD, Moore MR, Goldberg A. Tetraethyl-lead poisoning. *Lancet* 1972;2:12–15.
5. Gething J. Tetramethyl lead absorption: a report of human exposure to high level of tetramethyl lead. *Br J Ind Med* 1975;32:329–333.
6. Lehnert G, Mastall H, Szadkowski D, Schaller KH. Berufliche Bleibelastung durch Autoabgase in Großstadtstraßen. *Dtsch Med Wochenschr* 1970;95: 1097–1099.
7. Maruna RFL, Maruna H. [Lead level in taxi drivers as characterized by the urinary excretion of delta aminolevulinic acid. Report on lead poisoning preventive measures in the Vienna area in various occupational and other groups] [German]. *Wien Med Wochenschr* 1975;125:615–620.
8. Millar JA, Thompson GG, Goldberg A, Barry PS, Lowe EH. δ-Aminolevulinic acid dehydrase activity in the blood of man working with lead alkyls. *Br J Ind Med* 1972;29:317–320.
9. Seshia SS, Rajani KR, Boeckx RL, Chow PN. The neurological manifestations of chronic inhalation of leaded gasoline. *Dev Med Child Neurol* 1978;20:323–334.
10. Schmidt D, Sansoni B, Kracke W, Dietl F, Bauchinger M, Stich W. Die Bleibelastung der Münchner Verkehrspolizei. *Münch Med Wochenschr* 1972;114:1761–1763.
11. Stevens CP, Feldhake CJ, Kehoe RA. Isolation of triethyllead-ion from liver after inhalation of tetraethyllead. *J Pharmacol Exp Ther* 1960;128:90–94.
12. Schwartz BS, Bolla KI, Stewart W, Ford DP, Agnew J, Frumkin H. Decrements in neurobehavioral performance associated with mixed exposure to organic and inorganic lead. *Am J Epidemiol* 1993;137:1006–1021.
13. Burns CB, Currie B. The efficacy of chelation therapy and factors influencing mortality in lead intoxicated petrol sniffers. *Aust N Z J Med* 1995;25:197–203.
14. Eyl TB. Methyl mercury poisoning in fish and human beings. *Clin Toxicol* 1971;14:291–296.
15. Rivers JB, Pearson JE, Schultz CD. Total and organic mercury in main fish. *Bull Environ Contam Toxicol* 1972;8:257–267.
16. Swensson A, Ulfarsson V. Toxicology of organic mercury compounds used as fungicides. *Occup Health Rev* 1963;15:5–11.
17. Hamada R, Osame M. Minamata disease and other mercury syndromes. In: Chang LW, ed. *Toxicology of metals*. Boca Raton, FL: CRC Press, 1996:337–352.
18. Pierce PE, Thompson JF, Likosky WH, Nickey LN, Barthel WF, Hinman AR. Alkyl mercury poisoning in humans. *JAMA* 1972;220:1439–1442.
19. Somjien GG, Herman SP, Klein R, et al. The uptake of methyl mercury (^{203}Hg) in different tissues relates to its neurotoxic effects. *J Pharmacol Exp Ther* 1973;187:602–611.
20. Kershaw TG, Dhahir PH, Clarkson TW. The relationship between blood levels and dose of methylmercury in man. *Arch Environ Health* 1980;35:28–36.
21. Kojima K, Fujita M. Summary of recent studies in Japan on methyl-mercury poisoning. *Toxicology* 1973;1:43–62.
22. Amin-Zaki L, Elhassani S, Majeed MA, Clarkson TW, Doherty RA, Greenwood MR. Studies of infants postnatally exposed to methylmercury. *J Pediatr* 1974;85:81–84.
23. Boffetta P, Merler E, Vainio H. Carcinogenicity of mercury and mercury compounds. *Scand J Work Environ Health* 1993;19:1–7.
24. Clarkson T, Magos L, Cox C, et al. Tests of efficacy of antidotes for removal of methylmercury in human poisoning during the Iraq outbreak. *Pharmacology* 1981;218:74–83.
25. Gerhardsson L, Skerfving S. Concepts on biological markers and biomonitoring for metal toxicity. In: Chang LW, ed. *Toxicology of metals*. Boca Raton, FL: CRC Press, 1996:81–110.
26. Garcia Vargas GG, Cebrian ME. Health effects of arsenic. In: Chang LW, ed. *Toxicology of metals*. Boca Raton, FL: CRC Press, 1996:423–438.
27. Dangerous properties of industrial materials report Nov/Dec. 1988;8(6):8–16.
28. Jones CC. Nickel carbonyl poisoning. *Arch Environ Health* 1973;26:245–248.
29. Sundermann FW, Kincaid JF. Nickel poisoning. Studies on patients suffering from acute exposure of vapors of nickel compounds. *JAMA* 1954;1565:889–894.
30. Costa M. Mechanisms of nickel genotoxicity and carcinogenicity. In: Chang LW, ed. *Toxicology of metals*. Boca Raton, FL: CRC Press, 1996:245–252.
31. Kasprzak KS, Sunderman FW Jr. Metabolism of nickel-carbonyl-^{14}C. *Toxicol Appl Pharmacol* 1969;15:295–303.
32. Sunderman FW Jr. The treatment of acute nickel carbonyl poisoning with sodium diethyldithiocarbamate. *Ann Clin Res* 1971;3:182–185.
33. Sunderman FW, Sunderman FW Jr. Nickel poisoning: VIII. Dithiocarb: a new therapeutic agent for persons exposed to nickel carbonyl. *Am J Med Sci* 1958;236:26–31.
34. *MMWR Morbid Mortal Wkly Rep* 1991;40:280–281.
35. Wax P, Dockstader L. Tributyltin use in interior paints: a continuing health hazard. *Clin Toxicol* 1995;33(3):239–241.
36. Sittig M. *Handbook of toxic and hazardous chemicals*. Park Ridge, NJ: Noyes Publications, 1981.
37. Penninks A. In: Dayan AD, ed. *Immunotoxology of metals and immunotoxicology*. New York: Plenum Publishing, 1990:191–207.
38. Sharma RP, Dugyala RR. Effects of metals on cell-mediated immunity and biological response modulators. In: Chang LW, ed. *Toxicology of metals*. Boca Raton, FL: CRC Press, 1996:785–796.

CHAPTER 90

Alkali Metals: Sodium, Potassium, and Lithium

Edward P. Krenzelok

SOURCES AND PRODUCTION

Owing to their highly reactive nature, sodium, potassium, and lithium are not present in their elemental form in nature. Sodium is manufactured by the electrolysis of a molten mixture of the chloride salts of sodium and calcium (1). Potassium production relies on the thermal reduction of potassium chloride with elemental sodium (1). Elemental lithium is manufactured by electrolysis of dry lithium chloride (2). In addition to its elemental forms, sodium is available as an amalgam with mercury, which is said to be less reactive (3). Sodium and potassium are produced also as a combination alloy [NaK-78 (78% K)] containing both of the alkali metals (3–5).

All three of the metals are found in innumerable organic and inorganic salts and compounds. In their elemental forms, they are relatively soft ductile metals with a silver appearance (1,3). Specimens that appear to be a different color may be coated with highly reactive oxide compounds and should be disposed of properly or used only with extreme caution (5). Sodium, potassium, and lithium must be stored under airtight anhydrous conditions to prevent oxidation, which is a catalyst for reactivity. Sodium should be stored under oil and potassium under xylene (4–6). Lithium should be stored under kerosene or other inert petroleum products (7). The synonyms for sodium, potassium, and lithium are found in Table 90-1.

SITES, INDUSTRIES, AND BUSINESSES ASSOCIATED WITH EXPOSURE

Sodium, potassium, and lithium have a multitude of occupational applications (Table 90-2), and the salts of sodium and potassium are ubiquitous in the food chain. They are extremely important in a number of industrial processes. Combined with their highly reactive nature, the potential for human exposures and toxic sequelae is significant. Most occupational exposures to sodium and potassium occur when they are exposed to air and moisture through improper storage or while they are being used under improper precautionary measures. Elemental lithium is slightly less reactive than are sodium and potassium under normal conditions. Occupational exposures are more likely to result from the volatilization of lithium during welding or brazing processes or during the extraction of lithium from ore. Human exposures may result in two toxic insults: thermal burns generated from an exothermic reaction and burns from caustic chemicals produced during the reaction (8).

TABLE 90-1. Sodium, potassium, and lithium synonyms

Sodium	Potassium
Elemental sodium	Elemental potassium
Na	K
Natrium	Potassium, metal
Sodium, metal	CAS 7440-09-7
CAS 7440-23-5	UN 2257
UN 1428	NIOSH/RTECS TS 6460000
NIOSH/RTECS VY 0686000	STCC 49 164 45
OHM-TADS 7216885	
STCC 49 164 56	

Lithium
Elemental lithium
Li
Lithium, metal
CAS 7439-93-2
UN 1415
NIOSH/RTECS OJ 5540000

CAS, Chemical Abstracts Service; NIOSH, National Institute for Occupational Safety and Health; OHM-TADS, Oil and Hazardous Materials Technical Assistance Data System; RTECS, Registry of Toxic Effects of Chemical Substances; STCC, standard transportation commodity code.

TABLE 90-2. Industrial applications of sodium, potassium, and lithium

Sodium	
Chemical	Detergent production
	Polymerization catalyst
	Chemical production
	Caustic soda
	Sodium peroxide
	Sodium cyanide
Electronic	Photoelectric cells
Metal	Titanium purification
	Hardened metal alloys
Nuclear	Heat exchange medium with K in nuclear reactors
Potassium	
Chemical	Condensation, polymerization, and reduction catalyst
	Synthesis of organic chemicals
Nuclear	Heat exchange medium with Na in nuclear reactors
Solar	Heat transfer medium in solar collectors
Lithium	
Aeronautics	Solid-propellant rocket mixtures
Chemical	Batteries
	Organic synthesis
	Hydrogen production
Electronic	Vacuum tubes
Metal	Scavenger in metal manufacture
	Welding and brazing fluxes
	Self-fluxing brazing alloys
	Degasifier, deoxidizer, desulfurizer
Nuclear	Coolant or heat exchanger in nuclear reactors
Petroleum	Lubricants

SODIUM

Sodium has an autoignition temperature of 115°C, which suggests that it will not ignite at normal room temperatures (3). However, after the sodium is removed from its protective oil shroud, it is exposed to ambient air and moisture, which results in the oxidation of sodium and the external deposition of oxides and sodium hydroxide (3). These substances are hygroscopic, which results in the accumulation of more moisture and intensifies the production of oxides and hydrogen gas, ultimately producing autoignition at room temperature. As the sodium bursts into flame, it produces an intense yellow flame fueled by the continuous production of hydrogen during the combustion process (3,6). Depending on the conditions, the ignition process may range from spontaneous combustion to a violent explosive reaction.

A variety of occupational situations may produce hazardous conditions that terminate in a toxic exposure to sodium (6,9). Sodium should be used only in rooms that are warm and sufficiently dehumidified, as cold or unheated rooms may contain significant ambient moisture. Sodium should be stored in rust-free metal or glass containers (9). If a glass container is used, it should be stored in an external metal container so that if the glass breaks, the spill is contained (9).

Cutting sodium at room temperature is acceptable only if both the sodium and the knife blade are coated with mineral oil to prevent the formation of external oxidation products (9). Failure to follow these precautionary guidelines may lead to oxidation, resulting in autoignition of the sodium cake. Weighing sodium is another potentially hazardous situation. The metal can be removed from its protective oil environment for short periods to be weighed if the procedure is performed in a low-humidity environment (9). It is best to weigh it in a beaker containing an inert hydrocarbon to prevent the occurrence of oxidation.

When minor spills of most chemicals occur, a commonplace reaction is to wipe them up with absorbent materials, such as paper or cloth towels. This practice is extremely hazardous, as the absorbent material retains the oil and exposes small sodium fragments to air, which may produce spontaneous combustion of the absorbent material.

Carelessness and lack of awareness about the reactive nature of sodium are responsible for the majority of toxic exposures. Exhaustive lists of other substances that react violently with sodium have been published (6,10,11).

POTASSIUM

Potassium is the most reactive of the alkali metals and has the potential for autoignition at room temperature (3). As potassium becomes exposed to air and moisture, highly reactive superoxides are deposited on the potassium cake (3,6,11). Even minute amounts of superoxides can detonate the potassium, producing a violent and explosive reaction that results in the spattering of the potassium particles, affecting a large surface area and potentially several individuals. Potassium burns with a purple flame (3). The potassium and the superoxides react with a variety of organic and inorganic compounds (6,10,11).

Because potassium is even more reactive than sodium, greater care must be exercised during potassium's use. It cannot be stored in aluminum containers because it reacts with aluminum and forms potassium carbonate, which may corrode the container and lead to accidental exposures (6). Old potassium (identified by an external coating of yellow to orange potassium superoxide) should not be used for any application, as even minimal contact may lead to autoignition (6). Reactions may occur when potassium is cut under other than ideal conditions. Many hydrocarbons, such as kerosene, react violently with potassium. It should be cut only using forceps and anhydrous xylene (6).

LITHIUM

Lithium is less reactive than are sodium and potassium, and autoignition, although still a problem, is less of a hazard. However, if lithium is divided finely and exposed to air and moisture, autoignition can occur at room temperature. Lithium reacts violently when exposed to water. If exposed to air at or near its melting point (180.5°C) during an industrial process, lithium ignites spontaneously (6,7). When lithium burns, it produces an intense white flame (12).

SODIUM, POTASSIUM, AND LITHIUM FIRES

Alkali metal fires are extremely dangerous because of their explosive nature and the potential to inhale the corrosive metallic oxide by-products of combustion. As with all fires, they must be extinguished as expeditiously as possible. Alkali metal fires are classified as class D, which means that conventional extinguishers containing water, carbon dioxide, sodium bicarbonate, carbon tetrachloride, or soda acid must not be used (3,10). These agents accelerate the fire: Halogenated hydrocarbons and carbon dioxide provide a source of combustible carbon. Sand should not be placed on potassium fires, because it produces a violent reaction (3). Class D fire extinguishers limited to those containing sodium carbonate (soda ash), sodium chloride, or graphite should be used (3,8,10,11,13). Large quantities of sodium, potassium, or lithium should not be stored in areas where sprinkler systems are installed, as water is an explosive accelerant in these fires.

CLINICAL TOXICOLOGY

Burns are the primary sequelae associated with exposure to elemental sodium, potassium, and lithium. The burns are a consequence of the reaction of the elemental metals with the ambient environment or chemicals. Most commonly, the alkali react with moisture and produce a pronounced exothermic reaction and the evolution of metallic hydroxides (8). The other feature to consider is the explosive nature of the reaction, which may cause the alkali to become airborne projectiles embedding in the skin or subcutaneous tissue (8).

Dermal exposure occurs when the alkali explodes. Heat will produce thermal burns; metal hydroxides will produce liquefaction necrosis; and the embedded particles will be transformed slowly into the corrosive hydroxide salt, liberating heat and causing further thermal trauma in the process (8,14). This cascade of events will continue until the source of sodium, potassium, or lithium is exhausted or removed through surgical debridement. Ocular exposures also may occur owing to the spattering and explosive force associated with the reactions. The same exothermic and caustic processes can be expected to occur.

Toxic oxide, hydroxide, and carbonate salts evolve during the combustion process (10,15). As aerosolized particles of approximately 1 μm, they are respirable, can be deposited throughout the lower bronchial tree, and owing to their irritant properties, can produce pulmonary edema (15–17).

MANAGEMENT OF TOXICITY

The basic management of all poisoning emergencies rests on the foundation of providing life support measures and decontamination of affected patients (Table 90-3). Normal external decontamination procedures for exposure to alkali include the mandatory removal of any contaminated clothing, because the alkali impregnated in the clothing no longer is immersed in a protective hydrocarbon and is dangerously exposed to the air and any water with

TABLE 90-3. Basic management of dermal exposures to sodium, potassium, and lithium

Terminate exposure.
Provide life support.
Perform external decontamination of the patient:
- Avoid the use of water.
- Ensure that caregivers protect themselves from exposure.
- Remove contaminated clothing and store it in noncombustible containers in a covering of mineral oil, avoiding the use of water.
- Remove elemental metal fragments imbedded in the skin using dry metal forceps—immediately place in safe medium.
- Irrigate wounds with large volumes of water only after they have been debrided.

Treat the resultant external burns according to the standard of care.

which it may come into contact, as when it is inadvertently used for irrigation purposes. Water irrigation is contraindicated and *should not* be used to decontaminate an affected area, because these elemental metals react violently with water.

Those caring for victims with a dermal or an ocular exposure must protect themselves from the reactive nature of the elemental metals. Protective eyewear, gowns, and dry surgical gloves must be worn. Care must be taken not to drop alkali fragments carelessly in the ambulance, in the corridor leading to the emergency department, or in the treatment suite. The alkali should be handled only with dry forceps and never touched, even if gloves are being worn. All existing portions of the alkali must be placed into the appropriate medium to prevent additional reactions. Sodium debris can be placed in isopropyl alcohol containing no more than 2% water (11); normal 70% isopropyl alcohol contains too much water and is not acceptable. Mineral oil is a suitable medium for sodium. Potassium specimens are extremely unstable and may react even in mineral oil. If available, pure *tert*-butyl alcohol can be used to store potassium (6). Other alcohols, such as ethanol and methanol, even in absolute forms, should not be used (6). "Dry" xylene is acceptable as a medium for potassium storage (6). Ideally, lithium should be placed under kerosene (7).

After removal of an affected patient's clothing, the affected area should be covered with mineral or even cooking oil to prevent further exposure to air and moisture (8,18). This action may prevent oxidation and the exothermic reaction and avoid hydrolysis to the corrosive hydroxide. Even with the occlusive use of oil, water in the tissues may serve to catalyze the reaction of alkali fragments embedded in the skin. Potassium reactivity may not be hindered even with the application of oil.

If the alkali metal is embedded in the skin, the area must be debrided surgically, as the reactivity will not cease until the source is exhausted or removed (8). The removed fragments must be placed immediately into the nonreactive medium appropriate to that specific alkali metal to prevent further reactivity and subsequent harm to the patient and those providing patient care. Only after all evidence of the elemental metal is removed is irrigation of the area with water permissible in a manner consistent with the treatment of alkali burns (5,8).

The treatment of ocular burns should follow the same guidelines and precautions. The decontamination procedure should be performed as expeditiously as possible, because the eye is exquisitely sensitive to alkaline insults, and an important safeguard is to institute irrigation therapy as soon as the alkaline debris is removed.

REFERENCES

1. Patty FA. Alkaline materials. In: Patty FA, ed. *Industrial hygiene and toxicology.* New York: John Wiley and Sons, 1963:859–869.
2. Stokinger HE. The metals—lithium. In: Clayton GD, Clayton FE, eds. *Patty's industrial hygiene and toxicology.* New York: John Wiley and Sons, 1981:1728–1740.
3. Meyer E. *Chemistry of hazardous materials.* Englewood Cliffs, NJ: Prentice-Hall, 1977:156–161.
4. Birch NJ, Karim AR. Potassium. In: Seiler HG, Sigel H, eds. *Handbook on toxicity of inorganic compounds.* New York: Marcel Dekker Inc, 1988:543–547.
5. Birch NJ. Sodium. In: Seiler HG, Sigel H, eds. *Handbook on toxicity of inorganic compounds.* New York: Marcel Dekker Inc, 1988:625–629.
6. Bretherick L. *Handbook of reactive chemical hazards,* 2nd ed. Worcester: Billing and Son, 1984:1024–1031, 1045–1049, 1087–1095.
7. *Toxic and hazardous industrial chemicals safety manual.* Tokyo: The International Technical Information Institute, 1985:303.
8. Clare RA, Krenzelok EP. Chemical burns secondary to elemental metal exposure: two case reports. *Am J Emerg Med* 1988;6:355–357.
9. Hawkes AS, Hill EF, Sittig M. Useful hints for sodium handling in the laboratory. *J Chem Educ* 1953;30:467–470.
10. Sax NI. *Dangerous properties of industrial materials,* 6th ed. New York: Van Nostrand–Reinhold, 1984:2267–2268, 2406–2407.
11. *Toxic and hazardous industrial chemicals safety manual.* Tokyo: The International Technical Information Institute, 1982:425–426, 465–466.
12. Browning E. *Toxicity of industrial metals,* 2nd ed. New York: Appleton-Century-Crofts, 1969:200.
13. National Fire Protection Association. Lithium. *Fire protection guide on hazardous materials,* 8th ed. Quincy, MA: National Fire Protection Association, 1984:49.
14. Temple AR. Corrosive-alkaline. In: Rumack BH, ed. *Poisindex,* vol 60. Denver: Micromedex, 1997.
15. Busch RH, McDonald KE, Briant JK, Morris JE, Graham TM. Pathologic effects in rodents exposed to sodium combustion products. *Environ Res* 1983;31:138–147.
16. Proctor NH. Setting health standards: threshold limit values. In: Proctor NH, Hughes JP, Fischman ML, eds. *Chemical hazards of the workplace.* New York: Van Nostrand–Reinhold, 1989:3–9.
17. Allen MD, Greenspan BJ, Briant JK, Hoover MD. Generation of Li combustion aerosols for animal inhalation studies. *Health Phys* 1986;51:117–126.
18. Stewart CE. Chemical skin burns. *Am Fam Physician* 1985;31:149–157.

CHAPTER 91
Reactive Metals

John B. Sullivan, Jr.

Many metals, in their elemental state, are highly reactive with air or water and explode, combust, and release hazardous by-products in addition to their intrinsic toxicity (1). Metals having these characteristics are lithium, potassium, sodium, cadmium, zinc, aluminum, tin, magnesium, cesium, rubidium, thorium, titanium, uranium, plutonium, and zirconium (Table 91-1) (see Chapter 90).

Metals that are combustion hazards in a solid state are cesium, rubidium, sodium, lithium, and potassium (Table 91-2). Metals that are explosive and combustible when mixed with air as a dust include aluminum, beryllium, titanium, magnesium, and cadmium (1,2). Hazards related to these reactive metals are derived from their inherent toxicity, high degree of explosivity and flammability when exposed to water or air, and toxic by-products of their reactions.

ALKALI METALS

The alkali metals of sodium, potassium, and lithium are highly reactive. These three metals are used extensively in industry and have multiple commercial applications. The alkali metals exhibit general chemical reactivity characteristics, including reacting violently with water and generating hydrogen gas, which combusts or explodes, thereby intensifying a fire; possibly combusting spontaneously on contact with air; reacting with halogenated hydrocarbons to further combustion; and reacting with carbon dioxide. Their by-products of combustion are highly toxic and extremely caustic.

Sodium and potassium are much more reactive than is lithium. When lithium burns, it does so with an intense white flame and generates lithium oxide. If water is applied to burning lithium, an explosive reaction occurs, owing to generation of highly flammable hydrogen gas. Lithium also reacts with nitrogen gas (2).

Sodium, used in numerous synthetic processes, can ignite spontaneously in air at room temperature. When exposed to air, it becomes gray-white, owing to the deposition of a coating of sodium hydroxide and sodium oxide. Sodium hydroxide absorbs moisture from the air, which can lead to combustion of the metal (2). On contact with water, sodium violently decomposes and rapidly generates explosive hydrogen gas and sodium hydroxide. It burns with a yellow flame in air to form sodium oxide and burns in pure oxygen to form sodium peroxide (2). Sodium oxides are strong irritants to eyes, mucous membranes, and the respiratory tract.

TABLE 91-1. Reactive metals

Metal	Physiochemical properties and reactivity
Aluminum (Al)	Atomic weight, 26.98; atomic number, 13; MP, 660.37°C. Pure Al is a silver-white metal with high thermal conductivity and corrosion resistance. It is flammable in dust state, powder, or flakes. Dust suspended in air can explode. Al dust in contact with carbon tetrachloride can explode. When mixed with water, burning Al generates explosive hydrogen gas.
Antimony (Sb)	Atomic weight, 121.75; atomic number, 51; MP, 630.74°C. The explosive form of Sb contains small amounts of halogens. It is a poor thermal conductor. It is a blue-silver, brittle metal and burns with a blue flame. In molten conditions, Sb will react with water and release hydrogen, which then reacts with the Sb to form toxic stibine vapors. When heated, it releases toxic stibine fumes and stibine oxide.
Beryllium (Be)	Atomic weight, 9.012; atomic number, 4; MP, 1,278°C. Very light metal. Metal powder can be explosive in air. Dust can produce acute and chronic pulmonary injury.
Boron (B)	Atomic weight, 10.81; atomic number, 5; MP, 2,079.9°C. B sublimes at 2,550°C. Amorphous B is used in pyrotechnic flares and burns with a green flame. It is used as an ignition source in rockets.
Cadmium (Cd)	Atomic weight, 112.41; atomic number, 48; MP, 320.9°C. This soft, bluish-white metal is easily cut. Metal dusts of Cd mixed with air can be explosive. Cd dust inhalation can cause acute and chronic pulmonary disease.
Cerium (Ce)	Atomic weight, 140.12; atomic number, 58; MP, 799°C. A very abundant iron-gray rare earth metal. Decomposes rapidly in hot water and slowly in cold water. Pure Ce can ignite if scratched. Ce is used in "self-cleaning" ovens, glass manufacturing, glass polishing, carbon-arc lighting, and in nuclear industry.
Cesium (Cs)	Atomic weight, 132.90; atomic number, 55; MP, 28.4°C. Cs is a silvery, soft metal and a very alkaline element. It has a high affinity for O_2. Cesium hydroxide is the strongest base known. It is used in atomic clocks and rocket propulsion and is a highly reactive metal with air (pyrophoric) or water. Cs reacts explosively with cold water, generates hydrogen, and burns without a flame. It is very caustic to tissue and will produce rapid tissue necrosis on contact.
Lithium (Li)	Atomic weight, 6.941; atomic number, 3; MP, 180.54°C. Li is a soft silvery metal that is very lightweight and floats in hydrocarbon solvents. It reacts with water to evolve hydrogen. Li requires an ignition source owing to absorption of heat and hydrolysis by Li metal. The pure metal does not react spontaneously in air. Li reacts with O_2 in air at 400°F (200°C) to form lithium oxide. It combines directly with nitrogen to form lithium nitride. At its melting point, Li ignites and burns with a very intense, white flame. Burning Li reacts violently and explosively with water to form lithium hydroxide. Li burns in air, nitrogen, and carbon dioxide.
Magnesium (Mg)	Atomic weight, 24.305; atomic number, 12; MP, 648.8°C. Mg is a light, silver-white metal. In dust form, it can explode on contact with an ignition source. Mg chips and ribbons ignite easily. Water applied to burning Mg will cause an explosive reaction owing to the release of hydrogen gas.
Potassium (K)	Atomic weight, 39.09; atomic number, 19; MP, 63.25°C. This silver-white metal is more reactive than sodium. It reacts explosively on contact with water and generates hydrogen and potassium hydroxide. To prevent reaction in air, K is stored in a hydrocarbon, such as kerosene. K burns in air at room temperature with a purple flame, producing K_2O and K_2O_2. It forms superperoxide on contact with pure O_2. The potassium superperoxide can detonate on contact with organic solvents and organic matter.
Plutonium (Pu)	Atomic weight, 244; atomic number, 94; MP, 641°C. The isotope ^{239}Pu has a half-life of 24,900 years. Pu is a product of nuclear reactions involving uranium. It is extremely hazardous, owing to its emission of α particles. Pu is absorbed by bone marrow and is warm to the touch, owing to its intense α decay. The metal releases enough heat to boil water. It can cause tissue necrosis on contact.
Rubidium (Rb)	Atomic weight, 85.46; atomic number, 37; MP, 38.89°C. Rb is a soft, silver-white metal with high degree of electropositivity. It is the second most alkaline element. Rb ignites spontaneously in air, reacts violently with water, and liberates hydrogen, which combusts. In reaction with water, Rb forms caustic hydroxides that can cause tissue necrosis on contact.
Ruthenium (Ru)	Atomic weight, 101.07; atomic number, 44; MP, 2,310°C. This hard, white metal does not react with cold or hot acids; however, Ru explodes when mixed with potassium chlorates. It is used as a metal hardener.
Sodium (Na)	Atomic weight, 22.98; atomic number, 11; MP, 97.81°C. Na is a waxy-appearing, silver metal. When exposed to air, Na becomes coated with a gray layer of sodium hydroxide and sodium oxide, which can absorb moisture, thus causing combustion. Na can ignite spontaneously in room air and at room temperature. Exposure to water produces an explosive combustion, releasing hydrogen gas.
Strontium (Sr)	Atomic weight, 87.62; atomic number, 38; MP, 769°C. Sr is stored in kerosene to prevent oxidation. It is a silvery metal that turns yellow in air, forming an oxide. Metal dust in air spontaneously ignites. Sr salts are used in pyrotechnics to produce a crimson color. ^{90}Sr is a product of nuclear fallout, with a half-life of 28 years, and is a radiologic health hazard.
Sulfur (S)	Atomic weight, 37.06; atomic number, 16; MP, 112.8°C. S is a light-yellow, brittle solid that can take a crystalline form. S is a component of black gunpowder. Its dust in air can ignite and explode.
Tellurium (Te)	Atomic weight, 127.60; atomic number, 52; MP, 449.5°C. Te is used as an ingredient of blasting caps. It burns with a blue-green flame, forming dioxides. Toxicity is manifested by peripheral neuropathy, seizures, tremor, coma, liver damage, and kidney damage. Gases produce pulmonary irritation. Exposed individuals can develop garliclike breath, sweat, and urine odors.
Thorium (Th)	Atomic weight, 232.04; atomic number, 90; MP, 1,750°C. Th is a source of nuclear fuel. This metal is silver-white and soft in a pure state and pyrophoric in a dust state. It is commonly used in mantles and portable gas lighters and burns with a bright, white light.
Titanium (Ti)	Atomic weight, 47.88; atomic number, 22; MP, 1,660°C. When pure, Ti is a lustrous white metal that burns in both air and nitrogen. It resists the corrosive effects of acids. Ti is stronger and lighter than steel. Titanium tetrachloride is used in incendiary munitions and produces thick smoke when exposed to moisture in air.
Uranium (U)	Atomic weight, 238; atomic number, 92; MP, 1,132°C. U is a heavy, silver-white metal. It is pyrophoric in a dust state in air. U is dissolved by acid but not by alkalis.
Yttrium (Y)	Atomic weight, 88.9; atomic number, 39; MP, 1,522°C. This silvery metal ignites in air in its dust state. Yttrium oxide, the most common form of the metal, is used in color television tubes to impart the color red.
Zinc (Zn)	Atomic weight, 65.38; atomic number, 30; MP, 419.58°C. Zn dust can ignite in air and produce white fumes of zinc oxide.
Zirconium (Zr)	Atomic weight, 91.22; atomic number, 40; MP, 1,852°C. Zr is a gray-white lustrous metal. In a dust state, it can ignite spontaneously in air. It is used in nuclear reactors, explosive primers, flash bulbs, and lamp filaments and as an alloy with steel in surgical instruments.

MP, melting point.

TABLE 91-2. Explosive and flammable metals in nondust form

Potassium: ignites at room temperature, violet flame, more reactive than Na, produces H_2 gas with water
Sodium: ignites at room temperature, yellow flame, generates H_2 gas on water exposure
Lithium: intense white flame, generates H_2 gas when exposed to water while burning, less reactive than Na or K
Cesium: explodes on contact with water, generates H_2 gas, combusts in air
Cerium: ignites if scratched, decomposes in hot water
Sodium–potassium alloy: explosive with water, CO_2, halogenated hydrocarbons, and air
Rubidium: ignites in air
Plutonium: ignites in air

Potassium is a silver-white metal that is more reactive than sodium (2). Potassium ignites spontaneously in room air at room temperatures. It burns with a violet flame. This combustion releases toxic potassium oxide and potassium peroxide. Potassium explodes on contact with liquid bromine. It reacts violently with water in an explosive manner to form potassium hydroxide and hydrogen gas. On contact with pure oxygen, potassium forms superperoxide, which hydrolyzes both to oxygen and hydrogen peroxide and to KOH. The superoxide of potassium reacts explosively with organic solvents and other organic matter.

CESIUM AND CERIUM

Cesium is one of the most reactive of all metals and combusts on contact with air. It reacts explosively with cold water, generating combustible hydrogen gas. A highly caustic metal, it causes necrosis of tissue on contact. It burns without a visible flame (1). Cerium ignites if scratched and can decompose rapidly in hot water.

SODIUM-POTASSIUM ALLOY

A metal alloy of sodium-potassium forms a very unstable compound and is an effective heat exchange medium in nuclear reactors (2). This alloy reacts violently with air, water, halogenated hydrocarbons, and CO_2. Sodium-potassium alloy in contact with organic matter creates an explosive combination.

RUBIDIUM AND PLUTONIUM

Other pyrophoric metals that ignite spontaneously in air are rubidium and plutonium (1). Rubidium reacts violently with water, forming caustic by-products that can cause tissue necrosis on contact. Rubidium can be liquid at room temperature and is a soft, silver-white metal. It forms four oxides: Rb_2O, Rb_2O_2, RB_2O_3, and Rb_2O_4. Rubidium is ionized easily, and both cesium and rubidium are considered for use in "ion engines" for space travel. Naturally occurring rubidium contains ^{87}Rb, a β-particle emitter with a half-life of 5×10^{11} years.

Plutonium is a by-product of uranium use in nuclear reactors, with the most important isotope being ^{239}Pu (half-life, 24,900 years) (1). Plutonium is absorbed specifically by bone marrow and produces radiologic toxicity by intense α-particle emissions (1). As a metal, it can produce enough heat to boil water. Plutonium is a highly dangerous radiologic hazard. It is highly reactive and can cause necrotic damage to tissues and dermal burns (1).

TABLE 91-3. Hazardous properties of magnesium, zirconium, titanium, aluminum, and zinc

Pure forms of metal dust or fine metal particles are explosive.
Explosive properties diminish once the metal oxide forms.
Each is highly reactive with water, causing release of hydrogen (depending on the purity of the metal).
Exothermic reactions proceed to spontaneous combustion.
The powdered forms of each should be labeled as *flammable*.
Fires are extinguished by inert gases.

METAL DUST

The powdered or dust forms of pure thorium, sulfur, aluminum, strontium, magnesium, titanium, uranium, beryllium, yttrium, zinc, and zirconium can ignite and explode spontaneously in air (1,2). Table 91-3 lists some of the hazardous properties of these metals. The combustion hazard of these dusts is diminished greatly if the metals are not in a pure state. Formation of metal oxide coating around the metal reduces the hazard. Combustion also depends on metallic particle size and then dispersion in air.

MAGNESIUM

Magnesium dust is explosive when mixed with air. Solid magnesium burns with an intense white flame. Water directly applied to flaming magnesium produces an explosive reaction. Burning magnesium produces irritating magnesium oxide fumes that can injure the airways and lungs seriously. Magnesium is a very light metal used to reduce weight in machines and metal parts. It burns with an intense flame and heat. Water and magnesium generate hydrogen; therefore, water should not be used to extinguish magnesium fires because explosion can occur (2).

ALUMINUM

Aluminum dust is highly explosive when mixed with air and on contact with an ignition source (1,2). Aluminum also is highly flammable. Burning aluminum reacts with water, forming aluminum oxide and generating explosive hydrogen gas; reacts with CO_2 and halon fire extinguishers; and produces oxides and nitrides of the metal. The presence of the oxide forms a protective barrier on the metal's surface.

TITANIUM

In a pure state, titanium ignites in air as a dust. It burns also in nitrogen. It is very resistant to the corrosive effects of acids and alkalis (1).

Titanium tetrachloride ($TiCl_4$) reacts with water or with moisture in air to form an irritating, corrosive, thick smoke. Its hydrolysis products include hydrochloric acid, titanium hydroxide, $Ti(OH)_4$, and $TiOCl_2$. All are irritants of the respiratory tract and skin. Titanium dust is flammable and explosive both in fine particulate metal form and in bulk form. Burning titanium reacts with CO_2 and halon fire extinguishers. Burning titanium reacts with water to produce explosive hydrogen gas and produces titanium oxides and nitrides (1,2).

ZINC

Zinc metal dust is flammable and is an explosive hazard when mixed with air. It reacts slowly with water to generate explosive hydrogen gas and forms only the oxide, not the nitride, of the metal. Burning zinc reacts chemically with halon and CO_2 gas extinguishers (1,2).

ZIRCONIUM

Zirconium metal dust is extremely flammable and can cause explosions. It burns with a brilliant flame, forming oxides and nitrides of the metal. Burning zirconium also reacts with halon and CO_2 fire-extinguishing agents (1,2).

REFERENCES

1. Weast R, Astle M, Beyer W, eds. *CRC handbook of chemistry and physics.* Boca Raton, FL: CRC Press, 1986.
2. Meyer E. *Chemistry of hazardous materials.* Englewood Cliffs, NJ: Prentice-Hall, 1977.

CHAPTER 92
Acrylamides

Marianne Cloeren

CHEMICAL AND PHYSICAL PROPERTIES

Acrylamide ($CH_2CHCONH_2$; Chemical Abstracts Service registry number 79-06-1) is an odorless white crystalline solid at room temperature. Synonyms are *propenamide, acrylic amide,* and *akrylamid.* Acrylamide is a vinyl monomer produced from the hydration of acrylonitrile and sulfuric acid (84.5%) followed by neutralization. It is stable in solution and is soluble in polar solvents, such as water, ethanol, and acetone. Table 92-1 lists the general chemical and physical properties of acrylamide (1–3).

Acrylamide polymer has a wide range of applications. The major use of acrylamide monomer, a skin irritant and neurotoxin, is in the production of polymer, which is believed to be nontoxic (4,5). Acrylamide has two major functional groups—an amide group conjugated with a vinyl group—and it undergoes reactions at both of these groups.

TABLE 92-1. Physical and chemical properties of acrylamide

Appearance	White crystalline solid
Odor	None
Molecular formula	$CH_2 = CHCONH_2$
Molecular weight	71.08
Melting point	84.5°C
Boiling point	125°C at 25 mm Hg
Density	1.222 g/mL at 30°C
Heat of polymerization	19.8 kcal/mol

Adapted from refs. 1 and 7.

$$\underset{\beta}{CH_2} = \underset{\alpha}{CH}-\overset{O}{\overset{||}{C}}-NH_2$$

It reacts easily at the β position with hydroxy, amino, and thiol groups, but its most important reaction from an industrial standpoint is vinyl-type polymerization.

$$-(CH_2-\underset{\underset{CONH_2=}{|}}{CH})-_{\chi}$$

In the industrial polymerization of acrylamide, solutions of 8% to 30% acrylamide monomer are placed in a reactor vessel with one component of a redox system (e.g., sodium bromate–sodium sulfite) while the other component is added gradually. Metal ions sometimes are used as cocatalysts (4). Then the gelatinous solid polyacrylamide, which is impermeable to water, is poured out, washed and dried, cut up, ground, and sold as the granulated solid polymer (6).

SITES, INDUSTRIES, AND BUSINESSES ASSOCIATED WITH EXPOSURES

Monomeric acrylamide first was produced in Germany in 1893, was patented in the United States in 1935 by the Rohm and Haas Company, and first was produced commercially in the 1950s by American Cyanamid Company (7). There are three major U.S. manufacturers of acrylamide, which have a production capacity of more than 215 million pounds per year (8). Acrylamide monomer production has been estimated at 15 to 20 million pounds in 1966, 40 million in 1973, and 86 million in 1983 (7,8). Industry projections for 2000 put U.S. production at more than 95 to 100 million pounds.

Acrylamide polymers first were used as flocculators (used to separate solids from aqueous solution) in sewage and wastewater treatment and in some mining operations. This is still their major use, but acrylamide has many other applications, and the list is growing rapidly. Polyacrylamide long has been used in the paper and pulp industry to strengthen paper and board. It is used in the treatment of drinking water and in the oil industry to help to bring oil in a well to the surface. Acrylamide polymers break oil-in-water emulsions, dissipate fog, and stabilize soil. A major use of acrylamide is as a grouting agent; the liquid monomer, together with a catalyst and a cross-linking agent, is pumped into soil, clay, or stone walls of excavations, where it polymerizes to produce a watertight seal. It is used in this way in the construction of dams, foundations, tunnels, roadways, and sewer systems. In biomedical research, polyacrylamide gels are used for chromatography and electrophoresis. Other applications are in photography, metal coatings, ceramics, plastics, paints, adhesives, and binders and in the textile industry (dyes, sizing, and permanent press fabrics) (1,4,9). The National Institute for Occupational Safety and Health estimated in 1976 that 20,000 U.S. workers were exposed potentially to acrylamide (7). Table 92-2 lists industries associated with exposure to acrylamide.

Approximately 50 cases of human acrylamide intoxication have been reported in the literature, all occupationally related except for one Japanese family of five poisoned by contaminated well water (7,10). Although acrylamide polymer is used widely, the polymer is nontoxic and poses a health risk only from the small amount of monomer allowed to contaminate it (up to 2% in some applications) (4,5). All cases of occupational intoxication reported thus far occurred in workers involved in the polymer-

TABLE 92-2. Industries associated with potential exposure to acrylamide

Acrylamide manufacture
Adhesive tape manufacture
Ceramics plants
Construction (waterproofing of dams, sewers, roads, tunnels)
Flocculator production
Metal coating operations
Mining
Oil wells
Paint factories
Paper making
Synthetic fiber manufacture
Textile mills (in sizing, dyes, and permanent press fabrics)

ization of monomeric acrylamide (7), either in factories producing polymers (6,11) or during grouting operations (12,13).

CLINICAL TOXICOLOGY

Routes of Exposure, Absorption, Metabolism, and Elimination

Acrylamide is very soluble in water, is absorbed easily, and follows all routes of absorption except inhalation, which has not been examined closely. It has similar neurotoxicity whether administered orally, intravenously, intraperitoneally, subcutaneously, intramuscularly, or dermally in aqueous solution (14,15). Dermal contact and ingestion have been the major routes of exposure in humans, but no data are available regarding the possible contribution of inhalation of airborne acrylamide. Garland and Patterson (6) suggested that inhalation is an unimportant route of acrylamide exposure, as the monomer is heavy and forms no dust; they noted that no cases of acrylamide poisoning occurred at the factories they visited, where skin protection was enforced rigidly.

Studies of radionuclide-labeled acrylamide administered intravenously to rats showed that it was distributed within a few minutes throughout the total body water. Its serum concentration then decreased exponentially, with a half-life of less than 2 hours. Although freely distributed, the bulk was bound to tissues and circulating proteins, especially hemoglobin. At 1 day after injection, the highest levels of free and protein-bound radiolabel were found in whole blood, with decreasing levels found in kidney, liver, brain, spinal cord, and sciatic nerve. By 14 days after injection, the free radiolabel had disappeared, but the protein-bound radiolabel remained at 25% of its day-1 level, except in whole blood, where it remained at 100% of its day-1 level (16,17). This persistence of tissue-associated radiolabel may represent either protein binding or incorporation of metabolic fragments of acrylamide into proteins (18).

The major route of biotransformation of acrylamide is conjugation with glutathione, a reaction that appears to be detoxifying. After enzymatic and nonenzymatic reaction with glutathione, acrylamide is excreted eventually in the urine as *N*-acetyl-*S*-(3-amino-3-oxypropyl)cysteine. Acrylamide inhibits the enzyme activity of glutathione-*S*-transferase *in vitro* and *in vivo*; thus, it may inhibit its own detoxification via this route (16,18).

Acrylamide also undergoes biotransformation via the microsomal cytochrome P-450 system, as evidenced by increased clearing of acrylamide in homogenates from animals whose cytochrome P-450 levels have been elevated by pretreatment with phenobarbital (19); however, delay of acrylamide-induced neuropathy by pretreatment with phenobarbital shown in one study (19) has not been reproduced (16,20); in another study, the opposite effect was shown (21).

Sign, Symptoms, and Syndromes

GENERAL TOXICOLOGY

Acrylamide monomer has been recognized as a potent neurotoxin since the 1950s, when it first was produced commercially. After several poorly documented cases of neurotoxicity in workers handling acrylamide, numerous animal studies have confirmed its neurotoxicity. Although its neurologic effects predominate, weight loss is a consistent finding in animal studies, and the loss is not due to reduced food intake, as acrylamide-intoxicated animals gained less weight than did control rats fed to match the intake of the study rats (22). Weight loss has been described also in human cases (6,11). In addition, acrylamide causes a contact dermatitis, which may be the only sign of acrylamide exposure but often precedes development of neurologic symptoms (6,11–13,23,24).

NEUROTOXICITY

Acrylamide is best known for its peripheral (motor and sensory) polyneuropathy; however, it also affects the central and autonomic nervous systems. Acrylamide neuropathy falls into the category of "dying-back polyneuropathies," characterized by degeneration of axons proceeding distally to proximally and affecting fibers in both the peripheral and central nervous systems.

ACUTE TOXICITY

Human Cases. Only one episode of acute acrylamide poisoning has been reported in humans; it probably occurred over several days of exposure. Igisu et al. (10) described a family in Japan poisoned by acrylamide after it leached into their well water from nearby sewer-grouting work. The family used the well water for bathing, cooking, and drinking. Acrylamide subsequently was measured at 400 parts per million in the well water (a level that, when fed to rats daily, caused paralysis in 24 days) (14). Symptoms appeared some 3.5 weeks after the sewer work occurred. The symptoms in three adults, who were affected more severely than were the two children, were gait disturbance, delirium, and hallucinations (visual only in two; visual, auditory, and tactile in one). All three had slurred speech, two had horizontal nystagmus, and one had urinary retention. Initial examination revealed no sensory deficit, weakness, or decreased deep tendon reflexes; however, these findings developed in all three patients 2 to 4 weeks later, after mental status had returned to normal. Electroencephalography on initial presentation showed only excessive sleepiness. Blood hematology and chemistry test results were normal. At the time that sensory deficits appeared, motor nerve conduction tests showed decreased velocity in all three patients. The three adults had recovered within 4 months.

Of the two children, a 13-year-old boy was affected more than the 10-year-old, with drowsiness and truncal ataxia but no other findings on examination. He had recovered within 2 weeks. The 10-year-old had only peculiar behavior, which lasted only 3 days. The difference in effect in the children may be related to lower cumulative dose (they were at school during the day) or may be due to the relative protection of youth shown in some animal studies (25,26).

Table 92-3 lists the signs and symptoms of acute acrylamide poisoning in an exposed family. An interesting point about the aforementioned family is that none of the patients demonstrated signs of dermatitis (seen consistently in occupational cases),

TABLE 92-3. Signs and symptoms of acute acrylamide poisoning in a Japanese family

Patient	Mother	Father	Grandmother	Son	Daughter
Age (yr)	40	42	65	13	10
Initial presentation					
Ataxia	+	+	+	+	–
Hallucinations	+	+	+	–	–
Disorientation	+	+	+	–	–
Slurred speech	+	+	+	–	–
Nystagmus	–	+	+	–	–
Drowsiness	–	–	+	+	–
Later findings					
Decreased sensation	+	+	+	–	–
Paresthesias	+	+	–	–	–
Absent deep tendon reflexes	+	–	–	–	–

Adapted from ref. 10.

despite some probable contribution of dermal exposure through bath water. Likely, ingestion of acrylamide played a greater role in these cases than in the occupational cases.

Animal Experiments. Acute toxicity of acrylamide in cats was studied in 1958 by Kuperman (15), who found that the development of neurotoxicity was independent of the route of absorption and that the effects were cumulative if the toxin was given in divided doses; therefore, the same total dose was required to produce a given effect. The effects in cats were primarily ataxia and tremor, which were reversible when acrylamide was discontinued. Kuperman (15) also found that very high doses caused convulsions and death.

In 1964, McCollister et al. (14) studied the toxicity of acrylamide in various animals. They found the median lethal dose for a single oral dose to be 150 to 180 mg per kg in rats, guinea pigs, and rabbits and 100 to 200 mg per kg in cats and monkeys. One monkey given a total of 200 mg per kg in two divided doses was unable to stand on day 3 but had enough strength to crawl. It died the same day, and pathology showed congestion of lungs and kidneys and focal necrosis in the liver. Histologic examination of the liver showed congestion of the sinusoids, with fatty degeneration and necrosis. The kidneys showed degeneration of the convoluted tubules and glomeruli. Peripheral nerves were not examined, but no central nervous system pathology was seen. Signs of toxicity in rats, cats, and monkeys were, progressively, stiffness or weakness of the hindquarters (or both), loss of ability to control the hindquarters, urinary retention, ataxia of the forelimbs, and inability to stand. McCollister verified Kuperman's finding that the effects depended on the cumulative dose and were independent of route of absorption.

CHRONIC TOXICITY

Human Cases. Approximately 50 cases of acrylamide poisoning in humans have been reported in the literature (7). All these cases, with the exception of the previously discussed Japanese family, occurred over weeks to months in an occupation requiring handling of the monomer in the course of polymerization. Typically, a dermatitis occurred first and, in some patients, this may be the only symptom. Patients described peeling skin and red or blue discoloration of the skin where contact with acrylamide occurred (usually hands and arms). They also described excessive sweating, especially of the palms and soles. Gait disturbance usually follows or is concomitant with the skin changes, and then paresthesias, numbness, and weakness in the distal extremities are seen. Sometimes slurred speech and overflow incontinence occur, owing to neurogenic bladder. Weight loss is possible. Physical examination is notable for truncal ataxia, variable sensory deficits, distal weakness, absent deep tendon reflexes, and sometimes distal small muscle wasting. On cessation of exposure, all patients improved, but most required several months to return to baseline, and some had not recovered fully after 1 year (7,13). Table 92-4 lists the signs and symptoms of chronic acrylamide intoxication in the six patients (typical cases) described by Garland and Patterson (6); these six patients worked at three different factories producing flocculators.

Fullerton (27) examined the nerves of patients 1, 4, and 5 in the Garland and Patterson study (6) during recovery from acrylamide intoxication and found disproportionate slowing of conduction distally in muscle fibers and decreased sensory action potentials. Histologic examination of the sural nerve of the patient exposed most recently to acrylamide (2.5 months) showed some axonal degeneration, decreased density of large fibers, and evidence of nerve regeneration.

Animal Experiments. Numerous studies have examined chronic acrylamide toxicity in animals. Such intoxication predominantly produces a peripheral neuropathy. Signs appear distally initially and slowly progress proximally, as is typical of the dying-back polyneuropathies. Animals develop hindlimb unsteadiness, with loss of upper and lower deep tendon reflexes (28); this progresses to gross ataxia, then paralysis, and finally complete paralysis; bladder distention also is common (29). Hindlimb signs appear before forelimb signs. Reaction to painful stimuli is preserved even when the animals are paralyzed (28,30). Cessation of exposure always is followed by improvement and usually complete recovery, although it may take months. An anamnestic response has been noted; animals become more vulnerable to later repeat doses than they were originally (29,31). Kaplan and Murphy (31) suggested that this response may be due to reinjury of nerves that have regenerated only partially.

Electrophysiologic studies on acrylamide-intoxicated animals show no abnormalities until symptoms are present and then show a small reduction in nerve conduction velocity (30). In severely intoxicated animals, nerve conduction velocity is reduced 20% to 50% in distal regions (26,30,32). Hindlimbs are more affected than are forelimbs (30), and both velocity and amplitude reduction are more marked in sensory conduction than in motor conduction (32). The reduction in maximal nerve conduction velocity is thought to be secondary to degeneration of the largest-diameter, fastest-conducting nerve fibers (9). The early demise of large long axons has been confirmed by quantitative histologic studies (26,28,33).

At first, histopathologic studies in animals were unrewarding. The early light-microscopical studies did not look at peripheral nerves and found no central nervous system abnormalities (14,15). In 1966, Fullerton and Barnes (26) established acrylamide toxicity as a dying-back neuropathy by showing degeneration of the distal axons of long peripheral nerves.

Studies of baboons confirmed distal axonal degeneration in large-diameter nerves and showed some paranodal changes thought to be due to Schwann cell response to degeneration axons (28).

TABLE 92-4. Signs and symptoms of chronic acrylamide poisoning in six factory workers

	1	2	3	4	5	6
Age	19	23	30	56	59	57
Exposure (wk)	6	12	12	8	60	4
Excessive sweating	+	+	—	+	+	—
Peeling skin	+	+	—	+	—	—
Difficulty walking	+	—	—	—	—	—
Paresthesias	—	+	—	+	+	+
Weight loss	+	—	—	—	—	—
Lethargy, fatigue	+	—	+	+	+	+
Slurred speech	+	—	—	+	—	—
Decreased sensation	+	+	+	+	+	+
Temperature	—	+	—	+	—	—
Vibration	+	—	+	—	—	+
Pinprick	—	+	—	—	—	—
Light touch	—	+	—	—	—	—
Position	—	—	+	—	—	—
Positive Romberg's sign	+	+	+	—	+	+
Absent deep tendon reflexes	+	+	+	+	+	+
Muscle weakness	+	+	+	+	+	+
Muscle wasting	+	—	—		—	+
Other	[a]	—	—	[b]	—	—
Time to recovery (mo)	>6	8	? ("quick")	>6	?	>4

[a]Tremors.
[b]Urinary incontinence.
Adapted from ref. 6.

Electron microscopy allowed more detailed examination of affected nerves. Prineas (34) discovered that an increase in distal axonal neurofilaments preceded degeneration and that small axons in the spinal gray matter and axons in the gracile nucleus were affected along with large peripheral nerves. The earliest detectable morphologic changes in acrylamide-intoxicated cats were found by Schaumburg et al. (35) to occur in the pacinian corpuscles in the toe pads. First, filopod axon processes were lost, axolemmas disappeared, and axoplasm was phagocytosed by inner core cells. These changes were found before any clinical signs of toxicity. The next changes were degeneration of adjacent primary annulospiral endings of muscle spindles in hindfoot muscles, then degeneration of secondary muscle spindle endings of the motor nerve terminals supplying nearby extrafusal muscle fibers. Accumulation of neurofilaments occurred in these sensory and motor terminals as early degeneration began. Degeneration proceeded proximally and was accompanied by axonal Schwann cell ingrowths and swollen paranodal regions. Unmyelinated fibers were found to be relatively resistant; however, Post and McLeod (33,36) found involvement of unmyelinated nerves, with larger-diameter fibers degenerating more than the smaller fibers. They also showed that the sympathetic and parasympathetic nervous systems are damaged by acrylamide in the same way as is the peripheral nervous system.

Similar, although less marked, changes have been found in the central nervous system, in the gracile nucleus and fasciculus gracilis (34), in the cerebellar vermis (37), in the pineal gland (38), and in the distal ends of spinal cord fibers (34).

Chronic intoxication of rats with acrylamide reveals evidence of regeneration of nerve fibers, even in animals still receiving acrylamide in their diet (26). Regenerating nerve fibers were seen also in a sural nerve taken from a patient who had acrylamide poisoning and evidence of regeneration at the time of exposure (27). Although regeneration occurs in the presence of acrylamide, it is impaired (39,40). This impaired regeneration was studied by Griffin et al. (40), who found that [^{3}H]leucine was incorporated normally into sensory ganglia during regeneration but that the radioactivity was carried less rapidly beyond the crush injury zone than in controls. They noted that the radiolabel accumulated in abnormal growth sprouts and believed that the cause of delayed transport was this trapping of protein, not a primary defect in fast axonal transport.

The biochemical event (or events) responsible for the distal retrograde degeneration seen in acrylamide poisoning has not been determined, but recent studies have investigated the possibility that degeneration is caused by a perturbation in energy metabolism in the axon (41–46). Other studies have assessed axonal transport, especially alterations in retrograde axonal transport, which conceivably could disrupt biofeedback to the perikaryon regarding metabolic needs at the distal end (18,47). Other hypotheses argue for primary axon damage by local toxic action (35) or for metabolic damage to the perikaryon, rendering it unable to meet the metabolic demands of the distal axon (18,34,35). Elucidation of the biochemical mechanisms of acrylamide neurotoxicity may lead to treatment of similar distal retrograde neuropathies seen in some natural diseases, such as amyotrophic lateral sclerosis, Werdnig-Hoffmann's disease, and Friedreich's ataxia.

Acrylamide Analogs

Some attention has been paid to analogs of acrylamide, in the hope that studying them may shed light on the biochemical mechanisms of neurotoxicity. Several analogs were found to be neurotoxic, but none appeared more so than acrylamide. Reduction of the double bond or deletion of the nitrogen atom was found to eliminate neurotoxicity. The acrylyl moiety (CH_2CHCO^-) was found to be essential for neurotoxicity, and no relation was found between reactivity with sulfhydryl groups and neurotoxicity (18). *N*-Hydroxymethylacrylamide, *N*,*N*-diethylacrylamide, *N*-methylacrylamide, and *N*-isopropylacrylamide all caused some neurotoxicity at doses higher than those required for acrylamide (16,20,48–50). All these and several non-neurotoxic analogs were metabolized by glutathione and by microsomal enzymes (51). The neurotoxic analogs had negligible breakdown to acrylamide; thus, their neurotoxicity is not secondary to acrylamide itself (16). One analog—methylene-bis-acrylamide—was not neurotoxic but caused weight loss (20). As yet, no data have been published in regard to human poisonings with analogs of acrylamide.

Teratogenicity and Reproductive Effects

In rodent studies, acrylamide crosses the placenta to reach significant concentrations in the fetus, causing neurotoxic effects (tibial and optic nerve degeneration) in the neonates at levels that were nontoxic to the mother. The lowest observed effect level for developmental toxicity in mice was 20 mg per kg per day.

Acrylamide affects reproductive ability by causing decreased copulatory performance in male rats, decreased fertility in male mice, and degeneration of testicular epithelial tissue in mice. The lowest observed effect level and no-observed-effect level for reproductive effects in mice were 2.0 and 0.5 mg per kg per day, respectively. Acrylamide also causes dominant lethal effects by loss of total embryos implanted per litter and by increased resorption of embryos (8).

Carcinogenicity

Acrylamide studies of rats and mice have shown increased incidence of benign and malignant tumors, qualifying acrylamide as an animal carcinogen. Although the very limited epidemiologic data (52–57) do not show any increased mortality from cancer in humans exposed to acrylamide, the American Conference of Governmental Industrial Hygienists has assigned acrylamide an A2 rating (suspected human carcinogen), and the U.S. Occupational Safety and Health Administration is implementing stricter standards for workplace exposure to reduce the risk of cancer (53).

Management of Toxicity

DIAGNOSIS

Clinical examination should focus on the skin and on the neurologic system. No laboratory evaluation of blood or urine has proved useful in diagnosing or monitoring acrylamide intoxication. Suspicion of acrylamide poisoning, if such poisoning is occupational, warrants removal of affected individuals from the job and investigation of worksite conditions. Abnormal sensory and motor nerve conduction tests may be helpful in documenting deficits and monitoring recovery; however, what should be kept in mind is that in acute or subacute intoxication, these tests may not show abnormal results until many days after the initial presentation.

Although no routine laboratory tests are helpful in diagnosing acrylamide intoxication, some experimental methods have been suggested. Poole et al. (54) detected acrylamide in nerve tissue homogenates from intoxicated animals using electron-capture gas chromatography. Bailey et al. (55) suggested monitoring acrylamide exposure by determination of *S*-(2-carboxyethyl)cysteine in hydrolyzed hemoglobin; acrylamide exposure causes formation of a covalently bound reaction product with cysteine residues in hemoglobin, with a dose-response relationship between acrylamide dose and production of hemoglobin adduct.

TREATMENT

No treatment is available for acrylamide intoxication. Most patients gradually recover after cessation of exposure. Patients may be more susceptible to repeat injury from acrylamide if they return to an exposure situation before complete recovery. No reliable data address the considerations of when (or whether) patients should return to an exposure-related job.

REFERENCES

1. Hawley GG, ed. *The condensed chemical dictionary,* 10th ed. New York: Van Nostrand–Reinhold, 1981:16.
2. MacWilliams DC. In: *The Kirk-Othmer concise encyclopedia of chemical technology.* New York: John Wiley and Sons, 1985:22–23.
3. Rom WN, ed. *Environmental and occupational medicine.* Boston: Little, Brown and Company, 1983:603.
4. Spencer PS, Schaumburg HH. A review of acrylamide neurotoxicity: I. Properties, uses and human exposures. *Can J Neurol Sci* 1974;1:143–150.
5. McCollister DD, Oyen F, Rowe VK. Toxicologic investigations of polyacrylamides. *Toxicol Appl Pharmacol* 1965;7:639.
6. Garland TO, Patterson MWH. Six cases of acrylamide poisoning. *BMJ* 1967;4:134–138.
7. National Institute for Occupational Safety and Health. *Criteria for a recommended standard—occupational exposure to acrylamide.* DHEW (NIOSH) publication no. 77–112. Cincinnati: National Institute for Occupational Safety and Health, 1976.
8. Dearfield KL, Abemathy CO, Ottley MS, Brantnet JH, Hayes PF. Acrylamide: its metabolism, developmental and reproductive effects, genotoxicity, and carcinogenicity. *Mutat Res* 1988;195:45–77.
9. LeQuesne PM. Acrylamide. In: Spencer PS, Schaumburg HH, eds. *Experimental and clinical neurotoxicology.* Baltimore: Williams & Wilkins, 1980:309–325.
10. Igisu H, Goto I, Kawamura Y, Kato M, Izumi K, Kuroiwa Y. Acrylamide encephaloneuropathy due to well water pollution. *J Neurol Neurosurg Psychiatry* 1975;38:581–584.
11. Davenport JG, Farrell DF, Sumi SM. "Giant axonal neuropathy" caused by industrial chemicals: neurofilamentous axonal masses in man. *Neurology* 1976;26:919–923.
12. Auld RB, Bedwell SF. Peripheral neuropathy with sympathetic over-activity from industrial contact with acrylamide. *Can Med Assoc J* 1967;96:652–654.
13. Kesson CM, Baird AW, Lawson DH. Acrylamide poisoning. *Postgrad Med J* 1977;53:16–17.
14. McCollister DD, Oyen F, Rowe VK. Toxicology of acrylamide. *Toxicol Appl Pharmacol* 1964;6:172.
15. Kuperman AS. Effects of acrylamide on the central nervous system of the cat. *J Pharmacol Exp Ther* 1958;123:180–192.
16. Edwards PM. Distribution and metabolism of acrylamide and its neurotoxic analogues in rats. *Biochem Pharmacol* 1975;24:1277–1282.
17. Hashimoto K, Aldridge WN. Biochemical studies on acrylamide, a neurotoxic agent. *Biochem Pharmacol* 1970;19:2591–2604.
18. Miller MS, Spencer PS. The mechanisms of acrylamide axonopathy. *Annu Rev Pharmacol Toxicol* 1985;25:643–666.
19. Kaplan ML, Murphy SD, Gilles FH. Modification of acrylamide neuropathy in rats by selected factors. *Toxicol Appl Pharmacol* 1973;24:564–579.
20. Edwards PM. Neurotoxicity of acrylamide and its analogues, and effects of these analogues and other agents on acrylamide neuropathy. *Br J Ind Med* 1975;32:31–38.
21. Srivastava SP, Seth PK, Das M, Mukhtar H. Effects of mixed-function oxidase modifiers on neurotoxicity of acrylamide in rats. *Biochem Pharmacol* 1985;34:1099–1102.
22. Gipon L, Schotman P, Jennekens FGI, Gispen WH. Polyneuropathies and CNS protein metabolism: I. Description of acrylamide syndrome in rats. *Neuropathol Appl Neurobiol* 1977;3:115.
23. Pegum JS, Medhurst FA. Contact dermatitis from penetration of rubber gloves by acrylamide monomer. *BMJ* 1971;2:141–143.
24. Lambert J, Matthieu L, Dockx P. Contact dermatitis from acrylamide. *Contact Dermatitis* 1988;19:65.
25. Suzuki K, Pfaff LD. Acrylamide neuropathy in rats. *Acta Neuropathol* 1973;24:197–213.
26. Fullerton PM, Barnes JM. Peripheral neuropathy in rats produced by acrylamide. *Br J Ind Med* 1966;23:210–221.
27. Fullerton PM. Electrophysiologic and histologic observations on peripheral nerves in acrylamide poisoning in man. *J Neurol Neurosurg Psychiatry* 1969;32:186.
28. Hopkins A. Effect of acrylamide on the peripheral nervous system of the baboon. *J Neurol Neurosurg Psychiatry* 1970;33:805–816.
29. Spencer PS, Schaumburg HH. Review of acrylamide neurotoxicity: II. Experimental animal neurotoxicity and pathologic mechanisms. *Can J Neurol Sci* 1974;1:152–169.
30. Leswing RJ, Ribelin WE. Physiologic and pathologic changes in acrylamide neuropathy. *Arch Environ Health* 1969;18:23.
31. Kaplan ML, Murphy SD. Effect of acrylamide on rotarod performance and sciatic nerve beta-glucuronidase activity of rats. *Toxicol Appl Pharmacol* 1972;22:259.
32. Hopkins AP, Gilliatt RW. Motor and sensory conduction velocity in the baboon: normal values and changes during acrylamide neuropathy. *J Neurol Neurosurg Psychiatry* 1971;34:415–426.
33. Post EJ, McLeod JG. Acrylamide autonomic neuropathy in the cat: 1. Neurophysiological and histological studies. *J Neurol Sci* 1977;33:353.

34. Prineas J. The pathogenesis of dying-back neuropathies: II. An ultrastructural study of experimental acrylamide intoxication in the cat. *J Neuropathol Exp Neurol* 1969;28:598–621.
35. Schaumburg HH, Wisniewski HM, Spencer PS. Ultrastructural studies of the dying-back process: 1. Peripheral nerve terminal and axon degeneration in systemic acrylamide intoxication. *J Neuropathol Exp Neurol* 1974;33:260–284.
36. Post EJ, McLeod JG. Acrylamide autonomic neuropathy in the cat: 2. Effects on mesenteric vascular control. *J Neurol Sci* 1977;33:375.
37. Ghetti B, Wisniewski HM, Cook RD, Schaumburg HH. Changes in the CNS after acute and chronic acrylamide intoxication. *Am J Pathol* 973;70: 78A(abst).
38. Schmidt RE, Plurad SB, Clark HB. Acrylamide induced sympathetic autonomic neuropathy causing pineal degeneration. *Lab Invest* 1987;56:505–517.
39. Morgan-Hughes JA, Sinclair S, Durston JHJ. The pattern of peripheral nerve regeneration induced by crush in rats with severe acrylamide neuropathy. *Brain* 1974;97:235.
40. Griffin JW, Price DL, Drachman DB. Impaired axonal regeneration in acrylamide intoxication. *J Neurobiol* 1977;8:355.
41. Schotman P, Gipon L, Jennekens FGI, Gispen WH. Polyneuropathies and CNS protein metabolism: II. Changes in the incorporation rate of leucine during acrylamide intoxication. *Neuropathol Appl Neurobiol* 1977;3:125.
42. Schotman P, Gipon L, Jennekens FGI, Gispen WH. Polyneuropathies and CNS protein metabolism: III. Changes in protein synthesis rate induced by acrylamide intoxication. *J Neuropathol Exp Neurol* 1978;37:820.
43. Brimijoin WS, Hammond PJ. Acrylamide neuropathy in the rat: effects on energy metabolism in the sciatic nerve. *Mayo Clin Proc* 1985;60:3–8.
44. Howland RD. Biochemical studies of acrylamide neuropathy. *Neurotoxicology* 1985;6:7–16.
45. Sharma RP, Obersteiner EJ. Acrylamide cytotoxicity in chick ganglia cultures. *Toxicol Appl Pharmacol* 1977;42:149.
46. Johnson EC, Murphy SD. Effect of acrylamide intoxication on pyridine nucleotide concentration and functions in rat cerebral cortex. *Biochem Pharmacol* 1977;26:2151.
47. Miller MS, Miller MJ, Burks TF, Sipes IG. Altered retrograde axonal transport of nerve growth factor after single and repeated doses of acrylamide in the rat. *Toxicol Appl Pharmacol* 1983;69:96–101.
48. Tanii H, Hashimoto K. Neurotoxicity of acrylamide and related compounds in rats: effects on rotarod performance, morphology of nerves and neurotubulin. *Arch Toxicol* 1983;54:203–213.
49. Barnes JM. Observations on the effects on rats of compounds related to acrylamide. *Br J Ind Med* 1970;27:147–149.
50. Hashimoto K, Sakamoto J, Tanii H. Neurotoxicity of acrylamide and related compounds, and their effects on male gonads in mice. *Arch Toxicol* 1981;47: 179–189.
51. Tanii H, Hashimoto K. Studies on in vitro metabolism of acrylamide and related compounds. *Arch Toxicol* 1981;48:157–166.
52. Sobel W, Bond GG, Parsons TW, Brenner FE. Acrylamide cohort mortality study. *Br J Ind Med* 1986;43:785–788.
53. *Federal Register* 1989 Jan 19;54(12):2674.
54. Poole CF, Sye WF, Zlatkis A, Spencer PS. Determination of acrylamide in nerve tissue homogenates by electron-capture gas chromatography. *J Chromatogr* 1981;217:239–245.
55. Bailey E, Farmer PB, Bird I, Lamb JH, Peal JA. Monitoring exposure to acrylamide by the determination of *S*-(2-carboxyethyl)cysteine in hydrolyzed hemoglobin by gas chromatography mass spectrometry. *Anal Biochem* 1986;157:241–248.
56. McLean JD, Mann JR, Jacoby SA. A monitoring method for determining acrylamide in an industrial environment. *Am Ind Hyg Assoc J* 1978;39:247.
57. Collins JJ, Swaen SMH, Marsh GM, Utidjian HMD, Caporossi JC, Lucas LJ. Mortality patterns among workers exposed to acrylamide. *J Occup Med* 1989;31:614–617.

CHAPTER 93
Isocyanates

Karen K. Phillips and John M. Peters

Since the early 1950s, U.S. manufacturers have used isocyanates primarily as starting materials in the manufacture of a variety of plastic products, including rigid and flexible polyurethane foams, urethane-based coatings (e.g., paints and electrical wire insulation), and elastomers and spandex fibers. The main health effects of isocyanates involve the lungs, but other organ systems may be affected. Most reported toxic effects have been due to toluene diisocyanate (TDI) because of its widespread use. Although slightly different in their properties, other isocyanates cause similar problems under appropriate conditions.

USES OF ISOCYANATES

TDI [Chemical Abstracts Service (CAS) no. 26471-62-5] is a combination of 2,4-TDI (CAS no. 584-84-9) and 2,6-TDI (CAS no. 91-08-7), usually found in an 80:20 mixture of the isomers. TDI is required for the manufacture of flexible foam used in a variety of products, including mattresses, upholstery cushions, automobile seats, and packaging materials. Methylene diphenyl diisocyanate (MDI) has replaced TDI in the production of rigid foams because it is less hazardous, owing to its lower volatility. Rigid foam is used as insulation in home refrigerators and ovens, whereas spray-in foam is used for railroad cars, truck trailers, and boats. As protective coatings, polyurethanes are applied to electrical wiring, for which their insulating properties are valuable. They are used as two-part paints and floor, concrete, and wood finishes, for which their hardness and durability are advantageous. Aircraft, truck, and other coatings often are composed of diisocyanate prepolymer systems.

Isocyanates are used also as adhesives and as elastomers in automobile bumpers, printing rolls, liners for mine and grain elevator chutes, shoe soles, coated fabrics, and spandex fibers. MDI is used as part of a no-bake binder system for casting molds in foundries. Other diisocyanates, such as hexamethylene diisocyanate (a common component of paints), naphthalene diisocyanate, isophorone diisocyanate, polymethylene polyphenyl isocyanate, and dicyclohexyl methane diisocyanate (hydrogenated MDI), also have commercial uses.

The representative trade names for isocyanate products are Centari, Desmodur, Hylene, Imron, Isonate, Mondur, Nacconate, Niax, and Rubinate.

Methyl isocyanate is used in the manufacture of carbamate pesticides. The 1984 Bhopal, India, tragedy, in which more than 2,000 people died and 100,000 were affected, was due to the release of methyl isocyanate into the surrounding community.

SYNTHESIS OF ISOCYANATES AND POLYURETHANE

Isocyanates are readily reactive compounds because of their chemical configurations. They contain —N=C=O groups, which react with active hydrogens in such compounds as water, acids, and alcohols but can react also with themselves to form dimers or other polymers. Uncontrollable polymerization and heat formation occur when mixed with bases, such as caustic soda and tertiary amines (1).

Isocyanates are manufactured from the reaction of primary aliphatic or aromatic amines, such as 2,4- and 2,6-toluenediamine (TDA), and phosgene in a solvent, such as mono- or dichlorobenzene or xylene. This reaction occurs rapidly to form hydrogen chloride and an intermediate, which is converted to TDI on heating. TDI is a colorless to pale yellow liquid with a sharp, pungent odor.

In the manufacture of polyurethane foams, isocyanate (part A) typically is added to polyether or polyester polyols along with combustion-retarding agents, catalysts, and blowing agents (part B or resin) to form polyurethane. The addition of water causes the generation of carbon dioxide gas with subsequent foam formation. Without the addition of water, the polyurethane mixture can be used as a coating material. Commercially, polyurethane adhesives and coatings may be available as two-component systems that react together and must be mixed just prior to use or as one-component systems that require reaction with oxygen or moisture for curing after application.

CLINICAL TOXICOLOGY

A National Institute of Occupational Safety and Health (NIOSH) survey in 1983 estimated that 280,000 workers in the United States potentially are exposed to diisocyanates (2). Exposure to isocyanates can occur anywhere, from the initial manufacture of the isocyanates to their final use in the production of foams and other polyurethane products. Exposure can occur also from the application of polyurethane paints and coatings, from the handling and machining of foams, and from combustion of these materials (Table 93-1) (3).

Inhalation of isocyanates as vapors or aerosols is the main risk to the health of exposed workers. Dermal contact also may expose involved workers to the effects of isocyanates. TDI and hexamethylene diisocyanate, the more volatile isocyanates, cause problems at room temperature, whereas the less volatile isocyanates, MDI and naphthalene diisocyanate, are less likely to cause respiratory problems except when heated or inhaled as an aerosol. Hydrogenated MDI rarely causes respiratory sensitization even when heated but seems to elicit more dermal reactions. Of considerably less importance than isocyanates in causing health effects are the additives or solvents used in the production of polyurethane. Such catalysts as metal salts (e.g., organotin compounds) or tertiary amines may be used. Combustion-retarding agents and blowing agents also may be added to the preparation, are usually organic phosphates or phosphonates, and may contain chlorine or bromine. Methylene chloride or chlorofluorocarbons have been used as blowing agents in the manufacture of polyurethane foams (4).

Exposure to isocyanates is likely to be higher in the initial steps of polyurethane and other isocyanate-using productions than at the end. TDI exposures in the flexible polyurethane foam industry are higher on foam lines, in the maintenance department, and in research and development, where exposure to raw TDI is more likely than in the finishing areas (5).

Although most exposure occurs during the manufacture and use of isocyanates, finished products may contain some residual amounts of unreacted monomers, which may be released in small amounts (1). The application of polyurethane coatings, such as paints and varnishes, can cause exposure to diisocyanates. Single-component coatings exist in a prepolymerized form and so are less likely to be inhaled than are two-component products that contain unreacted isocyanates. Exposure has been demonstrated also from handling and machining polyurethane foam. Although reversal of dimerization can occur at high temperatures, thermal decomposition products of polyurethanes consist mainly of carbon monoxide, benzene, toluene, nitrogen oxides, hydrogen cyanide, acetaldehyde, acetone, propene, carbon dioxide, alkenes, and water vapor (4).

TABLE 93-1. Occupations associated with isocyanate exposure

Adhesive workers	Painters
Aircraft builders	Plastic foam makers
Appliance makers	Plastic molders
Boat makers	Polyurethane foam makers
Cushion makers	Rubber workers
Foam blowers	Shipbuilders
Insulation workers	Ship welders
Isocyanate workers	Textile processors
Lacquer workers	Upholstery workers
Life preserver makers	Varnishers
Mine tunnel coaters	Wire-coating workers

Mechanism of Action Causing Toxicity

A variety of mechanisms have been proposed to explain the toxicity of isocyanates. Immunologically, both humoral [mediated by immunoglobulin E (IgE)] and cellular mechanisms have been evaluated. Isocyanates are low-molecular-weight agents that are highly reactive with amino groups and that can haptenize readily with plasma proteins, producing neoantigens. IgE-mediated hypersensitivity mechanisms appear possible in the etiology of isocyanate-induced asthma, especially when symptoms occur immediately after exposure. Investigators have demonstrated isocyanate-specific IgE antibodies in the sera of exposed workers. The prevalence, however, of these antibodies approximates 20% in some studies, suggesting that this may not be the major mechanism of isocyanate asthma. Furthermore, specific IgE antibodies have been detected in the sera of exposed, asymptomatic individuals (6). Epidemiologic studies also have failed to show a correlation between isocyanate asthma and atopy, further indicating that the disease probably is not entirely IgE-mediated. A possible role of cellular mechanisms has been shown through the production of a leukocyte inhibitory factor by lymphocytes from sensitized individuals (3). Bronchoalveolar lavage and bronchial biopsies show the presence of T lymphocytes and eosinophils, suggesting that cellular immune responses play a role in the etiology (7). Research indicates that late-onset reactions to TDI and the associated airway responsiveness may be caused by airway inflammation (8).

TDI has been found also to suppress the increase of intracellular cyclic adenosine monophosphate by the β-agonist isoproterenol in peripheral blood lymphocytes, which is indicative of a pharmacologic mechanism of action (9). Research data suggest that isocyanates may cause nonspecific inhibition of a variety of membrane receptors and enzyme systems. Both immunologic and nonimmunologic mechanisms appear to be involved (10). Although much research has been directed toward the mechanism of isocyanate-induced disease, the complete pathophysiology remains unknown.

Signs, Symptoms, and Syndromes

Isocyanates cause varied effects, owing to exposure. TDI can act as a direct irritant to mucous membranes, skin, and the respiratory system. It can act also as a sensitizer capable of causing such adverse effects as TDI-induced asthma and bronchial hyperreactivity to nonspecific agents, and it can cause lung function decline in individuals not sensitive to the specific isocyanate.

RESPIRATORY EFFECTS

The principal patterns of respiratory response to TDI are (i) chemical bronchitis (after high doses); (ii) isocyanate asthma and nonspecific bronchial hyperreactivity (symptomatic variable airflow obstruction in sensitized subjects); (iii) acute nonspecific airway disease (acute asymptomatic deterioration in lung function during a work shift); (iv) chronic nonspecific airway disease (chronic deterioration in lung function with prolonged low levels of exposure); and (v) hypersensitivity pneumonitis (3).

Chemical Bronchitis. Acute exposure to isocyanates can cause respiratory and mucous membrane irritation. Such symptoms as eye, nose, and throat burning or irritation with rhinitis, laryngitis, or bronchitis may occur on inhalation. Cough with chest pain or tightness also may occur, frequently at night. Transitory changes in lung function may develop. High exposures may result in chemical pneumonitis and pulmonary edema. Changes in lung function seem to improve within 1 to 2 years in most cases, although they may persist. Chronic bronchitis also has been reported to be more frequent in workers exposed to high concentrations or exposed repeatedly to low concentrations of TDI (11).

Isocyanate Asthma. Asthma occurring from exposure to isocyanates in a polyurethane manufacturing plant first was recorded in 1951 by Fuchs and Valade (12). Patients with isocyanate asthma present clinically with symptoms of wheezing, cough, and shortness of breath, often at night; these symptoms improve on weekends and vacations, when patients are removed from the exposure source. Possible predisposing factors for isocyanate asthma include exposure to large or multiple isocyanate spills and upper respiratory tract infections, although usually an explanation is lacking (13). Some estimates maintain that 5% of exposed workers develop clinically apparent asthma owing to isocyanate sensitization, although values of up to 30% have been reported, depending on exposure levels and criteria used to define sensitivity (3). Isocyanates have been found to be the most common cause of occupational asthma (7).

Although varying periods of isocyanate exposure (1 day to years) may exist before the development of asthma, isocyanate asthma more often develops within the first few months of exposure. The duration and concentration of isocyanate exposure triggering sensitivity are unknown. Exposure to even low levels of isocyanate can cause asthma. Once an affected individual is sensitized, exposure to even smaller amounts can produce asthmatic episodes. Sudden death has occurred in sensitized subjects inadvertently exposed to relatively low concentrations of TDI (3). Workers who are found to be sensitized to isocyanates must be removed to jobs in which no further isocyanate exposure will occur. Many patients with occupational asthma due to TDI continue to have persistent asthma months or years after removal from exposure (14). In some subjects, the asthma may progress even if they no longer are exposed.

Workers who develop isocyanate asthma also may exhibit hypersensitivity to other environmental allergens. This nonspecific bronchial hyperreactivity does not always accompany specific sensitivity to isocyanates. Nonspecific hyperreactivity cannot be predicted from the presence of atopy or from the initial degree of airflow obstruction (15). Like isocyanate asthma, nonspecific hyperreactivity can disappear over time. It may persist, however, for prolonged periods after cessation of exposure to isocyanates. Decreases in isocyanate sensitivity and nonspecific hyperreactivity have occurred after removal from exposure but appeared again on reexposure.

Asthma due to isocyanate sensitization can be of immediate, late, or dual onset. Smooth-muscle contraction is thought to be the mechanism for immediate asthmatic responses induced by isocyanates, because such responses quickly reverse after bronchodilator administration or spontaneously (16). By contrast, bronchodilators do not prevent late asthmatic responses induced by isocyanates. Asthmatics without a history of exposure to isocyanates—even those with methacholine sensitivity—do not respond to TDI inhalation challenge, indicating an isocyanate-specific response. Prednisone has been shown to prevent both late asthmatic reactions and the associated increase in airway responsiveness. Prednisone has been found also to have no effect on the early component in those with dual responses. Elevated levels of inflammatory cells are found in TDI-sensitive individuals experiencing late or dual asthmatic episodes but not in those experiencing only immediate reactions. Late asthmatic reactions to TDI and the associated increase in airway responsiveness may be linked to an acute inflammatory process in the airways of sensitized subjects.

Paggiaro et al. (17) studied 114 subjects with asthma induced by TDI. Bronchial provocation with TDI elicited immediate responses in 24 subjects, late responses in 50, and dual responses in 40 subjects. Those with dual responses had a longer duration of symptoms and a greater prevalence of airway obstruction with a lower mean forced expiratory volume in 1 second (FEV_1). A methacholine challenge was performed on 27 subjects: Those with dual responses showed nonspecific bronchial hyperresponsiveness greater than that in those with only late or early responses. Mapp et al. (18) found bronchial hyperreactivity diagnosed by positive methacholine inhalation challenge to occur in TDI asthmatics with dual or late, but not immediate, responses. In addition, six workers with a clinical history suggestive of TDI sensitivity had initial methacholine challenges that were negative but, 8 hours after a TDI inhalation challenge, developed positive methacholine responses (19). Cross-reactivity to other diisocyanates by challenge testing has been seen in some people who have TDI asthma but no history of previous exposure to diisocyanates other than TDI.

In one study, only one-fourth of the subjects with isocyanate asthma recovered completely within 10 months after exposure ended (14). In those who recovered, methacholine responsiveness returned to normal, indicating that airway hyperresponsiveness is not a predisposing factor for the occurrence of isocyanate-induced asthma. Some subjects with early or dual responses totally recovered, whereas some with dual responses lost only their immediate reactions, becoming late responders. None with only late responses recovered.

Production of allergic skin sensitization of guinea pigs and mice is possible with solutions of TDI. Dermal contact with TDI may result in respiratory tract hypersensitivity, as has been shown in guinea pigs (3).

MDI has been reported also to cause asthma and hypersensitivity pneumonitis (20,21). Only a small proportion of patients demonstrate IgE antibodies to MDI-protein conjugates. Likely, most isocyanates react similarly and eventually will be shown to cause respiratory problems much like those associated with TDI.

Acute Nonspecific Airway Disease. Several studies have shown that workers exposed to TDI experience asymptomatic airflow obstruction during the course of a work shift (3). The degree of this acute change is correlated with long-term changes in pulmonary function and severity of exposure. Exposure to low levels of TDI has been shown to cause a dose-related acute loss of pulmonary function. At the same dose, chronic deterioration in FEV_1 has been seen. Therefore, some researchers have proposed that excessive long-term changes in lung function may be predicted from the daily change in individuals, which may provide a means of identifying susceptible subjects.

Chronic Nonspecific Airway Disease. A dose-response relationship has been demonstrated between prolonged low levels of exposure to isocyanates and chronic deterioration in lung function. Wegman et al. (22) found that exposure to low levels of isocyanates in a polyurethane manufacturing plant produced a dose-response decrease in FEV_1 when exposed for more than 2 years to 0.002 parts per million (ppm) of TDI. Groups of workers exposed to higher concentrations had larger average annual decrements in FEV_1 than those exposed to lower concentrations. Subjects showing the largest acute responses are likely to show the greatest chronic changes. These effects were seen in subjects exposed to levels of TDI below the existing permissible exposure limit.

Diem et al. (23) prospectively studied a plant manufacturing TDI to evaluate the respiratory function of its workers. Personal air samples showed frequent excursions of TDI exceeding 0.02 ppm. After 2 years, no exposure-related decline in pulmonary function occurred. Over 5.5 years, those who spent at least 15% of their time working in an environment with at least 0.005 ppm TDI showed a greater decline in FEV_1 than did other subjects. Nonsmokers had an annual excess loss of 38 mL of FEV_1, equal to a total loss of 1.5 L over a 40-year working lifetime. Smoking and TDI effects on lung function were found not to be additive. Current or previous smokers experienced no effect. The potential exists for long-term declines in pulmonary function in workers exposed to low levels of isocyanates.

Hypersensitivity Pneumonitis. Hypersensitivity pneumonitis or extrinsic allergic alveolitis has been linked to isocyanate exposure. Generally, symptoms of hypersensitivity pneumonitis include fever, chills, malaise, dyspnea, and a nonproductive cough. Chest radiography results may show diffuse patchy infiltrates or discrete nodules or may be normal even in symptomatic subjects. Pulmonary function testing may show a restrictive pattern and impaired diffusion capacity. Steroids have been shown to be effective in treating the illness, but further exposure must be avoided to prevent recurrence.

Pulmonary opacities resulting from exposure to diisocyanates also have been reported, accompanied by airflow obstruction (3). In one case, acute asthma followed hypersensitivity pneumonitis in a worker challenged with MDI in the laboratory. Exposure to TDI also has been reported to cause chronic restrictive pulmonary disease (1).

OTHER EFFECTS

Direct exposure to solutions of isocyanates is irritating to the skin and mucous membranes and may cause contact dermatitis. Erythema, edema, and blistering are possible. Exposure to aerosols may cause ocular irritation, rhinitis, and sore throat.

Neurologic symptoms, including a feeling of drunkenness, numbness, and loss of balance, have been described as occurring immediately after a single severe exposure to TDI by firemen in a burning polyurethane foam factory, with some symptoms persisting up to 4 years (24). They also reported nausea, vomiting, and abdominal pain, which were transitory. Whether these complications resulted from the neurotoxic effects of isocyanates, hypoxia from respiratory reactions, or other simultaneous chemical exposure is not known.

Carcinogenesis

In animal studies, commercial-grade TDI given by gavage has produced tumors in rats and mice in a dose-response relationship. After contact with water, TDI is converted to TDA, which is carcinogenic to both mice and rats (3). This action may explain the carcinogenicity by gavage. 2,4-Diaminotoluene, the hydrolysis product of 2,4-TDI, caused similar tumors when tested in rats and mice (1).

The International Agency for Research on Cancer determined the presence of sufficient evidence for the carcinogenicity of TDI to experimental animals but inadequate evidence to determine its carcinogenicity to humans (1). However, in the absence of adequate data in humans, a reasonable approach is to regard chemicals lacking sufficient evidence of carcinogenicity in animals as if they represented a carcinogenic risk to humans. NIOSH recently released information classifying TDI and TDA as potential occupational carcinogens (25). Teratogenesis and reproductive effects have not been studied in animals or human populations.

Management of Toxicity

CLINICAL EXAMINATION

Medical history may reveal symptoms of cough, shortness of breath, nocturnal wheezing, and chest pain in workers with respiratory symptoms due to isocyanates. Symptoms may worsen with continued TDI exposure. Depending on the type of respiratory response elicited, physical examination may reveal pulmonary wheezes, coarse rales, or a normal lung examination result. Irritation of mucous membranes may be present, including redness and swelling. Dermal reactions consisting of mild irritation to erythematous blisters may be seen.

LABORATORY DIAGNOSIS

Specific IgE antibodies to monofunctional isocyanates have been reported in sensitized workers, but specific IgE antibodies to diisocyanate conjugates have not been identified (3). In one study, *p*-tolyl monoisocyanate conjugated to human serum albumin was used to identify specific IgE antibodies in three of four subjects sensitized to TDI but was not found in exposed but nonsensitized subjects (9). A dose-response relationship appeared to exist between exposure concentration and number of individuals with a positive titer. Others have found that only 0% to 16% of sensitized subjects had specific IgE antibodies to tolyl monoisocyanate. Specific IgE antibodies have been exhibited also in exposed workers without asthma (6).

SPECIAL DIAGNOSTIC TESTS

Spirometry testing may reveal either normal pulmonary function or airway obstruction in subjects with isocyanate asthma. On inhalation challenge, immediate, late, or dual asthmatic reactions may develop, defined as a 20% decrease in FEV_1. Challenge testing may be indicated in carefully selected cases, although the risk is apparent. A diagnosis of isocyanate asthma usually can be made without the need to perform such a challenge. Isocyanate asthma may be diagnosed if the worker has reversible airflow obstruction associated with exposure to low levels of isocyanates. The doses of TDI used for inhalation challenges do not cause immediate or late bronchoconstriction in normal subjects or in asthmatic subjects not sensitized to TDI, even if they have hyperresponsive airways (26).

TREATMENT

Immediate treatment of direct contact with eyes or mucous membranes should include irrigation with saline or water. Skin should be washed with soap and water and then with alcohol. Inhalation requires immediate removal of the exposed individual to fresh air. Ingestion of TDI requires administering large quantities of water and inducing vomiting in conscious patients.

Bronchodilators are useful in ameliorating immediate asthmatic episodes. Theophylline partially inhibits both the immediate and late reactions of asthma induced by TDI but does not affect the increase in airway responsiveness, apparently affecting a bronchoconstrictor component of the late asthmatic reaction rather than the inflammatory component (27). Prednisone or high-dose inhaled beclomethasone is useful in preventing both late asthmatic episodes and the increase in nonspecific bronchial hyperreactivity induced by TDI. Obviously, individuals with diagnosed isocyanate asthma must be removed from further exposure.

BIOLOGICAL MONITORING

Medical surveillance should be provided to all workers exposed to diisocyanates in the workplace. Preplacement examinations, including recording a comprehensive medical and work history with special emphasis on preexisting respiratory conditions and smoking experience, should be performed (24). A physical examination with emphasis on the respiratory system, chest radiography, and baseline spirometry should be included. The worker also must be judged fit to use a respirator. Annual periodic examinations consisting of interim medical and work histories, a physical examination, and spirometric assessments before and after the work shift or work week should be performed. If medical conditions that are found could be aggravated directly or indirectly by exposure to diisocyanates (e.g., respiratory allergy, chronic upper or lower respiratory irritation, or chronic obstructive pulmonary disease), affected workers should be counseled about the increased risk from working with these substances. If evidence of sensitization is found, provisions must be made to remove such workers from further exposure.

Preplacement assessment has not been shown to be useful in predicting which employees will develop TDI-induced lung disease. Atopy and asthma unrelated to isocyanates do not predispose to isocyanate asthma. Not all subjects who have specific sensitivity to TDI have increased nonspecific bronchial hyperreactivity. Isocyanates in low concentrations have no effect on hyperreactive airways. Therefore, methacholine testing is not likely to identify those who will develop TDI asthma (28). Baseline methacholine testing is similar in subjects who develop immediate, dual, or late responses.

The available evidence indicates that serial measurement of the FEV_1 is a useful means of identifying acute and long-term effects of isocyanates in a workforce. Musk et al. (3) demonstrated a correlation between acute and chronic effects of TDI, which may provide a way of identifying individuals who are at risk of developing long-term declines in FEV_1. An annual FEV_1 decrement of 0.020 L in an adult nonsmoker would be anticipated from aging alone. Some researchers have suggested that all subjects should have preemployment measurements and subsequent measurements at least annually or more often if symptoms arise. Work shift decrements of 0.3 L or greater and annual decrements of 5% or 0.2 L should be cause for evaluation and more frequent testing, because these decrements may be associated with eventual chronic airflow obstruction or may be representative of asthma, which may become intractable.

ENVIRONMENTAL MONITORING

The NIOSH criteria document defines occupational exposure to diisocyanates as exposure to airborne levels exceeding one-half the recommended time-weighted average occupational exposure limit or in excess of the recommended ceiling limit (24). Adherence to all provisions of the standard is required at this level, including periodic medical examinations, respiratory protection, and personal monitoring.

Environmental monitoring of the workplace in which diisocyanates are present should be conducted annually or after any process changes, to determine whether exposure is present. If exposure is found, personal monitoring is used to calculate each employee's occupational exposure to diisocyanates. Area and source monitoring may be used to supplement personal monitoring. Samples from each operation in each work area and each shift should be taken at least once every 6 months. Records of environmental exposures applicable to involved employees must be included in their respective medical records.

Air levels of TDI can be measured by a variety of methods (3). The Marcali method and its derivatives, also called *wet colorimetric methods*, are the oldest and have been the reference for newer methods. They involve collecting air samples in a midget impinger by bubbling workplace air through an acid absorption medium. The intensity of the colored derivative is measured spectrophotometrically.

Tape methods, or *dry colorimetric methods*, for measuring isocyanates were developed initially by Reilly. Dry colorimetric methods are based on color-forming reactions that occur when chemically impregnated paper tape is exposed to air containing isocyanates. After monitoring, the tape is passed through a reflectance meter for quantification.

Chromatographic methods (gas chromatography, thin-layer chromatography, and high-performance liquid chromatography) are the most sensitive for measuring and distinguishing between isocyanates, but they are technically difficult and expensive. The current NIOSH-approved analytic method forms urea derivatives that can be measured quantitatively by high-performance liquid chromatography with ultraviolet spectrometric detection (1).

OCCUPATIONAL EXPOSURE LIMITS

The current U.S. Occupational Safety and Health Administration permissible exposure limit for TDI is 0.02 ppm (0.14 mg per cubic meter) (29). The American Conference of Governmental Industrial Hygienists' (30) threshold limit value for TDI is 0.005 ppm (0.036 mg per cubic meter) as an 8-hour time-weighted average, whereas the short-term exposure limit value is 0.02 ppm (0.14 mg per cubic meter).

Substitution should be the first approach for protecting workers. If not possible, engineering controls, such as enclosure, ventilation, or process automation, should be considered. However, in special cases, such as in the case of spills or accidents for which this is not practical, personal protective equipment must be used to prevent skin and eye contact. Rubber, polyvinyl chloride, or other materials resistant to penetration by diisocyanates should be used. Workers should wear face shields with goggles, gloves, aprons, suits, boots, and suitable respiratory equipment. While engineering controls are being installed, type C supplied-air respirators with full face pieces should be used in areas where the recommended safe exposure limits are likely to be exceeded. Safety showers and eyewash stations should be readily available at operations involving TDI and TDA.

REFERENCES

1. International Agency for Research on Cancer. Some chemicals used in plastics and elastomers. *IARC Monogr Eval Carcinog Risks Hum* 1986;39:287–323.
2. National Institute for Occupational Safety and Health Alert, March 1996. *Request for assistance in preventing asthma and death from diisocyanate exposure.* Cincinnati: US Department of Health and Human Services, Public Health Service, Center for Disease Control, National Institute for Occupational Safety and Health, 1966:1.
3. Musk AW, Peters JM, Wegman DH. Isocyanates and respiratory disease: current status. *Am J Ind Med* 1988;13:331–349.
4. Woolrich PF. Polyurethanes and polyisocyanurates. In: Cralley LV, Cralley LJ, eds. *Industrial hygiene aspects of plant operations*, vol 1. New York: Macmillan, 1982:423–439.
5. Rando RJ, Abdel-Kader H, Hughes J, Hammad YY. Toluene diisocyanate exposures in the flexible polyurethane foam industry. *Am Ind Hyg Assoc J* 1987;48:580–585.
6. Butcher BT, O'Neil CE, Reed MA, Salvaggio JE. Radioallergosorbent testing with *p*-tolyl monoisocyanate in toluene diisocyanate workers. *Clin Allergy* 1983;13:31–34.
7. Bernstein, JA. Overview of diisocyanate occupational asthma. *Toxicology* 1996;111:181–189.
8. Chan-Yeung M. Occupational asthma. *Chest* 1990;98(Suppl):148s–161s.
9. Chan-Yeung M, Lam S. Occupational asthma. *Am Rev Respir Dis* 1986;133: 686–703.
10. Bernstein IL. Isocyanate-induced pulmonary diseases: a current perspective. *J Allergy Clin Immunol* 1982;70:24–31.
11. McKerrow CB, Davies HJ, Jones AP. Symptoms and lung function following acute and chronic exposure to tolylene diisocyanate. *Proc R Soc Med* 1970; 63:376–378.

12. Fuchs S, Valade P. Etude clinique et experimentale sur quelques cas d'intoxication par le desmodur T (diisocyanate de tolylene 1-2-4 et 1-2-6). *Arch Mal Prof* 1951;12:191–196.
13. Banks DE, Butcher BT, Salvaggio JE. Isocyanate-induced respiratory disease. *Ann Allergy* 1986;57:389–396.
14. Mapp CE, Corona PC, Fabbri L. Persistent asthma due to isocyanates. *Am Rev Respir Dis* 1988;137:1326–1329.
15. Lam S, Wong R, Yeung M. Nonspecific bronchial reactivity in occupational asthma. *J Allergy Clin Immunol* 1979;63:28–34.
16. Fabbri LM, Boschetto P, Zocca E, et al. Bronchoalveolar neutrophilia during late asthmatic reactions induced by toluene diisocyanate. *Am Rev Respir Dis* 1987;136:36–42.
17. Paggiaro PL, Innocenti A, Bacci E, Rossi O, Talini D. Specific bronchial reactivity to toluene diisocyanate: relationship with baseline clinical findings. *Thorax* 1986;41:279–282.
18. Mapp CE, Di Giacomo GR, Omini C, Broseghini C, Fabbri LM. Late, but not early, asthmatic reactions induced by toluene-diisocyanate are associated with increased airway responsiveness to methacholine. *Eur J Respir Dis* 1986;69:276–284.
19. Mapp CE, Dal Vecchio L, Boschetto P, De Marzo N, Fabbri LM. Toluene diisocyanate–induced asthma without airway hyperresponsiveness. *Eur J Respir Dis* 1986;68:89–95.
20. Zammit-Tabona M, Sherkin M, Kijek K, Chan H, Chan-Yeung M. Asthma caused by diphenylmethane diisocyanate in foundry workers. *Am Rev Respir Dis* 1983;128:226–230.
21. Malo JL, Zeiss CR. Occupational hypersensitivity pneumonitis after exposure to diphenylmethane diisocyanate. *Am Rev Respir Dis* 1982;125:113–116.
22. Wegman DH, Peters JM, Pagnotto L, Fine LJ. Chronic pulmonary function loss from exposure to toluene diisocyanate. *Br J Ind Med* 1977;34:196–200.
23. Diem JE, Hones RN, Hendrick DJ, et al. Five-year longitudinal study of workers employed in a new toluene diisocyanate manufacturing plant. *Am Rev Respir Dis* 1982;126:420–428.
24. US Department of Health, Education and Welfare/National Institute for Occupational Safety and Health. *Criteria for a recommended standard: occupational exposure to diisocyanates.* DHEW/NIOSH publication no. 78-215. Washington: US Government Printing Office, 1978.
25. National Institute for Occupational Safety and Health. *Toluene diisocyanate (TDI) and toluenediamine (TDA): evidence of carcinogenicity.* DHHS publication no. (NIOSH) 90–101; current intelligence bulletin no. 53. Cincinnati: US Department of Health and Human Service, Centers for Disease Control, 1990.
26. Paggiaro P, Bacci E, Talini D, et al. Atropine does not inhibit late asthmatic responses induced by toluene-diisocyanate in sensitized subjects. *Am Rev Respir Dis* 1987;136:1237–1241.
27. Mapp C, Boschetto P, Dal Vecchio L, et al. Protective effects of anti-asthma drugs on late asthmatic reactions and increased airway responsiveness induced by toluene diisocyanate in sensitized subjects. *Am Rev Respir Dis* 1987;136:1403–1407.
28. Mapp CE, Boschetto P, Dal Vecchio L, Fabbri LM. Occupational asthma due to isocyanates. *Eur Respir J* 1988;3:273–279.
29. Occupational Safety and Health Administration. Rules and regulations, 29 *CFR* 1910.1000, Table Z-1. Washington: Government Printing Office.
30. American Conference of Governmental Industrial Hygienists. *Threshold limit values for chemical substances and physical agents and biological exposure indices.* Cincinnati: American Conference of Governmental Industrial Hygienists, 1996:35.

CHAPTER 94

Acrylates, Methacrylates, and Cyanoacrylates

Sue Sundstrom, Barbara Scolnick, and John B. Sullivan, Jr.

The main acrylic compounds in use are acrylates, methacrylates, and cyanoacrylates (Fig. 94-1). Exposure to these monomers and polymers occurs in plastic manufacturing, printing, dentistry, surgery, implants in patients' bodies, and in manicurists and the cosmetics industries. Because of their use in medicine, these materials have been subject to a great deal of study for pharmacologic, toxicologic, and biocompatibility considerations. The experience of the last 50 years clearly indicates that these chemicals are extremely useful; however, concerns have emerged regarding their toxicity.

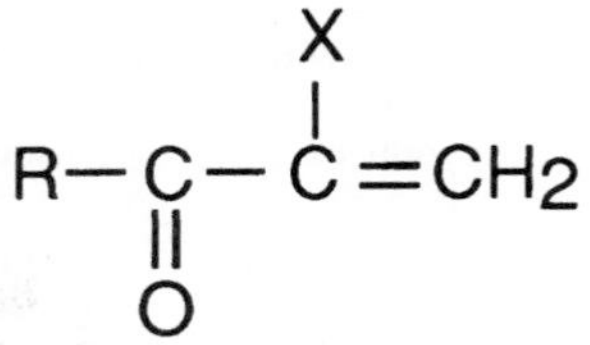

$$R-\underset{\underset{O}{\|}}{C}-\overset{\overset{X}{|}}{C}=CH_2$$

X= H: Acrylates
X= C≡N: Cyanoacrylates
X=CH_3: Methacrylates

Figure 94-1. The main acrylic compounds.

SOURCES AND PRODUCTION

Acrylic compounds commonly are used for their reactive and cross-linking properties. Acrylic resins are derivatives of acrylic acid, are malleable when heated, and can be formed into desired shapes. The term *thermoplastic* is applied to such plastic compounds. Acrylic resin monomers are either acrylic acids or methacrylic acids and their esters; cyanoacrylic acid and esters; acrylamides; and acrylonitrile. Monomers are polymerized either by heating or by ultraviolet (UV) light. Initiators, accelerators, and catalysts are added to speed up the process of polymerization. Polymers of great variability can result from polymerization of various monomers, from tough plastics to clear rubbers, and such polymers have been used extensively.

Commercially, the most important monomer is methylmethacrylate (MMA), and the polymethyl methacrylate (PMMA) polymer has unique characteristics. It transmits light well at wavelengths of 360 to 1,000 nm (whereas wavelengths of visible light are 400 to 700 nm). A tough, hard plastic that is weather- and moisture-resistant, PMMA is thermoplastic so that when heated beyond its glass transition temperature, it is bent or molded easily into complex shapes. Often, it is recognized by its brand names of Plexiglas or Lucite.

The commercial history of these monomers dates from the 1930s. Although Redtenbacker had described the production of acrylic acid by oxidizing acrolein in 1843, it was Otto Rohm's doctoral thesis in 1901 that described the tough, clear plastic prepared from polymers of ethylmethacrylate (1). In 1909, he and Otto Haas began a company to manufacture "organic glass," which was first used in creating safety glass. Rohm & Haas Germany and Rohm & Haas USA remain major producers.

The monomers are derived from basic petrochemicals. Since 1970, a propylene oxidation process has been used. It involves the oxidation of propylene to acrolein and subsequent oxidation of acrolein to acrylic acid (2).

All the monomers of commercial interest are liquids with a pungent odor, and all have a tendency for "spontaneous" polymerization and must be handled with care. They usually are stabilized with minimal amounts of inhibitors. The inhibitors used most frequently are hydroquinone or monomethylether of hydroquinone. For most applications, inhibitors do not have to be removed but, if necessary, they can be removed with ion exchange resins. Washed, uninhibited monomers are not stable and should be used promptly. In any case, monomers always should be used within 1 year. The chemical formulas and synonyms of some of the commercially important monomers of the acrylic acid series are summarized in Table 94-1.

The liquid monomers are polymerized in one of several processes: bulk, solution, emulsion, or suspension. The ensuing polymer is sheet plastic, liquid, or powder. The lower-molecular-

TABLE 94-1. Names and formulas of common acrylates

Compound	Synonyms	Formula	CAS no.
Acrylic acid	Propene acid Acroleic acid	$C_3H_4O_2$	79-10-7
Ethyl acrylate	Acrylic acid Ethyl ester	$C_5H_8O_2$	140-88-5
Methyl acrylate	Acrylic acid Methyl ester	$C_4H_6O_2$	96-33-3
Methacrylic acid	—	$C_4H_6O_2$	79-41-4
Methylmethacrylate	Methacrylic acid Methyl ester	$C_5H_8O_2$	80-62-6

CAS, Chemical Abstracts Service.

weight esters are soluble in aromatic hydrocarbons; those of higher molecular weight are soluble in aliphatic hydrocarbons. Polymerization can be initiated in a heat-curing process, requiring addition of heat; in a UV process, which requires the addition of a chemical that absorbs UV light into the system; or in a cold-curing process, which requires a chemical accelerator to start the polymerization (3).

SITES, INDUSTRIES, AND BUSINESSES ASSOCIATED WITH EXPOSURE

Acrylates are used in paints, paper, adhesives, textiles, building materials, automotive components, toys, leather, printing, optics, cosmetics, dentistry, and medicine and as oil additives.

Paints

Acrylic esters undergo polymerization with water to form emulsion polymers. When the emulsion, such as paint or adhesive, is applied to a surface, the water evaporates, leaving a tough film. The acrylate polymers form a coating that is resistant to water, sunlight, and weather. They are known as *latex paints*.

Paper

Emulsions of acrylic polymers are coated onto paper to render it more water-resistant and receptive to ink. They can be added also to paper pulp to render the paper resistant to grease and oil.

Adhesives

Acrylic emulsions are used as resin adhesives on envelopes, labels, and decals. Sealants are used also for bathtub caulk, baseboard seams, and glazing. Cyanoacrylates are used to form high-strength bonding glues, nail adhesives, and surgical tissue adhesives.

Textiles

Methyl acrylate is used primarily as a co-monomer with acrylonitrile in the preparation of acrylic fibers. Such fibers generally contain 85% acrylonitrile.

Building Materials

PMMA sheets are used in building panels, bathroom fixtures, and plumbing. As a glazing, PMMA is used for bank teller windows, police cars, enclosures for swimming pools, domes for tennis courts, skylights, and telephone booths.

Automotive Components

PMMA is used for dials, instrument panels, medallions, taillights, and backup lights on automobiles.

Toy Industry

High-performance colorful methacrylates are used extensively in the toy industry.

Oil Additives

Long-chain polymethacrylates are used as additives to increase the viscosity of automobile oils.

Leather

Emulsion acrylate polymers bind to leather to improve appearance, prevent cracking, and add scuff resistance.

Cosmetics

Ethyl acrylate has been used as a fragrance additive in some soaps and creams at levels of 0.001% to 0.01%. It smells somewhat like pineapple. Some reports have identified it in the volatile component of fresh pineapple. This is the only natural source of any acrylate (4).

Printing

"Solventless technology" in printing involves a system of synthetic resins, acrylate monomers, and UV light. When UV light is shown on the system, the monomers almost instantly bind and cross-link the polymers, causing curing. These monomers are more complex than are the low-molecular-weight traditional acrylates and are known as *multifunctional acrylic monomers* (MFAs). The most common are pentaerythritol triacrylate (PETA), trimethylolpropane triacrylate (TMPTA), and 1,6-hexanediol diacrylate (HDODA) (Fig. 94-2).

Dentistry

In 1946, PMMA began to be used in denture bases, the portion of the denture that rests in the mouth and retains the artificial teeth. The most common resin used is a liquid-powder type, wherein the liquid monomer is combined with the powder polymer into a doughlike consistency, is packed into a mold that conforms to the patient's mouth, and is cured by heat curing, UV light, or cold curing. Another use in dentistry is as filling material when combined with inorganic materials to form composite resins (5).

Medicine

MMA monomer [$CH_2 = C(CH_3)COOCHH_3$] is a highly volatile chemical with a characteristic odor. MMA is a widely used monomer commonly applied as bone cement in orthopedic and dental procedures. MMA resins are used to repair cranial defects and in plastic surgery. The major use of MMA, however, is found in orthopedics. In 1959, Sir John Charnley revolutionized hip replacement surgery by using cold-cured PMMA as a bony cement to anchor metallic hip prostheses (6). Although refinements have been made over the ensuing years, the basic system of cold curing the MMA monomer liquid and a polymer powder remains the same. In the operating room, the orthopedist kneads the mixture into the proper rubbery consistency and injects it into the joint. After extensive use in the United Kingdom in the

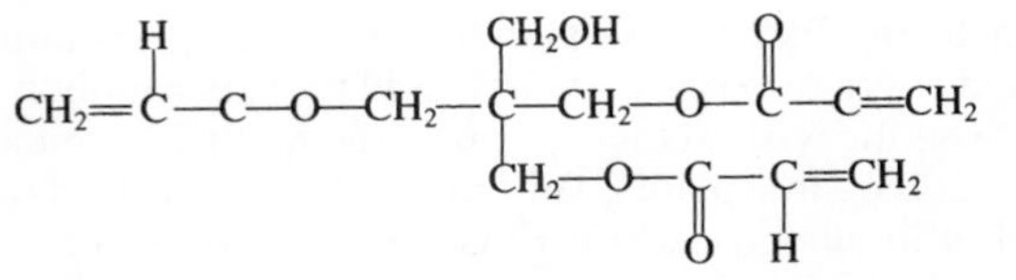

$CH_2{=}C(H){-}C{-}O{-}CH_2{-}C(CH_2OH)(CH_2{-}O{-}C(=O){-}C(H){=}CH_2){-}CH_2{-}O{-}C(=O){-}C{=}CH_2$

Pentaerythritol triacrylate (PETA)

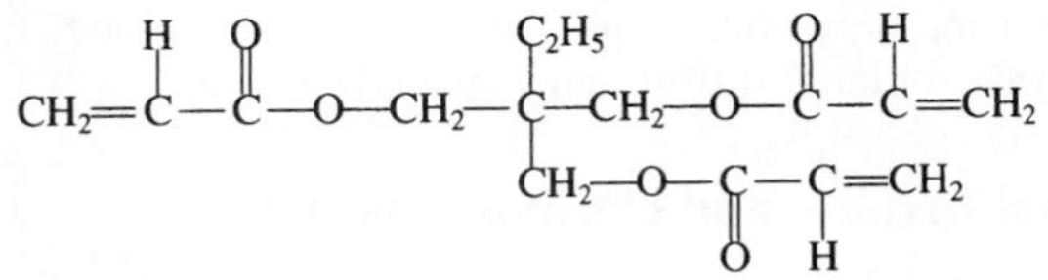

$CH_2{=}C(H){-}C(=O){-}O{-}CH_2{-}C(C_2H_5)(CH_2{-}O{-}C(=O){-}C(H){=}CH_2){-}CH_2{-}O{-}C(=O){-}C(H){=}CH_2$

Trimethylolpropane triacrylate (TMPTA)

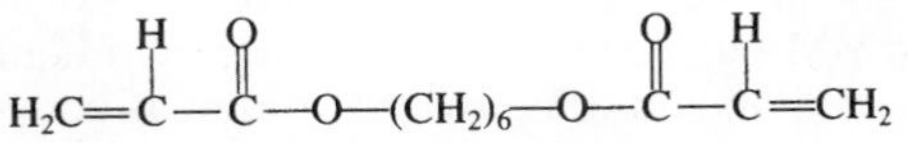

$H_2C{=}C(H){-}C(=O){-}O{-}(CH_2)_6{-}O{-}C(=O){-}C(H){=}CH_2$

1,6-Hexanediol diacrylate (HDODA)

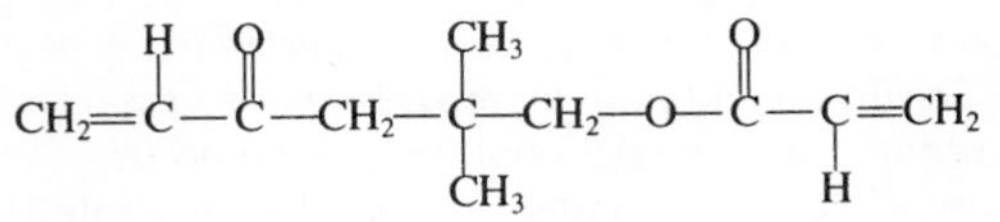

$CH_2{=}C(H){-}C(=O){-}CH_2{-}C(CH_3)_2{-}CH_2{-}O{-}C(=O){-}C(H){=}CH_2$

Neopentylglycol diacrylate (NPGDA)

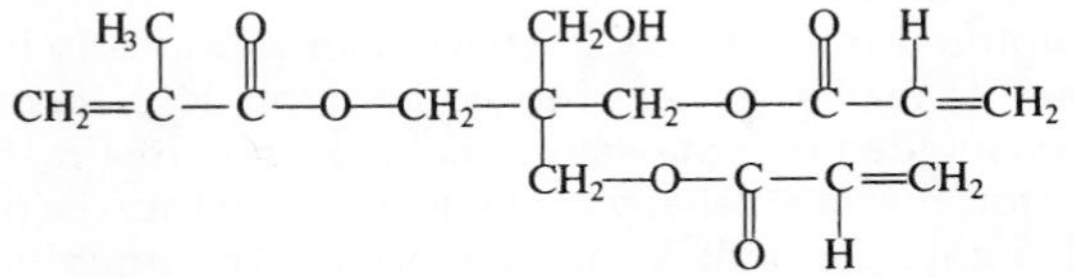

$CH_2{=}C(H_3C){-}C(=O){-}O{-}CH_2{-}C(CH_2OH)(CH_2{-}O{-}C(=O){-}C(H){=}CH_2){-}CH_2{-}O{-}C(=O){-}C(H){=}CH_2$

Trimethylolpropane trimethylacrylate (TMPTMA)

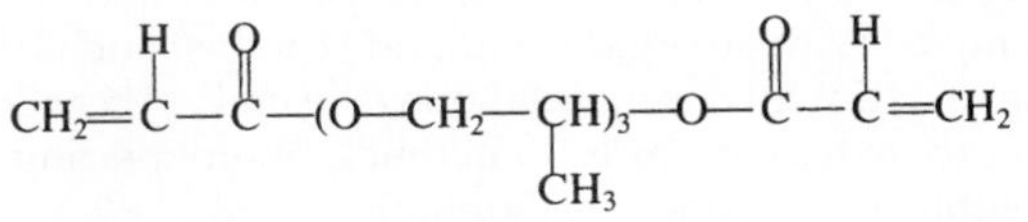

$CH_2{=}C(H){-}C(=O){-}(O{-}CH_2{-}CH(CH_3))_3{-}O{-}C(=O){-}C(H){=}CH_2$

Tripropyleneglycol diacrylate (TRPGDA)

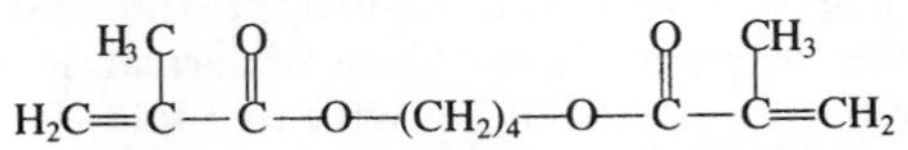

$H_2C{=}C(H_3C){-}C(=O){-}O{-}(CH_2)_4{-}O{-}C(=O){-}C(CH_3){=}CH_2$

Tetraethyleneglycol dimethacrylate (TTEGDMA)

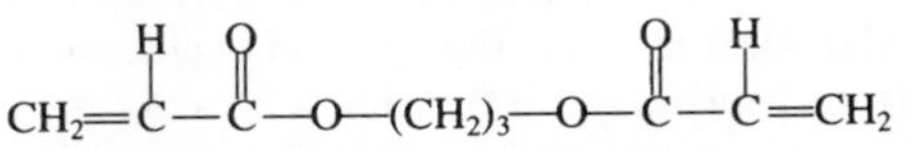

$CH_2{=}C(H){-}C(=O){-}O{-}(CH_2)_3{-}O{-}C(=O){-}C(H){=}CH_2$

Triethyleneglycol diacrylate (TREGDA)

Figure 94-2. Structure of multifunctional acrylic monomers.

1960s, bony cement was approved in the United States in 1969. Currently, 140,000 total joint replacements are performed annually (7).

Optics

The concept of replacing eyeglasses with lenses in direct contact with the cornea was conceived in the 1800s but was delayed because glass obviously was not suitable. After World War II, Ridley, an ophthalmologist, noted that fragments of air fighter canopies constructed of PMMA were tolerated well in the eyes of injured pilots (8). This led to its use in contact lenses. "Hard contact lenses" still are made of polymethacrylate. The hydrophobic nature of PMMA causes problems with comfort. A newer acrylic polymer is based on the monomer 2-hydroxyethyl methacrylate. When the methyl group is replaced with a hydroxyethyl (C–C–OH) group, the monomer becomes hydrophilic and can absorb a great deal of water, although it does not dissolve in water. This is the monomer used for soft contact lenses.

CLINICAL TOXICOLOGY

Routes of Exposure

Exposure to MMAs, acrylates, and cyanoacrylates occurs primarily by skin contact, inhalation, and eye contact. Ingestion of these compounds in their liquid monomeric form also can occur. These compounds primarily are irritants, although cases of allergy and hypersensitivity are reported for some products.

Metabolism

In humans undergoing total hip replacement (THR) surgery, both MMA and methacrylic acid were found in the circulation (9). Methacrylic acid as the coenzyme A ester is a normal intermediate in the catabolism of valine. In rats, more than 80% of an administered dose of ^{14}C-labeled MMA is respired as carbon dioxide within 5 to 6 hours (10). This finding supports the idea that MMA is metabolized via intermediate metabolism and the citric acid cycle. Thus, the metabolites are not likely to be dangerous reactive particles.

The acrylates behave differently. Studies using rats have found that methyl acrylate and ethyl acrylate are hydrolyzed enzymatically by plasma and homogenates of rat liver, lungs, and kidneys (11). However, the acrylates' ester also reacted with glutathione *in vitro* and decreased tissue nonprotein sulfhydryl groups *in vivo*. The carboxylase inhibitor triorthotolyl phosphate potentiated the toxicities of the acrylates. This finding implies that carboxylesterases are important in the detoxification of acrylates. Competition must exist between the glutathione conjugation system and carboxylesterases. The conjugation system could result in dangerous alkylating agents (12).

General Toxicity

All the liquid monomers have a pungent corrosive odor and are irritating to mucous membranes in high concentration. Most of the monomers are severe eye irritants. Methacrylates tend to be less irritating than are acrylates. If a liquid monomer from either series inadvertently is splashed in the eye, the eye should be irrigated with copious amounts of water.

In 1954, Fisher (13) reported allergic eczematous dermatitis affecting the hands of dentists who worked with the liquid methacrylate. Patch test results were positive, and the condition cleared when the monomer was avoided.

In the late 1960s, outbreaks of dermatitis were associated with artificial acrylic nails. Some of these cases were extreme, with onycholysis, nail dystrophy, and eczema around the nail bed. The U.S. Food and Drug Administration received sufficient complaints from consumers that, after litigation on July 3, 1974, the district court in Chicago issued an injunction prohibiting the further manufacture of a product called *Long Nails*, which contained an MMA monomer (14).

In 1971, Pegum and Medhurst (15) reported the case of an orthopedic surgeon who developed an allergic contact dermati-

TABLE 94-2. Median lethal inhalational concentration (LC_{50}) and median lethal dose (LD_{50}) for common acrylates

Route	Species	Compound	Dose (LD_{50} or LC_{50})
Oral	Rabbit	Methyl acrylate	7 mL/kg
Oral	Rabbit	Ethyl acrylate	4–6 mL/kg
Oral	Rabbit	Butyl acrylate	7–10 mL/kg
Oral	Rat	Methyl acrylate	8 mL/kg
Oral	Rat	Ethyl acrylate	14.8 mL/kg
Inhalation	Rat	Methyl acrylate	1,000 ppm
Inhalation	Rat	Methylmethacrylate	4,000 ppm

tis from bony cement. This case marked the first discovery that the monomer readily passes through rubber gloves. In the 1970s, as polyfunctional acrylic monomers began to find extensive use in UV-polymerizing systems, reports of contact dermatitis came from the printing trade (16–18).

The MFAs used most widely—PETA, TMPTA, and HDODA—are irritants and allergens. The aforementioned reports demonstrate that an individual can have a patch test result that is negative for MMA exposure (the most frequently tested) yet be allergic to other acrylates. Any estimate of the incidence of skin reactions is difficult. Spiechowicz (19) reported that after 2 to 14 years' exposure, 10% of dental technicians develop MMA sensitization.

All acrylates should be handled with minimal skin contact. If an already sensitized individual must continue to be exposed, heavy-gauge rubber or polyvinyl chloride gloves should be used.

Early toxicologic studies of acrylates were performed by Deichmann (20) in 1941, by Spealman et al. (21) in 1945, and by Treon et al. (22) in 1949. These researchers established the oral median lethal dose and the median lethal inhalational concentration in the guinea pig, rabbit, and rat. The results are summarized in Table 94-2. When toxic quantities of acrylates were absorbed, the animals developed accelerated respiration, followed by motor weakness, decreased respiration, and finally, coma.

Reports appearing in the literature cited severe hypotension occurring in patients undergoing THR surgery (23–26). Occasionally, cardiac arrest and patient death occurred (27,28). This phenomenon has been studied extensively, but its actual cause remains unknown. Some investigators have implicated fat and bone marrow emboli caused by reaming the femoral cavity. Others have questioned the heat effect from exothermic polymerization, and many believe that the residual monomer is toxic (29,30).

Mir et al. (30) studied the effects on blood pressure, heart rate, electrocardiography, and respiration in anesthetized dogs after intravenous administration of methacrylic acid and 12 of its esters. They found that all agents decreased heart rate, increased respiratory rate, produced electrocardiographic changes, and affected blood pressure by causing hypotension, hypertension, or a biphasic response. The same investigators perfused isolated rabbit heart with solutions containing methacrylate esters at concentrations of 1:1,000, 1:10,000, and 1:100,000 and found significant reduction in cardiac rate and force of contraction (31).

The question for patients is whether free MMA in the circulation ever reaches concentrations that are toxic. In THR, in which exposure is greatest, venous blood can reveal MMA levels of 1 mg per dL (32). Clinically, MMA is being used extensively and, for the moment, the profession is approving it cautiously.

No case reports have implicated any acrylate as a cardiovascular toxin in any occupationally exposed population. Only a few epidemiologic studies have addressed occupational exposure to methacrylates. In 1976, the National Institute for Occupational Safety and Health studied 91 workers in five plants manufacturing PMMA sheets, where the average 8-hour time-weighted average exposure was 4 to 49 parts per million (ppm) (33). These individuals were compared with 43 nonexposed workers at the same plants. The authors found no effect over the work shift in blood pressure, pulse, or symptoms. A few unexpected differences that were found may be statistical "red herrings" or may be significant. The high-exposure group had different mean values for glucose, cholesterol, albumin, and bilirubin and had more frequent complaints referable to the nervous system than did the control group.

Dermal Toxicity and Dermal Exposure

Contact dermatitis and allergic dermatitis in occupational exposures are problems associated with handling of acrylates and methacrylates. Those exposed are dental technicians, dentists, surgeons, nurses, and painters. Denture materials used by dental technicians contain MMA in the form of a monomer. Hydroquinone is added as an inhibitor, and dimethyl-*p*-toluidine is added as an accelerator. Ethylene glycol dimethyl acrylate is a cross-linking agent that is added, and dibutyl phthalate, which comes in both liquid and powder form, is added as a plasticizer. The powder form contains MMA polymers, colorants, and benzoyl peroxide as a catalyst. The liquid and powder are mixed in a vessel and, at this point, skin contact and inhalational contact can occur.

Methacrylates and acrylates can readily penetrate the latex gloves used in mixing these components. Some systems of mixture avoid skin contact by allowing the powder and liquid to be mixed in a closed system (34).

Sculptured artificial acrylic nails is another industry in which exposure to methacrylates and acrylates can occur. Sculptured nails are molded into the natural nail. The bonding material in kits for this purpose usually contains powdered acrylic polymer with benzoyl peroxide as an accelerator. The liquid acrylate monomer contains a stabilizer, such as hydroquinone, resorcinol, or dimethyl-*p*-toluidine or *p*-dimethyl amino chlorobenzene (35). Polymerization occurs when the polymer and the monomer are mixed with an organic peroxide catalyst and an accelerator. The material then is molded onto the nail and is allowed to harden at room temperature. Sometimes, photobonding is used, which requires exposure to UV radiation.

As acrylates and MMAs are allergens, the incidence of contact dermatitis in this industry is high. As the nail grows, further applications of acrylic are used to fill in approximately every 2 weeks, allowing further exposure. Cases of dermatitis and paresthesia have been reported along with nail fold dermatitis. Patch testing has demonstrated allergic contact dermatitis from exposure to the ingredients of these mixtures.

Clinical presentations include fingertip dermatitis, nail fold dermatitis, nail dystrophy, paresthesias, and eyelid and neck dermatitis (36). Three kinds of sculptured acrylic nails are available: (i) acrylate monomers and polymers that polymerize at room temperature with an organic peroxide catalyst and an accelerator; (ii) sculptured acrylic nails that are photobonded with UV radiation, catalyzing the polymerization; and (iii) cyanoacrylate nail preparations. Cyanoacrylates are used in glues and as a surgical tissue adhesive to provide high bond strength. Cyanoacrylates are used as contact adhesives for metal, glass, rubber, plastics, and textiles and to bind tissues for wound healing.

Two chemical facts significantly reduce the allergenic properties of cyanoacrylates: They polymerize rapidly when in contact with traces of water, and they bind immediately to keratin on the skin's surface, thus preventing contact with dermal immune cells. However, cases of contact allergy from exposure to cyanoacrylates are reported. Cyanoacrylates now are known to be contact allergens that can cause contact dermatitis and nail dystrophy.

TABLE 94-3. Clinical presentations of cyanoacrylate dermal injury

Fingertip dermatitis	Paresthesias
Nail fold dermatitis	Eyelid dermatitis
Subungual pain	Neck dermatitis
Paronychial pain	Infections
Nail dystrophy	

Bonded acrylic sculptured nails also can cause prolonged paresthesias of fingertips. This condition probably is due to the acrylate monomer that penetrates through the nail bed before polymerization occurs with UV radiation.

Manicurists whose hands are constantly exposed to acrylate materials are at risk for developing signs and symptoms of injury (Table 94-3). Rubber gloves are inadequate in protecting against penetration of acrylate monomers. A type of glove called *4-H* and made in Denmark has been demonstrated to be protective against acrylate monomers (36).

Eyelid and facial dermatitis can be caused by airborne dust of polymerized resins or by exposure to vapors and acrylate or methacrylate dust. Because acrylic nails have been implicated in transmission of infections, health care workers should be cautioned.

Nail lacquer also contains a thermoplastic resin—toluene sulfonamide–formaldehyde resin—which improves adhesion of the lacquer to the nail plate and provides hardness. It is a known allergen in cosmetics (37). Acrylate nail lacquer does not cure completely and allows monomers to remain nonpolymerized, thus providing a source of a sensitizing agent (37).

Allergic contact dermatitis from cyanoacrylates has been described with both glues and adhesives used for metal, glass, textiles, and artificial nails. Facial and skin dermatitis from cyanoacrylates has been seen in workers whose occupations expose them to ethylcyanoacrylate monomers (38). Periorbital eczema and orofacial edema has been described in hair stylists exposed to ethylcyanoacrylate adhesives (39). Such periorbital facial dermatitis has been shown to recur on reexposure in the worksite.

To be a sensitizer, a molecule must fulfill two conditions: Its chemical and physical properties must facilitate skin penetration and come into contact with immune cells, and its chemical reactivity toward nucleophilic residues of protein should be high to allow covalent bonds to form (39). Heretofore, many thought that the cyanoacrylates would be trapped in the keratin layers of the upper skin and would not be able to penetrate deeply enough to come into contact with immune cells. Many case studies and patch testing have now disproved that theory. When cyanoacrylates come into contact with water, they instantly polymerize, just as when they come into contact with the skin; however, in thin areas of skin, such as the eyelids, they may be able to penetrate because the skin is very thin (0.5 mm) as compared to other areas of the face (approximately 2 mm).

Neurotoxicity

Reports in the Russian literature suggest that MMA causes vague central nervous system symptoms, such as fatigue, headache, and loss of appetite (34,40). These studies suffer from lack of a control group. The 1976 study by the National Institute for Occupational Safety and Health found that complaints of dizziness, shakiness, and drowsiness were more common in the exposed group (46%) than in the control group (23%) (33). Innes and Tansay (41) studied the effect of MMA vapors on the electroencephalograms and neuronal discharge rates of rat brains. At a concentration of 400 ppm, four times the threshold limit value, MMA monomer vapor produced a rapid, reversible reduction, as compared to control animals, in neuronal discharge rates in the lateral hypothalamus and ventral hippocampus of rats.

MMA has been implicated as a peripheral neurotoxin, owing to reports of allergic dermatitis that have highlighted the finger and palmar paresthesias accompanying skin breakdown (42). The paresthesias often take 2 to 3 months to heal after the skin has recovered. Seppalainen and Rajaniemi (43) studied nerve conduction velocities of 20 dental hygienists and 18 control subjects: As compared to levels in the controls, dental technicians had significantly slower distal sensory conduction velocities from digits 1, 2, and 3 on the right hand and from the radial aspects of digits 2 and 3 on the left hand. Findings are considered to represent mild axonal degeneration in the area with the closest and most frequent contact with MMA.

Episodes of peripheral neuropathy and paresthesias have been reported in medical personnel after they handled acrylic bone cements. Acrylic bone cements, including MMA monomer, readily penetrate rubber gloves and can dissolve plastic and synthetic rubber compounds. Allergic contact dermatitis has occurred after such exposures. Reports of paresthesia affecting fingers of medical personnel exposed to acrylates and methacrylates have lasted for months after discontinuation of contact. MMA is a known skin sensitizer, and reports cite contact dermatitis that has developed in dental personnel, orthopedic surgeons, and other medical personnel handling these compounds while wearing rubber gloves. Paresthesias may accompany the dermatitis. MMA decreased the amplitude of the actual potential in peripheral nerves.

Chronic Toxic Effects on Metabolism

Borzelleca et al. (44) administered ethyl acrylate and MMA to rats at doses of 6 to 2,000 ppm for 2 years. The highest level (2,000 ppm) of ethyl acrylate was accompanied by a definite decrease in weight in the female rats over the course of the study.

Tansay et al. (45) found that the body weight of rats receiving daily 8-hour exposures to 116 ppm MMA vapor for 3 months was lower than that of controls. These authors found also that individual oxygen consumption measurements for exposed rats were 45% increased over those for controls. Necropsy revealed neither gross nor microscopical pathology to the heart, gastrointestinal tract, or liver.

One study (46) demonstrated that animals exposed to MMA and ethylmethacrylate increased their sleeping time. Unclear is whether this effect involved the enzymes or the central nervous system.

Tansay et al. (47) found that MMA vapors produce transient slowing of the small bowel in rats and dogs. *In vitro* studies of isolated guinea pig ileum demonstrated prompt inhibition of contraction when the intestine was bathed in a solution containing methacrylate esters (48).

The significance of these studies on occupationally exposed humans is unclear. Anecdotally, many dental students working with MMA complain of nausea and anorexia (49). An operating room nurse who developed a generalized hypersensitivity to bony cement complained of anorexia that lasted several hours after each THR case (50). McLaughlin et al. (51) reported that during three THRs, the concentration of the monomer vapor in the operating room never exceeded 280 ppm. This concentration was measured within 15 seconds after the cement was mixed. It dropped quickly to 50 ppm in 2 minutes and to approximately 2 ppm within 6 minutes, where it remained constant for 11 minutes (51).

Respiratory Effects

The same properties that render acrylic compounds ideal for polymerization processes and cross-binding also contribute to their sensitizing properties. Contact hypersensitivity to acrylic compounds has been known since the 1940s (52). Respiratory disease caused by acrylates first was reported in 1985; since then, such diseases have been diagnosed in many other patients with respiratory symptoms after exposure. Skin-prick tests with MMA and polyethylene glycol diethyl methacrylate have been performed on patients, as have tests with cyanoacrylates, and have been found to be positive in some cases.

Specific diagnosis of asthma was based on provocation challenge testing in an inhalation chamber. The tests were considered positive on a fall exceeding 15% in peak expiratory flow immediately or on a fall of 20% in a delayed manner. Cases of patients with respiratory disease linked to methacrylates have been documented (52). A 48-year-old atopic woman exposed to methacrylates developed respiratory distress at work, presenting with rhinorrhea and nasal stuffiness. Methacrylate challenge caused a 24% fall in her peak expiratory flow. Another patient, a 46-year-old woman, worked 20 years as a dental technician and developed paresthesias, but no dermatitis, of both hands. She developed chest tightness that subsided while she was away from work. She also had a positive response to methacrylate inhalation, but results of a skin-prick test were negative.

Although methacrylates are well-known dermal contact sensitizers and can elicit positive skin test results, bronchial provocation test results do not indicate that individuals have developed an immunoglobulin E–mediated response to methacrylates. The low-molecular-weight acrylates and methacrylates have not yet been shown to cause a specific immunoglobulin E–mediated reaction.

Another series of case reports noted that asthma occurred in association with exposure to cyanoacrylate-based adhesives in five patients and after exposure to MMA in another patient (53). Inhalational testing provoked a 42% fall in one patient's forced expiratory volume in 1 second 15 hours after the challenge. Such findings suggest that acrylates are causes of asthma in a nonspecific inflammatory mechanism rather than through an immunoglobulin E–mediated immediate hypersensitivity mechanism. Other cases of MMA and asthma and respiratory complaints have been identified in the literature, particularly with the use of bone cement and in orthopedic procedures (54,55).

Teratogenic Effects

No case reports or epidemiologic studies of humans have addressed the issues of acrylates as teratogens. However, results from several different animal studies have been both positive and negative. Singh et al. (56) treated pregnant rats with intraperitoneal injections of monomers of five methacrylate esters on days 5, 10, and 15 of gestation. On day 20 of gestation, these rats were sacrificed, as were those in a control group that had received intraperitoneal injection of cottonseed oil, water, or saline. At one or more of the doses used, each compound produced some or all of the following effects: resorption, gross skeletal malformations, fetal death, and decreased fetal size. This study has been criticized for using intraperitoneal exposure. Murray et al. (57) exposed Sprague-Dawley pregnant rats to inhaled ethyl acrylate for 6 hours per day on days 6 to 15 of gestation at doses 0, 50, and 150 ppm. They found no effect at 50 ppm but, at 150 ppm, they noted maternal toxicity marked by decreased body weight and decreased food consumption. McLaughlin et al. (51) exposed pregnant mice to MMA vapor at a concentration of 1,330 ppm on days 5 to 15 for 2 hours per day and found no evidence of fetal toxicity. Merkle and Klimish (58) exposed pregnant Sprague-Dawley rats by inhalation to *n*-butyl acrylate at 0, 25, 135, or 250 ppm for 6 hours per day on gestation days 7 to 16. At 135 and 250 ppm after implantation, deaths were increased, but no teratogenic response was found.

Carcinogenic Effects

Polymerized acrylates and methacrylates are presumed to be innocuous materials except for any residual monomer. The one exception is the possible oncogenic role of PMMA when used in implants. After Oppenheimer et al. (59) placed subcutaneous implants in Wistar rats, 11 of the 25 rats developed sarcomas. Similar results have been found by other investigators, some of whom defined the term *solid-state oncogenesis* for the induction of tumors by solid materials in experimental animals at the implantation site. Seemingly, the physical properties of the foreign body are more important than is the chemical nature.

The literature regarding solid-state carcinogenesis was reviewed by Williams and Roaf (60), who concluded that PMMA appears to be safe in humans. Assuming 25 years for induction of cancers in humans, we should now be seeing the rising tide of malignancies from early THR surgeries. However, no reports of malignant degeneration around hip replacement implant sites exist.

The liquid monomers, both older monofunctional and newer multifunctional acrylates, have been subject to much study in animal experiments. DePass et al. (61) studied the dermal oncogenic potential of acrylic acid, ethyl acrylate, and butyl acrylate by painting them on the dorsal skin of mice three times weekly for their entire lifetimes. These authors used a negative control of acetone and a positive control of 3-methylcholanthrene. They found no carcinogenic activity of any of these acrylates.

The same investigators studied dermal oncogenic potential of some newer acrylates used in photocurable coatings with the same experimental system. Mice showed the development of tumors: 8 and 6 tumors, respectively, as compared with 34 tumors in those in the positive anthracene control group and 0 tumors in the mice in the acetone group (62).

The Celanese Corporation studied eight MFAs in dermal tests conducted with C3H/Hej mice (63). Fifty animals were treated twice weekly for 80 weeks with a concentration determined to be only minimally irritating. Five of these MFAs—TMPTA, trimethylolpropane trimethylacrylate, HDODA, tripropyleneglycol diacrylate, and tetraethyleneglycol dimethacrylate—showed no increase in tumors. Three—PETA, triethyleneglycol diacrylate, and tetraethyleneglycol diacrylate—showed an increased number of tumors. Tetraethyleneglycol diacrylate caused severe skin damage and skin tumors. PETA and triethyleneglycol diacrylate showed increased numbers of skin cancers and, disturbingly, induced an increased incidence of lymphomas in treated animals.

The National Toxicology Program studied MMA exposure by the oral route in F344/N rats and B6C3F1 mice and found no induction of tumors (64). This organization studied ethyl acrylate by oral administration to mice and rats (65). Fifty male and female mice were fed ethyl acrylate in doses of 100 mg per kg of body weight and 200 mg per kg of body weight five times weekly for 103 weeks. Significant increases of squamous cell papillomas and carcinomas of the stomach were noted in both species.

Miller et al. (66) studied ethyl acrylate by inhalation in mice and rats. Groups of 105 female and male mice (B6C3F1) and rats (Fischer 344) were exposed to ethyl acrylate at concentrations of 25, 75, and 225 ppm for 6 hours per day, 5 days per week for 27 months. No increased incidence of tumors was found in the

TABLE 94-4. Exposure limits for common acrylates

Compound	ACGIH TLV	OSHA PEL
Acrylic acid	10 ppm	None
Ethyl acrylate	5 ppm	25 ppm
Methyl acrylate	10 ppm	10 ppm
Methacrylic acid	20 ppm	None
Methylmethacrylate	100 ppm	100 ppm

ACGIH, American Conference of Governmental Industrial Hygienists; OSHA, U.S. Occupational Safety and Health Administration; PEL, permissible exposure limit; TLV, threshold limit value.

exposed groups. In the most highly exposed groups, the mean body weight was lower, and nonneoplastic lesions of the olfactory mucosa were noted in both species.

Summarizing the data, the International Agency for Research on Cancer concluded that evidence is sufficient to consider ethyl acrylate as a carcinogen in experimental animals. With respect to methyl acrylate and *n*-butyl acrylate, the agency found evidence to be inadequate, and they did not evaluate the data for the MFAs (4).

Recently, a study of Rohm & Haas plant workers exposed to both ethyl acrylate and MMA reported a significant excess of colorectal cancers (standardized mortality ratio, 1.67; 52 observed/31.2 expected) (K. Maher, L. De Fonso, *unpublished data*, 1984). A standardized mortality ratio study, conducted from 1951 to 1981, of 2,671 men who were exposed to MMA at two American Cyanamid plants found no excess incidence of cancer (67).

EXPOSURE LIMITS

Table 94-4 summarizes the exposure limits for common acrylates recommended by the American Conference of Governmental Industrial Hygienists for threshold limit values based on an 8-hour day, 40-hour work week. These limits are mandated by the U.S. Occupational Safety and Health Administration for permissible exposure limits (68). The American Conference of Governmental Industrial Hygienists has established a 100-ppm threshold limit value for MMA monomer. The current Occupational Safety and Health Administration standard for MMA is 100 ppm over an 8-hour work shift (410 mg per cubic meter).

SUMMARY

The acrylates, methacrylates, and cyanoacrylates are exceedingly useful chemicals. Nonetheless, they also are strong skin sensitizers and are irritating to the skin, eyes, and via their pungent odor, the nasal passages (69). Their chronic toxicity has not been evaluated fully. The newer MFAs and ethyl acrylate have been implicated in the development of cancer in some test rodents.

REFERENCES

1. Glavis FS, Woodman JF, Rohm & Haas Co. Methacrylate compounds. In: Stander A, ed. *Kirk-Othmer encyclopedia of chemical technology,* 2nd ed, vol 13. New York: John Wiley and Sons, 1967:331–363.
2. Kine BB, Novak RW, Rohm & Haas Co. Methacrylic polymers. In: Grayson M, ed. *Kirk-Othmer encyclopedia of chemical technology,* 3rd ed, vol 15. New York: John Wiley and Sons, 1981:377–398.
3. Kine BB, Novak RW, Rohm & Haas Co. Acrylic polymers. In: Grayson M, ed. *Kirk-Othmer encyclopedia of chemical technology,* 3rd ed, vol 1. New York: John Wiley and Sons, 1978:386–408.
4. International Agency for Research on Cancer. Some chemicals used in plastics and elastomers. *IARC Monogr Eval Carcinog Risks Hum* 1985;39:81–98.
5. Combe EC. Acrylic dental polymers: formulation and synthesis. In: Bever MB, ed. *Encyclopedia of material science and engineering,* vol 1. Cambridge, MA: MIT Press, 1986:51–56.
6. Charnley J. Anchorage of the femoral head prosthesis to the shaft of the femur. *J Bone Joint Surg Br* 1960;42:28.
7. Wijn JR, van Mullen PJ. Biocompatibility of acrylic implants. In: Williams D, ed. *Biocompatibility of clinical implant materials,* vol 2. Boca Raton, FL: CRC Press, 1981:99–126.
8. Ridley H. Intraocular lenses: recent development in surgery of cataract. *Br J Ophthalmol* 1952;36:113.
9. Crout HG, Corkill JA, James ML, Ling RSM. Methylmethacrylate metabolism in man. *Clin Orthop Rel Res* 1979;141:90–95.
10. Bratt H, Hathaway HDE. Fate of methyl methacrylate in rats. *Br J Cancer* 1977;36:114–119.
11. Silver EH, Murphy SD. Potentiation of acrylate ester toxicity by prior treatment with the carboxylesterase inhibitor triorthotolyl phosphate (TOTP). *Toxicol Appl Pharmacol* 1981;57:208–219.
12. Delbressine LPC, Seutter-Berlage F, Seulter E. Identification of urinary mercapturic acids formed from acrylate methacrylate and crotonate in the rat. *Xenobiotica* 1981;11:241–247.
13. Fisher AA. Allergic sensitization of the skin and oral mucosa to acrylic denture materials. *JAMA* 1954;156:238.
14. Fisher AA, Franks A, Glick H. Allergic sensitization of the skin and nails to acrylic plastic nails. *J Allergy* 1957;28:84.
15. Pegum JS, Medhurst FA. Contact dermatitis from penetration of rubber gloves by acrylic monomer. *BMJ* 1971;2:141.
16. Nethercott JR. Skin problems associated with multifunctional acrylic monomers in ultraviolet curing inks. *Br J Dermatol* 1978;98:541–552.
17. Emmett EA. Contact dermatitis from polyfunctional acrylic monomers. *Contact Dermatitis* 1977;3:245–248.
18. Nethercott JR, Jakubovic HR, Pilger G, Smith JW. Allergic contact dermatitis due to urethane acrylate in ultraviolet cured inks. *Br J Ind Med* 1983;40:241–250.
19. Spiechowicz E. Experimental studies on the effect of acrylic resin on rabbit skin. *Berufsdermatosen* 1971;19:132–144.
20. Deichmann W. Toxicity of methyl, ethyl and *n*-butyl methacrylate. *J Ind Hyg Toxicol* 1941;23:343.
21. Spealman CR, Main RJ, Haag HB, Larson PS. Monomeric methyl methacrylate. *Ind Med* 1945;14:292–298.
22. Treon JR, Sigman H, Wright H, Kitzmiller KV. The toxicity of methyl and ethyl acrylate. *J Ind Hyg Toxicol* 1949;31:317–326.
23. Phillips H, Cole PV, Lettin AW. Cardiovascular effects of implanted acrylic bone cement. *BMJ* 1971;3:460.
24. Cohen CA, Smith TC. The intraoperative hazard of acrylic bone cement: report of a case. *Anesthesiology* 1971;35:547.
25. Gresham GA, Kuczmski A. Cardiac arrest and bone cement. *BMJ* 1970;3:465.
26. Hyland J, Robbins RHC. Cardiac arrest and bone cement. *BMJ* 1970;4:176.
27. Kepes ER, Underwood PS, Becsey L. Intraoperative death associated with acrylic bone cement. *JAMA* 1972;222:576.
28. Herndon JH, Bechtol CO, Crikenberger DP. Fat embolism during total hip replacement: a prospective study. *J Bone Joint Surg Am* 1974;56:1350.
29. Feith R. Side effects of acrylic cement implanted into bone. *Acta Orthop Scand Suppl* 1975:161.
30. Mir GN, Lawrence WH, Autian J. Toxicological and pharmacological actions of methacrylate monomers: III. Respiratory and cardiovascular functions of anesthetized dogs. *J Pharm Sci* 1974;63:376.
31. Mir GN, Lawrence WH, Autian J. Toxicological and pharmacological actions of methacrylate monomers: I. Effects on the isolated perfused rabbit heart. *J Pharm Sci* 1973;62:778.
32. Homsy CA, Tullos HS, Anderson MS, Differante NM, King JR. Some physiological aspects of prosthesis stabilization with acrylic cement. *Clin Orthop* 1972;83:317.
33. Cromer J, Kronoveter K. *A study of methyl methacrylate exposures and employee health.* Publ. no. DHEW (NIOSH) 77–119. Washington: Government Printing Office, 1976:1–43.
34. Blagodatin VM, Golova IA, Blagodatkina NK, et al. Issues of industrial hygiene and occupational pathology in the manufacture of organic glass [in Russian]. *Gig Tr Prof Zabol (Russ)* 1976;14:11–14.
35. Murer A, Poulsen O, Tuchsen F, Roed-Petersen J. Rapid increase in skin problems among dental technician trainees working with acrylates. *Contact Dermatitis* 1995;33:106–111.
36. Freeman S, Lee M, Gudmundsen K. Adverse contact reactions to sculptured acrylic nails: full case reports and a literature review. *Contact Dermatitis* 1995;33:381–385.
37. Kanerva L, Lauerma A, Jolanki R, et al. Methylacrylate: a new sensitizer in nail lacquer. *Contact Dermatitis* 1995;33:203.
38. Bruze M, Bjorkner B, Lepoittevin J. Occupational allergic contact dermatitis from ethylcyanoacrylate. *Contact Dermatitis* 1995;32:156–159.
39. Tumb R, Lepoittevin J, Durepaire François, et al. Ectopic contact dermatitis from ethylcyanoacrylate instant adhesives. *Contact Dermatitis* 1993;28:206–208.
40. Karpov BD. The effect of small concentrations of methyl methacrylate vapors on the inhibition and stimulation process of the cortex of the brain. *Trad Lenigr Sanit Gig Med Inst (Russ)* 1953;14:43–48.
41. Innes DL, Tansay MF. Central nervous system effects of methyl methacrylate vapor. *Neurotoxicity* 1981;2:515–522.
42. Blair FI, Fisher AA, Salvati EA. Contact dermatitis in surgeons from methylmethacrylate bone cement. *J Bone Joint Surg Am* 1975;57:547.

43. Seppalainen AM, Rajaniemi R. Local neurotoxicity of methylmethacrylate among dental technicians. *Am J Ind Med* 1984;5:471–477.
44. Borzelleca JF, Larson PS, Hennigar GR, Huf EG, Crawford EM, Smith RB. Studies of chronic oral toxicity of monomeric ethyl acrylate and methyl methacrylate. *Toxicol Appl Pharmacol* 1964;6:29–36.
45. Tansay MF, Kendall FM. Update on the toxicity of inhaled methylmethacrylate vapor. *Drug Chem Toxicol* 1979;2:315–330.
46. Autian J. Structure toxicity relationships of acrylic monomers. *Environ Health Perspect* 1975;2:141–152.
47. Tansay MF, Martin JS, Benhagen S, Sandin WE, Kendall FM. GI motor inhibition associated with acute exposure to methylmethacrylate vapor. *J Pharm Sci* 1977;66:613–618.
48. Mir GN, Lawrence WH, Autian J. Toxicological and pharmacological actions of methacrylate monomers: II. Effects on isolated guinea pig ileum. *J Pharm Sci* 1973;62:1258–1261.
49. Tansay MF, Benhagem S, Probst S, et al. The effects of methylmethacrylate vapor on gastric motor function. *J Am Dent Assoc* 1974;89:372–376.
50. Scolnick B, Collins J. Systemic reaction to methylmethacrylate in an operating room nurse. *J Occup Med* 1986;28(3):196–198.
51. McLaughlin RE, Reger SI, Barkalow BS, Allen MS, Di Fazio CA. Methylmethacrylate: a study of teratogenicity and fetal toxicity of the vapor in the mouse. *J Bone Joint Surg Am* 1978;60(30):355–358.
52. Sabonius B, Keskinen H, Tuppurainen M. Occupational respiratory disease caused by acrylates. *Clin Exp Allergy* 1993;23:416–424.
53. Lozewicz S, Davison AG, Hopkirk A, et al. Occupational asthma due to methyl methacrylate and cyanoacrylates. *Thorax* 1985;40:836–839.
54. Pickering C, Bainbridge D, Birtwistle IH, Griffiths DL. Occupational asthma due to methylmethacrylate in an orthopedic theatre sister. *BMJ* 1986;292:1362–1363.
55. Scolnick B. Systemic reaction to methylmethacrylate in an operating room nurse. *J Occup Med* 1986;28(3):196–198.
56. Singh AR, Lawrence WH, Autian J. Embryonic fetal toxicity and teratogenic effects of a group of methacrylate esters in rats. *J Penet Res* 1972;51:1632–1638.
57. Murray JS, Mille RR, Deacon TR, et al. Teratological evaluation of inhaled ethyl acrylate in rats. *Toxicol Appl Pharmacol* 1981;60:106–111.
58. Merkle J, Klimisch HR. *n*-Butyl acrylate: prenatal inhalation toxicity in the rat. *Fundam Appl Toxicol* 1983;3:443–447.
59. Oppenheimer BS, Oppenheimer ET, Stout AP, Danishefsky I. Malignant tumors resulting from embedding plastics in rodents. *Science* 1953;118:305.
60. Williams DF, Roaf S, eds. *Implants in surgery*. London: WB Saunders, 1973:274.
61. DePass LR, Fowler EH, Meckley DR, Weill CS. Dermal oncogenicity bioassays of acrylic acid, ethylacrylate, and butyl acrylate. *J Toxicol Environ Health* 1984;14:115–120.
62. DePass LR, Maronpot RR, Weil CS. Dermal oncogenicity bioassays of monofunctional and multifunctional acrylates and acrylate based oligomers. *J Toxicol Environ Health* 1958;16:55–60.
63. Andrews LS, Clary JJ. Review of the toxicity of multifunctional acrylates. *J Toxicol Environ Health* 1986;19:149–164.
64. Chan PC. *National toxicology program technical report on the toxicology and carcinogenesis studies of methylmethacrylate in F344/N rats and B6C3F1 mice.* US Department of Health and Human Services, NIH publ. no. 86-2570 NTP TR 314. Washington: Government Printing Office, 1985.
65. Carcinogenesis studies of ethylacrylate (CAS no. 140-88-5) in F344/N rats and B6C3F mice (gavage studies). National Toxicology Program technical report series no. 259, US Department of Health and Human Services, Public Health Service. NIH publ. no. 83-2515. Bethesda, MD: National Institutes of Health, 1983.
66. Miller RR, Young RJ, Kociba DG. Chronic toxicity and oncogenicity bioassay of inhaled ethylacrylate in Fischer 344 rats and B6C3F1 mice. *Drug Chem Toxicol* 1985;8:1–42.
67. Collins JJ, Page LC, Caporossi JC, Utidijian HM, Saipher JN. Mortality patterns among men exposed to methyl methacrylate. *J Occup Med* 1989;31:41–46.
68. US Occupational Safety and Health Administration. Occupational safety and health standards, subpart Z—toxic and hazardous substances, 29 *USC* 17 C1910.1000; 31: Washington: Government Printing Office, 1976:8303.
69. Cooke FW. Acrylics as biomedical materials In: Bever MB, ed. *Encyclopedia of material science and engineering,* vol 1. Cambridge, MA: MIT Press, 1986:59–65.

CHAPTER 95
Formaldehyde

John J. Clary and John B. Sullivan, Jr.

Formaldehyde has been manufactured commercially for nearly 100 years and presently is produced worldwide. Common names for formaldehyde include *BFV, Fannoform, Formalith, Formol, Fyde, Ivalon, Lysoform, Morbicid,* and *Superlysoform.* Generic names include *formaldehyde, formaldehyde gas, formaldehyde solution, formalin, formalin 40, formalin 100%, formic aldehyde, methaldehyde, methanal, methyl aldehyde, methylene glycol,* and *methylene oxide.*

Pure formaldehyde is a colorless gas that condenses and forms a liquid at high vapor pressure. Formaldehyde also exists in powdered and liquid states, the latter usually taking the form of an aqueous solution. Liquid formaldehyde, which has a boiling point of –19°C and a melting point of –118°C, is miscible with water, acetone, benzene, diethyl ether, chloroform, and ethanol (1). Trioxane, the cyclic trimer of formaldehyde, is a solid used as a fuel source, as it burns easily.

SOURCES, PRODUCTION, AND USES

Formaldehyde (HCHO) production is reported in terms of formalin, which is a 37% aqueous solution and the most common chemical form of formaldehyde. Formalin contains methanol at a concentration of 0.5% to 15.0% to prevent polymerization of formaldehyde to cyclic trimers or to paraformaldehyde. Formalin is a slightly acidic, clear solution with a strong, pungent odor. Formaldehyde is available also as its linear low-molecular-weight homopolymer, paraformaldehyde, or as a cyclic trimer, trioxane (1).

Formaldehyde is produced by the oxidation of methanol with air in the presence of a silver or an iron oxide–molybdenum oxide catalyst. The bulk of formaldehyde in the United States is used for plastics and resin manufacture. Urea-formaldehyde resins, which are used primarily as adhesives in the manufacture of particle board, medium-density fiberboard, and hardwood plywood account for more formaldehyde than do any other resins. Phenolic resins also use formaldehyde. Phenolic resins are used principally as adhesives in water-resistant plywood and as binders in fiberglass insulation. Polyacetal resins, produced from formaldehyde or its trimer, trioxane, are used as unreinforced thermoplastic resins in a variety of applications in which they can replace metals in mechanical working parts (e.g., automobiles, trucks, consumer articles, plumbing, industrial machinery, and appliances) (2,3).

Formaldehyde is used for the production of chemical intermediates. An example of this is the manufacture of acetylenic chemicals. This synthesis involves the reaction of two molecules of formaldehyde with acetylene to produce 2-butyne-1,4-diol, which then is hydrogenated to 1,4-butanediol (3).

Formaldehyde, the simplest aldehyde, is a chemical building block in both nature and industry. It has been used widely for many years as an embalming agent and a tissue preservative in hospitals, pathology laboratories, and funeral homes (1). Inhalational and dermal contact is possible during these uses.

Formaldehyde or chemicals that are formaldehyde generators, such as hexamethylenetetramine (HMT), have been used in preserving foods (especially fish) and in cosmetics, paints, and other industrial applications. Hence, dermal exposure to formaldehyde is possible also from cosmetics and personal health care products and from occupational uses of formaldehyde (Table 95-1).

Humans have been exposed to formaldehyde for millions of years. It is found as a natural component in fruits, vegetables, meats, and fish. For example, apples have 1.7 to 22.3 parts per million (ppm) formaldehyde, bread crust has 10 ppm of formaldehyde, and low levels are found in beverages with the exception of some fruit juices. A normal diet in the United States is thought to contain approximately 10 to 20 mg formaldehyde per day, which is found predominantly in bound form in foods. Table 95-2 lists some reported levels of formaldehyde in various

TABLE 95-1. Potential occupational exposure to formaldehyde

Anatomists	Glass etchers
Agricultural workers	Glue and adhesive makers
Bakers	Hexamethylenetetramine workers
Biologists	Hide preservers
Botanists	Histology technicians
Crease-resistant textile finishers	Ink makers
Deodorant makers	Lacquerers and lacquer makers
Disinfectant makers	Medical personnel
Disinfectors	Mirror workers
Dress shop workers	Oil well workers
Dressmakers	Paper makers
Drug makers	Particle board workers
Dye makers	Pentaerythritol workers
Electrical insulation makers	Photographic film makers
Embalmers	Plastic workers
Embalming fluid makers	Resin workers
Ethylene glycol makers	Soil sterilizers and greenhouse workers
Fertilizer makers	Surgeons
Fireproofers	Tannery workers
Formaldehyde resin makers	Taxidermists
Formaldehyde production workers	Textiles workers
Foundry workers	Varnish workers
Fumigators	Wood preservative workers
Fungicide workers	
Fur processors	

foods and beverages (4). Although analytic methods used and information on physical state (bound or free) will vary among different studies, the table illustrates how widespread is formaldehyde in the American diet. The normal level of formaldehyde in drinking water is very low (approximately 20 parts per billion). The level of formaldehyde in meat and fish consumed depends on the cooking or processing methods used, with smoked fish having levels in excess of 1,000 ppm. Formaldehyde is produced through the browning reaction during baking.

Environmentally, the air humans breathe contains formaldehyde from many sources, but the primary source outside the workplace is by-products produced during the combustion of organic and fossil fuels (coal, oil, wood, and natural gas). The motor vehicle is the biggest contributor to ambient formaldehyde air levels, especially in cities. The normal ambient level is 0.01 to 0.03 ppm (5). Formaldehyde vapor concentrations in mobile homes and other home environments may have concentrations typically ranging from 0.1 to 0.5 ppm. The average level in standard homes is approximately 0.070 ppm formaldehyde (6).

HMT, a formaldehyde generator, is used as a drug to prevent urinary infections. Mandelamine, a combination of HMT and an organic acid, is given at a rate of 4 g per day. HMT breaks down in an acid environment to ammonia and formaldehyde. A partial breakdown of HMT occurs in the acidic stomach, but approximately 70% of the HMT is absorbed from the gastrointestinal (GI) tract and transported in the blood to the kidney, where it is excreted into the acidic urine (because of the organic acid added to HMT). HMT then breaks down in the urine and releases formaldehyde, which is effective in reducing bacterial growth. Antibiotics are the treatment of choice for urinary bacterial infections, but HMT is prescribed for long periods to prevent urinary infections. Because of the partial HMT breakdown in the stomach, apparently an individual receiving standard HMT treatment would be exposed to approximately 1,000 mg formaldehyde per day in the GI tract (7).

Formaldehyde is a normal metabolite in animals and humans, being an integral part of one-carbon metabolism. Formaldehyde produced by the body is a source of methyl units that are transferred via tetrahydrofolate into the one-carbon pool. The average blood level of formaldehyde in both exposed (2 ppm) and unexposed animals and humans is approximately 2.5 ppm (8). It can be assumed that formaldehyde is present in all aqueous body fluids, owing to its water-soluble nature. This widespread distribution in the body is supported by measured formaldehyde levels (1.5 to 15.0 mg per kg) in various tissues (9).

TABLE 95-2. Level of formaldehyde in foods

Food source	Formaldehyde content (mg/kg)
Dairy	
Milk	0.3–3.3
Yogurt	0.3–3.3
Butter	0.1
Cheese	0.3–1.2
Eggs	0.2–1.2
Yolks	5.5
Provolone cheese	3.14–56.84
Fruit	
Apples	1.7–22.3
Pears	6.0–38.7
Grapes	2.9–3.3
Tomatoes	5.7–16.7
Breads and cereals	
Crust, crumb	
Method of baking	
Straight	2.0–9.9
Sponge	2.0–9.8
No time	1.7–8.6
Preferment	1.4–10.2
Vegetables	
Carrots	0.3–10.0
Cucumber	2.3
Cauliflower	6.6
Cabbage	4.7–5.3
Radish	3.7–4.4
Spinach	3.3–25.0
Onions	13.3–26.3
Meat and fish	
Raw sausage	
Filling	2.0–30.6
Skin	34.0–214
Raw marine fish	6.5–13.6
Raw freshwater fish	0.7–0.8
Fresh haddock	20
Kipper	50–1,000
Raw meat	
Beef	0.7–3.4
Veal	0.7–3.4
Pork	0.7–3.4
Mutton	0.7–3.4
Chicken	2.3–5.7
Smoked foods	
Wurst	1.26
Herring	0.65
Meats[a]	Trace
Vacuum-packed meats	0.7–2.8
Smoked bacon	
Inner layer	0.8–11.5
Outer layer	3.5–52.0
Smoked ham, outer layer	224–267
Boiled smoked sausage	0.7–32.2
Smoked marine fish	3.5–20.0
Smoked freshwater fish	1.5–8.8
Other	
Maple syrup	Up to 2
Beer	0.009
Soy bean	Trace–0.1

[a]Calabrian sausage, smoked pork fat, speck, lard, Hungarian salami, puriser.

It is estimated that the level of free formaldehyde is 1% to 2% of the total formaldehyde tissue level (9). Free formaldehyde tissue levels of 0.3 to 4.8 μg per kg have been reported (10).

Metabolic data support the concept that the body produces and uses formaldehyde in essential metabolic processes. With the normal metabolic pathways, the body can detoxify formaldehyde rapidly from exogenous sources. The small amount of exogenous formaldehyde that comes from occupational exposure and diet is less than 1% of normal metabolic production of formaldehyde by the body. This very small contribution of exogenous formaldehyde to the body pool corroborates that formaldehyde is not a systemic, developmental, or genotoxic hazard.

The lack of *in vivo* genotoxicity, systemic toxicity, and tumors at sites other than that of contact in rodent inhalational studies is supported by the fact that formaldehyde is found throughout the body as a normal metabolite. The normal metabolic process produces, distributes, and uses a daily loading of formaldehyde many times higher than the formaldehyde from all exogenous sources combined, even under maximum dietary and workplace exposure. It is widely recognized that exogenous formaldehyde (10 to 20 mg from food and 10 mg from occupational exposure over 8 hours at 0.75 ppm) has no impact on normal body levels of formaldehyde (11).

CLINICAL TOXICOLOGY

Absorption, Metabolism, and Excretion

Formaldehyde is absorbed readily from the respiratory and oral tracts and, to a much lesser degree, from the skin (1). It is the simplest aldehyde and reacts readily with macromolecules, such as proteins and nucleic acids. Inhalational exposure has been reported to result in almost complete absorption. Dermal absorption due to contact with formaldehyde-containing materials (e.g., textiles, permanent-press clothing, cosmetics, or other materials) is of a low order of magnitude.

As a normal metabolite of the body, formaldehyde is involved in methylation reactions through the tetrafolate mechanism. Normal blood levels of formaldehyde in humans and animals are approximately 2.5 ppm (2.5 mg per L). Formaldehyde is metabolized rapidly and has a half-life in blood of approximately 1.5 minutes (11). This half-life is based primarily on other primate data, although available human data are consistent with this observation of a very short half-life. Data from other species suggest that the half-life of formaldehyde is fairly similar in many species (Table 95-3). Formaldehyde's normal blood levels and short half-life, coupled with the assumption that the levels of water-soluble formaldehyde in the blood are in equilibrium with the body fluids pool, lead to a calculation that an adult human body normally produces and metabolizes

TABLE 95-3. Median lethal dose values for formaldehyde in various species

Species	Route	LD_{50}	Study
Rat	Oral	800	Smyth et al. (1941)
	Subcutaneous	420	Skog (1950)
	Intravenous	87	Langecker (1954)
Mouse	Subcutaneous	300	Skog (1950)
Rabbit	Dermal	270	Lewis and Tatkin (1980)
Guinea pig	Oral	260	Smyth et al. (1948)

LD_{50}, median lethal dose.

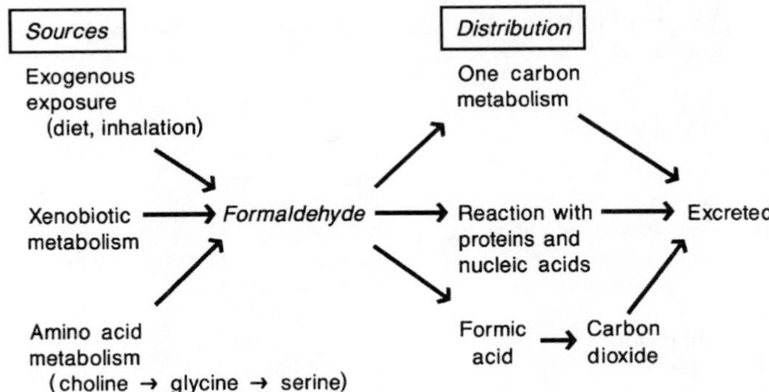

Figure 95-1. Sources and fate of formaldehyde in the body.

(detoxifies or uses) more than 50,000 mg of endogenous formaldehyde daily. It has been calculated that an adult human liver will metabolize 22 mg formaldehyde per minute (or 1,320 mg per hour) directly to carbon dioxide (4). Although this level is slightly more than one-half of the value calculated previously, it does not take into account metabolic incorporation into the one-carbon pool or the binding of formaldehyde that would occur.

Formaldehyde is found in the biosynthesis of some amino acids, purine, and thymidine. It either is converted to carbon dioxide by the formate pathway and exhaled or is incorporated into the one-carbon pool (12). Radioactivity after exposure to ^{14}C-formaldehyde is found throughout the body and supports the concept of rapid incorporation and metabolism. Figure 95-1 shows an overview of the general metabolic production and fate of formaldehyde in the body. The body's high endogenous production and use of formaldehyde are important in understanding the potential action of formaldehyde in the body and are consistent with the idea that formaldehyde is not a systemic toxin. Exogenous exposure is so low, as compared with endogenous production, that measured formaldehyde levels in the blood and tissues do not change after either inhalational exposure (15 ppm) or ingestion of foods containing high levels of formaldehyde (11). Conversion of formate to carbon dioxide is a rate-limiting step in the direct breakdown of formaldehyde in primates, including humans. The rodent, on the other hand, is much more efficient in the conversion of formate to carbon dioxide; as a result, demonstrating formate buildup in a rodent is very difficult. Formate accumulation can be observed in humans or primates under certain conditions (e.g., oral ingestion of high levels of methanol that is metabolized to formaldehyde). Formaldehyde normally is converted and excreted as carbon dioxide in the air, as formic acid in the urine, or as one of many breakdown products from one-carbon pool metabolism. As a result of rapid absorption by both the oral and inhalational routes and of its rapid metabolism, little or no formaldehyde is excreted unmetabolized. In rats exposed to ^{14}C-formaldehyde by inhalation, 40% of the radiolabel was excreted in the air and 20% in the urine and feces, whereas 40% remained in the carcass.

Routes of Exposure

DERMAL CONTACT

The use of formalin solutions in hospitals, pathology laboratories, and funeral homes to fix or preserve tissues can lead to both dermal and inhalational exposure (13). Low levels of dermal exposure are possible also in the general population from the use of cosmetics and personal health care products containing formaldehyde as a preservative (14). Dermal exposure in the workplace can occur if involved individuals handle solid paraformaldehyde or liquid formaldehyde products or materials that generate formaldehyde, such as trioxane. Permanent-press clothing is treated with formaldehyde resin systems, and some reports have cited dermal exposure to formaldehyde from these garments. However, the residual formaldehyde levels in clothing have been reduced significantly over the last few years (15).

INHALATION

Formaldehyde is a gas at room temperature, and exposure by inhalation can occur. Low concentrations of airborne formaldehyde are always found in the ambient air, primarily as a result of burning organic fuels (14). In 1978, the amount of formaldehyde generated from automobile exhaust in the United States was estimated to be 660,000,000 pounds per year. Concentrations found in the air under certain conditions can be relatively high (up to several hundred parts per billion) in areas such as unvented parking garages or tunnels with slowly moving traffic (1).

Inhalational exposure to formaldehyde can be found in the workplace wherever formaldehyde or formaldehyde resin systems are used. Polyacetal resins (plastic made from formaldehyde) can release formaldehyde vapors during the heating phase of the molding process. The use of formaldehyde generators, such as HMT and trioxane, also can produce formaldehyde vapors. Resin systems are used as glues in the manufacturing of wood products, such as furniture and paneling, and also could release measurable formaldehyde vapors. In addition, formaldehyde resin systems are used in several textile applications, such as the manufacture of carpets and permanent-press clothing (15).

Urea formaldehyde foam was injected into walls of homes in the past to reduce air leakage and heating costs. Under certain conditions, where installation was faulty, this led to an excess release of formaldehyde vapors into such homes. Owing to the controversy surrounding this application, this material currently is not used in the United States for retrofitting homes.

Cigarette smoking is also a source of airborne formaldehyde. The smoking of a cigarette will produce up to 50 μg of formaldehyde. The side stream of tobacco smoke is reported to contain up to 40 ppm of formaldehyde (1).

ORAL ROUTE

The potential for exposure by the oral route also exists. Many foods have measurable levels of formaldehyde. Foods that are either smoked or grilled can have as much as 1,000 ppm formaldehyde. Formaldehyde also is very common in such foods as fruits (apples, tomatoes, etc.), dairy products, and vegetables and in baked goods. Agents that release formaldehyde, such as HMT, sometimes are used both as a food preservative and as a drug. As stated earlier, the most common drug use of HMT is for urinary tract infections; normal use of this drug can release up to 4,000 mg of formaldehyde into the body (7). Oral exposure is possible also from the use of certain personal care products (mouthwashes, toothpaste, etc.) in which formaldehyde is used as a preservative (14). Formaldehyde exposure in drinking water is thought to be extremely low, although some reports claim that plastic fittings used in plumbing may release some formaldehyde into the water (1).

Signs, Symptoms, and Syndromes

The subject of potential health effects from formaldehyde exposure has been controversial for years (16,17). Acute local effects secondary to exposure, such as mucous membrane irritation, ocular irritation, and dermatitis, are well known. Controversial health effects include systemic reactions, such as immunologic alterations, cancer, and sensitization (16–18). Health effects secondary to chronic exposure to low concentrations of formaldehyde vapors have been associated with multiple medical complaints (19–21). Much debate has centered around low-level exposure to formaldehyde in the home and occupational environment and around subsequent health complaints.

Symptoms of eye irritation, throat irritation, fatigue, headache, and nausea at environmental air concentrations between 0.1 and 1.0 ppm (18–22) have been reported, but exposure between 0.8 and 1.0 ppm appears to be the threshold for respiratory symptoms and ocular irritation (23–28). However, in many cases, these complaints cannot be related directly to formaldehyde but to indoor air pollution in general, or they cannot be reproduced in similar studies.

Exposure to airborne formaldehyde results in a clear, nonlinear dose response in animal and humans. At low airborne levels, mucociliary defense mechanisms prevent formaldehyde from penetrating the mucociliary blanket and reaching nerve endings or tissue. Exposure to airborne formaldehyde at low levels (ranging up to approximately 0.8 ppm) is not noticed because of the body's normal mucociliary defense mechanism (29).

Human sensory response to formaldehyde has been evaluated under many different conditions. These conditions can be divided into three general study types: controlled chamber studies, workplace studies, and environmental complaint–type studies. All have advantages and disadvantages. The controlled chamber studies, in which exposure levels are controlled carefully, are the best to establish dose-response correlation with sensory irritation. No confounding factors (e.g., the presence of other chemicals or dust or changes in exposure levels during the observation period) are found in controlled studies. In most controlled studies, nonacclimatized individuals are used. This may be a drawback, but such subjects usually are more sensitive than are acclimatized individuals. Some individuals can develop a tolerance to the sensory irritation potential of formaldehyde.

These controlled chamber studies demonstrate that eye irritation is the first sign of sensory irritation in nonacclimatized subjects as the formaldehyde concentration is increased. The threshold for slight eye irritation is near 1.0 ppm. This eye response serves as a warning of exposure and helps to prevent upper respiratory tract irritation, which is seen at higher concentrations. No effect on pulmonary function was seen in any of these studies with exposure limited to formaldehyde (up to 3.0 ppm) and not to other confounding factors, such as dust.

In an early human controlled study (25), blink rate was found to increase statistically at formaldehyde concentrations in excess of 1.7 ppm, and the average irritation threshold was between 1 and 2 ppm. The response was greater if the exposure was intermittent rather than continuous, demonstrating some tolerance. In another early study (22), a small decrease in the mucus flow rate was reported by some subjects when exposed to 0.25, 0.42, or 1.6 ppm but not when exposed to 0.83 ppm. The lack of a dose response calls the significance of this observation into question. Fifteen of 16 subjects reported slight discomfort in the form of eye irritation on exposure to 0.83 ppm formaldehyde.

In an eye irritation study (23), approximately one-half of the volunteers were rejected either because they reported eye irritation from clean air (air movement) or because they were unresponsive in the test system. At formaldehyde levels of less than 1.0 ppm, the reported eye irritation was not significantly different from that attributed to clean air. At 1.0 ppm, 20 of 27 reported slight to moderate eye irritation.

In a 1987 study (24) of 19 nonsmoking subjects, nasal flow resistance was observed at exposure to 3.0 ppm but not less. Four of the 19 subjects reported eye irritation at concentrations of 1.0 ppm. Odor was detected by 4 of 9 subjects at 0.5 ppm. No significant decrement in pulmonary function or increase in bronchial reactivity to methacholine was noted at concentrations of 3.0 ppm.

The average subjective response to irritation at 1.0 and 2.0 ppm was described as mild (present but not annoying). At 3.0 ppm, eye irritation was classified as moderate (annoying). Many other controlled chamber studies in the 1980s reached similar conclusions about pulmonary function and sensory tract irritation (23–28). A very few isolated cases of respiratory sensitization in humans have been reported, although no respiratory sensitization has been demonstrated in any animal species (30–34).

The association between asthma and formaldehyde has been investigated. Being very water soluble, formaldehyde is absorbed mainly in the upper airway and thus usually does not reach the lower bronchial or alveolar areas in the lungs. Investigations involving individuals with asthma or symptoms of wheezing thought to be exacerbated by formaldehyde have demonstrated that vapor concentrations up to 3 ppm did not cause bronchospasm (22–28,35–42).

Both asthmatics and nonasthmatics experience upper respiratory tract irritation but no lower airway effects. Some researchers have suggested that certain individuals may be more sensitive to formaldehyde than is the average person and therefore may respond to formaldehyde by exhibiting bronchial asthma–like symptoms. This response should not be considered true respiratory sensitization (43–45).

The only reported effects on lower airways were studies in which dust from wood or urea formaldehyde foam insulation was present (46). Particles could carry formaldehyde into the lung, whereas gaseous formaldehyde by itself is trapped in the nasal mucus. The controlled chamber studies, with no confounding dust exposure, did not report any lower airway effects. These studies control and actually measure the air levels of formaldehyde, so accurate correlation of effects with exposure can be made. This is very important if the exposure level is to be used to relate exposure to human response. Because of the environmentally controlled nature of the chamber studies, distractions such as are found in the workplace are minimized, and individuals tend to be more responsive than would be someone in the workplace.

Airborne levels in excess of 4 to 5 ppm formaldehyde generally are intolerable (47). Skin contact with formaldehyde solutions (more than 2%) can cause skin rashes (13). Skin sensitization (allergic contact dermatitis, a type IV allergy) also can be caused by formaldehyde (13). These characteristic responses are the only known effects of formaldehyde exposure in humans.

Formaldehyde solutions (more than 2%) are dermal irritants (13). Concentrated formaldehyde solutions can be corrosive to the eye and can cause chemical burns to the skin in animals and in humans. The dermal sensitization potential of formaldehyde has been estimated to be as high as 5% in the general population (13). Dermal sensitization in animals also has been demonstrated adequately. In summary, formaldehyde is a dermal, eye, and respiratory irritant in humans and is a skin sensitizer.

ANIMAL STUDIES

Chronic Inhalation. Animal experiments have demonstrated that at repeated exposure levels exceeding 2 ppm cytotoxicity (in which the mucociliary defense mechanisms are saturated), cell proliferation, and tissue damage can ensue (29,48–50). High levels of inhalational exposure (15 ppm) have resulted in the production of squamous cell carcinomas in the nasal cavity (site of tissue damage) in rats and mice (49) but not in the hamster exposed to up to 10 ppm (29). In an earlier inhalational study in which mice were exposed for 1 hour per day, 3 days per week for up to 64 weeks at 0, 40, 80, and 120 ppm formaldehyde, no treatment-related tumors were noted (51). The squamous cell carcinomas in the rat are postulated to be related to tissue damage caused by high levels of airborne formaldehyde (Table 95-4).

TABLE 95-4. Incidence of squamous cell carcinomas in Fischer 344 rats and B6C3F1 mice exposed to formaldehyde vapor

	Dose (ppm)							
	0		2.0		5.6		14.3	
	M	F	M	F	M	F	M	F
Rat	0	0	0	0	1	1	51[a]	52[a]
Mouse	0	0	0	0	0	0	2[b]	0

[a]Statistically significant in life-table test for positive trend with dose ($p < .0167$) and life-table comparison of control group versus 14.3 ppm.
[b]Not statistically significant by life-table analysis or by Fischer's exact test.
Note: Number of tumor-bearing animals. Number of nasal cavities examined was between 115 and 120 for males and females of each species.
Adapted from Kerns WD, Donofrio DJ, Pavkov, KL. The chronic effects of formaldehyde in rats and mice: a preliminary report. In: Gibson JE, ed. *Formaldehyde toxicity.* New York: Hemisphere Publishing, 1983.

The response in rats to airborne formaldehyde has been studied in detail, and an understanding of the mechanism by which formaldehyde causes these tumors in rats has been evolving (16). Formaldehyde acts only at the site of contact (i.e., the nasal cavity for airborne formaldehyde) (52). Formaldehyde does not reach the lower respiratory tract in the rat studies, even at concentrations of 15 ppm. In the nasal cavity of rats, high local levels of formaldehyde cause tissue damage, produce more single-stranded DNA (as formaldehyde will react only with single-stranded DNA), and increase cellular proliferation (rapid replacement of damaged cells). This rapid proliferation of cells at levels of more than 2 ppm formaldehyde in rats diminishes the efficiency of the normal DNA repair mechanism, such that there is less time during which the normal DNA repair mechanisms can operate. A mutated cell that could produce a tumor and normally would be repaired may slip by the very efficient repair mechanism and eventually produce a tumor (53). Continuous cell proliferation appears necessary to produce a tumor response in rats (53). Numerous animal studies support a level at which no adverse health effects are observed. A no-observed-effect level in rats for cell proliferation, tissue damage, and nasal tumors has been demonstrated at concentrations of 2 ppm (16,48,49,52,53).

Formaldehyde is weakly genotoxic *in vitro*, but *in vivo* tests fail to demonstrate activity. This *in vivo* response is not unexpected considering the high body burden and turnover of endogenous formaldehyde.

DNA-protein cross-links have been used as a measure of the dose to the target tissue in rodent and primate experiments. These DNA cross-links are formed when formaldehyde reaches the nuclei of the target nasal epithelial cells. The rate is related directly to the concentration of free formaldehyde in the nuclei of target nasal cells. This information has been used to assist in relating the dose necessary to produce nasal tumors in primates to the effect levels in rats. The first thing noted is a very strong nonlinear response relating cell proliferation with DNA cross-links (formaldehyde binding to DNA). Species differences also were noted in binding (picomoles per milligram DNA per parts per million), the rat being approximately eight times more sensitive than is the monkey on a parts-per-million basis. The monkeys are approximately two times more sensitive than are humans (picomoles per milligram DNA per parts per million). This suggests that the rat is far more sensitive (approximately 14 times) than are humans to the same airborne concentration as far as DNA cross-links are concerned. The rat appears to over-predict the tumor potential in the nasal cavity in humans on the basis of airborne parts per million. This prediction is supported by the lack of a demonstrated cancer response in humans exposed to formaldehyde in the workplace (54). Squamous cell carcinomas in the nasal cavity are rare in humans.

DNA-protein cross-links do not accumulate with repeated exposure to formaldehyde. This suggests that the cross-linking is repaired readily, by the next day in most cases (55).

Teratogenesis. Potential teratogenicity has been studied in rodents after exposure to formaldehyde. In a study in which pregnant mice received formaldehyde by gavage at several doses (the highest dose resulting in death to several of the pregnant mice), no evidence of any treatment-related malformation was observed (56). Another study exposing rats to 10 ppm formaldehyde for 6 hours per day during the organogenesis period (6 to 15 days) showed no evidence of treatment-related malformations (57). The results are consistent with the lack of systemic toxicity suggested by the high normal production and metabolism of formaldehyde in the body.

Earlier animal studies that addressed the chronic and carcinogenic potential of formaldehyde were feeding studies using HMT. Formaldehyde and ammonia are the breakdown products of HMT in the acid environment of the stomach. These studies were conducted to support the use of HMT as a food preservative (58,59). In these feeding studies, no treatment-related tumors or effects on the stomach were reported in rats and mice (up to 5% in drinking water for 1 to 2 years) or in dogs (52 days at 600 or 1,250 ppm in feed). The breakdown of HMT in the stomach is incomplete and would result in a formaldehyde level in the stomach of approximately 30% of the ingested HMT levels. The remainder of the HMT is thought to be absorbed intact from the GI tract. This is the basis for using HMT as a drug to prevent urinary infections; the absorbed HMT does not generate formaldehyde until it reaches the acid environment of the urine.

More recent studies assess the effects of formaldehyde or formalin (which also contains methanol) in drinking water. In a rat study, nonneoplastic lesions (erosion or ulcers, hyperplasia, deep gastric pits) and benign tumors (squamous cell papilloma) were reported in the forestomach of treated rats (60). No malignant treatment-related tumors were noted at any site. Because of technical shortcomings, this study is of limited value but does demonstrate that the forestomach, the site of contact, is a target organ in oral studies.

In a second study conducted in Japan, early deaths and nonneoplastic lesions (erosion and ulcers) in both the glandular stomach and forestomach were observed primarily at a concentration of 0.5% formaldehyde in the drinking water (61). Squamous cell hyperplasia was seen only in the forestomach at the 0.5% level; no papillomas or other types of treatment-related tumors were found at any treatment level. All rats receiving 0.5% formaldehyde died before the end of the 24-month study period. The level of no observed treatment-related effects was 0.02% (200 ppm).

In a third study conducted in the Netherlands, histologic lesions in the high-dose group (ulcers and hyperplasia) were noted in the forestomach and in the glandular stomach (62). Atrophic gastritis was seen in the glandular stomach only at the high dose. No treatment-related tumors (including papillomas) were seen at any site or test level, again demonstrating the lack of direct systemic effects. The middose (25 mg per kg) was at the level of no adverse effect.

An oral study concluded that formaldehyde is a multipotential carcinogen on the basis of a reported increase in leukemia and malignant GI tract tumors (stomach and intestinal tumors combined) (63). Lack of information about time to tumor, absence of statistics, the combination of tumors from different sites, and the lack of historical tumor data pose many questions concerning this conclusion. This study's results are not consistent with results in earlier studies covering the same dose range and species. Normal metabolism of formaldehyde also supports the lack of systemic effects. The lack of reported nonneoplastic lesions creates difficulty in determining whether the forestomach is the target organ in this study. One Japanese study (61) had a top dose twice as high as the Italian study (64), and the Dutch study (62) used a top dose similar to that in the Italian study (64). No treatment-related tumors were reported in either the Japanese or Dutch study (61,62).

Feed treated with formaldehyde has been given to cattle, sheep, swine, and poultry (64–78). Formaldehyde reacts with protein in the feed to form a formaldehyde-protein complex that decrease the digestibility and limits the availability of formaldehyde. In some cases, an increase in the growth rate was noted, indicating improved feed use. In other cases, a decrease in the rate of weight gain was observed. No suggestion of any potential toxicity was reported.

HUMAN EPIDEMIOLOGIC STUDIES

Because nasal tumors have been seen in animal studies, more than 30 epidemiologic studies have investigated different human populations exposed to formaldehyde. The workers' exposure to formaldehyde in many of these studies was higher than the present U.S. Occupational Safety and Health Administration (OSHA) permissible exposure limit (PEL). Many workers had worked with formaldehyde for more than 20 years, and the time from first exposure to the end of the study period (latency) was at least 20 years. A review of these studies by an expert panel concluded that "for no malignancy in man is there convincing evidence of a relationship with formaldehyde exposure" (79). No specific tumor site or tumor type has been identified in humans exposed to formaldehyde.

The two largest occupational studies of formaldehyde-exposed workers demonstrates that formaldehyde exposure does not cause lung cancer in humans. The largest such study of formaldehyde-exposed workers was conducted by the National Cancer Institute in the United States and covered ten industrial plants involving 26,561 workers (80). To be included in the study, a worker had to have first been exposed to formaldehyde 20 or more years earlier. The exposures were divided into three groups—less than 0.5 ppm, 0.5 to 5.5 ppm, and more than 5.5 ppm formaldehyde. When the issue of lung cancer was evaluated in more detail, no significant correlation with intensity, duration, peak exposure, or cumulative exposure to formaldehyde was found. The authors concluded that the data in this study provided little evidence that mortality from cancer is associated with formaldehyde exposure. No history of smoking was recorded. The National Cancer Institute and the University of Pittsburgh reanalyzed these data and reported the results of their studies in the scientific literature (81–83). With each reanalysis of these studies, they reached the same conclusion: Formaldehyde does not cause cancer.

The second of these large studies, conducted in the United Kingdom by the Medical Research Council, involved six facilities with 7,680 workers (84). To be included in the study, a worker had to have first been exposed to formaldehyde in the workplace 20 or more years earlier. The exposures were divided into four groups—less than 0.1 ppm, 0.1 to 0.5 ppm, 0.6 to 2.0 ppm, and more than 2.0 ppm formaldehyde. The authors of this study and an updating study concluded that there was "no definite indication of this excess of lung cancer being clearly related to formaldehyde exposure" (84,85). No history of smoking was collected in either study. Both the larger epidemiologic studies show less than an expected rate of nasal cancer in exposed workers (80,84).

In the most recent published study of potential formaldehyde exposure and lung cancer, foundry workers were evaluated, and an increase in lung cancer was observed (86). This study was different from earlier studies of occupationally exposed groups, as the researchers evaluated all the cofactors that might be associated with the lung cancer noted in this population. A history of smoking was recorded. The study demonstrated that the increase in lung cancer found in foundry workers was due to smoking and silica exposure. Although formaldehyde exposure was high in this study, no association was found between formaldehyde exposure and deaths from malignant or nonmalignant diseases of the respiratory tract (including the lung). The 30-plus epidemiologic studies failed to demonstrate any consistent pattern of response associated solely with formaldehyde exposure and any cancer in humans. There are no reports of teratogenic effects in humans after formaldehyde exposure.

Management of Toxicity or Exposure

TREATMENT

Skin. Formaldehyde will enter the skin and cause allergic dermatitis. Contact urticaria has been reported in several cases. Skin exposure, primarily to solutions of formaldehyde, may cause dermal sensitization in some individuals. Generally, a formaldehyde solution of 2% or greater will cause skin irritation. This condition should be treated as a burn to prevent or minimize irritation. There is no indication that formaldehyde will cause photoirritation.

Ingestion. Ingestion of concentrated solutions of formaldehyde may cause severe gastric irritation and sloughing of the gastric epithelium, with gastric bleeding. Ingestion of high amounts of formaldehyde will cause blood levels of formaldehyde to increase, and metabolic acidosis may occur from the formation of formic and lactic acid. Hemodialysis is efficacious just as in methanol poisoning and should be considered if metabolic acidosis occurs. The lack of effects of formaldehyde in humans exposed to low levels by the oral route is supported by formaldehyde's use as a drug and the daily ingestion of formaldehyde in foods.

Inhalation. Exposure to airborne formaldehyde results in a clear, nonlinear dose response in animals and humans. Exposure exceeding approximately 1 ppm will produce a transient sensory irritation (eye, nose, and throat) (16). Higher levels produce severe upper respiratory tract irritation and cough. Exposure to airborne levels in excess of 6 ppm (in which the mucociliary defense mechanisms are saturated) may result in cytotoxicity or reversible tissue damage. Removal from exposure is the recommended treatment. However, no systemic effects have been demonstrated clearly in animals or humans after repeated exposure by any route. This observation is supported by the lack of an exogenous formaldehyde effect on the normal body formaldehyde burden.

Ocular Exposure. Solutions of formaldehyde may damage the conjunctiva and cornea. Affected eyes should be flushed immediately with water for 15 minutes if solutions of formaldehyde enter the eye.

LABORATORY DIAGNOSIS

A positive patch test result indicates an allergic hypersensitivity type IV skin reaction (21). An open skin test using less than 1% to 2% formalin will demonstrate immunologic contact urticaria by showing a wheal-and-flare response. Intradermal tests of formaldehyde for type I allergies are useless in humans. If radioimmunoassay testing for formaldehyde were developed, it would be useful to demonstrate whether asthma or respiratory complaints are due to formaldehyde allergy. There is no evidence of a type IV reaction involved in respiratory allergies to formaldehyde. Pulmonary function tests may be useful, although only small transient effects have been noted after high levels of exposure to formaldehyde or mixed exposures. Hyperactive airway syndrome has been demonstrated in standard tests using methacholine and histamine challenge, but these tests are of limited value in evaluating formaldehyde exposure, as do bronchial provocation tests (21).

Blood levels of formaldehyde and urinary formic acid have been suggested as tests to measure exposure biologically. Because of the high natural body production of formaldehyde, neither of these indicators is of any value in assessing formaldehyde exposure. They would be useful, however, if very high oral ingestion had taken place.

BIOLOGICAL MONITORING

No useful biological monitoring method has been developed for formaldehyde. Blood formaldehyde levels and urinary formate have been suggested as biological indicators of exposure, but the high normal body burden of formaldehyde (blood, 2.5 ppm) and complete, rapid metabolism render these tests useless as biological monitors.

ENVIRONMENTAL MONITORING

Several methods are available for collecting and measuring airborne formaldehyde. Sampling is accomplished with a bubbler, impinger, solid sorbent, or passive dosimeter. Concentrations are determined by colorimetric, polarographic, high-performance liquid chromatographic, gas chromatographic, or direct (electrochemical, colorimetric, infrared, or photoionization) instruments. The most passive technique is based on an impinger with 1% sodium bisulfite that uses chromotropic acid to develop color. The reported limit of detection of this method is 0.02 ppm, but the technique is sensitive to 0.01 ppm. The American Industrial Hygienists Association's *Occupational Exposure and Work Practice Guidelines for Formaldehyde*, published in 1989, details analytic methods, including limitations (49).

OCCUPATIONAL AND ENVIRONMENTAL REGULATIONS

The PEL for formaldehyde was set by OSHA as the level at which humans may be exposed to formaldehyde for 8 hours per day, 5 days per week, without adverse health effects. Prior to July 1992, the PEL for formaldehyde was 1 ppm as a time-weighted average of 8 hours and, since July 1992, the PEL has been 0.75 ppm as a time-weighted average. An OSHA formaldehyde medical standard also was established (Table 95-5).

Exposure to airborne formaldehyde at low levels (ranging up to approximately 0.8 ppm) produces no symptoms and is not noticed because of the body's normal mucociliary defense mechanism (29). This defense mechanism prevents formaldehyde from reaching nerve endings and tissues. If airborne levels exceed 1 ppm, a sensory irritation is noticed in humans (23–28). Sensory irritation consists of a watering and burning sensation of the eyes and irritation of the nose and throat. This sensory irritation serves as an exposure warning. Respirators have been

TABLE 95-5. Current occupational exposure limits

Country	TWA	STEL	Date
United States			
OSHA	0.75 ppm	2.0 ppm	1993
ACGIH	0.3 ppm	0.3 ppm	1993
Australia	1.0 ppm	2.0 ppm	1991
Belgium	1.0 ppm	2.0 ppm	1991
Denmark	0.3 ppm	—	1991
Finland	1.0 ppm	—	1991
France	2.0 ppm	—	1991
Germany	0.5 ppm	—	1993
Japan	0.5 ppm	—	1991
Netherlands	1.0 ppm	2.0 ppm	1986
Russia	0.5 ppm	0.5 ppm	1991
United Kingdom	2.0 ppm	2.0 ppm	1992

ACGIH, American Conference of Governmental Industrial Hygienists; OSHA, U.S. Occupational Safety and Health Administration; STEL, short-term exposure limit; TWA, time-weighted average.

shown to prevent inhalation of formaldehyde if levels exceed the PEL. The best control is adequate ventilation in cases in which exposure may approach or exceed the PEL. OSHA has established an action level of 0.5 ppm in which more frequent monitoring and other actions are required to ensure that a person's exposure remains at a level less than the PEL.

REFERENCES

1. National Research Council. *Formaldehyde and other aldehydes.* Washington: National Academy Press, 1981.
2. Gerberich HR, et al. Formaldehyde. In: Kirk RE, Othmer DF, eds. *Encyclopedia of chemical technology,* 3rd ed, vol 11. New York: John Wiley and Sons, 1985:231–250.
3. International Agency for Research on Cancer. Some industrial chemicals and dyestuffs. *IARC Monogr Eval Carcinog Risks Hum* 1982;29:345–389.
4. Owen BA, Dudney CS, Tan EL, Easterly CE. Formaldehyde in drinking water: comparative hazard evaluation and an approach to regulation. *Regul Toxicol Pharmacol* 1990;11:220.
5. US Environmental Protection Agency. *Urban air toxic monitoring program. GRAI* 1992;2.
6. Stock TH, Mendez SR. A survey of typical exposure to formaldehyde in Houston area residents. *Am Ind Hyg Assoc* 1985;46:313–317.
7. *Physicians' desk reference,* 49th ed. Montvale, NJ: Medical Economics Company, 1995.
8. Heck Hd'A, Casanova-Schmitz M, Dodd PB, et al. Formaldehyde concentrations in the blood of humans and Fischer-344 rats exposed to formaldehyde under controlled conditions. *Am Ind Hyg Assoc J* 1985;46:1–3.
9. Heck Hd'A. Biochemical toxicity of inhaled formaldehyde. *CIIT Activities* 1982;2:3.
10. Hileman B. Formaldehyde: assessing the risk. *Environ Sci Technol* 1984;18: 216(abst).
11. Cascieri TC, Clary JJ. Formaldehyde-oral toxicity assessment. *Comments Toxicol* 1992;4:295–304.
12. International Agency for Research on Cancer. Wood dust and formaldehyde. *IARC Monogr Eval Carcinog Risks Hum* 1995;62:294–301.
13. Maibach H. Formaldehyde: effects on animal and human skin. In: Gibson JE, ed. *Formaldehyde toxicology.* New York: Hemisphere Publishing Company, 1983:166–174.
14. Hart RW, Terturro A, Neimeth L. Consensus workshop in formaldehyde. *Environ Health Perspect* 1984;58:323–381.
15. Code of Federal Regulations 29, Part 1910–1926. Washington: Government Printing Office, 1987.
16. Clary JJ. Risk assessment for exposure to formaldehyde. In: Gibson JE, ed. *Formaldehyde toxicity.* New York: Hemisphere Publishing Company, 1983: 284–294.
17. Bardana EJ, Montanaro A. The formaldehyde fiasco: a review of the scientific data. *Immunol Allergy Pract* 1987;9:11–24.
18. Main DM, Hogan TJ. Health effects of low-level exposure to formaldehyde. *J Occup Med* 1983;25:896–900.
19. Bracken MJ, Leasa DJ, Morgan WKC. Exposure to formaldehyde: relationship to respiratory symptoms and function. *Can J Public Health* 1985;76:312–316.
20. Kilburn KH, Warshaw R, Boylen CT, et al. Pulmonary and neurobehavioral effects of formaldehyde exposure. *Arch Environ Health* 1985;40:254–260.
21. Imbus HR. Clinical evaluation of patients with complaints related to formaldehyde exposure. *J Allergy Clin Immunol* 1985;76:831–840.
22. Anderson I. Formaldehyde in the indoor environment—health implications of setting standards. In: Franger PO, Valbjorn O, eds. *Proc First International Indoor Climate* 1979;66–87.
23. Bender JR, Mullin LS, Graepel GJ, Wilson WE. Eye irritation response of humans to formaldehyde. *Am Ind Hyg Assoc J* 1983;44:463–465.
24. Kulle TJ, Sauder LR, Hebel JR, Green DJ, Chatham MD. Formaldehyde dose-responses in healthy nonsmokers. *J Air Pollut Contr Assoc* 1987;39:919–924.
25. Weber-Tschopp A, Fischer T, Grand JE. Reizuirkungen des formaldehyde (HCHO) auf den Menschen. *Arch Occup Environ Health* 1977;39:207–218.
26. Schacter NE, Tosun T, Beck GJ. A study of respiratory effects from exposure to 2 ppm formaldehyde in healthy subjects. *Arch Environ Health* 1986;41: 229–239.
27. Sauder LR, Wong SC, Uehara CF, Nadel JA, Boushey HA. Acute pulmonary response to formaldehyde exposure in healthy nonsmokers. *J Occup Med* 1986;28:420–424.
28. Green DJ, Sauder LR, Kulle TJ, Bascom R. Acute response to 3.0 ppm formaldehyde in exercising healthy nonsmokers and asthmatics. *Am Rev Respir Dis* 1987;135:1261–1286.
29. Starr T, Gibson JE, Barrow CS, et al. Estimating human cancer risk from formaldehyde: critical issues. In: *Formaldehyde: analytical chemistry and toxicology.* Washington: American Chemical Society, 1983:299–334.
30. Hendrick DJ, Rando RJ, Lane DJ, Morril MJ. Formaldehyde asthma: challenge exposure levels and fate after five years. *J Occup Med* 1982;24:893–897.
31. Hendrick DJ, Lane DJ. Occupational formalin asthma. *Br J Ind Med* 1977;34: 11–18.
32. Burge PS, Harries MG, O'Brien IM, Patchett PA. Occupational asthma due to formaldehyde. *Thorax* 1985;40:255–260.
33. Gorski P, Krakowiak A. Does formaldehyde-induced asthma exist? *Med Pr* 1992;43:187–190.
34. Nordman H, Keskinen H, Tuppurainen M. Formaldehyde asthma—rare or overlooked? *J Allergy Clin Immunol* 1985;75:91–99.
35. Sheppard D, Eschenbacher WL, Epstein J. Lack of bronchomotor response to up to 3 ppm formaldehyde in subjects with asthma. *Environ Res* 1984;35: 133–139.
36. Alexanderson R, Kolmodin-Hedman B, Hedenstierna G. Exposure to formaldehyde: effects on pulmonary function. *Arch Environ Health* 1982;37:279–284.
37. Frigas E, Filley WV, Reed CE. Bronchial challenge with formaldehyde gas: lack of bronchoconstriction in 13 patients suspected of having formaldehyde-induced asthma. *Mayo Clin Proc* 1984;59:295–299.
38. Witek TJ, Schachter EN, Tosun T, Beck GJ, Leaderer BP. An evaluation of respiratory effects following exposure to 2.0 ppm formaldehyde in asthmatics: lung function, symptoms and airway reactivity. *Arch Environ Health* 1987;42:230–237.
39. Uba G, Pachorek D, Bernstein J, et al. Prospective study of respiratory effects of formaldehyde among healthy and asthmatic medical students. *Am J Ind Med* 1989;15:91–101.
40. Harving H, Korsgaard J, Pederson OF, Molhave L, Dahl R. Pulmonary function and bronchial reactivity in asthmatics during low-level formaldehyde exposure. *Lung* 1990;168:15–21.
41. Saunder LR, Green DJ, Chatham MD, Kulle TJ. Acute pulmonary response of asthmatics to 3.0 ppm formaldehyde. *Toxicol Ind Health* 1987;3:569–578.
42. Day JH, Lees REM, Clark RT, et al. Respiratory response to formaldehyde and off-gas of urea formaldehyde foam insulation. *Can Med Assoc J* 1984;131:1061.
43. Dykewicz MS Patterson R, Cugell DW, Harris KE, Wu AF. Serum IgE and IgG to formaldehyde-human serum albumin: lack of relation to gaseous formaldehyde exposure and symptoms. *J Allergy Clin Immunol* 1991;7:48–57.
44. Grammar LC, Harris KE, Cugell DW, Paterson R. Evaluation of a worker with possible formaldehyde-induced asthma. *J Allergy Clin Immunol* 1993;92:29–33.
45. Grammar LC, Harris KE, Shaughnessy MN, et al. Clinical and immunologic evaluation of 37 workers exposed to gaseous formaldehyde. *J Allergy Clin Immunol* 1990;86:177–181.
46. Frigas E, Filley WV, Redd CE. Asthma induced by dust from urea-formaldehyde foam insulating material. *Chest* 1981;79:706–707.
47. American Industrial Hygienists Association. *Occupational exposure and work practice guidelines for formaldehyde.* American Industrial Hygienists Association, 1989.
48. Rusch GM, Clary JJ, Rhinehart WE, Bolte HF. A 26-week inhalation toxicity study with formaldehyde in the monkey, rat, and hamster. *Toxicol Appl Pharmacol* 1983;68:329–343.
49. Kerns WD, Pavkov KL, Donofrio DJ, Grallo EJ, Swenberg JA. Carcinogenicity of formaldehyde in rats and mice after long-term inhalation exposure. *Cancer Res* 1983;43:4382.
50. Feron VJ, Woutersen RA. Role of tissue damage in nasal carcinogenesis. In: Feron VJ, Basland MC, eds. *Nasal carcinogenesis in rodents: relevance to human health risk. Proceedings of the TNO-CIVO/NYU Symposium, Veldhoven, Netherlands, October 24–28, 1988.* 1988:76.
51. Horton AW, Russell T, Stemmer KL. Experimental carcinogenesis of the lung. Inhalation of gaseous formaldehyde or an aerosol of coal tar by C3H mice. *J Natl Cancer Inst* 1963;30:31–43.
52. Clary JJ. Formaldehyde risk analysis. In: Turoski V, ed. *Formaldehyde analytical chemistry and toxicology.* Washington: American Chemical Society, 1985: 341–356.
53. Monticello TM, Miller FJ, Morgan KT. Regional increase in rat nasal epithelial cell proliferation following acute and subchronic inhalation of formaldehyde. *Toxicol Appl Pharmacol* 1991;111:409–421.

54. Connolly RB, Andjelkovich A, Casanova M, et al. Multidisciplinary, iterative examination of the mechanism of formaldehyde carcinogenicity: the basis for better risk assessment. *CIIT Activities* 1995;15:1–10.
55. Casanova M, Morgan KT, Gross EA, Moss OR, Heck Hd'A. DNA-protein crosslinks and cell replication at specific sites in the nose of F344 rats exposed subchronically to formaldehyde. *Fundam Appl Toxicol* 1994;23:525–536.
56. Marks TA, Worthy WC, Staples RE, et al. Influence of formaldehyde and sonacide (potentiated acid glutaraldehyde) on embryo and fetal development in mice. *Teratology* 1980;22:51–58.
57. Robinson, et al. *A teratological study of inhaled formaldehyde in the rat.* Bio-Research Laboratories Ltd., project no. 81581. Sponsored by the Formaldehyde Council of Canada, 1985.
58. Della Porta G, Colnaghi MI, Parmiani G. Non-carcinogenicity of hexamethylenetetramine in mice and rats. *Food Cosmet Toxicol* 1968;6:707.
59. Hurni H, Ohder H. Reproduction studies with formaldehyde and hexamethylenetetramine in beagle dogs. *Food Cosmet Toxicol* 1977;11:459.
60. Takahashi M, Hasegawa R, Furukawa F, Toyoda K, Sato H, Hayashi Y. Effects of ethanol, potassium metabisulfite, formaldehyde and hydrogen peroxide on gastric carcinogenesis in rats after initiation with *n*-methyl-*n*'-nitro-*n*-nitroguanidine. *Jpn J Cancer Res (Gann)* 1986;77:118.
61. Tobe T, Naito K, Kurokawa Y. Chronic toxicity study on formaldehyde administered orally to rats. *Toxicology* 1989;56:79.
62. Til HP, Woutersen RA, Feron VJ, Hollanders VHM, Falke HE. Two-year drinking water study of formaldehyde in rats. *Food Chem Toxicol* 1989;27:77–87.
63. Soffritti M, Maltoni C, Maffei F, Biagi R. Formaldehyde: an experimental multipotential carcinogen. *Toxicol Ind Health* 1989;5:699.
64. Faichney GJ, Davies HL. The effect of formaldehyde treatment of peanut meal in concentrate diets on the performance of calves. *Aust J Agric Res* 1972;23:167.
65. Faichney GJ, Davies HL. The performance of calves given concentrate diets treated with formaldehyde. *Aust J Agric Res* 1973;24:613.
66. Gupta NK, Gupta BN. Effect of feeding formaldehyde-treated groundnut-cake on the growth and nutrient utilization in karan Swiss calves. *Indian J Anim Sci* 1984;54:1065.
67. Sharma HR, Ingalls JR. Comparative value of soybean, rapeseed and formaldehyde-treated rapeseed meals in urea-containing calf rations. *Can J Anim Sci* 1973;53:273.
68. Lindsay JA. The digestion of barley-based diets by cattle: the effect of level of feeding of three diets containing different amounts of formaldehyde-treated soybean meal. *Aust J Agric Res* 1983;34:809.
69. Reis PJ, Tunks DA. Evaluation of formaldehyde-treated casein for wool growth and nitrogen retention. *Aust J Agric Res* 1969;20:775.
70. Langlands JP. Wheat as a survival ration for sheep: I. The digestion of wheat and formaldehyde treated wheat. *Aust J Exp Agric Anim Husbandry* 1973; 13:341.
71. Barry TN. The effect of feeding formaldehyde treated casein to sheep on nitrogen retention and wool growth. *N Z J Agric Res* 1972;15:107.
72. Faichney GJ. The effect of formaldehyde treatment of a casein on the growth of ruminant lambs. *Aust J Agric Res* 1971;22:453.
73. Faichney GJ. Digestion by sheep of concentrated diets containing formaldehyde-treated peanut meal. *Aust J Agric Res* 1972;23:859.
74. Faichney GJ. The effect of formaldehyde treatment of a casein supplement on urea excretion and on digesta composition in sheep. *Aust J Agric Res* 1974;25:599.
75. Faichney GJ, Weston RH. Digestion by ruminant lambs of a diet containing formaldehyde-treated casein. *Aust J Agric Res* 1971;22:461.
76. Florence E, Milner DF. Determination of free and loosely protein-bound formaldehyde in the tissues of pigs fed formalin-treated skim milk as a protein supplement. *J Sci Food Agric* 1981;32:288.
77. Kowalezyk J, Otwinowska A. A note on the digestibility of rations containing formaldehyde treated rapeseed oilmeal in pigs. *Roczniki Nauck Rolniczych* 1976;97:93.
78. Nitsan Z, Bruckental I. Effect of treating soybean meal with formaldehyde on the activity of enzymatic inhibitors and on protein utilization in the chick. *J Anim Sci* 1975;44:998.
79. Universities Associated for Research and Education in Pathology. Epidemiology of chronic occupational exposure to formaldehyde: report of the ad hoc panel on health aspects of formaldehyde. *Toxicol Ind Health* 1988;4:77–90.
80. Blair A, Stewart P, O'Berg M, et al. Mortality among industrial workers exposed to formaldehyde. *J Natl Cancer Inst* 1986;76:1071–1084.
81. Blair A, Stewart P, Hoover RN. Mortality from lung cancer among workers employed in formaldehyde industries. *Am J Ind Med* 1990;17:683.
82. Marsh GM, Stone RA, Henderson VL. Lung cancer mortality among industrial workers exposed to formaldehyde: a poison regression analysis of the National Cancer Institute study. *Am Ind Hyg Assoc J* 1992;53:681–691.
83. Blair A, Stewart PA. Comments on the Sterling and Weinkam analysis of data from the National Cancer Institute formaldehyde study. *Am J Ind Med* 1994;25:603–606.
84. Acheson ED, Gardner MJ, Pannett B, et al. Formaldehyde in the British chemical industry—an occupational cohort study. *Lancet* 1984;1:611–616.
85. Gardner MJ, Pannett B, Winter PD, Cruddas AM. A cohort study of workers exposed to formaldehyde in the British chemical industry: an update. *Br J Ind Med* 1993;50:827–834.
86. Andjelkovich DA, Jansen DB, Brown MH, Richardson RB, Miller FJ. Mortality of iron foundry workers: IV. Analysis of a subcohort exposed to formaldehyde. *J Occup Med* 1995;37:826–837.

CHAPTER 96
Aldehydes

Donna L. Dehn and John B. Sullivan, Jr.

Aldehydes are highly reactive chemical compounds not only synthesized for industrial use but occurring naturally within mammals and the environment (1,2). Aldehydes are irritants, particularly the low-molecular-weight and halogen-substituted aldehydes. Inhalation of aldehyde vapors can cause chemical bronchitis, pneumonitis, and pulmonary edema. In general, the toxicity of aldehydes decreases with increasing molecular weight, whereas the presence of a double bond in aliphatic aldehydes considerably enhances their toxicity. Higher-molecular-weight, complex aldehydes are used in fragrances and occasionally may sensitize. Dialdehydes are uncommon in industry, but they might be expected to be more reactive on the basis of their chemistry. Aromatic or substituted aromatic groups that replace hydrogen on the aliphatic chain of aldehydes usually do not add to the toxicity of aldehydes (3,4).

Aldehydes are characterized by the presence of the formyl (CHO) functional group. Although the construction industry is their principal consumer, aldehydes are also important to agriculture and to the garment, pharmaceutical, and rubber industries. Higher-molecular-weight aldehydes are used as flavors and fragrances in essential oils and perfumes (3).

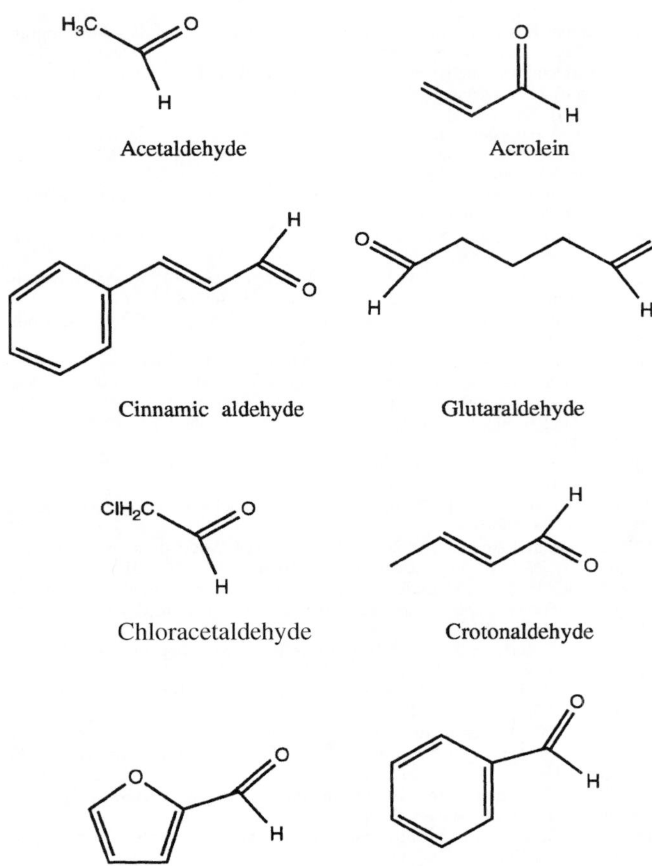

Figure 96-1. Chemical structure of various aldehydes.

Aldehydes that cause health problems because of their irritating, toxic, or immunologic effects include acetaldehyde, acrolein, cinnamaldehyde, formaldehyde, and glutaraldehyde. Other aldehydes that may pose some minor problems include butyraldehyde, chloroacetaldehyde, crotonaldehyde, and furfural. Acrolein, crotonaldehyde, and formaldehyde appear to be more toxic than is acetaldehyde (3–5).

ACETALDEHYDE

Acetaldehyde (acetic aldehyde, ethanol, ethyl aldehyde, CH_3CHO), a volatile, colorless, flammable liquid (Fig. 96-1), is a highly reactive compound that undergoes condensation, addition, and polymerization reactions. It may polymerize in air, under high temperatures, or with acids, bases, or metals. When mixed with air, it reacts to form corrosive acetic acid and highly unstable, explosive peroxides (6). Its physical and chemical properties are listed in Table 96-1. It is produced commercially for use as a chemical intermediate to manufacture acetic acid and many other chemicals (7). It is used also in the manufacture of such products as plastics, synthetic phenolic and urea resins, disinfectants, drugs, dyes, and explosives. In flavorings, it imparts orange, apple, and butter flavors and is added to milk products, fruit juices, candy, and soft drinks at up to 0.047%. It is found also in perfumes, photographic chemicals, rubber accelerators, antioxidants, varnishes, vinegar, and yeast (8,9).

Acetaldehyde is a naturally occurring compound. It is a product of most hydrocarbon oxidations, is a normal intermediate product in the respiration of higher plants, and occurs in traces in all ripe fruits and may form in wine and other alcoholic beverages after exposure to air (1). It is formed also in the body during normal metabolism and, to a large extent, as an oxidative metabolite of ethanol by the enzyme alcohol dehydrogenase (10). It is a highly reactive, freely diffusible molecule that can be found in the peripheral blood of patients abusing alcohol (11,12) in concentrations much higher than those in control populations.

The National Institute of Occupational Safety and Health (NIOSH) estimated that 14,000 workers could be exposed to acetaldehyde in a manufacturing or industrial setting (or both) (13). Environmental exposure occurs through ingestion of food containing acetaldehyde, consumption of coffee, or smoking of cigarettes. It is a major component in the gas phase of tobacco smoke; the acetaldehyde content of cigarette smoke from a single cigarette is up to 1 mg, of which 20 μg per minute has been estimated to reach the blood circulation within the lung (6). It occurs in the atmosphere partly as a consequence of wood combustion (forest fires, residential wood burning) and incomplete combustion of fuels (14–17). Residential burning of wood in the United States accounts for approximately 99 million pounds of acetaldehyde emissions annually. Fireplace emissions range from 0.083 to 0.2 g per kg of wood burned (6). Contributions to daily acetaldehyde production and release into the environment occur from automobile emissions, which can exceed 100 mg of acetaldehyde per mile (18).

Acetaldehyde is classified as a mild eye and mucous membrane irritant and, at high concentrations, causes narcosis in animals (3,4,19). Low to moderate air concentrations of acetaldehyde [50 to 200 parts per million (ppm)] cause eye irritation and upper respiratory discomfort. High blood concentrations can cause dyspnea and central nervous system depression. Acetaldehyde is toxic to the cilia of the respiratory epithelium and may represent a major cause of damage by cigarette smoke. Its irritant potential in the workplace usually is not a great problem, because it is perhaps only one-tenth as strong an irritant as is formaldehyde (3,4,9,20,21). If liquid acetaldehyde contacts skin for a prolonged period, it may cause erythema and burns. Repeated contact may result in dermatitis due to either primary irritation or sensitization.

In vitro cellular studies demonstrated that acetaldehyde produces cross-linking of DNA and induction of sister chromatid

TABLE 96-1. Chemical and physical parameters of various aldehydes

Parameter	Acetaldehyde	Acrolein	Cinnamic aldehyde	Glutaraldehyde	Chloroacetaldehyde	Crotonaldehyde	Furfural	Benzaldehyde
CAS no.	75-07-0	107-02-8	104-55-2	111-30-8	107-20-2	4170-30-3	98-01-1	100-52-7
Molecular weight	44.1	56.1	132.15	100.1	78.5	70.1	96.1	106.03
BP (°C @ 760 mm Hg)	21	53	246	187–189	85	104	161.8	179
MP (°C)	–123.5	–87	–7.5	100	43–50	–76.5	–36.5	–26
Density (g/mL)	0.788 @ 16°C	0.8621 @ 0°C	1.048 @ 25°C	—	—	—	1.1563 @ 25°C	1.043 @ 25°C
Solubility (mg/L)	1,000	208,000	—	—	—	150,000 @ 20°C	86.000 @ 25°C	6.950 @ 25°C
VD	1.5	1.94	4.6	3.4	—	2.41	—	3.6
VP (mm Hg)	740 @ 20°C	210 @ 20°C	1 @ 76.1°C	17 @ 20°C	100 @ 20°C	19 @ 20°C	2 @ 20°C	1 @ 26°C
IP (eV)	10.22	10.13	—	—	10.61	9.73	9.21	—
UEL (%)	60.0	31	—	—	—	15.5	19.3	13.5
LEL (%)	4	2.8	—	—	—	2.1	2.1	2.15
FP (°C)	–36	–26	71	Nonflammable	87.7		60	62
Henry's law constant (atm-m³/mol)	—	4.40E-06	—	—	2.00E-05	1.94E-05	3.70E-06	2.67E-05
K_{oc}		24	—	—	39	6.2	—	34–150
Bioconcentration factor		0.6–344	—	—	1	0.74	—	4.2–7.8

BP, boiling point; CAS, Chemical Abstracts Service; FP, flash point; IP, ionization potential; K_{oc}, partition coefficient; LEL, lower explosive limit; MP, melting point; VD, vapor density; VP, vapor pressure; UEL, upper explosive limit.

TABLE 96-2. Exposure guidelines, criteria, and standards for various aldehydes

Parameter	Acetaldehyde	Acrolein	Cinnamic aldehyde	Glutaraldehyde	Chloroacetaldehyde	Crotonaldehyde	Furfural	Benzaldehyde
Air								
OSHA PEL (ppm)	200	0.1		None	C 1	2	5 (skin)	
(mg/m^3)	360	0.25		None	C 3	6	20	
NIOSH STEL								
ACGIH TLV (ppm)	100	0.1		C 0.2	C 1	2	2 (skin)	
(mg/m^3)	180	0.23			C 3.2	5.7	7.9	
IDLH (ppm)	2,000	0		C 0.82	45	50	100	
Drinking water								
MCL (µg/L)								
Secondary MCL (mg/L)								
Health advisory (mg/L)								
Ambient water quality criteria								
HH/F&W (µg/L)		3.2E+02						
AF chronic, 4-d avg. (µg/L)		2.1E-01						
AF acute, 1-h avg. (µg/L)		6.8E + 1						
Other								
Oral RfD (mg/kg/day)		2.0E-02			Data inadequate	Under review	3.0E-03	1.0E-01
Inhalational RfC (mg/m^3)		2.0E-05					5.0E-02	
Carcinogen classification								
EPA weight of evidence		C				C		
IARC	2B	3				3	3	

ACGIH, American Conference of Governmental Industrial Hygienists; AF, criteria for the protection of aquatic life in freshwater resources; C, ceiling value that is not to be exceeded at any time; EPA, U.S. Environmental Protection Agency; HH/F&W, criteria for the protection of human health based on ingestion of 2 L of water and 0.65 g of fish per day from a surface water source; IARC, International Agency for Research on Cancer; IDLH, immediately dangerous to life and health; MCL, federally enforceable maximum contaminant limit for drinking water; NIOSH, National Institute of Occupational Safety and Health; RfC, reference concentration; RfD, reference dose, a provisional estimate of the daily exposure likely to be without appreciable risk of deleterious effects during a lifetime; OSHA, U.S. Occupational Safety and Health Administration; PEL, permissible exposure limit as a time-weighted average over an 8-hour workday in a 40-hour work week; REL, recommended exposure limit (time-weighted average concentration for up to a 10-hour workday in a 40-hour work week); secondary MCL, advisory level based on aesthetic concerns (taste, odor, staining); Skin, potential for dermal absorption, prevent skin exposure; STEL, short-term exposure limit (a 15-minute time-weighted average exposure that should not be exceeded at any time during a workday); TLV, threshold limit value as a time-weighted average for an 8-hour workday in a 40-hour work week.

exchanges, especially late in the G_1 phase of the cell cycle, after repeated or continuous exposure (22–27). Acetaldehyde has been shown to be toxic to cilia and chromosomes in plant and lower animal systems. The International Agency for Research on Cancer (IARC) has found sufficient evidence for carcinogenicity in animals. Acetaldehyde increased the incidence of squamous cell carcinomas and adenocarcinomas in the nasal mucosa in rats of both genders and laryngeal carcinomas in hamsters of both genders through inhalation. It was found also to enhance the incidence of respiratory tract tumors induced by benzo(a)pyrene in hamsters of both genders. Adequate data are not available to evaluate the carcinogenicity of acetaldehyde in humans, although anecdotal data for workers in an aldehyde plant showed an increased cancer incidence. The IARC has classified acetaldehyde as a 2B carcinogen, indicating that it is possibly carcinogenic to humans (28).

In addition to acetaldehyde's capacity to cross-link DNA by chemically reacting with nucleic acid bases, it may cross-link proteins by reacting primarily with lysine groups to form Schiff bases. Recent evidence suggests that the combination of acetaldehyde with albumin is an example of a hapten-carrier complex that can serve as an antigen, inducing antibodies to the hapten even when a nonimmunogenic self-protein such as rabbit serum albumin is used in immunizing rabbits (29). The titer and incidence of these antibodies appear to be increased in chronic alcoholics (30–32). Whether environmental or industrial exposure to acetaldehyde can similarly induce antibodies against acetaldehyde has not yet been studied.

New employees who may be exposed to acetaldehyde should be examined prior to and periodically after beginning work, with careful attention given to the eyes, skin, and respiratory system. Protective garments should be worn by workers to prevent skin and eye contact. Natural rubber products should be avoided for personal protection, as acetaldehyde causes decomposition of rubber (13). For accidental exposures, eye wash and shower equipment should be provided in work areas.

The occupational exposure limits for acetaldehyde in different countries vary between 25 and 200 ppm, which is roughly equivalent to concentrations of 46 to 360 mg per cubic meter of air. Table 96-2 presents exposure guidelines, criteria, and standards for acetaldehyde. Acetaldehyde has a reportable quantity of 1,000 pounds under the Comprehensive Environmental Response, Compensation, and Liability Act on the basis of aquatic toxicity as assigned by section 311(b)(4) of the Clean Water Act (33). It is a listed waste under the Resource Conservation and Recovery Act (RCRA) and therefore must be managed according to federal or state hazardous-waste regulations (34). Acetaldehyde is exempted under the federal Food, Drug, and Cosmetic Act from tolerances for pesticide chemicals. The U.S. Food and Drug Administration (FDA) regulates acetaldehyde as a direct food additive in the form of a synthetic flavoring substance and generally recognizes this chemical as safe (35).

The primary fate of acetaldehyde released to the environment is volatilization to the atmosphere, with subsequent degradation through photolysis and reaction with hydroxyl radicals. Its atmospheric half-life is 1 to 2 hours. Acetaldehyde is degraded by aerobic and anaerobic microorganisms and degrades readily in soil and water. It does not sorb to soil and readily leaches to groundwater. Its half-life in water is between 2 and 20 days. It is not expected to bioaccumulate because it is biodegraded easily.

ACROLEIN

Acrolein (acrylaldehyde, propenal, allyl aldehyde, ethylene aldehyde, aqualin, CH_2=CHCHO) is a three-carbon, unsaturated, highly reactive, highly volatile aldehyde at room temperature (see Fig. 96-1). Acrolein's extreme reactivity is attributed to the conjugation of a carbonyl group with a vinyl group within its structure. It has a piercing, disagreeable, acrid odor and is very water-soluble (36).

The bulk of acrolein is produced as an intermediate in the synthesis of acrylic acid and its esters. It is used in the manufacture of pharmaceuticals, perfumes, food supplements, and resins. It is used also as a biocide, a fungicide, an algaecide for water treatment, and an herbicide. It was used as a component of military poison gases during World War I. It occurs as a metabolite of glycerol, alkyl formate, and alkyl alcohol (37).

Emissions of acrolein occur at industrial facilities that produce or use it. Environmental exposure occurs primarily through inhalation of acrolein released to the air. It is a major component of wood, cotton, polyethylene, and cigarette smoke (38–42) and of diesel fuel exhausts and photochemical smog (43–45). High air concentrations are combustible (14).

Acrolein is a severe pulmonary irritant and lacrimating agent. It is ciliastatic and capable of causing direct tissue damage similar to that reported for formaldehyde (46–48). Owing to its high aqueous solubility and high chemical bioreactivity, acrolein has a relatively short half-life and exerts its greatest effects on the upper and lower respiratory tract (49,50). It is thought to be a significant contributor to smoke-induced inhalation, injury, and death.

The toxic effects of acrolein exposure include sensory irritation, enzymatic inhibition, elevated liver alkaline phosphatase levels, protein synthesis inhibition, weight loss, and death (51). Acrolein is a suspected carcinogen because of its 2,3-epoxy metabolite and its weak mutagenic activity in the *Salmonella* screen (46,52). On the basis of the overall evidence, the U.S. Environmental Protection Agency (EPA) classified acrolein as a group C carcinogen, as limited animal evidence of carcinogenicity exists (53). The IARC classified it as a group 3 agent, unclassifiable as to carcinogenicity in humans (54). Acrolein is also a weak sensitizer and may elicit asthma-type reactions. Some indications suggest that acrolein may possess immunotoxic potential. At air concentrations of 20 ppm, acrolein can induce pulmonary edema rapidly. In other organ systems, acrolein is believed to cause tissue damage by the mechanism of release of toxic oxygen radicals via activation of the arachidonic acid cascade, by binding to sulfhydryl groups, and by protein damage (55–57). Acrolein induces lacrimation. Lacrimation-inducing agents in general are known to be powerful skin irritants, and acrolein exposure causes painful dermatitis and chemical burn injury on longer exposure (58).

The NIOSH lists an acrolein concentration of 2 ppm as immediately dangerous to life and health (IDLH) (59). The U.S. Occupational Safety and Health Administration (OSHA) permissible exposure limit (PEL) for acrolein is 0.1 ppm, owing to its irritating effects. The EPA has derived a provisional oral reference dose (RfD) for acrolein based on a 90-day rat study, without listing a target organ for toxicity (60). An inhalational reference concentration (RfC of 0.00002 mg per cubic meter) is provided in the EPA's Integrated Risk Information System. This system is an online database updated by the EPA whenever new information becomes available (61). An RfC is a concentration of a contaminant in air (milligrams of acrolein per cubic meter of air) that is likely to be without appreciable risk of deleterious effects. The RfC is based on a subchronic rat inhalational study in which squamous metaplasia and neutrophilic infiltration of nasal epithelium were noted (61). Table 96-2 presents other exposure guidelines, criteria, and standards for acrolein.

Acrolein is a hazardous waste under the RCRA and must be managed according to federal or state hazardous-waste regulations (34). The National Response Center must be notified if a release of its reportable quantity of 1 pound occurs (62). Acrolein is classified as a list B pesticide and is a restricted-use ingredient for pesticides under the Federal Insecticide, Fungicide and Rodenticide Act Registration Standard (63). The FDA has set a 0.6% limitation for its use in food starch (5).

Owing to acrolein's high reactivity, transfer between environmental media is limited. Acrolein is sorbed weakly by soil, as indicated by an experimentally determined partition coefficient (K_{oc}) value (a measure of soil sorption) of 24 (64). Biodegradation may occur, but the compound is toxic to microorganisms, which limits its effectiveness. Acrolein reacts with surface water in a reversible hydration reaction. Its half-life in water ranges between several hours to several days (65). It also will volatilize from surface water, and its high vapor pressure indicates that volatilization is its primary fate when released to the environment. Once in the atmosphere, it may photodissociate or react with hydroxyl radicals and ozone. Atmospheric residence time is less than 1 day (66). Bioconcentration is not anticipated because of its high water solubility and extreme reactivity.

CINNAMIC ALDEHYDE

Cinnamic aldehyde (cinnamaldehyde, cinnamal, β-phenylacrolein, and 3-phenylpropenal, $C_6H_5CH{=}CHCHO$) is an aromatic aldehyde (see Fig. 96-1) and a yellow, oily combustible liquid. It is a constituent of cinnamon, with a burning taste responsible for the typical odor and flavor of the spice.

Cinnamic aldehyde is a common ingredient in household products, such as deodorizers, detergents, soaps, and cosmetics. It is used frequently as a flavoring agent in mouthwashes, dentifrices, cough mixtures, throat lozenges, candy, soft drinks, chewing gum, ice cream, baked goods, condiments, and meats. Cinnamic aldehyde and related chemicals present in cinnamon are used extensively in perfumes, hair tonics, and lotions (67).

It is a strong skin irritant and has been reported to be a sensitizer and an urticariogenic agent in most atopic and nonatopic individuals. Delayed contact dermatitis caused by this substance has been described by many investigators (67–72). As a perfume ingredient, cinnamaldehyde is considered an allergen (68,73–77). This aromatic aldehyde has been implicated in occupational dermatitis in bakers, confectioners, and chemists (78). Cinnamic aldehyde in dentifrices may produce irritating, stinging sensations and allergic cheilitis and stomatitis (79–84). Cinnamic alcohol and aldehyde in perfume, facial tissue, and sanitary napkins can produce allergic dermatitis. Because of its presence in such an extensive number of products, cinnamic aldehyde is one of the more common causes of contact urticaria (both nonimmunologic and immunologic) and may even produce a delayed systemic, eczematous contact dermatitis (85–87). Once sensitization to cinnamon occurs, cross-reactions may occur with balsam of Peru, balsam of Tolu, cassia oil, patchouli oil, and benzoin (88,89). Usually, the cinnamon oil used commercially is obtained from *Cinnamonum cassia*. As much as 68% of the oil consists of cinnamic aldehyde. Powdered cinnamon contains only approximately 1% of the aldehyde and is not an irritant under ordinary circumstances.

Cinnamic aldehyde has been shown to possess antifungal activity (90–92). Cinnamic aldehyde, benzaldehyde, and various aliphatic aldehydes all inhibit protein synthesis in a variety of *in vitro* systems (93–99).

Cinnamic aldehyde was classified as a list C pesticide, but it no longer is an active ingredient of any registered pesticide product. Therefore, the EPA characterized it as canceled. The FDA generally considers cinnamic aldehyde to be safe (35).

GLUTARALDEHYDE

Glutaraldehyde [glutaric dialdehyde, 1,5-pentanedial, $HCO(CH2)_3CHO$] is an aliphatic dialdehyde with a molecular weight three times that of formaldehyde (see Fig. 96-1). It is a clear, colorless, oily liquid that is nonflammable (36). It polymerizes readily and is available most frequently as a 50% aqueous solution.

In a buffered alkaline solution (pH, 7.5 to 8.5), it is a highly effective microbicidal agent (sporicidal, bactericidal, viricidal, fungicidal) (99–107). Alkaline glutaraldehyde is used widely in cold sterilization of medical, surgical, and dental equipment and instruments and for home sterilization of artificial kidney machines (105,106,108). Alkaline glutaraldehyde is used also as a biocide in contaminated water, cooling towers, and air conditioners. In the United States, glutaraldehyde is the second most commonly used aldehyde after formaldehyde (109).

Glutaraldehyde vapors are an irritant to bronchial and laryngeal mucous membranes, and prolonged exposure could produce localized edema and other symptoms suggestive of an allergic response. Occupational exposure to health care workers is common. Recent reports have implicated glutaraldehyde exposure as a cause of occupational asthma (109–112). It has been reported to cause asthma in endoscopy personnel exposed to glutaraldehyde cleaning solutions (108–116).

Glutaraldehyde is a known sensitizer, and case reports of occupational contact dermatitis from glutaraldehyde have been described (108–116). Sensitization has occurred mainly through its use as a cold sterilizing solution in hospitals and dental and medical clinics, where personnel may be exposed to activated glutaraldehyde in concentrations of 0.13% to 2%. Activated glutaraldehyde buffered to a pH of 7.5 to 8.5 is reported to be an irritant stronger than inactivated glutaraldehyde solutions, which have weak acidity.

The NIOSH recommended a ceiling limit for glutaraldehyde of 0.2 ppm (59). Other occupational exposure guidelines are listed in Table 96-2. NIOSH studies in hospital environments with cold sterilization using glutaraldehyde solutions demonstrated airborne glutaraldehyde concentrations of 0.4 ppm. A 2% glutaraldehyde sterilizing solution can produce airborne concentrations that exceed 0.2 ppm if proper hood ventilation is not provided when the solution is left uncovered. Containment of vapors and prevention of skin contact are important industrial hygiene principles to help to avoid sensitization of the skin and respiratory irritation or asthma. Proper skin protection and ventilation controls must be provided. Neoprene or butyl rubber gloves are protective, but latex rubber gloves are less so. Concomitant sensitization to rubber components and formaldehyde, appears to be common, and a tendency for hand eczema associated with glutaraldehyde appears to persist even when known sources of exposure to glutaraldehyde are avoided.

Glutaraldehyde was classified as a list B pesticide, and manufacturers are performing studies for registration (13). The FDA has approved glutaraldehyde as an indirect food additive and it is used as a component of adhesives (117).

CHLOROACETALDEHYDE

Chloroacetaldehyde (C_2H_3ClO), a liquid with an irritating odor, is used as a fungicide and a tree bark remover (see Fig. 96-1). It can be released to the environment during its use or in emissions from facilities that manufacture it. Owing to its strong irritant properties, the liquid can cause eye and skin burns after splash exposure. Exposure to the vapors can produce irritation of eyes, skin, and airway. High concentrations of the vapor can cause pulmonary edema. Chloroacetaldehyde has an IDLH level of 45 ppm (59). It has a ceiling threshold limit value of 1 ppm (3 mg per cubic meter). Other exposure guidelines are listed in Table 96-2.

Chloroacetaldehyde is a hazardous waste under the RCRA and must be managed according to federal or state hazardous-waste regulations (34). The National Response Center must be notified in the event of a release of its reportable quantity of 1,000 pounds (62).

Based on its vapor pressure, chloroacetaldehyde is expected to be in the vapor phase in the atmosphere. Reaction with hydroxyl radicals is expected to be its primary fate, and an atmospheric half-life of 2 days or less has been estimated. If it is released to water, volatilization should be its primary fate, as it does not bioaccumulate (on the basis of its estimated bioconcentration factor) and it does not undergo chemical oxidation in water (13). Its fate in soil depends on environmental conditions; in moist soil, it should be fairly mobile (as indicated by its K_{oc} and Henry's law constant); in dry soil, it would volatilize readily. Other physical and chemical properties are listed in Table 96-1.

CROTONALDEHYDE

Crotonaldehyde ($CH_3CH{=}CHCHO$; see Fig. 96-1) is a liquid that has a strong, irritating odor and is very flammable (8). Commercial use favors the *trans*-isomer, and its largest single use is in the manufacture of *n*-butanol (118). Similar to other halogenated aldehydes, it is emitted to the atmosphere during its production and use; from the combustion of wood; from gas and diesel engine exhaust; from turbine exhaust; from tobacco smoke; and from polymer combustion (17).

Owing to the potent irritant properties of crotonaldehyde, eye and skin contact with the liquid can result in severe burns. Its vapors are highly irritating to the eyes, mucous membranes, and respiratory system. Clinical cases of sensitization have occurred. Crotonaldehyde vapors may produce pulmonary edema at high concentrations.

The chemical has an OSHA PEL of 2 ppm (6 mg per cubic meter). Other occupational exposure guidelines are listed in Table 96-2. Health effects data for crotonaldehyde are under EPA review for developing an oral RfD (61). Crotonaldehyde has been found to be mutagenic in one or more strains of *Salmonella typhimurium* (119). The EPA has classified crotonaldehyde as a group C carcinogen, indicating that it is a possible human carcinogen; however, evidence in animals is limited, and human data are either inadequate or lacking (61). The IARC has classified it as a group 3 agent, indicating that it is unclassifiable as to its carcinogenicity in humans (54).

Crotonaldehyde has been designated as a hazardous substance under section 311(b)(2)(A) of the Federal Water Pollution Control Act (120) and as a toxic pollutant pursuant to section 307(a)(1) of the Clean Water Act; as such, it is subject to effluent limitations (121). The National Response Center must be notified on release of a reportable quantity of 100 pounds. It is classified as a hazardous waste under the RCRA and must be managed according to federal or state hazardous-waste regulations. Crotonaldehyde is regulated under section 8(d) of the Toxic Substances Control Act (TSCA), which requires submission of unpublished health and safety studies to the EPA (122), and under section 4 of the TSCA, which has testing consent orders and export notification requirements (123).

As with other aldehydes, crotonaldehyde degrades rapidly in the atmosphere through reaction with hydroxyl radicals. It has a typical half-life of 10 to 12 hours. In water, crotonaldehyde can degrade by reaction with oxidants and can volatilize to the atmosphere. It will react in soils in a manner similar to that of chloroacetaldehyde. Initial studies indicate that crotonaldehyde may biodegrade under both aerobic and anaerobic conditions, but insufficient data exist to determine reliably the importance of this mechanism. The estimated bioconcentration factor (see Table 96-1) indicates that bioaccumulation is not of concern (13).

FURFURAL

Furfural ($C_5H_4O_2$; see Fig. 96-1) is a colorless, oily liquid used in refining of lubricating oils, gas oils, diesel fuels, vegetable oils, resins, and other organic materials (118). It is an aromatic, heterocyclic aldehyde used in the production of insecticides, fungicides, and germicides (118) and as a reagent in analytic chemistry. It is produced from a variety of agricultural by-products, including corncobs; oat, rice, and cottonseed hulls; bagasse; and paper mill waste.

Furfural is a skin, eye, and mucous membrane irritant. Although the vapor is a potent irritant, the liquid has a relatively low volatility so that inhalation of significant quantities by workers is unlikely. Exposure of workers to air concentrations of from 2 to 14 ppm caused complaints of eye and throat irritation and headache (118). The liquid is irritating to the skin, and contact can cause dermatitis.

Its OSHA PEL is 5 ppm (20 mg per cubic meter), with a "skin" notation, which indicates its irritating properties. Its IDLH level is 100 ppm (NIOSH). The EPA has established a chronic oral RfD of 0.003 mg of furfural per kg body weight per day. This RfD is based on a level of lowest observed adverse effect of 11 mg per kg body weight per day derived from a subchronic oral study of rats in which mild hepatocellular vacuolization was observed (61). A provisional inhalational RfC of 0.05 mg per cubic meter is based on a study in which nasal cavity degeneration of hamsters was found with intermittent inhalational exposure (60). The IARC has classified furfural as a group 3 agent, indicating that it is unclassifiable as to its carcinogenicity in humans (54). Table 96-2 lists occupational and environmental exposure guidelines.

Furfural is a hazardous waste under the RCRA and must be managed according to federal or state hazardous-waste regulations (34). The National Response Center must be notified in the event of release of its reportable quantity of 5,000 pounds (62). It is regulated under section 8(d) of the TSCA, which requires submission of unpublished health and safety studies to the EPA (122). The FDA has approved furfural as an indirect food additive (117). It is exempted under the Federal Insecticide, Fungicide and Rodenticide Act from requirement of a tolerance when used as an inert ingredient in pesticide formulations (124).

As with other aldehydes, furfural is expected to be predominantly in the vapor phase in the atmosphere, where it degrades through reaction with hydroxyl radicals, with a typical half-life of one-half day. Reaction with nitrate radicals during the night also may be an important degradation process. Photochemical degradation in the atmosphere may occur. In water, furfural will undergo microbial degradation, with acclimation increasing the rate of removal and increased concentrations decreasing the rate of removal. Bioconcentration is not anticipated. The chemical does not sorb to soil, should leach readily, and should volatilize slowly, as indicated from its Henry's law constant (see Table 96-1) (13).

BENZALDEHYDE

Benzaldehyde ($C6H_5CHO$; see Fig. 96-1) is the simplest aromatic aldehyde. It is a colorless or yellowish liquid found in oil of bitter almond, preservatives, and biologicals and has been reported to cause contact urticaria. Benzaldehyde is found in dyes, pharmaceuticals, perfumes, and flavoring agents.

Among the higher aliphatic aldehydes, propionaldehyde is used primarily as a chemical intermediate in the production of 1-propanol, propionic acid, and trimethylolethane. Butyraldehydes are used as chemical intermediates in the production of 1-butanol, 2-butanol, 2-ethyl-1-hexanol, and a wide variety of specialty chemicals.

From a rat subchronic study in which forestomach lesions and kidney toxicity were observed (61), the EPA established a chronic oral RfD of 0.1 mg of benzaldehyde per kg body weight per day based on a no-observed-effect level of 200 mg per kg body weight per day. Benzaldehyde was classified as a list C pesticide, but it no longer is an active ingredient of any registered pesticide product; hence, the EPA has characterized it as canceled (13).

As with other aldehydes, benzaldehyde is expected to be predominantly in the vapor phase in the atmosphere, where it degrades through reaction with hydroxyl radicals and has a typical half-life of slightly longer than 1 day. It exists also as aerosol particulates that can be transferred to soil or water through wet deposition. In both water and soil, the primary removal process is biodegradation. Volatilization from soil and water may occur, and leaching is anticipated from soil to groundwater (as indicated by its K_{oc} in Table 96-1). Bioconcentration is not anticipated (13).

REFERENCES

1. Schauenstein E, Esterbauer E, Zollner H. *Aldehydes in biological systems. Their natural occurrence and biological activities.* London: Pion Ltd, 1977:205.
2. SRI International. *Class study report. Aldehydes.* Menlo Park, CA: SRI International, 1978.
3. Steinhagen WH, Barrow CS. Sensory-irritation structure—activity study of inhaled aldehydes in B6C3F1 and Swiss-Webster mice. *Toxicol Appl Pharmacol* 1984;72:495–503.
4. Raffle PAB, Lee WR, McCallum RJ, Murray R. *Hunter's diseases of occupations. Aromatic and aliphatic compounds: aldehydes, ketones, ethers, acetals.* Boston: Little, Brown and Company, 1987:321–326.
5. Brabec MJ. Aldehydes and acetals. In: Clayton GD, Clayton FE, eds. *Patty's industrial hygiene and toxicology: Vol 2A, Toxicology.* New York: Wiley, 1981:2621–2669.
6. Guerin MR. Chemical composition of cigarette smoke. In: Gori GB, Bock FG, eds. *A safe cigarette?* Banbury Reports vol 3. Cold Spring Harbor, NY: Cold Spring Harbor Laboratory, 1980.
7. Hester AS, Hemmler K. Chemicals from acetaldehyde. *Ind Engl Chem* 1959;51:1424–1430.
8. Sitting M. *Handbook of toxic and hazardous chemicals and carcinogens,* 2nd ed. Park Ridge, NJ: Noyes Publications, 1981:21.
9. International Agency for Research on Cancer. Allyl compounds, aldehydes, epoxides and peroxides. *IARC Monogr Eval Carcinog Risks Hum* 1985;36: 101–132.
10. Lindrios KO. Acetaldehyde—its metabolism and role in the actions of alcohol. In: Israel Y, Glaser FB, Kalart H, Popram RE, Schmidt W, Smart RG, eds. *Research advances in alcohol and drug problems.* 1978:1111–1176.
11. Lynch C, Lim CK, Thomas M, Peters TJ. Assay of blood and tissue aldehydes by HPLC analysis of their 2,4-dinitrophenylhydrazine adducts. *Clin Chim Acta* 1983;130:117–122.
12. Kozsten MA, Matsuzaki S, Feinman L, Leiber CS. High blood acetaldehyde levels after ethanol administration. *N Engl J Med* 1975;292:386–389.
13. Hazardous Substance Data Base. On-line, MEDLARS. Bethesda, MD: National Library of Medicine, 1997.
14. Salem H, Cullumbine H. Inhalation toxicities of some aldehydes. *Toxicol Appl Pharmacol* 1960;2:183–187.
15. Harke H-P, Boors A, Frahm B, Peters H, Schultz C. The problem of passive smoking. Concentration of smoke constituents in the air of large and small rooms as a function of number of cigarettes smoked and time. *Int Arch Arbeitsmed* 1972;29:323–339.
16. Jermini C, Weber A, Grandjean E. Quantitative determination of various gas-phase components of the side-stream smoke of cigarettes in the room air as a contribution to the problem of passive smoking. *Int Arch Occup Environ Health* 1976;36:169–181.
17. Graedel TE. *Chemical compounds in the atmosphere.* New York: Academic Press, 1979:440.
18. Lipari F, Swarin SJ. Determination of formaldehyde and other aldehydes in automobile exhaust with an improved 2,4-dinitrophenylhydrazine method. *J Chromatogr* 1982;247:297–306.
19. Proctor NH, Hughes J, Fischman M. *Chemical hazards of the workplace.* Philadelphia: JB Lippincott Co, 1988.
20. Auerback C, Moutschen-Dahmen M, Moutschen J. Genetic and cytogenetical effects of formaldehyde and related compounds. *Mutat Res* 1977;39: 317–362.
21. Fishbein L, Flamm WG, Falk HL. *Chemical mutagens.* New York: Academic Press, 1970:211–212.
22. Lambert B, He SM. DNA and chromosome damage induced by acetaldehyde in human lymphocytes in vitro. Living in a chemical world. *Ann N Y Acad Sci* 1988;534:369–376.
23. He SM, Lambert B. Induction and persistence of SCE-inducing damage in human lymphocytes exposed to vinyl acetate and acetaldehyde in vitro. *Mutat Res* 1985;158:201–208.
24. Hemminki K, Suni R. Sites of reaction of glutaraldehyde and acetaldehyde with nucleosides. *Arch Toxicol* 1984;35:186–190.
25. Norppa H, Tursi F, Pfüffli P, Müki-Paakanen J, Jürventaus H. Chromosome damage induced by vinyl acetate through in vitro formation of acetaldehyde in human lymphocytes and Chinese hamster ovary cells. *Cancer Res* 1985;45:4816–4821.
26. Obe G, Ristow H. Mutagenic cancerogenic and teratogenic effects of alcohol. *Mutat Res* 1979;65:229–259.
27. Obe G, Natarajan AT, Meyers M, Den Hertog A. Induction of chromosomal aberrations in peripheral lymphocytes of human blood in vitro and of SCEs in bone-marrow cells of mice in vitro by ethanol and its metabolite acetaldehyde. *Mutat Res* 1979;68:291–294.
28. International Agency for Research on Cancer. Some fumigants, the herbicides 2,4-d and 2,4,5-t, chlorinated dibenzodioxins and miscellaneous industrial chemicals—overall evaluations of carcinogenicity. *IARC Monogr Eval Carcinog Risks Hum* 1987;15(Suppl 7):1–42.
29. Fleisher JH, Lung CC, Meinke GC, Pinnas JL. Acetaldehyde-albumin adduct formation: possible relevance to an immunologic mechanism in alcoholism. *Alcohol Alcohol* 1988;23:133–141.
30. Lin RC, Lumeng L, Sheshidi S, Kelly T, Proud D. Protein-acetaldehyde adducts in serum of alcoholic patients. *Alcohol Clin Exp Res* 1990;14:438–443.
31. Niemela O, Klajner F, Orrego H, Vidins E, Blendis L, Israel Y. Antibodies against acetaldehyde modified protein epitopes in human alcoholics. *Hepatology* 1987;7:1210–1214.
32. Hoerner M, Behrens UJ, Warner T, Lieber CS. Humoral immune response to acetaldehyde adducts in alcoholic patients. *Res Commun Chem Pathol Pharmacol* 1986;54:3–12.
33. Federal Water Pollution Control Act, 40 *CFR* 117.3. *Determination of reportable quantities for hazardous substances.* 1989.
34. Resource Conservation and Recovery Act, 40 *CFR* 261.33. *Identification and listing of hazardous waste, protection of the environment.* 1994.
35. Food, Drug and Cosmetic Act, 21 *CFR* 182.60. *Substances generally regarded as safe, food and drugs.* 1993.
36. Sax NI, Lewis RJ Sr, eds. *Hawley's condensed chemical dictionary,* 11th ed. New York: Van Nostrand–Reinhold, 1987.
37. Izard C, Liberman C. Acrolein. *Mutat Res* 1978;47:115–138.
38. Hales CA, Barkin PW, Jung W, et al. Synthetic smoke with acrolein but not HCl produces pulmonary edema. *J Appl Physiol* 1988;64:1121–1133.
39. Morikawa T. Acrolein. Formaldehyde and volatile fatty acids from smoldering combustion. *J Combust Toxicol* 1976;3:135–151.
40. US Department of Health, Education, and Welfare. *Smoking and health. Report of the Advisory Committee to the Surgeon General of the Public Health Service* (USPHS publ. no. 1103). Washington: US Department of Health, Education, and Welfare, 1964.
41. Ayer HE, Yeager DW. Irritants in cigarette smoke plumes. *Am J Public Health* 1982;72:1283–1285.
42. Newsome JR, Norman V, Keith CH. Vapor phase analysis of tobacco smoke. *Tobacco Sci* 1965;9:102–110.
43. Pattle RE, Burgess F, Sinclair K, Edington JAG. The toxicity of fumes from a diesel engine under four different running conditions. *Br J Ind Med* 1957;14:47–52.
44. Altshuler AP, McPherson SP. Spectrophotometric analysis of aldehydes in the Los Angeles atmosphere. *J Air Pollut Control Assoc* 1963;13:109–111.
45. Kane LE, Alorie Y. Sensory irritation to formaldehyde and acrolein during single and repeated exposures in mice. *Am Ind Hyg Assoc J* 1977;38:509–522.
46. Denine EP, Robbins SL, Kensler CJ. The effects of acrolein inhalation on the tracheal mucosa of the chicken. *Toxicol Appl Pharmacol* 1971;19:416.
47. Kensler CJ, Battista SP. Components of cigarette smoke with ciliary-depressant activity. Their selective removal by filters containing activated charcoal granules. *N Engl J Med* 1963;269:1161.
48. Beauchamp RO Jr, Morgan KT, Kilgerman AD, Andelkobich DA, Heck HA. A critical review of the literature on acrolein toxicity. *CRC Crit Rev Toxicol* 1985;14:309–380.
49. Egle JL Jr. Retention of inhaled formaldehyde, propionaldehyde and acrolein in the dog. *Arch Environ Health* 1972;25:119–124.
50. Leikauf GD, Leming LM, O'Donnell JR, Doupnik GA. Bronchial responsiveness and inflammation in guinea pigs exposed to acrolein. *J Appl Physiol* 1989;66:171–178.
51. Astray AL, Jakab GL. The effects of acrolein exposure on pulmonary antibacterial defenses. *Toxicol Appl Pharmacol* 1983;67:49–54.

52. National Toxicology Program. *Review of current research related to toxicology,* NTP-82-040. Washington: National Toxicology Program, 1982.
53. Agency for Toxic Substances and Disease Registry. *Toxicological profile for acrolein (draft).* Atlanta: US Department of Health and Human Services, Public Health Service, ATSDR, 1989.
54. International Agency for Research on Cancer. Dry cleaning, some chlorinated solvents and other industrial chemicals. *IARC Monogr Eval Carcinog Risks Hum* 1995;63.
55. Dawson JR, Norbeck K, Anundi I, Maldeus P. The effectiveness of *N*-acetylcysteine in isolated hepatocytes against the toxicity of paracetamol, acrolein and paraquat. *Arch Toxicol* 1984;55:11–15.
56. Grundfest CC, Chang J, Newcombe D. Acrolein: a potent modulator of lung macrophage arachidonic acid metabolism. *Biochim Biophys Acta* 1982;713: 149–159.
57. Zitting A, Heinomen T. Decrease of reduced glutathione in isolated rat hepatocytes caused by acrolein, acrylonitrate and the thermal degradation products of styrene copolymers. *Toxicology* 1980;17:333–341.
58. *Hazardous chemicals data book,* 2nd ed. Park Ridge, NJ: G. Weiss Noyes Data Corporation, 1986:52.
59. National Institute of Occupational Safety and Health. *Pocket guide to chemical hazards.* US Department of Health and Human Services publ. no. 94-116. Washington: Government Printing Office, 1994.
60. US Environmental Protection Agency. *Health effects assessment summary tables FY-1995 annual,* EPA/540/R-95/036. Washington: Office of Solid Waste and Emergency Response, 1995.
61. National Library of Medicine. *Integrated risk information system.* MEDLARS online. Bethesda, MD: National Library of Medicine, 1997.
62. Resource Conservation and Recovery Act Designation, Reportable Quantities and Notification, Protection of the Environment: 40 *CFR* 302.4 (section IV.D.3.b), 1994.
63. Protection of the Environment, Pesticide Registration and Classification Procedures: 40 *CFR* 152.175, 1991.
64. Howard PH. *Handbook of environmental fate and exposure data for organic chemicals,* vol 1. Chelsea, MI: Lewis Publishers, 1989.
65. Bowmer KH, Higgins ML. Some aspects of the persistence and fate of acrolein herbicide in water. *Arch Environ Contam Toxicol* 1976;5:87–96.
66. Atkinson R, Aschmann SM, Pitts JN. Kinetics of the gas-phase reactions of OH radicals with a series of α,β-unsaturated carbonyls at 200 + 2K. *Int J Chem Kinet* 1983;15:75–81.
67. Collins TW, Mitchell JC. Aroma chemicals. Reference sources for perfume and flavor ingredients with special reference to cinnamic aldehyde. *Contact Dermatitis* 1975;1:43.
68. Calnan CD. Cinnamon dermatitis from ointment. *Contact Dermatitis* 1976; 2:167.
69. Aretander S. *Perfume and flavor chemicals (aroma chemicals),* vols 1 and 2. Montclair, NJ: S Aretander, 1969.
70. Bonnevie P. Some experiences of wartime industrial dermatoses. *Acta Derm Venereol* 1948;28:231–237.
71. Fisher AA. *Contact dermatitis,* 2nd ed. Philadelphia: Lea & Febiger, 1973.
72. Fisher AA. Dermatitis due to cinnamon and cinnamic aldehyde. *Cutis* 1975;16:383.
73. Rudzki E, Grzywa Z. Two types of contact urticaria and immediate reactions to patch-test allergens. *Dermatologica* 1978;157:110.
74. Schorr WF. Cinnamic aldehyde allergy. *Contact Dermatitis* 1975;1:108.
75. Ogier M, Duverneuil G. Dermites allergiques a l'aldéhyde cinnamique. *Arch Mal Prof Med Trav Secur Soc* 1977;38:835.
76. Hjorth N. Eczematous allergy to balsams, allied perfumes and flavoring agents. *Acta Derm Venereol* 1961;41(46):1–216.
77. Mathias CGT, Chappler RR, Maicbach HI. Contact urticaria from cinnamic aldehyde. *Arch Dermatol* 1980;116:74.
78. Malten KE. Four bakers showing positive patch tests to a number of fragrance materials which can be used in flavors. *Acta Derm Venereol (Stockh)* 1979;59:117.
79. Magnusson B, Wilkinson DS. Cinnamic aldehyde in toothpastes: 1. Clinical aspects and patch tests. *Contact Dermatitis* 1975;1:70.
80. Kirton V, Wilkinson DS. Sensitivity to cinnamic aldehyde in a toothpaste: 2. Further studies. *Contact Dermatitis* 1975;1:70–77.
81. Drake TE, Maibach HI. Allergic contact dermatitis and stomatitis caused by cinnamic aldehyde flavored toothpaste. *Arch Dermatol* 1976;112:202.
82. Anderson KE. Contact allergy to toothpaste flavors. *Contact Dermatitis* 1978;4:195.
83. Miller J. Cheilitis from sensitivity to oil of cinnamon present in bubble gum. *JAMA* 141;116:131–132.
84. Laubach JL, Malkinson FD, Ringiose, EJ. Cheilitis caused by cinnamon (cassia) oil in toothpaste. *JAMA* 1953;152:404–405.
85. Fisher AA. Systemic eczematous "contact-type" dermatitis medicamentosa. *Ann Allergy* 1966;24:415.
86. Kern AB. Contact dermatitis from cinnamon. *Arch Dermatol* 1960;81:599.
87. Leifer W. Contact dermatitis due to cinnamon: recurrence of dermatitis following oral administration of cinnamon oil. *Arch Dermatol* 1951;64:53.
88. Nearing H, van Ketel WG. Allergy from spices used in Indonesian cooking. Presented at the International Symposium on Contact Dermatitis, Gentofte, Denmark, 1974.
89. Bullerman LW, Liew FY, Seier SA. Inhibition of growth and aflatoxin production by cinnamon and clove oils. Cinnamic aldehyde and eugenol. *J Food Sci* 1977;42:1107–1109.
90. Kurita N, Miyaji M, Kurane R, Takahara Y, Ichimura K. Antifungal activity and molecular orbital energies of aldehyde compounds from oils of higher plants. *Agric Biol Chem* 1981;45:945–952.
91. Kurita N, Miyaji M, Kurane R, Takahara Y. Antifungal activity of components of essential oils. *Agric Biol Chem* 1981;45:945–952.
92. Moon KH, Pack MY. Cytotoxicity of cinnamic aldehyde on leukemia L1210 cells. *Drug Chem Toxicol* 1983;6:521–535.
93. Petterson EO, Ronning W, Nome O, Oftebro R. Effects of benzaldehyde on protein metabolism of human cells cultivated in vitro. *Eur J Cancer Clin Oncol* 1983;19:935–940.
94. Guidotti GG, Loreti L, Ciaranfi E. Studies on the antitumor activity of aliphatic aldehydes: I. The mechanism of inhibition of amino acid incorporation into protein of Yoshida ascites hepatoma cells. *Eur J Cancer Clin Oncol* 1965;1:23–32.
95. Sessa A, Scalabrino G, Arnaboldi A, Perin A. Effects of aliphatic aldehyde metabolism on protein and thiol compounds in rat liver and hepatoma induced by 4-dimethyl-aminoazobenzene. *Cancer Res* 1977;37:2170–2176.
96. Ciaranfi E, Loreti L, Borghetti A, Guidotte GG. Studies on the anti-tumor activity of aliphatic aldehydes: II. Effects on survival of Yoshida ascites hepatoma-bearing rats. *Eur J Cancer Clin Oncol* 1965;1:147–151.
97. Dornish JM, Patterson EO, Oftebro R. Synergistic cell inactivation of human NHIK 3025 cells by cinnamaldehyde in combination with *cis*-diaminedichloroplatinum(II). *Cancer Res* 1988;48:938–942.
98. Gorman SP, Scott EM, Russell AD. A review: antimicrobial activity, uses and mechanism of action of glutaraldehyde. *J Appl Bacteriol* 1980;48:161–190.
99. Snyder RW, Cheatle EL. Alkaline glutaraldehyde: an effective disinfectant. *Am J Hosp Pharmacol* 1965;22:321–327.
100. Stonehill AA, Knop S, Borick PM. Buffered glutaraldehyde: a new chemical of sterilizing solution. *Am J Hosp Pharmacol* 1963;20:458–465.
101. Borick PM, Donershine FH, Chandler VL. Alkylized glutaraldehyde: a new antimicrobial agent. *J Pharmacol Sci* 1984;53:1273.
102. Pepper RE, Chandler VL. Sporicidal activity of alkaline alcoholic saturated dialdehyde solutions. *Appl Microbiol* 1963;11:384.
103. Blough HA. Selective inactivation of biological activity of myxoviruses by glutaraldehyde. *J Bacteriol* 1966;92:226.
104. O'Brien HA, Mitchell JD, Haberman S, Rowan DF, Winford TE, Pellet J. The use of activated glutaraldehyde as a cold sterilizing agent for urological instruments. *J Urol* 1966;95:429.
105. Sabel FL, Hellman A, McDade MJ. Glutaraldehyde inactivation of virus in tissue. *Appl Microbiol* 1969;17:645.
106. Dabrowa N, Landau JW, Newcomer VD. Antifungal activity in vitro. *Arch Dermatol* 1972;105:555.
107. Boucher RMG. Potentiated acid 1,5-pentanedial—a new chemical sterilizing and disinfecting agent. *Am J Hosp Pharmacol* 1974;31:546.
108. Meeks CH, Pembleton WE, Hench ME. Sterilization of anesthesia apparatus. *JAMA* 1967;199:276.
109. Nicewicz JT, Murphy DMF, Welsh JP, Sualli H. Occupational asthma caused by glutaraldehyde exposure. *Immunol Allergy Pract* 1986;8:272.
110. Benson WG. Exposure to glutaraldehyde. *J Soc Occup Med* 1984;34:63–64.
111. Corrado OJ, Osman J, Davies, RJ. Asthma and rhinitis after exposure to glutaraldehyde in endoscopy units. *Hum Toxicol* 1986;5:325–328.
112. Norback D. Skin and respiratory symptoms from exposure to alkaline glutaraldehyde in medical services. *Scand J Work Environ Health* 1988;14: 366–371.
113. Ballantyne B, Berman B. Dermal sensitizing potential of glutaraldehyde: a review of recent observations. *J Toxicol Cut Ocul Toxicol* 1984;3:251–262.
114. Nethercott JR, Holness DL, Page E. Occupational contact dermatitis due to glutaraldehyde in health care workers. *Contact Dermatitis* 1988;193–196.
115. Nethercott JR, Holness DL. Contact dermatitis in funeral service workers. *Contact Dermatitis* 1988;18:263–267.
116. Berdazzi F, Melino M, Alagna G, Geronesi S. Glutaraldehyde dermatitis in nurses. *Contact Dermatitis* 1986;14:319–320.
117. Federal Food, Drug and Cosmetic Act, 21 *CFR* 175.105. *Food and drugs indirect food additives: adhesives.* 1993.
118. Dunlop AP. Furfural and other furan compounds. In: Standen A, ed. *Kirk-Othmer encyclopedia of chemical technology,* 2nd ed, vol 10. New York: Wiley-Interscience, 1966:237–251.
119. National Research Council. *Drinking water and health.* Washington: Safe Drinking Water Committee, National Academy of Sciences, 1977.
120. Federal Water Pollution Control Act, 40 *CFR* 116.4. *Protection of the environment, designation of hazardous substances.* 1987.
121. Federal Water Pollution Control Act, 40 *CFR* 401.15. *General provisions, toxic pollutants.* 1987.
122. Toxic Substance Control Act, 40 *CFR* 716.120, section 8(d). *Protection of the environment.* Health and Safety Data Reporting. 1994.
123. Toxic Substance Control Act, 40 *CFR* 799.5000. *Protection of the environment.* Testing Consent Order. 1994
124. Food, Drug and Cosmetic Act, 40 *CFR* 180.1001(d). *Tolerance and exemptions from tolerances for pesticide chemicals in or on raw agricultural commodities.* 1996.

CHAPTER 97

Biological Hazards, Biotoxins, and Toxigenic Fungi

Jacek Dutkiewicz, John B. Sullivan, Jr., and James Seltzer

Biological hazards consist of microorganisms, nonviable components of microorganisms, viruses, algae, protozoa, pollen, spores, chemical substances derived from microorganisms, and products from arthropods and mammals (Tables 97-1, 97-2) (1). The most common biological contaminants identified indoors are fungi and bacteria, usually present in the form of a biological aerosol or organic dust. Besides the adverse health potential of the microorganisms themselves, potential adverse health effects exist from exposure to the aerosolized chemical by-products of such microorganisms, such as endotoxins, β-1,3-glucans, mycotoxins, and volatile organic agents.

Biological exposures are common in many occupations, particularly agriculture (Table 97-3). Nonoccupational exposures occur via biological aerosols generated from contaminated ventilation systems, contaminated water supplies, and moisture-damaged building materials that allow for microbial growth and amplification.

Illness and diseases caused by or associated with biological agents and their chemical by-products include such allergy-mediated diseases as asthma, rhinitis, allergic conjunctivitis, hypersensitivity pneumonitis (HP), and allergic dermatitis; such nonallergic inflammatory conditions as pneumonitis, mucous membrane irritation, chronic bronchitis, non-allergy-mediated asthma (reactive airways), and contact dermatitis; infections caused by pathogens; such constitutional signs and symptoms as cough, headache, fatigue, myalgia, fever, and arthralgias.

BIOLOGICAL AEROSOLS AND AEROBIOLOGY

The term *biological aerosol* refers to viable and nonviable airborne particles of microbial origin and their chemical by-products that are disseminated into the air from a contaminating source by airflow or physical disturbance. Biological aerosols are basically organic dusts (Tables 97-4 through 97-7). Such aerosols contain organically derived particles that vary widely in shape and size, including microorganisms, spores, and chemical substances (Figs. 97-1, 97-2).

Factors that determine the growth, amplification, and adverse health potential of biological agents are ambient conditions, nutrient sources, microbial source, dissemination, aerodynamic particle size, pathogenicity, electrostatic charges on particles, biological aerosol concentration, and nature of the particle's surface (2).

TABLE 97-1. Biological hazard categories

Microbial factors	Toxin-producing or allergenic bacteria and fungi that grow on plant and animal surfaces as well as on different organic and inorganic synthetic materials; can be inhaled together with dusts or droplet aerosols and cause inflammatory reactions of the respiratory tract
Plant factors	Plant toxins (alkaloids, glycosides), volatile oils, aeroallergens (pollen), contact allergens that cause dermatitis, and allergenic or toxic dusts that are released during the processing of plant materials (e.g., tea dust, wood dust, buckwheat dust, cotton dust)
Animal factors	Toxin- and venom-producing animals (mites, ticks, spiders, stingrays, snakes) or allergens of animal origin (mite and insect particles, feather, dander, epithelial cells, hair, urine, feces, powdered enzymes) that may cause respiratory symptoms, conjunctivitis, or dermatitis

Ambient Conditions

Temperature, light, relative humidity, wind, and airflow both outdoors and indoors affect growth and dissemination of microorganisms. Some microorganisms, such as *Legionella pneumophila, Actinomycetes,* and *Micropolyspora faeni*, grow best at temperatures in excess of 50°C (122°F). High relative humidity (greater than 70%) will enhance fungal and bacterial growth as well as growth of dust mites. The outdoor air is also a source of biological contaminants that can be carried indoors.

Nutrient Sources

The prime nutrient sources for microbial growth are organic material and moisture. Fungi and bacteria can grow and amplify in damp soil, moist hay, animal feed, dead plants, building materials containing cellulose, cellulose insulation, gypsum board liner, wallpaper, and carpeting. Stagnant water is a prime nutrient source for microbial growth. Dust and dirt in ventilation systems are other nutrient sources.

Aerodynamic Particle Size

The diameter of a particle determines its airborne behavior. Particle aerodynamics are related to the size, shape, and density of a particle. For a spherical particle, the aerodynamic behavior is related directly to diameter. For elliptic or cylindric particles, the smallest diameter more accurately represents a particle's aerodynamic behavior. Larger particles fall faster than do smaller particles, and thus sampling that depends on gravity will overestimate large particles and underestimate smaller particles. Particles that are no larger than 10 μm in diameter are respirable.

Particle Surface and Electrostatic Charge

Particles may be hydrophobic or hydrophilic, thus determining their ease of adsorption on moist surfaces. Charged particles will be attracted to oppositely charged surfaces.

Biological Aerosol Concentration

Biological aerosol concentration is related directly to the exposure to, and thus the dose of, the contaminant. The makeup of the concentration will also influence a biological aerosol's health hazard. In general, high concentrations of biological aerosols in the respirable range present high health hazards. Biological aerosol concentrations are expressed in terms of colony-forming units (CFU) per cubic meter of air. Airborne concentrations between 1×10^4 and 1×10^9 are considered high and pose health risks.

Pathogenic Microorganisms

Until recently, at least 193 microbial agents were considered to pose significant risks owing to their pathogenicity (Tables 97-8,

TABLE 97-2. Common biological aerosol components

Source	Airborne unit	Examples	Health effects	Principal indoor sources
Bacteria	Organisms	*Legionella*	Pneumonia	Cooling towers
	Spores	*Thermoactinomyces*	Hypersensitivity pneumonitis	Hot-water sources; hot, damp surfaces
	Products	Endotoxin	Fever, chills	Stagnant water reservoirs
		Proteases	Asthma	Industrial processes
		Peptidoglycans	—	—
Fungi	Organisms	*Aspergillus* spp.	Hypersensitivity pneumonitis	Damp environmental surfaces
	Spores	*Alternaria* spp.	Asthma, rhinitis	Outdoor air, damp surfaces
	Chemical by-products	*Fusarium* spp.	Systemic infection	Bird droppings
		Cladosporium spp.	Asthma, rhinitis	Outdoor air
		Glucans	Cancer	Damp surfaces
		Aldehydes, ketones	Headaches, mucous membrane irritants	Damp surfaces
		Mycotoxins	—	—
Protozoa	Organisms	*Naegleria*	Infection	Contaminated water reservoirs
	Antigens	*Acanthamoeba*	Hypersensitivity pneumonitis	Contaminated water reservoirs
Viruses	Organisms	Influenza	Respiratory infection	Human hosts
Algae	Organisms	*Chlorococcus*	Asthma, rhinitis	Outdoor air
Plants	Pollen	Ambrosia (ragweed)	Asthma, rhinitis	Outdoor air and indoor air
Arthropods	Feces	*Dermatophagoides* (mites)	Asthma, rhinitis	Indoor air and dusts
	Insect parts	—	—	—
Mammals	Skin scales	Horses	Asthma, rhinitis	Horses
	Excreta	Cats	Asthma, rhinitis	Cats

Adapted from Seltzer J. Biologic contaminants. *Occup Med* 1995;10(1):1–26.

97-9) and opportunities for occupational exposure (1). This group of agents included 27 species of viruses, 38 species of bacteria, 28 species of fungi, 4 species of lower plants other than fungi, and 23 allergenic agents associated with vertebrate animals (1). Many new, important biological hazards have been identified and, at present, this group totals more than 250 agents. Table 97-10 provides a summary of biological safety levels for handling infectious agents.

Two main immunopathologic reactions are caused by biological exposure: type I and type IV hypersensitivity reactions. Antigen exposure is required for the development of both. The initial (primary) response on exposure to antigen generally results in subclinical (no symptoms or signs of illness) sensitization. Subsequent exposure to the same antigen may result in further subclinical sensitization (secondary or anamnestic response) and, in many, repeated exposure eventually produces some form of hypersensitivity illness. The level at which an exposure induces an immunologic response or causes disease depends on a number of factors, including the nature of the antigen, the concentration of antigen, the manner in which the antigen is presented to the immune system, the current state of health of the exposed individual, and such intervening factors as medications, which might alter the immune response.

TYPE I (IMMEDIATE) HYPERSENSITIVITY REACTION

Immediate hypersensitivity develops when a genetically predisposed individual is exposed to antigen, resulting in the sensitization of lymphocytes and the subsequent production of immunoglobulin E (IgE) specific for the offending antigen. IgM and IgG may also be produced, but generally it is the specific IgE bound to mast cells and basophils that, when combined with a sensitizing antigen, results in the degranulation of these cellular elements and the release of histamine and such other mediators of inflammation as leukotrienes.

Allergic rhinitis, conjunctivitis, asthma, and eczema represent the most common manifestations of immediate IgE hypersensitivity. Upper airway allergy affects 20% to 30% of the U.S. population (3). Asthma affects 14 to 15 million American people, making asthma the most common chronic illness in children in the United States (4). Occupational asthma accounts for as much as 15% of the prevalence of asthma (5). The prevalence of atopic dermatitis (allergic eczema) ranges somewhere between 1% and 2% (6).

Atopic dermatitis (eczema) usually presents as an itchy, erythematous, papulosquamous rash involving the hands, wrists, face, and extensor surfaces of the extremities. If upper airways, lower airways, or skin is involved in an individual, it is likely that another organ system will also be involved. Urticaria, angioedema, and anaphylaxis (generalized immediate hypersensitivity reaction) can result from this type of immunologic reaction.

TYPE IV (CELL-MEDIATED) HYPERSENSITIVITY

Cell-mediated hypersensitivity develops when lymphocytes are exposed to antigen presented by specialized cells such as tissue macrophages. Lymphocytes elaborate antigen-specific factors, which sensitize mast cells. On reexposure to antigen, the mast cells release vasoactive substances and inflammatory mediators, creating a cascade of increased vascular permeability, inflammation, attraction of sensitized helper T cells, and presentation of antigen by macrophages, and the further release of cytotoxic and chemotactic cytokines. Recruitment of lymphocytes and inflammatory cells (i.e., neutrophils, basophils, and monocytes) to the areas of antigen exposure results in further release of inflammatory mediators and inflammation, in addition to the cell-mediated (through elaborated cytokines) cytotoxicity—hence, the term *cell-mediated immunity*. Contact dermatitis is a classic example of type IV hypersensitivity (6). The clinical disorder has acquired the label *allergic contact dermatitis* to distinguish it from irritant dermatitis, wherein the offending agent causes skin damage directly. Plants of the *rhus* family (e.g., poison oak and poison ivy, *Primula obconica*, and chrysanthemums) can induce a delayed-type hypersensitivity reaction.

Allergic contact dermatitis usually presents with an acute, pruritic, erythematous, patchy vesicular rash at the areas of contact with the contact allergen. A variation of allergic contact dermatitis results from airborne contact with certain plants (e.g., composite family members ragweed, feverfew, marsh elder, and sneezeweed). This dermatitis may mimic atopic dermatitis or a photosen-

TABLE 97-3. Occupations in which biological exposures are possible

Occupation	Possible exposures
Farmers and agricultural industries	Organic dusts; allergenic or toxic bacteria and fungi; allergenic or toxic substances of plant origin (toxalbumins, lectins); animal allergens (dander, hair, feather, excreta); allergenic or biting insects (e.g., mites and ticks)
Gardeners and orchard workers	Contact allergens and toxins of plant origin, pollen, and mites
Foresters and wood-processing workers	Allergenic fungi; contact allergens of lichens and liverworts; allergens and toxins of trees (pollen, terpin oils, resins); allergenic and toxicogenic caterpillars; respirable wood dust
Fishing and seafood producers	Venomous sponges, coelenterates, fish, and snakes; airborne protein allergens of sponges, sea-squirts, crustaceans, clams, squids (cephalopods), and fish
Bakers	Antigens originating from wheat and flour and from microorganisms and arthropods associated with grain; major allergens causing baker's asthma: probably flour additives, such as fungal enzymes (α-amylase from *Aspergillus oryzae*, cellulase from *Aspergillus niger*), soybean lecithin, and powdered yeasts (*Saccharomyces cerevisiae*)
Cooks and salespersons in food stores	Contact allergens of plant and animal origin
Laboratory and health care workers	Protein allergens from laboratory animals; powdered enzymes used as drugs or reagents; natural rubber latex proteins; zoonosis from infectious agents
Pharmaceutical workers and pharmacists	Powders of plant and animal origin containing allergens (mainly enzymes) and toxins (alkaloids, glycosides)
Personal care workers (cosmetologists, hairdressers, podiatrists)	Respiratory allergens in human hair, dander, nail dust; allergens of dermatophytic fungi (*Trichophyton rubrum, Trichophyton mentagrophytes*); infectious agents (e.g., bacteria, fungi, and tinea)
Veterinarians, zookeepers, and taxidermists	Animal allergens; zoonotic infections
Biotechnology workers	Bacterial endotoxins released during processing of cultures of gram-negative bacteria; proteolytic enzymes of *Bacillus subtilis* used in production of biological detergents; *Bacillus thuringiensis* toxin released during production of bacterial insecticide; *Aspergillus niger* proteins released during production of citric acid
Textile industry	Endotoxin produced by gram-negative bacteria or plant fibers (cotton, flax, hemp); immunotoxic substances (e.g., tannin) in cotton itself; allergens of the silkworm and in animal hairs
Printers and workers in occupations where air must be humidified	Endotoxin-producing gram-negative bacteria (e.g., *Pseudomonas* species, *Cytophaga allerginae*); immunogenic microorganisms (thermophilic actinomycetes, fungi, amebae of the species *Naegleria gruberi*) that can develop in humidifiers and are dispersed into air, causing "humidifier fever," hypersensitivity pneumonitis, or asthma
Sewage workers	Endotoxin or enterotoxin produced by gram-negative bacteria, causing respiratory illness, asthma
Collecting, sorting, and recycling domestic waste (including composting)	Large quantities of microorganisms and biotoxins, which may cause respiratory and gastrointestinal disorders; at particular risk: individuals collecting garden waste, those manually sorting garbage, and compost workers who may be exposed to large amounts of allergenic molds (in particular *Aspergillus fumigatus*) and thermophilic actinomycetes
Miners	Mycotoxin-producing or allergenic fungi developing in mine shafts; allergenic mites
Librarians, archivists, and art renovators	Allergenic or toxicogenic fungi and bacteria growing on moist books, paintings, sculptures, and other objects
Solderers	Fumes of colophony (rosin, product of pine resin), which may be a cause of asthma
Machine operators	Oil mist polluted with toxins produced by bacteria and fungi that develop in cutting oil emulsions (a hazard that could be prevented by application of safe and effective biocides to oil emulsions)

sitivity eruption. Although patch testing with extracts from these plants remains the mainstay of identifying offending allergens for a given individual, great care must be taken in the application and interpretation of patch tests, because irritant substances that are part of the plant can contaminate even commercial extracts.

Cell-mediated immunity directed against viral antigens also appears to play a role in the development of some cases of autoimmune disease. Guillain-Barré syndrome frequently develops after a viral infection or after vaccination against virus. In the animal model analogous to Guillain-Barré syndrome, experimental autoimmune neuritis, transfer of the disease occurs with CD4+ T cells that react with myelin protein P_2; complement-fixing antibodies (humoral immunity) may also play a role (7,8).

A frequently studied experimental autoimmune disease animal model, experimental allergic encephalomyelitis, has demonstrated the role of cell-mediated immunity. The human equivalent, acute disseminated postinfectious encephalomyelitis, has been associated with recent viral infections (i.e., rubella, mumps, measles, and varicella). Suggestions for possible pathologic mechanisms include shared epitopes between host cells and virus and viral infection that renders central nervous system cells more susceptible to attack by the cell-mediated immune system (9).

Hypersensitivity Pneumonitis. HP (extrinsic allergic alveolitis) is a type IV immune-mediated disease caused by the inhalation of biological aerosols and organic dusts. The predominant identifiable agents causing HP are biological, although chemicals can also produce the disease. Cases have occurred in which either the contaminated material is suspected but the agent has not been identified or the clinical disease exists in the absence of an identifiable cause. Many cases are occupational in origin, probably because many of the antigens producing the disease are not found commonly in relatively high concentrations in nonoccupational settings.

HP may occur after inhalation of organic dust or exposure to thermophilic actinomycetes, a variety of fungi, or endotoxins. A variety of causative microbiological organisms and aeroallergens can be isolated from contaminated air-cooling and ventilation systems in buildings or home environments. Airborne fungi such as *Alternaria, Aspergillus, Cladosporium, Fusarium*, and *Penicillium* can contaminate such ventilation systems.

HP can be acute, subacute, or chronic. The acute phase is dominated by fever and respiratory and constitutional symptoms. Acute symptoms, including cough, sweating, fever, anorexia, myalgia, arthralgias, headache, nausea, and vomiting, begin 4 to 8 hours after exposure to an offending antigen. In the acute phase, if exposure is terminated, signs and symptoms abate in 7 to 10 days. The chronic and more serious form of disease can develop after repeated exposures. The presence of serum-precipitating antibodies aids in the diagnosis.

Physical examination of the chest usually reveals diffuse rales, and chest radiography may show fluffy, patchy, coalescing

TABLE 97-4. Concentrations of dust-borne microorganisms in the air of different working environments (CFU/m³)

Environment	Total microorganisms	Gram-negative bacteria	Fungi
Farming			
Handling of hay	8.4×10^4–1.4×10^7	ND	8.0×10^4–1.6×10^6
Handling of corn	ND	ND	9.3×10^5–1.2×10^8
Silo opening	1.5×10^5–4.4×10^9	ND	1.0×10^4–1.2×10^7
Cattle farms	5.2×10^4–2.0×10^5	9.4×10^3	1.3×10^4
Swine farms	1.7×10^4–1.4×10^6	8.4×10^3–7.5×10^4	2.0×10^2–3.0×10^4
Poultry farms	1.7×10^5–1.8×10^7	6.3×10^3–4.5×10^5	5.0×10^2–9.1×10^4
Industry			
Grain stores	1.3×10^5–1.3×10^6	5.9×10^4–5.5×10^5	7.4×10^3–4.5×10^4
Grain mills	2.2×10^4–1.9×10^5	7.8×10^3–1.2×10^5	2.6×10^3–1.2×10^4
Malt-house	5.4×10^5	1.4×10^5	1.8×10^4
Herb processing	9.4×10^4–6.3×10^5	5.0×10^3–5.8×10^4	1.7×10^4–1.1×10^5
Citrus fruit store	ND	ND	3.3×10^4–7.7×10^8
Poultry processing	3.0×10^4–1.3×10^6	1.0×10^3–9.1×10^4	3.0×10^2–2.0×10^4
Tobacco processing	1.5×10^3–1.1×10^4	ND	1.4×10^3–1.0×10^4
Sawmills, furniture	3.1×10^3–6.5×10^5	1.0×10^2–2.2×10^4	1.7×10^2–6.5×10^5
Wood chip processing	2.7×10^2–3.8×10^5	3.7×10^3–7.0×10^3	2.7×10^2–3.8×10^5
Cotton mills	1.3×10^5–1.4×10^6	5.0×10^3–1.1×10^5	1.8×10^4–8.1×10^4
Waste processing			
Sewage treatment	ND	1.0×10^1–1.0×10^5	ND
Compost plants	ND	7.0×10^1–9.6×10^4	1.0×10^2–1.5×10^6

CFU, colony-forming units; ND, no data.
Courtesy of Dr. Barbane Ochalska, Krakow, Poland.

infiltrates in both lung fields. Spirometry usually shows a parallel reduction in forced vital capacity and forced expiratory volume over 1 second. A restrictive defect with reduced diffusing capacity is found, as is hypoxemia occasionally. In addition, an early (immediate-phase) asthmatic type of reaction may be seen in those with pigeon protein or pituitary snuff HP. Leukocytosis with a leftward shift is common, and eosinophilia sometimes occurs. Although symptoms and laboratory abnormalities usually clear within 72 hours, lung auscultation abnormalities may persist for days or weeks.

The insidious or chronic form of HP presents as a very gradual and progressive development of dyspnea, cough, malaise, and weight loss. This form usually is associated with prolonged exposure to small amounts of antigen. Between episodes, chest radiography may show evidence of interstitial fibrotic disease. Some affected individuals, over a period of years, will progress to end-stage interstitial pulmonary fibrosis, sometimes dying from their lung disorder. Pulmonary function tests reveal a persistent restrictive defect and the concomitant changes seen in the acute form.

The chronic phase of HP is manifested by the presence of noncaseating pulmonary granulomatous disease and progressive intrapulmonary fibrosis. The disease process involves both bron-

TABLE 97-5. Concentrations of bacterial endotoxins in organic dusts and in the air of different working environments

Environment	Concentration in dust (μg/g) parts per million	Concentration in air (μg/m³)
Farming		
Grain harvesting	ND	0.01–102.40
Silo opening	87.2	0.16–8.85
Cattle-hay farms	440.0–980.0	18.0–34.0
Swine farms	5.0–100.0	0.12–1.20
Poultry farms	10.9–120.0	0.13–1.42
Industry		
Grain stores and mills	22.5–500.0	54.9
Rice production	21.2	0.49
Peanut shelling	22.6	ND
Herb processing	200.0–400.0	4.0–756.8
Poultry processing	186.8	0.63–0.92
Sawmills	ND	0.24–4.00
Furniture factories	ND	0.0012–0.3500
Wood chip processing	ND	1.23–40.00
Cotton mills	40.3–780.0	0.001–0.600
Cotton gin	ND	0.20–2.00
Waste processing		
Sewage treatment	195.0	0.10–0.78
Compost plants	7.0–870.0	0.001–0.042

ND, no data.

TABLE 97-6. Concentrations of mycotoxins in organic dusts and in the air at different working environments

Mycotoxin and environment	Concentration in dust (μg/g) parts per million	Concentration in air (μg/m³)
Aflatoxins		
Peanut processing	0.25–0.41	0.0004–0.0720
Handling of corn	0.013–0.190	ND
Grain stores	0–0.0005	ND
Zearalenone		
Grain stores	0.02–0.10	Up to 0.15
Silo opening	0	ND
Secalonic acid D (SAD)		
Grain stores	0.0005–0.0200	ND
Handling of corn	0.3–4.5	ND
Deoxynivalenol		
Grain stores	0.0005–0.0200	ND
Silo opening	0.1–0.2	ND

ND, no data.

TABLE 97-7. Concentrations of the animal protein allergens in the air of occupational settings

Place and allergen	Concentration (μg/m³)
Egg processing plant: egg white components	
Ovalbumin	50.0
Ovomucoid	10.7
Lysozyme	2.0
Cow sheds	
Bovine epithelial antigen	0.04–9.50
Laboratory animal facilities: urinary allergens	
Different animal species	0.054–50.600
Rat urinary allergen	0–50.0
Rat epithelial allergen	0–40.0

Determinations were made with chemical and immunochemical methods (enzyme-linked immunosorbent assay inhibition test, radioallergosorbent test inhibition assay).

chioles and alveoli. Uncommonly, an intermediate form of HP occurs, with characteristics of both the acute and chronic forms.

As exposure to offending antigen continues, symptoms worsen. The chest radiograph usually is normal in mild cases but, with more intense exposure, can take on a ground-glass appearance. Granulomas appear as opacities on chest radiography, usually in the middle and lower lung fields, sparing the costophrenic angle. Chest radiographic abnormalities do not correlate with severity of symptoms. Pulmonary function tests may show restrictive defects, impaired gas exchange, and an increased residual volume–total lung capacity ratio (10). The diagnosis of HP depends on presence of the preceding criteria. Many affected individuals will demonstrate precipitating IgG antibodies (precipitins) in their serum. Most laboratories offer an HP precipitins panel, testing for the most common of the offending antigens. If a different environmental antigen is suspected, prepared material from the contaminated source can be tested against serum from those affected. However, the presence of precipitating antibody is not diagnostic, as more than 50% of individuals who are not ill yet who are repeatedly exposed to the same antigen will demonstrate precipitins (11).

High-resolution computed tomography scans of the lungs are more sensitive than is routine chest radiography for detecting interstitial fibrosis and may be useful when the routine chest radiograph is negative or nondiagnostic. Occasionally, lung biopsy may be necessary. If HP is present, the biopsy may show granulomas and interstitial fibrosis.

Fogelmark et al. (12) found that inhaled β-1,3-glucans, components of the cell wall of many fungi and *Actinomycetes*, in conjunction with bacterial endotoxin can induce histologic changes in the lungs of guinea pigs that resemble HP, whereas neither agent did so when inhaled individually. Combinations of biohazardous materials such as those found in organic dusts may facilitate the induction of some human illnesses caused by immune or nonimmune mechanisms of inflammation.

Another disease entity, termed *humidifier fever*, is characterized by fever, chills, myalgia, and malaise, but absent pulmonary symptoms. Symptoms arise within 4 to 8 hours after exposure and generally abate within 24 hours.

Airway inflammation of a nonimmunopathologic origin, edema, and bronchiolar narrowing can be caused by biological aerosol exposure. Rhinorrhea, sneezing, and ocular irritation also are associated with biological aerosol exposure. One study identified 16 genera of fungi, of which 80% were of respirable

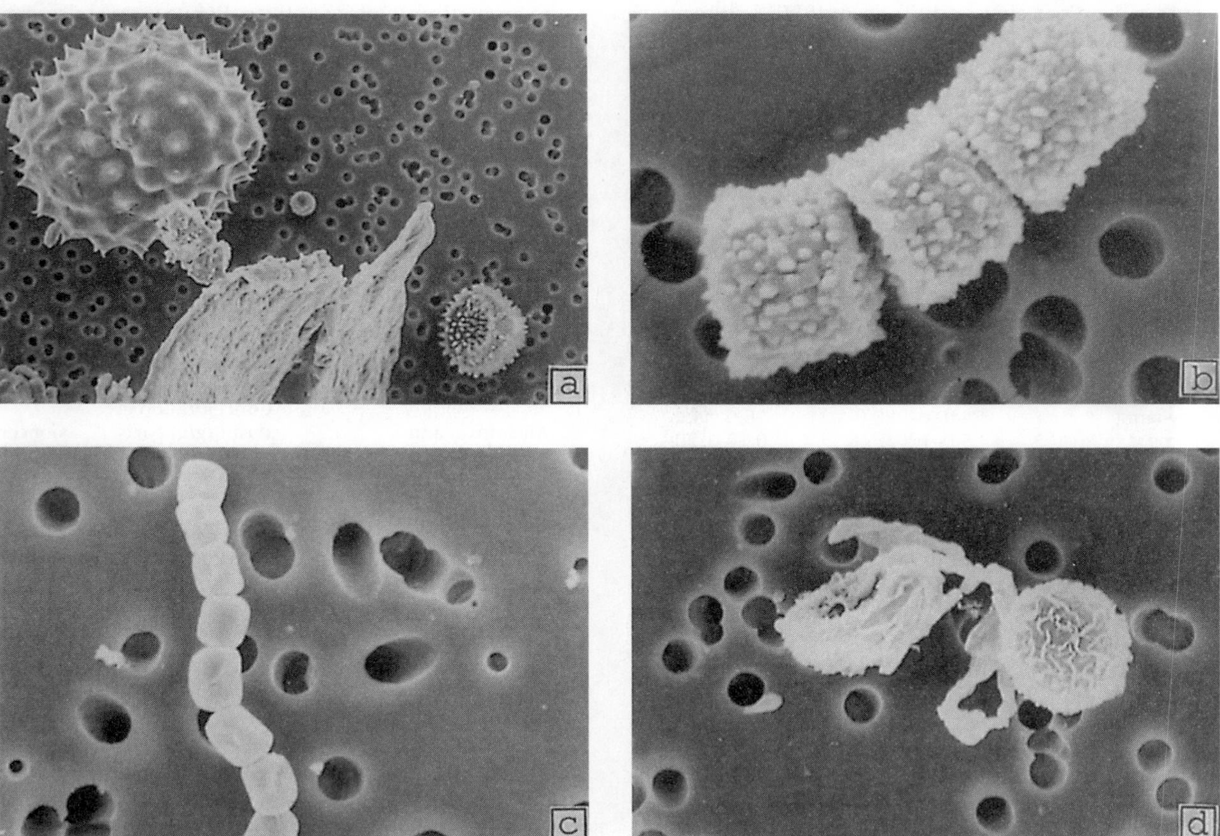

Figure 97-1. Organically derived particles contained in biological aerosols.

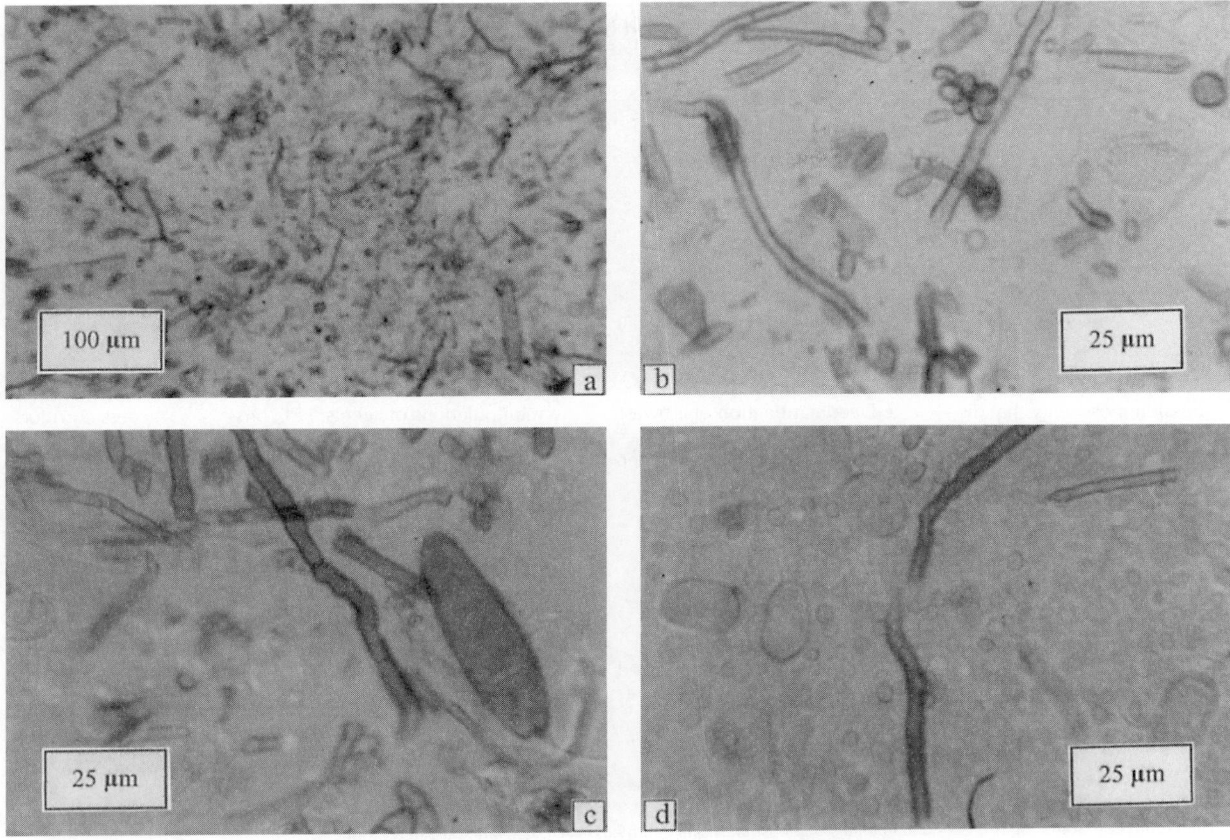

Figure 97-2. Organically derived particles contained in biological aerosols.

TABLE 97-8. Minimal human infective viral dose in volunteers

Viral agent	Inoculation route	Dose[a]
Measles virus	Intranasal spray	0.2[b]
Rhinovirus	Nasal drops	≤1
Venezuelan encephalitis virus	Subcutaneous	1[c]
West Nile fever virus	Intramuscular	1[d]
Parainfluenza 1 virus	Nasal drops	≤1.5
Poliovirus 1	Ingestion	2[b,e]
Rubella virus	Pharyngeal spray	≤10[b]
Coxsackie A21 virus	Inhalation	≤18
Rubella virus	Subcutaneous	30[b]
Adenovirus	Conjunctival swab	≤32
Rubella virus	Nasal drops	60[b]
Adenovirus 7	Nasal drops	≤150
Respiratory syncytial virus	Intranasal spray	≤160–640
Influenza A2 virus	Nasopharyngeal	≤790
SV-40 virus	Nasopharyngeal	10,000

[a]Median infectious tissue culture dose.
[b]Children.
[c]Guinea pig infective unit.
[d]Mouse infective unit.
[e]Plaque-forming unit.
Note: Illness was present after all inoculations except poliovirus, rubella virus (nasal drops), adenovirus (nasal drops), and simian virus SV-40; in these four, there was serologic conversion.
Adapted from Wedum et al., 1972:1558. Reprinted with permission from Plog BA, ed. *Fundamentals of industrial hygiene*, 4th ed. Itasca, IL: National Safety Council, 1996.

size (13). The fungi *Cladosporium* and *Aspergillus* made up 75% of respirable particulates of fungi identified in this study.

ALLERGIC BRONCHOPULMONARY MYCOSIS AND ASPERGILLOSIS

Whereas IgE-mediated reactions to fungal allergens are well documented, other immunologic reactions can produce an unusual form of asthma or sinusitis in some individuals. The pulmonary form of this disease, an allergic bronchopulmonary mycosis, is most commonly found in association with *Aspergillus* species, particularly *A. fumigatus*, and is called allergic bron-

TABLE 97-9. Infectious doses of selected diseases or agents for 25% to 50% of volunteers

Disease or agent	Inoculation route	Dose (no. of organisms)
Scrub typhus	Intradermal	3
Q fever	Inhalation	10
Tularemia	Inhalation	10
Malaria	Intravenous	10
Syphilis	Intradermal	57
Shigella flexneri	Ingestion	180
Anthrax	Inhalation	≤1,300
Typhoid fever	Ingestion	10^5
Cholera	Ingestion	10^8
Escherichia coli	Ingestion	10^8
Shigellosis	Ingestion	10^9

Adapted from Wedum et al., 1972:1558. Reprinted with permission from Plog BA, ed. *Fundamentals of industrial hygiene*, 4th ed. Itasca, IL: National Safety Council, 1996.

TABLE 97-10. Summary of recommended biological safety levels for infectious agents

BSL	Agents	Practices	Safety equipment (primary barriers)	Facilities (secondary barriers)
1	Not known to cause disease in healthy adults	Standard microbiological practices	None required	Open bench-top sink required
2	Associated with human disease; hazard is from autoinoculation, ingestion, mucous membrane exposure	BSL-1 practice plus • Limited access • Biohazard warning signs • "Sharps" precautions • Biological safety manual defining any necessary waste decontamination or medical surveillance policies	Class I or II BSCs or other physical containment devices used for all manipulations of agents that cause splashes or aerosols of infectious materials; PPE; laboratory coats; gloves; face protection as needed	BSL-1 plus autoclave available
3	Indigenous or exotic agents with potential for aerosol transmission; possibility that disease will have serious or lethal consequences	BSL-2 practice plus • Controlled access • Decontamination of all waste • Decontamination of laboratory clothing before laundering • Baseline serum	Class I or II BSCs or other physical containment devices used for all manipulations of agents; PPE; protective laboratory clothing; gloves; respiratory protection as needed	BSL-2 plus • Physical separation from access corridors • Self-closing, double-door access • Exhausted air not recirculated • Negative airflow into laboratory
4	Dangerous or exotic agents that pose high risk of life-threatening disease; aerosol-transmitted lab infections; or related agents with unknown risk for transmission	BSL-3 practices plus • Clothing change before entering facility • Shower on exit • All material decontaminated on exit from facility	All procedures conducted in class III BSCs or class I or II BSCs in combination with full-body, air-supplied, positive-pressure personnel suit	BSL-3 plus • Separate building or isolated zone • Dedicated supply and exhaust, vacuum, and decontamination systems • Other requirements as outlined in text

BSC, biological safety cabinet; BSL, biological safety level.
Reprinted with permission from Plog BA, ed. *Fundamentals of industrial hygiene,* 4th ed. Itasca, IL: National Safety Council, 1996.

chopulmonary aspergillosis (ABPA). ABPA can present at any age. Patients afflicted with ABPA often have labile, steroid-dependent asthma, and those who develop symptoms before age 30 often have other associated allergic disease (e.g., allergic rhinitis, atopic dermatitis) (14). Classically, ABPA presents with attacks of asthma accompanied by pulmonary infiltrates and, at times, atelectasis, thick mucous plugs in the shape of the bronchi, eosinophilia, fever, chest pain, malaise, and hemoptysis. As these attacks progress, the asthma may become more refractory, and central bronchiectasis and sometimes upper lobe fibrosis may develop. *Aspergillus* mycelia can be found growing in, but not invading, the bronchi. The results of skin testing for sensitivity to *A. fumigatus* are positive for both immediate and late-phase (6 to 8 hours postexposure) hypersensitivity. Total serum IgE often is very high (exceeding 1,000 ng per mL). Other features are precipitating *A. fumigatus*–specific IgG antibodies, peripheral eosinophilia (also seen in mucus), and elevated serum IgE and IgG levels (by enzyme-linked immunosorbent assay technique) as compared to asthmatics with immediate hypersensitivity to *A. fumigatus* but not having ABPA (15,16). Because ABPA can also present with mild asthma, no asthma, or simply pulmonary infiltrates out of proportion to the clinical picture, making the diagnosis accurately requires a good understanding of the five stages of the disease, the varied clinical presentations, and factors that influence the results of laboratory tests. These findings all suggest that types I, III (immune complexes), and IV immunologic reactions play a role in the pathogenesis of ABPA and other allergic bronchopulmonary mycoses.

Allergic fungal sinusitis is reported infrequently but can easily be missed. It has been most frequently reported with *Aspergillus.* Patients present with chronic sinusitis that is refractory to antibiotic therapy but responsive to systemic steroid therapy. Mucus evacuated from affected sinuses is very thick and contains eosinophils, Charcot-Leyden crystals, and *A. fumigatus* hyphae (Fig. 97-3). However, there is no evidence of invasion of the mucosa (17,18).

Specific immunologic reactions to antigens can result in illnesses that are not classified easily as specific immediate or delayed types of hypersensitivities. These often present with features of more than one of the four types of immunologic reactions. Specific IgG, in conjunction with lymphocytes, is thought

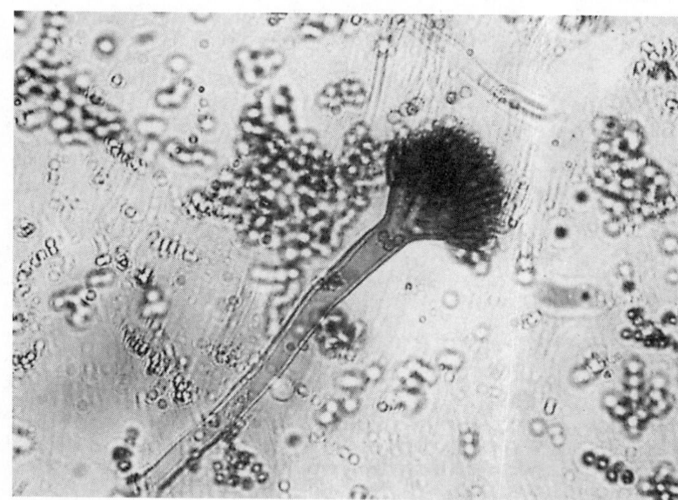

Figure 97-3. *Aspergillus fumigatus* (1,500×).

to play a role in the development of a form of asthma, allergic bronchopulmonary mycosis, which is unusually refractory to treatment.

FUNGAL BIOHAZARDS

Fungal biohazards are characterized as infectious or noninfectious. However, noninfectious fungi can become a health hazard if they contaminate an environment by overgrowth and aerosolization. Species of molds that contaminate foods, compost, grain, silage, tobacco, peanuts, fruits, wood, and building materials produce allergens and chemical by-products that can cause respiratory disease via inhaling of organic dusts that are generated. The majority of these hazardous species belongs to the genera *Aspergillus, Penicillium, Absidia, Alternaria, Cladosporium, Cryptostroma, Fusarium, Mucor, Rhizopus,* and *Stachybotrys* (19–21).

Noninfectious health effects of fungi on the respiratory system are due to allergenic response mediated through specific antibodies or sensitized cells or through non-immune-mediated inflammation (19–21). Illness occurring in an individual after inhalation of organic dust containing large amounts of spores, fungi, and their chemical by-products is due to stimulation of inflammation.

Among the chemical by-products are glucans, mycotoxins, and volatile organic chemicals (VOCs) (20–31). *Glucans* are polyglucose compounds found as structural components of the fungal cell wall. β-1,3-glucans are suspected of causing inflammation of the airways when inhaled. *Mycotoxins* are metabolites or natural products of various fungi that can be toxic to various organ systems, such as the gastrointestinal tract, kidneys, immune system, central nervous system, and heart, depending on the specific compound, dose, and route of exposure. Mycotoxin production depends on temperature and moisture conditions. Certain building materials containing cellulose are a nutrient source for mycotoxin-producing fungi. Disagreeable odors produced indoors by contaminating fungi are the result of such VOCs as alcohols, esters, aldehydes, ketones, acids, and other low-molecular-weight substances.

Aspergillus fumigatus, a common gray-greenish mold that occurs in large numbers on different materials such as compost, silage, wood, tobacco, and inorganic dusts, is both an infectious pathogen and a cause of allergic illness (32–36). *A. fumigatus* spherical spores measuring 2.0 to 3.5 μm are formed on columnar conidial heads (see Fig. 97-3). Inhalation of dust massively laden with the spores can cause HP, asthma, pulmonary mycosis (aspergillosis), and organic dust toxic syndrome (ODTS). This fungus also produces tremorgenic mycotoxins that pose a risk for sawmill workers (37). *A. flavus* and *A. parasiticus* produce aflatoxins, one of which (aflatoxin B_1) is a hepatic carcinogen.

Aspergillus clavatus has been identified as an agent of malt worker's disease, whereas *A. versicolor, A. flavus,* and *A. terreus* have been implicated in the etiology of farmer's lung disease (19,21). *A. flavus,* a producer of aflatoxins, grows on corn and peanuts and is present in airborne dust from these products (38,39). *A. niger* antigens have been implicated in the causation of bronchospasm in biotechnology workers in whom sensitization was confirmed by the radioallergosorbent test (40). Fungal extracts contain many different antigenic protein mixtures. For example, *A. fumigatus, Cladosporium herbarum,* and *Alternaria alternata* contain 60 different protein antigens (40).

The genus *Penicillium* comprises more than 150 species of blue or green molds forming characteristic, brushlike conidiophore heads that can be widely distributed on decomposing organic matter and in air polluted with organic dusts. Penicillium species have been described as causative agents of asthma, HP, suberosis from moldy cork, cheese worker's disease, illness due to exposure to moldy fuel chips, and disease of wood cutters (19,21,41).

Other allergenic or toxic molds include *Eurotium rubrum* (synonym, *A. umbrosus*), implicated in the etiology of farmer's lung disease in Scandinavia; *Cryptostroma corticale*, described as an agent of maple bark disease; *Rhizopus nigricans*, which causes respiratory disease in wood trimmers; and species of the genera *Cladosporium* and *Alternaria*, which are considered to be frequent causes of allergic rhinitis and asthma (19,41,42).

Airborne Fungal Biohazards and Health Effects

The American Conference of Governmental Industrial Hygienists recommends that indoor air fungal spore concentrations determined by viable collection techniques generally should not exceed 50% of outdoor concentrations. Kozak et al. (43) found that total indoor air fungal spore counts in uncontaminated homes in Southern California rarely exceeded 1,000 CFU per cubic meter, and these values were significantly lower in homes where air-conditioning was used. The most prevalent fungi found in the contaminated homes were *Cladosporium* (all homes), *Penicillium* (91% of homes), non-spore-forming mycelia (90%), and *Alternaria* (87%).

Because only viable fungal spores grow on culture media and the presence of fast-growing fungi can compete more effectively for nutrients, culture may underestimate the actual biological fungal mass present in a contamination site. One study involving six indoor investigations recommends that any airborne concentration of fungi in excess of 500 CFU per cubic meter be investigated further. However, comparison to outdoor levels is essential (44).

Other studies that compared outdoor to indoor fungal concentrations concluded that a maximum of 300 CFU per cubic meter of nontoxigenic and nonpathogenic microorganisms (fungi or bacteria or both) should be typical in an environment in which normal, nonimmunocompromised people dwell (45). Also, with the exception of *Cladosporium,* this study recommended that no one microorganism should individually contribute more than 50 CFU per cubic meter to the total biological environmental load. The study further recommends that levels exceeding 300 CFU per cubic meter warrant further investigation (45).

Important indoor fungal pathogens for immunocompromised hosts are *Aspergillus* species, *Mucoraceae* species, and *Cryptococcus neoformans. Aspergillus* and *Mucoraceae* (*Rhizopus, Rhizomucor, Absidia,* and *Mucor* species) can be isolated from the soil of potted plants. *C. neoformans* degrades bird urine and can be found in some bird cages (45).

Building dampness and fungal contamination are associated with increased respiratory symptoms in adults and children (46–48). A relationship between symptoms of workers and IgE and IgG antibodies from indoor fungus-contaminated buildings has been discovered (49,50). Workers reporting upper airway irritation, fatigue, headache, and respiratory symptoms temporally related to work in a particular building were more likely to have at least one positive IgE antibody test (50). In a study involving schoolteachers, a clear association was found between the presence in teachers of serum IgE specific to *Penicillium* species and symptoms (49).

Counting and culturing airborne fungi to characterize an environment may not provide accurate assessment of the true fungal indoor biomass. Other tests being developed to estimate biomass include quantification of ergosterol from fungal cell walls and propagules and 3-hydroxy fatty acids (a biomarker of endotoxin) in dust and building materials (51–54). Measuring biochemical indicators as a marker of fungal biomass helps to overcome the errors inherent in culturing. Thus, the fungal sterol ergosterol has been used to estimate fungal biomass but is variably present in spores of fungi commonly found indoors (53). Ergosterol is a membrane sterol, and living mycelia contain a fixed amount per unit of cell membrane. Thus, studies have attempted to provide a relationship between ergosterol and the dry weight of mycelia. For example, for *Aspergillus* and *Penicillium*, this ergosterol value ranges from 1.4 to 6.0 μg per milligram of mycelia (53).

The average ergosterol-to-spore relationship may be a more reliable method of estimating indoor fungal biomass. One study that examined airborne spores determined that the amount of ergosterol per spore was related to spore size (53). However, the amount of ergosterol per spore varied widely among species. This one study detected 1.0 μg of ergosterol per milligram of spores, with an interspecies variability of 25% (53). But ergosterol detection does not provide any information on fungal species present, and species characterization remains critical to determining health hazards.

Ergosterol and 3-OH fatty acids have been measured in house dust to estimate the level of fungal contamination and endotoxin present (50). The common assay used to detect endotoxin is a *Limulus*-based bioassay, which depends on the ability of endotoxin to activate proteolytic enzymes from horseshoe crab amebocytes and thus measure activity and not biomass (51). With this technique, gram-negative bacterial biomass can be estimated instead by measuring the relative distribution of 3-OH fatty acids. Also, because 3-OH fatty acids differ among species of gram-negative bacteria, the bacteria can be characterized by such an assay. Finally, measurement of 3-OH fatty acids determines the presence of lipopolysaccharide in endotoxin, even if the endotoxin is biologically inactive.

Because fungi also contain bioactive chemicals (β-1,3-glucans and mycotoxins), the detection of ergosterol may be beneficial in better characterizing health risks (51). Thus, gas chromatography-mass spectrometry has been adapted to the analysis of 3-OH fatty acids and ergosterol combined in dust, to assist in determining indoor fungal and gram-negative bacterial biomass (51).

The ergosterol content in building materials has been examined to afford an estimate of the fungal contamination level (52). The ergosterol content of house dust has been reported to be 0.7 to 45.0 μg per gram (52). For *Aspergillus, Penicillium, Fusarium, Rhizopus, Cladosporium, Candida*, and *Alternaria*, the ergosterol content has ranged from 0.4 to 14.3 μg per milligram of dry mycelia (52). The ergosterol content of indoor air has been reported to be in the range of 0.01 to 194.0 nanograms per cubic meter (52). In one study, the ergosterol content of contaminated building materials ranged from 0.017 to 68.0 μg per gram of dry mass material.

The use of fungal mass biomarkers is promising, but more research is necessary to validate findings.

Biologically Active Fungal Chemical Products

Many fungi produce biologically active chemicals, such as β-1,3-glucans, mycotoxins, and VOCs, which can be health hazards. Airborne β-1,3-glucans, a cell wall polyglucose, has been associated with respiratory symptoms, headache, fatigue, pulmonary function decrements, and airway inflammation (31,55). Studies show that the amounts of glucans in fungi can differ significantly depending on the species. For example, the amount of β-1,3-glucan is much higher for *Stachybotrys* than for *Penicillium* and *Aspergillus* (55). Of significance, β-1,3-glucan is present in both living and dead spores and can thus persist in the environment when a fungal biomass is killed. Glucan levels in *Stachybotrys* spores were all shown to be greater than 500 ng per 10^6 spores, with a maximum value of 39,330 ng per 10^6 spores (55).

Among collectors of compostable waste, airborne exposure levels of glucans ranged from 10.8 to 36.4 ng per cubic meter (31). In the same study, endotoxin airborne levels ranged from 0.1 to 1.2 ng per cubic meter. Those collecting unsorted waste were exposed to glucan airborne levels of 2.0 to 13.7 ng per cubic meter and endotoxin levels of 0.3 to 1.2 ng per cubic meter (31).

Glucan levels between 0.01 to 100.0 ng per cubic meter have been associated with respiratory inflammation in people without a previous history of reactive airways (27,28). Children have had asthmatic symptoms with average glucan airborne levels of 42 ng per cubic meter (27). Symptoms decreased when levels declined to 1.4 ng per cubic meter. Airborne glucan concentrations of 10 ng per cubic meter have been recommended as a threshold for health concerns (27,28). Thus, fungi present health hazards in the form of both viable cells and chemical by-products. Identifying these microbial contaminants within buildings and other indoor sites is possible, but interpreting the results of such identification studies is difficult.

Both fungi and bacteria are known to enhance the release of histamine, which may play a role in such inflammatory events as bronchospasm (56). Gram-positive and gram-negative bacteria trigger basophil histamine release in leukocyte suspensions from normal individuals (56). This response might be due to peptidoglycans in bacteria cell walls.

Volatile chemicals released from one fungus (*Trichoderma viride*) caused histamine release from human bronchoalveolar cells (57). The fungus was grown on wallpaper paste agar, and the generated volatile organic agents were collected and found to contain 2-methyl-1-propanol, 3-methyl-1-butanol, 2-methyl-1-butanol, and 1-pentanol. Results showed that these volatile agents interacted with human airway cells and caused cytotoxic mediator release (57).

Airborne fungi and bacteria may activate leukocytes to produce oxidative stress (58). Different fungi and bacterial species are able to induce the production of reactive oxygen metabolites in human leukocytes. Such reactive oxygen metabolites are toxic to the microorganism and surrounding tissues (58,59).

Airborne spores of *Streptomyces* species isolated from contaminated homes stimulated macrophages to produce tumor necrosis factor–α (TNF-α) and interleukin-6 and induced expression of nitric oxide synthetase with subsequent nitric oxide production (60). The study also examined whether other fungal strains found indoors, such as *Penicillium, Cladosporium, Aspergillus, Stachybotrys*, and *Candida*, could induce production of proinflammatory cytokines or activate nitric oxide production in macrophages. Besides *Streptomyces*, only high levels of *Stachybotrys, Candida*, and *Cladosporium* stimulated nitric oxide production. High levels of *Penicillium* and *Cladosporium* increased production of TNF-α, as compared to the level in controls, whereas *Streptomyces* easily produced increased TNF-α and interleukin-6 (60). Nitric oxide production and cytokines play a role in airway inflammation and host defense. *Streptomyces* also induced a marked increase in reactive oxygen metabolites in human polymorphonuclear leukocytes. *Streptomyces* spores are 1 μm in diameter and thus can penetrate into lower airways to reach alveoli (60).

Another study investigated whether exposure to indoor fungi influenced T-cell differentiation in children (61). Results showed that a group of children living in heavily contaminated homes (as compared to children living in a less contaminated dwelling) had a larger number of CD3+ T cells expressing CD45RO, which is a marker expressed on antigen-experienced

T cells. The children in the more contaminated homes also had a lower mean CD4:CD8 ratio than did controls. The study included a 1-year follow-up period and reported total and specific IgE. As compared to controls, children in more contaminated homes were found to have higher numbers of CD3+ T cells expressing CD45RO markers. Levels of total IgE and IgE specific to dust mites and cat antigens were higher in the more contaminated group, but these differences were not statistically significant (60). The altered distribution of lymphocyte populations between the two groups is consistent with chronic stimulation and differentiation of lymphocytes because, on exposure to antigen that a T cell is programmed to recognize, the CD45A marker changes to CD45RO, indicating a T-cell lymphocyte with memory that can aid B cells in humoral immune responses (60). Thus, children living in more fungus-contaminated homes are chronically exposed to fungi, which might induce chronic lymphocyte stimulation. The study indicated that further research was necessary to clarify the nature of the responsible fungal antigens or toxins (60).

Yeast cell wall preparations were demonstrated to be able to activate complement and stimulate production of superoxide anion, production of leukotriene B_4, production and release of TNF-α, and phagocytosis in a dose-related manner (59,62). Yeasts can activate macrophages and enhance oxidative metabolism and phagocytosis in alveolar macrophages. *C. albicans*, living and dead, can release arachidonic acid and its metabolites. Yeast cell wall preparations from *Pichia fabianii, Candida sake, Trichosporon capitatum, Rhodotorula glutinis*, and *Cryptococcus laurentii* activated complement and stimulated superoxide anion and leukotriene B_4 production (62).

These immunoreactive findings may have health implications. Indoor building materials that are water damaged usually are colonized by both fungi and bacteria. The most common fungi that colonize water-damaged building materials are *Stachybotrys atra* and *Penicillium* and *Aspergillus* species. Studies using the *Limulus* lysate assay of water extracts from moisture-damaged building materials reveal high contents of gram-negative endotoxins in the range of 17 ng per mL of *Escherichia coli* lipopolysaccharide equivalents (63). β-1,3-glucans also were found in high content. In addition, water damaged gypsum liners contained satrotoxin, a mycotoxin, in the range of 17 ng per mL of water extract material.

Water-damaged building materials colonized by fungi and bacteria are sources of biological aerosols that can cause illness indoors. In addition to fungal antigens, health hazards include peptidoglycans, endotoxins, β-1,3-glucans, lipoglycans, teichoic acids, and mycotoxins. These biotoxins can stimulate inflammatory responses and exhibit immunomodulating properties.

Studies of water-damaged gypsum liners of walls and ceilings demonstrated that liners were heavily contaminated by fungus and bacteria and contained bioactive and toxic compounds, several of which were immunoreactive (63). These findings indicate that water-damaged building materials can be sources of bioactive agents that might be the cause of symptoms associated with the quality of some indoor air. Scanning electron microscopy and transmission electron microscopy of moisture-damaged gypsum liner reveals the presence of hyphae, conidiophores, conidia, and bacteria (Figs. 97-4, 97-5). Samples from 9 of 11 sites with a history of water damage contained conidia, recognized as a *Stachybotrys* species, as the dominant organism present, ranging from 10^3 to 10^5 conidia per square centimeter (see Fig. 97-4) (63).

Areas of indoor contamination may be recognized as dark-staining spots on wallboards, which can be seen on the interior

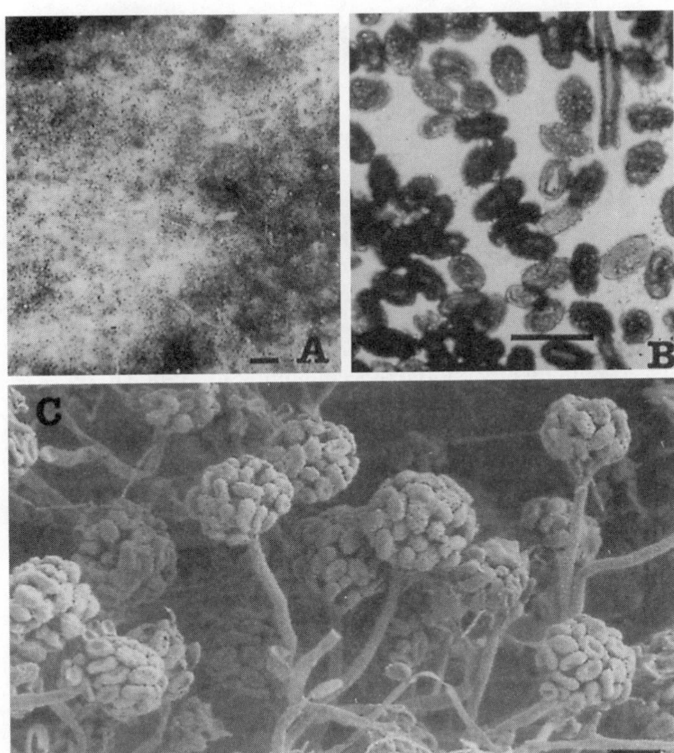

Figure 97-4. Analysis of moisture-damaged gypsum liner by scanning electron microscopy and transmission electron microscopy shows presence of hyphae, conidiophores, conidia, and bacteria.

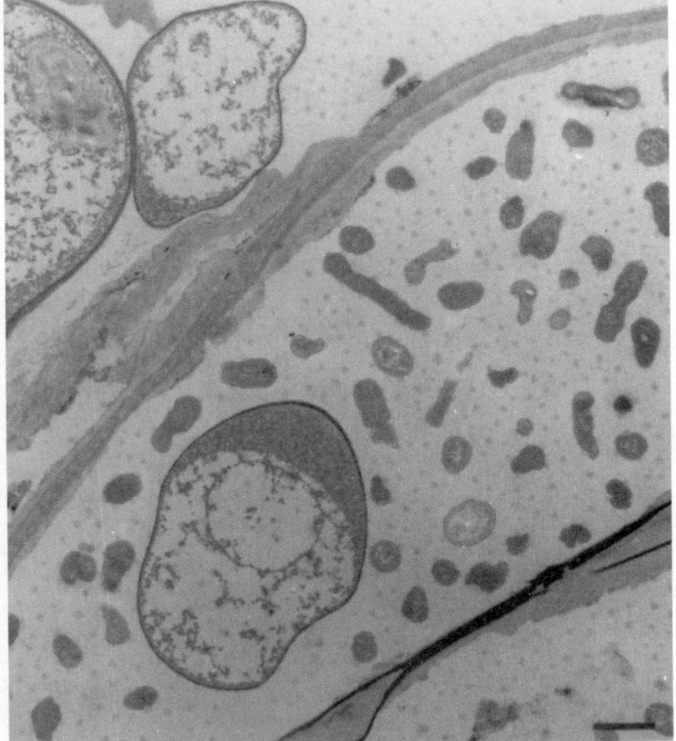

Figure 97-5. Analysis of moisture-damaged gypsum liner by scanning electron microscopy and transmission electron microscopy shows presence of hyphae, conidiophores, conidia, and bacteria.

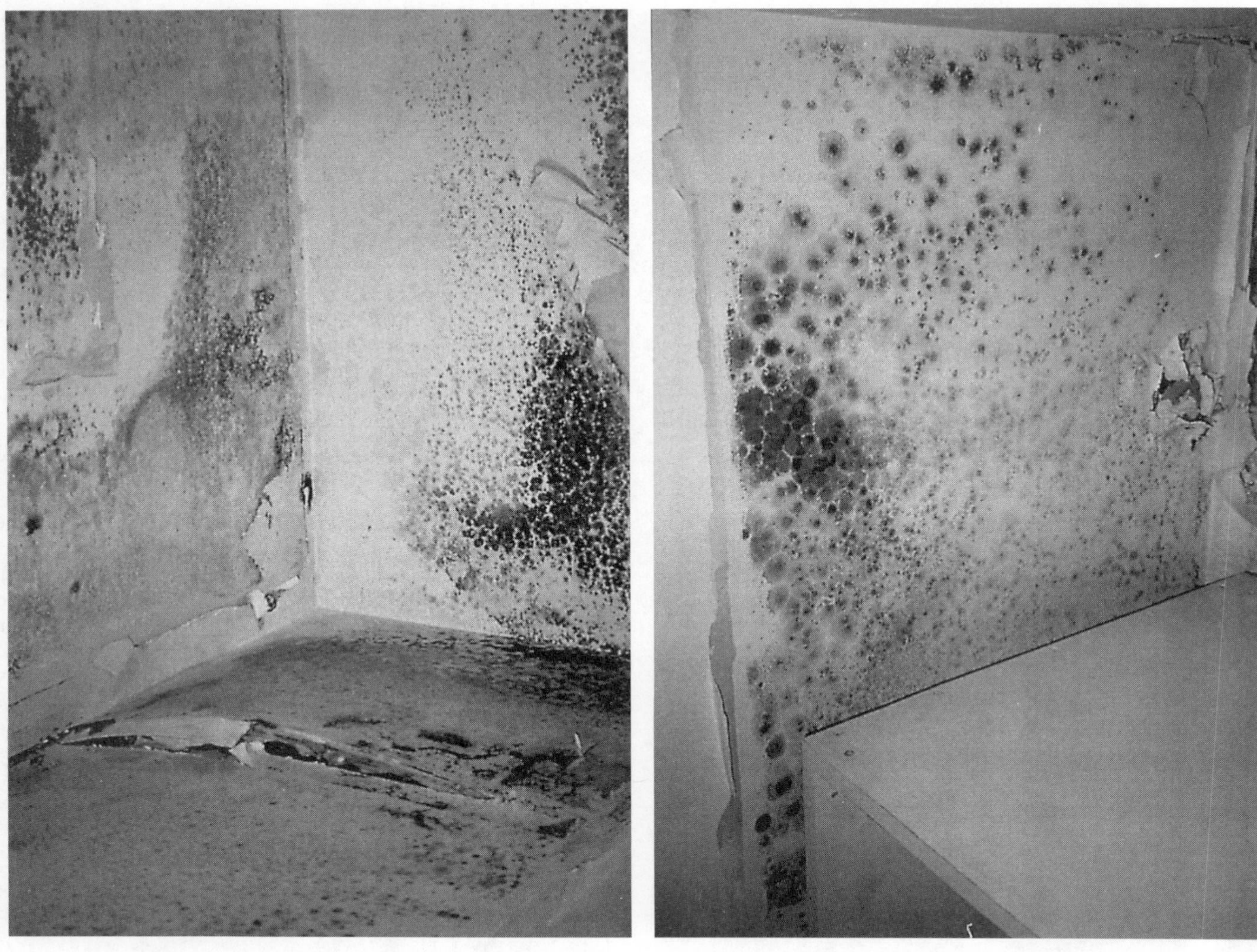

Figure 97-6. Areas of indoor contamination by fungus evidenced by dark-staining spots on wallboards, which can be seen on the interior of wallboards or on the inside of the indoor structure.

of wallboards or on the inside of the indoor structure, remaining invisible to the eye (Fig. 97-6).

Analysis of contaminated indoor sites has identified endotoxins, β-1,3-glucan, and mycotoxins in building materials (Table 97-11). *Limulus* lysate activity for endotoxins and for β-1,3-glucans are 10 to 100 times higher in building materials exhibiting water damage than in dry and non-water-damaged sites (63). Analysis of satrotoxin content in these materials showed that satrotoxin-G and satrotoxin-H were present in the moisture-damaged and contaminated area but not in the non-moisture-damaged area. Satrotoxin-G and satrotoxin-H were found in concentrations of 17 μg per gram of material (63). Verrucarol also was found.

Of note, the high contents of the endotoxins, β-1,3-glucans, and satrotoxins were located in the same area as was the heavy colonization of *Stachybotrys* species (63). The study also showed that the water-damaged gypsum board contained high concentrations of thermotropic, psychrotrophic, and mesophilic bacteria—100 times more than was found in samples from the nondamaged board. Sixteen taxa of molds were detected in different building materials and the genes and species were identified (63). Among these were *Penicillium, Aspergillus, Chaetomium, Cladosporium, Mucor, Paecilomyces,* and *Stachybotrys* species. Fifty-nine aerobic bacterial strains were isolated from the water-damaged gypsum board and from the nondamaged dry areas. However, the bacterial flora was more diverse and more expansive in the moisture-damaged areas than in the nondamaged board. Interestingly, in the moisture-damaged board, the flora was dominated by endotoxins containing gram-negative bacteria and rapidly growing *Mycobacterium* species (63).

Methanol extracts of the gypsum board were assayed for cell-line toxicity using the feline fetus lung cell line. Assays of satrotoxin-G and satrotoxin-H were performed by methanol extracts of building materials using high-performance liquid chromatography. Toxicity to boar spermatozoa was tested also. Results showed that the methanol extract of the moisture-damaged areas was 200 times more toxic to rabbit skin and feline lung cells than was the extract of the non-water-damaged sites, and the same methanol extract contained toxic materials that paralyze the motility of boar spermatozoa at very low concentrations (63). The feline fetus lung cell lines are very sensitive to mycotoxins, including satrotoxin-G and satrotoxin-H, T-2 toxin, Verrucarain-A, ochratoxin, and roridin. In this assay, the paralysis of boar spermatozoa, which are insensitive to satrotoxin and other mycotoxins, may indicate the presence of an unknown toxin.

TABLE 97-11. Endotoxin, β-D-glucan, and satrotoxin in the indoor building materials of a children's day-care center

Sample material	Amount (μg/g⁻¹) of toxins[a]		
	Endotoxin[b]	β-D-glucan[c]	Satrotoxin[d]
Day-care center			
Water-damaged gypsum board liner	17	210	17
Water-damaged gypsum board liner	2.3	14.0	
Water-damaged mineral wool	8.0	2.5	
Ceiling coating paper (randomly chosen)	4.2	41.0	
Settled dust from floor collected during demolition	0.17	0.50	
Mineral wool (randomly chosen)	0.1	<0.1	<1
Gypsum board liner (not water-damaged)	0.41	0.40	
Reference materials			
Pure culture (dry) of fungus (*Paecilomyces variotii* 95/111)	0.01	127.00	
Hay dust sampled from cow shed	27.0	1.9	

[a]The average difference between duplicate samples was ±5%.
[b]Endotoxin was measured as *Limulus* activity expressed as micrograms of *Escherichia coli* B lipopolysaccharide equivalents.
[c]β-D-glucan was measured as *Limulus* activity and expressed as micrograms of curdlan (β-1,3-glucan) equivalents.
[d]Satrotoxin was measured by high-performance liquid chromatography, using purified satrotoxin (G and H) as a standard.
Adapted from ref. 63.

Toxigenic Fungi and Mycotoxins

The presence of toxigenic fungi contaminating indoor building materials has escalated concerns about the possible causative relationship of mycotoxins to illness. Mycotoxins are low-molecular-weight cyclic toxins produced by a large variety of fungi, the most common being *Penicillium, Aspergillus, Fusarium,* and *Stachybotrys* (Tables 97-12, 97-13). Species of *Stachybotrys* and *Fusarium* produce macrocyclic trichothecenes, which inhibit protein synthesis and affect cellular membranes, nucleic acids, and T-cell and B-cell activity. *Fusarium* produces the trichothecenes T-2 toxin, deoxynivalenol, and diacetoxyscirpenol. *Fusarium* species also produce zearalenone, a mycotoxin with estrogenic effects. *Aspergillus versicolor* and *Penicillium* strains also produce mycotoxins such as sterigmatocystin, which is a hepatotoxin, and the nephrotoxin ochratoxin A. Aflatoxin B_1, a hepatic carcinogen, is produced by *Aspergillus flavus.*

TABLE 97-12. Mycotoxins

Diacetoxyscirpenol	Aflatoxin B_1, B_2, G_1, G_2, M_1
Sterigmatocystin	Ochratoxin A
Tannins	Satrotoxin F, G, H
T2-toxin	Verrucarin J
Deoxynivalenol	Roridin E
Fumonisin	Citrinin
Zearalenone	Roquefortine
Stachybotrys toxins	Patulin
Mycophenolic acid	Rubratoxin B

TABLE 97-13. Mycotoxins

Ochratoxin A	A group of isocoumarin derivatives found in cereals, beans, peanuts, and rice; produces immunosuppression, including lymphocytopenia and depletion of lymphoid cells; both cell mediated and humoral immunity affected by toxin in animal models
Citrinin	Found in wheat, rye, oats, and barley; immunostimulatory in the mouse model
Cyclopiazonic	Found in corn, peanuts, millet, and cheese
Patulin	Found in apple juice and moldy feeds, which can cause hemorrhagic lesions and ulceration; variable immunodepressive effects
Secalonic acid-D	Reduces lymphocyte counts in mice but increases white blood cell counts and neutrophil counts
Wortmannin	A metabolite of *Penicillium* and *Fusarium*; observed to cause necrosis of spleen, lymph nodes, and gastrointestinal tract–associated lymphoid tissue in animals receiving doses in a purified form; at lower than lethal levels, causes depression of a number of immune functions in animal models
Trichothecenes	Composed of more than 60 sesquiterpenoids that are potent protein synthesis inhibitors; include vomitoxin (deoxynivalenol, T-2 toxin nivalenol, and diacetoxyscirpenol); cause damage to actively dividing bone marrow cells in lymph node, spleen, thymus, and intestinal mucosa as a result of acute exposure to trichothecene mycotoxins; immunosuppressive and immunostimulatory; increase susceptibility to *Candida, Cryptococcus, Mycobacterium, Listeria, Salmonella,* and herpes simplex virus type 1 infections (particularly T-2 toxin and diacetoxyscirpenol); impair cell-mediated immunity in animal models; toxic for alveolar macrophages; depressed alveolar macrophage phagocytosis and response in swine after T-2 toxin inhalation
Fumonisin B_1	Produced by *Fusarium moniliforme*; causative agent of equine leukoencephalomalacia and porcine pulmonary edema

Stachybotrys chartarum (also referred to as *S. atra*) has received attention owing to its presence in cases of indoor contamination in which illness has occurred. The contamination by *S. chartarum* indoors and its production of toxins has been studied in a variety of building materials (63). Mycotoxins produced by *S. chartarum* cause adverse reactions in animals, who display such symptoms as irritation of the eyes, skin, and mucous membranes, necrosis of the skin, organ hemorrhages, and immunotoxicity.

S. chartarum produces *Stachybotrys* toxin and satrotoxins. Human stachybotryotoxicosis is controversial and has been described to include dermatitis, cough, rhinitis, irritation of mucous membranes, fever, headaches, and fatigue (64,65). However, these clinical symptoms are difficult to directly relate to *Stachybotrys*. Humans can be exposed to mycotoxins via ingestion of contaminated materials, but inhalation of airborne toxins has been considered a possible route of exposure (66).

Studies have examined the growth of *Stachybotrys chartarum* and its toxin production on building materials rich in cellulose in relative humidity ranging from 78% to 100% (67). *S. chartarum* is considered to be a tertiary wall colonizer that follows after growth of *Penicillium, Aspergillus,* and *Cladosporium* species. *Stachybotrys chartarum* forms spores at between 2° and 40°C, with a moisture requirement varying from 85% to 95% to allow germination, and a relative humidity of 91% to 96% to support growth and sporulation. Strains of *S. chartarum*–producing toxins have been isolated from cellulose-based agricultural materials and building materials.

High airborne CFU counts (as high as 18,000 CFU per cubic meter) have been found in indoor environments where *S. char-*

tarum contamination exists (68). However, the vast majority of these spores of *Stachybotrys* present in the air may not be viable, and culturing them is difficult. *Stachybotrys chartarum* growth on culture media can also be inhibited by species of *Penicillium*; therefore, plating of culture media for such slow-growing fungi should include CMA media.

Because mycotoxins have been found in aerosolized spores of *S. chartarum* (69), building materials—wallpaper, gypsum board, pine panel, paper, and insulating material—have also been studied for their potential nutrient source for *Stachybotrys* growth and mycotoxin production. Toxin production in these materials was verified by cytotoxicity testing (67). Wallpaper, hay, and building materials that absorb water were found to be sources of *Stachybotrys* growth. *Stachybotrys* grew on wallpaper, pine panels, and paper at a relative humidity range of 78% to 100% and on gypsum board liner and straw at a relative humidity range of 84% to 100%. No growth was seen in the insulating material in this study. *Stachybotrys* toxins were detected also in wallpaper.

Trichothecene mycotoxins identified were satrotoxin-G and satrotoxin-H and were cytotoxic in the test assay. *S. chartarum* produces other trichothecenes such as verrucarins and roridins. Trichothecenes consist of more than 60 sesquiterpenoids, which are potent protein synthesis inhibitors. Acute exposure to trichothecene mycotoxins causes damage to actively dividing bone marrow cells in the lymph node, spleen, thymus, and intestinal mucosa. Trichothecenes are immunosuppressive and immunostimulatory and include vomitoxin (deoxynivalenol, T-2 toxin, nivalenol, and diacetoxyscirpenol). Exposure to the trichothecenes, particularly T-2 toxin and diacetoxyscirpenol, increases susceptibility to infections from *Candida, Cryptococcus, Mycobacterium, Listeria*, and *Salmonella* species and from herpes simplex virus type 1. Trichothecenes impair cell-mediated immunity in animal models. They have toxicity for alveolar macrophages, and inhalation of T-2 toxin in swine results in depressed alveolar macrophage phagocytosis and response.

Health complaints registered by occupants in water-damaged buildings in which evidence of fungal contamination exists with the isolation of *Stachybotrys* have led to speculation that the illness described might be secondary to mycotoxins (23–25). Investigations of the health complaints among employees of water-damaged office buildings have been conducted in which *Stachybotrys atra* was isolated in bulk samples (26). Occupants of water-damaged buildings contaminated by heavy growth of *Stachybotrys* have complained of respiratory illnesses, neurobehavioral changes, skin and mucous membrane irritation, low-grade fever, and conjunctivitis. Thus, questions have arisen as to whether mycotoxins might have been the causative agents. A case-control study of infants in moisture-damaged building environments associated with toxigenic fungi exposure reported the infants' development of pulmonary hemosiderosis and hemorrhage (70). However, a review of the data revealed shortcomings in these studies (70a). Reviewers concluded that the evidence did not substantiate the relationship between pulmonary hemosiderosis and *Stachybotrys* or any causal connection with fungi (70a). These findings led to a revision of the New York Department of Health guidelines on fungal remediation reflecting that *Stachybotrys* was not unique among fungal contamination.

In studies of water-damaged buildings, fungi other than *Stachybotrys* often are found, including *Aspergillus, Penicillium, Fusarium, Acremonium*, and *Tritirachium* species, all of which are capable of producing mycotoxins. Of concern, though, is that *Stachybotrys* spores may contain high concentrations of mycotoxins (66). Mycotoxin production by *S. chartarum* depends on the specific mold, moisture, and temperature. Also, aerosolized conidia and conidiophores of *Stachybotrys* contain trichothecene mycotoxins (69). An analysis of extracts from filter collections of spores showed that trichothecene mycotoxins were present in aerosolized respirable conidia.

Most isolates of *S. chartarum* produce macrocyclic trichothecenes and trichoverroids such as Verrucarin-J, roridin-E, and satrotoxins-F, -G, and -H (71). A study in which dust samples were screened from the air ventilation system of office buildings affected by the so-called sick building syndrome showed evidence of trichothecene mycotoxins with a detection limit of 0.4 to 4.0 ng per mL of dust (72). Nonetheless, the isolation of a toxigenic fungus from an indoor environment does not prove exposure to mycotoxins or that health problems are due to mycotoxins.

Although airborne exposure to trichothecene mycotoxins has been suggested, this mechanism has yet to be proved to be the etiology of disease. However, studies have demonstrated that mycotoxins can be present in the conidia of *Stachybotrys* and also present in the dust of contaminated ventilation systems, so inhalational hazards exist. Dust samples collected from ventilation systems of a fungus-contaminated building studied extracts of 14 different fungal species cultured under laboratory conditions and analyzed for the presence of trichothecene mycotoxins (72). All dust extracts contained trichothecenes at concentrations detectable by high-pressure liquid chromatography. Trichothecene mycotoxins detected in these dust samples included T-2 toxin, roridin, T-2 tetraol, and diacetoxyscirpenol. The study detected similar mycotoxins from extracts of the fungi, thus connecting the presence of these fungi to the dust samples, providing direct evidence for the presence of trichothecene mycotoxins in dust samples collected from previously contaminated ventilation systems. However, in all these studies, multiple other factors such as the presence of VOCs derived from fungus and the presence of glucans, which are immunoreactive compounds, were not ruled out as confounding factors.

As mentioned, *Stachybotrys chartarum* is not alone in its production of mycotoxins. Thirty-seven percent of isolates of 503 damp and fungus-contaminated dwellings in Glasgow and Edinburgh, Scotland, were screened for cytotoxicity against the human embryonic diploid fibroblast lung cell line (73). Thirty-seven percent of the isolates of the genus *Penicillium* showed toxicity to these cell lines (73). Individuals in these dwellings reported constitutional symptoms, respiratory symptoms, headaches, fever, and fatigue. In the study of the molds found to produce mycotoxins, the penicillia were by far the greatest in number. Other isolates identified include *Aspergillus fumigatus* and *Cladosporium*.

Of some concern is that mycotoxins are stable in the environment even when fungi that produce them are dead. Thus, efforts to detect toxins might be preferred over culturing techniques. Methods used to measure mycotoxins have included gas chromatography–mass spectrometry, thin-layer chromatography, and high-pressure liquid chromatography. Cell culture–based cytotoxicity assays have also been used. Mycotoxin detection based on the inhibition of protein synthesis has been described (73). A rapid, inexpensive, and sensitive quantitative assay to assess mycotoxin presence in an environment is needed. Airborne exposure to toxigenic fungi can be estimated on the basis of culturing or spore-counting results; however, as demonstrated, *Stachybotrys chartarum* does not compete well with *Penicillium* species and other molds in culture media. Also, culturing may underestimate the concentration of mycotoxins because of the presence of nonviable spores or conidia in aerosolized samples. Spores that cannot germinate and are not viable still can contain trichothecene mycotoxins. Trichothecenes inhibit protein translocation processes in living cells, and thus an assay based on protein synthesis can be used to detect mycotoxins. Translation inhibition–based assays have been developed (73) that have shown that T-2 toxin, satrotoxin-G, and deoxynivalenol inhibit the translation of messenger RNA (74).

Whether fungi produce mycotoxins depends on a number of factors, including available nutrients and ambient conditions (75). Conversely, failure to identify mycotoxins in the culturing of mold spores does not confirm that mycotoxins were not present in the environment, because nonviable fungi (unable to grow in culture) may contain mycotoxins. Additionally, as noted earlier, some toxigenic molds, such as *Stachybotrys*, may not be detected by viable culture techniques because of their growth characteristics relative to other, more common fungi.

Whereas the effects of ingested mycotoxins on humans and animals are well described, much less is known about adverse health effects from the inhalation of mycotoxins. The potential inhalation of mycotoxins from contaminated dust and aerosolized conidia exists, but usually only low levels of mycotoxins are found in organic dusts. Nevertheless, evidence indicates that the levels of airborne aflatoxins and some other mycotoxins (secalonic acid D) may be relatively high in some occupational dust–polluted areas in which peanuts and corn are processed (76,77). Mycotoxins have also been associated with fine, respirable fractions of vegetable dusts (78). Autrup et al. (79) detected aflatoxin B_1 in the blood of the workers producing animal feed and estimated a mean level of exposure of 64 pg of aflatoxin B_1 per kg per day.

Although the presence of mycotoxins in residences and occupational environments raises questions of health concerns, speculation remains as to whether such exposure results in mycotoxin-induced disease (80,81). While mycotoxin-induced immunomodulation is a consideration in human exposure cases (82), the role of inhaled mycotoxins in the induction of human illness remains unproven and controversial. However, cause-and-effect evidence exists for production of the syndrome of pulmonary mycotoxicosis when mycotoxins are inhaled. This syndrome is similar to ODTS with the exception that acute diffuse pneumonia with infiltrates is a hallmark of pulmonary mycotoxicosis. ODTS develops in farm workers exposed to dense clouds of mold spores (including *Penicillium* and *Fusarium*) while cleaning out moldy silage (83). Some researchers have tried to link inhaled mycotoxins to chronic fatigue, sick building syndrome, and the development of cancer, but most of the supporting evidence is anecdotal or inconsistent. However, the role of aflatoxins in the development of cancer from high-dose occupational inhalation exposures (moldy peanuts or corn) has been well documented (76,84).

Aflatoxins

Aflatoxins are produced by *A. flavus* and *A. parasiticus*. They are hepatotoxins and hepatocarcinogens and exert immunomodulating effects. Aflatoxins adversely effect cell-mediated immunity in animal models (85). Aflatoxin B_1 poses a threat to the poultry industry in causing depression of delayed hypersensitivity and depression of self-mediated immunity. Cases of lung cancer and cancer of the colon have been described in people who were occupationally exposed to aflatoxin-contaminated peanut meal and to purified aflatoxin.

Volatile Organic Compounds from Fungi

Fungal contamination indoors generates low-molecular-weight, often odorous metabolites (alcohols, aldehydes, ketones, organic acids, sulfur compounds), which are released in large amounts into the air by the action of molds decomposing organic matter. As much as 1,400 to 4,000 mg per cubic meter of VOCs can be emitted from spoiled foods, and as many as 93 VOCs were identified in compost from household waste (86). Auger et al. (87) have suggested that fungal VOCs may cause chronic fatigue and other symptoms occurring in the inhabitants of sick houses. If adverse health effects can be linked to large amounts of airborne VOCs, waste-handling workers may be at risk (31,86).

Exposure to VOCs in waste-handling facilities has been identified to be three times higher than at landfill sites, with detected air concentrations measuring up to 3,000 μg per cubic meter (88). Adsorbent tube collection of VOCs revealed the following compound groups: aliphatic branched and unbranched hydrocarbons, cyclic hydrocarbons, aromatic hydrocarbons, esters, ethers, organic acids, aldehydes, ketones, alcohols, heterocyclic compounds, polyaromatic hydrocarbons, chlorinated hydrocarbons, and sulfur compounds (88).

ENDOTOXINS

Endotoxins are high-molecular-weight, heat-stable lipopolysaccharides consisting of a characteristic lipid component, the lipid A, covalently bound to a heteropolysaccharide. They are present in the outer membrane of gram-negative bacteria as heteropolymers with proteins and phospholipids and could easily be released to the surrounding dusty environment in the form of membrane disks measuring 30 to 50 nm (89). The inhaled particulate endotoxin activates alveolar macrophages and induces the release of inflammatory mediators causing fever (interleukin-1), bronchoconstriction (leukotriene C_4, prostaglandin F_2, thromboxane A_2, platelet-activating factor), and influx of neutrophils and platelets to the lung (90–93). The effects of endotoxin inhalation include endothelial alterations and increased pulmonary capillary permeability (91,94).

A correlation has been found between the concentration of endotoxins in airborne cotton dust and a decrease of forced expiratory volume over 1 second in exposed persons (90). Similar effects of endotoxins were observed in poultry farmers (95), pig farmers (96,97), brewery workers (98), and animal feed industry workers (99–101).

Respiratory exposure to endotoxins contained in aerosolized dusts can result in an acute inflammatory pulmonary response. Endotoxins on respirable particulate matter can penetrate deeply into areas such as bronchioles and alveoli. An endotoxin produces an inflammatory response once it comes into contact with pulmonary epithelium and pulmonary macrophages. Alone it has no direct toxic activity. Mediators of inflammation are released by macrophages and neutrophils that exert direct effects on the distal pulmonary tract. Clinically, exposure to endotoxins can produce acute fever, cough, dyspnea, and wheezing. Chronic exposure may result in reactive airways.

According to the International Committee on Occupational Health, clinical effects of endotoxins depend on exposure: Airborne levels of 1,000 ng per cubic meter can incite pneumonitis, whereas levels of 0.001 μg per cubic meter produce airway inflammation (102). Acute bronchoconstriction occurs at 100 to 200 ng per cubic meter, and mucous membrane irritation may occur at endotoxin levels of 20 to 50 ng per cubic meter. It was experimentally proved that endotoxins strongly stimulate the reaction of lung cells to respirable glucan (12) and fungal spores (103), potentiating their pathogenic effects.

ORGANIC DUSTS

Organic dusts represent a wide variety of microorganisms, antigens, particles, pollens, spores, and other biologically active components that can be inhaled. ODTS presents with a clinical picture similar (but not identical) to that of HP (104). Malaise,

TABLE 97-14. Fungi and actinomycetes isolated from airborne grain dust (1×10^3–10^6 CFU/m^3)

Alternaria spp.	*Saccharomonospora viridis*
Aspergillus candidus	*Saccharopolyspora rectivirgula*
Aspergillus flavus	*Streptomyces* spp.
Aspergillus fumigatus	*Thermoactinomyces* spp.
Aureobasidium, yeast	*Thermomonospora curvata*
Cladosporium spp.	*Verticillium* spp.
Eurotium spp.	*Wallemia* spp.
Penicillium spp.	

CFU, colony-forming units.

myalgia, fever, chills, dry cough, dyspnea, headache, and nausea occur 4 to 8 hours after exposure to high levels of organic dusts containing biological contaminants. Symptoms typically begin the first day of the work exposure week, often resolve as the week progresses, and recur the first day of the next workweek (assuming constant exposure). ODTS findings may vary from this "Monday fever" pattern when endotoxin exposure is either constant (e.g., residential) or irregular (e.g., exposure at the workplace or at locations other than one's own home).

ODTS differs from HP in that the pulmonary symptoms are less pronounced; chest radiographs usually do not show infiltrates; lung function may demonstrate transient, mild, reversible airway disease (even in nonasthmatics)—in contrast to restrictive disease—along with normal gas exchange; serum precipitins are absent and the cellular infiltrate is neutrophilic, not lymphocytic; and pulmonary granulomas do not develop. Progressive lung disease, even with repeated antigen exposure, is rare, with the exception of byssinosis, an ODTS-like disorder that develops in cotton workers in correlation with airborne endotoxin levels (94).

Organic dust frequently contains not only gram-negative bacteria and endotoxin but mold, mycotoxins, and other biological contaminants. Fungi have been recovered from bronchioalveolar lavage fluid (105) and open lung biopsy (83) in patients with ODTS, and glucans present in the cell wall of fungi and *Actinomycetes* have been implicated as the causative agents. Because Malmberg et al. (106) found no correlation between endotoxin levels in organic dust and febrile reactions, they proposed that spores from mold and the actinomycetes themselves could be causing these reactions.

Airborne microorganisms or biological contaminants contained in organic dust may alter the function of alveolar macrophages (107). The common event in organic dust exposure is inflammation and alveolitis, with an influx of various inflammatory cells to the epithelial surface of the airway. The alveolar macrophage is the first cell to phagocytose inhaled organic dusts after an exposure. One study demonstrated that microbial by-products were able to attract macrophages and polymorphonuclear leukocytes directly in a dose-dependent manner and can stimulate release of chemotactic factors from inflammatory cells (107). Tables 97-14 through 97-16 list some of the fungi and bacteria found in airborne grain dusts and their concentrations.

TABLE 97-15. Bacterial taxa consistently isolated from airborne grain dust

Gram-negative spp., rods
- *Enterobacter agglomerans*
- *Pseudomonas corrugata*
- *Pseudomonas diminuta*
- *Pseudomonas fluorescens*
- *Pseudomonas glycosyles*
- *Pseudomonas maltophilia*
- *Pseudomonas marginalis*
- *Pseudomonas testosteroni*

Gram-positive spp.
- Rods
  - *Bacillus licheniformis*
  - *Bacillus subtilis*
- Coccal rods
  - *Curtobacterium* spp.
- Cocci
  - *Micrococcus* spp.
  - *Staphylococcus cohnii*
  - *Staphylococcus epidermidis*
  - *Staphylococcus xylosus*

Adapted from ref. 131.

INFECTIOUS DISEASES

Microbial pathogens can be transmitted indoors via respiratory droplets or aerosol droplets that harbor microorganisms. One infectious agent from an environmental source is *Legionella* bacteria, which can be transmitted by a contaminated ventilation system or hot-water system, including showers and spas. *Legionella* pneumonia is a common form of community-acquired infection. The incidence in the United States is approximately 12 per 100,000 each year. Hot water in whirlpools, spas, water faucets, shower heads, and cooling towers of ventilation systems are common *Legionella* sources.

Tuberculosis infections can be acquired by airborne routes. Risk of infectious disease transmission increases with poor indoor air quality. Crowding, moisture damage, and inadequate ventilation help to disseminate infectious microorganisms.

Nontuberculous mycobacteria are recognized as causes of opportunistic infections in immunocompromised individuals. Nontuberculous mycobacteria, the most common isolate being *N. nycigebucyn*, have been detected in ice and public drinking water samples (108). Thus, water may be a route of infection or colonization of these mycobacterial species. Nontuberculous mycobacteria have emerged as a major cause of opportunistic infection in acquired immunodeficiency syndrome (AIDS) patients, the main organism being *Mycobacterium avium*, and such infections are second to AIDS wasting syndrome as a cause of death in these patients (108). In this study, nontuberculous mycobacteria were isolated from 38% of all drinking water samples from a wide geographic area, thus identifying a potential serious environmental source of opportunistic infection (108).

Infections secondary to building sites became recognized with the advent of Legionnaire's disease in 1976. This disease was traced to aerosolization of the bacteria from cooling towers, humidifiers, and evaporative condensers within buildings. The incubation period for *Legionella* pneumonia is 5 to 6 days. The *Legionella* organism is present in soils, and its dissemination from ventilation and cooling systems can be controlled by using a biocide in the cooling system. Another disease associated with the *Legionella* bacterium is Pontiac fever. This disease was described in an epidemic of 144 cases in Michigan in 1968.

Other agents of infection that can be transmitted within indoor air environments include a variety of viruses, bacteria, fungi, and rickettsial organisms. The rickettsia *Coxiella burnetii*, which causes Q fever, has been discovered in ventilation systems in proximity to housing facilities for infected sheep, goats,

TABLE 97-16. Fungi found in airborn grain dust

Sample	Concentration (CFU/m³)				
	Total No.	*Penicillium*	*Cladosporium*	*Alternaria*	*Verticillium*
Barley harvest					
Inside combine	1.4×10^5	2.1×10^3	1.0×10^5	2.1×10^4	2.1×10^3
In field downwind	2.7×10^5	0	8.7×10^4	1.1×10^5	2.7×10^3
Wheat harvest					
Outside combine	9.2×10^6	0	2.2×10^6	4.9×10^6	0
Inside combine	3.3×10^4	0	1.6×10^4	1.5×10^4	0
In grain store	3.7×10^5	9.3×10^4	5.9×10^4	1.8×10^5	0
By dresser	8.3×10^5	3.3×10^5	3.3×10^5	8.3×10^4	0
Stored grain					
Moving old wheat	3.6×10^5	3.6×10^5	9.5×10^2	9.6×10^2	0
Milling	2.7×10^5	2.2×10^3	5.9×10^3	4.0×10^4	0

CFU, colony-forming units.
Adapted from ref. 131.

or other animals. Q fever can manifest as fever, chills, headache, myalgia, pneumonia, hepatitis and, occasionally, endocarditis.

A variety of other febrile and coryza-related illnesses can be associated with recirculation of stale air or contaminated air. Outbreaks of febrile illness related to indoor environments have been documented in a variety of studies. An outbreak of febrile illness in Knoxville, Tennessee, in 1981 involved 40% of 325 office workers in a seven-story building. The individuals experienced headaches, myalgia, fever, chills, cough, or wheezing. A temporal relationship was observed between starting the heating, ventilation, and cooling (HVAC) system and the onset of symptoms in these individuals.

Another illness in 1982 was identified in Washington, DC, among the occupants of a large office building. Twelve of 41 employees experienced headache, myalgia, chest tightness, fever, chills, or nausea while within the work environment and relief on weekends. Numerous microorganisms were isolated from the HVAC system.

HP, humidifier fever, and other allergic manifestations of disease that have included symptoms of fever, chills, myalgia, and headache have been identified since the 1970s. Most of these outbreaks have been attributed to thermophilic actinomycetes, a variety of fungi, and endotoxins. Sources of the microbial contamination were mainly contaminated ventilation systems and air-handling units. The infectious agents can be divided into three major subgroups: (i) human sources, (ii) animal sources, and (iii) environmental sources.

Human Sources of Infectious Agents

Human sources of infectious agents include pathogenic bacteria, viruses, and infectious fungi. Hepatitis A, B, and C are examples of viral infectious agents. Other important agents include *Mycobacterium tuberculosis*, rubella virus, respiratory syncytial virus, herpes simplex virus, influenza viruses, *Salmonella* and *Staphylococcus aureus*, *Streptococcus pneumonia*, *Haemophilus influenzae*, *E. coli*, and *Klebsiella pseudommas* (109,110). *Helicobacter pylori*, a bacterium causing gastric ulcer, has recently been implicated as an occupational hazard for medical workers performing gastroendoscopy (111).

Animal Sources of Infectious Agents (Zoonoses)

Zoonotic diseases are transmitted from animals to humans. They are primarily occupational in origin (112). This group comprises approximately 50 agents indigenous to domestic and wild mammals and birds. Workers in occupations resulting in increased exposure to these zoonotic agents include farmers, animal breeders, laboratory workers, veterinarians, forestry workers, and workers processing animal carcasses and products (meat, skins, hair, feathers). Viruses (Orf, foot-and-mouth disease, vesicular stomatitis, Newcastle disease, rabies, and other viruses), bacteria (*Coxiella burnetii*, *Chlamydia psittaci*, *Leptospira interrogans*, *Brucella abortus*, *B. suis*, *B. melitensis*, *Francisella tularensis*, *Bacillus anthracis*, *Listeria monocytogenes*, *Erysipelothrix rhusiopathiae*, *Mycobacterium bovis*, etc.), fungi (*Trichophyton verrucosum*, *T. mentagrophytes*), and protozoans (*Toxoplasma gondii*) are commonly implicated (112).

Recent additions to this list of agents causing occupational zoonoses have been hemorrhagic fever viruses, Junin virus, *Sin Nombre*, and Hantavirus (Hantaan and Puumala viruses) transmitted from rodents to agricultural and laboratory workers, mainly in Asia, Europe, and South America (113); the gram-negative bacterium *Campylobacter jejuni*, transmitted from poultry to farmers (114); and *Streptococcus suis*, transmitted from pigs to farmers (115).

Also being considered are two other potential zoonotic hazards for animal breeders: transmission of prions that cause bovine spongiform encephalopathy ("mad cow disease"), which, in humans, may lead to contraction of Creutzfeldt-Jakob disease (116), and agents that cause chronic lymphocytic leukemias and low-grade non-Hodgkin's lymphomas, diseases very common among animal farmers (117). Although these threats are not proved, they certainly raise concern.

Many zoonotic agents of occupational concern are transmitted by invertebrates. Tick-borne encephalitis virus and the spiral bacterium *Borrelia burgdorferi*, which causes Lyme disease, pose a well-documented occupational risk for forestry workers (118–120), whereas the transmission by trombiculid mites of an agent of scrub typhus (*Rickettsia tsutsugamushi*) presents a risk for agricultural workers in Asia (121).

Vector-borne parasites pose a threat for agricultural workers and fishers, particularly those working in paddy rice fields, in warm climatic zones. The most important of these disease-causing agents are *Plasmodium* protozoans, transmitted by mosquitos and causing malaria; liver flukes of the genus *Schistosoma*, transmitted by water snails and causing systemic schistosomiasis and cercarial dermatitis; and the nematode *Onchocerca volvulus*, transmitted by blackflies of the genus *Simulium* in central Africa and causing river blindness (122,123).

American cutaneous leishmaniasis is an anthropozoonosis caused by a protozoan, *Leishmania*, the vector of which is the insect

Phlebotomus (124). This protozoan disease affects humans and wild and domestic animals in hot, undeveloped areas of the world. American cutaneous leishmaniasis is characterized by parasitization of mononuclear phagocytic cells and cutaneous lesions at the point of parasite inoculation. Leishmaniasis manifests different grades of severity and has a high incidence. The disease follows two epidemiologic patterns: epidemic outbreaks associated with deforestation via zoonosis of wild animals and zoonosis from domesticated animals (usually dogs, horses, and rodents) (124). Transmission occurs via a bite by *Phlebotomus* (*Psychodopygus, Lutzomyia*) species, which hide in dark, humid places during the hot daylight hours and are active at night. Only the female is hematophagous. Bites occur on uncovered areas of skin, inoculating the protozoa. The incubation phase lasts 1 to 12 months, during which the parasite multiplies as mastigote forms. Leishmanial lesions appear to herald the disease. The area of American cutaneous leishmaniasis incidence extends from south of the United States to north Argentina (124). Dogs and horses are the only animals that display infection, and treatment is with antimonials (124).

Environmental Sources of Infectious Agents

Environmental sources of infectious agents include viruses, bacteria, and protozoa present in sewage, water, and geophilic fungi (125). Important agents include *L. pneumophila*, nontuberculous mycobacterium, *Cryptosporidium, Giardia lamblia, Salmonella, Shigella, Blastomyces, Histoplasma*, and *Coccidioides*. The gram-negative bacterium *Legionella pneumophila* grows in water at the temperature range of 20° to 50°C and can cause legionellosis in workers maintaining water systems at power plants and on oil-drilling platforms and in immunocompromised patients exposed to contaminant sources (126,127). The related species *Legionella longbeachae*, recovered from potting soils in Australia, may pose a potential hazard for gardeners and plant-keepers (128).

The yeastlike geophilic fungi (*Coccidioides immitis, Histoplasma capsulatum, Sporothrix schenckii*, and *Blastomyces dermatitidis*) present in soil, decayed wood, and other vegetable matter may cause mycoses in agricultural workers, gardeners, woodworkers, miners, construction workers, and archeologists (129). Fungi of human pathogenic importance are (i) *anthropophilic* fungi (those able to grow only on humans, for which infection transmission occurs from person to person), (ii) *zoophilic* fungi (transmissible from animals to humans and cause of diseases in animals that can be transmitted to humans), and (iii) *geophilic* fungi (species whose natural habitat is soil and decomposing organic matter and that, under some conditions, may cause disease in humans) (130).

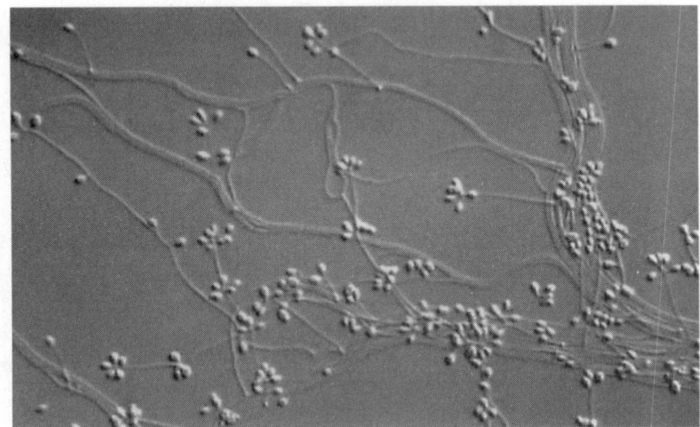

Figure 97-8. *Sporothrix schenckii.*

Geophilic and zoophilic fungi are known to cause skin disease in farmers. Among zoophilic fungi that cause skin infections are *Trichophyton* species (*T. mentagrophytes, T. erinacei, T. verrucosum, T. equinum, T. quinckeanum, T. simii, Microsporum canis, M. persicolor, M. equinum, M. nanum, M. gallinae*). Farmers can be infected in the work environment from cattle, horses, and sheep. Infections of *Microsporum canis* have occurred from a cat (Fig. 97-7). Other geophilic (soil) fungi of clinical importance are *Microsporum gypseum, M. flavum*, and *Sporothrix schenckii* (130). Sporotrichosis, a fungal skin infection caused by *Sporothrix schenckii* (Fig. 97-8), is a risk for gardeners, florists, and foresters. A case of lymphocutaneous sporotrichosis among moss producers has been described (130). *Acremonium, Fusarium*, and *Aspergillus* sometimes are cultured from nail infections (130).

Yeast fungi can also cause infections. One of the best-known to do so is *Candida albicans* (Fig. 97-9). High concentrations of *Candida* are found in manured soil (130). *Candida* species are also normal flora of the mouth, gastrointestinal tract, and vagina and also colonize the skin in some instances. Factors that lead to occupational infection by *Candida* are working with wet hands, working under high temperatures, and handling material having a high sugar content (130). Blastomycosis is caused by the geophilic fungus *Blastomyces dermatitidis* (Fig. 97-10). Blastomycosis may be transferred to humans from dogs, cats, and horses (130). Thus, it is both a geophilic and a zoophilic infectious disease.

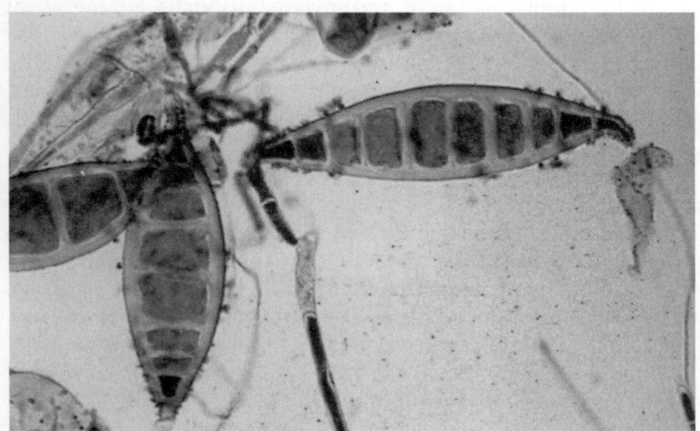

Figure 97-7. *Microsporum canis* infection transmitted by a cat.

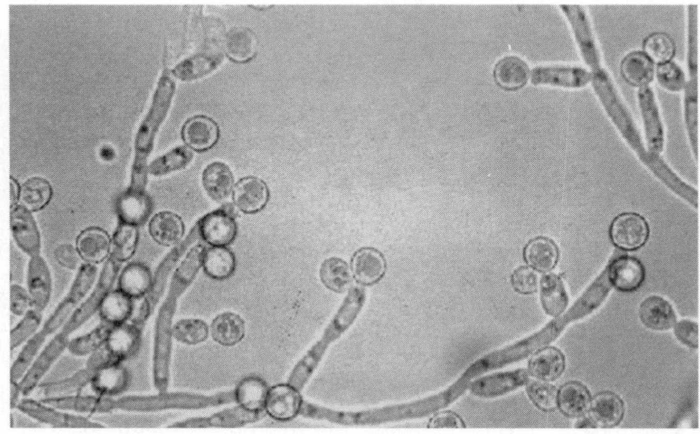

Figure 97-9. *Candida albicans.*

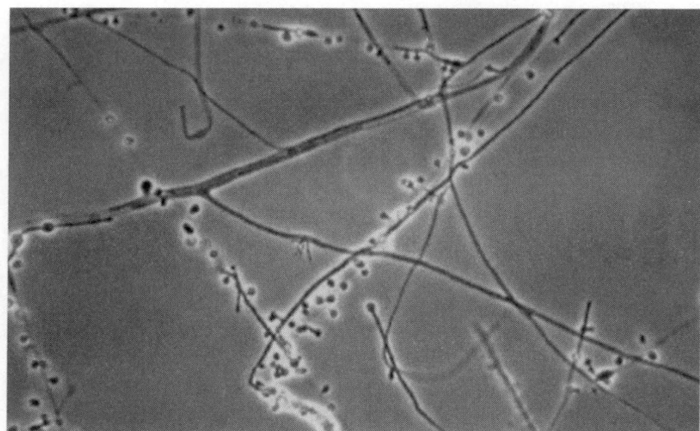

Figure 97-10. The geophilic fungus *Blastomyces dermatitidis.*

Respiratory disorders, often associated with fever, are common among agricultural workers during silo unloading, hay making, handling of grain, and work in animal confinement buildings, which are associated with exposure to high concentrations of organic dusts (more than 10 mg per cubic meter), endotoxins (more than 1.0 μg per cubic meter), and microorganisms (more than 10^5 CFU per cubic meter) (131).

The incidence of work-related symptoms (dyspnea, cough, chest tightness, chills, fever) in people exposed during such jobs has been estimated to be as high as 40% to 75% of the total working population (132,133). Farmers showing symptoms of ODTS or HP have been exposed during work to significantly higher amounts of airborne microorganisms than have those who are asymptomatic (134).

The prevalence of respiratory symptoms may be high also in industry workers processing certain plant and animal materials and in laboratory animal care workers (133–137). Airborne allergenic or toxic biohazards may be a cause of HP (allergic alveolitis, granulomatous pneumonitis), allergic rhinitis, asthma, byssinosis, ODTS (toxin fever, grain fever, silo unloader's syndrome, inhalation fever, toxic pneumonitis), humidifier fever, chronic bronchitis (136–140), and disorders related to sick buildings. Disease symptoms are thought to be caused by inflammatory reactions of lung cells to inhaled biological agents (138). The process usually begins with the activation of alveolar macrophages, which release cytokines and chemotoxins attracting neutrophils and platelets, which, in turn, secrete other inflammatory mediators. Other pathogenic pathways include activation of complement, sensitization of T lymphocytes, and mast cell activation by the interaction of mast cell–bound IgE and specific antibody in allergic asthma.

Dermatitis can be caused by allergic reactions to factors in organic dusts (urticaria, contact dermatitis, and eczema) and by local inflammatory reactions to toxic plant contact (dermatitis phytogenes) or to bites of insects, mites, and ticks.

INSECTS AND DUST MITES

In addition to pollens and molds, a frequent component of house dust is the dust mite, an arachnid that grows readily at moderate temperatures and high relative humidity (e.g., 25°C and relative humidity in excess of 60%) (141). In addition to water, its other major nutrient is human skin scale. Consequently, dust mite allergen can most frequently be found in the dust in bedroom and bathroom carpets; in bedding, pillows, and mattresses; and in upholstered furniture.

Although several different types of dust mites can be found in house dust, the major contributing species are *Dermatophagoides pteronyssinus* and *Dermatophagoides farinae* and their respective major allergens, *Der p* I and *Der f* I. These major allergens are found predominantly in fecal particles but can also be found in the mite bodies. Guidelines for the significance of dust mite concentrations in house dust have been derived from studies showing that certain threshold levels will predict the risk of sensitization in predisposed individuals. Clear-cut dose-response relationships for dust mite allergen are much less clear, as is the case for most allergens that we measure in the air.

Many factors affect the sensitized individual response to allergen, including his or her current state of health and recent exposures to relevant allergens, which may already have resulted in increased sensitivity or reactivity. Allergen measurement guidelines derive from studies correlating house dust allergen levels with asthma development or symptoms. Recommended guidelines for the dust mite allergen *Der p* I/g or *Der f* I/g of dust are as follows (141,142):

Low:	<2 μg per gram of dust
Significant:	2 to 10 μg per gram of dust
High:	>10 μg per gram of dust

Insect allergens from moths, midges, houseflies, crickets, locusts, fleas, and beetles have been associated with inhalant allergy. However, cockroach is the only insect that has been carefully studied. Although many species of cockroaches exist, the most commonly found species worldwide associated with the production of IgE is *Blattella germanica* (German cockroach). Two major allergens have been identified for *B germanica*: *Bla g* I and *Bla g* II. Two other allergenic species commonly found are *Periplaneta americana* (American cockroach) and *Blattella orientalis* (Oriental cockroach). Significant antigenic cross-reactivity can be demonstrated between cockroach species. Concentrations of cockroach antigen typically are very low in suburban homes (less than 1 unit *Bla g* II per gram of dust) and quite high in urban crowded housing (greater than 10 units *Bla g* II per gram of dust), paralleling the prevalence of cockroach sensitization and asthma in suburban versus crowded urban environments (143,144). These data suggest that cockroach antigen levels of less than 1 unit of *Bla g* II per gram of dust are not likely to sensitize and that concentrations exceeding 10 units *Bla g* II per gram of dust are likely to trigger asthma in cockroach-sensitive asthmatics and to sensitize those who are genetically predisposed.

ANIMAL PROTEINS

Although many animal allergens clearly induce specific IgE and produce allergic hypersensitivity, to date, a readily available assay for indoor assessment of animal antigen levels has been developed only for the cat. Cat allergens can be found in most homes, even those that are not currently housing a cat indoors. Suggested levels for the predominant allergen in cats, *Fel d* I/g dust, are as follows (145):

Low:	<1 μg per gram of dust
Moderate:	1 to 8 μg per gram of dust
High:	>8 μg per gram of dust

Levels of *Fel d* I as low as 2 μg per gram of dust may be a risk factor for sensitization (146).

BACTERIA

For indoor environments, the American Conference of Governmental Hygienists has suggested a maximum total bacterial concentration of 1,000 CFU per cubic meter as indicative of poor air quality (147). *Staphylococcus* species, *B. subtilis,* and *Micrococcus* predominate and originate from human skin scales and respiratory secretions. Excessive quantities of these bacteria indoors may indicate overcrowding or inadequate ventilation. In agricultural environments, dust may contain greater than 1×10^5 CFU per cubic meter of bacteria.

Legionella species frequently contaminate water reservoirs indoors and must be present in high concentrations and in the presence of a relevant human illness to be of clinical significance. Serotyping can assist with establishing a cause-and-effect link between *Legionella* present in the environment and disease. Because of its potential for causing pneumonia, concentrations of this contaminant in water sources should be kept to a minimum.

When large quantities of gram-negative bacteria are found in the presence of illness patterns that may be associated with endotoxins, assaying for endotoxins is indicated. If endotoxins are found in quantities of at least 100 times background levels, cause and effect are likely (147). A finding of any pathologic bacteria, such as *Pseudomonas* or thermophilic actinomycetes, indicates contamination.

VIRUSES

Because viral illnesses are so common and because most viral illnesses are spread by close airborne (respiratory secretions) or contact transmission, indoor assessment for the presence of viruses rarely is undertaken. Airborne transmission by contaminated HVAC systems has been established for a few outbreaks of viral illness [e.g., measles (148,149), varicella (150), and influenza (151)].

Animals residing indoors have been identified as vectors for human illness: For instance, African green monkeys may transmit Marburg viral disease (152), and rodents have been known to transmit Hantavirus (153) and Lassa fever (154). However, overcrowding and inadequate ventilation (inadequate clearing of aerosolized microbes) remain the most likely factors facilitating viral infection. The presence of susceptible populations (e.g., young children, the elderly, and those who are immunosuppressed) also increases the likelihood of infection.

PROTOZOA

Pathogenic protozoa can be found in numerous environmental sources. Indoor sources are rare but, when found, indicate contamination. Two protozoan genera have been associated with building-related illness: *Acanthamoeba* species and *Naegleria* species. Other protozoa that cause human disease are *Entamoeba histolytica, Giardia lamblia, Cryptosporidium* species, *Entamoeba polecki, Balantidium coli, Blastocystis hominis*, and *Trypanosoma cruzi* (Chagas' disease).

Cryptosporidium has received much attention as a cause of diarrhea from contaminated water sources. *Cryptosporidium* develops in the gastrointestinal tract of vertebrates through its life cycle. Other similar protozoa include *Eimeria, Isospora*, and *Cyclospora*. *Cryptosporidium parvum* is zoonotic, lacking host specificity among mammals, and is spread from animals to humans and from humans to humans. Generally, species isolated from one class of vertebrates are not infectious for animals of another class. This is not the case with *Cryptosporidium parvum* though. *Cryptosporidium parvum* is prevalent in young calves worldwide, which animals serve as a reservoir (155).

Cryptosporidium is a protozoan parasite, and the illness cryptosporidiosis begins with ingestion of the reproductive oocyst in contaminated drinking water. The protozoon then continues its life cycle in the gastrointestinal tract. *Cryptosporidium* can be transmitted via the oral-fecal route, by food handlers, and by children in day-care centers. Cryptosporidiosis can be caused by 10 to 25 oocysts that invade systemically. The disease lasts 2 to 10 days, and symptoms include abdominal cramping, fever, and diarrhea. The disease may also manifest as chronic diarrhea. Immunosuppressed individuals, children, and the elderly are more susceptible to cryptosporidiosis than are other populations.

Clinical cryptosporidiosis presents with watery, mucoid diarrhea. Dehydration is common. Abdominal cramping, fever, nausea, and vomiting occur. Diagnosis requires laboratory tests to detect the parasite or specific antigens in bodily fluids. Immunofluorescent assays and enzyme immunoassays are available to detect antigens and oocysts. Immunocompromised individuals are at high risk from infection. Also, extraintestinal sites (e.g., pulmonary system and gallbladder in AIDS patients) might be involved.

Sources of *Cryptosporidium* include human and animal waste in runoff water or other waste streams. Oocyst density in water may be increased by storms or heavy rains and snow that wash through watershed land contaminated with sewage and animal waste.

Cryptosporidium removal from drinking water is more difficult than is removal of *Giardia* because the organism is smaller, has a lower sedimentation rate, and is resistant to chlorination. Decreased water turbidity and filtration of particles less than 15 μm in diameter correlate with detection of *Cryptosporidium* in water supplies. Detecting *Cryptosporidium* in water supplies can be difficult, and ingestion of only a few oocysts is necessary to cause illness. Oocysts (0.003 to 4.74 oocysts per L) have been found in 6% to 87% of untreated surface waters sampled and in 4% to 40% of drinking water samples (0.002 to 0.015 oocysts per L). Aside from supportive care, no treatment is known.

Giardiasis begins with the ingestion of cysts in contaminated water or food. These cysts are triggered to become encysted by the acidic gastric pH of stomach fluids. The trophozoite stage is killed by the acidic pH of the stomach. Usually, the trophozoite will emerge in the duodenum and divide and colonize the small intestines, bile duct, and gallbladder. The incubation period is approximately 2 weeks. Clinical signs and symptoms consist of diarrhea, weakness, weight loss, dehydration, nausea, abdominal cramps, flatulence, fever, vomiting, belching, greasy stools, and abdominal distention. Treatment consists of rehydration plus metronidazole or quinacrine. *Giardia* are fairly resistant to water chlorination.

Cyclospora cayetanensis (cyanobacterium) was first recognized to cause human infections in 1977. *Cyclospora* is a parasite usually transmitted to humans by the fecal-oral route via oocysts. An outbreak was reported in South Carolina in 1996 (9) in association with consumption of raspberries (156). The incubation period is 1 week and may be followed by gastrointestinal symptoms and watery diarrhea. The *Cyclospora* oocyst measures 8 to 10 μm in diameter, twice the size of *Cryptosporidium* oocysts. The infection is treated with a 7-day course of trimethoprim-sulfamethoxazole.

GRAM-NEGATIVE BACTERIA

Numerous gram-negative bacteria of plant origin represent potential respiratory hazards as a source of endotoxins and allergens. The most well known among them is the epiphytic species *Pantoea agglomerans* (synonyms: *Erwinia herbicola, Enterobacter agglomerans*) (157,158). Bacteria belonging to this species are yellow-chromogenic, facultatively anaerobic, fermentative rods with peritrichous flagella (Fig. 97-11). They grow on a variety of plants and plant products and are common on grain and on cotton, in grain and cotton dusts (146,159,160), and in the air of grain stores and cotton mill carding rooms (161). *Pantoea agglomerans* produces endotoxins that have been identified as a cause of acute byssinosis symptoms (162) and allergens that may be a cause of allergic alveolitis or asthma (158,163,164).

Other gram-negative species that occur commonly in organic dusts and represent a potential risk for exposed persons belong

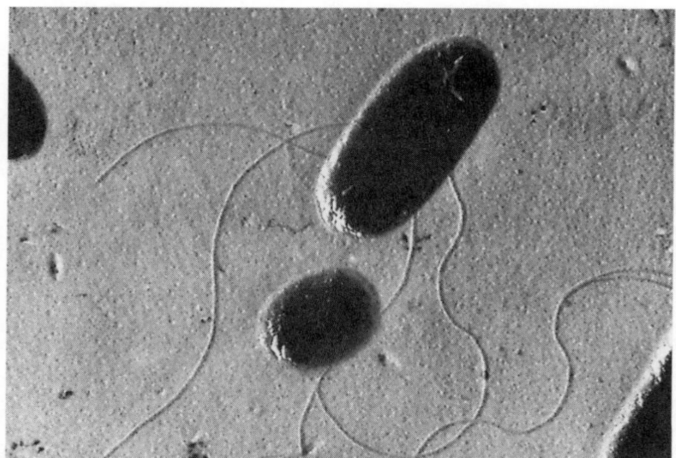

Figure 97-11. *Erwinia herbicola*, also known as *Enterobacter agglomerans* (30,000×). (Courtesy of Dr. B. Ochalska, Laboratory of Electron Microscopy, School of Medicine, Krakow, Poland.)

to the following genera: *Pseudomonas, Klebsiella, Alcaligenes, Acinetobacter, Citrobacter,* and *Enterobacter* (157–159,161,165). Droplet aerosol from humidifiers and sewage may contain toxins of *Cytophaga allerginae, Pseudomonas, Flavobacterium, Klebsiella, Enterobacter, Citrobacter, Acinetobacter, Serratia,* and *Aeromonas hydrophila* (158,166–168). Oil mist in machine industry settings contains numerous gram-negative bacteria, mainly of the genus *Pseudomonas* (169), which may cause respiratory disease in exposed workers (170).

THERMOPHILIC ACTINOMYCETES

Actinomycetes are a group of gram-positive bacteria that resemble fungi because they produce mycelium and spores. Actinomycete spores are present in biological aerosols of agricultural and waste-composting environments. The spores of actinomycetes are of three types: arthrospores, aleuriospores, and endospores. Spore production and release into air is required in order for a health hazard to exist. Spore aerosolization is enhanced by physical disturbance. The microorganism is found as a contaminant in moisture-damaged buildings. Airborne spores of various actinomycete species (*Saccharopolyspora rectivirgula, Micropolyspora faeni, Thermoactinomyces vulgaris,* and *Streptomyces albus*) can cause allergic alveolitis (171). *Streptomyces* species stimulate pulmonary macrophages and cause release of inflammatory mediators.

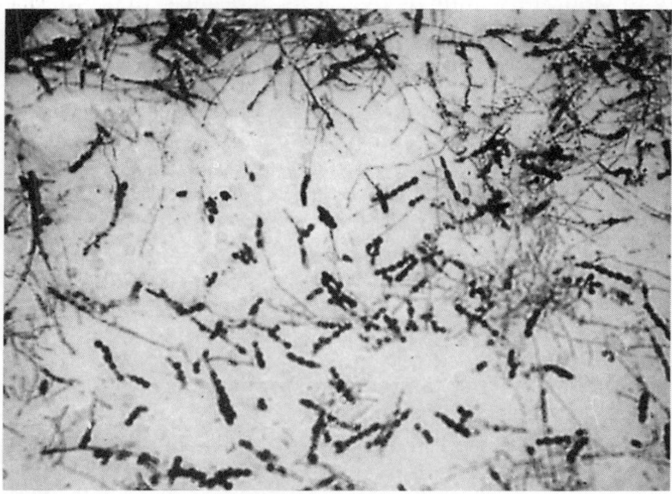

Figure 97-12. *Micropolyspora faeni* (1,500×).

The actinomycete *Saccharopolyspora rectivirgula* (synonyms: *Micropolyspora faeni, Faenia rectivirgula*) has been identified as a main source of the allergen causing farmer's lung disease, a form of HP. The organisms grow in the form of branching filaments (Fig. 97-12), chains of small spherical spores (0.7 to 1.3 μm in diameter). They develop in damp, self-heating plant materials such as hay. During handling of moldy hay, large amounts of spores are released into the air and, after inhalation by an individual, the spores may initiate cell-mediated or precipitin-mediated allergic reaction in the lung.

Thermoactinomyces vulgaris and *Thermoactinomyces thalpophilus* are other thermophilic species involved in the etiology of farmer's lung disease. The spores are formed singly, directly on filaments. The biological features of these organisms are similar to those of *S. rectivirgula.* The relative species *Thermoactinomyces sacchari* has been identified as a cause of bagassosis, the form of HP caused by inhalation of dust from bagasse (extracted sugar cane).

BASIDIOMYCETOUS FUNGI

Spores of rust (*Puccinia graminis*) and of smuts (*Ustilago, Tilletia*) are considered to be important aeroallergens that may be a cause of rhinitis, asthma, and conjunctivitis in farmers, millers, workers of granaries, and other exposed persons.

PLANT ALLERGENS AND PLANT DUST

Mucous membrane irritation or conjunctivitis can be caused by biological aerosols. Systemic reactions can be induced by stings or bites of venomous animals such as spiders, ray fish, and snakes.

Wind-borne pollen grains measure 14 to 60 μm in diameter and are found in variable concentrations outdoors, depending on the season. At times, pollen may be found indoors from passive infiltration and, less often, from entrainment in HVAC systems. Although the onset of seasonal allergic rhinitis symptoms has been associated with levels as low as 20 grass pollen grains per cubic meter, the many variables that determine exposure, sensitivity, and clinical response do not permit establishment of a threshold level for induction of symptoms and, hence, risk.

The flower pollens of grasses, weeds, and trees are well-known aeroallergens that may cause allergic rhinitis (pollinosis), asthma, and airborne dermatitis in sensitive persons. Symptoms of pollinosis are observed during flowering season in a wide range of urban and rural populations, but it is assumed that these aeroallergens pose a significant risk to certain professionals whose occupations afford them increased exposure (i.e., farmers, orchard workers, gardeners, greenhouse workers, florists, botanists) (172). The concentration of pollen in the air is greatly influenced by weather conditions. Solomon (173) reported a threshold level of 20 grains of Bermuda grass pollen per cubic meter of air for the induction of allergy symptoms in a sensitized individual. However, even lower levels may trigger allergy symptoms in a highly sensitive individual or one who has been primed by exposure to other relevant allergens.

A number of cultivated and wild growing plants produce toxins (alkaloids, glycosides, toxalbumins, photosensitizing substances, volatile oils, resins) and allergens. These may affect gardeners, farmers, herb processors, pharmacists, cooks, and salespersons by direct skin contact or by air, causing dermatitis or respiratory irritation. The best-known allergenic plants include bean, celery, capsicum, carrot, and okra (*Hibiscus esculentus*), various decorative plants (tulips, hyacinth, chrysanthemum, buttercups, *Scilla, Euphorbia, Dieffenbachia, Laportea, Ficus benjamina*, etc.), common rue (*Ruta graveolens*), castor bean (*Rici-*

nus communis), soapwort (*Saponaria officinalis*), vanilla, and poison ivy (*Toxicodendron radicans*) (174,175). Colophony (rosin), a solid substance obtained by distillation of pine resin and used as a solder flux or as an additive to glues and other products, can cause occupational asthma in electronics workers exposed to soldering fumes and contact dermatitis in other workers (176). Latex proteins from sap of rubber trees (e.g., *Hevea brasiliensis*) may cause dermal or systemic allergy in health care workers who wear gloves containing this substance.

The pathogenic effects of the dusts released from crushed or pulverized plant materials may be due to the associated microbial antigens and to specific allergens of plant origin. Various allergic disorders (asthma, rhinitis, conjunctivitis, urticaria) have been observed in workers exposed to dusts from tea, coffee, rice, herbs, and buckwheat; to "Maiko" dust from the tuberous root of devil's tongue (*Amorphophallus konjac*), cultivated in Japan; to powdered plant tissues used as drugs (psyllium, ipecac, isphagula); and to plant proteases (papain, bromelain) (177,178). Respirable dust from esparto grass (*Stipa tenacissima*) causes stipatosis, a specific form of HP (179). Recently, the possible role of the tannin component of cotton in evoking respiratory symptoms from exposure to cotton dust has been suggested (180).

Wood dust exposure appears to be linked to the occurrence of adenocarcinoma of the nasal sinuses. The incidence of this disease is approximately 1,000-fold greater in woodworkers than in other people (181). Exposure to dust from certain woods may cause dermatitis, rhinitis, conjunctivitis, and asthma (182). The greatest risk for asthma is posed by exotic woods and western red cedar (*Thuja plicata*), which contains plicatic acid, a low-molecular-weight allergen (182). Other allergenic woods include walnuts, locusts, and pines.

ARTHROPODS

Allergenic particles of the processed prawn (*Nephrops norvegicus*) and snow crab (*Chionoecetes opilio*) may cause hypersensitivity lung disease in exposed workers producing seafood (183). Occupational asthma has also been reported in individuals preparing feed for aquarium fishes from dried small crustaceans *Daphnia* species and *Artemia salina* (184).

Ticks (*Ixodidae, Argasidae*) and certain species of spiders (*Latrodectus*) and mites (*Dermanyssus gallinae, Ornithonyssus bacoti, Pyemotes ventricosus, Neotrombicula autumnalis, Leptotrombidium akamushi*) may cause local inflammatory reactions (184,185). Allergens of acarid mites (*Acarus siro, Tyrophagus putrescentiae, Lepidoglyphus destructor, Glycyphagus domesticus*) feeding on stored products (hay, grain) may cause respiratory and nasal symptoms in exposed farmworkers (186). Pest mites feeding on plants (*Tetranychus urticae, Panonychus ulmi*) cause allergy in agricultural workers, gardeners, orchard workers, and pest control unit workers (185,187). The latter category of workers may be additionally sensitized to predatory arthropods (e.g., the mite *Phytoseiulus persimilis*) that are reared for biological pest control (187). Two species of pyroglyphid mites—*Dermatophagoides pteronyssinus* and *Dermatophagoides farinae*—live in indoor environments, particularly homes, and feed on human dander. They can reach high concentrations in carpets and bedding, especially in the presence of excessive moisture. Sensitized individuals can develop respiratory and skin allergy to the potent allergens found in mite feces and mite bodies (188).

Contact with allergenic particles of insect origin (poisonous hairs, body fragments, excreta, feces) may cause asthma, rhinitis, conjunctivitis, and dermatitis in exposed laboratory workers (mainly entomologists), foresters, silk producers, granary workers, and farmers (184). The gypsy moth (*Lymantria dispar*), Douglas fir tussock moth (*Orgyia pseudotsugata*), silkworm (*Bombyx mori*), cochineal insects (*Dactylopius coccus*), midges (*Chironomidae*), locust (*Locusta migratoria*), mealworm (*Tenebrio molitor*), cockroaches (*Periplaneta, Blattella*), and grain weevil (*Sitophilus granarius*) are potent sensitizers (177,178,184,189,190). Bee keepers are at risk of allergy to bee venom and hive particles (191).

INVERTEBRATE ANIMALS

Contact with poisonous sponges, coelenterates, and bryozoans may cause skin inflammation or systemic reaction in fishers, sailors, divers, and swimmers. The respiratory disease of oyster breeders in Japan known as *Hoya asthma* is caused by allergens of sea-squirts (*Ascidiacea*) growing on oysters that become airborne during the process of the opening of shells (192). Aerosolized proteins of clams and squids cause respiratory allergy in seafood production workers (193). People inhaling the airborne dust from pearl-oyster shells during the manufacturing of ornaments may develop constitutional symptoms and HP (194).

VERTEBRATE ANIMALS

Contact with antigens or venoms present in the slime of fish and frogs may cause allergy in exposed persons (fishers, cooks, laboratory workers) (195). Sailors, fishers, divers, and swimmers are threatened by the sting of poisonous fish and the bite of poisonous sea snakes (*Hydrophiidae*), whereas agricultural workers in tropical regions and zoologists are endangered by the bite of terrestrial poisonous snakes (196). Inhalation exposure to fish proteins may cause asthma and HP in factory workers (197).

Inhalation of the allergenic particles of bird origin (droppings, feather) may cause respiratory disorders in bird breeders and in workers of poultry-processing plants (198). The well-known form of HP called *bird fancier's lung* is most common among breeders of pigeons and budgerigars, but also occurs in people who have contact with hens, ducks, turkeys, and wild birds (199,200). The incidence of this disease among poultry breeders in many countries is between 2% and 6% (200,201). The workers of egg-processing plants that produce whole egg powder, egg yolk powder, and liquid egg white can develop asthma owing to exposure to high concentrations of the airborne egg allergens present (202,203).

Farmers who breed domestic animals (e.g., cows, pigs, horses), veterinarians, workers of zoological gardens exposed to exotic mammals (e.g., lions, elephants), and owners of pets (e.g., dogs, cats, rabbits, rats) may develop allergic symptoms from inhalation of airborne particles of animal dander, hair, urine, feces, milk, and saliva (187,189,203,204). A particular risk exists with laboratory animals (e.g., rats and mice) that produce potent, high-molecular-weight (22- to 75-kD) protein allergens. Male rats pose the greatest risk as they are capable of releasing large amounts (up to 20 ng per minute) of a strong urinary allergen that has been identified as α_2-euglobulin and described as *Rat n* I (188). Laboratory animal allergens can occur in high concentrations in the air of animal facilities (205–208).

It is estimated that 11% to 30% of all laboratory animal care workers have a syndrome called *laboratory animal allergy*, characterized by rhinitis, asthma, conjunctivitis, or dermatitis (206). Other workers at risk for developing allergy from animal protein are pharmaceutical and laboratory workers exposed via inhalation to powdered enzymes (e.g., pepsin, trypsin, pancreatin) and candy workers exposed to proteins from dried milk (189,207). Furriers, tanners, and wool processors also are exposed to antigens in animal hair (188). A skin allergy due to contact with meat and cheese (protein dermatitis) has been observed in butchers, in workers of meat and dairy packaging plants, and in cooks. Allergic dermatitis after contact with amniotic fluid has been described in veterinarians.

REFERENCES

1. Dutkiewicz J, Jabłoński L, Olenchock SA. Occupational biohazards: a review. *Am J Ind Med* 1988;14:605–623.
2. Patterson WB, Craven DE, Schwartz DA, Nardell EA, Kasmer J, Noble J. Occupational hazards to hospital personnel. *Ann Intern Med* 1985;102:658–680.
3. Evans R III. Epidemiology and natural history of asthma, allergic rhinitis, and atopic dermatitis. In: Middleton E Jr, Reed CE, Ellis EF, Adkinson NF Jr, Yunginger JW, Busse WW, eds. *Allergy: principles and practice*, 4th ed. St Louis: Mosby, 1993:1109–1136.
4. Centers for Disease Control and Prevention. Asthma mortality and hospitalization among children and young adults—United States, 1990–1993. *MMWR Morb Mortal Wkly Rep* 1996;45:350–353.
5. Blanc P. Occupational asthma in a national disability survey. *Chest* 1987;92:613–617.
6. Askenase PW. Effector and regulatory mechanisms in delayed-type hypersensitivity. In: Middleton E Jr, Reed CE, Ellis EF, Adkinson NF Jr, Yunginger JW, Busse WW, eds. *Allergy: principles and practice*, 4th ed. St Louis: Mosby, 1993:362–389.
7. Pestronk A. Chronic immune polyneuropathies and serum antibodies. In: Rolak L, Harati Y, eds. *Neuroimmunology for the clinician*. Boston: Butterworth-Heinemann, 1997:Ch 13.
8. Rostami A, Sater R. Guillain-Barré syndrome. In: Rolak L, Harati Y, eds. *Neuroimmunology for the clinician*. Boston: Butterworth-Heinemann, 1997:Ch 11.
9. Zweiman B, Lissak RP. Cell-mediated immunity in neurologic diseases. *Hum Pathol* 1986;16:234.
10. Rose C. Hypersensitivity pneumonitis. In: Haber P, Schenker M, Balmes J, eds. *Occupational and environmental respiratory disease.* St Louis: Mosby, 1996: Ch 14.
11. Flaherty DK, Barboriak JJ, Emanuel D, et al. Multilaboratory comparison of three immunodiffusion methods used for the detection of precipitating antibodies in hypersensitivity pneumonitis. *J Lab Clin Med* 1974;84:298–306.
12. Fogelmark BF, Sjöstrand M, Rylander R. Pulmonary inflammation induced by repeated inhalations of β(1,3)-D-glucan and endotoxin. *Int J Exp Pathol* 1994;75:85–90.
13. Bukenya GB, Nsungwa JL, Makanga B, Salvator A. Schistosomiasis mansoni and paddy-rice growing in Uganda: an emerging new problem. *Ann Trop Med Parasitol* 1994;88:379–384.
14. McCarthy DS, Pepys J. Allergic bronchopulmonary aspergillosis—clinical immunology I: clinical features. *Clin Allergy* 1971;1:261.
15. Greenberger PA, Patterson R. Application of enzyme-linked immunosorbent assay (ELISA) in diagnosis of allergic bronchopulmonary aspergillosis. *J Lab Clin Med* 1982;99:288.
16. Greenberger PA, Liotta JL, Roberts M. The effects of age on isotopic antibody responses to *Aspergillus fumigatus*: implications regarding in vitro measurements. *J Lab Clin Med* 1989;114:278.
17. Katzenstein A-LA, Sale SR, Greenberger PA. Allergic *Aspergillus* sinusitis: a newly recognized form of sinusitis. *J Allergy Clin Immunol* 1983;72:89–93.
18. Katzenstein A-LA, Sale SR, Greenberger PA. Pathologic findings in allergic *Aspergillus* sinusitis: a newly recognized form of sinusitis. *Am J Surg Pathol* 1983;7:439.
19. Lacey J, Dutkiewicz J. Biological aerosols and occupational lung disease. *J Aerosol Sci* 1994;25:1371–1404.
20. Rylander R, Jacobs RR, eds. *Organic dusts: exposure, effects and prevention.* Boca Raton, FL: Lewis Publishers, 1994.
21. Lacey J, Crook B. Review: fungal and actinomycete spores as pollutants of the workplace and occupational allergens. *Ann Occup Hyg* 1988;32:515–533.
22. Millner PD, Olenchock SA, Epstein E, et al. Biological aerosols associated with composting facilities. *Compost Sci Util* 1994;2(4):6–55.
23. Johanning E, Biagini R, Hull D, et al. Health and immunology study following exposure to toxigenic fungi (*Stachybotrys chartarum*) in a water-damaged office environment. *Int Arch Occup Environ Health* 1996;68:207–218.
24. Hodgson M, Morey P, Leung W, et al. Building-associated pulmonary disease from exposure to *Stachybotrys chartarum* and *Aspergillus versicolor*. *J Occup Environ Med* 1998;40(3):241–249.
25. Fung F, Clark R, Williams S. *Stachybotrys*, a mycotoxin-producing fungus of increasing toxicologic importance. *Clin Toxicol* 1998;36(172):79–86.
26. Sudakin D. Toxigenic fungi in a water-damaged building: an intervention study. *Am J Ind Med* 1998;34:183–190.
27. Rylander R. Airborne (1,3)-β-D-glucan and airway disease in a day-care center before and after renovation. *Arch Environ Health* 1997;52(4):281–285.
28. Rylander R. Airway responsiveness and chest symptoms after inhalation of endotoxin of (1,3)-β-D-glucan. *Indoor Built Environ* 1996;5:106–111.
29. Skorska C, Mackiewicz B, Dutkiewicz J, et al. Effects of exposure to grain dust in Polish farmers: work-related symptoms and immunologic response to microbial antigens associated with dust. *Ann Agric Environ Med* 1998;5:147–153.
30. Mackiewicz B. Study on exposure of pig farm workers to biological aerosols: immunologic reactivity and health effects. *Ann Agric Environ Med* 1998;5:169–175.
31. Thorn J, Beijer L, Rylander R. Airways inflammation and glucan exposure among household waste collectors. *Am J Ind Med* 1998;33:463–470.
32. Clark CS, Rylander R, Larsson L. Levels of gram-negative bacteria, *Aspergillus fumigatus*, dust and endotoxin at compost plants. *Appl Environ Microbiol* 1983;45:1501–1505.
33. Huuskonen MS, Husman K, Järvisalo J, et al. Extrinsic allergic alveolitis in the tobacco industry. *Br J Ind Med* 1984;41:77–83.
34. Halweg H, Krakówka P, Podsiadlo B, Owczarek J, Ponahajba A, Pawlicka L. Studies on the pollution of air with fungal spores on selected working posts in a paper mill [in Polish]. *Pneumonol Pol* 1978;46:577–585.
35. Jäppinen P, Haahtela T, Liira J. Chip pile workers and mould exposure. *Allergy* 1987;42:545–548.
36. Dutkiewicz J, Olenchock SA, Sorenson WG, et al. Levels of bacteria, fungi and endotoxin in bulk and aerosolized corn silage. *Appl Environ Microbiol* 1989;55:1093–1099.
37. Land CJ, Rask-Andersen A, Lundström H, Werner S, Bardage S. Tremorgenic mycotoxins in conidia of *Aspergillus fumigatus*. In: Samson RA, Flannigan B, Flannigan ME, Verhoeff AP, Adan OCG, Hoekstra ES, eds. *Health implications of fungi in indoor environments.* Amsterdam: Elsevier Science, 1994:307–315.
38. Hill RA, Wilson DM, Burg WR, Shotwell OL. Viable fungi in corn dust. *Appl Environ Microbiol* 1984;47:84–87.
39. Hayes RB, van Nieuwenhuize JP, Raatgever JW, Ten Kate FJW. Aflatoxin exposures in the industrial setting: an epidemiological study of mortality. *Food Chem Toxicol* 1984;22:39–43.
40. Topping M, Scarisbrick D, Luczynska C, et al. Clinical and immunological reactions to *Aspergillus niger* among workers at a biotechnology plant. *Br J Ind Med* 1985;42:312–318.
41. Dutkiewicz J. Bacteria, fungi and endotoxin in stored timber logs and airborne sawdust in Poland. In: Llewellyn GC, O'Rear CE, eds. *Biodeterioration research 2.* Washington: Plenum Publishing, 1989:533–547.
42. Eduard W, Sandven P, Levy F. Serum IgG antibodies to mold spores in two Norwegian sawmill populations: relationship to respiratory and other work-related symptoms. *Am J Ind Med* 1993;24:207–222.
43. Kozak PP Jr, Cummins LJ, Gillman SA. Endogenous mold exposure: environmental risk to atopic and nonatopic patients. In: Gammage RB, Kay SV, eds. *Indoor air and human health*. Chelsea, MI: Lewis Publishers, 1985:149–170.
44. Reynolds S, Streifel A, McJilton C. Elevated airborne concentrations of fungi in residential and office environments. *Am Ind Hyg Assoc J* 1990;51(11):601–604.
45. Robertson L. Monitoring viable fungal and bacterial biological aerosol concentrations to identify acceptable levels for common indoor environments. *Indoor Built Environ* 1997;6:295–300.
46. Summerbell R, Staib F, Dales R, et al. Ecology of fungi in human dwellings. *J Med Vet Mycol* 1992;30[Suppl 1]:279–285.
47. Dales R, Burnett R, Zwanenburg H. Adverse health effects among adults exposed to home dampness and molds. *Am Rev Respir Dis* 1991;143:505–509.
48. Wan G, Li C. Dampness and airway inflammation and systemic symptoms in office building workers. *Arch Environ Health* 1999;54(1):58–63.
49. Meyer H, Larsen F, Jacobi H, et al. Sick building syndrome: association of symptoms with serum IgE specific to fungi. *Inflamm Res* 1998;47[Suppl 1]:S9–S10.
50. Malkin R, Martinez K, Marinkovich V, et al. The relationship between symptoms and IgG and IgE antibodies in an office environment. *Environ Res* 1998;76:85–93.
51. Saraf A, Larsson L, Burge H, Milton D. Quantification of ergosterol and 3-hydroxy fatty acids in settled house dust by gas chromatography–mass spectrometry: comparison with fungal culture and determination of endotoxin by a *Limulus* amebocyte lysate assay. *Appl Environ Microbiol* 1997;63(7):2554–2559.
52. Pasanen A, Yli-Pietila K, Pasanen P, et al. Ergosterol content in various fungal species and biocontaminated building materials. *Appl Environ Microbiol* 1999;65(1):138–142.
53. Miller J, Young J. The use of ergosterol to measure exposure to fungal propagules in indoor air. *Am Ind Hyg Assoc J* 1997;58:39–43.
54. Macnaughton S, Jenkins T, Alugupalli S, White D. Quantitative sampling of indoor air biomass by signature lipid biomarker analysis: feasibility studies in a model system. *Am Ind Hyg Assoc J* 1997;58:270–277.
55. Fogelmark B, Rylander R. (1,3)-β-D-Glucan in some indoor air fungi. *Indoor Built Environ* 1997;6:291–294.
56. Norn S. Microorganism-induced or enhanced mediator release: a possible mechanism in organic dust–related diseases. *Am J Ind Med* 1994;25:91–95.
57. Larsen F, Clementsen P, Hansen M, et al. Volatile organic compounds from the indoor mould *Trichoderma viride* cause histamine release from human bronchoalveolar cells. *Inflamm Res* 1998;S5–S6:1023–3830.
58. Ruotsalainen M, Hyvarinen A, Nevalainen A, Savolainen K. Production of reactive oxygen metabolites by opsonized fungi and bacteria isolated from indoor air, and their interactions with soluble stimuli, fMLP or PMA. *Environ Res* 1995;69:122–131.
59. Wakshull E, Brunke-Reese D, Lindermuth J, et al. PGG-glucan, a soluble β-(1,3)-glucan, enhances the oxidative burst response, microbicidal activity, and activates and NF-kB-like factor in human PMN: evidence for glycosphingolipid β-(1,3)-glucan receptor. *Immunopharmacology* 1999;41:89–107.
60. Hirvonen M, Nevalainen A, Makkonen N, et al. Induced production of nitric oxide, tumor necrosis factor, and interleukin-6 in RAW 264.7 macrophages by streptomycetes from indoor air of moldy houses. *Arch Environ Health* 1997;52(6):426–432.
61. Dales R, Miller D, White J, et al. Influence of residential fungal contamination on peripheral blood lymphocyte populations in children. *Arch Environ Health* 1998;53(3):190–195.
62. Sorenson W, Shahan T, Simpson J. Cell wall preparation from environmental yeasts: effect on alveolar macrophage function in vitro. *Ann Agric Environ Med* 1998;5:65–71.
63. Andersson M, Nikulin N, Kolgalg U, et al. Bacteria, molds and toxins in water-damaged building materials. *Appl Environ Microbiol* 1997;63(2):387–393.

64. Austwick P. Human mycotoxicosis: past, present and future. *Chem Ind* 1984;6:547–555.
65. Croft W, Jarvis B, Yatawara C. Airborne outbreak of trichothecene toxicosis. *Atmosphere Environ* 1986;20:549–552.
66. Sorenson WG, Gerberick GF, Lewis DM, Castranova V. Toxicity of mycotoxins for the rat pulmonary macrophage *in vitro*. *Environ Health Perspect* 1986;66:45–53.
67. Nikulin M, Pasanen A, Berg S, Hintikka E. *Stachybotrys atra* growth in toxin production in some building materials and fodder under different relative humidities. *Appl Environ Microbiol* 1994;60(9):3421–3424.
68. Hunter C, Grant C, Flanagan B. Moulds in buildings, the air spora of domestic dwellings. *Int Biodeterioration* 1988;24:81–101.
69. Sorenson W, Frazer B, Jarvis B, Simpson J, Robinson V. Trichothecene mycotoxins in aerosolized conidia of *Stachybotrys atra*. *Appl Environ Microbiol* 1987;53(6):1370–1375.
70. Dearborn D. Update: pulmonary hemorrhage/hemosiderosis among infants—Cleveland, Ohio. *MMWR Morb Mortal Wkly Rep* 1997;46:33–35.
70a. Centers for Disease Control and Prevention. *Morb Mortal Wkly Rep* 2000; 49:180–184.
71. Jarvis B, Lee Y, Comezoglu N. Trichothecenes produced by *Stachybotrys atra* from Eastern Europe. *Appl Environ Microbiol* 1986;52(5):915–918.
72. Smoragiewicz W, Cossette B, Boutard A. Trichothecene mycotoxins in the dust of ventilation systems in office buildings. *Int Arch Occup Environ Health* 1993;65:113–117.
73. Lewis C, Smith J, Anderson J, et al. The presence of mycotoxin-associated fungal spores isolated from the indoor air from the damp, domestic environment and cytotoxic to human cell lines. *Indoor Environ* 1994;3:323–330.
74. Yike I, Allan P, Sorenson W. Highly sensitive protein translation assay for trichothecene toxicity in airborne particulates: comparison with cytotoxicity assays. *Appl Environ Microbiol* 1999;65(1):88–94.
75. Sorenson WG. Mycotoxins. Toxic metabolites of fungi. In: Murphy JW, et al., eds. *Fungal infection and immune responses*. New York: Plenum Publishing, 1993:469–491.
76. Sorenson WG, Jones W, Simpson J, Davidson JI. Aflatoxin in respirable airborne peanut dust. *J Toxicol Environ Health* 1984;14:525–533.
77. Ehrlich KC, Lee LS, Ciegler A, Palmgren MS. Secalonic acid D: natural contaminant of corn dust. *Appl Environ Microbiol* 1982;44:1007–1008.
78. Sorenson WG, Peach MJ, Simpson JP, Olenchock SA, Taylor G. Size range of viable fungi particles from aflatoxin-contaminated corn aerosols. In: Dosman JA, Cotton DJ, eds. *Focus on grain dust and disease*. New York: Academic Press, 1980:527–536.
79. Autrup JL, Schmidt J, Autrup H. Exposure to aflatoxin B_1 in animal-feed production plant workers. *Environ Health Perspect* 1993;99:195–197.
80. Sorenson WG. Health impact of mycotoxins in the home and workplace: an overview. In: Llewellyn GC, O'Rear CE, eds. *Biodeterioration research 2*. Washington: Plenum Publishing, 1989:201–215.
81. Jesenska Z. Micromycetes and mycotoxins in the working environment. *Prog Ind Microbiol* 1993;28:198–207.
82. Pestka J, Bondy G. Mycotoxin induced immune modulation. In: Dean J, Lester M, Munson A, Kimber I, eds. *Immunotoxicology and immunopharmacology*, 2nd ed. New York: Raven Press, 1994:Ch 9.
83. Emanuel DA, Wenzel FJ, Lawton BR. Pulmonary mycotoxicosis. *Chest* 1975;67:293–297.
84. Sorenson WG, Simpson JP, Peach MJ III, et al. Aflatoxin in respirable corn dust particles. *J Toxicol Environ Health* 1981;7:669–672.
85. Lester M, Dean J, Munson A, Kimber I, eds. *Immunotoxicology and immunopharmacology*, 2nd ed. New York: Raven Press, 1994.
86. Poulsen OM, Breum NO, Ebbehøj N, et al. Sorting and recycling of domestic waste. Review of occupational health problems and their possible causes. *Sci Total Environ* 1995;168:33–56.
87. Auger PL, Gourdeau P, Miller JD. Clinical experience with patients suffering from a chronic fatigue–like syndrome and repeated upper respiratory infections in relation to airborne molds. *Am J Ind Med* 1994;25:41–42.
88. Kiviranta H, Tuomainen A, Reiman M, Laitinen S, Nevalainen A, Liesivuori J. Exposure to airborne microorganisms and volatile organic compounds in different types of waste handling. *Ann Agric Environ Med* 1999;6:39–44.
89. Dutkiewicz J, Tucker J, Burrell R, et al. Ultrastructure of the endotoxin produced by gram-negative bacteria associated with organic dusts. *System Appl Microbiol* 1992;15:474–485.
90. Rylander R. The role of endotoxin for reactions after exposure to cotton dust. *Am J Ind Med* 1987;12:687–697.
91. Buick JB, Lowry RC, Magee TRA. Isolation, enumeration, and identification of gram-negative bacteria from flax dust with reference to endotoxin concentration. *Am Ind Hyg Assoc J* 1994;55:59–61.
92. Burrell R, Lantz RC, Hinton DE. Mediators of pulmonary injury induced by inhalation of bacterial endotoxin. *Am Rev Respir Dis* 1988;137:100–105.
93. Burrell R. Immunomodulation by bacterial endotoxin. *Crit Rev Microbiol* 1990;17:189–208.
94. Castellan RM, Olenchock SA, Kinsley KB, Hankinson JL. Inhaled endotoxin and decreased spirometric values. An exposure-response relation for cotton dust. *N Engl J Med* 1987;317:605–610.
95. Thelin A, Tegler Ö, Rylander R. Lung reactions during poultry handling related to dust and bacterial endotoxins levels. *Eur J Respir Dis* 1984;65:266–271.
96. Heederik D, Brouwer R, Biersteker K, Boleij JSM. Relationship of airborne endotoxin and bacteria levels in pig farms with the lung function and respiratory symptoms of farmers. *Int Arch Occup Environ Health* 1991;62:595–601.
97. Donham K, Haglind P, Peterson Y, Rylander R, Belin L. Environmental and health studies of farm workers in Swedish swine confinement buildings. *Br J Ind Med* 1989;46:31–37.
98. Carvalheiro MF, Marques Gomes MJ, Santos O, et al. Symptoms and exposure to endotoxin among brewery employees. *Am J Ind Med* 1994;25:113–115.
99. Olenchock SA, Lenhart SW, Mull JC. Occupational exposure to airborne endotoxins during poultry processing. *J Toxicol Environ Health* 1982;9:339–349.
100. Smid T, Heederik D, Mensink G, Houba R, Boleij JSN. Exposure to dust, endotoxin and fungi in the animal feed industry. *Am Ind Hyg Assoc J* 1992;53: 362–368.
101. Smid T, Heederik D, Houba R, Quanjer PH. Dust- and endotoxin-related acute lung function changes and work-related symptoms in workers in the animal feed industry. *Am J Ind Med* 1994;25:877–888.
102. Dillion H, Heinsohn P, Miller D. *Field guide for the determination of biological contaminants in environmental samples*. Fairfax, VA: AIHA Publications, 1996.
103. Shahan TA, Sorenson WG, Lewis DM. Superoxide anion production in response to bacterial lipopolysaccharide and fungal spores implicated in organic dust toxic syndrome. *Environ Res* 1994;67:98–107.
104. Von Essen S, Robbins RA, Thompson AB, Rennard SI. Organic dust toxic syndrome: an acute febrile reaction to organic dust exposure distinct from hypersensitivity pneumonitis. *Clin Toxicol* 1990;28(4):389–420.
105. Emanuel DA, Marx JJ, Ault B, et al. Organic dust toxic syndrome (pulmonary mycotoxicosis)—a review of the experience in central Wisconsin. In: Dosman JA, Cockcroft DW, eds. *Principles of health and safety in agriculture*. Boca Raton, FL: CRC Press, 1989:72–75.
106. Malmberg P, Rask-Andersen A, Lundhom M, Palmgren U. Can spores from molds and actinomycetes cause an organic dust syndrome reaction? *Am J Ind Med* 1990;17:109–110.
107. Milanowski J, Sorenson W, Dutkiewicz J, Lewis D. Chemotaxis of alveolar macrophages and neutrophils in response to microbial products derived from organic dust. *Environ Res* 1995;69:59–66.
108. Covert T, Rodgers M, Reyes A, Stelma G. Occurrence of nontuberculous mycobacteria in environmental samples. *Appl Environ Microbiol* 1999;65(6): 2492–2496.
109. Sewell DL. Laboratory-associated infections and biosafety. *Clin Microbiol Rev* 1995;8:389–405.
110. Molinari JA. Hepatitis C virus infection. *Dent Clin North Am* 1996;40:309–325.
111. Chong J, Marshall BJ, Barkin JS, et al. Occupational exposure to *Helicobacter pylori* for the endoscopy professional: a seroepidemiological study. *Am J Gastroenterol* 1994;89:1987–1992.
112. Hubbert WT, McCulloch WF, Schnurrenberger PR, eds. *Diseases transmitted from animals to man*, 6th ed. Springfield, IL: Charles C Thomas Publisher, 1975.
113. Ellis BA, Mills JN, Childs JE. Rodent-borne hemorrhagic fever viruses of importance to agricultural workers. *J Agromed* 1995;2(4):7–44.
114. Ellis A, Irwin R, Hockin J, Borczyk A, Woodward D, Johnson W. Outbreak of *Campylobacter* infection among farm workers: an occupational hazard. *Can Commun Dis Rep* 1995;21(17):153–156.
115. Bartelink AK, Van Kregten E. *Streptococcus suis* as threat to pig-farmers and abattoir workers. *Lancet* 1995;346:1707.
116. Almond JW, Brown P, Gore SM, et al. Creutzfeldt-Jakob disease and bovine spongiform encephalopathy: any connection? *BMJ* 1995;311:1415–1421.
117. Amadori D, Nanni O, Falcini F, et al. Chronic lymphocytic leukaemias and non-Hodgkin's lymphomas by histological type in farming-animal breeding workers: a population case-control study based on job titles. *Occup Environ Med* 1995;52:374–379.
118. Neubert U, Munchhoff P, Volker B. *Borrelia burgdorferi* infections in Bavarian forest workers. *Ann N Y Acad Sci* 1988;539:476–479.
119. Nakama H, Muramatsu K, Uchikama K, Yamagishi T. Possibility of Lyme disease as an occupational disease—seroepidemiological study of regional residents and forestry workers. *Asia Pac J Public Health* 1994;7:214–217.
120. Dutkiewicz J. Arachnids as risk factors in occupational exposure [in Polish]. *Wiad Parazytol* 1995;41:253–266.
121. Nishimura S, Asakura K, Nishinari T, Takno K. Study on tsutsugamushi disease in Honjyo area in Akita prefecture. *Ann Agric Environ Med* 1994;1:169.
122. Dossou-Yovo J, Doannio J, Riviere F, Duval J. Rice cultivation and malaria transmission in Bouake city (Cote d'Ivoire). *Acta Trop* 1994;57:91–94.
123. Narain K, Mahanta J, Dutta R, Dutta P. Paddy field dermatitis in Assam: a cercarial dermatitis. *J Commun Dis* 1994;26:26–30.
124. Neto J, Basso G, Cipoli A, Kadre L. American cutaneous leishmaniasis in the state of Sao Paulo, Brazil—epidemiology in transformation. *Ann Agric Environ Med* 1998;5:1–6.
125. Clark CS. Potential and actual biological-related health risks of wastewater industry employment. *J Water Poll Contr Fed* 1987;59:999–1008.
126. Fraser DW, Deubner DC, Hill DI, Gilliam DK. Nonpneumonic, short-incubation-period legionellosis (Pontiac fever) in men who cleaned a steam turbine condenser. *Science* 1979;205:690–691.
127. Castellani PM, Greco D, Cacciottolo JM, Vassalo A, Grech A, Bartlett CLR. Legionnaires' disease on an oil drilling platform in the Mediterranean: a case report. *Br J Ind Med* 1987;44:645–646.
128. Ruehlemann SA, Crawford GR. Panic in the potting shed. The association between *Legionella longbeachae* serogroup 1 and potting soils in Australia. *Med J Aust* 1996;164:36–38.
129. Howard DH. The epidemiology and ecology of blastomycosis, coccidioidomycosis and histoplasmosis. *Zentralbl Bakteriol Mikrobiol Hyg [A]* 1984;219–227.
130. Spiewak R. Zoophilic and geophilic fungi as a cause of skin disease in farmers. *Ann Agric Environ Med* 1998;5:97–102.
131. Swan J, Crook B. Airborne microorganisms associated with grain handling. *Ann Agric Environ Med* 1998;5:7–15.

132. Warren CPW, Manfreda J. Respiratory systems in Manitoba farmers: association with grain and hay handling. *Can Med Assoc J* 1980;122:1259–1264.
133. Donham KJ, Haglind P, Peterson Y, Rylander R. Environmental and health studies in swine confinement buildings. *Am J Ind Med* 1986;10:289–293.
134. Kotimaa MH, Terho EO, Husman K. Airborne moulds and actinomycetes in the work environment of farmers. *Eur J Respir Dis* 1987;[Suppl 152]:91–100.
135. Beeson ME, Dewdney JM, Edwards RG, Lee D, Orr RG. Prevalence and diagnosis of laboratory animal allergy. *Clin Allergy* 1983;13:433–443.
136. Bryant DH, Boscato LM, Mboloi PN, Stuart MC. Allergy to laboratory animals among animal handlers. *Med J Aust* 1995;163:415–418.
137. Rylander R, Haglind P. Airborne endotoxins and humidifier disease. *Clin Allergy* 1984;14:109–112.
138. Rylander R. Organic dusts and lung disease: the role of inflammation. *Ann Agric Environ Med* 1994;1:7–10.
139. Rylander R, Persson K, Goto H, Yuasa K, Tanaka S. Airborne β-1,3-glucan may be related to symptoms in sick buildings. *Indoor Environ* 1992;1:263–267.
140. Norbäck D, Edling C, Wieslander G. In: Samson RA, Flannigan B, Flannigan ME, Verhoeff AP, Adan OCG, Hoekstra ES, eds. *Health implications of fungi in indoor environments.* Amsterdam: Elsevier Science, 1994:229–239.
141. Platts-Mills TAE, Heymann PW, Chapman MD, Smith TF, Wilkins SR. Mites of the genus *Dermatophagoides* in dust from the houses of asthmatic and other allergic patients in North America: development of a radioimmunoassay for allergen produced by *D. farinae* and/or *D. pteronyssinus*. *Int Arch Allergy Appl Immunol* 1985;77:163–165.
142. Luczynska CM, Li Y, Chapman MD, Platts-Mills TAE. Measurements using cascade impactor, liquid impinger, and a two-site monoclonal antibody assay for *Fel d* I. *Am Rev Respir Dis* 1990;141:361–367.
143. Pollart S, Smith TF, Morris EC, et al. Environmental exposure to cockroach allergens: analysis with monoclonal antibody–based enzyme immunoassays. *J Allergy Clin Immunol* 1991;87:505–510.
144. Gelber LE, Seltzer LM, Bouzoukis JK, et al. Sensitization and exposure to indoor allergens as risk factors for asthma among patients presenting to hospital. *Am Rev Respir Dis* 1993;147:573–578.
145. Dust Mite Task Force, International Association of Allergy and Immunology. Dust mite allergens and asthma—a worldwide problem. *J Allergy Clin Immunol* 1989;83:416–427.
146. Wood R, Eggleston P, Lind L, et al. Antigenic analysis of household dust samples. *Am Rev Respir Dis* 1988;137:358–363.
147. American Conference of Governmental Industrial Hygienists. *Guidelines for the assessment of biological aerosols in the indoor environment.* Cincinnati: American Conference of Governmental Industrial Hygienists, 1989.
148. Riley EC. The role of ventilation in the spread of measles in an elementary school. *Ann N Y Acad Sci* 1980;353:25–34.
149. Bloch AB, Orenstein WA, Ewing WM, et al. Measles outbreak in a pediatric practice: airborne transmission in an office setting. *Pediatrics* 1985;75:676–683.
150. Couch RB. Viruses and indoor air pollution. *Bull N Y Acad Med* 1981;57:907–921.
151. Moser MR, Bender TR, Margolis HS, et al. An outbreak of influenza aboard a commercial airliner. *Am J Epidemiol* 1979;110:1–6.
152. Simpson DH. *Marburg and Ebola virus infection. A guide for their diagnosis, management and control.* Offset publ. no. 36. Geneva: World Health Organization, 1977.
153. Centers for Disease Control and Prevention. Update: outbreak of Hantavirus infection—southwestern United States, 1993. *MMWR Morb Mortal Wkly Rep* 1993;42:495–496.
154. Mertens PE, Patten R, Baum JJ, Moath TP. Clinical presentation of Lassa fever cases during the hospital epidemic at Zorzor, Liberia, March–April 1972. *Am J Trop Med Hyg* 1973;22:780–784.
155. Bednarska M, Bajer A, Sinski E. Calves as a potential reservoir of *Cryptosporidium parvum* and *Giardia* spp. *Ann Agric Environ Med* 1998;5:135–138.
156. Centers for Disease Control and Prevention. Outbreaks of *Cyclospora cayetanensis* infection—United States, 1996. *MMWR Morb Mortal Wkly Rep* 1996;45:549–551.
157. Dutkiewicz J. Exposure to dust-borne bacteria in agriculture: I. Environmental studies. *Arch Environ Health* 1978;33:250–259.
158. Dutkiewicz J. Bacteria and their products as occupational allergens. *Pneumonol Alergol Pol* 1992;60[Suppl 2]:14–21.
159. Dutkiewicz J. Microbial hazards in plants processing grain and herbs. *Am J Ind Med* 1986;10:300–302.
160. DeLucca AJ II, Godshall MA, Palmgren MS. Gram-negative bacterial endotoxins in grain elevator dusts. *Am Ind Hyg Assoc J* 1984;45:336–339.
161. Haglind P, Lundholm M, Rylander R. Prevalence of byssinosis in Swedish cotton mills. *Br J Ind Med* 1981;38:138–143.
162. Burrell R. Immunotoxic reactions in the agricultural environment. *Ann Agric Environ Med* 1995;2:11–20.
163. Kuś L. Clinical and experimental studies on allergic alveolitis due to exposure to antigens present in grain dust [in Polish]. *Med Wiejska* 1980;15:73–80.
164. Dutkiewicz J, Kuś L, Dutkiewicz E, Warren CPW. Hypersensitivity pneumonitis in grain farmers due to sensitization to *Erwinia herbicola*. *Ann Allergy* 1985;54:65–68.
165. Milanowski J. An attempt to identify causative agents of allergic alveolitis in selected group of patients, with the use of microbiologic and immunologic methods [in Polish]. *Pneumonol Pol* 1988;56:100–105.
166. Liebert CA, Hood MA, Deck FH, Bishop K, Flaherty DA. Isolation and characterization of a new *Cytophaga* species implicated in work-related lung disease. *Appl Environ Microbiol* 1984;48:936–943.
167. Rylander R, Lundholm M, Clark CS. Exposure to aerosols of microorganisms and toxins during handling of sewage sludge. In: *Proceedings of the International Conference on Biohazards of Sludge Disposal in Cold Climates, Calgary, 1982.* 1982:69–78.
168. Laitinen S, Kangas J, Kotimaa M, et al. Workers' exposure to airborne bacteria and endotoxins at industrial wastewater treatment plants. *Am Ind Hyg Assoc J* 1994;55:1055–1060.
169. Travers-Glass SA, Griffin P, Crook B. Bacterially contaminated oil mists in engineering works: a possible respiratory hazard. *Grana* 1991;30:404–406.
170. Bernstein DI, Lummus ZL, Santilli G, Siskosky J, Bernstein IL. Machine operator's lung. A hypersensitivity pneumonitis disorder associated with exposure to metalworking fluid aerosols. *Chest* 1995;108:636–641.
171. Reponen T, Gazenko S, Grinshpun A, et al. Characteristics of airborne actinomycetes spores. *Appl Environ Microbiol* 1998;64(10):3807–3812.
172. Blanco C, Carrillo T, Quiralte J, Pascual C, Martin-Esteban M, Castillo R. Occupational rhinoconjunctivitis and bronchial asthma due to *Phoenix canariensis* pollen allergy. *Allergy* 1995;50:277–280.
173. Solomon WR. Aerobiology of pollinosis. *J Allergy Clin Immunol* 1984;74:449–461.
174. Axelsson IG. Allergy to *Ficus benjamina* (weeping fig) in nonatopic subjects. *Allergy* 1995;50:284–285.
175. Ueda A, Manda F, Aoyama K, et al. Immediate-type allergy related to okra (*Hibiscus esculentus* Linn) picking and packing. *Environ Res* 1993;62:189–199.
176. Burge PS. Occupational asthma due to soft soldering fluxes containing colophony (rosin, pine resin). *Eur J Respir Dis* 1982;63[Suppl 123]:65–77.
177. Fuchs E. Industrial allergens as cause of obstructive pulmonary diseases [in German]. *Schweiz Med Wochenschr* 1982;112:185–192.
178. Kobayashi S. Different aspects of occupational asthma in Japan. In: Frazier CA, ed. *Occupational asthma.* New York: Van Nostrand, 1980:229–244.
179. Gamboa PM, de Las Marinas MD, Antepara I, Jauregui I, Sanz MM. Extrinsic allergic alveolitis caused by esparto (*Stipa tenacissima*). *Allergol Immunopathol (Madr)* 1990;18:331–334.
180. Rohrbach MS. Modulation of alveolar macrophage function by condensed tannin. *Am J Ind Med* 1994;25:97–99.
181. Wills JH. Nasal carcinoma in woodworkers: a review. *J Occup Med* 1982;24: 526–530.
182. Woods B, Calnan CD. Toxic woods. *Br J Dermatol* 1976;94[Suppl 13]:1–97.
183. Malo JL, Cartier A. Occupational reactions in the seafood industry. *Clin Rev Allergy* 1993;11:223–240.
184. Wirtz RA. Allergic and toxic reactions to nonstinging arthropods. *Annu Rev Entomol* 1984;29:47–70.
185. Gordon S, Tee RD, Nieuwenhuijsen MJ, Lowson D, Harris J, Newman-Taylor AJ. Measurement of airborne rat urinary allergen in an epidemiological study. *Clin Exp Allergy* 1994;24:1070–1077.
186. Iversen M, Hallas TE. Storage mite allergy in farming. *Ann Agric Environ Med* 1995;2:27–30.
187. Dyne D, Campion K, Griffin P. Occupational allergy among workers producing arthropods for organic pest control purposes. *Ann Agric Environ Med* 1996;3:33–36.
188. Pope AM, Patterson R, Burge H, eds. *Indoor allergens.* Washington: National Academy Press, 1993.
189. Novey HS, Bernstein L, Mihalas LS, Terr AI, Yunginger JW. Guidelines for the clinical evaluation of occupational asthma due to high molecular weight (HMW) allergens. Report of the Subcommittee on the Clinical Evaluation of Occupational Asthma due to HMW Allergens. *J Allergy Clin Immunol* 1989; 84:829–833.
190. Etkind PH, O'Dell TM, Canada AT, Shama SK, Finn AM, Tuthill RW. The gypsy moth caterpillar: a significant new occupational and public health problem. *J Occup Med* 1982;24:659–662.
191. Bousquet J, Menardo JL, Michel FB. Allergy in beekeepers. *Allergol Immunopathol (Madr)* 1982;10:395–398.
192. Ohtsuka T, Tsuboi S, Katsutani T, et al. Results of 29-year study of hoya (seasquirt) asthma in Hatsukaichi, Hiroshima prefecture. *Arerugi* 1993;42:214–218.
193. Desjardins A, Malo JL, L'Archeveque J, Cartier A, McCants M, Lehrer SB. Occupational IgE-mediated sensitization and asthma caused by clam and shrimp. *J Allergy Clin Immunol* 1995;96:608–617.
194. Jäger J, Liebetrau G, Pielesch W, Bergmann L, Baur X. Pearl oyster dust as the cause of exogenous allergic alveolitis [in German]. *Pneumologie* 1991; 45:884–886.
195. Holtz J, Frechelin E, Noel B, Savolainen H. A case of frog allergy: antigenic skin protein. *Int Arch Allergy Immunol* 1993;101:299–300.
196. Kizer KW. Marine envenomations. *J Toxicol Clin Toxicol* 1984;21:527–555.
197. Douglas JD, McSharry C, Blaikie L, Morrow T, Miles S, Franklin D. Occupational asthma caused by automated salmon processing. *Lancet* 1995;346:737–740.
198. Petro W, Bergmann KC, Heinze R, Müller E, Wuthe H, Vogel J. Long-term occupational inhalation of organic dust—effect on pulmonary function. *Int Arch Occup Environ Health* 1978;42:119–127.
199. Molina C, Brun J, Tourreau A, Godefroid JM, Aiache JM. Respiratory disorders in poultry breeders [in French]. *Rev Franc Mal Respir* 1974;2:849–866.
200. Choy AC, Patterson R, Ray AH, Roberts M. Hypersensitivity pneumonitis in a raptor handler and a wild bird fancier. *Ann Allergy Asthma Immunol* 1995;74:437–441.
201. Bernstein DI, Smith AB, Moller DR, et al. Clinical and immunologic studies among egg-processing workers with occupational asthma. *J Allergy Clin Immunol* 1987;80:791–797.
202. Virtanen T, Vilhunen P, Husman K, Happonen P, Mäntyjärvi R. Level of airborne bovine epithelial antigen in Finnish cowsheds. *Int Arch Occup Environ Health* 1988;60:355–360.

203. Reijula K, Virtanen T, Halmepuro L, Anttonen H, Mäntyjärvi R, Hassi J. Detection of airborne reindeer epithelial antigen by enzyme-linked immunosorbent assay inhibition. *Allergy* 1992;47:203–206.
204. Edwards RG, Beeson ME, Dewdney JM. Laboratory animal allergy: the measurements of airborne urinary allergens and the effects of different environmental conditions. *Lab Anim* 1983;17:235–239.
205. Lewis DM, Bledsoe TA, Dement JM. Laboratory animal allergies. Use of the radioallergosorbent test inhibition assay to monitor airborne allergen levels. *Scand J Work Environ Health* 1988;14[Suppl 1]:74–76.
206. Eggleston PA, Ansari AA, Adkinson NF Jr, Wood RA. Environmental challenge studies in laboratory animal allergy. *Am J Respir Crit Care Med* 1995; 151:640–646.
207. Bernaola G, Echechipia S, Urrutia I, Fernandez E, Audicana M, Fernandez de Corres L. Occupational asthma and rhinoconjunctivitis from inhalation of dried cow's milk caused by sensitization alpha-lactalbumin. *Allergy* 1994; 49:189–191.
208. Ohman JL Jr, Hagberg K, MacDonald MR, Jones RR Jr, Paigen BJ, Kacergis B. Distribution of airborne mouse allergen in a major mouse breeding facility. *J Allergy Clin Immunol* 1994;94:810–817.

CHAPTER 98

Organophosphate and Carbamate Insecticides

Tareg A. Bey, John B. Sullivan, Jr., and Frank G. Walter

Pesticides are chemicals used to destroy pests and weeds and to control plant diseases. They include the following use categories: insecticides (arthropods), acaricides (mites), fungicides (mildew), herbicides (weeds), algaecides (algae), piscicides (fish), avicides (birds), rodenticides (rats), molluscicides (snails, slugs), and nematocides (worms) (1,2).

Insecticides can be categorized into four different groups: (i) synthetic organic insecticides, including chlorobenzene derivatives (dichlorodiphenyltrichloroethane), cyclodienes (chlordane, aldrin, dieldrin), benzene hexachlorides (lindane), carbamates, and organophosphates; (ii) inorganic chemical-type insecticides, such as arsenic, thallium, and cyanide compounds; (iii) biological insecticides, such as pheromones, insect-specific bacteria, and viruses; and (iv) insecticides from botanical sources, such as nicotine and pyrethrin (1,2).

Organophosphorus compounds have been in existence since 1854 but were not recognized as having toxic potential until the 1930s (2). The first organophosphate insecticide, tetraethylpyrophosphate (TEPP), was developed in Germany as a substitute for the botanical insecticide nicotine, which was in short supply before and during the second World War. After this, the chemical warfare nerve agents tabun and sarin were developed. Sarin was used in a 1995 terrorism incident in Japan (3,4). Although TEPP is an effective insecticide, its highly toxic profile and the fact that it can be inactivated rapidly by hydrolysis in the presence of moisture left researchers looking for stabler compounds. In 1944, parathion and its oxygen analog, paraoxon, were developed. Parathion has been recognized as one of the organophosphates used most widely, owing to its insecticidal activity and physiochemical profile, including low volatility, stability in water, and mild alkalinity. Despite parathion's popularity, its potential for toxicity has led to the development and use of less hazardous compounds.

Other applications of organophosphates include their use as phosphorothiate defoliants, phosphoglycine herbicides, and fire retardants. The beneficial activities of these substances do not depend on their anticholinesterase activity (2).

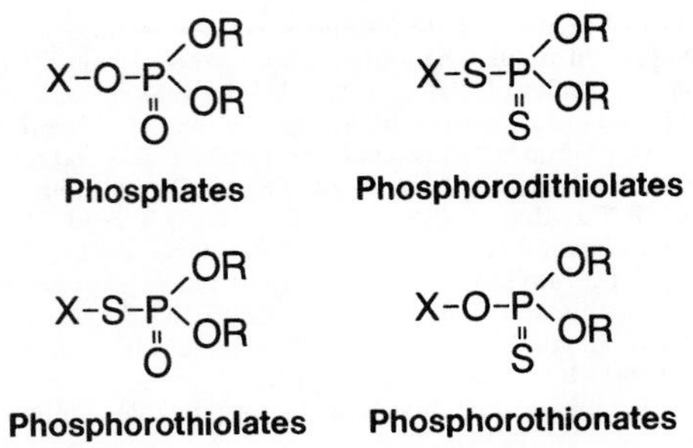

X-O-P(=O)(OR)(OR) — Phosphates

X-S-P(=S)(OR)(OR) — Phosphorodithiolates

X-S-P(=O)(OR)(OR) — Phosphorothiolates

X-O-P(=S)(OR)(OR) — Phosphorothionates

Figure 98-1. Basic structures of organophosphates. X, miscellaneous structure of the organophosphate; R, alkyl structure. (Adapted from Minton W, Murray V. A review of organophosphate poisoning. *Med Toxicol* 1988;3:350–375.)

ORGANOPHOSPHATES

Organophosphate insecticides are esters, amides, or thiol derivatives of phosphoric, phosphonic, phosphorothioic, or phosphonothioic acids (2). Both organophosphates and carbamates inhibit acetylcholinesterase (AChE) enzymes in tissues, blood, and plasma. The basic chemical structures of organophosphates are shown in Figure 98-1. A listing of commercial organophosphates is provided in Table 98-1.

CARBAMATES

Carbamates are represented by monomethyl-carbamates, which are esters of carbamic acid (Table 98-2) (5). The basic *N*-methyl structure of carbamate insecticides is shown in Figure 98-2. Carbamates used as insecticides and nematocides are highly toxic owing to carbamylation of AChE enzymes. Besides their role as insecticides, carbamates are employed as fungicides, herbicides, and nematocides (Table 98-3).

Toxicity of carbamate fungicides and herbicides is related to the aromatic moiety on the herbicides and the benzimidazole moiety on fungicides rather than to the carbamate portion of the molecule.

EXPOSURE SOURCES

Exposure to organophosphate and carbamates is attributable to three basic sources:

- *Agriculture*: Exposure that originates from agricultural activity, including people not working in agriculture
- *Structures*: Exposure that originates from pesticide applications to buildings and residential areas by regulated pest control companies
- *Accident or intention*: Exposure from home use

Global estimates of acute pesticide morbidity and mortality are based solely on mathematical models and outbreak investigation. The estimated number of global cases of pesticide poisonings has risen from 500,000 per year in 1972 to 25 million per year in 1990. These data were calculated in the absence of regular worldwide surveillance (6).

In California, the Department of Pesticide Regulations is responsible, under existing state laws and delegation by the U.S. Environmental Protection Agency (EPA), for registering all pesticides prior to sale for use. California's pesticide regulatory program is the most comprehensive in the world.

The Toxic Exposure Surveillance System data compiled by the American Association of Poison Control Centers annually reports human exposures to chemical compounds. A total of

TABLE 98-1. Cross reference for some of the cholinesterase-inhibiting organophosphate pesticide trade names

Trade name	Chemical name	Trade name	Chemical name
Aflix	Formothion	Exothion	Endothion
Afos	Mecarbam	Filariol	Bromophos ethyl
Agrisil	Trichloronate	Folidol E-605	Parathion
Agritox	Trichloronate	Folidol M	Methyl parathion
Agrothion	Fenitrothion	Folithion	Fenitrothion
Alkron	Parathion	Fostion MM	Dimethoate
Alleron	Parathion	Frumin Al	Disulfoton
Amiphos	DAEP	Fujithion	DMCP
Anthio	Formothion	Fyfanon	Malathion
Anthon	Trichlorfon	Gardentox	Diazinon
Appex	Gardona+	Garrathion	Carbophenothion
Asuntol	Coumaphos	Gusathion M	Azinphos-methyl
Azodrin	Monocrotophos	Guthion	Azinphos-methyl
Basudin	Diazinon	Hercules AC527	Dioxathion
Baymix	Coumaphos	Karbofos	Malathion
Bayrusil	Diethquinalphione	Klimite 40	TEPP
Baytex	Fenthion	Korlan	Ronnel
Baythion	Phoxim	Lebaycide	Fenthion
Betasan	Bensulide	Malamar	Malathion
Bidrin	Dicrotophos	Malaspray	Malathion
Bilobran	Monocrotophos	Maretin	Naphthalaphos
Birlane	Chlorfenvinphos	Meldane	Coumaphos
Bladafume	Sulfotepp	Menite	Mevinphos
Bladen	Parathion	Metasystox	Demeton methyl
Borinox	Trichlorfon	Metasystox-R	Oxydemeton-methyl
Bromex	Naled	Metron	Methyl parathion
Carbicron	Dicrotophos	Mintacol	Paraoxon
Carfene	Azinphos-methyl	MLT	Malathion
Cidial	Phenthoate	Mocap	Prophos
Citram	Amiton	Morphotox	Morphothion
Co-Ral	Coumaphos	Murfotox	Mecarbam
Corothion	Parathion	Muscatox	Coumaphos
Cygon	Dimethoate	N-2790	Dyfonate
Cythion	Malathion	Nankor	Ronnel
Dagadip	Carbophenothion	Neguvon	Trichlorfon
Dalf	Methyl parathion	Neragan	Bromphos Ethyl
Daphene	Dimethoate	Nialate	Ethion
Dasanit	Fensulfothion	Niram	Parathion
Dazzel	Diazinon	Nitrox	Methyl Parathion
Dedevap	Dichlorvos	No Pest	Dichlorvos
De-Fend	Dimethoate	Novathion	Fenitrothion
De-Green	DEF	Nuvacron	Monocrotophos
Delnav	Dioxathion	Nuvanol	Fenitrothion
Diazajet	Diazinon	Ortho Phosphate Defoliant	DEF
Diazide	Diazinon	Orthophos	Parathion
Diazol	Diazinon	Panthion	Parathion
Dibrom	Naled	Parathene	Parathion
Di-Captan	Dicapthon	Parawet	Parathion
Dimecron	Phosphamidon	Patron M	Methyl parathion
Dimethogen	Dimethoate	Perfekthion	Dimethoate
Dipterex	Trichlorfon	Pestan	Mecarbam
Di-Syston	Disulfoton	Pestox III	Schradan
Disyston S	Oxydisulfoton	Phosdrin	Mevinphos
Dithione	Sulfotepp	Phosfene	Mevinphos
Dursban	Chlorpyrifos	Phoskit	Parathion
Dylox	Trichlorfon	Phosphopyran	Endothion
E-605	Parathion	Phosvit	Dichlorvos
Easy Off-D	Folex	Phytosol	Trichloronate
Ectoral	Ronnel	PT-270	Chlorpyrifos
Ekatin	Thiometon	Rabon	Gardona+
Ekatin M	Morphothion	Rampart	Phorate
Ektafos	Dicrotophos	Rawetin	Naphthalaphos
Elsan	Phenthoate	Resistox	Coumaphose
Emmatos	Malathion	Rhodiatox	Parathion
Entex	Fenthion	Rogor	Dimethoate
Equinno-Aid	Trichlorfon	Rolate	Imidan
Ethyl parathion	Parathion	Roxion	Dimethoate
Etilon	Parathion	Ruelene	Crufomate
Etrolene	Ronnel	Ruphos	Dioxathion

(continued)

TABLE 98-1. *(continued)*

Trade name	Chemical name	Trade name	Chemical name
Sapecron	Chlorfenvinphos	Thiocron	Amidthion
Solverex	Disulfoton	Thiodemeton	Disulfoton
Soprathion	Parathion	Thiophos	Parathion
Spectracide	Diazinon	Thiotepp	Sulfotepp
Stathion	Parathion	Tiguvon	Fenthion
Sumithion	Fenitrothion	Timet	Phorate
Supona	Chlorfenvinphos	Trichlorophon	Trichlorfon
Systox	Demeton	Trimetion	Dimethoate
Sytam	Schradan	Trinox	Trichlorfon
Tamaron	Monitor	Trithion	Carbophenothion
Tanone	Phenthoate	Trolene	Ronnel
Tartan	Cyanthoate	Tugon	Trichlorfon
Task	Dichlorvos	Valexon	Phoxim
Tekwaisa	Methyl parathion	Vapona	Dichlorvos
Terracur P	Fensulfothion	Vaponite	Dichlorvos
Tetrachlorvinphos	Gardona	Vapotone	TEPP
Tetraethylpyrophosphate	TEPP	Viozene	Ronnel
Tetram	Amiton	Volaton	Phoxim
Tetron	TEPP	Zithiol	Malathion
Thimet	Phorate	Zolone	Phosalone

84,346 human exposures to pesticides were reported in 1995, of which 13 resulted in death, including 7 suicides (7).

Organophosphates and carbamates are available as emulsified concentrates or wettable powder formulations for reconstitution as liquid sprays and are available also as granules for soil application. A limited number are available as fogging formulations, smokes, impregnated resin strips for indoor use, or animal or human pharmaceutical preparations.

Agricultural pesticides are delivered mainly in two ways: land-based application and aerial spraying. In land-based delivery, generally the pesticide concentrates are mixed and loaded into tractor-powered or knapsack sprayers. For tractor spraying, the concentrated pesticide is diluted after loading; for knapsack sprayers, it is loaded from large drums as a premixed, diluted solution, thereby reducing the need to handle the concentrate.

Newer methods of application include ultra-low-volume-controlled droplet applicators that produce small drops from a spinning disc. The objective is to use less pesticide and to target crops more accurately, but the active chemical is much more concentrated than in conventional spraying and, in practice, has a greater potential for human toxicity.

A more effective means of application is the aerial spraying method using either helicopters or fixed-wing aircraft. The chemicals used are in a higher concentration; therefore, particular attention should be given to the possibility of an accidental human or environmental exposure. Specific environmental factors related to this dispersion method include (i) winds that spread organophosphates in open areas; (ii) temperature variations in hot climates, where volatility may increase and lead to high vapor concentrations; (iii) rain that could increase the spread of or area covered by the chemicals; (iv) fluvial and tidal flow, which will affect waterborne spread and contamination; and (v) residues remaining on crops and in soil.

MECHANISM OF TOXIC ACTION

Organophosphates and carbamates inhibit the enzyme AChE; hence, they are called *anticholinesterase* agents. Normally, acetylcholine (ACh)—the chemical neurotransmitter at ganglionic, parasympathetic, and neuromuscular synaptic junctions—is hydrolyzed into acetic acid and choline by the enzyme AChE. This four-step process requires only 80 microseconds, rendering AChE one of the fastest-metabolizing mammalian enzymes (8).

When AChE is inhibited, the accumulated ACh stimulates nicotinic and muscarinic receptors in the peripheral and central nervous system (9). Signs and symptoms of organophosphate and carbamate toxicity are due to overstimulation of muscarinic and nicotinic receptor sites by excess ACh, leading to eventual exhaustion of the receptor sites (Table 98-4). The anionic subsite of AChE, thought to attract the quaternary nitrogen of the substrate, may be misnamed because it contains, at most, one negative charge (9,10). Modeling of ACh suggests that the quaternary ammonium ion is bound not to a negatively charged "anionic" site but rather to a deep and narrow "active site gorge" that penetrates halfway into the enzyme (10).

The last step in the four-step process of inactivating AChE by organophosphates is irreversible. In this final step of the "aging" process of reacting with AChE, an alkyl group is split from the phosphorylated serine group at the active AChE site (8,11). An "aged" AChE cannot be reactivated by an oxime antidote. The inactivation of AChE by organophosphates and by carbamates leads to depressed activity of the enzyme in neuronal and non-neuronal tissues, such as in red blood cells (RBCs) and serum. As opposed to that of organophosphates, carbamate binding to AChE is spontaneously reversible. The aging process of the enzyme AChE and the rapidity of toxic signs and symptoms are dependent on physicochemical properties of the organophosphate and other host-related factors. With soman, for example, the aging process takes only 2 minutes. The knowledge of the aging half-time is important for therapeutic and prognostic considerations. With a rapidly aging agent, affected individuals most likely will respond less favorably to oxime reactivators and may have a prolonged course requiring intense supportive care measures.

Organophosphate compounds can be classified also as direct and indirect AChE inhibitors. Direct inhibitors are effective without further metabolic modification, whereas indirect inhibitors undergo biotransformation in the body to be effective (9). The insecticide dichlorvos is a direct inhibitor and parathion is

TABLE 98-2. Cross reference for some of the cholinesterase-inhibiting carbamate pesticide trade names

Trade name	Chemical name	Trade name	Chemical name
A363	Matacil	Mercaptodmethur	Mesurol
Ambush	Aldicarb	Metalkamate	Bufeneath
Aminocarb	Matacil	Methiocarb	Mesurol
Aphox	Pirimicarb	Metmercaptron	Mesurol
Arprocarb	Baygon	Minacide	Promecarb
B-37344	Mesurol	Mos 78	Mobam
Bay 39007	Baygon	MXMC	Mesurol
Bay 44646	Matacil	NC6897	Ficam
Bay 70142	Carbofuran	NIA 10242	Carbofuran
Bay 9010	Baygon	Nudrin	Methomyl
Bendiocarb	Ficam	OMS 716	Promecarb
Blattenex	Baygon	Ortho 5353	Bufencarb
Bux	Bufencarb	PHC	Baygon
Carbamult	Promecarb	Pirimor	Pirimicarb
Carbanolate	Banol	PP 062	Pirimicarb
Carpolin	Carbaryl	Propoxur	Baygon
Carzol	Formetanate (hydrochloride)	Ravyon	Carbaryl
CIBA 8353	Dioxacarb	Romate	Dichlormate
Curaterr	Carbofuran	Rowmate	Dichlormate
D-1221	Formetanate (hydrochloride)	Schering 34615	Promecarb
D-1410	Oxamyl	Schering 36056	Formetanate (hydrochloride)
Dicarol	Formetanate (hydrochloride)	Sendran	Baygon
Dowco 139	Mexacarbate	Septene	Carbaryl
Draza	Mesurol	Sevin	Carbaryl
Elocron	Dioxacarb	Sirmate	Dichlormate
ENT 27164	Carbofuran	Snip	Dimetilan
Ent 27300	Promecarb	Sok	Banol
EP 316	Promecarb	Suncide	Baygon
EP 332	Formetanate (hydrochloride)	Temik	Aldicarb
Famid	Dioxacarb	Tendex	Baygon
FMC 10242	Carbofuran	Tricarnam	Carbaryl
Furadan	Carbofuran	UC 21149	Aldicarb
G-13332	Dimetilan	UC 22463	Dichlormate
G-22870	Dimetilan	UC 7744	Carbaryl
Hexavin	Carbaryl	UC 9880	Promecarb
IPMC	Baygon	Unden	Baygon
Karbaspray	Carbaryl	Vydate	Oxamyl
Lannate	Methomyl	Yaltox	Carbofuran
Maz	Mexacarbate	Zectron	Mexacarbate
MCA-600	Mobam		

an indirect inhibitor of the AChE (9). Direct inhibitors usually have an onset of action faster than that of indirect inhibitors. Organophosphates that require metabolism to a toxic intermediate, such as parathion, malathion, and dimethoate, may present with delayed clinical toxicity.

Dimethoate, an agricultural pesticide, is an indirect-acting anticholinesterase. It is converted in the liver to active metabolites (12). Phosphorothioates, like dimethoate, require metabolic oxidation of the phosphorus-sulfur (P=S) bond before producing toxicity. Owing to this oxidation step, these substances can exhibit a slower onset of symptoms as compared to compounds possessing a direct-acting P=O bond (12). Dimethoxon, an active metabolite of dimethoate, is thought to be 75 to 100 times more potent than dimethoate for the inhibition of rat brain cholinesterase (12). Phosphorothioates are lipophilic, concentrate in the body fat, and are released over a relatively long period. This phenomenon may be responsible for the reappearance of acute clinical effects observed in an acute exposure after therapy.

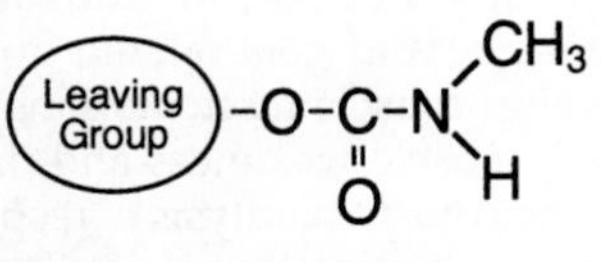

Figure 98-2. Basic structure of *N*-methyl carbamate insecticides.

Cholinesterase inhibition by carbamates in humans is labile, has a short duration, and is reversible. Also, cumulative AChE inhibition does not occur (5). The degradation of carbamates in humans occurs by hydrolysis, oxidation, and conjugation with end products of phenols, amines, or alcohols (5). The main route of excretion is urinary. Delayed neurologic damage, as seen with acute organophosphate poisoning, does not occur with carbamates (5).

PHARMACOLOGY OF CHOLINESTERASE ENZYMES

Vertebrates have two different enzymes that hydrolyze ACh. The enzyme AChE terminates the action of ACh at the synaptic cleft (13,14). AChE is present in the RBCs and the nervous tissue. The other cholinesterase is present in plasma and is called *butyrylcholinesterase* (BChE) or *pseudocholinesterase* (plasma cholinesterase) (13). BChE hydrolyzes the muscle relaxant succinylcholine. The physiologic function of BChE and RBC AChE is not yet understood (13,14), but inhibition of the activity of erythrocyte AChE is reasonably well correlated with the severity of poi-

TABLE 98-3. Uses of carbamates

- Carbamate insecticides
  - Alanycarb
  - Aldicarb
  - Aldoxycarb
  - Aminocarb
  - Bendiocarb
  - Benfuracarb
  - Butocarboxim
  - Carbaryl
  - Carbofuran
  - Carbosulfan
  - Cloethocarb
  - Dimetilan (BSI name)
  - Fenothiocarb
  - Fenoxycarb
  - Formetanate
  - Furathiocarb
  - Mecarbam
  - Methomyl
  - Nitralicarb
  - Oxyamyl
  - Pirimicarb
  - Promecarb
  - Propoxur
  - Thiodicarb
  - Thiofanox
- Carbamate herbicides and fungicides
  - Asulam
  - Barban
  - Benomyl
  - Carbendazim
  - Carbetamide
  - Chlorbufam
  - Chlorpropham
  - Desmidipham
  - Diallate
  - Dichlormate
  - EPTC
  - Molinate
  - Pebulate
  - Phenmedipham
  - Propamocarb
  - Propham
  - Terbucarb
  - Thiobencarb
  - Thiophanate-ethyl
  - Thiophanate-methyl
  - Triallate
  - Vernolate
- Dithiocarbamate fungicides
  - Thiurams
    - Disulfiram
    - Methiram
    - Thiram
  - Dimethyldithiocarbamates
    - Ferbam
    - Ziram
  - Unsaturated alkyldithiocarbamates
    - Ethylenebisdithiocarbamates
      - Mancozeb
      - Maneb
      - Nabam
      - Zineb
    - Propylenebisdithiocarbamates

soning (11). Usually, erythrocyte AChE inhibition overestimates the effect in the nervous system (14). BChE (plasma cholinesterase) is the most sensitive to inhibitors and is not correlated as well with toxicity (14,15).

The sites and types of synapses affected by organophosphates and carbamates relate to specific pathophysiologic effects in poisoned patients. The clinical signs and symptoms of organophosphate and carbamate poisoning can be divided into two groups on the basis of receptor pharmacology (2): nicotinic signs and symptoms and muscarinic signs and symptoms. A more anatomic classification given by Koelle (8) described four classes of cholinergic fibers:

- Sympathetic
- Parasympathetic
- Motor fibers to skeletal muscles
- Fibers within the central nervous system

Accumulation of excessive amounts of ACh at a muscarinic or nicotinic receptor site causes characteristic toxic responses. Excitatory (bronchospasm) or inhibitory (vasodilatory) responses occur at the muscarinic receptors (M receptors). At the nicotinic receptors (N receptors), the effect is first excitatory (a muscle fasciculation) and then inhibitory (muscle paralysis) (8).

The M receptors are G-protein coupled, and their activation is followed by a second messenger response. The N receptors, in contrast, are ligand-gated ion channels, and their activation causes an immediate increase in Na^+ and K^+ permeability (8). The difference in the susceptibility and rapidity of receptor response may explain why nicotinic effects are seen before muscarinic effects in organophosphate poisoning.

TABLE 98-4. Clinical effects of acetylcholinesterase inhibitors (acetylcholine excess)

Receptor site of action	Physiologic effects
Muscarinic effects	
Sweat glands	Sweating
Pupils	Constricted pupils
Lacrimal glands	Lacrimation
Salivary glands	Excessive salivation
Bronchial tree	Bronchospasm
Gastrointestinal	Pulmonary edema; cramps, vomiting, diarrhea
Cardiovascular	Bradycardia; PR, QRS, QT prolongation; ventricular dysrhythmias; torsades de pointes, atrioventricular dissociation, idioventricular rhythms
Ciliary body	Blurred vision
Bladder	Urinary incontinence
Nicotinic effects	
Striated muscle	Fasciculations; cramps; weakness, twitching, paralysis; respiratory depression and respiratory distress, respiratory arrest, cyanosis
Sympathetic ganglia	Tachycardia; elevated blood pressure; cardiac dysrhythmias
Central nervous system effects	Anxiety, confusion, restlessness; ataxia; convulsions; insomnia; coma; absent reflexes; respiratory and circulatory depression

CLINICAL TOXICOLOGY

Toxicity from organophosphates and carbamates is divided into acute, chronic, and long-term effects. Toxicity is based on the particular compound, concentration, amount absorbed, route of absorption, and types of receptor sites that are stimulated excessively (muscarinic and nicotinic). The rapidity and sequence of muscarinic effects due to organophosphate and carbamate poisoning depend on the route of exposure, the toxicity of the compound, and the prior status of AChE activity (8). Prior exposures may lower the level of enzyme activity and thus increase the risk of toxicity.

Acute Toxicity of Organophosphates

Organophosphates are absorbed readily through the skin either from direct contact or from contaminated clothes. In accidental exposures to airborne cholinesterase-inhibiting insecticides, the first effects usually are ocular and respiratory. These effects include miosis, ocular pain, congestion of the conjunctivae, spasm of the ciliary muscle, dimness of vision, and rhinorrhea. Respiratory symptoms include dyspnea and chest tightness. These initial signs and symptoms may be followed by bronchoconstriction and excessive tracheobronchial secretions. Individuals who ingest organophosphate compounds usually present with complaints related to the gastrointestinal tract, such as anorexia, nausea, vomiting, abdominal cramps, and diarrhea. In patients with percutaneous local exposure to liquid or airborne organophosphate compounds, localized excessive sweating and muscular fasciculations may be the earliest manifestations.

Nicotinic effects of organophosphate and carbamate poisons are more likely to prove immediately life-threatening because of the respiratory depressant effects (16). Initial manifestations of AChE blockade at myoneural junctions in skeletal muscle include muscle fatigue and generalized muscular weakness. Patients may develop muscle fasciculations or muscle twitchings. Subsequently, muscle weakness and paralysis occur and are followed by apnea due to paralysis of respiratory muscles. In untreated patients, these nicotinic effects, together with bron-

TABLE 98-5. Samples of organophosphate insecticides

Common name	Chemical name
High toxicity	
TEPP	Tetraethylpyrophosphate
Parathion	O,O-diethyl O-*p*-nitrophenyl phosphorothioate
Phosdrin	Dimethyl-O-(1-methyl-2-carbomethoxyvinyl phosphate)
Disyston	Dimethyl S-(4-oxo-1,2,3,-benzotriazinyl-3-methyl phosphorodithioate)
Intermediate toxicity	
Ronnel	O,O-dimethyl O-(2,4,5-tri-chlorophenyl) phosphorothioate
Coumaphos	Diethyl-O-(3-chloro-4-methyl-7-coumarinyl) phosphorothioate
Chlorpyrifos (dursban)	O,O-diethyl-O-(3,5,6-trichloro-2-pyridyl) phosphorothioate
Trichlorfon	Dimethyl trichlorohydroxy-ethyl phosphonate
Low toxicity	
Malathion	Dimethyl-S-(1,2-bis-carbo-ethyl) phosphorodithioate
Diazinon	Diethyl-O-(2-isopropyl-6-methyl-4-pyrimidyl) phosphorothioate
Dichlorvos, DDVP	O,O-dimethyl-O-2,2-dichlorovinyl phosphate

choconstriction and excessive tracheobronchial secretions, can produce a rapidly fatal course.

Central nervous system clinical toxicity due to organophosphate poisoning encompasses a wide clinical spectrum. In carbamate poisonings, the central nervous system signs are not as prominent as those produced by organophosphates. In the less severe forms of poisoning, confusion, ataxia, slurred speech, and loss of tendon reflexes can occur. With more severe involvement, patients develop Cheyne-Stokes respirations, generalized convulsions, coma, and central respiratory paralysis. Medullary vasomotor and other cardiovascular centers also may be affected, causing potentially lethal disruption of cardiorespiratory function (16).

Organophosphate compounds differ with respect to their toxicity to humans and their distribution in various commercial products (Table 98-5). The most toxic organophosphate compounds are agricultural insecticides, such as parathion and disyston. Malathion and diazinon, organophosphates frequently used in household insecticide sprays, have much lower toxicity.

Evaluation of patients with organophosphate poisoning should focus on identifying the severity of toxicity for the purposes of therapy. The organophosphate-containing diluent of many pesticides possesses a typical kerosenelike odor. Patients who have consumed such compounds frequently demonstrate this odor. Contamination of the skin and clothes with organophosphate-containing liquid also gives rise to the typical hydrocarbon odor and systemic toxicity via dermal absorption.

Toxicity of organophosphate and carbamate poisoning relates to the excessive stimulation of muscarinic and nicotinic receptor sites by excess ACh, with subsequent receptor exhaustion. However, the clinical syndrome can have different manifestations, depending on the age of the patient, dose, and nature of the pesticide. Also, those who are occupationally exposed may have decreased AChE activity and, therefore, are at risk for toxicity caused by lower-dose exposures.

Mild organophosphate poisoning may present with a syndrome of headache, nausea, vomiting, abdominal cramps, and diarrhea. Patients with moderate organophosphate poisoning may present with generalized muscle weakness, skeletal muscle fasciculations, dysarthria, miosis, excessive secretions, shortness of breath, chest tightness, and dyspnea. Severely poisoned patients may present with seizures, coma, miotic pupils, fasciculations, skeletal muscle paralysis, pulmonary edema, and respiratory failure.

Certain features of organophosphate poisoning may occur also in other disease states. In some patients, for instance, symptoms arising from oral ingestion may be mistaken for an episode of gastroenteritis. Patients with muscle weakness may simulate Guillain-Barré syndrome, especially those patients with diazinon and chlorpyrifos poisoning who may present with a predominance of nicotinic manifestations. The small-sized pupils erroneously may suggest opiate poisoning or even pontine infarction. Excessive tracheobronchial secretions and bronchospasm may mimic an attack of acute bronchial asthma (16,17).

Certain organophosphates may inhibit plasma cholinesterase or RBC cholinesterase selectively after an acute exposure. Mevinphos has been known to depress plasma cholinesterase selectively more than RBC cholinesterase after an acute exposure (18). In a few clinical cases managed by the authors, phosmet has depressed RBC cholinesterase selectively more than plasma cholinesterase. Chlorpyrifos exposure in anecdotal pediatric cases also has depressed plasma cholinesterase selectively. Dimethoate, a phosphorotrithioate, selectively depressed RBC cholinesterase in one clinical case. Erythrocyte AChE is more sensitive to inhibition by dimethoate than is plasma pseudocholinesterase (19).

Pediatric patients (and, occasionally, adult patients) may present with a predominance of nicotinic effects manifesting mainly neuromuscular weakness. This neuromuscular weakness can be overlooked in a small child, who may appear very quiet and still. In children, normal or abnormal muscle tone should be confirmed. Noteworthy is the fact that tachycardia and generalized tonic-clonic seizures are seen frequently in pediatric pesticide exposures and rarely are reported in adult poisoning unless a massive exposure has occurred (20).

Acute Toxicity of Carbamates

Signs and symptoms of carbamate toxicity appear within minutes of absorption and are determined by excessive stimulation of muscarinic and nicotinic receptor sites. However, the toxicity of carbamates is more readily reversible as compared to organophosphates. Carbamate insecticides do not readily cross the blood–brain barrier (5). Most carbamate-associated deaths occur by suicide. In the majority of acute poisonings, cholinergic symptoms subsided in a short period. RBC cholinesterase reflects the degree of carbamate inhibition.

Occupational and Chronic Exposure

Occupational exposure to organophosphates and carbamates occurs mainly in agricultural workers who mix and apply pesticides or who work with crops containing pesticide residues. Illness can occur from any of these exposures and may be insidious, rendering the diagnosis difficult. Exposure in occupational settings is primarily inhalational or dermal.

Cholinesterase values can be used to monitor exposed workers; however, the range of normal plasma and RBC cholinesterase values varies greatly. Occupational exposures to organophosphates can result in a decline in cholinesterase values, which might be 50% lower than the "normal" upper limits yet remain greater than the normal lower limits. This decline can be accompanied by mild to moderate symptoms of toxicity that can include nausea, headache, dizziness, blurred vision, abdominal pain, vomiting, chest tightness, and shortness of breath. Symptoms may be present for several months before the syndrome is identified. One study of field workers exposed to

TABLE 98-6. Laboratory techniques for plasma and red blood cell acetylcholinesterase activity

Laboratory method	Procedure	Normal values
Electrometric (Michel)	Plasma and red cells are incubated with acetylcholine for 1 h. The drop of the pH is due to the formation of acetic acid and is directly proportional to the cholinesterase activity.	Plasma, 0.53–1.24 pH units; red blood cells, 0.57–0.98 pH units
Titrimetric (pH stat)	Plasma and red cells are incubated with acetylcholine for 3 min, and the acid formed is titrated with a base. The amount of base used is directly proportional to the cholinesterase activity.	Plasma, 3.6–6.8 mM/mL/min; red blood cells, 11.1–16.0 mM/mL/min
Colorimetric (Ellman)	Plasma and red cells are incubated for 10 min with acetylthiocholine, and the resultant thiocholine produces a yellow color in the presence of 5:5-dithiobid-(2-nitrobenzoic acid). The concentration of the yellow complex is directly proportional to the amount of cholinesterase present.	Plasma, 5.8–16.6 M-SH/mL/3 min
Gas chromatographic (Cramer)	Plasma and red cells are reacted for 30 min with a compound similar to acetylcholine. The product formed, dimethyl butanol, is quantitated using a gas chromatograph.	Plasma, 2.1–4.6 mM/mL/min; red blood cells, 8.1–11.8 mM/mL/min

pesticides has shown that a 30% decrease in RBC cholinesterase can be associated with symptoms of moderate organophosphate toxicity (21). This same study indicated that a rise in plasma cholinesterase of 15% to 20% occurred after discontinuation of a significant exposure. This rise in plasma cholinesterase is consistent with the rapid rate of recovery of the enzyme in plasma (21).

A continued increase in plasma cholinesterase after discontinuation of exposure helps to confirm intoxication further. RBC cholinesterase values should be monitored until they stabilize before affected individuals are returned to work. RBC cholinesterase normally varies 10% (21). A less than 10% increase in RBC cholinesterase over a previous value is not indicative of poisoning (21), whereas a greater than 10% increase of RBC cholinesterase suggests regeneration of enzyme and a toxic effect. Workers who experience long-term exposure to organophosphates may have chronically depressed cholinesterase values yielding a falsely low baseline on medical surveillance (22).

Laboratory Diagnosis

The laboratory diagnosis of organophosphate poisoning is based on depression of plasma and RBC cholinesterase activity. Routine laboratory tests usually are unremarkable, with a few notable exceptions. Hyperglycemia and glucosuria occasionally have been observed (23). The increase in serum glucose is believed to be secondary to the release of catecholamines from the adrenal medulla, which is activated by hyperactivity of the sympathetic ganglia (23). Hypokalemia also has been noted occasionally and is speculated to be secondary to an alteration of the distribution of potassium between intracellular and extracellular membranes, which is presumed to be due to increased circulating catecholamines (24,25).

Leukocytosis, both with and without a leftward shift, was a common finding in studies of anticholinesterase poisoning (23). This is presumed to be due to demargination from increased circulating catecholamines. Elevated serum amylase secondary to pancreatic injury from parasympathetic overstimulation and hypersecretion has been observed (26). Proteinuria also has been noted (26).

Regarding essential prerequisites to accurate diagnosis, clinicians should know the potential limitations of cholinesterase assays and the utility of a "therapeutic test" in equivocal cases of organophosphate poisoning. Although not routinely available in most clinical laboratories, RBC cholinesterase activity estimation is the most specific diagnostic test for organophosphate poisoning. Four methods are used commonly to quantitate plasma and RBC AChE activities: the electrometric (Michel), the titrimetric (pH stat), the colorimetric (Ellman), and the gas chromatographic (Cramer) methods (Table 98-6).

Most organophosphates inhibit both plasma and RBC cholinesterase, although, as noted, a few exceptions have been reported to suppress either plasma or RBC cholinesterase preferentially (Table 98-7). Clinicians should order tests of both RBC and plasma cholinesterase activity levels. Although the RBC cholinesterase activity assay is more reflective of the true level of inhibition, the assay may not be readily available. Thus, plasma cholinesterase activity level may be a helpful guide if RBC cholinesterase assays are unavailable or require days for results to be confirmed.

In most cases, the depressed cholinesterase activity levels correspond to the severity of poisoning. Thus, symptomatic patients frequently have a more than 50% depression of serum cholinesterase. Cholinesterase activity levels that are 20% to 50% of normal (preexposure) often signify mild poisoning, whereas values of 10% to 20% of normal (preexposure) usually indicate moderately severe poisoning, and less than 10% cholinesterase activity points to severe poisoning (Table 98-8) (26). However, this correlation proves valid only in the initial stage of acute poisoning. Moreover, for most affected patients, a preexposure cholinesterase level is not available. The very wide normal range of cholinesterase activity is an average for a population and so is of little help in specific patients without a preexposure value. A greater degree of inhibition occurs in patients with repeated exposures; in them, depressed values may persist even after symptomatic recovery.

In severe poisoning, serum cholinesterase may not normalize for 4 weeks or more after the exposure. RBC cholinesterase activity may require 90 to more than 120 days to return to normal. Although a normal erythrocyte cholinesterase activity effectively

TABLE 98-7. Organophosphates and selective inhibition of acetylcholinesterase

Organophosphate	Selected cholinesterase inhibition
Phosdrin	Plasma cholinesterase
Phosmet	Red blood cell cholinesterase
Chlorpyrifos	Plasma cholinesterase
Dimethoate	Red blood cell cholinesterase

Note: These organophosphates may depress selectively the activity of either red blood cell or plasma cholinesterase in clinical situations.

TABLE 98-8. Summary of specific antidote treatment for acute organophosphate poisoning

Level of poisoning	Clinical features	Red cell cholinesterase (percentage normal)
Subclinical	No symptoms or signs	>50%
Mild	Tiredness, dizziness, headache, nausea, vomiting, diarrhea, abdominal pain, salivation, wheezing	20–50%
Moderate	Symptoms of mild poisoning plus weakness, inability to walk, muscle fasciculations, dysarthria, miosis	10–20%
Severe	Symptoms of moderate poisoning plus coma, flaccid paralysis, cyanosis, pulmonary edema, and respiratory distress; marked miosis with loss of pupil reflexes	<10%

From Minton W, Murray V. A review of organophosphate poisoning. *Med Toxicol* 1988;3:365. Reprinted with permission.

rules out severe organophosphate poisoning in most cases, evaluation of lowered values often is problematic. Moderately severe symptoms may occur, for instance, even in patients whose erythrocyte cholinesterase activity is only 33% inhibited (21). Another limitation stems from reliance on a laboratory normal range of cholinesterase activity to evaluate a given patient's status. As the normal range is wide, patients with baseline "high" normal values may have less than 50% of cholinesterase activity—a value within the normal range—and still be symptomatic.

Depression of serum cholinesterase activity may occur also in other diseases: parenchymal liver disease, viral hepatitis, cirrhosis, hepatic congestion due to cardiac failure, and metastatic carcinoma. Low cholinesterase activity values may occur in patients with malnutrition, acute infections, anemia, myocardial infarction, and dermatomyositis (Table 98-9). In approximately 3% of the general population, low cholinesterase levels occur owing to a genetic variant. Also, plasma cholinesterase with a normal RBC cholinesterase can be found in patients who are pregnant or who are taking birth control pills (27–29). In pregnancy, the plasma cholinesterase values have been known to fall well below the lower limits of normal values (27).

TABLE 98-9. States affecting cholinesterase activity

Cholinesterase	State
Plasma	
Low	Parenchymal liver disease, hepatic metastases
	Malnutrition (protein or thiamine)
	Chronic debilitating conditions
	Acute infections
	Some anemias
	Myocardial infarction
	Pregnancy
	Birth control pills
Normal	Uncomplicated obstructive jaundice
	Myasthenia gravis
	Hyperthyroidism
	Asthma
	Hypertension
	Epilepsy
	Diabetes mellitus
Raised	Nephrotic syndrome
Red cell	
Raised	Reticulocytosis due to anemias, hemorrhage, and treatment of megaloblastic-pernicious anemias

Note: A plasma cholinesterase may be reduced in debilitated patients with these conditions.
Adapted from W Minton, V Murray. A review of organophosphate poisoning. *Med Toxicol* 1988;3:363.

MANAGEMENT OF TOXICITY

Clinical management should be directed at decontamination followed by antidotal therapy with atropine and pralidoxime. Attention should be directed to controlling seizures, secretions, respiratory compromise, and cardiac dysrhythmias.

In patients who do not exhibit clear-cut features of organophosphate poisoning, clinicians may find the effect of atropine or pralidoxime (or both) useful for confirming the diagnosis (14). Because patients with organophosphate poisoning with muscarinic symptoms usually are resistant to atropine, a small dose of 0.5 to 1.0 mg of atropine given parenterally prior to pralidoxime administration often does not result in characteristic anticholinergic effects, such as tachycardia or mydriasis. However, if such signs develop soon after a small dose of atropine is administered, patients (i) have not been exposed to organophosphates, (ii) may have a very mild form of poisoning, or (iii) may have a predominance of effects. Intravenous injection of 500 mg to 1 g of pralidoxime aids by increasing muscle strength and ameliorating fasciculations.

Optimum management of organophosphate poisoning demands more than the administration of specific antidotes. To ensure a favorable outcome, clinicians also must pay attention to decontamination measures, provide adequate cardiorespiratory support, treat convulsions, and prevent specific complications. Finally, monitoring of seriously toxic patients is essential, as signs and symptoms of poisoning can recur when antidotal therapy is stopped prematurely.

Decontamination

Decontamination begins by removal of contaminated clothing and washing of affected patients with copious amounts of water and soap. Damage to the skin may lead to increased absorption of the poison. Contaminated or potentially contaminated clothing must be placed in plastic bags. Emergency care personnel should wear disposable gloves during the decontamination procedure. Frequently overlooked contaminated sites are hair and nails.

Ocular exposure not only may cause severe discomfort to the patient but may create confusion during the course of treatment. When organophosphate-containing aerosols or vapors directly affect the eyes, patients develop a severe degree of miosis that may last hours or days despite systemic therapy (18). Large amounts of sterile saline (up to 1 L per eye) should be used for 10 to 15 minutes to flush the chemical from the eyes. If saline is not available, clean tap water may be used.

In patients who have ingested organophosphate compounds either accidentally or with suicidal intent, the state of consciousness should be assessed carefully prior to gastric evacuation. As many of these pesticides have a solvent diluent, pulmonary aspiration with subsequent pneumonitis can occur. Gastrointestinal decontamination of unabsorbed poison is accomplished with activated charcoal. In patients who are unconscious, a nasogastric or orogastric tube should be inserted and gastric lavage should be performed. Appropriate precautions should be taken to protect the airway, such as placing the patient in the lateral decubitus position or performing intubation.

Cardiac Dysrhythmias

QT prolongation and torsades de pointes with ventricular dysrhythmias have been reported in organophosphate poisoning (30,31). Sinus bradycardia, asystole, atrioventricular dissociation, idioventricular rhythms, multifocal premature ventricular contractions, and prolongation of PR, QRS, and QT intervals have been observed (30,31). The etiology of these cardiac problems probably is multifocal: excess ACh, metabolic acidosis, autonomic dysfunction, electrolyte derangements, and repolarization problems. Clinical management should take into account the possibility of these dysrhythmias and conduction abnormalities. Dysrhythmias and sudden death have been reported several days after an acute poisoning episode (30,31). Cardiac monitoring is essential, and 12-lead electrocardiographs should be examined for prolongation of intervals, dysrhythmias, and early repolarization. Owing to the late occurrence of dysrhythmias, cardiac monitoring is warranted for several days after an acute, serious poisoning. Patients with organophosphate toxicity are susceptible to cardiac arrest due to bradyasystolic rhythms or ventricular fibrillation. Hypoxia and a direct toxic effect often result in a hyperirritable myocardium.

Respiratory Compromise and Respiratory Arrest

Appropriate respiratory support not only proves immediately life-saving but critically influences the outcome of organophosphate poisoning. Patients with severe poisoning may have pulmonary edema owing to the hyperstimulation of muscarinic receptors in the lungs. Without appropriate respiratory support, atropine may lead to ventricular fibrillation in hypoxic, acidotic patients. Adequate control of the airway, with proper ventilation to correct acidosis and restore tissue oxygenation as soon as possible, is important to reduce the hazards of ventricular ectopy. Depending on the degree of respiratory distress, patients may require a combination of atropine, airway suctioning with or without tracheal intubation, or positive airway pressure and mechanical ventilation. After restoration of adequate respiratory function, cardiovascular support frequently necessitates expansion of blood volume prior to the use of inotropic agents, such as dopamine. Severely poisoned patients often are hypovolemic, owing to emesis and diarrhea.

Additionally, atropine does not block nicotinic receptors; thus, a fully atropinized patient may succumb to respiratory arrest, owing to nicotinic receptor exhaustion. The skeletal muscle neurojunctions are nicotinic; thus, muscle paralysis can occur even with full atropinization.

Convulsions

Convulsions may arise as an effect of the poisoning, of cerebral hypoxia, or of the presence of another poison. In patients whose convulsions stem from cerebral hypoxia, improved cardiopulmonary function is essential prior to controlling the acute episode with anticonvulsants. In addition to optimum cerebral perfusion, intravenous diazepam can control seizures (up to 20 mg in adults, administered slowly until seizures stop). For children younger than 12 years, diazepam, 0.1 to 0.2 mg per kg, can be used. Lorazepam may be used at the dose of 0.03 to 0.05 mg per kg, up to a maximum of 4 mg every 6 hours. In all cases, patients should be watched carefully for hypotension and respiratory depression, both of which are especially likely to occur in such patients. The use of diazepam in organophosphate poisoning has been shown to improve mortality and morbidity in animal studies, independent of its anticonvulsant effects (16).

Pharmacotherapy

Pharmacologic treatment of organophosphate poisoning relies on concurrent or sequential administration of atropine and the cholinesterase "reactivator" pralidoxime. Although atropine counters the muscarinic and some central nervous system manifestations of organophosphate compound poisoning, pralidoxime reverses both the muscarinic and nicotinic effects.

Atropine

Owing to the fact that atropine is a tertiary amine, it crosses the blood–brain barrier and antagonizes ACh at central muscarinic receptors. However, atropine does not inhibit the action of ACh at the nicotinic receptors. Additionally, atropine has no effect on skeletal muscle weakness or respiratory failure and may have no effect on seizures or unconsciousness.

The concept of proper dosing of atropine is important. The end point of atropine therapy is to dry secretions (32). For adults, the recommended dose is 0.5 to 2.0 mg of the drug every 10 to 15 minutes intravenously until full atropinization occurs.

Atropine dose should be titrated to the point of drying secretions. Heart rate and pupillary size are not useful parameters in atropinizing poisoned patients. For example, miosis from direct ocular exposure to military war nerve gas is relatively unresponsive to atropine (5,32). For a child younger than 12 years, an initial intravenous atropine dose of 0.05 mg per kg is followed by a maintenance dose of 0.02 to 0.05 mg per kg, repeated every 10 to 30 minutes until cholinergic signs are reversed (33). Because absolute dose and frequency of atropine administration will depend on how severely an affected child is poisoned, titrating the amount of atropine to whatever level is required, rather than titrating to a specific dose, is appropriate to control cholinergic signs (33). Atropine also is fairly effective by the intramuscular route, although its anticholinergic effects ensue more promptly after intravenous administration.

Tachycardia is a nonspecific sign, and dilated (or even unequal) pupils have occurred, although rarely, in organophosphate poisoning. Cholinesterase inhibition may cause either bradycardia or tachycardia, depending on such factors as resting vagal tone and whether organophosphate toxicity produces predominantly muscarinic effects (bradycardia) or nicotinic effects (tachycardia) via sympathetic ganglia. An initially normal or slow pulse rate increasing after introduction of atropine usually indicates anticholinergic effect. Similarly, baseline normal or small-sized pupils that subsequently dilate on anticholinergic administration indicates atropinization.

Atropine administration should not be terminated suddenly if a patient has been treated for days. Instead, progressively increasing intervals should be used between successive doses while the patient is monitored for return of cholinergic features, such as miosis, excessive lacrimation or salivation, or depressed respiration. In many patients, such signs may prove fairly subtle and include recurrence of small-airway obstruction (wheezing) and rales. Such patients may, in fact, require further anticholinergic drug administration.

The decision to stop administration of atropine depends on a patient's clinical condition. In general, however, experts advise that occupational exposure with dermal contact or inhalation (or both) may necessitate full atropinization for at least 12 to 24 hours after thorough dermal decontamination is ensured. In patients who have ingested the poison, atropinization for several days may be essential, with a potential for administration of many grams of atropine. Also, patients exposed to toxic doses of fat-soluble organophosphates, such as fenthion, should be atropinized for 3 to 4 days to prevent recurrence of symptoms. Two laboratory

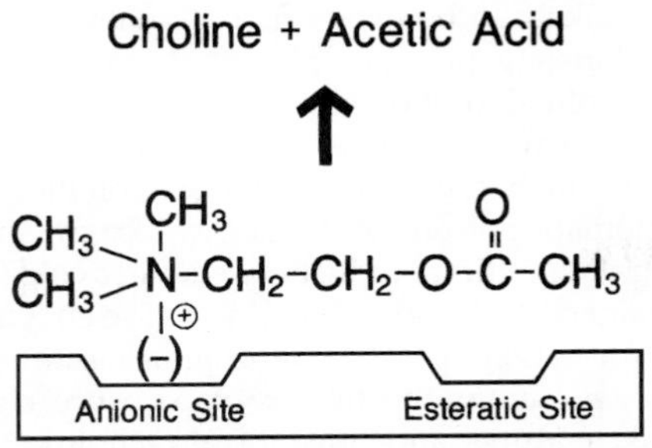

Choline + Acetic Acid

$(CH_3)_3N^{+}-CH_2-CH_2-O-C(=O)-CH_3$

(-)

Anionic Site Esteratic Site

Figure 98-3. Pralidoxime. Cholinesterase reactivating oxime used in the treatment of organophosphate poisoning.

estimations—rising levels of blood cholinesterase activity and elimination of organophosphate metabolites from patients' urine—may help in reducing atropine dosage.

Patients with significant exposure to organophosphate compounds usually demonstrate a large degree of tolerance to atropine. Hence, despite frequent administration of very large doses, atropine toxicity rarely occurs in such patients. Occasionally, however, in mildly poisoned patients given excessively large doses of atropine, such symptoms and signs as delirium, hyperpyrexia, and muscle fasciculations may occur. Mild degrees of atropinization merely prove discomforting to patients and do not require specific treatment.

Oximes

Severe degrees of organophosphate poisoning, especially in patients demonstrating muscle fasciculations and neuromuscular weakness, mandate use of pralidoxime chloride (PAM) (Fig. 98-3). PAM is efficacious in such patients through a combination of three major biochemical effects. Of these, the most important is cleavage of the phosphate bond from cholinesterase, which reactivates the cholinesterase enzyme. In addition, pralidoxime also may react directly with and detoxify the organophosphate molecule and has been said to possess an anticholinergic "atropinelike" effect by decreasing the need for atropine due to cholinesterase regeneration. Unlike atropine, however, pralidoxime administration reactivates cholinesterase enzyme at neuromuscular junctions and postganglionic autonomic neurons. Thus, pralidoxime helps to counter muscular weakness in such sites as thoracic muscles, alleviating respiratory dysfunction. Although pralidoxime is a quaternary ammonium compound and presumably does not cross into the central nervous system, it has been shown to mediate a beneficial effect in the central nervous system and should, therefore, be tried (16).

Pralidoxime should be administered regardless of the type of organophosphate involved. The effectiveness of pralidoxime depends on the length of the postexposure period prior to pralidoxime administration and the specific organophosphate compound involved. For optimum effects, pralidoxime should be administered immediately after poisoning. Reactivating inhibited AChE becomes difficult with time, owing to a process known as *aging* (also termed the *Straver reaction*). The organophosphorus moiety on the inhibited enzyme becomes dealkylated, which prevents reaction with the oxime. The rate of aging varies greatly among the different organophosphorus compounds. In patients administered the drug more than 36 hours after exposure, significant reactivation of cholinesterase may not occur. However, pralidoxime should be administered in these late cases in the hope of obtaining some effect. In some cases, pralidoxime has reversed toxicity of diazinon and chlorpyrifos successfully days after exposure. Treatment also proves effective in poisoning due to other cholinesterase inhibitors, such as TEPP and mevinphos. Studies have shown that toxic organophosphate levels can continue for days, requiring days of continuous intravenous infusions of pralidoxime (34).

In adult patients with normal renal function, the usual initial dose of pralidoxime is 1 to 2 g as an intravenous infusion, preferably given over 15 to 30 minutes (35,36). The drug should be diluted in 100 mL of normal saline. The initial bolus of pralidoxime should be followed by a continuous infusion of the drug at a rate of 500 mg per hour in adults.

The minimum effective plasma level of pralidoxime is 4 μg per mL. In an adult, pralidoxime levels fell below 4 μg per mL at 1.5 to 2.0 hours after a 1-g intravenous bolus of pralidoxime (35,36). This means that with an 8-hour intermittent bolus regimen for an adult patient, pralidoxime levels would be therapeutic for 1.5 hours and nontherapeutic for 6.5 hours (35,36).

Rapid intravenous injection of pralidoxime has produced tachycardia, laryngospasm, muscle rigidity, and transient neuromuscular blockade. Hypertension also has been reported (35,36). In a study involving seven organophosphate-poisoned children, between 15 and 50 mg per kg of pralidoxime was used as a loading dose and between 9 and 19 mg per kg per hour was administered as a continuous infusion (37).

In severely poisoned patients, an initial combination of atropine and pralidoxime may prove more effective. Serial determination of plasma or RBC cholinesterase also may help in judging the efficacy of pralidoxime administration.

In most patients, few side effects occur with therapeutic doses of pralidoxime. Adverse effects include excitement, mania, confusion, tachycardia, dizziness, headache, blurred vision, impaired accommodation, diplopia, muscle weakness, and rigidity. Excessively rapid administration of pralidoxime also may cause temporary worsening of cholinergic manifestations, an effect possibly related to the moderate anticholinesterase activity of oximes by binding to cholinesterase prior to regenerating its activity. Rarely, acute hypersensitivity reactions may occur after pralidoxime therapy.

Although pralidoxime currently is the oxime used most commonly in humans, such other oximes as obidoxime, trimedoxime, and asoxime have been shown to have potent enzyme-reactivating properties (38–40). Unlike pralidoxime, obidoxime is able to cross the blood–brain barrier and reactivate brain cholinesterases; however, this capability may not confer additional benefits over peripheral cholinesterase reactivators. Work with asoxime suggested that it has fewer side effects than does pralidoxime (40). Asoxime, also termed *HI-6*, has demonstrated efficacy against soman, a military nerve agent (40). Asoxime also has been shown to be effective and to have fewer side effects in treating humans with poisonings from commercial insecticide (40). Additionally, it produced clinical improvement before RBC cholinesterase values rose, thus indicating a direct pharmacologic effect (40).

Carbamates and the Use of Pralidoxime

Organophosphates and carbamates have similar modes of action and similar toxic effects. Despite these similarities, pralidoxime is not as popular for treating carbamate poisonings as it is for organophosphate poisonings. Reasons for this include the fact that carbamates are generally shorter-acting and that 2-PAM is thought to have a potential additive inhibitory effect on cholinesterase in carbamate poisoning.

No reported evidence in humans indicates that pralidoxime is unsafe as adjunctive therapy with atropine in a critically ill, carbamate-poisoned patient. In fact, published cases have cited effective pralidoxime therapy in carbamate-poisoned patients

(41,42). One author used pralidoxime effectively to treat a patient in cholinergic crisis with profound weakness and fasciculations. The patient ultimately proved to be poisoned with carbaryl.

COMPLICATIONS

The most frequent complications of organophosphate poisoning are aspiration pneumonia, chemical pneumonitis due to aspiration, complications of multiple seizures, and target organ effects of hypoxemia. Vigorous respiratory management, therefore, is crucial in all patients with organophosphate poisoning. Another complication that can occur is a recurrence of anticholinesterase signs and symptoms in severe poisoning cases. Respiratory arrest days after therapy can occur in such cases.

Delayed and Long-Term Effects

Delayed effects of organophosphate toxicity include neuropathy and ocular disease (43–49). Long-term consequences include chronic neurologic sequelae and neurobehavioral toxicity (50–53).

The delayed neurologic sequelae of organophosphates are termed *organophosphorus-induced delayed neuropathy* (OPIDN) (43,44). The neuropathy target esterase seems to play a major role in the etiology of OPIDN (44). The function of the neuropathy target esterase is not known. Protein kinase–mediated phosphorylation of cytoskeleton proteins of nerve cells also is linked to the development of OPIDN (45).

This OPIDN commences peripherally and proceeds proximally. Symptoms include lower-extremity paresthesias that may progress to weakness and ataxia, with occasional progression of symptoms to the arms (46–49). In the classic presentation, these symptoms usually occur 6 to 21 days after an acute nonlethal exposure. The early administration of pralidoxime and atropine does not seem to prevent this complication. In general, long-term recovery has been slow, with symptoms persisting for months to years.

Recently, several publications report findings in human populations of an increased incidence of myopia and a more advanced visual disease syndrome (Saku disease) (54). This disease was correlated with increasing use of organophosphates in agriculture. What remains to be established is whether ocular testing for individuals working with these agents will be used in the future for biological monitoring and risk assessment.

Prognosis

Severely poisoned, untreated patients usually die within 24 hours after complications occur. Severely poisoned, treated victims may succumb to complications after a period of days. In all other cases, provided cerebral hypoxia and multiorgan system failure have been prevented or treated successfully, clinicians can expect total symptomatic recovery within days to weeks (and occasionally months in severe cases).

PREVENTION OF EXPOSURE

In view of their potentially serious toxicity, organophosphate compounds necessitate strict adherence to certain precautions for those exposed at the workplace, especially for agricultural workers. Mandatory measures include adherence to strict personal hygiene, thorough cleansing of contaminated clothes, wearing of protective gloves and clothing at all times, and limiting of dermal contact.

In persons likely to be exposed continually or frequently to organophosphates (e.g., organophosphate mixers, loaders, and applicators), evaluation of baseline plasma and RBC cholinesterase levels may prove helpful. Assessment of intermittent levels also may be useful, because cholinesterase inhibition often occurs before symptomatic poisoning. Workers whose cholinesterase values demonstrate significant reductions should avoid further exposure and await normalization of cholinesterase enzyme activity.

Patients for whom prior cholinesterase estimates are not available may present with a history of exposure, cholinesterase inhibition–like features, and "low normal" cholinesterase levels. Such patients should return to work only after repeat plasma cholinesterase estimates are performed 3 to 5 days later. If significant exposure has occurred, repeat plasma cholinesterase levels will increase by 15% to 20%.

REGULATION OF PESTICIDES

The U.S. Federal Insecticide, Fungicide, and Rodenticide Act (FIFRA), enacted in 1947, remains the primary statute regulating pesticide manufacturing, use, and distribution. The FIFRA was amended in 1972, 1975, and 1978. The EPA has been responsible for regulation of pesticide use since 1970.

U.S. pesticide regulation first occurred under the Insecticide Act of 1910. This early act was a consumer protection measure against mislabeling and distribution of ineffective pesticides. The FIFRA eventually replaced this act. Pesticides also are regulated by the EPA under the following acts:

- Federal Environmental Pesticide Control Act
- Resource Conservation Recovery Act of 1972
- Comprehensive Environmental Response, Compensation, and Liability Act (Superfund)
- Toxic Substances Control Act
- Clean Water Act
- Safe Drinking Water Act

A pesticide is defined in the FIFRA as "any substance or mixture of substances intended for preventing, destroying, repelling, or mitigating any pest, and . . . any substance or mixture of substances intended for use as a plant regulator, defoliant, or desiccant." Pesticides include insecticides, fungicides, herbicides, rodenticides, desiccants, disinfectants, defoliants, and nematocides. The FIFRA requires that all pesticides sold or distributed be registered with the EPA. Once they are registered, the FIFRA classifies the use of a pesticide as general or restricted. The application and use of pesticides are tightly controlled by the EPA under FIFRA regulations.

The FIFRA prohibits the sale of unregistered pesticides, the production of pesticides by unregistered manufacturers, the use of adulterated pesticides, and the use of a pesticide in a manner inconsistent with its labeling. The EPA has the authority to enforce the FIFRA by legal sanctions, including civil penalties, criminal fines, injunctions, product seizure, and termination of product sales or recalls. When evidence indicates that a particular pesticide may be a significant health hazard, the appropriate regulatory agency or agencies can take any of the following actions (51):

- Issuance of permissible exposure limits for the workplace
- Cancellation of registration and withdrawal of the product from the market
- Placement of restrictions on use or application of the compound
- Setting of tolerance limits for pesticide residues on foodstuffs
- Establishment of maximum permissible contamination levels for the pesticides in drinking water

In addition to regulating pesticide use and application, the FIFRA requires that the pesticide manufacturer be registered with the EPA. The EPA, under agreement with the U.S. Food and Drug Administration, establishes pesticide tolerances for raw foods and produce. Pesticides that might be considered food additives are controlled by the EPA under the Food, Drug, and Cosmetic Act. Once a pesticide is discarded, it becomes a hazardous waste and then falls under regulation by the Resource Conservation and Recovery Act rather than by the FIFRA.

The 1978 amendment to the FIFRA allows manufacturers of pesticides to obtain a waiver on submission of data demonstrating efficacy of their product, except when the product has a direct relation to or effect on public health. In addition, the 1978 amendment allows for public disclosure of the safety and health data regarding pesticide regulation. The 1978 amendment also transfers to states the responsibility to enforce pesticide use regulations if they can demonstrate that they possess the means to do so. The EPA reserves the right to revoke any state's responsibility for pesticide regulation if that state is unable or unwilling to enforce the regulations.

REFERENCES

1. Al-Saleh IM. Pesticides: a review article. *J Environ Pathol Toxicol* 1994;13:151–161.
2. Marrs TC. Organophosphate poisoning. *Pharmacol Ther* 1993;58:51–66.
3. Morita H, Yanagisawa N, Nakajima, et al. Sarin poisoning in Matsumoto. *Lancet* 1995;346:290–293.
4. Okumura T, Nobukatsu T, Ishimatsu S, et al. Report on 640 victims of the Tokyo subway sarin attack. *Ann Emerg Med* 1996;28:129–135.
5. Machemer LH, Pickel M. Carbamate insecticides. *Toxicology* 1994;91:29–36.
6. Levine RS, Doull J. Global estimates of acute pesticide morbidity and mortality. *Rev Environ Contam Toxicol* 1992;129:29–50.
7. Litovitz TL, Felberg L, White S, et al. 1995 Annual report of the American Association of Poison Control Centers Toxic Exposure Surveillance System. *Am J Emerg Med* 1996;14:487–531.
8. Koelle GB. Pharmacology of organophosphates. *J Appl Toxicol* 1994;14:105–109.
9. Jeyaratnam J, Maroni M. Organophosphorus compounds. *Toxicology* 1994; 91:15–27.
10. Sussman JL, Harel M, Frolow F, et al. Atomic structure of acetylcholinesterase from *Torpedo californie*: a prototypic acetylcholine-binding protein. *Science* 1991;253:872–879.
11. Mason J, Waine E, Stevenson A, et al. Aging and spontaneous reactivation of human plasma cholinesterase activity after inhibition by organophosphorus pesticides. *Hum Exp Toxicol* 1993;12:556–559.
12. Sanderson D, Edson E. Toxicological properties of the organophosphate insecticide dimethioate. *Br J Ind Med* 1964;21:52–64.
13. Chatonnet A, Lockridge O. Comparison of butyrylcholinesterase and acetylcholinesterase. *Biochem J* 1989;260:625–634.
14. Lotti M. Cholinesterase inhibition: complexities in interpretation. *Clin Chem* 1995;41:1814–1818.
15. Nouira S, Abroug F, Elatrous S, et al. Prognostic value of serum cholinesterase in organophosphate poisoning. *Chest* 1994;106:1811–1814.
16. McDonough J, Jaax N, Crowley R, et al. Atropine and/or diazepam therapy protects against soman-induced neural and cardiac pathology. *Fundam Appl Toxicol* 1989;13:256–276.
17. Fisher J. Guillain-Barré syndrome following organophosphate poisoning. *JAMA* 1977;238:1950.
18. Coye M, Barnett P, Midtling J, Velasco A, et al. Clinical confirmation of organophosphate poisoning of agricultural workers. *Am J Ind Med* 1986;10:399–409.
19. Hayes W. *Pesticides studied in man*. Baltimore: Williams & Wilkins, 1982: 2884–435.
20. Zwiener RJ, Ginsburg CM. Organophosphate and carbamate poisoning in infants and children. *Pediatrics* 1988;81:121–126.
21. Midtling JE, Barnett PG, Coye MJ, et al. Clinical management of field worker organophosphate poisoning. *West J Med* 1985;142:514.
22. Ames RG, Brown SK, Mengle DC, Kahn E, Stratton JW, Jackson RJ. Cholinesterase activity depression among California agricultural pesticide applicators. *Am J Ind Med* 1989;15:143–150.
23. Mellar D, Fraser I, Kruger M. Hyperglycemia in anticholinesterase poisoning. *Can Med Assoc J* 1981;124:745–747.
24. Mackey C. Anticholinesterase insecticide poisoning. *Heart Lung* 1982; 11:479–484.
25. Hui K. Metabolic disturbances in organophosphate insecticide poisoning [letter]. *Arch Pathol Lab Med* 1983;104:154.
26. Haubenstock A. More on the triad of pancreatitis, hyperamylasemia and hyperglycemia. *JAMA* 1983;249:1563.
27. Hayes M, Van Der Westhuizen N, Gelfand M. Organophosphate poisoning in Rhodesia. *S Afr Med J* 1978;53:230–234.
28. Robson N, Robertson I, Whittaker M. Plasma cholinesterase changes during the puerperium. *Anesthesia* 1986;41:243–249.
29. Whittaker M, Charlier AR, Ramaswamy S. Changes in plasma cholinesterase isoenzymes due to oral contraceptives. *J Reprod Fertil* 1971;26:373–375.
30. Ludomirsky A, Klein H, Sarelli P, et al. Q-T prolongation and polymorphous ("torsade de pointes") ventricular arrhythmias associated with organophosphorus insecticide poisoning. *Am J Cardiol* 1982;49:1654–1658.
31. Brill D, Maisel A, Prabhu R. Polymorphic ventricular tachycardia and other complex arrhythmias in organophosphate insecticide poisoning. *J Electrocardiol* 1984;17(1):97–102.
32. Dunn MA, Sidell FR. Progress in medical defense against nerve agents. *JAMA* 1989;262:649–652.
33. Mortensen ML. Management of acute childhood poisonings caused by selected insecticides and herbicides. *Pediatr Clin North Am* 1986;33:421–445.
34. Willems J, Bisschop H, Verstraete A. Cholinesterase reactivation in organophosphorus poisoned patients depends on the plasma concentrations of the oxime pralidoxime methylsulfate and of the organophosphate. *Arch Toxicol* 1993;67:79–84.
35. Waser PG, Alioth-Streichenberg CM, Hopff WH, et al. Interaction of obidoxime with sarin in aqueous solution. *Arch Toxicol* 1992;66:211–215.
36. Thompson DF, Thompson GD, Greenwood RB, et al. Therapeutic dosing of pralidoxime chloride. *Drug Intell Clin Pharmacol* 1987;21:590–593.
37. Farrar HC, Wells TG, Kearns GL. Use of continuous infusion of pralidoxime for treatment of organophosphate poisoning in children. *J Pediatr* 1990;116: 658–661.
38. Kassa J. Comparison of efficacy of two oximes (HI-6 and obidoxime) in soman poisoning in rats. *Toxicology* 1995;101:167–174.
39. Das Gupta S, Ghosh AK, Moorthy MV, et al. Comparative studies of pralidoxime, trimedoxime, obidoxime and diethyxime in acute fluostigmine poisoning in rats. *Pharmazie* 1982;37:605.
40. Kusic R, Jovanovic D, Randjelovic S, et al. HI-6 in man: efficacy of the oxime in poisoning by organophosphorus insecticides. *Hum Exp Toxicol* 1991;10:113–118.
41. Burgess J, Bernstein J, Hurlbut K. Aldicarb poisoning. *Arch Intern Med* 1994;154:221–224.
42. Ekins B, Geller R. Methomyl-induced carbamate poisoning treated with pralidoxime chloride. *West J Med* 1994;161(1):68–70.
43. Wu SY, Casida JE. Subacute neurotoxicity induced in mice by potent organophosphorus neuropathy target esterase inhibitors. *Toxicol Appl Pharmacol* 1996;139:195–202.
44. Pope CN, Tanaka D, Padilla S. The role for neurotoxic esterase (NTE) in the prevention and potentiation of organophosphorus-induced delayed neurotoxicity (OPIDN). *Chem-Biol Interact* 1993;87:395–406.
45. Abou-Donia MB. The cytoskeleton as a target for organophosphorus ester–induced delayed neurotoxicity (OPIDN). *Chem Biol Interact* 1993;87:383–393.
46. Lotti M, Becker CE, Aminoff MJ. Organophosphate polyneuropathy: pathogenesis and prevention. *Neurology* 1984;34:658–662.
47. Gordon JJ, Inns RH, Johnson MK, et al. The delayed neuropathic effects of nerve agents and some other organophosphorus compounds. *Arch Toxicol* 1983;52:71–82.
48. Senanayake N, Johnson MK. Acute polyneuropathy after poisoning by a new organophosphate insecticide. *Med Intell* 1982;306:155–159.
49. Cherniack M. Organophosphorus esters and polyneuropathy. *Ann Intern Med* 1986;104:264–266.
50. Savage E, Keefe T, Mounce L, et al. Chronic neurological sequelae of acute organophosphate pesticide poisoning. *Arch Environ Health* 1988;43:38–45.
51. Rosenstock L, Keifer M, Daniel W, et al. Chronic central nervous system effects of acute organophosphate pesticide intoxication. *Lancet* 1991;338: 223–227.
52. Steeland K, Jenkins B, Ames R, et al. Chronic sequelae to organophosphate pesticide poisoning. *Am J Public Health* 1994;84:731–736.
53. Yokoyama K, Shunichi A, Murata K. Chronic neurobehavioral effects of Tokyo subway sarin poisoning in relation to post-traumatic stress disorder. *Arch Environ Health* 1998;53(4):249–256.
54. Dementi B. Ocular effects of organophosphates: a historical perspective of Saku disease. *J Appl Toxicol* 1994;14:119–129.

CHAPTER 99
Organochlorine Pesticides

Mark D. Van Ert and John B. Sullivan, Jr.

Chlorinated hydrocarbon pesticides include DDT, DDE, and DDD; hexachlorocyclohexane (HCH) and isomers, including lindane (γ-HCH); cyclodiene compounds; chlordecone, kelevan, and mirex; toxaphene; and dicofol and methoxychlor (Table 99-1). The general toxicity of chlorinated hydrocarbon insecti-

TABLE 99-1. Organochlorine pesticides

DDT
DDE
DDD (Rothane)
Aldrin
Dieldrin
Endrin
Endosulfan
Isobenzan (telodrin)
Chlordane
Heptachlor
Hexachlorocyclohexane (technical-grade)
Lindane (γ-hexachlorocyclohexane)
Chlordecone (Kepone)
Kelevan
Mirex (Dechlorane)
Dicofol (Kelthane)
Methoxychlor (Marlate)
Toxaphene

cides is central nervous system (CNS) stimulation or depression, depending on the compound and dose. Cyclodienes, HCHs, and toxaphene pesticides inhibit chloride influx in the CNS induced by gamma-aminobutyric acid (GABA) and thus interfere with GABA receptor function (1,2). This mechanism of inhibition is consistent with the clinical symptoms of CNS excitation and seizures seen in acute toxicity from organochlorine pesticides. In general, aldrin, dieldrin, lindane, toxaphene, endrin, and chlordane exposures via the oral, dermal, or inhalational route can cause seizures, muscle tremors, confusion, agitation, and coma as common manifestations.

DDT, DDE, AND DDD

DDT [dichlorodiphenyl trichloroethane or 1,1,1-trichloro-2,2-bis(*p*-chlorophenyl) ethane] was widely used for controlling insects, particularly those that carried typhus and malaria. Technical DDT is a mixture of three forms: *p,p*'-DDT, *o,p*'-DDT, and *o,o*'-DDT. These analogs of DDT are odorless, white crystalline solids. DDE [dichlorodiphenyl-dichloroethylene, 1,1-dichloro-2,3-bis(*p*-chlorophenyl) ethylene] and DDD [1,1-dichloro-2,2-bis(*p*-chlorophenyl) ethane] are minor contaminants found in technical DDT (3). DDT is no longer used as a pesticide in the United States. However, it is still used widely in other areas of the world for the control of insect disease vectors.

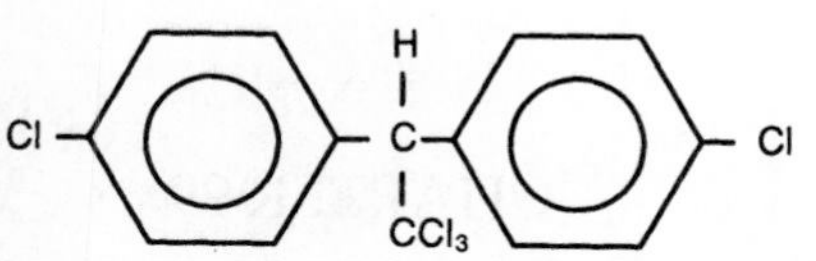

Cl–C₆H₄–C(H)(CCl₃)–C₆H₄–Cl

Chemical formula	$C_{14}H_9Cl_5$
Chemical name	*p,p'*-DDT
Synonyms	1,1,1-trichloro-2,2-bis(*p*-chlorphenyl) ethane; dichlorodiphenyl trichloroethane,4,4' DDT
Trade names	Genitox, Anofex, Detoxen, Pentachlorin, Dicophane, Chlorophenothane

Figure 99-1. DDT. (From ref. 3, with permission.)

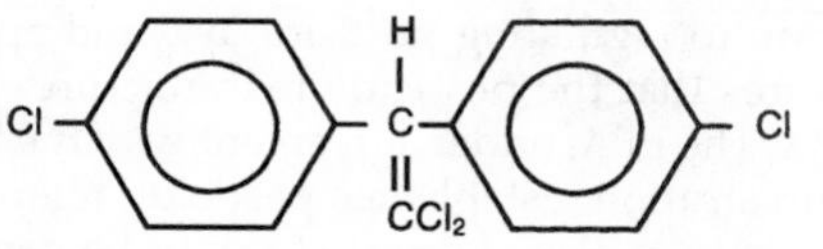

Chemical formula	$C_{14}H_8Cl_4$
Chemical name	*p,p'*-DDE
Synonyms	DDT dihydrochloride; dichlorodiphenyldichloroethylene; 1,1-dichloro-2,2-bis(*p*-chlorophenyl) ethylene

Figure 99-2. DDE. (From ref. 3, with permission.)

Chemical and Physical Properties

Chemical structures of DDT, DDE, and DDD are shown in Figures 99-1 through 99-3. Technical DDT is formed by condensing chloral hydrate with chlorobenzene in the presence of sulfuric acid (3). DDT was first synthesized in 1874, and its insecticide properties were discovered in 1939 (3). In 1972, the U.S. Environmental Protection Agency (EPA) banned the use of DDT except in cases of public health emergencies. Peak usage of DDT in the United States occurred in 1963, when 80 million kg of DDT was applied to agricultural areas (3).

Human Exposure to DDT, DDE, and DDD

Despite being banned in the United States in 1972, DDT still is used heavily in other areas of the world for control of disease-transmitting insects. Questions regarding DDT use remain unanswered: (i) Does DDT or its metabolites cause human cancer? (ii) Does the bioaccumulation of DDT, DDE, and DDD pose some unknown health effect to future generations? (iii) Does the persistence of DDT and its metabolites in the environment pose environmental health risks to animals and humans? DDT persists for long periods after soil application and is converted to DDE, which persists even longer. DDT, DDE, and DDD may leach into water supplies from soil and crops. DDT and DDE bioaccumulate up the food chain (3,4).

DDT and its primary metabolites, DDE and DDD, have been found at hazardous-waste sites on the National Priority List in the United States. DDT and its metabolites are ubiquitous in the environment and are constantly being transformed and redistributed. Volatilization of DDT and DDE account for losses from soil and water (3,4). DDD is less volatile than either DDT or DDE. DDT, DDE, and DDD are highly lipid soluble and thus concentrate in human and animal adipose tissue. The long envi-

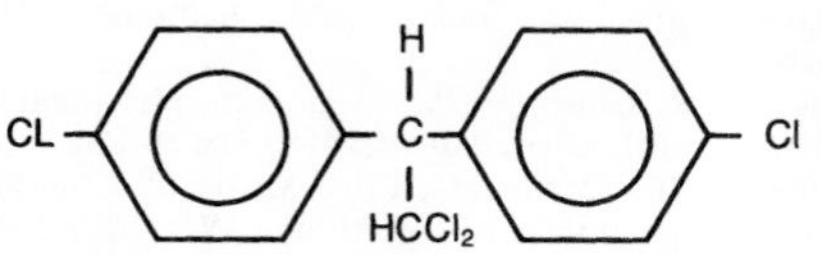

Chemical formula	$C_{14}H_{10}Cl_4$
Chemical name	*p,p'*-DDD
Synonyms	1,1-bis(4-chlorophenyl)-2,2-dichloroethane; 1,1-dichloro-2,2-bis(*p*-chlorophenyl) ethane
Trade names	DDD; Rothane; Dilene

Figure 99-3. DDD. (From ref. 3, with permission.)

TABLE 99-2. Regulations applicable to DDT, DDE, or DDD

Agency	Description	Value
Federal and international agencies, regulations		
WHO	Conditional acceptable daily intake in food	0.005 mg/kg
WHO	Evidence of human carcinogenicity	ND
OSHA	TWA	1 mg/m^3
EPA	Maximum contaminant level in drinking water	NA
EPA	Reportable quantity	1 lb (proposed)
EPA	Listing as a hazardous-waste substance	ND
EPA	Listing as toxic pollutant	ND
	Listed in RCRA Appendix IX for groundwater monitoring	ND
EPA	TSCA chemical substance inventory	ND
EPA	Recommended action levels for sum of residues	
	Range	0.05 (grapes, tomatoes) to 3.0 (carrots) ppm
	Most fruits and vegetables	0.1–0.5 ppm
	Eggs	0.5 ppm
	Grains	0.5 ppm
	Milk	0.05 ppm
	Meat	5 ppm
EPA	Reference dose (oral)	5.0×10^{-4} mg/kg/day
	Potency factor (oral, inhalation)	3.4×10^{-1} mg/kg/day (DDT, DDE) 2.4×10^{-1} mg/kg/day (DDD)
FIFRA	Most uses canceled in 1972	
Federal agencies, guidelines		
NIOSH	IDLH	ND
	TWA (air and skin)	1 mg/m^3
ACGIH	TWA	1 mg/m^3
NAS	Suggested no-adverse-response level (SNARL)	ND
	7-day	ND
	24-hour	ND
EPA	Ambient water quality criteria to protect human health	2.85 μg/L (DDT) ND (DDD and DDE)
EPA	Carcinogenic classification	B2[a]
	Water and fish and shellfish ingestion	0.0024 ng/L (DDT) (risk level corresponding to 10^{-7}) 2.6×10^{-6} μg/L for concentrations $<1 \times 10^3$ μg/L (DDD)
	Fish and shellfish consumption only	0.0024 ng/L (DDT) (risk level corresponding to 10^{-7})
State environmental agencies, regulations and guidelines		
	Drinking water quality standards for DDT in several states	
Alabama		No special or state rule
Alaska		No special or state rule
Arizona		No special or state rule
California		No special or state rule
Colorado		No special or state rule
Delaware		No special or state rule
Connecticut		No special or state rule
Florida		No special or state rule
Georgia		No special or state rule
Hawaii		No special or state rule
Idaho		No special or state rule
Illinois		50 μg/L
Indiana		No special or state rule
Iowa		No special or state rule
Kansas		0.42 μg/L (DDT) 2.4×10^{-5} μg/L (DDE) 2.4×10^{-5} μg/L (DDD)
Kentucky		No special or state rule
Maine		0.83 μg/L
Maryland		No special or state rule
Massachusetts		No special or state rule
Minnesota		1.0 μg/L
Mississippi		No special or state rule
Missouri		No special or state rule
Montana		No special or state rule
Nebraska		No special or state rule
Nevada		No special or state rule
New Hampshire		No special or state rule

(continued)

TABLE 99-2. *(continued)*

Agency	Description	Value
New Mexico		No special or state rule
New York		No special or state rule
North Carolina		No special or state rule
Ohio		No special or state rule
Oklahoma		No special or state rule
Oregon		No special or state rule
Rhode Island		No special or state rule
South Carolina		No special or state rule
South Dakota		No special or state rule
Tennessee		No special or state rule
Texas		No special or state rule
Utah		No special or state rule
Vermont		No special or state rule
Virginia		No special or state rule
West Virginia		No special or state rule
Wisconsin		No special or state rule
	Acceptable ambient air concentrations of DDT in several states	
Connecticut		5 $\mu g/m^3$ (8 h)
Kansas		2.381 $\mu g/m^3$ (DDT) (annual)
		2.4×10^{-5} $\mu g/kg$ (DDE) (guideline)
		2.4×10^{-5} $\mu g/L$ (DDD) (guideline)
Nevada		0.04 $\mu g/m^3$ (8 h)
Pennsylvania (Philadelphia)		1.8 $\mu g/m^3$ (DDT) (1 yr)
		1.8 $\mu g/m^3$ (DDE)
Virginia		16 $\mu g/m^3$ (24 h)

ACGIH, American Conference of Governmental Industrial Hygienists; EPA, U.S. Environmental Protection Agency; FIFRA, Federal Insecticide, Fungicide, and Rodenticide Act; IDLH, immediately dangerous to life and health; NAS, National Academy of Sciences; NA, not applicable; ND, no data; NIOSH, National Institute for Occupational Safety and Health; OSHA, U.S. Occupational Safety and Health Administration; TSCA, U. S. Toxic Substances Control Act; TWA, time-weighted average; WHO, World Health Organization.
[a]EPA weight-of-evidence classification scheme for carcinogens: A, human carcinogen—sufficient evidence from human epidemiologic studies; B1, probable human carcinogen—limited evidence from epidemiological studies and adequate evidence from animal studies; B2, probable human carcinogen—inadequate evidence from epidemiologic studies and adequate evidence from animal studies; C, possible human carcinogen—limited evidence in animals in the absence of human data; D, not classified as to human carcinogenicity; and E, evidence of noncarcinogenicity.
Adapted from ref. 3, with permission.

ronmental half-life of these compounds, coupled with their lipophilic properties, results in bioaccumulation.

Photooxidation and biodegradation of DDT can occur in air, soil, and water. DDT and DDE are slowly degraded to CO_2 and hydrochloric acid by solar radiation (3,4). Environmental concentrations of DDT, DDE, and DDD worldwide have tended to remain relatively constant despite continued widespread application, owing to their continuous biological oxidation by ultraviolet light (4).

The loss of DDT from soils is primarily through volatilization, water runoff, and chemical transformation. Some biodegradation occurs by aerobic and anaerobic microorganisms. Aerobic metabolism results in a conversion of DDT to DDE. Anaerobic conditions result in conversion of DDT to DDD. DDT conversion to DDE is slower than its conversion to DDD. The DDE and DDD metabolites of DDT are resistant to further transformation, and the half-life estimates for biodegradation of DDT in soil range from 2 to 15 years (3,4). Human exposures occur mainly through diet via bioaccumulation up the food chain and from breastfeeding.

Low levels of DDT and its metabolites will continue to be present in the environment because other countries are still applying it. Because of the partitioning of DDT and DDE into human breast milk, breast-fed infants will receive DDT and DDE from the mother. Exposure to DDT and its metabolites by inhalation is negligible.

Distribution of DDT in the Environment

DDT and its analogs are detected by gas chromatography–mass spectrometry in both environmental samples and human tissues. DDE, the primary metabolite of DDT, commonly is found in samples of human adipose tissue.

Regulations relating to DDT and its analogs are presented in Table 99-2. DDT, DDE, and DDD are also listed in the Toxic Chemicals Substance Section 313 of the Emergency Planning and Community Right to Know Act of 1986 Superfund Amendment Reauthorization Act (SARA Title III).

Airborne concentrations of DDT have been found to range from 1.4 to 1,560 ng per cubic meter and DDE from 1.9 to 131 ng per cubic meter (3). Since the ban on DDT use was enacted, air concentrations have been declining. Over the period 1974 to 1975, the arithmetic mean DDT air concentration decreased from 11.9 to 7.5 ng per cubic meter (3). Air samples collected in the Gulf of Mexico in 1977 showed a DDT range of 0.010 to 0.078 ng per cubic meter (3).

The U.S. National Soils Monitoring Program has followed the soil pattern concentration of DDT since its banning. DDT and DDE residues in soils have been steadily declining since 1972. In 1970, soil DDT concentrations averaged 0.18 parts per million (ppm), decreasing to 0.02 ppm by 1972 (3).

The concentrations of DDT and DDE also declined in foods between 1965 to 1975.

The median concentration of DDT and DDE in water samples in the United States is approximately 1 part per trillion (ppt) (3). Industrial effluents have shown concentrations of 10 ppt of DDT, DDE, and DDD. Overall, the concentrations of DDT and its residues appear to be decreasing in the environment since 1972.

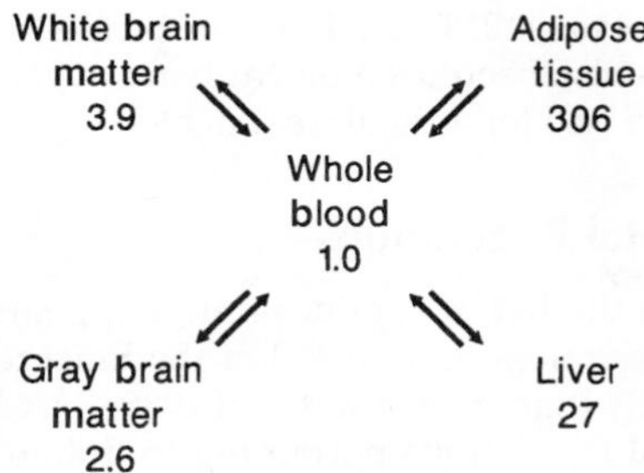

Figure 99-4. Relationship of the distribution of DDT and related chemicals among blood and certain tissues in humans. (From ref. 21, with permission.)

Absorption, Metabolism, and Excretion

DDT and its metabolites, DDE and DDD, are found in samples of human blood, adipose tissue, human breast milk, umbilical cord blood, and placental tissue (5–13). However, there is no correlation between the concentrations in human tissues and environmental concentrations. Higher ratios of DDD or DDT to DDE may indicate recent exposure, as DDT and DDD have shorter half-lives (3). Concentrations of DDT in fatty tissue are 300 times higher than those in blood (3). The partitioning of DDT among tissues as compared to blood demonstrates the high lipid solubility of the compound (Fig. 99-4). Due to the fact that DDT and DDE are stored in fatty tissues and are released slowly from these sites, making a correlation between concentrations in tissues and the time of exposure is difficult.

Environmental exposure concentrations are lower than any dose that will have identifiable health effects. A decline in human tissue concentrations of DDT has occurred since 1972 (4). The estimated daily dietary intake of DDT declined from 0.24 mg per person per day in 1970 to 0.008 mg per person per day in 1973 (4). The World Health Organization (WHO) established an acceptable dietary intake of DDT as 0.005 mg per kg per day and, from 1965 to 1970, the dietary intake of DDT declined to 0.0007 mg per kg per day (4).

The metabolism of DDT, DDE, and DDD has been studied in humans and other animal species (Fig. 99-5). Chronic oral ingestion of DDT induces the hepatic microsomal mixed-function oxidase system (3,4). Humans excrete DDT more slowly than do animals. Also, it is estimated that if all human DDT exposure were terminated, 10 to 20 years would pass before all DDT was removed from human tissue (4). However, DDE, with its longer half-life, will persist for many years beyond this (4).

Clinical Toxicology of DDT

Volunteers given DDT orally have developed symptoms of gait disturbance, malaise, fatigue, headache, nausea, tremors, and vomiting, depending on the dose. Test doses were 750 mg, 1,000 mg, or 1,500 mg of DDT (3). All subjects recovered from their symptoms within 24 hours. Ingestion of DDT, either accidentally or intentionally, can result in similar symptoms. Exposure to large oral doses of DDT can result in excitability, tremors, and convulsions. This neurologic effect probably is a result of interference with sodium and potassium conductance across cell membranes. Other health effects at high exposure concentrations of DDT are irritation of the mucous membranes, nose, throat, and mouth, nausea, and headache.

Carcinogenesis and Immunotoxicity

No information exists on the immunotoxic effects of DDT or its metabolites in humans. Although immunologic effects in animals have been documented, extrapolating these findings to the human condition has been difficult. Even though DDT has produced liver nodules in mice, several other studies in animals have not demonstrated carcinogenesis. No evidence reveals that DDT or its metabolites are human carcinogens. Further, no information establishes a causal relationship between DDT, DDE, and DDD concentrations in blood and fat or other tissues in relation to specific health effects.

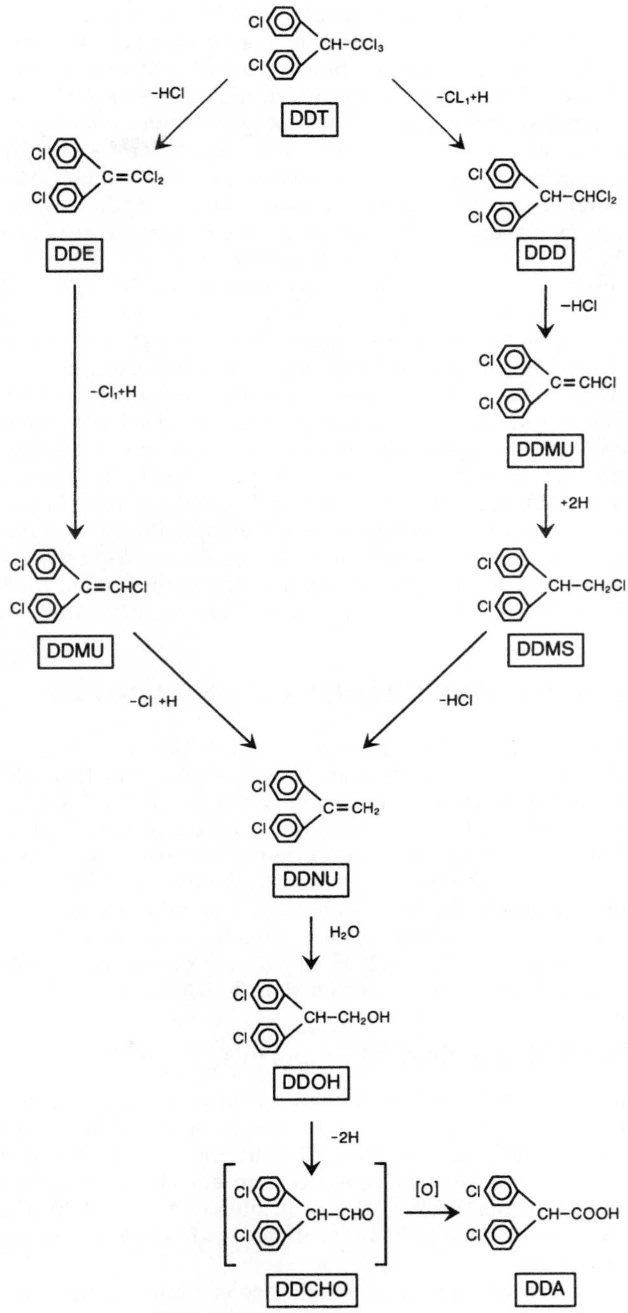

The International Agency for Research on Cancer has reviewed the literature on the carcinogenicity of these compounds and has found no convincing evidence of the carcinogenic risk of DDT and DDE in humans, although evidence of DDT carcinogenicity in the mouse model was found. In a large, multicenter prospective study, plasma levels of DDE and poly-

Figure 99-5. Metabolism of DDT. (From ref. 3, with permission.)

chlorinated biphenyls were measured in 240 women who subsequently were given a diagnosis of breast cancer (14). This study was triggered by the observation that breast cancer rates vary by up to fivefold across the globe. In addition, it has been observed that the daughters of women who migrate from a country with a low incidence of breast cancer to a country with a high incidence acquire the breast cancer rate of their new country. Many researchers have interpreted these epidemiologic data as being supportive of the hypothesis that breast cancer rates are strongly linked to environmental and lifestyle factors.

Because hormonal activity is associated with the organochlorine chemicals, a working hypothesis was proposed that linked these "environmental estrogens" with breast cancer rates. Hunter et al. (14) did not demonstrate a link between the median level of DDE and breast cancer risk. The median level of DDE was lower in case subjects than among control subjects. Similar data were found with polychlorinated biphenyl levels. These results were consistent with the data published by Krieger et al. in 1994 (15). An editorial in the *New England Journal of Medicine* stated, "The results of Hunter et al., along with those of other studies, should reassure the public that the weakly estrogenic organochlorine compounds such as [polychlorinated biphenyls], DDT, and DDE are not a cause of breast cancer" (16).

HEXACHLOROCYCLOHEXANE AND LINDANE

HCH, sometimes misnamed *benzene hexachloride*, was applied widely through the 1960s and 1970s. Discovered in 1825, HCH was used as a smoke munition in World War I. The insecticide properties of HCH were discovered in 1942. Owing to its chemical structure, various isomeric forms of HCH exist (Fig. 99-6), the best known of these being γ-HCH or lindane. Technical-grade lindane consists of several isomers: α, β, γ, and δ. The toxicity of these isomers, in terms of their effectiveness in controlling insects, is inequitable, γ-HCH being more potent than α-HCH, and α-HCH being more effective than β-HCH (17).

Chemical and Physical Properties

Eight isomers of HCH are known, and all have the empirical formula of $C_6H_6Cl_6$ and a molecular weight of 290.8. The isomeric mixture of HCH is a brown–off-white powder with a musty odor and is soluble in acetone, benzene, and chlorinated hydrocarbon solvents. HCH is almost insoluble in water (18). The γ isomer or lindane is heat-stable and can vaporize without decomposition.

HCH is manufactured by ultraviolet photochlorination of benzene (17). Technical-grade HCH consists of an isomeric mixture of α (70%), β (7%), γ (5%), δ (5%), and others (5%). Fractional crystallization of the γ-HCH isomer yields a 99.8% product of γ-HCH called *lindane* (17). Production of lindane was terminated in 1976 in the United States. Lindane has been available as an emulsifiable concentrate, liquids, powders, gas, pressurized liquids, aerosol sprays, and granules. Besides its past use as an insecticide, lindane still is used as a scabicide for humans and animals. It has also been used on fruit and vegetable crops, for seed treatment, and for animal treatment.

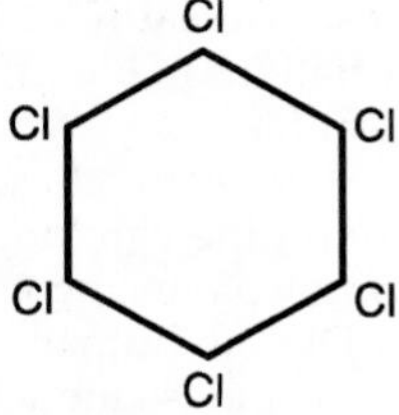

Figure 99-6. Hexachlorocyclohexane (α, β, γ, δ isomers).

Environmental Regulations

Lindane is on the list of chemicals that appears in the Toxic Chemicals Substances Section 313 of the Emergency Planning and Community Right to Know Act of 1986 (SARA Title III). The environmental regulations pertaining to lindane are summarized in Table 99-3.

Human Exposure

Exposure to lindane and other HCH isomers occurs from occupational and environmental sources via dermal contact, inhalation, or ingestion. Lindane and the other HCH isomers can reach the environment through their use as pesticides and during production of the product. HCH can be detected in air, soil, aquatic organisms, and water. Most human exposures occur through the ingestion of plants, animals, and dairy products. α-, β-, γ-, and δ-HCH isomers have been detected at a number of hazardous-waste sites. Lindane has been detected at waste sites in surface water at a mean concentration of 0.5 parts per billion (ppb) and in the soil around these sites at a concentration of 11 ppb (2). The β isomer of HCH has been found in surface water around hazardous-waste sites at a mean concentration of 2.89 ppb and in soil at these sites at a mean concentration of 150 ppb. The δ isomer has been detected at hazardous-waste sites at a mean concentration of 31 ppb and in the soil around these sites at a concentration of 6.6 ppb (18).

Release of lindane into the air has occurred through its application as a pesticide. Release of lindane into surface water occurs from surface runoff or from deposition of the chemical through rain and other forms of precipitation. Low concentrations of lindane have been detected in samples of water runoff in a variety of cities around the United States. Lindane movement in the environment occurs via leaching from soil into groundwater, adsorption to particles in the soil, and volatilization into the atmosphere. An important consideration pertaining to the release of lindane from soil into surface water is the relative content of the organic matter versus clay in the soil. Soil with a higher organic content will adsorb lindane and reduce leaching. Lindane in the soil is degraded primarily by microorganisms. Depending on the isomer, either anaerobic or aerobic conditions will be most conducive to biodegradation (18).

Lindane released into surface water can bioconcentrate in aquatic organisms. The other isomers of HCH, as well as lindane, bioconcentrate up through the food chain. Owing to its lipophilic nature, lindane concentrates in adipose tissue. Very little biodegradation of the HCH isomers occurs.

Monitoring of lindane and other HCH isomers in ambient air in the United States during the period 1970 to 1972 has shown a mean concentration of 0.9 ng per cubic meter in a ten-state area (18). A maximum lindane concentration of 11.7 ng per cubic meter was reported in the same study. Other monitoring that has been performed at a variety of locations in the United States has shown γ-HCH to be present at concentrations of 0.1 to 7.0 ng per cubic meter (18). However, there were no detectable concentrations in rural areas. During a heavy period of pesticide usage in 1972 to 1974, atmospheric concentrations of lindane were as high as 9.3 ng per cubic meter (18).

In global monitoring of HCH isomers, air samples in the world's remote areas range from 1.1 to 2.0 ng per cubic meter in air and 3.1 to 7.3 ng per L in water (18). Water concentrations of lindane evaluated at numerous areas across the United States have mea-

TABLE 99-3. Regulations and guidelines applicable to hexachlorocyclohexane

Agency	Description	Value
International agencies		
Oral		
WHO	Acceptable daily intake	0.0–0.01 mg/kg
	Allowable tolerances (γ-HCH) range	0.05 mg/kg (potatoes) to 2 mg/kg (lettuce)
	Most fruits and vegetables	0.5 mg/kg
WHO	Guideline for drinking water	0.003 mg/L
Other		
IARC	Carcinogenic classification	Group 3[a]
	α-HCH	
	β-HCH	
	γ-HCH	
National agencies		
Regulations		
Oral		
EPA	Tolerances (γ-HCH) range	0.01 ppm (pecans) to 7 ppm (meat fat)
	Most fruits and vegetables	1 or 3 ppm
EPA	Maximum contaminant level in drinking water (lindane)	0.004 mg/L
FDA	Permissible level in bottled water (lindane)	0.004 mg/L
	Action levels (lindane)	
	Most fruit and vegetables	0.5 ppm
	Cereals	0.1 ppm
	Milk	0.3 ppm
Inhalation		
OSHA	Permissible exposure limit, TWA for lindane (skin)	0.5 mg/m^3
Other		
EPA	Reportable quantity lindane	1 lb
	Extremely hazardous substance	
	Threshold planning quantity for lindane	1,000/10,000 lb
	Listing as toxic waste: discarded commercial products, off-specification species, container residues, and spill residues of lindane. Listing as a hazardous waste constituent. General pretreatment regulations for existing and new sources of pollution.	
	Maximum concentration of contaminants; toxicity (lindane)	0.4 mg/L
	TSCA chemical substance inventory (all isomers)	
	General permits under the National Pollutant Discharge Elimination System	
Guidelines		
Oral		
EPA	Maximum contaminant level goal, proposed, for lindane	0.0002 mg/L
	Health advisories for lindane	
	1-day	1.2 mg/L
	10-day	1.2 mg/L
	Longer-term	
	Adult	0.12 mg/L
	Child	0.033 mg/L
	Lifetime	0.2 μg/L
EPA	Ingestion of water and aquatic organisms	
	α-HCH	0.92–92.0 ng/L
	β-HCH	1.63–163.0 ng/L (risk, 10^{-7}–10^{-5})
	γ-HCH	1.86–186.0 ng/L (risk, 10^{-7}–10^{-5})
	Technical-grade HCH	1.23–23.0 ng/L (risk, 10^{-7}–10^{-5})
	Ingestion of aquatic organisms only	
	α-HCH	1–310.0 ng/L (risk, 10^{-7}–10^{-5})
	β-HCH	5.47–547.0 ng/L (risk, 10^{-7}–10^{-5})
	γ-HCH	6.25–625.0 ng/L (risk, 10^{-7}–10^{-5})
	Technical-grade HCH	4.14–414.0 ng/L (risk, 10^{-7}–10^{-5})
NAS	Suggested no-adverse-effect level for lindane	
	7-day	0.5 mg/L
	24-hour	3.5 mg/L
Inhalation		
ACGIH	Threshold limit value	
	TWA for lindane (skin)	0.5 mg/m^3
NIOSH	IDLH level (all isomers)	1,000 mg/m^3
Other		
EPA	Carcinogenic classification	
	α-HCH	Group B2[b]
	β-HCH	Group C[b]
	γ-HCH	Group B2/C[b,c]
	δ-HCH	Group D[b]

(continued)

TABLE 99-3. Regulations and guidelines applicable to hexachlorocyclohexane

Agency	Description	Value
	Technical-grade HCH	Group B2[b]
	Reference dose, oral (γ-HCH)	3×10^{-4} mg/kg/day
	$q_1{}^{*d}$ (oral)	
	α-HCH	6.3 $(mg/kg/day)^{-1}$
	β-HCH	1.8 $(mg/kg/day)^{-1}$
	γ-HCH	1.3 $(mg/kg/day)^{-1}$
	Technical-grade HCH	1.8 $(mg/kg/day)^{-1}$
	$q_1{}^{*d}$ (inhalation)	
	α-HCH	6.3 $(mg/kg/day)^{-1}$
	β-HCH	1.8 $(mg/kg/day)^{-1}$
	Technical-grade HCH	1.8 $(mg/kg/day)^{-1}$

ACGIH, American Conference of Governmental Industrial Hygienists; EPA, U.S. Environmental Protection Agency; FDA, U.S. Food and Drug Administration; HCH, hexachlorocyclohexane; IARC, International Agency for Research on Cancer; IDLH, immediately dangerous to life and health; NAS, National Academy of Sciences; NIOSH, National Institute for Occupational Safety and Health; OSHA, U.S. Occupational Safety and Health Administration; TSCA, U.S. Toxic Substances Control Act; TWA, time-weighted average; WHO, World Health Organization.

[a]IARC weight-of-evidence classification scheme for carcinogens: Group 1, carcinogenic to humans—sufficient evidence from human epidemiologic studies; Group 2A, probably carcinogenic to humans—limited evidence from human epidemiologic studies; Group 2B, probably carcinogenic to humans, inadequate data from human epidemiologic studies and sufficient evidence from animal studies; Group 3, cannot be classified as to its carcinogenicity in humans.

[b]EPA weight-of-evidence classification scheme for carcinogens: A, human carcinogen—sufficient evidence from human epidemiologic studies; B1, probable human carcinogen—limited evidence from epidemiological studies and adequate evidence from animal studies; B2, probable human carcinogen—inadequate evidence from epidemiologic studies and adequate evidence from animal studies; C, possible human carcinogen—limited evidence in animals in the absence of human data; D, not classified as to human carcinogenicity; and E, evidence of noncarcinogenicity.

[c]The EPA Office of Drinking Water and the Office of Pesticide Programs are considering γ-HCH (lindane) as Group C for regulatory purposes pending review.

[d]$q_1{}^*$ represents the upper-bound estimate of the low dose of the dose-response curve, as determined by the multistage procedure. The $q_1{}^*$ can be used to calculate an estimate of carcinogenic potency, the incremental excess cancer risk per unit of exposure (usually milligrams per liter of water, milligrams per kilogram of food per day, and grams per cubic meter of air).

Adapted from ref. 3, with permission.

sured between 10 and 319 ppt (18). Lindane is detected in approximately 10% of urban water runoff samples in cities across the United States in concentrations ranging from 0.052 to 0.1 ppt (18).

Given the widespread, but low, environmental concentrations of HCH isomers and their bioconcentration up the food chain, the most important human exposure at the present time is through ingestion of food products, mainly meats and dairy products. HCH isomers have been detected in dairy products, meats, fish, poultry, fruits, oils, fats, leafy vegetables, sugar, and other foods. To a lesser degree, other human exposures occur from the ingestion of drinking water that contains small concentrations of lindane. Previous estimates by the U.S. Department of Health, Education, and Welfare on the average daily intake of lindane have varied from 3 μg per day to a low of 0.22 μg per day (18).

In workers involved in the production of technical HCH and lindane, serum and adipose tissue concentrations of HCH isomers during production increase with exposure time (14,16–18). Human serum concentrations of HCH have been reported in the following ranges: α-HCH, 10 to 273 μg per L; β-HCH, 17 to 760 μg per L; and γ-HCH, 5 to 188 μg per L (17). A significant increase in β-HCH concentrations in the serum of chronically exposed workers was apparent (17). β-HCH adipose concentrations were 300 times greater than serum concentrations (17).

No documented adverse health effects among employees involved in lindane production have been noted as compared to control populations (18,19). Nonetheless, workers who directly handled HCH, as well as exposed nonhandlers, complained of headache, paresthesias, giddiness, malaise, tremors, apprehension, loss of sleep, confusion, vomiting, decreased libido, and impaired memory (20). The total HCH in the serum of those workers ranged from 0.143 to 1.152 μg per L (20). Serum concentrations of HCH are related to the degree and duration of exposure, with β-HCH accumulating more than the other isomers and accounting for nearly 30% of the total HCH serum concentrations (20).

Lindane and other HCH isomers have been detected in the blood and adipose tissue of the general public in a variety of countries (5–13,21–27). Lindane blood concentrations were found to be highest in people in the age group 41 to 60 years (18). The National Human Adipose Tissue Survey conducted in 1982 demonstrated that β-HCH was detected in 87% of samples collected, ranging in concentrations from 19 to 570 ng per gram of tissue (18). In autopsy surveys conducted between 1970 and 1975, β-HCH was present in more than 90% of human adipose tissue samples at a level of 300 ppb (18,21). Reports indicate that the median level of β-HCH in the United States has fallen from a level of 140 ppb to 80 ppb (18). Although the median concentration in human adipose tissue has diminished, the chemical still is detected in virtually 100% of the general population (5–13,21–27).

Factors influencing the body concentration of lindane include age, dietary habits, and location of the country in which the person lives. Higher levels of lindane and other HCH isomers are found in nonvegetarians. Studies of human breast milk have demonstrated HCH isomers in 82% of samples at a mean concentration of 81 ppb and a range of 0 to 480 ppb (18,23,28,29).

Gas chromatography–mass spectrometry methods can detect lindane and HCH isomers at the parts-per-billion level. Although methods are available that can detect and quantify concentrations of HCH isomers, correlating these concentrations with environmental concentrations or toxic effects remains impossible.

Despite the fact that HCH isomers can be detected in blood, serum, urine, and adipose tissue in the general population, the concentration in these tissues does not correlate with adverse health effects. Mean serum concentrations of total HCH in subjects have been reported to be 0.27 ppm for those who did not handle the product and 0.6 ppm for those who directly handled the product (20). Of the total HCH evaluated by assay in the serum of these individuals, 60% to 100% was in the form of the β-HCH isomer. The serum concentrations were reported as follows: 0.07 to 0.72 ppm of β-HCH, 0.004 to 0.18 ppm α-HCH, 0.0 to 0.17 ppm for lindane, and 0.0 to 0.16 ppm for δ-HCH (20). The investigators reported that handlers of HCH, as well as those

TABLE 99-4. Summary of hexachlorocyclohexane (HCH) occupational exposure

Study group	Total HCH	β-HCH	α-HCH	γ-HCH	δ-HCH
	Occupational exposure, serum concentrations (ppm)				
Controls (mean)	0.05 (0–0.37)	0.029 (0–0.1)	0.022 (0–0.26)	0.007 (0–0.01)	0
Handlers (mean)	0.60 (0.20–1.15)	0.41 (0.16–0.72)	0.10 (0.024–0.18)	0.06 (0.01–0.17)	0.04 (0–0.16)
Nonhandlers (mean)	0.266 (0.08–0.66)	0.207 (0.065–0.5)	0.0412 (0.004–0.16)	0.016 (0–0.04)	0.0017 (0–0.022)
		Occupational exposure, adipose tissue concentrations (mg/kg)			
Controls		0.3–2.4	0.01–0.2	0–0.1	
Workers		18–103 (45.6 ± 24.4)	1–15 (5.8 ± 5)	0–11 (3.2 ± 3.1)	
				Occupational exposure to lindane (γ-HCH)	
				Blood conc. (ppb)	**Air conc. (mg/m^3)**
Nonproduction workers				0.93 (0.3–2.5)	9–49
Production workers with no skin contact, Group I				4.6 (1.9–8.3)	31–1,800
Production workers with no skin contact, Group II				4.1 (1.0–8.9)	11–1,170
Production workers with no skin contact, Group III				30.6 (6.0–93)	11–1,170

Adapted from refs. 17, 20, and 31.

who were not directly exposed, had complained of facial paresthesias, headaches, dizziness, malaise, vomiting, tremors, confusion, and impaired memory (20). Serum levels were measured also in maintenance workers who periodically visited the worksite. Serum concentrations in these workers were much lower than in those workers who were occupationally exposed. Liver functions among the exposed workers were not statistically significantly different from those in controls (30). Table 99-4 summarizes HCH serum and adipose tissue concentrations in various occupational situations (17,23,31).

In one study, exposure levels of α-HCH were 0.002 to 1.99 mg per cubic meter, of β-HCH were 0.001 to 0.38 mg per cubic meter, and of lindane or γ-HCH were 0.004 to 0.15 mg per cubic meter. The mean blood levels of 57 workers measured 0.5 μg of α-HCH, 0.9 μg of β-HCH, and 0.7 μg of γ-HCH per L (17). The accumulation of β-HCH isomer has been demonstrated to increase in a linear fashion with the duration of exposure. Adipose concentrations in samples from autopsies have ranged from 0.03 to 0.47 ppm for total HCH and 0.04 to 0.57 ppm for β-HCH (24).

Animal studies have shown various distribution patterns of HCH isomers, the γ- and β-HCH isomers being stored primarily in the fatty tissues (32). The distribution of lindane also was highest in the fatty tissue, followed by brain, kidney, muscle, lungs, heart, spleen, liver, and blood. Lindane has a propensity to accumulate in the brain more than does β-HCH (18). Lindane also induces hepatic mixed-function oxidase systems, increasing its own metabolism. This process may minimize or reduce the accumulation of lindane in tissues (18).

Lindane has been detected in blood and CNS tissue of autopsied infants who have died after total body application of a 1% lotion (33). Initial blood concentrations of lindane were 206 ppb and declined to 1.0 ppb in 25 days. Brain concentrations were threefold that of blood in this report (33).

The accumulations of lindane in adipose tissue occur across the placenta and to newborns through breast milk (34–37). Concentrations of lindane in human breast milk were found to be five to seven times higher than concentrations in the maternal blood or in umbilical cord blood. Older women tend to harbor higher lindane concentrations of HCH and lindane in placental and umbilical cord blood than do younger women (34–36). Also noteworthy is that lindane concentrations increased in maternal blood during delivery and that, during pregnancy, higher concentrations were found in fetal blood and fetal tissue as well as placenta and amniotic fluid as compared to maternal fat tissue (34–36).

Metabolism of Lindane

The primary metabolites of lindane are chlorophenols and chlorobenzenes (Fig. 99-7) (30). Chlorinated metabolites in the urine have been found in lindane production workers. The major metabolite is trichlorophenol, which accounted for approximately 58% of lindane metabolites identified in the urine (18). Other metabolites are dichlorophenols, tetrachlorophenols, hexachlorobenzene, tetrachlorocyclohexanol, and pentachlorocyclohexene. Pentachlorophenol has also been identified as a urinary metabolite in humans after occupational exposure (18).

Clinical Toxicology of Lindane and Isomers

Human exposure that results in toxic health effects can occur by inhalation, dermal absorption, and via the gastrointestinal tract. Most studies of acute lindane inhalational poisoning have focused on anecdotal cases of home exposure from the use of vaporized lindane (37). Irritation of the eyes, throat, and upper airway may occur after short-term exposure to lindane vapors. Further reports of effects secondary to inhalation of lindane have included various blood dyscrasias: anemia, leukopenia, leukocytosis, granulocytopenia, granulocytosis, eosinophilia, thrombocytopenia, increased bone marrow megakaryocytes, and decreased bone marrow megaloblastoid erythroid series (37,38). Aplastic anemia and pancytopenia have also been reported to occur after lindane exposure (18,37,38).

Kashyap (27) reported statistically significant elevations in hepatic enzymes in 19 occupationally lindane-exposed individ-

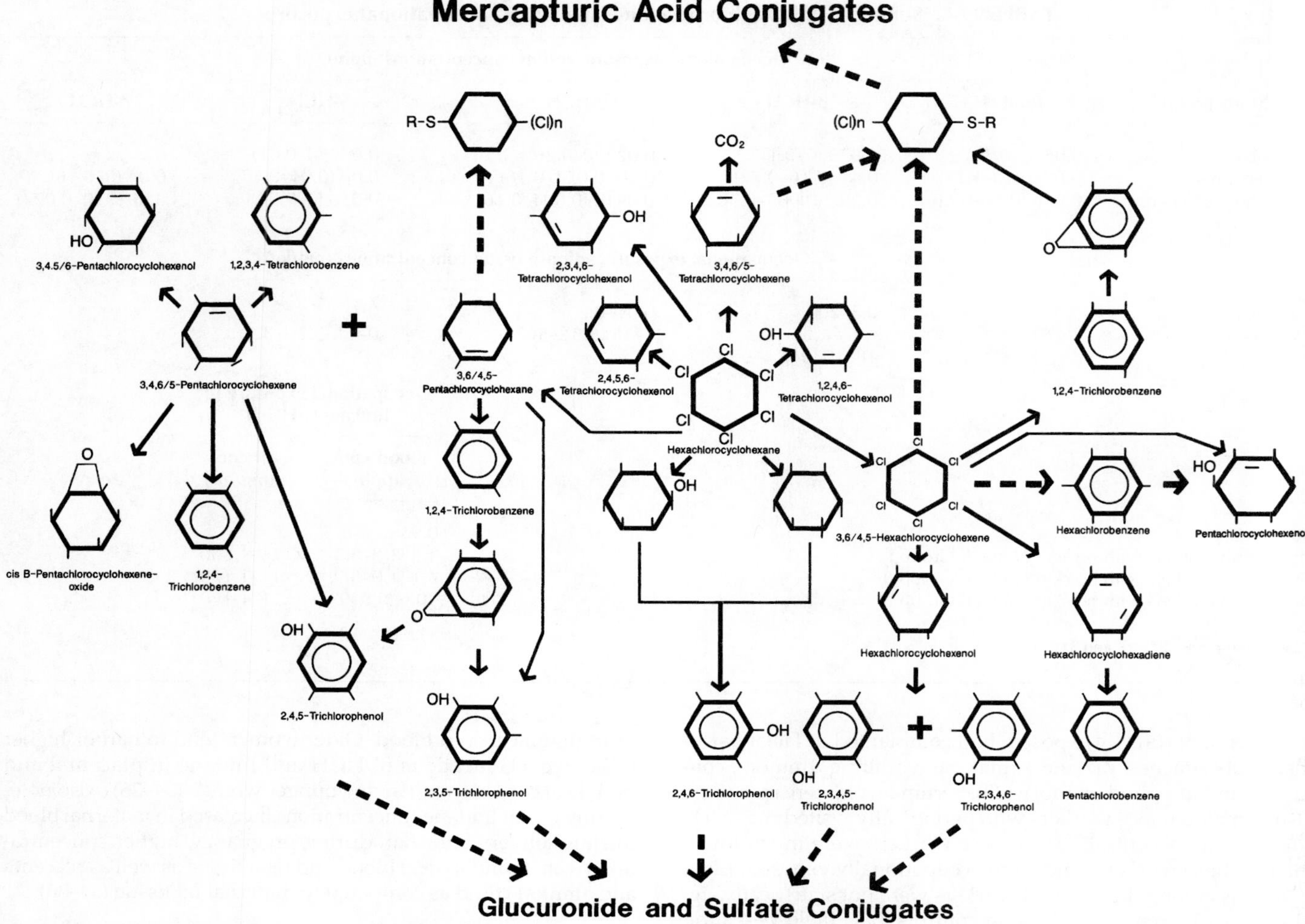

Figure 99-7. Proposed metabolism of γ-hexachlorocyclohexane. (From ref. 18, with permission.)

uals. These individuals were exposed to technical-grade HCH for 10 years in a production plant (27). The same study also reported a significant increase in the concentrations of serum immunoglobulin M. Other symptoms of exposed workers included facial paresthesias, headaches, and dizziness.

INGESTION OF LINDANE

From the 1950s through 1960s, some children experienced acute toxic effects from oral ingestion of lindane tablets used in vaporizers. Acute oral toxicity in animals manifests as ataxia, coma, and death. Acute ingestion in humans consists of abdominal pain, nausea, vomiting, excitability, seizures, muscle tremors, hyperreflexia, and coma. Rhabdomyolysis, myoglobinuria, and leukocytosis have been observed (39). Animal studies of oral dosing of lindane and technical-grade HCH have been reported to cause fatty degeneration and necrosis of the liver (18). No immunotoxic effects of HCH isomers have been detected in humans. Likewise, no studies have proved reproductive effects or carcinogenicity of the isomers of HCH in humans. In animal studies, the isomers of HCH as well as technical-grade HCH have been shown to produce liver cancer in rats and mice (18).

DERMAL ABSORPTION OF LINDANE

Most cases of lindane toxicity via dermal absorption have resulted from its use as a topical scabicide. Seizures and deaths in infants have been reported after topical application of 1% lindane lotion in large amounts (33,38). Lindane blood concentrations 46 hours after application of a 1% topical lotion to treat scabies in an infant who developed postapplication seizures were 0.10 μg per L (40). This high concentration compares to a mean blood concentration of 0.005 μg per L in most children treated with the 1% lotion. In this case, peak concentrations of lindane occur 6 hours after dermal application. Inappropriate application of excessive amounts of lindane ointment (1% scabicide) to the skin can result in clinical symptoms, including seizures (40).

Dermal absorption of organochlorine pesticide depends on the amount applied, surface area of application, breaks in the normal dermal barrier, and conditions that cause the compound to be removed from the skin, such as volatilization and dilution (41). Delayed absorption of such organochlorine pesticides as lindane, dieldrin, and aldrin has been demonstrated by the prolonged urinary excretion of these compounds up to 120 hours after dermal application (41).

NEUROTOXIC EFFECTS OF LINDANE

The neurotoxic effects of lindane exposure include seizures, headaches, dizziness, tremors, ataxia, facial paresthesias, giddiness, and coma. The mechanism of lindane neurotoxicity is believed to be inhibition of GABA-mediated neurotransmission (1,2). In the limbic system, lindane acts directly to increase excitability of neurons (42). Lindane accelerates kindling seizures, which is the sequence of changes that results from repetitive stimulation (42).

CHLORDANE AND HEPTACHLOR

Chlordane and heptachlor have been extensively used in the United States as termiticides and have been heavily applied to soils in both urban and rural settings. Its persistence in the environment is one reason that chlordane is so effective. Owing to its extensive application, chlordane can be detected in the indoor air of homes 10 to 15 years after termite treatment. It is estimated that approximately 50 million people have been exposed to chlordane in the United States, principally in the home environment (43).

Many foods contain chlordane, because it bioaccumulates up the food chain. Chlordane's persistence in soil can lead to oral and dermal exposure from ingestion of crops or from ingestion of treated soil.

In the United States, chlordane has been used almost exclusively as a termiticide by foundation injection or liquid application techniques in home environments (43). More than 200 million pounds of chlordane have been applied to the soil in the United States (43).

Chlordane is commonly detected in the groundwater runoff of hazardous-waste sites. As a component of indoor air in home environments, the chemical usually is present on dust particles and in a vapor phase. After application to the soil, chlordane can continue to be released into the indoor air of a home for years. Generally, if this is occurring, air concentrations of chlordane may exceed the National Academy of Sciences' (NAS) standard of 5 μg per cubic meter (44,45).

Production and Use of Chlordane

Chlordane, heptachlor, endrin, aldrin, dieldrin, endosulfan, and isobenzan are members of the cyclodiene class of organochlorine compounds (Fig. 99-8). Chlordane is produced by the chlorination of chlordene, which in turn is the product of the Diels-Alder reaction of hexochlorocyclopentadiene with cyclopentadiene (43). On April 14, 1988, the EPA canceled the registration and use of chlordane for commercial production, delivery, and sale in the United States.

Chemical Structure and Physical Properties

Technical-grade chlordane is a mixture of at least 50 different compounds, the major constituents being *cis-* and *trans*-chlordane, heptachlor, *cis-* and *trans*-nonachlor, and α-, β-, and γ-chlordane. Hexachlorocyclopentadiene is also a constituent (46). Seventy percent of commercial preparations comprise α- and β-chlordane (43). Of chlordane's two main isomers, *trans-* and *cis*-chlordane, the latter is more abundant (Fig. 99-9).

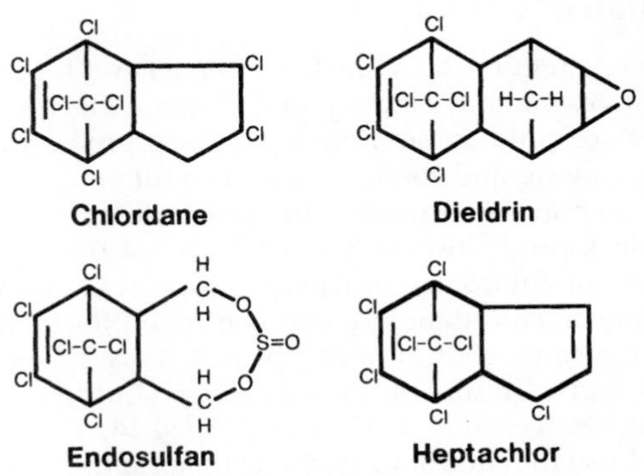

Chlordane

Dieldrin

Endosulfan

Heptachlor

Figure 99-8. Cyclodienes.

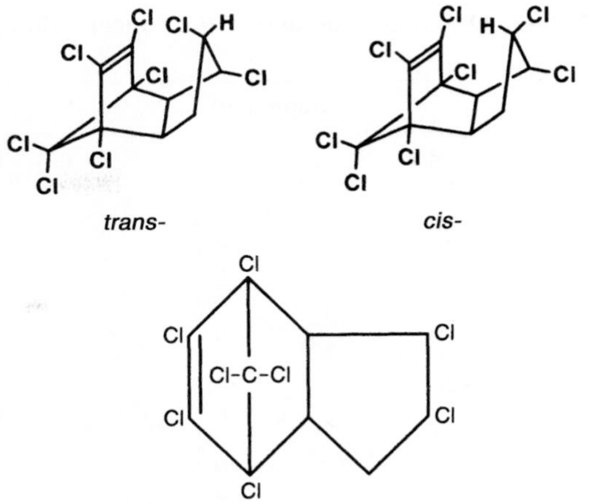

trans-

cis-

Chemical formula	$C_{10}H_6Cl_8$
Chemical name	1,2,4,5,6,7,8,8-Octachloro-2,3,3a,4,7,7a-hexahydro-4,7-methano-1H-indene
Synonym	1,2,4,5,6,7,8,8-Octachloro-3a,4,7,7a-tetrahydro-4,7-methanoindan
Trade names	Chlordan; Velsicol 1068; Octachlor; Termicide C-100

Figure 99-9. Chlordane. (From ref. 43, with permission.)

The individual components of the chlordane solution usually are solids. Pure chlordane, a viscous brown liquid (as a technical product), has a molecular weight of 409.76 (43). The individual isomers have different melting points and boiling points. Chlordane is miscible with hydrocarbon solvents.

Exposure Sources

Chlordane was used previously to treat crops and to control termites. It is identified at 46 of 1,117 hazardous-waste sites on the National Priority List in the United States (43).

The majority of exposures to chlordane occur in the home environment owing to prior application of chlordane as a termiticide. Chlordane has been detected in the indoor air of a home up to 15 years after treatment of the home for termites (44,45). It is estimated by the EPA that more than 80 million people in the United States live in homes that have been treated with cyclodiene termiticide agents such as chlordane (43). This probably is an underestimation, because foods and food sources also contain chlordane, which bioaccumulates and produces further exposure in humans as they consume the affected food.

Chlordane and other organochlorines have been detected in surface groundwater, in drinking water, and in urban runoff water (Tables 99-5, 99-6) (43). Chlordane concentrations in surface water generally are in the low nanogram-per-liter range (ppb).

Chlordane also is detected in soil, particularly around the outside walls of treated homes in concentrations ranging from less than 1 ppb to approximately 141 ppm (45–47). Persons involved in the manufacturing of chlordane also are likely to experience high-exposure incidents.

Chlordane bioconcentrates in marine animals via contamination of water. In soil, chlordane adsorbs to organic materials (43). Owing to the fact that it does adsorb to organic materials and volatilizes slowly, chlordane does not appreciably leach from soil. Depending on the type of soil, chlordane will be present to a lesser or greater extent. Sandy soils and soils that contain a

TABLE 99-5. Drinking water and serum concentrations of organochlorine pesticides and metabolites in samples from individuals who use well water

Water (ppt)				Serum (ppb)		
HCH	Dieldrin	HCB	b-HCH	*p,p*'-DDE	Dieldrin	*p,p*'-DDT
ND	<20	ND	ND	14.5	ND	<2.0
ND	<20	0.4	0.9	24.0	ND	2.0
ND	<20	0.3	<0.7	8.6	ND	ND
ND	<20	0.3	<0.7	17.0	<1.0	3.4
ND	<20	0.5	1.8	31.5	1.2	3.3
ND	<20	<0.2	0.8	22.0	ND	<2.0
ND	<20	<0.2	<0.7	6.8	<1.0	ND
ND	ND	0.3	<0.7	21.5	ND	2.0
ND	ND	0.8	1.1	11.0	ND	ND
ND	<20	<0.2	0.9	17.2	<1.0	<2.0
		0.3	<0.7	32.0	<1.0	<2.0
		0.4	0.9	12.3	<1.0	<2.0
		0.3	0.6	11.5	ND	<2.0
		0.3	ND	7.0	ND	<2.0
		0.4	<0.7	18.0	ND	2.3
		0.3	<0.7	14.7	ND	<2.0
		<0.2	0.9	17.2	<1.0	<2.0
		0.3	0.7	9.7	ND	<2.0
		0.5	0.8	26.7	ND	2.3
		<0.2	<0.7	7.1	ND	ND
		0.7	1.2	31.6	1.4	4.6
		0.3	1.5	17.0	<1.0	<2.0
		0.4	0.7	20.8	ND	<2.0
		0.4	ND	10.8	<1.0	<2.0
		0.3	ND	3.4	ND	<2.0
		0.6	<0.7	12.9	ND	<2.0

HCB, hexachlorobenzene; HCH, hexachlorocyclohexane; ND, not detected.
Reprinted from ref. 24, with permission.

small amount of organic materials retain chlordane less than do soils having a high organic content (43).

Chlordane is degraded in air by photooxidation. α-Chlordane is a photo-by-product of chlordane. Chlordane does not degrade rapidly in water.

Chlordane concentrations in the air of houses in urban areas range from less than the detectable limit (i.e., less than 0.1 ng per cubic meter) to 200 ng per cubic meter (45–47). Rural air concentrations of chlordane range from 0.1 to 0.8 ng per cubic meter (43). As compared to the outdoor air, chlordane concentrations in indoor air are much higher. Indoor air concentrations in houses treated with chlordane range from 0.8 to 600,000 ng per cubic meter (43–45). Indoor air sampling in previously treated homes demonstrated concentrations of γ-chlordane, α-chlordane, and *trans*-nonachlor. However, these concentrations were all lower than the 5-μg-per-cubic-meter guideline proposed by the NAS for indoor levels of chlordane.

Biological Monitoring

Biological monitoring of chlordane is via detection of chlordane or its metabolites in such human tissues and fluids as blood, adipose tissue, brain, liver, kidney, milk, and urine. Total chlordane residue levels appear to be higher in fat and liver than in the blood (47). However, attempting to correlate tissue levels with environmental levels is difficult owing to the bioaccumulative effects of chlordane.

Oxychlordane has been detected in concentrations ranging from 0.002 to 0.005 mg per L in human breast milk in a random sampling (48). In a Finnish study of human milk samples, chlordane residues averaged 0.41 mg per kg of milk fat (49). Other studies have indicated that *trans*-chlordane concentrations in skin lipids may be a biomarker of recent exposure and that oxychlordane concentration in skin lipids might be a better biomarker of previous exposure (50).

Other studies have shown that total chlordane residues in blood were between 3 and 16 times higher in persons employed as pesticide applicators and were 1.5 to 10 times higher in residents of contaminated areas in which houses had been treated with chlordane for termites (51). Other studies have shown a positive correlation between the length of exposure to airborne chlordane in treated homes and the concentration of chlordane in human milk fat (52).

Environmental Contamination and Regulation of Chlordane

Chlordane is regulated by the Clean Water Act for industrial point sources such as electroplating, steam electric production, asbestos production, timber products processing, metal finishing, paving and roofing, paint formulating, ink formulating, gum and wood processing, pesticide production, and carbon black production (43). On March 6, 1978, registration for all uses of chlordane on fruit products was discontinued (43). However, chlordane use was continued for treatment of homes for termite control until April 14, 1988, when the EPA canceled registrations for chlordane-containing termiticide products. Between July 1, 1983, and April 14, 1988, the only approved use for chlordane in the United States was for subterranean termites; for this usage, chlordane was applied as a

TABLE 99-6. Drinking water and serum concentrations of organochlorine pesticides and metabolites in samples from individuals who use city water

Water (ppt)				Serum (ppb)		
HCH	Dieldrin	HCB	b-HCH	*p,p'*-DDE	Dieldrin	*p,p'*-DDT
30	<20	0.7	5.8	68.4	ND	<2.0
68	<20	ND	ND	15.0	<1.0	ND
42	<20	0.7	0.9	7.4	ND	ND
<4	ND	<0.2	<0.7	ND	10.1	ND
ND	ND	ND	<0.7	10.9	ND	ND
ND	<20	0.4	0.8	16.8	ND	<2.0
ND	<20	0.4	1.0	20.0	0.9	<2.0
ND	<20	0.5	1.7	21.3	ND	ND
ND	<20	0.3	<0.7	17.6	ND	<2.0
ND	<20	0.9	1.1	36.1	<1.0	ND
		0.5	1.6	27.2	4.6	2.0
		0.7	1.7	22.0	1.9	4.7
		0.3	3.1	25.0	<1.0	3.0
		0.5	1.7	16.4	1.7	2.2
		0.3	0.8	14.2	<1.0	<2.0
		0.3	<0.7	23.9	<1.0	<2.0
		0.3	0.7	7.1	<1.0	<2.0
		<0.2	<0.7	3.9	ND	ND
		0.3	ND	24.3	<1.0	<2.0
		0.3	1.0	16.6	ND	<2.0
		0.4	<0.7	66.7	1.2	4.2
		0.3	ND	5.0	ND	ND
		0.2	ND	5.4	ND	ND
		0.7	0.8	21.0	ND	2.0
		0.4	<0.7	9.9	ND	<2.0
		0.4	0.8	19.0	<1.0	<2.0
		<0.2	<0.7	10.4	ND	<2.0
		<0.2	1.3	43.1	<1.0	3.4
		0.3	<0.7	12.6	ND	ND
		0.7	<0.7	20.7	ND	5.5
		1.1	1.0	20.6	1.3	3.5
		0.4	1.3	17.0	1.0	2.6
		0.5	0.8	10.6	ND	<2.0

HCB, hexachlorobenzene; HCH, hexachlorocyclohexane; ND, not detected.
Reprinted from ref. 24, with permission.

liquid that was poured or injected around the foundation of buildings. Regulatory guidelines for chlordane are shown in Table 99-7.

Although chlordane still is produced for export, its use in the United States now is prohibited by law, and it no longer is imported into the United States.

Chlordane is stable in the atmosphere and can be transported long distances. In water, it adsorbs to sediments and also volatilizes into the atmosphere. Partitioning of chlordane into sediment is correlated with the organic content of the sediment. Thus, where the organic content of suspended sediments in water is high, chlordane concentrations from release sites will increase.

Chlordane bioconcentrates in marine and fresh-water fish. It also bioconcentrates in aquatic plants. In soil, chlordane generally remains in the top 20 cm of most soils for years. Sandy soils and soils with smaller amounts of organic content retain chlordane less well than do soils that are of high clay content and high organic content.

In the atmosphere, chlordane is degraded by photolysis and oxidation. The *trans*-chlordane isomer degrades photochemically more readily than does the *cis*-chlordane isomer, and the *trans-cis* ratio of chlordane transported over long distances in the atmosphere changes from approximately 1 in the winter to 0.5 in the summer (53).

Chlordane persists for more than 20 years in some soils, and chlordane residues in excess of 10% of the initially applied amount have been found 10 years after that initial application (54). Only a few microorganisms capable of biodegrading chlordane have been isolated, and most studies indicate that chlordane does not biodegrade rapidly in soils.

Urban air concentrations range from below detection limits to 58 ng per cubic meter. Rural background concentrations range from 0.01 to 1.0 ng per cubic meter (43). Indoor air concentrations of treated homes may exceed 1 μg per cubic meter. Chlordane injected into the soil or poured around the foundation of a house can vaporize into the indoor air of that residence, indicating that it passes through cracks or ventilation ducts and possibly through the concrete (45,55). Studies also indicate that concentrations of chlordane in treated homes can be higher in the lower level and basement areas of homes (56). Basement concentrations of chlordane have been found to be three to ten times higher than in the living areas. After misapplication of chlordane, living area samples show concentrations of 3.28 μg per cubic meter, with 40% of samples in one study exceeding 5 μg per cubic meter (57).

On April 14, 1988, the EPA terminated the use of termiticide products containing chlordane and forbade the sale or commercial use of those products within the United States.

TABLE 99-7. Regulations applicable to chlordane

Agency	Description	Value
Federal and international agencies		
WHO	Guidelines for drinking water	0.3 μg/L
WHO	Residue tolerances for sum of α and γ isomers and oxychlordane	0.02–0.5 mg/kg
WHO	Acceptable daily intake	0–0.001 mg/kg/body wt
Regulations		
OSHA	Permissible exposure limit (8-h workday)	0.5 mg/m^3
EPA	Reportable quantity (released to the environment)	1 lb
NAS	Recommended maximum indoor concentration in homes	5 $μg/m^3$
	Threshold planning quantity	1,000 lb
Guidelines		
Air		
ACGIH	Threshold limit value (TLV) (8-h workday)	0.5 mg/m^3
STEL		2 mg/m^3
NRC	Interim guideline for military housing	5 $μg/m^3$
EPA	Inhalation	1.3 mg/kg/day
Water		
EPA	Health advisories	
	1-day (10-kg child)	0.06 mg/L
	10-day (10-kg child)	0.06 mg/L
	Longer-term (10-kg child)	0.5 μg/L
	Longer-term (70-kg adult)	2 μg/L
	Maximum contaminant level goal (proposed)	0 mg/L
	Ambient water quality criteria for the following lifetime increased cancer risk levels	
	With ingestion of water, fish, and shellfish	
	10^{-5}	4.6 ng/L
	10^{-6}	0.46 ng/L
	10^{-7}	0.046 ng/L
	With ingestion of fish and shellfish only	
	10^{-5}	4.8 ng/L
	10^{-6}	0.48 ng/L
	10^{-7}	0.048 ng/L
Other		
EPA	q_1*[a] (oral)	1.3 mg/kg/day
	RfD[b] (oral)	5×10^{-5} mg/kg/day
	PADI (oral)	5.0×10^{-5} mg/kg/day
	Group B2 cancer ranking (probable human carcinogen)	
	Designated as a hazardous waste (no. U036)	
State regulations and guidelines		
	Acceptable ambient air concentration	
Connecticut		2.5 $μg/m^3$ (8-h avg)
Kansas		1.19 $μg/m^3$ (annual avg)
Kentucky		0.05 $μg/m^3$ (8-h avg)
Massachusetts		0.068 $μg/m^3$ (24-h avg)
Nevada		0.012 $μg/m^3$ (8-h avg)
New York		1.7 $μg/m^3$ (1-yr avg)
Pennsylvania (Philadelphia)		0.35 $μg/m^3$ (1-yr avg)
Virginia		8.0 $μg/m^3$ (24-h avg)
	Acceptable drinking water concentrations	
Arizona		0.5 μg/L
California		0.55 μg/L
Illinois		3 μg/L
Kansas		0.22 μg/L
Maine		0.55 μg/L
Minnesota		0.22 μg/L
New Jersey		0.5 μg/L

ACGIH, American Conference of Governmental Industrial Hygienists; EPA, U.S. Environmental Protection Agency; NAS, National Academy of Sciences; NRC, National Research Council; OSHA, U.S. Occupational Safety and Health Administration; STEL, short-term exposure limit; TLV, threshold limit value; WHO, World Health Organization.

[a] *q_1** represents the upper-bound estimate of the low dose of the dose-response curve, as determined by the multistage procedure. The q_1* can be used to calculate an estimate of carcinogenic potency, the incremental excess cancer risk per unit of exposure (usually milligrams per liter of water, milligrams per kilogram of food per day, and grams per cubic meter of air).

[b] *RfD* represents an estimate (with uncertainty spanning perhaps an order of magnitude) of the daily exposure of the human population to a potential hazard that is likely to be without risk of deleterious effects during a lifetime. The RfD is operationally derived from the no-observable-adverse-effect level (from animal and human studies) by a consistent application of uncertainty factors that reflect various types of data used to estimate RfDs and an additional modifying factor, which is based on a professional judgment of the entire database on the chemical. The RfDs are not applicable to nonthreshold effects such as cancer.

Adapted from Agency for Toxic Substances and Disease Registry. *Toxicological profile for chlordane.* Atlanta: US Department of Health and Human Services, Public Health Service, ATSDR, 1989, with permission.

Clinical Toxicology of Chlordane

Chlordane can be absorbed systemically via oral, inhalational, and dermal routes. Acute chlordane poisoning has been reported (58–62). Animals that have been given fatal doses of chlordane exhibit symptoms of dyspnea, depressed respirations, tremors, convulsions, coma, and death. In human cases of acute chlordane ingestion, convulsions, muscle tremors, increased excitability, confusion, and coma are common (58–62). Symptoms usually begin within an hour of acute ingestion of this liquid, with manifestations of confusion followed by convulsions. Once absorbed, chlordane has a high distribution into adipose tissue. Human poisonings involving chlordane have also shown elevation of white blood cell count, pneumonias (probably secondary to aspiration), and hepatic and renal damage (58–62). Treatment is symptomatic.

SUBACUTE AND CHRONIC EXPOSURE TO CHLORDANE

Retrospective cohort mortality studies of workers in chlordane-manufacturing industries and pesticide applicators have shown no increase in mortality rates and no increase in a specific cause of death that could be attributed to chlordane exposure (63–65).

One study examined cause-specific mortality among workers occupationally exposed to chlordane or heptachlor and demonstrated no overall excess of death from cancer even in workers who were studied for 20 or more years after entry into the industry (64). Another study that examined the mortality of a cohort of 3,827 men licensed to apply pesticides in Florida showed an excess mortality from lung cancer among pesticide applicators (66). However, this study did not account for such other risk modifiers as smoking.

A retrospective mortality study of workers employed at organochlorine pesticide–manufacturing plants examined the mortality of workers employed in the manufacture of several different organochlorine hydrocarbons for use as pesticides (65). This study concluded that the standardized mortality ratio for all causes of death in each cohort was below the expected level.

Blood dyscrasias such as megaloblastic anemia and bone marrow depression have been associated with chlordane exposure in case reports (67,68). However, these case reports also identified exposures to pesticides other than chlordane, and no definitive study has indicated that chlordane is causative of blood dyscrasias.

Investigations into the health status of people living in private residences previously treated with chlordane have been undertaken (69). However, the study population was self-selected, thus indicating a bias toward involving those concerned about chlordane or who believed that they had experienced health problems related to chlordane (69). Occupational exposure to chlordane has not been associated with abnormal liver function tests or renal effects (43).

In individuals who have ingested chlordane, nausea, vomiting, abdominal pain, and diarrhea occur very early. Autopsies of individuals who have died after chlordane ingestion show inflammation of the mucosa of the upper gastrointestinal tract (43).

In animal studies of acute oral exposure to chlordane, evidence exists of hepatic microsomal enzyme induction and alteration in the activities of mitochondrial enzymes (43). Histochemical and morphological alterations in the liver also were seen.

HEMATOLOGIC EFFECTS

Anecdotal reports claim an association between blood dyscrasias and a number of the organochlorine pesticides including chlordane, lindane, and DDT (67,68). Case reports have described thrombocytopenic purpura, acute disseminated hemorrhages, aplastic anemia, hemolytic anemia, anemia, and megaloblastic anemia in individuals exposed to chlordane and heptachlor in residential environments or in professional settings in which these materials were used (69). However, confounding factors include exposure of the reported individuals to numerous other chemicals; hence, the case reports are insufficient to implicate chlordane as the sole etiologic agent for blood dyscrasias.

Studies from chlordane manufacturing showed no hematotoxic changes in workers exposed to chlordane (70). Likewise, no hematologic effects have been observed in animal models exposed to technical chlordane (71).

IMMUNOTOXICITY

Immune alterations in humans exposed to chlordane aerosols in the home or workplace for 3 days to 15 months have been reported (72). This same study also showed impaired lymphocyte proliferative responses to mitogens. However, confounding exposure factors were not eliminated.

In animal immune studies, reduced thymus weights have been observed in female rats but not male rats exposed to 28.2 mg of inhaled chlordane per cubic meter for 8 hours daily, 5 days per week, for 28 days (71). However, changes in thymus weight were not observed in female rats exposed to lower doses. Other animal studies in which chlordane was administered orally have demonstrated depressed cell-mediated immunity manifested by depressed hypersensitivity reactions and depressed mixed lymphocyte culture reactivity (73,74). Some animal studies show that chlordane interferes with cell-mediated immune proliferative responses of lymphocytes in monkeys (75).

TABLE 99-8. Residues of organochlorine compounds in human fat (mg/kg) in the United Kingdom, 1976–1977

	β-HCH	Total HCH	Heptachlor epoxide	Dieldrin (HEOD)	*p,p'*-DDE	*p,p'*-DDT	Total DDT[a]	HCB	PCB
Arithmetic mean	0–31	0.33	0.03	0.11	2.1	0.21	2.6	0.19	0.7
Range[b]	T–1.2	T–1.2	T–0.12	T–0.49	0.03–15	T–2.4	0.04–17	0.02–3.2	T–10
Standard error of mean	0.01	0.01		0.01	0.12	0.01	0.15	0.01	0.05
Median value	0.29	0.31		0.09	1.7	0.17	2.1	0.15	0.7
Geometric mean	0.24	0.27		0.09	1.5	0.15	1.9	0.15	0.6
95% Confidence interval	0.22–0.27	0.24–0.29		0.08–0.10	1.3–1.7	0.14–0.1 7	1.6–2.1	0.14–0.17	0.5–0.6

HCB, hexachlorobenzene; HCH, hexachlorocyclohexane; PCB, polychlorinated biphenyl.
[a]Total DDT was calculated by adding to the *p,p'*-DDT found as such the *p,p'*-DDT-equivalent of the *p,p'*-DDE and *p,p'*-TDE.
[b]T is less than 0.01 (less than 0.1 for PCB).
Note: Results obtained in 236 subjects older than 5 years.
Reprinted from ref. 26, with permission.

TABLE 99-9. Concentration of organochlorine insecticides in samples of adipose tissue and liver

Adipose						Liver		
Lindane	Heptachlor epoxide	Dieldrin	*p,p'*-DDT	*p,p'*-DDE	Total equiv. DDT	Dieldrin	*p,p'*-DDE	Total equiv. DDT
0.12	0.008	0.16	0.36	2.18	2.79	0.030	0.16	0.18
0.21	0.014	0.25	0.28	1.88	2.38	0.050	0.16	0.18
0.05	0.005	0.14	0.14	0.36	0.54	0.040	0.05	0.06
0.11	0.008	0.18	0.42	2.50	3.21	0.026	0.15	0.17
0.06	0.006	0.13	0.19	1.15	1.47	0.024	0.12	0.13
0.07	0.009	0.25	0.35	1.95	2.52	0.025	0.08	0.10
0.12	0.009	0.21	0.44	2.10	2.78	0.035	0.19	0.21
0.10	0.004	0.05	0.10	0.08	0.19	0.007	0.01	0.01
0.13	0.030	0.50	0.35	2.66	3.31	0.081	0.12	0.13
0.16	0.013	0.23	0.58	2.32	3.17	0.041	0.13	0.14
0.09	0.005	0.10	0.35	1.51	2.03	0.014	0.20	0.22

Reprinted from ref. 21, with permission.

CARCINOGENESIS

Retrospective studies reveal no evidence that links carcinogenesis with exposure to chlordane (76,77). Nonetheless, an association between chronic exposure to chlordane in treated homes and an increased risk of skin neoplasms and leukemia has been suggested (69,78). The EPA considers data from laboratory animal studies sufficient to classify chlordane in the group B-2 category—that is, as a probable human carcinogen.

REPRODUCTIVE, GENOTOXIC, AND DEVELOPMENTAL EFFECTS

No data are available regarding the developmental effects in humans after exposure to chlordane. Chlordane has been tested for mutagenicity in several systems, with mostly negative results. In terms of reproductive effects, studies on humans after exposure to chlordane are limited. One study compared to control populations indicated that the incidence rates of unspecified ovarian and uterine disease were significantly elevated in women exposed to chlordane vapors in their homes as compared to the rates among control populations (78). However, this study has serious limitations.

Absorption, Metabolism, and Excretion

Human samples of adipose tissue and plasma have been assayed for the presence of organochlorine pesticides (Tables 99-8, 99-9). Because these chemicals are found commonly in human adipose tissue and plasma (in approximately 80% of the U.S. population), associating these chemicals' presence with disease is difficult. Chlordane and its metabolites can be detected in a variety of human biological tissues such as blood, brain (Table 99-10), adipose tissue, liver, breast milk (Table 99-11), kidneys, and urine. However, no information currently available correlates concentrations found in these tissues with environmental chlordane concentrations or with human health effects.

In cases of intoxication, chlordane concentrations of the blood and other tissues have been found to be highly elevated. Blood chlordane concentrations of 3.4 mg per L were associated with seizures in one child (59). The half-life of chlordane in this case was 8 days as compared to other reports of 21 days. The urinary excretion of chlordane continued up to 130 days after ingestion (59). On the basis of this and other cases, the seizure threshold for chlordane is believed to be between 2 and 4 mg per L in serum.

Chlordane is well absorbed by the oral, dermal, and inhalational routes. Blood and tissue concentrations of chlordane and chlordane metabolites will increase with the duration of exposure. Information on the absorption and distribution of chlordane comes from acute oral exposures in humans from accidental or suicidal ingestions.

Chlordane concentrates in the fatty tissues and is excreted very slowly. After a massive chlordane ingestion by a 59-year-old man, which resulted in his death, concentrations of chlordane were measured in several tissues (62). In this case, fat tissue contained 22 μg of chlordane per gram of tissue; brain contained 23.3 μg per gram; kidneys, 14.1 μg per gram; liver, 59.9 μg per gram; and spleen, 19.2 μg per gram. In a child who drank technical-grade chlordane, the concentration in adipose tissue was measured. One-half hour after the exposure, the chlordane concentration was approximately 3.1 mg per kg of fat tissue, which peaked at 35 mg per kg of fat 8 days after ingestion (79).

Values for the concentration of the metabolite of chlordane, oxychlordane, in human adipose tissue have ranged from 0.03 to 0.5 mg per kg of fat tissue, with an average concentration of 0.11 to 0.19 mg per kg (80). The usual chlordane metabolites found in humans are heptachlor, oxychlordane, and heptachlor epoxide (Fig. 99-10).

One excretion route of metabolites of chlordane is through breast milk. Oxychlordane, *trans*-nonachlor, and heptachlor epoxide have been identified in human breast milk. *Trans*-nonachlor has been reported to be present in human breast milk in concentrations of 0.027 to 0.210 μg per mL, heptachlor epoxide in concentrations of 0.001 to 0.067 μg per mL, and oxychlordane in concentrations of 0.011 to 0.160 μg per mL.

TABLE 99-10. Mean concentrations of organochlorine insecticides in human brain tissues

	Dieldrin (ppm)		Total equivalent DDT (ppm)	
	White matter	Gray matter	White matter	Gray matter
Arithmetic mean	0.009	0.006	0.033	0.025
Standard deviation	0.002	0.001	0.005	0.004
Geometric mean	0.0061	0.0047	0.0023	0.020
Confidence limits (*p* = .05)	0.0047–0.0080	0.0037–0.0059	0.018–0.031	0.015–0.026

Reprinted from ref. 21, with permission.

TABLE 99-11. Mean values of samples taken at different times during breast feeding (pesticide levels in parts per million of whole milk)

Samples	Prefeeding mean ± SD (range)	Postfeeding mean ± SD (range)	Random mean ± SD (range)
Urban			
No. samples	43	42	45
% Lipid	2.7 ± 1.6 (0.3–9.7)	4.8 ± 1.8 (0.7–8.6)	3.3 ± 1.6 (0.8–7.9)
HCH	0.006 ± 0.004 (0.001–0.016)	0.010 ± 0.006 (0.002–0.025)	0.007 ± 0.005 (0.001–0.027)
γ-HCH	0.001 ± 0.002 (0.000–0.007)	0.001 ± 0.002 (0.000–0.009)	0.001 ± 0.002 (0.000–0.006)
Dieldrin	0.010 ± 0.008 (0.002–0.038)	0.012 ± 0.008 (0.002–0.041)	0.007 ± 0.005 (0.002–0.024)
DDE	0.023 ± 0.013 (0.005–0.067)	0.039 ± 0.019 (0.011–0.077)	0.029 ± 0.022 (0.006–0.127)
DDT	0.011 ± 0.009 (0.002–0.033)	0.017 ± 0.011 (0.003–0.051)	0.010 ± 0.008 (0.002–0.037)
Total DDT	0.036 ± 0.020 (0.008–0.096)	0.060 ± 0.028 (0.015–0.136)	0.042 ± 0.030 (0.009–0.179)
Rural			
No. samples	42	42	53
% Lipid	2.8 ± 1.3 (0.3–5.9)	4.8 ± 1.5 (0.7–9.2)	2.6 ± 1.3 (0.3–6.2)
HCH	0.006 ± 0.003 (0.001–0.015)	0.009 ± 0.004 (0.002–0.024)	0.006 ± 0.003 (0.002–0.019)
γ-HCH	0.000 ± 0.001 (0.000–0.003)	0.001 ± 0.002 (0.000–0.003)	0.000 ± 0.001 (0.000–0.002)
Dieldrin	0.006 ± 0.004	0.009 ± 0.006	0.008 ± 0.005

HCH, hexachlorocyclohexane.
Reprinted from ref. 29, with permission.

The elimination half-life has been reported to be 21 days in one study, 34 days in another, and 88 days in yet another study (62,79,81). Only small amounts of chlordane are excreted in the urine after ingestion. The fat-serum partition ratio for chlordane in exposed workers was found to be 660:1 (82).

ALDRIN AND DIELDRIN

Aldrin and dieldrin are cyclodiene pesticides that are chemically related. Aldrin is rapidly converted to dieldrin in the environment, and their toxicities are similar. Aldrin and dieldrin were used from the 1950s through the 1970s but were still manufactured through 1990. Both have been used in agricultural settings for control of disease vectors such as insects and as a soil insecticide. Dieldrin has also found use in the past as a veterinary dip for sheep. The use of both of these chemicals was banned in 1975; the manufacture of dieldrin was terminated in 1987 and that of aldrin in 1990.

Aldrin is prepared by the Diels-Alder reaction using hexachlorocyclopentadiene. Dieldrin is prepared by the oxidation of aldrin with an organic acid or hydrogen peroxide and a tungsten oxide catalyst. The insecticide dieldrin contains 85% 1,2,3,4,10,10-hexachloro-6,7-epoxy-1,4,4a,5,6,7,8,8a-octahydro-1,4-endo,exo-5,8-dimethanonaphthalene, or HEOD (83).

Exposure Sources

Aldrin is readily converted to dieldrin in the environment. Dieldrin is persistent and resists biodegradation, and thus bioaccumulates throughout the food chain. Aldrin readily volatilizes from soil. Dieldrin, however, volatilizes more slowly because it adsorbs to soil. In soil, aldrin is converted to dieldrin by epoxidation. Aldrin and dieldrin do not leach to appreciable degrees into groundwater.

Human exposure to aldrin and dieldrin has occurred through dermal and inhalational routes during pesticide application. However, owing to the persistence and bioaccumulation of these chemicals, human exposure also occurs through the food chain.

Air and drinking water are minor exposure sources. A study of U.S. drinking water samples revealed that fewer than 17% contained dieldrin, with very low concentrations of 4 to 10 ng per L of water (84).

Because aldrin is converted to dieldrin, soil concentrations of dieldrin are higher than those of aldrin. Dietary exposure to aldrin and dieldrin is the most significant source of exposure for the general population, and food is the main source of the human adipose tissue concentration of dieldrin in humans (Tables 99-12 through 99-16) (84).

Infants are the population at greatest risk from aldrin and dieldrin exposure in the diet. The concentration of dieldrin in breast milk is another factor that places infants at risk of exposure. Breast milk is one of the major excretion routes for organochlorine compounds, and exposure to infants from human milk sources can be significant (28,29). Dieldrin has been found in the breast milk of 80% of nursing mothers sampled (84). Transplacental transfer is possible, and concentrations in fetal tissue probably occur. Placental-fetal transfer of aldrin and dieldrin has also been documented (34–36).

Homes treated for termite control with aldrin and dieldrin are another source of exposure. Indoor air in these homes contains aldrin in varying concentrations, depending on the sampling. In one study, the aldrin concentration ranged between 77 and 102 ng per cubic meter within the first 7 days of treatment and fell to a low of 36 ng per cubic meter by 1 year after treatment (84). The concentration in crawl spaces of treated homes was much higher.

Chemical and Physical Forms

The chemical structures of cyclodienes aldrin and dieldrin are depicted in Figure 99-11.

Absorption, Metabolism, and Excretion

Aldrin and dieldrin can be absorbed by inhalational, dermal, and gastrointestinal routes. Rapid conversion of aldrin to the dieldrin epoxide takes place once absorption has occurred. Aldrin rarely is found in blood or tissue owing to this rapid conversion.

Dieldrin is stored in the fat and, during such periods of stress as weight loss and high fever, can be mobilized to the plasma, where it can be metabolized. The half-life of dieldrin in humans is 266 days (84). A correlation has been found between dieldrin concentrations in human breast milk and the pesticide treatment of homes. The distribution of dieldrin between blood and tissue of humans is shown in Figure 99-12. In human volunteers ingesting dieldrin, dieldrin concentrations in blood and fat tissue increased

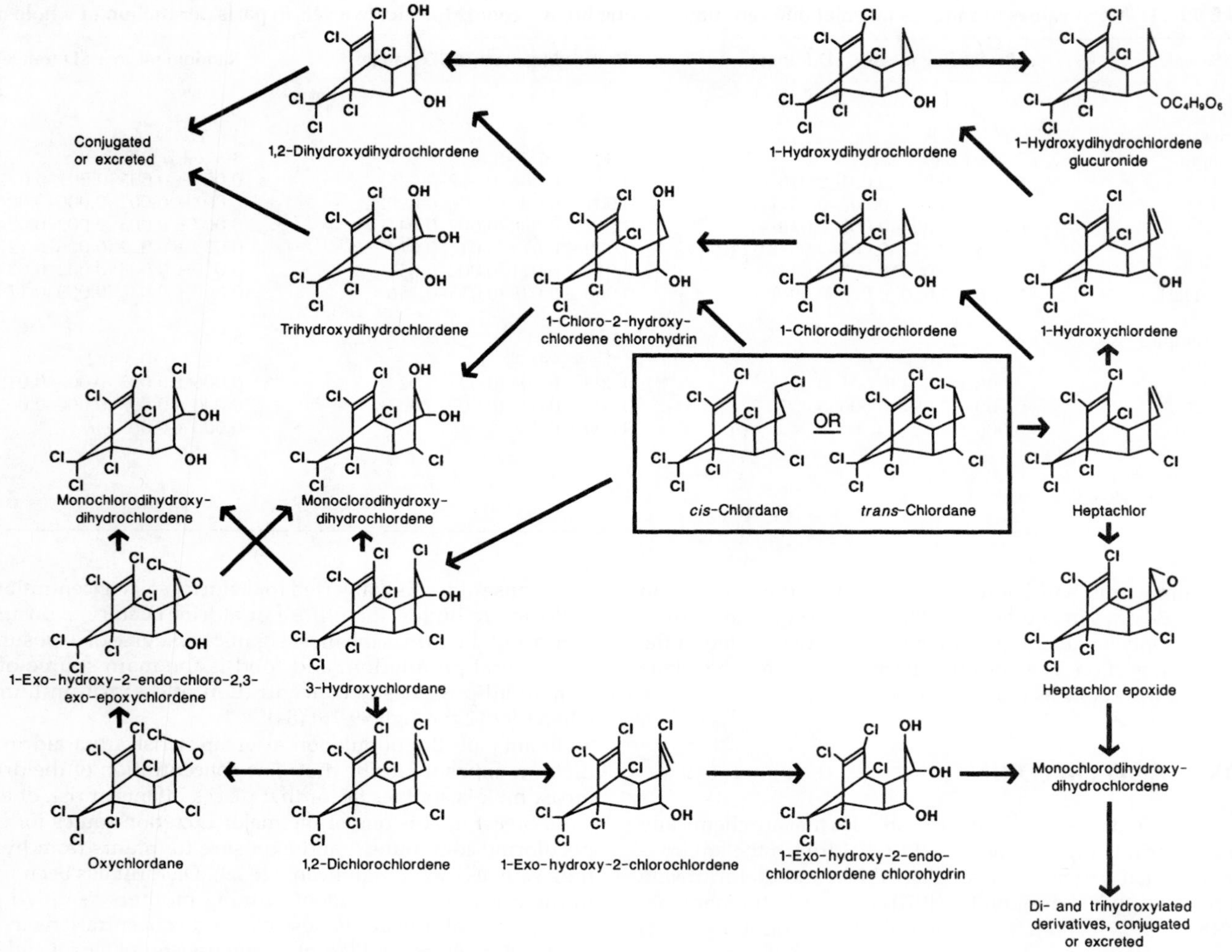

Figure 99-10. Metabolic pathways of chlordane. (From A Nomeir, N Hajjar. Metabolism of chlordane in mammals. *Rev Environ Contam Toxicol* 1987;100:1–22, with permission.)

in a dose-related fashion, the fat tissue–blood ratio being 136:1 (84). In this same study, after dieldrin administration was terminated, the biological half-life decreased exponentially and was approximately 369 days, with a range of 141 to 592 days. The biotransformation of aldrin to the dieldrin epoxide occurs primarily in the liver (Fig. 99-13). Ackerman (85), in 1980, noted that the concentration of dieldrin in humans reaches a constant concentration and that the amount ingested and absorbed equals the amount metabolized and excreted after a period. With the increasing concentration of dieldrin in the liver, the rate of metabolism increases.

The biological half-life of dieldrin in the blood of workers who were occupationally exposed was estimated to be approximately 266 days in reports in which the subjects were studied for 3 years after an occupational exposure (86,87). Hunter and Robinson (86) reported an estimated half-life of 369 days for dieldrin.

Clinical Toxicology

The clinical toxicology of aldrin and dieldrin can essentially be ascribed to dieldrin, as aldrin is rapidly metabolized to dieldrin after its absorption in the human body. Once aldrin has been converted, dieldrin is distributed extensively into tissue spaces and accumulates in adipose tissue. Dieldrin is metabolized hepatically, and metabolites are excreted in bile and feces. Major toxicity involves the CNS. Toxic exposure produces tremors, giddiness, hyperexcitability, seizures, and coma (88). Dieldrin inhibits GABA neurotransmission in a manner similar to that of other cyclodiene pesticides.

In animal studies, the median lethal dose for species of all laboratory animals ranged from 40 to 70 mg of aldrin per kg of body weight and 40 to 90 mg of dieldrin per kg of body weight (84). Also in animal studies, it was determined that weight loss resulted in immobilization of dieldrin from the fat stores, increased the blood levels peripherally, and produced toxic manifestations. No deaths have been reported from human intoxication during the manufacture of aldrin or dieldrin. Most deaths occur as a result of intentional or accidental exposure to concentrated amounts of the pesticides.

In occupational settings, aldrin and dieldrin have produced symptoms of headache, dizziness, ataxia, and muscle twitching (84). Occupational exposure to aldrin and dieldrin in pesticide workers showed that the average dieldrin blood level of those studied over a 4-year period was 0.035 µg per mL (87). Sprayers and pesticide applicators in India showed symptoms of intoxication that included headache, tremors, and seizures (84).

The mechanism of action of dieldrin in the CNS is at the level of the synapse, causing increased neuronal excitability. Evidence indicates that dieldrin produces impairment of memory and emotional disturbances in humans, which may be due to the effect of the chemical on the limbic system. In general, the cyclodiene insec-

TABLE 99-12. Individual donor information (urban)

	Average residue levels (ppm)				
HCH	γ-HCH	Dieldrin	DDE	DDT	Total DDT
0.003	0.002	0.013	0.012	0.021	0.034
0.002	0.003	0.011	0.010	0.013	0.024
0.002	Tr	0.008	0.009	0.017	0.027
0.002	0.001	0.009	0.017	0.011	0.030
0.009	Tr	0.013	0.033	0.020	0.057
0.005	0.005	0.017	0.026	0.019	0.048
0.010	0.002	0.024	0.026	0.007	0.036
0.009	0.007	0.011	0.019	0.021	0.042
0.009	0.001	0.008	0.024	0.007	0.034
0.002	Tr	0.005	0.023	0.005	0.031
0.015	0.001	0.015	0.055	0.029	0.090
0.008	Tr	0.009	0.020	0.004	0.026
0.012	0.001	0.009	0.046	0.022	0.073
0.016	0.001	0.024	0.057	0.028	0.092
0.007	Tr	0.005	0.014	0.005	0.021
0.012	0.003	0.015	0.041	0.013	0.059
0.011	0.003	0.011	0.044	0.037	0.086
0.004	Tr	0.007	0.026	0.008	0.037
0.006	Tr	0.010	0.047	0.015	0.067
0.006	Tr	0.012	0.029	0.007	0.039
0.007	0.002	0.012	0.050	0.012	0.068
0.010	Tr	0.005	0.039	0.014	0.057
0.005	0.002	0.008	0.034	0.027	0.065
0.006	Tr	0.003	0.023	0.006	0.032
0.003	0.001	0.024	0.024	0.014	0.041
0.010	0.001	0.007	0.029	0.009	0.041
0.004	0.001	0.003	0.012	0.003	0.016
0.005	0.001	0.007	0.036	0.013	0.053
0.004	Tr	0.007	0.034	0.010	0.048
0.003	0.001	0.002	0.011	0.004	0.016
0.017	Tr	0.012	0.073	0.027	0.108
0.006	Tr	0.004	0.025	0.006	0.034
0.012	Tr	0.007	0.039	0.011	0.054
0.011	Tr	0.009	0.041	0.009	0.055
0.007	Tr	0.003	0.016	0.005	0.023
0.007	Tr	0.003	0.037	0.006	0.047
0.010	Tr	0.008	0.034	0.012	0.050
0.011	Tr	0.005	0.025	0.007	0.035
0.013	Tr	0.007	0.043	0.009	0.057
0.007	0.004	0.005	0.024	0.006	0.033
0.006	Tr	0.003	0.022	0.004	0.029
0.010	Tr	0.005	0.034	0.009	0.047
0.008	0.001	0.008	0.022	0.007	0.032
0.008	Tr	0.021	0.028	0.008	0.039
0.004	Tr	0.006	0.013	0.004	0.018

HCH, hexachlorocyclohexane; Tr, trace amount.
Reprinted from ref. 29, with permission.

ticides mimic the action of picrotoxin: Dieldrin has been shown to bind to the picrotoxin receptor in rodent brain synaptosomes (89).

No evidence of hepatic injury was noted in exposed individuals manifesting serum concentrations of dieldrin (range, 4 to 350 ppb) (87). Hepatic enzyme activity levels were found to be normal in 233 pesticide applicators exposed occupationally to aldrin, dieldrin, endrin, and kelodrin for 4 to 12 years (87). Studies have concluded that long-term exposure to aldrin and dieldrin do not produce liver disease detectable by enzyme elevation or hepatic enzyme induction. Blood concentrations of dieldrin are normally lower than 10 ng per mL. Concentrations between 10 and 100 ng per mL probably are indicative of overexposure (90). Dieldrin blood concentrations from 100 to 200 ng per mL indicate significant and potentially serious exposure. Concentrations exceeding 200 ng per mL may be associated with toxic effects.

Carcinogenesis

The available data on aldrin and dieldrin are inadequate to establish a clear relationship between these compounds and cancer in humans. However, malignant tumors of the liver have been observed in animal studies involving these chemicals (91). Mortality studies of workers engaged in the manufacturing of aldrin, dieldrin, and endrin revealed excess cancer incidence.

Environmental Regulations of Aldrin and Dieldrin

The WHO recommends the following guidelines for aldrin and dieldrin concentrations:

- Food (extraneous residue limit): 0.02 to 0.2 mg per kg of product

TABLE 99-13. Mean levels of organochlorine pesticides in milk of individual donors exposed to indoor air concentrations of organochlorine pesticides (values expressed in nanograms per gram of whole milk)

Donor no.	No. of sample	HCH	γ-HCH	Chlordane	Heptachlor	Heptachlor epoxide	Dieldrin	DDE	DDT	Total DDT
1	4	12	1	2	Tr	3	14	27	8	38
2	6	15	2	2	Tr	3	14	50	5	61
3	7	3	2	32	Tr	2	10	15	3	20
4	6	4	1	2	Tr	2	9	18	3	23
5	2	13	4	3	Tr	7	26	104	23	139
6	6	7	1	2	Tr	3	21	28	6	37
7	6	10	2	2	1	5	10	33	5	42
8	1	5	1	2	Tr	1	19	40	5	50
9	3	5	1	1	Tr	2	19	17	3	22
10	14	15	1	4	2	11	13	48	10	63
11	4	9	1	1	1	2	7	17	4	23
12	7	5	1	3	1	2	9	18	5	25
13	4	8	Tr	2	1	2	8	16	3	21
14	4	4	1	8	Tr	3	16	44	8	57

HCH, hexachlorocyclohexane; Tr, trace amount.
Reprinted from ref. 23, with permission.

- Food (maximum residue limit): 0.02 to 0.1 mg per kg
- Drinking water: 0.03 μg per L
- Acceptable daily intake: 0.1 μg per kg of body weight (sum of aldrin and dieldrin)

The Occupational Safety and Health Administration established an 8-hour time-weighted average (TWA) atmospheric permissible exposure limit for aldrin of 0.25 mg per cubic meter and for dieldrin of 0.25 mg per cubic meter, with a skin notation for each compound (OSHA 1985).

In 1974, the EPA suspended all use of aldrin and dieldrin, and all food uses were canceled in 1975 (84). Specific precautions regarding the termiticide use of aldrin and dieldrin were instituted in 1981, and a label improvement program was initiated to reduce potential risk due to the possibility of misapplication in termiticide use. Label changes indicated precautions concerning application of these chemicals near water supplies, heating ducts, and intake ducts in dwellings and around structures having crawl spaces underneath (84). New labels also warned against annual applications (84).

Effluent limitations of zero discharge were established by the EPA in 1986, under the National Pollutant Discharge Elimination System, for both existing and new sources. Tolerances for residues of aldrin and dieldrin in or on various raw agricultural commodities are set at 0, 0.02, 0.05, or 0.1 ppm under section 408 of the Pesticide Residue Amendment to the Federal Food, Drug and Cosmetic Act as administered by the EPA. Aldrin (Waste Number P004) and dieldrin (Waste Number P037) are listed as hazardous wastes under the Resource Conservation and Recovery Act.

Aldrin and dieldrin are listed as toxic pollutants under section 307 of the Federal Water Pollution Control Act. They are regulated as hazardous substances with a reportable quantity of 1 pound (0.454 kg) for each, under section 102 of the Comprehensive Environmental Response, Compensation, and Liability Act for releases from vessels and facilities.

The American Conference of Governmental Industrial Hygienists has adopted TWA threshold limit values for exposure to aldrin and dieldrin of 0.25 mg per cubic meter. The American Conference of Governmental Industrial Hygienists' recommendation includes a "skin" notation to indicate the potential for absorption of the compound by the dermal or airborne route or by direct contact. The TWA limit for aldrin was chosen to prevent hepatic injury and to maintain the dieldrin load at a sufficiently low level to prevent systemic poisoning.

The National Institute for Occupational Safety and Health has recommended a permissible exposure limit for both aldrin and dieldrin of 0.25 mg per cubic meter and has recommended the designation of 100 mg of aldrin per cubic meter and 450 mg of dieldrin per cubic meter as those concentrations that are immediately dangerous to life or health.

TABLE 99-14. Dieldrin levels in donors for whom aldrin was the most recent pesticide used in the home

	Dieldrin levels (ng/g whole milk) in months after treatment[a]							
Donor no.	2 mo	3 mo	4 mo	5 mo	6 mo	7 mo	8 mo	9 mo
2	26	9	12	14	11	14		
6			19	21	26	31	21	8
9						16	24	16

[a]Note decline in concentration over time.
Reprinted from ref. 23, with permission.

TABLE 99-15. Chlordane levels in one breast-milk donor exposed to home pesticide spraying

Sample no.	Sampling time relative to treatment	Chlordane (ng/g whole milk)
1	3 days prior	Tr
2	1 week after	63
3	3 weeks after	66
4	7 weeks after	64
5	11 weeks after	26
6	15 weeks after	2
7	19 weeks after	2

Tr, trace amount (<1 ng/g).
Reprinted from ref. 23, with permission.

TABLE 99-16. Hexachlorobenzene, heptachlor, and heptachlor epoxide levels in breast milk of an individual after home application of pesticides (values expressed in nanograms per gram of whole milk)

Sample no.	Sampling time relative to treatment	HCH	Heptachlor	Heptachlor epoxide
1	3 months prior	3	—	1
2	2 months prior	8	Tr	4
3	1 month prior	7	Tr	3
4	1 day after	6	13	2
5	3 days after	22	2	4
6	1 week after	18	Tr	8
7	2 weeks after	17	Tr	8
8	3 weeks after	13	2	13
9	4 weeks after	22	3	29
10	5 weeks after	23	4	29
11	7 weeks after	21	2	21
12	9 weeks after	18	1	16
13	12 weeks after	17	Tr	7
14	15 weeks after	9	Tr	3

HCH, hexachlorocyclohexane; Tr, trace amount.
Reprinted from ref. 23, with permission.

The NAS has issued a health advisory for a level of 0.0031 ppb for chronic exposure in drinking water. The drinking water equivalent level for dieldrin is 2 μg per L and the draft drinking water equivalent level for aldrin is 0.9 μg per L. On the basis of estimates of carcinogenic potential, a level of 0.02 μg per L of drinking water corresponds to a cancer risk level of 1×10^{-5}.

In 1980, the EPA established a National Ambient Water Quality Criterion of 0.074 μg of aldrin per L and of 0.071 μg of dieldrin per L for human health (84). This was founded on a 1:1,000,000 risk for cancer and was based on estimates for the ingestion of contaminated water and contaminated organisms in the water. The International Agency for Research on Cancer in 1987 classified aldrin and dieldrin in group 3, as a possible human carcinogen, on the basis of limited evidence in animals as human data are lacking (84). Aldrin is also listed as a probable human carcinogen on the weight of experimental evidence under the EPA Proposed Guidelines for Carcinogen Risk Assessment released in 1984 (84). Evidence of the carcinogenicity of this substance from animal studies appears sufficient, although human studies have been inadequate. Dieldrin also is classified by the EPA as a probable human carcinogen, with sufficient evidence in animals and inadequate evidence in humans.

Aldrin	Dieldren
1,2,3,4,10,10-Hexachloro-1,4,4a,5,8,8a-hexahydro-exo-1,4-endo-5,8-dimethanonaphthalene (HHDN)	3,4,5,6,9,9-Hexachloro-1a,2,2a,3,6,6a,7,7a-octahydro 2,3,3,6-dimethanonaphth[2,3-b]-oxirene (HEOD)
Compound 118, Octalene, Aldrec, Aldrex, Drinox	Compound 497, Octalox, Panoram D-31, Alvit, Dieldrex, Quintox
$C_{12}H_8Cl_6$	$C_{12}H_8Cl_6O$

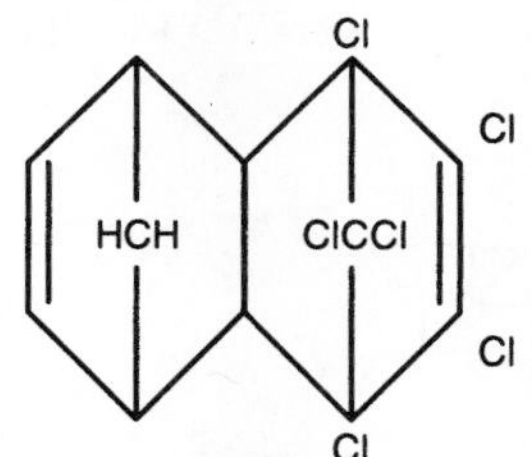

Figure 99-11. Chemical structures of aldrin and dieldrin. (From ref. 84, with permission.)

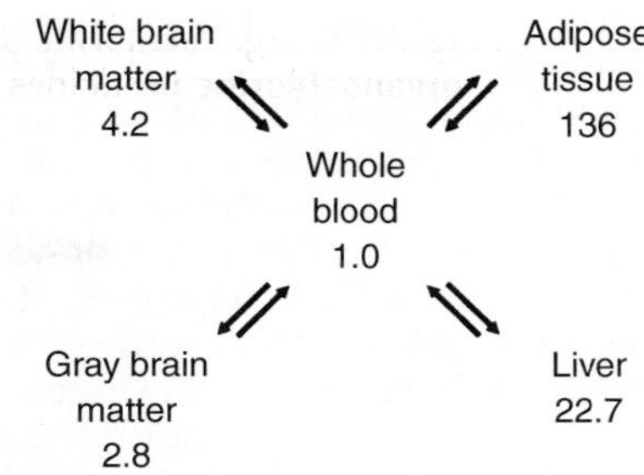

Figure 99-12. Relationship of the distribution of dieldrin among blood and certain tissues in humans. (From ref. 21, with permission.)

ENDRIN

Endrin, a stereoisomer of dieldrin, is a cyclodiene organochlorine pesticide with a formula of $C_{12}H_8Cl_6O$ and a molecular weight of 380.93. The technical product is approximately 85% endrin. Endrin, a white, crystalline solid introduced in 1951, is one of the most toxic of the cyclodiene compounds and produces dizziness, seizures, tremors, and confusion in acute toxic-

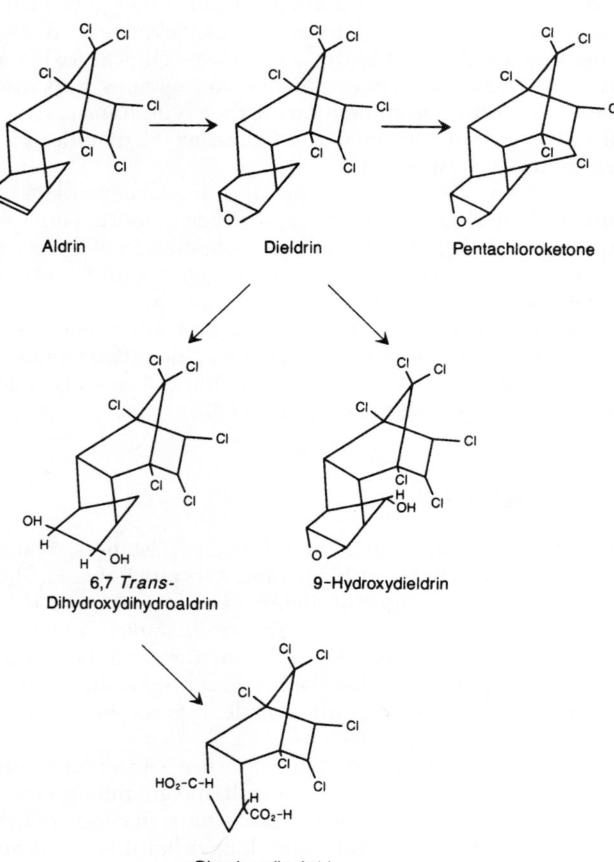

Figure 99-13. Metabolism of aldrin and dieldrin. (From ref. 84, with permission.)

ity (92). Toxicity has also been associated with hyperthermia and decerebrate rigidity (46).

Endrin is rapidly metabolized in animals and humans and does not accumulate in human tissues after exposure. In animals, endrin is metabolized to water-soluble compounds and is excreted mainly in the feces. The threshold limit value of endrin is 0.1 mg per cubic meter, which was set to prevent systemic toxicity. The short-term exposure limit for endrin is 0.3 mg per cubic meter. Endrin is toxic to animals in oral overdose studies (90). The half-life of endrin is 2 to 6 days. Endrin and a metabolite, anti-12-hydroxyendrin, can be found in the stool of humans. Anti-12-hydroxyendrin can also be found in the urine of occupationally exposed individuals and can be used as a biological monitoring marker. Endrin has not been found to be carcinogenic or teratogenic or to cause reproductive effects in animals studied.

An outbreak of endrin poisoning from contaminated food in Pakistan in 1984 resulted in a 10% mortality rate from seizures (92). Seizures occurred within 2 hours after the contaminated food was ingested and, in some instances, status epilepticus occurred. Endrin serum concentrations in these individuals ranged from 1.5 to 49.4 ppb. Nonfatally affected patients recovered within a few days.

ISOBENZAN

Isobenzan (telodrin) is a cyclodiene compound with a formula of $C_9H_4Cl_8O$ and a molecular weight of 411.79 (46). The technical product is greater than 95% isobenzan. The compound, a light brown crystalline powder, is soluble in other organic solvents although insoluble in water. It was produced between the years 1958 to 1965 and had limited agricultural use (90). Little is known about the human toxicology of isobenzan. Available human data indicate that this substance's clinical toxicologic effects are related to CNS stimulation and seizures, as is true of other organochlorine compounds. Other symptoms associated with isobenzan include headaches, dizziness, irritability, paresthesias, and drowsiness (46).

Exposure of the general population to isobenzan has been limited. Clinical cases of seizures have been reported after serious exposures (90). A mean blood concentration of 0.023 ng of isobenzan per mL (range, 1.017 to 0.030 ng per mL) was found in nine workers who experienced intoxication.

Isobenzan is well absorbed by the gastrointestinal tract. It accumulates in adipose tissue and has one identified metabolite, telodrin lactane. Isobenzan also crosses the placenta. Its biological half-life is reported to be 2.8 years (90).

ENDOSULFAN

Endosulfan (see Fig. 99-8) is a mixture of two isomers, α- and β-endosulfan. Introduced in 1956, it has a formula of $C_9H_6Cl_6O_3S$ and a molecular weight of 406.95 (46). Its common names include *benzoepin*, *cyclodane*, *malix*, *thimul*, *thiosulfan*, and *thionex*. The α isomer constitutes 70% of the mixture and the β isomer approximately 30% (46). Endosulfan is a brownish, crystalline powder that smells like sulfur dioxide. It is soluble in organic solvents and insoluble in water.

The primary source of human exposure is through residues on food and on tobacco (93). Endosulfan contamination is not widespread in the environment. The β isomer of endosulfan has a higher affinity for soil and thus a longer half-life in the environment. The soil half-life of the α isomer is 60 days, whereas the half-life of the β isomer is 900 days (93). Both isomers resist photodegradation.

Clinical toxicologic effects have been described in cases of ingestion and occupational exposures. After ingestion of endosulfan, symptomatology begins within a few hours, and death has been reported within 2 hours (93,94). The clinical syndrome consists of vomiting, agitation, pulmonary edema, seizures, dyspnea, and cyanosis (94). Occupational exposure has been associated with anxiety, headaches, dizziness, stupor, confusion, and seizures.

CHLORDECONE, KELEVAN, AND MIREX

The chemical formula for mirex is $C_{10}Cl_{12}$, which has a molecular weight of 545.51 (Fig. 99-14) (95). Mirex is a white, crystalline solid that melts at 485°C. It is insoluble in water but soluble in benzene, carbon tetrachloride, and xylene. It is a very stable compound in the environment and bioaccumulates up the food chain.

Introduced in 1955, mirex once was used extensively for the control of fire ants in the southern United States (95). The EPA began phasing out the use of mirex for this purpose in the mid-1970s. The substance has been detected in fat samples collected in geographic areas known to have been treated with the chemical (46). Mirex has also been used as a fire retardant, under the name *dechlorane*, in plastics, rubber, paint, paper, and electrical products (95). Most of the mirex produced between 1959 and 1975 was used in the United States.

Human environmental exposures to mirex occurred from food ingestion and from contaminated soil. Mirex is excreted in human breast milk. Adipose tissue concentrations ranging from 0.16 to 6.0 mg per kg of fat have been found in autopsy samples from persons residing in the southeastern United States (95). The mean blood concentration of mirex in pregnant women in Mississippi was 0.5 µg per L. Mirex resists metabolism in humans and animals. Cases of human poisoning have not been reported. Mirex was not fetotoxic in animal studies and was not a teratogen. It crosses the placenta in animal studies and is carcinogenic in mice and rats.

Chlordecone (Kepone) is a tan to white solid having a chemical formula of $C_{10}Cl_{10}O$ and a molecular weight of 490.61 (Fig. 99-15) (46). It is soluble in acetone and less soluble in benzene and similar petroleum solvents. Technical-grade chlordecone is 88% to 99% pure, with minor contamination by hexachlorocyclopentadiene (96).

Chlordecone production began in 1965 but was terminated in July 1975 after its manufacturing plant had been in operation for 16 months (46). No effective occupational control of chlordecone exposure had been determined, and workers were being excessively contaminated. The clinical syndrome of chlordecone toxicity was insidious, and its onset involved some weight loss, tremor of the muscles of the upper extremities, muscle weakness, abnormal eye movements, slurring of speech, mental status changes, chest pain, arthralgias, dermatitis, and abnormal liver function tests (46,97). After manufacturing of chlordecone was initiated, blood levels of this substance in residents of the community in close proximity to the plant were found to be as

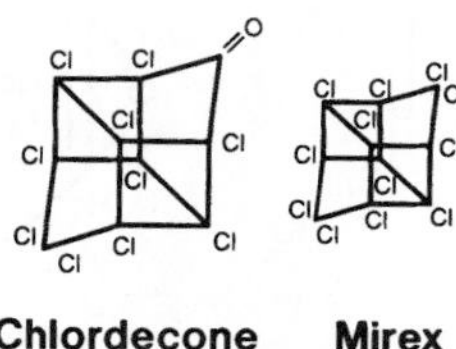

Figure 99-14. Chlordecone and mirex.

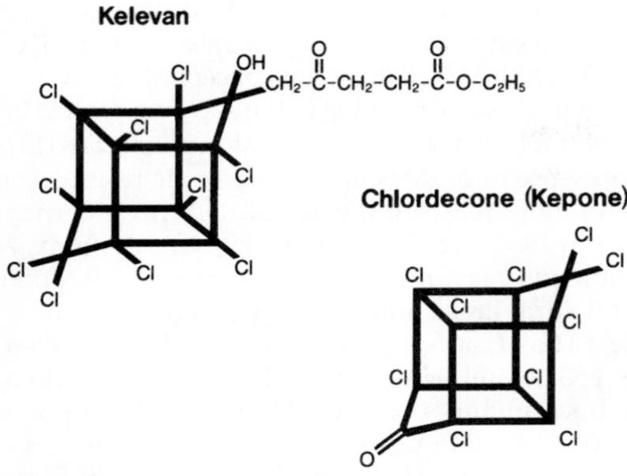

Figure 99-15. Kelevan and chlordecone (Kepone).

high as 0.033 ppm (46,97,98). Chlordecone is a known neurotoxin and can produce peripheral neuropathy.

Chlordecone is environmentally very stable. Human exposure to chlordecone has occurred via food residues owing to its bioaccumulation. It is excreted in human breast milk. Occupational exposure occurred in its production plant in 1975, with large amounts of chlordane contaminating the surrounding environment. Chlordecone blood concentrations in workers exhibiting health effects averaged 2.53 mg per L (98). Those exposed workers who were not ill had average blood concentrations of 0.60 mg per L. Chlordecone's half-life ranges from 63 to 148 days. Cholestyramine was found to enhance gastrointestinal elimination of this toxin in exposed individuals.

Chlordecone and kelevan are chemically related pesticides. Kelevan (Despirol, Elevat), a condensation product of chlordecone and ethyl levulinate (96), is a solid white powder with a molecular weight of 634.79 (see Fig. 99-15). Technical-grade kelevan is 94% to 98% pure, with minor contamination by chlordecone. Once absorbed by animals or humans, it is metabolized to chlordecone.

TOXAPHENE

Toxaphene, introduced in 1948, is a mixture of chlorinated bicyclic terpenes (chlorinated camphenes) containing 67% to 69% chlorine. Toxaphene is a yellow, waxy solid with a chemical formula of $C_{10}H_{10}Cl_{18}$ (Fig. 99-16). It is well absorbed dermally and via the gastrointestinal tract. Environmentally, toxaphene vaporizes from soil but can be adsorbed to soil with a half-life of up to 12 years. Toxaphene bioaccumulates in aquatic organisms (99). It is soluble in organic solvents but insoluble in water. In the environment, toxaphene is photodegraded by ultraviolet light and, in soil, is degraded by the action of bacteria (99).

Clinical toxicity from toxaphene occurs from occupational exposures and ingestion of the product. Cases of poisoning have manifested as seizures and respiratory depression (96). In occupational settings, inhalation of the product has been associated with decreased pulmonary function and dyspnea. Toxaphene exposure has resulted in death in some instances. Symptoms occur within 30 minutes to a few hours after ingestion. The main clinical manifestations of toxicity are convulsions, hyperthermia, tremors, and confusion (46).

Toxaphene is considered to be a potential human carcinogen, whereas in mice and rats it is a proved carcinogen. The threshold limit value is 0.5 mg per cubic meter, with a notation warning against dermal contact.

Figure 99-16. Toxaphene.

DICOFOL AND METHOXYCHLOR

Dicofol is a chlorinated hydrocarbon pesticide used mainly as an acaricide on grain crops (Fig. 99-17). The chemical's generic name is 1,1-bis(*p*-chlorophenyl)-2,2,2-trichloroethanol, and it is marketed as Kelthane, Acarin, and Mitigan. Dicofol has a molecular weight of 370.5 and is a white solid with a melting point of 79°C. The technical product is a light brown, viscous oil with a density of 1.45. Dicofol is insoluble in water but soluble in most aliphatic and aromatic solvents. It is highly lipophilic. This chemical is hydrolyzed by alkali to dichlorobenzophenone and chloroform (46).

Dicofol is manufactured by the chlorination of bis(4-chlorophenyl)carbinol. It is registered for use on vegetables, fruits, and a variety of field crops and is used widely in nurseries and greenhouses. It is relatively stable, although when heated or in contact with strong acids, it decomposes to hydrogen chloride, the vapors of which may cause acute health problems. The chemical is also structurally similar to DDT (46).

Dicofol is stable in the environment after application. Residues decrease rapidly, but trace amounts of the chemical can be found in soil up to a year after application. Human toxicity information is limited, as human exposures have demonstrated very little clinical toxicity. Animals given toxic doses have symptoms referable to CNS stimulation.

Methoxychlor [1,1,1-trichloro-2,2-bis(*p*-methoxyphenyl) ethane], having the chemical formula $C_{16}H_{15}C_{13}O_2$, has a molecular weight of 345.65 (see Fig. 99-17) (46). It is marketed as Marlate. The compound is a clear crystal in its pure state and a gray powder in its technical state (46). It was first introduced in 1945 as a wettable powder, dust, and concentrate. Like dicofol, methoxychlor has a low order of animal toxicity but, in sufficient doses, can produce seizures. Human volunteers ingesting up to 2 mg per kg per day for 8 weeks showed no health effects. In humans, dermatitis may occur from contact with either dicofol or methoxychlor. No cases of systemic intoxication from methoxychlor have been reported in humans.

Figure 99-17. Methoxychlor (Marlate) and dicofol (Kelthane).

ORGANOCHLORINE PESTICIDE CONCENTRATIONS IN HUMAN TISSUES

The period from the 1950s to 1970s witnessed heavy use of many organochlorine pesticides. The concentration of DDT in human adipose tissue during this time averaged approximately 5 ppm (24). At the same time, the adipose concentrations of DDT and DDE in combination averaged 15 ppm (24). After the ban on DDT was issued, a gradual reduction of adipose tissue concentrations of both DDT and DDE occurred. By the late 1960s, the average concentration ranged from 1 to 2 ppm of DDT and approximately 9 ppm for all DDT- and DDE-related pesticides (24).

Because pesticides had been used extensively throughout southern Florida, the presence of organochlorine pesticides in the serum of 59 female residents of Dade County, Florida, was surveyed and compared with pesticide content in the drinking water (24). Ten organochlorine pesticides and their metabolites were analyzed in this monitoring program: HCH, β-HCH, heptachlor, oxychlordane, heptachlor epoxide, *trans*-nonachlor, DDE, dieldrin, *o,p*'-DDT, and *p,p*'-DDT. In the subjects, HCH, β-HCH, *p,p*'-DDE, dieldrin, and *p,p*'-DDT were detected. Serum concentrations of most of these organochlorine compounds were in the parts-per-billion range (see Table 99-6). For all five compounds detected in the subject pool, each was undetectable in at least some subjects and ranged to various maximum concentrations as follows: HCH to 1.1 ppb, β-HCH to 5.8 ppb, DDE to 68.4 ppb, dieldrin to 10 ppb, and DDT to 5.5 ppb. When subjects were compared with individuals who consumed well water as opposed to city water, no significant difference in serum levels of organochlorine pesticide metabolites was noted (see Table 99-7) (24).

Organochlorine pesticide residues were studied in human adipose tissue in the United Kingdom between the years 1976 and 1977. These samples were taken from adipose tissue during autopsies on 236 individuals older than 5 years (26). The ranges of these compounds in adipose tissue were as follows: β-HCH ranged from undetectable to 1.2 mg per kg; heptachlor epoxide, from lower limits of detection to 0.12 mg per kg; dieldrin, from undetectable to 0.49 mg per kg; DDE, from 0.03 to 15 mg per kg; DDT, from 0.04 to 17 mg per kg; and total chlorinated biphenyls, from undetectable to 10 mg per kg (26). The concentrations of these organochlorine compounds were similar to those observed in other studies carried out in the 1960s. Results of the 1976 and 1977 study in the 236 subjects and the organochlorine pesticide residues found in human fat are summarized in Table 99-8.

Other studies performed in the 1960s in autopsy samples showed mean concentrations of dieldrin of 0.0061 ppm in the white matter of the brain, gray matter concentrations of 0.0047 ppm, liver concentrations of 0.03 ppm, and fatty tissue concentrations of 0.17 ppm (21). Figures 99-4 and 99-12 depict the distribution of DDT and dieldrin, respectively, in blood and other tissues in humans, as prepared from this study (21). Dieldrin has a greater tendency to be stored in liver and brain tissue relative to adipose tissue, as compared with DDT-related compounds. Concentrations of organochlorine pesticides typically found in adipose tissue, liver, and brain tissue are shown in Tables 99-9 and 99-10 (21).

Assays for oxychlordane metabolites were conducted in adipose tissue samples collected from postmortem examination and surgical procedures in the 1960s and 1970s (80). In 27 specimens, oxychlordane concentrations ranged from 0.03 to 0.40 ppm (80).

Isomers and metabolites of a variety of organochlorines—including *p,p*'-DDT, *o,p*'-DDT, *p,p*'-DDE, β-HCH, dieldrin, and heptachlor epoxide—have been found in persons who have had no occupational exposure. Serum pesticide concentrations in the parts-per-billion range were detected by Morgan and Lin (13) in a population studied between 1967 and 1973. These concentrations were compared with various clinical chemistries in more than 2,600 subjects (13). DDT and DDE serum concentrations were found to be higher in those subjects living in the southern United States. No evidence was found of abnormal hematologic studies (13).

The presence of organochlorine pesticide residue concentrations in human breast milk was studied in western Australia from 1979 to 1980 (see Table 99-11) (29). In this study, 267 samples of human breast milk were supplied by 140 donors from urban and rural areas and were analyzed for organochlorine pesticides. The organochlorine pesticides detected were aldrin, lindane, HCH, dieldrin, and DDT. Aldrin and lindane were found in trace amounts, whereas DDT-related compounds measuring 0.078 to 0.046 ppm were found. The levels of HCH ranged from 0.025 to 0.008 ppm and of dieldrin ranged from 0.005 to 0.009 ppm. A comparison of this study's results with those of a previous study conducted from 1970 to 1971 showed that, except for dieldrin concentrations (which were increasing), organochlorine pesticide concentrations in human breast milk were decreasing. The Australian government imposed controls on the use of organochlorine pesticides in western Australia in 1971. During the years 1978 to 1979, a decrease in pesticide concentrations was documented in most countries in which limitations had been placed on the use and application of chlorinated pesticides in the environment. Endeavors to correlate the pesticide concentrations in human tissues and the use of pesticides or the exposure to pesticides have been unsuccessful. The results of the 1979 to 1980 Australian study demonstrate that restricting the use of organochlorine pesticides reduces the human tissue content of these pesticides. Individual information on samples from the urban donors of human breast milk in this 1979 to 1980 study are shown in Table 99-12 (29).

Indoor air concentrations of organochloride pesticides, particularly chlordane, contribute to the total body burden of the residues found in humans (47). Sampling and analysis of indoor air for chlorinated pesticides has revealed low concentrations of chlordane and nonachlor (44,45). Concentrations of γ-chlordane, α-chlordane, and *trans*-nonachlor were found in the various homes sampled. In one study, 12 homes were sampled from November 1985 to October 1986 (45). The outdoor air concentrations of chlordane and *trans*-nonachlor were very low, the average outdoor air concentration of γ-chlordane being 0.5 ng per cubic meter (45). In contrast, the indoor air concentration of γ-chlordane ranged from 29 ng per cubic meter and averaged seven times higher than the outdoor air concentration. Interestingly, in this study, homes in which the windows were closed versus those in which windows were open did not show substantially different concentrations of indoor air (45). These homes had been treated with subsurface slab injection of chlordane for termites. Large cracks in the foundation probably were responsible for the high concentration of chlordane in indoor air (45).

Another 1985 study correlated home treatment with organochlorine pesticides to the presence of such pesticides in human breast milk (23). Fourteen subjects supplied breast milk in this study and answered questions regarding treatment of their houses with organochlorine pesticides. Most houses had been treated with applications of heptachlor and aldrin. This study concluded that a connection existed between the concentrations of pesticides and other metabolites in human breast milk and the use of such pesticides for spraying inside or outside the home (23). The mean concentrations of the organochlorine pesticides found in human breast milk from these donors are shown in Table 99-13. The subjects were chosen from among those whose houses had been recently treated with organochlorine pesticides. Table 99-14 indicates the concentrations of dieldrin in breast milk donors and the decline in dieldrin concentrations months after the application of dieldrin in the home environment (23). Table 99-15 shows chlordane concentrations in one of the subjects (expressed as nanograms per gram of whole breast milk) relative to the time of chlordane treatment in the subject's house. Table 99-16 shows concentrations of HCH, heptachlor, and heptachlor epoxide relative to treatment times in the home environment (23). These data demonstrate that spraying of homes with organochlorine pesticides is related to increased concentrations of pesticides in human breast milk (23).

The occupational permissible exposure limit of chlordane is 500 μg per cubic meter for a 40-hour work week. The NAS in 1979 considered this concentration to be unacceptable in the home environment because of continuous exposure 24 hours per day and recommended a concentration of chlordane of 5 μg per cubic meter as acceptable in the home environment (44). The NAS also recommended a concentration of 2 μg per cubic meter for heptachlor in homes (44).

Chlordane was measured in 474 family housing units at seven U.S. Air Force installations from the 1980 to 1981 (44). Chlordane had been used in these homes for treatment of termites by subsurface slab injection or exterior application, and 86% of these homes had chlordane air concentrations of less than 3.5 μg per cubic meter, whereas 12% had concentrations between 3.5 and 6.5 μg per cubic meter, and 2% had indoor air concentrations exceeding 6.5 μg per cubic meter (44).

REFERENCES

1. Gant DB, Eldefrawi ME, Eldefrawi AT. Cyclodiene insecticides inhibit GABA receptor–regulated chloride transport. *Toxicol Appl Pharmacol* 1987;88:313–321.
2. Lawrence LJ, Casida JE. Interactions of lindane, toxaphene and cyclodienes with brain-specific t-butylbicyclophosphorothionate receptor. *Life Sci* 1984;35:171–178.
3. Agency for Toxic Substances and Disease Registry. *Toxicological profile for* p,p'*-DDT,* p,p'*-DDE,* p,p'*-DDD*. Atlanta: US Department of Health and Human Services, Public Health Service, ATSDR, December 1989.
4. Coulston F. Reconsideration of the dilemma of DDT for the establishment of an acceptable daily intake. *Regul Toxicol Pharmacol* 1985;5:332–383.
5. Saxena MC, Siddiqui MKJ, Seth TD, Krishna Murti CR. Organochlorine pesticides in specimens from women undergoing spontaneous abortion, premature or full-term delivery. *J Anal Toxicol* 1981;5:6–9.
6. Mattison DR. Pesticides in human breast milk: changing patterns and estimates of cancer risk. Presented at the thirty-eighth annual meeting, San Antonio, TX, March 20–23, 1991.
7. Curtie RA, Kadis VW, Breitkreitz WE, Cunningham GB, Bruns GW. Pesticide residues in human milk, Alberta, Canada—1966–70, 1977–78. *Pestic Monit J* 1979;133:52–55.
8. Griffith FD, Blanke RV. Pesticides in people: blood organochlorine pesticide levels in Virginia residents. *Pestic Monit J* 1975;8:219–224.
9. Polishuk ZW, Ron M, Wassermann M, Cucos S, Wassermann D, Lemesch C. Pesticides in people: organochlorine compounds in human blood plasma and milk. *Pestic Monit J* 1977;10:121–129.
10. Radomski JL, Deichmann WB, Rey AA, Merkin T. Human pesticide blood levels as a measure of body burden and pesticide exposure. *Toxicol Appl Pharmacol* 1971;20:175–185.
11. Radomski JL, Astolfi E, Deichmann WB, Rey AA. Blood levels of organochlorine pesticides in Argentina: occupationally and nonoccupationally exposed adults, children and newborn infants. *Toxicol Appl Pharmacol* 1971;20:186–193.
12. Dale WE, Curley A, Hayes WJ Jr. Determination of chlorinated insecticides in human blood. *Ind Med Surg* 1967;36(4):275–280.
13. Morgan DP, Lin LI. Blood organochlorine pesticide concentrations, clinical hematology and biochemistry in workers occupationally exposed to pesticides. *Arch Environ Contam Toxicol* 1978;7:423–447.
14. Hunter DJ, Hankinson SE, Laden F, et al. Plasma organochlorine levels and the risk of breast cancer. *N Engl J Med* 1997;337(18):1253–1258.
15. Krieger N, Wolff MS, Hiatt RA, et al. Breast cancer and serum organochlorines: a prospective study among white, black, and Asian women. *J Natl Cancer Inst* 1994;86:589–599.
16. Safe SH. Xenoestrogens and breast cancer. *N Engl J Med* 1997;337(18):1303–1304.
17. Baumann K, Angerer J, Heinrich R, Lehnert G. Occupational exposure to hexachlorocyclohexane, part I. *Int Arch Occup Environ Health* 1980;47:119–127.
18. Agency for Toxic Substances and Disease Registry. *Toxicological profile for hexachlorocyclohexane.* Atlanta: US Department of Health and Human Services, Public Health Service, ATSDR, December 1989.
19. Baumann K, Behling K, Brassow HL, Stapel K. Occupational exposure to hexachlorocyclohexane, part 3. *Int Arch Occup Environ Health* 1981;48:165–172.
20. Nigam SK, Karnik AB, Majumder SK, et al. Serum hexachlorocyclohexane residues in workers engaged at a HCH manufacturing plant. *Int Arch Occup Environ Health* 1986;57:315–320.
21. de Vlieger M, Robinson J, Crabtree AN, van Dijk MC. The organochlorine insecticide content of human tissues. *Arch Environ Health* 1968;17:759–767.
22. Pines A, Cucos S, Ever-Hadani P, Ron M. Some organochlorine insecticide and polychlorinated biphenyl blood residues in infertile males in the general Israeli population of the middle 1980s. *Arch Environ Contam Toxicol* 1987;16:587–597.
23. Stacey CI, Tatum T. House treatment with organochlorine pesticides and their levels in human milk—Perth, Western Australia. *Bull Environ Contam Toxicol* 1985;35:202–208.
24. Barquet A, Morgade C, Pfaffenberger CD. Determination of organochlorine pesticides and metabolites in drinking water, human blood serum, and adipose tissue. *J Toxicol Environ Health* 1981;7:469–479.
25. Dale WE, Curley A, Cueto C Jr. Hexane extractable chlorinated insecticides in human blood. *Life Sci* 1966;5:47–54.
26. Abbott DC, Collins GB, Goulding R, Hoodless RA. Organochlorine pesticide residues in human fat in the United Kingdom 1976–7. *BMJ* 1981;283: 1425–1428.
27. Kashyap SK. Health surveillance and biological monitoring of pesticide formulators in India. *Toxicol Lett* 1986;33:107–114.
28. Takahashi W, Saidin D, Takei G, Wong L. Organochloride pesticide residues in human milk in Hawaii, 1979–80. *Bull Environ Contam Toxicol* 1981;27:506–511.
29. Stacey CI, Perriman WS, Whitney S. Organochlorine pesticide residue levels in human milk: Western Australia, 1979–1980. *Arch Environ Health* 1985;40: 102–108.
30. Brassow HL, Baumann K, Lehnert G. Occupational exposure to hexachlorocyclohexane, part 2. *Int Arch Occup Environ Health* 1981;48:81–87.
31. Milby TH, Samuels AJ, Ottoboni F. Human exposure to lindane: blood lindane levels as a function of exposure. *J Occup Med* 1968;10:584–587.
32. Ramachandran M, Banerjee M, Grover A, Zaidi S. DDT and HCH residues in the body fat and blood samples from some Delhi hospitals. *Ind J Med Res* 1984;80:590–593.
33. Davies JE, Dedhia HV, Morgade C, Barquet A, Maibach HI. Lindane poisonings. *Arch Dermatol* 1983;119:142–144.
34. Saxena MC, Siddiqui MKJ, Bhargava AK, Krishna Murti CR, Kutty D. Placental transfer of pesticides in humans. *Arch Toxicol* 1981;48:127–134.
35. Saxena MC, Siddiqui MKJ. A comparison of organochlorine insecticide contents in specimens of maternal blood, placenta, and umbilical cord blood from stillborn and live-born cases. *J Toxicol Environ Health* 1983;11:71–79.
36. Roncevic N, Pavkov S, Galetin-Smith R, et al. Serum concentrations of organochlorine compounds during pregnancy and the newborn. *Bull Environ Contam Toxicol* 1987;38:117–124.
37. Morgan DP, Stockdale EM, Roberts RJ, Walter AW. Anemia associated with exposure to lindane. *Arch Environ Health* 1980;35:307–310.
38. Berry DH, Brewster MA, Watson R, Neuberg RW. Untoward effects associated with lindane abuse [Letter]. *Am J Dis Child* 1987;14:125.
39. Jaeger U, Podczeck A, Haubenstock A, et al. Acute oral poisoning with lindane-solvent mixtures. *Vet Hum Toxicol* 1984;26:11–14.
40. Pramanik AK, Hansen RC. Transcutaneous gamma benzene hexachloride absorption and toxicity in infants and children. *Arch Dermatol* 1979;115: 1224–1225.
41. Feldmann RJ, Maibach HI. Percutaneous penetration of some pesticides and herbicides in man. *Toxicol Appl Pharmacol* 1974;28:126–132.
42. Joy RM, Albertson TE. Lindane and limbic system excitability. *Neurol Toxicol* 1985;2:193–214.
43. Agency for Toxic Substances and Disease Registry. *Toxicological profile for chlordane.* Atlanta: US Department of Health and Human Services, Public Health Service, ATSDR, 1994.
44. Wright CG, Leidy RB. Chlordane and heptachlor in the ambient air of houses treated for termites. *Bull Environ Contam Toxicol* 1982;28:617–623.
45. Anderson DJ, Hites RA. Chlorinated pesticides in indoor air. *Environ Sci Technol* 1988;22:717–720.
46. Hayes WJ. Chlorinated hydrocarbon insecticides. In: *Pesticides studied in man.* Baltimore: Williams & Wilkins, 1982:172–283.
47. Mussalo-Rauhamaa H. Partitioning and levels of neutral organochlorine compounds in human serum blood cells and adipose tissue and liver tissue. *Sci Total Environ* 1991;103:159–175.
48. Barnett R, D'Ercole A, Cain J, et al. Organochlorine pesticide residues in human milk samples from women living in northwest and northeast Mississippi, 1973–1975. *Pestic Monit J* 1979;13:47–51.
49. Mussalo-Rauhamaa H, Pyysalo H, Antervo K. Relation between the content of organochlorine compounds in Finnish human milk and characteristics of the mothers. *J Toxicol Environ Health* 1988;25:1–19.
50. Sasaki K, Kawasaky Y, Sekita K et al. Disposition of β-hexachlorocyclohexane, *p,p*-DDT and *trans*-chlordane administered subcutaneously to monkeys (*Macaca fascicularis*). *Arch Environ Contam Toxicol* 1992;22:25–29.
51. Wariishi M, Nishiyama K. Observations on the progress of chlordane contamination in humans by blood and sebum analysis. *Arch Environ Contam Toxicol* 1989;18:501–507.
52. Taguchi S, Yakushiji T. Influence of termite treatment in the home on chlordane concentration in human milk. *Arch Environ Contam Toxicol* 1988;17:65–72.

53. Oehme M. Dispersion and transport paths of toxic persistent organochlorines to the arctic levels and consequences. *Sci Total Environ* 1991;106:43–53.
54. Beeman R, Matsumara F. Metabolism of *cis*- and *trans*-chlordane by soil microorganism. *J Agric Food Chem* 1981;29:84–89.
55. Wallace L. Comparison of risk from outdoor and indoor exposure to toxic chemicals. *Environ Health Perspect* 1991;95:7–13.
56. Anderson D, Hites R. Indoor air: spacial variations of chlorinated pesticides. *Atmosphere Environ* 1989;23:2063–2066.
57. Fensk ER, Sternbach T. Indoor air levels of chlordane in residences in New Jersey. *Bull Environ Contam Toxicol* 1987;39:903–910.
58. Barnes R. Poisoning by the insecticide chlordane. *Med J Aust* 1967;1(19):972–973.
59. Aldrich FD, Holmes JH. Acute chlordane intoxication in a child. *Arch Environ Health* 1969;19:129–132.
60. Derbes VH, Dent JH, Forrest WW, Johnson MF. Fatal chlordane poisoning. Council on Pharmacy and Chemistry. *JAMA* 1955;158:1367–1369.
61. Dadey JL, Kammer AG. Chlordane intoxication. *JAMA* 1953;153:723–726.
62. Kutz FW, Strassman SC, Sperling JF, Cook BT. A fatal chlordane poisoning. *J Toxicol Clin Toxicol* 1983;20:167–174.
63. Wang HH, MacMahon B. Mortality of pesticide applicators. *J Occup Med* 1979;21:741–744.
64. Wang HH, MacMahon B. Mortality of workers employed in the manufacture of chlordane and heptachlor. *J Occup Med* 1979;21:745–748.
65. Ditraglia D, Brown DP, Namekata T, Iverson N. Mortality study of workers employed at organochlorine pesticide manufacturing plants. *Scand J Work Environ Health* 1981;7:140–146.
66. Blair A, Grauman DJ, Lubin JH, Fraumeni JF. Lung cancer and other causes of death among licensed pesticide applicators. *J Natl Cancer Inst* 1983;71:31–37.
67. Furie B, Trubowitz S. Insecticides and blood dyscrasias: chlordane exposure and self-limited refractory megaloblastic anemia. *JAMA* 1976;235:1720–1722.
68. Mendeloff AI, Smith DE. Clinicopathologic conference: exposure to insecticides, bone marrow failure, gastrointestinal bleeding, and uncontrollable infections. *Am J Med* 1955;(August):274–284.
69. Epstein S, Ozonoff D. Leukemias and blood dyscrasias following exposure to chlordane and heptachlor. *Teratog Carcinog Mutagen* 1987;7:527–540.
70. Fishbein W, White J, Isaacs H. Survey of workers exposed to chlordane. *Ind Med Surg* 1964;10:726–727.
71. Khasawina A, Hardy C, Clark G. Comparative inhalation toxicity of technical chlordane in rats and monkeys. *J Toxicol Environ Health* 1989;28:327–347.
72. McConnachie P, Zahalsky A. Immune alterations in humans exposed to the termiticide technical chlordane. *Arch Environ Health* 1992;47:295–301.
73. Barnett J, Holcomb D, Menna J, et al. The effect of prenatal chlordane exposure on specific anti-influenza cell-mediated immunity. *Toxicol Lett* 1985;25:229–238.
74. Barnett J, Soderberg L, Menna J. The effect of prenatal chlordane exposure on delayed hypersensitivity response of balb/c-mice. *Toxicol Lett* 1985;25:173–183.
75. Chuang L, Liu Y, Killam K, et al. Modulation by the insecticides heptachlor and chlordane of the cell mediated immune proliferative responses of the rhesus monkeys. *In Vivo* 1992;6:29–32.
76. Brown D. Mortality of workers employed at organochlorine pesticide manufacturing plants—an update. *Scand J Work Environ Health* 1992;18:155–161.
77. Cantor K, Blair A, Everett G, et al. Pesticides and other agricultural risk factors for non-Hodgkin's lymphoma among men in Iowa and Minnesota. *Cancer Res* 1992;52:2447–2455.
78. Menconi S, Clark J, Langenberg P, et al. A preliminary study of potential human health effects in private residences following chlordane applications for termite control. *Arch Environ Health* 1988;43:349–352.
79. Curley A, Garretson L. Acute chlordane poisoning: clinical and chemical studies. *Arch Environ Health* 1969;18:211–215.
80. Biros FJ, Enos HF. Oxychlordane residues in human adipose tissue. *Bull Environ Contam Toxicol* 1973;10:257–260.
81. Olanoff L, Bristow W, Cololough J. Acute chlordane intoxication. *J Toxicol Clin Toxicol* 1983;20:291–306.
82. Garretson L, Guzelian PS, Blanke R. Subacute chlordane poisoning. *J Toxicol Clin Toxicol* 1984;22:565–571.
83. Hunter CG, Robinson J. Pharmacodynamics of dieldrin (HEOD), part 1. *Arch Environ Health* 1967;15:614–626.
84. Agency for Toxic Substances and Disease Registry. *Toxicological profile for aldrin/dieldrin.* Atlanta: US Department of Health and Human Services, Public Health Service, ATSDR, May 1989.
85. Ackerman L. Humans—overview of human exposure to dieldrin residues in the environment and current trends of residue levels in tissue. *Pestic Monit J* 1980;14:64–69.
86. Hunter CG, Robinson J. Pharmacodynamics of dieldrin (HEOD): ingestion by human subjects for 18 to 24 months and postexposure for eight months. *Arch Environ Health* 1969;18:12–21.
87. Jager K. *Aldrin, dieldrin, endrin and telodrin—an epidemiological and toxicological study of long-term occupational exposure.* New York: Elsevier Science, 1970:121–131.
88. Patel TB, Hy B, Rao VN. Dieldrin poisoning in man: a report of 20 cases observed in Bombay State. *BMJ* 1958;19:919–922.
89. Bloomquist JR, Soderlund DM. Neurotoxic insecticides inhibit GABA-dependent chloride uptake by mouse brain vesicles. *Biochem Biophys Res Commun* 1985;133:37–43.
90. Jong de G. Long-term health effects of aldrin and dieldrin. *Toxicol Lett* 1991;[Suppl]:1–206.
91. Ribbens PH. Mortality study of industrial workers exposed to aldrin, dieldrin and endrin. *Int Arch Occup Environ Health* 1985;56:75–79.
92. Rowley D, Rab M, Hardjotanojo W, Liddie J. Convulsions caused by endrin poisoning in Pakistan. *Pediatrics* 1987;79(6):928–934.
93. World Health Organization. *Endosulfan: environmental health criteria 40.* Geneva: World Health Organization, 1984.
94. Shemesh Y, Bourvine A, Gold D, Bracha P. Survival after acute endosulfan intoxication. *J Toxicol Clin Toxicol* 1988;26:265–268.
95. World Health Organization. *Mirex: environmental health criteria 44.* Geneva: World Health Organization, 1984.
96. World Health Organization. *Kelevan: environmental health criteria 66.* Geneva: World Health Organization, 1986.
97. Taylor J. Neurological manifestations in humans exposed to chlordecone: follow-up of results. *Neurotoxicology* 1985;6:231–236.
98. World Health Organization. *Chlordecone: environmental health criteria 43.* Geneva: World Health Organization, 1984.
99. World Health Organization. *Camphechlor: environmental health criteria 45.* Geneva: World Health Organization, 1984.

CHAPTER 100
Fumigants

John A. Lowe and John B. Sullivan, Jr.

Fumigants are pesticides that exist as gases or vapors at specified temperatures and pressures (generally room temperature and ambient pressures). Fumigation is used to control a variety of pests, including insects in stored grain products, wood-destroying insects, and nematodes or fungi in soil (1). The advantages of fumigation are the speed with which it works, its ability to reach places that sprays cannot reach (i.e., within building materials or deep within soil), and the possible lower cost as compared to that of repeated spraying. Disadvantages are the need for specialized equipment and the requirement of training to use fumigants safely (2). Fumigants span several different classes of chemicals; however, nearly all the chemicals used as fumigants are highly toxic, both to pest species and to nontarget organisms (Table 100-1). Chemicals formerly used as fumigants are carbon tetrachloride, carbon disulfide, and hydrogen cyanide. Other chemicals with important commercial uses as fumigants [e.g., 1,2-dibromo-3-chloropropane (DBCP); ethylene dibromide (EDB); 1,3-dichloropropene (1,3-D); methyl bromide; and aluminum phosphide] have been associated with significant chronic and acute health effects in humans and laboratory animals. Carbon tetrachloride and methyl bromide potentially affect stratospheric ozone and the ability of the atmospheric ozone layer to protect the earth's surface from ultraviolet radiation.

Many fumigants epitomize the balance of economic benefits and estimated health risks associated with chemical use. Classic examples of this balance include such chemicals as EDB and DBCP, which have served vital roles in increasing crop yields by controlling soil-borne nematodes. Use of these compounds has resulted in potential widespread exposures of humans through groundwater contamination in agricultural areas and, in the case of DBCP, adverse effects in workers. EDB and DBCP have been demonstrated to be carcinogens in laboratory animals; hence, they represent a potential human cancer risk. The estimated cancer risk associated with these chemicals in groundwater has significantly influenced decisions to prohibit their use in agriculture in the United States. Over time, greater reliance has been placed on methyl bromide as a soil and object fumigant. However, production and use of methyl bromide eventually will cease by the early twenty-first century, principally owing to its ozone-depleting effects. Ultimately, the loss of methyl bromide presents an opportunity to move away from heavy reliance on a single chemical that has discouraged an in-depth

TABLE 100-1. Selected chemicals used in fumigation

Chemical	Uses	Status
Aluminum phosphide	Grain fumigant	Still in use
Calcium cyanide	Rodent control; beehive fumigant	Very limited uses
Carbon disulfide	Rodent control; soil fumigant	Early fumigant, no longer used
Carbon tetrachloride	Grain fumigant	Use suspended by EPA due to toxicity
Chloropicrin	Soil fumigant; warning agent	Still in use
Dibromochloropropane	Soil fumigant	Use suspended by EPA due to toxicity and groundwater contamination
1,3-Dichloropropene	Soil fumigant	Use suspended by EPA due to toxicity
Ethylene dibromide	Soil, grain, commodity, "spot" fumigant	Use suspended by EPA due to toxicity and groundwater contamination
Ethylene dichloride	Grain fumigant	Use suspended by EPA due to toxicity
Ethylene oxide	Medical instrument sterilizer	Still in use
Methyl bromide	Soil, commodity, structural fumigant	Still in use
Sulfuryl fluoride	Structural fumigant	Still in use

EPA, U.S. Environmental Protection Agency.

understanding of the soil dynamics of various crop systems. Significant research in alternative crop protection methods has been spurred by the impending loss of methyl bromide.

FUMIGATION METHODS

Fumigants afford a practical solution to control of insects and other pests within an enclosure. A good fumigant has several specific properties. The chemical must be volatile and be able to penetrate deeply into soil, stored products or, in the case of structural fumigants, building materials in which pests are located. The chemical must be toxic to pests but should not be corrosive or phytotoxic after use. The chemical must desorb readily from treated food products and not leave behind toxicologically significant or phytotoxic residues. Soil fumigants also should desorb or degrade readily prior to planting (1,3).

Fumigation can be performed under almost any circumstances that allow the forming of an enclosed space. However, the principal classes of fumigant use are space fumigation of commodities or commodity-processing equipment, soil fumigation, and fumigation for structural pest control.

Space Fumigation

Space fumigation often is performed within standing fumigation chambers or by enclosing the commodity with gas-proof sheeting. A fumigation chamber consists of three elements: (i) a system for introducing the fumigant into the chamber, (ii) a chamber into which the commodity to be fumigated is loaded, and (iii) an exhaust ventilation system for removing the fumigant from the chamber. A great variety of fumigant delivery and ventilation systems are possible; these provide different levels of exposures and potential hazards to the fumigation workers. For example, liquid fumigants, such as ethylene dichloride or carbon tetrachloride, could be introduced into a space by volatilization from a heated pan. This method could result in inhalational exposures and dermal contact with the fumigant as the material is poured. More sophisticated delivery systems include closed systems, in which the fumigant is metered into the chamber from sealed containers or compressed gas cylinders. These systems serve to reduce potential exposures to fumigants. Phosphine, used as a grain fumigant, is introduced into stockpiled grain as tablets of aluminum or magnesium phosphide. The tablets may be metered into the grain as it is poured into a silo or are introduced into stockpiles that then are covered with polyethylene tarpaulins. The moisture in the grain slowly hydrolyzes the solid compound, liberating phosphine gas over a period of several hours. Handling the solid compound is relatively safe as long as it is kept dry, as the hydrolysis reaction is exothermic and phosphine has a flash point of 100°C. Exposure to phosphine occurs by inhalation, most often after tarpaulin removal or opening of enclosures to ventilate grain prior to transport.

Soil Fumigation

Soil fumigation normally involves injecting liquid fumigant into the soil to depths from 6 inches to 3 feet, depending on the crop and pest to be controlled, through tubing attached to a set of shanks that are pulled through the soil. The shanks are mounted on a tool bar attached either to a wheeled or track-laying tractor. The treated soil then is sealed by a roller or cultipacker drawn by the fumigant rig or by a second tractor (in the case of such low-volatile fumigants as DBCP, EDB, or 1,3-D). Application rates of these compounds range from 5 to 15 gallons per acre for row crops and from 40 to 60 gallons per acre prior to establishing orchards or vineyards.

Fumigation techniques differ when methyl bromide is used. Methyl bromide is injected into the soil at rates of 200 to 325 pounds per acre. Immediately after fumigation with the chemical, the soil is sealed with a polyethylene sheet drawn over the soil by the fumigant rig. Employees shovel soil over the edges of the tarp to slow the dissipation of this highly volatile compound into the air.

DBCP, EDB, and 1,3-D are liquids at ambient conditions and are loaded into tanks on the fumigant rig from a nurse truck stationed at the edge of the field. Typically, loading is performed through closed systems using quick-disconnect, dry-break couplers and gasoline or electric pumps. The tractor tanks may be vented either to open air or into the shanks. Depending on the number and capacity of tractor tanks and application rates, fumigant loads are delivered every 45 minutes to 2 hours of application. The actual loading process requires from 5 to 15 minutes. Methyl bromide is a gas at ambient conditions and is injected into the soil through a closed system from a compressed gas cylinder.

Structural Fumigation

Structural fumigation generally is performed using gas-proof tarpaulins that are not impermeable but hold the desired fumigant concentration inside the structure for a required period. Prior to draping a structure with tarpaulins, the fumigator determines the structure volume and calculates the required fumigant dose; inspects the structure and roof for possible leak points (attached buildings, tunnels, vents or drains connecting to the outside or other buildings, roof vents, and television antennas);

shuts off gas valves; removes furnishings, foods, and personal items as required; clears shrubbery away from the walls; pads sharp edges, corners, and projections to protect the tarpaulins from tearing; and wets the soil around the perimeter of the structure to prevent migration of the gas. Tarpaulins then are carried up to the roof and are draped over the structure. The tarpaulin edges are rolled and clamped together with steel clothespins. During draping, the fumigant delivery hose and several fans are placed inside the structure. The tarpaulin edges are sealed at the bottom of the structure with sand snakes (long canvas tubes filled with sand). Secondary locks, designed to enclose a doorknob and prevent its operation, are placed on all doors.

After inspecting the integrity of the tarpaulin draping and checking the location of all workers, the fumigant and warning agents are introduced into the structure. The fumigant, typically methyl bromide or sulfuryl fluoride, is dispensed from a compressed gas cylinder through a heated manifold. The fumigant dose, in total pounds introduced, is measured by the loss of weight in the cylinder. Application rates of methyl bromide typically range from 1.5 to 3.0 pounds per 1,000 cubic feet of structure volume, providing concentrations calculated to range from 6,000 to 12,000 parts per million (ppm). Owing to the hazards associated with such high concentrations, structural fumigants are used in conjunction with a warning agent, typically chloropicrin. Chloropicrin can be introduced by hand by pouring into a shallow pan a few minutes prior to introduction of the fumigant. Many fumigants registered for structural use are formulated with 1% to 3% chloropicrin, which then is introduced along with the fumigant.

ASSESSMENT OF EXPOSURES TO FUMIGANTS

The potential pathways of human exposure for fumigants are inhalational exposure of workers and off-site individuals, skin and eye contact with liquids, which produces burns or irritation, and ingestion of groundwater that has been tainted by soil fumigants or treated commodities.

Space Fumigation

Studies of fumigant use on stored commodities, primarily with methyl bromide, indicate that large variations can exist in fumigation worker exposure. In California Department of Food and Agriculture studies involving air monitoring of methyl bromide use in fumigation chambers, personal exposures ranged from 0.2 to 33.4 ppm, based on sample durations of 3 to 20 minutes (sampling was performed only during work activities at the chamber). Area sampling performed during these studies in work areas located 50 feet or further from fumigation chambers indicated that methyl bromide concentrations were 1.0 ppm or less (4,5).

Work activities that potentially bring workers into contact with fumigants include (i) introducing the fumigant into the chamber or draped commodity, (ii) ventilating the remaining fumigant from the commodity, and (iii) opening the chamber door and removing the commodity from the fumigation chamber. Exposures fluctuate, depending on several factors, including chamber volume, number of fumigations performed per period, duration allowed for ventilation of the commodity, and fumigant dosage applied to the commodity. However, the highest-level exposures appear to be associated with opening the chamber door after fumigation and removing the commodity (4,5).

Soil Fumigation

Studies of methyl bromide fumigation in greenhouses in Belgium indicated that peak exposures could range from 100 to 1,000 ppm (duration unspecified). Work practices were reported to be more primitive than those in the United States, with workers pulling tarpaulins over fumigated soil by hand instead of using a fumigation rig to lay them down automatically. Such protective measures as wetting the soil and better coordinating activities between the tractor driver and tarpaulin installers reduced concentrations to approximately 100 ppm. One study reported that tarpaulin removal from the soil could result in peak exposures as high as 200 ppm and that tilling the soil several days after application produced concentrations of up to 15 ppm (6,7).

Several studies have evaluated worker exposures associated with methyl bromide–chloropicrin used as a soil fumigant. Several of these studies have been performed by the California Department of Food and Agriculture. Fumigant formulations used in the applications typically contained 67% methyl bromide and 33% chloropicrin. Types of workers monitored were drivers and "copilots" on the fumigant rig and shovelers sealing the edges of the tarpaulins. Concentrations of methyl bromide as great as 8.3 ppm and of chloropicrin as great as 0.18 ppm were found in air samples ranging from 30 to 45 minutes in duration. Most exposures to methyl bromide have not exceeded 5 ppm. Observation of work practices indicated that workers spent approximately one-half of a workday fumigating, with the balance spent driving to and from worksites or maintaining equipment. Exposures of tarpaulin removal operations were not monitored in these studies (8–10). However, one Connecticut case reported that nursery workers removing tarpaulins days after fumigation with methyl bromide experienced symptoms. Four field workers developed fatigue and lightheadedness, and three workers noted progressive respiratory, gastrointestinal, and neurologic symptoms. The acute systemic symptoms improved over several days, but later-onset neuropsychiatric symptoms persisted for several weeks. Exposure monitoring data were not available to compare symptoms with methyl bromide concentrations in air. This incident raised the possibility of an increased risk of toxicity associated with methyl bromide fumigation during a cool season (11).

One study reports an episode of acute symptoms in individuals residing near a field treated with methyl bromide and chloropicrin. This episode appeared to occur during times of low wind, atmospheric inversions, and elevated air temperatures (which also possibly represented warmer soil temperatures). The most frequent symptoms reported included headache, eye and throat irritation, and dizziness. Reports of these symptoms dropped off rapidly with distance from the site. In a field study of off-site movement of fumigants in Southern California, 30-minute air samples collected at the edge of the field showed methyl bromide concentrations between 0.3 and 0.4 ppm and concentrations of chloropicrin between 0.01 and 0.08 ppm immediately after fumigation. These concentrations typically declined over time. However, studies evaluating ambient concentrations under warm inversion conditions, as seen with the reported acute exposure incidents, have not been performed (12).

Beginning in 1993, the state of California implemented use practices that include buffer zones to mitigate unacceptable exposure of the general public to methyl bromide. Air dispersion modeling was used to calculate the size of the buffer zones, with validation through the collection of air-monitoring data. Field monitoring during warmer summer conditions was thought to represent worst-case conditions, because emissions would be greater under warmer soil conditions (as emissions are governed by adsorption and diffusion through soil gas). However, higher air concentrations may occur during winter months, owing to stabler atmospheric conditions. Monitoring studies conducted during winter months in 1997 showed that downwind air concentrations ranged from 0.082 to approximately 1 ppm [24-hour time-weighted average (TWA)] at the buffer zone distance. Off-site air concentrations exceeded a target level of 0.21 ppm (24-hour TWA) for protection of the public, developed by the California Department of Pesticide Regulation (memorandum to Paul H. Gosselin, Department of Pesticide Regulation Director, July 18, 1997: http://www.cdpr.ca.gov/docs/dprdocs/empm/mebr.htm).

Factors that could affect volatilization of fumigants from soil include soil temperature, moisture, and porosity; physical and chemical properties of the fumigant (e.g., vapor pressure, diffusion coefficient, and Henry's law constant); and the application rate. Some studies have reported that increasing the application rate also increases mobility of methyl bromide in soil. Higher application rates appear to result in increased methyl bromide concentrations in air. Soil porosity also influences fumigant mobility. Porosity in soil is reduced by soil moisture and clay content. Hence, fumigants have lower mobility in wet or clay soils. Soil temperature increases the volatility and, hence, the diffusivity of fumigants in soil (13–16). Emissions of fumigants from soil then would be highest under conditions of high application rates, high soil moisture, high clay content, and high soil temperatures. However, more recent studies have shown that elevated concentrations could be associated also with stable atmospheric conditions in the winter, when soil temperatures and emissions would be anticipated to be lower.

Exposures to DBCP, EDB, and 1,3-D have been evaluated also in studies performed by the California Department of Food and Agriculture. Generally, inhalational exposures of EDB and 1,3-D were lower than those of methyl bromide, owing to the lower vapor pressure of these compounds. Eight-hour TWA exposures to 1,3-D of 21 applicators applying Telone (Dow Chemical Company, 92% 1,3-D) and D-D [Shell Chemical Company, 50% 1,3-D and 30% 1,2-dichloropropane (or 1,2-D)] soil fumigants ranged from 0.07 to 3.61 ppm, with a mean of 0.71 ppm. Eight-hour TWA exposures to 1,2-D ranged from 0.003 to 0.44 ppm, with a mean of 0.17 ppm. Short-duration exposures during loading or repair operations were highly variable, ranging from 0.02 to 41.9 ppm (17). Eight-hour TWA exposures of 21 applicators applying EDB ranged from 0.001 to 4.3 ppm, with a mean of 0.73 ppm. Short-duration exposures during loading or repair operations ranged from nondetected to 2 ppm (18).

Groundwater Contamination

Greater focus has been given to soil fumigants as contaminants of groundwater. In 1979, wells near a pesticide-manufacturing facility near Lathrop, CA, were found to contain traces of DBCP at concentrations of up to 68 parts per billion (ppb). An expanded study of water samples from 262 wells in several California counties detected concentrations of DBCP ranging from 0.1 to 39.2 ppb in 92 water samples (19). At the time of the study, DBCP use had been suspended in California as a result of spermatotoxic effects observed in manufacturing workers and carcinogenicity in laboratory animals, and the California Department of Food and Agriculture was considering reregistering this fumigant with special requirements for reducing exposures. However, after the finding of groundwater contamination, the state of California elected to suspend use of DBCP permanently. Suspension of all use nationwide by the U.S. Environmental Protection Agency (EPA) followed shortly.

After the finding of DBCP in groundwater, attention turned to structurally similar compounds, such as EDB, 1,2-D, and 1,3-D. In 1983, EDB was detected in concentrations of up to 0.38 ppb in samples of 15 of 137 California wells, resulting in suspension of its use nationwide by the EPA (20). In 1982, 1,2-D was detected in well water at concentrations ranging from 0.4 to 16.0 ppb (21). 1,3-D has not been detected in groundwater, probably due to its more rapid hydrolysis and degradation in soil (22). Methyl bromide has not been evaluated as a groundwater contaminant.

Structural Fumigation

Structural fumigation potentially poses worker and public health hazards greater than those of other fumigant uses. From 1977 to 1984, 16 persons have died in California from unauthorized entry into structures undergoing fumigation with methyl bromide (23,24). Neurobehavioral evaluation of both soil and structural fumigators handling methyl bromide and sulfuryl fluoride indicate that even low levels of methyl bromide exposure could produce slight neurotoxic effects (25).

Monitoring of atmospheres inside structures undergoing fumigation with methyl bromide had shown that concentrations can range from 5,000 to 12,000 ppm. Exposure to such concentrations is rapidly fatal; hence, chloropicrin is added as a warning agent. Chloropicrin concentrations during fumigation range from 1 to 10 ppm. Chloropicrin is a respiratory and skin irritant and a tear producer. A concentration of 15 ppm in air for 1 minute was considered intolerable, as was a concentration of 7.5 ppm for 10 minutes (23,24). The lowest reported concentration producing irritation was 1.3 ppm. An odor threshold of 1.1 ppm was reported. A concentration range of 0.3 to 3.7 ppm produced "closing of the eyelids according to individual sensitivity." Much of these data, still being cited in the 1980s, were produced during and after World War I. Also, it is not known how test concentrations were verified analytically (23,24).

Fatalities from unauthorized entry into structures fumigated with methyl bromide have occurred despite the apparent presence of odorous or irritating concentrations of chloropicrin. Some individuals may possess a greater tolerance to the effects of chloropicrin, and intoxication with drugs or alcohol may blunt an individual's perception of odor or irritation. Given the high toxicity of methyl bromide, the current use of chloropicrin may not be sufficiently irritating to deter an individual from remaining in the toxic atmosphere for a length of time sufficient to cause incapacitation and inability to escape. Fumigators are reluctant to use increased dosages of chloropicrin, as it may render a structure uninhabitable by creating objectionable odors or irritation to the occupants. As chloropicrin is less volatile than is methyl bromide, it can sorb readily to interior surfaces and later slowly desorb into the structure atmosphere once fumigation is completed (23,24).

Worker exposure to methyl bromide during removal of tarpaulins after fumigation have ranged from 1.5 to 57.0 ppm, measured over durations of 10 to 53 minutes (23,24). These exposures periodically exceed occupational exposure standards. Peak exposures occurred during the first few moments during tarpaulin removal; 500 to 2,500 ppm methyl bromide can remain inside a structure at 24 hours after injection (23,24). Concentrations exceeding 100 ppm can persist up to 20 minutes after tarpaulin removal (23,24).

CLINICAL TOXICOLOGY

Halogenated Aliphatic Hydrocarbons

The chemicals DBCP, EDB, and 1,3-D (DCP) are halogenated short-chain aliphatic hydrocarbons and have been used in the past as soil fumigants for the control of plant-parasitic nematodes (EDB also having had some use in fumigation of milling machinery). These chemicals no longer are used in fumigation, owing to carcinogenicity observed in laboratory animals. DBCP and EDB have been shown also to be spermatotoxic in laboratory animals, and DBCP has been shown to be spermatotoxic in humans.

1,2-DIBROMO-3-CHLOROPROPANE

The effects of DBCP on male reproductive function observed in humans in the late 1970s were shown in laboratory animals as early as 1961 (26), which created controversy about the effectiveness of pesticide regulatory programs in detecting and mitigating health hazards. Although all use in the United States was suspended in 1979, groundwater contamination associated with DBCP use remains an environmental problem.

DBCP has been produced and used since the 1950s; however, the effects of this chemical on human health were not recognized until 1977 after studies of testicular function in DBCP production workers in California (27,28). These studies had confirmed workers' concerns about apparent infertility by demonstrating azoospermia or severe oligospermia in 14 of 25 workers studied. Similar reductions in sperm count were observed in workers performing soil fumigations. These studies have shown a dose-response relationship for DBCP-induced spermatotoxicity. Reductions in sperm production are accompanied also by elevations in serum follicle–stimulating and –luteinizing hormones and reductions in spermatogenic cells in the seminiferous vesicles (29,30). Follow-up studies of DBCP-exposed workers have shown that, after exposure ceases, recovery of sperm production does not occur or is impeded greatly in cases in which exposure has produced a complete absence of spermatogenesis. In cases in which spermatogenesis was inhibited only partially, complete recovery appears to occur a few months after exposure ceases (28,31,32). Exposure studies of pineapple workers performed by the National Institute for Occupational Safety and Health monitored both sperm counts and breathing-zone concentrations in air and indicated that sperm counts did not vary over exposures ranging from 0 to 1.8 ppm. The Institute concluded that 1 ppm in air had no observable effects on male fertility (33).

Animal studies have shown that the kidneys and the testes are primary target organs of DBCP in acute, subacute, and chronic exposure situations (26,34). Studies of the mode of action have revealed conflicting results, with DBCP producing depletion of glutathione in different organs but with toxicity not always being correlated with glutathione depletion (35,36). The lowest-observed-effect level in male rats from chronic oral exposure (for 8 months) in one study was reported to be 0.05 mg per kg, with 0.005 mg per kg being reported as a no-observed-effect level. This same study reported that both 0.5 and 5.0 mg per kg were gonadotoxic and produced functional disturbances in the liver and kidneys (37). Dose-related histopathologic changes of the nasal turbinates, including focal hyperplasia, squamous metaplasia, and loss of cilia, were detected in male and female rats exposed to 0, 1, 5, and 25 ppm DBCP in air, 6 hours per day, 5 days per week for 13 weeks (38). Limited studies suggest that DBCP is not teratogenic in rats at doses up to 50 mg per kg but does produce some maternal toxicity (39).

DBCP is considered to be a potent mutagen with microsomal activation in the Ames assay. It has induced sister-chromatid exchanges in Chinese hamster ovary cells and has produced increased frequency of chromosomal aberrations in sperm of exposed workers. In a cancer bioassay performed by the National Cancer Institute, technical-grade DBCP (with 16 impurities) given by gavage to rats and mice produced squamous cell carcinomas of the forestomach in both species. The TWA doses in rats were 0, 15, and 29 mg per kg per day; in male mice, 0, 114, and 219 mg per kg per day; and in female mice, 0, 110, and 209 mg per kg per day. The excess lifetime cancer risk based on the male rat data from this study is 7.8×10^{-6} per μg of DBCP per L of drinking water. In two different inhalation bioassays, mice or rats exposed to DBCP concentrations of 0, 0.6, or 3.0 ppm in air for 6 hours per day, 5 days per week, over 103 to 104 weeks developed alveolar and bronchial adenomas and carcinomas and tumors of the nasal cavity. DBCP is considered to be a complete carcinogen, producing tumors close to the site of administration.

ETHYLENE DIBROMIDE

EDB has been used extensively as a fumigant since 1948. Its volatility and versatility, based on chemical and biocidal properties, led to its use as a soil sterilant, as a spot fumigant of grain-milling machinery, and as a control agent in fighting grain, fruit, and vegetable infestations. In 1977, the EPA began a review of EDB's pesticidal uses, which eventually led to its cancellation for most agricultural applications. Disposal of EDB and contamination of water supplies remain major environmental concerns.

EDB is substantially more toxic than is DBCP. Acute dermal exposure produces painful local inflammation, swelling, and blistering. The liver appears to be a principal target organ for EDB toxicity. The mechanism of action of EDB appears to involve its conversion to reactive metabolites that become irreversibly bound to macromolecules, including DNA. Metabolism of EDB involves an oxidative pathway (cytochrome P-450) and a conjugation pathway (glutathione-*S*-transferases). Oral administration of EDB to rats has been shown to deplete glutathione levels in the liver through this metabolic pathway and, over time, to decrease the activity of glutathione-*S*-transferases. When glutathione levels are sufficiently depleted, EDB reactive metabolites apparently are free to inhibit the transferases and to interact with other macromolecules.

EDB has been studied for mutagenic potential by a variety of *in vitro* and *in vivo* test systems. EDB has consistently mutagenic potential in both bacterial assays and *in vitro* assays using eukaryotic cells. EDB caused an increase in unscheduled DNA synthesis in cultured mammalian cells (40–42) and single-strand DNA breaks in *in vitro* cultured cells (43) and in *in vivo* rat liver cells (44).

Numerous studies have shown that EDB is carcinogenic in laboratory animals. The National Cancer Institute (45) administered TWA doses of 27 and 29 mg per kg per day to male rats and 26 and 28 mg per kg per day to female rats by gavage for 49 and 61 weeks for the low- and high-dose groups, respectively. High treatment-related mortality prompted the early termination of the study (planned for 110 weeks) and alterations of the dosing regimen, resulting in similar TWA dosages for high- and low-treatment groups. Significant increased incidences of squamous cell carcinomas of the stomach (both genders), hepatocellular carcinomas and neoplastic nodules of the liver (females), and hemangiosarcomas of the circulatory system (males) were observed on histologic examination. The stomach tumors developed after a short latency period and were observed to metastasize to multiple sites. Male and female B6C3F1 mice received TWA doses of 44 or 77 mg per kg per day by gavage for 53 weeks and were observed for their lifetimes. The incidence of squamous cell carcinomas and alveolar-bronchiolar adenomas of the lung was increased significantly over the controls in all the mice. As in the rat bioassay, no tumors were observed in the controls, and high treatment-related mortality prompted dosing regimen alterations (45).

Fischer 344 rats and B6C3F1 mice of both genders were exposed to EDB vapors at 0, 10, or 40 ppm, 6 hours per day, 5 days per week, for their life spans. The incidence of nasal cavity carcinomas and adenocarcinomas in the rats of both genders and alveolar-bronchiolar carcinomas in female rats and mice of both genders was increased significantly over the incidence in controls. Chronic inhalation of EDB was associated also with circulatory system hemangiosarcomas in both genders of rats (high-dose only), mammary gland fibroadenomas of female rats, mammary gland adenocarcinomas of female mice, subcutaneous fibrosarcomas of female mice, and tunica vaginalis mesotheliomas of male rats (46). In a chronic inhalation study of experimental design identical to the U.S. National Toxicology Program (NTP) study (with B6C3F1 mice only), Stinson et al. (47) reported an elevated incidence of nasal cavity carcinomas in the female mice exposed to 40 ppm EDB. Both genders had dose-related epithelial hyperplastic lesions of the nasal cavity. Histologic and pathologic examinations were conducted only on the nasal cavity.

Wong et al. (48) exposed Sprague-Dawley rats of both genders by inhalation to 0 or 20 ppm EDB for 7 hours per day, 5 days per week, for 18 months. Incidences of splenic hemangiosarcomas and adrenal gland tumors of both genders, subcutaneous mesenchymal tumors in males, and mammary gland tumors in females were increased significantly over the incidences in controls.

Epidemiologic investigations of exposed workers have not revealed increased cancer incidences associated with EDB. Mortality studies of workers occupationally exposed to EDB found that neither total deaths nor total malignancies of individuals exposed to EDB exceeded the control rate. The studies are inconclusive, owing to their small cohort size; to lack of, or poorly characterized, exposure concentrations; or to concurrent exposure to other potential or known carcinogens (49).

1,2-DICHLOROPROPANE AND 1,3-DICHLOROPROPENE

Cis- and *trans-*1,3-D are components of the pre-plant soil fumigants Telone and D-D. 1,3-D is acknowledged as the nematocidal component of these pesticides, with the dichloropropane representing an inactive impurity in the formulation (application rates for D-D generally were twofold greater than application rates for Telone). Dichloropropane shares similarities in toxicity with the other halogenated aliphatic compounds but generally is less toxic than is either EDB or 1,3-D.

Exposures to 1,2-D result in injury to the liver and kidneys. The literature has reported a few cases of adverse effects from acute exposure; however, other data regarding human exposures to 1,2-D are very limited. Subacute inhalation exposures of 1,2-D at 1,000 ppm caused fatalities in dogs, rats, and guinea pigs. Severe liver damage was characteristic of the animals that had died. Exposures to 400 ppm for 7 hours per day, 5 days per week, for 128 to 140 exposures produced no effects in rats, with the exception of a decrease in weight gain. However, this exposure to a group of CH-strain mice produced fatalities in some animals and hepatomas in others (50). More recent studies have evaluated the subchronic toxicity of 1,2-D as it is formulated in D-D. Rats and mice were exposed to 5, 15, and 50 ppm for 6 hours per day, 5 days per week, for up to 12 weeks. The only compound-related effect observed was slight enlargement of hepatocytes. The major confounder to this study was the presence of 1,3-D, which produces similar toxicity at lower doses (51).

The NTP sponsored a 2-year cancer gavage bioassay in rats and mice. Male rats were administered 62 and 125 mg per kg 5 days per week; female rats were administered 125 and 250 mg per kg 5 days per week; and male and female mice were administered 125 and 250 mg per kg 5 days per week. Low survival was observed in the high-dose female rats and female mice groups. Dose-related hepatocellular adenomas were observed in male and female mice. Nonsignificant increases in hepatocellular adenocarcinomas were observed in both genders. The incidence of benign tumors was combined with the incidence of carcinomas for purposes of judging carcinogenicity in mice. Dose-related mammary gland adenocarcinomas were observed in female rats; however, 1,2-D did not produce carcinogenicity in male rats. Carcinogenicity observed in female rats may have been associated with toxic doses of 1,2-D compromising metabolic or endocrine functions. The carcinomas in the female rats were observed to be nonmetastatic, nonanaplastic, or noninvasive and were judged by some pathologists as fibroadenomas. This study concluded the absence of evidence of carcinogenicity in male rats, equivocal evidence of carcinogenicity in female rats, and some evidence of carcinogenicity in mice (52).

1,2-D is considered to be weakly mutagenic in bacterial strains as compared with other halogenated hydrocarbons, such as 1,3-D. Mutagenicity is not enhanced by greatly metabolic activation (53).

Metabolism of 1,2-D in the rat results in the formation of a mercapturic acid conjugate excreted largely in the urine. Proposed reactive intermediates include 1,2-epoxopropane; this intermediate is suspected of being responsible for the mutagenic effects of 1,2-D (54). Glutathione pathways are seen as detoxification mechanisms, and liver and kidney toxicity at high concentrations may be due to saturation of these pathways (51).

Few acute toxicity studies of 1,3-D are available. However, a study with D-D reported an oral median lethal dose of 300 mg per kg in the mouse and 140 mg per kg in the rat. The animals exhibited hyperexcitability, followed by tremors, incoordination, depression, and respiratory distress. Other effects observed were fatty degeneration of the liver and hemorrhage of the lungs. The 4-hour median lethal dose in the rat was estimated to be 1,000 ppm. The effects from acute inhalation exposure included severe pulmonary edema and alveolar hemorrhage (55). D-D was shown also to be a severe eye and skin irritant. Confirmation of this is found in reports of occupational exposures of agricultural workers, which are predominantly eye and skin injuries.

Torkleson and Oyen (56) investigated the effects of repeated inhalation exposure to 1,3-D. Initial subacute studies involving rats and guinea pigs exposed to 11 or 50 ppm demonstrated gross evidence of liver and kidney injury. Subchronic studies were performed also with rats, rabbits, and guinea pigs subjected to exposures to 1 or 3 ppm for 125 to 130 times over a period of 185 days. Male rats exposed to 3 ppm exhibited cloudy swelling of the renal tubular epithelium. Female rats exhibited slight but statistically significant increases in their liver-to-body weight ratio. The 1-ppm concentration appeared to be a no-observed-effect level. This study is significant in that it was the basis for the threshold limit value (TLV) recommended for 1,3-D by the American Conference for Governmental Industrial Hygienists (56).

One study exhibited a carcinogenic response with Telone in both rats and mice (57). F344 rats of each gender were given Telone in corn oil by gavage at doses of 0, 25, and 50 mg per kg per day three times weekly. No increased mortality occurred in treated animals. Elevated incidence of the following tumors was observed at the highest dose tested: (i) forestomach squamous cell papillomas in males and females; (ii) forestomach squamous cell papillomas and carcinomas combined in males; and (iii) liver neoplastic nodules in males. The increased incidence of forestomach tumors was accompanied by a positive trend for forestomach basal cell hyperplasia in male and female rats of both treated groups (25 and 50 mg per kg per day). B6C3F1 mice of each gender were given Telone II in corn oil by gavage at doses of 0, 50, and 100 mg per kg per day three times weekly for 104 weeks. A total of 50 mice of each gender were used for each dose group. Owing to excessive mortality in control male mice from myocardial inflammation approximately 1 year after the initiation of the study (a time at which neoplastic lesions would not be expected to occur), conclusions pertaining to oncogenicity were based on both concurrent control data and on available NTP historical control data. Elevated incidence of the following tumors was observed either at the highest dose level tested or at both dose levels tested: (i) forestomach squamous cell papillomas or papillomas and carcinomas combined in males and females, and squamous cell carcinomas in females; (ii) urinary bladder transitional cell carcinomas in males and females; and (iii) lung adenomas, and adenomas and carcinomas combined in males and females (57).

Groups of 50 male and 50 female B6C3F1 mice and Fischer 344 rats were exposed to 0, 5, 20, or 60 ppm technical-grade 1,3-D (i.e., Telone II, 0, 21, 84, or 251 mg per cubic meter assuming 25°C and 760 mm Hg; 49.5% *cis*- and 42.6% *trans*-1,3-D, 0.7% 1,2-D, 2% epoxidized soybean oil, and a 5.2% mixture of hexanes and hexadienes) for 6 hours per day, 5 days per week, for 2 years. In the mice, exposure-related changes were observed in the urinary bladder and in the nasal tissue in both genders exposed to 60 ppm and in the females exposed to 20 ppm after 2 years of treatment. The urinary bladders of both genders of mice had hyperplasia characterized by diffuse, uniform thickening of the transitional epithelium. Both genders of mice also had compound-related microscopic changes in the nasal tissue characterized by hypertrophy and hyperplasia of the respiratory epithelium or degeneration of the olfactory epithelium. Histopathologic examination revealed exposure-related effects in the nasal tissues of both male and female rats exposed to 60 ppm for 24 months. These effects included unilateral or bilateral decreased thickness of the olfactory epithelium due to degenerative changes, erosions of the olfactory epithelium, and fibrosis beneath the olfactory epithelium. No lesions of the respiratory tract were found after 6 or 12 months of treatment. In mice, the lowest observed adverse effect level (LOAEL) is identified as 20 ppm for hypertrophy and hyperplasia of the nasal respiratory epithelium. The no observed adverse-effect level (NOAEL) in mice is 5 ppm for hypertrophy and hyperplasia of the nasal respiratory epithelium and for epithelial hyperplasia and inflammation of the urinary bladder. In rats, the LOAEL is 60 ppm and the NOAEL is 20 ppm for the effects on the nasal olfactory epithelium (58).

Evidence that the nasal region of the respiratory tract is the critical target organ in laboratory animals for 1,3-D is provided by other studies (59). However, this effect has not been of primary concern for adverse effects to workers. 1,3-D is metabolized by conjugation with glutathione and is excreted primarily as a mercapturic acid conjugate. This urinary metabolite has been detected in workers exposed to 1,3-D vapor during fumigation. Applicator exposure was studied using personal air monitoring of 1,3-D and monitoring of urinary excretion of the mercapturic acid metabolite and the excretion of the renal tubular enzyme, *N*-acetylglucosaminidase (NAG). Urinary excretion of the metabolite correlated well with exposure to 1,3-D. Four workers (of 15 studied) had clinically elevated activity of NAG in any of their urine collections after baseline. Nine workers showed greater than 25% increases in NAG excretion as compared to baseline. Dichloropropene air exposure products of more than 700 mg per minute per cubic meter or excretion of the metabolite of more than 1.5 mg per day distinguished abnormally high daily excretion of NAG. These data demonstrate a relationship between air exposure and dose and a possible subclinical nephrotoxic effect in workers handling 1,3-D (60).

Methyl Bromide

Methyl bromide is an odorless, volatile liquid that rapidly disperses and penetrates rubber and clothes. It has a TLV of 5 ppm, with a skin notation to indicate the potential of dermal absorption. The concentration immediately dangerous to life and health (IDLH) is 2,000 ppm, and at this concentration, methyl bromide produces pulmonary edema, seizures, and death.

Methyl bromide is particularly hazardous because it has practically no odor and causes no immediate irritation of the nose or respiratory tract, even at highly toxic concentrations. More than 300 cases of systemic poisonings and 60 fatalities attributable to methyl bromide have been reported in the literature. Acute exposure to high concentrations produces rapid narcosis and death from respiratory failure. If death does not result, the most consistent response is lung irritation or pulmonary edema (or both).

Neurotoxicity also occurs from exposure to methyl bromide. Early symptoms include headache and nausea and vomiting and are followed by tremors, twitching, and seizures. The onset of neurologic effects from acute exposure may be delayed from 1 to 36 hours, complicating the diagnosis. The onset of neurologic effects shortens when acute exposure episodes are superimposed on chronic exposure. Signs and symptoms of chronic exposure include those from acute exposure plus visual and hearing disorders, numbness or tingling in the extremities, incoordination, ataxia, and loss of consciousness. Psychological symptoms have been associated with chronic exposure and include loss of initiative, depressed libido, personality changes, hallucinations, and an intolerance to alcohol (61).

Studies with laboratory animals confirm the neurotoxicity observed in humans. In one study, rats and rabbits were exposed to 65 ppm methyl bromide for 7.5 hours per day, 4 days per week, for 4 weeks. In rabbits, this exposure produced hindlimb paralysis, decreased nerve conduction velocity, and decreased magnitude of the eye-blink response (62). Neuropathic effects were not demonstrated in rats at these exposures. These studies confirm earlier studies demonstrating neurotoxicity in rabbits but not rats. Neurotoxic effects were investigated in rabbits exposed to lower concentrations for longer durations. An exposure concentration of 27 ppm for 7.5 hours per day, 4 days per week, for 8 months produced no neurologic effects in rabbits (63). Soil and structural fumigators underwent a neurologic examination in a cross-sectional occupational exposure study (64). Most of the structural fumigators used both methyl bromide and sulfuryl fluoride. More symptoms were reported in those in the exposed groups than in those of the reference population. On several behavioral tests, those in the exposed group did not perform as well as did referents (including tests of cognitive function, reflexes, and sensory and visual effects). Although this study suggested mild neurologic effects of exposure to methyl bromide, drawing any conclusions between exposure and effect is difficult because of the confounding factors, including prescription or recreational drug or alcohol use and a lack of an exposure history. However, review of some of the air-monitoring data used to assess fumigator exposure suggests that these effects associated with the observed neurobehavioral effects may be slightly underestimated. TWA airborne concentrations may not be of great value in characterizing adverse effects from methyl bromide exposures in the workplace; these exposures appear to be intermittent and of relatively short duration.

Methyl bromide has been shown to produce mutations in *Salmonella* strains sensitive to alkylating agents and to *Escherichia coli* both with and without addition of a metabolic activation system (65–67). Methyl bromide was mutagenic also in a modification of the standard *Salmonella* assay employing vapor phase exposure (68,69).

Methyl bromide was administered by gavage to groups of 10 male and female Wistar rats. Animals were administered doses of 0, 0.4, 2.0, 10.0, or 50.0 mg per kg per day of bromomethane in arachis oil for 5 days per week for 13 weeks, at which time the experiment was terminated. An apparent dose-related increase in diffuse hyperplasia was observed in the forestomach (69). These results subsequently were questioned (70; S. Schatzow, memorandum to D. Clay, November 9, 1984). A panel of NTP scientists reevaluated the histologic slides and concluded that the lesions were hyperplasia and inflammation rather than neoplasia. The NTP is testing methyl bromide for carcinogenicity (71).

In the NTP study, target organs of toxicity included the brain, bone (sternum), heart, and nose. In the brain, a statistically significant increase was seen in the incidence of cerebellar degeneration, myocardial degeneration, chronic cardiomyopathy, and olfactory epithelial necrosis and metaplasia in the nasal cavities in the animals exposed to 100 ppm for 6 hours per day, 5 days per week. A concentration of 100 ppm was considered to be an LOAEL for toxicity in multiple organs, whereas an NOAEL was considered to be 33 ppm (71). In a chronic inhalation study conducted by Reuzel et al. (72,73), a concentration of 90 ppm for 6 hours per day, 5 days per week produced decreased kidney and brain weights in male and female rats. Microscopical evaluation revealed that the nose, the heart, and the esophagus and forestomach were the principal targets of methyl bromide toxicity in this study. An LOAEL of 3 ppm for nasal effects was established from these data.

Available epidemiologic data are inadequate for evaluating the carcinogenicity of methyl bromide in humans. A prospective mortality study was reported for a population of 3,579 white male chemical workers. The men, employed between 1935 and 1976, were potentially exposed to DBCP, 2,3-dibromopropyl phosphate, polybrominated biphenyls, DDT, and several brominated organic and inorganic compounds (74). Overall mortality for the cohort and for several subgroups was less than expected. Of the 665 men exposed to methyl bromides (the only common exposure to organic bromides), 2 died from testicular cancer, as compared with the 0.11 expected. This finding may be noteworthy because testicular cancer usually is associated with a low mortality rate. Therefore, cancer cases could be more numerous than were thought on the basis of mortality. The authors noted that drawing definitive conclusions as to causality was difficult because of the lack of exposure information and the likelihood that subjects were exposed to many brominated compounds.

Acute toxic exposure to methyl bromide can result in initial symptoms of headache, nausea, vomiting, vertigo, myalgia, ataxia, diplopia, and decreased vision (75). These symptoms may be delayed for hours before onset and may not appear for up to 24 hours. Because it is heavier than air, methyl bromide constitutes a hazard in confined spaces. Exposure to methyl bromide occurs mainly by inhalational and dermal routes. Dermal toxicity can range from local dermatitis to vesicle formation and serious burns, depending on the level of exposure. Prolonged skin contact may occur because of absorption by clothing, particularly leather.

Low-level chronic exposure can result in neurologic symptoms consisting of weakness, tremors, paresthesias, ataxia, decreased reflexes, dysarthria, dysmetria and dysdiadochokinesia, seizures, and status epilepticus (75). Both acute and chronic exposures can result in behavioral toxicity manifested by psychosis, delirium, hallucinations, aggression, and mania. Cases of homicidal ideation and acute psychosis have been described after serious exposures (76). Reports of coma, seizures, and hepatic damage resembling Reye's syndrome have occurred (75).

Ophthalmologic toxicity consists of decreased vision, diplopia, lacrimation, disturbance of accommodation, and scotomas. Optic nerve damage with optic neuropathy has been reported (76). The neurologic lesions and ophthalmologic changes may last weeks or may be permanent.

The neurotoxicity of methyl bromide depends on the exposure concentration and duration. Short-term high exposure can produce abnormal reflexes, ataxia, visual changes, and muscle weakness (75,76). Tremor, paresthesias, and peripheral neuropathy may occur after extended exposures (75,76). Neurobehavioral evaluation of methyl bromide applicators indicated significant impairment in behavioral test results as compared with those of controls (75,76).

Methyl bromide is the chemical of choice for soil and commodity fumigation, for quarantine treatment requirements, and for structural pest control. Under the Clean Air Act, methyl bromide was declared an ozone-depleting compound in 1993, and its production and importation will be phased out by 2001. Methyl bromide is a significant ozone-depleting substance; recent scientific evidence estimates that bromine from this material is at least 50 times more effective at destroying ozone than is chlorine from chlorofluorocarbons on a per-molecule basis. The established scientific consensus maintains that the amount of methyl bromide produced by agricultural and other anthropogenic sources has a significant impact on stratospheric ozone. This activity potentially disrupts the natural balance of the atmosphere, increases the amount of hazardous ultraviolet radiation that reaches the earth's surface, and creates a potential impact on human health and the environment, including agricultural crops (77).

Methyl bromide has been used over the past three decades in pest control; in many cases, it has been the only treatment for control of agricultural or structural pests. No alternatives are available for many uses of methyl bromide. The potential alternative treatments include cold treatment, heat treatment, controlled atmospheres, irradiation, biocides, pest-free zones, and modification of host suitability through crop breeding. The potential exists for complete restructuring of the farming and marketing systems developed during the past 30 years if methyl bromide is lost as a key component of this system. That restructuring could include a broader understanding of soil-borne pest complexes that translate into development of effective, economical pest management systems. If this new information and technical advances are transferred efficiently to methyl bromide users, the combination will constitute a model with broad applications for the future of pest control (77,78).

Sulfuryl Fluoride

Sulfuryl fluoride (SO_2F_2, sulfuric oxyfluoride) is a colorless and odorless nonflammable gas with a TLV of 5 ppm and an IDLH level of 1,000 ppm. It is sold under the name *Vikane7*. The chemical is a strong irritant of the respiratory system, mucous membranes, eyes, and skin. Exposure routes are inhalation and dermal contact, although skin absorption is minimal.

Sulfuryl fluoride is a neurotoxin and produces central nervous system depression and paresthesias (79). Symptoms after toxic exposure begin with nausea, vomiting, abdominal pain, and mucous membrane irritation. Serious exposure can result in bronchospasm and paresthesias. As a result, sulfuryl fluoride is shipped as a compressed gas.

After fumigation, affected foods may be left with a high residual content of this gas. It is nonirritating but, when heated, gives off toxic and corrosive vapors, including hydrofluoric acid.

Animal studies show that high-dose toxicity is characterized by seizures and respiratory arrest. Animals exposed to low doses of sulfuryl fluoride exhibit parasympathetic stimulation with vomiting, diarrhea, lacrimation, salivation, and abdominal cramps (80). Pulmonary edema and cardiovascular collapse may follow. Toxicity is thought to involve release of free fluoride ions that bind calcium. Plasma fluoride concentrations may help to establish a diagnosis in death cases.

Chloropicrin

Chloropicrin (trichloronitromethane, nitrochloroform) is a colorless, oily liquid fumigant for cereals and grains and is used as a warning agent in structural fumigation with methyl bromide.

This powerful irritant and lacrimator has a TLV of 0.1 ppm. Its IDLH concentration is 4 ppm. Owing to its strong irritating properties, exposure produces eye irritation, pulmonary irritation, and dermatitis. More serious exposure can cause pulmonary edema, coma, hepatic necrosis, renal damage, and cardiac necrosis (81).

The irritant properties of chloropicrin have been studied in animals using the RD_{50} value, which is the air concentration of the chemical that elicits a 50% decrease in the respiratory rate of the animals studied. The RD_{50} of chloropicrin was 9 ppm, as compared to that of ammonia, which was 303 ppm (81). Exposure to chloropicrin vapors produces intense irritation and lacrimation. One report cited a home that was treated with chloropicrin and produced respiratory illness in the family and a pet dog. The dog developed bronchitis and pneumonia; the family members developed cough, sinus irritation, and inflammation of the oropharynx. Chloropicrin concentrations ranged up to 48 ppb in certain areas of the house (81).

In animals studies, chloropicrin vapors produced ulceration of the olfactory epithelium and necrosis of lung tissue. Human toxicity after inhalation of chloropicrin can be manifest by pulmonary and mucous membrane irritation and pulmonary edema (81).

Aluminum and Zinc Phosphide

Aluminum and zinc phosphide compounds are used to produce phosphine gas and are employed extensively as grain fumigants. Phosphine is generated by the action of water or acid on aluminum or zinc phosphide. Phosphine gas is colorless and has a TLV of 0.3 ppm, a short-term exposure limit of 1 ppm, and an IDLH level of 200 ppm. Clinical toxicology of phosphine poisoning involves early symptoms of headache, dizziness, nausea, vomiting, dyspnea, and cough. Severe poisoning cases have resulted in pulmonary edema, ataxia, coma, and myocardial necrosis (82,83).

Miscellaneous Fumigants

Hydrogen cyanide (HCN), often generated from calcium cyanide, has been used in vertebrate pest control (i.e., fumigation of rodent burrows) and in space fumigation. It has been used to fumigate mills, warehouses, and greenhouses and to fumigate commodities under gas-proof sheets. HCN toxicity in humans occurs by inhibition of the enzyme cytochrome oxidase, blocking the use of oxygen and producing respiratory arrest. HCN has an almond odor but poor warning properties (i.e., it does not provide an indication of overexposure by the presence of odor). HCN now has only limited use as a fumigant.

Carbon disulfide has been used in soil fumigation and fumigation of rodent burrows. CS_2 vapor is explosive, igniting spontaneously on contact with sparks or at temperatures exceeding 147°C. CS_2 is also highly neurotoxic in humans. It no longer is in use as a fumigant, owing to its toxicity and explosion hazards.

Carbon tetrachloride has been used in conjunction with EDB and ethylene dichloride as a grain fumigant. The EPA has suspended use of this compound owing to its severe hepatotoxicity in humans and its carcinogenicity in laboratory animals.

CONCLUSION

As stated, fumigants exemplify the balance between economic benefit and protection of public and worker health. Such soil fumigants as methyl bromide, DBCP, EDB, and Telone and D-D have been seen as important elements in control of plant-parasitic nematodes. Historically, as use of one chemical was suspended, uses of the others have increased. Suspension of the use of all these chemicals has led to the use of very low-volatility organophosphorus and carbamate compounds, such as fenaminophos (Nemacur) and carbofuran (Furadan), for control of nematodes. Use of these chemicals, both of which are highly toxic cholinesterase inhibitors, results in an interesting trade-off in which potential long-term chronic health hazards, such as carcinogenicity (found in laboratory animals), are replaced with known acute toxicity (and possible long-term neurotoxicity) hazards. The human health and environmental risks associated with fumigant chemicals in general have led to research in alternate pest control technologies that rely less on chemicals.

Such chemicals as DBCP and EDB no longer are in use, not because of the significant hazards to workers but because of the low and theoretic cancer risk posed from ingestion of groundwater contaminated with parts-per-billion concentrations. The utility of such trade-offs between long-term potential protection of public health and short-term worker risks and potential economic harm have not been analyzed sufficiently. In some cases, such as methyl bromide, the economic benefits and lack of suitable alternatives have outweighed the hazards so that this highly toxic material remains in use while the use of less toxic compounds (e.g., DBCP, Telone) has been suspended.

REFERENCES

1. Wilbur DA, Mills RB. Stored grain insects. In: Pfadt RE, ed. *Fundamentals of applied entomology.* New York: Macmillan, 1978.
2. 2. Mallis A, ed. Handbook of pest control, 8th ed. Cleveland: Mallis Handbook & Technical Training Co.
3. University of California. *Study guide for agricultural pest control advisers on nematodes and nematocides.* Division of Agricultural Sciences publ. no. 4045. Sacramento, CA: University of California, 1976.
4. Maddy KT, Schneider F, Lowe J, Alcoser D, Fredrickson AS. *Monitoring environmental levels of methyl bromide during commodity fumigation.* California Department of Food and Agriculture report no. HS-1078. Sacramento, CA: California Department of Food and Agriculture, 1983.
5. Maddy KT, Lowe J, Fredrickson AS. *Inhalation exposure of commodity handlers to methyl bromide in Yolo County, California, October 1983.* California Department of Food and Agriculture report no. HS-1186. Sacramento, CA: California Department of Food and Agriculture, 1984.
6. Maddy KT, Richmond D, Lowe J, Fredrickson AS. *A study of the inhalation exposure of workers to methyl bromide during preplant soil fumigations (shallow injections) in 1980 and 1981.* California Department of Food and Agriculture report no. HS-900. Sacramento, CA: California Department of Food and Agriculture, 1982.
7. Maddy KT, Gibbons D, Richmond DM, Fredrickson AS. *A study of the inhalation exposure of workers to methyl bromide and chloropicrin during preplant soil fumigations (shallow injections) in 1982—a preliminary report.* Sacramento, CA: California Department of Food and Agriculture report no. HS-1076. California Department of Food and Agriculture, 1984.
8. Maddy KT, Gibbons D, Richmond DM, Fredrickson AS. *Additional monitoring of the inhalation exposure of workers to methyl bromide and chloropicrin during preplant soil fumigation (shallow injection) in 1983.* California Department of Food and Agriculture report no. HS-1175. Sacramento, CA: California Department of Food and Agriculture, 1984.
9. Herzstein J, Cullen MR. Methyl bromide intoxication in four field-workers during removal of soil fumigation sheets. *Am J Ind Med* 1990;17:321–326.
10. Roosels D, Van Den Oever R, Lahaye D. Dangerous concentrations of methyl bromide used as a fumigant in Belgian greenhouses. *Arch Occup Environ Health* 1981;48:243–250.
11. Van Den Oever R, Roosels D, Lahaye D. Actual hazard of methyl bromide fumigation in soil disinfection. *Br J Ind Med* 1982;39:140–144.
12. Goldman LR, Mengle D, Epstein DM, Fredson D, Kelly K, Jackson RJ. Acute symptoms in persons residing near a field treated with the soil fumigants methyl bromide and chloropicrin. *West J Med* 1987;147:95–98.
13. Abdalla N, Raski D, Lear B, Schmitt RV. Distribution of methyl bromide in soils treated for nematode control in replant vineyards. *Pestic Sci* 1974;5:259–269.
14. Goring CA. Physical aspects of soil in relation to the action of soil fumigants. *Ann Rev Phytopathol* 1967;5:285–318.
15. Kolbezen MJ, Munnecke DE, Wilbur WD, Stolzy LH, Abu El-Haz FS, Szuszkiewics TE. Factors that affect deep penetration of field soils treated with methyl bromide. *Hilgardia* 1974;42:465–492.
16. Munnecke DE, Van Gundy SD. Movement of fumigants in soil: dosage, responses and differential effects. *Ann Rev Phytopathol* 1979;17:405–429.
17. Maddy KT, Edmiston S, Lowe J, Fredrickson AS. *Exposures of agricultural employees to 1,2-dichloropropane and 1,3-dichloropropene (Telone and D-D) in*

California. California Department of Food and Agriculture report no. HS-1161. California Department of Food and Agriculture, 1984.
18. Maddy KT, Edmiston S, Meinders DD, Fredrickson AS, Margetich S. Potential exposure of loader/applications to ethylene dibromide (EDB) during pre-plant soil fumigation in California in 1983, California Department of Food and Agriculture report no. HS-1148. Sacramento, CA: California Department of Food and Agriculture, 1984.
19. Peoples SA, Maddy KT, Cusick W, Jackson T, Cooper C, Fredrickson AS. A study of samples of well water collected from selected areas in California to determine the presence of DBCP and certain other pesticide residues. *Bull Environ Contam Toxicol* 1980;24:611–618.
20. Smith C, Margetich S, Fredrickson AS. *A survey of well water in selected counties of California for contamination by EDB in 1983.* California Department of Food and Agriculture report no. HS-1123. Sacramento, CA: California Department of Food and Agriculture, 1983.
21. Cohen D, Bowes G. *Water quality and pesticides: a California risk assessment program,* vol 1. Sacramento, CA: State Water Resources Control Board.
22. Maddy KT, Fong HR, Lowe JA, Conrad D, Fredrickson AS. A study of well water in selected California communities for residues of 1,3-dichloropropene, chloroallyl alcohol and 49 organophosphate or chlorinated hydrocarbon pesticides. *Bull Environ Contam Toxicol* 1982;29:354–359.
23. Maddy KT, Gibbons DB, Lowe JA. *Evaluation of chloropicrin as a warning agent and employee exposure to methyl bromide and chloropicrin during structural fumigation.* Presented at the American Industrial Hygiene Conference, Montreal, Quebec, Canada, May 31–June 5, 1987 (abst 181).
24. Maddy KT, Lowe JA, Gibbons DB, O'Connell LP, Richmond DM, Fredrickson AS. *Studies of methyl bromide and chloropicrin used as structural fumigants in California: I. Evaluation of chloropicrin as a warning agent. II. Employee exposure to methyl bromide and chloropicrin. III. Penetration of methyl bromide in plastic food storage bags.* California Department of Food and Agriculture report no. HS-1352. Sacramento, CA: California Department of Food and Agriculture, 1984.
25. Anger WK, Moody L, Burg J, et al. Neurobehavioral evaluation of soil and structural fumigators using methyl bromide and sulfuryl fluoride. *Neurotoxicology* 1986;7:137–156.
26. Torkleson TR, Sadek SE, Rowe VK, et al. Toxicologic investigations of 1,2-dibromo-3-chloropropane. *Toxicol Appl Pharmacol* 1961;3:545–559.
27. Whorton D, Krauss RM, Marshall S, Milby TH. Infertility in male pesticide workers. *Lancet* 1977;2:1259–1261.
28. Whorton D, Milby TH, Krauss RM, Stubbs HA. Testicular function in DBCP exposed pesticide workers. *J Occup Med* 1979;21:161–166.
29. Biava CG, Smuckler EA, Whorton D. The testicular morphology of individuals exposed to dibromochloropropane. *Exp Mol Pharmacol* 1978;29:448–458.
30. Engnatz DG, Ott MG, Townsend JC, Olson RD, Johns DB. DBCP and testicular effects in chemical workers: an epidemiological survey in Midland, Michigan. *J Occup Med* 1980;22:727–732.
31. Lantz GD, Cunningham GR, Huckins C, Lipshultz LI. Recovery from severe oligospermia after exposure to dibromochloropropane. *Fertil Steril* 1981;35: 46–53.
32. Whorton MD, TH Milby. Recovery of testicular function among DBCP workers. *J Occup Med* 1980;22:177–179.
33. National Institute for Occupational Safety and Health. *A recommended standard for occupational exposure to dibromochloropropane.* DHEW (NIOSH) publ. no. 78-115. Cincinnati: US Department of Health, Education, and Welfare, National Institute for Occupational Safety and Health, 1978.
34. Kluwe WM. Acute toxicity of 1,2-dibromo-3-chloropropane in the F344 male rat: I. Dose-response relationships and differences in routes of exposure. *Toxicol Appl Pharmacol* 1981;59:71–83.
35. Kato K, Sato K, Matano O, Goto S. Alkylation of cellular macromolecules by reactive metabolite intermediates of DBCP. *J Pestic Sci* 1980;5:45–53.
36. Kluwe WM. Acute toxicity of 1,2-dibromo-3-chloropropane in the F344 rat: II. Development and repair of the renal, epididymal, testicular and hepatic lesions. *Toxicol Appl Pharmacol* 1981;59:84–95.
37. National Research Council. *Drinking water and health,* vol 6. Washington: National Academy of Sciences Press, 1986:321.
38. National Toxicology Program. *Carcinogenesis bioassay of 1,2-dibromo-3-chloropropane (CAS no. 96-12-8) in F344 rats and B6C3F1 mice (inhalation study).* NTP technical report series no. 206, NIH publ. no. 82-1762. Washington: US Department of Health and Human Services, National Toxicology Program, 1982.
39. Ruddick JA, Newsome WH. A teratogenicity and tissue distribution study on dibromochloropropane in the rat. *Bull Environ Contam Toxicol* 1979;27:181–186.
40. Meneghini R. Repair replication of opossum lymphocyte DNA: effect of compounds that bind to DNA. *Chem Biol Interact* 1974;8:113–126.
41. Perocco P, Prodi G. DNA damage by haloalkanes in human lymphocytes cultured in vitro. *Cancer Lett* 1981;13:213–218.
42. Williams GM, Laspia MF, Dunkel VC. Reliability of the hepatocyte primary culture/DNA repair test in testing of coded carcinogens and noncarcinogens. *Mutat Res* 1982;97(5):359–370.
43. Sina JF, Bean CL, Dysart GR, Taylor VI, Bradley MO. Evaluation of the alkaline elution/rat hepatocyte assay as a predictor of carcinogenic/mutagenic potential. *Mutat Res* 1983;113(5):357–391.
44. Nachtomi E, Sarma DSR. Repair of rat liver DNA in vivo damaged by ethylene dibromide. *Biochem Pharmacol* 1977;26:1941–1945.
45. National Cancer Institute. *Bioassay of 1,2-dibromoethane for possible carcinogenicity, CAS no. 106-93-4.* NCI Carcinogenicity technical report series no. 86, PB-288-428. Washington: Government Printing Office, 1978.
46. National Toxicology Program. *Carcinogenesis bioassay of 1,2-dibromomethane in F344 rats and B6C3F1 mice (inhalation study).* NTP-80-28, NIH publ. no. 82-1766. Washington: US Department of Health and Human Services, National Toxicology Program, 1982.
47. Stinson SF, Reznik GR, Ward JM. Characteristics of proliferative lesions in the nasal cavities of mice following chronic inhalation of 1,2-dibromoethane. *Cancer Lett* 1981;12:121–129.
48. Wong LCK, Winston JM, Hong CB, Plotnick H. Carcinogenicity and toxicity of 1,2-dibromoethane in the rat. *Toxicol Appl Pharmacol* 1982;63:155–165.
49. Ott MG, Scharnweber HC, Langner RR. Mortality experience of 161 employees exposed to ethylene dibromide in two production units. *Br J Ind Med* 1980;37:163–168.
50. Heppel LA, Neal PA, Highman B, Porterfield VT. Toxicology of 1,2-dichloropropane (propylene dichloride): I. Studies on effects of daily inhalation. *J Ind Hyg Toxicol* 1946;28:1–8.
51. Parker CM, Coate W, Voelker R. Subchronic inhalation toxicity of 1,3-dichloropropene/1,2-dichloropropane (D-D) in mice and rats. *J Toxicol Environ Health* 1982;9:899–910.
52. National Toxicology Program. *Toxicology and carcinogenesis studies of 1,2-dichloropropane (propylene dichloride) (CAS no. 78-87-5) in F344/N rats and B6C3F1 mice (gavage studies).* NTP-TR-263, NCI publ. no. 86-2652. Washington: US Department of Health and Human Services, National Toxicology Program, 1986.
53. DeLorenzo F, Silengo L, Cortese R. Mutagenicity of pesticides containing 1,3-dichloropropene. *Cancer Res* 1977;37:1915.
54. Jones AR, Gibson I. 1,2-dichloropropane: metabolism and fate in the rat. *Xenobiotica* 1980;10:835–846.
55. Hine CH, Anderson HH, Moon HD, Kodama JK, Morse M, Jacobson NW. Toxicology and safe handling of CBP-55 (technical 1-chloro-3-bromo-propene-1). *AMA Arch Ind Hyg Occup Med* 1953;7:118–136.
56. Torkelson TR, F Oyen. The toxicity of 1,3-dichloropropene as determined by repeated exposure of laboratory animals. *Am Ind Hyg Assoc J* 1977;38:217–223.
57. National Toxicology Program. *Toxicology and carcinogenesis studies of Telone II in F344/N rats and B6C3F1 mice.* Technical report series no. 269. Washington: US Department of Health and Human Services, 1985.
58. Lomax LG, Stott WT, Johnson KA, Calhoun LL, Yano BL, Quast JF. The chronic toxicity and oncogenicity of inhaled technical-grade 1,3-dichloropropene in rats and mice. *Fundam Appl Toxicol* 1989;12:418–431.
59. Stott WT, Young JT, Calhoun LL, Battjes JE. Subchronic toxicity of inhaled technical grade 1,3-dichloropropene in rats and mice. *Fundam Appl Toxicol* 1988;11:207–220.
60. Osterloh JD, Wang R, Schneider F, Maddy KT. Biological monitoring of dichloropropene: air concentrations, urinary metabolite and renal enzyme excretion. *Arch Environ Health* 1984;44:207–213.
61. Alexeeff GV, Kilgore WW. Methyl bromide. *Res Rev* 1982;88:102–153.
62. Anger WK, Setzer JV, Russo JM, Brightwell WS, Wait RG, Johnson BL. Neurobehavioral effects of methyl bromide inhalation exposures. *Scand J Work Environ Health* 1981;7(Suppl 4):40–47.
63. Russo JM, Anger WK, Setzer JV, Brightwell WS. Neurobehavioral assessment of chronic low-level methyl bromide exposure in the rabbit. *J Toxicol Environ Health* 1984:14:247–255.
64. Voogd CE, Knaap AGAC, Van der Heijden CA, Kramers PG. Genotoxicity of methylbromide in short-term assay systems. *Mutat Res* 1982;97:233.
65. Moriya M, Ohta T, Watanabe K, Miyazawa T, Kato K, Shirasu Y. Further mutagenicity studies on pesticides in bacterial reversion assay systems. *Mutat Res* 1983;116(3):185–216.
66. Kramers PGN, Voogd CE, Knaap AGAC, Van der Heijden CA. Mutagenicity of methyl bromide in a series of short-term tests. *Mutat Res* 1985;155(1):41–47.
67. Djalali-Behzad G, Hussain S, Osterman-Golker S, Segerback D. Estimation of genetic risks of alkylating agents: VI. Exposure of mice and bacteria to methyl bromide. *Mutat Res* 1981;84(1):1–10.
68. Simmon VF, Tardiff RG. The mutagenic activity of halogenated compounds found in chlorinated drinking water. Water Chlorination, Environ Impact Health Eff Proc Conf, 1978;2:417–431.
69. Danse LHDC, van Velsen FL, Van der Heijden CA. Methylbromide: carcinogenic effects in the rat forestomach. *Toxicol Appl Pharmacol* 1984;72:262–271.
70. US Environmental Protection Agency. *Chemical hazard information profile, draft report, methyl bromide.* Rev February 20, 1985. Washington: US Environmental Protection Agency, 1985.
71. National Toxicology Program. *Toxicology and carcinogenesis studies of methyl bromide (CAS no. 74-83-9) in B6C3F1 mice (inhalation studies).* NTP TR 385, NIH publ. no. 91-2840. Washington: US Department of Health and Human Services, 1990.
72. Reuzel PGJ, Kuper CF, Dreef-van der Meulen HC, Hollanders VMH. *Chronic (29-month) inhalation toxicity and carcinogenicity study of methyl bromide in rats.* Report no. V86.469/221044. TNO, EPA/OTS doc. no. 86-8700001202. Washington/Delft, Netherlands: Netherlands Organization for Applied Scientific Research, Division for Nutrition and Food Research, 1987.
73. Reuzel PGJ, Dreef-van der Meulen HC, Hollanders VMH, Kuper CF, Feron VJ, van der Heijden CA. Chronic inhalation toxicity and carcinogenicity study of methyl bromide in Wistar rats. *Food Chem Toxicol* 1991;29(1):31–39.
74. Wong O, Brocker W, Davis HV, Nagle GS. Mortality of workers potentially exposed to organic and inorganic brominated chemicals, DBCP, TRIS, PBB, and DDT. *Br J Ind Med* 1984;41:15–24.
75. Shield L, Coleman T, Markesbery W. MB intoxication: neurological features including simulation of Reye's syndrome. *Neurology* 1977;27:959–962.

76. Chavez C, Hepler R, Straatsma B. Methyl bromide optic atrophy. *Ann J Ophthalmol* 1985;99:715–719.
77. US Environmental Protection Agency. *Methyl bromide phaseout.* [Website: http://www.epa.gov/ozone/mbr/mbrqa.html.] Washington: US Environmental Protection Agency, Stratospheric Protection Division, 1998.
78. Methyl Bromide Research Task Force. *Alternatives to methyl bromide: research needs for California.* Report of the Methyl Bromide Research Task Force to the Department of Pesticide Regulation and the California Department of Food and Agriculture, September, 1995. Sacramento, CA: California Department of Food and Agriculture, 1995.
79. Taxay E. Vikane inhalation. *J Occup Med* 1966;8:425–426.
80. Scheuerman E. Suicide by exposure to sulfuryl fluoride. *J Forensic Sci* 1986;31(3):1154–1158.
81. Teslaa G, Kaiser M, Biederman L, Stowe C. Chloropicrin toxicity involving animal and human exposure. *Vet Hum Toxicol* 1986;28(4):323–324.
82. Proctor PN, Hughes J, Fishman M. *Chemical hazards of the workplace,* 2nd ed. New York: JB Lippincott Co, 1988.
83. Sittig M. *Handbook of toxic and hazardous chemicals.* Park Ridge, NJ: Noyes Publications, 1981.

CHAPTER 101

Herbicides

Alvin C. Bronstein and John B. Sullivan, Jr.

Herbicides include a broad, diverse group of chemical compounds. These substances are classified according to their mechanism of action on plants. For many herbicides, these mechanisms remain unknown. The structure and activity relationships of the better-known herbicides in regard to plants are summarized in Table 101-1 (1). Commonly used herbicides are listed in Table 101-2. Herbicide exposure most commonly occurs as a result of occupational accidents, intentional ingestions, or low-level chronic exposures that may last for years (2). Table 101-3 lists occupational exposure limits of select herbicides.

CHLOROPHENOXY HERBICIDES

Sources and Production

Chlorophenoxy herbicides include 2,4-dichlorophenoxyacetic acid [2,4-D; Chemical Abstracts Service (CAS) number 94-75-7]; 2,4,5-trichlorophenoxyacetic acid (2,4,5-T; CAS number 93-76-5); 2-methoxy-3,6-dichlorobenzoic acid (Dicamba; CAS number 1918-00-9); 2-methyl-4-chlorophenoxyacetic acid (CAS number 94-74-6); 2-(2,4,5-trichlorophenoxy)-propionic acid (CAS number 93-72-1); and others. The group members, substituted organic acids, have similar biochemical properties (Fig. 101-1). These compounds usually contain from one to three chlorine atoms substituted on the organic acid serving as the base molecule. These acid backbones may include acetic, propionic, or butyric acid. Some may also have a methyl substitution as part of the chlorophenoxy portion. The chlorophenoxy herbicides usually are manufactured in the form of metal salts, alkylamine salts, or esters to produce materials of low volatility (2). This minimizes their possible spread to nontargeted plants growing nearby.

Chlorophenoxy herbicides are used extensively to control broadleaf weeds and woody plants in cereal crops, sugarcane, turf pastures, and noncrop lands (3). These herbicides are plant growth regulators. They function by acting as synthetic auxins or plant hormones, and they cause plant growth reactions similar to 12 naturally occurring indole auxins (4). The rapid growth interferes with nutrient transport and destroys the plant. The plants may develop high levels of nitrates or cyanide before wilting (2).

TABLE 101-1. Herbicide actions on plants

Inhibition of photosynthesis
- Anilides
- Benzimidazoles
- Biscarbamates
- Pyridazinones
- Triazinediones
- Triazines
- Triazinones
- Uracils
- Substituted ureas
- Quinones
- Hydroxybenzonitriles

Inhibition of amino acid synthesis
- Glyphosate
- Sulfonylureas
- Imidazolinones
- Bialophos
- Glufosinate

Production of photobleaching
- Bipyridyliums (paraquat and diquat)
- *p*-Nitrodiphenyl ethers
- Oxadiazoles
- *N*-phenylimides

Inhibition of lipid synthesis
- Aryloxphenoxy alkanoic acids
- Cyclohexanediones

Inhibition of cellulose synthesis
- Dichlorbenil

Inhibition of cell division
- Phosphoric amides
- Dinitroamilines

Inhibition of carotenoid synthesis and interference with protection against photooxidation
- Pyridazinones
- Phenoxybenzamides
- Fluoridone
- Difunone
- 4-Hydroxypyridines
- Amitrole

Inhibition of folate synthesis
- Asulam

Adapted from ref. 1.

The most widely known compounds are 2,4-D and 2,4,5-T. 2,4-D ($Cl_2CH_3OCH_2COOH$; molecular weight, 221.0 D) is a white to yellow crystalline, odorless powder. Its melting point is 280°F (140.5°C), giving off a slight phenolic odor. The boiling point is 160°C at 0.4 mm Hg. It is a noncombustible solid soluble

TABLE 101-2. Herbicides

Acrolein (Magnacide-H)
Barban
Dicamba
2,4-Dichlorophenoxy acetic acid (2,4-D)
Diquat
Glyphosate (Round-Up, Kleen-Up)
Metachlor
Nitrophenols (Dinosebs)
Paraquat
Propham
Substituted ureas (Diuron)
Terbutryne
Tetradifon
2,4,5-Trichlorophenoxy acetic acid (2,4,5-T)

TABLE 101-3. Occupational exposure levels

RTECS no.	(Prime) Name	CAS no.	TWA	STEL (C)	IDLH value (mg/m^3)
AG6825000	2,4-D	94-75-7			
ACGIH TLV			10 mg/m^{3,a}		
OSHA PEL			10 mg/m^3		
NIOSH REL			10 mg/m^3		100 mg/m^3
AJ8400000	2,4,5-T	93-76-5			
ACGIH TLV			10 mg/m^{3,a}		
OSHA PEL			10 mg/m^3		
NIOSH REL			10 mg/m^3		250 mg/m^3
DW1960000	Paraquat	4685-14-7			
ACGIH TLV			0.5 mg/m^3, total dust 0.1 mg/m^3, respirable particulate		
OSHA PEL			0.5 mg/m^3, respirable dust		
NIOSH REL			0.1 mg/m^3, respirable dust		1 mg/m^3
JM5685000	Diquat	2764-72-9			
ACGIH TLV			0.5 mg/m^{3,a}, inhalable particulate 0.1 mg/m^{3,a}, respirable particulate		
OSHA PEL			—		
NIOSH REL			0.5 mg/m^3		
SM6300000	Pentachlorophenol	87-86-5			
ACGIH TLV			0.5 mg/m^{3,b}		
OSHA PEL			0.5 mg/m^3		
NIOSH REL			0.5 mg/m^3		2.5 mg/m^3
DD6475000	Benomyl	17804-35-2			
ACGIH TLV			0.84 ppm^a 10 mg/m^{3,a}		
OSHA PEL			15 mg/m^3, total dust 5 mg/m^3, respirable fraction		
NIOSH REL			—		
NO8750000	Ferbam	14484-64-1			
ACGIH TLV			10 mg/m^{3,a}		
OSHA PEL			15 mg/m^3, total dust		
NIOSH REL			10 mg/m^3		
JO1225000	Disulfiram	97-77-8			
ACGIH TLV			2 mg/m^{3,a}		
OSHA PEL					
NIOSH REL			2 mg/m^3		800 mg/m^3
JO1400000	Thiram	137-26-8			
ACGIH TLV			1 mg/m^{3,a}		
OSHA PEL			5 mg/m^3		
NIOSH REL			5 mg/m^3		
AS1050000	Acrolein	107-02-8			
ACGIH TLV			0.1 ppm 0.23 mg/m^3	0.3 ppm; NIC: 0.1 ppm^a 0.69 mg/m^3; NIC: 0.23 mg/m^{3,a}	
OSHA PEL			0.1 ppm 0.25 mg/m^3		
NIOSH REL			0.1 ppm 0.25 mg/m^3	0.3 ppm 0.8 mg/m^3	100 mg/m^3
—	Organic compounds (e.g., Sn)	—			
ACGIH TLV			0.1 mg/m^{3,a}	0.2 mg/m^{3,a}; skin^c	
OSHA PEL			0.1 ppm		
NIOSH REL			0.1 mg/m^3		2 ppm

ACGIH, American Conference of Governmental Industrial Hygienists; CAS, Chemical Abstracts Service; IDLH, immediately dangerous to life and health; NIC, notice of intended changes; NIOSH, National Institute for Occupational Safety and Health; OSHA, U.S. Occupational Safety and Health Administration; PEL, permissible exposure limit; REL, recommended exposure limit; RTECS, Registry of Toxic Effects of Chemical Substances; STEL (C), short-term exposure limit ceiling; TLV, threshold limit value; TWA, time-weighted average.
[a]Not classifiable as a human carcinogen. Data are inadequate to classify the agent in terms of its carcinogenicity in humans or animals (or both).
[b]Animal carcinogen. The agent is carcinogenic in experimental animals at a relatively high dose, by route of administration, at site, by histologic type, or by mechanism not considered relevant to worker exposure. Available epidemiologic studies do not confirm an increased risk of cancer in exposed humans. Available evidence suggests that the agent is not likely to cause cancer in humans except under uncommon or unlikely routes or levels of exposure.
[c]*Skin* indicates danger of cutaneous absorption.

in water and hydrocarbon solvents. 2,4-D may be found in flammable liquids, such as hydrocarbon solvents (e.g., xylene). The herbicidal effects of 2,4-D originally were noted in 1942 (4). Registered as a broadleaf weed herbicide, 2,4-D is classified as a plant growth regulator. More than 60 million pounds are used in the United States annually (3).

2,4,5-T ($Cl_3C_6H_2OCH_2COOH$; molecular weight, 255.5 D) is a colorless to tan, odorless solid with a melting point between 154° and 155°C (309.2° and 311°F). 2,4,5-T is synthesized from the intermediate compound 2,4,5-trichlorophenol (TCP). During TCP manufacture, TCP has the ability to react with itself to produce 2,3,7,8-tetrachlorodibenzo-*p*-dioxin (TCDD). TCDD is one of a

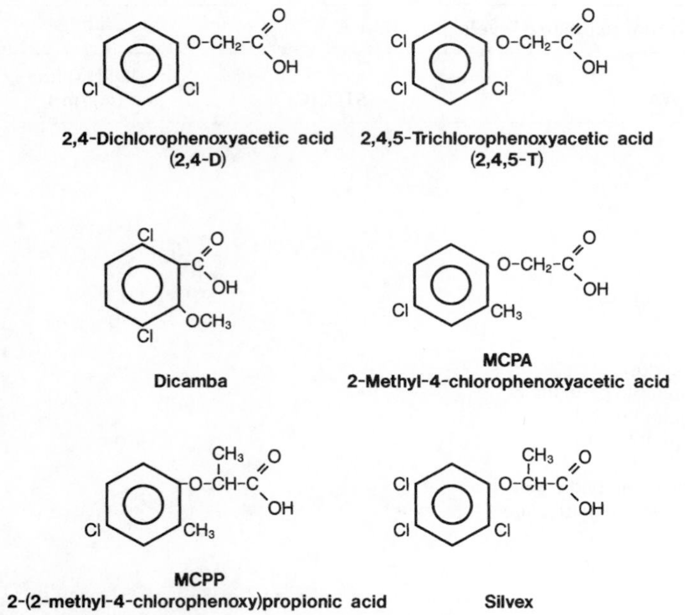

2,4-Dichlorophenoxyacetic acid (2,4-D) **2,4,5-Trichlorophenoxyacetic acid (2,4,5-T)**

Dicamba **MCPA 2-Methyl-4-chlorophenoxyacetic acid**

MCPP 2-(2-methyl-4-chlorophenoxy)propionic acid **Silvex**

Figure 101-1. Phenoxy acid herbicides.

family of compounds known collectively as *dioxins*. These compounds are produced as by-products during the synthesis of many organic chemicals. Dioxins are contaminants of 2,4,5-T and hexachlorophene synthesis (5). In addition, dioxins are released in emissions from coal-burning power plants, from diesel exhaust, and from the incomplete burning of chlorine waste, such as polyvinyl chloride plastic and polychlorinated biphenyls. These compounds also are produced naturally in small amounts by volcanoes and forest fires (5). TCDD is the best studied of approximately 75 dioxin compounds (5). The dioxins, along with related compounds—the furans (polychlorinated dibenzofurans), polychlorinated biphenyls, and polybrominated biphenyls—have been associated in both animal and human epidemiologic studies with an increased risk of cancer and other symptoms, such as chloracne (2,5,6). Dioxins bioaccumulate in the food chain, so human exposure usually results from consumption of fish, meat, and dairy products (5). Current herbicide-manufacturing processes are designed to remove dioxin contaminants.

The most notorious use of chlorophenoxy herbicide compounds occurred during the Vietnam War (from January 1962 to September 1971). The need for defoliants prompted the use of a variety of herbicide compounds and mixtures. Because of rushed production methods, dioxin contaminants were not removed uniformly during the synthesis process. To avoid clogging problems in the spraying apparatus, the various agents were shipped in color-coded drums. The 50:50 mixture of the *n*-butyl esters of 2,4,-D and 2,4,5-T was shipped in 55-gallon drums marked with an orange stripe. This herbicide mixture came to be known as *Agent Orange*. Other defoliants used in that context included Agent White (2,4-D) and Agent Blue (cacodylic acid, an arsenical compound: $C_2H_7AsO_2$). Because of its dioxin risk, 2,4,5-T was banned in the United States by the U.S. Environmental Protection Agency (EPA) in 1979. Millions of pounds of 2,4-D still are used annually in the United States.

Sites, Industries, and Businesses Associated with Exposures

The most common sources of exposure are found in the manufacture or application of these herbicide compounds. Skin absorption is the major route of exposure for herbicide applicators. Dermal exposure levels are 4 to 50 times greater than those of the inhalational route (7). The potential exists for civilian population exposure near chlorophenoxy herbicide application sites.

Clinical Toxicology

Chlorophenoxy herbicides appear to demonstrate similar pharmacokinetic profiles (8). 2,4-D and 2,4,5-T have been investigated intensively in animal and human studies. Rapid and almost complete absorption occurs after an oral dose (6,9–12). Differences exist among amine, salt, and ester formulations of 2,4-D and 2,4,5-T. The amine and salt compounds are hydrolyzed and absorbed rapidly (6,10). The ester preparations of 2,4-D demonstrate lower plasma concentrations (9). These compounds are highly bound to plasma proteins (8). Once absorbed, the chlorophenoxy herbicides are distributed widely throughout the body. The major organs of deposition are the kidneys, liver, gastrointestinal (GI) tract, and the central and peripheral nervous systems.

Oral absorption follows first-order kinetics (12,13). This is estimated in humans to be between 1% and more than 27% per hour (10,14). In humans, almost all of a 2,4-D oral dose is absorbed within 24 hours (15). Peak plasma concentrations are reached at between 4 and 24 hours in humans (6,9,10,12). In one study, six human volunteers received 5 mg per kg (e.g., 350 mg per 70 kg in adults) of 2,4-D orally. The average peak plasma concentration was 35 mg per L at 24 hours. The mean plasma half-life of 2,4-D in this study was 33 hours (10).

Elimination of 2,4-D is rapid. 2,4-D metabolites other than conjugates have not been detected in human urine (10). During the 4 days after ingestion by the six subjects mentioned, 77% of the dose was eliminated unchanged in the urine (10). All remained asymptomatic.

In another study, five male adult human volunteers ingested a single oral dose of 5 mg per kg of 2,4-D. No detectable clinical effects were noted. The average plasma half-life of 2,4-D was calculated to be 11.6 hours, with a mean urine half-life of 17.7 hours. Eighty-three percent of the ingested oral dose was excreted as the parent compound, and 12.8% of the oral dose was excreted in the urine as an acid-labile conjugate (12,15).

The chlorophenoxy herbicides demonstrate first-order elimination kinetics that are dose-dependent, similar to those of salicylates (7,13). Plasma half-lives range from 10 to 20 hours and may increase to 80 to 120 hours with large, acute poisonings (7). Members of this herbicide group have relatively small volumes of distribution (Vd) (3). Like salicylates, the Vd increases with increasing dose. Reflecting this dose-dependent Vd, chlorophenoxy acid herbicide tissue concentrations increase disproportionately with increasing dose as compared to plasma concentrations. Therefore, increasing the body burden increases the apparent Vd of the chlorophenoxy herbicides. No evidence suggests bioaccumulation (15).

The mean lethal human dose of 2,4-D is approximately 28 g (13,16). Pharmacokinetic studies by Young and Haley (17) of a 30.22-kg woman ingesting a 1-dL mixture of 2,4-D and Dicamba in an acute overdose attempt revealed that the Vd was 10.2 L (0.338 L per kg) for 2,4-D and 23.4 L (0.774 L per kg) for Dicamba. In human volunteers, at a dose of 5 mg per kg, the Vd of 2,4-D is approximately 0.1 L per kg (range, 0.098 to 0.104 L per kg) (10).

Workers exposed to an air concentration of 2,4,-D at 0.1 to 0.2 mg per cubic meter had urine concentrations ranging from 3 to 14 mg per L (18). Various studies have found workers to have urinary 2,4-D concentrations ranging from 0.2 to 8.2 mg per L (16).

SIGNS, SYNDROMES, AND SYMPTOMS FROM TOXIC EXPOSURE

Acute Toxicity. Acute chlorophenoxy herbicide toxicity presents a clinical picture of gastroenteritislike symptoms, including nausea, abdominal pain, GI hypermotility, and diarrhea (sometimes bloody) (2). These compounds have an irritant effect on mucous membranes. Elevations may occur in hepatic enzymes, such as lactate dehydrogenase (LDH) and aspartate aminotransferase (AST). Delayed fever of sudden onset may occur with ingestion (19). At higher doses, muscular and neurologic problems develop (2). Skeletal muscle myotonia (stiff legs, muscle twitching, and spasms) (19); muscle fibrillation; myoglobinuria (18); and rhabdomyolysis may be observed. Central nervous system (CNS) depression, ataxia, miosis, diminished coordination, and paralysis leading to coma are the major CNS findings. Tachycardia is a frequent finding along with the potential for other cardiac dysrhythmias. In one study of chlorophenoxy herbicide overdose patients, 7 of 27 patients developed hypotension (19). Pulmonary edema and hyperventilation have been reported (19–21). Albuminuria and hemoglobinuria have been seen, which may reflect glomerular or tubular injury (20). Acute renal failure secondary to rhabdomyolysis has occurred after poisoning with 2-(2-methyl-4-chlorophenoxy) propionic acid (MCPP) (21) or 2,4-D (19). Metabolic acidosis has been reported in severe cases (19,22). Ingestion of 2,4-D has been reported to produce hypocalcemia in association with hypophosphatemia and renal failure (23). Hyperkalemia also has been observed (20,21,24). Thrombocytopenia rarely has been seen (21,23). Death usually is due to peripheral vascular collapse (2).

Delayed onset of paresthesias and protracted polyneuropathy have been reported as being due to poisoning with herbicide mixtures containing chlorophenoxy compounds. Onset may be delayed for up to a month (25). A polyneuritis-type picture has been reported consisting of decreased vibratory and proprioceptive sensation with decreased deep tendon reflexes in the presence of superficial reflexes (2). Peripheral neuropathies may be seen in acute poisoning survivors or in subacute cases (26,27).

Major target organs are the central nervous and cardiovascular systems (22). Electrocardiogram abnormalities, including flattening or inversion of the T wave, have been reported. Hervonen et al. (28) found reversible damage to the endothelial cells of the blood–brain barrier in rats exposed to 2,4-D. Dudley and Thapar (29) reported autopsy findings in a 76-year-old white man with senile dementia who died 6 days after acute 2,4-D ingestion. Widespread plaques of acute perivascular demyelination and perivascular petechial hemorrhage without cellular infiltration were described. Single intraperitoneal doses of 200 mg per kg in rats produced reversible inhibition of cerebral electrical activity with direct attack on the reticular system. Electroencephalographic changes were seen as early as 24 hours after dosing (30).

Goldstein and Jones (31) were the first to report the development of peripheral neuropathy with electromyographic abnormalities in three cases after heavy 2,4-D ester dermal exposure. Symptomatology persisted. Recovery was still incomplete several years after exposure. A 39-year-old male farmer who sustained excessive exposure to 2,4-D while spraying crops developed a primary sensory peripheral neuropathy 4 days after exposure (32). Electromyographic and peroneal nerve conduction study results were within normal limits. Symptoms diminished, but the patient continued to experience intermittent numbness of the hands after prolonged use.

Concentrated solutions of 2,4-D (greater than 12%) have been shown to cause severe skin burns in rats and rabbits (33,34). In animal studies, topical application of a 24% solution of 2,4-D amine over a 3-week period produced ulcerative dermatitis, decreased body weight, and increased kidney size. A 12% solution of 2,4-D resulted in minimal skin changes. The dermal effect was thought to be due to a direct effect of the 2,4-D, as both the 12% and 24% solutions had a pH of 10. Additionally, at necropsy, the test animals revealed no neuropathologic changes (22,34).

Various authors have reported fatal human poisonings with 2,4-D and its congeners (11,22,34). As stated, the mean adult estimated lethal dose of 2,4-D is 28 g (13,16). Two thousand milligrams of 2,4-D given intravenously produced no symptoms in a patient terminally ill with coccidiomycosis (35); 3,600 mg has caused serious side effects, including fibrillary twitching of the mouth and both upper extremities and generalized hyporeflexia (36). Ingestion of 500 mg over 3 weeks produced no definable symptoms (37), whereas an intentional ingestion of 80 mg per kg caused death in a 23-year-old college student.

Postmortem 2,4-D blood concentrations of 720 mg per L were reported in a 64-year-old white woman who was found comatose and died of pulmonary edema 12 hours after hospital admission (38). In another report, a 26-year-old man ingested 360 mL of Ortho Weed B-Gone M (dimethylamine salts of 2,4-D, 10.8%, and MCPP (11.6%; 77.6% inert ingredients); Dexol (chlorpyrifos, 6.7% in petroleum distillates, 76.8%); and a few granules of warfarin, 0.025%. The patient died approximately 30 hours after admission after four episodes of bradycardia, hypotension, and asystole. Other findings included hyperkalemia, thrombocytopenia, hypocalcemia, and hypophosphatemia. The postmortem concentration of 2,4-D was 389.5 g per mL and of MCPP was 235.5 g per mL.

Chronic Toxicity. Neurotoxicity, chloracne, and hepatic dysfunction are the primary problems reported secondary to chronic exposure to 2,4-D. Chronic neurologic toxicity is due most likely to a direct neurotoxic effect of the chlorophenoxy herbicides (30). TCDD (dioxin) contamination may be responsible for other long-term and neurologic problems as well. Disorders of liver function, such as porphyria, have been reported in chronic occupational exposure cases (39).

Chloracne. The most common finding in individuals exposed to TCDD has been chloracne (40). In severely contaminated individuals, chloracne can persist for years after exposure (41). Chloracne consists of comedones, cysts, pustules, and abscesses. Hepatic dysfunction, peripheral neuropathy, fat metabolism disorders, elevated serum cholesterol, and porphyria cutanea tarda are the other findings associated most frequently with TCDD exposure in industrial settings (42). Zack and Suskind (40) studied 129 workers exposed to TCDD after a trichlorophenol processing plant explosion in Nitro, WV, in 1949. All 129 employees developed chloracne. No increased frequency of malignancies was found in this group after a 30-year follow-up. Symptoms reported after TCDD exposure included chloracne; severe pain in muscles of upper and lower extremities, shoulders, and thorax; fatigue; nervousness; vertigo; decreased libido; and cold intolerance. Liver impairment, demonstrated by increased prothrombin times, was observed (40). Over time, the symptoms may clear to some degree. Aches and pains in the lower extremities and back, nervousness, fatigue, and dyspnea may continue (40). In a later study of 204 exposed and 163 nonexposed workers, chloracne persisted in 55.7% of those in the exposed group. A positive association was found with GI tract ulcers, but no increased risk of cardiovascular disease, hepatic disease, renal disease, central or peripheral nervous system problems, or malignancies were found (43). In a related study focusing on workers with and without chloracne, the mean duration of chloracne was found to be 26 years. Increased γ-glutamyl transferase concentrations were found in the chloracne group. Abnormal sensory findings also were present in the chloracne group (44).

TCDD has been associated with soft-tissue sarcoma, Hodgkin's disease, non-Hodgkin's lymphoma, gastric cancer, nasal cancer, and liver cancer in various studies (45–56). Rats, mice, and hamsters exposed to TCDD have developed histiocytic lymphomas, fibrosarcomas, and tumors of liver, skin, lung, thyroid, tongue, hard palate, and nasal turbinates (56,57). Initiating or promoting carcinogenesis may be functions of TCDD (58–64).

Fingerhut et al. (3) conducted a retrospective study of a cohort of 5,172 workers occupationally exposed to TCDD during production of various chemicals contaminated with TCDD. TCDD serum concentrations were measured in 253 workers. Mortality from all cancers was increased significantly in the cohort. Cancer mortality from stomach, liver, and nasal tumors and from Hodgkin's disease and non-Hodgkin's lymphoma was not significantly different from expected mortality rates in the overall cohort. In a subcohort of 1,520 workers with more than 1 year of exposure and more than 20 years' latency since TCDD exposure, mortality was increased significantly from all cancers, specifically from soft-tissue sarcomas and respiratory tract cancers. Confounding variables, such as smoking and exposure to other industrial chemicals, could not be excluded as other potential causes of the cancer mortality rates. Mean TCDD serum concentration adjusted for lipids was 233 pg per gram of lipid (range, 2,000 to 3,000). This compared to 7 pg per gram for unexposed individuals. The mean TCDD concentration for 119 workers with 1 year of exposure or more was 418 pg per gram, with exposure having occurred 15 to 37 years earlier (3).

Although this study had multiple potential pitfalls, the data indicate probable human risk from TCDD exposure (63). On the basis of this study, the lifetime risk from TCDD-induced soft-tissue sarcoma approximates 2 per 1,000. This risk is far greater than the commonly accepted lifetime risk of 1 per 100,000 or 1 per million from exposure for the general public to potential carcinogens (63).

Multiple studies have been conducted of soft-tissue sarcoma incidence among Vietnam veterans (65). A case-control study including 217 cases of soft-tissue sarcoma and 599 controls found that Vietnam veterans with higher estimated Agent Orange exposure appeared to be at greater, although not statistically significant, risk for the development of soft-tissue sarcomas (66). An earlier hospital-based case-control study of 234 Vietnam veterans and 13,496 patients in the comparison group failed to find a significant association of soft-tissue sarcomas and previous military service in Vietnam (67). Other studies failed to confirm earlier reports of an association between exposure to chlorophenoxy herbicides and the risk of malignant lymphomas, specifically Hodgkin's and non-Hodgkin's lymphoma from Agent Orange exposure in Vietnam veterans (68–70).

Studies of Vietnam veterans in which the cohort was formed from participants in so-called Operation Ranch Hand failed to show an increased risk of cancer (71,72). The U. S. Air Force has been conducting a 20-year study to determine the health effects on Air Force veterans of Operation Ranch Hand (71). These veterans were responsible for spraying chlorophenoxy herbicides (including Agent Orange) during the Vietnam War. Most of the herbicides were sprayed from fixed-wing aircraft, but herbicides were applied also from helicopters, trucks, and riverboats and with hand applicators. The cohort consisted of 995 veterans who flew application aircraft, maintained aircraft and spray equipment, or handled bulk quantities of TCDD-contaminated herbicides for 1 year or longer. This cohort was studied and compared to a group of 1,200 Vietnam veterans who were not exposed directly. Several differences were found. Those in the Ranch Hand group had alkaline phosphatase concentrations averaging 98 units per L, as compared with the control group's average concentration of 90 units per L ($p < .01$). No prevalence differences were found in verified skin or systemic malignancies. Those in the Ranch Hand cohort had elevated serum TCDD concentrations as compared to those in the comparison group. The median Ranch Hand TCDD concentration was 12.4 parts per trillion (ppt) as compared to 4.2 ppt in the controls. Of the Ranch Hand group, nonflying enlisted personnel had the highest TCDD concentrations at 23.6 ppt, as compared to pilots at 7.3 ppt. No chloracne was found in those in either the Ranch Hand or the control group (71). An earlier study of Vietnam and non-Vietnam veterans found that the mean serum TCDD level was approximately 4.0 ppt for both groups. This study also suggested that TCDD exposure was higher in Vietnam veterans whose jobs involved handling of herbicides (73).

In a related study, the noncombat mortality in a group of 1,261 Ranch Hand veterans was compared to that in a control group of 19,101 Air Force veterans primarily involved in cargo missions. No significant difference in the all-cause standardized mortality ratio was found after adjustment for age, rank, and occupation (72).

Other studies have examined the possible association between phenoxy herbicide exposure and the risk of developing malignant lymphomas in Vietnam Veterans. A more recent case-control study of 329 lung cancer cases in Vietnam veterans correlated with Agent Orange exposure failed to find an increased risk of lung cancer associated with Vietnam service (74).

In 1971, sludge waste from a hexachlorophene manufacturing plant was mixed with waste oil and sprayed for dust control on dirt roads in residential, recreational, and commercial areas of eastern Missouri near St. Louis (75). By February 1986, 28 separate sites had been found to have TCDD soil concentrations of 1 part per billion (ppb) or more. Using 155 unexposed subjects as controls, Hoffman et al. (75) studied 154 exposed mobile home park residents where the soil TCDD concentration ranged from 1 to 2,200 ppb. The exposed residents demonstrated increased frequency of anergy, minor abnormalities in T-cell T4:T8 ratios of less than 1.0, and abnormal T-cell function, suggesting a possible association of long-term TCDD exposure with alterations in cell-mediated immunity. Peak urinary uroporphyrin levels were greater than 13 mg per gram of creatinine in 16.3% of the exposed cohort as compared to 7.5% in the controls. Mean urinary uroporphyrins were 9.6 mg per gram of creatinine versus 8.4 mg per gram of creatinine in those in the unexposed control group. The exposed residents experienced paresthesias of the hands and feet and headaches more than did the controls. Neuropsychological testing failed to find significant differences between the two groups (75).

Seveso, Italy (approximately 20 miles north of Milan), was the site of a TCDD release over a residential area in 1976. More than 37,000 people may have been exposed to dioxins as a result. No deaths were reported secondary to acute poisoning. Determining etiology of symptoms was confounded by concomitant exposure to release of other compounds. Chloracne appeared almost exclusively in children and young people; most cases resolved spontaneously. Transient lymphopenia and impaired liver function were observed. Subclinical peripheral nerve impairment was observed in 16 of 156 victims with chloracne at 6 years after the dioxin release. No cases of peripheral neuropathy were observed in this group of 156. Long-term epidemiologic studies of the exposed populations are continuing, with special emphasis to define any mutagenic or carcinogenic effects (76).

MANAGEMENT OF TOXICITY

Clinical Examination. Acutely exposed patients should be removed from the source of the exposure and decontaminated as the exposure and condition warrant (77). Rescue personnel should wear appropriate gloves, boots, and goggles. Special attention should be directed to the respiratory system, with monitoring of airway, breathing, and circulatory status. Supplemental oxygen and intravenous fluids should be begun as necessary.

Chronically exposed patients require a complete toxicologic history and physical examination, with special attention to the neurologic system. A comprehensive occupational history should be obtained.

Alkaline diuresis has been proposed to enhance the elimination of 2,4-D (78). Affected patients should be monitored for the development of metabolic acidosis, hyperthermia, seizures, coma, hyperventilation, tachycardia, electrocardiographic abnormalities, vasodilatation, diaphoresis, hypoxia, myotonia, hyperkalemia, myoglobinuria, hepatic dysfunction, or renal failure. Severe hypoxia associated with hyperventilation and normal P_{CO_2} may result from the uncoupling of oxidative phosphorylation.

Treatment

Enhanced Elimination. Various techniques have been advocated to enhance the elimination of the chlorophenoxy herbicides. Because of the relatively low pK_a (3.3) of the chlorophenoxy herbicides, alkaline diuresis may be theoretically helpful. As always, the risk versus benefit of alkaline diuresis must be gauged. Attempts to increase urine volume beyond 100 to 150 mL per hour increase the risk of complications from fluid overload but increase clearance only minimally. Prior to any alkaline diuresis therapy, hydration status should be documented to ensure that affected patients are well hydrated. Alkaline diuresis should not be attempted in the face of renal failure or impaired renal function. The usual method for alkaline diuresis is administration of a loading dose of sodium bicarbonate in the range of 1 to 2 mEq per L. This usually equates to two to three ampules (88 to 132 mEq). The necessity for coadministration of potassium is controversial. Probably more important is to maintain normal potassium status rather than arbitrarily loading affected patients with potassium. This usually can be accomplished by administration of 20 to 40 mEq of potassium chloride as needed in a crystalloid solution, such as 5% dextrose in water. Adequate urine output should be maintained. Optimal urine pH should be kept in the 7.5 to 8.0 range. Overly aggressive alkalinization should be avoided, as should excessive alkalinization of affected patients. Close monitoring of serum and urine pH is required.

Adequate alkalemia should be maintained via administration of additional sodium bicarbonate. A dose of 1 to 2 mEq per kg of sodium bicarbonate periodically, based on pH measurements, usually will maintain the alkalemia. Potassium chloride should be administered as needed to maintain normokalemia. Cautious administration of diuretics, such as furosemide or mannitol, may be required to maintain adequate diuresis. Renal function and serum electrolytes need careful, frequent monitoring (79). Serum and urine pH, intake and output, and electrolyte status should be recorded every hour. Pulmonary and CNS status should be monitored to avoid development of impending heart failure or pulmonary or cerebral edema with fluid overload. Alkaline diuresis should not be attempted in patients who have evidence of pulmonary edema or in those with renal failure.

Supportive therapy is the mainstay of treatment for acute chlorophenoxy herbicide poisoning. Forced alkaline diuresis for acute poisoning has been advocated, as the chlorophenoxy herbicides are organic acids with a measured pK_a of 3.3 (78). Prescott et al. (78) reported that the renal clearance of 2,4-D increased from 0.14 mL per minute at a urine pH of 5.1 to 5.1 mL per minute at pH 8.3. Flanagan et al. (19) reported the positive effect of alkaline diuresis in a series of 41 patients acutely poisoned with chlorophenoxy herbicides and ioxynil (4-hydroxy-3,5-di-iodobenzonitrite). Plasma half-lives were reduced to less than 30 hours with alkaline diuresis. Alkaline diuresis has been recommended in cases of severe poisoning with coma, acidemia, or total chlorophenoxy herbicide concentrations greater than 0.5 g per L. The 2,4-D pK_a in this study was reported as 2.6 (19).

Rhabdomyolysis is treated with aggressive intravenous fluid therapy to prevent renal insufficiency. Urinary alkalinization is not necessary. Input and output status should be assessed closely.

Laboratory Diagnosis. Patients exposed to chlorophenoxy herbicides require a full biochemical profile, including hepatic enzymes [aspartate aminotransferase (AST), alanine aminotransferase (ALT), γ-glutamyl transpeptidase (GGT), and LDH]; electrolytes; glucose; blood urea nitrogen; creatinine; serum aldolase; creatinine phosphokinase; complete blood count; and urinalysis. Baseline electrocardiography and continuous monitoring should be performed because of high probability of cardiac dysrhythmias. Cardiac dysrhythmia should be treated with standard advanced cardiac life support protocols.

Chronically exposed patients also require a thyroid profile and vitamin B_{12} and folate determinations to assist in the differentiation of other neurologic diseases. A computed axial tomographic scan or magnetic resonance imaging of the brain and electroencephalography may be necessary to rule out other possible CNS disease states. Electronystagmography and electromyelography studies should be undertaken in cases or suspected cases of peripheral neuropathies. Serum or adipose tissue measurements of TCDD may be performed to estimate exposure.

Special Diagnostic Tests. Concentrations of 2,4-D and other chlorophenoxy herbicides in various fluids may be measured with ultraviolet spectrophotometry, high-performance liquid chromatography (16,80), or flame-ionization or electron-capture gas chromatography (80). The latter two methods appear to be more sensitive and specific (16). Chlorophenoxy concentrations in blood have ranged from 58 to 1,220 mg per L in fatal acute overdoses (80). Measuring exposure to dioxin is difficult because of its extremely low concentrations in adipose tissue. It can be measured using gas chromatography–mass spectrometry. Usually it is measured as picograms per gram of serum lipid.

Adipose tissue sampling or serum measurements for TCDD are the most reliable methods by which to estimate an affected individual's TCDD exposure and body burden. Adipose tissue sampling has been viewed as the most accurate index of TCDD body burden. Recent use of TCDD determinations in the blood lipid component may prove as reliable as the more invasive adipose tissue sampling (81). Preliminary data in Vietnam veterans revealed via adipose tissue sampling that a TCDD blood concentration of 15 pg per gram of fat was associated with heavy exposure, with a correlation coefficient (r) of +0.89.

Thirty-nine of the aforementioned Missouri residents either exposed to soil TCDD concentrations of 20 to 100 ppb for 20 or more years or exposed for 6 months or more to soil concentrations of more than 100 ppb underwent adipose tissue sampling for TCDD (75). Their values were compared to those of 57 unexposed controls with adipose tissue sampling obtained during surgical procedures. The mean TCDD concentration in the exposed individuals was 17.0 ppt (range, 2.8 to 750 ppt) as compared with a median value of 6.4 (range, 1.4 to 20.2 ppt) in the controls (82). From this study, the half-life of TCDD in humans was estimated to be between 5 and 8 years (82).

Environmental Monitoring

Air samples for 2,4-D air concentration determinations should be analyzed by high-pressure liquid chromatography with an ultraviolet detection method, using National Institute for Occupational Safety and Health (NIOSH) analytic method 5001.83.

The U.S. Occupational Safety and Health Administration (OSHA) established a permissible exposure limit (PEL) for inhalational exposure to 2,4-D at 10 mg per cubic meter (83). The PEL for 2,4,5-T also is 10 mg per cubic meter. The NIOSH recommended exposure limit (REL) for 2,4-D is 10 mg per cubic meter and for 2,4,5-T is 10 mg per cubic meter. The immediately dangerous to life or health (IDLH) air concentration value for 2,4-D is 500 mg per cubic meter, whereas that for 2,4,5-T is 250 mg per cubic meter.

The American Conference of Governmental Industrial Hygienists (ACGIH) 1997 threshold limit value (TLV) time-weighted average (TWA) for 2,4-D is 10 mg per cubic meter. The ACGIH TLV TWA for 2,4,5-T is 10 mg per cubic meter. This organization has issued no short-term exposure limit (STEL) value for either compound. Both chemicals carry the *A4* notation by their TLVs. The *A4* designation signifies that a substance is not classifiable as a human carcinogen. Data are inadequate to classify the agent in terms of its carcinogenicity in humans or animals (or both) (83). The International Agency for Research on Cancer (IARC) classifies chlorophenoxy herbicides in group 2B, or possibly carcinogenic to humans (84).

PARAQUAT

Sources and Production

Paraquat (1,1'-dimethyl-4,4'-dipyridyl; $C_{12}H_{14}N_2$) is a bipyridyl compound (CAS number 4685-14-7). It was marketed first in 1962 as a broad-spectrum, nonselective, contact herbicide and desiccant (Fig. 101-2) after having been described first by Weidel and Rosso in 1882 (85). Paraquat's redox properties were published in 1933. It has been used as a redox indicator under the name of *methyl viologen* since 1933. A yellow solid with a faint ammonialike odor, its molecular weight is 257.2 D, and its boiling point at 760 mm Hg is 175° to 180°C (347° to 356°F). Paraquat is corrosive to metals and decomposes under ultraviolet light (85). It is a restricted-use herbicide in the United States.

Diquat (1,1'-ethylene-2,2'-dipydylium ion; $C_{12}H_{14}N_2$; CAS number 2764-72-9) is a paraquat analog having properties similar to paraquat's but causing a human toxicologic presentation different from that of paraquat. Diquat forms a monohydrate that is a colorless to yellow crystalline substance and has a melting point between 335° to 340°C (635° to 644°F). Its molecular weight is 186.26 D. Diquat usually is compounded for spraying as diquat dibromide [6,7-dihydrodipyrido(1,2-a:2',1'-c)pyrazidinium dibromide; $C_{12}H_{12}N_2Br_2$]. Its melting point is between 335° and 340°C; its molecular weight is 344.07 D. Diquat does not produce the pulmonary fibrosis seen in paraquat poisoning.

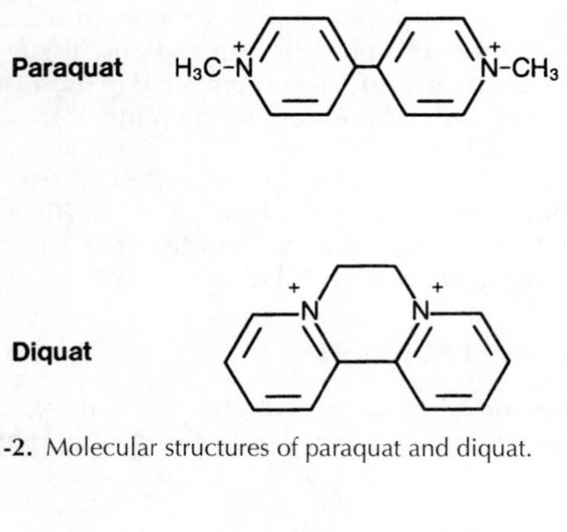

Paraquat H_3C-N^+ ... N^+-CH_3

Diquat

Figure 101-2. Molecular structures of paraquat and diquat.

Zeneca Agrochemicals manufactures the following products containing paraquat either alone or in combination: Gramoxone, Starfire, and Cyclone for sale in the United States. Paraquat is sold as Secatutto in Italy, as Preglox in Japan, as Gramonol in Holland, and as Spray Seed in Australia (86). The most common paraquat formulation is a 20% solution (200 mg per 100 cc). Manufacturers' directions usually recommend dilution at approximately 40 times to a 0.5% weight-per-volume paraquat ion solution (85). Other application procedures suggest a 100 to 200 times dilution for a spray solution. Inhalational poisonings may produce low toxicity because pulmonary absorption is low, as most of the aerosolized particles are larger than 5 mm in diameter and, therefore, are nonrespirable (i.e., do not reach the alveolar barrier) (85,87).

Sites, Industries, and Businesses Associated with Exposure

Paraquat may be applied using hand-held knapsack sprayers or vehicles (all-terrain vehicles, farm tractors, and high-cycle tractors) with attached spray booms. It may be applied also via aerial spraying (85). Skin exposure is thought to be the most significant route of occupational exposure (85). The most common sources of exposure occur in the manufacture or application of these compounds. The highest risk exists for contamination from spills and splashes during mixing, loading, and maintenance activities. The potential exists for exposure of civilian populations near application sites.

Clinical Toxicology

Paraquat is highly corrosive to tissue. It is absorbed poorly after inhalation but is extremely toxic if ingested (88). After paraquat ingestion, edema, burns, or ulceration may be seen in the mucosa of the mouth, pharynx, esophagus, stomach, and intestines (89). Death usually occurs within 48 hours of ingestion of 50 mg per kg; at lower doses, death may be delayed for several weeks (88). Toxicity is due to the bipyridyl compound's pulmonary accumulation, when it accepts an electron and forms a free radical (2). Paraquat ion is transported actively into pulmonary cells. Pulmonary edema or fibrosis is the sequela of lung uptake (87,89). Lipid peroxidation ensues, and nicotinamide adenine dinucleotide phosphate is depleted (88). Centrizonal hepatic necrosis, proximal renal tubule damage, myocardial damage, and skeletal muscle damage with focal necrosis may be seen. Pancreatic damage and CNS injury may occur. Pulmonary fibrosis usually begins 2 to 14 days after poisoning. With large ingestions (more than 20 mg per kg), pulmonary edema may be seen. Paraquat oxidation produces superoxide (free radical oxygen) ions, which cause mucous membrane lesions and secondary necrosis of the GI tract, liver, pancreas, renal tubules, and adrenal glands by lipid peroxidation.

Paraquat is excreted unchanged in the urine. Paraquat renal elimination is greater than the glomerular filtration rate in individuals with normal creatinine clearance. Paraquat does not appear to bioaccumulate. In animal models, low intravenous or subcutaneous doses are excreted rapidly in the urine (90–93). In the canine model, paraquat is not metabolized (94).

Intravenous paraquat infusions at 30 to 50 mg per kg produced rapid urinary excretion at clearance rates in excess of the glomerular filtration rate, signifying paraquat elimination by active secretion. Doses of 20 mg per kg produced renal failure. The kinetics could be described by a three-compartment model with the lungs as a slow uptake compartment. Paraquat doses high enough to cause renal failure did not produce peak lung concentrations until 15 hours after ingestion. This outcome means that initiation of paraquat removal by hemoperfusion in the first 12 to 15 hours should be helpful. Some have proposed that within the first 24 hours, humans who have ingested paraquat and have urinary paraquat concentrations of more than 10 mg per mL and lower creatinine clearance values should receive hemodialysis or hemoperfusion. Other studies disagree.

Oral ingestion of paraquat (all dilutions) has an average mortality rate of 33% to 50%. Mortality from an ingestion of the 20% solution may approach 78% (87). Potential exists for fatality from as little as one mouthful of a 20% solution. Death may be due either to circulatory failure at 3 days after ingestion or progressive irreversible pulmonary fibrosis at 5 to 31 days after ingestion.

The minimum lethal human dose is approximately 35 mg per kg (87,95). A mouthful (approximately 20 mL) produces a dose of 55 mg per kg in the average 70-kg adult. A study of 28 paraquat oral poisoning victims reported that one mouthful produced 6 of 12 deaths (50%) from pulmonary fibrosis at 5 to 31 days after ingestion; 11 to 12 (92%) died from circulatory failure within 48 hours after ingesting more than one mouthful (87,95).

The kinetics of paraquat poisoning in humans are similar to those in the canine model, with the peak plasma concentration attained by 2 hours after ingestion (96,97). Plasma concentrations decline quickly as the ion is distributed to the tissues. This fact obviously has implications for treatment, as any modality, such as charcoal hemoperfusion, must be initiated within this time frame if it is to be effective.

Absorption of paraquat is believed to take place in the small intestine. In rats and dogs, paraquat plasma concentrations are proportional to the amount of paraquat in the small intestine. Such medications as propantheline were administered to dogs to decrease gastric emptying time. This resulted in decreased paraquat plasma concentrations (94). Conversely, drugs that increase emptying time increase plasma concentrations. Food in the stomach or GI tract may decrease paraquat plasma concentrations. Lung and kidney paraquat concentrations continue to rise even after plasma concentrations seem to stabilize. Lung paraquat accumulation is an energy-dependent process that follows zero-order (saturable) kinetics. This system can be blocked by metabolic inhibitors, such as cyanide and iodoacetate.

Plasma paraquat concentrations have a predictive value with regard to survival. Patients whose plasma concentrations do not exceed 2.0, 0.6, 0.3, 0.16, and 0.1 mg per L at 4, 6, 10, 16, and 24 hours, respectively, are likely to survive (98,99). Plasma paraquat concentrations greater than 5 mg per L usually are fatal. In one study of ten cases in Crete, all patients with paraquat concentrations exceeding 5 mg per L died (100). In the same study, two patients with paraquat levels of 2.7 (approximately 41 hours after ingestion) and 2.8 mg per L (approximately 6 hours after ingestion) did not survive.

Paraquat crosses the placenta. Fetal concentration is four to six times that of the mother's. The fetus appears to tolerate maternal paraquat poisoning while it is dependent on the placental circulation and if the gestational age is less than 30 weeks. After that, birth and exposure to atmospheric oxygen result in signs of paraquat poisoning (100,101). Poor late-gestation survival may be due to the fact that type II pneumocytes appear between 28 and 32 weeks of gestation (100).

SIGNS, SYNDROMES, AND SYMPTOMS FROM TOXIC EXPOSURE

The severity of paraquat poisoning symptoms depends on the dose consumed. Most human fatalities are the result of suicide. Individuals consuming large amounts of paraquat usually die within a few days from cardiovascular collapse, whereas those consuming less usually succumb many days to weeks later of irreversible pulmonary fibrosis (87,95,102).

Two phases of paraquat pulmonary toxicity have been described. In phase I, type I and type II alveolar epithelial cells are destroyed (102). Alveolitis with extensive pulmonary destruction occurs. Pulmonary edema may develop with the infiltration of polymorphonuclear leukocytes into the lung tissue. Phase II is marked by extensive intraalveolar and interalveolar fibrosis. Normal alveolar architecture is destroyed and replaced by fibrous tissue. Gas exchange is impeded severely, leading to hypoxia and death.

Paraquat ion exposure may cause injuries to the nails, skin, eyes, and nose. These injuries result from exposure to the extremely irritating concentrated solutions prior to dilution. Paraquat produces a strong irritant action on various types of epithelial tissues. It can cause dryness, erythema, blistering, irritation, and ulceration and fissuring of the skin (103–105). Inhalation may cause epistaxis. Contact dermatitis has been reported after topical exposure. It is thought that paraquat diluted according to manufacturers' recommendations is unlikely to cause skin burns unless spray-soaked clothing is worn for prolonged periods. In one study, 15 consecutive occupational cases of a single skin or eye exposure to paraquat solutions caused only local lesions; no systemic effects were detected in affected patients (106).

Localized discoloration or a transverse white band of discoloration affecting the nail plate may be seen in spray operators (103–105). Transverse ridging and furrowing of the nail may progress to an irregular nail deformity and subsequent nail loss. Once exposure stops, normal nail growth usually returns.

Ocular exposure to paraquat concentrate may cause corneal and conjunctival inflammation. Inflammation may develop gradually and progress to maximal damage over a 12- to 24-hour period. Corneal opacification may occur. Frank corneal ulceration and lacrimal duct stenosis has been reported (105). Miosis may be present. Sometimes the severity of these injuries goes relatively unnoticed until symptoms have progressed to corneal scarring and opacification.

Paraquat can be absorbed through the skin. Local and systemic toxicity has been reported after dermal exposure, which may produce local irritation, burns, or systemic effects.

Three stages of paraquat poisoning have been described (87,89,102):

1. *Group 1 (mild poisoning)*: Ingestion of less than 20 mg paraquat ion per kg of body weight. Patients may be asymptomatic or experience vomiting and diarrhea. Transient decrement in the carbon monoxide diffusing capacity and vital capacity may be seen. Complete recovery usually occurs.
2. *Group 2 (moderate poisoning)*: Ingestion of 20 to 40 mg paraquat ion per kg of body weight. Vomiting and diarrhea are followed by generalized symptomatology of systemic toxicity. All patients will develop pulmonary fibrosis. Renal and hepatic failure may be present. Most patients will expire, but death may be delayed for 2 to 4 weeks.
3. *Group 3 (severe poisoning)*: Ingestion of more than 40 mg paraquat ion per kg of body weight. Nausea, vomiting, and diarrhea with marked oropharyngeal and esophageal ulceration are followed by failure of multiple organs (cardiac, respiratory, hepatic, renal adrenal, pancreatic, and CNS). Cardiotoxicity signs may include ventricular arrhythmias, hypotension, or cardiorespiratory arrest. Mortality usually is 100%, with death occurring usually in the first 24 hours after ingestion.

Initial symptoms of paraquat ingestion include burning of the mouth, throat, chest, and abdomen. Giddiness, headache, fever, myalgia, bloody diarrhea, and abdominal pain may be present. Urinalysis may show proteinuria, hematuria, or pyuria. Acute tubular necrosis may develop.

MANAGEMENT OF TOXICITY

Treatment of paraquat or diquat poisoning is difficult and may be ineffective. Use of absorbents, such as activated charcoal or fuller's earth, may blunt the paraquat absorption (88). Obtaining a clear history of the circumstances of the ingestion is vital in assessing victims of paraquat poisoning. The history should quantify the interval between ingestion and admission, circumstances of poisoning (accidental versus suicidal), exact name of paraquat or diquat compound and other ingredients, such as solvent vehicles, amount ingested and route, vomiting after ingestion, and time of last meal.

Clinical Examination. Acutely exposed patients should be removed from the source of the exposure and decontaminated as the exposure and condition warrant. Rescue personnel should wear appropriate gloves, boots, and goggles (107).

Chronically exposed patients require the recording of a complete toxicologic history and physical examination, with special attention given to the pulmonary system. A comprehensive occupational history also should be obtained. Areas of skin or eye exposure should be flushed copiously with water. Skin should be monitored for abrasions, inflammation, and the development of secondary infection.

Treatment. Urinary paraquat excretion is 20 to 50 times greater than plasma concentrations (108). Patients with normal renal function after ingestion have a paraquat clearance higher than creatinine clearance. This is due to active tubular secretion and nonionic diffusion additive to the glomerular filtration rate. Paraquat is not reabsorbed from the renal tubules; thus, forced diuresis does not enhance paraquat elimination. Forced diuresis still is advocated, because it may reduce the concentration of paraquat in the renal tubules.

To maximize chances for paraquat removal, GI decontamination should be initiated as soon as possible after paraquat ingestion and should be instituted on any suspicion of ingestion. Either fuller's earth or bentonite usually is used. If neither is available, activated charcoal may be used, as it has been shown to absorb paraquat almost as efficiently as fuller's earth or bentonite. Desorption of paraquat from the activated charcoal–paraquat complex as it passes through the GI tract is a theoretic (but not confirmed) disadvantage of the use of charcoal (102). Hypercalcemia may occur after the use of fuller's earth (109).

The activated charcoal dose for adults is 30 to 100 g; for children younger than age 12, it is 15 to 30 g or 1 to 2 g per kg. Bentonite clay USP (7% suspension) is administered to adults at 100 to 150 g and to children younger than age 12 at 2 g per kg. The dose for fuller's earth (30% suspension) is 100 to 150 g for adults and 2 g per kg for children younger than 12 years.

If less than 1 hour has passed since ingestion of paraquat, gastric lavage should be performed with a large-bore tube (102). The efficacy of gastric lavage probably is highest in the first hour after ingestion. Because of the high morbidity and mortality associated with paraquat poisoning, the decision to institute gastric lavage more than 1 hour after ingestion must be made on a case-by-case basis. After lavage, one of the aforementioned absorbents should be instilled via lavage tube. Doses may be repeated at 2- to 4-hour intervals. Bowel sounds and signs of GI perforation, hemorrhage, or ileus should be monitored. Magnesium sulfate or sorbitol may be used as a cathartic with the first absorbent (109). Hypermagnesemia has been reported after repeated administration of magnesium-containing cathartics in poisoned patients with normal renal function (110). Multiple dosing with cathartics is not recommended, as large fluid and electrolyte shifts are possible with catharsis.

Supplemental oxygen should not be given, as this increases paraquat pulmonary toxicity. Late stages of poisoning may require oxygen as pulmonary fibrosis develops. Hemodialysis is not effective in treating paraquat or diquat poisoning (111,112). Charcoal hemoperfusion has not been shown to reduce paraquat morbidity or mortality (102). A theoretic benefit is seen in clearing blood paraquat if hemoperfusion can be instituted during the first 2 hours after the poisoning. Neither hemoperfusion nor hemodialysis has been shown to be effective in reducing paraquat or diquat body burden (111,112). Pharmacokinetic data indicate a marked rebound effect from tissue on plasma paraquat levels. Thus, prolonged hemodialysis or hemoperfusion has been advocated by some authors (100). Lung transplantation has not been successful either, because the transplanted lung develops paraquat toxicity or other comorbidity factors (102,113,114).

Major prognostic indicators include route of administration (inhalation usually less severe than oral); ingested amount; time of last meal (as food delays absorption and neutralizes paraquat); gastric lesions; renal failure; and plasma paraquat concentrations.

Diquat ingestion, like that of paraquat, damages multiple organ systems. The clinical pattern is different even though diquat and paraquat share common mechanisms of toxicity. Infarction and purpura of the brainstem appear to be specific to diquat poisoning (115,116). Pontine purpura has been reported in three of seven adults who died from diquat ingestion (115,116). Potentially toxic diquat ion doses are in the range of 35 to 105 mL of the 20% solution. Diquat poisoning is characterized by GI tract injury, including burns to the oral mucosa, acute tubular necrosis, and bronchopneumonia. Paralytic ileus is seen more frequently in diquat than in paraquat ion poisoning. Pulmonary fibrosis is not seen in diquat ion poisoning, as diquat is not transported actively by lung tissue. Inhalation may produce nonspecific respiratory distress symptoms. Diquat produces cataracts in rats and dogs but, to date, not in humans. Treatment is similar to that of paraquat ion poisoning. Prompt initiation of charcoal hemoperfusion may be beneficial in minimizing tissue distribution and uptake by target organs.

Laboratory Diagnosis. Patients exposed to paraquat or diquat require the recording of a full biochemical profile, including hepatic enzymes (AST, ALT, GGT, and LDH), electrolytes, glucose, blood urea nitrogen, creatinine, serum aldolase, complete blood count, arterial blood gases, chest radiograph, and urinalysis. Chronically exposed patients also require a thyroid profile, vitamin B_{12}, and folate determination to assist in differentiation of other neurologic diseases.

Special Diagnostic Tests. The dithionite test is a rapid, semiquantitative colorimetric urine test that may be performed to detect paraquat (117). To 1 volume, add 0.5 volume 1% sodium dithionite (sodium hydrosulfite), add 1 normal sodium hydroxide. After 1 minute, the color should change: A deep blue reflects paraquat or diquat, with a urinary concentration of less than 0.5 mg per L. Positive or negative controls should be run (117). Urinary diquat is signified by the color green. In either case, the deeper the color, the higher is the relative paraquat or diquat concentration and the worse is the prognosis.

Paraquat may be measured via spectrophotometry, gas chromatography, high-performance liquid chromatography, or radioimmunoassay techniques. Radioimmunoassay is the sensitive and specific procedure. Plastic containers are used for urine and plasma samples (102). Plasma paraquat levels are important prognostic indicators. Plasma levels that exceed 5 mg per L invariably indicate a fatal outcome (102).

Medical information about paraquat poisoning and urine and plasma sample analysis for paraquat is available 24 hours per day, 7 days per week through the Zeneca Emergency Information Network [1-800-327-8633 (1-800-FASTMED)].

Paraquat Exposure Limits

The OSHA-established PEL for inhalation exposure to paraquat respirable dust is 0.5 mg per cubic meter (83). To prevent skin absorption, skin exposure should be prevented or reduced to the extent necessary in the workplace through the use of gloves, coveralls, goggles, or other appropriate personal protective equipment, engineering controls, and work practices.

The ACGIH TLV TWA are 0.5 mg per cubic meter of total dust as the cation and 0.1 mg per cubic meter of respirable dust as a fraction of the cation. No STEL has been established. The NIOSH REL TWA is 0.1 mg per cubic meter of respirable dust. The IDLH value is 1 mg per cubic meter. The NIOSH analytical method is 5003. The NIOSH REL for paraquat, either respiratory or skin exposure, is 0.1 mg per cubic meter. An IDLH concentration has been established at 1.5 mg per cubic meter.

The ACGIH TLV TWA for paraquat respirable sizes is 0.1 mg per cubic meter. No ACGIH STEL value exists (83). The OSHA and ACGIH TLV TWA for diquat is 0.5 mg per cubic meter (83).

GLYPHOSATE

Glyphosate (*N*-phosphonomethyl glycine) is an organophosphorus herbicide that does not inhibit cholinesterase function. It is marketed under a variety of trade names (Round-Up, Touchdown, Bronco, Network, and Kleen-Up). Glyphosate inhibits plant amino acid synthesis and has the chemical formula shown in Figure 101-3. The commercial product is formulated in water at concentrations between 0.5% and 5%. Concentrated Round-Up is sold as a 41% concentration prior to its final dilution as a 1% solution. Glyphosate usually is formulated with a 15% concentration of the nonionic tallow amine surfactant polyoxyethyleneamine (118). This surfactant aids in emulsifying the glyphosate. The toxicity of the Round-Up product has been attributed to both the glyphosate herbicide and to the surfactant (103,119). Uncoupling of oxidative phosphorylation has been proposed as the mechanism of toxicity for glyphosate (120). The toxicity of the surfactant has been reviewed and includes vomiting, diarrhea, hemolysis of red blood cells, hypotension, altered mental status, and pulmonary edema (121). Further study of the mechanism of both glyphosate and the surfactant is required.

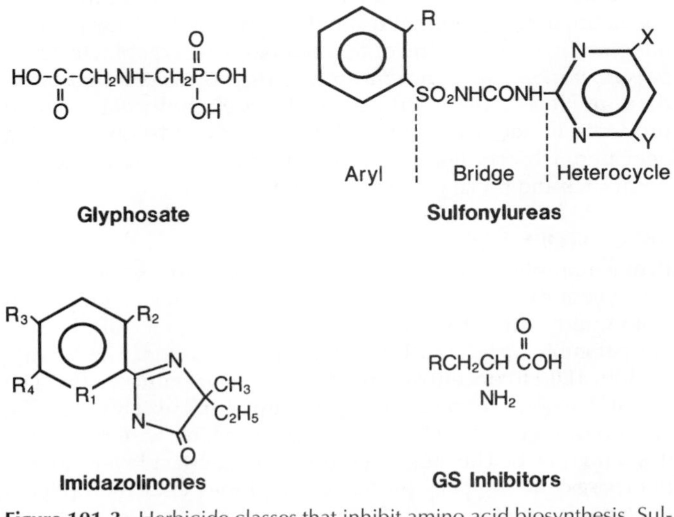

Glyphosate   Sulfonylureas (Aryl, Bridge, Heterocycle)

Imidazolinones   GS Inhibitors

Figure 101-3. Herbicide classes that inhibit amino acid biosynthesis. Sulfonylureas: R equals carboxymethyl, carboxyethyl, chloro, chloroethoxy; X + Y equals methoxy, chloro, methylethoxy. Imidazolinones: R_1 equals C or N; R_2 equals carboxy or carboxymethyl; R_3 equals H or phenylcarbon; R_4 equals H, ethyl, methyl, or phenylcarbon. GH inhibitors: R equals $CH_3POOHCH_2$, $CH_3SONHCH_2$, cyclic $CH_2NHCOCOH$. (From Duke S. Overview of herbicide mechanisms of action. *Environ Health Perspect* 1990;87:263–271.)

Clinical manifestations of ingestion of the product include pharyngitis, vomiting, diarrhea, abdominal pain, hepatic damage, leukocytosis, hypotension, renal damage with oliguria, and erosions of the esophagus, oropharynx, and stomach (103). Ocular exposure can cause conjunctivitis. Inhalation of the mist of the product can cause respiratory irritation. Other dermal contact has caused dermatitis and mild chemical burns. Glyphosate is poorly absorbed from both the GI tract and the skin. In a retrospective study, Tominack et al. (122) described a clinical toxic syndrome after ingestion of a mouthful or more as follows: hypotension, shock, oral esophageal and GI mucosal injury, pulmonary edema, oliguria or anuria, metabolic acidosis, leukocytosis, and fever.

As most poisoning from the product occurs by ingestion, clinical management is directed at controlling potential massive GI fluid loss and renal failure. Vomiting is common after ingestion; therefore, inducing emesis is unnecessary. Also, because the product is caustic to the esophagus, inducing emesis is not recommended. Administration of 30 g of activated charcoal may aid in adsorption of glyphosate and the surfactant. Aspiration of the product can produce pulmonary injury with pulmonary edema, so the airway must be protected. Intravenous rehydration is crucial to maintaining blood pressure and urine output.

Round-Up concentrate contains 41% glyphosate, and Kleen-Up contains up to 5% of the base herbicide. No PEL has been established for glyphosate or the surfactant.

FUNGICIDES AND BIOCIDES

Fungicides and biocides commonly are used in a variety of products to prevent the growth of microorganisms, such as bacteria and fungi. Fungicides are mixed into many types of paints and other products in which the growth of bacteria and fungi is undesirable. Fungicides and biocides are used also on vegetables and fruits. As a group of compounds, fungicides are diverse (Table 101-4) and include inorganic compounds, organometals, nitrobenzene, and phenol derivatives.

Pentachlorophenol

PRODUCTION, USES, AND SOURCES

Pentachlorophenol has been used extensively throughout the United States as a wood preservative and fungicide. Its most common use was as a wood preservative for telephone poles. The compound is produced by the chlorination of phenol in the presence of a catalyst. Commercial-grade pentachlorophenol is at least 86% pure and contains contaminants of other polychlorinated phenols, such as polychlorinated dibenzodioxins and polychlorinated dibenzofurans (123). Pure pentachlorophenol is a white organic solid with needlelike crystals (124). Impure pentachlorophenol (the form usually found at hazardous-waste sites) is dark gray to brown dust, beads, or flakes (125). Heating pentachlorophenol produces a sharp, characteristic phenolic odor, although very little odor is present at room temperature.

TABLE 101-4. Fungicides and biocides

Acrolein
2,3-Dichloro-1,4-naphthaquinone
Dithiocarbamates
  Ferbam
  Maneb
  Thiram
  Zineb
  Ziram
Formaldehyde
Inorganic metals
  Copper sulfate
Karathane (crotonic acid)
Organometals
  Bis(tributyltin) oxide
  Cyclohexylhydrostannane (plictran)
  Methylmercury
  Triethyltin
  Trimethyltin
  Triphenyltin
Pentachloronitrobenzene
Pentachlorophenol
Thiabendazoles
  Benomyl
  Thiabendazole
  Thiophanate methyl

Eighty percent of U.S. consumption of pentachlorophenol and its sodium salt (sodium pentachlorophenate) was as a wood preservative. It was registered for use as an insecticide, fungicide, acaricide, and herbicide and as a disinfectant. It also was used as an antifouling agent in paint. Although once widely used as an herbicide, it was banned in 1987 for these and other uses and for over-the-counter sales (126). Pentachlorophenol now is a restricted-use compound. It still is used in industry as a wood preservative for power poles, railroad ties, cross arms, and fence posts. Most commercial lumber produced in the United States still is treated with sodium pentachlorophenate to control fungal growth and sap stain (127). Pentachlorophenol no longer is used for wood-preserving solutions, insecticides, fungicides, or herbicides available for home use (124).

Owing to its extensive use throughout the United States, pentachlorophenol has been found in a variety of air, water, and soil samples. In 1983, production of pentachlorophenol totaled 45 million pounds (126). According to the EPA's toxic chemical release inventory, land and water releases between 1987 and 1993 totaled almost 100,000 pounds (126). The most widespread releases emanated from wood-preserving, explosives, and various chemical industries in many states. The EPA lists Arizona, Georgia, Nevada, Oregon, and Washington as the top five states experiencing land and water releases. The largest releases were from a military munitions plant in Nevada (126). Pentachlorophenol is a very stable compound and is not hydrolyzed or oxidized easily. However, it does undergo photooxidation by sunlight and can be biotransformed by soil microorganisms (124). Human exposure to pentachlorophenol is common and occurs through ingestion of contaminated water and food and from breathing of contaminated air. Pentachlorophenol is detected frequently in human biological media, such as plasma, blood, and urine.

EXPOSURE

Exposure to pentachlorophenol occurs in occupational settings and through environmental contamination sources. Some human exposure from indoor air pollution sources of pentachlorophenol occurs because the wood structure of affected homes may have been treated previously with the compound as a preservative. Pentachlorophenol is detected in adipose tissue, human milk, blood, and urine. On the average, the U.S. population has been shown to have urine concentrations of pentachlorophenol of approximately 5 ppb (123). Occupational exposure to pentachlorophenol as a wood preservative may yield urine concentrations that approximate 120 ppb.

Analyses of blood and urine samples from 6,000 persons in 64 communities within the United States were conducted between 1976 and 1980 (123). Pentachlorophenol was one of the compounds detected in 79% of urine samples collected in this survey. The level of pentachlorophenol in these urine samples was between 6 and 193 ppb. Blood concentrations of pentachlorophenol also varied, depending on severity of exposure. Individuals occupationally exposed to pentachlorophenol or using pentachlorophenol-treated materials have blood concentrations ranging from 83 to 57,600 ppb (123). Most affected individuals assessed in the federal study were involved in construction of log homes that were treated previously with pentachlorophenol (123). The adipose concentration of pentachlorophenol was shown in 1973 to be a mean of 26.3 g per kg in the general U.S. population (123). Dietary intake of pentachlorophenol occurs through contaminated food products. In a 1976 survey, pentachlorophenol was found also in drinking water supplies at a mean concentration of 0.07 g per L, the maximum concentration being 0.7 g per L (123).

Another survey of drinking water supplies detected pentachlorophenol between the ranges of 1 and 12 g per L in eight cities (123). Food and water supplies are common environmental sources of human intake of pentachlorophenol.

Indoor pentachlorophenol air concentrations can be particularly high in log homes or older homes that have been pretreated with the compound as a preservative. In air samples taken in log homes, pentachlorophenol has been found in the range of 7 to 8 ppb. Pentachlorophenol-treated wood products are another source of indoor air concentrations of this substance. In older homes, pentachlorophenol has been found by the EPA to range from 0.5 to 10.0 g per cubic meter (123). Higher concentrations at these levels of pentachlorophenol in treated wood have ranged from 34 to 104 g per cubic meter (123).

Human exposure to pentachlorophenol occurs by inhalation, ingestion, and the dermal route. Most occupational exposures have involved pest control applicators, carpenters, electrical power workers, and those in trades or professions that bring them in close contact with pentachlorophenol-treated wood products. Other at-risk populations include individuals living near pentachlorophenol-manufacturing sites and waste disposal sites and those who work in lumber mills.

REGULATORY ASPECTS

Pentachlorophenol is on the list of chemicals that appear in the toxic chemicals section (no. 313) of the Emergency Planning and Community Right to Know Act of 1986. The OSHA PEL is 0.5 mg per cubic meter as a TWA with a skin notation. The NIOSH lists an IDLH concentration of 150 mg per cubic meter. The ACGIH recommends a TLV of 0.5 mg per cubic meter. The National Academy of Sciences' safe drinking water guide is 0.021 mg per L. The suggested no-adverse-effect levels are 6 g per L in a child, 7 g per L of a technical-grade pentachlorophenol in an adult, and 9 g per L of commercial-grade pentachlorophenol in an adult. The EPA has listed pentachlorophenol as a hazardous waste and as a priority toxic pollutant.

PHYSICAL AND CHEMICAL CHARACTERISTICS

The molecular formula of pentachlorophenol is C_6Cl_5OH. It is a light-brown solid having a pungent odor and a melting point of 187°C. Pentachlorophenol is known also as *PCP, penchlorol,* and *Dowicide EC-7.* Pentachlorophenol is incompatible with strong oxidizers.

CLINICAL TOXICOLOGY AND HEALTH EFFECTS

Once absorbed, pentachlorophenol is highly protein-bound. Most of the compound undergoes glucuronide conjugation. A small amount is dechlorinated oxidatively to tetrachlorohydroquinone, which has been used as an occupational exposure marker. Elimination half-lives vary from 10 hours in acute exposure to 19 to 20 days in chronically exposed workers. The protein binding of pentachlorophenol may cause conformational changes in various enzymes involved in the cytochrome system, thus inhibiting oxidative phosphorylation (127).

In general, pentachlorophenol produces irritation of the eyes, nose, throat, and mucous membranes. Inhalation of pentachlorophenol compounds is a common mode of exposure. Deaths have occurred after acute inhalation (123). Inhalation produces irritation of the upper respiratory tract, coughing, and symptoms of bronchitis with chest tightness. Inhalational exposure also can produce cardiac effects of tachycardia. Ingestion of pentachlorophenol can result in abdominal pain, nausea, and vomiting with systemic absorption. Among the target organs for toxicity are the liver, kidneys, hematopoietic system, pulmonary system, and CNS. Pulmonary inhalation of high concentrations can result in pulmonary edema and death (123).

Cases of aplastic anemia have been associated with pentachlorophenol exposure (123). Pentachlorophenol-induced liver toxicity in humans has occurred in herbicide sprayers (123). Fatty infiltration of the liver and central lobular congestion with hepatocellular accumulation of fat have been noted. Also, elevation of liver enzymes has been seen after chronic dermal exposure to pentachlorophenol (123). Kidney effects secondary to exposure to pentachlorophenol also have been noted, as have increased incidents of proteinuria and hematuria.

Ocular and dermal exposure to pentachlorophenol can produce serious damage. Corneal injury can occur from splashes to the eye. Vapors of pentachlorophenol can produce ocular irritation, and the chemical can induce dermatitis, inflammation of the skin, desquamation, and hair loss (123).

The neurotoxicity of pentachlorophenol also has been recognized. Neurotoxicity usually occurs only after massive exposure. Hyperthermia, probably due to uncoupling of oxidative phosphorylation, has been observed. No report of peripheral neuropathy secondary to exposure has been issued. Lethargy and cerebral edema have occurred after short-term, high-level exposures to pentachlorophenol. These effects have been accompanied by seizures, coma, delirium, and hyperthermia.

No evidence of human immunotoxic effects from pentachlorophenol has been documented; however, animal studies have shown immunotoxic effects. No evidence supports reproductive toxicity or developmental effects secondary to human exposure to pentachlorophenol. However, an increase in the frequency of chromosomal aberrations has been seen in the peripheral lymphocytes of workers who are occupationally exposed to this compound (123).

Pentachlorophenol is well absorbed by the inhalational, dermal, and GI routes. The half-life of elimination of pentachlorophenol from plasma was found to be approximately 30 hours in human volunteers. Also, in the same study, 74% of a pentachlorophenol dose administered to human volunteers was eliminated as the parent compound, and 12% was eliminated as a glucuronide metabolite within 168 hours (123). Pentachlorophenol elimination is thought to follow first-order kinetics, with some enterohepatic recirculation after ingestion.

TREATMENT

No specific treatment for pentachlorophenol exposure exists. Removal of affected individuals from the exposure source and supportive care are the mainstays of treatment. Forced diuresis is not indicated (127).

2,3-Dichloro-1,4-Naphthoquinone

2,3-Dichloro-1,4-naphthoquinone (dichloronapthoquinone) is marketed under the trade names Algistat, Compound 604, Dichlone, Phygon, and Phygon XL. It has a molecular formula of $C_{10}H_4Cl_2O_2$ and a molecular weight of 227.04. Vapor density is 7.8 (density of air, 1.0). This compound is insoluble in water and moderately soluble in organic acids. It is a fungicide and algicide used for foliage and textiles and for seed disinfectant. It decomposes slowly in soil and water and may be stable enough to bioaccumulate up the food chain. A very irritating dust, this compound is considered to be moderately toxic by ingestion and is a skin, ocular, and mucous membrane irritant. CNS depression has been reported after substantial exposure. Thermal decomposition products include chlorine gas. Carcinogenicity data regarding 2,3-dichloro-1,4-naphthoquinone are inconclusive (128).

Thiabendazole Fungicides

The thiabendazole class of fungicides comprises heterocyclic derivatives of the parent thiabendazole (Fig. 101-4). These compounds include benomyl, thiabendazole, and thiophanate methyl. Three compounds of this class—benomyl, thiabendazole, and thiophenate-methyl—have been used extensively for the treatment of human and veterinary helminthiasis. Thiabendazole and its congeners produce many biochemical changes in susceptible nematodes: inhibition of mitochondrial fumarate reductase, reduced glucose transport, and uncoupling of oxidative phosphorylation. Inhibition of microtubule polymerization by binding to β-tubulin is the primary action of this drug class. The selective toxicity of these agents stems from the fact that specific, high-affinity binding to parasite β-tubulin occurs at much lower concentrations than does mammalian protein binding (129).

BENOMYL

Benomyl is a benzimidazole carbamate systemic fungicide. It is a white crystalline solid with a chemical formula of $C_{14}H_{18}N_4O_3$. It has been used widely as a fungicide for fruits and vegetables.

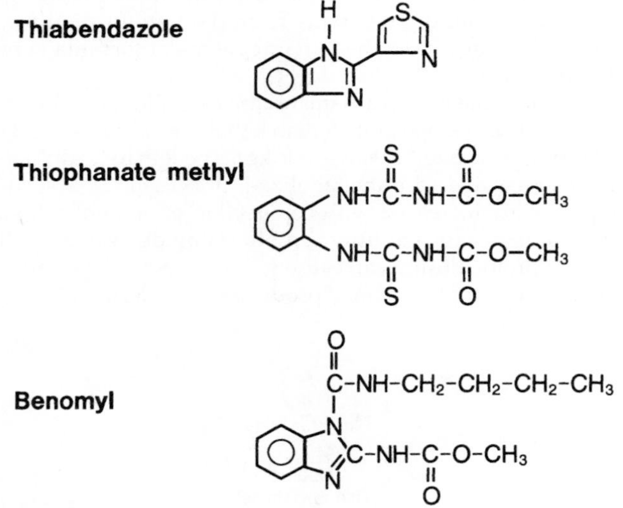

Figure 101-4. Thiabendazole fungicides.

Human health effects are related to its dermal irritant effects. On contact with the skin, it can produce erythema and edema (130). Benomyl also may cause eye and respiratory tract irritation. It does not inhibit acetylcholinesterase; therefore, this fungicide does not cause a cholinergic poisoning syndrome. Treatment is symptomatic and supportive.

The ACGIH TLV TWA is 0.84 parts per million (ppm) (10 mg per cubic meter) with an A4 designation. The OSHA PEL TWA is 15 mg per cubic meter as total dust and 5 mg per cubic meter as respirable fraction. No NIOSH REL exists for benomyl. The NIOSH analytical methods are 0500 (total dust) and 0600 (respirable particulates).

THIABENDAZOLE

Thiabendazole has the formula of $C_{10}H_7N_3S$ and is a white odorless powder used as an anthelmintic and fungicide (130). Thiabendazole contains a thiazole ring at position 2. Given orally, it is active against a wide range of GI tract nematodes, such as hookworm, roundworm, pinworm, and threadworm. Thiabendazole is absorbed rapidly in the GI tract and readily through the skin as a fungicidal agent. Oral thiabendazole incites the following adverse effects: nausea, dizziness, diarrhea, abdominal discomfort, drowsiness, headache, and vertigo. Acute oral overdoses may result in seizures, hyperexcitability, hypotension, bradycardia, renal toxicity, and hepatic toxicity. Hypersensitivity reactions include rashes, conjunctivitis, erythema multiforme, Stevens-Johnson syndrome, and angioedema. Because of its high relative side effects and toxicity, its use as a human drug has declined (131).

THIOPHANATE METHYL

Thiophanate methyl is a colorless crystalline solid. It has a molecular formula of $C_{12}H_{14}N_4O_4S_2$ and is water soluble (130). On contact with this compound, dermatitis consisting of swelling, erythema, and itching may ensue (130).

Dithiocarbamates

Dithiocarbamates include ferbam, thiram, methamsodium, ziram, sulfallate, anobam, maneb, nabam, and zineb (132). Dithiocarbamates find use mainly as fungicides, although some of these compounds are used as herbicides, and at least one—methamsodium—is used as a nematocide (132). The well-known drug disulfiram (Antabuse) is tetraethylthiuram, a dithiocarbamate compound used to treat alcoholism. Many of the dithiocarbamates can interact with ethanol and cause an Antabuse-like reaction (133). Most of our understanding of this class of compounds stems from data about disulfiram. Dithiocarbamates have the general chemical formula shown in Figure 101-5.

In general, the dithiocarbamates are of moderate to low toxicity (132). The average oral median lethal dose value is 2,523 mg per kg (range, 285 to 7,500 mg per kg). The less toxic dithiocarbamates are excreted unmetabolized in feces (132). Poisoning symptoms are increased with coingestion of ethanol. All such compounds produce antithyroid effects by decreasing iodine uptake. Chronic dosing can cause goiter. These compounds are also dermal irritants that may produce severe dermatitis.

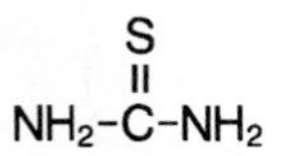

S
II
NH_2-C-NH_2

Thiourea
(Thiocarbamide)

Figure 101-5. Thiocarbamate fungicides—general structure.

FERBAM

Ferbam is a dithiocarbamate fungicide with the trade name of Cormate or Fermacide. It has a molecular formula of $C_9H_{18}N_3S_6Fe$ and a molecular weight of 416.5 D (130). Ferbam is used to control diseases in fruit and tobacco crops, conifers, ornamentals, nuts, and vegetables. Some specific target diseases include apple scab, cedar apple rust, peachleaf curl, tobacco blue mold, and cranberry diseases. This fungicide does not tend to persist in the environment and is degraded by soil microbes within approximately 28 days. Toxicologic data about this compound are limited. However, it is a chemical irritant to the eyes, skin, and mucous membranes and has a potential to produce kidney damage.

The OSHA PEL for this chemical is 15 mg per cubic meter (as total dust). The ACGIH TLV TWA is 10 mg per cubic meter; it is designated A4, not classifiable as a human carcinogen. The NIOSH REL is 10 mg per cubic meter. The IDLH value is 800 mg per cubic meter (83). The IARC classifies ferbam as a group 3 compound (unclassifiable as to carcinogenicity in humans) (134).

THIRAM

Thiram (tetramethylthiuram disulfide) is a general-use fungicide with a formula of $C_6H_{12}N_2S_4$ and molecular weight of 240.44 D (130). It takes the form of colorless crystals and is formulated as a powder and dust for application as a seed treatment. The dithiocarbamates can produce systemic toxic reactions of a disulfiram-like reaction if absorbed concurrently with ethanol. Other reported systemic toxicity includes nausea, vomiting, abdominal pain, hyperexcitability, and weakness (130). Thiram can produce contact dermatitis, but this response is not very common (135). Thiram has been used in the rubber industry as a vulcanizing agent.

It is insoluble in water but soluble in organic solvents and is decomposed after exposure to acids. In addition to being used as a fungicide, it has been used as an accelerator in the rubber industry and as an antioxidant. Thiram is a degradation product of both ferbam and ziram (136). Human exposure occurs via inhalation or skin exposure to dusts, sprays, mists, or aerosolized forms of the product.

Toxic exposure to thiram produces irritation of the eyes, mucous membranes, and skin. Erythema and urticarial reactions can occur after dermal exposure to thiram. Allergic contact dermatitis also can occur (136).

Thiram (Tetrathiuram) is metabolized by the liver to carbon disulfide. Environmentally, thiram can be degraded to carbon disulfide, hydrogen sulfide, and dimethylamine, all of which are toxic by-products. Thiram may produce hepatic toxicity once it is absorbed systematically (136). Other toxic manifestations of thiram include nausea, dizziness, headache, confusion, diarrhea, and flaccid paralysis (136). Death has occurred after ingestion. Thiram can produce GI focal necrosis.

The OSHA PEL TLV TWA is 5 mg per cubic meter. The ACGIH TLV TWA is 1.0 mg per cubic meter, with an A4 designation (83). No ACGIH ceiling or STEL limit has been set. The NIOSH REL TWA is 5 mg per cubic meter, and the IDLH value is 100 mg per cubic meter. The NIOSH analytical method for thiram is 5005. The IARC classifies thiram as a group 3 compound (unclassifiable as to carcinogenicity in humans) (137). The permitted residue tolerance level as a fungicide on vegetables and fruits is 7 mg per kg (136).

ZIRAM

Ziram (zinc dimethyldithiocarbamate) has a formula of $C_6H_{12}N_2S_4Zn$, and is an odorless powder with a molecular weight of 305.8 D (130). The human toxic hazard is mainly due to airborne dust, as it has negligible vapor pressure. Ziram is an irritant of the eyes, upper airway, and mucous membranes.

Ingestion can produce localized necrosis of the GI tract (130). Owing to its irritant properties, ziram can produce respiratory irritation and distress on inhalation of dust. Ziram is classified in IARC group 3 (138).

Acrolein (Acrylaldehyde)

Acrolein (CH_2CHCHO) is a potent herbicide and biocide used to control weeds, algae, and plant growth in irrigation canals and water drainage areas. Acrolein is a clear to yellowish liquid with a pungent odor and is very irritating to the eyes, skin, and mucous membranes. This liquid is used to make other chemicals and pesticides and is found in some livestock feeds and pesticides. Small amounts of acrolein can be formed and can enter the air when organic matter, such as trees and other plants (including tobacco) and fuels (e.g., gasoline and oil), are burned (139). Exposure occurs mainly by inhalation or dermal-ocular liquid contact by accidental splash. Acrolein is marketed under a variety of trade names, including Magnacide and Magnacide-H. Human exposure can result in severe dermatitis and burns to the skin, eyes, and mucous membranes. The EPA lists acrolein as a hazardous material and restricts its use as a pesticide. It is used in the production of glycerine and in the synthesis of other chemicals. Acrolein is incompatible with oxidizers, ammonia, and alkalis.

Routes of exposure to acrolein are by inhalation, dermal contact, and ingestion. It is a highly volatile liquid with an extremely irritating vapor that is flammable and forms explosive mixtures in air. The basic product comes as 92% acrolein by weight in a cylinder connected to a nitrogen gas pressurized delivery system. Acrolein is a highly reactive aldehyde and readily polymerizes with generation of heat. Improper handling or storing of the product can create a hazard that can result in a polymerization reaction, release of heat, and rupturing of the container. Contamination with air, oxidizers, ammonia, or alkalis can initiate a violent polymerization reaction.

Acrolein products used as biocides contain nitrogen, which excludes air and prevents polymerization reactions. Hydroquinone is added to help to inhibit oxygen-initiated polymerization. Acrolein readily binds to sulfhydryl groups and is a general cell poison. It will kill aquatic wildlife if the water concentration is not controlled. The permissible water concentration to protect aquatic life is 21 g per L on a chronic basis and 68 g per L on an acute basis. The product is forced from its container by pressurized oxygen-free N_2 and is introduced directly into canal water to form a "wave" that slowly moves in the direction of water flow, killing all plant life that it contacts.

Acrolein vapor and liquid are potent irritants. Owing to its highly irritating vapor and lacrimator action, humans cannot tolerate vapor concentrations of 0.1 to 1.0 ppm for even short periods. Acute human exposure to high levels (10 ppm) can cause death (140). Pulmonary irritation occurs at levels ranging from 0.17 to 0.43 ppm. The acrolein odor threshold is 0.2 ppm (140). Splash exposures to the liquid concentrate produce rapid ocular and skin damage. Skin injury from the concentrate can produce edema, erythema, and second-degree burns. Inhalation of the vapor or liquid will produce respiratory irritation, mucous membrane irritation, difficulty in breathing, and pulmonary edema. Any splash exposure should be irrigated immediately with water for 15 to 20 minutes.

Chronic acrolein inhalational exposure causes generalized respiratory tract symptoms, including upper and lower respiratory tract irritation. To date, no human reproductive effects have been documented. Acrolein has been reported to cause birth defects in rats when it is injected directly into the embryo (139). No human data are available regarding the possible human carcinogenic effects of acrolein.

TABLE 101-5. Health effects resulting from vapor concentrations of acrolein

Vapor concentration	Exposure	Effect
0.25 ppm	5 min	Moderate irritation
1 ppm	2–3 min	Ocular and nose irritation
5.5 ppm	1 min	Intolerable
153 ppm	10 min	Can be fatal

The EPA recommends that the concentration of acrolein in water should not exceed 320 g per L (0.32 ppm) to protect human health (139). Vapor concentrations of acrolein produce health effects as shown in Table 101-5. Personal protective equipment, including eye, skin, and respiratory protection, should be used when working with acrolein.

The OSHA PEL is 0.1 ppm or 0.25 mg per cubic meter. The 1997 ACGIH TLV TWA also is 0.1 ppm or 0.25 mg per cubic meter. The ACGIH ceiling STEL [STEL (C)] is 0.3 ppm (or 0.69 mg per cubic meter), with a notice of intended changes of 0.1 ppm (or 0.23 mg per cubic meter). Acrolein is classified by the ACGIH as A4 (83). The NIOSH RELs are TWA, 0.1 ppm or 0.25 mg per cubic meter, and STEL (C), 0.3 ppm or 0.8 mg per cubic meter. The NIOSH analytical method is 2501 for acrolein and 2539 for aldehyde. The IDLH value is 2 ppm. Acrolein is classified in group 3 by the IARC (141).

Organotin Compounds

Organotin compounds are used widely as biocidal agents, plastic stabilizers, and chemical process catalysts. These compounds, which do not occur naturally, are formed from the synthesis of tetravalent tin atoms and various organic moieties (142). Organotins may be found as di-, tri-, or tetraalkyl tin forms (143). Typical organotins are triethyltin, dibutyltin, tributyltin, and triphenyltin. Examples are triethyltin iodide, dibutyltin chloride, tributyltin chloride, triphenyltin acetate, and bis(tributyltin) oxide. Organotin compounds are used mainly as biocides. Organotin compounds are used also as additives in many products and processes that require preservation, such as wood, leather, paper, paint, and textiles.

Higher dialkyltin compounds are used as stabilizers for plastics or as fungicides. The lower trialkyltins are used as fungicides, molluscicides, insecticides, and miticides. Trimethyltin (TMT) is formed as a by-product during the production of dimethyltin (DMT). The synthesis of DMT from inorganic tin and methyl chloride produces 88% DMT, 8% TMT, and 4% monomethyltin. TMT evaporates more rapidly than do the other two compounds, rendering it easily inhaled and, therefore, a high toxicity risk. Other than as a by-product in chemical synthesis, TMT is not used for commercial applications (144). The tetraorganotins, although of little commercial utility by themselves, are important compounds because they are used as intermediates in the synthesis for many of the industrially important mono-, di-, and triorganotins. The tetraalkyltins are used also as catalysts for olefin polymerization (145). Tetraalkyltin compounds are relatively inert; they are converted in the body to trialkyltins. Tributyltin, triphenyltin, and tetraorganotin are incompatible with strong oxidizers.

Tin and lead occupy the same periodic table group; therefore, tin and lead and their respective organic compounds may present a similar pattern of organ injury (113). Organotin compounds produce a variety of poisoning symptoms. In general, the symptoms are irritation of the eyes, mucous membranes, throat, and skin. Some of the organotins are hepatotoxic. In animal studies, monoalkyltin compounds, such as methyltin trichloride and ethyltin trichloride, have caused hepatomegaly, bile duct inflammation, and renal fatty degeneration. Trialkyltin compounds easily cross the blood–brain barrier, producing acute neurotoxicity symptoms that include headache, dizziness, photophobia, tremors, hyperexcitability, muscle weakness, and flaccid paralysis. Respiratory paralysis also may be seen.

Trialkyltins and tetraalkyltins (due to their *in vivo* conversion to trialkyltins) are considered the most toxic of the alkyltin group (113,142,144,146). TMT and triethyltin produce clinically distinct syndromes (144). Triethyltin clinical features consist of increased intracranial pressure, paralysis, and generalized tonic-clonic seizures. Neurologic symptoms include severe headache, vertigo, photophobia, psychic disturbances, and other visual system abnormalities. Systemic symptoms reported are abdominal pain and vomiting, urinary retention, and psychic disturbances on ingestion. Persistent neurologic sequelae include diminished visual acuity, focal anesthesia, flaccid paralysis, incontinence, and cerebral edema. Autopsy findings have revealed diffuse intramyelinic edema in the brain (144). TMT toxicity is characterized by limbic system and cerebellar dysfunction, hearing loss, and to a lesser degree, a mild sensory disturbance (144,147).

Tributyltin is registered with the EPA as a biocide in paint. It is used for mildew and fungicide control in exterior paint. Tributyltin oxide is found in both solid and liquid forms. Human exposure can occur from inhalation and from skin absorption. Exposure to tributyltin can produce irritation of the eyes and throat, conjunctivitis, and mucous membrane irritation. Dermal contact with a solution or solid can produce chemical burns (110). Animal studies indicate that tributyltin produces immunosuppression, anemia, and weight loss. Human health effects from tributyltin include mucous membrane irritation; irritation of the eyes, nose, and throat; and cough. Tributyltin as a fungicide is to be used in exterior paints only.

Triphenyltin is a hepatotoxin and, in some occupational exposures, has produced hepatic damage with hepatomegaly and elevated liver enzymes. Triphenyltin is also a dermal irritant and can produce other effects, such as headache, nausea, vomiting, and blurred vision on toxic exposure.

By themselves, tetraalkyltin compounds are relatively inert. After ingestion, these compounds are converted to trialkyltins and produce trialkyltin poisoning with neurotoxicity symptoms and respiratory failure (148). Toxicity from tetraalkyltins may be delayed for 20 to 40 days after a single ingestion, probably owing to the time necessary to convert the tetraalkyltins to trialkyltins (149).

All the organotin compounds, especially tributyltin and dibutyltin, can produce severe dermal chemical burns. Intense itching, inflammation, and erythema can occur on exposure. The lesions that develop generally are diffuse and erythematous and heal quickly after exposure is terminated. Exposure to the eyes can produce lacrimation, conjunctivitis, and conjunctival edema.

MECHANISM OF ACTION

Organotin compounds interfere with several mitochondrial enzyme systems and uncouple oxidative phosphorylation (142,150). Dialkyltins inhibit the function of α-ketoacid oxidases, which in turn decreases mitochondrial oxygen use, thus increasing pyruvate concentrations (113). This inhibition and acute toxicity are blocked by administration of British anti-Lewisite (148). Triethyltin is the most potent known inhibitor of oxidative phosphorylation (143). This trialkyltin compound's inhibition of oxidative phosphorylation is not blocked by British anti-Lewisite. The effectiveness of triorganotin compound inhibition of oxidative phosphorylation, in descending order, is tributyltin, tripropyltin, triphenyltin, and TMT (151).

In rats, exposure to TMT compounds produces a syndrome of tremor, aggression, and seizures. Morphologic changes, including limbic and sensory CNS necrosis, also have been described (152). Allen et al. (152) fed rats experimental diets contaminated with 99% pure triethyltin at a concentration of 8 ppm. Neurobehavioral changes (aggression, shaking, and clonic convulsions) consistent with TMT poisoning became evident on day 22. Microscopical brain analysis revealed pronounced limbic system damage characterized by neuronal cell necrosis of the hippocampal formation and pyriform cortex, amygdaloid nuclei, and olfactory tuberculum. The greatest necrosis occurred in the hippocampal formation and pyriform cortex, and the least was seen in the amygdaloid nuclei and olfactory tuberculum. The spinal cord revealed slight vacuolation-degeneration of ventral horn motor neurons. Peripheral nervous system damage was evidenced by minimal wallerian-type degeneration of the sciatic nerve. In rat studies, triethyltin inhibited incorporation of ^{32}P into brain phospholipids (153). TMT neurotoxicity in mice may be due to alterations in neuronal adenosine triphosphatase systems or interference with ion transport, causing lesions in the limbic system (154). Neuronal cell lesions and degeneration of spinal cord ventral horn cells may be responsible for peripheral neurotoxicity; wallerian-type axonal degeneration also is possible.

The organotin compounds are known to produce immunotoxic properties in animals. An increased susceptibility to infection was found in guinea pigs receiving triphenyltin (155). Decreased lymphopoiesis was reported. The animals also showed decreases in the weight of thymus, spleen, and lymph nodes and a decrease in B-cell lymphocyte proliferation. Rats given oral tributyltin oxide showed decreases in the lymphoid organ weight, such as the thymus and spleen, a decrease in white blood cell count, and decreased lymphocyte counts. Human immunologic effects have not been reported.

CASE STUDIES

Besser et al. (144) reported on six patients with acute TMT intoxication. Six workers became poisoned after inhaling TMT while cleaning a tank used in the manufacture of DMT. Organotin 24-hour urine measurements were obtained at various intervals on each patient. Maximal organotin concentrations (range, 445 to 1,580 ppb) were reached within 4 to 10 days after exposure. Monitoring of 16 asymptomatic workers revealed mean urine concentrations of 36 ppb. Symptom severity correlated with the maximal urinary concentrations. Limbic system clinical signs included disorientation, confabulation, retrograde and anterograde amnesia, aggressiveness, hyperphagia, and disturbances of sexual behavior. Complex partial seizures and intermittent rhythmic delta activity arising from one or both temporal lobes were seen on electroencephalography. Cerebellar dysfunction ranged from mild gaze-evoked nystagmus to severe ataxia. Hearing loss varied from 15 to 30 dB. Paresthesias of the lower extremities, with mild slowing of sensory nerve conduction without loss of reflexes, was observed. One worker with episodes of altered consciousness and generalized seizure activity required mechanical ventilation. He expired on day 13. Attempts were made to increase urinary excretion in these patients with D-penicillamine and plasmapheresis, but these therapies were not successful.

Gross autopsy findings revealed tracheobronchitis, pneumonia, pulmonary edema, fatty degeneration of the liver, and shock kidneys. Neuropathologic findings consisted of swollen perikarya, eccentric or pyknotic nuclei, loss of Nissl substance, and cytoplasmic inclusions with a dense core and light halo. Temporal cortex nerve cell necrosis also was seen. Electron microscopy revealed cytoplasmic lamellated inclusions, termed *zebra bodies*, and many vacuoles and granulomembranous particles surrounded by trilaminar membranes. The finding of zebra bodies reflected an increase in brain lysosomal activity. These changes were most prominent in the amygdala and, to a lesser degree, in the temporal cortex, basal ganglia, and pontine nuclei. A marked loss of Purkinje cells occurred in the cerebellar cortex. These findings were similar to those from the rat studies with TMT.

TMT has produced hyperexcitability, neurologic and behavioral changes, and seizures in some animal studies. Kreyberg et al. (156) reported a case of a 48-year-old woman who died 6 days after consuming wine contaminated with an unknown amount of TMT (156). Within the first 3 hours after the ingestion, she became restless with episodes of unresponsiveness. After the first 3 hours, she became agitated and developed fecal incontinence. On hospital admission, she demonstrated hypokalemia and a leukocytosis. Metabolic acidosis and hepatotoxicity followed. By 72 hours, she developed multiorgan failure with disseminated intravascular coagulation. Renal function remained intact. The patient required ventilatory support and expired on day 6 from multiorgan failure.

Results of chemical analysis of the wine and the patient's urine were positive for TMT. Pathologic analysis revealed chromatolysis of the neurons of the brain spinal cord and spinal ganglia. Acute neuronal necrosis was observed in the fascia dentata of the hippocampus and in the spinal ganglia. Necrosis was seen also in the pyramidal cell layer of the hippocampus, in the cerebral cortex basal ganglia, and in the Purkinje cell layer of the cerebellum. The investigators believed that some of these latter changes may have been due to an anoxic episode shortly before death. Electron microscopy revealed marked accumulation of lysosomal dense bodies and disorganization of the granular endoplasmic reticulum in the neurons. These findings are similar to those of experimental TMT poisoning. Cytoplasmic zebra bodies were not present.

TREATMENT

No specific treatment for organotin poisoning is available. Treatment is primarily symptomatic and supportive. CNS function should be monitored and treated accordingly. Hepatic and renal function should be followed closely. Dermal, ocular, and mucous membrane irritation and burns are possible.

ORGANOTIN EXPOSURE LIMITS

The ACGIH TLV TWA of organotin is 0.1 mg per cubic meter and the STEL (C) is 0.2 mg per cubic meter. Both these limits carry the "skin" notation, signifying the potential significant contribution to overall exposure by the cutaneous route, including mucous membranes and the eyes, either by contact with vapors or, probably more significantly, by direct skin contact with the substance. Organotin is designated as class A4, not classifiable as a human carcinogen, as data are inadequate for classifying the agent in terms of its carcinogenicity in humans or in animals (or in both) (83). The OSHA PEL TWA is 0.1 mg per cubic meter; no STEL value is listed. The NIOSH REL TWA is 0.1 mg per cubic meter (skin) (83). The NIOSH analytical method is 5504.

REFERENCES

1. Duke S. Overview of herbicide mechanisms of action. *Environ Health Perspect* 1990;87:263–271.
2. Smith EA, Oehme FW. A review of selected herbicides and their toxicities. *Vet Hum Toxicol* 1991;33:596–608.
3. Fingerhut MA, Halperin WE, Marlow BS, et al. Cancer mortality in workers exposed to 2,3,7,8-tetrachlorodibenzo-*p*-dioxin. *N Engl J Med* 1991;324:212–218.
4. Stevens JT, Summer DD. Herbicides. In: Hayes WJ Jr, Laws ER Jr, eds. *Handbook of pesticide toxicology, vol 3: classes of pesticides.* San Diego: Academic Press, 1991:1317–1408.
5. US Department of Health and Human Services. *ASTDR case studies in environmental medicine: dioxin toxicity.* Monograph 7. Washington: US Department of Health and Human Services, Government Printing Office, 1990.
6. Erne K. Distribution and elimination of chlorinated phenoxyacetic acids in animals. *Acta Vet Scand* 1966;7:240–256.
7. Libich S, To JC, Frank R, Sirons GJ. Occupational exposure of herbicide applicators to herbicides used along electric power transmission line of right-of-way. *Am Ind Hyg Assoc J* 1984;45:56–62.
8. Arnold EK, Beasley VR. The pharmacokinetics of chlorinated phenoxyacid herbicides: a literature review. *Vet Hum Toxicol* 1989;31:121–125.
9. Bjorklund NE, Erne K. Toxicological studies of phenoxyacetic herbicides in animals. *Acta Vet Scand* 1966;7:364–390.
10. Kohli JD, Khanna RN, Gupta BN, Dhar MM, Tandon JS, Sirca KP. Absorption and excretion of 2,4-dichlorophenoxyacetic acid in man. *Xenobiotica* 1974;4:97–100.
11. Gehring PJ, Betso JE. Phenoxy acids: effects and fate in mammals. *Ecol Bull (Stockh)* 1978;27:122–133.
12. Sauerhoff MW, Braun WH, Blau GE, LeBeau JE. The fate of 2,4-dichlorophenoxyacetic acid (2,4-D) following oral administration. *Toxicol Appl Pharmacol* 1976;37:136–137.
13. Piper WN, Rose JQ, Leng ML, Gehring PJ. The fate of 2,4,5-trichlorophenoxyacetic acid (2,4,5-T) following oral administration to rats and dogs. *Toxicol Appl Pharmacol* 1973;26:339–351.
14. Gehring PJ, Kramer CG, Schweta BA, Rose JQ, Rowe VK. The fate of 2,4,5-trichlorophenoxyacetic acid (2,4,5-T) following oral administration to man. *Toxicol Appl Pharmacol* 1973;26:352–361.
15. Sauerhoff MW, Braun WH, Blau GE, Gehring PJ, Bergstrom R. The fate of 2,4-dichlorophenoxyacetic acid (2,4-D) following oral administration to man. *Toxicology* 1977;8:3–11.
16. Baselt RC, Cravey RH. *Disposition of toxic drugs and chemicals in man,* 3rd ed. Chicago: Year Book Medical Publishers,1989:262–264.
17. Young JF, Haley TJ. Pharmacokinetic study of a patient intoxicated with 2,4-dichlorophenoxy acid and 2-methoxy-3,6-dichlorobenzoic acid. *Clin Toxicol* 1977;11:489–500.
18. Kolmodin-Hedman B, Akerblom M. Field application of phenoxy acid herbicides. In: Tordoir WF, van Heemstra EAH, eds. *Field worker exposure during pesticide application.* New York: Elsevier Science, 1980:73–77.
19. Flanagan RJ, Meredith TJ, Ruprah M, Onyon LJ, Liddle A. Alkaline diuresis for acute poisoning with chlorophenoxy herbicides and ioxynil. *Lancet* 1990;335:454–458.
20. Friesen EG, Jones GR, Vaughan D. Clinical presentation and management of acute 2,4-D oral ingestion. *Drug Safety* 1990;5:155–159.
21. Meulenbelt J, Zwaveling JH, van Zoonen P, et al. Acute MCPP intoxication: report of two cases. *Hum Toxicol* 1988;7:289–292.
22. Osterloh J, Lotti M, Pond SM. Toxicologic studies in a fatal overdose of 2,4-D, MCPP, and chlorpyrifos. *J Anal Toxicol* 1983;7:125–129.
23. Kancir CB, Andersen C, Olesen AS, et al. Marked hypocalcemia in a fatal poisoning with chlorinated phenoxy acid derivatives. *Clin Toxicol* 1988;26:257–264.
24. Keller T, Skopp G, Wu M, et al. Fatal overdose of 2,4-dichlorophenoxyacetic acid (2,4-D). *Forens Sci Int* 1994;65:13–18.
25. O'Reilly JF. Prolonged coma and delayed peripheral neuropathy after ingestion of phenoxyacetic acid weed-killers. *Postgrad Med J* 1984;60:76–77.
26. Berwick P. 2,4-Dichlorophenoxyacetic acid poisoning in man. *JAMA* 1970;214:1114–1117.
27. Wells WDE, Wright N, Yeoman WB. Clinical features and management of poisoning with 2,4-D and mecoprop. *Clin Toxicol* 1981;18:273–276.
28. Hervonen H, Elo HA, Ylitalo P. Blood-brain barrier damage by 2-methyl-4-chlorophenoxyacetic acid herbicide in rats. *Toxicol Appl Pharmacol* 1982; 65:23–31.
29. Dudley AW, Thapar NT. Fatal human ingestion of 2,4-D, a common herbicide. *Arch Pathol* 1972;94:270–275.
30. Desi I, Sos J, Olasz J, Sule F, Markus V. Nervous system effects of a chemical herbicide. *Archiv Environ Health* 1962;4:101–108.
31. Goldstein NP, Jones PH. Peripheral neuropathy after exposure to an ester of dichlorophenoxyacetic acid. *JAMA* 1959;171:1306–1309.
32. Berkley MC, Magee KR. Neuropathy following exposure to dimethylamine salt of 2,4-D. *Arch Intern Med* 1963;111:351–352.
33. Mattson JL, Johnson KA, Albee RR. Lack of neuropathologic consequences of repeated dermal exposure to 2,4-dichlorophenoxyacetic acid in rats. *Fundam Appl Toxicol* 1986;6:175–181.
34. Kay JH, Palazzolo BS, Calandra MD. Subacute dermal toxicity of 2,4-D. *Arch Environ Health* 1965;11:648–651.
35. Nielsen K, Kaempe B, Jenson-Holm J. Fatal poisoning in man by 2,4-dichlorophenoxyacetic acid (2,4-D): determination of the agent in forensic materials. *Acta Pharmacol Toxicol* 1965;22:224–234.
36. Seabury JH. Toxicity of 2,4-dichlorophenoxyacetic acid for man and dog. *Arch Environ Health* 1963;7:202–209.
37. Curry AS. Twenty-one uncommon cases of poisoning. *BMJ* 1962;1:687–698.
38. Smith RA, Lewis D. Suicide by ingestion of 2,4-D: a case history demonstrating the prudence of using GC/MS as an investigative rather than a confirmatory tool. *Vet Hum Toxicol* 1987;29:259–261.

39. Bleiberg J, Wallen M, Brodkin R, Applebaum IL. Industrially acquired porphyria. *Arch Dermatol* 1964;89:793–797.
40. Zack JA, Suskind RS. The mortality experience of workers exposed to tetrachlorobenzodioxin in a trichlorophenol process accident. *J Occup Med* 1980;22:11–14.
41. Mary G. Tetrachlorodibenzodioxin: a survey of subjects ten years after exposure. *Br J Ind Med* 1982;39:128–135.
42. Oliver RM. Toxic effects of 2,3,7,8-tetrachloro-1,4-dioxin in laboratory workers. *Br J Ind Med* 1975;32:49–53.
43. Suskind RR, Hertzberg VS. Human health effects of 2,4,5-T and its toxic contaminants. *JAMA* 1984;251:2372–2380.
44. Moses M, Lilis R, Crow KD, et al. Health status of workers with past exposure to 2,3,7,8-tetrachlorodibenzo-*p*-dioxin in the manufacture of 2,4,5-trichlorophenoxyacetic acid: comparison of findings with and without chloracne. *Am J Ind Med* 1984;5:161–182.
45. Hardell L, Sandstrom A. Case-control study: soft tissue sarcomas and exposure to phenoxyacetic acids or chlorophenols. *Br J Cancer* 1979;39:711–717.
46. Eriksson M, Hardell L, Adami HP. Exposure to dioxins as a risk factor for soft tissue sarcoma: a population-based case-control study. *J Natl Cancer Inst* 1990;82:486–490.
47. Eriksson M, Hardell L, Berg N, Moller T, Axelson O. Soft-tissue sarcomas and exposure to chemical substances: a case referent study. *Br J Ind Med* 1981;38:27–33.
48. Hardell L, Eriksson M. The association between soft tissue sarcomas and exposure to phenoxyacetic acids: a new case-referent study. *Cancer* 1988;62:652–656.
49. Hardell L, Bengtsson NO. Epidemiologic study of socioeconomic factors and clinical findings in Hodgkin's disease, and reanalysis of previous data regarding chemical exposure. *Br J Cancer* 1983;48:217–225.
50. Hardell L, Eriksson M, Lenner P, Lundgren E. Malignant lymphoma and exposure to chemicals, especially organic solvents, chlorophenols and phenoxy acids: a case-control study. *Br J Cancer* 1981;43:169–176.
51. Woods JS, Polissar L, Severson RK, Heuser LS, Kulander BG. Soft tissue sarcoma and non-Hodgkin's lymphoma in relation to phenoxyherbicide and chlorinated phenol exposure in western Washington. *J Natl Cancer Inst* 1987;78:899–910.
52. Persson B, Dahlander A, Fredriksson M, Brage HN, Ohlson CG, Axelson O. Malignant lymphomas and occupational exposures. *Br J Intern Med* 1989:516–520.
53. Axelson O, Sundell L, Andersson K, Edling C, Hogstedt C, Kling H. Herbicide exposure and tumor mortality: an updated epidemiologic investigation on Swedish railroad car workers. *Scand J Work Environ Health* 1980;6:73–79.
54. Thiess AM, Frentzel-Beyme R, Link R. Mortality study of persons exposed to dioxin in a trichlorophenol-process accident that occurred in the BASF AG on November 17, 1953. *Am J Med* 1982;3:179–189.
55. Hardell L, Johansson B, Axelson O. Epidemiological study of nasal and nasopharyngeal cancer and their relation to phenoxy acid or chlorophenol exposure. *Am J Ind Med* 1982;3:247–257.
56. Kociba R, Keyes D, Beyer J, et al. Results of a two-year chronic toxicity and oncogenicity study of 2,3,7,8-tetrachlorodibenzo-*p*-dioxin in rats. *Toxicol Appl Pharmacol* 1978;46:279–303.
57. Rao MS, Subbarao V, Prasad JD, Scarpelli DG. Carcinogenicity of 2,3,7,8-tetrachlorodibenzo-*p*-dioxin in the Syrian golden hamster. *Carcinogenesis* 1988;9:1677–1679.
58. Smith AH, Pearce NE, Fisher DO, Giles HJ, Teague CA, Howard JK. Soft tissue sarcoma and exposure to phenoxyherbicides and chlorophenols in New Zealand. *J Natl Cancer Inst* 1984;73:1111–1117.
59. Wiklund K, Holm L. Soft tissue sarcoma risk in Swedish agricultural and forestry workers. *J Natl Cancer Inst* 1986;76:229–234.
60. Pearce NE, Sheppard RA, Smith AH, Teague CA. Non-Hodgkin's lymphoma and farming: an expanded case-control study. *Int J Cancer* 1987;39:155–161.
61. Wiklund K, Dich J, Holm LE. Risk of malignant lymphoma in Swedish pesticide appliers. *Br J Cancer* 1987;56:505–508.
62. Olsen JH, Jensen OM. Nasal cancer and chlorophenols. *Lancet* 1984;2:47–48.
63. Hardell L, Bengtsson N, Jonsson V, Ericksson S, Larsson L. Aetiological aspects on primary liver cancer with special regard to alcohol, organic solvents and acute intermittent porphyria—an epidemiological investigation. *Br J Cancer* 1984;50:389–397.
64. Bailar JC. How dangerous is dioxin? *N Engl J Med* 1991;324:260–262.
65. The Selected Cancers Cooperative Study Group. The association of selected cancers with service in the US military in Vietnam: II. Soft-tissue and other sarcomas. *Arch Intern Med* 1990;150:2485–2492.
66. Kang H, Enzinger FM, Breslin P, Feil M, Lee Y, Shepard B. Soft tissue sarcoma and military service in Vietnam: a case-control study *J Natl Cancer Inst* 1987;79:693–699.
67. Kang HK, Weatherbee L, Breslin PP, Lee Y, Shepard BM. Soft tissue sarcomas and military service in Vietnam: a case comparison group analysis of hospital patients. *J Occup Med* 1986;28:1215–1218.
68. Dalager NA, Kang HK, Burt VL, Weatherbee L. Hodgkin's disease and Vietnam service. *Ann Epidemiol* 1995;5:400–406.
69. Dalager NA, Kang HK, Burt VL, Weatherbee L. Non-Hodgkin's lymphoma among Vietnam veterans. *J Occup Med* 1991;33:774–779.
70. The Selected Cancers Cooperative Study Group. The association of selected cancers with service in the US military in Vietnam: I. Non-Hodgkin's lymphoma. *Arch Intern Med* 1990;150:2473–2483.
71. Wolfe WH, Michalek JE, Miner JC, et al. Health status of Air Force veterans occupationally exposed to herbicides in Vietnam: I. Physical health. *JAMA* 1990;264:1824–1831.
72. Michalek JE, Wolfe WH, Miner JC. Health status of Air Force veterans occupationally exposed to herbicides in Vietnam: II. Mortality. *JAMA* 1990; 264:1832–1836.
73. Centers for Disease Control Veterans Health Studies. Serum 2,3,7,8-tetrachlorodibenzo-*p*-dioxin levels in US Army Vietnam-era veterans. *JAMA* 1988;260:1249–1254.
74. Mahan CM, Bullman TA, Kang HK, Selvin S. A case-control study of lung cancer among Vietnam veterans. *J Occup Environ Med* 1997;39:740–747.
75. Hoffman RE, Stehr-Green PA, Webb KB, et al. Health effects of long-term exposure to 2,3,7,8-tetrachlorodibenzo-*p*-dioxin. *JAMA* 1986;255:2031–2038.
76. Reggiani G. Medical problems raised by the TCDD contamination in Seveso, Italy. *Arch Toxicol* 1978;40:161–188.
77. Bronstein AC, Currance PL. *Emergency care for hazardous material exposures*, 2nd ed. St. Louis: Mosby, 1994:292–295.
78. Prescott LF, Park J, Darrien I. Treatment of severe 2,4-D and mecoprop intoxication with alkaline diuresis. *Br J Clin Pharmacol* 1979;7:111–116.
79. Morgan DP. *Recognition and management of pesticide poisonings*, 4th ed. Washington: US Government Printing Office, 1989:63–67.
80. Fraser AD, Isner IF, Perry RA. Toxicologic studies in a fatal overdose of 2,4-D, mecoprop, and dicamba. *J Forensic Sci* 1984;29:1237–1241.
81. Kahn PC, Gochfeld M, Nygren M, et al. Dioxins and dibenzofurans in blood and adipose tissue of Agent Orange–exposed Vietnam veterans and matched controls. *JAMA* 1988;259:1661–1667.
82. Patterson DC, Hoffman RE, Needham LL, et al. 2,3,7,8-Tetrachlorodibenzo-*p*-dioxin levels in adipose tissue of exposed persons in Missouri. *JAMA* 1986; 256:2683–2686.
83. American Conference of Governmental and Industrial Hygienists. *TLVs and other occupational exposure values—1997.* CD-ROM version. Cincinnati: American Conference of Governmental and Industrial Hygienists, 1997.
84. International Agency for Research on Cancer. Chlorophenoxy herbicides. *IARC Monogr Eval Carcinog Risks Chem Man* 1987;41[Suppl 7]:156.
85. Hart TB. Paraquat—review of safety in agricultural and horticultural use. *Hum Toxicol* 1987;6:13–18.
86. Zeneca Agrochemicals. Principal products [on-line], 1998. *http://www.zeneca.com/zagro/herb.htm#gramox.*
87. Smith LL. Mechanism of paraquat toxicity in lung and its relevance to toxicity. *Hum Toxicol* 1987;6:31–36.
88. Bismuth C, Garnier R, Baud FJ, Muszynzki J, Keyes C. Paraquat poisoning—an overview of the current status. *Drug Safety* 1990;5:243–251.
89. Vale JA, Meredith TJ, Buckley BM. Paraquat poisoning: clinical features and immediate general management. *Hum Toxicol* 1987;6:41–47.
90. Hawksworth GM, Bennett PN, Davies DS. Kinetics of paraquat elimination in the dog. *Toxicol Appl Pharmacol* 1981;57:139–145.
91. Kurisaki E, Sato E. Tissue distribution of paraquat and diquat after oral administration in rats. *Forensic Sci Int* 1979;14:165–170.
92. Daniel JW, Gage JC. Absorption and excretion of diquat and paraquat in rats. *Br J Ind Med* 1966;28:133–136.
93. Murray RE, Gibson JE. Paraquat disposition in rats, guinea pigs and monkeys. *Toxicol Appl Pharmacol* 1974;27:283–291.
94. Bennett PN, Davies DS, Hawkesworth GM. In vitro absorption studies with paraquat and diquat in the dog. *Br J Pharmacol* 1976;58:284.
95. Bismuth C, Garnier R, Dally S, Fournier PE. Prognosis and treatment of paraquat poisoning: a review of 28 cases. *J Clin Toxicol* 1982;19:461–474.
96. Rose MS, Lock EA, Smith LL, Wyatt I. Paraquat accumulation tissue and species specificity. *Biochem Pharmacol* 1976;25:419–423.
97. Rose MS, Smith LL. Tissue uptake of paraquat and diquat. *Gen Pharmacol* 1977;8:173–176.
98. Proudfoot AT, Stewart MS, Levitt T, Widdop B. Paraquat poisoning: significance of plasma-paraquat concentrations. *Lancet* 1979;2:330–332.
99. Scherrmann JM, Houze P, Bismuth C, Bourdon R. Prognostic value of plasma and urine paraquat concentration. *Hum Toxicol* 1987;6:91–93.
100. Tsatsakis AM, Perakis K, Koumantakis E. Experience with acute paraquat poisoning in Crete. *Vet Hum Toxicol* 1996;38:113–117.
101. Talbot AR, Fu CC. Paraquat intoxication during pregnancy: a report of 9 cases. *Vet Hum Toxicol* 1988;30:12–17.
102. Pond SM. Manifestations and management of paraquat poisoning. *Med J Aust* 1990;152:256–259.
103. Hearn CED, Keir W. Nail damage in spray operators exposed to paraquat. *Br J Ind Med* 1971;28:399–403.
104. Joyce M. Ocular damage caused by paraquat. *Br J Ophthalmol* 1969;53:688–690.
105. Karai I, Nakano H, Horiguchi S. A case of lacrimal duct stenosis due to a herbicide paraquat. *Jpn J Ind Health* 1981;23:552–553.
106. Hoffer E, Taitelman U. Exposure to paraquat through skin absorption: clinical and laboratory observations of accidental splashing on healthy skin of agricultural workers. *Hum Toxicol* 1989;8(6):483–485.
107. National Institute for Occupational Safety and Health. *Pocket guide to chemical hazards.* DHHS publ. no. (PHS) 94-116. Cincinnati: National Institute for Occupational Safety and Health, 1994:240.
108. Bismuth C, Scherrmann, Garnier R, Baud FJ, Pontal PG. Elimination of paraquat. *Hum Toxicol* 1987;6:63–67.
109. Meredith TJ, Vale JA. Treatment of paraquat poisoning in man: methods to prevent absorption. *Hum Toxicol* 1987;6:49–55.

110. Smilkstein MJ, Smolinske SC, Kulig KW, et al. Severe hypermagnesemia due to multiple-dose cathartic therapy. *West J Med* 1988;148:208–211.
111. Proudfoot AT, Prescott LF, Jarvie DR. Haemodialysis for paraquat poisoning. *Hum Toxicol* 1987;6:69–74.
112. Edith CG, Pond SM. Failure of haemoperfusion and haemodialysis to prevent death in paraquat poisoning. *Med Toxicol* 1988;3:64–71.
113. Matthew H, Logan A, Woodruff MFA, et al. Paraquat poisoning. Lung transplantation. *BMJ* 1968;1:759–763.
114. Kalmolz S, Veith FJ, Mollenkopf F, et al. Single lung transplantation in paraquat intoxication. *N Y State J Med* 1984;84:81–85.
115. Powell D, Pond SM, Allen TB, Portale AA. Hemoperfusion in a child who ingested diquat and died from pontine infarction and hemorrhage. *J Toxicol Clin Toxicol* 1983;20(5):405–420.
116. Vanholder R, Colardyn F, DeReuck J, Praet M, Lameire N, Ringoir S. Diquat intoxication. Report of two cases and review of the literature. *Am J Med* 1981;70:1267–1271.
117. Braithwaite RA. Emergency analysis of paraquat in biological fluids. *Hum Toxicol* 1987;6:83–86.
118. Menkes D, Temple W, Edwards I. International self-poisoning with glyphosate-containing herbicides. *Hum Exp Toxicol* 1991;10:103–107.
119. Temple WA, Smith NA. Glyphosate herbicide poisoning experience in New Zealand. *N Z Med J* 1992;105:173–174.
120. Talbot AR, Shiaw MH, Huang JS, et al. Acute poisoning with a glyphosate-surfactant herbicide (Round-Up): a review of 93 cases. *Hum Exp Toxicol* 1991;10:1–8.
121. Bartnik F, Kunstler K. Biological effects, toxicology, and human safety. In: Falbe, ed. *Surfactants in consumer products—theory, technology, and application.* New York: Springer-Verlag, 1987:475–499.
122. Tominack RL, Yang GY, Tsai WJ, et al. Taiwan National Poison Center survey of glyphosate-surfactant herbicide ingestions. *J Toxicol Clin Toxicol* 1991;29:91–109.
123. Agency for Toxic Substances and Disease Registry. *Toxicological profile for pentachlorophenol (update).* Atlanta: Department of Health and Human Services, Public Health Service, 1994.
124. Agency for Toxic Substances and Disease Registry, Department of Health and Human Services, Public Health Service. ToxFAQs—pentachlorophenol [on-line monograph], 1995. *http://astdr1.astdr.cdc.gov:8080/trfacts51.html*
125. Agency for Toxic Substances and Disease Registry, Department of Health and Human Services, Public Health Service. Public health statement: pentachlorophenol [on-line monograph], 1989. *http://astdr1.astdr.cdc.gov:8080/ToxProfiles/phs8919.html*
126. Environmental Protection Agency Office of Ground Water and Drinking Water. Consumer factsheet on pentachlorophenol [on-line monograph], 1998. *http://www.epa.gov/orgwdw000/dwh/c-soc/pentachl.html*
127. US Department of Health and Human Services. *ATSDR case studies in environmental medicine: pentachlorophenol toxicity.* Monograph 23. Washington: US Department of Health and Human Services, Government Printing Office, 1990.
128. Lewis RJ. *Hazardous chemicals desk reference,* 3rd ed. New York: Van Nostrand–Rheinhold, 1993:425.
129. Lacey E. The role of the cytoskeletal protein, tubulin, in the mode of action and mechanism of drug resistance to benzimidazoles. *Int J Parasitol* 1988;18:885–936.
130. Hayes W. *Pesticide studies in man.* Baltimore: Williams & Wilkins, 1982:75–111.
131. Tracy JW, Webster LT. Drugs used in the chemotherapy of helminthiasis. In: Hardman JG, Gilman AG, Limbird LE, eds. *Goodman and Gilman's the pharmacological basis of therapeutics,* 9th ed. CD-ROM version. New York: McGraw-Hill, 1996.
132. Edwards IR, Ferry DG, Temple WA. Fungicides and related compounds. In: Hayes WJ Jr, Laws ER Jr, eds. *Handbook of pesticide toxicology, vol 3: classes of pesticides.* San Diego: Academic Press, 1991:1409–1470.
133. Eneanya DI, Bianchine JR, Duran DO, et al. The actions and metabolic fate of disulfiram. *Ann Rev Pharmacol Toxicol* 1981;21:575–579.
134. International Agency for Research on Cancer. Ferbam [14484-64-1]. *IARC Monogr Eval Carcinog Risk Chem Hum* 1987;12[Suppl 7].
135. Webb PK, Gibbs SCM, Mathias CT, et al. Disulfiram hypersensitivity and rubber contact dermatitis. *JAMA* 1979;241:2061.
136. Dalvi R. Toxicology of thiram (tetramethylthiuram disulfide)—a review. *Vet Hum Toxicol* 1988;30:480–482.
137. International Agency for Research on Cancer. Thiram [137-26-8]. *IARC Monogr Eval Carcinog Risk Chem Hum* 1991;53:104.
138. International Agency for Research on Cancer. Ziram [137-30-4]. *IARC Monogr Eval Carcinog Risk Chem Hum* 1991;53:423.
139. Agency for Toxic Substances and Disease Registry. *Toxicological profile for acrolein.* Atlanta: US Public Health Service, Department of Health and Human Services, ATSDR 1989.
140. US Environmental Protection Agency. *Integrated risk information system on acrolein.* Cincinnati: Environmental Criteria and Assessment Office, Office of Health and Environmental Assessment, Office of Research and Development, 1993.
141. International Agency for Research on Cancer. Acrolein [107-02-8]. *IARC Monogr Eval Carcinog Risk Chem Hum* 1995;63:337.
142. Attahiru US, Iyaniwura TT, Adaudi AO, Bonire JJ. Acute toxicity studies of tri-*N*-butyltin and triphenyltin acetates in rats. *Vet Hum Toxicol* 1991;33:554–556.
143. Clarkson TW. Inorganic and organometal pesticides. In: Hayes WJ Jr, Laws ER Jr, eds. *Handbook of pesticide toxicology, vol 3: classes of pesticides.* San Diego: Academic Press, 1991:497–583.
144. Besser R, Krämer G, Thümler R, et al. Acute trimethyltin limbic-cerebellar syndrome. *Neurology* 1987;37:945–950.
145. Seiler HG, Sigel H, Sigel A, eds. *Handbook on the toxicity of inorganic compounds.* New York: Marcel Dekker Inc, 1988:699.
146. Barnes JM, Stoner HB. Toxic properties of some dialkyl and trialkyl tin salts. *Br J Ind Med* 1958;15:15–22.
147. Feldman RG, White RF, Eriator II. Trimethyltin encephalopathy. *Arch Neurol* 1993;50:1320–1324.
148. Barnes JM, Stoner HB. The toxicology of tin compounds. *Pharmacol Rev* 1959;11:211–231.
149. Cremer JE. The biochemistry of organotin compounds. The conversion of tetraethyltin into triethyltin in mammals. *Biochem J* 1958;68:685–692.
150. Aldridge WN. The influence of organotin compounds on mitochondrial functions. In: Zuchermann JJ, ed. *Organotin compounds, new chemistry applications.* Washington: American Chemical Society, 1976:186–196.
151. Stockdale R, Dawson AP, Selwyn MJ. Effects of trialkyltin and triphenyltin compounds on mitochondrial respiration. *Eur J Biochem* 1970;15:342–351.
152. Allen SL, Simpson MG, Stonard MD, et al. Induction of trimethyltin neurotoxicity by dietary administration. *Neurotoxicology* 1994;15:651–654.
153. Rose MS, Aldridge WN. Triethyltin and the incorporation of (^{32}P) phosphate into rat brain phospholipids. *J Neurochem* 1996;13:103–108.
154. Chang LW. Neuropathology of trimethyltin: a proposed pathogenetic mechanism. *Fundam Appl Toxicol* 1986;6:217–232.
155. Verschuuren HG, Kroes R, Vink HH, Van Esch GJ. Short-term toxicity studies with triphenyltin compounds in rats and guinea pig. *Food Cosmet Toxicol* 1966;4:35–45.
156. Kreyberg, S, Torvik A, Bjørneboe W, Wiik-Larsen, Jacobsen D. Trimethyltin poisoning: report of a case with postmortem examination. *Clin Neuropathol* 1992;11:256–259.

CHAPTER 102
Fungicides and Biocides

Scott D. Phillips

Fungicides and biocides prevent the growth of such microorganisms as bacteria and fungi. They are used on a variety of vegetable and fruit crops and in paints and other products in which the growth of bacteria and fungus is undesirable. They are a diverse group of compounds (Tables 102-1 through 102-3) and include inorganic compounds, organometals, imidazoles, substituted benzenes, phenol derivatives, and several other substances.

Fungicides and biocides are divided into different categories on the basis of their mode of application. Soil fungicides are applied to the soil as liquids, powders, or granules. Foliar fungicides are applied to the plant above the ground to provide a protective barrier against fungi. Dressing fungicides, applied after the crop has been harvested, prevent fungus development on the stored crop.

Fungicides and biocides also may be described by their mode of action. *Protective fungicides* are applied to protect plants from the development of fungi. This can be accomplished by killing spores (*sporicidal fungicides*) or by acting as a *foliar fungicide* on the plant surface to create a hostile environment for the growth of the fungus. *Curative fungicides* may be used after plants have become infested, attacking and destroying the developing mycelium in the epidermis of the plant. After a plant has become symptomatic, an *eradicating fungicide* may be needed to kill mycelium and new spores. These penetrate the plant to the subdermal level (1).

The ideal fungicide would be characterized by the following properties: (i) low toxicity to animals or humans; (ii) little or no toxicity to the plant, despite ability to penetrate the plant; (iii) ability to penetrate spores and mycelium; and (iv) limited biodegradation on the plant surface under certain environmental conditions (wind, rain, sunlight, humidity). Although newer fungicides have less systemic toxicity to humans, only unusual fungicides incorporate all these properties.

Certain fungicides are suggested to be responsible for the majority of oncogenic risk (80%) among pesticides (2). This risk

TABLE 102-1. Common organic fungicides and biocides

- Substituted aromatics
  - Chloroneb
  - Chlorothalonil
  - Dichloran
  - Hexachlorobenzene
  - Pentachloronitrobenzene
  - Pentachlorophenol
  - Sodium pentachlorophenate
  - Tecnazene
- Benzimidazoles
  - Benomyl
  - Carbendazim
  - Fuberidazole
  - Imazalil
  - Terrazole
  - Thiabendazole
  - Thiophanate-methyl
- Oxathiins
  - Carboxin
  - Oxycarboxin
- Dithiocarbamates
  - Butylate
  - Cyclohexylamine sulfate
  - Sodium methyldithiocarbamate (metamsodium)
  - Metiram
  - Thiram
- Metallobisdithiocarbamates
  - Ferbam
  - Nabam
  - Ziram
- Ethylene bisdithiocarbamates
  - Mancozeb
  - Maneb
  - Trimanzone
  - Zineb
- Thiocarbonates
  - Sodium tetrathiocarbonate
- Dicarboximides
  - Captafol
  - Captan
  - Folpet
  - Iprodione
- Benzenoids
  - Metalaxyl
- Triazines
  - Ametryn
  - Atraton
  - Atrazine
  - Cyanazine
  - Desmetryn
  - Dyrene (anilazine)
  - Isomethiozin
  - Metribuzin
- Triazoles
  - Amitrole
  - Bitertanol
  - Diniconazole
  - Etridazole
  - Flutriafole
  - Hexaconazole
  - Isazophos
  - Paclobutrazole
  - Penconazole
  - Propiconazole
  - Tebuconazole
  - Tebuthiuron
  - Triadimefon
  - Triadimenol
  - Tricyclazole
  - Uniconazole
- Piperazine
  - Triforine
- Antibiotics
  - Cycloheximide
  - Iturin A
  - Streptomycin
  - Validamycin
- Dinitrophenols
  - Dinocap (crotonic acid)
- Quinones
  - Dichlone
- Aliphatic nitrogens
  - Dodine
- Cinnamic acid derivatives
  - Dimethomorph

has not been characterized adequately. Most fungicides result in positive mutation assays and are cytotoxic to eukaryotic cells. This is due to similarities of the common bacteria used and fungal cell walls (3). Almost 90% of fungicides are animal carcinogens. Little is known of the true risk of cancer to humans.

SUBSTITUTED AROMATICS

Substituted aromatics generally show halogenation of aromatic rings (Fig. 102-1). Fungicides included in this group are chloroneb, chlorothalonil, dichloran, hexachlorobenzene, pentachloronitrobenzene (PCNB), pentachlorophenol (PCP), and tecnazene.

Chloroneb

Chloroneb is used for soil treatment among crops, including cotton, beans, soybeans, and turf grass. It is available as a wettable powder for treatment of soil and has limited applicability for use as a seed treatment. Chloroneb is a systemic fungicide primarily taken up by roots and concentrates in the roots and lower portions of the plant, providing a fungistatic effect against invasion (4). The fungitoxicity of chloroneb is related to its inhibition of DNA polymerization (5).

TABLE 102-2. Common inorganic fungicides and biocides inorganic metals

- Boron calcium
- Cadmium-calcium-copper-zinc-chromate complex
- Cadmium chloride
- Cadmium sulfate
- Copper acetate
- Copper ammonium carbonate
- Copper carbonate
- Copper chloride
- Copper hydroxide
- Copper lime dust
- Copper oxychloride
- Copper oxylate
- Copper potassium
- Copper silicate
- Copper sulfate
- Cupric oxide
- Cuprous oxide
- Mercuric chloride (corrosive sublimate)
- Mercuric oxide (yellow oxide of mercury)
- Mercury sublimate
- Sulfur
- Tribasic (Bordeaux mixture)

Chloroneb exhibits a low oral toxicity to most species. No poisonings have been reported in humans. The oral lethal dose in humans is estimated to be between 5 and 15 g per kg, or roughly 1 quart in a 70-kg person. Chloroneb is absorbed and metabolized to 2,5-dichloro-4-methoxyphenol in both free and conjugated forms and is excreted primarily in the urine (6).

TABLE 102-3. Common organometals fungicides and biocides

- Organometals
  - Bis(tributyltin) oxide
  - Cadmium subacetate
  - Cadmium succinate
  - Copper acetate
  - Copper linoleate
  - Copper naphtholate
  - Copper oleate
  - Copper phenyl salicylate
  - Copper quinolinolate
  - Copper resinate
  - Cyclohexylhydrostannane (plictran)
  - Fenbutin oxide
  - Ferric ammonium salt of methane arsenic acid
  - Ferric methane arsonate
  - Mercury acetate
  - Mercury acetyl acetone
  - Mercury benzoate
  - Mercury pentachlorophenate
  - Mercury propionate
  - Mercury quinolinolate
  - Methoxyethyl mercury acetate
  - Methoxyethyl mercury chloride
  - Methoxymercury chloride
  - Methylmercury hydroxide
  - Methylmercury nitrile
  - Phenylaminocadmium dilactate
  - Phenylmercuric acetate
  - Tributyltin
  - Triethyltin
  - Trimethyltin
  - Triphenyltin (fentin hydroxide)
- Miscellaneous organic fungicides
  - Paraformaldehyde

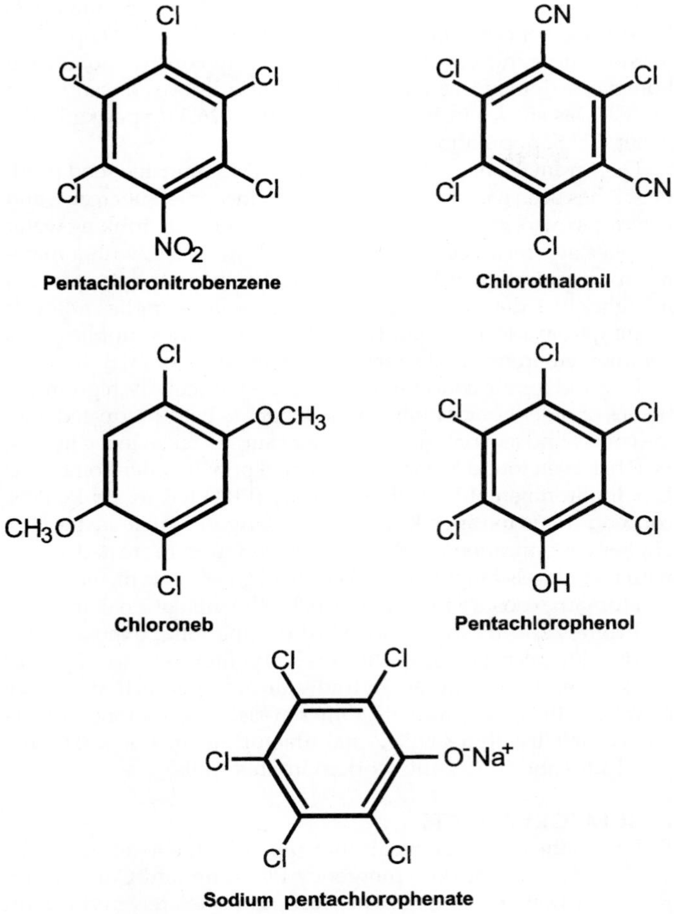

Pentachloronitrobenzene

Chlorothalonil

Chloroneb

Pentachlorophenol

Sodium pentachlorophenate

Figure 102-1. Substituted aromatics.

Chlorothalonil

Chlorothalonil is an organochlorine fungicide used to control fungal diseases in vegetables, fruits, turf, and ornamental plants. It has found additional use in controlling fruit rot in cranberry bogs and can be incorporated into paints to prevent mildew.

The compound has limited toxicity to mammals; however, very high doses may result in incoordination, rapid breathing, vomiting, hyperactivity, and bleeding. Airborne concentrations may result in irritation of the mucous membranes. The typical oral median lethal dose (LD_{50}) for rats is greater than 10,000 mg per kg. Current animal toxicity studies have demonstrated some kidney enlargement at doses of 60 parts per million (ppm) (7). No evidence has reported long-term reproductive toxicity, except at doses toxic to mothers. Establishing carcinogenicity for this fungicide is difficult; however, it is considered a potential human carcinogen, with effects on kidney, ureter, and bladder in experimental animals (8). The effects on rodent kidneys is due to the formation of dithiols and trithiols from the action of renal β-lyase on cysteine *S*-conjugates. These appear to derive from the glutathione conjugates of chlorothalonil (9).

A study in mice found that high-dose exposures for 2 years resulted in four stomach tumors in female mice only (9). The researchers concluded that the tumors were related to irritation from the compound itself. They hypothesized that tumors demonstrated in the rodent forestomach are due to the progression from cytotoxicity to hyperplasia to neoplasia (9). As humans lack the rodent forestomach organ, these data are not applicable to people. No cases of human poisoning have been reported. However, it would be advisable to consider treating a significant exposure to this fungicide as one would treat exposures to other substituted aromatic fungicides.

Dichloran

Dichloran is a broad-spectrum fungicide used on a variety of fruit and vegetable crops. It is available as a wettable or dry-application powder or dust and is available under the trade names Allisan and Clortran. Frequently, it is found as a mixture with other pesticides. Absorption occurs with this product, which has a typical half-life in humans of less than 27 hours.

Dichloran is metabolized to dichloroaminophenol, which has been known to uncouple oxidative phosphorylation. As with other fungicides in this category, this activity results in excessive heat production and related metabolic complications. These effects could include liver injury, hyperpyrexia, corneal opacities, and possibly, methemoglobinemia. A human study was performed with daily dosages of approximately 10 mg per day for 3 months in 20 adult male subjects. No observable adverse effects were determined (7). The estimated LD_{50} in rats is approximately 730 mg per kg. Toxicologically, ingestions should be managed in a manner similar to management of exposures to other compounds in this category of fungicides (10).

Hexachlorobenzene

Hexachlorobenzene is a chlorinated hydrocarbon fungicide used primarily as a seed treatment, especially on wheat. It has found use in the control of bunt. This fungicide is included for historical interest only, as it has been banned from use in the United States.

Its acute toxicity is low with single exposures in limited amounts. The LD_{50} for rats is in the neighborhood of 10,000 mg per kg. The American Conference of Governmental Industrial Hygienists (ACGIH) threshold limit value (TLV) and time-weighted average (TWA) for hexachlorobenzene is 0.02 mg per cubic meter.

Porphyria cutanea tarda developed in people who consumed hexachlorobenzene-contaminated flour in Turkey. An epidemic of an estimated 3,000 cases of porphyria cutanea tarda ensued from this consumption, which led to withdrawal of hexachlorobenzene from the market in 1959. However, cases of hexachlorobenzene-related porphyria cutanea tarda continued to be reported until 1961 (11). Recovery from the porphyria typically followed termination of exposure, although persistent effects were reported (12). In addition to the extensive morbidity, a mortality rate of 10% was associated with this condition. Follow-up studies some 20 years after hexachlorobenzene exposure demonstrated that some people reportedly were still experiencing ill effects (13). Daily intake of the compound from the contaminated wheat has been estimated to range from 50 to 200 mg per day. Those persons exposed also exhibited other signs of illness, including skin changes (typical of porphyria cutanea tarda), hepatomegaly, and hypertrichosis. The increased growth of hair, principally on the face of children affected during this epidemic, led to the term *monkey children*. The skin abnormality in this outbreak was termed *pema yara* ("pink sore").

Pentachloronitrobenzene

PCNB is an organochlorine fungicide used to treat seed and soil at the time of planting. It is used for a variety of vegetable and field crops, including lettuce, cotton, and tomatoes and on turf grass. Its compound is also known as *quintozene*. This fungicide may be used in combination with insecticides; however, the use of most products containing PCNB has been canceled in the United States.

Allergic contact dermatitis has been reported in patients repeatedly exposed (12). With heavy exposure, methemoglobinemia may occur. The estimated lethal dose for humans is 500 to 5,000 mg per kg, with an oral LD_{50} in rats of 1,500 mg per kg. Reproductive effects were noted in mice and rats at doses that approached the lethal level. Evaluating the carcinogenicity of this compound has been difficult as, in earlier studies examining PCNB, the tested compounds were found to contain hexachlorobenzene and other contaminants. When rodents were fed doses of 464 mg per kg by stomach tube, liver tumors were reported to develop.

Absorption is limited in mammals and some animal species; however, when PCNB was administered to monkeys, it was absorbed rapidly from the gastrointestinal (GI) tract and metabolized rapidly by the liver with biliary excretion. The elimination half-life is believed to be approximately 4 days through slow biliary excretion.

Depending on its manufacturer, PCNB can include such impurities as hexachlorobenzene, pentachlorobenzene, and tetrachloronitrobenzene.

Pentachlorophenol

PCP has been used extensively as a preservative of wood and as a fungicide throughout the United States. Its fungicidal activity was discovered in 1936 as a timber preservative (14). Its most common use was as a wood preservative for telephone poles. The compound is produced by the chlorination of a phenol in the presence of a catalyst. Commercial-grade PCP is at least 86% pure and contains contaminants of other polychlorinated phenols, such as polychlorinated dibenzodioxin and polychlorinated dibenzofurans (15). Pure PCP is a white organic solid with needle crystals. Impure PCP is dark gray to brown and is produced as a dust or as flakes. Heating PCP produces a sharp, pungent phenolic odor. Little odor is present at room temperature.

Eighty percent of U.S. consumption of PCP in the past was as a wood preservative. It was registered for use as an insecticide, fungicide, acaricide, herbicide, and disinfectant. Formerly, it was used also as an antifouling agent in paint. PCP is now a restricted-use compound and is no longer used as a wood-preserving solution or as a fungicide available for home use.

Owing to the extensive use of PCP throughout the United States, it has been found in air and various water and soil types. A very stable compound, it is not hydrolyzed or oxidized easily. However, it does undergo photooxidation by sunlight and can be biotransformed by soil microorganisms.

EXPOSURE SOURCES

Exposure to PCP occurs in occupational settings and through environmental contamination sources. Some human exposure occurs from indoor air pollution, because the wood structure of a home may have been treated previously with PCP as a preservative. PCP is detected in adipose tissue, human milk, blood, and urine. On average, the U.S. population has been shown to have urinary PCP concentrations of approximately 5 parts per billion (ppb) (15). In those who are exposed occupationally to PCP in its use as a wood preservative, urine concentrations approximate 120 ppb.

Analyses of blood and urine samples from 6,000 persons in 64 communities within the United States were conducted between 1976 and 1980 (15). PCP was one of the compounds detected in 79% of urine samples collected in this survey, the level of PCP ranging between 6 and 193 ppb. Blood concentrations of PCP also varied depending on the exposure. Individuals occupationally exposed to PCP or using PCP-treated materials have blood concentrations that range from 83 to 57,600 ppb (15). Most of these individuals were involved in construction of log homes previously treated with PCP. The adipose concentration of PCP was shown in 1973 to be a mean of 26.3 μg per kg in the general U.S. population (15).

Dietary intake of PCP occurs through contaminated food products. It has been used as an herbicide on pineapple, sugarcane, and rice crops. Also, in a 1976 survey, PCP was found in drinking water supplies at a mean concentration of 0.07 μg per L, with a maximum concentration of 0.7 μg per L (15). Another survey conducted in eight cities detected PCP in drinking water supplies at levels ranging from 1 to 12 μg per L (15). Food and water supplies are a common environmental source of human intake of PCP.

PCP indoor air concentrations can be particularly high in log homes or older homes built of wood that has been pretreated with the compound as a preservative. In air samples taken in log homes, PCP has been found to range from 7 to 8 ppb. In older homes, the U.S. Environmental Protection Agency (EPA) has found PCP air concentrations to range from 0.5 to 10.0 μg per cubic meter (15). Higher concentrations of PCP have been found in treated wood, with these levels ranging from 34 to 104 μg per cubic meter (15).

Human exposure to PCP occurs by the inhalational and dermal routes and by ingestion. Most occupational exposure has occurred to pest control applicators, carpenters, electrical power workers, and any workers in trades or professions that involve contact with wood products. Other at-risk populations include individuals living near PCP-manufacturing sites or waste disposal sites and those who work in lumber mills.

REGULATORY ASPECTS

PCP is on the list of chemicals that appear in the toxic chemicals section (no. 313) of the Emergency Planning and Community Right to Know Act of 1986. The Occupational Safety and Health Administration (OSHA) permissible exposure limit (PEL) is 0.5 mg per cubic meter as a TWA, with a skin notation. The National Institute of Occupational Safety and Health (NIOSH) lists 150 μg per cubic meter as the concentration that is immediately dangerous to life and health (IDLH). The ACGIH recommends a TLV of 0.5 mg per cubic meter. The National Academy of Sciences' safe drinking water guide is 0.021 mg per L. The suggested no-adverse-effect level is 6 μg per L in a child, 7 μg per L of a technical-grade PCP in an adult, and 9 μg per L of commercial-grade PCP in an adult. PCP is listed by the EPA as a hazardous waste and a priority toxic pollutant.

CLINICAL TOXICOLOGY

The molecular formula of PCP is C_6Cl_5OH. It is a light brown solid and has a pungent odor and a melting point of 187°C. PCP (also known as *penchlorol* and *Dowicide EC*) is incompatible with strong oxidizers.

In general, PCP produces irritation of the eyes, nose, throat, and mucous membranes. Inhalational exposure to PCP compounds is a common mode of exposure. Deaths have occurred after acute inhalation of PCP (15). Inhalation of PCP produces irritation of the upper respiratory tract, coughing, and symptoms of bronchitis with chest tightness. Such exposure also can produce cardiac effects of tachycardia. The ingestion of PCP can result in abdominal pain, nausea, and vomiting with systemic absorption. Target organs for toxicity include the liver, kidneys, hematopoietic system, pulmonary system, and the central nervous system (CNS). Pulmonary inhalation of high concentrations can result in pulmonary edema and death (15).

Cases of aplastic anemia have been associated with PCP exposure (15). PCP-induced liver toxicity in humans has occurred in herbicide sprayers. Fatty infiltration of the liver and central lobular congestion with hepatocellular accumulation of fat has been noted. Also, elevation of liver enzymes has been seen after chronic dermal exposure to PCP (15). Kidney effects secondary to exposure to PCP have been noted also, along with increased incidence of proteinuria and hematuria.

Corneal injury can occur from splashes to the eye, and vapors of PCP can produce ocular irritation. PCP also can induce dermatitis, inflammation of the skin, desquamation, and hair loss (15).

Neurotoxicity of PCP can occur after massive exposure. Hyperthermia, probably due to uncoupling of oxidative phosphorylation, has been observed. No report has cited peripheral neuropathy secondary to exposure. Lethargy and cerebral edema have occurred after short-term, high-level exposures to PCP. These effects have been accompanied also by seizures, coma, delirium, and hyperthermia.

No evidence of human immunotoxic effects from PCP has been documented. However, animal studies have shown immunotoxic effects. Although no evidence substantiates reproductive toxicity or developmental effects secondary to human exposure to PCP, an increase in the frequency of chromosomal aberrations has been seen in the peripheral lymphocytes of workers occupationally exposed to PCP (15).

PCP is well absorbed by the inhalational, dermal, and GI routes. Once absorbed, it is highly protein bound. The compound undergoes glucuronide conjugation, and a minor amount undergoes oxidation to tetrachlorohydroquinone, which can be used as a biomarker of PCP exposure. The half-life of elimination of PCP from plasma was found to be 30 hours in human volunteers (15). Also, in the same study, 74% of the PCP dose administered to human volunteers was eliminated as the parent compound, and 12% was eliminated as a glucuronide metabolite within 168 hours (15). PCP elimination is believed to be first order, with some enterohepatic recirculation after ingestion.

Benomyl

Terrazole

Thiabendazole

Fuberidazole

Carbendazim

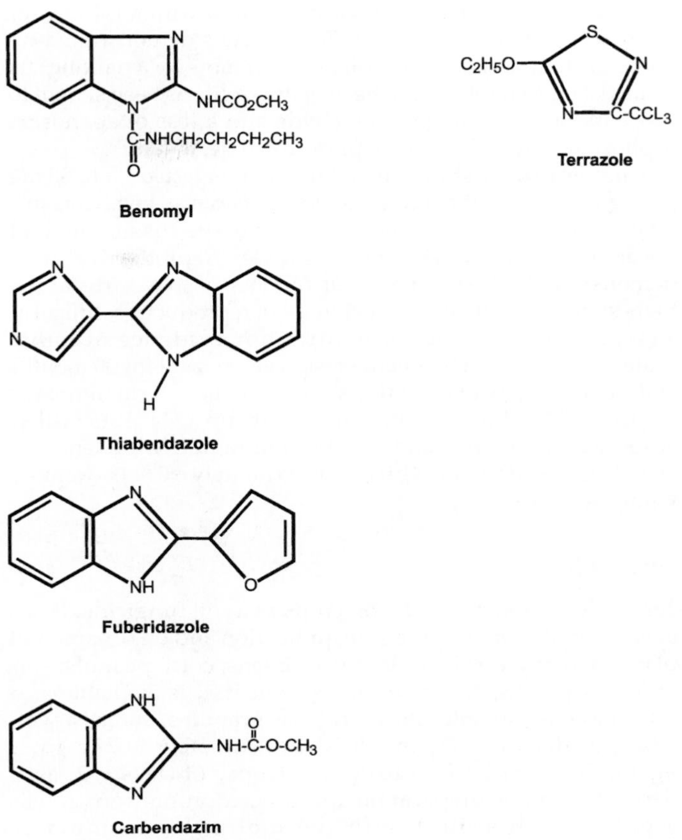

Figure 102-2. Thiabendazoles.

THIABENDAZOLES

The thiabendazole class of fungicides comprises heterocyclic derivatives of the parent thiabendazole compound (Fig. 102-2). These compounds include benomyl, thiabendazole, thiophanate-methyl, mebendazole, and albendazole. Mebendazole and albendazole have been used to treat human and veterinary helminthiasis. Thiabendazole and its congeners produce many biochemical changes in susceptible nematodes: inhibition of mitochondrial fumarate reductase, reduced glucose transport, and uncoupling of oxidative phosphorylation. Inhibition of microtubule polymerization by binding to α-tubulin is the primary action of this drug class. The selective toxicity of these agents stems from the fact that specific, high-affinity binding to parasite α-tubulin occurs at much lower concentrations than does mammalian protein binding.

Benomyl

Benomyl, a white crystalline solid benzimidazole carbamate with a formula $C_{14}H_{18}N_4O_3$, is a systemic fungicide that has selective toxicity to microorganisms and invertebrates. It is especially active against earthworms. It finds use against a wide range of fungal diseases in the agricultural industry, including field crops, fruits, nuts, and turf. According to the World Health Organization, because benomyl lacks significant toxicity, it is rated as a class 0, meaning that it is unlikely to present any acute hazard during its normal use (16). In fact, the LD_{50} in rats was found to be in excess of 10,000 mg per kg per day using a 50% wettable powder formulation. However, this substance is known to be irritating to the skin and can result in allergic skin reactions.

Rats fed diets of up to 150 mg per kg per day in a 2-year study found no toxic effects (12). However, dogs fed similar doses exhibited evidence of increased liver function abnormalities. Certain animals given high doses developed liver cirrhosis after a 2-year feeding program (12). A three-generation rat study demonstrated no difference in reproductive or lactational differences at doses of 150 mg per kg per day orally (12). Mixed results have been found in rats fed between 62 and 150 mg per kg per day. When benomyl was administered by stomach tube on days 7 to 16 of pregnancy, birth defects were noted (17). A 2-year feeding study that fed albino rats diets of up to 2,500 mg per kg per day found no significant adverse effects.

Benomyl is absorbed rapidly, is broken down to carbendazim and butyl isocyanate, and is eliminated. The parent compounds are noted to be absent within 6 hours, with no evidence of residue in muscle or fat stores (12). Carbendazim and benomyl have similar toxicologic properties and produce dermal irritant effects. On skin contact, benomyl produces erythema and edema. It is also a mucous membrane irritant. However, the metabolite is not a skin sensitizer (18). Some reports have cited impaired ciliary function in dogs after exposure. The beat frequency is markedly reduced, and mitochondrial swelling is found in the ciliary cell (19). The ACGIH TLV/TWA for benomyl is 0.84 ppm, or 10 mg per cubic meter. The OSHA PEL/TWA is 15 mg per cubic meter as a total dose.

Imazalil

Imazalil is a systemic fungicide used to control a wide range of fungi in fruits and vegetables. It is a yellow or brown crystalline powder soluble in organic compounds and is available as an emulsifiable concentrate, water-soluble powder, and soluble liquid.

Imazalil is a moderately toxic compound with a rat LD_{50} of approximately 300 mg per kg. Test animals demonstrated no goose flesh, muscular incoordination, tremors, or vomiting. Its principal effect has been on the liver. Imazalil has been shown to cause induction of malondialdehyde and a loss of adenosine triphosphate and glutathione prior to cell death (20).

Chronic toxicity studies in animals that ingested up to 80 mg per kg for 3.5 months did not affect appearance, behavior, survival, food consumption, urinalysis, or tissue consumption of the animals (21). A three-generation rodent reproductive study demonstrated a trend to a lower number of live births at the highest doses, with no other evidence of reproductive difficulty. Also, neither fetal abnormalities nor evidence of lethal mutagenic effects were noted. Rats given imazalil for 30 months at doses of 5 mg per kg per day showed no increase in tumors as compared to those in the control group (21). Imazalil is absorbed, distributed, and metabolized rapidly in rodent species. It is a sulfate, of which approximately 90% is excreted within 96 hours.

Terrazole

Terrazole is used primarily on crops as a soil fungicide. It has been used also on turf as a soil application and on ornamental plants. Other crops include cotton, beans, corn, peanuts, sorghum, soybeans, sugar beets, and wheat. It is available as a dust and emulsifiable concentrate, as granules, and as a wettable powder. The LD_{50} in rats is approximately 1,077 mg per kg and includes an EPA toxicity category of class 1, 2, or 3, depending on its preparation and concentration. Terrazole is a pale yellow liquid with the molecular formula of $C_5H_5C_3N_2OS$.

Acute toxicity in animals includes ataxia, hyperreactivity, and asthenia. A study that fed terrazole orally to dogs at diet levels of up to 1,000 ppm for 3 months revealed decreased spleen–to–body weight ratios and decreased weight gain, increased serum liver enzymes, increased liver weight, and cholestasis (22). Human toxicity is not reported in the medical literature; however, the estimated acute toxicity is believed to be fairly low.

Thiabendazole

Thiabendazole has a formula of $C_{10}H_7N_3S$ and is a white odorless powder used as an anthelmintic and fungicide (23). Thiabendazole is a systemic benzimidazole fungicide used to control fruit and vegetable diseases, such as mold rot, blight, and stain. It is active also against Dutch elm disease. The rat LD_{50} is approximately 3,000 to 3,500 mg per kg.

Thiabendazole is used in humans as an oral drug for treatment of nematodes, such as hookworms, roundworms, pinworms, and threadworms. As a drug, it is absorbed rapidly via the GI tract. It also is absorbed readily through the skin as a fungicidal agent. Ingestion of thiabendazole incites adverse effects of nausea, dizziness, diarrhea, abdominal discomfort, drowsiness, headache, and vertigo. Acute oral overdoses may result in seizures, hyperexcitability, hypotension, bradycardia, renal toxicity, and hepatic toxicity (24). Hypersensitivity reactions include rashes, conjunctivitis, erythema multiforme, Stevens-Johnson syndrome, and angioedema (24).

In a rat-feeding study, 200 mg per kg per day was administered for 2 years, with little or no effect noted (13). Dogs fed similar doses for a 2-year period exhibited few effects other than occasional attacks of vomiting and persistent anemia. Other species have shown few symptoms (12). When pregnant rats were fed diets of 200 mg per kg on day 11 of pregnancy, offspring were noted to have skeletal defects. When similar doses were administered on day 12 of pregnancy, the young were noted to have absent tails and cleft palates. Two-year feeding studies conducted with rats demonstrated no evidence of cancer related to thiabendazole.

Common side effects reported in patients taking thiabendazole medicinally include anorexia, nausea, vomiting, dizziness, occasional diarrhea, parietes, drowsiness, and headache (25).

Thiophanate-Methyl

Thiophanate-methyl, a colorless crystalline solid with a molecular formula of $C_{12}H_{14}N_4O_4S_2$, is water soluble (23). On contact, this compound can cause dermatitis consisting of swelling, erythema, and itching (23).

CARBOXANILIDES (CARBOXIN, OXATHIINS)

Carboxanilides are systemic fungicides used in the prevention or control of fungal infections (Fig. 102-3). Their uses include the control of smut, rot, and blight on cereal grains, cotton, and vegetables. They have been used also to control "fairy rings" on turf. These rings are the annular appearance of mushrooms on the surface as the mycelia grows beneath the ground.

Carboxin

Carboxin is a systemic fungicide that is sold under the trade names of Cadan, Padan, Sanvex, Thiobel, and Vegetox. These compounds have limited toxicity, with nausea, vomiting, and headache being reported after exposure. Data regarding human exposure are lacking; however, an adolescent who ingested treated seeds developed nausea, vomiting, and headache within 1 hour, with resolution of symptoms in 2 hours. Details about the amount ingested, treatment, and coingestants are not clear (26). No animal evidence suggests that carboxin has clinically significant reproductive, teratogenic, mutagenic, or carcinogenic effects.

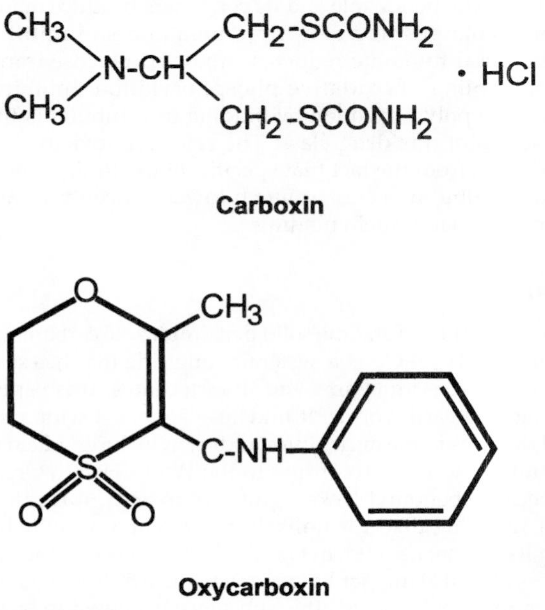

Carboxin

Oxycarboxin

Figure 102-3. Oxathiins.

Rats have been reported to excrete almost an entire dose within 24 hours, primarily in the urine (27). The principal metabolite is carbon sulfoxide (known also as *oxycarboxin*), which is active. Carboxin has limited absorption in both rats and rabbits and does not accumulate in tissues (26). Other metabolites include carboxin sulfone, hydroxycarboxin, and carbon dioxide.

Current exposure guidelines have set the no-observed-effect level (NOEL) at 10 mg per kg per day. In a 70-kg adult, this would represent 700 mg per day. The oral LD_{50} in rats is 2,000 mg per kg, and the dermal limit is more than 16,000 mg per kg based on carbon sulfoxide (27). Chickens are far more resistant to toxicity, having an oral LD_{50} of 24,000 gm per kg (13). On the basis of animal data and very limited human information, this fungicide would have limited toxicity.

Oxycarboxin

Oxycarboxin, like carboxin, is a systemic fungicide. Its foliar application is used to control rust on carnations and geraniums in greenhouses only. It is available as an emulsifiable concentrate and as a wettable powder. Initially, it was described and used as a seed treatment. Typically, it is applied at 1.5 to 4.0 pounds per acre. The toxicologic profile is that of carboxin, which is limited.

DITHIOCARBAMATES

Dithiocarbamates find use mainly as fungicides, although some of these compounds are used as herbicides and nematocides (Fig. 102-4) (23). This class of fungicides includes ziram, ferbam, thiram, methamsodium, sulfallate, anobam, maneb, nabam, and zineb. Methamsodium is used as a nematocide. In addition, disulfiram (triethylthiuram, Antabuse) is related structurally to this class of fungicides and inhibits acetaldehyde dehydrogenase, creating the disulfiram effect.

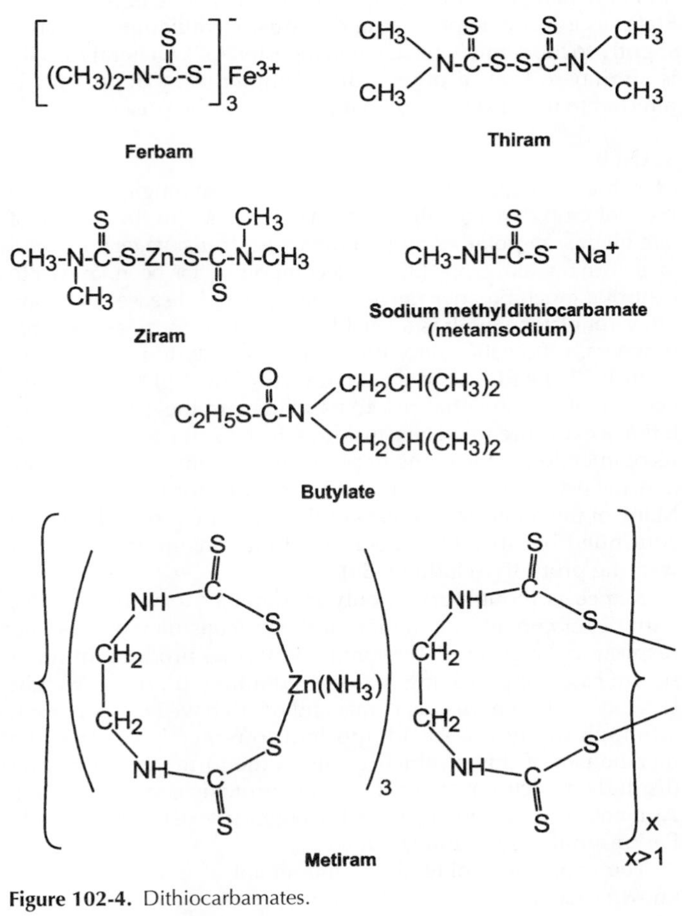

Ferbam

Thiram

Ziram

Sodium methyldithiocarbamate (metamsodium)

Butylate

Metiram

Figure 102-4. Dithiocarbamates.

The toxicity of dithiocarbamates is increased by coingestion of ethanol. These compounds also produce antithyroid effects by decreasing iodine uptake. Workers using thiram fungicides have experienced typical disulfiramlike symptoms that include nausea, vomiting, headache, diaphoresis, and thirst when disulfiram is consumed with alcohol. This class of fungicides also has some irritant-type properties, and hemolysis has been reported.

Typically, these substances are absorbed poorly; however, after limited absorption, all the dithiocarbamates are metabolized to carbon disulfide. Like that of carbon disulfide, thiram poisoning has resulted in peripheral neuropathies.

Thiram

Thiram (tetramethylthiuram disulfide) is a general-use fungicide with a formula of $C_6H_{12}N_2S_4$ and a molecular weight of 240.44 D (23). Thiram is insoluble in water but soluble in organic solvents. It is decomposed after exposure to acids (24). In addition to its use as a fungicide, it has been used as an accelerator in the rubber industry and as an antioxidant. Thiram is a degradation product of both ferbam and ziram (28,29). It takes the form of colorless crystals and is formulated as a powder and as a dust for application as a seed treatment.

The dithiocarbamates can produce systemic toxic reactions of a disulfiramlike reaction if absorbed concurrently with ethanol. Other systemic toxicity reported includes nausea, vomiting, abdominal pain, hyperexcitability, and weakness (23). Thiram also can produce contact dermatitis, but this is not very common. Thiram has been used in the rubber industry as a vulcanizing agent and has been associated with dermatitis (28).

Human exposure occurs via inhalational or skin exposure to dusts, sprays, mists, or aerosolized forms of the product. The OSHA workplace exposure limit is 5 mg per cubic meter as a TLV/TWA. The ACGIH TLV is 1.0 mg per cubic meter. Its carcinogenicity classification is A4, meaning that it is not a human carcinogen. The IDLH value is 100 mg per cubic meter. The residue tolerance level as a fungicide on vegetables and fruits is 7 mg per kg (29).

Toxic exposure to thiram produces irritation of eyes, mucous membranes, and the skin. Erythema and urticarial reactions can occur after dermal exposure to thiram. Allergic contact dermatitis also can occur (29).

Thiram is metabolized by the liver to carbon disulfide (see Chapter 109). Environmentally, thiram can be degraded to carbon disulfide, hydrogen sulfide, and dimethylamine, all of which are toxic by-products. Thiram also may produce hepatotoxicity once systemically absorbed (29). Other toxic manifestations of thiram include nausea, dizziness, headache, confusion ataxia, vomiting, diarrhea, and flaccid paralysis (29). Death has occurred after ingestion. Thiram can produce GI focal necrosis.

Metallobisdithiocarbamates

Fungicides in the metallobisdithiocarbamate group derive their names from the attached metal. Ferbam contains iron (Fe) and ziram contains zinc. These fungicides are similar to the ethylene bisdithiocarbamates. They may cause irritation and inhibit alcohol dehydrogenase.

FERBAM

Ferbam is a dithiocarbamate fungicide marketed under the trade names Cormate and Fennacide. It has a molecular formula of $C_9H_{18}N_3S_6$ and a molecular weight of 416.5 D (23). Ferbam is used to control diseases of fruit, tobacco, conifers, nuts, ornamental plants, and vegetables. This fungicide does not tend to persist in the environment and is degraded by soil microbes within 28 days of application. It is an irritant chemical to the eyes, skin, and mucous membranes and has a potential to produce kidney damage. The OSHA PEL for a TWA is 15 mg per cubic meter (total dust). The ACGIH recommends a TLV of 10 mg per cubic meter, with a short-term exposure limit (STEL) of 20 mg per cubic meter for 15 minutes. The IDLH value is 800 mg per cubic meter.

ZIRAM

Ziram (zinc dimethyldithiocarbamate) has a formula of $C_6H_{12}N_2S_4Zn$ and is an odorless powder with a molecular weight of 305.8 D (23). The human toxic hazard is mainly due to airborne dust, because it has negligible vapor pressure, but reports are limited. Ziram is an irritant of the eyes, upper airway, and mucous membranes. Ingestion can produce localized necrosis of the GI tract (23). Due to its irritant properties, ziram can produce respiratory irritation and distress on inhalation of dust (30). It is classified by the International Agency for Research on Cancer as a group 3 agent (i.e., unclassifiable as a human carcinogen).

Ethylene Bisdithiocarbamates

The ethylene bisdithiocarbamate (EBDC) fungicides include maneb, mancozeb, nabam, trimanzone, and zineb (Fig. 102-5). These fungicides have been known to cause irritation of the mucous membranes and, in the case of maneb and zineb, are thought to be responsible for some cases of allergic skin conditions. A major concern with the EBDC fungicides, including maneb, is ethylene thiourea (ETU), which is present both as a contaminant and as a breakdown product of these pesticides. Its breakdown can be accelerated by heating this product, such as the cooking of foods that have been treated with this pesticide.

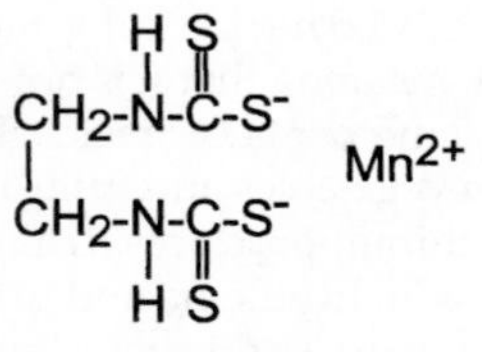

Maneb

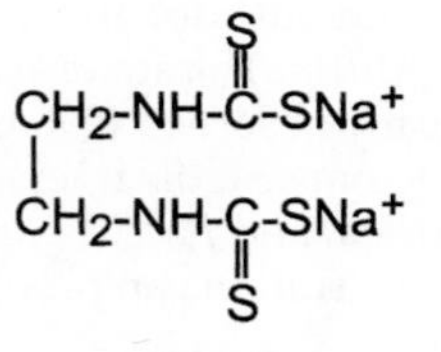

Nabam

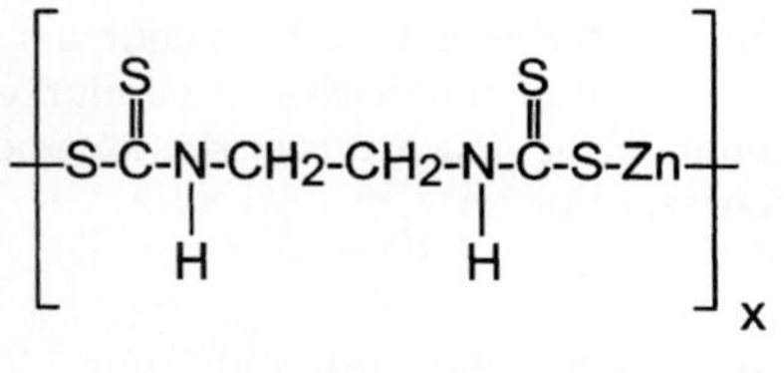

Zineb

Figure 102-5. Ethylene bisdithiocarbamates.

This metabolite was reported to result in goiter and hyperthyroid in animals. In addition to the goitrogenic effect of EBDCs, concern for cancer of the thyroid and an Antabuse like reaction have been reported. Tests in animals have suggested an increased number of stillborn offspring, and fetal abnormalities of the eye, ear, body wall, CNS, and musculoskeletal system in animals have been reported (31).

Nabam has the greatest water solubility and absorbability of this category of fungicides. Maneb is only moderately water-soluble, with mancozeb and zineb having limited water solubility. Unlike the dithiocarbamate fungicides, the EBDC compounds do not inhibit aldehyde dehydrogenase and thus do not result in Antabuse like reactions.

MANCOZEB

The uses of mancozeb are similar to those of other EBDC fungicides. Mancozeb is applied to a wide variety of crops. Its uses include treatment of crops for potato blight, leaf spot, and rust on ornamental plants. It is found also in use as a seed treatment for cotton, potatoes, corn, sorghum, peanuts, and some cereal grains (32,33). Mancozeb is actually a combination of two other EBDC fungicides, maneb and zineb (34).

Mancozeb, like any other fungicide, is available as a dust, as a liquid, as a dispersible granule, as a wettable powder, and as a ready-to-use formulation (35). It has a very low order of acute toxicity to mammals. (See later discussion of the acute toxicity of maneb.) It is compounded with zineb.

ZINEB

Zineb also is a generally used fungicide of the EBDC classification. It has found uses in the protection of fruit and vegetable crops. Reportedly, this product can be formed by the combination of nabam and zinc sulfate (36). It is available in the United States as a wettable powder and in dust formulations. Zineb is slightly to moderately toxic when ingested (37). General toxicity is similar to that of other EBDC fungicides. (The reader is referred to the next section on maneb for further discussion.)

MANEB

Maneb is a manganese-containing general-use fungicide used to prevent crop damage (38). Its primary uses are in the control of late blights on potatoes and on tomatoes, fruits, vegetables, and some ornamental crops (35). This compound has been known to control a much broader range of plant-related diseases than any other fungicide (36). It is available in granular form, as wettable powders, as flowable concentrates, and as ready-to-use formulas.

In 1987, the EPA conducted a review of the EBDC fungicides because of the potential risk to handlers and the general population's exposure to dietary residues. In 1992, the special review recommended the wearing of protective clothing by applicators and the establishment of a 24-hour reentry for these workers. Many of the home garden uses of these products have been discontinued because of the concern that consumers were not wearing protective clothing (39).

Maneb is thought to be only moderately toxic to humans, with development of irritation of the mucous membranes and respiratory tract on direct contact with this product. In more severe cases of poisoning, nausea, vomiting, diarrhea, weight loss, headache, confusion, coma, and death have been reported, although rarely (5). Also important to remember is that the metabolism of this product results in the formation of carbon disulfide, which possesses its own neurotoxic capabilities (40). As maneb contains manganese, the potential exists for a possible Parkinson-like syndrome to develop.

The main metabolite and contaminant of maneb is ETU, a known rodent teratogenic. Poisoning produces a high incidence

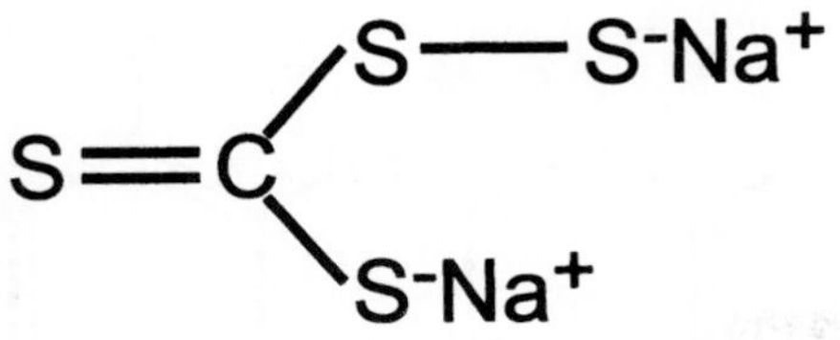

Figure 102-6. Sodium tetrathiocarbonate.

of skeletal malformations, and defects in the closing of the neural tube have been reported (41). ETU has been shown to be teratogenic in both rats and hamsters but not in mice (9).

All the EBDC pesticides are classified as probable human carcinogens by the EPA, owing to the formation of ETU during their metabolism (39). The formation of ETU appears to be dose-related and increases the incidence of liver tumors in mice and dose-related malignant thyroid tumors in rats.

SODIUM TETRATHIOCARBONATE

Sodium tetrathiocarbonate is an interesting fungicide, insecticide, nematicide, and soil fumigant (Fig. 102-6). It acts through its conversion to carbon disulfide and is used in the treatment of grape *Phylloxera* and root-rot diseases. In the United States, it is limited geographically to the citrus and grape crops of the West Coast and Arizona. In addition to carbon disulfide, it degrades to carbonate and sulfate in the soil, thus providing nutrition to plants.

This product is available under the name of Enzone and has limited toxicity. It is known to cause mucous membrane irritation but does not cause dermal sensitization (35). It has caused cutaneous burns and, when inadvertently mixed with acids, may release hydrogen sulfide or carbon disulfide gas (see Chapter 109).

DICARBOXIMIDES

Dicarboximides form a group of fungicides that are chloralkylthiodicarboximide compounds (Fig. 102-7). These agents were registered by the EPA between 1949 and 1962. Captan is used on many crops; however, folpet is used only as a preservative in paints. All domestic licensed indications for captafol were withdrawn by the EPA in 1987, owing to the findings of oncogenicity in laboratory animals. All these substances are listed as group B2 carcinogens by the EPA (42).

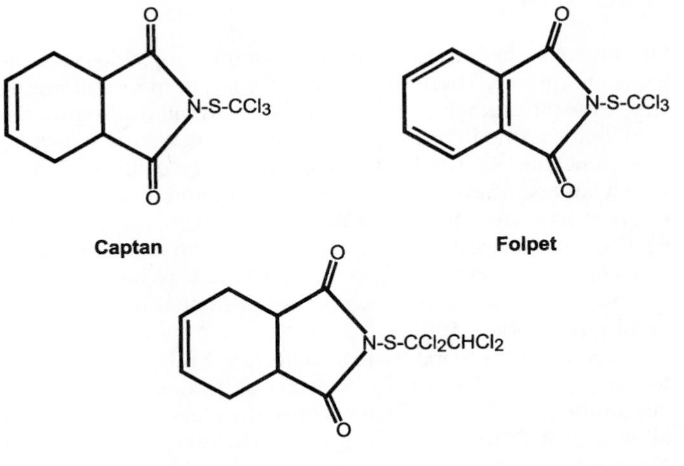

Figure 102-7. Dicarboximides.

Captafol

Captafol is a broad-spectrum fungicide belonging to the sulfanilamide group. It is used widely as a contact fungicide on a variety of fruit and vegetable crops. It also is used in the lumber and timber industries and as a seed protectant. Captafol is available as a dust; in flowable, wettable, and dispersible forms; or in a suspension.

The LD_{50} in rats is approximately 6,500 mg per kg, which places this compound in EPA class 4. In other words, the word *caution* must be printed on the label.

Acute allergic reactions have been reported in humans (4,35). Dogs fed diets of 100 or 300 mg per kg per day have developed vomiting, diarrhea, anemia, weight loss, and growth deficiencies. Other studies of chronic use of Captafol of up to 300 mg per kg have demonstrated increased organ weights with no evidence of histopathology or histopathologic abnormalities, blood chemistry abnormalities, or abnormalities of the liver enzymes (9,10). No reproductive abnormalities are noted in rats fed up to 1,000 mg per kg. When rhesus monkeys were fed diets of 6.25 to 25.0 mg per kg per day from days 22 to 32 of gestation, no teratogenic effects were noted (43).

When Captafol is combined with acids, chloride vapors may emanate. These include some organic chlorides, which have been known to decompose to phosgene. The possible oral lethal dose for humans may be between 0.5 and 5.0 grams per kg for a 70-kg adult (5). Ingestion of Captafol is known to cause vomiting and diarrhea and irritant signs and symptoms of the GI tract. The major metabolite is tetrahydrophthalimide.

Workers who have sprayed Captafol, including farmers, have developed erythematous dermatitis, which is believed to be a photodermatitis. In a study of 133 workers exposed to Captafol, 23% gave a history suggesting contact dermatitis. Typically, this is an irritant dermatitis, although allergic contact dermatitis has been reported (44). Other less common findings included hypertension, edema, proteinuria, and anemia (23). The ACGIH exposure regulation is a TLV/TWA of 0.1 mg per cubic meter of skin.

Captan

Captan is another dicarboximide, a nonsystemic fungicide used to control diseases primarily in fruit crops. It is available also for home use and for agricultural production. The major use of captan is in the apple industry; 50% of apple acreage is treated with captan. It is applied to apples after the harvest, during the packaging and shipping process. Other common uses include its application to almond and strawberry crops, and other less common uses include its incorporation into such materials as canvas, leather, wallpaper paste, paints, and plastics. More than 300 registered pesticide products contain captan. The ACGIH TLV/TWA is 5 mg per cubic meter.

Typically, captan is available in dust and powder forms and generally is a toxicology class 3 or 4 pesticide. The typical rat LD_{50} ranges from approximately 8,000 to 15,000 mg per kg. The lowest dose reported to cause death in humans was 1,071 mg per kg (13). A study in mice maintained on a diet of 50 mg per kg over three generations has found no reproductive abnormalities and normal fertility, litter size, and growth of the young.

With mixed reports of teratogenicity in rats, rabbits, hamsters, and dogs, captan is thought not to result in birth defects.

Evidence in rodent models suggests that captan may result in GI and renal tumors. These tumors have appeared at doses of approximately 300 mg per kg. Because of this, captan is classified by the EPA as a probable human carcinogen. In one study, workers exposed to high concentrations of captan in air (approximately 5 mg per cubic meter) experienced irritant symptoms of the eyes and skin.

Captan is absorbed rapidly in the GI tract. It is metabolized rapidly in residues found primarily in the urine. After absorption, captan reacts readily with thiol-containing compounds (45). Its typical half-life in animals ranges from 12 to 18 hours. Captan interacts with sulfhydryl groups within fungi to produce thiophosgene. Other effects include inhibition of RNA polymerase in bacteria and the inhibition of decarboxylation (46).

Folpet

Folpet is a protective leaf fungicide. It no longer is sold in the United States but previously had been used on fruit, vegetables, and ornamental crops. This fungicide inhibits cell division of a variety of microorganisms. The oral toxicity for rats is approximately 10 g per kg, and it has been known to cause skin, mucous membrane, and eye irritation when inhaled.

A 1-year chronic oral feeding study in dogs at doses of 10 to 120 mg per kg per day demonstrated slight decreases in cholesterol, total protein, and albumen in the high-dose groups. However, no organ weight changes or histopathologic findings were believed to be associated with folpet. An eight-generation reproductive study in rats found a NOEL of 34.5 mg per kg per day when the agent was administered parenterally (47). Folpet demonstrates a dose-dependent increase in adenocarcinomas of the duodenum in CD-1 mice given doses of 142 to 1,700 mg per kg per day.

An *in vitro* study evaluating folpet's stability in human blood found a half-life of approximately 1 minute. Folpet is degraded rapidly to phthalimide and, ultimately, to phthalic acid and ammonia (47).

Treatment after Dicarboximide Exposure

Treatment for ingestion of any of the dicarboximides is similar. Initial removal of the patient from exposure and decontamination with copious amounts of fresh water or soap and water are recommended for cutaneous exposures. Significant ingestion should be treated by gastric lavage and activated charcoal.

BENZENOIDS

Metalaxyl is a benzenoid fungicide sold under the trade names Ridomil, Apron, Delta-Coat AD, and Subdue 2E (Fig. 102-8). It is a systemic fungicide used in mixtures on tropical crops, in soil treatments, and as a seed treatment for the control of mildew. Its major uses are found in protecting tobacco, ornamental crops, conifer trees, and turf applications (48). It is available as an emulsifiable concentrate, as granules, and as flowable and wettable powders. Metalaxyl is considered generally as a relatively nontoxic fungicide. A 12-hour restricted-entry provision is required after application. The agent's NOEL, based on an increased serum alkaline phosphatase, is 6.25 mg per kg per day based on dog studies.

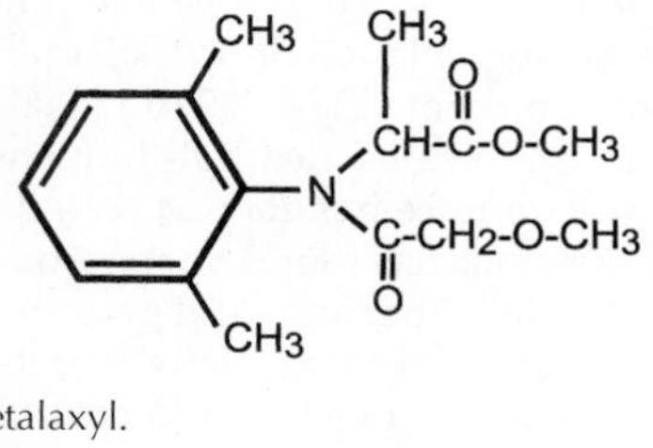

No evidence of reproductive, teratogenic, mutagenic, or oncogenic effects has been reported. Data regarding humans are limited.

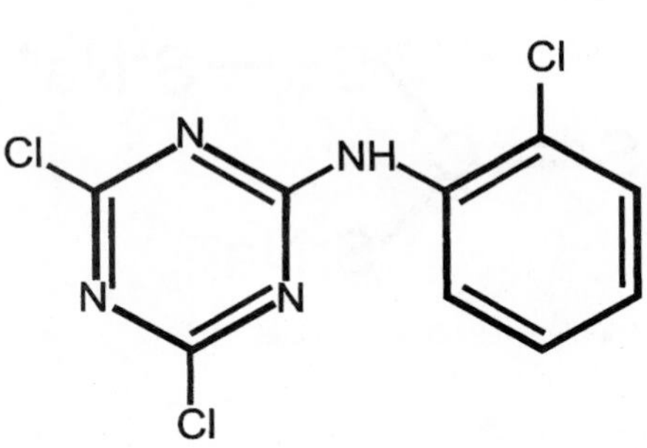

Figure 102-8. Metalaxyl.

Figure 102-9. Dyrene (anilazine).

TRIAZINES: DYRENE (ANILAZINE)

Dyrene represents the triazine class of fungicides (Fig. 102-9). Dyrene's activity is due to its alkylation of fungal enzymes (5). However, despite this particular mechanism of action, dyrene is found to have limited ability to result in sensitization, with the exception of mild irritation. Limited skin irritation has occurred after prolonged contact (5), as has sensitization during patch testing. A chronic feeding study of rats over a 2-year period at 5,000 ppm found no evidence of toxicity (5).

Reports citing acutely poisoned animals have included symptoms of vesiculation, muscle spasms, and congestion of lung, liver, and kidneys (5). Mixed data are available regarding the association of cancer with the triazine fungicides (49).

The product appears to be well absorbed orally and has been found to react with sulfhydryl groups. After this conjugation, it is excreted in the urine and feces (6).

TRIAZOLES

Substances in the triazole group are systemic fungicides used on fruits and grains. These fungicides are known to inhibit ergosterol biosynthesis, which results in disrupted cell wall synthesis. Some have termed these agents *ergosterol biosynthesis–inhibiting fungicides* (EBIFs). The EBIF agents induce cytochrome P-450, which has been shown to enhance the oxidation of certain organophosphate insecticides to their respective oxon products. EBIF agents also result in increased detoxification via oxidative dearylation and esterolytic cleavage. This may be important when multiple exposures have occurred, such as in an applicator or farm worker (50).

Hyperactivity secondary to the effects of EBIFs is attributable to the agents' effect on CNS catecholamines, particularly dopamine (51). This has been reported in laboratory animals after exposure to triadimefon and triadimenol but was not observed with the other triazole fungicides. The occurrence of hyperactivity and CNS stimulation could be anticipated after human exposure (52).

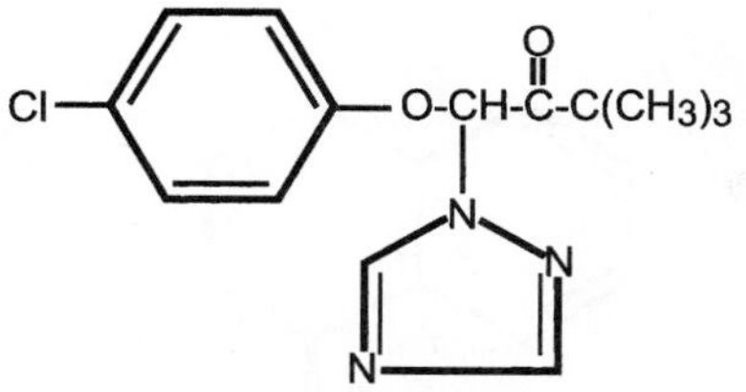

Figure 102-10. Triadimefon.

Triadimefon

Triadimefon (Fig. 102-10) is a systemic fungicide used for control of powdery mildew on cereals, fruits, grapes, and vegetables. It is available under the names of Amiral, Bay MEB 6447, and Bayleton. It has found use also for control of rust diseases on cereals, coffee, seed grasses, sugarcane, and pineapple and for control on turf and ornamental plants. Triadimefon is available in dry, flowable, emulsifiable concentrates, in granules, and as a wettable powder.

Triadimenol

Triadimenol is a triazole systemic fungicide used in seed treatment to control smut and bunt of wheat. Specific trade names include Bayfidan, Baytan 30, and Vydan. It is used also on vegetables, ornamental plants, coffee, tobacco, bananas, and other crops. It is available as an emulsifiable concentrate, a flowable agent, a granule, a seed dressing, water-dispersible granules, a water-oil emulsion, and a wettable powder. Common seed treatments include wheat, barley, oats, rye, and corn.

PIPERAZINE: TRIFORINE

The piperazine class is represented by triforine (Fig. 102-11). Triforine is a systemic fungicide used for control of mildew, rusts, rot, and scab. It is applied to nuts, cereal, fruit, and ornamental and vegetable crops. It has low toxicity to certain beneficial insects, such as bees, and limited toxicity in humans. Sold under the trade names of Brolly, Denarin, Funginex, Nimrod T, and Saprol, triforine is applied frequently in a mixture with other pesticides. Little information is available on its acute or chronic effects on people; however, the animal study data suggest that little toxicity would be expected from this product alone.

The acute oral LD_{50} in rats is in excess of 16,000 mg per kg. Triforine is absorbed and metabolized rapidly by rodents (53). Studies have not found this compound to be a reproductive hazard or to be teratogenic, mutagenic, or oncogenic (54). Triforine is available as a wettable powder and as a dispersible concentrate.

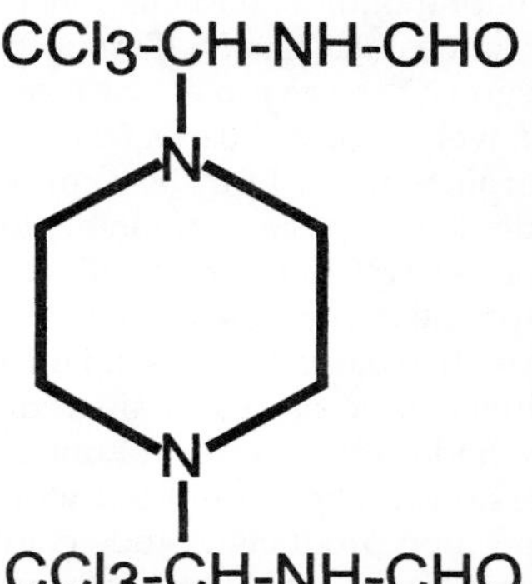

Figure 102-11. Triforine.

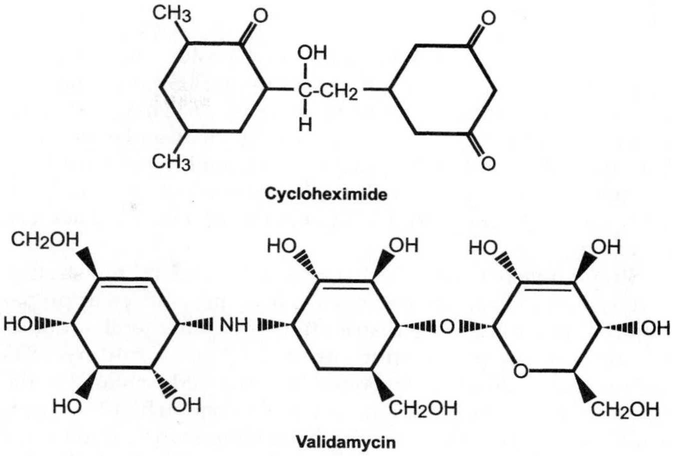

Cycloheximide

Validamycin

Figure 102-12. Antibiotics.

ANTIBIOTICS

Some antibiotics are used as fungicides and are represented by cycloheximide, iturin-A, validamycin, and streptomycin (Fig. 102-12).

Cycloheximide

Cycloheximide is an inhibitor of protein synthesis. The product is available as a wettable powder and, on occasion, is combined with other fungicides. No known reports of human toxicity exist with this product; however, it has been toxic to rats and less so to dogs and monkeys. Findings after poisonings include excessive salivation, bloody diarrhea, tremors, CNS excitation, coma, and death. In an animal study, hydrocortisone increased the rate of survival in poisoned rats (34). High concentrations have been shown to have certain adverse reproductive effects, including effects on fertility in rodent species.

An interesting aspect of cycloheximide is that it has been shown to inhibit the cytotoxicity of paclitaxel (Taxol). Taxol is a form of hormonal therapy used for patients with breast and other cancers. It was found that cycloheximide reduces cytotoxicity due to paclitaxel by preventing cells from entering mitosis, which is a prerequisite for paclitaxel-induced cytotoxicity (55).

Iturin-A

Iturin-A is a cyclic lipopeptide produced by the bacterium *Bacillus subtilis*. Iturins in general have been used to treat human fungal infection (56,57). These fungicides have found efficacy against microflora in tests of treated seeds. Iturin-A, which is related to the antibiotics bacillomyxin and mycosubtilin, may be used in the future for seed treatment. The iturins have strong antifungal properties and low mammalian toxicity. Today, no data are available regarding acute toxicity in humans from iturin-A exposures. However, the mouse LD_{50} by intravenous administration was 65 mg per kg (58).

Streptomycin

Streptomycin is a well-known aminoglycoside antibiotic and fungicidal agent. Streptomycin binds to the 30S ribosomal subunit, inhibiting bacterial protein synthesis. Toxic manifestations may be constitutional symptoms and ototoxicity and nephrotoxicity typical of aminoglycosides. Occasional hypersensitivity reactions, including anaphylaxis, have been reported. As with other aminoglycoside antibiotics, neuromuscular blockade has occurred.

Streptomycin is absorbed poorly after oral administration and is, therefore, given medicinally as an intramuscular preparation. It possesses wide distribution after parenteral administration but low penetration into the CNS. Streptomycin is approximately 36% protein bound. It is excreted primarily in the urine by glomerular filtration, and its elimination half-life is typically 2 to 3 hours. Patients with renal failure who exhibit signs and symptoms of significant toxicity may require hemodialysis for removal of this compound.

DINITROPHENOLS

Dinocap is in the dinitrophenol class of fungicides (Fig. 102-13). Dinocap, also known as *karathane* or *crotonic acid*, is a contact fungicide used to control fungi and is used also as an agaricide. Trade names include Arathane, Caprane, Caproyl, and Mildex. In 1985, the EPA initiated a special review of products containing dinocap, a review that was undertaken because laboratory results indicated rabbit birth defects and chronic reproductive effects (59). The special review, completed in 1990, resulted in the EPA's requirement of a variety of measures to reduce exposure to mixers and applicators. Requirements include the wearing of protective suits, goggles, and face shields; the use of enclosed vehicles for apple cutters; the wearing of a protective hood or wide-brimmed hat during mist-blower or air-blast applications; the wearing of protective suits on leaving an enclosed vehicle; the removal of applicators' contaminated protective equipment, clothing, and shoes; soap-and-water showering before leaving affected premises; and a teratogenicity warning statement on product labels.

Dinocap was registered in the late 1950s and has been used widely since that time on a variety of fruit, vegetable, and ornamental crops. Apples are the major crop on which dinocap is used (approximately 90%) (60). It is available as a dust, as a liquid concentrate, and as a wettable powder. Dinocap is moderately toxic by ingestion and has limited dermal absorption, although with significant ingestion or inhalation, irritant symptoms may develop (61).

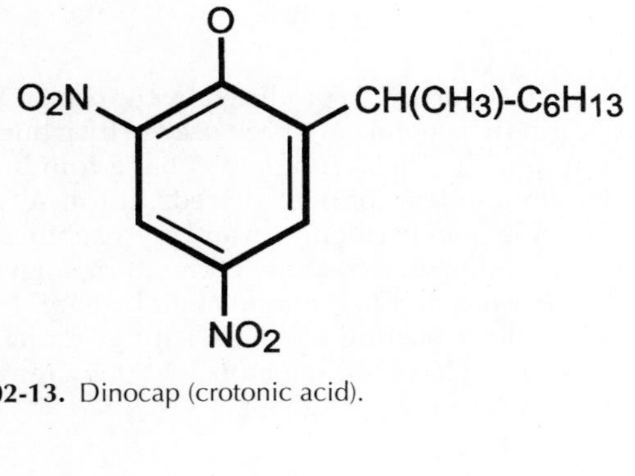

Figure 102-13. Dinocap (crotonic acid).

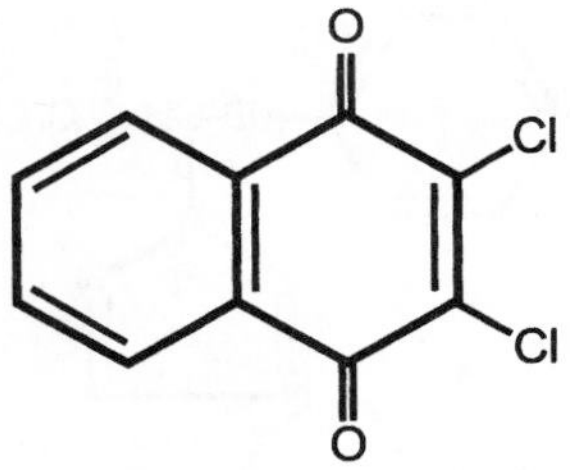

Figure 102-14. Dichlone.

QUINONES

Dichlone, a quinone also known as *chloranil*, is a yellow to colorless crystal material used as a fungicide against seed decay (Fig. 102-14). It is sold under the names of Quintar and Phygon. It is used also to treat diseases in fruit and vegetable crops. 2,3-Dichloro-1,4-naphthoquinone is marketed under the trade names Compound 605, Phygon, and Algistat. It has a molecular formula of $C_{10}H_4Cl_2O_2$ and a molecular weight of 227.04 D.

The fungicide dichlone is used for foliage and textiles and as a seed disinfectant. This compound decomposes slowly in soil and water and may be stable enough to bioaccumulate up the food chain. It has a vapor density of 7.8 (as compared to that of air, which is 1.0). Dichlone is considered to be moderately toxic by ingestion and has irritant properties affecting the skin, eyes, and mucous membranes. It also can produce CNS depression, and it is a very irritating dust (61).

Dichlone exerts relatively low toxicity in both animals and humans (5). The product is absorbed poorly from the GI tract; however, with significant exposure, eye irritation, CNS depression (including coma, vomiting, and diarrhea), and abnormalities in liver function test results may be expected. In addition, methemoglobinemia is theoretically possible, based on the chemical structure of this compound. For patients displaying evidence of signs or symptoms suggestive of methemoglobinemia, treatment with oxygen and methylene blue should be considered. The LD_{50} for rats is approximately 6,950 mg per kg, but no workplace standards have been established for this compound. Some of the toxicity of the naphthoquinone compounds has been postulated to be related to redox cycling of the one-electron reduction reactions, which generates reactive oxygen intermediates and consumes intracellular glutathione (62). Dichlone carries the EPA toxicity class designation of 3 and is a known animal carcinogen (63).

2,3-DICHLORO-1,4-NAPHTHOQUINONE

2,3-Dichloro-1,4-naphthoquinone (dichloronapthoquinone), sold under the trade names of Algistat, Compound 604, Dichlone, Phygon, and Phygon XL, has a molecular formula of $C_{10}H_4Cl_2O_2$ and a molecular weight of 227.04 D. Vapor density is 7.8 (as opposed to that of air, which is 1.0). The compound is insoluble in water and is moderately soluble in organic acids. It is a fungicide and an algaecide used for foliage and textiles and as a seed disinfectant. This compound decomposes slowly in soil and water and may be stable enough to bioaccumulate up the food chain. A very irritating dust, this compound is considered to be moderately toxic by ingestion and is a skin, eye, and mucous membrane irritant. CNS depression has been reported with large exposures. Thermal decomposition products include chlorine gas. Carcinogenicity data regarding 2,3-dichloro-1,4-naphthoquinone are inconclusive.

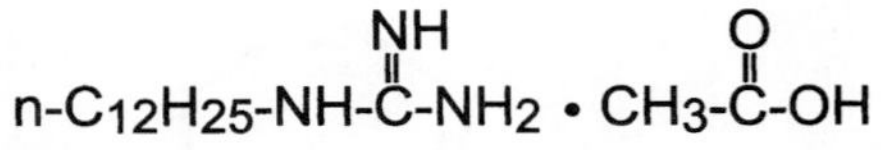

$$n\text{-}C_{12}H_{25}\text{-}NH\text{-}\overset{NH}{\overset{\|}{C}}\text{-}NH_2 \cdot CH_3\text{-}\overset{O}{\overset{\|}{C}}\text{-}OH$$

Figure 102-15. Dodine.

ALIPHATIC NITROGENS

Dodine is a contact surfactant with an antifungicidal activity (Fig. 102-15). It is available as a wettable powder and in other formulations. In the United States, this fungicide is available under the trade names of Carpene, Curitan, Cyprex, Efuzin, and others. Dodine is used to control scab on apples, pears, and pecans and for several other foliar diseases of cherries, strawberries, and peaches. In addition to being used for its fungicidal activity, it is used also as an industrial biocide and preservative.

Because of its acute and severe eye injury on exposure, dodine is considered to be a highly toxic material. It occupies an EPA toxicity class of 1 based on eye irritation (35). Chronic toxicity studies conducted with rats demonstrate reduced food consumption in male animals only. A 1-year feeding study in dogs revealed histologic changes of the thyroid, which indicated some stimulation of that organ. No teratogenic, mutagenic, or carcinogenic effects have been noted. Notice is available regarding human toxicity.

CINNAMIC ACID: DIMETHOMORPH

Dimethomorph is a representative of this class of fungicides (Fig. 102-16). Dimethomorph is a systemic fungicide used also as a wood preservative to control downy mildew in certain vines and to control blight on potatoes (64). It is sold under the names Acrobat, Forum, CME 151, and others. This product is available as a wettable powder, a dispersible concentrate, and a suspension concentrate. Dimethomorph is slightly toxic to mammals, with an LD_{50} in rats of approximately 3,900 mg per kg.

Acute toxicity has demonstrated that it is not irritating to mucous membranes and is not sensitizing to guinea pigs in skin testing (54). Studies on dimethomorph have not found developmental, mutagenic, or carcinogenic activity after exposure. No evidence of human toxicity has been reported.

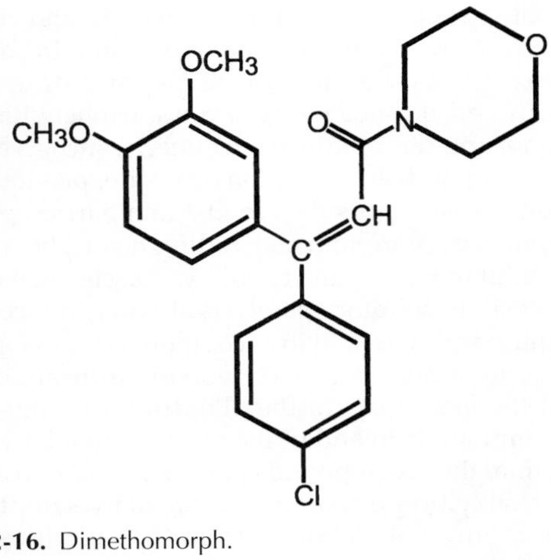

Figure 102-16. Dimethomorph.

MISCELLANEOUS FUNGICIDES

Hexachlorobutadiene

Hexachlorobutadiene (HCBD) is a chlorinated hydrocarbon fungicide. No specific human toxicologic information is available about this agent; however, animals are asymptomatic at an air level of 0.13 ppm, whereas levels of 1.3 ppm could produce some reversible symptoms. Others report that mucous membrane irritation has occurred with exposures that have exceeded 250 ppm (37). Higher exposures have resulted in dyspnea, bronchitis, and pulmonary hemorrhage in animals. The ACGIH TLV/TWA is 0.21 mg per cubic meter.

Currently, HCBD is encountered most commonly in the United States as a by-product in the chlorination of various hydrocarbon products. It is absorbed rapidly through the skin and GI tract of animals. Agricultural workers exposed to 30 mg per cubic meter of HCBD have reported some CNS depression (65). Current liver disease also has been reported in agricultural workers with similar exposure (65). Animal studies have demonstrated renal tubular necrosis in rats given a dose of 50 mg of HCBD per kg intraperitoneally. The exact nature of this injury is not known. The chronic ingestion of 20 mg per kg per day for a 2-year study in rats demonstrated an increase in renal tubular adenomas and adenocarcinomas, with some atelectasis to lungs (37).

Acrolein (Acrylaldehyde)

Acrolein (CH_2CHCHO) is a potent herbicide and biocide used to control weeds, algae, and plant growth in irrigation canals and water drainage areas. Acrolein is a clear to yellowish liquid with a pungent odor. Exposure occurs mainly by inhalation or contact of the liquid by accidental splash (66). Human exposure can result in severe dermatitis and burns to the skin, eyes, and mucous membranes. The EPA lists acrolein as a hazardous material and restricts its use as a pesticide.

Acrolein is used also in the production of glycerin and in the synthesis of other chemicals. It is incompatible with oxidizers, ammonia, and alkalis. Acrolein is a highly volatile liquid, the vapor of which is flammable and forms explosive mixtures in air. The basic product comes as 92% acrolein by weight in a cylinder connected to a nitrogen gas–pressurized delivery system. Acrolein is a highly reactive aldehyde and readily polymerizes with generation of heat. Improper handling or storage of the product can create a hazard that can result in a polymerization reaction, release of heat, and rupturing of the container. Contamination with air, oxidizers, ammonia, or alkalis can initiate a violent polymerization reaction. The OSHA PEL for this agent is 0.1 ppm (0.25 mg per cubic meter). The ACGIH TLV also is 0.1 ppm, and the STEL is 0.3 ppm (0.69 mg per cubic meter). The IDLH concentration is 2.0 ppm (66).

Acrolein readily binds to sulfhydryl groups and is a general cell poison. It will kill aquatic wildlife if the water concentration is not controlled. The permissible water concentration to protect aquatic life is 21 μg per L on a chronic basis and 68 μg per L on an acute basis (66). To protect human health, the concentration of acrolein in water should not exceed 320 μg per L (66). The product is ejected from its container by pressurized oxygen-free nitrogen gas directly into canal water to form a "wave" that slowly moves in the direction of water flow, killing all plant life as it makes contact.

Owing to acrolein's highly irritating vapor and lacrimating action, humans cannot tolerate vapor concentrations of 0.1 to 1.0 ppm for even short periods. Splash exposures to the liquid concentrate can produce rapid ocular and skin damage. Skin injury from the concentrate rapidly can produce edema, erythema, and second-degree burns. Inhalation of the vapor or liquid will produce respiratory irritation, mucous membrane irritation, difficulty in breathing, and pulmonary edema. Human exposure to high airborne concentrations of 10 ppm can result in death. Pulmonary irritation occurs at levels ranging from 0.17 ppm to 0.43 ppm. The odor threshold is 0.2 ppm.

Any splash exposure should be irrigated immediately with water for 15 to 20 minutes. Personal protective equipment, including, eye, skin, and respiratory protection, should be used in working with acrolein.

Acrolein has been reported to cause birth defects in rats when injected directly into the embryo. To date, no human reproductive effects have been documented. No human data are available regarding the possible human carcinogenic effects of acrolein.

The ACGIH classifies acrolein as A4, not classifiable as a human carcinogen. The NIOSH-recommended exposure limits are as follows: TWA, 0.1 ppm or 0.25 mg per cubic meter; and STEL (C) (ceiling limit that should not be exceeded at any time), 0.3 ppm or 0.8 mg per cubic meter. Acrolein is classified by the International Agency for Research on Cancer as a group 3 agent (i.e., unclassifiable as to its carcinogenicity in humans).

Paraformaldehyde

Paraformaldehyde is used as a fumigant and as a soil fungicide, in preplant application or in furrows during the planting of barley or oats. A polymer of formaldehyde, it typically is 8 to 100 monomer units long. The latter is released slowly in the soil after application. Paraformaldehyde is available as flakes or powders. It is used also in the dental profession as lozenges and as a paste. Concentrations for those uses are very small and pose no risk to human health (67).

Like formaldehyde, paraformaldehyde may be irritating to the mucous membranes if concentrations are sufficient. GI irritation occurs after ingestion, with nausea, vomiting, abdominal pain, and diarrhea. Systemic acidosis may occur. Coma and seizures have been reported after large exposures (68).

ORGANOTIN COMPOUNDS

Organotin compounds are used widely as biocidal agents, plastic stabilizers, and chemical process catalysts. Organotins are formed from the synthesis of tetravalent tin atoms and various organic moieties. Typical organotins are triethyltin, dibutyltin, tributyltin, and triphenyltin (fentin hydroxide) (Fig. 102-17). Examples include triethyltin iodide, dibutyltin chloride, tributyltin chloride, triphenyltin acetate, and bis(tributyltin) oxide. Besides being used as biocides, organotin compounds are used as additives in many products and processes that require preservation, such as wood, leather, paper, paint, and textiles.

Higher dialkyltin compounds are used as stabilizers for plastics or as fungicides. The lower trialkyltins are used as fungicides, molluscicides, insecticides, and miticides.

Trimethyltin (TMT) is formed as a by-product during the production of dimethyltin (DMT). The synthesis of DMT from inorganic tin and methyl chloride produces 88% DMT, 8% TMT, and 4% monomethyltin. TMT evaporates more rapidly than do the other two compounds, rendering it easily inhaled and, therefore, a high toxicity risk. Other than as a by-product in chemical synthesis, TMT is not used for commercial applications. The tetraorganotins, although of little commercial utility by themselves, are important compounds, as they are used as intermediates in the synthesis of many of the industrially important mono-, di-, and triorganotins. The tetraalkyltins also are used as catalysts for olefin polymerization. Tetraalkyltin compounds are relatively inert. They are converted in the body to trialkyltins. Tributyltin, triphenyltin, and tetraorganotin are incompatible with strong oxidizers.

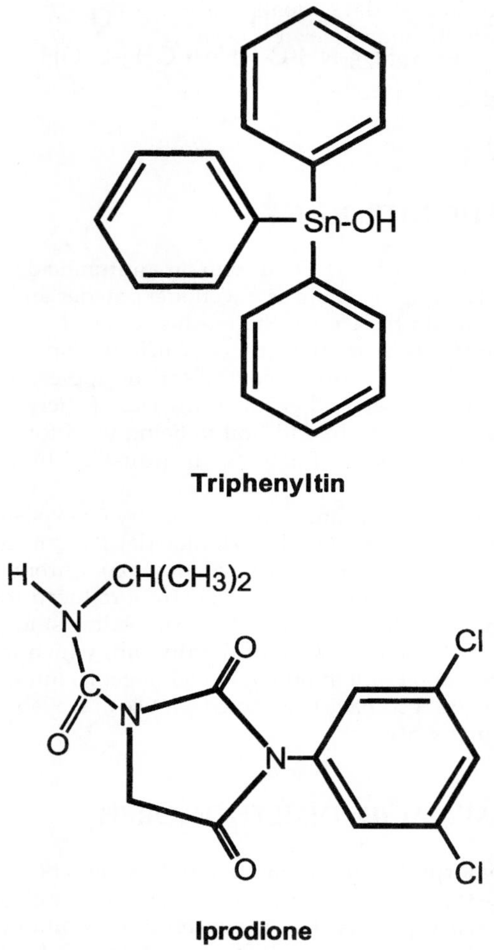

Sn-OH

Triphenyltin

H CH(CH3)2 N O Cl C N N O O Cl

Iprodione

Figure 102-17. Organometals.

General Toxicology

In general, the organotin compounds produce irritation of the eyes, mucous membranes, throat, and skin. Some of the organotins are hepatotoxic. Such monoalkyltin compounds as methyltin trichloride and ethyltin trichloride in animal studies have caused hepatomegaly, bile duct inflammation, and renal fatty degeneration. Triphenyltin is a hepatotoxin and, in some occupational exposures, has produced hepatic damage with hepatomegaly and elevated liver enzymes. Triphenyltin is also a dermal irritant and can produce other effects, such as headache, nausea, vomiting, and blurred vision on toxic exposure. Trialkyltin compounds easily cross the blood–brain barrier, producing acute neurotoxicity symptoms, including headache, dizziness, photophobia, tremors, hyperexcitability, muscle weakness, and flaccid paralysis. Respiratory paralysis also may be seen.

Trialkyltins and tetraalkyltin compounds (owing to tetraalkyltin compounds' *in vivo* conversion to trialkyltins) are considered the most toxic of the alkyltin group (69–72). Tetraalkyltin compounds in and of themselves are relatively inert. After ingestion, these compounds are converted to trialkyltins, producing trialkyltin poisoning: neurotoxicity symptoms and respiratory failure (73). Toxicity from tetraalkyltins may be delayed for 20 to 40 days after a single ingestion. This is probably owing to the time necessary to convert the tetraalkyltins to trialkyltins (74).

All the organotin compounds, especially tributyltin and dibutyltin, can produce severe dermal chemical burns. Intense itching, inflammation, and erythema can occur on exposure. The lesions that develop are generally diffuse and erythematous and heal quickly after exposure is terminated. Exposure to the eyes can produce lacrimation, conjunctivitis, and conjunctival edema.

Organotin compounds interfere with several mitochondrial enzyme systems and uncouple oxidative phosphorylation (70,75). Dialkyltins inhibit the function of α-ketoacid oxidases. This inhibition, which decreases mitochondrial oxygen use and thus increases pyruvate concentrations (69), is blocked by administration of British anti-Lewisite, as is acute toxicity (73). Triethyltin is the most potent known inhibitor of oxidative phosphorylation (76), but this trialkyltin compound's inhibition of oxidative phosphorylation is *not* blocked by British anti-Lewisite. The effectiveness of triorganotin compounds, in descending order, in inhibiting oxidative phosphorylation is as follows: tributyltin, tripropyltin, triphenyltin, trimethyltin (77).

Neurotoxicity

TMT and triethyltin produce clinically distinct neurotoxic syndromes (71). The clinical features of triethyltin toxicity are increased intracranial pressure, paralysis, and generalized tonic-clonic seizures. Neurologic symptoms include headache, vertigo, photophobia, psychic disturbances, and other visual system abnormalities. Reported systemic symptoms are abdominal pain and vomiting, urinary retention, and neurobehavioral symptoms on ingestion. Persistent neurologic sequelae include diminished visual acuity, focal anesthesia, flaccid paralysis, incontinence, and cerebral edema. Autopsy findings have revealed diffuse intramyelinic edema in the brain (71).

TMT toxicity is characterized by limbic system and cerebellar dysfunction, hearing loss, and to a lesser degree, a mild sensory disturbance (71,78). In rats, exposure to TMT compounds produces a syndrome of tremor, aggression, and seizures. Morphologic changes, including limbic and sensory CNS necrosis, also have been described. Allen et al. (79) fed rats experimental diets contaminated with 99% pure triethyltin at a concentration of 8 ppm. Neurobehavioral changes (aggression, shaking, and clonic convulsions) consistent with TMT poisoning became evident on day 22. Microscopical brain analysis revealed pronounced limbic system damage characterized by neuronal cell necrosis of the hippocampal formation and pyriform cortex, amygdaloid nuclei, and olfactory tuberculum. The greatest necrosis was in the hippocampal formation and pyriform cortex, and the least was seen in the amygdaloid nuclei and olfactory tuberculum. The spinal cord revealed slight vacuolation-degeneration of ventral horn motor neurons. Peripheral nervous system damage was evidenced by minimal wallerian degeneration of the sciatic nerve. In rat studies, triethyltin inhibited incorporation of ^{32}P into brain phospholipids (80). TMT neurotoxicity in mice may be due to alterations in neuronal adenosine triphosphatase systems or interference with ion transport, causing lesions in the limbic system (81). Neuronal cell lesions and degeneration of spinal cord ventral horn cells may be responsible for peripheral neurotoxicity. Wallerian axonal degeneration also is possible.

Immunotoxicity

The organotin compounds are known also to have immunotoxic properties in animals. An increased susceptibility to infection was found in guinea pigs receiving triphenyltin (82). Decreased lymphopoiesis was reported. The animals also showed decreases in the weight of thymus, spleen, and lymph nodes and demonstrated a decrease in T-cell–dependent antibody response and B-cell lymphocyte proliferation of between 60% and 80%. In addition, TMT affected cellular immunity and was shown to incite an 80% decrease in T-lymphocyte proliferation from mitogen stimulation (83).

Tributyltin oxide also has been shown to exert immunotoxic effects in animal species. Rats orally fed tributyltin oxide showed decreases in the lymphoid organ weight, such as the thymus and spleen, and a decrease in white blood cell count. Delayed hypersensitivity reactions, decreased T-cell lymphocyte proliferation in response to mitogen, and decreased host resistance also were observed. Immunologic effects in humans have not been reported.

Organotin Toxicity Examples

Bresser et al. (71) reported six patients with acute TMT intoxication. Six workers became poisoned after inhaling TMT while cleaning a tank used in the manufacturing of DMT. Organotin 24-hour urine measurements were obtained at various intervals from each patient. Maximal organotin concentrations (range, 445 to 1,580 ppb) were reached within days 4 to 10 after exposure. Monitoring of 16 asymptomatic workers revealed mean urinary concentrations of 36 ppb. Symptom severity correlated with the maximal urinary concentrations. Limbic system clinical signs included disorientation, confabulation, retrograde and anterograde amnesia, aggressiveness, hyperphagia, and disturbances of sexual behavior. Complex partial seizures and intermittent rhythmic delta activity arising from one or both temporal lobes were seen on electroencephalography. Cerebellar dysfunction ranged from mild gaze-evoked nystagmus to severe ataxia. Hearing loss varied from 15 to 30 dB. Paresthesias of the lower extremities with mild slowing of sensory nerve conduction without loss of reflexes was observed. One worker with episodes of altered consciousness and generalized seizure activity required mechanical ventilation. He expired on day 13. Attempts were made to increase urinary excretion in these patients by using D-penicillamine and plasmapheresis, but these therapies proved unsuccessful.

Gross autopsy findings revealed tracheobronchitis, pneumonia, pulmonary edema, fatty degeneration of the liver, and shock kidneys. Neuropathologic findings consisted of swollen perikarya; eccentric or pyknotic nuclei; loss of Nissl substance; and cytoplasmic inclusions with a dense core and light halo. Temporal cortex nerve cell necrosis also was seen. Electron microscopy showed cytoplasmic lamellated inclusions termed *zebra bodies* and many vacuoles and granulomembranous particles surrounded by trilaminar membranes. The finding of zebra bodies reflected an increase in brain lysosomal activity. These changes were most prominent in the amygdala and, to a lesser degree, in the temporal cortex, basal ganglia, and pontine nuclei. A marked loss of Purkinje cells occurred in the cerebellar cortex. These findings were similar to those in the rat studies with TMT (71).

TMT has produced hyperexcitability and neurologic and behavioral changes in animals and has resulted in seizures in some animal studies. Kreyberg et al. (84) reported a case of a 48-year-old woman who died 6 days after consuming wine contaminated with an unknown amount of TMT. Within the first 3 hours after the ingestion, she became restless and experienced episodes of unresponsiveness. After the 3 hours, she became agitated and developed fecal incontinence. On hospital admission, she demonstrated hypokalemia and leukocytosis. Metabolic acidosis and hepatotoxicity followed. By 72 hours, she developed multiorgan failure with disseminated intravascular coagulation.

Renal function remained intact. The patient required ventilatory support and expired on day 6 from multiorgan failure.

Chemical analyses of the wine and the patient's urine were positive for TMT (84). Pathologic analysis revealed chromatolysis of the neurons of the brain, spinal cord, and spinal ganglia. Acute neuronal necrosis was observed in the fascia dentata of the hippocampus and in the spinal ganglia. Necrosis also was seen in the pyramidal cell layer of the hippocampus, the cerebral cortex basal ganglia, and the Purkinje cell layer of the cerebellum. The investigators thought that some of these latter changes may have been due to an anoxic episode shortly before death. Electron microscopy revealed marked accumulation of lysosomal dense bodies and disorganization of the granular endoplasmic reticulum in the neurons. These findings are similar to those noted on experimental TMT poisoning. Cytoplasmic zebra bodies were not present (84).

Organotin Occupational Exposure Levels

The ACGIH TLV/TWA is 0.1 mg per cubic meter (A4, not classifiable as a human carcinogen). The STEL(C) is 0.2 mg per cubic meter (also A4). Both limits carry the skin notation, signifying the potential significant contribution to the overall exposure by the cutaneous route, including mucous membranes and eyes, either by contact with vapors or, probably more significantly, by direct skin contact with the substance. Data are inadequate to classify the agent in terms of its carcinogenicity in humans or animals (or both). The OSHA PEL/TWA is 0.1 mg per cubic meter. No STEL value is listed. The NIOSH recommended exposure limit TWA is 0.1 mg per cubic meter (with a skin notation). The NIOSH analytical method is 5504.

Tributyltin

Tributyltin is registered with the EPA as a biocide in paint and is used for mildew and fungicide control in exterior paint only. Tributyltin oxide is available in both solid and liquid forms. Human exposures can occur from inhalation and from skin absorption. Exposure to tributyltin can produce irritation of the eyes and throat, conjunctivitis, and mucous membrane irritation. Dermal contact with a solution or solid can produce chemical burns (85). Animal studies indicate that tributyltin produces immunosuppression, anemia, and weight loss.

A report from the Centers for Disease Control and Prevention indicates that a person who was exposed to tributyltin oxide as a biocide in paint developed health effects after the rooms of her apartment were painted with paint containing this biocide. Her symptoms included mucous membrane irritation, headache, epistaxis, cough, nausea, and vomiting. The paint contained 25% bis(tributyltin) oxide (86).

Management

The specific treatment for organotin poisoning is primarily symptomatic and supportive. CNS function should be monitored and treated accordingly. Hepatic and renal function should be studied closely. Dermal, ocular, and mucous membrane irritation and burns are possible.

REFERENCES

1. Kramer W. Fungicides and bactericides. In: Buchel KH, ed. *Chemistry of pesticides.* New York: John Wiley and Sons, 1983:227–321.
2. National Academy of Sciences. *Regulating pesticides in food. The Delaney paradox.* Report of the Committee on Scientific and Regulatory Issues Underlying Pesticide Use Patterns and Agricultural Innovation. Washington: National Academy Press, 1987.
3. Lukens RJ. *Chemistry of fungicidal action.* New York: Springer-Verlag, 1971.
4. Worthing CR, Walker SB, eds. *The pesticide manual—a world compendium,* 7th ed. Levenham, Suffolk, UK: The Levenham Press Ltd, 1983:115.
5. Gosselin RE, et al. *Clinical toxicology of commercial products,* 5th ed. Baltimore: Williams & Wilkins, 1994.
6. Menzie CM. *Metabolism of pesticides, an update.* US Department of the Interior, Fish and Wildlife Service, Special Scientific Report, Wildlife No. 184. Washington: US Government Printing Office, 1974:103.
7. US Environmental Protection Agency. *Recognition and management of pesticide poisonings,* 4th ed. EPA-540/9-88-001. Washington: US Environmental Protection Agency, 1989:94.
8. Sweet DV, ed. 1987 *Registry of toxic effects of chemical substances microfiche.* Cincinnati: National Institute for Occupational Safety and Health, 1997.
9. Wilkerson CF, Killeen JC. A mechanistic interpretation of the oncogenicity of chlorothalonil in rodents and an assessment of human relevance. *Reg Toxicol Pharmacol* 1996;24:69–84.
10. Rumack BH, Rider PK, Gelman CR, eds. *POISINDEX7 System,* vol 95. Englewood, CO: MicroMedix, Inc.
11. Schmidt R. Cutaneous porphyria in Turkey. *N Engl J Med* 1960;263:397.
12. Edwards IR, Ferry DG, Temple WA. Fungicides and related compounds. In: Hayes WJ Jr, Laws ER Jr, eds. *The handbook of pesticide toxicology, vol 3: classes of pesticides.* New York: Academic Press, 1991.
13. National Library of Medicine. *Hazardous substance data bank.* Bethesda: TOXNET, 1992.
14. Cline RE, Hill RH, Phillips DL, Needham LL. Pentachlorophenol measurements in body fluids of people in log homes and workplaces. *Arch Environ Contam Toxicol* 1989;18:475–481.
15. Agency for Toxic Substances and Disease Registry. ATSDR Toxicological profile for pentachlorophenol. Atlanta: US Department of Health and Human Services, Public Health Service, ATSDR, 1994.
16. World Health Organization. *Environmental health criteria 148: benomyl.* Geneva: World Health Organization, 1993.
17. Cummings AM, Ebron-McCoy MT, Rodgers JM, Barbee BD, Harris ST. Developmental effects of methyl benzimidazole carbomate following exposure during early pregnancy. *Fundam Appl Toxicol* 1992;18:288–293.
18. Food and Agricultural Organization of the United Nations. *Pesticide residues in food—1983: Evaluations. FAO plant production and protection.* Paper 61. Geneva: World Health Organization, 1983.
19. Kucera SP, Swann JM, Kennedy JR, Schultz TW. The effects of benomyl and its breakdown products carbendazim and butyl isocyanate on the structure and function of tracheal ciliated cells. *J Environ Sci Health* 1995;B30:779–799.
20. Nakagawa Y, Tayama K. Acute hepatoxic potential of imazalil fungicide in rats. *Bull Environ Contam Toxicol* 1997;58:402–407.
21. Food and Agricultural Organization of the United Nations. *Pesticide residues in food—1997. FAO plant production and protection.* Paper 10 [Supplement]. Geneva: World Health Organization, 1977.
22. Borzelleca JF, Egle JL Jr, Hennigar GR, et al. A toxicologic evaluation of 5-ethoxy-3-trichloromethyl-1,2,4-thiadiazole (ETMT). *Toxicol Appl Pharmacol* 1980;56:164–170.
23. Hayes W. *Pesticide studies in man.* Baltimore: Williams & Wilkins, 1982:75–111.
24. American Society of Hospital Pharmacists. *American hospital formulary service—drug information.* Bethesda: American Society of Hospital Pharmacists, 1991.
25. Gilman AG, Goodman LS, Gilman A, eds. *Goodman and Gilman's The pharmacological basis of therapeutics,* 6th ed. New York: Macmillan, 1980:10–27.
26. US Environmental Protection Agency. *Carboxin health advisory.* Washington: Office of Drinking Water, 1987.
27. Food and Drug Administration. *The FDA surveillance index.* Springfield, VA: Bureau of Foods, Department of Commerce, National Technical Information Service, 1986.
28. Wilson HT. Rubber dermatitis: an investigation of 106 cases of contact dermatitis caused by rubber. *Br J Dermatol* 1969;81:175–179.
29. Dalvi R. Toxicology of thiram (tetramethylthiuram disulfide)—a review. *Vet Hum Toxicol* 1988;30:480–482.
30. Proctor J, Fischman N. *Chemical hazards of the workplace,* 2nd ed. Philadelphia: JB Lippincott Co, 1988.
31. Occupational Health Services, Inc. *MSDS for maneb.* Secaucus, NJ: Occupational Health Services, Inc, 1991.
32. Berg GL, ed. *Farm chemicals handbook.* Willoughby, OH: Meister Publishing , 1988.
33. Hayes WJ Jr, Laws ER Jr, eds. *Handbook of pesticide toxicology, vol 3: classes of pesticides.* New York: Academic Press, 1991.
34. Morgan DP. *Recognition and management of pesticide poisonings,* 3rd ed. Washington: US Government Printing Office, 1982.
35. Meister RT, ed. *Farm chemicals handbook.* Willoughby, OH: Meister Publishing, 1992.
36. Harding WC. *Pesticide profiles: 1. Insecticides and miticides.* Bulletin 267. Baltimore: Cooperative Extension Service, University of Maryland, 1979.
37. Clayton GD, Clayton FE, eds. *Patty's industrial hygiene and toxicology, vol 2: toxicology, 3rd ed.* New York: John Wiley and Sons, 1991.
38. US Environmental Protection Agency. *Guidance for the registration of pesticide products containing maneb as the active ingredient.* Washington: Office of Pesticides and Toxic Substances, US Environmental Protection Agency, 1988.

39. US Environmental Protection Agency. Ethylene bisdithiocarbamates (EBDCs): notice of intent to cancel and conclusion of special review. *Federal Register* 1992;57(41):7434–7530.
40. Hallenback WH, Cunningham-Burns KM. *Pesticides and human health.* New York: Springer-Verlag, 1985.
41. Shepard TH. *Catalog of teratogenic agents,* 5th ed. Baltimore: Johns Hopkins University Press, 1996.
42. Quest JA, Fenner-Crisp PA, Burnam W, et al. Evaluation of the carcinogenic potential of pesticides: 4. Chloralkylthiodicarboximide compounds with fungicidal activity. *Reg Toxicol Pharmacol* 1993;17:19–34.
43. World Health Organization/FAO. *1966 Evaluation of some pesticide residues in food.* Rome: FAO, 1970.
44. Stoke, JC. Captafol dermatitis in the timber industry. *Contact Dermatitis* 1979;5:284–292.
45. National Research Council. *Drinking water and health, vol 1.* Washington: National Academy Press, 1977:661.
46. White-Stevens R, ed. *Pesticides and the environment,* vol 1. New York: Marcel Dekker Inc, 1971:16.
47. US Environmental Protection Agency. *Pesticide fact sheet no. 215: Folpet.* Washington: US Environmental Protection Agency, Office of Pesticides and Toxic Substances, Office of Pesticide Programs, June 1987.
48. Kimmel EC, Casida JE, Ruzo LO. Formamidine insecticides and chloroacetanilide herbicides: distributed anilines and nitrobenzenes as mammalian metabolites and bacterial mutagens. *J Agric Food Chem* 1986;34:157–161.
49. Sathiakumar N, Delzell E. A review of epidemiologic studies of triazine herbicides and cancer. *Crit Rev Toxicol* 1997;27:599–613.
50. Ronis MJ, Badger TM. Toxic interactions between fungicides that inhibit ergosterol biosynthesis and phosphorothioate insecticides in the male rat and bobwhite quail (*Colinus virginianus*). *Toxicol Appl Pharmacol* 1995;130:221–228.
51. Walker QD, Mailman RB. Triadimefon: neurotoxicity expressed by inhibition of the dopamine transporter. *Toxicologist* 1995;13:214(abst).
52. Crofton KM. A structure-activity relationship for the neurotoxicity of triazole fungicides. *Toxicol Lett* 1996;84:155–159.
53. Occupational Health Services, Inc. *OHS Database. MSDS for triforine.* Secaucus, NJ: Occupational Health Services, Inc, 1994.
54. Shell Agriculture. *Dimethomorph: the new protection against oomycete fungi.* Princeton, NJ: 1994.
55. Liebmann J, Cook JA, Teag D, Fisher J, Mitchell JB. Cycloheximide inhibits the cytotoxicity of paclitaxel (Taxol). *Anticancer Drugs* 1994;5:287–292.
56. Delcambe L, Peypoux F, Guinand M, Michel G. Iturin and iturinic acid. *Rev Ferment Ind Aliment* 1976;36:147–151.
57. Klich MA, Arthur KS, Lax AR, Bland JM. Iturin A: a potential new fungicide for stored grain. *Mycopathologia* 1994;127:123–127.
58. Berdy J, ed. *CRC handbook of antibiotic compounds,* vol 1. Boca Raton, FL: CRC Press, 1980:381.
59. US Environmental Protection Agency, Office of Pesticide Programs. Suspended, canceled, and registered pesticides: dinocap—special review, 50 *CFR* 1119. *Federal Register* 1990 Feb.
60. US Environmental Protection Agency. *Pesticide fact sheet no. 65: dinocap.* Washington: US Environmental Protection Agency, Office of Pesticide Programs, 1978.
61. Sacks NI. *Dangerous properties of industrial materials,* 6th ed. New York: Van Nostrand–Reinhold, 1984.
62. Babich H, Palace MR, Borenfreund E, Stern A. Naphthoquinone cytotoxicity to bluegill sunfish BF-2 cells. *Arch Environ Contam Toxicol* 1994;27:8–13.
63. National Institute for Occupational Safety and Health. *Registry of toxic effects of chemical substances.* CD-ROM version. Denver: Micromedics, Inc, 1991.
64. Royal Society of Chemistry Information Systems. *The EGRO chemicals handbook,* 3rd ed. Surrey, UK: UNWIN Brothers Ltd, 1994.
65. Parmeggiani L, ed. *Encyclopedia of occupational health and safety,* 3rd ed, vol 1. Geneva: International Labour Office, 1983:1041–1042.
66. Sittig M. *Handbook of toxic and hazardous chemicals.* Park Ridge, NJ: Noyes Publications, 1981.
67. Council on Dental Therapeutics. The use of root canal filling materials containing paraformaldehyde: a status report. *J Am Dent Assoc* 1987;114:95.
68. Parfit K, ed. Martindale: the complete drug reference guide, 32nd ed. London: The Pharmaceutical Press, 1999.
69. Matthew H, Logan A, Woodruff MFA, et al. Paraquat poisoning, lung transplantation. *BMJ* 1968;1:179–763.
70. Attahiru US, Iyaniwura TT, Adaudi AO, Bonire JJ. Acute toxicity studies of tri-*N*-butyltin and triphenyltin acetates in rats. *Vet Hum Toxicol* 1991;33:554–556.
71. Bresser R, Kramer G, Thumler R, et al. Acute trimethyltin limbic-cerebellar syndrome. *Neurology* 1987;37:945–950.
72. Barnes JM, Stoner HB. Toxic properties of some dialkyl and trialkyl tin salts. *Br J Ind Med* 1958;15:15–22.
73. Barnes JM, Stoner HB. The toxicology of tin compounds. *Pharmacol Rev* 1959;11:211–231.
74. Cremer JE. The biochemistry of organotin compounds. The conversion of tetraethyltin into triethyltin in mammals. *Biochem J* 1958;68:685–692.
75. Aldridge WN. The influence of organotin compounds on mitochondrial functions. In: Zuchermann JJ, ed. *Organotin compounds, new chemistry applications.* Washington: American Chemical Society, 1976:186–196.
76. Clarkson TW. Inorganic and organometal pesticides. In: Hayes WJ Jr, Laws ER Jr, eds. *Handbook of pesticide toxicology, vol 2: classes of pesticides.* San Diego: Academic Press, 1991:497–583.
77. Stockdale R, Dawson AP, Selwyn MJ. Effects of trialkyltin and triphenyltin compounds on mitochondrial respiration. *Eur J Biochem* 1970;15:342–351.
78. Feldman RG, White RF, Eriator II. Trimethyltin encephalopathy. *Arch Neurol* 1993;50:1320–1324.
79. Allen SL, Simpson MG, Stonard MD, et al. Induction of trimethyltin neurotoxicity by dietary administration. *Neurotoxicology* 1994;15:651–654.
80. Rose MS, Aldridge WN. Triethyltin and the incorporation of (^{32}P) phosphate into rat brain phospholipds. *J Neurochem* 1996;13:103–108.
81. Chang LW. Neuropathology of trimethyltin: a proposed pathogenetic mechanism. *Fundam Appl Toxicol* 1986;6:217–232.
82. Verschuuren HG, Kroes R, Vink HH, Van Esch GJ. Short-term toxicity studies with triphenyltin compounds in rats and guinea pig. *Food Cosmet Toxicol* 1966;4:35–45.
83. Descotes J. *Immunotoxicology of drugs and chemicals.* New York: Elsevier Science, 1986.
84. Kreyberg S, Torvik A, Bjorneboe W, Wiik-Larsen, Jacobsen D. Trimethyltin poisoning: report of a case with postmortem examination. *Clin Neuropathol* 1992;11:256–259.
85. Smilkstein MJ, Smolinske SC, Kulig KW, et al. Severe hypermagnesemia due to multiple-dose cathartic therapy. *West J Med* 1988;148:208–211.
86. The Selected Cancers Cooperative Study Group. The association of selected cancers with service in the US military in Vietnam: I. Non-Hodgkin's lymphoma. *Arch Intern Med* 1990;150:2473–2483.

CHAPTER 103
Pyrethrins

Raquel L. Gibly and John B. Sullivan, Jr.

SOURCES AND PRODUCTION

Pyrethrins have been used as insecticides for centuries (1). They are esters of pyrethric and chrysanthemumic acids, which are obtained from the flowers of the *Chrysanthemum cinerariaefolium* and related species. The active ingredients are extracted by grinding the flowers into a powder, which contains 1% to 3% active material, or by extraction with a solvent such as alcohol, naphtha, or kerosene (2).

In the purified form, pyrethrins contain carbon, hydrogen, and oxygen. There are six similar esters (Table 103-1) (3). They are viscous, nonpolar liquids that decompose easily in the presence of acid, alkali, and ultraviolet light (1). Pyrethrins are extremely photosensitive (1).

Pyrethroids are synthetic, photostable analogs of the pyrethrins. They are neurotoxic compounds exhibiting broad-spectrum insecticidal activity with low-order mammalian toxicity (4). More than 1,000 pyrethroids have been synthesized, many of which consist of optical (*R/S* or *D/L*) and geometric (*cis/trans*) isomers (4,5). The isomers often are mixed together and posses very different biological activities and strengths. Many pyrethroids have been modified structurally to include nitrogen, sulfur, and halogen moieties (1). These physical and chemical modifications allow the pyrethroids to exhibit biological activity greater than that of the natural pyrethrins. Factors increasing pyrethroid activity and toxicity are lower temperature (6), halogenation, and stereospecificity (i.e., *cis* isomers are usually more toxic than are *trans* isomers) (7).

The synthetic pyrethroids are divided into two types, depending on the presence or absence of a cyano-group at the α-carbon of the phenoxybenzyl moiety. The type I pyrethroids lack the α-cyano group and are less volatile than are the type II pyrethroids, which possess the α-cyano group. The α-cyano group gives the type II pyrethroids higher insecticidal activity and greater photostability (Table 103-2) (4).

TABLE 103-1. Names and structures of the six pyrethrin esters

Common name	Formula	CAS number	Structure
Cinerin I	$C_{20}H_{28}O_3$	25402-06-6	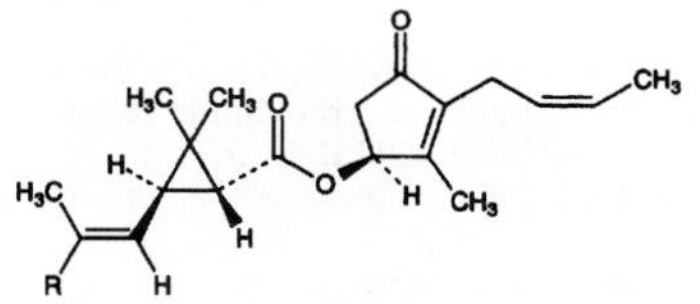 Cinerin I R = CH_3
Cinerin II	$C_{21}H_{28}O_5$	121-20-0	Cinerin II R = $COOCH_3$
Jasmolin I	$C_{21}H_{30}O_3$	4466-14-2	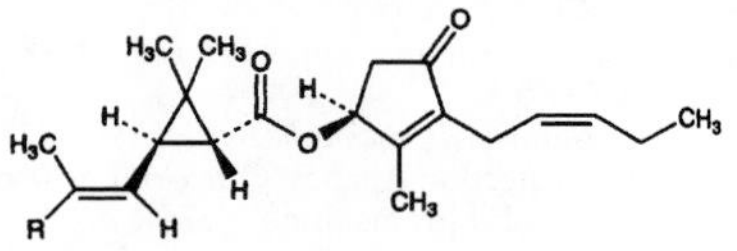 Jasmolin I R = CH_3
Jasmolin II	$C_{22}H_{30}O_5$	1172-63-0	Jasmolin II R = $COOCH_3$
Pyrethrin I	$C_{21}H_{28}O_3$	121-21-1	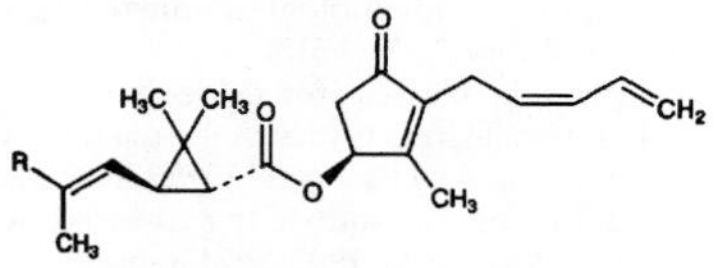 Pyrethrin I R = CH_3
Pyrethrin II	$C_{22}H_{28}O_5$	121-29-9	Pyrethrin II R = $COOCH_3$

CAS, Chemical Abstracts Service.
Adapted from ref. 3.

OCCUPATIONAL AND ENVIRONMENTAL EXPOSURE SOURCES

Pyrethrins and pyrethroids are found ubiquitously in fungicides, ixodicides, and insecticides. Pyrethrins are available as purified extracts (20% to 25% pyrethrins) and as a refined grade (60% active ingredients) (2). They are highly diversified products and can be marketed as liquids, powders, creams, solutions, and vapor bombs. Pyrethrins are used commercially, in household products, and for agriculture (8,9). They are the product used most widely in insecticide sprays and are found in more than 2,000 commercially available sprays and powders (Table 103-3) (2,8,10).

Pyrethroids were introduced first in the 1950s and are believed to be more environmentally stable than pyrethrins (9). They are more selective than pyrethrins and, therefore, can be used more safely and are less toxic toward mammals (2,11). They have remarkably high killing activity (e.g., deltamethrin), rapid paralytic activity (e.g., prallethrin), vapor action at room temperature (e.g., empenthrin), and photostability (e.g., cypermethrin), rendering them more effective as insecticides than are the pyrethrins (9,11).

Pyrethrins and pyrethroids often are mixed with a synergist that increases their stability and insecticidal effectiveness and may add to their toxic and biological effects (2). One of the more common synergists is piperonyl butoxide (PBO). Others include sesame oil derivatives (sesamin, sesamolin); MGK-264; piperonyl cyclonene; *n*-octyl sulfoxide of isisafrole; *n*-propyl isome; *N,N*-diethyl-m-toluamide (DEET); and *N*-isobutylundecylenamide (2,12). Some of the synergists are inhibitors of the hepatic microsomal enzymes (e.g., PBO, MGK-264), thereby decreasing the metabolism of the pyrethrins and increasing their toxicities (13). Others may enhance dermal absorption of the products (e.g., DEET) or increase central nervous system toxicity (e.g., MGK-264, DEET). Mixing with cholinesterase inhibitors (organophosphates and carbamates) also will increase the toxicity of some pyrethroids (9). When in spray forms, the pyrethrins and pyrethroids usually are mixed with petroleum distillates or hydrocarbons.

CLINICAL TOXICOLOGY

Routes of Exposure

Exposure routes most commonly were noted to be dermal and inhalational, with dermal exposure believed to be the leading route (14). Dermal exposure usually occurred secondary to wiping away sweat with contaminated hands, gloves, and sleeves; from hand-mixing the chemicals before spraying or applying them; and from sloppy handling of the chemicals. Inadequate clothing protection also was a common problem (14). No significant absorption of pyrethroids or pyrethrins has been observed to occur through intact skin (7,9). Ocular exposure can occur by contact with contaminated clothing or hands or by direct exposure. Accidental and intentional ingestions have been reported.

Distribution

The highest concentrations of pyrethroids are found in body fat, which is consistent with its high lipid solubility. Other tissues in which pyrethroids are concentrated include skin, liver, kidneys, adrenal glands, biliary tract, and brain tissue (15). Tissue residuals generally are low, with no significant bioaccumulation. Tissue concentrations, from highest to lowest, are as follows: liver, ovary, skin, kidney, blood, lung, spleen, muscle, and brain (11).

Metabolism

Pyrethroids have been noted to be metabolized rapidly and to leave very low tissue residuals (11,16). No significant bioaccumulation has been noted (11). They are absorbed poorly from

TABLE 103-2. Names and structures of the pyrethroids

Common name	Trade name	Formula	CAS number	Structure
Noncyano pyrethroids (type I)				
Allethrin I	Pynamin, Pyresyn	$C_{19}H_{26}O_3$	584-79-2	Allethrin I R = CH_3
Allethrin II	ENT-17510	$C_{20}H_{26}O_3$	497-92-7	Allethrin II R = $COOCH_3$
Barthrin	—	$C_{18}H_{21}ClO_4$	70-43-9	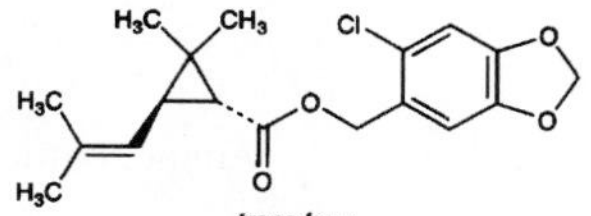 *trans*-form
Bifenthrin	Brigade, Talstar, Capture	$C_{23}N_{22}ClF_3O_2$	82653-04-3	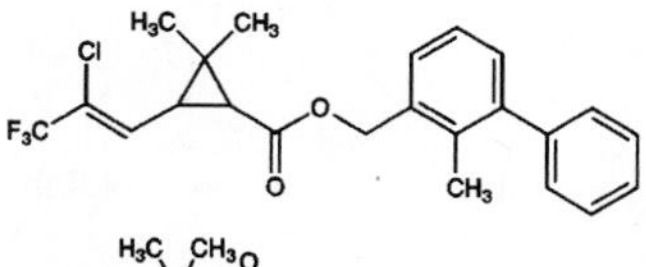
Bioresmethrin	Resbuthrin, Biobenzyfuroline	$C_{22}H_{26}O_3$	28434-01-7	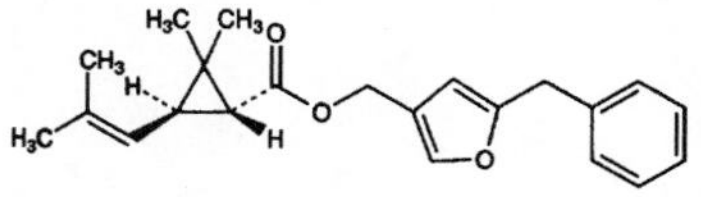
Cyclethrin	—	$C_{21}H_{28}O_3$	97-11-0	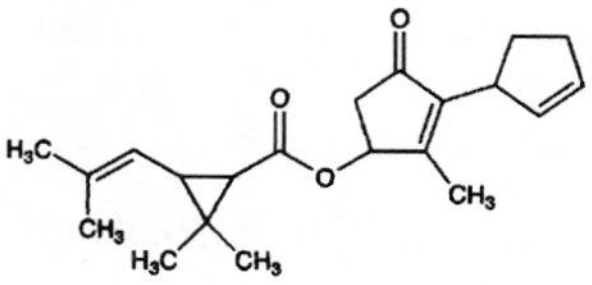
Fluvalinate	Mavrik	$C_{26}H_{22}ClF_3N_2O_3$	69409-94-5	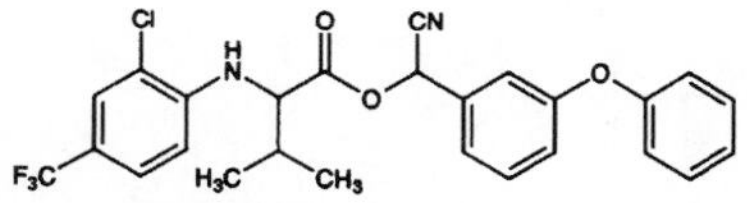
Permethrin	Ambush, Dragnet, Nix	$C_{21}H_{20}Cl_2O_3$	52645-53-1	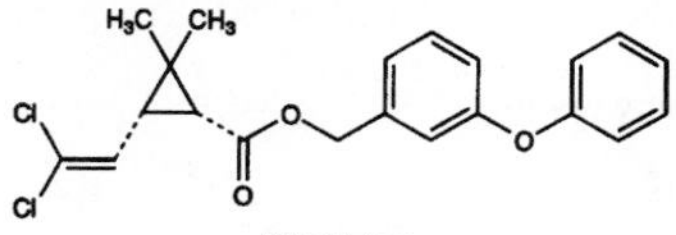 (1R-*cis*)-form
Phenothrin	Sumithrin	$C_{23}H_{26}O_3$	26002-80-2	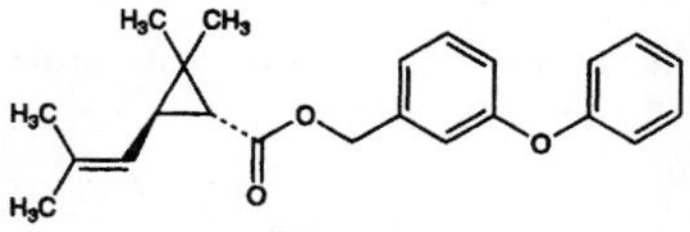 (1R-*trans*)-form
Pyrethrosin	—	$C_{17}H_{22}O_3$	28272-18-6	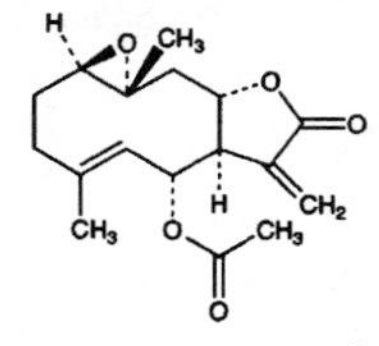
Tefluthrin	Force, Forza, Comet RP	$C_{17}H_{14}ClF_7O_2$	79538-32-2	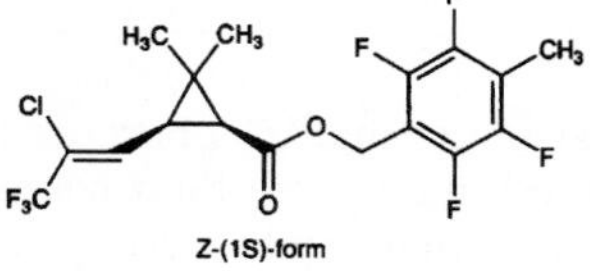 Z-(1S)-form
Tetramethrin	Neo-Pynamin	$C_{19}H_{25}NO_4$	7696-12-0	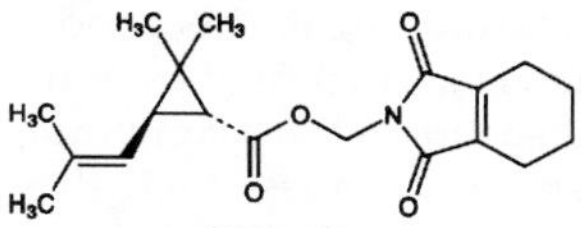 (1R-*trans*)-form

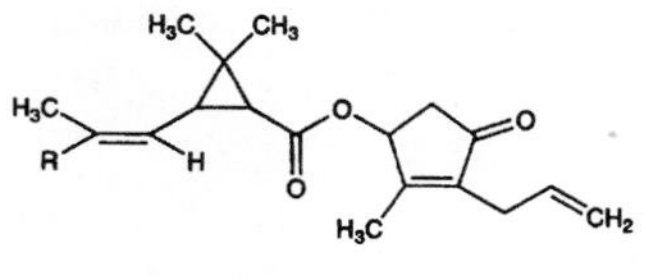

(continued)

TABLE 103-2. *(continued)*

Common name	Trade name	Formula	CAS number	Structure
α-Cyano pyrethroids (type II)				
Cyfluthrin	Baythroid	$C_{22}H_{18}Cl_2FNO_3$	68359-37-5	(1R,3R,αR)-form
Cyhalothrin	Grenade	$C_{23}H_{19}ClF_3NO_3$	68085-85-8	(Z)-(1S)-*cis*-form
Cypermethrin	Ammo, Barricade, Cyperkill	$C_{22}H_{19}C_{12}NO_3$	52315-07-8	*cis*-form
Cyphenothrin	Forte, Gokliaht	$C_{24}H_{25}NO_3$	39515-40	*cis*-form
Deltamethrin	Butox, Decis, K-Othrine	$C_{22}H_{19}Br_2NO_3$	52918-63-5	
Fenpropathrin	Danitol, Meothrin, Rody	$C_{22}H_{23}NO_3$	39515-41-8	
Fenvalerate	Pydrin, Pyridin, Sumicidin	$C_{25}H_{22}ClNO_3$	51630-58-1	
Flucythrinate	Cybolt, Guardian, Pay-Off	$C_{26}H_{23}F_2NO_4$	70124-77-5	
Tralomethrin	Saga, Scout, Tracker, Tralox	$C_{22}H_{19}Br_4NO_3$	66841-25-6	

CAS, Chemical Abstracts Service.
Adapted from ref. 3.

the gastrointestinal tract because they are highly lipophilic and prefer to remain with their solvent. These products often are found unchanged in the feces.

Pyrethroids are metabolized extensively in the liver to carbon dioxide via a mixture of ester hydrolysis, oxidation, and conjugation reactions. *Trans* compounds are eliminated more rapidly and generally are less toxic than are the *cis* formulations (13). Sunlight causes rapid ester cleavage, epoxidation, oxidation, and hyperperoxidation, all of which degrade and inactivate the compounds (17,18). They often are excreted as glycine, sulfate, glucuronide, or glucoside conjugates (11).

Higher toxicity has been noted in newborn animal models, primarily as a result of their immature hepatic degradation systems and their decreased ability to perform oxidation and ester hydrolysis (11). Bioactivation has been noted with several pyrethroids (e.g., tralomethrin, tralocythrin).

Elimination

In the adult mammal and human, pyrethroids are excreted from the body rapidly and completely (Table 103-4) (11,15,17,19–23). Both urinary and fecal routes are used, with 40% to 60% of elimination occurring via the urine and 30% to 50% occurring via the feces (15). Rates of excretion vary with the compound but, on the whole, 90% of elimination of these compounds occurs within 24 to 48 hours (11). This rapid initial

TABLE 103-3. Common products containing pyrethrins

Product	Manufacturer	PYR	PBO	PH/D
Alleviate Food Plant Fogging Spray (oil base)	Fairfield American	1.25	5.0	93.6
Arab Flea and Tick Spray Mist	Federal Chemical	0.05	0.25	—
Arab Ant and Roach Spray	Federal Chemical	0.10	0.52	98.8
Black Flag Flea and Tick Killer Rug & Room Spray	Boyle-Midway	—	0.68	—
Bonide Garden Dust for Vegetable Flowers	Bonide	0.03	—	—
Carson Pesticidal Shampoo	Carson Chemicals Inc.	—	0.05	0.5
Purge II Concentrated Aerosol Insect Killer	Cline-Beckner, Inc.	1.0	2.0	13.6
Purina Animal Shampoo	Ralston	0.07	0.75	—
Purina Cattle Lice-Chek	Ralston	7.6	—	56.7
Purina Dairy Spray	Ralston	0.06	0.48	99.4
Purina Roach, Ant, and Spider Spray	Ralston	0.05	0.1	58.6
Purina Tomato and Vegetable Dust	Ralston	0.05	0.5	—
Pyrenone Crop Spray (oil base)	Fairfield American	6.0	6.0	24
Pyrenone Food Plant Fogging Insecticide	Fairfield American	0.5	5.0	94.5
Pyrin-aid Liquid (kills lice)	Columbia Medical	0.2	2.0	—
Raze Ant and Roach Spray	ABCO, Inc	0.05	0.125	91.6
Real-Kill Automatic Indoor Fogger	Realex Corp.	0.3	—	14.2
Rid-a-Bird 1100	Rid-A-Bird	11	—	11
Roberts House and Garden Aerosol	Roberts Labs	0.35	—	0.46
Science Rose and Floral Spray	Science Products	0.02	0.2	0.2

PYR, pyrethrin content (%); PBO, piperonyl butoxide content (%); PH/D, petroleum hydrocarbons/distillates content (%).
Note: This list represents examples of products on the market and is not all-inclusive.
Adapted from ref. 10.

clearance rate is followed by a much slower rate of clearance (weeks) for the remaining 10% (7).

Organ System and Laboratory Abnormalities

Pyrethroid and pyrethrin exposures have not been noted to cause abnormalities in the heart, liver, or kidneys or in the menstrual cycle (16). They have not been noted to inhibit any enzymes directly (11). Increases in plasma noradrenaline and guanosine 3',5'-cyclic monophosphate may occur in pyrethroid poisonings with severe intoxication and have been noted to occur in animal studies associated with type II pyrethroid poisoning, particularly when choreoathetotic writhing is present (16). No abnormalities have been noted in testosterone, thyroxine, serum transaminases (serum glutamic-oxaloacetic transaminase and serum glutamic-pyruvic transaminase), blood glucose, or plasma electrolytes in pyrethrin factory workers (24).

TABLE 103-4. Examples of rates of pyrethroid degradation and excretion

Product	Soil	Water	Plants	Excretion[a]
Cyhalothrin	22–82 d		40 d	3 d = equilibrium between ingestion and excretion
Deltamethrin	>8 wk		1.1 wk	2–4 d
Fenvalerate	15–90 d	4–15 d	8–14 d	99% at 6 d
Cypermethrin	2–4 wk	2 wk		50–65% at 48 h
Permethrin	28 d	6–24 h	10 d	12 d
d-Phenothrin	1–2 d		<1 d	3–7 d
Resmethrin	98% in 16 d	47 min		

[a]For the parent compound; metabolites may be present for longer periods.
Adapted from refs. 15, 17, and 19–23.

Plasma or red blood cell cholinesterase is not inhibited. No mutagenicity, change in fertility, or birth defects have been seen with these agents (7).

Axonal degeneration has been seen only with administration of near-lethal dosages of both type I and type II pyrethroids. Discontinuation of the compounds was associated with axonal repair (25).

Mechanisms of Action

The pyrethrins are neurotoxic chemicals that slow the gate kinetics of the sodium channel at the nerve membrane. This slowing interferes with both opening and closing of the sodium channel, causing the channel to remain open for a longer period and allowing greater influx of sodium into a cell (26). Increased cellular sodium causes hyperexcitability of the entire nervous system. The type I pyrethroids cause repetitive discharges that manifest as tremors and jerking activities. The type II (α-cyano) pyrethroids cause a more continuous depolarization that eventually can lead to total blocking of neuronal impulses and prolonged membrane depolarization (27). Interaction of the pyrethroids at the sodium channel seems to be a reversible process, with spontaneous reactivation of these channels occurring as pyrethroid metabolism leads to dissociation of the parent compound from the channels. The rapid rate of detoxification of the pyrethroids explains the rapid disappearance of symptoms (25).

The type II pyrethroids have been shown also to inhibit the chloride channel function at the γ-aminobutyric acid receptors by forming an ionophore complex at the picrotoxin-binding site (6,7,27,28). This inhibition may cause seizure activity.

Pyrethroids have been hypothesized to affect calcium regulation by direct inhibition of calcium uptake. The type I analogs influence the calcium–adenosine triphosphatase systems, whereas the type II analogs affect the calcium–magnesium–adenosine triphosphatase systems (7,27). Pyrethroids are hypothesized also to affect nicotinic receptors (7).

TABLE 103-5. Diagnostic criteria for occupational acute pyrethroid poisoning

Poisoning suspected
- Abnormal facial sensations
- Miliary papules, contact dermatitis
- No significant systemic symptoms or signs

Mild acute poisoning
- Skin signs or symptoms as noted in preceding list
- Significant systemic symptoms (e.g., dizziness, headache, nausea, anorexia, fatigue)
- Listlessness, vomiting, or increased stomal secretions
- Results in sick leave for more than 1 day

Moderate acute poisoning
- Aggravation of foregoing systemic signs and symptoms
- Mild disturbances of consciousness
- Muscular fasciculations

Severe acute poisoning
- Foregoing symptoms and signs
- Convulsions, coma, or pulmonary edema

Note: Poisoning assumes verified exposure within 2 days prior to onset of symptoms and reasonable exclusion of other diseases.
Reprinted from ref. 29, with permission.

Signs, Symptoms, and Syndromes

Pyrethroids and pyrethrins are considered highly insecticidal but of low-order toxicity to mammals and humans (1,5,7,11). Adverse effects usually consist of mild allergic reactions to inhalational or dermal exposure (8).

One-half of the patients allergic to ragweed exhibit cross-reactivity with pyrethrins because ragweed and *Chrysanthemum* are of the same botanical genus (8,9). The most common allergic manifestations include dermatitis, rhinitis, asthma, hypersensitivity pneumonitis, and anaphylactoid and anaphylactic reactions (8). The frequency of reactions to pyrethroids in human subjects by patch testing has been noted to be 2.6% for allergic reactions and 1.7% for irritant reactions (4).

Dermal symptoms usually occur within 2 to 4 hours of exposure. They include rashes, blistering, and paresthesias. Chronic exposure can cause erythematous, rough, itchy skin. Facial exposure can cause pain, lacrimation, photophobia, congestion, and edema of the conjunctivae and eyelids (29). Dermal symptoms can be exacerbated by sweating and washing with warm water (5).

Inhalational exposure commonly occurs secondary to spraying against the wind, cleaning sprayer-nozzle stoppages with the mouth and hands, being in close proximity to someone who is spraying, and being in the proximity of airborne pyrethroids or pyrethrins without benefit of personal protective gear (29). Most commonly, upper respiratory symptoms include stuffy nose, scratchy throat, sneezing, and edema of the oral and laryngeal tissues. Lower respiratory symptoms include cough, wheezing, shortness of breath, hypersensitivity, pneumonitis, bronchospasm, and pulmonary edema (7,9,11). One death has been reported in an asthmatic, associated with an inhalational exposure to pyrethroids (8). No death has been reported as a result of professional exposure (11).

Ingestive symptoms occur within 10 minutes to 1 hour and consist of epigastric pain, nausea, and vomiting. Erosive gastritis has occurred. Deaths have been reported after intentional ingestions (29).

A study of pyrethroid sprayers showed that 26.8% of people exposed at an occupational level manifest symptoms. The most common symptoms were abnormal facial sensations, dizziness, headache, fatigue, nausea, and decreased appetite (14). Mild pyrethroid poisoning as an occupational diagnosis was exhibited by 0.31% of the sprayers (Table 103-5). All the people in whom this syndrome was diagnosed recovered within 4 days (14).

Moderate poisoning should be suspected when the symptoms of mild poisoning progress to include a change in mental status and muscular fasciculations in large muscle groups of the extremities. The majority of affected patients recover in 1 to 6 days. In severely poisoned patients, increased secretions, pulmonary edema, and hypotension create difficulty in differentiating between pyrethroid and organophosphate toxicity. Analysis of plasma or red blood cell pseudocholinesterase levels may be helpful.

In cases of severe toxicity, coma and seizures may occur. Seizures may be frequent and recurrent, up to 10 to 30 times daily during the first week of poisoning (29). They gradually will decrease, and total recovery usually is expected in 2 to 4 weeks (5,29). Deaths have occurred in patients with severe, uncontrolled seizures (29).

The symptoms of pyrethroid exposure can be divided into two syndromes, depending on the group of pyrethroids. The T (tremor) syndrome is caused by the type I, non-cyano-containing pyrethroids and is characterized by tremor, increased sensitivity to external stimuli, and hyperthermia (11). The type II α-cyano pyrethroids cause the more severe CS (choreoathetotic, salivation) syndrome characterized by salivation, choreoathetotic movements, increased startle response, and tonic-clonic seizures. Some pyrethroids (i.e., fenpropathrin, cyphenothrin) exhibit a mixed picture.

Long-term effects have not been noted in mammals (7). Chronic exposure in pyrethrin factory workers has been shown to produce no serious long-term changes (24).

Management of Toxicity or Exposure

The pyrethrins and pyrethroids have no specific antidotes, and treatment consists of decontamination and supportive care. If ingestion is suspected, emesis, gastric aspiration, and lavage should be considered. Hydrocarbons often are mixed with the pyrethrin products, and care should be exercised in orogastric decontamination when hydrocarbons are involved. Pyrethroids are highly lipophilic and will adsorb well to activated charcoal. Charcoal is recommended (if not otherwise contraindicated secondary to coingested agents or associated gastric injury). Because pyrethroids undergo enterohepatic recirculation, repeat-dose activated charcoal has been suggested if symptoms are severe and protracted (1).

For dermal exposure, decontamination of the body and hair should be performed by washing thoroughly at least two times with soap and water (9). Clothing should be washed as well, although in an army study of permethrin-impregnated clothing, ten washings reduced the amount of pyrethroid impregnated in the clothing by only 50% (30). The results of this study suggest that discarding contaminated clothing may be necessary. Vitamin E has been used successfully as a topical treatment for paresthesias occurring after dermal exposure (9). Vitamin E, mineral oil, benzocaine, and creams containing vitamins A and D, when used prior to exposure, also have been found to be effective in preventing the onset of symptoms (11).

Ocular exposure demands immediate and copious irrigation with a stream of water or normal saline for a minimum of 10 minutes (5).

Rhinitis can be treated with oral antihistamines and decongestants (9). Bronchospasm has been reported and should be treated with bronchodilators. Anaphylactic reactions should be treated with diphenhydramine (Benadryl), epinephrine, steroids, and bronchodilators as needed. Close airway supervision may be necessary, with intubation as indicated. Atropine has been used effectively to combat the salivation caused by type II pyrethroids, but this treatment has not been shown to affect mortality (11). The need for more than 10 mg of atropine in these patients should prompt suspicion of a concurrent exposure to an organophosphate (29).

Muscle spasms, cramping, and fasciculations may occur. Muscle relaxants, such as methocarbamol and diazepam, sometimes have been found useful for reducing musculoskeletal symptoms (11).

Neurologic symptoms, such as paresthesias and various abnormal sensations, may be minor or may be severe, as in a seizure. Seizures may be prolonged, and their control may prove difficult. They should be treated aggressively with high-dose benzodiazepines; up to 3 mg per kg has been needed in animal studies (9,28). Diazepam (Valium) has been most effective in the treatment of type II symptoms (6), probably because benzodiazepines such as diazepam work at the γ-aminobutyric acid receptor (27). Barbiturates have not been found to be as efficacious as Valium, and phenytoin use in this situation is questionable (9,11,28).

All persons with severe poisoning should be admitted to the hospital for close respiratory and airway monitoring. Diazepam should be given immediately at the onset of neuromuscular symptomatology (5).

Associated Toxicities

When many of the halogenated pyrethrins (e.g., deltamethrin, fenpropathrin, permethrin) are heated to decomposition, toxic fumes of NO_x, CL^-, and CN^- gas are released (30). These exposures should be treated appropriately.

Pyrethrins almost never are packaged alone, and toxicities associated with accompanying agents must be considered. Hydrocarbon, organophosphate, carbamate, and other synergistic agents may cause inhalational, gastric, and neurologic symptoms. These always must be considered in a pyrethroid poisoning. Inert ingredients, as listed on the product label, usually are confidential products known only to the manufacturer and may or may not have toxic effects (12).

PBO is one of the most commonly used synergists. It has little pesticide activity but increases the effectiveness of the pyrethroids. Acute oral ingestion or dermal exposure has not been shown to be toxic and should not produce significant symptomatology (9,12). At very high levels, PBO has exhibited a dose-dependent toxic effect, causing hepatocellular carcinoma (12).

SPECIALIZED PRODUCT INFORMATION

If a clinically significant exposure has occurred, the local emergency medical services system should be activated. Product information, including manufacturer's name and phone number, often is listed on a product label or packaging. A local or regional poison center should be able to help to identify the contents of a suspect product and explain toxicities and recommended treatments for exposure. The National Pesticide Telecommunications Network has a hot line for pesticide information. The network can be reached Monday through Friday between the hours of 6:30 a.m. and 4:30 p.m. Pacific Standard Time at 1-800-858-7377 or 1-800-858-7378.

MEDICAL MONITORING

Medical monitoring in the workplace should include a preplacement examination to identify preexisting medical conditions—especially dermal, neurologic, or pulmonary diseases—that may be exacerbated by exposure to pyrethroids. People with open dermal lesions and asthma are especially susceptible to reactions from dermal or inhaled pyrethroids, respectively. People with central and peripheral nervous system diseases should not be exposed to pyrethroids (5). Periodic health examinations should follow to detect the symptoms of early exposure-related health effects. If exposure-related effects are noted, occupational exposure should be reduced, and improvement in work practices, personal protection, and work environment (ventilation, etc.) should be considered. Performance of specific examinations, such as electroneuromyography, may be necessary. Affected persons should not be allowed to return to work until symptoms resolve and postexposure examination and testing results are within normal limits (5).

BIOLOGICAL AND OCCUPATIONAL MONITORING

Most pyrethrin and pyrethroid residues can be detected after extraction via gas chromatography with electron-capture detection, gas chromatography with mass selective detection, or high-performance liquid chromatography with ultraviolet detection (15,17,18). Extractions can be obtained from most substances, most commonly tissue samples, soil, grains, food, air, and clothing. Minimal detectable limits can be as low as 0.005 mg per kg.

Urinary detection of pyrethrins and their metabolites can be performed via gas chromatography with a detection limit of 0.05 mg per L (5). Biological exposure indices have not yet been recommended for urinary metabolites.

OCCUPATIONAL AND ENVIRONMENTAL REGULATIONS

Information about each of the more than 2,000 pyrethrin products is not available; however, as many of the compounds are isomers and have similar mechanisms of action, generalizations can be made (11). Using pyrethrum as a prototype, the following workplace standards have been established: The threshold limit value time-weighted average and the U.S. Occupational Safety and Health Administration permissible exposure limits are 5 mg per cubic meter, and the value that is considered immediately dangerous to life and health is 5,000 mg per cubic meter. No short-term exposure limit, ceiling limit, or odor threshold is available (32).

Very few human data for pyrethrin exposure limits are available. Overall, the no-observed-adverse-effect limit and lethal dose in 50% of animals studied are from experimental data in mammal studies and are considered relatively high, allowing a large margin of safety for human exposure. The lethal dose in 50% of animals studied and the no-observed-adverse-effect limits of teratogenicity, fetal mutagenicity, and fertility also have been studied in animals: Very high milligram-per-kilogram levels are needed to cause effects (Table 103-6) (5,7,11,15,17–23,31–33).

TABLE 103-6. Examples of exposure data and median lethal dose for pyrethrins and pyrethroids

Common name	LD_{50} (mg/kg)		LC_{50} (mg/m^3)	NOAEL[a]			
	Oral	Dermal	Inhalational	General	Oncologic	Reproductive	Other
Pyrethrin esters	50						TLV, PEL = 5 $LDL_{0\ (h\text{-}oral)}$ = 1,000 mg/kg $LDL_{0\ (child\text{-}oral)}$ = 750 mg/kg
Allethrin	310		>1,500	5–50 mg/$kg_{(d)}$	2,000 mg/kg diet		
Cyfluthrin	$300_{(m)}$		200	50 mg/kg			
Cyhalothrin	$37_{(m)}$	200–2,000		50 mg/kg	7.2 mg/kg	7.5 mg/kg	
Cypermethrin	251	219–4,000		7.5 mg/kg	70 mg/kg	100 mg/kg diet	
Deltamethrin	121			1 mg/$kg_{(d)}$	50 mg/kg diet	10 mg/kg	
Fenpropathrin	49	$2,000_{(b)}$					
Fenvalerate	451	$2,500_{(b)}$		7.5 mg/kg	1,000 mg/kg		NOAEL teratogenic, 50 mg/$kg_{(m)}$
Permethrin	410	500 mg/$d_{(b)}$	685 mg/m^3	20 mg/kg			NOAEL teratogenic, 225 mg/kg
d-Phenothrin	>5,000	>5,000	>3,760 mg/m^3			7–8 mg/kg	NOAEL teratogenic, 3,000 mg/$kg_{(m)}$
Resmethrin	>5,000			10 mg/$kg_{(d)}$	5,000 mg/kg		NOAEL inhalational, 100 mg/m^3
Telfluthrin	35	200					
Tetramethrin	$1,000_{(m)}$	$>2,000_{(b)}$	49 mg/m^3			500 mg/kg	NOAEL teratogenic, 1,000 mg/kg

$_{(b)}$, rabbit; $_{(d)}$, dog; $_{(h)}$, human; LC_{50}, median lethal concentration; LD_{50}, median lethal dose; LDL_0, lethal dose (lowest) for 0% of the population; $_{(m)}$, mouse; NOAEL, no-observable-adverse-effect limit; PEL, permissible exposure limit; TLV, threshold limit value.

[a]If data from multiple species were available, the most conservative estimates were chosen.

Note: Species is rat unless otherwise indicated.

Adapted from refs. 7, 15, 17–23, 31–33.

EXPOSURE CONTROL

Personal protective gear and adequate personal hygiene seem to be the best means of protection against occupational exposure to pyrethrins. Long-sleeved clothing, gloves, goggles, and face masks should be worn. Workers also must be instructed in proper spraying and handling techniques so as not to contaminate themselves or nearby workers. Frequent monitoring for symptoms in the workplace and removal from exposure with the onset of any symptoms of clinical toxicity should be performed routinely.

ENVIRONMENTAL FATE

Environmental degradation rates of the pyrethrins are fairly complete. Degradation occurs relatively quickly (in days to weeks) (see Table 103-4). No significant long-term accumulation has been noted.

REFERENCES

1. Valentine WM. Pyrethrin and pyrethroid insecticides. *Vet Clin North Am Small Anim Pract* 1990;20(2):375–382.
2. Gosselin RE. Therapeutics index—pyrethrum. In: Gosselin RE, Smith RP, Hodge HC, eds. *Clinical toxicology of commercial products,* 5th ed. Baltimore: Williams & Wilkins, 1984:352–354.
3. Budavari S, O'Neil MJ, Smith A, et al., eds. *The Merck index,* 12th ed. Whitehouse Station, NJ: Merck and Co, 1996.
4. Lsi P. Sensitization risk of pyrethroid insecticides. *Contact Dermatitis* 1992; 26:349–350.
5. He F. Synthetic pyrethroids. *Toxicology* 1994;91:43–49.
6. Narahashi T, Carter DB, Frey J, et al. Sodium channels and $GABA_A$ receptor-channel complex as targets of environmental toxicants. *Toxicol Lett* 1995;82:239–245.
7. Bradbury SP, Coats JR. Comparative toxicology of the pyrethroid insecticides. *Rev Environ Contam Toxicol* 1989;108:133–177.
8. Wax PM, Hoffman RS. Fatality associated with inhalation of a pyrethrin shampoo. *Clin Toxicol* 1994;32(4):457–460.
9. Mack RB. He came, he saw, he conquered—pyrethrin insecticide exposure. *N C Med J* 1989;50(9):509–511.
10. Braddock J. Trade name index. In: Gosselin RE, Smith RP, Hodge HC, eds. *Clinical toxicology of commercial products,* 5th ed. Baltimore: Williams & Wilkins, 1984:vi–735.
11. Miyamoto J, Kaneko H, Tsuji R, et al. Pyrethroids, nerve poisons: how their risks to human health should be assessed. *Toxicol Lett* 1995;82:933–940.
12. Grossman J. What's hiding under the sink: dangers of household pesticides. *Environ Health Perspect* 1995;103(6):550–554.
13. Dorman DC, Beasley VR. Neurotoxicology of pyrethrin and pyrethroid insecticides. *Vet Hum Toxicol* 1991;33(3):238–243.
14. Chen S, Zhang Z, He F, et al. An epidemiological study on occupational acute pyrethroid poisoning in cotton farmers. *Br J Ind Med* 1991;48:77–81.
15. World Health Organization. *Cypermethrin.* Environmental health criteria 82. Geneva: World Health Organization, 1989.
16. He F, Sun J, Han K, et al. Effects of pyrethroid insecticides on subjects engaged in packaging pyrethroids. *Br J Ind Med* 1988;45:548–551.
17. *Permethrin health and safety guide* (no. 33). Geneva: World Health Organization, 1989.
18. *Tetramethrin health and safety guide* (no. 31). Geneva: World Health Organization, 1989.
19. *Deltamethrin health and safety guide* (no. 30). Geneva: World Health Organization, 1989.
20. *Fenvalerate health and safety guide* (no. 34). Geneva: World Health Organization, 1989.
21. *Cyhalothrin and lambda-cyhalothrin* (no. 38). Geneva: World Health Organization, 1990.
22. d-*Phenothrin health and safety guide* (no. 32). Geneva: World Health Organization, 1989.
23. *Resmethrins health and safety guide* (no. 25). Geneva: World Health Organization, 1989.
24. Gombe S, Ogada TA. Health of men on long-term exposure to pyrethrins. *East Afr Med J* 1988;65(11):734–742.
25. Aldridge WN. An assessment of the toxicological properties of pyrethroids and their neurotoxicity. *Toxicology* 1990;21(2):89–104.
26. Song JH, Narahashi T. Modulation of sodium channels of rat cerebellar Purkinje neurons by the pyrethroid tetramethrin. *J Pharmacol Exp Ther* 1996;277:445–453.
27. Coats JR. Mechanisms of toxic actions and structure-activity relationships for organochlorine and synthetic pyrethroid insecticides. *Environ Health Perspect* 1990;87:255–262.
28. Gammon DW, Lawrence LJ, Casida JE. Pyrethroid toxicology: protective effects of diazepam and phenobarbital in the mouse and the cockroach. *Toxicol Appl Pharmacol* 1982;66:290–296.

29. He F, Wang S, Liu L, et al. Clinical manifestations and diagnosis of acute pyrethroid poisoning. *Arch Toxicol* 1989;63:54–58.
30. Snodgrass HL. Permethrin transfer from treated cloth to the skin surface: potential for exposure in humans. *J Toxicol Environ Health* 1992;35:91–105.
31. Sax NI, Lewis RJ. *Dangerous properties of industrial materials*, 7th ed. New York: Van Nostrand–Reinhold, 1989.
32. *Poisondex: toxicologic management—pyrethrins*, vol 89. Englewood, CO: MicroMedix, Inc, 1974–1996:7.3–7.7.
33. *Allethrins health and safety guide* (no. 24). Geneva: World Health Organization, 1989.

CHAPTER 104

Ethylene Oxide and Propylene Oxide

John B. Sullivan, Jr.

SOURCES, PRODUCTION, AND USES

Ethylene oxide, used widely as a gas sterilization agent, is a highly reactive biocide and fumigant. Owing to its highly reactive nature, it is an ideal intermediate from which other chemicals are developed. It is estimated that the annual U.S. production of ethylene oxide is between 6 and 7 billion pounds, which makes it one of the most prolifically produced chemicals in the United States (1).

Ethylene oxide has been produced commercially since the 1920s. Besides being a primary sterilization gas for medical equipment, it is used extensively as an intermediate chemical in the production of other compounds such as ethylene glycol (2,3). More than 99% of commercially produced ethylene oxide is used for manufacturing other products: Some 70% is used to manufacture ethylene glycol. The remainder is used in producing nonionic surface-active agents for detergents and industrial surfactants; ethanolamines for cosmetics and detergents; glycol ethers for coatings, fuel additives, brake fluids, and inks; diethylene and triethylene glycol for manufacturing polyester resins, drying natural gas, and for emulsifiers, plasticizers, and lubricants; and polyethylene glycols (3,4).

Less than 5% of the ethylene oxide that is produced is used in the health care industry for sterilization purposes. For this application, ethylene oxide is mixed with chlorofluorocarbons (Freon) or carbon dioxide and is sold in gas cylinders. It has been used also as a fumigant and a biocide in warehouses, granaries, and ship cargoes.

Ethylene oxide is very effective for sterilizing materials that are heat-sensitive. The vapor of ethylene oxide penetrates paper, cellophane, fabrics, rubber, polyethylene, and polyvinyl chloride. It is used to sterilize a great variety of hospital products, including surgical equipment (e.g., bronchoscopes, endoscopes), syringes, gloves, plastic goods such as catheters, tubing, other instruments, medications, implantable devices, and prosthetic devices.

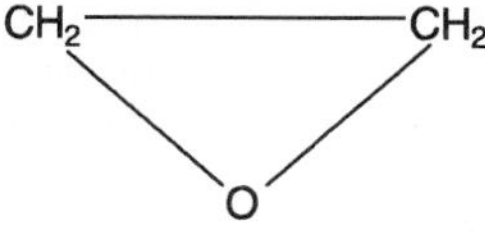

Figure 104-1. Ethylene oxide.

CHEMICAL FORMS AND REACTIVITY

Ethylene oxide (1,2-epoxyethane, oxirane, dihydrooxirene, dimethylene oxide) is the simplest epoxide (C_2H_4O), having a molecular weight of 44.06 D (Fig. 104-1). It is a clear, colorless liquid below its boiling point of 10°C (51.3°F), whereas at higher temperatures it is a colorless gas. Ethylene oxide gas has an odor very similar to that of ether at approximately 700 parts per million (ppm), which makes it easily recognizable. It is heavier than air, having a vapor density of 1.49 (as compared to that of air, which is 1.0). A 3% ethylene oxide vapor in air is combustible and can result in explosions in a confined space. It is also explosive when heated or in the presence of alkali metal hydroxides and catalytic surfaces. Dilution of ethylene oxide with 23 volumes of water renders it nonflammable.

Owing to the fact that it is heavier than air, ethylene oxide can disperse along the floor to ignition sources. To reduce the explosion hazard of ethylene oxide, it is mixed with inert gases such as carbon dioxide or halocarbons such as Freon. Used as a sterilizing agent, it is prepared in mixtures of 10% ethylene oxide and 90% carbon dioxide or 12% ethylene oxide and 88% Freon.

Ethylene oxide is readily mixable with water, alcohol, and organic solvents (3). It is an alkylating agent and binds irreversibly with organic molecules such as amino acids, histidine, hemoglobin, and nucleoproteins (3). Owing to its high degree of reactivity with organic molecules, it is a very effective fungicide for treatment of soil and plants (3). Ethylene oxide will violently polymerize if contaminated with aqueous alkalis, amines, mineral acids, metal oxides, and metal chlorides. Violent decomposition will occur at temperatures exceeding 800°F. Hazardous products of decomposition are hydrochloric acid and carbon dioxide. Ethylene oxide will also alkylate sulfhydryl groups, amino groups, carboxyl groups, and hydroxyl groups of proteins (4).

SITES, INDUSTRIES, AND BUSINESSES ASSOCIATED WITH EXPOSURE

Persons at risk from ethylene oxide exposure are hospital sterilization workers and workers who produce and use ethylene oxide in the chemical industry. Owing to its high solubility in porous plastics, residual amounts of ethylene oxide can de-gas from products after sterilization and constitute an exposure risk for hospital personnel (5). It is estimated that more than 75,000 health care workers in the United States are exposed to ethylene oxide (1).

Given the fact that ethylene oxide is very well controlled within the industrial environment and also owing to its known flammability and explosive hazards, exposures to ethylene oxide are not very common. In contrast, in the health care industry, because the use of pure ethylene oxide is uncommon, exposures probably are more frequent. Health care workers are exposed during de-gassing from porous plastics and to residual gas from sterilization procedures (6). These exposures are usually low level, but exposures to bursts of higher ethylene oxide concentrations can occur on opening of sterilizer doors.

Hospital sterilization procedures require that the gas be retained in a pressurized sterilization unit long enough to penetrate all items within the unit. The sterilization environment must be properly humidified to assist penetration of polyethylene plastic wrappings and to allow ethylene oxide gas to diffuse into small pores and cracks. After the passage of an adequate sterilization time, the ethylene oxide gas is evacuated from the sterilizer chamber. Appropriate aeration time is necessary after sterilization procedures to allow de-gassing of ethylene oxide from plastic items. All plastic and rubber items must be allowed to aerate for safe release of residual ethylene oxide. Removal of residual ethylene oxide from a sterilization chamber is also necessary to avoid workers' exposure.

Sterilizers using the 12% ethylene oxide and 88% Freon (12/88) mixture usually operate under a pressure of 10 pounds per square inch (7). Negative-pressure sterilization uses 100% ethylene oxide and helps to reduce the risk of ethylene oxide exposure because a negative-pressure process reduces leaks around sterilizer seals, gaskets, and pressure-relief valves. In addition, with a negative-pressure process, no connection valve is present by which ethylene oxide gas is introduced into the chamber, as the ethylene oxide cylinder is punctured once it is inside the closed unit. However, 100% ethylene oxide cylinders are a hazard, and their storage remains a problem. Also, negative-pressure sterilizers do not have the capacity of the positive-pressure sterilizer units. Because 100% ethylene oxide is an explosion and flammability hazard, most hospital sterilizers typically are pressurized and use the 12/88 mixture (7). In a given facility, the design of sterilizers and engineering and administrative controls that are in place will determine personnel exposure risks.

Basic sterilizers operate through four phases (7):

1. Air evacuation, humidification, and introduction of ethylene oxide into the sterilizer chamber
2. Dwell period during which sterilization occurs (usually 2.5 hours at 130°F for non–heat degree–sensitive items and 5 hours at 100°F for heat degree–sensitive items)
3. Evacuation of ethylene oxide from the chamber via a vacuum pump
4. Aeration period of 12 hours to allow de-gassing of ethylene oxide residue from items sterilized

Some more sophisticated sterilizer units incorporate into the aeration cycle an allowance for articles to remain in the chamber, making their transfer to a different area unnecessary.

POTENTIAL HUMAN EXPOSURE SITUATIONS

As stated, exposure to ethylene oxide occurs mainly in health care workers who perform job-related sterilization procedures. Exposure scenarios include the following (7):

High-level, acute exposure to several hundred or thousand parts per million could occur secondary to a sudden release from an ethylene oxide cylinder. Each cylinder may contain from 100 to several thousand grams of ethylene oxide. Releases can occur at cylinder connecting points or during the process of connecting to supply lines or from accidents. High-level exposure to sterilizer workers may also occur from leaks around sterilizer gaskets in pressurized procedures or from faulty pressure relief valves during purging of sterilizer chambers.

Opening the sterilizer door at the completion of the sterilization process can expose a worker to air concentrations that meet or exceed the excursion limit of 5 ppm of ethylene oxide. Normally, an evacuation cycle helps to eliminate residual ethylene oxide; however, despite this cycle, some ethylene oxide usually remains. Escape of the hot gases into the room after the sterilizer door is opened can diffuse ethylene oxide throughout the room. Local exhaust ventilation usually helps to eliminate excess ethylene oxide gas. Normally, the residual ethylene oxide is removed from the sterilizer via a vacuum pump and released into a sewer drain. Plumbing codes require an air gap at this discharge point to prevent siphoning of liquid back up into the drainage system. This plumbing gap is a (potentially significant) point of exposure of gas back into the atmosphere of the surrounding area. Residual ethylene oxide de-gasses from sterilized products, particularly plastics. Removal of such products from the sterilizer and transport of the load to the aerator is another source of exposure that can exceed or meet the excursion limit.

Exposure to a few parts per million of ethylene oxide, which might meet or exceed the time-weighted average (TWA), is the most common scenario and results from opening sterilizer doors (probably the source of greatest exposure risk), transporting de-gassing sterilized items, and cleaning the inside of a sterilizer.

CLINICAL TOXICOLOGY

Exposures may occur owing to faulty ventilation, poor aeration of items, or faulty evacuation of ethylene oxide. Ethylene oxide is a recognized neurotoxin. Also, owing to its highly reactive epoxide structure, it has mutagenic and carcinogenic potential. Another health hazard of ethylene oxide results from the fact that it is highly explosive when mixed with air in concentrations greater than 3% by volume (4). Ethylene oxide is unstable when mixed with acids or alkalis. Mixing ethylene oxide with an inert gas such as carbon dioxide or Freon decreases its explosiveness (4).

The health effects of ethylene oxide can be divided into the following broad categories: acute toxic, chronic toxic, carcinogenic, mutagenic, and reproductive effects (Table 104-1).

Signs, Symptoms, and Syndromes

ACUTE TOXICITY

Acute exposures to ethylene oxide of more than 300 ppm in either the gas or liquid form have caused significant health effects (6). The earliest effects of acute inhalational exposure are ocular irritation, nausea, vomiting, and headache. The etherlike odor is not detectable until the concentration reaches approximately 700 ppm, an extremely high exposure level. Thus, an individual who notices the odor has experienced a potentially serious toxic exposure. Later symptoms include respiratory irritation and, if the exposure is sufficiently high, pulmonary edema. Syncope, seizures, dizziness, and slurring of speech can also ensue. Delayed symptoms include ataxia, fatigue, and weakness.

Solutions of ethylene oxide have vesicant actions and can produce injury to the eye or skin on contact. Dermal irritation and burns are most likely to occur when the solution is in contact with the skin through clothing (8). Ethylene oxide in liquid form will easily penetrate rubber, leather, and other clothing.

TABLE 104-1. Ethylene oxide toxicity

Acute and chronic effects	Long-term sequelae
Ocular irritation and corneal injury	Peripheral neuropathy
Nausea	Mutagenicity risk
Vomiting (periodic and prolonged)	Carcinogenicity risk
Dizziness	Hypersensitivity
Seizures	Reproductive effects
Syncope	Chromosomal aberrations
Ataxia	Cataract formation
Urticaria (type I IgE)	Neurotoxic effects
Contact dermatitis	Paresthesias
Pulmonary edema	Distal extremity weakness
Pneumonitis	Peripheral neuropathy
Peripheral neuropathy	Neurobehavioral disturbances
Fatigue	Ataxia
Nystagmus	Seizures

The liquid also produces ocular injury and irritation after splash exposure. Injury to the cornea can occur, as can chemical burns to the skin and blister formation. Ingestion of the liquid can produce severe gastritis and hepatic damage.

Dermal effects after ethylene oxide exposure include burns, blistering, vesicle formation, contact dermatitis, and allergic urticarial rashes. Dermal contact with ethylene oxide has resulted in vesicular eruptions in workers who are exposed to 1% ethylene oxide in water (9). Patch testing with ethylene oxide demonstrated a delayed hypersensitivity reaction to approximately 100 ppm of ethylene oxide (9). The most common dermal reaction to ethylene oxide gas is a severe irritant reaction or burn, with vesicular eruptions occurring in 6 to 12 hours.

Sterilized items can retain ethylene oxide residues that may produce effects via direct skin contact or from de-gassing. Adequate aeration of sterilized items is imperative to ensure that residues of ethylene oxide do not come into contact with humans (8).

Ethylene oxide is an established peripheral neurotoxin. It impairs both sensory and motor function and can result in muscular atrophy. Human cases of peripheral neuropathy have been described. Neuropathies can occur after a one-time acute exposure or after chronic exposure to ethylene oxide.

Seizures, coma, respiratory failure, and vomiting were observed in animals as an effect of ethylene oxide exposure in concentrations ranging from 200 to 700 ppm (10). Repeated exposures of animals to ethylene oxide also resulted in peripheral neuropathies affecting lumbosacral nerves (10). In most animal species studied, the range of ethylene oxide concentrations that produced neurotoxic effects was 100 to 200 ppm (10). Other neurologic manifestations include fatigue, dizziness, syncope, convulsions, and behavioral disturbances (10).

Vomiting may be periodic, occurring approximately every 30 minutes after an acute exposure (10). The vomiting and nausea can be prolonged and last for days. Coma and somnolence can occur also after an acute exposure to ethylene oxide. These symptoms would occur at concentrations of several hundred parts per million, but they might also be associated with exposures to very high concentrations of the vapor or of the liquid in confined spaces (10).

CHRONIC TOXICITY

Target Organ Effects. Repeated exposures to ethylene oxide can result in symptoms similar to those seen in acute exposures: headache, dizziness, vomiting, nausea, ocular irritation, respiratory irritation, fatigue, nystagmus, ataxia, and slurred speech (10). Repeated exposures to ethylene oxide also can result in a delayed allergic contact dermatitis (8).

Chronic exposure can produce sensitization, which has been reported to result in type I immunoglobulin E reactions (5). Manifestations of such reactions include anaphylaxis, periorbital edema, facial erythema, and urticarial rashes. Dermatologic effects from ethylene oxide result from its vesicant action and ability to sensitize the skin.

Nerve biopsies conducted in individuals with peripheral neuropathy after ethylene oxide exposure have demonstrated axonal degeneration (10). Exposure to ethylene oxide on a repeated basis can also produce certain behavioral effects such as disorientation, aggression, and some irrational behavior (10,11). A report of cognitive changes associated with chronic ethylene oxide exposure in workers demonstrated impaired memory, increased irritability, clumsiness, and episodes of falling (11). After exposure ceased, these symptoms improved over a period of months but did not disappear. Environmental monitoring in this report indicated an average ethylene oxide concentration of 2.4 ppm (11). Ethylene oxide concentrations adjacent to the sterilizing area where the individuals worked were 4.2 ppm (11).

Other studies of health care workers chronically exposed to ethylene oxide in normal sterilization operations indicate the occurrence of neuropsychological effects and cognitive disorders (12,13). These employees had detected the odor of ethylene oxide during operation of equipment, and ethylene oxide air concentrations had not been routinely monitored (12,13). Sampling in breathing zones demonstrated concentrations of 15 ppm during these operations and up to 250 ppm in breathing zone areas for some locations during other monitoring periods (12,13). These studies indicated that low-level exposure to ethylene oxide can result in dysfunctional personality and cognitive disorders.

Peripheral neuropathy after prolonged exposure to ethylene oxide is associated with paresthesias of the distal extremities, weakness of the distal extremities, and fatigue (4). It also is associated with decreased pinprick sensation in fingers and toes and decreased vibratory sensation. Nerve conduction studies have been consistent with sensorimotor polyneuropathies (4).

The chronic and long-term effects of ethylene oxide are mainly neurologic manifestations. Mutagenicity, reproductive toxicity, and carcinogenicity are possible. The extreme reactivity of ethylene oxide with nucleoproteins and amino acids gives it carcinogenic and mutagenic potential (3).

Carcinogenicity. Animal studies have demonstrated that ethylene oxide is a carcinogen at levels of less than 50 ppm (1). Incidences of mononuclear cell leukemia were significantly increased in a dose-related fashion in female rats exposed to ethylene oxide (1). In male rats, the frequency of mononuclear cell leukemia, peritoneal mesothelioma, and cerebral glioma increased in a dose-related fashion (1).

Mortality studies in ethylene oxide production workers have not been able to conclude beyond doubt that ethylene oxide exposure was associated with human malignancies; however, it is considered suspect as a cause of malignancies. A study of ethylene oxide production workers in Sweden was conducted from 1961 through 1977 (2). These workers experienced variable exposures to ethylene oxide depending on where they were employed in the production facility. However, ethylene oxide was not the only agent to which these workers may have been exposed; other chemical exposures occurred through the production of ethylene oxide by a chlorohydrin process that began with ethylene and produced ethylene chlorohydrin as an intermediate (2). Ethylene dichloride and bis(2-chloroethyl)ether were by-products of the process and are carcinogens. Ethylene chlorohydrin is also a mutagen. This study found an excess of malignancies, among them leukemia and gastrointestinal tumors (2).

Another epidemiologic study conducted in 1979 suggested that ethylene oxide was associated with an excess of hematopoietic cancers in Swedish workers (6). Two cases of leukemia were reported among 230 workers in this study, and an earlier report cited two cases of leukemia among 241 ethylene oxide production workers who were followed up from 1960 through 1977 (6). A recent updating of this cohort included the reporting of a third group of 355 production workers among whom a few more cases of leukemia were reported (6). In contrast to these Swedish reports, other studies in larger groups found no excess leukemia deaths among workers potentially exposed to ethylene oxide.

On the basis of earlier reports that linked risk of leukemia with ethylene oxide exposure, another mortality study was published in 1981 that examined 767 men with a 5-year history of exposure to ethylene oxide in a production plant between the years 1955 and 1977 (14). No deaths from leukemia were observed, and no excess mortality was noted as compared with the general population (14). This 1981 study did show an excess death rate from pancreatic cancer and Hodgkin's disease. In 1986, Hogstedt et al. (15) published a cancer mortality report on

733 ethylene oxide–exposed workers. Among these workers were eight cases of leukemia and six cases of stomach cancer. The researchers suggested that the study indicated a relationship between low-level ethylene oxide exposure and cancer (14).

Animal studies have shown ethylene oxide to be a carcinogen by any route of administration and in multiple species of animals. Leukemia, brain cancer, and mesothelioma have been induced in animals in inhalational studies. Consideration of these studies in conjunction with human epidemiologic studies points to ethylene oxide exposure as a potential cause of hematopoietic cancers and cancer in other organs in humans. The International Agency for Research on Cancer has issued a statement that ethylene oxide is probably carcinogenic to humans.

Mutagenicity. Ethylene oxide is a mutagen for bacteria and human lymphocytes and produces chromosome damage in both experimental animals and humans (1). Unscheduled DNA synthesis, a measure of the repair of DNA damage, in germinal cells is increased with increasing doses of ethylene oxide in mice exposed to 300 or 500 ppm for 8 hours per day, 5 days per week, for 1 week (16). Studies of humans experiencing symptoms of ethylene oxide exposure have shown increased chromosomal aberrations.

The frequency of sister chromatid exchanges (SCEs) and chromosomal aberrations has been studied in animals exposed to ethylene oxide (1). The frequency of SCEs is an indication of chromosomal damage and was found to increase in a dose-related fashion (1) and with duration of exposure (2). In animals exposed to 50 ppm, SCEs occurred 1.8 times more frequently than in the unexposed controls (1). In those animals exposed to 100 ppm, SCEs were 3.1 times more frequent than in controls (1).

Owing to the fact that ethylene oxide is a strong alkylating agent, mutagenicity and chromosomal damage studies have been conducted also after human exposures (17,18). SCEs have been investigated as a tool for detecting potential mutagenicity. An SCE is the visual manifestation of a four-stranded exchange in the DNA. The number of such exchanges in chromosomes is a measure of exposure to an agent that produces DNA damage through formation of covalent adducts or disturbance of the bases. Increases in SCEs may occur after exposure to mutagens or carcinogens. Although SCEs are not accepted as absolute quantitations or predictors of health effects, they are useful for probing potential health problems.

Individuals working in sterilization areas of hospitals were monitored for SCEs in cultured lymphocytes and were compared with control SCE levels (17). Environmental monitoring of the worksite of these individuals showed ethylene oxide concentrations of 36 ppm in the air (17). Concentrations of ethylene oxide as low as 50 ppm in ambient air for 4 hours have been shown to produce mutagenic effects in mice (17,18). For individuals who developed mild symptomatology secondary to ethylene oxide in the workplace, chromosomal damage via increased SCEs was demonstrated and persisted for as long as 8 weeks after the last known exposure to ethylene oxide (17). In health care workers exposed to ethylene oxide, a statistically significant increase in SCEs occurred in workers in sterilizing areas who were most heavily exposed (17). The studies were controlled for subject age and smoking habits, and subjects were divided into low- and high-exposure groups. The workers were exposed to ethylene oxide for brief periods, but those with the highest exposure exhibited a significant increase in mean SCEs per lymphocyte (17).

Another assessment of the mutagenicity of ethylene oxide was conducted in factory workers exposed to ethylene oxide at concentrations of 0.5 to 1.0 ppm (19). In this study, ethylene oxide was shown to elevate unscheduled DNA synthesis significantly and to increase chromosomal aberrations in peripheral lymphocytes (19).

TABLE 104-2. Reproductive and mutagenic toxicity of ethylene oxide

Unscheduled DNA synthesis
Sister chromatid exchange
Chromosomal aberrations
Functional sperm abnormalities
Spontaneous abortions

Reproductive Effects. Ethylene oxide has been shown to be a reproductive toxin in male and female animals (1). It induces dominant chromosomal lethal mutations in germinal cells. However, experimental studies have indicated that ethylene oxide has had no adverse effects on reproduction in animals exposed to 100 ppm (3).

Ethylene oxide exposure of hospital staff has been related to an increased incidence of spontaneous abortions (1,20). The frequency of spontaneous abortions among the exposed individuals was 16.7%, as compared with a 5.6% frequency among the nonexposed control subjects. Animal and human studies demonstrating chromosomal mutations and spontaneous abortions corroborate the reproductive toxicity of ethylene oxide. Table 104-2 summarizes mutagenic and reproductive effects.

Management of Toxicity

Eyes that have been exposed to ethylene oxide should be flushed immediately with copious amounts of water. Contact lenses should not be worn by anyone working with ethylene oxide. Ocular examinations should include evaluation of the cornea and adjacent tissue for injury.

Any exposed skin site should be washed immediately with copious amounts of water. All contaminated clothing should be removed, and contaminated leather shoes or other leather articles must be discarded. Skin should be examined for burns, erythema, and blisters, which may not be apparent for 6 to 12 hours. Dermal exposure should be treated as a chemical burn. Bleb formation may occur with desquamation. Healing takes 3 to 4 weeks. Injured areas may exhibit residual brown pigmentation for weeks to months. Pure liquid ethylene oxide can produce frostbite.

The person who experiences inhalational exposure should be moved to an area of fresh air and adequate ventilation. Medical management is symptomatic care. Syncope, seizures, pulmonary insult, and dermal and ocular injury should be considered. Seizures and pulmonary edema can occur. As for all exposures, the person's clothing may be contaminated and should be removed.

Ethylene oxide liquid ingestion will produce gastrointestinal distress with vomiting. Management is symptomatic.

ENVIRONMENTAL MONITORING AND REGULATIONS

Owing to the multiple health risks associated with ethylene oxide exposure, the Occupational Safety and Health Administration (OSHA) in 1984 lowered the permissible exposure limit (PEL) from 50 to 1 ppm and established an action level of 0.5 ppm, based on an 8-hour TWA (16). The action level is the level above which employers must initiate certain activities to protect and monitor workers, as set forth in the OSHA ruling (16). This 1984 standard provided for methods of exposure control, monitoring of employee exposures, personal protective measures, record keeping, signs and labels, medical surveillance, and emergency procedures (16).

The reduction of the PEL from 50 to 1 ppm by OSHA was based on risk assessment studies that concluded that an excess cancer risk existed at the 50-ppm TWA for occupational exposures. By reducing the PEL to 1 ppm, OSHA projected that there would be a 98% reduction in cancer mortality risk (16).

In 1988, OSHA issued regulations adopting a short-term exposure limit (STEL) of 5 ppm averaged over a sampling period of 15 minutes (21). This new regulation also established exposure monitoring and training programs for workers in whom exposure exceeded this 5-ppm STEL. In addition, the new ruling required warning signs on products capable of releasing ethylene oxide to the extent that an employee might be exposed above the STEL, and it ordered that such exposure areas be identified per the regulations (21). In the 1988 ruling, OSHA addressed the health effects to employees whose 8-hour TWA never exceeded 1 ppm but who could be exposed to several short-term releases of ethylene oxide in excess of 5 ppm. Establishing such an excursion limit would further reduce the dose of ethylene oxide and, consequently, the cancer risk (16).

Workers at risk for violation of the excursion limit are engaged in such activities as loading and unloading sterilizers, changing ethylene oxide tanks or sterilizer equipment, collecting samples from ethylene oxide processes, and disconnecting piping from a railroad tank car (21). These types of activities might expose an employee to high short-term concentrations of ethylene oxide. Owing to this fact, OSHA requires monitoring of employees for potential short-term exposure whose activities are associated with operations that are most likely to produce exposures in excess of the 5-ppm excursion limit for each work shift, for each job classification, in each work area (Table 104-3) (21). These monitoring requirements are based on the combination of scenarios involving the PEL, the action level, and the excursion limit (21). According to OSHA, the 8-hour TWA action level of 0.5 ppm largely determines monitoring requirements.

The final regulatory limits on ethylene oxide can be summarized as follows: 8-hour TWA PEL, 1 ppm (16); 8-hour TWA action level, 0.5 ppm (16); and excursion limit (determined as a 15-minute TWA), 5 ppm (21).

Exposure Control

ENVIRONMENTAL CONTROL

OSHA regulates occupational exposure of ethylene oxide using PELs and required monitoring, engineering, and work practice controls (see Table 104-3). All employees exposed to ethylene oxide must be monitored, and access to areas using ethylene oxide must be restricted to authorized personnel. In addition, an emergency warning system must be in place to warn employees of sudden ethylene oxide releases.

OSHA requires that hazard warning signs be posted in areas where ethylene oxide exposure may occur. Regulated areas must be demarcated by signs carrying the following legend (16):

- Danger
- Ethylene oxide
- Cancer hazard and reproductive hazard
- Authorized personnel only
- Respirators and protective clothing may be required to be worn in this area

The intent of OSHA is to warn employees who may not know that they are entering an area that is regulated and where exposure to ethylene oxide may exceed the PEL. Warning signs are also necessary in areas where temporary exposure hazards may exist, such as during maintenance or equipment repair, when ethylene oxide leak could occur.

OSHA also requires that the following label be affixed to every ethylene oxide cylinder (16):

TABLE 104-3. Ethylene oxide monitoring requirements of OSHA, 1988

Exposure	Required monitoring
Below action level and at or below the excursion limit	No monitoring required
Below action level and above excursion limit	Monitor STEL four times per year; no TWA monitoring required
At or above level, at or below the TWA, and at or below the excursion limit	Monitor TWA exposures two times per year
At or above the action level, at or below the TWA, and above the excursion limit	Monitor TWA exposures two times per year and monitor STEL four times per year
Above the TWA and at or below the excursion limit	Monitor TWA exposures four times per year
Above the TWA and above the excursion limit	Monitor TWA exposures four times per year; monitor excursion limit exposures four times per year

OSHA, U.S. Occupational Safety and Health Administration; STEL, short-term exposure limit; TWA, time-weighted average.
Adapted from ref. 21.

- Caution
- Contains ethylene oxide
- Cancer and reproductive hazard

Emergency warning alarms are required to alert employees of an unexpected, significant release of ethylene oxide into the environment. OSHA does not further define such an emergency release. Presumably, such a release would be sudden and would violate PELs.

One of the primary methods by which ethylene oxide exposure is controlled is through ventilation. Local exhaust ventilation should be placed at certain points that best control releases of the gas into the work environment, such as above sterilizer doors and at drain sites. Adequately functioning door and drain ventilation is critical to controlling employee exposure to gas releases during sterilizer operation. Cylinders should be stored under a ventilation hood.

Because ethylene oxide odors are detected at air concentrations of approximately 700 ppm, odor detection indicates a high-level exposure. Ten nonrecirculating air exchanges per hour is standard for ethylene oxide areas. Respiratory protection is required for cylinder or filter changing or in maintenance areas. The goal of OSHA's standard is to control emission sources and to establish respiratory protection as a secondary antiexposure method.

Because ethylene oxide is a flammable liquid, and vapors can be explosive when mixed with air, cylinders must be stored in cool, well-ventilated areas away from ignition sources, oxidizers, alkalis, acids, and acetylide-forming metals such as copper, silver, mercury, and their alloys. A written emergency plan must also be developed for the workplace. Regulations regarding ethylene oxide control are detailed in OSHA's final standard, "Occupational Exposure to Ethylene Oxide" (16).

PERSONAL PROTECTION

Ethylene oxide exposure is reduced by the use of technical and engineering controls. Nonetheless, the use of personal protective devices, such as respirators and special clothing, is required by OSHA to limit exposures in the following situations (16):

- During intervals required to install or implement engineering and work practice controls

- In such work operations as maintenance and repair activities and chamber cleaning and in other situations in which work practice controls are not feasible
- In situations in which work practice controls are not sufficient to reduce exposures to or below PELs or excursion limits
- In emergency situations

OSHA requires employers to provide respirators to employees at no cost. Only air-supplied, positive-pressure, full face–piece respirators are approved for protection against ethylene oxide, and these must be jointly approved by the National Institute of Occupational Safety and Health and the Mine Safety and Health Administration, which mandate proper instruction and respirator fit testing to provide maximum protection against ethylene oxide exposure.

Protective, impermeable clothing (e.g., gloves, garments, face shields) is required in areas where eye or skin contact with ethylene oxide gas or liquid might occur. Protective clothing that becomes wet with liquid ethylene oxide may be a flammable hazard and may ignite. Any clothes splashed with ethylene oxide should be immediately removed under a shower. Splash-proof eye protection is mandatory in areas where ethylene oxide liquid is used or stored (16).

MEDICAL SURVEILLANCE

Employers are required by OSHA standards to have a medical surveillance program in place for all employees who are or will be exposed to ethylene oxide at or above the action level (0.5 ppm TWA) for at least 30 days per year, without regard to respirator use (16). All medical evaluations must be performed by or under the supervision of a licensed physician. OSHA requires inclusion of the following provisions in the medical surveillance program (16):

- Medical and work histories, with special emphasis directed to symptoms related to the pulmonary, hematologic, neurologic, and reproductive systems and to the eyes and skin
- Physical examination, with particular emphasis given to the pulmonary, hematologic, neurologic, and reproductive systems and to the eyes and skin
- Complete blood count to include at least a white cell count (including differential cell count), red cell count, hematocrit, and hemoglobin
- Any laboratory or other test that the examining physician deems necessary by sound medical practice
- If requested by the employee, pregnancy testing or laboratory evaluation of fertility as deemed appropriate by the physician

In certain cases, to provide sound medical advice to the employer and the employee, the physician must evaluate situations not directly related to ethylene oxide. For example, employees with skin diseases may be unable to tolerate wearing protective clothing. In addition, those with chronic respiratory diseases may not tolerate the wearing of negative-pressure (air-purifying) respirators. Additional tests and procedures that will help the physician to determine which employees are medically unable to wear such respirators should include an evaluation of cardiovascular function, a baseline chest radiograph (to be repeated at 5-year intervals), and a pulmonary function test (to be repeated every 3 years). The pulmonary function test should include measurement of the employee's forced vital capacity (FVC) and forced expiratory volume at 1 second (FEV_1). It also should include calculation of the ratios of FEV_1 to FVC and measured FVC and measured FEV_1 to expected values, corrected for variation due to age, gender, race, and height.

The employer is required to make the prescribed tests available at least annually to employees who are or will be exposed at or above the action level for 30 or more days per year; more often than specified if recommended by the examining physician; and on the employee's termination of employment or reassignment to another work area. Although little is known about the long-term consequences of high short-term exposures, the close monitoring of such affected employees seems prudent in light of existing health data. The employer shall provide physician-recommended examinations to any employee exposed in emergency condition. Likewise, the employer shall make available medical consultations, including physician-recommended examinations, to employees who believe they are experiencing signs or symptoms of exposure to ethylene oxide.

The employer is required to provide the physician with the following information: a copy of the applicable OSHA standard and its appendices; a description of the affected employee's duties as they relate to the employee exposure level; and information from the employee's previous medical examinations that is not readily available to the examining physician. Making this information available to the physician will aid in his or her evaluation of the employee's health in relation to assigned duties and fitness to wear personal protective equipment when required.

The employer also is required to obtain a written opinion from the examining physician, outlining the results of the medical examinations; the physician's opinion as to whether the employee has any detected medical conditions that would place the employee at increased risk of material impairment of his or her health from exposure to ethylene oxide; any recommended restrictions on the employee's exposure to ethylene oxide or on the use of protective clothing or equipment (e.g., respirators); and a statement that the employee has been informed by the physician of the results of the medical examination and of any medical conditions that require further explanation or treatment. This written opinion must not reveal specific findings or diagnoses unrelated to occupational exposure to ethylene oxide, and a copy of the opinion must be provided to the affected employee. The purpose of requiring the examining physician to supply the employer with a written opinion is to provide the employer with a medical basis that will aid in the determination of initial placement of an employee and in assessment of an employee's ability to use protective clothing and equipment.

OSHA requires that the hazards of ethylene oxide exposure be communicated to the employee. This is accomplished via (i) warning labels and warning signs in designated areas and attached to ethylene oxide cylinders, (ii) material safety data sheets, and (iii) training and information for employees exposed at or above the action level of 0.5 ppm TWA. This training and information must be provided annually and must include an explanation of the OSHA ethylene oxide standard as well as the health hazards of ethylene oxide.

The OSHA standard requires that accurate records be kept regarding employee exposures, personal monitoring data, equipment used, and methods (16,21). These records must be accessible to employees on request. Employees are required to retain employee medical records and exposure records for the period of employment plus 30 years.

Environmental Monitoring

Monitoring of employees' exposure to ethylene oxide is mandatory. Sampling frequencies are guided by the information in Table 104-3. Environmental monitoring must be performed initially to assess typical exposure concentrations for each work shift (7). Two types of monitoring are available: active sampling of air concentrations and personal passive dosimetry (7).

Active sampling includes charcoal tube adsorption, gas sampling bags, impingers, and detector tubes. Portable ethylene oxide gas analyzers also are available. Descriptions of sampling methods are included in the OSHA standards (16).

The purpose of environmental monitoring is to portray accurately typical workplace exposures, which requires sampling workers with the highest exposure risks (7). All monitoring—active and passive—must meet OSHA's accuracy requirements of ±25% at 1 ppm and ±35% below 1 ppm (7). Passive monitoring is performed by personal dosimetry badges worn by employees. These badges, which must be developed before results can be quantified, are designed to indicate the amount of ethylene oxide absorbed. Personal dosimeters have an advantage over active sampling in terms of cost and reduced complexity (22). However, conflicting data exist regarding the ability of passive dosimetry accurately to meet OSHA's regulations of a 1-ppm PEL and a 0.5-ppm action level (23). Passive dosimeters that meet OSHA's monitoring standards have been designed (23). Errors in passive dosimetry monitoring can occur owing to interference when the dosimeter is worn in direct sunlight or is worn for less than 8 hours (23). In addition, the capacity of the dosimeter can be exceeded by concentrations of ethylene oxide greater than 9.9 ppm (23).

REFERENCES

1. Landrigan PJ, Meinhardt TJ, Gordon J, et al. Ethylene oxide: an overview of toxicologic and epidemiologic research. *Am J Ind Med* 1984;6:103–115.
2. Hogstedt C, Rohlen O, Berndtsson BS, Axelson O, Ehrenberg L. A cohort study of mortality and cancer incidence in ethylene oxide production workers. *Br J Ind Med* 1979;36:276–280.
3. Sheikh K. Adverse health effects of ethylene oxide and occupational exposure limits. *Am J Ind Med* 1984;6:117–127.
4. Gross JA, Haas ML, Swift TR. Ethylene oxide neurotoxicity: report of four cases and review of the literature. *Neurology* 1979;29:978–983.
5. Leitman SF, Boltansky H, Alter HJ, Pearson FC, Kaliner MA. Allergic reactions in healthy plateletpheresis donors caused by sensitization to ethylene oxide gas. *N Engl J Med* 1986;315:1192–1196.
6. Austin SG, Sielken RL. Issues in assessing the carcinogenic hazards of ethylene oxide. *J Occup Med* 1988;30:236–245.
7. Ethylene oxide control technology: I. Occupational exposure. In: Healthcare Hazardous Materials Management, Plymouth Meeting, PA, vol 3, September 1990.
8. Taylor JS. Dermatologic hazards from ethylene oxide. *Cutis* 1977;19:189–192.
9. Shupack JL, Anderson SR, Romano SJ. Human skin reactions to ethylene oxide. *J Lab Clin Med* 1981;98:723–729.
10. Golberg L, Phil D. Neuropharmacologic and neurotoxic effects. In: Golberg L, Phil D, eds. *Hazard assessment of ethylene oxide*. Boca Raton, FL: CRC Press,1986.
11. Crystal HA, Schaumburg HH, Grober E, Fuld PA, Lipton RB. Cognitive impairment and sensory loss associated with chronic low-level ethylene oxide exposure. *Neurology* 1988;38:567–569.
12. Estrin WJ, Bowler RM, Lash A, Becker CE. Neurotoxicological evaluation of hospital sterilizer workers exposed to ethylene oxide. *J Toxicol Clin Toxicol* 1990;28:1–20.
13. Klees JE, Lash A, Bowler RM, Shore M, Becker CE. Neuropsychologic "impairment" in a cohort of hospital workers chronically exposed to ethylene oxide. *J Toxicol Clin Toxicol* 1990;28:21–28.
14. Morgan RW, Claxton KW, Divine BJ, Kaplan SD, Harris VB. Mortality among ethylene oxide workers. *J Occup Med* 1981;23:767–770.
15. Hogstedt C, Aringer L, Gustavsson A. Epidemiologic support for ethylene oxide as a cancer-causing agent. *JAMA* 1986;255:1575–1578.
16. Occupational Safety and Health Administration. Code of federal regulations. Occupational exposure to ethylene oxide: final standard—no. 29 *CFR*, 1910. *Federal Register* 1984 June 22;49:122.
17. Yager J, Hines C, Spear R. Exposure to ethylene oxide at work increases sister chromatid exchanges in human peripheral lymphocytes. *Science* 1983; 219:1221–1223.
18. Garry VF, Hozier J, Jacobs D, Wade RL, Gray DG. Ethylene oxide: evidence of human chromosomal effects. *Environ Mol Mutagen* 1979;1:375–382.
19. Pero RW, Widegren B, Hogstedt B, Mitelman F. *In vivo* and *in vitro* ethylene oxide exposure of human lymphocytes assessed by chemical stimulation of unscheduled DNA synthesis. *Mutat Res* 1981;83:271–289.
20. Hemminki K, Mutanen P, Saloniemi I, Niemi ML, Vainio H. Spontaneous abortions in hospital staff engaged in sterilizing instruments with chemical agents. *BMJ* 1982;285:1461–1463.
21. Occupational Safety and Health Administration. Code of federal regulations. Occupational exposure to ethylene oxide: final standard—29 *CFR*, 1910. *Federal Register* 1988 April 6;53:66.
22. Puskar MA, Hecker LH. Field validation of passive dosimeters for determination of employee exposures to ethylene oxide in hospital product sterilization facilities. *Am Ind Hyg Assoc J* 1989;50:30–36.
23. Puskar MA, Nowak JL, Hecker LH. Generation of ethylene oxide permissible exposure limit data with on-site sample analysis using the EO self-scan passive monitor. *Am Ind Hyg Assoc J* 1990;51:273–279.

CHAPTER 105
Aromatic Solvents

John B. Sullivan, Jr., and Mark D. Van Ert

Aromatic solvents are benzene derivatives with high vapor pressures and low boiling points that increase with increasing molecular weight. These solvents possess high vapor densities and are not very water soluble. Most of these compounds are used as starting chemicals or intermediate chemicals for synthesis of other organic compounds. Aromatic solvents are used also in myriad occupations and industries, in paints, lacquers manufacturing, resins, pharmaceuticals, printing, glues and adhesives, degreasing operations, electronics, and rubber manufacturing (1).

Commonly used aromatic compounds include toluene, benzene, xylene, styrene, ethylbenzene, monochlorobenzene (MCB), and trimethylbenzene (Fig. 105-1). Benzene is discussed in a separate chapter (see Chapter 59).

Most commercial aromatic solvents have a boiling point not much lower than 0°C or higher than 200°C (1). If the boiling point of a solvent is too high and the vapor pressure too low, separating the solvent from the material it is used to dissolve would be difficult. Therefore, most organic solvents are liquid at room temperature.

Aromatic solvents are characterized by nonpolarity and high lipid solubility. These solvents frequently are used in mixtures in occupational settings, such as combinations of toluene, benzene, styrene, ethylbenzene, trimethylbenzene, and xylene. Naphthalene, although an aromatic compound, is not a solvent; rather, it is a white, crystalline solid used as a repellent for moths, and it volatilizes easily.

Aromatic solvents are derivatives of coal and petroleum refining. When coal is heated in the absence of air, it is broken down into volatile compounds consisting of coal gas and coal tar. The residue of this process is termed *coke*.

The distillation of coal tar results in the production of aromatic compounds such as benzene, toluene, xylenes, phenols, cresols, and naphthalene. Aromatic compounds can also be produced by catalytic processes in which aliphatic hydrocarbons are employed at high temperatures and high pressures to dehydrogenate the compounds and form cyclic structures of the aromatic hydrocarbons.

FACTORS INVOLVED IN SOLVENT TOXICITY

Exposure to aromatic solvents occurs through contact with vapor or liquid, the main routes of absorption being pulmonary and dermal. The toxicity of a solvent relates to a combination of its physiochemical properties, inherent toxicity, metabolites, and clinical pharmacokinetics. For solvents, such as benzene and styrene, metabolites are the primary toxins. Toxicity factors can be summarized as follows:

- Toxic nature of parent compound
- Toxic nature of metabolites
- Target organs and target tissues
- Interaction with other solvents or drugs

Toluene

Ethylbenzene

Styrene

o-Xylene

m-Xylene

p-Xylene

Monochlorobenzene

1,2-Dichlorobenzene

1,3-Dichlorobenzene

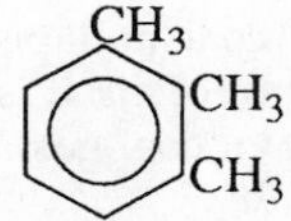

1,2,4-Trichlorobenzene

1,3,5-Trimethylbenzene

1,2,4-Trimethylbenzene

1,2,3-Trimethylbenzene

Figure 105-1. Common aromatic solvents.

- Influence of prior disease states
- Exposure (dose, duration, intensity)
- Solvent physiochemical characteristics (vapor pressure, vapor density, reactivity)
- Routes of exposure [pulmonary, dermal, gastrointestinal (GI)]

Solvent Vapor Pressure and Vapor Hazard Index

The vapor pressure of a solvent is an important health aspect that is directly related to its airborne concentration and, therefore, to its potential for exposure and toxicity. This concept is known as the *vapor hazard index* (VHI) of a solvent.

Vapor pressure is defined as the force per unit area exerted by molecules of a vapor that is in equilibrium with a liquid or solid (2). Vapor pressure is expressed in terms of millimeters of mercury in relation to atmospheric pressure (1 atm = 760 mm Hg) and directly relates to the concentration of solvent in the breathing zone of exposed individuals. The vapor pressure of a solvent obeys the same physical laws as do other gases: $P_v = nRt/V$, where P_v = vapor pressure (expressed as millimeters of mercury); n = moles; V = gas volume (expressed as cubic meters); R = gas constant (6.236×10^{-5}); and t = absolute gas temperature (in degrees Kelvin).

Rearrangement of this formula yields an equation that allows for calculation of the vapor concentration from the vapor pressure of a gas that is in an equilibrium state:

$$P_v = \frac{nRt}{V} = \frac{CRt}{MW} = x(\text{atm})(2 \times 10^{-6})$$

where C = concentration (expressed as millimeters per cubic meter); MW = molecular weight (expressed in daltons); x = concentration [expressed as parts per million (ppm)]; *atm* = 760 mm Hg.

The vapor hazard ratio of solvents can be compared by this method to help to determine the potential of human exposure. The formula expresses the vapor pressure in terms of an equilibrium state, or worst-case scenario, as would be achieved in a closed environment. Solvents or chemicals with the same threshold limit value (TLV) or permissible exposure limit (PEL) may present two distinctly different health hazards owing to their different vapor pressures. Such a relationship is expressed by the VHI of the individual chemicals. Two related examples of VHI follow:

Chemical A: TLV = 0.02 ppm
Vapor pressure = 0.00014 at 25°C
Chemical B: TLV = 0.02 ppm
Vapor pressure = 0.00001 at 25°C

Rearranging this equation allows for a calculation of the saturated vapor concentration in parts per million of a vapor in an equilibrium state (V_{peq}):

$$V_{peq} = P_v \times \frac{1 \times 10^6}{\text{atm}}$$

The equilibrium vapor pressure, as calculated using the preceding formula, can be used to calculate the VHI:

$$\text{VHI} = \frac{\text{Equilibrium vapor pressure (ppm)}}{\text{TLV (ppm)}}$$

The greater the VHI, the greater is the potential hazard for inhalation and dermal contact (1).

$$\text{Chemical A: } V_{peq} = \frac{(1.4 \times 10^{-4})(1 \times 10^6)}{760 \text{ mm Hg}} = 0.184 \text{ ppm}$$

$$\text{Chemical B: } V_{peq} = \frac{(1 \times 10^{-5})(1 \times 10^6)}{760 \text{ mm Hg}} = 0.0132 \text{ ppm}$$

$$\text{Chemical A: VHI} = \frac{0.184 \text{ ppm}}{0.02 \text{ ppm}} = 92$$

$$\text{Chemical B: VHI} = \frac{0.0132 \text{ ppm}}{0.02 \text{ ppm}} = 6.6$$

Chemical B would present less of a hazard than chemical A in terms of vapor exposure:

$$\text{VHI}\left(\frac{\text{chemical A}}{\text{chemical B}}\right) = \frac{92}{6.6} = \frac{13.9}{1}$$

Dose, Exposure, and Target Organ Toxicity

The predominant target organs for aromatic solvents are the nervous system, liver, kidneys, skin, lungs, and mucous membranes of the airways and eyes. Benzene's main target organ is the hematopoietic system. Target organ toxicity of solvents can be categorized as neurologic (peripheral, central, neurobehavioral); hepatic; renal; dermal (contact and allergic); pulmonary (acute and chronic bronchitis, bronchial hyperresponsiveness, airway irritation, and mucous membrane inflammation); upper airway (mucous membrane irritation, vocal cord irritation); and ocular toxicity (irritation).

Clinical effects of exposure depend on the inherent toxicity of the solvent, the exposure concentration, absorbed dose, length of exposure, toxic metabolites, preexisting medical conditions, and route of exposure. Exposure to multiple solvents is a common occupational hazard.

Owing to the vapor hazards of aromatic solvents, inhalation is the most common route of exposure. However, dermal absorption via contact with vapors or liquids can contribute to or cause toxicity. Chemicals that have the potential for dermal absorption or for dermal toxicity are labeled with a "skin" notation by the American Conference of Governmental Industrial Hygienists (ACGIH) (3).

TABLE 105-1. Summary of aromatic solvent toxicity

Acute exposure	Chronic exposure
Dizziness	Fatigue
Euphoria	Headache
Confusion	Nausea
Agitation	Neurobehavioral disturbances
Syncope	Cerebral atrophy
Cardiac dysrhythmias	Confusion
Coma	Dementia
Ocular irritation	Cognitive decline
Respiratory irritation	Memory loss
Headache	Cerebellar signs
Liver damage	Ataxia
Renal damage	Neuropsychological damage
	Liver damage
	Renal damage

Aromatic solvents vary with respect to skin penetration. Factors that increase skin penetration include injury, high moisture content, surface area of exposure, anatomic part, and duration of contact. Other important factors directly relating to increased absorbed dose of a solvent exposure are physical exercise and respiratory rate. Physical exercise and increased respirations will result in an increased absorbed dose of solvent vapors. Coingestion of ethanol inhibits the metabolism of some solvents and will result in higher blood levels. Coexposure to other solvents will result in competition for enzymatic sites and decrease metabolism of solvents. These factors influence the results of biological monitoring and toxicity.

Solvents may produce acute, reversible neurotoxic changes or permanent neuropathology, again depending on the solvent, dose, exposure time, and metabolism. Table 105-1 summarizes the acute and chronic effects of aromatic solvent exposure. Acute inhalational exposure to high airborne concentrations can produce dizziness, syncope, confusion, euphoria, respiratory irritation, and in some instances, coma (4,5). Acute and chronic exposure to toxic concentrations from inhalational solvent abuse may cause neurobehavioral disturbances, cerebral atrophy, cerebellar dysfunction, dementia, and permanent neuropsychological dysfunction. Such is the case with toluene (4,5).

Toxic neuropathy due to aromatic solvent exposure is confined primarily to the central nervous system (CNS). Only isolated case reports indicate the potential for peripheral neuropathy. The term *toxic encephalopathy* is used to describe permanent residual neurocognitive defects and neurologic impairment. Some limited evidence reveals that aromatic solvents also can cause peripheral neuropathy. However, occupational exposure is usually to a mixture of solvents and, therefore, relating clinical effects to a specific agent can be difficult.

Organic solvents tend to be lipophilic, thus favoring distribution to tissues high in lipid content, such as the brain and liver. In general, the more lipid solvents are metabolized to more polar metabolites, which reduces their ability to penetrate across biological membranes. Overall, solvent metabolism involves two phases by the cytochrome P-450–dependent monooxygenase system: The first phase consists of introduction of a polar group or unmasking of a polar group by oxidative, reductive, or hydrolytic reaction. The second phase consists of conjugation with glucuronic acid, sulfate, or glutathione. The liver is the main metabolic organ, but other sites of P-450 metabolism are the kidneys, lung, skin, olfactory epithelium, and nasal epithelium.

Excretion of unchanged solvent occurs mainly via the lungs. Excretion of metabolites occurs primarily in the urine. In some instances, volatile metabolites are exhaled by the lungs. More lipid solvents exhibit multiple phases of elimination: a rapid removal from the blood to lipid compartments and then a slow elimination phase from lipid storage sites.

DIAGNOSTIC APPROACH TO SOLVENT NEUROTOXICITY

Diagnosing a neurologic disease caused by solvent exposure requires obtaining a careful history inclusive of occupational and environmental exposures and performing a neurologic examination and tests to confirm the suspected diagnosis. The neurologic examination should note specific signs and symptoms related to mental status, motor tone and function, strength, sensory function, gait, posture, reflexes, cranial nerve functions, cognition, speech functions of the cortex, the basal ganglia, the midbrain, the brainstem, and the spinal cord. Aside from the usual clinical laboratory tests and biological markers of exposure, specific neurologic tests from which to select include neurophysiologic assessments [nerve conduction studies and electromyography (EMG)], electroencephalography (EEG), evoked potentials, neuroimaging, and neuropsychological tests. Neurologic tests reported to be abnormal in cases of solvent toxicity include the electroencephalograph, cerebral blood flow studies, magnetic resonance imaging (MRI) and computed tomography (CT) scans, nerve conduction velocities (NCVs) and EMG, evoked potentials, and neuropsychological tests (6–10). However, some published studies suffer from a lack of controls and fail to show an association between chronic low-level solvent exposure and neurotoxicity (11–14).

Neuropsychological Testing

Chronic occupational exposure to organic solvents has been reported in some studies to result in abnormal neuropsychological effects, referred to as the *solvent syndrome* (6–15). However, there is disagreement regarding the verification of this solvent syndrome (5,11,15–26). Studies have failed to demonstrate an association or dose-response relationship between chronic low-level exposure to organic solvents and a psychoorganic brain syndrome (11). Those studies that support a low-level exposure solvent-induced psychoorganic syndrome have been criticized for their lack of controls, multiple unaccounted-for environmental exposures, retrospective nature of the study, and lack of objective evidence of CNS neurologic damage (4). One controlled study of individuals with a diagnosis of toxic encephalopathy from chronic solvent exposure did not demonstrate, by CT scanning, any difference in cerebral atrophy between patients and controls (26).

However, most published studies of the solvent-induced psychoorganic syndrome have relied on neuropsychological testing, which is generally accepted as being more sensitive for detecting early behavioral dysfunction caused by CNS neurotoxins as compared to routine neurologic examinations, MRI, and CT scanning (27,28). Although experts widely accept that neuropsychological methods are sensitive indicators of brain dysfunction, many variables and confounding factors must be taken into account: cultural differences, premorbid status, prior disabilities, demographic variables, age, alcohol use, education, prior intellectual function, mood changes, personality, drug use and abuse, and head injury (27,28). These variables have a strong influence on the outcome of neuropsychological testing.

To be of value, neuropsychological studies must be performed by a qualified neuropsychologist experienced in testing patients with neurotoxic exposures. An appropriate testing battery must be used that is sufficiently sensitive and specific to detect the effects of neurologic toxins. Properly performed neuropsychological testing must characterize a patient's preexisting neurocognitive status and provide evidence of the presence of psychiatric disorders, depression, stress, and premorbid cognitive state.

Neuropsychological impairments secondary to toxic exposure may involve the following functional areas, which can be tested by appropriate methods (29): attention, function, visuospatial skills, learning, short-term memory, mood, fluency (verbal or visual), motor abilities, adjustment, and intelligence. Published studies linking low-level solvent exposure with abnormal neuropsychological test findings suggest that chronic low-level exposures in occupational settings are associated with cognitive changes, abnormal reaction times, short-term memory problems, and abnormal visuospatial functions. Verbal and nonverbal reasoning seem not to be affected (28). However, whereas most authorities agree that acute intoxication from high levels of organic solvents can cause toxic encephalopathy, dizziness, confusion, headache, CNS depression, lethargy, and incoordination, the effects of low-level chronic exposure remain controversial. Because of the continued controversy surrounding the psychoorganic syndrome and chronic solvent exposure, the World Health Organization proposed a categorization relating to the degree of impairment (Table 105-2) (4).

Solvent neurotoxicity must also be discerned from other neurologic diseases. For example, Alzheimer's disease is associated with decline in language abilities, visuospatial skills, and memory function (30). Patients with solvent-induced neurotoxicity may also demonstrate visuospatial difficulties and memory deficits. However, Alzheimer's disease is associated with language dysfunction, whereas solvent neurotoxicity is not. In addition, individuals with chronic neurotoxicity secondary to solvent exposure tend to remain the same or improve over time once the exposure has terminated. In contrast, patients with Alzheimer's disease generally will show neuropsychological decay over time (30). Solvent-toxic individuals may have problems with attention and tracking as well as visuospatial processing and short-term memory. This is consistent also with an Alzheimer's diagnosis. However, retention of language, writing, and reading skills is more clearly indicative of solvent toxicity than of Alzheimer's disease.

The intelligence quotient (IQ) of an individual can be affected after toxic exposure to a solvent and in Alzheimer's disease. However, with solvent exposure, IQ deterioration terminates after discontinuation of exposure, whereas in Alzheimer's disease, IQ deterioration can continue. Intact reading and writing abilities favor solvent-induced neurotoxicity. Progression of cognitive decline in the absence of exposure favors a diagnosis of dementia such as Alzheimer's disease. Once solvent exposure is terminated, cognitive function usually remains stable or improves in patients with solvent-induced neurotoxicity.

TABLE 105-2. World Health Organization solvent impairment categories

Type 1	Complaints of nonspecific symptoms only, which are reversible if exposure is terminated.
Type 2A	Sustained personality or mood change symptoms not reversible on discontinuation of exposure.
Type 2B	Intellectual function impairment with objective signs and evidence of impairment on neuropsychological tests. Possible presence of minor neurologic signs that are not reversible.
Type 3	Dementia and marked global deterioration in intellectual function and positive neurologic signs that are poorly reversible and nonprogressive once exposure ends.

Adapted from ref. 4, with permission.

Neurophysiologic Testing

EMG and nerve conduction studies are used to evaluate peripheral nerve functions. EMG is employed to assess motor function and the integrity of the motor neuron, its axon, and the muscle cells it supplies. Before EMG results become abnormal, denervation of the motor unit must occur (4,29). EMG is a sensitive tool for detecting ongoing or previous axonal degeneration.

NCVs test the integrity of nerve fibers, cell body, and axon and its myelin sheath and can localize areas of impaired function (axonal dysfunction, demyelination, myopathy, or nerve atrophy). NCVs are sensitive to nerve demyelination changes but are insensitive to quantifying axonopathies. NCVs may remain normal if only a few fibers continue to conduct at velocities (4). Both EMG and NCV results may be normal in the early phases of a toxic peripheral neuropathy.

ELECTROENCEPHALOGRAPHY

EEG provides real-time monitoring of the brain's electrophysiologic activity (4,29). Brain dysfunction may appear as an asymmetry of EEG patterns, changes in wave amplitude, frequencies, and wave patterns. Some toxic solvent exposures can cause the EEG results to become abnormal. Neurodegenerative diseases may first appear with a normal EEG outcome; then, as the disease progresses, abnormal EEG slowing occurs (29). However, EEG generally is not sufficiently specific for diagnosing neurotoxic diseases.

NEUROIMAGING

Neuroimaging techniques include CT and MRI as the two standard methods by which to image CNS anatomic structures. Other, less frequently used methods are single-photon emission computed tomography (SPECT), positron emission tomography (PET), and magnetic resonance spectroscopy.

CT and MRI have limited use in detecting neurotoxicity caused by solvents except in cases of high-dose exposure such as with intentional toluene inhalational abuse (4,29). CT and MRI of toluene abusers have revealed neuropathologic changes such as diffuse cerebral atrophy, cerebellar atrophy, brainstem atrophy, and loss of gray–white matter differentiation (4). However, in cases of low-level chronic occupational solvent exposure, CT has not proved capable of discerning healthy control subjects from individuals with symptoms (26).

SPECT scanning has been reported to have value in assessing neurotoxic effects of chemicals (31,32). Other researchers have reported no significant advantage of SPECT scanning in such cases (33). SPECT imaging reflects regional cerebral blood flow by measuring the uptake of a radiopharmaceutical (^{99m}Tc hexamethyl propyleneamine oxine) in blood and brain tissue. SPECT measures dynamic brain functioning by determining the metabolic process that removes radiolabeled tracers from blood. Thus, SPECT scanning remains a potential tool for assessing neurotoxicity but must be used and interpreted in light of other findings.

PET scanning also demonstrates cerebral function and elucidates CNS changes that are functional as opposed to anatomic. PET is expensive and requires specialized equipment. PET scanning may eventually become of diagnostic value in neurotoxic exposure diagnosis, but more studies of this method are required. PET tracers include ^{15}O-labeled water (for assessing cerebral blood flow), ^{18}F-fluorodeoxyglucose (for evaluating brain metabolism), and ^{18}F-fluorodopa (for assessing levels of dopamine receptor) (4).

EVOKED POTENTIALS

Evoked potentials are electrical cortical responses produced by the stimulation of specific afferent pathways and recorded through the scalp from the brain's surface. They are used to assess the integrity of CNS sensory pathways, and their use is limited in diagnosing neurotoxicity. Evoked potentials represent the integrity of electrical manifestations through multisynaptic pathway activity within the CNS and, thus, they can be used to screen the integrity of the synapses in the CNS (4,29). They include auditory evoked potentials, visual evoked potentials (VEPs), and somatosensory evoked potentials (SEPs). Currently, evoked potentials should be viewed as a limited screening tool for assessing the integrity of the receptor-to-cortex pathway.

VEPs examine the integrity of the optic system pathway from the optic nerve to the geniculate nuclei up to the calcarine cortex, following stimuli to the retina. Two forms exist: flash VEPs and pattern-shift VEPs. Each eye is tested separately. Normal latency is approximately 100 milliseconds (P100 peak).

Brainstem auditory evoked potentials are used to study neurodegenerative disease of the brainstem and demyelinating diseases such as multiple sclerosis. Noise stimuli are used to activate cranial nerve VIII pathways.

SEPs are assessed by stimulation of peripheral nerves, and findings are recorded over the sensory cortex via the dorsal column of the spinal cord to brainstem, thalamus, and cortex. Neurotoxins that affect peripheral nerves can cause these readings to be abnormal.

The use of evoked potentials as a diagnostic tool for neurotoxicity is limited, and results must be interpreted in light of other findings. Abnormal evoked potentials have been found in toluene-related toxic exposures involving inhalational abuse (34).

RESPIRATORY IRRITATION AND INFLAMMATORY EFFECTS OF AROMATIC SOLVENTS

The respiratory toxicity of solvents depends on the chemical and physical nature of the solvent, the concentration of the solvent inhaled, and the additive effects of solvents in mixtures. Respiratory toxicity is most apparent with high-level exposures. However, studies show that pulmonary injury is not limited to high-dose exposure but can occur at concentrations of multiple solvents below the U.S. Occupational Safety and Health Administration (OSHA) PELs (35).

Most solvents, including the aromatic solvents, are mucous membrane irritants and thus are irritants of the upper and lower respiratory tract. Tests of sensory irritation have demonstrated the irritant nature of toluene, xylene, ethylbenzene, and styrene (36,37). Studies performed in animals under controlled chamber conditions showed a qualitative correlation for eye, nose, and throat irritation experienced by humans from vapors of common solvents (36,37). However, these solvents were mixtures of aliphatic compounds and alcohols.

Both upper and lower respiratory symptoms have been reported in cases of individuals exposed to low-level volatile organic solvents. However, most case reports have included multiple solvents and thus have multiple confounding factors. Although it is generally accepted that high-level aromatic solvent exposure produces CNS effects and may also result in pulmonary toxicity, studies are showing that low-level exposures also can result in respiratory symptoms such as shortness of breath, cough, and chest tightness. Apparently, mixtures of volatile organic solvents tend to have additive effects.

In animal studies, the upper respiratory tract mucosae of rats showed inflammatory cell infiltration in the nasal cavity, trachea, and larynx when the rats were exposed to low concentrations of a mixture of paraffins, naphthenes, and alkyl aromatic hydrocarbons (38). Further low-level exposure of rats to xylene caused alterations in pulmonary membrane structures (39).

That both high-level and low-level exposure to aromatic solvents can cause bronchial hyperresponsiveness is documented in published case reports. Bronchial hyperresponsiveness is a reversible airway obstruction after physical, chemical, or pharmacologic stimuli. Its clinical presentation includes wheezing, cough, and shortness of breath on exercise or inhalation of cold air and irritants. Bronchial hyperresponsiveness may be present as a preexisting condition in individuals without respiratory symptomatology. Evidence points to an inflammatory process as the basis or underlying pathophysiologic mechanism of bronchial reactivity, which results in smooth-muscle contraction, airway edema, and stimulation of the nervous system, which in turn leads to symptoms (40).

Airway hyperresponsiveness as an acquired condition resulting from exposure to airborne irritants is substantiated by evidence. Bronchial reactivity has been defined as a 20% declination in the forced expiratory volume over 1 second (FEV_1). Some individuals have bronchial hyperresponsiveness yet can be asymptomatic and still have a 20% declination of their FEV_1 on methacholine challenge (40). Evidence for acquired airway responsiveness from irritant exposure comes from experimental studies, case reports, and epidemiologic studies (5).

Cellular changes described in bronchoalveolar lavage fluid from patients who demonstrate bronchial hyperresponsiveness include an increased number of desquamated epithelial cells, activated inflammatory cells, mast cells, and macrophages (41). Also, increased concentrations of inflammatory mediators are found in bronchoalveolar lavage fluid, indicating activation of these immune cells. Studies have shown that blood interleukin-8 production is increased in chemical workers with bronchitis symptoms (41). In these cases, bronchitis was diagnosed as productive cough after waking up, during smoking, or during the winter season. Chronic bronchitis was diagnosed if these complaints were present on most days for at least 3 months in the year for at least 2 successive years. The blood interleukin-8 level was significantly higher in workers with respiratory symptoms of the acute and chronic bronchitic variety as compared to workers without those symptoms. Once a person has developed reactive airways, exposure to a variety of unrelated airborne irritants may trigger symptoms (42–45). However, bronchial hyperresponsiveness is not the equivalent of reactive airways dysfunction syndrome (RADS). First described by Brooks et al. (46) in 1985, RADS is considered to be a subset of irritant-induced asthma. Since then, the American College of Chest Physicians has defined RADS as follows (47):

- A documented absence of preceding respiratory complaints
- Onset of symptoms after a single exposure incident or accident
- Exposure to a gas, smoke, fume, or vapor with irritant properties present in high concentrations
- Onset of symptoms within 24 hours after the exposure and persistence of symptoms for at least 3 months
- Symptoms simulating asthma
- Evidence of airflow obstruction on pulmonary function tests and presence of bronchial hyperresponsiveness
- Absence of other pulmonary disease

Evidence from case reports, human studies, and animal toxicologic studies indicates that low-level chronic exposure to respiratory irritants, including volatile organic solvents, can result in acquired bronchial hyperresponsiveness or hyperreactive airways (48). Experimental studies and case reports provide evidence that temporary increases in airway hyperresponsiveness occur after low-level irritant exposure and that persistent asthma can occur after episodes of higher-level irritant exposure. However, the results of epidemiologic studies are conflicting. Whereas population-based epidemiologic studies suggest that occupational solvent exposure can be associated with respiratory symptoms, impaired pulmonary function, and respiratory diseases, many of these studies have suffered from the lack of appropriate controls, which limits their applicability (5,35).

Most consistent information on the respiratory effects of solvents comes from acute high-dose exposures or from acute and chronic exposures to selected solvents. However, individuals exposed to low-level solvent vapors report higher rates of airway irritation, chest tightness, cough, and respiratory symptoms. One study performed on healthy adults in a chamber showed that toluene at a concentration of 100 ppm caused irritation of the eyes and nose but had no effect on pulmonary function (49).

Alkylbenzenes are irritants of the respiratory tract (50). In a controlled exposure study of a mixture of 22 common organic solvents, mucous membrane irritation was shown to occur in the upper airway in healthy subjects at total airborne concentrations of 5 mg per cubic meter (51). Further chamber studies investigated the effects of low-level solvent mixtures on FEV_1 and showed a decline in FEV_1 among subjects who had preexisting bronchial hyperreactivity at concentrations of 25 mg per cubic meter but found no influence on the FEV_1 at concentrations of 2.5 mg per cubic meter (48). Airborne concentrations of 25 mg per cubic meter can commonly be found in the occupational and work environments. Case studies and controlled human studies thus support the conclusion that volatile organic compounds at low-level exposure concentrations can act as bronchial irritants in the work or home environment.

A recent study suggests that long-term solvent exposure may be a cause of sleep apnea (52). Digital oximetry performed on solvent-exposed printers with neurobehavioral complaints who were also nonsmokers showed a significant occurrence of nocturnal oxygen desaturation as compared to unexposed controls. Airborne solvent concentrations did not violate TLVs (52). The clinical significance of this effect remains unknown.

Volatile organic solvents as a group are sensory irritants. The sensory irritation effects of alkylbenzenes, halogenated benzenes, and halogenated alkylbenzenes have been evaluated by investigating the reflexively induced decrease in respiratory rate in mice. It was found that the potencies of alkylbenzenes increase with increasing length of the alkyl chain (53). Studies have shown that exposure to a mixture equal to a total airborne load of 25 mg per cubic meter produces neutrophil influx into the nasal passages, indicating inflammation. The studies showed a statistically significant increase in inflammatory cells immediately after a 4-hour exposure to the volatile organic chemicals and 18 hours after the exposure (54). This 25-mg-per-cubic-meter total volatile organic chemical concentration is considered to be low level and representative of what is found in new homes, office buildings, and spaces with poor indoor air quality. These levels are below OSHA PELs of any one individual chemical found.

Solvents previously were not thought to be able to cause asthma or to act as pulmonary sensitizers. However, a variety of respiratory diseases caused by solvent exposures have been described in the medical literature. Reported postexposure respiratory outcomes have included both restrictive and obstructive processes, including asthma (50). Volatile organic solvents all have the potential to produce mucous membrane irritation. Chemical substances that are reactive and bind to tissues covalently cause irritation. Also, relatively nonreactive substances that bind to tissues physically and reversibly can cause irritation. Nonreactive-type volatile organic compounds predominate in low concentrations in many indoor contaminant situations (55).

Irritation reflects a stimulation of mucous membrane tissues, particularly in the upper airways. The nerves in the airways that mediate irritation also mediate mechanically and thermally induced irritation symptoms and sensations. An important property is that of temporal summation, whereby the longer a stimulus lasts, the longer will be the sensation of irritation.

Xylenes are an excellent example of an irritating volatile organic chemical. They also produce effects on the CNS and local irritating effects on the eye, nose, and throat (56). In one case report in a small community hospital, 15 people were affected 1 hour after 1 L of liquid xylene was discarded down a laboratory sink. Symptoms reported included headache, nausea, dizziness, and vomiting in addition to eye, nose, and throat irritation (57). Also, neurobehavioral symptoms were reported.

Evidence in case reports, clinical series, and animal toxicologic studies indicate that low levels of volatile organic solvent mixtures can produce upper airway and lower airway irritation and airway hyperreactivity or asthma. Adequate evidence exists that an inflammatory process in the airway wall is the underlying pathophysiologic mechanism of bronchial hyperresponsiveness and asthma. Medical evidence has accumulated that adequately demonstrates that reactive airways or asthma symptoms can be initiated by a low- or moderate-level exposure to an irritant substance (58). Generally, the clinical presentation is that of a patient who has no preceding respiratory complaints or asthma signs or symptoms (but in whom asymptomatic bronchial hyperresponsiveness or a preexisting bronchial hyperresponsiveness may be resident) who develops reactive airways or asthma for the first time after experiencing an irritant exposure that may last only a few minutes or hours, several days, or weeks (58). The irritant is generally in a vapor form but can take the form of particulates or fumes. The exposure levels causing these asthmalike symptoms need not be massive but can be moderate or low level. Respiratory symptoms can develop abruptly or evolve slowly over days or weeks. Initially, upper respiratory symptoms predominate, with eye, nose, and throat irritation and laryngeal symptoms. The individual may develop what seems to be an increased sensitivity to many and varied nonspecific irritants while removed from the exposure source (58). These manifestations have been termed *bronchial irritability* or *bronchial hyperresponsiveness* and include symptoms of coughing, choking, wheezing, and chest tightness occurring after many and varied nonspecific low-level irritant exposures (58).

In one study that examined in a workplace the effects of volatile organic compounds on pulmonary function tests, 42 patients with a history of industrial exposure to organic solvents and pulmonary symptomatology were investigated. Pulmonary function tests were performed, followed by methacholine challenge. Forty-two percent of the patients had significantly abnormal methacholine stimulation tests, whereas only 10% to 15% of these patients had abnormal initial screening spirometry (59). These data show that exposure to volatile organic solvents is associated with bronchial hyperreactivity that is not commonly detected by initial screening spirometry, and so methacholine challenge testing is required in individuals with unexplained respiratory symptomatology and a history of exposure to volatile organic solvents (59). Also, such mucosal irritation can disrupt vocal cord mechanisms (60).

A recent case series reported symptoms of respiratory irritation, breathing difficulties, headache, and nausea among a group of individuals exposed to a collective total volatile organic solvent load (61). In this study, the airborne concentrations of the solvents were well below OSHA PELs. The employee whose problems appeared most clearly to be related to the solvent exposure in the building was a 50-year-old woman who was experiencing persistent hoarseness and episodic shortness of breath and in whom new-onset asthma and new-onset vocal cord dysfunction (based on video laryngoscopy) were diagnosed. This woman was unable to reenter the building without exacerbation of her symptoms. She improved after months of asthma therapy and treatment aimed at vocal cord dysfunction and eventually returned to work.

Another study examined the effect of 32 different volatile organic solvents detected in the air of a printing shop, all of which were present in concentrations lower than regulatory standards. Workers exhibited signs and symptoms of eye, nose, throat, and airway irritation as well as neurobehavioral symptoms (62).

DERMAL ABSORPTION AND TOXICITY

Dermal absorption of alkylbenzenes is a potential route of toxicity. Dermal absorption of a solvent is related to such variables as concentration of the solvent; duration of exposure; the condition, thickness, and vascularity of the skin; and the surface area exposed (63,64). Injury, burn, or rashes will increase solvent absorption. Another important variable that dictates absorption of volatile organic chemicals is the hydration status of the skin. The more hydrated the skin is, as from perspiration or immersion in water, the more chemical absorption is facilitated across the dermal barrier. In addition, increased skin temperature will enhance skin absorption, owing to increased blood flow through the skin.

Absorption variabilities depend also on the anatomic location. The palms of the hands and soles of the feet, for instance, present a dermal barrier to absorption as compared to other parts of the body such as the scalp, neck, or abdomen and scrotal area. Studies have shown that combinations of solvents or multiple solvents in aqueous media have a greater chance of being more readily absorbed than does a pure solvent (59).

Dermal absorption can represent a significant exposure route for some organic solvents and may represent from 30% to 90% of the total daily intake of organic solvents from aqueous media. The absorption of toluene, styrene, xylene, and ethylbenzene across human skin has been studied (Table 105-3) (63,64).

The absorption of toluene across the skin is slow and, in solution, was found to be proportional to the concentration of toluene that came in contact with the skin (63,65). The dermal absorption rate of liquid toluene was 14 to 23 mg per square centimeter per hour in subjects studied. Ethylbenzene demonstrated similar dermal absorption rates depending on the concentration that came in contact with the skin (64). The dermal absorption of liquid styrene was found to be 9 to 15 mg per square centimeter per hour and was linear to the concentration of styrene. The rate of absorption of liquid xylene ranged from 4 to 10 mg per square centimeter per hour.

BIOLOGICAL EXPOSURE INDICES

Biological exposure indices (BEIs) serve as a reference intended to evaluate potential health hazards of chemicals. They represent the level of a metabolite likely to be found in the urine or

TABLE 105-3. Dermal absorption of aromatic solvents

Solvent	Rate	Reference
Toluene (liquid)	14–23 mg/cm^2/h	(63)
Xylene (liquid)	4.5–9.6 mg/cm^2/h	(63)
Xylene (liquid, hand)	2 µg/cm^2/min	(143)
Styrene (liquid)	9–15 mg/cm^2/h	(63)
Styrene (liquid, hand)	0.06 mg/cm^2/h	(165)
Aqueous styrene solution	40–180 µg/cm^2/h	—
Ethylbenzene (liquid, hand)	22–33 mg/cm^2/h	(64)
Aqueous ethylbenzene	118–215 µg/cm^2/h	—

TABLE 105-4. Aromatic solvent biological exposure indices

Solvent	Urine	Blood	Time	BEI
Toluene	Hippuric acid		End of shift	2.5 g/g creatinine
		Toluene	End of shift	1 mg/L
Styrene	Mandelic acid		End of shift	800 mg/g creatinine
			Prior to next shift	300 mg/g creatinine
	Phenylglyoxylic acid		End of shift	240 mg/g
			Prior to next shift	100 mg/g
		Styrene	End of shift	0.55 mg/L
			Prior to next shift	0.02 mg/L
Xylene	Methyl hippuric acids		End of shift	1.5 g/g creatinine
Ethylbenzene	Mandelic acid		End of shift at end of work week	1.5 g/g creatinine

BEI, biological exposure index.

blood of a healthy worker exposed to chemicals to the same extent as an inhalational TLV exposure. BEIs do not represent a clear distinction between hazardous and nonhazardous exposures. They are influenced by biological variability of individuals. BEIs apply to 8-hour exposure, 6 days per week, and should not be used to determine the presence of adverse effects or for diagnosing an occupational exposure illness.

In some cases, exposure to aromatic organic solvents can be verified by detection of metabolic products in urine or blood (Table 105-4). Coexposure to ethanol or other solvents can decrease the urinary metabolite excretion and increase the blood levels of solvents. Thus, these factors must be considered in biological monitoring interpretation. Physical activity also influences excretion of metabolites by increasing vapor absorption.

TOLUENE

Toluene is an alkylbenzene derived from crude oil and coal tar during petroleum refining. It is formed by attaching one methyl group to benzene (see Fig. 105-1). Toluene is a common component of gasoline, adhesives, paints, inks, and solvents.

Physiochemical Properties

Toluene (methylbenzene) has a molecular formula of $C_6H_5CH_3$ and a molecular weight of 92.15 D. It has a sweet odor and is flammable. The boiling point of toluene is 110.6°C, and its vapor pressure is 22 mm Hg at 20°C. It autoignites at 480°C. Toluene's odor threshold in air is 8 ppm (Table 105-5).

TABLE 105-5. Physiochemical properties of toluene

Synonyms	Methylbenzene, phenylmethane
Molecular formula	$C_6H_5CH_3$
Molecular weight	92.15 D
Physical state	Colorless liquid
Boiling point	110.6°C
Density (20°C)	0.8669 g/L
Odor	Sweet
Odor threshold	
In air	8 ppm
In water	0.04–1.00 ppm
Vapor pressure (25°C)	28.4 mm Hg
Autoignition	480°C
Conversion factor	1 ppm = 3.75 mg/m^3
Explosive limits	
Lower limit	1.3%
Upper limit	7%

Sources, Production, and Uses

Approximately 10% to 11% of the toluene produced in the United States is isolated as toluene, with the remaining 90% being used to formulate gasoline (66). Nonisolated toluene is employed in a mixture with benzene and xylene (BTX) and is added to gasoline to improve octane rating. Isolated toluene is used in solvents, cleaning agents, paints, adhesives, inks, and other commercial chemical products. Toluene also finds use as a starter chemical for the synthesis of such other organic chemicals as urethanes, polyurethane foams, inks, and trinitrotoluene.

Toluene is regulated by the Resource Conservation and Recovery Act as a hazardous waste. Industrial wastes that contain solvents may not be disposed of on land if the extract of this waste contains more than 0.33 mg per L of toluene (66). Also, wastewater containing greater than 1.12 mg per L of toluene may not be land disposed (40 *CFR* 268.41).

Human exposure to toluene occurs from inhalation during occupational use, airborne levels in the home, inhalational abuse of paints containing toluene, and from other sources of environmental release. Toluene is a common indoor air contaminant that averages approximately 30 µg per cubic meter of air (66).

The largest exposure source of toluene is in the production and use of gasoline, which contains 5% to 7% toluene by weight. Large amounts of toluene are introduced into the environment yearly through the use of gasoline and through its production and petroleum refinement processes.

Other environmental sources of toluene are the disposal of solvents in home wastewater, industrial discharges, land disposal of solvents, petroleum wastes, and tobacco smoking. Toluene can volatilize from solvent mixtures, paints, and other products used in the home and occupational settings. Ambient air concentrations of toluene vary in their ranges depending on location (Table 105-6). The main source of toluene in the atmosphere is the use of gasoline.

The presence of toluene in water supplies is generally less than 3 µg per L (66). Toluene commonly contaminates both water and soil in the vicinity of waste sites or chemical and industrial sources that use or produce toluene. Concentrations in the water of such sites range between 7 and 20 µg per L, and concentrations in soil may approximate 70 µg per kg (66). Toluene released into water rapidly volatilizes into the air.

Environmental Fate and Transport

Toluene tends to vaporize into the atmosphere from surface water or soil. After toluene is released into soil, volatilization of more than 90% of the toluene released usually occurs within 24 hours, depending on the environmental circumstances (e.g., tem-

TABLE 105-6. Median toluene levels in ambient air

Air sampled	No. of samples	Daily mean (ppb)	Concentration (μg/m³)
Remote	225	0.049	0.18
Rural	248	0.35	1.3
Suburban	958	0.195	0.731
Urban	2,519	2.883	10.81
Indoor	101	8.4	31.5
Workplace	80	0.865	3.24

From ref. 66, with permisison.

perature and humidity) and the type of soil (67). Toluene is soluble in water and can be transported from soil by water runoff, depending on the soil's organic content, as toluene has a higher affinity for soil with an excess of organic matter and is more easily released from soils that have low organic matter content.

Toluene can bioaccumulate in aquatic organisms owing to its lipophilic properties. However, an organism's metabolism limits toluene's ability to bioaccumulate. The highest toluene levels are found in organisms that have a limited ability to metabolize (e.g., crabs) (66). Biodegradation is rapid in both the soil and the atmosphere. Atmospheric toluene is degraded to cresol and benzaldehyde. The primary degradation process in the atmosphere is a reaction with hydroxyl radicals. The atmospheric half-life of toluene is approximately 13 hours (68).

Owing to the miscibility of toluene with water, the rate of aqueous biodegradation is somewhat slower than atmospheric biodegradation. Biodegradation in water occurs mainly through the action of microorganisms; toluene's half-life in this setting ranges between 13 and 54 days. The presence of sulfate enhances aqueous toluene biodegradation (66). Soil biodegradation of toluene by bacteria is mainly by *Pseudomonas* and *Achromobacter* species in two phases: The first phase degrades to benzoic acid, whereas the second phase cleaves the aromatic ring to produce Krebs cycle intermediates.

Exposure Sources

Human exposure to toluene occurs mainly from inhalation. Calculations show that given an average concentration of toluene of 32 μg per m³ in the indoor air of homes and an inhalation rate of air at 20 m³ per day, a person can absorb 320 μg per day if only 50% of the inhaled toluene is absorbed (66). Tobacco smoke contributes 1,000 μg of toluene or more per day to the indoor environment.

The OSHA has set a PEL of 200 ppm as a time-weighted average (TWA) for toluene in the work environment. This PEL was recently increased from 100 ppm after a legal decision by the U.S. Supreme Court.

Toluene concentrations found in the indoor air of houses are attributable to volatilization of toluene from paints, solvents, glues, adhesives, environmental tobacco smoke, and other materials used within the home environment. Tobacco smoke is a significant source of toluene within the home environment, as approximately 80 to 100 μg of toluene is released per smoked cigarette.

The National Academy of Sciences has developed a methodology by which to calculate acceptable concentrations of solvents in drinking water. This methodology was incorporated into the U.S. Environmental Protection Agency's (EPA's) suggested no-adverse-response levels. These levels are the highest concentrations of a chemical that produce no observed adverse effect from chronic dosing in animals or humans. The figures are divided by a safety factor to obtain what is termed an *acceptable daily intake.* To calculate the acceptable concentration of a chemical in water, the acceptable daily intake is divided by the volume of water consumed by the average person, either adult or child. The EPA has reported concentrations of toluene in surface water sources ranging from 1 to 2,000 μg per L (66). The daily intake of toluene from drinking water generally is quite small and would be a negligible source of toluene absorption in most cases. Although drinking water contamination by toluene is generally less than 0.1 μg per L, EPA surveys have found levels exceeding 0.1 μg per L. Assuming the ingestion of 2 L of water per day, water intake would contribute a total daily dose of 0.3 to 0.5 μg of toluene (66).

Exposures to toluene also could occur near waste sites or from contaminated water or soil at hazardous-waste sites. Calculating the human exposure to toluene secondary to such waste sites depends on the pathways of migration into air, water, and soil and the human intake of these materials. In situations such as this, exposure occurs primarily via the inhalational and dermal absorption routes.

Absorption, Metabolism, and Excretion

In humans, toluene is absorbed from the respiratory tract and GI tract and through the skin. Owing to the lipophilic nature of this compound, the concentration in lipid tissues can be very high. The metabolism of toluene is depicted in Figure 105-2. Toluene's metabolic products are cresol (less than 1%) and the intermediate metabolite, benzaldehyde. Benzaldehyde then is metabolized to benzoic acid, which is conjugated with glycine to form hippuric acid (69–73). In humans, up to 75% of inhaled toluene is metabolized to hippuric acid and excreted in the urine within 12 hours

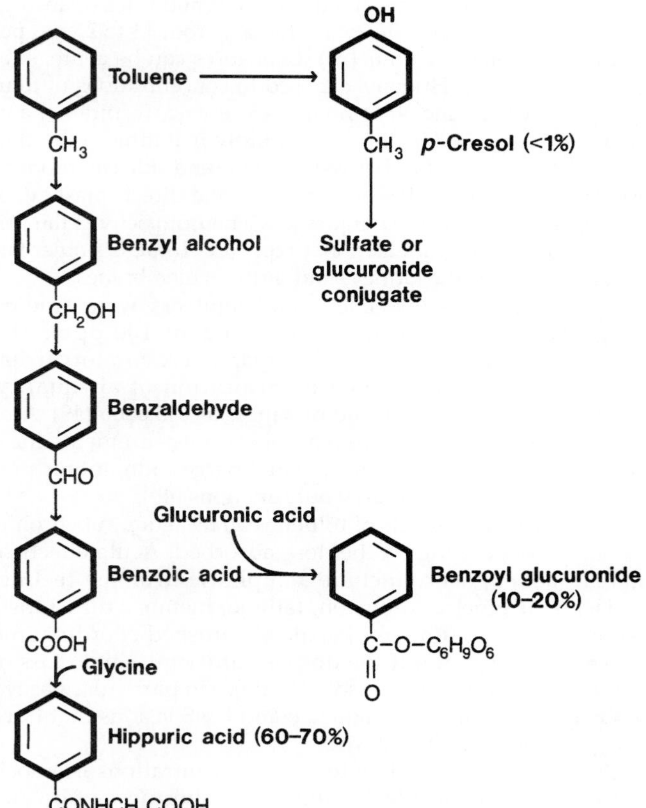

Figure 105-2. Metabolism of toluene in humans.

TABLE 105-7. Toluene health effects

Acute	Brainstem atrophy
CNS depression	Optic neuropathy
Coma	Decreased visual acuity
Agitation	Severe cognitive impairment
Delirium	Oculomotor abnormalities
Euphoria	Corticospinal tract dysfunction
Chronic	Deafness
Permanent CNS impairment	Hyposmia
Tremors	CNS demyelination
Ataxia	Neurobehavioral abnormalities
Cerebral atrophy	Renal tubular acidosis
Cerebellar atrophy	

CNS, central nervous system.

of exposure. The remainder of the toluene is excreted unchanged, with a small percentage being excreted as a sulfate or glucuronide of cresol. The metabolism and excretion of toluene are rapid, occurring within 12 hours of exposure. The half-life of toluene in adipose tissue of humans has ranged from 0.5 to 3 days.

Dermal absorption of toluene ranges from 14 to 23 mg per square centimeter per hour (74) (see Table 105-3). Absorbed toluene is quickly distributed to lipid-containing, highly vascular tissues: the CNS (particularly white matter), bone marrow, liver, kidneys, and nervous tissues.

Clinical Toxicology

Human toxicity from toluene exposure occurs primarily by the inhalational and dermal routes, although ingestion is another absorption route (Table 105-7) (75). Toluene is well absorbed by the lungs (76). It also is absorbed dermally, and rates of absorption have been studied and found to vary from 14 to 23 mg per square centimeter per hour (76). Exposures can be acute, subchronic, or chronic. Humans exposed to concentrations of toluene of between 200 and 800 ppm may experience respiratory and ocular irritation (76,77). Toluene is mildly irritating to the skin and eyes. Chronic contact between toluene and skin can produce irritation in animal models and humans, and direct splashing of the eyes may cause corneal injury. CNS neurotoxicity is the primary concern in toxic inhalational exposure. Toluene's other target organs include the kidneys and mucous membranes.

Controlled exposure effects on volunteers were studied using toluene concentrations of 40, 60, or 100 ppm. The exposed individuals experienced ocular and respiratory irritation along with a perceived deterioration of air quality, enhanced odor, headache, and dizziness at 100 ppm (49). Also at exposures of 100 ppm, psychological measurements indicated decrements in vigilance, visual perception, motor performance, and ability to carry out functions (49).

The toxic health effects of toluene can be acute, subchronic, or chronic, depending on the dose absorbed. Acute effects of inhalational exposure include a euphoric drunken feeling, headache, dizziness, confusion, fatigue, memory difficulties, disturbed equilibrium and balance, disturbed coordination, nausea, vomiting, and if the dose is sufficiently high, loss of consciousness. Inhalational solvent abuse in particular has led to permanent neurologic sequelae and CNS lesions that have been described on CT and MRI.

Chronic exposure to low toluene concentrations is associated with fatigue, headache, dizziness, shortness of breath, cough, throat irritation, nausea, and other constitutional symptoms. Disturbance of vestibuloocular responses has been demonstrated in subjects exposed to concentrations of toluene ranging from 103 to 140 ppm for more than 2 hours while doing light work (78). Color vision has also been shown to be impaired by occupational exposure to toluene (79).

Because of the accumulation of toluene in the CNS's anatomic areas, symptoms can last hours beyond an exposure. Such impairments may be cognitive or involve coordination, motor control, intention tremor, and gait disturbances. Common features in chronic toluene sniffers include euphoria, hallucinations, coma, ataxia, convulsions, cognitive impairment, and diplopia (80).

NEUROTOXICITY

Acute inhalational exposure to high concentrations of toluene vapor causes CNS depression, syncope, euphoria, delusions, acute excitation, and dizziness. Chronic exposure to high toluene vapor concentrations can result in permanent neuropsychological and CNS damage. Severe and persistent neurotoxicity can be a result of chronic toluene inhalation and chronic toluene abuse. Optic neuropathy, hearing loss, cerebellar ataxia, and cognitive dysfunction have all been described. Neuroimaging studies show that CNS white matter changes due to toluene toxicity appear to be irreversible.

Ataxia, tremors, visual impairment, diffuse cerebral atrophy, cerebellar atrophy, and brainstem atrophy occurred after intentional inhalational toluene abuse (81). Decreased vision and ataxia have been described in individuals chronically inhaling toluene-containing solvents (82). Optic neuropathy is manifest as decreased visual acuity but normal pupillary reactions along with associated cerebellar signs. Improvement in vision has occurred after discontinuation of toluene exposure. Rosenberg et al. (81) reported neurotoxicity in chronic toluene abusers that was characterized by severe cognitive impairment, cerebellar ataxia, corticospinal tract dysfunction, oculomotor abnormalities, tremor, deafness, and hyposmia. MRI of the CNS in toluene vapor abusers has demonstrated multifocal CNS involvement and diffuse CNS demyelination (83). The clinical presentation of these individuals included neurobehavioral, cerebellar, brainstem, and pyramidal tract abnormalities. Autopsy findings in those who have died from toluene inhalation revealed diffuse myelin pallor in the deep white matter of the cerebral hemispheres and the cerebellum. In these autopsies, diffuse demyelination of the subcortical white matter and axonopathy of the peripheral and central nervous systems were demonstrated (81).

A strong correlation exists between the concentrations of toluene in alveolar air and concentrations in the blood, so that inhalational exposure to toluene can result in rapid transfer across the alveolar capillary membrane and into the blood. In humans, toluene is distributed between plasma and red cells at a 1 to 1 ratio (84). The penetration of the red cell by toluene allows more of this compound to be transported to target organ sites, including the CNS. Toluene has a predilection to concentrate in lipid tissues. Autoradiographic studies in animals demonstrate that after inhalation of toluene, high levels are found in adipose tissue, bone marrow, nerves, spinal cord, brain white matter, and kidneys, and radioactivity was observed at lower levels in the blood, kidney, and liver (85).

The systemic and anatomic distribution of toluene, particularly in the CNS, has been studied (86). In rats, labeled toluene was detected in all brain regions and in the blood and liver. Maximum concentrations were obtained 10 minutes after inhalation, the greatest concentration being found in the medulla and pons, followed (in descending order) by the midbrain, cerebellum, thalamus, frontal cortex, hippocampus, caudate, and hypothalamus (86). The medulla, pons, and midbrain had the highest concentration of toluene.

In the human brain, toluene has a greater affinity for the lipid-rich areas of the white matter (e.g., brainstem) than for the gray matter. In autopsies, the hippocampus and cerebellum had lower brain-to-blood toluene ratios than did the spinal cord, midbrain, medulla oblongata, and pons (87).

Toluene concentrations in individual brain regions are eliminated in an exponential manner, such that almost no toluene remains detectable at the end of 4 hours. Toluene appears to have an affinity for the brainstem regions, medulla, and pons region owing to their high lipid content and regional blood flow differences. Of interest, toluene metabolites have not been detected in the brain (81,82,84–87). Such results correlated to clinical studies indicate that low-level exposure that results in neurologic symptoms such as dizziness, incoordination, and other CNS effects does so because of the rapid toluene buildup in the specific anatomic CNS regions of the brain, with levels reaching their maximum within 10 minutes after inhalational exposure.

Other neurologic findings that have been permanent or, in some cases, partially reversible in inhalational toluene abusers include cerebellar ataxia, intention tremor, ocular dysmetria, pyramidal tract dysfunction, and cognitive impairment. The anatomic regional distributions of toluene help to explain these clinical manifestations.

Organ concentrations of toluene in the case of a human who abused the compound by inhaling it have been described (Table 105-8) (87). The mean ratios of the brain region–to–blood toluene concentration were highest in the brainstem region in areas such as the pons and medulla oblongata. These were followed by the midbrain, thalamus, caudate, putamen, hypothalamus, and cerebellum. The lowest ranges were in the hippocampus and cerebral cortex. Because white matter is enriched with myelin and, therefore, contains more lipid than does gray matter, more toluene concentrates in white matter rather than gray matter. Cerebral cortex and hippocampal areas, which are composed of gray matter, demonstrate the lowest concentrations of toluene (87). Thus toluene, once it passes the blood–brain barrier, is distributed according to the lipid content in the CNS anatomic regions. In other human autopsy cases, toluene concentrations have been documented in the various tissues and fluids (Table 105-9) (88).

TABLE 105-8. Regional brain distribution of toluene in a human autopsy case

Sample	Toluene concentration (µg/g)	Ratio (brain–blood)
Brain region		
Cerebral cortex	8.18	1.76
Hippocampus	6.86	1.47
Caudate-putamen	8.71	1.87
Thalamus	8.93	1.91
Hypothalamus	9.51	2.04
Corpus callosum	12.40	2.66
Midbrain	10.78	2.31
Pons	10.20	2.18
Medulla oblongata	10.42	2.23
Cerebellum	7.03	1.51
Cervical spinal cord	11.00	2.35
Blood		
Femoral vein	4.61	—
Thoracic cavity	4.67	—

Adapted from ref. 87, with permission.

TABLE 105-9. Toluene concentrations in various fluids and tissues of human death case

Samples	Concentration (µg/g)
Blood	27.6
Heart	62.6
Liver	433.5
Lung	27.4
Kidney	23.0
Brain	85.3
Spleen	30.0
Pancreas	88.2
Skeletal muscle	27.2
Cerebrospinal fluid	11.1
Fat	12.2
Small gastric content	38.2
Stomach content	1,071.5
Urine	2.1

Adapted from ref. 88, with permission.

NEUROIMAGING AND ELECTROPHYSIOLOGIC PATHOLOGY OF TOLUENE TOXICITY

MRI in toluene abusers reveals diffuse cerebellar atrophy, cerebral atrophy, and atrophy of the brainstem, with decreased differentiation between gray and white matter and increased periventricular white matter signal intensity on T2-weighted images (34). Toluene abuse also is associated with cerebellar and cerebral atrophy on CT scans. Other radiologic findings on CT scans include widening of the cerebellar and cerebral sulci and basal cisterns and enlargement of the ventricular system. Neurologic lesions on MRI and CT scanning correlate with impairments on psychological tests in toluene abusers.

Neuropathologic changes correlated with MRI or CT scanning in toluene abuse patients include diffuse cerebral demyelination, diffuse cerebellar demyelination, demyelination of subcortical white matter, degeneration and gliosis of ascending and descending long fiber tracts and nerves of the corpus callosum, and atrophy of the cerebrum, cerebellum, and corpus callosum (89). Necropsy showed myelin pallor in deep periventricular white matter, with axonal and neuronal loss combined with demyelination. EEG abnormalities are reported in some cases (90).

Individuals exposed to long-term low concentrations of toluene as compared to controls showed abnormal VEPs (90). Toluene exposure was determined in this study by measuring toluene in blood and hippuric acid and *o*-cresol levels in urine.

CARDIOTOXICITY

Cardiotoxicity (e.g., cardiac dysrhythmias), as is seen in toxic exposures to such other solvents as the chlorinated solvents, is not commonly observed in human exposures to toluene. However, animal studies involving chronic dosing of toluene intraperitoneally and subcutaneously have demonstrated atrial fibrillation and ventricular ectopy (75).

HEMATOTOXICITY

A decreased leukocyte count has been observed in dogs exposed acutely to 700 ppm of toluene (75). This and other hematologic effects (e.g., thrombocytopenia) have been observed in other animal studies after the animals' exposure to toluene. A report from the National Toxicology Program in 1989 stated that exposure to toluene concentrations of up to 1,200 ppm for 2 years or less had no hematopoietic systemic effects on mice or rats (75). Human occupational exposure studies also have not demonstrated hematologic effects (77). Previous investigations linking toluene to hematotoxicity failed to account for coexposures to other solvents.

HEPATOTOXICITY

In most studies of human exposure to toluene, hepatic damage has not been observed (77,91,92). Likewise, in animal studies conducted by the National Toxicology Program, toluene was not observed to be hepatotoxic; the studies were conducted in mice over a 2-year period, and the mice were exposed to toluene doses of 1,200 ppm (75). Nonetheless, some clinical reports of acute reversible liver damage after inhalational abuse of toluene have been published (75,92–94). Other cases of single-dose, massive exposure have resulted in coma but no demonstrated liver injury.

Occupational studies of exposed workers have failed to demonstrate a consistent pattern of liver injury or hepatic enzyme elevation (75,91–93). In most occupational studies, other solvents are involved and present a confounding factor.

Occupational studies of painters exposed to a wide variety of solvents, including toluene, have demonstrated elevation of hepatic enzymes (94). Biopsies revealed liver histopathologic findings of steatosis and enlarged portal tracts with fibrosis and necrosis (94).

RENAL TOXICITY

Toluene can cause nephrotoxicity in two forms: acute renal failure after massive ingestions and distal renal tubular acidosis (95–100). Clinical reports state that excess proteinuria, abnormal liver function test results, interstitial nephritis, and glomerulonephritis have also been related to toluene exposure (95–100). Nephrotoxic effects that have been documented in chronic toluene abusers include hematuria, proteinuria, and type 1 renal tubular acidosis (92,93,101–105). In contrast, animal studies have been conflicting: In some studies, renal toxicity has been observed, whereas in others, it has not.

Workers exposed to more than 100 ppm of toluene for 6.5 hours demonstrated no significant increase in urinary excretion of β_2-microglobulin, a sensitive indicator of distal renal tubular damage. Other workers exposed to toluene levels of 80 to 107 ppm as well as other solvents did not exhibit increased urinary excretion of β_2-microglobulin (105).

Chronic toluene inhalational abuse can result in a normal anion gap metabolic acidosis with hypokalemia, hypophosphatemia, and hyperchloremia. This type of acidosis was first described in association with glue sniffing and is termed *type I renal tubular acidosis* (102). Renal tubular acidosis is a derangement in the capacity of distal renal tubules to maintain a hydrogen ion gradient and usually is reversible within a few days once exposure to toluene ceases, although reversal of this disorder may require several weeks (103). Treatment ranges from observation to administration of sodium bicarbonate and potassium, depending on the severity of the acidemia and electrolyte loss (103). Patients with metabolic acidosis after toluene inhalational abuse have also exhibited associated hypokalemic muscular weakness and paralysis with neuropsychiatric manifestations (106).

TERATOGENICITY, MUTAGENICITY, AND REPRODUCTIVE EFFECTS

Animal studies have shown developmental effects secondary to toluene exposure (107–109). Developmental effects have been demonstrated also in pregnant women exposed occupationally to solvents, including toluene, and in pregnant women as a result of solvent abuse (109). However, determining whether the toluene was actually causative is difficult, because these women were exposed to multiple solvents as well as to drugs and medications.

Children with microcephaly, minor craniofacial and limb anomalies, CNS defects, attention disorders, developmental delay, learning disorders, and language deficits were born to mothers who abused toluene by inhalation during pregnancy (108,109). Whether these congenital defects and conditions are secondary to toluene abuse alone remains unclear. However, exposure to organic solvents in general may have some embryotoxic effect. The term *fetal solvent syndrome* has been applied to such conditions.

Reproductive effects associated with toluene exposure have included an increased spontaneous abortion rate among women exposed to an average of 88 ppm of toluene (110), changes in gonadotropic hormone levels, and decreased levels of luteinizing hormone, follicle-stimulating hormone, and testosterone after exposures to increasing levels of toluene (from 8 to 111 ppm) (111,112).

Toluene has an adverse effect on the developing fetus in animal studies. Neonates born to women who were chronic inhalational abusers of toluene have exhibited renal tubular acidosis at birth that resolved within a few days (94,113). Increased risks of CNS defects, anomalies, and developmental delays are suggested in some studies, but these studies have been retrospective and were compromised by multiple confounding factors (113,114).

Studies examining the incidence of sister chromatid exchange frequencies and chromosomal aberrations in workers occupationally exposed to toluene have been reported (115–117). These studies indicated an increased frequency of sister chromatid exchanges. However, the relevance of these findings is unclear, as workers in the studies experienced multiple other chemical exposures.

CARCINOGENICITY

Toluene is considered to be noncarcinogenic, as no human epidemiologic studies indicate that toluene exposure increases the risk of carcinogenesis. Animal studies also have not demonstrated carcinogenic effects of toluene. Retrospective mortality studies of humans occupationally exposed to toluene have included exposures to other chemicals.

IMMUNOTOXICITY

No human data exist to indicate that toluene is an immunotoxicant. Animal studies involving mice exposed to toluene in drinking water for 28 days (105 ng of toluene per kg of body weight per day) showed a decrease in thymus weights, mixed lymphocyte culture response, antibody plaque-forming cell response, mitogen-stimulated lymphocyte proliferation, and presence of interleukin-2 (118).

Biological Monitoring

Hippuric acid is used as a biological marker for occupational exposure to toluene (see Table 105-4). Minor toluene metabolites are *o*-cresol, *p*-cresol, and phenol. The minor metabolites are conjugated with either sulfate or glucuronic acid and are excreted in the urine (70–73).

Individual variations with respect to metabolism of toluene and the correlation of occupational exposure to toluene and urinary excretion of hippuric acid and cresol metabolites can occur, especially if there is coexposure to other solvents or ethanol (72,119). Ethnic variations in toluene metabolism also are seen (119). Owing to this variability of metabolism among individuals, the biological monitoring of hippuric acid and other metabolite excretions is merely a qualitative indication of exposure and not a quantitative indication of toluene toxicity.

Studies performed in occupational settings have indicated that both hippuric acid and *o*-cresol excretion are related to the environmental concentration of toluene and workers' exposure, if excretion is corrected for creatinine and urine specific gravity (77). The correlation coefficient was stronger for hippuric acid (0.88 and 0.84) than it was for *o*-cresol (0.63 to 0.62) (69).

The urinary excretion of hippuric acid is a reliable biological indicator of low-level toluene exposure. At exposures below the TLVs of toluene, urinary concentrations of hippuric acid and *o*-cresol may increase (69).

The presence of ethanol will decrease the metabolic clearance of toluene (120–123). Propranolol and cimetidine do not affect toluene metabolism (121). Blood concentrations of toluene have been shown to increase in exposed workers during shifts and to correlate with the air concentrations (124).

The combination of ethanol and toluene increases the hepatotoxicity of toluene, owing to inhibition of metabolism. Human studies indicate that even low ethanol blood levels inhibit toluene metabolism (70). Even a single alcoholic drink produces this metabolic inhibitory effect. Hippuric acid excretion was decreased by an ethanol dose of 0.32 g per kg (69). A source of error in the biological monitoring of toluene can be introduced by dermal absorption (125).

Toluene interferes with benzene metabolism and its hematopoietic toxicity (126). The toxicity of benzene depends on its metabolism to myelotoxic and clastogenic by-products. Benzene is metabolized to phenol first, by P-450 monooxygenases in the liver, and then to hydroquinone. Final benzene toxic metabolites are benzoquinones and semiquinone radicals, which are produced by bone marrow myeloperoxidase action on hydroquinone (127). Both the P-450 enzyme system and myeloperoxidase enzymes are inhibited by toluene to the degree that coexposure to both benzene and toluene inhibits benzene metabolism and immunotoxicity in mice. Evidence of this protective effect has also been found in humans (74,83,128,129).

Regulatory Aspects

The OSHA PEL TWA is 200 ppm, with a 15-minute ceiling of 300 ppm. The ACGIH, in 1996, recommended a TLV of 50 ppm with no designated short-term exposure limit (STEL). The ACGIH 15-minute ceiling limit is 150 ppm. The recommended BEI in urine for hippuric acid is 2.5 g per gram of creatinine at a work shift's end. The National Institute of Occupational Safety and Health (NIOSH) recommends a TLV of 100 ppm, with a 10-minute ceiling of 200 ppm. The toluene vapor concentration that is considered immediately dangerous to life and health (IDLH) is 2,000 ppm. The EPA recommends a maximum concentration level in water of 1 mg per L.

XYLENE

Xylene (dimethylbenzene) is a commonly used aromatic solvent with three isomeric forms: *ortho*-, *meta*-, and *para*-xylene (see Fig. 105-1). Xylenes are one of the highest-volume chemicals produced and used by industry. A mixture of all three isomers is termed *xylol*. Xylene is a sweet, clear liquid solvent, the vapors of which can be very irritating to eyes, nose, throat, skin, and mucous membranes (130). It is flammable, volatile, and soluble in alcohol and organic liquids but relatively insoluble in water.

Physiochemical Properties

Physiochemical properties of xylene are listed in Table 105-10. Each isomeric form of xylene is a colorless liquid that is highly volatile.

TABLE 105-10. Physiochemical properties of xylenes

	o-Xylene	*m*-Xylene	*p*-Xylene
Physical state (20°C; 101.3 kPa)	Colorless liquid	Colorless liquid	Colorless liquid
Boiling point (°C; 101.3 kPa)	144.4	139.1	138.3
Melting point (°C; 101.3 kPa)	−25.2	−47.9	13.3
Relative density (25°/4°C)	0.876	0.860	0.857
Vapor pressure (kPa at 20°C)	0.66	0.79	0.86
Flash point (°C) (closed cup)	30	25	25
Saturation % in air (101.3 kPa)	1.03 (32%)	1.03 (28%)	1.03 (27%)
Explosion limits (vol% in air)	1.0–6.0	1.1–7.0	1.1–9.0
Autoignition temp (°C)	465	525	525
Octanol–water partition coefficient (log P)	3.12	3.2	3.15
Solubility in water (mg/L)	142	146	185

Adapted from World Health Organization. *Xylenes*. Environmental health criteria 190. Geneva: World Health Organization, 1997.

Sources, Production, and Uses

Mixed xylene isomers (*m*-, *o*-, and *p*-isomers) are widely used as solvents. The physical and chemical properties of each isomeric form are similar (127). All mixed commercial xylene produced by catalytic processing of petroleum is a combination of 20% *o*-xylene, 44% *m*-xylene, and 20% *p*-xylene, and also contains 15% ethylbenzene (130). Xylene is produced also from coal tar, which yields an isomer mixture of 45% to 70% *m*-xylene, 23% *p*-xylene, 1% to 15% *o*-xylene, and 6% to 10% ethylbenzene (130).

Commercial xylene often is contaminated with other organic compounds such as ethylbenzene, toluene, benzene, trimethylbenzene, phenol, thiophene, and pyridine. The volumes of these contaminants are very minor, making up less than a fraction of 1% (130).

Xylene is used in paints, inks, dyes, varnishes, and glues. Both xylene and xylol are used by histology technicians for tissue preparation. Xylene, toluene, and benzene (BTX) are blended into gasolines. Xylene is used as a solvent vehicle for pesticides and in manufacturing epoxy resins, coatings, fabrics, perfumes, and insect repellents. Seventy percent of xylene is used to produce ethylbenzene (130).

The xylene isomers are used as chemical intermediates in the synthesis of other compounds. *m*-Xylene is used to produce isophthalic acid, *m*-toluic acid, and isophthalonitrile (130). Isophthalic acid is used to make polyesters. *o*-Xylene is used to manufacture phthalic anhydride for plasticizers, terephthalic acid for polyesters, isophthalic acid, vitamins, and pharmaceuticals (130). *p*-Xylene is a chemical intermediate for synthesizing dimethyl terephthalate and terephthalic acid for polyesters and for vitamins and pharmaceuticals. *p*-Xylene and *o*-xylene are also components of insecticides (130).

Environmental Fate and Transport

Owing to low vapor pressures, volatilization is the main process that governs xylene transport and environmental behavior. Xylenes readily volatilize from ground and water sources into the atmosphere, where they are quickly transformed by photooxidation via hydroxy radicals (130). Xylenes are relatively stable to oxidation and hydrolysis in water. Biodegradation of xylenes occurs in surface soils but is a slow process (130).

Xylene can occasionallybe detected degassing from landfill disposal hazardous-waste sites. Average air levels detected have ranged from 0.86 mg per cubic meter for *o*-xylene (0.20 ppm) to 3.6 mg per cubic meter for *m*-xylene (0.83 ppm) and 1.2 mg per cubic meter for *p*-xylene (0.28 ppm) (130).

Xylenes are introduced into groundwater by releases of fuel oil, gasoline, and industrial spills; leaking storage tanks; and leaching from disposal waste sites. Xylene isomers have been detected in leachate at concentrations of 10 to 4,400 μg per L for hazardous-waste sites and from 3.7 to 38.0 μg per L for domestic landfills (130).

Xylene readily partitions from water and soil into the atmosphere, with a half-life of 5.6 hours at a depth of 1 m (130). Spills into soil result in both volatilization and soil leaching. As the organic content of the soil increases, the residence time of xylene increases (130). Xylene tends to adsorb to highly organic soil. In subsurface soils with a low organic content, xylene will be more quickly transported to groundwater. Xylene moves through unsaturated soil faster than through polar substances and water.

Exposure Sources

Because xylenes are ubiquitous in the environment, exposure to xylene can occur both in and out of an occupational setting. Xylenes are detected in the atmosphere, soils, surface waters, sediments, rain, drinking water, aquatic organisms, human blood, urine, and expired alveolar air (130).

Xylenes do not occur naturally in the environment. Their presence is due to releases from industrial sources, automobile exhaust, petroleum refining, commercial uses, and general solvent volatilization, spills, and waste disposal. Individuals are exposed to xylene while pumping gas. This compound can enter the soil and groundwater after releases of gasoline, fuel oil, and other xylene-containing solvent mixtures. Surface releases result in rapid volatilization into the atmosphere.

Tobacco smoke contains xylene, which can be detected in the blood of smokers (131). The breath level of xylene is twofold higher in smokers as compared to nonsmokers (132). Indoor environmental levels of xylene in 350 residences studied were 3 parts per billion (ppb) for *m*-xylene and *p*-xylene and 1 ppb for *o*-xylene (133). Blood xylene levels in nonoccupationally exposed individuals ranged from 0.074 to 0.78 ppb for *m*-xylene and *p*-xylene and 0.044 to 0.30 ppb for *o*-xylene (134).

Absorption, Metabolism, and Excretion

Xylene is absorbed via the inhalational, dermal, and GI routes. Inhalation of xylene vapors is a common occupational exposure route, and urinary metabolites increase as the level of respiratory exposure increases. Approximately 60% of inhaled xylene is absorbed (135).

The kinetics of *m*-xylene have been studied in humans (135–138). Physical exercise results in increased absorption of solvent vapors through increased rate of ventilation. One study examined 18 healthy male volunteers and carried out controlled studies of *m*-xylene vapor exposure (138). The results showed that the concentration of xylene in blood samples increased with physical activity. Alveolar air concentrations of xylene were increased 40% over baseline after exposure to 30 ppm during exercise (139).

Xylene is a GI irritant and a mucous membrane irritant. GI absorption occurs after ingestion, and urinary metabolites can be detected.

Dermal xylene absorption is low as compared to respiratory tract absorption (see Table 105-3). Liquid xylene penetrates hand skin at a rate of 2 μg per square centimeter per minute (140). Other studies demonstrate dermal absorption rates varying from 4.5 to 9.6 mg per square centimeter per hour (63). Dermal absorption of xylene increased with prolonged immersion in liquid and is increased by a factor of three if the dermis is damaged (140,141).

Xylene is very soluble in blood and lipid-containing tissue. Thus, its distribution depends on blood flow to organs and tissue lipid content. Organs with high blood perfusion will receive more xylene. Adipose tissue has a slow continuous xylene uptake lasting beyond termination of an exposure. Thus, the potential exists for adipose tissue accumulation of xylene in chronic exposure (142). During exercise, xylene appears to be shunted to subcutaneous tissues and adipose stores.

Xylene CNS levels approximate those of blood, the concentration in the brain being approximately 40% of that of arterial blood (135). Studies in animals indicate that the rate of rise of blood xylene is correlated with CNS rise of xylene and acute symptoms. Accumulation of xylene in the brains of rats is both time and concentration dependent.

The biotransformation of xylene through side chain oxidation and aromatic oxidation results in metabolites of methylbenzyl alcohols, methylbenzaldehyde, and methylbenzoic acids (toluic acids) (143). Methylbenzoic acids are conjugated with glycine to form methyl hippuric acids, the main urinary metabolites of xylene. A minor (1% to 4%) metabolic pathway of xylene metabolism is aromatic ring hydroxylation, which forms xylenol (143).

In summary, less than 5% of xylene is excreted unchanged in exhaled air, approximately 95% is excreted as methyl hippuric acid metabolites, and 1% to 4% is excreted as xylenol metabolites (Fig. 105-3).

Aromatic compounds are metabolized via the P-450 mixed-function microsomal enzyme system in the endoplasmic reticulum of the liver. The coingestion of ethanol will inhibit the metabolism of xylene (136). Ethanol inhibits oxidation of both the aromatic ring and the alkyl side chain, probably through a direct inhibitory effect on microsomal oxidation by ethanol. Xylene blood concentrations increase up to twofold after ethanol ingestion, indicating inhibition of metabolism (136). Liver necrosis and steatosis have been reported after xylene exposure (137).

Despite the fact that ethanol decreases xylene metabolism by 50%, the urinary excretion of 2,4-xylenol, a minor xylene metabolite, was not decreased by ethanol (136). The ingestion of moderate doses of ethanol has increased blood xylene concentrations twofold. Coingestion of ethanol and xylene also results in a decrease in methyl hippuric acid excretion in the urine. The ratio of 2,4-xylenol to methyl hippuric acid was significantly increased with the combination of alcohol ingestion and xylene exposure.

Xylene clearance is mainly renal, and 36% is excreted by the end of a work period in which exposure occurs, whereas 70% to 80% of xylene metabolites are excreted within 24 hours of exposure termination (143). Coexposure to other solvents affects xylene metabolism (144). Exposure to both methyl ethyl ketone and xylene results in approximately a 50% increase in blood xylene concentrations. Also, urinary excretion of methyl hippuric acid decreases, indicating competition for enzyme metabolism (144). Coexposure to trichloroethylene, ethylbenzene, and toluene also inhibits xylene metabolism (145). Increased use of the minor aromatic ring hydroxylation pathway occurs when other solvents compete with P-450 enzyme pathway metabolism.

Clinical Toxicology

Exposure to xylene is common as it is a constituent of paints and glues and is used as a general solvent in many processes and products. Owing to its high vapor pressure, most exposures to xylene and its isomers are by inhalation.

Death has been reported in an individual who was exposed to paint solvents containing primarily xylene, the estimated atmospheric concentrations being 10,000 ppm (146). Autopsy of

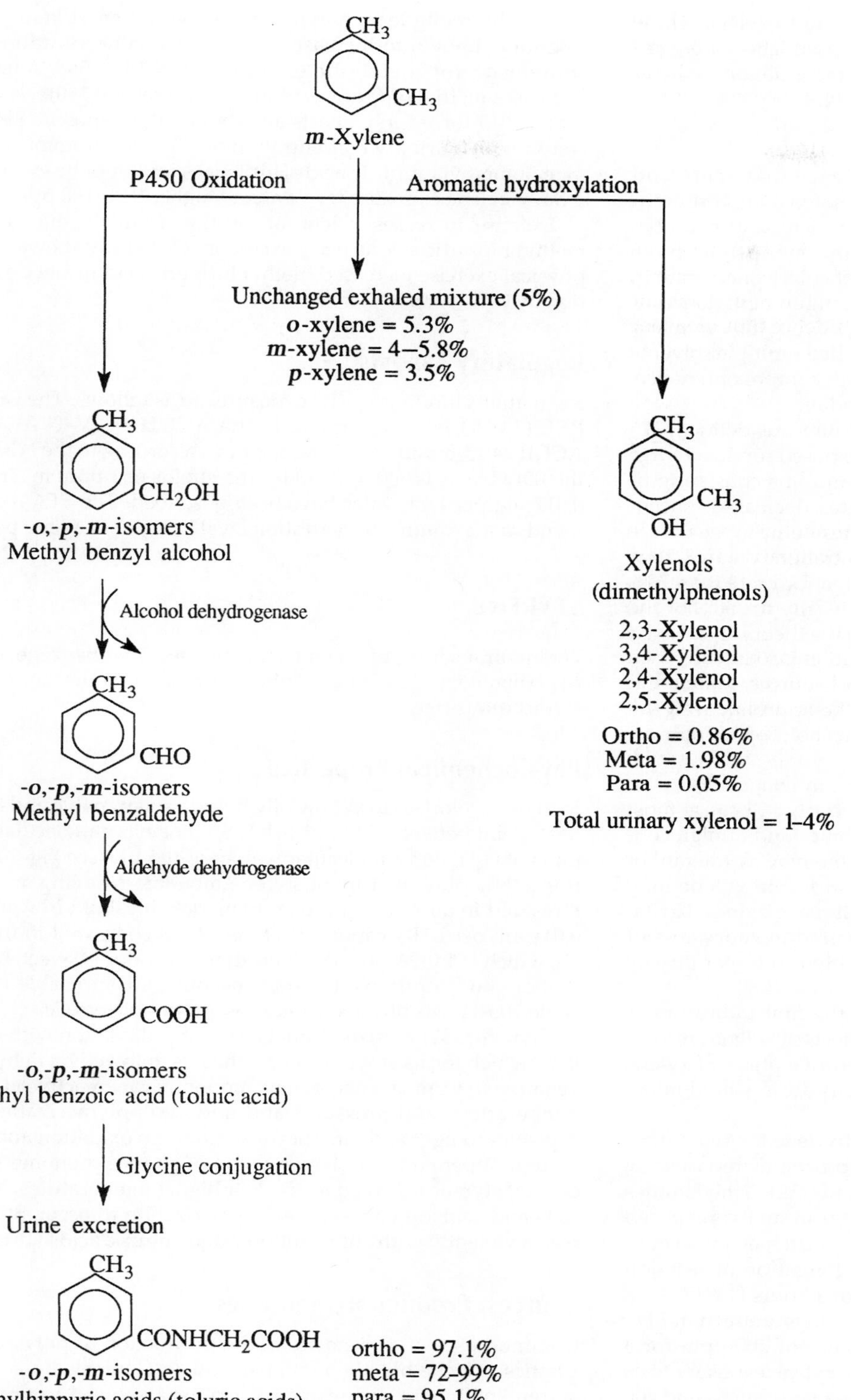

Figure 105-3. Xylene metabolism.

this individual demonstrated severe pulmonary congestion with hemorrhage and pulmonary edema. Data in animal models suggest that *p*-xylene might be more toxic than the other xylene isomers.

OCULAR AND PULMONARY SYSTEM EFFECTS

Nose and throat irritation from xylene has been reported at 200 ppm for 3 to 5 minutes and 100 ppm for 1 to 7.5 hours per day for 5 days (130). Chronic occupational exposure to unspecified or unknown concentrations of xylene vapors has been associated with difficulty breathing and impaired pulmonary function (147,148). Nose and throat irritation has been reported with increased prevalence by workers who are exposed chronically to xylene vapors at a geometric mean TWA concentration of 14 ppm (56).

A wide body of literature exists showing upper airway, throat, eyes, and nose irritation caused by acute inhalational exposure to xylene at varying concentrations (56,130). Such adverse respiratory effects are noted also in animal models after acute and intermediate inhalational exposure to xylene. These effects include decreased respiration, increased labor of breathing, respiratory irritation, pulmonary edema, pulmonary hemorrhage, and pulmonary inflammation (130).

NEUROTOXICITY

Case reports and studies provide evidence that acute and chronic inhalational exposure to xylene or solvent mixtures containing xylene are associated with neurotoxicity and neurobehavioral changes. Neurologic signs and symptoms have included headache, nausea, dizziness, difficulty concentrating, impaired memory, slurred speech, ataxia, fatigue, agitation, confusion, tremors, and noise sensitivity (57,130,149,150). In many of these case reports, exposures have included multiple solvents in which xylene was involved as the main component; hence, confounding factors compromise such studies.

In one study in which the xylene exposure was defined, 175 workers in a Chinese factory who were exposed for an average of 7 years reported neurobehavioral symptoms consisting of headache, anxiety, forgetfulness, nightmares, decreased concentration, and decreased grasp (149). These employees were exposed to mixed xylene airborne concentrations on an 8-hour TWA of 21 ppm, in which xylene accounted for more than 70% of the total exposure and *m*-xylene specifically for 50% of the exposure. Animal studies lend support to the theory that mixed xylene isomers are neurotoxic after inhalation (130).

The odor threshold of xylenes depends on the isomer. On average, the odor threshold appears to be approximately 1.0 ppm. *m*-Xylene has an airborne odor threshold of 3.7 ppm, *o*-xylene 0.17 ppm, and *p*-xylene 0.47 ppm.

Xylene vapors have a sweet odor that, in conjunction with irritation of the airways and respiratory tract, will cause most individuals to note the presence of the compound at high concentrations and to avoid it. Individuals who may be tolerant of the odor or who remain in the area of airborne xylene may develop headaches, nausea, vomiting, fatigue, dizziness, irritability, insomnia, a drunken feeling, impaired memory, loss of coordination, and unsteady gait, in addition to upper airway and ocular irritation (149–151).

Neurobehavioral symptoms may be the first indication of low-level xylene intoxication. The CNS effects of xylene are excitatory and occur mainly during the absorptive phase of xylene exposure, whereas a depressive effect occurs during the elimination phase of xylene exposure (151).

Subjects exposed to 690 ppm of mixed xylene for 15 minutes experience dizziness, but this same symptom was reported by only one of six persons exposed to 460 ppm (152). Other studies showed no impairment in performance tests in subjects exposed to 299 ppm for 70 minutes (153) or at 396 ppm in men for 30 minutes (154,155). Some studies report prolongation of reaction times in exposure to xylene at 100 ppm for 4 hours (155).

Increased theta waves over occipital regions are seen in EEG results in subjects exposed to xylene peaks of 200 ppm for 4 hours (150). Other researchers report that xylene exposure for 6 hours for 6 to 9 days with levels fluctuating between 64 and 400 ppm produced impairment in balance and reaction time (156,157). Peripheral neuropathy has been associated with xylene exposure, but no biological or chemical mechanism has been established, although it is thought that xylene interrupts fast axonal transport (158).

Biological Monitoring

Assays of blood and alveolar air can detect xylene, and its metabolites can be detected in urine. Blood levels of xylene can be affected by coexposure to other solvents. Coexposure to toluene, trichloroethylene, ethylbenzene, methyl ethyl ketone, or alcohol is known to increase xylene blood concentrations by competing for metabolic enzymes (144,145,159). Aspirin decreases methyl hippuric acid urinary excretion (160).

The BEI for xylene reflects an 8-hour TWA exposure period resulting in a urinary concentration of 1.5 g per gram of creatinine of methyl hippuric acid. This level should not be exceeded if daily xylene exposure levels are no higher than 100 ppm.

Exercise increases xylene absorption from the lungs and methyl hippuric acid urinary excretion. One study showed that physical exercise increased methyl hippuric acid urinary excretion by 24% (138).

Regulatory Aspects

Regulations limiting xylene exposure are as follows: The OSHA PEL (TWA) is 100 ppm, as is the ACGIH TLV-TWA. The ACGIH's 15-minute STEL is 150 ppm. According to the NIOSH, the IDLH level is 900 ppm. Odor thresholds of 1 ppm in air and 0.017 mg per L of water have been described. The EPA recommends a maximum concentration level in water of 10 mg per L.

STYRENE

The natural source of styrene (cinnamene, vinyl benzene, ethenyl benzene, phenylethene, phenylethylene) is the sap of the styracaceous tree.

Physiochemical Properties

Styrene, a colorless to yellow oily liquid, is flammable and has a flash point between 73° and 141°F. Styrene has a molecular formula of C_8H_8 and a molecular weight of 104.1 D (see Fig. 105-1). It is a 99% pure mixture of styrene monomers having an odor threshold in air of 0.32 ppm and an odor threshold in water of 0.011 mL per L. Its vapor density is 3.6 (as compared to that of air, which is 1.0). At low concentrations, its odor is sweet, but at higher concentrations, the odor becomes disagreeable (161). Table 105-11 lists physiochemical properties of styrene.

Styrene is synthesized from benzene by alkylation with ethylene, which forms ethylbenzene, which is followed by dehydrogenation to form xylene. Styrene monomers are reactive at high temperatures and pressures and undergo polymerization on exposure to light and air. They also undergo oxidation and formation of peroxides. Polymerization of styrene monomers can occur if styrene is heated to 150°F or higher temperatures. Metal salts and acids can also cause polymerization to occur. Styrene reacts violently with chlorosulfonic and sulfuric acids (161).

Sources, Production, and Uses

Common uses of styrene are in the production of polystyrene plastics, styrene-butadiene rubber, and acrylonitrile-butadiene-styrene polymers and resins. Styrene is also used to produce styrene-butadiene latex protective coatings and in the formation of polyesters and copolymer resins.

Environmental Fate and Transport

Most styrene that is released to the environment volatilizes into the atmosphere. However, styrene can also contaminate soil and groundwater. Investigations report that between 87% and 95% of styrene in landfill soil is converted to carbon dioxide within 16 weeks (162). Various fungi and bacteria grow on styrene, thus indicating that it is biodegradable.

TABLE 105-11. Physiochemical properties of styrene

Molecular weight	104.14 D
Molecular formula	C_8H_8
Autoignition temperature	490°
Explosiveness range	1.1–6.1% by volume in air
Solubility	Slight in water
	Miscible in alcohol, ether, methanol, acetone, carbon disulfide
Specific gravity	0.9045 (25/25°C)
Boiling point	145.2°C
Vapor pressure (mm Hg)	
−1.6°C	1
20°C	4.5
25°C	6.1
33°C	10
66°C	50
Volume in saturated air	8,026 ppm
Conversion factors	1 ppm = 0.00426 mg/dL
	1 mg/L of vapor = 234.7 ppm
Partition coefficients	
Water/air	4.38
Blood/air	32
Oil/blood	130
Oil/air	4,160

Studies show that styrene rapidly volatilizes from shallow bodies of water, with 50% being lost in 1 to 3 hours (162). However, only 26% of styrene is volatilized from a soil depth of 1.5 cm within 31 days. Within 30 hours of a release into soil, 9% of styrene is adsorbed to minerals and organic soil (162).

Styrene is rapidly biodegraded by microorganisms in aerobic environments, but this rate of biodegradation slows when styrene concentrations are low in water or aquifers and in low-pH environments (162). Aerobic microorganisms in soil convert styrene to 2-hydroxyphenylacetic acid and styrene oxide, which then are biodegraded further. The mineralization of styrene in soil is proportional to its concentration.

Exposure Sources

Styrene exposure can occur during the manufacturing of plastics, polymers, and styrene-butadiene rubber and during its use as a solvent and in resins. Exposure to styrene also can occur in boat building and manufacturing of fiberglass-reinforced plastics. Use of a variety of styrene-containing products (e.g., paints, waxes, polishes, adhesives, cleaners, putty, varnishes) can result in exposure. In addition, environmental tobacco smoke and automobile exhaust contain styrene.

Styrene is detectable in air at vapor concentrations of 0.32 ppm. Aldehydes and peroxides can form from styrene when it is exposed to air, increasing its disagreeable odor. The vapors of styrene are very irritating.

Styrene is detected in the blood of nonoccupationally exposed individuals, indicating the potential environmental exposure sources (163). Styrene can also migrate from polystyrene plastics into packaged foods, which represent a possible source of styrene ingestion (164).

Absorption, Metabolism, and Excretion

Styrene is absorbed via respiratory, dermal, and GI routes. Systemic absorption of styrene via respiration is increased with increasing physical activity. Uptake is five to six times greater during heavy physical labor (165). From 60% to 70% of inhaled styrene is absorbed in humans, and 85% of this inhaled styrene is eliminated in the urine as mandelic acid and phenylglyoxylic acid metabolites (see later). Only 1% to 3% of styrene is exhaled unchanged. Styrene has dose-dependent kinetics (166). A BEI is based on the urinary excretion of mandelic acid (see Table 105-4).

Dermal absorption of styrene is considered to be minimal. However, skin absorption does occur and rates have been determined for both vapor and liquid (see Table 105-3) (63,167). Percutaneous absorption of styrene is increased if skin is injured.

Absorbed styrene is first metabolized by hepatic cytochrome P-450 enzymes to styrene-7,8-oxide, which is considered to be the main toxic metabolite, even more toxic than styrene. Styrene and styrene oxide are metabolized further by the liver as well as by the kidney, intestines, lungs, and skin. Styrene oxide is metabolized to phenylethylene glycol by microsomal epoxide hydrolase and, subsequently, to its two major metabolites, mandelic acid (85%) and phenyl glyoxylic acid (10%) (166,168,169). Up to 90% of absorbed styrene is excreted as urinary metabolites (Fig. 105-4) (170,171). A minor metabolic pathway involving phenylethylene glycol and mandelic acid is metabolism to benzoic acid, which then is conjugated with glycine to form hippuric acid.

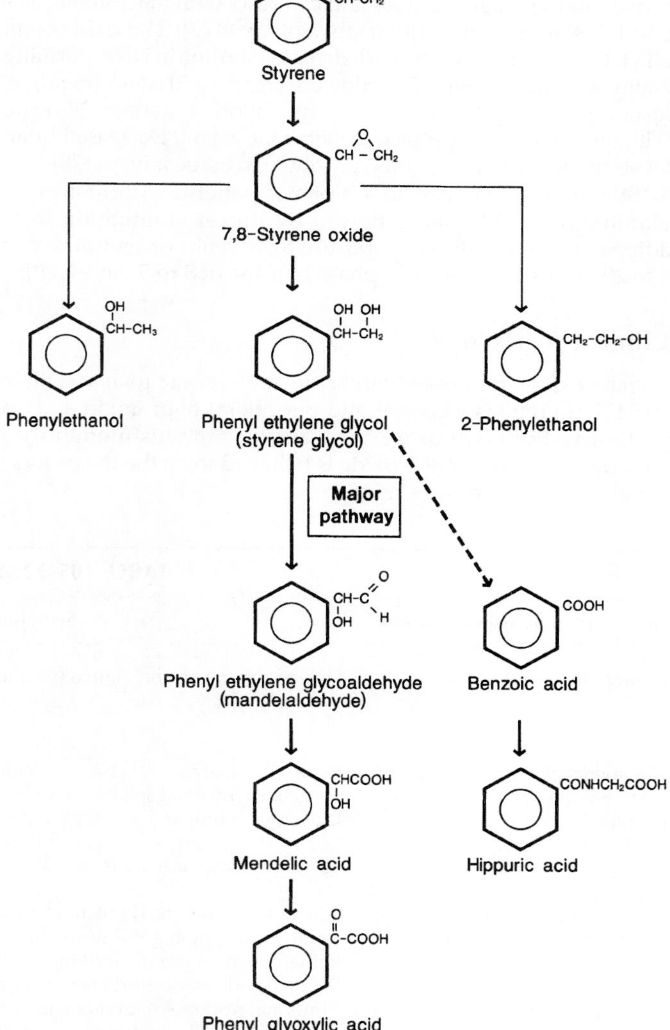

Figure 105-4. Metabolism of styrene.

Styrene dermal absorption has been studied using the urinary excretion of mandelic acid as a marker. The rate of absorption of liquid styrene across the dermal barrier was 9 to 15 mg per square centimeter per hour. The rate of aqueous solution absorption was 40 to 180 µm per square centimeter per hour, and the absorption from solution was linear with the concentration (63,64,165,167).

The metabolism of styrene is inhibited by ethanol as well as other solvents. Styrene metabolism is suppressed by coexposure to toluene. Acute alcohol ingestion inhibits P-450 enzymatic metabolism of styrene. Chronic ethanol ingestion will increase metabolism via induction of hepatic microsomal oxidizing enzymes, with increased formation of styrene-7,8-oxide (172). Coexposure to trichloroethylene or to toluene will inhibit styrene metabolism (173). Animal models indicate that ethanol and styrene coexposure decreases levels of brain glutathione (174). The major metabolite of styrene found in the urine is mandelic acid. The excretion of mandelic acid in the urine appears to be linearly related to exposure to styrene up to 150 ppm (175). Investigations have shown that the summation of mandelic acid and phenylglyoxylic acid in the urine correlates with total exposure to styrene.

Other minor metabolites of styrene metabolism are 4-vinyl phenol, phenylethylene glycol, phenylethanol, and hippuric acid (175). Styrene toxicity is believed to be related to styrene-7,8-oxide, which is four times as toxic as styrene (176). Styrene-7,8-oxide is formed in the brain and liver and can react with macromolecules and DNA to disrupt cellular physiology (177). The oxide is an alkylating agent and reacts with deoxyguanosine in DNA, forming 7-alkylguanine. Styrene-7,8-oxide also reacts with deoxycytidine, forming *N*-3-alkylcytosine. The conjugation of styrene-7,8-oxide with glutathione is a protective metabolic action. Decreased brain levels of glutathione can thus contribute to tissue injury (178).

Styrene is eliminated in a biphasic pattern, with first rapid elimination from blood followed by slower elimination from adipose tissue. Studies of exposure to styrene concentrations of 3 to 20 ppm show a second-phase half-life of 3 to 5 days (179).

Clinical Toxicology

Styrene exposure causes both acute and chronic toxicity (Table 105-12). Styrene is a central and peripheral neurotoxin and an irritant to the respiratory tract and to mucous membranes (166,168,169). Styrene-7,8-oxide is believed to be the major toxic metabolite that produces injury.

Acute toxic effects of styrene include mucous membrane irritation, respiratory irritation, headache, dizziness, decreased attention span, nausea, vomiting, impaired memory, and fatigue. Styrene is a neurotoxin with adverse effects on both the central and peripheral nervous systems.

Exposure of volunteers to styrene vapors of up to 375 ppm for up to 1 hour resulted in eye irritation and nasal irritation along with burning of the skin and face (180). In the same study, vapors of 50 to 115 ppm caused subjects to report strong odors but produced no signs and symptoms. At the 375-ppm level, some subjects reported difficulties in manual dexterity and balance and feelings of inebriation, especially after 60 minutes of exposure. Individuals exposed to much higher concentrations of styrene reported ocular irritation, throat irritation, drowsiness, vertigo, CNS depression, and unsteadiness of gait (169).

The health effects of styrene are dose related. Mild complaints consist of mucous membrane irritation, headache, nausea, vertigo, and fatigue. Workers exposed to between 4 and 165 ppm also expressed more complaints of depression, tinnitus, ocular irritation, and dizziness (181).

Chronic exposure to styrene has produced neurobehavioral symptoms with complaints of attention deficit, memory problems, fatigue, paresthesia, and muscle weaknesses (166,182). Workers exposed to styrene vapors of 3 to 251 ppm for a median duration of 7 years were compared with unexposed controls. Neurologic examination showed no evidence of peripheral neuropathy or encephalopathy in these exposed individuals as compared to controls. Neurobehavioral assessments involving intelligence, reaction time, short-term memory, and personality also demonstrated no differences between exposed and unexposed control subjects (183).

Other workers exposed chronically to styrene in industry have reported symptoms of excessive tiredness, difficulty concentrating, nausea, and memory disturbances. Styrene concentrations in their environment ranged from less than 20 to more than 150 ppm (182).

NEUROTOXIC MANIFESTATIONS

Neurophysiologic studies indicate that styrene is a central and peripheral neurotoxin. Abnormal EEG reaction times and NCVs have been found in workers who were exposed to styrene and reported neurobehavioral and neurologic symptoms. Reviews of EEG studies in populations of workers confirmed that exposure to high levels of styrene produce quantitative EEG changes. However, many of these workers were exposed to multiple

TABLE 105-12. Styrene neurotoxicity

Target organ or assessment tool	Symptoms	Concentration	Reference
Neurobehavioral effects	Depression, headache, difficulty concentrating, memory deficit, fatigue	20–150 ppm	182
		4–165 ppm	181
		30 ppm	195
		>50 ppm	196
Electroencephalographic effects	Dose-related abnormal changes, including excessive diffuse theta-wave activity, bilateral spike and wave discharge, local slow waves	5–125 ppm	184–186
Peripheral neuropathy	Prolonged motor and sensory conduction velocities	5–125 ppm	186
		3–63 ppm	186,188
	32 workers with urinary mandelic acid >250 mg/L	<40 ppm	189–191
		<50 ppm	
Evoked potentials effects	Somatosensory evoked potential abnormalities after 5–22 years' exposure	140–570 mg/m^3	187
Autonomic nervous system	Electrocardiographic R-R disturbance	22 ppm	188
	Urinary mandelic acid <420 mg/g creatinine		
Balance equilibrium	Balance and sway disturbance on posturography after 6–15 years' exposure		192,193
Hearing	Abnormal response to audiometric tests		179
Color vision	Impairment of blue-yellow and red-green vision		194

other solvents, which introduces confounding factors (184). Nonetheless, dose-dependent EEG changes—diffuse and localized theta waves, increased beta activity in central and rostral hemispheres, and increased fast- and slow-wave activity—have been reported (185,186).

Evoked potential studies comparing styrene-exposed workers to unexposed controls indicated that SEPs, especially peripheral and cortical SEPs, showed prolonged latencies (187).

Neurophysiologic studies involving motor conduction velocities and NCVs in styrene-exposed workers exhibited significantly slower sensory conduction velocities and NCVs. These workers were exposed to a range of 3 to 63 ppm, and mandelic acid and phenylglyoxylic acid metabolites in the urine were monitored. These results suggest that styrene has effects on faster myelinated fibers in the peripheral nervous system (188).

The fact that styrene is a peripheral neurotoxin has been confirmed in nerve conduction studies. However, exposure to less than 100 ppm has not been associated with peripheral neuropathy (183). Other reports have cited increased frequency of peripheral neuropathologic alterations in nerve conduction studies of radial and peroneal nerves in workers exposed to styrene monomers (186,189).

The relationship between styrene exposure and NCVs was investigated in 32 exposed workers and a control group (190). This study demonstrated a dose-response relationship between urinary mandelic acid concentration and ulnar and peroneal motor distal latencies. Those workers with urinary mandelic acid concentrations greater than 250 mg per L had significantly longer latencies than did those whose urinary concentrations did not exceed 250 mg per L. Airborne styrene concentrations were reported to be less than 40 ppm. However, some high concentrations (117 ppm and 94.8 ppm) were noted.

Sensory conduction defects also were found in other workers with chronic styrene exposure, some of whom were exposed to concentrations of less than 50 ppm of styrene (191). As the concentration of styrene increased to between 50 and 100 ppm, the incidence of sensory conduction defects increased. Up to 71% of subjects studied showed defects when styrene concentrations exceeded 100 ppm. Cessation of exposure resulted in improved conduction velocities. Thus, termination of exposure can improve the neuropathologic signs and symptoms of chronically exposed workers.

Styrene adversely affects balance and equilibrium (192,193). Exposed styrene workers (as compared to unexposed controls) were assessed for balance, sway, and changes in hearing. Abnormal findings in speech and cortical response to audiometric tests were noted in 7 of 18 workers (192,193). The exposed group also showed significant balance disturbance on testing. Further studies suggest that styrene interferes with the cerebellar inhibition of the vestibulooculomotor system (169). Other research has revealed impairment of color vision in exposed workers (194). In these subjects, blue-yellow vision was affected, although red-green vision loss has also been reported (194).

As mentioned, neuropsychological abnormalities have been detected in individuals exposed chronically to styrene. Impairment of short-term memory has been noted in individuals exposed to styrene levels of approximately 30 ppm for up to 5 years (195). Other studies have confirmed similar findings in neuropsychological tests involving short-term memory. Neuropsychological tests administered include simple reaction time, choice reaction time, and digit span. The combined urinary metabolites of mandelic acid and phenylglyoxylic acid measured at the end of the work shift were determined to be 575 mg per gram of creatinine (195). When compared to unexposed controls, the exposed individuals showed significant detriments of short-term memory and simple and choice reaction times.

Likewise, workers exposed to airborne styrene concentrations in excess of 50 ppm have demonstrated decrements on neuropsychological tests (including short-term memory tests) as compared to those who were exposed to less than 50 ppm (196).

Other studies have examined neurobehavioral changes in individuals exposed to 12 ppm of styrene. Symptoms included fatigue and memory problems and, among those subjects with higher exposures, headache, irritability, and difficulty in concentrating also were observed. In this study, no differences on neurobehavioral testing were noted between the groups at this airborne concentration (197). It must be emphasized that in *all* studies of neurobehavioral and neuropsychological testing, exposure to multiple solvents can be a confounding factor.

Autonomic nervous system disruption has been demonstrated at airborne styrene concentrations of 22 ppm and mandelic acid urinary concentrations of less than 420 mg per gram of creatinine (188). This disturbance was seen in the R-R electrocardiographic interval (CV_{R-R}), which is a method by which to check autonomic nervous system function in the hypothalamus and brainstem.

MECHANISM OF NEUROTOXICITY

The mechanism by which styrene causes neurotoxicity is unknown, but it is thought that the styrene-7,8-oxide probably plays a role because of its highly reactive alkylating features. Investigators have shown that specific regions of the brain are affected by styrene, with astrogliosis in the sensory motor cortex and hippocampus that persist for months after exposure has been terminated (198). Investigations have shown increased concentrations of glial cell protein markers as an indicator of brain injuries. Exposure of cultured cells to styrene oxide increased concentrations of extracellular calcium and decreased intracellular concentrations of glutathione and adenosine triphosphate (199). Styrene also interferes with the activity of the dopaminergic system and causes a decrease in dopamine levels in the striatum and tuberoinfundibular system of exposed animals at vapor concentrations of 750 ppm (200).

Biological Monitoring

Styrene easily crosses the blood–brain barrier into the CNS and, therefore, blood levels alone will not accurately reflect toxic effects.

The peak urinary excretion of mandelic acid occurs at approximately 4 to 8 hours after styrene exposure. Mandelic acid has a half-life in urine of 7.8 hours after exposure to between 50 and 200 ppm, and phenylglyoxylic acid has a urinary half-life of 8.5 hours (201).

Current ACGIH BEIs for styrene exposure are listed in Table 105-4. The concentration of urinary mandelic acid should not exceed 300 mg per gram of creatinine at the beginning of a work shift or 800 mg per gram of creatinine at the end of a shift. The sum of mandelic acid and phenylglyoxylic acid more accurately reflects exposure and should not exceed 1,000 mg per gram of creatinine at the end of a work shift. Phenylglyoxylic acid also is used as biological marker of exposure, but this acid is unstable unless the urine is frozen immediately; otherwise, the levels will decrease owing to decarboxylation.

Because coexposure to ethanol, toluene, or xylene can result in decreased mandelic acid excretion, detection of stereochemically different enantiomers of styrene metabolites (as opposed to ethylbenzene metabolites) is recommended (202). Mandelic acid produced by styrene metabolism is racemic, composed of *R*- and *S*-enantiomeric forms, whereas mandelic acid produced by ethylbenzene metabolism occurs only in the *R*-enantiomeric form (202).

Styrene metabolism also produces specific mercapturic acids, termed *M1* and *M2*, and correlations have been identified between the urinary excretion of these mercapturic acids and BEIs (203). Styrene is metabolized by hepatic cytochrome P-450 enzymes to two enantiomeric forms—*R*–styrene oxide and *S*–styrene oxide—which can covalently bind to macromolecules. Styrene oxide metabolism follows two pathways: hydrolysis to styrene glycol or conjugation with glutathione. Glutathione conjugation of styrene oxide enantiomers (*R*- and *S*-) results in urinary excretion of distinctive *N*-acetyl-*S*-C1-phenyl-2-hydroxyethyl-*S*-cysteine (M1) and *N*-acetyl-*S*-C2-phenyl-2-hydroxyethyl-L-cysteine (M2) metabolites, with two diastereoisomer forms: M1-*S*, M1-*R* and M2-*S*, M2-*R* (203).

In an exposure study in which the mean airborne styrene concentration was 112 mg per cubic meter (44 to 228 mg per cubic meter), M1 and M2 mercapturic acid urine concentrations proved to be a reliable parameter of exposure. Workers with a urinary mandelic acid concentration of 200 mg per L excrete a total M1 plus M2 concentration between 0.8 and 2.0 mg per gram of creatinine. Some authors have suggested that the stereochemically selective enantiomers are responsible for the toxic mutagenic potential of styrene (204).

Regulatory Aspects

Regulatory limits for styrene have been established as follows: The OSHA PEL standard for exposure to styrene monomers is 100 ppm, with a ceiling value of 200 ppm (15-minute TWA) and an acceptable exposure of 600 ppm for 5 minutes in any 3-hour period. The ACGIH recommends a TLV-TWA of 50 ppm and a STEL of 100 ppm. The ACGIH TLV-TWA is 50 ppm (215 mg per cubic meter), and the STEL is 100 ppm (425 mg per cubic meter). The NIOSH recommended exposure limit (10-hour TWA) is 50 ppm; the STEL, 100 ppm; and the IDLH, 700 ppm.

In storage, styrene monomer vapors may form polymers. Consequently, the Hazardous Materials Transportation Act designates styrene monomers in quantities of 1,000 pounds or more as a hazardous material for transportation purposes. Any styrene monomer is considered to be a flammable liquid and requires such labeling.

CHLOROBENZENE

The chlorobenzenes are aromatic compounds formed by the addition of between one and six atoms of chlorine directly to the benzene ring. This chlorination process can result in 12 different compounds subdivided as follows: MCB; three isomeric forms each of di-, tri-, and tetrachlorobenzenes; pentachlorobenzene; and hexachlorobenzene (Table 105-13) (205). Substitution of chlorine on the aromatic ring is indicated as follows: 1-monochlorobenzene, 1,2-dichlorobenzene, 1,2,3-trichlorobenzene, 1,2,3,4-tetrachlorobenzene, and 1,2,3,4,5-pentachlorobenzene (see Fig. 105-1).

Physiochemical Properties

With the exception of MCB, 1,2-dichlorobenzene, 1,3-dichlorobenzene, and 1,2,4-trichlorobenzene, which are colorless liquids used as solvents in intermediate chemicals and chemical processes, chlorobenzenes are white, crystalline solids at room temperature. The water solubility of chlorobenzenes decreases with increasing chlorination. The flammability of these compounds is low, and the octanol-water partition coefficients are moderate to high and increase with increasing chlorination. The vapor pressures of these compounds is low to moderate and decreases with increasing chlorination (205).

Commercially used chlorobenzenes are contaminated with a variety of isomers. Pure MCB can contain as much as 0.05% benzene and 0.1% dichlorobenzenes. Technical-grade 1,2-dichlorobenzene can contain up to 19% of other dichlorobenzenes (205).

TABLE 105-13. Chlorobenzene compounds derived by chlorination

Compound	Abbreviated chemical name	Molecular formula
Monochlorobenzene	MCB	C_6H_5Cl
1,2-Dichlorobenzene	1,2,-DCB	$C_6H_4Cl_2$
1,3-Dichlorobenzene	1,3,-DCB	$C_6H_4Cl_2$
1,4-Dichlorobenzene	1,4,-DCB	$C_6H_4Cl_2$
1,2,3-Trichlorobenzene	1,2,3-TCB	$C_6H_3Cl_3$
1,2,4-Trichlorobenzene	1,2,4-TCB	$C_6H_3Cl_3$
1,3,5-Trichlorobenzene	1,3,5-TCB	$C_6H_3Cl_3$
1,2,3,4-Tetrachlorobenzene	1,2,3,4-TeCB	$C_6H_4Cl_4$
1,2,3,5-Tetrachlorobenzene	1,2,3,5-TeCB	$C_6H_4Cl_4$
1,2,4,5-Tetrachlorobenzene	1,2,4,5-TeCB	$C_6H_2Cl_4$
Pentachlorobenzene	PeCB	C_6HCl_5
Hexachlorobenzene	HxCB	C_6H_6Cl

MCB's odor can be described as mild to somewhat sweet and aromatic. It is a colorless, flammable liquid that reacts violently with oxidizers. Vapors can form dangerously explosive mixtures with air, because MCB is highly reactive and its vapors are heavier than air. MCB vapors can travel along floors to ignition sources. The vapor density of MCB is 3.88 (as compared to that of air, which is 1). When heated, toxic combustion products include chlorine gas.

Sources, Production, and Uses

MCB and dichlorobenzenes are produced by direct chlorination of benzene using a Lewis acid catalyst such as ferric chloride (205). Trichlorobenzenes are obtained from the chlorination of dichlorobenzenes, and tetrachlorobenzenes are produced by adding chlorine to trichlorobenzenes. The tetrachlorobenzenes are precursors of pentachlorobenzene. MCB makes up 70% of the world production of all chlorobenzenes (205).

The chlorobenzenes are used as intermediates in the synthesis of pesticides and other chemicals. MCB is used as an intermediate in the manufacture of chloronitrobenzenes, diphenyloxide, DDT, and silicones. It is also a solvent used with methylene diisocyanate; for adhesives; in polishes, waxes, and pharmaceutical products; and with natural rubber.

1,2-Dichlorobenzene is used as a solvent for organic materials, in drain cleaners, in the manufacture of 3,4-dichloroaniline, as a solvent carrier for the production of toluene diisocyanate, and in the manufacture of dyes, fumigants, and insecticides. 1,3-Dichlorobenzene is used as a fumigant and an insecticide. Table 105-14 lists the uses of various other chlorobenzene compounds (205).

Environmental Fate and Transport

Chlorobenzenes as a chemical family can persist in soil for several months, in air for 3.5 days, and in water for 1 day or less. Chlorobenzenes released into water environments will evaporate from water to the atmosphere.

Henry's law constant, the soil sorption constant (K_{oc}), and the octanol-water (K_{ow}) constant predict movement and fate in the environment. The distribution from water to air will decrease with increasing chlorination of the compound. Ninety-six percent of MCB is released to the atmosphere from aquatic environments (206). In other studies, 99% of MCB, 1,2-dichlorobenzene, 1,4-dichlorobenzene, and 1,2,4-trichlorobenzene evaporated from water solutions within 4 hours (205).

TABLE 105-14. Chlorobenzene uses

Compound	Uses
MCB	Intermediate in the manufacture of chloronitrobenzenes, diphenyl oxide, DDT, and silicones; as a process solvent for methylene diisocyanate, adhesives, polishes, waxes, pharmaceutical products, and natural rubber; as a degrading solvent
1,2-DCB	In the manufacture of 3,4-dichloroaniline; as a solvent for a wide range of organic materials and for oxides of nonferrous metals; as a solvent carrier in the production of toluene diisocyanate; in the manufacture of dyes; as a fumigant and insecticide; in degreasing hides and wool; in metal polishes; in industrial odor control; in cleaners for drains
1,3-DCB	As a fumigant and insecticide
1,4,-DCB	As a moth repellent, general insecticide, germicide, space deodorant; in the manufacture of 2,5-dichloroaniline and dyes; as a chemical intermediate; in pharmaceutical products; in agricultural fumigants
1,2,3-TCB	As a chemical intermediate; otherwise, same as those for 1,2,4-TCB
1,2,4-TCB	As an intermediate in the manufacture of herbicides; dye carrier, dielectric fluid; solvent; heat-transfer medium
1,3,5-TCB	Solvent for products melting at high temperatures; coolant in electrical insulators; heat-transfer medium, lubricant, and synthetic transformer oil; termite preparation and insecticide; in dyes
1,2,3,4-TeCB	Component in dielectric fluids; in the synthesis of fungicides
1,2,3,5-TeCB	Not available
1,2,4,5-TeCB	Intermediate for herbicides and defoliants; insecticide; moisture-resistant impregnator; electric insulation; in packing protection
1,2,4,5-TeCB	Formerly in a pesticide used to combat oyster drills; chemical intermediate

Adapted from ref. 205, with permission.

The half-life of chlorobenzenes released into aquatic environments is 100 days, with the majority being released to the atmosphere and the remainder being present in lake outflows and sediments (207). Some studies report that up to 50% of MCB evaporated from sandy soil having a low organic content over a 21-day period and that 50% of 1,4-dichlorobenzene and 1,2,4-trichlorobenzene were degraded or unaccounted for, indicating that they may have leached into groundwater (208).

Because of their chemical structure, the chlorobenzenes are environmentally persistent. Photochemical reactions and microbial degradation are the most likely path for their removal and biotransformation. Soils rich in organic matter and aquatic sediments will adsorb these compounds. 1,2-Dichlorobenzene and 1,2,4-trichlorobenzene are especially persistent in the environment, with half-lives from 1 day in rivers to 10 days in lakes and 100 days in groundwater (209).

Atmospheric chlorobenzenes are degraded by sunlight. They can also be adsorbed onto particulates that can be removed by precipitation.

Dichlorobenzenes, trichlorobenzenes, and pentachlorobenzenes are resistant to microbial degradation in soil and produce chlorophenol degradation by-products. The highly chlorinated chlorobenzenes are not very reactive compounds and disappear slowly from the environment via photolysis, hydrolysis, and oxidative reactions. However, photodegradation occurs slowly.

The half-life of 1,4-dichlorobenzene under artificial sunlight irradiation is estimated to be 115 hours (205). Reductive dechlorination is the photochemical reaction involving chlorobenzenes. The biodegradation of chlorobenzenes has been reported in various studies using soil, sediment, and sewage sludge (205).

Bioaccumulation of chlorobenzenes by aquatic organisms is reflected by the octanol-water partition coefficient. Uptake from water by aquatic organisms increases with increasing chlorination, which increases the chlorobenzenes' lipid solubility. Also, the adsorption of chlorobenzenes onto soil organic matter increases with increasing chlorination. Biomagnification up the food chain has not been studied.

In summary, chlorobenzenes move preferentially from water to the atmosphere but, in waters containing large amounts of organic materials, chlorobenzenes may be retained by the organic material and move into the aquatic environment. The concentration in sediments in aquatic environments is high—at least 1,000 times higher than the concentration found in water. Thus, soils rich in organic matter are major environmental sinks for the chlorobenzenes.

Exposure Sources

Exposure sources of chlorobenzenes are ambient outdoor air with mono-, di-, and trichlorobenzene concentrations ranging from the low microgram-per-cubic-meter range up to 100 µg per cubic meter (205). Concentrations of chlorobenzenes in the indoor air are similar to those in the ambient outdoor air but, occasionally, indoor air concentrations may be found to be higher. Tables 105-15 and 105-16 summarize select indoor and outdoor concentrations of chlorobenzenes.

TABLE 105-15. Chlorobenzenes in indoor air

Compound	Location	Concentration (µg/m^3)
MCB	Urban office, United States	1.8–3.2
	Greensboro, NC	Median 0.09
	Baton Rouge–Geismar, LA	Median 2.1
	Houston, TX	Median 5.5
1,2-DCB	Personal air samples	
	Los Angeles, CA, February	0.4
	Los Angeles, CA, May	0.3
	Contra Costa, CA, June	0.6
1,3-DCB	Netherlands, postwar homes	Median <0.6
	Netherlands, <6-year-old homes	Median <0.6
	Rotterdam, Netherlands	Median <0.6
1,4-DCB	Netherlands, postwar homes	Median 2
	Netherlands, <6-year-old homes	Median <0.6
	Rotterdam, Netherlands	Median <0.6
1,3-DCB, 1,4-DCB	Personal air samples	
	Elizabeth/Bayonne, NJ, fall	45
	Elizabeth/Bayonne, NJ, summer	50
	Elizabeth/Bayonne, NJ, winter	71
	Los Angeles, CA, February	18
	Los Angeles, CA, May	12
	Contra Costa, CA, June	5.5
1,2,3-TCB	Netherlands, postwar homes	Median <0.8
	Netherlands, <6-year-old homes	Median <0.8
	Rotterdam, Netherlands	Median <0.8
TeCBs	Love Canal, NY, house basements	0.03–20.0
PeCB	Love Canal, NY, house basements	Trace–0.49

Adapted from ref. 205, with permission.

TABLE 105-16. Chlorobenzenes in outdoor air

Compound	Location	Concentration (μg/m³)
MCB	U.S. cities	
	Newark, NJ	0.5
	Elizabeth, NJ	0.4
	Camden, NJ	0.3
1,2-DCB	U.S. cities	
	Los Angeles, CA, February	0.2
	Los Angeles, CA, May	0.8
	Contra Costa, CA, June	0.07
	Elizabeth/Bayonne, NJ	0.17
	Canadian cities	
	Montreal	0.0
	Toronto	0.02
1,3-DCB	Germany; city and environs (Bochum)	3.7
1,4-DCB	Northern Italy, various towns	<5
1,2,4-TCB	U.S. cities	
	Los Angeles, CA	0.05
	Phoenix, AZ	0.02
	Oakland, CA	0.02

Adapted from ref. 205, with permission.

Absorption, Metabolism, and Excretion

Chlorobenzenes are readily absorbed from the GI and respiratory tracts. Chlorobenzenes are distributed into highly perfused tissues and accumulate in lipid tissues. Lipid accumulation is greatest for the more highly chlorinated chlorobenzene compounds.

Chlorobenzenes are metabolized by microsomal oxidation to form arene oxide intermediates and then further to their corresponding chlorophenols, which are excreted in the urine as mercapturic acids after conjugation with glutathione or as glucuronic acid or sulfate conjugates. A small percentage are eliminated unchanged in expired air or feces (205).

MCB is metabolized to an arene oxide and then to phenolic compounds and mercapturic acid. The major MCB urinary metabolites are 4-chlorocatechol and 4–chlorophenol–mercapturic acid. 2-Chlorophenol, 3-chlorophenol, 4-chlorophenol, and 3-chlorocatechol are minor metabolites of MCB. The availability of glutathione and conjugation of the catechol and chlorophenol metabolites play an important role in the production of metabolites of MCB. Saturation of glutathione conjugation is thought to be important in the manifestation of toxic effects of MCB exposure (210).

A minor metabolite of 1,4-dichlorobenzene is 2,5-dichloroquinol. Mercapturic acids and catechols are not formed during metabolism of 1,4-dichlorobenzene in animals (205). Dichlorophenol is detected in the urine of workers exposed to 1,4-dichlorobenzene in amounts ranging from 10 to 230 mL per L (205).

Metabolic products of trichlorobenzenes proceed through arene oxides and form trichlorophenols, with minor metabolites including trichlorocatechols and mercapturic acids. Tetrachlorobenzenes are slowly metabolized to tetrachlorophenols, with arene oxides as metabolic intermediates (205). Mercaptotrichlorophenols and trichlorophenol are metabolites of tetrachlorophenols in animal models. Tetrachlorophenols are primarily metabolized to pentachlorophenol by oxidation or to 2,3,4,5-tetrachlorophenol via the arene oxide intermediate.

Clinical Toxicology

Occupational exposure data are available from case reports and reveal many confounding variables, including dose, exposure duration, and coincident exposures to other solvents. Case reports of MCB occupational exposure cite headaches, lethargy, and ocular and upper respiratory tract irritation as common symptoms after chronic exposure.

Reports of worker exposure to 1,2,-dichlorobenzene have offered conflicting accounts of hematologic disorders, including anemia and leukemias, after long-term inhalational exposure. However, a cross-sectional epidemiologic study of workers exposed to 1,2-dichlorobenzene demonstrated no evidence of hematologic effects at mean levels of 90 mg per cubic meter (215 ppm) (205). Chromosomal aberrations consisting of single and double breaks in peripheral leukocytes were reported in laboratory workers exposed to 1,2-dichlorobenzene vapors as compared to unexposed laboratory personnel (211). Of all the white blood cells analyzed, approximately 9% of the exposed cells contained aberrations, as compared with only 2% of the control group's cells. However, a confounding factor was the lack of a determination of exposure concentrations in air.

CNS depression, excitation, and seizures are possible after ingestion of liquid chlorobenzenes. Inhalation of high concentrations of MCB has produced CNS depression, seizures, muscular twitching, cyanosis, and cardiac arrhythmias. The compound is toxic by inhalation and by absorption through skin. MCB is also irritating to mucous membranes and the respiratory tract. Repeated exposures to the skin can produce dermatitis.

Irritation of the eyes and mucous membranes in humans occurs at approximately 200 ppm, at which level the odor threshold has been greatly exceeded. Hence, the odor threshold and irritative phenomena are insufficient to provide a protective warning about exposure.

Regulatory Aspects

The OSHA PEL as a TWA for MCB is 75 ppm. The NIOSH IDLH value is 2,400 ppm. The ACGIH has recommended a TLV-TWA for chlorobenzene of 10 ppm and has proposed that this compound be designated an A3 (animal) carcinogen.

ETHYLBENZENE

Ethylbenzene, a colorless, liquid solvent, is an irritant of the skin, mucous membranes, and eyes. At high concentrations, it can produce CNS depression in both humans and animals. The OSHA PEL for ethylbenzene is 100 ppm.

Physiochemical Properties

Ethylbenzene (phenylethane) has a molecular formula of $C_6H_5(C_2H_5)$ (see Fig. 105-1). Its physiochemical properties are summarized in Table 105-17. It is a highly volatile liquid aromatic solvent with a vapor pressure of 7 mm Hg (20°C). Its odor threshold is approximately 20 to 100 ppb. Ethylbenzene is a fire and explosion hazard; it reacts violently with oxidizing materials.

Sources, Production, and Uses

Ethylbenzene is found as a natural component of petroleum oil and refined petroleum products. It is formulated also by the alkylation of benzene with ethylene. Gasoline can contain up to 20% ethylbenzene. Ethylbenzene's high vapor pressure allows it to volatilize quickly into the atmosphere from release sources.

Ethylbenzene is a by-product of incomplete combustion of natural materials and is found in tobacco smoke and by-products of vehicle exhaust.

TABLE 105-17. Physiochemical properties of ethylbenzene

Physical state	Colorless, flammable liquid
Molecular weight	106.16 D
Boiling point	136.2°C
Autoignition	432°C
Flash point	18°C
LEL	6.7%
Henry's constant	6.6×10^{-3} (20°C)
Odor threshold	20–100 ppb (aromatic gasoline odor)
Solubility	Miscible in ethyl ether, ethanol, organic solvent
Organol-water constant (K_{ow})	3.15
Specific gravity	0.866
Vapor density	3.66 (air = 1)
Vapor pressure (20°C)	7 mm Hg

LEL, lowest explosive level.

Ethylbenzene is used in the chemical industry. It is produced by the Friedel-Crafts alkylation of benzene with ethylene, using an aluminum chloride catalyst. Most ethylbenzene is used as an intermediate chemical in the production of styrene (212). Among its other uses are as a general solvent in paint thinners, as a degreaser for paints and inks, and as a solvent in paints and lacquers. It is used also in the rubber and chemical manufacturing sectors.

Environmental Fate and Transport

The main environmental fate of ethylbenzene is volatilization into the atmosphere. Only small amounts of environmental ethylbenzene are found in water and soil, where it is slowly biodegraded. Ethylbenzene has low water solubility (152 mg per L at 20°C) and high vapor pressure (1.24 kPa at 20°C) (212).

Ethylbenzene is biodegradable in aquatic systems and soil. Soil bacteria metabolize ethylbenzene as a carbon source. Microbial oxidative degradation involves hydroxylation of the aromatic ring to 2,3-dihydroxy-1-ethylbenzene by soil bacteria. The biodegradation half-life is 2 days to 2 weeks (212). Ethylbenzene also undergoes aquatic anaerobic degradation by microorganisms in the presence of nitrates. Ethylbenzene undergoes atmospheric oxidation rapidly via photochemically produced free radicals. The atmospheric half-life ranges from 1 hour to a few weeks.

Exposure Sources

Mean concentrations of ethylbenzene in the atmosphere range from 0.74 to 100.0 µg per meter in urban areas, industries being the principal release points. Rural atmospheric concentrations are usually less than 2 µg per cubic meter (212). Industrial water concentrations up to 15 µg per L have been reported, whereas nonindustrial surface water contains less than 0.1 µg of ethylbenzene per L. Concentrations of ethylbenzene in uncontaminated groundwater are less than 0.1 µg per L. Higher concentrations have been found in contaminated groundwater from hydrocarbon releases, industrial facility releases, and waste disposal. Ethylbenzene is found also in effluents from wastewater and sewage treatment plants. Concentrations of ethylbenzene are elevated in urban areas owing to industrial releases.

The EPA studied ethylbenzene air concentrations in public buildings and found concentrations as high as 387 µg per cubic meter (90 ppb), which declined to 39 µg per cubic meter (9 ppb) several months after the buildings were completed (212). Ethylbenzene is emitted from carpet adhesives at a mean concentration of 6.4 µg per cubic meter, which corresponds to an emission rate of 77 ng per minute per square meter. Ethylbenzene is a common volatile organic chemical found in indoor building sites and new office buildings at levels ranging from 7.0 to 11.8 µg per cubic meter, as compared to 1.8 µg per cubic meter in the outdoor air (213,214).

Indoor air concentrations of ethylbenzene in randomly selected Canadian residences were studied in 1986, and mean concentrations were 6.46 µg per cubic meter in winter, 8.15 µg per cubic meter in spring, 4.35 µg per cubic meter in summer, and 13.97 µg per cubic meter in autumn (215).

Ethylbenzene also is contained in mainstream tobacco smoke, and blood concentrations of ethylbenzene can be measured in smokers as well as nonsmokers exposed to sidestream tobacco smoke (131). Combustion sources, including tobacco smoke, gasoline vapors, and other combustion products, contain ethylbenzene and increase human exposures to ethylbenzene.

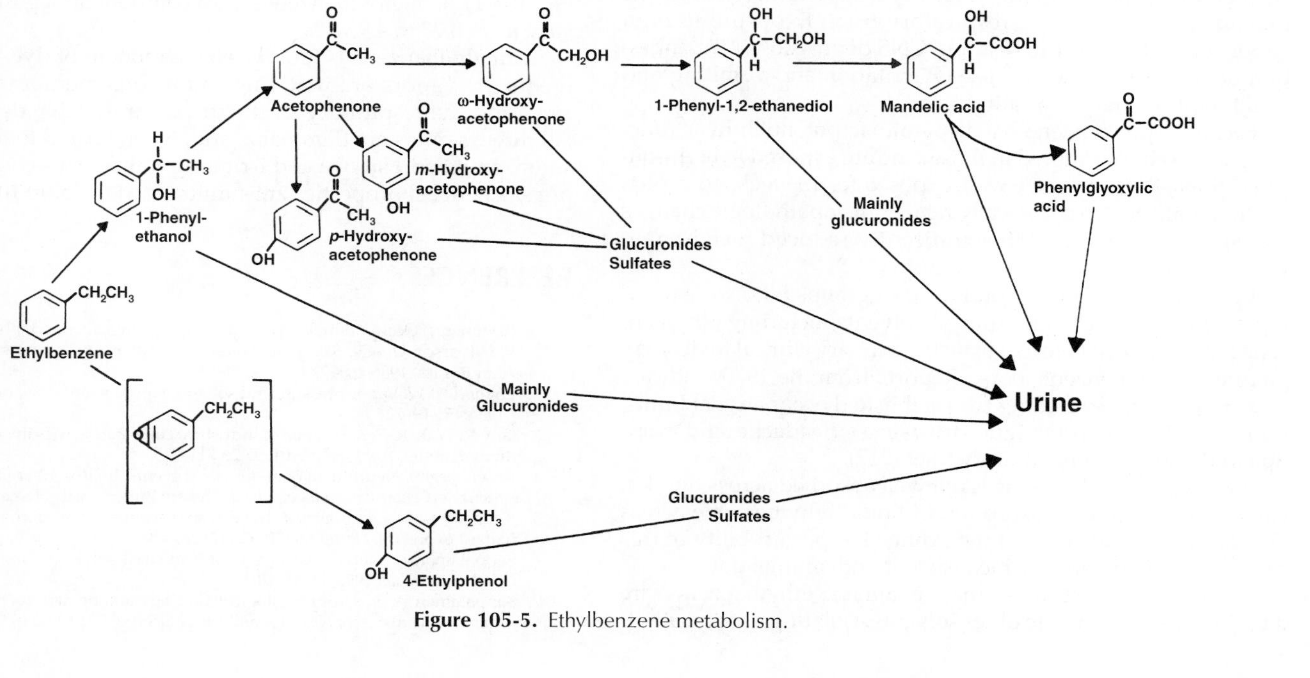

Figure 105-5. Ethylbenzene metabolism.

TABLE 105-18. Physiochemical properties of trimethylbenzene isomers

Property	1,3,5-Trimethylbenzene	1,2,3-Trimethylbenzene	1,2,4-Trimethylbenzene
Physical state	Colorless liquid	Colorless liquid	Colorless liquid
Molecular weight	120.19 D	120.19 D	120.19 D
Gasoline	1.32 wt%	0.73 wt%	4.9 wt%
Odor threshold			
In water	0.027 mg/L (0.00024–0.062 mg/L)	—	—
In air	0.1–1.0 mg/m^3	0.1–1.0 mg/m^3	0.1–1.0 mg/m^3
Vapor density	4.15	4.15	4.15
Specific gravity (20°C)	0.865	0.89	0.88
Conversion factor	1 ppm = 5 mg/m^3	1 ppm = 5 mg/m^3	1 ppm = 5 mg/m^3
Solubility	Miscible with ether, alcohol benzene; insoluble in water	Miscible with ether, alcohol benzene; insoluble in water	Miscible with ether, alcohol benzene; insoluble in water
Autoignition	1,022°F	878°F	959°F

Absorption, Metabolism, and Excretion

Ethylbenzene is readily absorbed via the inhalational, dermal, and GI routes. After systemic absorption, high concentrations are found in lungs, adipose tissue, kidneys, liver, and GI tract in those animals studied. Metabolism in animals is not the same as that in humans.

The metabolic transformation of ethylbenzene is shown in Figure 105-5. The main metabolic pathways involve oxidation of the side chains, and the main metabolites of ethylbenzene in humans are mandelic acid (64%) and phenylglyoxylic acid (25%) (171,216). Ethylbenzene is metabolized by the microsomal cytochrome P-450 enzyme system. The elimination half-life of ethylbenzene has been shown to vary from a few hours to 1 to 2 days, which is in agreement with the elimination of other volatile organic compounds, which have relatively resident times in the human body (216).

Clinical Toxicology

Ethylbenzene is absorbed via inhalation, ingestion, and dermal exposure, with dermal absorption in the range of 22 to 33 mg per square centimeter per hour (see Table 105-3) (64). Mucous membrane irritative effects from ethylbenzene occur at exposure to approximately 200 ppm.

Ethylbenzene possesses the potential to incite both acute and chronic toxic effects. Acutely, its vapors are an irritant to the mucous membranes and respiratory tract. Exposure to high vapor concentrations can result in CNS depression (217). Ingestion of ethylbenzene can cause GI irritation and vomiting and result in pulmonary aspiration.

Because ethylbenzene has hepatotoxic potential, liver functions should be monitored in those who are exposed to high concentrations. Rats and mice were exposed for 13 weeks to vapors of ethylbenzene. No chronically related histopathologic changes were observed and only insignificantly reduced weight gain was seen at an exposure of 1,000 ppm (212).

Epidemiologic studies conducted in groups who were occupationally exposed to mixtures of solvents including ethylbenzene have not been able to isolate the primary clinical toxicology picture of ethylbenzene alone. Reports from the 1970s indicate that at exposures exceeding the established occupational limits, human subjects report fatigue, drowsiness, headache, and irritation of the eyes and respiratory tract (217).

As a vapor, ethylbenzene is not well absorbed across the skin barrier. Although the absorption of liquid ethylbenzene across skin has been studied, data regarding skin permeability of this compound in humans are inconsistent with animal data.

Because most studies that evaluate ethylbenzene are designed also to evaluate other solvents, isolating data on ethylbenzene is difficult. Hence, little information is available on the long-term clinical toxic effects and the dose response or dose effect of ethylbenzene in humans.

Biological Monitoring

The determination of mandelic acid levels in urinary samples is a biomarker of exposure to ethylbenzene. A value of 1.5 g of mandelic acid per gram of creatinine is the post–work shift urinary level recommended as a BEI by the ACGIH (see Table 105-4). Measurement of phenylglyoxylic acid also is suggested for use as a biomarker (218).

Regulatory Aspects

The ACGIH TLV-TWA is 100 ppm (434 mg per cubic meter) and the STEL, 125 ppm (453 mg per cubic meter). The NIOSH's IDLH is 2,000 ppm.

TRIMETHYLBENZENE

Trimethylbenzenes are represented by the isomeric forms 1,2,3-trimethylbenzene (hemimellitene), 1,2,4-trimethylbenzene (pseudocumene), and 1,3,5-trimethylbenzene (mesitylene) (see Fig. 105-1). Trimethylbenzenes are a component of gasoline and vary from 0.73 to 4.9 wt%.

Trimethylbenzene is found as a component of dyes and pigments. Its vapors are irritating to mucous membranes, skin, eyes, and the respiratory tract and can cause CNS depression. All three isomers are flammable and, when heated to decomposition, emit acrid smoke and irritating fumes. This compound's physiochemical properties are summarized in Table 105-18.

REFERENCES

1. Juntunen J. Occupational solvent poisoning: clinical aspects. In: Riihimaki V, Ulfvarson U, eds. *Safety and health aspects of organic solvents.* New York: Alan R. Liss, 1986:265–279.
2. Popendorf W. Vapor pressure and solvent vapor hazards. *Am Ind Hyg Assoc J* 1984;45:719–726.
3. Guy R, Potts R. Penetrations of industrial chemicals across the skin—a predictive model. *Am J Ind Med* 1993;23:711–719.
4. Rosenberg N. Neurotoxicity of organic solvents. In: Rosenberg N, ed. *Occupational and environmental neurology.* Boston: Butterworth-Heinemann, 1995.
5. Kennedy S. Acquired airway hyperresponsiveness from nonimmunogenic irritant exposure. *Occup Med* 1992;7(2):287–300.
6. Seppalainen A. Neurotoxic effects of industrial solvents. *Electroencephalog Clin Neurophysiol* 1973;34:702–703.
7. Seppalainen A. Neurophysiological findings among workers exposed to organic solvents. *Acta Neurol Scand* 1982;66[Suppl 92]:109–116.

8. Mutti A, Cavatorta A, Lommi G, et al. Neurophysiological effects of long-term exposure to hydrocarbon mixtures. *Arch Toxicol* 1982;5:120–124.
9. Hagstadius S, Risberg J. Regional cerebral blood flow in subjects occupationally exposure to organic solvents. In: *Neurobehavioral methods in occupational health*. Oxford: Pergamon Press, 1983.
10. Arlien-Soborg P, Henriksen L, Gade A, et al. Cerebral blood flow in chronic toxic in-house painters exposed to organic solvents. *Acta Neurol* 1982;66:34–41.
11. Bolla K, Schwartz B, Agnew J, et al. Subclinical neuropsychiatric effects of chronic low level solvent exposure in U.S. paint manufacturers. *J Occup Med* 1990;32:671–677.
12. Errebo-Knudsen EO, Olsen F. Organic solvents and presenile dementia (the painters' syndrome). A critical review of the Danish literature. *Sci Total Environ* 1986;48:45–67.
13. Triebi G, Claus D, Csuzda I, et al. Cross-sectional epidemiological study on neurotoxicity of solvents in paints and lacquers. *Int Arch Occup Environ Health* 1988;60:233–241.
14. Errebo-Knudsen, Olsen F. Solvents and the brain: explanation of the discrepancy between the number of toxic encephalopathy reported (and compensated) in Denmark and other countries. *Br J Ind Med* 1987;44:71–72.
15. Maizlish NA, Langolf GD, Whitehead LW, et al. Behavioral evaluation of workers exposed to mixtures of organic solvents. *Br J Ind Med* 1985;42:579–590.
16. Baker EL, Smith TJ, Landrigan PJ. The neurotoxicity of industrial solvents: a review of the literature. *Am J Ind Med* 1985;8:207–217.
17. Flodin U, Edling C, Axelson O. Clinical studies of psychoorganic syndromes among workers with exposure to solvents. *Am J Ind Med* 1984;5:287–295.
18. Gregersen P, Angelso B, Nielson TE, Norgaard B, Uldal C. Neurotoxic effects of organic solvents in exposed workers: an occupational, neuropsychological and neurological investigation. *Am J Ind Med* 1984;5:201–225.
19. Morrow LA, Ryan CM, Goldstein G, Hodgson MJ. A distinct pattern of personality disturbance following exposure to mixtures of organic solvents. *J Occup Med* 1989;31:743–746.
20. Seppalainen AM, Lindstrom K, Martelin T. Neurophysiological and psychological picture of solvent poisoning. *Am J Ind Med* 1980;1:31–42.
21. Seppalainen AM. Neurophysiological aspects of the toxicity of organic solvents. *Scand J Work Environ Health* 1985;11:61–64.
22. Valciukas JA, Lilis R, Singer RM, Glickman L, Nicholson WJ. Neurobehavioral changes among shipyard painters exposed to solvents. *Arch Environ Health* 1985;40:47–52.
23. Gregersen P, Stigsby B. Reaction time of industrial workers exposed to organic solvents: relationship to degree of exposure and psychological performance. *Am J Ind Med* 1981;2:313–321.
24. Crossen JR, Wiens AN. Wechsler memory scale—revised: deficits in performance associated with neurotoxic solvent exposure. *Clin Neuropsychol* 1988;2:181–187.
25. Grasso P, Sharbratt M, Davies DM, Irvine D. Neurophysiological and psychological disorders and occupational exposure to organic solvents. *Food Chem Toxicol* 1984;22:819–852.
26. Orbaek P, Lindgren M, Olivecrona H. Computed brain tomography and psychometric test performances in patients with solvent induced chronic toxic encephalopathy and healthy controls. *Br J Ind Med* 1987;44:175–179.
27. Rasmussen K, Jeppesen HJ, Sabroe S. Psychometric tests for assessment of brain function after solvent exposure. *Am J Ind Med* 1993;24:553–565.
28. Neuropsychological toxicology of solvents. In: Hartman DE, ed. *Neuropsychological toxicology identification and assessment of human neurotoxic syndromes.* New York: Pergamon Press, 1988.
29. Feldman R. In: *Occupational and environmental neurotoxicology.* Philadelphia: Lippincott-Raven Publishers, 1999.
30. White RF. Differential diagnosis of probable Alzheimer's disease and solvent encephalopathy in older workers. *Clin Neuropsychol* 1987;1:153–160.
31. Callender T, Moreno L, Subrainanian K, et al. Three-dimensional brain metabolic imaging in patients with toxic encephalopathy. *Environ Res* 1993;60:295–319.
32. Fincher C, Chang T, Harrell E, et al. Comparison of single photon emission computed tomography findings in cases of healthy adults and solvent-exposed adults. *Am J Ind Med* 1997;31:4–14.
33. Triberg G, Lang C. Brain imaging techniques applied to chemically solvent-exposed workers—current results and clinical evaluation. *Environ Res* 1993;61:239–250.
34. Rosenberg N, Spitz M, Filley C, et al. Central nervous system effects of chronic toluene abuse—clinical, brainstem evoked response and magnetic resonance imaging studies. *Neurotoxicol Teratol* 1988;10:489–495.
35. Shenker M, Jacobs J. Organic solvents. In: Harber P, Schenker M, Balmes J, eds. *Occupational and environmental respiratory disease.* St. Louis: Mosby, 1996.
36. De Ceaurriz JC, Micillino JC, Bonnet P, Guenier JP. Sensory irritation caused by various industrial airborne chemicals. *Toxicol Lett* 1981;9:137–143.
37. Hellquist H, Irander K, Edling C, Odkvist L. Nasal symptoms and histopathology in a group of spray-painters. *Acta Otolaryngol* 1983;96:495–500.
38. Riley A, Collings A, Browne N, Grasso P. Response of the upper respiratory tract of the rat to white spirit vapour. *Toxicol Lett* 1984;22:125–131.
39. Silverman D, Schatz R. Pulmonary microsomal alterations following short-term, low-level inhalation of *p*-xylene in rats. *Toxicology* 1991;65:271–281.
40. Jansen D, Timens W, Kraan J, et al. Symptomatic bronchial hyperresponsiveness and asthma. *Respir Med* 1997;91:121–134.
41. Keman S, Willemse B, Tollerud D, et al. Blood interleukin-8 production is increased in chemicals workers with bronchitic symptoms. *Am J Ind Med* 1997;32:670–673.
42. Seltzer J, et al. Effects of the indoor environment on health. *Occup Med* 1995;10(1).
43. Damgard G. Mechanisms of activation of the sensory irritant receptor by airborne chemicals. *Toxicology* 1991;21(3):183–208.
44. Farley J. Inhaled toxicants and airway hyper-responsiveness. *Annu Rev Pharmacol Toxicol* 1992;32:67–88.
45. Bascom R, Kesavanathan J, Swift D. Human susceptibility to indoor contaminants. *Occup Med* 1993;10(1):119–132.
46. Brooks SM, Weiss MA, Bernstein IL. Reactive airways dysfunction syndrome (RADS): persistent asthma syndrome after high-level irritant exposures. *Chest* 1985;58:376–384.
47. Alberts WM, doPico G. Reactive airways dysfunction syndromes 3. *Chest* 1996;109:1618–1626.
48. Harving H, Dahl R, Molhave L. Lung function and bronchial reactivity in asthmatics during exposure to volatile organic compounds. *Am Rev Respir Dis* 1991;143:751–754.
49. Andersen I, Lundquist G, Molhave L, et al. Human response to controlled levels of toluene in 6-hour exposures. *Scand J Work Environ Health* 1983;9:405–418.
50. Nielsen G, Alaire Y. Sensory irritation, pulmonary irritation, respiratory stimulation by airborne benzene and alkylbenzenes: prediction of safe industrial exposure levels in correlation with their thermodynamic properties. *Toxicol Appl Pharmacol* 1982;65:459–477.
51. Molhave L, Bach B, Pedersen O. Human reactions to low concentrations of volatile organic compounds. *Environ Int* 1986;12:167–175.
52. Laire G, Viaene M, Veulemans H, Masschelein R, Nemery B. Nocturnal oxygen desaturation, as assessed by home oximetry, in long-term solvent-exposed workers. *Am J Ind Med* 1997;32:656–664.
53. Nielsen G. Mechanisms of activation of the sensory irritant receptor by airborne chemicals. *Crit Rev Toxicol* 1991;21(3):183–208.
54. Koren H, Graham DE, Devlin RB. Exposure of humans to volatile organic mixture: III. Inflammatory response. *Arch Environ Health* 1992;47(1):39–44.
55. Cain W. Irritation and odor as indicators of indoor air pollution. *Occup Med* 1995;10(1):133–145.
56. Uchida Y, Nakatsuka H, Ukai H, et al. Symptoms and signs of workers exposed predominantly to xylenes. *Int Arch Occup Environ Health* 1993;64:597–605.
57. Klancke D, Johansen M, Vogt R. An outbreak of xylene intoxication in a hospital. *Am J Ind Med* 1982;3:173–178.
58. Brooks S. Occupational asthma. In: Weiss E, Stein M, eds. *Bronchial asthma: mechanisms and therapeutics,* 3rd ed. Boston: Little, Brown and Company, 1993.
59. Jones K, Brautbar N. Reactive airway disease in patients with prolonged exposure to industrial solvents. *Toxicol Ind Health* 1997;13(6):743–750.
60. Sataloff R. The impact of pollution on the voice. *Otolaryngol Head Neck Surg* 1992;106(6):701–706.
61. Lunch R, Kipen H. Building-related illness and employee lost time following application of hot asphalt roof: a call for prevention. *Toxicol Ind Health* 1998;14(6):857–868.
62. Belum J, Anderson I, Molhave L. Acute and subacute symptoms among workers in the printing industry. *Br J Ind Med* 1982;39:70–75.
63. Dutkiewicz T, Tyras H. Skin absorption of toluene, styrene and xylene by man. *Br J Ind Med* 1968;25:243.
64. Dutkiewicz T, Tyras H. A study of skin absorption of ethylbenzene in man. *Br J Ind Med* 1967;24:330–332.
65. Brown HS, Bishop DR, Rowan CA. The role of skin absorption as a route of exposure for volatile organic compounds (VOCs) in drinking water. *Am J Public Health* 1984;74:479–484.
66. Agency for Toxic Substances and Disease Registry. *Toxicological profile for toluene*. Atlanta: US Department of Health and Human Services, Public Health Service, ATSDR, 1994.
67. Thibodeaux L, Hwang S. Land farming of petroleum wastes: modeling the emissions problem. *Environ Progr* 1982;1:42–46.
68. Hoshino M, Alimoto H, Okyda M. Photochemical oxidation of benzene, toluene and ethylbenzene initiated by hydroxyl radicals in gas phase. *Bull Chem Soc Jpn* 1978;51:718–724.
69. De Rosa E, Bartolucci GB, Sigon M, et al. Hippuric acid and orthocresol as biological indicators of occupational exposure to toluene. *Am J Ind Med* 1987;11:529–537.
70. Hasegawa K, Shiojima S, Koizumi A, Ikeda M. Hippuric acid and *o*-cresol in the urine of workers exposed to toluene. *Int Arch Occup Environ Health* 1983;52:197–208.
71. Angerer J. Occupational chronic exposure to organic solvents: XII. *o*-Cresol excretion after toluene exposure. *Int Arch Occup Environ Health* 1985;56:323–328.
72. De Rosa E, Brugnone F, Bartolucci GB, et al. The validity of urinary metabolites as indicators of low exposures to toluene. *Int Arch Occup Environ Health* 1985;56:135–145.
73. Andersson R, Carlsson A, Nordqvist MB, Sollenberg J. Urinary excretion of hippuric acid and *o*-cresol after laboratory exposure of humans to toluene. *Int Arch Occup Environ Health* 1983;53:101–108.
74. Medinsky M, Schlosser P, Bond J. Critical issues in benzene toxicity and metabolism: the effect of interactions with other organic chemicals on risk assessment. *Environ Health Perspect* 1994;102[Suppl 9]:119–124.
75. Low LK, Meeks JR, Mackerer CR. Health effects of the alkylbenzenes: toluene. *Toxicol Ind Health* 1988;4:49–75.
76. Carlsson A. Exposure to toluene uptake, distribution and elimination in man. *Br J Work Environ Health* 1982;8:43–55.
77. Tahti H, Karkkainen S, Pyykko K, et al. Chronic occupational exposure to toluene. *Int Arch Occup Environ Health* 1981;48:61–69.

78. Hyden D, Larsby B, Anderson H, et al. Impairment of visuovestibular interaction in humans exposed to toluene. *Autorhinolaryngology* 1983;45:262–269.
79. Zavalic M, Mandic Z, Turk R, et al. Quantitative assessment of color vision impairment in workers exposed to toluene. *Am J Ind Med* 1998;33:297–304.
80. Feldman R. Toluene. In: *Occupational and environmental neurotoxicology.* Philadelphia: Lippincott-Raven Publishers, 1999.
81. Rosenberg NL, Kleinschmidt-DeMasters BK, Davis KA, Hormes JT. Toluene abuse causes diffuse central nervous system white matter changes. *Ann Neurol* 1988;23:611–614.
82. Keane JR. Toluene optic neuropathy. *Ann Neurol* 1978;4:390.
83. Purcell K, Cason G, Gargas M, et al. In vivo metabolic interactions of benzene and toluene. *Toxicol Lett* 1990;52:141–152.
84. Lam C, Galen T, Boyd J, et al. Mechanism of transport and distribution of organic solvents in blood. *Toxicol Appl Pharmacol* 1990;104:117–129.
85. Bergman K. Application and results of whole body autoradiography in distribution studies of organic studies. *Crit Rev Toxicol* 1979;12:59–118.
86. Gospe S, Calaban M. Central nervous system distribution of inhaled toluene. *Fund Appl Toxicol* 1988;11:540–545.
87. Ameno K, Kiriu T, Fuke C, Ameno S, Shinohara T, Ijiri I. Regional brain distribution of toluene in rats and in a human autopsy. *Arch Toxicol* 1992; 66:153–156.
88. Ameno K, Fuke C, Setsuko A, Takahiro K, Kazuhiko S, Ijiri I. A fatal case of oral ingestion of toluene. *Forensic Sci Int* 1989;41:255–260.
89. Xiong L, Matthes J, Li J, Jinkins R. MR imaging of "spray heads": toluene abuse via aerosol paint inhalation. *J Am Soc Neuroradiol* 1993;14:1195–1199.
90. Vrca A, Bozicevic D, Karacic V, et al. Visual evoked potentials in individuals exposed to long-term low concentrations of toluene. *Arch Toxicol* 1995; 69:337–340.
91. Klockars M. Solvents and the liver. In: Riihimaki V, Ulfvarson U, eds. *Safety and health aspects of organic solvents.* New York: Alan R. Liss, 1986:139–154.
92. Hayden JW. Toxicology of toluene (methylbenzene): a review of current literature. *Clin Toxicol* 1977;11:549–559.
93. Cohr KH, Stokholm J. Toluene—a toxicologic review. *Scand J Work Environ Health* 1979;5:71–90.
94. Dossing M, Arlien-Soborg P, Petersen L, Ranek L. Liver damage associated with occupational exposure to organic solvents in house painters. *Eur J Clin Invest* 1983;13:151–157.
95. Batlle D, Sabatini S, Kurtzman N. On the mechanism of toluene-induced renal tubular acidosis. *Nephron* 1988;49:210–218.
96. Kamijima M, Nakazawa Y, Yamakawa M, et al. Metabolic acidosis and renal tubular injury due to pure toluene inhalation. *Arch Environ Health* 1994; 49(5):410–413.
97. Ng T, Ong S, Lam W, et al. Urinary levels of proteins and metabolites in workers exposed to toluene. *Int Arch Occup Environ Health* 1990;62:43–46.
98. Gupta R, van der Meulen J, Johny K. Oliguric acute renal failure due to gluesniffing. *Scand J Urol Nephrol* 1991;25:247–250.
99. Guzelian P, Mills S, Fallon H. Liver structure and function in print workers exposed to toluene. *J Occup Med* 1988;30(10):791–796.
100. Taverner D, Harrison D, Bell G. Acute renal failure due to interstitial nephritis induced by "glue-sniffing" with subsequent recovery. *Scot Med J* 1988;33:246–247.
101. Taher SM, Anderson RJ, McCartney R, Popovtzer MM, Schrier RW. Renal tubular acidosis associated with toluene "sniffing." *N Engl J Med* 1974;290: 765–768.
102. Moss AH, Gabow PA, Kaehny WD, et al. Fanconi's syndrome and distal renal tubular acidosis after glue sniffing. *Ann Intern Med* 1980;92:69–70.
103. Voigts A, Kaufman CE. Acidosis and other metabolic abnormalities associated with paint sniffing. *South Med J* 1983;76:443–452.
104. Goodwin TM. Toluene abuse and renal tubular acidosis in pregnancy. *Obstet Gynecol* 1988;71:715–718.
105. Nielsen HK, Krusell L, Baelum J, et al. Renal effects of acute exposure to toluene. *Acta Med Scand* 1985;218:317–321.
106. Bennett RH, Forman HR. Hypokalemic periodic paralysis in chronic toluene exposure. *Arch Neurol* 1980;37:673.
107. Lindbohm M, Taskinen H, Salimen M, et al. Spontaneous abortions among women exposed to organic solvents. *Am J Ind Med* 1990;17:449–463.
108. Hersh JH, Podruch PE, Rogers G, Weisskopf B. Toluene embryopathy. *J Pediatr* 1985;106:922–927.
109. Holmberg PC. Central nervous system defects in children born to mothers exposed to organic solvents during pregnancy. *Lancet* 1979;2(8135):177–179.
110. Ng T, Foo S, Yoong T. Risk of spontaneous abortion in workers exposed to toluene. *Br J Ind Med* 1992;49:804–808.
111. Svensson B, Nise G, Erfurth E, et al. Hormone status in occupational toluene exposure. *Am J Ind Med* 1992;22:99–107.
112. Svensson B, Nise G, Erfurth E, et al. Neuroendocrine effects in printing workers exposed to toluene. *Br J Ind Med* 1992;49:402–408.
113. Lindeman R. Congenital renal tubular dysfunction associated with maternal sniffing of organic solvents. *Acta Pediatr Scand* 1991;80:882–884.
114. Wilkins-Haug L, Gabow P. Toluene abuse during pregnancy: obstetric complications and perinatal outcomes. *Obstet Gynecol* 1991;77:504–509.
115. Maki-Paakkanen J, Husgafvel-Pursiainen K, Kalliomak PL, Tuominen J, Sorsa M. Toluene-exposed workers and chromosome aberrations. *J Toxicol Environ Health* 1960;6(4):775–781.
116. Haglund U, Lundberg I, Zech L. Chromosome aberrations and sister chromatid exchanges in Swedish paint industry workers. *Scand J Work Environ Health* 1980;6:291–298.
117. Forni A, Pacifico E, Limonta A. Chromosome studies in workers exposed to benzene or toluene or both. *Arch Environ Health* 1971;22:373–378.
118. Hsieh G, Sharma P, Parker R. Immunotoxicological evaluation of toluene exposure via drinking water in mice. *Environ Res* 1989;49:93–103.
119. Baelum J, Andersen IB, Lundqvist GR, et al. Response of solvent-exposed printers and unexposed controls to six-hour toluene exposure. *Scand J Work Environ Health* 1985;11:271–280.
120. Inoue O, Seiji K, Watanabe T, et al. Possible ethnic difference in toluene metabolism: a comparative study among Chinese, Turkish, and Japanese solvent workers. *Toxicol Lett* 1986;34:167–174.
121. Wallen M, Naslund H, Nordqvist B. The effects of ethanol on the kinetics of toluene in man. *Toxicol Appl Pharmacol* 1984;76:414–419.
122. Dossing M, Baelum J, Hansen SH, Lundqvist GR. Effect of ethanol, cimetidine and propranolol on toluene metabolism in man. *Int Arch Occup Environ Health* 1984;54:309–315.
123. Howell S, Christian J, Isom G. The hepatotoxic potential of combined toluene–chronic ethanol exposure. *Arch Toxicol* 1986;59:45–50.
124. Baelum J, Molhave L, Hansen S, Dossing M. Hepatic metabolism of toluene after gastrointestinal uptake in humans. *Scand J Work Environ Health* 1993;19:55–62.
125. Konietzko H, Keilbach J, Drysch K. Cumulative effects of daily toluene exposure. *Int Arch Occup Environ Health* 1980;46:53–58.
126. Aitio A, Pekari K, Jarvisalo J. Skin absorption as a source of error in biological monitoring. *Scand J Work Environ Health* 1984;10:317–320.
127. Andrews L, Lee E, Witmer C. Effects of toluene on the metabolism, disposition and hemopoietic toxicity of [^{3}H] benzene. *Biochem Pharmacol* 1977; 26:293–300.
128. Inoue O, Seiji K, Watanabe T, et al. Mutual metabolic suppression between benzene and toluene in man. *Int Arch Occup Environ Health* 1988;60:15–20.
129. Plappert U, Barthel E, Seidel H. Reduction of benzene toxicity by toluene. *Environ Mol Mutagen* 1994;24:283–292.
130. Fay M, Eisenmann C, Diwan S, de Rosa C. ATSDR evaluation of health effects of chemicals: V. Xylenes: health effects, toxicokinetics, human exposure and environmental fate. *Toxicol Ind Health* 1998;14(5):571–781.
131. Harjimiragha H, Ewers U, Brockhaus A, et al. Levels of benzene and other volatile aromatic compounds in the blood of nonsmokers and smokers. *Int Arch Occup Environ Health* 1989;61:513–518.
132. Wallace L, Pellizzari E, Hartwell T, et al. The California team study: breath concentrations and personal exposures to 26 volatile compounds in air and drinking water of 188 residents of Los Angeles, Antioch, and Pittsburg, CA. *Atmos Environ* 1988;22:2141–2163.
133. Wallace L, Pellizzari E, Hartweel T, et al. Concentrations of 20 volatile organic compounds in air and drinking water of 350 residents of New Jersey compared with concentrations in their exhaled breath. *J Occup Med* 1986;28:603–608.
134. Ashley D, Bonin M, Cardinali F, et al. Determining volatile organic compounds in human blood from a large sample production by using purge and trap gas chromatography–mass spectrometry. *Anal Chem* 1992;64:1021–1029.
135. Riihimaki V, Savolainen K. Human exposure to *m*-xylene kinetics and acute effects on the central nervous system. *Ann Occup Hyg* 1980;23:411–422.
136. Riihimaki V, Savolainen K, Pfaffli P, Pekari K, Sippel HW, Laine A. Metabolic interaction between *m*-xylene and ethanol. *Arch Toxicol* 1982;49:253–263.
137. Lundberg I, Hakansson M. Normal serum activities of liver enzymes in Swedish paint industry workers with heavy exposure to organic solvents. *Br J Ind Med* 1985;42:596–600.
138. Riihimaki V, Pfaffli P, Savolainen K. Kinetics of *m*-xylene in man. Influence of intermittent physical exercise and changing environmental concentrations on kinetics. *Scand J Work Environ Health* 1979;5:232–248.
139. Lapere S, Tardif R, Brodeur J. Effects of various exposure scenarios on the biological monitoring of organic solvents in alveolar air. *Int Arch Occup Environ Health* 1993;64:569–580.
140. Engstrom K, Husman K, Riihimake V. Percutaneous absorption of *m*-xylene in man. *Int Arch Occup Environ Health* 1977;39:181–189.
141. Riihimaki V, Pfaffli P. Percutaneous absorption of solvent vapors in man. *Scand J Work Environ Health* 1978;4:73–85.
142. Engerstrom K, Bjurstrom R. Exposure to xylene and ethylbenzene: II. Concentration in subcutaneous adipose tissue. *Scand J Work Environ Health* 1978;4:195–203.
143. Kawai T, Mizunuma K, Yasugi T. Urinary methylhippuric acid isomer levels after occupational exposure to a xylene mixture. *Int Arch Occup Environ Health* 1991;63:69–75.
144. Kiira J, Riihimaki V, Engstrom K. Coexposure of man to *m*-xylene and methyl ethyl ketone. Kinetics and metabolism. *Scand J Work Environ Health* 1988;14:322–327.
145. Sato A, Endoh K, Kaneko T, Johanson G. Effects of consumption of ethanol on the biological monitoring of exposure to organic solvent vapors: a simulation study with trichloroethylene. *Br J Ind Med* 1991(1);48:548–556.
146. Morley R, Eccleston D, Douglas C, et al. Xylene poisoning: a report on one fatal case and two cases of recovery after prolonged unconsciousness. *BMJ* 1970;3:442–443.
147. Roberts F, Lucas E, Marsden E, et al. Near-pure xylene causing reversible neuropsychiatric disturbance [Letter]. *Lancet* 1988;2:273.
148. Hipolito R. Xylene poisoning in laboratory workers: case reports and discussion. *Lab Med* 1980;11:593–595.

149. Langman J. Xylene: its toxicity, measurement of exposure levels, absorption, metabolism and clearance. *Pathology* 1994;26:301–309.
150. Feldman R. Xylene. In: *Occupational and environmental neurotoxicology*. Philadelphia: Lippincott-Raven Publishers, 1999.
151. Laine A, Savolainen K, Riihimaki V. Acute effects of *m*-xylene inhalation on body sway, reaction times, and sleep in man. *Int Arch Occup Environ Health* 1993;65:179–188.
152. Carpenter C, Kinkead E, Geary D, et al. Petroleum hydrocarbon toxicity studies: V. Animal and human response to vapors of mixed xylenes. *Toxicol Appl Pharmacol* 1975;33:553–558.
153. Gamberale F, Annwall G, Hultengren M. Exposure to xylene and ethylbenzene: III. Effects on central nervous functions. *Scand J Work Environ Health* 1978;4:204–211.
154. Hastings L, Cooper G, Burg W. Human sensory response to selected petroleum hydrocarbons. *Adv Mod Environ Toxicol* 1986;6.
155. Dudek B, Gralewicz K, Jakubowski M, et al. Neurobehavioral effects of experimental exposure to toluene, xylene and their mixture, POL. *J Occup Med* 1990;3:109–116.
156. Savolainen KN, Riihimaki V. An early sign of xylene effect on human equilibrium. *Acta Pharmacol Toxicol* 1981;48:279–283.
157. Savolainen KN. Combined effects of xylene and alcohol on the central nervous system. *Acta Pharmacol Toxicol* 1980;46:366–372.
158. Ruitjen M, Hooisma J, Brons J. Neurobehavioral effects of long-term exposure to xylene and mixed organic solvents in shipyard painters. *Neurotoxicology* 1994;15:613–620.
159. Tardif R, Lapare S, Plaa G. Effect of simultaneous exposure to toluene and xylene on their respective biological exposure indices in humans. *Int Arch Occup Environ Health* 1991;63:279–284.
160. Campbell L, Wilson H, Sammuel A. Interactions of *m*-xylene and aspirin metabolism in man. *Br J Ind Med* 1988;45:127–132.
161. Chemical review: styrene. *Danger Prop Ind Mat Rep* 1988;8:10–44.
162. Hong Fu M, Alexander M. Biodegradation of styrene in samples of natural environments. *Environ Sci Technol* 1992;26:1540–1544.
163. Ashley D, Bonnin M, Cardinali F, McCraw JM, Wooten JV. Blood concentrations of volatile organic compounds in nonoccupationally exposed U.S. population and in groups with suspected exposure. *Clin Chem* 1994; 40:1401–1404.
164. Murphy P, MacDonald A, Lickly T. Styrene migration from general-purpose and high-impact polystyrene into food stimulating solvents. *Food Chem Toxicol* 1992;39(3):225–232.
165. Engstrom J, Bjurstrom R, Astrand I. Uptake, distribution and elimination of styrene in man: concentration in subcutaneous adipose tissue. *Scand J Work Environ Health* 1978;4:315–323.
166. Bond J. Review of the toxicology of styrene. *Crit Rev Toxicol* 1989;3:227–249.
167. Berode M, Droz P, Guillemin M. Human exposure to styrene: VI. Percutaneous absorption in human volunteers. *Int Arch Occup Environ Health* 1985; 55:331–336.
168. Pahwa R, Kalra J. A critical review of the neurotoxicity of styrene in humans. *Vet Hum Toxicol* 1993;35:516–520.
169. Feldman R. Styrene. In: *Occupational and environmental neurotoxicology*. Philadelphia: Lippincott-Raven Publishers, 1999.
170. Leibman K. Metabolism and toxicity of styrene. *Environ Health Perspect* 1975;11:115–119.
171. Bardodej Z, Bardodejova E. Biotransformation of ethylbenzene, styrene and alpha methyl styrene in man. *Am Ind Hyg Assoc J* 1970;31:206–209.
172. Cerny S, Mraz J, Flek J. Effect of ethanol on the urinary excretion of mandelic acid and phenylglyoxylic acids after human exposure to styrene. *Int Arch Occup Health* 1990;62:243–247.
173. Ikeda M, Hirayama T. Possible metabolic interaction of styrene with organic solvents. *Scand J Work Environ Health* 1978;4:41–46.
174. Coccini T, Di Nucci A, Tonini M. Effects of ethanol administration on cerebral non-protein sulfhydryl content in rats exposed to styrene vapour. *Toxicology* 1996;106:115–122.
175. Guillemin MP, Berode M. Biological monitoring of styrene: a review. *Am Ind Hyg Assoc J* 1988;49:497–505.
176. Ohtsuji H, Ikeda M. The metabolism of styrene in the rat and the stimulatory effect of phenobarbital. *Toxicol Appl Pharmacol* 1991;18:321–328.
177. Parke D. Activation mechanisms to chemical toxicity. *Arch Toxicol* 1987;60:5–15.
178. Trenga C, Kunkel D, Eaton D. Effects of styrene oxide on rat brain glutathione. *Neurotoxicology* 1991;12:165–168.
179. Engstrom J. Styrene in subcutaneous adipose tissue after experimental and industrial exposure. *Scand J Work Environ Health* 1978;4:119–120.
180. Stewart R, Dodd H, Baretta B. Human exposure to styrene vapor. *Arch Environ Health* 1968;16:656–662.
181. Geuskens R, Vander Klaauw M, et al. Exposure to styrene and health complaints in the Dutch glass reinforced plastic industry. *Ann Occup Hyg* 1992; 36:47–57.
182. Matikainen E, Forsman-Gronholm L, Pfaffli P. Nervous system effects of occupational exposure to styrene: a clinical and neurophysiological study. *Environ Res* 1993;61:84–92.
183. Triebig G, Lehrl S, Weltle D, et al. Clinical and neurobehavioral study of acute and chronic neurotoxicity of styrene. *Br J Ind Med* 1989;46:799–804.
184. Rebert C, Hall T. The neuroepidemiology of styrene: a critical review of representative literature. *Crit Rev Toxicol* 1994;24[Suppl 1]:S57–S106.
185. Seppalainen A, Harkonen H. Neurophysiological findings among workers occupationally exposed to styrene. *Scand J Work Environ Health* 1976;3:140–146.
186. Rosen I, Haeger-Aronsen B, Rehnstrom S. Neurophysiological observations after chronic styrene exposure. *Scand J Work Environ Health* 1978; 4:184–194.
187. Stetkarova I, Urban P, Prochazka B. Somatosensory evoked potentials in workers exposed to toluene and styrene. *Br J Ind Med* 1993;50:520–527.
188. Murata K, Araki S, Yokoyama K. Assessment of the peripheral, central and autonomic nervous system function in styrene workers. *Am J Ind Med* 1991;20:775–784.
189. Lilis R, Lorimer W, Diamond S. Neurotoxicity of styrene in production and polymerization workers. *Environ Res* 1978;15:133–138.
190. Yuasa J, Reiko K, Eguchi T, et al. Study of urinary mandelic acid concentration and peripheral nerve conduction among styrene workers. *Am J Ind Med* 1996;30:41–47.
191. Cherry N, Gautrin D. Neurotoxic effects of styrene; further evidence. *Br J Ind Med* 1990;47:29–37.
192. Ledin T, Odkvist L, Moller C. Posturography findings in workers exposed to industrial solvents. *Acta Otolaryngol* 1989;107:357–361.
193. Moller C, Odkvist L, Larsby B. Otoneurological findings in workers exposed to styrene. *Scand J Work Environ Health* 1990;16:189–194.
194. Fallas C, Fallas J, Maslar DP. Subclinical impairment of color vision among workers exposed to styrene. *Br J Ind Med* 1992;49:679–682.
195. Jegaden D, Amann D, Simon J. Study of the neurobehavioral toxicity of styrene at low levels of exposure. *Int Arch Occup Environ Health* 1993;64:527–531.
196. Letz R, Mahoney F, Hershman D. Neurobehavioral effects of acute styrene exposure in fiberglass boat builders. *Neurotoxicol Teratol* 1990;12:665–668.
197. Floden U, Ekberg K, Angersson L. Neuropsychiatric effects of low exposure to styrene. *Br J Ind Med* 1989;46:805–808.
198. Rosengren L, Haglid K. Long-term neurotoxicity of styrene. A quantitative study of glial fibrillary acidic protein (GFA) and S-100. *Br J Ind Med* 1989;46:316–320.
199. Dypbukt J, Costa L, Manzo L. Cytotoxic and genotoxic effects of styrene-7,8-oxide in neuradrenergic PC-12 cells. *Carcinogenesis* 1992;13:417–424.
200. Romanelli A, Falzoi M, Mutti A. Effects of some monocyclic aromatic solvents and their metabolites on brain dopamine in rabbits. *J Appl Toxicol* 1986;6:431–436.
201. Ikeda M, Imamura T, Hayaskh M, Tabuchi T, Hara I. Evaluation of hippuric acid, phenylglyoxylic acid, and mandelic acid in urine as indices of styrene exposure. *Int Arch Arbeitsmed* 1974;32:93–101.
202. Drummond L, Coldwell J, Wilson H. The metabolism of ethylbenzene and styrene to mandelic acid: stereochemical considerations. *Xenobiotica* 1989; 19:199–207.
203. Ghittori S, Maestri L, Imbriani M, et al. Urinary excretion of specific mercapturic acids in workers exposed to styrene. *Am J Ind Med* 1997;31:636–644.
204. Sinsheimer J, Chen R, Das S, et al. The genotoxicity of enantiomeric aliphatic epoxides. *Mutat Res* 1993;298:197–206.
205. World Health Organization. *Chlorobenzenes other than hexachlorobenzenes*. Environmental health criteria 128. Geneva: World Health Organization, 1991.
206. Lu P, Metcalf R. Environmental fate and biodegradability of benzene derivatives as studied in a model aquatic ecosystem. *Environ Health Perspect* 1975;10:269–284.
207. Schwarzenbach R, Giger W, Hoehn E, et al. Behavior of organic compounds during infiltration of river water to ground water. *Field Stud Environ Sci Technol* 1983;17:472–479.
208. Wilson J, Enfield C, Dunlap W, et al. Transport and fate of selected organic pollutants in a sandy soil. *J Environ Qual* 1981;10(4):501–506.
209. Zoeteman B, Harmsen K, Linders J, et al. Persistent organic pollutants in river water and ground water of the Netherlands. *Chemosphere* 1980;9:231–249.
210. Sullivan T, Boren G, Carlson G, et al. The pharmacokinetics of inhaled chlorobenzene in the rat. *Toxicol Appl Pharmacol* 1983;71:194–203.
211. Zapata-Gayon C, Zapata-Gayon N, Gonzales-Angulo A. Clastogenic chromosomal aberrations in 26 individuals accidentally exposed to orthodichlorobenzene vapors in the National Medical Center in Mexico City. *Arch Environ Health* 1982;37(4):231–235.
212. World Health Organization. *Ethylbenzene*. Environmental health criteria 186. Geneva: World Health Organization, 1996.
213. Wallace L, Pellizzari E, Hartwell T, et al. The TEAM study: personal exposure to toxic substances in air, drinking water and breath of 400 residents of New Jersey, North Carolina, and North Dakota. *Environ Res* 1987;43:290–307.
214. Wallace L, Pellizzari E, Leaderer B. Emissions of volatile organic compounds from building materials and consumer products. *Atmosph Environ* 1987;21(2):385–393.
215. Fellin P, Otson R. Seasonal trends of volatile organic compounds (VOCs) in Canadian homes. In: *Proceedings of the sixth conference on indoor air quality and climate*, vol 2. 1993:117–122.
216. Pellizzari E, Wallace L, Gordon S. Elimination kinetics of volatile organics in humans using breath measurements. *J Expo Analyt Environ Epidemiol* 1992;2:341–355.
217. Toxicology update: ethylbenzene. *J Appl Toxicol* 1992;12(1):69–71.
218. Inoue O, Seiji K, Kudo S, et al. Urinary phenylglyoxylic acid excretion after exposure to ethylbenzene among exposed Chinese workers. *Int J Occup Environ Health* 1995;1:1–8.

CHAPTER 106
Solvents and Chemical Intermediates

Kimberlie A. Graeme and John B. Sullivan, Jr.

SOLVENT CHARACTERISTICS: PROTIC AND APROTIC

Solvents can be subdivided into the general categories of protic and aprotic, depending on their reactivity. Aprotic solvents have strong ionizing powers, are able to dissolve ionic reagents (which often are inorganic chemicals), and promote dissociation of organic molecules. Aprotic solvents such as dimethylformamide (DMF) and dimethyl sulfoxide (DMSO) dissolve both organic and inorganic compounds but, during the dissolution of these compounds, these solvents leave the anionic portions unencumbered and highly reactive for further chemical reactions.

Water and alcohol are protic solvents, because they contain hydrogen that is attached to oxygen or nitrogen and they are acidic in nature. Protic solvents strongly solvate anions, and these anions, as bases or nucleophiles, usually are the important components of an ionic reagent. Thus, protic solvents can drastically lower the reactivity of compounds.

Table 106-1 lists identifying characteristics and occupational exposure limits of several solvents and reactive intermediary compounds discussed in this chapter. Figure 106-1 depicts the chemical structures of these solvents.

BUTYL MERCAPTANS

Butyl mercaptans ($C_4H_{10}S$) possess a strong, disagreeable, skunklike or rotten-egg odor. Butyl mercaptans exist in four isomeric forms: (i) isobutyl mercaptan, (ii) *n*-butyl mercaptan, (iii) sec-butyl mercaptan, and (iv) *tert*-butyl mercaptan.

Isobutyl Mercaptan

Isobutyl mercaptan [$CH_3CH(CH_3)CH_2SH$; 2-methyl-1-propanethiol] is a flammable liquid that reacts with oxidizing materials. Central nervous system (CNS) effects have been demonstrated in animal models. Isobutyl mercaptan is an irritant that is absorbed after ingestion or inhalation (1).

n-Butyl Mercaptan

n-Butyl mercaptan [$CH_3(CH_2)_3SH$; thiobutyl alcohol] is a colorless, flammable liquid that is prepared by reacting *n*-butylene and hydrogen sulfide with a catalyst or by passing vapors of butanol and hydrogen sulfide over a catalyst (1). *n*-Butyl mercaptan is used as a solvent, in the production of pesticides, and as an odorant.

In animals, CNS depression, ataxia, weakness, tremors, anorexia, and ocular and mucous membrane irritation have been reported. *n*-Butyl mercaptan is known to be an ocular and mucous membrane irritant. The strong, objectionable sulfhydryllike odor generally limits significant exposures; however, systemic toxicity has been reported (1).

Accidental exposure of seven workers for 1 hour at concentrations 5 to 50 times the U.S. Occupational Safety and Health Administration permissible exposure limit (PEL) resulted in sweating, nausea, vomiting, headache, dizziness, muscular weakness, malaise, confusion, and coma (1). *n*-Butyl mercaptan does not appear to be mutagenic. The American Conference of Governmental Industrial Hygienists has set a threshold limit value of 0.5 parts per million (ppm), and the Occupational Safety and Health Administration PEL is 10 ppm. The odor threshold is 0.001 to 0.001 ppm. The level that is considered immediately dangerous to life and health (IDLH) is 2,500 ppm (2,3).

DIMETHYLFORMAMIDE

DMF, which is used in the manufacturing of polyurethane products and in the pharmaceutical industry, is well absorbed by the skin and also by inhalation of vapors and is metabolized by the liver. DMF [$(CH_3)_2NCHO$] is a colorless liquid with an unpleasant taste and an ammonia odor. The odor threshold ranges from 0.12 to 0.15 mg per cubic meter (4). DMF is a stable, hygroscopic compound, which means that it easily absorbs water from the atmosphere. As such, DMF must be stored under dry nitrogen. It reacts readily with alkyl aluminums, carbon tetrachloride, halogenated hydrocarbons, and strong oxidizing agents, which can result in explosions and fire (4). Table 106-2 lists the physiochemical properties of DMF.

TABLE 106-1. Occupational exposure limits for select solvents and intermediates

Solvent	Description	OSHA PEL	ACGIH TLV	IDLH
Isobutyl mercaptan	Colorless; skunklike odor	10 ppm TWA (35 mg/m^3)	0.5 ppm TWA (1.8 mg/m^3)	—
n-Butyl mercaptan	Colorless to yellow; skunklike odor	10 ppm TWA (35 mg/m^3)	0.5 ppm TWA (1.8 mg/m^3)	2,500 ppm
Dimethylformamide	Colorless to pale yellow; aminelike odor	10 ppm TWA (30 mg/m^3)	10 ppm TWA (30 mg/m^3)	3,500 ppm
Naphtha (coal tar)	Colorless to reddish brown; aromatic odor	100 ppm TWA (400 mg/m^3)	400 ppm TWA (1,590 mg/m^3)	10,000 ppm
Petroleum naphtha	—	500 ppm	—	20,000 ppm
Nitroethane	Colorless and oily; fruity odor	100 ppm TWA (310 mg/m^3)	100 ppm TWA (307 mg/m^3)	—
Nitromethane	Colorless and oily; disagreeable odor	100 ppm TWA (250 mg/m^3)	100 ppm TWA (250 mg/m^3)	—
2-Nitropropane	Colorless and oily; pleasant, fruity odor	25 ppm TWA (90 mg/m^3)	10 ppm TWA (36 mg/m^3)	—
Pyridine	Colorless to yellow; nauseating, fishlike odor	5 ppm TWA (15 mg/m^3)	5 ppm TWA (16 mg/m^3)	3,600 ppm
Stoddard solvent	Colorless; kerosenelike odor	500 ppm TWA (2,900 mg/m^3)	100 ppm TWA (525 mg/m^3)	—
Turpentine	Colorless; characteristic odor	100 ppm TWA (560 mg/m^3)	100 ppm TWA (556 mg/m^3)	—

ACGIH, American Conference of Governmental Industrial Hygienists; IDLH, immediately dangerous to life and health; OSHA, U.S. Occupational Safety and Health Administration; PEL, permissible exposure limit; TLV, threshold limit value; TWA, time-weighted average.
From http://www.cdc.gov/niosh.

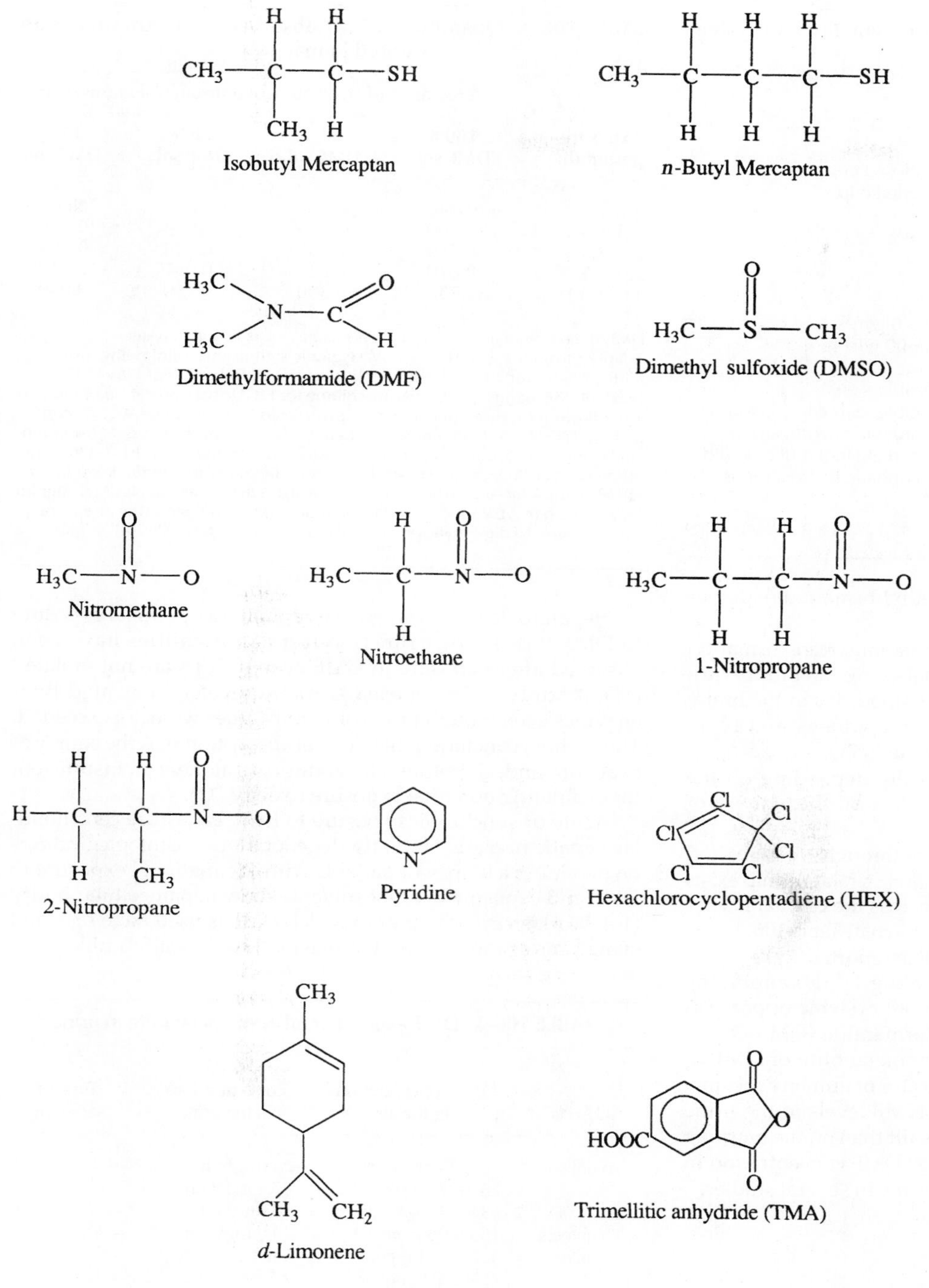

Isobutyl Mercaptan

n-Butyl Mercaptan

Dimethylformamide (DMF)

Dimethyl sulfoxide (DMSO)

Nitromethane

Nitroethane

1-Nitropropane

2-Nitropropane

Pyridine

Hexachlorocyclopentadiene (HEX)

d-Limonene

Trimellitic anhydride (TMA)

Figure 106-1. Chemical structures of some solvents and their reactive intermediary compounds.

Sources, Production, and Uses

DMF is produced by reaction carbon monoxide with dimethylamine. DMF is used as a solvent for vinyl-based and polar polymers (e.g., polyvinyl chloride and polyacrylonitrile) and in the manufacture of films, acrylic fibers, and coatings (e.g., polyurethane lacquers for clothing and accessories made of synthetic leather). DMF also is used in the production of pharmaceuticals and pesticides (4). DMF is a universal solvent owing to its water solubility and high dielectric constant. Because it is hepatotoxic, it is not used as an untransformed solvent in pharmaceutical or cosmetic products. It is shipped in tank trucks, containers, and steel drums. Seals for these containers are made of material that does not react with DMF, such as polytetrafluoroethylene or polyethylene.

Environmental Fate

DMF is stable in the atmosphere. In aqueous solutions, it undergoes hydrolysis at a neutral pH. DMF has high water solubility and a low *n*-octanol-water partition coefficient, meaning that it can leach into groundwater. It is biodegraded by bacteria in the environment. Low concentrations of DMF can be found in effluent waters from sewage treatment plants or from municipal sewage treatment systems (4).

Absorption, Metabolism, and Excretion

DMF is readily absorbed through the skin, respiratory system, and gastrointestinal tract (4,5). Only a small amount is excreted unchanged in the urine. The majority of DMF is metabolized to

TABLE 106-2. Physiochemical properties of dimethylformamide

Property	Value
Melting point (°C)	–60.5
Boiling point (°C)	153
Flash point (°C)	58 (closed cup) 67 (open cup)
Autoignition temperature (°C)	445
Density at 25°C [specific gravity (g/mL)]	0.9445
Relative vapor density	2.51
Vapor pressure (mm Hg) at 25°C	3.7
Explosive limits in air at 20°C	
Lower limit	2.2 (70 g/m³)
Upper limit	16 (500 g/m³)
n-Octanol-water partition coefficient	0.13
Solubility in water	Miscible
Solubility in organic solvents	Miscible with ether, ketones, aromatic hydrocarbons, and ethanol, but not with aliphatic hydrocarbons

Adapted from ref. 4, with permission.

TABLE 106-3. Quantities of DMF absorbed in *in vitro* studies on excised human skin

	Percentage of DMF absorbed through skin (mg/cm²)			
Exposure period (h)	100% DMF sol.	60% DMF sol.	30% DMF sol.	15% DMF sol.
0.5	0.046	ND	ND	ND
1.0–1.5	7.400	0.035	0.013	0.006
2.0–2.5	20.550	0.087	0.048	0.009
3.0–3.5	40.810	0.222	0.097	0.017
4.0–4.5	51.730	0.300	0.160	0.069

DMF, dimethylformamide; ND, not detectable; sol., solution in water.
Adapted from ref. 4; Bortsevich SV. Hygienic significance of dimethylformamide penetration through the skin [Russian]. *Gig Tr Prof Zabol* 1984;11:55–57.; Maxfield ME, Barnes JR, Azar A, Trochimowicz HT. Urinary excretion of metabolite following experimental human exposures to DMF or to DMAC. *J Occup Med* 1975;17:506–511.; Kimmerle G, Eben A. Metabolism studies of *N,N*-dimethylformamide. II. Studies in persons. *Int Arch Arbeitsmed* 1975;34:127–136.; Kimmerle G, Eben A. Metabolism studies of N,N-dimethylformamide. I. Studies in rats and dogs. *Int Arch Arbeitsmed* 1975;34:109–126.; Krivaneck ND, McLaughlin M, Fayweather WE. Monomethylformamide levels in human urine after repetitive exposure to dimethylformamide vapor. *J Occup Med* 1978;20:179–182.

a demethylated product (*N*-hydroxymethylformamide) and *N*-acetyl-*S*-(*n*-methylcarbamoyl) cysteine.

The absorption, distribution, and metabolic transformation of DMF has been studied in animal models. After an intraperitoneal dose in rats, 4% is recovered in the blood, 1% in the brain, heart, lung, stomach, intestines, spleen, and kidneys, and 1% to 3% in the liver, adipose tissues, and muscle (6,7).

DMF and ethanol interact metabolically depending on the dose of DMF. DMF has an inhibitory effect on the activity of alcohol dehydrogenase.

In humans, absorption of DMF occurs through the skin, and DMF appears to enhance its own penetration. A relationship exists between the amount of DMF absorbed across the dermal barrier and the DMF concentration in water, as shown in Table 106-3.

The main human metabolite of DMF is reported to be DMF-hydroxy (4,5). In male volunteers inhaling DMF vapors, the metabolite *n*-acetyl-*S*-(*n*-methylcarbamoyl) cysteine appears in the urine. *N*-hydroxymethyl-*n*-methylformamide (DMF-OH or NMF) is identified as the main urinary metabolite of DMF in humans and is a sensitive biological indicator of human exposure. In the case of occupational exposures, NMF levels in the urine usually are greater at the end of a work shift than on the morning after the exposure. Table 106-4 correlates DMF concentration in the air with NMF concentrations in the urine in several studies.

Clinical Toxicology

Cases of acute DMF toxicity are reported secondary to splashing of DMF over the body or to contact with skin that occurred owing to lack of protective measures, with subsequent dermal absorption. Symptoms appear from hours to days after exposure and include epigastric pain, dizziness, nausea, anorexia, vomiting, fatigue, alcohol intolerance, and skin irritation (4). Elevated liver function tests return to normal within 2 to 3 weeks. Long-term exposure produces eye irritation, headache, anorexia, gastrointestinal upset, and signs of toxic hepatitis, with elevation of liver enzymes. Table 106-5 summarizes the findings in DMF occupational exposure studies.

Alcohol intolerance among workers exposed to DMF has been reported. Symptoms include facial flushing, dizziness, nausea, chest tightness, dyspnea, and cardiac palpitations occurring within 24 hours of DMF exposure and alcohol ingestion. These episodes lasted for approximately 2 hours (8).

Hepatotoxicity also is associated with occupational exposure to DMF (9,10). Liver function test abnormalities have been observed after exposure to DMF even if PELs are not violated (11). A study of 75 exposed workers revealed elevated liver enzymes even though threshold limit values were not exceeded. The authors concluded that dermal absorption was the source of exposure and, therefore, air monitoring alone was insufficient for evaluating potential exposure toxicity (11).

Acute or subchronic exposure to DMF can cause centrilobular hepatic necrosis and fatty degeneration. Histologic findings on obtaining a biopsy of patients with occupational exposure to DMF and exposure to other solvents show hepatocellular injury (10). Workers in industries in which DMF is used have reported symptoms of anorexia, abdominal pain, and disulfiramlike reac-

TABLE 106-4. DMF exposure and NMF metabolite in urine

Subjects	DMF concentrations in the air	NMF concentrations in the urine	Time of sampling
4 Volunteers	78 ± 24 mg/m³, [a]	24 mg/24 h	—
	261 ± 75 mg/m³, [a]	97.4 mg/24 h	—
	63 ± 12 mg/m³, [b]	30 mg/24 h	—
4 Volunteers	159 ± 96 mg/m³, [a]	44.8 mg/24 h	—
4 Volunteers	32.4 ± 2.1 mg/m³, [a, c]	5 mg/24 h	—
8 Volunteers	26.4 ± 0.9 mg/m³, [b]	2.5 mg/24 h	—
22 Workers	13 mg/m³, [b]	20–40 mg/g creatinine	Postshift samples
9 Workers	15.4 mg/m³, [b]	0.4–19.6 mg/24 h	—
85 Workers	30–150 mg/m³, [c]	0.104–0.224 mg/mL	—
23 Workers	>30 mg/m³, [b]	20–40 mg/24 h	—
30 Workers	14.0–86.3 mg/m³, [b]	12.0–188.3 mg/g creatinine	In different work areas 4 h after work shift

DMF, dimethylformamide; NMF, *N*-methylformamide.
[a]Single inhalational exposure to DMF (2, 4, or 6 h/d).
[b]Repeated inhalational exposure to DMF (6, 7, 7.5 h/d).
[c]Dermal absorption.
Adapted from ref. 4, with permission.

TABLE 106-5. Studies on workers with long-term DMF exposures

Number of exposed subjects	Number of nonexposed controls	Length of exposure (yr)	DMF exposure (mg/m³)	Urinary NMF	Hepatotoxicity	Alcohol intolerance	Other effects
22	28	5	1–47 (usually <30; gloves worn)	20–63 mg/g creatinine	—	+	Not reported
11	—	3	3–15	0.4–20.0 mg/24 h	—	+ (6)	Not reported
28	29	3–5	30–60	Not reported	—	Not reported	Reports of eye and respiratory tract irritation; no hematologic changes
115	67	1.0–1.5	30–150 with higher peaks + skin exposure	Not reported	+ (a few among 29)	Not reported	Reports of gastrointestinal tract or cardiovascular and ovarian disturbances
177	—	3–5	10–30	Not reported	—	Not reported	Reports of cardiovascular disturbances

DMF, dimethylformamide; NMF, *N*-methylformamide.
Adapted from ref. 4, with permission.

tions after ingesting alcohol (11). In these workers, chronic exposure to DMF resulted in mildly increased hepatic enzymes and steatosis, without inflammation or fibrosis on biopsy of the liver. After removal from exposure, the symptoms of these individuals resolved within 16 months (10). Animal studies have demonstrated that DMF is hepatotoxic (12–16).

The International Agency for Research on Cancer evaluated the carcinogenicity of DMF and concluded that limited evidence points to DMF carcinogenicity in humans and that the evidence for DMF carcinogenicity in experimental animals is inadequate. In its overall evaluation, the International Agency for Research on Cancer placed DMF in group 2B, meaning it is possibly carcinogenic to humans. The PEL for DMF is 10 ppm (as a time-weighted average). The IDLH level is 3,500 ppm.

In humans, acute exposure is associated with gastrointestinal upset, abdominal pain, nausea and vomiting, elevated liver enzymes, hepatitis, dermatitis, and irritation of the skin, eyes, and upper respiratory tract (15–17). Liver damage can be produced by single, large exposures or by repeated small exposures. In 1986, a small outbreak of hepatitis occurred in polyurethane fabric coaters who were exposed to DMF. Workers presented with abdominal pain, nausea, anorexia, jaundice, dizziness, and headache. Death ensued in some workers. Centrilobular and midzonal hepatic necrosis with regeneration and diffuse macrovesicular and microvesicular steatosis were seen on histologic examination (9). On further investigation, 62% of asymptomatic workers were found to have elevated alanine aminotransferase (ALT) and aspartate aminotransferase (AST) levels, with an AST/ALT ratio of less than 1. Elevated direct bilirubin and alkaline phosphatase levels were less frequently observed. The elevations in AST and ALT improved gradually over months to years after DMF exposure ceased (9). A case of fulminant hepatic failure and death after an acute ingestion of DMF has been reported (18).

Facial flushing, dizziness, anxiety, palpitations, and blurred vision may occur after DMF-exposed workers consume ethanol (8,9,19–21).

In animals, DMF does not appear to be genotoxic or carcinogenic. Recent concern over possible testicular cancer in leather workers exposed to DMF has arisen, but epidemiologic studies are inconsistent (22).

Although a urine test that measures monomethylformamide (a urinary metabolite of DMF) exists, correlation between exposure to DMF and the amount of monomethylformamide in a spot urine sample is not well established (9). The current recommended biological exposure index is 40 mg NMF per gram of creatine in a urine sample collected at the end of a work shift (23).

DIMETHYL SULFOXIDE

DMSO [$(CH_3)_2SO$] is a polar solvent that alters the stratum corneum barrier of the skin and facilitates dermal absorption of other substances. The only approved U.S. Food and Drug Administration use for DMSO is in the treatment of interstitial cystitis. It also has been used topically to treat inadvertent extravasation of chemotherapeutic agents (24). Although ocular injury and cataract formation are reported with dermal and ocular exposure in experimental animals, most recent animal studies report hepatic and renal protective effects of DMSO.

Production and Uses

DMSO is prepared by oxidation of dimethyl sulfide with nitrogen oxide. It is used as a solvent for sulfur dioxide and acetylene. DMSO is used also in organic reactions, as a hydraulic fluid, and as antifreeze. Its use has been recommended as a topical antiinflammatory agent. It finds use in veterinary medicine, as an analytic agent, and in other industries, for cleaners, pesticides, and paint stripping.

Clinical Toxicity

Overall, DMSO has little toxicity. It may actually protect the liver from injury produced by hepatotoxins. Guinea pigs that received DMSO treatment 10 hours after inhalational halothane demonstrated less hepatic necrosis than did control animals (25). Rats receiving DMSO 10 hours after oral chloroform was administered demonstrated significantly less hepatic and renal injury than did control animals (25). Further, rats treated with DMSO and other nephrotoxins (e.g., *N*-(3,5-dichlorophenyl) succinimide or cisplatin) demonstrated less nephrotoxicity than did control rats given the nephrotoxins alone (2,26). Hamsters treated with DMSO 1 hour after diphenylamine administration demonstrated less renal papillary necrosis than did control animals that received diphenylamine alone (3).

Toxic effects in humans are minimal: nausea, skin rashes, eye irritation, respiratory tract irritation, and a garlicky odor on the body and on a person's breath if absorbed. Human exposures have not resulted in ocular toxicity. The use of DMSO to protect against toxin-induced renal and hepatic injury has not been substantiated in humans.

DMSO has demonstrated mutagenic activity in some bacterial strains by Ames testing. In contrast, some animal studies indicate that DMSO may be protective against toxin-induced mutagenicity (27,28).

DMSO easily penetrates the dermis, carrying other dissolved chemicals into the systemic circulation. This substance is reported to cause anaphylaxis and urticaria. Photophobia and color vision disturbances have also been described after exposure. Splash exposures to the skin and eyes should be irrigated with water. For ingested DMSO, vomiting is not recommended, to avoid aspiration. Dermal irritation and dermal burns can occur on exposure if not irrigated. Cases of systemic contact dermatitis have been reported after intravesical DMSO treatment for interstitial cystitis (29).

Aside from its dermal penetration, DMSO exhibits other properties including antiinflammatory activity, diuresis, cholinesterase inhibition, and free radical scavenging activity. DMSO finds veterinary use in a 90% gel for topical treatment of joint and muscle pains. In addition, DMSO (60% weight per volume) is available in combination with a steroid as an otic medication for dogs (30).

Chest pains have been reported after DMSO use. Cardiovascular effects of DMSO are vasodilation and tachycardia. Tachycardia has been seen in patients given a 10% DMSO solution intravenously (31). Hypotension also was noted in this case.

A garlicky breath odor appears after intravenous or topical dosing of DMSO, owing to a sulfone metabolite. Reports of dyspnea and exacerbations of asthma symptoms have been reported after DMSO use. Other adverse health effects include headache, dizziness, and sedation. Also, agitation has been noted in patients receiving intravenous DMSO (31). One elderly patient who received intravenous DMSO therapy for 3 weeks on a daily basis reported development of confusion, lethargy, and disorientation during the third week of therapy. He also experienced dysarthria and hypoactive reflexes. After therapy was discontinued, these symptoms continued for another 8 days (32).

DMSO has been known to release histamine from mast cells. Hence, it can worsen asthma and produce urticaria and other allergic-type reactions.

NAPHTHA

Naphtha is a general solvent that is produced in two forms: a petroleum distillate or a coal tar naphtha. They are used as solvents for oils, paints, lacquers, varnishes, rubber cement, degreasing, agrochemicals, dry cleaning, and industrial cleaning.

Petroleum naphtha is a colorless liquid containing benzene and aliphatic hydrocarbons. It is used as a solvent for oils, lacquers, paints, rubber cement, dry cleaning, and degreasing. Petroleum naphtha vapor is a CNS depressant and an irritant of the mucous membranes and respiratory tract. Exposure to high concentrations of the vapor can produce headache, dizziness, nausea, and shortness of breath. Dermal contact to vapor or liquid can produce dermatitis. The PEL for petroleum naphtha is 500 ppm.

Coal tar naphtha is a light yellow liquid that boils at between 110° and 190°C. It is a general solvent for a variety of uses and is a CNS depressant. Coal tar naphtha is a mixture of aromatic hydrocarbons, including toluene, xylene, cumene, and benzene.

Exposure to coal tar naphtha vapors or liquid produces symptoms similar to those incited by other aromatic hydrocarbons, such as CNS depression, dermal irritation, potential hepatotoxicity, and renal toxicity (33). The presence of benzene in coal tar naphtha can be a hazard for bone marrow depression and other toxic effects if exposure is high enough. Clinical toxicity consists of dizziness, irritation of mucous membranes and eyes, and dermatitis after exposure. The overall toxicity of coal tar naphtha is similar to its individual aromatic hydrocarbon components. The PEL for coal tar naphtha is 100 ppm. The IDLH level for both naphthas is 10,000 ppm.

High-flash aromatic naphtha is a solvent consisting primarily of nine-carbon aromatic molecules, especially ethyltoluene and trimethylbenzene (34). It is formed by catalytic reforming, a refining process that converts naphthenes to aromatics by dehydrogenation to make higher-octane gasoline blending components (34,35).

In rabbit studies, naphthas are mild to moderate eye irritants and dermal irritants (33). Irritating properties may be due to phenol, which is present in raw naphtha. Dermal effects include erythema, edema, fissuring, eschar formation, exfoliation, and desquamation (33). In rats, ingestion is associated with CNS depression, atonia, tremors, and reddened lungs on necropsy (33). Mice and rats exposed by inhalation exhibit ocular irritation, lacrimation, respiratory distress, and alopecia (33). Rats injected with naphtha in the tail vein developed severe hemorrhagic pneumonitis without hepatic damage; however, naphtha injected into the portal vein produced significant hepatic necrosis (36).

Formulations of naphtha have produced nephrotoxicity (e.g., renal cortical tubular degeneration) in experimental animals (37). Rats exposed to high-flash aromatic naphtha for 90 days revealed no evidence of permanent neurotoxicity (34). Inhalation of near-lethal levels of high-flash aromatic naphtha results in fetal mortality, reduced weight, and cleft palate in offspring of mice (35).

The toxicity of petroleum naphtha and coal tar naphtha is similar to the toxicity produced by individual components of naphthas. CNS depression, dizziness, possible hepatotoxicity and nephrotoxicity, and irritation of the mucous membranes, respiratory tract, and skin (e.g., dermatitis) may be seen (33,37). Intravenous injection of naphtha can produce pleuritic chest pain, dyspnea, hypoxemia, hemoptysis, hemorrhagic pneumonitis, and pulmonary edema (38–40). Subcutaneous injection is associated with sterile abscess formation (39).

STODDARD SOLVENT

Stoddard solvent is named after W.J. Stoddard for his work with petroleum distillates in the dry-cleaning industry. The solvent is a colorless, flammable liquid with a gasoline odor (41). Stoddard is a petroleum distillate in a commonly used solvent. It is a mixture of C_7 through C_{12} hydrocarbons consisting of three major groups (41):

- Paraffins: linear and branched alkanes comprising 30% to 50% of the mixture
- Cycloalkanes: cycloparaffins or naphthenes, comprising 30% to 40% of the mixture
- Aromatic hydrocarbons, comprising 10% to 20% of the mixture

Stoddard solvent is a blend of different treated oil fractions, the composition of which varies depending on the process of production. Table 106-6 shows the various formulations of Stod-

TABLE 106-6. Formulations of Stoddard solvent (percentage)

Hydrocarbons	White spirits 2	White spirits 3	Stoddard solvent (regular)	Stoddard solvent (140 flash)	Stoddard solvent
Alkanes (paraffins)	61.0	62.8	30–50 (48 average)	60.8	34.9
n-Nonane	13.3	1.9			
n-Decane	10.0	9.1			
Methylnonanes	7.9				
2,6-Dimethyloctane	4.1				
n-Undecane	2.4	17.5			
Dodecanes		11.6			
Terdecanes		2.7			
Others	23.3				
Cycloalkanes (cycloparaffins)	27.3		30–40 (38 average)	35.7	
Monocycloparaffins	13.7			24.5	34.9
Trimethylcyclohexane	7.2				
tert-Butylcyclohexane	4.0				
n-Butylcyclopentane	1.3				
n-Butylcyclohexane	1.2				
Other cycloparaffins	13.1			11.2	
Dicycloparaffins					5.0
Tricycloparaffins					0.4
Acenaphthenes					0.4
Aromatics	11.7	17.0	10–20 (14.1 average)	3.40	
Alkybenzenes			14.0	3.03	22.0
Dimethylethylbenzenes	3.0				
n-Propylbenzene	2.0				
Thyltoluenes	1.2				
1,2,4-Trimethylbenzene	0.9				
Other aromatics	4.6				1.1
Other benzenes					
Indans/tetralins			0.1	0.07	1.8
Indenes			<1	0.3	0.1
Naphthalenes					0.2
Acenaphthalenes					0.3
Tricyclic aromatics					0.1

Adapted from ref. 41, with permission.

dard solvent, which has a mean molecular weight of 144 D (range, 135 to 145). Its odor threshold is 0.9 ppm (5.1 mg per cubic meter). It is insoluble in water but soluble in other solvents such as alcohol, benzene, ether, chloroform, and carbon disulfide. Its vapor pressure is 4.0 to 4.5 mm Hg at 25°C. Stoddard solvent boils at between 150° and 200°C.

White spirits, which sometimes is used erroneously as a synonym for Stoddard solvent, contain hydrocarbons between C_7 and C_{11}. The types of white spirits differ on the basis of the percentages of the alkane carbon content. A solvent that is similar to Stoddard solvent is naphtha, which is a term applied to petroleum distillates consisting of 70% to 80% C_9 aromatics and 20% to 30% C_8 or C_{10} aromatics. In contrast, Stoddard solvent is only 10% to 20% aromatic. The term *naphtha* also applies to petroleum distillates containing C_5 through C_{13} aliphatic hydrocarbons.

Table 106-7 provides the physiochemical properties of Stoddard solvent. Solvents that are sometimes confused with Stoddard solvent are mineral spirits and benzine. Benzine differs from Stoddard solvent in that it contains C_5 through C_9 hydrocarbons and has a boiling point between 154°C and 204°C. Mineral spirits have a distillation range of 136° through 277°C. Stoddard solvent sometimes is considered a subset of mineral spirits.

Uses

Stoddard solvent is present in paints, paint thinners, lacquers, varnishes, agrochemicals, photocopier toners, printing inks, silicone compounds, metal degreasers, adhesives, fabric waterproofing solutions, herbicides, insecticides, pesticides, dry-cleaning solutions, and household and industrial cleaning fluids. It is used for the extraction of fats and oils and to process synthetic yarns.

Absorption, Metabolism, and Excretion

Inhalation is the principal route of exposure to Stoddard solvent. Dermal exposure occurs, but absorption is limited. Ingestion also can occur and can produce aspiration pneumonia. Stoddard solvent is metabolized by the liver and excreted by the lungs and kidneys.

Metabolic products of Stoddard solvent exposure have been identified as 1,2,4-trimethylbenzene and 3,4-dimethylhippuric acid (42).

In animals, Stoddard solvent lowers the myocardial threshold to catecholamines and can cause dysrhythmias; however, dysrhythmias have not been reported in humans (41). Inhalational exposures produced incoordination, tremors, clonic spasms, and death. In rats, but not dogs, long-term exposure to Stoddard solvent is associated with kidney damage.

Environmental Fate and Transport

The environmental fate and transport of Stoddard solvent depends on the individual hydrocarbon components and their activity within the environment. Lower-molecular-weight

TABLE 106-7. Physiochemical properties of Stoddard solvent

Property	Information
Molecular weight	144 (mean); 135–145 (range)
Color	Clear, colorless
Physical state	Liquid
Boiling point	154–202°C
Density at 20°C	0.78 g/mL
Odor	Similar to kerosene
Odor threshold	0.9 ppm (5.1 mg/m^3)
Solubility	
Water	Insoluble
Organic solvent(s)	Absolute alcohol, benzene, ether, chloroform, carbon tetrachloride, carbon disulfide
Partition coefficients	
Log K_{ow}	3.16–7.06
Log K_{oc}	2.85–6.74
Vapor pressure at 25°C	4.0–4.5 mm Hg
Autoignition temperature	37.8°–60.0°C
Flash point	38°–43°C
Flammability limits (% volume in air at 25°C)	0.9–6.0
Conversion factors	1 mg/L = 174.60 ppm
At 25°C and 760 mm	1 ppm = 5.73 mg/m^3
At 25°C	1 ppm = 5.77 mg/m^3
Explosive limits	
Lower limit	0.9%
Upper limit	6.0%

K_{oc}, soil sorption constant; K_{ow}, *n*-octanol-water partition coefficient.
Adapted from refs. 48 and 49, with permission.

alkanes and the aromatics can volatilize easily and also undergo photodegradation in the atmosphere. The higher-molecular-weight alkanes and cycloalkanes may be adsorbed to organic matter in the soil. Also, the higher-molecular-weight aromatics may dissolve in surface waters more easily.

Clinical Toxicology

Stoddard solvent is detected by its odor at vapor concentrations of less than 1 ppm. However, olfactory fatigue can occur within minutes. Thus, the odor-warning properties are insufficient to provide adequate protection to prevent serious exposures.

SIGNS, SYMPTOMS, AND SYNDROMES

Acute inhalational exposure can cause nose, throat, and eye irritation, as well as nervous system toxicity headache including, dizziness, visual disturbances, confusion, tiredness, and feelings of inebriation. At high concentrations, coma can occur. After ingestion of Stoddard solvent, aspiration is associated with chemical pneumonitis, pulmonary edema, pulmonary emphysema, pneumothorax, pleuritis, pleural effusion, empyema, and pneumatoceles (43,44).

Slowed reaction times and attention deficits were noted in house painters exposed to Stoddard solvent (45). Memory deficits, fatigue, inebriation, and subtle changes in color vision have been reported. Chronic exposure is associated with headaches, fatigue, intermittent inebriation, and memory deficits that generally resolve with removal from exposure. Liver damage has been reported in house painters exposed to mixtures of solvents, including Stoddard solvent; however, a causal relationship has not been firmly established.

Stoddard solvent is also a cutaneous irritant, causing acute dermatitis with vesicle formation, ulcerations, crusting, erythema, and desquamation. Dermal effects may be secondary to dehydrating and defatting actions or due to irritant contact dermatitis. Ulcerative and erythematous lesions on the genitals and buttocks were seen when Stoddard solvent was used as a dry-cleaning solvent for coveralls that were worn before adequate drying and often without undergarments (43). The lesions resolved with the application of saline compresses and 1% hydrocortisone cream. Long-term exposure has been associated with dermatitis characterized by drying, cracking, and reddening of the skin. Conjunctivitis may be seen after ocular exposure.

Stoddard solvent has not been associated with human cancer and is not classified by the International Agency for Research on Cancer.

Protective clothing is recommended and self-contained breathing systems are indicated for work in areas of highly concentrated Stoddard solvent. Patients who have ingested Stoddard solvent should not be encouraged to vomit, because aspiration carries the risk of severe pulmonary damage. Activated charcoal administration is recommended. After ocular and dermal exposure, contaminated clothing should be removed and the eyes and skin should be flushed for at least 15 minutes.

EPIDEMIOLOGIC AND ANIMAL STUDIES

The clinical toxicity of Stoddard solvent has been studied in animals and in humans. Cardiovascular effects of Stoddard solvent have been studied in individuals exposed to 2,500 mg of vaporized solvent per cubic meter (476 ppm), containing 83% aliphatic and 17% aromatic components, for 30 minutes and showed no electrocardiographic changes or changes in cardiac output, alveolar ventilation, or heart rate at rest or during exercise (44).

An epidemiologic retrospective cohort study showed no changes in blood pressure in painters exposed to unspecified various solvents for between 4 and 42 years (45). Animal studies have not demonstrated cardiac pathology on 90-day continual exposure to high concentrations (1,271 mg per cubic meter) of vaporized mineral spirits, the composition of which was similar to Stoddard solvent (41).

Nausea has been reported in workers who use Stoddard solvent, but volunteers exposed to 610 mg per cubic meter for 6 hours reported no nausea (46). Hematologic effects have been less well documented, yet causal relationships have not been verified. Studies of individuals exposed to a variety of solvents showed some decreased red blood cell counts and increased platelets as compared to others without contact. However, these studies are confounded and do not delineate Stoddard solvent in particular as the primary exposure (47). No hematologic effects were seen in animals exposed to high concentrations of vaporized Stoddard solvent. Studies of humans exposed for 6 hours to 610 mg of vaporized solvent per cubic meter, having a composition similar to Stoddard solvent, showed no change in liver enzyme functions (46). The same study showed that there were no changes in renal function, urine albumen level, or β_2-microglobulins in the urine as compared to preexposure levels.

Stoddard solvent has not proved to be particularly neurotoxic at high concentrations. Human subjects exposed for 30 minutes to vaporized Stoddard solvent at 0, 600, 1,800, and 2,400 mg per cubic meter exhibited no dose-related changes in hand-eye coordination, reaction time, decision making, or visuomotor skill coordination. However, a statistically significant change was observed in hand-eye coordination and visuomotor tests at 600 mg per cubic meter as compared to control values (48). Minor neurologic effects of dizziness were seen in test subjects in a 15-minute exposure to 2,700 mg of Stoddard solvent per cubic meter (49). In other studies, perceptual speed, numeric abilities, manual dexterity, reaction time, and short-term memory were not altered by a 30-minute exposure to white spirits at 625 mg per cubic meter followed by 30 minutes at 1,250 mg per cubic meter and then 30 minutes at 1,875 mg per cubic meter, up to a total dose of 2,500 mg per cubic meter for another 30 minutes (50). Epidemiologic studies and case reports have described neurologic health effects secondary to exposure to Stoddard solvent, but these were retrospective studies, exposure concentrations were not measured, and other solvents were involved as confounding or contributing cofactors. Thus, a cause-and-effect relationship cannot be determined.

In humans, no change in respiratory rate occurred when subjects were exposed to 2,400 mg per cubic meter (457 ppm) for 30 minutes (48). Upper airway irritation was noted in one of six subjects exposed to 2,700 mg of completely vaporized Stoddard solvent per cubic meter for 15 minutes per day for 3 days (49). One case report tells of a man who, for more than 1 year, soaked his hands in Stoddard solvent at work without protection and developed glomerulonephritis (51). Humans exposed to high concentrations of vaporized solvent (600 mg to 1,800 mg per cubic meter) showed no signs of ocular irritation, but individuals exposed to 2,400 mg per cubic meter demonstrated ocular irritation as measured by the eye blink rate (48).

REFERENCES

1. Gobbato F, Terribile PM. Toxicologic properties of mercaptans. *Folia Med* 1968;51:329–341.
2. Rankin GO, Beers KW, Nicoll DW, et al. Effects of dimethyl sulfoxide on N-(3,5-dichlorophenyl)succinimide (NDPS) and NDPS metabolite nephrotoxicity. *Toxicology* 1995;100(1–3):79–88.
3. Lenz SD, Carlton WW. Decreased incidence of diphenylamine-induced renal papillary necrosis in Syrian hamsters given dimethyl sulfoxide. *Food Chem Toxicol* 1991;29:409–418.
4. World Health Organization. *Dimethylformamide*. Environmental health criteria 114. Geneva: World Health Organization, 1991.
5. Mraz J, Nohova H. Absorption, metabolism and elimination of *N,N*-dimethylformamide in humans. *Int Arch Occup Environ Health* 1992;64:85–92.
6. Scailteur V, Lauwerys R. Dimethylformamide (DMF) hepatotoxicity. *Toxicology* 1987;43:231–238.
7. Scailteur V, Hoffmann E, Buchet J, et al. Study on in vivo and in vitro metabolism of dimethylformamide in male and female rats. *Toxicology* 1984;29:222–234.
8. Yonemoto J, Suzuki S. Relation of exposure to dimethylformamide vapor and the metabolite methylformamide in urine of workers. *Int Arch Occup Environ Health* 1980;46(1):59–165.
9. Redlich CA, Beckett WS, Sparer J, et al. Liver disease associated with occupational exposure to the solvent dimethylformamide. *Ann Intern Med* 1988;108:680–686.
10. Redlich CA, West AB, Fleming L, Ture LD, Cullen MR, Riely CA. Clinical and pathological characteristics of hepatotoxicity associated with occupational exposure to dimethylformamide. *Gastroenterology* 1990;99:748–757.
11. Fiorito A, Larese F, Molinari S, Zanin T. Liver function alterations in synthetic leather workers exposed to dimethylformamide. *Am J Ind Med* 1997;32:255–260.
12. Stula EF, Krauss WC. Embryotoxicity in rats and rabbits from cutaneous application of amide-type solvents and substituted ureas. *Toxicol App Pharmacol* 1977;41:35–55.
13. Llewellyn GC, Hastings WS, Kimbrough TD, Rea FW, O'Rear CE. The effects of dimethylformamide on female Mongolian gerbils, *Merions unguiculatus*. *Bull Environ Contam Toxicol* 1974;11:467–473.
14. Hurtt ME, Placke ME, Killinger JM, Singer AW, Kennedy GL Jr. 13-Week inhalation toxicity study of dimethylformamide (DMF) in cynomolgus monkeys. *Fundam App Toxicol* 1992;18:596–601.
15. Perbellini L, Brugnone F, Grigolini L, Cunegatti P, Tacconi A. Alveolar air and blood dichloromethane concentration in shoe sole factory workers. *Int Arch Occup Environ Health* 1977;40:241–247.
16. Fleming LE, Shalat SL, Redlich CA. Liver injury in workers exposed to dimethylformamide. *Scand J Work Environ Health* 1990;16:289–292.
17. Wang JD, Lai MY, Chen JS, et al. Dimethylformamide induced liver damage among synthetic leather workers. *Arch Environ Health* 1991;46:161–166.
18. Nicolas F, Rodineau P, Rouzioux JM, et al. Fulminant hepatic failure in poisoning due to ingestion of T 61, a veterinary euthanasia drug. *Crit Care Med* 1990;18:573–575.
19. Lyle WH, Spence TW, McKinneley WM, Duckers K. Dimethylformamide and alcohol intolerance. *Br J Ind Med* 1979;36:63–66.
20. Chivers CP. Disulfiram effect from inhalation of dimethylformamide [Letter]. *Lancet* 1978;1980:573–575.
21. Cox NH, Mustchin CP. Prolonged spontaneous and alcohol-induced flushing due to the solvent dimethylformamide. *Contact Dermatitis* 1991;24:69–70.
22. Testicular cancer in leather workers—Fulton County, New York. *MMWR Morbid Mortal Wkly Rep* 1989;38:105–114.
23. American Conference of Governmental Industrial Hygienists. *Documentation of the threshold limit values (TLVs) and biological exposure indices (BEIs)*. Cincinnati: American Conference of Governmental Industrial Hygienists, Technical Information Office, 1992.
24. Lebredo L, Barrie R, Woltering EA. DMSO protects against Adriamycin-induced tissue necrosis. *J Surg Res* 1992;53:62–65.
25. Lind RC, Gandolfi AJ. Late dimethyl sulfoxide administration provides a protective action against chemically induced injury in both the liver and the kidney. *Toxicol Appl Pharmacol* 1997;142:201–207.
26. Jones MM, Basinger MA, Field L, Holscher MA. Coadministration of dimethyl sulfoxide reduces cisplatin nephrotoxicity. *Anticancer Res* 1991; 11:1939–1942.
27. Hakura A, Mochida H, Yarnatsu K. Dimethyl sulfoxide (DMSO) is mutagenic for bacterial mutagenicity tester strains. *Mutat Res* 1993;303:127–133.
28. Hrelia P, Scotti M, Morotti M, et al. Dimethyl sulfoxide as modifier of the organospecific mutagenicity of metronidazole in mice. *Teratog Carcinog Mutagen* 1990;10:263–271.
29. Nishimura M, Takano Y, Toshitani S. Systemic contact dermatitis medicamentosa occurring after intravesical dimethyl sulfoxide treatment for interstitial cystitis. *Arch Dermatol* 1988;124:182–183.
30. Luery N, Rohrbaugh T, Cupit G. Dimethyl sulfoxide toxicity. *Drug Intell Clin Pharm* 1984;18:591–592.
31. O'Donnell J, Burnett A, Sheehan T, et al. Safety of dimethyl sulfoxide. *Lancet* 1981;1:498.
32. Bond G, Curry S, Dahl D. Dimethyl sulfoxide induced encephalopathy. *Lancet* 1989;1:1134–1135.
33. McKee RH, Biles RW, Kapp RW, Hinz JP. The acute toxicity of coal liquefaction derived materials. *J Appl Toxicol* 1984;4:198–205.
34. Douglas JF, McKee RH, Cagen SZ. A neurotoxicity assessment of high-flash aromatic naphtha. *Toxicol Ind Health* 1993;9:1047–1058.
35. McKee RH, Wong ZA, Schmitt S. The reproductive and developmental toxicity of high-flash aromatic naphtha. *Toxicol Ind Health* 1990;6(3–4):441–460.
36. Bratton L, Haddow EJ. Ingestion of charcoal lighter fluid. *J Pediatr* 1975;87: 633–636.
37. Rocskay AZ, Robins TG, Schork MA, Echeverria D, Proctor SP, White RE. Renal effects of naphtha exposure among automotive workers. *J Occup Med* 1993;35:617–622.
38. Wason S, Greiner PT. Intravenous hydrocarbon abuse. *Am J Emerg Med* 1986;4:543–544.
39. Vaziri ND, Smith PJ, Wilson A. Toxicity with intravenous injection of naphtha in man. *Clin Toxicol* 1980;16:335–343.
40. Vaziri ND, Jeminson-Smith P, Wilson AF. Hemorrhagic pneumonitis after intravenous injection of charcoal lighter fluid. *Ann Intern Med* 1979;90:794–795.
41. Agency for Toxic Substances and Disease Registry. *Toxicological profile for Stoddard solvent*. Atlanta: US Department of Health and Human Services, Public Health Service, ATSDR, 1995.
42. Fukaya Y, Saito I, Matsumoto T, et al. Determination of 3,4-dimethylhippuric acid as a biological monitoring index for trimethylbenzene exposure and transfer printing workers. *Int Arch Occup Environ Health* 1994;65:295–297.
43. Nethercott JR, Pierce JM, Likwornick G, Murray AH. Genital ulceration due to Stoddard solvent. *J Occup Med* 1980;22:549–552.
44. Astrand I, Kilbom A, Ovrum P. Exposure to white spirit: I. Concentration in alveolar air and blood during rest and exercise. *Scand J Work Environ Health* 1975;12:15–30.
45. Hane M, Axelson O, Blume J, et al. Psychological function changes among house painters. *Scand J Work Environ Health* 1977;3:91–99.
46. Pedersen L, Cohr K. Biochemical pattern and experimental exposure of humans to white spirit: I. The effects of a six hour single dose. *Active Pharmacol Toxicol* 1984;55:317–324.
47. Beving H, Tornling G, Olsson P. Increased erythrocyte volume in car repair painters and car mechanics. *Br J Ind Med* 1991;48:499–501.
48. Hastings L, Cooper G, Burg W. Human sensory response to selected petroleum hydrocarbons. In: McFarland H, Holsworth C, MacGregor J. *Advances in modern environmental toxicology: 6. Applied toxicology of petroleum hydrocarbons*. Princeton: Princeton Scientific Publishers, 1984.
49. Carpenter C, Kankead E, Jeary D, et al. Petroleum hydrocarbon toxicity studies: III. Animal and human response to vapors of Stoddard solvent. *Toxicol Appl Pharmacol* 1975;32:282–297.
50. Gamberalli F, Annwall G, Hultengren M. Exposure to white spirit: II. Psychological functions. *Scand J Work Environ Health* 1975;1:31–39.
51. Daniell W, Couser W, Rosenstock L. Occupational solvent exposure and glomerulonephritis: a case report and review of the literature. *JAMA* 1988;259:2280–2283.

CHAPTER 107

Solvents and Chemical Intermediates: Alcohols, Ketones, Esters, and Ethers

Daniel A. Spyker and John B. Sullivan, Jr.

Alcohols, ketones, ethers, and esters have multiple uses as solvents and as intermediate chemicals in the synthesis of other compounds. Tables 107-1 through 107-4 summarize the toxicity of many of these commonly used compounds.

ALCOHOLS

Alcohols have the general chemical formula of R-OH, where *R* is an alkyl or substituted alkyl group. Alcohols are classified as primary, secondary, or tertiary according to the number of hydrogen atoms bonded to the carbon atom containing the hydroxyl (–OH) group (Fig. 107-1). Phenols are an exception in that the alcohol group is attached directly to a benzene ring. Table 107-1 summarizes the health hazards of common alcohols.

Alcohols may be aliphatic or aromatic (aryl). The prefix *iso* means "a branching of the carbon chain." Alcohols containing two hydroxyl groups are called *glycols*. Alcohols undergo numerous chemical reactions that involve the O–H bond or the C–O bond. The physiochemical behavior of alcohols with a small hydrocarbon group is similar to that of water, whereas alcohols with large alkyl groups tend to behave more like the larger alkyl structure.

Uses

Alcohols are used in a variety of industrial and commercial processes as solvents and chemical intermediates. The uses of specific alcohols are addressed in the sections devoted to those compounds. The toxicity of alcohols varies as a function of their systemic absorption, volatility, and production of toxic metabolites.

Absorption, Metabolism, and Excretion

Ethanol is completely and rapidly absorbed after it is ingested. It distributes in total body water (60% for men, 48% for women) with a volume of distribution of 600 mg per kg and is eliminated by saturable hepatic metabolism. The maximum rate of ethanol metabolism is approximately 24 mg per dL per hour (75 to 175 mg per kg per hour), and the process is half-saturated at a blood level of 9 mg per dL. A blood alcohol level of 100 mg per dL increases the likelihood of a motor vehicle accident by 7-fold, and a level of 150 mg per dL increases the likelihood by 25-fold. Automobile accidents increase dramatically when the blood alcohol concentration rises to 50 mg per dL (0.05%) or more.

Figure 107-2 shows the principal metabolic pathway for ethanol. Most ethanol (90%) is oxidized, and the 10% that remains unchanged is excreted by the lungs and kidneys. Oxidation occurs principally in the liver, forming acetate as a metabolite by the following enzyme systems, which enter the Krebs cycle:

- Peroxidase-catalase system, associated with the microsomes
- Microsomal ethanol-oxidizing system on the endoplasmic reticulum (main path induced in alcoholics; as much as doubled)
- Alcohol dehydrogenase (ADH) pathway located in the cell cytosol (principal pathway)

ADH is a zinc-containing enzyme and uses nicotinamide adenine dinucleotide (NAD) as an H^+ acceptor. The H^+ is transferred from ethanol to NADH. The excess of reducing equivalents increases redox potential (NADH/NAD) and leads to many of the adverse metabolic effects of alcoholism.

Isopropanol

Isopropanol (2-propanol, isopropyl alcohol) is a clear, colorless, flammable aliphatic alcohol (see Fig. 107-1). It is completely miscible with water and organic solvents such as ethanol, acetone, chloroform, and benzene (1). Isopropanol has been widely substituted for ethanol in industrial processes (including food processing) and generally is a relatively safe solvent. It is widely available to the general public as rubbing alcohol (70% isopropanol) but is used also in paints, paint thinner, paint remover, inks, fuels, cleaners, disinfectants, coatings, dyes, cements, and medications and as a deicer. It is used in the production of acetone, as a preservative, as a food flavoring, and in extractions and purification of natural products such as animal and vegetable oils, gums, resins, waxes, and flavorings. Isopropanol undergoes chemical reactions typical of secondary alcohols and reacts violently with strong oxidizing agents.

ENVIRONMENTAL FATE AND TRANSPORT

Once released into the environment, isopropanol is transferred among water, soil, and air owing to its high volatilization. Transport from the atmosphere back to the soil or water can occur through precipitation. In the atmosphere, isopropanol is degraded by hydroxy radicals. Residence time in the atmosphere has been calculated to be 1.4 to 2.3 days (1). Following isopropanol's reaction with hydroxy radicals, subsequent reactions produce peroxyacetyl nitrate, formaldehyde, methyl nitrate, and formic acid. The *n*-octanol-water partition coefficient (log K_{ow}) is 0.14, and the compound is highly biodegradable; therefore, no bioaccumulation occurs (1).

ABSORPTION, METABOLISM, AND ELIMINATION

The metabolism and elimination of isopropanol is shown in Figure 107-3. Because isopropanol is highly water soluble, it is distributed rapidly throughout the body after it is ingested. Isopropanol is absorbed rapidly from the GI tract and distributes in total body water (500 to 700 mL per kg) (2). The kidney excretes 25% to 50% unchanged, and the balance is metabolized by ADH to acetone, which frequently is found in the blood, alveolar air, and urine of humans after ingestion. It has also been found in spinal fluid at levels similar to those in the blood (3).

Acetone is more slowly eliminated than is isopropanol, and acetone levels typically exceed isopropanol levels a few hours after absorption. Although acetone may contribute to CNS depression, long-term sequelae are not generally attributed to either isopropanol or acetone toxicity. After isopropanol's inhalation, the acetone-isopropanol ratio in blood decreases with increasing isopropanol concentrations, indicating saturation of the oxidative metabolic pathway. Volunteers who drank isopropanol have shown a total urinary excretion of 2% of the ingested dose.

Endogenous formation of isopropanol has been found at autopsy in individuals who were not previously exposed. It is thought that isopropanol results from the reduction of acetone by liver ADH in the presence of high concentrations of acetone and high NADH/NAD ratios. These conditions are found in such situations as diabetes, starvation, chronic alcoholism, and severe dehydration (4,5).

TABLE 107-1. Alcohols

Chemical name	Chemical formula	Toxicity	Regulatory limits
Allyl alcohol	CH_2OH	Colorless, flammable liquid. Incompatible with oxidizers. Used as a fungicide and herbicide in past and in preparation of acrolein and glycerol. An eye, skin, and respiratory tract irritant. Can cause dermal and ocular burns on contact; hence, contact with skin or eye should immediately be decontaminated with water. Can be absorbed through skin or inhaled.	OSHA PEL = 2 ppm; IDLH level = 150 ppm
n-Butyl alcohol (*n*-butanol)	C_4H_9OH	Colorless, flammable liquid having a very strong, disagreeable odor. Used as a solvent for lacquers and also in manufacturing of plastics and cement. Incompatible with oxidizing agents. A strong irritant of mucous membranes, eyes, skin, and respiratory tract. Possible causative agent in CNS depression if in high concentrations in air.	OSHA PEL = 100 ppm; ACGIH TLV(ceiling) = 50 ppm; IDLH level = 8,000 ppm
sec-Butyl alcohol	$CH_3CH_2CHOHCH_3$	Colorless, flammable liquid having a strong, disagreeable odor. Also known as *2-butanol.* Used as a solvent for paint removing and in polishing and cleaning materials; also used in synthesis of methyl ethyl ketone. Incompatible with strong oxidizing agents. At high concentrations in air, possible cause of narcosis and CNS depression. A strong irritant of mucous membranes, eyes, and respiratory tract.	OSHA PEL = 150 ppm: ACGIH TLV = 100 ppm; IDLH level = 10,000 ppm
tert-Butyl alcohol (*n*-propanol)	$(CH_3)_3COH$	Colorless, flammable liquid having a disagreeable odor. Used in manufacturing of plastics and esters and as intermediate in formulating other chemicals. High concentrations in air possible cause of CNS depression and irritating to eyes, throat, and mucous membranes. Mild chemical burns possible from contact of the liquid with skin.	OSHA PEL = 100 ppm, ACGIH TLV = 100 ppm; IDLH level = 8,000 ppm
Isobutyl alcohol	$(CH_3)_2CH_2OH$	Colorless, flammable liquid used in paint removers and as a general solvent. Used also in manufacture of esters. An irritant of skin, eyes, and mucous membranes.	OSHA PEL = 100 ppm; ACGIH TLV = 50 ppm; IDLH level = 8,000 ppm
Cyclohexanol	$C_6H_{11}OH$	Colorless, thick liquid with odor of camphor. Used as solvent for ethyl cellulose and other resins, in manufacture of soap, and in manufacture of adipic acid, which is used in nylon production; used also in plastic manufacturing. Incompatible with strong oxidizers. An irritant of eyes, skin, and mucous membranes; can produce CNS depression at high air concentrations.	OSHA PEL = 50 ppm; ACGIH TLV = 50 ppm; IDLH level = 3,500 ppm
Diacetone alcohol	$(CH_3)_2C(OH)CH_2CO\,H_3$	Flammable liquid used as solvent for cellulose esters, pigments, oils, and fats; also used in hydraulic brake fluids and as an antifreezing agent. Incompatible with strong oxidizers and alkaline substances. On exposure, skin irritation and irritation of eyes, mucous membranes, and respiratory tract produced. At higher concentrations in air, CNS depression possible.	OSHA PEL = 50 ppm; ACGIH TLV = 50 ppm; IDLH level = 2,100 ppm
Dibutylaminoethanol	$(C_4H_9)_2NCH_2OH$	Colorless, flammable liquid. An irritant of eyes, skin, and mucous membranes.	No OSHA PEL established; ACGIH TLV-TWA = 2 ppm, with a skin notation
Diethylaminoethanol	$(C_2H_5)_2NCH_2CH_2OH$	Colorless, flammable liquid. Used as a chemical intermediate in production of numerous compounds and such products as detergents, cosmetics, textile finishing agents, and pharmaceuticals. Incompatible with strong oxidizing agents and acids. An irritant of eyes, mucous membranes, skin, and respiratory tract. Can also produce nausea and vomiting.	OSHA PEL = 10 ppm; ACGIH TLV = 10 ppm; IDLH level = 500 ppm
Ethyl alcohol (ethanol)	C_2H_5OH	Colorless, very volatile, flammable liquid. Used in grain alcohol, wines, and other alcoholic consumption beverages; also used in chemical synthesis of many other compounds. A general solvent used in many processes such as the manufacturing of pharmaceutical agents. Used also as a general solvent in perfumes, cosmetics, adhesives, inks, and preservatives, and as a fuel and antifreeze. Common, well-known intoxication states possible after ingestion.	OSHA PEL = 1,000 ppm
β-Chloroethyl alcohol (ethylene chlorhydrin)		Flammable, colorless liquid having an odor like ether. Used in production of ethylene glycol and ethylene oxide; also used as a solvent for cellulose acetates and esters, resins, waxes, and ethers. Used in chemical reactions in which hydroxyethyl groups must be introduced into organic compounds. In cleaning industry, used to remove tar from clothing. Also used as general solvent and for fabric dying. Incompatible with strong oxidizing agents and alkaline substances. An irritant of skin, eyes, and mucous membranes; a hepatotoxin whose metabolites are chloroacetaldehyde and chloroacetic acid; also a renal toxin. Irritation to eyes, mucous membranes, and respiratory tract and nausea and vomiting possible after toxic exposure to vapors. Headache, hypotension, cardiovascular collapse, and coma possible after low-level exposure.	OSHA PEL = 5 ppm; ACGIH TLV = 1 ppm; ACGIH ceiling value = 1 ppm, with a skin notation; IDLH level = 10 ppm
Furfuryl alcohol (furfural alcohol, 2-furanmethanol)	$C_4H_3OCH_2OH$	Colorless liquid. Used as a starting monomer in production of furan resins or furan polymers; also used as a solvent for cellulase ethers, esters, resins, and dyes, as well as in manufacturing of resin compounds. Incompatible with strong acids and strong oxidizing agents, which can lead to rapid polymerization; liquid turns dark in air. Irritating to respiratory tract, mucous membranes, and eyes. Possible cause of CNS depression if high concentrations in air.	OSHA PEL = 50 ppm; ACGIH TLV = 10 ppm, with a skin notation; IDLH level = 250 ppm
Isoamyl alcohol (fusel oil, 3-methyl-1-butanol)	$(C_2H_5)_2CHOH$	Colorless, flammable liquid. Used in manufacture of lacquers, paint, varnishes, paint removers, cements, perfumes, pharmaceuticals, rubber, and plastic; also used in production of isobutyl esters. Irritating to skin and eyes; mildly irritating to mucous membranes, respiratory tract, and skin. CNS depression possible at high air concentrations. On ingestion, can produce narcosis, headache, vomiting, weakness, and CNS depression.	OSHA PEL = 100 ppm; ACGIH TLV = 100 ppm; IDLH level = 8,000 ppm

(continued)

TABLE 107-1. *(continued)*

Chemical name	Chemical formula	Toxicity	Regulatory limits
Isopropyl alcohol (isopropanol)	$CH_3CHOHCH_3$	Colorless, flammable liquid. Widely used in cosmetics and as a solvent in perfumes and many other commercial processes. Incompatible with strong oxidizing agents. Possibly irritating to eyes, mucous membranes, and respiratory tract. At high concentrations, possible cause of CNS depression on inhalation. GI bleeding, CNS depression, and hypotension possible after ingestion.	OSHA PEL = 400 ppm; ACGIH TLV = 400 ppm; IDLH level = 20,000 ppm
Isooctyl alcohol (isooctanol)	$C_7H_{15}CH_2OH$	Clear liquid. Used as raw material for surfactants, as an antifoaming agent, and as a solvent; used in formation of phthalate esters, maleate esters, and adipate esters, which in turn are used to form plastics.	ACGIH TLV-TWA = 50 ppm, with a skin notation
Methyl alcohol (methanal)	CH_3OH	Colorless, flammable liquid. Used in many organic syntheses such as formation of formaldehyde, ethylene glycol, ethyl amines, pesticides, and methacrylates; also used as antifreeze. Metabolic acidosis with an anion gap, owing to formation of toxic metabolites of formaldehyde and formic acid, most common toxic manifestation of ingestion.	OSHA PEL = 200 ppm; ACGIH TLV = 200 ppm, with a skin notation; IDLH level = 25,000 ppm
Methyl cyclohexanol	$CH_3C_6H_{10}OH$	Slightly yellow, flammable liquid having slight odor of coconuts. Used as a solvent for lacquers and as an antioxidant in lubricants. Incompatible with strong oxidizing agents. Irritation to eyes, skin, and mucous membranes possible from exposure to vapors. Easily detected at airborne concentration of 500 ppm, a concentration that can produce irritant effects.	OSHA PEL = 100 ppm; ACGIH TLV = 50 ppm; IDLH level = 10,000 ppm
Methyl amyl alcohol (methyl isobutyl carbinol)	$CH_3CHOHCH_2CH(CH_3)_2$	Colorless, flammable liquid. Used as a solvent, in manufacturing and formulation of brake fluid, and as an intermediate in synthesis of other organic compounds. An irritant of eyes and mucous membranes at high concentrations; can produce CNS depression.	OSHA PEL = 25 ppm; ACGIH TLV = 25 ppm; IDLH level = 2,000 ppm
N-propyl alcohol (1-propanol)	CH_3CH_2OH	Clear, flammable liquid used in lacquers, cosmetics, cleaners, polishers, polishing agents, and pharmaceuticals; also used as an antiseptic agent. Incompatible with strong oxidizing agents. An irritant of the eyes, skin, and mucous membranes and, in high concentrations in air, can produce CNS depression. Also can produce CNS depression after ingestion, and is thought to be more toxic than isopropyl alcohol. Not very irritating to the skin.	OSHA PEL = 200 ppm; ACGIH TLV = 200 ppm; IDLH level = 4,000 ppm

ACGIH, American Conference of Governmental Industrial Hygienists; CNS, central nervous system; GI, gastrointestinal; IDLH, immediately dangerous to life and health; OSHA, U.S. Occupational Safety and Health Administration; PEL, permissible exposure limit; TLV, threshold limit value; TWA, time-weighted average.

The elimination of isopropanol from humans follows first-order kinetics. It appears to have a half-life of 2.5 to 3 hours. As acetone is formed, levels decline slowly over approximately 30 hours. In nonalcoholics, the half-life of isopropanol appears to be nearly 6.4 hours, with the acetone reaching a maximum concentration in the blood 30 hours after ingestion (3).

CLINICAL TOXICOLOGY

Clinical toxicity occurs after isopropanol is ingested or used as rubbing alcohol (via skin absorption) (2,6). Isopropanol is absorbed rapidly after inhalation or ingestion and can be absorbed dermally. The compound is a central nervous system (CNS) depressant and is believed to be twice as active as ethanol in producing a longer duration of coma owing to its slower metabolism and to the contribution of acetone to CNS depression. Death can occur from respiratory depression and coma. Large ingestions can cause hypotension, shock, and cardiac arrest. Hyperglycemia and elevated cerebrospinal fluid proteins have also been observed after overdose.

Oral ingestion produces gastritis, nausea, vomiting, abdominal pain, and gastrointestinal (GI) hemorrhage. Tachycardia and hypothermia have occurred in conjunction with hypotension, coma, and death. Coma has been reported secondary to sponge bathing from isopropanol absorption through the skin (6).

Although ingestion generally is considered to represent the greatest hazard, the use of isopropanol, with or without water, in a sponge bath to lower fever has led to coma in infants and adults, owing to dermal absorption.

Isopropanol can be removed by hemodialysis. Hypotension is considered to be an indicator of a poor outcome.

1-Propanol

1-Propanol is a colorless, flammable liquid that is volatile at room temperature and normal atmospheric pressure. Its chemical structure is depicted in Figure 107-1. It mixes easily with water and organic solvents. Exposure can occur through ingestion or inhalation.

Entry of 1-propanol into the environment is mainly through emissions into the atmosphere during its production and storage, use, or disposal. 1-Propanol is metabolized rapidly in the atmosphere by reaction with hydroxy radicals. It also is biodegradable aerobically and anaerobically. Hence, it usually does not accumulate in the environment. The bioconcentration factor of 1-propanol is 0.7, which means that it does not bioaccumulate (K_{ow}, 0.34) (7).

1-Propanol is found in fuel oils. It is used mainly as a solvent and is a carrier for natural products such as flavoring, vegetable oils, resins, waxes, and gums. It also is used as a solvent for such synthetic polymers as lacquers and cellulose esters and for polyvinyl chloride (PVC) adhesives (7). 1-Propanol is used in the polymerization of acrylonitrile, in the dying of wool, in printing inks, and in antiseptic preparations, cosmetics, lotions, soaps, and nail polishes. Other uses include degreasing agents, brake fluid, and such polishing compounds as window cleaners and floor polishes.

ABSORPTION, METABOLISM, AND EXCRETION

Ingested or inhaled 1-propanol is absorbed and distributed rapidly. It is metabolized by ADH to propionic acid and may enter the Krebs cycle. Oxidation is the rate-limiting step of 1-propanol metabolism. The affinity of 1-propanol for ADH and the other microsomal oxidizing enzymes is much higher than that of alcohol or ethanol (7).

TABLE 107-2. Esters

Chemical name	Chemical formula	Toxicity	Regulatory limits
n-Amyl acetate	$CH_3COOC_5H_{11}$	Clear, flammable liquid with a bananalike odor. Irritation of mucous membranes, eyes, and throat possible on exposure to vapors. CNS depression also possible after exposure.	OSHA PEL = 100 ppm; ACGIH TLV = 100 ppm; IDLH level = 4,000 ppm
Sec-amyl acetate (α-methylbutyl acetate, banana oil)	$C_7H_{14}O_2$	Clear, flammable liquid. An irritant of mucous membranes, eyes, and skin and, in high concentrations, possible producer of CNS depression.	OSHA PEL = 125 ppm; ACGIH TLV = 125 ppm; IDLH level = 9,000 ppm
Isoamyl acetate (amyl acetate, banana oil, pear oil)	$CH_3C(O)CH_2(CH_3)C_2H_5$	Colorless, flammable liquid. An irritant of mucous membranes, eyes, and throat and, at high concentrations, possible producer of CNS depression.	OSHA PEL = 100 ppm; ACGIH TLV = 100 ppm; IDLH level = 3,000 ppm
Iso-*n*-butyl acetate	$CH_3CH_2CH_2CH_2OCOCH_3$	Clear, flammable liquid with a pleasant fruity odor. One of four isomers of the butyl acetates. Used as a solvent for nitrocellulose, resins, waxes, fats, and oils and in the manufacture of lacquer, plastics, and perfumes. Irritating to mucous membranes and eyes and, in high concentrations, possible producer of CNS depression.	OSHA PEL = 100 ppm; ACGIH TLV = 150 ppm; IDLH level = 10,000 ppm
sec-Butyl acetate (2-butanol acetate)	$CH_3CH_2CH(CH_3)OCH_3$	Clear, flammable liquid with a fruity odor. Used as a solvent for lacquers and paper coatings; also used as a solvent for nitrocellulose and nail enamels. At high air concentrations, a CNS depressant. Can produce irritation of mucous membranes, eyes, and respiratory tract.	OSHA PEL = 200 ppm; ACGIH TLV = 200 ppm; IDLH level = 10,000 ppm
Isobutyl acetate	$(CH_3)_2CHCH_2OCOCH_3$	Colorless, flammable liquid. Used as a solvent and flavoring agent; also used as a solvent for nitrocellulose and in perfumes. Can produce CNS depression in high air concentrations. Can produce mucous membrane and eye irritation.	OSHA PEL = 150 ppm; ACGIH TLV = 150 ppm; IDLH level = 7,500 ppm
tert-Butyl acetate	$(CH_3)_3COCOCH_3$	Colorless, flammable liquid having a pleasant odor. Used as a gasoline additive and as a solvent. An irritant of eyes and mucous membranes. Possible CNS depressant.	OSHA PEL = 200 ppm; ACGIH TLV = 200 ppm; IDLH level = 8,000 ppm
n-Butyl acrylate (butyl ester)	$CH_2{=}CHCOOC_4H_9$	Colorless, flammable liquid. A monomer used in the production of polymers for solvent coatings, adhesive, paints, and binders. An irritant of mucous membranes and eyes; on ocular exposure in animals, can produce corneal damage and necrosis. Also an irritant of respiratory tract.	ACGIH TLV = 10 ppm
2-Ethoxyethyl acetate (cellosolve acetate, glycol monoethyl ether acetate)	$C_2H_5OCH_2OCOCH_3$	Colorless, flammable liquid. Used as a solvent for nitrocellulose and resins. In high concentrations, can produce CNS depression and is an irritant to eyes and mucous membranes.	ACGIH TLV = 5 ppm
Ethyl acetate	$CH_3COOC_2H_5$	Clear, flammable liquid having a pleasant odor. Used as a solvent for lacquers and as an artificial perfume agent. Can produce irritation of eyes, mucous membranes, and respiratory tract. In high concentrations, can produce CNS depression.	OSHA PEL = 400 ppm; ACGIH TLV = 400 ppm; IDLH level = 10,000 ppm
Ethyl acrylate	$CH_2{=}CHCOOC_2H_5$	Clear, flammable liquid. Used as a monomer in manufacture of polymer resins and in production of paints and plastics. Irritating to eyes, mucous membranes, and skin; may produce skin sensitization. Vapors possibly very irritating at 4–5 ppm. Odor detectable at concentrations of <1 ppm in the air.	ACGIH TLV = 5 ppm
Ethyl formate (formic acid ethyl ester)	$HCOOC_2H_5$	Colorless, flammable liquid having a fruity odor. Used as a solvent for cellulose nitrate and acetate; also used as a solvent for oils and greases and as a fumigant. Irritant of eyes and mucous membranes; can cause CNS depression. Incompatible with nitrates, strong oxidizers, and strong acids.	OSHA PEL = 100 ppm; ACGIH TLV = 100 ppm; IDLH level = 8,000 ppm
2-Ethylhexyl acrylate	$H_2C{=}CHC(O)OCH_2CH(C_2H_5)(CH_2)_3$	Colorless, flammable liquid used to produce latex paint, plastics, and protective coatings. Irritating to skin and mucous membranes; can produce skin sensitization.	No TLV established
Ethyl methacrylate [Plexiglas (when in polymeric form)]	$CH_2{=}C(CH_3)COOC_2H_5$	Clear, flammable liquid. Used to make polymers of Plexiglas and, in polymerized form, is nontoxic; however, monomers are irritants of skin, eyes, mucous membranes, lungs.	
sec-Hexyl acetate	$CH_{15}O_2$	Clear, flammable liquid having a pleasant fruity odor. Used as a solvent in spray lacquers and for cellulose esters and resins. Incompatible with strong alkalis, acids, oxidizing agents. Irritating to mucous membranes, respiratory tract, eyes.	ACGIH TLV = 50 ppm; OSHA PEL = 50 ppm; IDLH level = 4,000 ppm
Isopropyl acetate (2-propyl acetate)	$CH_3COOCH(CH_3)_2$	Flammable liquid solvent. Irritant of eyes, mucous membranes, and lungs and, in high air concentrations, possible producer of CNS depression. Incompatible with strong oxidizing agents, strong alkalis, acids.	OSHA PEL = 250 ppm; ACGIH TLV = 250 ppm; IDLH level = 16,000 ppm
2-Methoxyethyl acetate		Clear, flammable liquid used in lacquer industry, printing, and photographic film and in coatings and adhesives. Mild irritant of mucous membranes and eyes. Can produce CNS depression in high concentrations.	ACGIH TLV = 5 ppm

(continued)

TABLE 107-2. *(continued)*

Chemical name	Chemical formula	Toxicity	Regulatory limits
Methyl silicate (tetramethoxysilane)	$Si(OCH_3)_4$	Clear liquid used in ceramics industry for coating and closing pores and as a bonding agent; used to coat television tubes. An eye and respiratory irritant. VP = 12 mm Hg (25°C). Producer of corneal irritation (possibly) at 200–300 ppm; corneal lesions and ulcerations at >1,000 ppm.	ACGIH TLV = 1 ppm (6 mg/m³); STEL = 5 ppm (30 mg/m³)
Ethylsilicate (tetraethylorthosilicate)	$Si(OCH_2H_4)_4$	Colorless, flammable liquid having a pleasant odor. Insoluble in water. Used as a rocket propellant, fuel ignition promoter; in production of cases and molds. Heat-resistant adhesive. Hydrolyzed by water to ethanol and silicic acid. Produces explosive mixtures of vapor and air at elevated temperatures. Irritating to eyes and respiratory tract. Can cause dermatitis. VP = 1 mm Hg (20°C).	OSHA PEL = 25 ppm (110 mg/m³); ACGIH STEL = 40 ppm (170 mg/m³); IDLH level = 2,000 ppm
Methyl formate (formic acid methyl ester)	$HCOOCH_3$	Colorless, flammable liquid having ethyl ether odor. Used in combination with other solvents for cellulose nitrate, for oils and greases; also used as a fumigant. Explosive mixtures formed by vapor and air at normal temperatures. Can be adsorbed via inhalation, ingestion, and skin. Irritant and CNS depressant effects at high vapor concentration. VP = 400 mm Hg (16°C).	OSHA PEL = 100 ppm (250 mg/m³); ACGIH STEL = 150 ppm (375 mg/m³); IDLH level = 5,000 ppm
Ethyl formate (formic acid ethyl ester)	$HCOOC_2H_5$	Colorless, flammable liquid having aromatic odor. Solvent for cellulose nitrate and for oil and greases. Vapor levels of 330 ppm irritating to eyes and mucous membranes. Causes CNS depression in animals. Forms explosive vapor mixtures with air at normal temperatures. VP = 40 mm Hg (31.6°C).	OSHA PEL = 100 ppm (300 mg/m³); ACGIH STEL = 150 ppm (450 mg/m³); IDLH level = 8,000 ppm
n-Propyl nitrate	$CH_3(CH_2)_2NO_3$	Clear to yellow liquid having sickening odor. Used as rocket propellant and ignition promoter. Irritant of eyes and mucous membranes; yellow skin discoloration on contact; methemoglobinemia. Explosion hazard on heating.	OSHA PEL = 25 ppm (110 mg/m³); ACGIH TLV = 40 ppm (170 mg/m³); IDLH level = 2,000 ppm
Butyl formate	$HCOO(CH_2)_3CH_3$	Flammable, colorless liquid. Solvent for cellulose compounds and resins. Explosive hazard in vapor formation at normal temperatures. Ocular and respiratory irritant. VP = 40 mm Hg (31.6°C).	

ACGIH, American Conference of Governmental Industrial Hygienists; CNS, central nervous system; IDLH, immediately dangerous to life and health; OSHA, U.S. Occupational Safety and Health Administration; PEL, permissible exposure limit; STEL, short-term exposure limit; TLV, threshold limit value; VP, vapor pressure.

TABLE 107-3. Common ketones

Chemical name	Chemical formula	Toxicity	Regulatory limits
Acetone (dimethyl ketone)	CH_3COCH_3	Colorless, flammable liquid having a sweet odor. Highly volatile. Vapors explosive in air. Absorbed via lungs, skin, and GI tract. Airway irritant, CNS narcotic by inhalation and dermal absorption. VP = 181.72 mm Hg (20°C).	OSHA PEL = 750 ppm
Methyl *n*-butyl ketone (MBK)	$CH_3COCH_2CH_2CH_2CH_3$	Colorless liquid solvent. Highly volatile. Metabolism produces neurotoxic metabolite (2,5-hexanedione).	OSHA PEL = 100 ppm; IDLH level = 1,600 ppm
Methyl ethyl ketone (MEK)	$CH_3COCH_2CH_3$	Colorless, highly flammable, volatile liquid solvent having acetone odor. Forms explosive vapor mixture with air. Absorbed via lungs, skin, and GI tract. Can cause coma and metabolic acidosis.	OSHA PEL = 200 ppm (590 mg/m³); IDLH level = 3,000 ppm
Methyl isobutyl ketone (MIBK)	$CH_3COCH_2CH(CH_3)_2$	Clear, flammable liquid having sweet odor. Occurs naturally in certain foods. Solvent for lacquers and flavoring agent. Respiratory tract irritant, eye irritant, CNS depressant. Vapor density = 3.45 (air = 1.00).	OSHA PEL = 410 mg/m³
Isophorone	$C_9H_{14}O$	Component of an essential oil solvent for resins and polymers, fats, oils. Absorbed by oral, dermal, and inhalational routes. Eye and mucous membrane irritant; causes headache, dizziness.	OSHA PEL = 4 ppm
Cyclohexanone	$C_6H_{10}O$	Clear to pale-yellow liquid having sweet odor. Solvent and degreaser. Used in production of nylon and solvent in paints and lacquers; also solvent for cellulose and acetate resins. Eye, nose, and throat irritation at high vapor concentrations. Vapor density = 3.4 (air = 1.0). Causes narcosis and CNS depression in animals; eye contact with liquid possible cause of corneal injury.	OSHA PEL = 50 ppm (200 mg/m³)

CNS, central nervous system; GI, gastrointestinal; IDLH, immediately dangerous to life and health; OSHA, U.S. Occupational Safety and Health Administration; PEL, permissible exposure limit; VP, vapor pressure.

TABLE 107-4. Ethers

Chemical name	Chemical formula	Toxicity	Regulatory limits
Ethyl ether	$C_2H_5OC_2H_5$	Colorless, highly flammable liquid having characteristic ether odor. Anesthetic gas. Solvent for cellulose, fats, oils, gums, waxes, resins. Forms explosive peroxides in air or sunlight. Vapor density = 2.56.	OSHA PEL = 400 ppm (1,200 mg/m³); IDLH level = 19,000 ppm
Methyl ether	CH_3OCH_3	Colorless gas with ether odor. Vapor density = 1.62. 50% mixture with air has unpleasant, suffocating odor response.	
Isopropyl ether	$(CH_3)_2CHOCH(CH_3)_2$	Colorless, highly flammable liquid having ether odor. Anesthetic agent. Forms explosive peroxide in air. Ocular irritant at 800 ppm; incites dermatitis. Vapor density = 2.4.	
Dichloroisopropyl ether	$[ClCH_2C(CH_3)H]_2O$	Colorless liquid. Fire and explosion hazard. Can penetrate skin and cause toxicity and death; renal and liver toxin. Vapor density = 6.0.	
Vinyl ether	CH_2:CHOCH:CH_2	Colorless, volatile, highly flammable liquid that forms explosive peroxide. Anesthetic agent. Hepatotoxin on prolonged exposure. Vapor density = 2.4.	

IDLH, immediately dangerous to life and health; OSHA, U.S. Occupational Safety and Health Administration; PEL, permissible exposure limit.

In an animal model, the half-life of 1-propanol was 45 minutes. 1-Propanol can be eliminated through expired air or in the urine. In humans, the urinary excretion is approximately 2% of the dose. Few reports exist of adverse health effects from exposure to 1-propanol, and its toxicity appears to be low via the dermal, oral, or respiratory inhalational route of exposure. Acute effects of ingestion of 1-propanol are intoxication and narcosis, similar to the effects of ethanol, although 1-propanol appears to be at least two to four times as intoxicating as ethanol.

1-Propanol is oxidized to propionaldehyde by ADH. This is followed by conversion to propionic acid, which is formed also from the metabolism of odd-chain fatty acids. Hence, propionic acid occurring from the oxidation of 1-propanol can form coenzyme A, and enter the Krebs cycle (7).

CLINICAL TOXICOLOGY

Case reports of acute poisoning with 1-propanol indicate that it is similar to ethanol and can produce coma and respiratory depression (7). Patch testing indicates that occupational exposure and inclusion of this compound in cosmetics may cause allergic reactions (8).

Methanol

Methanol (methyl alcohol) is known as *wood alcohol* and is used widely as an industrial and household solvent. Methanol has caused poisonings by inhalation and skin absorption as well as by ingestion, resulting in severe metabolic acidosis. Owing in part to the variation in methanol toxicity among species, the human toxicity was not fully recognized until the 1920s.

ABSORPTION, METABOLISM, AND EXCRETION

Methanol has approximately one-third the intoxicating effect of ethanol, but hepatic metabolism via ADH produces highly toxic formic acid (formate). Methanol is metabolized slowly to formaldehyde, but conversion to formic acid ensues rapidly, and formic acid concentrations correlate well with a high anion gap metabolic acidosis and ocular toxicity (Fig. 107-4).

CLINICAL TOXICOLOGY

After methanol ingestion, toxicity may be delayed from 12 to 24 hours as the compound undergoes metabolism to toxic metabolites. Visual disturbances, ranging from decreased acuity to blindness, occur early. Other symptoms include headache, dizziness, and a decreased level of consciousness. In severe cases of toxicity, individuals develop coma and seizures. Early in the course after methanol ingestion, abdominal pain and vomiting occur. An anion gap metabolic acidosis with an osmolar gap is a hallmark of methanol toxicity. Toxicity may occur after methanol doses of 0.21 mL per kg.

Imaging scans of severely poisoned patients have demonstrated lesions in the putamen and globus pallidus (9,10). Such lesions can result in a parkinsonian syndrome with hypophonia, tremors, rigidity, and bradykinesia.

In 1978, 372 patients were poisoned by ingesting an 82% methanol and 18% isopropanol mixture that was mistakenly substituted for their methylated spirits. Visual disturbance was noted in 27% (102 of 372 patients), and mortality was 5% (18 of 372). Of the 102 patients with visual disturbances, 29 were blind (4 of whom remained so), 65 reported blurring of vision (44 with pupil or fundus changes), and 10 had dilated pupils (two nonreactive).

MANAGEMENT OF TOXICITY

Methanol is metabolized first by ADH to formaldehyde, which then is metabolized rapidly by ADH to formic acid (see Fig. 107-4). Formic acid (formate) is the toxic metabolite responsible for methanol poisoning. Management is directed at preventing further metabolism of methanol to formic acid and eliminating the methanol and metabolic acids by dialysis (11). Although methanol-poisoned patients who are severely acidotic and comatose have a high mortality, both the severe acid–base disturbances and the toxic levels of formic acid can be effectively managed with hemodialysis combined with antidotal agents that inhibit ADH and, thus, the formation of formic acid (12).

ADH is the metabolic site of action of antidotal treatment (blockade of the toxic synthesis) for methanol and ethylene glycol toxicity, by either ethanol or by the competitive ADH inhibitor 4-methylpyrazole (4-MP) (see Fig. 107-4) (12,13). Synthesis of formic acid is essentially blocked by a blood ethanol level of 130 mg per dL. This blood ethanol level can be achieved by administering a loading dose of ethanol in dextrose followed by a maintenance dose to keep the blood level at approximately 130 mg per dL. The loading dose and maintenance dosing of ethanol are described in Table 107-5.

The drug 4-MP (fomepizole) is a competitive ADH inhibitor and an effective antidote for methanol and ethylene glycol poisoning. The concentration at which 4-MP inhibits 50% of ADH is 0.1 μmol per L (14). The drug is used intravenously and orally and is eliminated by Michaelis-Menten kinetics. Therapeutic blood levels are 8.2 to 24.6 mg per L. An intravenous loading dose of 15 mg per kg is followed by 10 mg per kg every 12 hours for four doses, then 15 mg per kg every 12 hours until levels of methanol or ethylene glycol are less than 20 mg per dL (see Table 107-5) (14).

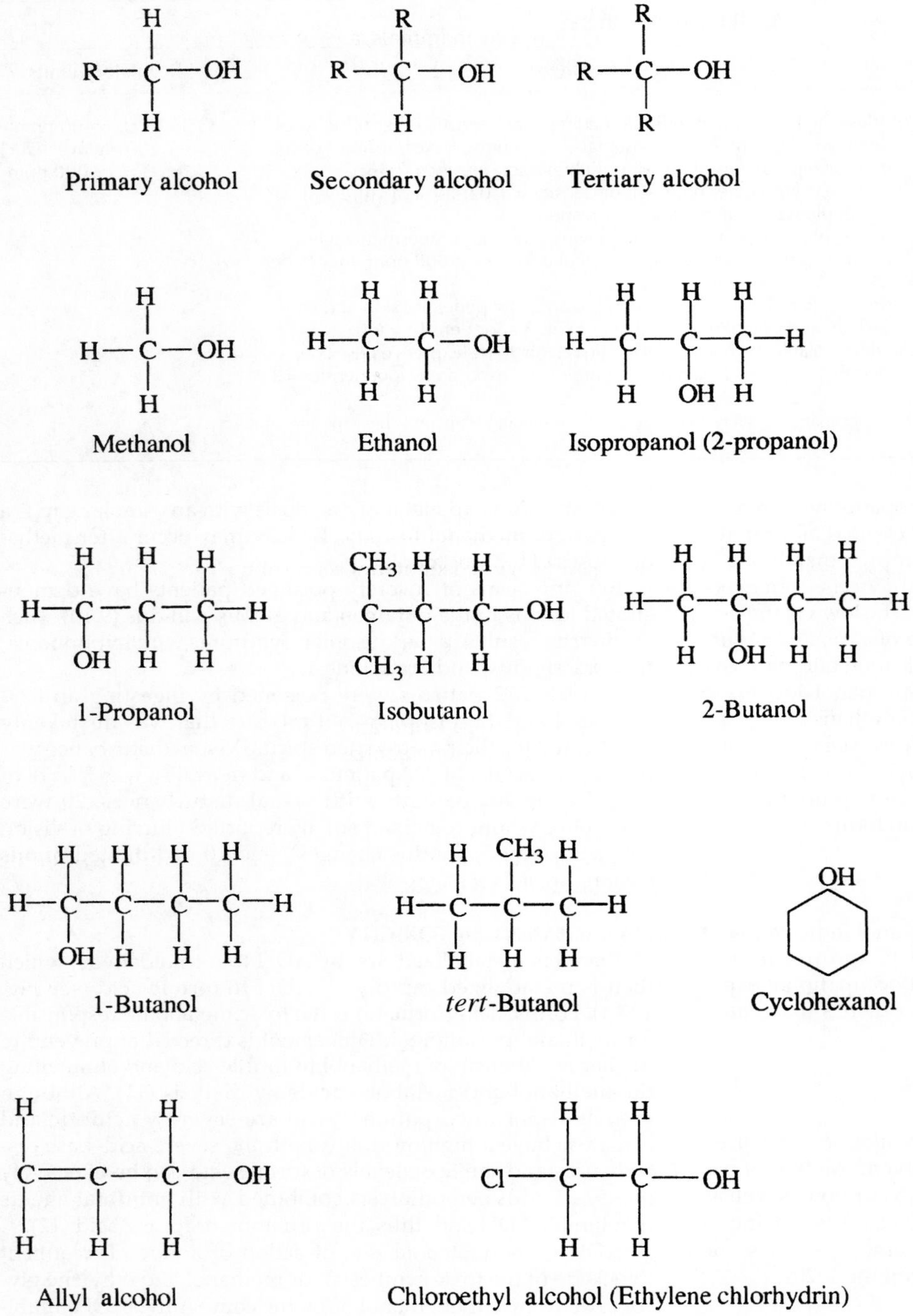

Primary alcohol
Secondary alcohol
Tertiary alcohol
Methanol
Ethanol
Isopropanol (2-propanol)
1-Propanol
Isobutanol
2-Butanol
1-Butanol
tert-Butanol
Cyclohexanol
Allyl alcohol
Chloroethyl alcohol (Ethylene chlorhydrin)

Figure 107-1. Chemical structure of various alcohols.

The drug is administered as a slow intravenous infusion over 30 minutes. Table 107-6 shows 4-MP dosing during dialysis.

Although clinical data are limited, folate or folinic acid (leucovorin, citrovorum factor) commonly is given during the first 24 hours and is believed to hasten formate metabolism to carbon dioxide and water.

1-Butanol

1-Butanol (butyl alcohol) (see Fig. 107-1) is a colorless liquid having a rancid, sweet odor and an odor threshold of 3.08 mg per cubic meter. It is used as an ingredient in perfumes and flavors; for extraction of flavoring materials, vegetable oils, and perfumes; and as a solvent. It also is used as a flavoring agent in foods (15).

1-Butanol can be found in many environments and has been detected in indoor air with a mean concentration of 5 parts per billion (ppb) and a range of 0.7 to 26.0 ppb (16).

ABSORPTION, METABOLISM, AND EXCRETION

1-Butanol is readily absorbed through the skin, lungs, and GI tract. Its metabolism is mainly via ADH. The general population is exposed to 1-butanol through food and beverages and via occupational exposures. 1-Butanol is rapidly metabolized by ADH to its corresponding acid.

Toxic manifestations after oral ingestion or inhalation of 1-butanol are similar to those associated with alcohol intoxication, including narcosis and CNS depression. Exposure to 1-butanol vapors produces irritation of the nose and throat, headache, dizziness, and drowsiness. Such vapors also can damage the super-

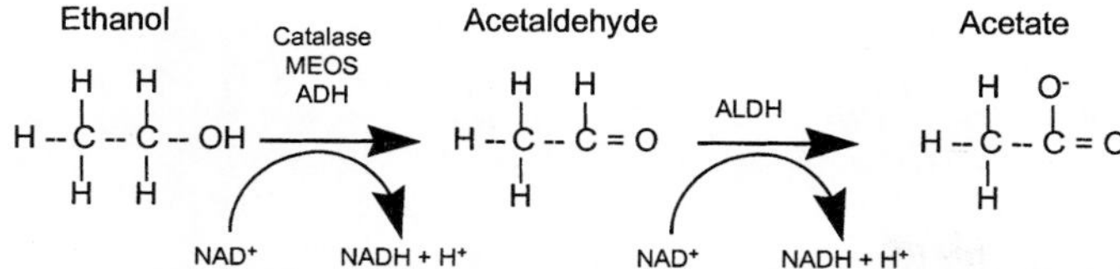

Figure 107-2. Ethanol metabolism. ADH, alcohol dehydrogenase; ALDH, aldehyde dehydrogenase; MEOS, microsomal ethanol-oxidizing system; NAD, nicotinamide adenine dinucleotide; NADH, nicotinamide adenine dinucleotide (reduced form).

ficial layers of the cornea. Contact dermatitis can result from 1-butanol skin contact (15).

CLINICAL TOXICOLOGY

Case reports of occupational exposure indicate burning and itching of the eyes, swelling of the eyelids, and eye redness after exposure to vapors. Blurring of vision, lacrimation, and photophobia have been observed. Repeated, long, high-dose inhalation may result in pathologic changes in the lungs. Also, high-level exposures may result in liver and kidney damage.

2-Butanol

2-Butanol (*sec*-butyl alcohol) is a flammable, colorless liquid having a sweet odor (see Fig. 107-1). Its odor threshold is 7.69 mg per cubic meter [2.5 parts per million (ppm)] (15). Its vapor is 2.6 times denser than is air. 2-Butanol occurs as a natural product of fermentation of carbohydrates.

2-Butanol is used mainly as a chemical intermediate for conversion into methyl ethyl ketone. It also is used for extraction of fish protein concentrates; as a solvent in lacquers, enamels, vegetable oils, gums, and resins; and in hydraulic brake fluids, cleaning compounds, polishes, and oils.

In animal models, 2-butanol is oxidized to methyl ethyl ketone (15). Excessive exposure to 2-butanol vapors can result in headache, dizziness, drowsiness, and narcosis.

tert-Butanol

tert-Butanol occurs as a colorless liquid or a white crystalline solid having a camphorlike odor (see Fig. 107-1). The odor threshold is 144.7 mg per cubic meter (47 ppm). It is soluble in water, and its K_{ow} is 0.37. Its vapor is 2.6 times denser than air (15).

tert-Butanol is used as a solvent, a dehydrating agent, and an intermediate chemical in the manufacture of other chemicals. It is biodegradable and does not bioaccumulate.

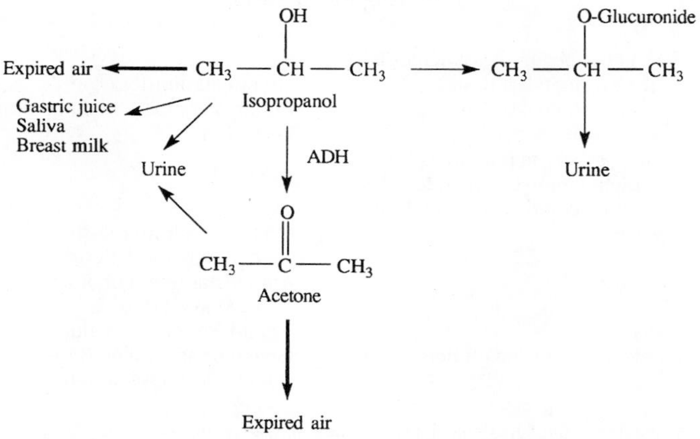

Figure 107-3. Isopropanol metabolism. ADH, alcohol dehydrogenase.

tert-Butanol is not a substrate for ADH enzymes. It is metabolized slowly by mammals, and its metabolic routes are believed to be direct conjugation of the hydroxyl group with glucuronic acid and oxidation of alkyl substituents (15). Twenty-four percent of the dose is eliminated in the urine as the glucuronide, and 10% can be excreted in the breath and urine as acetone (15). *tert*-Butanol appears to be mild irritating to the skin; otherwise, little human toxicity is documented. Animals exposed to *tert*-butanol vapors manifest restlessness, irritation of mucous membranes, ataxia, and narcosis.

Isobutanol

Isobutanol (2-methyl propanol) is a flammable, colorless liquid having a sweet odor similar to that of amyl alcohol (see Fig. 107-1). Its K_{ow} is 0.83, and its vapor is 2.6 times heavier than air (15). It is a natural product of fermentation reactions.

The major use of isobutanol is in the manufacture of isobutyl acetate, which is employed in lacquers. Isobutanol is used as a solvent in paint and varnish removers, as a plasticizer, and in the manufacture of isobutyl esters. It also is used in perfumes and as a flavoring agent. Isobutanol is one of the three main alcohols in fusel oil and can be found in some alcoholic beverages. It is found also in fruits, coffees, ciders, and cheeses.

Isobutanol is easily biodegraded and does not bioaccumulate. Because it is readily biodegradable, it may pose an indirect hazard for aquatic biota, because it may help lead to aquatic oxygen depletion. Isobutanol is absorbed via the skin, lungs, and GI tract and is metabolized by ADH to isobutyric acid (15).

Very few data are available on isobutanol's clinical toxicity in humans. Dermal exposure can cause erythematous lesions of the skin. Anecdotal case histories of individuals exposed in enclosed spaces indicate transient vertigo, nausea, vomiting, and headache. Eye irritation, blurred vision, and superficial corneal vacuolization have been described after excessive exposures in enclosed environments (15).

Cyclohexanol

Cyclohexanol, the chemical formula of which is $C_6H_{11}OH$, is a colorless, viscous liquid used as a solvent for oils and resins and in the manufacture of plastics, soaps, and cellulose (see Fig. 107-1). Cyclohexanol vapors cause irritation of the upper airway, eyes, nose, and throat and, in high concentrations, can produce narcosis. Humans exposed to airborne concentrations of 100 ppm for 3 to 5 minutes experience throat, eye, and nose irritation.

KETONES

Ketones are organic compounds containing a carbonyl (C=O) group attached to two carbon atoms (R–CO–R') (Fig. 107-5). Common commercial ketones include acetone, methyl ethyl ketone (MEK), methyl-*n*-butyl ketone (MBK), methyl isobutyl ketone (MIBK), cyclohexanone, and isophorone (see Table 107-3). The extensive industrial use of ketones reflects low production costs, excellent solvent properties, moderate vapor pressure, and miscibility with other liquids.

Ketones occur naturally in certain food products. Throughout the ages, they have served to provide pleasant aromas and food flavoring and therapeutic remedies for illness. Naturally occurring ketones are found in animal secretions and extracts of plants and as by-products of bacterial fermentation. Essential oils, oleoresins, waxes, and spices from plants are plant ketones.

Ketones are chemically formed by the *oxo reaction*, which is defined as a reaction among an olefin, carbon monoxide, and

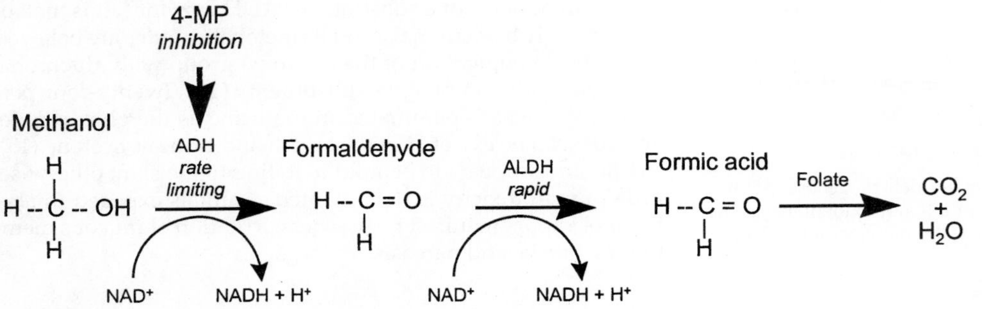

Figure 107-4. Methanol metabolism. ADH, alcohol dehydrogenase; ALDH, aldehyde dehydrogenase; 4-MP, 4-methylpyrazole; NAD, nicotinamide adenine dinucleotide; NADH, nicotinamide adenine dinucleotide (reduced form).

hydrogen to form saturated aldehydes and ketones. (The term *oxo* derives from the German word *oxierung*, meaning "ketonization." Terms such as *hydroformylation*, *carboxylation*, and *formylation* have replaced the term *oxo reaction*.) Another method by which ketones form is by oxidation of secondary alcohols.

Ketones can be subdivided into the following chemical categories (Table 107-7): aliphatic, cyclic, aromatic, and mixed (monobasic and dibasic) ketones, hydroxyketones, diketones, and quinones. They may take their names from the alcohols from which they are derived or may be named for the acid that may be oxidized.

The properties of ketones are attributable both to the carbonyl group and to the additional number, size, and kinds of structures and substitutes on the carbonyl group. Ketones display the following properties:

- All ketones up to C_{11} are neutral, volatile liquids.
- Ketones above C_{11} are solids under ambient conditions.
- Ketones have agreeable odors.
- All ketones, except those with a high number of carbon atoms, are soluble in water, with solubility decreasing as the carbon number increases.
- Most ketones are soluble in alcohol or ether.
- The specific gravity of ketones rises uniformly to 0.83 as molecular weight rises.

The C=O group determines the chemical behavior of ketones, which are easily reduced to form secondary alcohols. Ketones are generally stable and do not combine with alcohols or NH_3 as do aldehydes. They also do not reduce alkaline solutions of metals and do not readily undergo polymerization as do aldehydes. They combine with hydroxylamine to form ketoximes; react with hydrazine to form hydrazone; and react with semicarbazine to form semicarbizone. In the presence of H_2SO_4 or HCl, ketones undergo a cyclic trimerization. When oxidized, ketones decompose to two acids. Finally, they react with HCN to form cyanohydrins.

Acetone

Acetone (dimethyl ketone, 2-propanone, CH_3COCH_3) is a colorless, highly flammable, volatile liquid having a sweet odor and a molecular weight of 58.078 D (see Fig. 107-5). The physiochemical properties of and regulations that apply to acetone are listed in Table 107-8. The highly volatile acetone has a vapor pressure of 181.72 mm Hg at 20°C and can be explosive when mixed with air. It is completely miscible with water and organic solvents.

Acetone and the other ketones are used widely as solvents in the production of lubricating oils, in the dyeing and celluloid industries, and as chemical intermediates in a number of synthetic processes. Acetone is a powerful solvent and will dissolve fats, oils, waxes, greases, resins, dyes, and cellulose derivatives. It will dissolve many times its own volume of acetylene gas and so is used to store this gas in compressed cylinders (17).

Acetone also undergoes numerous chemical reactions and thus is an intermediate for the formation of various chemical products.

ENVIRONMENTAL FATE AND TRANSPORT

Reaction with hydroxy radicals and photolysis are the two main transformations that determine the atmospheric fate of acetone. Acetone's half-life in the atmosphere is estimated to be 22 days (18). Acetone is released to the environment from natural and anthropomorphic processes. Plants and trees are the main natural sources of acetone emissions. Acetone also is produced endogenously in the body and is exhaled from the lungs (19). It

TABLE 107-5. Alcohol dehydrogenase competitive inhibitors

Ethanol	
Loading dose	10 cc/kg in dextrose solution (10%) administered intravenously over 20–30 min
Maintenance dose	$\left[\frac{(125\ mg/kg/h^{a})(kg)}{750\ mg/mL^{b}}\right] \times 10 =$ mL of 10% ETOH in dextrose solution per h to maintain a blood level of 130 mg/dL
4-Methylpyrazole	
Loading dose	15 mg/kg IV slowly over 30 min
Maintenance dose	10 mg/kg IV q12h × 4 doses 15 mg/kg IV q12h until levels <20 mg/dL

[a]Density of ethanol (ETOH).
[b]Average metabolic rate for ethanol, range = 75–175 mg/kg/h.

TABLE 107-6. 4-Methylpyrazole dosing in patients requiring hemodialysis

Dose at the beginning of hemodialysis	
If <6 h since last dose	Do not administer dose
If ≥6 h since last dose	Administer next scheduled dose
Dosing during hemodialysis	Dose q4h
Dosing at time hemodialysis is completed (time between last dose and the end of hemodialysis)	
<1 h	Do not administer dose at the end of hemodialysis
1–3 h	Administer one-half of next scheduled dose
>3 h	Administer next scheduled dose
Maintenance dosing off hemodialysis	Give next scheduled dose 12 h after last dose administered

Adapted from Orphan Medical, Inc., Minnesota, with permission.

TABLE 107-7. Ketone classes

Aliphatic
- Acetone (dimethyl ketone or 2-propanone)
- Methylacetone (methyl ketone)
- Chloroacetone
- Dichlorotetrafluoroacetone
- Trichlorotrifluoroacetone
- Dichlorotetrafluoroacetone
- 1,1,3-Trichlorotrifluoroacetone
- Pentafluoromonochloroacetone
- Hexafluoroacetone
- Methyl ethyl ketone (2-butanone, MEK)
- Methyl isopropyl ketone (3-methyl-butanone-2, MIPK)
- Methyl *n*-propyl ketone (2-propanone, MPK)
- Methyl *n*-butyl ketone (2-hexanone, MBK)
- Methyl isobutyl ketone (4-methyl-2-pentanone, MIBK, henone)
- Methyl isoamyl ketone (MIAK)
- Pentoxone (4-methoxy-4-methyl-pentanone-2)
- Methyl hexyl ketone (2-octanone)
- Kiethyl ketone (3-pentanone, DEK, proprionone)
- Ethyl amyl ketone (EAM, 5-methyl-heptanone-3)
- Di-*n*-propyl ketone (4-heptanone, butyrone)
- Diisobutyl ketone (2,6-dimethyl-4-heptanone, DIBK, valerone)
- Isobutyl heptyl ketone (2,6,8-trimethyl-nananone-4, IBHK)
- Mesityl oxide (4-methyl-3-penten-2-one, MO)

Cyclic
- Cyclohexanone (nadone)
- Isophorone
- Methyl cyclohexanone (methylanon)
- 2-Cyclohexylcyclohexanone

Aromatic
- Acetophenone (methyl phenyl ketone, acetylbenzene)
- Benzophenone (diphenyl ketone)
- *p*-Chlorobenzophenone (4-chlorobenzophenone)
- 4-Dodecycloxy-2-hydroxybenzophenone (DOBP)
- 2-Hydroxy-4-methoxy-5-sulfobenzophenone (UV-2-284)
- Dibenzyl ketone (phenyl α-methylstyryl ketone, dypnone)
- Fenchone (*d*-1,3,3-trimethyl-2-norcamphanone)
- Hercosol (mixture of terpene ketones such as fenchone, camphor, and dipentene)

Mixed
- *Monobasic ketonic acids*: contain both a carbonyl group and a carboxylic acid group and react like a ketone and an acid. Subdivided into α- or 1-, β- or 2-, and γ- or 3-ketonic acids
  - α-Ketoacid (1-ketoacid, pyroracemic acid, propaneone)
    - Pyruvic acid
  - β-Ketoacid (2-ketoacid, β-ketobutyric acid)
    - β-Acetoacidic acid
  - γ-Ketoacid (3-ketoacid, γ-ketovaleric acid)
    - Levulinic acid
- *Dibasic ketonic acids*: contain one carbonyl group and two carboxylic acid groups
  - Mesoalic acid
  - Oxaloacetic acid
  - Acetone dicarboxylic acid
  - Dihydroxy tartaric acid
  - Diaceto succinic acid
  - Acetone dicarboxylic acid

Hydroxy ketones: have both a carbonyl group and at least one –OH group
- Acetol (acetyl alcohol, hydroxyacetone)
- Propinyl carbinol (hydroxymethyl ketone)
- Acetoin (acetylmethylcarbinol)
- β-Acetyl ethyl alcohol
- Methylacetonylcarbinol
- Methyl γ-hydroxypropyl ketone (5-pentanol-2-one)
- Diacetone (diacetone alcohol, 4-hydroxy-4-methyl-2-pentanone)
- Dihydroxyacetone (DHA)
- Benzoin (phenylbenzoyl carbinol)

Diketones: three types—α- or 1,2-; β- or 1,3-; and γ- or 1,4-diketone—represented by the formula R-CO-COR; where R and R' are alkyl, aryl, or hetracyclic groups
- α-Diketone (1,2-diketone)
  - Diacetyl
  - 2,3-Pentonedime
  - Methylethyl glyoxal
  - Diphenyl glyoxal
  - Biacetyl (2,3-butanedione)
  - Acetyl proprionyl
  - Benzil (diphenyl diketone)
  - Anisil
  - Furil
- β-Diketone
  - 2,4-Pentanedione
- γ-Diketone (1,4-diketone)
  - 2,5-Hexanedione

Quinones: exist as *ortho*- or *para*-, but not as *meta*-, positions
- Quinone (1,4-benzoquinone)
- 2,5-Diphenyl-*p*-benzoquinone (DPQ)
- Tetramethyl-1,3-cyclobutanedione
- Benzil (dibenzoyl)
- Kojic acid (2-hydroxymethyl-5-hydroxy-γ-pyrone)

is released into the environment through vehicle exhaust, wood burning, pulping of wood, polyethylene combustion, petroleum production, and the use of solvents. Acetone is a common compound found in hazardous-waste sites.

Ambient air concentrations of acetone are low, being less than 1 ppb in remote areas (less than 0.001 ppm). In urban areas of the United States, the mean concentration of acetone has been determined to be 6.9 ppb. Concentrations in indoor air are slightly higher than in outdoor air (8.0 ppb versus 6.9 ppb) (Table 107-9) (20). Acetone is also detected in seawater and in rivers and other bodies of water in the low parts-per-billion range. Thus, general populations are exposed through contamination of water and ambient air. Painters, workers in the chemical production industry, and those who use solvents containing acetone have the highest exposure.

Acetone leaches easily in soil and, therefore, can move into groundwater from landfills and other release sites. Organic compounds with ambient vapor pressures exceeding 1×10^{-4} mm Hg exist entirely in the vapor phase (21). Acetone has a very high vapor pressure of 181.72 mm Hg at 20°C and will exist exclusively in the vapor phase in the atmosphere.

Adsorption of acetone to sediments and suspended solids and water is insignificant, although the liquid is readily miscible with water. In low-water-content solids, acetone adsorbs strongly to the clay component by hydrogen bonding (17). Adsorption to soil depends on the relative humidity, increasing humidity serving to decrease the adsorption. Acetone volatilizes readily from water sources into the atmosphere. The low log of the K_{ow} value of –0.24 indicates that bioconcentration is insignificant. Studies have indicated that acetone is easily biodegradable by microorganisms in the soil.

Acetone is produced endogenously by all humans. Acetone exposure occurs by inhaling air containing acetone or by drinking water or ingesting food that contains acetone.

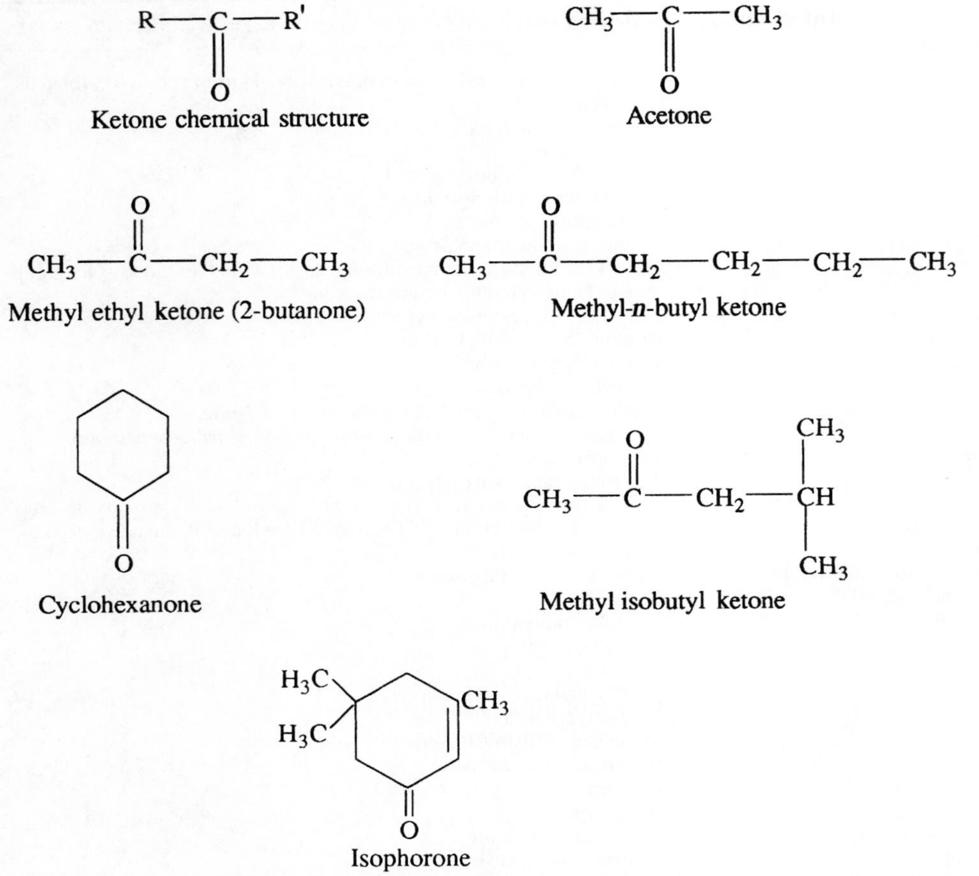

R—C(=O)—R'

Ketone chemical structure

CH_3—C(=O)—CH_3

Acetone

CH_3—C(=O)—CH_2—CH_3

Methyl ethyl ketone (2-butanone)

CH_3—C(=O)—CH_2—CH_2—CH_2—CH_3

Methyl-*n*-butyl ketone

Cyclohexanone

CH_3—C(=O)—CH_2—CH(CH_3)—CH_3

Methyl isobutyl ketone

H_3C H_3C CH_3 O

Isophorone

Figure 107-5. Chemical structure of various ketones.

ABSORPTION, METABOLISM, AND EXCRETION

Acetone is rapidly absorbed from the lungs and the GI tract and across the skin. The application to human skin of cotton soaked in acetone can result in significant blood acetone levels, alveolar air levels, and urinary concentrations (17). Blood levels of acetone rise according to the exposure dose without reaching a steady state, indicating continuous absorption and distribution. Being highly water soluble, acetone is widely distributed to those tissues and organs having a high water content. Metabolism of acetone takes place mainly in the liver and involves gluconeogenetic pathways (Fig. 107-6).

Acetone is initially oxidized to acetol by acetone monooxygenase, then to methylglyoxal by acetol monooxygenase. Methylglyoxal is converted to glucose directly or to D-lactate. In addition, acetol can be converted to 1,2-propanediol, which can form either L-lactate or D-glucose or can degrade to acetate and formate. The toxic activity of acetone does not appear to be due to its metabolites.

The metabolism of fat *in vivo* produces acetone, with levels reaching 10 to 70 mg per dL in diabetic ketoacidosis. At levels of less than 100 mg per dL, the half-life is approximately 4 hours; the kidneys excrete approximately 30%, respiration accounts for nearly 20%, and the balance is metabolized. At higher blood levels, the elimination half-life increases to 30 hours or so.

CLINICAL TOXICOLOGY

Acetone is well absorbed through the lung, skin, and GI tract. It has irritating effects on the nose, throat, trachea, and lungs. Irritation has been reported with exposures to acetone greater than 900 ppm (22,23). Human volunteers exposed to 100 ppm for 6 hours have experienced irritating effects. Also, prolonged exposures result in olfactory fatigue to the odor.

The neurologic depressant effects of acetone are well described. Patients have become comatose after hip casts, the setting fluid of which contained acetone, were applied, indicating acetone's rapid dermal absorption. Such individuals experienced headache, dizziness, weakness, and difficulty talking. The breath of these individuals smelled strongly of acetone. Most of these case reports date back to the 1940s and 1950s.

Neurologic and neurobehavioral effects have been documented in human volunteers tested under controlled laboratory conditions of acetone exposure. These effects include lethargy, weakness, headache, delayed visual reaction time, and other subjective symptoms. In the setting of extremely high airborne concentrations of acetone, narcosis can occur. The narcotic effects of acetone occur after oral and inhalational exposures.

Liquid acetone can cause degenerative changes in the skin after direct exposure. Cases of acute contact dermatitis after handling acetone have been described (24).

Ocular toxicity has been observed in animals after direct instillation of acetone into the eye, which can result in corneal burns, edema, and necrosis.

Methyl-*n*-Butyl Ketone

MBK (*n*-hexanone) is a clear, colorless solvent that is highly volatile and has the odor of acetone (see Fig. 107-5). MBK is a neurotoxic metabolite of the oxidation of *n*-hexane, and both *n*-hexane and MBK are metabolized to a common neurotoxic intermediate, 2,5-hexanedione (Fig. 107-7).

The capacity for aliphatic alkanes or monoketones to produce peripheral neuropathies depends on the presence of an alkane chain of at least six carbons that can form a metabolic intermediate of a γ-diketone from the parent compound

TABLE 107-8. Physiochemical properties of and regulations applicable to acetone

Molecular weight	58.08
Physical state	Colorless liquid
Melting point	–95.35°C
Boiling point	56.2°C at 1 atm
Density	
At 20°C	0.78998 g/mL
At 25°C	0.78440 g/mL
At 30°C	0.78033 g/mL
Odor	Mildly pungent and aromatic
Odor threshold	
Water	20 ppm (wt/vol)
Air (absolute)	13–20 ppm (vol/vol)
100% Odor recognition	100–140 ppm
Solubility	
Water at 20°C	Completely miscible
Organic solvent(s)	Soluble in benzene and ethanol
Partition coefficients	
Log K_{ow}	–0.24 (recommended value)
Log K_{oc}	0.73 (estimated)
Vapor pressure at 20°C	181.72 mm Hg
Henry's law constant at 25°C	4.26×10^{-5} atm-m³/mol
Autoignition temperature	465°C
Flash point (closed cup)	–20°C
Flammability limits in air at 25°C	
Lower limit	2.15%
Upper limit	13.0%
Conversion factor in air at 25°C	1 ppm = 2.374 mg/m³
Explosive limits in air (vol/vol)	
Lower limit	2.6%
Upper limit	12.8%
Regulations, air	
OSHA PEL TWA	750 ppm (1,780 mg/m³)
OSHA STEL	1,000 ppm (2,400 mg/m³)
Guidelines, air	
ACGIH TLV TWA	750 ppm (1,780 mg/m³)
ACGIH STEL	1,000 ppm (2,380 mg/m³)
NIOSH REL TWA	250 ppm (590 mg/m³)
Other guidelines	
EPA RfD (oral)	0.1 mg/kg/day
Carcinogen classification	D

ACGIH, American Conference of Governmental Industrial Hygienists; EPA, U.S. Environmental Protection Agency; K_{oc}, soil sorption constant; K_{ow}, octanol-water constant; NIOSH, National Institute for Occupational Safety and Health; OSHA, U.S. Occupational Safety and Health Administration; PEL, permissible exposure limit; REL, recommended exposure limit; RfD, reference dose; STEL, short-term exposure limit; TLV, threshold limit value; TWA, time-weighted average.

(25,26). Neurotoxicity of the toxic metabolite is related to the spacing of its functional groups in the ketone structure. Ketones such as MEK and MIBK cannot form γ-diketones owing to their chemical structures and, therefore, are not neurotoxic. Also, aliphatic alkanes such as propane, butane, and pentane are less neurotoxic and cannot form such intermediate metabolites; therefore, they do not produce peripheral neuropathies.

ABSORPTION, METABOLISM, AND EXCRETION

Inhalation is the primary route of absorption of MBK, and it is very efficient. Approximately 85% of an inhaled dose of MBK is absorbed on inhalation, as compared to 20% absorption of an inhaled dose of *n*-hexane vapor. This is due to the relatively low blood-air partition coefficient of *n*-hexane as opposed to MBK (25).

Peripheral neuropathy can occur after ingestion or inhalation of or dermal exposure to MBK. Dermal absorption in volunteers exposed to MBK ranged from 4.8 to 8.0 µg per square centimeter

TABLE 107-9. Acetone levels in the troposphere and urban, rural, and remote areas

Location	Monitoring year	Concentration in parts per billion (vol/vol)
U.S. outdoor[a]	1980–1986	6.9
Indoor air of a newly constructed office building, Portland, OR[b]	1987–1988	12.1–28.1
Point Barrow, AK[c]	1984–1985	0.47
Troposphere (lower)[d]	1984–1985	0.12

[a]From ref. 20.
[b]Hodgson A. *J Air Waste Manage Assoc* 1991;41:1461–1468.
[c]Cavanagh L. *Environ Sci Technol* 1969;3(3):251–257.
[d]Arnold F. *Nature* 1986;321:505–507.

per hour (27). Protective gloves and other dermal barriers help to reduce toxicity by reducing dermal absorption.

The distribution of MBK correlates with the lipid content of tissues. It readily crosses the blood–brain barrier. Tissues with high blood perfusion (e.g., kidney, spleen, brain, and muscles) also receive high doses of MBK, whereas more time is required for saturation and equilibration to occur in adipose tissue. Thus, the kidney, spleen, brain, liver, and muscles receive early distribution of MBK, with equilibration to the less perfused adipose tissues. Elimination half-life from adipose tissue is slower than that from other tissues, and the metabolites of MBK accumulate in adipose tissue and are gradually released.

MBK metabolism occurs in the liver and in other tissues such as the brain (see Fig. 107-7). 2-Hexanol, a metabolite of MBK, may be responsible for the narcotic effects on the brain, whereas the metabolite 2,5-hexanedione is responsible for peripheral neuropathy.

After oral ingestion of MBK by human volunteers, 40% was metabolized and exhaled as carbon dioxide, reaching a peak concentration 4 hours after ingestion. Urinary excretion of MBK was maximal between 24 and 48 hours after ingestion. Twenty-five percent of an oral dose was excreted in the urine during the first 8 days after an exposure (25). Thus, chronic exposure to MBK leads to accumulation of the neurotoxic metabolite in tissues and in the blood. Urinary metabolites of MBK include 2-hexanol, 5-hydroxy-2-hexanone, 4,5-dihydroxy-2-hexanone, and 2,5-hexanedione (25).

Chronic exposure to ethanol, to phenobarbital, and to MEK will increase urinary excretion of 2,5-hexanedione. Thus, it appears that MEK induces the enzyme systems that metabolize MBK, leading to increased formation of the neurotoxic metabolite 2,5-hexanedione. However, MEK also inhibits a step in the metabolic pathway of the formation of 4,5-dihydroxy-2-hexanone, which serves to increase both the blood and urine concentrations of the neurotoxic metabolite. Levels of 2,5-hexanedione can be detected in the urine and blood of people who are not exposed to MBK, suggesting that an endogenous metabolic source exists, probably from environmental pollutants (28).

CLINICAL TOXICOLOGY

Exposure to MBK occurs during its production, petroleum refining, and its use in industries. *n*-Hexane and MBK often are mixed with other chemicals such as toluene, benzene, and acetone, and exposure to these mixtures can occur through exposure to products in which they are used—glues, inks, paints, paint thinners, and laminates. Thus, simultaneous exposures to *n*-hexane, MBK, and other volatile solvents is possible.

Clinical toxicity of MBK is a result of chronic exposure, which can produce neuropathologic signs and symptoms at lower

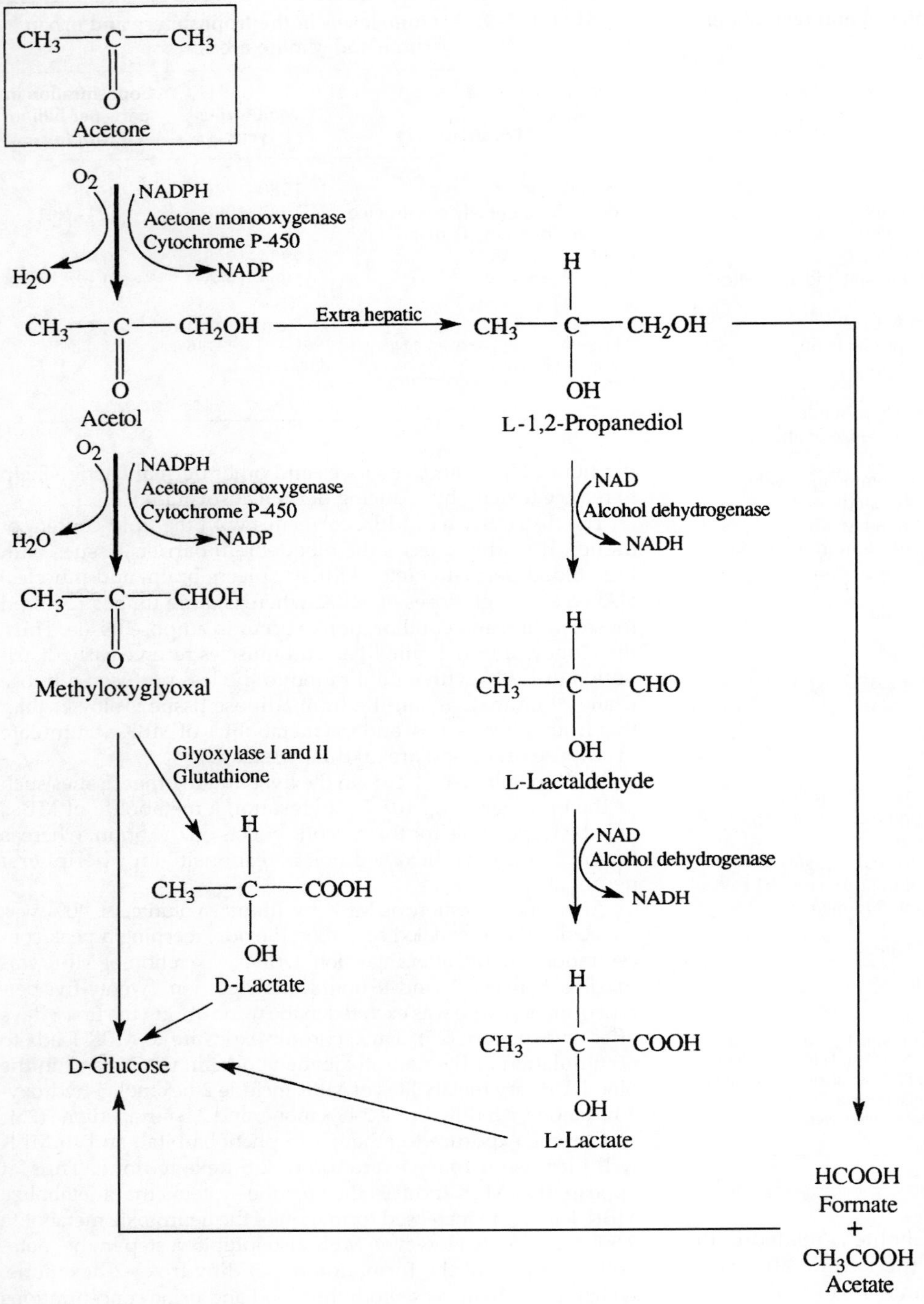

Figure 107-6. Metabolic pathways for acetone. NAD, nicotinamide adenine dinucleotide; NADH, nicotinamide adenine dinucleotide (reduced form); NADP/NADPH, nicotinamide adenine dinucleotide phosphate.

exposure concentrations and sooner than occurs with *n*-hexane (29). The syndrome is characterized by painless sensorimotor polyneuropathy beginning several weeks to months after continual exposure (30,31). Following cessation of exposure, a period of continued worsening symptoms occurs before stabilization. Such a course reflects the covalent binding of the toxic metabolite to neurofilaments, with interference and impairment of axonal transport mechanisms. Weight loss may occur as an early symptom. Neuropathy begins in the hands and feet, with loss of small-fiber sensation to light touch, pinprick, and temperature and sparing of large-fiber sensation such as position and vibration. An axonal polyneuropathy with multifocal axonal degeneration and multiple axonal swellings may be demonstrated on electrophysiologic studies. A biopsy specimen can demonstrate neurofilament accumulation at perinodal areas and thinning of the myelin sheath, a finding typical of a "dying-back" neuropathy (25). Extreme fatigue, weight loss, and muscle atrophy ensue and can progress even after cessation of exposure. Weakness and atrophy of distal muscles may extend proximally in severe cases. Occasionally, individuals who are severely intoxicated may experience involvement of respiratory muscles and truncal weakness. Vibratory and position sense are impaired only with severe toxicity.

Blurred vision is a common symptom reported initially in exposed individuals. Ophthalmologic evaluations in patients expressing ocular toxicity reveal constricted visual fields, optic nerve atrophy, and retrobulbar neuritis. Macular degeneration and deficits in color discrimination have also been reported (25).

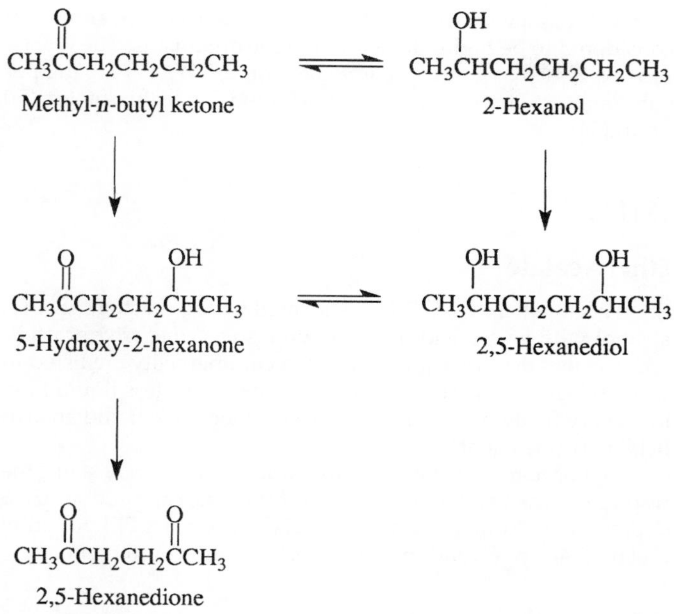

$CH_3CCH_2CH_2CH_2CH_3$ ⇌ $CH_3CHCH_2CH_2CH_2CH_3$

Methyl-*n*-butyl ketone — 2-Hexanol

$CH_3CCH_2CH_2CHCH_3$ ⇌ $CH_3CHCH_2CH_2CHCH_3$

5-Hydroxy-2-hexanone — 2,5-Hexanediol

$CH_3CCH_2CH_2CCH_3$

2,5-Hexanedione

Figure 107-7. Methyl-*n*-butyl ketone metabolism.

Nerve conduction studies show slowing of motor conduction velocities and increased distal latencies in the nerves studied (e.g., the median ulnar, tibial, and peroneal nerves). Such abnormalities in nerve conduction studies have been seen up to 1.5 years after exposure (25). Thus, prognosis depends on the duration of the exposure and the intensity of the exposure. Electromyographic studies reveal muscle denervation from the motor neuropathy. Also, visual evoked potentials may be affected, as are sensory evoked potentials. Individuals exposed to MBK may also show neuropsychological changes, with neurobehavioral test results confirming motor function impairment.

Neuroimaging studies can be useful, but no neuroimaging studies have been reported in individuals in whom clinical toxicity from MBK has been diagnosed (25).

Although it is more efficiently absorbed, MBK exerts fewer acute CNS effects than does 2-hexane. Exposure to ethanol and MBK has an additive acute depressant effect on the CNS, probably owing to the competition of 2-hexanol and ethanol for the alcohol dehydrogenase enzyme. Chronic exposure to ethanol will induce the cytochrome P-450 mixed-oxidase enzyme system and enhance the metabolism of MBK, thus producing an increased amount of the neurotoxic 2,5-hexanedione. The neurotoxic effects of simultaneous exposure to *n*-hexane and MBK are additive (25,26).

Recovery from MBK toxicity may occur, although such residual disabilities as atrophy and muscle weakness may persist.

BIOLOGICAL MONITORING

Biological monitoring of 2,5-hexanedione can be used as a marker of exposure. 2,5-Hexanedione can be detected in the blood of human volunteers after exposure to MBK vapors at concentrations greater than 50 ppm. In one study, exposure of volunteers to MBK vapors at concentrations of 100 ppm for 4 hours did not result in detectable levels of urinary metabolites including 2,5-hexanedione (25). Thus, a biological exposure index for MBK has not been established.

REGULATORY CONTROLS

The U.S. Occupational Safety and Health Administration (OSHA) has established a permissible exposure limit (PEL) for MBK of 100 ppm. The American Conference of Governmental Industrial Hygienists (ACGIH) has set a threshold limit value (TLV) of 5 ppm with a skin notation. The odor threshold of MBK is 0.076 ppm, and the level that is considered immediately dangerous to life and health (IDLH) is 1,600 ppm.

Methyl Ethyl Ketone

MEK (2-butanone) is a clear, colorless, volatile, and highly flammable liquid having an odor of acetone (see Fig. 107-5). It is partially soluble in water but completely miscible with several organic solvents. MEK forms explosive peroxides on prolonged storage. It also forms explosive mixtures with the atmosphere.

ENVIRONMENTAL FATE AND TRANSPORT

In the atmosphere, MEK is rapidly photodecomposed. It does not bioaccumulate, as exhibited by its bioconcentration factor of 0.5 (32). MEK is photochemically decomposed rapidly in the atmosphere. Volatilization of MEK from a variety of building materials and other products can contribute to air pollution both indoors and outdoors. Levels of less than 3 μg per cubic meter (1 ppb) have been found in minimally polluted air, and 131 μg per cubic meter (44.5 ppb) has been measured in heavily polluted air (17). In indoor air, mean values of MEK reported are 8 μg per cubic meter, with 38 μg per cubic meter as a maximum value (32).

MEK is a minor component of gasoline. Other environmental sources include tobacco smoke. MEK is also naturally present in many different food products.

ABSORPTION, METABOLISM, AND EXCRETION

Absorption of MEK occurs through the skin and lungs and via ingestion. It is absorbed rapidly through the skin, and vapors of MEK can be found in exhaled air within 3 minutes after its application to the skin (Fig. 107-8) (32). Absorption is slower on dry skin than on moist skin; MEK has been detected in the exhaled air within 30 seconds after application to moist skin versus 10 to 15 minutes after application to dry skin. Percutaneous penetration of MEK is calculated to be 0.46 μg per square centimeter per minute for dry skin and 0.59 μg per square centimeter per minute for moist skin (32).

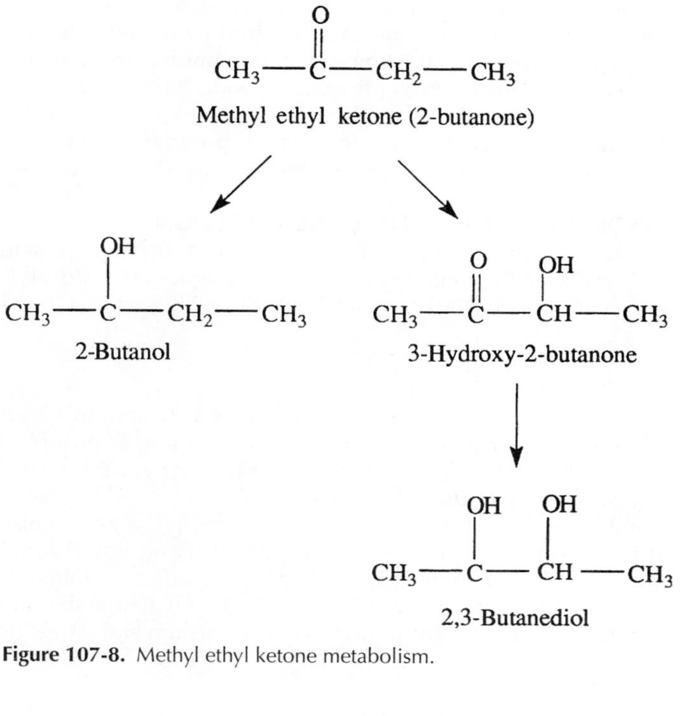

$CH_3—C—CH_2—CH_3$

Methyl ethyl ketone (2-butanone)

$CH_3—C—CH_2—CH_3$

2-Butanol

$CH_3—C—CH—CH_3$

3-Hydroxy-2-butanone

$CH_3—C—CH—CH_3$

2,3-Butanediol

Figure 107-8. Methyl ethyl ketone metabolism.

The solubility and distribution of MEK are similar for all tissues. Uptake and distribution of MEK from the lungs can occur in approximately 3 minutes. MEK readily penetrates to highly vascularized tissues, with a half-life that varies from 0.8 to 23.0 minutes (33).

MEK vapors are rapidly transported via the lungs into the bloodstream, and excretion occurs back through exhaled air. Concentrations in the blood and, subsequently, in the urine correlate with environmental exposure. Exercise increases the MEK level in the blood in those persons who are environmentally exposed. A correlation exists between occupational and environmental levels of MEK and the amount excreted in the urine of exposed individuals (33).

MEK is a metabolic end product of natural gas that contains methane 88%, ethane 5%, propane 5%, and isobutane 2% (32). Metabolites of MEK include 2-butanol and 3-hydroxy-2-butanone, which is metabolized to 2,3-butanediole and then to carbon dioxide in water. MEK is identified as a normal constituent of human metabolism. Both the MEK parent compound and its metabolites are excreted by the lungs and kidneys. Only 3% of an absorbed dose is secreted unchanged in the exhaled air of volunteers after exposure, and 3-hydroxy-2-butanone is detected. The levels of the metabolites 2-butanol and 2,3-butanediole do not appear to correlate with exposure.

CLINICAL TOXICOLOGY

Oral ingestion of MEK has caused coma and metabolic acidosis. Short-term inhalational exposure to concentrations of 270 ppm for 4 hours per day had little effect on neurobehavioral manifestations: Exposure to 90 to 270 ppm for up to 4 hours per day caused subjects to underestimate times. Other studies have found no significant behavioral effects. In some cases, dermatitis has been reported from prolonged dermal contact.

MEK is present in some solvent mixtures containing hexane and thus may contribute to hexane neurotoxicity.

Methyl Isobutyl Ketone

MIBK (4-methyl-2-pentanone) is a clear liquid having a sweet odor and an odor threshold of 0.4 ppm, or 1.64 mg per cubic meter (see Fig. 107-5) (34). It is moderately water soluble. MIBK occurs naturally in foods and as a flavoring agent. It is also a component of polyurethane lacquers and paint solvents. It is used as a solvent for extraction and in the manufacture of methyl amyl alcohol. Owing to its presence in foods, whether naturally or as an additive, the general population is exposed to MIBK. Ambient air concentrations for general population exposure have been found to range from 0.1 to 0.2 mg per cubic meter (34).

ABSORPTION, METABOLISM, AND EXCRETION

MIBK is absorbed via inhalation or ingestion or through the skin and is widely distributed systemically throughout the body. It is metabolized extensively to metabolites that are excreted in the urine.

CLINICAL TOXICOLOGY

The principal health effects of MIBK toxicity are respiratory tract irritation, ocular irritation, and CNS depression. Exposure to airborne levels of 2.4 to 100.0 ppm (10 to 410 mg per cubic meter) can produce irritation of the eyes, nose, throat, and mucous membranes (34). Headache, nausea, and vertigo can occur also at these concentrations. Both in vapor form and liquid form, MIBK is an irritant of the skin and eyes. CNS effects manifest as headaches, nausea, and narcosis. MIBK is highly flammable and should be kept away from sources of combustion and flame. Its vapor density is 3.45 times that of air.

MIBK has a very short half-life in the environment and is not considered to be highly toxic for aquatic organisms. The OSHA PEL expressed as a time-weighted average (TWA) is 410 mg per cubic meter. The ACGIH TLV is 205 mg per cubic meter (50 ppm) (34).

ESTERS

Ethyl Acetate

Ethyl acetate ($CH_3COOC_2H_5$) is formed by the reaction of ethyl alcohol with acetic acid. It is known also as *ethyl ester* or *acidic ether.* (Esters that are commonly used commercially are listed in Table 107-10.) Ethyl acetate is a flammable, colorless liquid having a very fruity odor. It is used as a lacquer solvent and an artificial perfume agent.

Ethyl acetate is irritating to the mucous membranes and the respiratory tract and, in higher concentrations, can produce CNS depression in humans and in animals. The OSHA PEL for ethyl acetate is 400 ppm, and the IDLH concentration is 400 ppm.

2-Ethoxyethyl Acetate

2-Ethoxyethyl acetate (ethylene glycol monoethyl acetate, cellosolve acetate) is a flammable, colorless liquid that is used as a solvent for nitrocellulose and resins and is incompatible with oxidizing agents, alkalis, and nitrates. This compound is very irritating to the mucous membranes, eyes, and respiratory system. In high air concentrations, it can produce CNS and respiratory depression. The ACGIH has recommended a TLV of 5 ppm with a skin notation, owing to potential skin absorption of the compound.

n-Amyl Acetate

n-Amyl acetate ($CH_3CCOC_5H_{11}$) (amyl acetate, pear oil) is a clear, colorless, flammable liquid having a bananalike odor. Its three isomers are *n*-amyl acetate, *sec*-amyl acetate, and isoamyl acetate. The amyl acetates in general are used as solvents and as flavoring. They also are used in the manufacturing of furniture polish, photographic film, artificial glass, celluloid, lacquers, artificial leathers, and artificial silk.

TABLE 107-10. Esters in common commercial use

Methyl acetate	Ethyl stearate
Ethyl acetate	Ethyl phenyl acetate
n-Propyl acetate	Ethyl benzoate
n-Butyl acetate	*n*-Amyl acetate
Isobutyl acetate	Isoamyl acetate
sec-Butyl acetate	Butyl acetate
tert-Butyl acetate	Isopropyl acetate
n-Pentyl acetate	Vinyl acetate
Isopentyl acetate	Methyl silicate
Hexyl acetate	Ethyl silicate
Cyclohexyl acetate	*n*-Propyl nitrate
Methylcyclohexyl acetate	Methyl formate
Benzyl acetate	Ethyl formate
Phenyl acetate	Butyl formate
Ethyl formate	Allyl formate
Ethyl acetate	Cyclohexyl formate
Ethyl propionate	Methylcyclohexyl formate
Methyl propionate	Benzyl formate
Ethyl *n*-butyrate	Ethyl oxalate
Ethyl *n*-valerate	Polyesters

They are incompatible with strong oxidizing agents, alkalis, and nitrates. The vapors of all the amyl acetate isomers form explosive mixtures in air. In general, amyl acetates cause irritation to the eyes and mucous membranes and can cause dermatitis. In high air concentrations, the amyl acetates can produce CNS depression.

Methyl Acetate

Methyl acetate is formed by a reaction of methanol with acetic acid, sulfuric acid being the catalyst. It is used as a solvent for nitrocellulose, oils, and fats; in plastics and artificial leather; and in the production of perfumes, coloring agents, and lacquers. Methyl acetate is flammable, and its vapor forms explosive mixtures with air.

Methyl acetate is an eye and mucous membrane irritant. Its vapors can cause headache, vertigo, lacrimation, eye irritation, drowsiness, and dyspnea. The OSHA PEL is 20 ppm (610 mg per cubic meter), the ACGIH short-term exposure limit (STEL) is 250 ppm (760 mg per cubic meter), and the IDLH level is 10,000 ppm.

n-Propyl Acetate and Isopropyl Acetate

n-Propyl acetate ($CH_3COOC_3H_7$) and isopropyl acetate [$CH_3COOCH(CH_3)_2$] are flammable liquids, the vapors of which form explosive mixtures with air at normal temperatures. Both esters are eye and respiratory irritants in vapor concentrations of 200 ppm. They serve as solvents for nitrocellulose in the production of lacquers and are used in the plastics industry.

Butyl Acetate Esters

Among the butyl acetate esters are butyl acetate ($CH_3COOC_4H_9$), *sec*-butyl acetate ($CH_3COOC_4H_9$), *tert*-butyl acetate [$(CH_3)_3COH$], and isobutyl acetate ($C_9H_9COOCH_3$). Butyl acetate is used commonly in the production of nitrocellulose lacquers, vinyl resins, artificial leather, photographic film, and perfumes. These esters are irritants to the eyes and respiratory tract.

Propionate Esters

The propionate esters include methyl propionate ($C_2H_5COOH_3$), ethyl propionate ($C_2H_5COOC_2H_5$), and butyl propionate ($C_2H_5COOC_5H_{11}$). Propionates are used in the production of lacquers and perfumes. They are all flammable liquids. Methyl, ethyl, and butyl propionates can form explosive or flammable airborne concentrations at room temperatures. Amyl propionate vapors can be flammable in hot environments.

Formate Esters

Among the formate esters are methyl formate ($HCOOCH_3$), ethyl formate ($HCOOC_2H_5$), butyl formate [$HCOO(CH_2)_3CH_3$], and allyl formate ($HCOOCH_2CH{:}CH_2$). Methyl formate is a flammable liquid that forms explosive vapor mixtures with air. It has irritant and CNS depressant toxic effects. Routes of absorption are via the skin and inhalation. Animal toxicity consists of convulsions, dyspnea, and coma. Humans may experience narcosis, irritation of airways, dyspnea, and euphoria when exposed to methyl formate vapors. The OSHA PEL is 100 ppm (250 mg per cubic meter), the ACGIH STEL is 150 ppm (375 mg per cubic meter), and the IDLH level is 5,000 ppm.

Ethyl formate is a colorless, flammable liquid having an aromatic odor and is used as a solvent for cellulose nitrate, oils, and greases. It also has been used as a fumigant. Its vapors form explosive mixtures with air at normal temperatures. Workers exposed to vapors of 330 ppm reported experiencing eye and mucous membrane irritation. It causes CNS depression in animal toxicity studies. The OSHA PEL is 100 ppm (300 mg per cubic meter), the ACGIH STEL is 150 ppm (450 mg per cubic meter), and the IDLH level is 8,000 ppm.

Butyl formate is a flammable, colorless liquid, the vapors of which form explosive mixtures with air at normal temperatures. It is an ocular and respiratory irritant.

Allyl formate is highly toxic to animals and causes hepatic damage. It has a mustard odor.

Phthalates

Phthalates, or phthalic acid esters, are used frequently as plasticizers. Two such plasticizers are di-*n*-butyl phthalate (DBP) and diethylhexyl phthalate (DEHP). Phthalate acid esters are the most widely used plasticizers for the production of PVC. Phthalates can be released to the environment during production and distribution, manufacturing, disposal, or use as a plasticizer in products.

DI-*n*-BUTYL PHTHALATE

DBP is a phthalic acid ester with a molecular formula of $C_{16}H_{22}O_4$ and a molecular weight of 278.4. It is known also as *butyl phthalate* or *dibutyl phthalate*. An oily, colorless liquid having a mild aromatic odor, DBP has a vapor pressure of 1.0×10^{-5} mm Hg at 25°C. Its density at 20°C is 1.047. Phthalic acid esters form colloidal dispersions in water.

DBP is used mainly as a plasticizer for nitrose, cellulose, polyvinyl acetate, and PVC. It is one of the most commonly used plasticizers in cellulose film, present in the nitrocellulose coating (35). DBP appears also in cosmetics and perfumes and finds use as an antifoaming agent, a lubricant, a skin emollient, and a plasticizer in nail polish and hair sprays.

In the environment, DBP is moderately adsorbed to soil but also forms complexes with water-soluble fulvic acid, which increases its mobilization. Owing to DBP's low vapor pressure, volatilization into the atmosphere is very low. DBP is biodegradable in surface waters, with a half-life ranging from 1 to 14 days. It is also photooxidized, having a half-life in air of 7 hours to 3 days. It is biodegraded both aerobically and anaerobically. Owing to the log K_{ow} of 4.3 to 4.8, DBP is expected to bioaccumulate. However, it is metabolized by some aquatic organisms.

DBP can be detected in the atmosphere in a variety of locations: in rainwater, surface water, urban runoff water, sewage treatment plants, and sediments in soils. Atmospheric concentrations have ranged from 3 to 18 ng per cubic meter in residential and populated areas to a low of 0.1 to 1.0 ng per cubic meter in clean environments in isolated areas (36). DBP is found also as a component of one of the volatile chemicals in indoor air. In one study, the concentration of DBP was 2.85 mg per cubic meter, whereas in another survey of 125 homes in California, the median concentration of DBP in indoor air during the daytime was 240 ng per cubic meter (36).

DBP has been noted in certain foods, particularly in plastic-wrapped foods such as snacks and biscuits, chocolates, butter, and margarine, reflecting the impact of plastic packaging on the DBP content of foods.

Absorption, Metabolism, and Excretion. DBP is absorbed slowly through the human skin but rapidly through the GI tract. In animals, DBP is metabolized by esterases by hydrolysis to produce mono-*n*-butyl phthalate. This and other metabolites are excreted in the urine as glucuronide conjugates.

Clinical Toxicology. Ingestion of DBP can produce acute toxicity consisting of nausea, vomiting, dizziness, headache, lacrimation, photophobia, and conjunctivitis. Case reports also indicate renal injury with hematuria and obsolete crystaluria.

Dermatitis has been reported after exposure to DBP, with evidence of positive patch testing. Dermal exposure in cosmetic use has resulted in pruritus and erythema of the skin. Neurologic symptoms have been reported after workplace exposure to DBP and to other phthalate esters (37). Neurologic symptoms consisted of extremity pain, spasms, and numbness. Symptoms were noted to develop after 6 to 7 years of employment in the exposure industry. Polyneuritis also was noted in some individuals (37).

Other studies have noted neurologic signs and symptoms developing in occupationally exposed individuals. These symptoms consisted of paresthesias of the limbs that became more continuous with increasing exposure. Excessive perspiration and vasomotor instability also were present and indicated autonomic dysfunction in some workers. Neurologic examination revealed polyneuropathy in 57% of the workers exposed to phthalates. Other workers developed painful sensitivity of the skin and feet with decreased vibratory sensation. Sensory neu–ropathy has been observed in those with long-term exposure.

DIETHYLHEXYL PHTHALATE

DEHP [di(2-ethylhexyl)phthalate] is an oily, yellow liquid at room temperature and normal atmospheric pressures. Its log K_{ow} is 3 to 5. DEHP forms colloidal dispersions in water and is miscible with most organic solvents. Like other phthalates, DEHP has been found in a wide variety of soils, plants, and animals over a widespread geographic area. It has been in use since 1949 (38).

DEHP tends to grade into organic-rich soil or sediment, owing to its K_{ow}. Its solubility in water is low. It is photodegraded in the atmosphere and has a half-life of less than 1 day. It also is aerobically degraded in soil, sludge, sediment, and water, whereas anaerobic degradation is slower. DEHP is highly lipophilic and tends to bioaccumulate in lipid substances. Thus, it can be found in aquatic organisms such as fish and shellfish. It also is found widely as an environmental contaminant in air, precipitation, water, sediment, soil, aquatic organisms, and the like. Residues can be detected in foods and in humans.

Absorption, Metabolism, and Excretion. After its absorption, DEHP is hydrolyzed to monoethylhexyl phthalate. In animal studies, radiolabeled DEHP had an elimination-phase half-life of 4.5 to 9.0 minutes in one study and of 22 minutes in another study (38).

Clinical Toxicology. Ingestion of 5 to 10 g of DEHP produced mild gastric disturbances and diarrhea in subjects. Occupational exposure studies revealed signs of polyneuropathy in workers at PVC-processing plants in the U.S.S.R. However, these workers also were exposed to other compounds, including tricresyl phosphate (TCP), a known neurotoxin. A case of occupational asthma due to DEHP has been reported in a PVC-processing plant (38).

Dimethyl Ester

Dimethyl ester, also known as *dimethyl sulfate* (DMS), is an odorous, oily liquid used as an alkylating agent. Its chemical formula is shown in Figure 107-9. DMS has a slightly onionlike odor and a vapor density of 4.35 times that of air. Its vapor pressure is 0.8 mm Hg at 25°C. It mixes with polar organic solvents and aromatic hydrocarbons but is only slightly soluble in water and in aliphatic hydrocarbons (Table 107-11). DMS is hydrolyzed in moist air or cold water, the hydrolytic products being monomethyl sulfate and methanol. DMS is a strong methylating agent. Its major use is as an alkylating agent such as for the alkylation of phenols and amines (39).

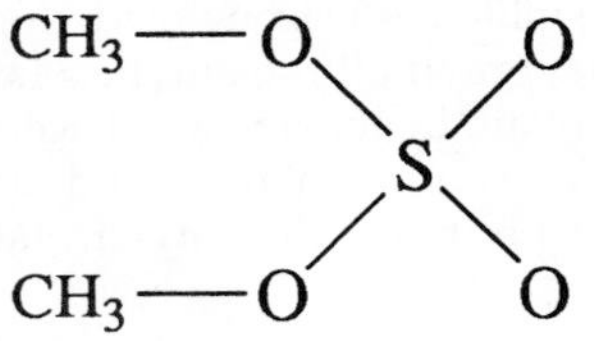

CH_3—O, CH_3—O, S, O, O

Dimethyl sulfate (dimethyl ester)

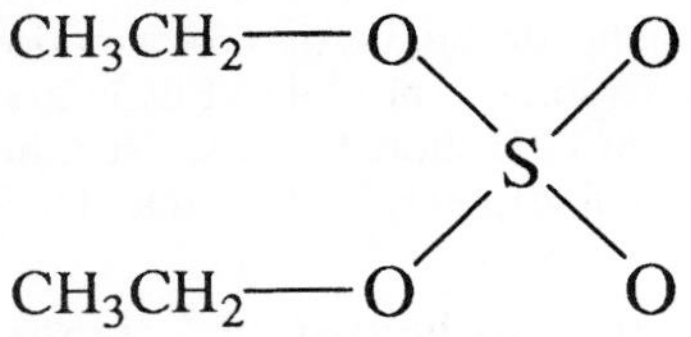

CH_3CH_2—O, CH_3CH_2—O, S, O, O

Diethyl sulfate (diethyl ester)

Figure 107-9. Chemical structure of dimethyl and diethyl sulfate.

ABSORPTION, METABOLISM, AND EXCRETION

DMS is absorbed dermally, via the respiratory tract, and orally. It appears from studies that DMS does not equilibrate throughout the body but breaks down in organs that it contacts first, owing to its alkylating abilities. Concentrations of methanol have been found in animal models given doses of DMS (39). DMS alkylates nucleic acids.

CLINICAL TOXICOLOGY

DMS is highly toxic; inhalation to 97 ppm for 10 minutes has been fatal (38). Its low odor warning potential makes it a hazardous chemical in enclosed spaces. Airborne concentrations exceeding 5 mg per cubic meter (1 ppm) can cause ocular irritation. Acute inhalational exposure can result in convulsions, delirium, coma, pulmonary edema, renal and hepatic failure, and cardiac injury. Pulmonary fibrosis has been reported. In fatal cases of occupational exposure, severe damage occurs to the respiratory epithelium and mucosa of the upper airways and lungs.

Oral ingestion of DMS has resulted in fatalities. It also causes irritation of the throat and mouth and increased salivation.

TABLE 107-11. Physiochemical properties of dimethyl sulfate

Molecular weight	126.13
Boiling point	188°C (with decomposition)
Melting point	–32°C
Flash point	83°C
Vapor density	4.35
Specific gravity (liquid density; at 20–24°C)	1.33
Vapor pressure (at 25°C)	0.106 kPa (0.8 mm Hg)
Water solubility	28 kg/m^3 (2.8 g/dL; with hydrolysis)
Octanol-water partition coefficient (log K_{ow})	–4.26

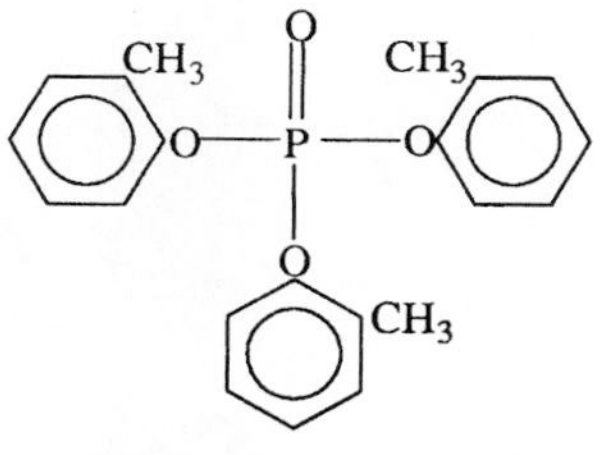

Tri-*o*-cresyl phosphate (TOCP)

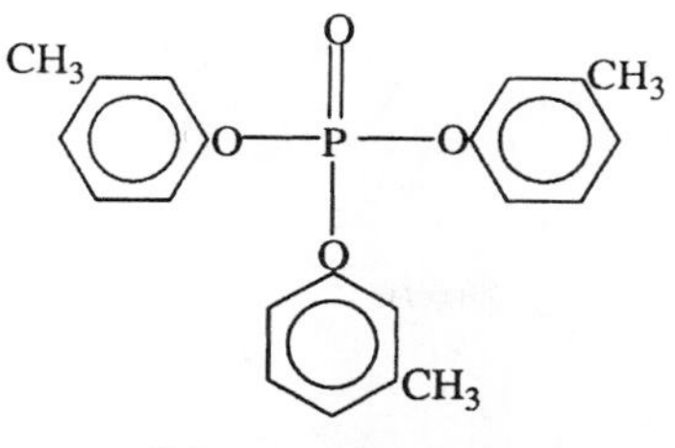

Tri-*m*-cresyl phosphate

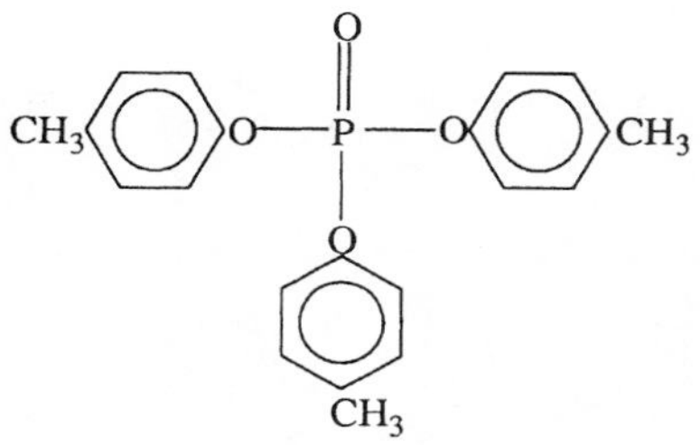

Tri-*p*-cresyl phosphate

Figure 107-10. Chemical structure of the tricresyl phosphates.

Edema of the airway with asphyxiation may follow oral ingestion. A case of sudden-onset glottic edema and death 24 hours after oral ingestion has been reported (38).

Dermal contact results in delayed onset of burns, despite immediate irrigation with water. Corneal ulceration and inflammation of eyes and eyelids with photophobia can occur after ocular exposure.

Lung cancer may be a concern in long-term exposure to DMS. DMS induces genotoxic effects in test systems and has been demonstrated to be carcinogenic in animal models. At present, DMS is considered by the International Agency for Research on Cancer (IARC) to be a probable carcinogen in humans. Therefore, it should be assumed to be a human carcinogen and adequately controlled in terms of exposure.

Diethyl Sulfate

Diethyl sulfate, also known as *sulfuric acid diethyl ester,* is formed from ethanol and sulfuric acid (see Fig. 107-9). It is used as a dye-setting agent and in carbonless paper. It also is used for producing agricultural chemicals and as an ethylating agent. Its vapor density is 5.3 (air, 1.0) and its vapor pressure is 0.1 mm Hg at 20°C. Diethyl sulfate is a clear liquid having a peppermint odor. It is insoluble in hot water, and it decomposes rapidly into monoethyl sulfate and alcohol.

Vapors of diethyl sulfate can produce eye, skin, and upper respiratory tract irritation, nausea, and vomiting. The IARC classifies the vapors as group 2A, a probable human carcinogen.

Tricresyl Phosphate

TCP has three isomers: tri-*o*-cresyl, tri-*m*-cresyl, and tri-*p*-cresyl phosphate (Fig. 107-10). The isomeric mixture of TCP is a nonexplosive, nonflammable, colorless liquid having a slightly aromatic odor. Commercial TCP is a mixture of its three isomers. The *ortho* isomer (TOCP) is a colorless liquid, the *meta* isomer (TMCP) is a colorless half-solid, and the *para* isomer (TPCP) is a colorless crystalline solid; all have a slightly aromatic odor. Table 107-12 lists the physiochemical properties of these three isomers.

PRODUCTION, SOURCES, AND USES

TCP is used as a plasticizer in vinyl plastic manufacturing, as a flame retardant, as a solvent for nitrocellulose, as an additive to lubricants that must undergo extreme pressure, and as a nonflammable fluid in hydraulic systems (40). The manufacture of fire-resistant hydraulic brake fluids and lubricants creates a growing use for these organic phosphate esters.

TCP has low water solubility and, when released into the environment, can be found in water and sediments near release sites. TCP can be biodegraded in the environment with hydrolysis to orthophosphates and phenolic components (40). It also can be found in the atmosphere located next to industrial sites. Concentrations of 70 ng per cubic meter have been detected in some locations, but monitoring of production sites in the United States has revealed levels of 2 ng per cubic meter (40).

TRI-*o*-CRESYL PHOSPHATE

Of the three TCP isomers, TOCP is the most neurotoxic to humans. Its metabolism is shown in Figure 107-11. The toxicity of commercial products of TCP depends on the concentration of the *ortho* isomer.

TABLE 107-12. Physiochemical properties of tricresyl phosphate isomers

Physical properties	Tricresyl phosphate (mixtures of isomers)	Tri-*o*-cresyl phosphate	Tri-*m*-cresyl phosphate	Tri-*p*-cresyl phosphate
Physical state	Liquid	Liquid	Half-solid	Crystalline solid
Color	Colorless	Colorless	Colorless	Colorless
Odor	Very slightly aromatic	Very slightly aromatic	Very slightly aromatic	Very slightly aromatic
Melting or freezing point (°C)	−33	11	25.6	77.78
Boiling point or range (°C)	241–255 (4 mm Hg) 190–200 (0.5–10.0 mm Hg)	410 (760 mm Hg)	260 (15 mm Hg)	244 (3.5 mm Hg)
Specific gravity (density)	1.160–1.175 (25°C); 1.165	1.1955	1.150	1.237
Refractive index	1.553–1.556 (25°C); 1.556 (20°C)	1.5675	1.5575	—
Viscosity (cSt)	60.0 (25°C); 4.0 (100°C)	—	—	—
Flash point (°C)	257	—	—	—
Vapor pressure (mm Hg)	1×10^{-4} (20°C)	10 (265°C)	—	—
Henry's law constant	1.128×10^{-6} atm-m^3/mol	—	—	—
Solubility in water (mg/L)	0.36; 0.34 ± 0.04	—	—	0.074
Octanol-water partition coefficient (log K_{ow})	5.11; 5.12	—	—	—

Adapted from ref. 40, with permission.

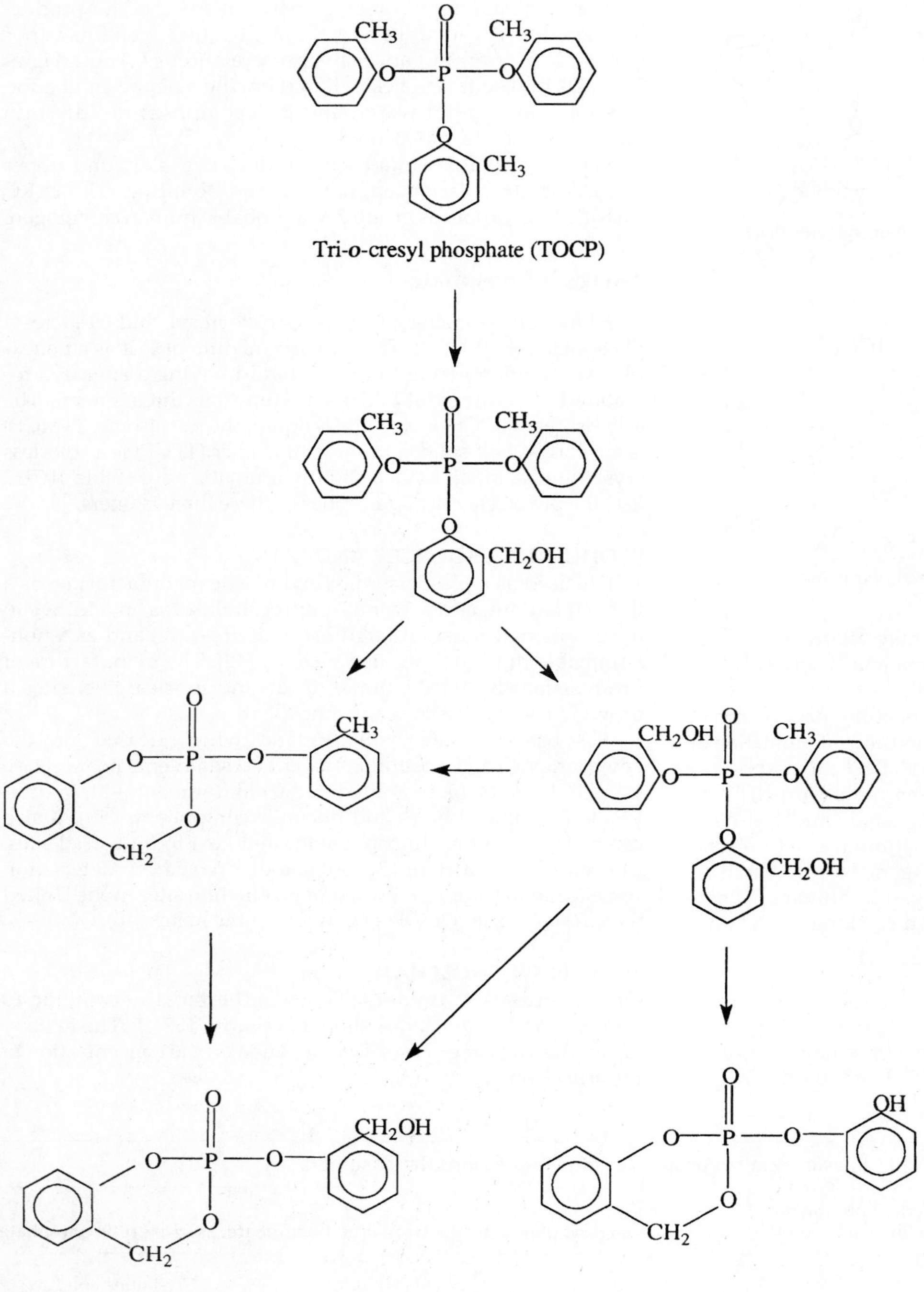

Tri-*o*-cresyl phosphate (TOCP)

Figure 107-11. Metabolism and cyclization of tri-*o*-cresyl phosphate.

TOCP produces delayed neurotoxicity of the central and peripheral nervous systems. Major epidemic outbreaks of TOCP poisoning have occurred worldwide and can be traced back to 1898 but have occurred as recently as 1980 (41).

The ingestion of TOCP by populations has been associated with outbreaks of polyneuropathy, including bilateral foot and wristdrop. Fifty thousand people were poisoned by a substitute for ethanol called *ginger jake,* which was proved to contain approximately 2% TOCP and which caused paralysis (42). Other epidemic outbreaks involving TOCP and neurotoxicity have been reported from the ingestion of contaminated flour, contaminated water, contaminated alcoholic beverages, and contamination of cooking oils. Ingestion of lubricant oils containing TOCP has been reported to produce severe neurointoxication, including GI symptoms and delayed cholinergic crisis (43).

Severity of signs and symptoms does not always appear to be proportional to the dose. Initial symptoms are gastrointestinal, with nausea and vomiting, sometimes abdominal pain, and diarrhea. These symptoms are transient, lasting a few hours to a few days. Initial GI symptoms are followed by a latent period of 3 to 28 days after an acute exposure, before onset of neurotoxicity. Neurotoxic symptoms begin with cramping pains in the calves and paresthesias in the feet and hands. This is followed by painful neuritis and weakness of the lower extremities, an unsteady gait and impaired balance. Crampy pains may persist for days to weeks while paralysis progresses. Muscle weakness spreads from the feet to the hands, and patients may have wrist-drop, total loss of muscular strength in the hands, and weakness in the elbows. Bilateral footdrop with complete loss of muscular power from the ankle to the toes is common.

Most of the neurologic abnormalities are noted in the lower extremities. In extreme cases of poisoning, truncal weakness may be observed. A few weeks after the onset of paralysis, rapid muscle wasting may be observed. This wasting involves the muscles of the feet, calves, thighs, and hands. Changes seem to be most evident in the small-muscle groups. Ankle and knee reflexes are affected. The ankle reflexes may be absent first whereas the knee reflexes remain normal, but knee reflexes are lost later.

In severe cases, hyperreflexia of the knee may be seen, indicating upper motor neuron involvement. Such involvement can include pyramidal signs near the third week after exposure. Reflexes continue to exhibit hyperreflexia with increased muscle tone of the limbs. A Babinski response may be observed in such cases.

Some authors have stated that sensory disturbances from TOCP poisoning do not occur. However, others have noted loss of pinprick and temperature sensations and interference of vibratory sensation. Cranial nerves are not involved.

The muscle weakness can progress over several weeks to months. The neurosensory changes regress slowly depending on the seriousness of the poisoning. Muscle strength begins to return gradually in people who are only mildly poisoned. Muscular improvement begins with sensation, then improved muscle strength in the hands, followed eventually by muscle strengthening in the lower extremities. Individuals with pyramidal tract signs may recover poorly because of the seriousness of their poisoning.

In cases of epidemic outbreaks of TOCP poisoning, many individuals have been left totally incapacitated. Patients have shown signs and symptoms of the disease 18 years after the poisoning occurred (40). In the mildest cases of residual disease, patients may have slight muscle weakness in the ankles, whereas those most severely affected may have footdrop, muscle atrophy, and pyramidal signs such as spasticity, ankle clonus, and positive Babinski signs. Usually, residual symptomatology is confined to the lower extremities, with weakness and muscle atrophy. Histopathologic evaluations of muscle biopsies have shown marked degenerative changes in the anterior horn cells of the spinal nerves. Degeneration of peripheral nerves has been described. Major disabilities can be expected if upper motor neurons are involved and the patient shows evidence of pyramidal signs and upper motor neurotoxicity with spasticity.

No specific antidote is available. Atropine and pralidoxime have been used to counteract cholinergic effects.

Signs and symptoms have been reported also from the ingestion of 0.15 g of an isomeric mixture of TCP. Humans appear to be particularly sensitive to TOCP. The pure *ortho* isomer and isomeric mixtures of TCP are considered to be major human health hazards; no level is safe for ingestion.

Tri-*n*-Butyl Phosphate

Tri-*n*-butyl phosphate (TBP) is a colorless, odorless, nonflammable, nonexplosive liquid. Its chemical structure is shown in Figure 107-12, and its physiochemical properties are listed in Table 107-13. TBP is thermally unstable and decomposes at temperatures below its boiling point (289°C), where it splits into butene and phosphoric acid. TBP does not occur naturally in the environment.

It is used as a solvent for cellulose esters, lacquers, and natural gums and as a primary plasticizer in the manufacture of plastics and vinyl resins. It is used also as an antifoaming agent (44).

TBP can be released into the environment from landfill sites or from plastics disposed in sites. It is found widely in air, water, sediment, and aquatic organisms in low concentrations. The biodegradation of TBP is slow. Ambient air concentrations range from nondetectable up to 41.4 ng per cubic meter, the highest concentrations being found near manufacturing facilities. TBP levels of up to 111 ng per gram of biological and aquatic organisms have been found (44). Adipose tissue from autopsies of humans who were not occupationally exposed to TBP show its presence in at least one subject, at a level of 9 ng per gram. Exposure of the gen-

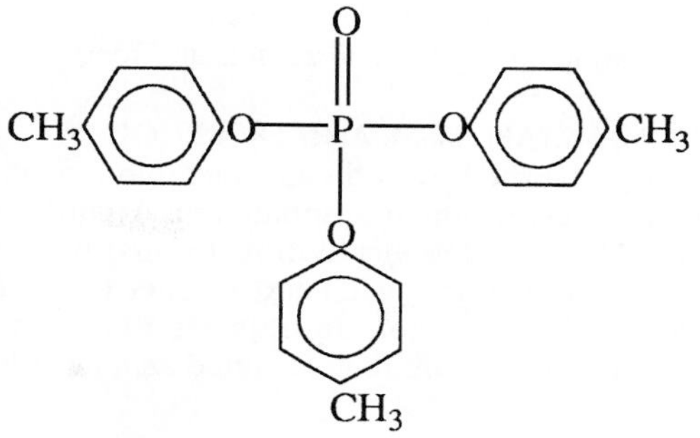

Triphenyl phosphate (TPP)

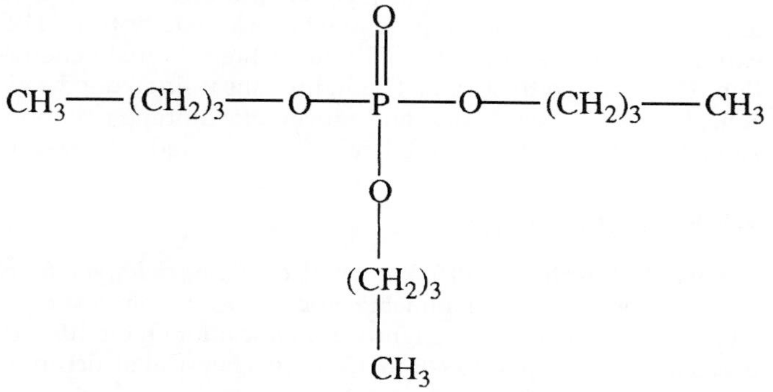

Tri-*n*-butyl phosphate (TBP)

Figure 107-12. Chemical structure of triphenyl and tri-*n*-butyl phosphate.

TABLE 107-13. Physiochemical properties of tri-*n*-butyl phosphate

Physical state	Colorless, odorless liquid
Melting point	–80°C
Boiling point	289°C (with decomposition) 150°C (1.33 kPa)
Flash point	193°C ; 166°C ; 146°C
Relative density	
At 25°C	0.973–0.983
At 20°C	0.978
Vapor pressure	
At 150°C	973 Pa
At 100°C	133 Pa
At 25°C	9 Pa
Solubility in organic solvents	Miscible with organic solvents
Solubility in water	
At 4°C	1,012 mg/L
At 25°C	0.422 mg/L
At 50°C	2.85×10^{-4} mg/L
Octanol-water partition coefficient (log K_{ow})	4.00

Adapted from ref. 40, with permission.

eral population occurs through drinking contaminated water and ingesting contaminated aquatic organisms and food.

ABSORPTION, METABOLISM, AND EXCRETION

TBP is readily absorbed from the GI tract. No information is available on its absorption after inhalation. According to animal studies, TBP is metabolically transformed by oxidation, which produces carboxylic acids and ketones (45). After oxidation occurs, the alkyl compounds are removed as glutathione conjugates and are then excreted as *n*-acetylcysteine derivatives.

CLINICAL TOXICOLOGY

TBP enters the body by dermal penetration and ingestion. Inhalation causes respiratory irritation. Workers exposed to TBP at concentrations in the air of 15 mg per cubic meter report nausea and headaches. No cases of delayed neurotoxicity from TBP exposure have been reported. TBP has a high dermal penetration. The reported toxicity of TBP in humans is limited to headache, nausea, and skin, eye, and mucous membrane irritation. Animal studies fail to suggest that TBP is a delayed neurotoxin.

Triphenyl Phosphate

Triphenyl phosphate (TPP), known also as the *triphenyl ester of phosphoric acid*, is a nonflammable, nonexplosive, colorless crystalline substance having a slightly aromatic odor (Table 107-14). It has a log K_{ow} equal to 4.6 to 476.0. Its chemical structure is shown in Figure 107-12.

TPP decomposes at 600°C, producing aromatic hydrocarbons, naphthalene, biphenyl, phenanthrene, and anthracene, as well as oxygenated aromatic compounds such as phenol, dibenzyl furans, diphenyl ethers, and phosphoric oxides.

PRODUCTION, SOURCES, AND USES

TPP does not occur naturally in the environment. It has been used as a flame retardant in phenolics and phenolene oxide base resins for the manufacture of electrical and automotive components and as a nonflammable plasticizer in cellulose acetate for photographic films (46). TPP is a component of hydraulic fluids and lubricant oils. Other uses are as a noncombustible substitute for camphor in celluloid; for lacquers and varnishes; and as a plasticizer in vinyl automotive upholstery.

TPP has been found widely in air, water, sediment, and aquatic organisms at low concentrations. Ambient air concentrations in rural areas have ranged from 0.5 to 1.4 ng per cubic meter and, in urban areas, from 0.9 to 4.1 ng per cubic meter (46).

CLINICAL TOXICOLOGY

Exposure to humans occurs by ingestion of contaminated drinking water, aquatic organisms, or other contaminated foodstuffs. Occupational exposures occur in manufacturing industries, automotive and aircraft facilities, and hydraulic fluids handling. Airborne levels of 0.008 to 29.600 mg per cubic meter have been detected in the air at TPP manufacturing sites (46). Levels in aquatic organisms range from 2 to 150 ng per gram. No evidence points to a connection between neurologic disease and TPP. No abnormalities were found in workers exposed to TPP vapor, mist, or dust of the TWA of 3.5 mg per cubic meter for an average of 7.4 years (47).

TABLE 107-14. Physiochemical properties of triphenyl phosphate

Physical state	Colorless crystalline solid
Odor	Very slightly aromatic
Melting point	49°–50°C; 49°C; 49.2°C
Boiling point	245°C (11 mm Hg); 220°C (5 mm Hg); 234°C (5 mm Hg); 370°C
Relative density	1.185–1.202 (25°C)
Flash point	220°C; 225°C
Vapor pressure	
At 150°C	0.15 mm Hg
At 200°C	1.90 mm Hg
At 193.5°C	1.0 mm Hg
Henry's law constant	$1.8–3.6 \times 10^{-7}$ atm-m^3/mol
Solubility in organic solvents	Soluble in benzene, chloroform, ether, acetone; moderately soluble in ethanol
Solubility in water	1.9 mg/L; 0.73 mg/L; 2.1 mg/L (± 0.1)
Octanol-water partition coefficient (log K_{ow})	4.63; 4.61; 4.76

Adapted from ref. 46, with permission.

ETHERS

Ethers have the basic formula of R–O–R''. If R and R' are different, the compound is called a *mixed ether*, which frequently is made up of different alcohols. Phenols also form ethers, such as methylphenyl ether (anisole): C_6H_5–O–CH_3. In thioethers, a sulfur atom links two groups (R–S–R''). Examples of thioethers are diethylsulfide (C_2H_5–S–C_2H_5) and methylethylsulfide (CH_3–S–C_2H_5). Some commercially important ethers are listed in Table 107-15. Table 107-4 summarizes toxic properties of select ethers. Some properties of ethers are as follows:

- Lower-molecular-weight ethers (methyl, ethyl, isopropyl, vinyl, ethyl isopropyl, and vinyl isopropyl) are volatile, flammable liquids that are lighter than water and have a flash point that is lower than normal room temperature.
- Ethers are relatively chemically inert.
- Ethers form substitution products with chlorine and bromine.
- Ethers decompose when heated with strong acids, yielding esters.
- Dimethyl ether is a gas (as opposed to a volatile liquid).
- On prolonged storage in the presence of air or in sunlight, ethers form explosive peroxide mixtures.
- Except for chloromethyl ethers and glycidyl ethers, the ethers generally produce CNS narcosis as their toxic effect.

TABLE 107-15. Commercialy important ethers

Allyl ether	Glycol ethers
Anisole	Buaiacol
Butyl ether	Hexyl ether
Bis-(phenoxyphenyl) ether	Hydroquinone ethers
Butyl vinyl ethers	Isopropyl ether
Cellulose ethers	Isopropyl vinyl ether
Chlorinated phenyl ethers	Methyl ether
Chloromethyl ether	Methyl ethyl ether
Dichloroethyl ether	Methyl isopropyl ether
Chlorotrifluoroethyl methyl ether	Methyl propyl ether
Dichloroisopropyl ether	Methyl-*tert*-butyl ether
Diphenyl ether	Phenetole
Ethyl butyl ether	Vanillin
Ethyl vinyl ether	Vinyl ether
Eugenol	Glycidyl ethers

Ethyl Ether

Ethyl ether ($C_2H_5OC_2H_5$), also known as *diethyl ether,* is a colorless liquid having a sweet odor and a vapor pressure of 440 mm Hg; hence, it is highly volatile. Its vapor density is 2.56 (as compared to that of air, which is 1.00). It is used as a solvent and formerly was used as an anesthetic gas. Ethyl ether is explosive when mixed with air, which creates one of its main hazards.

Acute vapor inhalation produces drowsiness, apathy, depression, anorexia, and loss of consciousness. Chronic exposure can produce drowsiness, dizziness, headache, and irritability. Nasal irritation has occurred at exposures of 200 ppm.

The OSHA PEL for ethyl ether is 400 ppm (1,210 mg per cubic meter). The ACGIH TLV is identical to this limit. The ACGIH also has set a 15-minute STEL of 500 ppm.

Methyl Ether

Methyl ether (CH_3OCH_3), or dimethyl ether, is a colorless gas having an etherlike odor. Its vapor density is 1.62 (air, 1.00). A mixture of 50% methyl ether with air provides a highly unpleasant odor. It is used as a refrigerant, an aerosol dispersate, an anesthetic agent, a rocket propellant, and a cold-weather gasoline starter.

Isopropyl Ether

Isopropyl ether is a colorless liquid used as a solvent and a chemical intermediate. It has a chemical formula of $(CH_3)_2CHOCH(CH_3)_2$. Most exposures generally occur by inhalation. It is a mild irritant of the eyes and mucous membranes and, at high concentrations in animal models, has produced narcosis. Humans exposed to 800 ppm for 5 minutes reported irritation of the eyes, nose, and throat.

Vinyl Ether

Also known as *divinyl ether, ethenyloxyethene,* and *divinyl oxide,* vinyl ether has a chemical formula of $CH_2{:}CHOCH{:}CH_2$. It is produced by the action of sodium hydroxide on dichloroethyl ether. Prolonged exposure to this highly volatile, colorless, and highly flammable liquid can cause hepatotoxicity. Its vapor pressure is 430 mm Hg (20°C) and its vapor density 2.4 (air, 1.0).

Chloromethyl Ethers

Chloromethyl ethers ($ClCH_2OCH_3$) have received much attention as causes of excess cases of respiratory cancer among exposed workers (35,48). Animal studies show that inhaled bis-chloromethyl ether (BCME) is a more potent pulmonary carcinogen than is chloromethyl methyl ether (CMME). CMME vapors undergo rapid hydrolysis in air, as opposed to the more stable BCME vapors. Therefore, BCME inhalation is inferred to be the chloromethyl ether most likely to be responsible for pulmonary cancer in human exposures. The respiratory cancers attributable to chloromethyl ether exposure share certain features (35,48):

- Exposed groups exhibit excess rates of respiratory cancer but not other cancer types.
- Cancers tend to occur at earlier-than-usual ages, especially among nonsmokers.
- Small-cell cancers with a predominance of oat-cell types are the most common histologic types seen.
- Studies report a dose-response relationship.
- The mean elapsed time from first exposure to diagnosis is 13 years.

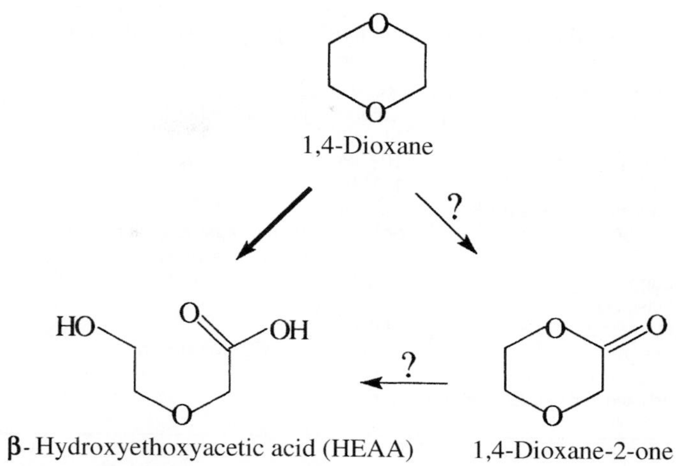

1,4-Dioxane

?

HO OH

?

β-Hydroxyethoxyacetic acid (HEAA) 1,4-Dioxane-2-one

Figure 107-13. Suspected metabolism of 1,4-dioxane.

Studies report a relative lung cancer risk in exposed workers of 5.0 as compared to unexposed workers and a risk of 7.6 as compared with an external population. The OSHA classifies CMME and BCME as probable human carcinogens. The ACGIH lists BCME as a confirmed human carcinogen. The IARC and the U.S. Environmental Protection Agency list both as human carcinogens.

Airborne concentrations of CMME in excess of 100 ppm and exposure to the liquid can cause eye irritation. High-level inhalation is irritating to the lungs and can cause pulmonary edema. BCME has more acute toxicity than does CMME.

Dioxane

Dioxane (*p*-dioxane; 1,4-dioxane; 1,4-diethylene dioxide; 1,4-diethyleneoxide) is a colorless liquid ether having a faint alcohol or ethyl ether odor (Fig. 107-13). Its molecular formula is $C_4H_8O_2$, and its molecular weight is 88.12 D. Dioxane is formed by dimerizing ethylene oxide or by dehydrating ethylene glycol.

Dioxane is heavier than air (vapor density, 3.0; air, 1.0) and very flammable, forms explosive peroxides, and may flash back along a vapor trail. It can pose an explosion hazard when exposed to ignition sources. Owing to its flammability and explosive hazards, any spill or release of dioxane must be handled with caution. Because of its high degree of reactivity, vapors of dioxane can form explosive peroxide mixtures with air.

The flammability limits of dioxane in air range from 1.97% to 22.5% by volume. When heated, toxic vapors are generated. Dioxane vapors are heavier than air and consequently travel along lower areas to ignition sources to produce flashback or explosion. Also, owing to the fact that dioxane has a vapor pressure three times that of air, the chemical may reside in confined spaces below surface level. Dioxane's physiochemical properties are listed in Table 107-16.

PRODUCTION, USES, AND SOURCES

1,4-Dioxane finds extensive use as a solvent for organic compounds and is found in many consumer products (e.g., lacquers, plastics, varnishes, paints, dyes, oils, fats, greases, waxes). It is used commonly as a solvent for resins and oils. Technical-grade 1,4-dioxane is more than 99.9% pure but can contain bis(2-chloroethyl)ether impurities (49). 1,4-Dioxane persists in the environment and does not biodegrade readily but may be subject to photochemical oxidation.

TABLE 107-16. Physiochemical properties of dioxane

Molecular weight	88.10
Physical state	Colorless, flammable liquid
Melting point	11.8°C
Boiling point	101.1°C
Density (20°C)	1.0329
Vapor pressure (20°C)	30 mm Hg
Solubility	Soluble in water, organic solvents, oils, aromatic hydrocarbons
Log K_{ow}	–0.27
Flash point	12°C
Ignition temperature	180°C
Reactivity	Forms explosive peroxides in air

Adapted from ref. 49, with permission.

ABSORPTION, METABOLISM, EXCRETION

Dioxane can be absorbed after inhalational or dermal exposure. Dermal absorption occurs but to a much lesser extent than absorption via other routes. Dioxane is metabolized mainly to β-hydroxyethoxyacetic acid (HEAA), in which form approximately 85% of dioxane is excreted into the urine (49). Hepatic mixed-function oxidase enzymes probably catalyze the reaction that forms HEAA. At high doses of dioxane, the metabolism to HEAA is saturated.

Another proposed metabolite of dioxane is 1,4-dioxane-2-one (DeRosa) (see Fig. 107-13). However, whether 1,4-dioxane is first metabolized to HEAA, which can cyclize to 1,4-dioxane-2-one, or the parent is metabolized directly to 1,4-dioxane-2-one remains unanswered.

Inhalational studies of volunteers exposed to 50 ppm dioxane for 6 hours showed that HEAA accounted for more than 99% of the dioxane dose (50). The plasma concentration of dioxane in this study reached 10 µg per mL at 3 hours after exposure, 2.5 µg per L at 5 hours, and 4 µg per L at 6 hours. The elimination half-life was 2.7 hours, with a plasma clearance of 75 mg per minute.

CLINICAL TOXICOLOGY

Dioxane is heavier than water and thus sinks when mixed with water. It produces an irritating vapor. Workers should avoid contact with both the liquid and the vapor. They should be provided with appropriate personal protective equipment when working with dioxane. Owing to its flammability, dioxane may explode if ignited in an enclosed area.

Dioxane has a pleasant odor that reaches an air threshold of recognition at 170 ppm. This odor recognition threshold allows for dioxane to be detected before acute toxic effects occur. However, chronic exposure can result in serious health effects. Irritation from dioxane vapors occurs at somewhere between a 0.1% and 3.0% vapor concentration, which can produce CNS depression and, if the exposure continues, pulmonary edema and death.

Renal and hepatic injury can occur after toxic exposure to dioxane. Dioxane is an acute health hazard and is highly toxic by inhalational, dermal, and GI routes. Lethal concentrations for humans can occur at 470 ppm.

Owing to its mild odor, which serves as a warning to exposure at the odor threshold level, workers may be exposed to chronically high concentrations without knowing that they are being exposed. Workers exposed to high vapor concentrations of dioxane experience mucous membrane irritation; ocular, nasal, and pulmonary irritation; drowsiness; headache; nausea; vomiting; and hepatic and renal damage (49). Acute exposure to dioxane can result in confusion, ataxia, drowsiness, convulsions, renal and hepatic damage, and pulmonary edema. Skin

Allyl glycidyl ether

Isopropyl glycidyl ether

Phenyl glycidyl ether

***n*-Butyl glycidyl ether**

Diglycidyl ether

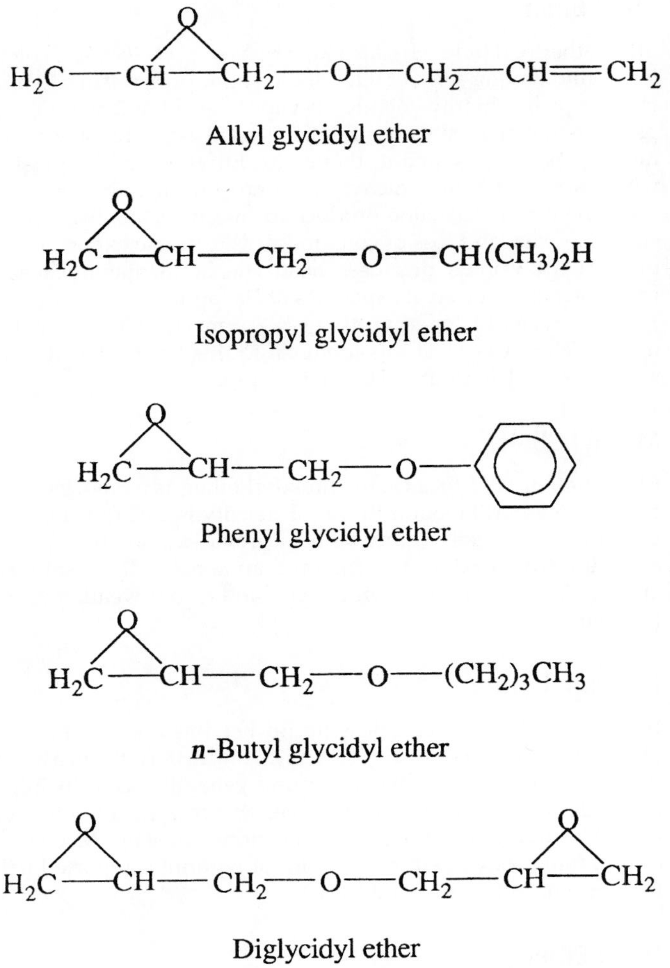

Figure 107-14. Chemical structure of various glycidyl ethers.

contact with vapor or liquid (which is a defatting agent) can result in dermatitis. Dioxane is absorbed dermally.

Exposures of the eye, which can lead to corneal damage, must be flushed immediately with water. Likewise, any clothing that becomes contaminated with dioxane should be removed and contaminated skin irrigated with soap and water. Because of the poor warning properties of the vapor threshold of dioxane, illness in exposed individuals may be delayed.

In animals, kidney injury, liver injury, progressive weakness, depression, incoordination, coma, and death are seen. In guinea

TABLE 107-17. Glycidyl ethers

Diglycidyl ether
n-Butyl glycidyl ether
Phenyl glycidyl ether
Resorcinol glycidyl ether
Allyl glycidyl ether
Octyl decyl glycidyl ether
Isopropyl glycidyl ether
Triglycidyl glycerol ether
Triethylene glycol glycidyl ether
o-Cresol glycidyl ether
Butanediol diglycidyl ether
Diethylene glycol diglycidyl ether

TABLE 107-18. Physiochemical properties of glycidyl ethers

	Isopropyl glycidyl ether	Phenyl glycidyl ether	*n*-Butyl glycidyl ether	Diglycidyl ether
Physical state	Colorless liquid	Colorless liquid	Colorless liquid	Colorless liquid
Odor	—	—	Irritating odor	Irritating odor at >5 ppm
Vapor pressure	0.4 mm Hg (25°C)	0.01 mm Hg (20°C)	3.2 mm Hg (25°C)	0.09 mm Hg (25°C)
Flash point	33°C	120°C	54.4°C	64°C
Molecular weight	116	150	130	130
Boiling point	137°C	245°C	164°C	220–260°C
Specific gravity	0.92	1.11	0.91	1.26
OSHA PEL	50 ppm (240 mg/m^3)	10 ppm (60 mg/m^3)	50 ppm (270 mg/m^3)	0.5 ppm (2.8 mg/m^3)
IDLH level	1,500 ppm	—	3,500 ppm	85 ppm
Vapor density (air = 1.0)	—	4.37	3.78	3.78

IDLH, immediately dangerous to life and health; OSHA, Occupational Safety and Health Administration; PEL, permissible exposure limit.

pigs, rabbits, and cats, intravenous dioxane results in degeneration of liver cells and convoluted tubule cells of the kidneys. Studies in cats demonstrate narcotic effects, loss of equilibrium, increased salivation, and lacrimation. Fatty livers and pulmonary edema, with respiratory failure and inflamed respiratory tracts, are reported on necropsy.

In 1933, five cases of fatal industrial poisoning from dioxane occurred at a synthetic textile factory in England. Toxicity ensued after inhalational exposure. Fatal illnesses occurred without warning, and workers died within 5 to 8 days of exposure. Workers presented with eye and upper airway irritation, coughing, pulmonary edema, anorexia, abdominal pain, nausea, vomiting, hepatomegaly, back pain, renal failure, uremia, drowsiness, vertigo, headache, coma, and death. Autopsies revealed pulmonary and cerebral edema, centrilobular hepatic necrosis, and hemorrhagic nephritis.

GENOTOXICITY AND CARCINOGENICITY

Carcinogenicity testing has shown that high-dose dioxane can produce hepatocellular carcinomas or adenomas of the liver and squamous cell carcinoma of the nasal passages of certain animals (49). Studies of genotoxicity are inconsistent. Human epidemiologic studies have not demonstrated a causal association between industrial dioxane exposure and tumor formation.

REGULATORY CONTROLS

The IDLH concentration of dioxane is 200 ppm. The OSHA PEL for dioxane is 100 ppm with a skin notation. The National Institute of Occupational Safety and Health has suggested a ceiling of 1 ppm for 30 minutes. The TLV for dioxane is 25 ppm with a short-term inhalation limit of 100 ppm for 16 minutes. The ACGIH suggests a TLV of 25 ppm and recommends a STEL of 100 ppm.

Glycidyl Ethers

Glycidyl ethers have a 2,3-epoxy propyl (epoxy propoxy radical) group with an ether linkage to another organic moiety (Fig. 107-14). Important glycidyl ethers are listed in Table 107-17. Most glycidyl ethers are liquids, although a few are solids. The physiochemical properties of select glycidyl ethers are listed in Table 107-18. Monoglycidyl and diglycidyl ethers are used on a limited basis as intermediates for resins, ethers, and esters and as diluents for epoxy resins and stabilizers for chlorinated compounds, vinyl resins, and rubber. Glycidyl ethers have a low vapor pressure and a strong irritating odor. They are used in epoxy resin systems as reactive diluents to decrease the polymer viscosity.

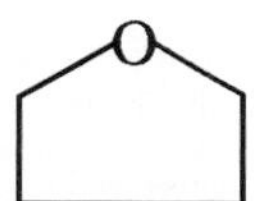

Figure 107-15. Chemical structure of tetrahydrofuran.

Glycidyl ethers are irritating to the respiratory tract, eye, and skin. Prolonged skin contact may cause burns. Contact allergic reactions have been reported (51). Acute exposure from an *n*-butyl glycidyl ether spill has been described (52). In this incident, workers experienced CNS and GI effects. Allyl glycidyl ether forms DNA adducts (53).

Isopropyl Glycidyl Ether

Isopropyl glycidyl ether (see Fig. 107-14) is a reactive diluent for epoxy resins. Exposure to the vapors causes irritation, sensitization, and dermatitis. Diglycidyl ether inhalation causes severe irritation of the eyes, respiratory tract, and skin. Hematopoietic toxic effects have been seen in animals. It is a solvent for epoxy resins and an intermediate in the production of esters and ethers.

Phenyl Glycidyl Ether

Phenyl glycidyl ether is a colorless liquid with respiratory irritant properties. Liver necrosis is seen in animal exposure models at 15 to 22 ppm. Mutagenic activity is seen in bacteria. Used as a solvent for halogenated compounds, it is a mucous membrane, skin, and eye irritant. Exposed workers have developed dermatitis and skin burns. Contact allergic dermatitis has been reported.

n-Butyl Glycidyl Ether

n-Butyl glycidyl ether ($C_7H_{14}O_2$) is a colorless liquid with an irritating odor. Adverse health effects in humans have not been reported, although in animal models this compound produces CNS depression and eye and skin irritation. Animals exposed to *n*-butyl glycidyl ether vapor have experienced lacrimation and breathing difficulty. Pneumonitis also is seen in animal inhalation models.

Diglycidyl Ether

Diglycidyl ether is a colorless liquid ($C_6H_{10}O_3$) having an irritating odor at levels exceeding 5 ppm. Hematopoietic abnormali-

TABLE 107-19. Physiochemical properties of and regulations applicable to tetrahydrofuran

Molecular weight	72.1
Specific gravity	0.89
Vapor pressure	114 mm Hg (15°C)
Color	Colorless
Odor	Acetonelike
OSHA PEL	200 ppm (590 mg/m^3)
ACGIH STEL	250 ppm (735 mg/m^3)
IDLH level	20,000 ppm

ACGIH, American Conference of Governmental Industrial Hygienists; IDLH, immediately dangerous to life and health; OSHA, U.S. Occupational Safety and Health Administration; PEL, permissible exposure limit; STEL, short-term exposure limit.

ties are seen in animal models after dermal application or inhalation. This ether is a solvent for epoxy resins. It can cause irritation of skin, eyes, and the respiratory tract. Diglycidyl ether is very injurious to skin in animal studies. Humans should use precautions to avoid dermal, ocular, and respiratory exposure.

Tetrahydrofuran

Tetrahydrofuran (THF, diethylene oxide) $[(C_2H_4)_2O]$ is a colorless, liquid, four-carbon cyclic ether that is soluble in ethyl alcohol, ethyl ether, and water (Fig. 107-15). It is used as a solvent in glues, paints, varnishes, inks, and wetting and dispersing agents for textile processing. It also is a solvent for resins. THF forms explosive peroxides when exposed to air. Explosions of THF can occur on contact with lithium-aluminum alloys. The physiochemical properties of THF and regulations limiting its use are listed in Table 107-19.

THF enhances the toxicity of other compounds (i.e., solvent effect) by stimulating their rapid absorption. It further inhibits a number of cytochrome P-450–dependent mixed-function oxidase enzymes, especially the P-450 CYP2E1 isoenzyme complex. THF also forms peroxides. These mechanisms may account for, or contribute to, hepatotoxicity.

THF is embryotoxic in pregnant mice and causes uterine atrophy in nonpregnant mice. Subchronic toxicity of rodents exposed to THF vapors includes CNS toxicity (e.g., narcosis and ataxia) and increased liver weights with mild centrilobular hepatomegaly.

The primary concerns in human exposure to THF are CNS depression and hepatotoxicity. THF vapors are ocular and skin irritants. Exposed individuals have reported experiencing severe headaches.

REFERENCES

1. World Health Organization. *2-Propanol*. Environmental health criteria 103. Geneva: World Health Organization, 1990.
2. Martinez T, Jaeger R, De Castro J, Thompson MW, Hamilton MF. A comparison of the absorption and metabolism of isopropyl alcohol by oral, dermal and inhalation routes. *Vet Hum Toxicol* 1986;28:233–236.
3. Natowicz M, Donahue J, Gorman L, et al. Pharmacokinetic analysis of a case of isopropanol intoxication. *Clin Med* 1985;31:326–328.
4. Davis P, Dal-Cortivo L, Maturo J. Endogenous isopropanol: forensic and biochemical implications. *J Anal Toxicol* 1984;8:209–212.
5. Lewis G, Laufman A, McAnally B. Metabolism of acetone to isopropyl alcohol in rats and humans. *J Forensic Sci* 1984;29:541–549.
6. Lewin G, Oppenheimer P, Wingert W. Coma from alcohol sponging. *J Am Coll Emerg Phys* 1977;6:165–167.
7. World Health Organization. *1-Propanol*. Environmental health criteria 102. Geneva: World Health Organization, 1990.
8. Ludwig E, Hausen B. Sensitivity to isopropyl alcohol. *Contact Dermatitis* 1977;3:240–244.
9. Rosenberg N. Methylmalonic acid, methanol, metabolic acidosis and lesions of the basal ganglia. *Ann Neurol* 1987;22:96–97.
10. Aquilonius S, Bergstrom K, Enoksson P, et al. Cerebral computed tomography in methanol intoxication. *J Comput Assist Tomogr* 1980;4:425–428.
11. Osterloh J, Pond S, Grady S, Becker C. Serum formate concentrations in methanol intoxication as a criterion for hemodialysis. *Ann Intern Med* 1986; 104:200–203.
12. Jacobsen D, McMartin K. Antidotes for methanol and ethylene glycol poisoning. *Clin Toxicol* 1997;35(2):127–143.
13. Bergerdon R, Cardinal J, Geadah D. Prevention of methanol toxicity by ethanol therapy. *N Engl J Med* 1982;9:1528.
14. Shannon M. Toxicology reviews: fomepisole—a new antidote. *Pediatr Emerg Care* 1998;14(2):170–172.
15. World Health Organization. *Butanols—4 isomers: 1-butanol, 2-butanol, tert-butanol, isobutanol*. Environmental health criteria 65. Geneva: World Health Organization, 1987.
16. Connor T, Theiss J, Hanna H, et al. Genotoxicity of organic chemicals frequently found in the air of mobile homes. *Toxicol Lett* 1985;25:33–40.
17. Agency for Toxic Substances and Disease Registry. *Toxicological profile for acetone*. Atlanta: US Department of Health and Human Services, Public Health Service, ATSDR, 1994.
18. Meyrahn H, Pauly J, Schneider W, et al. Quantum yield for the photodissociation of acetone in the air and an estimate for the life time of acetone in the lower troposphere. *J Atmosph Chem* 1986;4:277–291.
19. Conkle J, Camp B, Welch B. Trace composition of human respiratory gas. *Arch Environ Health* 1975;30:290–295.
20. Shah J, Singh H. Distribution of volatile organic chemicals in outdoor and indoor air. *Environ Sci Technol* 1988;22:1381–1388.
21. Eisenreich S, Looney B, Thornton J. Airborne organic contaminates in the Great Lakes' ecosystem. *Environ Sci Technol* 1981;15(1):30–38.
22. Ross D. Acute acetone intoxication involving eight male workers. *Ann Occup Hyg* 1973;16:73–75.
23. Raleigh R, McGee W. Effects of short, high-concentration exposure to acetone as determined by observation in the work area. *J Occup Med* 1972;14:607–610.
24. Tosti A, Bardazzi F, Ghetti P. Unusual complication of sensitizing therapy for alopecia aneata. *Contact Dermatitis* 1988;18:322.
25. Feldman R. Hexane and methyl-*n*-butyl ketone. In: Feldman RG, ed. *Occupational and environmental neurotoxicology*. Philadelphia: Lippincott–Raven Publishers, 1999.
26. Rosenberg N. Neurotoxicology of organic solvents. In: Rosenberg N, ed. *Occupational and environmental neurology*. Boston: Butterworth–Heinemann, 1995.
27. DiVincenzo G, Hamilton M, Kaplan C, et al. Studies on the respiratory uptake and excretion and the skin absorption of methyl-*n*-butyl ketone in humans and dogs. *Toxicol Appl Pharmacol* 1978;44:539–604.
28. Perbellini L, Pezzoli G, Brugnone F. Biochemical and physiological aspects of 2,5-hexanedione: endogenous or exogenous product? *Int Arch Occup Environ Health* 1993;65:49–52.
29. Krasavage W, O'Donoghue J, DeVincinco G. The relative neurotoxicity of methyl-*n*-butyl ketone, *n*-hexane and their metabolites. *Toxicol Appl Pharmacol* 1980;52:433–441.
30. Ruth J. Odor thresholds and irritation levels of several chemical substances: a review. *Am Ind Hyg Assoc J* 1986;47:A142–151.
31. Patel JM, Gordon WP, Nelson SD, Leibman KC. Comparison of hepatic biotransformation and toxicity of allyl alcohol and [1,1-2H2]allyl alcohol in rats. *Drug Metab Dispos* 1983;11:164–166.
32. World Health Organization. *Methyl ethyl ketone*. Environmental health criteria 143. Geneva: World Health Organization, 1993.
33. Myasaka M, Kumai M, Koizumi A, et al. Biological monitoring of occupational exposure to methyl ethyl ketone by means of urinalysis for methyl ethyl ketone itself. *Int Arch Occup Environ Health* 1982;50:131–137.
34. World Health Organization. *Methyl isobutyl ketone health and safety guide*. Health and safety guide no. 58. Geneva: World Health Organization, 1991.
35. Maher K, DeFonso L. Respiratory cancer among chloromethyl ether workers. *J Natl Cancer Inst* 1987:89(5):839–843.
36. World Health Organization. *Di-n-butylphthalate*. Environmental health criteria 189. Geneva: World Health Organization, 1997.
37. Milkov L, Aldyrova M, Popova T, et al. Health status of workers exposed to phthalate plasticizers in the manufacture of artificial leather and films based on PVC resins. *Environ Health Perspect* 1973;3:175–178.
38. World Health Organization. *Diethylhexyl phthalate*. Environmental health criteria 131. Geneva: World Health Organization, 1992.
39. World Health Organization. *Dimethyl sulphate*. Environmental health criteria 48. Geneva: World Health Organization, 1985.
40. World Health Organization. *Tricresyl phosphate*. Environmental health criteria 110. Geneva: World Health Organization, 1990.
41. Vasilescu C, Florescu A. Clinical and electrophysiological study of neuropathy after organophosphorus compound poisoning. *Arch Toxicol* 1980;43:305–315.
42. Morgan J. The Jamaica ginger paralysis. *JAMA* 1982;248:1864–1867.
43. Goldstein D, McGuigan M, Ripley B. Acute tricresyl phosphate intoxication in childhood. *Hum Toxicol* 1988;7:179–182.
44. World Health Organization. *Tri-n-butyl phosphate*. Environmental health criteria 112. Geneva: World Health Organization, 1991.
45. Suzuki T, Sasaki K, Takeda M, et al. Metabolism of tributyl phosphate in male rates. *J Agric Food Chem* 1984;32:603–610.
46. World Health Organization. *Triphenyl phosphate*. Environmental health criteria 111. Geneva: World Health Organization, 1991.

47. Sutton W, Therhaar C, Miller F, et al. Studies on the industrial hygiene and toxicology of triphenyl phosphate. *Arch Environ Health* 1960;1:45–58.
48. Gowers D, DeFonso L, Schaffer P, et al. Incidence of respiratory cancer among workers exposed to chloromethyl ethers. *Am J Epidemiol* 1993;137(1):31–42.
49. DeRosa C, Wilbur S, Holler J, et al. Health evaluation of 1,4-dioxane. *Toxicol Ind Health* 1996;12(1):1–43.
50. Young J, Braun W, Rampy L. Pharmacokinetics of 1,4-dioxane in humans. *J Toxicol Environ Health* 1977;3:507–520.
51. Dooms-Goossens A, Bruze M, Buysse L, Fregert S, Grunberger B, Stals H. Contact allergy to allyl glycidyl ether present as an impurity in 3-glycidyl-oxypropyltrimethyoxysilane, a fixing additive in silicone and polyurethane resins. *Contact Dermatitis* 1995;33:17–19.
52. Lawless E. Effects of *n*-butyl glycidyl ether exposure. *J Soc Occup Med* 1979; 29:142–143.
53. Plena K, Sergerback D, Schweda E. DNA adduct formation by allyl glycidyl ether. *Carcinogenesis* 1996;17:1465–1471.

CHAPTER 108
Glycol Ethers

Gary R. Krieger and John B. Sullivan, Jr.

The glycol ethers are a group of organic solvents that are widely used in both industrial and household products. Although numerous glycol derivatives exist, the most commonly studied and evaluated are the E-series and P-series compounds. The E series comprises the family of ethylene glycol ethers (EGEs), whereas the P series contains the propylene glycol ethers. The E-series compounds are most frequently encountered by consumers and workers and are considered more toxic than are the P-series compounds. Hence, considerable research as been focused on the monoalkyl ethers of ethylene glycol (EG) (1–5).

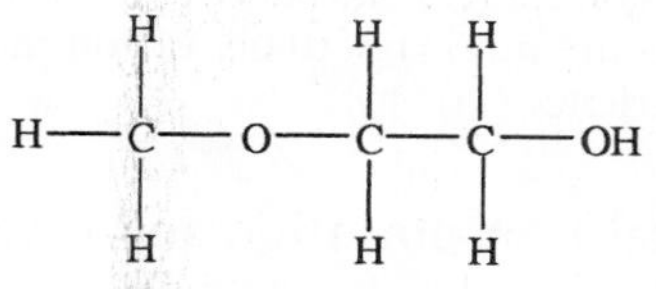

2-Methoxyethanol
(2-ME, ethylene glycol monomethyl ether, methyl cellosolve)

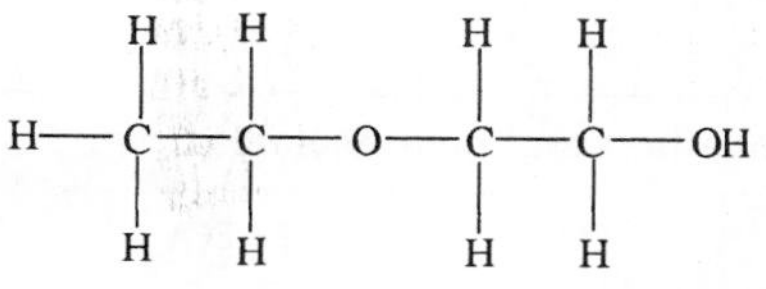

2-Ethoxyethanol
(2-EE, ethylene glycol monoethyl ether, cellosolve)

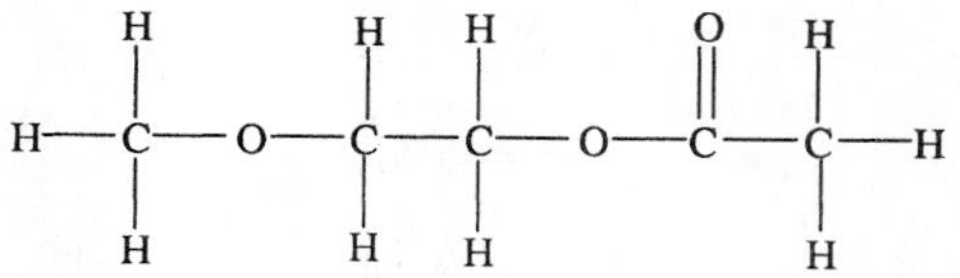

2-Methoxyethyl Acetate
(2-MEA, ethylene glycol monomethyl ether acetate, methyl cellosolve acetate)

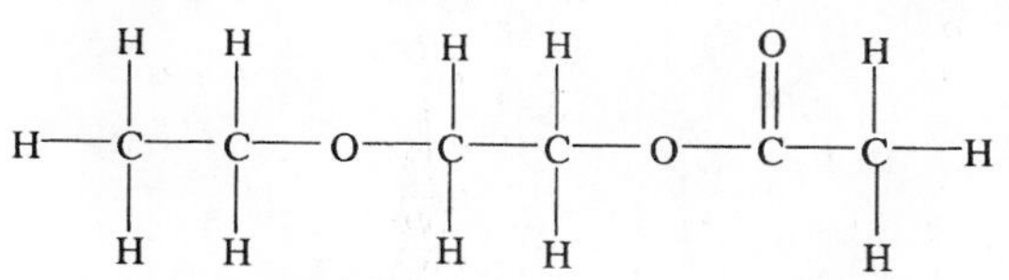

2-Ethoxyethyl Acetate
(2-EEA, ethylene glycol monoethyl ether acetate, cellosolve acetate)

Figure 108-1. Chemical structures for glycol ethers.

Considerable concern has been expressed regarding the human toxicology of the EGEs. However, the environmental risks appear to be low, as these compounds are neither persistent nor bioaccumulative in the environment, and they demonstrate minimal toxicity to aquatic organisms (5).

The family of EG monoalkyl ethers is represented by the formula $R_1OCH_2CH_2OR_2$, where R_1 represents an alkyl group and R_2 represents either a hydrogen or an acetate (Fig. 108-1). Discussions of glycol ethers commonly refer specifically to ethylene glycol monomethyl ether [EGME, or 2-methoxyethanol (2-ME)] and ethylene glycol monoethyl ether [EGEE, cellosolve, or 2-ethoxyethanol (2-EE)]. The acetates of these two compounds make up the other two members of this family of glycol ethers: ethylene glycol monomethyl ether acetate (EGMEA, or 2-MEA) and ethylene glycol monoethyl ether acetate (EGEEA, or 2-EEA).

Ethylene glycol monobutyl ether (EGBE, butyl cellosolve, or 2-butoxyethanol) is a glycol ether used as a solvent and viscosity-decreasing agent in hair dyes, hair colors, other hair products, and cosmetics. Among other glycol ethers are diethylene glycol mono-*n*-butyl ether (DGBE) and triethylene glycol ethers.

ETHYLENE GLYCOL ETHERS

Sources, Uses, and Production

2-ME and 2-EE are produced by the reaction of ethylene oxide with methylmethanol or ethanol. They also can be manufactured by alkylation of EG with dimethyl sulfate or diethyl sulfate. The acetates of these compounds are prepared by esterifying the individual glycol ether with acetic acid chloride or acetic acid anhydride (2).

Glycol ethers have a number of commercial product uses (Table 108-1). Their physiochemical characteristics make them ideal for use in coatings, resins, lacquers, metal cleaners, paints, detergents, polishes, hydraulic fluid, and deicers. 2-ME is a jet fuel deicer: JP-4 jet fuel contains 0.1% to 0.2% 2-ME as a deicing agent, and JP-5 uses 0.15% diethylene glycol, or diethylene glycol monomethyl ether, as a deicer. Diethylene glycol is used in the manufacture of printed circuit boards and as an intermediate in the formation of plasticizers, inks, coatings, and dyeing applications.

EGMEA is an intermediate for plasticizers. 2-EE is a chemical intermediate for EGEEA production and is a solvent for coatings and in cleaning and for printing ink formulations. EGEEA is a solvent used for coating applications, automobiles, machinery, equipment, appliances, and metals.

The glycol ethers have an important function in paints and coatings and generally make up less than 10% of the final product. These ethers help to keep other components of paints and coatings in solution. Glycol ethers also enhance the coalescing properties of a product and improve penetration and bonding qualities of paints and coatings.

Exposure to glycol ethers can occur through inhalation and skin contact in the use or manufacture of printing inks that contain such compounds. Cleaning agents and such other solvents as spot removers, carburetor cleaners, metal cleaners, and glass cleaners can contain glycol ethers in generally less than a 5% concentration.

Butoxyethanol (EGBE) is a clear liquid that is soluble in water and most organic solvents and is prepared by the reaction of ethylene oxide with butyl alcohol or by alkylation of EG with

TABLE 108-1. Uses of ethylene glycols and acetates

Compound	Uses
Ethylene glycol monomethyl ether (EGME, 2-ME)	As a solvent for many purposes: cellulose esters, dyes, resins, lacquers, varnishes and stains; as a perfume fixative; as a jet fuel deicing additive
Ethylene glycol monomethyl ether acetate (EGMEA, 2-MEA)	In photographic films, lacquers, textile printing; as a solvent for waxes, oils, various gums and resins, cellulose acetate, nitrocellulose
Ethylene glycol monoethyl ether (EGEE, 2-EE)	As a solvent for nitrocellulose, natural and synthetic resins; as a mutual solvent for the formulation of soluble oils; in lacquers, the dyeing and printing of textiles, varnish removers, cleaning solutions, products for the treatment of leather; as an antiicing additive for aviation fuels
Ethylene glycol monoethyl ether acetate (EGEEA, 2-EEA)	As a blush retardant in lacquers; as a solvent for nitrocellulose, oils, and resins; in wood stains, varnish removers, products for the treatment of textiles and leathers
Butoxyethanol [ethylene glycol monobutyl ether (EGBE)]	As a solvent for resins, viscosity-decreasing agent, hair dyes, cosmetics, varnishes, waxes, polishes, hydraulic brake fluid
Diethylene glycol mono-*n*-butyl ether (DGBE)	In hard surface cleaners and paints
Diethylene glycol *n*-butyl acetate (DGBA)	In paints and cleaners

dibutyl sulfate. Butoxyethanol is used as a solvent and as a viscosity-decreasing agent in hair dyes, other hair products, and cosmetics. More than 740 products contain butoxyethanol, and many of these are for household use. Butoxyethanol is also a solvent in resins, varnishes, hydraulic fluids, floor polishes, floor waxes, and cleaning agents for upholstery, glass, and leather. It is used as a defoaming agent in the manufacture of paper and paper board and is a solvent in polysulfide polymer-polyepoxide resins and in sanitizing solutions.

Physiochemical Properties

The EGEs have physical and chemical properties that enhance their use in an industrial setting. Generally, the EGEs have an inoffensive odor, low evaporation rates, and favorable solubility characteristics in water and other organic solvents. Hence, they frequently are found in paints, resins, and lacquers (1). The physiochemical properties of selected glycol ethers are listed in Table 108-2.

Exposure Sources

Most human exposure to glycol ethers occurs in occupational settings. For example, glycol ethers and their acetates are extensively used in the semiconductor industry (Table 108-3). Studies have evaluated the possible link to adverse reproductive outcomes and EGE exposure (6–10). Two glycol ethers, diethylene glycol dimethyl ether and EGMEA, have been linked with increases in spontaneous abortions in semiconductor workers (7,8,10). The current occupational exposure guidelines (permissible exposure limits) established by the U.S. Occupational Safety and Health Administration for 2-ME and 2-EE are 25 ppm and 200 ppm, respectively. However, owing to the intense scrutiny surrounding the EGEs, changes of standards would not be unexpected.

Models used to estimate exposure to glycol ethers from the use of paint, coating, stains, dyes, and inks containing these products and their acetates indicate that peak exposure values greater than 30 ppm, with values averaging greater than 5 ppm for 1 hour, can occur when these products contain more than 20% glycol ethers (3).

Ingestion of commercial and household products containing glycol ethers occurs but is relatively uncommon in poison control center experience (1).

Environmental Transportation and Fate

Environmental exposure to glycol ethers results from their release into the atmosphere from volatilization, from manufacturing releases and effluents, and from other general commer-

TABLE 108-2. Physiochemical properties of select glycol ethers and their acetates

Property	EGME	EGMEA	EGEE	EGEEA	EGBE
Molecular formula	$C_3H_8O_2$	$C_5H_{10}O_3$	$C_4H_{10}O_2$	$C_6H_{12}O_3$	$C_5H_{12}O_2$
Color	Clear liquid	Clear liquid	Clear liquid	Clear liquid	Clear
Molecular weight	76.1	118.1	90.1	132.2	118.18
Specific gravity (25°/4°C)	0.962	1.007	0.926	0.975	0.890–0.906
Evaporation rate (butyl acetate = 1.0)	0.62	0.30	0.41	0.2	0.1
Boiling point (°C)	124.2	144.5	135.0	156.3	171–172
Freezing point (°C)	–85	–65.1	–100	–61.7	<–40
Vapor pressure (mm Hg at 25°C)	9.7	2.0–3.7	5.75	2.8	0.88
Flash point (°C)	39	49	43	52	60
Autoignition temperature (°C)	285	392	235	379	238
Flammability limits (vol% in air)	1.8–14.0	1.5–12.3	1.70–15.60	1.7	1.10–12.70
Water solubility (wt%)	Miscible	Miscible	Miscible	23 mg/100 g at 20°C	Miscible
Vapor density (air = 1.0)	2.6	4.1	3.1	4.6	
Volume in saturated air (ppm at 25°C)	12,800	2,600–4,900	7,600	3,700	
Conversion factors					
Milligrams per cubic meter at 25°C (760 mm Hg = 1 ppm)	3.11	4.83	3.69	5.41	
Parts per million at 25°C (760 mm Hg = 1 mg/m³)	0.32	0.21	0.27	0.19	
Explosive limits (%)					
Lower limit	2.5	1.1	1.8	1.7	
Upper limit	19.8	8.2	14		

EGBE, ethylene glycol monobutyl ether (2-butoxyethanol); EGEE, ethylene glycol monoethyl ether (2-EE); EGEEA, ethylene glycol monoethyl ether acetate; EGME, ethylene glycol monomethyl ether (2-ME); EGMEA, ethylene glycol monomethyl ether acetate.

TABLE 108-3. Exposure to glycol ethers within the semiconductor industry in the United States (mg/m³)

	2-EEA			2-ME			2-MEA		
Sampling data	No. of samples	Range	Mean + SD	No. of samples	Range	Mean + SD	No. of samples	Range	Mean + SD
Personal (TWA)	96	0.0054–2.7000	0.27 ± 0.43	6	0.12–3.11	0.68 ± 1.18	16	ND	0.048 ± 0.000
Personal (short-term)	21	0.0054–97.2000	15.23 ± 29.20	1	NA	80.0	1	NA	82.0
Area (TWA)	128	0.0054–9.7200	0.27 ± 0.86	4	0.093–2.490	0.72 ± 1.18	20	ND	0.048 ± 0.000
Area (short-term)	10	0.027–81.000	8.42 ± 25.49	1	NA	80.9	1	NA	87.0

2-EEA, ethylene glycol monoethyl ether acetate; 2-ME, ethylene glycol monomethyl ether; 2-MEA, ethylene glycol monomethyl ether acetate; NA, not applicable; ND, not detectable; SD, standard deviation; TWA, time-weighted average.
Note: Analytical limit of detection: 2-EEA, 0.0054 mg/m³; 2-ME, 0.093 mg/m³; and 2-MEA, 0.048 mg/m³.
Adapted from ref. 37, with permission.

cial uses. Because glycol ethers have low vapor pressure and high water solubility, they can accumulate in environmental media such as soil. However, they undergo rapid hydrolysis and oxidation and, therefore, do not bioaccumulate. Studies show that sludge can digest these compounds, with 90% degradation of 2-EE after 5.5 days (3).

2-ME serves as a substrate for anaerobic methane fermentation and is digested by anaerobic sludge. Therefore, under aerobic conditions, 2-ME and 2-EE and their acetates will degrade readily to carbon dioxide in water by the action of microorganisms. 2-ME is degraded by sludge via anaerobic mechanisms. Because of this ready biodegradation, bioaccumulation up the food chain is unlikely to occur. EGEs are not persistent in the aquatic environment (5).

Absorption, Metabolism, and Excretion

The glycol ethers are rapidly absorbed by the dermal, inhalational, and oral routes. Exposure via multiple routes is possible, particularly in an occupational setting, where both dermal and inhalational exposure could occur simultaneously.

Dermal absorption can be a significant exposure route (11–14). Experimental dermal absorption rates have been studied for 2-ME, 2-EE, and butoxyethanol (Table 108-4). Dermal absorption depends on the molecular weight of the compound, a decrease in absorption being a function of increasing molecular weight (2-ME being heavier than 2-EE which, in turn, is heavier than butoxyethanol). A tenfold difference in measured percutaneous absorption is found between 2-ME and butoxyethanol. However, one study demonstrated significant butoxyethanol uptake via dermal exposure using a 100% solution and a 2-hour exposure (12).

Gastrointestinal absorption of glycol ethers is rapid. One case report describes a blood concentration of 432 mg of butoxyethanol per L 1 hour after the ingestion of a household cleaner containing 12.7% butoxyethanol (15).

Respiratory absorption of glycol ethers is significant: More than 50% of both 2-EE and butoxyethanol are absorbed via this route. Also, pulmonary absorption increases linearly with increasing respiratory rate, and thus physical activity will increase absorption during airborne exposure. A linear relationship among exposure, workload, and urinary excretion of acetates (milligrams of acetate per gram of creatinine) at the end of work shifts has been demonstrated (16–18).

Data obtained by patch testing in humans demonstrated only minimal signs of irritation and hypersensitivity reactions to 10% butoxyethanol exposure under occlusion for 24 hours, despite a finding of dermal hypersensitivity in animals (19). Dermal uptake for EGs in the vapor phase is between 5% and 10% of the exposure; hence, vapor exposure constitutes a potential dermal absorption hazard but contributes little to overall systemic absorption (18).

The metabolism of the monoalkyl ethers of EG is via the alcohol dehydrogenase enzyme, which transforms the parent compounds into alkoxyacetic acids (16,20). Ethanol has been demonstrated to inhibit the metabolism of glycol ethers competitively (21). This observation has potential clinical significance, as the toxicity of the parent compound appears to be substantially less than that of the acid metabolite. Humans exposed to acetates of glycol ethers will first hydrolyze them to the corresponding glycol ether and then reconvert this ether to the acetate in the metabolic process. Although the enzyme systems differ, an interesting analogous situation has been observed with the active metabolites of benzene and competitive interaction with toluene (22,23).

Nonoxidative metabolism of butoxyethanol via conjugation with long-chain fatty acids has been demonstrated in rats (24).

TABLE 108-4. Dermal absorption of select glycol ethers

	Skin absorption (mg/cm²/h)		
Glycol ether	Duggard et al.[a]	Walter and Scott[b]	Leber[c]
Ethylene glycol monomethyl ether (2-ME)	2.82	1.66	2.2
Ethylene glycol monoethyl ether (2-EE)	0.80	0.13	—
Ethylene glycol butyl ether (2-BE)	0.20	0.03	—
Ethylene glycol monoethyl ether acetate (2-EEA)	0.80	—	—
Triethylene glycol monomethyl ether (TGME)	—	—	0.034
Triethylene glycol monoethyl ether (TGEE)	—	—	0.024
Triethylene glycol monobutyl ether (TGBE)	—	—	0.022

[a]Adapted from Duggard PH, Walker M, Mawdsley SJ, Scott RC. Absorption of some glycol ethers through human skin in vitro. *Environ Health Perspect* 1984;57:193–197.
[b]Adapted from Walter M, Scott R. Report to Chemical Manufacturers Association 1987.
[c]Adapted from ref. 44.

The biological significance of butoxyethanol conjugation with fatty acids is unknown.

The primary urinary metabolite of the EGEs is an alkoxyacetic acid derivative, but a minor pathway exists through formation of EG to oxalic acid (25). One study demonstrated that, in silk-screen workers exposed, the excretion of urinary calcium increased in relationship to urinary alkoxyacetic acid load. The tendency to form renal stones was 2.4-fold higher among those exposed to EGEs in this study (25). The highest urinary alkoxyacetic acid load was also associated with increased excretion of glucosaminoglycans, which might reflect the toxicity of the EGEs (25).

Absorbed butoxyethanol is metabolized via alcohol dehydrogenase to butoxyacetaldehyde first and then by aldehyde dehydrogenase to butoxyacetic acid, which is excreted in the urine.

In the metabolism of glycol ethers, methoxyacetic acid and methoxyacetyl glycine are the primary metabolites. The elimination half-life of 2-methoxyacetic acid in humans is reported to be approximately 77 hours. Humans hydrolyze EGEEA to 2-EE first, which then is reconverted to the ethoxyacetic acid metabolite and excreted in the urine. Twelve days after termination of exposure to glycol ethers, the ethoxyacetic acid metabolite has been found in the urine of occupationally exposed persons (25). Activation of the minor metabolic pathway that converts EGEs to EG has been speculated to result in oxaluria in acute ingestions, as has been described in some case reports (26,27).

Clinical Toxicology

The toxicities of the EGEs and their acetates can be subcategorized as acute, chronic, reproductive, and mutagenic.

REPRODUCTIVE TOXICITY

The reproductive toxicology of glycol ethers has been studied in a variety of laboratory animals. After continuous dosing of 2-ME, male reproductive toxicity in animal models has been seen, consisting of testicular damage and changes in sperm motility, morphology, and concentration (3). Embryotoxicity and developmental effects have also been shown to be associated with administration of 2-ME in animal models (3). 2-EE has been demonstrated to incite embryologic toxicity, resulting in fetal wastage and skeletal and vascular abnormalities (3,28). The teratogenic effects of 2-EE and 2-ethoxyethanol acetate have been studied in animal models, in which a significant increase in the incidence of such major malformations as ventral wall defects of the aorta with the pulmonary artery, and minor abnormalities in skeletal variants have been exhibited (3,28).

MUTAGENICITY

Mutagenicity studies on 2-EE and 2-ME have demonstrated mixed results. Sister chromatid exchanges and chromosomal aberrations have been noted after exposure to certain doses of 2-EE. No statistically significant increase in chromosomal aberrations was seen in rats after exposure by inhalation to 2-ME (3).

ACUTE TOXICITY

Acute toxic effects fall into three general categories: central nervous system (CNS), hematologic, and renal and metabolic. Among the CNS effects are agitation, encephalopathy, and coma. The onset of coma may be rapid owing to quick gastrointestinal absorption of EGEs. Hematotoxicity consists of hemolysis, hemoglobinuria, decreased erythrocyte counts, and hypocellular bone marrow. Renal and metabolic toxic effects include metabolic acidosis and renal tubular degeneration. Metabolic acidosis has been reported in a few cases of oral ingestion of EGEs (26,27). This acidosis generally resolves within 24 hours with supportive care. A minor metabolic pathway to EG has been suggested.

Significant species-specific differences exist in the toxicity of EGEs, particularly the hemolytic effects, which are more pronounced in mice, rats, and rabbits. For example, metabolism of butoxyethanol to butoxyacetic acid is required to cause hemolysis in animals, and blockade of alcohol dehydrogenase will prevent this hemolysis. Humans appear to be resistant to butoxyethanol-induced hemolysis.

Acute ingestion of glycol ethers has been reported to result in coma and death, with pathologic findings of acute hemorrhagic gastritis, liver necrosis, and kidney necrosis (including renal tubular necrosis). Nonfatal cases of 2-ME ingestion have resulted in agitation, confusion, nausea, cyanosis, and metabolic acidosis. In another case report, ingestion of just more than an ounce of 2-EE caused dizziness, unconsciousness, and metabolic acidosis.

CHRONIC TOXICITY

The toxic effects of chronic exposure to glycol ethers are neurologic, hematologic, and reproductive. Studies in the semiconductor industry and a metaanalysis of similar studies culled from a review of 559 articles indicate that adverse reproductive outcomes may be a significant problem with chronic workplace EGE exposure of sufficient magnitude (6–10). Consideration of these potential toxic effects may incite a reevaluation of exposure limits for both women and men.

Chronic neurologic toxicity consists of personality changes, lethargy, memory problems, dizziness, headache, lack of concentration, tremor, dysarthria, hyperreflexia, ataxia, increased muscle tone, and balance disturbance. Neurotoxicity has also been reported after high vapor exposure.

Case reports of subacute exposure to 2-ME described in the microfilm industry have cited reversible neurobehavioral and hematopoietic effects (29). Hemotoxicity, consisting of bone marrow depression involving erythroid and myeloid cell lines, also is demonstrated in animals exposed to EGEs (30). The microfilm case report mainly involved occupational exposure to 2-ME and low levels of propylene glycol monomethyl ether and methyl ethyl ketone. Symptoms consisted of depression, irritability, and fatigue. Laboratory findings consisted of a reduced red blood cell count, leukopenia, and macrocytic anemia. The personal breathing zone exposure to 2-ME as a time-weighted average was determined to be 18.2 to 57.8 parts per million (ppm). Methyl ethyl ketone exposure measured 1 to 5 ppm, and propylene glycol measured 4.2 to 12.8 ppm. These exposures occurred over an 8-month period, and the hematologic effects reversed after 2 to 3 months once exposure ceased (29). Other case reports have revealed hematopoietic and neurobehavioral effects in workers chronically exposed to 2-ME. Reports dating from 1938 have described lethargy, fatigue, and leukopenia in chronically exposed workers (30–32).

More recent studies have also noted hematologic changes and bone marrow biopsy changes in workers chronically exposed to glycol ethers (33,34). However, confounding factors included multiple exposure to other solvents, among them aromatic, aliphatic, and halogenated hydrocarbons. Another study in seven workers exposed to glycol ethers in offset printing revealed no peripheral blood smear alterations, although evidence of bone marrow injury was discovered by biopsy in three of the seven workers who were studied (33). These bone marrow biopsies demonstrated areas of stromal injury with myeloid hypoplasia.

Some researchers have investigated the immune response of workers exposed to a mixture of organic solvents, including 2-ME and 2-EE, as compared with the response of a control group of healthy individuals (35). Mean exposures to 2-ME and 2-EE were 6.1 and 4.8 mg per cubic meter, respectively. Mean blood levels also were obtained in these studies: 40.1 μg per dL for 2-ME and 2.0 μg per dL for 2-EE . However, other solvents such as butanol, isobutanol, toluene, *m*-xylene, 2-butanone, and 2-hexanone were present. This study noted decreased levels of helper T cells and CD4 cells and increased levels of natural killer cells and human B lymphocytes. CD8 suppressor cell levels were normal (35).

Other health concerns for human exposure to glycol ethers include developmental toxicity and testicular toxic effects (36,37). These adverse effects are noted in both short-term and long-term exposures. The glycol ethers have similar testicular and developmental toxicities in animal species studied by all routes of exposure. Epidemiologic studies of male employees in the manufacturing of 2-ME have demonstrated no leukopenia or anemia, but decreases in the white blood cell count and testicular size were noted in exposed workers.

In other studies, workers exposed to 2-EE had significantly lower average sperm counts than did controls. The reproductive effects of 2-ME and 2-EE have also been studied in shipyard workers (34,36). In these studies, of 94 painters examined, 10% were found to have anemia and 5% had granulocytopenia (34). None of these effects as noted in the control subjects (34). In 73 painters from a population of 153, an increased prevalence of oligospermia and azoospermia and a lower sperm count were noted as compared to controls (36).

Biological Monitoring

After exposure to 2-ME and 2-EE, their metabolites, methoxyacetic acid, and ethoxyacetic acid are detected in the urine of exposed humans. Hazard concerns extend to dermal exposure, as skin absorption of these toxins is rapid. Systemic absorption of vapors is enhanced by increased physical activity and increased respiration.

SPECIFIC ETHYLENE GLYCOL ETHERS

Butoxyethanol

Butoxyethanol is a solvent for resins, varnishes, hydraulic fluids, floor polishes, floor waxes, upholstery, glass cleaners, and leather cleaners. Dermal absorption of butoxyethanol in animals and humans increases as a function of time and is enhanced by an occlusive dressing over the skin. Dermal absorption across abdominal skin from humans has been calculated to be 0.20 mg per square centimeter (14).

Butoxyacetic acid is the major metabolite of butoxyethanol (16,20). Butoxyethanol metabolism is inhibited by pretreatment of animals with pyrazole, which causes a significant increase in the half-life of butoxyethanol and a decrease in its systemic clearance (20). Also, pyrazole decreases the maximum plasma concentration and half-life of butoxyacetic acid. Pyrazole inhibits alcohol dehydrogenase and aldehyde dehydrogenase and protects animals against butoxyethanol-induced hemolytic anemia (20). Thus, it appears that the metabolism of butoxyethanol to butoxyacetic acid is required for hematotoxicity to occur. Also, the presence of ethanol competes with butoxyethanol for alcohol dehydrogenase and aldehyde dehydrogenase enzymes, and alcohol decreases the elimination of butoxyethanol.

Toxicologic studies in animals show that butoxyethanol has hematotoxic, hepatotoxic, and renal toxic effects (38). Decreased erythrocyte counts, decreased hemoglobin, increased erythrocyte fragility, and hemolysis have been seen in animal models of butoxyethanol poisoning. Renal toxicity included increased blood urea nitrogen concentrations. Focal necrosis of hepatocytes has been observed in animal studies of acute toxicity (38).

Dermal penetration of butoxyethanol has resulted in hematotoxicity, renal toxicity, and hepatotoxicity (38). Both butoxyethanol and its metabolite, butoxyacetic acid, are potent hematotoxins in animal studies. Also, studies with butoxyethanol conducted in human promyelocytic cell lines have concluded that butoxyethanol is a potent hematopoietic toxin (38). Mutagenicity studies, including the Ames test, sister chromatid assays, unscheduled DNA synthesis, and chromosomal aberrations, point mutations, and forward mutations in Chinese hamster ovary cells, suggest that butoxyethanol is not a mutagen (38).

Studies of finger dermal absorption conducted in five male human volunteers who were nonoccupationally exposed to undiluted butoxyethanol for 2 hours demonstrated no evidence of skin irritation. However, small fissures in the skin were noted within a few hours after the exposure, and a drying effect on the hands was confirmed. Erythematous reactions were observed around the fissures within 1 to 2 days.

The half-life of butoxyethanol ranges from 0.6 to 4.8 hours, and 17% of the absorbed dose is excreted in the urine (11). Other dermal absorption studies in adult men who were exposed for 2 hours to 50 ppm of butoxyethanol demonstrated that the dermal uptake of butoxyethanol accounted for 75% of the total uptake during whole-body exposure to butoxyethanol vapor (39). In contrast, a physiologically based pharmacokinetic model demonstrated that no more than 15% to 27% of the total uptake of butoxyethanol by humans experiencing whole-body vapor exposure can be attributed to dermal absorption (40).

The metabolism of inhaled butoxyethanol was studied in male volunteers with no history of occupational exposure (16). These subjects were allowed to engage in light physical exercise while being exposed to 20 ppm of butoxyethanol in a chamber. Concentrations of butoxyethanol increased rapidly in the blood and reached a plateau within 1 to 2 hours. No butoxyethanol was detected in the blood 2 to 4 hours after the exposure. The amount of butoxyacetic acid excreted was 41% of the butoxyethanol uptake. No toxicity was noted in the study's subjects (16).

In another study involving women with weekly exposure averaging 0.65 ppm of butoxyethanol, an 8.30-hour half-life was calculated (38). Two subjects who inhaled 200 ppm of butoxyethanol for two 4-hour periods separated by a 30-minute break excreted large amounts of butoxyacetic acid in their urine. One other excreted only trace amounts. All subjects experienced irritation of the nose and throat and ocular and taste disturbances. One subject experienced a severe headache for 24 hours (38).

In another study of four subjects exposed to 100 ppm of butoxyethanol vapors for two 4-hour periods separated by a 30-minute break, vomiting occurred in one subject and a headache was experienced by another subject. Two adult men exposed to an average concentration of 113 ppm butoxyethanol experienced nasal and ocular irritation, a metallic taste, nasal discharge, and increased abdominal gas.

Studies of skin irritation from and sensitization to butoxyethanol in human subjects revealed no evidence of skin sensitization to a 10% aqueous butoxyethanol solution. Other investigations for skin sensitization using patch testing in humans also have failed to supply evidence of induction of sensitization or photosensitization reactions in subjects (38).

Clinical signs and symptoms in individuals exposed to butoxyethanol vapors of 3 to 5 ppm included headache, sore throat, nosebleeds, ocular irritation, throat irritation, chest tightness, and coughing. Respiratory symptoms have been noted in other individuals, as have asthma, respiratory irritation, and abnormal baseline pulmonary functions (38). One study showed a difference in the lymphocyte subpopulations in workers exposed to butoxyethanol, with changes in lymphocyte population between experimental control groups (35).

The risk of hemolysis in humans exposed to butoxyethanol was assessed using a physiologically based pharmacokinetic model to describe the disposition of 2-butoxyethanol and butoxyacetic acid, its major metabolite in humans (41). Humans are less susceptible to the hemolytic effects of the butoxyacetic acid metabolite as a result of exposure to butoxyethanol. Another study showed that butoxyacetic acid did not cause hemolytic effects when incubated with the red blood cells of humans (42). Thus, butoxyethanol appears to cause hemolysis in animals but not in humans.

Diethylene Glycol Mono-*n*-butyl Ether

DGBE is a solvent used in consumer products including art products, surface cleaners, and paints. Its acetate ester is diethylene glycol *n*-butyl acetate (DGBA), which also is used in paints. Exposure to DGBE occurs dermally and to DGBA by inhalation. DGBA, once absorbed, is metabolized back to DGBE. In animal studies, DGBA is absorbed through the skin of rats *in vivo* and has not been shown to be genotoxic or mutagenic. It also has not been demonstrated to be a systemic toxin or reproductive toxin. Inhalational studies of 18 ppm of DGBE in animals reported no adverse effects (43).

Triethylene Glycol Ethers

Triethylene glycol ethers include triethylene glycol monomethyl ether, triethylene glycol monoethyl ether, and triethylene glycol monobutyl ether. Triethylene glycol ethers are absorbed more slowly through the skin with decreasing rates of dermal absorption with increasing molecular wieght (44).

ETHYLENE GLYCOL

EG is a clear, colorless, odorless, sweet-tasting, viscous liquid. It has a low vapor pressure and, therefore, does not present an inhalational risk.

EG finds common use as an antifreeze and in hydraulic fluids. It is used also as a solvent and can be found in products such as inks, polishes, adhesives, and sometimes, pesticides. Serious toxicity follows ingestion of EG, with its hallmarks metabolic acidosis, coma, seizures, and renal failure.

Environmental Exposure Sources

EG finds its way into the environment from waste streams and when used for deicing. Contamination of groundwater may occur from its use as a deicer.

Absorption, Metabolism, and Excretion

EG is a highly toxic substance after its ingestion and metabolism. It is absorbed via the lungs and dermally, but less so than through the gastrointestinal tract. Owing to its low vapor pressure, it does not present an inhalational hazard.

EG has a volume of distribution similar to that of ethanol and methanol, or approximately 600 mL per kg. Its half-life is approximately 2.5 hours in serum.

EG is metabolized by the liver to a series of toxic metabolites (Fig. 108-2). Some of these metabolites have much longer half-lives than does the parent compound. The rate-limiting metabolic step for EG is action by alcohol dehydrogenase, which converts the EG to glycolaldehyde.

Clinical Toxicology

The metabolites of EG produce its toxicity. Ingestion of toxic amounts of EG can result in CNS depression, ataxia, nystagmus, seizures, and coma. Ingestion may also be associated with nausea and vomiting. Cardiotoxicity may occur, along with hypocalcemia due to deposition of calcium oxalate crystals in tissues. Many of these effects likely will occur within minutes, although they may be delayed up to 12 hours after EG's ingestion.

The hallmark of EG toxicity is metabolic acidosis with an elevated anion and osmolal gap. EG does not result in ketosis. Ingestion can incite renal failure. After EG ingestion, a state of intoxication similar to alcohol intoxication may occur, which is attributable to the presence of unmetabolized EG and its aldehyde metabolites.

Metabolic acidosis generally occurs within 24 to 72 hours after the ingestion. Acute renal failure and hyperkalemia may occur due to calcium oxalate crystal deposition in the kidneys. Along with CNS depression, coma, seizures, and cerebral edema may occur. Some patients have developed pulmonary edema within 72 hours of ingestion.

The extreme metabolic acidosis of EG is caused by the accumulation of glycolic and glyoxylic acids, which results in an elevated anion and osmolal gap (see Fig. 108-2). Hypocalcemia may also result in tetany. Renal failure may occur between 24 and 72 hours after EG ingestion and may be permanent, although in most cases, renal function recovers.

EG poisoning should be suspected from metabolic findings and the presence of oxalate crystals in the urine. Generally, toxicity is associated with EG levels greater than 50 mg per dL. At least eight intermediate metabolites have been identified from EG metabolism, with the toxic organic acids being glycolic, glyoxylic, and oxalic acids. Special laboratory procedures are necessary to identify EG.

Owing to the metabolism of EG by alcohol dehydrogenase, ethanol is used as an antidote to prevent further metabolism to this compound's toxic acid metabolites. Both EG and ethanol compete for alcohol dehydrogenase and aldehyde dehydrogenase enzymes. 4-Methylpyrazole (fomepizole), another alcohol dehydrogenase competitor, is now available for treating EG poisoning. The goals of therapy are as follows:

- Competitive inhibition of the alcohol dehydrogenase enzyme site by ethanol or 4-methylpyrazole
- Reversal of metabolic acidosis by use of intravenous sodium bicarbonate
- Consideration of hemodialysis to remove both EG and toxic acid metabolites
- Management of electrolyte abnormalities, hypoglycemia, hyperkalemia, and hypocalcemia

Table 107-5 provides information on the proper loading and maintenance doses for alcohol and for 4-methylpyrazole in EG poisoning. Antidotal therapy consists of administration of either ethanol or 4-methylpyrazole if EG concentrations are greater than 20 mg per dL (45–50).

Thiamine and pyridoxine are B-complex vitamins that have been recommended for administration to patients with EG toxicity, to aid in metabolizing the toxin along nontoxic pathways (see Fig. 108-2). Pyridoxine is administered intravenously at one dose of 1 mg per kg daily until poisoning is resolved or in a dose of 100 mg per day. Owing to the fact that both pyridoxine and thiamine can be removed by hemodialysis, redosing is important after hemodialysis. Thiamine is administered as a dose of 1 mg per kg daily (or 100 mg intravenously) until poisoning is resolved.

4-Methylpyrazole is an inhibitor of the alcohol dehydrogenase enzyme and is replacing ethanol as antidotal therapy for

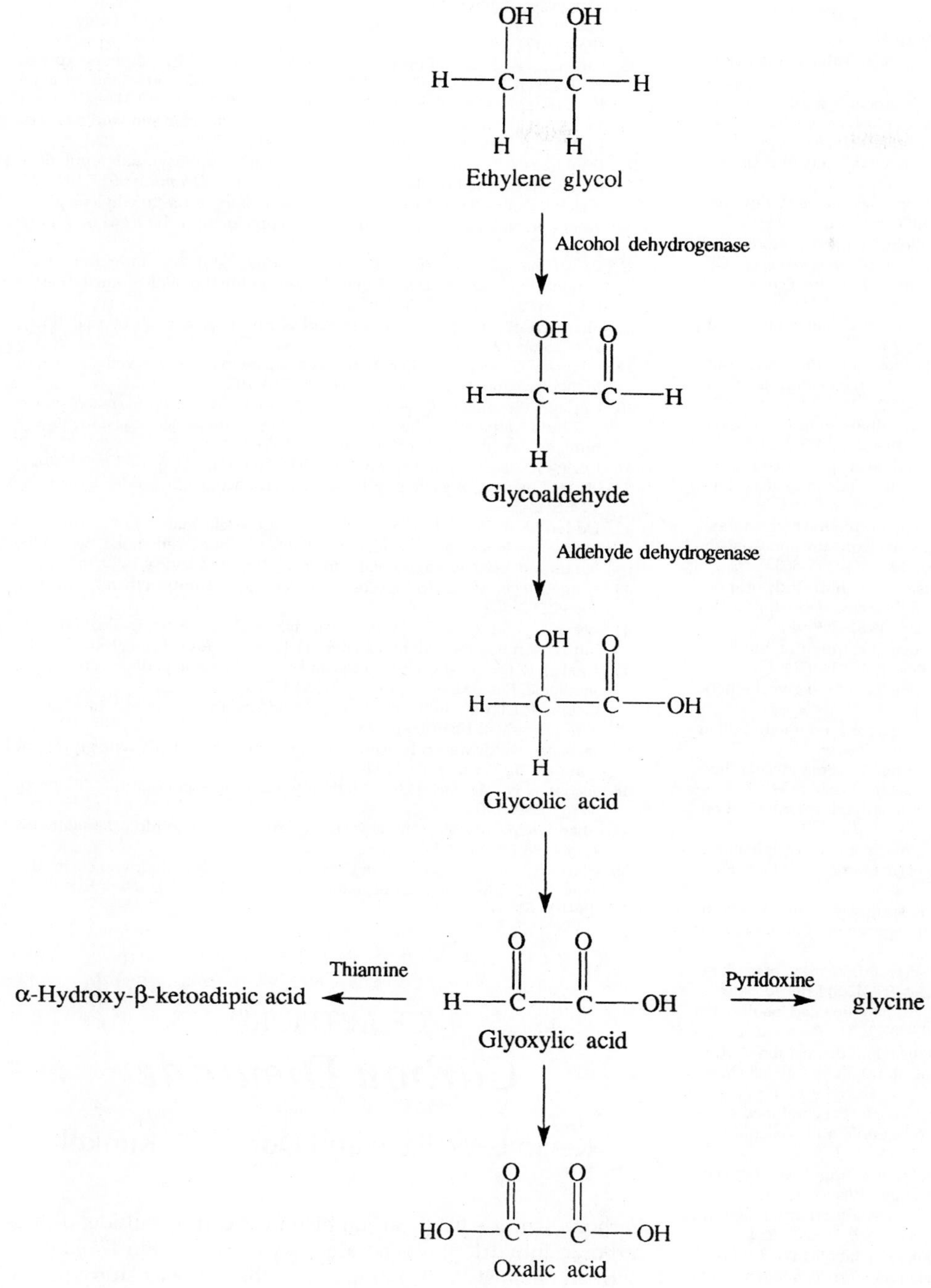

Figure 108-2. Ethylene glycol metabolism.

EG poisoning and methanol poisoning (48–50). 4-Methylpyrazole has an affinity for alcohol dehydrogenase that is 8,000 times greater than the affinity of ethanol and can prevent the metabolism of EG to its metabolic toxins. This inhibitor has a volume of distribution between 600 and 1,000 mL per kg. Its therapeutic concentration in the serum is 8 to 25 mg per L. Concentrations exceeding 15 mg per L provide complete inhibition of alcohol dehydrogenase (50). 4-Methylpyrazole is metabolized via the P-450 mixed-function oxidase system by the liver, and elimination follows Michaelis-Menten kinetics. Table 107-6 provides the dosing schedule for 4-methylpyrazole in EG poisoning with and without hemodialysis.

4-Methylpyrazole is administered intravenously and is supplied as a 1.5-mL vial with a concentration of 1 g per mL. A loading dose of 15 mg per kg is administered, followed by doses of 10 mg per kg every 12 hours for a total of four doses. The dose then is increased to 15 mg per kg every 12 hours until the EG concentration is less than 20 mg per dL. The dose should be administered by slow intravenous infusion over 30 minutes. Adverse effects secondary to 4-methylpyrazole administration include headache, nausea, and dizziness. Vomiting and abdominal pain have also been described.

During therapy with 4-methylpyrazole, forced diuresis is recommended to enhance elimination of unmetabolized glycol in the urine, particularly if hemodialysis is not performed. Once EG metabolism is prevented by 4-methylpyrazole, the only elimination route is through the urine. Therefore, a turnover of approximately 600 mL per kg (volume of distribution), which, in a 70-kg individual, would be 42 L of urine, would be required to ensure elimination of EG.

REFERENCES

1. Browning RG, Curry SC. Clinical toxicology of ethylene glycol monoalkyl ethers. *Hum Exp Toxicol* 1994;13(5):325–335.
2. US Department of Health and Human Services, National Institute for Occupational Safety and Health, Centers for Disease Control. *Occupational exposure to ethylene glycol monomethylether, ethylene glycol ethylether, and their acetates.* Cincinnati: National Institute for Occupational Safety and Health, 1991.
3. World Health Organization. *2-Methoxyethanol, and their acetates*. Environmental health criteria 115. Geneva: World Health Organization, 1990.
4. European Chemical Industry, Ecology and Toxicology Centre. *The toxicology of glycol ethers and its relevance to man: Technical report no. 17. An updating of ECETOC technical report no. 4.* Brussels: European Chemical Industry, Ecology and Toxicology Centre, 1985; updated 1995.
5. Staples CA, Boatman RJ, Cano ML. Ethylene glycol ethers: an environmental risk assessment. *Chemosphere* 1998;36(7):1585–1613.
6. McMartin KI, Chu M, Kopecky E, Einarson TR, Koren G. Pregnancy outcome following maternal organic solvent exposure: a meta-analysis of epidemiologic studies. *Am J Ind Med* 1998;34(3):288–292.
7. Correa A, Gray RH, Cohen R, et al. Ethylene glycol ethers and risks of spontaneous abortion and subfertility. *Am J Epidemiol* 1996;143(7):707–717.
8. Schenker MB, Gold EB, Beaumont JJ, et al. Association of spontaneous abortion and other reproductive effects with work in the semiconductor industry. *Am J Ind Med* 1995;28(6):639–659.
9. Cordier S, Bergeret A, Goujard J, et al. Congenital malformation and maternal occupational exposure to glycol ethers. Occupational Exposure and Congenital Malformations Working Group. *Epidemiology* 1997;8(4):355–363.
10. Swan SH, Beaumont JJ, Hammond SK, et al. Historical cohort study of spontaneous abortion among fabrication workers in the Semiconductor Health Study: agent-level analysis. *Am J Ind Med* 1995;28(6):751–769.
11. Johanson G, Boman A, Dynesius B. Percutaneous absorption of 2-butoxyethanol in man. *Scand J Work Environ Health* 1988;14(2):101–109.
12. Johanson G. Aspects of biological monitoring of exposure to glycol ethers. *Toxicol Lett* 1988;43(1–3):5–21.
13. Oiohi G, Wegman D. Transcutaneous ethylene glycol monomethyl ether poisoning in the work setting. *J Occup Med* 1978;20:675–676.
14. Dugard P, Walker M, Mawdsley S, et al. Absorption of some glycol ethers through human skin in vitro. *Environ Health Perspect* 1984;57:193–197.
15. Gijsenbergh F, Jenco M, Veulemans H, et al. Acute butylglycol intoxication: a case report. *Hum Toxicol* 1989;8:243–245.
16. Johanson G, Kornbord H, Naslund P, et al. Toxicokinetics of inhaled 2-butoxyethanol (ethylene glycol monobutyl ether) in man. *Scand J Work Environ Health* 986;12:594–602.
17. Groesenken D, Veulemans H, Masschelein R. Respiratory uptake and elimination of ethylene glycol monoethyl ether in experimental human exposure. *Br J Ind Med* 1986;43:544–549.
18. Brooke I, Cocker J, Delic J, et al. Dermal uptake of solvents from the vapour phase: an experimental study in humans. *Ann Occup Hyg* 1998;42(8):531–540.
19. Greenspan A, Reardon R, Gingell R, Rosica K. Human repeated insult patch test of 2-butoxyethanol. *Contact Dermatitis* 1995;33:59.
20. Ghanayem B, Burka L, Sanders J, et al. Metabolism and disposition of ethylene glycol monobutylether (2-butoxyethanol) in rats. *Drug Metab Dispos* 1987;15:478–484.
21. Morel G, Lambert A, Rieger B, Subra I. Interactive effect of combined exposure to glycol ethers and alcohols on toxicodynamic and toxicokinetic parameters. *Arch Toxicol* 1996;70(8):519–525.
22. Inoue O, Seiji K, Watanabe T, et al. Mutual metabolic suppression between benzene and toluene in man. *Int Arch Environ Health* 1988;60:15–20.
23. Medinsky M, Kenyon E, Schlosser P. Benzene: a case study in parent chemical and metabolite interactions of toxicology. *Toxicology* 1995;105:225–233.
24. Kaphalia B, Ghanayem B, Ansari G. Nonoxidative metabolism of 2-butoxyethanol via fatty acid conjugation in Fischer 344 rats. *J Toxicol Environ Health* 1996;49(5):463–479.
25. Laitinen J, Liesivuori J, Savolainen H. Urinary alkoxyacetic acids and renal effects of exposure to ethylene glycol ethers. *Occup Environ Med* 1996; 53(9):595–600.
26. Nitter-Hauge S. Poisoning with ethylene glycol monomethyl ether: report of two cases. *Acta Med Scand* 1970;188:227–280.
27. Rambourg-Schepens M, Buffet M, Bertault R, et al. Severe ethylene glycol butyl ether poisoning—kinetics and metabolic pattern. *Hum Toxicol* 1988; 7:187–189.
28. Andrew F, Hardin B. Developmental effects after inhalation exposure of gravid rabbits and rats to ethylene glycol monoethyl ether. *Environ Health Perspect* 1984;57:13–23.
29. Cohen R. Reversible subacute ethylene glycol monomethyl ether toxicity associated with microfilm production: a case report. *Am J Ind Med* 1984;6:441–446.
30. Ghanayem B. Metabolic and cellular basis of 2-butoxy-ethanol-induced hemolytic anemia in rats and assessment of human risk in vitro. *Biochem Pharmacol* 1989;38:1679–1684.
31. Greenberg L, Payers M, Goldwater L, et al. Health hazards in the manufacture of "fused collars": I. Exposures to ethylene glycol monomethyl ether. *J Ind Hyg Toxicol* 1938;20:134–147.
32. Parsons C, Parsons M. Toxic encephalopathy and "granulopenic anemia" due to volatile solvents in industry: report of two cases. *J Ind Hyg Toxicol* 1938;20:124–133.
33. Cullen M, Rado T, Waldron J. Bone marrow injury in lithographers exposed to glycol ethers and organic solvents used in multicolor offset and ultraviolet curing printing processes. *Arch Environ Health* 1983;38(6):347–354.
34. Welch L, Cullen M. Effects of exposure to glycol ethers in shipyard painters: III. Hematologic effects. *Am J Ind Med* 1988;14:527–536.
35. Denkhaus W, Steldern D, Botzenhardt U, et al. Lymphocyte subpopulations in solvent exposed workers. *Int Arch Occup Environ Health* 1986;57:109–155.
36. Welch L, Schrader S, Turner T, et al. Effects of exposure to ethylene glycol ethers on shipyard painters: II. Male reproduction. *Am J Ind Med* 1988; 14:509–526.
37. Paustenbach D. Assessment of the developmental risk resulting from occupational exposure to selected glycolethers within the semiconductor industry. *J Toxicol Environ Health* 1988;23:29–75.
38. Final report on the safety assessment of butoxyethanol. *J Am Coll Toxicol* 1996;15(6):462–526.
39. Johanson G, Boman A. Percutaneous absorption of 2-butoxyethanol vapor in human subjects. *Br J Ind Med* 1991;48:788–792.
40. Corley R, Bormett G, Ghanayem B. Physiologically based pharmacokinetics of 2-butoxyethanol and its major metabolite, 2-butoxy acetic acid in rats and humans. *Toxicol Appl Pharmacol* 1994;129:61–79.
41. Corley R. Assessing the risk of hemolysis in humans exposed to 2-butoxyethanol using a physiologically based pharmacokinetic model. *Occup Hyg* 1996;2:45–55.
42. Udden M, Patton C. Hemolysis and decreased deformability of erythrocytes exposed to butoxy acetic acid, a metabolite of 2-butoxyethanol: I. Sensitivity in rats and resistance in normal humans. *J Appl Toxicol* 1994;14(2):91–96.
43. Gingell R, et al. Toxicology of diethylene glycol butyl ether. *Occup Hyg* 1996;2:293–302.
44. Leber A, Scott R, Hodge M, et al. Triethylene glycol ethers. Evaluations of in vitro absorption through human dermis. *J Am Coll Toxicol* 1990;9:507–515.
45. Chabali R. Diagnostic use of anion and osmolal gaps in pediatric emergency medicine. *Pediatr Emerg Care* 1997;13:204–210.
46. Gabow P, Clay K, Sullivan J. Organic acids in ethylene glycol intoxication. *Ann Intern Med* 1986;105:16–28.
47. Jacobsen D, McMartin K. Antidotes for methanol and ethylene glycol poisoning. *Clin Toxicol* 1997;35:127–143.
48. Jacobsen D, McMartin K. 4-Methylpyrazole—present status. *Clin Toxicol* 1996;34:379–381.
49. Shannon M. Toxicology reviews: fomepizole—a new antidote. *Pediatr Emerg Care* 1998;14(2):170–172.
50. Harry P, Turcant A, Bouachour G, et al. Efficacy of 4-methylpyrazole in ethylene glycol poisoning: clinical and toxicokinetic aspects. *Hum Exp Toxicol* 1994;13:61–64.

CHAPTER 109

Carbon Disulfide

Kevin L. Wallace and Donald B. Kunkel

Carbon disulfide (CS_2, carbon bisulfide, carbon sulfide, dithiocarbonic anhydride) was accidentally discovered in 1796 by the German chemist W. A. Lampadius while he was studying the action of pyrites on carbon. In the first half-century after its discovery, the compound was used in medicine to treat a variety of diseases and was used experimentally as an anesthetic agent before the introduction of chloroform.

Recognizing the remarkable organic solvent properties of carbon disulfide (gums, resins, waxes, sulfur, phosphorus, iodine, bromine, camphor), industry began to use CS_2 in 1851 as a phosphorus solvent in the manufacture of matches, and its use rapidly spread to such endeavors as the refining of paraffins and petroleum and the extraction of plant and animal oils. Major use of CS_2 began in Europe in the middle and later nineteenth century with, first, the discovery of the "cold" vulcanization process for rubber manufacture and, second, the development of the viscose rayon industry, in which, on an international scale, CS_2 continues to play an important role.

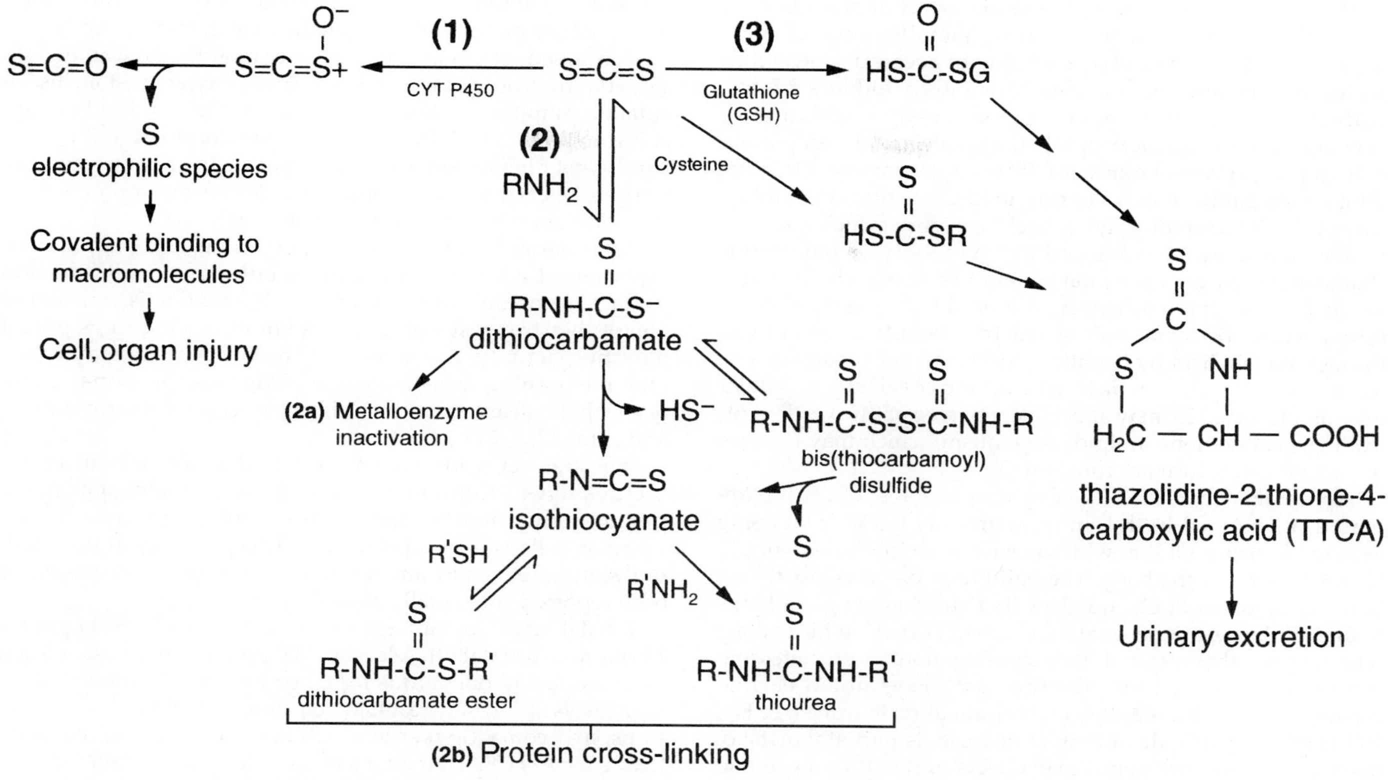

Figure 109-1. Major pathways of carbon disulfide metabolism: (1) oxidative metabolism by hepatic cytochrome P-450 (CYT P-450), resulting in the generation of reactive species capable of causing cell and organ injury; (2) dithiocarbamate adduct formation, resulting in (a) direct effects on metalloenzyme activity and (b) protein cross-linking; (3) reductive conversion via glutathione and cysteine moieties to metabolites (e.g., TTCA) that undergo renal elimination.

Cold vulcanization of rubber involved the dipping of thin strips of rubber into a solution of sulfur monochloride and CS_2. This process softened the rubber and made possible the manufacture of thin sheets of rubber. These rubber sheets then were used in the production of surgical gloves, balloons, and contraceptives. Cold vulcanization often was conducted in small, poorly ventilated workshops. This process was abandoned after several decades owing to unequivocal evidence of severe toxic effects of CS_2 in this work environment. Cold vulcanization was not used in the United States to any great extent.

USES

CS_2 is used as a chemical intermediate for rayon, cellophane, carbon tetrachloride, xanthogenates, soil disinfectants and herbicides, carbonyl sulfide, adhesives, and other compounds (1). It finds uses as a solvent for phosphorus, selenium, bromine, iodine, fats, and resins and in the manufacturing of electronic vacuum tubes and optical glass. It also is used as a fumigant for commodities and in space fumigation, as a cleaning and extraction solvent in metal treatment and plating (e.g., gold and nickel), as a corrosion inhibitor, as a polymerization inhibitor for vinyl chloride, as an agent in removal of metals from wastewater, as a regenerator for transition metal sulfide catalysts in instant color photography, and as a veterinary anthelmintic (1).

PHYSIOCHEMICAL PROPERTIES

CS_2 (chemical structure: S=C=S) is a colorless liquid with a sweet (pure) or foul (commercial-grade) odor. It is highly flammable and has a vapor density of 2.63 (air = 1.00). In addition, CS_2 is highly soluble in organic solvents and only slightly soluble in water. CS_2 readily vaporizes (vapor pressure, 400 mm Hg), and the odor threshold is 0.11 parts per million (ppm).

ABSORPTION, METABOLISM, AND EXCRETION

CS_2 is absorbed by vapor inhalation, ingestion, or skin contact [thereby warranting a skin notation by the U.S. Occupational Safety and Health Administration (OSHA)]. After absorption via inhalation, free CS_2 in animal models reaches steady-state concentrations in plasma within 15 minutes of exposure and approaches a plateau in red blood cells (RBCs) within 2 hours. CS_2 in blood has been shown to be bound predominantly (90%) to RBCs (2), and RBC transport is believed to be an important factor in the movement of CS_2 from lungs to tissue and vice versa. Accumulation of CS_2 in human adipose tissue with repeated or prolonged exposure is expected, based on the demonstration of a slow [half-life ($t_{1/2}$) of 68 hours] as well as a fast ($t_{1/2}$ of 6 hours) phase of elimination in viscose production workers (3).

Toxic mechanisms of action may follow two basic pathways (Fig. 109-1) (3). First, CS_2 is known to react directly with amines and thiols and to interfere with their cellular functions. This reaction may, in turn, lead to the formation of dithiocarbamate metabolites capable of inactivating metalloenzymes (e.g., dopamine α-hydroxylase) by chelation of necessary metal ions such as copper and zinc and to the formation of dithiocarbamate adducts, which, after undergoing successive oxidation or decomposition to an electrophile (isothiocyanate), can participate in protein cross-linking (4). It has been proposed that the thiol-amine pathway may contribute to CS_2-induced neurotoxicity of the "filamentous, dying-back" category, which is similar to that caused by *n*-hexane and methyl-*n*-butyl ketone and is characterized by accumulation of neurofilaments within axonal swellings. A second mechanism, responsible for observed hepatotoxicity, is the formation of reactive intermediates of CS_2 through metabolism by hepatic cytochrome P-450 pathways to reactive sulfur species, which, in turn, bind covalently to cellular macromolecules. CS_2 may affect liver enzyme pathways directly, leading to alterations in lipid metabolism, which may have an impact on cardiovascular function (5).

Approximately 8% to 20% of an absorbed dose of CS_2 is eliminated unchanged by the lung, with only 0.5% or so being excreted in urine. Of that which is absorbed, 50% to 90% of CS_2 is metabolized in the body. The half-life in blood is less than 1 hour. Metabolism of CS_2 involves its reduction via glutathione to thiazolidine-2-thione-4-carboxylic acid (TTCA), which, along with several other metabolites (including inorganic sulfates and thiourea) generated by the other pathways noted earlier, accounts for the vast majority of its elimination in urine (see Fig. 109-1) (6). The drug disulfiram (Antabuse) is partially metabolized to CS_2, and the neurotoxic effects of disulfiram use and overdose may reflect CS_2 toxicity (7).

CLINICAL TOXICOLOGY

The medical toxicology of CS_2 can occur via inhalation, dermal contact, and ingestion. Toxicity is may be acute or chronic.

Acute Toxicity

The acute effects of CS_2 are summarized in Table 109-1 (8). Exposure to CS_2 vapors for hours can result in irritation of the eyes, mucous membranes, and upper airway. Ocular irritation is a frequent complaint of those occupationally exposed. CS_2 often is used in combination with H_2S in the viscose rayon industry, and both are ocular irritants. Lacrimation may be induced by this CS_2 and H_2S combination (9). Direct ocular exposures may result in immediate discomfort and conjunctival inflammation (10).

Continued recurrent exposure over months can lead to nausea, vomiting, headache, dizziness, irritability, confusion, disorientation, tinnitus, vertigo, insomnia, syncope, and pulmonary abnormalities (9). Hallucinations, behavioral irritability, and hand tremor have been seen after exposure to unknown concentrations of CS_2 over a 2-month period. These symptoms fully abated when exposure was terminated (11).

After dermal contact with CS_2, erythema and pain may be experienced with lesser exposures, but more significant skin contact may result in full-thickness burns. CS_2 is considered one of the strongest skin irritants known owing to its potent defatting activity. Anesthesia of the contact site may ensue after the burning sensation passes. Skin absorption may cause headache, nausea, vomiting, dizziness, cardiac dysrhythmias, and coma (2).

Ingestion of CS_2 in a volume of 15 mL has been fatal in adults. Victims have exhibited a variety of neurologic (spasmodic tremor, convulsions, coma), cardiovascular (cyanosis, cardiovascular collapse), and pulmonary (dyspnea, respiratory failure) signs after significant ingestions (9). Ingestions have rarely been reported and usually are suicidal in nature.

Inhalation of CS_2 vapors in a concentration of 4,800 ppm for 1 hour may be fatal (9). A level of 500 ppm has been established as immediately dangerous to life or health (12). Inhalation of high levels of CS_2 may result in delirium, hallucinations, convulsions, and coma. Spyker et al. (8) have reported on the acute toxic effects of CS_2 in air after a massive leak from a railroad tank car, resulting in airborne CS_2 concentrations of 20 ppm at a site distant from the incident.

TABLE 109-1. Symptoms of 27 patients acutely exposed to airborne carbon disulfide

Symptom	Subjects	
	Number	Percentage
Headache	16	59
Slight	8	30
Moderate	6	21
Severe	2	7
Nausea	14	52
Vomiting	1	4
Burning of throat, lips, or skin	11	40
Dizziness	16	59
Shortness of breath or chest pain	4	15
Impotence	2	7

Reprinted from ref. 8, with permission.

Chronic Toxicity

CS_2 exposure for months to years can result in the symptoms listed in Table 109-2. Prominent symptoms include neurotoxicity, hypertension, neurobehavioral disturbances, and ophthalmologic toxicity.

NEUROTOXICITY

Numerous hypotheses concerning the mode of action of CS_2 on nerve tissue have been suggested to explain the widespread effects of this solvent on central and peripheral nervous sys-

TABLE 109-2. Carbon disulfide chronic exposure toxicity

Neurologic	Ocular
Headache	Microaneurysms
Dizziness	Retinopathy with hemorrhages
Vertigo	Choroidal circulation problems
Irritability	Retinal nerve damage
Loss of libido	Damage to retinal vessels
Impotence	Decreased visual acuity
Sleep disturbance	Color vision disturbance
Nightmare	Central scotomas
Fatigue	Dyschromatopsia
Memory problems	Cardiac
Difficulty concentrating	Hypertension
Paresthesias	Angina
Gait problems	Syncope
Muscular weakness	
Myalgia	
Painful neuritis	

Adapted from Aaserud O, Homemren J, Ivedt B, et al. Carbon disulfide exposure and neurotoxic sequelae among viscose rayon workers. *Am J Ind Med* 1990;18:25–37.

tems. In addition to basic concepts already mentioned, various authors have debated the effects of CS_2 on catecholaminergic and dopaminergic systems, its possible interference with vitamin B_6 (pyridoxine) metabolism, the possible effects of free sulfur and free radical formation in the metabolism of CS_2, the role of neurofilament reactive adduct formation and subsequent cross-linking in the pathogenesis of distal axonopathy and, interestingly, whether neurotoxic effects might reflect only vascular damage caused by this agent (4,13).

The focus of earlier reports of CS_2 toxicity among workers was the observation of bizarre behavioral patterns, with many unfortunate victims of CS_2 relegated to European insane asylums in the nineteenth century. Among the more noticeable symptoms recorded were (i) extreme irritability and uncontrollable anger accompanied by rapid mood changes, including mania and suicidal tendencies; (ii) marked memory defects; (iii) severe insomnia and constant bad dreams; and (iv) interference with sexual functions in individuals who were younger than is normal for loss of libido (14). In addition, episodes of facial flushing, headache, and palpitations were described in rubber workers who consumed ethanol after exposure to CS_2 and other thiuram compounds (15); these unsuspected and unintentional effects of thiuram-ethanol interaction ultimately led to clinical trials of disulfiram in the treatment of chronic alcoholism (16).

Although behavioral and cognitive dysfunctions accounted for the great majority of reports of chronic and subacute exposure-related findings in earlier reports, later reports and studies involving perhaps lesser exposure levels have tended to focus on extrapyramidal, cerebellar, and peripheral nerve dysfunction. An excellent study of 21 workers in the United States who were exposed to CS_2 as a fumigant for grain revealed evidence of atypical parkinsonism, cerebellar signs, hearing loss, and sensory changes (17). Of the group studied, 80% exhibited cogwheel rigidity, 71% displayed decreased movement, 48% had resting tremors, and 52% had intention tremors (17). Peripheral sensory shading was detected in 62%, and 44% had abnormal nerve conduction study results.

Reports of overt CS_2-induced polyneuropathy continue to be issued from countries in which the regulation of workplace air quality has not yet become subject to rigorous government standards. More than half (53%) of recently studied workers from the fiber-cutting department of a Taiwanese rayon plant, where fixed air concentrations of CS_2 had previously been noted to range from 150 to 300 ppm, had polyneuropathy as assessed by physical examination (18). In addition, although the vast majority of workers from the relatively low-exposure (15 to 100 ppm) spinning areas of the plant had no overt clinical symptoms, they, like their fiber-cutting coworkers, underwent electrophysiologic studies that, in comparison to test results in matched controls, revealed significant reductions in nerve conduction in a pattern consistent with primary distal axonopathy. Data from the same study also support a dose-response relationship between severity of neuropathy and CS_2 exposure (18).

Although better hygienic practices have markedly reduced reports of neurotoxicity in the workplace, concern has been expressed over prolonged exposures at even low levels of CS_2 in workplace air, with evidence that ambient CS_2 concentrations of less than 20 ppm may cause subtle peripheral neuropathic changes over several years of worker exposure (19). Interestingly, in contrast to some evidence supporting the irreversibility of CS_2-induced neuropathology, a recently reported study in Japanese rayon workers having an estimated time-weighted average (TWA) exposure to CS_2 ranging between 2.3 and 17.0 ppm suggests the possibility of recovery (based on improved nerve conduction study results) after removal from exposure (20).

CARDIOTOXICITY

Cohort studies, including the initial demonstration by Tiller et al. (21), have shown an increased incidence of cardiovascular disease among CS_2 workers; and a epidemiologic critique of the literature has reconfirmed this association (22). An increased incidence of atherosclerosis in workers has been suggested, although causal mechanisms are not well understood (23). One extensive study of exposed workers suggests that the increased risk of cardiac death in CS_2 workers may not be due to atherosclerotic disease but rather, based on a closer relationship between mortality and recent exposure than between mortality and total exposure, may be due to a direct and reversible cardiotoxic or thrombotic effect (24). Further support for a reversible, dose-dependent effect is found in a study of Finnish rayon workers in whom the mortality from ischemic heart disease was observed to decline from a fivefold excess to control rates after a preventive program was established that lowered exposure levels to less than 10 ppm (25).

Effects of exposure that may contribute to CS_2-induced cardiovascular disease have been demonstrated in animals and humans and include hypertension and atherogenic disturbances in the serum lipid profile (26,27). A recent study in German rayon workers who were exposed to levels estimated to range from less than 0.2 to 66.0 ppm (median, 4.0 ppm) over a period of 4 to 220 months (median, 66 months), however, found no significant differences between exposed and control groups with respect to blood pressure, low-density lipoproteins, high-density lipoproteins, triglycerides, blood glucose, and fibrinolytic activity (28).

OCULAR TOXICITY

Severe, acute CS_2 intoxication and significant chronic CS_2 exposure are both known to result in optic nerve damage resembling optic neuritis. Chronic CS_2 exposure also affects choroidal microvascular circulation, and the observation of delayed choroidal filling has been considered essential for the diagnosis of chronic CS_2 intoxication. Reports of retinal pathology characterized by microvascular aneurysms and hemorrhages seem to be limited to those involving viscose rayon workers; vascular or microvascular effects have been either minor or absent in other groups of exposed workers (11,29–31). Additionally, discrete pigmentary changes of the posterior pole have been described (30).

In severe poisonings, a central scotoma with impaired red-green discrimination may be detected, suggesting an impairment in the receptivity of the ganglion cells or demyelination of optic nerve fibers (32). Central scotomas, decreased visual acuity, and dyschromatopsia are described (31).

REPRODUCTIVE EFFECTS

Numerous studies of the potential effects of CS_2 on reproductive function have been conducted and have used such end points as spermatogenesis, serum follicle-stimulating hormone and luteinizing hormone levels, and libido. A 1981 study of U.S. CS_2 workers failed to document impaired semen quality, but this report has been criticized because of relatively short durations of exposure (33,34). A more recent European case-control study of 116 male viscose rayon workers having a median duration of employment of 4.5 years also failed to demonstrate an effect on fertility or semen quality (35).

OTHER ORGAN SYSTEM EFFECTS

CS_2 can alter hepatic microsomal enzyme systems, with the potential of interfering with drug metabolism. Other toxic hepatic effects have not been demonstrated. Scant data exist to implicate CS_2 as a renal toxin. Chronic cough has been described in viscose rayon workers, but the presence of other irritants, including hydrogen disulfide, in the work setting weakens any causal association with pulmonary disease. In addition to those mentioned earlier, effects on endocrine function have been thought to include corticosteroid effects, impairment of thyroid function, and possible diabetogenic changes (13). However, a recent case-control study examining 117 viscose rayon workers failed to demonstrate—after adjustment for age, alcohol use, smoking habits, body mass index, and stress level—any association between cumulative CS_2 exposure and serum thyroxine, luteinizing hormone, follicle-stimulating hormone, prolactin, and testosterone levels (36). CS_2 is not classified as a carcinogen by authoritative agencies, including the International Agency for Research on Cancer.

Overall, factors that continue to plague the epidemiologic study of the health effects of CS_2 include the lack of adequate past exposure data (or a reliable method of translating exposure data into acquired disease risk) and the presence of multiple confounders, including other chemicals (e.g., hydrogen sulfide) and lifestyle-related determinants such as smoking and alcohol consumption (26).

Treatment

Treatment of CS_2 exposures consists of removal from exposure and, in the case of acute toxic exposure, decontamination of eye, skin, or gastrointestinal tract and supportive care. No antidote for this compound is known.

ENVIRONMENTAL AND BIOLOGICAL MONITORING

Ambient CS_2 can be collected by charcoal tube method and analyzed after toluene desorption by gas chromatography with flame-photometric detection (37). Urinary TTCA is considered a reliable marker of CS_2 exposure, and its direct measurement by high-performance liquid chromatographic assay appears to be far superior to the older, nonspecific iodine-azide test for urinary metabolites resulting from recent exposure to CS_2 in the workplace (38,39). A pre–work shift spot urine TTCA value of 0.95 mmol of CS_2 per mole of creatinine has been proposed as a sensitive and reliable indicator of recent CS_2 exposure at an 8-hour TWA level of 10 ppm (3). Elevation of RBC concentrations of spectrin dimers, cross-linked by CS_2 or its metabolites in a manner similar to that involving neurofilaments, may serve as a longer-term biological marker of CS_2 exposure and has been shown in animals to be proportional to both time and dose of exposure, with detection occurring before the development of clinical or morphologic neurotoxicity (40).

REGULATORY CONSIDERATIONS

The OSHA permissible exposure limit is 20 ppm (12 mg per cubic meter) in air as an 8-hour TWA, with a short-term exposure limit of 30 ppm (36 mg per cubic meter) (41). A 30-minute TWA exposure concentration of 100 ppm is allowed but should not be exceeded. The level considered to be immediately dangerous to life and health is 500 ppm (41).

OSHA had previously issued limits in 1989 that instituted a lowering of the permissible exposure limit to 4 ppm, but these revised limits were vacated by the Eleventh Circuit Court of Appeals on July 7, 1992. The National Institute for Occupational Safety and Health has recommended an 8-hour TWA of 1 ppm (3 mg per cubic meter) and a short-term exposure level of 10 ppm (30 mg per cubic meter). Both OSHA and the National Institute for Occupational Safety and Health have added the skin notation. *Occupational exposure* to CS_2 is defined as exposure exceeding an action level of 1.5 mg per cubic meter. CS_2 is considered both a hazardous substance and a hazardous waste by the U.S. Environmental Protection Agency (42).

The American Conference of Governmental Industrial Hygienists threshold limit value (8-hour TWA) is 10 ppm. CS_2 has an odor threshold of 0.11 ppm.

REFERENCES

1. US Department of Labor, Occupational Safety and Health Administration. Industrial exposure and control technologies for OSHA-regulated hazardous substances (part 1 of 4): carbon disulfide. Doc. no. PB89-210199. Washington: US Occupational Safety and Health Administration, 1989:366–369.
2. Lam CW, Di Stefano V. Characteristics of carbon disulfide binding in blood and to other biological substances. *Toxicol Appl Pharmacol* 1986;86:235–242.
3. Riihimaki V, Kivisto H, Peltonen K, Helpio E, Aitio A. Assessment of exposure to carbon disulfide in viscose production workers from urinary 2-thiothiazolidine-4-carboxylic acid determinations. *Am J Ind Med* 1992;22(1):85–97.
4. Graham DG, Amarnath V, Valentine WM, Pyle SJ, Anthony DC. Pathogenetic studies of hexane and carbon disulfide neurotoxicity. *Crit Rev Toxicol* 1995;25(2):91–112.
5. Rojas MM, Oehme FW. A review of the acute effects of carbon disulphide on lipid liver metabolism. *Vet Hum Toxicol* 1982;24:337–342.
6. Baselt RC, Cravey RH, eds. *Disposition of toxic drugs and chemicals in man*, 4th ed. Chicago: Year Book Medical Publishers, 1995:120–121.
7. Rainey JM. Disulfiram toxicity and carbon disulfide poisoning. *Am J Psychiatry* 1977;134:371–378.
8. Spyker DA, Gallanosa AG, Suratt PM. Health effects of acute carbon disulfide exposure. *J Toxicol Clin Toxicol* 1982;19:87–93.
9. van Hoorne M, de Douck A, de Bacquer D. Epidemiological study of eye irritation by hydrogen sulfide and/or carbon disulfide in viscose rayon workers. *Ann Occup Hyg* 1995;39:307–315.
10. van Hoorne M, de Douck A, de Bacquer D. Epidemiological study of the systemic ophthalmological effects of carbon disulfide. *Arch Environ Health* 1996;51:188.
11. Braceland F. Mental symptoms following carbon disulfide absorption and intoxication. *Ann Intern Med* 1942;16:246–261.
12. US Department of Health and Human Services, National Institute for Occupational Safety and Health. *NIOSH pocket guide to chemical hazards.* DHHS (NIOSH) publ. no. 90-117. Cincinnati: National Institute for Occupational Safety and Health, 1990:60.
13. Seppalainen AM, Haltia M. Carbon disulfide. In: Spencer PS, Schaumburg HH, eds. *Experimental and clinical neurotoxicology.* Baltimore: Williams & Wilkins, 1980:356–373.
14. Davidson M, Feinleib M. Carbon disulfide poisoning: a review. *Am Heart J* 1972;83:100–114.
15. Williams EE. Effects of alcohol on workers with carbon disulfide. *JAMA* 1937;109:1472.
16. Martensen-Larsen O. Treatment of alcoholism with a sensitizing drug. *Lancet* 1948;2:1004.
17. Peters HA, Levine R, Matthews CG, Chapman LJ. Extrapyramidal and other neurologic manifestations associated with carbon disulfide fumigant exposure. *Arch Neurol* 1988;45:537–540.
18. Chu C, Huang C, Chen R, Shih T. Polyneuropathy induced by carbon disulphide in viscose rayon workers. *Occup Environ Med* 1995;52:404–407.
19. Johnson BL, Boyd J, Burg JR, Lee ST, Xintaras C, Albright BE. Effects on the peripheral nervous system of workers' exposure to carbon disulfide. *Neurotoxicology* 1983;4:53–66.
20. Hirata M, Ogawa Y, Goto S. A cross-sectional study of nerve conduction velocities among workers exposed to carbon disulphide. *Med Lav* 1996; 87(1):29–34.
21. Tiller JR, Schilling RSF, Morris JN. Occupational toxic factor in mortality from coronary heart disease. *BMJ* 1968;4:407–411.
22. Kristensen TS. Cardiovascular diseases and the work environment. *Scand J Work Environ Health* 1989;15:245–264.
23. Kruppa K, Hietanen E, Klockars M, et al. Chemical exposures at work and cardiovascular morbidity. *Scand J Work Environ Health* 1984;10:381–388.
24. Sweetnam PM, Taylor SWC, Elwood PC. Exposure to carbon disulphide and ischaemic heart disease in a viscose rayon factory. *Br J Ind Med* 1987;44:220–227.
25. Nurminen M, Hernberg SL. Effects of intervention on the cardiovascular mortality of workers exposed to carbon disulphide: a 15-year follow-up. *BMJ* 1985;42:32–35.
26. van Hoorne M, de Bacquer D, Debacker G. Epidemiological study of the cardiovascular effects of carbon disulphide. *Int J Epidemiol* 1992;21:745–752.
27. Antove G, Kazakova B, Spasovski M, et al. Effect of carbon disulphide on the cardiovascular system. *J Hyg Epidemiol Microbiol Immunol* 1985;29:329.
28. Drexler H, Ulm K, Hubmann M, et al. Carbon disulphide: III. Risk factors for coronary heart diseases in workers in the viscose industry. *Int Arch Occup Environ Health* 1995;67:243–252.

29. Sugimoto K, Goto S, Taniguchi H. Ocular fundus photography of workers exposed to carbon disulfide: a comparative epidemiological study between Japan and Finland. *Int Arch Occup Environ Health* 1977;39:97–101.
30. de Laey JJ, de Rouck A, Priem H, van Hoorne M. Ophthalmological aspects of chronic CS_2 intoxication. *Int Ophthalmol* 1980;3:51–56.
31. Grant WM, Schuman JS. *Toxicology of the eye: effects on the eyes and visual system from chemicals, drugs, metals, minerals, plants, toxins and venoms*, 4th ed. Springfield, IL: Charles C Thomas Publisher, 1993:318–323.
32. Raitta CR, Teir H, Tolonen M, Nerminen M, Helpio E, Malmstrom S. Impaired color discrimination among viscose rayon workers exposed to carbon disulfide. *J Occup Med* 1981;23:189–192.
33. Meyer CR. Semen quality in workers exposed to carbon disulfide compared to a control group from the same plant. *J Occup Med* 1981;23:435–439.
34. Schrag SD, Dixon R. Occupational exposures associated with male reproductive dysfunction. *Am Rev Pharmacol Toxicol* 1985;25:567–592.
35. van Hoorne M, Comhaire F, de Bacquer D. Epidemiological study of the effects of carbon disulfide on male sexuality and reproduction. *Arch Environ Health* 1994;49(4):273–278.
36. van Hoorne M, Vermeulen A, de Bacquer D. Epidemiological study of endocrinological effects of carbon disulfide. *Arch Environ Health* 1993;48(5):370–375.
37. National Institute for Occupational Safety and Health. *Manual of analytical methods*, 3rd ed. Cincinnati: National Institute for Occupational Safety and Health, 1984.
38. Cox C, Shane S, Hee Q, Tolos W. Biological monitoring of workers exposed to carbon disulfide. *Am J Ind Med* 1998;33:48–54.
39. Ghittori B, Maestri L, Contardi I, et al. Biological monitoring of workers exposed to carbon disulfide (CS_2) in a viscose rayon fibers factory. *Am J Ind Med* 1998;33:478–484.
40. Valentine WM, Graham DG, Anthony DC. Covalent cross-linking of erythrocyte spectrin by carbon disulfide in vivo. *Toxicol Appl Pharmacol* 1992;121:71–77.
41. Agency for Toxic Substances and Disease Registry. *Toxicological profile for carbon disulfide*. Atlanta: US Department of Health and Human Services, Public Health Service, ATSDR, 1996:161.
42. Sittig M. *Handbook of toxic and hazardous chemicals and carcinogens*, 2nd ed. Park Ridge, NJ: Noyes Publications, 1985.

CHAPTER 110

n-*Hexane and 2-Hexanone*

Lorne K. Garrettson

SOURCES AND PRODUCTION

The two common, six-carbon, aliphatic compounds *n*-hexane and 2-hexanone have the same neurotoxic metabolite, 2,5-hexanedione. *n*-Hexane is used as a solvent in glues, adhesives, and cements. 2-Hexanone (methyl-*n*-butyl ketone, MBK) is also a commonly used solvent (Table 110-1).

Both compounds are nonionized, flammable, volatile liquids at ambient temperature and pressure. *n*-Hexane has a chemical formula of C_6H_{14} and a molecular weight of 86.20 D. Its vapor density is 2.97 (air = 1.00). Hexane is flammable and explosive when exposed to heat. Its vapor is flammable in air at concentrations between 1.2% and 7.7%. 2-Hexanone is a colorless, flammable liquid with a chemical formula of $C_6H_{12}O$ and a molecular weight of 100.16 D (Fig. 110-1, Table 110-2). 2-Hexanone has a vapor density of 3.0 (air = 1.0).

n-Hexane is a component of crude oil and is manufactured by distillation.

TABLE 110-1. Uses and users of *n*-hexane and 2-hexanone

Uses	Users
Glues, rubber glues	Shoemakers
Cleaners	Furniture makers
Paint and lacquer solvents	Industrial painters
Seed oil extraction (soy, flax, safflower)	Hobbyist using rubber glues
Grinding with diamond dust	Precision industrial grinders
	Adhesive tape manufacturers
	Glue sniffers

$$H_3C-CH_2-CH_2-CH_2-CH_2-CH_3$$

n-hexane

$$CH_3-\overset{O}{\overset{\|}{C}}-CH_2-CH_2-CH_2-CH_3$$

2-Hexanone
(methyl-*n*-butyl ketone)

Figure 110-1. Chemical formulas for *n*-hexane and 2-hexanone.

EXPOSURE SOURCES

Exposure has primarily occurred from inhalation. Worker exposure to *n*-hexane may occur during the production or application of glues and adhesives. Reports from Japan and the United States have linked peripheral neuropathy with *n*-hexane exposure when glues were used in shoe and furniture manufacture (1,2). Epidemics of weakness due to exposure to 2-hexanone were seminal in initiating the studies that identified the toxic metabolite. Cases came from an Ohio plant in which coated fabrics were being made (3,4). A similar cluster of cases of polyneuropathy was reported in spray painters repainting a dam (5).

These epidemics were associated with exposures to the two different compounds, but the clinical findings were the same. The saga of discovery of the relationship between these compounds and a common disease caused by a common toxic metabolite has been reviewed (Fig. 110-2) (6). The neurotoxic metabolite is 2,5-hexanedione (7).

CLINICAL TOXICOLOGY

Routes of Exposure

Inhalation is the primary route of exposure. Exposures that occur in an enclosed place are more dangerous owing to the high vapor density and high vapor pressures of both *n*-hexane

TABLE 110-2. Common names and chemical names

Chemical name	Common names
n-Hexane (CAS no. 110-54-3)	Dipropyl
	Hexane
	Hexyl hydride
	Skellysolve B
2-Hexanone (CAS no. 591-78-6)	Methyl butyl ketone (MBK)
	2-Oxohexane
	Ketone, butyl methyl
	Methyl-*n*-butyl ketone (MBK, MnBK)
	Propylacetone
	Hexan-2-one

CAS, Chemical Abstracts Service.

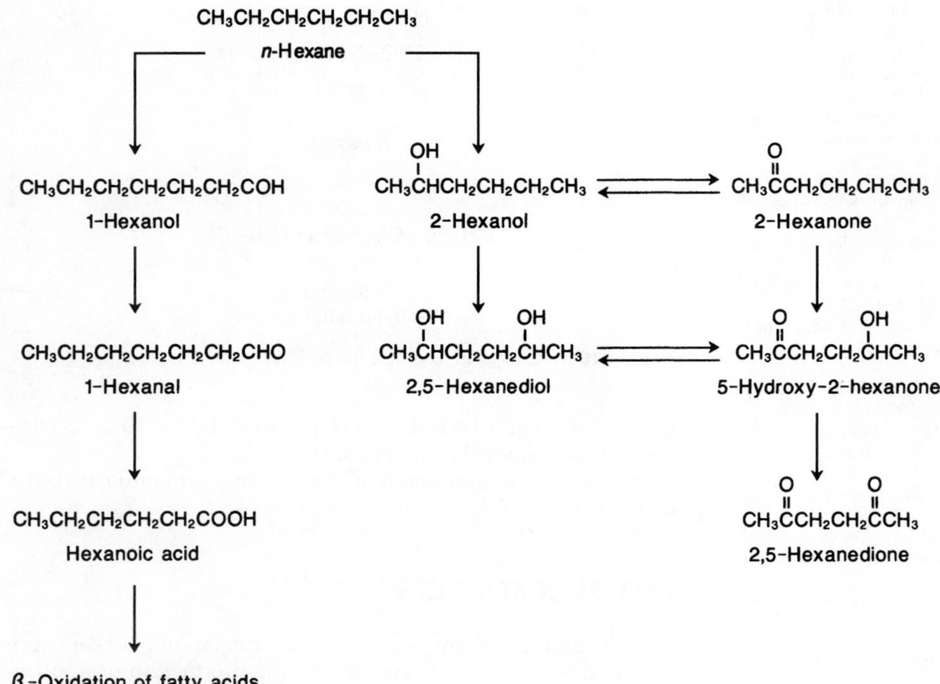

Figure 110-2. Metabolism of *n*-hexane.

and 2-hexanone. However, dermatologic exposure can lead to skin irritation, and absorption may contribute to chronic exposure and polyneuropathy. Ingestion has rarely been reported.

Absorption, Metabolism, and Excretion

Both compounds are readily absorbed from the lungs. Systemic absorption from dermal exposure has not been well studied.

Both compounds are metabolized by the liver to a common toxic metabolite, 2,5-hexanedione (see Fig. 110-2), which is a direct neurotoxin (8,9). An apparent high degree of specificity exists for the toxic effect of this compound, as related metabolites of similar solvents have no similar toxicity. 2,5-Hexanedione is a γ-diketone. Other diketones (α, β, δ) do not produce neurotoxicity.

The proposed mechanisms of action have been reviewed (10). Current evidence supports the concept that adducts are formed which lead to cross-linkages between neurofilaments. These cross-linkages lead to the axonal swellings seen on microscopy and, ultimately, to distal degeneration of the nerve.

The metabolite is reduced to the corresponding 2,5-hexanediol or to 5-hydroxy-2-hexanone. Compounds with a hydroxyl group are conjugated with glucuronide and eliminated in the urine. 2,5-Hexanedione can be found in the urine of workers as a marker of occupational exposure.

Renal clearance of *n*-hexane has been measured and found to be 2 L per minute (11). Elimination of the parent compounds is primarily by metabolism, and very little is exhaled unchanged. The toxic metabolite, 2,5-hexanedione, is the principal metabolite. Other minor metabolites have been identified, but none has been found to be toxic.

Signs, Symptoms, and Syndromes

ACUTE TOXICITY

Acute exposure to *n*-hexane vapor produces upper airway irritation, drowsiness, central nervous system (CNS) depression, confusion, and giddiness. 2-Hexanone vapor produces ocular and upper airway irritation. Brief exposures to high vapor concentrations of approximately 5,000 parts per million (ppm) of 2-hexanone can produce drowsiness and CNS depression.

CHRONIC TOXICITY

After chronic exposure to large amounts of these solvents, a syndrome of sensorimotor polyneuropathy may occur. Although motor findings predominate, diminished vibratory sensation has been observed (12). Studies of cardiac electrophysiology suggest that parasympathetic nerves may be affected (13). Maculopathy and diminished color discrimination were common among workers in one study of an *n*-hexane–exposed group (14). Loss of memory or other cognitive effects of these compounds have not been reported after industrial exposure. The potential for CNS effects at workplace levels of exposure is supported by the finding of alteration in evoked potentials in workers (15). More recently, two cases of parkinsonism have been reported in individuals with chronic, urinary excretion–documented exposure to *n*-hexane (16,17). Positron emission tomography revealed abnormalities in the caudate nucleus and putamen. No teratogenic or carcinogenic effects of these compounds are known.

Management of Toxicity

An accurate history is essential to determine whether a person has been exposed to one of the offending agents. Proof of the exposure may require a review of the products used at a worksite and assessment of the work environment by an industrial hygienist.

Patients may report weakness, muscle cramps, numbness, and paresthesias such as the feeling of tingling, burning, and freezing. Impotence may occur (Table 110-3).

The physical examination should examine all muscle groups for weakness. Peripheral muscles are affected first, with more proximal weakness after more prolonged exposure. Muscle stretch reflexes are absent distally in areas of weakness. Atrophy of the hand muscles has been reported. Hyperhidrosis may occur. All sensory modalities may be affected, including touch and proprioception. Patients should be assessed for cerebellar

TABLE 110-3. Clinical presentation of *n*-hexane neurotoxicity

Extremity paresthesias
Muscle cramping
Distal muscle weakness
Blurred vision
Tinnitus
Fatigue
Loss of muscle stretch reflexes
Sensory impairment
Muscle atrophy
Parkinsonism

signs and tremor. Visual acuity and peripheral vision changes have not been reported, whereas blurred vision has. Tinnitus may occur. Signs of parkinsonism should be sought.

The differential diagnosis of weakness in workers includes exposure to tri-*o*-cresyl phosphate, although patients with this intoxication are less likely to demonstrate sensory loss, and muscle stretch reflexes remain normal even with debilitating weakness. Other compounds causing peripheral nerve injury include carbon disulfide, lead, arsenic, acute or chronic exposure to organophosphates, acrylamide, toluene, styrene, and ethylene oxide.

The patient must be removed from all future exposure. Physical therapy should be initiated to maintain full range of motion until reinnervation occurs. Recovery is slow, as the regeneration of axon fibers must take place. Complete recovery of strength may not occur.

MEDICAL AND ENVIRONMENTAL MONITORING

Nerve conduction studies will be abnormal after clinical weakness has become apparent. Fast fibers are affected at lower levels of exposure than are slow fibers (15,18). Nerve conduction velocity is correlated with clinical severity. Velocities are more profoundly reduced in the peripheral axon (19). The action potential amplitude was observed to be reduced in one group of patients even when the conduction velocity was within normal limits. This finding may be useful in early detection (20). Studies of exposed workers have shown depression in the amplitude of several peaks in the visual evoked response. Auditory evoked potentials show prolongation of peak V latency and central conduction time. The amplitude of the electroretinogram has been found to be reduced in *n*-hexane workers (21). Documentation that these compounds are the cause of the peripheral neuropathy requires a biopsy of a peripheral nerve (sural). The findings expected are of perinodal axonal swellings that consist of neurofilaments. Loss of myelinated fibers does not necessarily occur (22). Retraction of the myelin sheaths and focal demyelination may be seen (Figs. 110-3, 110-4) (23,24).

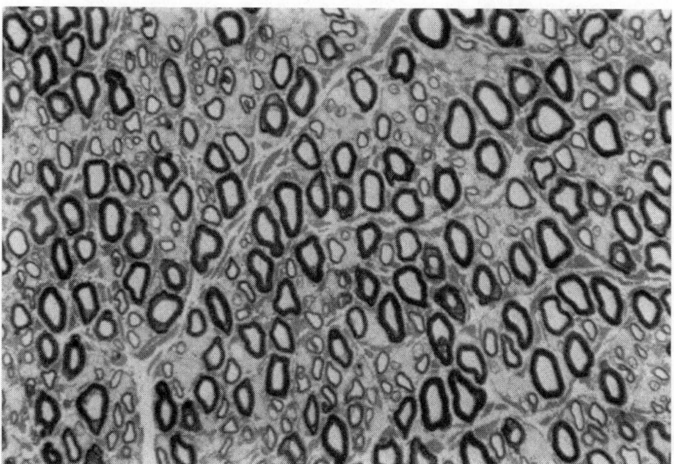

Figure 110-3. Normal sural nerve.

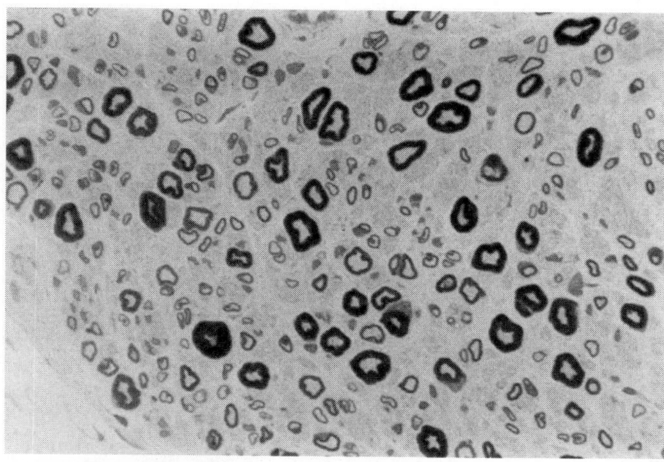

Figure 110-4. Histologic section of sural nerve, obtained by biopsy, showing loss and thinning of large fibers from toxic neuropathy caused by *n*-hexane.

n-Hexane and 2-hexanedione can be assayed in blood by some laboratories. However, such assays have little utility in acute illness, as clearance of the compounds is rapid (11).

Determination of the urinary 2,5-hexanedione concentration documents the level of exposure (25). Normal values for 2,5-hexanedione are less than 10 µg per L, the current limit of detection. Urinary concentrations of 2,5-hexanedione in exposed workers may exceed 200 µg per L, although it should not exceed 5 mg per L (26). The measurement of 2,5-hexanedione in the urine after 8 hours of environmental exposure correlates well with active air sampling of the workplace (27).

Levels of exhaled *n*-hexane correlates well with urinary excretion of 2,5-diketohexane and environmental *n*-hexane and may be preferred in some industrial situations (28).

Passive dosimeters are as effective as active air sampling and may be used for assessment of the exposure of workers to *n*-hexane and 2-hexanone (26).

OCCUPATIONAL AND ENVIRONMENTAL REGULATIONS

For *n*-hexane, the U.S. Occupational Safety and Health Administration recommended a time-weighted average (TWA) exposure of not more than 50 ppm (180 mg per cubic meter) for an 8-hour day, although the permissible exposure limit is 500 ppm. The National Institute of Occupational Safety and Health (NIOSH) uses a recommended exposure limit of 50 ppm for a 10-hour day (29). The American Conference of Governmental Industrial Hygienists (ACGIH) suggests an 8-hour TWA of 50 ppm and an excursion limit of three times this value for a maximum of 30 minutes (Table 110-4).

The ACGIH has assigned a biological exposure index for urinary 2,5-hexanedione of 5 mg per gram of creatinine at the end of an 8-hour workday.

For 2-hexanone, the U.S. Occupational Safety and Health Administration threshold limit value TWA permissible exposure limit is 100 ppm for an 8-hour exposure day. NIOSH gives 1 ppm as the recommended exposure limit for a 10-hour day.

TABLE 110-4. Occupational and environmental regulations

Compounds	TLV-TWA	Excursion limits	IDLH (NIOSH)
n-Hexane	50 ppm , 8-h d (OSHA) 500 ppm, 8-h d PEL (OSHA) 50 ppm, 10-h d REL (NIOSH) 50 ppm, 8-h d REL (ACGIH)	3 × the TLV for 30 min (ACGIH)	110 ppm
2-Hexanone	100 ppm, 8-h d PEL (OSHA) 1 ppm, 10-h d REL (NIOSH) 5 ppm, 8-h d REL (ACGIH)	3 × the TLV for 30 min (ACGIH)	1,600 ppm

ACGIH, American Conference of Governmental Industrial Hygienists; IDLH, immediately dangerous to life and health; NIOSH, National Institute of Occupational Safety and Health; OSHA, U.S. Occupational Safety and Health Administration; PEL, permissible exposure limit; REL, recommended exposure limit; TLV, threshold limit value; TWA, time-weighted average.

The ACGIH sets 5 ppm as the TWA for an 8-hour day. The excursion limit is three times this value for a 30-minute period (see Table 110-4).

EXPOSURE CONTROLS

For both compounds, wetted clothing should be removed immediately, and wetted skin should be washed immediately. When the environmental concentration of *n*-hexane is less than 500 ppm or of 2-hexanone (a more irritating compound) is more than 10 ppm, the use of a supplied-air respirator is recommended by NIOSH. At a concentration exceeding 25 ppm, the respirator must be operable in a continuous-flow mode. At more than 50 ppm, such a respirator must be used with a tightly fitting mask.

REFERENCES

1. Yamamura Y. *n*-Hexane polyneuropathy. *Folia Psychiatr Neurol Jpn* 1969; 23:45–50.
2. Herskowitz A, Ishii N, Schaumburg H. *n*-Hexane neuropathy: a syndrome occurring as a result of industrial exposure. *N Engl J Med* 1971;285:82–85.
3. Billmaier D, Allen N, Craft B, Williams N, Epstein S, Fontaine R. Peripheral neuropathy in a coated fabrics plant. *J Occup Med* 1974;16:665–671.
4. Allen N, Mendell JM, Billmaier DJ, Fontaine RE, O'Neil J. Toxic polyneuropathy due to methyl *n*-butyl ketone. *Arch Neurol* 1975;32:209–218.
5. Mallov JS. MBK neuropathy among spray painters. *JAMA* 1976;235:1455–1457.
6. Couri D, Milks MM. Hexacarbon neuropathy: tracking a toxin. *Neurotoxicology* 1985;6:65–72.
7. DeCaprio AP. Molecular mechanisms of diketone neurotoxicity. *Chem Biol Interact* 1985;54:257–270.
8. DiVincenzo GD, Kaplan CJ, Dedinas J. Characterization of the metabolites of methyl *n*-butyl ketone, methyl isobutyl ketone, and methyl ethyl ketone in guinea pig serum and their clearance. *Toxicol Appl Pharmacol* 1976;36:511–522.
9. Spencer PS, Schaumburg HH. Feline nervous system response to chronic intoxication with commercial grades of methyl *n*-butyl ketone, methyl isobutyl ketone, and methyl ethyl ketone. *Toxicol Appl Pharmacol* 1976;37:301–311.
10. Graham DG, Amarnath V, Valentine WM, Pyle SJ, Anthony DC. Pathogenetic studies of hexane and carbon disulfide neurotoxicity. *Crit Rev Toxicol* 1995;25:91–112.
11. Filser JG, Peter H, Bolt HM, Fedtke N. Pharmacokinetics of the neurotoxin *n*-hexane in rat and man. *Arch Toxicol* 1987;60:77–80.
12. Bachman MO, de Beer Z, Myers JE. *n*-Hexane neurotoxicity in metal can manufacturing workers. *Occup Med* 1993;43:149–154.
13. Murata K, Araki S, Yokoyama K, Yamashita K, Okajima F, Nakaaki K. Changes in autonomic function as determined by ECG R-R interval variability in sandal, shoe and leather workers exposed to *n*-hexane, xylene and toluene. *Neurotoxicology* 1994;15:867–876.
14. Raitta CH, Seppalainen AM, Huuskonen MS. *n*-Hexane maculopathy in industrial workers. *Albrecht von Graefes Arch Klin Exp Ophthalmol* 1979;209:99–110.
15. Huang C-C, Chu N-S. Evoked potentials in chronic *n*-hexane intoxication. *Clin Electroencephalogr* 1989;20:162–168.
16. Pezzoli G, Barbieri S, Ferrante C, Zecchinelli A, Foa V. Parkinsonism due to *n*-hexane [Letter]. *Lancet* 1989:2:874.
17. Pezzoli G, Antonini A, Barbieri S, et al. *n*-Hexane-induced maculopathy in parkinsonism: pathogenetic hypotheses. *Mov Disord* 1995;10:279–282.
18. Yokoyama K, Feldman RG, Sax DS, Salzsider BT, Kucera J. Relation of distribution of conduction velocities to nerve biopsy findings in *n*-hexane poisoning. *Muscle Nerve* 1990;13:314–320.
19. Oge AM, Yazici J, Boyaciyan A, et al. Peripheral and central conduction in *n*-hexane polyneuropathy. *Muscle Nerve* 1994;17:1416–1430.
20. Pastore C, Marhuenda D, Marti J, Cardona A. Early diagnosis of *n*-hexane-caused neuropathy. *Muscle Nerve* 1994;17:981–986.
21. Seppalainen AM, Raitta C, Huuskonen MS. Hexane induced changes in visual evoked potentials and electroretinograms of industrial users. *Electroencephalogr Clin Neurophysiol* 1979;47:492–498.
22. Towfighi J, Gonatas N, Pleasure D, Cooper H, McCrea L. Glue sniffer's neuropathy. *Neurology* 1976;26:238–243.
23. Saida K, Mendell JR, Weiss HS. Peripheral nerve changes induced by methyl *n*-butyl ketone and potentiation by methyl ethyl ketone. *J Neuropathol Exp Neurol* 1976;35:207–225.
24. Krobkin R, Asbury AK, Sumner A, Nielsen SL. Glue-sniffing neuropathy. *Arch Neurol* 1975;32:158–162.
25. Dawai T, Mizunuma K, Yasugi T, Uchida Y, Ikeda M. The method of choice for the determination of 2,5-hexanedione as an indicator of occupational exposure to *n*-hexane. *Int Arch Occup Environ Health* 1990;62:403–408.
26. American Conference of Governmental Industrial Hygienists. *The 1995–1996 TLV for chemical substances and physical agents and biological exposure indices.* Cincinnati: American Conference of Governmental Industrial Hygienists, 1995.
27. Bartolucci GB, Perbellini L, Gori GP, Brugnone F, Chiesura-Corona P, DeRosa E. Occupational exposure to solvents: field comparison of active and passive samplers and biologic monitoring of exposed workers. *Ann Occup Hyg* 1986;30:295–306.
28. Periago JF, Morente A, Villanueva M, Luna A. Correlation between concentrations of *n*-hexane and toluene in exhaled and environmental air in an occupationally exposed population. *J Appl Toxicol* 1994;14:63–67.
29. National Institute of Occupational Safety and Health Pocket Guide. Cincinnati: NIOSH, 1994.

CHAPTER 111
Asbestos

John P. Holland and Dorsett D. Smith

SOURCES AND PRODUCTION

Common Names

Asbestos is the commercial designation given collectively to a group of six distinct types of natural mineral fibers. It is subdivided into two groups, serpentine and amphibole. The only fiber in the serpentine group is chrysotile (commonly known as *white asbestos*). The five amphibole fibers are crocidolite (blue asbestos), amosite (brown asbestos), tremolite, actinolite, and anthophyllite.

Chemical Forms

All types of asbestos are hydrated magnesium silicates. Each fiber type has its own general chemical form and crystalline structure but, even for fibers of a specific type, the percentages of major chemical components vary. Differing amounts of metals may also be found in asbestos, including iron, chromium, cobalt, manganese, and nickel. These are either incorporated into the crystalline structure or are contaminants from surrounding minerals that cannot easily be removed.

Chrysotile contains approximately 40% each of magnesium oxide and silica but very little iron oxide (1%). Crocidolite and amosite contain more iron oxides (20% to 44%) and silica (49% to 53%) but little magnesium oxide (0% to 7%). Tremolite, actinolite, and anthophyllite also contain large amounts of silica (51% to 60%) but are intermediate in their content of magnesium oxide (15% to 34%) and iron oxides (0% to 15%) (1,2).

The general chemical formula of chrysotile is $[Mg_3Si_2O_5(OH)_4]$, which makes it chemically similar to micas and kaolinites. However, chrysotile has a fibrous structure that is not found in these other minerals. General chemical formulas for the amphibole fibers are as follows: crocidolite $[Na_2(MgFe^{+++}Fe^{++})Si_8O_{22}(OH)]$, amosite $[(MgFe^{++})_7Si_8O_{22}(OH)_4]$, tremolite $[Ca_2(MgFe^{++})_5Si_8O_{22}]$, actinolite $[Ca_2(MgFe^{++})_5Si_8O_{22}(OH)_2]$, and anthophyllite $[(MgFe^{++})_7Si_8O_{22}(OH)_2]$ (3).

Although they are relatively resistant to degradation by chemicals and heat, asbestos fibers dissolve to various degrees in strong acid and alkali solutions. Asbestos fibers are not flammable but, when heated to temperatures in excess of 800°F (427°C), amphiboles tend to lose the water incorporated in their crystalline structure and become very brittle, whereas chrysotile keeps its flexibility at such temperatures (1–3).

Physical Forms

Asbestos particles found in natural mineral deposits do not have fixed dimensions but form as parallel aggregations of long crystalline fibrils or fibers. In natural mineral formations, these fibers can be up to several centimeters long. They are very brittle and, when stressed, break easily into shorter lengths. In its preparation for commercial use, asbestos-containing rock is crushed mechanically and cleaned in a process called *milling*. This results in an infinite variety of sizes of commercial asbestos fibers; most are less than 50 μm long, and many are shorter than 1 μm (1).

SERPENTINE GROUP

Chrysotile is the only fiber type in the serpentine group. It also is the only asbestos fiber that is curly and often is found in intertwined bundles. The crystalline structure of chrysotile consists of parallel sheets of silica and magnesium hydroxide (i.e., brucite), which give the appearance of overlapping scrolls in cross section (Fig. 111-1).

The basic structural unit of chrysotile is the fibril, which is a curved sheet of brucite that forms into a scroll or tube. Chrysotile fibrils have a fixed diameter of 0.02 to 0.04 μm, which makes them the thinnest fiber found in nature. (By comparison, the diameters of a cotton fiber and a human hair are 10 and 40 μm, respectively.) In nature, these chrysotile fibrils usually are found bunched together to form a chrysotile fiber with a typical diameter of 0.75 to 1.50 μm.

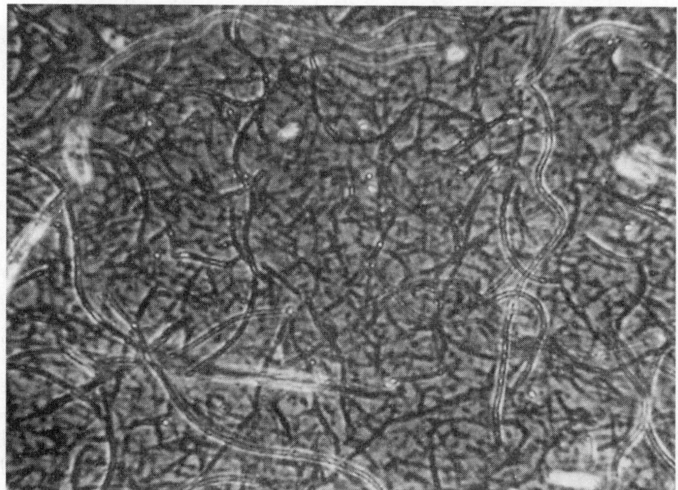

Figure 111-1. Chrysotile fibers (magnification, 300×).

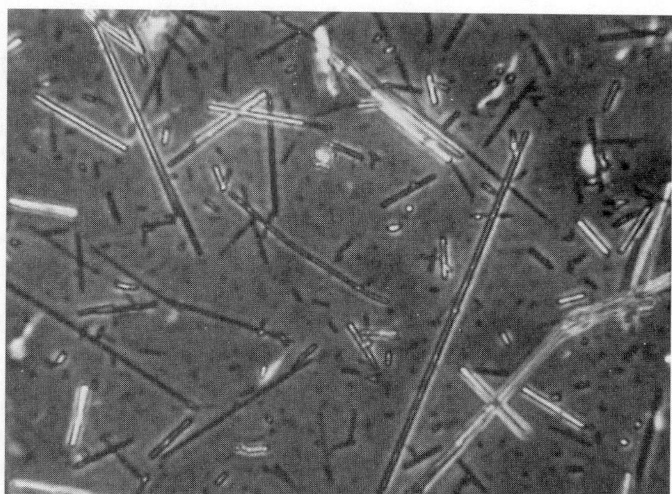

Figure 111-2. Amosite fibers (magnification, 300×).

Serpentine fibers derive their name from serpentine rocks, in which they are found. Asbestos forms when very hot liquid supersaturated with minerals invades fissures in serpentine rock and then slowly cools and crystallizes into veins. In natural formations, chrysotile often is found with quartz micas, fosterite, brucite, and feldspar, so commercial formulations may be contaminated with these materials (1,3).

AMPHIBOLE GROUP

All the amphiboles have a straight, needlelike shape and are found in nature stacked in parallel rows. In crystalline structure, the amphiboles are parallel chains of silica tetrahedra in which are incorporated varying amounts of different metal ions, giving each type its unique chemical form (Figs. 111-2, 111-3).

Amphiboles do not have a true fibril structure but are formed as parallel plates of crystalline material that can shear apart to form fibers of various diameters. The thinnest amphibole fibers are 0.1 to 0.2 μm, but more typical diameters are 1.5 to 4.0 μm.

Amphibole asbestos is formed by forces of heat and pressure rearranging and recrystallizing materials in existing mineral formations. Crocidolite and amosite are found in sedimentary rocks called *banded ironstones*. Tremolite, actinolite, and anthophyllite deposits are found as pockets in igneous, metamorphic, or sedimentary rocks. In natural mineral formations, the amphibole fiber types often are mixed with iron oxides and quartz, so commercial formulations can be contaminated with these materials (1,3). Asbestos is found in numerous common locations (Table 111-1).

HUMAN EXPOSURE

Asbestos Production

Commercial asbestos is obtained from asbestos-bearing rocks mined in open-pit or underground mines. The rock then is crushed, and asbestos fibers are separated and washed in a process known as *milling*. The commercial asbestos fibers are shipped in bags. In the past, these bags often were constructed of woven jute, which allowed fibers to escape, but today they are made of impervious paper or plastic.

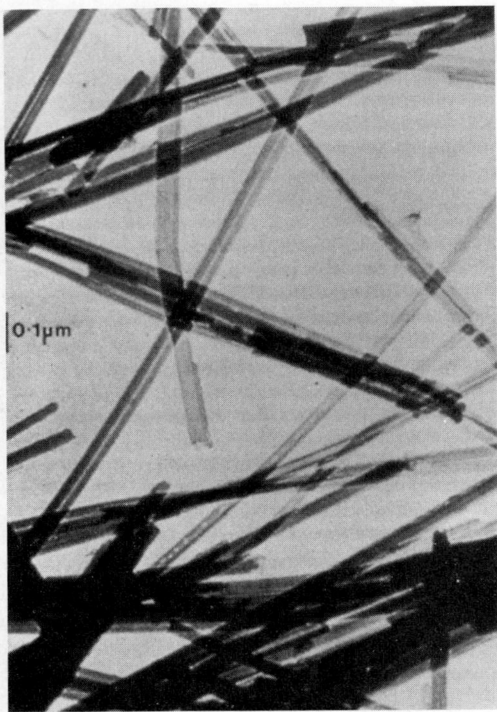

Figure 111-3. Amosite asbestos fibers (magnification, 400×). Fibers, by definition, are 5 mm long, with length-to-width aspect ratio of 3:1.

In recent years, the former Soviet Union has been the largest producer of asbestos, with most of the product being used in the former Eastern bloc countries. Historically, most of the asbestos mined in North America has been chrysotile; 90% of this has come from Canada, especially from large mines in Quebec. Approximately 95% of all asbestos used in the United States has been chrysotile, and most of this has come from Quebec's mines. In the past in the United States, chrysotile was mined in smaller amounts in Arizona, California, Vermont, and other states but is no longer produced in significant quantities. South Africa has been the third largest producer of asbestos worldwide and has produced most of the crocidolite and amosite used in the United States; some crocidolite from Australia also was used in this country.

TABLE 111-1. Sites and businesses linked with asbestos exposure

Mining and milling of asbestos
Manufacture of
- Cement pipe
- Cement panels and flooring
- Pipe and boiler insulation
- Electrical insulation
- Gaskets and fittings
- Roofing, wallboard, and siding materials
- Composite floor and ceiling tiles
- Friction products
- Fireproof clothing
- Chemical filters
- Paper and plastics

Insulation work
General construction
Shipbuilding and shipwrecking
Locomotive repair
Building demolition
Power plants
Marine engine rooms
Chemical plants
Automobile repair
Building maintenance

Reprinted from ref. 1, with permission.

Worldwide consumption of commercial asbestos peaked in the early 1970s at 6 million tons per year. (The annual U.S. consumption at that time was approximately 1.6 million tons.) Commercial use has dropped since then, but it is estimated that more than 30 million tons of asbestos have been used in the United States during the twentieth century, and much of this is still in existing structures and manufactured items.

The only other fiber types used in large quantities in the United States have been crocidolite and amosite. Tremolite and actinolite have little commercial importance but may be found as contaminants in other types of commercially used asbestos. Tremolite is sometimes found also in small amounts in industrial talc, vermiculite, and sandstone. Anthophyllite has little commercial importance in North America but is found in exposed natural deposits in Finland (1,3).

Commercial Uses

The physical properties of asbestos make it a unique and commercially useful material. These properties include resistance to degradation by heat and chemicals, strength, durability, and a fibrous structure (which allows it to be made into cloth or felt and to act as a good binder in ceramic materials).

Asbestos has been used extensively in the industrialized world since the exploitation of large commercial deposits, beginning in Quebec in the 1860s and South Africa in the 1890s. Asbestos has more than 3,000 commercial uses, the most important of which are listed in Table 111-1. The commercial use of asbestos has been widespread in the construction of buildings, ships, power plants, chemical plants, and other industrial facilities.

The largest single use of asbestos has been as a binder in cement pipes and cement panels. Asbestos has also been used extensively in all types of insulation and fireproofing, including pipe and boiler insulation (in which loose asbestos fibers mixed with water formerly were applied often as a "mud") and spray-on fireproofing on ceilings and exposed structural beams. Asbestos has been incorporated into a variety of building products including house siding, wallboard, and floor and ceiling tiles.

Asbestos cloth has been used in fire-resistant clothing and fire and welding blankets. When pressed into a felt, asbestos is used in pipe gaskets, and it also is used as a binder in plastics and paper. As a filtering material, asbestos has been used in gas masks and a variety of chemical processes, such as in the membranes of hydrolytic cells in chlorine production plants. Finally, asbestos has been used extensively in friction products such as automobile brake shoes (1,4).

Other Occupational and Environmental Exposure Sources

OCCUPATIONAL EXPOSURES

In the United States, millions of individuals have had significant workplace exposures to asbestos since the beginning of the twentieth century, with the most extensive exposures occurring in the three decades during and after World War II. Limited information is available on historical levels of asbestos exposure for U.S. workers. It is estimated that in the early part of the twentieth century, asbestos exposures in some industries exceeded 100 fibers per cubic centimeter of air, whereas exposures of 10 fibers per cubic centimeter of air were common among insulators and other highly exposed workers during and after World

War II. These historical levels are 100 to 1,000 times higher than the current U.S. Occupational Safety and Health Administration (OSHA) permissible exposure level (PEL) for asbestos of 0.1 fiber per cubic centimeter of air (1,5–7).

Historically, workers in the United States who had the highest asbestos exposures were in mining and milling, primary manufacturing (i.e., use of asbestos as a raw material to make products such as concrete pipe or floor tiles), and insulation trades (including those in both general construction and shipbuilding). The next highest exposures were for workers in secondary manufacturing [i.e., incorporating asbestos-containing materials (ACMs) into manufactured items] and construction and shipbuilding workers who were not insulators.

In the United States, the shipbuilding and construction industries have included the largest cohorts of workers with heavy asbestos exposures: It is estimated that in shipyards alone, more than 1 million workers have experienced significant exposure. In both these industries, insulators have had twice the rate of asbestos-related diseases as compared with workers in other trades.

At the other end of the spectrum, workers whose only exposure to asbestos was in changing automobile brake shoes containing asbestos have shown no increased incidence of any asbestos-related disease. The reason for this is unclear, although one theory suggests that high heat from friction on the brake shoe transforms the asbestos into a nontoxic material that does not cause disease. Nonetheless, the same OSHA standards apply for asbestos exposures in all types of industries (1,7).

By the mid-1960s, it was apparent that asbestos was a serious health hazard that could cause asbestosis, lung cancer, and mesothelioma. Workplace regulation of asbestos exposure has become increasingly more stringent in the United States since passage of the OSHA Act of 1970. In 1994, OSHA lowered the PEL for asbestos in workplace air to its current level of 0.1 fiber per cubic centimeter of air. Table 111-2 shows the historical recommended and legally mandated occupational exposure limits for asbestos in the United States since 1946 (7,8).

Since the 1970s, commercial use of asbestos has declined steadily, whereas use of industrial respirators and changes in production processes have increased, all of which has resulted in markedly reduced worker exposures. Spray-on applications of asbestos for insulation or fireproofing, as well as a number of other uses of asbestos, have been completely banned in the United States by the Environmental Protection Agency (EPA). In 1990, the EPA enacted an Asbestos Phase-out Rule to eliminate the importation, manufacture, or processing of the vast majority of all asbestos products in the United States over a period of years (9,10).

TABLE 111-2. History of U.S. exposure standards for asbestos

Organization issuing standard	Year[a]	PEL/TLV[b]
ACGIH	1946	5 mp/ft^3
ACGIH	1968	12 f/cm^3 (2 mp/ft^3)
Department of Labor	1969	12 f/cm^3
OSHA	1971	5 f/cm^3
OSHA	1976	2 f/cm^3
OSHA	1986	0.2 f/cm^3
OSHA	1994	0.1 f/cm^3

ACGIH, American Conference of Governmental Industrial Hygienists; f/cm^3, fibers per cubic centimeter; mp/ft^3, million particles per cubic foot of air; OSHA, U.S. Occupational Safety and Health Administration; PEL, permissible exposure limit (mandatory, issued by OSHA); TLV, threshold limit value (advisory, issued by the ACGIH).
[a]Year OSHA PEL went into effect (year of final rule) or TLV was issued by the ACGIH.
[b]PELS and TLVs are for 8-hour time-weighted average exposures.
Adapted from refs. 7 and 9.

Heavy, unprotected asbestos exposures now are rare in the United States and in most developed countries. Because most epidemiologic studies of asbestos-related disease are based on occupational groups who have experienced heavy exposures before 1970, the risk estimates derived from these studies do not reflect the health risks for similar jobs today.

However, because diseases caused by asbestos often have latency periods of 10 to 40 years or longer, many workers who were heavily exposed in the past will continue to develop asbestos-related diseases in the coming decades. Asbestos present in existing structures, plants, ships, and equipment also will remain a potential hazard for workers who demolish, repair, or refurbish them. In addition, asbestosis and other asbestos-related diseases may continue to be significant problems in many rapidly industrializing third world countries where occupational exposures are not well controlled (4,5).

Epidemiologic studies of asbestos have generally focused on cumulative lifetime exposure as the most important risk factor for asbestos-related diseases. These exposure estimates for individuals are based on either years worked in specific job categories multiplied by estimated exposures for these jobs or asbestos fiber counts from lung tissue specimens. Exposure estimates based on work history can be inaccurate because historical data on exposure levels and fiber mix seldom are known and probably vary greatly over the working life of an individual. Retrospective studies also often lack good work histories. Basing exposure estimates on fiber counts of lung tissue specimens also has limitations (see the section Deposition and Clearance of Asbestos Fibers) (5).

The differential toxic effects of specific fiber types have been investigated in many studies. These studies have focused on groups whose lifetime exposures appeared to be predominantly to a single fiber type, such as chrysotile miners in Quebec, gas-mask assemblers in England (who worked primarily with crocidolite), and those living near anthophyllite outcroppings in Finland. Typically, these studies have found crocidolite to be most toxic in causing asbestos-related diseases; amosite has intermediate toxicity, and chrysotile is least toxic.

However, recent studies suggest that the supposedly "pure" forms of asbestos seem to be contaminated with small amounts of other fiber types. Such contamination is a confounding factor that makes difficult the drawing of conclusions about unique effects of a specific fiber type. For example, chrysotile from one mine in Quebec, which was previously believed to be pure, has been found to contain small amounts of tremolite, which may be a major cause of toxicity for this material (5).

ASBESTOS EXPOSURES IN BUILDING OCCUPANTS

Since the 1980s, there has been public concern about health risk from exposures to low levels of airborne asbestos among occupants in schools and other public buildings. Asbestos has been used extensively in these buildings since World War II for boiler and pipe insulation, spray-on insulation, and fireproofing for ceilings and structural beams and as a component in wallboard, floor tiles, and ceiling tiles. An estimated 20% of all buildings in the United States have some ACM, which is defined by both the EPA and OSHA as any material containing more than 1% asbestos (9,11).

Asbestos found in buildings is a health hazard only if it is friable (that is, if it is capable of easily releasing asbestos fibers into the air). In buildings, ACMs that have the highest potential for being friable include sprayed-on decorative ceilings and sprayed-on insulation on structural beams or walls. Other types of ACMs in buildings, such as that found in formed thermal insulation, floor tiles, or wallboard, generally is not friable unless the material has been cut, ground, or otherwise damaged or if it has deteriorated so that asbestos fibers can be released (10).

Surveys of airborne asbestos fibers in public buildings and schools known to contain asbestos found mean levels of 0.0004 to 0.0010 fiber per cubic centimeter of air even when damaged ACM was present. These levels of exposure are 100 to 200 times lower than the OSHA PEL and up to 5,000 times lower than the heavy asbestos exposures experienced before 1970 by those worker cohorts that have been the subjects of most epidemiologic studies of asbestos-related disease (see the section, Low-Level Asbestos Exposures and Public Policy) (11).

In contrast, there is evidence that custodians and other maintenance workers in buildings with ACM can experience significant asbestos exposures. Four studies of school custodians in Boston, New York City, Wisconsin, and California found that 11% to 33% had asbestos-related changes on chest radiographs, including pleural plaques and interstitial fibrosis (12–15). Although these studies all had methodological flaws, the findings do suggest that many school maintenance workers had significant asbestos exposures, at least before the 1970s. Building maintenance tasks with the highest potential for asbestos exposure include asbestos removal, drywall demolition or repair, repair of boiler insulation, work above dropped ceilings, and work on lighting or ventilation systems (16).

ASBESTOS EXPOSURES IN OUTDOOR AMBIENT AIR

Asbestos fibers can be found in the outdoor ambient air in all industrialized and urban areas. These fibers come from a variety of sources including worn or damaged asbestos-containing building materials, demolished buildings, worn automobile brake shoes, and improper disposal of asbestos wastes. In some areas, asbestos also enters the atmosphere from weathering of natural rock formations or surface wastes of mines. Levels of asbestos found in ambient atmosphere in industrialized areas in the United States are very low (typically less than 0.0001 fiber per cubic centimeter of air) and are not considered significant health risks (17).

ASBESTOS IN DRINKING WATER AND FOOD

Asbestos is found in very low concentrations as a normal contaminant in drinking water in many areas of the United States. Much of this contamination comes from water passing over natural formations of asbestos-containing rock, and some may come from asbestos cement pipes. Asbestos fibers also are found in trace amounts as a contaminant in some processed foods. These exposures to asbestos fibers in drinking water and food are not considered significant health risks (18).

CLINICAL TOXICOLOGY

Routes of Exposure

INHALATION

Inhalation of asbestos fibers is the only significant route of exposure leading to adverse health effects. Asbestos appears to exert its effect either by direct contact with lung tissue (as a possible basis for carcinogenesis) or by stimulating an acute and chronic inflammatory reaction in lung tissue (as in asbestosis). Asbestos in the lungs does not become absorbed into the blood, so there is no true systemic effect, although fibers can mechanically penetrate and migrate through lung tissue and can enter the lymphatic system in the lungs.

INGESTION

The primary source of ingestion of asbestos fibers is from inhaled asbestos that is captured in respiratory mucus and then swallowed. Trace amounts of asbestos are ingested also in drinking water and food. Most authorities believe that ingestion of asbestos fibers does not lead to adverse health effects. Asbestos fibers in the gastrointestinal tract have been found to penetrate the gastrointestinal mucosa, especially about the cecum. However, these ingested asbestos fibers are not systemically absorbed, and they do not appear to stimulate an inflammatory reaction, cancer, or any other adverse effect. A metaanalysis of studies of colon cancer and asbestos exposure found no convincing evidence that exposure to asbestos increased the risk for colon cancer (19,20).

SKIN CONTACT AND OTHER ROUTES OF EXPOSURE

Asbestos fibers have no adverse effects on contact with the eyes, intact skin, or wounds, and asbestos is not absorbed through the skin. Proper safety practices for working with asbestos do include protective clothing to keep asbestos fibers off the skin and clothes, but this is to avoid carrying fibers out of the workplace where they may later be reentrained in the air and inhaled. No routes of exposure to asbestos other than inhalation appear to cause adverse health effects.

Deposition and Clearance of Asbestos Fibers

DEPOSITION IN THE LUNG

As with any inhaled particles, the pattern of initial deposition of asbestos fibers in the lungs is determined by particle size and shape, the principles of aerodynamics (i.e., the settling time of fibers and airflow dynamics), and the physical structure and protective mechanisms of the respiratory system. A *fiber* is defined as a particle with a length-to-diameter ratio of more than 3:1. The settling time of fibers is inversely related to the square of its diameter. For a typical asbestos fiber 5 μm long and 1 μm in diameter, the settling time in still air is approximately 4 hours. Air turbulence from a person walking into a room can reentrain settled asbestos fibers into the air, so that free asbestos particles in an area should be assumed to be airborne by persons entering that space.

When asbestos is inhaled, many larger fibers more than 10 to 20 μm long are filtered out in the upper airways or collide with the walls of the conducting airway walls in the lungs, where they are captured in the respiratory mucus. These fibers then are removed from the lung by the mucociliary elevator and are coughed up or swallowed. Occasionally, fibers up to 100 μm long are seen in the lungs, especially if they are draped over a branch point of conducting airways in a saddlelike effect. Due to their aerodynamic properties, asbestos fibers less than 10 μm long are more likely to stay in the center of the air stream and eventually reach the alveoli (21,22).

CLEARANCE AND PERSISTENCE OF FIBERS IN THE LUNGS

Asbestos fibers deposited in the alveoli can undergo a variety of fates. Some fibers penetrate the alveolar walls and enter the interstitial fluid, where they may be cleared by the lymphatic drainage and deposited in the perihilar lymph nodes. Other fibers, especially amphiboles, may penetrate the lung parenchyma and enter the pleural space or the peritoneal space (via the diaphragm). The fibers that remain in place in the alveoli can become engulfed by respiratory macrophages with varying results.

Chrysotile appears to be more susceptible to degradation by respiratory macrophages than do amphiboles, which may explain why chrysotile is the least toxic of the asbestos fiber types. This also explains why chrysotile is found in smaller amounts in lung tissue autopsy specimens than are amphibole fibers, even though most asbestos exposures in the United States probably involve chrysotile.

Amphibole fibers longer than 10 μm are not easily degraded by macrophages and tend to persist in the alveoli. Some of these larger fibers become partially engulfed by macrophages but are not degraded. Instead, the macrophage dies, leaving a brown, iron-containing, proteinaceous coating about the fiber; this is known as an *asbestos body* and can be seen on light microscopy of lung tissue or sputum after iron staining has been performed. Asbestos bodies found in sputum, bronchoscopy washings, or lung tissue specimens do indicate prior asbestos exposure but cannot be reliably used to determine the degree of exposure or to diagnose asbestos-related disease.

The numbers, sizes, and types of asbestos fibers deposited in the lung have been studied extensively in specimens from autopsy and open lung biopsy. This involves treating the lung tissue with a chemical that dissolves the tissue but leaves the asbestos fibers intact. Fibers then are counted using standard techniques, with results reported as the numbers and types of fibers per gram of dried lung. The numbers and types of asbestos fibers present can be used as a rough estimate of cumulative asbestos exposure. This technique has been used extensively to study dose-response relationships for asbestos-related diseases. One problem with this technique is that fiber counts from lung tissue are likely to underrepresent a person's cumulative exposure to chrysotile as compared to their exposure to amphiboles, as chrysotile fibers are much more easily cleared from the lung by alveolar macrophages than are amphiboles. Asbestos fibers can be found in bronchial washings obtained by bronchoscopy, but estimating the amount of asbestos deposited in the lung using this technique is difficult.

A background level of asbestos appears to exist in the lungs of the general population in the United States, measuring less than 1 million fibers per gram of dried lung (or fewer than 100 asbestos bodies per gram of wet lung). Individuals with a history of occupational asbestos exposure generally have at least three times this number of fibers in the lungs, whereas those persons with asbestosis have more than 100 times the background level, as illustrated in Table 111-3 (23–25). Using this method for estimating cumulative exposure, the dose-response relationship between asbestos exposure and disease appears to be strong for asbestosis and lung cancer but less strong for mesothelioma (for which only a small increase in fiber burden may exist in patients as compared to that in a nonexposed population).

As stated previously, reliance on fiber counts in lung tissue to estimate exposures presents some problems, as amphiboles are more persistent in the lung than are chrysotile fibers. Chrysotile fibers in the alveoli have a greater tendency either to dissolve or to be removed by macrophages, possibly because, with time, magnesium leaches out of the fibers, which may make them more susceptible to degradation. In addition, the extent to which asbestosis is related to acute reactions to chrysotile fibers, which then are cleared, and to chronic reactions to persistent amphibole fibers is uncertain (4,5,25–28).

TABLE 111-3. Asbestos fiber counts in lung tissue correlated with exposure setting and disease state

Exposure setting and disease state	Amosite and crocidolite (fibers/g dry lung × 10^6)		Chrysotile and tremolite (fibers/g dry lung × 10^6)	
	Range	Mean	Range	Mean
Occupational groups	Shipyard and insulation workers[a]		Chrysotile mining and milling[b]	
Asbestosis	1.0–100.0	26	50–1,200	110
Mesothelioma	0.07–35.00	0.7	50–2,200	290
General public, no disease[c]	0.0–0.3	0	0.00–0.25	0.4

[a]These shipyard and insulation workers from Vancouver, British Columbia, were exposed primarily to crocidolite and amosite but also had some chrysotile exposures (23).
[b]These chrysotile milling and mining workers from Quebec had no significant amphibole exposures except for tremolite found as a natural contaminant in the chrysotile ore (23).
[c]Analysis of autopsy specimens from persons in Vancouver, British Columbia, who had no known history of occupational asbestos exposures (24).
Adapted from refs. 23 and 24.

Signs, Symptoms, and Syndromes from Exposure

TARGET ORGAN TOXICITY

The only target organ affected acutely by asbestos is the lung, although no clinical effects are noted from acute asbestos exposures. However, recent research suggests that, within weeks after asbestos fibers are inhaled into the lungs, an asymptomatic inflammatory reaction does occur at the level of the terminal bronchioles and alveoli (5). This is the first stage of a reaction that may lead to asbestosis (see the section, Asbestosis) (5).

All chronic adverse health effects from asbestos are related to fibers being inhaled in the lungs. The target organs affected chronically are the lungs (asbestosis and lung cancer), pleura (malignant mesothelioma, benign pleural effusion, pleural plaques, pleural thickening), pericardium (benign effusion), and peritoneum (mesothelioma).

Recently, controversy among some researchers has centered on whether asbestos can be a causative factor for clinically significant small-airways disease and therefore a contributing factor for development of chronic obstructive pulmonary disease (COPD). Studying this issue is difficult, because workers with asbestos-related diseases also have a history of being heavy smokers, and smoking is a well-known cause of COPD. However, several well-controlled studies have not found any evidence that asbestos contributes to small-airways disease or COPD (4).

No convincing evidence exists that links asbestos with any adverse effects on other target organs. Although asbestos exposure has been implicated as a cause of other types of cancers, particularly colon cancer and laryngeal cancer, no clear association has been found (see the section, Carcinogenesis) (4).

ASBESTOSIS

Epidemiology. All types of asbestos fibers can cause asbestosis, but the amphiboles, especially crocidolite, are more potent or toxic than are exposures to equivalent amounts of chrysotile. Although it is clear that higher doses impart a greater risk, the exact nature of the dose-response relationship and differences in toxicity by fiber types are difficult to determine because of inherent problems in both epidemiologic and pathologic studies of the issue. Smoking does increase the risk of developing asbestosis, perhaps in part because it leads to decreased clearance of asbestos fibers from the lung (5).

Pathophysiology. Asbestosis is an interstitial fibrosis of the lung parenchyma due to asbestos exposure; it is a form of pneumoconiosis, as are silicosis and coal workers' pneumoconiosis. This is a nonmalignant disease that occurs only after heavy and prolonged asbestos exposures.

The typical latency period between first exposure to asbestos and diagnosis is usually more than 20 years, but this depends greatly on the person's cumulative dose. Some researchers have published reports of workers with extremely heavy exposures in the early 1900s who developed asbestosis after as few as 5 years from time of first exposure. In contrast, for the cohort of insulators studied by Selikoff (who all had at least 20 years of heavy asbestos exposure during and after World War II), the latency periods between first exposure and clinically apparent asbestosis were typically 20 to 30 years. The evidence suggests that for persons with even lower cumulative asbestos exposures, especially those first exposed after the mid-1960s, the latency period between first exposure and clinically apparent asbestosis may be 40 years or longer (5).

The primary lesion of asbestosis is fibrosis around the terminal bronchiole, which then extends to the adjacent alveoli. This appears to be caused by an inflammatory response to asbestos fibers deposited in the alveoli and probably is mediated by respiratory macrophages. Asbestos fibers in the alveolar spaces stimulate both acute and chronic inflammatory responses. Within several weeks after deposition of asbestos fibers in the alveoli, an acute inflammatory response occurs in which respiratory macrophages attempt to digest the fibers with varying results. In this process, macrophages release various chemical mediators that stimulate an infiltrate of neutrophils and eosinophils and also induce formation of fibrous tissue (28,29).

Fibers less than 5 μm long, and especially chrysotile, are readily digested by the macrophages. However, larger amphibole fibers are not as easily dissolved or readily digested; they tend to persist in the alveoli and apparently stimulate a chronic antiinflammatory response. Fibrous tissue forms about the alveoli, inhibiting passive diffusion of oxygen from the alveolar space into the pulmonary capillaries (resulting in ventilation-perfusion abnormalities). As fibrosis becomes more extensive, the lung contracts and loses elasticity. However, asbestos does not appear to cause obstructive lung disease in these individuals.

In approximately one-third of those who develop asbestosis, the disease progresses to severe pulmonary fibrosis. In these cases, the diffuse fibrosis and contraction of lung tissue constricts the pulmonary vasculature, causing pulmonary hypertension, which often leads to death from right-sided heart failure. The two-thirds of asbestosis patients in whom severe pulmonary fibrosis does not develop may experience very little limitation in their daily activities, especially as they tend to be an older group that already has cut back on vigorous physical activities. Persons with milder exposures to asbestos are not likely to progress. No effective preventive measures or treatments for asbestosis are known (5,30).

Individuals with advanced asbestosis are more susceptible to pulmonary infections, possibly owing to altered lung anatomy and mechanics. Lung cancer is the most common cause of death among those with asbestosis. In addition, strong evidence suggests that development of asbestosis may be a necessary condition for the development of asbestos-related lung cancer (see the sections, Lung Cancer and Carcinogenesis) (4,5,31).

Clinical Presentation. The first symptoms of asbestosis are dyspnea with exertion and reduced exercise tolerance. These early effects may be overlooked or interpreted as normal changes of aging, as they usually occur when individuals are in their fifties or sixties and are no longer engaging in vigorous physical exertion. Other manifestations include cough and inspiratory rales in the lung bases.

Sputum production is not a manifestation of asbestosis itself but frequently is seen because many with asbestosis also have COPD due to smoking and are more susceptible to lung infections. Finally, chest pain due to asbestosis is not common but may be related to lung cancer or mesothelioma, which are significant risks for those with asbestos exposures heavy enough to have caused asbestosis (5).

The two-thirds of asbestosis patients who do not progress to severe pulmonary fibrosis may experience little practical limitation on normal activities. For those whose disease does progress, dyspnea with exertion worsens and may lead to dyspnea at rest, clubbing of the fingers, and cyanosis. If severe pulmonary fibrosis develops, signs of pulmonary hypertension and right-sided heart failure are seen (5,30).

Diagnostic Tests. With asbestosis, the earliest physiologic changes to be detected are reduced forced vital capacity (FVC), lung volumes, lung compliance, and lung diffusing capacity (32). Decreased oxygen saturation of arterial blood on maximal exercise is a later finding that suggests advanced disease; this is diagnosed by analyzing arterial blood from an indwelling arterial catheter during exercise stress testing. As the disease progresses, decreased oxygen saturation of arterial blood can be seen at rest. Asbestos does not appear to cause obstructive lung disease, so the ratio of FVC to forced expiratory volume over 1 second may remain normal unless other disease processes are present (33,34).

Chest radiographic abnormalities consistent with asbestosis may be seen either before or after abnormalities in lung function tests are noted. Typical findings include evidence of parenchymal interstitial fibrosis, first noted as small opacities in the periphery of the lung, especially in the lung bases. This may progress to more diffuse opacification of the lung parenchyma. Asbestos-related pleural changes may also be seen on radiography, but these are disease processes separate from asbestosis (5,32).

A standard rating system has been developed by the International Labor Organization (ILO) for interpreting chest radiographic changes of asbestosis and other pneumoconioses. This system uses standardized scales to rate the extent of parenchymal fibrosis as well as asbestos-related pleural changes (35). The National Institute of Occupational Safety and Health certifies physicians who interpret chest radiographs using the ILO criteria; those who pass the certification examination are designated as *B-readers*. Interpretation of chest radiographs by a B-reader is required by the OSHA medical surveillance standard for asbestos and is considered the standard of care for diagnosing asbestos-related diseases (7).

Although the intent of the ILO criteria is to promote consistency in interpreting chest radiographs, a great deal of variation still exists among B-readers in interpreting normal versus mild changes of asbestosis on chest radiographs. Interpretation of these borderline cases presents a major problem in evaluating the validity and significance of epidemiologic and clinical studies and is also often a contentious issue in litigation.

Treatment and Prevention. No effective treatment is known for asbestosis once it has developed. The only effective preventive measure is to keep large quantities of asbestos fibers out of the lungs, as individuals with low cumulative exposures (less than 5 fiber-years) do not appear to develop this disease.

Whether those with objective evidence of asbestosis should be restricted from working around asbestos remains controversial. Some studies suggest that once asbestosis has started, further inhalation of asbestos fibers causes acute inflammatory reactions that can worsen the disease. However, in the United States, individuals with asbestosis probably do not need to be removed from work with asbestos as long as proper protective equipment and work practices are used, as these measures should effectively prevent workers from inhaling asbestos fibers (4,7).

LUNG CANCER

Epidemiology. Several studies have shown an increased incidence of lung cancer, or bronchogenic carcinoma, in groups of workers with moderate to heavy asbestos exposure. All fiber types are associated with this disease, but crocidolite is most toxic, followed by amosite and chrysotile. Approximately

130,000 persons die of lung cancer in the United States annually, and nearly 5% of these cases are attributed at least partially to asbestos exposure, whereas cigarette smoking accounts for at least 85%. A dose-response relationship appears to exist for cumulative asbestos exposures that are moderate to heavy, but this may not hold true at very low doses (36–40).

Cigarette smokers who have also had heavy cumulative asbestos exposure have a combined lung cancer risk greater than expected for each exposure alone. Selikoff's study of insulators with 20 years of heavy asbestos exposure found that, as compared to nonsmokers with no asbestos exposures, the relative risks for lung cancer in the asbestos-exposed workers were 5.0 for nonsmokers and 50 to 84 for cigarette smokers. This was compared to other studies of non-asbestos-exposed persons in whom the relative risk for lung cancer was 11.0 for cigarette smokers as compared to nonsmokers (1,36,41).

Previous theories maintained that very low cumulative exposures to asbestos presented a real, although small, risk for developing lung cancer. However, a significant amount of evidence now exists that indicates that asbestos-related lung cancer occurs only after very large cumulative asbestos exposures. Several studies suggest that lung cancer due to asbestos exposure occurs only in the presence of asbestosis, suggesting that this may be a type of scar cancer (25,36,37).

The threshold dose (i.e., cumulative asbestos exposure) needed to develop lung cancer from asbestos exposure appears to be the same as that required for the development of asbestosis—that is, a cumulative exposure of 5 fiber-years. This would require 50 years of exposure at the current OSHA PEL of 0.1 fiber per cubic centimeter of air. Persons with cumulative exposures below this level may not be at any actual increased risk for lung cancer (42–45).

Pathophysiology. Lung cancer related to asbestos exposure appears to be histologically the same as lung cancer caused by cigarette smoking, radiation, or chemical carcinogens. The latency period for lung cancer is generally 20 to 30 years. Lung cancer begins in the lung parenchyma and invades locally, often blocking airways and eroding into blood vessels, thus leading to hemoptysis. Metastatic spread also occurs throughout the lung and to other parts of the body, especially to the spine or brain.

The reasons for the greatly increased risk of lung cancer from combined exposure to asbestos and cigarette smoking are not clear. Smoking itself is the most common cause of lung cancer. Cigarette smoke also inhibits ciliary function in the lung epithelium, inhibiting clearance of asbestos from the lung and possibly increasing the risk of lung cancer from asbestos.

In the period during and after World War II, when many U.S. workers had their heaviest asbestos exposures, the prevalence of cigarette smoking among blue collar workers was approximately 80%. Because lung cancer caused by asbestos and cigarette smoking look the same histologically, attribution of the cause of lung cancer is often a contentious issue in litigation in the United States. In Germany and the United Kingdom, lung cancer is legally attributed to asbestos if asbestosis is also present (5,41).

Clinical Presentation. The presenting symptoms of lung cancer can vary. Chest pain, chronic cough, hemoptysis, and decreased exercise tolerance may reflect local extension about the airways. In some cases, subtle neurologic symptoms due to metastases to the brain may be the presenting sign (5).

Diagnostic Tests. The diagnosis usually is first suspected on the basis of an abnormal chest radiograph. No screening tests exist that can effectively diagnose lung cancer at an early enough stage to effect improved survival. Neither periodic chest radiographs nor sputum cytologic testing has been useful in screening high-risk populations.

Computed tomography (CT) scans and magnetic resonance imaging can sometimes detect small lesions not seen on chest radiographs. Although these tests can be useful in establishing the diagnosis of lung cancer, they have not been evaluated as screening tools. Tissue biopsy via bronchoscopy or thoracotomy usually is obtained to confirm the diagnosis. The presenting finding may also be a pleural effusion that may or may not contain malignant cells (5).

Treatment and Prevention. At the time of diagnosis, lung cancer usually is too advanced for successful curative treatment, although palliative treatment often is initiated. Although improvements have been made in the treatment of lung cancer in recent years, the long-term survival rates are still low after surgical resection and treatment with chemotherapy or radiation therapy. The only proved preventive measures are to keep asbestos fibers out of the lungs and to avoid cigarette smoking.

MESOTHELIOMA

Mesothelioma is another type of malignancy associated with asbestos exposure. Asbestos is the only known cause for this tumor in the United States, and a history of significant asbestos exposure is found in 80% of cases; the causative agent in the other 20% of cases is unknown. Residents of the Cappadocia region of Turkey have a high incidence of mesothelioma from exposures to erionite (a mineral fiber similar to asbestos) in the soil and rock outcroppings, but such exposures do not occur in the United States (46).

The latency period for mesothelioma is 40 or more years from first asbestos exposure. A strong dose-response relationship appears to exist between the cumulative asbestos exposure and mesothelioma, and all fiber types have been associated with this tumor. As with asbestosis and lung cancer, crocidolite is most toxic, followed by amosite and chrysotile. However, the evidence suggests that chrysotile is associated with mesothelioma only after very high cumulative exposures and when this material is highly contaminated with amphiboles (especially fibrous tremolite). Smokers are at no increased risk for mesothelioma as compared with nonsmokers (46).

Many studies of worker groups with heavy asbestos exposures have found increased risks for mesothelioma. Cohorts of asbestos insulators with historically high cumulative asbestos exposures have been shown to have death rates of 7% to 10% from mesothelioma. However, mesotheliomas have also been reported in persons with moderately low asbestos exposures. Mesotheliomas have developed in family members of asbestos workers (in whom the primary exposure was apparently asbestos fibers carried home on the workers' clothes) and in persons living near crocidolite mines in South Africa (in whom the primary exposures were from wind-borne fibers in the environment). However, studies have not shown increased risk for mesothelioma in groups with very low-dose asbestos exposures, such as are seen in the general urban environment or to occupants of buildings containing asbestos (26,46).

Studies show that persons exposed primarily to chrysotile will develop mesotheliomas only after very high cumulative exposures. Research suggests that in most of these individuals, mesotheliomas have actually been caused by exposure to the amphibole fiber tremolite. Tremolite has been found as a natural contaminant in much chrysotile asbestos, including the chrysotile mined in Quebec, which historically has been the most common type of asbestos used in the United States. Studies of workers in the chrysotile mining and milling industry in Quebec have found that those workers who developed mesothelioma all had lung asbestos fiber counts at least twice the lowest cumulative exposure required to produce asbestosis. This indicates that very heavy exposures to chrysotile and to fibrous tremolite were required to produce mesothelioma (47).

Pathophysiology. Mesotheliomas appear to be initiated by asbestos fibers that have migrated through the lung parenchyma to the pleural surfaces or through the diaphragm to the peritoneum. Presumably, a chronic irritation from these fibers stimulates malignant cell growth. Experiments with rodents show that when asbestos is injected into the pleural space, it is a complete carcinogen with both initiating and promoting properties (4,48).

As the tumor grows, it further expands in the pleural and peritoneal spaces but does not metastasize. Portions of the lung parenchyma and pulmonary vasculature may become compressed or entrapped in the tumor, leading to reduced air exchange and pulmonary hypertension. Death may be due to respiratory or cardiac failure or to general debilitation from the tumor. Survival is usually less than 1 year after diagnosis (46).

Clinical Presentation. The first symptoms of mesothelioma are those associated with pleural irritation, such as chest pain and dyspnea. In contrast to lung cancer, hemoptysis is not common, as airways are not eroded. The diagnosis often is first suggested by a chest radiograph showing a pleural effusion or a mass; half of these show calcifications. Chest radiographic evidence of interstitial fibrosis (indicating asbestosis) or pleural thickening is seen in approximately 20% of cases at diagnosis.

Pleural effusions due to mesothelioma may not be attributed initially to this disease, as malignant cells are not always seen in pleurocentesis fluid. CT and magnetic resonance imaging scans may be useful in establishing the presence of a mass. A tissue biopsy obtained by thoracotomy or laparotomy usually is necessary to confirm the diagnosis, as needle biopsy specimens often are inadequate. Even after adequate tissue is obtained, the histologic interpretation often is difficult and may be confused with inflammatory reactions, exuberant mesothelial hyperplasia, or metastatic cancer (46,49,50).

Treatment and Prevention. No effective treatment is known for mesothelioma, and death usually occurs within 1 year after diagnosis. Chemotherapy and surgical resection may prolong survival in a few select cases but generally have limited usefulness. Radiation therapy may be useful for pain relief. The only effective preventive measure is avoidance of significant asbestos exposure (46).

NONMALIGNANT PLEURAL DISEASES

Epidemiology. Nonmalignant pleural changes are the fourth major type of health effect caused by asbestos. These include benign pleural effusions, pleural thickening, pleural plaques, and rounded atelectasis.

Pathophysiology. The cause of nonmalignant pleural changes is not clear but is presumed to be related to irritation effects from asbestos fibers that migrate through the lung parenchyma to lodge in the pleura. Benign pleural effusions are seen in a small number of workers. The diagnosis is made if there is a history of significant asbestos exposure and all other causes of effusion have been ruled out. Symptoms, which are seen in only one-third of cases, include dyspnea and pleuritic pain. Most effusions resolve spontaneously (51).

Pleural thickening related to asbestos is most often seen in the lower lobes and can be unilateral or bilateral. Histologically, asbestos-related pleural thickening may not be distinguishable from pleural thickening due to other causes such as lung infections. Rounded atelectasis occurs when pleural fibrosis entraps adjacent lung parenchyma; on chest radiography, this sometimes is mistaken for a tumor (52).

Pleural plaques form as discrete confluent patches of fibrohyaline tissue on the pleural surfaces of the chest wall or diaphragm and, occasionally, the pericardium. They may become calcified. Pleural plaques are considered pathognomonic signs of asbestos exposure and are the most common diagnostic test finding related to asbestos exposure (53).

The dose-response relationships and the relative toxicity of fiber types are not as well defined for these nonmalignant pleural conditions as for other asbestos-related diseases. Whether smokers are at increased risk for these problems remains unclear (31,51).

Clinical Presentation. In the past, all of these pleural changes were regarded as markers of asbestos exposure that probably had no functional significance. However, recent studies suggest that extensive diffuse pleural thickening, with or without pleural plaques, can produce significant restrictive lung disease leading to dyspnea with exertion, or even at rest, and reduced exercise capacity, even in those without significant asbestosis. Few other clinical manifestations may be seen (31).

Diagnostic Tests. Nonmalignant pleural diseases usually are first suspected on the basis of chest radiographic findings. Pleural plaques noted on chest radiography may be subtle and can be confused with old rib fractures or pleural fat pads. On a standard posteroanterior chest radiograph, a plaque covering the anterior of the chest, known as an *en face plaque*, may not be identified easily and can be mistaken for a parenchymal infiltrate or tumor. Oblique and lateral radiographic views often reveal such plaques well and are obtained routinely by some clinicians evaluating asbestos-related disease. CT scans can more accurately differentiate plaques from fat pads and lesions in the lung parenchyma (5,32).

Depending on the extent of involvement, lung function tests may show restrictive disease with decreases in FVC, residual capacity, and measurements of lung compliance. However, diffusing capacity should be normal unless there is concomitant parenchymal fibrosis due to asbestosis. Exercise testing may also be useful in determining to what extent restrictive impairment is due to pleural disease versus parenchymal fibrosis related to asbestosis (5,31,32,34,53).

Treatment and Prevention. No effective treatments are known for these nonmalignant pleural diseases. In addition, the only reliable preventive measure is keeping asbestos fibers out of the lungs.

TERATOGENESIS

Asbestos has not been implicated as a teratogen. Asbestos fibers are not absorbed into the blood, and they do not cross the placenta.

CARCINOGENESIS

Asbestos does cause lung cancer and malignant mesothelioma (see earlier). Some studies have suggested that asbestos exposure is associated also with cancers of the larynx, colon, kidney, pancreas, ovary, and eye, and with lymphomas. However, no convincing evidence exists to associate asbestos with increased rates of any of these cancers.

The potential association between asbestos exposure and colon cancer has been evaluated in more that 30 epidemiologic studies. Most of these studies, and a recent metaanalysis on the topic, found no increased risk for colon cancer associated with asbestos exposures (19,20). Some studies have shown a slightly increased risk of laryngeal cancer from asbestos exposure, but this was insignificant when compared with the much larger attributed risks for this cancer from alcohol consumption and smoking (20,54).

Recognition by the general medical community that all forms of asbestos caused lung cancer occurred after publication of the seminal work of Selikoff in 1965 (55). Studies by Wagner (56) in South Africa and others in Great Britain in the 1960s suggested that exposure to crocidolite was strongly associated with the development of mesotheliomas. Amosite also was incriminated as a cause of mesotheliomas in 1972. It now is generally recognized that the majority of mesotheliomas are probably due to amphibole exposures (57).

Determining the mechanisms of asbestos-related carcinogenesis has been the subject of extensive research over the last 30 years. The role of different mechanisms of asbestos-related cell injury and tumor initiation is unresolved. Asbestos fibers may incite tumor formation either through indirect mechanisms (e.g., formation of active oxygen species or growth factors) or by fiber-induced direct interference with cell division (58).

Asbestos is unique among the carcinogens in that most mutagens are genotoxic and cause abnormalities or evidence of DNA damage when assayed by the Ames test. Asbestos is not mutagenic according to the Ames test but is genotoxic when a sensitive human-hamster hybrid cell is used. We now know that asbestos fibers cause point mutations and large deletions of chromosomes in normal cells. Recent studies using high-resolution time-lapse microscopy have demonstrated that long asbestos fibers interfere with chromosome distribution during cell division, causing genomic changes such as chromosomal deletions, translocations, and aneuploidy (59). These genomic changes lead to cell transformation and neoplastic progression. Such chromosomal changes have been found in asbestos-related mesotheliomas and lung cancers.

Asbestos as a carcinogen has been associated with lengthy latency periods from initial exposure to the development of cancer. Asbestos, like various other carcinogens, causes genetic changes in the cell that occur over a long period. A series of oncogenic mutations must occur before the actual tumor develops and, presumably, the greater number of mutations required or the length of time required to produce these mutations explains the long latency period from asbestos exposure to the development of an asbestos-related neoplasm.

Asbestos fibers are taken up by inflammatory cells such as pulmonary macrophages in the lung, and these inflammatory cells in turn release cytokines as well as active oxygen species. The chronic production of transforming growth factor, insulin-like growth factor II, and other cytokines such as platelet-derived growth factor is responsible for recruitment of inflammatory cells. Mesothelial cells may produce these cytokines by an autocrine loop, which, in turn, perpetuates the inflammatory response (60). Asbestos-induced cell proliferation in both epithelial cells and mesothelial cells via growth factors is important to tumor cell initiation, promotion, and progression (61). This may be a secondary effect of active oxygen species generation, or the cytokines may incite other direct effects on mutagenesis and genetic changes in cells. This is an area of current research.

Asbestos is primarily a cytotoxin, meaning that it causes changes in the genetic makeup of a cell. Another purported mechanism of cell and genome damage is thought to be related to the propensity of long asbestos fibers to invoke a chronic inflammatory reaction, which then evokes the recruitment of cell-damaging cytokines and inflammatory products. Numerous investigators have noted that active oxygen species are produced when asbestos is placed in a medium with cultured lymphocytes. The critical target molecule for reactive oxygen species is DNA (62). A variety of antitoxic enzymes such as superoxide dismutase inhibit asbestos-related cytotoxicity. Free iron catalyzes the formation of the highly toxic hydroxyl radical (OH) from superoxide anion (O_2^-) and hydrogen peroxide (H_2O_2) through the Harber-Weiss reaction. Only minute quantities of free iron are necessary for catalytic enhancement of this reaction. Iron chelation inhibits the formation of free radicals in cell culture and indicates that iron seems to be a critical and necessary cofactor in asbestos-induced cytotoxicity, liquid preoccupation, and DNA breakage (63).

Chrysotile asbestos contains relatively little iron (approximately 2% to 3% in the average sample), whereas crocidolite asbestos, which generally is considered to be the most carcinogenic form of asbestos, contains up to 36% iron by weight. It has been reported that individuals who consume excessive amounts of iron are at increased risk of developing cancer. Iron appears to be toxic and, when asbestos fibers are phagocytized, abnormal release of iron may occur that is not controlled by the proteins involved in normal iron metabolism. Administration of the antioxidant enzyme catalase to rats during inhalation of asbestos fibers can ameliorate inflammation, lung damage, and pulmonary fibrosis or asbestosis. It seems plausible that asbestos fiber iron content relates to its carcinogenicity. In fact, the evidence that asbestos-related cytotoxicity is inhibited by antitoxin enzymes and iron chelation indicates a strong biological contribution of active oxygen species and the secondary role of iron content in asbestos fibers to asbestos's toxic effects, which may have future clinical implications.

The majority of studies on asbestos-related cytotoxicity have been conducted with models of human or animal mesothelial cells in culture. Bronchial epithelial cells appear to be more resistant to the genotoxic and cytotoxic effects of asbestos. This finding correlates with clinical epidemiologic studies, which have shown a relatively low incidence of asbestos-related lung cancers in heavily exposed nonsmokers with asbestosis. Asbestos acts primarily as a cocarcinogen and promoter. Although cigarette smoke is the primary cocarcinogen with asbestos, very little information is available regarding the role of other cocarcinogens in the workplace in the induction of asbestos-related lung cancers. A variety of other carcinogens probably play an important role in the induction of asbestos-related lung cancers.

The dose required for production of an asbestos-related lung cancer must be high enough to produce asbestosis, as asbestos-related lung cancers are not seen in most clinical studies unless there is coexistent asbestosis (42). This is true also in the animal model. Thus, there appears to be a threshold dose for lung cancer and that threshold dose is the dose below which asbestosis does not develop.

The information on asbestos and mesothelioma suggests that a relatively low dose of amphibole asbestos is required for the production of a mesothelioma. This dose probably is approximately 5 fiber-years of exposure (which is equivalent to 3 to 4 months of employment in an area of heavy exposure in a shipyard during World War II or to 50 years of exposure at the current OSHA PEL for asbestos). Once the exposure has occurred, some of the asbestos fibers migrate to the pleura. The experimental animal data suggest that it is the longer, thinner fibers, primarily fibers less than 0.1 μm in diameter, that are most mesotheliogenic. Once trapped in the pleural space, these fibers generate reactive oxygen species and produce chronic cytotoxicity. A series of mutations then occur over a period of many years, probably at least 20 to 30 years, before the actual mesothelioma is produced, after which time these malignant tumor cells multiply slowly.

Once the malignant cell has begun to multiply, probably another 20 years pass before mesothelioma is diagnosed in the affected individual. This is supported by epidemiologic data from a metaanalysis of 1,690 cases of mesothelioma, in which 99% of cases had a latent period of more than 15 years and 95% had a latent period of greater than 20 years (64). Epidemiologic studies indicate that the earliest exposures are most likely to be causative and, therefore, statistical methods of latency analysis are useful in determining which exposures are most likely to cause a mesothelioma.

The latest wrinkle in the causation of human mesotheliomas has been the recent evidence of an important role for simian virus 40 (SV40). This virus is native to the rhesus monkey and normally grows in monkey kidney cells without causing cytopathic changes. It gained entry into the human population through contamination of polio vaccines (oral and inactivated Salk vaccines) between 1956 and 1963. Parenteral adenovirus vaccines contaminated with SV40 were used by the military and some civilian populations between 1957 and 1960. The viral contamination was not discovered until 1960. Initial studies suggested that it was harmless, but more recent data by Pass et al. (65) in 1994 indicate that this virus is found in approximately 60% of mesotheliomas. Most of these patients had some exposure to asbestos. SV40 immortalizes itself in human mesothelial cells, but these cells are not oncogenic unless additional DNA alterations occur. Asbestos may induce DNA alterations and so may act as a cocarcinogen. Asbestos also facilitates transfection of other mesothelioma cells by SV40. The toxicologic implications of these data suggest that a certain subpopulation of humans may be at increased risk for development of a mesothelioma based on infection with SV40. A possible explanation for the high numbers of mesotheliomas diagnosed in the 1990s may be SV40 infection.

BIOLOGICAL MONITORING

Biological monitoring is not conducted for asbestos. Blood and urine tests are not useful because asbestos is not absorbed systemically, and no good biochemical marker of acute or chronic exposure exists.

ENVIRONMENTAL MONITORING

Sampling Methods

Asbestos fibers are measured in ambient air using standardized monitoring methods specified by OSHA and the EPA. Such monitoring involves pumping a measured volume of air through a piece of filter paper fixed in a container worn by individual workers (personnel monitoring) or placed in a specific area (area monitoring). Asbestos surveys of buildings involve bulk samples taken from materials that might contain asbestos or wipe samples of settled dust (7).

Fiber Counting and Identification

The number of fibers captured on a filter or in a bulk sample can be counted under a phase-contrast light microscope using standardized techniques approved by OSHA. Fibers are counted only if they are larger than 5 μm and have a length-to-diameter ratio greater than 3:1. Individuals conducting asbestos fiber counts to meet OSHA regulations must take a formal training course and become certified (7).

The limit of resolution of light microscopes is approximately 0.3 μm. Electron microscopes can identify much smaller fibers, and some researchers suggest that 90% of all asbestos fibers are of this smaller size. One study that used both standard light microscopy and transmission electron microscopy to analyze air samples obtained during bagging of asbestos found that light microscopy detected only 0.6% of all crocidolite fibers, 16.9% of all amosite fibers, and 1.6% of all chrysotile fibers that were counted using transmission electron microscopy (66). This has important implications in studying asbestos-related disease, as some researchers suggest that fibers less than 0.3 μm in diameter and more than 5 μm long (which are not detectable using light microscopy) may have high potential for causing disease.

Almost all epidemiologic studies and government regulations involve or are based on asbestos counts using light microscopy. Much confusion has been created by trying to draw clinical and epidemiologic correlations among exposure data obtained by standard light microscopy, because the small fibers found at the same light-microscopy level vary greatly in terms of asbestos type and industrial process.

The asbestos fiber type can be determined by specialized techniques such as electron microscopy or x-ray dispersion analysis of samples. Although this is not required by OSHA, it is important in epidemiologic research. Airborne concentrations of asbestos are reported either as being of mixed fiber types or by the percentages of each type of fiber. Because both types of reporting are found in the research literature, comparison of findings between studies can be difficult.

EXPOSURE LIMITS AND REGULATIONS

Occupational Exposure Limits

The current OSHA PEL for asbestos is 0.1 fiber per cubic centimeter of air as an 8-hour time-weighted average. The OSHA also requires the employer to ensure that no employee is exposed beyond the excursion limit of 1.0 fiber per cubic centimeter of air averaged over a 30-minute sampling period (7).

The American Conference of Governmental Industrial Hygienists' 1996 threshold limit values for asbestos were 0.2 fiber per cubic centimeter of air for crocidolite, 0.5 fiber per cubic centimeter of air for amosite, and 2.0 fibers per cubic centimeter of air for chrysotile (8).

The OSHA requires that employers institute a medial surveillance program for all employees exposed to asbestos fibers at or above either the PEL or the excursion limit. The OSHA asbestos standard specifies the frequency, content, procedures, and quality requirements for these medical examinations. Such medical surveillance examinations must include a standardized medical history and exposure questionnaire, a physical examination, spirometry (FVC and forced expiratory volume over 1 second), and periodic posteroanterior chest radiographs interpreted by a B-reader. Baseline, annual, and exit examinations are required. Procedures for reporting results, record-keeping requirements, and quality control measures are specified by the standard, which should be reviewed before these examinations are carried out (7).

Environmental Regulations

The EPA regulates commercial, construction, and manufacturing activities that may cause the release of asbestos fibers into the atmosphere. This organization also regulates the disposal of asbestos. Although it does have legal authority to regulate asbestos exposures to students in schools and to other occupants of public buildings, the EPA has not established any legal exposure limits for these situations. However, the OSHA PEL for asbestos applies to persons who work as employees in such buildings (7,9,10).

Since 1984, the EPA has required that asbestos surveys be conducted on all school buildings, although the agency has never set any PELs for airborne asbestos in schools or other buildings. Initially, the EPA provided little guidance regarding what should be

TABLE 111-4. Estimated lifetime cancer deaths from exposures to different levels of mixed asbestos fibers[a]

Exposure setting	Level of exposure (f/cm^3)	Duration of exposure (yr)	Cumulative exposure (fiber-yr)	Estimated deaths from asbestos-related diseases per million persons exposed		
				Total	Lung cancer	Mesothelioma
Occupational exposures						
High-exposure trades in shipyards before 1972	10	20	200	200,000	—	—
Workers in asbestos cement manufacturing in 1980s	0.5	40	20	8,200	5,100	3,100
	0.5	20	10	5,300	2,600	2,700
Environmental exposures						
Students in schools containing asbestos[b]						
Higher level	0.003	6	0.018	15	1.9	13.2
Lower level	0.001	6	0.006	5	0.6	4.4
Occupants in buildings containing asbestos[b]						
Higher level	0.002	20	0.04	40	—	—
Lower level	0.0002	20	0.004	4	—	—
Ambient air in urban areas	0.0001	80	0.008	40	—	—

[a]Risk estimates are taken from quantitative risk assessments provided by Weill and Hughes (68), and the Health Effects Institute (11) and the U.S. Occupational Safety and Health Administration; estimates are for cancer deaths attributed to asbestos exposure and assume that exposed persons did not use respiratory protection.
[b]Higher and lower exposure levels are representative of levels found in U.S. schools and building surveys (11,68).
Adapted from refs. 11 and 68.

done if asbestos were found in a school. By the late 1980s, after many school districts had removed asbestos from school buildings, studies showed that levels of airborne asbestos fibers inside school buildings were sometimes actually higher after the ACM had been removed (9,10). Some reports estimate that the removal of asbestos from U.S. schools could cost $160 billion, yet whether such removal would result in any meaningful reduction in health risk for the public remains controversial (67).

These considerations led to the current EPA recommendation that ACM that is not damaged or potentially friable is best managed by leaving it in place and possibly encapsulating it in plastic. The EPA does recommend that ACM that is damaged or otherwise potentially friable should be repaired or removed from buildings according to procedures established by OSHA (for removal and repair) and EPA (for disposal). These procedures must also be followed for all repairs and remodeling that involves ACM and when a building containing ACM is demolished (10).

No federal government agency regulates asbestos exposures to individuals in their own homes, but some local governments do have regulations to control how homeowners can remove asbestos from their homes. It is now common practice for purchasers of commercial and residential real estate to require as a condition of sale inspections of buildings for asbestos, even though this seldom is a legal requirement.

Those wishing to remove asbestos materials from a building should be aware that strict OSHA guidelines exist for workers who remove or repair asbestos. Such repair or removal should be performed by certified asbestos workers who have been trained in methods of handling asbestos that prevent worker exposure and contamination of the environment. The OSHA, EPA, and equivalent local agencies should be consulted for details. Before disturbing ACMs, individuals wishing to remove asbestos from their own homes should consult with their local health department or EPA office for advice on proper procedures. The disposal of asbestos-containing wastes must be conducted according to EPA guidelines (7,10).

Low-Level Asbestos Exposures and Public Policy

Since the mid-1980s, great public concern has been generated about the risks to occupants of buildings that contain asbestos. Surveys of schools and other public buildings containing ACM have generally found very low levels of airborne asbestos: Several building surveys found mean exposure levels of 0.0004 to 0.0010 asbestos fiber per cubic centimeter of air (11). Several asbestos risk assessments suggest that health risks from such very low asbestos exposures are minimal (67).

Weill and Hughes (68) estimated that schoolchildren exposed to airborne asbestos at levels typically found in schools (i.e., 0.00024 fibers per mL of air) had very small health risks from these asbestos exposures, especially as compared with risks that are commonly encountered in everyday life. These authors estimated that for 1 million students exposed to asbestos in schools (at the level of 0.001 fiber per cubic centimeter of air), a lifetime risk of 0.6 deaths from lung cancer and 4.4 deaths from mesothelioma would be attributable to this asbestos exposure (68). Table 111-4 summarizes risk estimates from asbestos exposures both for occupants of buildings containing asbestos and for workers with higher historical asbestos exposures. Table 111-5 compares

TABLE 111-5. Estimated risks from asbestos exposures in schools and other common risk situations[a]

Cause of death	Estimated annual deaths per million persons exposed
Long-term smoking	1,200
Bicycling accident (for 10- to 14-year-old children)	14
Accident during high school football play	10
Consumption of 4 tbsp peanut butter per day	8
Aircraft accident	6
Whooping cough vaccination	1–6
Exposure in schools to mixed-fiber asbestos at 0.001 $fiber/cm^3$ [b]	0.02–0.37[c]

[a]Based on estimates from multiple risk assessments performed by different researchers, as summarized by Weill and Hughes (68).
[b]Defined as 6 years of exposure before age 15, with 0.001 $fiber/cm^3$ used as the best estimate of exposure levels found in U.S. schools.
[c]Annual death rates were calculated from estimates of lifetime excess lung cancer and mesothelioma deaths attributed to such asbestos exposure in schools.
Adapted from ref. 68.

the risk for asbestos exposures in schoolchildren to other common risks encountered in everyday life. These tables illustrate that health risks from asbestos exposures are estimated to be extremely low to occupants of schools and other buildings that contain asbestos.

Epidemiologic studies of worker cohorts with historically heavy asbestos exposures are the basis for most dose-response calculations for asbestos-related disease. Most asbestos risk assessments, including those by Weill and Hughes (68), use such historical data and linear-extrapolation, nonthreshold models to estimate the risks for low-level asbestos exposures. Such models assume that there is no lower threshold dose for asbestos-related cancers. Some researchers maintain that there is a threshold effect for asbestos-related cancers, which suggests that very low-level asbestos exposures may not pose significant health risks for society even if millions of persons are exposed (67). However, the linear nonthreshold models, which may be more conservative, continue to be used by OSHA and the EPA as the basis for establishing exposure limits and regulating asbestos.

CHANGING PATTERNS OF ASBESTOS-RELATED DISEASES

In U.S. workers exposed to asbestos before the mid-1970s (when exposures often were higher than current levels), asbestos-related diseases probably will continue to be diagnosed well into the first several decades of the twenty-first century. Because workers first exposed in the 1960s or later will have lower cumulative asbestos exposures, those who develop asbestos-related diseases will have longer latency periods and may develop clinically apparent disease only 40 or more years after their first exposure.

Workers' asbestos exposures have declined dramatically since the 1970s, owing primarily to OSHA and EPA regulations. Because of this, asbestosis and asbestos-related lung cancer may eventually become rare diseases for U.S. workers, as evidence suggests that development of both of these diseases requires a threshold of 5 fiber-years of cumulative asbestos exposure.

The risk for mesothelioma development is dose-dependent, although some risk for mesothelioma attaches to even relatively small cumulative exposures (at least to amphiboles). Due to markedly decreased asbestos exposures in workers since the 1970s, the incidence rates for this tumor should decline dramatically in the United States in the coming decades. However, because a large proportion of U.S. buildings contain asbestos, some future mesothelioma risk will continue for workers and others exposed to lower levels of asbestos when repairing or demolishing ACM in such structures.

Similar decreases in all types of asbestos-related diseases will probably be seen in the future in Canada, Western Europe, and similar developed countries, which, like the United States, have strictly enforced occupational health regulations. In contrast, for many newly industrializing countries, especially in Asia, the use of asbestos is growing, and regulations to protect workers from asbestos exposures do not exist or are not enforced. In those parts of the world, it is possible that rather than declining, rates of asbestos-related diseases will actually increase in the next century.

REFERENCES

1. Selikoff IJ, Lee DH. *Asbestos and disease*. New York: Academic Press, 1978:34–50.
2. Pooley FD. Asbestos mineralogy. In: Antman K, Aisner J, eds. *Asbestos-related malignancy*. Orlando, FL: Grune & Stratton, 1987:3–27.
3. Morgan WK, Seaton A, eds. *Occupational lung diseases*, 2nd ed. Philadelphia: WB Saunders, 1984:323–376.
4. Mossman BT, Gee JB. Asbestos-related diseases. *N Engl J Med* 1989;320: 1721–1730.
5. Becklake MR, Case BW. Fiber burden and asbestos-related lung disease: determinants of dose-response relationships. Am J Respir Crit Care Med 1994;150:1488–1492.
6. Davis JM, McDonald C. Low level exposure to asbestos: is there a cancer risk? *Fr J Ind Med* 1988;45:505.
7. US Code of Federal Regulations no. 29 *CFR*, 1910.1001. Asbestos. Washington: US Government Printing Office, 1996.
8. *Threshold limit values and biological exposure indices for 1996*. Cincinnati, OH: American Conference of Governmental Industrial Hygienists, 1990.
9. US Environmental Protection Agency. *EPA report to Congress: study of asbestos-containing materials in public buildings.* Washington: US Environmental Protection Agency, 1988:5.
10. US Environmental Protection Agency. *Managing asbestos in place: a building owner's guide to operations and maintenance programs for asbestos-containing materials.* Washington: US Environmental Protection Agency, Office of Pesticides and Toxic Substances, 1990.
11. Health Effects Institute—Asbestos Research. *Asbestos in public and commercial buildings: a literature review and synthesis of current knowledge.* Cambridge, MA: Health Effects Institute—Asbestos Research, 1991.
12. Oliver LC, Sprince NL, Greene R. Asbestos-related disease in public school custodians. *Am J Ind Med* 1991;19:303–316.
13. Levin SM, Selikoff IJ. Radiographic abnormalities and asbestos exposure among custodians of the New York City Board of Education. In: Landrigan PJ, Kazemi H, eds. *The third wave of asbestos disease: exposure to asbestos in place. Public health control.* New York: New York Academy of Sciences, 1991:530–539.
14. Anderson HA, Hanrahan LP, Higgins DN, Sarow PG. A radiographic survey of public building maintenance and custodial employees. *Environ Res* 1992;59:159–166.
15. Balmes JR, Duponte A, Cone JE. Asbestos-related disease in custodial and building maintenance workers from a large municipal school district. In: Landrigan PJ, Kazemi H, eds. *The third wave of asbestos disease: exposure to asbestos in place. Public health control.* New York: New York Academy of Sciences, 1991:540–549.
16. CONSAD Research Corporation. *Economic analysis of the proposed revisions to the OSHA asbestos standards for construction and general industry.* OSHA J-9-F-8-0033. Washington: US Department of Labor, 1990.
17. McDonald JC. Health implications of environmental exposure to asbestos. *Environ Health Perspect* 1985;62:319–328.
18. National Research Council, Committee on Nonoccupational Health Risks of Asbestiform Fibers. *Asbestiform fibers: nonoccupational health risks*. Washington: National Academy Press, 1984.
19. Edelman DA. Exposure to asbestos and the risk of gastrointestinal cancer: a reassessment. *Br J Ind Med* 1988;45:75–82.
20. Weiss W. The lack of causality between asbestos and colorectal cancer. *J Occup Environ Med* 1995;37:1364–1373.
21. Wright GW. The pulmonary effects of inhaled inorganic dust. In: Clayton GD, Clayton EC, eds. *Patty's industrial hygiene and toxicology*, 3rd ed. New York: John Wiley and Sons, 1981:165–202.
22. Timbrell V, Bevan NE, Davies AS, Munday DE. Hollow casts of lungs for experimental purposes. *Nature* 1970;225:9708.
23. Churg A, Wright JL. Fibre content of lung in amphibole- and chrysotile-induced mesothelioma: implications for environmental exposure. *IARC Sci Publ* 1989;90:314–318.
24. Churg A, Wiggs B. Fiber size and number in workers exposed to processed chrysotile asbestos, chrysotile miners and the general public. *Am J Ind Med* 1986;9:143–152.
25. Churg A. Current issues in the pathologic and mineralogical diagnosis of asbestos-induced disease. *Chest* 1983;84:275–280.
26. Bignon J, Jaurand MC. Asbestos fiber toxicity and lung disease. In: Gee JB, ed. *Occupational lung disease*. New York: Churchill Livingstone, 1984: 5171.
27. Craighead JE, Abraham JL, Churg A, et al. The pathology of asbestos-associated diseases of the lungs and pleural cavities: diagnostic criteria and proposed grading schema. *Arch Pathol Lab Med* 1982;106:544–596.
28. Rom WN, Bitterman PB, Rennard SI, Cantin A, Crystal RG. Characterization of the lower respiratory tract inflammation of nonsmoking individuals with interstitial lung disease associated with chronic inhalation of inorganic dusts. *Am Rev Respir Dis* 1987;136:1429–1434.
29. Robinson BW, Rose AH, James A, Whitaker D, Musk AW. Alveolitis of pulmonary asbestosis: bronchoalveolar lavage studies in crocidolite- and chrysotile-exposed individuals. *Chest* 1986;90:396–402.
30. Gaensler EA. Progression of asbestos. *Chest* 1987;91:305(abst).
31. Smith DD. *Asbestos-related pleural disease: questions in need of answers. Clin Pulm Med* 1994;1:289–300.
32. American Thoracic Society. Medical Section of the American Lung Association: the diagnosis of nonmalignant diseases related to asbestos. *Am Rev Respir Dis* 1986;134:363–368.
33. Smith DD, Agostoni PG. The discriminatory value of the $P(A\text{-}a)O_2$ during exercise in asbestos exposed workers. *Chest* 1989;95:52–55.
34. Agostoni P, Smith DD, Schoene RB, Robertson HT, Butler J. *Evaluation of breathlessness in asbestos workers*. *Am Rev Respir Dis* 1987;135:812–816.

35. International Labour Office. *Guidelines for the use of ILO international classification of radiographs of pneumoconioses.* Occupational Safety and Health Series no. 22 (rev). Geneva: International Labour Organization1980.
36. McDonald JC, McDonald AD. Epidemiology of asbestos-related lung cancer. In: Antman K, Aisner J, eds. *Asbestos-related malignancy.* Orlando, FL: Grune & Stratton, 1987:57–79.
37. Berry G, Newhouse ML. Mortality of workers manufacturing friction materials using asbestos. *Br J Ind Med* 1983;40:1–7.
38. Gardner MJ, Winter PD, Pannett B, Powell CA. Follow-up study of workers manufacturing chrysotile asbestos cement products. *Br J Ind Med* 1986; 43:726–732.
39. Ohlson CG, Hogstedt C. Lung cancer among asbestos cement workers: a Swedish cohort study and a review. *Br J Ind Med* 1985;43:397–402.
40. Thomas HF, Benjamin IT, Elwood PC, Sweetnam PM. Further follow-up of workers from an asbestos cement factory. *Br J Ind Med* 1982;39:273–276.
41. US Surgeon General. *The health consequences of smoking: cancer and chronic lung disease in the workplace.* Washington: US Department of Health and Human Services, 1985:19–96.
42. Churg A. Lung asbestos content in long-term residents of a chrysotile mining town. *Am Rev Respir Dis* 1987;134:125–127.
43. Cordier S, Lazar P, Brochard P, Bignon J, Ameille J, Proteau J. Epidemiologic investigation of respiratory effects related to environmental exposure to asbestos inside insulated buildings. *Arch Environ Health* 1987; 42:303–309.
44. Kuschner M. The effects of MMMF on animal systems: some reflections on their pathogenesis. *Ann Occup Hyg* 1987;31:791–797.
45. Kipen HM, Lilis R, Suzuki Y, Valciukas JA, Selikoff IJ. Pulmonary fibrosis in asbestos insulation workers with lung cancer: a radiological and histopathological evaluation. *Br J Ind Med* 1987;44:96–100.
46. Antman KH, Corson JM. Benign and malignant pleural mesothelioma. *Clin Chest Med* 1985;6:127–140.
47. Churg A. Chrysotile, tremolite, and malignant mesothelioma in man. *Chest* 1993;3:621–628.
48. Stanton MF, Wrench C. Mechanisms of mesothelioma induction with asbestos and fibrous glass. *J Natl Cancer Inst* 1972;48:797–821.
49. Grant DC, Seltzer SE, Antman KH, Finberg HJ, Koster K. Computed tomography of malignant pleural mesothelioma. *J Comput Assist Tomogr* 1983;7: 626–632.
50. Craighead JE. Current pathogenetic concepts of diffuse malignant mesothelioma. *Hum Pathol* 1987;18:544–557.
51. Robinson BW, Musk AW. Benign asbestos pleural effusion: diagnosis and course. *Thorax* 1981;36:896–900.
52. Stephens M, Gibbs AR, Pooley FD, Wagner JC. Asbestos induced diffuse pleural fibrosis: pathology and mineralogy. *Thorax* 1987;42:583–588.
53. Smith DD. Plaques, cancer, and confusion. *Chest* 1994;105:8–9.
54. Chan CK, Gee JB. Asbestos exposure and laryngeal cancer: an analysis of the epidemiologic evidence. *J Occup Med* 1988;30:34–27.
55. Selikoff IJ, Churg J, Hammond E. The occurrence of asbestosis among insulation workers in the United States. *Ann N Y Acad Sci* 1965;132:139.
56. Wagner JC. The discovery of the association between blue asbestos and mesotheliomas and the aftermath. *Br J Ind Med* 1991;48:399–403.
57. Mossman BT. Mechanisms of asbestos carcinogenesis and toxicity: the amphibole hypothesis revisited. *Br J Ind Med* 1993;50:673–676.
58. Mossman BT, Kamp DW, Weitzman SA. Mechanisms of carcinogenesis and clinical features of asbestos-associated cancers. *Cancer Invest* 1996;14(5): 466–480.
59. Jensen CG, Jensen LCW, Rieder CL, Cole RW, Ault JG. Long crocidolite asbestos fibers cause polyploidy by sterically blocked cytokinesis. *Carcinogenesis* 1996;17:2013–2021.
60. Walker C, Everitt J, Barrett JC. Possible cellular and molecular mechanisms for asbestos carcinogenicity. *Am J Ind Med* 1992;21:253–273.
61. Warheit DB, Driscoll KE, Oberdoerster G, et al. Symposium overview: contemporary issues in fiber toxicology. *Fund Appl Toxicol* 1995;25:171–183.
62. Moyer VD, Cistulli CA, Vaslet CA, Kane AB. Oxygen radicals and asbestos carcinogenesis. *Environ Health Perspect* 1994;102:131–136.
63. Chao CC, Aust AE. Effect of long-term removal of iron from asbestos by desferrioxamine B on subsequent mobilization by other chelators and induction of DNA single-strand breaks. *Arch Biochem Biophys* 1994; 308:64–69.
64. Lanphear BP, Buncher CR. Latent period for malignant mesothelioma of occupational origin. *J Occup Med* 1992;34:718–721.
65. Pass HI, Kennedy RC, Carbone M. Evidence for and implications of SV40-like sequences in human mesotheliomas. In: De Vita VT, Hellman S, Rosenberg SA, eds. *Important advances in oncology.* Philadelphia: Lippincott-Raven Publishers, 1996:89–108.
66. Gibbs GW, Hwang CY. Dimensions of airborne asbestos fibres. In: *Biological effects of mineral fibres.* IARC symposium. Lyon: International Agency for Research on Cancer, 1980:69–77.
67. Mossman BT, Bignon J, Corn M, Seaton A, Gee JB. Asbestos: scientific developments and implications for public policy. *Science* 1990;247:294–301.
68. Weill H, Hughes JM. Asbestos as a public health risk: disease and policy. *Annu Rev Public Health* 1986;7:171–192.

CHAPTER 112
Man-Made Mineral Fibers

Thomas W. Hesterberg, Robert Anderson, William B. Bunn III, Gerald R. Chase, and Georgia A. Hart

Synthetic vitreous fibers (SVFs; also known as *man-made vitreous fibers* or *MMVF*) are a class of insulating materials that are used widely in residential and industrial settings. *SVF* is a generic term for fibrous, inorganic substances that have an amorphous, glassy (vitreous) composition and are made primarily from glass, rock, slag, or clay. The three general categories of SVFs are fiberglass, mineral wool, and refractory ceramic fibers (RCFs) (Fig. 112-1).

Since the initial development of the first SVFs in the late 1800s, large numbers of people have worked with these materials in various occupational settings, including manufacture, installation, and demolition. In some situations, SVF materials can release fine, airborne dust particles, some of which are small enough to be respirable. Thus, workers may be exposed to SVF fibers by dermal contact or by inhalation. Because the lung contains a very large surface area of relatively unprotected tissue, an understanding of the potential health effects of any airborne, respirable material is important, especially in the workplace where exposure could be long-term. Fibrous particles having long, thin geometry present a special problem to the respiratory tract: Because fibers are thin, they can penetrate into the deep lung and, because they are long, mobile lung cells may have difficulty in removing them. Therefore, many studies have been, and continue to be, conducted on the biological activity of SVFs. National and international agencies and organizations have reviewed these studies and have suggested maximum exposure levels to airborne fibers.

MATERIAL CHARACTERISTICS

Because of their physical characteristics, SVFs have become some of the world's most useful and beneficial man-made materials. SVFs do not burn, rot, or absorb moisture or odors. They do not directly support the growth of mold or bacteria. However, microbes can grow in insulation or filtration materials that have become clogged with pollutants (which provide a food source) and remain wet for a prolonged period. SVFs are dimensionally stable and have high tensile strength. Because of these

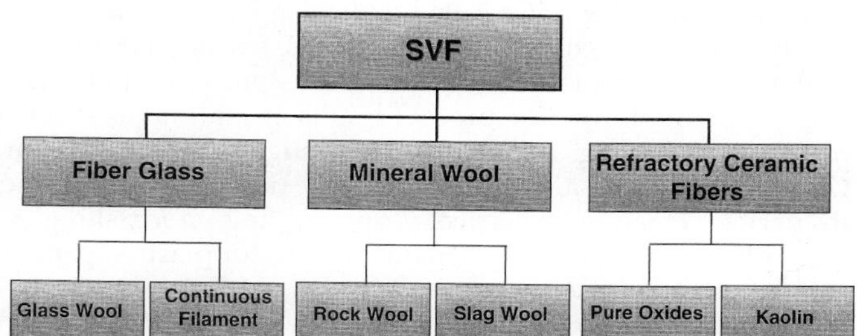

Figure 112-1. Three classes of synthetic vitreous fibers (SVF). Fiberglass is classified further into glass wool and continuous filament (also called *textile fiber*). Mineral wool is further classified as rock wool and slag wool. Refractory ceramic fiber can be divided into fibers made from pure oxides and fibers made from kaolin derived from clay.

characteristics, SVFs can help to control heat flow, absorb acoustic energy, filter impurities from gases and liquids, and with a vapor barrier, control condensation. Owing to their fibrous configuration, SVF products can trap large volumes of air, which makes them effective and lightweight thermal insulators. Also owing to the fibrous configuration, fiberglass is a highly efficient filter medium with substantial particle-trapping capacity. Hence, SVFs not only reduce the consumption of fossil fuels for heating; they also reduce the air pollution that results from burning fuels to provide heat (1).

For human health considerations, an especially important attribute of SVF fibers is that they do not split longitudinally as do asbestos fibers. Because asbestos fibers tend to split longitudinally, over time in the lung, the numbers of long, thin asbestos fibers can actually increase, resulting in increasing lung irritation even after exposure to asbestos has stopped. In contrast, SVFs tend to break transversely into shorter segments, which the lung can clear more readily than it can long fibers. Phagocytic lung cells (alveolar macrophages) are able to engulf these shorter segments and carry them to the upper airways, where they are carried by the ciliary motion of the airway epithelium up to the throat, are swallowed, and eventually are eliminated.

SYNTHETIC VITREOUS FIBER TYPES

Fiberglass

Production of fiberglass began in the 1930s, with materials manufactured in the two basic forms that still predominate today: wool fibers and textile fibers (2). Glass wool fibers are produced by spinning or blowing molten glass consisting of silicon, aluminum, boron, calcium, sodium, and other inorganic oxides (3). Glass wool was developed originally for use in residential insulation and furnace filters. Today, it is used widely to control noise as well as temperature. The current major uses of glass wool are in commercial and residential thermal insulation, noise-control (acoustic) products, linings for air-handling ducts, pipe insulation, air filters, roof insulation, and insulation for automobiles, aircraft, mobile homes, refrigerators, domestic cooking appliances, and a wide variety of other appliances and equipment. For thermal and acoustic applications, the nominal diameter of fibers ranges from 1 to 8 µm. For air filtration media, the nominal diameter of fibers ranges from 1 to 5 µm.

Glass wool fibers are also manufactured in the submicrometer diameter range and are known in this form as *glass microfibers*. In the United States, glass microfiber production constitutes less than 1% of total fiberglass production. Glass microfiber generally is used in high-technology products, such as high-efficiency particulate air filters, specialty filter papers, battery components, and aerospace insulation.

Glass textile fibers, also called *continuous filament*, differ from glass wool in that textile fibers are drawn or extruded from holes in the base of a container in a continuous process, rather than being spun or blown. The process results in continuous strands or filaments having diameters in the range of 3.5 to 25.0 µm. Glass textile fibers are most commonly used in curtains and draperies, screening, electrical yarns, roofing paper, shingles, and industrial fabrics and as reinforcement for plastics, papers, rubber, and other materials.

Mineral Wool

Mineral wools include rock or stone wool and slag wool. These wools were first produced in Europe in 1840 (4). Commercial production began in the United States in 1897. Mineral wool production peaked in the 1950s, at which time glass wool began to capture more of the insulation market. In Europe, more rock and stone wool is produced than slag wool, whereas in the United States, the reverse is true.

Mineral wools are produced by melting raw materials and centrifuging and drawing or blowing the molten matter into the desired fibrous form. Because the fibers are cooled quickly after formation, the fibers remain noncrystalline (vitreous). As a result of this processing, mineral wools generally contain a very high ratio of nonfibrous particles, or *shot*. Shot particles have little insulating capacity and do not contribute to the product's utility. After formation, the materials are sprayed with lubricating oils and binders to reduce dustiness and fiber breakage.

Rock or stone wools are typically produced from molten igneous rock that is rich in calcium and magnesium. Slag wool is produced from the slag by-products of metal smelting. The slag is essentially a calcium aluminum silicate containing varying amounts of iron and magnesium. The composition of slag fibers varies with the source of the slag used.

Mineral wool applications are very similar to those of glass wool—thermal insulation, including fire protection, and acoustic insulation. Much of the mineral wool produced is used for blown-in insulation in attics and side walls. Another popular use of mineral wool is in the manufacture of decorative and acoustic ceiling tiles for commercial buildings.

Refractory Ceramic Fiber

RCF, commercialized in the 1960s, is a relatively new material compared to the other SVFs. RCF is formulated to help control heat flow in high-temperature, industrial situations. All RCFs are blends of alumina and silica and other refractory oxides (5). Various RCF types are produced for different industrial applications. The three general categories of RCFs are (i) kaolin clay-based products, for which the clay is obtained by mining; (ii) blends of alumina, silica, and refractory metal oxides (e.g., chromous and zirconia oxides); and (iii) high-purity products that are a blend of purified alumina and silica and other materials. RCFs are produced by spinning molten mixtures of their components. Fiber diameters range from 1.2 to 3.5 µm. Fiber length varies from very long down to micrometer size (3).

Applications vary for RCFs, but all are used in high-temperature, industrial environments. RCF blankets are used as furnace and kiln liners, as backup insulation to refractory brick, as soaking pit covers, and in annealing welds. Loose RCF is used as a filler in packing voids and in expansion joints. Custom-molded shapes of RCF are used widely in metal molding, in catalytic converters, and as combustion chamber liners in industrial furnaces (3,6).

HEALTH EFFECTS

Skin Irritation

SVFs may irritate the skin of some workers who are engaged in manufacturing, fabricating, or installing SVF products. This skin irritation (itching and possible inflammation) is a mechanical reaction to sharp, broken ends of fibers that rub or become embedded in the outer layer of the skin and does not appear to be an allergic (hypersensitivity) response. Skin reactions are associated more often with fibers of large diameter (greater than 5 µm) than with fibers of fine diameter. Typically, irritation does not persist and can be relieved by washing exposed skin gently with warm water and mild soap.

Some individuals may be more sensitive than others to skin irritation from SVF, and a relatively small number of unusually sensitive individuals may be forced to seek other employment. The vast majority of SVF workers, however, can control skin irritation by following appropriate work practices and using proper personal protective equipment (discussed later in the section, Safety Precautions) (7).

Upper Respiratory Tract Irritation

If large amounts of airborne fine fiber are released during manufacture or handling of SVF products, and improper work practices permit inhalation of the fibers, some workers may experience temporary upper respiratory irritation (scratching or burning sensations in the nose or throat). The irritation consists of a nonspecific, temporary respiratory condition, usually manifested by coughing or wheezing. Similar to skin irritation, upper respiratory irritation is mechanically induced by sharp fibers and does not appear to be an allergic reaction. The irritation subsides soon after the worker is removed from exposure and should have no further impact on his or her health and well-being. However, when handling SVFs, workers should use appropriate respiratory protection, as discussed in the next section (4).

Safety Precautions

Occupational health professionals recommend three levels of precautions for protecting people when they are manufacturing or handling SVF materials. First, whenever feasible, SVF products should be engineered and designed to limit their release of airborne dust. Second, manufacturing processes and controls should be used to minimize airborne dust in the work environment. Third, when handling or installing SVFs, people should wear approved respiratory protection and clothing that covers the skin as much as possible (e.g., long-sleeved shirts and long pants). These precautions effectively reduce airborne SVF exposure and prevent skin and upper respiratory irritation (8,9).

EPIDEMIOLOGIC STUDIES

Tens of thousands of workers have been employed in manufacturing SVFs in the 150 years since SVFs were developed. Various groups of these workers have been and still are the subject of epidemiologic studies. In these studies, researchers look for unusual patterns of diseases or symptoms among SVF workers and review all causes of death. They focus especially on incidences of lung cancer, mesothelioma (cancer of the pleural membranes that cover the lungs and line the chest cavity), and nonmalignant respiratory disease.

Fiberglass and Mineral Wool Mortality Studies

Two major mortality studies have been conducted on large groups of individuals engaged in the production of either glass or mineral wool, one in Europe (10,11) and the other in the United States (12–24). A third, more limited study, was conducted on Canadian fiberglass production workers (15,16).

For the European study, researchers surveyed the mortality of almost 25,000 workers (2,836 deaths) in 13 European SVF factories, including 11,852 fiberglass production workers and 10,115 mineral wool production workers through 1982 (10) and updated through 1990 (11) for most plants (4,521 deaths). The researchers found an overall mortality excess among the SVF workers, with the excess particularly evident among workers with less than 1 year of employment. Among the causes of death that were more numerous were malignant neoplasms, mental disorders, cardiovascular diseases (in particular, ischemic heart disease), respiratory diseases, digestive diseases (in particular, cirrhosis of the liver), and external causes. Simonato et al. (10) reported an "excess of lung cancer among rock wool–slag wool workers employed during an early technological phase before the introduction of dust-suppressing agents," and concluded that "fiber exposure, either alone or in combination with other exposures, may have contributed to the elevated risk." In the latest update, the researchers concluded that "the ensemble of these results is not sufficient to conclude that the increased lung cancer risk is related specifically to MMVF [i.e., SVF]: however, insofar as respirable fibres were a significant component of the ambient pollution of the working environment, they may have contributed to the increased risk" (11). For glass wool workers, the report stated that the findings "indicate some excess of lung cancer, clearly reduced once local adjustment factors are applied to national mortality rates, and with no relation to duration of employment nor time since first employment" (10). No anomalies were found for the continuous glass filament workers, but the total number of workers studied is rather small. Five mesotheliomas have been identified by death certificate, one in the glass wool subcohort and four in the rock wool and slag wool subcohort (two from a location in which asbestos was processed). No clear increased risk of mesothelioma has been identified, although the researchers have concluded that "the possibility of such increase is suggested by the results." The authors reported no association between employment in the SVF industry and mortality from other cancers or from nonmalignant respiratory diseases (10,11). A nested case-control study of lung cancer deaths in the rock wool and slag wool subcohort has been initiated.

For the U.S. study, Enterline et al. (12) conducted a comprehensive mortality review of almost 17,000 U.S. workers, many with SVF exposure of up to 40 years, at 17 U.S. fiberglass and mineral wool manufacturing plants (14,800 fiberglass workers in 11 plants and 1,846 mineral wool workers in 6 plants). The original report, made available in 1982, covered the mortality statistics from the 1940s to the end of 1977. The same group of workers was followed through 1982, with additional analyses available in June 1987 (12) and updated again through 1985 (13). The mineral wool subcohort has been enlarged and updated through 1989 (11). The update also included an enhancement and update of potential workplace exposures. An analogous update is under way for the fiberglass workers.

As with the European study, the U.S. study found a higher overall mortality rate among SVF workers as compared to local and national mortality. For deaths due to cancer or nonmalignant respiratory disease, the study reported essentially negative data for glass wool and glass textile production workers, but positive evidence existed for fine glass and mineral wool production workers (using local mortality rates on data from 1960 through 1982). The standard mortality ratio (or actual deaths in the test population divided by expected deaths based on the local population) for all causes was 102.5 for glass wool and glass textile workers and 112.3 for mineral wool workers. The standard mortality ratios for lung cancer deaths were 103.7 in the glass wool and glass textile cohort and 138.7 in the mineral wool cohort. The researchers concluded that "[e]ither there was something unusual about the way mineral wool workers were selected for employment or something in their environment had an extraordinary effect on their health" (12). However, the researchers point out, the data are not consistent with a causal relationship because the excesses in mineral wool and glass microfiber deaths were not directly related to duration of exposure; in fact, for mineral wool exposure, the relationship was inverse (longer exposure was associated with less mortality). The number of deaths from mesothelioma in the study cohort is considered to be within the expected range for the general population.

In the update through 1985 (13), a small but statistically significant excess in respiratory cancer deaths was reported for workers employed in glass wool and mineral wool plants. The mortality of the group of workers classified as having worked with finer-diameter fibers is not discussed in this update. Considering the cumulative evidence for respiratory cancer and all factors that might support a relationship in the 1985 update, the researchers concluded that the evidence of an association appeared "somewhat weaker" than in the 1982 update (12,13). In the update through 1989 (14) for the rock wool and slag wool workers, the pattern of findings was generally consistent with findings observed in previous updates; no consistent evidence remains of an association between lung cancer or nonmalignant respiratory diseases and any of the respirable fiber measures considered.

Although the authors regarded the respiratory cancer findings for glass textile (continuous filament) and glass wool workers as essentially negative, they agree with other occupational health investigators that the relationship between work and health in the SVF industry should continue to be explored.

The third and more limited mortality study was conducted on 2,557 male workers at a Canadian glass wool plant through 1977 (15) and was updated through 1984 (16). The authors reported a statistically significant excess in mortality due to lung cancer among the fiberglass production workers. They concluded that the interpretation of this finding was difficult because no relationship existed between the excess of lung cancer and the length of time since first exposure to the fiberglass production environment (15,16).

Fiberglass and Mineral Wool Morbidity Studies

Morbidity studies, which investigate disease occurrence among living workers, are extremely useful in assessing the potential risk of nonmalignant disease. In the most widely cited SVF morbidity study, Weill et al. (17,18) reported on the respiratory health of 1,089 workers who were currently employed during 1979 and 1980 at five fiberglass and two mineral wool plants in the United States. For each worker, the researchers conducted a respiratory questionnaire and lung function test and evaluated a chest radiograph. They found the study populations to be generally healthy, with no respiratory symptoms and no detected adverse lung functions related to the fiber exposure. A low incidence of small lung opacities was observed in the chest radiographs (opaque areas sometimes observed in the lungs of workers in potentially dusty trades). In summarizing their findings, Weill et al. (17,18) noted that, in general, "the minimal evidence of respiratory effects detected in the investigation, which cannot, at present, be considered clinically significant, is encouraging concerning the question of potential health effects of exposure to MMVF [i.e., SVF]" (17,18). The study has been updated and enlarged to include more than 1,400 workers employed in the late 1980s, with more than 300 comparison (control) workers (19). The authors concluded that the "results indicate no adverse clinical, functional, or radiographic signs of effects of exposure to MMMFs in these workers."

Refractory Ceramic Fiber Morbidity Studies

Although many studies have been conducted on fiberglass- and mineral wool–exposed workers, only one known published report is found in the medical literature on the health effects of occupational exposure to RCFs (20). RCF is a relatively new material, and approximately 32,000 people in the United States are involved in its manufacture, distribution, installation, conversion, and end use (21). Between 1987 and 1992, a retrospective cohort and nested case-control study evaluated chest radiographs from 652 workers involved in the manufacture of these fibers, for plausibility of a causal relationship between exposure to RCF and chest radiographic changes. The researchers reported an association between exposures to RCF and the occurrence of pleural plaques. The nested case-control study confirmed that asbestos exposure did not account for the observed association. Among the RCF workers, no significant increase was seen in parenchymal changes consistent with interstitial fibrosis. Another investigation has been under way in Europe, but results have not been published. As with the investigation of other fibers, these studies address the respiratory morbidity of RCF using pulmonary function tests, chest radiographs, and questionnaires. Although a mortality study has been considered, the relatively small number of exposed workers, short total duration of production, and confounding past asbestos exposure all provide significant challenges for such a study (22).

ANIMAL TOXICOLOGIC STUDIES

Two categories of whole-animal studies have been used in the study of fiber toxicology: Implantation studies artificially inject fibers into the body cavities of laboratory animals, whereas inhalational studies expose laboratory animals to airborne fibers by inhalation.

Animal Implantation Studies

Implantation studies artificially expose laboratory animals to fibers by injection into the pleural (chest) cavity or peritoneal (abdominal) cavity or by instillation into the trachea (23–25). Implantation studies have the advantage of being faster and considerably less expensive than inhalational studies because animals can be dosed quickly with high levels of fibers using a minimum of equipment. However, these studies have several drawbacks. Because implantation is not a natural exposure route, it bypasses the natural defenses of the respiratory tract. Organ doses can be much higher than those that could be achieved by inhalation, and biological responses may therefore be nonspecific to the test fiber and simply a result of organ overload. Distribution of fibers in the tissues (especially with intratracheal instillation) can be uneven, simultaneously creating areas of extreme concentration and areas of no exposure. Additionally, implantation techniques can expose internal tissues to fibers that are too large to enter the lung normally by inhalation.

When implanted into laboratory animals, high concentrations of any fibrous material have been observed to cause adverse biological effects if that material is at least moderately durable and contains fibers longer than 10 μm. Other characteristics of the fibers, such as chemical composition and surface microfeatures, appear to play little or no role in determining fiber toxicity in implantation experiments (25).

The high pathogenicity of SVFs observed in implantation studies does not parallel results from human epidemiologic or animal inhalational studies. In rat studies, intrapleural injection of glass fibers with diameters of less than 1.5 μm induced cancer and scarring of the lung (25), but inhalation of two different glass wool compositions produced only transient inflammation of the lung (26). Smith et al. (27) exposed rats and hamsters to RCF, either by implantation (intraperitoneal injection) or by inhalation. In the injection group, half of the hamsters died immediately, and 20% of the surviving hamsters and 83% of the rats developed abdominal tumors (mostly mesotheliomas). In the inhalation group, neither the rats nor the hamsters developed any permanent lung or pleural damage. Davis et al. also exposed rats to RCF either by intraperitoneal injection or by inhalation (28,29). In contrast to the Smith study, the Davis study reported a low incidence of tumors in both the injection and inhalational groups of rats.

Implantation experiments are based on introducing large amounts of fiber into animals by artificial means that bypass normal body defenses. The circumstances of actual exposure are totally different in humans. For these reasons, and because the toxicology induced by implantation of fibers into rodents does not parallel the findings from inhalational studies, implantation studies are not valid for risk assessment or for concluding anything about the human health hazard associated with the inhalation of airborne SVFs. On the other hand, implantation studies have provided useful information on the mechanisms of fiber toxicity. For example, long fibers (longer than 10 to 20 μm) are most active in implantation as well as in cell culture studies, so scientists have hypothesized that biological activity is directly associated with fiber length.

Animal Inhalational Studies

The animal inhalation model is currently the only valid laboratory method for assessing the hazard to humans of exposure to airborne SVFs. Before 1989, a number of rodent inhalational studies evaluated the biological effects of the different types of SVFs. Seven studies of fiberglass (27,29—35) and three of mineral wool (27,32,34) were negative for fibrosis and tumorigenesis. Two studies of RCF produced differing results: One study reported fibrosis and tumorigenesis (28), whereas the other reported neither fibrosis nor tumors in rats and only 2% mesotheliomas in hamsters (27).

These earlier studies were limited by the technology of the time: They typically used relatively short test fibers [e.g., in two studies, more than 70% of test fibers were shorter than 10 μm (32,33)]. The data on fiber numbers and dimensions in aerosols and lung burdens often were incomplete. In addition, whole-body rather than nose-only inhalational exposure was used. Nonetheless, these earlier studies contributed to advances in technology that permitted more accurate assessments of the biological effects of fibers in later inhalational studies.

In the late 1980s and 1990s, a new generation of rodent inhalational studies of SVFs was initiated at the Research and Consulting Co. (RCC), Füllinsdorf, Switzerland, to test thoroughly the biological effects and lung biological persistence of representatives of each class of SVF. Seven long-term and several short-term studies have been completed, and two more are currently in progress (36–43). For each of these studies, test fibers were prepared by new size-separation methods so that they had small dimensional ranges and approximate average dimensions of 1 × 20 μm. An aerosolization system was used that creates uniform high concentrations of airborne fibers without destroying the biologically important long thin fiber geometry. A nose-only inhalational exposure system was used in which each rat or hamster inhaled fresh fiber aerosol that had not been affected by the exhalation of other animals (44). To simulate occupational exposure, animals were exposed 6 hours per day, 5 days per week. Aerosol and lung fibers were evaluated (counted, measured, and chemically and morphologically analyzed) at regular intervals using scanning electron microscopy. Pathologic findings (macroscopic and microscopical) were evaluated at regular intervals by veterinary pathologists.

The RCC studies include two basic protocols: chronic inhalational studies that evaluate thoracic fibrogenesis and tumorigenesis during and after a long-term exposure of 1.5 to 2.0 years and short-term inhalational studies that evaluate fiber biological persistence in the lung (fiber numbers, morphology, and chemistry) during 1 year of "recovery" after a 5-day exposure. Two

TABLE 112-1. Fibrosis and tumor findings in rodent studies involving inhalational exposure to man-made mineral fibers

Fiber type	Test fiber	Fibrosis	Lung tumors	Mesothelioma
Asbestos	Amosite	+	+	+
	Crocidolite	+	+	+
	Chrysotile	+	+	+
Refractory ceramic	RCF1	+	+	+
Rock wool	MMVF21	+	–	–
Slag wool	MMVF22	–	–	–
Stone wool	MMVF34	–	–	–
Glass wool	MMVF10	–	–	–
	MMVF11	–	–	–
E glass	MMVF32	+[a]	+[b]	+[b]
475 Glass	MMVF33	±[b]	–[a]	±[a]

MMVF, man-made vitreous fiber; RCF, refractory ceramic fiber.
[a]Results from Davis JMG, Unpublished results from the Institute of Occupational Medicine, Edinburgh, Scotland.
[b]Preliminary results; study still in progress (35). Although the preliminary results from an ongoing study indicate that this fiber can induce lung disease at high doses, five previous chronic inhalational studies and one current study have shown no lung disease resulting from exposure to this fiber.

species—rats and hamsters—are being tested. In these studies, numerous controls and measurements ensure that exposures are uniform and comparable for each of the different SVF compositions. Three types of asbestos (chrysotile, crocidolite, and amosite) have been included in these studies. Lifetime exposure to 10 mg per cubic meter of asbestos induced early pulmonary fibrosis and tumors, thus demonstrating the responsiveness of the rodent chronic inhalational model to known human carcinogenic fibers.

In the RCC chronic studies, test SVFs having similar dimensions but different compositions have induced different biological effects (Table 112-1). Biological effects approximately parallel fiber biological persistence in the lung. Fiber compositions that are more lung-persistent would accumulate during a chronic exposure and persist longer after termination of exposure and would, therefore, cause more lung irritation than compositions that dissolve or fragment transversely into shorter segments. Differences in biological effects could also be related to fiber surface reactivity (36–43).

FIBERGLASS

In the 1970s and 1980s, seven different rodent inhalational studies reported no tumorigenesis for several forms of fiberglass (27,30–35). More recently, researchers at RCC conducted a multidose chronic study of two fiberglass insulation wools (901 glass, coded *MMVF10*, and CertainTeed insulation glass, coded *MMVF11*) in rats (26). Exposure was for 2 years, and the maximum dose was 30 mg per cubic meter (approximately 250 fibers longer than 5 μm per cubic centimeter). As in the earlier studies, fiberglass did not induce fibrosis or tumors, whereas crocidolite asbestos induced both types of lung disease (26). The same two fiberglass products and crocidolite asbestos also were tested in a biological persistence study conducted at RCC (41). In the fiberglass-exposed rats, the numbers of long fibers per lung declined more rapidly than the numbers of short fibers per lung, suggesting that the long fibers were fragmenting transversely and contributing to the short-fiber pool. In contrast, the numbers of long crocidolite asbestos fibers per lung declined more slowly than did the short fibers, demonstrating that long crocidolite fibers were more biologically persistent in the rat lung than were long glass fibers.

Infante et al. (45) disagree with the conclusions drawn by Hesterberg et al. (26) regarding the carcinogenicity of these two fiberglass products as demonstrated in the rat chronic inhalational study. The main argument of Infante et al. (45) is that the maximum dose of 30 mg per cubic meter (approximately 250 fibers longer than 5 μm per cubic centimeter) was insufficient to test the carcinogenicity of fiberglass thoroughly. However, midway through the chronic study, this dose and a lower dose caused a failure of lung clearance mechanisms, indicating lung overload, which is evidence that the maximum tolerated dose (MTD) was attained or even exceeded (46). Results from a subchronic inhalational study provided even further evidence that the MTD was attained (46). Furthermore, in parallel RCC rat chronic inhalation studies, RCF1 at an equivalent aerosol concentration induced fibrosis and elevated the incidence of cancer (36,37).

A new chronic inhalational study being conducted at RCC currently is using hamsters to compare the biological effects of amosite asbestos and two forms of fiberglass—901 insulation wool and a durable fiber composed of 475 glass (42). The durable 475 glass is used primarily in high-efficiency air filtration media. Exposures of the three fiber types were similar in average dimensions (roughly 1 μm × 20 μm) and in concentrations (250 to 320 fibers longer than 5 μm per centimeter). As in the previous RCC study with rats, 901 insulation wool induced no permanent lung changes in hamsters during the 18-month exposure period. However, 475 fiberglass induced minimal lung fibrosis and one tumor, a mesothelioma. Amosite asbestos also induced fibrosis, but an earlier and more severe case than that induced by 475 glass, and a low to moderate incidence of mesothelioma. These findings are preliminary and subject to change because the study is still in progress (42).

The current hamster study provides the first known published report of permanent lung damage in a laboratory animal after inhalation of a fiberglass composition. Davis et al. (Institute of Occupational Medicine, Edinburgh, Scotland; unpublished report of a study in progress) observed fibrosis and pulmonary tumors in rats exposed by inhalation to another durable glass microfiber composition, E glass (which is no longer produced in the United States or Europe as a microfiber). However, in contrast to the RCC hamster study, the Davis study found no fibrosis and no thoracic cancer in the 475 glass–exposed rats.

The durable 475 fiberglass used in the RCC hamster study is the same composition that tested negatively for fibrosis and tumorigenesis in five earlier rodent inhalational studies involving rats and hamsters (27,32–35). Explanations for the positive results found in the current RCC hamster study but not in the previous studies could include exposure techniques (current study uses nose-only exposure, whereas previous studies used whole-body exposure), fiber size (the previous test fibers typically had shorter average lengths), and fiber aerosolization techniques (current study uses nondestructive lofting techniques that preserve the length of the longer fibers). The 475 glass aerosol in the Davis study was higher in concentration than that used in the RCC study. However, the Davis study used whole-body exposure, which could have resulted in a lower lung burden than that achieved in the RCC study; lung burdens have not yet been analyzed for the Davis study. The Davis study also involved rats, which could be less sensitive to 475 glass than are hamsters.

In the current RCC hamster study, toxicity somewhat parallels lung biological persistence of fibers (42). After 12 months of exposure, the number per lung of fibers longer than 20 μm was seven to eight times higher for high-dose amosite than for 475 glass, which was three to four times higher than for 901 glass. Lung deposition was equivalent for the two glass fiber types and for high-dose amosite asbestos. Thus, the greater lung accumulation of long fibers of amosite as compared with the fiberglass products and of 475 glass as compared with 901 glass suggests that the glass fibers (901 in particular) are clearing from the lung more rapidly than is amosite. In agreement with previous findings, these data once again link fiber length and biological persistence to toxicity.

MINERAL WOOL

Before 1990, three inhalational studies reported no fibrosis or tumors as a result of chronic exposure to mineral wool (27,32,34). A recent study conducted at RCC exposed rats by nose-only inhalation to two different compositions of mineral wool—MMVF21 (rock wool) and MMVF22 (slag wool)—in three concentrations, the maximum of which was 30 mg per cubic meter (approximately 250 fibers per cubic centimeter), for 6 hours per day, 5 days per week, for 24 months. Test fibers were size-selected to have average dimensions of approximately 1 μm × 20 μm. As in the previous inhalational studies of mineral wool, neither test fiber was tumorigenic. However, in the RCC study, the rock wool–exposed rats developed minimal fibrosis late in the inhalational period (39).

REFRACTORY CERAMIC FIBERS

Two inhalation studies of RCFs were published before 1990, with conflicting results. Davis et al. (28) reported 5% pulmonary fibrosis and 17% pulmonary tumors in rats after 8 months of RCF inhalation. However, Smith et al. (27) reported RCF-associated fibrosis but no tumors in rats and no fibrosis and only one mesothelioma in hamsters. Aerosol doses in these studies were 95 and 200 fibers per cubic centimeter, respectively.

In the more recent RCC studies, rats and hamsters were exposed for 6 hours per day, 5 days per week to a maximum dose of 30 mg per cubic meter (200 to 250 fibers longer than 5 μm per cubic centimeter) of RCF. As in the other RCC studies, test fibers were size-selected to have average dimensions as close as possible to 1 × 20 μm. Rats were exposed to one of four different types of RCFs, and hamsters were exposed only to kaolin-based RCF. Both studies included positive (chrysotile asbestos) and negative (filtered air) controls. Rats exposed to RCF developed lung fibrosis, pulmonary tumors (13% in the kaolin-based RCF group), and pleural mesothelioma (1.6%) (36). Hamsters exposed to RCF developed lung fibrosis but no lung cancers, and 42 of 112 animals developed mesotheliomas (38%) (40,47). The RCC study presents a striking difference between rat and hamster responses to the same test fiber. The high rate of mesotheliomas in hamsters (38%) as compared to rats (1.6%) and the lack of lung cancer in hamsters opens questions of species-related differences and which species, if either, is representative of humans.

Cell Culture Studies

A number of *in vitro* studies have shown that fiber toxicity to cultured cells is related directly to fiber length and perhaps indirectly to fiber diameter (26,48–52). Some researchers reported that chemical composition was associated with the *in vitro* toxicity of fibers (53), whereas others have found no relationship between *in vitro* toxicity and fiber composition (52). SVFs induce neoplastic transformation (50,54) and genetic damage to cells in culture (55,56). Some investigators suggest that an assortment of cell culture tests could be used as part of a battery of short-term screening tests to assess the toxic and tumorigenic potential of SVFs (51,57). After nearly two decades of research, such a battery has still not been validated.

However, *in vitro* studies have contributed much to a better understanding of the molecular mechanisms of fiber-induced lung injury. Recently, a number of studies have focused on the role of inflammatory cells (macrophages and other leukocytes) in fiber-induced lung injury. In their critical role of lung defense, inflammatory cells inactivate and clear foreign agents and recruit more inflammatory cells from the blood stream into the lung. During this process, inflammatory cells release biologically destructive factors, such as reactive oxygen species and proteolytic enzymes, that not only destroy microbes but also injure lung cells [reviewed by Warheit et al. (58)]. These cellular activities are mediated at least in part by cytokines, chemical messengers released by cells that activate or attract other cells.

In vitro studies have helped to fill in the gaps of knowledge on fiber-induced pathogenesis at the cellular and molecular levels. By studying cells that either were exposed to fibers *in vitro* or were exposed *in vivo* before being cultured, scientists have determined some of the cytokines that are active and what they do. Soon after an irritant particle such as crocidolite asbestos is deposited in the lung, a cytokine called *tumor necrosis factor-α* (TNF-α) appears in the lung fluid and is followed by a large increase in the numbers of inflammatory cells in the lung (59). *In vitro*, TNF-α is released by cultured macrophages that have been exposed to crocidolite asbestos. TNF-α stimulates other cultured lung cells to release chemoattractant cytokines called *macrophage inflammatory proteins* (MIPs). MIPs induce macrophages and other inflammatory cells to migrate *in vitro* along the MIP concentration gradient. (*In vivo*, this would be toward the source of the irritant.) Thus, several *in vitro* researchers have offered a mechanistic model of fiber-induced lung damage as follows: Fibers stimulate macrophages to release TNF-α, which stimulates other lung cells to release MIPs, which recruit more inflammatory cells to the irritant in the lung. The activated inflammatory cells, in an attempt to destroy foreign invaders, release biologically destructive agents that also injure lung tissue. Repair and cell proliferative responses to injury ensue. If the initiating fibers are biologically persistent (i.e., the lung is unable to remove or inactivate them), the cascade continues and expands and could result in increasing lung injury, repair mechanisms, and possibly, permanent lung damage such as fibrosis or even tumorigenesis (58).

STUDIES OF FIBER BIOLOGICAL PERSISTENCE AND BIOTRANSFORMATION

In Vivo Studies

Biological persistence of fibers in the lung is the ability of fibers to persist in the lung after they have been inhaled. *Biotransformation* is any change in dimension, composition, or surface morphology that occurs in a fiber during lung residence. Researchers have only recently begun to scrutinize the mechanisms of fiber biological persistence and biotransformation and their roles in lung injury. The simple model offered in the past was that fibers that

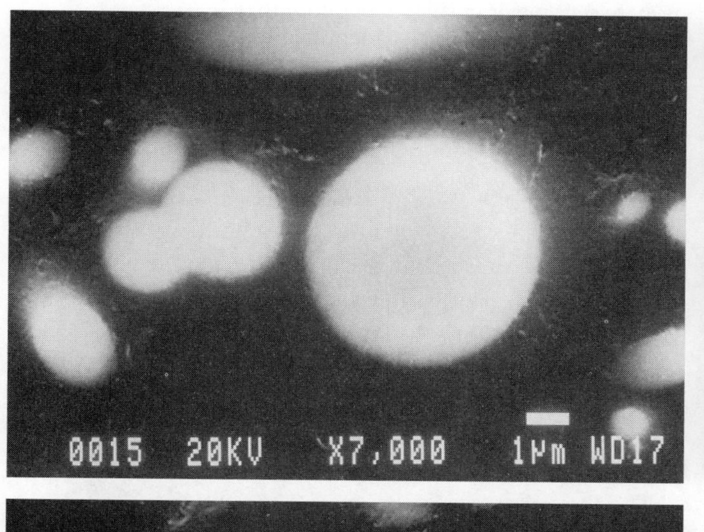

A

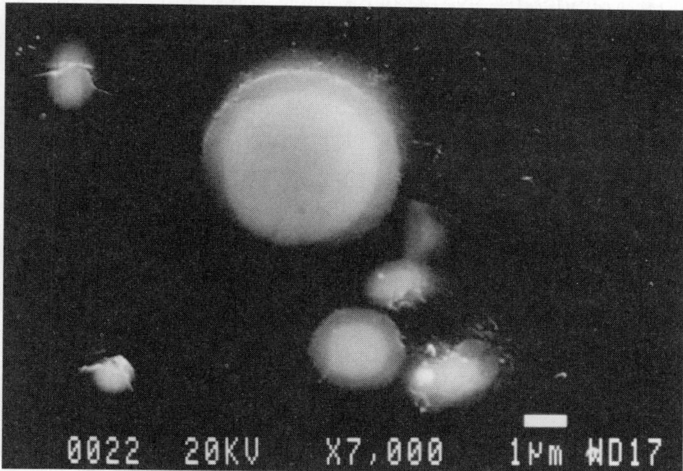

B

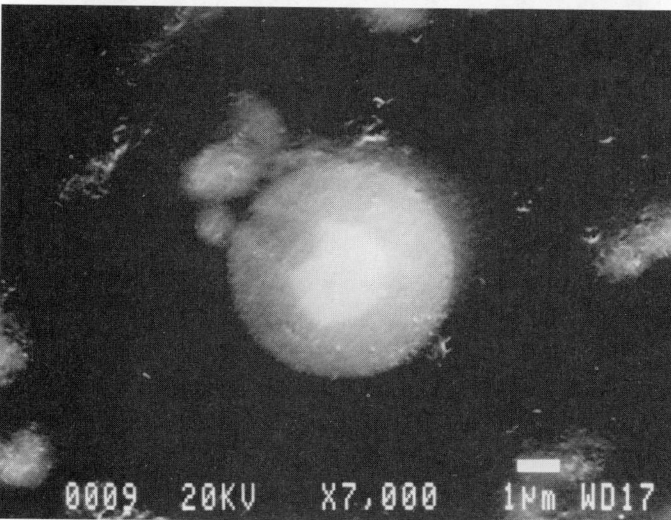

C

Figure 112-2. Fiber persistence. Fibers were incubated in simulated lung fluid in a continuously flowing *in vitro* system for 500 h, then removed, cut in cross section, and examined using electron microscopy at 7,000×. Rock wool (**A**) showed no visible dissolution; slag wool (**B**) has a small, leached outer core, demonstrating a moderate rate of incongruent dissolution; and 901 insulation fiberglass (**C**) has a very large, leached outer core, demonstrating a rapid rate of incongruent dissolution (66).

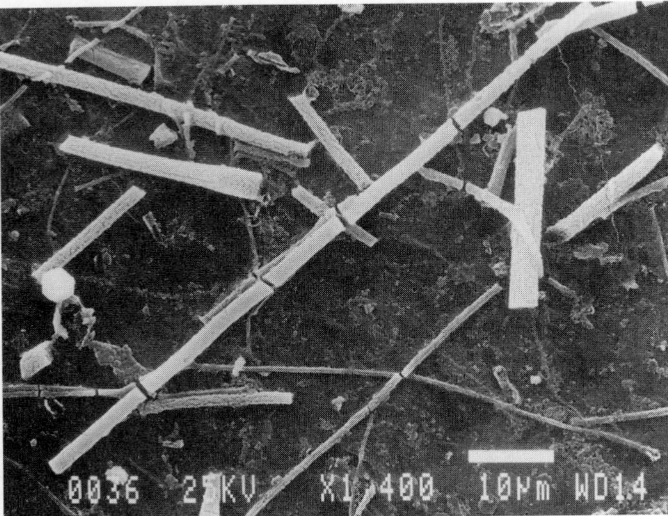

Figure 112-3. Transverse fragmentation of fiberglass. 901 glass insulation fibers were incubated in simulated lung fluid in a continuously flowing *in vitro* system for 500 h and then were removed and viewed under the electron microscope at 1,400×. The central fiber shows transverse fragmentation into segments that are 10–20 μm long. Segmentation is believed to be enhanced by leaching. Short segments clear from the lung much more readily than do long fibers.

enter the lung and rapidly dissolve are innocuous, and those that do not rapidly dissolve are pathogenic. The situation appears to be more complex than this, however. In his recent fiber inhalational study in rats, Davis et al. (unpublished report) note the strikingly greater pathology of E glass as compared to 475 glass and point out that 475 glass, although innocuous in this study, cleared slowly from the lungs of rats in a previous study. Davis cautions that the concept of biological persistence must be broader than the simple, visible retention of fibers in the lung. Although 475 glass was detectable in the rat lung for long periods, it underwent marked changes in chemistry owing to leaching. This is also true of 901 glass fibers (MMVF10), which were innocuous but cleared at the same rate as did rock wool fibers (MMVF21), which caused fibrosis in the rat lung (41); 901 glass fibers underwent chemical changes due to leaching, whereas rock wool did not.

In Vitro Studies

A closer look into the molecular mechanisms of biotransformation is provided by *in vitro* studies that measure the deterioration of fibers in simulated lung fluids (60–63). In these studies, a physiologic saline solution is passed through a cartridge that contains two filters sandwiching a fiber sample. The eluent from the system is analyzed for dissolved fiber components, and the rate of dissolution is determined (dissolution constant, or K_{dis}). *In vitro* dissolution studies have demonstrated widely varying dissolution rates for different fiber compositions. Examples of some *in vitro* dissolution rates at neutral pH are less than 1 ng per square centimeter of surface per hour for crocidolite asbestos; 8 ng per square centimeter of surface per hour for RCF; and 140 to 260 ng per square centimeter of surface per hour for glass insulation fibers (64). Some new stone wool insulation fibers have even higher dissolution rates (at pH 4.5) of more than 400 ng per square centimeter of surface per hour (65).

In vitro studies have also identified two different types of dissolution: Fibers can dissolve congruently (i.e., all components dissolve at approximately the same rate) or noncongruently (i.e., certain components dissolve more rapidly than others, leaving a

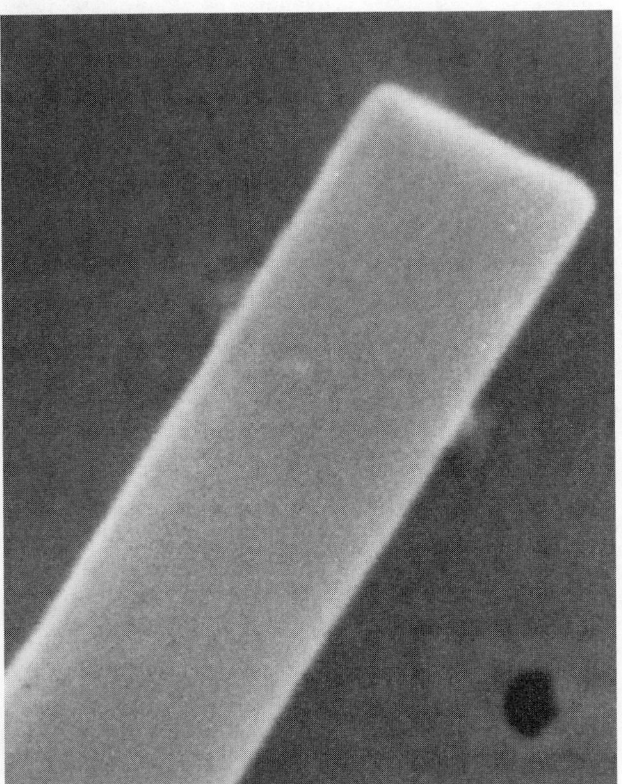

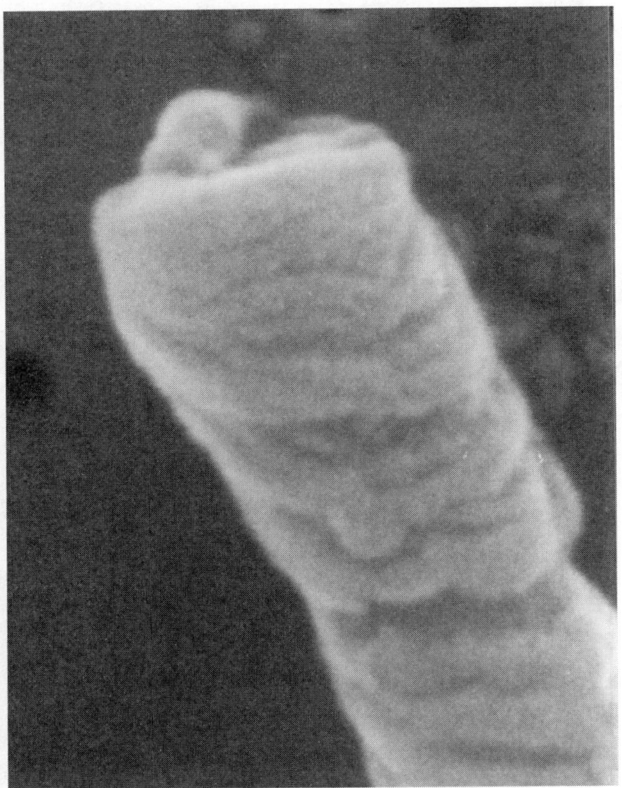

Figure 112-4. Fibers after 6 months in the rat lung. Rock wool fibers (**A**) showed no surface deterioration, whereas slag wool (**B**) showed much surface deterioration. Electron micrographs, 52,000× (66).

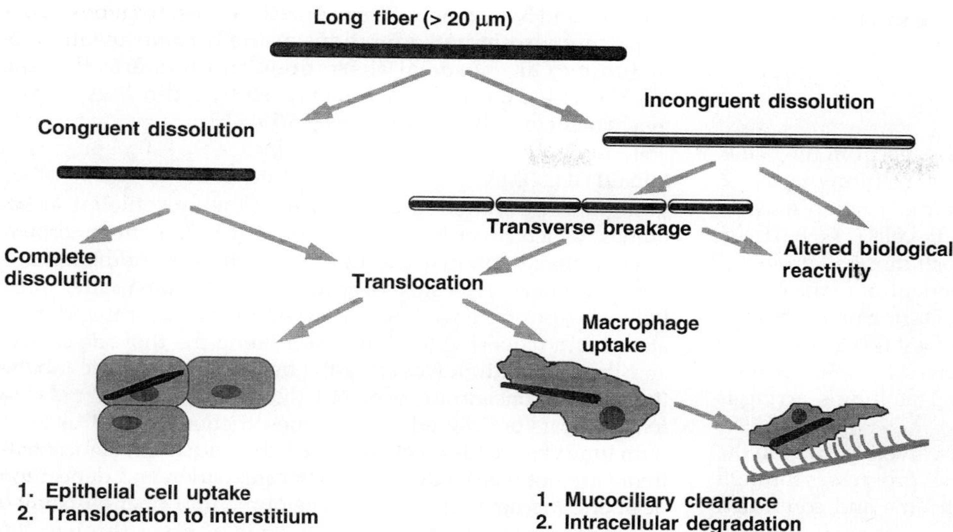

Figure 112-5. Determinants of fiber biological persistence. Fibers longer than 20 μm that are inhaled into the lower lung cannot be removed by phagocytic, mobile lung cells (macrophages). They may dissolve into smaller fibers or undergo leaching and fragment into shorter segments, both of which can be translocated out of the lung. Long fibers that do not leach or dissolve remain in the lung and continue to cause irritation.

depleted fiber residuum; also called *leaching*). Fibers from the inhalational studies were subjected to *in vitro* dissolution for 500 hours and then were sectioned and viewed with electron microscopy. In the electron micrographs in Figure 112-2, note that the three fiber types depicted show varying proportions of core versus periphery, exhibiting varying degrees of leaching. For rock wool, which was fibrogenic in rat studies, 100% of the core is intact and no leaching is seen. In contrast, slag wool and 901 glass, both of which were innocuous in rat studies, have approximately 90% and 50% of their cores intact, indicating moderate and rapid leaching, respectively (see Fig. 112-2) (66). Whereas congruent dissolution can lead to the total dissolution and disappearance of fine fibers, incongruent leaching can weaken the infrastructure of the fiber and thereby trigger transverse fragmentation, resulting in short fiber segments that are biologically less active and are more readily removed from the lungs by phagocytic cells. Relatively rapid *in vitro* leaching and transverse fragmentation have been demonstrated with glass insulation wool *in vitro*, as seen in Figure 112-3 (66). Leaching-induced changes in fiber chemistry could also have an impact on the biological reactivity of the fiber surface. The leached fiber residuum of the innocuous MMVF11 fiberglass (Fig. 112-4), while still retaining a fibrous geometry, presents a very altered surface to the lung environment and thus could have a very different effect on lung cells than the intact, original fiber. In contrast, the unaltered surface of the fibrogenic MMVF21 rock wool fiber (see Fig. 112-4) may retain whatever biological activity it originally possessed.

In vitro rates of biotransformation (dissolution or leaching and fragmentation) roughly parallel *in vivo* lung clearance rates (66). Thus, fibers that undergo rapid biotransformation may be less toxic and less likely to cause lung tumors because their altered dimensions or chemistry enhances their clearance and may also decrease their biological reactivity. These relationships are illustrated in Figure 112-5.

MECHANISMS OF FIBER-INDUCED PATHOGENICITY

Lung Deposition

Size and shape determine whether a fiber is respirable. These two factors plus specific gravity (density) determine where in the lung the fiber will deposit. *Aerodynamic diameter* is a term that combines all three of these characteristics (size, shape, and density). The aerodynamic diameter of a fiber is equivalent to the diameter of a sphere with a specific gravity of 1 that settles in air at the same rate as the fiber and is determined by the following formula:

$$D_A = 1.3^{1/2} d^{5/6} L^{1/6}$$

where D_A = aerodynamic diameter; p = density; d = diameter; and L = length). From this formula, it can be seen that fiber diameter is more important than length in determining the aerodynamic diameter of a fiber and, hence, the lung depth to which it will penetrate. Fibers with an aerodynamic diameter greater than 12 μm are not likely to reach the deep lung in humans.

Once the fiber reaches the target area of the deep lung (bronchioles and alveoli), fiber length affects lung clearance (longer fibers translate to reduced clearance) and also translocation into the lung interstitium and into the mesothelial membranes (pleura) on the outer surface of the lung. Fibers longer than 5 μm and less than 1.5 μm in diameter have the greatest potential to reach the target areas of the lung and pleura (67). Fibers longer than 20 μm may be too long to be removed from the lung by alveolar macrophages.

Although fiber aerodynamic diameter controls the entry and final site of deposition in the lung, fiber durability is the critical basis for the accumulation of a lung burden of fibers. For example, crocidolite asbestos, which belongs to the more durable amphibole class of asbestos, accumulates in human lungs in quantities that correlate with cumulative exposure, whereas chrysotile asbestos, a less durable asbestos type, does not. Other factors that may affect the intrapulmonary fate of fibers are their rigidity, their surface properties, and the architecture of their ends (smooth, grainy, spicule-shaped edges, etc.) (68).

Inflammatory Response

The initial response to deposition of foreign agents, including fibers, into the bronchioalveolar region is inflammation (alveolitis), which is initiated by lung macrophages. Activated macrophages migrate to the site of fiber deposition and phagocytize the fibers. Individual macrophages appear to engulf short fibers completely, but several macrophages may fuse as they engulf longer fibers. The very long fibers may frustrate complete ingestion by a single macrophage or groups of macrophages, resulting in the release of a variety of cell messengers, reactive oxygen species, and proteases from the macrophages. The cell messengers signal the influx and activation of more macrophages and other inflammatory cells.

Fibrosis

Biologically destructive agents that are released from lung cells during inflammation attack the lung walls, resulting in tissue necrosis. A primary player in this tissue destruction may be active oxygen species liberated by phagocytic cells (57,69). Tissue injury stimulates tissue repair processes, including cell proliferation and deposition of collagen (a component of extracellular matrix) by fibroblasts within the lung wall. During prolonged tissue repair processes, normal lung morphology is destroyed and is replaced by scar tissue that is characterized by an accumulation of collagen in the lung interstitium. This lung scarring is called *lung fibrosis*.

Fibrosis originates in the bronchioles (or alveolar ducts in the rat) where they join with the alveoli. Fibrosis progresses through the lung parenchyma (inner layer). With time and continued irritation, the fibrotic lesions coalesce into larger areas that ultimately replace large portions of the lung with scar tissue. Fibrotic scarring can also occur in the mesothelial membranes (pleura) that enclose the lungs and line the thoracic cavity. Fibrotic lesions in the lung and surrounding membranes reduce the efficiency of gas exchange, leaving the individual with an excess of carbon dioxide and a deficit of oxygen. Lung fibrosis resulting from inhalation of asbestos (asbestosis) is a progressive disease for which, currently, no effective treatment is known.

Neoplastic Tissue Response

Numerous human epidemiologic and rodent inhalational studies have demonstrated that inhalation of asbestos fibers induces thoracic cancers. Asbestos can induce cancer in two sites, the lung epithelium (bronchogenic carcinoma, or lung cancer) and the mesothelial membranes (pleura) surrounding the lungs (mesothelioma) (70,71). Very recently, rodent inhalational studies demonstrated for the first time that chronic inhalation of some durable SVF types (RCF, E glass microfibers) at MTD (300-fold greater than typical worker exposure) could also be associated with fibrosis and thoracic cancers (43). Preliminary results indicate that, when produced as microfibers, 475 durable glass at an MTD may also induce mesothelioma in hamsters (43).

LUNG CANCER

Lung cancer could develop as a by-product of the chronic fibrosis that results from the chronic lung irritation and inflammation caused by durable lung fibers. This mechanism would require that the fiber be very biologically persistent in the lung. In fibrosis, scar tissue replaces the normal architecture of the lung parenchyma, and portions of lung epithelium can become isolated and entrapped within the scar tissue. Chronic inflammation stimulates tissue repair, which includes epithelial cell proliferation. These conditions create a milieu similar to that reported in studies of scar cancer in the past. The sequestered pulmonary epithelium apparently is more susceptible to the development of carcinoma. The scarcity of lung cancer in nonsmokers and the enhanced lung cancer risk in asbestos workers who are or were smokers suggest that tobacco smoke is a crucial factor in the development of fiber-related lung cancers (72). In the absence of a history of cigarette smoking, the role of asbestos in the development of lung cancer would probably be limited to the bronchioalveolar region and be associated with or preceded by advanced fibrosis.

A second possible mechanism of asbestos-induced carcinogenesis is a direct genotoxic effect, as suggested by cell culture studies. Several studies have shown that concentrations of asbestos and SVFs that induce neoplastic transformation of cells in culture also induce mutations at the chromosomal level, including chromosomal aberrations and numeric changes (56,73). Thus, inorganic fibers may act by a direct genotoxic mechanism to induce neoplasms (56,73).

MESOTHELIOMA

Malignant mesothelioma is cancer of the mesothelial membranes, which cover the internal organs and line the inner surfaces of the abdominal and thoracic cavities. Mesothelioma is rare in humans. Asbestos-associated mesotheliomas after inhalational exposure have been observed in the visceral and parietal pleura (covering the lungs and lining the thoracic cavity) and the pericardium (covering the heart). After chronic inhalation of high concentrations of RCF, 42% of hamsters but only 1% to 3% of rats developed thoracic mesotheliomas (36,37,40). As with lung cancer, the mechanisms of fiber induction of mesothelioma are not well understood. After inhalation and deposition of fibers, the next step in the development of fiber-associated mesothelioma may be the translocation of fibers through the lung wall into the pleural membranes. This could happen only with fibers that are biologically persistent and of translocatable sizes and compositions. Subsequent steps may involve the development and advancement of pleural fibrosis in the same way that lung fibrosis is theorized to be a mechanism in the development of lung cancer. As with lung cancer mechanisms, a second potential mechanism of mesothelioma development would be direct genotoxicity of the fibers in the pleural space. Lechner et al. (73) have shown that chromosomal aberrations are associated with asbestos-induced transformation of human mesothelial cells in culture.

Summary of Mechanisms

Although not completely understood, the mechanisms of fiber-induced biological effects are believed to include the following: (i) Inhaled fibers enter the deep lung; (ii) fibers resist lung clearance and degradation mechanisms; (iii) fibers are translocated into the lung interstitium and, possibly, also the pleural membranes; (iv) fibers stimulate the cellular release of inflammatory mediators; and (v) the mediators initiate fibrosis and epithelial cell proliferation. In addition, fibers may also induce neoplastic changes directly in the genetic material of the cell. These factors are critically affected by the target-organ dose (lung deposition); fiber size, shape, and durability; and, possibly, fiber surface area and reactivity. Also affecting the potential pathogenesis are other factors that compromise pulmonary health, including previous or current disease or exposure to toxic cofactors such as cigarette smoke, other dusts, or industrial fumes. It is important to note that lung defense mechanisms can be overwhelmed by extreme experimental exposure concentrations, resulting in lung injury that is not specific to the particle type. In the RCC rodent studies, the MTDs were at least 300 times greater than fiber aerosols typically experienced by SVF workers (74). At overload concentrations, lung injuries can be induced by innocuous dusts that, at normal exposure levels, would be cleared from the lung before they were able to accumulate sufficiently to inflict injury.

OCCUPATIONAL EXPOSURE TO AIRBORNE FIBERS

Industrial Hygiene Studies

Each year, industrial hygienists analyze more than 1,000 occupational exposure samples in at least 20 SVF manufacturing plants in

North America and Europe. Air samples are also taken during SVF insulation installation and in buildings where SVF insulation and air filtration products are in use. In the United States, the National Institute for Occupational Safety and Health (NIOSH) sets standards for sampling and analyzing various categories of airborne particulates (75). The World Health Organization (WHO) also sets standards that are generally recognized worldwide.

To determine the mass concentration of total airborne dust, a measured volume of air is drawn through a specialized preweighed filter. The mass of the deposited dust sample is determined and reported as milligrams of airborne particles per cubic meter of air [NIOSH method 0500 (75)]. This measurement does not provide any information about the characteristics of the particles and is, by itself, inadequate for determining health risk, especially where airborne dust is likely to contain fibers. For example, a high-mass concentration consisting mostly of large nonfibrous particles might not be as great a threat to respiratory health as a low-mass concentration consisting of respirable fibers. Therefore, NIOSH method 7400 and the WHO reference method established procedures for microscopically determining the number of respirable fibers per cubic centimeter of air (75,76).

Synthetic Vitreous Fiber Exposure Levels

In general, exposure to SVFs during manufacture, installation, and final use has been very low or undetectable. In SVF manufacturing workplaces, airborne fiber exposures have typically been less than 0.2 fiber per cubic centimeter, with total particulate matter less than 1.0 mg per cubic meter (61). During installation of fiberglass, fiber exposures averaged less than 0.5 fiber per cubic centimeter, with a range of 0 to 20 fibers per cubic centimeter, and total particulate matter averaged less than 4.2 mg per cubic meter, with a range of 0.04 to 114.00 mg per cubic meter.

Air samples were analyzed from a number of public buildings in which fiberglass air filters were in use or in which fiberglass insulation had been installed; these analyses demonstrated no significant fiberglass exposure to the building occupants (77,78). In another study, air samples were collected at various intake and exhaust points of the air ducts of a large office complex before changing the fiberglass air filters and at the exhaust 23 days after installation of the new filters. Analyses of these samples using electron microscopy indicated a very low initial fiber release after installation that rapidly decreased to below the level of detection (Manville Corporation, unpublished industrial hygiene survey data, 1987).

Airborne concentrations of dust and fibers in U.S. mineral wool plants are generally higher than in U.S. glass wool facilities. Average fiber concentrations ranged from 0.01 to 1.40 fibers per cubic centimeter in mineral wool plants, as compared with 0.1 to 0.3 fiber per cubic centimeter in glass wool plants. Total particulate matter ranged from 0.05 to 23.60 mg per cubic meter in the mineral wool plants and 0.09 to 8.48 mg per cubic meter in glass wool plants (79).

Exposures during application or installation are also typically higher for mineral wool products than for similar glass wool products. These levels are directly related to the methods of installation and the engineering controls and work practices that have been instituted to limit exposure.

Industrial hygiene monitoring data obtained on a regular basis at locations where RCF products are manufactured show that exposures are generally less than 1.0 fiber per cubic centimeter and often lower than 0.2 fiber per cubic centimeter. During installation of RCF products, exposures can be 1 to 5 fibers per cubic centimeter or higher if appropriate engineering controls and work practices are not followed (Manville Corporation, unpublished industrial hygiene surveys data, 1985 through 1988).

Occupational Exposure Limits

Currently, no regulations are in place that specifically limit SVF exposure. In the United States, the Occupational Safety and Health Administration classifies SVFs as nuisance dusts. Permissible exposure limits for respirable and total nuisance dusts have been established at 5.0 and 15.0 mg per cubic meter, respectively. NIOSH has recommended a fiber-based exposure limit of 3.0 fibers per cubic centimeter for fibers less than 3.5 μm in diameter and more than 10 μm long. Several SVF manufacturers have recommended exposure limits of 1.0 to 2.0 fibers per cubic centimeter for fiberglass, mineral wool, and RCF. Because recent rodent inhalational studies have reported an association between lung disease and chronic exposure to high levels of RCF and some durable fiberglass products (e.g., E glass and perhaps also 475 glass) (5,8; Hesterberg et al., 1997), it is wise to reduce SVF dusts—especially those containing durable fibers—to the lowest practicable level and to require that respiratory protection be used until additional information is available that will permit an adequate risk assessment of each fiber type (1,8).

Occupational Exposure to Other Compounds

To accurately assess the toxicologic potential of a substance in the workplace, all other substances present in the environment must be considered. Many SVF products contain an assortment of chemical binders and lubricating oils. In addition to SVF dusts, workers can be exposed to an array of other substances, including formaldehyde, phenol, ammonia, urea, crystalline silica, asbestos, polycyclic aromatic hydrocarbons, and asphalt. The potential cumulative effects of exposure to all these materials must be considered in any operation to develop a sound plan for employee and environmental health and safety.

EVALUATION OF SYNTHETIC VITREOUS FIBERS

International Agency for Research on Cancer Evaluation

In 1971, the International Agency for Research on Cancer (IARC) initiated a program by which to evaluate data regarding the carcinogenic risk of chemicals to humans. In this program, scientists have been asked to write and critically evaluate a series of monographs on individual chemicals. The IARC generally appoints a special working group of scientists to evaluate the data for a class of chemical agents. Before the group meets, several members of the group are appointed to review data that fall in their respective fields of expertise; for example, laboratory researchers review animal and *in vitro* experiments and epidemiologists review human studies. Under IARC procedures, after review, the IARC may classify an agent as one of the following:

- *Group 1*: sufficient evidence of human carcinogenicity
- *Group 2A*: probably carcinogenic to humans
- *Group 2B*: possibly carcinogenic to humans
- *Group 3*: not classifiable as to human carcinogenicity
- *Group 4*: probably not carcinogenic to humans

In 1987, the IARC appointed a working group of 20 scientists to evaluate the carcinogenic risk of exposure to SVFs. Even though the human studies were extensive, the group judged the data available at that time to be inadequate for establishing the carcinogenicity of glass wool. The agency did, however, designate glass wool in group 2B. This classification was based in large part on reports that artificial implantation of some types of glass fibers caused tumors in laboratory animals. Continuous filament (glass textile) was designated as IARC group 3. The IARC classified rock wool as group 2B, on the basis of limited evidence in experimental animals and limited evidence in humans. Likewise, slag wool was classified as group 2B, on the basis of inadequate evidence in animals and limited evidence in humans. As was noted earlier in this chapter, no data from human studies are available by which to evaluate RCF for carcinogenicity. Nonetheless, the IARC designated RCF as a group 2B substance on the basis of studies using laboratory animals (80).

International Program on Chemical Safety Evaluation

In 1977, the thirtieth World Health Assembly requested the director-general of WHO to devise long-term strategies for controlling and limiting the impact of chemicals on human health and the environment. In January 1979, the sixty-third session of the WHO executive board endorsed a plan of action and joined with other international organizations to establish the International Program on Chemical Safety (IPCS), which became operational in April 1980.

The IPCS is a joint venture of the United Nations Environment Program, the International Labor Organization, and WHO. Its main objectives are to investigate the effects of chemicals on human health and the environment and to disseminate the findings. The IPCS program supports the development of standardized methods for epidemiology, laboratory experimentation, and risk assessment (including extrapolation of experimental data to human risk), so that findings from international sources can be compared. Methods and findings are published in a WHO monograph series (80).

Under the IPCS program, a task group was assembled in 1987 to finalize the environmental health criteria document on man-made mineral fibers (i.e., SVFs). The SVF task group considered health risks for both occupational exposure and the general population, for neoplastic and nonneoplastic lung diseases, and for dermatitis. Subgroups were formed to discuss separately the human epidemiologic data and animal experimental data. The subgroups prepared a report of findings and conclusions and submitted this to the IPCS. In 1988, the WHO published the report as environmental health criteria 77, "Man-Made Mineral Fibres" (80).

On the basis of available data (no epidemiologic data being available for RCF), the report did not find any quantitative human risks associated with SVF exposure. The report noted the possibility of transient effects of skin and upper respiratory irritation, as discussed earlier. Considering all results of animal studies, the IPCS task group concluded that an increased risk of lung cancer in some sectors of the SVF industry is biologically plausible and recommended protective equipment to guard against a potential elevation in lung cancer risk for workers engaged in activities in which elevated airborne exposure levels are possible.

For SVF in general, the IPCS report stated, "[T]he overall picture indicates that the possible risk of lung cancer among the general public is very low, if there is any at all, and should not be a cause for concern if the current low levels of exposure continue" (80).

OCCUPATIONAL HEALTH CONSIDERATIONS

Prevention and Protection

Whenever there exists a potential for employees to be exposed to substances that either are known to be harmful or have not been completely evaluated, the first step is to minimize exposure to the lowest practicable level. In SVF occupational settings, modifications to the product design can sometimes reduce the amount of dust that it releases during manufacture or installation. Exhaust ventilation can remove dusts at their points of origin. Appropriate work practices can also limit the amount of dust generated; for example, vacuum cleaning is better than dry-sweeping with a broom or with compressed air. SVF workers can further protect themselves by wearing safety glasses or goggles to prevent eye exposure, long-sleeved shirts and long pants to minimize skin exposure, and respiratory protection to minimize dust inhalation. A careful evaluation of the workplace should be conducted to determine the appropriate devices to be used in an individual situation (8,17).

Monitoring Exposure and Health

Whenever employees are exposed to potentially harmful substances, a program should be established to monitor their exposure levels and health routinely. First, exposure ranges and averages should be determined for each operation or task. Next, the appropriate type of personal protective equipment should be determined for each task. A medical surveillance program should be established, including a review of general health, occupational history, physical examination, clinical chemistries and blood count, pulmonary function testing, a baseline chest radiograph, and other testing as indicated by the occupational history. For SVF workers, the focus should be on respiratory and dermatologic health. Exposure and health monitoring should continue on a regular basis (e.g., yearly) or whenever processes or products change. Findings should be reviewed regularly, both for individuals and groups (1,8).

HEALTH EFFECTS SUMMARY

SVFs are extremely useful products, serving human needs for insulation and filtration for more than a century. SVF products can be grouped into three basic classes: various fiberglass types, mineral wools, and RCFs. To aid us in better understanding the potential health effects of occupational exposure to these substances, SVFs continue to be evaluated in laboratory experiments, epidemiologic analyses of SVF workers, and industrial hygiene studies that measure human exposure. In these studies, the primary concern is human respiratory health in SVF workplaces.

Currently, the only relevant laboratory method for assessing the potential hazard of SVFs to human respiratory health is the animal inhalational model. In rodent inhalational studies, asbestos induced fibrosis and thoracic cancer, thus validating this model with a known human carcinogen (which is also a naturally occurring fiber). In these studies, glass insulation wools and slag wool produced no permanent injury, even after 2 years of exposure to high concentrations (at least 300-fold the concentrations to which human SVF workers typically are exposed). In recent rodent inhalational studies, two durable SVF compositions were associated with permanent lung injury: rock wool (MMVF21) induced fibrosis late in the study, and RCF induced fibrosis and tumorigenesis. Preliminary results from another, in-progress study suggest that a third durable fiber, E glass microfiber, may also induce fibrosis and tumorigenesis in rats. Preliminary results suggest that a fourth relatively durable fiber, 475 glass, induces fibrosis and, possibly, mesothelioma in hamsters but not in rats. Thus, the rodent inhalational studies demonstrate a broad range of biological effects for the different SVFs. Rodent inhalational studies also demonstrate a very broad range in lung clearance rates among various fiber compositions: Lung clearance of 90% of long fibers requires more than 3 years for asbestos, 1 year for RCF, 2 to 3 months for fiberglass insulation wools, and 3 weeks for HT stone wool. These results demonstrate that SVFs not only differ in important ways from asbestos, but they also differ greatly among themselves, indicating that SVF types should not be lumped together but should be evaluated individually.

The biological effects of fibers have also been investigated in animal implantation and *in vitro* cell culture models. However, for several reasons, these models are not useful for human hazard assessment: Most notably, neither of these models provides toxicity results that parallel findings from human epidemiologic or animal inhalational studies. When artificially implanted into the body cavities of rodents, almost any composition of long, thin fibers can induce fibrosis and tumors. However, implantation bypasses the natural defenses and can easily achieve organ doses vastly in excess of that which would be possible through the normal exposure route, inhalation. *In vitro* cell culture systems also do not include host defense mechanisms and are typically too brief to model differences in fiber biological persistence.

Large epidemiologic studies of SVF have been conducted for a number of years and continue to be updated. The two largest studies are the Marsh-Enterline study in the United States and the Saracci study in Europe. Neither study has associated increased pulmonary morbidity or mortality with exposure to fiberglass. A small excess in morbidity exists among mineral wool workers, but the excess does not show a dose-response relationship and it does not correlate with length of employment in the mineral wool industry.

Industrial hygiene studies conducted in SVF manufacturing plants typically demonstrate low exposures to airborne fibers. However, industrial hygiene studies conducted in the field during installation of SVF products indicate that some individual situations can result in high occupational exposures to fibers. One example is the blow-in installation of SVF products. In these situations, respiratory protection, enhanced work practices, and application of engineering controls are appropriate and prudent.

The potential health effects of SVFs have been reviewed by scientific panels, such as the IARC and IPCS. In 1987, the IARC designated fiberglass, mineral wools, and RCF as group 2B (possible) carcinogens based on limited or inadequate evidence from animal studies (largely from implantation studies) and human epidemiology. In the IPCS review (1988), the absence of disease in the vast majority of workers exposed to fiberglass during the last 50 years suggests that fiberglass products pose "little, if any, health risk to humans." Much has been learned since these critical reviews were conducted, and much more research is needed to evaluate better which fibers are pathogenic to the respiratory tract and why. New research is being planned. Broadened updates of the U.S. (Marsh-Enterline) mortality study are already under way, including further review of potential confounders. In addition to conducting and updating the RCF morbidity study, the RCF industry in 1984 initiated the largest respiratory health surveillance program for production workers in the world, and initial study of that database has begun. Additional rodent inhalational studies are also in planning or under way for a variety of SVF compositions. *In vitro* modeling of fiber degradation in simulated lung fluid continues to contribute to an expanding database. *In vitro* cell culture studies continue to contribute to the molecular mechanisms of cell interactions with fibers. A world that depends on energy will always need insulation to help to conserve fuels and filters to prevent air pollution from the byproducts of fuel consumption. This research will help to ensure that safe SVF products are available for these vital functions.

REFERENCES

1. Chase G, Anderson R. *Health and safety aspects of fiberglass*. Denver, CO: Manville Corporation, 1986:22.
2. Pundsack FL. Fiber glass—manufacture, use, and physical properties. In: LeVee WN, Schulte PA, eds. *Occupational exposure to fiberglass*. US Department of Health, Education, and Welfare (NIOSH) publ. no. 76151; National Technical Information publ. no. PB258869. Cincinnati: National Institute for Occupational Safety and Health, 1976:11–18.
3. Boyd DC, Thompson DA. Glass. In: Grayson M, Mark HF, Othmer DF, Overberger CG, Seaborg GT, eds. *Kirk-Othmer encyclopedia of chemical technology*, 3rd ed, vol 11. New York: John Wiley and Sons, 1980:807–880.
4. Mohr JG, Rowe WP. *Fiberglass*. New York: Van Nostrand–Reinhold, 1978.
5. Arledter HF, Knowles SE. Ceramic fibers. In: Battista OA, ed. *Synthetic fibers in papermaking*. New York: Interscience, 1964:185–244.
6. Dement JM. Environmental aspects of fibrous glass production and utilization. *Environ Res* 1975;9:295–312.
7. Possick PA, Gillin GA, Key MM. Fiberglass dermatitis. *Am Ind Hyg Assoc J* 1970;31(1):12–15.
8. Chase G, Anderson R. *Health and safety aspects of refractory ceramic fibers*. Denver, CO: Manville Corporation, 1988.
9. Parmeggiani L, ed. *Encyclopedia of occupational health and safety*, 3rd ed, vol 1. Geneva: International Labor Office, 1983.
10. Simonato L, Fletcher AC, Cherrie J, et al. International Agency for Research on Cancer. Historical cohort study of SVF production workers in seven European countries: extension of the followup. *Ann Occup Hyg* 1987;31:603–623.
11. Boffetta P, Saracci R, Ferro G, et al. *IARC historical cohort study of man-made vitreous fibre production workers in seven European countries—extension of the mortality and cancer incidence follow-up until 1990.* IARC internal report 95/003. Geneva: World Health Organization, 1995.
12. Enterline PE, Marsh GM, Henderson V, Callahan C. Mortality update of a cohort of U.S. manmade mineral fibre workers. *Ann Occup Hyg* 1987;31:625–656.
13. Marsh GM, Enterline PE, Stone RA, Henderson MS. Mortality among a cohort of U.S. manmade mineral fiber workers: 1985 followup. *J Occup Med* 1990;32:594–604.
14. Marsh G, Stone R, Youk A, et al. Mortality among United States rock wool and slag wool workers: 1989 update. *J Occup Health Safety Aust N Z* 1996;12(3):297–312.
15. Shannon HS, Hayes M, Julian JA, Muir DCF, Walsh C. Mortality experience of glass fibre workers. *Br J Ind Med* 1984;41:35–38.
16. Shannon HS, Hayes M, Julian JA, Muir DCF. Mortality experience of Ontario glass fibre workers—extended followup. *Ann Occup Hyg* 1987;31:657–662.
17. Weill H, Hughes JM, Hammad YY, Glindmeyer HW III, Sharon G, Jones RN. Respiratory health in workers exposed to manmade vitreous fibers. *Am Rev Respir Dis* 1983;128:104–122.
18. Weill H, Hughes JM, Hammad YY, Glindmeyer HW III, Sharon G, Jones RN. Respiratory health of workers exposed to SVF. In: *Biological effects of manmade mineral fibres*, vol 1. Proceedings of a WHO/IARC conference. Copenhagen: World Health Organization, 1984:387–412.
19. Hughes JM, Jones RN, Glindmeyer HW, Hammad YY, Weill H. Follow up study of workers exposed to man made mineral fibres. *Br J Ind Med* 1993; 50(7):658–667.
20. Lockey J, Lemasters G, Wiot J. Refractory ceramic fiber exposure and pleural plaques. *Am J Respir Crit Care Med* 1996;154(5):1405.
21. Thermal Insulation Manufacturers' Association. *Health and safety aspects of man-made vitreous fibers*, part IV. Stamford, CT: Thermal Insulation Manufacturers' Association, Inc, 1990.
22. Bunn WB, Hesterberg T, Versen R. The health effects of fiberglass and refractory ceramic fiber. Glass Technology, 1989.
23. Pott F, Ziem U, Mohr U. Lung carcinomas and mesotheliomas following intratracheal instillation of glass fibres and asbestos. In: *Proceedings of the Sixth International Pneumoconiosis Conference, Bochum, Federal Republic of Germany, 20–23 September 1983*, vol 2. Geneva: International Labour Office, 1984:746–756.
24. Pott F, Schlipkoter HW, Ziem U, Spurny K, Huth F. New results from implantation experiments with mineral fibres. In: *Biological effects of manmade mineral fibres,* vol 2. Proceedings of a WHO/IARC conference. Copenhagen: World Health Organization, 1984:286–302.
25. Stanton JF, Layard M, Tegeris A, et al. Relation of particle dimension to carcinogenicity in amphibole asbestoses and other fibrous minerals. *J Natl Cancer Inst* 1981;67:965–975.
26. Hesterberg TW, Hart GA, Bunn WB. *In vitro* toxicology of fibers: mechanistic studies and possible use for screening assays. In: Warheit D, *Fiber toxicology.* New York: Academic Press, 1993:139–170.
27. Smith DM, Ortiz LW, Archuleta RF, Johnson NF. Long-term health effects in hamsters and rats exposed chronically to manmade vitreous fibers. *Ann Occup Hyg* 1987;31:731–754.
28. Davis JMG, Addison J, Bolton RE, Donaldson K, Jones AD, Wright A. The pathogenic effects of fibrous ceramic aluminum silicate glass administered to rats by inhalation or peritoneal injection. In: *Biological effects of manmade mineral fibres*, vol 2. Proceedings of a WHO/IARC conference. Copenhagen: World Health Organization, 1984:303–322.
29. Davis JMG. A review of experimental evidence for the carcinogenicity of manmade vitreous fibers. *Scand J Work Environ Health* 1986;12[Suppl 1]:12–17.
30. Gross P, de Treville RTP, Cralley LJ, Granquist WT, Pundsack FL. The pulmonary response to fibrous dusts of diverse compositions. *Am Ind Hyg Assoc J* 1970;31:125–132.

31. Lee KP, Barras CE, Griffith FD, Waritz RS, Lapin CA. Comparative pulmonary responses to inhaled inorganic fibers with asbestos and fiberglass. *Environ Res* 1981;24:167–191.
32. Wagner JC, Berry GB, Hill RJ, Munday DE, Skidmore JW. Animal experiments with MMM(V)F—effects of inhalation and intrapleural inoculation in rats. In: *Biological effects of manmade mineral fibres,* vol 2. Proceedings of a WHO/IARC conference. Copenhagen: World Health Organization, 1984:209–233.
33. McConnell EE, Wagner JC, Skidmore JW, Moore JA. A comparative study of the fibrogenic and carcinogenic effects of UICC Canadian chrysotile B asbestos and glass microfibre (JM 100). In: *Biological effects of manmade mineral fibres,* vol 2. Proceedings of a WHO/IARC conference. Copenhagen: World Health Organization, 1984:234–252.
34. LeBouffant L, Daniel H, Henin JP, et al. Experimental study on long-term effects of inhaled SVF on the lung of rats. *Ann Occup Hyg* 1987;31:765–790.
35. Muhle H, Pott F, Bellmann B, Takenaka S, Ziem U. Inhalation and injection experiments in rats to test the carcinogenicity of SVF. *Ann Occup Hyg* 1987;31:755–764.
36. Mast RW, McConnell EE, Anderson R, et al. Studies on the chronic toxicity (inhalation) of refractory ceramic fiber in male Fischer 344 rats. *Inhal Toxicol* 1995;7:425-467.
37. Mast R, McConnell EE, Hesterberg TW, et al. A multiple dose chronic inhalation study of size-separated kaolin refractory ceramic fiber in male Fischer 344 rats. *Inhal Toxicol* 1995;7:469–502.
38. Bunn WB, Bender J, Hesterberg T, Chase GR, Konsen J. Recent studies of man-made vitreous fibers. *J Occup Med* 1993;35(2):101–113.
39. McConnell EE, Kamstrup O, Musselman R, et al. Chronic inhalation study of size-separated rock and slag wool insulation fibers in Fischer 344/N rats. *Inhal Toxicol* 1994;6(6):571–614.
40. McConnell EE, Mast RW, Hesterberg TW, et al. Chronic inhalation toxicity of a kaolin-based refractory ceramic fiber (RCF) in Syrian golden hamsters. *Inhal Toxicol* 1995;7:503–532.
41. Hesterberg TW, Miller WC, Musselman RP, Kamstrup O, Hamilton RD, Thevenaz P. Biopersistence of man-made vitreous fibers and crocidolite in rat lung following inhalation. *Fund Appl Toxicol* 1996;29:267–279.
42. Hesterberg TW, Axten C, Hadley J, et al. Chronic inhalation study of fiber glass and amosite asbestos in hamsters: twelve-month preliminary results. *Environ Health Perspect* 1997;105[Suppl 5]:1223–1229.
43. Hesterberg TW, Chase G, Axten C, et al. Biopersistence of synthetic vitreous fibers and amosite asbestos in the rat lung following inhalation. *Toxicol Appl Pharmacol* 1998; 262–275.
44. Bernstein DM, Thevenaz P, Fleissner H, Anderson R, Hesterberg T, Mast R. Evaluation of the oncogenic potential of man-made vitreous fibers: the inhalation model. *Ann Occup Hyg* 1995:39(5):661–672.
45. Infante PF, Schuman LD, Dement J, Huff J. Commentary: fibrous glass and cancer. *Am J Ind Med* 1994;26:559–584.
46. Hesterberg TW, McConnell EE, Miller WC, et al. Use of lung toxicity and lung particle clearance to estimate the maximum tolerated dose (MTD) for a fiberglass chronic inhalation study in the rat. *Fund Appl Toxicol* 1996;32:31–44.
47. Rossiter CE, Chase GR. Statistical analysis of results of carcinogenicity studies of synthetic vitreous fibers at Research and Consulting Co, Füllinsdorf, Switzerland. *Br J Ind Med* 1995;39(5):759–769.
48. Chamberlain M, Brown RC, Davies R, Griffiths DM. *In vitro* prediction of the pathogenicity of mineral dusts. *Br J Exp Pathol* 1979;60:320–327.
49. Tilkes F, Beck EG. Comparison of length dependent cytotoxicity of inhalable asbestos and manmade mineral fibres. In: Wagner JC, ed. *Biological effects of mineral fibres* (IARC Scientific publ. no. 30). Lyon: International Agency for Research on Cancer, 1980:475–483.
50. Hesterberg TW, Barrett JC. Dependence of asbestos and mineral dust-induced transformation of mammalian cells in culture on fiber dimension. *Cancer Res* 1984;44:2170–2180.
51. Hart GA, Newman M, Bunn WB, Hesterberg TW. Cytotoxicity of refractory ceramic fibers to Chinese hamster ovary cells in culture. *Toxicology* 1992; 6(4):317–325.
52. Hart GA, Kathman LM, Hesterberg TW. *In vitro* cytotoxicity of asbestos and man-made vitreous fibers: roles of fiber length, diameter and composition. *Carcinogenesis* 1994;15:971–977.
53. Ririe DG, Hesterberg TW, Barrett JC, Nettesheim P. Toxicity of asbestos and glass fibers for rat tracheal epithelial cells in culture. In: Beck EG, Bignon J, eds. In vitro *effects of mineral dusts*, vol G3. NATO ASI Series. Berlin: Springer, 1985:177–184.
54. Poole A, Brown RC, Rood AP. The *in vitro* activities of a highly carcinogenic mineral fibre—potassium octatitanate. *Br J Exp Pathol* 1986;67:289–296.
55. Sincock A, Seabright M. Induction of chromosome changes in Chinese hamster cells by exposure to asbestos fibres. *Nature* 1925;257:56–58.
56. Oshimura M, Hesterberg TW, Tsutsui T, Barrett CJ. Correlation of asbestos-induced cytogenetic effects with cell transformation of Syrian hamster embryo cells in culture. *Cancer Res* 1984;44:5017–5022.
57. Mossman BT, Sesko AM. *In vitro* assays to predict the pathogenicity of mineral fibers. *Toxicology* 1990;60(1–2):53–61.
58. Warheit DB, Hansen JF, Yuen IS, Kelly DP, Snajdr SI, Hartsky MA. Inhalation of high concentrations of low toxicity dusts in rats results in impaired pulmonary clearance mechanisms and persistent inflammation. *Toxicol Appl Pharmacol* 1997;145:10–22.
59. Driscoll KE. The toxicology of crystalline silica studied *in vitro*. *Appl Environ Hyg* 1995;10(12):1118.
60. Klingholz R, Steinkopf B. The reactions of SVF in a physiological model fluid and in water. In: *Biological effects of manmade mineral fibres,* vol 2. Proceedings of a WHO/IARC conference. Copenhagen: World Health Organization, 1984:60–86.
61. Leineweber JP. Solubility of fibres *in vitro* and *in vivo*. In: *Biological effects of manmade mineral fibres,* vol 2. Proceedings of a WHO/IARC conference. Copenhagen: World Health Organization, 1984:87–101.
62. Law B, Bunn WB, Hesterberg TW. Dissolution of natural mineral and man-made vitreous fibers in Karnovsky's and formalin fixatives. *Inhalation Toxicol* 1991;3:309–321.
63. Law B, Bunn WB, Hesterberg TW. Solubility of polymeric organic fibers and man-made vitreous fibers in Gambles solution. *Inhalation Toxicol* 1990;2:321–339.
64. Zoitos B, Rouyer-Archer E, De Meringo A, et al. *In vitro* measurement of fiber dissolution rate. *Inhal Toxicol* 1997;9:525–540.
65. Knudsen T. New type of stone wool (HT fibres) with a high dissolution rate at pH = 4.5. *Glastech Ber Glass Sci Technol* 1996;69(10):331–337.
66. Hesterberg TW, Miller WC, Hart GA, Bauer J, Hamilton RD. Physical and chemical transformation of synthetic vitreous fibers in the lung and *in vitro*. *J Occup Health Safety Aust N Z* 1996;12(3):345–355.
67. Stober W. Dynamic shape factors of nonspherical aerosol particles. In: Mercer TT, Morrow PE, Stober W, eds. *Assessment of airborne particles*. Springfield, IL: Charles C Thomas Publisher, 1972.
68. Lippman M. Review asbestos exposure indices. *Environ Res* 1988;46:86–106.
69. Hansen L, Mossman BT. Generation of superoxide (O_2) from alveolar macrophages exposed to asbestiform and nonfibrous particles. *Cancer Res* 1987; 47:1681–1686.
70. Demy NG, Adler H. Asbestos and malignancy. *Am J Roentgenol* 1967; 100:597.
71. McDonald JC, Becklake MR, Gibbs GW, McDonald AD, Rossiter DE. The health of chrysotile asbestos mine and mill workers of Quebec. *Arch Environ Health* 1974;38:61.
72. Selikoff IJ, Churg, J, Hammond, EC. The occurrence of asbestosis among insulation workers in the United States. *Ann N Y Acad Sci* 1965;132:139.
73. Lechner JF, Tokiwa T, Yeager H Jr, Harris CC. Asbestos-associated chromosomal changes in human mesothelial cells. In: Beck EG, Bignon J, eds. In vitro *effects of mineral dusts*. Berlin: Springer-Verlag, 1985.
74. Hesterberg TW, Hart GA. A comparison of human exposures to fiber glass with those used in a recent rat chronic inhalation study. *Regul Toxicol Pharmacol* 1994;20:S35–S46.
75. *NIOSH manual of analytical methods,* 3rd ed. Atlanta: US Department of Health and Human Services, Public Health Service, Centers for Disease Control.
76. World Health Organization. *Reference methods for measuring airborne manmade mineral fibres*. WHO/EURO Technical Committee for Monitoring and Evaluating Airborne SVF. Copenhagen: World Health Organization, 1985.
77. Balzer JL, Cooper WC, Fowler DP. Fiberglass-lined air transmission systems: an assessment of their environmental effects. *Am Ind Hyg Assoc J* 1971;32:512–518.
78. Cholak J, Schafer L. Erosion of fibers from installed fiber glass ducts. *Arch Environ Health* 1971;22:220–229.
79. Esmen N. *Estimation of employee exposures to total suspended particulate matter and airborne fibers in insulation installation operations*. Pittsburgh: University of Pittsburgh, 1980.
80. World Health Organization. *Manmade mineral fibres*. Environmental health criteria 77. *IARC Monogr Eval Carcinog Risks Hum* 1988;43:59–171.

CHAPTER 113
Polycyclic Aromatic Hydrocarbons

Ken Kulig and Steven Pike

Polycyclic aromatic hydrocarbons (PAHs) are scientifically important because several members of this class are prototypical human carcinogens and have been studied extensively for their mechanisms of carcinogenic action. Benzo[a]pyrene (BaP) diol-epoxide adducts, for example, have recently been discovered to bind covalently to several guanine positions of the bronchial epithelial cell DNA p53 gene (1), where cancer mutations are known to occur from exposure to cigarette smoke. This finding has provided the precise genotoxic mechanism of cancer causation by tobacco smoke, which had eluded scientists for many years. Future mechanistic research such as this may provide great insight as to how other PAHs, as well as other classes of

TABLE 113-1. Emission sources

Source	Benzo[a]pyrene emissions (tons/yr)	Percentage of total
Wood-burning fireplaces, etc.	25	2.8
Coal refuse fires	310	34.7
Residential furnaces	300	33.6
Coke production	170	19.0
Mobile sources, gasoline	11	1.2
Forest and agricultural refuse burning	11	1.2
Open refuse burning	11	1.2
Vehicle disposal open burning	25	2.8

From the U.S. Environmental Protection Agency, *Preferred standards path report for polycyclic organic matter.* Durham, NC: U.S. Environmental Protection Agency, Office of Air Quality Planning and Standards, Strategies Air Standards Division, 1974, as adapted from Baum EJ. *Polycyclic hydrocarbons and cancer: 1. Occurrence and surveillance of polycyclic aromatic hydrocarbons.* Orlando: Academic Press, 1978.

chemicals, cause cancer in humans and may help us to identify those persons at risk from a specific exposure.

SOURCES OF EXPOSURE

PAHs are ecologically important because they are common byproducts of combustion processes, and most people are exposed to them regularly in our air, water, and food (Tables 113-1 through 113-4). The burning of fossil fuels, wood, coal, and waste constitutes the main human source of PAHs emitted into the atmosphere (see Table 113-1). Diesel exhaust contains significant quantities of PAHs.

PAHs are found in charbroiled meats, smoked foods, tobacco products, roasted coffee, tea, peanuts, and even vegetables and fruit (see Table 113-4). Plants may synthesize PAHs or absorb them via water, air, or soil. PAHs are found in coal tar, which may be used therapeutically in both prescription and over-the-counter treatments of skin disorders such as psoriasis or dandruff (2).

Humans are exposed occupationally and from common exposure sources daily (see Table 113-2). PAHs are commonly found in water (3) and soil (4) from either man-made or natural sources (see Table 113-3). They are released into the atmosphere from natural processes such as volcanoes and forest fires. They

TABLE 113-2. Environmental sources

Exposure category	Benzo[a]pyrene
Cigarette smoking, unfiltered (1 pack/d)	0.7 μg/d
Cigarette smoking, filtered (1 pack/d)	0.4 μg/d
Airline cockpits (prior to nonsmoking regulations)	
Transatlantic	0.093 μg/m³ (8-h TWA)
Domestic	0.138 μg/m³ (8-h TWA)
Coke-oven workers	
Topside	18 μg/m³ (8-h TWA)
Side and bench	7 μg/m³ (8-h TWA)
Roof tarring	14 μg/m³
Sidewalk tarring	78 μg/m³
Restaurant workers	0.8 μg/day
	0.03–0.14 μg/m³

TWA, time-weighted average.
Adapted from Bridbord K, Finlea JF, Wagoner JK, Moran JB, Caplan P. Human exposure to polynuclear aromatic hydrocarbons. In: Freudenthal RI, Jones PW, eds. *Carcinogenesis: 1. Polynuclear aromatic hydrocarbons: chemistry, metabolism, and carcinogenesis.* New York: Raven Press, 1976.

TABLE 113-3. Soil and water benzo[a]pyrene concentrations (μg/kg)

Source	Benzo[a]pyrene (mg/kg)
Forest	≤1,300[a]
Nonindustrial sites	≤127
Towns and vicinities	≤939
Near traffic (soils only)	≤2,000
Near oil refinery	200,000
Near airport	785
Contaminated by coal tar pitch	685,000
Remote areas	10–20

[a]Seldom exceeding 10–20 mg/kg in remote areas.
From the World Health Organization, *Certain polycyclic aromatic hydrocarbons and heterocyclic compounds: 3. Monograph on the evaluation of carcinogenic risks of the chemical to man.* Geneva: International Agency for Research on Cancer, WHO, 1973, as adapted by Baum EJ. *Polycyclic hydrocarbons and cancer: 1. Occurrence and surveillance of polycyclic aromatic hydrocarbons.* Orlando: Academic Press, 1978.

may travel great distances and settle in remote regions of the earth that are relatively uncontaminated by urban pollution. PAHs and metabolites readily cross the placenta and are also excreted in breast milk. Virtually all humans are exposed to PAHs on an ongoing basis from birth until death (5–7).

Workers at risk for the highest exposure to PAHs include aluminum workers, asphalt workers, coal gas workers, carbon black workers, chimney sweeps, fishers (coal tar on nets), graphite electrode workers, machinists, mechanics, printers, road workers, steel foundry workers, tire and rubber manufacturers, and anyone who works with creosote (e.g., railroad workers and farmers).

Large concentrations of PAHs exist as waste deposits throughout developed countries where gas for lighting and heating was manufactured from coal or oil. These plants were in common operation from the mid-1800s until the early 1950s, at which time they were phased out by the introduction of interstate natural gas pipelines. An estimated 1,000+ such plants existed throughout the United States before World War II, most of these concentrated in the Midwest and East (8). The major classes of chemicals associated with gas plant wastes are PAHs, phenolics, volatile organic hydrocarbons, various inorganic sulfur and nitrogen species, and to a lesser extent, trace metals. Epidemiologic studies in gas workers report an increased incidence of cancers, particularly of the lung (9,10).

Table 113-3 lists some concentrations of BaP that have been detected in soil and water in various geographic locations. Surface water concentrations are reported to range from 0.6 to 114.0 ng per L (11).

CLINICAL TOXICOLOGY

PAHs, also called *polynuclear hydrocarbons, polynuclear aromatic hydrocarbons,* or *polycyclic organic matter,* are compounds that contain three or more fused, unsaturated carbon rings (Fig. 113-1). Approximately 100 such compounds are known. They have relatively high molecular weights, exist in solid form at room temperature, and commonly are found as condensates on particles or surfaces. They are practically insoluble in water but are soluble in organic solvents. PAHs entering the atmosphere condense when hot combustion gases cool and form very small particles that can be adsorbed onto existing particles.

PAHs almost always occur as mixtures in which the components may be synergistic. Some PAHs are initiators but not promoters, whereas others are promoters but not initiators. Because BaP is

TABLE 113-4. Polycyclic aromatic hydrocarbons in food (mg/kg dried material)

Source	Benzo[a]pyrene	Chrysene	Benzanthracene
Cereals	0.25–0.84	0.80–14.5	0.4–6.8
Salad	2.8–5.3	5.7–26.5	4.6–15.4
Spinach	7.4	28.0	16.1
Tomatoes	0.22	0.5	0.3
Refined oils and fats	0.9–15.0	0.5–129.0	0.5–13.5
Broiled meat and fish	0.2–162.0	0.5–25.4	0.2–31.0
Smoked meat and fish	0.2–107.0	0.3–123.0	0.02–189
Roasted coffee	0.1–4.0	0.6–19.1	0.5–14.2
Tea	3.9–21.3	4.6–6.3	—

From Grimmer G. Carcinogenic hydrocarbons in the human environment. *Dtsch Aptoth Ztg* 1968;108:529; Shabad LM, Cohan YL. Contents of benzo(a)pyrene in some crops. *Arch Geschwulstforsch* 1972;40:237; and the World Health Organization. *Certain polycyclic aromatic hydrocarbons and heterocyclic compounds: 3. Monograph on the evaluation of carcinogenic risks of the chemical to man.* Geneva: International Agency for Research on Cancer, WHO, 1973, as adapted by Baum EJ. *Polycyclic hydrocarbons and cancer: 1. Occurrence and surveillance of polycyclic aromatic hydrocarbons.* Orlando: Academic Press, 1978.

the most intensely studied PAH in both animals and humans, it often is used as a predictor of the toxicity of a mixture. This, however, may not be consistently reliable. Because of the mixture phenomenon, most of the following discussion focuses on the toxicity of PAH mixtures. Characteristics of a particular PAH may not always be true of other PAHs, however. This is especially true of metabolism, which is critical to the ultimate toxicity of a PAH.

Toxicokinetics

The biological activation of PAHs into reactive metabolites is a key factor in their toxicity. Binding of PAH metabolites to DNA is believed to be the mechanism of PAH-induced carcinogenesis. Understanding the processes involved may allow an understanding of which individuals are most at risk for developing cancer from exposure. Complicating this attempt, however, is the fact that the results of animal research, primarily involving rodents administered the maximum tolerated dose, may not be analogous to human exposure outcomes and mechanisms. For example, biological activation of PAHs occurs primarily in the liver. Therefore, oral exposure would be expected to create quantitatively greater amounts of toxic metabolites than would other routes of exposure, as first-pass metabolism via the portal circulation would be greater. Therefore, oral exposure may not be analogous to inhalational or dermal exposure. As a general rule, animal research provides valuable information that allows risk assessment estimates, but one should not assume that findings can be directly extrapolated to humans. Epidemiologic studies, studies in human tissue culture, and mechanistic studies must be considered also.

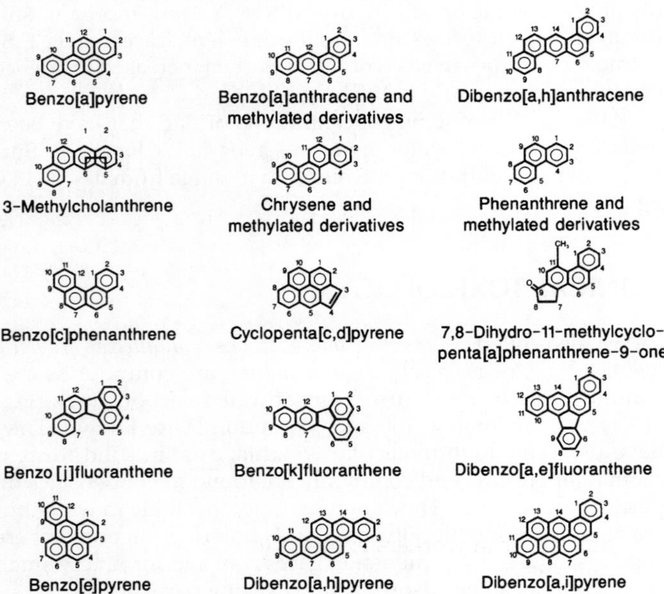

Figure 113-1. Chemical structures of common polycyclic aromatic hydrocarbons.

Absorption of PAHs in humans is inferred by measuring metabolites, primarily 1-hydroxypyrene, in urine (12,13). Absorption in animal models can be determined by collecting urine and excreta or by harvesting organs and measuring metabolites or radiolabeled material (14–19). Collectively, the data demonstrate some absorption after inhalational, dermal, or oral exposure. The percentage absorbed varies among studies and is difficult to assess accurately for several reasons. The vehicle in which the PAHs are found may be important (20). PAHs found on the surface of airborne particulate matter are not well absorbed, whereas the same dose in the lungs not bound to particulate matter may be better absorbed (21,22). Airborne exposure usually involves simultaneous dermal and, perhaps, oral exposure too. Human studies also must take into account diet, smoking, exposure to combusted fossil fuels and wood, and other non-workplace-related sources.

Data concerning the distribution of absorbed PAHs in humans is notably lacking. In a variety of rodent exposed to PAHs by various routes of exposure, radiolabeled BaP seems to distribute primarily to the gastrointestinal (GI) tract, lung, liver, testes, and kidneys (14,23,24). The distribution to the GI tract may reflect significant bile concentrations and, perhaps, enterohepatic recirculation. Not all PAHs have identical distribution patterns, and some are apparently more lipophilic than others (25). Many are distributed to the fetus, although levels may be ten times lower than in the mother.

Metabolism of PAHs occurs primarily (but not solely) in the liver by the P-450 mixed-function oxidase system (26–31). Aryl hydrocarbon hydrolase, the primary cytochrome P-450 isoenzyme that biologically activates BaP, is inducible by other PAHs and, possibly, other substances (32,33). This property may be inherited and may determine, at least in part, genetic susceptibility to PAH-induced carcinogenesis (e.g., from cigarette smoking).

The wide variability in potency of the enantiomeric forms of diol-epoxides led Jerina et al. (34,35) to propose the bay region

TABLE 113-5. Acute toxicity of various PAHs: median lethal dose (mg/kg)

PAH	Oral		Subcutaneous		Intravenous	
	Rat	Mouse	Rat	Mouse	Rat	Mouse
7,12-Dimethylbenzanthracene	327	340	—	—	54	—
Benzanthracene	—	—	—	—	—	10
Chrysene	—	—	—	—	—	—
Benzo[a]pyrene	—	—	50	—	—	—
Phenanthrene	—	700	—	—	—	56
Anthracene	—	—	—	—	—	—
Pyrene	—	—	—	—	—	—
Naphthalene	1,780	—	—	969	—	100
Acenaphthylene	—	—	—	—	—	—
Benzo[j]fluoranthene	—	—	—	—	—	—
Benzo[k]fluoranthene	—	—	—	—	—	—
Benzo[b]fluoranthene	—	—	—	—	—	—
Benzo[ghi]perylene	—	—	—	—	—	—
Benzo[c]phenanthrene	—	—	—	—	—	—

PAH, polycyclic aromatic hydrocarbon.
From the Tatken RL, Lewis RJ Sr, eds. *National Institute of Occupational Safety and Health registry of toxic effects of chemical substances.* Cincinnati: U.S. Department of Health and Human Services, Public Health Service, Centers for Disease Control and Prevention, National Institute for Occupational Safety and Health, 1983.

theory to assist us in understanding the mechanism of carcinogenicity from PAHs. The bay region is the space between the aromatic rings of the PAH molecule, such as that between carbon 10 and 11 in BaP (see Fig. 113-1). This theory predicts that epoxides located on saturated angular rings in the bay region of a PAH should be highly reactive and, therefore, the presence of bay regions would predict mutagenicity (36).

PAH metabolites include multiple arene oxides, phenols, and quinones, which then are converted to dihydrodiols (via epoxide hydrolase) and phenol-diols. The dihydrodiols may be converted to diol-epoxides. Most metabolites are conjugated to glucuronides and sulfates, which then are excreted in the bile or urine. DNA adducts may be measured in a variety of biological media after an individual has been exposed (37–40).

The excretion of PAHs and their metabolites is primarily through urine and bile. 1-Hydroxypyrene is the most commonly measured urinary metabolite (12,38,39,41). Excretion onset is rapid in most models tested. In one rat model using [^{14}C]-BaP by inhalation, excretion of fecal radioactivity composed 96% of the dose (12). Excretion half-lives were 22 and 28 hours in feces and urine, respectively.

Clinical Effects

Few published reports address the acute toxicity of PAHs in either humans or animals. In general, the acute toxicity of PAHs increases as the molecular weight increases and with increasing side-chain alkyl substitution on the aromatic nucleus. In animals, the acute toxicity of oral or dermal exposure is relatively low, based on experiments in mice and rats. The median lethal doses for specific PAHs are relatively high (Table 113-5). In cases of human exposure to PAHs, acute symptoms often are due to coexposures such as to irritant gases.

The noncarcinogenic effects of PAHs after chronic exposure involve primarily the pulmonary, GI, renal, and dermatologic systems. Gupta et al. (42), in 1993, evaluated respiratory function in 667 workers in a rubber factory and correlated it with BaP air levels and with duration of employment. Workers with the highest estimated dose demonstrated a statistically significant decrease in pulmonary function and radiographic abnormalities, including pleural effusions, patch opacities, and bronchiovascular markings. Symptoms included cough, dyspnea, throat irritation, chest pain, and hematemesis. Coexposures were not investigated.

Some evidence indicates that PAH exposure accelerates atherosclerosis (43). This would be particularly relevant to cigarette smoking, a known risk factor for arterial disease. Use of anthracene laxatives has been associated with melanosis of the colon and rectum (44). Hepatic hyperplasia and injury have been described in rodent models but not in humans (32,45–47). Likewise, renal injury may be seen in a rodent model but not in humans (48). Both humoral and cellular immunity have been depressed by PAHs *in vitro* and in a variety of animal models (49–53). Rats fed dimethylbenzanthracene at doses between 50 and 300 mg per kg have developed agranulocytosis, anemia, lymphopenia, pancytopenia, and testicular degeneration (54). In mice, thymic degeneration, impaired thyroid development, general wasting, and immunosuppression have been observed at doses of 3-methylcholanthrene in excess of 150 mg per kg (55,56). In a mouse model, levels of the brain neurotransmitters dopamine and norepinephrine have been found to be depressed after exposure to BaP (57). The decrease in fecundity in women who smoke cigarettes is believed to be secondary to PAH exposure (58,59).

The mutagenic and carcinogenic effects of PAHs and metabolites after chronic exposure remain the primary toxicities and areas of research interest. Large numbers of animal studies have clearly demonstrated the potent carcinogenicity of specific PAHs. As little as a few micromoles of BaP were sufficient to cause cancer in less than 6 months in mice that were repeatedly dosed (60). Skin-painting studies in a variety of animal models have demonstrated the ability of benz[a]anthracene and indeno[1,2,3-c,d]pyrene to induce skin tumors, and these therefore are considered to be complete carcinogens (both initiators and promoters) (61–66). Anthracene, fluoranthene, fluorene, phenanthrene, and pyrene do not act as complete carcinogens.

Epidemiologic studies have demonstrated increased mortality from cancer in workers exposed to PAH mixtures (67–71). Concomitant exposure to other potentially carcinogenic materials often occurred in these studies. Human exposure to diesel exhaust is of particular interest, given the vast numbers of humans so exposed. Epidemiologic studies to date have suggested a small increased risk of cancer in workers exposed to diesel exhaust (72–78). A significant problem in these types of epidemiologic studies is the fact that exposure is almost always to mixtures (79).

REGULATORY ISSUES

The U.S. Department of Health and Human Services (DHHS) has determined that benz[a]anthracene, benzo[b]fluoranthene, benzo[j]fluoranthene, benzo[k]fluoranthene, BaP, dibenz[a,h]anthracene, and indeno[1,2,3-c,d]pyrene are known animal carcinogens. The International Agency for Research on Cancer has determined that benz[a]anthracene and BaP are probably carcinogenic to humans; benzo[a]fluoranthene, benzo[k]fluoranthene, and indeno[1,2,3-c,d]pyrene are possibly carcinogenic to humans; and anthracene, benzo[g,h,i]perylene, benzo[e]pyrene, chrysene, fluoranthene, fluorene, phenanthrene, and pyrene are not classifiable as to their carcinogenicity to humans. The U.S. Environmental Protection Agency has determined that benz[a]anthracene, BaP, benzo[b]fluoranthene, benzo[k]fluoranthene, chrysene, dibenz[a,h]anthracene, and indeno[1,2,3-c,d]pyrene are probable human carcinogens and that acenaphthylene, anthracene, benzo[g,h,i]perylene, fluoranthene, fluorene, phenanthrene, and pyrene are not classifiable as to human carcinogenicity.

The current air-level workplace standards for PAH mixtures include the following:

- American Conference of Governmental Industrial Hygienists time-weighted average: 0.2 mg per cubic meter for benzene-soluble coal tar pitch fraction
- Occupational Safety and Health Administration permissible exposure limit: 0.2 mg per cubic meter for benzene-soluble coal tar pitch fraction
- National Institute for Occupational Safety and Health: 0.1 mg per cubic meter for coal tar pitch volatile agents

For a more complete listing of specific PAHs, with specific agencies' classifications and recommendations for exposure limits (including state regulations), the reader is advised to contact the Agency for Toxic Substances and Disease Registry or to refer to each PAH's published toxicologic profile (80).

The American Conference of Governmental Industrial Hygienists has not currently recommended a biological exposure index for PAHs. The Environmental Protection Agency's proposed maximum contaminant level goal for BaP is 0.2 parts per billion. The U.S. Food and Drug Administration has not established a standard governing the PAH content of food.

REFERENCES

1. Denissenko MF. Preferential formation of benzo[a]pyrene adducts at lung cancer mutational hotspots in P53. *Science* 1996;274:430–432.
2. van Schooten F-J. Coal tar therapy: is it carcinogenic? *Drug Safety* 1996;6(Dec 15):374–377.
3. Neff JM. *Polycyclic aromatic hydrocarbons in the aquatic environment: sources, fates and biological effects*. London: Applied Science Publishers, 1979.
4. Shabad LM, Cohan YL, Ilnitsky AP, Khesina AYA, Shcherbak NP, Smirnov GA. The carcinogenic hydrocarbon benzo(a)pyrene in the soil. *J Natl Cancer Inst* 1971;47:1179–1191.
5. Edwards NY. Polycyclic aromatic hydrocarbons (PAHs) in the terrestrial environment—a review. *J Environ Qual* 1983;12(4):427–441.
6. Graef W, Diehl H. The natural normal levels of carcinogenic polycyclic aromatic hydrocarbons and the reasons therefore. *Arch Hyg Bakteriol* 1996;150:49.
7. Mastrangelo G. Polycyclic aromatic hydrocarbons and cancer in man. *Environ Health Perspect* 1996;104:1166–1170.
8. Environmental Research and Technology Inc, Koppers Company Inc (for the Utility Solid Waste Activities Group, Superfund Committee, Washington, DC). *Handbook on manufactured gas plant sites*. Pittsburgh: Edison Electric Institute, 1984.
9. Doll R, Fisher REW, Gammon EJ, et al. Mortality of gas workers with special reference to cancers of the lung and bladder, chronic bronchitis and pneumoconiosis. *Br J Ind Med* 1965;22:1–12.
10. Doll R, Vessey MP, Beasley RWR, et al. Mortality of gas workers—final report of a prospective study. *Br J Ind Med* 1972;29:394–406.
11. Sawicki E, Corey RC, Dooley AE, et al. Tentative method for spectrophotometric analysis for benzo(a)pyrene in atmospheric particulate matter. *Health Lab Sci* 1970;7[Suppl 8]:68–71.
12. Becher G, Bjorseth A. Determination of exposure to polycyclic aromatic hydrocarbons by analysis of human urine. *Cancer Lett* 1983;17:301–311.
13. Van Rooij JGM, Van Lieshout EMA, Bodelier-Bade MM, et al. Effect of the reduction of skin contamination on the internal dose of creosote workers exposed to polycyclic aromatic hydrocarbons. *Scand J Work Environ Health* 1993;19:200–207.
14. Wolff MS, Herbert R, Marcus M, et al. Polycyclic aromatic hydrocarbon (PAH) residues on skin in relation to air levels among roofers. *Arch Environ Health* 1989;44(3):157–163.
15. Weyand EH, Bevan DR. Benzo(a)pyrene disposition and metabolism in rats following intratracheal instillation. *Cancer Res* 1986;46:5655–5661.
16. Weyand EH, Bevan DR. Benzo(a)pyrene metabolism *in vitro* following intratracheal administration. In: Cooke M, Dannis AJ, eds. *Polynuclear aromatic hydrocarbons: a decade of progress*. Columbus: Battelle Press, 1988:913–923.
17. Weyand EH, Bevan DR. Species differences in disposition of benzo(a)pyrene. *Drug Metab Dispos* 1987;15:442–448.
18. Yamazaki H, Kakiuchi Y. The uptake and distribution of benzo(a)pyrene in rat after continuous oral administration. *Toxicol Environ Chem* 1989;24(1/2):95–104.
19. Yang JJ, Roy TA, Mackerer CR. Percutaneous absorption of anthracene in the rat: comparison of *in vivo* and *in vitro* results. *Toxicol Ind Health* 1986;2:79–84.
20. Kawamura Y, Kamata E, Ogawa Y, et al. The effect of various foods on the intestinal absorption of benzo-a-pyrene in rats. *J Food Hyg Soc Jpn* 1988; 29(1):21–25.
21. Cresia DA, Poggenburg JK, Nettesheim P. Elution of benzo(a)pyrene from carbon particles in the respiratory tract of mice. *J Toxicol Environ Health* 1976;1:967–975.
22. Seto H. Determination of polycyclic aromatic hydrocarbons in the lung. *Arch Environ Contam Toxicol* 1993;24:498–503.
23. Bevan DR, Weyand EH. Compartmental analysis of the disposition of benzo(a)pyrene in rats. *Carcinogenesis* 1988;9(11):2027–2032.
24. Bartosek I, Guaitani A, Modica R, et al. Comparative kinetics of oral benz(a)anthracene, chrysene and triphenylene in rats: study with hydrocarbon mixtures. *Toxicol Lett* 1984;23:333–339.
25. Busbee DL, Normal JO, Ziprin RL. Comparative uptake, vascular transport and cellular internalization of aflatoxin B1 and benzo(a)pyrene. *Arch Toxicol* 1990;64(4):285–290.
26. Panthanickal A, Marnett LJ. Arachidonic acid–dependent metabolism of (±)-7,8-dihydroxy-7,8-dihydrobenzo[a]pyrene to polyguanylic acid-binding derivatives. *Chem Biol Interact* 1981;33:239–252.
27. Hall M, Grover PL. Differential stereoselectivity in the metabolism of benzo(a)pyrene and anthracene by rabbit epidermal and hepatic microsomes. *Cancer Lett* 1987;38:57–64.
28. Moteith DK, Novotny A, Michalopoulos G, et al. Metabolism of benzo(a)pyrene in primary cultures of human hepatocytes: dose-response over a four-log range. *Carcinogenesis* 1987;8:983–988.
29. Kapitulnik J, Levin W, Lu AYH, et al. Hydration of arene and alkene oxides by epoxide hydrase in human liver microsomes. *Clin Pharmacol Ther* 1977;21:158–165.
30. Kiefer F, Cumpelik O, Wiebel FJ. Metabolism and cytotoxicity of benzo(a)pyrene in the human lung tumour cell line NCI-H322. *Xenobiotica* 1988;18:747–755.
31. Petridou-Fischer J, Whaley SL, Dahl AR. In vivo metabolism of nasally instilled benzo(a)pyrene in dogs and monkeys. *Toxicology* 1988;48(1):31–40.
32. Kemena A, Norpoth KH, Jacob J. Differential induction of the monooxygenase isoenzymes in mouse liver microsomes by polycyclic aromatic hydrocarbons. In: Cooke M, Dennis AJ, eds. *Polynuclear aromatic hydrocarbons: a decade of progress. Proceedings of the tenth international symposium*. Columbus: Battelle Press, 1988:449–460.
33. Robinson JR, Felton JS, Levitt RC, et al. Relationship between "aromatic hydrocarbon responsiveness" and the survival times in mice treated with various drugs and environmental compounds. *Mol Pharmacol* 1975;11:850–865.
34. Jerina DM, Daly JW. Oxidation at carbon. In: Parke DV, Smith RL, eds. *Drug metabolism*. London: Taylor and Francis Ltd, 1976.
35. Jerina DM, Lehr RE, Yagi H, et al. Mutagenicity of benzo(a)pyrene derivatives and the description of a quantum mechanical model which predicts the ease of carbonium ion formation from diolepoxides. In: DeSerres FJ, Fouts JR, Bend JR, Philpot RM, eds. In vitro *metabolic activation and mutagenesis testing*. Amsterdam: Elsevier/North-Holland Biomedical, 1976.
36. Weis LM. Bay or baylike regions of polycyclic aromatic hydrocarbons were potent inhibitors of gap junctional intercellular communication. *Environ Health Perspect* 1998;106:17–22.
37. Ross J, Nelson G, Erexson G, et al. DNA adducts in rat lung, liver and peripheral blood lymphocytes produced by i.p. administration of benzo[a]pyrene metabolites and derivatives. *Carcinogenesis* 1991;12(10):1953–1955.
38. Popp W. DNA single strand breakage, DNA adducts, and sister chromatid exchange in lymphocytes and phenanthrene and pyrene metabolites in urine of coke oven workers. *Occup Environ Med* 1997;54:176–183.

39. Santella RM, Hemminki K, Tang D-L, et al. Polycyclic aromatic hydrocarbon–DNA adducts in white blood cells and urinary 1-hydroxypyrene in foundry workers. *Cancer Epidemiol Biomarkers Prev* 1993;2:59–62.
40. Weyand EH, LaVoie EJ. Comparison of PAH: DNA adduct formation and tumor initiating activity in newborn mice. *Proc Annu Meet Am Assoc Cancer Res* 1988;29:A390(abst).
41. Granella M, Clonfero E. Urinary excretion of 1-pyrenol in automotive repair workers. *Int Arch Occup Environ Health* 1993;65:241–245.
42. Gupta P, Banerjee DK, Bhargave SK, et al. Prevalence of impaired lung function in rubber manufacturing factory workers exposed to benzo(a)pyrene and respirable particulate matter. *Indoor Environ* 1991;2:26–31.
43. Hough JL, Baired MB, Sfeir GT, et al. Benzo(a)pyrene enhances atherosclerosis in white carneau and show racer pigeons. *Arterioscler Thromb Vasc Biol* 1993;13:1721–1727.
44. Badiali D, Marcheggiano A, Pallone F, et al. Melanosis of the rectum in patients with chronic constipation. *Dis Colon Rectum* 1985;28:241–245.
45. Danz M, Hartmann A, Otto M, et al. Hitherto unknown additive growth effects of fluorene and 2-acetylaminofluorene on bile duct epithelium and hepatocytes in rats. *Arch Toxicol Suppl* 1991;14:71–74.
46. Yoshikawa T, Ruhr LP, Flory W, et al. Toxicity of polycyclic aromatic hydrocarbons: III. Effects of beta-naphthoflavone pretreatment on hepatotoxicity of compounds produced in the ozonation of NO_2-nitration of phenanthrene and pyrene in rats. *Vet Hum Toxicol* 1987;29:113–117.
47. Ambs S. Acute and chronic toxicity of aromatic amines studied in the isolated perfused rat liver. *Toxicol Appl Pharmacol* 1996;139:186–194.
48. Rigdon RH, Giannukos NJ. Effect of carcinogenic hydrocarbons on growth of mice. *Arch Pathol* 1964;77:198–204.
49. Szczeklik A, Szczeklik J, Galuscka Z, et al. Humoral immunosuppression in men exposed to polycyclic aromatic hydrocarbons and related carcinogens in polluted environments. *Environ Health Perspect* 1994;102(3):302–304.
50. Hahon N, Booth JA. Coinhibition of viral interferon induction by benzo[a]pyrene and chrysotile asbestos. *Environ Res* 1986;40(1):103–109.
51. Blanton RJ, Lyte M, Myers MJ, et al. Immunomodulation by polyaromatic hydrocarbons in mice and murine cells. *Cancer Res* 1986;46:2735–2739.
52. Blanton RH, Myers MJ, Bick PH. Modulation of immunocompetent cell populations by benzo(a)pyrene. *Toxicol Appl Pharmacol* 1988;93:267–274.
53. Zhao ZH, Ho W, Shiu J-H, et al. Effects of benzo(a)pyrene on the humoral immunity of mice exposed by single intraperitoneal injection. *Chin J Prevent Med* 1990;24(4):220–222.
54. Philips FS, Steinberg SS, Marquardt H. *In vivo* cytotoxicity of polycyclic hydrocarbons. In: Loomis TA, ed. *Pharmacology and the future of man: 2. Toxicological problems. Proceedings of the fifth international congress on pharmacology, San Francisco, CA, July 23–28, 1972.*1973:75–88.
55. Malmgren RA, Bennison BE, McKinley TW Jr. Reduced antibody titers in mice treated with carcinogenic and cancer chemotherapeutic agents. *Proc Soc Exp Biol Med* 1952;79:484–488.
56. Yasuhira K. Damage to the thymus and other lymphoid tissues from 3-methylcholanthrene, and subsequent thymoma production, in mice. *Cancer Res* 1964;24:558–569.
57. Dasgupta PS, Lahiri T. Alteration of brain catecholamines during growth of benzo(a)pyrene induced murine fibrosarcoma. *Neoplasma* 1992;39(3):163–165.
58. Weinberg CR, Wilcox AJ, Baird DD. Reduced fecundability in women with prenatal exposure to cigarette smoking. *Am J Epidemiol* 1989;129:1072–1078.
59. Wilcox AJ, Baird DD, Weinberg CR. Do women with childhood exposure to cigarette smoking have increased fecundability? *Am J Epidemiol* 1989; 129:1079–1083.
60. Rigdon RH, Neal J. Relationship of leukemia to lung and stomach tumors in mice fed benzo(a)pyrene. *Proc Soc Exp Biol* 1969;130:146–148.
61. Alexandrov K, Rojas-Moreno M. In vivo DNA adduct formation by benzo(a)pyrene in mouse and rat epidermal and dermal fibroblasts after topical application of an initiating dose of benzo(a)pyrene. *Arch Geschwulstforsch* 1990;60(5):329–340.
62. Albert RE, Miler ML, Cody TE, et al. Cell kinetics and benzo[a]pyrene-DNA adducts in mouse skin tumorigenesis. *Prog Clin Biol Res* 1991;369:115–122.
63. Cavalieri EL, Rogan E, Cremonesi P, et al. Tumorigenicity of 6-halogenated derivatives of benzo[a]pyrene in mouse skin and rat mammary gland. *J Cancer Res Clin Oncol* 1988;114:10–15.
64. Levin W, Wood AW, Yagi H, et al. Carcinogenicity of benzo(a)pyrene 4, 5–7, 8–11, and 9,10-oxides on mouse skin. *Proc Natl Acad Sci U S A* 1976;73:243.
65. Moen BE. Assessment of exposure to polycyclic aromatic hydrocarbons in engine rooms by measurement of urinary 1-hydroxypyrene. *Occup Environ Med* 1996;53:692–696.
66. Moen BE. Assessment of exposure to polycyclic aromatic hydrocarbons during fire fighting by measurement of urinary 1-hydroxypyrene. *Occup Environ Med* 1997;39:515–519.
67. Lloyd JW. Long-term mortality study of steelworkers: V. Respiratory cancer in coke plant workers. *J Occup Med* 1971;13:53–68.
68. Mazumdar S, Redmond C, Sollecito W, Sussman N. An epidemiological study of exposure to coal tar pitch volatiles among coke oven workers. *J Air Pollut Cont Assoc* 1975;25:382–389.
69. Redmond CK, Ciocco A, Lloyd JW, Rush HW. Long-term mortality study of steelworkers: VI. Mortality from malignant neoplasms among coke oven workers. *J Occup Med* 1972;14:621–629.
70. Redmond CK, Strobino BR, Cypress RH. Cancer experience among coke by-product workers. *Ann N Y Acad Sci* 1976;271:102–115.
71. Hammond EC, Selikoff IJ, Lawther PL, Seidman H. Inhalation of benzpyrene and cancer in man. *Ann N Y Acad Sci* 1976;271:116–124.
72. Bhatia R, Lopipeto P, Smith AH. Diesel exhaust exposure and lung cancer. *Epidemiology* 1998;9:84–91.
73. Garshick E, Schenker MB, Muñoz A, et al. A case-control study of lung cancer and diesel exhaust exposure in railroad workers. *Am Rev Respir Dis* 1987;135:1242–1248.
74. Boffetta P, Stellman SD, Garfinkel L. Diesel exhaust exposure and mortality among males in the American Cancer Society prospective study. *Am J Ind Med* 1988;14:403–415.
75. Garshick E, Schenker MB, Muñoz A, et al. A retrospective cohort study of lung cancer and diesel exhaust exposure in railroad workers. *Am Rev Respir Dis* 1988;137:820–825.
76. Boffetta P, Harris RE, Wynder EL. Case-control study on occupational exposure to diesel exhaust and lung cancer risk. *Am J Ind Med* 1990;17:577–591.
77. Steenland K, Silverman DT, Hornung RW. Case-control study of lung cancer and truck driving in the Teamsters Union. *Am J Public Health* 1990;80:670–674.
78. Steenland K, Silverman DT, Zebst D. Exposure to diesel exhaust in the trucking industry and possible relationships with lung cancer. *Am J Ind Med* 1992;21:887–890.
79. Samet JM. What can we expect from epidemiologic studies of chemical mixtures? *Toxicology* 1995;105:307–314.
80. Agency for Toxic Substances and Disease Registry. *Toxicological profile for polycyclic aromatic hydrocarbons*. Atlanta: US Department of Health and Human Services, Public Health Service, ATSDR, 1995.

CHAPTER 114

Creosote, Coal Tar, and Coal Tar Pitch

John B. Sullivan, Jr.

SOURCES AND USES

Creosote exists in two forms: wood creosote and coal tar creosote (1). Wood creosotes are derived from beech wood and from resin in leaves of the creosote bush. Wood creosote contains phenol, phenolic compounds, cresols, guaiacols, and xylenols. It ranges from colorless to pale yellow and has a smoky odor.

Wood creosote has been used as a disinfectant, a laxative, and an expectorant. Phenol, *p*-cresol, and guaiacols are the primary constituents of wood creosote, with the xylenols, methylated guaiacols, and trimethylphenols accounting for the remaining minor components (Table 114-1). The creosote bush resin contains phenolic compounds (nordihydroguaiaretic acid), which make up approximately 80% to 90% of the total resin, and flavonoids, which account for approximately 5% to 10% of the weight of the dry leaves.

Coal tar creosote is a by-product of coal tars that are generated by carbonization of bituminous coal in the production of coke or natural gas. It is heavier than water and has a boiling range beginning at approximately 200°C. Coal tar creosote is 85% polycyclic aromatic hydrocarbons (PAHs) and 2% to 17% phenolic compounds. This oily liquid is a dark yellowish green to brown color. Coal tar creosotes are constituted mainly of aromatic hydrocarbons, anthracene, naphthalene, and phenanthrene.

Coal tar pitch, produced during the distillation of coal tar, is a shiny, dark brown residue and contains PAHs along with their methyl and polymethyl derivatives and heteronuclear compounds (Table 114-2).

Creosotes, particularly coal tar creosote, have been employed as wood preservatives for more than 100 years. Creosote is used as waterproofing for log homes, railroad ties, telephone poles, marine pilings, and fence posts. It prevents algae growth on marine pilings. It has also been used as an insecticide or animal dip and as a fungicide.

TABLE 114-1. Major components of wood creosote

Compound	Relative percentage
o-Cresol	3.22
p-Cresol	13.60
Dimethylhydroxycyclopentenone	0.50
4-Ethylguaiacol	6.36
4-Ethyl-5-methylguaiacol	0.21
Guaiacol	23.76
3-Methylguaiacol	1.85
4-Methylguaiacol	1.29
5-Methylguaiacol	19.01
6-Methylguaiacol	0.31
Methylhydroxycyclopentenone	0.23
Phenol	14.45
4-Propylguaiacol	0.45
2,3,6-Trimethylphenol	0.48
2,4,6-Trimethylphenol	0.40
Unknown	1.31
2,3-Xylenol	0.70
2,4-Xylenol	2.80
2,5-Xylenol	0.68
2,6-Xylenol	1.04
3,4-Xylenol	0.70
3,5-Xylenol	2.94

Adapted from ref. 1.

POTENTIAL HUMAN EXPOSURE SOURCES

Workers in the wood-preserving industry have been exposed to coal tar creosote for years. Human exposure is via direct contact with the skin or through inhalation. Children may be exposed by playing with discarded creosote. Creosote has been identified in 33 of the 1,430 hazardous-waste sites listed in the U.S. Environmental Protection Agency's National Priority List. Microbial biodegradation in soil is the primary process of environmental transformation (1).

ENVIRONMENTAL FATE AND TRANSPORT

Creosotes are complex mixtures, and environmental contamination can occur from point source uses or from production facilities. Naphthalene, phenanthrene, acenaphthene, dibenzofuran, fluorene, and 2-methylnaphthalene have been found in water as a result of creosote environmental contamination. Creosotes are viscous and, therefore, their movement through soil is physically limited. Phenols, heterocyclic compounds, and PAHs have low water solubility and strongly sorb to soil particles. They can be transported through the environment into groundwater and aquifers. Owing to the viscous nature of creosotes, coal tar, and coal pitch, these compounds usually remain physically nonpartitioned in the environment, although PAHs and the heterocyclic compounds can migrate in groundwater. PAHs can be taken up by plant roots.

Biodegradation of creosote components occurs in soil and in aquatic environments. *Pseudomonas* bacteria degrade quinoline and phenol-type compounds in creosote. Biotransformation of the phenolic components of creosote occurs under anaerobic conditions in groundwater and soil. High-molecular-weight PAHs, however, are resistant to much of the biological degradation.

Bioaccumulation of benzo[a]pyrene, anthracene, chrysene, and phenanthrene has been discovered in snails and mussels in aquatic environments around creosote-treated pilings and contaminated water.

CLINICAL TOXICOLOGY

Among cohorts of workers exposed to coal tar pitch during aluminum production, a significant increase in mortality from brain cancer was noted. Other studies have found increased mortality from lung cancer in coke plant workers (2,3). Overall, the occupational exposure to coal tar creosotes and coal tar pitch is associated with an increased incidence of cancers (4–6). Case reports and other occupational studies associate exposure to creosote with the development of skin cancer. Cancer of the scrotum has also been associated with long-term coal tar creosote exposure.

Dermal and Ocular Injury

Creosotes, particularly coal tar creosotes, can cause acute skin burns and irritation. They also are photosensitizers. The components of creosote can be dermally absorbed. Interestingly, coal tar has been used to treat psoriasis.

Burns and irritation of the skin are common clinical manifestations of exposure to coal tar creosote. Phototoxic skin reactions occur after exposure to this creosote and absorption of ultraviolet A light by chemicals in the skin, whereas the usual sunburn is produced by ultraviolet B light. Symptoms of phototoxicity are erythema, skin peeling, and folliculitis. Coal tar creosote also can produce other noncancerous skin lesions such as squamous cell papilloma.

Beechwood creosote also is irritating to skin and other tissues. Direct ocular exposure can cause burns and irritation. Allergic dermatitis occurs, manifested by erythematous and vesicular lesions. Allergies to the creosote bush have also been reported.

Acute Systemic Toxicity

Deaths due to multiorgan failure have been reported to occur within 30 hours of creosote ingestion (7). Individuals who have ingested leaves of the creosote bush containing nordihydroguaiaretic acid have become clinically toxic. One individual ingesting a compound known as *chaparral capsules* developed aspiration pneumonia, jaundice, fatigue, anorexia, and pruritus after taking the product for approximately 2 months (8). Liver enzymes and the total bilirubin level were elevated in this patient. Liver biopsy demonstrated acute hepatitis and hepatic necrosis (9).

Beechwood creosote is used therapeutically in some countries as an expectorant–cough suppressant. Acute ingestions of large amounts have resulted in oropharyngeal hemorrhages and ulceration and gastrointestinal hemorrhages. In reported deaths, hepatic necrosis has been observed.

A 60-year-old woman who had ingested capsules containing beechwood creosote for nearly 10 months developed flulike symptoms with jaundice and liver failure. Liver biopsy showed acute necrosis, lobular collapse, and nodular regeneration with portal inflammation and bioduct proliferation.

Renal failure has been noted after acute ingestion of fatal doses of coal tar creosote. The pathologic diagnosis at autopsy was acute tubular necrosis.

Respiratory effects include restrictive and obstructive deficits exhibited on pulmonary function tests.

Mutagenicity and Genotoxicity

Coal tar is genotoxic, as evidenced by sister chromatid exchanges in lymphocytes and DNA adducts that occur after coal tar exposure. These adducts are mainly of the PAH-DNA type. The mutagenicity of coal tar creosote is due to the PAH

TABLE 114-2. Polycyclic aromatic hydrocarbons in coal tar pitch

Polycyclic aromatic hydrocarbons
Naphthalene
Benzo[b]thiophene
Quinoline
2-Methylnaphthalene
1-Methylnaphthalene
Biphenyl
2-Ethylnaphthalene
Dimethylnaphthalene
Methylbiphenyl
Acenaphthene
Naphthonitrile or azaacenaphthylene
Dibenzofuran
Fluorene
Methylacenaphthene
Methyldibenzofuran
9,10-Dihydroanthracene
9,10-Dihydrophenanthrene
Methylfluorene
1,2,3,4-Tetrahydroanthracene
Dibenzo[bd]thiophene
Phenanthrene
Anthracene
Acridine
Phenanthridine
Carbazole
Methylphenanthrene, methylphenanthracene
4H-Cyclopenta[def]phenanthrene
Methylcarbazole
2-Phenylnaphthalene
Dihydropyrene or isomer
Fluoranthene
Azafluoranthene, azafluorpyrene
Phenanthro[4,5-bcd]thiophene
Pyrene
Benzonaphthofuran
Benzacenaphthene or isomer
Benzo[lmn]phenanthridine
Benzo[kl]xanthene
Mathylfluoranthene, mathylfluorpyrene
4H-Benzo[def]carbazole
Benzo[a]flourene
Benzo[c]fluorene or isomer
Methylbenzonaphthofuran or isomer
Methylpyrene or isomer
Methylazapyrene or isomer
Methylbenzofluorene
Dihydrochrysene or isomer
Dimethylfluoranthene, dimethylfluorpyrene
Trimethylfluoranthene, trimethylfluorpyrene
Benzo[b]naphtho[2,1-d]thiophene
Benzo[c]phenanthrene
Benzo[ghi]fluoranthene
Dimethylbenzonaphthofuran
Benzo[b]naphtho[1,2-d]thiophene
Dibenzoquinoline or isomer
Tetrahydrochrysene or isomer
Benzo[a]naphtho[2,3-d]thiophene
Benz[a]anthracene
Chrysene
11H-Benzo[a]carbazole
Naphthacene
Methylbenzonaphthothiophene
Methylbenz[a]anthracene or isomer
Tetramethylfluoranthene or isomer
7H-Benzo[c]carbazole
5H-Benzo[b]carbazole
Methylbenzophenanthridine or isomer
Dimethylbenzo[cdf]carbazole
Methylchrysene or isomer
Dimethylbenz[a]anthracene or isomer
11H-Benz[bc]aceanthrylene or isomer
4H-Cyclopenta[def]chrysene or isomer
Binaphthalene or isomer
4H-Cyclopenta[def]triphenrylene or isomer
Phenylphenanthrene or isomer
Dihydrobenzofluoranthene or isomer
Dimethylchrysene or isomer
Dibenzophenanthridine or isomer
Biquinoline
Benzo[j]fluoranthene
Benzo[b]fluoranthene
Benzo[k]fluoranthene
Dibenzonaphthofuran or isomer
Azabenzopyrene or isomer
Benzo[e]pyrene
Benzo[a]pyrene
Perylene
Methylbenzofluoranthene or isomer
4H-Naphtho[1,2,3,4-def]carbazole or isomer
Dibenzofluorene or isomer
Dihydroindenopyrene or isomer
Methylbenzopyrene or isomer
6-Dibenzo[cg]phenanthrene or isomer
Dimethyldibenzonaphthofuran or isomer
11H-Cyclopenta[ghi]perylene or isomer
Dimethylbenzopyrene or isomer
11H-Indeno[2,1,7-cde]pyrene or isomer
Dinaphthothiophene
Dibenzophenanthridine or isomer
Dibenzonaphthothiophene
Dibenzocarbazole
Dibenzo[bg]phenanthrene or isomer
Benzo[g]chrysene or isomer
Dimethylbenzofluoranthene or isomer
Dibenzoacridine or isomer
Benzo[c]chrysene or isomer
Dibenz[aj]anthracene
Indenopyrene or isomer
Methyldibenzophenanthrene, methyldibenzophenanthracene
Methylbenzophenanthrothiophene
Dibenz[ac]anthracene
Dibenz[ah]anthracene
Trimethylbenzofluoranthene or isomer
Dimethyldibenzophenanthrene, dimethyldibenzophenanthracene
Benzo[b]chrysene
Picene
Benzo[ghi]perylene
Benzo[a]naphthacene or benzo[a]pentacene
Anthanthrene
Methyl indenopyrene or isomer

Adapted from ref. 1.

components and, therefore, exposure to PAHs from any source may produce these findings. The metabolites of PAHs may also be present in the urine of smokers and so can be a confounding factor in determining whether coal tar creosote exposure is excessive.

METABOLISM, EXCRETION, AND BIOLOGICAL MARKERS OF EXPOSURE

Most of the compounds that have been studied in creosotes and coal tars for their kinetics are PAHs. Detection of PAHs and analysis of metabolites of PAHs can be accomplished in the urine of exposed individuals. A metabolite of coal tar creosote, 1-hydroxypyrene, can be assayed in the urine from workers who handle creosote (10,11). Concentrations of 1-hydroxypyrene ranging from 1 to 40 µg per gram of creatinine were found in urine samples in workers.

PAHs are ever-present in the environment and, therefore, the direct detection of PAH metabolites may not be specific for exposure to creosotes. Also, although PAHs form DNA adducts that can be measured in biological fluids after creosote exposure, PAH-DNA adducts are not specific for creosote.

REFERENCES

1. Agency for Toxic Substances and Disease Registry. *Toxicological profile for creosote.* Atlanta: US Department of Health and Human Services, Public Health Service, ATSDR, 1996.
2. Landrigan P. Health risk of creosotes. *JAMA* 1993;269(10):1309.
3. Karlehagen S, Anderson A, Ohlson C. Cancer incidents among creosote exposed workers. *Scand J Work Environ Health* 1992;19(1):26–29.
4. Spinelli J, Band P, Svirshev L. Mortality in cancer incidents in aluminum reduction plant workers. *J Occup Med* 1991;33(11):1150–1155.
5. Mazumdar S, Redmond C, Sollecito W. An epidemiological study of exposure to coal tar pitch volatiles among coke oven workers. *J Air Pollut Control Assoc* 1975;25(4):382–389.
6. Armstrong B, Tremblay C, Baris D. Lung cancer mortality and polynuclear aromatic hydrocarbons: a case cohort study of aluminum production workers in Arvida, Quebec, Canada. *Am J Epidemiol* 1994;139(3):250–262.
7. Bowman C, Muhleman M, Walters E. A fatal case of creosote poison. *Postgrad Med J* 1984;60:499–500.
8. Gordon D, Rosenthal G, Hart J. Chaparral ingestion: the broadening spectrum of liver injury caused by herbal medications. *JAMA* 1995;273(6):489–490.
9. Alderman S, Kailas S, Goldfarb S. Cholestatic hepatitis after ingestion of chaparral leaf: confirmation by endoscopic retrograde cholangiopancreatography and liver biopsy. *J Clin Gastroenterol* 1994;19(3):242–247.
10. Jongeneelen F, Anzion R, Leijdekkers C. 1-Hydroxypyrene in human urine as a biological indicator of exposure to polycyclic aromatic hydrocarbons in several work environments. *Ann Occup Hyg* 1988;32:34–43.
11. Jongeneelen F, Anzion R, Scheepers T. 1-Hydroxypyrene in human urine after exposure to a coal tar derived product. *Int Arch Occup Environ Health* 1985;57:47–55.

CHAPTER 115

Phenols and Phenol Derivatives

Donna L. Dehn and John B. Sullivan, Jr.

Phenol and phenol derivatives are widely used in a variety of industrial, agricultural, and pharmaceutical products. Phenols are characterized by the presence of a hydroxy group on an unsaturated benzene ring (Fig. 115-1). They do not dehydrate or form ketones, which require an H–COH linkage, but they do hydrogen-bond to one another. Phenol derivatives such as chlorophenols (pentachlorophenol), methylphenols (cresols), nitrophenols (dinitrophenol), and hydroxyphenols are commercially important and are similar in structure to phenols, with direct substitutions of the benzene ring.

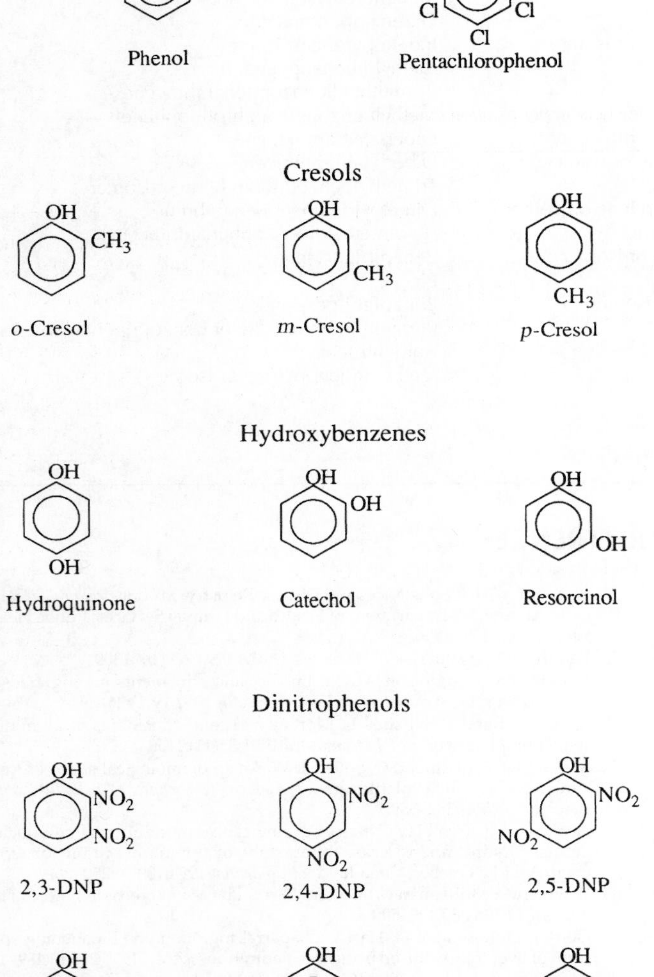

Figure 115-1. Chemical structure of phenol and phenol derivatives. DNP, dinitrophenol.

The structure-activity relationships of phenol and its derivatives vary widely. However, phenolic compounds all share some local anesthetic properties, are central nervous system (CNS) depressants, and are corrosive on direct contact. Because of their direct inhibition of cellular whereas dihydroxy phenol compounds behave as local irritants. Dinitrophenol (DNP) uncouples oxidative phosphorylation. The toxicologic properties of phenol derivatives are very similar to those of phenol, although some may be more toxic and reactive (1).

PHENOL

Phenol, also known as *carbolic acid, monohydrobenzene, oxybenzene, phenic acid, phenyl alcohol, phenyl hydrate,* and *phenyl hydroxide,* has one –OH group directly bonded to a benzene ring (see Fig. 115-1). It is colorless or white as a pure solid. On exposure to air or to light, phenols turn pinkish to reddish (2,3). The physiochemical properties of phenol and its derivatives are listed in Tables 115-1 through 115-3.

Sources, Uses, and Production

Phenol is obtained from petroleum as a naturally occurring compound by the oxidation of toluene and by cumene hydroperoxidation (4,5). The largest single use of phenol is for the production of phenolic resins (e.g., phenol-formaldehyde resins), which are used in the plywood adhesive, construction, automotive, and appliance industries. In the United States, approximately half of the phenol used is applied in the housing and construction industries in the form of phenolic resins that serve as binders in insulation materials, chipboard, and triplex. The second most common usage of phenol is in the manufacture of bisphenol A and caprolactam. Bisphenol A, in turn, is used to produce epoxy resins, and caprolactam is used in the manufacture of nylon. Phenol also finds use in the manufacture of

TABLE 115-1. Physiochemical parameters of hydroquinone, catechol, and resorcinol

Parameter	Hydroquinone	Catechol	Resorcinol
CAS no.	123-31-9	120-80-9	108-46-3
Molecular weight	110.10	110.11	110.10
Boiling point (°C at 760 mm Hg)	285.0	245.5	280.0
Melting point (°C)	170	105	109–111
Density (g/mL)	1.332 at 15°C	1.344 at 20°C	1.272 at 20°C
Solubility (mg/L)	73,300 at 25°C	44,000 at 25°C	900,000 at 25°C
Vapor density	3.81	3.79	3.79
Vapor pressure (mm Hg)	6.7×10^{-4} at 25°C	0.003 at 20°C	3.84×10^{-4} at 25°C
Ionization potential	7.95	ND	8.63
Explosive limits			
Upper limit (%)	—	—	—
Lower limit (%)	—	1.4	1.4
Flash point (°C)	165.0	127.2	127.2
Henry's law constant (atm-m³/mol)	1.32×10^{-9}	8.10×10^{-11}	—
K_{oc}	—	72	—
Bioconcentration factor	40	3	—

CAS, Chemical Abstracts Service; K_{oc}, soil sorption constant; ND, no data.

TABLE 115-2. Physiochemical parameters of the dinitrophenols

Parameter	2,3-DNP	2,4-DNP	2,5-DNP	2,6-DNP	3,4-DNP	3,5-DNP	DNP Mixture
CAS no.	66-56-8	51-28-5	329-71-5	573-56-8	577-71-9	586-11-8	25550-58-7
Molecular weight	184.1	184.1	184.1	184.1	184.1	184.1	184.1
Boiling point (°C at 760 mm Hg)	—	Sublimes	—	—	—	—	—
Melting point (°C)	144	112–114	108	63–64	134	122–123	—
Density (g/mL)	1.681 g/cm^3	1.683 g/cm^3	—	—	1.672 g/cm^3	—	—
Solubility (mg/L)	2,200 at 35°–36°C	5,600 at 18°C; 790 at 35°–36°C	385 at 20°C; 680 at 35°–36°C	—	160 at 35°–36°C	—	Soluble in alcohol, ether, benzene, and chloroform
Vapor density	—	—	—	—	—	—	—
Vapor pressure (mm Hg)	—	—	—	—	—	—	—
Ionization potential	—	—	—	—	—	—	—
Explosive limits							
Upper limit (%)	—	Explosive solid	—	Moderate explosion hazard when exposed to heat	—	—	Severe explosion hazard when dry
Lower limit (%)	—	Explosive solid	—	Moderate explosion hazard when exposed to heat	—	—	Severe explosion hazard when dry
Flash point (°C)	—	—	—	—	—	—	—
Henry's law constant (atm-m^3/mol)	—	2.82×10^{-7}	6.61×10^{-7}	—	—	—	—
K_{oc}	—	—	—	—	—	—	—
Bioconcentration factor	—	Log K_{ow} = 2.36	—	—	—	—	—

CAS, Chemical Abstracts Service; DNP, dinitrophenols; K_{oc}, soil sorption constant; K_{ow}, *n*-octanol-water partition coefficient.

numerous other organic compounds including herbicides (2,4-diphenoxyacetic acid), pharmaceuticals, cresols, xylenols, and aniline and alkyl phenols. An additional 12% to 15% of the total phenol used is related to automotive applications.

Phenols are also applied in the manufacture and production of industrial organic compounds, dyes, plastics, adhesives, preservatives, barn deodorants, explosives, fertilizers, coke, illuminating gas, lampblack, paints, paint removers, rubber, asbestos products, textiles, perfumes, and Bakelite. It is used also in caustics, fuel-oil sludge inhibitors, and solvents and in the petroleum, leather, paper, soap, toy, and agricultural industries.

Phenol has found use as a germicidal agent, as it is bacteriostatic in a concentration of approximately 0.2%, bactericidal in concentrations exceeding 1%, and fungicidal in concentrations of at least 1.3%. It has been used in drugs and pharmaceutical preparations as an anesthetic and an antiseptic. It is a component (0.1% to 4.5%) of various liquids, gels, ointments, and lotions (including phenolated calamine lotion), throat sprays, gargles, and lozenges. In the preparation of many medications, phenol is used as a preservative (4,5). The U.S. Food and Drug Administration has approved phenol's use as an indirect food additive for purposes of preserving foods and as a component of adhesives (6).

TABLE 115-3. Physiochemical parameters of phenol, pentachlorophenol, and the cresols

			Cresol		
Parameter	Phenol	Pentachlorophenol	*o*-Cresol	*p*-Cresol	*m*-Cresol
CAS no.	108-95-2	87-86-5	95-48-7	106-44-5	108-39-4
Molecular weight	94.11	266.32	108.14	108.14	108.14
Boiling point (°C at 760 mm Hg)	181.8	309	190.95	201.9	202
Melting point (°C)	40.9	191	30.944	34.739	12.22
Density (g/mL)	1.0545 at 45°C	—	1.0273 at 20°C	1.0178 at 20°C	1.0336 at 20°C
Solubility (mg/L)	93,000 at 25°C	14 at 20°C	31,000 at 25°C	24,000 at 25°C	23,500 at 25°C
Vapor density	3.24	932	—	—	—
Vapor pressure (mm Hg)	0.3513 at 25°C	1.1×10^{-4} at 20°C	0.299 at 25°C	0.11 at 25°C	0.138 at 25°C
Ionization potential	8.47	NA	8.98	8.97	8.98
Explosive limits					
Upper limit (%)	8.6	NA	—	—	—
Lower limit (%)	1.7	NA	1.4	1.1	1.1
Flash point (°C)	85	—	80	80	80
Henry's law constant (atm-m^3/mol)	3.33×10^{-7}	2.75×10^{-6}	1.20×10^{-6}	7.92×10^{-7}	8.65×10^{-7}
K_{oc}	9–135	53,000	22	49	20
Bioconcentration factor	1.4–5.7	770	18	18	35

CAS, Chemical Abstracts Service; K_{oc}, soil sorption constant; NA, not available.

The U.S. Environmental Protection Agency (EPA) estimates that annual production volume of phenol may exceed 3.5 billion pounds (7). In 1992, it was estimated that fewer than 10 million pounds per year were imported (8). In 1994, more than 700 industries registered its use in compliance with Section 313 of the Emergency Planning and Community Right-to-Know Act of 1986 (9). Approximately 320,000 workers may be exposed to phenol in a variety of industrial activities and, because of the presence of phenol in consumer products, consumers have the potential for exposure as well (7).

Physiochemical Properties

Phenol has a chemical formula of C_6H_5OH and a molecular weight of 94.1. Pure phenol is a crystalline solid with a melting point of 43°C and boiling point of 182°C (4). Phenol is an acidic compound with a pK_a of 9.994 in aqueous solutions (4). The most important physiochemical characteristics of phenol are its acidity and reactivity, both of which are attributable to the proximity of a hydroxy group with the resonance structure of an aromatic ring. This structure imparts a high electrophilic substitution reactivity.

Phenol is very highly soluble in most organic solvents (alcohol, chloroform, ether, ethyl acetate, ethanol, carbon disulfide) (10–12) and, at temperatures exceeding 64°C, is entirely soluble in water (12). Solutions of phenol are stable for 24 hours under normal conditions (2). Phenol is moderately volatile at room temperature. It occurs naturally in animal wastes and is produced by decomposition of organic wastes.

Phenol is not very volatile. Consequently, most toxic effects occur from dermal and oral exposure. It has a distinctive odor that is somewhat acrid. The odor threshold of phenol is 7.9 parts per million (ppm) in water and 0.05 ppm in air.

Phenol's chemical properties are determined by its resonance stabilization and the phenolate ion. Its pK_a of 9.994 indicates that it acts as a weak acid. It is incompatible with strong oxidizers such as calcium hypochlorite, chlorine, and bromine (13). Oxidation results in various products such as dihydroxy- and trihydroxybenzenes and quinones. Because phenol is readily oxidized, it is suitable as an antioxidant, functioning as a radical-trapping agent (12).

Exposure Sources

Environmental contamination by phenol is principally due to its manufacture and use in various chemical processes. Phenol is produced as a result of burning wood and automobile exhaust. It is found in numerous hazardous-waste sites on the U.S. National Priority List.

Phenol enters the environment from natural sources such as coal tar as well as chemical wastes from industries that manufacture resin, plastics, adhesives, rubber, iron, steel, and aluminum and from pulp mills and wood treatment facilities (5). Natural sources of phenol in water are animal wastes and decomposition of organic wastes. Phenol contamination of groundwater occurs secondary to leaching from contaminated soil after spills of phenol and hazardous releases.

Phenol is found in surface water, groundwater, drinking water, and rain water as well as urban runoff water and water in and around hazardous-waste sites. The concentrations of phenol can be as high as 1 part per billion (ppb) in uncontaminated groundwater (5). Phenol is found in higher concentration in bodies of water and water sources that receive discharge from industrial sites.

Another source of phenol is the mainstream smoke from tobacco products. The concentrations of phenol released into the environment in this sidestream smoke ranges from 100 to 420 μg per cigarette (4).

Environmental exposure of humans to phenol occurs primarily in industrial settings or in areas that have a significant concentration of phenol in the environment. Human exposure from phenol occurs from ingestion of drinking water from contaminated sources, ingestion of phenol-containing products, use of phenol-containing medicinal agents, and from sidestream tobacco smoke. Phenol is used heavily within the pulpwood industry, and so this is one of the more common occupational exposure sites. Exposure and absorption of phenol is mainly via dermal or gastrointestinal pathways.

Industries and occupations associated with phenol exposure are pharmaceuticals and the iron and steel, leather-tanning, aluminum-forming, electrical, organic- and plastic-manufacturing, paint and ink formulation, and rubber industries. Phenol-containing medicinal uses include mouthwashes, throat lozenges, phenol-containing ointments, nose and eardrops, analgesic rubs, and antiseptic lotions (5).

Environmental Fate and Transport

Phenol is formed during the natural decomposition of organic matter (14). It also is a photooxidation product of benzene and is produced in the atmosphere from benzene emissions. It may be released to the environment as air emissions and wastewater discharges from refuse combustion, brewing, foundries, wood pulping, plastics manufacturing, lacquer manufacturing, glass fiber manufacturing, leather tanning, iron and steel manufacturing, and petroleum refining, as a result of its production and use (14,15). Wood smoke contains high concentrations of phenol and would be expected to be a major source of phenol in the atmosphere during the winter (16). Wood smoke also contributes to phenol detected in smoked foods (17). Phenol is found in gasoline and diesel engine exhaust (18) and in cigarette smoke (15). It is released from organic waste decomposition and the thermal decomposition of resins (19,20).

As a vapor in air, phenol has a short half-life of approximately 12 to 15 hours, but it persists in water for much longer (4,5). The biodegradation of phenol in water can range from 1 to 9 days. It also is photochemically oxidized, and its photooxidation half-life is approximately 19 hours (5). Peroxyl radicals are produced as a photodegradation product of phenol. Phenol in soil generally degrades very quickly. Mean ambient air concentrations of phenol have been found to be 30 parts per trillion in urban and suburban atmospheres (5). Phenol does not concentrate or bioconcentrate in aquatic organisms to any significant degree.

The transport and movement of phenol in the environment are affected by the pH of the environment or the medium in which phenol is present, as phenol's pK_a indicates that it will exist in a partially dissociated state in water and in moist soil (5). Phenol is biodegradable in water sources if the concentration is not high enough to produce significant inhibition of degradation by microorganisms. In fact, phenol may degrade in less than 1 day in surface waters (5). The degradation of phenol is slower in salt water as compared to fresh water.

Absorption, Metabolism, and Excretion

Phenol is readily absorbed from all routes of entry: inhalational, dermal, and gastrointestinal (4,5). Absorption of phenol in both liquid and vapor form occurs through the skin, although higher concentrations of phenol in solution (greater than 10%) act to denature epidermal protein, which then can retard the rate of absorption (4,5,21). Absorption efficiency through the skin is approximately equal to that via inhalation.

Once absorbed, phenol is rapidly distributed to all tissues. Conjugation with glucuronic acid and sulfate represents major metabolic pathways for phenol detoxification (4,5). Phenyl sulfate is the major metabolite in oral administration of phenol to rats; however, increasing the phenol dose changes the major metabolite to phenyl glucuronate as saturation of the sulfation process occurs (22). Conjugation of phenol appears to be species-specific, as the pig has limited ability for phenol sulfation and the cat lacks the ability to produce phenyl glucuronate. Humans metabolize phenol primarily as phenyl sulfate (two-thirds of which is excreted in the urine within 24 hours) and phenyl glucuronide (23). Phenol sulfation occurs in a variety of tissues, and the location of first-pass metabolism depends on the route of entry.

Urinary excretion is the major route of elimination in both test animals and humans. Rate of excretion varies with the dose and route of entry (24). Minor amounts of unchanged phenol may be excreted in exhaled air. Its half-life in humans, as determined from human volunteers, is approximately 3.5 hours (25).

Prolonged skin contact with concentrated phenol can result in burns, necrosis, slow absorption, and a prolonged half-life. One such case involving 90% phenol spilled over 3% of an individual's body surface area resulted in a half-life of 13.9 hours owing to prolonged absorption (26).

Once absorbed systemically, phenol is rapidly excreted in the urine as free phenol or as a conjugate of phenol. It is found normally in human urine in subjects with no known exposure (4,5). However, a correlation exists between the urinary phenol concentrations and the exposure of humans to phenol and the amount that is absorbed (4). Owing to the fact that phenol is rapidly excreted within 1 to 2 days after an exposure, the presence of phenol in the urine can be used as a marker of recent exposure. Studies of phenol dermal absorption in volunteers demonstrated that 13% of an applied dose in solution was absorbed within 30 minutes (5). Eighty percent of this dose was recovered in the urine within 24 hours. As the concentration of phenol solution is increased, the dermal permeability of phenol increases. High concentrations of phenol destroy the skin barrier and, in some cases, may retard absorption.

Four major urinary metabolites of phenol exist: (i) phenol glucuronide, (ii) phenol sulfate, (iii) 1,4-dihydroxybenzene glucuronide, and (iv) 1,4-dihydroxybenzene sulfate (4). Dehydroxylation of phenol is catalyzed by the cytochrome P-450 microsomal monooxygenate system. The sulfate and glucuronide conjugation of phenol varies depending on the animal.

Clinical Toxicology

Health effects from phenol exposure range from mucous membrane irritation, dermal injury, and burns to systemic toxicity with hypotension, cardiac dysrhythmias, and coma, depending on exposure, dose, and route of absorption (Table 115-4).

Air concentrations of phenol vapors below the permissible exposure limit (PEL) of 5 ppm are not associated with health effects, although the odor of phenol is noticeable. Air concentrations that exceed the PEL of 5 ppm are associated with irritation of mucous membranes (8 ppm) (4). The clinical toxicity caused by phenol is similar regardless of the route of absorption. Owing to its low odor threshold of 0.05 ppm in air, phenol can be detected long before it becomes a vapor hazard.

Fatalities have occurred within 10 minutes after 25% of a body surface area liquid exposure to phenol (5). Death has occurred after intentional oral ingestion of phenol. Systemic effects from oral ingestion of phenol include gastrointestinal irritation, vomiting, diarrhea, gastrointestinal bleeding, and cardiac dysrhythmias. Application of concentrated solutions of phenol to the skin can result in skin necrosis, inflammation, and edema at the site of exposure. Animal studies indicate that exposure to 0.5 mL per square centimeter is sufficient to cause skin irritation (26–28).

TABLE 115-4. Phenol's toxic effects

Skin	Neurologic system
Burns	Ataxia
Dark discoloration	Coma
Irritation	Confusion
Necrosis	Muscle tremors
Cardiac system	Seizures
Atrial fibrillation	Syncope
Hypotension	Vertigo
Tachycardia	Gastrointestinal system (ingestion)
Ventricular dysrhythmias	Diarrhea
Metabolic system	Esophageal burns
Acidosis	Gastrointestinal bleeding
	Vomiting
	Renal system
	Dark green urine
	Nephritis
	Hepatic system
	Elevated enzymes

The concentration of phenol is important in determining dermal absorption, skin injury, and systemic toxicity. Phenol is a denaturant, and skin exposure can result in severe burns and systemic toxicity, depending on the concentration. Cardiac dysrhythmias are reported in clinical cases of individuals after both oral ingestion and dermal application of phenol solution, particularly concentrated solutions (21,26,28). Elevated liver enzymes have been demonstrated in individuals with phenol toxicity. Animal studies indicate neurologic toxicity such as tremors, convulsions, coma, and ataxia after dermal or oral exposure (26–28).

Dermal absorption of phenol depends on concentration, surface area of contact, duration of contact, skin occlusion, temperature of the skin (increased absorption with increased temperature), and condition of the skin (Table 115-5) (21). Phenol easily penetrates the human dermal barrier to be systemically absorbed and can produce serious toxicity via solutions that come into contact with the skin or by vapor contact (21,26–29). Urinary excretion of phenol occurs within 30 minutes of dermal contact.

Ventricular ectopy has occurred after application of solutions of 6 mL containing 40% phenol (2.4 g of phenol) to the skin (26,28). High concentrations of phenol, such as 40% or more, denature the dermis and coagulate keratin, causing the underlying skin to become hyperemic. This can result in an increased systemic absorption of phenol (21,26).

Clinical cases involving 90% phenol spilled over 3% of the body surface area have been associated with confusion, vertigo, hypotension, ventricular ectopy, atrial fibrillation, dark green urine, blue-black dermal discoloration, dermal swelling, hypalgesia, and hypesthesia of the contaminated area 4 hours after exposure (27). This case resulted in high systemic (21.6 μg per L) and urinary phenol concentrations (13,416 mg per gram of creatinine) associated with a prolonged half-life of elimination of 13.9 hours, representing continued dermal absorption or extensive tissue distribution. The patient had been decontaminated with water. Skin discoloration still was present 4 months later (27).

TABLE 115-5. Dermal absorption for phenol (21)

Dermal absorption	
2.5 g/L	0.079–0.300 mg/cm^2/h
5 mg/L	0.181–0.047 mg/cm^2/h
10 g/L	0.300–0.048 mg/cm^2/h

DERMAL INJURY AND DECONTAMINATION

Prolonged cutaneous exposure may result in ochronosis, a discoloration of collagenous tissue. After repeated low-grade exposure, persons experience redness, itching, and burning during the development of contact dermatitis. Depigmentation of the skin can occur in workers exposed to phenolic compounds for approximately 6 months. The onset may be preceded by mild erythema and pruritus until leukoderma appears months after initial exposure. Recovery may take several months or years but is complete.

Phenol is rapidly absorbed via the skin and, depending on concentration and skin area involved, systemic effects or death can occur in minutes to hours. High phenol concentrations, prolonged skin contact time, large exposed surface areas, and site occlusion are high-risk factors for serious and life-threatening toxicity. Thus, rapid skin decontamination is crucial to help prevent absorption, serious toxicity, and death. However, decontamination techniques have been controversial.

Studies conducted using various skin decontamination procedures demonstrated that increased absorption of phenol can occur after water is used as a decontaminant, but water frequently is all that is available (27). The use of water is believed to help spread and enlarge the surface area of phenol contact with skin. However, other studies demonstrate that copious irrigation of exposed skin with water removes significant amounts of phenol (30).

The threshold concentration for human skin damage from phenol is 1.5% (31). Phenol chemically alters the stratum corneum and significantly impairs the capacity of the skin to prevent penetration. Increasing the concentration of phenol increases the permeability coefficient more than severalfold (31). The permeability coefficient for a 5% phenol solution is 50-fold higher than for a 1% solution (31).

The decontaminant that was found to prevent phenol absorption and systemic toxicity best is 50% solution of polyethylene glycol (PEG-300 or PEG-400) (28,30,31). Another effective decontaminating solution studied was a combination of PEG-400 and industrial methylated spirits (30–33). Swabbing phenol-contaminated skin with either PEG-300 or PEG-400 was effective at reducing dermal burns and systemic toxicity in all studies (27,30–32). Swabbing a small, exposed site with isopropyl alcohol also is effective as a decontaminant for small surface areas (32). Studies support the claim that decontamination is beneficial to survival.

Thus, recommendations for managing a contaminated patient are (i) removal of contaminated clothing, (ii) immediate irrigation with copious water and soap, (iii) swabbing of the skin with cotton swabs soaked with PEG-300 or PEG-400 for a minimum of 10 to 20 minutes, and (iv) medical observation for medical complications (see Table 115-5). The speed of decontamination is essential in preventing dermal burns and systemic toxicity from phenol.

IMMUNOTOXICITY

No immunotoxic effects in humans are known secondary to phenol exposure. In addition, no developmental, reproductive, or genotoxic effects are known to occur secondary to phenol exposure in humans. Phenol is not a human carcinogen. The National Cancer Institute has reported cancer in laboratory animals secondary to phenol exposure, although its carcinogenic effects in animals have been equivocal. Phenol is a tumor promoter when applied to the skin and might be a complete carcinogen (initiator and promoter) in mice (5).

RENAL TOXICITY

Renal toxicity has been reported in laboratory animals. Phenol is nephrotoxic to humans and animals, especially after chronic exposure. Animal studies show a direct toxic effect on renal parenchyma. Humans have experienced nephritis after toxic dermal exposure (34).

CARDIOTOXICITY

Ingestion or dermal absorption of phenol can cause cardiac dysrhythmias and death from ventricular ectopy (26–28). A case report described a 52-year-old woman who was mistakenly administered 1 ounce of 89% phenol as a preoperative medication. She developed hypotension, ventricular dysrhythmias, seizures, metabolic acidosis, esophageal burns, coma, and respiratory arrest 30 minutes after the ingestion (27).

MUTAGENICITY

Data from bacterial and yeast studies provide conflicting results on the mutagenicity of phenol. Some researchers report negative results with *Salmonella typhimurium* both with and without metabolic activation (35,36), whereas others report phenol-induced mutation in the *Salmonella* strain TA1538 in the presence of activation (37). The National Toxicology Program evaluated phenol for mutations in *Drosophila melanogaster* and found negative results at all concentrations tested either through injection (5,250 ppm) or feeding (2,000 ppm) (38); earlier research had found an increase in lethal mutations after *in vitro* exposure to phenol and implantation into host larvae. Exposure of rainbow trout (*Salmo gairdneri*) to phenol resulted in significant chromosomal aberrations in gill and kidney tissue (39). *In vitro* studies of the effects of phenol exposure on various mammalian (Chinese hamster) cells provided positive, negative, and inconclusive results (40–42). Phenol has not been reported to cause any teratogenic effects (43).

CARCINOGENICITY

Skin application of phenol results in the promotion of skin tumors in strains of mice specially inbred for sensitivity to tumor development; however, this appears to be associated with irritation and subsequent skin hyperplasia (44). The International Agency for Research on Cancer considers phenol not classifiable as to its carcinogenicity (group 3) owing to inadequate data. The EPA has classified phenol in group D, which indicates that it is not classifiable as to human carcinogenicity because no human carcinogenicity data exist and animal data are inadequate (45).

Biomarkers of Exposure

Phenol may be detected in biological samples (urine and blood) if exposure is suspected. Colorimetric methods for the determination of free phenol in urine are available, although all phenols combine for a positive reaction, and normal urine often is positive. Elevated urinary phenol excretion is not a specific indication of exposure. In addition, a large range of normal urine values, from 0.5 to 81.5 mg per L, exist, which limits the usefulness of this value as an accurate index of occupational exposure (46). Gas chromatography–flame ionization detection of total phenol in urine has a detection limit of 0.5 μg per L (47). Gas chromatography–mass spectrometry detection is possible after hydrolysis of glucuronide and sulfate conjugates with sulfuric acid and derivation with propanoic anhydride to form a large molecule having ions characteristic for positive identification. The detection limit is reported to be 10 μg per L (48).

Normal phenol levels in blood are 0 to 4 mg of free phenol, 0.1 to 2.0 mg of conjugated phenol, and 0.15 to 7.96 mg of total phenol per dL of blood. The American Conference of Governmental Industrial Hygienists has established a biological exposure index for phenol of 250 mg per gram of creatinine for end-of-shift urine samples.

TABLE 115-6. Exposure guidelines, criteria, and standards for phenol and phenol derivatives

Parameter	Phenol	Pentachlorophenol	Cresol			2,4-DNP	Hydroquinone	Catechol	Resorcinol
			o-Cresol	*p*-Cresol	*m*-Cresol				
Air									
OSHA PEL									
(ppm)	5 (skin)	0.5 (skin)	5 (skin)	5 (skin)	5 (skin)	—	—	None	None
(mg/m^3)	19	—	22	22	22	—	2	—	—
NIOSH REL									
(ppm)	5	0.5 (skin)	2.3	2.3	2.3	—	—	5	10
(mg/m^3)	19	—	10	10	10	—	2	20	45
NIOSH STEL									
(ppm)	15.6	—	—	—	—	—	—	—	20
(mg/m^3)	60	—	—	—	—	—	—	—	90
ACGIH TLV									
(ppm)	5	0.5 (skin)	5 (skin)	5 (skin)	5 (skin)	—	—	5 (skin)	10
(mg/m^3)	19	—	22	22	22	—	2	23	45
IDLH									
(ppm)	—	—	250	250	250	—	50	—	—
(mg/m^3)	—	2.5	—	—	—	—	—	—	—
Drinking water									
MCL (μg/L)	—	0.001	—	—	—	—	—	—	—
Secondary MCL (mg/L)	—	0.03	—	—	—	—	—	—	—
Health Advisory (mg/L)	—	—	—	—	—	—	—	—	—
AWQC									
HH/F&W (μg/L)	3,500	1.01×10^3	—	—	—	70	—	—	—
AF, chronic (4-d avg) (μg/L)	600	1.3×10^1	—	—	—	2.3×10^2	—	—	—
AF, acute (1-h avg) (μg/L)	3,400	2.2×10^1	—	—	—	1.15×10^2	—	—	—
Other									
Oral RfD (mg/kg/d)	6.0×10^{-1}	3.0×10^{-2}	5.0×10^{-2}	5.0×10^{-3}	5.0×10^{-2}	2.0×10^{-3}	4.0×10^{-2}	—	—
Inhalational RfC (mg/m^3)	—	—	—	—	—	—	—	—	—
Carcinogen classification	—	—	—	—	—	—	—	—	—
EPA weight of evidence	D	B2	—	—	—	—	—	—	—
IARC	3	2B	—	—	—	—	group 3	group 3	group 3

ACGIH, American Conference of Governmental Industrial Hygienists; AF, criteria (either chronic or acute) for the protection of aquatic life in freshwater resources; AWQC, ambient water-quality criteria; DNP, dinitrophenol; EPA, U.S Environmental Protection Agency; HH/F&W, criteria for the protection of human health based on ingestion of 2 L water and 0.65 g fish per day from a surface water source; IARC, International Agency for Research on Cancer; IDLH, immediately dangerous to life and health; MCL, federally enforceable maximum contaminant limit for drinking water; NIOSH, National Institute of Occupational Safety and Health; OSHA, U.S. Occupational Safety and Health Administration; PEL, permissible exposure limit as a TWA over an 8-h workday in a 40-h work week; REL, recommended exposure limit (TWA concentration for up to a 10-h workday in a 40-h work week); RfC, inhalation reference concentration that is likely to be without appreciable risk of deleterious effects over a lifetime; RfD, reference dose, a provisional estimate of the daily exposure that is likely to be without appreciable risk of deleterious effects during a lifetime; secondary MCL, advisory level based on aesthetic concerns (taste, odor, staining); skin, notation indicating potential for dermal absorption and caution to prevent skin exposure; STEL, short-term exposure limit (a 15-minute TWA exposure that should not be exceeded at any time during a workday); TLV, threshold limit value as a TWA for an 8-h workday in a 40-h work week; TWA, time-weighted average.

Biological Exposure Limits

The U.S. Occupational Safety and Health Administration PEL for phenol is 5 ppm as a time-weighted average for up to a 10-hour work shift (with a skin notation). The American Conference of Governmental Industrial Hygienists recommends a threshold limit value–time-weighted average of 5 ppm and a biological exposure index for total phenol in urine of 250 mg per gram of creatinine at the end of a work shift (see Table 115-5).

Environmental Controls and Regulations

Table 115-6 list the occupational and environmental regulations for phenol and phenol derivatives. Phenol is designated as *Poison B* by the Department of Transportation, and phenol containers must be labeled *poison* for shipping (49). The National Fire Protection Agency has rated phenol as a *3* for health, indicating that short exposure could cause serious temporary or residual injury that requires protection from all bodily contact; a *2* for flammability, which indicates that it must be heated before ignition will occur and that water can be used to extinguish fires because the material can be cooled below its flash point; and a *0* for reactivity, which indicates that phenol is normally stable and does not react with water.

Phenol has been designated as a hazardous substance under section 311(b)(2)(A) of the Federal Water Pollution Control Act (50) and as a toxic pollutant designated pursuant to section 307(a)(1) of the Clean Water Act and is subject to effluent limitations (51). The National Response Center must be notified if a release of its reportable quantity of 1,000 pounds or 454 kg occurs (52). It is a hazardous waste under the Resource Conservation and Recovery Act (RCRA) and must be managed according to federal and state hazardous-waste regulations (53). The EPA recently added phenol to the list of chemicals subject to section 4 of the Toxic Substances Control Act, which requires testing consent orders and export notification requirements.

The U.S. EPA RfD/RfC Work Group has established a chronic oral reference dose (RfD) of 0.6 mg of phenol per kg of body weight per day, on the basis of a no-observed-adverse-effect level of 60 mg per kg of body weight per day from a developmental study in which reduced fetal body weights of rats were observed after phenol exposure. An oral RfD is an estimate of the daily intake that is likely to be without appreciable risk of deleterious effects if ingested over a lifetime. The health effects data for phenol have been determined to be inadequate for derivation of an inhalational reference concentration (RfC). An RfC is a concentration of a contaminant in air (milligrams of phenol per cubic meter of air) that is likely to be without appreciable risk of deleterious effects if inhaled over a lifetime. RfDs and RfCs that have been peer-reviewed and verified by the U.S. EPA RfD/RfC Work Group are listed in the EPA's Integrated Risk Information System (IRIS). IRIS is an online database that is updated by the EPA whenever new information becomes available (45). Provisional, unverified RfDs and RfCs are listed in the EPA's Annual Health Effects Assessment Summary Tables, which are limited to chemicals that have undergone review but have not met with a high-quality agency-wide consensus (54).

Engineering controls are the most effective way of reducing exposure. Such controls include enclosing operations and providing local exhaust ventilation. When possible, automatically pumping liquid phenol from drums or storage containers to processing containers will help to avoid skin contact (55). Under all circumstances in which skin contact with phenol is possible, protective clothing, including gloves and a face shield, should be worn. Clothing should be of a material that is impervious to phenol (e.g., neoprene, polyethylene, or rubber). Under conditions in which airborne concentrations exceed 20 mg per cubic meter, a full-face respiratory device also is required.

Phenol is weakly sorbed by soil, as indicated by experimentally determined soil sorption coefficient (K_{oc}) values, ranging between 9 and 135 for generic soil types to 700 for clay soils (56–59). Phenol should readily leach to groundwater. Based on its pK_a, phenol exists in a partially dissociated state in moist soil, and it is assumed that its transport and reactivity could be affected by pH (60). Its vapor pressure (see Table 115-6) and low adsorptivity to soil indicate that volatilization from dry soil may occur (60). Studies by Jury et al. (61) indicate that phenol has an effective volatilization half-life from soil of between 15 and 30 days. Radiolabeled phenol was rapidly released from soil; after 1 day, half the label was found in the air phase (61).

Phenol is susceptible to chemical degradation mechanisms in the soil-groundwater system. It is sensitive to indirect photolysis, which can occur on the soil surface (62). Reaction with molecular oxygen, resulting in carbon monoxide formation, has been demonstrated in sterile soils (63). Simple hydrolysis (reaction with water) does not take place rapidly in the environment. An aqueous hydrolysis rate constant of 8.2 to 8.5×10^{-9} cubic meters per mole per second has been experimentally determined (64). Phenol can also be oxidized in oxygen-rich water, especially if iron or copper species are present to act as catalysts (65). Photooxidation to carbon dioxide in aerated, near-surface water was detected under experimental conditions (65–67). Typical half-lives in fresh water range from 19 to 100 hours (60).

Biodegradation appears to be the primary removal process in the environment. Numerous studies have shown that microorganisms in the environment easily degraded phenol under aerobic conditions to carbon dioxide (65,66,68–70) and that phenol is less readily degraded under anaerobic conditions to carbon dioxide or methane (71,72). Intermediates in the biodegradation process include benzoate, catechol, *cis-cis*-muconate, succinate, and acetate (72,73). Acclimation of populations of microorganisms is rapid. Several types of microorganisms can use phenol as their sole source of carbon (74), but this is concentration-dependent. At concentrations exceeding 100 mg per L, microorganisms may be inhibited or killed. Rate studies have been carried out, but the prediction of biodegradation rate constants for specific environments remains questionable (66).

Phenols degrade rapidly in sewage, soil, fresh water, and seawater. Under aerobic conditions in sewage, biodegradation is rapid, typically 90% in an 8-hour period; in soils, complete biodegradation occurs in 2 to 5 days; in fresh water, complete biodegradation occurs in less than 1 day; and in seawater, a half-life of 9 days has been observed (60). Under anaerobic conditions, degradation is slower and microbial adaptation periods lag (75).

Phenol does not bioconcentrate in aquatic organisms. Its measured or estimated bioconcentration factors range between 1.4 and 5.7 (76,77) and indicate no potential for bioaccumulation.

Phenol may be detected in air through the collection of samples on an impinger, the filter of which is impregnated with sodium hydroxide solution. Sorbent tubes (Tenax, silica gel) can also be used. Sorbent tubes are also useful for collecting samples from water and solid wastes. Air samples can be analyzed by gas chromatography in combination with flame ionization detection to obtain a detection limit between 1 and 4 µg per cubic meter (78,79) or with high-performance liquid chromatography in combination with ultraviolet detection to obtain detection limits as low as 0.2 µg per cubic meter (80). Phenol in water and soil can be analyzed by gas chromatography in combination with mass spectrometry to detect concentrations as low as micrograms per liter or micrograms per kilogram, respectively (81).

PENTACHLOROPHENOL

Once one of the most widely used biocides, pentachlorophenol (PCP) now is regulated as a restricted-use pesticide by the EPA. Formerly, it was widely used as a fungicide, herbicide, molluscicide, algicide, disinfectant, antifouling agent, and wood preservative.

Sources, Uses, and Production

The most commonly used abbreviations for pentachlorophenol are *PCP* and *penta*. Among the many synonyms and trade names are pentachlorophenate, Dowcide 7, Durotox, Lauxtol, Weedone, and Triox (51).

Most of the lower-chlorinated phenols (mono-, di-, tri-, and tetrachlorophenol) are used as chemical intermediates in the manufacturer of PCP. PCP is formed by direct chlorination of phenol with chlorine gas in the presence of a catalyst at temperatures rising to 200°C. Technical-grade PCP contains polychlorinated dibenzodioxins and dibenzofurans. These other compounds formed during PCP production are isomers of hexa-, hepta-, and octachlorodibenzo-*p*-dioxins and furans (commonly termed *dioxins* and *furan*).

PCP is a commercially important and widely used compound to protect timber products from fungal rot and wood-boring insects. As a wood preservative, it is commonly applied as a 0.1% solution in mineral spirits, No. 2 fuel oil, or kerosene or as a 5% solution in the pressure treatment of lumber (82). It also is used as a defoliant, an herbicide, and a pesticide. As an herbicide, it is restricted to nonagricultural uses (driveways, ditches, roadways). Because of the contamination of PCP products with dioxins and furans, pesticides containing PCPs are no longer available for over-the-counter sale in the United States and may be purchased and used only by certified applicators (83).

Physiochemical Properties

At 20°C, PCP is a white to light brown crystalline solid or orange-tan powder. PCP (2,3,4,5,6-PCP) has a chemical formula of C_6Cl_5OH; its structure is shown in Figure 115-1. Table 115-3 lists its physiochemical properties. PCP is soluble in alcohol, ether, and benzene and has a solubility in water of 24 mg per L at 20°C (84). Its odor threshold in water is 0.857 mg per L at 30°C, and its vapor pressure is 0.00011 mm Hg. PCP is incompatible with strong bases, acid chlorides, and acid anhydrides, and it reacts with strong oxidizing agents (85). It forms salts with alkaline metals.

Exposure Sources

Workers in occupations that use PCP have the highest potential for exposure through direct handling of raw material and freshly treated wood. The general public may be exposed through handling wood that has been treated with PCP solutions. Treated wood will "bleed"—that is, PCP on the interior of the wood will move to the surface, where it is available for direct contact, may evaporate into the air, or can leach into water. Farm animals ingest PCP through chewing and licking outdoor wood structures. Humans can be exposed through ingestion and bathing with contaminated household water (84,86).

PCP can be detected in human blood, urine, breast milk, adipose tissue, and cerebrospinal fluid. The average PCP level in the urine of a nonoccupationally exposed population was 4.9 ppb, as compared to 119.9 ppb in those who were occupationally exposed (87). Multiple studies have found PCP to be present in human biological samples, linking the subjects to some source of exposure (Table 115-7) (88–95). By comparing daily intake of PCP to tissue concentrations, the following bioconcentration ratios were developed from levels found in various human tissues (84): liver, 5.7; brain, 3.3; blood, 1.4; spleen, 1.4, and adipose tissue, 1.0. PCP has also been found in human breast milk at a concentration of 0.03 to 2.8 µg per kg (93). In human tissues removed at autopsy, PCP has been detected in all tissues at a range of 0.007 µg per gram of adipose tissue to 4.14 µg per gram of testicular tissue (94), and levels of 420 ppb have been found in blood and urine of people living in log homes.

Environmental Fate and Transport

PCP may enter the environment through emissions and discharge from manufacturing plants, from use of the chemical in a final product, or through volatilization from treated wood. It is discharged into water from nonpoint and point sources and from soil to water by runoff and leaching from spills and treated products.

PCP is stable to oxidation and hydrolysis but undergoes rapid photooxidation by sunlight. It is metabolized by microorganisms, animals, and plants, and it bioaccumulates up the food chain to some extent. PCP adsorbs to acidic soils more than to alkaline or neutral soils.

In wastewater, PCP adsorbs to sludges and concentrates. PCP that volatilizes into the atmosphere can be transported back to soil and water via precipitation. Atmospheric PCP is chemically transformed via radical oxidation photolysis (84). Volatilization is not a significant transport mechanism under ambient conditions.

Adsorption of PCP onto soil and sediments depends on the organic content and is controlled by soil pH. As soil organic content increases, the amount of PCP adsorption increases. PCP adsorbs to soil under acidic pH conditions but is mobile under alkaline and neutral pHs (84). The compound has a pK_a of 4.74. A decrease in sorption occurs as the pH rises from 5 to 7, although a slight increase in sorption occurs with increasing organic matter (96). No accurate prediction can be made of K_{oc} from the octanol-water partition coefficient (K_{ow}) because of the strong dissociation of PCP and the uncertain effects of pH on the value of K_{ow}. If PCP dissociates in soil, little volatilization would occur because of its low vapor pressure and low value of Henry's law constant, but water solubility would increase, as would the mobility to groundwater. Maximum soil adsorption occurs at a pH of 4.6 to 5.1.

Photolysis and hydrolysis (no hydrolyzable functional groups) do not appear to be significant processes for removal of PCP from soil. PCP will biodegrade in soil with a half-life of weeks to months, depending on the microbial population, temperature, and PCP concentration. Ultimately, it undergoes complete biodegradation, as all carbons are converted to carbon dioxide (97).

TABLE 115-7. Pentachlorophenol in human samples

Biological sample	Population	Reference
Urine		
4.9 ppb	General Florida population	87
119.9 ppb	Boat builders, sprayers, carpenters	87
1,100–5,910 ppb	Japanese pest control operators	88
10–50 ppb	Nonoccupational exposure	88
1,802 ppb	Occupational exposure	89
40 ppb	Nonoccupational exposure	89
14 ppb	Median concentration in urine samples from 197 children	90
22 µg/L (mean; range, 4–60 µg/L)	Patients (n = 16) with neurologic symptoms	91
69 ppb (mean)	Log home dwellers	95
6.3 ppb (max. level, 193 ppb)	National Human Adipose Tissue Monitoring Survey, 6,000 persons (blood and tissue) in United States 1976–1980	92
Cerebrospinal fluid: 0.75 µg/L (mean; range, 0.24–2.03 µg/L)	Patients (n = 16) with neurologic symptoms	91
Human breast milk: 0.03–2.8 µg/kg	West German population	93
Adipose tissue: 0.007 µg/g (ppm)	Autopsy samples	94
Blood		
420 ppb (mean)	Log home dwellers	95
83–57,600 ppb	Workers with exposure to pentachlorophenol	95

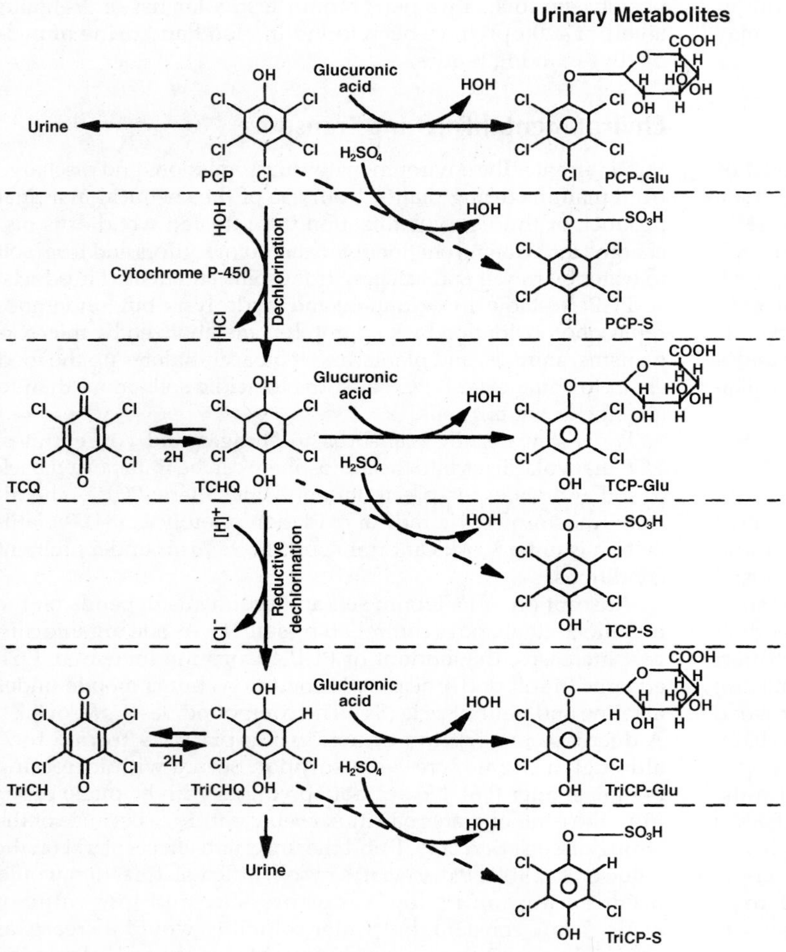

Figure 115-2. Proposed metabolism of pentachlorophenol. PCP, pentachlorophenol; PCP-Glu, pentachlorophenol-β-glucuronide; PCP-S, pentachlorophenylsulfate; TCHQ, tetrachloro-p-hydroquinone; TCP-Glu, tetrachlorophenol-β-glucuronide; TCP-S, tetrachlorophenylsulfate; TCQ, tetrachloroquinone; TriCHQ, trichloro-p-hydroquinone; TriCP-Glue, trichlorophenyl-β-glucuronide; TriCP-S, trichlorophenylsulfate; TriCQ, trichloro-p-quinone. (From ref. 84, with permission.)

PCP is moderately persistent in water, with a half-life between 20 and 200 days, and is eliminated mainly by biodegradation near the surface. It is degraded by sunlight in surface water, but it also binds to sediments and suspended particulates. It does not evaporate to a significant degree. It will bioaccumulate to a moderate degree in aquatic organisms and domestic animals (through the drinking of contaminated surface water).

Slightly less than half of the PCP released to the environment will end up in soil, approximately 45% in aquatic sediments, 5% in water, and nearly 1% in air. Monitoring for PCP in the environment is similar to that described for phenol.

Absorption, Metabolism, and Excretion

PCP is absorbed by the inhalational, oral, and dermal routes of exposure. Exposure to PCP is ubiquitous from environmental sources, and concentrations can be found in all human tissues (see Table 115-7). The liver, kidneys, plasma proteins, brain, spleen, and adipose tissue are major sites of PCP deposition. However, accumulation usually is uncommon. PCP is excreted rapidly and mainly unchanged in urine, as the parent compound (82%) and as the PCP glucuronide (13%) (98). As has been mentioned, PCP is detected in a variety of human tissues, particularly human fat. PCP levels in human adipose tissue range from 4 to 250 ppb. The half-life of PCP in humans is 27 to 36 hours. Small amounts of PPC in the parts-per-billion range generally are detected in blood and urine of the general population from numerous environmental sources, among which the ingestion of contaminated food accounts for the majority. The metabolism of PCP is depicted in Figure 115-2.

Clinical Toxicology

Human exposure to PCP is by inhalation, dermal exposure, and ingestion, and all three routes result in significant systemic absorption and toxicity (Table 115-8). Oral absorption of PCP is rapid, and a half-life of 1.3 hours has been calculated (98). PCP is absorbed across the skin and appears to be absorbed to a greater extent when in an oily rather than an aqueous solution. One study showed that 62% of PCP in diesel oil solution penetrated the skin, whereas only 16% of an aqueous solution penetrated the skin (99). PCP binds to plasma proteins, which affects

TABLE 115-8. Manifestations of acute pentachlorophenol toxicity

Abdominal pain
Anorexia
Convulsions
Dermal irritation and chloracne
Diaphoresis
Fatigue
Hyperthermia (uncouples oxidative phosphorylation)
Muscular spasm
Renal tubular dysfunction
Respiratory tract inflammation

its distribution systemically; it has been demonstrated that 95% of PCP in plasma is protein-bound (98).

Minimal risk levels (MRLs) for PCP have been calculated for oral ingestion (MRL = 0.005 mg per kg per day) based on a lowest-observable-adverse-effect level (LOAEL) of 5 mg per kg per day (84). The intermediate MRL has been calculated to be 0.001 mg per kg per day based on an LOAEL of 1.2 mg per kg per day, related to an increase in the serum enzyme levels of alkaline phosphatase and serum glutamic-pyruvic transaminase in rats, which may indicate hepatotoxicity (84). Chronic MRLs have not been calculated for human exposures.

Fatal human exposures to PCP have been associated with hyperthermia. Other clinical manifestations are sweating, abdominal symptoms, muscle spasms, anorexia, and fatigue (99). PCP uncouples oxidative phosphorylation, thus interfering with cellular metabolism and resulting in hyperthermia. The toxicity of PCP is enhanced in the presence of hydrocarbon solvents such as fuel oils. Such solvents may allow more efficient absorption.

PCP vapor can cause upper respiratory tract inflammation and bronchitis, symptoms that have been noted in workers chronically exposed to PCP at high levels (100). Hematologic effects secondary to PCP exposure have been reported to include aplastic anemia, red cell aplasia, and hemolytic anemia (101,102). Such hematologic pathologic findings have been seen in animals exposed to technical-grade PCP but not in animals exposed to pure PCP. Therefore, the hematotoxicity of PCP in humans may be secondary to contaminants.

Hepatotoxicity is manifested by elevation of liver enzymes. Centrilobular hepatic necrosis has been seen after both fatal and nonfatal PCP exposures, as has fatty infiltration of the liver (100). However, these hepatic effects may also be due to the impurities or contaminants present in technical-grade PCP and not to the pure PCP.

Human cases of PCP exposure have been marked by renal dysfunction, impairment of glomerular filtration, and tubular dysfunction. These effects have been reversible (103). PCP can be irritating to the eyes, nose, throat, and skin. Dermal exposures have been associated with chloracne (104). Other case reports of PCP exposure indicate both central and peripheral nervous system toxicity. However, much of this neurologic toxicity is probably due to the hyperthermic response from uncoupling of oxidative phosphorylation in the mitochondria and presents as lethargy, tachypnea, tachycardia, delirium, convulsions, possible coma, and cerebral edema (105). PCP does not appear to be a primary CNS toxin.

Immunopathologic effects, genotoxicity, and adrenal dysfunction as a result of PCP exposure are controversial. Although prolonged exposure has been reported to result in changes in endocrine gland function and immune dysfunction, the evidence supporting such changes is sparse. Gerhard et al. (106) have linked adrenal dysfunction to reproductive disorders in women after long-term exposure to PCP and wood preservatives. However, this brief report was presented in a letter and did not consider confounding factors and contaminants of technical-grade PCP.

Evidence of immune dysfunction is lacking. Animal data indicate that technical-grade PCP may affect immune function, but this may be an effect of impurities, since the immunosuppression seen with technical-grade PCP is not seen with pure-grade PCP (107,108). Nonetheless, other tests in which human lymphocytes were exposed *in vitro* to both technical- and pure-grade PCP indicate immunotoxic effects on T-cell response and humoral immune activity (109). PCP may not have the same effects *in vivo*. Immunotoxicity studies in animals and *in vitro* human tests do not appear to have a biological significance in terms of increased risk of infection or cancer.

The teratogenicity of PCP has been investigated in a number of animal studies, none of which indicated a positive relationship between PCP and teratogenic effects. PCP does not cross the placental barrier, and so observed fetal toxicity may be a reflection of maternal toxicity. PCP has not been determined to have mutagenic effects in test systems, although some indication that PCP has clastogenic potential is available.

The EPA has classified PCP as a B2 compound, which means that it is a probable human carcinogen, based on statistically significant increases in the incidences of hepatocellular adenomas and carcinomas, adrenal medulla and malignant pheochromocytomas, and hemangiosarcomas and hemangiomas in both genders of a specific strain of mice using two different PCP preparations (110). In 1991, the International Agency for Research on Cancer classified PCP as possibly carcinogenic (group 2B), there being sufficient evidence in experimental animals but inadequate evidence in humans (111).

Dermal Decontamination

PCP is absorbed quickly across the dermal layer and can injure the skin. Because dermal absorption may lead to systemic toxicity, decontamination is critical. Recommendations for managing a contaminated patient are similar to those for phenol contamination: (i) removal of contaminated clothing, (ii) immediate irrigation of the skin with copious soap and water, (iii) swabbing of the skin with cotton soaked with PEG-300 or PEG-400 for a minimum of 10 to 20 minutes, and (iv) medical observation for medical complications. Although no direct evidence indicates that PEG will prevent PCP dermal absorption, the application of PEG is reasonable given the physiochemical similarities between PCP and phenol. The speed of decontamination is essential in preventing dermal burns and systemic toxicity.

Biomarkers of Exposure

PCP is excreted mainly unmetabolized in the urine, and therefore its presence in urine can be used as an exposure biomarker. The urinary metabolite tetrachloro-*p*-hydroquinone has also been proposed as a biomarker of exposure to PCP (see Fig. 115-2) (112).

Environmental Controls and Regulations

Tables 115-6 and 115-9 list occupational and environmental regulations applicable to PCP. PCP has a maximum contaminant limit (MCL) of 0.001 μg per L, which is associated with a lifetime individual risk of less than 1×10^{-6}. MCLs are federally enforceable limits for contaminants in drinking water that are based on health goals, treatment techniques, and cost. The MCL uses the MCL goal (MCLG), a nonenforceable health goal, to determine the standard. The MCLG for PCP is 0 μg per L; because of the potential for carcinogenic effects, the MCL is set equal to the practical quantitation limit (0.001 mg per L) (113–115). Secondary MCLs are nonenforceable and establish concentrations for contaminants that may affect the aesthetic qualities (e.g., taste and odor) of drinking water. The proposed secondary MCL for PCP is based on adverse taste (116).

The EPA has established a chronic RfD of 0.03 mg per kg of body weight per day based on a no-observed-adverse-effect level of 3 mg per kg of body weight per day. This level was determined from a chronic oral feeding study in which pathologic changes in liver and kidney were observed (110).

The National Fire Protection Agency has rated PCP as a 3 for health, indicating that short-term exposure could cause serious temporary or residual injury that requires protection from all bodily contact; an 0/2 for flammability, which indicates that PCP

TABLE 115-9. Environmental regulations applicable to pentachlorophenol

Agency	Regulatory class	Limits and date enacted
OSHA	PEL (TWA)	Skin, 0.5 mg/m^3 (1989)
IARC	Carcinogenic classification	Group 2Ba (possible human carcinogen) (1991)
WHO	Drinking water guideline	10 μg/L (1984)
ATSDR	Acute oral MRL based on developmental defects in rats	0.005 mg/kg/d
	Intermediate MRL based on increased hepatic enzymes	0.001 mg/kg/d
EPA	RfD with uncertain factor of 100 based on rat liver and kidney pathology	0.03 mg/kg/d
	Carcinogen classification	B2 (probable human carcinogen)
	Section 313 Toxic Chemicals Subject to Emergency Planning and Right to Know Act of 1986	1986
	Restricted use and sale of pesticide products containing pentachlorophenol	1987

ATSDR, Agency for Toxic Substances and Disease Registry; EPA, U.S. Environmental Protection Agency; IARC, International Agency for Research on Cancer; MRL, minimal risk level; OSHA, U.S. Occupational Safety and Health Administration; PEL, permissible exposure limit; RfD, reference dose; TWA, time-weighted average; WHO, World Health Organization.

is a nonflammable compound but that poisonous gases may be produced in a fire; and a 0 for reactivity, which indicates that phenol is normally stable and does not react with water.

PCP has a reportable quantity of 10 pounds under the Comprehensive Environmental Response, Compensation, and Liability Act, based on aquatic toxicity as assigned by section 311(b)(4) of the Clean Water Act (117). It is a listed waste under the RCRA and must be managed according to federal and state hazardous-waste regulations. Under the Federal Insecticide, Fungicide, and Rodenticide Act registration standard, it is a list B pesticide (118).

As with all products containing phenol, engineering controls are the safest way to reduce or eliminate potential exposures. Protective clothing should be worn when handling PCP. Because PCP in oily solutions degrades natural rubber, the use of nitrile or polyvinyl chloride gloves for worker protection is recommended (119).

CRESOLS

Cresols are isomeric substituted phenols, with methyl groups at the *ortho* (*o*-), *meta* (*m*-), and *para* (*p*-) positions. Commercial cresol is called *cresylic acid* and contains all three isomeric forms and a small fraction of xylene and phenol. Table 115-10 lists the constituents of cresylic acid.

TABLE 115-10. Constituents of cresylic acid

Constituent	Percentage by volume
m- and *p*-Cresol	0–1
2,4- and 2,6-Xylenols	0–3
2,3- and 3,5-Xylenols	10–20
3,4-Xylenols	20–30
C_9-phenols	50–60

Sources, Uses, and Production

Commercial cresol is a mixture of three isomers, but repeated fractional distillation and crystallization or double distillation separates out *o*-cresol. *m*-Cresol and *p*-cresol can then be separated out by treatment with sulfuric acid and subsequent steam hydrolyzation and distillation (120,121). Commercial cresol or crude cresol is refined from petroleum and coal tar or synthetically prepared by toluene sulfonation or oxidation (120–123). Cresols generally are manufactured as a mixture of *o*-, *m*-, and *p*-cresols in the following percentages: 20% *o*-cresol, 40% *m*-cresol, 30% *p*-cresol, and 10% phenol and xylenols (120,121).

Cresols also are found as natural compounds formed as metabolites of microbial activity and excreted in the urine of mammals (120,121). They occur naturally in various plant lipids and oils from jasmine, cassia, Easter lily, ylang-ylang, and *Yucca gloriosa* flowers, peppermint, eucalyptus, and camphor (120,121). Cresols are found in environmental tobacco smoke, fly ash from coal and wood combustion, and emissions from the incineration of vegetable materials. In addition, they are a product of combustion and are released to the atmosphere during forest fires and volcanic activity (120–125). They can be produced in the atmosphere from the reaction of toluene with hydroxyl radicals (123–125).

Cresols are used in making synthetic resins, in ore flotation, as a textile scouring agent, in degreasing compounds and paintbrush cleaners, as additives to lubricating oils, as a fumigant, in disinfecting solutions, in photographic developers, and in explosives (120,121). They also are used as a solvent and disinfectant and as an intermediate chemical for a variety of deodorizers and odor-enhancing compounds, pharmaceuticals, fragrances, dyes, antioxidants, pesticides, and resins. *o*-Cresol is used as an additive to phenol-formaldehyde resins. *p*-Cresol is used to formulate antioxidants and to make lubricating oils, motor oils, rubbers, polymers, elastomers, and food products. It is used also as an intermediate in the production of fragrances. *m*-Cresol is used in the production of herbicides and insecticides, antioxidants, and fragrances. Mixtures of *m*- and *p*-cresol are used as disinfectants in wood preservatives. Crude cresols are used as wood preservatives.

Cresols are produced as metabolic intermediates in the degradation process of phenols by microorganisms in the soil. Tricresyl phosphate and diphenyl cresyl phosphate are produced by *m*- and *p*-cresol mixtures and are employed as flame-retardant plasticizers, for fire-resistant hydraulic fluids, and as additives for lubricants and oil filters (120,121).

Physiochemical Properties

Cresol has the chemical formula of $CH_3C_6H_4OH$ and exists as the isomeric substituted phenols (2-methyl, 4-methyl, and 3-methyl phenol), with methyl groups at the *ortho*, *meta*, and *para* positions relative to the hydroxy group (see Fig. 115-1). Cresols are similar to phenol in their physiochemical behavior and undergo electrophilic substitution reactions at vacant *ortho* and *para* positions. They undergo condensation reactions with aldehydes, ketones, and dienes (120,121).

Commercial cresol is a colorless liquid that turns brown on exposure to air or light. The individual isomers cover a range of colors and forms. *o*-Cresol is a white, crystalline solid or yellow liquid, *m*-cresol is a colorless to yellowish liquid, and *p*-cresol is a crystalline solid or yellowish liquid. The isomeric mixture is a colorless to yellowish liquid (120,121).

Cresols have a phenollike odor. The density of the three isomers is 3.7 relative to air; hence, vapors will seek out low-lying areas where they can accumulate. Table 115-3 lists the physiochemical properties of cresol and its isomers.

Exposure Sources

Human exposure to cresols occurs from inhalation of contaminated air, from ingesting contaminated drinking water or contaminated food, or from dermal contact with contaminated products or the direct solid or liquid material. Occupational exposure occurs among workers in processes that use cresol compounds.

The major source of cresols in the environment is industrial effluents or spills. However, cresols are emitted from motor vehicles burning petroleum-based fuels, during the burning of wood and cigarettes, from coal-fired and petroleum-fueled electricity-generating plants, and from facilities that process animal manure (122–125). Cresol release into the atmosphere also occurs from fires, volcanic activity, and human production.

Environmental Fate and Transport

The environmental fate and transport of cresols is similar to that of other phenolic compounds. Owing to the volatility of cresols, they move from water or soil into the atmosphere. The vapor pressure of cresols ranges from 0.13 to 0.31 mm Hg; compounds with values in excess of 0.0001 mm Hg are in vapor phase. The vapor pressure of cresols is such that they would exist as an atmospheric gas in the vapor phase but would be removed during precipitation because they are highly water-soluble [as shown by the octanol-water partition coefficient (10 g K_{ow} = 1.95)]. Cresols degrade by reaction with atmospheric radicals, primarily hydroxyl and nitrate, with half-lives of approximately 1 day (120,121).

Cresols are not strongly sorbed to soils but, as with other phenolic compounds, the pH of the soil strongly influences sorption (126). Mobility from soil to groundwater and degradation by soil microorganisms appears to be the dominant fate of cresols in soil. Biodegradation appears to be the primary mechanism of cresol degradation in aerobic waters, the half-life being between 1 and 7 days (127,128).

Cresols are short-lived in the atmosphere. Reactions with hydroxyl groups and nitrate radicals determine the fate of atmospheric cresols, their half-lives during daylight hours ranging from 3 to 5 hours (121). Transformation products of cresols from atmospheric reactions are pyruvic acid, acetaldehyde, formaldehyde, peroxyacylnitrate, and nitrocresols. Nitrate radicals are formed in the atmosphere owing to reactions of nitrogen oxide with ozone and are photochemically decomposed rapidly by sunlight. Therefore, reactions of nitrate radicals with cresol vapors are significant during nighttime hours, and the half-life of cresols is only minutes (121).

Photolysis, hydrolysis, and oxidation by photolytic activities play a minor role in the transformation of cresols in water. Cresols sorb to soils with a high clay content and a high pH. Cresol volatilization occurs from highly contaminated soil sources. Cresols in water partitioned by their sorption to solids and sediments may bioaccumulate in aquatic organisms. However, the bioconcentration factors of cresols (see Table 115-6) indicate that very little biomagnification up the food chain occurs.

Biodegradation of cresols in soil and water is an important transformation process, and photochemical reactions involving cresols occur in the upper few millimeters of the soil's surface (121). Cresols degrade rapidly in aerobic biodegradation processes, but degradation is much slower under anaerobic conditions or aerobic conditions in salt water (128). Chemical oxidation and photolysis are minor removal processes.

Monitoring for cresols in the environment is similar to that for phenol. The rate of biodegradation of the cresols increases from the *para* to *meta* to *ortho* isomers. Biodegradation results in formation of hydroxylation products followed by ring-opening reactions. Higher temperatures and nutrient sources increase the biodegradation of cresols.

Absorption, Metabolism, and Elimination

Cresols are absorbed through the respiratory system, the gastrointestinal tract, and intact skin. Cresols are absorbed more efficiently across skin than is phenol, which can lead to rapid onset of toxic effects (129). Animal studies showed that 70% of cresol doses were absorbed within 6 hours (130). Metabolic conversion of cresols is via glucuronic acid conjugation and sulfate conjugation. Minor metabolic pathways include ring hydroxylation (121). At normal pHs (pH 7.0 to 7.4), the conjugated metabolites are ionized, thus reducing their renal reabsorption and increasing their urinary excretion. Cresols undergo enterohepatic circulation and are excreted in bile and then reabsorbed from the intestine. However, renal elimination is the primary route of excretion (121). Humans normally excrete approximately 50 mg of *p*-cresol in the urine daily (131). *p*-Cresol is produced endogenously from tyrosine by anaerobic bacteria in the gastrointestinal tract.

Clinical Toxicology

The clinical toxicology of cresols is similar to that of phenols (Table 115-11). Cresols are powerful irritants and are readily absorbed through all exposure routes. Ingestion of cresols can result in mouth and throat burns, vomiting, abdominal pain, coma, hypotension, methemoglobinemia, hemolysis, renal failure, and death (132,133). In one case, coma occurred within 2 hours of ingestion of 250 mL of a 50% cresol solution (132). In another case, hypotension occurred within 12 hours of ingestion of 45 mL cresol, followed by death in 4 days from pulmonary edema (133).

Acute ingestion has been associated with cardiovascular collapse, coma, ventricular fibrillation, sudden death, renal failure, and hemolytic anemia. Pulmonary edema and pulmonary hemorrhage have also occurred. Death has occurred within 30 minutes after massive cresol ingestion. Case reports describe coma, dyspnea, hypotension, and methemoglobinemia (133,134).

Dermal exposure can cause skin necrosis, discoloration, and scarring, followed by systemic toxicity. A 1-year-old child who was dermally exposed to 20 mL of cresol affecting 7% of the body's surface experienced a coma within 5 minutes and death within 4 hours (135). Autopsy revealed hemorrhagic edema with centrilobular and midzonal hepatic necrosis, renal tubular necrosis, and cerebral edema.

TABLE 115-11. Manifestations of cresol toxicity

Abdominal pain	Microvascular hemolysis
Cardiac arrest	Premature ventricular contractions
Coma	Renal failure
Fatty degeneration of the kidney	Renal tubular necrosis
Fatty degeneration of the liver	Tachycardia
Glomerulonephritis	Throat and mouth irritation and burns
Hemoglobinuria	Ventricular fibrillation
Hemolytic anemia	Vomiting
Methemoglobinemia	

TABLE 115-12. Cresol dermal exposure cases and systemic toxic effects

Exposure source (reference)	Effects
15% BSA burns from falling into vat (154)	Anuria 36 h after exposure; coma 9 d after admission; death 10 d after event from cardiac failure
Hand immersion in 6% cresylic acid solution for 5–6 h (155)	Eye burning, facial pain, facial paralysis
Thirteen cases of burns varying between 0.5% and 10% BSA and of varying depth, treated by immediate water flushing of site (156)	Skin necrosis; no deaths
Fifty-year-old individual exposed to cresol mixture; burn area immediately irrigated with water (157)	Dermal burn, dizziness, vomiting, skin site numbness, oliguria, skin discoloration; recovered in 27 d

BSA, body surface area.

Occupational exposure to cresol is usually through dermal contact, which can result in burns followed by rapid absorption of cresol and symptoms of acute toxicity. Small burns should not be ignored, as they can result in significant systemic absorption of cresols (Table 115-12). Skin can become erythematous, inflamed, and discolored within minutes of exposure.

Overall treatment is mainly supportive, targeted to the organ systems involved. Individuals with glucose-6-phosphate dehydrogenase deficiency will be at increased risk of developing hemolytic anemia on exposure to cresols.

DERMAL DECONTAMINATION

Because cresols can rapidly penetrate the skin after direct contact, decontamination should be immediate and should include (i) removal of contaminated clothing, (ii) immediate irrigation with copious soap and water, (iii) swabbing of the skin with cotton soaked with PEG-300 or PEG-400 for a minimum of 10 to 20 minutes, and (iv) medical observation for medical complications. The speed of decontamination is essential in preventing dermal burns as well as systemic toxicity from cresol.

Although no direct evidence indicates that PEG will prevent cresol dermal absorption, the evidence for such effects after phenol exposure is incontrovertible, and phenol and cresol compounds are physiochemically similar. In addition, the solubility of cresol indicates that it will preferentially move into water. Workers who use cresols or solutions containing cresols must wear protective clothing.

TERATOGENICITY AND MUTAGENICITY

Cresols do not appear to be teratogenic, although fetotoxic effects have been seen at maternally toxic doses in animals (121). Cresol may be mutagenic, although various assays provide different results, as do assays on individual isomers. For example, *o*-cresol and *p*-cresol are positively mutagenic in Chinese hamster ovary cells in *in vitro* assays but not in human fibroblasts, whereas in *in vivo* tests of mice, all isomers provided negative results.

Environmental Controls and Regulations

The EPA has evaluated available data to derive oral RfDs and inhalational RfCs for these isomers. A provisional RfD of 0.005 mg per kg of body weight per day for *p*-cresol has been published by the EPA (120). The IRIS database provides a chronic RfD of 0.05 mg per kg of body weight per day for both *o*- and *m*-cresol. These values both are based on a 90-day subchronic exposure study of rats that showed decreased body weights and neurotoxicity (120). Data were inadequate to derive inhalational RfCs for any isomer (120).

Both *o*- and *m*-cresol are listed wastes under the RCRA and must be managed according to federal and state hazardous-waste regulations. Under the Federal Insecticide, Fungicide, and Rodenticide Act, *m*-cresol is a list D pesticide. None of the isomers is regulated by the Toxic Substances Control Act. Other occupational and environmental regulations and guidelines for cresols are listed in Table 115-6.

HYDROXYPHENOLS

Three hydroxyphenol (dihydroxybenzene) isomers are known—hydroquinone (*p*-dihydroxybenzene), catechol (*o*-dihydroxybenzene), and resorcinol (*m*-dihydroxybenzene)—each having the molecular formula $C_6H_4(OH)_2$ (see Fig. 115-1). Table 115-1 lists the physiochemical properties of each isomer. All the isomers are colorless crystals that darken or redden on exposure to air or light, especially when moist. All three isomers have similar uses: as a photographic reducer and developer; as an antioxidant for fats and oils; as an inhibitor of polymerization; as a stabilizer in paints, varnishes, motor fuels, and oil; and as an antifungal preservative. Resorcinol in concentrations up to 10% is used also in medication for the treatment of acne, ringworm, psoriasis, eczema, seborrheic dermatitis, and other cutaneous lesions.

Hydroquinone

Hydroquinone is a white, crystalline chemical in its pure state and is highly soluble in water. The main property of hydroquinone is its reducing-agent capacity, in which it is reversibly oxidized to semiquinone and quinone (136). Quinone is a more toxic compound.

SOURCES, USES, AND PRODUCTION

Hydroquinone both is commercially produced and occurs naturally in the environment as a by-product of plants and animals. It is found in a nonvolatile extract of coffee beans (136). When released environmentally, owing to its high water solubility, hydroquinone will be found in the water phase. Hydroxylation of phenols to hydroquinone is reported to occur in nature and as a metabolite in the biodegradation of substituted phenols.

Hydroquinone is used as a photographic developer, in graphic arts, and for x-ray films (136). It is used also in the manufacture of rubber antioxidants and as a food antioxidant such as in stabilized vitamin A, vitamin D, vitamin E, beta-carotene, and antibiotics. It is a chemical intermediate for production of other chemicals. Hydroquinone is found in cosmetics and is used as a depigmenting agent and for hair dyeing. As a natural compound, it is found in roasted coffee and the leaves of various berries, such as blueberry, cranberry, or bearberry.

Hydroquinone is produced through the oxidation of aniline to quinone and the reduction of quinone to hydroquinone or through the hydroxylation of phenol with 70% hydrogen peroxide in the liquid phase with a soluble acid catalyst (136). It is a light tan to gray crystal that darkens on exposure to air and light. It reacts with strong oxidizers and alkalis and is an explosion hazard when exposed to heat.

PHYSIOCHEMICAL PROPERTIES

Hydroquinone is also known as *1,4-benzenediol*, p-*benzenediol*, *benzohydroquinone*, and p-*hydroxyphenol*. It has a molecular weight of 110.11, and its physical state consists of odorless, long white needles. It is combustible when heated and has a vapor density of 3.81 (as compared to air, with a vapor density of 1.00). It is highly soluble in water and is soluble in most polar organic solvents such as ethyl alcohol acetone, methylisobutylketone, 2-ethylhexanone, and ethylacetate. It is a reducing agent with a pK_1 of 9.9 and a pK_2 of 11.6. Hydroquinone undergoes a reversible reduction-oxidation (redox) change from hydroquinone to semiquinone and to quinone. Hydroquinone is oxidized by many oxidants including nitric acid, halogen persulfates, and metal salts. It also reacts with molecular oxygen. Its vapor pressure is 1.8×10^{-5} mm Hg at 25°C and its log K_{ow} is 0.59.

EXPOSURE SOURCES

Exposure to hydroquinone can occur from developing black and white films and from use of certain cosmetics and other products containing hydroquinone. Cosmetic concentrations of 0.1% to 5.0% have been reported (137). Exposure to hydroquinone can also occur when this compound is used as a skin-depigmenting agent. In 1982, the U.S. Food and Drug Administration issued a notice of proposed rule, allowing for the use of hydroquinone as a skin lightener in over-the-counter preparations at concentrations between 1.5% and 2.0% (136).

Hydroquinone is a product of environmental tobacco smoke, with amounts ranging from 110 to 300 µg per cigarette (136). Hydroquinones are also found in food samples such as wheat germ, coffee beans, yogurt, and diet colas (136).

Exposure to hydroquinone in an occupational setting can be in either its solid crystalline form or in solution. It has a low vapor pressure and can be oxidized by the presence of moisture to form quinone, which is even more volatile and more toxic than its parent compound. In certain commercial settings, hydroquinone can be found in airborne concentrations. The occupational exposure limit for quinone is 2 mg per cubic meter (136).

ENVIRONMENTAL FATE AND TRANSPORT

Hydroquinone biodegradation is related to pH, temperature, and aerobic or anaerobic environmental conditions. Pure cultures of microorganisms have been shown to use hydroquinone as a carbon source. Hydroquinone is readily degraded by photodegradation (136). It does not bioaccumulate, as indicated by its log K_{ow} of 0.59.

ABSORPTION, METABOLISM, AND EXCRETION

Oral absorption of hydroquinone is rapid, but the rate of hydroquinone permeability through the skin is slow (136). The absorption of hydroquinone through skin depends on the concentration of exposure, the length of exposure, and the vehicle in which it is dissolved. *In vivo* human data indicate dermal absorption of 3 µg per square centimeter per hour (138). Fifty-seven percent of a total dermal dose of radiolabeled hydroquinone applied to volunteers was excreted in the urine after 5 days.

After oral administration, wide distribution occurs in animals, most of the compound being localized in the kidney and liver, but less than 2% of the total dose was present after 48 hours (136). Other animal studies show that binding in the thymus bone marrow and white blood cells also occurs and that the route of administration can influence the profile of distribution.

Hydroquinone is transformed metabolically by phase II metabolism to water-soluble conjugates, with recovery of very little of the parent compound (0.25% to 7.00%) as parabenzoquinone. However, large amounts of hydroquinone-monoglucuronide and hydroquinone-monosulfate (more than 90%) appear in the urine (139). Hydroquinone, once absorbed systemically and distributed, is excreted mainly (90%) as a form of water-soluble metabolites. Such extensive metabolism may signify that the metabolites, not the parent compound itself, are responsible for toxicity.

The covalent binding properties and oxidative properties of hydroquinone are postulated toxic mechanisms. The *p*-benzosemiquinone radical and *p*-benzoquinone radical also may contribute to toxicity (136).

Oxidized hydroquinone metabolites may covalently bind to cell proteins, macromolecules, and alkylate glutathione, interfering with enzyme systems and altering nucleic acids. The metabolite benzoquinone, reacting with glutathione, forms conjugates that then can be transformed to cysteine conjugates, which are thought to mediate renal cellular toxicity through acylation or oxidation mechanisms involving redox cycling (140).

CLINICAL TOXICOLOGY

Reports of the effects of hydroquinone ingestion have listed the following clinical manifestations: vomiting, abdominal pain, tachycardia, seizures, tremors, dyspnea, cyanosis, coma, loss of reflexes, and death (136).

In long-term dermal exposures, hydroquinone products act as bleaching agents and inhibit the production of melanin. Prolonged dermal use of concentrations greater than 5% can cause ochronosis and depigmentation (141,142). Cases of leukodermia after use of creams containing 2% hydroquinone have been reported, as has sensitization to hydroquinone. Occupational dermal exposure can cause depigmentation of skin in photographic developers. This is particularly so if the material is spilled into gloves that become occlusive, allowing long-term contact of the chemical with the skin.

Exposure of the eyes to quinone vapors and hydroquinone dust can cause ocular damage consisting of irritation, light sensitivity, lacrimation, injury to the corneal epithelium, and corneal ulceration (136). Chronic exposure to hydroquinone dust can cause green-brown corneal staining, corneal opacity, and brown to black conjunctival staining. It also may result in some loss of vision owing to opacification of the cornea. The corneal discoloration, distortion, and opacification is attributable to hydroquinone dust that oxidizes to brown benzoquinone in the eye. Concentrations of 10 to 30 mg per cubic meter have been reported to result in keratitis and discoloration of the eye, noted as a brownish stain in the conjunctiva. Ocular irritation has been reported in dust exposures of 2.25 mg per cubic meter, with marked irritation at 13.50 mg per cubic meter (136). Some researchers have reported cases of corneal pigmentation among those persons occupationally exposed to hydroquinone dust. Inflammation and discoloration of the cornea and conjunctiva have occurred after daily exposures to 0.05 to 14.40 mg of hydroquinone dust per cubic meter for at least 2 years (136).

Systemic toxicity has occurred from exposure to hydroquinone or quinone vapors (136). An increase of respiratory symptoms in workers exposed to hydroquinone and its derivatives has been reported, and exposed workers had a higher prevalence of cough and pulmonary function decrements as compared to nonexposed groups (143,144). Hydroquinone may induce dyspnea and reversible airway obstruction in exposed workers.

Catechol and Resorcinol

Catechol is produced several different ways: by treatment of salicylaldehyde with hydrogen peroxide, by fusion of *o*-phenolsulfonic acid with alkali, by treatment of guaiacol with hydrobromic acid to cleave the methyl ether group, or by the heating of *o*-chlorophenol with a solution of sodium hydroxide at high temperatures. It also is a natural compound found in tannins, in the mycorrhiza of pine, in the leaves and branches of oak and willow, and in onions and crude beet sugars. Resorcinol is produced commercially by fusion of the sodium salt of *m*-benzenedisulfonic acid with sodium hydroxide, followed by acidification.

ABSORPTION, METABOLISM, AND EXCRETION

Catechol is rapidly absorbed from the gastrointestinal tract, as is resorcinol. These compounds are also absorbed in the respiratory tract. Catechol is metabolized by oxidation with polyphenol oxidase to *o*-benzoquinone or is conjugated with acids and excreted in urine. Very little is excreted in the urine as free catechol. Resorcinol is metabolized in a similar fashion and is excreted in a free and conjugated state.

CLINICAL TOXICOLOGY

Catechol is more toxic than is phenol. It induces CNS depression and a rise in blood pressure due to peripheral vasoconstriction. Resorcinol acts in a similar manner, although it is less toxic than catechol.

Chronic dermal exposure to any of the hydroxyphenols has resulted in dermatitis. Continued application of resorcinol for medicinal purposes can cause itching, edema, corrosion, and loss of the outer layers of skin. Methemoglobinemia can occur from subacute and chronic exposure to any of the hydroxyphenols.

Environmental Fate and Transport of Hydroxyphenols

The environmental fate and transport of hydroxyphenols in the environment are similar to those of other phenolic compounds. The vapor pressure of these compounds is such that they exist in the vapor phase in the atmosphere and degrade rapidly by reaction with hydroxy radicals. Biodegradation in soils and groundwater is the major removal process for these compounds. They should not sorb to or volatilize from soil. None of the isomers would be expected to sorb to sediments, hydrolyze, volatilize, or bioconcentrate in aquatic organisms. Monitoring for hydroxyphenols in the environment is similar to that for phenol.

Environmental Regulations for Hydroxyphenols

The EPA has not derived a chronic RfD for catechol or resorcinol. A provisional RfD is available for hydroquinone and is listed in Table 115-6. Other occupational and environmental regulations and guidelines for the hydroxyphenols also are listed in Table 115-6.

DINITROPHENOL

DNP is used in the synthesis of dyes, picric acid (explosive), picramic acid, wood preservatives, and insecticides, as a photographic developer (diaminophenol dihydrochloride), and as a pH indicator. Six isomeric forms of DNP exist.

Sources, Uses, and Production

DNP and its isomers are produced by heating phenol with dilute sulfuric acid and then supplying nitrates while keeping the temperature lower than 50°C (145). 2,3-DNP, 2,5-DNP, and 3,4-DNP are prepared by nitrating *m*-nitrophenol.

Commercial DNP, which is a mixture of 2,3-, 2,6-, and mainly 2,4-DNP isomers, is used in the synthesis of dyes, picric acid, picramic acid, and wood preservatives and as a developing agent. It is also used in the manufacturing of explosives and insecticides and as a pH indicator. 2,4-DNP is used as an insecticide, acaricide, and fungicide. DNPs are used in the manufacture of herbicides, fungicides, and styrene.

Physiochemical Properties

DNPs are yellow solids. The six isomeric forms are 2,3-DNP, 2,4-DNP, 2,5-DNP, 2,6-DNP, 3,4-DNP, and 3,5-DNP (see Fig. 115-1). Its molecular weight is 184.1 (145).

Exposure Sources

DNPs are released to the environment during their manufacture and use. Hazardous-waste sites may contain DNPs. These compounds also are formed atmospherically via the reaction of benzene with oxides of nitrogen (146). DNPs can be released into water supplies and surface water from point or distributive sources. Application of pesticides containing 2,4-DNP are a source of soil and water contamination. Vehicle exhaust contains DNPs (146). Therefore, soil along roadways may be found to contain DNPs. Combustion of hazardous waste can also be a source of DNPs into the air.

Environmental Fate and Transport

Most of the information regarding DNPs in the environment is related to 2,4-DNP. Owing to the vapor pressure of 2,4-DNP (1.49×10^{-5} mm Hg at 18°C), it will exist partly in a vapor phase and partly in the particulate phase in the atmosphere. DNPs can be detected in precipitation, which can also be a source of physical removal from the atmosphere.

Soil loss of DNPs due to volatilization is insignificant, and mobility and movement of the DNPs through soils decrease with increased acidity, increased clay content, or increased organic content of the soil. Increased mobility of DNPs in soil of increased alkalinity and water occurs because of the creation of the ionized form of the compound, which is more water-soluble (145). DNPs are predominantly in their ionic forms in most natural water, owing to their pK_a of 4.09. Increases in the organic content and in the amount of clay in soil and a decrease in the soil's pH would increase the amount of DNPs absorbed to soil by increasing the un-ionized form of DNP. Thus, movement and absorption of DNPs from water to solids would be more significant in natural waters that are more acidic or have a higher organic matter or clay content (145).

Bioaccumulation of the DNPs is not expected to be significant in aquatic organisms, as estimated from the K_{ow} (145). As just stated, the leaching of DNP from soils depends on the chemical nature of the soil.

The photodegradation of DNPs in water is very slow and is not an important process in DNP's environmental fate. 2,4-DNP is biodegraded by microorganisms such as *Pseudomonas* species and other microorganisms (145). The biodegradation by organisms in pure culture, though, does not reflect actual environmental conditions in which mixed microorganisms reside and present a different challenge for biodegradation of DNPs. Biodegradation of 2,4-DNP occurs under aerobic conditions with mixed microorganisms in sludge and enriched sewage or sediment from waste lagoons, aeration lagoons, and settling ponds (145).

Absorption and Metabolism

The proposed metabolic pathway for 2,4-DNP is shown in Figure 115-3. After DNP poisoning, the compounds found in the urine include 2,4-DNP, 2-amino-4-nitrophenol, 4-amino-2-nitrophenol, and 2,4-diaminophenol. In the case of fatal occupational exposures to 2,4-DNP, the urine was found to contain 2.08 g of 2,4-DNP per L and 50 mg of 2-amino-4-DNP per L (147). Most information that we have regarding 2,4-DNP

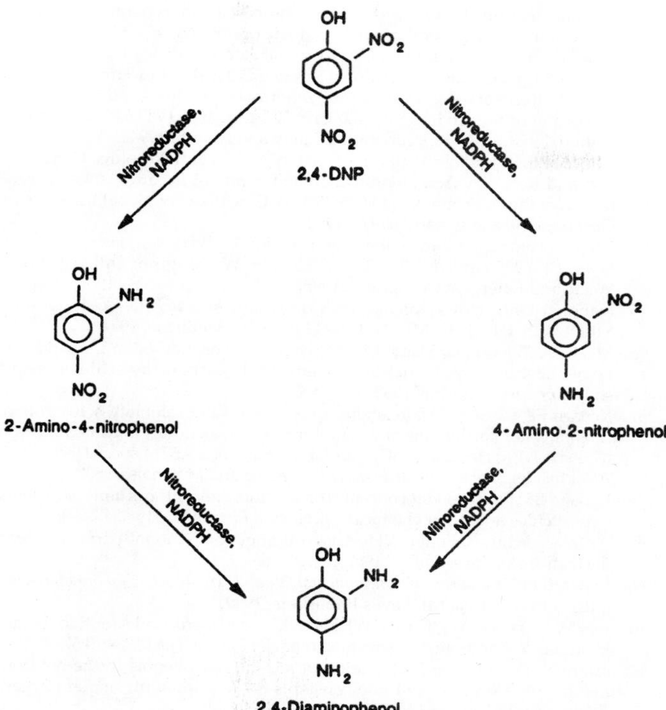

Figure 115-3. Proposed metabolism of dinitrophenol (DNP). NADPH, nicotinamide adenine dinucleotide phosphate. (From ref. 145, with permission.)

metabolism has been gleaned from animal studies. 2,4-DNP and its metabolites have been detected in blood and biological samples of blood, urine, and tissues from humans. The predominant compounds found in blood and urine are the unchanged 2,4-DNP and 2-amino-4-nitrophenol and smaller amounts of 4-amino-nitrophenol.

Clinical Toxicology

The DNPs are yellow solids, and inhalational exposure (except to DNP dusts) would be rare. Fatalities from DNP toxicity were reported in the munitions industry in the early 1900s in individuals exposed to airborne vapors and dust. Deaths were associated with hyperthermia, sweating, and respiratory distress. Convulsions often preceded death. Studies from the 1940s of workers exposed to 2,4-DNP dust in U.S. chemical plants also reported hyperthermia, sweating, and fatigue, and reported some deaths (147). Other reports from the 1930s describe granulocytopenia-related deaths secondary to DNP exposure (148).

Oral ingestion of DNP has been associated with deaths with clinical manifestations of hyperthermia, hyperpnea, chest pain, tachycardia, hypotension, and coma. Most of these cases were described in the 1930s. Agranulocytosis cases were reported in the 1940s after patients had ingested 2,4-DNP or its sodium salt. In the 1940s, 2,4-DNP had been used for dietary weight reduction therapy. Individuals who ingested 5.7 mg per kg per day of 2,4-DNP for 2 weeks have been reported to experience agranulocytosis (149). Other oral ingestions of DNP of at least 2 mg per kg per day have also been associated with agranulocytosis.

Cataracts were noted in a small number of patients who orally ingested 2,4-DNP. Doses ranged from 1.86 to 4.29 mg per kg per day, with rapid development of cataracts while the individual was taking the medication or after cessation of ingestion. The cataracts were bilateral and progressed to total blindness (150,151).

2,4-DNP induces hyperthermia due to an elevation of the basal metabolic rate. Such increased metabolic rates have been documented in animal models (152).

Hearing impairment has also been associated with the ingestion of DNP dating from the 1930s. Neurologic manifestations have included headache, weakness, and dizziness in individuals ingesting 2,4-DNP. Cases of peripheral neuritis have occurred after dosing for 4 to 10 weeks but abated when ingestion was discontinued.

Very few studies exist regarding skin-related health effects in humans or animals after exposure to DNPs, but solutions of DNP can cause yellow discoloration of the skin. The lowest dermal dose that caused death in guinea pigs was 350 mg per kg of a 20% solution, and the lowest dose that caused 100% mortality was 700 mg per kg in guinea pigs exposed dermally to 1,000 mg per kg of 2,4-DNP for 4 hours (153). Applications of a 3% 2,4-DNP solution in 95% ethanol to the ears of rabbits showed no skin irritation (153). Mild erythema and irritation was shown on the bare skin of the abdomen in the same animal study. However, dermal absorption might be a serious route of systemic absorption. Another clinical toxicologic consideration after exposure to DNP is methemoglobinemia.

Environmental Controls and Regulations

Table 115-6 lists the environmental regulations of DNPs. The EPA lists DNPs as hazardous air pollutants under the Clean Air Act. An MRL of 0.01 mg per kg per day has been derived for acute oral exposure to 2,4-DNP, based on an LOAEL of 1.2 mg per kg per day in humans. The EPA lists a chronic RfD of 0.002 mg per kg per day for 2,4-DNP, based on an LOAEL of 2 mg per kg per day (145).

REFERENCES

1. James RC. Toxic effects of organic solvents. In: Williams PL, Burson JL, eds. *Industrial toxicology, safety and health applications in the workplace.* New York: Van Nostrand–Reinhold, 1985.
2. Windholz M, ed. *The Merck index,* 10th ed. Rahway, NJ: Merck and Company, 1983.
3. American Conference of Governmental Industrial Hygienists. *Documentation of threshold limit values.* Cincinnati: American Conference of Governmental Industrial Hygienists, 1991.
4. Bruce RM, Santodonato J, Neal MW. Summary review of the health effects associated with phenol. *Toxicol Ind Health* 1987;3:535–569.
5. Agency for Toxic Substances and Disease Registry. *Production, import, use and disposal. Toxicological profile for phenol.* Atlanta: US Department of Health and Human Services, Public Health Service, ATSDR, 1989.
6. National Institute for Occupational Safety and Health. Federal Food, Drug and Cosmetic Act. Food and drugs indirect food additives: adhesives, 21 *CFR* 175.105. Cincinnati: National Institute for Occupational Safety and Health, 1993.
7. US Environmental Protection Agency. Testing consent order for phenol, final consent agreement and order; direct final rule. *Federal Register* 1997 Jan 17:62(12):2607–2611.
8. Kavaler AR. *Chem Market Rep* 1993;232(11):49.
9. National Library of Medicine. *Toxic chemicals release inventory for 1994.* On-line MEDLARS. Bethesda, MD: National Library of Medicine, 1997.
10. Sax N, Lewis R, eds. *Hawley's condensed chemical dictionary,* 11th ed. New York: Van Nostrand–Reinhold, 1987.
11. Lide DR, Frederikse HPR, eds. *CRC handbook of chemistry and physics,* 76th ed. Boca Raton, FL: CRC Press, 1995.
12. World Health Organization. *Phenol.* Environmental health criteria 161. Geneva: World Health Organization, 1994.
13. Sax NI, ed. *Dangerous properties of industrial materials,* 7th ed. New York: Van Nostrand–Reinhold, 1989.
14. Hubble BR, Stetter JR, Gebert E, Harkness JBL, Flotard RD. Experimental measurements from residential wood-burning stoves. *Proceedings of the International Conference on Residential Solid Fuels: environmental impacts and solutions, 1981.*
15. Graedel TE, ed. *Chemical compounds in the atmosphere.* New York: Academic Press, 1978.
16. Hawthorne SB, Miller DJ, Langenfield JJ, Krieger MS. PM-10: high volume collection and quantitation of semi- and nonvolatile phenols, methoxylated phenols, alkanes, and polycyclic aromatic hydrocarbons from winter urban

air and their relationship to wood smoke emissions. *Environ Sci Technol* 1992;26(11):2251–2262.

17. Potthast K. Dark smoking at high smokehouse temperatures. *Fleischwirtschaft* 1982;62:1578–1582.
18. Harley A, Cass GR. Modeling the concentrations of gas-phase toxic organic air pollutants: direct emissions and atmospheric formation. *Environ Sci Technol* 1994;28(1):88–98.
19. US Environmental Protection Agency. *Treatability manual.* EPA 600/2-82-001A. Washington: Office of Solid Waste and Emergency Response, 1981.
20. Peters GT, Cowell FS. Effects of stream order and season on mineralization of [^{14}C] phenol in streams. *Hydrobiologia* 1989;174:79–87.
21. Baranowska-Dutkiewicz B. Skin absorption of phenol from aqueous solutions in men. *Int Arch Occup Environ Health* 1981;49:99–104.
22. Koster HJ, Halsema J, Scholtens E, Knippers M, Mulder GJ. Dose-dependent shifts in the sulfation and glucuronidation of phenolic compounds in the rat *in vivo* and in isolated hepatocytes. The role of saturation of phenolsulfotransferase. *Biochem Pharmacol* 1981;30(18):2569–2575.
23. Capel ID, Milburn P, Williams RT. Monophenyl phosphate, a new conjugate of phenol in the cat. *Biochem Soc Trans* 1974;2:305–306.
24. US Environmental Protection Agency. *Ambient water quality criteria document: phenol.* EPA 440/5-80-066. Washington: Office of Water Regulations and Standards, Criteria and Standards Division, 1980.
25. Piotrowski JK. Evaluation of exposure to phenol, absorption of phenol vapor in the lungs and through the skin and excretion of phenol in urine. *Br J Ind Med* 1971;28:172–178.
26. Warner MA, Harper JV. Cardiac dysrhythmias associated with chemical peeling with phenol. *Anesthesiology* 1985;62:366–367.
27. Bentur Y, Shoshani O, Tabak A, et al. Prolonged elimination half-life of phenol after dermal exposure. *Clin Toxicol* 1998;36(7):707–711.
28. Horch R, Spilker G, Stark G. Phenol burns and intoxications. *Burns* 1994; 20(1):45–50.
29. Lewin JF, Cleary WT. An accidental death cause by the absorption of phenol through skin. A case report. *Forensic Sci Int* 1982;19:177–179.
30. Conning DM, Hayes JM. The dermal toxicity of phenol: an investigation of the most effective first-aid measures. *Br J Ind Med* 1970;27:155–159.
31. Brown VKH, Box VL, Simpson BJ. Decontamination procedures for skin exposed to phenolic substances. *Arch Environ Health* 1975;30:1–6.
32. Hunter D, Timerding B, Leonard R, McCalmont T, Schwartz E. Effects of isopropyl alcohol, ethanol and polyethylene glycol/industrial methylated spirits in the treatment of acute phenol burns. *Ann Emerg Med* 1992;21:11–15.
33. Pullin TG, Pinkerton MN, Johnston RV, Kilian DJ. Decontamination of the skin of swine following phenol exposure: a comparison of the relative efficacy of water versus polyethylene glycol/industrial methylated spirits. *Toxicol Appl Pharmacol* 1978;43:199–206.
34. Coan ML, Baggs RB, Dosmann HB. Demonstration of direct toxicity of phenol on kidney. *Res Commun Chem Pathol Pharmacol* 1982;36:229–239.
35. Epler JL, Rao TK, Guerin MR. Evaluation of feasibility of mutagenic listing of shale oil products and effluents. *Environ Health Perspect* 1979;30:179–184.
36. Haworth S, Lawlor T, Mortelmans K, Speck W, Zeiger E. *Salmonella* mutagenicity test results for 250 chemicals. *Environ Mutagen* 1983;1[Suppl]:3–142.
37. Gocke E, King MT, Eckhart K, Wild D. Mutagenicity of cosmetic ingredients licensed by the European Communities. *Mutat Res* 1981;90:91–109.
38. Woodruff RC, Mason JM, Valencia R, Zimmering S. Chemical mutagenesis testing in *Drosophila*. Results of 53 coded compounds tested for the National Toxicology Program. *Environ Mutagen* 1985;7:677–702.
39. Al-Sabti K. Frequency of chromosomal aberrations in the rainbow trout, *Salmo gairdneri*, exposed to 5 pollutants. *J Fish Biol* 1985;26(1):13–20.
40. Wangenheim J, Bolcsfoldi G. Mouse lymphoma L5178Y thymidine kinase locus assay of 50 compounds. *Mutagenesis* 1988;3(3):193–205.
41. Bohrman JS, Burg JR, Elmore E, et al. Interlaboratory studies with the Chinese hamster V79 cell metabolic cooperation assay to detect tumor-promoting agents. *Environ Mol Mutagen* 1988;12(1):33–51.
42. McGregor DB, Brown A, Cattanach P, et al. Responses of the L5178Ytk+/tk- mouse lymphoma cell forward mutation assay: 3. 72 Coded chemicals. *Environ Mol Mutagen* 1988;12:85–154.
43. Minor JL, Becker BA. A comparison of the teratogenic properties of sodium salicylate, sodium benzoate and phenol. *Toxicol Appl Pharmacol* 1971;19:373.
44. Boutwell RK, Bosch DK. The tumor-promoting action of phenol and related compounds for mouse skin. *Cancer Res* 1959;19:413–424.
45. National Library of Medicine. *Integrated risk information system.* On-line MEDLARS. Bethesda, MD: National Library of Medicine, 1997.
46. Pekari K, Vainotalo S, Heikkila P, Palotie A, Luotamo M, Riihimake V. Biological monitoring of occupational exposure to low levels of benzene. *Scand J Work Environ Health* 1992;18:317–322.
47. National Institute for Occupational Safety and Health. Method 8305-Phenol, Method 8303-1-Pentachlorophenol. In: *NIOSH manual of analytical methods,* 3rd ed. Cincinnati: National Institute for Occupational Safety and Health, 1985.
48. Pierce WM, Nerland DE. Qualitative and quantitative analyses of phenol, phenylglucuronide and phenylsulfate in urine and plasma by gas chromatography mass spectrometry. *J Anal Toxicol* 1988;12:344–347.
49. US Department of Transportation. *Emergency response guidebook: guide for hazardous materials incidents.* Washington: US Department of Transportation, 1993.
50. National Institute for Occupational Safety and Health. Federal Water Pollution Control Act. Protection of the environment: designation of hazardous substances, 40 *CFR* 116.4. Cincinnati: National Institute for Occupational Safety and Health, 1987.
51. National Institute for Occupational Safety and Health. Federal Water Pollution Control Act. General provisions: toxic pollutants, 40 *CFR* 401.15. Cincinnati: National Institute for Occupational Safety and Health, 1987.
52. National Institute for Occupational Safety and Health. Resource Conservation and Recovery Act. Designation, reportable quantities and notification: protection of the environment, 40 *CFR* 302.4 (section IV.D.3.b). Cincinnati: National Institute for Occupational Safety and Health, 1994.
53. National Institute for Occupational Safety and Health. Resource Conservation and Recovery Act. Identification and listing of hazardous waste: protection of the environment, 40 *CFR* 261.33. Cincinnati: National Institute for Occupational Safety and Health, 1994.
54. US Environmental Protection Agency. *Health effects assessment summary tables FY-1995 annual.* EPA/540/R-95/036. Washington: Office of Solid Waste and Emergency Response, 1995.
55. National Library of Medicine. *Toxic chemical release inventory facts.* On-line MEDLARS. Bethesda, MD: National Library of Medicine, 1997.
56. Means JC, Wood SG, Hassett JJ, Banwart WL. Sorption of amino- and carboxy-substituted polynuclear aromatic hydrocarbons by sediments and soils. *Environ Sci Technol* 1982;16:93–98.
57. Kenaga EE, Goring CAI. Relationship between water solubility, soil sorption, octanol-water partitioning and concentrations of chemicals in biota. In: Eaton JG, Parrish PR, Hendrikcs AC, eds. *Aquatic toxicology.* ASTM special tech. publ. 707. Philadelphia: American Society for Testing and Materials, 1980.
58. Kenaga EE. Predicted bioconcentration factors and soil sorption coefficients of pesticides and other chemicals. *Ecotoxicol Environ Saf* 1980;4:26–38.
59. Artiola-Fortuny J, Fuller WH. Adsorption of some monohydroxybenzene derivatives by soils. *Soil Sci* 1982;133:18–26.
60. Howard PH. *Handbook of environmental fate and exposure data for organic chemicals,* vol 1. Chelsea, MI: Lewis Publishers, 1989.
61. Jury WA, Spencer WF, Farmer WJ. Behavior assessment model for trace organics in soil: 3. Application of screening model. *J Environ Qual* 1984;13:573–579.
62. Tratnyek PG, Holgne J. Oxidation of substituted phenols in the environment: a QSAR analysis of rate constants for reaction with singlet oxygen. *Environ Sci Technol* 1991;25:1596–1604.
63. Conrad R, Seiler W. Characteristics of abiological carbon monoxide formation from soil organic matter, humic acids, and phenolic compounds. *Environ Sci Technol* 1985;19(9):1165–1169.
64. Shetiya RS, Rao KN, Shatnar J. OH radical rate constants of phenols using *p*-nitrosodimethylaniline. *Ind J Chem* 1976;14A:575–578.
65. Callahan MA, et al. *Water-related environmental fate of 129 priority pollutants,* vols 1 and 2. EPA-440/4-79-029a and -029b. Washington: US Environmental Protection Agency, Office of Water Planning and Standards, 1979.
66. Scow K, Goyer M, Payne E, et al. *An exposure and risk assessment for phenol.* Washington: US Environmental Protection Agency, Office of Water Regulations and Standards, 1980.
67. Kawaguchi H. Photocatalytic decomposition of phenol in the presence of titanium dioxide. *Environ Technol Lett* 1984;5:471–474.
68. Chesney RH, Sollitti P, Rubin HE. Incorporation of phenol carbon at trace concentrations by phenol-mineralizing microorganisms in fresh water. *Appl Environ Microbiol* 1985;49:15–18.
69. Boyd SA, Shelton DR, Berry D, Tiedje JM. Anaerobic biodegradation of phenolic compounds in digested sludge. *Appl Environ Microbiol* 1983;46:50–54.
70. Newfield RD, Mack JD, Strakey JP. Anaerobic phenol biokinetics. *J Water Pollut Control Fed* 1980;52:2367–2377.
71. Tschech A, Fuchs G. Anaerobic degradation of phenol by pure cultures of newly isolated denitrifying pseudomonads. *Arch Microbiol* 1987;148(3):213–217.
72. Fedorack PM, Hrudey SE. Nutrient requirements for the methanogenic degradation of phenol and *p*-cresol in anaerobic draw and feed cultures. *Water Res* 1986;20(7):929.
73. Krug M, Ziegler H, Straube G. Degradation of phenolic compounds by the yeast *Candida tropicalis* HP-15: 1. Physiology and growth and substrate utilization. *J Basic Microbiol* 1985;25(2):103–110.
74. Tibbles BJ, Baecker AAW. Effects and fate of phenol in simulated landfill sites. *Microb Ecol* 1989;17(2):201–206.
75. Baker MD, Mayfield CI. Microbial and nonbiological decomposition of chlorophenols and phenol in soil. *Water Air Soil Pollut* 1980;13:411–424.
76. Mackay D. Correlation of bioconcentration factors. *Environ Sci Technol* 1982;16:274–278.
77. Veith GD, Kosian P. Estimating bioconcentration potential from octanol-water partition coefficients. In: *Physical behavior of PCBs in the Great Lakes.* Ann Arbor, MI: Ann Arbor Science Publishers, 1983.
78. Russell JW. Analysis of air pollutants using sampling tubes and gas chromatography. *Environ Sci Technol* 1975;9(13):1175–1178.
79. Katz M, ed. Tentative method of analysis for determination of phenolic compounds in the atmosphere with the 4-amino antipyrine method. In: *Methods of air sampling and analysis,* 2nd ed. Washington: American Public Health Association, 1977.
80. Kuwata K, Uebori M, Yamazaki Y. Determination of phenol in polluted air as *p*-nitrobenzene azophenol derivative by reversed phase high performance liquid chromatography *Anal Chem* 1980;52(6):857–860.
81. US Environmental Protection Agency. *Test methods for evaluating solid waste—physical/chemical methods,* 3rd ed. EPA report no. SW-846. Washington: Office of Solid Waste and Emergency Response, 1986.
82. Morgan DP. *Recognition and management of pesticide poisonings,* 4th ed. EPA 540/9-88-001. Washington: Office of Pesticides and Toxic Substances, 1988.

83. National Library of Medicine. *Hazardous substance data base.* On-line MEDLARS. Bethesda, MD: National Library of Medicine, 1997.
84. Agency for Toxic Substances and Disease Registry. *Toxicological profile for pentachlorophenol.* Atlanta: US Department of Health and Human Services, Public Health Service, ATSDR, 1994.
85. National Institute for Occupational Safety and Health. *Pocket guide to chemical hazards.* NIOSH publ. no. 94-116. Washington: US Government Printing Office, 1994.
86. Hattemer-Frey HA, Travis CC. Pentachlorophenol: environmental partitioning and human exposure. *Arch Environ Contam Toxicol* 1989;18:482–489.
87. Cranmer M, Freal J. Gas chromatographic analysis of pentachlorophenol in human urine by formation of alkyl esters. *Life Sci* 1970;9:121–128.
88. Bevenue A, Beckman H. Pentachlorophenol: a discussion of its properties and its occurrence as a residue in human and animal tissues. *Residue Rev* 1967;19:83–134.
89. Bevenue A, Wilson J, Cassarett L, et al. A survey of pentachlorophenol content in human urine. *Bull Environ Contam Toxicol* 1967;2:319–332.
90. Hill R, To T, Holler J, et al. Residues of chlorinated phenols and phenoxy acid herbicides in the urine of Arkansas children. *Arch Environ Contam Toxicol* 1989;18:469–474.
91. Jorens P, Janssens J, Tichelen W, et al. Pentachlorophenol concentrations in human cerebrospinal fluid. *Neurotoxicology* 1991;12:1–7.
92. Murphy R, Kutz F, Strassmen S. Selected pesticide residues or metabolites in blood and urine specimens from a general population. *Environ Health Perspect* 1983;48:81–86.
93. Gerbefugi I, Korte F. Pentachlorophenol contamination of human milk supplies. *Chemosphere* 1983;12:1055–1060.
94. Wagner S, Durand L, Inman R, et al. Residues of pentachlorophenol and other contaminants in human tissues—analysis by electron captive gas chromatography and electron captive negative ion mass spectrometry. *Arch Environ Contam Toxicol* 1991;21:596–606.
95. Cline R, Hill R, Phillips O, Needham L. Pentachlorophenol measurements in body fluids of people in log homes and workplaces. *Arch Environ Contam Toxicol* 1989;18:475–481.
96. Choi J, Aomine S. Adsorption of pentachlorophenol by soils. *Soil Sci Plant Nutr* 1974;20:135–144.
97. Valo R, Apajalahti J, Salkinoja-Salonen K. Studies on the physiology of microbial degradation of pentachlorophenol. *Appl Microbiol Biotechnol* 1985;21:313–319.
98. Braun W, Blau G, Chenoweth M. The metabolism/pharmacokinetics of pentachlorophenol in man, and a comparison with a rat and monkey. In: Deichmann W, ed. *Toxicology and occupational medicine.* New York: Elsevier Science, 1979.
99. Hortsman S, Rossner A, Kalman D, et al. Penetration of pentachlorophenol in tetrachlorophenol through human skin. *J Environ Sci Health* 1989;A24:229–242.
100. Klemmer H, Wong L, Sato N, et al. Clinical findings in workers exposed to pentachlorophenol. *Arch Environ Contam Toxicol* 1980;9:715–725.
101. Rugman F, Cosstick R. Aplastic anemia associated with organochlorine pesticide: case reports and review of evidence. *J Clin Pathol* 1990;43:98–101.
102. Roberts H. Pentachlorophenol associated aplastic anemia, red cell aplasia, leukemia and other blood disorders. *J Fla Med Assoc* 1990;77(2):86–90.
103. Begley J, Reichtert A, Siesemen A, et al. Association between renal function test and pentachlorophenol exposure. *Clin Toxicol* 1977;11:97–106.
104. O'Malley M, Carpenter A, Sweeney M. Chloracne associated with employment in the production of pentachlorophenol. *Am J Ind Med* 1990;17:411–421.
105. Gray R, Gilliland R, Smith E, et al. Pentachlorophenol intoxication: report of a fatal case with comments on the clinical course and pathologic anatomy. *Arch Environ Health* 1985;49:161–164.
106. Gerhard I, Derner M, Runnebaum B. Prolonged exposure to wood preservatives produces endocrine and immunologic disorders in women. *Am J Obstet Gynecol* 1991;165:487–488.
107. Kerkvliet N, Brauner J, Matlock J. Humoral immunotoxicity of polychlorinated diphenyl ethers, phenoxyphenols, dioxins and furans present as contaminants of technical grade pentachlorophenol. *Toxicology* 1985;36:307–324.
108. Kerkvliet N, Brauner J, Baecher-Steppan L. Effects of dietary technical pentachlorophenol exposure on T-cell, macrophage, and natural killer cell activity in C57BL/6 mice. *Int J Immunopharmacol* 1985;7:239–247.
109. Lang D, Mueller-Ruchholtz W. Human lymphocyte reactivity after *in vitro* exposure to technical and analytical grade pentachlorophenol. *Toxicology* 1991;70:271–282.
110. Schwetz BA, Quast JF, Keelev PA, Humiston CG, Kociba RJ. Results of 2-year toxicity and reproduction studies on pentachlorophenol in rats. In: Rao KR, ed. *Pentachlorophenol: chemistry, pharmacology and environmental toxicology.* New York: Plenum Press, 1978.
111. International Agency for Research on Cancer. Occupational exposures in insecticide application and some pesticides. *IARC Monogr Eval Carcinog Risks Hum* 1991;53:5–586.
112. Reigner B, Rigod J, Tozer T. Simultaneous assay of pentachlorophenol and its metabolite, tetrachlorohydroquinone, by gas chromatography without derivation. *J Chromatogr Biomed Appl* 1990;98:111–124.
113. *Federal Register* 1991 Jan 30:56:3600.
114. *Federal Register* 1991 Jul 1:56:30266.
115. *Federal Register* 1989 May 22:54:22062.
116. *Federal Register* 1991 Jan 30:56:3526.
117. National Institute for Occupational Safety and Health. Federal Water Pollution Control Act. Determination of reportable quantities for hazardous substances, 40 *CFR* 117.3. Cincinnati: National Institute for Occupational Safety and Health, 1989.
118. *Federal Register* 1989 May 25:54:22706.
119. Silkowski JB, Horstman SW, Morgan MS. Permeation through five commercially available glove materials by two pentachlorophenol formulations. *J Am Ind Hyg Assoc* 1984;45(8):501–504.
120. Agency for Toxic Substances and Disease Registry. *Toxicological profile for cresols:* o-*cresol,* p-*cresol,* m-*cresol, draft.* Atlanta: US Department of Health and Human Services, Public Health Service, ATSDR, 1990.
121. World Health Organization. *Cresols.* Environmental health criteria 168. Geneva: World Health Organization, 1995.
122. Giabbai M, Cross W, Chian E, Dewall F. Characterization of major and minor organic pollutants in wastewaters from coal gasification processes. *Int J Environ Anal Chem* 1985;20:113–129.
123. Leone J, Flagan R, Grosjean D, Seinfeld J. An outdoor smog chamber and modeling study of toluene $-NO_x$ photooxidation. *Int J Chem Kinet* 1985;17(2):177–216.
124. Grosjean D. Atmospheric reactions of orthocresol: gas phase and aerosol products. *Atmosphere Environ* 1984;18:1641–1652.
125. Grosjean D. Reactions of *o*-cresol and nitrocresol with NO_x in sunlight and with ozone-nitrogen dioxide mixtures in the dark. *Environ Sci Technol* 1985;19(10):968–974.
126. Namkoong W, Loehr RC, Malina JF. Kinetics of phenolic compounds removal in soil. *Hazard Waste Hazard Mat* 1988;5(4):321–328.
127. Faust BC, Holgne J. Sensitized photooxidation of phenols by fulvic acid in natural waters. *Environ Sci Technol* 1987;21:957–964.
128. Brown S, Grady C. Biodegradation kinetics of substituted phenolics: demonstration of a protocol based on electrolytic respirometry. *Water Res* 1990;24(7):853–862.
129. Roberts M, Anderson R, Swabrick J. Permeability of human epidermis to the phenolic compounds. *J Pharm Pharmacol* 1977;29:677–683.
130. Hinz R, Lorence C, Hodson C, et al. Percutaneous penetration of para-substituted phenols in vitro. *Fundam Appl Toxicol* 1991;17:575–583.
131. Renwick A, Thakrar A, Lawrie C. Microbial amino acid metabolites and bladder cancer—no evidence of promoting activity in man. *Hum Toxicol* 1988;7(3):267–272.
132. Arthurs F, Wise C, Coles G. Poisoning by cresols. *Anesthesia* 1977;32:642–643.
133. Chan T, Mak L, Ng R. Methemoglobinemia, Heinz bodies and acute massive intravascular hemolysis in lysol poisoning. *Blood* 1971;38:739–744.
134. Minami M, Katzumata M, Tomoda A. Methemoglobinemia with oxidized hemoglobins and modified hemoglobins found in bloods of workers handling aromatic compounds and in those of man who drank cresol solution. *Biomed Biochem Acta* 1990;49(2–3):5327–5333.
135. Green M. A household remedy misused—fatal cresol poisoning following cutaneous absorption (a case report). *Med Sci Law* 1975;15:65–66.
136. World Health Organization. *Hydroquinone.* Environmental health criteria 157. Geneva: World Health Organization, 1994.
137. Cosmetic Ingredient Review Expert Panel. Cosmetic ingredient review: final report on the safety assessment of hydroquinone and pyrocatechol. *J Am Coll Toxicol* 1986;5(3):123–165.
138. Bucks D, McMaster J, Guy R, et al. Percutaneous absorption of hydroquinone in humans, effective 1-dodecylazacycloheptan-2-one (azone) and 2-ethylhexyl ester, 4-dimethylamino (benzoic acid) (escalol 507). *J Toxicol Environ Health* 1988;24:279–289.
139. Devincenco Z, Hamilton M, Reynolds R, et al. Metabolic fate and disposition of (C^{14}) hydroquinone given orally to Sprague-Dawley rats. *Toxicology* 1984;33:9–18.
140. Lau S, Hill B, Highet R, et al. Sequential oxidation and glutathione addition to 1,4-benzoquinone: correlation of toxicity with increased glutathione substitution. *Mol Pharmacol* 1988;34:829–836.
141. Fidlay G, de Beer H. Chronic hydroquinone poisoning of the skin from skin lightening cosmetics. A South African epidemic of ochronosis of the face in dark skin individuals. *S Afr Med J* 1980;57:187–190.
142. Fisher A. Can bleaching creams containing 2% hydroquinone produce leukodermia? *J Am Acad Dermatol* 1982;7:134.
143. Shoudat D, Neukrich F, Brochard P, et al. Allergy and occupational exposure to hydroquinone and to methionine. *Br J Ind Med* 1988;45:376–380.
144. O'Brien PJ. Molecular mechanisms of quinone cytotoxicity. *Chem Biol Interact* 1991;80:1–41.
145. Agency for Toxic Substances and Disease Registry. *Toxicological profile for dinitrophenols.* Washington: US Department of Health and Human Services. Public Health Service, ATSDR, 1995.
146. Nojima K, Kawaguchi A, Ohya T, et al. Studies on photochemical reaction of air pollutants: identification of nitrophenols in suspended particulates. *Chem Pharm Bull (Tokyo)* 1983;31:1047–1051.
147. Gisclard J, Woodward M. 2,4-dinitrophenol poisoning: a case report. *J Ind Hyg Toxicol* 1946;28:47–51.
148. Goldman A, Haber M. Acute complete granulopenia with death due to dinitrophenol poisoning. *JAMA* 1936;107:2115–2117.
149. Hoffman A, Butt E, Hickey N. Neutropenia following aminopyrine. *JAMA* 1934;102:1213–1214.
150. Horner W, Jones R, Boardman W. Cataracts following dinitrophenol: preliminary report of three cases. *JAMA* 1935;105:108–110.

151. Horner W. Dinitrophenol and its relation to formation of cataracts. *Arch Ophthalmol* 1942;27:1097–1121.
152. Dominguez S, Menkel J, Fairbrother A. The effect of 2,4-dinitrophenol on the metabolic rate of bobwhite quail. *Toxicol Appl Pharmacol* 1993;123(2):226–233.
153. Spencer H, Rowe V, Irish D. Toxicological studies on laboratory animals of certain alkyl dinitrophenols used in agriculture. *J Ind Hyg Toxicol* 1948;30:10–25.
154. Carson J. Report on three extensive industrial chemical burns. *BMJ* 1959; 1:827–829.
155. Klinger M, Norton J. Toxicity of cresylic acid containing solvent. *US Navy Med Bull* 1945;44(2):438–439.
156. Ma S, Ma C, Lynn R. Clinical studies of 83 cases of chemical burns [in Chinese]. *Chin J Dermatol* 1982;15(1):9–10.
157. Wu H, Quan Y. Case report of an acute renal failure complicated by cresol burns [in Chinese]. *Chin J Prev Med* 1984;18:145–149.

CHAPTER 116

Uranium, Plutonium, and Transuranium Radionuclide Hazards

George L. Voelz, Charles E. Stewart, and John B. Sullivan, Jr.

BIOLOGICALLY IMPORTANT PARTICLE–EMITTING NUCLIDES

The onset of the nuclear era has created concerns about a special class of α particle–emitting elements: uranium and man-made nuclides called the *transuranium elements*. The transuranium elements consist of those with atomic weights greater than 92. Of these, plutonium is the most important. Owing to their high rate of emission of α particles, the transuranium elements are radiologic poisons.

The elements of the periodic table from atomic number 89 (actinium) through atomic number 103 (lawrencium) are chemically similar to the lanthanide (rare earth) series of the periodic table (atomic numbers 58 through 71). Because of this similarity, elements 89 through 103 are called the *actinide series*. Elements beyond the actinide series have different properties and are referred to as *transactinide elements*. The elements above uranium (atomic number 92), from atomic number 93 through atomic number 105, are termed *transuranium elements* (Table 116-1).

TABLE 116-1. Transuranium elements

Name	Symbol	Atomic no.
Neptunium	Np	93
Plutonium	Pu	94
Americium	Am	95
Curium	Cm	96
Berkelium	Bk	97
Californium	Cf	98
Einsteinium	Es	99
Fermium	Fm	100
Mendelevium	Md	101
Nobelium	No	102
Lawrencium	Lr	103
Rutherfordium	Rf	104
Neilsbohrium	Ns	105

Many different isotopes of the same element may be unstable and seek greater stability by decay. Nuclear instability results from either neutron or proton excess. Isotopes attempting to reach stability by emitting radiation are termed *radionuclides*. Radionuclides have multiple mechanisms of decay: α emission, β decay, positron emission, electron capture, and isomeric transition. In α emission, an α particle with a 2^+ charge is emitted that consists of two protons and two neutrons, resulting in a decrease in atomic mass. The mass and charge of α particles are so great that they can travel only a few centimeters in air and cannot penetrate paper. α Emitters are hazardous only if they are internalized by ingestion, inhalation, or injection.

Many of the transuranic elements have half-lives so short that they were discovered only through nuclear reactions. Their short half-lives ensured that they could not have lasted from the time of their original creation.

In nuclear reactors, the quantity and kind of transuranic elements produced depends on the type of reactor and how long the fuel element has been in the reactor. Quantities are described in terms of weight or activity (curies or becquerels). A curie, the unit of radioactive decay, named in honor of Madame Marie Curie, is defined as that quantity of radionuclide that is disintegrating (decaying) at a rate of 37 billion disintegrations per second (3.7×10^{10} per second).

The radioactive energy delivered to biological tissues depends on two factors (1): the number of radioactive decay events per unit of time from the radioactive material source, and the amount of energy released by each transformation that occurs. Two methods exist to express energy delivered per unit weight of tissue. The term *rad* was devised for measuring the absorbed dose of energy. The *erg* has historically been used to describe energy delivered by ionizing radiation. One hundred ergs of energy deposited in 1 g of tissue equals 1 rad:

$$1 \text{ rad} = \frac{100 \text{ ergs}}{1 \text{ g tissue}}$$

Rads do not distinguish the kind of radiation dose delivered: α, β, γ. The rad has been replaced by the international unit, the *gray* (Gy): 1 Gy = 100 rads. Thus, another term, *rems*, was devised to reflect a "relative biological effectiveness" (RBE), which is the difference in delivered effectiveness of one form of ionizing radiation over another:

$$\text{rems} = \text{rads} \times \text{RBE}$$

An international unit termed the *sievert* (Sv) has now replaced the rem: 1 Sv = 100 rem.

Spent, high-burn-up nuclear fuel produces the major plutonium radionuclides (Table 116-2). *Burn-up* is the term that describes how much usable, fissionable material has actually undergone fission, described in megawatt-days per ton of fuel. There are two ways to describe the persistence of these radionuclides. The first is the time it takes for their radioactivity to decrease by a factor of 1,000 or the time for their radioactivity to

TABLE 116-2. Plutonium isotopes: half-lives and distribution by weight in spent fuel

Radionuclide	Percentage of weight	Half-life (yr)
^{239}Pu	60	24,100
^{240}Pu	22	6,540
^{241}Pu	12	14
^{242}Pu	4.5	3.8×10^5
^{238}Pu	1.5	88

TABLE 116-3. Transuranium isotopes in reactor fuel 150 days after removal from reactor

Element	Radionuclide	Half-life	Radioactive decay	Curies/MW-yr
Neptunium	$^{239}_{93}Np$	2.33 d	β^-	0.6
Plutonium	$^{238}_{94}Pu$	88 yr	α	94.0
Plutonium	$^{239}_{94}Pu$	24,100 yr	α	11.0
Plutonium	$^{240}_{94}Pu$	6,540 yr	α	16.0
Plutonium	$^{241}_{94}Pu$	14 yr	β^-	3,850.0
Americium	$^{241}_{95}Am$	432 yr	α	6.7
Curium	$^{242}_{96}Cm$	163 d	α	503.0
Curium	$^{244}_{96}Cm$	18 yr	α	84.0

decrease by a factor of 1 million. For a factor of 1,000, 10 half-lives of radioactive decay are required; for a factor of 1 million, 20 half-lives of radioactive decay are required (1). For ^{239}Pu, 10 half-lives equals 241,000 years, and 20 half-lives equals 482,000 years. The second method for describing biologically toxic persistence of these radionuclides is the average life of an atom. For any atom, this is described as the half-life ($t_{1/2}$) divided by 0.693. For ^{239}Pu, this would be as follows:

$$\frac{24{,}400 \text{ years}}{0.693} = 34{,}776 \text{ years}$$

Thus, one can envision the enormous time frames involved in plutonium contamination and persistence in the environment.

^{238}U and ^{235}U nuclides of natural uranium provide the original source for the generation of all plutonium nuclides. This is described by the nuclide generation reaction (n,γ), which means that a neutron is captured and a γ-ray is emitted. The other reaction in the generation of radionuclides is radioactive decay with the emission of β particles (β^-), which means that within the nucleus, a neutron is converted to a proton (1).

The production of other transuranic radionuclides in nuclear reactors is related to fuel burn-up and the nature of the reactor. In light-water reactor fuel, the transuranic radionuclides that are found 150 days after fuel rods are removed from the reactor and after high burn-up are listed in Table 116-3.

Although ^{239}Pu is the dominant radionuclide in percentage of weight after 150 days, it is not dominant in terms of radioactivity (curies). All relationships in curie strength among transuranic radionuclide species change with time. For example, gradually over 70 years and beyond, ^{241}Pu converts into ^{241}Am, an α particle emitter, so that by then the number of curies in a transuranic mixture of ^{241}Am is actually greater than the total number of curies of ^{238}Pu and ^{240}Pu combined. The production of selected transuranic radionuclides is shown in Figures 116-1 through 116-3, and select decay schemes are shown in Figures 116-4 through 116-7.

$$^{238}_{92}U \xrightarrow[(n,\gamma)]{} {}^{239}_{92}U \xrightarrow[t_{1/2}\ 23.5\ \text{min}]{\beta^-} {}^{239}_{93}Np \xrightarrow[t_{1/2}\ 2.33\ \text{d}]{\beta^-} {}^{239}_{94}Pu \xrightarrow[n,\gamma]{}$$

$$^{240}_{93}Pu \xrightarrow[n,\gamma]{} {}^{241}_{94}Pu \xrightarrow[n,\gamma]{} {}^{242}_{94}Pu \xrightarrow[n,\gamma]{} {}^{243}_{94}Pu$$

Figure 116-1. Reaction from uranium 238 to production of plutonium radionuclides.

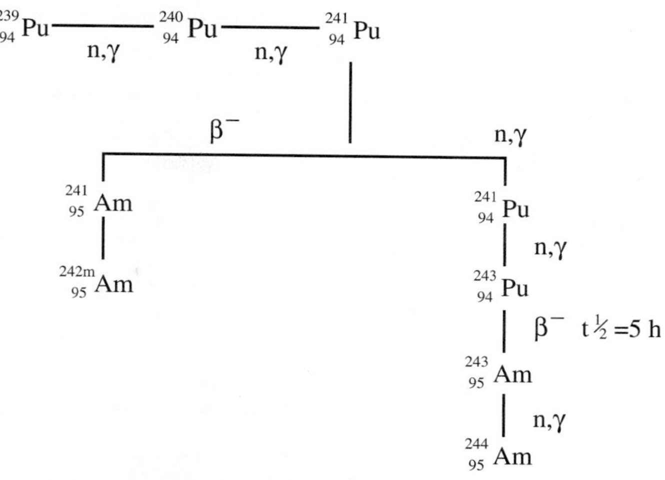

Figure 116-2. Production of americium radionuclides.

URANIUM

Sources and Forms

Uranium as found in nature (U_{nat}) is a radioactive element that contains three isotopes: 99.27% by weight ^{238}U, 0.72% ^{235}U, and less than 0.01% ^{234}U. U_{nat} is widely distributed in small quantities throughout the earth's crust, in water, and in a variety of minerals. The discovery of uranium dates to 1789 when it was found in pitchblende ores. Uranium was the element in which radioactivity was first discovered in 1896 by Becquerel. It is found in varying amounts in rocks and sediments of the earth's crust. Uraninite is a blackish form that is the most common deposit found. Coffinite is a hydrous uranium silicate also associated with deposits found naturally. Brannerite, uranium titanate, is a component of some black ore deposits. Yellow oxidized uranium is less important. Original sources of uranium included the Colorado Plateau and the Belgian Congo, as well as Bear Lake area pitchblende deposits. Canada, the United States, and South Africa are the world's major sources of uranium, but deposits exist in other countries also.

^{238}U is the long-lived parent ($t_{1/2}$ = 4.5 billion years) of the uranium series (Table 116-4). Minerals and ores of U_{nat} contain daughter products such as ^{230}Th, ^{226}Ra, and many nuclides with shorter half-lives, formed during radioactive decay throughout the series. In the natural state, these nuclides often are present by weight in proportion to their radioactive half-life, a condition termed *radioactive equilibrium*. Because of its long half-life, ^{238}U itself has a very low level of radioactivity, and its principal hazard comes from chemical toxicity rather than radiation.

Three isotopes of uranium are essential to the development of nuclear fuels and nuclear explosives: ^{238}U and ^{235}U, found in U_{nat}, and ^{233}U ($t_{1/2} = 1.62 \times 10^5$ years), which is not found in nature or as a product of a uranium decay series. ^{235}U is the key isotope for nuclear reactions. The basic nuclear reaction involv-

$$^{241}_{95}Am \xrightarrow[(n,\gamma)]{} {}^{242}_{95}Am \xrightarrow[t_{1/2}\ 16\ \text{h}]{\beta^-} {}^{242}_{96}Cm$$

$$^{243}_{95}Am \xrightarrow[(n,\gamma)]{} {}^{244}_{95}Am \xrightarrow[t_{1/2}\ 26\ \text{min}]{\beta^-} {}^{244}_{96}Cm$$

Figure 116-3. Production of curium radionuclides.

α-Particle emitters

$$^{237}_{93}\text{Np} \longrightarrow {}^{233}_{91}\text{Pa} \qquad t_{1/2} = 2.2 \times 10^{6}\ \text{yr}$$

β-Particle emitters

$$^{236}_{93}\text{Np} \xrightarrow{\beta^-} {}^{236}_{94}\text{Pu} \qquad t_{1/2} = 22\ \text{h}$$

$$^{238}_{93}\text{Np} \xrightarrow{\beta^-} {}^{238}_{94}\text{Pu} \qquad t_{1/2} = 2.1\ \text{d}$$

$$^{239}_{93}\text{Np} \xrightarrow{\beta^-} {}^{239}_{94}\text{Pu} \qquad t_{1/2} = 2.33\ \text{d}$$

Figure 116-4. Neptunium radionuclide decay.

ing ^{235}U is fission, the process of the disintegration of a heavy nucleus into two or three lighter nuclei (fission products) with the concomitant release of tremendous amounts of energy (8×10^{17} ergs per g). The loss of mass of the original material appears as energy, the amount expressed by Einstein's famous equation $e = mc^2$. This nuclear reaction is the basis of the explosive, thermal, and radioactive power of the atomic bomb.

All uranium isotopes have unstable nuclei, and ^{238}U and ^{235}U are the parents of complicated decay chains that produce α and β emissions. Both of these eventually decay into stable lead isotopes. However, before that occurs, ^{238}U passes through ^{226}Ra.

^{235}U is the key to nuclear fission reactions. Although its natural presence is only 0.71%, ^{235}U undergoes fission with slow neutrons so readily that a self-sustaining fission chain reaction can occur in a nuclear reactor. ^{238}U, although more abundant than ^{235}U, will not in itself undergo fission with slow neutrons, but it does capture neutrons to produce plutonium (^{239}Pu):

$$^{238}_{92}\text{U} \xrightarrow[\text{n},\,\gamma]{} {}^{239}_{92}\text{U} \xrightarrow{\beta^-} {}^{239}_{92}\text{Np} \xrightarrow{\beta^-} {}^{239}_{92}\text{Pu}$$

^{239}Pu is also very fissionable and is used as a concentrated form of nuclear fuel and as a nuclear explosive. The nuclear conver-

α-Particle emitters

$$^{236}_{94}\text{Pu} \longrightarrow {}^{232}_{92}\text{U} \qquad t_{1/2} = 92\ \text{yr}$$

$$^{238}_{94}\text{Pu} \longrightarrow {}^{234}_{92}\text{U} \qquad t_{1/2} = 92\ \text{yr}$$

$$^{239}_{94}\text{Pu} \longrightarrow {}^{235}_{92}\text{U} \qquad t_{1/2} = 24{,}000\ \text{yr}$$

$$^{240}_{94}\text{Pu} \longrightarrow {}^{236}_{92}\text{U} \qquad t_{1/2} = 6{,}580\ \text{yr}$$

$$^{242}_{94}\text{Pu} \longrightarrow {}^{238}_{92}\text{U} \qquad t_{1/2} = 5 \times 10^{5}\ \text{yr}$$

β-Particle emitters

$$^{241}_{94}\text{Pu} \longrightarrow {}^{241}_{95}\text{Am} \qquad t_{1/2} = 14\ \text{yr}$$

$$^{243}_{94}\text{Pu} \longrightarrow {}^{243}_{95}\text{Am} \qquad t_{1/2} = 5\ \text{h}$$

Figure 116-5. Plutonium radionuclide decay.

α-Particle emitters

$$^{241}_{95}\text{Am} \longrightarrow {}^{237}_{93}\text{Np} \qquad t_{1/2} = 475\ \text{yr}$$

$$^{243}_{95}\text{Am} \longrightarrow {}^{239}_{93}\text{Np} \qquad t_{1/2} = 10^{4}\ \text{yr}$$

β-Particle emitters

$$^{242}_{95}\text{Am} \longrightarrow {}^{242}_{96}\text{Cm} \qquad t_{1/2} = 16\ \text{h}$$

$$^{244}_{95}\text{Am} \longrightarrow {}^{244}_{96}\text{Cm} \qquad t_{1/2} = 26\ \text{min}$$

Figure 116-6. Americium radionuclide decay.

sion of ^{238}U into ^{239}Pu can be performed in a "breeder" nuclear reactor, in which more new fissionable material than that consumed in initiating the chain reaction is produced. Owing to the nuclear reactor conversion of ^{238}U to ^{239}Pu, natural uranium can supply most fissionable nuclear fuels. Thus, the rare ^{235}U can be concentrated to use as a fuel or explosive. ^{233}U, the third isotope of importance for fission reactions, is produced by irradiating natural thorium (^{232}Th) with neutrons:

$$^{232}_{90}\text{Th} \xrightarrow[\text{n},\,\gamma]{} {}^{233}_{90}\text{Th} \xrightarrow{\beta^-} {}^{233}_{91}\text{Pa} \xrightarrow{\beta^-} {}^{233}_{92}\text{U}$$

Breeder reactors are used to convert thorium into usable nuclear fuels.

The principal use of uranium is as fuel for nuclear power reactors. Nearly 43 million kg of uranium per year are mined to produce ^{235}U-rich fuel rods for these reactions. The waste product of this production, depleted uranium, has been used for armor-piercing bullets (depleted uranium rounds).

A wide variety of chemical forms of uranium may be encountered. The three that will be most commonly found in industry are yellowcake uranium, uranium oxide (U_3O_8), and uranium hexafluoride (UF_6). Yellowcake is the semirefined product from the milling of uranium and contains more than 80% uranium oxide.

Metabolic uranium is a lustrous, silvery metal with a melting point of 1,132°C. It is malleable, ductile, and highly chemically reactive. The lustrous metal exposed to air will become coated by a dull black oxide. The metal crystallizes in an orthorhombic form that is stable at room temperatures. The metal can also be pyrophoric and combines with halides, oxygen, gaseous hydrogen, nitrogen, carbon dioxide, and carbon monoxide. Uranium reacts directly with water but is not attacked by alkalis. It dissolves readily in acids, producing U^{3+} and U^{4+}. Uranium ions have four different oxidation states in aqueous solution:

U^{3+}	red
U^{4+}	green
UO_2^{+}	unstable (liberates H_2 from H_2O)
UO_2^{2+}	yellow

α-Particle emitters

$$^{242}_{96}\text{Cm} \longrightarrow {}^{238}_{94}\text{Pu} \qquad t_{1/2} = 162\ \text{d}$$

$$^{244}_{96}\text{Am} \longrightarrow {}^{240}_{94}\text{Pu} \qquad t_{1/2} = 19\ \text{yr}$$

Figure 116-7. Curium radionuclide decay.

TABLE 116-4. Isotopes present in natural uranium

Isotope	Abundance (%)	Half-life (yr)
^{238}U	99.300	45×10^8
^{235}U	0.700	8×10^8
^{234}U	0.005	2×10^5

Uranium oxides are UO_2, UO_3, UO, U_2O_5, and U_3O_8. Uranium carbides are UC (uranium monocarbide), UC_2 (dicarbide), and U_2C_3 (sesquicarbide). Uranium metal reacts with nitrogen to yield nitrides: UN, U_2N_3, and UN_2. Uranium nitrides and uranium carbides are semimetallic and, when ignited in air, convert to U_3O_8. The nitrides and carbides also react with water.

Uranium ore is mined both by open-pit and by underground mining techniques. Raw ores contain between 0.1% and 1.0% natural uranium. Aside from the usual hazards of mining, uranium mines contain radon and daughter products of radon disintegration. An increased incidence of lung cancer occurs in uranium miners from inhalation of this radioactive by-product of uranium but not from the uranium itself. Likewise, most external γ-radiation in uranium mines comes from the disintegration products of uranium rather than from uranium itself.

Airborne uranium compounds are the main pathway for occupational exposure hazards in milling uranium. The dust by-product of crushing operations is ore dust, whereas yellowcake dust is a by-product of the drying and packaging operations.

The next step in enriching uranium with ^{235}U is to convert the yellowcake to fluoride and then to separate $^{235}UF_6$ from $^{238}UF_6$. Two different processes are used to separate the two isotopes. The United States enriches ^{235}U by the gaseous diffusion process at the Department of Energy facilities. After the enriched UF_6 is obtained, the uranium is converted back to uranium oxide powder, which is used to produce pellets or weapons parts. For commercial use, the final product has 0.9% to 5.0% ^{235}U for commercial applications and up to 90% ^{235}U for military applications.

During these operations, inhalation of dusts may occur during processing of the yellowcake, removal of ash after the purification phase, any maintenance activities, or loading UF_6 in or out of the various processes. The dusts may contain yellowcake, uranium disintegration products, UF_4, UO_2, UO_3, uranyl fluoride (UO_2F_2), or UF_6. When exposed to air, UF_6 will react with moisture to form uranyl fluoride and hydrofluoric acid. Inhalation of hydrofluoric acid is a major toxic hazard in uranium processing.

Classification of uranium compounds according to their solubility and transportability between organs of the body and excretion from the body is useful for understanding the compounds' potential toxic effects (Table 116-5). Scott (2) divided uranium compounds into three classes: highly transportable (biological half-life of days), moderately transportable (biological half-life of weeks to months), and slightly transportable (biological half-life of months to years) (2). Highly transportable uranium compounds include UF_6, $UO_2(NO_3)_2$, sulfates, and carbonates. In the moderately transportable class are UO_3, UF_4, UCl_4, and nitrates. The slightly transportable compounds are UO_2, U_3O_8, oxides, hydrides, and carbides. Scott (2) also noted that subjecting some compounds to high temperatures tends to decrease their rate of transportability.

TABLE 116-5. Transportability of uranium compounds

Highly transportable	Moderately transportable	Slightly transportable
UF_6	UF_4	UO_2
UO_3	UO_3	UO_3O_8
$UO_2(NO_3)_2$	UO_2	Uranium oxides
UF_4	UO_3O_8	Uranium hydrides
Uranium sulfates	Uranium nitrates	Uranium carbides
Uranium carbonates		

Uses of Uranium and Exposure Potentials in the Uranium Industry

The principal use of uranium is as fuel for the 410 nuclear power reactors in the world and for nuclear-powered submarines (3). Most reactors require a higher content of ^{235}U in the uranium fuel rods than is found in U_{nat}. The uranium industry processes U_{nat} to provide appropriate fuel rods. As mentioned, uranium production is approximately 43 million kg per year (4).

Other industrial uses of uranium are limited. It is used as an intensifier in photography, in dry copying ink, as a colorant in ceramics, and as ballast. Uranium also is used as an additive to dental porcelain to provide a more natural fluorescent appearance.

Because nuclear fuel is the major product of uranium, the uranium fuel-manufacturing process is of interest (Fig. 116-8). It consists of mining uranium ore, milling ore to yellowcake, converting yellowcake to UF_6, enriching the ^{235}U in the UF_6, and then fabricating uranium oxide fuel pellets (5). Each of these steps is accomplished at different plant facilities and locations. The process thus involves packaging and shipping of the intermediate products to the next facility.

Production of the volatile UF_6 involves sampling and preparing the yellowcake feed, converting it to fluoride, and purifying the product. Inhalation of dusts occurs mainly in emptying and refilling yellowcake drums, removing ash waste after the purification phase, and performing maintenance jobs throughout the facilities. The dust may contain yellowcake, uranium daughters, UF_4, UO_2, UO_3, and uranyl fluoride (UO_2F_2). The product, UF_6, if released in air, reacts with moisture to form UO_2F_2 and hydrofluoric acid.

Uranium fuel fabrication consists of converting enriched UF_6 to uranium dioxide powder, which is used to produce uranium pellets. The pellets are placed into the fuel pins or rods used in nuclear reactors. Inhalation of gases or dusts is the major exposure potential in fuel fabrication.

Depleted Uranium

The term *depleted uranium* (DU) signifies that ^{235}U has been removed and that it is essentially all ^{238}U (natural uranium). DU is a by-product of uranium enrichment processes and is used in armor-piercing projectiles by the military owing to its hardness, pyrophoric reactions, density, and strength; as counterweights by the aircraft industry; and as radiation shielding by power industries. The potential of radiation exposure from DU is small as it emits α particles that do not penetrate human skin. However, taken internally as shrapnel, it irradiates tissues and carries the risk of uranium nephrotoxicity. This issue currently is being researched on wounded Gulf War veterans.

DU is two and a half times denser than lead on a weight-to-weight basis. This density makes DU military projectiles smaller than those made of lead but with the same mass and less air resistance, thus providing higher velocity, maximum

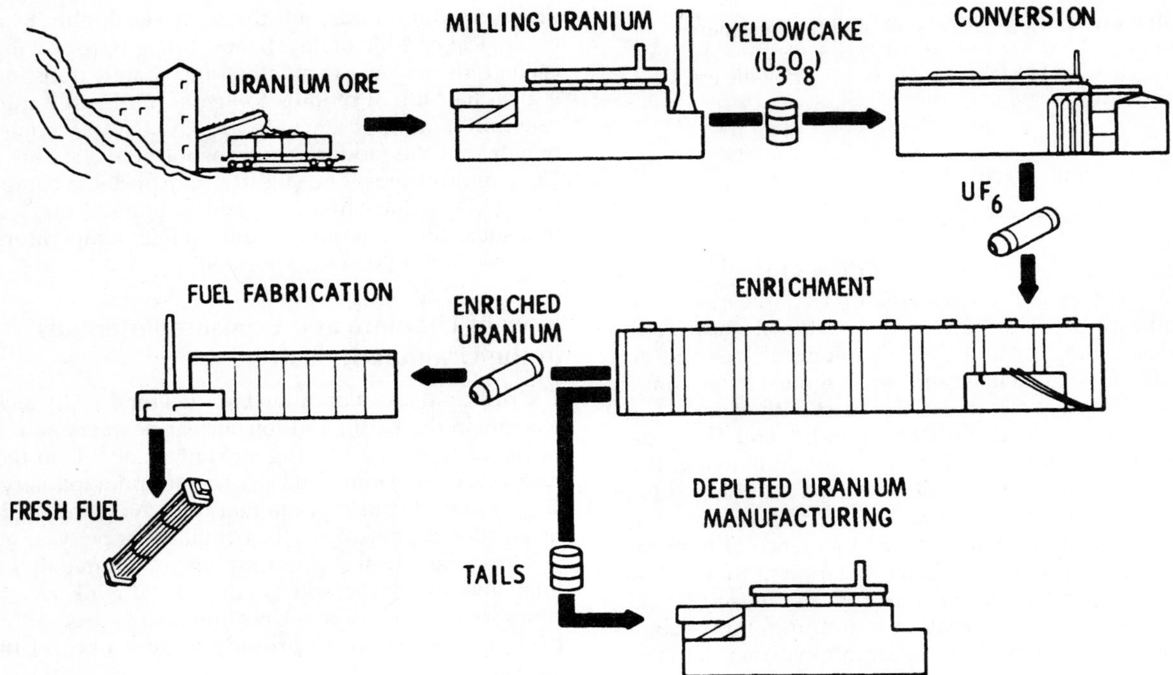

Figure 116-8. Uranium fuel manufacturing.

penetrative power, and extended range. DU weapons concentrate a larger amount of weight on a smaller spot of armor, thus making them armor piercing. However, the major mechanisms of DU weapons' penetrative power are the pyrophoric reactions, which allow such weapons to melt their way through armor.

Absorption and Metabolism

Inhalation of uranium particles is the most common route of occupational exposure. Uptake can occur by ingestion, but uptake via the human gastrointestinal (GI) tract is low; the best value for drinking water is judged to be 1.4% of the soluble uranium present (6). A recent extensive review confirms that a reasonable central estimate of GI uptake of uranium in adult humans may be approximately 101.5%, but uptake may be less than 0.1% or as high as 506.0% under some conditions (7). Soluble uranium compounds are absorbed also through skin. In experimental animals, sufficient amounts could be absorbed through skin to cause severe uranium poisoning and death (7). Some uranium compounds cause mild to moderate skin irritation.

Particle size and chemical solubility in body fluids determine the absorption rate of uranium particles from the lung. A general idea of this uptake rate, redistribution to other organs, and excretion in urine can be obtained from the compound classification by transportability described earlier (see Table 116-5). Long-term inhalational experiments with UO_2 in dogs showed a lung clearance half-life of 340 days (8). In humans, biological half-lives for uranium oxide exposures have been estimated to be as long as 1,470 days (9). On average, however, a biological half-life of approximately 15 days is commonly cited (10), but this value obviously varies with different compounds. For example, after inhaling UF_6 particles, humans during the first day excrete in urine approximately 73% of the solubilized uranium from the lung, with a biological half-life of approximately 4 hours, and another 10% with a half-life of 1.3 days (11). In a second stage of slower excretion, a biological half-life of approximately 6 days is estimated by the second day or later.

Once absorbed into the blood, uranium is principally passed through the kidney. In one study, from 50% to more than 80% of intravenously administered uranium was excreted in urine within 24 hours in most people (12). From excretion data after an accidental inhalational exposure of soluble uranium particles, Chalabreysse (13) estimated that approximately 80% of the absorbed uranium was excreted during the first 24 hours. In reviewing the literature, Durbin (14) concluded that approximately 70% of uranium taken up in the blood is excreted in the urine during the first day. A significant percentage of uranium retained in the body is deposited in the kidney. Dog and rat experiments indicate that approximately 5% to 10% of the absorbed dose is present in the kidneys and is eliminated with a half-life of 2.2 days, and the remainder is eliminated with a half-life of 103 days (14–16).

Very little uranium is present in feces (less than 0.1% to approximately 0.3% of intravenous doses administered in humans) (12). After inhalation, particles brought out of the lung by mucociliary clearance will be swallowed and will add to the quantity of uranium found in feces.

Deposition in bone is the most important long-term storage site in the body for uranium introduced in soluble form. The process of deposition by ionic exchange processes and involving the entire bone volume rather than surfaces was described by Neuman et al. in 1953 (17). Donoghue et al. (18) estimated that uranium deposited in bone accounted for approximately 85% of that absorbed and metabolized. Some portion of this deposition has a very long biological half-life: The International Commission on Radiological Protection (19) describes a biokinetic model for uranium in bone in which fractions of 0.200 and 0.023 are transferred to mineral bone and retained there with half-lives of 20 and 5,000 days, respectively. Substantial uncertainties remain as to the long-term retention of uranium in bone and soft tissues, despite numerous studies on its metabolic behavior in laboratory animals and more limited studies in humans. A full discussion of this subject, including biokinetic data and dose coefficients, is available in International Commission on Radiological Protection publications (20–22).

Health Effects and Clinical Management

ACUTE TOXICITY

Biological hazard from uranium exposures may occur from chemical toxicity, radiation dose, or both. This fact, together with the complex chemical forms, isotopic mixtures, and metabolic pathways, gives rise to an interesting toxicologic puzzle, but it can be greatly simplified for clinical management. As regards acute toxicity, chemical toxicity of the kidney is clearly the most important effect from soluble forms of uranium (23).

Approximately 60% of uranium absorbed into the blood is transported in the form of a bicarbonate complex, and 40% is bound to plasma proteins. The uranyl-bicarbonate complex is filtered out of the blood by the renal glomerulus and is passed into the tubules. The pH of urine decreases in the tubules, resulting in dissociation of the complex and release of the reactive uranyl ion. Nephrotoxicity results primarily from damage to the tubular epithelium, which allows leakage of glucose, protein, amino acids, and enzymes into the urine. In high doses (more than 6 mg uranium per kg), glomerular damage may also occur, causing decreased renal blood flow and a decreased glomerular filtration rate.

The kidney responds to toxic levels of uranium within 24 to 48 hours after exposure. The changes become progressively more severe over approximately a 5-day period. The damaged tubular epithelium regenerates quickly as the uranium concentration is reduced.

Large accidental intakes of U_{nat} in industrial accidents have been summarized (12). In more than 40 workers with acute uranium exposures, the estimated total systemic uptake of uranium largely ranged from approximately 1 to 3 mg, although in one case, the estimated uptake was in excess of 15 mg. Initial uranium excretion rates in urine ranged from approximately 0.15 to more than 6.00 mg per L. Apparently none of the workers sustained permanent injury as a result of internal exposure to uranium.

The effects of UF_6 exposures were impressively displayed in a 1944 accident involving 21 workers (24). One individual died in 15 minutes due to severe steam burns and the effects of UF_6 and its degradation products, hydrogen fluoride and uranium oxyfluoride. Another worker died 70 minutes after exposure due to progressive respiratory distress. Most of the other 14 persons requiring hospitalization had corrosive irritation of the eyes, skin, and respiratory tract but were well enough to be released in 48 hours. Three more seriously exposed individuals were retained for observation for 10 to 14 days owing to pulmonary edema and nephrotoxicity. The peak urinary uranium excretion values in these three patients ranged from 0.15 to 0.50 mg per L. All three persons experienced some urine volume suppression for 3 days, and albumin, red cells, and casts were found in their urine. In one of these patients, mild elevation of blood urea and nonprotein nitrogen was seen for 3 weeks after the accident. Two of the three individuals with acute toxicity were examined 38 years later (25). No physical changes related to their exposure and no uranium deposition were detected. An observation from these cases and other exposed workers suggests that the pulmonary edema may have slowed the absorption of uranium from the lungs and lengthened its biological half-life (9,20). Human data on acute poisoning from uranium are insufficiently adequate to allow estimation of a median lethal dose (LD_{50}). Systemic doses of 0.1 to 0.3 mg per kg of soluble uranium have not caused any deaths in humans. The animal (dog, rat) LD_{50} dose is approximately 1 to 2 mg per kg (26).

CHRONIC AND LONG-TERM TOXIC EFFECTS

The search for acute and chronic effects from uranium in animals and humans spans a long history starting in 1824. This history is brilliantly recorded by Hodge (27). The early studies of humans were made from approximately 1860 into the early 1900s, during which time uranium was administered as a therapeutic agent for diabetes and other diseases. Toxic effects recorded were neither consistent nor specific.

Exposure conditions in uranium work areas during the early 1940s were dusty and dirty. Stannard (28) indicates that they were "some of the worst conditions of exposure with the largest number of persons exposed of any section of the Atomic Bomb Project." For a decade after World War II, potential occupational exposures increased markedly with expansion of the industry. Fortunately, industrial hygiene controls also improved. Now, after some 50 years of operations of the nuclear industry, the evidence for chronic effects in workers still is not consistent or specific. The chief potential effects are considered to be chronic effects on the kidney for soluble compounds and radiogenic lung cancer for inhaled particles with low solubility in body fluids. Radiogenic bone cancer is also a concern for soluble compounds of enriched uranium.

Uranium toxicity in the kidney is the basis for the limits for occupational exposure to soluble, nonenriched uranium (29). Only a few studies on renal tubular dysfunction in chronically exposed workers have been conducted. Dounce et al. (30) reported increased tubular enzyme catalase in the urine of 46 exposed chemical workers, but the results were not controlled for differences in urinary concentration. Clarkson and Kench (31) measured increased excretion of total amino-nitrogen and some individual amino acids in 18 exposed workers. Thun et al. (32) found low-level β_2-microglobulinuria and aminoaciduria in 39 uranium mill workers. The clinical significance of these findings, if any, is unclear. The potent uranium nephrotoxicity demonstrated in animal experiments has not resulted in identified clinical problems in workers with chronic occupational exposures (32).

Inhalation of poorly solubilized uranium particles results in a radiologic risk to the lung. Other target organs for radiation effects are tracheobronchial lymph nodes, bone, bone marrow, and kidney. It has generally been estimated that the radiation risk does not exceed the chemical nephrotoxicity for soluble uranium until the enrichment is 5% to 8% ^{235}U by weight, but the relative risk between chemical and radiation risks continues to be an open question (28,29,33).

Results of epidemiologic studies of workers (34–42) have been variable and have not resolved the issue of chemical versus radiation risks. Checkoway et al. (40) found a slight excess of lung cancer in white male employees from a facility that produces enriched uranium. A radiation dose-response relationship was found for lung cancer, but the rate ratios were imprecise owing to the small number of cases in the analysis. Also, the influence of smoking could not be taken into account. Cookfair et al. (38) found an increased relative risk for lung cancer in workers with a cumulative lung dose of 20 rads or more from inhaled uranium, but only among those workers who were older than 45 years when first exposed. Other studies have not demonstrated increased risks of lung cancer due to uranium. However, Waxweiler et al. (39) found a significantly increased risk for nonmalignant respiratory disease in uranium mill workers.

Archer (35,37) found a significant excess of lymphatic and hematopoietic tissue cancers other than leukemia (four cases observed versus one expected) in a preliminary study of uranium mill workers. Thus far, this finding has not been confirmed by other studies.

None of these studies has reported a significant excess risk of kidney disease. Waxweiler et al. (39) observed 6 deaths from chronic nephritis as compared with an expected 3.6 deaths, which was not a statistically significant increase.

In an excellent review of human studies, the BEIR-IV Committee on the Biological Effects of Ionizing Radiation found "little convincing epidemiological evidence that serious renal disease has occurred in human populations as a result of chronic low-level exposure nor of increased rates of malignant tumors" (26). Considering the exposure conditions in the industry during and after World War II, one might consider this conclusion as reassurance that the hazards of uranium have not been underestimated. Under current industrial hygiene and radiation protection standards and practice, the health risks from uranium in industry should be extremely low.

Management of Toxicity

No specific clinical findings are ordinarily associated with uranium exposure. In the exceptional case of accidental inhalation of high concentrations of uranium hexafluoride, signs and symptoms of pulmonary edema from hydrogen fluoride will dominate the clinical course. Significant irritation of the eyes and skin from the fluoride ion may also be present after such exposure.

Monitoring of accidental uranium exposures and its effects on the kidney is accomplished by measurement of the uranium excreted in the urine and abnormalities in the clinical urinalyses. Glucose and albumin in urine are among the most sensitive indicators of kidney damage (23). Henge-Napoli et al. (43) have found urinary excretion of γ-glutamyltransferase to be the most sensitive indicator. These various indicators of renal injury can be assessed within a few hours of exposure to dose levels of at least 0.1 mg of uranium per kg (23).

Daily urine samples should be collected after large accidental exposures (23,44), and collection should continue for at least 2 weeks. The collection of 24-hour urine samples whenever possible is advantageous. These samples will be used for measuring uranium excretion and for clinical urinalysis. Bacterial degradation of glucose and other constituents of urine can be prevented by the addition of sodium azide to the sample or by immediate cooling of the sample to 5°C. If analysis for amino acids or enzymes is to be performed later, freezing the sample at –40°C is advisable. Quantitative measurement of glucose and protein in the urine is preferable to the usual qualitative analyses. Quantitative measurement of glucose and protein in the serum should also be performed. Serum creatinine and creatinine clearance studies are needed to assess glomerular function. Clearance tests may underestimate filtration rate if tubular injury is present.

The many methods used to measure uranium in urine and other sample matrices were extensively reviewed recently by Wessman (45). Fluorometry is the most widely used method in monitoring and bioassay, but it also is the most inaccurate and least reliable method owing to interferences. Mass spectrometry and α spectrometry are the most accurate and reliable methods and produce the most isotopic information.

Direct or *in vivo* measurements over the chest are often superior to urine excretion data in evaluating depositions, and this is the best method available to assess the inhalation of insoluble material. Palmer (46) described the performance of high-purity germanium planar detectors used in chest counting. The sensitivity for a 1-hour count is approximately 1.6 mg of U_{nat} at a 99% confidence level. Sensitivity for phoswich detectors is approximately 4 mg and, for NaI(Tl) detectors, is somewhat less, approximately 8 mg. The sensitivity will vary with the isotopic mixture of uranium to be counted, being better with material enriched with ^{235}U and ^{234}U.

For acute uranium nephrotoxicity, oral doses or infusions of sodium bicarbonate are administered to maintain an alkaline urine (44,47), which should be monitored frequently by pH measurements. Alkaline urine prevents dissociation of the uranium-bicarbonate complex and thus protects the renal tubular epithelium from exposure to the reactive uranyl ion. Forcing fluids to increase urinary output is desirable.

The use of chelation drugs for acute uranium exposures—a controversial practice, as evidenced in the literature—was reviewed by Lincoln and Voelz (44). Limited animal research indicates that the LD_{50} can be raised by a factor of two to three through the immediate administration of chelating drugs, such as calcium disodium–ethylenediaminetetraacetic acid ($CaNa_2$-EDTA) and diethylenetriamine pentaacetic acid (DTPA) (48–50). Chelation must begin within 4 hours of the exposure to be effective and is most effective if given within a few minutes of the exposure. Some authors have advised against the use of chelation because precipitation of uranium in the kidney may cause additional damage, although support for this concern has not been presented. Soviet research indicates that chelating agents can significantly reduce the risk of acute uranium injury to kidneys (50). A Soviet drug preparation known as *trimephacin* was found to be more effective than DTPA in their studies and has been adopted in the Soviet Union as an antidote for uranium intoxication. No cases of uranium exposure have been reported as being treated with chelation in the Western world. The current Investigational New Drug agreement with the U.S. Food and Drug Administration for the use of DTPA does not include uranium on the list of radionuclides approved for treatment. The use of chelating agents seems quite improbable for acute uranium exposures, especially given the need for immediate administration. Its place, if there is one, is in the event of an exposure so high that it is judged to be life-threatening.

Exposure Standards

Current occupational guidelines using derived air concentrations for insoluble uranium compounds is 0.6 Bq per cubic meter. For highly soluble uranium compounds, the derived air concentration value is 20 Bq per cubic meter. These air limits are based on radiation protection guidelines for workers of 0.05 Sv (5 rem) per year. For occupational emergency use, a 1980 review in the United Kingdom recommended emergency standards of 3, 2, and 1 Bq per cubic meter for 10-, 30-, and 60-minute exposures, respectively (29).

PLUTONIUM

Sources and Forms

Plutonium was discovered by G. T. Seaborg and colleagues in 1941 (51). It is a man-made transuranium metal produced by neutron bombardment of uranium and is produced in quantity in nuclear reactors from natural uranium:

$$^{238}_{92}U(n,\gamma)\ ^{239}_{92}U \xrightarrow[t_{1/2}\,=\,23.5\ \text{min}]{} {}^{239}_{93}Np \xrightarrow[t_{1/2}\,=\,2.3\ \text{d}]{} {}^{239}_{94}Pu$$

^{239}Pu was used in the atomic bomb that destroyed Nagasaki and is formed in large quantities in nuclear reactors. The production of ^{239}Pu is inevitable anytime a nuclear chain reaction is maintained by neutrons and ^{238}U is present. An intermediate product in the nuclear sequence of ^{238}Pu production is neptunium

(^{239}Np), another transuranium element. ^{239}Np is fissionable, but only with fast neutrons. ^{239}Pu decays by α particle emission and has a half-life of 24,100 years (20).

Of the 15 isotopes of plutonium, the most common is ^{239}Pu, which is an α emitter. The use of the word *plutonium* in this chapter refers specifically to ^{239}Pu. From 1941 to 1945, only scant quantities of this metal were available for evaluation, and its hazards were essentially unknown. In January 1944, an allocation (11 mg) for health effects research was made from the first small production of plutonium. By 1945, the United States had made kilogram quantities of plutonium, and small amounts were diverted for toxicologic studies of the metal (51). Our knowledge about the biochemistry, dosimetry, and biology of plutonium has increased enormously in the 57 years since its discovery. Plutonium has received much attention as an explosive element in nuclear weapons. One pound of plutonium is equivalent to approximately 10 million kilowatt-hours of heat energy.

Plutonium has been referred to in the news media as the "most poisonous substance known to man." This perception has contributed to intense discussions about the use of plutonium in spacecraft, as a weapon of terrorism, and the possibility of accidental dispersion during various operations of the nuclear fuel industry. Indeed, "what might happen" if everything goes wrong causes considerable confusion in the public mind in these discussions.

Plutonium has a silvery appearance, is chemically reactive, and melts at 639.5°C. It exists in five valence states in aqueous solution:

Pu^{3+}	blue/lavender
Pu^{4+}	yellow/brown
PuO_2^{1+}	pink
PuO_2^{2+}	pink/orange (unstable in solution)
PuO_6^{5-} or PuO_5^{3-}	green

Plutonium forms binary compounds with oxygen (PuO and PuO_2) and with halides (PuF_3, PuF_4, PuCl, $PuBr_3$, PuI_3), with carbon, nitrogen, and silicon (PuC, PuN, $PuSi_2$), and with oxyhalides (PuOCl, PuOB4, PuOI).

Experimental studies in rodents and dogs during 1944 and 1945 sought to discover the acute, lethal, and subacute effects of plutonium (52). These studies also examined uptake pathways and distribution in the body, effects in organs, and the mechanisms of excretion. Over the subsequent 50 years, thousands of workers have studied the effects of plutonium in a variety of animal species in universities and commercial, national, and military laboratories throughout the world. No single summary could do justice to this monumental mass of technical work, but Stannard (52) has written nearly 2,000 pages covering the results of research on most of the internal emitters. Thompson (53) summarizes four decades of research about the effects of plutonium and other radionuclides in dogs (53).

Interestingly enough, despite common perceptions, plutonium was found to be less acutely "toxic" to humans than botulinus toxin, diphtheria toxin, curare, or strychnine (54). Unfortunately, many of the early studies involved rats, mice, dogs, and rabbits. The data were often contradictory because different species metabolize plutonium differently, and injected results of injected plutonium studies were inappropriately extrapolated to inhaled plutonium effects.

Absorption and Metabolism

The health risks from plutonium are present only when it is deposited in the body. The α particle emitted by plutonium has a very short range (3 to 4 cm in air, less than 50 μm in tissue), and it cannot burn or penetrate the skin. Particles of plutonium itself do not pass through intact skin into the body. Skin wounds contaminated with plutonium are a potential entry portal to the body, especially for workers in glove boxes in which high levels of plutonium are handled.

Absorption into the body through inhalation or contaminated wound is the main pathway for internal deposition of plutonium. The most frequent pathway is by inhalation of tiny plutonium particles. Ingestion is a third pathway, but the absorption rate via this route is very low. In adults, the GI tract uptake is only 10^{-5} (1 part per 100,000) for relatively insoluble plutonium oxide and 5×10^{-4} for soluble plutonium compounds (22). In persons younger than 1 year, the absorption may be up to ten times greater than in the adult.

The absorption, distribution, and excretion of inhaled plutonium by humans is markedly influenced by its chemical form. Plutonium nitrate, a soluble chemical form, is absorbed at a fast rate (days) and is labeled a *type F* (fast) uptake. Plutonium oxide, especially if fired at high temperatures, is absorbed slowly (years) and is a *type S* (slow) uptake. Other chemical forms, such as plutonium fluoride, are absorbed at an intermediate rate (weeks) and are described as *type M* (moderate) uptakes. If the chemical form is unknown, the dosimetry model used for calculating radiation doses applies the type M parameters as default values.

Particle size determines the deposition and lung clearance rates of inhaled plutonium particles. Small particles (1 μm or less) are likely to be deposited and retained in the bronchioles and alveoli, where there is very little lung clearance. Accidents involving exposure to smoke, fumes, or fine aerosols may be suspected to contain small particles. Larger particles (10 μm or larger) are more likely formed from cutting and machine tools. These particles are more likely to be deposited in larger bronchi where mucociliary clearance takes place.

Although originally thought to be a bone-seeking radionuclide, plutonium presents a higher risk to the respiratory tract. The principal hazard of plutonium is the inhalation of fine particulate matter with resulting deposition in the respiratory tract (55,56). A highly simplified model suggests that when PuO_2 is deposited in the pulmonary system, 40% of it is eliminated within the first day through the GI tract. Another 40% of it is eliminated through the GI tract with a 500-day half-life, 5% goes into the blood stream with a 500-day half life, and 15% goes into the tracheobronchial lymph nodes with a 500-day half life. Of the amount deposited in the lymph nodes, 90% is released into the blood stream with a 1,000-day half-life. Of the plutonium that goes into the blood stream, approximately 45% is deposited in bone, 45% is deposited in the liver, and the rest is either excreted or deposited in other organs (55,56). These numbers vary widely among individuals, especially in relation to the chemical form and particle size of the plutonium.

Lung cancer, especially in smokers, is the major health risk from inhaled plutonium. The risk depends on the amount of plutonium deposited in the lung. U.S. workers who have been exposed to plutonium have not demonstrated a statistically significant increase in lung cancer (51), because the exposures have apparently been too small. A retrospective cohort study of 1,479 male workers at Russia's Mayak Production Association observed a statistically significant association of lung cancer mortality and α particle radiation (57). The doses in the Russian subjects were much higher than in the U.S. workers. In a dose range lower than 30 Sv (3,000 rem), the association was described in terms of a linear nonthreshold function. Lifetime lung cancer risk in this dose range is 1.21×10^{-2} Sv^{-1}, or approximately a 1% risk of lung cancer from plutonium per sievert (100 rem). The current radiation dose limit for occupational exposures (0.05 Sv, or 5 rem, per year for both external and internal radiation exposures) is incurred with an internal deposition of approximately 0.5 μg of plutonium over the course of a lifetime.

An independent lung cancer case-control study of workers from the same Russian facility observed a lung threshold dose of approximately 0.80 Gy (1,600 rem) (57). The data from this study are satisfactorily described by either linear-quadratic or quadratic models. Confounding by smoking may account for some of the marked differences between these two studies: Adjustment for smoking risk appears to have been taken into account better within the case-control study. The association of lung cancer with plutonium deposition in the lung is clear from both these Russian studies, but the correct shape of the dose-response curve and the presence or absence of a threshold remains unclear. The dose-effect relationship is assumed to be linear without a threshold for purposes of setting radiation protection standards and making lung dose calculations.

After very high experimental depositions of plutonium in dogs' lungs, death from pulmonary fibrosis was observed within a few months to a year or more after exposure. In Russian workers with high plutonium intakes, plutonium pneumosclerosis, a roentgenographic diagnosis of fibrosis (graded from I to III) seen in the upper and middle lung lobes, has been diagnosed (58). Vital capacity was reduced by 15% to 50%, but clinical manifestations of obstructive impairment were not observed. Pulmonary fibrosis is a late effect of high plutonium exposures, usually occurring years after initial exposure. The plutonium lung doses ranged from 5 Gy (100 Sv; 10,000 rem) for grade I cases up to 17 Gy (340 Sv, 34,000 rem) for grade III cases. The plutonium depositions for these cases were 18.5 kBq (500 nCi) to 70.0 kBq (1,900 nCi), respectively (58).

The plutonium contamination of wounds, usually tiny puncture wounds or small cuts or abrasions of the hand, have caused less than 25% of occupational exposures, although some of the larger occupational uptakes have occurred through contaminated wounds. This mode of exposure leads to absorption directly into the blood and lymph at a rate that depends on the chemical form of the plutonium. The main uptake occurs in liver and bone. Regional lymph nodes also are involved. Unless there is an associated inhalational exposure, the dose to the lung is very low.

The systemic uptake and distribution of plutonium by blood from entry sites, whether lung or contaminated wounds, is transported mostly (approximately 90%) to bone and liver. In bone, the initial deposition occurs on the bone surface, especially the endosteum. Dog experiments demonstrated increased risk of bone tumors (especially osteogenic sarcomas) and lesser risk of liver or bile duct cancers. Excess bone tumors have not been observed after inhalation of $^{239}PuO_2$ but are the most common cause of delayed death in dogs inhaling $^{238}PuO_2$ (53). The ^{238}Pu isotope has greater solubility owing to its high specific activity, and hence it is transported to bone more quickly than is ^{239}Pu.

Management of Plutonium Contamination

A useful general reference for treatment of many internal emitters, including plutonium, is the report published by the National Council on Radiation Protection and Measurements (10). Although it was published almost 20 years ago, the material is still highly relevant, and almost no new therapies in this field have been devised since then.

ON-SITE MANAGEMENT

Emergency responders must assure that adequate breathing and circulation are present. Plutonium exposures usually do not involve serious physical injuries, and so the need for life-saving treatment is unlikely. In the event that cardiopulmonary resuscitation is needed in a person who also has high external contamination levels on the face, as determined by health physicists at the facility, use of a mechanical respirator is advisable.

All cases of plutonium exposure will require some level of external decontamination—usually clothing, hands, or face. Monitoring should be done with α survey instruments by a health physicist or technician familiar with the special requirements of α monitoring. Clothing is removed. Skin is washed with soap and detergent. For contamination of a large skin area, a shower is the best procedure. Repeat monitoring is conducted between washings. In some cases, hair clipping may be necessary. A washcloth or sanitary pad, not scrub brushes, should be used for gentle scrubbing. If detergents are not fully effective, use of household bleach (sodium hypochlorite) in full strength may be more successful on tougher skin areas, but a 1:4 dilution with water is recommended for use on sensitive skin, face, around eyes, or wounds. If internal uptake of plutonium is possible, the external decontamination procedures should be completed as quickly as possible so as to get on with evaluation and possible treatment. The first goal of skin decontamination is to remove the transportable (loose) contaminants. Fixed contaminants can be left for additional decontamination later.

WOUND DECONTAMINATION

Most frequently, contaminated wounds are small cuts or punctures of the hand. Evaluation of the level of contamination requires the use of a wound counter and an operator familiar with the equipment and its calibration procedure. Use of an α survey instrument can be misleading. Any moisture, blood, or tissue over the area being counted is sufficient to block detection of the α radiation. Wound counters, unlike α survey instruments, are designed to detect more penetrating photons that will be present. Treatment decisions are based on the amount of plutonium present in the wound. As a general rule, any wound with suspect contamination should be immediately rinsed with running tap water or saline irrigation. Use of a pulsating water jet stream may be helpful. If the wound counter still indicates activity, a decision must be made as to whether the radioactivity is located in the wound or on nearby external skin areas. Use of a thin metal sheet with a small open aperture placed over the wound area may be helpful in locating the main site of the contamination.

If the activity in the wound is less than 74 Bq (2 nCi), more than careful wound cleansing usually is not necessary. If the activity is between 74 Bq (2 nCi) and 370 Bq (10 nCi), wound excision may be undertaken if it is located such that no functional impairment will result from the surgery. The procedure is elective, and the decision includes the wishes of the patient. Wounds contaminated with more than 370 Bq (10 nCi) of plutonium should be excised, if possible. If the location of the wound raises questions of potential functional impairment, the services of an experienced surgeon and time to set up the wound counter at the hospital should be sought rather than rushing into the procedure in an emergency room or occupational medicine office. In any event, use of chelation therapy, as explained later, should be started as soon as a decision for wound excision is made.

INHALATIONAL EXPOSURE

The most difficult part in the management of inhalational exposures is likely to be the early decision regarding whether treatment is necessary. *In vivo* chest (lung) counts and measurement of plutonium excretion in urine are the two principal methods for obtaining quantitative exposure data. Lung counters are not highly sensitive in detecting plutonium itself, but their much better detection capability for americium (^{241}Am) often is useful. Americium is another transuranium element always present as a low percentage of the total radioactivity present in plutonium contamination cases. The Am-Pu ratio of the specific material involved in the exposure is measured so that the plutonium deposition can be calculated from the americium data. A problem with these sensitive counters shortly after an accident is the difficulty of determining whether the activity is on the skin or inside the chest. The importance of getting this type of measurement in the first few hours is overrated, but no time should be wasted in arranging for these counts before the important initial medical treatment decisions are made.

Urine samples measured for plutonium are the principal and most sensitive method of estimating the deposition of plutonium in the body. Urine levels reflect the plutonium concentration in the blood. The blood level soon after an inhalation depends on how soluble the inhaled plutonium particles are. After inhalation of high-fired insoluble plutonium oxide, the urinary excretion may be below minimum detection levels or at a low level for weeks to months before it begins to rise. Thus, early urine sample results may be misleading. Furthermore, the collection of a 24-hour sample plus a long processing time means that urine sample results will not be available at the time of early decision making. However, this information becomes very valuable in the days to come, when further decisions on treatment must be made. Twenty-four-hour urine samples should be collected each day for the first several days after an accidental exposure to evaluate the initial excretion pattern. Fecal samples are collected by some caregivers in the first days after an accident for plutonium analysis, but sample collection, analysis, and interpretation are difficult and seldom contribute much to patient care.

The immediate objective is to reach a decision regarding whether to treat the patient by chelation, preferably within the first 3 hours after exposure. The decision will be made on the basis of the circumstances of the accident, the length of exposure time, plutonium air concentrations in the room at the time of the accident, levels of contamination in the accident area, levels of contamination on the patient's clothing and skin, and early nose swipe results. In a plutonium facility, the health physicists and technicians are trained to take nose swipes immediately from individuals potentially exposed to contaminated air. The anterior chamber of each nostril is swiped with a separate moistened cotton-tipped swab. The swabs then are placed in separate clean containers, are dried, and then are counted for α activity. Levels of 500 disintegrations per minute (dpm) or less suggest a relatively low contamination level that does not require treatment. Persons with 2,000 dpm or higher in each nostril are good candidates for treatment. A gross disparity between the counts from the right and left nares—say 50 on one side and 2,000 on the other—suggests that the contamination may have come from nearby facial contamination or a contaminated finger. Less weight is given to such results. An obstructed nasal passage from a severely deviated septum or polyps may also cause such unequal findings. Results from nasal swipes taken 1 hour or more after the accident are not trustworthy as a result of possible nose blowing, snuffling water in the shower, and normal clearance from the anterior nares.

Irrigation of the mouth, nose, and nasopharynx is not normally performed in treating inhalation cases. Any contaminated material in these areas will be swallowed in the normal course of events and evacuated with feces. Because of the very low uptake from the GI tract, the passage of this material through it does not add significantly to the internal deposition.

Lung Lavage. Lavage of the lung bronchi has shown some therapeutic promise in animal studies for treating very high-level exposures. Dogs treated by lung lavage after the inhalation of insoluble radioactive particles have exhibited reductions of approximately 25% to 50% of the lung load (average, 44% in eight dogs) after five lavages of both right and left lungs. Radiation pneumonitis and early deaths were prevented in 75% of the treated dogs as compared to untreated dogs. In baboons, 60% to 90% of the lung burden of plutonium oxide was removed by ten pulmonary lavages. This treatment should be reserved for high doses of insoluble particles that might produce radiation pneumonitis or fibrosis. Persons who have inhaled high-fired plutonium oxide particles in excess of 1,000 nCi, might be suitable candidates for lavage therapy.

Lung lavage requires cooperation by a team of specialists who are experienced in this form of therapy. To date, it has been used only once in a human after inhalation of plutonium, with limited success. Physicians should bear in mind that the risk of the procedure, although small, is immediate, whereas potential late effects (e.g., such as lung cancer) from the radiation dose to the lung would occur many years later.

Chelation Therapy. Several chemical compounds are known to enhance the elimination of metals from the body by chelation, a process by which organic compounds exchange less firmly bonded ions for inorganic ions (metallic compounds) to form a relatively stable nonionized ring complex. This soluble complex is excreted in urine. Chelation therapy is most effective when it is begun immediately after exposure (within 3 hours, if possible), while the majority of metallic ions remains in extracellular fluids, before their incorporation into cells. Treatment at later times, even days or a few weeks later, may still be useful, but it will not be nearly as effective as when given in the first few hours after exposure.

The chelating agent of choice to treat plutonium exposures is DTPA. Data from persons treated with DTPA within approximately 3 hours of exposure indicate that approximately 60% or more of soluble forms of plutonium are removed. DTPA does not cross cell membranes, so it does not effectively chelate intracellular material. DTPA also is not effective for inhaled insoluble plutonium particles. Insoluble particles remain primarily in the lung initially, and only tiny amounts of plutonium are present in the blood and extracellular fluids soon after exposure. Because solubility of inhaled plutonium is unknown in the first hours after an accident, giving DTPA as a therapeutic trial often is necessary. Its effectiveness is determined by the quantity of plutonium excreted in urine during the following 24 hours.

Two forms of DTPA used clinically are the calcium salt (CaDTPA) and the zinc salt (ZnDTPA). CaDTPA is approximately ten times more effective than ZnDTPA (at least in rats) when given promptly after inhalational exposure to plutonium. Thus, CaDTPA is generally preferred for use during the first day or two after inhalational exposure or in the setting of contaminated wounds. After that, ZnDTPA is, for all practical purposes, as effective as CaDTPA. ZnDTPA is recommended for longer-term treatment and for use in pregnant women because it has less toxicity resulting from the loss of vital trace metals from the body.

The recommended dose of DTPA is 1 g delivered once daily, which may be repeated on 5 successive days each week. The daily dose should not be fractionated. It can be given either intravenously or by aerosol inhalation. Intravenous administration of 1 g DTPA diluted in 250 mL of normal saline or 5% glucose in water over 15 to 30 minutes has been the traditional procedure. An alternate procedure—1 g diluted in 10 to 20 mL of normal saline and injected intravenously by syringe over 5 minutes—is preferred by some physicians. In either case, care should be taken to avoid extravasation outside the vein. Aerosol administration is accomplished with 1 g CaDTPA (1:1 dilution with water or saline) placed in a nebulizer.

No serious toxicity in humans has been reported as a result of more than 600 CaDTPA and 1,000 ZnDTPA administrations in recommended doses. Long-term, low-dose administrations in one patient (1 g CaDTPA per week) caused no adverse effects after 4 years. CaDTPA binds and causes excretion of trace metals, such as zinc and manganese. Reduction of these two metals apparently accounts for the toxicity seen after high doses in animal experiments. Doses exceeding 2,000 mol per kg can produce severe lesions of the kidneys, intestinal mucosa, and liver in animals. The clinical human dose range is 10 to 30 mol per kg. Teratogenesis and fetal death have occurred in mice when similarly high doses are given throughout gestation.

DTPA is not to be used in minors. A blood count and clinical urinalyses should be obtained before the drug is administered. Blood pressure and pulse should be monitored during drug infusion. Significant leukopenia, thrombocytopenia, or impaired kidney function are contraindications to DTPA use. DTPA treatment should be discontinued if diarrhea occurs.

Both CaDTPA and ZnDTPA are approved as investigational new drugs in the United States. A specific treatment protocol and follow-up reports are required under the terms of the investigational new drug agreement. For physicians having a potential need for these drugs, DTPA can be requested from the Oak Ridge Associated Universities, REACTS Center, Oak Ridge, TN 37831-0117 (phone: 423-576-3131).

OTHER TRANSURANIUM ELEMENTS

The transuranic elements other than plutonium were discovered from mid-1942 through 1970, when element 105 (proposed name, *nielsbohrium*) was discovered. All these elements, from americium (atomic number 95) through element 105, were discovered in nuclear reaction processes. Many have very short half-lives.

Curium

Curium (atomic number 96) was named after Marie and Pierre Curie. Curium was the third transuranium element to be discovered by Seaborg, James, and Ghiorso in 1944 as a result of helium-ion bombardment of ^{239}Pu. The isotope ^{242}Cm has a half-life of 163 days, and ^{244}Cm has a half-life of 26 minutes. Production of ^{242}Cm and ^{244}Cm is from americium isotopes (see Fig. 116-3). ^{247}Cm has a half-life of 16 million years, and ^{249}Cm has a half-life of 350,000 years. The serial production of Cm isotopes is as follows:

$$^{214}Cm \xrightarrow[n,\gamma]{} {}^{245}Cm \xrightarrow[n,\gamma]{} {}^{246}Cm \xrightarrow[n,\gamma]{} {}^{247}Cm \xrightarrow[n,\gamma]{} {}^{248}Cm$$

^{248}Cm is also the α decay daughter ^{252}Cf. Curium metal melts at 1,340°C and exists in aqueous solution as Cm^{3+} predominantly. Compounds of CmO_2, CmF_4, Cm_2O_3, CmF_3, CmC_1, and $CmBr_3$, CmI_3 have been prepared.

Americium

Americium (atomic number 95) was the fourth transuranium element to be discovered. The isotope ^{241}Am was identified in 1944 as a result of successive neutron capture reactions by plutonium isotopes (see Fig. 116-2). ^{241}Am has a half-life of 433 years, and ^{243}Am has a half-life of 7,370 years. Americium is a silver-white reactive metal with a melting point of 1,176°C. The element exists in four oxidation states in aqueous solution:

Am^{3+}	salmon
Am^{4+}	pink-red
AmO_2^{+}	yellow
AmO_2^{2+}	light tan

AmO_2^{+} is unstable and forms Am^{3+} and AmO_2^{2+}. Am^{4+} is unstable in solution unless in the form of a fluoride. Important oxide compounds are americium dioxide (AmO_2) and americium trioxide (Am_2O_3). Americium forms halides (AmF_2, AmF_3, AmF_4, $AmCl_2$, AmI_2, and AmI_3). ^{241}Am is present in plutonium as a decay product from ^{241}Pu and in amounts that increase as the plutonium ages.

Neptunium

Neptunium (atomic number 93) has a silvery appearance and is chemically reactive with five oxidation states in solution:

Np^{3+}	pale purple
Np^{4+}	yellow green
NpO_2^{+}	green/blue
NpO_2^{2+}	pale pink
NpO_6^{5-} or NpO_5^{3-}	green

Neptunium forms trihalides and tetrahalides (NpF_3, NpF_4, $NpCl_3$, $NpCl_4$, $NpBr_3$, and NpI_3) and various oxides, including Np_3O_8 and NpO_2. ^{237}Np isotope (half-life, 2.2×10^6 years) is a byproduct of nuclear reactors. Trace quantities are found in nature.

Neptunium radionuclides are produced in the nuclear reaction of uranium to plutonium. The Fermi series of reactions that produce neptunium radionuclides can proceed from ^{235}U or from ^{238}U:

$$^{238}U \xrightarrow[n,\gamma]{} {}^{239}U \xrightarrow[t_{1/2} = 23.5\text{ min}]{\beta^-} {}^{239}Np \xrightarrow[t_{1/2} = 2.33\text{ d}]{\beta^-} {}^{239}Pu$$

$$^{235}U \xrightarrow[n,\gamma]{} {}^{236}U \xrightarrow[n,\gamma]{} {}^{237}U \xrightarrow[t_{1/2} = 6.75\text{ d}]{\beta^-} {}^{237}Np \xrightarrow{n,\gamma} {}^{238}Np$$

$$\xrightarrow[t_{1/2} = 2.10\text{ d}]{\beta^-} {}^{238}Pu \xrightarrow[n,2n]{} {}^{236}Np \xrightarrow[t_{1/2} = 22\text{ h}]{\beta^-} {}^{236}Pu$$

^{239}Np is fissionable, but only with fast neutrons. Neptunium radionuclide decay patterns are shown in Figure 116-4.

Berkelium

Berkelium (atomic number 97) was discovered in 1949 by Seaborg, Thompson, and Ghiorso as the fifth transuranium element, produced by cyclotron bombardment of ^{241}Am with helium atoms. Berkelium has two oxidation states in aqueous solution: Bk^{3+} (green-yellow) and an unstable Bk^{4+} (yellow). Oxides include BkO_2 and Bk_2O. Halides are BkF_3, BkF_4, $BkCl_3$, $BkBr_3$, and BkI_3. ^{249}Bk has a half-life of 314 days and is produced by neutron bombardment of ^{244}Cm.

Californium

Californium (atomic number 98) is the sixth transuranium element, discovered in 1950 by helium bombardment of ^{242}Cm. ^{249}Cf, with a half-life of 352 years, is produced as the β-decay product of ^{249}Bk:

$$^{249}Bk \xrightarrow[(n,\gamma)]{} {}^{250}Bk \xrightarrow{\beta^-} {}^{250}Cf \xrightarrow[(n,\gamma)]{} {}^{251}Cf \xrightarrow[(n,\gamma)]{} {}^{252}Cf$$

In an aqueous solution, californium exists mainly as Cf^{3+} (green). Oxides include CfO_2 and Cf_2O_3. Halides include CfF_3, $CfCl_3$, $CfBr_2$, $CfBr_3$, and CfI_3. The metal californium is very volatile.

Einsteinium

Einsteinium (atomic number 99) was named after Albert Einstein and discovered in 1952 from the debris of a thermonuclear explosion. The isotope ^{253}Es has a half-life of 20.5 days, ^{254}Es has a half-life of 276 days, and ^{255}Es has a half-life of 38.3 days. Einsteinium is an even more volatile metal than is californium. In aqueous solution, it exists as Es^{3+} (green). Solid compounds of einsteinium include Es_2O_3, $EsCl_3$, EsOCl, $EsBr_2$, $EsBr_3$, EsI_2, and EsI_3.

Fermium

Fermium (atomic number 100), named after Enrico Fermi, was the eighth transuranium element to be discovered, in 1953, as debris in a thermonuclear explosion. The isotope identified was ^{255}Fm, originating from the β particle decay of ^{255}U. ^{257}Fm has the longest half-life, 80 days. In aqueous solution, fermium exists as Fm^{3+}.

Mendelevium

Mendelevium (atomic number 101), named after Dimitri Mendeleer, is the ninth transuranium element, discovered in 1955 after bombardment of ^{253}Es with helium. The isotope ^{256}Md was produced, which decays to ^{256}Fm, which itself decays with a half-life of 1.5 hours.

Nobelium

Nobelium (atomic number 102) was named after Alfred Nobel and is the tenth transuranium element, discovered in 1958. The first isotope was ^{254}No, with a half-life of 55 seconds.

Lawrencium

Lawrencium (atomic number 103) is the eleventh transuranium element and was discovered in 1961. The isotope produced by bombardment of californium with boron ions was ^{258}Lr, which has a half-life of 5 seconds. ^{256}Lr has a longer half-life of 35 seconds. The 3+ state appears to be the only stable oxidation state of lawrencium in aqueous solution.

Elements 104 and 105

Element 104, the first transactinide element, was discovered by the bombardment of ^{249}Cf with ^{12}C ions to produce $^{257}104$ and $^{259}104$. ^{248}Cm was bombarded with ^{18}O ions to form $^{261}104$. Half-lives were 4, 3, and 70 seconds, respectively. These isotopes are characterized by α particle emission during decay. Element 104 was named *rutherfordium* (Rf) after Lord Ernest Rutherford.

Element 105 is the second transactinide element. It was discovered in 1970 and decayed with α particle emissions with a half-life of 2 seconds. The isotope $^{260}105$ was prepared at Berkeley from reaction of ^{14}N ions on ^{249}Cf and has been identified as an α emitter. The name *nielsbohrium* (Ns) was proposed.

REFERENCES

1. Gofman J. *Radiation and human health.* San Francisco: Sierra Club Books, 1981.
2. Scott LM. Environmental monitoring and personnel protection in uranium processing. In: Hodge HC, Stannard JN, Hursh JB, eds. *Uranium-plutonium-transplutonic elements.* New York: Springer-Verlag, 1973:271–306.
3. Anonymous. World list of nuclear power plants. *Nuclear News* 1988;69–88.
4. Walton H. *Uranium industry annual 1987 preliminary data.* Presented to the U.S. Council for Energy Awareness Fuel cycle 88 conference, April 1988.
5. Stoetzel GA, Moore RH, Fisher DR, Quilici DG, McCormack WD, Hoenes GR. *Occupational exposures to uranium: processes, hazards and regulations.* Rep. no. PNL-3341 USUR-01. Springfield, VA: National and Technical Information Service, 1981.
6. Wrenn ME, Durbin PW, Howard B, et al. Metabolism of ingested U and RA. *Health Phys* 1985;48:601–633.
7. Leggett RW, Harrison JD. Fractional absorption of ingested uranium in humans. *Health Phys* 1995;68:484-498.
8. Yulie CL. Animal experiments. In: Hodge HC, Stannard JN, Hursh JB, eds. *Uranium-plutonium-transplutonic elements.* New York: Springer-Verlag, 1973:165–196.
9. West CM, Scott LM. Uranium cases showing long chest burden retention—an update. *Health Phys* 1969;17:781.
10. National Council on Radiation Protection and Measurements. *Management of persons accidentally contaminated with radionuclides.* NCRP rep. 65. Washington: National Council on Radiation Protection and Measurements Publications, 1980.
11. Beau PG, Chalabreysse J. Knowledge gained from bioassay data on some metabolic and toxicological features of uranium hexafluoride and of its degradation products. *Radiat Protect Dos* 1989;26:107–112.
12. Hursh JB, Spoor NL. Data on man. In: Hodge HC, Stannard JN, Hursh JB, eds. *Uranium-plutonium-transplutonic elements.* New York: Springer-Verlag , 1973:197–239.
13. Chalabreysse J. Etudes et resultats d'examens effectues à la suite d'une inhalaton de composess dits solubles d'uranium naturel. *Radioprot* 1970;5:305–310.
14. Durbin PW. Metabolic models for uranium. In: *Biokinetics and analysis of uranium in man.* F1-F65. U.S. Uranium Registry rep. no. USUR-05-HEHF-47. Springfield, VA: National Technical Information Service, 1984,
15. Morrow PE, Leach LJ, Smith FA, et al. *Acute effects of inhalation exposure to uranium hexafluoride and patterns of deposition.* Rep. no. NUREG/CR-1045. Springfield, VA: National Technical Information Service, 1980.
16. Wrenn ME, Lipsztein J, Bertelli L. Pharmacokinetic models relevant to toxicity and metabolism for uranium in humans and animals. *Radiat Protect Dos* 1989;26:243–248.
17. Neuman WF, Tishkoff GH. The deposition of uranium in bone. In: Voegtlin C, Hodge HC, eds. *Pharmacology and toxicology of uranium compounds.* National Nuclear Energy Series. New York: McGraw-Hill, 1953:1911–1991.
18. Donoghue JK, Dyson ED, Hislop JS, Leach AM, Spoor NL. Human exposure to natural uranium: a case history and analytical results from some postmortem tissues. *Br J Ind Med* 1972;29:81–89.
19. International Commission on Radiological Protection. *Individual monitoring for intakes of radionuclides by workers: design and interpretation.* ICRP publ. no. 54. *Ann ICRP* 1988;19:209–236.
20. International Commission on Radiological Protection. Dose coefficients for intakes of radionuclides by workers. ICRP publ. no. 68. *Ann ICRP* 1994;24(4):1–83.
21. International Commission on Radiological Protection. Age-dependent dose to members of the public from intake of radionuclides: 3. Ingestion dose coefficients. ICRP publ. no. 69. *Ann ICRP* 1995;25(1):1–74.
22. International Commission on Radiological Protection. Age-dependent doses to members of the public from intake of radionuclides: 5. Compilation of ingestion and inhalation dose coefficients. ICRP publ. no. 72. *Ann ICRP* 1996;26(1):1–91.
23. Diamond GL. Biological consequences of exposure to soluble forms of natural uranium. *Radiat Protect Dos* 1989;26:23–33.
24. Howland JW. Studies in human exposure to uranium compounds. In: *Pharmacology and toxicology of uranium compounds,* vol 2. New York: McGraw-Hill 1949:993–1017.
25. Moore RH, Kathren RL. A World War II uranium hexafluoride inhalation event with pulmonary implications for today. *J Occup Med* 1985;27:753–756.
26. National Academy of Science/National Research Council. Uranium. In: *Health risks of radon and other internally deposited alpha-emitters.* BEIR-IV, Committee on the Biological Effects of Ionizing Radiation. Washington: National Academy Press, 1988:276–302.
27. Hodge HC. A history of uranium poisoning (1824–1942). In: Hodge HC, Stannard JN, Hursh JB, eds. *Uranium-plutonium-transplutonic elements.* New York: Springer-Verlag, 1973:5–68.
28. Stannard JN. Uranium and man. In: *Biokinetics and analysis of uranium in man.* D1-D26. U.S. Uranium Registry rep. no. USUR-05 HEHF-47. Springfield, VA: National Technical Information Service, 1984:D3.
29. Spoor NL, Harrison NT. *Emergency exposure levels for natural uranium.* National Radiographical Protection Board rep. no. NRPB-R1111. Harwell, England: National Radiographical Protection Board, 1980:15.
30. Dounce AL, Roberts E, Wills JH. Catalasuria as a sensitive test for uranium poisoning. In: Voegtlin C, Hodge HC, eds. *Pharmacology and toxicology of uranium compounds,* vol 1. New York: McGraw-Hill, 1949:889–950.
31. Clarkson TW, Kench JE. Urinary excretion of amino acids by men absorbing heavy metals. *Biochem J* 1952;62:361–271.
32. Thun MJ, Baker DB, Steenland K, Smith AB, Halperin W, Berl T. Renal toxicity in uranium mill workers. *Scand J Work Environ Health* 1985;11:83–90.
33. Morrow PE. Biokinetics and toxicology of uranium. In: *Biokinetics and analysis of uranium in man.* D1-E27. U.S. Uranium Registry rep. no. USUR-05 HEHF-47. Springfield, VA: National Technical Information Service, 1984.
34. Wagoner JK, Archer VE, Carroll BE, el al. Cancer mortality patterns amongst U.S. uranium miners and millers, 1950 through 1962. *J Natl Cancer Inst* 1964;32:787–801.
35. Archer VE, Wagoner JK, Lundin FE. Cancer mortality among uranium mill workers. *J Occup Med* 1973;15:11–14.

36. Poledak AP, Frome EL. Mortality among men employed between 1943 and 1947 at a uranium processing plant. *J Occup Med* 1981;23:169–178.
37. Archer VE. Health concerns in uranium mining and milling. *J Occup Med* 1981;23:502–505.
38. Cookfair DL, Beck WL, Shy C, Lushbaugh CC, Sowder CL, Lung cancer among workers at a uranium processing plant. In: *Epidemiology applied to health physics.* CONF-830101. Springfield, VA: National Technical Information Service, 1983:398–406.
39. Waxweiler JK, Archer VE, Roscoe RJ, Watanabe A, Thun MJ. Mortality patterns among a retrospective cohort of uranium mill workers. In: *Epidemiology applied to health physics.* CONF-830101. Springfield, VA: National Technical Information Service, 1983:428–435.
40. Checkoway H, Pearce N, Crawford-Brown DJ, Cragle DL. Radiation doses and cause-specific mortality among workers at a nuclear materials fabrication plant. *Am J Epidemiol* 1988;127:255–266.
41. Dupree EA, Cragle DL, McLain RW, et al. Mortality among workers at a uranium processing facility, the Linde Air Products Company ceramics plant, 1943–1949. *Scand J Work Environ Health* 1987;13:100–107.
42. Burr WW. Human experience and epidemiology. In: *Biokinetics and analysis of uranium in man.* H1-H21. US Uranium Registry rep. no. USUR-05 HEHF-47. Springfield, VA: National Technical Information Service, 1984.
43. Henge-Napoli MH, Rongier E, Ansoborlo E, Chalabreysse J. Comparison of the in vitro and in vivo dissolution rates of two diuranates and research on an early urinary indicator of renal failure in humans and animals poisoned with uranium. *Radiat Protect Dos* 1989;26:113–117.
44. Lincoln TA, Voelz GL. Management of persons accidentally exposed to uranium compounds. In: Ricks RC, Fry SA, eds. *The medical basis for radiation preparedness: II. Clinical experience and follow-up since 1979.* New York: Elsevier Science, 1990:221–230.
45. Wessman RA. An overview of the radiochemical analysis of uranium. In: *Biokinetics and analysis of uranium in man.* JA-J57. U.S. Uranium Registry rep. no. USUR-05 HEHF-47. Springfield, VA: National Technical Information Service, 1984.
46. Palmer HE. In vivo counting of uranium. In: *Biokinetics and analysis of uranium in man.* I1-I29. U.S. Uranium Registry rep. no. USUR-05 HEHF-47. Springfield, VA: National Technical Information Service, 1984.
47. MacNider WDB. The inhibition of the toxicity of uranium nitrate by sodium carbonate, and the protection of the kidney acutely nephropathic from uranium from the toxic action of an anesthetic by sodium carbonate. *J Exp Med* 1916;23:171–187.
48. Catsch A. Die Wirkung einger Chelatbidner auf die akute Toxicitat von Uranylnitrat. *Klin Wachr* 1959;37:657–666.
49. Catsch A. *Radioactive metal mobilization in medicine.* Springfield, IL: Charles C Thomas Publisher, 1964:9, 57, 105–106.
50. Ivannikov AT. *On medicative application of complexing agents in the case of uranium intoxication.* Central Scientific Institute of Information and Technical Research on Nuclear Science and Technology. Moscow: TsNIIatominform, 1987:3–15.
51. Voelz GL. Health considerations for workers exposed to plutonium. *Occup Med* 1991;6(4):681–694.
52. Stannard JN. *Radioactivity and health: a history.* DOE/RL/01830-T59. Richland, WA: Battelle Pacific Northwest Laboratory, 1988.
53. Thompson RC. *Life span effects of ionizing radiation in the beagle dog.* Rep. no. PNL-6822. Richland, WA: Battelle Pacific Northwest Laboratory, 1989.
54. Stannard JN. Plutonium toxicology and other toxicology. In: Jee WSS, ed. *The health effects of plutonium and radium.* Salt Lake City: JW Press, 1976:363–372.
55. Cohen BL. Hazards from plutonium toxicity. *Health Phys* 1977;32:359–379.
56. Koshurnikova NA, Bolotnikova MG, Ilyin LA, et al. Lung cancer risk due to exposure to incorporated plutonium. *Radiat Res* 1998;149:366–371.
57. Tokarskaya ZB, Okladnikova ND, Belyaeva ZD, Drozhko EG. Multifactorial analysis of lung cancer dose-response relationships for workers at the Mayak nuclear enterprise. *Health Phys* 1997;73:899–905.
58. Tokarskaya ZB, Okladnikova ND, Belyaeva ZD, Drozhko EG. The influence of radiation and nonradiation factors on the lung cancer incidence among the workers of the nuclear enterprise Mayak. *Health Phys* 1995;69:356–366.

CHAPTER 117
Latex

Donald W. Kautz and John B. Sullivan, Jr.

SOURCES AND PRODUCTION

Natural rubber latex (NRL) is a milky fluid produced by lactiferous cells within the phloem of the *Hevea brasiliensis* tree. NRL contains carbohydrates, lipids, phospholipids, proteins, and *cis*-1,4-polyisoprene. Chemically, latex is a complicated arrangement of highly anastomosed cells that synthesize the *cis*-1,4-polyisoprene. The isoprene subunit is the backbone of the biomolecules that compose NRL. NRL contains a wide range of proteins and polypeptides to which exposed individuals may develop allergic reactions.

Rubber trees require 8 to 10 years to reach maturity before they can be tapped for natural latex. Approximately 150 adult trees will produce nearly 100 g of solid natural latex per week. This will make approximately 10 pairs of surgical gloves, or 1,500 pairs per acre of trees. NRL products are used in a wide range of medical applications owing to the unique combination of strength, flexibility, elasticity, tear resistance, and barrier qualities of natural rubber.

Latex is also a general term sometimes used for a material's coating properties. For example, in the paint industry, the name *latex paint* is used for many types of both oil- and water-based paints, despite the fact that there is no NRL in latex paint.

During World War II, natural rubber use escalated and eventually supplied 100% of the market. Today, natural rubber supplies approximately 35% of the market. Synthetic rubber has replaced natural rubber in many arenas. Also, the addition of chemical additives to rubber products has greatly expanded the market application of rubber. Additives used in the vulcanization process include accelerators, curing agents, antioxidants, retardants, and other agents that can cause dermatitis.

LATEX ALLERGY: PREVALENCE AND INCIDENCE

Allergy to latex products such as surgical gloves is a growing medical problem (1–5). At a minimum, approximately 3% of hospital-based physicians and nurses may be affected, and higher rates have been reported in surgical units. Other estimates, based on skin test results, give a higher prevalence of latex allergy, ranging from 10% to 17% among health care workers and 40% to 65% in children with myelodysplasia (spina bifida) (6–9). Others note that health care and rubber industry workers were affected by latex allergies at a rate of approximately 11% (4).

Direct contact with the rubber may not be necessary for the initiation of a latex reaction, indicating that at least some antigens may be aerosolized. Antigen may even be carried on syringe needles from the rubber stoppers of multiple-use vials.

Allergic reactions typically are local and may be delayed or immediate. Systemic reactions can be potentially fatal and include asthma and anaphylaxis. Latex-allergic patients are at risk in the health care setting, as the latex proteins can be absorbed in the glove powder and then aerosolized.

More than 15 immunoglobulin E (IgE)-binding polypeptides have been identified in individuals with latex sensitivity or from pooled sera of sensitized patients (6). Proteins described include 14-, 20-, and 27-kD proteins. The 14-kD protein is referred to as a *rubber elongation factor* and may be a major NRL allergen (10). However, NRL is a complex source of antigens, and research has demonstrated great variation in the antigen content of both NRL and latex glove extracts (11).

Severe and sometimes fatal anaphylactic reactions to latex have raised awareness of the risks to those exposed. In the 1980s, the U.S. Food and Drug Administration (FDA), noting a number of deaths from anaphylaxis, issued an alert regarding latex allergies. Since that time, published reports have estimated that 5% to 10% of physicians and nurses working in surgical areas and operating rooms are sensitized to latex gloves (7,9,12).

The total amount of protein that can be eluted from latex gloves varies widely, depending on the method used for extraction and measurement (11,13–15). Studies show that IgE antibodies in sera from sensitized individuals bind to several of the proteins extracted from latex gloves (11). Such studies, though, fail to detect lower-molecular-weight or higher-molecular-weight proteins that could serve as antigens (11). One study showed that at least six antigens present in NRL bind IgE (16). Such studies suggest that the natural proteins could be altered during manufacturing of gloves and also other rubber products, creating neoantigens. Allergens are also found in final products that are not found in NRL (11,16). The different methods of antigen detection—immunoblotting, immunoelectrophoresis, and radioimmunoelectrophoresis—may account for some of the antigen differences found in latex gloves. However, the total protein content of latex gloves and allergenicity are unrelated (11). Thus, total protein determinations are an ineffective method of screening or monitoring for the allergen content of latex gloves.

CLINICAL REACTIONS TO LATEX

Clinically significant reactions to latex can be divided into hypersensitivity reactions and nonallergic contact dermatitis (Table 117-1). Immediate hypersensitivity reactions can range from contact urticaria and asthma to anaphylaxis. In general, when large numbers of cases are reviewed, health care workers having latex allergies present mainly with hand eczema and allergic contact dermatitis (3,4). Many patients with latex allergy have a history of atopy.

Predisposing factors to latex allergy are hand eczema, allergic rhinitis, asthma, and allergic conjunctivitis in individuals exposed to latex. Also, glove powder binds latex proteins that can then be aerosolized, allowing significant aeroallergen exposure (4).

Type I Hypersensitivity

The major reaction to latex proteins are type I IgE-mediated. This reaction occurs as a response to inoculation or inhalation of the latex antigen in sensitized patients. The reaction can range from contact urticaria to asthma to fatal anaphylaxis. A person previously sensitized by any latex product might experience respiratory symptoms when inflating a child's balloon, or at the dentist's office if a rubber dam is used. The antigen in the IgE-mediated response is one or more latex proteins or polypeptides. Whether the protein antigen is intrinsic to latex or is a by-product that modifies the natural product is unclear. Another form of IgE-mediated allergic reaction from latex is contact urticaria. However, the dermatitis picture caused by latex can be highly variable, ranging from urticaria and eczema to keratosis, purpura, or achromia (3).

TABLE 117-1. Clinical reactions to natural rubber latex

Condition	Features
Irritant contact dermatitis	This condition is a result of direct skin injury that causes inflammation at the site of contact. Initial signs and symptoms are erythema, skin edema, itching, and burning. Chronic exposure can result in dry skin, fissuring, cracked skin, and papules. Lesions usually are isolated to glove contact areas. However, lesions may occur at distant sites owing to transfer of antigen. Risks are related also to chemicals being present, excessive powder, prolonged glove use, and occlusion.
Type I hypersensitivity	This condition is immunoglobulin E-mediated and may range from dermal contact urticaria to generalized urticaria, asthma, and anaphylaxis. This reaction is caused by the proteins contained in natural rubber latex.
Type IV hypersensitivity	This condition is T lymphocyte–mediated and is a delayed hypersensitivity reaction. Dermal lesions appear as clusters of erythematous, painful vesicles. Chronic exposure can lead to skin thickening and fissuring.

Type IV Hypersensitivity

Type IV latex hypersensitivity is a T cell–mediated immunologic reaction initiated by contact-sensitizing chemicals or protein allergens present in rubber. Additives include chemical sensitizers such as mercaptobenzothiazoles and carbamates. No symptoms occur during the initial sensitization period. The acute reaction occurs in 48 to 96 hours after exposure and usually involves vesicular skin eruptions of the hands or areas contacted. Chronic dermatitis can occur from prolonged and repeated exposure, resulting in skin that is dry, cracked, fissured, and thickened. These symptoms may extend beyond the boundary of the gloves.

Contact Dermatitis

Contact dermatitis is a common clinical reaction to latex products. Hand eczema is the most common dermatitis seen. The origin of the eczematous forms of latex reactions can be allergic or irritative (3). Eczematous lesions are diverse and may be sharply limited, giving an indication of the object or garment that has caused the dermatosis (glove, boot, mask, glasses, etc.). In other cases, the lesions are dispersed without precise limits. All clinical phases of eczema can be observed (erythema, papules, vesicles, scabs). Lesions may be found not only in the area of contact but also elsewhere, such as the eyebrows, genitalia, face, or flexion areas of the arms and legs, simulating atopy. In these cases, the lesions may be transferred by the hands to areas distant from direct contact with the allergen (17). However, the possible existence of aeroallergens has been documented (18).

Keratosis appears mainly on the palmar and plantar surfaces of the hands and feet, respectively. The lesions graduate from slight dryness with light scaling to the intense keratotic forms, with cracks simulating palmus plantar keratosis, psoriasis, and mycotic keratosis. These clinical forms are attributable to the action of an allergen on a specific area of the skin.

Hydroquinone and its derivatives are among the numerous substances that can cause leukoderma. These substances once were used commonly in the rubber industry as stabilizers; today, their use is less frequent.

Asthma

Latex-associated occupational asthma has been described (18,19). Diagnosis was made on the basis of a skin test response to latex in the presence of work-related respiratory symptoms, spirometry changes, and methacholine changes related to workplace exposure. Two of the workers examined were glove inspectors, and one worked in quality control. A fourth worker had findings suggestive of occupational asthma, but no workplace allergen could be identified. Therefore, the responsible antigen in these workers is likely to be in the latex solution itself. The route of sensitization was unclear, although one suspected route was airborne powder (cornstarch) that contained latex proteins (19). Studies indicate that cornstarch binds to aerosolized latex proteins, creating a significant aeroallergic NRL exposure, especially in medical centers. Asthmatic symptoms did not demonstrate as high a correlation with positive skin tests.

AT-RISK POPULATIONS

A careful history should be obtained from every patient before he or she undergoes any procedure involving contact with latex. The medical history, especially unexplained allergic or anaphylactic reactions during a medical procedure, may indicate sensitization. Contact dermatitis is the most frequent symptom. Respiratory tract symptoms are the second most common manifestation.

People who have a history of only mild latex-glove eczema rarely experience anaphylactic events. However, a history of severe or worsening latex glove–induced eczema, urticaria, or work-related conjunctivitis, rhinitis, asthma, or urticaria may indicate allergic sensitization and increased risk for more severe reactions in the future.

Powdered gloves normally contain a much higher level of protein that can be absorbed by the powder and transferred to the skin. When gloves are removed, the powder is aerosolized. When the next set of gloves is donned before the wearer washes his or her hands, the powder remains, so that allergens from the old powder and from the new are combined, thus increasing exposure.

With increasing use of latex, a concomitant increase in systemic and serious reactions has been noted. Populations at greatest risk of developing latex allergy include (i) health care workers, (ii) workers at plants that manufacture latex products, (iii) children with spina bifida, (iv) children or adults who have undergone multiple surgical procedures, and (v) workers who experience other occupational exposures.

The large percentage of children with spinal bifida with both atopy and NRL allergy suggests the possibility of a neuroimmunologic abnormality underlying these disorders (14). Preliminary reports correlating the risk of latex sensitization in children with spina bifida with the number of previously undergone major medical procedures raises the alternate possibility that the presumed excess of cases among this group is attributable to the children's very early and high level of exposure.

An allergic, atopic history appears to increase the risk of specific latex hypersensitivity, as does frequent latex exposure. Sussman and Beezhold (2) reported that 57% of the patients sensitized to latex gloves had a background of rhinitis, bronchial asthma, eczema, or food allergy.

Glove exposure appears to have a significantly greater correlation to the development of latex allergy than does contact with any other source of latex (9). Only 63% of symptomatic, test-positive allergic patients noted improvement on using powder-free gloves, demonstrating the reduced latex protein content in powder-free gloves but emphasizing that powder-free latex gloves are still allergy-inciting and should be avoided by allergic persons (7).

The risk for NRL allergy among health care workers appears to vary with the frequency and intensity of exposure. Among the most exposed (operating room) personnel, prevalence rates are higher, but other employees, such as housekeepers, also appear to have substantial rates of sensitization.

The diagnosis of NRL allergy should be expected in high-risk patients and in anyone who has a history of urticaria, angioedema of the lips when inflating balloons, or itching, burning, or urticaria when donning gloves. A history of adverse reactions to barium enema examinations or urticaria or other systemic symptoms incited by exposure to latex devices should raise suspicions.

TESTING FOR LATEX HYPERSENSITIVITY

Testing for latex IgE hypersensitivity has greatly improved with the advent of immunoassays. Scratch tests were performed initially but, in 1989, were replaced by skin-prick tests. For scratch testing, 7- to 10-mm scratches were made on the forearm with a sterile lancet, followed by application of 1-cm pieces of various brands of latex gloves used by the patients and 1-cm pieces of dried NRL. Cornstarch and talc reactions also were tested by placing a pinch of each on the scratch. Positive reactions after 20 minutes were graded as 2+ (erythema and wheal) and 3+ (erythema and wheal with pseudopods) at generated response.

Skin-Prick Testing

Skin-prick testing (SPT) has been used extensively for diagnosing NRL allergy. The method involves extracting elutable proteins by cutting 1 g of glove material into small pieces and soaking the pieces at room temperature in 5 mL of physiologic saline for 15 minutes.

In Europe, a standardized commercial NRL allergen for SPT became available in 1995. Nonstandardized allergens are available, but their sensitivity is questionable. In the United States, no standardized allergen is available, but work is under way to remedy this.

One study suggests that the larger the SPT response to the latex skin-test solution, the more likely patients are to report severe symptoms on exposure to latex (17). Results of latex SPT may therefore predict the severity of the clinical response to latex exposure. The study results showed that the information from the SPT was useful in advising high-risk patients as to the extent of precautions that must be taken to avoid such exposure and in determining the likely need for such patients to carry a syringe preloaded with epinephrine. When a reliable history cannot be obtained, the SPT response provides important health information and may allow health care providers to minimize patient risk by avoiding use of latex-containing products (17).

Reinheimer and Ownby (20) defined a positive SPT as more than 2 cm of erythema in the presence of a negative saline control. A positive intradermal test was defined as a wheal larger than 0.5 cm and more than 2.0 cm of erythema (20).

Jaeger et al. (18) found a good correlation (82%) between latex IgE radioallergosorbent test (RAST) and the latex skin-prick test, as revealed in a subgroup of 45 subjects. Some believe that the prick test is not very accurate; these researchers do not recommend prick tests for high-risk patients such as those with spina bifida (21).

TABLE 117-2. Foods containing allergens associated with natural rubber latex[a]

High	Low or undetermined
Avocado	Apricot
Banana	Cherry
Chestnut	Grape
Papaya (papain)	Grasses
Moderate	Hazelnut
Apple	Mugwort
Carrot	Mustard
Celery	Passion fruit
Fig	Pear
Kiwi	Peanut
Melons	Pepper
Potato	Pineapple
Peach	Ragweed
Tomato	Rye
	Soybean
	Strawberry
	Walnut
	Wheat

[a]Grouped according to their degree of association with natural rubber latex.

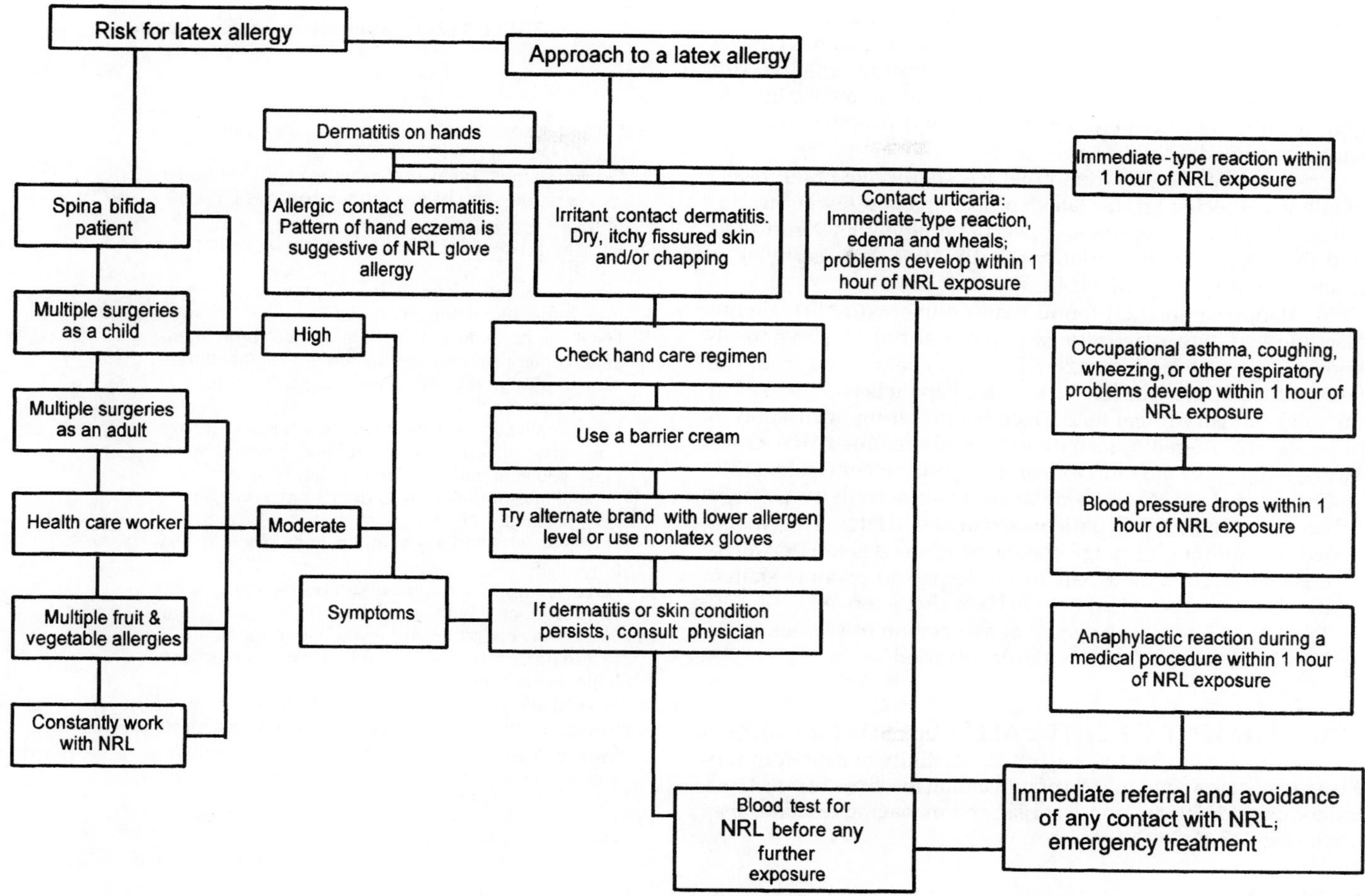

Figure 117-1. Management of latex allergies. NRL, natural rubber latex.

Radioallergosorbent Test

The presently available FDA-approved RAST uses a blood sample from a suspected NRL-sensitized individual and measures specific IgE antibodies against NRL allergens. This method is available from Pharmacia and Upjohn. The RAST appears to hold the best promise for the future of latex allergy testing.

Source material is from NRL without any treatment and consists of sap collected in saline. Activity is demonstrated with four major latex proteins (14 kD, 18 kD, 46 kD, and 110 kD) and six minor proteins (15 kD through 128 kD). The RAST clinically agrees with skin testing in 84% of cases. The method has a sensitivity of 75% and a specificity of 94%.

AlaSTAT Assay

AlaSTAT assay is an enzyme-linked immunometric assay that uses liquid-phase polymerized allergens and monoclonal antibodies to measure specific IgE. Ligand-labeled latex antigen matrix and individual serum samples are mixed in ligand-coated tubes and allowed to incubate. This permits any latex-specific IgE to bind to the latex matrix. A multivalent antiligand then is added, which creates a bridge between the IgE latex matrix and the ligand-coated tube. Next, the unbound IgE is removed by washing. Horseradish peroxidase–labeled monoclonal anti-IgE then is added to the tubes, incubated, and washed. A chromogenic substrate is added, and color development is terminated after 15 minutes. The resulting color is directly related to the amount of latex-specific IgE, which is interpolated from a standard curve (20).

CROSS-REACTIVITY AMONG LATEX, OTHER PLANTS, AND FOODS

Coincident IgE-mediated allergies to latex and multiple fruits or vegetables have been documented (22–26). *In vivo* and *in vitro* investigations of clinical specificity have produced complex patterns of allergenic cross-reactivity that suggest shared or common antigenic components among botanically unrelated plants. Although the details of the clinical association of latex and food allergies await further study, documentation of food allergies known to coexist with latex sensitivities may be useful for identifying the risks of latex exposure for some patients.

The high coincidence among symptoms elicited by latex, chestnut, and banana is unexplained by mere random association (22–24). An important correlation exists among SPT, RAST, and HR results against latex and chestnut, which suggests cross-reactivity. The total inhibition of chestnut RAST by a latex extract suggests the presence of a common allergen in latex and chestnut that is responsible for the symptomatology.

The existence of cross-reactivity among latex, avocado, chestnut, and banana through RAST inhibition has been demonstrated (23). Rodriguez's study (23) suggested that the three foods and latex share common antigenic determinants. Other fruits that show lower association rates with latex (kiwi, papaya, and fig) might also share some epitopes. Latex is an important allergen that shares antigenic determinants with various fruits that are not botanically related, a fact that has clinical consequences. If latex shares epitopic symptomatology with other fruits, the associated food sensitivities in a certain geographic area could depend on the type and proportion of the fruits consumed.

Crisi and Belsito (24) found that RASTs revealed high levels of allergen-specific IgE for latex and banana and lower but significant levels for avocado and peach. Of note, they also found that the RAST for latex allergy shortly after the anaphylactic reaction to SPT was equivocal.

Vandenplas et al. (25) found that a nurse with NRL allergy also showed skin reactivity to papain, although she had no known exposure to this enzyme, which is extracted from the latex of the papaya tree (*Carica papaya*). Papain is widely used in the food industry (meat tenderizer, beer clearing agent) and in pharmaceutical agents as a natural (herbal) treatment of necrotic ulcers, a digestive aid, and a cleaning agent for contact lenses.

Delbourg et al. (26), in a similar study, showed that an allergy to banana often occurs in patients sensitized to latex. They maintained that although the IgE-mediated responses to latex allergens is well documented, banana allergens and epitopes shared by these two allergens had not yet been characterized.

Table 117-2 shows the degree of association of various fruits and vegetables linked with NRL sensitization.

MANAGEMENT OF LATEX ALLERGIES

Management is a combination of preventing reactions in sensitized individuals, identifying those at risk, and managing reactions that occur (Fig. 117-1) (27–29).

Food and Drug Administration Guidelines for Health Professionals

As regards latex allergies, the FDA recommends certain guidelines to health professionals, including the following (27): When obtaining a general history from a patient, questions about latex sensitivity should be included (Table 117-3). For surgical and radiologic patients, spina bifida patients, and health care workers, this recommendation is especially important. Questions about itching, rash, or wheezing after wearing latex gloves or inflating a toy balloon may be useful. Charts of patients with positive histories should be flagged.

If latex sensitivity is suspected, the use of devices made with alternative materials, such as nitrile, vinyl, or plastic, should be considered. For example, a health professional could wear a nonlatex glove over the latex glove if the patient is sensitive. If both the health professional and patient are sensitive, a latex middle glove could be used. (Note that latex gloves labeled *hypoallergenic* may not always prevent adverse reactions.)

Whenever latex-containing medical devices are used, especially when the latex comes in contact with mucous membranes, the physician must be alert to the possibility of an allergic reaction. If an allergic reaction does occur and latex is suspected, the patient must be advised of a possible latex sensitivity and should consider giving permission to undergo a RAST test and evaluation.

Patients must be advised to tell health professionals and emergency personnel about any known latex sensitivity before undergoing medical procedures. The physician should consider advising patients with severe latex sensitivity to wear a medical identification bracelet.

The FDA is also asking health professionals to report incidents of adverse reactions to latex or other materials used in medical devices.

TABLE 117-3. Latex allergy questionnaire

Question	Yes	No
1. Do you have (or do you think you have) an allergy to natural latex or rubber?		
2. Do your hands "break out" when you put on rubber gloves or after you have worn these gloves for some time?		
3. Do your lips swell or tingle when you blow up balloons?		
4. Have you experienced vaginal or penile swelling or discomfort after using a condom?		
5. Have you had unusual swelling or discomfort after (a) a rectal or pelvic examination, (b) vaginal ultrasonography, (c) prostatic ultrasonography, or (d) a barium enema?		
6. Do your allergies or asthma worsen when you are in a hospital or other place where rubber gloves are worn?		
7. Have you ever had an allergic reaction to local or general anesthesia during a dental procedure, surgery, or childbirth?		
8. Have you ever had a systemic allergic reaction (anaphylaxis)?		
9. Have you ever experienced skin or respiratory problems associated with your job?		
10. How many operations have you had in the past, including dental surgeries and obstetric and gynecologic procedures?		
11. Are you allergic to any fruits or vegetables? Are any of your family members allergic to fruits or vegetables? Do any of you have hay fever or an animal allergy?		
12. Have you had any unexplained allergies after being treated at a health care facility?		
13. Do you work in the latex manufacturing industry?		
14. How often to you wear latex rubber gloves? __Very seldom __ Once per week __ Often __ Daily		

Latex Avoidance Procedures for Health Care Workers

Programs to educate health care workers in the care of latex-sensitive patients should be developed. These should include educational programs for patients and their families in the care and precautions that should be taken to prevent latex exposure (Table 117-4).

By touching any latex object, the health care worker can transmit the allergen by hand to the patient. Care should be

TABLE 117-4. Latex allergy guidelines for health care facilities

- Form a multidisciplinary latex allergy awareness committee.
- Develop a uniform policy for handling latex sensitization and allergic reactions.
- Develop a comprehensive standard questionnaire for patients and employees for detecting undiagnosed or confirmed latex allergy. This questionnaire should be part of the new employee orientation.
- Clarify in writing from manufacturers or distributors the latex rubber content of all products used in the facility. Set up a uniform system to update and disseminate this information.
- Develop carts carrying latex-free emergency equipment and adequate substitute devices. Cover such carts to prevent aerosolized glove powders from settling on the equipment.
- Develop and disseminate educational materials.
- Monitor the quality of the program.
- Educate personnel on the risks of latex allergy.
- Purchase latex-free gloves on recommendations of employee health and infection control personnel. Hypoallergenic gloves are *not* suitable as a substitute.

TABLE 117-5. Responsibilities in the care of the latex-sensitive surgical patient

- Assess all patients for latex sensitivity. Use a medical history questionnaire.
- Identify latex-allergic patients by using an allergy bracelet, flagging records, and posting a sign on the door (or some other means) to ensure that staff is aware of the allergy.
- Notify all hospital sections involved with the operation so that proper equipment and presurgical prophylaxis (if necessary) can be initiated.
- Remove all latex items from the patient's operating room and immediate holding area. Clean the operating room completely.
- Ensure that all personnel in contact with the patient are aware of the latex precaution.
- Secure the list of nonlatex alternatives and prepare ahead for the patient's needs.
- Schedule a latex-sensitive patient as the first case of the day.
- Mark the patient's operating room cart and the operating room doors for latex allergy.
- Avoid contact with all latex products during preoperative care.
- Ensure that examination gloves used in the room are synthetic, not latex.
- Use a cotton dressing to prepare the extremity that will be used to monitor blood pressure, to minimize exposure to the latex tubing.
- Use a stopcock rather than rubber ports to add medication to intravenous lines. Remove rubber stoppers to draw up medications. Use nonlatex catheter equipment.
- Instruct the scrub nurse to maintain a latex-free environment throughout the procedure.
- Communicate with the postanesthesia staff prior to the patient's arrival, to maintain the latex-free environment.
- Perform all procedures on children with spina bifida in a latex-free environment.

TABLE 117-6. Protocol for care of patients with confirmed or suspected latex allergy

- Medical staff should discuss with the patient the need for him or her to wear a medical bracelet alerting personnel to the risk of latex allergy.
- The patient's medical charts must be labeled to avoid the inadvertent introduction of latex products into the patient's room. Rooms should also be marked as latex-free, especially for the sensitized patient, as the mere removal of gloves can aerosolize powder that may cause an anaphylactic reaction.
- A clear notation must be made in the medical record of how a diagnosis or suspected diagnosis was made. Include any history or questionnaire.
- Examination gloves used in the room in which a latex-sensitive patient is receiving care should be nonlatex, whether or not the gloves actually come in contact with the patient. Hypoallergenic gloves should be considered latex-containing.
- Prepackaged kits and trays that contain latex products must not be used.
- Three-way stopcocks are placed in intravenous lines for the administration of medications (i.e., no latex injection ports).
- Rubber medication stoppers and intravenous rubber injection ports should not be used. If a rubber stopper is on a medication vial, it must first be removed rather than drawing through the stopper, which places latex on the needle.
- An educational plan should be developed to familiarize the staff, patient, and his or her family about latex allergies and precautions.
- A system should be established for reviewing all suspected reactions to natural rubber latex and monitoring the effectiveness of latex avoidance procedures.
- Patients with suspected latex sensitization should be referred to a physician for evaluation (enzyme-linked immunosorbent assay).
- Patients who have developed systemic symptoms or anaphylaxis should carry injectable epinephrine (0.3 cc) as emergency medication at all times.
- Patients in a high-risk group who have not exhibited symptoms of latex allergy should nonetheless have limited exposure to latex products when possible.

taken to keep the powder from the gloves away from the patient, because the powder can serve as a carrier for latex proteins. Therefore, to reduce the possibility of the latex protein becoming airborne, one must exercise care in not snapping gloves on and off; a better alternative is the use of powderless or nonlatex gloves. A readily available master list of latex-free devices and products should be kept and updated as necessary.

Latex-sensitive patients should be protected from unintended exposures in the same manner as are drug-sensitive patients. Some methods include a *latex-sensitive* alert notice worn on a wrist band, door or bed signs, flagging of records, or latex alert tags on hospitalized patients' garments (Tables 117-5, 117-6). Patients with any latex allergy should be encouraged to wear medical alert bracelets, necklaces, or tags, regardless of the severity of their reactions, as the allergic reaction may convert from a local to a systemic reaction.

Workers in private offices, clinics, and hospitals must be cognizant of possible risks to latex-sensitive patients and health care personnel. All products and medical procedures that come in intimate patient contact or are used by health care personnel must be reviewed for possible latex content. A readily available master list of items that are safe for sensitive patients may help to avoid unintended exposures.

Patients with myelomeningocele (spina bifida) should be referred for elective surgical procedures to centers in which latex-free surgical suites are available. Other patients with a history suggesting a high risk of anaphylaxis should be evaluated and appropriately tested before surgery, with recommendations to be made on a case-by-case basis.

Health care personnel who show signs of latex contact dermatitis or latex hypersensitivity should be encouraged to avoid continued exposure to natural latex products and to use either synthetic latex or nonlatex substitutes. Because the natural history of this condition is still unclear, however, some individuals have become anaphylactic-sensitive over time.

Patients and health care workers who are at risk should be cautioned about the risk of repeated reactions in situations of latex exposure, to include exposures both in the hospital and outside the medical environment.

Manufacturers are working on processes to remove proteins from latex. Some have created hypoallergenic gloves. However, a Department of Health and Human Services–FDA four-policy letter states that the term *hypoallergenic* is inconsistent and misleading with respect to latex-containing products. Such a labeling claim may put latex-sensitive users at risk for a serious adverse reaction.

The FDA believes that latex in devices poses a significant health risk to some patients and that the patients and their health care providers should be informed of its presence. Legislation has been recommended to put the following labeling into effect: "This product contains natural rubber latex." In light of the manufacturers' inability to keep the proteins out of latex either by removal or inactivation, the strategy of protection, substitution, and avoidance appears to be the only solution.

CONCLUSION

Enforcement by the U.S. Occupational Safety and Health Administration of the Centers for Disease Control and Prevention's universal precautions, latex gloves are being worn at a significantly higher rate, accounting for an increase in latex allergies. In addition, it has been suggested that inferior gloves on the market are subjecting people to higher concentrations of proteins in latex gloves. Many latex alternatives are available, and health care facilities, with the aid of infection control personnel, should begin to substitute these alternative products for latex-containing products, to ensure that barrier requirements are met safely and with the lowest risk possible.

Safe and effective means of testing for latex hypersensitivity are readily available. These tests will confirm IgE-mediated allergies and thus will help to prevent anaphylactic episodes.

REFERENCES

1. Aamir J, Safadi H, Manselik J, et al. A guinea pig model of hypersensitivity to allergy of natural rubber latex fractions. *Int Arch Allergy Immunol* 1996;110:187–194.
2. Sussman G, Beezhold D. Allergy to latex rubber. *Ann Intern Med* 1995;122(1): 43–46.
3. Conde-Salazar L. Rubber dermatitis. *Dermatol Clin* 1990;8(1):49–55.
4. Taylor JS, Praditsuwan P. Latex allergy: review of 44 cases including outcome and frequent association with allergic hand eczema. *Arch Dermatol* 1996;132:265–271.
5. Slater JE, Monsrello LA, Shaer C, Hosinger RW. Type 1 hypersensitivity to rubber. *Ann Allergy* 1990;65(5):411–414.
6. Hamann C. Natural rubber latex protein sensitivity in review. *Am J Contact Dermat* 1993;4:4–21.
7. Arellano R, Bradley J, Sussman G. Prevalence of latex sensitization among hospital physicians occupationally exposed to latex gloves. *Anesthesiology* 1992;77:905–908.
8. Yassin M, Lierl M, Fischer T, et al. Latex allergy in hospital employees. *Ann Allergy* 1994;72:245–249.
9. Lagier F, Vervloet D, Lhermet I, et al. Prevalence of latex allergy in operating room nurses. *J Allergy Clin Immunol* 1992;90:319–322.
10. Czuppon A, Chen Z, Rennert S, Engelke T, et al. The rubber elongation factor of rubber trees (*Hevea brasiliensis*) is the major allergen in latex. *J Allergy Clin Immunol* 1993;92:690–697.
11. Alenius H, Makinen-Kiljunen S, Turjanmaa K, Palosuo T, Reunala T. Allergen and protein content of latex gloves. *Ann Allergy* 1994;73:315–320.
12. Turjanmaa K. Incidence of immediate allergy to latex gloves in hospital personnel. *Contact Dermatitis* 1987;17:270–275.
13. Slater J, Chabra S. Latex antigens. *J Allergy Clin Immunol* 1992;89:673–678.
14. Alenius H, Palosuo T, Kelley K, et al. IgE reactivity to 14-kD and 27-kD natural rubber proteins in latex allergic children with spina bifida and other congenital abnormalities. *Int Arch Allergy Immunol* 1993;102:61–66.
15. Jones R, Scheppmann D, Heilman D, Yunginger J. Prospective study of extractable latex allergen contents of disposable medical gloves. *Ann Allergy* 1994;73:321–325.
16. Alenius H, Turhanmaa K, Palosuo T, et al. Surgical latex gloves allergy—characterization of rubber protein allergens by immunoblotting. *Int Arch Allergy Appl Immunol* 1991;96:376–380.
17. Hadjiliadis D, Banks D, Tarlo SM. Toronto: the relationship between latex skin-prick test responses and clinical allergic responses. *J Allergy Clin Immunol* 1996;97(6):1202–1206.
18. Jaeger D, Kleinhans D, Czuppon A, Baur X. Latex-specific proteins causing immediate-type cutaneous, nasal, bronchial, and systemic reactions. *J Allergy Clin Immunol* 1992;83(3):759–768.
19. Tarlo S, Wong L, Roos J, Booth N. Occupational asthma caused by latex in a surgical glove manufacturing plant. *J Allergy Clin Immunol* 1990;85(3):626–631.
20. Reinheimer G, Ownby D. Prevalence of latex-specific IgE antibodies in patients being evaluated for allergy. *Ann Allergy Asthma Immunol* 1995;74:184–187.
21. Moneret-Vautrin DA, Laxenaire M-C. Routine testing for latex allergy in patients with spina bifida is not recommended [Letter]. *Anesthesiology* 1991;391.
22. Blanco C, Carrillo T, Castillo R, Quiralte J, Cuevas M. Latex allergy: clinical features and cross-reactivity with fruits. *Ann Allergy* 1994;73:309–314.
23. Rodriguez M, Vega F, Garcia M, et al. Hypersensitivity to latex, chestnut, and banana. *Ann Allergy* 1993;70:31–34.
24. Crisi G, Belsito D. Contact urticaria from latex in a patient with immediate hypersensitivity to banana, avocado and peach. *Contact Dermatitis* 1993; 28:247–248.
25. Vandenplas O, Vandezande L-M, Halloy J-L, Delwiche J-P, Jamart J, Looze Y. Association between sensitization to natural rubber latex and papain. *J Allergy Clin Immunol* 1996;97(6):1421–1424.
26. Delbourg MF, Guillox L, Moneret-Vautfin DA, Ville G. Hypersensitivity to banana in latex-allergic patients. Identification of two major banana allergens of 33- and 37-kD. *Ann Allergy Asthma Immunol* 1996;76:321–326.
27. Gelb L. FDA medical alert: allergic reactions to latex-containing medical devices. US Department of Health and Human Services, Food and Drug Administration. *Public Health Sci* March 29, 1991;MDA91-1.
28. Position statement: latex allergy—an emerging healthcare problem. Latex Hypersensitivity Committee. *Ann Allergy Asthma Immunol* 1995;75:19–21.
29. Merguerian P, Klein R, Graven M, Rozycki A. Intraoperative anaphylactic reaction due to latex hypersensitivity. *Urology* 1991;37(4):301–303.

APPENDIX
Toxic Exposures and Environmental Health Resources

John B. Sullivan, Jr., Gary R. Krieger, Jude T. McNally, and Theodore G. Tong

The following resources are available to provide information for professionals and the public on toxic exposures and environmental health:

- Government agencies and institutions
- Poison control centers
- Environmental health consultants
- Physician consultants
- Professional organizations
- Internet sites
- Journals

GOVERNMENT AGENCIES AND INSTITUTIONS

U.S. Environmental Protection Agency (EPA)

EPA, general number for information: 202-260-2090
Operator assistance in directing call to the appropriate division

Office of Water: 800-426-4791 (hotline)
Groundwater, drinking water, wastewater management, wetlands, watersheds, oceans

Resource Conservation and Recovery Act (RCRA), Superfund (CERCLA) Emergency Planning and Community Right-to-Know (EPCRA): 800-535-0202; http://www.epa.gov/epaoswer/hotline
Identification, treatment, and storage of hazardous wastes.
Cleanup of hazardous wastes, oil spill program

Toxic Chemical Release Inventory System (EPA): 800-535-0202
Information about which chemicals are used, stored, released by companies

Toxic Substances Control Act (TSCA): 202-554-1404
Includes PCBs and asbestos

Safe Water Drinking Act (SDWA): 800-426-4791
Pollution: 202-260-1023
Prevention information clearinghouse

Indoor air quality: 800-438-4318
Chlorofluorocarbons (CFC) regulations: 800-296-1996
Stratospheric ozone

Asbestos: 800-368-5888
Small business assistance

Agency for Toxic Substances and Disease Registry (ATSDR)

ATSDR Information Center: 404-639-6300 (general information); 888-422-8737
1600 Clifton Road NE
Mailstop E-29

Atlanta, GA 30333
General ATSDR information resource

Public Information

Envir-O-Phone: 1-800-320-APIE
Public information on the environment 8:30 a.m.–5:30 p.m. (Eastern Standard Time, Mon–Fri); public questions about environmental issues

National Institute of Occupational Safety and Health

NIOSH information service: 800-356-4674
Technical specialist or NIOSH publications

Respiratory Disease

Lungline/National Jewish Hospital: 800-222-5864
Information on lung disease; to schedule an appointment or learn more about programs

Metals

Centers for Disease Control and Prevention: 404-639-2510 (general number); 888-232-6789 (publications)
Lead poisoning prevention

National Lead Information Center: 800-LEAD-FYI
Provides documents and publications, HUD lead inspection

Pesticides

National Pesticide Telecommunications Network (NPTN): 800-858-7378; http://ace.orst.edu/info/nptn/
Open 7 a.m.–7 p.m. (6:30 a.m.–4:30 p.m. Pacific Standard Time). Assistance with the following topics: pesticides, recognition and management of pesticide poisoning, toxicology of pesticides, environmental chemistry of pesticides

Sterilants, Disinfectants, Antimicrobial Products

National Antimicrobial Information Network (NAIN): 800-447-6349; 800-858-PEST (7378); http://ace.orst.edu/info/nain/
Oregon State University
323 Weniger Hall
Corvallis, OR 97331-6502
Service provides information on the following topics: antimicrobial products, disinfectants, sterilants, regulations and registration, interpretation of labels and permitted uses

Radon

National Safety Council Radon hotline: 800-SOS-RADON
Information on radon

Indoor Air Quality

American Society of Heating, Refrigerating and Air Conditioning Engineers, Inc. (ASHRAE): 404-636-8400
1791 Tullie Circle, NE
Atlanta, GA 30329-2305
Sets ventilation standards for acceptable indoor air quality (ASHRAE Standard 62-1989). Supplies technical information to professionals, products, and handbooks on energy efficiency, heating, ventilation, and air conditioning. Publishes the *ASHRAE Journal*

Center for Building Performance and Diagnostics: 412-268-2350
Department of Architecture
Carnegie-Mellon University
5000 Forbes Avenue
Pittsburgh PA 15213
Provides answers to questions and consultation on solar energy design, energy-related building performance, energy conservation, systems integration, and air quality. Center conducts seminars and workshops and distributes publications.

National Air Duct Cleaners Association (NADCA): 202-737-2926; 202-347-8847 (fax)
1518 K Street, NW, Ste 503
Washington, DC 20005
Publishes standards and guides (NADCA Standard 1992-01) relating to mechanical cleaning of nonporous air conveyance systems. NADCA offers a certifying examination for its members.

U.S. Environmental Protection Agency (EPA): 800-438-4318
Indoor Air Division
Indoor Air Quality Information Clearinghouse
PO Box 37133
Washington, DC 20013-7133

Office of Air and Radiation
401 M Street SW
Washington, DC 20460

North American Insulation Manufacturers Association (NAIMA): 703-684-0084; 703-684-0427 (fax)
44 Canal Plaza, Ste 310
Alexandria, VA 22314
Represents manufacturers of flexible duct liners and ductboard. The organization has produced guidelines for proper fabrication, installation, and maintenance of their members' products. Provides fibrous glass duct construction standards

Sheet Metal and Air Conditioning Contractor's National Association (SMACNA): 703-803-2980
4201 Lafayette Center Drive
Chantilly, VA 20151
Standards and guides governing the fabrication and installation of heating, ventilation and air conditioning (HVAC) systems (HVAC Duct Construction Standard—Metal and Flexible)

National Air Filtration Association (NAFA): 202-628-5328; 202-638-4833 (fax)
1518 K Street, NW, Ste 503
Washington, DC 20005
Members include air filter sales and service companies. NAFA developed the Certified Air Filtration Specialist program to recognize professionals knowledgeable in the technical aspects of air filtration. Certified individuals must pass an examination on air filtration principles, methods, and application. Provides guides to air filtration and publishes *NAFA Guide to Air Filtration*. A listing of members in your area can be obtained by calling.

Reproductive Toxicology

Teratogen Exposure Registry and Surveillance (TERAS): 617-732-7510
Department of Pathology

Brigham and Women's Hospital
75 Francis Street
Boston, MA 02115

TERAS is a network of geneticists and pathologists studying human embryos and fetuses exposed to teratogens. TERAS maintains information networks for consultation and evaluations.

MotherRisk Program: 416-813-6780
Hospital for Sick Children
555 University Avenue
Toronto, Ontario M5G1X8

The MotherRisk Program counsels callers about the safety of an exposure to drugs, chemicals, or radiation during pregnancy or breast feeding. The team of physicians and information specialists gives advice on whether medications, x-rays, or chemicals in the work environment will harm the developing fetus or breast-fed baby. Genetic counseling is available from the Genetic Department of the Hospital for Sick Children.

POISON CONTROL CENTERS

Poison control centers provide 24-hour-a-day consultation, collect data, and provide professional and public education about poisons and toxic exposures. The American Association of Poison Control Center (AAPCC) establishes criteria by which poison control centers are certified. AAPCC-designated centers include a medical director who is board-certified in medical toxicology; a managing director who is a registered nurse, pharmacist, or physician; and poison information specialists who are registered nurses or pharmacists and are certified by the AAPCC as poison information specialists. Specialists complete a training program approved by the medical director and are certified by the AAPCC by an examination.

The Canadian Association of Poison Control Center (CAPCC) maintains similar standards, and its members may join as associate members of the AAPCC. Other foreign institutions may join the AAPCC as an associate institutional member.

American Association of Poison Control Center

AAPCC: 202-362-7217; 202-362-8377 (fax); AAPCC@aol.com (E-mail)
3201 New Mexico Avenue NW, Ste 310
Washington, DC 20016
Executive Director: Toby Litovitz, MD

AAPCC-Designated Poison Control Centers

Akron Regional Poison Center: 216-379-8562 (emergency phone); 800-362-9922 (OH only); 216-379-8446 (TTY); 216-258-3066 (administrative phone); 216-379-8447 (fax)
1 Perkins Square
Akron, OH 44308

Alabama Poison Center: 800-462-0800 (emergency phone); 205-759-7994 (fax); fisher3@aol.com *or* jfisher@ua1vm.ua.edu (E-mail)
408-D Paul Bryant Drive
Tuscaloosa, AL 35401
AAPCC-Certified Regional Poison Center

Anchorage Poison Control Center: 907-261-3193 (emergency phone); 907-261-3633 (administrative phone); 907-261-3645 (fax)
Providence Hospital Pharmacy
PO Box 196604
Anchorage, AK 95516-6604

Arizona Poison and Drug Information Center: 520-626-6016 (emergency phone); 800-362-0101 (emergency phone, AZ only); 520-626-7899 (administrative phone); 520-626-2720 (fax); mcnally@tonic.pharm.arizona.edu (E-mail)
Arizona Health Sciences Center, Room 1156
1501 N Campbell Avenue
Tucson, AZ 85724
AAPCC Certified Regional Poison Center

Arkansas Poison and Drug Information Center: 800-376-4766 (emergency phone); 501-686-5540 (administrative phone); 501-686-7357 (fax); poison@poison.uams.edu (E-mail)
University of Arkansas for Medical Sciences
4301 West Markham-Slot 522-2
Little Rock, AR 72205

Blodgett Regional Poison Center: 800-POISON-1 (emergency phone); 800-356-3232 (TTY); 616-774-7851 (administrative phone); 616-774-7204 (fax); johntres@delphi.com (E-mail)
1840 Wealthy SE
Grand Rapids, MI 49506-2968
AAPCC Certified Regional Poison Center

Blue Ridge Poison Center: 804-924-5543 *or* 800-451-1428 (emergency phone); 804-924-5308 (administrative phone); 804-243-6335 (fax)
UVA Health System
PO Box 800774
Charlottesville, VA 22908-0774
AAPCC Certified Regional Poison Center

California Poison Control System—Fresno/Madera: 800-876-4766 (emergency phone); 559-622-2300 (administrative phone); 559-622-2322 (fax)
9300 Valley Children's Place, MB15
Madera, CA 93638-8762
AAPCC Certified Regional Poison Center

California Poison Control System—Sacramento: 800-876-4766 (emergency phone) *or* 800-342-9293 (emergency phone, northern CA only); 916-227-1400 (administrative phone); 916-734-7796 (fax)
2315 Stockton Boulevard
Room 1024, House Staff Facility
Sacramento, CA 95817
AAPCC Certified Regional Poison Center

California Poison Control System—San Diego: 619-543-6000 (emergency phone) *or* 800-876-4766 (emergency phone, 619 area code only); 619-543-3666 (administrative phone); 619-692-1867 (fax); amanoguerra@ucsd.edu (E-mail)
UCSD Medical Center
200 West Arbor Drive
San Diego, CA 92103-8925
AAPCC Certified Regional Poison Center

California Poison Control System—San Francisco: 800-523-2222 (emergency phone); 415-206-5480 (fax)
San Francisco General Hospital
1001 Potrero Avenue, Building 80, Room 230
San Francisco, CA 94110

Cardinal Glennon Children's Hospital Regional Poison Center: 314-772-5200, 800-366-8888, *or* 800-392-9111(emergency phone); 314-772-8300 (administrative phone); 314-577-5355 (fax); mthompson@ssmhcs.com (E-mail)
1465 S Grand Boulevard

St. Louis, MO 63104
AAPCC Certified Regional Poison Center

Carolinas Poison Center: 704-355-4000 *or* 800-84-TOXIN (800-848-6946) (emergency phone); 704-355-4051 (fax); wahoo@med.unc.edu (E-mail)
1012 S Kings Drive, Ste 206
Charlotte, NC 28232-2861
AAPCC Certified Regional Poison Center

Central New York Poison Control Center: 315-476-4766 *or* 800-252-5655 (emergency phone); 315-464-7078 (administrative phone); 315-464-7077 (fax)
SUNY Health Science Center
750 E Adams Street
Syracuse, NY 13210

Central Ohio Poison Center: 614-228-1323 *or* 800-682-7625 (emergency phone); 614-228-2272 (TTY); 614-722-2635 (administrative phone); 614-221-2672 (fax)
700 Children's Drive
Columbus, OH 43205-2696
AAPCC Certified Regional Poison Center

Central Pennsylvania Poison Center: 800-521-6110 *or* 717-531-6111 (emergency phone); 717-531-8955 (administrative phone); 717-531-6932 *or* 717-531-7057 (fax)
University Hospital
Milton S. Hershey Medical Center
Hershey, PA 17033-0850
AAPCC Certified Regional Poison Center

Central Texas Poison Center: 800-POISON1 (800-764-7661) (emergency phone); 813-724-7408 (fax)
Scott & White Memorial Clinic & Hospital
2401 S 31st Street
Temple, TX 76508

Children's Hospital of Michigan Poison Control Center: 313-745-5711 *or* 800-764-7661 (emergency phone); 313-745-5335 (administrative phone); 313-745-5493 (fax); Scsmoli@CMS.CC.Wayne.edu (E-mail)
Harper Professional Office Building
4160 John R, Ste 425
Detroit, MI 48201
AAPCC Certified Regional Poison Center

Children's Hospital of Wisconsin Poison Center: 414-266-2222 (emergency phone) *or* 800-815-8855 (emergency phone, WI only); 414-266-2820 (fax)
PO Box 1997
Milwaukee, WI 53201

Cincinnati Drug & Poison Information Center and Regional Poison Control System: 513-558-5111 (emergency phone) *or* 800-872-5111 (emergency phone, OH only); 800-253-7955 (TTY); 513-558-0230 (administrative phone); 513-558-5301 (fax)
PO Box 670144
Cincinnati, OH 45267-0144
AAPCC Certified Regional Poison Center

Connecticut Poison Control Center: 800-343-2722 (emergency phone, CT only); 203-679-1991 (fax)
University of Connecticut Health Center
263 Farmington Avenue
Farmington, CT 06030
AAPCC Certified Regional Poison Center

Finger Lakes Regional Poison Center: 716-275-3232 (emergency phone) *or* 800-333-0542; 716-273-4155 (administrative phone); 716-244-1677 (fax); dljc@troi.cc.rochester.edu (E-mail)
Box 777
University of Rochester Medical Center
601 Elmwood Avenue, Box 321, Room G-3275
Rochester, NY 14642
AAPCC Certified Regional Poison Center

Florida Poison Information Center—Jacksonville: 800-282-3171 (emergency phone; FL only) *or* 904-549-4465; 904-244-4063 (administrative phone); 904-549-4063 (fax); schauben.pcc@mail.health.ufl.edu (E-mail)
University Medical Center
University of Florida Health Science Center, Jacksonville
655 West 8th Street
Jacksonville, FL 32209
AAPCC Certified Regional Poison Center

Florida Poison Information Center—Miami: 800-282-3171 (emergency phone, FL only); 305-585-5250 (administrative phone); 305-545-9762 (fax); rweisman@mednet.med.miami.edu (E-mail)
University of Miami, Jackson Memorial Hospital
1611 NW 12th Avenue
Urgent Care Center Building, Room 219
Miami, FL 33136

Florida Poison Information Center and Toxicology Resource Center Tampa General Hospital: 800-282-3171 (emergency phone, FL only); 813-254-7044 (administrative phone); 813-253-4443 (fax); sven.normann@ashp.com (E-mail)
PO Box 1289
Tampa, FL 33601
AAPCC Certified Regional Poison Center

Georgia Poison Center: 404-616-9000 (emergency phone) *or* 800-282-5846 (emergency phone, GA only); 404-616-9287 (TDD); 404-616-9237 (administrative phone); 404-616-6657 (fax); lopez_g@mercer.edu (E-mail)
Hughes Spalding Children's Hospital
Grady Health Systems
80 Butler Street SE
PO Box 26066
Atlanta, GA 30335-3801
AAPCC Certified Regional Poison Center

Greater Cleveland Poison Control Center: 888-231-4455 (emergency phone, toll-free) *or* 216-231-4455; 216-844-1573 (administrative phone); 216-844-3242 (fax)
11100 Euclid Avenue
Cleveland, OH 44106

Hawaii Poison Center: 808-941-4411 (emergency phone); 808-535-7921 (administrative phone); 808-973-8085 (fax)
1319 Punahou Street
Honolulu, HI 96826

Hennepin Regional Poison Center: 800-222-1222 *or* 612-347-3141 (emergency phone); 612-904-4691 (TTY); 612-337-7387 (pet line); 612-337-7474 (TDD); 612-347-3144 (administrative phone); 612-904-4289 (fax); deb.anderson@co.hennepin.mn.us (E-mail)
Hennepin County Medical Center
701 Park Avenue
Minneapolis, MN 55415
AAPCC Certified Regional Poison Center

Hudson Valley Poison Center: 800-336-6997 *or* 914-366-3030 (emergency phone); 914-366-3031 (administrative phone); 914-366-1400 (fax)
Phelps Memorial Hospital Center
701 N Broadway
North Tarrytown, NY 10591
AAPCC Certified Regional Poison Center

Illinois Poison Center: 800-942-5969 (emergency phone); 312-906-6136 (administrative phone); 312-803-5400 *or* 312-993-0779 (fax)
222 S Riverside Plaza, Ste 1900
Chicago, IL 60606

Indiana Poison Center: 317-929-2323 (emergency phone) *or* 800-382-9097 (emergency phone, IN only); 317-929-2335 (administrative phone); 317-929-2337 (fax); jmowry@mhi.com (E-mail)
Methodist Hospital of Indiana
I-65 and 21st Street
PO Box 1367
Indianapolis, IN 46206-1367
AAPCC Certified Regional Poison Center

Iowa Poison Control Center: 800-272-6477 *or* 800-222-1222 (emergency phone); 319-356-2600 (administrative phone); 319-356-4545 (fax)
2720 Stone Park Boulevard
Sioux City, IA 51104

Kentucky Regional Poison Center of Kosair's Children's Hospital: 502-589-8222 (emergency phone) *or* 800-722-5725 (emergency phone, KY only); 502-629-5326 *or* 502-629-7264 (administrative phone); 502-629-7277 (fax)
Medical Towers South, Ste 572
PO Box 35070
Louisville, KY 40232-5070
AAPCC Certified Regional Poison Center

Lehigh Valley Hospital Poison Prevention Program: 610-402-2536 (administration phone); 610-402-2696 (fax)
17th and Chew Streets
PO Box 7017
Allentown, PA 18105-7017

Long Island Regional Poison Control Center: 516-542-2323 (emergency phone); 516-739-2066 *or* 516-542-6317 (administrative phone); 516-739-2070 (fax)
Winthrop University Hospital
259 First Street
Mineola, NY 11501
AAPCC Certified Regional Poison Center

Louisiana Drug and Poison Information Center: 800-256-9822 (emergency phone, LA only) *or* 318-362-5393 (emergency phone); 318-342-1710 (administrative phone); 318-342-1744 (fax); pydick@alpha.nlu.edu (E-mail)
Northeast Louisiana University
Sugar Hall
Monroe, LA 71209-6430
AAPCC Certified Regional Poison Center

Maine Poison Control Center: 207-871-2950 (emergency phone) *or* 800-442-6305 (emergency phone, ME only); 207-871-2664 (administrative phone); 207-871-6226 (fax)
Maine Medical Center
Department of Emergency Medicine
22 Bramhall Street
Portland, ME 04102

Maryland Poison Center: 410-706-7701 (emergency phone) *or* 800-492-2414 (emergency phone, MD only); 410-706-7184 (administrative phone)
University of Maryland School of Pharmacy
20 N Pine Street
Baltimore, MD 21201
AAPCC Certified Regional Poison Center

Massachusetts Poison Control System (also serves Rhode Island): 617-232-2120 *or* 800-682-9211 (emergency phone); 617-735-6089 (TDD); 617-738-0032 (fax)
300 Longwood Avenue
Boston, MA 02115
AAPCC Certified Regional Poison Center

McKennan Poison Control Center: 605-336-3894 *or* 800-952-0123 (emergency phone); 605-322-2818 (fax)
Box 5045
800 E 21st Street
Sioux Falls, SD 58118-5045

Medical College of Ohio Poison and Drug Information Center: 419-383-3897 (emergency phone) *or* 800-589-3897 (emergency phone, 419 area code only); 419-381-2818 (fax)
3000 Arlington Avenue
Toledo, OH 43614

Mid-America Poison Control Center: 913-588-6633 (emergency phone) *or* 800-332-6633 (emergency phone, KS only); 913-588-2350 (fax)
University of Kansas Medical Center
3901 Rainbow Boulevard, Room B-400
Kansas City, KS 66160-7231

Middle Tennessee Poison Center: 615-936-2034 (emergency phone, local) *or* 800-288-9999 (emergency phone, regional); 615-322-0157 (TDD); 615-936-0760 (administrative phone); 615-936-2046 (fax)
The Center for Clinical Toxicology
Vanderbilt University Medical Center
1161 21st Avenue South
501 Oxford House
Nashville, TN 37232-4632
AAPCC Certified Regional Poison Center

Mid-Iowa Poison and Drug Information Center: 515-241-6254 (emergency phone) *or* 800-362-2327 (emergency phone, IA only); 515-241-8211 (administrative phone); 515-241-5085 (fax)
Variety Club Poison and Drug Information Center
Iowa Methodist Medical Center
1200 Pleasant Street
Des Moines, IA 50309

Mississippi Regional Poison Control Center: 601-354-7660 (emergency phone); 601-984-1675 (administrative phone); 601-984-1676 (fax)
University of Mississippi Medical Center
2500 North State Street
Jackson, MS 39216-4505

National Capitol Poison Center: 202-625-3333 (emergency phone); 202-362-8563 (TTY); 202-362-3867 (administrative phone); 202-362-8377 (fax)
3201 New Mexico Avenue, NW, Ste 310
Washington, DC 20016
AAPCC Certified Regional Poison Center

New Hampshire Poison Information Center: 603-650-8000 (emergency phone), 603-650-5000 (emergency phone, 11 p.m.–8 a.m.), *or* 800-562-8263 (emergency phone, NH only);

603-650-6318 (administrative phone); 603-650-8986 (fax); 1.courtemanche@dartmouth.edu (E-mail)
Dartmouth-Hitchcock Medical Center
One Medical Center Drive
Lebanon, NH 03756

New Jersey Poison Information and Education System: 800-POISON1 (800-764-7661) (emergency phone); 201-926-7443 (administrative phone); 201-926-0013 (fax); toxdoc@IBM.net (E-mail)
201 Lyons Avenue
Newark, NJ 07112
AAPCC Certified Regional Poison Center

New Mexico Poison and Drug Information Center: 505-843-2551 (emergency phone) *or* 800-432-6866 (emergency phone, NM only); 505-277-4261 (administrative phone); 505-277-5892 (fax); troutman@medusa.unm.edu (E-mail)
University of New Mexico
Health Science Center Library, Room 125
Albuquerque, NM 87131-1076
AAPCC Certified Regional Poison Center

New York City Poison Control Center: 212-340-4494 *or* 212-POISONS (emergency phone); 212-689-9014 (TDD); 212-447-8154 (administrative phone); 212-447-8223 (fax)
NYC Department of Health
455 First Avenue, Room 123
New York, NY 10016
AAPCC Certified Regional Poison Center

North Dakota Poison Information Center: 701-234-5575 (emergency phone) *or* 800-732-2200 (emergency phone, ND, MN, and SD only); 701-234-6062 (administrative phone); 701-234-5090 (fax)
MeritCare Medical Center
720 4th Street North
Fargo, ND 58122

North Texas Poison Center: 800-POISON1 (800-746-7661) (emergency phone); 214-590-5008 (fax)
Texas Poison Center Network at Parkland Memorial Hospital
5201 Harry Hines Boulevard
PO Box 35926
Dallas, TX 75235
AAPCC Certified Regional Poison Center

Northeast Ohio Poison Education and Information Center: 800-362-9922 (emergency phone, OH only); 216-489-1267 (fax)
1320 Timken Mercy Drive NW
Canton, OH 44708

Oklahoma Poison Control Center: 405-271-5454 (emergency phone) *or* 800-764-7661 (emergency phone, OK only); 405-271-1816 (fax)
940 NE 13th Street, Room 3N118
Oklahoma, OK 73104

Oregon Poison Center: 503-494-8968 (emergency phone) *or* 800-452-7165 (emergency phone, OR only); 503-494-7799 (administrative phone); 503-494-4980 (fax); lastname@OHSU.EDU (E-mail)
Oregon Health Sciences University
CB550 3181 SW Sam Jackson Park Road
Portland, OR 97201
AAPCC Certified Regional Poison Center

Palmetto Poison Center: 800-922-1117 (emergency phone); 803-777-7909 (administrative phone); 803-777-6127 (fax); Metts@phar2.pharm.scarolina.edu (E-mail)
College of Pharmacy
University of South Carolina
Columbia, SC 29208

Pittsburgh Poison Center: 412-681-6669 (emergency phone); 412-692-5600 (administrative phone); 412-692-5793, -5868, *or* -7497 (fax); Krenzee@CHPLINK.EDU (E-mail)
3705 Fifth Avenue
Pittsburgh, PA 15213
AAPCC Certified Regional Poison Center

The Poison Center: 402-955-5555 (emergency phone, Omaha) *or* 800-955-9119 (NE, WY) *or* 800-955-9119 (national); 402-955-5467 (administrative phone); 402-390-3049 (fax)
8200 Dodge Street
Omaha, NE 68114
AAPCC Certified Regional Poison Center

The Poison Control Center: 215-386-2100 *or* 800-722-1222 (emergency phone); 215-590-2003 *or* 215-386-2066 (administrative phone); 215-590-4419 (fax)
3600 Sciences Center, Ste 220
Philadelphia, PA 19104-2641
AAPCC Certified Regional Poison Center

Regional Poison Control Center: 205-939-9201, 205-939-9202, 205-933-4050 (emergency phone), *or* 800-292-6678 (emergency phone, AL only); 205-939-9720 (administrative phone); 205-939-9245 (fax)
The Children's Hospital of Alabama
1600 7th Avenue South
Birmingham, AL 35233-1711
AAPCC Certified Regional Poison Center

Regional Poison Prevention Education Center: 814-949-4197 (administrative phone); 814-949-4872 (fax)
Mercy Regional Health System
2500 Seventh Avenue
Altoona, PA 16602

Rhode Island Poison Center: 401-444-5727 (emergency phone); 401-444-5906 (administrative phone); 401-444-8062 (fax)
593 Eddy Street
Providence, RI 02903
AAPCC Certified Regional Poison Center

Rocky Mountain Poison and Drug Center: 303-739-1123 *or* 800-332-3073 (emergency phone, CO), 800-525-5042 (emergency phone, MT), *or* 800-446-6179 (emergency phone, NV); 303-739-1127 (TTY); 303-739-1100 (administrative phone); 303-739-1119 (fax)
8802 E 9th Avenue
Denver, CO 80220-6800
AAPCC Certified Regional Poison Center

Samaritan Regional Poison Center: 602-253-3334 (emergency phone) *or* 800-362-0101 (emergency phone, AZ only); 602-495-4884 (administrative phone); 602-256-7579 (fax); richardt@samaritan.edu (E-mail)
1111 E McDowell Road, Ancillary 1
Phoenix, AZ 85006
AAPCC Certified Regional Poison Center

Southern Poison Center, Inc.: 901-528-6048 (emergency phone) *or* 800-288-9999 (emergency phone, TN only); 901-448-6800 (administrative phone); 901-448-5419 (fax); pchyka@utmeml.utmem.edu (E-mail)
847 Monroe Avenue, Ste 230

Memphis, TN 38163

South Texas Poison Center: 800-POISON1 (800-764-7661) (emergency phone, TX only); 210-567-5762 (administrative phone); 210-567-5718 (fax)
University of Texas Health Science Center
146 Forensic Science Center
San Antonio, TX 78284-7849

St. Luke's Poison Center: 712-277-2222 *or* 800-352-2222 (emergency phone); 712-279-3710 (administrative phone); 712-279-1852 (fax); kalinl@stlukes.org (E-mail)
St. Luke's Regional Medical Center
2720 Stone Park Boulevard
Sioux City, IA 51104

Texas Poison Control Network at Amarillo: 800-764-7661 (emergency phone); 806-354-1630 (administrative phone); 806-354-1667 (fax)
PO Box 1110
1501 S Coulter
Amarillo, TX 79175

Texas Poison Control Network at Galveston: 409-765-1420 (emergency phone, Galveston) *or* 800-764-7661 (emergency phone, TX only); 409-772-3917 (fax); mellis@mspo1.med.utmb.edu (E-mail)
Southeast Texas Poison Center
The University of Texas Medical Branch
301 University Boulevard
Galveston, TX 77555-1175
AAPCC Certified Regional Poison Center

University of Wisconsin Hospital Regional Poison Center: 800-815-8855 (emergency phone); 608-262-7537 (administrative phone); 608-263-9424 (fax); lc.vermeulen@hosp.wisc.edu (E-mail)
E5/238 CSC
600 Highland Avenue
Madison, WI 53792

Utah Poison Control Center: 801-581-2151 (emergency phone) *or* 800-456-7707 (emergency phone, UT only); 801-581-7504 (administrative phone); 801-581-4199 (fax); barbara.crouch@hsc.utah.edu (E-mail)
410 Chipeta Way, Ste 230
Salt Lake City, UT 84108
AAPCC Certified Regional Poison Center

Vermont Poison Center: 802-658-3456 (emergency phone); 802-847-3456 (administrative phone); 802-656-4802 (fax); ruphold@moose.uvm.edu (E-mail)
Fletcher Allen Health Care
111 Colchester Avenue
Burlington, VT 05401

Virginia Poison Center: 804-828-9123 (emergency phone, Richmond) *or* 800-552-6337 (emergency phone, VA only); 804-828-4780 (administrative phone); 804-828-5291 (fax); sliner@gems.vcu.edu (E-mail)
401 N 12th Street
Virginia Commonwealth University
Richmond, VA 23298-0522

Washington Poison Center: 206-526-2121 (emergency phone) *or* 800-732-6985 (emergency phone, WA only); 206-517-2394 (emergency TDD) *or* 800-572-0638 (TDD, WA only); 206-517-2350 (administrative phone); 206-526-8490 (fax)
155 NE 100th St, Ste 400
Seattle, WA 98125
AAPCC Certified Regional Poison Center

West Texas Regional Poison Center: 800-764-7661 (emergency phone, TX only); 915-534-3800 (administrative phone); 915-534-3809 (fax)
4815 Alameda Avenue
El Paso, TX 79905

West Virginia Poison Center: 800-642-3625 (emergency phone, WV only); 304-347-1212 (administrative phone); 304-348-9560 (fax)
3110 MacCorkle Avenue SE
Charleston, WV 25304
AAPCC Certified Regional Poison Center

Western New York Regional Poison Control Center: 716-878-7654, -7655, -7856, -7857 (emergency phone); 716-878-7857 (fax); daq11537@ov.chob.edu (E-mail)
Children's Hospital of Buffalo
219 Bryant Street
Buffalo, NY 14222

Other Countries

AUSTRALIA

Victorian Poisons Information Centre: 011-61-3-6113-1126 (emergency phone); 011-61-3-9345-5333 (administrative phone); 011-61-3-9349-1261 (fax)
Royal Children's Hospital
Flemington Road
Parkville, Victoria 3052
Australia

BRAZIL

Centro de Informacao Toxicologica do Rio Grande do Sul: 011-55-51-223-6110 (emergency phone)
Rua Domingos Crescencio 132-80 Andar
90650-090-Porto Alegre-RS-Brasil

CANADA

BC Drug and Poison Information Centre: 800-567-8911 *or* 604-682-5050 (emergency phone); 604-682-2344, ext. 2126 (administrative phone); 604-631-5262 (fax); daws@dpk.bcca (E-mail)
1081 Burrard Street
Vancouver, BC
Canada V6Z 1Y6

IWK Grace Poison Information Centre
5850 University Avenue
PO Box 3070
Halifax, Nova Scotia B3F 3G9
Canada

Ontario Regional Poison Control Centre: 416-813-5900 (emergency phone); 800-268-9017 (emergency phone, Ontario only); 416-813-6474 (administrative phone); 416-813-7489 (fax)
The Hospital for Sick Children
555 University Avenue
Toronto, Ontario M5G 1X8
Canada

Poison and Drug Information Service: 800-332-1414 (emergency phone; Alberta only) *or* 403-670-1414
Foothills Hospital
1403 29th Street, NW
Calgary, Alberta T2N 2T9
Canada

Poison Information Centre: 800-565-8161 (emergency phone, Prince Edward Island) *or* 902-428-8161 (emergency phone, Nova Scotia); 902-428-8132 (administrative phone); 902-428-3213 (fax)
1 WK Children's Hospital
PO Box 3070
5850 University Avenue
Halifax, Nova Scotia
Canada B3J3G9

Quebec Poison Control Center: 418-656-8090 (emergency phone); 418-654-2731 (administrative phone); 418-654-2747 (fax)
2705 Boulevard Laurier, J782
Sainte-Foy, Quebec
Canada G1V 4G2

NEW ZEALAND

New Zealand National Poisons Information Centre: 011-64-3-474-7000 (emergency phone); 011-64-3-479-7248 (administrative phone); 011-64-3-477-0509 (fax)
National Toxicology Group
University of Otago Medical School, Dunedin School of Medicine
Gt King Street
PO Box 913
Dunedin, New Zealand

Veterinary Poison Centers

The National Animal Poison Control Center (NAPCC) is a division of the American Society for the Prevention of Cruelty to Animals (ASPCA). The emergency hotline is staffed by specially trained veterinary toxicologists.
National Animal Poison Control Center: 800-548-2423
2001 South Lincoln Avenue
Urbana, IL 61801

ENVIRONMENTAL HEALTH CONSULTANTS, PHYSICIAN CONSULTANTS, AND CERTIFIED INDUSTRIAL HYGIENISTS

American Industrial Hygiene Association

The American Industrial Hygiene Association (AIHA) publishes a listing of certified industrial hygienists by state every 6 months in the *AIHA Journal*. The AIHA can assist with locating qualified consultants specializing in the following areas: asbestos, biological monitoring, ergonomics, indoor air quality, chemistry, noise control, radiologic control, lead, air pollution, safety, water pollution, toxicology, ventilation, and training and education.

AIHA: 703-849-8888 (administrative phone); 703-207-3561 (fax)
2700 Prosperity Avenue, Ste 250
Fairfax, VA 22031-4307

American College of Occupational and Environmental Medicine

The American College of Occupational and Environmental Medicine (ACOEM) maintains a list of physicians who specialize in occupational and environmental health and medical toxicology and who are willing to perform consultations and patient evaluations.

ACOEM Headquarters Office: 847-228-6850 (administrative phone); 847-228-1856 (fax); http://www.acoem.org (Web site)
35 West Seegers Road
Arlington Heights, IL 60005

American College of Medical Toxicology

The purpose of the American College of Medical Toxicology (ACMT) is to advance the science, study, and practice of medical toxicology by fostering the development of medical toxicology in its provision of emergency, consultation, forensic, legal, community, and industrial services; and by otherwise striving to advance and elevate the science, study, and practice of medical toxicology. The college was formerly known as the American Board of Medical Toxicology (ABMT). The ABMT offered specialty certification in medical toxicology at a time when the American Board of Medical Specialties (ABMS) did not recognize subspecialty certification in toxicology. When the ABMS approved formal recognition of medical toxicology as a subspecialty in September 1992, the ABMT discontinued its function as a certifying body. It was reincorporated in September 1993 as the American College of Medical Toxicology, a specialty society providing support and representation for medical toxicologists. Active members of the ACMT are physicians who have been certified by the ABMT or by the Sub-Board in Medical Toxicology of the ABMS (or both).

ACMT: 717-558-7846 (administrative phone)
777 East Park Drive
PO Box 8820
Harrisburg, PA 17105-8820

American Academy of Clinical Toxicology

The American Academy of Clinical Toxicology (AACT) is a professional organization dedicated to the scientific pursuit of fostering knowledge and education in clinical toxicology.

AACT: 717-558-7847 (administrative phone)
777 East Park Drive
PO Box 8820
Harrisburg, PA 17105-8820

Association of Occupational and Environmental Clinics

The Association of Occupational and Environmental Clinics (AOEC) maintains a list of clinics that accept referrals and perform evaluations of individuals with toxic or hazardous exposures. For location of clinics, call 888-422-8737.

AOEC Headquarters: 202-347-4976 (administrative phone); 202-347-4950 (fax)
1010 Vermont Avenue NW #513
Washington, DC 20005

INTERNET SITES

Toxicology and Environmental Health

The Extension Toxicology Network (EXTOXNET)
http://ace.orst.edu/info/extoxnet/ghindex.html

Pesticide Information and Toxicity
Medscape
http://www.medscape.com/
Provides access for clinicians to National Library of Medicine databases (TOXLINE and Medline)

Occupational Safety and Health Administration (OSHA)
http://www.osha.gov/
Occupational health standards, office sites, government regulations concerning hazardous materials and individual toxic substances

National Institute of Occupational Safety and Health (NIOSH)
http://www.cdc.gov/niosh/homepage.html
NIOSH databases such as Agricultural Safety Database, Chemical Hazards, Registry of Toxic Effects of Chemical Substances

National Pesticide Telecommunications Network (NPTN)
http://ace.orst.edu/info/nptn/
Pesticides; recognition and management of pesticide poisoning; toxicology of pesticides; environmental chemistry of pesticides

National Antimicrobial Information Network (NAIN)
http://ace.orst.edu/info/nain/
Antimicrobial products; disinfectants; sterilants; regulations and registration; interpretation of labels and permitted uses

Arizona Poison Information Center
http://www.pharmacy.arizona.edu
General Web site
http://www.pharmacy.arizona.edu/centers/poisoncenter/index.html

Florida Poison Information Center (FPIC)
http://www.pediatrics.med.miami.edu/FPIC/index.html

FPIC/Other Poison Centers
http://www.pediatrics.med.miami.edu/FPIC/links.html

Poison Prevention Web Site
http://www.ipl.org/youth/poisonsafe

American Association of Poison Control Centers
http://www.nlu.edu/aapcc

HyperTox Web: Clinical Toxicology and Pharmacology
http://www.newcastle.edu.au/department/md/htas/toxi0002.htm
http://www.newcastle.edu.au/department/md/htas/clintox.htm

Toxikon Multimedia Project
http://toxikon.er.uic.edu/

Karolinska Institute Library: Poisoning
http://www.mic.ki.se/Diseases/c21.613.html

TOXLINE
http://www.medscape.com/medscape/public/announcements/toxlinesearch.html

U.S. National Library of Medicine Toxicology and Environmental Health Information Program (TEHIP)
http://www.nlm.nih.gov
Consumer health information

U.S. Health and Human Services Office
http://www.healthfinder.gov
General health topics for consumers

FOOD AND DRUG ADMINISTRATION (FDA)

FDA: Consumer Magazine
http://www.fda.gov/fdac/default.htm

FDA Home Page
http://www.fda.gov/default.htm
For professionals and consumers

FDA: Information for Consumers
http://www.fda.gov/opacom/morecons.html

Food Safety and Natural Toxins

Center for Food Safety and Nutrition
http://vm.cfsan.fda.gov

FDA *Bad Bug Book*
http://vm.cfsan.fda.gov/~mow/intro.html
Foodborne pathogenic microorganisms and natural toxins from USDA, CDC, and NIH

Food Risks: International Food Information Council
http://ificinfo.health.org/brochure/lesson5.htm

CENTERS FOR DISEASE CONTROL (CDC)

CDC Home Page
http://www.cdc.gov/cdc.html

CDC Documents
http://www.cdc.gov/search.htm

CDC Foodborne Illnesses
http://www.cdc.gov/health/foodill.htm

World Health Organization
http://www.who.ch

Agency for Toxic Substances and Disease Registry (ATSDR)
http://atsdr1.atsdr.cdc.gov:8080

Material Safety Data Sheets
http://www.ilpi.com/msds/index.chtml#internet

POISONOUS PLANTS

Cornell University
http://www.ansci.cornell.edu/plants.html

Arizona Poison Information Center (plants)
http://www.pharmacy.arizona.edu
http://www.pharmacy.arizona.edu/centers/poisoncenter/plants/plant.html *or* search under Arizona Poison and Drug Center for plants

Arizona Poison Information Center (envenomations)
http://www.pharmacy.arizona.edu
http://www.pharmacy.arizona.edu/centers/poisoncenter/critters/venom.html

Australian "Critters"
http://www.usyd.edu.au/su/anaes/envenomation.html

HERBALS AND PHYTOMEDICINE

Botanical.com Home Page
http://www.botanical.com/index.html

American Botanical Council
http://www.herbalgram.org

Agricultural Research Service Databases
http://www.ars-grin.gov/

National Institute of Health, Office of Alternative Medicine
http://altmed.od.nih.gov

Herb Encyclopedia
http://www.wic.net/waltzark/herbenc.htm

National Center for Environmental Assessment (EPA)

http://www.epa.gov

EPA Superfund World Wide Web Site
http://www.epa.gov/superfund

JOURNALS

Environmental Health

Annals of Agricultural and Environmental Medicine
Annals of the ICRP (International Commission on Radiological Protection)
Applied Radiation and Isotopes
Archives of Environmental Contamination and Toxicology
Archives of Environmental Health
Aviation Space and Environmental Medicine
Biological Trace Element Research
Biomedical and Environmental Sciences
Bulletin of Environmental Contamination and Toxicology
Chemosphere
Ecotoxicology and Environmental Safety
Environmental and Molecular Mutagenesis
Environmental Health Perspectives
Environmental Research
Health Physics
Industrial Health
International Archives of Occupational and Environmental Health
International Journal of Food Microbiology
International Journal of Occupational Medicine and Environmental Health
Journal of Environmental Pathology, Toxicology, and Oncology
Journal of Environmental Science and Health, Part B: Pesticides, Food Contaminants, and Agricultural Wastes
Journal of Exposure Analysis and Environmental Epidemiology
Journal of Occupational and Environmental Medicine
Journal of Radiation Research
Journal of the Air and Waste Management Association
Journal of Toxicology and Environmental Health
Journal of Trace Elements in Medicine and Biology
Journal of Vector Ecology
Microbiological Research
Molecular Ecology
Mutagenesis
Neurotoxicology
Occupational and Environmental Medicine
Radiation and Environmental Biophysics
Research Report/Health Effects Institute
Reviews on Environmental Health
Scandinavian Journal of Work, Environment, and Health
Science of the Total Environment
Studies in Human Ecology
WHO Regional Publications, European Series

Occupational Medicine

American Industrial Hygiene Association Journal
American Journal of Industrial Medicine
Annals of Occupational Hygiene
Archives of Environmental Health
European Journal of Applied Physiology and Occupational Physiology
Industrial Health
International Archives of Occupational and Environmental Health
International Journal of Occupational Medicine and Environmental Health
Journal of Occupational and Environmental Medicine
Occupational and Environmental Medicine
Occupational Health and Safety
Occupational Medicine
Scandinavian Journal of Work, Environment, and Health

Toxicology

Adverse Drug Reactions and Toxicological Reviews
Annual Review of Pharmacology and Toxicology
Archives of Environmental Contamination and Toxicology
Archives of Toxicology
Archives of Toxicology, Supplement
Bulletin of Environmental Contamination and Toxicology
Chemical Research in Toxicology
Critical Reviews in Toxicology
Drug and Chemical Toxicology
Ecotoxicology and Environmental Safety
Experimental and Toxicologic Pathology
Food and Chemical Toxicology
Human and Experimental Toxicology
Immunopharmacology and Immunotoxicology
Journal of Analytical Toxicology
Journal of Applied Toxicology
Journal of Biochemical and Molecular Toxicology
Journal of Environmental Pathology, Toxicology, and Oncology
Journal of Toxicology and Environmental Health
Journal of Toxicology, Clinical Toxicology
Neurotoxicology
Pharmacology and Toxicology
Reproductive Toxicology
Reviews of Environmental Contamination and Toxicology
Toxicologic Pathology
Toxicological Sciences
Toxicology
Toxicology and Applied Pharmacology
Toxicology and Industrial Health
Toxicology Letters
Toxicon
Veterinary and Human Toxicology

Subject Index

Note: Numbers followed by *f* indicate figures, numbers followed by *t* indicate tables.